Contents in Brief

YOUR GUIDE TO
DAVIS ADVANTAGE FOR
BASIC NURSING

Build a successful foundation for your
NURSING EDUCATION
CLASS | CLINICAL | EXAMS | NCLEX®

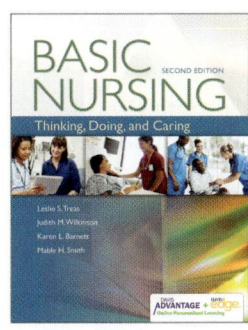
+
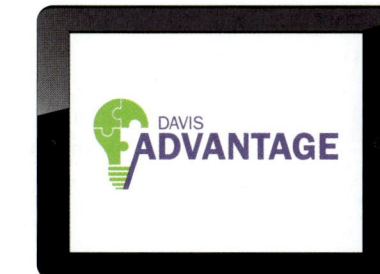
+
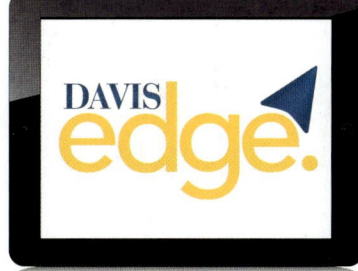

LEARNING

Your text provides the foundational knowledge to teach you to think like a nurse from the very first day.

APPLYING

Davis Advantage provides a personalized learning experience that helps you make the connections and apply your knowledge to master must-know concepts.

ASSESSING

Davis Edge's online quizzing evaluates your mastery of course material and builds your test-taking skills.

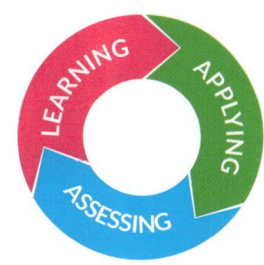

DAVIS ADVANTAGE **BASIC NURSING**

combines your text with Online Personalized Learning and Quizzing to help you master this challenging, but essential foundational content.

YOUR JOURNEY TO
FUNDAMENTALS
SUCCESS BEGINS HERE!

Don't miss all of the resources waiting online to make learning easier...and save you time. Follow the instructions on the inside front cover to use the access code to unlock **Davis Advantage for Basic Nursing** today.

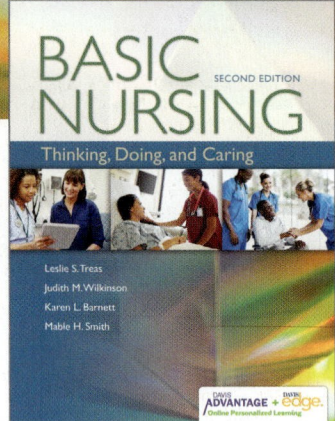

LEARNING

STEP #1

Build a solid foundation and learn how to think like a nurse from the very first day.

Basic Nursing provides a comprehensive approach to care and prepares you for the real world of nursing practice.

Two types of **case studies** illustrate key points and bring concepts to life through examples of real-world nursing care.

Caring for the Nguyens

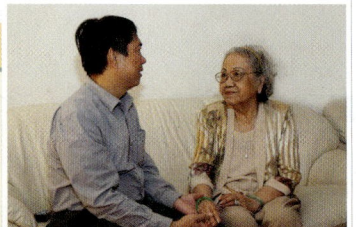

Mai Nguyen, the 76-year-old mother of Nam Nguyen, has been experiencing blurred vision and decreased visual acuity. A local ophthalmologist diagnosed bilateral cataracts and has recommended cataract removal in the left eye, with insertion of an intraocular lens. He told Mai Nguyen to schedule the surgery "at your convenience" and explained that the surgery would be performed on an outpatient basis. The ophthalmologist gave Mai Nguyen the following list of activities to prepare for the surgery:

- Schedule a date for your surgery. My receptionist will set up a time for your surgery. All surgeries are performed at Western Medical Center Same-Day Surgery Department.
- Please arrange to be seen by your primary care provider 1 to 2 weeks prior to the surgery to receive clearance for surgery.
- Make an appointment with the Preoperative Center at Western Medical Center Same-Day Surgery Department 1 to 2 days before surgery.
- Arrange to have a ride to and from the surgery.

A. What preoperative testing is Mrs. Nguyen likely to undergo? Explain your rationale.

B. The preoperative list states that the client must be seen by the primary care provider to receive clearance for surgery. Why is this an essential part of the preoperative period?

C. What theoretical knowledge do you need to perform preoperative teaching for Mai Nguyen? How could you obtain that information? Be specific about your sources.

D. What content would you include in N[...] preoperative teaching?

E. The ophthalmologist has planned ane[...] sedation. What factors, if any, might ke[...] from receiving this form of anesthesia[...] information do you need to answer t[...]

Go to Davis Advantage, Resources, Ch[...]
the Nguyens—Suggested Responses.

Meet Your Patient

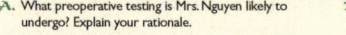

Nishad Singh is a 68-year-old man who came to the emergency department (ED) with sudden onset of rectal bleeding. He tells the ED nurse, "I've been real tired and dragging for several months. This morning I felt a little worse than usual. When I went to the bathroom, there was a lot of blood. I've never had that before, and it scared me. I've had to go to the bathroom a couple times this morning, and it's all blood." The ED nurse collects the following data:
BP: 138/88 mm Hg
Pulse: 104 beats/min and regular
Respiratory rate: 20 breaths/min
Temperature: 36.7°C (98.0°F)
Oxygen saturation: 98%

The ED nurse assesses that Mr. Singh is mildly anxious. His breath sounds are clear, but his abdomen is tender in the left lower quadrant. The nurse draws blood to be sent to the lab. While they are waiting for the lab results, Mr. Singh tells the nurse, "My stomach is cramping down low, and I need to go to the bathroom." She provides him with a bedpan. He passes approximately 200 mL of bright red blood with a small amount of fecal material. He becomes sweaty and light-headed after the BM.

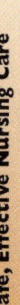

Surgical Team Communication

Key Concepts: Perioperative Nursing, Preoperative Care, Intraoperative Care, Postoperative Care

SENC Competency: *Provide goal-directed, client-centered care*
Eliciting each patient's values, preferences, and expressed needs as part of the focused nursing history will assist you in providing goal-directed, client-centered care. You can then communicate patient values, preferences, and expressed needs to other members of the healthcare team to assure patient-centered care with sensitivity and respect for the diversity of individual patients.

SENC Competency: *Collaborate with the interdisciplinary healthcare team*
To provide for effective collaboration within nursing and interdisciplinary teams, nurses must engage in open communication, mutual respect, and shared decision to ensure safe and effective patient care. Two-minute briefings just before surgery, led by the attending surgeon using a standardized format, have been found to improve communication and reduce delays and wrong-site surgery (Lee, 2016). Surgical briefings encourage team members to talk when there is no problem, so they are more likely to speak up when they have misgivings when problems occur (Berger, Greenberg, & Bilimoria, 2015).

Think Like a Nurse questions check your understanding while developing your critical-thinking and clinical-reasoning skills.

Think**Like a Nurse** 40-3

Which, if any, of the preceding nursing diagnoses would be most appropriate for Mr. Singh (Meet Your Patient)? Do not use the potential complications in Table 40-2. Explain your reasoning.

Safe and Effective Nursing Care boxes illustrate how to provide safe, quality care to patients.

Applying the Full-Spectrum Nursing Model

PATIENT SITUATION

Recall Nishad Singh (Meet Your Patient). He is a 68-year-old man who came to the emergency department (ED) with sudden onset of rectal bleeding. He had been "tired and dragging for several months." The ED nurse identified nursing diagnoses of Mild Anxiety, Pain, and Risk for Bleeding. Preoperatively, his vital signs were as follows:

BP: 138/88 mm Hg
Pulse: 104 beats/min and regular; 120 beats/min; 134 beats/min
Respiratory rate: 20 breaths/min
Temperature: 36.7°C (98.0°F)
Oxygen saturation: 98%

THINKING

1. *Theoretical Knowledge:*
   a. What is a left hemicolectomy? If you do not know the answer, consult an appropriate reference.
   b. What does "metastasis to the liver" mean? If you do not know the answer, consult an appropriate reference.
2. *Critical Thinking (Inquiry):*
   a. Why might Mr. Singh have needed a colostomy instead of having his transverse colon reconnected to the remaining lower colon or rectum? State the reference you used to answer this question.
   b. Why do you think Mr. Singh has a colostomy above the level of the umbilicus and not lower down in his abdomen? State the reference you used to answer this question.

DOING

3. *Practical Knowledge:* Mr. Singh returned from surgery with knee-high antiembolism stockings.
   a. You notice that the stockings have slid down and become wrinkled between his knees and ankles. After you straighten them and pull them up, the tops reach to about 7.6 cm (3 in.) below Mr. Singh's knees. What does this probably mean, and what should you do?
   b. Which of the following instructions should you give when delegating care of Mr. Singh's antiembolism stockings to the nursing assistant? (Mr. Singh's stockings have closed toes.)
   ▪ Remove the stockings and bathe and dry the legs every 8 to 12 hours.
   ▪ Massage the legs after removing Mr. Singh's stockings.

CARING

5. *Self-Knowledge:*
   a. If you were assigned to care for Mr. Singh today, what aspect of care would you feel best prepared [to provide?] Explain your thinking.
   b. What aspect of Mr. Singh's care would you be most uncomfortable providing? Explain your thinking.
6. *Ethical Knowledge:* You want to provide culturally competent care. What is the first thing you will need [to do] in order to address Mr. Singh's cultural needs? Review Chapter 15 if you need to.

Clinical Reasoning: Applying the Full-Spectrum Nursing exercises reinforce the concepts of thinking, doing, and caring to help you develop your clinical decision-making skills, while you apply what you are learning to real patients.

♥ iCare 40-1

Perioperative Care

▪ Perioperative nursing is a specialized area of nursing with specific, established standards of care. A caring nurse strives to integrate those standards into the nursing process and to apply standards to each patient in a caring manner.

▪ Caring nurses ensure that a person is cognitively and psychologically prepared for surgery.

▪ Caring nurses advocate for patients. An example is stopping the line and placing a HOLD on surgery when a person identifies an error or a risk in a process or in the surgical procedure. This exhibits *200% accountability* and embraces *high reliability* behaviors. You can do this by saying to others, *"I have a concern"; "We need to stop and verify"; "I am uncomfortable proceeding";* or even stronger language: *"I cannot send Ms. Brown until the surgeon comes back up and reviews her surgical procedure with her again; she clearly does not understand."*

KEY POINT: *Preventing errors and "never events" is everyone's responsibility.*

---

iCare highlights the role of caring in nursing and demonstrates how a nurse provides safe and effective care in a particular situation.

✚ An unconscious client is usually positioned on his side to help maintain an open airway. This decreases the likelihood of aspirating mucus or saliva by allowing it to drain out instead of back into the throat. Elevating the superior arm on a pillow allows for good chest expansion so the patient can breathe deeply and expand the lungs fully.

Safety icons alert you to important aspects of safe care to avoid potential hazardous or high-risk issues.

Over 230 step-by-step procedures with rationales teach you how to perform and master essential nursing skills.

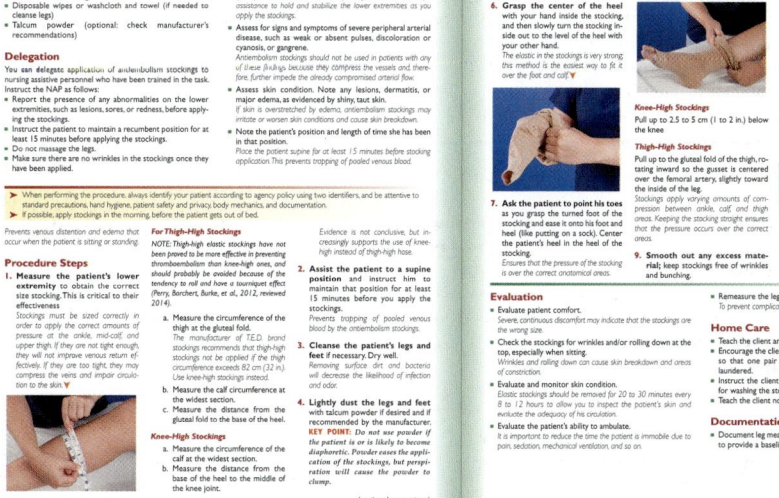

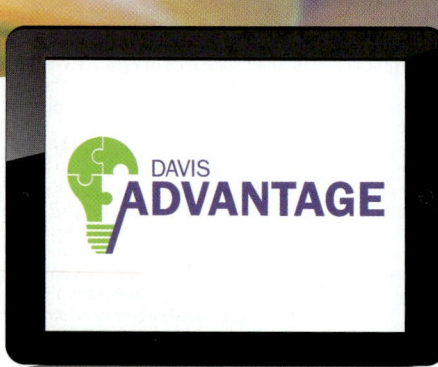

APPLYING

STEP #2

Make the connections and apply your knowledge with Online Personalized Learning.

Quiz yourself on how well you understand key fundamentals nursing concepts. Based on your performance, you will receive a Personalized Learning Plan with engaging videos and interactive activities. You'll know exactly where you need to focus your studies until you've mastered the concepts and are ready to apply them in class, clinical, and practice.

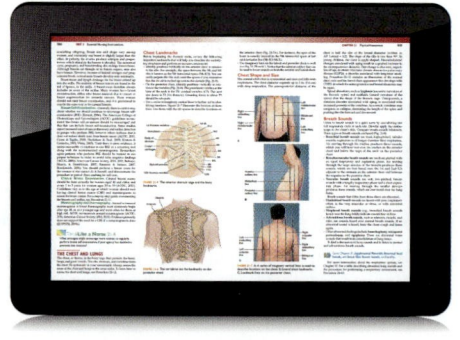

A FREE ebook version of your text, available with each new printed book, makes studying and reviewing easier, anytime, anywhere. Use the access code on the inside front cover.

Assignments

DISPLAY: ALL ACTIVE COMPLETED

Fundamentals | Student Name | Start Date: 09/01/17 | End Date: 12/31/17

Perioperative Nursing

Reading Assignment: Chapter 40 · View eBook · Due Date: 12/31/2017 · Start

Urinary Elimination

Reading Assignment: Chapter 29 · View eBook · Due Date: 12/31/2017 · Start

---

Pre-Assessment for Perioperative Nursing

Question 2 of 2

The nurse is caring for a client who had a colon resection for removal of a cancerous tumor. On the surgical unit, which postoperative actions are important for complication prevention? *Select all that apply.*

- ☐ Ambulate routinely as ordered.
- ☐ Monitor vital signs regularly.
- ☐ Teach the patient about the type of tumor removed.
- ☐ Assess the drainage from the surgical site.
- ☐ Assist the patient to turn, breathe deeply, and cough every 2 hours.

Submit

Each assignment is mapped to a specific chapter in the text. Begin by reading from your printed text or from the integrated ebook.

Pre-Assessment Results

The below results show your areas of strength and weakness. Your results have been added to your Personalized Learning Plan.

Basic Nursing

Topic	Pre-Assessment	
Perioperative Nursing	👎	Start

View PLP

Following your reading, take the **Pre-Assessment quiz** to evaluate your understanding of the content. Based on the results, a **Personalized Learning Plan** is mapped to your needs and guides you on a path to success.

Perioperative Nursing

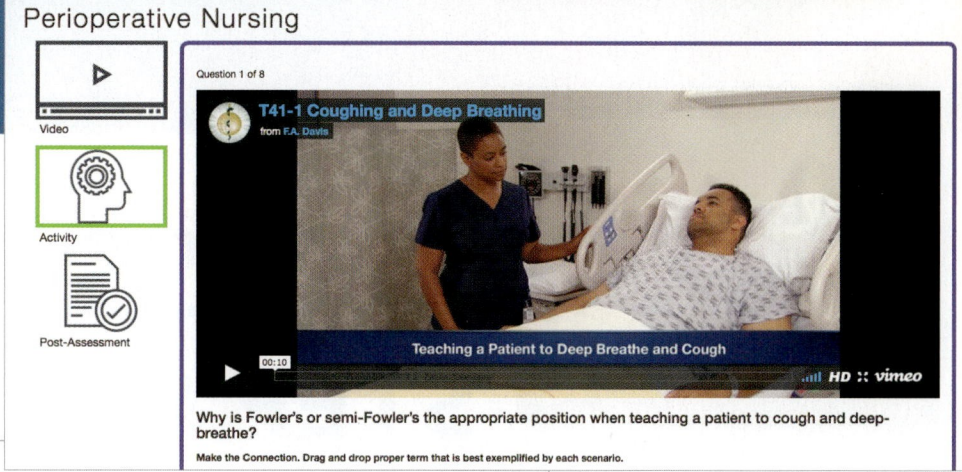

Video

Activity

Post-Assessment

Question 1 of 8

T41-1 Coughing and Deep Breathing
from F.A. Davis

Teaching a Patient to Deep Breathe and Cough

00:10

HD :: vimeo

Why is Fowler's or semi-Fowler's the appropriate position when teaching a patient to cough and deep-breathe?

Make the Connection. Drag and drop proper term that is best exemplified by each scenario.

Perioperative Nursing

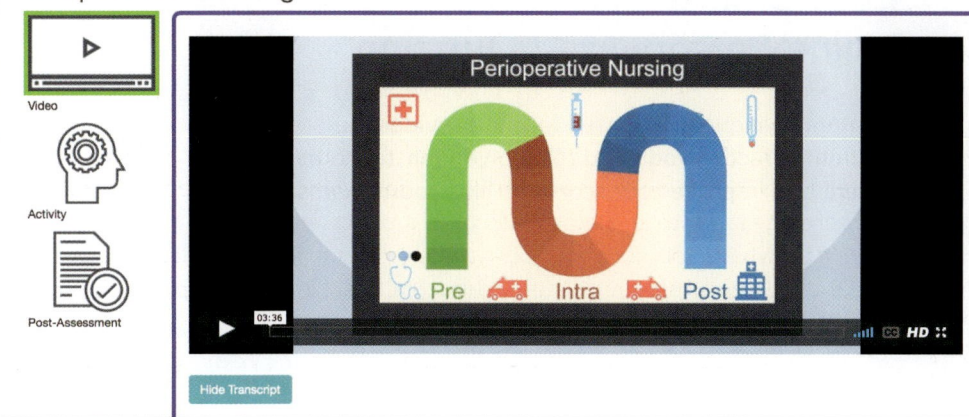

Video

Activity

Post-Assessment

Perioperative Nursing

Pre   Intra   Post

03:36

HD

Hide Transcript

Animated mini-lecture videos present key concepts in a way that makes the content more memorable and understandable, while **interactive learning activities** help you apply and expand your knowledge.

Post-Assessment for Perioperative Nursing

Question 1 of 1

The nurse has a new order to apply antiembolism stockings. At what point should that occur?

○ During surgery

● **Prior to surgery**

○ In the PACU

○ Upon discharge

Submit

After working through the animated mini-lecture video and activity, a **Post-Assessment** quiz tests your mastery. The results feed into your Personalized Learning Plan, where your instructor is able to view them.

Post-Assessment for Perioperative Nursing

Results

You answered 5 out of 5 correctly.

Try Again   View PLP

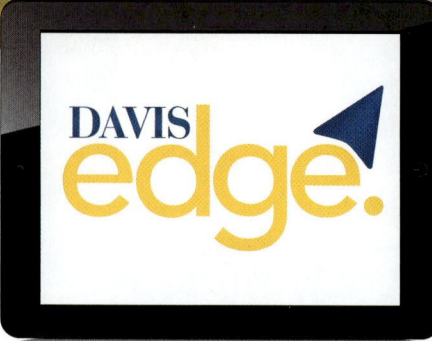

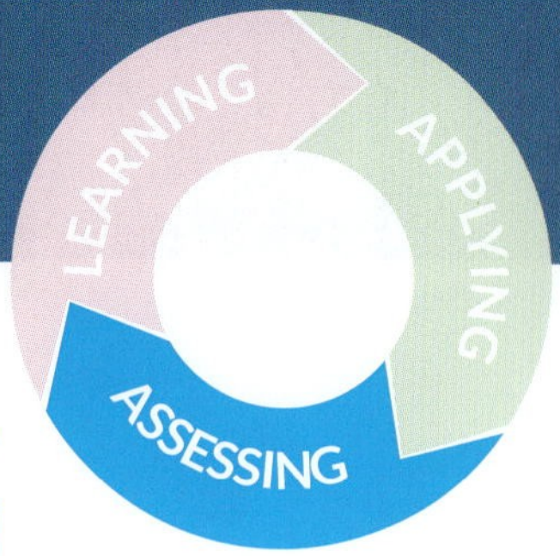

ASSESSING

STEP #3

Study Smarter, Not Harder with Online Personalized Quizzing

An interactive question-based format provides the additional practice you need to help you master course content and improve your scores on classroom exams.

Quizzing assignments are made by your instructor. Or, **create your own practice quizzes** on topics you'd like to focus on.

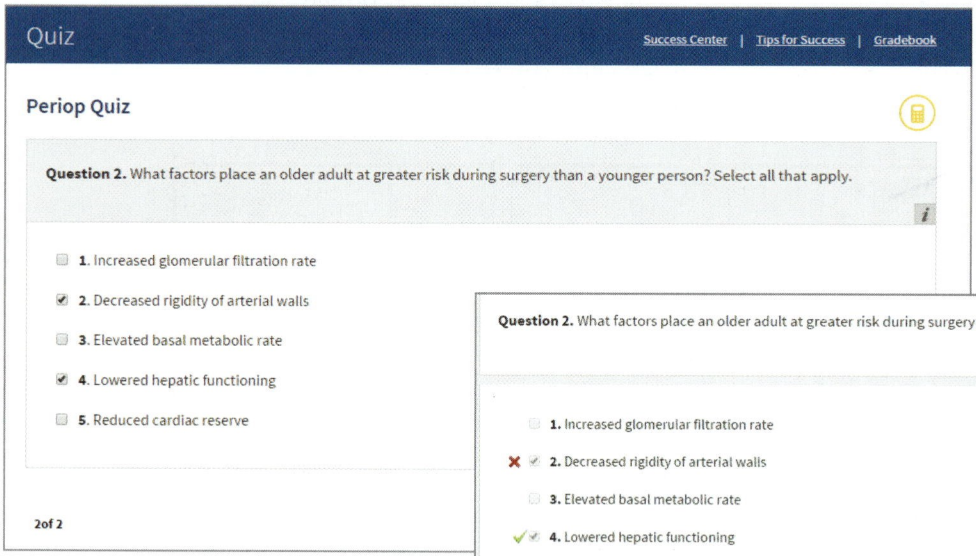

Quiz

Success Center | Tips for Success | Gradebook

Periop Quiz

Question 2. What factors place an older adult at greater risk during surgery than a younger person? Select all that apply.

i

- ☐ 1. Increased glomerular filtration rate
- ☑ 2. Decreased rigidity of arterial walls
- ☐ 3. Elevated basal metabolic rate
- ☑ 4. Lowered hepatic functioning
- ☐ 5. Reduced cardiac reserve

2of 2

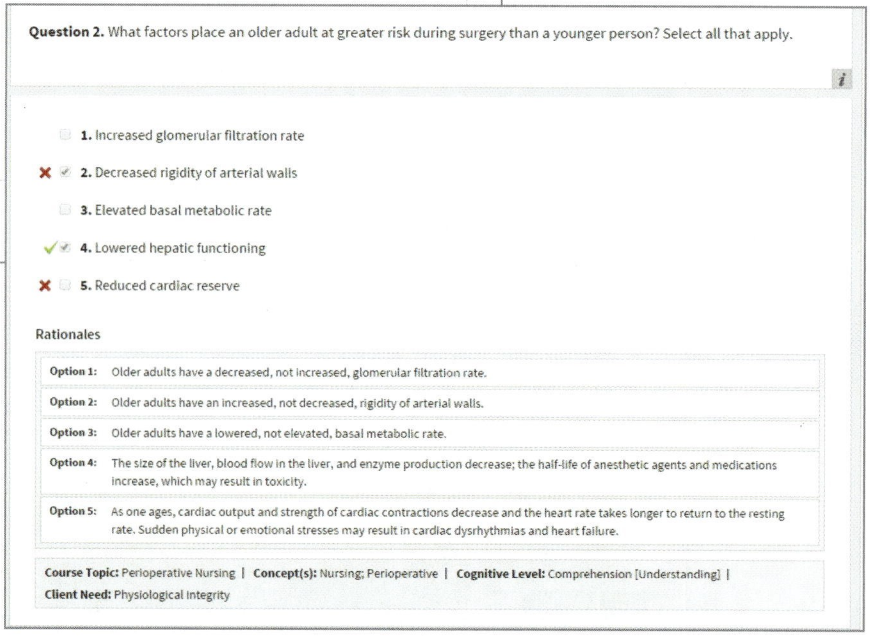

Question 2. What factors place an older adult at greater risk during surgery than a younger person? Select all that apply.

i

- ☐ 1. Increased glomerular filtration rate
- ✗ ☑ 2. Decreased rigidity of arterial walls
- ☐ 3. Elevated basal metabolic rate
- ✓ ☑ 4. Lowered hepatic functioning
- ✗ ☐ 5. Reduced cardiac reserve

Rationales

Option 1:	Older adults have a decreased, not increased, glomerular filtration rate.
Option 2:	Older adults have an increased, not decreased, rigidity of arterial walls.
Option 3:	Older adults have a lowered, not elevated, basal metabolic rate.
Option 4:	The size of the liver, blood flow in the liver, and enzyme production decrease; the half-life of anesthetic agents and medications increase, which may result in toxicity.
Option 5:	As one ages, cardiac output and strength of cardiac contractions decrease and the heart rate takes longer to return to the resting rate. Sudden physical or emotional stresses may result in cardiac dysrhythmias and heart failure.

Course Topic: Perioperative Nursing | **Concept(s):** Nursing; Perioperative | **Cognitive Level:** Comprehension [Understanding] |
Client Need: Physiological Integrity

Immediate feedback with rationales for correct and incorrect responses enhance critical thinking and help you build your knowledge base. Many questions also include test-taking tips that show you how to analyze questions and reduce your test-taking anxieties.

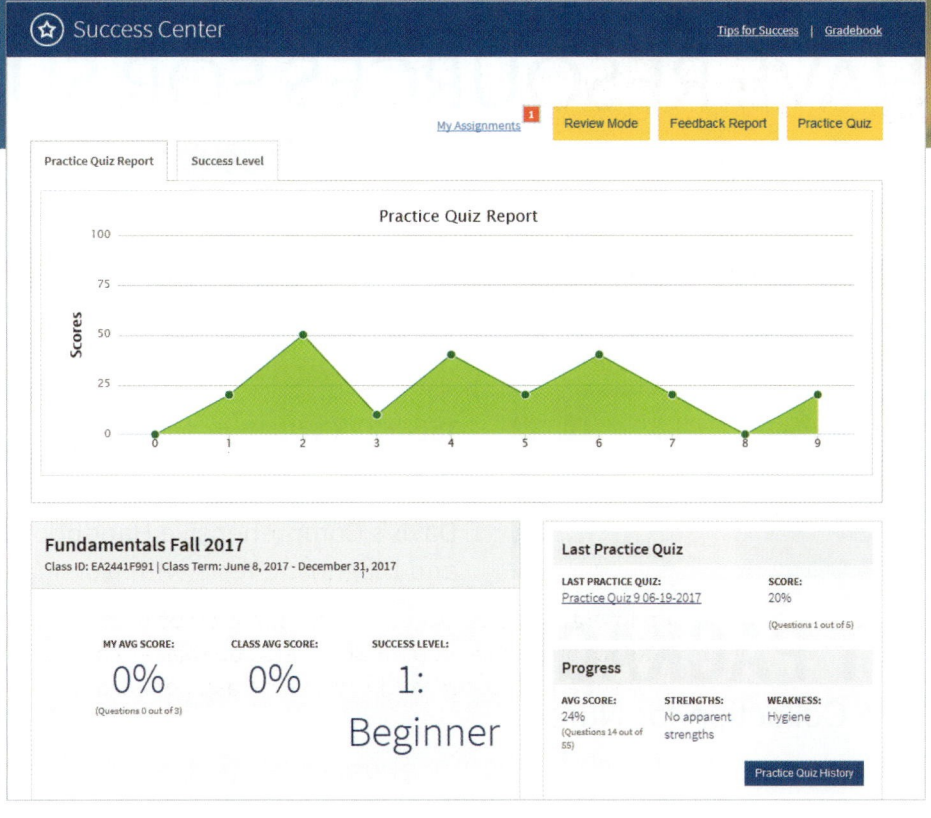

Your **Success Center** offers a snapshot of your progress and identifies your strengths and weaknesses. The **Feedback Report** drills down to show your performance in individual content areas. It's easy to create new practice quizzes that focus on your areas of weakness or to select the topics or concepts you want to study.

Feedback Report

Create Practice Quiz On Weak Areas   Course Topic ▼

Strengths and Weaknesses will appear for a specific course topic or concept once you have answered a minimum of 10 questions in that area. Select to view by Course Topic or Concept from the drop down box above. Choose 'Create quiz on weak areas' above to begin creating a new quiz based on all weak areas.

Course Topic ⬍	Strength / Weakness ⬍	Number of Questions Answered ⬍	Success Level ⬍	Create Quiz
Fluid and Electrolyte Balance	● Progressing	14	1: Beginner	Create Practice Quiz
Acid-Base Balance	● Needs More Practice	10	1: Beginner	Create Practice Quiz

GET STARTED

by using the access code in the inside front cover to unlock **Davis Advantage for Basic Nursing** today!

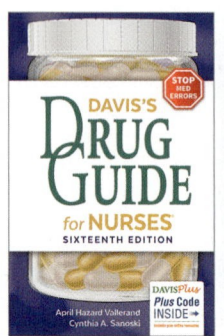
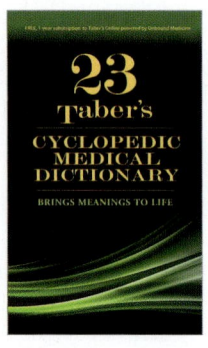
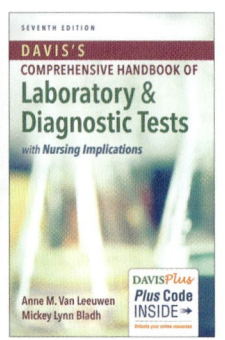
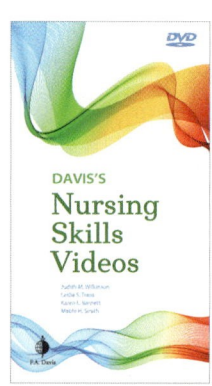
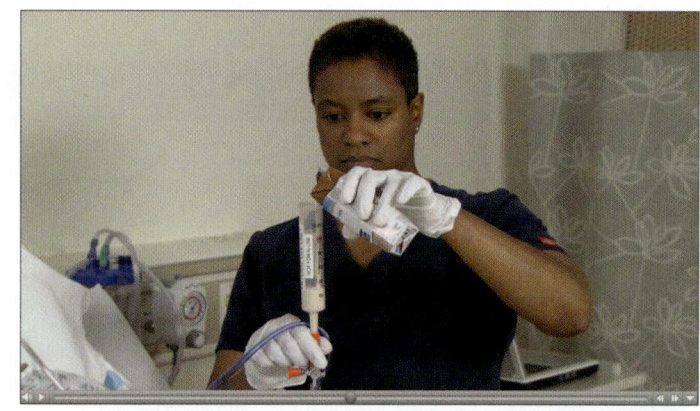
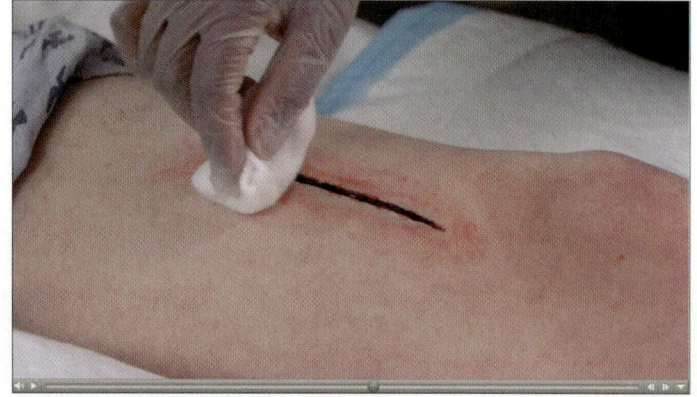

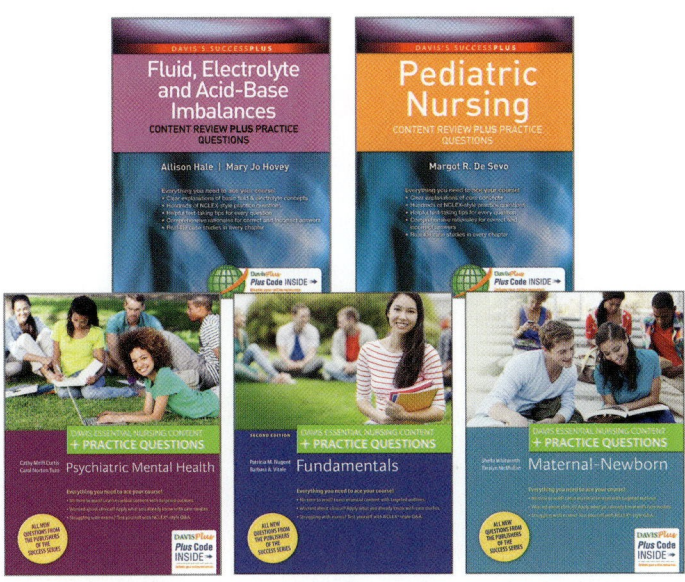
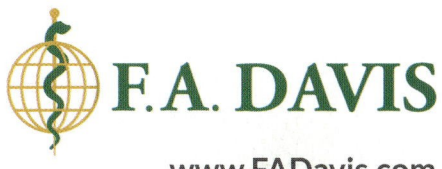

BASIC NURSING

SECOND EDITION

Thinking, Doing, and Caring

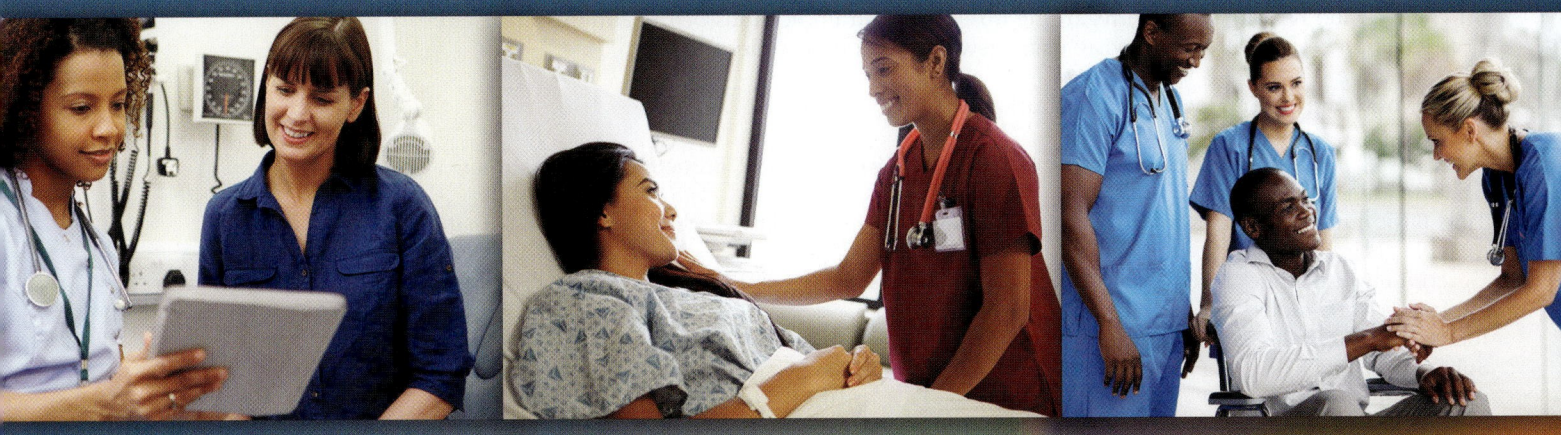

Leslie S. Treas, PhD, RN, CPNP-PC, NNP-BC

Judith M. Wilkinson, PhD, ARNP

Karen L. Barnett, DNP, RN

Mable H. Smith, PhD, JD, MN, NEA-BC

F.A. Davis Company • Philadelphia

F. A. Davis Company
1915 Arch Street
Philadelphia, PA 19103
www.fadavis.com

Last digit indicates print number: 10 9 8 7 6 5

Publisher, Nursing: Lisa B. Houck
Content Project Manager II: Julia L. Curcio
Electronic Project Managers: Jacki Albertini and Eric Van Osten
Design and Illustrations Manager: Carolyn O'Brien

As new scientific information becomes available through basic and clinical research, recommended treatments and drug therapies undergo changes. The author(s) and publisher have done everything possible to make this book accurate, up to date, and in accord with accepted standards at the time of publication. The author(s), editors, and publisher are not responsible for errors or omissions or for consequences from application of the book, and make no warranty, expressed or implied, in regard to the contents of the book. Any practice described in this book should be applied by the reader in accordance with professional standards of care used in regard to the unique circumstances that may apply in each situation. The reader is advised always to check product information (package inserts) for changes and new information regarding dose and contraindications before administering any drug. Caution is especially urged when using new or infrequently ordered drugs.

Library of Congress Cataloging-in-Publication Data

Names: Treas, Leslie S., author. | Wilkinson, Judith M., 1946- author. | Barnett, Karen L., author. | Smith, Mable H., author.
Title: Basic nursing : thinking, doing, and caring / Leslie S. Treas, Judith M. Wilkinson, Karen Barnett, Mable H. Smith.
Description: 2nd edition. | Philadelphia, PA : F. A. Davis Company, 2017. | Includes bibliographical references and index.
Identifiers: LCCN 2017034667| ISBN 9780803659421 (alk. paper) | ISBN 0803659423 (alk. paper)
Subjects: | MESH: Nursing Care—methods | Nursing Assessment | Nurse's Role
Classification: LCC RT49 | NLM WY 100.1 | DDC 610.73—dc23 LC record available at https://lccn.loc.gov/2017034667

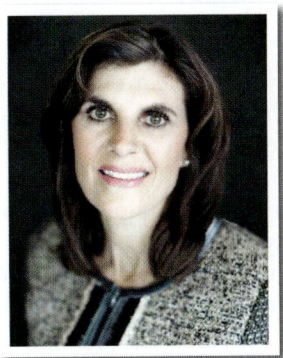

Leslie S. Treas, PhD, RN, CPNP-PC, NNP-BC

Dr. Leslie Treas, one of the founders and former Vice-President, Research and Development of Assessment Technologies Institute ™, LLC (ATI), demonstrated leadership and expertise forecasting and directing the design and development of ATI product testing and educational product line at the formation of the company. In this role, Dr. Treas planned and implemented norming, test validation, and standard-setting studies to support data-driven product development, creating tests with sound psychometric properties. Under her management, ATI produced a series of NCLEX®-style remediation materials in print, video, and online formats. She has conducted clinical and educational research, publishing in peer-reviewed journals of health and education.

Dr. Treas was involved in the start-up of a continuing education company for nurses, physicians, and allied health professionals, serving as Director of Education and Accreditation, AcaMedic Institute™, LLC.

Dr. Treas earned a BSN from Pennsylvania State University and an MSN degree with emphasis in maternal–child health at the University of Kansas. She obtained a PhD from the University of Kansas in the Educational Psychology and Research Department with dual areas of study of testing and measurement and nursing education. Her primary area of clinical expertise is the care of sick newborns in the NICU and labor and delivery settings in the clinical role of a neonatal nurse practitioner. Dr. Treas obtained dual pediatric and neonatal nurse practitioner certifications at the Cleveland Metropolitan General Hospital, an affiliate of Case Western University.

Her journal and textbook publications have featured various clinical topics ranging from care of neonatal patients to education-based areas related to nursing licensure preparation and prediction, critical thinking, and others. Dr. Treas has also written articles geared toward new graduate readers, addressing contemporary issues involving role change, employment, and communication. She is also the co-author of the F.A. Davis text, *Fundamentals of Nursing: Theory, Concepts & Application* as well as *Basic Nursing: Concepts, Skills & Reasoning*.

Dr. Treas has presented papers at annual conferences for Sigma Theta Tau, National Association of Associate Degree Nurses, National Association of Neonatal Nurses, American Association of Colleges of Nursing, National Conference on Professional Nursing Education and Development, and the Association for the Advancement of Educational Research, to name a few.

She has test-writing expertise; she is a former test-item writer for the National Certification Examination for Pediatric Nurse Practitioners and Nurses as well as the National Certification Corporation for Neonatal Nurse Practitioner Exam.

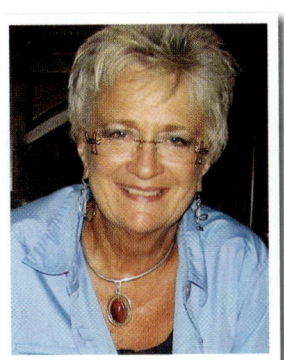

Judith M. Wilkinson, PhD, ARNP

Dr. Judith Wilkinson taught fundamentals of nursing for 22 years and, more recently, has taught graduate-level courses in theory, research, and health policy. She also developed and taught for many years an LPN-to-RN transition course. She has given numerous presentations and provided consultation and faculty development workshops for nursing and other schools—primarily in the areas of critical thinking and nursing ethics, but also in standardized nursing languages, teaching strategies, testing, evaluation, and curriculum.

She obtained her PhD in Nursing from the University of Kansas School of Nursing, and master's degrees in Education and Nursing from the University of Missouri–Kansas City School of Nursing. Her basic nursing degree is an ADN from Johnson County Community College, followed by a BSN from Graceland College. Her master's thesis was a seminal work in moral distress, which was presented at the International Nursing Research Conference in Edmonton, Alberta. She was granted a National Endowment for the Humanities fellowship to study nursing ethics, and a Nurses' Educational Fund (Isabel Hampton Robb) scholarship for her nursing doctoral study. Her dissertation was a historical study of nursing ethics and was nominated for the University of Kansas Argersinger Dissertation Award.

Dr. Wilkinson's broad clinical background includes emergency, critical care, medical-surgical (float), and obstetric nursing. While engaged in full-time teaching, she also maintained certification in inpatient obstetric nursing; her advanced practice license is in nursing care of women.

Her other publications include F.A. Davis's *Fundamentals of Nursing*; a nursing process text and a nursing diagnosis handbook (each having been published in multiple editions); a maternal–newborn care planning book (as a co-author); and journal articles on the topics of curriculum, critical thinking, and nursing ethics. Over the years, she has contributed chapters to several textbooks and authored many ancillary materials, including test banks, learning modules, and review modules.

Dr. Wilkinson is a Member of the American Nurses Association, the National League for Nursing, Sigma Theta Tau, and the Organization for Associate Degree nursing, in which she serves as an OADN Foundation board member.

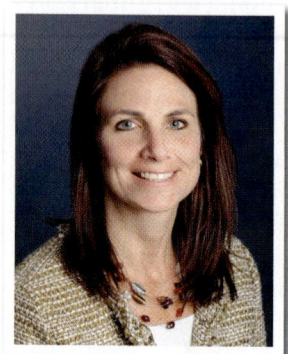

Karen L. Barnett, DNP, RN

Dr. Karen L. Barnett has been a nurse for more than 25 years and has held various positions in nursing, including patient care, administration, and education. Most recently, Dr. Barnett serves as Assistant Dean of Undergraduate Studies for the College of Nursing at the University of Massachusetts, Dartmouth Campus. Prior to that, she was the Dean of Health Sciences at St. Vincent's College in Bridgeport, Connecticut. She has served on the faculty of Norwalk Community College and Southern Connecticut State University. Dr. Barnett's area of clinical expertise is critical care, medical-surgical, and cardiac-telemetry. While engaged in full-time teaching, she continued to maintain clinical competence in her role as nursing supervisor at an acute care community hospital. Dr. Barnett earned a Bachelor's of Science in Nursing from Southern Connecticut State University and a Master's of Science in Nursing degree with a focus in nursing administration from Sacred Heart University. She earned a Doctor of Nursing Practice degree from the Francis Payne Bolton School of Nursing at Case Western Reserve University in 2010 with a focus in nursing education leadership. Dr. Barnett is a member of the American Nurses Association, Connecticut Nurse Association, National League for Nursing, and Sigma Theta Tau International Nursing Honor Society. She was honored with a Nightingale Award for Excellence in Nursing in 2013. Research interests include student learning outcomes, simulation as a learning tool, and critical thinking/clinical judgment. Dr. Barnett has contributed to chapters in several textbooks and authored other ancillary material including test banks and concept maps.

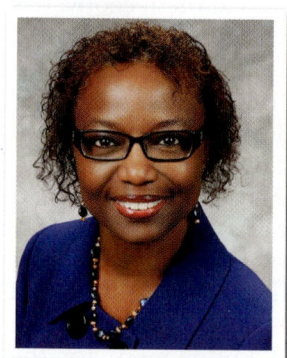

Mable H. Smith, PhD, JD, MN, NEA-BC

Dr. Mable Smith has an extensive background in academia, administration, and clinical practice. She is the currently the Dean of the College of Nursing and Public Health at South University. Dr. Smith was also the founding Dean of the Colleges of Nursing at Roseman University of Health Sciences, Nevada and Utah. She has been in education for more than 25 years and has taught at all academic levels, including undergraduate courses in professional nursing, leadership and management, role transition. legal/ethical aspects of practice, healthcare policies, and adult health/critical care nursing. She has developed and taught graduate level courses in theoretical foundations, research, healthcare finance, trends and issues, and role of the nurse educator. She has published and presented in numerous arenas on legal and ethical issues in nursing education and in nursing/healthcare. Her publications have appeared in leading refereed journals, and she authored the book *The Legal, Ethical and Professional Dimension of Nursing Education*, currently in its second edition.

In addition to the academic environment, Dr. Smith is a Lt Col in the U.S. Air Force Reserves. She is the Chief, Nursing Services at the 413th ASTS, Warner Robins, Georgia.

Dr. Smith earned a BSN from Florida State University (FSU) and an MN from Emory University, with an emphasis in education. She obtained a PhD in Higher Education Administration and JD from FSU. Dr. Smith has served on the faculties of Florida A&M University, Old Dominion University, and the University of South Mississippi. Her primary areas of clinical expertise is adult health/medical-surgical nursing. Dr. Smith is a member of the American Nurses Association, The American Association of Nurse Attorneys, and American College of Healthcare Executives. She was honored by the National Association of Women Business Owners as a *Women of Distinction* for her contributions to the education field in southern Nevada and was named a Healthcare Headliner by *In Business Las Vegas*, one of southern Nevada's premier business publications. She is also a Robert Wood Johnson Executive Nurse Fellow Alumna.

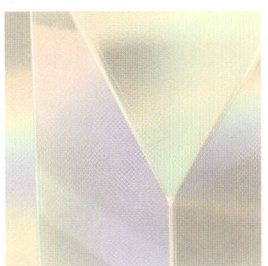

We dedicate this book to:

■ The creative, dedicated nurse educators, who give so much of themselves to help prepare their students for providing quality care across the full spectrum of nursing.

■ Nursing students, as they strive to acquire the knowledge, skills, and attitudes that they must transfer to their imminent practice.

■ Practicing nurses, who struggle with daily realities to promote and maintain health and to provide comfort and care during illness and at end of life.

The health of the nation depends on all of us.

—Leslie S. Treas

—Judith M. Wilkinson

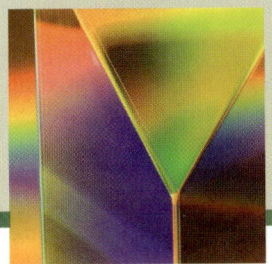

Preface

We chose our book title carefully. We used *basic nursing* in the title because this text and fundamental courses are truly that: the basis for all that follows. In that sense, and because this basic, fundamental content will be used throughout the nurse's career, we believe it is—or should be—the most important course students take. We want them to say, "Everything I need to know, I learned in fundamentals—all I needed to know about how to think, what to do, and how to care" (at a basic level). You will see those themes integrated throughout each chapter.

We have kept the same open, user-friendly, easy-to-read style that students have been telling us they love in the previous edition and in our other fundamentals products.

ORGANIZATION

Our chapters are self-contained and rich in cross-references so that teachers and students can use them in any order that fits their needs.

Optional Chapters—We anticipate this text will be used as a reference throughout the student's career—and we intended it to be comprehensive but not overwhelming. To that end, we have included two complete chapters on Davis*Advantage*: Chapter 45, Nursing Informatics, and Chapter 46, Holistic Nursing. We recognize that curricula differ—that, for example, many schools cover nursing informatics in another course and do not need that chapter in a basic nursing text. However, for those who do need it, the complete chapter is online.

Within-Chapter Organization—Content within each chapter is generally organized into two major sections: Theoretical Knowledge: Knowing Why, and Practical Knowledge: Knowing How. There is some overlap in these concepts because the two types of knowledge are interdependent. We have made the general distinction because many nursing programs begin with content learned in supporting prerequisite classes and then layer on additional Theoretical Knowledge to explain the rationale for nursing actions and activities (Practical Knowledge). This distinction also affords more flexibility in teaching fundamentals. For example, it is useful to teachers who believe students are more motivated when they present first the concrete (Practical Knowledge), and then the abstract (Theoretical Knowledge); it is equally useful for those who teach from the theoretical to the practical.

Procedures (Nursing Skills) and Clinical Insights—These are placed at the end of the chapter for two reasons: (1) So they do not interrupt the logical flow of content when the student is studying didactic material, and (2) So they will be easier to locate when the student is looking for a particular procedure.

FEATURES

The chapters have numerous pedagogical features to facilitate student learning. These features include:

- *Learning Outcomes*—These focus the student's study and provide repetition to facilitate retention of material.

- *Interactive Approach*—The text is written in an engaging style that speaks directly to the student. Critical-thinking and recall questions are integrated throughout the content to break chapters up into small, manageable segments and maintain interest. They also occur in the clinical reasoning exercises in each chapter and in other activities on Davis*Advantage*.

- *Caring for the Nguyens*—This opening feature in the *Clinical Reasoning* section is an ongoing case study that appears in every chapter. It allows students to become familiar with a single family and to experience vicariously the continuity of care they may encounter in outpatient settings. As with all exercises, response sheets are provided on Davis*Advantage*.

- *Key Concepts List and Concept Map*—The key concepts are the umbrella concepts for the chapter—right after the opening features. We listed them to help students begin to use concepts to organize content in their memory. In the section About the Key Concepts we explain how those concepts relate to or can be used to organize chapter content. On the last page of each chapter is a Concept Map, which shows the relationships among the key concepts and many subordinate, related chapter concepts.

- *Meet Your Patient*—This opening feature in each chapter introduces one or more patients, as you might see in "real life" nursing. It is used throughout the chapter to illustrate theoretical points and to make the content come alive. These patients are often followed in the Think Like a Nurse questions found throughout the chapter.

- *New for Second Edition. Example Problems*—New to this edition are graphic-driven, content-rich example problems that are tied to key concepts within the chapter. The need-to-know information is attractively displayed with an easy-to-use and easy-to-remember format.

- *Knowledge Checks*—These questions provide opportunity for students to test their recall of the material presented in the text. Answers are provided on Davis*Advantage*.

- *Critical-Thinking Activities*—Thought-provoking questions (Think Like a Nurse) are interspersed within each chapter to allow the student to synthesize content and explore personal beliefs. Suggested responses are found on Davis*Advantage*.

- *Safe, Effective Nursing Care Competencies*—We have introduced competencies for nurses providing safe, effective patient and family care. To remind students that these competencies have practical implications, many of the chapters have a Safe, Effective Nursing Care box, providing an example of how a competency is expressed in practice.

- *What if . . .*—Procedures include a section to aid students in knowing what to do in special situations that require decisions during a procedure. For example, what if you perform a fingerstick to monitor blood glucose, and the monitor shows a very unusual result or an error message? What should you do? We provide the answer. What if's are placed after the procedure steps so they will not distract from the steps while the student learns the procedure.

- *Toward Evidenced-Based Practice Boxes*—In every chapter, we describe research related to the chapter topic and pose critical-thinking exercises for students to examine these findings. The concept of evidence-based practice is introduced in Chapter 6 (Planning Interventions), further explained in Chapter 8 (Theory, Research, & Evidence-Based Practice), and mentioned frequently in other chapters as well.
- *Care Plans*—Seventeen care plans integrating NANDA International, NIC, and NOC are found in the book and on Davis*Advantage*. They are based on case studies that allow students to see the nursing process in action. Evidence-based rationales are provided for interventions.
- *Care Maps*—Care Maps associated with each care plan allow visual learners to grasp the connection between the phases of the nursing process. They also provide an alternative method of care planning.
- *Teaching: Self-Care Boxes*—Self-care boxes are like the traditional "teaching boxes" but focus on equipping patients to perform self-care.
- *Home Care Boxes*—These provide guidelines for safely modifying care for delivery in the home. Many of the procedures also have a Home Care section for adapting the procedure in the patient's home.
- *Complementary & Alternative Modalities (CAM) Boxes*—Included in several chapters, these describe a complementary therapy related to the chapter topic or present research concerning a complementary therapy (e.g., intercessory prayer in the spirituality chapter).
- *Clinical Reasoning Section: Applying the Full-Spectrum Nursing Model*—These clinically-based exercises guide students to safely practice their clinical reasoning skills, and at the same time reinforce the full-spectrum model concepts of thinking, doing, and caring introduced in Chapter 2 and integrated throughout the book.
- *Diagnostic Testing Boxes*—These are found in applicable chapters. We believe it is more meaningful to place the diagnostic test information near the related content rather than in an isolated chapter. If students need a more comprehensive reference, we recommend a diagnostic testing book.
- *Knowledge Maps*—These are a type of concept map found on Davis*Advantage* for each chapter. They are maps of chapter content. Rather than demonstrating relationship among chapter concepts, the maps show the relationships among the various topics covered in the chapter.
- *Concept Maps*—These are found at the end of each chapter in the book. They visually demonstrate the relationship among chapter key concepts and subconcepts. This is especially useful to visual learners.
- *PICOT Boxes*—We have added this feature to most chapters to facilitate the skill of inquiry, especially as it relates to evidence-based practice.

THEMES

The following themes are integrated and stressed throughout this text, some of them in every chapter:

- *Critical Thinking, Clinical Reasoning, and the Full-Spectrum Model of Nursing.* In addition to the critical-thinking questions and exercises, we promote critical thinking by often presenting content in an inductive manner, or by posing a question to the student (e.g., "What would happen if . . . ?"). The full spectrum model of nursing is a comprehensive approach to care that uses critical thinking in all aspects of care. It is not rigidly overlaid on each chapter. Because students cannot focus on everything at once, different parts are stressed at different times. Sometimes the discussion asks, "What theoretical knowledge do you need to . . . ?" In other instances, they might be asked, "What biases do you have that might interfere with . . . ?" The full-spectrum model is reinforced in every chapter, as well as in the feature Clinical Reasoning: Applying the Full-Spectrum Nursing Model, which requires students to use the model concepts of thinking, doing, and caring.
- *Nursing Process.* Chapter 2 explains the relationship between nursing process, critical thinking, and clinical reasoning; Chapters 3 through 7 make up a comprehensive presentation of the nursing process, which is presented as reflexive rather than linear. The Practical Knowledge sections are organized according to the nursing process phases; and the procedures all have assessment and evaluation components. In addition, many of the questions and exercises provide opportunity for using the nursing process.
- *Safety Features.* Safety is a central focus in nursing and healthcare. To emphasize and help students remember important aspects of safe care, we have safety points marked with an icon and shading for high visibility. This book also includes an entire chapter, Chapter 23, Safety.
- *Caring.* Caring is an important dimension of nursing, as caring is what matters to patients and families. Therefore, we have added brand-new iCare boxes in this book that feature ways nurses can show caring and compassion in patient care. Additionally, caring passages in the text are highlighted with an icon to call attention to the integration of caring into nursing practice. In addition, Chapter 1 provides historical examples of nursing as a caring profession. Chapter 8 describes the important caring theories. The case study introduces Watson's theory, and that theory is used throughout Chapter 8 to illustrate how theory is applied in nursing. As well, the Applying the Full-Spectrum Nursing Model features all have questions involving caring.
- *Safe, Effective Nursing Care.* To remind students of the knowledge (thinking), skills (doing), and attitudes (caring) needed to achieve the competencies for safe and effective nursing care, we have included new boxes based on competencies reflecting the full-spectrum nursing model. These boxes provide practical examples of how a competency is expressed (see Features).
- *Culture.* Cultural diversity is highlighted throughout the text in clinical scenarios, illustrations, and theoretical discussion. Chapter 15 focuses on culturally sensitive nursing care. The Caring for the Nguyens opening scenario features a Vietnamese family; and ethnic variations are described, as applicable, in procedures.
- *Gerontology.* To allow for an in-depth discussion of aging and gerontology, provided by an expert on this topic, Chapter 10 is entirely devoted to the older adult developmental stage. Assessments and interventions specifically for the young-old, middle-old, oldest-old, and frail elderly are provided. We have also included interventions specific to older adults in clinical chapters where they apply (e.g., assessing for pain, in Chapter 31; variations for older adults in the health assessment procedures in Chapter 22). You will also find that many features and exercises use an older adult as the patient.
- *Developmental Stage.* Chapter 9 is devoted entirely to growth and development from conception through middle age. The Theoretical Knowledge section in most chapters devotes a portion to the discussion of the effects of the life span on the chapter topic. In addition, the procedures include variations for children and older adults.

- *Documentation.* All chapters include reference to documentation, where relevant. The procedures all have guidelines for documenting the procedure.
- *Informatics.* Chapter 45 is an excellent introduction to nursing informatics. Standardized languages and electronic care planning and documentation are interspersed throughout the book (e.g., in the nursing process and medications chapters). We also emphasize electronic documentation in Chapter 18. We encourage use of technology by providing students with links to other Web sites related to the chapter topic.
- *Contemporary Issues.* In Chapter 22, we include extensive information about bioterrorism, multi-drug resistant organisms, and emerging infectious diseases, and healthcare-related infections. Those topics are also included in Chapter 42 as relevant to Community Nursing; and in the Meet Your Nurse Role Model scenario in the informatics chapter). The safety chapter includes ways to assess for and cope with violence in the healthcare setting. Additionally, Chapter 36, Skin Integrity & Wound Healing, covers updated terminology for pressure injury.
- *NANDA-I, NIC, and NOC Standardized Languages.* Because these are important for electronic health records, the book includes a thorough discussion of these taxonomies in the nursing process and other chapters. NOC outcomes and NIC interventions are included in every clinical chapter. The Omaha System and the Clinical Care Classification are also used in the community and home health chapters.
- *Wellness.* Many examples and scenarios used in this text refer to people who are not ill. Chapter 11 emphasizes health, and Chapter 27 talks about the nurse's role in health promotion.
- *Spirituality.* Chapter 16 is one of the most extensive presentations of spiritual care available in a fundamentals text. Spirituality is integrated within various chapters in scenarios, examples, and exercises.
- *Delegation.* Delegation is introduced early, in the nursing process chapters, and is a thread woven through most chapters. All procedures have guidelines for delegating. Chapter 41, Leading & Managing, also discusses delegation.
- *ANA Standards.* Nursing and other healthcare standards (e.g., The Joint Commission, Medicare) are frequently referenced. Links to pertinent Web sites are given so students can keep up with changes to standards.
- *Ethics.* In addition to the comprehensive treatment in Chapter 45, ethical knowledge is an aspect of our full-spectrum model. As such, many of the critical-thinking exercises ask students to grapple with ethical issues. Good examples are found in Chapter 6 and in the Clinical Reasoning feature, Applying the Full-Spectrum Nursing Model, in every chapter.
- *Legal Issues.* Chapter 44 is devoted to legal issues that nurses face in their practice. Legal issues are integrated in many other chapters as well (e.g., licensing in Chapter 1, end-of-life legal considerations in Chapter 17).
- *Community and Home Nursing.* Chapter 42 is devoted exclusively to these topics. In other chapters, clinical scenarios and examples involve nurses in these settings; we include special feature boxes regarding these topics; and the procedures have sections for adapting skills to home care, where applicable.
- *Complementary Therapies.* Nursing is presented as holistic throughout. Chapter 46 (found on DavisAdvantage) is devoted exclusively to complementary and alternative therapies; and several chapters in the book (e.g., Chapter 15, Culture & Ethnicity) contain material and/or boxes related to this topic.

THE TEXT AS A RESPONSE TO CHANGE

This book was developed to address the needs of today's nursing students and in response to the following changes in nursing education and practice.

Changes in Students

- **Nontraditional Students.** Students range from traditional, younger students just out of high school to older, second-career students. Many have work or family responsibilities that compete with the time needed for classes and studying. To address this change, we have followed three principles of adult learning: Learning must be relevant, efficient, and meaningful to the person.
- **Variety in Learning Styles.** Students learn in different ways. To address this, we have used more than 1,400 photos and as many diagrams, care maps, concept maps, graphic displays for example problems to assist visual learners. To teach psychomotor skills, we have, in addition to step-by-step procedures, skills videos, and checklists that students can print out for practicing procedures or teachers to use in evaluations.

Because learning improves when content is meaningful to the learner, each chapter opens with a patient scenario or story of a practicing nurse. This story is woven throughout the chapter to provide context for theoretical information and to show how concepts are applied and how nurses think. We stress practical application throughout the text because adults want to apply knowledge in real-life circumstances. The Nguyen family case, which is introduced in Chapter 1 and continues throughout all chapters, is a prime example.

- **Reading Comprehension.** Whether because of changes in admission requirements, students having English as a second language, or other reasons, some schools are finding students' reading abilities to be on a lower level than in the past. We address this change by writing in an informal style, addressing the student directly ("you will . . ."). We have not made the content more superficial, but have made reading about it more inviting and user friendly.
- **The Technology Generation.** The newer generation of students is accustomed to using technology and multitasking. To hold their attention, in addition to our easy-to-read style, we have presented information in an interactive manner, and in relatively short segments interspersed with review questions and critical-thinking questions. For this same reason, the text frequently directs students to find related information on the DavisAdvantage Web site, and on the Internet.

The e-Edition of *Basic Nursing* lets student access their textbook from wherever the student has Internet access without having to lug around heavy books. Also available from the same authors is a set of skills videos that can be purchased on DavisPlus.

Changes in Curriculum

- **Concepts-Based Learning.** Even if a curriculum is not entirely concepts based, there is a trend to teaching and learning in a more concepts-based manner. We believe that all fundamentals books are, by nature, concepts based. That is, each chapter consists of the explication of one or two basic concepts. To assist instructors and students in adopting a more concepts-based approach, in each chapter we have listed the key concepts, included an explanation of their use (About the Key Concepts), made use of Example Problem graphics (e.g., urinary retention in Chapter 30), and included a Concept Map at the end of each chapter to illustrate the relationships among the key concepts and subconcepts in the chapter.

- **Teachers say they do not have enough time to "cover the content."** A concepts-based approach is one way to limit the amount of content that must be presented. See the preceding discussion. Another way to address this problem is to not re-teach material students have had in other classes. We provide, for example, just enough anatomy and physiology in each chapter to aid students who need to review A&P, or who are taking A&P concurrently with nursing courses. You should not need to "cover" it in class.
- **Some curricula have de-emphasized mental health**. Mental health may be taught in other (e.g., medical–surgical) clinical areas, without a separate mental health course in the curriculum. In response to pleas from educators, we include expanded mental health content and tools for psychosocial assessment. In addition to the usual concepts of self-concept and self-esteem, Chapter 13 includes basic assessments and interventions for the Example Problems of anxiety and depression, which students will encounter commonly in all areas, not just on mental health units. In Chapter 21, the communication chapter, we have excellent content on the nurse-patient relationship and communication techniques that mental health teachers find so essential. Chapter 12, Stress & Adaptation, includes information about defense mechanisms.
- **The curriculum does not include separate pharmacology, nutrition, ethics, or nursing process or leadership courses.** Because all nurses need grounding in these topics, we have provided extensive coverage of them. Chapter 25, Administering Medications, provides basic pharmacology information. Chapter 28, Nutrition, provides a foundation for understanding patients' nutritional needs. Chapter 43 is a comprehensive look at nursing ethics. Chapter 41 is a thorough presentation of leadership. We have, arguably, the most useful and thorough presentation of the nursing process available in a fundamentals text. These chapters, as well as most others, will be a valuable reference for students when they take other clinical nursing courses.

Changes in Nursing and Healthcare

- *The nursing role is increasingly complex, requiring management, decision-making, delegation, and supervision skills early in the career.*
  To address this change, the critical-thinking and clinical decision-making exercises, as well as the Nguyens feature, help students to develop clinical decision-making skills. Delegation is presented early, in the nursing process chapters, and stressed in the rest of the chapters as applicable. The procedures each contain a Delegation section. We have included a comprehensive discussion of leadership and management chapter.
- *Healthcare has moved increasingly from the hospital to the home and community.*
  To address this change, Chapter 1 discusses the history of nursing, as well as the contemporary healthcare delivery system. Chapter 42 discusses community and home nursing, and home and community care are integrated throughout the book (e.g., *Healthy People 2020* goals are cited). The procedures include home care adaptations, as well as patient teaching points that will enable patients and caregivers to assume more responsibility for care.
- *Nurses need to be critical thinkers and life-long learners.*
  The text is organized around a model of full-spectrum nursing, a comprehensive approach to care that uses critical thinking in all aspects of care. The model is reinforced in each chapter in the feature Clinical Reasoning: Applying the Full-Spectrum Nursing Model. Critical thinking is integrated throughout the text, both in discussion and in Think Like a Nurse exercises. Discussion of this model follows.

THE FULL-SPECTRUM MODEL OF NURSING

We believe that nursing knowledge is a fusion of theoretical knowledge, practical knowledge, self-knowledge, and ethical knowledge. To function at the highest level, nurses use critical thinking and the nursing process to blend thinking and doing to put caring into action. We refer to this blend as **full-spectrum nursing.** We have organized our learning package to reflect this philosophy. This model includes the major concepts of thinking, doing, and caring, patient situation, and patient outcomes. It is presented in Chapter 2 and referred to and used throughout the text.

THE LEARNING PACKAGE

This well-integrated and cross-referenced package contains both a text and the student and instructor resources on the Davis*Advantage* Web site. Also available from the same authors, for purchase to expand the learning package, are a comprehensive set of skills videos and a small *Pocket Nursing Skills* book (a handy review of skills to be used in the clinical setting).

Advantage

How students learn is evolving. In this digital age, we consume information in new ways. Online, we are spoon-fed information in bite-sized, dynamic chunks.

In order to meet the needs of today's learners, how faculty teach is also evolving. Classroom time is valuable for active learning. This approach makes students responsible for the key concepts, allowing faculty to focus on clinical application. Relying on the textbook alone to support an active classroom leaves a gap. *Davis Advantage for Basic Nursing* fills that gap with the following resources:

- **A Strong Core Textbook** that provides the foundation of knowledge that today's nursing students need to pass the NCLEX and enter practice prepared for success.
- **Online Student Tools** to learn and practice the content in an engaging, interactive format. **Pre-Assessment Quizzes** test students on their comprehension of a key topic and then give them a **Personalized Learning Plan** to work through that is based on their strengths and weaknesses. They are engaged in an interactive experience that uses multimedia content to help spark connections and bring concepts to life. Once students complete the interactive experience, **Post-Assessment Quizzes** assess their comprehension of the material.
- **Online Instructor Resources** create a dynamic classroom experience that is tailored to students' needs. Results from the pre-and-post-assessments are available to faculty, in aggregate or by student, and inform a **Personalized Teaching Plan** that faculty can use to deliver a targeted classroom experience. Faculty will know students' strengths and weaknesses *before* they come to class and can spend class time focusing on where students are struggling. Turn-key, easy to implement in-class activities are provided to help create an active, hands-on learning environment that helps students connect more deeply with the content. NCLEX-style questions from the **Instructor Test Bank** and **PowerPoint**

slides that correspond to the textbook chapters are referenced in the Personalized Teaching Plans.

- **Davis Edge** online quizzing assesses understanding, using an adaptive format with NCLEX-style questions. Faculty can set up a review and remediation system to take a constant pulse of classroom performance, with student results available in real-time to easily identify areas of weakness. Comprehensive rationales for all answer options are provided for students and explain why an answer is correct or incorrect.

The Textbook

The textbook contains all the theoretical and conceptual material typically present in a fundamentals text, presented in a clinically focused, user-friendly manner, and incorporating many examples. The nursing process is used as the model to organize the Practical Knowledge sections in most chapters.

Unit 1 focuses on how nurses think. It begins by showing the evolution of nursing: how our history relates to our present. Chapter 2 focuses on critical thinking, and Chapters 3 through 7 provide an extensive treatment of the nursing process. This unit prepares students to follow the organization of subsequent chapters and provides the thinking tools and processes they need to apply the content of the other chapters. Chapter 8 contains an overview of the processes of theory building, nursing research, and evidence-based practice as they relate to the nurse in practice.

Unit 2 is about the internal and external factors that affect an individual's health (e.g., life stage, health and illness status, stress, psychosocial health, family, culture, and spirituality). Internal factors are personal beliefs or attributes that influence how the client views health, healthcare, and nursing. A groundbreaking feature is Chapter 11, which describes the health–illness–wellness continuum in an experiential way, encouraging self-knowledge, personal growth, and affective learning of that content.

Unit 3 examines essential nursing interventions. We consider these skills essential because nurses use some of these skills in *all* areas of nursing, regardless of setting or patient diagnosis. The unit begins with documentation and includes communication, teaching, taking vital signs, physical assessment, asepsis, safety, hygiene, and medication administration.

Unit 4 concentrates on nursing care that supports physiological function. We examine broad categories of physiological function (e.g., nutrition, elimination, oxygenation) and discuss related nursing care. Most of these chapters make use of Example Problems to help focus on concepts-based learning and the importance of *nursing* problems and interventions.

Unit 5 looks at the context for nurses' work. This includes chapters on perioperative nursing, and home and community care, as well as the ethical and legal contexts for nursing work. In addition, we include, in the eBook, excellent chapters on nursing informatics (Chapter 45) and on holistic healing (Chapter 46).

HOW TO USE THIS LEARNING PACKAGE (FOR INSTRUCTORS)

You are fortunate to be working with students at perhaps the most formative point in their nursing education: the fundamentals course. We are certain that each of you will bring your own special style to the teaching of this most-important-of-all nursing course, and that you will find new and creative ways to use the many teaching and learning features we have provided. We hope your enjoyment of this new and improved learning package is equal to our pride in it.

We have also prepared for you a PowerPoint slide presentation and a test bank. You can use either or both to orient new teachers and students so they can easily navigate the entire learning package.

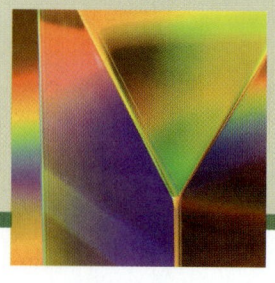

Contributors

The following contributors provided their knowledge and expertise in creating this learning package. We are grateful for their assistance.

Dr. Darlene Sperlazza-Anthony, DNP, MSN, APRN, FNP-BC
Assistant Professor of Nursing
South University, Online Nursing Program
Spirituality chapter

Dr. Lindsey Carlson, MSN, FNP-BC
Assistant Professor of Nursing
William Jewell College, School of Nursing
Skin Integrity & Wound Healing chapter

Dr. Susan Goncalves, DNP, MS, RN-BC
Assistant Professor
Sacred Heart University, College of Nursing
iCare Feature

Dr. Cherie Howk, PhD, FNP-BC
Assistant Professor of Nursing
South University, Online Nursing Program
Sexual Health chapter

Elaine F. Martin, PhD, RNC, FNP, PNP
Assistant Professor of Nursing
Southern Connecticut State University
Active Caring: Patient Experiences in Fundamentals of Nursing, 3rd edition

Alice C. Murr, BSN, RN (retired)
Nursing Author
Nursing Process chapters

Amando Okolo, JD, BSN, RN
Senior Regulatory Analyst
Accenture Health Practice
Legal Accountability chapter

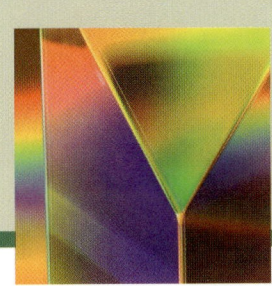

Contributors and Reviewers of Previous Treas and Wilkinson Textbooks

Jocelyn Amberg, MSN, RN
Albuquerque, New Mexico

Elizabeth M. Andal, PhD, PMHCNS-BC, FAAN
Bakersfield, California

Deborah A. Andris, MSN, APNP
Milwaukee, Wisconsin

Patrice Balkcom, RN, MSN
Milledgeville, Georgia

Karen Barnett, DNP, RN
New Haven, Connecticut

Barbara Bonenberger, RN, MNEd, CNE
Pittsburgh, Pennsylvania

Wanda Bonnel, PhD, RN
Kansas City, Kansas

Diane Breckenridge, RN, PhD, MSN
Philadelphia, Pennsylvania

Colette Dieujuste, RNC, MS
Boston, Massachusetts

Joyce Arlene Ennis, RN, MSN, ANP-BC
Waukesha, Wisconsin

Sally Flesch, BSN, MS, EdS, PhD
Moline, Illinois

Deborah L. Galante, RN, MSN, CNOR
Newark, Delaware

Deborah B. Hadley, RN, MSN, CNOR
Natchez, Mississippi

Linda K. Heitman, PhD, RN, ACNS-BC
Cape Girardeau, Missouri

Tracey Hopkins, BSN, RN

Gladys L. Husted, RN, PhD, CNE
Pittsburgh, Pennsylvania

Kathleen C. Jones, MSN, RN, CNS
Greeneville, Tennessee

Jeanie Krause-Bachand, EdD, MSN, RN
York, Pennsylvania

Janice Garrison Lanham, RN, MS, CCNS, FNP
Seneca, South Carolina

Dawn LaPorte, BSN, RN, CRRN
Salem, New Hampshire

Maureen McDonald, RN, MS
Brockton, Massachusetts

Laura Smith McKenna, DNSc, RN
Concord, California

Mary N. Meyer, RN, MSN
Kansas City, Kansas

Pamela S. Miller, MS, RN
Columbus, Ohio

Christine Ouellette, MS, NP
Quincy, Massachusetts

Linda Pasto, MS, RN, CNE
Dryden, New York

Carla E. Randall, RN, PhD
Lewiston, Maine

Debra L. Renna, MSN, CCRN
North Miami, Florida

Patsy M. Spratling, MSN, RN
Ridgeland, Mississippi

Lynn M. Stover, RN, BC, DSN, SANE
Morrow, Georgia

Mary Pat Szutenbach, PhD, RN, CNS
Denver, Colorado

Marcy Tanner, RN, MSN
Weatherford, Oklahoma

Pamela K. Weinberg, RN, MSN
Sumter, South Carolina

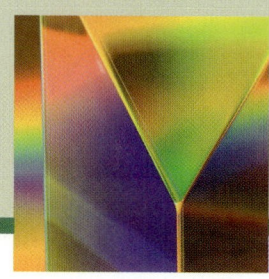

Acknowledgments

We wish to extend sincere thanks to the exceptional team who helped us create this learning package, and especially to the following people:

- **Lisa Houck,** Acquisitions Editor and friend, for her vision in helping to create this popular, new resource for nursing fundamentals where learners can conveniently access all need-to-know information in one book.
- **Julia Curcio,** Content Project Manager, for her skill in organizing and retrieving information and files, all the while churning out a mountain of work. She made our lives easier and kept the process moving smoothly.
- **Beth LoGiudice,** Developmental Editor, for keen eye for detail and amazing attitude, making this project an enjoyable endeavor.
- **Cathy Carroll,** Manager of Project and eProject Management, for her continued support of the fundamentals projects.

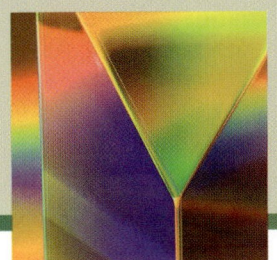

Contents

CHAPTER **13**

Psychosocial Health & Illness   **264**

CHAPTER **20**

Communicating & Therapeutic Relationships   476

CHAPTER **21**

Physical Assessment   499

CHAPTER **22**

Infection Prevention & Control   619

CHAPTER **23**

Safety   667

CHAPTER **24**

Hygiene   704

CHAPTER **25**

Administering Medications 771

Unit 4

Supporting Physiological Function 933

CHAPTER **29**

Bowel Elimination   1006

CHAPTER **30**

Urinary Elimination 1059

CHAPTER **31**

Sensory Perception 1122

CHAPTER **32**

Pain 1149

CHAPTER **33**

Activity & Exercise 1180

CHAPTER **36**

Skin Integrity & Wound Healing   1288

CHAPTER **37**

Oxygenation   1361

CHAPTER **38**

Circulation & Perfusion   1438

CHAPTER **39**

Fluids, Electrolytes, & Acid–Base Balance 1461

Unit 5

The Context for Nurses' Work 1527

CHAPTER **40**

Perioperative Nursing 1528

CHAPTER **41**

Leading & Managing 1584

Meet the Nguyens

$\mathcal{T}$hroughout this text, you will be applying what you have learned as you care for the Nguyen family. In Chapter 1 you will meet Nam Nguyen, a construction worker supervisor, who arrives at the Family Medicine Center for his first physical exam in more than 10 years. His knee pain has caused him to seek help because it affects his work. But as you will see, Nam will discover that he has other serious health problems that require him to be more vigilant about his health. As you read and work through the exercises in Caring for the Nguyens, you will also come to know Nam's wife, Yen Nguyen; his grandchild, Kim Phan; other members of his extended family; and his friends as they deal with health issues and life changes.

Your experience in caring for the Nguyens will show you that every patient comes to you with symptoms, but each person brings unique values, lifestyle, problems, and relationships to the encounter. From the Nguyens, you will learn what it means to care for the whole person and how to be a full-spectrum nurse.

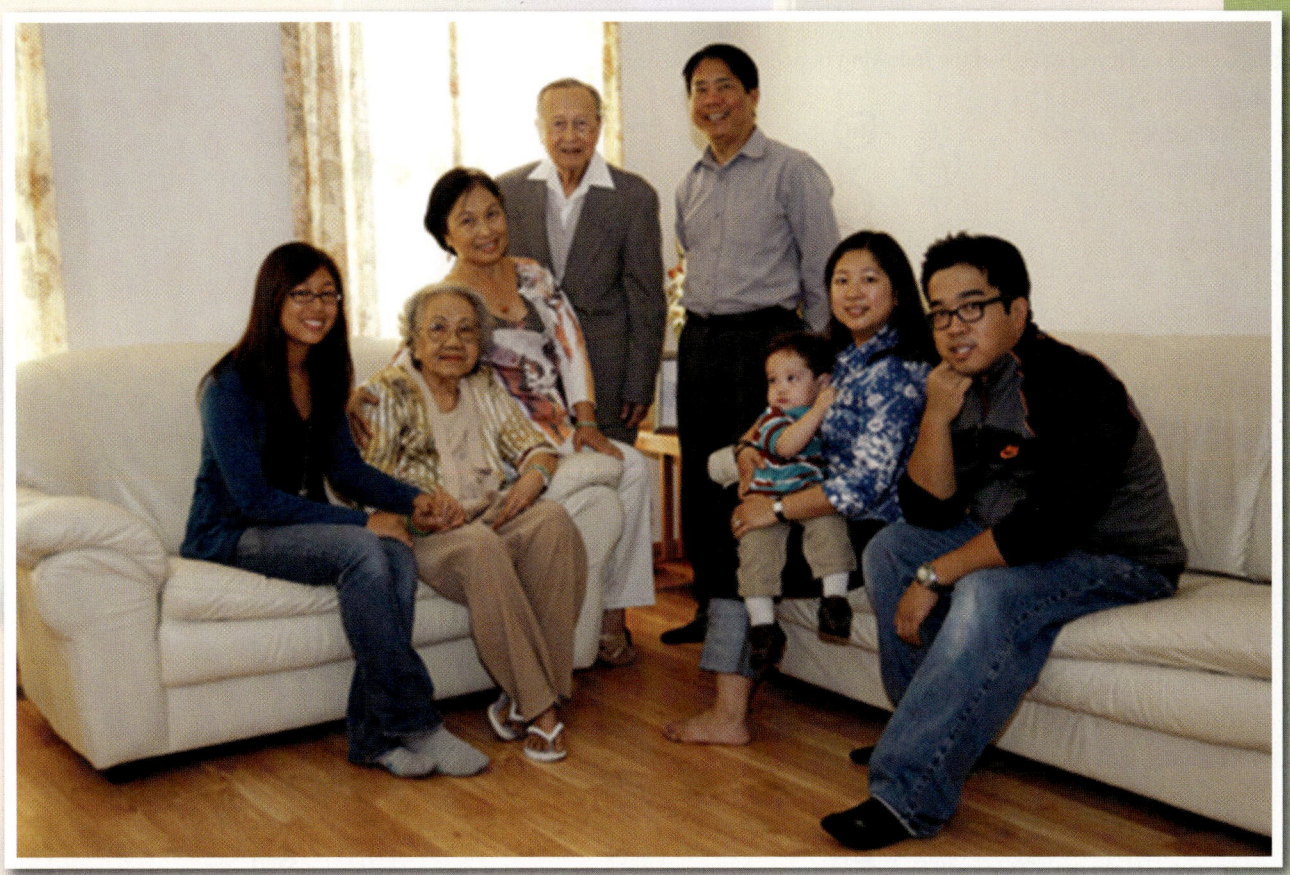

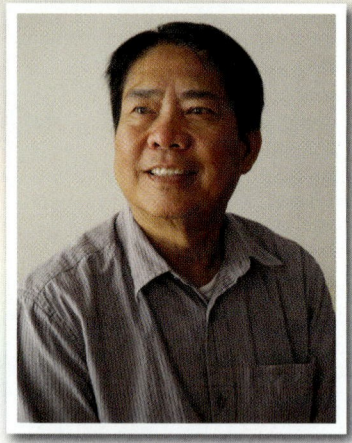

Mr. Nam Nguyen is a new patient at the Family Medicine Center. He arrives at the center for a scheduled physical exam and completes the following admission questionnaire:

Name: *Nam Nguyen*   Age: *56*

Marital Status   S   (M)   W   D   Partnered

If applicable, spouse/partner name: *Yen*

Occupation: *Construction supervisor*   Spouse/partner occupation: *Day-care teacher*

Does your spouse or partner have any healthcare problems? If so, please list:

High blood pressure

Do you have children? *Yes*   Ages? *30, 27, 22*

Please circle yes if you have had the following or no if you have not.

AIDS/HIV +	YES	(NO)	Headaches	YES	(NO)
Allergies	(YES)	NO	Heart Disease	YES	(NO)
Anemia	YES	(NO)	Hernia	(YES)	NO
Anorexia	YES	(NO)	Herpes	YES	(NO)
Anxiety	YES	(NO)	High Cholesterol	YES	(NO)
Arthritis	YES	(NO)	High Blood Pressure	YES	(NO)
Bleeding Disorder	YES	(NO)	Kidney Problems	YES	(NO)
Breast Problems	YES	(NO)	Liver Problems	YES	(NO)
Cancer	YES	(NO)	Abnormal Mammogram	(N/A) YES	NO
Chicken Pox	(YES)	NO	Menopause	(N/A)	YES	NO
Colon Disorder	YES	(NO)	Mononucleosis	YES	(NO)
COPD/Emphysema	YES	(NO)	Multiple Sclerosis	YES	(NO)
Depression	YES	(NO)	Osteoporosis	YES	(NO)
Diabetes	YES	(NO)	Pneumonia	YES	(NO)
Epilepsy/Seizures	YES	(NO)	Polio	YES	(NO)
Eye Problems	(YES)	NO	Prostate Problems	YES	(NO)
Gallbladder Disorder	YES	(NO)	Skin Problems	YES	(NO)
Stomach Problems/Ulcer	YES	(NO)	Stroke	YES	(NO)
Gout	YES	(NO)	Suicide Attempt	YES	(NO)
Gynecological Problems	YES	(NO)	Thyroid Problems	YES	(NO)
Sexually Transmitted Disease	YES	(NO)	Other	YES	(NO)

Please list your current medications and dosages. Also list over-the-counter and herbal products you use regularly.

Ibuprofen   *Ben-Gay Balm on knees*

MultiVitamin 1 per day

Acetaminophen

The Diagnosis

During the visit, the clinic nurse records the following information in Mr. Nguyen's chart:

Height	5 ft 4 in.
Weight	165 lb (75 kg)
BP	162/94 mm Hg
Pulse	84 beats/min
RR	20 breaths/min
Temp	98.2°F oral

Presenting Complaint: Patient states he is here to become established as a patient at the center and that he has not had a physical exam in more than 10 years. Wife accompanies. He is currently experiencing bilateral knee pain that is affecting his work performance. "I supervise construction workers. To check on things, I have to climb up and down ladders, lift things, and crawl around a lot." Has not missed any work but has been using increasing amounts of acetaminophen and ibuprofen "to get through the day." The medications provide only limited relief. States pain occurs daily even if not at work and is achy and dull. Feels best when he is off his feet. Desires pain relief and checkup. Explains that both parents have heart disease, his father had cancer, and his mother has diabetes. Wife expresses worry that he may be developing heart problems "because he's so tired after work and he gets short of breath easily."

The nurse explains to Nam that he will be seen by the nurse practitioner shortly. She asks him whether he would like his wife to be present for the exam. He answers yes.

Zach Miller, MSN, FNP-BC, is on duty at the center today. Zach has 10 years of experience as an RN in the emergency department and urgent care clinic. He has been a family nurse practitioner (FNP-BC) for 5 years. Zach enters the room and introduces himself to Mr. and Mrs. Nguyen. To begin the exam, Zach reviews the information Mr. Nguyen supplied on the admission form and then asks Nam about his family history.

Zach:	Are your parents still living?
Nam:	Yes, they're both alive. My father is 80 years old and my mother is 76.
Zach:	I'd like to hear a little more about your family history. Tell me about your father's cancer. How old was he when he was first diagnosed? Has he had treatment?

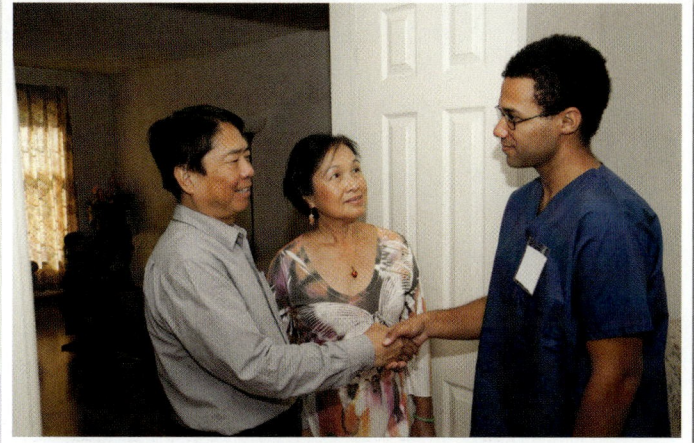

Nam:	He was probably about 60 when he first found out about it. I know he had some kind of surgery and takes medicines but I don't know the details. He seems all right though.
Zach:	Your father also has high blood pressure and heart disease. Please tell me a little more about that.
Nam:	My father and mother both have high blood pressure and heart disease. They both take medicines for their blood pressure. My father had a small heart attack about 10 years ago. My mother has never had a heart attack that I know of, but she sometimes has chest pain.
Zach:	Your mother also has diabetes?
Nam:	She's had that for a long time. A lot of people in my family have diabetes, especially on my father's side—but nobody in my mother's family. Yet my mother is the one with the diabetes!
Yen:	A lot of people in my family have diabetes too. But so far I'm okay, I think.
Zach:	Have you had a health exam lately, Mrs. Nguyen?
Yen:	Not in about a year, but I'm going to schedule an appointment here.

The Nguyens and Zach continue to review the health information. After reviewing the history and discussing current complaints, Zach performs a complete physical exam.

How Nurses Think

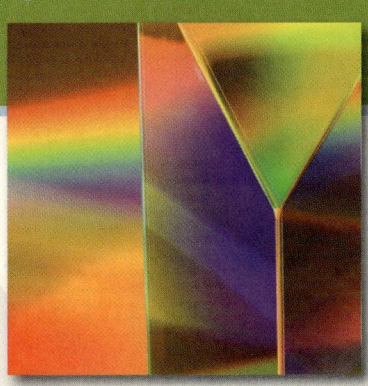

CHAPTER 1

Nursing Past & Present

Learning Outcomes

After completing this chapter, you should be able to:

➤ Define *nursing* in your own words.

➤ Discuss the transitions that nursing education has undergone in the last century.

➤ Differentiate between the various forms of nursing education.

➤ Explain how nursing practice is regulated.

➤ Give four examples of influential nursing organizations.

➤ Name and recognize the four purposes of nursing care.

➤ Describe the healthcare delivery system in the United States, including sites for care, types of workers, regulation, and financing of healthcare.

➤ Name nine expanded roles for nursing.

➤ Discuss issues related to healthcare reform.

➤ Delineate the forces and trends affecting contemporary nursing practice.

Key Concepts

Contemporary nursing education
Contemporary nursing practice
Healthcare delivery system
Nursing
Nursing history

Related Concepts

See the Concept Map at the end of this chapter.

Nurses Make a Difference . . .

Then & Now

Time: 1854, the Crimean Conflict (Russia). Place: Uskudar (Scutari), Turkey, across the Bosporus Strait from Constantinople (Istanbul).

The hospital in Scutari is several days' journey by ship from the battle in Crimea. The injured and dying lie on cots or on crowded floors filled with filth. There are few blankets; soldiers arrive muddy from battle and covered with crusted blood. Outside, the air is crisp, yet the barrack reeks of disease and death. For several weeks, the army physicians refuse to allow Florence Nightingale and her staff of 38 nurses to do any real nursing work. Meanwhile, the nurses review conditions and open windows to clear the fetid air. Next, they scrub all surfaces—ceiling to floor.

They bathe the wounded, sew bedclothes, and fashion bandages. As they prove their usefulness, they are allowed to dress wounds, feed the injured, and comfort those who are in pain or dying. They offer emotional care and encouragement and help write letters home. Within a few months, the mortality rate drops from 47% to 2% and morale improves immeasurably.

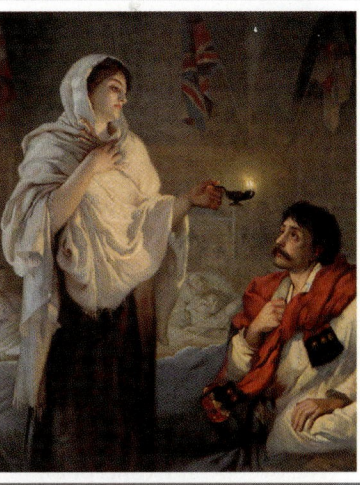

(Continued)

Nurses Make a Difference . . .(continued)

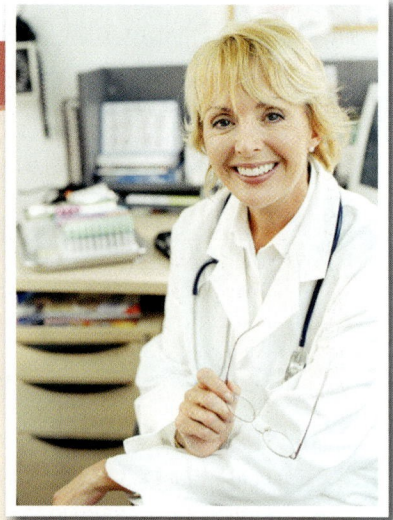

Time: 2017. Place: Your Local Hospital.

While standing at the bedside mixing an antibiotic solution, Susan listens to the ventilator cycle. She notes that her client has begun to trigger breaths on his own. In the background she hears the cardiac monitor sounds, which have become more irregular over the past hour. She mentally runs through her client assessment. "Why is his heart so irritable?" she wonders. She calls the lab and has the morning blood work results e-mailed to her. Susan notes that the potassium level is low (2.9 mEq/L). She notifies the provider of the lab results and the client's cardiac irritability, adding, "The client's potassium is low from the diarrhea he's had since we began the antibiotics." Together they develop a plan to administer intravenous (IV) potassium to raise the client's potassium level and to check the level every 8 hours. Several hours later, Susan documents on the computer that the *ectopy* (irregular heartbeat) has decreased to fewer than 2 beats/min.

Time: 2030. Place: A Local Home.

Yesterday, Mr. Samuels underwent cardiac surgery. He was discharged to his home this morning and is now under your care. As a home health nurse, your role is to assess his condition, provide skilled care, teach Mr. Samuels how to care for himself, instruct his family about his care, and coordinate any required additional services. Since discharge, you have been monitoring his condition remotely via telehealth technologies. Mrs. Samuels greets you at the front door. She tells you that her husband is in a lot of pain and that the chest drainage system is full. She looks frightened as she says, "When my father had cardiac surgery 25 years ago, he spent 4 days in the hospital. I don't understand why my husband got sent home so quickly." You explain that changes in technology and the healthcare system allow you to take care of clients in their own homes who would previously have been in the hospital. As you begin your assessments, you tell Mrs. Samuels, "After I've gathered more information, we'll make a plan for his care that will make all of us more comfortable."

In each of these scenarios, the nurses engaged in *full-spectrum nursing;* that is, they used their minds and their hands to improve the client's comfort and condition. Their actions exemplify caring. As the scenarios illustrate, nursing roles have changed over time, yet nursing remains a profession dedicated to care of the client.

Think **Like a Nurse 1-1**

The Institute of Medicine (IOM) (Greiner & Knebel, 2003) identified core competencies for healthcare providers (see the Safe, Effective Nursing Care box What Is Safe, Effective Nursing Care [SENC]?). These IOM competencies are the basis for the SENC competencies. You will see them used throughout this text. Which of these competencies did Florence Nightingale demonstrate? Explain your thinking.

ABOUT THE KEY CONCEPTS

The overarching concept for this chapter is of **nursing.** As you come to understand other key concepts (i.e., **nursing history, contemporary nursing education, contemporary nursing practice, healthcare delivery system**), you will grasp how nursing has evolved into today's contemporary nursing practice.

HISTORICAL CONTEXT OF NURSING

KEY POINT: *An understanding of the past can lend insight into the customs, values, and future of nursing.* When exploring history, it becomes apparent that societal beliefs about health and illness, Christianity, and the military had strong influences on the evolution and images of professional nursing.

Images of Nursing

As you think of each of the three scenarios at the opening of this chapter, what images of the scene and of the nurse do you see? Does each of these images reinforce nursing's legacy of caring? What is your image of yourself as a nurse? The following are images of the nurse that have developed throughout history—and that persist to a greater or lesser extent even now. To view a PechaKucha slide presentation, Soul of the Nurse, about the images of nursing, enter this URL into your browser: http://www.elizabethannrobinson.com/nurse-archetype/

Angel of Mercy This image grew out of the influence of religion and the risks inherent to the practice of nursing. Images of the angel-nurse are usually serene and content and include a halo or other religious symbol.

Battle-Ax The image of the nurse as a battle-ax emerged as science and philosophy grew popular during the 17th century and religious orders became less common. A more recent historical example is found in the 1975 film *One Flew Over the Cuckoo's Nest,* in which Nurse Ratched personifies the nurse as the battle-ax or torturer, treating her patients with cruelty and disdain.

Nurse as Professional The battle-ax image of an unprofessional nurse remained until it was transformed by Florence Nightingale (Fig. 1-1). Florence Nightingale kept meticulous notes and statistics that were used for advocating and obtaining

What Is Safe, Effective Nursing Care (SENC)?

Competencies: This table contains the IOM competencies and their parallels to safe, effective nursing care that a graduate nurse should be able to provide within the framework of the full-spectrum nursing model (see Chapter 2). To implement full-spectrum nursing, a nurse must demonstrate the model concepts (thinking, doing, and caring) that are aspects of every competency.

IOM Core Competencies	Safe, Effective Nursing Care (Thinking, Doing, Caring)
Provide patient-centered care ➤ Respect patients' differences, values, preferences, and expressed needs ➤ Relieve pain and suffering ➤ Coordinate continuous care ➤ Communicate and provide patient education ➤ Focus on health promotion and illness prevention	**Provide goal-directed, client-centered care** ➤ Establish mutual goals with clients ➤ Show respect for client values, religious beliefs, needs, and preferences ➤ Implement interventions to promote client comfort ➤ Provide client education to foster informed decisions and involvement in care and to facilitate postdischarge health
Work in interprofessional teams ➤ Collaborate, communicate, and jointly implement client care	**Collaborate with the interprofessional healthcare team** ➤ Function as an essential member of the healthcare team ➤ Develop a comprehensive plan of client care that includes members of the interprofessional healthcare team ➤ Evaluate client care from a holistic, multiteam approach
Employ evidence-based practice ➤ Integrate research with clinical expertise and patient values for optimal care ➤ Maintain knowledge of current research	**Validate evidence-based research to incorporate into practice** ➤ Incorporate evidence-based findings into client care ➤ Evaluate client outcomes using valid and reliable research tools
Apply quality improvement ➤ Identify and avoid care errors ➤ Design a framework that includes structure, process, and outcomes in relation to patient and community needs ➤ Evaluate the framework	**Provide safe, quality client care** ➤ Evaluate and use techniques/processes to avoid medical/nursing errors in the delivery of client care ➤ Design a "Thinking, Doing, Caring" framework that incorporates a holistic approach to client care ➤ Evaluate the framework, incorporating the structure, process, and outcomes components of quality improvement approaches
Utilize informatics ➤ Communicate, manage knowledge, mitigate error, and support decision making using information technology	**Embrace/incorporate technological advances** ➤ Use technology to deliver safe, effective care ➤ Remain current in information technology ➤ Communicate with technology support systems to ensure optimal client outcomes

Source: Greiner, A., & Knebel, E. (Eds.). (2003). *Health professions education: A bridge to quality.* Institute of Medicine (US) Committee on the Health Professions Education Summit. Washington, DC: National Academies Press. Retrieved from http://www.ncbi.nlm.nih.gov/books/NBK221528/

changes in healthcare. She used her political connections and social standing to return nursing to a respectable profession. The Nightingale School for Nurses was opened in 1860 and is considered the first official nursing program.

Naughty Nurse The image of the sexy, risqué nurse arose in the early part of the 20th century with burlesque shows and still persists today. For example, in many television programs such as *M*A*S*H* and, more recently, *Grey's Anatomy,* nurses are portrayed as sexy, mindless, irrelevant, or simply potential dates for bright and talented surgeons.

Military Image Throughout the last century (the 1900s), nurses were frequently portrayed in uniform providing support at the battlefield, and nurses are still often characterized as warriors fighting disease. The impact of wars has had positive influences on the development of nursing as a profession. Nurses took the lead in providing care to the sick, wounded, and dying soldiers in each of the following wars, which highlighted the need for nurses to be trained: American Civil War, Spanish-American War, World Wars I and II, and the Korean, Vietnam, Iraq, and Afghanistan conflicts.

Handmaiden Image This stereotype portrays the male physician in the dominant role, with the female nurse merely assisting the doctor or perhaps supporting the patient at the bedside. This image grew out of the nurse's early limited role in healing, from the legal and financial authority of physicians, and from the nurse's working position as an employee.

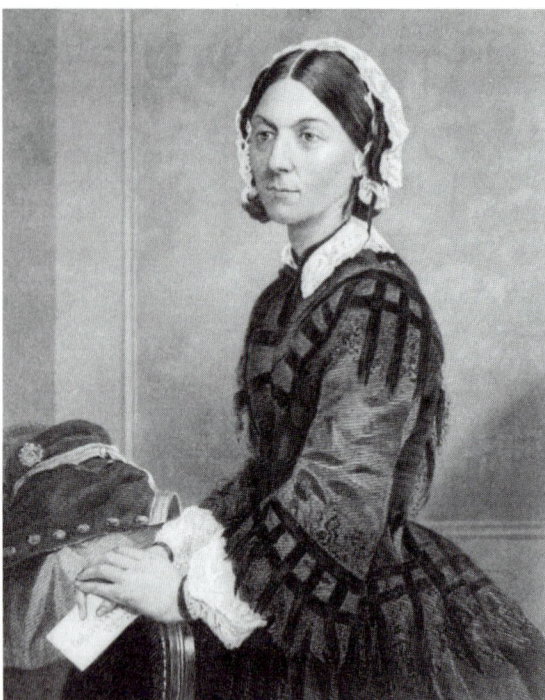

FIGURE I-I Florence Nightingale (1820–1910).

Nursing Today: Full-Spectrum Nursing

Nurses today are highly trained, well-educated, caring, and competent professionals. They are essential members of the healthcare team. The complexity of healthcare delivery requires that nurses use their critical thinking, communication, organizational, leadership, advocacy, and technical skills to ensure that patients receive safe and effective care.

Safe, Effective Nursing Care Nursing education emphasizes quality and safety so that students will be able to deliver safe, effective nursing care in their practice after graduation.

- *Nursing Practice.* The Institute of Medicine (Greiner & Knebel, 2003) has identified quality and safety competencies that all health professionals are expected to demonstrate in their practice (see the Safe, Effective Nursing Care box Quality Improvement Competency).
- *Nursing Education.* The Quality and Safety Education for Nurses (QSEN) project has identified competencies that students are expected to acquire before graduation (Cronenwett, Sherwood, Barnsteiner, et al., 2007). If you are interested in the QSEN competencies,

    Go to the QSEN Institute Web site at http://qsen.org/ competencies/pre-licensure-ksas/

- *Full-Spectrum Nursing and Safe, Effective Nursing Care.* To implement quality care using the full-spectrum nursing model (Chapter 2), we will refer to "safe, effective nursing care" competencies (see the Safe, Effective Nursing Care [SENC] boxes that appear in almost all chapters in this book).

Application of Knowledge, Skill, and Caring KEY POINT: *Nurses apply knowledge from the arts and sciences in their various roles to provide patient-centered care (Table 1-1).* Nurses use clinical judgment, critical thinking, and problem-solving as they care for patients. (You will learn more about full-spectrum nursing in the section in Chapter 2, What Is Full-Spectrum Nursing?) ✚ To be safe providers, nurses

must carefully consider their actions and think carefully about the patient, the treatment plan, the healthcare environment, the patient's support system, the nurse's support system and resources, and safety.

Clinical judgment involves observing, comparing, contrasting, and evaluating the client's condition to determine whether change has occurred. It also involves careful consideration of the client's health status in light of what is expected based on the client's condition, medications, and treatment. These actions, collectively known as the nursing process, are discussed in Chapters 3 through 7 and in each of the clinically focused chapters.

Critical thinking is a reflective thinking process that involves collecting information, analyzing the adequacy and accuracy of the information, and carefully considering options for action. Nurses use critical thinking in every aspect of nursing care. Critical thinking is discussed at length in Chapter 2 and applied in every chapter in this text.

Problem-solving is a process by which nurses consider an issue and attempt to find a satisfactory solution to achieve the best outcomes. You will often use problem-solving in your professional life. The nursing process (see Chapters 2 through 7) is one type of problem-solving process.

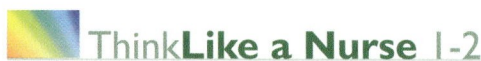

ThinkLike a Nurse 1-2

In the three scenarios of Nurses Make a Difference . . . Then & Now, what image of nursing predominates: thinking or doing?

CONTEMPORARY NURSING: EDUCATION, REGULATION, AND PRACTICE

As a student about to enter your new professional life, you need to realistically grasp the nature and demands of your chosen career. The remainder of this chapter discusses the current state of nursing, nursing education, and the trends affecting nursing. You will also be introduced to the healthcare delivery system.

How Is Nursing Defined?

As you have seen, there are many images of nursing. These images are only loosely based on fact and they sometimes conflict. They make it difficult for the public to know the reality of nursing—and they are confusing to nurses and to other members of the healthcare team. In addition, the constantly changing nature of nursing, healthcare, and society further complicates the definition of *nursing*. **KEY POINT:** *Therefore, it is important for nurses to articulate clearly, for themselves and for the public, what nursing is and what nurses do.* The following are the views of two important nursing organizations in answer to the question, "What is nursing?"

International Council of Nurses Definition

The International Council of Nurses (ICN) is an organization that represents nurses throughout the world. In 1973, ICN defined *nursing* as follows:

> The unique function of the nurse is to assist the individual, sick or well, in the performance of those activities contributing to health or its recovery (or to peaceful death) that he would perform unaided if he had the necessary strength, will or knowledge. (Henderson, 1966, p. 15)

In the decades since the adoption of that definition, nursing throughout the world has changed. Advances in healthcare have

Table 1-1 ➤ Roles and Functions of the Nurse

ROLE	FUNCTION	EXAMPLES
Direct care provider	Addressing the physical, emotional, social, and spiritual needs of the client	Listening to lung sounds Administering medications Patient teaching
Communicator	Using interpersonal and therapeutic communication skills to address the client needs, to facilitate communication in the healthcare team, and to advise the community about health promotion and disease prevention	Counseling a client Discussing unit staffing needs at a meeting Teaching about HIV prevention at a local school
Client/family educator	Assessing and diagnosing the teaching needs of the client, group, family, or community; planning how to meet those needs, implementing the teaching plan, and evaluating its effectiveness	Preoperative teaching Prenatal education for siblings Community classes on nutrition
Client advocate	Supporting clients' right to make healthcare decisions when they are able to voice their opinions and protecting them from harm when they are unable to make decisions	Helping a client explain to his family that he does not want to have further chemotherapy
Counselor	Using therapeutic communication skills to advise clients about health-related issues	Counseling a client on weight-loss strategies
Change agent	Advocating for change on an individual, family, group, community, or societal level that enhances health. The nurse may use counseling, communication, and educator skills to accomplish such change.	Working to improve the nutritional quality of the lunch program at a preschool
Leader	Inspiring others by setting an example of positive health, assertive communication, and willingness to improve	Florence Nightingale Walt Whitman Harriet Tubman
Manager	Coordinating and managing the activities of all members of the team	Charge nurse on a hospital unit (e.g., assigns patients to staff nurses)
Case manager	Coordinating the care delivered to a client	Coordinator of services for clients with tuberculosis
Research consumer	Applying evidence-based practice to provide the most appropriate care, to identify clinical problems that warrant research, and to protect the rights of research subjects	Reading journal articles Attending continuing education; seeking additional education

altered the type of care required by clients. To reflect these changes, the ICN has revised its definition of nursing, as follows:

Nursing encompasses autonomous and collaborative care of individuals of all ages, families, groups and communities, sick or well and in all settings. Nursing includes the promotion of health, prevention of illness, and the care of ill, disabled and dying people. Advocacy, promotion of a safe environment, research, participation in shaping health policy and in patient and health systems management, and education are also key nursing roles. (International Council of Nurses [ICN], 2010)

ThinkLike a Nurse 1-3

Look at the three scenarios of Nurses Make a Difference . . . Then & Now. What nursing actions did the nurses perform that are represented in the ICN definition of *nursing*?

American Nursing Association Definition

You can see similar changes in the approach of the American Nurses Association (ANA). In 1980, the ANA defined *nursing* as "the diagnosis and treatment of human responses to actual and potential health problems" (p. 2). Attempts to refine this definition have been difficult. Nurses are a widely varied group of people with varying skills. They perform activities designed to provide care ranging from basic to complex in a growing number of settings. Therefore, it is not easy to describe the boundaries of the profession.

In 2010, the ANA acknowledged five characteristics of registered nursing:

- Nursing practice is individualized.
- Nurses coordinate care by establishing partnerships (with persons, families, support systems, and other providers).
- Caring is central to the practice of the registered nurse.

- Registered nurses use the nursing process to plan and provide individualized care to their healthcare consumers.
- A strong link exists between the professional work environment and the registered nurse's ability to provide quality healthcare and achieve optimal outcomes. (ANA, 2010a, pp. 4–5)

The ANA now defines professional nursing as:

Nursing is the protection, promotion, and optimization of <u>health</u> and abilities, prevention of illness and injury, facilitation of healing, alleviation of suffering through the diagnosis and treatment of human response, and advocacy in the care of individuals, families, groups, communities, and populations. (ANA, 2015, p. 1)

Why Is a Definition Important?

Nursing organizations and leaders have pushed for accurate definitions to (1) help the public understand the value of nursing, (2) describe what activities and roles belong to nursing versus other health professions, and (3) help students and practicing nurses understand what is expected of them within their role as nurses. From history, you can tell that nursing has undergone tremendous change, from a role limited to providing kindness and support to full-spectrum nursing, which is based in science but still focuses on care and nurturing. Box 1-1 lists several additional definitions of nursing for you to consider.

As a student entering nursing, you can use definitions and descriptions to understand what is expected of you. To aid you in this task, refer to Table 1-1 and review the essential components of the nursing role. While in the clinical setting, you will observe nurses functioning in each of these capacities and identify the qualities listed in Box 1-2 that are essential for safe nursing practice

---

BOX 1-1 ■ What Is Nursing?

- I use the word *nursing,* for want of a better. It has been limited to signify little more than the administration of medicines and the application of poultices. It ought to signify the proper use of fresh air, light, warmth, cleanliness, quiet, and the proper choosing and giving of diet—all at the least expense of vital power to the patient. (Nightingale, 1876, p. 5)
- Events that give rise to higher degrees of consideration for those who are helpless or oppressed, kindliness and sympathy for the unfortunate and for those who suffer, tolerance for those of differing religion, race, color, etc.—all tend to promote activities like nursing which are primarily humanitarian. (Dock & Stewart, 1938, p. 3)
- Nursing has been called the oldest of the arts and the youngest of the professions. As such, it has gone through many stages and has been an integral part of societal movements. Nursing has been involved in the existing culture—shaped by it and yet helping to develop it. (Donahue, 1985, p. 3)
- Nurses provide care for people in the midst of health, pain, loss, fear, disfigurement, death, grieving, challenge, growth, birth, and transition on an intimate front-line basis. Expert nurses call this the privileged place of nursing. (Benner & Wrubel, 1989, p. xi)
- Nurses provide and coordinate patient care, educate patients and the public about various health conditions, and provide advice and emotional support to patients and their family members. (Bureau of Labor Statistics, U.S. Department of Labor, 2014b)

BOX 1-2 ■ Important Qualities for Nurses

Critical-Thinking Skills

Required Action: Monitor the client, note changes, and take actions to ensure safe and effective care.
Example: Call the provider to obtain a stronger pain medication for a client who, 2 hours after receiving pain medication, rates his pain 7 out of 10.

Caring and Compassion

Required Action: Show kindness, concern, and sincerity that convey to clients that you care about their well-being.
Example: Sit with and hold the hand of a client who has just been told that he has a terminal illness.

Detail Oriented

Required Action: Pay attention to details to prevent and identify potentially harmful errors in care.
Example: Seek clarification and correct a dosage that is written as 7 mg that should be 0.7 mg.

Organizational Skills

Required Action: Prioritize the needs of your client and meet the needs of the most critical clients first.
Example: Care for the postoperative client with difficulty breathing prior to performing a dressing change.

Speaking Skills

Required Action: Communicate correct and pertinent information to clients and members of the healthcare team.
Example: Teach the client how to perform a dressing change at home after discharge from the hospital.

Listening Skills

Required Action: Listen to clients' concerns; take verbal or telephone prescriptions from providers.
Example: The provider telephones you and gives you prescriptions to implement for your client.

Patience

Required Action: In stressful situations in the work environment, think clearly and take the correct actions.
Example: Remain calm when a client's condition deteriorates, provide the needed care, and transfer the client to the ICU.

Competence

Required Action: Obtain the knowledge and skills to ensure safe, quality client outcomes.
Example: Recognize that the correct dose for the drug is 0.10 mg rather than 10 mg.

Emotional Stability

Required Action: Develop the ability to cope with human suffering, emergencies, and other stresses.
Example: Provide care to a patient accused of child abuse and to the child who suffered severe head injuries.

Physical Stamina

Required Action: Perform physical tasks and endure long hours walking and standing.
Example: Assist another nurse to lift a 300-lb patient after working 10 hours of a 12-hour shift.

Source: Adapted from Bureau of Labor Statistics, U.S. Department of Labor. (2014b). Registered nurses. *Occupational outlook handbook, 2014–15 edition.* Washington, DC: Author.

KnowledgeCheck 1-1

What factors make it difficult to define *nursing*?
Based on the ICN definition of nursing, what does a nurse do?

Is Nursing a Profession, Discipline, or Occupation?

One strategy used to describe a field of work is to categorize it as a profession, a discipline, or an occupation.

Profession Although the term *profession* is freely used, a group must meet certain criteria to be considered a **profession** (see Table 1-2). Nursing appears to meet all criteria of a profession as defined by Starr (1982) and Miller, Adams, and Beck (1993).

Discipline To be considered a **discipline,** a profession must have a domain of knowledge that has both theoretical and practical boundaries. The **theoretical boundaries** of a profession are the questions that arise from clinical practice and are then investigated through research. The **practical boundaries** are the current state of knowledge and research in the field—the facts that dictate safe practice (Meleis, 1991). A case can be made that nursing is both a profession and a discipline:

- It is a scientifically based and self-governed *profession* that focuses on the ethical care of others.
- It is a *discipline*, driven by aspects of theory and practice. It demands mastery of both theoretical knowledge and clinical skills.

Occupation In spite of meeting criteria for both designations (profession and discipline), nursing is often described as an **occupation,** or job. Most physicians are in control of their practice environment, working conditions, and schedule. In contrast, most nurses are hourly wage earners. The employer, not the nurse, decides the conditions of practice and the nature of the work. Nevertheless, nurse practice acts do not prevent nurses from functioning more autonomously.

Rather than continuing to develop arguments to "prove" that nursing is a profession, the following actions might do more to improve the status of nursing:

- Standardizing the educational requirements for entry into practice
- Enacting uniform continuing education requirements
- Encouraging the participation of more nurses in professional organizations
- Educating the public about the true nature of nursing practice

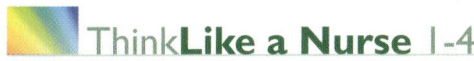

ThinkLike a Nurse 1-4

Evaluate the status of nursing. Is nursing a respected profession? Give examples to support your opinion.

How Do Nurses' Educational Paths Differ?

The transition into the nursing profession involves the concepts of formal and informal processes. **Formal education** consists of completing the initial and continuing education required for licensure. **Informal education** involves a gradual progression in skill and clinical judgment that allows the nurse to advance in the profession.

Formal Education

When the patient calls out "Nurse!," who can respond? To legally use the title *nurse*, a person must be a graduate of an accredited nursing education program and have successfully passed the National Council Licensure Examination (NCLEX®). Other personnel might respond to the patient's call, but they cannot legally be considered nurses. Students may enter nursing through two paths: as a practical nurse or as a registered nurse.

Practical and Vocational Nursing Education

Practical nursing education prepares nurses to provide basic care to clients under the direction of a registered nurse (RN) or primary care provider. Practical nurses are known as licensed practical nurses (LPNs) or licensed vocational nurses (LVNs). Educational programs for LPN/LVNs offer both classroom and clinical teaching and usually last 1 year. After completing the practical nursing education program, the student must pass the NCLEX-PN® exam.

Registered Nursing Entry Education

Currently, five educational pathways lead to licensure as a registered nurse (RN). Graduates of all these programs

Table 1-2 ▶ Nursing: Is It a Profession?	
STARR CRITERIA	**EXAMPLES IN NURSING**
The knowledge of the group must be based on technical and scientific knowledge.	■ Entry-level nursing education requires course work in basic and social sciences as well as humanities, arts, and general education. ■ Nursing education and practice are increasingly based on research from nursing and related fields.
The knowledge and competence of members of the group must be evaluated by a community of peers.	■ State regulatory bodies have defined the criteria that nurses must meet to practice, and they monitor members for adherence to standards.
The group must have a service orientation and a code of ethics.	■ Nursing is clearly focused on providing service to others. ■ The major professional organizations have developed ethical guidelines to guide the practice of nursing.

Source: Starr, P. (1982). The social transformation of American medicine. New York, NY: Basic Books.

must successfully complete the NCLEX-RN® exam to practice as RNs.

- **Diploma programs.** Hospital-based programs, modeled after the Nightingale Schools of Nursing apprenticeship style of learning, were the mainstay of nursing education until the 1960s. The typical program lasts 3 years and focuses on clinical experience in direct patient care. Since the 1960s, the number of diploma programs has steadily decreased. In 2014, only about 4% of nursing schools were diploma programs (National League for Nursing, 2014). These programs prepare 4% of new RN graduates (Robert Wood Johnson Foundation [RWJF], 2013).

- **Associate degree.** This type of program, conceptualized by Mildred Montag, emerged during the nursing shortage following World War II. Associate degree (AD) programs offered in community colleges accounted for 58% of all nursing programs in 2014 (National League for Nursing, 2014). Although the nursing component typically lasts 2 years, students are required to take numerous other courses in liberal arts and the sciences. ADN nurses are prepared to provide direct patient care.

- **Baccalaureate degree.** The course of study in baccalaureate programs lasts at least eight semesters. Students are prepared to address complex clinical situations, provide direct patient care, work in community care, apply research findings, and enter graduate education (Bureau of Labor Statistics, U.S. Department of Labor, 2014b). The goal of the Institute of Medicine (2011) is to increase the proportion of baccalaureate-prepared nurses to 80% by 2020. In 2014, only about 38% of nursing schools were baccalaureate programs (National League for Nursing, 2014). These programs prepare about 43% of new RN graduates (RWJF, 2013).

- **RN to BSN.** With the current trend to hire baccalaureate-prepared nurses, many ADN graduates enroll in programs to obtain the BSN degree. The number of RN-BSN graduates increased an estimated 86% from 2009 to 2013 (Health Resources and Services Administration, 2013). These programs prepare about 53% of new RN graduates (RWJF, 2013).

- **Master's entry.** The typical student in these programs has a baccalaureate degree in another field and has entered nursing as a second career. Programs usually are completed in 3 years of full-time study, with the first year devoted to basic nursing content. At the program's completion, the student is eligible to take the licensing exam and is awarded a master's degree in nursing.

- **Doctoral entry**. This is the most unusual entry pathway into nursing. The nursing doctorate (ND) path parallels the pathway through which physicians enter the healthcare field. This entry path has very limited enrollment.

Graduate Nursing Education

Graduate education prepares the RN for advanced practice, expanded roles, or research.

- **Master's degree programs** prepare RNs to function in a more independent and autonomous role, such as nurse practitioner, clinical specialist, nurse educator, or nursing administrator. These programs typically last 2 years or longer.

- **Doctoral programs** in nursing offer professional degrees. Typically, the student has completed a baccalaureate and master's degree before entry into a doctoral program. Doctoral degree programs in nursing offer one of the following:
  - Doctor of Nursing Practice (DNP)—a practice degree
  - Doctor of Nursing Science (DSN/DNSc)—a degree with a focus on research
  - Doctor of Philosophy (PhD)—a research-focused degree.

Other Forms of Formal Education

Advances in healthcare have a strong influence on nursing practice. Because nurses must keep current in their practice, you will be socialized to the concept of "nurses as lifelong learners." This means that you must engage in continuing education to enhance your intellectual and practical knowledge throughout your nursing career.

- **Continuing education** is designed to help you stay current in your clinical knowledge after graduation. Continuing education programs are available at work sites, at colleges and universities, through privately operated educational groups, on the Internet, and in professional journals. In many states, renewal of the nursing license requires successful completion of a specified number, and in some cases type of, continuing education courses. Your state board of nursing (SBN) will notify you about continuing education requirements, if any, when you receive your initial license. Thereafter, the SBN will notify you of any changes in the requirements, as regulations change frequently.

- **In-service education** is another form of ongoing education. It is offered at the work site and usually does not count toward meeting the continuing education requirement for license renewal. In-service education is typically institution specific (e.g., change in policies) or product specific (e.g., use of new equipment). It is designed to enhance your continuing competence in knowledge, skills, and attitudes.

Informal Education

Socialization is the informal education that occurs as you move into your new profession. It is the knowledge gained from direct experience, observation in the real world, and informal discussion with peers and colleagues. **KEY POINT:** *Professional socialization begins when you enter the educational program and continues as you gain expertise throughout your career.* Informal education complements formal education to create clinical competence.

Benner's Model

Patricia Benner (1984) described the process by which a nurse acquires clinical skills and judgment. It shows that expertise is a personal integration of knowledge that requires technical skill, thoughtful application, and insight. That is what we mean in this text when we use the term *full-spectrum nursing* as thinking, doing, and caring. Benner's process occurs in stages:

- *Stage 1: Novice.* This phase begins with the onset of education. The novice has little clinical experience and is task oriented and narrowly focused on "learning the rules."

- *Stage 2: Advanced beginner.* A new graduate usually functions at this level. An advanced beginner begins to focus on more aspects of a clinical situation, uses more facts, and recognizes abnormalities in situations. However, the nurse functioning at this level cannot readily attach meaning to the findings.

- *Stage 3: Competence.* Nurses achieve competence after 2 to 3 years of nursing practice in the same area. Competent performers have gained additional experience and are able to handle their patient load, deal with complexity, and prioritize situations. They are also more involved in their caregiving role and may be emotionally involved in the clinical choices made. Although competent nurses manage clinical care with mastery, they often do not fully grasp the overall scope and most important aspects.

- *Stage 4: Proficient.* The proficient nurse is able to quickly take in all aspects of a situation and immediately give meaning to the cluster of assessment data. Such nurses are a resource for less experienced nurses. Proficient nurses are able to see the "big picture" and can coordinate services and forecast needs. They are much more flexible and able to adapt to the nuances of various patient situations.

- *Stage 5: Expert.* Expert nurses are able to see what needs to be achieved and how to do it. They trust in and use their intuition while operating with a deep understanding of a situation, often recognizing a problem in the absence of its classic signs and symptoms. They are often consulted when others need advice or assistance.

Benner's model deals with the development of clinical wisdom and competence. Keep in mind that this progression is not automatic. Years of experience do not necessarily move a nurse through the stages. Instead, this model assumes that to improve in skill and judgment, you must also be attuned to each clinical situation. This requires an ability to take in information from a variety of sources and to notice subtle variations. Although expertise (stage 5) is a goal, not everyone can achieve this level.

Nursing Organization Guidelines

The ANA and other organizations are also involved in helping nurses to continue to improve their practice (e.g., by setting standards and articulating nursing values). For example, in the Code for Nurses, the ANA provides guidelines for how nurses should conduct themselves in their day-to-day practice. These guidelines describe acceptable and unacceptable behaviors and identify values to help improve your practice and participation in the profession. Box 1-3 presents values and behaviors essential to nursing practice. See Chapter 43 for further discussion of nursing values and the ANA Code for Nurses.

KnowledgeCheck 1-2

- Compare and contrast formal and informal education.
- Name and describe five educational pathways leading to licensure as an RN.

How Is Nursing Practice Regulated?

Laws, standards of practice, and guidelines from professional organizations regulate the practice of nursing.

Nurse Practice Acts In the United States, each state enacts its own nurse practice act—a compilation of laws that regulate the practice of nursing and direct a state board of nursing to oversee and regulate nursing practice. Although there are minor variations, each board of nursing is responsible for:

- Defining the practice of professional nursing. This definition usually includes the scope of practice (i.e., activities that nurses are expected to perform and, by implication, those they may not).
- Approving nursing education programs
- Establishing criteria that allow a person to be licensed as an RN or LPN/LVN

BOX 1-3 ■ Nursing Values and Behaviors

The nurse's primary concern is the good of the client.
Nurses must be competent.
Nurses demonstrate a strong commitment to service.
Nurses believe in the dignity and worth of each person.
Nurses constantly strive to improve their profession.
Nurses work collaboratively within the profession.

- Developing rules and regulations for guidance to nurses
- Enforcing the rules that govern nursing practice

KEY POINT: *To practice nursing, you must be licensed as a nurse by the state board of nursing.* All states require graduation from an approved nursing program and successful completion of the NCLEX. To receive licensure in another state, the nurse simply applies for licensure by endorsement (reciprocity) or follows the guidance of the mutual recognition model. For further details about licensing and the regulation of nursing practice, see Chapter 44.

Standards of Practice Nursing is also guided by **standards of practice,** which "describe a competent level of nursing care as demonstrated by the critical thinking model known as the nursing process" (ANA, 2015, p. 4). Standards are "authoritative statements of the duties that all registered nurses, regardless of role, population, or specialty, are expected to perform competently" (ANA, 2015, p. 3). Standards provide a guide to the knowledge, skills, and attitudes (KSAs) that nurses must incorporate into their practice to provide safe, quality care. They are also widely used by employers of nurses, professional organizations, and other professions.

As a student nurse, you will use the ANA standards to better define your nursing practice (Table 1-3). Practicing nurses use the standards to judge their own performance, develop an improvement plan, and understand employers' expectations. Employers may incorporate the standards into annual employee evaluation tools. Professional organizations use the standards to educate the public about nursing, to plan for continuing education programs for nurses, and to guide their efforts at lobbying and other advocacy activities for nurses. Finally, other health professionals read the standards of practice to examine the boundaries between nursing and their professions.

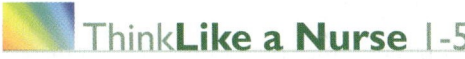 ThinkLike a Nurse 1-5

What additional information have you learned about nursing from your review of the ANA Standards of Practice?

What Are Some Important Nursing Organizations?

Numerous organizations are involved in the profession of nursing. Some of the most influential are discussed here.

American Nurses Association

The American Nurses Association (ANA) is the official professional organizations for nurses in the United States. The ANA was formed in 1911 from an organization previously known as the Nurses' Associated Alumnae of the United States and Canada. Originally this organization focused on (1) establishing standards of nursing to promote high-quality care and (2) working toward licensure as a means of ensuring adherence to the standards.

The ANA continues to promote the interests of the nursing profession and to update its standards. Representatives are elected from the local branches of the state organizations to bring their concerns to the national level. Local representatives:

- Track healthcare legislation
- Serve as liaisons with national government representatives
- Communicate the impact of enacted legislation on nursing in their area
- Develop and sponsor legislation expected to have a positive effect on nursing and patient care

The ANA publishes educational materials on nursing news, issues, and standards. The official publication is *The American Nurse.*

Table 1-3 ➤ American Nurses Association: Scope and Standards of Nursing Practice

STANDARDS OF CARE

Standard 1	Assessment	The registered nurse collects pertinent data and information relative to the healthcare consumer's health or the situation.
Standard 2	Diagnosis	The registered nurse analyzes the assessment data to determine actual or potential diagnoses, problems, and issues.
Standard 3	Outcome Identification	The registered nurse identifies expected outcomes for a plan individualized to the healthcare consumer or the situation.
Standard 4	Planning	The registered nurse develops a plan that prescribes strategies to attain expected, measurable outcomes.
Standard 5	Implementation	The registered nurse implements the identified plan.
Standard 5A	Coordination of Care	The registered nurse coordinates care delivery.
Standard 5B	Health Teaching and Health Promotion	The registered nurse employs strategies to promote health and a safe environment.
Standard 5C	Consultation	The graduate-level prepared specialty nurse or advanced practice registered nurse provides consultation to influence the identified plan, enhance the abilities of others, and effect change.
Standard 5D	Prescriptive Authority and Treatment	The advanced practice registered nurse uses prescriptive authority, procedures, referrals, treatments, and therapies in accordance with state and federal laws and regulations.
Standard 6	Evaluation	The registered nurse evaluates progress toward attainment of goals and outcomes.

STANDARDS OF PROFESSIONAL PERFORMANCE

Standard 7	Ethics	The registered nurse practices ethically.
Standard 8	Culturally Congruent Practice	The registered nurse practices in a manner that is congruent with cultural diversity and inclusion principles.
Standard 9	Communication	The registered nurse communicates effectively in all areas of practice.
Standard 10	Collaboration	The registered nurse collaborates with healthcare consumers and other key stakeholders in the conduct of nursing practice.
Standard 11	Leadership	The registered nurse leads within the professional practice setting and the profession.
Standard 12	Education	The registered nurse seeks knowledge and competence that reflects current nursing practice and promotes futuristic thinking.
Standard 13	Evidence-based Practice and Research	The registered nurse integrates evidence and research findings into practice.
Standard 14	Quality of Practice	The registered nurse contributes to quality nursing practice.
Standard 15	Professional Practice Evaluation	The registered nurse evaluates one's own and others' nursing practice.
Standard 16	Resource Utilization	The registered nurse utilizes appropriate resources to plan, provide, and sustain evidence-based nursing services that are safe, effective, and fiscally responsible.
Standard 17	Environmental Health	The registered nurse practices in an environmentally safe and healthy manner.

Source: American Nurses Association. (2015). *Nursing: Scope and standards of practice* (3rd ed.). Silver Spring, MD: Author.

National League for Nursing

Originally founded as the American Society of Superintendents of Training Schools for Nurses in 1893, the National League for Nursing (NLN) was the first nursing organization with a goal to establish and maintain a universal standard of education. The NLN:

- Sets standards for all types of nursing education programs
- Studies the nursing workforce
- Lobbies and participates with other major healthcare organizations to set policies for the nursing workforce
- Aids faculty development
- Funds research on nursing education
- Publishes the journal *Nursing Education Perspectives*

International Council of Nursing

The International Council of Nursing (ICN) represents more than 13 million nurses on a global scale. It is composed of a federation of national nursing organizations from more than 130 nations. The ICN aims to ensure quality nursing care for all by:

- Supporting global health policies that advance nursing and improve worldwide health
- Striving to improve working conditions for nurses throughout the world

National Student Nurses Association

The National Student Nurses Association (NSNA) represents nursing students in the United States. It is the student counterpart of the ANA. Like the ANA, this association is made up of elected volunteers who advocate on behalf of student nurses. Local chapters are usually organized at individual schools. The NSNA sponsors yearly conventions to address student concerns. It also publishes *Image,* a journal dedicated to nursing student issues.

Sigma Theta Tau International

Sigma Theta Tau International (STTI) is the international honor society for nursing. Membership includes the clinical, education, and nursing research communities and senior-level baccalaureate and graduate programs. The goal of this organization is to foster nursing scholarship, leadership, service, and research to improve health worldwide. The official publication of STTI is the *Journal of Nursing Scholarship.*

Specialty Organizations

Numerous specialty organizations have developed around clinical specialties, group identification, or similarly held values. The following are some examples:

- *Clinical specialty.* Association of periOperative Registered Nurses (AORN), Association of Nurses in AIDS Care (ANAC), Emergency Nurses Association (ENA)
- *Group identification.* National Organization for Associate Degree Nursing (NOADN), National Association of Hispanic Nurses (NAHN), American Assembly for Men in Nursing (AAMN)
- *Similar values.* Nurses Christian Fellowship (NCF), Nursing Ethics Network (NEN)

Nursing Practice: Caring for Clients

Look again at the definitions of *nursing* in this chapter (e.g., see Box 1-1). Notice that they all agree that nursing is about caring for clients. Research trends show that staffing and the education preparation of the nurse are related to client outcomes. Hospitals with a higher percentage of baccalaureate-prepared RNs reported lower client complications (e.g., lower levels of congestive heart failure mortality, decubitus ulcers, failure to rescue, and postoperative deep vein thrombosis) and shorter length of stay (Blegen, Goode, Park, et al., 2013). Similarly, smaller nurse-to-patient ratios (i.e., when each nurse cared for fewer patients) were related to positive patient outcomes, lower patient mortality, improved detection of predischarge infections, less nurse burnout, and higher job satisfaction for nurses (Aiken, Sloane, Cimiotti, et al., 2010; Penoyer, 2010; Unruh & Zhang, 2012).

Who Are the Recipients of Nursing Care?

The recipients of nursing care may be individuals, groups, families, or communities. They can be referred to as patients, clients, or persons.

- **Direct care** involves personal interaction between the nurse and clients (e.g., giving medications or teaching a client about a treatment).
- **Indirect care** is working on behalf of clients to improve their health status (e.g., ordering unit supplies or serving on an ethics committee).

A nurse may use independent judgment to determine the care needed or may work under the direct order of a primary care provider. As a nurse, you should view patients as active recipients of care. **KEY POINT:** *You should actively encourage clients to participate in decisions about their care and be collaborative members of their healthcare teams.*

What Are the Purposes of Nursing Care?

Nurses provide care to achieve the goals of health promotion, illness prevention, health restoration, and end-of-life care. Together these aspects of care represent a range of services that cover the health spectrum from complete well-being to death.

Where Do Nurses Work?

As a nurse you will have the opportunity to work in a variety of settings. During your education you will have assignments in many settings and clinical units that will allow you to see some of the options available to you after you obtain your nursing license. Approximately 61% of nurses work in hospitals. Others work in extended care facilities, providers' offices, ambulatory care, home health, correctional facilities, public health, the military, or schools (Bureau of Labor Statistics, U.S. Department of Labor, 2014b).

What Models of Care Are Used to Provide Nursing Care?

Nursing care is structured in various ways. The organization of the nursing team reflects the philosophy and beliefs of the institution, as well as the prevailing views on nursing. The structure of the team is often referred to as the *model of care.* The most common models include the following:

Case Method The **case method,** also called *total care,* is one-to-one care; one nurse provides all aspects of care for one patient during a single shift. In this method, the nurse and patient work more closely together, the patient's needs are quickly met, and the nurse has a greater degree of autonomy. Although this method may be satisfying for patients and nurses, high costs limit its widespread use. The case method is used mainly in intensive care, labor and delivery, and private duty care.

Functional Nursing In **functional nursing,** care is compartmentalized, with each task assigned to a staff member with the appropriate knowledge and skills. For example, the RN is in charge and performs complex treatments, the LPN/LVN may distribute medications, and the nursing assistant may give bed baths and make beds. This approach requires a clear understanding of what tasks each member may perform (scope of practice). Although this approach is economical and efficient, it can make it difficult for the nurse to have the "whole picture" of the patient (*fragmentation of care*).

Team Nursing The **team nursing** approach is efficient. It maintains the costs saving of functional nursing while seeking to limit fragmentation. In team nursing, a licensed nurse (RN or LPN/ LVN) is paired with a nursing assistant or nursing assistive personnel (NAP). The team is assigned to a group of patients. Teams led by RNs are assigned to high-acuity patients. Team nursing is popular during times of nursing shortages (Holt, 2011; King, Long, & Lisy, 2014).

Primary Nursing In **primary nursing,** one nurse manages care for a group of patients. The primary nurse assesses the patient and develops a plan of care. When she is at work, she provides care for the patients for whom she is responsible. In her absence, associate nurses deliver care and implement the plan developed by the primary nurse.

Differentiated Practice **Differentiated practice** recognizes that education and experience lead to differences in the care delivered by nurses. Each unit identifies the type of expertise needed by the patients and the nursing competencies required to deliver that care. Individual nurses put together a portfolio to demonstrate their competencies, and patients are assigned accordingly.

THE HEALTHCARE DELIVERY SYSTEM

The healthcare delivery system in the United States is a complex collection of patients, providers, facilities, vendors, and rules. The rest of this chapter is designed to help you gain a beginner's understanding of it. You will need to know the components of the system to understand the continuum of healthcare that patients receive, the providers involved in that care, and the factors that influence the type and amount of care that patients receive.

Where Is Healthcare Provided?

Patients can receive treatment in a variety of environments based on their needs. Hospitals, extended care facilities, ambulatory care centers, and home healthcare agencies are the most visible sites for delivery of healthcare. A patient who has been admitted to a healthcare facility is an **inpatient.** An **outpatient** is a person who receives treatment at a healthcare facility but does not stay overnight. Inpatient services occur in various hospital settings.

Hospitals

Hospitals are the most expensive and the most frequently used site for care. They provide a broad range of services to treat various injuries and disease processes (Fig. 1-2). Smaller hospitals offer basic services, whereas larger medical centers usually offer additional and specialty services. Basic services include inpatient beds, radiology, and laboratory services. Hospitals usually have an emergency department, diagnostic centers, and other units such as intensive care, medical, surgical, pediatrics, and maternal newborn. They employ a variety of healthcare providers to ensure the acute care needs of the patient are met around the clock. A patient's length of stay is limited to the amount of time that he requires 24-hour observation.

Extended Care Facilities

Extended care facilities provide care for clients for an extended period of time—usually longer than 1 month. As the

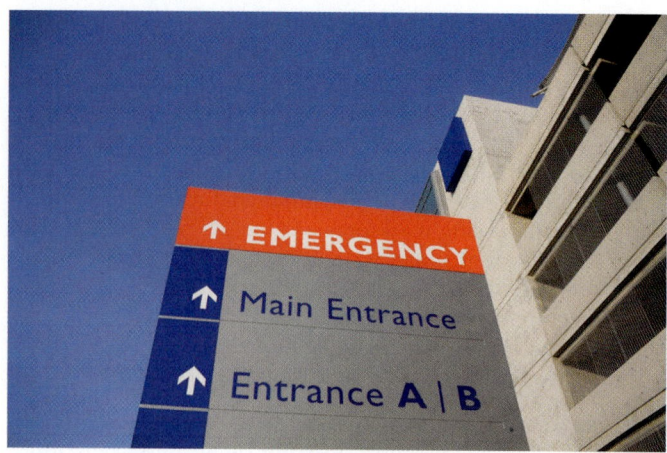

FIGURE 1-2 Emergency departments may be the primary source of healthcare for many individuals.

length of stay in hospitals has declined, extended care facilities have begun to deliver services that were previously provided in the hospital. Extended care is delivered in nursing homes, skilled nursing facilities (also known as convalescent hospitals), and rehabilitation facilities.

The distinction among extended care facilities is based primarily on whether they provide skilled or custodial care. **Skilled care** includes services of trained professionals that are needed for a limited period of time after an injury or illness (e.g., wound care, intravenous infusions). **Custodial care,** in contrast, consists of help with activities of daily living: bathing, dressing, eating, grooming, ambulation, toileting, and other care that people typically do for themselves (e.g., taking medications, monitoring blood glucose levels).

- **Nursing homes** provide custodial care for people who cannot live on their own but are not sick enough to require hospitalization. They may be permanent homes for people who require continual supervision to ensure their safety.
- **Assisted living facilities** were designed to bridge the gap between independence and institutionalization for older adults who have a decline in health status and cannot live independently. Residents of these facilities are able to perform self-care activities but require assistance with meals, housekeeping, or medications.
- **Rehabilitation centers** provide extended care and treatment for patients with physical and mental illness. Types of services include alcohol and drug rehabilitation, physical rehabilitation services for patients who have experienced traumatic injuries, and rehabilitation of patients after stroke or heart attack.

Ambulatory Care Centers

Same-day, cost-effective healthcare is offered at **ambulatory care centers.** They provide services for clients (outpatients) who are able to come and go from the facility for same-day or special services (e.g., same-day surgery, chemotherapy). Ambulatory centers may be connected to hospitals (Fig. 1-3).

Home Healthcare Agencies

Home healthcare agencies provide continuing care to patients after hospitalization in their home. Services are usually coordinated by a home health or visiting nurse service and include nursing care as well as various therapies and home assistance programs. Chapter 43 provides further discussion on home health nursing.

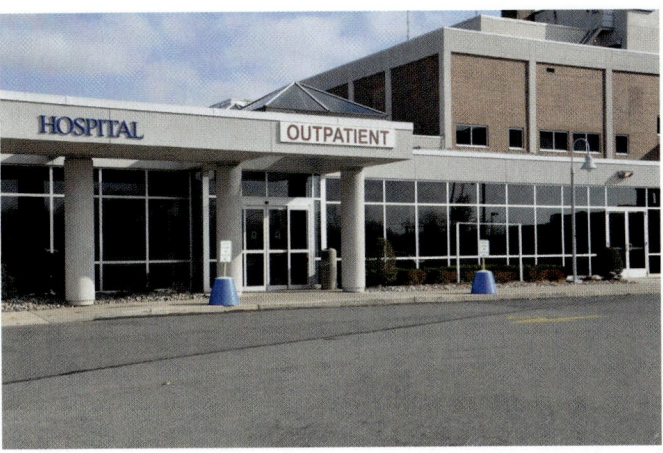

FIGURE 1-3 The shift to outpatient care is a cost-saving strategy.

Community or Public Health Centers

Community or public health centers are community-based centers that provide care for the community at large. Community health nurses provide services to at risk populations and devise strategies to improve the health status of the surrounding community (e.g., school-based programs to decrease teen pregnancies, healthcare for the homeless). **Community care** is a comprehensive term that describes the care provided to client groups at various sites, such as church, schools, shelters, workplaces, and public clinics. Chapter 43 provides further discussion on community healthcare.

Independent Living Facilities

Also known as retirement homes, **independent living facilities** are designed for seniors 55 years or older who (1) are independent in all aspects and (2) want to live in a community with other senior citizens. Living facilities range from apartment-style homes to smaller separate residential homes. Nurses may provide periodic health screening and health information.

How Is Healthcare Categorized?

Because the boundaries of care have become fluid, it is useful to look at the system in a different light. **KEY POINT:** *The complexity of care no longer is a predictor of where care will be delivered. Instead, regulators, finances, and the patient's support system dictate where a patient will be located in the system.* On a basic level, healthcare is categorized by the degree of complexity into primary, secondary, and tertiary services.

Primary Services

Primary services are directed toward keeping the patient well by preventing illness and promoting illness-prevention activities. At this level, general or primary care providers in offices, clinics, and diagnostic centers provide most of the care. Primary care focuses on health promotion and disease prevention. Activities include health education and immunizations for infectious diseases.

Nursing and Health Promotion In 1948, the World Health Organization (WHO) defined health as "a state of complete physical, mental, and social well-being and not merely the absence of disease or infirmity." The definition has not been amended since that time (WHO, 2006). Health-promotion

activities foster the highest state of well-being of the recipient of the activities. The following are examples:

- *Individual level*—Counseling a pregnant client about the importance of adequate prenatal nutrition to promote health for the client and baby
- *Group and family level*—Teaching about nutrition during pregnancy in family education programs
- *Community level*—Posting signs in grocery stores recommending the best foods for pregnant women
- *Societal level*—Working with international partners to establish worldwide prenatal nutrition standards

Nursing and Illness Prevention Illness prevention focuses on avoidance of disease, infection, and other comorbidities. Activities are targeted to minimize the risk of development of or exposure to disease. For example, pneumonia causes many deaths every year. Teaching the importance of hand hygiene is one nursing activity to decrease the risk of the spread of pneumonia. Good nutrition increases the person's resistance to the disease should exposure occur.

Secondary Services

Secondary services consist of services for early diagnosis and treatment of illness, disease, and injury. Historically, we have thought of this as hospital-based care, but increasingly these services are being performed in surgery centers, offices, and outpatient centers.

Nursing and Health Restoration Health restoration activities foster a return to health for those already ill. The nurse provides direct care to ill individuals, groups, families, or communities to restore their health. This nursing role includes addressing the physical, mental, spiritual, and social dimensions of client care.

Tertiary Services

Tertiary services refer to long-term rehabilitation services and care for the dying. Historically, these services were provided in extended care facilities. Now, however, many tertiary care services are provided in the home or in outpatient settings.

Nursing and End-of-Life Care Death is an inevitable destination on the journey of life. Nurses work with dying individuals, their family members and support persons, and organizations (hospice) that focus on the needs of the terminally ill to promote comfort, maintain quality of life, provide culturally relevant spiritual care, maintain dignity, and ease the emotional burden of death (see Chapter 17).

KnowledgeCheck 1-3

Recall the last time that you had a cold. Identify health-promotion, illness-prevention, and health-restoration activities for individuals, families, groups, and communities in relation to the common cold.

Who Are the Members of the Interprofessional Healthcare Team?

As a nurse, you will be part of an interprofessional healthcare team consisting of numerous professionals whose primary role is to ensure quality patient outcomes (Fig. 1-4). The composition of the team varies depending on the healthcare needs of the patient. Each provider's role in the health team is covered in the discussion that follows.

Physicians The team leader for an inpatient is typically a physician whose primary role is to make a medical diagnosis and outline the treatment plan. Physicians are licensed as medical doctors (MD) or doctors of osteopathy (DO). A physician

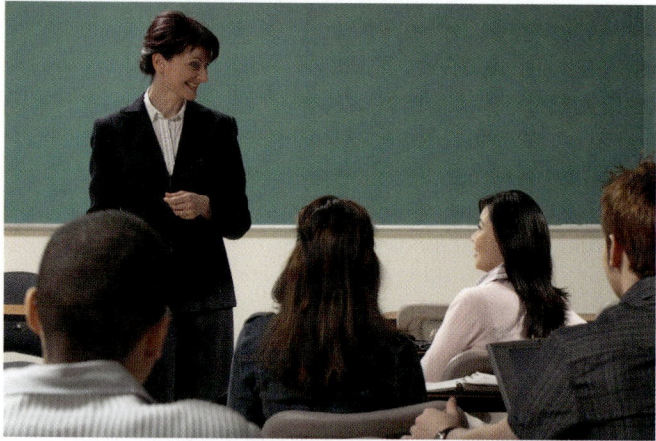

FIGURE 1-4 Quality patient outcomes require the collaboration of the entire healthcare team.

may work independently, as part of a medical group, or as an employee of a health facility. Physicians may provide care in an office setting, in the hospital, or in a variety of clinics or ambulatory sites. Physicians who provide only hospital care are known as *hospitalists*.

Nurse Practitioners Nurse practitioners (NPs) are licensed, independent practitioners with advanced education and training to provide medical and nursing care based on their specialty area. NPs engage in activities ranging from health promotion to caring for clients with acute or chronic healthcare problems.

Physician Assistants (PAs) PAs diagnose and treat certain diseases and injuries. Although many function in a fashion similar to nurse practitioners, they are not independently licensed. Therefore, they must practice under the supervision of a physician.

Registered Nurses (RNs) RNs use the treatment plan outlined by the medical provider to develop and implement holistic, continuous, and comprehensive nursing care to clients. RNs administer treatments and medications, provide education, and modify the nursing care plan based on patient responses to treatment.

Licensed Practical Nurses (LPNs) LPNs implement client care under the supervision of the RN. They can administer certain medications, provide non-complex care, and communicate client information to the RN.

Nursing Assistive Personnel (NAPs) NAP is an umbrella term that covers nursing assistants, aides, and technicians. NAPs provide custodial-type care under the direction of nurses and physicians in a variety of settings. Some NAPs introduce themselves to patients by stating, "I'm your nurse." Because they are not licensed nurses, they are making a false claim. Be sure to clarify your role and the NAP's role with all of your patients.

Pharmacists Pharmacists prepare and dispense medications and therapeutic solutions in hospitals, community pharmacies, and other healthcare settings. They also collaborate with nurses, physicians, and other health-team members to ensure the selection of safe and effective medications to be included in the treatment plan.

Therapists Allied healthcare providers are various therapists (e.g., physical therapists, occupational therapists) who focus on the rehabilitative needs of the patient. The goal of the rehabilitative team is to treat and maximize functioning and/or assist the patient to adapt to limitations.

How Is Healthcare Financed?

Payors for healthcare in the United States include individuals, individual private insurance, employment-based group private insurance, the government, and charitable sources.

Individuals

Until the latter half of the 20th century, physicians made house calls and clients paid either with cash or by trading goods and services. Today, we refer to payments made directly by individuals as *direct payment of services* and *out-of-pocket expenses*. Many of those without insurance cannot afford to pay the direct cost of services. Individuals with private or government insurance pay for services through **cost sharing** in the form of insurance premiums, insurance deductibles, copayments, costs above fixed payments, and noncovered services.
KEY POINT: *Although insurance does pay for a share of the costs, even consumers with insurance sometimes avoid or delay services because of high out-of-pocket expenses.*

Individual Private Insurance

Healthcare insurance is purchased to protect individuals from having to pay the costs associated with illness and hospitalization. The cost of seeking treatment in the emergency department is four times higher than that of an office visit to a provider (Ollove, 2015). The average annual cost of medical insurance premiums in 2015 was $6,251 for single coverage and $17,545 for family coverage (Henry J. Kaiser Family Foundation, 2015). Insurance is intended to protect persons from "medical bankruptcy" associated with the costs from a major medical event (Fig. 1-5).

A person with private insurance pays premiums to an insurance company. The insurance company then contracts with healthcare providers to deliver care to insured members at prearranged rates. Patients share in the cost of care through out-of-pocket expenses.

Employment-Based Private Insurance

Most private insurance in the United States is employment based and was developed in the United States during World War II when a labor shortage limited salary increases. Employers financed fringe benefits such as health insurance to attract and reward employees and to improve the health of employees. Healthy employees benefit employers because of reduced sick time and a full workforce.

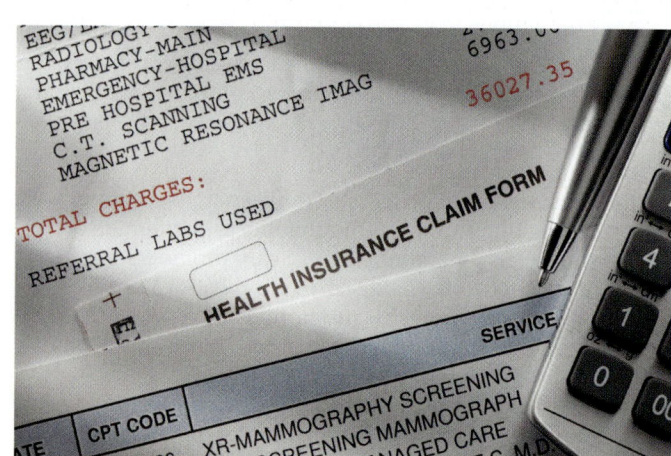

FIGURE 1-5 The high cost of healthcare is a barrier to early screening and prevention.

The employer pays all or a portion of the costs (e.g., premiums) for employment-based health insurance. The cost of health insurance premiums for employers continues to increase annually. Although the federal government subsidizes employer-based health insurance by not taxing health insurance and allowing employers to deduct these benefits as a business expense (Bodenheimer & Grumbach, 2016), employers are shifting more of the costs to employees (Blumberg & Holahan, 2014).

Government (Public) Financing

KEY POINT: *Government-funded programs are paid for with revenue from taxes on the citizenry. Programs include Medicare and Medicaid as well as children's, specialty, and categorical programs. They include federal, state, local, and jointly funded programs.*

Medicare Medicare is a federal insurance program created by Title XVIII of the Social Security Act of 1965. This act was designed for persons aged 65 years and older and later expanded to include younger people with permanent disabilities such as end-stage renal disease. Medicare financing comes from a payroll tax levied on employers and employees and from premiums paid by Medicare subscribers (patients). It provides only limited coverage for long-term care.

Medicaid Medicaid was developed under Title XIX of the Social Security Act of 1965 to provide access to healthcare services for individuals with low incomes and minimal resources. Medicaid is a joint federal and state endeavor; therefore, the eligibility criteria for Medicaid and the range of medical services offered vary from state to state.

Children's Health Insurance Program (CHIP) CHIP is a joint venture between the federal government and the states to provide health insurance to millions of children whose family income exceeds Medicaid eligibility criteria but cannot afford private insurance and are not covered under a parent's policy. CHIP's goal is to ensure that children have health insurance and can access healthcare, either through an expansion of Medicaid or the development of a separate program. The Affordable Care Act (ACA) extended CHIP's funding through fiscal year 2015 and authorized the program until 2019 (Medicaid.gov, 2015).

Specialty and Categorical Programs Categorical programs are designated by federal laws to provide access to healthcare for certain categories of people, such as immigrants or children in Head Start programs. Specialty programs target certain populations (e.g., Indian Health Service military personnel and dependents).

KnowledgeCheck 1-4

- Compare and contrast private and government-funded health insurance.
- How does being uninsured affect a person's health status?

Charitable Organizations

Charitable organizations are an increasingly important funding source for healthcare. Community agencies that are funded through networks such as the United Way, Salvation Army, and Red Cross provide important resources to children, poor families, the aged, and vulnerable populations, such as the homeless, mentally ill, and victims of violence. Charitable organizations provide direct services and cover the costs for some traditional health services.

How Are Supplies and Equipment Provided?

Suppliers are the companies and corporations who bring goods to the healthcare industry. Pharmaceutical companies and medical equipment suppliers are the largest suppliers. The costs associated with the research, development, and testing of pharmaceuticals and medical equipment are passed on to consumers in the form of higher prices, rising insurance premiums, and increased out-of-pocket expenses.

How Is Healthcare Regulated?

Regulators are governing bodies that exert influence or control over the healthcare system. They include accrediting (e.g., Accrediting Commission for Education in Nursing, Commission on Collegiate Nursing Education) and licensing agencies (boards of nursing) and legislators. The most prominent regulating body in the healthcare system is The Joint Commission. Reimbursement from government and insurance sources is dependent upon accreditation by The Joint Commission. Legislators can redefine eligibility criteria for government-funded health plans. The Affordable Care Act (ACA) that was signed into law in 2010 is an example of the impact of legislation on healthcare.

How Have Healthcare Reform Efforts Affected Care?

Healthcare reform has impacted not only access to care but also reimbursement rates for providers. A notable example is the shift in Medicare and insurance reform.

Medicare and Public Policy

When Medicare was initially created, health services were reimbursed using a **retrospective system.** In other words, Medicare paid hospitals based on the actual cost of providing services to individuals. With no cap on expenses, Medicare payments made to hospitals had increased from $3 billion in the early years of the program to $37 billion by 1983.

To slow the rising costs of healthcare, a **prospective reimbursement system** was created under the Social Security Amendment of 1983. Hospitals have since been reimbursed on a per-case, flat rate basis determined by patient groups having similar needs. These groups were called **diagnostic-related groups (DRGs).** If the patient's hospital costs were greater than the reimbursed ("set") amounts, the hospital lost money. If the costs were less than the rate set by Medicare, the hospital made a profit. Private insurance companies, following the lead of Medicare, reimbursed in the same manner.

The introduction of DRGs forced hospitals to consider new ways of delivering care and created a number of changes in patient care (e.g., decreased length of hospital stay, increase in rehabilitation care). For example, allowed length of stay for a postoperative hip replacement client has now decreased from 10 days to 4 days under the prospective payment system.

Managed Care

Managed care, designed to control healthcare costs, is a competitive approach to healthcare pricing. Managed care organizations (MCOs) contract with medical providers to provide services (1) at discounted rates, or (2) based on predetermined fixed payment per individual covered under the plan (capitation). Providers treat more clients to offset their discounted rates. The most common types of managed care plans follow.

Health Maintenance Organizations (HMOs) HMOs are a model of care based on **capitated** (per head) costs. Each

HMO primary care provider receives a predetermined, fixed amount each month regardless of whether the patient receives healthcare services or not. The primary care provider coordinates all care, including referrals to specialists. Providers often choose to be a part of an HMO because of the steady income it offers.

Preferred Provider Organizations (PPOs) The PPO has many of the features of an HMO, such as a network of providers who will provide healthcare at the established contracted rate. Compared with HMOs, PPOs allow patients to have more choice among providers, medications, and devices; however, the patient pays more in premiums and must choose from the list of in-network providers.

Point of Service (POS) The POS is a physician that the patient selects from a list of network physicians. This physician is the POS for treatment and referrals to in-network specialists. There is limited out-of-network coverage at a higher coinsurance and copay.

Integrated Delivery Networks (IDNs) IDNs combine providers, health facilities, pharmaceuticals, and services into one care system. Providers see only IDN patients, in IDN facilities, using IDN services and IDN-approved pharmaceuticals. In this linked system, patients can be readily moved among IDN services and providers.

What Are the Issues Related to Healthcare Reform?

The profound changes created by the transition of the healthcare system from a retrospective to a prospective fixed-rate payment system have created unprecedented leadership opportunities for nurse executives.

ANA Recommendations for Reform

The ANA document *ANA's Healthcare System Reform Agenda* (2008) includes several recommendations to redesign the healthcare system:

- Provide universal access to essential healthcare services for all citizens and residents.
- Establish health policies that support safe, effective, patient-centered, timely, efficient, and fair care based on outcomes research.
- Shift the priority from illness care to health promotion, and balance between high-tech treatment and community-based and preventive services.
- Establish a single-payer system for financing healthcare.

Work Redesign

Work redesign involves looking at the level of care required and the mix of personnel necessary to achieve the best patient outcomes. Out of this redesign, a concept known as the critical pathway emerged. A **critical pathway** is a multidisciplinary approach to care that sequences interventions over a length of stay for a given case type. Using the critical pathways model, the interprofessional team delivers care that yields the desired outcomes in the quickest manner to reduce the patient's length of stay. (See Chapter 5 for more information about critical pathways.)

Case management, another work redesign, is the coordination of care across the healthcare system. Many hospitals, home health agencies, and insurance companies employ nurse case managers to ensure that a patient receives efficient quality patient care using the most cost-effective resources. Typically, nurses manage patients with specific diagnoses throughout the system from outpatient to inpatient.

Is Healthcare a Right or a Privilege?

Underlying all healthcare reform is the fundamental question of whether healthcare is a right or a privilege. This question raises more questions. For example, if healthcare is a right of all citizens, should noncitizens be offered coverage? Moreover, what responsibility does an individual have to preserve her own health through lifestyle changes (e.g., not smoke)? Should extensive and/or expensive therapies be offered if they have little likelihood of preserving life? Finally, if you believe that healthcare should be affordable for all, are you willing to limit your salary and benefits to help control the costs of care? Are you willing to pay higher taxes? These fundamental questions were discussed during the debate on the Affordable Care Act. You will continue to hear them discussed further as universal healthcare continues to evolve.

KnowledgeCheck 1-5

- Do you view healthcare as a right or a privilege?
- What are factors that impact your view (draw on your self-knowledge to answer this question)?

How Do Providers and Facilities Ensure Quality Care?

As you learned previously, a number of accrediting bodies inspect healthcare organizations. These inspections are designed to ensure that patients receive safe, quality care. To promote safety, regulators establish a minimum competency level that must be met for accreditation to be granted. However, most healthcare organizations and professionals declare that their goal is to deliver *excellent* care rather than merely meeting minimum standards.

Continuous Quality Improvement Programs

Continuous quality improvement (CQI) programs (also called *total quality management,* or TQM) focus on quality (excellent) care as an ongoing goal rather than something that is periodically verified by audit or when a problem is identified.

Traditionally, quality *assurance* programs (not called quality *improvement*) consisted of **retrospective audit programs.** Material from the past (e.g., patient records) is reviewed for evidence of compliance with preselected criteria. For example, a nursing unit might set a goal of 100% compliance that nurses' notes will state the reason why any medication is held (not given).

If the QI auditors determine that the goal for compliance is not met, they will often launch a program to improve compliance (e.g., mandatory in-service education, adding labels in the medication administration records, and installing a computer-based medication system that prompts staff to document the reason for holding a medication). At a later date, a second audit is conducted to determine whether compliance has improved.

Another form of retrospective quality improvement is **peer review.** Colleagues review medical records or patient satisfaction data that reflect the care given by their peers. Peer review requires objective criteria; an open, honest professional dialogue; and a willingness to improve.

ANA Model for Quality Improvement

In 1975, the ANA developed a model for QI (then called *quality assurance,* or QA). This model is useful to understanding the CQI process (see the SENC box Quality Improvement Competency).

Quality Improvement Competency

Chapter Key Concept: Healthcare Delivery System

Competency: Provide Safe, Quality Care

Question. Based on work done by the Institute of Medicine, this textbook identifies quality improvement (QI) as a competency you should achieve during your nursing education. QI includes the ability to "evaluate and use techniques/processes to avoid medical/nursing errors" and to evaluate the framework used for care delivery, incorporating structure, process, and outcomes of the care. How do you think the staffing mix in a hospital might affect care quality?

Research. Recent research shows that when the proportion of RNs increases in an agency, quality of care rises and death and infection rates drop. Consider the following examples from *Critical Care* ("Low Hospital Staff Levels," 2007); Landon, Normand, Lessler, et al. (2006); Tourangeau, Doran, Hall, et al. (2007); and Yang, Hung, Chen, et al. (2012):

➤ Hospitals with higher proportions of RNs and baccalaureate-prepared RNs have lower patient death rates.

➤ Increasing the proportion of RNs on staff by 10% resulted in six fewer deaths per 1,000.

➤ Hospitals with adequate staffing had lower death rates.

➤ Hospitals with a higher proportion of RNs on staff performed better on a variety of performance measures.

➤ When the ratio of nurses to patients falls (e.g., from 1:6 nurses:patients to 1:4), risk for infection falls.

Think about it: How does the SENC competency of quality improvement relate to the chapter's key concept: healthcare delivery system?

FACTORS THAT INFLUENCE CONTEMPORARY NURSING PRACTICE

Factors that influence nursing practice include societal factors at large as well as factors within nursing and healthcare.

What Are Some Trends in Society?

In addition to our historical roots, nursing is influenced by trends in the economy—the growing number of older adults, increased consumer knowledge, legislation, the women's movement, and collective bargaining.

■ *Historically, in the United States, health insurance coverage was linked to full-time employment with health insurance benefits.* Thus when unemployment increased, so did the number of people without health insurance. People delayed seeking treatment or used the emergency department for healthcare. The Affordable Care Act (ACA) has expanded health insurance coverage for even the unemployed, resulting in a larger demand for care. More healthcare personnel, especially advanced practice nurses, are needed to meet this demand.

■ *The healthcare system employs an enormous number and variety of people.* If you consider that there are 3.1 million professionally active RNs, 914,720 active physicians (Kaiser Family Foundation, 2015), and more than 290,700 employed pharmacists (Bureau of Labor Statistics, 2014a), you begin to understand how large the healthcare system is when all other providers are added to the count.

The Growing Proportion of Older Adults in the United States

As people age, they experience more acute and chronic illnesses and a need for more medical and nursing care. In 2010, the growth rate for adults aged 65 years and older greatly outpaced the growth of the population, at 15% (40.3 million) compared with the country as a whole (9.7%) (U.S. Census Bureau, 2010a). In 2050, the population aged 65 and over is projected to be 83.7 million, almost double its estimated population of 43.1 million in 2012 (Ortman, Velkoff, & Hogan, 2014). At the same time, there are fewer younger people to provide care, which has significant implications for the healthcare system.

Changes in Healthcare Consumers

Historically, patients relied on the knowledge and decision making of the healthcare team. Now, however, consumers are demanding greater choice in the decisions that affect their health.

■ *Patients have access to vast amounts of health and medical information, particularly through the Internet* (e.g., Web sites such as WebMD and PubMed). Informed consumers tend to be active participants in discussions about their health problems and therapy options. Patients need to be taught which sites are valid for gathering information.

■ *Direct-to-consumer marketing is another form of health information* in which corporations advertise medications and therapies directed at the potential user (e.g., Internet, magazines, television). Clients may then request their healthcare providers to prescribe specific brand-name therapies. You need to educate and present balanced information to clients, particularly as it is appropriate for individual clients' conditions. You must also be comfortable with your knowledge and not be unduly persuaded by consumers who are relying on the latest fads. Your knowledge, standards of nursing practice, and communications with the healthcare team should be the foundation for making patient-related decisions.

Legislation

Consumer interest sometimes generates legislation that affects nursing care. Legislation directed at the confidentiality of patient records, treating patients who need emergency care, the patient's right to know (informed consent), and the patient's right to a dignified death (living will/advance directives) all govern the care that nurses render to patients. These acts are discussed further in Chapters 43 and 44.

The Women's Movement

Historically, only unmarried women were allowed to practice nursing. As the women's movement gained momentum, women were able to combine careers and family. Whereas women's careers were traditionally limited to teaching, clerical work, and nursing, the women's movement opened up more choices. As a result, nursing is just one of many options for a career for women. Societal views of nursing as a women's profession have also influenced the decisions of men to enter (or not enter) nursing (Fig. 1-6).

Collective Bargaining

Collective bargaining is a form of negotiating that allows nurses to seek better wages and working conditions as a group rather than individually. Not all states have collective bargaining groups for nurses. Collective bargaining has resulted in significant improvements in wages, benefits, and working

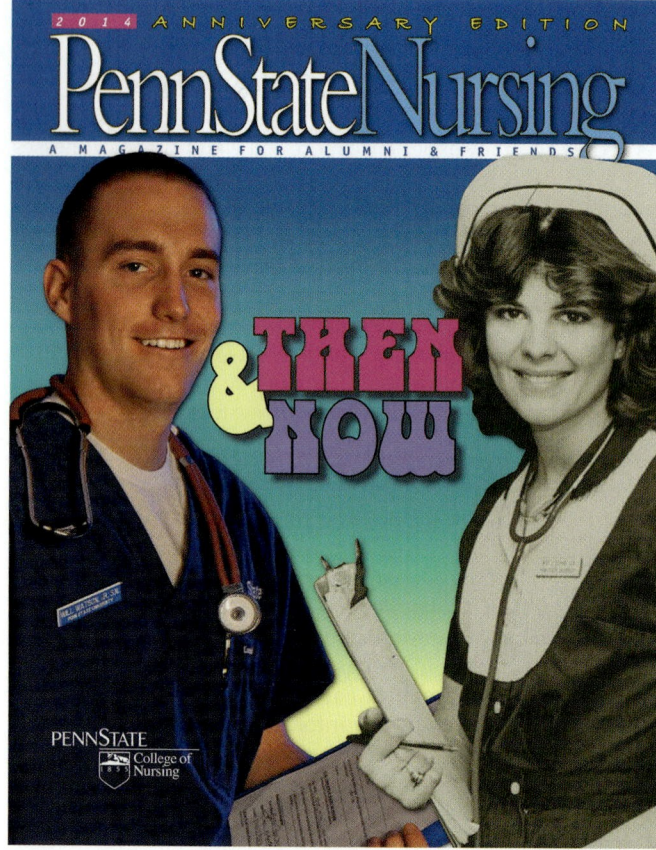

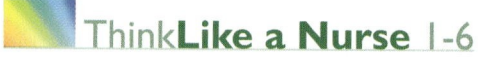
FIGURE 1-6   Nursing students: 2013 and 1983.

conditions for nurses as well as safer conditions for patients. These improvements have made nursing more attractive as a career choice.

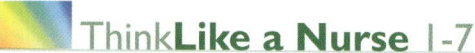
ThinkLike a Nurse 1-6

What effect do you think the women's movement has had on the number of women in the nursing workforce? Speculate on the ways in which women entering nursing might have been different before and after the women's movement.

What Are Some Trends in Nursing and Healthcare?

In addition to societal factors, trends in nursing and healthcare also affect contemporary practice.

Increased Use of Complementary and Alternative Medicine

The National Institutes of Health define healthcare treatments or services outside the traditional healthcare system as **complementary and alternative medicine (CAM).** They include medical systems such as homeopathy, naturopathy, chiropractic, and traditional Chinese medicine as well as specific treatments such as herbal medications, dietary changes, massage therapy, yoga, aromatherapy, prayer, and hypnotism. There is growing interest in CAM for various reasons, including costs of traditional care and increasing cultural diversity in the population. For a more extensive discussion,

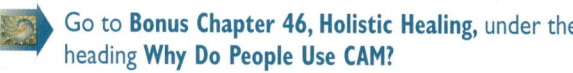
Go to **Bonus Chapter 46, Holistic Healing,** under the heading **Why Do People Use CAM?**

Expanded Variety of Settings for Care

Nearly 40% of registered nurses now work outside the hospital setting compared with 20% in 1980 (ANA, 2010b; Health Resources and Services Administration, 2013; Jonas & Kovner, 2011). As this trend continues, nurses must be prepared to function in alternative settings. This change requires entry-level education programs to prepare nurses for these types of work (Wilkinson, 1996). In the hospital, you have access to major resources (e.g., support personnel, consultation with other healthcare providers, medical records, diagnostic testing services). As more care is delivered in outpatient, community, or home settings, you must be prepared to function more autonomously and creatively.

Telehealth nursing is practiced in a variety of settings, including rural clinics, home healthcare, corrective facilities, and physician's offices, using communication devices such as the telephone or two-way video technology. As telehealth nursing continues to evolve, you will need to combine the use of technology with your nursing knowledge to safely care for patients remotely.

ThinkLike a Nurse 1-7

What is your nursing program doing to prepare you to work outside of the hospital setting?

Interest in Interprofessional Collaboration

Nursing has changed from a largely supportive role to one of increasing responsibility. This is due, in part, to the growing role of nursing in outpatient settings, the increasing complexity of care, consumer demands, and the increased use of technology. Healthcare leaders are finding that interprofessional teamwork is essential to providing safe, high-quality patient outcomes.

Collaboration is the process of joint decision making among independent parties involving joint ownership of decisions and collective responsibility for outcomes (Disch, Bellman, & Ingbar, as cited in Sterchi, 2007). However, in a relationship where there is a power imbalance, true collaboration can occur only if the more powerful parties are willing for it to occur. Physicians and nurses tend to have different values and to place different emphases on patient care (Gadkari, 2013). This may contribute to strained relationships and disagreements about a patient's plan of care, which may lead to undesired outcomes for patients. True collaboration occurs when institutions enforce the goal and give recognition to those who practice it.

On a typical day, a hospitalized patient may interact with six or more individuals who are involved in the plan of care. A primary cause of serious medical errors in healthcare facilities is communication failure, which often stems from lack of collaboration. To minimize these occurrences, healthcare providers are encouraged to use a standardized system of communication known as SBAR-R (Situation, Background, Assessment, Recommendation, and Readback) (see Chapter 20).

Expanded Career Roles for Nurses

Numerous **expanded roles** extend the traditional practice of the nurse. The roles may or may not be clinical.

Advanced Practice Nurses (APNs) RNs, usually with a master's degree, who work in expanded roles with a clinical focus are collectively termed *advanced practice nurses (APNs).*

- **Clinical Nurse Specialist (CNS)**—A nurse with advanced education and expertise in an area of clinical specialization

Toward Evidence-Based Practice

Research has shown that the single intervention—application of siderails—is not effective in preventing patient falls. These researchers have concluded that a multifactorial approach is needed.

Miake-Lye, I., Hempel, S., Ganz, D., et al. (2013). Inpatient fall prevention programs as a patient safety strategy: A systematic review [Supplement]. *Annals of Internal Medicine,* *158(5),* 390–396.

Research supports previous conclusions that fall prevention is multifaceted and expanded on required interventions. Successful programs included "leadership support, engagement of front-line staff in program design, guidance of the prevention program by a multidisciplinary committee, pilot-testing interventions, use of information technology systems to provide data about falls, staff education and training, and changes in nihilistic attitudes about fall prevention" (p. 390).

Spoelstra, S. L., Given, B. A., & Given, C. W. (2012). Fall prevention in hospitals: An integrative review. *Clinical Nursing Research, 21(1),* 92–112.

This study found that intervention programs that included a multiple approach to preventing patient falls were more effective than relying on a single intervention. Fall prevention programs should include staff education, fall-risk assessments, environmental assessments and modifications, alarm systems, and patient assistance with transferring and toileting.

Capezuti, E. E., Wagner, L., Brush, B., et al. (2007). Consequences of an intervention to reduce restrictive side rail use in nursing homes. *Journal of the American Geriatrics Society, 55(3),* 334–341.

This study of more than 700 nursing home residents at four sites found that routine use of siderails does not reduce the risk of bed-related falls.

Brush, B. L., & Capezuti, E. (2001). Historical analysis of siderail use in American hospitals. *Journal of Nursing Scholarship, 33(4),* 381–385.

This study examined the pattern of siderail use, the value attached to siderails, and attitudes about raising siderails over time. Initially, siderails were used for temporary protection of confused patients. Prior to the 1930s, nurses used direct observations to ensure patient safety. However, in the 1930s, nurse shortages, litigation against hospitals and nurses for fall-related injuries, and replacement of the open ward with semiprivate and private rooms promoted the use of siderails. Research has demonstrated that siderail-induced falls may occur and that sustained bedrest has negative physical and emotional consequences. Still, side-rail use remains the norm to promote patient safety.

1. What trends and factors currently affecting nursing might influence whether siderail use will change in the near future?

2. What additional information would you like to know before advocating for a change in siderail use?

 Go to Davis Advantage, Resources, Chapter 1, **Toward Evidence-Based Practice Suggested Responses.**

(e.g., cardiovascular, pulmonary, orthopedics). The CNS may provide direct patient care; consult on client care; engage in client, family, community, or staff teaching; and/or conduct research.

- **Nurse Practitioner (NP)**—A nurse with advanced education focused on providing primary care (comprehensive healthcare) to an age-group or within a specialty area. NPs may work independently or in practice with physicians. They assess, diagnose, and treat diseases and illnesses and prescribe medications and treatments.
- **Certified Registered Nurse Anesthetist (CRNA)**—A nurse with advanced education focused on providing anesthesia. Nurse anesthetists conduct preoperative screening and evaluation of patients, administer anesthesia during surgery, and evaluate patients' response to anesthesia in the postoperative period.
- **Certified Nurse Midwife (CNM)**—A nurse with advanced education focused on women's health, pregnancy, and delivery. A CNM provides prenatal care, performs uncomplicated deliveries, and provides postpartum care.

Professional and public reports (e.g., Tourangeau, Doran, Hall, et al., 2007) demonstrate high levels of patient satisfaction with APNs, comparable and at times superior patient outcomes over physician-provided care, better understanding of and compliance with treatment regimens, fewer hospitalizations, and greater cost-effectiveness when compared with physician providers. This positive reaction to APNs has resulted in increased acceptance and demand.

Non-Clinical Expanded Roles Expanded roles with other than a clinical focus include the following:

- **Nurse Researcher**—A nurse with advanced education at the master's or doctoral level who engages in research related to clinical practice, the discipline, or nursing education.
- **Nurse Administrator**—A nurse whose practice focuses on the management and administration of nursing care, health facilities, or health resources.
- **Nurse Educator**—A nurse with advanced education and expertise who teaches in the clinical or academic setting.
- **Nurse Informaticist**—A nurse with specialized education focused on the use of technology in healthcare and the incorporation of standardized languages and classifications into nursing practice.
- **Nurse Entrepreneur**—A nurse who has created an independent or innovative business. Entrepreneurs may serve as

consultants, administer a health-related business, or provide educational services.

KnowledgeCheck 1-6

Compare and contrast advanced practice clinical roles for nurses.

Increased Use of Nursing Assistive Personnel

Nursing assistive personnel (NAP) help nurses provide patient care. Common NAP roles include nurse aide, assistant, orderly, and technician. NAPs may perform simple nursing tasks (e.g., bathing, taking vital signs) under the direction of the licensed nurse. Some institutions even train NAPs for more complex tasks traditionally reserved for licensed nurses (e.g., inserting urinary catheters, giving certain medications). This redistribution of workload has prompted controversy about safety and quality of care.

Although it may be appropriate to allow the NAP to assume the simple tasks, this distances the licensed nurse from many aspects of direct patient care. The nurse retains ultimate responsibility for the patient yet must base important patient-care decisions on information obtained by the NAP. The nurse is able to use a higher level of critical thinking and a greater depth of knowledge and therefore should be able to gather more in-depth patient data.

As you progress through your program, you will notice that nurses often gather different information from a client than does someone without nursing experience. For example, after bathing an older adult, a NAP will be able to tell the nurse that there are no open areas on the skin. However, a nurse performing the same task would be able to do an extensive client assessment while giving the bath. The nurse would be able to assess the client's level of cognition (orientation to surroundings and self), tolerance for activity, breath sounds, heart sounds, bowel sounds, and condition of the skin. The nurse might also use the time during the bath to teach the client or gather information for discharge planning.

Influence of Nurses on Health Policy

Professional nursing organizations are actively involved in local, state, and national politics.

- The major professional organizations actively lobby and educate government officials about the role of nursing in healthcare.
- Nursing organizations sponsor legislation that promotes the interest of the profession and supports changes that positively influence health outcomes (e.g., safe staffing in hospitals, funding for nursing education, needle exchange programs to minimize the spread of infectious diseases).

As individuals, nurses should vote, lobby their elected representatives, and run for political office. Together, nurses represent the largest health professional group (more than 3.8 million); thus, when united as a voting block, they have strong political power. Many nurses organize local nursing groups to support candidates or legislation or run successful campaigns at local, state, and national levels.

Nurses also influence policy by serving on federal or state advisory panels. For example, nurse leaders serve on the National Advisory Council for Healthcare Research and Quality to provide a nursing voice on issues related to healthcare quality, safety, and evidence-based practice. You should consider all of these political activities as you move into the profession.

Divergence Between High-Tech and High-Touch

Advances in clinical knowledge and technology have contributed to improved care and a longer life for many patients who are critically ill (e.g., premature newborns and patients with advanced cardiovascular, pulmonary, or renal disease). This trend is in contrast to the concurrent trend toward holism and high-touch therapies, which often avoid technology. One of the challenges in healthcare is integrating these two divergent trends. For an excellent discussion of these colliding values, read *Holistic Health and Healing* by Mary Anne Bright (2002).

CLINICALREASONING

The questions and exercises in this section allow you to practice the kind of thinking you will use as a full-spectrum nurse. Critical-thinking questions usually have more than one right answer, so we do not provide "correct answers" for these features. It is more important to develop your nursing judgment than to just cover content. You will learn by discussing the questions with your peers. If you are still unsure, see the Davis Advantage chapter resources for suggested responses.

Caring for the Nguyens

Review the opening scenario in the front of the book. On Nam Nguyen's preliminary visit to the Family Medicine Center, he is examined by Zach Miller, MSN, FNP-BC.

A. How would you respond to Nam if he is concerned that he is being examined by someone who is "just a nurse"?

B. What factors might cause Mr. Nguyen to question care given by "a male nurse"?

 To explore learning resources for this chapter,

 Go to **www.DavisAdvantage.com** and find:

Answers and Suggested Responses for all questions in this chapter

Knowledge Map

References and Bibliography

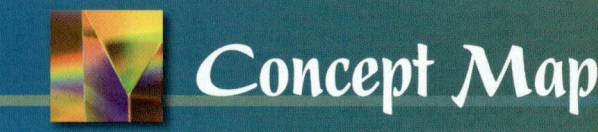

Concept Map

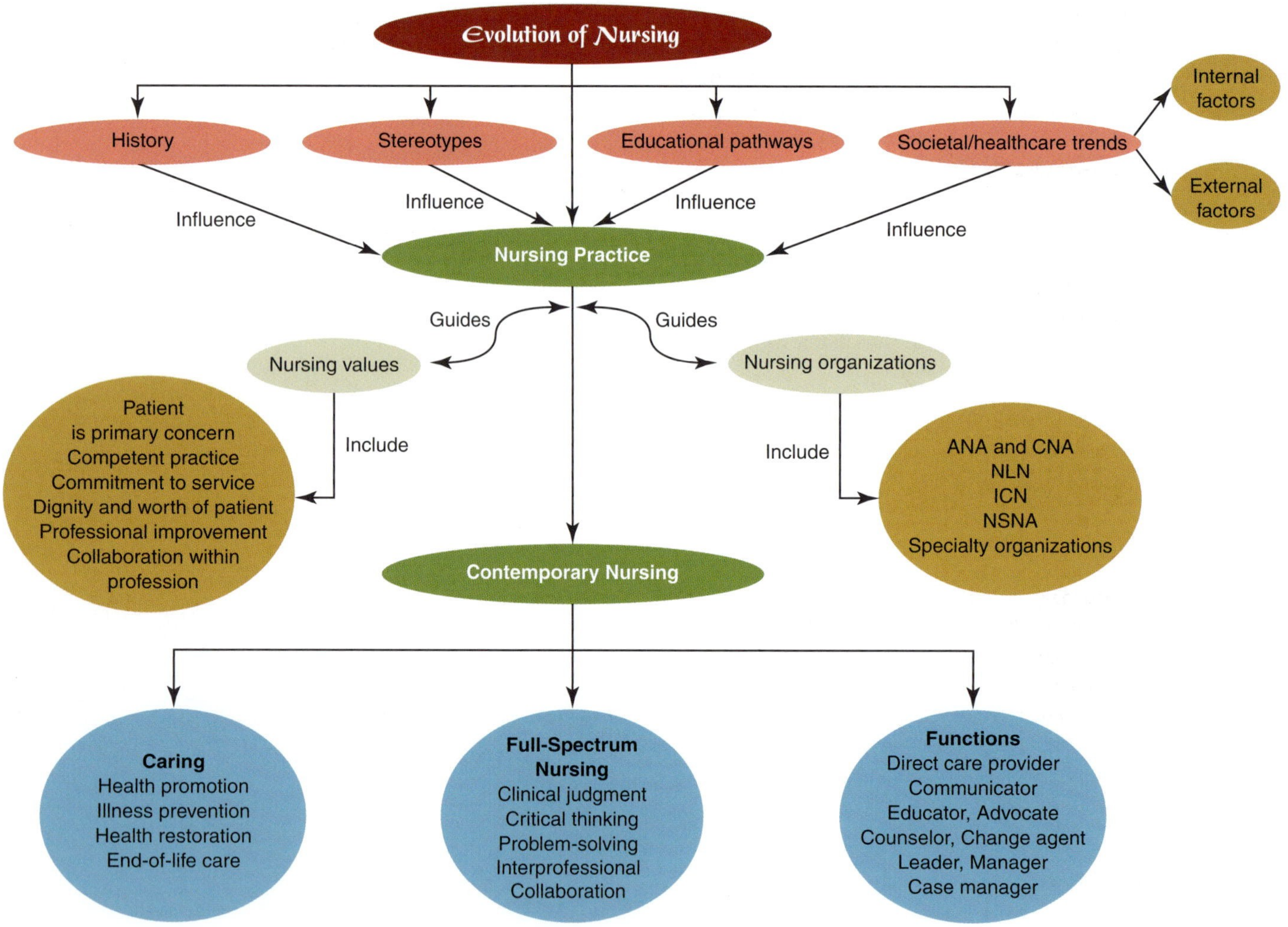

Evolution of Nursing

History   Stereotypes   Educational pathways   Societal/healthcare trends

Internal factors

External factors

Influence   Influence   Influence   Influence

Nursing Practice

Guides   Guides

Nursing values   Nursing organizations

Include   Include

Patient
is primary concern
Competent practice
Commitment to service
Dignity and worth of patient
Professional improvement
Collaboration within
profession

ANA and CNA
NLN
ICN
NSNA
Specialty organizations

Contemporary Nursing

Caring
Health promotion
Illness prevention
Health restoration
End-of-life care

**Full-Spectrum
Nursing**
Clinical judgment
Critical thinking
Problem-solving
Interprofessional
Collaboration

Functions
Direct care provider
Communicator
Educator, Advocate
Counselor, Change agent
Leader, Manager
Case manager

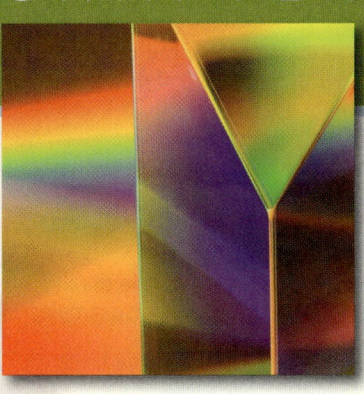
Critical Thinking & the Nursing Process

Learning Outcomes

After completing this chapter, you should be able to:

- ➤ Give one definition and one example of *critical thinking*.
- ➤ List and describe at least six critical-thinking skills.
- ➤ List and discuss seven attitudes of the critical thinker.
- ➤ Explain ways in which nurses use critical thinking.
- ➤ Describe the six overlapping and interdependent phases of the nursing process.
- ➤ Explain how critical thinking is used in the nursing process.
- ➤ List the four types of nursing knowledge discussed in this chapter.
- ➤ Name and describe the main concepts of the full-spectrum nursing model.
- ➤ Explain how the key concepts of nursing knowledge, nursing process, and critical thinking work together in full-spectrum nursing.

Key Concepts

Critical thinking

Full-spectrum nursing

Nursing knowledge

Nursing process

Related Concepts

See the Concept Map at the end of this chapter.

Explore Your Nursing Role

It's a pleasant Saturday afternoon, and you're meeting with an old friend whom you haven't seen in 2 years. She says, "I hear you've decided to become a nurse. What made you choose that? I don't think I could be around people who are sick and in pain. Hospitals are such sad places." To respond to her, you will need to consider your motivation for becoming a nurse and your beliefs about the profession.

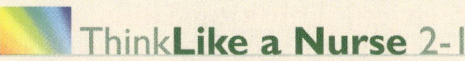Think**Like a Nurse** 2-1

How would you reply to her question?

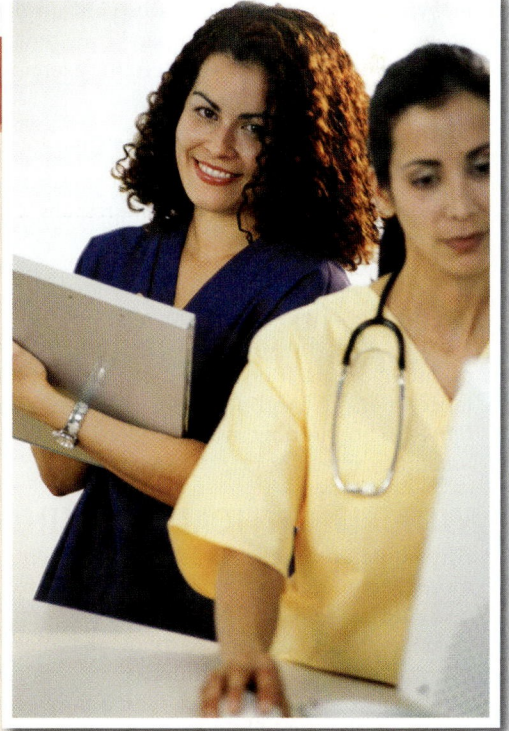

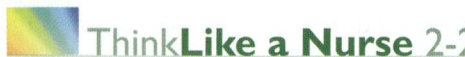

ThinkLike a Nurse 2-2

- What factors or persons influenced your decision to be a nurse?
- Of the possible answers you are considering, which answer best reflects your true feelings about your career choice? Why are the other answers not appropriate?
- What makes this situation similar to or different from your prior experiences?
- What's important in this situation?

If you are able to answer these questions, then you have used critical thinking to guide your decision making. You carefully considered a situation to arrive at a solution based on analysis of the data. That is vital when making important decisions. It is the kind of thinking you will use as a nurse.

TheoreticalKnowledge
knowing why

ABOUT THE KEY CONCEPTS

Keep the key concepts in mind as you read this chapter. They will give you the "hooks" on which you can "hang" the other details in the chapter. As you gain understanding of **critical thinking, nursing knowledge,** and **nursing process,** you will begin to see how they all work together in **full-spectrum nursing.**

WHAT DOES NURSING INVOLVE?

Chapter 1 introduced you to nursing roles, responsibilities, and activities and to the career of nursing. Throughout this text, you will learn much more. Thus, your view of nursing may change as you progress in your studies. To track your progress, you can later compare your developing view with the baseline you will establish in the exercises in this chapter.

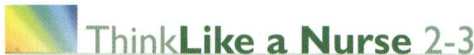

ThinkLike a Nurse 2-3

What is your image of nursing? List at least five attributes a nurse should have and at least five responsibilities that you consider to be part of nursing.

In the preceding exercise, you may have mentioned activities such as "gives medications" or "performs tests and treatments." And you were correct—partially. Nursing is activity oriented; that is, it involves *doing.* But don't forget the importance of *caring.* And now more than ever the emphasis is on *thinking.* So, another way to describe nursing is to say that *nursing involves thinking, doing, and caring.*

WHAT IS CRITICAL THINKING?

Any situation that requires critical thinking is likely to have more than one so-called right answer. For example, you do not need critical thinking to add 2 + 2 and come up with the answer. You simply know and follow the rules of addition. However, you *do* need critical thinking to work through more complex decisions and those in which the best answer is not so clear (e.g., "Should I buy a new car or a used one?").

There are many definitions of critical thinking because it is a complex concept and people think about it in different ways. Refer to the definitions in Box 2-1. Critical thinkers have intellectual skills that allow them to use their curiosity to

---

BOX 2-1 ■ Some Definitions of Critical Thinking

Highlight the important concepts in each of the definitions that follow. Then compare their similarities and differences.

A Simplistic (But Memorable) Definition

Critical thinking is "the art of thinking about your thinking while you are thinking in order to make your thinking better: more clear, more accurate, or more defensible" (Paul, 1990).

This definition tells us that we should reflect on the thinking process we are using to figure something out. For example:
- Why did I ask those particular questions?
- Do I have enough information to decide, or have I jumped to a conclusion?
- Have I considered all the possibilities?"

A Formal Definition (Study This One)

Critical thinking is a combination of reasoned thinking, an openness to alternatives, an ability to reflect, and a desire to seek truth.

Other Definitions

- ...the disciplined, intellectual process of applying skillful reasoning as a guide to belief or action. (Paul, Ennis, & Norris, 1996)
- ...careful and deliberate determination of whether to accept, reject, or suspend judgment. (Moore & Parker, 2015)
- ...reasonable and reflective thinking focused on deciding what to believe or do. (Ennis, 2011)
- ...(for clinical decision making in nursing), the ability to think in a systematic and logical manner with openness to questions and to reflect on the reasoning process used to ensure safe nursing practice and quality care. (Heaslip, 1992)
- ...disciplined, self-directed, rational thinking that supports what we know and makes clear what we don't know. (Wilkinson, 2012)
- The ideal critical thinker is well informed ... wise in judgments and decision making, logical ... uses sound reasoning, and is willing to consider valid alternatives. (American Philosophical Association, 1990)

---

their advantage, and they have critical attitudes that motivate them to use those skills responsibly.

What Are Critical-Thinking Skills?

Skills in critical thinking refer to the cognitive (intellectual) processes used in complex thinking operations such as problem-solving and decision making.

When planning nursing care, nurses gather information about the client (skill) and then **draw tentative conclusions about the meaning of the information (complex thinking process)** *to identify the client's problems. Then they think of several different actions they might take* **to help solve or relieve the problem.**

The following are examples of critical-thinking skills:
- Objectively gathering information on a problem or issue
- Recognizing the need for more information
- Evaluating the credibility and usefulness of sources of information
- Recognizing gaps in one's own knowledge

- Listening carefully; reading thoughtfully
- Separating relevant from irrelevant data and important from unimportant data
- Organizing or grouping information in meaningful ways
- Making inferences (tentative conclusions) about the meaning of the information
- Visualizing potential solutions to a problem
- Exploring the advantages, disadvantages, and consequences of each potential action
- Evaluating the credibility and usefulness of sources of information
- Recognizing differences and similarities among things or situations
- Prioritizing or ranking data as needed

What Are Critical-Thinking Attitudes?

Attitudes are not the same as intellectual skills. They are more like feelings and states of mind. Your attitudes and character determine whether you will use your thinking skills fairly and with an open mind. Without a critical attitude, people tend to use thinking skills to justify narrow-mindedness and prejudice and to benefit themselves rather than others. The following are some critical-thinking attitudes (Paul, 1990):

- **Independent thinking.** Critical thinkers do not believe everything they are told or just go along with the crowd. They listen to what others think and they learn from new ideas. They do not accept or reject an idea before they understand it. Nurses should challenge actions, practices, and policies having little logical support.
- **Intellectual curiosity.** Critical thinkers love to learn new things. They are inquisitive, exhibit an attitude of inquiry, and frequently think or ask, "What if . . . ?" "How could we do this differently?" "How does this work?" or "Why did that happen?"
- **Intellectual humility.** Critical thinkers are aware that they do not know everything. When they are unsure, they are not too proud or embarrassed to ask for help from mentors with wisdom, knowledge, skill, and ability. They reevaluate their conclusions or actions in light of new information and are willing to admit when they are wrong.
- **Intellectual empathy.** Critical thinkers try to understand the feelings and perceptions of others. They try to see a situation as the other person sees it.
- **Intellectual courage.** Critical thinkers consider and examine fairly their own values and beliefs as well as the beliefs of others, even when this is uncomfortable. They are willing to rethink, and even reject, previously held beliefs that are not well justified. Without intellectual courage, people become resistant to change.
- **Intellectual perseverance.** Critical thinkers don't jump to conclusions or settle for the quick, obvious answer. Important questions are usually complex, and critical thinkers give them serious thought and research, even when this takes a great deal of effort and time.
- **Fair-mindedness.** Critical thinkers try to make impartial judgments. They treat all viewpoints fairly, realizing that personal biases, customs, and social pressures can influence their thinking. They examine their own biases each time they make a decision.

Critical thinking can be used in all aspects of your life. Whenever you are trying to reach an important decision, reasoned action (critical thinking) is called for. Everyday uses of critical thinking might include deciding where you should live, choosing which nursing programs you should apply to, and deciding among several job offers. The rest of this chapter shows you why critical thinking is important to you in your chosen career, nursing.

KnowledgeCheck 2-1

- Define *critical thinking* in your own words.
- List five skills or attitudes that reflect critical thinking.

WHY IS CRITICAL THINKING IMPORTANT FOR NURSES?

Critical thinking helps you to know what is important about each patient's situation, when you need more information, and when you need help to make the best decision. Nurses use complex critical-thinking processes in every aspect of their work—that is, groups of thinking skills, such as problem-solving, decision making, and clinical reasoning (Table 2-1).

You should understand up front that it is not enough to just remember facts. It is impossible to learn, much less memorize, everything you need to know in nursing school. There is simply too much information. You will need to think conceptually and be a lifelong learner.

Nurses Deal With Complex Situations

Critical thinking is important for nurses because they deal with complicated situations. One example of a complex situation is that of caring for patients with **comorbidities** (more than one health problem occurring at the same time). Consider the following examples:

- **A healthy 9-year-old who fell and fractured his right arm; he has no comorbidities.** He would experience pain and discomfort, but with proper casting and time to heal the child would recover. While recovering, he may have to use his left hand to eat or limit the use of his injured arm. The child would likely be discharged home from the urgent setting in the care of his parent(s) or guardian(s). The nurse's primary interventions would be to teach the home caregivers how to provide care for the child.

- **An older adult who has fractured his right arm; he is also recovering from a stroke that limits the use of his left arm.** His experience would be quite different from that of the 9-year-old. A right-arm fracture would severely affect this person's ability to care for himself. The nurse would need to evaluate whether the adult requires care in the hospital or in a skilled-care facility and what support services he will need as he convalesces. In the inpatient setting, nursing interventions might initially include assisting the client with eating, bathing, and toileting.

Clients Are Unique

Critical thinking is important because each client is unique. Their differences (e.g., type of illness, cultural background, and age) make it impossible to provide rigid rules for all client care.

Individual Differences   Research-based care plans and protocols identify guidelines for providing care; however, nurses must evaluate and modify these guidelines to be sure they are appropriate for each client. Consider the following example: You may have been told to drink plenty of fluids when you have a cough to keep the secretions moist. Now imagine you are caring for a client in renal failure. Your client no longer urinates and may need dialysis. When she develops a persistent cough, should you encourage her to drink as much fluid as possible? Do you see how you could cause harm to a client by

Table 2-1 ➤ Complex Thinking Processes

The following are **complex thinking (reasoning) processes** that involve use of a combination of critical-thinking skills and attitudes:

PROCESS AND DEFINITION	DESCRIPTION/DISCUSSION
Problem-Solving: Identifying a problem and finding reasonable solutions to it.	Requires critical-thinking skills such as: ■ Organizing data ■ Identifying relevant and important data ■ Making inferences ■ Making decisions ■ Projecting consequences of actions ■ Applying theoretical knowledge to a specific patient context
Decision Making: Choosing the best action to take. In nursing, this is usually the action likely to produce the desired patient outcome.	■ Requires thinking skills such as making judgments (e.g., about what is important) and making choices ■ Important in problem-solving; however, many decisions are made that are not related to problem-solving.
Clinical Reasoning: Reflective, concurrent, creative thinking about patients and patient care.	■ **Reasoning** is logical thinking that links thoughts together to create meaning. ■ Nurses use **clinical reasoning** in the nursing process.

unthinkingly doing as you have been told? **KEY POINT:** *Nurses must always think, "How will that work for this client?" "How is this like or different from similar situations?"*

Multiple and Varying Concerns In addition to their health problems, patients are concerned about their families, their jobs, and so on. This means that a patient's response to therapy may not always be apparent nor be as expected. Nurses constantly use reasoning and reflection to assess patients, to decide what interventions to use, and to determine whether treatments worked. If the treatments did not work, they need to discover what could have been changed or done differently.

Client's Culture Ethnic and cultural differences affect a person's view of health and the healthcare system as well as his responses to health problems. Cultural beliefs influence how people define sickness, at what point they seek healthcare, what type of healthcare provider they see, and the type of treatment they consider acceptable. Critical thinking enables the nurse to assess the client's and family's cultural beliefs and adapt care so that it is culturally sensitive and responsive to their needs.

Client's Roles A client's *roles* also influence when, how, and why a person seeks healthcare. A single mother with young children may ask to be discharged from the hospital early to meet the needs of her family. Clients with extensive support from family or friends may be willing to take more time to convalesce when they are ill. Nurses take these things into consideration—for example, when determining why a nursing intervention was (or was not) successful.

Other Factors In addition, the following factors may influence how a person responds to illness or to healthcare intervention:

■ *Age.* Each of us was raised with beliefs, values, and knowledge that were strongly influenced by the prevailing views of our times.

■ *Personal bias.* Clients may have fixed beliefs about health and illness.

■ *Personality.* Individuals have unique personalities. This means that every person is different; all have individual ways of responding to stress, fear, illness, and pain. Some are hardy and show an attitude of strength and endurance and exhibit a high threshold to pain. Others are less tolerant and may outwardly express pain or other conditions associated with illness, hospitalization, and death.

■ *Previous experience with healthcare problems.* For example, a boy who has experienced a painful injection in the past may be terrified when he sees the nurse approach with a syringe.

Nurses Apply Knowledge to Provide Holistic Care

In addition to the uniqueness of clients, some aspects of nursing itself require that the nurse be a critical thinker:

■ *Nursing is an applied discipline.* Nurses deal with complex, ill-defined, and sometimes confusing problems—not well-defined, straightforward ones such as you find in a math book. This means that nurses must *apply* their knowledge, not merely memorize and regurgitate facts. **KEY POINT:** *To be a safe and competent nurse you must be able to* **apply** *your knowledge and skills in caring for patients.*

■ *Nursing uses knowledge from other fields.* Nurses use information from chemistry, physiology, psychology, social sciences, and other disciplines to identify and plan interventions for patient problems. Nursing plays an important role within a multidisciplinary approach to patient care.

■ *Nursing is fast paced.* Nurses often deal with demanding situations. A patient's condition may change hour to hour or even minute to minute, so knowing the routine may not be adequate. You will need critical thinking in order to respond appropriately under stress.

- *The scientific basis for patient care changes constantly.* Therefore, you must constantly update your knowledge and skills throughout your career. You will need to develop and refine your critical-thinking skills as well.
- *Critical thinking is linked to evidence-based practice,* which you will learn more about later in this book. Evidence-based practice is a research-based method for judging and choosing nursing interventions. The critical-thinking skill of identifying and checking your assumptions is an important aspect of the research process.

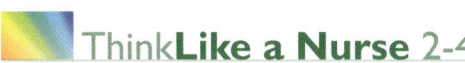

ThinkLike a Nurse 2-4

Write a short scenario (story) about a nurse that illustrates one of the reasons why nurses need to be critical thinkers.

A MODEL FOR CRITICAL THINKING

A **model** is a set of interrelated concepts that represent a particular way of thinking about something—much in the same way that the shape of a lens affects what you see. For example, you would look through a telescope to view a distant star. Looking at the star through reading glasses would give a different view. You will learn more about models in Chapter 8.

The critical-thinking model used throughout this book provides one way of making sense of critical thinking. This model organizes critical thinking into five major categories. Box 2-2 defines each category and provides questions to help you focus your thinking in clinical reasoning. You can use some of the questions when deciding what to think about and do; you can use others when analyzing a situation after it happens (reflecting). Figure 2-1 is a simpler representation of the model, relating it to the nursing process, which is introduced later in this chapter.

This model is not meant to be all inclusive; critical thinking is more than just considering the questions listed in Box 2-2. Use it as a guide when faced with clinical decisions or unfamiliar situations. It should help you to achieve good outcomes for your patients. The questions can help you to "think about your thinking" as you apply principles and knowledge from various sources to a patient problem. You do not need to ask yourself every question in every situation—just those that are relevant.

BOX 2-2 ■ Critical-Thinking Model

Contextual Awareness

- Deciding what to observe and consider
- An awareness of what's happening in the total situation, including values, cultural issues, interpersonal relationships, and environmental influences

Questions for Focusing Thinking

- What is going on in the situation that may influence the outcome?
- What factors may influence my behavior and that of others in this situation (e.g., culture, roles, relationships, economic status)?
- What about this situation have I seen before? What is new?
- Who should be involved in order to improve the outcome?
- What else was happening at the same time that affected me in this situation?
- What happened just before this incident that made a difference?
- What emotional responses influenced how I reacted in this situation?
- What changes in behavior alerted me that something was wrong?

Inquiry

- Based on credible sources
- Applying standards of good reasoning to your thinking when analyzing a situation and evaluating your actions

Questions for Focusing Thinking

- How do I go about gathering the information I need?
- What framework should I use to organize my information?
- Do I have enough knowledge to decide? If not, what do I need to know?
- Have I used a valid, reliable source of information (e.g., patient, other professionals, references)?
- Did I (do I need to) validate the data (e.g., with the client)?

- What else do I need to know? What information is missing?
- Are the data accurate? Precise?
- What's important and what's not important in this situation?
- Did I consider professional, ethical, and legal standards?
- Have I jumped to conclusions?

Considering Alternatives

Exploring and imagining as many alternatives as you can think of for the situation

Questions for Focusing Thinking

- What is one possible explanation for what is happening or what happened?
- What are other explanations for what is happening? What is one thing I could do in this situation?
- What are two more possibilities/alternatives?
- Are there others who might help me develop more alternatives?
- Of the possible actions I am considering, which one is most reasonable? Why are the others not as reasonable?
- Of the possible actions I am considering, which one is most likely to achieve the desired outcomes?

Analyzing Assumptions

Recognizing and analyzing assumptions you are making about the situation and examining the beliefs that underlie your choices

Questions for Focusing Thinking

- What have I (or others) taken for granted in this situation?
- Which beliefs/values are shaping my assumptions?
- What assumptions contributed to the problem in this situation?
- What rationale supports my assumptions?
- How will I know whether my assumptions are correct?
- What biases do I have that may affect my thinking and my decisions in this situation?

(Continued)

BOX 2-2 ■ Critical-Thinking Model—cont'd

Reflecting Skeptically and Deciding What to Do

Questioning, analyzing, and reflecting on the rationale for your decisions

Questions for Focusing Thinking

- What aspects of this situation require the most careful attention?
- What else might work in this situation?
- Am I sure of my interpretation of this situation?
- Why is (was) it important to intervene?
- What rationale do I have for my decisions?
- In priority order, what should I do in this situation and why?
- Having decided what was wrong/happening, what is the best response?
- What might I delegate in this situation?

- What got me started taking some action?
- What priorities were missed?
- What was done? Why was it done?
- What would I do differently after reflecting on this situation?

Sources: Model based on Brookfield, S. D. (1991). *Developing critical thinkers.* San Francisco, CA: Jossey-Bass; McDonald, M. E. (2002). *Systematic assessment of learning outcomes: Developing multiple-choice exams.* Boston, MA: Jones & Bartlett; Paul, R. W. (1993). *Critical thinking: What every person needs to survive in a rapidly changing world* (3rd ed.). Santa Rosa, CA: Foundation for Critical Thinking; Raingruber, B., & Haffer, A. (2001). *Using your head to land on your feet.* Philadelphia, PA: F. A. Davis; and Wilkinson, J. M. (2012). *Nursing process and critical thinking* (5th ed.). Upper Saddle River, NJ: Prentice Hall.

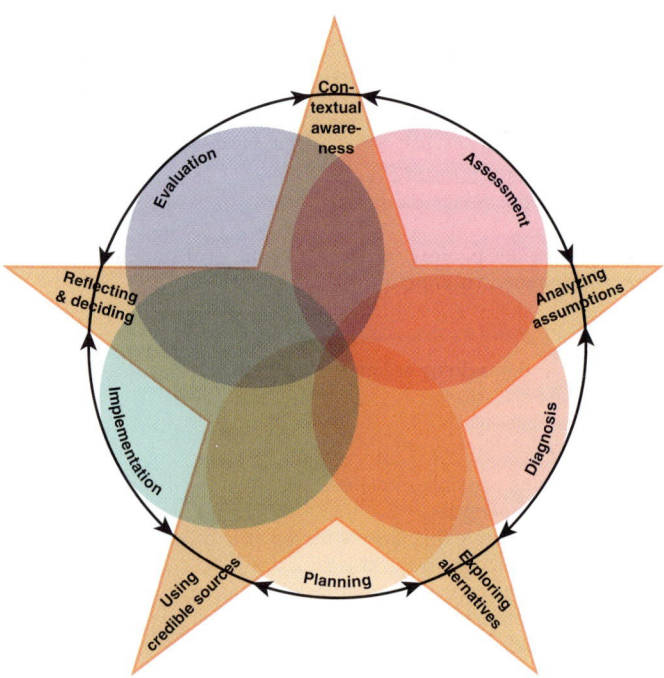

FIGURE 2-1 Model of critical thinking and the nursing process.

The processes do not occur sequentially, so you may jump back and forth between them.

Applying the Model: An Example

Let's apply the model to a familiar situation. Soon you will begin your clinical rotations if you have not already done so. Many students find this exciting yet somewhat intimidating.

✚ How could you use the five points of the critical-thinking star (Fig. 2-1) to approach your first clinical day so you will be well prepared and able to function safely?

Contextual Awareness One of the first things you need to consider is your usual response to new experiences. How do you react to change? What other tasks or assignments do you

have that will dictate the timing of your preparation? Have you had any previous experiences that will aid or hamper you in your preparation? As you consider these questions, you are addressing the star point of contextual awareness.

Using Credible Sources You need to gather accurate information about the clinical experience. Base your inquiry on *credible sources.* Consider these examples:

- Ask your instructor for guidance on how to best prepare.
- Consult a student who has successfully completed the same course.

You will also need accurate information about the clients who have been assigned to you. Use only *knowledgeable, reliable sources,* such as the following:

- The client's chart
- Certain Internet sites
- Nursing texts and journals (not popular, nonscholarly magazines, such as *Parents* magazine)

After you have more information, reexamine your response to the situation. You may find that you are feeling less anxious already! All of this is a part of *inquiry.*

Exploring Alternatives and Analyzing Assumptions Now that you know something about the clinical experience, you can plan your day. You need to consider alternatives and analyze your assumptions about the experience.

- What is expected of you?
- What do you expect from the experience?
- How should you approach your client?
- How will you introduce yourself?
- What skills do you have?
- How will you apply your skills to caring for your client?

Reflecting and Deciding After you have addressed these concerns, quickly review your preparation (*reflective skepticism*).

- Do you have enough information to feel comfortable in the situation?
- Have you left anything out?
- Do you need more information?

This was a demonstration of how you might apply the critical-thinking model to a real experience. In this example, you also used theoretical, practical, personal (self), and ethical knowledge, which are explained in the next section.

WHAT ARE THE DIFFERENT KINDS OF NURSING KNOWLEDGE?

Critical thinking does not occur in a vacuum. You must have something to think *about*—a knowledge base.

Theoretical Knowledge Each chapter in your text begins by presenting theoretical knowledge. **Theoretical knowledge**—knowing why—consists of information, facts, principles, and evidence-based theories in nursing and related disciplines (e.g., physiology and psychology). It includes research findings and rationally constructed explanations of phenomena. You will use it to describe your patients, understand their health status, explain your reasoning for choosing interventions, and predict patient responses to interventions and treatments.

Practical Knowledge Each chapter also provides the practical knowledge that enables you to apply your theoretical knowledge to caring for patients. **Practical knowledge**—knowing what to do and how to do it—consists of processes (e.g., decision process, nursing process, change process) and procedures (e.g., how to give an injection) and is an aspect of nursing expertise.

Self-Knowledge In addition to theoretical and practical knowledge, nurses use **self-knowledge,** or self-understanding. To think critically, you must be aware of your beliefs, values, and cultural and religious biases. This kind of knowledge helps you find errors in your thinking and enables you to tune in to your patients. You can gain self-knowledge by developing personal awareness—by reflecting (asking yourself), "Why did I do that?" or "How did I come to think that?"

Ethical Knowledge Finally, nurses use **ethical knowledge,** that is, knowledge of obligation, or right and wrong. Ethical knowledge consists of information about moral principles and processes for making moral decisions. Ethical knowledge helps you to fulfill your ethical obligations to patients and colleagues. Chapter 43 will help expand your ethical knowledge.

This text is organized using the concepts of practical knowledge and theoretical knowledge, as summarized in the following list:

Practical Knowledge:	Knowing What *(That is, knowing what to do and how to do it)*
Theoretical Knowledge:	Knowing Why *(That is, knowing why to do something)*

KnowledgeCheck 2-2

Think about the preceding discussion of the five points of the critical-thinking model and identify the actions that demonstrate use of each of the four types of knowledge.

PracticalKnowledge
knowing **how**

WHAT IS NURSING PROCESS?

Nursing process is a systematic problem-solving process that guides all nursing actions. It is the type of thinking and doing nurses use in their practice. In fact, the American Nurses Association (ANA) organizes its standards of care around the nursing process (ANA, 2015).

ThinkLike a Nurse 2-5

Practice your critical thinking. What questions should you ask about the last paragraph you have just read? For hints, look at Figure 2-1 and Box 2-2. An obvious first question might be, "Do I know what the ANA is and what it does?"

Nursing process has the following characteristics:

- **Useful in many settings.** Nurses apply nursing process, to well and ill clients alike, in many settings (e.g., homes, clinics, hospitals).
- **Goal directed and client centered.** The purpose of the nursing process is to help the nurse provide goal-directed, client-centered care.
- **Involves both thinking and doing.** Nurses must have good psychomotor and interpersonal skills, a sound knowledge base, and good judgment to use the nursing process effectively.
- **Not linear.** One step does not rigidly follow another. Instead, it is a *cyclical* process that follows a logical progression. The evaluation step requires you to begin again using all the other steps. You will find that you go back and forth between the steps, especially as you gain nursing experience.
- **Steps may be concurrent.** In addition to being cyclical, some of the steps may occur at the same time. For example, while inserting a urinary catheter (implementation), the nurse also observes the urine that returns through the tube (assessment).

What Are the Phases of the Nursing Process?

The nursing process consists of six phases (or steps): assessment, diagnosis, planning outcomes, planning interventions, implementation, and evaluation (Wilkinson, 2012). A model illustrating these phases is shown in Figure 2-2. Various experts

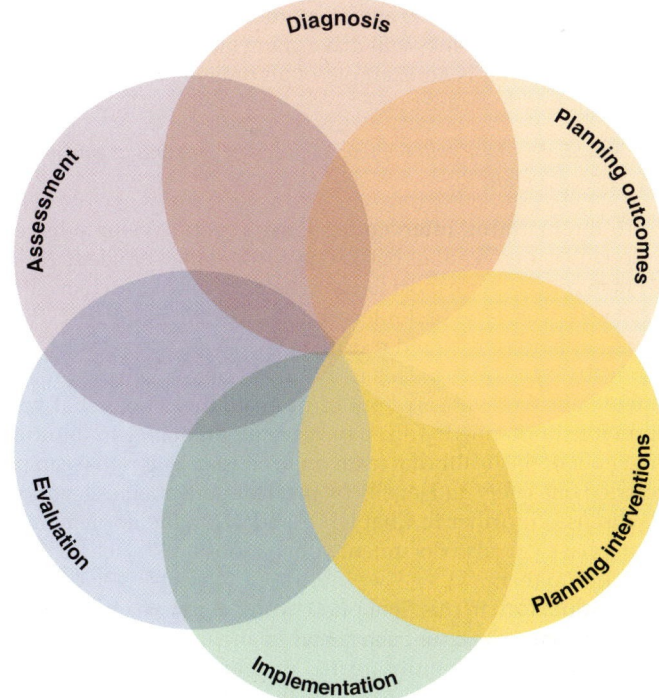

FIGURE 2-2 The phases of the nursing process.

organize the phases in different ways. Some have a four-step process that combines assessment and diagnosis into one phase that they call "assessment." Many have a five-step process, combining outcomes and interventions into one "planning" phase. There is no "right" way to do it, and experienced nurses do not use the steps separately. Your text presents them as distinct and separate only to make it easier for you to learn how the process works.

What follows is a summary of each nursing process phase. You will learn about them in more depth in Chapters 3 through 7.

Assessment   The first phase of the nursing process—the data-gathering stage—is assessment.

- **Multiple sources.** You will obtain information from many sources: the client via history or physical examination, the client record, other health professionals, the client's family or support system, and the professional literature.
- **Purpose of assessment.** You will use the data that you gather to draw conclusions about the client's health status.

Diagnosis   This is the second phase of the nursing process. In this step you will identify the client's health strengths and needs (usually stated in the form of a problem) based on careful review of your assessment data. The term *diagnosis* has been thought of as being medical, such as a diagnosis of cancer or diabetes. However, nursing diagnoses reflect the client's responses to actual or potential health problems and are different from medical diagnoses, as you will discover in Chapter 4.

Planning (Outcomes and Interventions)   The third and fourth steps both involve planning—planning outcomes and planning interventions. The end result of planning is a holistic nursing care plan, individualized to reflect the client's problems and strengths. A care plan is a written or electronic document containing detailed instructions for a client's nursing care. See Chapter 5 for more about goals and outcomes and Chapter 6 for more about interventions.

- In the **planning outcomes** step, you work with the client to decide goals for client care—that is, the client outcomes (or changes) you want to achieve through your nursing activities. These outcomes will drive your choice of interventions. The following is an example of an outcome statement you might find in a care plan:

  Nutritional status will improve as evidenced by a weight gain of 3 lb (1.4 kg) by July 1.

- In the **planning interventions** phase, you develop a list of possible interventions based on your nursing knowledge and then choose those most likely to help the client to achieve the stated goals. The best interventions are evidence-based, that is, supported by sound research.

Implementation   This is the action phase. During implementation you will carry out or delegate the actions that you previously planned. You may delegate an action to another member of the healthcare team only if it is an action that can be carried out safely and legally by that team member. Delegation is discussed further in Chapters 7 and 41. In the implementation phase you also document your actions and the client's responses to them.

Evaluation   In this final phase, you determine whether the desired outcomes have been achieved and judge whether your actions have successfully treated or prevented the identified health problems. You then modify the care plan as needed. For example, if a problem has been resolved, you delete it from the care plan; if outcomes have not been achieved, you determine why. It may be that a new intervention is needed. If so, you add it.

KnowledgeCheck 2-3

- List the six phases of the nursing process.
- In which stage does the nurse collect data?
- Which stage involves problem identification?
- What does the nurse do in the evaluation step?
- True or False: Nursing process phases must be used in order.

How Is the Nursing Process Related to Critical Thinking?

KEY POINT: *Critical thinking and nursing process are interrelated but not identical.*

- **We think critically about things other than patient care.** Nursing decisions that require critical thinking may not be related to the nursing process (e.g., deciding how many nurses are needed to staff the unit).
- **Some nursing activities do not require reflective critical thinking,** although they must be done skillfully (e.g., applying a cardiac monitor, inserting a urinary catheter).
- **Nursing process is essentially a problem-solving process.** As such, it is one of the *complex critical-thinking skills* (see Table 2-1). Complex thinking skills, such as the nursing process, make use of many different critical-thinking skills (see Box 2-2 and Fig. 2-1). The remainder of the chapter illustrates how nurses use critical thinking and nursing knowledge in each phase of the nursing process.

WHAT IS CARING?

Caring involves personal concern for people, events, projects, and things. It allows you to connect with others and to give help as well as receive it. One aspect of self-knowledge is to be aware of what and whom you care about. Knowing what the patient cares about reveals what is stressful for the patient, because only things that matter can create stress. Caring also enables the nurse to notice which interventions are effective.

- *Caring is always specific and relational for each nurse–person encounter.* A caring perspective highlights each person as unique and valued.
- *Caring is not an abstraction.* That is, you don't just care for "suffering humankind," but you respond compassionately to *this* patient's needs right now, in the moment, even if you are busy and tired.
- *Caring involves thinking and acting in ways that preserve human dignity and humanity.* It does not treat people as objects. For example, a caring nurse drapes a patient for privacy when inserting a urinary catheter. A caring nurse's actions are never routine or impersonal.

Caring has at least five components (see Table 2-2). Caring is the central concept in several nursing theories. You will learn more about those theories in Chapter 8.

WHAT IS FULL-SPECTRUM NURSING?

KEY POINT: Full-spectrum nursing *is a unique blend of thinking, doing, and caring.* Full-spectrum nursing is performed by nurses who fully develop and apply nursing knowledge, critical

Table 2-2 ➤ Five Components of Caring

CARING COMPONENT	DEFINITION	EXAMPLES
Knowing	Striving to understand what an event means in the life of the patient	Illness A new baby Loss of a loved one
Being With	Being emotionally present for the patient	Making eye contact Active listening
Doing For	Doing what the patient would do for himself if he could	Bathing Feeding Calling the patient's pastor
Enabling	Supporting the patient through coping with life changes and unfamiliar events	Hospitalization Birth of a premature infant
Maintaining Belief	Having faith in the patient's ability to get through the change or event and to find fulfillment and meaning (Swanson, 1990)	Adapting to a new colostomy Adapting to loss of a limb Cardiac rehabilitation

thinking, and the nursing process to patient situations. The purpose of full-spectrum nursing is to achieve safe, effective care and promote good patient outcomes.

What Concepts Are Used in the Full-Spectrum Nursing Model?

You have learned about the model for critical thinking. You are now prepared to learn about a model to explain the concept of *nursing*. You'll learn more about concepts in Chapter 8; for now, think of them as ideas. The four main concepts that describe full-spectrum nursing are *thinking, doing, caring,* and *patient situation* (or context) (Table 2-3).

When nurses think, they use the nursing knowledge that they have stored in their memory. In addition, they think about the patient situation, which they acquire through use of

the nursing process. **Situation,** or **context,** refers to the context for care, the patient's environment outside the care setting, relationships, resources available for patient care, and so on. Figure 2-3 is a simple, visual model of full-spectrum nursing. You can see that the concept's full model involves everything you have learned about in this chapter—critical thinking, nursing knowledge, and nursing process—but organized under the simple concepts of thinking, doing, caring, and patient situation.

Let's see how the model concepts work together for a full-spectrum nurse. They are all interrelated and overlapping, but we divide them into simple categories to help you understand and remember them. You can see that a full-spectrum nurse needs excellent thinking skills because there is so much to think *about* and so much to *do*.

Table 2-3 ➤ Full-Spectrum Nursing Concepts

THINKING	DOING	CARING	PATIENT SITUATION
Critical Thinking Enables you to fully use your knowledge and skills	**Practical Knowledge** Skills, procedures, and processes (including the nursing process)	**Self-Knowledge** Awareness of your values, beliefs, and biases	**Patient Data** Physical, psychosocial, spiritual
Theoretical Knowledge Principles, facts, theories; what you have to think with	**Nursing Process** *Assessment and Evaluation:* Everything you know about the patient including context *Planning and Implementation:* What you do for the patient	**Ethical Knowledge** Understanding your obligations; sense of right and wrong	**Patient Preferences, Context** Context for care, environment, relationships, culture, resources, supports

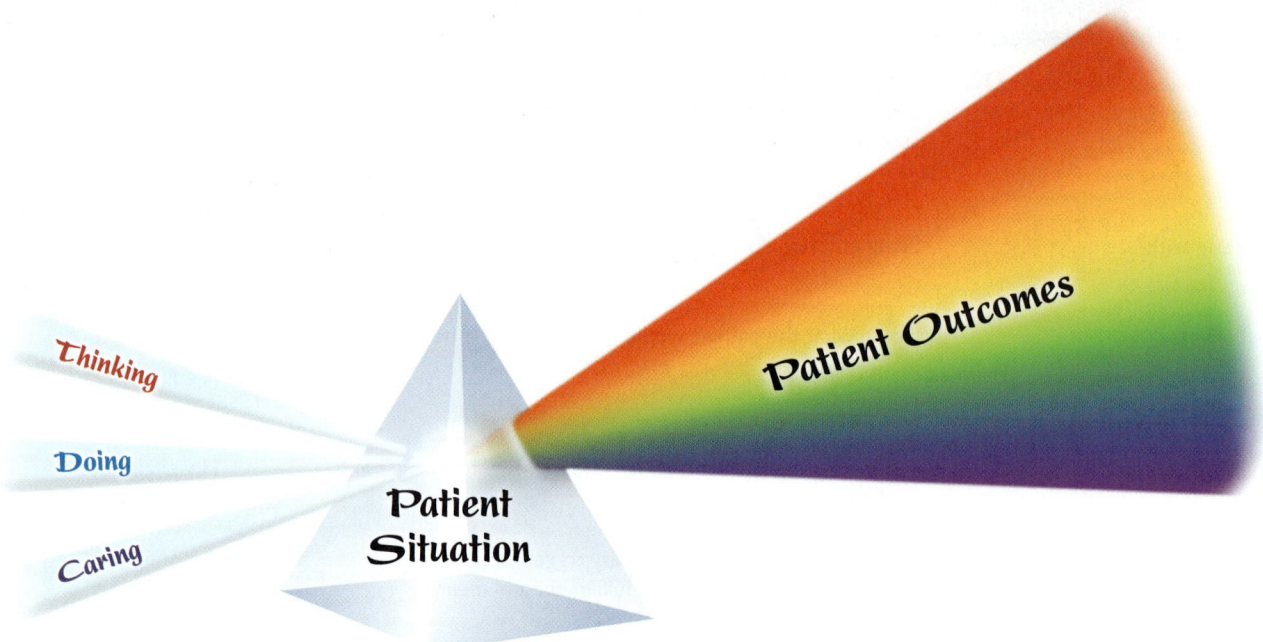

FIGURE 2-3 Model of full-spectrum nursing.

KnowledgeCheck 2-4

- What are the four main concepts of the full-spectrum model of nursing?
- Where do the four types of nursing knowledge fit into the full-spectrum model?
- What is the ultimate purpose of full-spectrum nursing?
- List all the characteristics of caring that you can remember.

How Does the Model Work?

The full-spectrum nursing model is used throughout this text, so it is important that you understand how it works. Nurses use critical *thinking* in all steps of the nursing process. They also apply critical thinking to the four kinds of nursing knowledge. When they are *doing* for the patient, *caring* motivates and facilitates the *thinking* and *doing*. The goal of all this is to have a positive effect on a patient's health outcomes.

The following patient situation illustrates how the four main dimensions of full-spectrum nursing work together. As you read, notice how the concepts overlap. For example, recall that nursing process and problem-solving are themselves complex critical-thinking skills. Also notice how the nurse uses critical thinking with nursing knowledge and the nursing process.

Patient Situation

When taking a patient's oral temperature, a nurse sees a glass of ice water on the overbed table. Realizing that a cold drink can reduce the accuracy of the temperature reading, she asks the patient, "How long has it been since you've taken a drink of water?" The patient tells her it was just a minute ago. The nurse is busy and tired, but she returns to take the patient's temperature again at a later time when it will be accurate.

Thinking

- *Theoretical knowledge.* The nurse realized that a cold drink can lower the patient's temperature. The nurse used interviewing principles to get more information from the patient.
- *Critical thinking.* The nurse recognized relevant information and identified the need for more data. She used the patient's answer to decide what to do. Being aware of context is an aspect of critical thinking. The context in this scenario includes the following: (1) The ice water was within the patient's reach and (2) the patient was physically capable of reaching it and had just taken a drink.

Doing

- *Practical knowledge.* The nurse used a psychomotor skill when she measured the patient's temperature to acquire more patient vital sign data. She used a communication process to question the patient.
- *Nursing process. (Assessment)* The nurse observed the glass of ice water on the table. The nurse asked, "How long has it been since you've taken a drink of water?" The nurse also observed the environmental data (e.g., ice water at the bedside). *(Implementation)* The nurse took the patient's temperature.

Caring

The scenario does not state this, but a caring nurse, even a very busy one, would not be annoyed with the patient for the inconvenience of having to return to take the temperature.

- *Self-knowledge* might include the nurse's awareness that she is tired and feeling irritable.
- *Ethical knowledge* would tell her that she has an obligation to get an accurate temperature from the patient rather than thinking, "Oh, I'll just estimate the reading a degree or two higher, as it doesn't matter that much."

As a full-spectrum nurse, you will apply thinking, doing, and caring to patient situations to help benefit patients and bring about good outcomes.

Toward Evidence-Based Practice

Catlett, S., & Lovan, S. (2011). Being a good nurse and doing the right thing: A replication study. *Nursing Ethics*, 18(1), 54–63.

The purpose of this qualitative study was to examine nurses' perceptions of what it means to be a good nurse and to do the right thing. Researchers used open-ended questions to interview nurse subjects. They identified four categories that related to being a good nurse and doing the right thing: (1) personal traits and attributes; (2) technical skills and management of care; (3) work environment and coworkers; and (4) caring and caring behaviors.

1. What examples of full-spectrum nursing can you see in the four categories identified?

2. Based on this abstract, which of the following questions might this study answer satisfactorily for you? Explain your reasoning.
   a. What is a good nurse?
   b. Did the nurse subjects demonstrate critical thinking?
   c. How did the nurse subjects describe a good nurse?

 Go to Davis Advantage, Resources, Chapter 2, **Toward Evidence-Based Practice Suggested Responses.**

CLINICALREASONING

The questions and exercises in this section allow you to practice the kind of thinking you will use as a full-spectrum nurse. Critical-thinking questions usually have more than one correct answer, so we do not provide "correct answers" for these features. It is more important to develop your nursing judgment than to just cover content. You will learn by discussing the questions with your peers. If you are still unsure, see the Davis Advantage chapter resources for suggested responses.

Caring for the Nguyens

Review the opening scenario of Nam Nguyen in the front of this book. Imagine you are the clinic nurse at the Family Medicine Center. Based on the information presented in the scenario, work through the following questions:

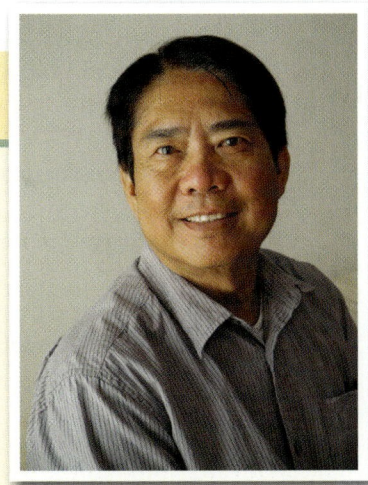

A. Patient Situation
   - Why is Mr. Nguyen at the clinic?
   - What are his wife's concerns?
   - Are they similar to or different from his?

B. Critical Thinking
   - How do I go about getting the data I need? What sources should I use?
   - Are my data congruent?
   - What is one possible explanation for what is happening in this situation?

C. Nursing Knowledge
   - What type of nursing knowledge (theoretical, practical, ethical, or self-knowledge) is needed to answer the following questions?

   - What health concerns does Mr. Nguyen have that should be addressed by the healthcare team?
   - What is the role of Zach Miller on the healthcare team?
   - What role will you play in the care of Mr. Nguyen?

D. Nursing Process
   - In what phase of the nursing process are you engaged when you are asking Mr. Nguyen about the reason for his visit?
   - What activities are involved in the diagnosis phase? In planning outcomes? In planning interventions?
   - Why would you not, at this point, be using the evaluation phase?

Applying the **Full-Spectrum Nursing Model**_____

PATIENT SITUATION

Mrs. Castillo has late-stage cancer and is not expected to live more than a few months. With chemotherapy, she could live perhaps a year or two more. She cannot decide what to do. She knows that the chemotherapy will have unpleasant side effects and will be very expensive, and she wants to protect her family from the emotional and financial hardships of a lingering illness. She is showing physical signs of anxiety and distress (e.g., increased heart rate, restlessness, tearfulness). You want to provide support for her decision, whatever it may be.

THINKING

1. *Theoretical Knowledge:* What theoretical knowledge do you need to help Mrs. Castillo?
2. *Critical Thinking (Contextual Awareness):* What details in the scenario represent "patient situation" or "context"?

DOING

3. *Practical Knowledge:*
   a. What practical knowledge do you need to help Mrs. Castillo?
   b. Which skills can you already perform? Which skills would you need to learn or review before caring for this patient?

CARING

4. *Ethical Knowledge:* Depending on Mrs. Castillo's decision, can you think of one ethical issue that might arise for you or members of her family later on?

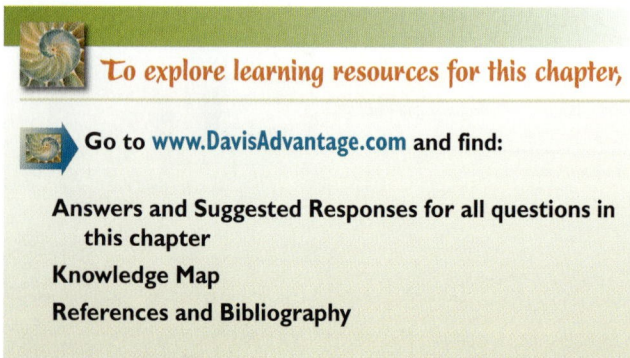

To explore learning resources for this chapter,

Go to **www.DavisAdvantage.com** and find:

Answers and Suggested Responses for all questions in this chapter
Knowledge Map
References and Bibliography

Concept Map

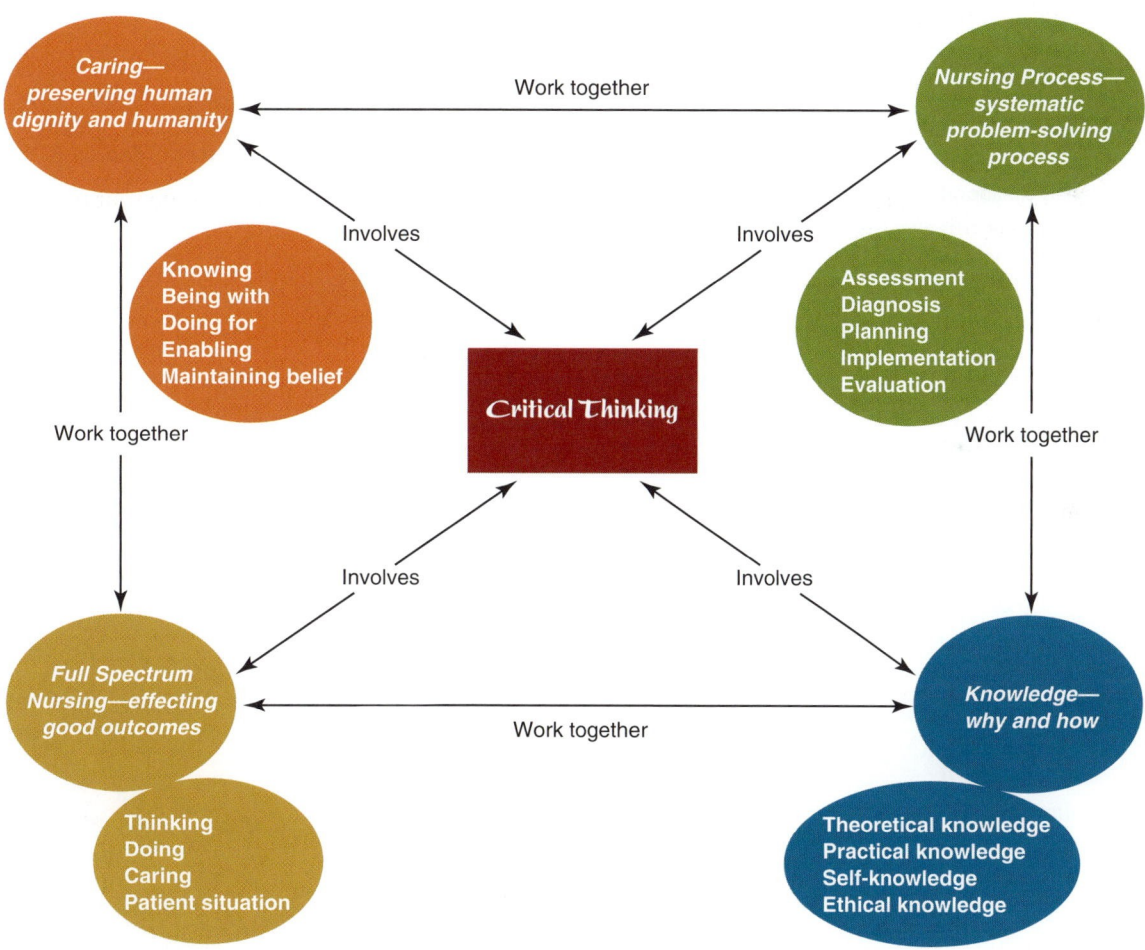

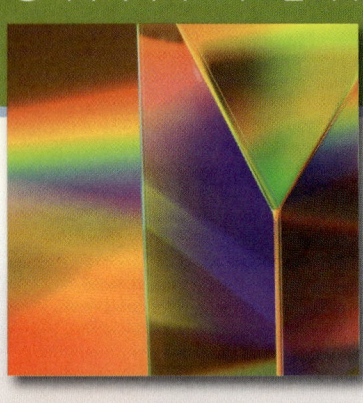

CHAPTER 3

Assessment

Learning Outcomes

After completing this chapter, you should be able to:

- Define *nursing assessment*.
- Explain how assessment is related to each of the other steps of the nursing process.
- Discuss the relationship between nursing process and collaborative care.
- Discuss professional standards affecting nursing process (e.g., American Nurses Association, The Joint Commission).
- Differentiate among four sources of data: subjective, objective, primary source, secondary source.
- Describe and differentiate among initial, ongoing, comprehensive, focused, and special needs assessment.
- Explain the importance of discharge planning assessment.
- Identify and describe at least four components of a nursing health history.
- Discuss how to prepare for and conduct an interview.
- Compare and contrast open-ended and closed questions.
- Describe circumstances in which you should validate data.
- Use nursing frameworks to organize data.
- State at least four guidelines for documenting data.
- Reflect critically about your assessments.

Key Concepts

Assessment
Data

Related Concepts

See the Concept Map.

Meet Your Patient

As the intake nurse in a community-based clinic, your role is to complete a comprehensive nursing assessment and initiate a plan of care for the clients. Your first client is a 24-year-old single woman, Sami, who is requesting clinic services for her general healthcare needs. Sami is Cuban American and lives alone in a one-bedroom apartment. She works as a fitness trainer at the local fitness club while attending college part-time. Her family lives across the state. Sami's earnings place her at the poverty level. She realizes that she must have healthcare to prevent health problems and to detect and receive treatment of illnesses should they arise. You will be asked to apply full-spectrum thinking to Sami's case throughout the chapter as you learn the concepts of assessment.

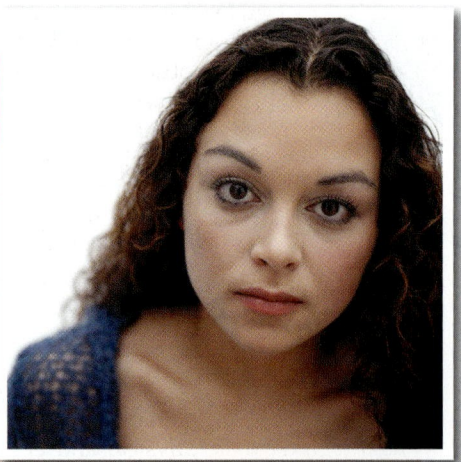

Theoretical Knowledge
knowing why

In this section, you will learn about the role of assessment in nursing process and collaborative care, about sources of data, and about various types of assessment.

ABOUT THE KEY CONCEPTS

Assessment is a key concept because it is integral to the nursing role. It is closely tied to another key concept: **data.** The related concepts in this chapter will help you understand the components of assessment and to see how they all fit together.

ASSESSMENT: THE FIRST STEP OF THE NURSING PROCESS

Assessment is the systematic gathering of information related to the physiological, psychological, sociocultural, developmental, and spiritual status of an individual, group, or community. Although various definitions exist, all definitions of assessment include the following features: collecting data, categorizing data, recording data, and using a systematic and ongoing process.

The purpose of assessment is to obtain data to allow you to help the patient. Data must be accurate and complete, because the remainder of the nursing process rests on this foundation. The facts, impressions, and contextual information obtained in your assessment become a part of the **patient database.** From this, you will develop a plan of care.

How Is Assessment Related to Other Steps of the Nursing Process?

Assessment is the first phase of nursing process. Assessment is related to other nursing process steps as follows (Fig. 3-1):

- *Diagnosis*—Assessment provides the data necessary for identifying the client's health problems and strengths.
- *Planning outcomes*—Data about the client's motivation, family, and available resources help you and the client formulate realistic goals.
- *Planning interventions*—Assessment data help you to choose the most effective interventions for the client.
- *Implementation*—As you perform nursing actions, you will also gather data by observing the client's responses to your interventions. For example: While helping a client ambulate, you might observe that she becomes short of breath. If this is new information, you might then identify a new nursing diagnosis such as Activity Intolerance.
- *Evaluation*—After performing interventions for existing diagnoses, you assess client responses. This *reassessment* provides the basis for changes in the care plan.

How Does Nursing Assessment Fit Into Collaborative Care?

Traditional medical assessments focus on identifying disease. As a nurse, you will focus on your clients' *responses* to illness, which include their physical and emotional responses and concerns, their understanding of the illness and how it affects their lives, and their ability to care for themselves. You will also use assessment with healthy clients to help them identify ways to maintain their current level of wellness and prevent illness.

Nurses and other healthcare professionals can access the database created from the nursing assessment findings to assist in decisions about the best course of treatment for the

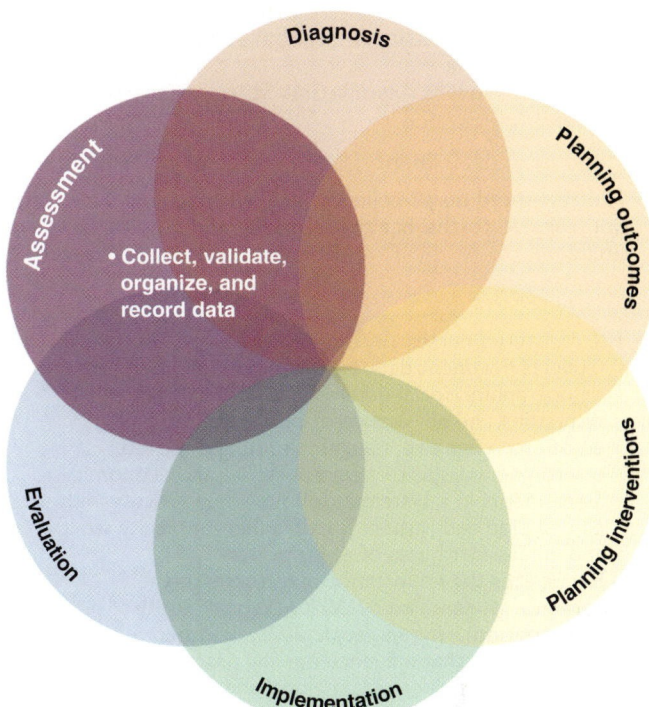

FIGURE 3-1 Nursing process: assessment phase.

client. In some settings, the nurse looks at the database and delegates or makes referrals to other professionals with expertise in a particular area of healthcare. This helps ensure that clients receive proper care by qualified individuals at the time it is needed.

Sami's case illustrates this. Sami has not had a gynecological (female) examination for 5 years. In the interview, she tells you that her mother has had breast cancer and that her sister is being treated for endometriosis. You ask first whether, because of any religious or other beliefs, Sami would be offended by an open discussion. Then you ask her about her sexual activity, assuring her that you will keep all information confidential. As a result of this interview, you encourage Sami to get a women's health examination as soon as possible. She agrees, and you refer her to a women's clinic, where she will be charged according to her ability to pay.

What Do Professional Standards Say About Assessment?

Complete, skillful, and timely assessment is an essential skill for nurses in all healthcare settings. Standards of governmental agencies, professional organizations, and accrediting bodies, such as the following, all address assessment.

- The American Nurses Association (ANA) in *Scope and Standards of Practice* (2015) (which applies to professional nurses [registered nurses RNs]) identifies assessment as a professional responsibility (Box 3-1).
- The National Council of State Boards of Nursing (NCSBN) in "Working With Others: A Position Paper" (2005, updated 2015) and the ANA and NCSBN in *Joint Statement on Delegation* (2005, updated 2015) assert that the RN may not delegate the function of assessment.
- The Joint Commission (TJC) in its standards for "Provision of Care, Treatment, and Services" (2015a, p. PC-1) identifies assessment as a core component of patient care. In agencies

BOX 3-1 ■ Professional Standards for Assessment

American Nurses Association Standards of Nursing Practice

Standard 1. Assessment

The registered nurse collects pertinent data and information relative to the healthcare consumer's health or the situation.

Competencies

The registered nurse:

- Collects pertinent data, including but not limited to demographics, social determinants of health, health disparities, and physical, functional, psychosocial, emotional, cognitive, sexual, cultural, age-related, environmental, spiritual/transpersonal, and economic assessments in a systematic and ongoing process with compassion and respect for the inherent dignity, worth, and unique attributes of every person.
- Recognizes the importance of the assessment parameters identified by WHO (World Health Organization), *Healthy People 2020*, or other organizations that influence nursing practice.
- Integrates knowledge from global and environmental factors into the assessment process.
- Elicits the healthcare consumer's values, preferences, expressed and unexpressed needs, and knowledge of the healthcare situation.
- Recognizes the impact of ones own personal attitudes, values, and beliefs on the assessment process.
- Identifies barriers to effective communication based on psychosocial, literacy, financial, and cultural considerations.
- Assesses the impact of family dynamics on healthcare consumer health and wellness.
- Engages the healthcare consumer and other interprofessional team members in holistic, culturally sensitive data collection.
- Prioritizes data collection based on the healthcare consumer's immediate condition, or the anticipated needs of the healthcare consumer or situation.
- Uses evidence-based assessment techniques, instruments and tools, available data, information, and knowledge relevant to the situation to identify patterns and variances.
- Applies ethical, legal, and privacy guidelines and policies to the collection, maintenance, use, and dissemination of data and information.
- Recognizes the healthcare consumer as the authority on their own health by honoring their care preferences.
- Documents relevant data accurately and in a manner accessible to the interprofessional team.

Source: American Nurses Association. (2015). *Nursing: Scope and standards of practice* (3rd ed.). Silver Spring, MD: Author.

in which there is an RN on staff, an RN must assess patients' needs for nursing care within 24 hours of inpatient admission (p. PC-7).

- TJC standards require agencies to provide evidence that:
  - Agency policy designates (1) when each patient is to be reassessed and (2) which disciplines can make which assessments (e.g., physical, psychological, and social needs; nutrition, hydration, and functional status).
  - All patients are assessed for pain, nutritional status, and risk for falls. (pp. PC-8–PC-9)

KnowledgeCheck 3-1

- What are the four features common to all definitions of assessment?
- How is a nursing assessment different from a medical assessment?

Can I Delegate Assessments?

Legally, a professional nurse must perform the assessment portion of the nursing process. **KEY POINT:** *Nurse aides or other nursing assistive personnel (NAP) and licensed practical nurses (LPNs) collect information such as vital signs, pain reports, and fingerstick blood glucose levels. However, it is the responsibility of the professional nurse to assign those tasks, validate the data collected, conduct the interview, and complete the physical assessment.* See Chapters 7 and 44 for a thorough discussion of delegation of tasks.

The following resources can guide you in deciding which caregivers are qualified to perform parts or all of an assessment:

- The ANA's *Scope and Standards of Practice* (2015)
- The ANA and NCSBN's *Joint Statement on Delegation* (2005, updated 2015) states that the RN may delegate components of care but cannot delegate the nursing process itself. The functions of assessment, planning, evaluation, and nursing judgment cannot be delegated. To find the complete joint statement and to access the ANA Web site for official position statements,

 Go to the NCSBN Web site at **https://www.ncsbn.org/**

- State *nurse practice acts*. Each state nurse practice act specifies which portions of the assessment can legally be completed by individuals with different credentials.
  - *Agency policies/procedures* will state which caregivers can collect and document specified data within that agency/facility.
  - *Accrediting agencies* such as The Joint Commission determine the highest priority patient safety issues and how best to address them.

ThinkLike a Nurse 3-1

Think about the following situation, and then answer the questions. Compare your ideas with those of other students; if you have any questions, consult your instructor.

Suppose you are a nurse in a healthcare setting where the policy states that nursing assistive personnel (NAP) can take vital signs (blood pressure, pulse, temperature, and respirations). You have a patient who is critically ill and whose condition is changing rapidly. Would you measure the vital signs or delegate the task to the NAP? Why or why not?

It is obvious from the preceding exercise that you must use good judgment when applying standards and policies and deciding when to delegate assessments.

Types of Data

Data can be categorized according to the source. The following will help you categorize data as you perform and document your assessment:

Subjective Data—What the Patient Says Also called *covert data,* or *symptoms data.* They consist of information communicated to the nurse by the client, family, or community. Subjective data:

- Reveal the perspective of the person giving the data, and include thoughts, feelings, beliefs, and sensations.

- Can be used to clarify objective data (e.g., "How did you get this scar?").
  You should know the following:
- Some people (e.g., infants, adults in mental illness) are unable to provide subjective data. Others can give subjective data, but their accuracy may be in question. For example, how credible is a diabetic patient's response that she complies with a diet and medication regimen when her A1c level is markedly elevated?
- For a given situation, the data you obtain from two or more people may not be the same. For example, people with insomnia often report getting much less sleep than their sleep partner says they do.

Objective Data—What Professionals Observe Also called *overt data,* or *signs data:*

- **Are gathered by physical assessment and from laboratory or diagnostic tests.**
- **Can be measured or observed by the nurse or other healthcare providers** (e.g., vital signs, urine output).
- **May be used to validate (check) subjective data.** For example, if you think a patient's report of dietary intake and insulin use is inaccurate, you would measure the blood sugar and ask for a dietary journal.
- **May be used to verify subjective information that seems accurate.** For example, Sami's subjective family history revealed significant risk factors for breast and cervical cancers, so you referred her for a gynecological exam. The results of the breast exam and Pap smear (a smear of cervical cells) provide objective data about these risk factors.

Primary Data are the subjective and objective information obtained directly from the client in what the client says or what you observe.

Secondary Data are obtained "secondhand," for example, from the medical record or from another caregiver. Table 3-1 provides further examples of types and sources of data.

KnowledgeCheck 3-2

During Sami's appointment at the women's clinic, she informs the nurse that her menstrual flow is very heavy and that she experiences severe abdominal cramping during menstruation. Sami's breast exam is normal. When the nurse sees the lab results (i.e., Pap smear result is normal, but hemoglobin level is low), she suspects that the heavy flow may be causing Sami's anemia. According to clinic protocol, birth control pills are prescribed to control Sami's heavy, painful periods and to provide contraception. Ongoing assessment will include visits every 6 months to evaluate Sami's response to hormone therapy and to monitor the anemia. State whether the following data are primary or secondary, subjective or objective:

- You see in Sami's health record that her breast exam was normal.
- Sami tells the nurse that she experiences cramping with her menstrual cycle.
- The nurse tells you that Sami is anemic.
- You check the result of the Pap smear in her electronic health record and see that it is normal.

Nursing Assessment Skills

Nurses collect data through the use of all their senses. Whether assessment is initial or ongoing, comprehensive or focused, you will use the skills of observation, physical examination, and interviewing.

Table 3-1 ➤ Examples of Data Types and Sources

Data Types

SUBJECTIVE DATA (CLIENT STATES)	OBJECTIVE DATA (NURSE OBSERVES)
"My throat hurts when I swallow."	White patches noted at the back of the throat and tonsillar area reddened and swollen
"Our children have no place to go after football games. That is why they get into so much trouble."	In a windshield survey, no public facility was open after football games to allow young people to socialize under supervision.

Data Sources

PRIMARY SOURCE (CLIENT STATES OR NURSE OBSERVES)	SECONDARY SOURCES (EVERYTHING ELSE)
"My heart feels like it's beating fast."	EKG report: Sinus tachycardia rate of 100 beats/min
"I am feeling short of breath at night."	In transfer report, nurse states client is on oxygen at night for dyspnea.

Observation refers to the deliberate use of all of your senses to gather and interpret patient and environmental data. Try to use the same sequence of observation at each patient contact. Observing systematically helps you be sure not to miss an assessment area. The CROP mnemonic (memory aid) in Box 3-2 may help.

Physical Assessment (or *physical examination*) produces mostly objective data, and makes use of the following techniques: inspection (visual examination), palpation (touch), percussion (tapping a body surface), direct auscultation (listening with the unaided ear), and indirect auscultation (listening with a stethoscope). All of these are described in detail in Chapter 21.

Interviewing is purposeful, structured communication in which you question the patient in order to gather subjective data for the nursing database (Fig. 3-2). The admission interview is structured and broad, but in ongoing assessment the interview may be informal, brief, and narrowly focused.

BOX 3-2 ■ CROP Mnemonic for Systematic Observing

Client—Look quickly for obvious signs of distress (e.g., pain, vomiting, crying).
Room—Scan room for safety hazards; look at machines and lines (e.g., ECG monitor, IV).
Observe—Observe/examine the client more thoroughly (e.g., breathing, dressings, odors).
People—Who are the people in the room; what are they doing?

KnowledgeCheck 3-3

Give at least two more examples of data you might obtain with each of your following senses. One example is provided for each.

- Touch (e.g., bladder distention)
- Vision (e.g., facial expression of pain)
- Smell (e.g., fecal odor)
- Hearing (e.g., bowel sounds)

Types of Assessment

KEY POINT: *Assessment can be broad and general or very specific. The type of assessment you do depends on the client's status.* In acute care settings, such as the emergency department, the assessments are rapid and focused on the presenting problem. In inpatient settings, you may perform an initial comprehensive assessment at admission and other, more focused assessments over time, according to the client's needs (see Fig. 3-2).

Initial and Ongoing Assessments

Assessments are said to be "initial" or "ongoing," depending on the time they are performed (e.g., one time on initial patient contact, or repeated at intervals). For a comparison of initial assessment and ongoing assessment, see Table 3-2.

Comprehensive Assessments

A **comprehensive assessment,** also called a *global assessment, patient database,* or *nursing database,* does the following:

- Provides holistic information about the client's overall health status.
- Enables you to identify client problems and strengths.

- Enhances your sensitivity to a patient's culture, values, beliefs, and economic situation.
- Uses the nursing skills of observation, physical assessment, and interviewing.

Focused Assessments

A **focused assessment** is performed to obtain data about an actual, potential, or possible problem that has been identified or is suspected. It focuses on a particular topic, body part, or functional ability rather than on overall health status (e.g., focused assessments of pain or nutrition).

- An *initial focused assessment* is used to follow up on client-reported symptoms or unusual findings discovered during the first exam.
- An *ongoing focused assessment* is used to evaluate the status of existing problems and goals.

ThinkLike a Nurse 3-2

- Give examples of each type of assessment (initial, ongoing, comprehensive, focused) using patients you have observed or cared for or your own personal experiences as a patient.
- Suppose you are the triage nurse at the community clinic in the Meet Your Patient scenario. What kind of assessment do you perform at Sami's first visit (initial, ongoing, comprehensive, focused)? What type will the care provider perform at the women's clinic?

Special Needs Assessments

A **special needs assessment** is a type of focused assessment that provides in-depth information about a particular area of client

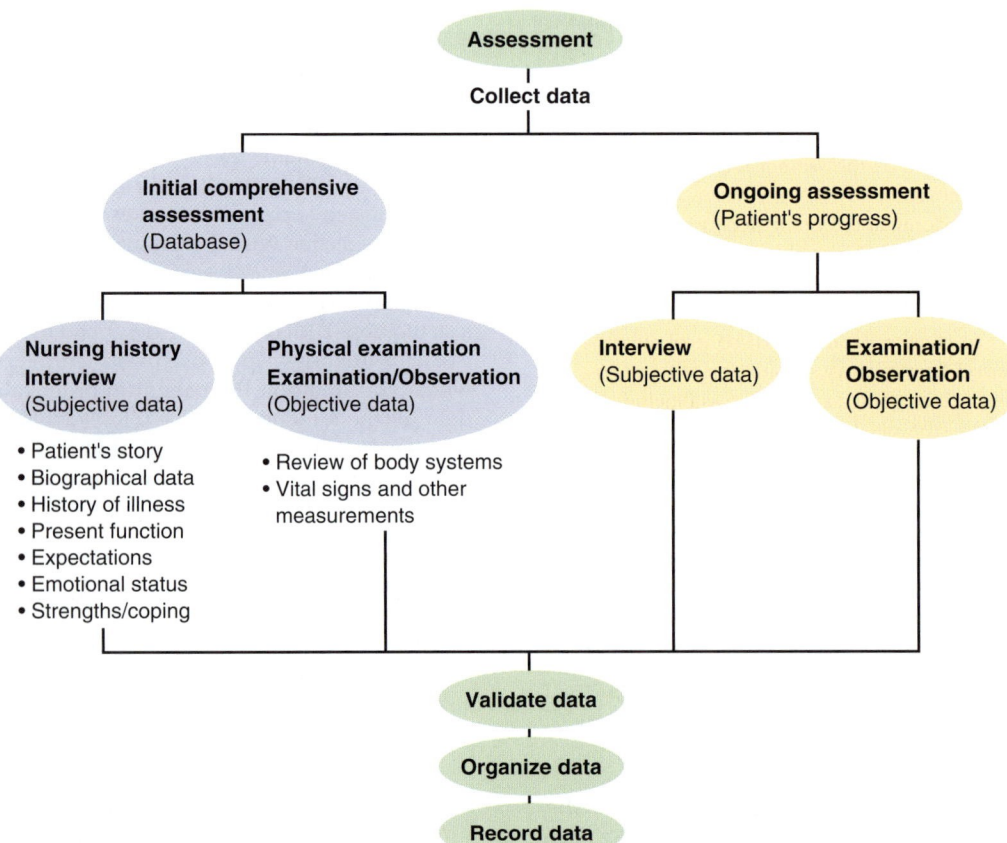

FIGURE 3-2 Overview of assessment content and methods.

Table 3-2 ➤ Initial Versus Ongoing Assessment		
	INITIAL ASSESSMENT	**ONGOING ASSESSMENT**
When Performed	■ Completed when the client first comes to the healthcare agency.	■ Performed as needed, at any time after the initial database is completed.
Purpose of Data	*Data:* ■ Is related to the person's reason for seeking nursing or medical assistance. ■ Provides guidance for care. ■ Helps determine need for further assessment.	*Data:* ■ Helps identify new problems. ■ Follows up on previously identified problems.
Discussion	■ A comprehensive assessment can be completed as the client's condition permits.	The data reflect the ever-changing state of the client. For example, vital signs may change rapidly, which is an important indicator of developing or resolving health problems.

functioning. It often involves using a specially designed form. Accrediting agency (e.g., The Joint Commission) standards may require certain special needs assessments (e.g., nutrition, pain). You may also perform a special needs assessment any time assessment cues suggest risk factors or problems for the client. The following are some special needs assessments:

- **Nutritional Assessment.** Perform a nutritional assessment when warranted by patient's needs or condition (i.e. malnourishment or new diabetes diagnosis). In addition to information about food intake, it includes information related to personal, psychosocial, and economic problems that may affect nutrition. See Chapter 28 for more information about nutritional assessments.
- **Pain Assessment.** Some accrediting agency (e.g., The Joint Commission) standards require pain screening for all patients during initial and ongoing assessments. A comprehensive pain assessment may be required for ongoing, unrelieved, or severe pain. See Chapter 32 for more information on pain assessments.
- **Cultural Assessment.** Awareness of cultural influences should guide your nursing care. For content included in a cultural assessment, see Chapter 15.
- **Spiritual Health Assessment.** Spiritual health assessment provides insight into how a client's spirituality is affected by current life events and health status—far more than merely asking about the client's religious preference. See Chapter 16 for detailed information on assessing spiritual health.
- **Psychosocial Assessment.** A psychosocial assessment typically includes data about family, lifestyle, usual coping patterns, understanding of the current illness, personality style, previous psychiatric disorders, recent stressors, major issues related to the illness, and mental status. See Chapters 13 and 21 for more details.
- **Wellness Assessment.** A wellness assessment includes data about spiritual health, social support, nutrition, physical fitness, health beliefs, and lifestyle, as well as a life-stress review. See Chapter 27 for a more detailed discussion of assessing wellness.
- **Family Assessment.** A family assessment provides a better understanding of the client's family-related health values, beliefs, and behaviors. Family assessment is discussed in Chapter 14.
- **Community Assessment.** A community assessment provides information about community demographics, health concerns, environmental risks, and community resources, norms and values, and points of referral. See Chapter 42 for more information about community assessments.

Functional Ability Assessment A functional ability assessment is a specific kind of special needs assessment. Health problems and normal aging changes often bring a decline in functional status. The Joint Commission (2015) requires a functional ability assessment for all patients "based on the patient's condition" (pp. PC-1–PC-8).

Functional ability is especially important in discharge planning, because future rehabilitation and palliative needs are derived from functional ability assessments. See the accompanying Focused Assessment box for questions to use when assessing activities of daily living (ADLs). The following three functional assessment tools are commonly used:

- **The Katz Index of ADL scale (1963).** This instrument is one of the best for assessing independent performance in very basic areas. It assigns one point for independence in each of the following areas: bathing, dressing, toileting, transfer, continence, and feeding (Wallace & Shelkey, revised 2012). To see the Katz scale, go to the ConsultGeri Web site at http://consultgerirn.org/uploads/File/trythis/try_this_2.pdf
- **Lawton Instrumental Activities of Daily Living (IADL) scale (1969).** The Lawton scale is particularly helpful in assessing a person's ability to independently perform the more sophisticated tasks of everyday life, such as shopping, planning and preparing meals, or paying bills. This scale is especially useful for older adults, who may begin to experience functional decline within 48 hours of hospital admission (Graf, 2008; Lawton & Brody, 1969). To see the Lawton scale, go to the ConsultGeri Web site at https://consultgeri.org/try-this/general-assessment/issue-23.pdf
- **The Karnofsky Performance Scale (Karnofsky & Burchenal, 1949).** This tool is used primarily in palliative care settings to assess functional abilities at the end of life. To see the scale, go to http://www.hospicepatients.org/karnofsky.html

ThinkLike a Nurse 3-3

Based on the data you have so far about Sami, consider the need to perform any of the special-purpose assessments. What is your rationale for using or not using a special needs assessment for her?

Questions for Assessing Independence in Activities of Daily Living

Mobility

Does the client require devices (e.g., cane, crutches) for support?

Transfer

Can the client get in and out of bed or chair without assistance?
    If not, how much help does the client need?

Feeding

Can the client feed self without assistance?
    If not, specifically what assistance does the client need (e.g., help with cutting meat)?

Bathing

Can the client perform a sponge bath, tub bath, or shower bath without help?
    If not, specifically what assistance does the client need?

Dressing

Can the client get all necessary clothing from drawers and closets and get dressed without help?
    If not, specifically what assistance does the client need?

Toileting

Can the client go to the bathroom, use the toilet, clean self, and rearrange clothing without help?
    If not, specifically what assistance does the client need?

Continence

Does the client independently control urination and bowel movements?
    If not, how often is the client incontinent of bladder or bowel?
    Does the client require an indwelling urinary catheter?

PracticalKnowledge
knowing **how**

In assessment, practical knowledge involves your skill in using structured and unstructured methods of data collection, as well as validating, organizing, and documenting your assessment findings.

INTERVIEWING TO OBTAIN A NURSING HEALTH HISTORY

Suppose that an elderly man is admitted with a fractured hip. The physician is interested in the cause of the fracture, the extent of the injury, and any preexisting medical problems that suggest the client is a poor surgical risk. As a nurse, you too would ask about the cause of the injury. However, you would also want to (1) know what effect the injury has on the man's ability to perform his everyday activities, and (2) identify his supports and strengths to begin planning

for his eventual discharge and self-care. **KEY POINT:** *So you see, the nursing health history covers some of the same topics as the medical history, but the rationale for the questions is different.*

Health history forms vary according to purpose among agencies (e.g., inpatient, clinic, surgery, medical, emergency room), but most include subjective data about the following components:

- Biographical data
- Chief complaint (reason for seeking healthcare)
- History of present illness
- Client's perception of health status and expectations for care
- Past health history (sometimes called *medical history*)
- Family health history
- Social history
- Medication history and device use
- Complementary/alternative modalities (CAM)
- Review of body systems and associated functional abilities

ThinkLike a Nurse 3-4

Most professional organizations identify assessment as a necessary skill for patient-centered care. In the full-spectrum model used in this book, the caring nurse is expected to use ethical knowledge to elicit patient values, preferences, and expressed needs as part of a clinical interview. Safe, effective care is an integral part of thinking, doing, and caring, as well. Where do you think these types of patient information fit into the preceding components of a nursing health history? Why?

Types of Interviews

Interviews may be directive or nondirective (see Table 3-3). A successful interview uses a combination of closed and open-ended questions.

- **Closed questions** are those that can be answered with "yes," "no," or other short, factual answers. They usually begin with *who, when, where, what, do (did, does),* and *is (are, were).*
- **Open-ended questions** specify a topic to be explored, but phrase it broadly to encourage the patient to elaborate. Use such questions when you want to obtain subjective data.

In nondirective interviewing, use broad, open-ended questions to guide the patient to talk about certain topics. From the answers to the broad questions, you can decide which topics to clarify or follow up with specific and closed questions. Part of the interview with Sami might have gone like this:

NURSE	When was your last physical examination? *(closed question)*
SAMI	I had a female exam about 5 years ago.
NURSE	What problems have you had in that area? *(open-ended question)*
SAMI	None, really.
NURSE	What about other women in your family? *(open-ended question)*
SAMI	Well, my mother had breast cancer about the same time that I went for my checkup. She's okay now though.
NURSE	Go on . . . *(open-ended question)*
SAMI	And my sister has been taking some pills for endometriosis. She hasn't been able to get pregnant because of that.

Table 3-3 ➤ Comparison of Directive and Nondirective Interviews		
	DIRECTIVE INTERVIEW	**NONDIRECTIVE INTERVIEW**
Characteristics	Nurse controls the topics.	Patient controls subject matter.
	Uses mostly **closed questions**	Nurse clarifies, summarizes, and questions.
		Uses mostly **open-ended questions**
Uses	Obtain factual, easily categorized information	Promote communication
	In emergency situation	Facilitate thought
		Build rapport
		Help patient to express feelings

NURSE   Are you sexually active? *(closed question)*
SAMI   Yes.
NURSE   Tell me about that. *(open-ended question)*

Your interviews will go more smoothly if you take time to prepare yourself, your patient, and the interview space before you begin asking questions.

HOW AND WHEN SHOULD I VALIDATE DATA?

Suppose a patient has told you that he has never had high blood pressure (BP), but you obtain an abnormal BP reading of 180/98 mm Hg. Would you record the 180/98 mm Hg reading, or would you:

- Check the BP in the patient's other arm?
- Wait a few minutes and take the reading again in the same arm?
- Retake the BP using a different sphygmomanometer?
- Compare the reading to previous entries in the chart?
- Ask another nurse to double-check your findings?

All of these are ways to **validate** (double-check) your data. Validating data helps to ensure that they are accurate, complete, and factual and that you have not jumped to conclusions.

Not all data must be validated; you should validate data under the following circumstances (Wilkinson, 2012):

- **Subjective and objective data do not agree, or do not make sense together.**
  Example: In the preceding situation, the subjective data item "never had high BP," but the objective data item, BP 180/98 mm Hg, is a high reading.
- **The patient's statements differ at different times in the interview.**
  Example: A patient tells you that he follows a low-cholesterol diet. However, when describing his usual daily food pattern, he includes eggs, a cheese sandwich, and a hamburger for dinner.
- **The data fall far outside normal range.**
  Example: A patient has no symptoms of infection or high fever, but you obtain an elevated oral temperature reading of 104°F (40°C). (Hint: Ask him whether he has just had something warm to drink.)
- **Factors are present that interfere with accurate measurement.**
  Example: The patient has very large arms, and there are no appropriately sized BP cuffs available. Therefore, because the BP will not be accurate you should take it again after you are able to obtain appropriate equipment.

Toward Evidence-Based Practice

Considine, J., & Currey, J. (2014). Ensuring a proactive, evidence-based, patient safety approach to patient assessment. *Journal of Clinical Nursing, 24,* 300–307.

These authors suggest that the most commonly used approaches to assessment (such as body systems) are not evidence based nor focused on patient safety. They posit the idea that if nurses were to use a "primary survey" approach for each patient assessment (both initial and follow-up), they would be more likely to detect changes in the patient's clinical status.

Further, they say that first responders universally evaluate a patient by means of assessing airway, breathing, circulation, and disability (neurological status). This is known in many countries as the "Primary Survey" and is a structured and systematic means of identifying and potentially correcting life-threatening conditions. The authors hypothesize that the primary survey approach has numerous advantages in promoting evidence-based nursing assessment and interventions. For example:

1. *Data are collected and documented according to clinical importance.* In assessing vital signs, respirations have a higher importance than temperature, contrary to the way vital signs are normally read (i.e., temperature, pulse, respirations).

2. *Data are collected in the form of a scored checklist.* This promotes consistency in symptoms evaluated, and produces evidence of change in patient condition by means of changes in physiological score values.

(Continued)

Toward Evidence-Based Practice—cont'd

3. *Rapid-response systems are devised to be activated when the patient meets certain predetermined criteria (such as abnormalities in vital signs or physiological scoring) documenting change in patient's condition and potentiating early intervention.*

1. The authors believe it is possible that if nurses use a primary survey approach for all assessments that changes in the patient's

condition would be detected sooner and early treatment could be implemented. Do you think they are correct? Explain your thinking.

 Go to Davis Advantage, Resources, Chapter 3, **Toward Evidence-Based Practice Suggested Responses.**

HOW CAN I ORGANIZE DATA?

Professional standards require systematic data collection (see Box 3-1). This means you collect and record data in predetermined categories, not just at random. Data in most initial (e.g., admission) assessments are already categorized by the agency's data-collection form. For ongoing assessments, you may need to provide your own organizing structure (framework or model). **KEY POINT:** *Because a* **framework** *represents a particular way of thinking about clients and health, it indicates which information is significant and guides you in deciding which patient data to observe.*

The major concepts of a model help you to cluster data and find patterns. If you don't understand what a framework is, refer to Chapter 8.

Nursing Models

Nurse theorists have developed many theories and models for thinking about nursing, clients, health, and the environment (see Chapter 8). These produce a holistic database that will help you to identify nursing rather than medical diagnoses. Table 3-4 identifies the major concepts of five models frequently used to structure nursing assessments. The concepts are the categories that you would use to gather and cluster data. **KEY POINT:** *ANA professional standards state that nursing data collection should be holistic.*

Nonnursing Models

Many agency assessment forms use a **body systems (medical) framework.** That model is useful for identifying medical problems, but it needs to be combined with other models (e.g., a nursing model or Maslow's model) to provide the holistic data you need to identify both nursing and medical problems.

Maslow's Hierarchy of Needs (Maslow, 1970; Maslow & Lowery, 1998) groups data according to human needs. It states that basic needs must be met before higher needs can be addressed. The following are Maslow's categories of needs, from most basic to highest:

- *Physiological.* Basic survival needs (e.g., oxygen, water, food, and shelter)
- *Safety and security.* The need to be safe and comfortable, including psychological security (e.g., safe from falls and treatment side effects)
- *Love and belonging.* The need for love and affection (e.g., family, social supports)
- *Esteem and self-esteem.* The need to feel good about oneself (e.g., body image, pride in achievements, admiration from others)

- *Cognitive.* The need for knowledge, understanding, and exploration
- *Aesthetic.* The need for symmetry, order, and beauty
- *Self-actualization.* The need to achieve one's potential; the need for growth and change (e.g., extent to which goals are achieved, role performance)

See Chapter 8 for a more complete discussion of Maslow's model.

HOW SHOULD I DOCUMENT DATA?

The ANA's *Scope and Standards of Practice* (2015) and The Joint Commission's *Hospital Accreditation Standards* (2015) emphasize the importance of complete, accurate, and timely patient records. Documentation of all assessment findings benefits both patients and nurses.

- It benefits patients by providing the basis for planning effective nursing care.
- It protects nurses by establishing that you actually performed the needed assessments. The nursing database is a permanent part of the client's record (a legal document). A malpractice suit may be filed years after you care for a patient, and the assumption in malpractice cases is "If it isn't documented, it wasn't done."

Guidelines for Recording Assessment Data

Follow these guidelines when recording assessment data:

- **Document as soon as possible** after you perform the assessment.
- **Write neatly, legibly, and in black ink** or record data electronically.
- **Use proper spelling and grammar.**
- **Use acronyms sparingly,** using only agency-approved abbreviations.
- **Write the patient's own words, when possible,** in quotation marks. If the comments are too long, summarize what the patient says (e.g., Patient states he is sleepy).
- **Record only the most important patient words.** If you record everything the patient says, your notes will contain irrelevant data and be too long. For example, write "Patient states, 'I hardly slept at all last night,'" even though what he actually said was, "I hardly slept at all last night. People kept waking me up, then I had to get up to go to the bathroom, and my wife called early this morning."
- **Use concrete, specific information** rather than vague generalities such as *normal, adequate, good,* and *tolerated well.*
- **Record cues, not inferences. Cues** are what the client says and what you observe. **Inferences** are judgments and

Table 3-4 ▸ Models for Organizing Data: Major Concepts

MODEL	MAJOR MODEL CONCEPTS
Gordon's Functional Health	Describes common patterns of behavior that can be functional or dysfunctional. Gordon intended the model for nursing assessment. The functional health patterns are major model concepts.

Health perception/health management	Self-perception/self-concept
Nutritional/metabolic	Sleep/rest
Elimination	Role/relationship
Activity/Exercise	Coping/stress tolerance
Cognitive/perceptual	Value/belief

MODEL	MAJOR MODEL CONCEPTS
The NANDA-International Nursing Diagnosis Taxonomy II	Consists of functional patterns and is a modified version of the Gordon model. Intended as a model for categorizing nursing diagnoses, not as a fully developed theory of nursing. The NANDA-I domains (categories) are:

Health Promotion	Sexuality
Nutrition	Coping/Stress Tolerance
Elimination and Exchange	Life Principles
Activity/Rest	Safety/Protection
Perception/Cognition	Comfort
Self-Perception	Growth/Development
Role Relationships	

Source: Adapted from *Nursing Diagnoses—Definitions and Classification 2018–2020.* © 2010 NANDA International, ISBN 978-1-62623-929-6. Used by arrangement with the Thieme Group, Stuttgart/New York.

MODEL	MAJOR MODEL CONCEPTS
The Roy Adaptation Model	Conceptualizes patients as adapting constantly to internal and external demands within a biological and psychosocial context. Using this model, you would look at the person's ability to achieve balance in the following "adaptive modes":

Activity and rest	Temperature regulation
Nutrition	Regulation of the senses
Elimination	Physical self-concept
Fluid and electrolytes	Personal self-concept
Oxygenation	Role function
Protection	Interdependence

Source: Adapted from Roy, C., & Andrews, H.A. (1991). *The Roy adaptation model: The definitive statement* (pp. 15–17). Norwalk, CT: Appleton & Lange; and Roy, C., & Andrews, H.A. (1999). *The Roy adaptation model* (2nd ed.). Norwalk, CT: Appleton & Lange.

MODEL	MAJOR MODEL CONCEPTS
Orem's Self-Care Model	Conceptualizes health as the ability to perform self-care. Using this model, you would gather data to identify the following universal self-care deficits that require nursing assistance:

Maintenance of a sufficient intake of air, water, and food

Maintenance of a balance between activity and rest

Maintenance of a balance between time alone and time with others

Provision of care associated with elimination processes and excrements

Prevention of hazards to human life, functioning, and well-being

Promotion of human functioning and development within social groups in accord with human potential, limitations, and desire to be normal (as determined by science, culture, and social values

Source: Adapted from Orem, D. E. (2001). *Nursing: Concepts of practice* (6th ed.). St. Louis, MO: Mosby.

interpretations about what the cues mean. When recording cues, you do not need to use words such as *appears* and *seems* (e.g., "incision seems red").

Cues	Inferences
Incision red, draining pus, edges separated.	Incision is infected.
Tearful. States that father died of a heart attack. Trembling.	Anxious about scheduled cardiac catheterization.
States, "I hate my mother. I wish I was dead."	Angry and suicidal.

Tools for Recording Assessment Data

Each organization has its own forms and formats for documenting initial and ongoing assessments. You will record data on a variety of documents, including nurses' notes and the following:

- **Graphic flow sheet.** Includes vital signs such as blood pressure, pulse, respirations, and temperature so trends over time can be seen clearly (Fig. 3-3).
- **Intake and output (I&O) sheet.** May be on the graphic sheet or separate. Has spaces for recording all types or intake (e.g., oral, intravenous) and output (e.g., urine, fluid from drainage tubes).
- **Nursing admission assessment.** Although agency forms differ in organization, all collect similar data as specified by The Joint Commission.
- **Nursing discharge summary.** This may be a part of the initial assessment form because data obtained at admission are used for discharge planning.
- **Special-purpose forms.** Examples are diabetic flow sheets and medication administration forms.
- **Electronic documentation.** In most facilities, initial data and ongoing assessment data are entered into a computer program for organization, shared communication, and easy retrieval (Fig. 3-4).

KnowledgeCheck 3-4

- Give an example of a closed question.
- Open-ended questions are most essential for which type of interview: directive or nondirective?
- Which data are most likely to need validation: laboratory data or subjective data?

REFLECTING CRITICALLY ABOUT ASSESSMENT

After gathering and recording patient data, use critical thinking to help you evaluate the quality of your assessment. See Chapter 2 for a review of critical thinking, as needed. The following are questions to guide your final judgments about your data.

1. Are my data complete?
   - Have I completed all areas of the assessment form?
   - Is there anything else I need to know to identify or rule out a nursing diagnosis?
   - Have I collected holistic data: physical, emotional, interpersonal, spiritual, and cultural?
2. How do I know the data are accurate?
3. Have I recorded data rather than conclusions (cues, not inferences)?
4. Did I validate any data that do not make sense? Do any of the data conflict with other data?
5. Did I record the data in clear, specific terms, using the patient's own words, when possible, for subjective data? Did I avoid vague terms such as "normal," "good," and "slept well"?
6. Have I followed up with in-depth special needs assessments when appropriate?
7. Have I included only relevant data, taking care to protect the client's privacy?

GRAPHICS

VITAL SIGNS RECORD

DATE	5/6/2014						
Days after Admission	0						
Operation	n/a						
TIME	0400	0800	1200	1600	2000	2400	0400

C	F							
40.0	104							
39.4	103							
38.8	102							
38.3	101							
37.7	100		X					
37.2	99			X	X	X		
36.6	98							
36.1	97						X	
35.5	96							
35.0	95							

		0400	0800	1200	1600	2000	2400	0400
PULSE			88	76	80	74			
RESPIRATIONS			16	14	18	16			
Blood pressure	Systolic		140	138	130	128			
	Diastolic		84	84	88	82			
HEIGHT & WEIGHT	5'5" 165 lbs							
TYPE OF DIET	Clear liquids							

Oral formula	150	450	400	1,000	
Blood					
I.V.	650	650	650	1,950	
Plasma					
Other					
TOTAL	800	1,100	1,050	2,850	

Drainage					
Urine	100	300	810	1,210	
Gastric aspiration	10	15	5	30	
Emesis					
Bowel movement					
Other					
TOTAL				1,240	
Initials				(sig)	
REGISTER NO.			WARD NO.		

PATIENT'S IDENTIFICATION (For typed or written entries give: Name–last, first, middle; grade; rank; rate; hospital or medical facility)

FIGURE 3-3 Graphic flow sheet.

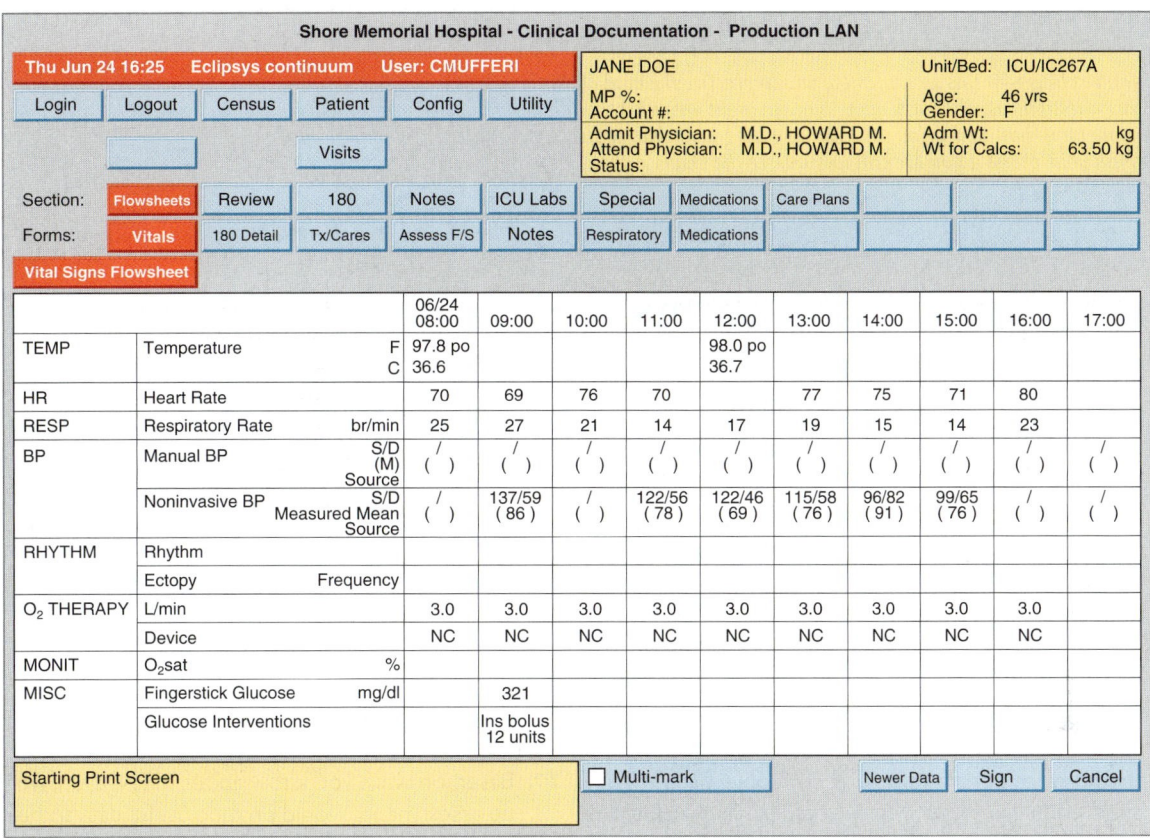

Shore Memorial Hospital - Clinical Documentation - Production LAN

Thu Jun 24 16:25	Eclipsys continuum	User: CMUFFERI	JANE DOE	Unit/Bed: ICU/IC267A

Login | Logout | Census | Patient | Config | Utility

Visits

MP %:
Account #:
Admit Physician: M.D., HOWARD M.
Attend Physician: M.D., HOWARD M.
Status:

Age: 46 yrs
Gender: F
Adm Wt: kg
Wt for Calcs: 63.50 kg

Section: Flowsheets | Review | 180 | Notes | ICU Labs | Special | Medications | Care Plans

Forms: Vitals | 180 Detail | Tx/Cares | Assess F/S | Notes | Respiratory | Medications

Vital Signs Flowsheet

			06/24 08:00	09:00	10:00	11:00	12:00	13:00	14:00	15:00	16:00	17:00
TEMP	Temperature	F	97.8 po				98.0 po					
		C	36.6				36.7					
HR	Heart Rate		70	69	76	70		77	75	71	80	
RESP	Respiratory Rate	br/min	25	27	21	14	17	19	15	14	23	
BP	Manual BP	S/D (M) Source	/ ( )	/ ( )	/ ( )	/ ( )	/ ( )	/ ( )	/ ( )	/ ( )	/ ( )	/ ( )
	Noninvasive BP	S/D Measured Mean Source	/ ( )	137/59 (86)	/ ( )	122/56 (78)	122/46 (69)	115/58 (76)	96/82 (91)	99/65 (76)	/ ( )	/ ( )
RHYTHM	Rhythm											
	Ectopy	Frequency										
O$_2$ THERAPY	L/min		3.0	3.0	3.0	3.0	3.0	3.0	3.0	3.0	3.0	
	Device		NC	NC	NC	NC	NC	NC	NC	NC	NC	
MONIT	O$_2$sat	%										
MISC	Fingerstick Glucose	mg/dl		321								
	Glucose Interventions			Ins bolus 12 units								

Starting Print Screen | ☐ Multi-mark | Newer Data | Sign | Cancel

FIGURE 3-4 Computer screen capture: assessment data.

8. During the interview:
   - Did I use therapeutic communication?
   - Did I ask too many questions or use too many closed questions?
   - How comfortable was I during the interview?
   - What cues and signals did I get from the client? Did I follow up on them?
9. During physical assessment, observation, and examination:
   - How did the client and significant others respond to me verbally and nonverbally?

- Did I pay attention to detail?
- Were my assessment techniques performed skillfully (palpation, percussion, auscultation, inspection)?

10. Did I have to repeat any area of assessment because I could not remember what I saw, heard, smelled, or felt?

If you have followed the recommended processes and reflected critically on your assessment, you should have the data necessary to create a holistic plan of care individualized to meet the client's needs.

CLINICALREASONING

The questions and exercises in this section allow you to practice the kind of thinking you will use as a full-spectrum nurse. Critical-thinking questions usually have more than one right answer, so we do not provide "correct answers" for these features. It is more important to develop your nursing judgment than to just cover content. You will learn by discussing the questions with your peers. If you are still unsure, see the Davis Advantage chapter resources for suggested responses.

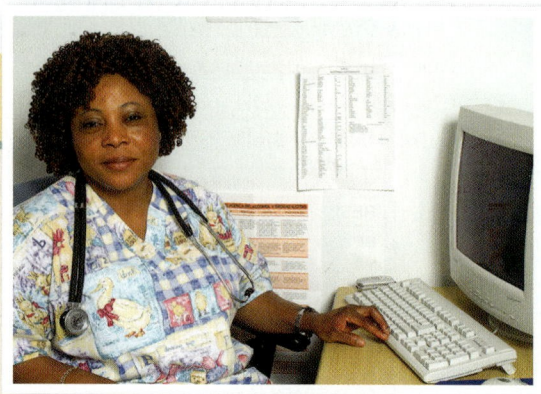

Caring for the Nguyens

Imagine you are the clinic nurse at the Family Medicine Center. Using the data in the opening scenario of Nam Nguyen in the front of the book, work through the following questions:

A. What type of assessment, comprehensive or focused, is being performed at this clinic visit? Explain your thinking.

B. Identify the types of data (e.g., subjective/objective, primary/secondary) that have been gathered so far. Give an example of each type.

C. How might you verify data that Mr. Nguyen provided on the intake sheet?

D. Based on what you know about Mr. Nguyen, what follow-up assessments would provide useful data to help with the care of Mr. Nguyen? Why would you make these assessments?

Applying the **Full-Spectrum Nursing Model**_____

PATIENT SITUATION

Review the case of your client Sami, introduced earlier in this chapter, and consider the following questions:

THINKING

1. *Theoretical Knowledge:* To care for Sami, what knowledge would you need that you do not already have? Can you list the URL for at least one online reputable source for this information?
2. *Critical Thinking:* The nurse asks Sami, "If you can't afford healthcare, couldn't you get a roommate to save some money on rent?" What are some critical-thinking questions you should ask yourself when reflecting on this question later?

DOING

3. *Practical Knowledge:* What practical knowledge will you, as the nurse, use in this scenario?
4. *Nursing Process:* What kind of assessment will you perform for Sami (e.g., comprehensive, focused, special needs, discharge)?

CARING

5. *Self-Knowledge*: In what ways are you similar to Sami? In what ways are you different?

To explore learning resources for this chapter,

 Go to www.DavisAdvantage.com and find:

Answers and Suggested Responses for all questions in this chapter

Knowledge Map

List of NANDA-I Diagnoses

References and Bibliography

Concept Map

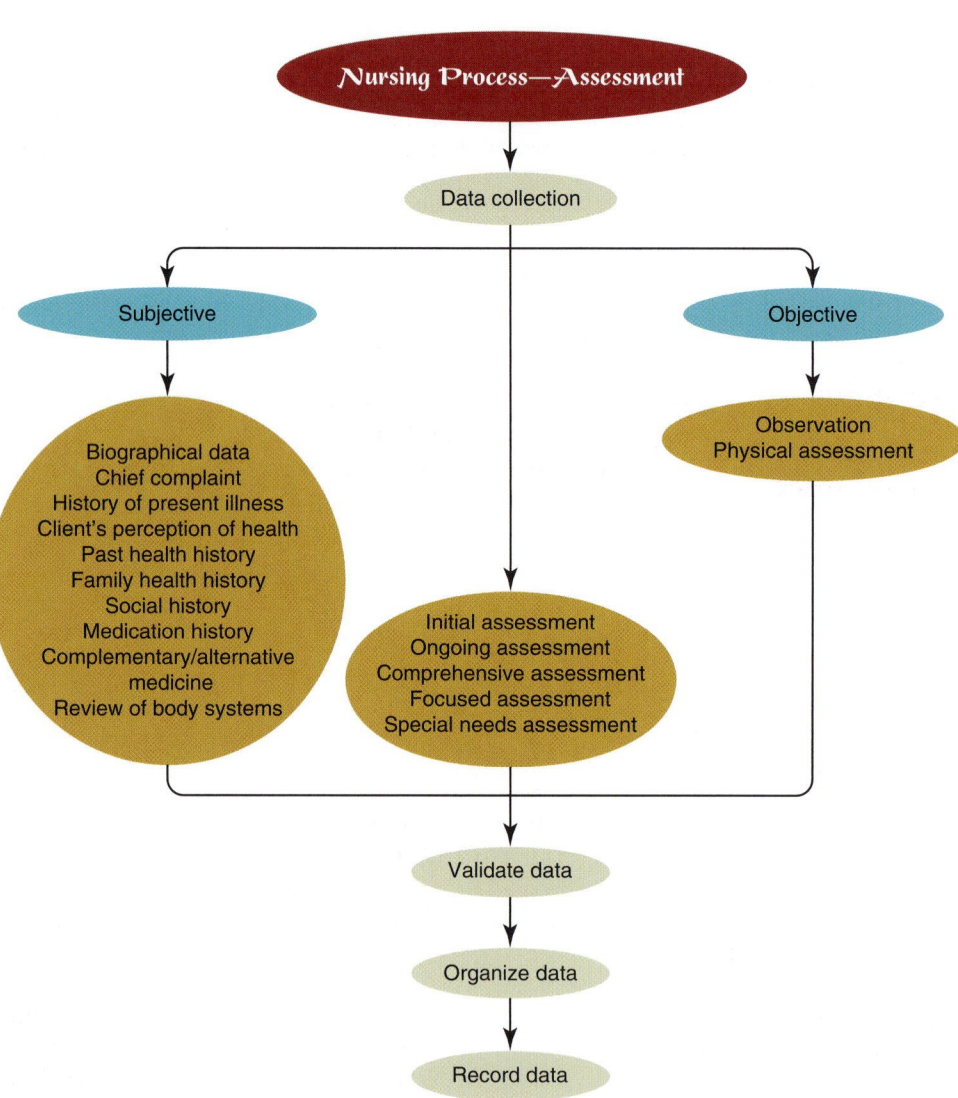

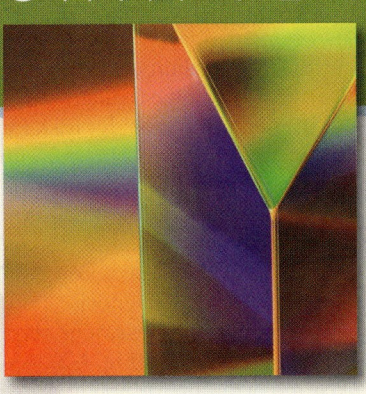

CHAPTER 4

Nursing Process: Diagnosis

Learning Outcomes

After completing this chapter, you should be able to:

➤ Define the following terms: *diagnosis, nursing diagnosis, diagnostic reasoning, diagnostic label, defining characteristics, related factors, risk factors, health problem.*

➤ Explain how nursing diagnosis is related to other phases of the nursing process.

➤ Differentiate between nursing diagnoses, medical diagnoses, and collaborative problems.

➤ Explain the differences between actual, risk, possible, syndrome, and wellness nursing diagnoses.

➤ Describe at least two frameworks for prioritizing nursing diagnoses.

➤ Describe errors of theoretical and self-knowledge that may occur in diagnostic reasoning.

➤ Use standardized nursing language to write nursing diagnoses.

➤ Use collaborative problem statements appropriately.

➤ Explain the relationship between nursing diagnoses and goals/interventions.

➤ State at least five criteria for judging the quality of a diagnostic statement.

Key Concepts

Diagnostic format

Diagnostic reasoning (diagnostic process)

Nursing diagnosis

Related Concepts

See the Concept Map at the end of this chapter.

Meet Your Patient

You will be admitting a client, Todd, from the emergency department (ED). According to the ED report, Todd's admitting medical diagnosis is chronic renal failure. He is married, 58 years old, and employed, and he has a long-standing history of type 2 diabetes mellitus (DM). During the past 3 days, he reports that he has developed swelling and decreased sensation in his legs and difficulty walking, which he describes as "slight loss of mobility." You have many questions concerning Todd's immediate and long-term needs, which include the following:

His medication regimen

His compliance with his diabetes treatment plan

The extent to which his family is involved

What laboratory tests have been completed

How severe his renal dysfunction has become

His safety needs

After you obtain necessary data, you need to organize and analyze them to form some initial impressions about

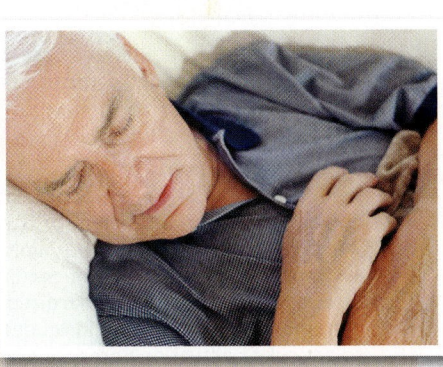

what they mean. For example:

- Admitting diagnosis is chronic renal failure; anticipate a problem with fluid balance.

- Decreased sensation in lower extremities; patient may have a mobility and a safety problem.

- Diabetes; Todd is at risk for Impaired Skin and Tissue Integrity.

- Diabetes and renal failure require complex treatment regimens and self-care: Is Todd managing his therapy effectively? If not, is it because he is not motivated to do so?

When Todd and his family arrive on your unit, you begin gathering comprehensive data. From that, you then make a list of Todd's health problems in order of priority. These actions illustrate the diagnosis phase of the nursing process.

Theoretical Knowledge
knowing **why**

KEY POINT: *Professional standards of practice (see Box 4-1), as well as many state nurse practice acts, identify diagnosing as the unique obligation of the professional nurse.* Although many nursing activities may be delegated, diagnosis cannot. Most state nurse practice acts limit the role of the licensed practical nurse/licensed vocational nurse (LPN/LVN) to gathering data that will be analyzed by the registered nurse (RN).

ABOUT THE KEY CONCEPTS

Nursing diagnosis is the single concept in this chapter that ties all the other concepts together. **Diagnostic reasoning,** also called *diagnostic process,* represents the thinking aspect of nursing diagnosis. The **diagnostic format,** or *diagnostic statement,* is the concrete product.

DIAGNOSIS: THE SECOND STEP OF THE NURSING PROCESS

Diagnosis is the phase in which you analyze the assessment data. Using critical-thinking skills, you identify patterns in the data and draw conclusions about the client's health status, including strengths, problems, and factors contributing to the problems. (*Note:* Involve the patient and family in this process to the extent possible.)

BOX 4-1 ■ Professional Standards for Diagnosing

American Nurses Association Standards of Nursing Practice

Standard 2. Diagnosis

The registered nurse analyzes assessment data to determine actual or potential diagnoses, problems, and issues.

Competencies

The registered nurse:
- Identifies actual or potential risks to the healthcare consumer's health and safety or barriers to health, which may include but are not limited to interpersonal, systematic, or environmental circumstances.
- Uses assessment data, standardized classification systems, technology, and clinical decision support tools to articulate actual or potential diagnoses, problems, and issues.
- Verifies the diagnoses, problems, and issues with the individual, family, group, community, population, and interprofessional colleagues.
- Prioritizes diagnoses, problems, and issues based on mutually established goals to meet the needs of the healthcare consumer across the health-illness continuum.
- Documents diagnoses, problems, and issues in a manner that facilitates the determination of the expected outcomes and plan.

Note: There are additional measurement criteria for advanced practice registered nurses.

Source: American Nurses Association. (2015). *Nursing: Scope and standards of practice* (3rd ed.). Silver Spring, MD: Author.

As you can see in Figure 4-1, diagnosis overlaps with the other nursing process steps. Most nurses actually begin diagnostic reasoning during the assessment phase. For example, you probably formed your initial impressions about Todd while still gathering data. On learning the medical diagnosis of chronic renal failure, you would immediately consider Risk for Imbalanced Fluid Volume. However, you would obtain more data before confirming and recording that as a nursing diagnosis; your tentative diagnostic conclusion actually leads you to collect more data: *Is he still producing urine? What is his oral intake? Does he demonstrate edema?* Do you see how you would move back and forth between assessment and diagnosis?

Diagnosis is critical because it links the assessment step, which precedes it, to all the steps that follow it (Fig. 4-2). Assessment data must be complete and accurate for you to make an accurate nursing diagnosis. **KEY POINT:** *The purpose of diagnosing is to identify the client's health status. Accuracy is essential because the diagnosis is the basis for planning client-centered goals and interventions.*

Terminology   The term **diagnosis,** as used in nursing, has four different meanings. Table 4-1 summarizes those terms and provides examples of how we use nursing diagnosis terminology in this text.

To see an alphabetical list of NANDA-I diagnoses,

 Go to Davis Advantage, Resources, Chapter 4, **Alphabetical List of NANDA-I Diagnoses.**

What Are the Origins of Nursing Diagnosis?

Before the 1950s, nurses assisted physicians by collecting data to help them diagnose and treat disease. Nursing care was thought of as a set of tasks and organized as a list of things to do. The term *nursing diagnosis* was first used in 1953 to differentiate

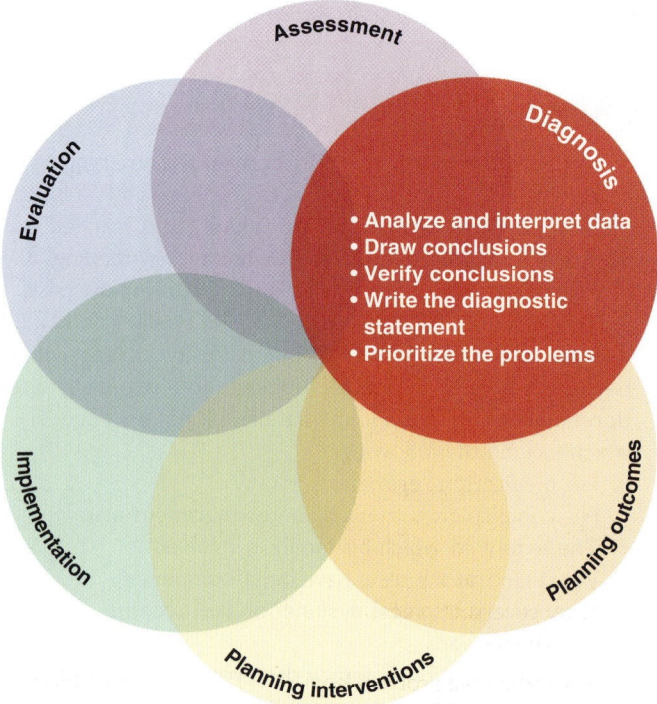

FIGURE 4-1 Nursing diagnosis: second phase of the nursing process.

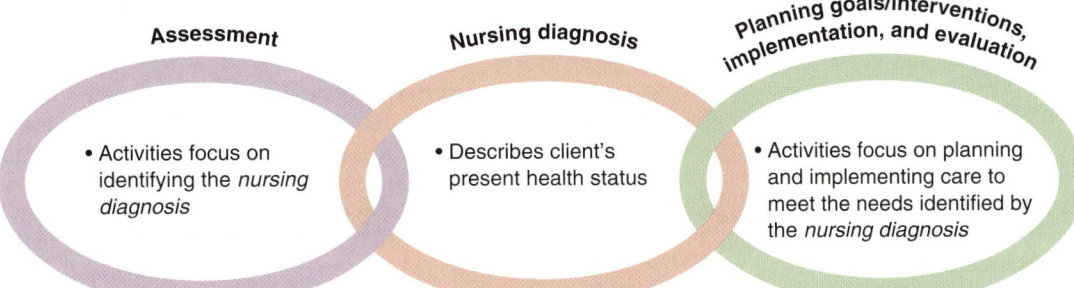

FIGURE 4-2 Diagnosis links the assessment phase to the rest of the nursing process.

nursing from medicine, when Fry (1953) stated that a nursing diagnosis identifies the client's needs for nursing rather than for medical care. Until the early 1970s, nursing diagnosis was not widely used in nursing practice, but two major events in 1973 spurred change:

- The First National Conference on Nursing Diagnosis was held (Gebbie & Lavin, 1975). A national task force was formed to begin developing a language to describe the health problems treated by nurses.
- The American Nurses Association's (ANA) *Standards of Nursing Practice* included nursing diagnosis as an expectation of professional nurses.

In 1980, the ANA published *ANA Social Policy Statement,* which characterized nursing as "the diagnosis and treatment of human response to actual or potential health problems" (ANA, 1980). As a result of this statement and the work of the nursing diagnosis task force, most state nurse practice acts began to designate nursing diagnosis as an exclusive responsibility of registered nurses. Nursing diagnosis is now widely used in nursing education and practice. **KEY POINT:** *The formal list of nursing diagnostic labels describes health problems that can be addressed by independent nursing actions and, in that sense, forms the body of knowledge that is unique to nursing.*

Since the first conference, the nursing diagnosis group has continued to meet every 2 years, and is now an international organization known as NANDA International, Inc. (NANDA-I). NANDA-I continues the work of refining diagnostic labels and reviewing nursing diagnoses submitted by individuals or nursing organizations. Diagnoses on the official list are approved for clinical use and further study. They do not represent a finished product, as many of the diagnoses are only partially substantiated by research.

KnowledgeCheck 4-1

- Why is the diagnosis step so critical to the other phases of the nursing process?
- Which two nursing organizations have been responsible for making diagnosis a part of the professional nursing role?

What Are Health Problems?

A **health problem** is any condition that requires intervention to prevent or treat disease or illness. After you identify a health problem, you must decide how to treat it: independently or in collaboration with other health professionals. **The answer determines whether it is a nursing diagnosis, a medical diagnosis,**

Table 4-1 ➤ Nursing Diagnosis Terminology

TERM AND EXISTING MEANINGS	TERMINOLOGY USED IN THIS BOOK	EXAMPLE
Diagnosis		
1. The second phase of the nursing process	1. Diagnosis	With Todd (Meet Your Patient) you used *diagnostic* reasoning to *diagnose* and list his problems. This is the *diagnosis phase* of the nursing process.
2. The reasoning process used in identifying patient problems and strengths	2. Diagnostic process, diagnostic reasoning or diagnosing	
Nursing Diagnosis		
1. The end product of the diagnostic reasoning process: a full diagnostic statement describing client health status. It contains both problem and etiology.	1. Nursing diagnosis, diagnostic statement	For Todd, you might have made a *nursing diagnosis* of Excess Fluid Volume secondary to renal failure. To write that statement, you would have used the NANDA-I *label* Excess Fluid Volume.
2. A standardized problem label from the NANDA-I taxonomy (e.g., Anxiety)	2. Label, NANDA-I label, problem label, diagnostic label	

or a collaborative problem. See Figure 4-3 for a comparison of these problem types.

Recognizing Nursing Diagnoses

A **nursing diagnosis** is

- A statement of client health status that nurses can identify, prevent, or treat independently.
- Stated in terms of **human responses** (reactions) to disease, injury, or other stressors.
- A human response that can be biological, emotional, interpersonal, social, or spiritual, and can be either a problem or a strength.

In 1990, NANDA officially defined nursing diagnosis as "a clinical judgment about individual, family, or community experiences/responses to actual or potential health problems/life processes. Nursing diagnosis provides the basis for selection of nursing interventions to achieve outcomes for which the nurse is accountable. Definition was approved at 9th conference, and amended in 2013" (NANDA International, 2016). **KEY POINT:** *This definition emphasizes the clinical judgment aspect of diagnosing.*

ThinkLike a Nurse 4-1

Imagine that you have been in an automobile accident. You have internal injuries and broken bones and will be hospitalized for at least 2 weeks, right before your final exams. What human responses (physical, emotional, interpersonal, social, spiritual) would you have?

Recognizing Medical Diagnoses

A **medical diagnosis** describes a disease, illness, or injury. Its purpose is to identify a pathology so that appropriate treatment can be given to cure the condition. Todd has two medical diagnoses: chronic renal failure and type 2 DM.

KEY POINT: *Except for advanced practice nurses, nurses cannot legally diagnose or treat medical problems.* Your assessment data can, however, be helpful in identifying disease states and in evaluating the effects of medical therapies (e.g., whether a medication relieves a patient's pain). You need to understand the pathophysiology of the patient's illness in order to know how to focus your assessments. The following are differences between medical and nursing diagnoses:

- **A medical diagnosis is more narrowly focused than a nursing diagnosis.**
- **You cannot predict a patient's nursing diagnoses just by knowing his medical diagnosis or pathology.** Nursing diagnoses are human responses, complex and unique to each person. A medical diagnosis, in contrast, remains the same as long as a particular injury or pathology is present. In the Meet Your Patient scenario, Todd's medical diagnosis of type 2 DM will not change because his body's inability to properly utilize glucose cannot change.
- **A medical diagnosis, disease, or pathological condition can have any number of nursing diagnoses associated with it.** For example, in response to his type 2 DM, Todd might have nursing diagnoses of Ineffective Health Management and Risk for Impaired Skin/Tissue Integrity (to name only two).
- **Clients with the same medical diagnosis may have different nursing diagnoses.** Another client with type 2 DM may not have a nursing diagnosis of Ineffective Health Management, but instead may have a diagnosis of Ineffective Denial because he simply cannot accept that he truly has diabetes.

Recognizing Collaborative Problems

Collaborative problems are "certain physiologic complications that nurses monitor to detect onset or changes in status. Nurses manage collaborative problems using physician-prescribed and nursing-prescribed interventions to minimize the complications of the events" (Carpenito-Moyet, 2010, p 24). They have the following characteristics:

- **All patients who have a certain disease or medical treatment are at risk for developing the same complications.** That is, the collaborative problems (complications) are determined by the medical diagnosis or pathology. Consider these examples:

  Because Todd has type 2 DM, he has the collaborative problem Potential Complication of type 2 DM: hyperglycemia and/or hypoglycemia. All other patients with type 2 DM also have those potential complications.

  All patients having surgery have the collaborative problem Potential Complication of surgery: infection.

- **A collaborative problem is always a *potential* problem.** Consider what would be needed if a risk for infection became an *actual* infection of a surgical incision. Could a nurse treat that independently?
- **If you can prevent the complication with independent nursing interventions alone, it is not a collaborative problem.**

See Figure 4-3 for an algorithm to help you differentiate nursing diagnoses from medical diagnoses and collaborative problems.

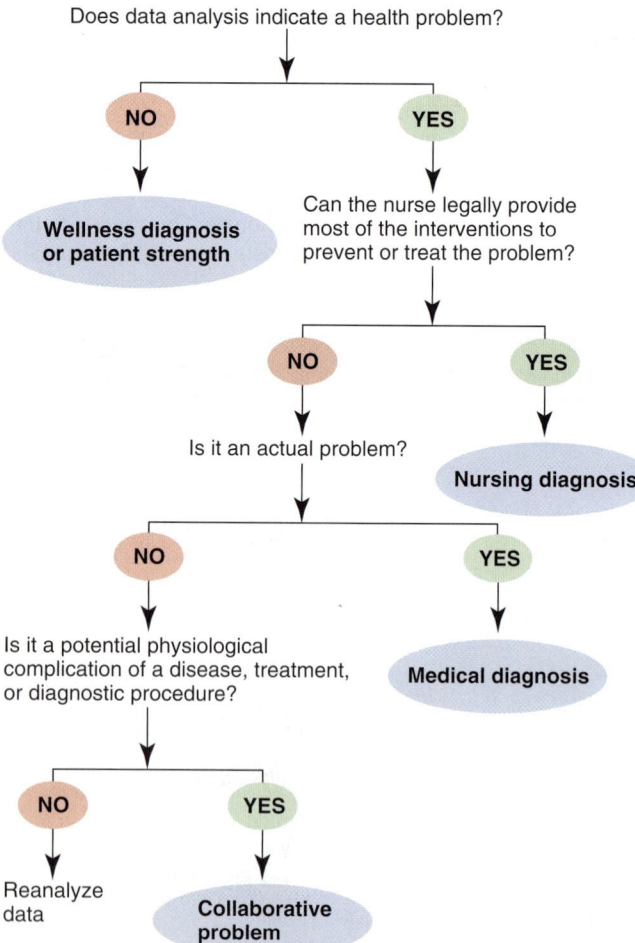

FIGURE 4-3 Algorithm for distinguishing among nursing, medical, and collaborative problems.

KnowledgeCheck 4-2

State whether each of the following represents a nursing diagnosis, medical diagnosis, or collaborative problem:

- After giving birth, all women are at risk for developing postpartum hemorrhage.
- A patient has signs and symptoms of appendicitis, which must be treated with surgery and antibiotics.
- A client is at risk for constipation because he postpones defecation and also does not consume enough dietary fiber and fluids.

Types of Nursing Diagnoses

You must determine the status, or type, of each nursing diagnosis. Is it an actual or potential (risk) problem, or is it a collaborative, wellness, or syndrome diagnosis? This is important because each status requires (1) different wording in the diagnostic statement and (2) different interventions. Figure 4-4 provides an algorithm for determining types of diagnoses. Table 4-2 compares diagnosis types.

KnowledgeCheck 4-3

- What are the five types of nursing diagnoses?
- Determine the type of nursing diagnosis for each of the following:
  a. Jane Thomas regularly engages in exercise but tells you she would like to increase her endurance.

b. Mrs. King has several of the signs and symptoms (defining characteristics) of the nursing diagnosis Ineffective Coping.
c. Alicia Hernandez seems anxious, but you are not sure whether she actually is. You would like to have more data in order to diagnose or rule out a diagnosis of Anxiety.
d. Charles Oberfeldt has no symptoms of constipation. However, he reports that he does not include many fiber-rich foods in his diet and drinks few liquids. In addition, he is now fairly inactive because of a back injury. These are all risk factors for a diagnosis of Constipation.

WHAT IS DIAGNOSTIC REASONING?

KEY POINT: Diagnostic reasoning *is the thinking process that enables you to make sense of data gathered during a comprehensive patient assessment. It is also known as diagnostic process.* In diagnostic reasoning, you will think critically to analyze and interpret data, draw conclusions about the patient's health status, verify problems with the patient, prioritize the problems, and record the diagnostic statements. This text presents diagnostic reasoning in separate steps so that it is easier to learn, but that is not the way it really occurs (see Fig. 4-5). Just as you now move back and forth between *assessing* and *diagnosing,* you will soon find yourself moving back and forth between the multiple steps of diagnostic reasoning

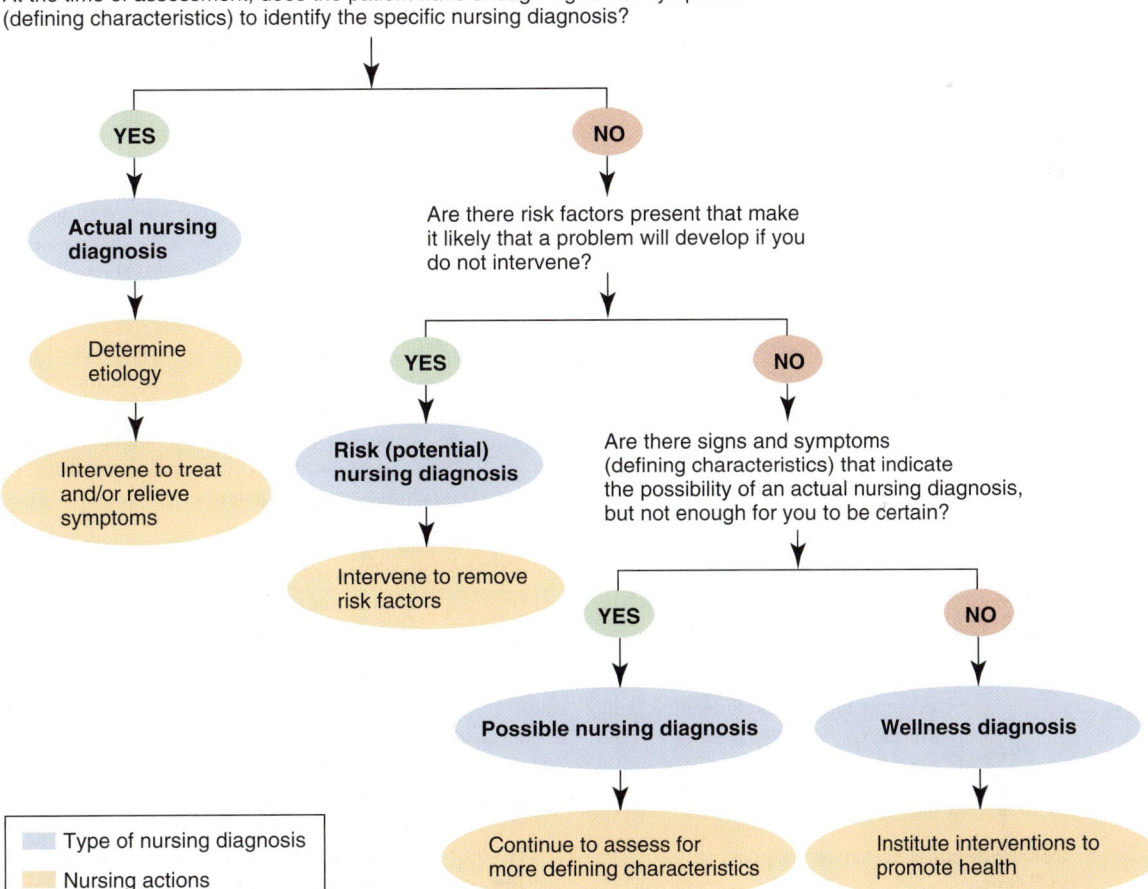

FIGURE 4-4 Algorithm for determining whether a diagnosis is an actual diagnosis, a risk (potential) diagnosis, a possible diagnosis, or a wellness diagnosis.

Table 4-2 ➤ Differentiating Problem Types: Medical, Collaborative, and Actual, Risk, Possible, Syndrome, and Wellness Nursing Diagnoses

DIAGNOSIS TYPE	DEFINITION AND CHARACTERISTICS	EXAMPLES
Medical Diagnosis	Describes a disease, illness, or injury. Its purpose is to identify a pathology so that appropriate treatment can be given.	Example: Todd (Meet Your Patient) has two medical diagnoses: chronic renal failure and type 2 DM.
Collaborative Problem	Determined by medical diagnosis or pathology and are potential events that nurses monitor to detect onset or changes in status. Managed by physician-prescribed and nursing-prescribed interventions to minimize the complications.	Example: Todd has type 2 DM, has the collaborative problem Potential Complication of type 2 DM: hyperglycemia and/or hypoglycemia. All other patients with type 2 DM also have those potential complications.
Actual Nursing Diagnosis: Problem Is Present	A problem response that exists at the time of the assessment. Signs and symptoms (cues) that are present.	Todd may have at least one actual nursing diagnosis (Impaired Walking or perhaps Impaired Physical Mobility), related to his lack of peripheral sensation; however, no signs and symptoms were given in the scenario to support that diagnosis.
Risk (Potential) Nursing Diagnosis: Problem May Occur	A problem response that is likely to develop in a vulnerable patient if the nurse and patient do not intervene to prevent it. No signs/symptoms of the problem, but the risk factors are present that increase the patient's vulnerability. The patient is more susceptible to the problem than others in the same or a comparable setting (e.g., one who is undernourished or who has a compromised immune system).	*Examples:* 1. Todd's loss of lower limb sensation is a risk factor for a diagnosis of Risk for Falls even though Todd has no symptoms or history of falling. 2. All surgical patients have at least some risk for developing infection, so do not routinely write Risk for Infection or Surgical Site Infection on every surgical care plan. Instead, write Potential Complication of surgery: infection (incision and systemic).
Possible Nursing Diagnosis: Problem May Be Present	Use when your intuition and experience direct you to suspect that a diagnosis is present, but you do not have enough data to support the diagnosis. The main reason for including this type of diagnosis on a care plan is to alert other nurses to continue to collect data to confirm or rule out the problem.	Todd has a symptom, "slight difficulty walking." This could indicate the diagnosis Impaired Physical Mobility, Impaired Walking, or Risk for Falls. You need more data about his difficulty walking to decide which mobility nursing diagnosis is appropriate. Or you might write a nursing diagnosis of Risk for Falls related to decreased sensation in both legs.
Syndrome Nursing Diagnosis: Several Related Problems Are Present	Represents a collection of nursing diagnoses that usually occur together. Use when you notice that the patient has more than one nursing diagnosis with the same etiology (cause, contributing factors).	The NANDA-I label Risk for Disuse Syndrome is used to represent all the complications that can occur as a result of immobility (e.g., pressure injury, constipation, stasis of pulmonary secretions, thrombosis, body image disturbance).
Patient Strengths	Data include history and observations obtained during assessment. Noticing the patient's strengths (what and who matters to the patient) helps support recovery and healing.	Todd might include his marital status, family involvement, religious activities, and steady employment
Wellness Nursing Diagnosis: No Problem Is Present	Describes health status, but does not describe a problem; can apply to an individual, family, group, or community. Use when the client is in transition from one level of wellness to a higher level. Two conditions must be present: 1. The client's present level of wellness is effective. 2. The client wants to move to a higher level of wellness.	Suppose that Todd tells you that he prays, participates in religious activities, and trusts in God, but he would like to feel even closer to God. He asks to meet with the minister from his church. You might make a diagnosis of Readiness for Enhanced Spiritual Well-Being.

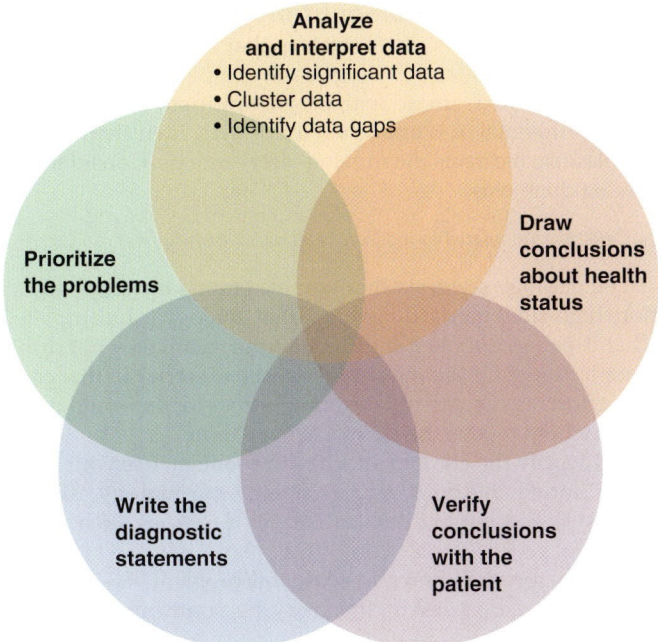

FIGURE 4-5 The process of diagnostic reasoning.

BOX 4-2 ▪ Recognizing Cues

The following may indicate cues:
1. **A deviation from population norms** (e.g., oral temperature of 103°F)
2. **Changes in usual behaviors in roles or relationships**
   Example: A previously successful student begins to skip classes. She stays up late partying and sleeps most of the day. Despite a previous close relationship with her parents, she barely talks to them when they contact her.
3. **Nonproductive or dysfunctional behavior**
   This may or may not be a change in behavior. It could be a long-standing dysfunctional behavior.
   Example: A man has been abusing alcohol for many years, even though it is causing many problems with his family and job and has begun to damage his liver.

Source: Adapted from Gordon, M. (1994). *Nursing diagnosis: Process and application* (3rd ed.). St. Louis, MO: Mosby.

Analyze and Interpret Data

To analyze and interpret data, follow three steps: (1) Identify significant data, (2) cluster cues, and (3) identify data gaps and inconsistencies.

Step 1. Identify Significant Data

Significant data (also called **cues**):
- Influence your conclusions about the client's health status.
- Usually are unhealthy responses.
- Draw on your theoretical knowledge (e.g., of anatomy, physiology, psychology).
- Are compared with standards and norms.
- One cue should alert you to look for others that might be related to it (forming a pattern).
  For example: Suppose you have noted that a woman's pulse rate is 110 beats/min. Is this an unhealthy response—a cue? Compare the rate with your theoretical knowledge—for example, the normal range for an adult pulse is 60 to 100 beats/min. This woman is a longtime cigarette smoker who also drinks a lot of coffee. These habits increase pulse rate, so 100 beats/min may be a normal finding for this client. See Box 4-2 for other indications of clues.

KnowledgeCheck 4-4
- What is a cue?
- What are three ways you can recognize a cue?

Step 2. Cluster Cues

A **cluster** is a group of cues that are related to each other in some way. The cluster may suggest a health problem. **KEY POINT:** *To help ensure accuracy, you should always derive a nursing diagnosis from data clusters rather than from a single cue.*

Consider this example: Alma was transferred to the hospital from a long-term care facility. Because of a CVA (cerebrovascular accident, or stroke), Alma can make sounds but cannot speak; because of joint contractures, she cannot use her hands and arms. Alma is frequently incontinent of urine and has been diagnosed with Overflow Urinary Incontinence. When a nursing student is assigned to care for Alma, the student looks for additional cues:

- The student notices that Alma is often incontinent after loud vocalizing.
- She sees a pattern in these cues: Alma is incontinent, cannot use her hands and arms, and cannot communicate in words but is vocalizing.
- The student changes the nursing diagnosis to Self-Care Deficit: Toileting related to immobility and inability to communicate the need to void.
- After the student provides a call device that fits under the arm, Alma is able to press the device and call the nurse when she needs to void.
- Alma is no longer incontinent of urine.

ThinkLike a Nurse 4-2

For each of the following cue clusters, decide whether the cues represent a pattern; that is, are all the cues related in some way? If so, explain how they are related. If not, state which cue does not fit.
a. Dry skin, abnormal skin turgor (more than 4 seconds), thirst, and scanty, dark yellow urine
b. Pain and limited range of motion in knees, uses walker, medical diagnosis of osteoarthritis
c. Hard, painful bowel movement about every 3 days; does not exercise regularly; eats very little dietary fiber; skin is dry.

Step 3. Identify Data Gaps and Inconsistencies

As you cluster and think about relationships among the cues, you will identify the need for data that were not previously apparent. In Think Like a Nurse 4-2, item (c), you have enough data to support a diagnosis of Constipation. However, you still need to identify factors contributing to the problem. You have two: lack of dietary fiber and lack of exercise. But you should also ask about other causes of Constipation. Does the patient postpone defecation? Does he have a history of relying on laxatives? How much fluid does he drink?

Data Gaps As another example, look again at Todd's (Meet Your Patient) data. Except for medical diagnoses, there are very few data. The following data gaps exist:

- His admitting diagnosis of chronic renal failure suggests the possibility of fluid imbalance; however, data needed to support that include decreased intake and output, dark urine, poor skin turgor, and complaints of thirst.
- Decreased sensation in his lower extremities certainly could create mobility or safety problems, but you need to know the degree of sensation loss and the exact meaning of "slight loss of mobility."

Inconsistencies Look for inconsistencies in the data. Suppose a client tells you, "I really don't eat much." However, she is 5 feet tall and weighs 190 pounds. This seems inconsistent because your theoretical knowledge tells you that obesity is usually caused by excessive intake of calories. You need more specific data, such as what she actually eats or whether she has any medical problems that might contribute to obesity (e.g., hypothyroidism).

Draw Conclusions About Health Status

After clustering cues and collecting any missing data, the next step is to begin drawing conclusions about the patient's health status—strengths as well as problems. You will need to make inferences and identify problem etiologies, as well as decide which type of problem the cue cluster represents (also see Table 4-2).

Step 1. Make Inferences

Making inferences is a critical-thinking skill. Recall that cues are facts (or data), whereas inferences are conclusions (judgments, interpretations) that are based on the data. An inference is not a fact because you cannot directly check its truth or accuracy. For example:

Fact:	Patient is crying. (You can observe that directly.)
	Patient is trembling. (You can observe that directly.)
Inference:	Patient is anxious. (You cannot observe anxiety, but you know that crying and trembling may be signs of anxiety.)

Some inferences are supported by more complete and reliable data than others. In the preceding example, suppose you said to the patient, "You seem upset. Can you tell me what's going on?" And the patient replied, "So much has been happening. I guess I'm just anxious about everything." Now you have enough data to support your inference, and you can be reasonably sure that it is accurate (valid).

KEY POINT: *Nursing diagnoses are inferences—and are only your reasoned judgment about a patient's health status. Try not to think of a diagnosis as being right or wrong but instead as being more accurate or less accurate. You can never construct a perfect diagnosis, but you must strive to make your diagnostic statements as accurate as possible to ensure that care is effective.*

KnowledgeCheck 4-5

- What are the possible conclusions you can draw about a client's health status (e.g., that no problem exists)?
- What is the difference between a cue and an inference?

Step 2. Identify Problem Etiologies

An **etiology** consists of the factors that are causing or contributing to a problem. Etiologies may be pathophysiological, treatment related, situational, social, spiritual, maturational, or environmental. It is important to correctly identify the etiology because it directs the nursing interventions. Consider this nursing diagnosis:

Constipation related to inadequate intake of dietary fiber

The etiology suggests that you encourage the client to eat more high-fiber foods. But what if that etiology is incomplete? What if you overlooked the fact that the client does not drink enough fluids? Or that he gets very little exercise? In that case, your efforts to increase intake of high-fiber foods would probably not help relieve the client's constipation.

To identify the etiology of a health problem, use your theoretical knowledge (e.g., of psychology, physiology, disease processes) and patient data to answer questions such as the following:

- What factors are known to cause this problem?
- What cues are present that may be contributing to this problem?
- How likely is it that these factors are contributing to the problem?
- Are these cues *causing* the problem, or are they merely *symptoms* of the problem?

KEY POINT: *An etiology is always an inference because you can never actually observe the "link" between etiology and problem.* For example, in the preceding Constipation diagnosis, you could measure (observe) the person's fiber intake. You could also observe infrequent, hard stools (Constipation). But you cannot observe that the lack of fiber is the cause of the Constipation. You have to infer that link based on your knowledge of normal elimination and your experiences with other patients.

ThinkLike a Nurse 4-3

- How would your nursing interventions be different for the following diagnoses?
  - a. Constipation related to lack of knowledge about laxative use
  - b. Constipation related to weak abdominal muscles secondary to long-term immobility

Verify Problems With the Patient

After identifying problems and etiologies, verify them with the patient. A diagnostic statement is an interpretation of the data, and the patient's interpretations may differ from yours. For example, if you have diagnosed Ineffective Breastfeeding related to lack of knowledge about breastfeeding techniques, you might verify it by saying, "It seems to me you are not sure how to position him and get him to latch on to your breast. Is that accurate?" The woman might confirm your diagnosis, or she might say, "No. I *do* know how to do it; I am just tired and a little nervous with you watching me." **KEY POINT:** *Think of nursing diagnoses as tentative, and be open to changing them based on new data or insights from the patient.*

Prioritize Problems

Up to this point, the diagnostic process has focused on identifying and validating health problems. **KEY POINT:** *However, clients often have more than one problem, so you must use* *nursing judgment to decide which to address first and which are safe to address later. This is* **prioritizing**.

- Prioritizing puts the problems in order of importance, but it does not mean you must resolve one problem before attending to another.
- You will usually prioritize problems as you are recording them.
- You can indicate the priority by designating each problem as high, medium, or low priority or by ranking all the problems in order from lowest to highest (e.g., 1, 2, 3, 4).
- Problem priority is largely determined by the theoretical framework that you use—for example, whether your criteria are human needs, problem urgency, future consequences, or patient preference.

Maslow's Hierarchy of Human Needs

Even though it is not a nursing framework, many nurses use Maslow's hierarchy to prioritize nursing diagnoses (Fig. 4-6). Maslow (1970) ranks human needs on eight levels, beginning with the most basic needs. In Maslow's model, basic needs must be met before a person can focus on higher needs; therefore, most nursing diagnoses fall at the cognitive and lower levels.

For further information on the Maslow theory, see Chapter 8.

 ## ThinkLike a Nurse 4-4

Prioritize the following nursing diagnosis labels (problems) based on the Maslow framework (see Fig. 4-6):

(1) Assign each diagnosis a high, medium, or low priority.
(2) Rank them in order of importance, with 1 being most important and 5 being least important.

_____ Ineffective Airway Clearance
_____ Ineffective Breathing Pattern
_____ Diarrhea
_____ Risk for Falls
_____ Impaired Memory

Problem Urgency

If you use problem urgency as your ranking criterion, you would rank problems according to the *degree of threat* they pose to the patient's life or to the *immediacy* with which treatment is needed. Assign:

High priority to problems that are life threatening (e.g., Ineffective Airway Clearance) or that could have a destructive effect on the client (e.g., Self-directed Violence)

Medium priority to problems that do not pose a direct threat to life but that may cause destructive physical or emotional changes (e.g., Ineffective Denial, Unilateral Neglect)

Low priority to problems that require minimal supportive nursing intervention (e.g., Ineffective Role Performance, mild Anxiety)

Future Consequences

When assigning priorities, also consider the possible future effects of a problem. Even if a problem is not life threatening and even if the patient does not see the problem as a priority, it may result in harmful future consequences for the patient. For example, suppose that Todd's (Meet Your Patient) physician prescribes a renal diet and insulin (instead of his previous oral medications) to treat the diabetes underlying his renal failure. Todd announces that he would like to go home to his job and family as soon as possible. He resists being taught about his medicines and how to administer his insulin. He admits neglecting to take his medication as prescribed in the past. You suspect that he has not been taking his medicines because he

Transcendence
of self; helping
others self-actualize

Self-actualization
Personal growth,
reaching potential

Aesthetic
Symmetry, order, beauty

Cognitive
Knowledge, understanding, exploration

Self-esteem
Pride, sense of accomplishment,
recognition by others

Love and belonging
Giving and receiving affection, meaningful
relationships, belonging to group(s)

Safety and security
Protection, emotional and physical
safety and security, order, law, stability, shelter

Physiological
Food, air, water, temperature regulation,
elimination, rest, sex, and physical activity

FIGURE 4-6 Maslow's hierarchy of human needs can be used for prioritizing problems.

is in denial about his health problems. Clearly his Ineffective Denial may lead to further problems with his treatment plan. You would assign high priority to this problem and address it before attempting to provide teaching for his nursing diagnosis of Deficient Knowledge (insulin).

Patient Preference

Give high priority to problems the patient thinks are most important, provided that this does not conflict with basic/survival needs or medical treatments. *Consider this example.* Mr. Amani has had major surgery within the past 24 hours. His priority is to obtain pain relief. He refuses to turn, deep-breathe, and cough (TDBC) because doing so causes pain. However, as his nurse, you realize that these activities are essential for preventing Ineffective Airway Clearance, so you cannot safely support Mr. Amani's priorities. You should provide pain medication before helping him TDBC. You would explain your actions and continue to emphasize the importance of TDBC. **KEY POINT:** *When you explain the importance of your priorities, patients often come to agree with them and cooperate more fully with interventions.*

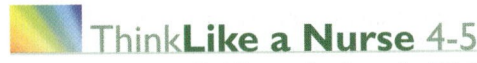 ## ThinkLike a Nurse 4-5

Suppose that on Todd's transfer from the ED (Meet Your Patient), you made the following nursing diagnoses for him. Using problem urgency as your criterion, assign each of these diagnoses a low, medium, or high priority.

- Risk for Imbalanced Fluid Volume secondary to renal failure
- Risk for Falls related to (r/t) decreased sensation and mobility in legs
- Deficient Knowledge (renal disease process) r/t new diagnosis of renal involvement secondary to type 2 DM

Computer-Assisted Diagnosing

Many institutions use computers for planning and documenting patient care. Some expert (knowledge-based) systems allow you to enter assessment data, and the computer program will then generate a list of possible problems. After you choose a problem label, the computer will provide a screen with the definition and defining characteristics of the problem so you can compare them with the actual patient data. After you "accept" the diagnostic label, you complete the problem statement by choosing etiologies from the next computer screen. For an example of a care planning screen, see Figure 6-4.

KnowledgeCheck 4-6

List the steps in the diagnostic process.

REFLECTING CRITICALLY ON YOUR DIAGNOSTIC REASONING

Diagnostic reasoning is complex and vulnerable to error. Therefore, after prioritizing your list of problems, you need to evaluate the list for accuracy. When using electronic health records, there is an even greater need for accuracy of nursing diagnoses. When diagnosing, you apply critical thinking to your theoretical and self-knowledge and to the patient data and situation (recall the full-spectrum nursing model in Chapter 2).

Critical thinking + Knowledge + Data = Statement of health status

Think About Your Theoretical Knowledge

The better your knowledge base, the better your diagnostic reasoning. Ask yourself the following questions:

- Is this diagnosis based on sound knowledge (e.g., of pathophysiology, psychology, nutrition, and other related disciplines)?
- Do I have sound knowledge about the defining characteristics (cues) associated with various nursing diagnoses?
- Do I feel reasonably sure I have interpreted the data correctly?
- Have I identified the problem type correctly—that is, can this problem be treated primarily by nursing interventions?

To avoid diagnostic error, build a good knowledge base and learn from your clinical experiences. These will help you to (1) recognize cues and patterns, (2) associate patterns with the correct problem, (3) gain confidence in your ability to reason, and (4) keep from relying too much on authority figures (Wilkinson, 2012).

Think About Your Self-Knowledge

Realize that your beliefs, values, and experiences affect your thinking and can be misleading. For example, imagine that a nurse in a labor and delivery unit believes it is important to be strong and uncomplaining, even when experiencing severe pain. When this nurse cares for a woman in early labor who cries out and complains of pain, the nurse sees it as a problem of either Anxiety or Ineffective Coping, not as a problem of Pain. Can you see how that changes the focus of the nurse's care? Ask yourself the following questions (Wilkinson, 2012):

What biases and stereotypes may have influenced my interpretation of the data?

- **Bias** is the tendency to slant your judgment based on personal opinion or unfounded beliefs, as the nurse did in the preceding example.
- **Stereotypes** are judgments and expectations about an individual based on the personal beliefs you have about a group when you have little or no actual experience with the group (e.g., men are unemotional; teenagers are irresponsible). You form stereotypes by making flawed assumptions.

Did I rely too much on past experiences? This is like stereotyping in that you draw conclusions about an individual based on what you know about people in similar situations. Consider, for example, a nurse who has cared for many first-time mothers (primiparas) during labor. Most of these women experienced moderate anxiety even during early labor. Now each time the nurse cares for a primipara, she expects to see anxiety, so she tends to identify cue clusters as Anxiety, failing to check for other explanations such as Pain or Deficient Knowledge.

Did I rely too much on the client's medical diagnosis, the setting, or what others say about the client instead of on the data? Medical diagnoses and statements from others can help you to think of possible explanations for your data, but they can also bias your thinking and prevent you from gathering your own data. For example, Ms. Grayson returned to the unit last evening after undergoing a total colectomy and colostomy. This morning, the night nurse reported, "Ms. Grayson is aware that she has cancer and she is coping well." However, while bathing Ms. Grayson, you begin to talk to her about her colostomy. She seems shocked. "I didn't know they did that! What's wrong with me?" As you answer her questions, you realize that she has been very groggy from the anesthesia and pain medication and may not recall or did not understand what was told to her about her surgery or diagnosis.

Think About Your Thinking

After reflecting on your knowledge, think about how you used the diagnostic process. Be sure your analysis of the data was thorough, that you have accurately identified the patient's problems, and that the problems are logically linked to the etiologies. Refresh your critiquing process by reviewing Box 4-3.

KnowledgeCheck 4-7

To help you fix them in your mind, list at least 10 questions to ask yourself when evaluating your diagnostic reasoning. Refer to Box 4-3 if you need help preparing this list.

PracticalKnowledge
knowing **how**

After you have completed the diagnostic reasoning process, the final activity in the diagnosis step is to record patient strengths and problem statements. Practical knowledge regarding nursing diagnosis involves selecting the correct problem labels and writing the diagnostic statements. The following section explains the need for standardized languages, explains how to

BOX 4-3 ■ Critiquing Your Diagnostic Reasoning Process

Data Analysis

Did you:
- Identify all the significant data (cues)?
- Omit any important cues from the cluster?
- Include unnecessary cues that may have confused your interpretation?
- Try more than one way of grouping the cues?
- Consider the patient's social, cultural, and spiritual beliefs and needs?
- Identify all the data gaps and inconsistencies?

Drawing Inferences and Interpretations of the Data

- Did you consider all the possible explanations for the cue cluster?
- Is this the best explanation for the cue cluster?
- Did you have enough data to make that inference?
- Did you look at patterns, not single cues?
- Did you look at behavior over time, not just isolated incidents?
- Did you jump to conclusions? Or did you take the time to carefully analyze and synthesize the data?

Critiquing the Diagnostic Statement (Problem + Etiology)

- Is the diagnosis relevant, and does it reflect the data?
- Does the diagnostic statement give a clear and accurate picture of the patient's problem or strength?

- When identifying the problem and etiology, did you look beyond medical diagnoses and consider human responses?
- Did you consider strengths and wellness diagnoses?
- Can you explain how the etiology relates to the problem—that is, how it would produce the problem response?
- Does the complete list of problems fully describe the patient's overall health status?

Verifying the Diagnosis

- Did the patient verify this diagnosis?
- When you verified the diagnosis, are you certain the patient understood your description of his health status?
- Did you obtain feedback from the patient, or did you merely assume that the patient agreed?
- Did you keep an open mind, realizing all diagnoses are tentative and subject to change as you acquire more data?

Prioritizing

- Considering the whole situation, what are the most important problems?
- What aspects of the situation require immediate attention?
- Did you consider patient preferences when setting priorities? If not, was there a good reason?

---

use the NANDA-I standardized terminology, and describes formats for diagnostic statements.

STANDARDIZED NURSING LANGUAGES

In order to communicate, people need a shared language. A **standardized language** is one in which the terms are carefully defined and mean the same thing to all who use them. One example is the periodic table for chemical elements. When a chemist in the United States writes Fe or Zn, chemists throughout the world know that she means iron or zinc. There is no confusion.

Nurses also need clear, precise, consistent terminology in their practice when referring to the same clinical problems and treatments. **Standardized nursing languages** are a comparatively recent attempt to bring such clarity to communication about nursing knowledge, thinking, and practice. A standardized nursing language can do the following:
- Support electronic health records.
- Define, communicate, and expand nursing knowledge.
- Increase visibility and awareness of nursing interventions.
- Facilitate research to demonstrate the contribution of nurses to healthcare and influence health policy decisions (Shever, 2011).
- Improve patient care by providing better communication between nurses and other healthcare providers and facilitating the testing of nursing interventions.

What Is a Classification System?

A **taxonomy** is a system for classifying ideas or objects based on characteristics they have in common. This requires use of a specific (standardized) vocabulary of terms for a particular topic in

accord with specific laws or principles (Lang, Hudgings, Jacox, et al., 1995). For example, the periodic table mentioned earlier classifies elements according to their atomic mass, number of protons, and so on. Medications are classified in various ways, such as according to their use (e.g., analgesics, antibiotics) or by the chemical nature of the drug (e.g., catecholamines, barbiturates), and so forth.

Classification Systems Used in Healthcare

Standardized classifications are created and used for various reasons. For example, point of service–level vocabularies are used for documenting and translating patient care information into electronic records.

The following classification systems are widely used in healthcare:
- The American Psychiatric Association's (APA) *Diagnostic and Statistical Manual of Mental Disorders (DSM-5)* (5th ed.) describes mental disorders (APA, 2013).
- The *International Statistical Classification of Diseases and Related Health Problems (ICD-10)* names and classifies medical conditions (World Health Organization, 2016).
- The *Current Procedural Terminology (CPT)* codes are used for reimbursement of physician services; they name and define medical services and procedures. CPT code updates are ongoing.

The following are classification systems recognized by the American Nurses Association (ANA) for describing nursing diagnoses (some describe outcomes and interventions as well):
- The *NANDA International (NANDA-I)* classification is based on identification of client problems and strengths obtained during assessment (see Chapter 3). The current taxonomy

includes more diagnostic labels, domains, and classes (NANDA-I, 2014) with etiologies, risk factors, and defining characteristics. Most chapters of this textbook use NANDA-I terminology.

- *The Clinical Care Classification (CCC)* uses a framework of care components to classify healthcare patterns (e.g., diagnoses and interventions). Specifically designed for clinical information systems, the CCC system facilitates nursing documentation at the point of care. See Chapter 42 for more information about CCC.

- *The Omaha System* consists of three interrelated components: the Problem Classification Scheme, the Intervention Scheme, and the Problem Rating Scale for Outcomes. It contains nursing diagnosis concepts, interventions, and outcomes. The Omaha System was designed to be computer compatible from the outset and is used across the continuum of healthcare settings. Refer to Chapter 42 for more information about the Omaha System.

- *Perioperative Nursing Data Set (PNDS).* This system is designed for use only in perioperative nursing (Petersen, 2011). Nursing diagnoses are focused on risk identification and safety within the perioperative environment (safety, physiological responses, behavioral responses, and health system factors). See Chapter 40 for more information about the PNDS.

- *International Classification for Nursing Practice (ICNP).* This system includes diagnoses, outcomes, and nursing actions The ICNP intends to provide a common language and comparison of nursing data across clinical populations, settings, geographic areas, and time (International Council of Nurses, 2015).

NANDA-I Taxonomy of Diagnostic Terminology

The NANDA-I taxonomy is not alphabetical. It classifies nursing diagnoses in a hierarchical system that helps us organize the concepts of concern for nursing. It categorizes nursing diagnoses (concepts) into 13 domains and 47 classes (NANDA-I, 2018).

- A **domain** is an area of activity, study, or interest (e.g., health promotion, nutrition).
- A **class** is a subdivision of a domain (e.g., health awareness is a class under health promotion; digestion is a class under nutrition).

In addition to being a classification system, the NANDA-I taxonomy provides a **standardized terminology,** or standardized language, to use when describing human responses. To see an alphabetical list of the terms in the NANDA-I standardized terminology for nursing diagnoses,

 Go to Davis Advantage, Resources, Chapter 4, **Alphabetical List of NANDA-I Diagnoses, 2018–2020.**

KEY POINT: *The terms contained in the NANDA-I taxonomy and the NANDA-I standardized terminology are the same. The difference is that the taxonomy organizes the words in a particular groupings; a terminology list does not.*

What Are the Components of a NANDA-I Nursing Diagnosis?

Each nursing diagnosis in the NANDA-I taxonomy has the following parts: diagnostic label, definition, defining characteristics, and either related factors or risk factors. You must consider all four parts when formulating a nursing diagnosis. Table 4-3 describes the diagnosis components.

KnowledgeCheck 4-8

- What are the components of a NANDA-I nursing diagnosis?
- What purpose does each part of the nursing diagnosis serve for directing the care of the client?

How Do I Know Which Label to Use?

During the diagnostic process, you will already have determined the general topic of the problem and perhaps even have some tentative problem labels in mind. For the following sections, you will need access to the NANDA-I labels, definitions, and so on, as well as to *Taxonomy II.* You can use either a NANDA-I handbook or a nursing diagnosis handbook.

1. ***First, identify the broad topic (or domain) that seems to fit the cue cluster.*** You can look at the NANDA-I taxonomy to see which domain the problem seems to fit. For example, suppose that after further assessment, you find that Todd (Meet Your Patient) has the following defining characteristics:

   Intake exceeds output
   Oliguria (low volume of urine)
   Generalized edema
   Recent rapid weight gain

   Which of the following NANDA-I domains are suggested by those cues?

   Nutrition   Self-Perception
   Elimination and Exchange   Activity/Rest

   The most logical domains would be the Nutrition domain and the Elimination and Exchange domain.

2. ***Narrow your search (to the class or most likely labels).*** In the NANDA-I taxonomy, after reading the definitions for the Nutrition domain and for the Elimination and Exchange domain, look at the classes in each.

   - *Nutrition.* Look at the *Hydration class.* All of the diagnosis labels there describe fluid balance. You can easily eliminate both "risk" labels because Todd has an actual problem (he has symptoms). Therefore, you must choose between Deficient Fluid Volume and Excess Fluid Volume. From this point, you simply compare Todd's cue cluster with the defining characteristics and definitions of those two labels and choose the best match.

   - *Elimination and Exchange.* Class 1 is *Urinary Function.* Because Todd has renal failure, you may think that his nursing diagnosis will be found in this class. However, you will see that none of the diagnoses in the *Urinary Function* class accurately represents Todd's defining characteristics. **KEY POINT:** *That is because renal failure is a pathology or disease, whereas you should be looking for Todd's responses to renal failure.*

3. ***Using a nursing diagnosis handbook, compare definitions and defining characteristics of the diagnostic labels with your cue cluster.*** You cannot know exactly what a diagnostic label means from the label name alone.

   Example: Suppose you have a patient who is not sleeping well at night. As a result, she is too tired to concentrate during the day. Which label would you use to describe this problem: Activity Intolerance, Fatigue, or Insomnia? You can answer that question only if you know the definition and defining characteristics of those labels.

   Not all of the defining characteristics need to be present for a diagnosis, but recall that the more data you have when

Table 4-3 ➤ Components of a NANDA-I Nursing Diagnosis

DEFINITION AND CHARACTERISTICS	EXAMPLES
Component: DIAGNOSTIC LABEL (title or name)	
■ A word or phrase that provides a name for the diagnosis ■ Represents a pattern of related cues and describes a problem or wellness response ■ Some labels include modifiers (also called descriptors) for time, age, and other factors	Disturbed Body Image Readiness for Enhanced Nutrition Acute, chronic, complicated, compromised, decreased deficient, delayed, disturbed, effective, excess, impaired ineffective
Component: DEFINITION	
■ Explains the meaning of the label ■ Distinguishes it from similar nursing diagnoses	For a patient with a sleep problem, would you label the problem Sleep Deprivation or Disturbed Sleep Pattern? The following definitions can help you to decide: ■ Sleep Deprivation: *Prolonged periods of time without sleep* ■ Disturbed Sleep Pattern: *Prolonged periods of time without sustained natural, periodic suspension of relative consciousness that provides rest*
Component: DEFINING CHARACTERISTICS	
■ Cues (signs and symptoms) that allow you to identify a problem or wellness diagnosis ■ A cluster of defining characteristics must be present in the patient data to use the problem label appropriately.	For the diagnosis Sleep Deprivation—Agitation, anxiety, fatigue, perceptual disorders For example, you cannot decide to use the Sleep Deprivation label merely by reading the definition. You must be sure the patient actually has some of the defining characteristics (above examples).
Component: RELATED FACTORS	
■ Related factors are the cues, conditions, or circumstances that cause, precede, influence, contribute to, or in some way show a patterned relationship with the problem (label). ■ Related factors can be pathophysiological, psychological, social, treatment related, situational, maturational, etc. ■ The list of related factors is not exhaustive. Factors other than those listed by NANDA-I could also be associated with the problem. ■ The problem may have more than one related factor. Human beings are complex, and their problems rarely have a single cause. ■ An individual patient's etiology will not include all the related factors that NANDA-I lists.	For Sleep Deprivation—Age-related sleep stage shifts, narcolepsy, overstimulating environment, prolonged discomfort For example, imagine the vast number of factors that might cause someone to have Chronic Low Self-Esteem.
Component: RISK FACTORS	
■ Risk factors function as the defining characteristics in potential (risk) diagnoses. ■ They are events, circumstances, or conditions that increase the vulnerability of a person or group to a health problem. ■ They can be environmental, physiological, psychological, genetic, or chemical. ■ Must be present to make the diagnosis, and they almost always form at least a part of the etiology of the diagnostic statement.	For the diagnosis Constipation— Habitually ignores the urge to defecate Abdominal muscle weakness Obesity Pregnancy

KEY POINT: *To help you remember:*
- *Related factors are similar to signs and symptoms (of actual problems).*
- *Risk factors are similar to etiologies (of potential problems).*

you make an inference, the more certain you can be that your inference is correct. For example, NANDA-I lists 15 defining characteristics for Ineffective Thermoregulation, including the following:

- Fluctuations in body temperature above and below normal range
- Cyanotic nailbeds
- Pallor
- Slow capillary refill
- Tachycardia

You could diagnose Ineffective Thermoregulation on the basis of the first defining characteristic alone, but you might be more certain of your diagnosis if some other cues were also present.

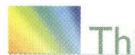 Think**Like a Nurse** 4-6

In the preceding example, what if the first defining characteristic (temperature fluctuations) were not present and you had only cyanotic nailbeds, pallor, and slow capillary refill as cues? Could you conclude that Ineffective Thermoregulation is causing those signs? What other explanations might there be for cyanotic nailbeds, pallor, and slow capillary refill?

WRITING DIAGNOSTIC STATEMENTS

KEY POINT: *A diagnostic statement consists of a problem and an etiology linked by a connecting phrase.*

Problem

- *Describes the client's health status* (or a human response to a health problem).
- *Identifies a response that needs to be changed.*
  - Use a NANDA-I label when possible, including descriptors (e.g., acute, imbalanced, impaired, ineffective, deficient, disturbed, risk-prone).
  - In alphabetical lists, you will see diagnosis labels arranged with the descriptor after the main word (e.g., Physical Mobility, Impaired). However, you should record diagnosis statements as you would say them, for example:
    Incorrect: Physical Mobility, Impaired r/t pain in left knee
    Correct: Impaired Physical Mobility r/t pain in left knee

Etiology

- *Contains one or more factors that cause, contribute to, or create a risk for the problem.*
  - Factors may include a NANDA-I label, defining characteristics, related factors, or risk factors.
- *Helps you individualize nursing care, because etiologies are unique to the individual.*

Suppose two patients have the following nursing diagnoses:
John: Anxiety r/t lack of knowledge of the treatment procedure
Janet: Anxiety r/t prior negative experiences and lack of trust in health professionals

The problem, Anxiety, has the same definition for both patients. They probably share some of the same defining characteristics, and you would use some of the same interventions for both John and Janet. However, to prevent anxiety from occurring or recurring, you would need to treat its cause.

To relieve John's anxiety, you would teach him what to expect from the impending procedure.

For Janet, you would need to (1) spend time building a relationship that demonstrates you can be trusted and (2) encourage her to talk about her fears and feelings.

- *The etiology directs the nursing interventions,* so include only factors that are influenced by nursing interventions.
- *Avoid using a medical diagnosis or treatment as an etiology* because you cannot write nursing orders to change it.

Connecting Phrase (related to)

- Most nurses use *related to* (r/t) to connect the problem and etiology, believing that the phrase *due to* implies a direct causal relationship.
- Because humans are complex, usually many factors combine to "cause" a problem, so it is nearly impossible to prove an exact cause. In fact, even if interventions eliminate the etiological factors, the problem might remain. For example, even if Janet begins to trust health professionals, she may become anxious for another reason.

Formats for Diagnostic Statements

A diagnostic statement should describe the client's health status as specifically as possible. The format varies depending on the type of problem you are describing.

One-Part Statement

Certain kinds of diagnostic statements need no etiology:

- **Syndrome Diagnosis**—A label that represents a collection of several nursing diagnoses

  Example: Disuse Syndrome

- **Wellness Diagnosis**—As a rule, this is a one-part statement beginning with the phrase Readiness for Enhanced. A wellness label does not describe a problem, so there is no etiology ("cause").

  Example: Readiness for Enhanced Nutrition

- **Very Specific NANDA-I Labels** —Some labels are so specific that they imply the etiology, or the only possible etiology is a medical diagnosis.

  Example: Latex Allergic Reaction

  It would be redundant to write *Latex Allergic Reaction r/t sensitivity to latex.* The etiology adds nothing to your understanding of the problem, and it suggests no interventions different from those suggested by the problem label.

Basic Two-Part Statement

Two-part statements can be used for actual, risk, and possible diagnoses. The format is:

Problem (NANDA-I label)   r/t   Etiology (related factors)

- **Actual diagnoses**—the etiology consists of related factors (e.g., *Nausea r/t anxiety*)
- **Risk diagnoses**—the etiology consists of risk factors (e.g., *Risk for Deficient Fluid Volume r/t excessive vomiting*)
- **Possible diagnoses**—the etiology consists of the patient's cues, which are not complete enough to diagnose (e.g., *Possible Constipation r/t patient's statement of no BM for 2 days*)

Basic Three-Part Statement

This is also called the **PES format** (problem, etiology, and symptom). Primarily for students, this method helps ensure that they have enough data to support the problem they have identified.

- The format is

  Problem r/t etiology as manifested by (AMB) signs or symptoms

- The connecting phrase can be either *AEB (as evidenced by)* or *AMB (as manifested by).*

- After the connector (*AMB*), this format adds the patient signs or symptoms that confirm the diagnosis.

*Constipation r/t inadequate intake of fluids and fiber-rich foods **AMB painful, hard stool and bowel movement every 3 or 4 days**.*

- You cannot use the PES format for risk nursing diagnoses, because patients "at risk" do not yet have symptoms.

Other Format Variations

"Specify" (Add to the problem label.) Some NANDA-I labels include the word "specify" (*e.g., Decisional Conflict [specify]*). That label is useful only if it describes the problem more specifically.

Example: Impaired Physical Mobility: Inability to maintain balance

"Secondary to" (Add to the etiology.) When the defining characteristics are vague (e.g., *chronic physical disability*) you may need to add a second part to the etiology, usually a disease or pathophysiology. Use the connector *secondary to* (symbolized as 2°).

*Example: Chronic Pain r/t chronic physical disability **2° rheumatoid arthritis**.*

The term *secondary to* makes clear that the nurse is not ultimately responsible for the pathophysiological part of the etiology.

Two-Part NANDA-I Label The first part describes a general response; the second part, following a colon, makes it more specific.

*Example: Imbalanced Nutrition: **Less Than Body Requirements** r/t . . .*

Adding Words to the NANDA-I Label **KEY POINT:** *The "rule" for adding words is first to try to make the statement specific or descriptive by writing a good etiology, using the PES format, or adding **secondary to**. If that does not fully describe the health status, add descriptive words to the problem label.* Does Impaired Bed Mobility mean that the patient cannot roll from side to side—or that she cannot move at all? You would need to add your own words to the label to make it more descriptive (e.g., *Impaired Bed Mobility: **Inability to turn self in bed** r/t weakness, secondary to low sodium level*).

Decide whether the clarifying words belong in the problem or in the etiology. For example, you may see a diagnosis of Acute Pain r/t surgical incision. However, surgical incision is a medical treatment and should not be used as the etiology. It would be better to write:

Example: Acute pain (abdominal incision) r/t turning and moving 2° abdominal surgery.

Unknown Etiology Sometimes you will not be able to identify the etiology. For example, you might diagnose a patient's Parental Role Conflict, but you may need more information to determine the cause. Perhaps there is an impending divorce; perhaps she has taken on the care of an elderly parent. In this case, you could write *Parental Role Conflict r/t unknown etiology*. Later, when you obtain more data, you will be able to complete the etiology.

Complex Etiology Some problems have too many etiological factors to list, or the etiology is too complex to explain in a brief diagnostic statement. Imagine the number of factors that might contribute to problems such as Disabled Family Coping.

For such problems you can replace the etiology with the phrase *complex factors* (e.g., *Disabled Family Coping r/t complex factors*).

Collaborative Problems

KEY POINT: *A collaborative problem is always a potential problem (e.g., a complication of a disease, test, or medical treatment).* The disease, test, or treatment is actually the etiology of the problem. You should not use the *problem + etiology* format because you cannot treat the etiology with independent nursing interventions. The focus of your interventions is monitoring for and preventing the complication. The word(s) following the colon represent the problem you are monitoring and trying to prevent.

Example: Potential Complication of thrombophlebitis: Pulmonary embolism

KnowledgeCheck 4-9

Write an example of each of the following six diagnostic statement formats, using the three listed components—mix and match:

> *Problem labels:* Anxiety, Pain (lower back)
> *Etiologies:* Unknown outcome of surgery; muscle strain and tissue inflammation
> *Cues:* Exhibits physical manifestations of anxiety (e.g., hands shaking); states pain is 9 on a scale of 1 to 10.

- Basic two-part statement
- Basic three-part statement
- Basic two-part statement, using "secondary to" (create your own disease/pathology)
- Statement with unknown etiology
- Possible nursing diagnosis
- Risk nursing diagnosis

How Does the Nursing Diagnosis Relate to Outcomes and Interventions?

The Problem Suggests Goals

The problem describes a health status that needs to be changed. The problem guides you in determining the patient outcomes for measuring this change. Consider the following diagnostic statement: Risk for Impaired Skin Integrity r/t complete immobility 2° spinal cord injury.

- **The goal, or outcome, is the opposite of the unhealthy response:** Skin will remain intact and healthy.
- **The goals suggest assessments** (a type of nursing intervention). For example, the diagnosis *Risk for Impaired Skin Integrity* tells you to monitor the patient's skin condition.
- **If the problem is not an accurate statement of health status, then your goals and resulting assessments will be wrong.** If you incorrectly identified the previous problem as *Impaired Physical Mobility 2° spinal cord injury*, then the goal would suggest that you monitor the patient's mobility. That nursing action would not improve the mobility and might cause you to miss a developing skin problem.

KEY POINT: *As a general rule, the problem suggests goals, and the etiology suggests interventions.*

The Etiology Suggests Interventions

In the preceding mobility example, you could not cure the spinal cord injury or restore the patient's ability to move about. However, you could provide some mobility by turning and repositioning the patient frequently. This would help prevent Impaired Skin Integrity. **KEY POINT:** *The aim of the nursing interventions is to remove or alter the factors contributing to the problem.*

REFLECTING CRITICALLY ABOUT DIAGNOSTIC STATEMENTS

Just as you critiqued your diagnostic reasoning process, you must reflect on the content, format, and meaning of your diagnostic statements. After you have written your diagnostic statements, use the criteria in Table 4-4 to judge their quality (Wilkinson, 2012).

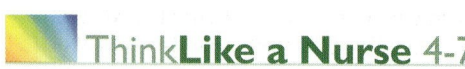

ThinkLike a Nurse 4-7

Rewrite the following diagnostic statement so it contains no legally questionable language. Use imaginary etiological factors if you need to. **Risk for Falls r/t lack of staff to assist with Ambulation**

Critiquing the NANDA-I System

Despite its potential benefits, some nurses have criticized the use of standardized language and the NANDA-I taxonomy in particular. However, try not to reject the idea of standardized language just because of a few problematic labels. You do not need to use the official NANDA-I labels exclusively. If you are uncomfortable with a label, change the wording to make it more useful, or write a completely new label. **KEY POINT:** *Remember, the point of a standardized language is to more clearly communicate the nature of the patient problem in nursing terms.*

Toward Evidence-Based Practice

Read about the following study, and then answer the questions at the end of the box.

Paans, W., Sermeus, W., Nieweg, R., et al. (2012). Do knowledge, knowledge sources and reasoning skills affect the accuracy of nursing diagnoses? A randomised study. *BMC Nursing 2012.* doi:10.1186/1472-6955-11-11

This randomized study was carried out in 11 hospitals to determine whether the knowledge sources and a predefined record structure affected the accuracy of nursing diagnoses. Possible determinants included the influence of the individual nurse's knowledge and critical-thinking skills. Researchers defined how knowledge is obtained and utilized in the following manner:

1. **Knowledge** is obtained through *knowledge sources* (acquired through the use of protocols, prestructured data sets or forms, and clinical pathways).
2. Additional factors are related to the nurse's cognitive abilities and ready knowledge.
3. **Ready knowledge** includes numerous factors, such as prior information the nurse may have about a particular patient's history, or her ability to interpret relevant patient data. Ready knowledge also includes that which the nurse has previously acquired either through

education or experience in similar patient situations. These latter factors require that the nurse has a disposition toward critical-thinking (e.g., open-mindedness, inquisitiveness, and maturity) and reasoning skills (e.g., deduction, analysis, inference, and evaluation).

Researchers concluded that use of a knowledge source (e.g., predefined record structure or protocols) resulted in significantly higher accuracy of the nursing diagnoses. It was also determined that almost half of the variance of diagnoses accuracy was explained by the use of a predefined record structure in addition to a nurse's age, and the reasoning skills of deduction and analysis.

---

1. Does this study reveal anything important about the process of arriving at accurate nursing diagnoses? Explain your reasoning.

2. Can you explain the difference between the use of knowledge sources and ready knowledge as it pertains to your nursing education?

3. From this report, could you reasonably infer that the use of a predetermined assessment/documentation format (e.g., PES) would improve the accuracy of your nursing diagnoses? If not, what else might be helpful?

Table 4-4 ➤ Reflecting Critically About Your Diagnostic Statements

GUIDELINE	DISCUSSION AND EXAMPLES
1. **In choosing a NANDA-I label, do not rely on the label definition alone.**	Compare patient data with defining characteristics and the label definition.
2. **Include both problem and etiology, with cause and effect stated correctly.** A quick check of this is to read your statement backward: "Etiology causes problem," and see whether it makes sense.	*Correct example:* Ineffective Breastfeeding r/t Deficient Knowledge (positioning infant at breast). *Read backward,* this statement says that deficient knowledge of positioning the infant "causes" Ineffective Breastfeeding. This makes sense. *Incorrect example:* Deficient Knowledge r/t Ineffective breastfeeding (incorrect positioning of the infant at breast). *Read backward* this statement says Ineffective breastfeeding causes deficient knowledge. This does not make sense.
3. **Be sure that the etiology does not merely restate the problem.**	*Incorrect example:* Impaired Physical Mobility r/t inability to walk *Correct example:* Risk for Impaired Skin Integrity (ulcers, infection) r/t diabetes mellitus
4. **Write the statement clearly.** The statement should give a clear picture of the client's health status, readily understood by other team members.	Avoid abbreviations and jargon. For example, do you know what this statement means? *Imp. Phys. Mobility (inability to get OOB w/o assist.) r/t muscle weakness and pain in LL*
5. **Write the statement concisely.**	A wordy statement is likely to be unclear.
6. **Be sure the statement is descriptive and specific.**	A vaguely stated problem and/or etiology cannot provide guidance for formulating goals and nursing interventions.
7. **State the problem as a patient response.** ▪ **A problem is not a patient need.** Avoid using the word "need" in describing a problem. ▪ **A problem is not a medical test, treatment, diagnosis, or equipment.** ▪ **A problem is not a nursing goal, a nursing problem, or a nursing action.**	A need may cause a problem, but it is not a human response. *Incorrect example:* Needs increased fluids related to . . . *Incorrect example:* Foley catheter in place
Nursing Goal—Prevent urinary tract infection.	*Correct example:* Risk for Urinary Tract Infection
Nursing Problem—Combative, hits caregivers.	*Correct example:* Risk for Other-Directed Violence
Nursing Action—Provide emotional support.	*Correct examples:* Anxiety, Grieving
8. **Use nonjudgmental language.** Look for phrases that may imply bias or criticism of a patient.	*Example:* Risk for Infection r/t poor hygiene and housekeeping
9. **Avoid legally questionable language.** Be alert for legal implications.	Look for phrases that seem to blame caregivers or patients or that refer negatively to patient care. *Example:* Risk for Falls r/t lack of staff to assist with ambulation

CLINICALREASONING

The questions and exercises in this section allow you to practice the kind of thinking you will use as a full-spectrum nurse. Critical-thinking questions usually have more than one correct answer, so we do not provide "correct answers" for these features. It is more important to develop your nursing judgment than to just cover content. You will learn by discussing the questions with your peers. If you are still unsure, see the Davis Advantage chapter resources for suggested responses.

Caring for the Nguyens

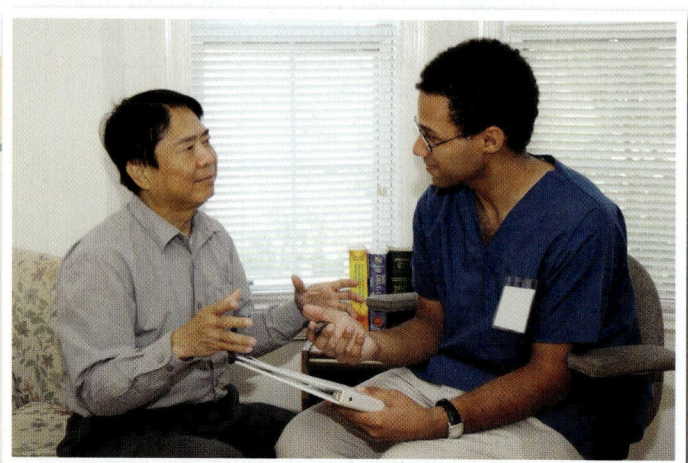

Review the opening scenario of Nam Nguyen in the front of this book. After the nurse practitioner completed the interview and physical examination of Mr. Nguyen, he listed the following diagnoses on the problem list:

Hypertension
Obesity
Musculoskeletal pain
Tobacco abuse
Family history of prostate cancer
Family history of cardiovascular disease
Family history of diabetes mellitus (DM)

A. What type of problem list does this one represent? How is it similar to or different from a problem list that you might generate?

B. Based on the data in the scenario, identify at least one actual, one potential, and one wellness diagnosis for Mr. Nguyen. Identify the NANDA-I labels and describe the cues that support your choices.

C. The nurse has identified Overweight as a problem for Mr. Nguyen.
- What information do you need in order to determine the etiology of this problem?
- Because you do not have that information, write a two-part diagnostic statement describing Mr. Nguyen's nutritional status.

D. Now rewrite the nutrition statement as a three-part statement, including the phrase *as evidenced by*.

E. The nurse has identified Acute Pain (knees) for Mr. Nguyen. If the pain were caused by a medical condition, like osteoarthritis, how would you write a two-part diagnostic statement to describe this health status?

 Go to Davis Advantage, Resources, Chapter 4, **Caring for the Nguyens Suggested Responses.**

Applying the **Full-Spectrum Nursing Model**_____

PATIENT SITUATION

Refer to the Meet Your Patient scenario near the beginning of this chapter. You have now admitted Todd from the ED.

THINKING

1. *Theoretical Knowledge:* What theoretical knowledge will you need to identify the collaborative problems and nursing diagnoses for Todd?
2. *Critical Thinking (Inquiry Based on Credible Sources):*
   a. What resources would you use to find out more about the pathophysiology of renal failure? How do you know the source is credible?
   b. When you are making your assessments of Todd, who is your best source of data? Why?

DOING

3. *Nursing Process (Diagnosis):*
   a. Write one collaborative problem for Todd. If you do not know the potential complications of chronic renal failure, look them up in a medical–surgical or pathophysiology textbook. Explain why you would not use a nursing diagnosis to describe the problem.
   b. After further assessment, you observe that Todd's skin is intact and without redness or lesions. Write a nursing diagnosis (problem and etiology) to describe your concerns about his skin.
   c. Based on Maslow's hierarchy of needs, which problem has the highest priority?

CARING

4. *Ethical Knowledge:* The scenario doesn't provide enough information for you to identify the ethical dimensions of Todd's care. However, based on what you already know about him, speculate about some things that might create ethical questions for you.

PATIENT SITUATION

5. *Patient Preferences:* Think critically about the patient's preferences and concerns. Suppose that Todd's main concern is not the same as the high-priority problem you identified. Speculate about some other concerns he might have. What else might he want to have resolved that could—for him—be more important than his chronic renal failure? Aside from his physical condition, what life concerns do you think Todd might have right now?

To explore learning resources for this chapter,

Go to **www.DavisAdvantage.com** and find:

Answers and Suggested Responses for all questions in this chapter

List of NANDA-I Diagnoses

Knowledge Map

References and Bibliography

Concept Map

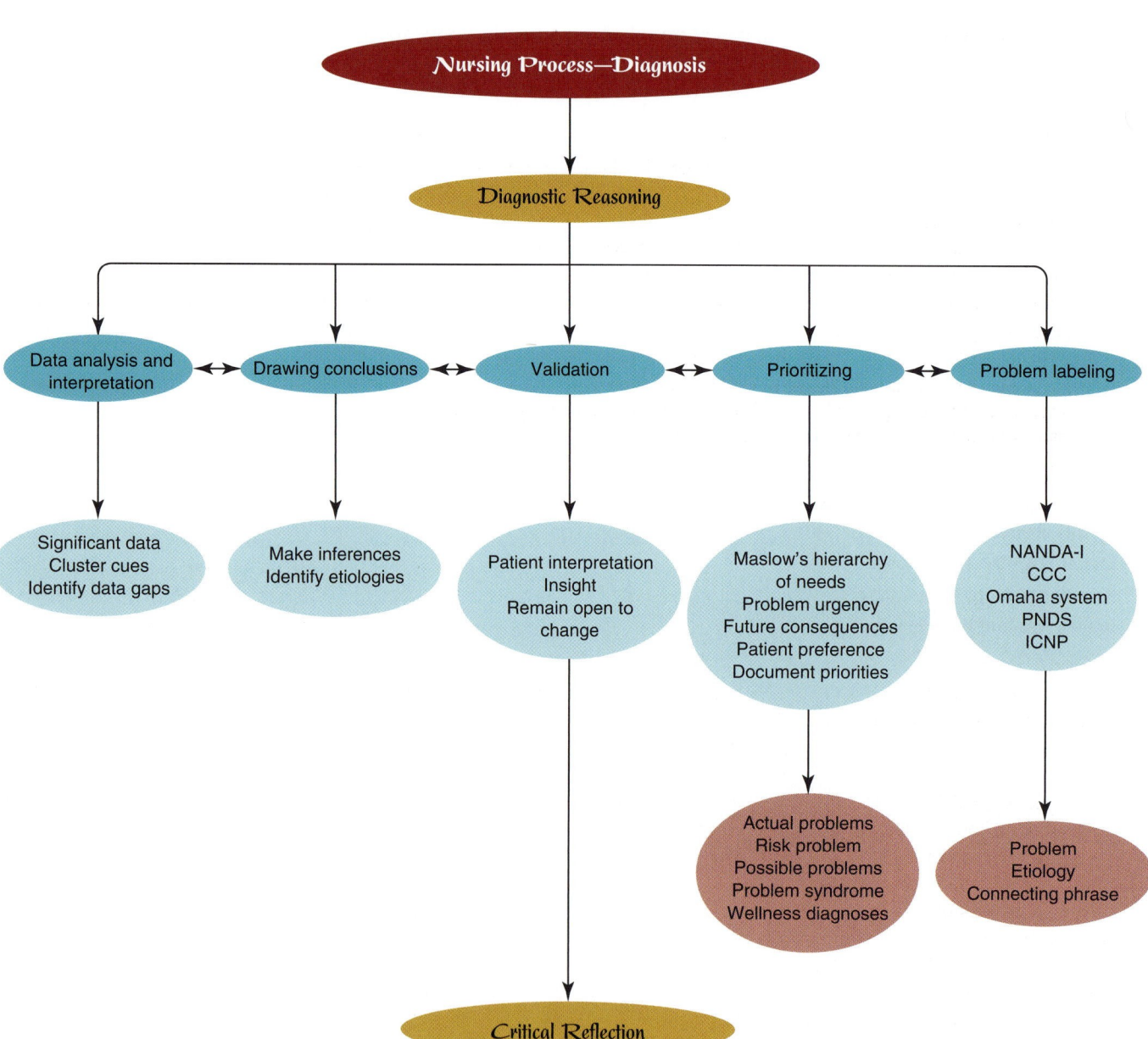

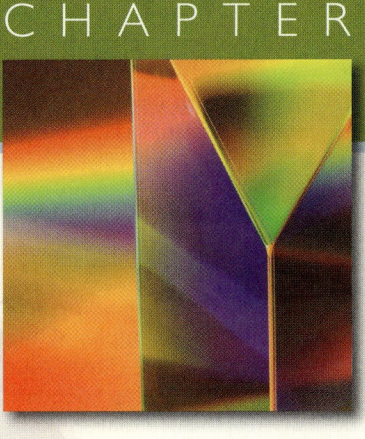

Planning Outcomes

Learning Outcomes

After completing this chapter, you should be able to:

➤ Describe formal, informal, initial, ongoing, and discharge planning.

➤ Identify patients who need a comprehensive, formal discharge plan.

➤ Describe the information contained in a comprehensive nursing care plan.

➤ Discuss the advantages and disadvantages of computerized care planning.

➤ Describe a process for writing an individualized care plan, making use of available standardized care-planning documents.

➤ Define the following terms: *goal, outcome, expected outcome,* and *nursing-sensitive outcome.*

➤ Differentiate between short-term and long-term goals.

➤ Explain how a goal is derived from a nursing diagnosis.

➤ Write appropriate goals for actual, risk, and possible nursing diagnoses.

➤ Use standardized terminology to state patient goals.

Key Concepts

Goals/Outcomes

Patient Care Plan

Planning

Related Concepts

See the Concept Map at the end of this chapter.

Meet Your Patient

Ben Ivanos has just been admitted to an orthopedic unit after a motorcycle accident. Mr. Ivanos is 24 years old and healthy; he takes no medications. He had surgical reduction of fractures and now has casts on both legs and a cast on one arm. He is receiving morphine sulfate intravenously via a patient-controlled analgesia (PCA) pump. Imagine that you are an orthopedic nurse and must plan care for Mr. Ivanos. You rank the following nursing diagnoses as highest priority:

1. Acute Pain secondary to musculoskeletal trauma (arms, legs, body) and muscle spasms
2. Risk for Peripheral Neurovascular Dysfunction secondary to casts/traction

You write the following desired outcomes (goals) on the care plan:

Goals for diagnosis

Demonstrates correct use of PCA pump.

Rates pain not higher than 4 on a scale of 1 to 10 at all times.

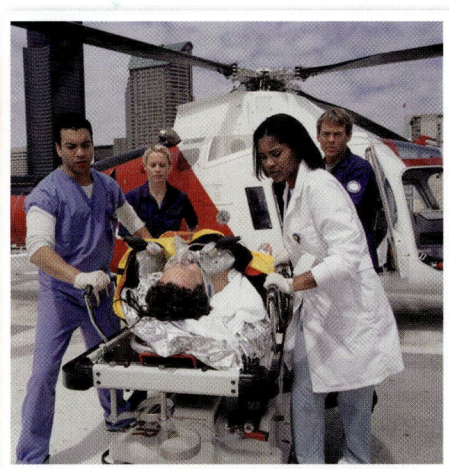

Goals for diagnosis 2

Peripheral pulses palpable

Fingers and toes warm

Fingers and toes without edema, pallor, or cyanosis

Capillary refill less than 3 seconds

These goals will guide you in choosing nursing interventions for relieving Mr. Ivanos's pain, preventing peripheral neurovascular dysfunction.

Theoretical Knowledge
knowing why

This text separates the process of planning outcomes from the process of planning interventions because, although related, they are distinctly different activities. This chapter (1) describes planning as a general process, (2) explains how to create a nursing care plan, and (3) discusses how to write patient goals/expected outcomes.

ABOUT THE KEY CONCEPTS

To help you understand and remember the content in this chapter, try to organize what you learn under the key concepts of **planning, goals** and **outcomes,** and **nursing care plans.** *Planning* is the broad umbrella term that covers the rest of the chapter concepts. In this chapter, you will learn how they are all related.

WHAT IS PLANNING?

The professional nurse is responsible for care planning and cannot delegate it. The end product of formal planning is a holistic plan of care that addresses the patient's unique problems and strengths. Box 5-1 lists American Nurses Association

(ANA) standards that specifically identify planning as the role of the registered nurse.

Planning can be formal or informal. **KEY POINT: Formal planning** *"is a conscious, deliberate activity involving decision making, critical thinking, and creativity" (Wilkinson, 2012).* During the planning phases, you:

- Work with the patient and family to derive desired outcomes from identified problems (e.g., nursing diagnoses).
- Identify nursing interventions to help achieve those outcomes.

KEY POINT: Informal planning *occurs while you are performing other nursing process steps.* For example, while performing neurovascular checks for Ben Ivanos (Meet Your Patient), you might discover that he is not obtaining adequate pain relief. What would you do? Any response in that scenario would require some planning.

How Is Planning Related to Other Steps of the Nursing Process?

Nursing process steps are overlapping and interdependent. To develop a plan of care with realistic goals and effective nursing orders, you:

- Must have accurate, complete *assessment* data.
- Need correctly identified and prioritized *nursing diagnoses.*

BOX 5-1 ■ American Nurses Association Standards of Nursing Practice for Outcomes and Planning

Standard 3. Outcomes Identification

The registered nurse identifies expected outcomes for a plan individualized to the healthcare consumer or the situation.

Competencies

The registered nurse:

Engages the healthcare consumer, interprofessional team, and others to identify expected outcomes.

Formulates culturally appropriate expected outcomes derived from assessments and diagnoses.

Uses clinical expertise and current evidence-based practice to identify health risks, benefits, costs, and/or expected trajectory of the condition.

Collaborates with the healthcare consumer to define expected outcomes integrating the healthcare consumer's culture, values, and ethical considerations.

Generates a time frame for attainment of expected outcomes.

Develops expected outcomes that facilitate coordination of care.

Modifies expected outcomes based on the evaluation of the status of the healthcare consumer and situation.

Documents expected outcomes as measurable goals.

Standard 4. Planning

The registered nurse develops a plan that prescribes strategies to attain expected, measurable outcomes.

Competencies

The registered nurse:

Develops an individualized, holistic, evidence-based plan in partnership with the healthcare consumer and interprofessional team.

Establishes the plan priorities with the healthcare consumer, family, and interprofessional team.

Advocates for responsible and appropriate use of interventions to minimize unwarranted or unwanted treatment and/or healthcare consumer suffering.

Identifies evidence-based strategies in the plan to address each of the identified diagnoses, problems, or issues. These strategies may include but are not limited to:

- Promotion and restoration of health,
- Prevention of illness, injury, and disease,
- Alleviation of suffering, and
- Supportive care.

Incorporates an implementation pathway that describes steps and milestones.

Identifies cost and economic implications of the plan.

Develops a plan that reflects compliance with current statutes, rules and regulations, and standards.

Modifies the plan according to the ongoing assessment of the healthcare consumer's response and other outcome indicators.

Documents the plan using standardized language or recognized terminology.

Note: There are additional standards for advanced practice nurses.

Source: American Nurses Association. (2015). *Nursing: Scope and standards of practice* (3rd ed.). Silver Spring, MD: Author.

- Must recognize that *goals/desired outcomes* flow logically from the nursing diagnoses.
- Should understand that by stating what is to be achieved, the goals suggest nursing interventions (written as nursing orders).

Figure 5-1 illustrates the relationship of planning outcomes to the other stages of the nursing process.

Initial and Ongoing Planning

- **Initial planning** begins with the first patient contact. It refers to the development of the initial comprehensive care plan, which should be written as soon as possible after the initial assessment.

    You may sometimes need to begin care planning even though the initial database is incomplete. For example, the patient may require emergency care before assessment is complete. In such a situation, make a preliminary plan with whatever information you have. You can complete and refine the plan when you are able to perform a more detailed assessment.

- **Ongoing planning** refers to changes made in the plan (1) as you evaluate the patient's responses to care or (2) as you obtain new data and make new nursing diagnoses. For example, nurses discovered that Ben Ivanos (Meet Your Patient) had not slept well during his first night in the hospital. They identified a new nursing diagnosis: Disturbed Sleep Pattern r/t unfamiliar environment, immobilization, and pain. They then developed a plan to address this problem. Ongoing planning allows you to decide which problems to focus on each day that you care for the patient.

Discharge Planning

Discharge planning is the process of planning for self-care and continuity of care after the patient leaves a healthcare setting. The purpose of discharge planning is to (1) promote the patient's progress toward health or disease management outside of facility care; and (2) reduce early readmissions to hospital care.

> *Example:* If the recommended length of stay for patients with surgical reduction of fractures is 2 days, then Ben Ivanos will still have casts on his arm and both legs when he leaves the hospital. Obviously, he will not be able to manage his own activities of daily living. What questions come to your mind when you think about how he will manage? Who will drive him home? Who will change his dressings? Take a moment now to jot down your ideas.

Ben Ivanos's case is not unusual. In the United States, outpatient surgeries and short hospital stays are the norm. Many patients are discharged despite ongoing need for nursing care and complex treatments. Therefore, nurses must prepare family members to perform tasks such as changing sterile dressings and monitoring IV medications. If family members are not available or if skilled nursing care is needed, arrangements must be made for home healthcare or transfer to a skilled nursing or rehabilitation facility. If appropriate care and services are not provided, the patient may experience delayed recovery or complications that require hospital readmission.

Comprehensive discharge planning involves collaboration. Ideally, it is done *with*, not *for*, the patient. In addition, a patient's postdischarge needs often call for the services of a multidisciplinary team (e.g., home care service personnel; physical therapists; social service; physicians; hospice) as well as members of the patient's family.

To learn more about the process of discharging patients from an institution, refer to the section Maintain Trust During Transitions in Chapter 11. Also see Procedure 11-4, Discharging a Patient From the Healthcare Facility.

Discharge Planning Begins at Initial Assessment

Because patients are in the surgery center or hospital for such a short time, discharge planning must begin at the initial assessment, which should include following patient data:

- Estimated date of discharge
- Physical condition and functional and self-care limitations
- Emotional stability and ability to learn
- Financial resources (e.g., personal finances, community resources such as nutrition assistance programs, Medicaid)
- Family or other caregivers available
- Caregiving responsibilities the patient may have for others
- Environment, both home and community (e.g., stairs, space for supplies and equipment, availability of transportation to healthcare services)
- Use of community services before admission

Written Discharge Plans

All patients need discharge planning. Sometimes it is enough to include discharge assessments and teaching as nursing orders on the patient's comprehensive care plan. For example, a middle-aged patient who has been hospitalized for deep vein thrombosis will be able to care for herself independently when she goes home. For this patient, you could simply write a nursing order to teach her about the side effects of the anticoagulant ("blood thinner") she will be taking at home.

In contrast, you will probably need a written, comprehensive discharge plan if the patient is an older adult or is likely to have one or more of the following (Bowles, Hanlon,

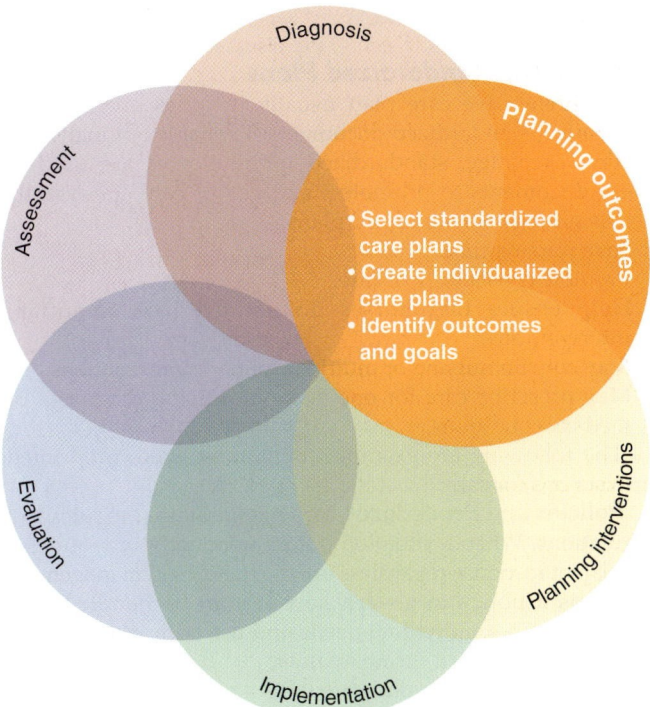

FIGURE 5-1 Nursing process phases: planning outcomes.

Diagnosis

Assessment

Planning outcomes

- Select standardized care plans
- Create individualized care plans
- Identify outcomes and goals

Evaluation

Implementation

Planning interventions

Holland, et al., 2014; NSW Department of Health, 2011; Reddick & Holland, 2015):

- *Personal characteristics that interfere with self-care, such as the following:*
  - Difficulty learning or a memory deficit
  - Emotional or mental illness
  - Poor mobility
  - Self-care deficits (e.g., dressing, feeding, bathing, toileting)
  - Incontinence
- *Disease or treatment characteristics; coexisting illness:*
  - Terminal illness
  - Complicated major surgery
  - Complex treatment regimen or more than three medications to continue at home
  - An illness with an expected long period of recovery
  - A newly diagnosed problem or multiple chronic health problems (e.g., diabetes, chronic pain)
  - Preexisting wound
  - Malnutrition
- *Social or family factors:*
  - Inadequate services available in the community
  - Inadequate financial resources
  - No family or significant others to help provide care

Discharge Planning for Older Adults

Older adults tend to have complex needs when discharged. Therefore, it is especially important to start discharge planning at the initial admission assessment. Functional abilities, cognition, vision, hearing, social support, and psychological well-being must be a part of the initial assessment so that you can identify needed services at discharge. A comprehensive discharge process should help older adults to achieve the following objectives:

- Maintain functional ability.
- Lengthen the time before rehospitalization (or between hospitalizations).
- Involve all concerned parties in decision making.
- Improve interagency communication (e.g., hospital to nursing home).
- Emphasize client and family involvement and interdisciplinary collaboration.

KnowledgeCheck 5-1

- What does the nurse do in the planning phases of the nursing process?
- What is the purpose of initial planning? Ongoing planning? Discharge planning?

NURSING CARE PLANS

The **comprehensive nursing care plan** (a type of *patient care plan*) is the central source of information needed to guide holistic, goal-oriented care to address each patient's unique needs. It specifies dependent, interdependent, and independent nursing actions necessary for a specific patient.

Why Is a Written Nursing Care Plan Important?

A well-written comprehensive care plan benefits the patient and the healthcare institution by doing the following:

- Ensuring that care is complete.
- Providing continuity of care.
- Promoting efficient use of nursing efforts.
- Providing a guide for assessments and charting.
- Meeting the requirements of accrediting.

What Information Does a Comprehensive Nursing Care Plan Contain?

Comprehensive care plans include directions for four different kinds of care and include both medical and nursing interventions:

- Basic needs and activities of daily living (ADLs)
- Medical/multidisciplinary treatment
- Nursing diagnoses and collaborative problems (nursing diagnosis care plan)
- Special discharge needs or teaching needs

What Documents Make Up a Comprehensive Nursing Care Plan?

You will use a variety of documents to create a care plan, to be discussed over the next few pages. In most healthcare organizations, caregivers use preprinted, standardized plans that can be adapted to meet individual needs.

Form for Client Profile and Basic Needs

Some essential client data either do not change or are used or updated often. This includes the client's:

- Profile (e.g., age, providers)
- Basic needs (e.g., for hygiene and elimination)
- Diagnostic tests and treatments (e.g., laboratory tests, radiology procedures)

To provide quick and easy access, such information is usually recorded on a standardized form and not organized according to medical or nursing diagnoses. These patient care summaries are often in electronic format but may be printed on cardstock (Kardex) and kept in a central location.

For clients who require more than routine attention to their basic needs, you may need to write a nursing diagnosis care plan. Examples include a client with no appetite and the nursing diagnosis Imbalanced Nutrition: Less Than Body Requirements, or an immobile client with the diagnosis Risk for Impaired Skin Integrity.

Preprinted, Standardized Plans

A comprehensive care plan usually includes one or more preprinted, standardized documents. To enable optimal information exchange, standardized terminologies are used in these documents to promote standards of care consistently across settings. Standardized plans:

- Save nursing time.
- Promote consistency of care.
- Help ensure that nurses do not overlook important interventions.
- May contain nursing or multidisciplinary interventions.
- May prescribe care for one or more nursing diagnoses or medical conditions.

The following are examples of standardized, preprinted instructions for care:

Policies and Procedures **Policies** are similar to rules and regulations. When a situation occurs frequently or requires a consistent response regardless of who handles it, management develops a policy to govern how it is to be handled. You should consider individual needs and use critical thinking to interpret policies in a caring manner.

Example: In some critical care units a patient is allowed one visitor for a few minutes each hour. Imagine, though, that a patient is expected to die soon and that his daughter has come from a distant state and brought her three children for one last visit. Would you tell the daughter to take the children in to see their grandfather? Would you insist that she follow the rule and send them in without her, one at a time?

Protocols Protocols cover specific actions usually required for a clinical problem unique to a subgroup of patients.

Example: Not every patient on a medical–surgical unit is at risk for falls, but many are. The nurse would therefore add a **falls protocol** to the care plan for a patient in that subgroup.

Protocols may be written for a particular medical diagnosis (e.g., seizure), treatments (e.g., administration of oxytocin to induce labor), or diagnostic tests (e.g., barium enema). They contain both medical and nursing orders.

Unit Standards of Care Unit standards of care describe the care that nurses are expected to provide for all patients in defined situations (e.g., all women admitted to a labor unit or all patients admitted to a critical care unit). Unit standards of care differ from nursing care plans in the following ways:

- They describe the *minimum* level of care rather than *ideal* care.
- They describe the care that nurses are expected to achieve given the institution's resources and the client population.
- They are not usually organized according to nursing diagnoses.
- They resemble a list of things to do (e.g., complete comprehensive assessment within 2 hours of admission) rather than detailed instructions for care.

ThinkLike a Nurse 5-1

- Think of some other defined situations for which unit standards of care might be useful.
- Suggest some other subgroups for which a protocol might be appropriate.

Standardized Nursing Care Plan Standardized (model) **nursing care plans** detail the nursing care that is usually needed for a particular nursing diagnosis or for all nursing diagnoses that commonly occur with a medical condition. Figure 5-2 is a standardized care plan for a single nursing diagnosis. Although similar to unit standards of care, model care plans are different in that they usually:

- Provide more detailed interventions than do unit standards of care.
- Are organized by nursing diagnosis.
- Include specific patient goals and nursing orders.
- Become a part of the permanent record.
- Describe ideal rather than minimum nursing care.
- Allow you to incorporate addendum care plans.
- Include checklists, blank lines, or empty spaces so that you can individualize goals and interventions.

KEY POINT: *Model care plans can be used as guides, but they do not address a client's individual, specific needs. For this reason, they may lead you to focus on the common, predictable problems and overlook an unusual—and perhaps more important—problem that the person is experiencing.*

Critical Pathways Critical pathways are outcomes-based, interdisciplinary plans that sequence patient care according to case type. They specify predicted patient outcomes for each day or, in some situations, for each hour (see Fig. 5-3). They describe the minimal standard of care required to meet the recommended length of stay for patients with a particular condition or *diagnosis-related group (DRG)* (e.g., postpartum, myocardial infarction).

KEY POINT: *An agency usually develops critical pathways for its most frequent case types or for situations in which standardized care can produce predictable outcomes.*

Integrated Plans of Care Integrated plans of care **(IPOCs)** are standardized plans that function as both care plan and documentation form. Many critical pathways are designed as IPOCs; however, IPOCs do not necessarily (1) organize care according to diagnosis, (2) describe minimal standards of care, or (3) specify a timeline for interventions and outcomes.

Individualized Nursing Care Plans

Nurses use individualized care plans to address nursing diagnoses unique to a particular client. These care plans reflect the independent component of nursing practice and, therefore, best demonstrate the nurse's critical thinking and clinical expertise.

Standardized plans do not address unusual problems and may not meet a patient's individual needs. Therefore, you often need to adapt the plan by adding the necessary nursing diagnoses, goals/outcomes, and nursing orders they do not include.

Example: A standardized plan for a client with a myocardial infarction would undoubtedly prescribe care for the nursing diagnosis Acute Pain and for the potential complication of Heart Failure. However, it might not address the needs of a person who is not complying with treatments because he is in denial about his illness (nursing diagnosis: Ineffective Denial).

You may sometimes include medical orders in a nursing diagnosis or collaborative problem care plan. For example, for a client with a nursing diagnosis of Deficient Fluid Volume, you might list the medical prescription for intravenously administered fluids in the Nursing Orders column.

Nursing Diagnosis:	*Nursing Orders:*
Deficient Fluid Volume r/t vomiting and diarrhea	Check skin turgor and mucous membranes q4hr Monitor urine output . . .

Medical Orders:
IV normal saline, 150 mL/hr

Special Discharge or Teaching Plans

A nursing plan of care may also contain one or more discharge or teaching plans. These are sometimes referred to as *special-purpose* or *addendum* care plans. You can address routine discharge planning and teaching needs by using standardized plans or by including teaching as part of the nursing orders on an individualized care plan.

Example: A care plan for the nursing diagnosis Acute Pain secondary to abdominal surgery might include the nursing order "Teach patient to splint incision when turning in bed."

Chapter 26 shows an example of a teaching plan for the diagnosis Deficient Knowledge.

Computer Plans of Care

Most healthcare organizations use electronic health records (EHRs), including *computer-generated care plans.* The computer stores standardized plans (e.g., for nursing diagnoses, medical diagnoses, or diagnosis-related groups [DRGs]). When you enter a diagnosis or a desired outcome, the computer generates a list of suggested interventions from which to choose. You can individualize them by choosing from checklists or typing in your own interventions and strategies.

PATIENT PLAN OF CARE - GENESIS MEDICAL CENTER - Davenport, Iowa

PAIN, ACUTE: Experience of an unpleasant sensory and emotional sensation for a duration of less than 6 months.
SIGNS & SYMPTOMS: Observed or reported (select at least 2)

☐ Change in BP   ☐ Restlessness   ☐ Grimacing   ☐ Crying
☐ Patients self-report of pain   ☐ Diaphoresis   ☐ Increased muscle tension   ☐ Change in pulse rate
☐ Change in respiratory pattern ☐ Whimpering   ☐ Whining

OUTCOME SCORING

RELATED FACTORS	OUTCOMES	ADM				DC	INTERVENTIONS
☐ Physical injuring agent ☐ Psychological injuring agent	4 Pain control behavior – Recognizes causal factors – Uses non-analgesic relief measures – Uses analgesics appropriately – Reports pain controlled 3 Pain level – Oral/facial expressions of pain – Change in respiratory rate, heart rate, BP – Restlessness – Reported pain 3 Comfort level – Reported satisfaction with symptom control – Expressed satisfaction with pain control – Reported physical well-being						☐ Pain management ☐ Analgesic administration ☐ Patient-controlled analgesic (PCA) assistance ☐ Analgesic administration: intraspinal ☐ Environmental management: comfort ☐ Anxiety reduction ☐ Transcutaneous electrical nerve stimulation (TENS) ☐ Heat/cold application ☐ Distraction ☐ Simple relaxation therapy ☐ Simple massage ☐ Developmental care ☐ Preparatory sensory information ☐ Positioning

Definition of scoring scales	1	2	3	4	5
Pain control— Personal actions to control pain	Never demonstrated	Rarely demonstrated	Sometimes demonstrated	Often demonstrated	Consistently demonstrated
Pain level— Severity of reported pain	Severe	Substantial	Moderate	Slight	None
Comfort level— Extent of physical and psychological ease	None	Limited	Moderate	Substantial	Extensive

Diagnosis _____

Date Initiated _____ RN Initials _____

Date Resolved _____

FIGURE 5-2 Computer printout of standardized care plan for a single nursing diagnosis using standardized language.

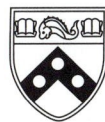

HOSPITAL OF THE UNIVERSITY OF PENNSYLVANIA

TOTAL LOWER JOINT (HIP/KNEE)
CLINICAL PATHWAY

ELIGIBILITY CRITERIA: All primary unilateral total hip or total knee
replacements

EXPECTED LOS: 3 Days   ADDRESSOGRAPH

CLINICAL KEYS:

1. Pain managed midpoint on painscale
2. Transfer to chair/commode with assistance POD 1; Ambulate in room, bathroom POD2
3. DVT precautions
4. Discharge plan completed by POD2
5. Patient verbalizes knowledge of hip or knee precautions
6. Knee motion 10 to 70 or better (TKA patients only)

	PACU	IMMED. POST-OP	POD 1	POD 2	POD 3-4
ASSESSMENTS	• NV checks with VS q1h × 4 • Pain • Effects of narcotics/ tolerance • 1 & 0 × 24hr • Pulse Ox q8 if on O2	• NV check / VS q 4hr → → • S/S DVT →	→ → → → • Pulse Ox × 1 on RA • Dsg/wound status q4	• NV check / VS q 8hr → → → • D/C pulse ox if O2 D/C • Dsg/wound status q8	→ → → → →
CONSULTS		• PT • PMR	→ (If not done already) → (If not done already)		
TESTS	• A/P hip X-ray (THA) • A/P knee X-ray (TKA)		• CBC	→ • INR (if on warfarin)	• A/P hip X-ray →
TREATMENTS	• O2	• D/C O2 if sat 94% • Incentive spirometry • Order walker (hip chair, elevated commode if needed) • Pneumatic compression device (ankle for knees, calf for hips)	→ → • D/C foley • Dressing change (1st dsg change by MD) →	→ → • Dressing change q day and pm →	→ → → →
MEDICATIONS	• PCA or epidural	→ • Anticoagulation	• IV heplock → • Consider conversion to oral pain meds	• D/C heplock → • D/C PCA/PCEA • PO pain meds	→
ACTIVITY	• Bedrest • Hip precautions if THA • CPM for total knee	→ → →	• OOB to chair BID → • Weight bear per order • Ambulate with assistive device	• OOB TID → → → → • PT ×2	→ → → → →
NUTRITION	• NPO	• NPO → ice → advance to full as tolerated	• Regular	→	→
EDUCATION / D/C PLANNING	• Deep breathing exercises	• Pain management • Initiate d/c plan	→ • Home vs rehab decision • Anticoagulation if indicated	→ • S/S wound infection • Medications • Activity level • D/C plan in place	→ → • Car transfer

Transfer to rehab when:	Discharge to home when:
1. Able to participate in care 2. Tolerating 2 physical therapy sessions 3. Not requiring IV pain medicine 4. Blood values are stable 5. Motivation is commensurate with projected functional status	1. Mobility and ADL's appropriate for degree of assistance at home and home environment 2. Appropriate assistive device and necessary adaptive equipment is used 3. Independent with hip/knee precautions 4. Independent with home exercise program or ongoing PT in the home or outpatient **IF D/C TO HOME, ENSURE APPROPRIATE CONSULTS TO ARRANGE HOME CARE FOLLOW-UP AND EQUIPMENT

FIGURE 5-3 Portion of a critical pathway.

Computer prompts help ensure that you consider a variety of actions and do not overlook common and important interventions. Current research supports that, overall, nurses' attitudes are favorable toward the use of EHR. In the past, nurses felt that because computerized planning required constant use of a step-by-step thinking process (linear thinking), it could stifle nursing intuition, insight, or expertise (Harmon, Fogle, & Roussel, 2015; Kossman & Scheidenhelm, 2008). Always look for creative approaches that might be more effective for a particular individual.

KnowledgeCheck 5-2

- In addition to care related to the patient's basic needs, what other types of information does a comprehensive care plan contain?
- How are critical pathways different from other standardized care plans?
- What is the main disadvantage of computerized and standardized care plans?

ThinkLike a Nurse 5-2

Suppose a nurse sees one of your student care plans and says to you, "You're wasting your time writing those things. We never use the nursing process in the real world." Take a few minutes to think about how you might respond.

Student Care Plans

You may have noticed that the care plans you see in clinical settings look different from the ones you create as a part of your clinical preparation. This is because student care plans are designed to help you learn and apply concepts from the nursing process, physiology, and psychopathology. For this reason, they may contain more detailed nursing orders as well as other information the instructor may require (e.g., information and data to support the nursing diagnoses). Some instructors may ask you to write **rationales** and cite references to support them. Rationales state the scientific principles or research that supports nursing interventions. Writing rationales helps ensure that you understand the reasons for your interventions. For an example of a student care plan,

 Go to Davis Advantage, Resources, Chapter 5, **Student Care Plan Example,** and **Care Map of Student Care Plan Example.**

Mind-Mapping Student Care Plans **Mind-mapping** is a technique for showing relationships between ideas and concepts in a graphical, or pictorial, way. A mind-mapped care plan uses shapes and pictures to represent the steps of the nursing process, as well as the patient's pathophysiology and other pertinent information. In nursing, the use of mind maps has been suggested (although not researched) for use in care planning (Mueller, Johnston, & Bligh, 2001; Kern, Bush, & McCleish, 2006). For an example of a care map, refer to the care plan and care map in Chapter 34.

PracticalKnowledge
knowing **how**

The rest of this chapter will help you learn how to apply your knowledge of the key concepts, goals, outcomes, patient care plan, and planning, as well as the many related concepts you have learned.

WHAT IS THE PROCESS FOR WRITING AN INDIVIDUALIZED NURSING CARE PLAN?

In this section, you will need to use your theoretical knowledge of concepts related to care planning (e.g., standardized care plans, protocols, individualized patient care plans). Writing an individualized nursing care plan follows in natural sequence from the assessment and diagnosis phases of the nursing process:

1. *Make a working problem list.* Suppose that after assessment you prioritized Ben Ivanos's (Meet Your Patient) problems as follows:

    Examples:

    A. Acute Pain secondary to musculoskeletal trauma (arms, legs, body) and muscle spasms

    B. Risk for Peripheral Neurovascular Dysfunction secondary to casts

    C. Self-Care Deficit (Total) r/t immobility secondary to casts, especially cast on dominant right arm

    D. Potential Complication of fracture: Delayed, union, malunion, or nonunion of bone

2. *Determine which problems can be managed with standardized care plans or critical pathways.*

    Example: Suppose that the hospital has a critical pathway for "Patient With Casts and/or Traction." It should contain assessments, outcomes/goals, and interventions for problems A and B.

3. *Individualize the standardized plan as needed.*

    Example: If the plan reads, "Perform neurovascular (NV) checks q_____," you would fill in the frequency of the NV checks according to Mr. Ivanos's needs.

4. *Transcribe medical orders to appropriate documents.*

    Example: You might write orders for pain medications on a special medication administration record. Or details about Mr. Ivanos's cast care might be recorded in a special section of the critical pathway.

5. *Write ADLs and basic care needs in the patient care summary (e.g., on the Kardex or in the electronic health record).*

    Example: For Ben Ivanos, you might note in the patient care summary that he requires a complete bed bath and help with eating.

6. *Develop individualized care plans for problems not addressed by standardized documents.*

    Example 1: For Ben Ivanos, you would need to write a plan for problems A and C. The critical pathway probably contains some outcomes and basic interventions for problem A (Acute Pain), but you might need to individualize them to make them more effective. If your unit had a Pain protocol, you would add it to Mr. Ivanos's care plan. If not, you would hand-write goals and interventions for the Pain diagnosis or insert them on the interactive page of the electronic record.

    Example 2: Problem C, Self-Care Deficit, would be partially addressed in the basic care section of Mr. Ivanos's patient care summary, but he has special needs. For example, he will need teaching and therapy to increase his ability to care for himself. So you would need to hand-write a plan for this nursing diagnosis.

KnowledgeCheck 5-3

Briefly describe a process for creating a comprehensive, individualized care plan that incorporates collaborative care and standardized planning documents.

PLANNING PATIENT GOALS/OUTCOMES

After assessment and diagnosis, the next step in individualized care planning is to formulate goals for improving or maintaining the patient's health status. **KEY POINT: Goals** *(also called* **expected outcomes, desired outcomes,** *or* **predicted outcomes)** *describe the changes in patient health status that you hope to achieve.* Although critical pathways describe the expected outcomes of multidisciplinary care, they do not provide a way to judge *nursing* effectiveness. **Nurse-sensitive outcomes** are those that can be influenced by nursing interventions. The rest of this chapter discusses individualized care planning and nurse-sensitive outcomes.

Importance of Goals The purposes of precise, descriptive, clearly stated goals/expected outcomes are to:

- Provide a guide for selecting nursing interventions by describing what you wish to achieve.
- Motivate the client and the nurse by providing a sense of achievement when the goals are met.
- Form the criteria you will use in the evaluation phase of the nursing process.

Nursing Responsibility Professional nurses are responsible for formulating goals/expected outcomes (see Box 5-1). If the client is not able to participate actively, the nurse acts on the client's behalf to develop client-centered goals. See the accompanying iCare box.

♥ iCare

The caring nurse formulates patient-focused goals.

- Remember that outcomes should state patient behaviors, not nursing activities.
- Example: If a patient outcome is to walk 10 feet unassisted with a walker by the end of the day, you might ask, "*At what time of the day do you like to walk?*" or "*At what time of day is it easier for you to walk?*"
- You should involve the patient as much as possible in goal setting, because goal achievement is more likely if the goals are realistic and important to the client.

How Should I Use the Terms *Goal* and *Outcome*?

Many nurses use the terms *goal* and *outcome* interchangeably. Some nurses use the term *goal* to mean a broad, nonspecific statement about the desired results of nursing activities. They use *outcomes* (and other outcome terms such as *expected outcomes*) to mean the more specific, observable responses that you would use to judge whether the goal has been met.

- **KEY POINT:** *When goals are stated as broad, specific statements, you must include both goals and expected outcomes on the care plan because a broad goal does not provide enough guidance for evaluating patient responses to care.*
- **KEY POINT:** *You must include expected outcomes on the care plan; however, use of broad goals is optional.*

Toward Evidence-Based Practice

Mello, B., Massutti, T., Longaray, V., et al. (2016, February). **Applicability of the Nursing Outcomes Classification (NOC) to the evaluation of cancer patients with acute or chronic pain in palliative care [Abstract].** *Applied Nursing Research, 29,* 12–18.

This small, prospective longitudinal study was carried out in Brazil to verify the clinical applicability of the Nursing Outcomes Classification (NOC) to the evaluation of cancer patients with a nursing diagnosis of Acute Pain or Chronic Pain. Data were collected with an instrument containing 8 NOC outcomes (e.g., Pain Level, Pain Control, Comfort Status, Client Satisfaction, Will to Live, Sleep, Vital Signs) and 19 NOC indicators (e.g., reported pain, length of pain episodes, personal and psychological well-being, pain regularly monitored, and actions to relieve pain or provide comfort).

Statistical differences were found between the first and last assessment indicating satisfaction in several of the indicators and outcomes, including the followings:

- Reported pain and length of pain episodes (in the *pain level* outcome)

- Social relationships (in the *personal well-being* outcome)
- Describes causal factors (in the *pain control* outcome)

Scores in *pain management* and *will to live* outcomes were consistently elevated. Scores on *personal well-being* outcome indicated that "patients and their families were satisfied with nursing interventions to manage patient pain and to promote physical and psychological well-being."

Conclusions: The researchers concluded that use of NOC outcomes with their indicators and interventions could be helpful to palliative care nurses in choosing the most effective methods of evaluating and minimizing cancer-related pain.

On the basis of this study, can you think of at least two additional conclusions you might realize from this study other than those listed here?

 Go to Davis Advantage, Resources, Chapter 5, **Toward Evidence-Based Practice Suggested Responses.**

In this text, we usually use the Nursing Outcomes Classification (NOC) terminology:

- The word *outcome*, used alone, means *any* patient response (positive or negative) to interventions (e.g., pain could become better or worse; both are outcomes).
- We use *goals, expected outcomes, desired outcomes,* or *predicted outcomes* when referring to desired (positive) patient responses.
- You can combine the broad goal and specific expected outcome into a single statement by writing *as evidenced by,* as in the following example:

Broad statement (goal)	Constipation relieved
Specific expected outcome (evaluation criteria)	Will have soft, formed bowel movement within 24 hours
Combined statement (goal + outcome)	Constipation will be relieved *as evidenced by* soft, formed bowel movement within 24 hours

How Do I Distinguish Between Short-Term and Long-Term Goals?

Short-term goals are those you expect the patient to achieve within a few hours or days. **Long-term goals** are changes in health status that you wish to achieve over a longer period—perhaps a week, a month, or longer. See Table 5-1 for a comparison of short-term and long-term goals.

KnowledgeCheck 5-4

Refer to Meet Your Patient at the beginning of the chapter. State whether each of Mr. Ivanos's goals was a short-term or long-term goal.

What Are the Components of a Goal Statement?

Every expected outcome/goal statement must have the following parts:

- **Subject.** The subject is understood to be the client, but it can also be a function or part of the client. You do not need to write "client." Assume the client is the subject; specify only if he is not.
    > *Example 1: Client[subject]* Will walk to the doorway with the help of one person by 12/13/18.
    > *Example 2: Lung sounds[subject]* will be clear to auscultation within 2 days after receiving antibiotics.

- **Action verb.** Use an action verb to indicate what activity the client will perform: what the client will learn, do, or say (e.g., Will *walk* to the doorway). Use concrete verbs (i.e., describing actions that you can see, hear, smell, feel, or measure), such as the following:

apply	explain	report
choose	eat	select
demonstrate	list	transfer

- **Performance criteria.** These describe the extent to which you expect to see the action or behavior, using concrete, observable terms. Specify:
    (a) How, what, when, or where something is to be done
    (b) Amount, quality, accuracy, speed, distance, and so forth
    > *Example:* [Client] Will walk *to the doorway* with the help of one person by 12/13/18.

- **Target time.** This is the realistic date or time by which the client should achieve the performance or behavior.
    > *Example 1:* [Client] Will walk to the doorway with the help of one person *by 12/13/18.*
    > *Example 2:* Other examples of target times are *by discharge, within 24 hours, at the next visit, each hour, at all times.*

    For risk (potential) nursing diagnoses, the desired outcome is that the problem will never occur. You can assume that the desired response should occur "at all times," but you may wish to schedule times for evaluating the outcome. For example:
    > *Nursing diagnosis:* Risk for Constipation r/t inadequate fluid intake
    > *Expected outcome:* Bowel movements will be of normal frequency and consistency.
    > *Target time:* At all times
    > *Evaluate:* Daily

- **Special conditions.** Special conditions describe the amount of assistance or resources needed or the experiences/treatments

Table 5-1 ➤ Comparison of Short-Term and Long-Term Goals			
	DEFINITION	**SITUATIONS FOR USE**	**EXAMPLES**
Short-Term Goals	▪ Can be achieved in a few hours or a few days.	▪ Acute care ▪ Day surgery ▪ Clinics; student assignments ▪ To focus on immediate needs ▪ To evaluate progress toward long-term goals	▪ 1) Describes pain as <3 on a 1–10 scale within 30 min after receiving analgesic. ▪ 2) Limits food intake to 1,500 calories per day.
Long-Term Goals	▪ Expected changes that occur over a week or more ▪ Optimal level of functioning, given health status and resources	▪ Home healthcare ▪ Extended-care facilities ▪ Rehabilitation centers ▪ Chronic illness ▪ To focus on conditions that are managed, not cured	1) Infant will double birth weight within 5 mo. 2) Within 3 mo after physical therapy treatments, will dress self except for buttons.

the client should have to perform the behavior. Include special conditions when it is important for other nurses to know them.

Example: [Client] Will walk to the doorway *with the help of one person* by 12/13/18.

KnowledgeCheck 5-5

In the following predicted outcomes, identify the subject, action verb, performance criterion, target time, and special conditions (if any). State which components are assumed, if any.

- (Client) will walk to the doorway with the help of one person by 12/13/18.
- After two teaching sessions, (client) will be able to identify which foods to avoid on a low-fat diet by 3/1/18.
- Bowel movements will be soft and formed and of usual frequency.
- Lungs clear to auscultation at all times.

How Do Goals Relate to Nursing Diagnoses?

Expected outcomes are derived directly from the nursing diagnosis. Therefore, they will be appropriate only if you identify the nursing diagnosis correctly. The problem clause of a nursing diagnosis (the clause on the left side in Table 5-2) describes the response or health status you wish to change. A desired outcome states the *opposite* of the problem and implies this response is what the interventions are intended to achieve (see Table 5-2).

ThinkLike a Nurse 5-3

Answer the following questions for Ben Ivanos's (Meet Your Patient) nursing diagnosis of Acute Pain secondary to musculoskeletal trauma and muscle spasms:

- What would be the opposite, healthy response to his problem?
- If the problem is prevented or solved, how will Mr. Ivanos look or behave? What will you be able to observe?
- What should Mr. Ivanos be able to do to demonstrate a positive change? How well, or how soon, should he be able to do it?

You might have said that the opposite response to pain would be absence of (or relief from) pain, but you couldn't really observe that. "Absence of pain" might serve as a broad goal statement. But how about more specific, observable expected outcomes? How would you show that Mr. Ivanos's pain was relieved?

Example: A few specific, observable behaviors that demonstrate absence of pain include the following: "Relaxed body posture, states pain is relieved, rates pain as less than 3 on a 1–10 scale."

Essential Versus Nonessential Goals

In general, the problem side of the nursing diagnosis suggests the goals, and the etiology suggests nursing interventions. You can also derive some goals from the etiology; however, **KEY POINT:** *the essential patient goals flow from the problem side of the nursing diagnosis (see the bold print in Table 5-3) because the problem side describes the unhealthy response you intend to change.*

Notice in Table 5-3 that the goals derived from the etiology may help resolve the problem, but they could also be achieved without improving the problem.

Example: Suppose that for a patient with Ineffective Airway Clearance you had written only the goals in regular type (in Table 5-3). If the patient achieves all three goals, you might think you could discontinue the interventions for Ineffective Airway Clearance. However, even a client who demonstrates all three of those responses still might not be coughing productively enough to clear the airways and still might not have clear lung sounds. Always observe the following rule:

KEY POINT: *For every nursing diagnosis, you must state one goal that if achieved would demonstrate resolution or improvement of the problem.*

Goals for Actual, Risk, and Possible Nursing Diagnoses

You will develop expected outcomes to promote, maintain, or restore health, depending on the status of the nursing diagnosis. See Table 5-4 for explanations and examples. Review Chapter 4 as needed.

Goals for Collaborative Problems

Recall that collaborative problems are physiological complications of diseases (e.g., diabetes) or medical treatments (e.g., cardiac catheterization) that nurses monitor to detect onset or changes in status. The desired outcome is always that the complication will not develop. They are not nurse-sensitive—they

Table 5-2 ▶ Comparison of Nursing Diagnoses and Goals

NURSING DIAGNOSIS (PROBLEM SIDE)	GOAL/EXPECTED OUTCOME
Problem response	Opposite of problem response
Present health status	Desired health status
Response that you hope to change	Response that you hope to achieve
Examples:	**Examples:**
Ineffective Airway Clearance ⟶	Lungs clear to auscultation
r/t ineffective cough secondary to incision pain ⟶	Coughs productively

Table 5-3 ➤ Deriving Goals and Nursing Activities From Nursing Diagnoses

NURSING DIAGNOSIS		GOALS/EXPECTED OUTCOMES		NURSING ACTIVITIES
Problem *Ineffective Airway* *Clearance* r/t	⟶	**Lungs clear to auscultation** **Coughs productively** **Respirations 12–20 breaths/min** **No pallor or cyanosis** **No dyspnea or shortness of breath (SOB)**	⟶	Teach deep breathing and coughing Auscultate lungs q4hr Assess respiratory rate, breathing, and skin color q4hr
Etiology: *Ineffective cough* *secondary to* *incisional pain*	⟶	Coughs forcefully/effectively Rates pain as <3 on 1–10 scale Splints incision while coughing	⟶	Teach to splint incision while coughing Turn, cough, and deep-breathe (TCDB) hourly Medicate for pain 30 min before TCDB

Table 5-4 ➤ Expected Outcomes for Various Problem Types

TYPE OF PROBLEM	EXAMPLE OF DIAGNOSIS	EXPLANATION OF DIAGNOSIS	EXAMPLE OF EXPECTED PATIENT OUTCOME	PURPOSE OF NURSING INTERVENTIONS
Actual Nursing Diagnosis	Constipation r/t inadequate dietary fiber and fluids	Symptoms of constipation present (e.g., no bowel movement [BM] × 3 days)	Will have normal, formed BM within 24 hr after receiving stool softener.	Resolution or reduction of problem; prevention of complications.
Risk (Potential) Nursing Diagnosis	Risk for Constipation r/t inadequate dietary fiber and fluids	Risk factors present (e.g., not drinking enough or eating adequate fiber)	Will have bowel function within normal limits for patient (e.g., daily BM with no need for stool softener or laxative).	Prevention and early detection of problem.
Possible Nursing Diagnosis	Possible Constipation r/t suspected inadequate intake of dietary fiber and fluids	Not enough data (e.g., no BM for 2 days, but no data on intake or on his usual bowel habits)	No patient goal. The *nursing* goal is "Confirm or rule out the problem."	Confirm or rule out problem.
Collaborative Problem	Potential Complication of abdominal surgery: ileus	Medical treatment creates risk for complication that is prevented by collaborative care.	None. Patient responses depend on collaborative care. The broad nursing goal is early identification of the problem.	Primarily detection; prevention is collaborative.
Wellness Diagnosis	Readiness for Enhanced Bowel Elimination	Bowel habits and dietary intake within normal limits, but fiber content and fluid intake can be improved.	Reports increased intake of dietary fiber and fluids; reports bowel functioning within normal limits.	Maintain or promote higher level of health.

do not result primarily from nursing interventions. Consider the following example:

> *Collaborative problem:* Potential Complication of abdominal surgery: Paralytic ileus (paralysis of the ileum of the small intestine)
>
> *Goal:* Patient will not develop paralytic ileus.

Suppose that 36 hours after surgery, the patient's bowel sounds are absent, his abdomen is distended and painful, and he begins vomiting. What could the nurse have done to prevent this situation? Can the nurse relieve the ileus and bring about return of peristalsis? Actually, there is very little that the nurse could do. The primary interventions are medical and, if there is obstruction, probably surgical. Therefore, it would not be appropriate to include a goal for this problem on a nursing care plan, because that would imply that nurses are primarily accountable for the outcome.

Collaborative goals are appropriate on multidisciplinary care plans and critical pathways. For collaborative problems, instead of patient outcomes you might wish to write a *nursing goal*, such as "Early detection of complication, should it occur." See Table 5-4.

How Do I Use Standardized Terminology for Outcomes?

In Chapter 4, you learned about the NANDA-I standardized terminology for nursing diagnoses. The American Nurses Association (ANA) has also approved several standardized vocabularies for describing client outcomes. The one used throughout most of this book is the **Nursing Outcomes Classification (NOC).**

The NOC is a standardized vocabulary of nursing-sensitive outcomes developed by a research team at the University of Iowa. In the NOC vocabulary, an **outcome** is "an individual, family, or community state, behavior, or perception that is measured along a continuum in response to nursing interventions" (Moorhead, Johnson, Maas, et al., 2013, p. 2). The NOC is appropriate for use in all specialty and practice areas.

Components of a NOC Outcome

Each NOC outcome consists of an outcome label, indicators, and a measurement scale.

- The **outcome label** (referred to as *the outcome*) is broadly stated (e.g., Decision Making, Concentration). It is neutral to allow for positive, negative, or no change in patient health status. Because NOC outcomes are linked to NANDA-I nursing diagnoses, you can use the NANDA-I/NIC/NOC "linkages" book to look up a nursing diagnosis and see the list of outcomes suggested for it (Johnson, Moorhead, Bulechek, et al., 2012).
- The **indicators** are the behaviors and states that you can use to evaluate patient status. In Table 5-5, the indicators are in the first column. The first one is "Identifies relevant information." This indicator means that Decision Making (the broad outcome) was being achieved. For each outcome, select the indicators that are appropriate to the patient. You can add to the list of indicators if necessary.
- For each outcome, NOC has a **measurement scale** (the numbers in Table 5-5) for describing patient status for each indicator, with 1 being least desirable and 5 the most desirable. During your initial assessment, you would have assigned the number that represents the patient's present health status. To form the "goal," you assign the scale number that the patient can realistically achieve after the

interventions. Using Table 5-5, you might assign the following numbers:

> (NOC Outcome) **Decision Making**
> *Goals (Indicators + measurement scale):*
> Identifies relevant information (4, mildly compromised)
> Identifies alternatives (4, mildly compromised)
> Identifies potential consequences of each alternative (5, not compromised)

KnowledgeCheck 5-6

Figure 5-2, a patient plan of care for Acute Pain, uses NOC language.

- What outcomes did the nurse choose for this patient?
- List two indicators for each of the outcomes.
- For which outcome does the nurse expect the highest level of functioning to occur after interventions? (Note that in this care plan the measuring scale has been applied to the outcomes rather than to the indicators.)

ThinkLike a Nurse 5-4

In Figure 5-2, what do you think the nurse expects to happen? Why do you think she ranked the outcomes this way?

Using NOC With Computerized Care Plans

Standardized language (e.g., NOC) is especially useful in computerized care systems. For example, the nurse could choose Circulation Status as a patient outcome; the program would then provide the definition and NOC indicators for Circulation Status. The nurse needs only to check the indicators that apply to the patient.

KEY POINT: *The computer does not think for you. You are responsible for deciding which outcomes and indicators to use for each patient and for identifying a target time.*

How Do I Write Goals for Groups?

- Community health goals are those you would use to specify and evaluate the health of groups, aggregates, or populations. They tend to emphasize health promotion, health maintenance, and disease prevention outcomes. For example, the U.S. Public Health Service has published broad, overarching goals for improving the health of the nation by a target date of 2020 (*Healthy People 2020,* 2010a, 2010b) to:
- Attain high-quality, longer lives free of preventable disease, disability, injury, and premature death.
- Achieve health equity, eliminate disparities, and improve the health of all groups.
- Create social and physical environments that promote good health for all.
- Promote quality of life, healthy development, and healthy behaviors across all life stages.

  NOC Outcomes can be used to write group goals in all settings, including home and community nursing.

- NOC *Community Health* includes outcomes, which are defined as "outcomes that describe the health, well-being, and functioning of a community or population" (Moorhead, Johnson, Maas, et al., 2013, p. 44.). Two examples are Community Competence and Community Risk Control: Lead Exposure.
- NOC *family* health outcomes describe the health of a family as a unit. Two examples are Family Coping and Family Health Status.

Table 5-5 ▸ Example of an NOC Outcome

Decision Making (0906)

Domain—Physiological Health (II)

Class—Neurocognitive (J)

Scale(s)—Severely compromised to Not compromised

Definition: Ability to make judgments and choose between two or more alternatives

DECISION MAKING	SEVERELY COMPROMISED	SUBSTANTIALLY COMPROMISED	MODERATELY COMPROMISED	MILDLY COMPROMISED	NOT COMPROMISED
Overall Rating					
Identifies relevant information.	1	2	3	4	5
Identifies alternatives.	1	2	3	4	5
Identifies potential consequences of each alternative.	1	2	3	4	5
Identifies needed resources to support each alternative.	1	2	3	4	5
Identifies time frame necessary to support each alternative.	1	2	3	4	5
Identifies sequence necessary to support each alternative.	1	2	3	4	5
Recognizes contradiction with others' desires.	1	2	3	4	5
Acknowledges social context of the situation.	1	2	3	4	5
Acknowledges relevant legal implications.	1	2	3	4	5
Weighs alternatives.	1	2	3	4	5
Chooses among alternatives.	1	2	3	4	5

Source: Moorhead, S., Johnson, M., Maas, M., et al. (2013). *Nursing outcomes classification (NOC)* (5th ed.). St. Louis, MO: Mosby/Elsevier.

For further explanation, see Chapters 14 and 42. Also search for Nursing Outcomes Classification on the Web or

 Go to the Center for Nursing Classification and Clinical Effectiveness (CNC) (Overview: Nursing Outcomes Classification [NOC]) Web site at http://www.nursing.uiowa.edu/cncce/nursing-outcomes-classification-overview

The Clinical Care Classification (CCC) system was first developed by Virginia Saba, a nurse-researcher, for use in home health nursing. It can now be used across all healthcare settings. In the CCC, you form goals by adding modifiers to the nursing diagnoses. This system has nursing diagnoses, such as Family Coping Impairment and Disabled Family Coping, that are clearly for family units. The CCC also includes a diagnosis specifically for communities: Community Coping Impairment. For a complete description of the CCC system,

 Go to the CCC Web site at http://www.sabacare.com/

The Omaha System was developed specifically for community health nursing. However, it can now be used across all healthcare settings. In this system, you must label all nursing diagnoses as *individual, family,* or *group.* You can write aggregate outcomes by specifying a *family* or *group* diagnosis and then creating a goal from it by using terms in a Problem Rating Scale for Outcomes, as in the following example:

Omaha Nursing Diagnosis:

Personal Hygiene. Family. Deficit (Actual Problem)

Present status	*Expected outcome*
Minimal knowledge of *family* personal hygiene	Adequate knowledge of *family* personal hygiene

For a complete description of the Omaha System and to see the Problem Rating Scale for Outcomes,

 Go to the Omaha System Web site at http://www.omahasystem.org/overview.html

How Do I Write Goals for Wellness Diagnoses?

Expected outcomes for wellness diagnoses describe behaviors or responses that demonstrate health maintenance or achievement of a higher level of health. For example, "Over the next year, [Mr. Needham] will continue to eat a balanced diet with more emphasis on including whole grains and fiber." By using the highest number (5) on the rating scale, you can use the NOC to write wellness outcomes. For example:

Nursing diagnosis: Readiness for Enhanced Nutrition

Expected outcome: Nutritional Status: (5) Not compromised

In addition, many NOC outcomes can be used with other diagnoses (e.g., Activity Tolerance, Child Development, Growth, Nutritional Status). See Chapter 27 or go to the NOC Web site for a complete list of wellness outcomes.

REFLECTING CRITICALLY ABOUT EXPECTED OUTCOMES/GOALS

After writing the expected outcomes for a client, use the full-spectrum nursing model to help you evaluate their quality. Use the following questions as a guide:

For Each Nursing Diagnosis:

1. **Is there at least one goal that, when met, would demonstrate problem resolution?** That is, does at least one goal flow from the problem clause?
2. **Do the predicted outcomes completely address the nursing diagnosis?** Review Table 5-3.

For Each Expected Outcome:

1. **Is the outcome appropriate for the nursing diagnosis?** If not, a new nursing diagnosis should be written rather than adding a not-quite-related goal to the existing plan.
2. **Is each outcome derived from only one nursing diagnosis?** That is, does it describe only one patient response?
3. **Is the outcome stated as a patient behavior, not a nurse activity?**

   Incorrect (nurse activity): Prevent skin irritation.

   Correct (patient response): Skin will not show signs of irritation.
4. **Is the outcome stated in positive terms?** As a rule, state what you intend to occur rather than what should not occur.

   Example: Say "incision dry" rather than "no incision drainage."

This is not always possible, especially for potential problems.

   Example: Write "No redness" (even though it is negative) not "Skin color normal," because "normal" is too vague.
5. **Is the outcome measurable or observable?**

   Correct: Explains the actions and side effects of Coumadin, by 8/11

   Incorrect: Understands the actions and side effects of Coumadin, by 8/11
6. **Are the performance criteria specific and concrete?** Avoid words such as *normal, sufficient, enough, more, less, adequate, increased.* Vague words can be interpreted differently by different people.
7. **Does each goal include all the necessary parts?**
8. **Is the expected outcome realistic and achievable by this patient, given the available resources?** Be sure to consider the patient's support system, financial status, available community services, and physical and mental status.
9. **Does the outcome conflict with the medical or other collaborative treatment plan?**

   Example: An outcome of "Ambulates to end of hall" would not be compatible with the medical treatment plan for a patient who is sleepy and lethargic from the side effects of medications.
10. **Do the patient, family, community, and nurse value the outcome?** When the nurse's goals conflict with the patient's, explore the patient's reasoning. Explain your reasoning to the patient and try to find a compromise or an alternative approach.
11. **Does the goal conflict with any religious or cultural values?** When a patient is "noncompliant," the reason may be that she values her cultural beliefs more than the caregiver's plan of care.

KnowledgeCheck 5-7

List at least eight questions you could ask to critically evaluate the quality of your goal/outcome statements.

CLINICALREASONING

The questions and exercises in this section allow you to practice the kind of thinking you will use as a full-spectrum nurse. Critical-thinking questions usually have more than one right answer, so we do not provide "correct answers" for these features. It is more important to develop your nursing judgment than to just cover content. You will learn by discussing the questions with your peers. If you are still unsure, see the Davis Advantage chapter resources for suggested responses.

Caring for the Nguyens

Review the opening scenario of Nam Nguyen at the front of this book. As the clinic nurse, you have written the following nursing diagnostic statement: Overweight r/t inappropriate food choices and serving size as evidenced by body mass index (BMI) of 28.5.

Write at least two short-term and two long-term goals for Mr. Nguyen based on this diagnostic statement. Remember that your goals must be realistic and take into account Mr. Nguyen's other health problems.

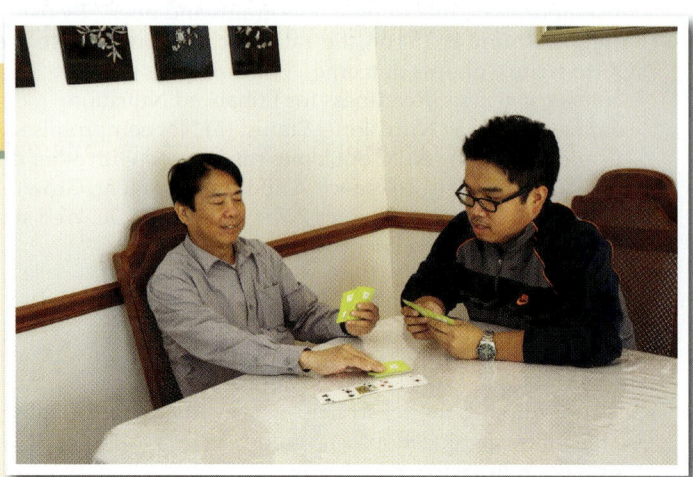

Applying the **Full-Spectrum Nursing Model**_____

PATIENT SITUATION

Ivan Benjamin has just been admitted to an orthopedic unit after an automobile accident. He was driving. Mr. Benjamin is 80 years old and has been living at home. He has the following preexisting comorbidities: type 2 diabetes and osteoarthritis. He has casts and traction on both legs and a cast on one arm. He is receiving morphine sulfate intravenously via PCA pump. Imagine that you are an orthopedic nurse and must plan care for Mr. Benjamin. The admitting nurse wrote the following diagnoses and goals on the plan of care.

NURSING DIAGNOSES

1. Acute Pain secondary to musculoskeletal trauma (arms, legs, body) and muscle spasms

2. Risk for Peripheral Neurovascular Dysfunction secondary to casts/traction

GOALS/EXPECTED OUTCOMES

- Demonstrates correct use of PCA pump.
- Rates pain not higher than 4 on a scale of 1 to 10 at all times.
- Peripheral pulses palpable
- Fingers and toes warm
- Fingers and toes without pallor or cyanosis
- No edema of fingers and toes
- Capillary refill less than 3 sec

THINKING

1. *Theoretical Knowledge:* What general theoretical knowledge will you need to care for this patient? Just identify the topics; limit the answer to about 150 words.
2. *Critical Thinking (Considering Alternatives):* Older adults are especially sensitive to certain medications, including morphine sulfate. What is one thing you could do to ensure Mr. Benjamin's safety while managing his acute pain?
3. *Critical Thinking (Inquiry):* List at least two more things you need to know about Mr. Benjamin in order to begin his discharge planning.

DOING

4. *Practical Knowledge:* What general practical knowledge will you need? What would you do to obtain this knowledge?
5. *Nursing Process:*
   a. *Diagnosis:* What is another nursing diagnosis you might want to assess for Mr. Benjamin?
   b. *Planning Goals:* On the care plan, rewrite the goals/expected outcomes for Acute Pain so that they will have all the required components. Assume that today's date is January 4.

CARING

6. *Self-Knowledge:* What beliefs, values, biases, or emotional responses might interfere with your ability to provide the best care to Mr. Benjamin?

CONTEXT

7. Think critically about the context. Is there anything in this situation that you have seen before? Identify any familiar elements. For example, you may have an elderly male relative, even if you have never cared for an 80-year-old patient before.

 To explore learning resources for this chapter,

 Go to www.DavisAdvantage.com and find:

Answers and Suggested Responses for all questions in this chapter

Lists of NIC Interventions and NOC Outcomes

List of NANDA-I Diagnoses

Knowledge Map

Student Care Plan Example

Care Map of Student Care Plan Example

References and Bibliography

Concept Map

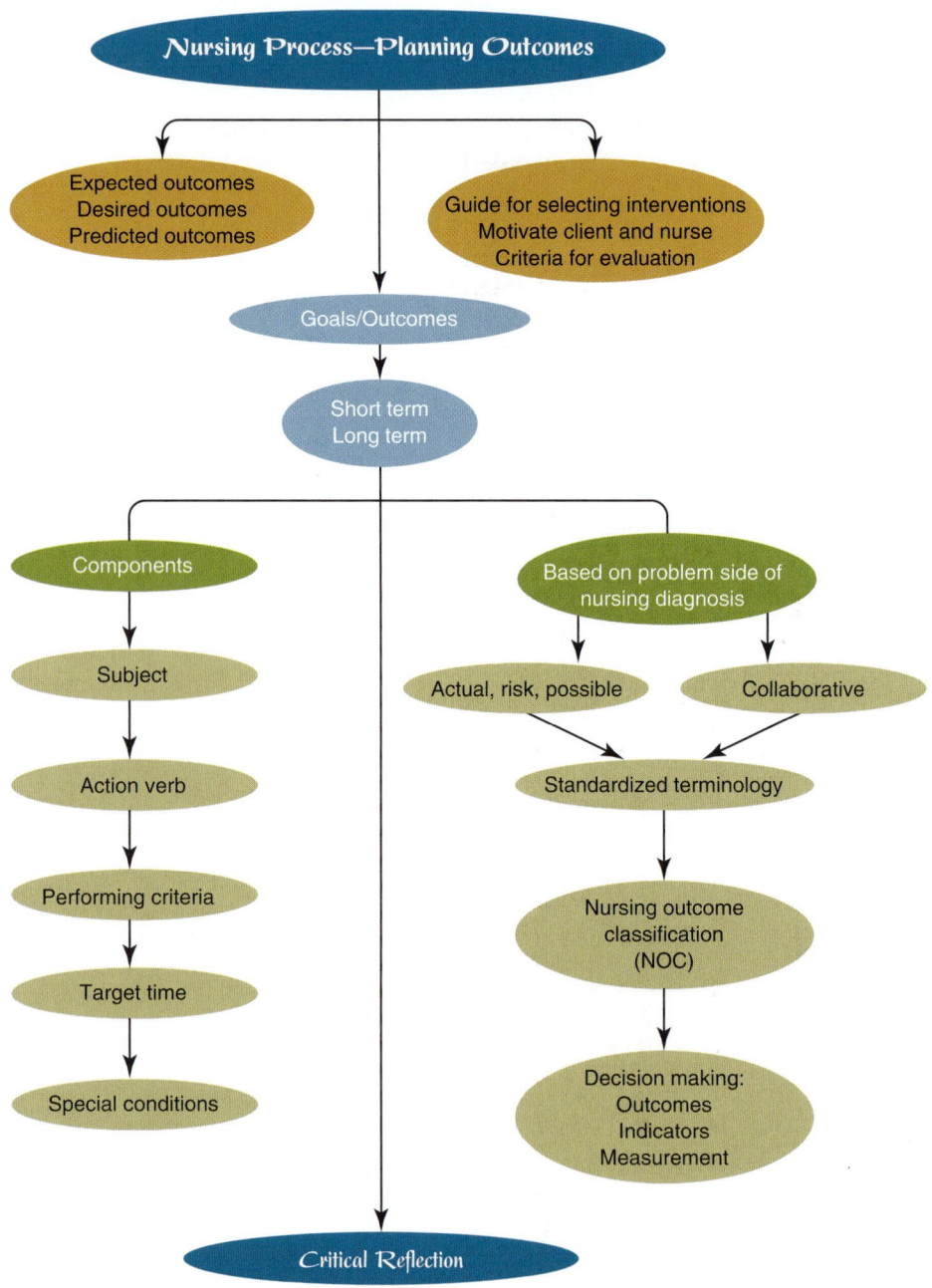

Nursing Process—Planning Outcomes

Expected outcomes
Desired outcomes
Predicted outcomes

Guide for selecting interventions
Motivate client and nurse
Criteria for evaluation

Goals/Outcomes

Short term
Long term

Components

Based on problem side of
nursing diagnosis

Subject

Actual, risk, possible

Collaborative

Action verb

Standardized terminology

Performing criteria

Nursing outcome
classification
(NOC)

Target time

Special conditions

Decision making:
Outcomes
Indicators
Measurement

Critical Reflection

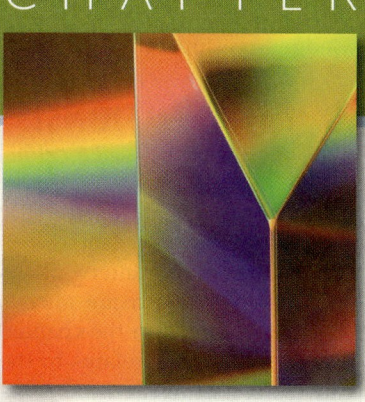

CHAPTER 6

Planning Interventions

Learning Outcomes

After completing this chapter, you should be able to:

➤ Define the term *nursing intervention*.

➤ Compare and contrast independent, dependent, and interdependent (collaborative) nursing interventions.

➤ Explain how theories, research, and evidence-based practice influence the choice of nursing interventions.

➤ Explain how nursing interventions are determined by problem status (i.e., as actual or potential problems).

➤ Explain how to use a standardized vocabulary for nursing interventions.

➤ Give an example of a standardized wellness (health promotion) intervention and one individualized nursing order for performing that intervention.

➤ Give an example of a standardized spirituality intervention and one individualized nursing order for performing that intervention.

➤ Write complete, detailed nursing orders, in correct format, for patients.

➤ Give examples of some questions for reflecting critically about nursing orders you have written.

➤ Describe a process for generating nursing interventions for a client.

Key Concepts

Evidence-based practice
Nursing interventions

Related Concepts

See the Concept Map at the end of the chapter.

Meet Your Patient

Ben Ivanos, whom you met in Chapter 5, was admitted after a motorcycle accident. He had surgery for fracture reduction on his legs and now has casts on both legs and one arm. For the past 3 days, he has been receiving narcotic analgesics for severe pain. He has a new nursing diagnosis today: Constipation related to immobility and decreased gastrointestinal (GI) motility secondary to narcotic analgesics. The nurse enters the diagnosis into an electronic care plan. In addition to a list of suggested assessments, the computer database generates the following list of suggested interventions:

1. Institute a program to establish a regular pattern of bowel movements.
2. Administer laxative or stool softener, as prescribed.
3. Administer enema.
4. Remove stool manually.
5. Encourage increased fluid intake, including warm liquids.
6. Instruct on and encourage a high-fiber diet.
7. Encourage a regular program of activity and exercise.

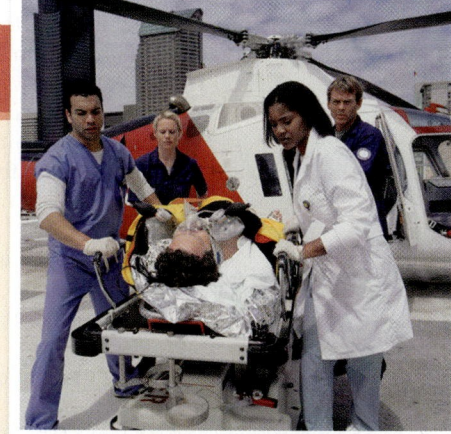

8. Perform manual reduction of rectal prolapse.

Which interventions should the nurse choose? Which can he eliminate, based on the information provided? You may not yet have enough nursing knowledge to be sure about your answers to these questions, but before you read on, try to think it through with the information and life experience available to you.

Mr. Ivanos's nurse eliminated interventions 1, 3, 4, 7, and 8. Take a few moments to see whether you can explain the nurse's reasons for deleting these interventions.

Theoretical Knowledge
knowing why

For the interventions eliminated in the Meet Your Patient scenario, compare your explanations with the following reasons given by the nurse:

- **1**—because it is useful for patients who are constipated as a result of irregular bowel habits, whereas Mr. Ivanos's problem is caused by immobility and narcotic side effects.
- **3 and 4**—because Mr. Ivanos's symptoms did not seem severe enough to warrant an enema or manual removal of stool.
- **7**—because it is not practical: Mr. Ivanos cannot exercise in his present condition.
- **8**—because it is not relevant: Mr. Ivanos does not have rectal prolapse.

The nurse chose the following interventions to include in the care plan:

- **2**—because it directly addresses the problem, Constipation.
- **5 and 6**—because they address the etiology of the problem: Fluid and fiber soften the stool and help to stimulate bowel activity.

The nurse also reasoned that because opioid analgesics cause constipation, it would be good to administer them less frequently to Mr. Ivanos if other satisfactory pain-relief measures could be found. So he added the following to the care plan:

- Assist to change position every 1–2 hours.
- Encourage distraction (e.g., watching TV, reading).
- Assist with relaxation and visualization techniques.
- Obtain medical prescription for nonnarcotic analgesics to enhance nonpharmacological pain-relief measures.
- Assess effectiveness of nonpharmacological interventions for pain.
- Give prescribed narcotic analgesics if other measures are ineffective.

The nurse knows people are often self-conscious or embarrassed about using a bedpan, especially in the presence of others. So he also added the following to the care plan:

- Encourage Mr. Ivanos to summon the nurse when he feels the urge to defecate (place call light within reach). If he does not, then ask at least every 4 hr whether he needs the bedpan.
- Provide privacy: Pull the bed curtain; turn on the TV or radio if he has a roommate; explain that you will leave the room and that he should call when he is ready for you to return; shut the door.

As you can see, to develop interventions to meet Mr. Ivanos's specific needs, the nurse needed to do more than just look at a list and follow physician orders. He thought critically about:

- His theoretical knowledge (of narcotics, bowel elimination, and psychological needs).
- His past experiences with similar patients.
- The patient situation (the data about Mr. Ivanos and the factors contributing to his problem).

By thinking of interventions to meet the client's specific needs, this nurse may prevent Mr. Ivanos's constipation from becoming worse.

ABOUT THE KEY CONCEPTS

As you study this chapter, try to think about how related concepts (such as theories, standardized language, and nursing orders) are linked to the key concepts of **evidence-based** practice and **nursing interventions.** This should help you understand and remember chapter material, as well as improve your ability to use your knowledge in caring for patients.

WHAT ARE NURSING INTERVENTIONS?

KEY POINT: **Nursing interventions** *are actions based on clinical judgment and nursing knowledge that nurses perform to achieve client outcomes.* This chapter uses the terms nursing *interventions, actions, measures, strategies,* and *activities* interchangeably except when referring to the Nursing Interventions Classification (NIC) standardized labels, which are always called *interventions.* The NIC is discussed later in the chapter. Figure 6-1 shows how planning interventions relates to the other phases of the nursing process. Nursing interventions include a broad range of activities:

- **Direct-care interventions** are performed through interaction with the client(s) (e.g., physical care, emotional support, and patient teaching).
- **Indirect-care interventions** are performed away from the client but on behalf of a client or group of clients e.g., (advocacy, managing the environment, consulting with other members of the healthcare team, and making referrals).

ThinkLike a Nurse 6-1

- Can you think of an example of a direct-care intervention?
- Can you think of an example of an indirect-care intervention?

Nurses work collaboratively with other healthcare providers. Interventions may be independent, dependent, or interdependent (collaborative).

Independent Interventions *Nurse A makes a nursing diagnosis of Anxiety related to deficient knowledge about barium enema; she writes a nursing order to teach the patient what to expect from the upcoming diagnostic test.*

- This is an **independent intervention**—one that registered nurses (RNs) are **accountable** for and are licensed to prescribe, perform, or delegate based on their knowledge and skills.
- It does not require a provider's order.
- Knowing how, when, and why to perform an activity makes the action **autonomous** (independent).
- Nurses prescribe and perform independent interventions in response to a nursing diagnosis. **KEY POINT:** *As a nurse, you are* **accountable** *(answerable) for your decisions and actions with regard to nursing diagnoses and independent interventions.*

Dependent Interventions *Nurse B reads a prescription in a patient's chart: "Give cephalothin sodium (Keflin) 1 g IV [through the intravenous line] before surgery, and then every 6 hours for 24 hours." She prepares and administers the medication.*

- This is a **dependent intervention**—one that is prescribed by a physician or advanced practice nurse but carried out by the nurse.
- Dependent interventions are usually prescriptions for diagnostic tests, medications, treatments, IV therapy, diet, and activity.
- In addition to carrying out medical prescriptions, you will be responsible for assessing the need for the prescription, explaining the activities to the patient, and evaluating the effectiveness of the prescription.

> *Example:* After giving the Keflin (an antibiotic), Nurse B observes that the patient has developed a rash. Suspecting an allergic reaction, she contacts the prescriber so that the medication can be changed.

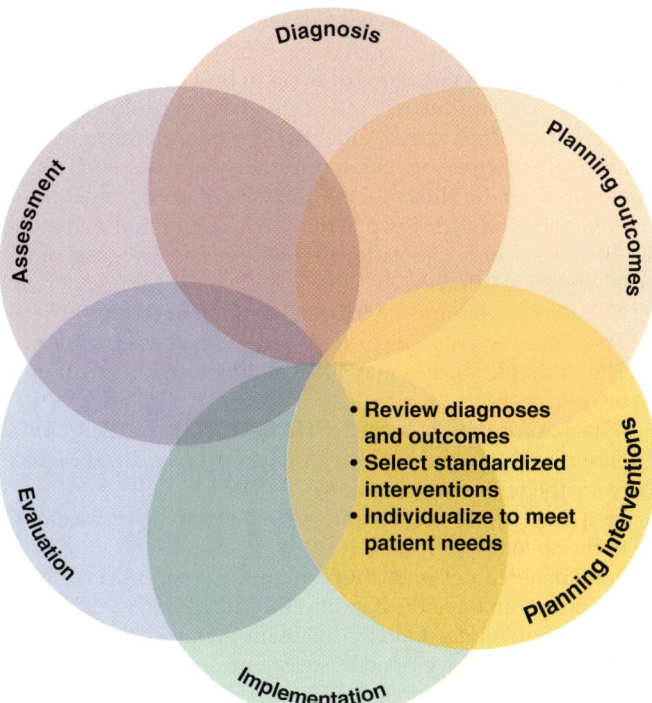

FIGURE 6-1   Nursing process phase: planning interventions.

Interdependent (Collaborative) Interventions   *Nurse C notes that a client newly diagnosed with diabetes has been seen by a dietitian, who taught and provided materials about a diabetic diet. The nurse observes the client's menu choices. She notes that the client is eating candy brought by visitors. She explains to the client how concentrated sugar affects his diabetes; she also communicates her assessments and teaching to the dietitian.*

- This is an **interdependent (collaborative) intervention—** one that is carried out in collaboration with other health team members (e.g., physical therapists, physicians).

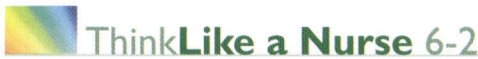 **ThinkLike a Nurse 6-2**

- What are some other examples of independent interventions?
- What are some other examples of dependent interventions?
- What are some other examples of interdependent interventions?

HOW DO I DECIDE WHICH INTERVENTIONS TO USE?

In addition to the ANA standards, a variety of theories, nursing research, and the client's problem status will all influence your choice of interventions.

American Nurses Association (ANA) Standards

To review ANA (2015a) standards of care related to planning interventions, refer to Box 5-1, Standard 4 in Chapter 5. Use the ANA standards to guide you in selecting interventions appropriate for the client's nursing diagnoses, collaborative problems, and desired outcomes.

   KEY POINT: *As a nurse, you will be responsible for choosing nursing interventions. You cannot delegate this responsibility to nursing assistive personnel.* As a rule, licensed practical/ vocational nurses (LPN/LVNs) give care according to a plan

created by the RN. The LPN/LVN contributes to the plan by providing data or by giving feedback about the effectiveness of the interventions. For more information about delegation, see Chapter 7.

How Do Theories Influence My Choice of Interventions?

A **theory** is a set of interrelated concepts (ideas) that describes or explains something—nursing, for example. Like a lens, a theory influences your perspective: what you notice, what you consider to be a problem, and how you define a problem— which in turn, more or less determines what you choose to do about the problem. For example, suppose a patient is pale and fidgeting and has sweaty palms and a rapid pulse.

- If you look at this person through the lens of *psychology* theory, your first thought might be that the patient is anxious. Your first intervention would probably be to assess for the cause of his anxiety.
- If you use a *physiology* lens, you might suspect pain. In that case, your first intervention might be to ask the patient whether he is having pain.

   To understand more about nursing theories, see Chapter 8.

How Does Nursing Research Influence My Choice of Interventions?

Although much nursing and medical practice is based on tradition, experience, and professional opinion, this is not an ideal basis for choosing an intervention. Ideally, a nurse should choose an intervention because of firm evidence that it is the best possible approach for the patient. Such interventions would be those that were developed from a sound body of scientific research.

   American Nurses Association (ANA) Standard 13 Regarding evidence, Standard 13 of the ANA Standards of Nursing Practice (ANA, 2015a, p. 77) states that the registered nurse:

- Uses current evidence-based nursing knowledge, including research findings, to guide practice.
- Incorporates evidence when initiating changes in nursing practice.
- Participates in the formation of evidence-based practice through research.
- Shares peer-reviewed research findings with colleagues to integrate knowledge into nursing practice.

   To see whether you have the most current ANA standards,

 Go to http://nursingworld.org/MainMenuCategories/ ThePracticeofProfessionalNursing/NursingStandards.aspxl

   Institute of Medicine (IOM) The purpose of the IOM core competencies is to employ evidence-based practice. This includes integrating clinical expertise with knowledge of current research (Greiner & Knebel, 2003). See the SENC box What Is Safe, Effective Nursing Care? in Chapter 1.

   SENC Competencies The Safe, Effective Nursing Care (SENC) competencies used in this text are similar to the IOM competencies. They require that the nurse:

- Validate evidence-based research to incorporate it into client care.
- Evaluate client outcomes using evidence-based research tools.

   See the Chapter 1 SENC box cited above to help you identify and bridge gaps between what is and what should be and to focus your work through the lens of quality and safety.

QSEN Competencies The Quality and Safety Education for Nurses (QSEN) competencies state that when you graduate from your nursing program, you should be able to differentiate clinical opinion from research and evidence summaries (Cronenwett, 2002; Cronenwett, Sherwood, Barnesteiner, et al., 2007).

What Is Evidence-Based Practice?

Evidence-based practice (EBP) is an approach that uses firm scientific data rather than anecdote, tradition, intuition, or folklore in making decisions about medical and nursing practice. In nursing, it includes blending clinical judgment and expertise, the best available research evidence, patient characteristics, and patient preferences. **KEY POINT:** *The goal of evidence-based practice is to identify the most effective and cost-efficient treatments for a particular disease, condition, or problem.* Steps in the EBP process include the following:

1. Formulating an answerable question about prevention, diagnosis, prognosis (likely outcome), and interventions. In Chapter 8, you will learn how to write a PICOT question to help you do this.
2. Conducting a systematic review of published evidence (research) to find studies that shed light on the desired topic.
3. Evaluating or grading the quality of the evidence obtained. Quality involves:
   - *Validity* (closeness to the truth),
   - *Applicability* (usefulness), and
   - *Impact* (extent of the effect).
   Figure 6-2 lists evidence from strongest to weakest.
4. Compiling and analyzing the data to prepare a structured report of the review.
5. Translating the evidence into guidelines for practice.
6. Integrating the guidelines and evidence with clinical expertise and the patient's preferences and characteristics.

A number of healthcare organizations and groups are devoted to compiling study results that provide evidence to use in formulating guidelines for medical and nursing practice. Online examples include the Joanna Briggs Institute and the Cochrane Database of Systematic Reviews. You will find such compiled information in clinical practice guidelines, evidence reports, and sometimes in local healthcare agency tools (e.g., clinical pathways and protocols). For more discussion on the importance of research and evidence-based nursing practice, see Chapter 8.

Types of Research-Based Support

Research-based support for an intervention includes single studies, critical pathways and protocols, clinical practice guidelines, systematic reviews of the literature, and evidence reports.

Single Studies It is not difficult to find individual studies that give you an idea of the effectiveness of an intervention. Research reports are available and are often interpreted and published in widely circulated nursing journals such as the *American Journal of Nursing (AJN)*, *Nursing,* and *Nursing Research,* as well as online sites. Keep in mind that single studies may not be reliable when choosing an intervention because of the following limitations:

- Not all interventions have been included in the study.
- There may be only one or two studies of an intervention.
- The available studies may have included only a small number of patients.

Critical Pathways and Protocols (also called *clinical pathways* and *collaborative care plans*) are standardized plans of care for the following situations:

- Frequently occurring conditions (e.g., total hip replacement) in the agency
- Similar outcomes and interventions are appropriate for all patients who have the condition

You should understand the following about critical pathways:

- They are tools developed by an organization for its own use.
- They are intended to guide best practice only at the local level.
- They may not be based on research.

Critical pathways have, at the very least, been developed on the basis of expert opinion and perhaps some research, so they do provide some guidance for interventions. See Chapter 5 for additional discussion and examples of critical pathways and protocols.

Evidence Reports are systematic reviews of clinical topics for the purpose of providing evidence for practice guidelines, quality improvement, and funding decisions. Evidence reports are usually developed by scientists rather than by clinicians, patients, and advocacy groups. One source of such reports is the Evidence-Based Practice Center (EPC) Program of the federal Agency for Healthcare Research and Quality (AHRQ). The EPC uses explicit grading systems to review studies and rank the strength of their evidence. For free access to online reviews,

 Go to the AHRQ Web site at http://www.ahrq.gov/research/findings/evidence-based-reports/index.html

Clinical Practice Guidelines Evidence reports often form the basis for developing clinical practice guidelines. **Clinical practice guidelines** are systematically developed statements to assist practitioners and patients in making decisions about appropriate healthcare for a particular disease or procedure. They are typically developed by clinicians, patients, and advocacy groups and are published by specialty organizations, universities, and government agencies. They form the basis for nursing interventions. The following are examples:

- *Joanna Briggs Institute (JBI) Database of Systemic Reviews and Implementation Reports:* "Family Involvement in Decision Making for People With Dementia in Residential Aged Care" (2013)
- National Guideline Clearinghouse (NCG): "Guideline Summary: Recommendations on Screening for Cognitive Impairment in Older Adults" (2016).

For years, relying on conventional wisdom and word of mouth, nurses tried to prevent pressure injuries with the nursing order "Massage skin over bony prominences." They reasoned

- Meta-analysis of randomized clinical trials
- Individual randomized clinical trials
- Individual cohort study
- Outcomes research
- Individual case-control study
- Case studies
- Expert opinion

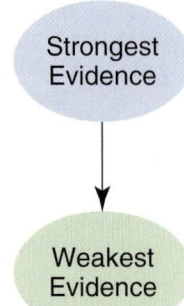

Strongest Evidence

Weakest Evidence

FIGURE 6-2 Hierarchy of research evidence.

that because poor circulation can contribute to the formation of pressure injuries, improving circulation to the area would prevent them. But as you can see in the example in Box 6-1, research-based guidelines show that massage may instead be harmful. This report would surely motivate you to remove this "standard" intervention from your practice.

KnowledgeCheck 6-1

- Explain how theory influences your choice of nursing interventions.
- Why does a clinical practice guideline provide better support for an intervention than does a single study?
- Why does a clinical practice guideline provide better support for an intervention than does an agency's critical pathway?

How Does Problem Status Influence Nursing Interventions?

Nursing interventions include activities for observation/ assessment, prevention, treatment, and health promotion. As you can see in Table 6-1, the status of the problem (i.e., whether it is a collaborative problem or an actual, potential, possible, or wellness nursing diagnosis) determines which types of activities are required (for a review of problem status, see Chapter 4).

A nursing intervention can be a preventive measure in one situation and a treatment in another. For example, you might

---

BOX 6-1 ■ Portion of a Clinical Practice Guideline on Pressure Injury Prevention

Note: This is not the complete practice guideline.

Assessment*

- Use a reliable and standardized tool for doing a risk assessment, such as the Braden Scale.
- Document risk assessment on admission to a facility and whenever the client's condition changes and based on patient care setting (e.g., acute care, every 24–48 hr)

Nursing Care Strategies and Interventions

- Keep patients off the reddened areas of skin. Repositioning schedules should be individualized. (Evidence Level I)
- Do not massage bony prominences. (Evidence Level I)
- Use pressure-reducing devices (static air, alternating air, gel, water mattresses). (Evidence Level II)
- Raise heels of bedbound clients off the bed; do not use donut-type devices. (Evidence Level III)
- Avoid hot water and soaps that are drying when bathing the elderly. Use body wash and skin protectant. (Evidence Level III)

---

*"Strength of evidence" is an AHRQ ranking (I to VI) of the amount and quality of research supporting the guideline. The best ranking is I.

Source: Agency for Healthcare Research and Quality (AHRQ), National Guideline Clearinghouse. (2003; updated 2012). Guideline summary. Pressure ulcer prevention. In *Evidence-based geriatric nursing protocols for best practice*. Retrieved from https://www.guideline.gov/content.aspx?id=43935-Section427

---

write the nursing order "Teach the importance of adequate fluids" to treat a patient with an actual diagnosis of Constipation or to help prevent the problem for a patient with a diagnosis of Risk for Constipation.

KnowledgeCheck 6-2

Review problem status (actual, potential, or possible nursing diagnosis; collaborative problem; or wellness diagnosis) in Chapter 4. For which type(s) of problem(s) would you write:

- Nursing orders for observation/assessments?
- Nursing orders for treatments?
- Nursing orders for health promotion interventions?
- Preventive nursing orders?

What Process Can I Use for Generating and Selecting Interventions?

As you can see from the case of Ben Ivanos (Meet Your Patient), several nursing measures might be effective for any one problem. The idea, of course, is to select those most likely to achieve the desired goals. Generating interventions requires you to use critical thinking. Consider the following example:

Example: You are caring for a hospice patient who has cancer and is dying. She has told you that she is experiencing significant pain, but also that she wants to spend her last hours with her husband and two daughters, who are staying with her.

Thinking critically about the hospice patient, you might reason as follows:

- "What did I learn in psychology class that might help me here?" (*Making interdisciplinary connections*)
- "If I give morphine to the patient, it should relieve her pain, but she will probably become drowsy." (*Predicting*)
- "I have used touch to relieve anxiety many times in similar situations; perhaps it will also help for this patient." (*Generalizing*)
- "Morphine does cause drowsiness, but there may be other pain relief measures that can help a bit." (*Explaining*)
- "The patient wants to spend quality time with her family before she dies. Because the morphine makes her drowsy, I should find out whether she wants me to give a smaller dose, perhaps along with some nonpharmacological comfort measures." (*Therapeutic judgment*)

A full-spectrum nurse takes such details into account before choosing an intervention. The sections that follow describe a process that will help you to select the best interventions (Wilkinson, 2012).

1. Review the Nursing Diagnosis

Choose strategies you expect will reduce or remove the etiological factors that contribute to actual problems (unhealthy responses) or that will reduce or remove risk factors for potential problems.

- **When it is not possible to change the etiology,** choose strategies to treat the patient's symptoms (the AMB part of a diagnosis, referred to in Chapter 4). For example, if the cause of pain is a surgical incision, you cannot "cure" the incision. Your nursing actions should focus on measures to relieve the pain.
- **When you do not know the etiology of the problem.** Some interventions may relieve a problem regardless of its cause. For example:

  When a client is anxious, it is helpful to approach him calmly regardless of the cause.

Table 6-1 ➤ Relationship of Problem Status to Intervention Type

PROBLEM STATUS	OBSERVATION	PREVENTION	TREATMENT	HEALTH PROMOTION
		Intervention Type		
Actual nursing diagnosis	To detect change in status (improvement, exacerbation of problem)	To help keep the problem from becoming worse	To relieve symptoms and resolve etiologies (contributing factors)	
Potential (risk) nursing diagnosis	To detect (1) progression to an actual problem or (2) an increase or decrease in risk factors	To remove or reduce risk factors in an effort to keep the problem from developing		
Possible nursing diagnosis	To obtain more data to confirm or rule out a suspected nursing diagnosis			
Collaborative problem	To detect onset of a complication for early physician notification	To implement nursing and medical orders to help prevent development of a complication	To implement nursing and medical orders for relieving or eliminating the underlying condition for which complications may develop	
Wellness diagnosis	To assess a client's wellness practices	To prevent specific diseases (e.g., giving immunizations)	Clients usually manage their own wellness treatment	To support a client's health promotion efforts and achieve a higher level of wellness

When a client has Constipation, it is always appropriate to assess the characteristics of the stool, regardless of the cause. Consider the nursing diagnosis and interventions for Mr. Ivanos in Figure 6-3.

Obviously, some people with constipation do not have pain. The pain-relief nursing order, which flows from the etiology of the problem, is specific to Mr. Ivanos's needs. Administering a stool softener and laxative, however, is a common strategy for constipation, whatever its cause. **KEY POINT:** *As a rule, standardized interventions (care common to all patients with a particular condition) flow from the problem side of a nursing diagnosis; individualized interventions, from the etiology.*

ThinkLike a Nurse 6-3

For the following nursing diagnoses, write one intervention to address the problem and one for the etiology of the problem:

- Ineffective Airway Clearance r/t thick secretions and decreased chest expansion secondary to dehydration and pain
- Self-Care Deficit: Bathing/Hygiene and Dressing/Grooming r/t fatigue secondary to disturbed sleep pattern

2. Review the Desired Patient Outcomes

Desired outcomes (goals) suggest nursing strategies that are specific to the individual patient. For example, Table 6-2 shows some goals and outcomes for Mr. Ivanos's Constipation diagnosis. For each goal on the care plan, column 3 answers the question "What intervention(s) will help to produce this patient response?" As you can see, there may be one or more interventions for each goal, and a single intervention may help to achieve more than one goal.

3. Identify Several Interventions or Actions

The next step is to think of several nursing activities that might achieve the desired outcomes. Don't try to narrow your list at this point; include unusual and creative ideas. To get started, ask yourself: For this nursing diagnosis, (1) What assessments/observations do I need to make? and (2) What do I need to do for the patient? Include both dependent and independent activities as appropriate.

You can refer to a standardized list of interventions (e.g., the NIC list on Davis Advantage) or choose interventions from standardized care plans and agency protocols. Alternatively, you can generate the interventions yourself based on your knowledge, experience, and use of nursing texts, journal articles, practice guidelines, and professional nurses.

4. Choose the Best Interventions for the Patient

The best interventions are those you expect to be most effective in helping to achieve client goals. When possible, choose interventions based on research and scientific principles. Use the following critical-thinking questions from the full-spectrum nursing model (in Chapter 2) to help you determine the best actions.

Contextual Awareness

- Is this intervention acceptable to the client (e.g., congruent with the patient's culture, values, and wishes)?
- Is this intervention culturally sensitive?
- What is going on in the patient's life (e.g., family, work) and health status (e.g., knowledge, abilities, resources, severity of illness) that could affect the success of the intervention?

Credible Sources

- Have I used valid, reliable sources of information to identify this intervention (e.g., patient, other professionals, best practice resources)?
- Did I consider professional, ethical, and legal standards?
- What is the research basis for this intervention, if any?

Considering Alternatives

- Is there adequate rationale for this intervention (e.g., principles, theory, facts)?
- Which action(s) is (are) most likely to achieve stated goals?

Analyzing Assumptions

- What beliefs, values, or biases do I have that may affect my thinking and choices?
- Do I feel any discomfort with this intervention?

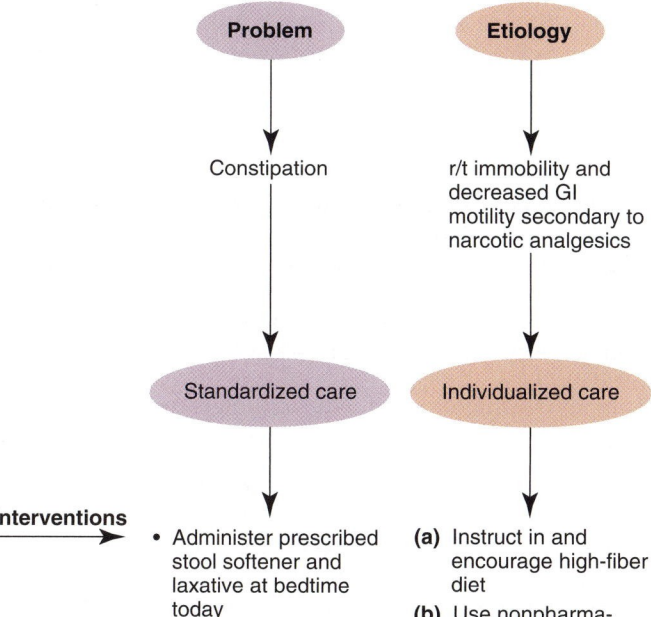

FIGURE 6-3 Nursing interventions flow from the nursing diagnosis.

Table 6-2 ➤ Interventions Flow From Desired Outcomes

1. **Will have bowel movement within 12 hours after receiving stool softener and laxative.**	A. **Administer prescribed stool softener and laxative at bedtime today.**
2. Will have daily soft, formed bowel movement during rest of hospital stay.	B. Instruct in and encourage high-fiber diet.
	C. Encourage increased fluid intake.
3. <u>Within 24 hours, will need narcotics to manage pain <2×/day.</u>	D. <u>Use nonpharmacological measures (e.g., distraction) to minimize need for narcotics.</u>
4. *Calls nurse when urge to defecate is felt; does not delay defecation.*	E. *Encourage Mr. Ivanos to summon the nurse when he feels the urge to defecate.*
	F. *Provide privacy (e.g., pull the bed curtain, turn on the TV, leave room).*

Discussion:

- Strategy A would help to achieve goal 1; but because the effects of these medications are short lived, it would do nothing to achieve goals 2 through 4.
- Strategies B and C both help to achieve goal 2.
- Strategy D (minimize narcotics), in contrast, directly addresses goal 3 and indirectly helps to achieve goal 2.
- Strategies E and F both directly address goal 4 and indirectly address goal 2.

Note: Dotted lines indicate indirect contribution to goal.

Reflecting Skeptically

- Are there other interventions I have overlooked?
- What might be the consequences of this intervention? Does it have any potential ill effects? If so, how will we manage them?
- Is this intervention feasible? For example, is it cost effective; can the patient or family manage it at home?
- How will the intervention interact with medical orders? For example, you cannot order "elevate head of bed" to facilitate breathing if there is a medical order to keep the patient flat.
- Do I have the knowledge and skills needed for the intervention, or do I need to consult with someone more qualified in this area?
- In priority order, what should I do in this situation and why?

5. Individualize Standardized Interventions

Practice guidelines, protocols, critical pathways, and even textbooks describe interventions that are appropriate for most people. However, they cannot take into account all the factors that contribute to a problem or that might affect the effectiveness of

Toward Evidence-Based Practice

Eilers, J., Harris, D., Henry, K., et al. (2015). Evidence-based interventions for cancer treatment–related mucositis: Putting evidence into practice. *Clinical Journal of Oncology Nursing, 18*(6), 80–96.

This article reviews evidence-based interventions for mucositis arising out of a large number of research studies and provides guidelines for nursing assessment and prevention interventions.

Mucositis is an inflammatory process of the membranous tissue lining the digestive tract. It is often associated with therapies prescribed for cancer-related effects such as nausea and vomiting and decreased neutrophils (a type of white blood cell). Mucositis increases the risk of bleeding and systemic infections caused by the breakdown of the protective mucosal barrier. Oral mucositis causes pain and changes in function (such as difficulty speaking and swallowing), necessitates restricted oral intake, and often results in the interruption of treatment.

Among the nursing and collaborative protocols for oral care deemed likely to be effective are the following:

- **Routine assessment and reporting** of changes in mouth (e.g., pain with swallowing, changes in the color or integrity of oral surfaces).

- **Consistent and frequent oral hygiene** (e.g., brushing and flossing twice a day, using alcohol-free mouthwashes).
- **Preventive and comfort-promoting interventions.** Sodium bicarbonate mouth rinses and topical cold applications (e.g., ice chips or lollipops) during chemotherapy infusions can promote comfort/reduce pain if ulceration is present.
- **Collaborative interventions** may include use of lactobacillus lozenges for comfort, or prophylactic chlorhexidine mouth rinses to reduce incidences of mucositis.
- **Patient teaching and self-management.**

This study also includes interventions for the treatment of mucositis (e.g., sucralfate), which were previously but no longer recommended.

1. Why is it important for a patient with mucositis to use alcohol-free mouthwash?

2. Why would you expect chlorhexidine mouth rinses to reduce mucositis?

3. When and what would you teach a person or caregiver about mucositis?

 Go to Davis Advantage, Resources, Chapter 6, **Toward Evidence-Based Practice—Suggested Responses.**

---

an intervention. You must always consider how an intervention can be used with a particular person. For example, after Ben Ivanos's nurse decided which of the computer-generated list of interventions to use, he adapted them to fit Ben's unique needs and preferences. **KEY POINT:** *Each person has unique needs and responds in unique ways.* Table 6-3 provides examples of standardized and individualized interventions for Mr. Ivanos.

KnowledgeCheck 6-3

Describe a five-step process for generating and choosing nursing interventions.

Computer-Generated Interventions

Most electronic care planning programs will generate a list of suggested interventions when you enter either a problem (nursing diagnosis, medical, collaborative) or an outcome (Fig. 6-4). You then choose the interventions appropriate for the patient (as in the case of Ben Ivanos) or type in nursing actions of your own. Computer prompts provide a wide range of interventions for your consideration. However, always look for other, perhaps more effective, strategies based on the patient data.

HOW CAN I USE STANDARDIZED LANGUAGE TO PLAN INTERVENTIONS?

As a review before reading this section, you may wish to read the discussion of standardized language in Chapter 4 (NANDA-I for nursing diagnoses) and in Chapter 5 (NOC for patient outcomes).

Recall that standardized nursing terminologies are important for electronic health records (EHR), for research, and for clear, precise, consistent communication among nurses and with other disciplines. The ANA (Sewall & Thede, 2012; Thede & Schwirian, 2013) recognizes 12 standardized vocabularies for recording and tracking the clinical care process. Those most commonly used for describing nursing interventions are the Nursing Interventions Classification (NIC), the Clinical Care Classification (CCC), and the Omaha System. NIC classifies only interventions; the CCC and the Omaha System also include nursing diagnoses and outcomes.

There is evidence reporting the successful integration and use in electronic health records for at least two standardized nursing terminology *sets* which contain terminology for nursing diagnoses, outcomes, and interventions (Tastan, Lunch, Keenan, et al., 2014).
1. NANDA-International, Nursing Interventions Classification, and Nursing Outcome Classification set (NANDA-I, NIC, NOC)
2. The Omaha System set

What Is the Nursing Interventions Classification?

Developed by a research team at the University of Iowa, the Nursing Interventions Classification (NIC) was the first comprehensive standardized classification of nursing interventions (McCloskey & Bulechek, 1992). The NIC (Bulechek, Butcher, & Dochterman, 2013) describes more than 500 direct- and indirect-care activities performed by nurses. The NIC (pronounced "nick") is versatile—appropriate for use in all

Table 6-3 ➤ Individualizing Nursing Actions for Ben Ivanos

STANDARDIZED INTERVENTIONS	INDIVIDUALIZED NURSING ORDERS
1. Encourage increased fluid intake.	1. Remind patient to drink a glass of water every hr; also keep ice and tea available at the bedside.
2. Instruct on and encourage a high-fiber diet.	2. Assist with menu choices to obtain more fiber; encourage family to bring fiber-rich crackers or bars, nuts, and fruits (e.g., pears, figs, prunes) from home for snacks.
3. Encourage distraction (e.g., watching TV, reading, listening to music).	3. Provide books from hospital library (he does not enjoy many TV programs); have family bring handheld electronics and headphones from home.
4. Give prescribed narcotic analgesics if other measures are ineffective.	4. Give prescribed oral narcotic every 4 hr if relaxation, visualization, and distraction are not effective. If orally administered analgesic is not effective, advise patient to administer IV morphine via patient-controlled analgesia pump.

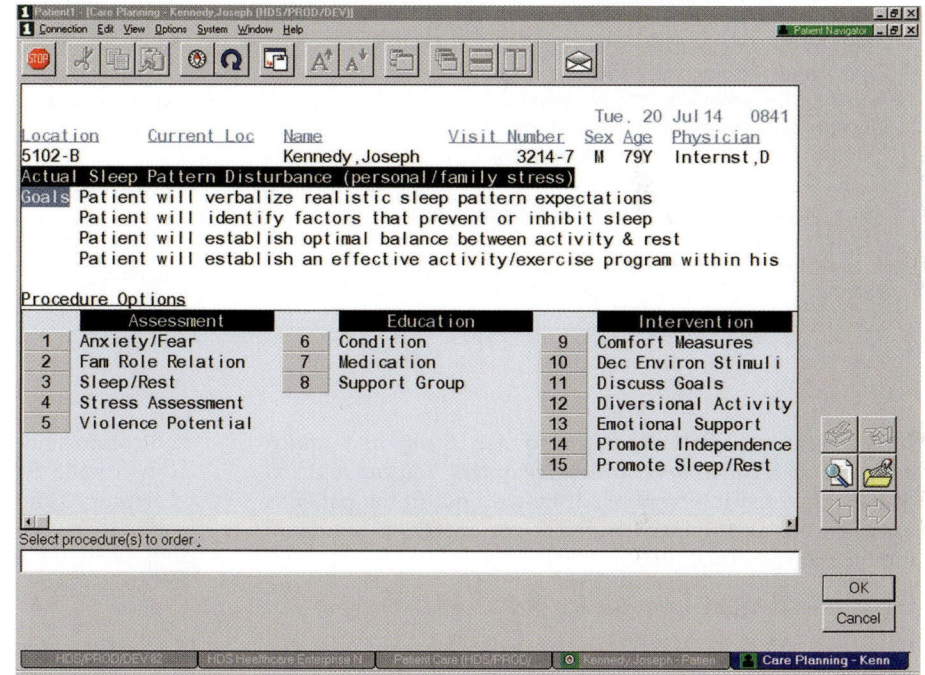

FIGURE 6-4 Computer care planning: When the nurse selects a nursing diagnosis of Sleep Pattern Disturbance, the computer database generates a list of suggested goals and "procedure options" (interventions); the nurse then chooses those best suited for the patient.

specialty and practice areas, including home health and community nursing.

Each NIC intervention consists of a label, a definition, and a list of the specific **activities** nurses perform in carrying out the intervention (Box 6-2). The **label,** usually consisting of two or three words, is the standardized terminology. The **definition** explains the meaning of the label. You are free to word the activities any way you choose in a care plan or client record. For a complete list of NIC intervention labels and definitions,

 Go to **NIC Interventions** on Davis Advantage.

Locating Appropriate NIC Interventions and Activities

NIC interventions are linked to NANDA-I nursing diagnoses and NOC outcome labels in a "linkages" book, *NOC and NIC Linkages to NANDA-I and Clinical Conditions,* referred to by most nurses as the NNN linkages book (Johnson, Moorhead, Bulechek, et al., 2012). In this book, you can look up a nursing diagnosis to see the list of outcomes suggested for it and the interventions for achieving each outcome. Refer to Box 6-3 for an example of interventions linked to the nursing diagnosis Risk for Aspiration.

Once you have chosen the interventions (based on your knowledge and judgment), you then choose the appropriate activities to carry out the intervention. As you might guess from looking at Box 6-2, you will probably never need to perform all of the activities for a client. Choose the best ones to fit the situation, the client, and the resources (e.g., supplies, equipment).

Using NIC in Electronic Care Plans

Standardized language is especially useful in computerized care systems. For any NIC intervention, the program will also list the more specific nursing activities, which you can individualize as nursing orders. **KEY POINT:** *Remember that you, not the computer, are responsible for choosing which interventions*

BOX 6-2 ■ NIC Intervention: Bathing

Definition

Cleaning of the body for the purposes of relaxation, cleanliness, and healing

Activities

Assist with chair shower, tub bath, bedside bath, standing shower, or sitz bath, as appropriate or desired.

Wash hair, as needed and desired.

Bathe in water of a comfortable temperature.

Use fun bathing techniques with children (e.g., wash dolls or toys; pretend a boat is a submarine; punch holes in bottom of plastic cup, fill with water, and let it "rain" on child).

Assist with perineal care, as needed.

Assist with hygiene measures (e.g., use of deodorant or perfume).

Administer foot soaks, as needed.

Shave patient, as indicated.

Apply lubricating ointment and cream to dry skin areas.

Offer hand washing after toileting and before meals.

Apply drying powders to deep skin folds.

Monitor skin condition while bathing.

Monitor functional ability while bathing.

Source: Bulechek, B. M., Butcher, H. K., & Dochterman, J. M. (Eds.). (2013). *Nursing interventions classification (NIC)* (6th ed., p. 91). St. Louis, MO: C.V. Mosby. Used with permission from Elsevier Science.

BOX 6-3 ■ NIC Interventions Linked to NANDA-I Diagnosis, Risk for Aspiration

Aspiration, Risk for

Vulnerable to entry of gastrointestinal secretions, oropharyngeal secretions, solids or fluids, into tracheobronchial passages, which may compromise health.

NICs Associated With Prevention of Aspiration

Airway Management	Medication Administration:
Airway Suctioning	Oral
Artificial Airway	Neurological Monitoring
Management	Positioning
Aspiration Precautions	Postanesthesia Care
Chest Physiotherapy	Respiratory Monitoring
Cough Enhancement	Resuscitation: Neonate
Dementia Management	Risk Identification
Enteral Tube Feeding	Sedation Management
Gastrointestinal	Self-Care Assistance
Intubation	Surveillance
Mechanical Ventilation	Swallowing Therapy
Management: Invasive	Tube Care: Gastrointestinal
Medication Administration:	Vomiting Management
Enteral	

Source: Johnson, M., Moorhead, S., Bulechek, G., et al. (2012). *NOC and NIC linkages to NANDA-I and clinical conditions* (3rd ed. p. 250). St. Louis, MO: C.V. Mosby. Used with permission from Elsevier Science.

to use for each patient, when to use them, and which activities to write as specific nursing orders. You can reject *all* of the suggested interventions if they do not fit the patient's unique needs and, in many systems, type or write in your own interventions and activities.

Standardized Languages for Home Health and Community Care

The NIC includes interventions applicable in all settings, including home health and community nursing. However, the following taxonomies were created specifically for community-based practice:

■ **The Clinical Care Classification (CCC),** previously called the *Home Healthcare Classification,* was developed for use in home healthcare (*Clinical Care Classification (CCC) System,* 2012; Saba, 1995). In addition to terminology for nursing diagnoses and outcomes, the CCC (Version 2.5) has more than 800 nursing interventions. For a complete description of the CCC system, see the nursing process section of Chapter 42 and

 Go to the CCC Web site at http://www.sabacare.com/

■ **The Omaha System** was developed for community health nurses to use in caring for individuals, families, and **aggregates** (community groups or entire communities) (Martin, 2005). In its present form, it is designed to communicate multidisciplinary practice for a broad spectrum of patients and levels of health. It includes terminology for diagnoses,

outcomes, and interventions. For a complete description of the Omaha System, see the nursing process section of Chapter 42 and

 Go to the Omaha System Web site at http://www.omahasystem.org/

KnowledgeCheck 6-4

■ Name and describe three standardized intervention vocabularies recognized by the ANA.

■ In the NIC system, what is the difference between interventions and activities?

Does Standardized Language Interfere With Holistic Care?

Some nurses have criticized standardized terminologies for focusing on illness and physical interventions. However, NIC, Omaha, and CCC do include interventions to address health promotion and cultural and spiritual needs. Using a common language should help rather than hinder your choice of interventions and make clear in health records that holistic techniques are appropriate as nursing interventions. For further discussion of holistic nursing care,

 Go to **Bonus Chapter 46, Holistic Healing,** in your Davis Digital Version of the textbook.

The sections that follow discuss interventions focused on wellness, spiritual needs, and culturally sensitive care.

Wellness Interventions When you are caring for a healthy client, the client is the primary decision maker. You will function mainly as a teacher and health counselor. Frequently, the nursing orders outline lifestyle modification or behavior changes the client wants to make, along with self-rewards to reinforce the behaviors. For example,

Specific behavior change: I will consume fewer than 1,400 calories per day for the next week.

Self-reward: I will reward myself with an evening out to hear my favorite band.

The NIC contains most of the wellness interventions you will need. However, they are not all grouped together in one class. Some examples are Decision-Making Support, Exercise Promotion, and Health Screening. For more information on using standardized languages to describe wellness interventions, see Chapter 27.

Spiritual Care Interventions NIC, CCC, and the Omaha System all include terminology to describe spiritual interventions. The following are just a few examples:

NIC: Spiritual Growth Facilitation, Religious Ritual Enhancement
CCC: Spiritual Care, Coping Skills
Omaha: Spiritual Support, Bereavement Support

Chapter 16 provides full discussion of standardized nursing interventions to address spiritual needs. As you will see, you could also use most of those interventions (e.g., Coping Skills) for other than spiritual problems.

Culturally Sensitive Care Except for the NIC Culture Brokerage intervention, there are no standardized interventions that are unique to culturally based needs. All standardized interventions will result in culturally sensitive care if they are delivered by a culturally competent nurse.

PracticalKnowledge
knowing **how**

WHAT ARE NURSING ORDERS, AND HOW DO I WRITE THEM?

Nursing orders are instructions that describe how and when nursing interventions are to be implemented. They are usually written on a nursing care plan. Other nurses and nursing assistive personnel (NAP) are responsible and accountable for implementing nursing orders.

ThinkLike a Nurse 6-4

Suppose you are caring for a patient 24 hours after a major surgery. You see the following order on the nursing care plan: Ambulate 24 hours postoperatively.
- When you care for the patient, how will you go about implementing this nursing order?
- What else do you need to know to effectively carry out this order?

Components of a Nursing Order

Did you have trouble answering the preceding questions? Even experienced nurses would, because the nursing order is incomplete. As you see from this example, nursing orders must be specific and detailed because many caregivers will use the care plan, and they all need to be able to interpret the orders correctly. A well-written nursing order, whether on paper or as an electronic care plan, contains the following components:

- **Date.** Indicate the date the order was written. Change the date each time you review or revise the order. Why do you think it is important to have the date?
- **Subject.** Nursing orders are instructions to nurses, so they are written in terms of *nurse* behaviors. It is understood that the subject of the order is "the nurse." Therefore, you do not actually need to write "the nurse" in your orders. For each order, think, but do not write, "The nurse will . . ." or "The nurse should . . ." This will help you to state the order properly so that it doesn't sound like a goal statement. **KEY POINT:** *Goals state* patient *behaviors; nursing orders state* nurse *behaviors.* For example:

Goal/expected Outcome	Nursing Order
[Patient] Drinks 100 mL fluid	[Nurse will] Offer 100 mL fluids (water or juice) per hour on the day shift

- **Action Verb.** This tells the nurse what action to take—what to do. Examples of action verbs are *assist, assess, auscultate, bathe, change, demonstrate, explain, give, teach,* and *turn.* The following nursing orders show the action verbs in italics:

  Teach the components of a healthy diet, 9/13, day shift.
  Offer 100 mL water every hour.
  Administer acetaminophen 500 mg orally at least 30 min before dressing change.

- **Times and Limits.** State when (e.g., which shift, what day), how often, and how long the activity is to be done. Consider the unit routines (e.g., visiting hours, mealtimes), the patient's usual rest times, scheduled tests and procedures (e.g., x-ray studies), and treatments (e.g., physical therapy). Specify exact times when needed. The following nursing orders show times and limits:

  Teach the components of a healthy diet *on 9/13, day shift.*
  Offer 100 mL water *every hour between 0700 and 1900.*
  Administer acetaminophen 500 mg orally *at least 30 min before dressing change.*

- **Signature.** The nurse who writes the order should sign it. A signature indicates that you accept legal and ethical accountability for your orders and allows others to know whom to contact if they have questions or comments. An electronic care plan may not require an actual signature. However, the name of the nurse who entered the intervention should be indicated in some manner.

KnowledgeCheck 6-5

List the five components of a nursing order.

Reflecting Critically About Nursing Orders

After writing the nursing orders, reflect on the interventions you have chosen. If you followed the process in the section What Process Can I Use for Generating and Selecting Interventions? you will already have thought critically and made some considered decisions as you were choosing the interventions and activities. The following are questions to guide your final judgments about the plan of care:

1. *Is the set of orders complete?* That is, do they address all aspects of the problem?
   - Do they address the etiology of the problem?

- If the etiology cannot be changed, do the orders focus on the symptoms of the problem?
- Have I considered physical, emotional, interpersonal, spiritual, and cultural needs?

2. *Is each order technically complete?* That is, does it contain all the required components?

3. *Are the orders clear, specific, and precise?* If you have included all the required components, the orders will usually provide specific enough directions (when, how often, etc.) to be useful to other nurses. Did you avoid vague language? Ask yourself, "Would all nurses interpret this order in the same way? Would they all do the same thing after reading it?"

   Example: An order to "Offer emotional support" is too general to offer direction for care. One nurse might think this means to ask the client about his family, another might sit quietly with the patient, and still another might use a therapeutic statement such as, "This must be difficult for you."

4. *Is the order individualized for this particular patient?* For example, even if you have written an order to "Offer 100 mL fluids every hr," it is better if you also make a note of the kinds of fluids the patient likes or can tolerate

5. *Are the orders concise?* Long, complex statements may be unclear. Keep the orders as brief as possible without sacrificing clarity and specificity

   Example: If the patient requires complex procedures (e.g., insertion of a urinary catheter), don't write the details of the procedure on the care plan. In some instances, you may want to write a remark such as "Refer to unit protocol." You will, however, need to write in the care plan any modifications to a procedure (e.g., "Do not use alcohol; client's skin is very dry").

6. *Which orders have priority?* Which nursing orders must be implemented immediately or at least as soon as possible? If you can, write them in priority order. In Chapter 4, you learned about frameworks for prioritizing nursing diagnoses (e.g., Maslow's hierarchy, problem urgency, future consequences, and patient preference). You can use those frameworks to help you prioritize nursing orders.

If you have followed the recommended processes and reflected critically on your interventions, you should have a holistic plan of care individualized to meet the client's needs.

CLINICALREASONING

The questions and exercises in this section allow you to practice the kind of thinking you will use as a full-spectrum nurse. Critical-thinking questions usually have more than one right answer, so we do not provide "correct answers" for these features. It is more important to develop your nursing judgment than to just cover content. You will learn by discussing the questions with your peers. If you are still unsure, see the Davis Advantage chapter resources for suggested responses.

Caring for the Nguyens

Recall that you have written the following nursing diagnosis for Mr. Nguyen:

Overweight related to inappropriate food choices and serving size, as evidenced by body mass index (BMI) of 28.5.

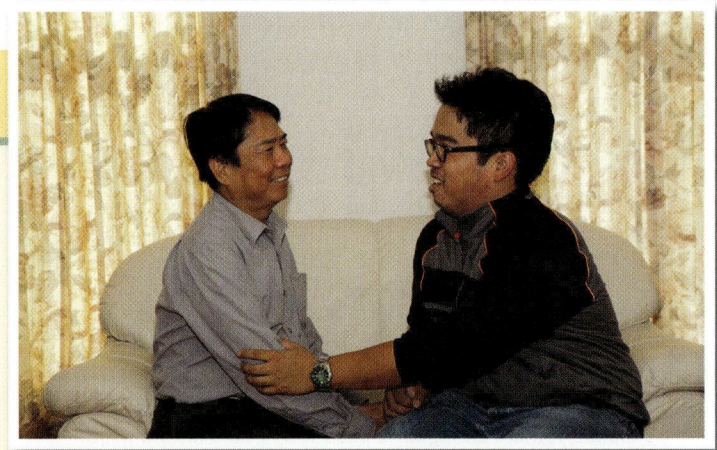

A. Based on the outcomes you wrote in Chapter 5, Planning Outcomes, identify four possible interventions to address the diagnosis and outcomes.

B. Review the interventions, and identify two that would be most appropriate for Mr. Nguyen given all of the information you have about his health status.

C. Write a nursing order for each of the two interventions you identified above.

Applying the **Full-Spectrum Nursing Model**_____

PATIENT SITUATION

Mr. Sanborn is a 65-year-old man who has come to the clinic for a complete physical checkup. He has no health complaints and his physical examination is negative except for a few minor changes associated with aging. During the interview, he tells you that he is gay, and that he has had the same partner for 5 years. On further questioning, he reveals that he has had numerous sex partners during his lifetime. He says, "I was wondering if I should be tested for HIV" and "Mike, that's my partner, says I ought to get a flu shot and maybe a hepatitis shot. What do you think?"

THINKING

1. *Theoretical Knowledge:* What principles and concepts do you need to know in order to help Mr. Sanborn today?
2. *Inquiry:* Which of those do you already know enough about, and which ones will you have to study further?

DOING

3. *Practical Knowledge:* What psychomotor and communication skills will you need in order to help Mr. Sanborn?
4. *Nursing Process (Assessment):* What further data do you need about Mr. Sanborn's sexual activity?
5. *Nursing Process (Planning Interventions):* What is one important nursing intervention for today?

CARING

6. *Self-Knowledge:* How do you feel about same-sex relationships? Would you be able to care for Mr. Sanborn effectively?
7. *Ethical Knowledge:* What does the ANA *Nursing Code of Ethics* (2015b) say about relationships to patients and the nature of patient health problems? For access to the 2015 *Nursing Code of Ethics,*

Go to http://www.nursingworld.org/MainMenuCategories/EthicsStandards/CodeofEthicsforNurses/Code-of-Ethics-For-Nurses.html

To explore learning resources for this chapter,

Go to **www.DavisAdvantage.com** and find:

Answers and suggested responses for all questions in this chapter

Lists of NIC Interventions and NOC Outcomes

List of NANDA-I Diagnoses

Knowledge Map

References and Bibliography

Concept Map

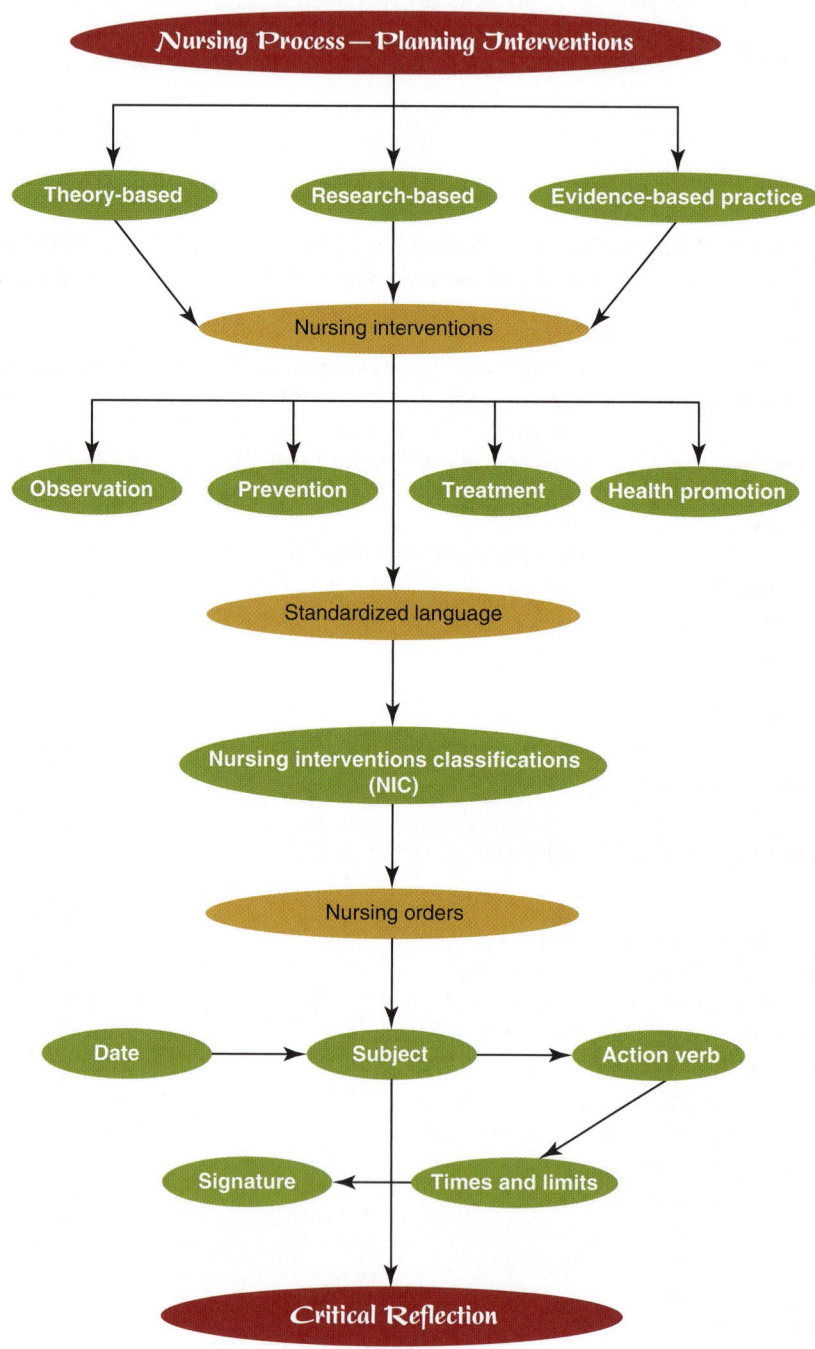

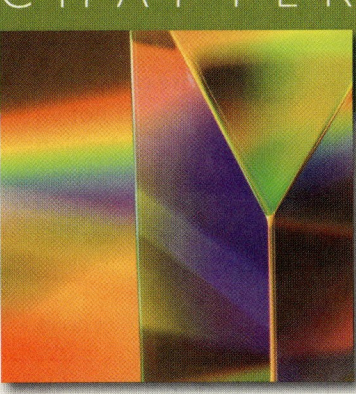

Implementation & Evaluation

Learning Outcomes

After completing this chapter, you should be able to:

➤ Define *implementation,* including a description of the three broad phases (doing, delegating, recording).

➤ Describe what nurses do in the implementation phase of the nursing process.

➤ Compare and contrast the terms *delegation* and *supervision.*

➤ Identify and describe the "five rights" of delegation.

➤ Explain how standards and criteria are used in evaluation.

➤ Explain how structure, process, and outcomes evaluation are related.

➤ Distinguish between ongoing, intermittent, and terminal evaluation.

➤ Describe a process for evaluating client health status (outcomes) after interventions.

➤ Describe a process for evaluating the effectiveness of a nursing care plan.

➤ List variables that may influence the effectiveness of a nursing intervention; state which ones the nurse can and cannot control.

➤ Discuss the importance of nurses' involvement in evaluating the quality of care in an organization.

Key Concepts

Evaluation

Implementation

Quality improvement

Related Concepts

See the Concept Map at the end of the chapter.

Meet Your Patients

Patient 1

Jeannette Wu is a very thin 80-year-old woman who is in the hospital after fracturing her hip. Her hip was surgically repaired 4 days ago, but because of her overall fragile health and some postsurgery confusion, her recovery is slower than usual. One of her nursing diagnoses is Self-Care Deficits (Bathing, Dressing, and Toileting) related to weakness, pain, alteration in cognitive functioning, and impaired mobility. Her nursing orders (NIC) include Self-Care Assistance: Bathing/Hygiene/Toileting. As the nurse is helping a nursing assistive personnel (NAP) with Mrs. Wu's bath, she notices a reddened area on Mrs. Wu's sacrum. Realizing that this may be the beginning of a pressure injury, the nurse examines the area carefully and notes a small skin excoriation (abrasion) in the area. She repositions Mrs. Wu to prevent further pressure on her sacrum. After finishing the bath, the nurse records her findings and enters on Mrs. Wu's care plan a nursing diagnosis of Impaired Skin Integrity related to mechanical forces (e.g. shearing forces, pressure, physical immobility), alteration in skin turgor, and pressure over bony prominence. She

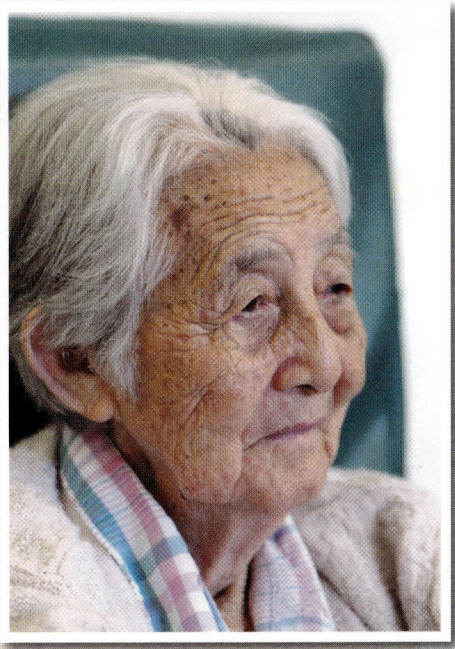

(Continued)

Meet Your Patients (continued)

writes appropriate nursing orders, including an order to observe skin over bony prominences every 4 hours, and then delegates to the NAP the task of turning and repositioning Mrs. Wu every 2 hours. The nurse also places Mrs. Wu on a pressure-relief mattress and obtains a foam cushion for her wheelchair.

Patient 2

Patsy Jimenez is a healthy 25-year-old woman with no medical problems. She eats a balanced diet but says she does not exercise much. She and the nurse have created a plan to help her increase her physical activity. Ms. Jimenez will try to walk for 30 minutes at least 5 days a week. Each week she is successful, she plans to reward herself with a movie

or a milkshake, which she usually avoids because of the fat content. The nurse would prefer that Ms. Jimenez not reward herself with food but respects the patient's decision and realizes that if it is to serve as motivation, the reward must be something that Ms. Jimenez values.

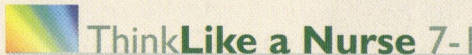 ThinkLike a Nurse 7-1

- For Jeannette Wu, which parts of the scenario illustrate *doing* by the nurse?
- For Jeannette Wu, which parts of the scenario illustrate *thinking* by the nurse?
- For Patsy Jimenez, who will be implementing (carrying out) the plan of care?

ABOUT THE KEY CONCEPTS

As you study this chapter, keep the concepts of **implementation, evaluation,** and **quality improvement** in mind. Everything in the chapter will relate to those concepts in some way, and you will begin to understand how they are related to each other and to your role as a nurse.

IMPLEMENTATION: THE ACTION PHASE OF THE NURSING PROCESS

Implementation involves action. Of course, it involves thinking, but the emphasis is on doing.

- During implementation, you perform or delegate planned interventions—that is, carry out the care plan.
- This phase ends when you document the nursing actions.
- Implementation evolves into evaluation as you document the resulting client responses (Fig. 7-1).

   KEY POINT: *In short, implementation is doing, delegating, and documenting.* For professional standards relating to implementation, see Box 7-1.

   As in all phases of the nursing process, think of the client as a collaborative partner. But be aware that clients vary in their ability and desire to participate. In the opening scenarios, for example, Mrs. Wu was able to participate very little, but Patsy Jimenez participated fully. When Mrs. Wu is less confused and better able to move about, the nurse will encourage her to help with her own bath.

How Is Implementation Related to Other Steps of the Nursing Process?

Nursing process phases are interdependent (see Fig. 7-1). Without the assessment, diagnosis, and planning steps, implementation would reflect only dependent functions, such as carrying out policies, protocols, and medical prescriptions. The autonomous nursing activities performed during implementation are built on the nurse's reasoning in the assessment, diagnosis, and planning steps.

- **Implementation overlaps with assessment.** Nurses use assessment data to individualize interventions Implementation

provides the opportunity to assess your patient at every contact. When performing an ongoing assessment, you are both implementing and assessing.

   Example: In Meet Your Patients, what data did the nurse obtain while bathing Mrs. Wu? What ongoing assessment was ordered for Mrs. Wu?

- **Implementation overlaps with diagnosis.** Nurses use data discovered during implementation to identify new diagnoses or to revise existing ones.

   Example: What new nursing diagnosis did the nurse make for Mrs. Wu after bathing her?

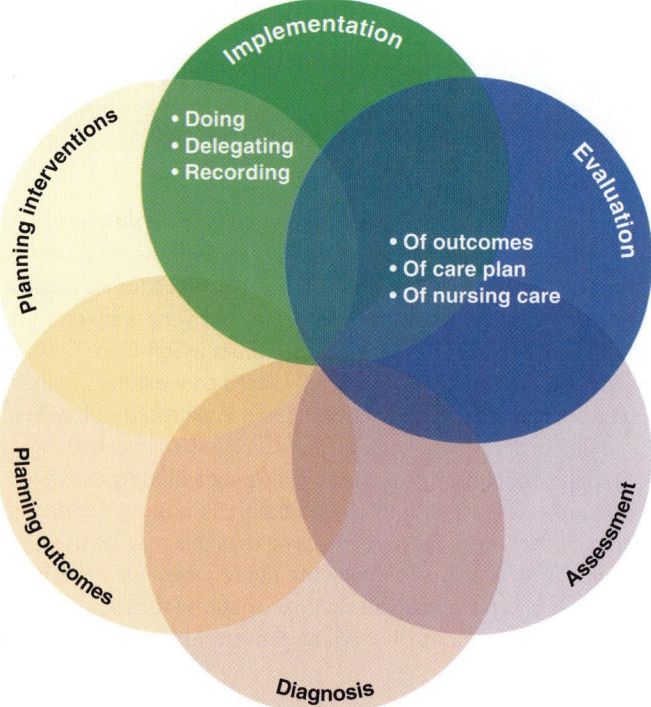

FIGURE 7-1 Nursing process phase: implementation and evaluation.

BOX 7-1 ■ ANA Standards of Practice for Implementation

Standard 5. Implementation

The registered nurse implements the identified plan.

Competencies

The registered nurse:
- Partners with the healthcare consumer to implement the plan in a safe, effective, efficient, timely, patient-centered, and equitable manner (IOM, 2010).
- Integrates interprofessional team partners in implementation of the plan through collaboration and communication across the continuum of care.
- Demonstrates caring to develop therapeutic relationships.
- Provides culturally congruent, holistic care that focuses on the healthcare consumer and addresses and advocates for the needs of diverse populations across the lifespan.
- Uses evidence-based interventions and strategies to achieve the mutually identified goals and outcomes specific to the diagnosis or problem.
- Integrates critical thinking and technology solutions to implement the nursing process to collect, measure, record, retrieve, trend, and analyze data and information to enhance nursing practice and healthcare consumer outcomes.
- Delegates according to the health, safety, and welfare of the healthcare consumer and considering the circumstance, task, direction or communication, supervision, evaluation, as well as the state practice act regulations, institution, and regulatory entities while maintaining accountability for care.
- Documents implementation and any modifications, including changes or omissions, of the identified plan.

Standard 5A: Coordination of Care

The registered nurse coordinates care delivery.

Competencies

The registered nurse:
- Organizes the components of the plan.
- Collaborates with the consumer to help manage health care based on mutually agreed upon outcomes.
- Manages a healthcare consumer's care in order to reach mutually agreed upon outcomes.
- Engages healthcare consumer in self-care to achieve preferred goals for quality of life.
- Assists the healthcare consumer in identifying options for care.
- Communicates with the healthcare consumer, interprofessional team, and community-based resources to affect safe transitions in continuity of care.
- Advocates for the delivery of dignified and holistic care by the interprofessional team.
- Documents the coordination of the care.

Standard 5B: Health Teaching and Health Promotion

The registered nurse employs strategies to promote health and a safe environment.

Competencies

The registered nurse:
- Provides opportunities for the healthcare consumer to identify needed healthcare promotion, disease prevention, and self-management topics.
- Uses health promotion and health teaching methods in collaboration with the healthcare consumer's values, beliefs, health practices, developmental level, learning needs, readiness and ability to learn, language preference, spirituality, culture, and socioeconomic status.
- Uses feedback and evaluation from the healthcare consumer to determine the effectiveness of the employed strategies.
- Uses technologies to communicate health promotion and disease prevention information to the healthcare consumer.
- Provides healthcare consumers with information about intended effects and potential adverse effects of the plan of care.
- Engages consumer alliance and advocacy groups in health teaching and health promotion activities for healthcare consumers.
- Provides anticipatory guidance to healthcare consumers to promote health and prevent or reduce the risk of negative health outcomes.

Standard 16. Resource Utilization

The registered nurse utilizes appropriate resources to plan, provide, and sustain evidence-based nursing services that are safe, effective, and fiscally responsible.

Competencies

The registered nurse:
- Assesses healthcare consumer care needs and resources available to achieve desired outcomes.
- Assists the healthcare consumer in factoring costs, risks, and benefits in decisions about care.
- Assists the healthcare consumer in identifying and securing appropriate services to address needs across the healthcare continuum.
- Delegates in accordance with applicable legal and policy parameters.
- Identifies impact of resource allocation on the potential for harm, complexity of the task and desired outcomes.
- Integrates telehealth and mobile technologies into practice to promote positive interactions between healthcare consumers and care providers.
- Uses organizational and community resources to implement interprofessional plans.
- Addresses discriminatory healthcare practices and the impact on resource allocation.

Source: American Nurses Association. (2015). *Nursing: Scope and standards of practice* (3rd ed., pp. 61–65, 82). Silver Spring, MD: Author.

- **Implementation overlaps with planning outcomes and interventions.** As you care for a client, you begin to know her better, and her unique needs become more apparent.
- **Implementation overlaps with evaluation.** When evaluating patient health status and progress toward goals, you will compare the responses you observe during implementation with the existing goals (which were written in the planning outcomes phase).

Preparing for Implementation

Implementation involves some preparation. Although the care plan will already have been developed in the planning stages of the nursing process, you should do some more planning just before implementing the plan, as explained in the following steps. Notice how important critical thinking and nursing knowledge are to this "doing" phase of the nursing process.

Check Your Knowledge and Abilities

Before beginning a nursing activity, review the care plan and reflect critically on the nursing and medical prescriptions.

- **Clarify orders.** As a nurse, you are obligated ethically and legally to clarify or question orders that you believe to be unclear, incorrect, or inappropriate.
- **Be sure you are qualified/authorized.** Is the action allowed by your state's nurse practice act, your facility's policies and procedures, and your job description? Is it allowed by your instructor or supervisor? Do you have the required knowledge, skill, and experience? Can you accept accountability for the outcomes of your action?
- **Be sure the action is safe, reasonable, and prudent.** Assess the patient to see whether the action is still indicated. Have you checked for contraindications, identified possible harmful patient responses, and minimized risks? Do you have a plan for what to do if something does not go as planned? Have you planned for safety, privacy, and comfort? Have you considered whether the action is ethical (Alfaro-LeFevre, 2007)?

KEY POINT: *If the answer to any of the preceding questions is no, then you must get help or advice from your instructor or supervisor.*

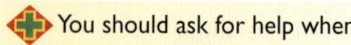 You should ask for help when:

- You do not have the knowledge or skill needed to implement an order (e.g., when administering an unfamiliar medication).
- You cannot perform the activity safely alone (e.g., helping an overweight, weak patient to ambulate).
- Performing the activity alone would cause undue stress for the patient (e.g., giving back care to a patient with multiple fractures).

Organize Your Work

You must work efficiently in order to control healthcare costs and to make the most of every patient contact. Think ahead about interventions you can perform at the same time. For example, while changing a dressing you might teach the patient about wound care at home. Many institutions have forms for scheduling your work, or you may need to write your own list of "things to do" in the order you need to do them. For example, you could make a form with a column for tasks you must accomplish and a column for each of your patients. In column 1 include information such as:

Room #
Name patient prefers

Admitting diagnosis
Significant others
Current health status (from report); does care plan need to be modified?
Basic care needs (e.g., hygiene, elimination, feeding, dressing, other)
Safety precautions
Medications
IVs
Tests & treatments today
Prioritized nursing diagnoses
Interventions that must be done today
New medical orders to implement
Teaching and counseling for today

Establish Feedback Points You cannot assume you will be able to carry out a nursing order in exactly the way it was written.

Example: Suppose the nursing order states, "Help to ambulate in the hall b.i.d [twice a day]." When you help the patient to stand, he becomes pale, dizzy, diaphoretic, and short of breath. Would you still carry out the order?

You must always be ready to alter the activity on the spot as the patient's responses demand. This means that you observe how the patient is responding to the activity as you perform care. Because this evaluation is done before the intervention is complete, we call it **feedback.** Feedback is not always verbal; it could be a change in vital signs, skin color, or level of consciousness, as in the example above. When organizing your work, identify points in each intervention where you want to pause for feedback

KEY POINT: *Notice how the concept of feedback relates to the concept of organization and how they both are related to the key concept, implementation.*

Prepare Supplies and Equipment Gather all the supplies and equipment you need before going to the patient's room. This allows you to work efficiently by eliminating the need to leave the room to obtain items you have overlooked.

Prepare the Patient

Before performing a nursing activity, identify and reassess the patient to make sure the activity is still necessary and the patient is physically and psychologically ready for the intervention.

- **Check Your Assumptions.** Don't assume that an intervention is still needed simply because it is written on the care plan.
  - *Example:* On postoperative day 6 after Jeannette Wu's surgery, the nursing assistant is preparing to give her a bed bath, as instructed on the care plan (Table 7-1, entry for December 18). However, Mrs. Wu has regained some of her strength, is alert and oriented, and is able to sit in a chair. So the nurse and the assistant agree that, with help, Mrs. Wu can bathe at the sink instead of requiring a complete bed bath.
- **Assess the Patient's Readiness.** To obtain the most benefit from an intervention, a client must be physically and psychologically ready.
  - *Example:* The hospital's critical pathway for hip fractures recommended a "help bath" on postoperative day 3 for Mrs. Wu. However, her physical condition indicated that she needed a bed bath on day 3. The nurse did not assume Mrs. Wu was ready to progress just because the critical pathway dictated it.

Table 7-1 ➤ Portions of the Care Plan for Jeannette Wu

Date: 12/16/18 Care Plan Before Implementation on Post-Op Day 4

NURSING DIAGNOSIS	DESIRED OUTCOMES	NURSING ORDERS	EVALUATION
12/16/18 Self-Care Deficits (Bathing/Hygiene, Dressing/Grooming, and Toileting) related to weakness, pain, alteration in cognitive functioning, and impaired mobility	By post-op day 6 (12/18/18) will assist with bath and oral hygiene.	■ Complete bed bath daily in a.m. ■ Give prescribed analgesic ½ hr before bath. ■ Assist with range-of-motion exercises.	

Date: 12/16/18 Care Plan After Implementation on Post-Op Day 4

NURSING DIAGNOSIS	DESIRED OUTCOMES	NURSING ORDERS	EVALUATION
12/16/18 Self-Care Deficits (Bathing/Hygiene, Dressing/Grooming, and Toileting) related to weakness, pain, alteration in cognitive functioning, and impaired mobility	By post-op day 6 (12/18/18) will assist with bath and oral hygiene.	■ Complete bed bath daily in a.m. (NAP). ■ Give Tylenol #3, tabs i by mouth, ½ hr before bath. ■ Assist with range-of-motion exercises tid (RN).	12/16/18 Too soon to evaluate.
12/16/18 Impaired skin integrity (sacrum) r/t pressure 2° immobility	*By 12/23/18, skin healed over sacrum; skin intact and normal color over all bony prominences.*	■ *Turn and reposition q2hr; do not place supine (NAP).* ■ *Observe skin over bony prominences q4hr (RN).*	12/16/18 Too soon to evaluate.

Date: 12/18/18 Care Plan After Implementation on Post-Op Day 6

NURSING DIAGNOSIS	DESIRED OUTCOMES	NURSING ORDERS	EVALUATION
12/16/18 Self-Care Deficits (Bathing/Hygiene, Dressing/Grooming, and Toileting) related to weakness, pain, and impaired mobility	By post-op day 6 (12/18/18) will assist with bath and oral hygiene.	■ Complete bed bath daily in A.M. ■ *12/18/18 NAP help with bath at sink daily in a.m. Patient can wash hands and face and perform oral hygiene.* ■ Give prescribed analgesic ½ hr before bath. ■ Assist with range-of-motion exercises tid (RN).	*12/18/18 Goal met. Sat in chair for help bath. Performed oral hygiene and washed hands and face.*
12/16/18 Impaired skin integrity (sacrum) r/t pressure 2° immobility	By 12/23/18, skin healed over sacrum; skin intact and normal color over all bony prominences.	■ Turn and reposition q2hr; do not place supine (NAP). ■ Observe skin over bony prominences q4hr (RN). ■ *Place in specialty bed (air fluidized/low-air-loss bed) to reduce shear and decrease moisture.* ■ *Provide foam padding for chair when out of bed.* ■ *Teach patient how to shift weight when up in chair.*	*12/18/18 Skin excoriation over sacrum is stable, not spreading, and appears to be healing. Skin over coccyx pink, (no longer red)*

- **Explain What You Will Do and What the Patient Will Feel.** Many interventions require the patient's participation or cooperation. ♥ **iCare** Caring nurses take time to explain because it helps to motivate the person and gives him the information he needs to participate. Knowing what to expect helps to relieve anxiety, enables the person to cope with unpleasant or painful sensations, and promotes a trusting relationship.
- **Provide Privacy.** This helps to assure psychological readiness and respects the patient's dignity.

KnowledgeCheck 7-1

- Why is it important to organize your work before implementing care?
- In addition to organizing your work, what other preparations should you make before implementing care?

Implementing the Plan: Doing or Delegating

After both you and the patient are prepared, it is time to act.

- Nursing actions include both those you do yourself and those you delegate to others.
- Interventions may be collaborative, independent, or dependent (see Chapter 6 if you do not recall the meaning of these terms).
- During implementation, you will coordinate and carry out both the nursing orders on the nursing care plan and the medical orders that relate to the patient's medical treatment.

What Knowledge and Skills Do I Need?

There is almost no limit to the number and kinds of nursing interventions you might perform.

- The *Nursing Interventions Classification (NIC)*, for example, lists more than 500 broad interventions (Bulechek, Butcher, Dochterman, et al., 2012).
- During implementation, you can expect to use all types of knowledge—theoretical, practical, personal, and ethical—as well as knowledge about the patient situation.
- You will also use various combinations of cognitive, psychomotor, and interpersonal skills to perform nursing activities (thinking, doing, caring).

  Example: When you are inserting an IV catheter, you need cognitive knowledge of sterile procedure, interpersonal skills to reassure the patient, and psychomotor skills to apply the tourniquet and insert the IV catheter.

ThinkLike a Nurse 7-2

Use the examples provided in the preceding paragraph to help you write a definition for each of the following terms:

- Cognitive skills
- Psychomotor skills
- Interpersonal skills

How Can I Promote Client Participation and Adherence?

Different interventions require differing levels of participation. However, even a nurse-initiated intervention, such as inserting a urinary catheter, goes more smoothly if the patient participates at least to the extent of holding still while you perform the procedure.

- **Many interventions depend almost entirely on the patient's adhering to the therapy.** In the case of Ms. Jimenez (Meet Your Patients), the intervention (walking for 30 minutes at least 5 days a week) depends entirely on the client.
- **People fail to follow therapeutic regimens for various reasons,** such as lack of understanding, cultural or religious objections, embarrassment, or hesitation to ask questions.
- **People need access to information that they can understand,** including knowledge of medical words, how their healthcare system works, and how to manage their disease.
- **You can promote cooperation with treatments and therapies by following these guidelines:**

  Provide Teaching such as the following:

- Assess the client's understanding of his illness and treatments.
- Provide essential and desired information in plain language.
- Keep instructions simple, clear, and as specific as possible.
- Ask the client to state in his own words key concepts about current health issues, decisions, and instructions you just discussed.
- Supply a written copy of instructions to the client and/or caregiver, taking into account cognitive abilities and readiness for additional information.
- Utilize pictures and other visual aids relevant to the client's medical condition and needs.

  Assess the Client's Supports and Resources You may find the following obstacles:

- People may not have enough money for treatments or medicine, even if they wish to follow the therapy.
- Some people cannot read or understand printed instructions.
- Some do not have family or friends to help with their care at home.
- The patient may not have transportation to the healthcare facility.

  Be Sensitive to the Client's Cultural, Spiritual, and Other Needs

- Keep in mind that shared decision making is a way to reach a goal, and the goal in patient care is to achieve outcomes that (1) matter most to the patient and (2) promote his health.
- Modify interventions as much as possible to reflect client preferences and beliefs.
- Incorporate benign alternative practices and preferences into client's care plan (e.g. food preference and preparation, folk remedies, family presence and decision making, use of significant spiritual rituals).

  Realize and Accept That Some Attitudes Cannot Be Changed Information alone will not change a person's behavior. For example, regardless of the effects of obesity on blood pressure, a client will not lose weight simply because you tell him it is important. The client must *want* to lose weight.

  Determine the Client's Main Concerns For example, you may be concerned that lack of exercise makes it difficult to regulate a client's blood sugar; the client's main concern may be that exercise makes her joints hurt.

  Help the Client Set Realistic Goals Clients usually more readily accept small, rather than drastic, behavioral or lifestyle changes. For example, perhaps a client with a child who has asthma cannot even imagine that she could stop smoking. But you may be able to convince her it would be better for her child if she would smoke outdoors rather than in the house or in the car.

  Talk Openly and Regularly About Adherence

- Let the client know you understand how difficult treatment can be and that others struggle with adherence as well.

- Offer information about support groups/resources that might be helpful.

What Should I Know About Collaborating and Coordinating Care?

For successful implementation, you need the skills of collaboration and coordination.

Collaboration As you have learned, **collaboration** simply means working with patients and other caregivers (e.g., physicians, therapists, nutritionists) to plan, make decisions, or perform interventions. Unlike delegated activities, true collaboration requires shared decision making. One of the competencies you must acquire is the ability to function on an interdisciplinary team. This means, in part, that you will learn to be assertive in discussions about patient care. At the same time, you need to recognize the differences in authority and power that exist on interdisciplinary teams and choose your communication style carefully

Coordination Coordinating care includes scheduling treatments and activities with other departments (e.g., laboratory, physical therapy, radiology). But it is more than that. Nurses are the professionals who have the most frequent and continuous contact with the patient, so they have the most complete picture of the person. You will be expected to read reports of other professionals, help interpret the results for the patient and family, and make sure that everyone sees the whole picture.

KnowledgeCheck 7-2

- What are some reasons that a client may not follow a recommended treatment regimen?
- List at least four things you could do to promote client participation in care or adherence to recommendations for treatment.

What Should I Know About Delegation and Supervision?

Delegation takes place when the registered nurse (RN), who holds the *authority* for nursing care delivery, transfers *responsibility* for the performance of a task to nursing assistive personnel (NAP) while retaining *accountability* for a safe outcome (American Nurses Association, 2012; Mueller & Vogelsmeier, 2013). When the nursing assistant accepts the *responsibility* for the delegated task, he or she has the *authority* to complete it as directed. As an RN, you will frequently delegate patient care activities to licensed vocational (or practical) nurses (LVN/LPNs) and NAPs.

Delegating Is Not the Same as Assigning You may *assign* tasks to other RNs (e.g., as a nurse in charge tasks making unit assignments for the day). However, this is not delegation because those RNs are accountable for the outcome of their activities. Remember, you can only delegate *down* in the chain of command.

You Cannot Delegate Nursing Care Decisions You can delegate only the responsibility for performing a defined activity in a particular situation.

> *Example:* Even though the nurse has delegated to the NAP the task of turning Mrs. Wu (Meet Your Patients) every 2 hours, it is *the nurse* who must assess her skin condition and take action if it does not improve.

Use NAPs Appropriately Nurses often find themselves in a difficult position of caring for more seriously ill patients

and using continually changing technologies. They must juggle these activities with overseeing delegated work. Many nurses are concerned that delegation could be a threat to patient safety. You will need to be vigilant and action-oriented regarding appropriate and well-supervised delegation. According to the American Nurses Association (ANA):

- Any nursing intervention that requires critical thinking or professional judgment cannot be delegated.
- In accordance with state nurse practice acts, the RN delegates and directs *specific tasks* to NAPs that are appropriate, safe, and resource efficient (ANA, 2007).
- Standard 15 of *Nursing: Scope and Standards of Practice* (3rd ed.) (ANA, 2015) states that the RN "delegates in accordance with applicable legal and policy parameters."

The Five Rights of Delegation

When deciding whether to delegate tasks, you should think critically about the five critical elements, or "five rights," of delegating. For a checklist to help with your decision, see Box 7-2.

KnowledgeCheck 7-3

- List the "five rights" of delegation.
- As an RN, how would you establish that a NAP is competent to perform a task?
- List at least three ways to help ensure that the NAP will understand clearly what she needs to do when you delegate a task.
- List at least three things you should do when providing supervision to an unlicensed caregiver.

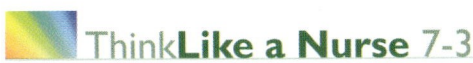 **ThinkLike a Nurse** 7-3

For your patient, Jeannette Wu:
- Which activity did the nurse delegate to someone else?
- What collaborative activities should the nurse consider?

Documenting: The Final Step of Implementation

After giving care, record the nursing activities and the patient's responses. Documentation is a mode of communication among health team members, and it provides the information you need to evaluate the patient's health status and the nursing care plan. For a thorough discussion of documenting, refer to Chapter 18.

Reflecting Critically About Implementation

During the implementation phase, perhaps more than at any other time, nurses combine **thinking** and **doing.** You should always be prepared to modify an activity based on the patient's responses. Afterward, when you have some time to reflect, you can think critically about what happened and why. Use the following questions or refer to the critical thinking model.

- What was done? Why was it done? What were the patient's responses?
- Did I forget to do anything?
- What was going on in the situation that may have influenced the outcome?
- What factors influenced my behavior (or others' behavior) in this situation?

BOX 7-2 ■ The Five Rights of Delegation—Checklist

Right Task (Can I delegate it?)

As a rule, you should delegate an activity only if it meets *all* of the following criteria (ANA, 2012; ANA/NCSBN, 2006; NCSBN, 2016):

- Delegable for a specific patient.
- Within the licensed nurse's scope of practice and the delegatee's job description.
- Permitted by the state's nurse practice act.
- Permitted by the agency's policies.
- Is performed according to an established sequence of steps and requires little or no modification from one situation to another.
- Does *not* require independent, specialized nursing knowledge, skills, or judgment.
- Is *not* health teaching or counseling.
- Does not endanger a client's life or well-being.

Right Circumstance (Should I delegate it?)

Before delegating, assess the patient to be certain that her needs match the abilities of the NAP or LPN. Consider patient safety:

- Is the patient setting appropriate?
- Is the patient's condition relatively stable?
- Can the patient perform self-care activities without extensive help?
- Are adequate resources available?
- Are there other factors to maintain safety?

Right Person (Who is best prepared to do it?)

The right person:

- Is delegating the task (the nurse must be competent to delegate).
- Will be performing the task (the NAP must be competent to do the task).
- Will receive the care (i.e., the severity of the patient's illness is considered).
- Has performed the task often or has worked with patients with similar diagnoses.
- Has a workload that allows time to do the task properly.

The facility:

- Has documented proof that the person has demonstrated competence. If evidence is lacking, you need to establish the NAP's competence (e.g., observe and evaluate his performance or ask the NAP, "How many times have you done this procedure?"

Right Direction/Communication (What does the NAP need to know?)

- **Explain exactly what the task is.** For example, "Empty the catheter bag, and measure the amount of urine using the clear, marked plastic container"—not just "Measure the urine."
- **Include specific times and methods for reporting.** For example, "Come tell me the patient's temperature every hour."

- **Explain the purpose or objective of the task.** For example, "Change Mrs. Wu's position every 2 hours to prevent bedsores; she is not able to turn by herself."
- **Describe the expected results or potential complications.** For example, "I have given her medications, so her temperature should be below 100°F by 0900. If not, let me know immediately."
- **Be specific in your instructions.** For example, "Let me know whether Mrs. Wu has any more red spots or broken skin areas when you turn her" not "Tell me what her skin looks like."
- **Be certain the delegatee (NAP) understands** the communication and that he or she cannot **modify the task** without first consulting the nurse.

Right Supervision/Evaluation (How will I follow up?)

As the RN, you are responsible for providing supervision and evaluating the outcomes. This includes the following:

- **Monitoring the NAP/LVN's work.** Does it comply with standards of practice and agency policy and procedures?
- **Intervening as needed.** Some NAPs receive little training, so you may need to demonstrate and receive return demonstrations of the NAP's ability to perform some activities.
- **Obtaining feedback from the patient.** Evaluate both the client's responses to the NAP interventions and the relationship with the NAP.
- **Obtaining feedback from the delegatee.** Provide both positive and negative feedback. If performance is not acceptable, speak privately with the NAP to explain the specific mistakes. Listen to the NAP's view of the situation.
- **Evaluating client outcomes.**
- **Ensuring proper documentation of the delegatee's actions.** Some agencies permit NAPs to record vital signs and other patient data. However, the RN is still responsible for seeing that all necessary data are recorded and that they are accurate.

Sources: American Nurses Association. (2012). *ANA's principles for delegation by registered nurses to unlicensed assistive personnel (UAP).* Silver Spring, MD: Author.

American Nurses Association (ANA) and the National Council of State Boards of Nursing (NCSBN). (2006). *Joint statement on delegation.* Retrieved from https://www.ncsbn.org/Delegation_joint_statement_NCSBN-ANA.pdf; National Council of State Boards of Nursing. (2016). National guidelines for nursing delegation. *Journal of Nursing Regulation,* 7(1), 5–14. Retrieved rom http://dx.doi.org/10.1016/S2155-8256(16)31035-3

- Did I communicate clearly to the patient?
- Did I convey respect and caring?
- What could I have delegated? What did I delegate that I should *not* have? Why?
- After reflecting on it, what would I do differently in this situation?

The following is an example of how reflection questions might be used in a clinical situation:

Situation: The nursing order read, "Assist to ambulate to the end of the hall . . ." However, the patient was able to walk only half that distance before becoming too weak to stand.

Question for Reflection: What was going on in the situation that may have influenced the outcome?

What Might Have Happened: Perhaps the patient was weak because he had not slept well the night before, or perhaps he had just completed a long, tiring session of physical therapy.

EVALUATION: THE FINAL STEP OF THE NURSING PROCESS

Evaluation, the final step of the nursing process, is a planned, ongoing, systematic activity in which you will make judgments about:

- The client's progress toward desired health outcomes.
- The effectiveness of the nursing care plan.
- The quality of nursing care in the healthcare setting.

How Is Evaluation Related to Other Steps of the Nursing Process?
Patient outcomes stated in the *planning outcomes* stage must be concrete, observable, and appropriate for the patient in order to be useful as evaluation criteria. Appropriate outcomes, in turn, depend on complete and accurate *assessment* data and *nursing diagnoses*. You will observe and evaluate client responses during *implementation* in order to make on-the-spot changes in activity. And, of course, *interventions* must be *planned* and *implemented* to produce the patient behaviors that you evaluate. **KEY POINT:** *Evaluation and the assessment step both involve data collection. The difference is in when you collect and how you use the data.*

- **Assessment data** are collected before interventions are performed to determine initial or baseline health status and to make nursing diagnoses.
- **Evaluation data** are collected after interventions are performed to determine whether client goals were achieved.

Why Is Evaluation Essential to Full-Spectrum Nursing?

The following are a few reasons:

- **The patient is the nurse's first priority.** The aim of all nursing activity is to achieve positive outcomes for patients. Evaluation lets you know whether your interventions are helping the patient as intended and guides your next action.
- **Evaluation helps nurses to conserve scarce resources.** Nursing time must be used wisely and efficiently. Evaluation allows you to discard interventions that are not working well and focus on more effective ones.
- **Professional standards of practice require evaluation.** See the ANA practice standards in Box 7-3.
- **The ANA Code of Ethics requires evaluation.** "Nurses have a responsibility to define, implement, and maintain standards of professional practice. Nurses must plan, establish, implement, and evaluate review mechanisms to safeguard patients, nurses, colleagues, and the environment" (ANA, 2014, Provision 4.3, p. 15).
- **The Joint Commission and other professional standards review organizations require evaluation.** These organizations use outcomes and performance measures to evaluate the quality of care in healthcare institutions. They conceptualize quality of care as the degree to which health services increase the likelihood of desired health outcomes.
- **Evaluation helps ensure nursing's survival.** Linking nursing interventions to achievement of client outcomes demonstrates the value of nursing. In today's competitive healthcare market, that is essential for ensuring continued funding for nursing services, education, and research.

Standard 6. Evaluation

The registered nurse evaluates progress toward attainment of goals and outcomes.

Competencies

The registered nurse:

- Conducts a holistic, systematic, ongoing, and criterion-based evaluation of the goals and outcomes in relation to the structure and processes and timeline prescribed in the plan.
- Collaborates with the healthcare consumer and others involved in the care or situation in the evaluation process.
- Determines, in partnership with the healthcare consumer and other stakeholders, the patient-centeredness, effectiveness, efficiency, safety, timeliness, and equitability (IOM, 2001) of the strategies in relation to the plan and attainment of outcomes. Other critieria (e.g., Quality and Safety Education for Nurses) may be used as well.
- Documents the results of the evaluation.

Source: American Nurses Association. (2015). *Nursing: Scope and standards of practice* (3rd ed., p. 66). Silver Spring, MD: Author.

♥ **iCare** ■ **Evaluation demonstrates caring and responsibility.** Without evaluation, you would not know whether your patient care was effective. Examining outcomes implies that you care about how your activities affect your clients.

How Are Standards and Criteria Used in Evaluation?

In a broad sense, evaluation is the systematic process of judging the quality or value of something (e.g., a car, a movie) by comparing it with one or more standards or criteria. **KEY POINT:** *For formal evaluation, however, you must decide in advance which standards and criteria you will use.* In nursing, standards are used to describe quality nursing care.

- **The ANA's standards of practice** are a good example of *broadly written standards* (see Boxes 7-1 and 7-3).
- **Criteria and competencies.** Notice that each of the ANA standards includes a set of measurement criteria, called competencies, to help describe the standard. Criteria are measurable or observable characteristics, properties, attributes, or qualities. They describe the specific skills, knowledge, behaviors, and attitudes that are desired or expected.
- **Patient goals and outcomes,** discussed in Chapter 5, are also examples of criteria. As you learned, criteria should be concrete and specific enough to serve as guides for collecting evaluation data. In addition, they should be reliable and valid.

Reliability A criterion is **reliable** if it yields the same results every time, regardless of who uses it. For example, suppose you measure a patient's temperature by (1) using an oral thermometer and (2) placing the back of your hand on the patient's forehead. Which method would probably give the same (or nearly the same) results every time? As you probably concluded, the oral thermometer is more reliable.

Validity A criterion is **valid** if it is really measuring what it was intended to measure. For example, fever is often used as a criterion for concluding that a person has an infection.

However, if used alone, it is not a valid indicator because (1) other conditions, such as dehydration, can cause a fever and (2) elevated temperature is not present in all infections. Validity of that criterion is increased when you use additional criteria (e.g., elevated white blood cell count, presence of signs of infection such as redness and pus).

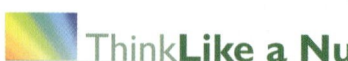

ThinkLike a Nurse 7-4

- The outcome "Patient will not complain of pain" by itself is not a valid criterion for measuring pain. Why? What would be a more valid criterion for pain?
- A criterion reads, "Measures client vital signs once per shift, or as ordered." For which of the following standards would it be valid (i.e., which conclusion could you draw if you knew that a nurse measured the vital signs once per shift or as ordered)?
Follows unit policies.
Performs skills accurately.

What Are the Types of Evaluation?

Evaluation is categorized according to (1) what is being evaluated (structures, processes, or outcomes) and (2) frequency and time of evaluation.

Evaluation of Structures, Processes, and Outcomes

Structures, processes, and outcomes all work together to affect care. However, each requires different criteria and methods of evaluation.

Structure Evaluation

- Focuses on the setting in which care is provided.
- Explores the effect of organizational characteristics on the quality of care.
- Requires standards and data about policies, procedures, fiscal resources, physical facilities and equipment, and number and qualifications of personnel.

The following are an examples of criteria for structure evaluation:

- At least one RN is present on each unit at all times.
- A resuscitation cart is available on each floor.

Process Evaluation

- Focuses on the manner in which care is given—the activities performed. As a rule, it does not describe the *results* of your activities.

   Example: Your instructor uses process evaluation to assess your clinical performance, that is, what you did and how well you did it.

- Explores whether the care was relevant to patient needs, appropriate, complete, and timely.

   Examples: Protects patient's privacy when performing procedures.

   Washes hands before each patient contact.

Outcomes Evaluation

- Focuses on observable or measurable changes in the patient's health status that result from the care given.
- Although structure and process are important to quality, the most important aspect is improvement in patient health status.
- Used in the evaluation step of the nursing process.

   Examples:

   Patient will walk, assisted, to end of hall by postoperative day three.

   Patient reports pain less than 4 on a scale of 1 to 10 within 1 hour after analgesic administration.

- Also used when evaluating quality of care in an organization. When used for that purpose, the criteria also state the percentage of clients expected to have the outcome when care is satisfactory.

   Example: Post-catheterization urinary tract infection does not occur.

   Expected compliance: 100% (Criterion would be met only if no patients developed a urinary tract infection after being catheterized.)

Ongoing, Intermittent, and Terminal Evaluation

Evaluation begins as soon as you have completed the first nursing activity and continues during each client contact until all goals are achieved or the client is discharged from nursing care. The client's status determines how often you evaluate.

   Examples:

   (1) After a patient undergoes surgery, you may measure vital signs every 15 minutes; as the patient nears discharge, you may evaluate once a day.

   (2) In long-term care settings, residents often have chronic health problems that require evaluation over an extended period of time. Care providers may participate in weekly care conferences to evaluate the resident's response to the current plan of care.

- **Ongoing evaluation** is performed while implementing care, immediately after an intervention, and at each patient contact.
- **Intermittent evaluation,** in contrast, is performed at specified times.

   Examples:

   Will rate pain as <3 on a scale of 1 to 10 *within 1 hr after medication.*

   Will lose 1 lb *per week* until weight of 125 lb is achieved.

- **Terminal evaluation** describes the client's health status and progress toward goals at the time of discharge. Most institutions have special discharge forms for terminal evaluation that also include instructions about medications, treatments, and follow-up care.

   KEY POINT: *As the nurse, you are responsible for drawing evaluative conclusions; however, you should use input from the patient, the family, NAPs, and other caregivers (see Box 7-3).*

ThinkLike a Nurse 7-5

For each of the following goals, when or how often should the nurse collect evaluation data?

- Will rate pain as <3 on a scale of 1 to 10 within *1 hr after medication.*
- By the second home visit, mother will demonstrate proper techniques for breastfeeding.

KnowledgeCheck 7-4

Explain what is evaluated in each of the following types of evaluation (i.e., the focus of each type of evaluation): structure, process, and outcomes.

1. In the Emergency Department, the time from patient sign-in to assessment by a healthcare worker will be less than 15 minutes.
2. A fire extinguisher is located in an accessible spot on each unit.
3. No patients with indwelling urinary catheters will develop urinary tract infection.

Toward Evidence-Based Practice

Read the following summary about a nurse-driven quality improvement project, and then answer the questions at the end of the box.

> Schelling, K., Palamone, J., Thomas, K., et al. (2015). **Reducing catheter-associated urinary tract infections in a neuro–spine intensive care unit.** *American Journal of Infection Control, 43*(8), 892–894.

A collaborative team (nurses, doctors, administrators, and infection patrol) at an academic medical center carried out a quality-improvement project. They discovered that patients in their neuro–spine intensive care unit (NSICU) had a higher rate of catheter-associated urinary tract infections than occurred in patients in the five other intensive care units in their institution. To understand and intervene in reducing the infection rate, a tracking and action plan was developed and implemented. Interventions included daily rounding to continually prompt conversations regarding catheter appropriateness and maintenance.

- Catheter Appropriateness: If even one of the agreed-upon indications was not met, the nurse asked the physician to order catheter discontinuation.

- Catheter Maintenance: The action plan included (1) changes in hand hygiene and glove changing protocol when nurses moved from one area of the body to another during routine care, (2) implementation of a new securement device, and (3) introduction of a bowel management program to reduce diarrhea prevalence.

Conclusions: Data outcomes revealed that the "catheter-associated urinary tract infection rate in this NSICU was reduced from 8.18 to 0.93 per 1,000 catheter-days and standardized infection ratio decreased from 2.16 to 0.37" (p. 893).

Considering the importance of nurses' involvement in evaluating the quality of care in an organization, answer the following questions:
1. What nursing process phases were in place for this study?

2. Does this study address structure, process, or outcomes?

 Go to Davis Advantage, Resources, Chapter 7, **Toward Evidence-Based Practice—Suggested Responses.**

How Do I Evaluate Patient Progress?

Evaluation does not "end" the nursing process. It merely provides the information you need to begin another cycle. After giving care, you compare patient responses with the desired outcomes and use that information to reflect critically on (1) the care plan and (2) each step of the nursing process as it applies to that patient. Figure 7-1 illustrates the relationship of the evaluation phase to the rest of the nursing process. When evaluating patient progress, you will review the desired outcomes, collect reassessment data, judge whether goals have been met, and record the evaluative statement.

Review Outcomes

The goals and indicators identified in the planning outcomes phase serve two purposes in evaluation:
- Suggest the kind of assessments you need to make
- Provide criteria by which to judge the data

Collect Reassessment Data

Assess client responses to the current interventions. To minimize confusion, assessments made for the purpose of evaluation are called **reassessments.** Reassessments are always **focused assessments** (see Chapter 3).

> *Example:* The nursing care plan lists the following goal: "By 8/24/18, will walk, unassisted, to the end of the hall without pallor or shortness of breath."

What kind of assessments would you make to know whether this goal has been met?

> *Answer:* You would observe the patient's skin color as he walked, count his respirations, and ask him whether he felt short of breath. You must question to clarify, for example, "Were you short of breath at any time? Were you short of breath by the time the walk was finished?"

ThinkLike a Nurse 7-6

In the example in the preceding paragraph, which aspects of critical thinking (in the full-spectrum nursing model in Chapter 2) did you use to decide what data you needed?

Goals can be cognitive, psychomotor, or affective, or they may refer to body appearance and function. The nature of the goal determines the kind of data you need to collect (see Table 7-2). As in the assessment phase, you will collect data from the client, family, friends, and health team members, as well as from the client's chart. **KEY POINT:** *The RN is responsible for evaluating goal achievement, even though someone else may have supplied the data.*

Judge Goal Achievement

Compare the reassessment data with the patient's goals. As always, get the patient's input: for example, does she think the goals have been achieved? Goals or outcomes can be judged to be one of the following:
- *Achieved.* The actual responses are the same as the desired outcome.
- *Partially achieved.* Some, but not all, of the desired behaviors were observed, or the desired response occurs only some of the time (e.g., the desired heart rate is <100 beats/min, a goal that is achieved except for one or two episodes a day when it is 120 beats/min).
- *Not achieved.* The desired response did not occur.

Record the Evaluative Statement

Professional standards require that you record your evaluations. (See ANA Standard 6, in Box 7-3.) You may write an evaluative summary in the nursing notes or on the care plan,

Table 7-2 ➤ Reassessments for Different Types of Goals

TYPE OF GOAL	INVOLVES	EXAMPLE OF GOALS	REASSESSMENT TECHNIQUES
Cognitive	Increases in patient knowledge	■ By 8/24/18 accurately describes schedule for taking medications. ■ By 8/25/18 correctly describes the procedure for pouring liquid medications.	Ask the person to repeat information or to apply new knowledge (e.g., to describe to you the schedule for taking her medications).
Affective	Changes in feelings, values, beliefs, and attitudes	■ By 8/24/18 expresses positive feelings for the newborn. ■ By 8/24/18 states he is only mildly anxious about changing his own dressing.	Observe client behavior reflecting values and beliefs; talk to the client about feelings and beliefs; observe nonverbal expression of feelings (e.g., laughing, crying).
Psychomotor	Patient's ability to perform skills	■ By 8/24/18 performs own dressing change, using proper aseptic technique. ■ By 8/24/18 measures liquid medication accurately.	Ask the person to demonstrate the new skill (e.g., change a dressing, measure a liquid medication).
Body appearance and function	Changes in body systems and functions	■ Heart rate will be 100 beats/min after ambulation to end of hall. ■ By 8/24/18 can dress self and fasten own zipper.	Observe functioning, examine the body, perform measurements, read laboratory reports (e.g., measure vital signs, observe skin color, assess for pain).

depending on agency procedures. An evaluative statement should include:

■ The conclusion about whether the goal was achieved
■ Reassessment data to support the judgment

  Example: An evaluative statement for a pain goal of "By 8/24/18 will notify nurse as soon as pain begins" might be the following:

8/25/18, 0100. Goal not met. Has not used call light at all this a.m. Restless and grimacing with movement during a.m. care. When asked, described pain as 8 on a scale of 1 to 10.

When using standardized outcomes (e.g., Nursing Outcomes Classification [NOC]) or electronic care plans, your evaluative statements may be different. In the NOC system, each outcome has a scale and indicators, numbered 1 through 5, which you can use to write goals (see Chapter 5).

  Example: A patient with a problem of decreased peripheral circulation might have this goal: "Circulation status not compromised."

Using standardized language from NOC, you might write a goal (*desired* status) of:

  Goal: Circulation Status: 5 (5 means "no deviation from normal range" in the NOC scale).

Each of the indicators could also be made into a goal by adding the desired scale numbers, as follows:

Systolic BP in expected range: 5
Diastolic BP in expected range: 5
Mean BP in expected range: 5

Evaluation statements are written exactly the same as goals, but the scale number describes the patient's *actual* status.

  Example: If on reassessment, the patient's blood pressure is quite low and he has orthostatic hypotension, the evaluative statement might be:

  Evaluative Statement: Circulation Status: 3 (3 means "moderately compromised" on this NOC scale).

Figure 7-2 is a computer screen showing the NOC outcome of Acceptance: Health Status. The Initial Scale shows the initial assessment; the Expected Scale is the goal; and the Outcome Scale is the evaluative statement after intervention and reassessment. Did the interventions achieve the desired effect or not?

KnowledgeCheck 7-5

Using the following outcomes and reassessment data, determine whether each goal has been met, partially met, or not met:

1. *Goal:* By 8/24/18, will walk, unassisted, to the end of the hall without pallor or shortness of breath.
   Reassessment data: 8/24/18. Walked, unassisted, to end of hall; states no shortness of breath, but skin color was noticeably pale.
2. *Goal:* By 8/24/18, will walk, unassisted, to the end of the hall without pallor or shortness of breath.
   Reassessment data: 8/23/18. Walked, unassisted, to end of hall. Skin color pink; respirations 14 breaths/min; no dyspnea observed; states no shortness of breath.
3. *Goal:* By 8/24/18, will walk, unassisted, to the end of the hall without pallor or shortness of breath.
   Reassessment data: 8/25/18. Walked halfway to end of hall before becoming pale and short of breath.

Evaluating Collaborative Problems

Because collaborative problems are the responsibility of the entire healthcare team, goals for collaborative problems are not included on the nursing care plan, and the evaluation process is slightly different. The desired outcome for all collaborative problems is that no complication will occur. To evaluate, you will compare the reassessment data with established norms and determine whether data are within an acceptable range.

■ **If the reassessment data are within normal limits,** this does not mean that the collaborative problem is resolved—only

Edit Outcome Progress   [X]

Outcome Definition

Name

| Acceptance: Health Status |

Initial Scale   On Date

| Limited   ▼ | | 06/24/2019 | [...]

Expected Scale   On Date

| Substantial   ▼ | | 07/24/2019 | [...]

Outcome progress

Outcome Scale   Encounter Date   Save

| Substantial   ▼ | | 07/30/2019 | [...]   Close

Explanation of Figure

Computer field	Nursing process terminology	Represents	Status recorded on computer
Initial scale	Initial assessment	*Actual* status *before* intervention	Limited acceptance of health status
Expected scale	Goal	*Desired* status *after* intervention	Substantial acceptance of health status
Outcome scale	Evaluative statement	*Actual* status *after* intervention	Substantial acceptance of health status

FIGURE 7-2 Computer screen showing outcome progress, using NOC.

that the complication has not occurred. As long as the patient has the medical condition (e.g., myocardial infarction), the collaborative problem (e.g., congestive heart failure) still exists.

- **If the data indicate the client's condition is worsening,** notify the medical provider.

See Chapter 4 if you need to review collaborative problems.

Evaluating and Revising the Care Plan

After evaluating patient progress, you will use your conclusions about goal achievement to decide whether to continue, modify, or discontinue the care plan.

Relate Outcomes to Interventions

Even when goals have been met, you cannot assume that the patient outcomes were a result of the nursing interventions. You need to use critical reflection to identify factors that might have supported or interfered with the effectiveness of an intervention. The variables can affect the ability of an intervention to produce the desired outcome:

- The client's ability and motivation to follow directions for treatment
- Availability and support from family and significant others
- Treatments and therapies performed by other healthcare team members
- Client failure to provide complete information during assessment
- Client's lack of experience, knowledge, or ability
- Staffing in the institution (ratio of licensed to unlicensed caregivers; number of patients for whom a nurse is responsible)
- Nurse's physical and mental well-being

Identifying these factors allows you to reinforce or change them. Remember, though, that you cannot control all the variables that might affect the success of an intervention.

Draw Conclusions About Problem Status

Whether you retain or remove a nursing diagnosis from the care plan depends on whether or not goals were met, as follows:

Goals met: If all goals for a nursing diagnosis have been met, you can **discontinue** the care plan for that diagnosis.

Goals partially met: If some outcomes are met and others not, you may **revise** the care plan for that problem.

Goals not met: You should **examine the entire plan and review all steps** of the nursing process to decide whether to revise the care plan.

Revise the Care Plan

To decide how to revise the care plan, you must review each step of the nursing process. You cannot just discontinue the ineffective interventions and try new ones. The interventions may not need to be changed at all. When goals have not been met, it may be due to errors in other steps of the nursing process.

1. *Review of assessment.* Review all initial and ongoing assessment data. Were the data complete, accurate, and validated as needed? If there are errors or omissions, or if there are changes in the client's condition, you may need to revise the care plan.
2. *Review of diagnosis.* Even if there were no assessment errors, you may need to revise or add new nursing diagnoses (e.g., if the problem status has changed, or if the diagnosis was inaccurate).
3. *Review of planning outcomes.* You will probably need to revise the outcomes if you have added new data or revised the nursing diagnosis. If assessment and diagnosis steps are satisfactory, perhaps the outcomes were unrealistic or had unrealistic target times.

4. *Review of planning interventions.* You will probably need to modify nursing orders (a) if you determine that interventions were not effective (e.g., they were unclear, incomplete, or not specific) or (b) if you have revised nursing diagnoses or outcomes.

5. *Review of implementation.* It could be that goals were not met because of a failure to implement the nursing orders or because of the manner in which they were implemented. Get input from the client, significant others, other caregivers, and the client records to find out what went wrong.

Reflecting Critically About Evaluation

After evaluating the patient's health status and the nursing care plan, reflect on your thinking during the evaluation process. That's right: Think about your thinking, not just about your actions (see critical thinking model from Chapter 2).

Inquiring

Is my evaluation statement clearly stated?
Were my information sources reliable?
Do I need any other data to validate my conclusion?

Noticing Context

What was going on either before or during evaluation that might have influenced my ability to gather data or draw conclusions?
What emotional responses influenced my conclusions about goal achievement?

Analyzing Assumptions

What biases do I have that may have affected my ability to reassess or evaluate goal achievement?

Reflecting Skeptically

Did I make evaluating a priority?
Did I schedule time for it, the same as I do for interventions?
KEY POINT: *The most common errors of evaluation are failing to:*
- *Evaluate systematically.*
- *Record the results.*
- *Use the reassessment data to examine and modify the care plan.*

It is relatively easy for most nurses to make a plan and take action. However, you will need determined effort to make time to *observe regularly and systematically* and *document the patient's responses* and include them in your actions. Only in that way can you be sure the care has met the client's needs.

Evaluating the Quality of Care in a Healthcare Setting

As a nurse, you will be involved in evaluating and improving the overall quality of nursing care in an organization or a geographic area. Applying quality improvement in healthcare is a core competency of all health professionals (ANA, 2015; Cronenwett, Sherwood, Barnsteiner, et al., 2007; Cronenwett, Sherwood, & Gelmon, 2009; Institute of Medicine, 2011). At a minimum, your documentation will provide data that regulatory agencies (e.g., The Joint Commission, state boards of nursing) use to determine whether nursing care meets nursing standards.

Quality Assurance Programs These are specially designed programs to promote excellence in nursing. Variations of quality assurance are quality improvement, continuous quality improvement, total quality management, and persistent quality improvement. Whatever the approach, the goal is

---

Safe, Effective Nursing Care (SENC)

Learning About the Outcomes of Care

Chapter Key Concepts: Evaluation, Quality Improvement (Thinking, Caring, Doing)

Competency: Provide safe, quality client care.

The SENC model of safe, quality care requires the nurse to:

- **Evaluate and use techniques/process to avoid nursing errors in the delivery of client care.**
  Example: You suspect that the incidence of central line infections has increased on your pediatric unit. You are in a unique position to identify problems in the patient populations for which you provide care. Before you can obtain a positive outcome, you must first be able to quantify the poor outcomes and then determine the cause of that outcome.

- **Design a "Thinking, Doing, Caring" framework that incorporates a holistic approach to client care.**
  Example of thinking: You have noticed a lot of variation in how different nurses provide central line care. Knowing that variation in treatment often leads to negative variations in outcomes, what data do you need to support your suspicions? What outcome must you measure? What root cause should be assessed? Now, how can you obtain data about those two factors? Potential sources for tracking outcomes data in your facility might include databases kept by quality improvement, safety, and/or infection control departments. Some patient care units also track quality measures.
  Example of doing and caring: Suppose you identified the rate of central line infections as the poor outcome and how central line dressing changes are performed as the problem in nursing practice. Your next steps would be to develop and implement an action plan that improves on the manner in which you are performing central line dressing care. Tracking the changes in nursing interventions and client responses is an essential part of doing and caring.

- **Evaluate the framework, incorporating the structure, processes, and outcomes components of quality improvement issues.**
  Example: Improving the quality of care is possible only by evaluating goals with clear measurements. Evaluation and reevaluations provide insight and provide a baseline against which practice changes and patient outcomes can be judged.

Source: Draper, D., Felland, L., Liebhaber, A., et al. (2008). *The role of nurses in hospital quality improvement* (HSC Research Brief No. 3). Retrieved from http://www.hschange.com/CONTENT/972/

---

to evaluate and improve the care provided in an agency or for a group of patients.

This chapter has described (1) outcomes evaluation of *client progress* and (2) process evaluation of the *effectiveness of the nursing care plan.* Quality improvement involves evaluation of *structures,* as well as outcomes and processes. All are important because structures (e.g., staffing, money) and processes (e.g., policies and procedures) affect patient outcomes. Adequate structures and processes do not guarantee desired patient outcomes; however, without them, it is very difficult to obtain good outcomes.

Example: A unit could be well staffed (structure) and follow infection-control procedures carefully (process), yet have a higher-than-average rate of urinary tract infections (outcome). One possible reason might be that most of the patients treated on that unit have compromised immune systems, making them especially susceptible to infection.

CLINICALREASONING

The questions and exercises in this section allow you to practice the kind of thinking you will use as a full-spectrum nurse. Critical-thinking questions usually have more than one right answer, so we do not provide "correct answers" for these features. It is more important to develop your nursing judgment than to just cover content. You will learn by discussing the questions with your peers. If you are still unsure, see the Davis Advantage chapter resources for suggested responses.

Caring for the Nguyens

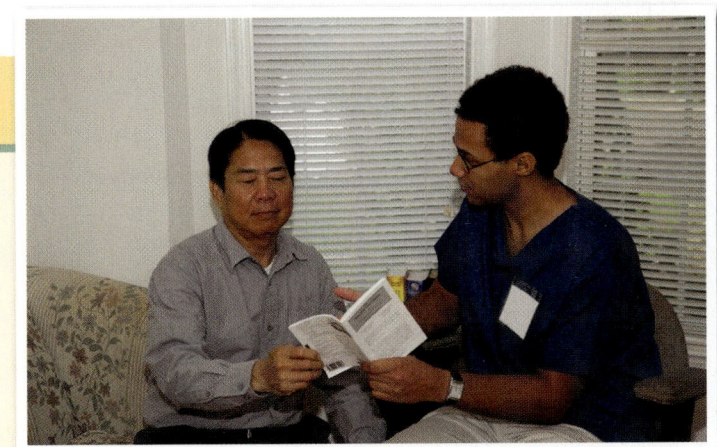

The following information is recorded on Mr. Nguyen's clinic health record:

9/1/18 Overweight related to inappropriate food choices and serving size, as evidenced by BMI of 28.5

Outcome: Will lose 5 lb by 10/15/2018

Interventions:

- Collect 3-day nutrition history 9/2/2018 through 9/4/2018.
- Have patient meet with clinic nurse for diet review and nutrition instruction 9/8/2018.
- Provide sample meal plans at 9/8/2018 instruction.
- Phone patient 9/22/2018 to discuss nutrition questions and review progress.
- Have patient return to clinic 10/15/2018 for follow-up visit.

A. What must you do before implementing each nursing intervention?

B. Identify at least two strategies that will help promote Mr. Nguyen's participation in and adherence to the plan.

C. How will you determine whether Mr. Nguyen has met his goal?

Applying the **Full-Spectrum Nursing Model**_____

Recall Jeannette Wu (Meet Your Patient) to answer the following questions about Mrs. Wu.

THINKING

1. *Theoretical Knowledge:*
   a. What facts and principles do you already know about the causes of pressure injury?
   b. Do you have enough information to provide interventions for Mrs. Wu's actual Impaired Skin Integrity? If not, what do you still need to find out?
2. *Critical Thinking (Inquiry):* What resource would be best to use to find out exactly what is meant by Mrs. Wu's diagnosis of Self-Care Deficit? Why?

DOING

3. *Practical Knowledge:* What do you know about positioning patients? How would you explain to the NAP about how to position Mrs. Wu "to prevent further pressure on her sacrum"?
4. *Nursing Process (Evaluation):*
   a. To evaluate Mrs. Wu's Impaired Skin Integrity problem, what reassessments would you make?
   b. To evaluate Mrs. Wu's Self-Care Deficit problem, what reassessments would you make? Who can or should make them? How often, or when, would you reassess?

CARING

5. *Self-Knowledge:* How comfortable would you be caring for Mrs. Wu, who is a frail older adult? What is one problem, not described in the scenario, that might arise?

To explore learning resources for this chapter,

Go to **www.DavisAdvantage.com** and find:

Answers and suggested responses for all questions in this chapter

Lists of NIC Interventions and NOC Outcomes

List of NANDA-I Diagnoses

Knowledge Map

References and Bibliography

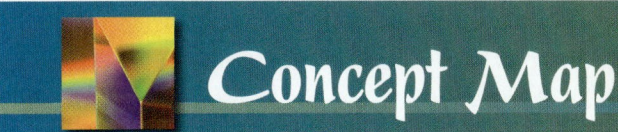

Concept Map

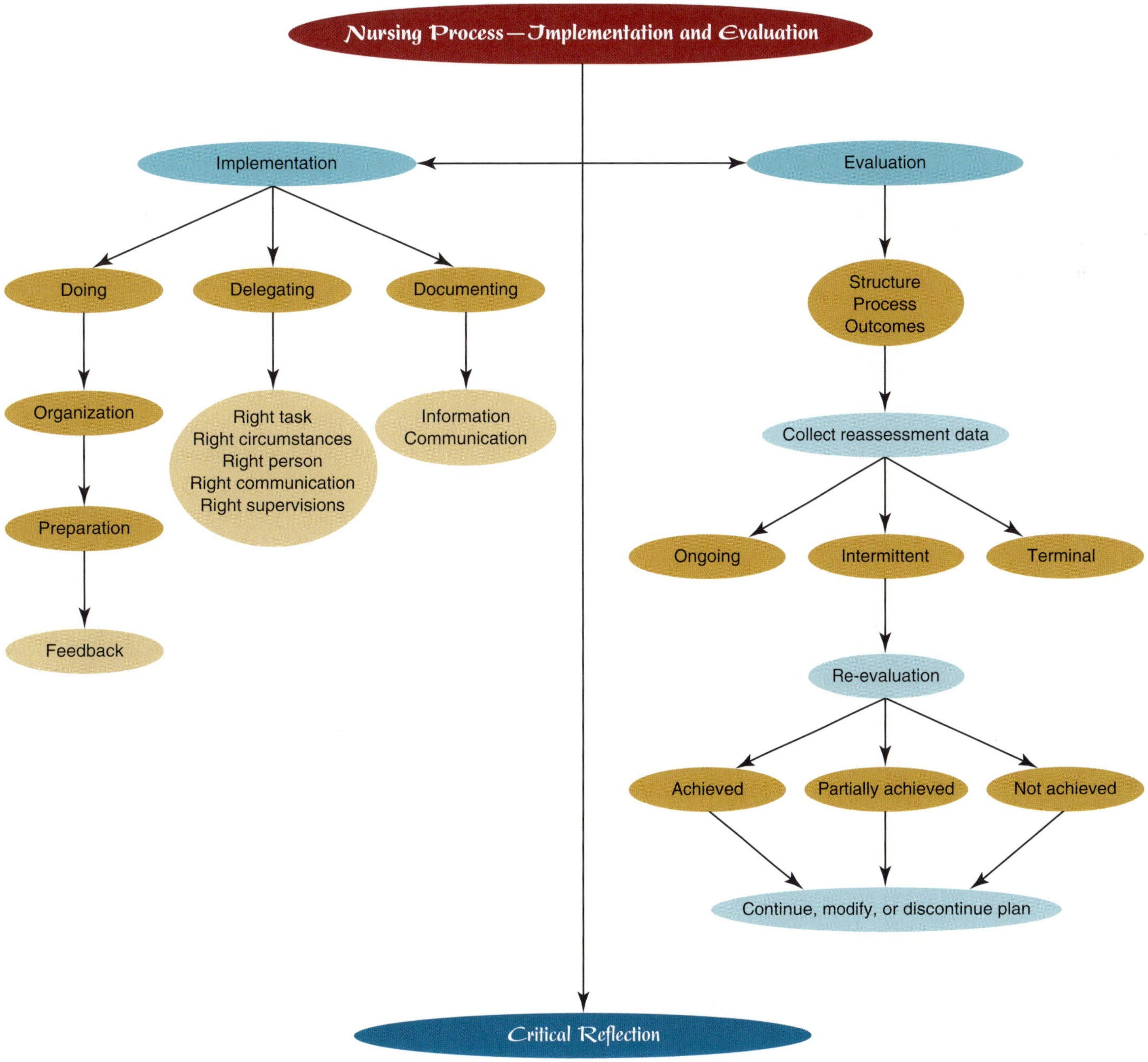

Nursing Process—Implementation and Evaluation

Implementation ⟷ **Evaluation**

Implementation branch

- **Doing**
  - Organization
  - Preparation
  - Feedback
- **Delegating**
  - Right task
    Right circumstances
    Right person
    Right communication
    Right supervisions
- **Documenting**
  - Information
    Communication

Evaluation branch

- Structure
  Process
  Outcomes
- Collect reassessment data
  - Ongoing
  - Intermittent
  - Terminal
- Re-evaluation
  - Achieved
  - Partially achieved
  - Not achieved
- Continue, modify, or discontinue plan

Critical Reflection

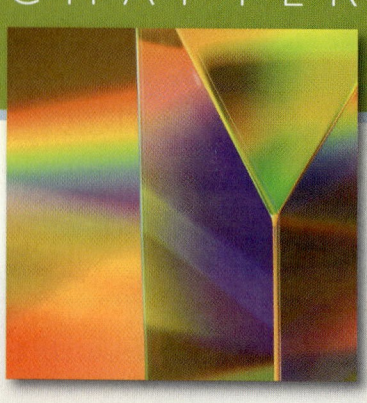

CHAPTER 8

Theory, Research, & Evidence-Based Practice

Learning Outcomes

After completing this chapter, you should be able to:

➤ Define *nursing theory*.

➤ Explain how the four building blocks (components) are used in developing a theory.

➤ List the four essential concepts in a *nursing* theory.

➤ List three ways in which you can use nursing theory.

➤ Name two prominent nurses who proposed theories of caring.

➤ Describe three non-nursing theories and their contributions to nursing.

➤ Discuss the significance of evidence-based nursing practice.

➤ Compare and contrast quantitative and qualitative nursing research.

➤ List three components of the research process and explain their importance.

➤ Name three priorities in the process of protecting research participants.

➤ Use the PICOT method to formulate a question for guiding a literature search.

➤ Discuss the process of analytic reading and explain its significance to the appraisal of research.

➤ Discuss how you might integrate nursing research into your nursing practice.

Key Concepts

Evidence-based practice

Nursing research

Nursing theory

Theory

Related Concepts

See the Concept Map at the end of this chapter.

Meet Your Patient

Imagine you are the charge nurse on the night shift at a long-term care facility. You hear the certified nursing assistant (CNA) and another person speaking loudly down the hall. You immediately go to see what has happened. You are startled by what you see. An older patient, Mr. Wilkey, is sitting on the bed of another patient, Mrs. Fredrickson, who is crying and shouting, "Get out! Get out!" Mr. Wilkey is tearful and looks frightened. He keeps repeating, "Where is Momma? Where is Momma?" The CNA is visibly upset and is grabbing at Mr. Wilkey in an effort to get him off the bed.

What are you going to do, and why do you think it will help? Don't be concerned if you don't think you know enough to answer this question. Before you read on, try to answer it based on the knowledge and experience that you *do* have.

One reaction might be to be upset with Mr. Wilkey and take him from the room immediately, explaining sternly that

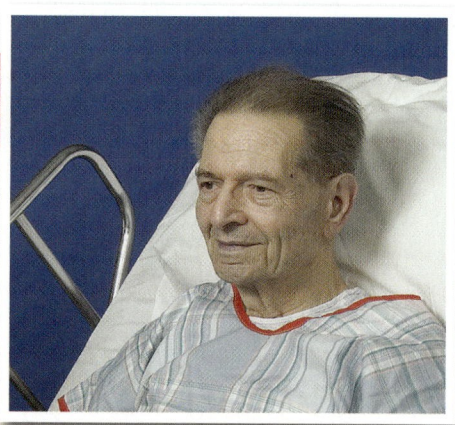

his behavior is not acceptable and he must stay in his room. Another possibility is to ask the CNA to calm Mrs. Fredrickson while you talk quietly to Mr. Wilkey and gently guide him out of the room, not rushing him. While you are talking to him, you might ask, "Who is Momma? What does she look like? Do you miss her?" By the time you lead him to his room, you might realize he is exhibiting stage II dementia. You infer that he probably woke up scared and confused and began looking for his long-dead mother. Seeing Mrs. Fredrickson, Mr. Wilkey thought he had found his mother and crawled into her bed.

This scenario demonstrates the powerful impact of nursing theory and research on your daily practice as a nurse. In the scenario:

- The first approach demonstrates **mechanistic nursing** (getting the tasks done).
- In the second approach, nursing behavior is based on **holistic nursing** (meeting the needs of the whole person).

ABOUT THE KEY CONCEPTS

The overall goal of this chapter is that you will understand the concepts of **nursing theory, nursing research,** and **evidence-based practice** well enough to see how they are related and how they form the foundations for patient care. You will learn about a related concept, *caring,* which is central to some theories and also to the full-spectrum nursing model in Chapter 2.

TheoreticalKnowledge
knowing **why**

This chapter introduces you to nursing theory and research and looks at them as the foundations for patient care. It emphasizes caring theory; however, in subsequent chapters you will find other theories that pertain to specific aspects of practice. For example, Chapter 9 uses developmental theories, Chapter 12 uses theories of self-esteem, and Chapter 14 makes use of family theories.

Think of full-spectrum nursing as a jigsaw puzzle (Fig. 8-1).

- *Practice, the first puzzle piece*—Initially, a nurse has an idea, which usually comes out of experiences in *practice.* Perhaps the idea is something simple, such as, "Why don't I slow down and spend more time with the patients' families? That would really help them."
- *Research, the second puzzle piece*—After seriously considering the idea, the nurse may decide it is worth investigating with *research.* The research question might be, "How does spending more time with family members affect the quality of care the patient receives?"
- *Theory, the third puzzle piece*—If the research supports the nurse's idea, she could then use the research findings to develop a *theory.* The nurse might even take the research results to nursing administrators to determine whether the theory could be put into practice in the organization— perhaps as a policy or in a standardized care plan. That would be the beginning of what is called a **clinical practice theory,** a theory that is immediately applicable in the clinical setting.

THE IMPORTANCE OF NURSING THEORY AND RESEARCH

Following are three classic examples that demonstrate how important theory and research are to you in your career as a nurse.

The Framingham Studies   The Framingham studies are a longitudinal, multidisciplinary research project (*longitudinal* means done over a long period of time). It consisted of several studies carried out over 50 years (from 1948 to 1998) to identify the health and healthcare practices of one community: Framingham, Massachusetts. The results of the various Framingham studies have influenced healthcare practices for diabetes mellitus, breast cancer, heart disease, osteoarthritis in older adults, and other disease entities. For example, there was a

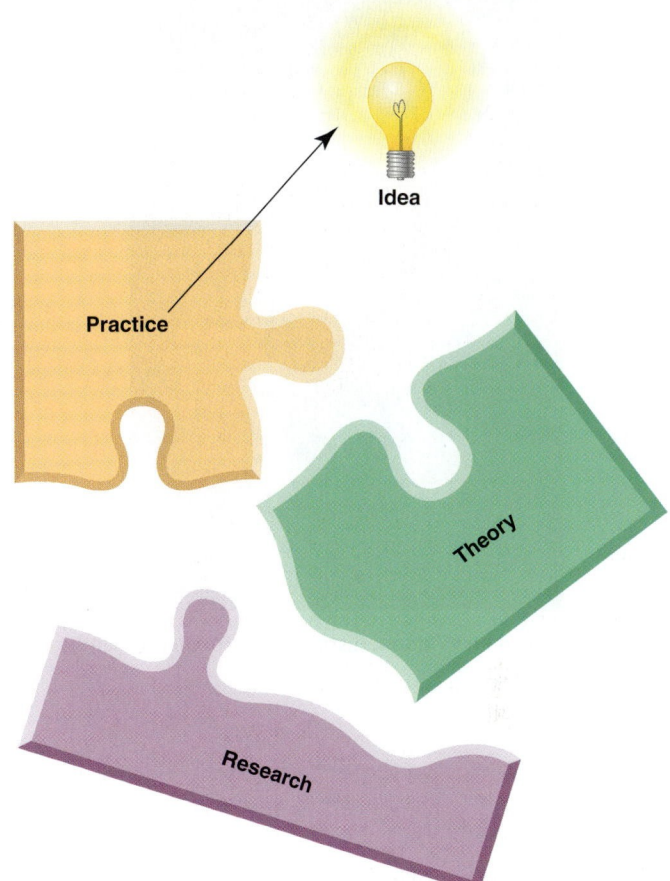

FIGURE 8-1 Practice, theory, and research are interrelated. A nurse has an idea, conducts research to test the idea, and finally develops a theory.

time when mammography was considered unreliable and unimportant in screening for breast cancer. The Framingham project changed that attitude and, as a result, improved the healthcare of women (Boston University, n.d.; National Heart, Lung, and Blood Institute, National Institutes of Health, 2015).

♥ **iCare** **Watson's Science of Human Caring** Dr. Jean Watson (Fig. 8-2) developed a nursing theory called the **Science of Human Caring** (Watson, 1988). This theory describes what *caring* means from a nursing perspective. It may not seem that nurses need to be taught how to care, but Dr. Watson and other nursing theorists found that they did. Before the so-called caring theorists, nurses were more mechanistic in the work they did, much like the first alternative for dealing with Mr. Wilkey (Meet Your Patient). A mechanistic nurse has a list of things to do, completes the list, and does nothing more. The "something more" often consists of caring behaviors, such as singing to a frightened child or taking the time to teach a new mother for the second time how to bathe her baby.

This is not to say that nurses didn't care about their patients before Watson. The point is that a *theory* can change the *focus* of nursing. Certainly Nightingale must have cared about the soldiers who were her patients. But what she wrote about and what she taught the nurses was a set of things to do. Nurses were valued for the tasks they performed in patient care. Caring theories demonstrate the value of the non–task oriented aspects of nursing.

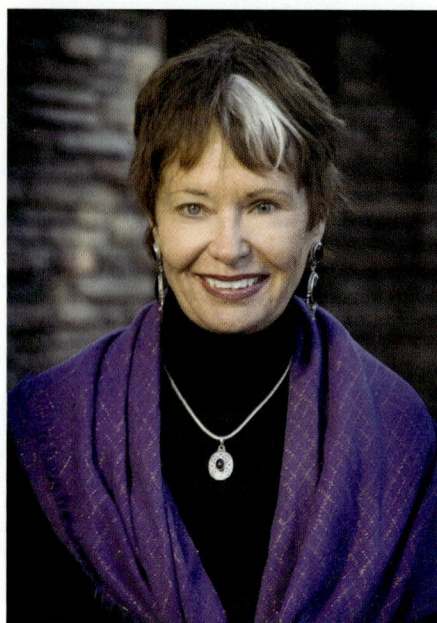

FIGURE 8-2 Dr. Jean Watson, distinguished professor and nursing theorist.

Benner's Novice to Expert Dr. Patricia Benner, in the book *From Novice to Expert* (1984), proposed a theory that should be of special interest to you. This theory, which is explained in Chapter 1, describes the progression of a beginning nurse to increasing levels of expertise. You are a **novice,** or a beginning nurse, simply because you are new to the nursing profession. Benner's theory provides the information necessary to understand how you learn and perform your nursing responsibilities. Benner's theory of caring is discussed later in this chapter.

KnowledgeCheck 8-1

- Compare mechanistic and holistic nursing. Select one of these concepts and describe a scenario in which it is used.
- Briefly describe the Framingham studies and list three diseases for which these studies influenced care.

NURSING THEORIES

Florence Nightingale (1859/1992) stated that nursing theories describe and explain what is and what is not nursing. That makes it helpful to learn them in the beginning of your nursing education. Before focusing on nursing theory, though, you need to learn a little more about theory in general. Exactly what *is* a theory? And how is a theory created?

A **theory** is an organized set of related ideas and concepts that helps us:

- Find meaning in our experiences (such as nursing).
- Organize our thinking around an idea (such as caring).
- Develop new ideas and insights into the work we do.

Stated simply, a theory answers the questions *What is this? And how does it work?* Although a theory is based on observations of facts, the theory itself is *not* a fact. A theory is merely a way of viewing phenomena (reality); it defines and illustrates concepts and explains how they are related or linked. **KEY POINT:** *Theories can be, and usually are, revised.*

What Are the Components of a Theory?

Theories are made up of assumptions, phenomena, concepts, definitions, and statements (or propositions). You can think of these as the building blocks of a theory.

Assumptions Ideas that we take for granted are called **assumptions.** In a theory, they are the ideas that the theorist or researcher presumes to be true and does not intend to test with research. For example, Watson assumed nursing had its own professional concepts and that one of them was caring. Assumptions may or may not be stated. For example, most nursing theorists assume but do not state that human beings are complex.

Phenomena Aspects of reality that you can observe and experience are called **phenomena.** Phenomena are the subject matter of a discipline (in that context, they are often called *phenomena of concern*). Think of phenomena as marking the boundaries *(domain)* of a discipline—making one discipline unique from another. For example, for pharmacists, the phenomena of concern are medications: their chemical composition and their effects on the body. For nurses, the phenomena of concern are human beings and, more specifically, their body-mind-spirit responses to illness and injuries. It may seem a subtle difference, but Watson's theory of caring gave us the words and ideas for describing the nursing phenomena of concern in terms of *human beings in their environments.*

Concepts A **concept** is a mental image of a phenomenon. Concepts represent observations or experiences. They are typically used to draw similarities, make distinctions among, organize, and categorize information, objects, or like ideas. For example, what does the word *fever* bring to mind? From your own experience with fever, you know the subjective feeling that fever produces. You have the theoretical knowledge that it is an elevated body temperature; you know the physiology of temperature regulation, so you know what is going on in the body. You may have the visual image of a thermometer or someone who is warm to the touch and possibly perspiring. The word *fever* is a symbol for all of those ideas and images. It is a concept.

Concepts range from simple to complex and from concrete to abstract. Simple, concrete concepts are those you can observe directly (e.g., height, gender). More abstract and complex concepts are those you observe indirectly (e.g., gender, nutritional status). Abstract concepts are those you must infer from many direct and indirect observations (e.g., self-esteem, wellness).

A theory usually contains several concepts. For example, Watson includes 10 "caring processes" in her original theory (Box 8-1). Each is a complex concept. She more recently refers to caring (carative) acts as *caritas.* This word comes from the Greek language, meaning "to cherish, to appreciate, and to give special, loving attention."

Definitions A **definition** is a statement of the meaning of a term or concept that sets forth the concept's characteristics or indicators—that is, the things that allow you to identify the concept. A definition may be general or specific.

- A **theoretical definition** refers to the conceptual meaning of a term (e.g., pain).
  - *Example:* Pain is an unpleasant sensory and emotional experience associated with actual or potential tissue damage.
- An **operational definition** specifies how you would observe or measure the concept (e.g., when doing research on pain).
  - *Example:* Pain is the patient's verbal statement that he is in pain.

BOX 8-1 ■ Watson's 10 Caring Processes

1. Forming a humanistic–altruistic system of values
2. Instilling faith and hope
3. Cultivating sensitivity to self and others
4. Forming helping and trusting relationships
5. Conveying and accepting the expression of positive and negative feelings
6. Systematically using the scientific problem-solving method that involves caring process
7. Promoting transpersonal teaching–learning
8. Providing for supportive; protective; and corrective mental, physical, sociocultural, and spiritual environment
9. Assisting with gratification of human needs
10. Sensitivity to existential–phenomenological forces

Source: Watson, J. (1988). *Nursing: Human science and human care. A theory of nursing* (NLN Publication No. 15-2236). New York, NY: National League for Nursing Press.

Statements Statements, or **propositions,** systematically describe the linkages and interactions among the concepts of a theory. The statements, taken as a whole, make up the theory. In Maslow's theory, for example, two concepts are *physiological needs* and *self-esteem needs.* An example of a statement in that theory would be the following: *"Physiological needs* must be met to an acceptable degree before a person can attempt to meet his *self-esteem needs."*

Paradigm, Framework, Model, or Theory?

In any discussion of nursing knowledge, you may hear the terms *paradigm, framework, model,* or *theory.* It may be difficult to differentiate between these terms because (1) they are so abstract, (2) they are defined differently by theorists, and (3) they are often used interchangeably in general conversation among nurses. As you progress in your career and education, you will need to pay careful attention to the similarities and differences among these terms. The following are some basic definitions:

A **paradigm** is the worldview or ideology of a discipline. It is the broadest, most global conceptual framework of a discipline. For example, the medical paradigm views a person through a lens that focuses on identifying and treating disease. This lens causes you to look in depth at the person's "parts" (e.g., cells, organs). The nursing paradigm views the person through a lens that focuses more broadly on the entire person and how he responds to isolated changes in his cells and organs. **KEY POINT:** *Paradigms are not theories; they are just "how we see things."*

A **conceptual framework** (also referred to as a *theoretical framework*) is a set of concepts that are related to form a whole or pattern. As a rule, frameworks are not developed using research processes and have not been tested in practice. Frameworks and models are broader and more philosophical than theories. Don't be concerned if you can't tell the difference between a theory and a theoretical framework. Experts don't always agree, either. Many theorists, for example, classify the early nursing theories (e.g., those presented in this chapter) as conceptual frameworks; others classify them as theories.

A **model** is a symbolic representation of a framework or concepts—a diagram, graph, picture, drawing, or physical model. The plastic body parts you have seen in anatomy class are three-dimensional models of the real human body. Figure 8-1 is a graphic model of the relationships between nursing practice, theory, and research. Some models are more complex.

A **conceptual model** (often used interchangeably with *conceptual framework*) is a model that is expressed in language—the symbols are words. In one sense, all models are "conceptual" because they all represent ideas. The full-spectrum model (see Fig. 2-3) is a conceptual model or framework.

For now, it is enough for you to remember that:

1. **KEY POINT:** *The terms* **theory, model,** *and* **framework** *all refer to a group of related concepts.*
2. The terms differ in meaning, depending on the extent to which the set of concepts has been used and tested in practice and on the level of detail and organization of the concepts.
3. A theory has a higher level of research, detail, and organization of concepts than do models and frameworks.

KnowledgeCheck 8-2

- Name the five building blocks of a theory.
- How is a *paradigm* different from a *theory?*

How Are Theories Developed?

As you learned in Figure 8-1, a theorist begins a theory with an idea that seems worth exploring. Then research is performed to see whether the ideas make sense. The validated ideas are used to develop the theory. Once the theorist has a research-based theory, she shares it with others, hoping to change nursing practice.

Theories are developed through a specific way of thinking called *logical reasoning* (Marriner-Tomey & Raile-Alligood, 2014). Generally, you can think of **reasoning** as connecting ideas in a way that makes sense. The purpose of **logical reasoning** is to develop an argument or statement based on evidence that will result in a logical conclusion. The most commonly used types of logical reasoning are inductive and deductive reasoning.

- **Inductive reasoning** is often used in the nursing process. If you walk into a person's room and note that the patient has a temperature of 101°F (38°C), a pulse of 104 beats/min, and respiration rate of 20 breaths/min, you could reasonably *induce* (conclude) that the person is ill. **KEY POINT:** *Induction moves from the specific to the general.* You gathered separate pieces of information, recognized a pattern, and formed a generalization. Remember induction by thinking, "INduction: I have specific data 'out there,' and I bring the data 'IN' to make the generalization" (Fig. 8-3).

- **Deductive reasoning** is the opposite of inductive reasoning. Deduction starts with a *general premise* and moves to a *specific deduction.* Suppose you receive a call from the emergency department stating they will be receiving a new patient with acute pyelonephritis (kidney infection). Because you know what is involved in the general premise (pyelonephritis), you deduce that the patient will probably have a fever and back pain. **KEY POINT:** *You have the "big picture" about what is true in general, and from that you can figure out logically what is likely to be true for a particular individual.*

Understanding logical thinking, even on this basic level, will help you understand the thinking that goes into both nursing theory and nursing research.

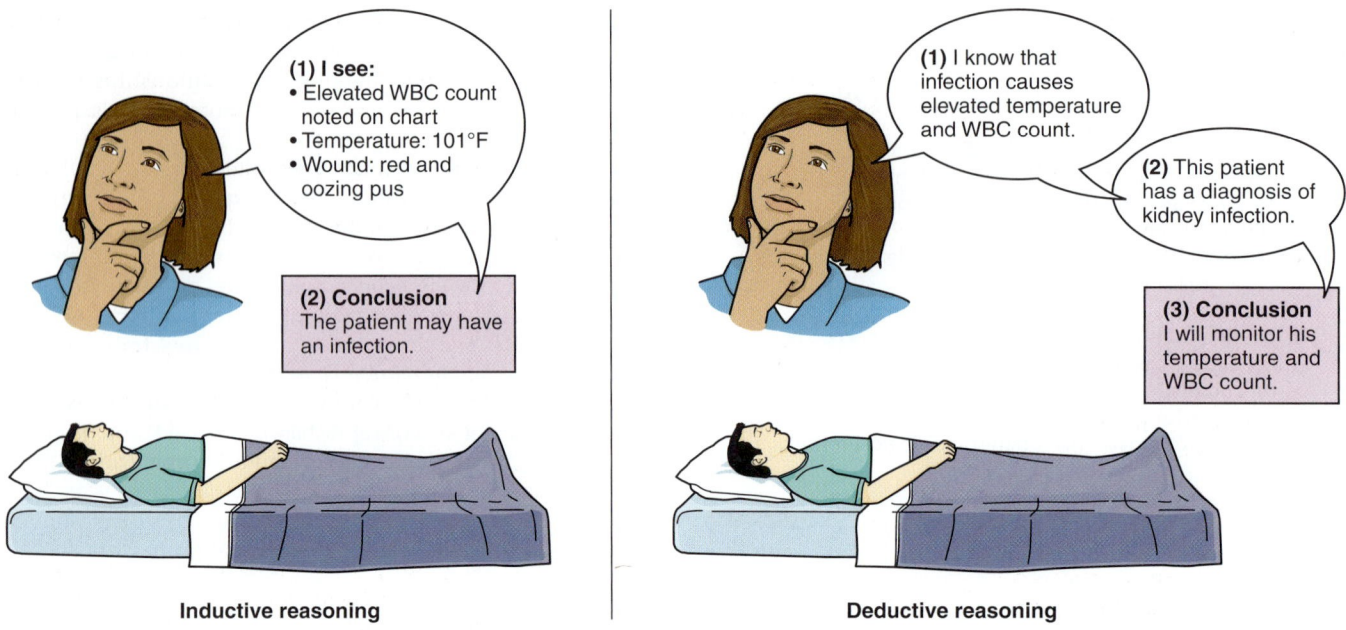

FIGURE 8-3 A comparison of inductive and deductive reasoning. Theorists and nurses in practice use both types of reasoning.

ThinkLike a Nurse 8-1

- Your patient is grimacing, groaning, and holding his hands over his abdominal incision. You induce that the patient is having incision pain. How could you be sure your induction is factual (true)?
- Earlier you deduced that your emergency department patient with pyelonephritis will have an elevated temperature and back pain. How confident are you that this is actually so? How could you be more certain your deduction is correct?

The preceding exercise should demonstrate that inductions and deductions are not "facts" or "truth," but rather that they point you in the direction to go in seeking truth (reality). Induction and deduction allow you to make connections between ideas when you are developing a theory. The more information you have to support your conclusions, the more confident you can be that they are correct.

What Are the Essential Concepts of a *Nursing* Theory?

Any nursing theory should address four basic concepts: **person, environment, health,** and **nursing** (Yura & Torres, 1975). These concepts are said to represent phenomena of concern for nursing. Notice this further divides the puzzle piece for nursing theory into four more pieces (Fig. 8-4).

A meaningful nursing theory defines those four puzzle pieces and explains how they are related to one another. Consider a theory that does not include the concept of person. Such a theory would not deal with the person's reaction to her health or lack of health. As a result, the person's learning needs, fears, family concerns, or discharge arrangements would not be considered. That sounds mechanistic, doesn't it?

Watson, in her science of human caring (1988), viewed the four basic concepts as follows: She explored the concept of *caring* as it relates to the person, environment, health, and nursing. Watson focused heavily on the *person* and the *nurse*. She talked about the "transpersonal" caring moments that exist

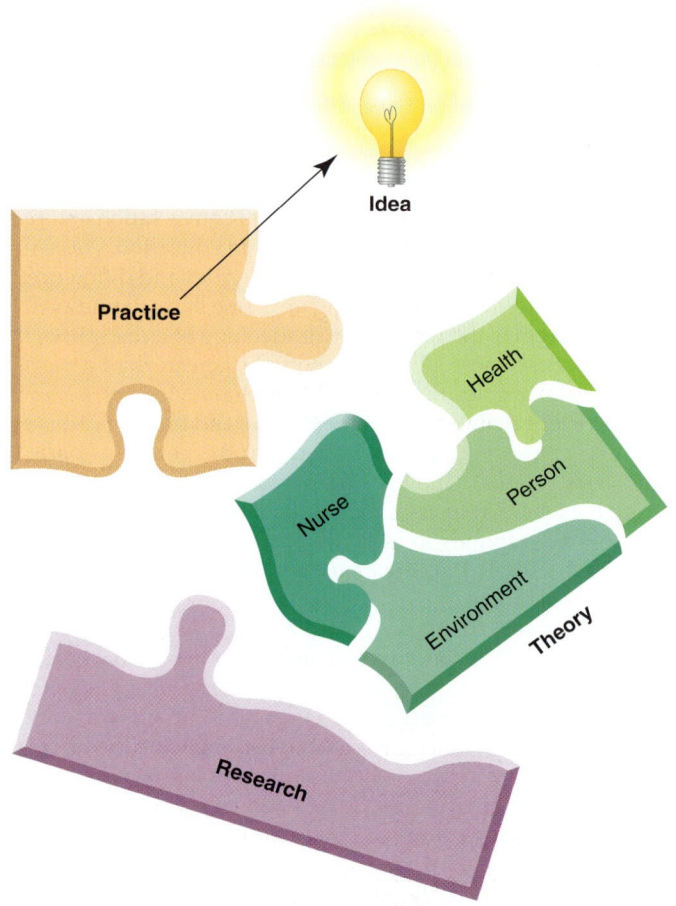

FIGURE 8-4 The four components of a nursing theory are person, nurse, health, and environment.

between the two. She presented the *environment* as another way to show caring: by keeping it clean, colorful, or quiet or including whatever promotes health for the person. All of the caring behaviors (see Box 8-1) listed in Watson's theory focus on improving the *health* of the person.

Observing nursing situations within the framework of the four components of nursing theory will help you understand the importance of each. This is very important because the finished puzzle reflects excellent (full-spectrum) nursing care.

ThinkLike a Nurse 8-2

Think of an experience you have had in clinical. Perhaps it was taking vital signs or bathing a confused patient. Describe how each of the four components of a nursing theory occurred in your clinical situation. Share your thinking with a classmate or coworker.

- Who was the *person(s)* involved (*person* refers to the patient or resident or the family and support persons)?
- What was the *environment*? A community center? A bathing room in a nursing home? The person's bedside in a hospital?
- What was the *health* condition of the person? For example, was the person seeking information for self-care? Critical? In pain? Ready for discharge?
- How was *nursing* involved? For example, was the nurse compassionate? Angry? Efficient? A novice or an expert?

KnowledgeCheck 8-3

- What are the four essential concepts in a nursing theory?
- What is the title of Dr. Watson's theory?
- Caring processes are critical to her theory. What is the purpose of the caring processes?

How Do Nurses Use Theories?

Nursing theories try to describe, explain, and predict human behavior. The case of Mr. Wilkey (Meet Your Patient) shows how the use of a certain theory might guide the nurse to more compassionate care. Think of a theory as a lens. You can see the stars more clearly if you look at them through a telescope than you can by using binoculars. Theories offer a way of looking at nursing, and in this way they affect your entire perspective. The theory you use influences what you look for, what you notice, what you perceive as a problem, what outcomes you hope to achieve, and what interventions you will choose.

In Nursing Practice

Nursing theories serve as a guide for assessment, problem identification, and nursing interventions. They help nurses communicate to others what it is that makes nurses unique and important to the interdisciplinary team.

Clinical practice theories very specifically guide what you do each day. They are limited in scope—that is, they do not attempt to explain all of nursing. A theory on human interaction can direct nurse–client communication; another theory provides a guide for teaching people how to be self-reliant. The following are other examples:

1. Nightingale's theory emphasized the importance of the environment in the care of patients. Her work affected the design and building of hospitals for decades.
2. Dr. Imogene Rigdon had the idea and developed a theory about bereavement of older women after noticing that older women handled grief differently from men and younger women (Rigdon, Clayton, & Dimond, 1987). Hospice organizations now use this theory to work with older women who have lost a significant other.
3. Nola Pender's theory (Pender, Murdaugh, & Parsons, 2015) on health promotion (see Chapter 27) is the basis for most health promotion teaching done by nurses.
4. Dr. Katharine Kolcaba (1994) developed a theory of holistic comfort in nursing that provides a more holistic view than earlier theories of pain and anxiety.

In Nursing Education

The theories used to guide program and curriculum planning in schools of nursing are frequently grand theories, such as Watson's theory of caring or Rogers's science of unitary human beings. A **grand theory** covers broad areas of concern within a discipline. A grand theory is usually abstract and does not outline specific nursing interventions. It tends to deal with the relationships between nurse, person, health, and environment.

An in-service education director in a nursing home may choose a **mid-range (or practice) theory** about comfort. Mid-range theories are narrower and more specific and can be used to create nursing protocols and procedures and design educational programs.

In Nursing Research

Researchers use theories and models as a framework for structuring a study. Theories provide a systematic way to define the questions to study, identify the variables to measure, and interpret the findings. For example, Kolcaba tested her statement that comfort interventions, as defined in her theory, would improve the health of the whole person.

Who Are Some Important Nurse Theorists?

As an educated nurse, you should have at least a basic understanding of the nurse theorists who have influenced nursing practice. The following three theorists, along with the caring theorists, are presented because of their historical significance. Their theories are simple and applicable to what you do every day as a nurse.

Florence Nightingale

As you learned in Chapter 1, Florence Nightingale revolutionized nursing. In the hospital in Scutari during the Crimean War, Nightingale's "idea" was that *more men would survive if they had a clean and healthy environment and nutritious food (so that the body could heal itself)*. That may not seem remarkable to you, but consider that the germ theory of infectious disease had not yet been identified.

Nightingale also was an outstanding researcher. She stayed awake late at night to keep records of what was happening at the hospital before and after she introduced her ideas (research). She used her research to develop her theory that a clean environment would improve the health of patients. Because of her theory and research, Nightingale dramatically reduced the death rate of the soldiers and changed the way the entire British Army hospital system was managed (Dossey, 1999).

Virginia Henderson

Virginia Henderson began her career as a U.S. Army nurse in 1918. She became a visiting nurse in New York City and then a teacher of nursing. Her pamphlet, *Basic Principles of Nursing Care,* was published in 1960 by the International Council of Nursing and has been translated into 20 languages.

While a nursing student at Walter Reed Army Hospital, Henderson began to question the mechanistic nursing care she was taught to give, as well as the fact she was expected to be the physicians' handmaiden. As a teacher of nursing, she came to recognize there were no clear descriptions of the purpose and function of nursing. She was the first nurse to identify that as a concern. Her idea was that *nurses deserve to know what it means to be a nurse.*

Henderson's 1966 book, *The Nature of Nursing,* described her theory of nursing's primary, unique function. She identified 14 basic needs that are addressed by nursing care (Box 8-2). Although the simple things on that list are commonplace today, they had not been identified as components of nursing care until Virginia Henderson did so. Henderson's (1966, p. 3) definition of nursing states that "the unique function of the nurse is to assist the individual, sick or well, in the performance of those activities contributing to health or its recovery (or to a peaceful death) that he would perform unaided if he had the necessary strength, will or knowledge. And do this in such a way as to help him gain independence as rapidly as possible." Through her work, Henderson defined what nursing was in the 20th century.

Hildegard Peplau

Hildegard E. Peplau was born in 1909 to immigrant parents in Pennsylvania. She was a psychiatric nurse who influenced the advancement of standards in nursing education, promoted self-regulation in nursing through credentialing, and was a strong advocate for advanced nursing practice.

Dr. Peplau's idea was that *health could be improved for psychiatric patients if there were a more effective way to communicate with them.* Again, you may feel this is an unnecessary theory because nurses communicate with patients all the time. But remember that in the early 1900s, actually talking to and developing a

personal relationship with psychiatric patients simply was not done. Psychiatric patients did not have the benefit of psychotropic drugs, so they were often agitated and extremely difficult to communicate with.

Peplau's research showed that developing a relationship with psychiatric patients does make their treatment more effective. She developed the theory of interpersonal relations, which focuses on the relationship a nurse has with the patient. This is a theory you use every day without even knowing it existed.

The Caring Theorists

It could be argued that the three leading caring theorists in nursing are Dr. Jean Watson, Dr. Patricia Benner, and Dr. Madeleine Leininger. We have been using Watson's ideas to illustrate principles and concepts of theory. In this section, we discuss Benner and Leininger.

Patricia Benner

♥ **iCare**   *Caring* is the central concept in Benner and Wrubel's *primacy of caring model.* The nurse's caring helps the client cope. Moreover, it offers opportunity for the nurse to connect with others and to receive as well as give help (Benner & Wrubel, 1989). Caring involves personal concern for persons, events, projects, and things. Therefore, it reveals what is stressful for a person (because if something does not matter to a person, it will not create stress) and provides motivation. Caring also makes the nurse notice which interventions are effective. This theory stresses that each person is unique, so that caring is always specific and relational for each nurse–person encounter.

In Chapter 1, we discussed another of Benner's theories. As a critical care nurse, she wanted to find out *what makes an expert nurse.* In this case, the idea took the form of a question. An example of an expert nurse, for her, was an intensive care unit (ICU) nurse who knew intuitively when it was time to extubate a critical patient. To discover what makes a nurse expert enough to know that and other critical information, Benner interviewed ICU nurses and, from her data, identified five stages of knowledge development and acquisition of nursing skills. As you may recall, the first level is that of a novice nurse (you). The others are advanced beginner, competent, proficient, and expert nurse (see Chapter 1 if you need to review).

Let's see whether this novice-to-expert theory addresses the four components of a nursing theory. *Person* and *nurse* are very clearly points of focus. Knowing the *nurse's* skill level (novice, advanced beginner, competent, proficient, or expert) provides for a logical way to match the nurse's skill with the patient's *(person)* acuity. This is the basis of the theory. The theory also indicates that the nurse contributes to the person's *health* according to her skill level. The *environment* is clearly stated as the ICU. Benner's theory does meet the criteria of the four concepts of a nursing theory, although as in most theories, some components are emphasized more than others.

Madeleine Leininger

Leininger is the founder of transcultural nursing and was the first nurse in the United States to earn a doctoral degree in cultural and social anthropology. Her theory focuses on caring as **cultural competence** (using knowledge of cultures and of nursing to provide culturally congruent and responsible care). Her idea came from working with children from diverse cultures who were under her care in a psychiatric hospital: *Would psychotherapy for children be more effective if delivered within the framework of the child's culture?* (See Marriner-Tomey & Raile-Alligood, 2014.)

BOX 8-2 ■ Virginia Henderson's List of Basic Needs

1. Breathe normally.
2. Eat and drink adequately.
3. Eliminate body wastes.
4. Move and maintain desirable posture.
5. Sleep and rest.
6. Select suitable clothes—dress and undress.
7. Maintain body temperature within normal range by adjusting clothing and modifying the environment.
8. Keep the body clean and well groomed and protect the integument.
9. Avoid dangers in the environment and avoid injuring others.
10. Communicate with others in expressing emotions, needs, fears, or opinions.
11. Worship according to one's faith.
12. Work in such a way that there is a sense of accomplishment.
13. Play or participate in various forms of recreation.
14. Learn, discover, or satisfy the curiosity that leads to normal development and health and use of the available health facilities.

Source: Marriner-Tomey, A., & Raile-Alligood, M. (2014). *Nursing theorists and their work* (8th ed.). St. Louis, MO: C.V. Mosby.

Leininger performed the research to confirm her idea that culturally competent care made a difference, and then she developed her theory. The theory includes all the puzzle pieces referred to throughout this chapter.

- *Person*—an individual with cultural beliefs that are specific to herself and that may differ from the beliefs of others. All human beings can feel concern for others, but ways of caring vary across cultures.
- *Nurse*—the professional who values the cultural diversity of the person and is willing to make cultural accommodations for the health benefit of the person. This requires specialized cultural knowledge.
- *Environment*—wherever the *nurse* and the *person* are together in the healthcare system
- *Health*—defined by the *person* and may be culturally specific in its definition.

You will learn more about Leininger's theory in Chapter 15. You may be thinking, "This is all about culture; what does that have to do with caring?" Leininger's theory brings together the cultures of the *person,* the *nurse,* and the *healthcare system* (indeed, there is a culture of healthcare, as you will discover in Chapter 15) to improve healthcare delivery and its effectiveness.

A nurse tells this true culture-care story. It is an example of applying a theory directly to the needs of an ill person:

As a young nurse, I was caring for a patient who was a monk. He had just had surgery, and he would not take any pain medication. He wanted to "offer the pain up to God." I believed the patient was jeopardizing his health, yet respected his right to live his beliefs. We worked out a compromise. The monk agreed to take pain medication every 8 hours (instead of the prescribed every 3 to 4 hours), and I made sure to attend to his ambulation, hygiene, and other needs during the times the medication was in effect.

Other Selected Nurse Theorists

You will find a list of selected nurse theorists and a brief description of their theories in Table 8-1.

KnowledgeCheck 8-4

Define in a brief conceptual form or title the nursing theory of each theorist listed below:
- Florence Nightingale
- Virginia Henderson
- Hildegard Peplau

How Do Nurses Use Theories From Other Disciplines?

Theory development is relatively new in nursing. Except for Nightingale (1859/1992), it was not until the mid-1950s that nursing leaders began to publish their theories about nursing. The profession relied heavily on the theories of other disciplines (you may hear these referred to as "borrowed" theories). Nurses still use knowledge from other disciplines as a part of their scientific knowledge base. The following sections discuss a few of the many theories used by other disciplines that, nevertheless, apply in nursing.

Maslow's Hierarchy of Basic Human Needs

One classic theory still used in most nursing education and practice settings is Maslow's hierarchy of needs (1970). Maslow observed that certain human needs are common to all people, but some needs are more basic than others. The lower-level (e.g., physiological) needs must be met to some degree before the higher needs (e.g., self-esteem) can be achieved (Fig. 8-5). For example, if you sit down to study but the room is cold, you will likely decide to put on a sweater or turn up the heat before you can focus on what you are learning. Nevertheless, a person may consciously choose to ignore a lower-level need in order to achieve a higher need. For example, the first responders at the World Trade Center on 9/11 and volunteer disaster workers for Hurricane Katrina in 2005 ignored their need for safety and security to help others (transcendence of self). In reality, most needs are not completely satisfied, nor completely unsatisfied.

KEY POINT: *Everyone has a dominant need, but it varies among individuals.* For example, a teenager may have a self-esteem need to be accepted by a group. A tobacco addict needs to satisfy her cravings for nicotine and will be less concerned with the long-term effects on health.

Physiological Needs Physiological needs, the most basic, are those that must be met to maintain life. They include the needs for food, air, water, temperature regulation, elimination, rest, sex, and physical activity. Most healthy adults meet their physiological needs through self-care. However, many of your nursing interventions will support patients' physiological needs.

Safety and Security Needs The needs for safety and security are the next priority. Safety and security may refer to either physical or emotional needs. *Physical safety and security* mean protection from physical harm (e.g., falls, infection, and effects of medications) and having adequate shelter (e.g., housing with sanitation, heat, and safety). *Emotional safety and security* involve freedom from fear and anxiety—feeling safe in the physical environment as well as in relationships. We need the security of a home and family. If there is an abusive husband, for example, the wife will spend most of her time and energy trying not to trigger episodes of violence or abuse. This leaves little attention for meeting self-esteem and other higher needs.

Love and Belonging Needs Needs for love and belonging are sometimes called social or affiliation needs. When they dominate, the person strives for meaningful relationships with others. Everyone has a basic need to love and be loved, give and receive affection, and have a feeling of belonging (e.g., in a family, peer group, or community). When these needs are not met, a person may feel isolated and lonely and may withdraw or become demanding and critical.

Self-Esteem Needs People who have begun to satisfy their need to belong may begin to feel the need for self-esteem. Self-esteem comes through a sense of accomplishment and recognition from others and brings confidence and independence. As we discuss in Chapter 13, illness can affect self-esteem by causing role changes (e.g., inability to perform one's job), or a change of body image (e.g., loss of a body part). When recognition cannot be obtained through positive behaviors, the person may resort to disruptive or irresponsible actions.

Self-Actualization Needs The highest level on Maslow's original hierarchy, self-actualization refers to the need to reach your full potential and to act unselfishly. At this level, a person develops wisdom and knows what to do in a variety of situations.

In his later work, Maslow identified two growth needs that must be met before reaching self-actualization (Maslow & Lowery, 1998):

Cognitive needs to know, understand, and explore

Aesthetic needs for symmetry, order, and beauty

Transcendence of Self Later research led Maslow to identify another even higher need (Maslow, 1971): the need for

Table 8-1 ➤ Selected Nurse Theorists

THEORIST	THEORY
Peplau, Hildegard E. 1952	Interpersonal relations model: Interpersonal communication can improve mental health.
Henderson, Virginia 1955	14 basic needs addressed by nursing care; definition of nursing; do for the patient what he cannot do for himself.
Abdellah, Faye G. 1960	21 nursing problems; deliver care to the whole person.
Orlando, Ida Jean 1961	Interpersonal process; nursing process theory.
Wiedenbach, Ernestine 1964	The purpose of nursing is to support and meet patients' needs for help. Nursing is a helping art.
Levine, Myra 1967, 1973	Conservation model; designed to promote adaptation of the person while maintaining wholeness, or health.
Johnson, Dorothy 1968, 1980	The behavioral system model: Incorporates five principles of systems thinking to establish a balance or equilibrium (adaptation) in the person. The patient is a behavioral system consisting of subsystems.
Rogers, Martha 1970	The science of unitary human beings focuses on the betterment of humankind through new and innovative modalities. Maintaining an environment free of negative energy is important.
Orem, Dorothea 1971	The self-care deficit nursing theory explains what nursing care is required when people are not able to care for themselves. The goal is to help the client attain total self-care.
King, Imogene 1971	First of two theories was the interacting systems framework, designed to explain the organized wholes within which nurses are expected to function, i.e., society, groups, and individuals. The first theory led to the theory of goal attainment, which focuses on mutual goal setting between a nurse and patient and the process for meeting the goals.
Neuman, Betty 1972	Neuman's systems model is based on general system theory (a non-nursing theory) and reflects the nature of living organisms as open systems.
Roy, Sr. Callista 1974	Adaptation model was inspired by the strength and resiliency of children. The model relates to the choices that people make as they adapt to illness and wellness.
Leininger, Madeleine M. 1978, 1984	Cultural care diversity and universality theory. Caring theory.
Newman, Margaret 1979	Theory of health as expanding consciousness describes nursing intervention as nonintervention, in which the nurse's presence helps patients recognize their own pattern of interacting with the environment.
Watson, Jean 1979	Caring theory. Nursing is an interpersonal process.
Parse, Rosemarie Rizzo 1981	Theory of human becoming focuses on the human-universe-health process and knowledge related to human becoming (or reaching one's potential).
Benner, Patricia, and Wrubel, Judith 1989	Primacy of caring model. Caring is central to the model and helps the client cope with stressors of illness. Knowledge is acquired in stages.

transcendence of self. This is the drive to connect to something beyond one's self and to help others realize their potential. Some people include spirituality at this level, which is also the basis for acts of self-sacrifice (e.g., donating a kidney so that another person can live).

Applying Maslow's Theory   The following example illustrates how you might use Maslow's theory when teaching patients. Suppose you have been assigned to teach your patient about how to care for her colostomy before her discharge. Because she speaks little English, you obtain materials in her

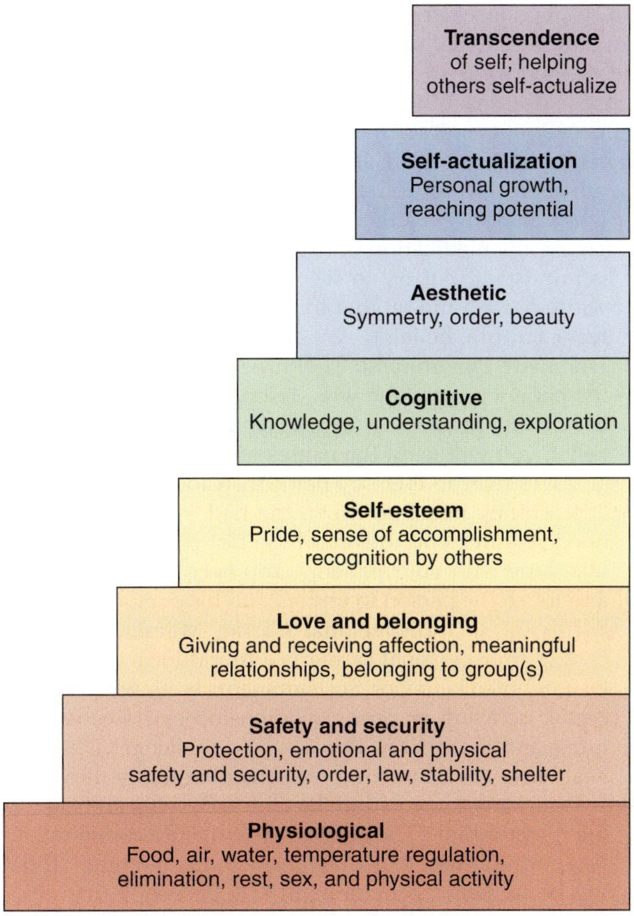

FIGURE 8-5 Maslow's hierarchy of human needs is a theory nurses use every day.

primary language, and you have arranged for an interpreter in case she has some questions you can't understand or answer. As you enter the room to begin teaching, you observe that she seems to be in a great deal of pain. What will you do?

Maslow's hierarchy of needs tells you that until the pain (a physiological need) is controlled, your patient cannot learn. (Maslow considered pursuit of knowledge a self-actualization need.) You arrange for pain medication to be administered and reschedule the teaching session. If you went ahead with the teaching, the experience would be for the sole purpose of crossing it off your list (remember mechanistic nursing?) rather than actually teaching.

Validation Theory

Validation theory (Feil, 2003) arises from social work and provides for a way to communicate with older people with dementia. The theory asks the caregiver to *go where the demented person is in his own mind.* For example, Mr. Wilkey (Meet Your Patient) is talking about his mother, who has been dead for many years. Learning of his mother's death would be a shocking and traumatic experience, which he would relive each time he heard the news. So instead of telling him that she is dead, you would *go where Mr. Wilkey is in his own mind* by asking him, for example, about the color of his mother's eyes, what songs she sings to him, or other personal questions that will likely stimulate meaningful conversation about his mother.

Stress and Adaptation Theory

Hans Selye (1993) developed the stress and adaptation theory. His was the forerunner of the many existing theories about stress. Selye's theory states that a certain amount of stress is good for people; it keeps them motivated and alert. However, too much stress, called *distress,* results in physiological symptoms and eventual illness. Does that happen to you at the end of the semester when you are distressed over the number of papers due and the difficulty of the tests for which you are studying? Generally, the human body will respond to distress with an illness, such as a cold, that will force the body to slow down or simply go to bed. Selye's theory is discussed more in Chapter 12.

Developmental Theories

Developmental theories look at stages through which individuals, groups, families, and communities progress over time. The following are some important examples:

- Erickson's psychosocial developmental theory (discussed in Chapter 9)
- Theories of family development (discussed in Chapters 13 and 14)
- Kohlberg's and Gilligan's theories of moral development (discussed in Chapters 9 and 44)

These theories are useful in nursing practice because they identify norms and expectations at various stages of development and help you identify activities and interventions that are appropriate for your client.

System Theory

Ludwig von Bertalanffy created system theory in the 1940s (von Bertalanffy, 1976). He intended it to be abstract enough to use for theory and research in any discipline. Today the understanding of systems has evolved to the point that many of the concepts are a part of our everyday language (e.g., healthcare system, body systems, information systems, family systems).

KEY POINT: *One of the premises of systems theory is that all complex phenomena, regardless of their type, have some principles, laws, and organization in common.* A **system** is made up of separate components (or **subsystems**), which constantly interact with one another and with other systems. For example, the cardiovascular and renal systems are subsystems of the body; the cells are subsystems of those systems. All of those systems and subsystems exchange processes and information with one another and with systems outside the body.

A system maintains some organization even though it is constantly facing internal and external changes. All systems have some common elements. For example, the goal (function) of any system is to process **input** (the energy, information, or materials that enter the system) for use within the system or in the **environment** (everything outside the system) or both. Other common elements include the following:

- **Output** is the product or service that results from the system's throughput. Examples of output are documents, money, cars, and nursing diagnoses.
- **Throughput** consists of the processes the system uses to convert input (raw materials) into output (products). Examples of throughput are thinking, planning, sorting, meeting in groups, sterilizing, hammering, and cutting.
- **Feedback** is information about some aspect of the processing that is used to monitor the system and make its performance more effective (e.g., evaluation in the nursing process: how the patient responded to the interventions).

- **Open systems** exchange information and energy freely with the environment. Open systems are capable of growth, development, and adaptation. Examples of open systems include people, body systems, hospitals, and businesses.
- **Closed systems** have fixed, automatic relationships among their components and little give-and-take with the environment. One example is a rock. A nursing example is a family that is isolated from the community and resists outside influences.

Several nursing theories have been built on system theory, for example, Johnson's (1968, 1980) behavioral system model, King's (1971) interacting systems framework, and the Neuman systems model (Neuman & Young, 1972), to name a few.

KnowledgeCheck 8-5

- Name four theories that nurses "borrow" from other disciplines.
- What are the five original levels of Maslow's basic human needs (not including cognitive needs, aesthetic needs, and transcendence)?

PracticalKnowledge
knowing **how**

Practical knowledge about theory means using theories to guide you in your use of the nursing process. Recall the lens metaphor.

- *Assessment.* In the assessment step of the nursing process, your theory concepts and principles tell you what to assess and provide the rationale for the assessments. Its major concepts serve as categories for organizing the data.
- *Diagnosis.* In the diagnosis step, your theory guides you in defining patient problems; in fact, it determines whether you will even recognize a cluster of cues as a problem.
- *Outcomes and Interventions.* The theory helps you to generate appropriate, achievable client outcomes; to choose effective nursing interventions; and to provide rationales for your actions.

There is no reason to read about theory unless you can apply the information. To show you how, this section applies caring theory to the planning of nursing interventions. Of course, you can use *any* theory for this purpose. We use caring theory because of the powerful and positive impact it can have on your nursing care. In reading this chapter, you should have become familiar with two well-known caring theories. Test your recall by writing the theorists' names and basic ideas. If you have difficulty, be sure to review the information about caring theorists before proceeding.

ThinkLike a Nurse 8-3

Write a paragraph describing a clinical experience in which you applied or observed one or both of the caring theories. Record your thinking on a piece of paper and be prepared to share it with your classmates. You may title it "My Experience in Caring."

Planning Theory-Based Interventions/Implementation

The Nursing Interventions Classification, or NIC (Bulechek, Butcher, Dochterman, et al., 2013), introduced in Chapter 6, is theory development in an early stage. Each of the standardized intervention labels (e.g., Exercise Promotion, Infection Control) is a concept, and defining or describing concepts is an important step in theory development. In this section, we use nine key concepts of Watson's caring theory to describe how a theory might influence your choice of nursing activities and approaches.

1. **Holistic Nursing Care.** Holistic nursing care allows nurses to examine the complete person and his context when making healthcare decisions. It goes beyond just giving the medication or dressing a wound. Physical care is important, but try to see nursing as giving care to the entire person and all that this entails (e.g., family, friends, fears, cultural beliefs).

2. **Honoring Personhood.** The three caring theorists believe the patient is someone who deserves to be honored for individuality in behavior as well as needs. If you accept that belief, you will learn the names of the people in your care and will refer to them by name instead of "Room 331," or "the kidney infection down the hall." Honoring personhood requires you to control the fast pace of nursing and take time with your patients. You need to look at, talk to, and touch the person to understand his personhood.

♥ **iCare   3. Transpersonal Caring Moments.** The concept of transpersonal caring is a moral ideal rather than a task-oriented behavior. Such moments occur when an actual caring occasion or caring relationship exists between the nurse and the person. This can be a challenge! The current healthcare environment moves people rapidly through the system. How can you find the time to develop authentic caring relationships? The first step is to make a commitment to be a caring nurse: to go to work with the thought, "Today I will be authentic [genuine, real] with the people in my care." Or you might think, "I will focus on creating transpersonal caring moments instead of rushed and harried interactions." As a student, you might think, "Today I will practice changing dressings or starting intravenous solutions." However, developing the ability to have transpersonal caring moments is just as important. Think back to Mr. Wilkey at the beginning of the chapter. Where did opportunities arise for transpersonal caring moments with him?

4. **Personal Presence.** Another phrase for being authentic and in the moment is *personal presence*. The concept of presence suggests that you, the nurse, are emotionally and physically *with* the person for the time you are there. You are not thinking about a medication you need to give or medical orders you need to get. If the person in the bed is fearful, you should be fully present, recognize the fear, and support the person experiencing it. Your support may take the form of answering simple questions or providing more in-depth education. It may simply be staying with the person for 2 or 3 minutes while quietly listening and holding her hand. As your psychomotor and nursing process skills become second nature to you, you will find it easier to remain in the moment.

5. **Comfort.** Some nurses think of comfort as the relief of pain, but it is much more. In Kolcaba's (1994) theory, comfort occurs in four contexts: physical, psychospiritual, social, and environmental. For example, is the person comfortable with you as the caregiver? Some women, especially from Middle Eastern or Asian cultures, are uncomfortable with male nurses as their caregivers. You must know and respect the person's cultural values. Other aspects to consider for a complex picture of comfort are whether

- The patient's modesty is being respected.
- There is too much or too little environmental stimuli.

- The room temperature is not too cold nor too warm.
- The patient needs more rest periods in order to heal.
- The patient needs someone to spend a transpersonal caring moment with him so he can express fears and anxiety.

6. **Listening.** Listening requires you to quiet your mind and truly listen with your mind and heart. The caring theorists also talk about listening from within yourself. Some call that *intuition.* Benner believes it is intuition that allows nurses to advance to expert-level practice.

7. **Spiritual Care.** Spiritual care is a critical aspect of holistic nursing care. You need to know what an individual's spiritual needs are and make appropriate plans to meet them. If the person does not want to talk about or deal with her spirituality, you will listen and follow her instructions. However, generally the opposite is true. People who are ill often want to talk about their spiritual needs, but they may be uncomfortable doing so. Helping someone to meet spiritual needs may be as simple as offering to call a clergy member or praying with the person who is sick. Chapter 16 provides more information about spiritual care.

♥ **iCare** 8. **Caring for the Family.** Nurses who base their practice on caring theories recognize the importance of including the family of the person who is receiving care. Nontraditional family structure is not a reason to withdraw support, even if it conflicts with your values. What about an older family member with dementia? This person deserves to know what is happening to his loved one even though he most likely will forget the information. If he does forget, patiently repeat what he needs to know. You will find more information about family care in Chapter 14.

9. **Cultural Competence.** This was discussed in the explanation of Leininger's cultural care theory. Also see Chapter 15 if you want more information.

Do you see the value of each of these nine abstract concepts? From them flow very real, concrete nursing actions that make a difference in the lives of patients. Understanding nursing theories and applying them throughout your career is essential to full-spectrum nursing care. To perform the essential clinical tasks of nursing within the framework of caring is the highest possible performance of the profession.

KnowledgeCheck 8-6

List and explain three ways to incorporate caring theory into your nursing care.

NURSING RESEARCH

You now have a good beginning (novice) grasp of the concepts in nursing theory. Remember the puzzle pieces (see Fig. 8-2)? A nurse has an idea, does research to determine whether the idea is a valid one, and then develops a nursing theory. It is now time to study the research piece of the puzzle.

TheoreticalKnowledge
knowing **why**

Were you aware of the research done in the field of caring before reading this chapter? Most novice nurses would not be. Remember the Framingham studies, which changed medical and nursing practice? Had you heard of that before you read about it in this book? Many people, including some nurses, do not realize that nurses do research. They think of nurses as people who work in hospitals, wear scrubs, and carry a stethoscope in their pocket. To be an effective professional nurse in the 21st century, you need to understand the basic principles of nursing research and their powerful impact on healthcare and the nursing profession. This section of the chapter is designed to show you what research is and how to incorporate it into your practice.

Definition Although there are many definitions of nursing research, this chapter defines **nursing research** as the systematic, objective process of analyzing phenomena of importance to nursing (Nieswiadomy, 2012). Its purpose is to develop knowledge about issues that are important in nursing. Nursing research encompasses all clinical practice arenas, nursing education, and nursing administration.

Evidence-Based Practice Example Nurse researchers currently are making important contributions to the evidence-based practice necessary for professional nursing. Consider this example: When you are in the clinical setting, you will notice that when a nurse discontinues an intravenous (IV) fluid infusion, she sometimes replaces it with a lock, or plug, to maintain a route for IV medications, even though the patient no longer needs the fluids. Not many years ago, she would periodically flush the plug with heparin to keep blood from clotting and blocking the IV catheter. But heparin is a drug, and it has side effects. Nurses and other professionals performed several studies to see whether saline (which has no side effects) would work just as well. Goode and colleagues (1996) performed a meta-analysis of those studies showing that saline was indeed just as effective, and it is now the standard of care in most institutions. (A **meta-analysis** combines and analyzes the data from several different studies.)

Why Should I Learn About Research?

The best reason for learning about research, of course, is that the ability to read and use nursing research enhances your ability to give quality patient care. A practical reason is that educational and practice standards require that you acquire a degree of research competence. Like theory, research affects you every day you are a nurse.

Full-spectrum nurses participate in research by doing the following:

- Identifying ideas that should be examined through the research process
- Assisting in, designing, and/or performing research
- Using research as a basis for their practice

ANA Standards

The position of the American Nurses Association (ANA) is that all nurses share a commitment to the advancement and ethical conduct of nursing science (ANA, 2015). The registered nurse integrates evidence and research findings into practice. Competencies of the ANA Standards of Professional Performance, Standard 13, Evidence-Based Practice and Research include the following competencies:

- "Identifies questions in the healthcare setting and practice that can be answered by nursing research.
- Promotes ethical principles of research in practice and the healthcare setting.
- Uses current evidence-based nursing knowledge, including research findings, to guide practice decisions.

- Incorporates evidence when initiating changes in nursing practice.
- Participates in the formulation of evidence-based practice through research.
- Shares peer-reviewed research findings with colleagues to integrate into nursing practice." (ANA, 2015, p. 77).

Educational Competencies

QSEN. Recall that the Quality and Safety Education for Nurses (QSEN) project has identified quality and safety competencies for nurses. One important competency is evidence-based practice: the ability to "integrate the best current evidence with clinical expertise and patient/family preferences and values for delivery of optimal healthcare" (Cronenwett, Sherwood, Barnsteiner, et al., 2007).

Institute of Medicine. The Institute of Medicine (IOM) core competencies for health providers are the basis for the Safe, Effective Nursing Care (SENC) competencies used in this text. See Chapter 1. The competencies related to research include the following:

IOM—Employ evidence-based practice.
SENC—Validate evidence-based research to incorporate in practice:
- Incorporate evidence-based findings into client care.
- Evaluate client outcomes using valid and reliable research tools.

What Is the History of Nursing Research?

The records Florence Nightingale kept while nursing soldiers in the Crimea were the beginning of formalized nursing research. As she developed schools of nursing throughout Britain and the United States, Nightingale urged her students to do clinical research. Yet because she had passed on to them the authoritarian tradition of her time, they were usually not prepared to perform it. Authority-style education does not promote intellectual inquiry or critical thinking, two characteristics essential for research. This is one reason nursing research was slow to develop, although this is rapidly changing now with nursing's professional commitment to evidence-based practice.

Nursing research is now supported by federal funds and private grants, and results are reported in a growing number of nursing (and other) research journals. Nurses present their research at national and international conferences and publish their results in national and international journals. The preparation of doctoral-level nurses with a strong background in research has enhanced the quality and diversity of nursing research.

How Are Priorities for Nursing Research Developed?

Nursing research provides evidence on which to base nursing care. Ideally, all nursing interventions should be validated through research to show their safety and effectiveness. Professional organizations, such as the ANA and specialty organizations (e.g., the Oncology Nursing Society), have established research priorities that will assist nursing to build a strong knowledge base in areas of importance to society. The National Institute of Nursing Research (NINR), a federally funded agency that is a part of the National Institutes of Health (NIH), periodically identifies research themes and priorities for funding.

KnowledgeCheck 8-7
- Define *nursing research*.
- According to the text, why has nursing research been slow to develop?

What Educational Preparation Does a Researcher Need?

At each level of educational preparation, nurses function in different roles in the research process.

Associate Degree and Diploma Nursing At this educational level, there are four research roles you can fulfill. You can (1) be aware of the importance of research to evidence-based practice, (2) help identify problem areas in nursing, (3) help collect data with a more experienced nurse researcher, and (4) use evidence-based practice in planning nursing interventions.

Baccalaureate Degree in Nursing If you are a baccalaureate-prepared nurse, you should be able to:
- Critique research for application to clinical practice.
- Identify nursing research problems and help implement research studies.
- Apply research findings to establish sound, evidence-based clinical practice.

Master's Degree in Nursing Nurses with graduate degrees should be able to:
- Analyze problems so that appropriately designed research can be used to solve the problem.
- Through clinical expertise, apply evidence-based practice to nursing care situations.
- Provide support to ongoing research projects.
- Conduct research for the purpose of assuring quality nursing care.

Doctoral Degree in Nursing or Related Field Doctorally prepared nurses are specifically educated to be nurse researchers. They are qualified to:
- Conduct nursing research.
- Serve as leaders in applying research results to the clinical arena.
- Develop ways to monitor the quality of nursing care being administered by nurses (adapted from ANA, 1981).
- In addition, they should disseminate their research findings via publications and conferences.

PracticalKnowledge
knowing **how**

No one expects you to have a sophisticated understanding of research at this point in your nursing career. However, you do need some basic practical knowledge, including information about the scientific method, types of research design, the research process, how to find practice-related research articles, how to identify researchable problems, and how to critique research reports.

How Do We Gain Knowledge?

Recall that in Chapter 2 you learned the different kinds of nursing knowledge: theoretical, practical, ethical, and self-knowledge. There are also various ways to *acquire* knowledge.

Trial and Error Plus Common Sense Suppose a patient has been medicated but is still in pain. You might try repositioning him. If that doesn't help, you might try distraction, visualization techniques, and perhaps various other measures. If visualization provides some relief, you would probably try that technique first when a similar situation occurs with another patient.

Authority and Tradition This means relying on an expert or doing what has always been done. For the patient with unrelieved pain, this would mean you might ask a more experienced nurse what to do. Or you could consult a procedure manual.

Intuition and Inspiration Intuition is a feeling about something—an inner sense. Nurses say, "I just had a feeling something was wrong with the patient, but I can't explain why." For the patient in pain, you might have a feeling that a complication was developing, that the pain was due to more than just ineffective pain medication. However, as a novice, you should always check with a more experienced nurse before acting on your intuition.

Logical Reasoning Using your knowledge and the facts available, you form conclusions (refer to the section How Are Theories Developed?). For the patient in pain, you might think, "My patient is 70 lb overweight, yet I administered only the standard dose of medication. Likely she needs a higher dose."

Scientific Method Research uses the scientific method (or scientific inquiry). **Scientific method** is the process in which the researcher, through use of the senses, systematically collects observable, verifiable data to describe, explain, or predict events. The goals of scientific inquiry are to find solutions to problems and to develop explanations of the world (theories). **KEY POINT:** *The scientific method has two unique characteristics that the other ways of gaining knowledge do not:*

1. *Objectivity,* or *self-correction.* This means the researcher uses techniques to keep her personal beliefs, values, and attitudes separate from the research process.
2. *The use of empirical data.* Researchers use their senses to gather empirical data *through* observation. They attempt to verify the information gathered through a variety of methods so that the research conclusions are based in reality rather than on the researcher's beliefs, biases, or hunches.

Box 8-3 summarizes the characteristics of the scientific method.

BOX 8-3 ■ Characteristics of the Scientific Method

Begins with an identified problem or need to be studied.
Uses theories, models, and conceptual themes that have been empirically tested.
Uses systematic, orderly methods to acquire empirical evidence to test theories.
Uses methods of control for ruling out other variables that might affect the relationships among the variables they are studying.
Avoids explanations that cannot be empirically tested.
Prefers to generalize the findings (knowledge) so that they can be applied in cases other than those in the study.
Uses built-in mechanisms for self-correction.

Source: Adapted from Wilson, H. S. (1992). *Introducing research in nursing* (2nd ed.). Redwood City, CA: Addison-Wesley Nursing.

What Are Two Approaches to Research?

The scientific method makes use of a variety of procedures and study designs intended to help ensure that the data collected will be reliable, relevant, and unbiased. You should recognize the two major categories of research design: *quantitative* and *qualitative.* Each category has within it several specific types of research methodologies; however, for now you need to understand only the basic differences (Table 8-2).

Quantitative Research

KEY POINT: *The main purpose of* **quantitative research** *is to gather data from enough* **subjects** *(people being studied), using sound sampling methods, to be able to generalize the results to a similar population.* **Generalizing results** means that you think, "What I found to be so for this sample group of people will probably be the same for all people who are similar" (e.g., "My findings for *this* group of women over age 40 in the United States will probably be useful for *all* women over age 40 in the United States"). In quantitative research, researchers carefully control data collection and are careful to maintain the objectivity of the process. Quantitative data are reported as numbers. The Framingham studies are a classic example of a quantitative study—actually of several quantitative studies.

Another classic example of quantitative nursing research is the Conduct and Utilization of Research in Nursing (CURN) project, which was intended to increase the use of research by direct-care nurses (Horsley, Cane, Crabtree, et al., 1983). Many of the protocols (procedures) developed from these studies are currently used with some modification. The following are some CURN protocol examples:

Clean intermittent catheterization
Intravenous cannula change
Distress reduction through sensory preparation
Preventing decubitus ulcers

Qualitative Research

Qualitative research focuses on the lived experience of people. It uses words, quotations from persons interviewed, observations, and other nonnumeric sources of data. The purpose is not to generalize the data but to share the experience of the person or persons in the study. There is no need for large numbers. A case study of one person can, for example, examine the lived experience, for example, of a 19-year-old, single mother of twins or a middle-aged woman with HIV.

The Nun Study, a long-term, multidisciplinary project, was designed to study aging and disability caused by Alzheimer's disease. Qualitative data included interviews with Catholic nuns, 75 to 102 years old, in a convent in Minnesota. Researchers also examined samples of writing from the nuns' diaries, reports, and letters.

KnowledgeCheck 8-8

- Define *quantitative research.* Name one study presented as an example in this chapter.
- Define *qualitative research.* Name one study presented as an example in this chapter.

What Are the Phases of the Research Process?

At the novice level, you will be using but not performing research. But in order to evaluate the research you read, you should have a general idea of the steps for conducting valid,

Table 8-2 ➤ Comparison of Quantitative and Qualitative Research

	QUANTITATIVE RESEARCH	QUALITATIVE RESEARCH
Data	Numerical data, e.g., questionnaires, number of incidents, or reactions to a medication.	Nonnumerical data; data may consist of words from interviews, observations, written documents, and even art or photos.
Persons studied	Large numbers of *subjects* so they can be generalized to other similar populations.	Often uses small numbers of *participants*; is not designed with the intent to generalize.
Hypothesis	Has a hypothesis.	No hypothesis, because it is the research of the "lived experience" of the person or persons being studied; study may be guided by research questions.
Environment	Can be a laboratory setting; needs to be a controlled environment.	Is often done in the "natural" setting, i.e., the person's home or work site.
Analysis	Objective data, tested with statistical methods.	Subjective data; identify themes; sometimes converted to numerical data (e.g., by counting categories).

reliable research. The research process is a problem-solving process, similar to but not the same as the nursing process. Different study designs require different steps, and you will find some variation in how different authors present the research process steps. However, in general, the steps include the following five phases:

1. Select and define the problem.
2. Select a research design.
3. Collect data.
4. Analyze data.
5. Use the research findings.

 ThinkLike a Nurse 8-4

Take 10 minutes to sit quietly and think about nursing research. Do you have an idea or a patient problem you would like to see investigated with a research project? If nothing comes to mind quickly, then ponder for a few moments more. Write the information on a sheet of paper. Take the time to do your best thinking. Then share what you have written with your instructor and other students.

- What would you like to have more information about in nursing? Explain why it is a problem or what brought about your idea.
- If you were the research assistant on a nursing research project on your topic, what one-sentence problem statement would you write regarding your research idea?
- What is the purpose of doing this research project? Why should it be done?

You may struggle with this assignment and wonder about its value to you, yet one of the most important things that nurses do is identify problems. Here is your chance to practice.

What Are the Rights of Research Participants?

Every nurse has a moral and legal responsibility to protect research participants from being harmed during the research process. Although research is crucial to the development of the profession, it should never be held in higher regard than the rights of the individuals being studied. The U.S. government, through the Department of Health and Human Services (USDHHS), has a complex set of standards that all researchers must follow.

Informed Consent

As a rule, **informed consent** must be obtained from every participant in a study. Consent is obtained by discussing what is expected of the participant, providing written information on the project to the participant, and obtaining the participant's written consent to be a subject. The following critical concepts are part of the informed consent:

- *Right to not be harmed.* The information given to the participant outlines the safety protocols of the study. If preliminary data indicate potential harm to the participant, the study must be stopped immediately.
- *Right to full disclosure* (e.g., of risks, benefits, payments, purpose of the research, whom to contact with questions and concerns).
- *Right to self-determination.* This refers to the right to say no. At any time in a study, the participant has the right to stop participating, for any reason.
- *Rights of privacy and confidentiality.* This includes the right to have one's identity protected, for example, by using codes instead of names. The researcher is responsible for protecting the raw data (e.g., questionnaires and taped interviews).

Institutional Review Boards

The mechanism for overseeing the ethical standards established by the USDHHS is the Institutional Review Board (IRB). Every federally funded hospital, university, or other healthcare facility has an IRB. It consists of healthcare professionals and people from the community who are willing to review and critique research proposals. The two main responsibilities of the IRB are (1) to protect the research participants from harm and (2) to ensure that the research is of value.

KnowledgeCheck 8-9

- List the phases of the research process.
- List four critical concepts that make up informed consent.

How Can I Base My Practice on the Best Evidence?

Recall from Chapter 6 that research provides the data for evidence-based practice. When there is a body of research on a topic, experts and professional groups evaluate the quality of the research reports and translate them into guidelines for practice. In your own evidence-based practice, you should use research findings and practice guidelines when they are available. When they are not, you will need to rely on the research reports themselves. Similar to the phases of research, the following steps should assist you in finding the best evidence for your own interventions:

Identify a Clinical Nursing Problem

Even as a novice nurse, you should be prepared to identify clinical problems for research. Identifying a clinical nursing problem comes from being alert and interested in what you are doing each day in your clinical setting. How do you think the temporal thermometer came into clinical use? Someone became frustrated with the discomfort patients experienced when temperatures were taken rectally. At the same time, there was a great deal of concern over the inaccuracy of axillary temperatures. Someone noticed the problem and wondered, "Is there a better way to do this?"

Common sources of clinical problems are experience, social issues, theories, ideas from others, and the nursing literature (Polit & Beck, 2016). Most of these sources are relevant whether you are identifying a problem for a research study or doing a literature search.

Experience As you go about your work, you will notice interventions that require a great deal of effort for the minimal good they do. You will wonder, "How could we do this better?" Or you may notice that outcomes for clients with a particular health problem are often not good. You will wonder, "How could we improve the care so the patient's health improves?" Another question might be, "Why do we do this procedure this way?" If you are curious about why things are done and about what might happen if changes were made, you will find plenty of problems—for example, problems in staffing, equipment, nursing interventions, or coordination among health professionals.

Social Issues You may be concerned about broader social issues that affect or require nursing care, such as issues of gender equity, sexual harassment, and domestic violence. You may be concerned about patients who do not have access to healthcare or about the health problems of a particular group or subculture.

Theories Recall that theories must be tested in order to be useful in nursing practice. You might want to suggest research to test a theory in which you are interested. If the theory is accurate, what behaviors would you expect to find, or what evidence would you need to support the theory?

Ideas From Others Your instructor may suggest a topic to research, or perhaps you might brainstorm with nurses or other students. Agencies and organizations that fund research often ask for proposals on certain topics (e.g., the ANA and the National Institute of Nursing Research).

Nursing Literature Read widely in your field of interest. You may identify clinical problems by reading articles and research reports in nursing journals.

- An article may stimulate your imagination and interest in a topic.
- You may notice a discrepancy in what staff nurses are doing and what the literature recommends.
- You may notice inconsistencies in the findings of two different studies on the same topic.
- You may read a study on a topic of interest to you (e.g., a technique for measuring blood pressure) and wonder whether the results would be the same if the study had been done in a different setting (e.g., a clinic instead of a hospital) or with a different population (e.g., healthy instead of ill people).

Formulate a Searchable Question

When you have found a topic of interest, the next step is to state it in such a way that you can find it in the vast amount of nursing literature that is published. Stated too broadly, the search may yield thousands of irrelevant results. Stated too narrowly, you may get no results. Using the acronym PICOT enables you to search efficiently by asking focused questions. The acronym stands for *P*atient or problem, *I*ntervention, *C*omparison interventions, *O*utcomes, and *T*ime. You may not always need a comparison intervention (C) or a time (T). See the PICOT box Skin Care for Pressure Injury in Frail Elderly Woman.

Search the Literature

Once you have stated your guiding question, the next step is to look for research articles related to the question (or problem statement). You may be thinking, "Where do I look for research articles?" As previously stated, evidence reports and practice guidelines may already exist for your clinical problem, so look first for those. If there are none, proceed to search for your topic in research reports in scientific journals.

Indexes and Databases

Obviously you need to go online or to a library and search a database or index for appropriate journal references. A **database** is an electronic bibliographic file that can be accessed online. The best database for you as a novice nurse is the Cumulative Index to Nursing and Allied Health Literature (CINAHL). This is a comprehensive database that includes nearly 3,000 nursing and allied health journals. Generally, you will be able to find in CINAHL whatever you are looking for in clinical nursing. Most university libraries have access to CINAHL and other indexes online. If you are an online user, it will be worth your time to get information from the library about conducting online searches. In the library, you will find the printed version of CINAHL in a set of large books in the reference section.

Once you have access to CINAHL, select words that relate to your topic (e.g., *dementia* or *nursing ethics*). The index or database will list journal articles related to the keywords. Sometimes you will get a large number of articles (more than 1,000) that contain that word or phrase. A PICOT question should help you narrow your search, but you may need to ask the librarian for assistance. It is beyond the scope of this chapter to provide detailed instructions for literature searches. For more information about literature databases,

Go to **Bonus Chapter 45, Informatics,** in your Davis Digital Version of the textbook.

KnowledgeCheck 8-10

Where can you go to use CINAHL?

Journals

It also is easy to search in a specific journal for articles. The title of a journal provides clues to its content. For example, critical care, oncology, orthopedics, and other specialty journals will have, obviously, articles specific to their own specialty. Looking for such journals is another way to do a casual search

PICOT

Skin Care for Pressure Injury in Frail Elderly Woman

Situation: An elderly, frail resident in an extended care facility experiences urinary incontinence. Her skin is reddened and beginning to break down at pressure points on her sacrum. Knowing that urine is harsh on the skin and moisture, pressure, friction, and shear can lead to skin breakdown, the nurse is concerned that the woman may be developing a pressure injury. She searches the literature for an evidence-based intervention that would be most effective.

	Sample Questions	Example
P—Patient population, or Problem	What is the medical diagnosis, nursing diagnosis, patient problem, symptom, situation, or need that requires an intervention? How would you describe a group of similar patients?	For patients with Impaired Skin Integrity (sacrum, perineum) related to urinary incontinence
I—Intervention, treatment, cause, contributing factor	Which intervention are you considering? Specifically, what might help the problem (improve the situation, etc.)?	Would applying a hydrocolloid dressing help?
C—Comparison intervention	What other interventions are being considered or used?	As compared with applying a gauze dressing after incontinent episodes
O—Outcome	What effect could the intervention realistically have? What do you hope to achieve?	To prevent or reduce sacral excoriation? Are there any undesired effects associated with the intervention?
T—Time	How often or when will the outcome be measured? How often or how long will the intervention or treatment be administered?	After incontinent episodes.

Searchable Question: Do _____(P) who are receive _____ (I) as compared _____(C) demonstrate _____(O) after _____(T)?

Example of Evidence: The American College of Physicians (Qaseem, Humphrey, Forciea, et al., 2015) published practice guidelines for risk assessment, prevention, and treatment of pressure injuries. Among other interventions, guidelines recommend using hydrocolloid dressings in patients with pressure injuries to promote healing by absorbing wound exudate and forming a protective surface around the wound. The evidence showed that hydrocolloid dressings are better than gauze for reducing wound size.

Practice Change: The nurse verified knowledge of skin care, including cleansing and applying barrier cream for the prevention and early treatment of pressure injuries in a woman at risk for skin breakdown.

Source: Qaseem, A., Humphrey, L. L., Forciea, M. A., et al. (2015, March 3). Treatment of pressure ulcers: A clinical practice guideline from the American College of Physicians. *Annals of Internal Medicine, 162*(5), 370–379. doi:10.7326/M14-1568

Adapted from: University of Southern California, Health Sciences, Los Angeles. (n.d.). Evidence based decision making, asking a good question (PICO). Retrieved from www.usc.edu/hsc/ebnet/ebframe/PICO.htm; Center for Evidence Based Medicine. (n.d.). Asking focused clinical questions. Retrieved from www.cebm.net/index.aspx?o=1036; Sacket, D. L., Richardson, W. S., Rosenberg, W., et al. (1997). *Evidence-based medicine: How to practice and teach EBM* (4th ed.). New York, NY: Churchill Livingstone; Stilwell, S., Fineout-Overholt, E., Melnyk, B. M., et al. (2010). Evidence-based practice, step by step: Asking the clinical question: A key step in evidence-based practice. *American Journal of Nursing, 110*(3), 58–61. doi:10.1097/01.NAJ.0000368959.11129.79

---

for articles of interest. Remember that it is up to you to identify whether the article is research, educational, or another form of information sharing.

- *Why use refereed journals?* You will find the highest quality research articles published in refereed journals. **Refereed journals** are scholarly journals (not popular magazines, such as *Men's Health* or *Fitness*) in which professionals with expertise in the topic review each article and then recommend whether it should be published. The easiest way to identify a refereed journal is to see whether it has an extensive editorial board listed in the front of the journal. Refereed journals have a high standard for publication, which makes the information you read more credible (and therefore more useful to your work). Two examples of refereed

nursing research journals are *Advances in Nursing Science* and *Nursing Research.*

- *How to identify a research article.* How can you tell whether the article you retrieve is a research article? Simply look for the steps in the research process described earlier in this chapter. For example, does the article have a problem statement and a purpose? Is there a section on the sample and site of the research? And so on.
- *Specialty journals.* If your focus is clinical practice, you should not overlook specialty journals, such as *Geriatric Nursing* or the *Journal of Gerontological Nursing,* if you really want information on, say, older adults with dementia. They are not research journals, but they generally have one or two research articles in each issue.

- *General interest journals.* If you do not have a specialty interest, review the *American Journal of Nursing, Nursing,* or *RN* for articles of general interest.

Evaluate the Quality of the Research

As mentioned previously, you may be fortunate enough to find clinical practice guidelines related to your topic. If so, the related research has already been evaluated by experts and should have a notation about the level of evidence supporting the guideline.

If no practice guidelines are available, you will need to critically appraise the individual research articles you find. You can do this by reading analytically and performing a careful appraisal of the research you read.

Analytic Reading

You cannot expect to do a complex critique of a research report at this stage of your education, or probably even on graduation from your basic education. However, you need to know enough to help you decide which articles are worthy of using in your practice. You will make that decision after you have examined the research to determine whether it is well done and meaningful to your work. Begin this process by learning to read analytically. **Analytic reading** occurs when you "begin asking questions of what you are reading so that you can truly understand it" (Wilson, 1992, p. 25). For questions to use when reading analytically, see Box 8-4.

Research Appraisal

Not all research is good research. Some published studies contain serious flaws, and you need to be able to recognize them. An effective strategy for conducting a research appraisal is to read the entire article, using the four analytic reading questions in Box 8-4 and making notes of questions you have. Then go back and evaluate the article section by section, thinking critically about each (Wilson, 1992).

- *Researcher qualifications* are an easy place to start. Was the researcher qualified as an expert on the study topic? Try to determine whether the author's credentials and background fit with the topic.
- *The title* should be concise and clear. Keywords in the title should provide clues to the research topic.

BOX 8-4 ■ Reading Analytically

When reading analytically, ask yourself the following questions:
1. **What is the book, journal, or article about as a whole?** That is, what is the theme and how is it developed?
2. **What is being said in detail, and how?** What are the author's main ideas, claims, and arguments? In a research article, you will find this mainly in the abstract and the conclusions.
3. **Is the book, journal, or article true in whole or part?** You must decide this for yourself. The strategies in the section Research Appraisal may help you to determine the truth of a research report.
4. **What of it?** Is it of any significance? Is there any way to use the information to improve patient care, to add to your education, or to enhance other areas of nursing?

- *The abstract* is a brief (perhaps 500 words) summary of the study. It should be interesting and usually describes at least the purpose, methods, sample, and findings of the study.
- *The introduction* should catch your interest and set the stage for the rest of the report. The introduction may contain the *review of the literature, theoretical (conceptual) framework, assumptions,* and *limitations.* At this stage of your expertise, you should primarily check that these are present; however, some explanation follows:
  - *Review of the literature* should be thorough and relevant. The references should logically pertain to the study topic and methods and consist primarily of research and theory articles. The references should support the researcher's variable definitions, methodology, and choices of data-collection tools and present background work on the topic being studied.
  - *Study assumptions should be clearly stated* to avoid confusion regarding the study. Recall that assumptions are beliefs that you "take for granted" as true but that have not been proven. For example, you assume that when people are in bed, they sleep; and you assume that study participants answer truthfully to the researcher's questions.
  - *Limitations of the study.* Every study has limitations or weaknesses. The author should admit openly the things that could not be controlled. For example, a study may test a population of people that would not generalize to other populations (e.g., testing only Caucasian students instead of testing a variety of students who represent the ethnic diversity of the university).
- *The purpose* should provide the reasons for doing the study. Ask the following to help you judge it: Will the study (1) solve a problem relevant to nursing, (2) present facts that are useful to nursing, or (3) contribute to nursing knowledge?
- *The problem statement* should appear early in the report, and it should be researchable; that is, it (1) is stated as a question, (2) involves the relationship between two or more variables, and (3) can be answered by collecting empirical data.
- *Definition of terms* is essential in a formal research report. However, it often is not included in a published article because of the lack of space.
- *The research design* indicates the plan for collecting data. As a novice, you probably cannot judge the adequacy of the design, but you should be sure the researcher names and describes it and discusses its strengths and weakness. The researcher should include an explanation of what was done to enhance the validity and reliability of the study. To oversimplify, **validity** means the study actually measures the concept it claims to measure. **Reliability** refers to the accuracy, consistency, and precision of a measure. That is, if someone else repeated the study using the same design, would they obtain similar results? For example, if you weighed the same item on a scale each day and obtained the same weight each time, you could say the scale is reliable—but a scale would not give you a valid measure of body fat.
- *Setting, population, and sample.* The researcher should identify the type of setting where the data was collected, describe the population and sample, and state the criteria that were used for choosing study participants. This section may also contain information about how informed consent was obtained.
- *Data-collection methods* answer the basic questions of what, how, who, where, and when. Data-collection instruments are the tools used to gather the data (e.g., questionnaires or a

laboratory instrument). The researcher should provide evidence (pilot tests, literature) that the tools used were reliable and valid.

- *Data analysis.* A quantitative report would include statistical analyses of the data, frequently in the form of tables and graphs. A qualitative report would include quotes from the participants. The analyses of both types of data are very specific and beyond the scope of this textbook.
- *Discussion of findings and conclusion* are the sections of a research report that you may find most interesting. They are the "So what was learned?" and "What it means" sections. The researcher should present all findings objectively and compare them with information found in the literature. The easiest errors for you to recognize with your present knowledge level are that the researcher:
  1. Generalizes beyond the data or the sample. For example, the sample may have been young adult women in a clinic setting, but the researcher might have suggested that the same intervention be used for all women in the clinic, regardless of age.
  2. Does not mention any limitations that might have influenced the results.
  3. Does not present findings in a clear, logical manner (i.e., you have trouble figuring out what the findings actually are).
- *Implications and recommendations* are the final pieces of the research critique. The implications are the "shoulds" of the research. In essence, the researcher says, "Now we know this fact; therefore, nurses should . . ." For example, "the research should be replicated with another population," or "the instrument should be revised and retested," or "this is how nurses could use the study intervention in their practice."

When you read a research article, examine it for each of the preceding items. Although you have limited knowledge and experience, every time you review an article thoroughly, you will learn more about the research process. As you learn, you will be better able to determine the quality of research you will accept as a basis for changing your nursing practice.

KnowledgeCheck 8-11

- Explain the difference between analytic reading and research appraisal.
- What are the parts of a PICOT question?

Integrate the Research Into Your Practice

True evidence-based practice requires that after discovering and critiquing the best available evidence, nursing expertise must be applied to see how the recommended interventions fit into the practice setting and whether they are compatible with patient preferences. If the intervention is to involve more than just an individual nurse, nurse managers must consider costs, barriers to change, facilitators for change, and staff education before deciding to implement the clinical practice guideline in their unit or hospital.

Research is more than just an exercise that nurses engage in to earn master's and doctoral degrees. The ultimate reason for conducting research is to establish an evidence-based practice or to gain greater understanding of a phenomenon. This means that nurses in practice have a responsibility for finding and using the credible, scientific research that others do. Remember the discussion of authority-based practice during Florence Nightingale's era? Even in the 21st century, much nursing practice is still based on authority and tradition. That is not acceptable for full-spectrum professional nurses. You must have reasons for what you do. Research can provide those reasons.

Although there are barriers (Box 8-5), you can use nursing research to enhance your practice by acting on the information in this chapter. Read and talk about research with your colleagues and instructors. Once you have a research-based idea clear in your mind, try it out in your clinical setting (with approval from the nurse manager or instructor). Then discuss it with others. You can learn to read and use research effectively, and then you can motivate others to do the same.

BOX 8-5 ■ Barriers to Using Research

Common reasons nurses *do not* use research as the basis for their practice (Nieswiadomy, 2012) include the following:
1. Lack of knowledge of nursing research
2. Negative attitudes toward research
3. Inadequate forums for disseminating research
4. Lack of support from the employing institution
5. Study findings that are not ready for the clinical environment

CLINICALREASONING

The questions and exercises in this section allow you to practice the kind of thinking you will use as a full-spectrum nurse. Critical-thinking questions usually have more than one right answer, so we do not provide "correct answers" for these features. It is more important to develop your nursing judgment than to just cover content. You will learn by discussing the questions with your peers. If you are still unsure, see the Davis Advantage chapter resources for suggested responses.

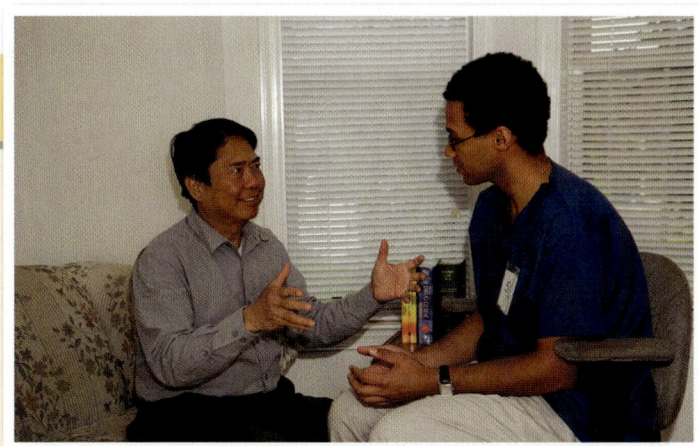

Caring for the Nguyens

Mr. Nguyen arrives at the clinic for a follow-up visit. As you may recall, he has been diagnosed with hypertension. At a previous visit, you wrote a nursing diagnosis of Obesity related to inappropriate food choices and serving size, as evidenced by a BMI of 28.5.

Today you have gathered the following intake data:

Blood pressure: 174/96 mm/Hg
Heart rate: 88 beats/min
Respiratory rate: 18 breaths/min
Temperature: 98.5°F
Weight: 175 lb

A. What observations can you make about today's data in comparison with his initial visit?

B. As part of the treatment plan for Mr. Nguyen, you have been asked to educate him about a diet to assist with weight loss and hypertension management. How would you determine the most appropriate diet to include in your treatment plan?

C. A number of sources recommend the DASH (Dietary Approaches to Stop Hypertension) eating plan. Go online and search for "Dietary Approaches to Stop Hypertension." Is there sufficient research to support incorporating this information into Mr. Nguyen's treatment plan? If so, describe the research and summarize the DASH eating plan.

Applying the **Full-Spectrum Nursing Model**_____

PATIENT SITUATION

You are caring for a 90-year-old patient in a long-term care facility. He is completely dependent for activities of daily living. In addition, he has been unresponsive, cannot swallow safely, and for many months has been receiving fluids and nutrition through a feeding tube. His adult grandson has recently discovered a living will, in which the patient had stated that he does not wish to be kept alive by "artificial means, including being tube fed." The grandson, John, insists that the patient's wishes be honored, but the patient's son (Mr. Lee) threatens a lawsuit if the caregivers discontinue the feedings. They argue loudly, and Mr. Lee yells to his son, "You just want him gone because you're in a hurry to get his money! You know you're getting the major part of it."

THINKING

1. *Theoretical Knowledge:* What facts are important to know in order to decide whether to stop the feedings?
2. *Critical Thinking (Analyzing Assumptions):* Without thinking too carefully about it, what is your first thought about what is causing the disagreement between Mr. Lee and his son, John? Examine your assumption. How certain are you it is true? What else might be going on in their lives to cause father and son to disagree on this issue?

DOING

3. *Nursing Process (Assessment):* In order to provide some information about the patient that might be helpful in restoring peace between Mr. Lee and John, what patient assessments should you make?

CARING

4. *Ethical Knowledge:* State one ethical issue involved in this case—or one moral problem that it would be present for you if you were involved in it.

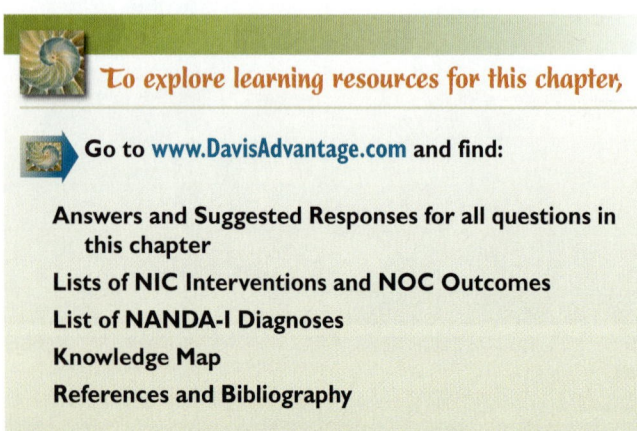

To explore learning resources for this chapter,

Go to www.DavisAdvantage.com and find:

Answers and Suggested Responses for all questions in this chapter

Lists of NIC Interventions and NOC Outcomes

List of NANDA-I Diagnoses

Knowledge Map

References and Bibliography

Concept Map

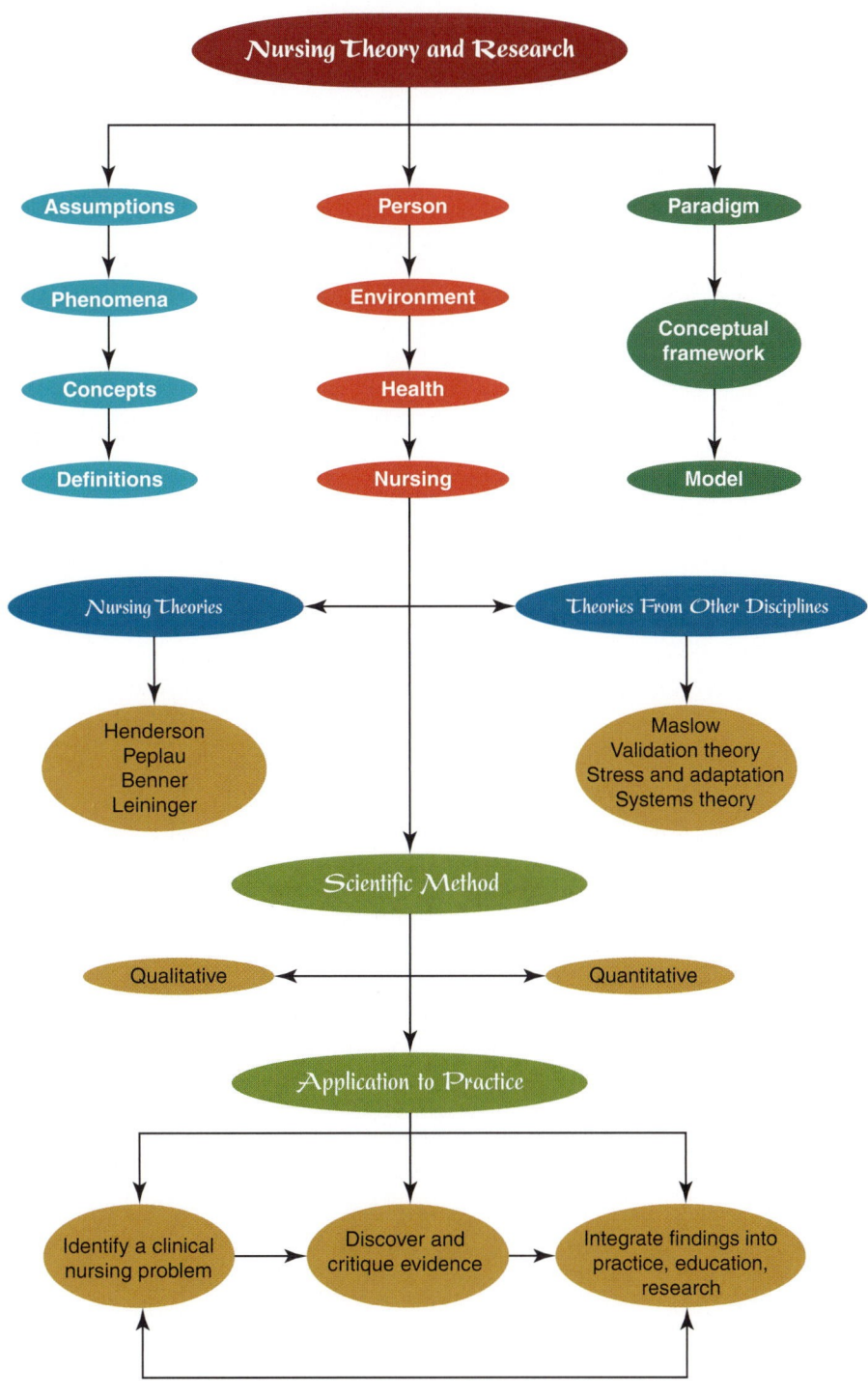

Factors Affecting Health

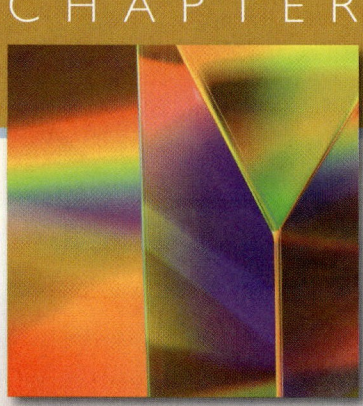

CHAPTER 9

Development: Infancy Through Middle Adulthood

Learning Outcomes

After completing this chapter, you should be able to:

➤ Discuss the principles of growth and development.

➤ Compare and contrast developmental task theory, psychoanalytic theory, cognitive theory, and the psychosocial theory of growth and development.

➤ Outline the major principles involved in moral and spiritual development.

➤ Identify conditions that influence growth and development at all ages.

➤ Discuss the cognitive and psychosocial challenges for each age-group, infant through middle age.

➤ Identify common health problems seen in each stage of development.

➤ Describe special assessments unique to each age-group.

➤ Discuss age-appropriate interventions for each age-group.

➤ Incorporate developmental principles into nursing care.

Key Concepts

Development
Growth
Stages

Related Concepts

See the Concept Map at the end of this chapter.

Example Problems

Abuse, neglect, and violence
Substance abuse

Meet Your Patients

At the end of your first clinical day on the pediatric unit, you reflect on your experiences. You provided care for the following three children who were diagnosed with pneumonia:

■ Tamika, a 3-year-old, lives with her grandparents. Her grandmother is present only during afternoon visiting hours because she must care for her husband, who suffers from numerous health problems.

■ Miguel, a 2-month-old, lives with his mother. Since his admission yesterday, Miguel's mother has stayed at his bedside and provided most of her son's care. Miguel's mother is 17 years old and is very concerned about her son's condition.

■ Carrie, a 13-year-old, lives with her parents. Both parents are able to visit only during evening visiting hours after they leave work.

You think back to another clinical day when you were assigned to care for Ms. Lowenstein, a middle-aged patient with pneumonia who lives alone.

Each of these patients is unique. Although they share the same medical diagnosis, their needs and your nursing care differ dramatically. These differences stem from a variety of factors, one of the most significant of which is each patient's developmental stage. Throughout the life span, human beings are in a constant process of physical, cognitive, and emotional change, whether or not it is visible to the eye.

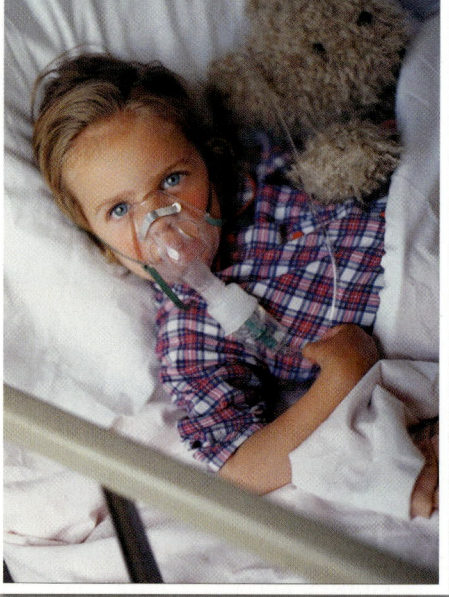

Theoretical Knowledge
knowing **why**

In this chapter, you will learn principles and theories of growth and development that can form the foundation for planning and delivering effective patient care. You will also find a discussion of normal growth and development across the life span. A fundamentals course or textbook can provide only a basic foundation covering infant and child development. For situations in which you need more in-depth or specialized knowledge, refer to a child development or pediatric nursing textbook.

ABOUT THE KEY CONCEPTS

Development refers to the process of adapting to one's body and environment over time, which is enabled by increasing complexity of function and skill progression. A few examples of development are a child who comes to recognize right from wrong, an adolescent who decides on a vocation, and an older adult who recognizes the nearness of death.

  Growth refers to physical changes that occur over time, such as increases in height, sexual maturation, or gains in weight and muscle tone. Growth is the physical aspect of development; the rest is behavioral.

  As you read this chapter, you will see how the key concept of **stages** is intertwined with the concepts of growth and development.

HOW DOES DEVELOPMENT OCCUR?

The Greek philosopher Heraclitus said, "Nothing is permanent but change." We readily see this truth in the dramatic physical, cognitive, and emotional growth that children undergo from one month to another, but it is true also for adults. **KEY POINT:** *Change is constant throughout the life span.*

  What has been the most important force in your becoming the person you are now: characteristics that you inherited from your parents or the environment in which you were raised? This is not an easy question to answer. For centuries, scientists have debated the effects of nature versus nurture on growth and development. **Nature** refers to genetic endowment, whereas **nurture** is the influence of the environment on the individual.

  The birth of a child can be compared to the planting of a tulip. Within the bulb is nearly everything it needs to sprout; but whether it reaches its full potential—that is, grows into a flowering plan—also depends on the environment. Is the soil rich in nutrients? Is there adequate sunshine? Water? Similarly, the joining of ovum and sperm forms chromosomes that determine appearance and characteristics and affect how the child will grow and develop. However, environmental factors, such as access to food, love and affection, healthcare, and education, also affect how the child develops and thrives throughout the life span.

Principles of Growth and Development

Important principles of growth and development include the following:

- **Growth and development usually follow an orderly, predictable pattern.** However, the timing, rate of change, and response to change are unique for each individual. For example, all children learn to sit before they walk. One child may learn to sit at 6 months of age and walk at 10 months, whereas another may first sit at 7 months and not walk until 15 months. Each of these children is developing in the same pattern, and both are progressing within a normal time frame

- **Growth and development follow a cephalocaudal pattern,** beginning at the head and progressing down to the chest, trunk, and lower extremities. The following are examples:

    Cephalocaudal growth—When an infant is born, the head is the largest portion of the body. In the first year, the head, chest, and trunk gain in size, yet the legs remain short. Growth of the legs is readily apparent in the second year.

    Cephalocaudal development—This is the tendency of infants to use their arms before their legs.

- **Growth and development proceed in a proximodistal pattern,** beginning at the center of the body and moving outward.

    Proximodistal growth—This occurs in utero, for example, when the baby's central body is formed before the limbs.

    Proximodistal development—The infant first begins to focus his eyes, then lifts his head, and later pushes up and rolls over. As the infant gains strength and coordination distally, he will crawl and later walk.

- **Simple skills develop separately and independently.** Later they are integrated into more complex skills. Many complex skills actually represent a compilation of simple skills. For example, feeding yourself requires the ability to find your mouth, grasp an object, control movement of that object, coordinate movement of the hand from the plate to the mouth, and swallow solid food.

- **Each body system grows at its own rate.** This principle is readily apparent in fetal development and the onset of puberty. In the years leading up to puberty, the cardiovascular, respiratory, and nervous systems grow and develop dramatically, yet the reproductive system changes very little. Puberty is a series of changes that lead to full development of the reproductive system and triggers growth in the musculoskeletal system.

- **Body system functions become increasingly differentiated over time.** Have you ever seen a newborn respond to a loud noise? The newborn's startle response involves the whole body. With maturity, the response becomes more focused, for example, covering the ears. An adult is often able to identify the location of the sound and distinguish the origin of the sound.

Theories of Development

Theories of development describe and explain patterns of development common to all people. Such theories provide a basis for clinical decision making. The needs of a 6-year-old differ from those of a 25-year-old or a 65-year-old, even though they may have the same medical diagnosis (e.g., asthma) or even the same nursing diagnosis (e.g., Anxiety). Understanding the tasks associated with a person's developmental stage assists you in assessing whether behaviors are as expected or whether they need further assessment. Knowledge of development also suggests specific interventions to support and encourage the person's developmental progress and health outcomes.

  Developmental theories divide the life span into stages. Each stage represents a period of time that shares common characteristics. Most theories also identify tasks that are usually accomplished in each stage. An understanding of the following key developmental theories is essential to full-spectrum nursing practice:

Developmental Task Theory

Robert Havighurst theorized that learning is a lifelong process. He believed a person moves through six life stages, each associated with a number of tasks that must be learned. Failure to master a task leads to imbalance within the individual, unhappiness, and difficulty mastering future tasks and interacting with others. Conceptually, a **developmental task** is "midway between an individual need and societal demand. It assumes an active learner interacting with an active social environment" (1971, p. vi). Table 9-1 presents the tasks associated with each stage of life. It is easy to evaluate whether a client has completed Havighurst's broadly written tasks, but the nonspecific time frame limits the theory's usefulness for assessing individuals for appropriate development.

ThinkLike a Nurse 9-1

Which stage in Havighurst's developmental task theory contains the most complex tasks and would be the most difficult to master? Why?

Psychoanalytic Theory

Sigmund Freud was a pioneer in the science of human development. Psychoanalytic theory was the foremost theory of early 20th-century psychotherapy. Freud developed his theory in the Victorian era, when societal norms were very strict; sexual repression and male dominance over female behavior were the cultural standard. Because of this, many of today's social scientists question whether the theory is relevant to life in the 21st century.

KEY POINT: *Freud's psychoanalytic theory focuses on the motivation for human behavior and personality development.* He believed that development is maintained by instinctual drives, such as libido (sexual instinct), aggression, and survival (Table 9-2) (Sadock & Sadock, 2014). Different drives predominate, depending on the age of the individual.

Table 9-1 ➤ Havighurst's Developmental Task Theory	
STAGE	**TASKS**
Infants and Toddlers	
Physical Development ■ Walking ■ Taking solid foods ■ Talking ■ Controlling bowel and bladder elimination ■ Learning sex differences and acquiring sexual modesty	*Cognitive and Social Development* ■ Acquiring psychological stability ■ Forming concepts; learning language ■ Getting ready to read
Preschool and School Age	
Physical Development ■ Learning physical skills necessary for ordinary games	*Cognitive and Social Development* ■ Building wholesome attitudes toward oneself as a growing organism ■ Learning to get along with age-mates ■ Learning masculine or feminine social role ■ Acquiring fundamental skills in reading, writing, and calculating ■ Developing concepts necessary for everyday living ■ Developing a conscience, morality, and a scale of values ■ Achieving personal independence ■ Acquiring attitudes toward social groups and institutions
Adolescents	
Physical Development ■ Accepting one's physique and using the body effectively	*Cognitive and Social Development* ■ Achieving new and more mature relations with age-mates of both sexes ■ Achieving masculine or feminine social role ■ Developing emotional independence from parents and other adults ■ Preparing for future marriage and family life ■ Preparing for a career ■ Acquiring values and an ethical system to guide behavior; developing an ideology ■ Aspiring to and achieving socially responsible behavior

Table 9-1 ➤ Havighurst's Developmental Task Theory—cont'd

STAGE	TASKS
Young Adults	
	Cognitive and Social Development
	■ Choosing a mate
	■ Achieving a masculine or feminine social role
	■ Learning to live with a partner
	■ Rearing children
	■ Managing a home
	■ Establishing an occupation
	■ Taking on community responsibilities
	■ Finding a compatible social group
Middle Adults	
Physical Development ■ Adjusting to the physiological changes of middle age	*Cognitive and Social Development* ■ Assisting teenage children to become responsible and happy adults ■ Achieving adult civic and social responsibility ■ Reaching and maintaining satisfactory performance in one's occupational career ■ Developing adult leisure-time activities ■ Relating oneself to one's spouse as a person
Older Adults (refer to Chapter 10)	

Adapted from: Havighurst, R. J. (1971). *Developmental tasks and education* (3rd ed.). New York, NY: Longman.

Table 9-2 ➤ Freud's Stages of Psychosexual Development

STAGE AND AGE	DESCRIPTION
Oral Birth–18 mo	The infant's primary needs are centered on the oral zone: lips, tongue, mouth. The need for hunger and pleasure is satisfied through the oral zone. Trust is developed through the meeting of needs. When needs are not met, aggression can manifest itself in the form of biting, spitting, or crying.
Anal 18 mo–3 yr	Neuromuscular control over the anal sphincter allows the child to have control over expulsion or retention of feces. This coincides with the child's struggle for separation and independence from caregivers. Successful completion of this stage yields a child who is self-directed, cooperative, and without shame. Conversely, the anal child exhibits willfulness, stubbornness, and need for orderliness.
Phallic 3–6 yr	The focus is on the genital organs. This coincides with the development of gender identity. Unconscious sexual feelings toward the parent of the opposite sex are common. Children emerge from this stage with a sense of sexual curiosity and a mastery of their instinctual impulses.
Latency 6–12 yr	Ego functioning matures, and sexual urges diminish. The child focuses his energy on same-sex relationships and mastery of his world, including relationships with significant others (teachers, coaches).
Genital 13–20 yr	Puberty causes an intensification of instinctual drives, particularly sexual. The focus of this stage is the resolution of previous conflicts and the development of a mature identity and the ability to form adult relationships.

In Freud's theory, the personality consists of the id, ego, and superego—different parts that develop at different life stages. Each factor, or force, has a unique function:

- The **id** represents instinctual urges, pleasure, and gratification, such as hunger, procreation, pleasure, and aggression. We are born with our id. It is dominant in infants and young children, as well as older children and adults who cannot control their urges.
- The **ego** begins to develop around 4 to 6 months of age, and is thought to represent reality. It strives to balance what is *wanted* (id) and what is *possible* to obtain or achieve.
- The **superego** is sometimes referred to as our conscience. This force develops in early childhood (aged 5–6) as a result of the internalization of primary caregiver responses to environmental events.
- The **unconscious mind** is composed of thoughts and memories that are not readily recalled but unconsciously influence behavior.

In the mid-1950s, Freud's daughter, the psychologist Anna Freud, identified a number of **defense mechanisms,** which she described as thought patterns or behaviors that the ego makes use of in the face of threat to biological or psychological integrity (Townsend, 2015). These defense mechanisms protect us from excess anxiety. All people use defense mechanisms to varying degrees. For a comprehensive discussion of defense mechanisms, see Chapter 12 and Table 12-1.

KnowledgeCheck 9-1

- According to Freud, which motivator of personality is based in reality?
- Which is referred to as our conscience?
- What is the purpose of defense mechanisms?

Cognitive Development Theory

Swiss psychologist Jean Piaget studied his own children to understand how humans develop **cognitive abilities** (i.e., the ability to think, reason, and use language). In this theory, cognitive development requires three core competencies:

- **Adaptation** is the ability to adjust to and interact with one's environment. To be able to adapt, one must assimilate and accommodate.
- **Assimilation** is the integration of new experiences with one's own system of knowledge.
- **Accommodation** is the change in one's system of knowledge that results from processing new information. For example, an infant is born with an innate ability to suck. Presented with the mother's nipple, the infant is able to assimilate the nipple to the behavior of sucking. If given a bottle, the infant can learn to accommodate the artificial nipple.

According to Piaget, cognitive development occurs from birth through adolescence in a sequence of four stages (see Table 9-3). A child must complete each stage before moving to the next. The rate at which a child moves through the stages is determined both by inherited intellect and the environment. Piaget does not address cognitive development after adolescence.

KnowledgeCheck 9-2

- According to Piaget, what core competencies are necessary for cognitive development?
- During which stage is the child the most egocentric?
- When does abstract thinking develop?

Psychosocial Development Theory

Erikson's theory of psychosocial development was introduced in the 1950s and is widely used in nursing and healthcare. He

Table 9-3 ➤ Piaget's Stages of Cognitive Development	
STAGE AND AGE	**CHARACTERISTICS OF DEVELOPMENT**
Sensorimotor Birth–2 yr	- Learns the world through the senses - Displays curiosity - Shows intentional behavior - Begins to see that objects exist apart and separate from self - Begins to see objects separate from self
Preoperational 2–7 yr	- Uses symbols and language - Sees himself as the center of the universe: egocentric - Thought based on perception rather than logic
Concrete operations 7–11 yr	- Operates and reacts to the concrete: What the child perceives is considered actual. - Egocentricity diminishes, can see from others' viewpoints - Able to use logic and reason in thinking - Able to conserve: To see that objects may change but recognizes them as the same (e.g., a tower of blocks is the same as a long fence of blocks)
Formal operations 11–adolescence	- Develops the ability to think abstractly: to reason, deduce, and define concepts in a logical manner - Some individuals cannot think abstractly, even as adults.

was strongly influenced by Freud but believed that personality continues to evolve throughout the life span. He hypothesized that individuals must master eight stages as they progress through life. Most people successfully move from stage to stage; however, a person can regress to earlier stages during times of stress or be forced to face tasks of later stages because of unforeseen life events (e.g., terminal illness). Failure to successfully master a stage leads to maladjustment. Erikson's eight stages include the following:

Stage 1: Trust Versus Mistrust (Birth to About 18 Months)

Stage 2: Autonomy Versus Shame and Doubt (About 18 Months to 3 Years)

Stage 3: Initiative Versus Guilt (3 to 5 Years)

Stage 4: Industry Versus Inferiority (6 to 11 Years)

Stage 5: Identity Versus Role Confusion (11 to 21 Years)

Stage 6: Intimacy Versus Isolation (21 to 40 Years)

Stage 7: Generativity Versus Stagnation (40 to 65 Years)

Stage 8: Ego Integrity Versus Despair (Over 65 Years)

 ## ThinkLike a Nurse 9-2

Review the case study in the Meet Your Patients section of the chapter. Based on what you know about theories of development, what kind of behavior would you anticipate from Carrie?

Moral Development Theory: Kohlberg

Lawrence Kohlberg (1968) studied the responses to moral dilemmas of 84 boys whose development he followed for a period of 20 years. From that data, Kohlberg hypothesized that a person's level of moral development can be identified by analyzing the rationale he gives for action in a moral dilemma.

In this theory, moral reasoning appears to be somewhat age related, and moral development is based on one's ability to think at progressively higher levels. Increased maturity provides some degree of higher-level thinking but does not guarantee the ability to function at the highest level.

Kohlberg described the following levels; each has two stages (1968, 1981; Waugh, 1978). Not all people are able to achieve the higher levels.

Level I. Preconventional

Stage 1—punishment–obedience orientation (right action is that which avoids punishment)

Stage 2—personal interest orientation (right action is that which satisfies personal needs)

Level II. Conventional

Stage 3—"good boy–nice girl" orientation (right actions are those that please others)

Stage 4—law-and-order orientation (right action is following the rules)

Level III. Postconventional, Autonomous, or Principled

Stage 5—legalistic, social contract orientation (right action is decided in terms of individual rights and standards agreed upon by the whole society)

Stage 6—universal ethical principles orientation (right action is determined by conscience and abstract principles such as the Golden Rule)

Moral Development Theory: Gilligan

Although all his research subjects were male, Kohlberg claimed that his sequence of stages applies equally to everyone. The validity of his theory for women has been sharply criticized, most prominently by Carol Gilligan (1982, 1993). To address the moral development of women, Gilligan proposed an alternative theory that incorporates the concepts of caring, interpersonal relationships, and responsibility. She described a three-stage approach to moral development:

- **Stage 1: Caring for Oneself.** The focus is on providing for oneself and surviving. The individual is egocentric in thought and does not consider the needs of others. When concerns about selfishness begin to emerge, the individual is signaling a readiness to move to stage 2.

- **Stage 2: Caring for Others.** The woman recognizes the importance of relationships with others. She is willing to make sacrifices to help others, often at the expense of her own needs. When she recognizes the conflict between caring for oneself and caring for others, she is ready to move to stage 3.

- **Stage 3: Caring for Self and Others.** This is the highest stage of moral development. Care is the focus of decision making. The woman carefully balances her own needs against the needs of others to decide on a course of action.

See Chapter 43 for more discussion of moral development.

Spiritual Development Theory

James Fowler, a minister, defined faith as a universal human concern and as a process of growing in trust. He noticed that his congregants had very different approaches to faith, depending on their age. Basing his studies on the work of Piaget, Erikson, and Kohlberg, he developed a theory of faith development, which includes a pre-stage (stage 0) and six stages of faith (Fowler, 1981).

Stages 0, 1, and 2 are closely associated with evolving cognitive abilities. In these stages, faith depends largely on the views expressed by the parents, caregivers, and those who have significant influence in the life of the person.

Stage 3 coincides with the ability to use **logic** and **hypothetical thinking** to construct and evaluate ideas. At this point, faith is largely a collection of conventional, unexamined beliefs. Fowler's studies demonstrated that approximately one-fourth of all adults function at this level or lower.

Stages 4, 5, and 6 represent increasing levels of refinement of faith. With each increase in level there is decreasing likelihood that an individual can attain this stage of development. Fowler found that very few people achieve stage 6.

The rest of this chapter describes the human life span as a series of developmental stages: physical, cognitive, and psychosocial. Development and common health problems are discussed for each stage. To simplify organization, nursing assessments and interventions to promote health are included with the discussion of each stage rather than in a single Practical Knowledge section.

THE GESTATIONAL PERIOD: CONCEPTION TO BIRTH

The time between conception and birth is called the **gestational period.** Human gestation (pregnancy) is calculated from the first day of the mother's last menstrual period and lasts approximately 40 weeks, or 280 days. Full discussions of pregnancy and childbirth are beyond the scope of a fundamentals text. If you need more information, refer to a maternal health textbook.

Fetal Physical Development During Gestation

Pregnancy is usually divided into three trimesters, each lasting about 13 weeks.

First Trimester The first 8 weeks is known as the **embryonic phase.** It begins when an egg that has been released from a woman's ovary unites with a sperm cell, usually in one of the woman's fallopian tubes. This is called **fertilization** (or conception).

- *First 7 days.* Continual cell division leads to the development of a tiny ball of cells called the **morula,** which travels toward the uterus for a period of about 7 days before implanting in the woman's uterus.
- *Upon implantation,* three primary germ layers begin to differentiate, and the **embryo** begins to resemble a tiny organism with a head and tail.
- *By week 4,* the brain, heart, and liver have begun to form, and tiny limb buds are present.
- *As early as 6 to 7 weeks,* you can hear the fetal heartbeat with a fetal ultrasound Doppler.
- *By the end of week 8,* all organs are formed, and the embryo is now called a fetus.

Second Trimester Rapid fetal growth and further development of the body systems characterize the second trimester. At approximately 16 to 20 weeks of pregnancy, the mother can feel her fetus move, a sensation called **quickening.** At the end of the second trimester, the fetus has all organs and body parts intact, which become more efficient during the last trimester. For example:

- The kidneys are intact and begin to produce urine, although they do not effectively concentrate urine until later in the third trimester.
- The lungs are formed, although they do not contain enough of the substance that keeps air sacs open after birth until later in the third trimester.

Third Trimester The fetus continues to grow in size and add subcutaneous fat. Body systems mature in preparation for extrauterine life. If born prematurely during this trimester, the newborn may be able to survive with intensive care. By week 37, the fetus is considered full term; birth after 41 weeks is considered post-term. A normal full-term baby weighs, on average, 5 lb 8 oz to 8 lb 13 oz (2,500 to 4,000 g) and is 20 in. (50 cm) long.

Maternal Changes During Pregnancy

A woman's health during pregnancy is essential for healthy, sustained growth and development of the fetus. It is important for young women to develop good health practices well before conception, including exercise, a balanced diet, smoking cessation, avoidance of alcohol, and regular dental checkups.

KEY POINT: *The growing fetus depends entirely on the health of the placenta for oxygen and nutrition.* Therefore, many of the physical changes that the woman experiences during pregnancy are for the purpose of increasing blood flow through the placenta to the baby.

- The heart of a pregnant woman typically enlarges slightly.
- Cardiac output increases significantly.
- The chest wall expands so that respiratory rate increases significantly.
- The woman increases her normal blood flow by about 30% by the 35th week of pregnancy.

First Trimester Menses typically cease. Hormone shifts occur, primarily in progesterone and estrogen. These cause many pregnant women to experience morning sickness, fullness in the pelvic area, breast enlargement and tenderness, urinary frequency, and fatigue.

Second Trimester The uterus enlarges and hyperpigmentation of the skin occurs, often creating a dark line from the umbilicus to the symphysis pubis and causing the nipples to darken. Other common changes include the mottling of the cheeks and forehead, swelling and bleeding of the gums, and "stuffiness" from swelling of the mucous membranes in the nose. The woman begins to feel the fetus moving and may experience mild contractions, called Braxton Hicks.

Third Trimester Fetal movement is the predominant feature of the latter period of pregnancy. The breasts begin to produce and secrete colostrum in preparation for lactation. Pressure from the enlarged fetus may cause shortness of breath and urinary frequency.

Psychosocial Challenges The birth of a child is a life-changing condition, so it is normal for women to feel ambivalent about pregnancy at first. However, these feelings usually resolve in the second trimester. The pregnant woman must adapt to changes in body image and role and expectations, concerns about sexuality and whether the partner is sexually satisfied, fears about labor and delivery, concern for the baby's health and safety, planning for care of the child after birth, financial pressures, and stresses involving employment during pregnancy.

Common Health Problems During Gestation

Blood circulating through the placenta carries nutrients and oxygen to the fetus and carries toxins and metabolic wastes away from the fetus. Other substances also cross the placenta, for example, **teratogens.**

Teratogens are substances that interfere with normal growth and development.

KEY POINT: *Because the brain and other vital organs develop rapidly during the first trimester, this is the time when the fetus is most vulnerable to teratogens, including the following:*

- *Alcohol* can cause birth defects, growth retardation, developmental delay, and impaired intellectual development.
- *Nicotine* interferes with the transport of oxygen to the fetus, contributing to premature birth, low birth weight, and learning disabilities.
- *Morphine, heroin, methadone, and other narcotics,* when used during pregnancy, cause the newborn to suffer from withdrawal at birth. Symptoms include tremors, restlessness, hyperactive reflexes, poor temperature control, vomiting and diarrhea, high-pitched cries, seizures, and sometimes death.
- *Cocaine, including crack, and methamphetamines* are highly addictive and potentially harmful to the fetus. Infants born to cocaine users and crack users are more likely to suffer from growth retardation and to have sleep disturbances, hyperactive reflexes, irritability, feeding difficulties, attention and behavioral disorders, and learning disabilities at school age. These infants are also more likely to die of **sudden infant death syndrome (SIDS),** the sudden, unexplained death of an infant (discussed in more detail in the next section).
- ✚ *Medications,* prescribed or over the counter, can have teratogenic effects. Examples include the acne medication isotretinoin (Accutane), tetracycline (Achromycin), phenytoin (Dilantin), and lithium (Lithobid). Pregnant women should check with their primary care provider before taking any medications or herbal remedies.

Effects of Maternal Age

- *Adolescence.* The risk for preterm birth, low birth weight, and fetal death is higher for babies born to adolescent mothers.
- *Over age 40.* The risk of fetal death is also higher for mothers over age 40 (Matthews, MacDorman, & Thoma, 2015).
- *Down syndrome.* The risk of conceiving a child with Down syndrome (trisomy 21) and other congenital anomalies increases for each year over the age of 35, but dramatically so after age 42.

Effects of Maternal Health

Maternal diseases, such as rubella, syphilis, and gonorrhea, although not common, can cause fetal blindness, deafness, or fetal loss.

- *Cytomegalovirus* (CMV) is a common flu-like viral infection in adults. If the mother acquires CMV during pregnancy, the fetus can suffer intrauterine growth retardation, poor brain growth, enlarged liver (hepatomegaly) with jaundice, irritation of the lung (pneumonitis), and bleeding problems.
- *Toxoplasmosis* can be transmitted to the unborn fetus through handling of contaminated cat litter.
- *Genital herpes* can be passed to the infant during delivery if the mother experiences an outbreak at that time.
- *Maternal diabetes* can result in low blood sugar after birth and can also have lasting effects on the fetus. Poor glucose control during pregnancy may lead to neural tube and heart defects, as well as **macrosomia** (large body size).

Effects of Maternal Nutrition

Appropriate, healthy weight management before conception contributes to fetal and maternal health. Appropriate maternal weight gain contributes to appropriate fetal birth weight and reduces the risk of fetal illness and infections (Fig. 9-1). The recommended average weight gain for a pregnancy is 25 to 35 pounds. The expected weight gain is higher for underweight women and lower for overweight women.

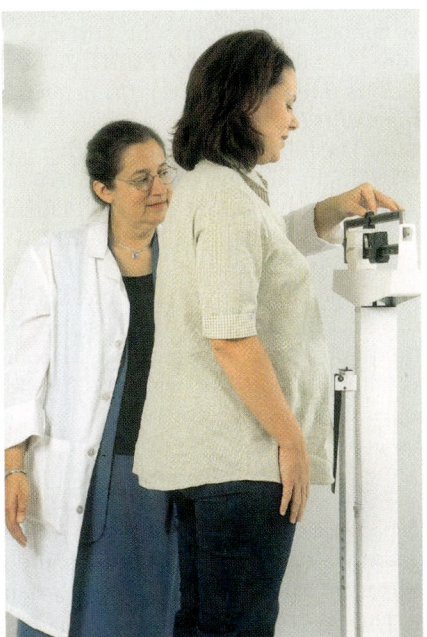

FIGURE 9-1 After establishing a baseline weight in early pregnancy, monitor for appropriate weight gain at each prenatal visit.

✚ *Folic acid deficiency* in the first weeks of pregnancy—typically before the woman even knows she is pregnant—is a risk factor for neural tube defects such as spina bifida. Neural tube defects occur during the first week of fetal development.

ASSESSMENT (Prenatal) NP

Routine prenatal visits and screenings usually take place monthly until 28 weeks, then every 2 weeks until 36 weeks, then weekly until birth. Vital signs, weight, fetal heart tones, nutritional status, and other measures of maternal–fetal well-being (following) should be assessed at each visit.

- *Common discomforts associated with pregnancy,* such as nausea, fatigue, and back pain
- *Preexisting conditions* (e.g., heart disease)
- *Medication use,* including over-the-counter (OTC) drugs; the use of alternative therapies, and other substances

Screening is also done for complications of pregnancy, such as the following:

- **Birth defects.** Women who are at higher risk for a fetus with a birth defect are those with advanced maternal age (over age 40), family history of congenital anomalies, maternal diabetes with insulin use, viral infection during pregnancy, and exposure to high levels of radiation. Blood markers and ultrasound screening are done to detect neural tube defects, abdominal wall defects, trisomy 21 (Down syndrome), and trisomy 18.
- **Gestational diabetes.** Screening for gestational diabetes is most often done between 24 and 28 weeks' gestation—earlier if there is a history of gestational diabetes with a previous pregnancy.
- **Group B streptococcus.** The Centers for Disease Control and Prevention (CDC), the American Academy of Pediatrics (AAP), and the American College of Obstetricians and Gynecologists (ACOG) recommend that pregnant women be screened for group B streptococcus between 35 and 37 weeks' gestation.

INTERVENTIONS (Prenatal) NP

KEY POINT: *One of the most important nursing interventions in promoting maternal and fetal health is to facilitate and teach the importance of early and continuing prenatal care.* Early prenatal care makes it possible to identify complications of pregnancy and to prevent some of the effects of maternal diseases such as diabetes. Each prenatal visit is an opportunity for patient education.

KEY POINT: *Maternal nutrition is important for a healthy baby. The mother's food intake should be well balanced.*

- *Vitamins and minerals.* Recommended dietary allowances of vitamins and minerals for a pregnant woman are 25% to 50% higher than for a nonpregnant woman.
- *Calories.* Pregnant women should increase their caloric intake by 10% to 15%.
- *Protein.* Inadequate protein affects formation of the placenta and fetal brain development.
- *Folic acid.* Increasing folic acid (also called folate) intake to 400 mcg daily reduces the risk of neural tube defects.

Women who are of childbearing age should follow these guidelines even before pregnancy. This will help achieve a national objective for the year 2020 of reducing the incidence of neural tube defects (U.S. Department of Health and Human

Services, 2010a). You can find this and other national goals for 2020 on the *Healthy People 2020* Web site:

 Go to http://www.healthypeople.gov/2020/topics-objectives/ topic/maternal-infant-and-child-health/objectives

Other teaching topics include the following:
Information regarding sexually transmitted diseases and vaginal infections
Information about urinary tract infections
Exercise patterns
Child care
Growth and development of the fetus
Potentially hazardous substances that should be avoided
Avoiding use of OTC medications without approval from the supervising provider
Self-care measures for common discomforts of pregnancy
Danger signs that alert the woman to call her care provider
Signs of impending labor; when to go to the birthing unit

KnowledgeCheck 9-3

- What are the most common health concerns to monitor in the gestational period?
- Identify at least four important topics for health teaching with the expectant mother.
- Why is early prenatal care so important?

NEONATAL PERIOD: BIRTH TO 28 DAYS

During the neonatal period (the first month of life), the newborn's primary task is to stabilize the body's major organ systems and adapt to life outside the uterus. Behaviors are primarily reflexive.

Physical Development of the Neonate

Growth   Following are characteristics of the normal full-term newborn:

- *Weight.* 5 lb 8 oz to 8 lb 13 oz. (2,500 to 4,000 g). Lower birth weights are seen with prematurity; higher birth weights are associated with gestational diabetes.
- *Length.* Between 18 and 22 in. (46 and 56 cm) (Fig. 9-2). The arms are slightly longer than the legs.
- *Head and skull.* At birth, the head is one-fourth the total body length; head circumference is 13 to 14 in. (33 to 35 cm). The head may appear asymmetrical for a few days because of molding during vaginal birth. The skull consists of six soft bones separated by sutures composed of cartilage (Fig. 9-3), with anterior and posterior **fontanels** (soft spots). The fontanels allow room to accommodate the rapid growth of the infant's brain during the first months of life.

Respirations   KEY POINT: *At birth, the most critical adaptation is the* **establishment of respirations.** Pressure on the baby's

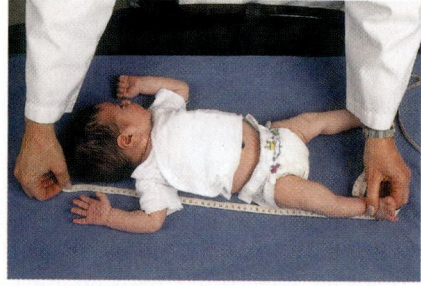

FIGURE 9-2 Measuring the length of a newborn.

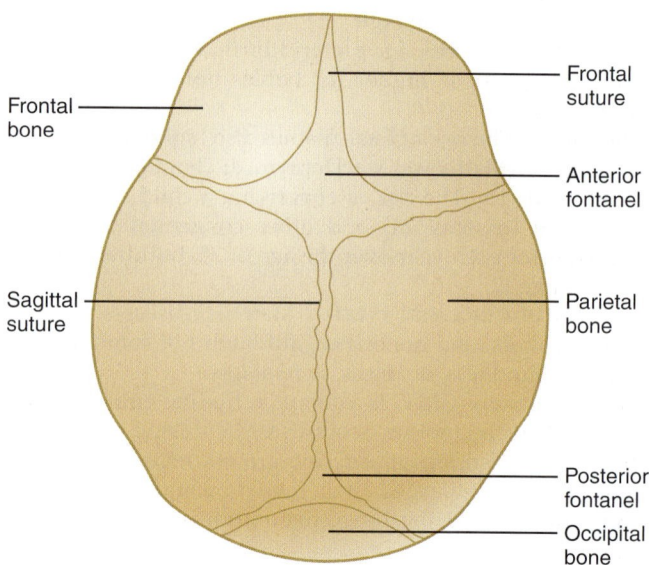

FIGURE 9-3 Sutures and fontanels of the newborn's skull.

chest during vaginal birth helps remove amniotic fluid from the lungs in preparation for breathing. The normal newborn's respirations are irregular, shallow, and 30 to 50 breaths/min, with brief periods of **periodic breathing** (pauses in breathing).

Cardiovascular System   The cardiovascular system must adapt to the change from placental blood flow and convert to independent circulation. The average heart rate of a newborn is 120 to 140 beats/min, with slightly lower rates at rest and higher rates with activity or crying. Poor peripheral circulation causes a bluish coloration of the hands and feet; this is normal and usually disappears within a few hours of birth.

Thermoregulation   The normal newborn's temperature should be close to that of an adult. Maintaining a normal body temperature is a critical task at birth, as the newborn chills easily. The newborn can produce adequate heat but cannot protect against heat loss. Heat may be lost by exposure to cool air temperatures, contact with cooler solid surfaces, or evaporation of moisture from the skin. **KEY POINT:** *To facilitate thermoregulation, it is important to keep the newborn warm and dry, with a cap on his head.*

Elimination   The following are normal characteristics:
- *Kidneys.* At birth, the kidneys produce 15 to 60 mL of urine per kilogram of body weight per day. During the first 24 hours, the infant voids 5 to 25 times. Newborns have limited ability to concentrate urine.
- *Bowel.* At birth, the newborn's lower intestine is filled with **meconium,** a sticky, greenish-black substance formed from amniotic fluid and intestinal secretions. Meconium is usually passed within 12 hours of birth, and the stool progressively changes in color to yellow.
- *Gastrointestinal system.* The full-term infant is able to swallow, digest, metabolize, and absorb proteins and simple carbohydrates. Stomach capacity varies from 30 to 90 mL. Normal colonic bacteria are established within a week of birth.

Epidermis and Dermis   The epidermis and dermis are very thin at birth and can be easily damaged. Infants are born with varying degrees of **vernix caseosa,** a cheese-like protective covering for the skin. **Milia,** tiny white spots, may be present on the newborn's face, and the area over the sacrum may show a darkly pigmented area called a **mongolian spot.** All such features disappear spontaneously.

Neuromuscular System   The neuromuscular system is not completely developed at birth, but the following **reflexes** (automatic responses) are present at birth. Selected reflexes are illustrated in Figure 9-4.

- **Rooting.** Rooting is elicited by stroking the infant's cheek with the nipple or finger. In response, the newborn turns his head toward the stimulus, opens his mouth, takes hold, and sucks. This reflex disappears by 3 to 4 months of age.
- **Sucking Reflex.** The sucking reflex is elicited by touching the infant's lips.
- **Swallowing Reflex.** The swallowing reflex is coordinated with sucking and usually occurs without gagging, coughing, or vomiting. This response is weak with prematurity or neurological defect.
- **Grasp Reflex.** The grasp reflex is triggered by placing a finger in the palm of the infant's hand (palmar) or at the base of the toes (plantar). The infant's fingers curl around the examiner's fingers, or the toes curl downward. The palmar reflex lessens by 3 to 4 months, and the plantar reflex lessens by 8 months.
- **Tonic Neck or Fencing Reflex.** The tonic neck reflex is elicited by rotating the infant's head to the left with the left arm and leg extended and the right arm and leg flexed. Turn the head to the right and the extremities assume the opposite posture. The response disappears by 3 to 4 months.
- **Moro or Startle Reflex.** This reflex is elicited by placing the infant on a flat surface and striking the surface to startle the infant. Symmetrical abduction and extension of the arms are expected as an indicator of overall neurological health. The fingers fan out and form a C with the thumb and forefinger. This response is absent by 6 months.
- **Stepping Reflex.** Elicit the stepping reflex by holding the infant vertically, allowing one foot to touch a surface (e.g., tabletop). The infant will simulate walking by alternating flexion and extension of the feet during the first 3 to 4 weeks of life.
- **Crawling Reflex.** The crawling reflex is noted by placing the infant on her abdomen. The newborn makes crawling movements with her arms and legs. This response should disappear by 6 weeks of age.
- **Babinski Reflex.** The Babinski reflex is elicited by stroking upward along the lateral aspect of the sole. A positive response occurs when the toes hyperextend and the great toe dorsiflexes. An infant who does not respond in this manner should undergo a neurological evaluation. This reflex disappears as the infant begins to walk or between 12 and 18 months.

Cognitive Development of the Neonate

In the first month of life, the neonate responds to stimuli in a reflexive manner. Piaget described this as stage 1 of the *sensorimotor phase*. But despite the newborn's limited voluntary abilities, the sensory functions are well developed.

Vision   At birth, the eyes are treated with antibiotics to prevent blindness caused by gonorrhea.

- After the ointment has been absorbed, the newborn begins to fixate on objects. During the first few weeks of life, the infant focuses on objects, following from side to side with his gaze.
- The infant has visual preferences for the human face, black-and-white contrasting patterns, and large objects.
- Some newborns appear cross-eyed because of undeveloped ocular muscle control; this normally resolves in 3 to 4 months.
- Eye color varies from dark to slate gray to pale blue.
- Because the lacrimal apparatus is not fully developed, the newborn does not produce tears until at least week 4 of life.

Hearing and Smell   Once the amniotic fluid drains from the ears, hearing is equivalent to that of an adult. Newborns react strongly to pungent odors by turning the head away

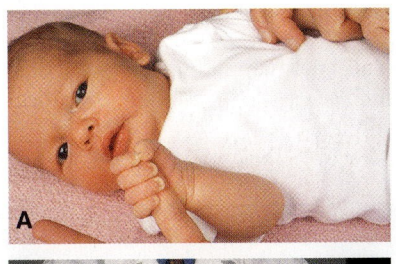
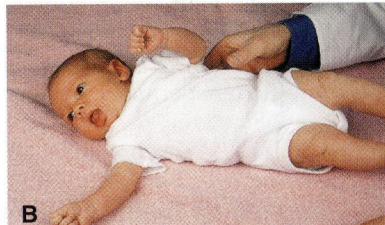
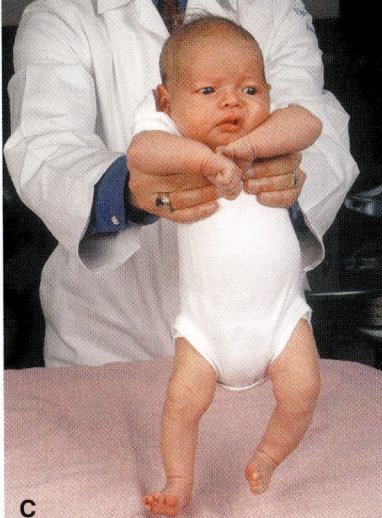
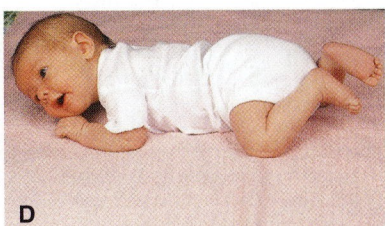

FIGURE 9-4 Several infant reflexes. (A) The palmar grasp reflex. (B) Tonic neck reflex. (C) Stepping reflex. (D) Crawling reflex.

from a smell and are able to distinguish their own mother's breast milk from that of other women. They will cry for their mother when her breasts are engorged and leaking.

Touch The newborn has a highly developed sense of touch, and his tactile sensation is surprisingly sophisticated, especially around the mouth, hands, and feet.

Psychosocial Development of the Neonate

The neonate calms when held or with other pacifying measures, such as a warm blanket, pacifier, and swaddling. Crying is the principal method for communicating a need or displeasure. Sometimes crying occurs simply because the neurological system is immature. Erikson identified the central developmental task of the first 18 months of life as developing a sense of trust. The neonate is completely dependent on her caretakers for all needs. Prompt responses to cries of discomfort create security and trust and promote **attachment,** emotional bonding between parent and child.

Common Health Problems of the Neonate

Respiratory Distress Respiratory distress is one of the most serious problems facing newborns. It occurs most commonly in infants born before the lungs mature but can also be caused by aspiration of meconium during the birthing process. Symptoms are pale or mottled skin, labored respirations, hypothermia, and flaccid muscle tone.

Birth Injuries Birth injuries may occur during the birthing process. The following are three examples:

- *Caput succedaneum,* edema of the scalp that crosses the suture lines, results from head compression against the cervix during labor. The fluid is reabsorbed in 1 to 3 days.
- *Fracture of the clavicle* occurs with breech presentation or as a result of difficulty delivering a large baby whose shoulder gets stuck behind the mother's pelvic bones. Often no intervention is needed except for careful handling and supporting the affected bone.
- *Birth asphyxia* is a serious and potentially permanent injury resulting from perinatal events, such as a *cord prolapse*

(compression of the umbilical cord), *placental abruption* (bleeding secondary to tear of the placenta), other interruption of the blood supply between the baby and placenta, or delay in infant respiration after birth.

Congenital Anomalies Congenital anomalies (birth defects) may be visible at birth or may become apparent in the neonatal period. Treatment may be initiated if appropriate. Congenital heart defects, fistulas, and cleft lip and palate, or inborn metabolic problems are some common birth defects.

Infectious Microorganisms Infectious microorganisms that do not cause illness in older babies can cause sepsis for newborns, especially those born prematurely. Pregnant women should be screened prenatally for sexually transmitted infections (STIs) and treatment initiated if possible. Newborns exposed to infections during the gestational period should be tested as soon as possible after birth.

Jaundice Within 48 to 72 hours after birth, the newborn's red blood cell (RBC) count normally begins to decrease. One byproduct of RBC destruction is **bilirubin,** a yellowish pigment. If the newborn is not successful in eliminating the excess bilirubin, **jaundice** develops, giving the newborn's skin a yellowish cast. If the bilirubin level becomes too high, the newborn can suffer neurological consequences as the pigment enters the brain. Sunlight breaks down bilirubin; thus phototherapy is a treatment of choice for jaundice.

Fetal Alcohol Syndrome Fetal alcohol syndrome may occur in infants of pregnant women addicted to alcohol. It is characterized by irregular facial features and cognitive deficits.

Mothers With Substance Addiction Newborns born to women who abuse substances during pregnancy are at risk for respiratory distress, behavioral abnormalities, and birth defects, as well as drug withdrawal.

ASSESSMENT (Neonate) NP

Physical assessment begins at birth. The initial assessment tool is the **Apgar scoring system** (see Table 9-4). Each category is scored at 1 and 5 minutes after birth. The 1-minute score indicates how well the baby tolerated the birthing process; the 5-minute score indicates how well the baby is

Table 9-4 ▶ Apgar Scoring			
CATEGORY	**0**	**I**	**2**
Breathing effort	Not breathing	Respirations slow (less than 30 breaths/min) or irregular	Infant cries well
Heart rate (by stethoscope)	None	Less than 100 beats/min	Greater than 100 beats/min
Muscle tone	Loose and floppy	Some muscle tone, weak flexion	Active motion, full flexion
Grimace response or Reflex irritability (response to stimulation such as mild pinch)	No reaction	Grimacing	Grimacing and cough, sneeze, or vigorous cry
Skin color	Pale blue	Pink with blue extremities	Entire body is pink

Source: Apgar score. (n.d.). Medline Plus, U.S. National Library of Medicine, National Institutes of Health. Retrieved from http://www.nlm.nih.gov/medlineplus/ency/article/003402.htm

adapting to the new environment. A high score indicates fetal well-being. Prematurity, neuromuscular disease, and maternal sedation during the birthing process are all factors that can lower the Apgar scores.

During the first 24 hours after birth, the nurse assesses the infant's transition to extrauterine life:

- *First 8 hours.* The infant alternately cries and appears interested in the environment.
- *Sleep stage.* The infant then enters the sleep stage, which lasts 2 to 4 hours. The heart and respiratory rates decrease and the infant is in a state of calm.
- *Alert stage.* After the sleep phase, the infant is alert and responsive. The heart and respiratory rates again increase.

Shortly after birth, newborns are screened for a variety of genetic disorders. Most states require screening for phenylketonuria (PKU) (an inborn error of metabolism), hypothyroidism, galactosemia, and sickle cell disease. You will also need to assess the following parameters:

Vital signs
Elimination (first urine and meconium)
Presence of congenital anomalies
Reflexes
Ability to breastfeed or take formula from a bottle
Skin integrity
Parent–infant attachment

INTERVENTIONS (Neonate) NP

The neonatal period is a time of transition. Feeding concerns and uncertainty about appropriate care are the primary reasons parents seek healthcare advice. Nursing interventions for the neonate are designed to smooth the transition to extrauterine life and help the neonate adjust to his new environment. Activities include the following:

- ✚ Thoroughly dry the neonate at birth and after bathing to prevent heat loss via evaporation. Also wrap the neonate in blankets and place her in her mother's arms or in a warmed crib.

- Assist the mother with breastfeeding or formula feeding. Often assistance is needed with the first few feedings as the newborn learns to latch on to the nipple.
- Teach parents the importance of providing warmth, nutrition, and a clean environment to prevent infection.
- Teach the caregivers about expected behavior, including crying, eating, and elimination.
- Provide circumcision care. **Circumcision** is surgical removal of the foreskin of the penis. Many male infants are circumcised a day or two after birth, although there is controversy over risks and benefits. The main reason most parents elect circumcision for their infant is social, so their child looks like other family members and peers. Parental consent is required for this procedure. Care of the site depends on the type of procedure. For all circumcisions, the nurse should observe and teach parents to observe for hemorrhage, swelling, or oozing (signs of infection).

INFANCY: 1 MONTH TO 1 YEAR OF AGE

The remainder of the first year is known as infancy. This is a time associated with dramatic physical changes and acquisition of numerous skills.

Physical Development of the Infant

Growth The full-term newborn:
- Loses approximately 8% to 10% of birth weight in the first days of life but will regain it by 2 weeks of age.

- Gains about 1½ pounds per month for the first 3 months.
- Doubles in birth weight by 5 months of age and triples by 1 year.
- Increases in length approximately 1 inch per month until 6 months of age; it then slows to 1 inch over the next 6 months.
- Increases head circumference by about 33% in the first year.

Eruption of Primary Teeth Eruption of teeth varies among children, but there is a distinct, predictable pattern for eruption. The first tooth typically appears between 6 and 8 months of age. First to appear are lower central incisors, followed by the upper central incisors.

Feeding Infants typically consume about 30 ounces of breast milk or formula per day by 4 months of age. Breastfeeding is recommended because it is considered the most complete nutritional source for infants up to 6 months of age. **KEY POINT:** *Breastfed infants have a lower incidence of food allergies, gastroenteritis, ear infections, and overweight in childhood, adolescence, and adulthood (Salone, Vann, & Dee, 2013). In addition, breast milk supplies immunoglobulins that help the infant to resist infection. However, if breastfeeding is not possible or acceptable to the parents, the nurse should support the parents' choice of method.*

Most infants are physiologically ready to take solid foods between 4 and 6 months of age, but adequate nutrition can be maintained with breast milk or formula for a full year. The choices of when to begin introducing solid foods and when to wean are often culturally determined.

Sleep Patterns Sleep patterns vary among infants. Generally, by 3 to 4 months the infant has developed a night pattern of sleeping and can sleep approximately 10 hours. Infants vary in the number and length of naps they take, but the total numbers of hours they sleep per day is about 15.

Motor Development Motor development follows a predictable pattern. Box 9-1 lists typical milestones.

BOX 9-1 ■ Milestones of Infant Development

- By age 3 months, infant can smile.
- By 5 months, rolls from abdomen to back.
- By 6 months, turns from back to abdomen.
- At 7 months, most can sit alone.
- At around 9 months, crawls on hands and knees.
- By 10 months, pincer grasp is well enough developed to pick up finger foods; and can move from a prone to sitting position.
- At 11 months, can "cruise"—walk holding on to furniture.
- By 12 months, many infants attempt their first independent steps.
- By 12 months, many can pick up objects and let them go, put objects into a container, and take them out again. Typically, can also find an object that has been hidden, and are beginning to use objects, such as cups and combs, correctly, as when "combing dolly's hair."
- By 12 months, typically responds to simple verbal requests and commands, such as "Stop!" or "No." May also use simple gestures such as waving bye-bye or shaking their head no, and may try to imitate adults' words.
- Psychosocial milestones include testing of caregivers to see what response is elicited by crying, refusals, and so on; anxiety with strangers; and strong preference for the primary caregiver (usually the mother).

Cognitive Development of the Infant

Piaget describes the infancy phase of cognitive development as the *sensorimotor phase*.

- Whereas the neonate responds in a reflexive manner, the infant makes major strides in motor development and is able to verbally interact with caregivers.
- An infant's visual acuity and color discrimination allow her to see and explore the environment.
- Hearing is becoming more discriminating, and infants please themselves by vocalizing with cooing, laughing, and repeating sounds they find pleasurable.
- By the 12th month, the infant is able to imitate sounds and understand simple words and may have a vocabulary of four or five simple words, such as "da-da."
- At this stage, infants learn by doing. They develop a simple sense of cause and effect, delighting in the fact that squeezing a ball, for example, causes it to squeak and repeating their experiment over and over again.

Psychosocial Development of the Infant

In infancy the central task remains the development of trust. The response of the caregivers in the neonatal phase has set the tone for ongoing interaction between caregivers and child. Continued prompt responses to discomfort, cuddling, and stimulating interaction provide the infant with a sense of trust in the world.

Freud refers to infancy as the *oral stage*. The infant receives pleasure in sucking and learns to quiet himself by oral stimulation such as eating, sucking on a pacifier, or placing his hand in his mouth. At 2 or 3 months of age, infants begin to smile in response to others. At about 9 months they interact more with their environment and socialize with others. They enjoy simple games, such as peek-a-boo and patty-cake.

Common Health Problems of the Infant

Common problems that cause distress for infants and their caregivers include the following:

Crying and Colic

Crying often alarms parents, but it is a form of communication for the infant and a normal infant reaction to discomfort, cold, or hunger. A healthy infant will have "fussy" periods each day that may last up to 1 to 2 hours. Extended crying may be a sign of **colic,** a term used to describe frequent episodes of abdominal pain. The infant is often inconsolable during these episodes. The cause is unknown, although you may hear several theories. Colic typically disappears at about 3 months of age.

Failure to Thrive

Infants depend on their caregivers for food, water, warmth, comfort, and love. An infant who is deprived of a comforting, responsive relationship with a mother or caregiver will not thrive even if supplied with adequate nutrition. The infant will fail to gain weight, be unable to meet age-appropriate developmental tasks, be malnourished, and may have difficulty interacting with others. This syndrome, known as **failure to thrive,** is exhibited, for example, in some infants in orphanages. Erikson believed the syndrome was proof of the essential nature of the trust versus mistrust stage. Notice, however, that failure to thrive can also stem from organic causes, such as disease or drug withdrawal.

Dental Caries

Dental caries (tooth decay) can develop even by the end of the first year in infants allowed to sleep with a bottle containing anything other than water. Caries are caused by pooling in the back of the mouth of fluids containing sugar, such as breast milk, formula, or juice. If you need more information about dental problems, see Chapter 24.

Example Problem: Abuse and Neglect

We have chosen abuse and neglect as a classic example of a problem of development because it is common and occurs in all developmental stages. You will read about it again and again in sections about other developmental stages, where we discuss how it manifests in those stages and suggest with appropriate nursing interventions.

The youngest children are the most vulnerable to maltreatment. In 2013, 52 states reported that more than one-quarter (27.3%) of victims were younger than 3 years. The rate was highest for children younger than 1 year (National Data Archive on Child Abuse and Neglect, 2013). Also refer to the accompanying Example Problem, Abuse, Neglect, and Violence and the SENC box.

Unintentional Injury

Automobile accidents are a major cause of death in infants, often because the child was not properly restrained. Falls, burns, choking, and drowning are other common causes of accidental injury and death in infants. As infants mature, they may attempt to climb from cribs onto chairs or tables or up or down ungated stairs. Their tendency to explore things with their mouths may lead to choking on small objects such as bottle caps, buttons, and parts of toys. If you require more information about infant safety, refer to Chapter 23.

Sudden Infant Death Syndrome (SIDS)

SIDS is the sudden death of a previously healthy infant with no explainable cause. Even postmortem examinations

---

Safe, Effective Nursing Care

Detecting and Preventing Abuse

Chapter-Related Concepts: Age-Specific Assessments, Age-Specific Interventions

Competency: Thinking, Doing, Caring

Thinking: Detection and prevention of abuse require collaborative efforts of the healthcare team. The goal of the collaborative approach is to reduce trauma to the victims during the investigation and assessment of the patient.

Doing: The team (comprising members from the Department of Child and Family Services [DCFS], law enforcement, state's attorney's office, medical personnel, and mental health counselors) employs a multidisciplinary approach in dealing with issues of child abuse.

Caring: The team approach decreases the number of interviews and invasive procedures a child must endure, thereby reducing the trauma that children face when they have been victims of sexual or physical abuse.

Think about it

Do you see how teamwork and collaboration relate to the key concepts of development and stage?

EXAMPLE PROBLEM: Abuse, Neglect, and Violence

Abuse may be physical, emotional, or sexual; neglect is also a form of abuse. These are all common problems in all developmental stages.

Infants
Abusive head trauma (formerly shaken-baby syndrome) caused by violent shaking of an infant; it can cause severe brain injury.

Toddlers, Preschoolers
Often detected in this stage as children come in contact with more people outside the home.

School-Age
School violence can be addressed through psychological counseling, weapons-screening devices, school-wide educational programs, and policies calling for the suspension or expulsion of students who are caught intimidating other children or participating in fights on school property.

Adolescents
Dating violence is widespread. It has serious short- and long-term effects. Many teens do not report it because they are afraid or embarrassed to tell friends and family.

Young Adulthood
Each year, over 10 million women and men in the United States experience physical violence by a current or former intimate partner.

Middle Adulthood
Intimate murder—Women aged 30 to 49 are the most vulnerable.

Intimate violence—Occurs more often in younger women.

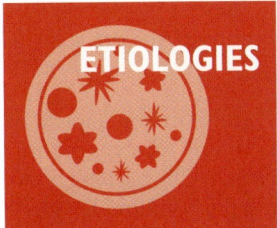

ETIOLOGIES

Large family size
Low income status
Low maternal education

Young maternal age
Single-parent household
Psychiatric disturbances

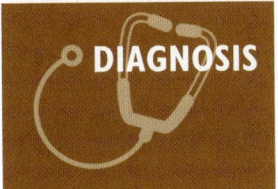

DIAGNOSIS

Self-esteem disturbance related to feeling guilty and responsible for being a victim.

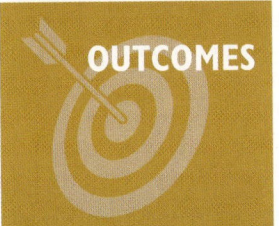

OUTCOMES

- Recognition of abuse relationship
- Healing of physical and psychological injuries
- Improved self-esteem

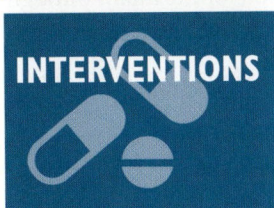

INTERVENTIONS

- Screen for risk factors associated with domestic abuse.
- Determine congruence of injury and the description of cause.

- Provide confidential information regarding domestic violence shelters.
- Monitor use of community resources.
- Refer to Procedure 9-1 at the end of this chapter.

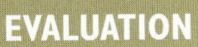

EVALUATION

- The patient will verbalize improved personal judgment of self-worth.

fail to reveal a cause of death. The peak incidence is usually around 3 to 4 months of age, although it may occur up to 12 months of age. An increased incidence is associated with prematurity, low birth weight, male gender, African American race, smoking in the household, swaddling, and putting an infant to sleep in the prone position (Fig. 9-5). Breastfeeding and offering a pacifier at naptime and bedtime are thought to be preventive measures (Alm, Wennergren, Möllborg, et al., 2015; Hauck, Thompson, Tanabe, et al., 2011).

ASSESSMENT (Infants) NP

The infant typically has regular appointments with the pediatrician or primary care provider until at least 6 months of age. As a rule, visits are timed to coincide with the immunization schedule at 2, 4, 6, and 12 months. At each visit, measure the infant's growth and development and compare against standards for height, weight, head circumference, and gross and fine motor skills.

The Denver Developmental Screening Test (Denver II) is a frequently used standardized test to assess development. The Denver II assesses four major areas: personal–social, fine motor skills, language, and gross motor skills. It requires specialized training to administer and evaluate.

✚ Be aware of factors that increase the risk for child abuse. Assess for abuse any time there is an injury that is not well explained by the parent's account of how it occurred. For further discussion about assessing for abuse, see Procedure 9-1.

INTERVENTIONS (Infants) NP

Nursing interventions for the infant focus on health promotion, safety, and growth and development.

Nutrition Teach parents about adequate nutrition, adding foods to the diet, and expected elimination patterns. If breastfeeding is not possible or is not the parents' method of choice, commercially prepared formulas fortified with vitamins and minerals are acceptable. Cow's milk should not be used during the first year of life because infants have difficulty digesting the fat, and cow's milk is low in iron.

Colic Provide information about using warmth, motion, and security to relieve colic. For example, swaddling

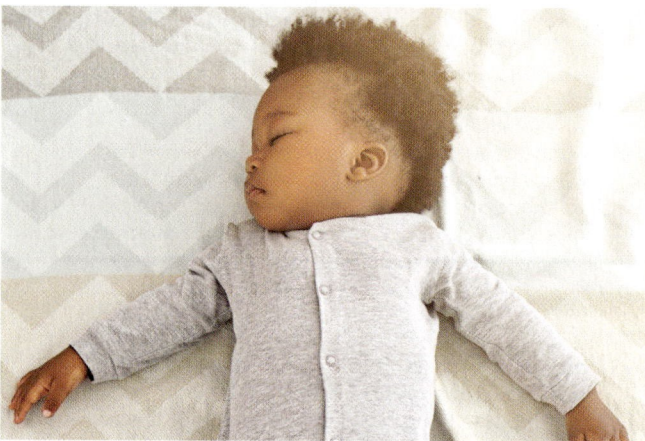

FIGURE 9-5 The Back to Sleep campaign teaches parents to place the infant in the supine position for sleeping.

the baby, cuddling him close to the parent's body, rocking him, placing him in a "kangaroo" pouch or a backpack, or placing him in a swinging chair are all interventions that may provide relief.

SIDS In accordance with recommendations in *Healthy People 2020*, teach parents to place infants on their backs to sleep. Research shows that this greatly decreases the risk for SIDS. Additional interventions are discussed in Chapter 23.

Car Seats Stress the importance of car seats. Under federal law, infants must be secured in an approved car seat (in the backseat) every time they are in a vehicle. Because of poorly developed musculoskeletal head support, infants should be placed in a rear-facing position until 2 years of age and until they reach the height and weight recommended by the seat manufacturer (American Academy of Pediatrics, 2011).

For more information about car seat restraints, refer to Chapter 23 and

Go to the American Academy of Pediatrics Web site at www.aap.org

Immunizations Immunizations are a major aspect of health promotion for the infant. The infant receives immunizations at 2, 4, 6, and 12 months. The CDC is no longer expressing a preference for administering the combined MMRV vaccine rather than two shots (MMR for measles, mumps, and rubella, and a separate one for varicella [chicken pox]). To see the CDC's optimal immunization schedule for children up to 6 years of age,

Go to the CDC Web site at http://www.cdc.gov/vaccines/ schedules/easy-to-read/child.html

Unintentional Injury ✚ Stress the importance of constant supervision. As the infant gains greater mobility, potential dangers (e.g., drowning, falls, burns) increase. To prevent drowning, infants should never be left unattended in sinks, shallow baths, or plastic wading pools, even for a few seconds. To prevent scalding, caregivers should not drink or carry hot foods or fluids while holding the baby.

Play Encourage sensory stimulation for the infant through parental interaction and age-appropriate toys.

Example Problem Interventions: Abuse ✚ Teach parents about the dangers of shaking a baby or picking him up by an arm or leg.

If you suspect abuse, you are legally responsible for reporting your observations. As a beginning student, it is best to first discuss your concerns and findings with your instructor or the nurse assigned to the client. Federal funds support a variety of home visit programs directed at high-risk mothers. Further information reporting abuse is included in Chapter 44, under Mandatory Reporting Laws, and in Procedure 9-1.

Think Like a Nurse 9-3

Recall the story of Miguel, a 2-month-old infant, in the Meet Your Patients scenario. How might a prolonged hospitalization affect his growth and development? What nursing actions would you take to offset developmental delays?

KnowledgeCheck 9-4

- Identify at least two reflexes present in the neonate.
- According to Erikson, what is the developmental stage of the infant?
- What teaching guideline is important in reducing the risk of SIDS?

TODDLERHOOD: AGES 1 TO 3 YEARS

The toddler period is from 12 to 36 months of age. This is a period of increased mobility, independence, and exploration. It is also the time of temper tantrums and negative behavior, stemming from the toddler's desire to gain autonomy.

Physical Development of the Toddler

- *Growth rate* for toddlers is much slower than it is in infancy.

  Weight. The average toddler gains 5 lb (2.3 kg) per year. By the second birthday the typical toddler weighs 27 lb (12.25 kg).

  Height. By the second birthday, the typical toddler is 34 in. (86 cm) tall. Length is added mainly in the legs.

  Head. Head circumference is equal to the chest circumference. Between 12 and 18 months, the anterior fontanel closes (see Fig. 9-3).

- *Respirations and heart rate* slow in comparison to infancy, but blood pressure increases.
- *The stomach* increases in size to accommodate larger portions. Toddlers typically eat about six times a day, in relatively small portions, and join the family at mealtimes. Most toddlers enjoy picking up food with their hands to feed themselves.
- *Physical ability to control the anal and urethral sphincters* develops between 18 and 24 months. However, the child is ready to toilet train when she can signal that her diaper is wet or soiled or is able to say that she would like to go to the potty. This usually occurs at about 18 to 24 months of age, but it is not uncommon for a child to be in diapers until 3 years of age (Chobey & George, 2008).
- *Gross motor skills* continue to be refined during toddlerhood. By 10 to 15 months, the toddler can walk using a wide stance. At the age of 24 months, many toddlers can walk up and down stairs one step at a time. At 30 months, he can jump using both feet. Before the age of 3, the toddler can stand on one foot and climb steps alternating feet.
- *Fine motor skills* also continue to be refined. By 15 months the toddler can not only grab small objects but can release objects as well. By 18 months he can throw a ball overhand (Fig. 9-6). The toddler uses his new motor skills and all five senses to explore his environment, and safety continues to be an important concern
- *Visual acuity* improves to 20/40 by the end of the toddler stage, and **strabismus** (crossed eyes) may still be seen transiently.
- *Hearing* should be fully developed by toddlerhood.

  Developmental milestones of toddlerhood are listed in Box 9-2.

Cognitive Development of the Toddler

During toddlerhood the child completes Piaget's *sensorimotor phase* and moves into the *preconceptual phase*. This is a time of rapid language development and increasing curiosity. The toddler is able to name many things and begins to recognize that different objects (such as a ball, a block, and a puzzle) may be named the same thing (toys). This is the beginning of categorization and concept development. In the preconceptual

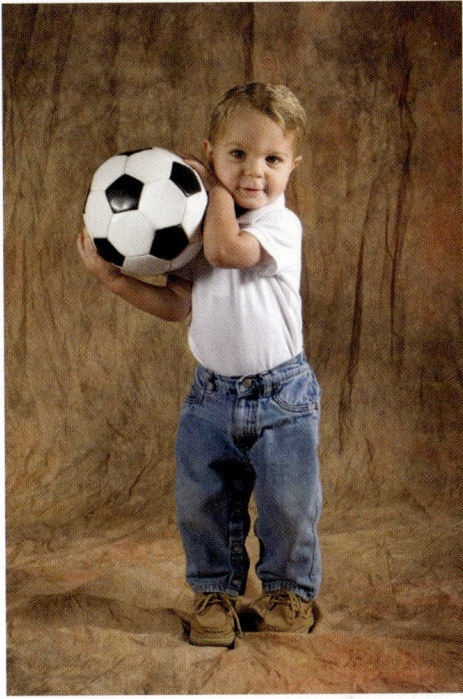

FIGURE 9-6 By 18 mo, the toddler can throw a ball overhand.

BOX 9-2 ■ Milestones of Toddlerhood

- The toddler can ride a tricycle, put simple puzzles together, build a tower of six to eight blocks, turn knobs, and open lids.
- Most toddlers can copy a circle or a vertical line.
- Not only can the toddler find an object that has been hidden in his view, but he can also actively search for and find a hidden object.
- By age 3, most toddlers are toilet trained. However, it is not abnormal for toddlers to continue to experience toileting problems well into the preschool period.
- Most toddlers can play matching games, sorting games, and simple mechanical games.
- Most toddlers have only a limited understanding of jokes and hyperbole; thus, if teased, "That balloon is so big, it might fly away with you," the child may become frightened and try to give the balloon away.
- Many toddlers can speak sentences of four or five words. However, some perfectly healthy toddlers do not yet speak, whereas others can speak in sentences of 10 or 11 words in length and even tell complex stories. If the toddler does speak, enunciation is good enough by the end of this period that strangers can usually understand what is said.
- Psychosocial milestones include the following: The toddler tolerates short separations from the primary caregiver, feels possessive of personal property, and openly expresses affection. Most toddlers object vehemently to changes in routine and may suffer regression following a move, change of school, or other upset.
- The toddler imitates adults, peers, and characters seen on television and videos and enjoys pretending to cook, iron, repair something broken, and mimicking other familiar adult tasks.
- In shared play, the toddler can understand the concept of "taking turns" and wait a short period of time for her turn.

phase, the child abandons trial and error and begins to solve problems by thinking. However, reasoning and judgment lag far behind. This discrepancy places the child at risk for accidents and injuries.

Psychosocial Development of the Toddler

The most important psychosocial developmental task for the toddler is to initiate more independence, control, and autonomy. Erikson refers to this stage as *autonomy versus shame and doubt.* To successfully negotiate this stage, the child must learn to see herself as separate from mother, tolerate separation from the parents, withstand delayed gratification, learn to control anal and urinary sphincters, and begin to verbally communicate and interact with others.

Toddlers exert their independence by saying no to parental requests or actions or by "throwing a tantrum" to protest a parental decision they don't like. This behavior is best understood as a necessary attempt to define boundaries and test parental limits; it may be far more challenging to parents who view it as stubbornness or naughtiness. A firm but calm parental response to such "misbehavior" allows toddlers to feel secure while exploring their boundaries.

Freud defined this phase as the *anal stage.* To Freud, a successful toilet-training experience accompanied by praise is necessary to becoming a well-functioning adult; difficulty in this phase leads to obsessive–compulsive behavior in adulthood. Contemporary theorists find this view somewhat narrow.

Common Health Problems of Toddlers

Unintentional Injury Drowning is the leading cause of accidental death in this age-group (Gholipour, 2014). Most drowning accidents result from unsupervised access to swimming pools or other water sources (bathtubs). Other common causes of injuries to toddlers are falls, accidents, burns and scalds, and choking. As toddlers gain increasing mobility, poisoning from household medications and toxic cleansers becomes a concern, as does access to knives, guns, and other dangers. For further discussion of safety concerns for toddlers, see Chapter 23.

Infections The most common infections are colds, ear infections, and tonsillitis. Other common infections include parasitic diseases, such as lice and tapeworms. The shorter and flatter eustachian tube in infants and toddlers increases their risk for multiple ear infections, which in turn increase the risk for hearing loss. Upper respiratory infections are common among toddlers for the following reasons:

- Toddlers no longer have the passive immunity acquired in utero.
- Because breastfeeding usually ends before the first birthday, most toddlers no longer receive maternal antibodies in breast milk.
- As toddlers enter into more public and social settings, they are exposed to more children. Those in day care and those who have school-age siblings are particularly at risk.

Immunization The CDC (2015a) recommendations for immunization are designed to protect infants and children early in life, when they are most vulnerable and before they are exposed to potentially life-threatening diseases. Vaccines should be administered at the recommended age; but if not done, a vaccine can be administered at a later well-child visit. Catch-up schedules and minimum intervals between doses for children whose vaccinations have been delayed are included

in the recommendations. The CDC updates the immunization schedules periodically. To see the CDC's optimal immunization schedule for children up to 6 years of age,

 Go to the CDC Web Site at http://www.cdc.gov/vaccines/schedules/easy-to-read/child.html

The CDC (2015a) immunization schedule for toddlers includes the following vaccines: hepatitis A, hepatitis B, *Haemophilus influenzae,* meningococcal conjugate, tetanus and diphtheria toxoids (Td), acellular pertussis (Tdap), pneumococcal pneumonia, inactivated poliovirus, varicella, measles/mumps/rubella (MMR), and rotavirus.

Delayed Toilet Training Although not strictly speaking a "health" problem, many parents are concerned about what they perceive as delayed toilet training. Physiologically, most children develop sphincter and neurological control by age 2, but there is more involved in successful toileting. Children must be able to unfasten their clothing and pull down their pants, use toilet paper effectively, dress again, and wash their hands before complete independence is reached. The child also must be able to sense the need to go to the bathroom, even when preoccupied with play activities, before it is "too late." Accidents are frequent and should be expected.

ASSESSMENT (Toddlers) NP

Children of this age are generally fearful of strangers. Thus, before beginning your assessment, you will need to establish rapport. To do so, you might engage the child in play—for example, by playing catch with a soft ball or asking the child to introduce you to the stuffed animal he may have brought along. This is a nonthreatening way to assess the toddler's language skills and motor development. Encourage parents to relieve their child's stress and anxiety by holding him during the exam and speaking to him in a calm and reassuring voice.

Toddlers need regular physical exams. At each office visit, assess the toddler for height, weight, and growth and development against standard growth charts and by comparing his skills against age-appropriate norms. Beginning at age 3, blood pressure should be checked at least once yearly and results recorded with age/gender/height percentile and reviewed with parents (National Heart, Lung, and Blood Institute, 2012).

INTERVENTIONS (Toddlers) NP

Health Teaching You cannot stress safety strongly enough to the parents. Teach them how to childproof the environment. Emphasize that increasing motor skills and dexterity allow the toddler to find many dangers, including stairways, windows, and electrical outlets. To prevent injury or death from such hazards, parents must provide constant supervision. They should use consistent, firm limits to help the toddler remain safe. Parents should also be vigilant about the toys they buy for their children in light of recent toy recalls because they contained lead and other toxic substances. Toys should be larger than the diameter of the trachea in order to avoid choking accidents. Plan ahead by teaching parents basic first aid and the choking rescue maneuver. Encourage parents to enroll in a basic life support class. You will find the choking rescue maneuver as well as a detailed list of safety measures for toddlers in Chapter 23.

Health Promotion Interventions At each wellness visit, reinforce the need for hand washing, tooth brushing, regular dental exams, and a balanced diet. This is also a time for additional immunizations and boosters. Oral health teaching should include information on brushing, fluoride, non-nutritive oral habits, and dental injury prevention (AAP, 2014). AAP recommends that children have a dental home by 1 year of age.

Methicillin-Resistant *Staphylococcus aureus* (MRSA) and Vancomycin-Resistant Enterococci (VRE) These organisms have put a spotlight on the threat posed by drug-resistant bacteria. **KEY POINT:** *Teach parents that antibiotics should not be used for simple colds and flu. Explain the importance of taking the entire prescription when an antibiotic must be prescribed, even if the child's symptoms resolve before all the medication has been taken.* These actions help prevent the development of drug-resistant strains of bacteria.

Remind parents that many over-the-counter cough and cold medicines are not safe for and may not been approved for use in children, regardless of how they are marketed. Parents should be certain that any over-the-counter medicines are truly safe for children.

KnowledgeCheck 9-5

- According to Erikson, what is the developmental stage of the toddler?
- What is the leading cause of accidental death in toddlers?

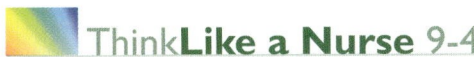 ThinkLike a Nurse 9-4

Recall the story of Tamika, a 3-year-old girl, in the Meet Your Patients scenario. Her grandmother, who is also caring for her ill husband, is raising Tamika. What concerns might that flag for you about the home environment?

PRESCHOOL STAGE: AGES 4 AND 5 YEARS

The preschooler is growing increasingly verbal and independent and is refining gross and fine motor skills. She is able to maintain separation from parents, use language to communicate needs, control bodily functions, and cooperate with children as well as adults. These skills prepare the child to enter school.

Physical Development of the Preschooler

Growth

- By 4 years of age, the average preschooler weighs about 36 lb (16.3 kg) and is 40 in. (1 m) tall.
- By age 5, the preschooler has gained an additional 5 lb (2.3 kg) and has grown 3 more in. (7.6 cm) in height.
- The proportions of head to trunk are somewhat closer, and the "pot belly" and exaggerated lumbar curve of toddlerhood gradually disappear.
- The average pulse rate is 90 to 100 beats/min, and respirations are 22 to 25 breaths/min.

Sensorimotor Development The preschooler has mature depth and color perception and 20/20 vision. Hearing is also mature. The preschooler continues to develop eye–hand coordination. At age 4, the child can hop, skip, and jump on one leg. Improvement in fine motor skills is most evident in artwork. Drawings become much more precise and detailed. The child is becoming independent in the ability to dress. Developmental milestones for preschoolers are listed in Box 9-3.

BOX 9-3 ■ Milestones of Preschool Development

- By age 5, most children can stand on one foot for 10 sec, skip, jump, hop on one foot or both feet together, climb play structures with ease, repeat simple dance steps, and begin to learn to skate.
- Most preschoolers can copy a triangle, square, and stick figure; print at least some letters; and use a fork and spoon.
- Most can dress and use the bathroom without assistance.
- Language abilities continue to be variable, but most preschoolers can tell stories, recall parts of a story told to them, and speak in sentences of more than five words. They can state their name, age, and address, and many can repeat their home phone number. A toddler who is not speaking intelligibly by age 4 requires evaluation.
- Preschoolers can count 10 or more objects, such as buttons or coins, and may be able to name several colors and shapes. They can compare big and small, long and short, and so on and often delight in completing simple mazes and "connect the dots" games.
- Preschoolers become increasingly aware of sex organ differences and curious about sexuality.
- Preschoolers may begin to ask about God, death, how babies are born, and other questions of a philosophical or scientific nature.
- Preschoolers typically can distinguish fantasy from reality and enjoy jokes and simple riddles.
- Psychosocial milestones include assertion of independence; pride in showing off skills, new toys and clothes, and prize possessions to friends; and a strong desire to socialize with peers.

Cognitive Development of the Preschooler

According to Piaget, the preschooler has entered the phase of *intuitive thought*. She is able to classify objects and continues to form concepts. She continues to use trial and error as a way to solve problems but increasingly uses thought to reason them out. Verbal skills expand dramatically during this phase, allowing the child to interact with more people. Preschool children are very interested in books, learning to read, and counting.

Preschoolers still lack the ability to reason formally and are unable to understand that two objects that appear different may in fact be the same (e.g., two balls of clay in two different shapes). They have a limited ability to tell time or understand the passage of time, and they may say "yesterday" in describing an event of several months ago. They also retain a strong belief in magic, monsters, and mythic figures such as Santa Claus. Preschoolers often have irrational fears—for example, of tigers lurking in the basement. Their fascination with powerful figures, such as dinosaurs and superheroes, is one way of coping with their feelings of powerlessness.

Psychosocial Development of the Preschooler

The preschooler is in Erikson's stage of *initiative versus guilt*, in which the child develops a conscience and readily recognizes right from wrong. The child becomes socially aware of others and develops the ability to consider other people's viewpoints. At this age, play is often used to teach life experiences.

The preschooler begins to fully express his personality and develop a self-concept (see Chapter 13 if you need to learn more about self-concept). He readily expresses likes and dislikes. Encouraging the child to participate in his favorite activities helps foster a positive self-concept (Fig. 9-7). Preschool children enjoy playing in small groups and use their language skills to facilitate imaginative play. Often elaborate stories, improvised costumes, and role-playing become part of the play experience. Many preschoolers have a best friend.

Freud identified the preschool years as the *phallic stage* of development. The child is aware of gender differences and often imitates the same-sex parent. He also develops an attraction to the opposite-sex parent and may feel jealousy toward the same-sex parent.

Common Health Problems of Preschoolers

The preschooler experiences health problems similar to those of the toddler.

Communicable Diseases Communicable diseases (e.g., respiratory infections, intestinal viruses, and parasites such as scabies and lice) remain a major health issue, especially as preschoolers start to come in contact with more children in play and structured preschool experiences. They interact more with playmates and are hands-on, so they can readily transmit viruses through direct contact and airborne vectors.

Poisoning Poisoning remains a significant risk for preschoolers. They use imitation as a way to learn about new things, so they may be predisposed to ingesting substances used by the adults in the house (e.g., prescription medicines and alcohol, or substances that appear similar).

Enuresis Parents of preschoolers may report a concern about bedwetting **(enuresis)**, especially in boys. The causes of enuresis are not fully understood, but it is known that in some children the bladder is simply unable to hold a full night's output of urine until later in childhood, whereas others lack the

neurological ability to waken in response to a full bladder. Most cases resolve spontaneously with only an occasional episode past age 6. In contrast, daytime wetting or soiling **(encopresis)** requires evaluation.

Example Problem: Child Abuse, Neglect, and Violence
Child abuse is often detected in toddlers and preschoolers when they come in contact with more people outside the home. Of the confirmed cases of abuse and neglect reported to Child Protective Services, more than half are under the age of 7. **KEY POINT:** *Child abuse can occur at any age, in any culture, and at any socioeconomic or education level.* The following are a few of the reasons why some people have difficulty meeting the demands of parenthood:

- **Parental characteristics:**
  Parents were themselves abused as a child.
  Parents or caregivers have unrealistic expectations of the child.
  Parent(s) have unmet emotional needs.
  Parents themselves exhibit immaturity or lack parenting knowledge.
  There are issues of difficulty in relationships.
  There is alcohol and/or drug addiction.
- **Characteristics of the child:**
  The child has a physical or mental disability.
  The child was born to unmarried parents.
  The child was unwanted.
- **Situational characteristics:**
  The living space may be crowded for the number of people it holds.
  There are the usual stresses of child care to contend with.
  The parents face employment pressures or unemployment.
  The family must cope with poor housing and frequent household moves.

For more information on child abuse, be sure to refer to the preceding section on Infancy, including the Example Problem: Abuse, Neglect, and Violence. Refer also to Procedure 9-1.

ASSESSMENT (Preschoolers) NP

Assessments for preschoolers should include the following:

Weight and Vital Signs Compare your findings with age-appropriate norms. Calculate and plot body mass index (BMI) at every well-child visit. To obtain a body mass calculator and information about BMI,

 Go to BMI—Body Mass Index at http://www.cdc.gov/nccdphp/dnpa/bmi/index.htm

Nutrition Assess for food preferences, habits, and amount eaten. The preschool child often has strong food preferences.

Sleep Habits Assess the numbers of hours slept, bedtime rituals, and problems with night awakenings. Preschoolers are generally very active but require adequate rest. This is also the time when children stop taking afternoon naps.

Vision Screening U.S. Preventive Services Task Force (USPSTF) (2014a) recommends vision screening for all children at least once between the ages of 3 and 5 years, to detect the presence of vision loss or its risk factors.

Dental Hygiene During the preschool years, all deciduous teeth have erupted. Therefore, dental hygiene is very important. At each visit, ask the child about tooth-brushing habits. If possible, have the child demonstrate how he brushes. The child should already have made at least one visit to a dentist by age 3. *Healthy People 2020* oral health goals include prevention and control of oral and craniofacial

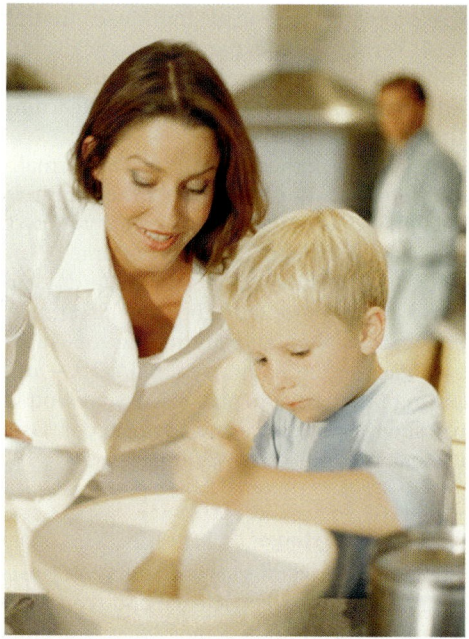

FIGURE 9-7 Preschoolers typically enjoy helping a parent in the kitchen.

diseases by providing access for all school-age children to fluoridated water, tooth sealants, and preventive oral care. For more information,

 Go to the *HealthyPeople 2020* Web site at http://www. healthypeople.gov/2020/topics-objectives/topic/oral-health

Safety Risks ✚ Assess for parent and child knowledge of hazards and precautions. Because the preschool child is mobile and involved in active play (e.g., riding a tricycle, crossing streets) accidents increase.

School Readiness A physical examination is required before the child enters school. This exam should include an assessment for *readiness*—whether the child has acquired skills, such as an ability to converse with adults; follow instructions; hold a pencil; and perform a variety of motor skills, such as jump, hop, and walk a straight line. Also review the immunization record. Several boosters and immunizations are due at this time, and any that have been missed must be administered before the child enters school. To see the CDC Catch-up Immunization Schedule,

 Go to the CDC Web site at http://www.cdc.gov/vaccines/schedules/hcp/imz/catchup.html

Assessments for Example Problem: Child Abuse, Neglect, and Violence At each visit, assess for risk factors for abuse and for subtle signs of actual abuse (see Procedure 9-1).

INTERVENTIONS (Preschoolers) NP

The preschool child is interactive and curious. Speak directly to the child, and include her in your teaching sessions. Teaching topics include the following:

- *Frequent hand washing to prevent the spread of disease.* Teach the child hand-washing technique, and encourage parents to model frequent hand washing.
- *Proper brushing and flossing of teeth.* Most preschoolers still need supervision while brushing their teeth.
- *Essentials of a balanced diet.* Encourage parents to offer a well-balanced diet and to instill healthy eating habits. By the age of 5 most children are willing to try new foods and are better able to sit during an entire meal. Generally, preschoolers eat half the food portion of that of an adult.
- *Importance of adequate rest.* The average preschooler requires at least 12 hours of sleep each night.

- ✚ *Hazard of stranger danger.* Increasing independence and mobility place preschoolers at risk for abduction. Teach the child to avoid talking to strangers and never to enter a stranger's home or car. This topic is explored in depth once the child enters school.

- ✚ *Importance of seat belts and car seats.* Current recommendations are to use booster seats for children weighing between 40 and 80 pounds and to continue using the seat until the child is at least 4 feet 9 inches tall.

KnowledgeCheck 9-6

- According to Erikson, what is the developmental stage of the preschooler?
- Identify at least two important assessments to make when providing care to a preschooler.

SCHOOL-AGE: AGES 6 TO 12 YEARS

The school-age child becomes more independent and confident, and places more importance on relationships outside the immediate family. Developmental milestones of the school-age period are summarized in Box 9-4.

Physical Development of the School-Age Child

Growth During the school-age years, the child grows about 2 in. (5 cm) taller and gains 4 to 7 lb (2.3 to 3 kg) per year. The child takes on a slimmer appearance, with longer legs and a lower center of gravity.

- *Musculoskeletal.* Muscle mass rapidly increases, and ossification of bones continues throughout this age. Strength and physical abilities rapidly improve, and the child gains more poise and coordination.
- *Brain and skull.* The brain and skull grow slowly, and facial characteristics mature.
- *GI system.* The gastrointestinal system matures and stomach capacity increases, although caloric demands decrease.
- *Immune system.* As the immune system develops, the school-age child begins to produce antibodies and antigens.
- *Gender comparisons.* Initially boys and girls vary little in size. Toward the end of this phase, marked differences become apparent. Girls grow rapidly in the latter school-age years, as puberty begins, and experience onset of puberty about 2 years before boys do.

Visual Acuity Visual acuity improves with age. By 6 years of age, distance visual acuity should be at least 20/30 in each eye with less than two lines' difference between the two eyes. Any child not meeting these criteria should be referred for a complete eye examination.

Dentition School-age children begin to lose their primary teeth (baby teeth) at about age 6 or 7, and the permanent teeth appear soon after. Their large size in relation to the remaining primary teeth and the child's jaw, as well as the gaps left by teeth not yet replaced, can make even the most beautiful children look somewhat awkward at this stage.

BOX 9-4 ■ Milestones of School-Age Development

- By age 7, most children can tie their own shoelaces; print their names; and perform self-care, such as bathing and feeding themselves. Many can even prepare simple meals.
- By age 8, improved fine motor skills allow the child to begin to write, learn to knit or crochet, and/or take up a musical instrument.
- By age 9, motor development approaches that of an adult.
- School-age children understand the concept of payment for work and the value of money.
- Fears of ghosts and monsters may continue through age 7 but give way to more realistic fears, such as of school failure or divorce of parents, by age 8 or 9.
- By age 6, the child has a vocabulary of 3,000 words and usually can read. By the end of the school-age period, the child can write complex compositions with appropriate grammar, spelling, and accurate description.
- Psychosocial development includes team play, peer friendships, and ability to look beyond family members for social support.

Cognitive Development of the School-Age Child

School-age children use their thought processes to experience actions and events. Piaget describes this as *concrete operations.*

- Concrete and systematic thinking
- Magical beliefs gradually replaced with a passion to understand how things really are
- Can see another person's point of view and develops an understanding of relationships
- Learns to classify objects according to similarities
- Enjoys learning by handling and manipulating objects
- Learns to tell time; gains an experiential understanding of the length of days, months, and years
- Reads independently; does numerical calculations without representative objects, such as fingers or beads
- By the end of this stage, is able to think through a task and understand it without actually performing the task

Psychosocial Development of the School-Age Child

Erikson describes this stage as a time of *industry versus inferiority.* During this stage, the child is able to work at more complex projects independently. Through participation in school, she is recognized for achievements and accomplishments. For the child to progress through this stage, the parent must provide praise for accomplishments. This recognition builds self-confidence. The child will develop a sense of inferiority and lack of self-worth if her accomplishments are met with a negative response.

Peers take on increasing importance, influencing the child's choices of what to eat, wear, and do. Friendships during the school-age years are usually with children of the same gender and may be intense but short-lived (Fig. 9-8). However, some children have one best friend throughout their childhood. In the later school-age years, friendships become more reciprocal, with each child recognizing the unique qualities of the other.

Common Health Problems of School-Age Children

School-age children are at risk for problems similar to those of preschoolers, including upper respiratory tract infections, parasitic infections such as scabies and lice, and dental caries. Although violence, bullying, smoking, and experimentation with alcohol, drugs, and sex are more common among adolescents, these problems are also seen toward the end of the

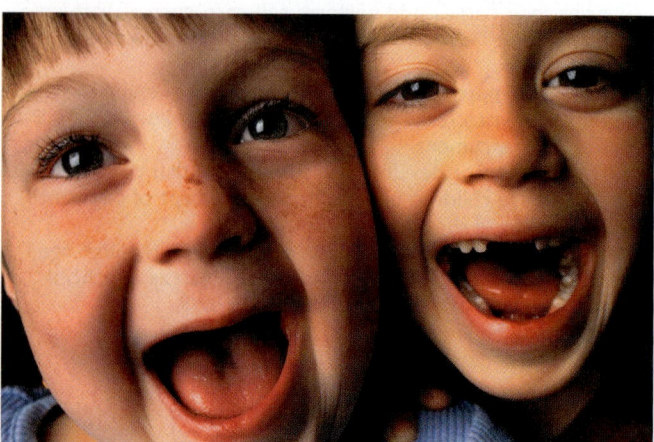

FIGURE 9-8 Same-gender friendships are important to school-age children.

school-age years. The presence of a gun in the home significantly increases the risk of accidental death, even in the school-age population.

Childhood Obesity

- **Obesity is a growing problem for preschoolers.** Despite recent declines in the prevalence among preschool-age children, obesity among school-age children is still too high. For children and adolescents aged 2 to 19 years, the prevalence of obesity has remained fairly stable at about 17% for the past decade and affects about 12.7 million children and adolescents (CDC, 2001, reviewed 2015; CDC, 2015c).
- **Nutrition and lifestyle are primarily responsible for this epidemic.** Children spend much less time playing outside than in past generations and more time watching television and playing video games, texting, and using social media. They consume more fast food and bigger portions and eat fewer vegetables. Thirty percent of all meals are taken outside the home and fast food contributes to 10% of overall calorie intake (American Heart Association, 2010).
- **As a result of the obesity epidemic, more children now have obesity-related diseases,** such as type 2 diabetes mellitus (type 2 DM), hyperlipidemia, and hypertension. **Type 2 DM** is an endocrine disorder characterized by insulin resistance: Insulin fails to effectively transfer glucose from the bloodstream into the body's cells. Treatment involves lifestyle changes and perhaps medication.

Childhood Asthma

Asthma, a chronic inflammatory disorder of the airways, is one of the most common chronic disorders in childhood, currently affecting an estimated 7.1 million children under 18 years. Of those, 4.1 million suffered from an asthma attack or episode in 2011 (American Lung Association, 2014). Asthma is one of the leading causes of school absenteeism and the third leading cause of hospitalization among children under the age of 15 years. Even in children who do not require emergency care, asthma can decrease attention span in school and make participation in school activities difficult. Social problems may occur, as children are often teased and stigmatized as being "wheezers" or "lazy."

Asthma has complex causes, including a strong genetic component, but poverty appears to play at least some role. Recent research has focused on indoor air allergens such as pet dander, dust mites, fungi or mold, and the decomposing corpses of cockroaches as significant triggers.

Unintentional Injuries in School-Age Children

School-age children experience fewer injuries than preschoolers because of their improved coordination and reasoning abilities. Nevertheless, they have a high incidence of fractures, sprains, strains, cuts, and abrasions. Falls are the most common form of nonfatal injury for children aged 6 to 12 years, whereas the leading cause of unintentional injury death is motor vehicle and traffic injury (CDC, 2012a). Injuries also occur from riding bicycles on the street, skiing, skateboarding, sledding, and playing sports.

Concussions are one of the most commonly reported injuries in children and adolescents who participate in sports and recreation activities. Although many concussions may be considered mild, they can result in health consequences such as impaired thinking, memory problems, and emotional or behavioral changes (U.S. Department of Health and Human Services, 2015).

If you would like more information about unintentional injuries, see Chapter 23.

ASSESSMENT (School-Age) NP

The school-age child should have a routine health maintenance visit every 1 or 2 years. Annual physical exams are scheduled for those who participate in sports. Allow time to meet with the child alone as well as time with the caregiver present. School-age children often have questions about puberty and the changes their bodies are undergoing. Private time with the child will allow you to explore these concerns in a private manner.

Nursing Interview The nursing interview should cover the following topics:

- **Nutrition.** Assess the child's eating patterns and the intake of key nutrients such as calcium, vitamin D, and iron.
- **Allergies.** Ask the child whether he ever experiences difficulty breathing or feels too tired to play. Ask about symptoms such clear nasal discharge, frequent sneezing, or watery eyes. Listen to breath sounds and observe for allergy symptoms.
- **Visual Acuity.** Ask about any eye screening. Because children do not complain about visual difficulties, the AAP recommends that children aged older than 5 years should be screened every 1 to 2 years (2012). Many school systems have regular vision screening programs that are carried out by professionals and properly trained volunteers. Screening can be done there quickly, accurately, and with minimal expense.
- **Dental Hygiene.** Interview the child to determine his knowledge of dental hygiene. Inspect the mouth for secondary teeth eruption according to expected patterns ands for tooth decay and gum disease.
- **Sleep Pattern.** Assess the child's sleep pattern. To remain healthy and function well at school, the school-age child needs 9 to 10 hours of sleep each night.
- **✚ Safety.** Determine the child's awareness of safety. Be sure to assess risk-taking behavior.

  Smoking—Has the child tried smoking? Does he have friends who are smoking?

  Substances—What is the child's experience with alcohol and drugs? Has he tried them? What does his peer group think about drinking and drugs?

  Sexual activity—Has he ever been sexually active? Does he have friends who are sexually active?

  Violence—Has the child engaged in fistfights or fights with knives or other weapons?

  Weapons—Is there a gun in the home? Does the child have access to it?

  Although these concerns are seen with greater frequency in adolescence, you should assess for them among school-age children.

BMI At each visit, asses the child's vital signs, height, weight, and developmental skills. After weighing the child, correlate your measurements with growth charts. The American Heart Association (2013) BMI classifications are as follows:

Overweight	At 85th percentile
Obese	At the 95th percentile or above

Visual Acuity should be at least 20/30 in each eye with less than two lines' difference between the two eyes. Any child not meeting these criteria should be referred for a complete eye examination.

Scoliosis Screening Scoliosis is an abnormal spinal curvature that affects primarily females. Screening is done in the preadolescent period, usually in the sixth grade. Refer to an orthopedic surgeon for evaluation and follow-up if an abnormal curvature is discovered.

Immunizations Review the immunization record. Although immunization against hepatitis B is recommended in infancy, many parents skip these immunizations. Several states require students to complete the hepatitis B series prior to entry into seventh grade. The child must begin the series at or before 12 years of age to complete it in time for seventh grade.

The CDC (2015a) recommends the following vaccines for school-age children: human papillomavirus; meningococcal; pneumococcal; influenza; hepatitis A; hepatitis B; inactivated poliovirus; measles, mumps, and rubella; varicella; and tetanus, diphtheria, and pertussis booster. To see this schedule,

 Go to the CDC, 2015 Recommended Immunization Schedule for Persons Aged 0 Through 18 Years at http://www.cdc.gov/vaccines/schedules/hcp/imz/child-adolescent.html

Also refer to the previous section Common Health Problems of Toddlers

INTERVENTIONS (School-Age) NP

The *Healthy People 2020* campaign focuses on preventing injury rather than treating illness. Your efforts in teaching will help promote those objectives. Use age-appropriate teaching materials and objectives.

Teaching for Safety

✚ To help prevent injury in the school-age child:

- Educate the child and parents on safety and the proper use of equipment and gear.
- Teach the child and parents to wear seat belts at all times when in a vehicle.
- Encourage parents to be firm about the use of helmets for bicycle safety.
- Stress that head injury is the most common cause of death in this group.
- For those who play sports, stress the importance of warming up before playing, using proper safety equipment and gear that is properly fitted, and avoiding overtraining.

Teaching About Nutrition and Exercise for Weight Loss

Counsel overweight and obese children about nutrition for weight loss and the importance of daily physical activity.

Teaching About Nutrition Encourage children to develop good eating habits by choosing nutritious foods and snacks. For example, encourage them to avoid junk foods, such as sodas, and to choose instead milk, calcium-fortified orange juice, or water. If the diet is severely restrictive and if it has none of the child's favorite foods, it is likely to fail. Focus on making small but permanent changes. Refer for further counseling, if indicated.

Teaching About Exercise
- *Recommend at least 60 minutes of enjoyable, moderate-intensity physical activities every day* that are developmentally appropriate

and varied (American Heart Association, 2013). If they don't have a full 60-minute activity break each day, encourage at least two 30-minute periods or four 15-minute periods.

- **KEY POINT:** *Explain how important exercise is to weight loss—diet alone will not achieve it for them.*
- *Exercise does not necessarily need to be structured.* For example, it might consist of family walks in the community, bike riding or skateboarding, or swimming in a neighborhood pool. Even table tennis requires more activity than watching television. The American Academy of Pediatrics recommends the following:

  Limit TV viewing and video game playing to 2 hours a day.
  Boys should take at least 11,000 steps daily.
  Girls should take at least 13,000 steps daily.

- Suggest parents buy a pedometer, if possible, so the child can track the number of steps.
- *Teach children about self-regulation of impulse control, decision-making skills, and social competence.* Making more informed choices could help reduce calorie intake and establish good physical activity habits early.
- **KEY POINT:** *The most effective programs for preventing obesity focus on children, rather than their parents. However, management of obesity does involve the whole family.* A child cannot make lifestyle changes if his environment remains the same. Parents can help by modeling healthy eating.
- *Recommend group-based or family-based counseling.* Many parents do not perceive that their child is overweight; of course they must come to recognize this if they are to cooperate with needed changes.
- *Work with the community to involve the schools in obesity prevention.* Many schools have removed soda from their campuses and are now offering healthy menus in their cafeterias. In addition, physical education in the schools has been mandated in many U.S. states.

Teaching About Diabetes

The parents and child must understand that diabetes involves dietary changes, weight loss, and exercise. Medications are required if the lifestyle changes are not sufficient to control blood sugar, but they cannot be relied on. You may need to refer the family to a nutritionist or diabetes counselor.

Teaching About Asthma

- *Teach parents and children about indoor environmental asthma triggers.* Examples are mold, cockroaches, pets, and nitrogen dioxide (a gas that is a byproduct of indoor fuel-burning appliances such as gas stoves, fireplaces, or wood stoves) (U.S. Environmental Protection Agency, last updated 2013).
- *Provide and help fill out, as necessary, an asthma action card* for the child to carry when away from home. An action plan should include (1) the child's asthma triggers, (2) instructions for asthma medicines, (3) what to do if the child has an attack, (4) when to call the doctor, and (5) emergency telephone numbers. You can obtain a Student Asthma Action Card by searching that title on the U.S. Environmental Protection Agency's Asthma home page:

 Go to http://www.epa.gov/asthma/

Teaching About Violence and Risk-Taking Behaviors

At the community health level, school violence can be addressed through psychological counseling, weapons-screening devices, school-wide educational programs, and policies calling for the suspension or expulsion of students who are caught intimidating other children or participating in fights on school property. The school-age period offers many opportunities to educate children about the hazards of smoking, drinking, and using drugs, which often contribute to violence.

Helping the Hospitalized Child

Help children express their fears and respond to specific needs. Hospitalized children may fear the unknown, the strange environment, and the strange professionals. They are afraid of tests and treatments (i.e., operations, needles) pain, and dying. They miss the comforts of home: their mother's cooking, their own room, and so on. They are bothered by separation from family and friends and by loss of control over their personal needs. You can help them in the following ways:

- Maximize their contact with outside friends and school.
- Minimize the adverse aspects of the hospital environment.
- Offer choices, when possible, to restore some sense of control (e.g., whether to have a tub bath or shower, or what they would prefer to eat for meals).
- Encourage parents to bring familiar items from home to personalize their space.
- Involve parents in their care and provide them accurate information so they can relieve children's anxieties.

KnowledgeCheck 9-7

- What important physical changes occur in the school-age group?
- According to Piaget, what is the cognitive developmental stage of the school-age child?

ADOLESCENCE: AGES 12 TO 18 YEARS

Adolescence marks the transition from child to adult. **Puberty** refers to the beginning of reproductive abilities. In this period of development, the child experiences progressive physical, cognitive, and psychological change.

Physical Development of Adolescents

Physical and hormonal changes are readily apparent during the adolescent years. Developmental milestones of adolescence are summarized in Box 9-5.

BOX 9-5 ▪ Milestones of Adolescent Development

- The adolescent reaches adult height and about 90% of peak bone density by the end of this period.
- Menarche occurs by age 14 in most girls, who develop adult primary and secondary sex characteristics by about age 16.
- Boys have developed adult primary and secondary sex characteristics by about age 17 to 19.
- Motor development is equal to that of adults.
- Maturation of the central nervous system allows formal operational thought processes, logic, and abstract reasoning.
- Psychosocial development includes the teen's increasing reliance on peers, ambivalent feelings toward family, anxiety over and/or preoccupation with sex and sexuality, and determination of sexual orientation.

Growth

- *Females* undergo a growth spurt between 9 and 14 years of age. Height increases 2 to 8 in. (5.1 to 7.6 cm) and weight gain varies from 15 to 55 lb (6.8 to 24.9 kg). By the onset of menstruation, girls have attained 90% of their adult height.
- *Males* undergo a growth spurt between 10 and 16 years. Height increases by 4 to 12 in. (10.2 to 30.5 cm) and weight increases by 15 to 65 lb (6.8 to 29.5 kg). Boys continue to grow until 18 to 20 years of age. Bone mass continues to accumulate until about age 20.
- *In both males and females,* the blood pressure and the size and strength of the heart increase. The pulse rate decreases. By the time of adolescence, blood values are that of the adult. Respiratory rate, volume, and capacity also reach the adult rates. By the end of the adolescent period, all vital organs reach adult size.

Onset of Puberty   The onset of puberty varies widely, but the sequences of these changes are standard (Tanner, 1962).

- *In females,* the time from the first appearance of breast tissue to full sexual maturation is 2 to 6 years. **Menarche** (first menstruation) occurs approximately 2 years after the beginning of puberty. The average age of menarche is 12 years, depending on racial group and body mass.
- *In males,* the onset of puberty occurs between 9 and 14 years of age. Throughout puberty, boys become more muscular, the voice deepens, and facial hair begins to grow and coarsen. It may take 2 to 5 years for the genitalia to reach adult size.
- *In both males and females,* hormonal changes are accompanied by increased activity of the sweat (apocrine) glands, and heavy perspiration may occur for the first time. For the same reason, the sebaceous glands become active, and the adolescent may experience acne.
- For more information about the changes in secondary sexual characteristics associated with puberty for males and females, see the tables in Procedures 21-17 and 21-18, respectively.

Cognitive Development of Adolescents

Piaget refers to adolescence as the period of *formal operations.* The adolescent develops the ability to think abstractly and is receptive to more detailed information. This opens the door to scientific reasoning and logic. She can now imagine what may occur in the future as well as the consequences of her own decisions. Although the adolescent has more refined cognitive abilities, adolescents may still lack judgment and common sense. These develop later through life experience.

Psychosocial Development of Adolescents

The major psychosocial task of the adolescent is to develop a *personal identity.* Teenagers shift their emotional attachment away from their parents and create close bonds among their peers (Fig. 9-9). This helps the teenager to further characterize the differences between himself and his parents. The adolescent often takes on a new style of dress, dance, music, or hairstyle; develops personal values; and begins to make choices about career and further education.

Group Acceptance   One of the strongest needs for teens is to feel accepted within a group of their own choosing. Acceptance on a sports team, into a club, or into a clique or gang increases the teen's sense of self-esteem. In contrast, unpopular teens feel alienated, resentful, and antagonistic and may

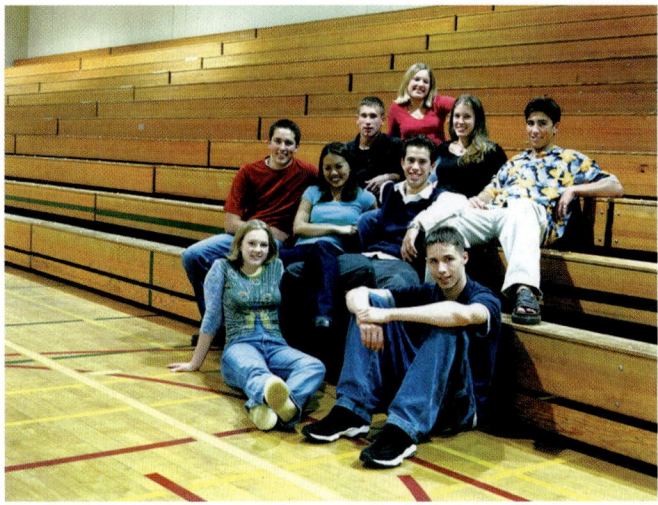

FIGURE 9-9 Teenagers create close bonds among their peers.

react with violence directed at themselves or others (Kingery, Erdley, & Marshall, 2011).

Tattoos and Piercings   Adolescents may engage in the trend of body art and piercings for a number of reasons, including a desire for social bonding, to look like their peers, and to commemorate a friend or loved one. In the 10-year period after the mid-1990s, the number of teens who had tattoos increased from 4.5% to 14%. The average age at time of tattooing is around 17 years. Body piercings, likewise, are not unusual. Both tattoos and piercings can cause skin infections and blood-borne diseases such as HIV and hepatitis. Some studies have reported a significant relationship between piercing and substance abuse, leading some to speculate that body piercing may serve as a marker of an at risk teen (Desai & Smith, 2011).

Emerging Sexual Orientation   Most adolescents have a sense of their emerging sexual orientation. Approximately 1.9% of people between 18 and 44 years of age identify themselves as homosexual and 1.1% as bisexual (CDC, 2014c). A higher percentage report having had same-sex intercourse at least once, but consider themselves heterosexual. Some youth are bisexual—that is, attracted somewhat equally to both males and females.

Common Health Problems of Adolescents

In the United States, 72% of all deaths among young people aged 10 through 24 years result from four causes: motor vehicle crashes (26%), other unintentional injuries (13%), homicide (15%), and suicide (16%). Many adolescents engage in behaviors that increase their likelihood of death of injury from these four causes: distracted driving (e.g., texting, eating), driving under the influence of alcohol or drugs, carrying a weapon, and using alcohol or other drugs. In a recent year, 25% of high school students reported having been in a physical fight (CDC, 2014b). Illnesses are responsible for less than one-fourth of deaths; cancer and heart disease are the most common.

Example Problem: Substance Abuse

Substance abuse is a major concern because it is widespread and because of the physical, mental, and spiritual toll it takes on teens, families, and communities. See the accompanying Example Problem: Substance Abuse. Also see Substance Abuse and Mental Illness in Chapter 12, as needed.

EXAMPLE PROBLEM: Substance Abuse

Definition
Regular use of drugs or other substances for purposes other than medical use that causes physical or psychological harm to the person.

Incidence
- In 2013, 36% of high-school seniors said they had used marijuana in the past year, compared with 30% in 2006.
- It is illegal to sell tobacco to minors, yet 9.5% of middle school students and 25.6% of high school students currently use some form of tobacco (American Lung Association, 2010; Substance Abuse and Mental Health Services Administration, 2008, updated 2015). Over 54% say they have tried a cigarette.
- Prescription and over-the-counter medications account for most of the top drugs abused by 12th graders in 2013.

- Abuse of prescription drugs is highest among young adults aged 18 to 25, with 5.9% reporting nonmedical use in the past month.

Possible Consequences
- Violence, sexual assault, rape, and alcohol/drug overdose
- Associated with risk-taking behaviors resulting in injury and death (e.g., automobile accidents, falls, drowning, suicide)
- Increased risks of cancer, high blood pressure, cirrhosis, epilepsy, and homicide
- Persons diagnosed with drug disorders are roughly twice as likely to have mood or anxiety disorders.
- Every year, 599,000 people are unintentionally injured while under the influence.
- **And more than 1,700 die.**

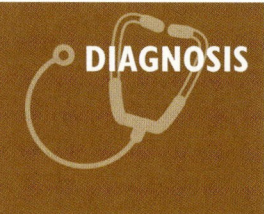

DIAGNOSIS

Nursing Diagnosis, Examples
- **Risk-Prone Health Behavior** r/t excessive alcohol, smoking, drug use.
- **Impaired Parenting** r/t alcohol abuse
- **Impaired Social Interaction** r/t substance abuse

- **Ineffective Role Performance** r/t changes in mental status secondary to substance abuse
- **Risk for Suicide** r/t to feelings of powerlessness

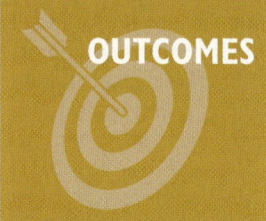

OUTCOMES

- Identifies emotional state that precipitates substance abuse.
- Uses available support groups and community resources.

- Commits to alcohol/drug and/or tobacco abstinence.

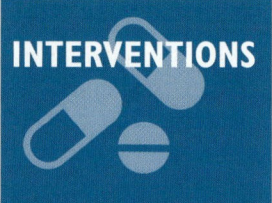

INTERVENTIONS

Assessment
- Assess for risk factors.
- Ask about drug, alcohol, and tobacco use.

Collaborating
- Make appropriate referrals or provide information on cessation programs.
- Discuss and plan for risk-reduction activities in collaboration with individual or group.
- If your assessment identifies drug or alcohol use, make appropriate referrals.

Teaching
- Discuss the effects of drugs, alcohol, and tobacco and the hazards associated with their use.

- Remind teens that the earlier a person begins using tobacco, the harder it is to break the addiction.
- Stress the unattractive physical effects, such as bad breath, stained teeth and fingers, and a long-term cough.
- Stress the expense and inconvenience of purchasing cigarettes and smokeless tobacco.
- Correct misinformation that smokeless tobacco products are safer than smoking.

EVALUATION

Patient will implement healthy lifestyle behaviors to promote alcohol/drug/tobacco elimination

Depression

Depression affects up to 8.5% of adolescents in the United States (Substance Abuse and Mental Health Services Administration, 2008, updated 2015) compared with 11% of the adult population. A government survey identifies an even higher percentage: During the 12 months preceding the survey, 28% of students nationwide had felt so sad or hopeless almost every day for more than 2 weeks in a row that they stopped doing some usual activities (CDC, 2014b).

Risk factors for adolescent depression include a family history of depression, cigarette smoking, stress, loss of a loved one, breakup of a romantic relationship, learning disorders, attention or behavioral disorders, chronic illnesses (e.g., diabetes), abuse, neglect, or other trauma such as natural disasters. If you would like more information about depression, see Chapter 13.

Suicide

Suicide is the third leading cause of death in teenagers. The CDC (2014b) estimates that 8% of high school students have attempted suicide. Twice as many adolescent girls as boys attempt suicide, but because boys tend to use more lethal methods, such as guns and hanging, they are more likely to die from the attempt. Risk factors include problems at school or in romantic or family relationships, low self-esteem, social isolation, substance abuse, and depression.

Eating Disorders

Although anorexia and bulimia create nutritional problems and manifest as eating disorders, they are psychiatric disorders that require medical and psychiatric intervention.

Anorexia Nervosa A person with **anorexia nervosa** dramatically restricts food intake and may exercise excessively in an attempt to lose weight. Anorexia is characterized by a distorted body image; often the person sees herself as fat in spite of being markedly thin. It is the third most common chronic illness among adolescents. It occurs predominately in, but is not limited to, high-achieving adolescent females from upper-middle-class backgrounds. Physical consequences include amenorrhea, bradycardia, low white blood cell count, anemia, infertility, and bone loss.

Eating disorders have the highest mortality of any mental illness: 5% to 10% of patients die within 10 years of developing anorexia nervosa. One in five dies by committing suicide (Arcelus, Mitchell, Wales, et al., 2011).

Bulimia Bulimia is another eating disorder seen in adolescent girls as well as in boys who participate in sports that require them to maintain a specific weight. **Bulimia** is characterized by binge eating followed by inappropriate mechanisms to remove the food that was consumed (usually inducing vomiting, using laxatives, or engaging in excessive exercise). Binge eating may occur every few days or as often as several times a day. People with bulimia frequently experience electrolyte imbalances, decayed teeth (from gastric acid exposure), or abdominal pain (from gastric overload or laxative use).

Overweight and Obesity

Overweight and obesity continue to be a concern during adolescence, partly because the incidence is so high. Moreover, overweight children are more likely to be overweight adults. Consider the following facts:

- *Today, about one in three American teens is overweight or obese,* nearly triple the rate in 1963 (American Heart Association, 2014, updated 2016).

- *Causes of teen obesity* are similar to those of childhood obesity: sedentary lifestyles, eating larger portions, eating fast foods, and substituting high-calorie, nutrient-poor snacks for balanced meals. Even school vending machines contain so-called junk foods such as soda, snack cakes, candy, and chips, although this is changing in some areas.
- *One-third of American children aged 4 to 19 years eat fast food daily.* The percentage is undoubtedly higher for adolescents, who eat fewer meals at home and have more freedom to choose their own foods. Food preferences are influenced by television and marketing strategies in other media; on children's television shows, most of the advertising is for foods of poor nutritional value.
- *Type 2 DM, hypertension, high cholesterol, and heart disease* are occurring with increasing frequency in adolescents, now that so many are affected by obesity. These diseases were previously seen mostly in adults.

Risky Sexual Behaviors

Sexual activity is common among teenagers. By age 13, 4% of girls and 10% of boys have had sexual intercourse. This tends to increase with age, with 35% of students (grades 9 through 12) being sexually active. About 15% of students have had sexual intercourse with four or more persons (CDC, 2014b).

Condom Use Almost two-thirds of sexually active high school students report having used a condom at most recent sexual intercourse. Child Trends (2013) reports that males are more likely to use condoms than are females, and black males are more likely to use condoms than are Hispanic males. The federal government's *HealthyPeople 2020* initiative has set a national goal to increase effective condom use among sexually active adolescents aged 15 to 19 years. Desired outcomes are to prevent pregnancy and provide barrier protection against disease.

Oral Sex Many adolescents engage in sexual behaviors other than vaginal intercourse. Between 2007 and 2010, 49% of males and 48% of females aged 15 to 19 years reported that they had engaged in oral sex with an opposite sex partner. This often occurs prior to initiating sexual intercourse (Child Trends, 2013). **KEY POINT:** *Oral sex does not put adolescents at risk of pregnancy; however, unless barrier precautions are taken, it can put them at increased risk of STIs (Child Trends, 2013).*

Social Media Social media may have a significant impact on the social and sexual well-being of adolescents. In many adolescents, self-regulation and judgment skills are not yet fully mature. This often leads to risky behaviors, especially on social network sites.

- *Online disinhibition effect.* This means that people more readily release personal and private information into the public domain than they would in face-to-face interactions. Adolescents can fall easy prey to this effect because of the anonymity social network sites provide.
- *Social network sites provide an attractive outlet for adolescents* during a time in development in which self-expression and validation are important. This expression may then translate into risky social and sexual behaviors.
- *"Sexting."* Adolescents may not directly reference sexual behavior but may partake in a practice known as "sexting": sending, receiving, or forwarding sexually explicit messages, photographs, images, or videos via the Internet, a cell phone, or another digital device. One survey found that 20% of adolescents between 13 and 19 years old have sent or posted a nude or semi-nude photo or video of themselves to another adolescent (Cookingham & Ryan, 2015).

- *Risky behaviors and sexual wellness.* We now believe that social media may be increasing risky sexual behaviors and decreasing overall social and sexual wellness in adolescents. They are the group at highest risk for contracting an STI because they are more likely to have concurrent sexual partners, multiple sexual partners, and a lack of consistent condom use.

Sexually Transmitted Infections (STIs) Approximately one in four U.S. teens has an STI. STIs, including HIV/AIDS, are a major health consequence associated with sexual activity and especially with unprotected sexual activity. **KEY POINT:** *A majority of adolescents mistakenly believe that condoms are a foolproof method of preventing STIs and HIV/AIDS.* Trichomonal and monilial infections and human papillomavirus (HPV) are common. Those and other STIs occur in both males and females and can have serious complications.

AIDS is a major cause of death worldwide, reaching epidemic proportions in some countries. It is transmitted primarily through genital, oral, or anal sexual activities but can also be transmitted in other ways (e.g., by sharing needles with an infected person). In 2010, the greatest number of new HIV infections (4,800) among men occurred in young black/African American males aged 13 to 24 years who have sex with males (MSM). Young black MSM accounted for 45% of new HIV infections among black MSM and 55% of new HIV infections among young MSM overall (CDC, 2014d). For more information about STIs, see Chapter 34.

Adolescent Pregnancy The birth rate for women in this age-group is 26.5 per 1,000 females. This is a record low for U.S. teens in this age-group, and a drop of 10% from 2012. Birth rates fell 13% for females aged 15 to 17 years and 8% for females aged 18 to 19 years. Still, the teen pregnancy rate in the United States is substantially higher than it is in other Western industrialized nations (CDC, 2015b). A similar percentage of teens are sexually active in the United States; however, consistency and effectiveness of condom use are lower.

Adolescents who become pregnant face physiological risks, such as bone density loss and iron-deficiency anemia, the interruption of progress in their own developmental tasks, and loss of educational opportunities. Teen mothers are less likely to complete high school and more likely to live in poverty than are other teens. They are less likely to be married, to receive prenatal care, and to gain appropriate weight, and more likely to smoke than are older mothers. This puts them and their babies at higher risk for complications of pregnancy and low-birth-weight infants.

Example Problem: Abuse, Neglect, and Violence

There is no age limit on abuse and neglect. One study of children aged 13 to adulthood reported that more than 9% of the nearly 1,000 subjects had substantiated maltreatment. Maltreatment included sexual abuse, physical abuse, emotional abuse, and neglect. Abuse may be linked to later violent crimes and illicit drug use. See the Example Problem: Abuse, Neglect, and Violence.

ASSESSMENT (Adolescents) NP

Adolescents should have a general health examination every 2 years. Communicating with adolescents can be challenging because they may feel the need to resist "authority," and may be hesitant to share information with adults. Attempt to establish rapport and reassure the teenager that you will maintain confidentiality. At these visits, you should assess for the common problems of adolescence, including abuse and neglect (see Procedure 9-1).

Obtain a Thorough Health History Obtain information in the following areas:

- *Medications and other drugs.* Be sure to ask about use of prescription and over-the-counter medications, tobacco, and recreational drugs. If any are being used, find out what, how much, and for how long.
- *Psychosocial profile.* Obtain a psychosocial profile focusing on health practices and behaviors. Assess the adolescent's ability to cope with stressors. **KEY POINT:** *A change in academic performance or lack of interest in school may indicate a problem such as depression.* Young adolescents may have difficulty in identifying and describing their emotional or mood states. Instead of saying how bad they feel, they may be irritable or act out by disobeying or misbehaving; they may sulk, be negative or grouchy, feel misunderstood, and get into trouble at school.
- *Peer relationships.* Assess the quality of the adolescent's peer relationships to assess risk for social isolation and to determine risk for school and/or gang-related violence.
- *Nutrition and body image.* Ask questions about body image in relation to the adolescent's nutritional status. Assess both overeating and undereating patterns, as well as intake of key nutrients such as protein, iron, calcium, and vitamin D.
- *Tattoos and piercings.* The tattoo or piercing may be in a concealed location, so ask about tattoos and piercings and ask to look at them during the visit. Discuss the risks of body art and modification.
- *Activity and exercise patterns.* If the adolescent engages in activities that increase the risk for injuries, ask about the use of protective equipment, such as helmets, mouth guards, and padding. If the adolescent reports no regular physical activity, assess his or her understanding of the benefits of exercise.
- *Sleep patterns.* Teens often get little sleep during school days and sleep late on weekends. Ask whether the teen feels refreshed after a night's sleep.
- ✚ *Safety.* Determine whether the adolescent wears a seat belt. Ask whether she is aware of the hazards of driving under the influence of drugs and alcohol or while texting and talking on the phone. Such distractions, including other teens in the car, can compete with the teen's focus on traffic and driving safety.
- *Sexual activity.* Determine whether the adolescent is sexually active. If so, ask about condom use.
- *Review all body systems,* keeping in mind changes or problems that are specific to the adolescent.

Perform a General Survey Complete a general survey after you have gathered the subjective data.

- Include vital signs, height, and weight. Follow with a head-to-toe physical exam.
- If you identify any problems in the course of the history and physical examination, actively involve both the adolescent and the parents in a plan of care.
- **Calculate the BMI** using a BMI calculator and BMI-for-age percentiles for children and teens. Adult calculators will not give accurate results for teens. The following are the CDC weight status categories:

Underweight	Less than 5th percentile
Healthy weight	5th to less than 85th percentile
At risk of overweight	85th to less than 95th percentile
Overweight	95th percentile or greater

To use the CDC BMI Percentile Calculator for Child and Teen,

Go to the CDC Web site at http://nccd.cdc.gov/dnpabmi/ Calculator.aspx

To see the CDC body mass index-for-age percentile charts for girls and boys aged 2 to 20,

 Go to the CDC Web site http://www.cdc.gov/growthcharts/

INTERVENTIONS (Adolescents) NP

When working with adolescents, your goal is to help the adolescent make informed decisions. Avoid scare tactics and encourage open discussion. Often a teenager will feel more comfortable asking a nurse or other health professional about sensitive topics than asking a parent. **KEY POINT:** *Reassure the adolescent that you will maintain confidentiality. However, if there is concern about suicide, explain that you are required to share this information with others. Provide mental health referrals immediately when an adolescent contemplates suicide.*

Focus your age-specific interventions on educating the teenager about common health problems and avoidance of injury and disease. Include the following topics:

Preventing and Treating Obesity

Help the patient to make small but permanent changes in eating and exercise. These usually work better than a series of extreme short-term diets and exercise plans that cannot be sustained. Gradual weight loss is the healthiest approach. Even for teens, parental involvement is important—not to police the eating, but to model healthy eating and physical activity.

Calorie Intake Reducing calorie intake is usually the easiest change to make. As a rule, avoid highly restrictive diets that forbid favorite foods. It is important to encourage strong support from parents and others involved in buying and preparing food and to teach the teen how to choose highly nutritious foods at school to replace junk foods and to limit fruit juices and sodas.

Physical Activity Stress the importance of regular physical activity. Some adolescents may be able to walk to school instead of driving or taking a bus. If this is not practical, involve the family in planning regular physical activities—for example, a long walk after dinner. Even mild exercise, such as shooting hoops or swimming, provides more activity than watching television or playing computer games. You might start with the following goals:

- *Limit television, phone, and video game use* to 1 or 2 hours a day. Discourage use before school, during homework, and late at night. Keep the television and other media off during family mealtimes.
- *Engage in 30 minutes of outdoor activity every day.* Some activity is better than none. Work up to an hour a day of more strenuous exercise.

Preventing Pregnancy and STIs

One of the *Healthy People 2020* national goals is to increase the percentage of adolescents who either abstain from sex or use condoms with hormonal intrauterine contraception. To see the *Healthy People 2020* objectives,

 Go to the *Healthy People 2020* Web site at http://www. healthypeople.gov/

Abstinence is the only 100% effective way to prevent pregnancy and STIs. However, if the adolescent is sexually active, explain that using condoms can greatly reduce, although do not eliminate, those risks. Be sure teens understand that STIs can be transmitted orally and anally, as well as vaginally, so it is important that they use a condom, regardless of the type of sexual activity.

A practice guideline from the AAP (2013) recommends that schools make condoms available for adolescents and, with community involvement, develop a comprehensive sequential sexuality education as a part of a K–12 health education program. Some parents may worry that sex education and condom availability encourage teenage sex but data show that making condoms available does not increase the rate of sexual activity.

Breast Self-Awareness

There is a trend toward promoting breast self-awareness, which educates patients about the normal feel and appearance of their breasts. For many patients, breast self-awareness also may include performing breast self-examinations. **Breast self-exam (BSE)** is a step-by-step approach that a woman can use to look at and feel her breasts. However, many guidelines no longer recommend BSE as a screening tool for breast cancer. Although it seemed promising when it was first introduced, studies have shown BSE does not offer the early detection and survival benefits of other screening tests (U.S. Preventive Services Task Force, 2015a). However, they both have the potential to alert the patient to changes in her breast and may lead to earlier detection of breast cancer.

Testicular Self-Exam (TSE)

Guidelines are not consistent regarding testicular self-exam (TSE).

- The U.S. Preventive Services Task Force (USPSTF) (2015b) recommends against routine screening of asymptomatic patients, stating that outcomes are not sufficiently improved to merit routine TSE.
- The American Cancer Society (ACS) recommends a testicular exam by a doctor as part of a routine cancer-related checkup but does not have a recommendation about regular testicular self-exams.

Nevertheless, some doctors recommend that all men examine their testicles monthly after puberty. If your patient chooses to perform TSE, advise him to perform the exam after a warm bath or shower (heat relaxes the scrotum, making it easier to find abnormalities).

Immunizations

For adolescents aged 13 to 17, none of the *Healthy People 2010* objectives for vaccinations were met. Fewer than half have current tetanus, diphtheria, and pertussis immunization. About double that number have been vaccinated for hepatitis B, measles, mumps, and rubella.

KEY POINT: *Recently, human papillomavirus (HPV) vaccine has been recommended for both males and females at age 11 to 12 years (Advisory Committee on Immunization Practices, 2014) so they are protected before ever being exposed to the virus.* HPV is a common virus; nearly 80 million people—about one in four—are currently infected in the United States. About 14 million people, including teens, become infected with HPV each year. HPV infection can cause cervical, vaginal, and vulvar cancers in women; penile cancer in men; and anal cancer and mouth/throat (oropharyngeal) cancer, as well as genital warts in both men and women.

Toward Evidence-Based Practice

Perry, R., Kayekjian, K., Braun, R., et al. (2011). Adolescents' perspectives on the use of text messaging service for preventive sexual health promotion. *Journal of Adolescent Health, 51*(3), 220–225.

This study investigated the perspectives of 26 adolescents (aged 15 to 20 years) regarding a preventive sexual health text messaging service. Participants reported that they generally enjoyed receiving health-related text messages that were relevant to and directly helpful in their daily lives. They stated that receiving the text messages helped to stimulate or guide positive discussions with peers about sexual health. Findings indicated that using text messaging to relay health information to teens was convenient for the participants, did not pose financial concerns for most, and generally created a greater sense of privacy than did traditional communication tools.

Kogan, S., Yu, T., Brody, T., et al. (2012). Integrating condom skills into family-centered prevention: Efficacy of the strong African American families–teen program. *Journal of Adolescent Health, 51*(2), 164–170.

In this study 16-year-old rural African American youths and their primary caregivers were randomly assigned to one of two groups that participated in a 5-week family skills training program.

- One group was given a condom skills unit along with the training intervention.
- The other, control group was not offered the condom skills unit as part of the intervention.

Findings indicated that the intervention with the condom skills unit was effective in reducing the frequency of unprotected intercourse and increasing condom efficacy among rural African American high school students. These results suggest that integrating condom skills education into a family-centered prevention programs is effective when caregivers' input on the issue is respected.

1. What important points does the first research study make pertaining to adolescent learning needs that you could use in your preventive healthcare teaching?

2. What implications do the findings from the research studies have on how you might provide preventive services to adolescents?

To see the national goals for 2020,

 Go to the *Healthy People 2020* Web site at http://www. healthypeople.gov/

For the recommended immunization schedule for adolescents,

 Go to the CDC Web site at http://www.cdc.gov/vaccines/ schedules/hcp/imz/child-adolescent-shell.html

Other Health Promotion Activities

Other nursing activities include promoting adolescent health and safety:

- *Rest.* Explain the importance of adequate rest. Teens need 8 hours of sleep a night for maximum performance in academics and sports.
- *Nutrition.* Stress the importance of adequate nutrition, including intake of 1,300 mg of calcium and 400 IU of vitamin D daily to reach maximum bone density during this critical period of rapid increase in growth and bone mass. Teach teens how to choose foods that include fruits, vegetables, cereal and grains, lean meats, chicken, fish, and low-fat dairy products and to avoid foods and drinks that are high in sugar, fat, or caffeine.
- *Dental hygiene.* Advise parents that the adolescent should have a preventive dental care visit at least once a year. Teach the teen to brush twice a day with a soft toothbrush and to floss daily.
- ✚ *Safety.* Remind teens to wear a seat belt when riding in the car and avoid distractions while driving (talking or texting on a cell phone, changing a radio station). Ask them *never* to drive under the influence of alcohol or drugs. Remind them to wear a helmet and protective gear for activities such as bicycling, in-line skating, and skateboarding. Teach the importance of sun safety (e.g., applying a sunscreen of at least SPF 15, avoiding tanning beds, wearing sunglasses when in the sun).

KnowledgeCheck 9-8

- According to Erikson, what is the developmental stage of the adolescent?
- Name two common health problems of adolescents.

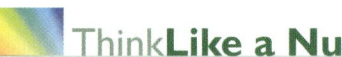 ThinkLike a Nurse 9-5

Recall Carrie, a 13-year-old girl, in the Meet Your Patients scenario. Carrie is hospitalized for pneumonia. What effect might this have on her behavior? As her nurse, how might you intervene?

YOUNG ADULTHOOD: AGES 19 TO 40 YEARS

Young adulthood is the time of transition to independence and responsibility. This is usually the healthiest stage of a person's life.

Physical Development of Young Adults

Maturation of the body systems is complete. Peak bone density is achieved for both females and males by age 25. Vision and hearing are typically acute. For women, the ages between 20 and 30 years are the optimal years for childbearing. For men, male hormone levels that surged in adolescence begin to slowly decrease and stabilize around age 24.

Cognitive Development of Young Adults

According to Piaget, learning continues throughout life but patterns of thinking do not alter after adolescence. In the *formal operations* phase, teenagers are able to think rationally, predict outcomes, and hypothesize about the future. At this point, thought processes and mental abilities are well established; the teen is able to think rationally, predict outcomes, and hypothesize about the future. All of this is true of young adults, as well.

Contemporary psychologists have proposed an additional and more complex stage of cognitive development called *post-formal operations*. In this phase, the young adult is able to accept contradictions and fine points in thinking. For example, the post-formal thinker recognizes that her opinion on a social controversy has aspects of two opposing viewpoints. She sees merit in both parts of the argument and is comfortable with the discrepancy.

Psychosocial Development of Young Adults

The transition to adulthood involves important life events, such as graduating from high school, entering college or starting a career, and leaving home and becoming self-sufficient. Young adults begin to explore options for intimate relationships, marriage or alternative relationships, and careers. Around age 30, most young adults experience a period of self-evaluation. This often results in a job, career, or relationship change.

- Erikson describes this period as the stage of *intimacy versus isolation.* Successful completion of this phase requires establishment of lasting friendships and associations.
- Freud described this phase of life as the *genital stage.* He believed that young adults are instinctively driven to form a sexually intimate relationship.

Common Health Problems of Young Adults

Young adults are generally active and in good physical health. Frequently seen health problems include STIs, unplanned pregnancies, traumatic injury, suicide attempts, substance abuse, domestic violence, obesity, diabetes, and hypertension. Unintentional injury is the leading cause of death in young adults (National Center for Health Statistics, 2015).

Sexually Transmitted Infections

Sexual experimentation often continues in this stage. Among those 15 to 44 years of age, nearly all have had penile-vaginal intercourse and most have had oral sex with an opposite-sex partner. More than one-third of women and 44% of men have had anal sex with an opposite-sex partner.

Twice as many women aged 25 to 44 (12%) reported same-sex contact in their lifetime, compared with men (5.8%). Six percent of men have had oral or anal sex with another man, and 11% of women have had a sexual experience with another woman (Chandra, Mosher, Copen, et al., 2012).

Some common STIs include chlamydia, genital warts (condyloma acuminata), gonorrhea, and genital herpes. The large majority of newly diagnosed cases (nearly 39%) of acquired immunodeficiency syndrome (AIDS) are among young adults (CDC, 2012b). For more information about STIs, see Chapter 34.

Example Problems: Abuse, Neglect, and Violence

Roughly 30,000 people a year die as a result of firearm injuries; most of these are suicides and homicides rather than accidental. This is a rate of about 1 death per 10,000 people. **Domestic**

violence (or intimate partner violence [IPV]) is the abuse of power and control within an intimate relationship, most often between spouses or domestic partners. The CDC recognizes four categories of IPV: physical violence, sexual violence, threat of physical or sexual violence, and psychological or emotional abuse. More often than not, the abuser is a spouse or domestic partner, but it is sometimes another family member.

Incidence More than 10 million women and men in the United States experience physical violence each year by a current or former intimate partner. At some time in their lifetime:

- Approximately 22.3% (one in five) of women have experienced severe physical violence from an intimate partner.
- Data from National Intimate Partner and Sexual Violence Survey also show that nearly 1 in 11 women (8.8%) has been raped by a current or former intimate partner.
- Approximately 9.2% of women and 2.5% of men have been stalked by an intimate partner (Breiding, Basile, Smith, et al., 2015).

Globally, one in every three women has been assaulted, coerced into sex, or otherwise abused at some point in her life (U.N. Women, 2016). Many victims do not report the abuse, so survey results vary.

Risk Factors Abuse occurs in all ethnic and socioeconomic groups. Factors associated with intimate partner violence include young age, low income status, pregnancy, young maternal age, low maternal education, large family size, mental health problems, alcohol or substance abuse by victims or perpetrators, separated or divorced status, single-parent household, and history of childhood sexual or physical abuse (Nelson, Bougatsos, & Blazina, 2012). Females 16 to 24 years of age are the most vulnerable to nonfatal violence. In the United States, women are 7 to 14 times more likely to be abused than are men. About 31% of female murder victims are killed by an intimate partner, compared with 3% of male victims. Refer to the Example Problem: Abuse, Neglect, and Violence.

Health Consequences Intimate partner violence has negative consequences for physical, sexual, and psychological health. Abuse victims can suffer acute and chronic pain, disability, damage to the eyes, sleep disorders, miscarriage, STIs, poor self-esteem, depression, anxiety, and even suicidal behavior.

Obesity

Obesity rates have increased to crisis level over the past 25 years. In the United States, two-thirds of adults are either overweight (BMI 25–29) or obese (BMI >30). With increased obesity rates, the incidences of type 2 DM and hypertension have grown dramatically among young adults

ASSESSMENT (Young Adults) NP

Young adults should have an annual physical examination, including assessment of physical health, mental health, and lifestyle. Be sure to assess nutrition, exercise, sleep, and use of tobacco, alcohol, and drugs. For women, the physical should include a pelvic exam.

Screening Screening for diabetes and hypertension is very important in the young adult, especially for those who are overweight or who have a family history cardiac disease.

The American Cancer Society (ACS) recommends a clinical breast examination at least once every 3 years.

The USPSTF (2015b) no longer recommends clinical testicular exams or monthly TSE. However, the ACS (n.d., revised 2015) recommends a testicular exam by a doctor as part of a routine cancer-related checkup, but does not have a recommendation about testicular self-exams.

Example Problem: Violence Screening IPV is common but often remains undetected, so the USPSTF recommends that clinicians screen women of childbearing age for abuse or domestic violence and provide or refer women who screen positive to intervention services (USPSTF, 2013). If there is any reason to suspect abuse, conduct a thorough assessment.

➕ If the patient discloses domestic violence, act immediately. Ask the patient whether she would like you to contact the agency's domestic violence advocate (if there is one). If not, provide contact information for community domestic violence programs. Patients are often fearful, isolated, and in real danger, but they may refuse help the first time it is offered.

For further information on assessing and reporting abuse, see Procedure 9-1. Also see the preceding Example Problem: Abuse, Neglect, and Violence and Mandatory Reporting Laws in Chapter 44.

INTERVENTIONS (Young Adults) NP

Nursing interventions for the young adult are similar to those for the adolescent. As a newly independent person, the young adult is establishing health patterns, including how she will interact with healthcare providers. Reinforce the teaching that was begun in the earlier age-group. Stress the importance of health promotion activities such as a Papanicolaou (Pap) test (to screen for cervical cancer) every 3 years for women between the ages of 21 and 30 (USPSTF, 2012).

Breast Cancer Prevention Breast cancer prevention starts with healthy habits.

Teach for risk reduction. Teach patients what they can do to reduce their breast cancer risk (e.g., limit alcohol and stay physically active).

Promote breast self-awareness. Tell the patient to be vigilant about breast cancer detection. If she notices any changes in her breasts, such as a new lump or skin changes, instruct her to consult their doctor.

Advise about mammograms. Women younger than 40 who have risk factors should ask their healthcare provider whether they need mammograms. Risk factors include personal and family history of breast cancer, having the first child late in the childbearing cycle, having the first menstrual period before age 12, and certain breast changes (e.g., cells that look abnormal under a microscope). Studies have shown no link between abortion or miscarriage and breast cancer.

Exercise Recommend to women that they engage in 2.5 hours a week of moderate-intensity, or 75 minutes a week of vigorous-intensity, aerobic physical activity. Increasing exercise to 300 minutes a week provides even more health benefits. They should also do muscle-strengthening activities that involve all major muscle groups performed on 2 or more days per week (U.S. Department of Health and Human Services, 2009, updated 2015).

KnowledgeCheck 9-9

- According to Erikson, what is the developmental stage of the young adult?
- What is the leading cause of death for this age-group?
- What gender-specific assessments should be emphasized with this age-group?

MIDDLE ADULTHOOD: AGES 40 TO 64 YEARS

The middle adult years are a time when people realize the difference between their early aspirations and their actual achievements.

Physical Development of Middle Adults

Physiological changes during the middle adult years include graying or thinning hair, decrease in elasticity of the blood vessels, and decrease in muscle tone, skin moisture and turgor, and gastrointestinal (GI) motility. A decrease in bone mass often causes a slight loss of height.

Menopause One of the principal changes that women experience in the middle adult years is **menopause,** the cessation of menstrual periods for at least 12 months. The ovaries no longer produce eggs on a cyclical basis, and reproductive ability is lost (although some women do become pregnant after not having menses for a year). The average age of menopause is 51 years. Most women experience a transition that takes place over many years.

Perimenopausal symptoms are related to a decline in estrogen levels and may precede menopause by as much as 5 to 7 years. These symptoms include hot flashes, a decrease in breast size, changes in the length of the menstrual cycle and menstrual flow, vaginal dryness, nighttime awakenings, and moodiness.

Andropause Men do not experience such a clear-cut transition, but many men do experience a transitional period known as andropause. **Andropause** is characterized by a decrease in testosterone production, a lower sperm count, and a need for more time to achieve an erection. Andropause does not result in an inability to reproduce but does limit reproductive abilities.

Cognitive Development of Middle Adults

Piaget theorized that the middle adult moves freely between formal operations, concrete operations, and problem-solving as the task demands. Middle adults are able to reflect on the past and anticipate the future. Creativity may reach its peak during this stage. Memory is intact, but reaction time begins to diminish because of a decrease in nerve impulses.

Psychosocial Development of Middle Adults

Erikson describes middle adulthood as a stage of *generativity versus stagnation. Generativity* is the process of guiding the next generation, or improving the whole of society. *Stagnation* occurs when development ceases: A stagnant middle adult cannot guide the next generation or contribute to society, or prepare adequately for the final life stage, old age.

Middle adulthood is a time of transition. This is often a time when children mature and leave the home. As a result, many middle adults and their children feel a need to redefine family roles.

Middle adults often complain of declining energy and competing demands as they raise children, care for aging parents, and work at the peak of their career (Fig. 9-10). These stressors in combination with visible signs of aging may produce a **midlife crisis**—a recognition that youth is over and that life is limited. Coping skills learned in earlier years are important predictors of how the middle adult reacts to these changes

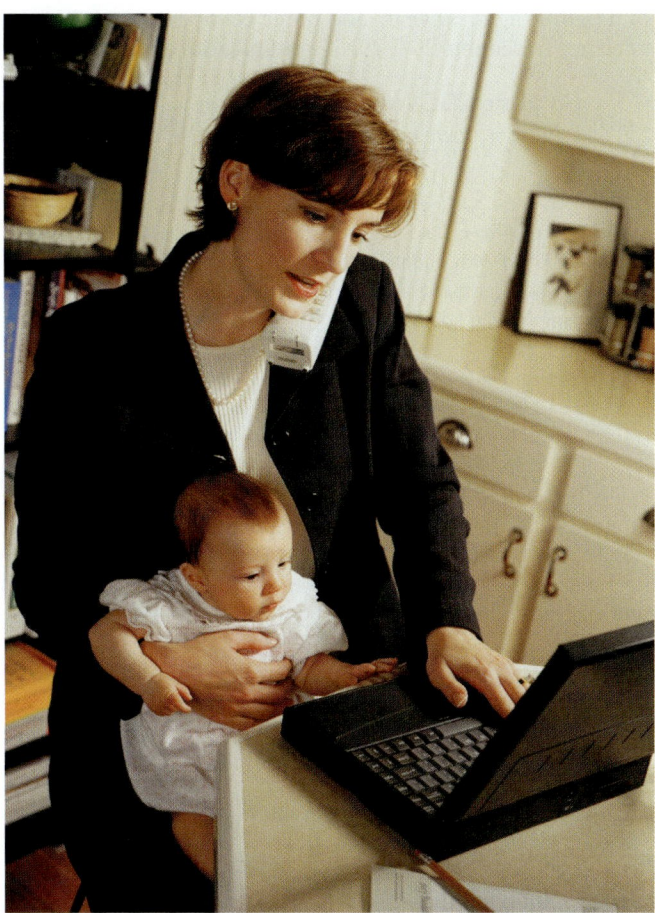

FIGURE 9-10 Middle adulthood is a time of competing demands.

Common Health Problems of Middle Adults

In the middle adult years, chronic diseases emerge as a major health problem. The most common chronic diseases are cancer, obesity, diabetes, hypertension, and cardiovascular disease. Many interventions for younger age-groups are directed at preventing the development of these chronic disorders.

Cancer The majority of cancer diagnoses occur in the middle and older adult years. Lung cancer remained the leading cause of cancer death, accounting for 27% (157,017) of the total cancer deaths in 2011. Rates for female breast and colorectal cancer have each declined slightly in recent years, but the number of deaths attributed to each has remained stable, with an average of approximately 41,000 and 53,000 annual deaths, respectively (CDC, 2014e). A man's risk of prostate cancer increases as he ages. Nearly 65% of prostate cancer occurs after the age of 65. Other factors that increase the risk of prostate cancer are family history, race (African American men have the highest rate), and possibly diet. There is some evidence that a diet high in animal fat may increase the risk.

Obesity As we have seen, obesity is a major health problem in all age-groups. It often triggers development of type 2 DM; hypertension; joint pain; and cardiovascular diseases, such as coronary artery disease, atherosclerosis, and venous insufficiency. Diet and exercise must be consistently used together to combat obesity. Ironically, obesity leads to a variety of problems that make it even harder to exercise.

Cardiovascular Disease Atherosclerotic plaque can develop in the peripheral vascular system, the heart, major vessels, or any combination of these areas. Cardiovascular disease (CVD) is the result of inadequately treated hypertension, ongoing weight gain or obesity, an aftermath of poorly controlled type 2 DM, and an outcome of a sedentary lifestyle. Hypertension (high blood pressure) is a complex disorder. As the elasticity of the vascular system declines with each passing year, the incidence of hypertension increases. If there is a strong family history of hypertension, the likelihood of needing treatment escalates sharply.

Except for age and family history, factors that increase the risk of hypertension are under the patient's control. They include excess weight, sedentary lifestyle, high sodium intake, high fat intake, smoking, and the ingestion of more than 1.5 ounces of alcohol per day. For further discussion of hypertension, see Chapter 19. Smoking and excess alcohol use are additional risk factors, as is long-term hormone replacement therapy for women. CVD is among the leading causes of death in the middle adult years.

Example Problem: Domestic Violence Women aged 30 to 49 are the most vulnerable to intimate murder, although younger women are more likely to experience nonfatal violence (U.S. Department of Justice, 2011). Also see Common Health Problems of Young Adults, as well as the Example Problem: Abuse, Neglect and Violence, preceding.

ASSESSMENT (Middle Adults) NP

Middle adults should undergo an annual physical exam. In addition to height, weight, BMI, and vital signs, the exam should include the following:

- *Lipid panel screening:* total cholesterol, triglycerides, high-density lipoprotein (HDL), low-density lipoprotein (LDL), and ratios
- *Blood glucose screening.*
- *Clinical breast and pelvic examination* for women. The American College of Obstetricians and Gynecologists (ACOG), ACS, and the National Comprehensive Cancer Network recommend that clinical breast examination be performed annually in women aged 40 years and older (ACOG, 2012, reaffirmed 2014; ACS, 2010, revised 2015). Women older than 30 should have a Pap test every 3 to 5 years based on health history and discussion with their primary care provider.
- *Annual or biannual mammogram* for women. The ACS recommends that women with average risk of breast cancer should undergo regular screening mammography starting at age 45 years. Women aged 45 to 54 years should be screened while women 55 years and older should transition to biennial screening or have the opportunity to continue screening annually. Women should have the opportunity to begin annual screening between the ages of 40 and 44 years if history warrants and should continue as long as a woman is in good health and is expected to live 10 more years or longer (Oeffinger, Fontham, Etzioni, et al., 2015).
- *Digital rectal exam for prostate evaluation* in men should be offered but not routinely done (ACS, n.d., revised 2015). An enlarged prostate can indicate either benign prostatic hypertrophy or prostate cancer. Serum prostate-specific antigen (PSA) level is a sensitive indicator of prostate disorders. Recommendations vary. Some caution against routine screening; however, the American Cancer Society says this test should be given beginning at age 45 to men who want to be screened and at age 40 for those who are at higher risk.

- *Annual eye exam.* Visual changes are common in this age-group and include the development of presbyopia (far-sightedness) and the onset of glaucoma and cataracts.
- *Colorectal cancer screening.* Regular screening is key to preventing colorectal cancer. The USPSTF (2014b) recommends screening for colorectal cancer using stool for occult blood testing and sigmoidoscopy or colonoscopy beginning at age 50 (or at age 40 for high-risk patients) until age 75 years. The frequency of repeat exams depends on the findings.
- *Osteoporosis screening* should be done at or prior to menopause for at risk women who elect it. Most guidelines recommend assessing all adults age 50 years or older for risk factors (e.g., smoking, low body weight) with bone density measurement (called a DEXA test) based on risk profile (Florence, Allen, Benedict, et al., 2013).

INTERVENTIONS (Middle Adults) NP

Care for middle adults focuses on identifying risk factors and promoting a healthy lifestyle. At each annual exam and at periodic health visits, you should discuss the hazards of alcohol and tobacco use, the importance of regular exercise, stress-management techniques, safety, and the benefits of a balanced nutritional intake. You will also need to add teaching topics and interventions if any chronic problem is discovered.

Nutrition For menopausal women, encourage daily intake of 1,200 mg of calcium and 600 IU of vitamin D, as well as regular weight-bearing exercise, to promote optimal bone density (Florence, Allen, Benedict, et al., 2013). There is growing consensus that even this amount may be too low. Many clinicians are prescribing higher doses, especially in cases of known deficiency.

Hormone Replacement Therapy (HRT) has been used extensively in the past, but recent studies have raised questions about the safety of hormone therapy to treat a naturally occurring phenomenon. HRT can relieve symptoms such as hot flashes and vaginal dryness. It may also protect against osteoporosis and age-linked eye disease. Some studies show that it may help prevent dementia; others show that it does not. However, the risks of HRT include heart disease, breast cancer, stroke, and blood clots.

The National Institutes of Health (2008) concludes that the risks of long-term combination hormone (estrogen and progestin) therapy outweigh the benefits for postmenopausal women. Advise women to consult their primary care provider about estrogen-alone therapy, bioidentical therapies, and certain natural remedies that can provide symptom relief.

Exercise Although the usual recommendation is for 60 minutes of exercise daily, and that amount brings the most health benefits, researchers now suggest that even smaller amounts of exercise can improve the quality of life for sedentary, overweight, or obese postmenopausal women. Even 30 minutes a day can improve social functioning and decrease limitations in work and other activities due to physical or emotional problems (U.S. Department of Health and Human Services, 2009, updated 2015).

Immunizations Review the patient's immunization record regularly. Middle adults often require periodic boosters, for example, for pertussis. Teach patients that annual influenza vaccination is recommended for all persons aged 6 months and older who do not have contraindications. Strongly encourage clients with respiratory problems to receive pneumonia vaccination as well. The CDC recommends that people aged 60 years and older get one dose of shingles vaccine. To see the CDC 2016 immunization schedule,

 Go to the CDC Web site at http://www.cdc.gov/vaccines/schedules/downloads/adult/adult-schedule-easy-read.pdf

KnowledgeCheck 9-10
- According to Erikson, what is the developmental stage associated with middle adulthood?
- Identify at least five appropriate topics for health teaching during middle adulthood.

PracticalKnowledge
knowing why

This section of the book focuses on using standardized nursing language for growth and development nursing diagnoses, patient outcomes, and interventions for patients in all age-groups. Age-group-specific assessments and interventions were discussed within each of the developmental stages in the preceding Theoretical Knowledge section.

Analysis/Diagnosis Although most NANDA-I diagnoses can be used for any age-group, the following NANDA-I diagnoses focuses specifically on growth and development. Risk for Delayed Development diagnoses for older adults are found in Chapter 10.

An example of a diagnosis you might write is Risk for Delayed Development r/t inadequate stimulation secondary to parental substance abuse.

Short-term illness does not usually lead to delays in growth and development. Such delays are more likely to be caused by family dysfunction, inadequate nutrition, or severe or long-term illness. Of course, patients you see for other problems may very well also be growth or developmentally delayed.

As with other diagnoses, Growth and Development diagnoses can, instead of being the problem focus, be defining characteristics or risk factors for other diagnoses. For example: Impaired Parenting r/t mother's chronic disability and evidenced by child's delayed growth.

Only one NANDA-I diagnosis specifically address growth and development; however, other NANDA-I diagnoses do address age-specific problems (e.g., Ineffective Breastfeeding).

Individualized Goals/Outcomes and Interventions for growth and development outcomes and interventions might include the following examples:

Diagnosis: Risk for Delayed Development
- *Goal:* The child will continue to meet developmental cognitive milestones as measured at the next well-child check.
- *Intervention (example):* Teach parent(s) 3 techniques they can use to stimulate the child's cognition.

PUTTING IT ALL TOGETHER

Recall 3-year-old Tamika, who is being raised by her grandmother and has been hospitalized with pneumonia (Meet Your Patients scenario). Tamika has been abandoned by her mother, who is addicted to heroin. You observe that Tamika is small for her age. For the following NANDA-I *nursing diagnosis* you might write:

- *Risk for Delayed Development r/t abandonment by mother, recent change in living status, and gestational heroin exposure as evidenced by underweight status and short stature*

- To address Tamika's diagnosis, you might use the following outcomes:
- *NOC outcome:* Child Development, 3 years
- *Individualized goal:* Tamika will achieve developmental milestones as demonstrated by (1) specified weight gain at next visit, (2) showing affection and bonding with grandmother, (3) grandmother's reports of adequate nutrition.

Because the grandmother is also caring for her ill husband, you may need to refer this family to community support services for ongoing help in the home and for nutritional services.

CLINICALREASONING

The questions and exercises in this section allow you to practice the kind of thinking you will use as a full spectrum nurse. Critical thinking questions usually have more than one correct answer, so we do not provide "correct answers" for these features. It is more important to develop nursing judgment than to cover content. You will learn by discussing these questions with your peers. If you are still unsure, see the Davis Advantage chapter resources for suggested responses.

Caring for the Nguyens

Review the scenario of Nam Nguyen in the front of this book. Answer the following questions based on that scenario.

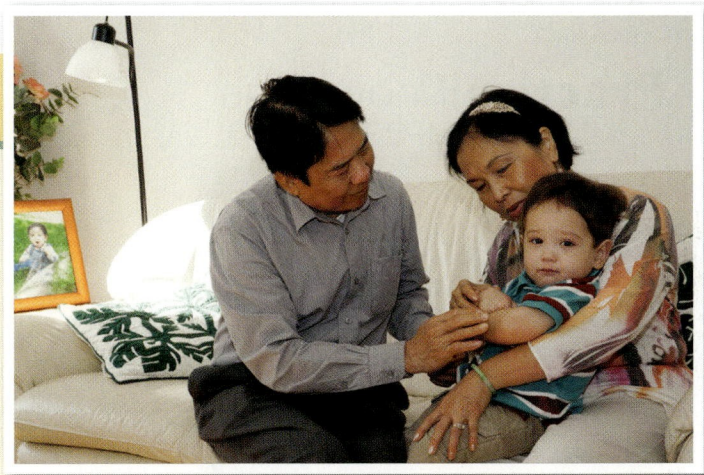

A. Evaluate Mr. Nguyen's physical health status in comparison with what is expected for someone in his age-group.

B. Mr. Nguyen and his wife are raising their 3-year-old grandson. What effect might this have on Mr. Nguyen's ability to accomplish his developmental tasks?

Applying the **Full-Spectrum Nursing Model**

PATIENT SITUATION

Lani Ettinger is a 30-year-old woman, married, with three school-age children. She has just had a mastectomy (removal of a breast) because her biopsy was positive for cancer. The surgery was uncomplicated, the cancer was removed at an early stage, and she is expected to recover completely. As you are helping her prepare to leave the hospital, she begins crying.

THINKING

1. *Theoretical Knowledge:* What are Havighurst's developmental tasks of young adulthood?
2. *Critical Thinking (Contextual Awareness):* Which of those developmental tasks is/are most likely to be affected by Lani's mastectomy and her emotional reaction to it?

DOING

3. *Nursing Process (Assessment):* When you see that Lani is crying, what do you need to do?

CARING

4. *Self-Knowledge:* Suppose Lani tells you, "My husband has gone to get the car, but when he was here, he didn't want to hug me or kiss me. I asked him if he will still love me and he didn't say anything. He was crying when he left." What would your feelings be about the husband? You do not need to speculate on exactly what he meant; just imagine what your initial feelings would be.

PracticalKnowledge
clinical application

One important aspect of developmental care across the life span is to identify abuse and intervene with patients who are being abused. You will find information on elder abuse in Chapter 10; however, the following procedure can be used for patients of all ages.

Keep in mind that if there is an injury, there is the possibility that it was inflicted. The flow chart depicted in Figure 9-11 and Procedure 9-1 will aid you in identifying cases of abuse.

PracticalKnowledge
procedures

Possible Abuse Flow Chart

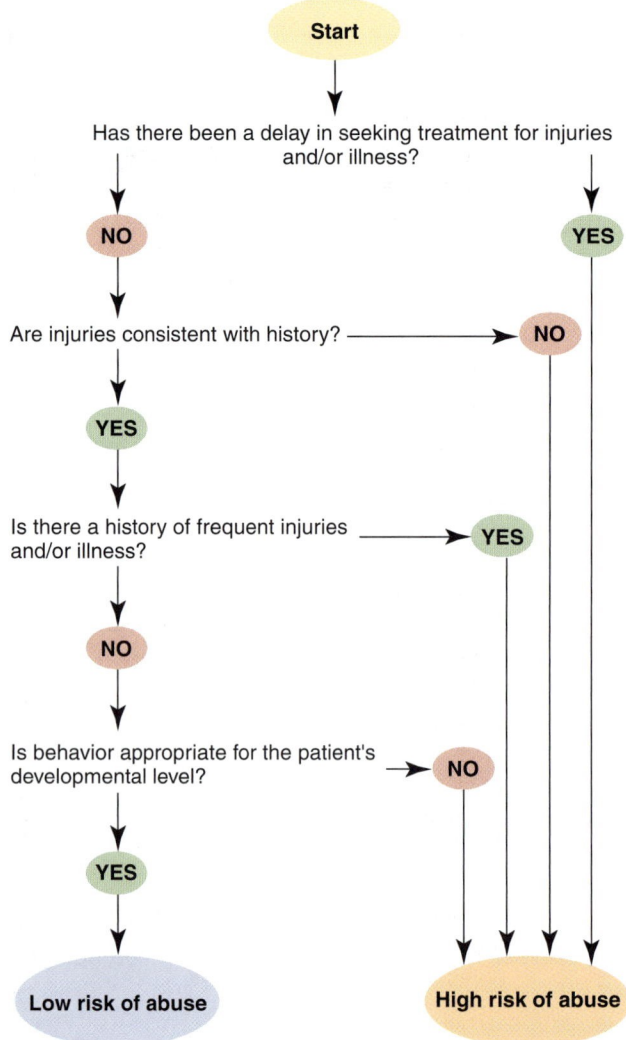

FIGURE 9-11 Possible Abuse Flow Chart.

Procedure 9-1 ■ Assessing for Abuse

➤ For steps to follow in *all* procedures, refer to the Universal Steps for All Procedures found on the page facing the inside back cover.

Pre-Procedure Assessment

■ If you suspect sexual abuse, request a forensic nurse or sexual assault nurse examiner (SANE) be present.
A forensic nurse and SANE are trained to identify findings that indicate abuse, to support the patient, and to handle the evidence to ensure validity in a court of law.

■ Assess for abuse routinely in elderly or vulnerable adults and women of childbearing age, and any time a child, dependent person, or spouse has an injury.

Although there is not a strong base of evidence to support screening, the Joint Commission requires that all patients be screened for abuse and domestic violence.

Delegation

KEY POINT: *Assessment is a nursing responsibility and cannot be delegated.*

➤ When performing the procedure, always identify your patient according to agency policy, using two identifiers, and be attentive to standard precautions, hand hygiene, patient safety and privacy, body mechanics, and documentation.

➤ *Note:* Privacy and confidentiality are extremely important for this procedure.

Procedure Steps

Obtain a Focused Health History

1. **Interview the patient and family members or caregivers separately.** If more than one caregiver is present, separate them for the interview as well.
An abused person may be afraid to talk with the abuser present. Victims have often been intimidated and will usually support the abuser's version of events. If two adults accompany a child, it may be that one of them is abusing both the partner and the child. To help rule that out, separate the caregivers to be certain that they tell the same story.

2. **Approach the subject in a non-threatening and caring manner.** For example, you might say, "The law requires us to ask about certain injuries. We are not accusing you of anything. I know you care about your child/parent/spouse and want to do everything possible for her health."

3. **Consider the patient's developmental and cognitive level** in assessing whether the story of how the injury occurred is consistent with the injuries.
The patient must be developmentally capable of performing an activity in a situation in which an injury occurred. *For example, an infant is not likely to have opened a medication bottle and taken pills; if a child cannot yet walk, it is not likely he reached up to pull a hot pan off the stove.*

4. **Observe the patient's behavior. Is it inconsistent with his developmental level?**
In the presence of the abuser, it is common for the victim to appear passive and withdrawn and avoid eye contact. The victim may exhibit anxiety or fear; may look to the parent or caregiver before answering questions; may be overly compliant; or may let the abuser answer the questions for him.

5. **Ask about the injury or incident.** Ask detailed questions about how and when the injury occurred or the illness began:
"When did this injury happen or when did you first begin to feel ill?" "How did you get this injury?" "What happened to you?" "What have you been doing to treat your symptoms since you first became ill?"
A delay of treatment of 12 to 18 hours may indicate abuse. If the details of the history of an injury change during the interview, the likelihood of abuse increases.

6. **Ask about past injuries or incidents:**
"Have you ever had similar injuries?" "Have you ever required emergency care in the past?"
Abusive behavior typically occurs over and over. If an injury is due to abuse, the patient would most likely have experienced abuse in the past and would have evidence of old injuries.

7. **Ask about the patient's usual diet:**
"What do you usually eat for breakfast? Lunch? Dinner? What kind of snacks do you have during the day?"
Neglect and abuse may be exhibited by an inadequate or inappropriate diet.

Assess for Sexual Abuse

8. **Ask directly whether the patient has been touched inappropriately** or forced to have sexual relations.
Whenever possible, question the patient directly so your question will not be misunderstood.

9. **Ask whether the patient has genitourinary symptoms:** "Have you had any burning or itching when you urinate? How about any vaginal discharge?"
In a child, genitourinary symptoms may indicate sexual abuse or neglect.

(continued on next page)

Procedure 9-1 ■ Assessing for Abuse (continued)

10. **Does the child display knowledge or interest in sexual acts** inappropriate to his or her age, or even seductive behavior?

11. **Does the child appear to avoid another person,** or display unusual behavior—either very aggressive or very passive?

12. **Does the victim display destructive behaviors,** such as alcohol or drug abuse, self-mutilation, or suicide attempts?

13. **Is the victim pregnant,** particularly if no intimate relationship is known or the victim is very young?

Assess for Psychological Abuse

14. **Ask parents or caregivers,** "Are there family members or friends who help you with problems?"
   Isolation is a risk factor for abuse. Parents or caregivers may not have the support they need.

15. **Ask the patient, "Whom do you talk to** when you are having problems?"
   An abuser will try to isolate the victim from family and friends over time. Ask questions to determine the relationship between the victim and family and friends.

16. **Ask, "Tell me how you feel about yourself."**
   An abuser demeans and degrades the victim so that the victim has a low self-worth and feels the "punishment" is deserved; conversely, the victim may desire the attention.

17. **Observe whether the child acts fearful,** shies away from touch, or appears to be afraid to go home.

18. **Ask, "Who manages the family finances,** and how are decisions made regarding spending?" (for adults)
   An abuser frequently controls all the finances and restricts the resources of

the victim. Abusers typically seek control of victims by fostering dependency and powerlessness.

Perform a Focused Physical Assessment

19. **If sexual abuse is suspected from the interview,** have a forensic nurse or sexual assault nurse examiner (SANE) present if possible.
   For any sexual examination, always have a witness in the room to protect the patient and the examiner.

20. **Assess the current injury and look for evidence** of previous injuries. Look for the following cues:
   a. Bruises that form an outline of a hand, cord loop, buckle, or belt
   *Injuries of different ages and multiple injuries may show a pattern of abuse. Be careful to assess the bruise accurately. Some home treatments may cause what looks like bruising. For example, **moxibustion** (includes such things as firmly rubbing a warm spoon down the affected area) is used in some Asian cultures.*
   b. Injuries that are inconsistent with the history of the injury and are of varying ages (e.g., bruises of different colors, cuts in various stages of healing)
   c. Obvious nonaccidental burns, such as burns to both feet and lower legs from immersion in hot water
   One method of abuse is to immerse the victim's hands or feet into scalding water. The resulting injury has a well-defined border and usually occurs on both extremities.
   d. Circular burns, possibly from cigarettes
   Burns at several locations on the body are signs of abuse.
   e. Bite marks
   f. Oral ecchymosis or injury from forced oral sex

Forced oral sex causes injuries to the mouth.
   g. Bruising at the crease above the eyelids, tense fontanel if the victim is an infant, hyphema, subconjunctival hemorrhage or retinal bleeding, detached retina, ruptured tympanic membrane
   KEY POINT: *Injuries to the head are common in abuse. Abusive head trauma (AHT, previously referred to as shaken-baby syndrome) is one of the most common and most serious injuries for a young child to sustain.*
   h. Bleeding or bruising of genitalia, poor sphincter tone, encopresis (poor bowel control) and bruises on inner thighs
   i. Positive culture for STI or positive pregnancy test
   STI, particularly in a child, can indicate sexual abuse.
   j. Bruises on wrists and ankles from being restrained
   Abused individuals may be tied or locked in a closet or other small space.
   k. Refer to the figure for typical features of injuries that may be nonaccidental:
   Injuries to both sides of the body
   Injuries to soft tissue
   Injuries in the "triangle of safety": ears, side of face, neck, and top of the shoulders
   Accidental injuries in the triangle of safety are unusual. Accidental injuries are usually over bony prominences. One suspicious patter is called the "swimsuit zone" on the trunk, breast, abdomen, genitalia, and buttocks ➤

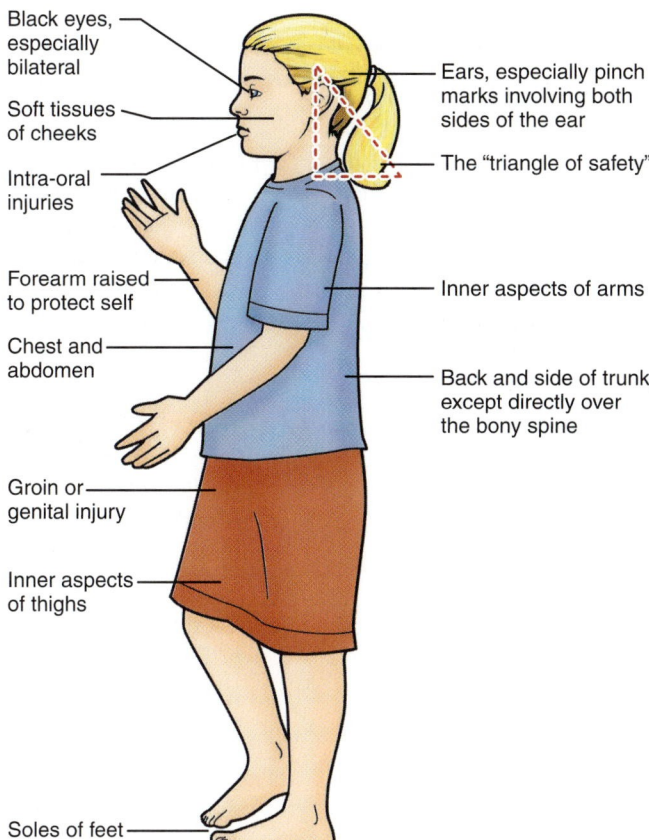

Black eyes, especially bilateral

Soft tissues of cheeks

Intra-oral injuries

Forearm raised to protect self

Chest and abdomen

Groin or genital injury

Inner aspects of thighs

Soles of feet

Ears, especially pinch marks involving both sides of the ear

The "triangle of safety"

Inner aspects of arms

Back and side of trunk, except directly over the bony spine

21. Assess whether injuries are consistent with the history.

If injuries are not consistent with the history, you must assume abuse.

22. Observe for signs of neglect:

- Malnutrition, such as a distended abdomen, or weight markedly below ideal body weight
- Excess body weight for height and age
- Poor hygiene, including oral hygiene
- Ingrown nails
- Untreated sores, pressure sores, or other medical conditions
- Matted hair
- Dehydration
- Confusion
- Clothing that is inappropriate for the weather, such as heavy, long-sleeved pants and shirts on hot days
- Periods of time a young child or frail, older adult is left alone without care or supervision

Signs of neglect occur because of long-term starvation or underfeeding, poor personal care, untreated sores or injuries, and inadequate

fluid intake. Neglect can also result in childhood obesity as a result of food of poor quality, erratic eating patterns, and poor supervision of the diet.

After the Examination

23. If the forensic nurse or primary care provider determines that abuse has occurred, follow legal procedures to ensure that all evidence is secured. If possible, have a forensic nurse and social worker work with the patient.

In situations in which violation of the law has occurred, strict procedures are essential to ensure that your findings can be used in a court of law and to protect yourself against legal liability.

24. Provide referrals, if appropriate, for the abused person, partner, family member, or caregiver to obtain assistance in escaping the abusive situation and/or stopping the abuse.

Resources are available to assist the abused individual and to assist the parent or caregiver to stop the abuse. Be aware of local and national resources.

25. Report concerns regarding abuse according to agency and state guidelines.

KEY POINT: *Suspected child and elder abuse must be reported to the appropriate agency, according to federal and state laws. Spousal abuse may be mandatory to report, depending on state law. The Joint Commission requires that all cases of possible abuse or neglect are immediately reported in the hospital.*

26. Treat physical injuries or refer to the primary care provider for medical care, as needed.

Detection and prevention of abuse require collaborative efforts of the healthcare team.

? What if . . .

- **My patient is a child? Are there any special assessments I should make or actions I should take?**

Follow steps 1 through 6 above, with these modifications:

NOTE: The interview is important in ruling out sexual abuse in children. Physical findings are often absent, even when the perpetrator admits to penetration of the child's genitalia. Most expert interviewers do not interview children younger than 3 years.

a. To assess for sexual abuse, ask whether the patient has been touched inappropriately:
   - *Child older than 2:* Ask about being touched in "private parts."
   - *Older child:* Ask a question such as, "Sometimes people you know may touch or kiss you in a way that you feel is strange or wrong. Has this ever happened to you?"
   - *Adolescent:* Ask, "Sometimes people touch you in ways you feel are wrong. This can be frightening, and it is wrong for people to do that to you. Has this ever happened to you?"

b. Ask the parent or caregiver:
   - "Has the child started wetting the bed or soiling himself?"

(continued on next page)

Procedure 9-1 ■ Assessing for Abuse (continued)

- "Does the child have fears that seem unreasonable?"

  Abuse may result in regression to former behaviors. Symptoms of sexual abuse in children may be general and nonspecific, such as sleep disturbances, bed-wetting, or excessive fears.

- "Has the child been masturbating or sexually acting out with other children?"

  A child who is sexually abused may exhibit inappropriate sexual behavior.

- "Has the child ever run away? If she leaves, does she go to somewhere safe?" "Is the child/adolescent sexually active?"

  An abused child may have feelings of low self-worth and may demonstrate risk-taking behavior, such as running away to places that are unsafe.

c. To assess for psychological abuse, ask the parent or caregiver:

- "Was the child a result of a planned pregnancy? What were the pregnancy, birth, and postpartum period like?"

  Risk factors for abuse include an unplanned pregnancy, complications during pregnancy, stressors (e.g., moving, illness, loss of job, divorce), a difficult pregnancy or birth, and lengthy stay in the neonatal intensive care unit.

- "How would you describe the child now?"

  An abusive parent may describe the child as a "problem child" who is always doing something wrong. The opposite is sometimes seen, when the child is "perfect."

- "How does the child's behavior compare with that of others in the family?"

  Determine whether the parent sees the child differently from siblings. This is a risk factor for abuse.

- "Has the child experienced physical or emotional problems in the past?"

  A history of physical or emotional problems may indicate abuse.

- "What are your expectations of the child's behavior (e.g., school performance, following instructions)?"

  The expectations of parents or caregivers who are more at risk to abuse a child may be that the child will "always be a problem" or will be a "perfect" son or daughter.

- "What form of discipline works best with the child?"

  Determine whether the parents or caregivers use physical or emotional punishment that may be abusive or disproportionate for the act or situation.

- "Do you have any history of depression, anxiety, difficulty coping with situations or everyday life, or other history of mental health problems?"

  Mental health disorders interfere with a person's ability to perceive others and situations in a realistic and appropriate way. When coping is compromised, the risk for abuse escalates.

d. Perform a physical assessment. Signs of physical abuse and neglect in children include the following:

- Bruises on head, face, ears, buttocks, and lower back that are inconsistent with the history of the injury and are of varying stages of healing (different colors)
- Hemorrhage of the eye, detached retina, ruptured eardrum

  Bruising may occur in different patterns. Children often have accidental bruises over bony areas, but usually not on the abdomen. Injuries to the head are common in abuse. The abusive head trauma (AHT) syndrome may cause detached

retina(s), hemorrhages, and subdural hematomas.

- Assess for abdominal pain and other nonspecific complaints.

  Abdominal pain may be a symptom of sexual abuse in children. Signs of sexual abuse may be general and nonspecific in children.

? What if . . .

- **My patient is an older adult? Are there any special assessments I should make or actions I should take?**

a. Ask the patient and caregiver:

- "Describe the patient's personal support network. Who visits the patient? How often does the patient have visitors?"

  As in spousal abuse, people who victimize older people often isolate the person from any support network.

- "Who is the patient's primary healthcare provider?"

  Multiple healthcare providers, or lack of a provider, can be an indication of abuse. The caregiver may bring the patient to a different physician with each injury or illness to avoid discovery.

- "Has the patient ever received the wrong dose of medication?"

  Getting the wrong medication or dosage of medication (especially oversedation) may indicate abuse or inability to provide safe care.

- "Who manages the patient's finances?"

  Financial abuse is a fairly common form of abuse in this population. Determine who has control of the older person's finances and makes the decisions regarding spending.

b. Ask the patient:

- "Do you feel safe in your home?"

  The patient who is being abused does not feel safe. Keep in mind that abandonment is a form of abuse.

■ "Tell me about your usual day." "Are you able to take care of yourself?" "Who helps you shower and dress?" "Do you require help with showering or dressing?" "Who is responsible for grocery shopping and cooking in your home?" "How do you get to your appointments or other places you want or need to go?" *To determine the patient's usual level of self-care.*

c. Observe for signs of self-neglect.

 What if . . .

■ **You feel that you are or the patient is in immediate danger?**

If the patient's or your safety is at risk, immediate intervention is required. You may need to secure the area (e.g., by closing the door), notify the in-house security officer, and then call the police.

Evaluation

■ Determine whether abuse may have occurred.
■ Ensure that appropriate agencies have been notified of the possible abuse.
■ Evaluate whether it is safe to let the patient leave the facility.

Patient Teaching

■ Inform the patient, parent, partner, and/or caregiver of local resources for prevention or intervention in situations of child, spousal, or elder abuse.
■ Inform the patient that abuse is suspected. Ask for her perceptions of the situation.
■ Emphasize to the patient that her safety is the primary concern.

Home Care

■ If potential abuse is identified in the home, follow agency and state legal guidelines.
■ If the patient's safety is at risk, immediate intervention is required. You may need to notify the police or call an ambulance. Be sure to carry a fully charged cell phone with you.
■ If you believe that you are at risk for harm (common in abusive situations), leave the setting before notifying the police.

Documentation

■ Follow legal requirements for documenting possible abuse, including disposition of potential evidence.
■ If possible, include pictures of the injuries in the charting, using a digital camera. Place a ruler or other common

object next to the injury for reference for a third party viewer.
Photos must be saved and stored in-house because of the requirement to protect confidentiality.

■ Chart all findings factually—do not add any interpretations. For example:

Do Chart:

4-year-old boy admitted with second-degree burns to both feet extending to midpoint of shins. Father says, "I put him in the bathtub and didn't realize how hot the water was."

Don't Chart:

4-year-old boy admitted with immersion burns to both feet extending to midpoint of shins, such as those found in abuse.

Practice Resource
Dembrow, M., Golden, A., Paulk, D., et al. (2007); USPSTF (2013).

 To explore learning resources for this chapter,

Go to www.DavisAdvantage.com and find:

Answers and Suggested Responses for all questions in this chapter
Lists of NIC Interventions and NOC Outcomes
List of NANDA-I Diagnoses
Knowledge Map
References and Bibliography

Concept Map

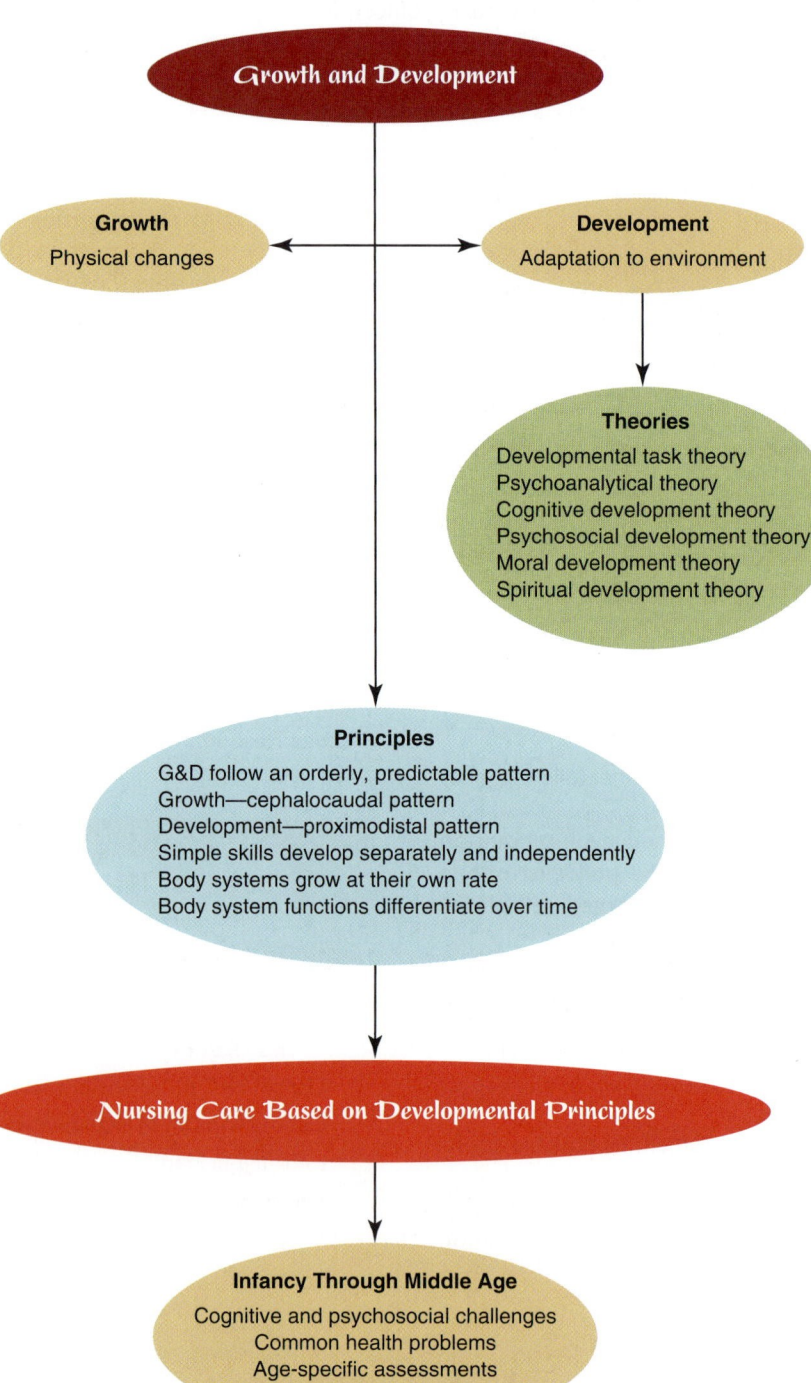

Growth and Development

Growth
Physical changes

Development
Adaptation to environment

Theories
Developmental task theory
Psychoanalytical theory
Cognitive development theory
Psychosocial development theory
Moral development theory
Spiritual development theory

Principles
G&D follow an orderly, predictable pattern
Growth—cephalocaudal pattern
Development—proximodistal pattern
Simple skills develop separately and independently
Body systems grow at their own rate
Body system functions differentiate over time

Nursing Care Based on Developmental Principles

Infancy Through Middle Age
Cognitive and psychosocial challenges
Common health problems
Age-specific assessments
Age-appropriate interventions

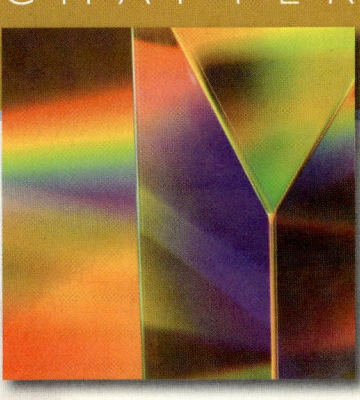

CHAPTER 10

Development: Older Adulthood

Learning Outcomes

After completing this chapter, you should be able to:

➤ Discuss the relationship of life expectancy and livable communities.

➤ Discuss the developmental challenges for each older adult age-group.

➤ Identify common health problems seen in each group and for all older adults.

➤ Describe any special assessments unique to each group of older adults.

➤ Discuss age-appropriate interventions for older adults and for each group.

➤ Incorporate developmental principles of aging into nursing care.

Key Concepts

Developmental changes

Functional status

Older adulthood

Related Concepts

See the Concept Map at the end of this chapter.

Example Problems

Dementia

Elder abuse

Frail elderly

Meet Your Patient

Ethel Higginbotham, an 80-year-old woman, is in the hospital with pneumonia. She lives alone. Her son tells you that she began to lose weight rapidly, complains of no appetite, and became withdrawn after the death of her husband. At a recent visit to her home, he found his mother confused, with a productive cough, and with small open lesions on her lower legs. This led to her hospitalization. Even though she is no longer receiving oxygen, you observe that she is very thin and weak, sleeps most of the time, and refuses to eat. "I just want to die," she tells you.

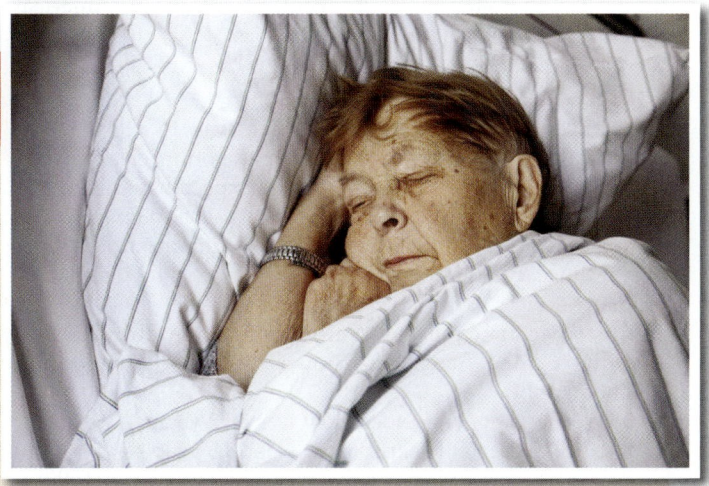

Theoretical Knowledge
knowing **why**

Why should you learn about older adults? One very important reason is that most of your patients are likely to be older adults. Half of all hospitalized patients are older adults. Moreover, because older adults are more likely to have disabilities and chronic health problems, they will likely make up a sizeable number of the patients you see in clinics, home care, and other settings as well. This chapter presents the most important topics and issues about aging.

ABOUT THE KEY CONCEPTS

You may have thought of **developmental stages** as something that applies mostly to children. However, as you learned in Chapter 9, developmental changes occur throughout life, even in **older adulthood.** You will learn how normal changes, as well as illness, can affect **functional status**—a major focus in caring for older adults.

PERSPECTIVES ON AGING

Older adulthood is the fastest growing age-group in developed nations. To understand this, you will need to look at some statistics from the U.S. Census Bureau (2008):

- In 1900, a mere 4.1% of the U.S. population was aged 65 or older.
- By 2013, life expectancy had increased, and older adults made up 14% of the population.
- By 2050, older adults are expected to represent 20% of the population.

This chapter examines aging from different angles. We will discuss the concepts of life expectancy, distribution of age-groups, life-span perspective, and percentage of total population. All of these topics require you to think about numerical descriptions of population characteristics.

Life Expectancy

The concept of life expectancy is one way to view aging. Around the world, people in developed countries are living longer and having fewer children. Life expectancy can be calculated in one of the two following ways. The following data from the U.S. Department of Health and Human Services illustrates those calculations (U.S. Department of Health and Human Services, 2015):

- **Life expectancy measured at birth** has risen dramatically in the United States, as shown by the following two statements:
  In 1900, average life expectancy was 49.2 years.
  In 2013, average life expectancy was 78.8 years.
- **Life expectancy measured at age 65** has risen, as the following two statements state:
  In 1900, a 65-year-old person could expect to live 11.9 more years.
  In 2013, a 65-year-old person could expect to live 19.3 more years.

This means that a baby born in 2013 could expect to live for nearly 79 years, whereas a person who was 65 years old in 2013 could expect to live another 19.3 years, to almost age 85. Those numbers reflect the average life expectancy for both sexes and all ethnic/racial groups. However, differences in life expectancy emerge when you examine sex and ethnic group data.

Gender Disparities The following differences emerge when taking gender into account:

- *Life expectancy at birth.* For infants born in 2013, the average total life expectancy for females is 81.4 years. For males it is only 76 years. This difference is especially noticeable in the 85-plus-year-old population, in which women greatly outnumber men (Population Reference Bureau, 2014).
- *Life expectancy measured at age 65* was nearly the same for men and women in 1900; however, women had a lead of about 5 years over men in 2013, narrowing the gap as men age. The longer a man lives, the longer he can expect to live.

Racial Disparities In 1900, race defined U.S. life expectancy at birth. As of 2013, the picture was less clear (as you can see in the following data from National Center for Health Statistics [2015]):

- *Life expectancy at birth:* Hispanic females had the highest life expectancy at birth but following closely behind were white females and black females. However, the life expectancy of black males at birth in 2013 was a little over 12 years less than Hispanic females.
- *Life expectancy at age 65:* Hispanic women led life expectancy with 22 years, followed closely by white women at 20.4 and black women at 19.4 years. Black men at age 65 had the lowest life expectancy at 16.1 years. Notice, though, that the gap for ethnicity decreases as a person ages:
  A black baby boy born in 2014 can expect to live to about age 75.
  A black man at age 65 in 2014 can expect to live another 16.1 years, to age 81.

The future population of older adults will be more ethnically and racially diverse, with minority groups (everyone except non-Hispanic, single-race whites) representing 54% of the population in 2050. The non-Hispanic white population—64% of the population in 2010—is projected to decrease and to compose only 46% of the total population in 2050. Latinos are projected to compose 30% of the population and blacks 15% in 2050 (U.S. Census Bureau, 2012).

Migration and Distribution of Age-Groups

In addition to life expectancy, in-migration and out-migration within countries and between countries contribute to the distribution of age-groups and the median age of a population. From 2013 to 2014, only 3% of older persons moved as opposed to 13% of the under-65 population. Most older movers (60%) stayed in the same county and 81% remained in the same state. Only 19% of the movers moved from out-of-state or abroad. In 2010, the median age (years):

Of the U.S. population	was	37.2
Of the state of Maine	was	42.7
Of the state of Utah	was	29.2

The median age of the population in the United States is increasing. In 2050, the median age of the U.S. population is expected to be 39 years.

Percentage of Total Population

Yet another way to view aging is by the *percentage of total population* each age-group represents. In the United States, older adults composed approximately:

4.1% of the population in 1900
14% of the population in 2013
20% of the population in 2050 (projected by the U.S. Census Bureau, 2008).

Age distribution of a population is often illustrated as a pyramid, with the youngest age-group (0–4) at the base and the oldest age-group (85+) at the peak, men on the left of the figure and women on the right. The shape of a population pyramid changes to rectangle in developed countries with fewer births and increased life expectancy. To view a population pyramid that illustrates the projected age distribution of the U.S. population in 2010, 2030, and 2050, see Figure 10-1. To see an animated pyramid,

 Go to the Web site http://www.pewresearch.org/next-america/age-pyramid/

Notice also that the percentage for centenarians almost doubles from 2030 to 2050. The Census Bureau reports the following in total number of centenarians (U.S. Census Bureau, 2011):

67,000 centenarians—actual total number in 2013
600,000 centenarians—projected total number in 2050

ThinkLike a Nurse 10-1

- What factors account for the overall increase in life expectancy?
- What effect will the distribution of the population by age within your state have on your nursing practice?

Refer to Figure 10-1 for the next three questions.

- In the 85-to-89 age-group in the 2030 data, what percentage of the population are men? What percentage are women?
- In the 85-to-89 age-group in the 2050 data, what percentage of the population are men? What percentage are women?
- In the 85-to-89 age-group, which group increases the most between 2030 and 2050: women or men?

Life-Span Perspective

Another way to view aging is from a *life-span perspective*. In this perspective, *genes* inherited at conception, *behaviors* expressed throughout a lifetime, and *environments* within which a person lives, works, and plays interact with each other over

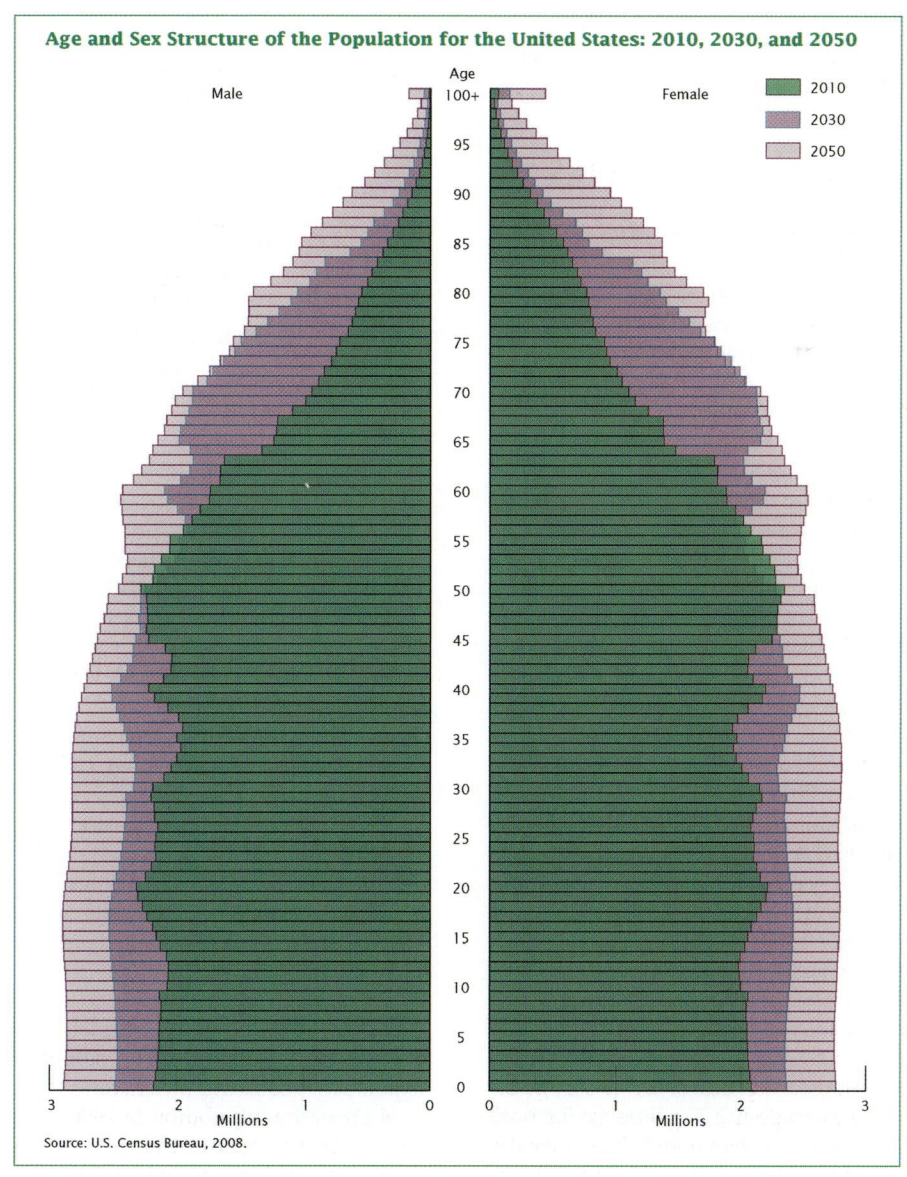

FIGURE 10-1 Age and Sex Structure of the Population for the United States: 2010, 2030, and 2050.

time. The cumulative effect of these interactions is seen in older adulthood.

Think of the genetic–behavior–environment interaction as a survival mechanism of aging. Attending to healthy behaviors (e.g., daily exercise) and avoiding unhealthy behaviors (i.e., tobacco use) is a lifelong process. A lifetime of positive health behaviors interacting with a healthful environment has the potential to shift effects of a harmful genetic trait—that is, a person may have the genetic trait for a particular disease but never show signs of the disease.

Remember the Nun Study discussed in Chapter 8? Some of the nuns demonstrated no symptoms of Alzheimer's disease during their lifetime, yet upon autopsy scientists discovered the typical neurological changes associated with Alzheimer's disease (Snowdon, 2003). The Nun Study results illustrate strong evidence of the power of behaviors and the environment over genes resulting in centenarians who are cognitively intact and asymptomatic for Alzheimer's disease.

 ThinkLike a Nurse 10-2

Plot your birth year on a timeline that extends in 10-year increments through your 65th and 100th years. What is the projected distribution of age and gender when you are an older adult? What genetic, environmental, and behavioral attributes will influence your life expectancy and state of health as an older adult?

AGING IN PLACE AND ALTERNATIVES

KEY POINT: *Contrary to popular belief, most older adults live independently (Chatterji, Byles, Cutler, et al., 2015).* **Aging in place** means that as they age, persons live in their own residences and receive supportive services for their changing needs rather than moving to another location or type of housing. Aging in place requires an age-friendly residence and an age-friendly or livable community that provides maximum accessibility, minimal barriers, and adequate resources and services to maintain independence for as long as possible.

Age-Friendly Residences Among the considerations for a safe and *age-friendly residence* are the following:

- Ground-level entry or no-step entry
- One-level living area
- Wide doorways to allow for assistive devices such as walkers and wheelchairs
- Lever-style door and faucet handles for easy grasp
- Grab bars, shower seats, and elevated toilet seat in bathrooms
- Kitchen appliances, cabinets, and surfaces no higher than 48 inches above the floor
- Shelves no more than 10 inches deep
- Adequate light in all areas inside and outside
- Walking areas free of clutter, including area rugs

Age-Friendly Communities Livable communities (also referred to as *age friendly*) emphasize older people's continuing participation in social, economic, cultural, spiritual and civic affair (Phillipson, 2015). To illustrate the need for elder-friendly communities, consider these facts about older adults in 2014 (U.S. Department of Health and Human Services, 2015):

- 8.4 million (18.6%) Americans aged 65 and older were in the labor force.
- Over 4.2 million people aged 65 and older (9.5%) were below the poverty level and another 2.5 million, or 5.6%, of older adults were classified as "near-poor" (between the poverty level and 125% of poverty level).
- 26% held a bachelor's degree or higher.

- 43% of noninstitutionalized people aged 65 and older assessed their health as excellent or very good.
- Many older adults spent at least 25% of their income on housing. This includes:
  81% (approximately) of older adults who owned their own homes, and
  19% of older adults who were renters.

Livable communities offer the following:

- Housing that is affordable and appropriate for all ages
- Supportive services and features
- Dependable and affordable transportation and housing
- Resources that facilitate individual independence and socialization of residents (AARP Public Policy Institute, 2015)
- Affordable and accessible health care
- Safe, low-crime environment
- Community engagement

Naturally Occurring Retirement Communities

When persons "age in place" within a specific apartment building or a community/street of single-family homes, that area is referred to as a **naturally occurring retirement community (NORC).** Persons within a NORC have aged together. More often than not, they have, over the years, developed access to services needed to maintain the highest quality of life for all within the NORC. When one neighbor needs assistance, others pitch in to help or to obtain help. The U.S. Administration on Aging provides competitive funding to support the development and maintenance of services within a NORC.

Retirement Communities

Some housing developments are planned specifically as **retirement communities.** They are planned to provide elder-friendly dwellings and environments for independent living and allow older adults to "downsize" into a house that has less than 2,000 square feet in single-level livable space. Purchase of a home in a retirement community usually includes, for an annual association fee, services such as home maintenance and repair; lawn care and trash removal; some home utilities; security; fire and theft insurance; recreational amenities (e.g., pool, golf); and planned activities. They usually have a minimum age restriction of 55, 60, or 62 for residents. Age restriction may be problematic if grandparents become the primary care providers for a grandchild.

Continuing Care Retirement Communities

Continuing care retirement communities (CCRCs), or *life care communities,* offer a wide range of living accommodations from residential living (e.g., cottages, cluster homes, apartments), assisted living, skilled nursing care, rehabilitation, and dementia care on a large campus-like setting. CCRCs also include many amenities, ranging from golf courses and indoor sport facilities to a full range of hobby and clubrooms and personal services. A CCRC is an example of aging in place, except that an older adult must first move to it. Therefore, in that sense it is not a NORC.

Entrance requirements include physical, mental, and financial health evaluations. Contracts may include lifetime care, time-specified care, or fee-for-service care. CCRCs are usually expensive, requiring an entrance fee and monthly fees that may increase with annual cost-of-living estimates. Depending on the contract, monthly fees may cover a set number of meals per month, transportation, housekeeping, unit maintenance, laundry service, health monitoring, some utilities, coordinated social activities, emergency call monitoring, and round-the-clock security. A health clinic is usually on site. Healthcare providers may include a registered nurse, nurse practitioner, physician, dentist, and physical therapist.

CCRCs vary by their affiliation (e.g., ethnic or religious group, university, corporation) and whether the living space is rented or purchased. University-affiliated CCRCs incorporate all aspects of academic life into the lives of residents and provide opportunities for cross-generation interactions on the CCRC and university campuses.

Assisted-Living Facilities

Assisted-living facilities (ALFs) are congregate residential settings that provide or coordinate personal services, 24-hour supervision and assistance (scheduled and unscheduled), activities, and health-related services. ALFs are *not* aging-in-place environments. State regulations and level of services do not allow residents to stay in an ALF when their needs become greater than the resources and services provided. ALFs are designed to do the following:

- Minimize the need to move
- Accommodate individual residents' changing needs and preferences
- Maximize residents' dignity, autonomy, privacy, independence, and safety
- Encourage family and community involvement (Total Living Choices, 2000–2015)

ALFs have multiple definitions and goals; they have no physical size, design, or model in common. ALFs might be self-standing or housed within a CCRC as one level of housing and service. Each ALF has its own culture, rules, norms, values, and rituals that are created by the residents. An ALF may have limitations such as reduced consumer choice, little flexibility, and an illusion of certainty.

Nursing Care Facilities (Nursing Homes)

Nursing care facilities, or **nursing homes,** provide skilled and unskilled nursing care for older adults and adults with disabilities. To understand the scope of nursing care facilities in the overall picture of aging, consider the following facts. In 2012:

- About 1.4 million residents lived in more than 16,000 U.S. nursing facilities.
- Of persons aged 65 and older, only 2.8% lived in nursing facilities; however, this rises to 10.2% for people over 85 years.
- Nearly 75% of residents are aged 75 or older; the median age is 83.2.
- Nearly half of the residents of nursing homes had dementia, and one-fifth had other psychological diagnoses.
- Women composed nearly 70% of the nursing home population (U.S. Census Bureau, 2012).
- Medicaid is the primary source of payment for most (65%) of the residents; Medicare pays for about 13%, primarily for short stays; and individual long-term care insurance or private sources pay for 22%.

KnowledgeCheck 10-1

- Approximately what percentage of people over age 65 live in nursing homes?
- What percentage of people over 85 years old live in nursing homes?
- Who has the longer life expectancy, women or men?

KnowledgeCheck 10-2

What is the difference between a retirement community and a continuing care retirement community (CCRC)?

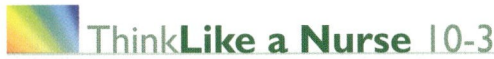

ThinkLike a Nurse 10-3

How elder friendly is the community in which you live?

THEORIES OF AGING

There is no single explanation for how the body ages, but four groups of physiological theories predominate. Despite wide debate on these theories, most scientists consider aging to be a combination of factors, including inherited traits and the cell's response to environmental stressors.

Wear-and-Tear Theory proposes that repeated insults and the accumulation of metabolic wastes eventually cause cells to wear out and cease functioning.

Genetic Theories of aging propose that cells have a preprogrammed, finite number of cell divisions. Therefore, the time of naturally occurring death is determined at birth. The genetic messages within the various cells specify how many times the cell can reproduce, thus defining the life of that cell.

Cellular Malfunction hypothesizes that a malfunction in the cell causes changes in cellular DNA, leading to problems with cell replication. The cellular malfunction can be the result of:

- A chemical reaction with the DNA (cross-linking theory)
- An abundance of free radicals that damage cells and impair their ability to function normally (free-radical theory)
- A buildup of toxins over time that causes cell death (toxin theory)

Autoimmune Reaction hypothesizes that cells change with age. Over time, the changes result in the immune system's perceiving some cells as foreign substances and triggering an immune response to destroy the cells.

STAGES OF OLDER ADULTHOOD

Most references use 65 years as the age when older adulthood begins. The stages of older adulthood are typically referred to as the *young-old* (ages 65 to 74), *middle-old* (ages 75 to 84) and *oldest-old* (age 85 and older). **KEY POINT:** *The fastest growing segment of older adults is the oldest-old, some of whom are the frail elderly and* **centenarians** *(people over 100 years old).* For more in-depth information about aging and older adults, refer to a life-span development or gerontology resource.

Young-Old: Ages 65 to 74

Physical and psychological adaptations to retirement are paramount in this age-group. At retirement, a person's usual social contacts and structure for daily activities may change markedly. A newly retired young-old adult may be searching for new interests outside of the previous work environment.

One key indicator of well-being is use of leisure time. On an average day, young-old persons spend most of their time (57%) watching television; 18% in solitary activities of reading, relaxing, and thinking; 11% socializing and communicating; 3% participating in sports, exercise, and recreation; and the remaining time in other activities, including travel (Federal Interagency Forum on Aging-Related Statistics, 2012).

By the time they reach age 65, many young-old persons are experiencing the effects of chronic illnesses that began in middle adulthood along with the effects of lack of time for self-care because of the demands and stressors of work present during middle adulthood. Retirement frees up time for the young-old to make up for these effects and focus on health-promoting behaviors to help prevent the decline of health as they age. However, young-old persons face barriers to health, such as the following:

- A lack of supplemental insurance for health screening or physicals that are not covered under Medicare
- Perception of self as "getting old"
- Changes in physical activity
- Being in a deconditioned state by not participating in exercise before retirement. There is some evidence that the amount of physical activity declines as early as age 63 for some and by age 70 for most people.

Middle-Old: Ages 75 to 84

The developmental challenge of middle-old persons is an increasingly solitary, sedentary lifestyle. This age-group spends one-fourth of their leisure time in the solitary activities of reading, relaxing, and thinking—more than their younger cohort. They spend only 2% of their time participating in sports, exercise, and recreation—less than their younger cohort (Federal Interagency Forum on Aging-Related Statistics, 2012). Without physical activity, the risk of disability associated with chronic conditions increases during the middle-old years.

Adapted physical activity (APA) programs are group exercise programs designed for persons with chronic conditions. APA programs are aimed at correcting a sedentary lifestyle and preventing disability secondary to the chronic condition. The focus of APA programs is on functional ability rather than treating existing disability, and they are beneficial throughout the older adult years. Even after critical incidents such as a stroke, APA programs prevent further disability, maximize function, increase quality of life, and curtail the effects of social isolation and depression (Taricco, Dallolio, Calugi et al., 2014).

Senior centers are beginning to offer APA programs as they update their programs for the active baby-boomer generation. Some health and fitness facilities may also offer senior health programs and books that illustrate adapted strategies for life-long walkers and marathon runners. Although physical activity declines in the middle-old group overall, older adults represent the fastest-growing segment of participants in competitive sports, with some 80-year-old finishers at road races such as the New York City Marathon.

Oldest-Old: Age 85 and Older

The developmental challenges of the oldest-old are sensory impairments, oral health problems, inadequate nutritional intake, and functional limitations. The following examples are from the Federal Interagency Forum on Aging-Related Statistics (2012):

- *Hearing.* Nearly half of older men and more than one-third of older women reported difficulty hearing. This was higher for the 85-plus age-group than for the young-old and the middle-old.
- *Vision.* 23% of the 85-plus age-group reported trouble seeing.
- *Edentulism.* 33% of those over 85 years old reported **edentulism** (having no natural teeth). This tends to be income related: 42% of older adults below the poverty line reported edentulism, whereas for those above the poverty line the incidence was only 22%.

- *Nutrition.* Edentulism compromises an already inadequate nutritional intake of older adults and fosters a diet of "soft" foods that may be higher in fats, carbohydrates, and calories. For the oldest-old, this occurs at a time when they need to decrease intake of these foods to combat obesity and counter decreased activity levels.
- *Functional limitations.* Ability to stoop/kneel, reach overhead, walk two or three blocks, and lift 10 pounds are common parameters for determining functional abilities of older adults. Thirty-eight percent of men in the oldest-old group reported they were unable to perform at least one of these activities. More than half of women in that group were unable to perform at least one activity. There were minimal to no differences across ethnic and racial groups.

Centenarians People aged 100 years and older **(centenarians)** are a subgroup of the oldest-old. It appears that surviving to an extreme old age is the result of favorable interactions between genetic composition, environment, and lifestyle (behaviors). The most significant factor may be the presence of a loved one in the life of the older adult. Their commitment to community is also linked to their longevity. One genetic variation of centenarians has been linked with longevity, but mapping the centenarian genome is essential to determine whether they do, in fact, carry a so-called longevity gene (Perls, 2006; Perls, Silver, & Lauerman, 1999).

Among the characteristics of centenarians are that 12% live independently and 90% are cognitively intact into their 90s.

Example Problem: Frail Elderly

The frail elderly make up another category of older adults based on the person's health status and vulnerability to a downward spiral in health in response to even a minor insult (e.g., a cold). See the box Example Problem: Frail Elderly.

KnowledgeCheck 10-3

- Name and give the age ranges of the four stages of older adulthood.
- Name and briefly describe four theories of aging.

DEVELOPMENTAL CHANGES OF OLDER ADULTS

Although not all people age at the same pace, there are predictable patterns of physical, cognitive, and psychosocial change. For example, it is common for older adults to have several, often chronic, health problems.

Physical Development of Older Adults

Although there is variation among individuals, patterns of change can be predicted in each body system. Table 10-1 presents an overview of changes seen with aging as well as corresponding areas for assessment.

Cognitive Development of Older Adults

Reaction time slows in older adults, and short-term memory declines; it takes longer to respond to a stimulus and to process incoming information. Thus, older adults learn new material more slowly. **KEY POINT:** *However, there is no loss of intelligence as a person ages.*

Memory Loss of short-term memory is more common than loss of long-term memory; thus, older adults may remember incidents from many years ago but may have trouble recalling what they did earlier in the day.

EXAMPLE PROBLEM: Frail Elderly

Definition of Frailty

As humans age, they are gradually less able to adapt to internal challenges (e.g., disease) and external environments (e.g., injury). Multiple systems are usually involved.

- **Frailty** is a syndrome (set of characteristics) that describes a heightened state of vulnerability for developing adverse health outcomes.
- **Frailty** is the point at which the human organism is believed to have its least capacity for survival and will fail in response to a minor internal or external insult. *Example: A frail older adult might die merely as a result of an upper respiratory infection (such as a cold).*

Characteristics of Frailty

Characteristics: To be considered frail, a person must have three or more of the following characteristics:

- Low level of physical activity
- Muscle weakness
- Slowed performance
- Fatigue or poor endurance

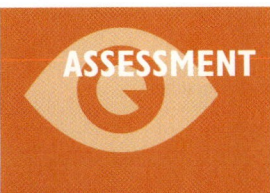

ASSESSMENT

Assess for:
- Weakness
- Ability to live independently, assistance needed to perform ADLs
- Impaired mental abilities

- Medical problems
- Psychosocial and behavioral factors (e.g., depression, caregiver problems, and housing)
- Other risk factors (e.g., smoking, underweight)

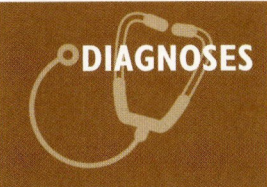

DIAGNOSES

- **Powerlessness** related to dependence on others
- **Risk for Injury** related to poor balance, confusion

Self-Care Deficits related to loss of mobility, fatigue, mental status changes

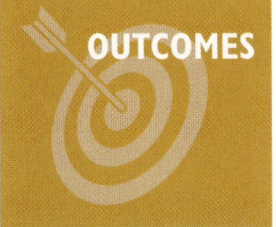

OUTCOMES

- Identifies normal changes, adapts routine, and reports alterations in ADLs and IADLs that are outside expected change for age

- Maintains independence longer and delays the aging process

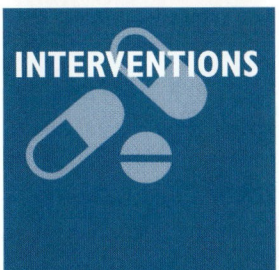

INTERVENTIONS

- Fall-preventive (moderate-intensity) group (Faber, Bosscher, Paw, et al., 2006)
- For the obese and frail, combined weight loss and exercise therapy (Villareal, Banks, Sinacore, et al., 2006)
- Internet access may maintain physical and cognitive status (Tomita, Mann, Stanton, et al., 2006).

- Teach and assist to keep the mind active (socializing, reading, puzzles, games).
- Arrange for care as needed, and teach caregivers how and when to seek profession help.
- Recognize and treat depression and other medical problems.
- Facilitate good nutritional status (Bartali, Semba, Frongillo, et al., 2006).

EVALUATION

Monitor for positive changes in functional ability and level of independence.

Evaluate changes in mobility, fatigue, or mental status.

- Physical health problems or medications may also affect memory.
- An active social life with complete engagement and participation in the community delays memory loss with aging (Ertel, Glymour, & Berkman, 2008).

- Regular mental exercises (e.g., crossword puzzles, conversation) appear to stimulate the brain and enhance memory.
- Other factors that slow memory loss are adequate sleep and rest, a nourishing diet, avoidance of drugs and alcohol, and adequate social stimulation.

Table 10-1 ➤ Age-Related Changes and Areas for Assessment

	NORMAL AGING CHANGE	AREAS FOR ASSESSMENT
Musculoskeletal	Decreased: muscle strength, body mass, bone mass, joint mobility Increased fat deposit	▪ Activity/exercise tolerance ▪ Joint pain, range of motion ▪ Gait, balance, posture, change in height ▪ Susceptibility to falls ▪ Ability to perform ADLs
Cardiovascular	Decreased cardiac output Increased peripheral resistance, systolic blood pressure	▪ Activity tolerance ▪ Blood pressure ▪ Orthostatic hypotension ▪ Arrhythmia
Respiratory	Decreased elasticity of chest wall, intercostals muscle strength, cough reflex Increased anteroposterior diameter of chest, rigidity of lung tissue	▪ Cough reflex ▪ Use of accessory muscles ▪ Gas exchange ▪ Mouth breathing
Gastrointestinal	Decreased saliva production, GI motility, gastric acid production	▪ Ability to chew ▪ Dentition ▪ Pattern of elimination ▪ Frequency/size of meals
Integumentary	Decreased skin elasticity, nail growth Increased dryness of skin, thinning of skin layers, nail thickening, hair thinning	▪ Susceptibility to hypo/hyperthermia ▪ Intact skin, bruising ▪ Dry skin ▪ Bathing pattern
Genitourinary	Decreased glomerular filtration rate, blood flow to kidneys, bladder capacity, vaginal lubrication, hardness of erection	▪ Continence ▪ Urgency, frequency, nocturia ▪ Hydration status ▪ Drug levels ▪ Sexual pattern
Nervous	Decreased nerve cells, neurotransmitters, REM sleep, blood flow to CNS	▪ Diminished reflexes ▪ Sleep pattern ▪ Depression
Endocrine	Decreased insulin release, thyroid function, estrogen and testosterone	▪ Change in weight ▪ Libido ▪ Energy level
Sensory	Decreased visual acuity (presbyopia or impaired near vision) and depth perception, tear production, pupil size, accommodation, acuity of smell and taste, hearing of high-frequency sound, sense of balance, changes in pain sensation Increased glare sensitivity, thickening of lens of the eye, changes in pain sensation Macular degeneration causing loss of central vision (not a normal change, but a common one)	▪ Adequate lighting ▪ Cerumen buildup ▪ Home safety ▪ Pain sensation ▪ Driving ability ▪ Environmental stimulation

Table 10-1 ➤ Age-Related Changes and Areas for Assessment—cont'd

	NORMAL AGING CHANGE	AREAS FOR ASSESSMENT
Cognition	Decreased short-term memory	▪ Memory changes
	Increased reaction time, information processing time	▪ Learning barriers
		▪ Adaptive coping
Personality	Increased cautiousness	▪ Sources of social support
	Retirement, widowhood, grandparenthood	▪ Social network

ADLs = activities of daily living; CNS = central nervous system; GI = gastrointestinal; REM = rapid eye movement.

Psychosocial Development of Older Adults

Rather than explaining how the body ages, psychosocial theories of aging attempt to explain the psychological and social adjustment associated with aging.

Disengagement Theory (1961) Cumming and Henry (1961) hypothesized that the older adult and society gradually and mutually withdraw or disengage from each other. Mandatory retirement, chronic illness, the deaths of relatives and friends, and poverty are among the factors that may contribute to this phenomenon. As interaction between the person and his world decreases there is (1) more time for reflection and (2) freedom from societal roles. Power transfers to younger members of society as the older adult withdraws. **KEY POINT:** *Disengagement is not the norm for the current generation of older adults in the United States, nor is it universally true for cultures that value older adults' advice as essential for family decision making.*

Activity Theory (1963) Activity theory posits that the individual should stay as active and engaged as possible to enjoy the highest life satisfaction (Fig. 10-2). On retirement, another activity, such as travel, sports, hobbies, or volunteering, replaces time spent at work. Havighurst's theory (1963) is the counterpart of disengagement theory. According to Havighurst (1971), the following are physical, cognitive, and social developmental tasks of older adults:

Adjusting to decreasing physical strength and health
Adjusting to retirement
Adjusting to a lower income
Adjusting to death of a spouse
Establishing an open affiliation with one's age-group
Adopting and adapting flexible social roles
Establishing satisfactory physical living arrangements

Psychosocial Development Theory (1963) Erikson's developmental theory (1963) identifies *ego integrity versus despair* as the task of the older adult. This stage of development has as its cornerstone the acceptance that one's life has had meaning and that death is a part of the continuum of life. This outlook allows a person to accept the inevitable changes in health and life circumstances. The basic virtue gained at this stage is wisdom. Recall that Erikson's theory is discussed in Chapter 9.

Psychosocial changes in this age-group are many and significant. The older adult must face multiple losses, such as the following:

▪ Death of a spouse or partner, family members, and friends
▪ Challenges to health and youthful vitality

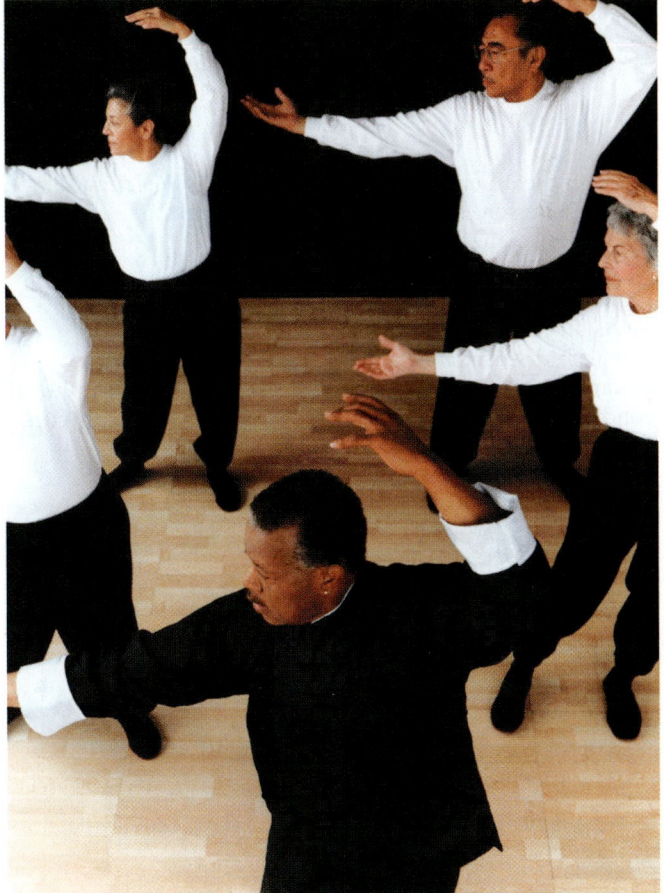

FIGURE 10-2 Many older adults are able to remain active and engaged well into their later years.

▪ Loss of independence and the ability to live at home without assistance

Cumulative losses often have a negative psychological affect on the older adult. Loss is discussed in detail in Chapter 17.

Common Health Problems of Older Adults

The 10 leading causes of death for older Americans are found in Box 10-1. **KEY POINT:** *Six of the seven leading causes of death among older adults are chronic diseases.* Prevalence of chronic conditions differs by race and ethnicity. For example,

BOX 10-1 ■ 10 Leading Causes of Death for Older Americans

The 10 leading causes of death for older Americans are as follow:

1. Heart disease
2. Cancer
3. Stroke
4. Chronic lower respiratory diseases
5. Alzheimer's disease
6. Diabetes mellitus
7. Influenza and pneumonia
8. Accidents
9. Kidney disease
10. Septicemia

Source: U.S. Department of Health and Human Services. (2015). *A profile of older Americans: 2014.* Washington, DC: Administration on Aging. Retrieved from http://www.aoa.acl.gov/Aging_Statistics/Profile/2014/docs/2014-Profile.pdf

consider the different prevalence in diabetes in older adults in 2010 (Caspersen, Thomas, Boseman, et al., 2012):

Non-Hispanic blacks	32.4%
Hispanics	30.5%
Non-Hispanic whites	19%
Asian Americans	8.4%

Heart disease, cancer, stroke, and diabetes are not only among the most common but are also the most costly health conditions. These are long-term illnesses that are rarely cured,

but many can be prevented or modified with therapeutic lifestyle changes.

Osteoporosis, a loss in bone mineral density that increases the risk of fracture, affects an estimated 10 million Americans. In advanced cases, bones become so porous that they fracture spontaneously, merely from the stress of bearing a person's weight. The risk for osteoporosis:

- Increases with age
- Is much greater for women (in part because of their decreased bone density compared with that of men, hormonal changes at menopause, and inadequate calcium intake)
- Is increased by cigarette smoking
- Is increased by moderate to heavy alcohol consumption
- Is increased by lack of weight-bearing exercise

Example Problem: Dementia

For an overview, see the box Example Problem: Dementia. To learn about distinguishing dementia from normal aging. see Table 10-2.

Polypharmacy

Polypharmacy, the use of multiple medications, is a risk factor for acute confusion, delirium, and depression in older adults. Continued growth in knowledge about the human genome has accelerated the field of **pharmacogenomics** (the discipline that blends pharmacology with genomics); therefore, the future of drug therapy for older adults will consider DNA variants and individual responses to medical treatments when developing customized drugs for certain subgroups. This technology is expected to increase the efficiency of the drug industry and result in cheaper, more effective drug therapies for older adults.

Table 10-2 ➤ Distinguishing the Changes of Typical Aging From Dementia

TYPICAL AGING	DEMENTIA
Independence in daily activities preserved	Dependent on others for key independent-living activities
Complains of memory loss but able to provide a good amount of detail regarding incidents of forgetfulness	May complain of memory problems only if specifically asked; cannot recall instances in which memory loss was noticed
Is more concerned about forgetfulness than are close family members	Close family members much more concerned about incidents of memory loss than patient
Recent memory for important events, affairs; conversations are intact	Significant decline in memory for recent events and ability to engage in conversation
Occasional difficulty finding words	Often has difficulty finding words; uses many pauses and substitutions
In familiar territory, may have to pause momentarily to remember way, but doesn't get lost	Gets lost in familiar territory while walking or driving, sometimes taking hours to eventually return home
Unwilling to learn how to operate new devices, but is able to operate common and familiar appliances	Unable to operate common and even familiar appliances; cannot learn to operate even simple new appliances
Maintains prior level of interpersonal social skills	Shows loss of interest in social activities; behaves inappropriately in social situations
Performs normally on mental status exams, taking into account education and culture	Abnormal performance on mental status exams; performance not explained by education or cultural factors

Source: Adapted from Differentiating normal aging and dementia [Tables]. (1996, November). Adapted from Agency for Healthcare Research and Quality (AHRQ), *Clinical practice guidelines* No. 19 (Publication #97-0702). Washington, DC: US Department of Health and Human Services. Retrieved from http://www.dartmouth-hitchcock.org/dhmc-internet-upload/file_collection/111609_aging_vs_dementia_table.pdf

EXAMPLE PROBLEM: Dementia

Dementia
Irreversible progressive decline in mental abilities; affects about one in five adults older than 70 years. **KEY POINT:** *Is not a normal result of aging—common, but not normal.*

Alzheimer's Disease
- The primary form of dementia
- Considered progressive
- Affects about half of adults aged 85 and older

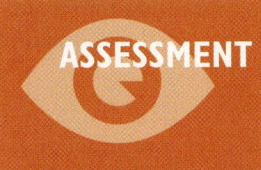
ASSESSMENT

To distinguish dementia from depression use one or more of the following mental status exams:
- **The "Sweet 16"**
  - Correlates highly with MMSE
  - 16 oral questions; easy to use
  - Tests for orientation, registration, sustained attention, and short-term memory (Fong, Jones, Rudolph, et al., 2010)

- **Mini Mental State Exam (MMSE)**
- **Ultrabrief screening:** Ask patient to recite the months of the year backward; then ask the day of the week (Fick, Inouye, Guess, et al. 2015)
Also refer to Table 10-2.

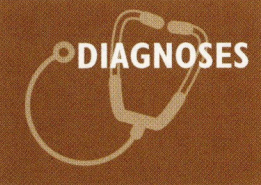
DIAGNOSES

- **Impaired Verbal Communication** related to irreversible, progressive decline in mental abilities

- **Fear** related to difficulty speaking and understanding

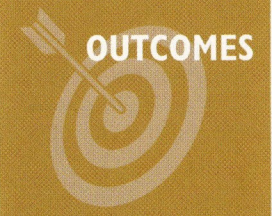
OUTCOMES

- Will not be fearful
- Carries out simple 2- and 3-word commands.

- Will be free from harm

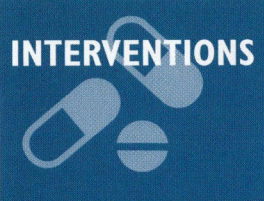
INTERVENTIONS

KEY POINT: *Realize that the patient's reality is distorted and he is behaving in the only way he is able.*
- Provide a safe environment.
- To facilitate communication:
  - Use simple, short sentences, containing one idea each.
  - Avoid vague comments.
  - If the patient doesn't understand, repeat your words *exactly.*
  - Also see Communicating with Persons with Cognitive Deficit, in this chapter.

- Promote cognitive function: Provide activities and materials that are engaging and involve some degree of cognitive processing (e.g., reading, playing board games, playing a musical instrument, dancing).
- Activities should be person-centered and appropriate for age-group.
- Orient the patient to reality.
- Use life review and reminiscence.
- Assist with or provide ADLs.
- Provide caregiver support.
- Emphasize and support social activities.

EVALUATION

- Monitor for physical, behavioral, emotional, and cognitive symptoms of fear (e.g., breathlessness, crying).

- Elicit feedback to ensure communications are understood.

For a step-by-step procedure for assessing mental status, see Procedure 21-16, Assessing the Sensory-Neurological System.

Depression

Medical problems can cause depression in older adults either directly or as a psychological reaction to the illness. Any chronic medical condition, particularly if it is painful, disabling, or life threatening, can lead to depression or make depression symptoms worse. In 2010, 16% of older women reported depressive symptoms compared with 11% of older men, numbers that have remained fairly stable for nearly a decade and may be related to appropriate antidepressant drug treatment for older adults (Federal Interagency Forum on Aging-Related Statistics, 2012).

Depression not only affects mood but also impacts energy, sleep, appetite, and physical health. Many of the symptoms of depression are similar to those of dementia (memory problems, sluggish speech and movements, and low motivation) so it may be difficult to tell the two apart. Symptoms of depression can also be the side effect of many commonly prescribed drugs, especially if the person is taking multiple medications. Older adults are more sensitive to mood-related side effects of prescription medication because, as they age, their bodies become less efficient at metabolizing and processing drugs.

Example Problem: Elder Abuse

Be alert for the following unique patterns of injury in older adults, as there a strong possibility of abuse (Lowry, 2012):

- Maxillofacial or dental trauma
- Subdural hematomas
- Periorbital and laryngeal trauma
- Rib fractures
- Upper extremity injuries
- A wasted and unkempt appearance

KEY POINT: *If you suspect abuse, your first priority is to assure the client is safe and cared for. Next, you must report the abuse.*

To learn to about elder abuse, see the box Example Problem: Elder Abuse.

Ageism

Ageism is age-based discrimination. Negative expectations for older adults can cloud nursing assessments, planning, and interventions. The National Institute on Aging and the National Library of Medicine (2015) developed a quiz to test your knowledge of aging. Take the quiz so that you can be prepared to best assist your older adult clients.

 Go to *What's Your Aging IQ? Online Quiz* at https://www.nia.nih.gov/health/publication/whats-your-aging-iq/about-booklet

KnowledgeCheck 10-4

- Name two age-related changes seen in older adults.
- According to Erikson, what is the developmental stage of the older adult?
- What are the top two causes of death among older adults?

PracticalKnowledge
knowing **how**

You would expect differences in functioning in older adults who are relatively healthy and those who have one or more illnesses. You will, of course, base nursing care on individual needs, not on a person's age category. However, in general, you would expect a patient's needs to be different at age 65 from what they would be at age 85. **KEY POINT:** *Remember, though, that an* **individual's** *health status and needs are affected by many more variables than just his or her age (e.g., chronic illness, stressors).*

ASSESSMENT NP

This section presents information to use in caring for all older adults, as well as separately for the young-old, the middle-old, the oldest-old, and the frail elderly.

Assessment for All Older Adults

Recommend to older adults that they have an annual physical and dental examination. The exam should include the same categories as in middle adulthood (see Chapter 9), as well as screening for mood, cognition, and ability to perform activities of daily living (ADLs) (e.g., bathing and dressing), and instrumental activities of daily living (IADLs) (e.g., shopping, doing laundry). Table 10-1 identifies the areas for physical assessment related to the aging process. Also see the Focused Assessment box Assessments for All Older Adults. **KEY POINT:** *Expect frequent changes to recommendations for screening exams (e.g., for breast, cervical and colon cancers).*

ThinkLike a Nurse 10-4

To determine whether Mrs. Higginbotham's pneumonia is resolving (Meet Your Patient), you are monitoring her vital signs. Her oral temperature is 98.9°F (37.2°C). What do you need to keep in mind when evaluating the meaning of this reading? Do you think this represents a fever?

Assessing Cognitive Status

Some tools for assessing mental status of older adults include the following. Also see the box Example Problem: Dementia.

- Mini Mental State Exam (MMSE) (2015)
- Ultrabrief screening: Ask the patient to recite the months of the year backward, and then ask the day of the week (Fick, Inouye, Guess, et al., 2015).
- Sweet Sixteen (Fong, Jones, Rudolph, et al., 2010)

Assessing Functional Status

Functional status is the ability to perform self-care and other ADLs and IADLs.

- **Activities of Daily Living.** You can use the Katz Index of Independence in Activities of Daily Living to rate a client's independence in bathing, dressing, toileting, transferring, continence, and feeding (Katz, Down, Cash, et al., 1970; "Katz Index of Independence," 2007). To use the Katz assessment tool,

 Go to https://consultgeri.org/try-this/general-assessment/issue-2

- **Instrumental Activities of Daily Living. IADLs** are the activities needed to maintain one's immediate environment, for example, shopping, using the telephone, housekeeping, managing money, preparing food, and managing one's medications. Loss of ability to perform IADLs frequently marks a need for assisted living, nursing home placement, or the aid of family or homemaker services to allow an older adult to age in place.

EXAMPLE PROBLEM: Elder Abuse

KEY POINT: *Like domestic violence, elder abuse is seen in all cultures and socioeconomic groups.*

Abuse Types—Abuse takes many forms.

Physical	Emotional	Sexual
Financial	Neglect	Abandonment

Risk Factors
KEY POINT: *Risk of abuse is higher for women and those with physical and cognitive vulnerabilities.*

Dependence on others	Health issues (physical or mental)	Isolation
Difficulty managing money	Being female	Substance abuse

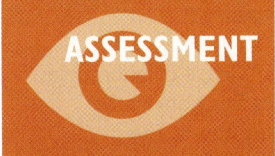

ASSESSMENT

- Assess older adults for abuse any time there is a possibility that an injury may have been inflicted rather than accidental.

- For a screening tool and a procedure to aid you in assessing for abuse, see Procedure 9-1.

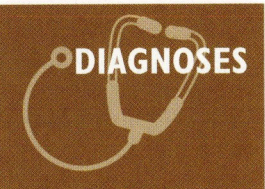

DIAGNOSES

- **Situational low self-esteem**

- **Risk for Injury** related to physical or psychological abuse

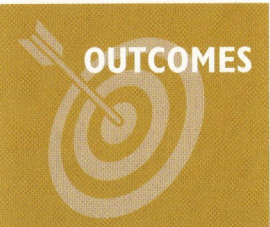

OUTCOMES

- Remains safe and free from physical and/or psychological harm
- Maintains dignity

- Verbalizes positive self-worth

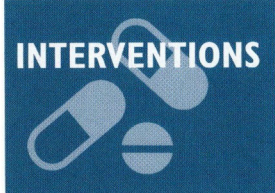

INTERVENTIONS

KEY POINT: *Prevention Is Key: Listen, Intervene, Educate.*
- Screen for risk factors associated with elder abuse.
- Observe for injuries indicative of elder abuse.

- Determine congruence of injury and the description of cause.
- Remove patient from dangerous situation.
- Notify appropriate authorities of suspected abuse.

OTHER

Stop Elder Abuse: REPORT IT.
- *Suspicion of elder abuse must be reported to adult protection services and/or the authority designated by law in each state to investigate and prosecute elder abuse.*
- *Call the police or 9-1-1 immediately if someone you know is in immediate, life-threatening danger.*

Elder Abuse Resources
- The National Center on Elder Abuse (NCEA) **(http://www.ncea.aoa.gov)**
- Clearinghouse on Abuse and Neglect of the Elderly (CANE) **(http://www.cane. udel.edu)**

Assessments for All Older Adults

➤ **Vital signs**—Be aware that the normal ranges for VS are slightly different for older adults (see Chapter 19). For example, the average body temperature is lower.

➤ **Height measurement**—Compare with previous height (as a screen for osteoporosis). Especially important past age 65.

➤ **Weight and body mass index (BMI),** calculated

➤ **Lipid panel screening**—total cholesterol, triglycerides, high-density lipoprotein (HDL), low-density lipoprotein (LDL), and ratios

➤ **Blood glucose screening**

➤ **Annual clinical breast examination**—for women aged 40 years and older (U.S. Preventive Services Task Force, 2009b, updated 2015).

➤ **Breast self-awareness**—Women should know how their breasts normally look and feel and report any breast changes to a health care provider right away. Breast self-exam is an option for women throughout their life span.

➤ **Biannual mammogram or thermography**—for women aged 55 and older. Screening should continue as long as a woman is in good health and is expected to live 10 more years or longer.

   Age alone is not a reason to stop having mammograms (American Cancer Society, n.d., last revised 2015). The U.S. Preventive Services Task Force (USPSTF) (2009b, updated 2015) does not recommend biannual mammograms after age 75. However, other guidelines recommend them even beyond age 80 or 85 if the woman is in good health (American College of Obstetricians and Gynecologists, 2011). Women should be educated about the benefits of mammography and the potential for false-positive results that may be followed by recommendations for further imaging or biopsies that are not actually needed.

➤ **Cervical cancer screening (Pap test)**—Women over age 65 who have had regular cervical cancer testing in the past 10 years with normal results should not be tested for cervical cancer. Once testing is stopped, it should not be started again. Women with a history of a serious cervical precancer should continue to be tested for at least 20 years after that diagnosis, even if testing goes beyond age 65.

➤ A woman who has had her uterus and cervix removed (a total hysterectomy) for reasons not related to cervical cancer and who has no history of cervical cancer or serious precancer should not be tested (American Cancer[0] Society, n.d., last revised 2015).

➤ **Colon cancer screening**—The USPSTF recommends screening for colorectal cancer using fecal occult blood testing, sigmoidoscopy, or colonoscopy in adults, beginning at age 50 years and continuing to age 75 years. Intervals for recommended screening strategies include the following:

➤ **Annual screening with high-sensitivity fecal occult blood testing.**

➤ **Sigmoidoscopy**—every 5 years, with high-sensitivity fecal occult blood testing every 3 years.

➤ **Screening colonoscopy**—every 10 years.

➤ **Screening CT colonographies,** or "virtual colonoscopies" are particularly safe for older adults as a noninvasive test that requires no sedation or anesthesia. The American Cancer Society considers CT colonography, as a first-line colon-cancer screening test, to be as effective as the traditional colonoscopy. However, the USPSTF (2009a, updated 2014) recommends against routine colorectal cancer screening for those aged 76 years and older.

➤ **Digital rectal exam (for males)** is done when patient conditions indicate to detect an enlarged prostate. Enlargement can indicate either benign prostatic hypertrophy or prostate cancer. It is no longer recommended for routine screening in men (USPSTF, 2012b, updated 2015).

➤ **Serum prostate-specific antigen (PSA) level** (for men) is a more sensitive indicator than is the digital rectal exam. Some guidelines encourage yearly screening for men over age 50; some caution against routine screening; others make decisions on an individual basis. The USPSTF recommends that, regardless of age, men without symptoms should not routinely have the PSA blood test to screen for prostate cancer (USPSTF, 2012b, updated 2015).

➤ **Eye exam**—every 2 years if there are no problems; otherwise annually, particularly if the older adult has chronic conditions such as hypertension, cardiovascular disease, or diabetes.

➤ **Bone-density scan**—recommended for all women aged 65 and older as a routine screening for osteoporosis. For women at increased risk for osteoporotic fractures (postmenopausal, tobacco smoking, history of fragility fractures, low body weight), screening should begin at age 60 years (National Guideline Clearinghouse, 2011). The test is also recommended for men older than age 70.

Assessing for Depression

For more information about depression in older adults, see the box Example Problem: Depression in Chapter 13. To assess for depression, you may wish to use the Geriatric Depression Scale (GDS), a 30-item questionnaire that screens for depression. It is tailored to the concerns that older adults face.

Assessment (Young-Old)

Your assessments of young-old patients should also include the following:

▪ *Daily routines, social interactions, and short- and long-term goals:* This helps determine the degree to which the person has adapted to retirement.

- *Level of fitness and the level of effort for physical activity:* This and the following point are essential to determine before beginning a program of routine exercise.
- *Chronic conditions:* How a chronic condition affects the client's ability to do regular physical activities safely, and to what extent
- *Barriers to exercise*
- *Client's self-confidence* in ability to maintain an exercise program

Assessment (Middle-Old)

It is critical that you assess the function, support system, social network, and mental health of the middle-old client.

> Observe for cues to triggers that the client is entering a spiral of vulnerability. For example, a decrease in an older adult's mobility and the use of an assistive device such as a cane may indicate prolonged inactivity associated with physiological changes. These may be associated with an unsteady or slow gait and slower response and reaction times—all resulting in deliberate, slow actions.

Thus begins a spiral of vulnerability: The older adult may become a victim of abuse, fall, and sustain an injury; the injury may require hospitalization, giving rise to the potential complications of infection and pressure injuries and the need for rehabilitation. The impact of this spiral of vulnerability is felt in psychological and financial costs to the client and society, as well as loss of client independence. It is easier to intervene and stop the spiral if cues are found early (Fig. 10-3).

Assessment (Oldest-Old)

The oldest-old need similar assessments as the middle-old. Keep in mind that assessments of physical, psychosocial, and cognitive abilities as well as social engagement and living conditions are crucial for the oldest-old. Psychosocial and environmental factors may be the cues for frailty when subtle physiological changes are not obvious.

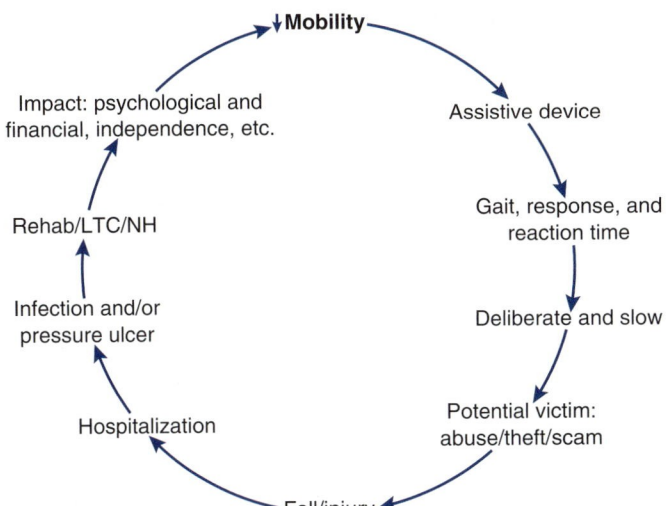

Assessment of the Middle-Old
Spiral of Vulnerability Example

FIGURE 10-3 A seemingly small event for a middle-old adult may trigger a spiral of vulnerability. (Courtesy of V. Rempusheski, PhD.)

Assessment (Example Problem: Frail Elderly)

It is important to assess for characteristics associated with frailty so that early interventions to prevent or slow the spiral of vulnerability are possible. See the box Example Problem: Frail Elderly, earlier in this chapter. Most are women, are more than 80 years old, and receive care from an adult child.

ANALYSIS/DIAGNOSIS (ALL OLDER ADULTS) NP

Although most NANDA-I diagnoses can be used for any age-group, the following diagnoses focus specifically on growth and development:

    Frail Elderly Syndrome
    Risk for Frail Elderly Syndrome
    Nutrition: Less than Body Requirements, Imbalanced
    Risk for Delayed Development

An understanding of age-related changes can help older adults identify normal changes, adapt their routine, and report alterations in ADLs and IADLs that are outside the expected changes for their age. Many such changes signal conditions that are treatable. Consider these examples:

- Frequent falls and loss of balance are not the result of normal age-related changes but could signal a neuropathology such as Parkinson's disease or early symptoms of dementia. They should be reported to a health-care provider.
- Urinary incontinence is not the result of usual age-related changes. It may signal a urinary tract infection, a prostate problem, excessive urogenital drying, or the need for in-home assistance.

OUTCOMES/EVALUATION (ALL OLDER ADULTS) NP

Nursing goals for all older adults should be to maintain the person's ability to function independently for as long as possible, arrange for appropriate care, and teach clients and caregivers how and when to call for professional help.

INTERVENTIONS/IMPLEMENTATION NP

As you know, interventions depend on the nursing diagnoses that you identify for each individual. This section presents interventions specific to each of the older-adult age-groups, as well as interventions that apply to all older adults. Also refer to Example Problem boxes for Frail Elderly, Dementia, and Elder Abuse.

Interventions (Young-Old)

Young-old adults may need support for positive retirement, identifying and overcoming barriers to health promotion, evaluating methods for introducing health promotion for positive long-term change, and describing short- and long-term benefits of health promotion (Wilson & Palha, 2007). Providing resources for social and civic engagement will help a new retiree reestablish a satisfying and rewarding retirement.

Physical Activity It is also important to teach and help the client plan for physical exercise. A sedentary lifestyle increases the risk of aging-related diseases and premature death. DNA changes occur partly as a result of stress and oxidative damage to cells. By reducing stress, exercise may reduce some of these oxidative changes and slow the aging process (Mundstock, Zatti, Louzada, et al., 2015). More research is needed.

The Centers for Disease Control and Prevention (2011, updated 2014) recommend the following activities for older adults:

- *Regular aerobic physical activity.* Engage in 150 minutes a week of moderate-intensity aerobic exercise. Alternatively, engage in 75 minutes a week of vigorous-intensity activity. Each episode of activity should last for at least 10 minutes, and the client should spread the exercise throughout the week. Additional benefits can be obtained by gradually increasing the amount of exercise (perhaps up to 300 minutes per week).
- *Muscle-strengthening activities.* Perform moderate- or high-intensity muscle-strengthening activities on 2 or more days a week. The weight-bearing and toning exercises should involve all major muscle groups.
- *Balance-promoting activities.* These are especially important for older adults at risk for falls.
- *Adapted physical activities.* Older adults with chronic conditions should to be as physically active as abilities and conditions allow. (The nurse should help them to make adaptations that allow them to do so or refer them to an exercise therapist.)

KEY POINT: *Some activity is better than none, and more is better than some.* Remind clients that doing some activity at least 3 days a week produces health benefits and helps avoid excessive fatigue. Some practical suggestions for exercising include the following:

- A brisk 15-minute walk twice a day, every day of the week would easily meet the minimum guidelines for aerobic activity.
- Muscle-strengthening activities can include use of exercise bands, handheld weights, digging, lifting and carrying as part of gardening, carrying groceries, and some yoga and tai chi exercises.

- Inactive older adults or those with a very low level of fitness should begin with 10 minutes of walking and increase minutes and intensity slowly with subsequent walks.

You can provide support for the client's exercise regimen by suggesting a range of choices and a list of community resources (e.g., parks, organizations, recreation centers). Also, teach the client how to walk, as needed, and safety considerations. Help the young-old adult institute self-monitoring methods to help her see her progress (e.g., a graph, a chart, a step counter) and reinforce personal progress, such as decreased fatigue and weight loss.

Interventions (Middle-Old)

Older adults who have maintained healthy behaviors throughout their lifetimes are likely to remain vital and actively engaged. However, the occurrence of a health crisis and even a short period of restrictive activity may lead to a decreased functional ability and the need for encouragement, support, and a planned program of limited activity progressing to optimal function for clients in this age-group.

Interventions (Oldest-Old)

The goal of interventions for the oldest-old is to ensure independence for as long as possible by maximizing function and preventing disability or loss of function. Broad interventions important for the oldest-old include the following:

- Supportive environments and conditions allow a person to function.
- Modified adapted activity is especially important for this age-group, including walking, flexibility exercises, yoga, tai chi, and water aerobics.
- Nutrition is an important focus, as well. Whole grains, dark green and orange vegetables and legumes, all types of fruits and vegetables, and fat-free and low-fat dairy products are among the food groups most needing inclusion in this age-group's diet to combat obesity and inactivity.

PICOT

Physical Activity and Well-Being of Older Adults

Situation

While caring for patients in the rehab unit, the nurse notes that there is a wide range of health among the elderly patients and that not all 75-year-old clients heal at the same rate.

PICOT Components

P	Population/patient	=	Older adults
I	Intervention/indicator	=	Regular exercise and physical activity
C	Comparator/control	=	No regular exercise, sedentary
O	Outcome	=	Improved well-being into aging
T	Time	=	None

Searchable Question\

Do _____ (P) who receive/are exposed to _____ (I) demonstrate _____ (O) as compared with _____ (C) during _____ (T)?

Example of Evidence

Advances in healthcare have increased the life span as well as the quality of life for many people. Physical fitness as a

younger adult may improve the physical and emotional well-being later in life. One of the specific goals of *Healthy People 2020* is to increase physical activity, with the expectation that it will slow the decline in physical functioning associated with age. This should help to improve the quality of life in later adulthood, promote faster recovery time, and, therefore, help decrease the dollars spent each year on medical care.

Practice Change

The nurse emphasizes to all her patients the importance of regular exercise and helps them think of ways they might incorporate more activity into their present routines. She also discusses with the unit manager the possibility of incorporating this nursing action into unit routines.

Source: Tahmaseb-McConatha, J., Volkwein-Caplan, K., & DiGregorio, N. (2011). Culture, aging and well-being: The importance of place and space. *International Journal of Sport & Society, 2*(2), 41–48.

Interventions/Implementation (Example Problem: Frail Elderly)

Prevention of frailty and care of the frail elderly are complex and specialized. Research supports some preventive measures that may give you some ideas for positive interventions. At least one study suggests that fall-preventive moderate-intensity group exercise programs have positive effects on older adults only *before* frailty occurs. The frail elderly do not appear to benefit (Faber, Bosscher, Paw, et al., 2006). Also see the box Example Problem: Frail Elderly for interventions.

Interventions for All Older Adults

For all interventions and interactions, always ask yourself, "Does this promote the client's dignity and self-esteem?"

Promoting Independence and Maintaining Functional Ability

The overall goals of nursing care of older adults are to maximize independent activity and enhance function. Often this will involve helping clients to adapt and develop new skills so they can continue to take part in activities they enjoy.

- *Focus on preserving the patient's functional abilities,* including both the ability and motivation to function in his environment. Consider any environmental modifications that might aid independence, including assistive technology.
- *Electronic technology* is increasingly being used to deliver care "remotely" and support older adults in their own homes. *Telehealth technologies* include electronic reminder systems, video conference visiting, and remotely controlled security sensors (Gellis, Kenaley, McGinty, et al., 2012; Stall, Nowaczynski, & Sinha, 2013; Young, Foster, Silander, et al., 2011).
- *Look for simple things you can do to promote better functioning.* For example, if the patient cannot see to sort his medications, you might try turning on more lights or having a brighter light installed.
- *Facilitate and encourage physical exercise* in order to help improve continence and help prevent further loss of mobility. Exercise also improves strength, balance, and endurance, and aids in falls prevention. Older adults who engage in progressive aerobic training can maintain their independence longer and delay the aging process, perhaps by as much as 10 years (Almeida, Khan, Hankey, et al., 2014).
- *Facilitate empowerment.* Many older adults are Internet savvy. You can empower them by suggesting Web sites that offer resources to help them understand and cope with the unknowns of their situation.

Promoting Cognitive Function

The National Institute for Health and Clinical Excellence (2006) identified a link between improving cognitive symptoms and ability to maintain day-to-day functioning for interventions to promote cognitive function, refer to the box Example Problem: Dementia.

✚ Teaching for Safety

Teach older adults about age-related changes and what these changes mean for their daily routine. For example, age-related changes diminish stamina, conditioning, reflexes, and the speed of processing information. Therefore, when multitasking and performing seemingly nonthinking physical activities, older adults need to be very purposeful in their actions and pay attention to the details of the task or activity. Failing to do so could result in missteps, injury, or exhaustion.

Illness Prevention

Although the risks of disease and disability increase with age, poor health need not always occur. Known prevention measures can help older adults avoid many illnesses and disabilities associated with chronic diseases. Stress the importance of a healthy lifestyle (e.g., healthy eating; regular physical activity; avoiding tobacco use; and screening for breast, cervical, and colorectal cancers).

Immunizations Health-promotion activities include teaching and facilitating immunizations for varicella, influenza, pneumonia, herpes zoster (shingles), and tetanus/diphtheria/pertussis. To see the Recommended Adult Immunization Schedule,

 Go to Recommended Adult Immunization Schedule, United States, 2016, at http://www.cdc.gov/vaccines/schedules/downloads/adult/adult-schedule.pdf

Communicating With Older Adults

Many normal changes of aging affect communication. For example, older adults tend to process information more slowly or may have sensory deficits. See the iCare box regarding personhood and dignity, in addition to the following,:

- *Check for sensory deficits at the beginning of your interaction.* Until you know there is no hearing deficit, look at the patient as you speak to allow for lip reading. But do not assume that all older adults are deaf or that they do not understand the meaning of your communication.
- *You will need to rely on body language more than usual.* Notice nonverbal communication, such as fidgeting, hand wringing, tearfulness, or quivering lips. Memory deficits make it difficult for some older adults to find the words to express what they mean.
- *Appropriate speech may be accompanied by inappropriate affect.* For instance, a client may speak coherently and make sense while telling you that she was able to walk to the bathroom today and then begin crying for no apparent reason. Nevertheless, the information about her ambulation may be credible.
- *Conversely, inappropriate affect and incoherent speech do not always indicate lack of understanding.* For example, a client may laugh appropriately at something funny but not be able to speak clearly or find the words to ask you what time it is.
- *Be aware that some older adults are confused at one time and not another.* A client may begin by giving you credible information, but as the conversation progresses, he may lose track of the topic or talk about something irrelevant. When a client seems confused, use focused assessment to determine his mental status. If you conclude that his communication is unreliable, you can always finish the talk later, when he is less confused.
- **KEY POINT:** *The ability to speak does not always reflect the person's ability to understand, and what the patient says may or may not match what she is feeling.*

Communicating With Persons With Cognitive Deficit

In addition to the normal changes of aging, many older adults have more severe problems with memory and at least one other cognitive ability (e.g., judgment, thinking, language, or coordination). Because of their decline in mental abilities, people with dementia have difficulty speaking and

♥ iCare 10-1

Caring Is Respecting Personhood and Dignity.

There are several ways you can demonstrate caring in patient interactions:

➤ Never call a person "sweetie" or "honey" or "dear." This sends a message that you think the person is not your equal.

➤ Ask, "What is your name?" and "How would you like to be addressed?"

➤ Provide eyeglasses, hearing aids, and dentures prior to engaging in conversation.

➤ Get to know the patient as a person (What work did they do? What are their likes/dislikes?).

➤ Encourage storytelling and reminiscing.

➤ Pull up a chair and sit down to speak with the person at eye level.

➤ Be present. Do not check your phone or take notes while conversing. Focus on what the person is saying.

➤ Try to respond to the person's feelings instead of the content of his words. This helps to reassure them. For example, if a woman is constantly searching for her husband, don't say, "Your husband is not here." Instead, say, "You must miss your husband," or "Tell me about your husband."

➤ Approach unhurriedly, do not rush an older adult and do not speak too rapidly.

➤ Allow the patient time to speak and express his or her concerns.

➤ If the person has difficulty finding the right word, supply it unless doing so upsets the person. This helps control frustration levels.

➤ If you do not understand what the patient is trying to say, ask him or her to point to it or describe it (e.g., "What does *abcd* look like?").

➤ Avoid providing care standing up, and especially with your back to the person.

➤ Provide privacy during bath time or when in the bathroom.

➤ Gently hold or pat the person's hand, offering comfort and reassurance.

understanding. In addition to the general approaches for all older adults, the following are some ideas to help you communicate with people with cognitive deficits:

- *Use simple, short sentences, with one idea at a time.* Ask, "Where does it hurt?" rather than, "Please describe the quality and location of your pain."

- *Avoid vague comments* (e.g., "I see," "Um-hmm," "Yes, yes, okay"). The patient will not be able to interpret these responses. Instead, echo the patient's comment and state your response directly and simply: "You are hungry. I will bring your lunch."

- *Repeat your words exactly if the patient doesn't understand what you say.* Under other circumstances, you usually rephrase your sentences when someone doesn't understand, but for patients with dementia, giving new information just adds to their confusion.

- *Try to understand that the patient's reality is distorted* and he is behaving in the only way he is able. When the patient is

conversing superficially and seems comfortable, it may seem he is competent.

Providing Caregiver Support

A diagnosis of dementia or a debilitating physical condition can be traumatic and devastating. Family members are often the primary caregivers (either through choice or necessity). Caregivers of any patient are more likely than noncaregivers to be at risk for depression, heart disease, high blood pressure, and other chronic illnesses, even death. Caring for a person with dementia puts them at even higher risk.

Most caregivers are also older adults who themselves have special needs. They often feel abandoned and unsupported, not only by services but also by family and friends. Exhaustion and despair can quickly follow. Supportive interventions such as the following can contribute to physical and psychological well-being, help maintain hope, and reduce caregiver burden (Brodaty, Woodward, Boundy, et al., & PRIME Study Group, 2014):

- Education about dementia
- Supportive counseling
- Psychotherapy
- Rapid support in crisis
- Support from other caregivers (respite)
- Faith-based spiritual assistance

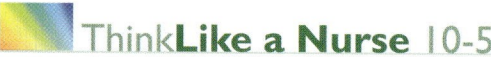

ThinkLike a Nurse 10-5

What factors contribute to a community of functionally active older adults?

PUTTING IT ALL TOGETHER

Recall Ethel Higginbotham, in the Meet Your Patient scenario. She is very thin and frail and refuses to eat. She says, "I just want to die." Do you feel ready to plan her care now?

You might diagnose Mrs. Higginbotham with Frail Elderly Syndrome. An appropriate *NOC outcome* would be Will to Live. An *individualized goal* might be "Mrs. Higginbotham will gain 1 pound and participate in at least one daily group activity by the first of next month." Interventions depend on the diagnosis and its etiology.

Mrs. Higginbotham will need care that helps her adjust to widowhood, provides adequate nutrition, and offers activities that provide interaction with others. *NIC interventions* appropriate for Mrs. Higginbotham are as follows: Coping Enhancement, Hope Inspiration, Self-Care Assistance, Spiritual Support.

Individualized interventions for Mrs. Higginbotham include grief counseling, nutritional support, and working with her and her family to determine whether it is appropriate for her to continue to live independently.

As a full-spectrum nurse, you should assess the developmental stage of each of your clients. In maternity and pediatric care, this is a routine part of nursing care. However, growth and development continue to be important throughout the life span. To assess growth and development you must gather data such as the client's age, height and weight, activities the client engages in, and the client's communication skills. You should also perform age-specific assessments such as those discussed in previous sections.

CLINICALREASONING

The questions and exercises in this section allow you to practice the kind of thinking you will use as a full-spectrum nurse. Critical-thinking questions usually have more than one correct answer, so we do not provide "correct answers" for these features. It is more important to develop your nursing judgment than to just cover content. You will learn by discussing the questions with your peers. If you are still unsure, see the Davis Advantage chapter resources for suggested responses.

Caring for the Nguyens

Nam Nguyen's father, Binh, is 80 years old and has multiple health problems. He has hypertension and heart disease. Although he had surgery for prostate cancer many years ago, the cancer has now metastasized. Because Binh's health was declining rapidly, Nam and Yen moved him and his wife, Mai, into their home last year. Both Nam and his wife work outside the home, so the elderly Mai cares for her husband as best she can during the day. Binh is too weak to get out of bed without help, and his wife is not strong enough to support him. She cooks for him, but he eats only a few bites, then pushes the plate away. Nam telephones today to say, "We can't take care of him safely at home any longer. Can you tell me how to get him admitted to a hospital or a nursing home?"

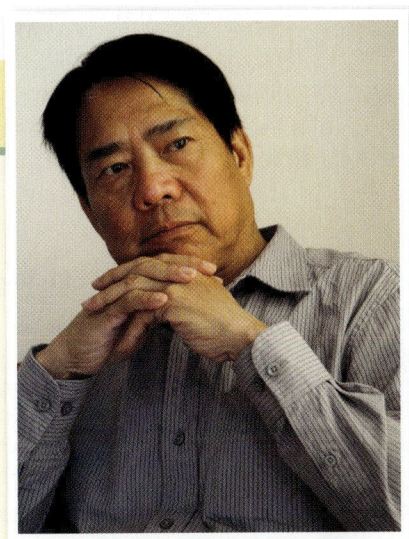

A. What other ideas do you have for helping the Nguyens to care or to find care for Binh other than placing him in a hospital or nursing home?

B. Nam's first concern seems to be about getting help for his father. What do you think his next concern will be?

C. What actual data do you have about Binh Nguyen's nutritional status?

D. What else do you need to know to fully assess Binh's nutritional status? If you do not know the answer to this, you will find some information in the Assessment sections of this chapter. For more complete information, refer to Screening for Nutritional Problems and in Focused Nutritional Assessment in Chapter 28.

E. Would you consider Binh Nguyen to be a frail elderly person? Why or why not?

Applying the **Full-Spectrum Nursing Model**

PATIENT SITUATION

Alvin Bell, 82 years old, was just discharged from the hospital following a myocardial infarction (heart attack). On your first home visit to supervise his medication regimen, you notice that the house looks as though it has not been cleaned in weeks. Piled on every flat surface, including the floor, is what appears to be months' accumulation of newspapers, magazines, and other clutter. Dishes are piled in the sink, apparently left there before his hospitalization. There is hardly any food in the cupboard. When you weigh Mr. Bell, you see that he has lost 3 pounds in the 3 days he has been home. He admits he has not been eating: "I'm not hungry, and it's too much trouble." As you talk with him, you learn that his wife died of cancer 7 months ago. He says, "I don't know what to do without her. I hate living alone. There doesn't seem to be much reason for going on." Mr. Bell is alert and oriented but talks and moves very slowly.

THINKING

1. *Theoretical Knowledge:*
   a. What do you know about depression in older adults? Do you have enough knowledge of that topic to be able to assess whether Mr. Bell is depressed? If not, what resources would you use to find out? (List specific resources; that is, give the URL, don't just say "the Internet"; give the name or author of the book, not just "my psych-nursing book.")
   b. You will also need to know whether it is normal for appetite to decrease in older adults, and what their calorie needs are compared with other age-groups. Where can you go to find this information?

2. *Critical Thinking (Considering Alternatives):*

   a. As you survey Mr. Bell's overall situation, what is your first impulse to improve his situation? What questions come to you?

   b. What community services might be helpful for Mr. Bell?

   c. How would you handle referrals? Would you leave a list of telephone numbers? Would you call the agencies yourself? Explain your thinking.

DOING

3. *Practical Knowledge:* In your physical examination of Mr. Bell, you find no old or recent bruises or other injuries. However, because he is depressed and losing weight, you wonder whether he is suffering neglect or financial abuse. What questions could you ask to find out?

CARING

4. *Self-Knowledge:* Think of one patient you have cared for who has something in common with Mr. Bell. Describe the way(s) in which they are alike.

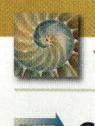

To explore learning resources for this chapter,

  Go to www.DavisAdvantage.com and find:

Answers and Suggested Responses for all questions in this chapter

Lists of NIC Interventions and NOC Outcomes

List of NANDA-I Diagnoses

Knowledge Map

References and Bibliography

Concept Map

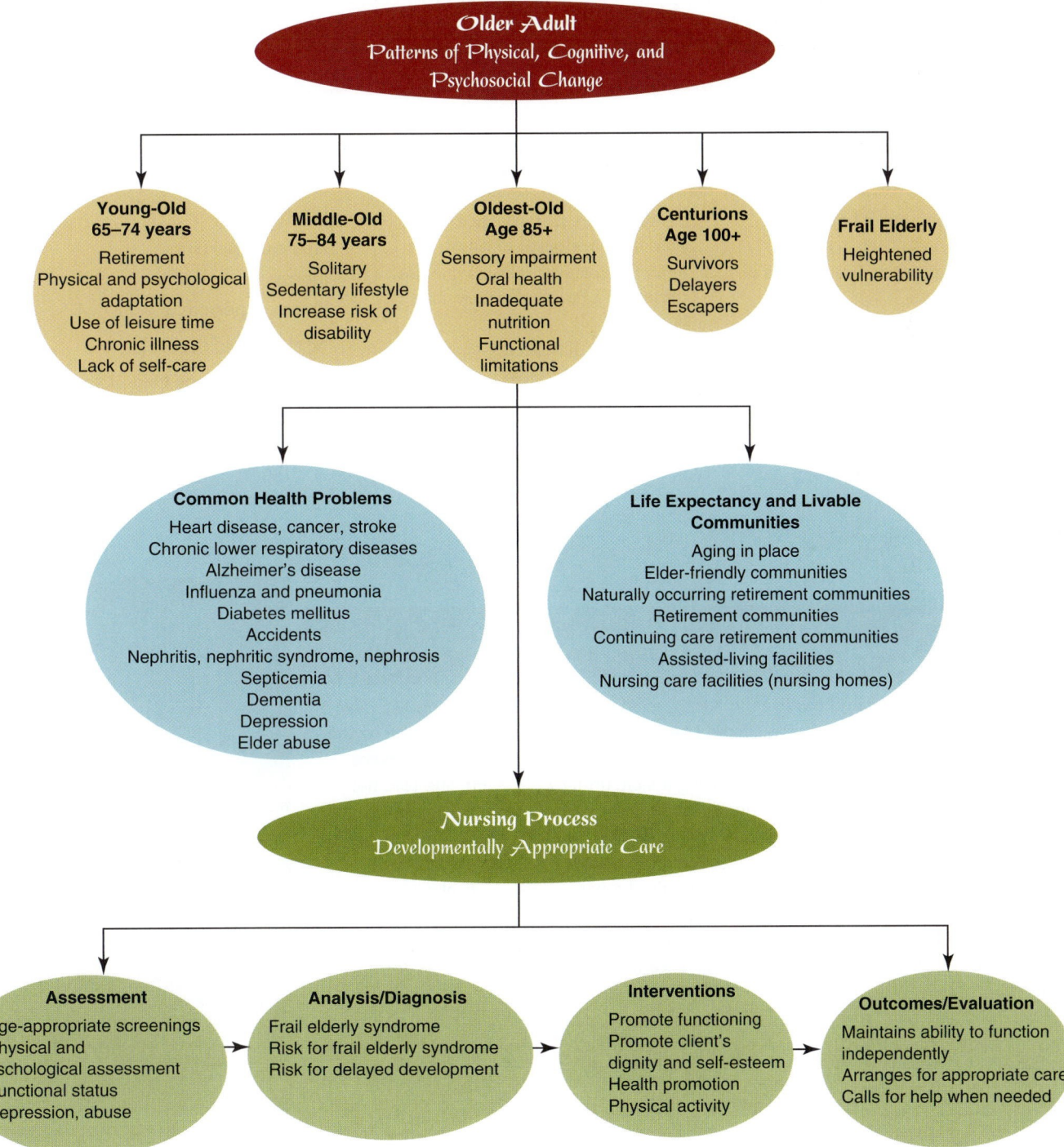

Older Adult
Patterns of Physical, Cognitive, and Psychosocial Change

**Young-Old
65–74 years**
Retirement
Physical and psychological adaptation
Use of leisure time
Chronic illness
Lack of self-care

**Middle-Old
75–84 years**
Solitary
Sedentary lifestyle
Increase risk of disability

**Oldest-Old
Age 85+**
Sensory impairment
Oral health
Inadequate nutrition
Functional limitations

**Centurions
Age 100+**
Survivors
Delayers
Escapers

Frail Elderly
Heightened vulnerability

Common Health Problems
Heart disease, cancer, stroke
Chronic lower respiratory diseases
Alzheimer's disease
Influenza and pneumonia
Diabetes mellitus
Accidents
Nephritis, nephritic syndrome, nephrosis
Septicemia
Dementia
Depression
Elder abuse

Life Expectancy and Livable Communities
Aging in place
Elder-friendly communities
Naturally occurring retirement communities
Retirement communities
Continuing care retirement communities
Assisted-living facilities
Nursing care facilities (nursing homes)

Nursing Process
Developmentally Appropriate Care

Assessment
Age-appropriate screenings
Physical and pschological assessment
Functional status
Depression, abuse

Analysis/Diagnosis
Frail elderly syndrome
Risk for frail elderly syndrome
Risk for delayed development

Interventions
Promote functioning
Promote client's dignity and self-esteem
Health promotion
Physical activity

Outcomes/Evaluation
Maintains ability to function independently
Arranges for appropriate care
Calls for help when needed

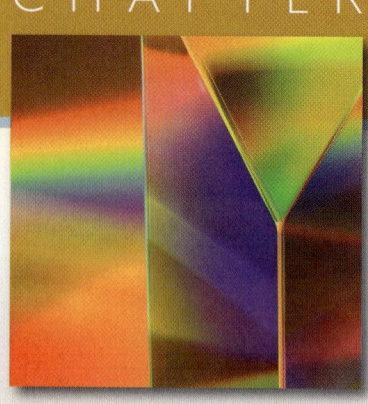

CHAPTER 11

Experiencing Health & Illness

Learning Outcomes

After completing this chapter, you should be able to:

➤ Explore the concepts of health and illness from a holistic perspective.

➤ Compare and contrast three models of health and illness.

➤ Describe the various ways that people experience health and illness.

➤ Identify factors that disrupt health.

➤ Describe the five stages of illness behavior.

➤ Differentiate between acute and chronic illness.

➤ Identify factors that influence individuals' responses to illness.

➤ Apply the concepts presented in this chapter to a variety of patient care situations.

➤ Explain what the concepts in this chapter mean to you as you work toward becoming a full-spectrum nurse.

Key Concepts

Health

Health experience

Illness

Illness experience

Related Concepts

See the Concept Map at the end of this chapter.

Meet Your Patient

Evelyn is 87 years old and has lived in a long-term care facility for the past 5 years. She suffers from congestive heart failure (CHF), hypertension, diabetes, macular degeneration resulting in near blindness, a severe hearing deficit, urinary incontinence, and immobility resulting from a hip fracture.

Evelyn was married nearly 60 years to Lloyd, who died 6 years ago. Evelyn has 5 children, 17 grandchildren, and 14 great-grandchildren. In these past few years, she has experienced the loss of her husband, home, vision, hearing, mobility, and bladder control. Despite these limitations, she keeps current in the lives of all of her extended family and friends.

She is the confidante of the facility staff and knows about their children, their romances, and the gossip around the institution. She is an avid Minnesota Twins fan and also keeps track of the televised high school basketball tournaments. Whenever there is an election, she makes sure that she votes. She "reads" every audio book she can get her hands

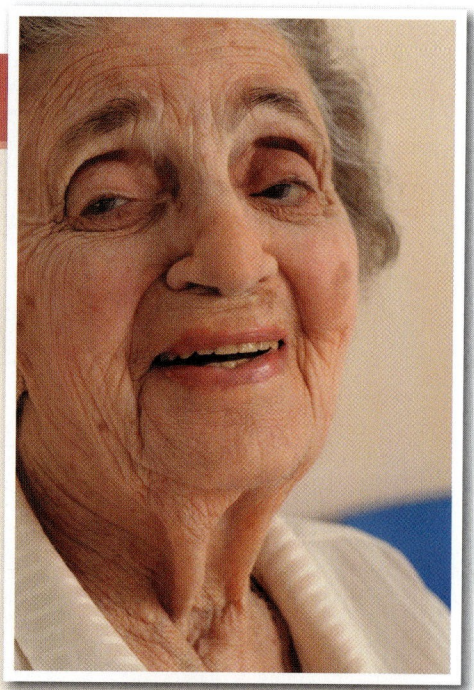

on. Recently, Evelyn was admitted to the hospital in severe CHF. She told her pastor, "I don't want to die yet. I'm having too much fun!"

Evelyn's situation is a far cry from what most people would picture as good health. However, as you consider the ideas of health presented in this chapter, you might conclude that in many ways she is a reasonably healthy person.

Theoretical Knowledge
knowing why

Every day there is something in the news about health or illness. Politicians talk about their desire to improve our health and reorganize healthcare. Schools want students to eat healthy foods, exercise, and receive regular immunizations. In an attempt to reduce health insurance claims, employers open on-site fitness centers and employ nurses and counselors to work with employees to improve employee health. Everyone says they want to be healthy.

As a nursing student, you have probably already cared for clients in various stages of health and illness. But have you ever considered what those terms mean? Our understanding of health and illness is influenced by our family, culture, health history, and a host of other factors. As you evolve as a nurse, you'll find that your understanding of these concepts evolves, too. We will examine some ways that you and your clients might define *health* and *illness* and some ways that full-spectrum nurses have come to understand these terms through their thinking, doing, and caring.

You may find this chapter a little different from other chapters in this book and other textbooks. That is because the goal of the chapter is not so much to help you learn facts about health and illness, but to understand how people experience them. Even the language of the chapter is designed for that purpose. Relax and flow with the chapter. Instead of agonizing over each detail, read it in a way that will help you see the "big picture."

ABOUT THE KEY CONCEPTS

You will need to understand the abstract concepts of **health** and **illness** to help you appreciate the **experience of health and illness** as lived by real, not abstract, people. Strive for an overview of factors that are disruptive to health and factors that nourish health. Understand the subconcepts of **hardiness** as it relates to patients, and of **healing presence** as it relates to your work as a nurse.

HOW DO WE UNDERSTAND HEALTH AND ILLNESS?

First let's examine the key concept, health. What is your image of health? Here are some ideas.

- **The "body beautiful."** Being a "picture of health" can depend on whether you were born in the right era—or in the right country. Styles of beautiful bodies come and go. For instance, much Indian, African, Greek, and European art portrays ideal women as well-rounded creatures. The perfect body view of health also denies the possibility of health to people who use wheelchairs, prosthetics, or even eyeglasses and hearing aids. Yet many full-spectrum nurses working with disabled clients would describe their clients as healthy.
- **Not having illness.** In describing healthy people, would you disqualify someone with a cold, dandruff, or athlete's foot? What about diabetes, heart disease, or cancer? Doing so would reflect another view of health: that is, not having illness. This view may be unfair because it restricts health only to those who do not have some kind of physical impairment.
- **Something you can buy.** Another popular concept is that health is something you can buy: exercise equipment, membership in a health club, medicine, liposuction, a coronary bypass, and so on. In this view, health does not come from within. It's something "out there" that is available if you have enough money or insurance.
- **Ideal physical and mental well-being.** Health can also be described as an ideal state of physical and mental well-being: something to strive for, but never to attain. Good health is never actually reached, because there is always something more to be achieved. Health is the goal itself, the end instead of one of the means to fulfilling life's purposes.
- **The ability of the soul to cope.** Theologian Jürgen Moltmann (1983) described health in a different way: "True health is the strength to live, the strength to suffer, and the strength to die. Health is not a condition of my body; it is the power of my soul to cope with the varying condition of that body" (p. 142). Similarly, author Robert Louis Stevenson wrote of health, "It is not a matter of holding good cards, it's playing a poor hand well." For more traditional definitions of health, refer to Box 11-1.

Nurses Understand Health and Illness as Individual Experiences

If you were the nurse caring for Evelyn (Meet Your Patient), would you understand health as a perfect body or the absence of disease? Probably not. **KEY POINT:** *Nurses understand health and illness as individual experiences, emerging from each patient's unique responses. The person with an illness rarely perceives the experience as a medical diagnosis. Instead, people describe their illness in terms of how it makes them* **feel.**

Think back to the last time you were ill. How did you feel? Did you feel pain, sadness, fatigue, loss? Did you feel overwhelmed? These responses are **disruptions** to health and, as such, constitute the lived experience of illness. **Lived experience** is unique to each patient: Just as Evelyn might describe herself as "raring to go," another patient who is 10 years younger and on half as many medications may

---

BOX 11-1 ■ What Do the Experts Say About Health?

- *The World Health Organization (WHO)* has defined health as "a state of complete physical, mental and social well-being and not merely the absence of disease or infirmity" (WHO, 1948).
- *Traditional Chinese medicine* considers health to be a balance between the opposite energy forces of *yin* and *yang*.
- *Ayurveda,* an ancient Indian medical system, describes health as the trinity of body, mind, and spiritual awareness (Sheinfeld-Gorin & Arnold, 2006).
- *Florence Nightingale* believed that health was prevention of disease through the use of fresh air, pure water, efficient drainage, cleanliness, and light (1859/1992).
- *Nursing theorist Jean Watson* (1979) believes that health implies at least three elements: (1) a high level of overall physical, mental, and social functioning; (2) a general adaptive–maintenance level of daily functioning; and (3) the absence of illness (or the presence of efforts that lead to its absence). To Watson, health is a matter of perception. Even a person with a terminal illness may be considered healthy if he has a high level of functioning, is coping with the diagnosis, and is actively making efforts to improve his status.

describe herself as "exhausted all the time" and "just wait-ing to die." In short, nurses honor the client's understanding of her state of being.

For many years nurses have recognized that, like Evelyn, some clients strive to maintain a state of optimal health even when coping with chronic and even terminal disease. Many experience this state as wellness: "a way of life oriented toward optimal health and well-being in which body, mind, and spirit are integrated by the individual to live more fully within the human and natural community" (Myers, Sweeney, & Witmer, 2000, p. 252). This perspective acknowledges the influence of attitude and lifestyle choices on the client's state of being. It also implies that nursing interventions in support of wellness are important not only for healthy clients but also for those who are experiencing disease, and even those facing death.

ThinkLike a Nurse 11-1

What qualities are essential to your own personal definition of *health*? How do you define *illness*?

KnowledgeCheck 11-1

- Provide at least two common definitions of *health*.
- Explain how full-spectrum nurses define *health* and *illness*.
- Define *wellness* in your own words.

Nurses Use Conceptual Models to Understand Health and Illness

You can use a variety of models to understand health and illness. Each emphasizes somewhat different aspects of these experiences. Nurses have found the following models particularly useful:

The Health–Illness Continuum

Most of us recognize that our health status changes frequently. For example: "Although today I feel pretty good and yesterday I was exhausted, I believe I was healthy on both of those days. I know that my exhaustion was related to staying up late enjoy-ing the company of good friends. My medical record states that I have diabetes and hypertension, but I keep both diseases in control. I take multiple medications, read food labels, exercise aerobically 5 days a week, and lift weights 3 days a week. Am I healthy, ill, or a health nut?"

The preceding example illustrates the varied and dynamic nature of human health. In an effort to describe this complex state, many theorists speak of a **health–illness continuum,** that is, they see health and illness as a graduated spectrum that cannot be divided—except arbitrarily—into parts. A person's position moves back and forth on the continuum with physio-logical changes, lifestyle choices, and the results of various therapies. As shown in Figure 11-1, the number 1 represents a state of being gravely ill, and the number 10 represents excel-lent health, or a person in peak form. Notice, however, that a client such as Evelyn (Meet Your Patient) may view herself at various points on this continuum according to how she feels on any particular day. In other words, the continuum is per-sonal and dynamic. Health changes over the course of time.

Dunn's Health Grid

Dunn (1959) created a health grid that plots a person's status on the health–illness continuum against environmental con-ditions (Fig. 11-2). Many nurses use this grid to help them

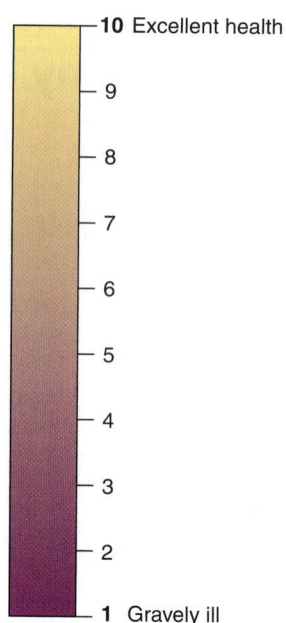

FIGURE 11-1 Over a lifetime, an individual moves up and down on the health–illness continuum.

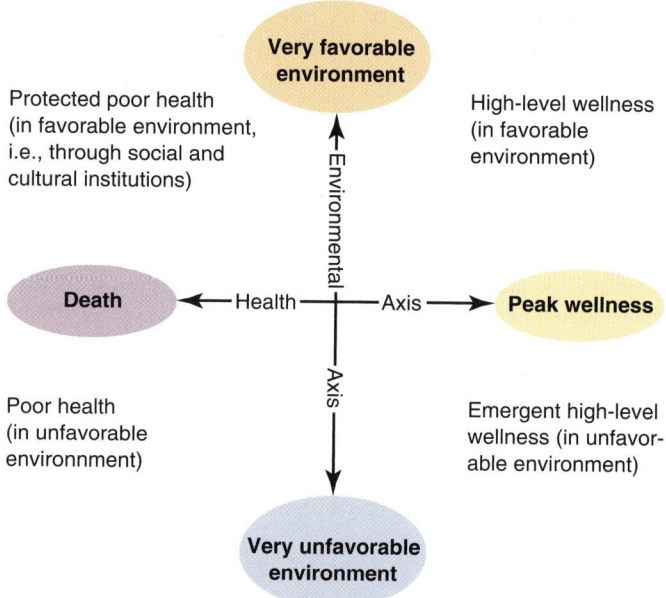

FIGURE 11-2 Dunn's health grid: Health is affected by an individual's status on the health–illness continuum as well as environmental conditions.

predict the likelihood that a client will experience a change in health status. For example, Evelyn (Meet Your Patient) has several health problems. On a scale of 1 to 10, an observer who does not know Evelyn well might rate her health as a 3. However, Evelyn has a positive outlook and tells her pastor, "I don't want to die yet. I'm having too much fun!" She also has excellent support from her friends, family, and the facil-ity staff. Clearly, Evelyn is in a favorable environment. This positive setting protects her from harm and provides a good quality of life. On Dunn's grid, Evelyn would probably fall in the area of "protected poor health."

Neuman's Continuum

Nursing theorist Betty Neuman (2002) views health as an expression of living energy available to an individual. The energy is displayed as a continuum with high energy (wellness) at one end and low energy (illness) at the opposite end (Fig. 11-3). The person is said to have varying levels of energy at various stages of life. When more energy is generated than expended, there is wellness. When more energy is expended than is generated, there is illness—possibly death. Although Evelyn (Meet Your Patient) has several clearly identified health problems, she is engaged in life and active with her family, friends, and long-term care facility staff. We might not all agree on where to place her on Neuman's continuum, but certainly her activity and energy counterbalance her physical frailty.

HOW DO PEOPLE EXPERIENCE HEALTH AND ILLNESS?

In envisioning health and illness as a continuum, full-spectrum nurses promote wellness regardless of the circumstances a client faces now or in the future. This approach requires the holistic understanding that health is multidimensional. The following are some of the many dimensions of health that we experience along the health–illness continuum.

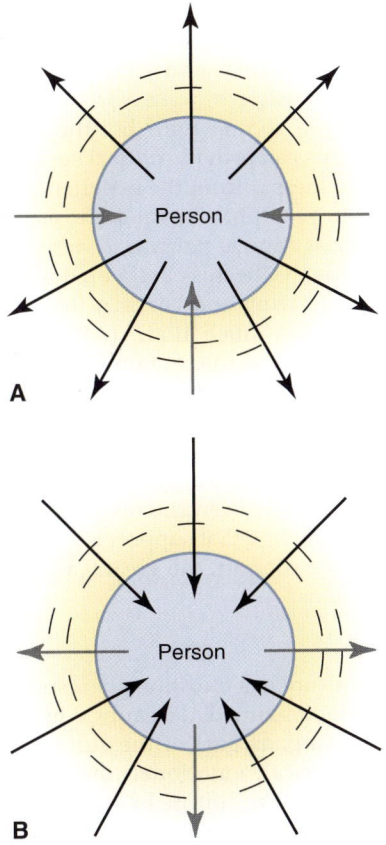

FIGURE 11-3 Neuman's continuum: a balance of input and output. (A) When energy output exceeds input, illness results. (B) Wellness occurs when more energy is generated than expended.

An understanding of these dimensions should broaden your concept of health.

Biological Factors

Although biological factors are not entirely within our control, most people consider them when they describe themselves as "well" or "ill." A healthy genetic makeup and freedom from debilitating age-related changes are certainly desired states and, along with gender, they tip the scale toward the wellness end of the health–illness continuum.

Genetic Makeup For example, the risk of breast cancer increases dramatically in women who have a family history of a mother, sister, or daughter with breast cancer. A genetic marker for this type of breast cancer has been discovered, indicating that some people inherit a tendency to develop breast cancer.

Gender Many diseases occur more commonly in one gender than in another. For example, rheumatoid arthritis, osteoporosis, and breast cancer are more common in women, whereas ulcers, color blindness, and bladder cancer are more common in men.

Age and Developmental Stage Age and developmental stage influence the likelihood of becoming ill. Certain health problems can be correlated to developmental stage. For example, more than 75% of new breast cancer cases are diagnosed in women older than age 50. As another example, adolescent boys have much higher rates of head injury and spinal cord injury than the general public because of their tendency to engage in risk-taking behaviors. For further discussion of growth and development, see Chapters 9 and 10 in this book.

- **Developmental influences on coping ability.** Developmental stage also influences a person's ability to cope with stressors that tend to move him toward the illness end of the continuum. Infants or children who are ill, frightened, or hurt have a limited repertoire of experiences, communication ability, and understanding to help them in their responses. As we progress through the stages of development, we develop understanding and skills to help us deal with illness.

- **Developmental influences on perceptions.** When disease, loss, or other disruptions occur at a younger age than expected, they change our perception of the event and may present a greater challenge to our coping skills than disruptions that are expected. For example, a child's death may seem more tragic than that of an older adult. It is important, though, not to discount the impact of disruptions that occur during the period of a person's life when they might be expected. For example, the death of a spouse is no less traumatic for an older adult than it would be for a young spouse. Losing someone with whom one has spent most of one's life is an incredible loss, whether or not it is "expected" at that stage of life.

Nutrition

Health requires nourishment, and the most obvious form of nourishment is food. The influence of diet on human health is undeniable: Nutrient-deficiency diseases, such as scurvy and night blindness, are unknown in people who consume a nutritious diet. In addition, many chronic diseases, such as type 2 diabetes mellitus and heart disease, are influenced by our diets. Nutrition appears to play at least a moderate role in a variety of other diseases, such as osteoporosis and some forms of cancer (Thompson & Manore, 2014). As more studies look at the protective properties of some foods (e.g., antioxidants) and the hazards of others (e.g., refined carbohydrates, *trans*-fatty acids), the phrase "You are what you eat" seems more accurate each day. Chapter 28 discusses nutrition in greater detail.

Physical Activity

Healthy people are usually active people. When they are unable to maintain previous levels of activity, people may perceive themselves as less healthy. Studies support the benefit of moderate physical activity in reducing the risk of chronic disease and promoting longevity (Thompson & Manore, 2014). As little as 30 minutes of gardening or 15 minutes of jogging on most days of the week can lead to these benefits. In addition, certain types of exercise have been shown to reduce the risk of specific diseases, such as osteoporosis and heart disease. For example, weight training has been shown to increase bone density and reduce the risk of osteoporosis in women older than age 40, and aerobic activity, such as walking, decreases the risk of heart disease. Physical activity is discussed more fully in Chapter 33.

Sleep and Rest

Sleep nourishes health. Most of the body's growth hormone, which assists in tissue regeneration, synthesis of bone, and formation of red blood cells, is released during sleep. Sleep is also important to mental health because it provides time for the mind to slow down and rejuvenate. In controlled studies, people kept awake for 24 hours experienced difficulty concentrating and performing routine tasks. With increasing levels of sleep deprivation, sensory deficits and mood disturbances occurred. Outside the laboratory, mild but chronic sleep deprivation is common, particularly among students, mothers of infants and young children, perimenopausal women, and people in pain. Sleep and rest are discussed in more detail in Chapter 35.

Meaningful Work

Many people find that work is a healthy way to cope with stressors. Psychologist Victor Frankl, who survived internment in a Nazi concentration camp, observed in *Man's Search for Meaning* (1959, 1962, 1984, 2004) that engaging in meaningful work promotes health and, even in the midst of horrific stressors, can defend against physical and mental breakdown. Many share the view of "meaningful work" offered by Morrie Schwartz in *Tuesdays With Morrie:* "You know what really gives you satisfaction? Offering others what you have to give. . . . [D]evote yourself to your community around you, and . . . to creating something that gives you purpose and meaning. You notice, there's nothing in there about a salary" (Albom, 43, 1997).

People also experience meaningful work as a dimension of wellness. For many people, volunteering, pursuing hobbies, and engaging in pleasurable activities can be forms of meaningful work. For example, some find that singing, playing a musical instrument, or listening to music is particularly healing. For others, it may be reading, painting, playing basketball, knitting, gardening, hiking in the wilderness, or even shopping. Being healthy is not all about denying yourself the pleasure of ice cream and French fries. Healthful activities can be fun, too. By supporting clients' life work, hobbies, and personal interests, you help them nourish their health in their unique way.

Lifestyle Choices

People who consider themselves healthy are usually those who make healthy lifestyle choices. They are aware of the threats to health created by smoking cigarettes, consuming alcohol, abusing drugs, engaging in unprotected sex, and other risky behaviors. Consider the following examples:

- **Tobacco.** Tobacco use increases recovery time from illnesses, injuries, and surgery. Smoking also increases the risk of cancer, respiratory diseases, diabetes, infertility, low-birth-weight babies, and perinatal death.
- **Alcohol.** Studies indicate that drinking a glass of red wine each day can reduce the risk of heart disease and slow bone loss. In contrast, excessive alcohol consumption damages the brain, liver, pancreas, intestines, and neurological system and can lead to malnutrition. It has also been implicated in several forms of cancer and in fetal alcohol syndrome in newborns. ✚ Finally, excessive alcohol consumption is implicated in about half of all motor vehicle accidents, falls, and other injuries.
- **Other Substances.** Substance abuse (e.g., of alcohol, illicit drugs, and prescribed drugs) is a risk factor in many diseases. Substance abuse leads to a deterioration in health, functioning, and relationships. For example, people who inject illegal drugs and share needles are at increased risk of hepatitis and HIV.

Personal Relationships

Living in a healthy family is an important dimension of wellness. Moreover, the family influences a person's view of himself as well or ill. Of the five pairs of families listed in Table 11-1, which family in each pair would you expect to experience a higher level of wellness?

When clients are coping with life-threatening disease, family relationships can provide critical sustenance and preserve optimal wellness during the experience. Weeks before his death from amyotrophic lateral sclerosis, a neurological disease, sociologist Morrie Schwartz stated, "It's become quite clear to me as I've been sick. If you don't have the support and love and caring and concern that you get from a family, you don't have much at all" (Albom, 91, 1997). You will learn more about the role of family in human health in Chapter 14.

When illness occurs, some people prefer to be totally independent, priding themselves on never asking for or accepting help. But the reality is that during times of disruption, support from others (e.g. family, friends, coworkers, pastors, counselors) is crucial. Knowing that support is available, and being willing to accept the support, can greatly affect a person's response to disruptions.

Culture

The healthcare culture has traditionally responded to illness with specific therapies aimed at treating a biophysical disorder, whereas nursing, as part of the culture of holism, responds to the physical, emotional, mental, and spiritual dimensions of illness. The culture of a region, neighborhood dynamics, a school or work environment, affluence or poverty, or a religious group can influence individual and family health. Culture affects the experience of illness in the following ways:

- **It influences health decisions, behaviors, perceptions, and view of self as well or ill.** For example, the cultural group

Table 11-1 ➤ Family Personal Relationships		
Which Family Would Likely Experience a Higher Level of Wellness?		
Family A: Places a high priority on health promotion	OR	**Family B:** Responds to health issues only in times of serious illness
Family C: Encourages adventure and risk taking	OR	**Family D:** Emphasizes caution in new situations
Family E: Is very open about expressing feelings and disagreements	OR	**Family F:** Squelches personal feelings to avoid conflict in the family
Family G: Views the family as capable and successful	OR	**Family H:** Views themselves as powerless victims
Family I: Teaches good negotiation skills and builds a network of family support while encouraging the development of independence	OR	**Family J:** Parents do not have a large repertoire of coping and communication skills to share with their children

may share health-promoting values, such as nutritious diet or regular physical activity. This is not to say that individuals can be "defined" by their culture. Some, either consciously or unconsciously, decide to break away from culturally conditioned responses.

- **It influences responses to illness.** For example, people who belong to certain religions may interpret illness as a punishment from God and may bear their symptoms stoically (i.e., hide their symptoms) to try to pay for their sins (retribution), while some members of other religions may believe that illness is a lesson we give ourselves to teach us something we need to learn for our spiritual evolution. If you need more information about the influence of culture on health and illness, see Chapter 15.

Religion and Spirituality

Clients' religious beliefs and practices can influence their healthcare choices. For some people, spiritual beliefs influence the mind–body connection to promote wellness and healing. A dramatic example is seemingly spontaneous recovery after a religious rite, as when a congregation member who can't walk undergoes a special rite or ceremony and then recovers enough to walk across the room. When healing is not possible because of terminal illness or external circumstances beyond our control, spiritual reserves can help maintain our view of ourselves as "well." You will learn more about the influence of spirituality on health in Chapter 16.

Environmental Factors

The environment can also nourish wellness. For institutionalized clients, establishing a little corner of the room that is uniquely theirs, with photos and other mementos, can be healing. Other clients may be soothed by the quiet of a chapel, a walk in a park, or even a trip to a shopping mall. Spending time in any place where they feel harmony and peace and draw strength can promote clients' health.

Environmental pollutants are a common cause of illness. For example, exposure to secondhand smoke causes an estimated 7,300 deaths from lung cancer among American non-smoking adults each year (Centers for Disease Control and Prevention [CDC], 2014). Carbon monoxide and lead poisoning, molds, radon, chemicals (e.g., insecticides), and other pollutants also cause serious disease. See Chapter 23 for more information about environmental pollutants.

Finances

It is often said that money doesn't buy happiness. Certainly, this is true. However, money does buy healthcare choices and access, and thus nourishes wellness. In the United States:

- Health insurance is often tied to employment or income level.
- Health insurance dictates which providers individuals have access to and what services are available to each person.

Even in countries with national health programs, such as Canada and some European countries, the standard care available may not include all the services or medications that a person desires. The same is true in the United States under government programs like Medicare.

People often do not take advantage of services that are available to them. Healthcare professionals may wonder why patients let things go so long before seeking help—or why they do not follow up with recommended treatment plans. **KEY POINT:** *A client's apparent lack of concern or lack of compliance to a treatment regimen may be, in reality, a problem of access to healthcare. One or more factors may keep people and families from getting the help that they need (e.g., distance from the resources, knowledge of available resources, trust in the available resources, financial status and lifestyle adjustments such as a change in employment).*

ThinkLike a Nurse 11-2

- In what ways could you improve your eating, exercise, and sleep habits?
- How might a hospitalized patient get away from the routine and find peace and harmony?

WHAT FACTORS DISRUPT HEALTH?

We spend much of our lives trying to maintain good health—eating, sleeping, keeping our bodies at a comfortable temperature—in general, tending to our high-maintenance bodily needs. It's a continual process because of the many disruptions to health we face. Not all disruptions are incapacitating, but all challenge our ability to function and enjoy our everyday lives, and they tend to move us toward the illness end of the health–illness continuum. What are **health disruptions?** Let's explore the concept by learning about some specific examples.

Physical Disease

Disease disrupts our lives in so many ways:

- It may reduce our ability to perform our life roles or to engage in activities we enjoyed before the illness.
- The diagnosis of a serious disease may bring shock, fear, anxiety, anger, or grief: Will I become disabled? How will I support my family? What did I do to deserve this?
- Physical illness may also cause clients to question the meaning and purpose of their lives, to become more inwardly focused, or to embrace life even more fully.

> When she first learned, of her diagnosis of breast cancer at age 36, Treya Killam Wilber wrote, "Strange things happen to the mind when catastrophe strikes. . . . I was so stunned that it was as if absolutely nothing had happened. A tremendous strength descended on me. . . . I was clear, present, and very determined" (Wilber, 2000).

Injury

Although injury can cause the same symptoms and emotions as disease, perhaps its most disruptive aspect is its suddenness. In *Still Me*, actor Christopher Reeve (*Superman* [1978]) described his thoughts in the first days after he recovered consciousness following his cervical spinal cord injury: "The thought that kept going through my mind was: 'I've ruined my life, and you only get one.' There's no counter you can go up to and say, 'I dropped my ice cream cone; could I please have another one?'. . . . Why isn't there a higher authority you can go to and say, 'Wait a minute, you didn't mean for this to happen to *me*'" (Reeve, 1998).

Mental Illness

Mental illness causes clients and families to experience a level of pain, suffering, and chronic sorrow that is difficult for healthy people to fully appreciate (Ahmann, 2013; Richardson, Cobham, McDermott et al., 2013). In addition, if the illness affects work ability, they experience loss of income and altered role relationships, along with the costs of various therapies.

Mental illness carries with it a stigma that may be diminishing slowly, but is highly visible to those who suffer from its effects. This stigmatization can also disrupt the health of family members. Families must adjust to a major upheaval in their lives as they experience the pain associated with the loss of a once promising child or relative to the spiral of mental illness (Townsend, 2014). Family members may also live in constant fear that their loved one will hurt herself or even commit suicide.

Pain

Whether mild or severe, temporary or long lasting, pain is a disruption. It's not that we can't live with pain—many people do, every day of their lives. However, pain disrupts the smooth operation of our lives; it can change personality, erode coping skills, and interfere with healthy communication. It's hard to concentrate on what we are trying to accomplish when pain is competing for our attention.

Pain that is easily remedied with over-the-counter medications or that is short lived serves only as a minor disruption. However, pain that is all encompassing permeates a person's entire existence. Sometimes that pain is physical; sometimes it is psychological. One young mother of a profoundly mentally disabled 14-year-old girl spoke of "hurting so bad that my bones hurt."

As you know, some of our nursing interventions inflict pain. We ask patients to turn, deep-breathe, and cough after surgery, even though it hurts—a *lot*! We put needles in them, catheterize them, and get them out of bed when they would rather sleep. We pull off tape. We invade their physical personal space. We ask them questions about personal things, such as their bowel movements. It is a challenge—but essential—to be a comforting, healing presence when we have to do things that cause discomfort.

Loss

Loss is a disruption that cuts to the core of who we are—whether the loss of a job, the end of a romantic relationship, the death of a loved one, or the loss of youth, beauty, functioning, or identity. Most of us cling to a unique identity, which usually does *not* include gaining weight or getting wrinkles and gray hair, let alone being a "patient" or losing major bodily functions. The resulting period of significant disintegration may continue until the person either finds a way to cope with the loss or succeeds in reinterpreting the loss in a meaningful way. Toward the end of her battle with cancer, Treya Killam Wilber lost her near vision. One way she coped with this loss was by replacing her passion for reading with sitting at her window contemplating the mountains beyond (Wilber, 2000).

Loss of Sense of Self Many have written about the indignities people suffered in concentration camps, including nakedness, exposure to human excrement, and being treated like children, incapable of thoughtful judgment (Bettelheim, 1979; Frankl, 1959, 1962, 1984, 2004; Valladares, 2001). Those three indignities are crucial threats to a person's sense of self. Sadly, patients in healthcare institutions may also suffer those indignities. Think how patients feel who have to don a hospital gown and allow their body to be exposed for various tests or procedures, or how it feels to lose control of bladder or bowel function. One woman who was paralyzed as the result of a lesion on her spine indicated that one of the toughest things she had to deal with was having her daughter give her enemas and clean her up as if she were a baby. ♥ **iCare** As healthcare providers, we may easily forget how humiliating such "routine procedures" may be for the patient. You can help relieve the disruption of disease and injury when you respect patients' dignity, provide for privacy, and allow them to make choices regarding their care.

Permanent Loss If temporary losses are difficult, what about those that are permanent? C. S. Lewis (1961) wrote about his response to the death of his wife: "I know that the thing I want is exactly the thing I can never get. The old life, the jokes, the drinks, the arguments, the lovemaking, the tiny, heartbreaking commonplace" (p. 22). As nurses, we would like to "fix" everything. Though we can't "fix" the holes that are left when a person suffers a loss, we can be open and sensitive to his heart's cry.

Impending Death

It is easy for most of us to ignore that we all have 100% chance of dying eventually and live as though death were only a remote possibility. Lifton and Olson (1974) state that during middle age, even without the presence of life-threatening illness, people tend to become more aware of the compelling reality of death: "One's life is suddenly felt to be limited. . . . It also becomes apparent that . . . there will not be time for all one's projects" (p. 63).

As a nurse, you will care for clients who are living in disruption of the shadow of death. Some may be aware of their condition; others may choose to deny it, ignore it, or "fight it to the end" by trying a series of conventional and alternative therapies. Caring for dying clients makes us painfully aware of our own frailty and is one of the most difficult experiences you will face as a nurse. Chapter 17 provides further discussion of loss, grieving, and dying.

Competing Demands

Even in the normal flow of life, there are many competing demands. Taken independently, they may be easy to handle. Taken together, the cumulative effect wears us down. In times of illness, the other competing demands continue. Children need to be cared for. Aging parents may need care. Bills still need to be paid. Job responsibilities press in. One man with depression reported, "[T]he whole thing bundled together—one caused the other, which caused more and it was just a degenerative loop. . . . [O]ne thing feeds another, which feeds another, and so forth until you just constantly go down" (Smith, 1992, p. 104).

Sometimes people ignore health issues because the competing demands are too great. Symptoms may even go unnoticed because attention is scattered in so many directions and there is not enough time and energy to research one's symptoms, schedule a doctor's appointment, or follow through with treatments.

When an illness is acute, such as a broken bone, the stress is usually bearable because it is usually lasts for a set amount of time. Bettleheim (1979) states, "The worst calamity becomes bearable if one believes its end is in sight" (pp. 3–4). But when the illness is chronic, the competing demands can take a heavy toll. One woman took care of her husband who lived at home, his breathing assisted by a ventilator. She recounted the overwhelming burden she felt when, after 2 years, he was "no better and no worse. This could go on forever!" Although people came in to help, she felt she had to maintain constant alertness in case something went wrong with his ventilator, and she still had to meet many other demands and challenges each day.

As nurses, we sometimes find it easy to criticize how people deal with their situations. But it is so important to realize that the short amount of time that you spend with someone in a hospital or clinic or in a home visit is only one tiny fragment of the cumulative experience that patients and their families experience, sometimes unrelentingly for years on end.

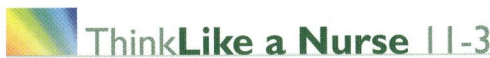

ThinkLike a Nurse 11-3

How might you assist your patient to maintain normalcy in spite of illness?

The Unknown

The following are examples of unknowns that patients experience:

- **Normal life changes.** Even normal life changes present challenges. For example, most parents bringing their first baby home from the hospital are in for plenty of surprises.
- **Anticipated life changes.** With some unknowns, there is time to investigate the potential problem and prepare. For example, if an expectant couple learns via amniocentesis (a prenatal test) that their child has a genetic defect, then during the remaining months of pregnancy they can read about the disorder and meet with other parents who have had children similarly affected.

- **Unexpected/sudden life changes.** However, injuries and illnesses can happen abruptly, with no chance to prepare for new realities. A woman described her experience of finding out she had cancer of the lung with metastasis: "It was on a . . . Friday—I got to feeling kind of bad—kind of like you had the flu or something, you know? . . . so I went to the doctor. . . . And . . . they started doin' tests on me—all kinds of tests—and found out I had cancer" (Smith, 1992, p. 107).

Imbalance

Our sense of justice tells us that when we are good, good things should happen. When we are bad, bad things should happen. The Buddhist concept of *karma* suggests that there is a fair balance between what one gives to life and what one receives. Thus, when we perceive that life has violated this rule, we experience the violation as a disruption and imbalance, as in these examples:

- **Death of a child.** Our sense of balance is perhaps most dramatically disturbed by the death of children. Such deaths are sometimes referred to as "out of order" because children (of any age) "should not" die before their parents.
- **Treatment failure.** Balance is also disrupted when patients, expecting that their painful and harrowing treatments "should" help them get better, do not get better. One young woman under treatment for advanced cancer described it like this: "It's just—you've been working hard . . . you're doin' what you're supposed to be doin' and focusing and all this and that—and your body is still not responding" (Smith, 1992, p. 111).

Have you seen the bumper sticker "Life is hard. And then you die"? Cynical perhaps, but most of us realize early in life that as much as we would like for everything to be fair, it is not going to happen. Knowing this intellectually, however, does not necessarily reduce the disruptive effect of the imbalance.

Isolation

How many times have you thought, "No one knows what I'm going through"? A sense of isolation or aloneness seems to accompany suffering. C. S. Lewis (1961) states, "You can't really share someone else's weakness, or fear, or pain" (p. 13). Vanauken (1977), in writing about the death of his young wife, reveals that it was not only suffering his loss, but having to go through the experience without her that made it so difficult: "Along with the emptiness . . . I kept wanting to tell her about it. We always told each other—that was what sharing was—and now this huge thing was happening to me, and I couldn't tell her" (p. 181).

The sense of aloneness reported by seriously ill clients is related in part to their actual physical separation from loved ones during treatments, hospitalizations, or clinic visits. But it also stems from their feeling that there is no one who is really "in their world." Having someone physically present does not necessarily remove the sense of aloneness:

When I lay here it's lonely—very, very lonely. Because [my daughter] can't just sit here and talk to me all the time. She's got wash to do, fold, and all that stuff. And then the kids to worry about. . . . The worst thing I've found about this whole disease is the loneliness. . . . Because your family can be with you and if they don't come and sit down and talk to you about different things, you're lonely. It's the loneliness that makes you sad inside. . . . It's like everybody's afraid . . . that maybe they're gonna catch what you got or something. (Smith, 1992)

KnowledgeCheck 11-2

Identify at least four factors that disrupt health.

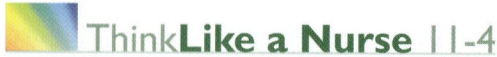

ThinkLike a Nurse 11-4

- What impact do disruptions have on your life?
- How could you apply the information about disruptions to the health of a community? To the health of a nation?

WHY DO PEOPLE EXPERIENCE ILLNESS DIFFERENTLY?

Why is it that people vary so greatly in terms of their response to life situations? Why do some people react to seemingly insurmountable problems with calmness and grace, while others fall apart over seemingly small disruptions? The human experience is too complex and interactive to fit it into neat little categories or derive a score for predicting how a person will respond to a given situation. There are several factors, however, that may influence an individual's responses to illness. We focus now on four such factors, beginning with the stages of illness behavior.

Stages of Illness Behavior

How people react to an illness depends in part on their illness stage. Suchman (1972) identified five stages of illness behaviors that people move through as they cope with disruptions to health, discussed in the following sections:

Experiencing Symptoms Symptoms are a signal that illness has begun. If the symptoms are recognizable, such as runny nose, sneezing, and a cough, you may identify the problem as a common cold and turn to previously used remedies. Common problems rarely progress beyond this stage. However, if the symptoms are unusual, severe, or overwhelming, you may progress to the next stage.

Sick Role Behavior When you have identified yourself as ill, you assume the sick role, which relieves you from normal duties, such as work, school, or tasks at home. In Western biomedical culture, the prevailing view is that sick persons are not responsible for their illnesses and that a curative process outside the person is needed to restore wellness. We believe that the sick person has a duty to try to get well, to seek healthcare, and to cooperate with the care providers (Cockerham, 2015). The severity of the symptoms and anticipated length of illness determine whether you will progress further along the stages of illness.

Seeking Professional Care To reach this stage, you must determine that you are ill and that professional care is required to treat the illness. Persons who seek professional care are asking for validation of their illness, explanations for their symptoms, appropriate treatment, and information about the anticipated length of illness. Healthcare professionals often bypass this stage, relying on themselves to identify and treat their own problem. This is not always the best course of action because it is difficult to be objective when examining yourself.

Dependence on Others When you accept the diagnosis and treatment of the healthcare provider, you typically also accept the need to depend on others. The severity of the illness and the type of treatment determine the extent of dependence. This may be limited to listening to the provider's instructions, filling the prescription, and following directions given in the office. However, illness that requires hospitalization is often associated with dependence on nursing staff and hospital personnel for activities of daily living, medications, and treatments. Some people easily make the transition to dependence; others remain as independent as possible even in the face of severe illness. Personal characteristics and values play a large role in determining how each of us will respond to the challenges of being dependent.

Recovery The final stage of illness is called **recovery.** The person gradually resumes independence and returns to normal roles and functioning. In minor illness, this is usually a return to the status quo. Severe illnesses may require a redefinition of optimum function. The greater the change in health status, the more difficult this transition will be. Learning to manage a chronic illness is the equivalent of a cure in an acute illness (Parsons, 1975). Both represent the recovery stage.

Safe, Effective Nursing Care

Chronic Illness and Self-Management Through Telehealth

Chapter Key Concepts: Health, Illness

Competency: Embrace/Incorporate Technological Advances

Background. Telehealth encourages patients to be in more control of their health and to take ownership of their condition (Pearce, 2012). Healthcare is transitioning to a focus on patient self-management. Telecommunication provides a strategy for self-management by empowering patients and helping them feel more secure in monitoring and managing their care. In chronic conditions there is a window of opportunity for remote monitoring to detect health changes sooner and to initiate earlier interventions (Kim, Kim, Kim, et al., 2012).

Scenario.
A patient with long-standing chronic obstructive pulmonary disease (COPD) frequently experiences exacerbations requiring hospital admission. Because the patient lives in a remote rural area he often delays seeking healthcare. At the last clinic visit, the nurse provided the patient with home-monitoring devices that connected him to telehealth services.

Think about it:
➤ What advantages can telehealth provide for a patient with chronic illness?
➤ How might telehealth increase the patient's self-care management of COPD?
➤ Discuss how informatics (specifically telehealth) can impact an individual's position on the health–illness continuum.

The Nature of the Illness

The nature of the illness (e.g., whether the illness is acute or chronic) affects the way persons react to disruptions and respond to illness.

Acute Illness An **acute illness** occurs suddenly and lasts for a limited amount of time. Acute illnesses, such as a cold, flu, or viral infection, may be minor and require no formal health-care. More serious acute illness, such as strep throat, may require a visit to a health provider for treatment or even hospitalization or surgery, as in cholecystitis (gallbladder inflammation secondary to gallstone formation) or pyelonephritis (infection of the kidney). Although hospitalization and surgery can be traumatic, in each case the person is expected to recover. In acute illness, a person may experience the disruptions of pain, competing demands, and the unknown. However, an end is in sight. Relief is expected.

Chronic Illness In contrast, **chronic illness** lasts for a long period of time, usually 6 months or more, often for a lifetime. Chronic illness requires the person to make life changes. These changes might be regular visits to the clinic or hospital, daily injections, or lifestyle modifications such as a low-fat diet or smoking cessation. Common chronic illnesses include AIDS, diabetes mellitus, rheumatoid arthritis, and hypertension. Because of the lengthy period of illness, people with chronic disease often experience periods of remission or exacerbation.

- A **remission** occurs when symptoms are minimal to none.
- An **exacerbation** ("flare-up") occurs when symptoms intensify.

Clients with chronic illness often complain about the unrelenting nature of their health problems. A person with chronic illness may experience virtually all of the disruptions identified earlier. Box 11-2 identifies some interesting facts about chronic conditions.

Hardiness

Why does one client who drinks, smokes, overeats, and avoids exercise live into his 90s, yet another client who "follows all the rules" dies of a sudden heart attack at age 39? Our bodies do not react to the same stressors in the same way. One factor that may contribute to this difference is the person's hardiness.

Will to Live Hardiness has been described as developing a very strong positive force to live—and enjoying the ride (Fig. 11-4)! A man with heart problems said, "I guess everybody that's in the situation, who has to fight to live, and has learned the mental wizardry of it, you know, to make yourself want to live on. But if you want to, you develop this—this very, very strong positive force to make it go" (Smith, 1992, p. 131). Seigel (1986) reported a study conducted by London researchers that revealed a 10-year survival rate of 75% "among cancer patients who reacted to the diagnosis with a 'fighting spirit'" compared with a 22% survival rate "among those who responded with 'stoic acceptance' or feelings of helplessness or hopelessness" (p. 25).

Adapting to Change Another aspect of hardiness is the willingness to draw on resources within oneself or from others to break out of old patterns of living when life situations change. When disruption hits, some people don't have the cognitive, communicative, creative, and spiritual resources they need to make life changes, and they just give up. Hardy individuals are willing to seek out information and take the initiative in dealing with life situations rather than sitting back and letting someone else control their lives. Ironically, some

---

BOX 11-2 ■ Facts About Chronic Conditions

- More than 90 million Americans live with chronic conditions.
- Chronic conditions account for about 70% of all deaths in the United States.

  - About 80% of older adults have at least one chronic condition; 50% have at least two.
  - Approximately 6% of adults older than age 65 have a diagnosable depressive illness.
- The top three risks factors for functional decline are cognitive impairment, depression, and disease burden.
- The largest declines in functional abilities are associated with arthritis of the hip or knee, sciatica, and chronic pulmonary diseases.
- Arthritis affects one in five U.S. adults; for more than 40% of those, arthritis limits their activities.
- About 35% of the adult population and 17% of children and adolescents aged 2 to 19 years are obese (CDC, 2015a, 2015b).
- In a large sample of Medicare beneficiaries, the following were the most frequent chronic physical conditions:

Hypertension (55%)	Depression (16%)
Hyperlipidemia (45%)	Alzheimer's disease/dementia (10%)
Arthritis (29%)	Emphysema, asthma, or COPD (11.2%)
Ischemic heart disease (27%)	Any cancer (other than skin cancer) (8%)
Diabetes (13.7%)	Atrial fibrillation (8%)
Chronic kidney disease (17%)	Osteoporosis (6%)
Heart failure (14%)	Stroke (4%)

Sources: Centers for Disease Control and Prevention. (2015a,). Adult obesity facts. Retrieved from http://www.cdc.gov/obesity/data/adult.html; Centers for Disease Control and Prevention. (2015b). Child obesity facts. Retrieved from http://www.cdc.gov/obesity/data/childhood.html; Centers for Medicare & Medicaid Services. (2014). *Chronic conditions among Medicare beneficiaries.* Baltimore, MD: Chart Book; Peikes, D., Chen, A., Schore, J., et al. (2009). Effects of care coordination on hospitalization, quality of care, and health care expenditures among Medicare beneficiaries. *JAMA, 301*(6), 603–618; Stuck, A. E., Walthert, J. M., Nikolaus, T., et al. (1999). Risk factors for functional status decline in community living elderly people: A systematic literature review. *Social Science and Medicine, 48*(4), 445–469; Wiktorsson, S., Runeson, B., Skoog, I., et al. (2010). Attempted suicide in the elderly: Characteristics of suicide attempters 70 years and older and a general population comparison group. *American Journal of Geriatric Psychology, 18*(1), 57.

---

people survive and thrive during times of adversity. Those who see themselves as hardy tend to approach disruptions with an "I can deal with this" attitude.

The Intensity, Duration, and Multiplicity of the Disruption

Everyone has limits. For healthcare providers, too many demands over too long a period of time can lead to *burnout,* a feeling of being overwhelmed and demoralized. For clients and their families, dealing with the cumulative effect of illness and other life disruptions can break down what might otherwise be effective coping skills. After reaching a breaking point, their responses may not be typical of what they usually have demonstrated.

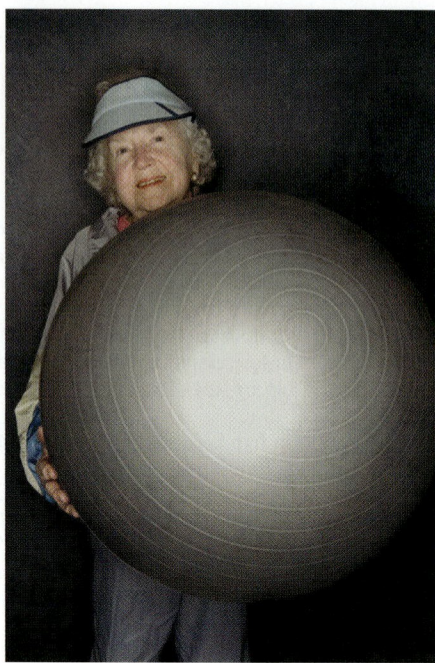

FIGURE 11-4 Hardiness has been described as developing a very strong positive force to live—and enjoying the fight!

KnowledgeCheck 11-3

- Identify the factors that affect how a person responds to the disruptions of illness.
- Define *hardiness*.

PracticalKnowledge
knowing **how**

In the preceding section, you learned how people experience health, wellness, and illness. In this section, you will learn how these concepts can be applied to your nursing practice.

USING THE NURSING PROCESS TO PROMOTE HEALTH

Throughout this textbook, you will learn to use the nursing process to help clients deal with a variety of health problems. But how does the nursing process relate to the broader aspects of health and illness described in this chapter? Overall, it involves helping clients—regardless of the type of health problem—to look within themselves to develop creative ways to deal with the realities they are facing.

Patients may fail to follow a proposed healthcare regimen if healthcare providers develop a plan of care that has no cultural or personal relevance for the patient (or family). Perhaps the plan does not consider the knowledge level of the patient or caregiver, or perhaps it is not feasible in terms of available support, time, energy, finances, or location. Patients may leave a hospital setting *against medical advice,* thereby endangering their chances of recovery. They may believe the treatment offered them will not help or that the illness is preferable to the proposed treatment. Noncompliance often occurs because the effort, inconvenience, or pain involved with a therapeutic plan of care is too much for them to handle.

Remember that people probably do not refuse to carry out a plan of care simply out of stubbornness, hostility toward healthcare providers, or wanton disregard for their own welfare. The challenge for nurses is to develop an individualized plan of care in collaboration with patients, based on mutual goals and respect.

ASSESSMENT NP

In looking at an individual's health status, it is easy to focus on the measurable aspects. Physical needs obviously are crucial, but competing issues may be present and cause the client to view the therapeutic interventions as irrelevant or even disruptive.

What Does It Mean to Communicate Care and Concern?

KEY POINT: *Obtaining data about the psychosocial, emotional, and spiritual aspects of health requires a level of communication that goes beyond a neat list of skills. Communicating*

Toward Evidence-Based Practice

Rodin, D., & Stewart, D. E. (2012). Resilience in elderly survivors of child maltreatment. *SAGE Open, 2*(2), 1–9.

This study of older adults was conducted to better understand the factors that contribute to resilience (positive adaptation of individuals, despite exposure to adversity) in the elderly population. In this qualitative study of nine survivors of childhood abuse, resilience was found to be high, despite earlier trauma and the subsequent challenges of old age. The authors found that active engagement in relationships and in valued activities were the most often mentioned contributors to resilience.

Jaser, S. S., & White, L. E. (2011). Coping and resilience in adolescents with type 1 diabetes. *Child: Care, Health and Development, 37*(3), 335–342.

Thirty adolescents between the ages of 10 and 16 with type 1 diabetes and their mothers completed questionnaires on

adolescents' coping strategy use, social competence, and quality of life. Greater use of coping strategies (such as problem-solving and emotional expression) was associated with higher social competence scores, better quality of life, and better metabolic control. Adolescents who reported a lack of coping strategies (instead using withdrawal or denial) reported lower social competence and poorer metabolic control of their diabetes.

How do the results of these studies apply to the concept of health as presented in this chapter?

Identify ways in which the methods and findings could be applied to other populations.

 Go to Davis Advantage, Resources, Chapter 11, **Toward Evidence-Based Practice Suggested Responses,** on DavisAdvantage.

genuine care, concern, and sensitivity comes from who you are as a person, not from assuming a professional persona (putting on your "nurse hat"). The following are aspects of high level communication:

Settling In Your initial approach to a patient creates a climate that determines the level of communication that takes place. The patient is probably in a new environment, and your tone, words, and facial expressions can bring comfort and ease. Nurses can be in new situations too, and taking a few moments to settle in to the situation can be helpful in establishing a therapeutic relationship and facilitating communication.

Attuning Being maximally attentive is another key factor in facilitating communication. Most people are hungry for someone to listen to them. Often listeners are so busy thinking about what they want to say that they fail to really listen. Try to focus on what the patient or family has to say instead of thinking ahead to what you want to ask next.

Acceptance Another vital aspect of communicating is acceptance—acceptance of appearance, lifestyles, ways of coping, and values. You might ask, "How can I be accepting when there are aspects of this person that go against my entire value system?" Accepting is not the same as "agreeing with." You can accept people as valued, creative, unique individuals despite their differences from your own ways of being. This view of acceptance does not mean that people should not be held accountable for their actions—for example, in cases of domestic violence and child abuse. It does mean, though, that in your role as a caregiver, you must convey an attitude of accepting the intrinsic value of life—in whatever forms that life takes.

Enjoying Perhaps even more difficult than accepting is the concept of enjoying. You will come into contact with a wide array of individuals, many of whom are different from people you have grown up around and have come to know and enjoy. A challenge for you is to broaden the repertoire of people you enjoy: to see and enjoy commonalities among individuals seemingly so different and to recognize and appreciate the pathos of suffering in the unique experience of each person.

How Can I Be a Better Communicator?

Settling in, attuning, respecting, and enjoying—certainly this is not a step-by-step process, but each aspect is vital to creating a climate for the openness and communication needed for assessment.

Take Time to Communicate You might argue that the healthcare environment does not allow time for such a high level of attentiveness. Consider, though, how much time is spent in delivering nursing care. As a full-spectrum nurse, you will assess patients continually while thinking, doing, and caring for your patients. In fact, the physical contact involved in carrying out nursing procedures seems to break down barriers of communication. Nurses hold a unique opportunity in "being with" individuals during difficult life situations; indeed, Benner and Wrubel (1989) state that expert nurses call this the "privileged place of nursing" (p. xi).

Identify the Patient's Main Concern One way to approach assessment, whether in the outpatient, acute care, long-term care, or home setting, is to ask the patient, "What is the biggest concern you are dealing with today?" You may have a plan of care that addresses areas that you know to be important, but it may fall far short of meeting your patient's needs if you have not addressed the concern that is fundamental to your patient.

Develop Your Observation Skills In addition to communicating, developing your observation skills will enable you to assess your patients more fully. Watching your patient's responses to you and your care; observing the presence or absence of visitors and the effect on your patients; and observing signs of religious or cultural practices that have significance all provide important information about your patient's strengths and needs.

KnowledgeCheck 11-4

Compare and contrast attuning, acceptance, and enjoying.

ANALYSIS/NURSING DIAGNOSIS NP

Several of the nursing diagnosis labels identified by NANDA-I relate to health issues discussed in this chapter. Some examples are Anxiety, Caregiver Role Strain, Deficient Knowledge, and Spiritual Distress. An analysis of your assessment data should also provide the information needed to describe related causal factors, such as:

- Spiritual Distress related to fear of impending death
- Situational Low Self-esteem related to loss of job secondary to frequent absences for chemotherapy

PLANNING OUTCOMES/EVALUATION NP

Goals and outcomes should be both realistic and valued by the patient and family. When you set goals in the broader dimension of health and illness (as in this chapter), it is much harder to be specific in describing expected outcomes and time frames. As a nurse, your role is to help the patient (or family member) envision acceptable outcomes and to set smaller, realistic goals so that the patient recognizes progress. For example, an older woman caring for a spouse with Alzheimer's disease may have a nursing diagnosis of Caregiver Role Strain related to care of spouse with dementia. Together you would establish acceptable goals and break them down into realistic steps. You also would identify outcomes to indicate that the caregiver actually experiences a reduction in strain, such as being able to sleep or having time to pursue meaningful activities.

PLANNING INTERVENTIONS/ IMPLEMENTATION NP

The ideal approach is to draw on patient and family strengths to help achieve the desired outcomes. In the preceding example of the older adult caregiver, you would discuss with her the options available to provide support, but she would identify which options were acceptable to her and her spouse. In the stress of illness, patients and families may not recognize the strengths and creative abilities that they bring to a situation. **KEY POINT:** *Part of the art of nursing is to envision strengths and potential in patients and families, just as an artful teacher might recognize a "spark" in a child and encourage that child to learn and grow.*

ThinkLike a Nurse 11-5

- How can you use the concepts of health when you are admitting a patient to a hospital setting? To a clinic? To an emergency department? To a rehabilitation or long-term care setting? In initiating home care?
- What questions can you ask or what observations can you make to help you gain information about individuals' health strategies, disruptions to health, and factors contributing to their responses to disruptions?
- How would you consider health concepts in planning for patients' discharge from healthcare settings?

How Can I Honor Each Client's Unique Health/Illness Experience?

As a nurse, you can be an instrument of healing in a hurtful world. However, being an instrument of healing does not come automatically with your nursing license. Nor does it allow you the luxury of learning a single approach and applying it to every client. It means you must cultivate a healing presence by listening and in addition by:

- Being maximally attentive
- Being aware of your own gifts and limitations of communication
- Being willing to learn from those in your care
- Recognizing and respecting others' ways of coping
- Enjoying others for who they are

♥ **iCare**   Patients may be impressed by your skill and knowledge and amazed by the healthcare technology used to diagnose and treat their illnesses. However, what they most often remember, perhaps through the rest of their lives, is that person who connected with them in a very special way. One man, quadriplegic for 26 years following a car accident in his teens, spoke of a senior nursing student who cared for him during his initial hospitalization. He said that after 26 years, he not only still remembered her but also still could sense the warmth of her caring presence.

During times of vulnerability, people seem acutely attuned to those who are helpful to them and also to those who slight them in hurtful ways, whether intentionally or not. What a challenge this creates for nurses! In this section, we discuss steps you can take to prepare yourself for responding to your clients in ways that are meaningful and healing to them.

Examine Life's Uncertainties

Wellness is a balancing act between living in the mostly known present and the mostly unknown future. Encourage your clients to make active decisions that positively affect their future. You do not have control over a drunk driver who sails across the median and hits you head-on, but you do have control over getting the brakes on your car fixed or wearing your seat belt. Likewise, you do not know whether you will develop cancer or heart disease, but you can take responsibility for learning and practicing prevention and detection of problems.

Making health-promoting lifestyle choices is important, but it cannot protect us from risk. Significant life experiences, such as getting married, having children, investing in friendships, venturing into business, and selecting a profession, all involve risk. Making a commitment to *anything* is a risk. Each person has a different "risk-comfort range." Some are willing to risk little, have fewer disappointments, and less sparkling achievements. To others, security is not as important, and they are comfortable taking greater risks.

In *A Severe Mercy*, Sheldon Vanauken (1977) writes about finding and losing a great love. He reasons: "The joy would be worth the pain—if, indeed, they went together. If there were a choice . . . between, on the one hand, the heights and the depths and, on the other hand, some sort of safe, cautious middle way, he, for one, here and now chose the heights and the depths" (p. 9). He did, indeed, find a great love, and when he lost his wife at an early age, he was able to accept their time together as one of his life's greatest blessings. As a nurse, you will face many uncertainties and dilemmas. You will certainly face new experiences and challenges, situations you thought you never would have to deal with. You will observe pain, suffering, and death. You may never understand the apparent unfairness of it all. But often life brings new meaning when it takes a different direction from the one planned. For example, a couple formerly embittered over their third miscarriage found joy in adopting two children with disabilities.

You will also be privileged to witness many joys. Some might even qualify as minor triumphs: a patient taking his first steps after major surgery, a pathology report that isn't as bad as feared, or even a peaceful death that brings closure to a grieving family. As you move from novice to expert, you may find that such witnessing causes you to stop questioning life's uncertainties and instead to start treasuring them.

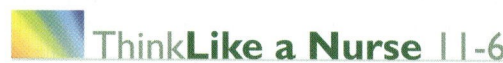

ThinkLike a Nurse 11-6

- What uncertainties have you struggled with?
- What approaches have proved effective for you in dealing with uncertainties?

Envision Wellness for Your Clients and Yourself

Wherever there is a dream, there is someone there to tell you it can't be done, or at least not by you. There is something to be said, however, for "envisioning" wellness for your clients and yourself. Remember Evelyn (Meet Your Patient)? If her nurses had labeled her as debilitated and close to death, how would that have affected her? In contrast, their acceptance of her vision of herself as well and full of life supports her and aids her healing. In the same way, think of how you view your own health. Is the life you envision for yourself characterized by zest and vigor? What are your family relationships like? What are your values? Does your work give meaning and purpose to your life? The wellness that you envision for yourself can be the blueprint for what you want to become. The skeptic in you might say, "What if I do everything that I know to do to maintain a healthy life but I still have a heart attack at 45?" As we have seen, life is full of uncertainties. That does not mean that you have to stop envisioning. Instead, use *flexible envisioning*, adjusting your goals and dreams to each new reality. Health does not mean always getting your first choice. Part of health is being able to dream a new dream, starting over if you need to, but always envisioning that there is something worth striving for.

Establish Trust at Your First Patient Contact

When patients are admitted to a hospital or ambulatory care facility, your role as a full-spectrum nurse is to support them in their transition from wellness to illness, in dealing with the unknown, and in adjusting to a new environment. The relationship and trust you establish in your first contact with patients can go a long way toward relieving their anxiety and preserving the energy needed for healing. Take time to get to know your client. Try to set a tone of caring, respect, and understanding.

You can make the transition smoother for patients if you are prepared. The following activities should be incorporated into your nursing care:

- **Prepare the room.** A room that is prepared for the client conveys a message of acceptance. Room preparation depends on the type of unit or facility, the client's needs, and the anticipated treatment. See Clinical Insight 11-1.

- **Greet the client.** Gather basic information ahead of time, such as name, diagnosis, and anticipated length of stay. Imagine how it might feel if you were a new patient and you heard the staff say, "Who's this? I didn't know we were getting another admit. How am I supposed to take care of this one, too?"
- **Introduce yourself to the client and family.** Explain who you are. Don't be afraid to tell a client that you are a nursing student. Many clients are aware that students have more time to spend with them.
- **Orient the client to the room and the unit.** Make sure the client knows how to use the bed, the call light, and any equipment that you expect him to use. Show the client the location of the restroom. If you will be measuring the client's intake and output, tell him so during your orientation. If the client is alert, he may be able to assist you with these measures. Remember that one of the disruptions associated with illness is anxiety about the unknown. If you tell your client what to expect, you help to minimize his anxiety.
- **Gather a health history.** In Chapter 3, you learned about assessment. Chapter 21 provides a step-by-step approach to physical assessment. Be sure to include in your health history the client's expectations and concerns.
- **Establish a relationship with the client.** Take time to get to know your client. Try to set a tone of caring, respect, and understanding.

For detailed directions on how to admit a client to a hospital unit, including orienting the client to the room and gathering a health history, see Procedure 11-1.

Provide a Healing Presence

♥ iCare   Part of what you do as a healing presence will never show up in a written care plan, but it may be the most important aspect of care that you have to offer. A statement by a young woman undergoing chemotherapy illustrates the difference a nurse's healing presence made:

> *The nursing care I got was in response to the physical symptoms I showed. If I was not feeling good, they were sympathetic with me, you know. . . . But it was nothing further than that. There was no exploration of feelings or anything like that.*
>
> *Some of them were—seemed to be very caring. [One nurse] . . . was just a really nice person. And I remember one time that I was throwing up dreadfully. . . . I rang for her and I said, 'I'm sorry,' and she was almost crying and she said, 'No, I'm sorry you have to do this—you must feel awful.' And she was just very empathetic with it, and I felt like, you know, I wasn't infringing upon her to make her empty my emesis basin or anything like that. (Smith, 1992, pp. 233–234)*

Maintain Trust During Transitions

Just as you help patients to transition into illness, your support is important in helping them transition to other units within the agency, other agencies, or home. As discussed in Chapter 5, planning for discharge begins with the admission assessment and continues until the patient is well enough to go home or is transferred to another unit or facility.

Handoffs and Transfers

Patients may transfer from one unit to another when their health status changes. For example, a patient on a general nursing unit may be transferred to an intensive care unit when he develops *sepsis* (a generalized, systemic infection that is often fatal). Patients may transfer from the hospital to a long-term care facility or rehabilitation center when they no longer require an acute care hospital or when their changed health status means that family members will not be able to care for him at home. A patient residing in a long-term care facility may be transferred to a hospital when he becomes acutely ill.

When the patient is transferred, he must adjust to a new environment, new routines, and new caregivers. This is yet another disruption for the patient and family. You can help by ensuring that the transition is smooth and that there is continuity of care. Ensure the patient's comfort and safety, provide for teaching needs, and communicate with the agency or unit sending or receiving the patient. The process at the time of transfer is similar. For detailed information on transfer reports (e.g., SBAR), see Chapter 18. Also refer to Procedures 11-2 and 11-3.

Discharge From the Healthcare Facility

As much as patients usually look forward to being discharged, this, too, is a disruption. Patients are discharged when the outcomes of care are met. However, they are often dependent on family members for care and treatments they cannot manage alone. Inability to assume self-care can be stressful and anxiety producing. **KEY POINT:** *Successful discharge planning must begin at first patient assessment on admission to the facility.* The same conditions that require a formal discharge plan frequently also indicate the need for referrals for posthospital care in the community. Review Discharge Planning in Chapter 5, as needed.

Procedures for discharge vary among agencies. There may be a discharge planner or case manager to coordinate the transition to another agency or to home, but often you will need to manage the discharge. You can help by communicating and coordinating care and services, and by teaching the patient and caregivers about the continuing care the patient needs (Figs. 11-5 and 11-6.) Also see Procedure 11-4 to learn more about discharging patients from a healthcare facility.

KnowledgeCheck 11-5

Explain how you can promote patient trust during admissions, transfers, and discharges.

Is a Healthy Life Attainable?

The concepts suggested in this chapter for ways to live a healthy life did not come from people who had easy lives. These themes were teased from literature, autobiographies, and interviews with people who were dealing with life situations that would be viewed as difficult from anyone's standpoint. However, in the midst of their circumstances, they were very much involved in *living*. Ripples or even waves of disruption or despair came into their lives, but through it all they evolved an overriding sense of a life worth pursuing. This can be true for you as a nurse and also for those privileged to be under your care.

As a nurse, you offer your personal health and strength to your patients and their families every day. If you barely have enough physical, emotional, and spiritual strength to manage your own stressors, you will not have much available to offer others who are depleted. This is why it is so important for you to nurture yourself in all aspects of your life, to balance learning how to care for others with caring for yourself, to develop yourself as a healing presence in this world.

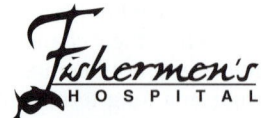

Discharge Assessment/Instructions

Date of Discharge	Time of Discharge	Mode of Discharge ☐ Ambulatory ☐ Wheelchair ☐ Stretcher ☐ Ambulance	Accompanied by:
Belongings sent with patient/family ☐ Yes ☐ No		Personal Medications sent with patient/family ☐ Yes ☐ No	
Temp	P	Discharge Destination ☐ Home ☐ AMA ☐ Facility_____ ☐ Home Health	Transfer Information Sent ☐ Yes ☐ No
R	BP		

Special Instructions

Patient Assessment and Health Status									
	Yes	**No**		**Yes**	**No**			**Yes**	**No**
Afebrile	☐	☐	Skin Intact	☐	☐	Hygiene		☐	☐
Able to live independently	☐	☐	Eating Well	☐	☐	Self-Care		☐	☐
Pain Controlled	☐	☐	Adequate Hydration	☐	☐	Assist		☐	☐
Oriented	☐	☐				Total Care		☐	☐
Appropriate Behavior	☐	☐				Adequate Elimination		☐	☐
Functions Independently	☐	☐							

Additional Comments:

Weight monitoring daily   Avoid all tobacco products

Instructions
Diet ☐ No Restrictions
Activity ☐ No Restrictions
Special Equipment/Treatment ☐ No Restrictions
Discharge Medications (Name, Amount, Special Instructions) ☐ No Meds   See Patient Education
Special Instructions/Discharge Summary **Call MD or go to the ER if symptoms worsen**

☐ Pt or Caregiver given instructions about and counseled on potential for drug-food interactions

Physician Follow-up Appointment	Outpatient Visit
Referral ☐ None Required	

I have received all personal belongings.
I have received a copy and understand the above Instructions.
I have received a copy of the Patient Education form.

	Patient Identification
_____ **Signature/Responsible Party**	
_____ **Physician/Nurse Signature Date**	

0916065

FIGURE 11-5 Discharge assessment/instructions.

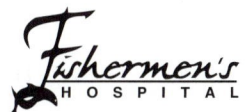

3301 Overseas Highway, Marathon, FL 33050 • Ph 305-743-5533 • Fax 305-743-3962

Allergies/Reactions	No known drug allergies ☐			IN-PATIENT Circle Y to continue or N to not continue and sign below to authenticate order.		AT DISCHARGE Circle Y to continue at same dose or N to not continue or document any changes in dose.		
MEDICATION NAME (Include Herbal, OTC, Vitamins)	**Dose / Route / Freq**	**Reason Taken**	**LAST DOSE DATE/TIME**	**Continue on Admission**		**Continue at home on same dose**		**Continue with the following changes:**
Patient takes no medication ☐								
				Y	N	Y	N	
				Y	N	Y	N	
				Y	N	Y	N	
				Y	N	Y	N	
				Y	N	Y	N	
				Y	N	Y	N	
				Y	N	Y	N	
				Y	N	Y	N	
				Y	N	Y	N	
				Y	N	Y	N	
				Y	N	Y	N	
				Y	N	Y	N	
				Y	N	Y	N	
				Y	N	Y	N	

Source-of-Medication list *(check all used):*
___ **Bottles/List**
___ **Patient/Family**
___ **Retail pharmacy**_____
_____
___ **MD office records**
___ **Previous discharge medical record**
___ **Medication Administration Record from**_____
_____
___ **Med Reconciliation Form**
Meds:
___ **Sent home with**_____
___ **Removed**
    Sent to Pharmacy for approval

New medications prescribed for patient discharge:

Meds	Dose / Route / Freq	Reason

ADMITTING NURSE SIGNATURE	DATE	DISCHARGE NURSE SIGNATURE	DATE

Patient Education Form

Page ____ of ____

FORM N-100, Rev. 12-07   White: Chart   Yellow: Patient

FIGURE 11-6 Patient education form.

CLINICALREASONING

The questions and exercises in this section allow you to practice the kind of thinking you will use as a full-spectrum nurse. Critical-thinking questions usually have more than one right answer, so we do not provide "correct answers" for these features. It is more important to develop your nursing judgment than to just cover content. You will learn by discussing the questions with your peers. If you are still unsure, see the Davis Advantage chapter resources for suggested responses.

Caring for the Nguyens

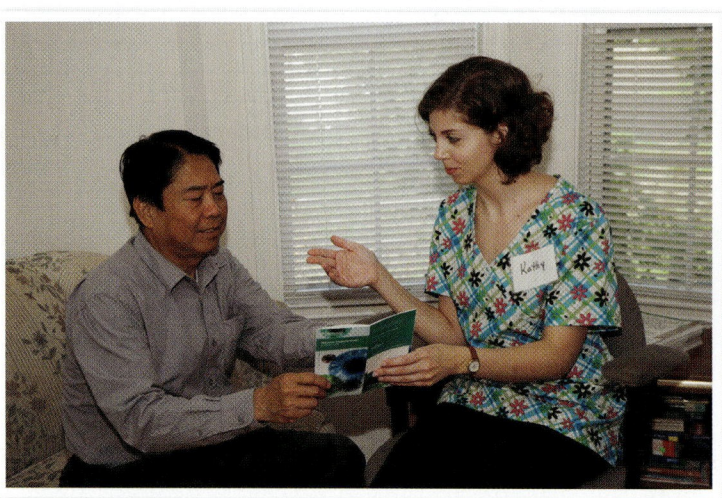

Nam Nguyen has recently been diagnosed with hypertension, obesity, and degenerative joint disease. He is struggling with these diagnoses. He tells his wife, Yen, "I feel so old now. These are the kind of things my parents are dealing with." At a clinic visit, Nam tells you, "It's hard to think of myself as sick. I've been depressed ever since Zach told me about his findings. Now he's asked me to get some lab work. I'm afraid he may find even more problems."

A. Identify the disruptions that Mr. Nguyen must deal with based on these diagnoses. Explain your reasons for choosing these disruptions.

B. How would you evaluate Mr. Nguyen's health status? Review the sections The Health–Illness Continuum and Dunn's Health Grid, as needed.

C. What kinds of activities could you suggest to Nam to improve his health status?

D. What stage of illness behavior is Mr. Nguyen exhibiting in regard to his recent medical diagnoses? (See the sections The Health–Illness Continuum and Dunn's Health Grid, earlier in this chapter.)

Applying the **Full-Spectrum Nursing Model**_____

PATIENT SITUATION

Recall Evelyn (Meet Your Patient). Evelyn is 87 years old and has lived in a nursing home for the past 5 years. She suffers from CHF, hypertension, diabetes, macular degeneration resulting in near blindness, a severe hearing deficit, urinary incontinence, and immobility resulting from a hip fracture. Despite these limitations, she keeps current in the lives of all of her family members and friends. At the nursing home, staff members confide in Evelyn and she knows about their children, their romances, and the gossip around the nursing home. Whenever there is an election, she makes sure that she gets to vote. She "reads" every audio book she can get her hands on.

Recently Evelyn was admitted to the hospital in severe CHF. When leaving the nursing home, she told her pastor, "I don't want to die yet. I'm having too much fun!" You notice that the papers from the nursing home do not contain an advance directive, and it was not mentioned in their report to you.

THINKING

1. *Critical Thinking (Considering Alternatives):*
   a. What are some possible reasons that there is no advance directive?
   b. Which of those seems most likely to you?
   c. How might you find out about the status of Evelyn's advance directive?

DOING

2. *Nursing Process (Nursing Diagnosis):* On the care plan from the nursing home, there were two nursing diagnoses:
   Urge Urinary Incontinence related to difficulty ambulating to bathroom
   Impaired Skin Integrity related to immobility and incontinence
   Which of these can you remove from the care plan for now? Explain your decision.

CARING

3. *Self-Knowledge:* The next day, despite aggressive treatment, Evelyn's condition worsens. She is not responding to verbal stimuli and her oxygen level is decreasing. There is discussion about putting her on a ventilator.

a. What would you be feeling?

b. If Evelyn has an advance directive that says "No ventilator," how would that change your feelings?

c. If there is an advance directive that says, "Do everything possible to keep me alive," how would that change your feelings?

Note: We are not asking you what you would do; rather, consider and describe how you would feel.

PracticalKnowledge: clinical application

Practical knowledge in this chapter means using the nursing process and skills to apply what you have learned about how people experience health, wellness and illness.

CLINICAL INSIGHTS

Clinical Insight 11-1 ➤ **Preparing the Room for a Newly Admitted Patient**

Delegation

As a general rule, these tasks can be delegated to nursing assistive personnel (NAPs). The nurse is responsible for evaluating and supervising, as well as for setting up special equipment (although the NAP may obtain it from storage).

Clean the Room

Agencies differ; however, it is common for the housekeeping department to clean the room and change the bed linens when a patient is discharged, so you should find the room ready for your preparations. The rest of these guidelines assume that fact.

Prepare the Bed

- Position the bed according to patient status. If the patient is ambulatory, put the bed in the lowest position and lock the wheels. If the patient will arrive on a stretcher, place the bed at stretcher height.
- If necessary, rearrange the furniture to allow easy access to the bed.
- Fold back the top linens to "open" the bed (see the figure).
  The patient may need to go to bed immediately, so it should be ready when she arrives.

Prepare Routine Supplies

- Most agencies have an admission pack containing a bath basin, soap, lotion, tissues, water pitcher, and drinking glass. Open it and put it in the room.
- Place a hospital gown on the bed and nonslip footwear by the bedside. Patients may choose to wear their own sleep clothing, though.

Prepare Equipment

You will need the following:

- A stethoscope, thermometer, and blood pressure cuff in the room for taking vital signs
- A scale for measuring and weighing the patient
- Bedpan and urinal if the patient is not ambulatory; possibly a bedside commode
- A clean-catch urine specimen container if laboratory work has not already been done
- Set up and check special equipment (e.g., oxygen, suction, cardiac monitor, pulse oximeter, IV pump).

Prepare the Environment

Turn on the lights and adjust the room temperature. Open or close curtains, as needed.

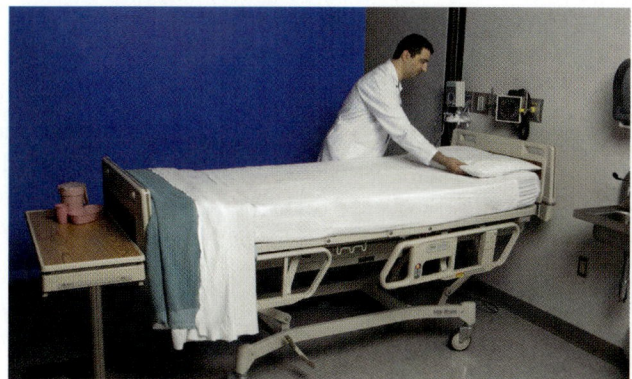

PracticalKnowledge
procedures

The procedures and the preceding clinical insight in this chapter will help you admit, transfer, and discharge patients in such a way that you can begin to establish trust at the very first contact.

Procedure 11-1 ■ Admitting a Patient to a Nursing Unit

➤ For steps to follow in *all* procedures, refer to the Universal Steps for All Procedures found on the page facing the inside back cover.

Equipment

- Identifying armband (if this has not been supplied in the admissions department)
- Patient's chart, including physician's orders and nursing admission record
- Thermometer, blood pressure cuff, and stethoscope
- Scales for height and weight
- Gown
- Admission pack (e.g., water pitcher, soap, comb, toothbrush, mouthwash, and facial tissues)
- Nursing care plan or clinical pathway, if one has already been made
- Hospital brochures, Patient Care Partnership, and other forms
- Admission assessment form

Delegation

A registered nurse is responsible for managing medical orders and assessing the patient's need for nursing care in all settings, although this may vary in some specifics according to hospital policy, the law, and regulations. Most other admission activities can be delegated to nursing assistive personnel (NAP) if the patient is stable.

Pre-Procedure Assessments

- Assess for signs of emotional and/or physical distress.
- Assess ability to ambulate and/or move.
- Assess ability to communicate and understand what is occurring.

➤ When performing the procedure, always identify your patient according to agency policy, using two identifiers, and be attentive to standard precautions, hand hygiene, patient safety and privacy, body mechanics, and documentation.

Procedure Steps

1. **Ensure placement of patient labels** (e.g., on the chart, at the bedside, outside the door).

2. **Introduce yourself to the patient and family.** Explain who you are. Don't be afraid to tell a client that you are a nursing student.
   Many clients are aware that students have more time to spend with them. Talking to the patient and family reassures them and provides information about the patient's level of consciousness and awareness, social relationships, and other data.

3. **Assist the patient into a hospital gown.**
   If the patient is able to stand, assist her into a gown before weighing her to obtain the most accurate weight.

4. **Measure height and weight** while the patient stands on a floor scale, if possible. If she is unable to stand, transfer her into the bed and measure her weight using a bed scale.
   Weigh in the same manner each time to ensure accuracy.

5. **Assist the patient into the bed.**
   Get the patient comfortable before continuing the admission to prevent overtiring her.

6. ✚ **Check the patient's identification band** to ensure the information, including allergies, is correct. Verify this information with the patient or family.
   Questioning the patient about allergies and verifying with the family will ensure that the information is accurate and documented on the wristband and the chart.

7. **Measure vital signs.**
   Measuring the vital signs before completing the rest of the admission ensures that you are aware of the patient's status. If the vital signs are abnormal, further assess the patient's condition before
   continuing. Report your findings to the admitting care provider.

8. **Complete the nursing admission assessment,** including health history and physical assessment. Be sure to include the patient's expectations and concerns. For inpatients, this must be completed within 24 hours after admission. All patients should be screened on admission for risk for pressure injuries. (Chapter 21 provides a step-by-step approach to physical assessment.)
   An admission assessment is needed to identify problems and establish a baseline. The Joint Commission requires that each patient have an admission assessment performed by a registered nurse.

9. ✚ **Check that the list of the patient's current medications** (created in the admitting department) is complete and accurate. Usually the patient's own medications are sent home with the family, or they may be sent to the pharmacy for storage.

It is important to know what medications the patient has been taking. The pharmacy will identify medicines from home when necessary. When medications are ordered and given during the patient's stay, they are compared to those on the list so any discrepancies can be resolved.

10. Orient the client to the room.
These actions ensure that the patient and family will be able to call for assistance if needed and increase the patient's and family's level of comfort and ability to function in the hospital setting. Remember that one of the disruptions associated with illness is anxiety about the unknown. If you tell your client what to expect, you help to minimize his anxiety.

   a. Make sure that the client knows how to use the bed, the call light, and any equipment that you expect him to use.

   b. Point out the location of personal care items.

   c. Show the client the location of the restroom.

   d. If you will be measuring the client's intake and output, tell him so during your orientation.
If the client is alert, he may be able to assist you with these measures.

11. Explain hospital routines, including use of siderails, meal times, and so on. Answer the patient's and family's questions.
Hospitalization takes away control of basic decisions. Knowing the routines and available choices increases patient and family comfort.

12. Verify with the patient all other admission data on the chart for completeness and accuracy.
Basic data such as name, address, marital status, name of admitting physician, admitting diagnosis, consent to treatment, and so on will usually be obtained in the admitting office. However, you will need to be sure all the admitting information is complete, and complete it if it is not.

13. Ask the patient whether he has an advance directive (e.g., power of attorney or living will). If so, place a copy in the hospital record. If not,

explain the purpose of the document and give the patient a form to fill out if he wishes to do so. (See Chapters 17 and 44 if you need more information about advance directives.)
Advance directives enable patients to indicate their preferences about treatments and prolonging life.

14. Advise the patient of his privacy rights under HIPAA. See that he has a written explanation of his privacy rights (see Chapter 44 as needed).

15. Inventory the patient's belongings. Encourage the family to take home valuable items and money. If that is not possible, arrange to have valuables placed in the hospital safe. Most agencies require money in excess of $5.00 to be sent home or to the cashier's office.
Patient belongings, including valuables, are frequently lost during hospitalization. Documenting the disposition of everything ensures being able to return the belongings to the patient upon discharge.

16. Complete or ensure that all admission orders have been completed (e.g., laboratory tests, medications, diet and fluid orders).
Unless it is an unscheduled admission, diagnostic tests are usually completed on an outpatient basis before admission to the hospital. However, there may still be some orders that need to be done immediately, while others can be delayed. Make sure the orders are completed in the most appropriate time frame.

17. Ensure patient comfort (e.g., positioning, pain, water at bedside).

18. Make one last safety check (i.e., call light within reach, bed in low position, siderails up as appropriate, equipment functioning properly).

19. Before leaving, ask if there is anything else you can do for the patient and family.

20. Initiate the care plan or clinical pathway.
Identifying the patient's priority problems enables the nurse to develop the most appropriate nursing orders.

? What if . . .

■ **The patient may be at risk for falls?**
Perform falls risk assessment as appropriate to the patient, and according to agency policy.
Falls are common in inpatient facilities, especially among older adults. If a patient has falls risk factors, risk reduction measures can be instituted.

■ **The patient has special care needs?**
When the patient has special needs, such as allergies, a nothing by mouth (NPO) order, or an intake and output order, post patient care reminders at the head of the bed or at the door to remind other care providers.

■ **The patient needs a more in-depth assessment in some areas?**
Perform special needs assessments as relevant to the care and condition of the patient (social situation, nutrition and hydration status, functional abilities, spiritual and cultural variables). If these are warranted, they must be completed within 24 hours after admission or prior to surgery.
In-depth assessment of these topics is not a part of all admission assessments, but should be done if the patient's condition warrants.

■ **The patient has a learning disability?**
If possible, preadmissions should be arranged for the patient and main caregiver. This allows more time to discuss issues of consent, alleviate anxiety, and set up links with a learning disability specialist or social worker. Whether or not this is possible, allow more time for the admission process.
Use short sentences, with one idea at a time.
Include the caregiver in the admission process, but encourage the patient to participate as much as possible.
Document the main caregiver and contact numbers.
Expect the patient to be anxious.
Include special communication and personal needs in the plan of care.

(continued on next page)

Procedure 11-1 ■ Admitting a Patient to a Nursing Unit (continued)

Give the patient hospital information with pictures, such as those given to children, if appropriate for her developmental level.

 ■ **The patient is an older adult?**

Ask all older adults if they have had any falls in the past year. If they report a fall, observe them as they stand up from a chair without using their arms, walk several paces, and return ("get up and go"). If they are steady, no further assessment is required. If there is unsteadiness or if the person reports more than one fall, further assessment is required.

The incidence and severity of fall-related complications rise steadily after age 60. Fall rates in nursing homes and hospitals are almost three times the rate for those living at home.

■ **The patient is a child?**

Use a friendly approach.

The first priority is to establish a trusting relationship with the child and parents to help relieve fears and anxiety. Children younger than 3 years may fear being separated from parents. Older children usually worry more about what is going to happen to them.

Explain the visiting and rooming-in policies to the parents.

Ask about the child's usual routine (e.g., toileting, bedtime rituals, favorite foods).

Speak to the child directly if she is old enough to understand.

Direct the family to the bathroom, playroom, television, and snack room, if those are available.

Encourage the parents to bring toys and other favorite items from home.

It helps the child feel more comfortable in the unfamiliar surroundings.

Documentation

■ Document all assessment findings on the admission database provided by the institution.
■ Document an admission note and any teaching or other interventions in the nursing notes or flow sheet (according to agency policy).

■ Recall that a discharge plan is created on admission. See Fig. 11-5 for an example.

Practice Resources

American Geriatrics Society (n.d.); The Joint Commission (2015); Michael, Y., Lin, J., Whitlock, E., et al. (2010); U.S. Preventive Services Task Force (2012).

Procedure 11-2 ■ Transferring a Patient to Another Unit in the Agency

➤ For steps to follow in *all* procedures, refer to the Universal Steps for All Procedures found on the page facing the inside back cover.

Equipment

■ Medical record or chart
■ Care plan
■ Patient's medications
■ Supplies for any ongoing treatments
■ Patient's belongings, clothes, and personal care articles
■ Standardized handoff form, if available
■ A utility cart, if belongings are numerous
■ Wheelchair or transfer cart

Delegation

If the patient's condition allows, you can delegate the physical transfer of the patient and have the NAP move the patient's belongings to the other room. However, as the nurse, you are responsible for obtaining and completing the necessary records, making the final assessment, and gathering and checking the medications. You must also give the handoff report to another nurse.

Pre-Procedure Assessment

■ Make a final, brief focused physical assessment.
■ Assess the patient's mobility and ability to assist.
■ Assess for emotional and/or physical distress (administer medications, as needed).
■ Assess the patient's ability to communicate and understand what is occurring.

➤ When performing the procedure, always identify your patient according to agency policy, using two identifiers, and be attentive to standard precautions, hand hygiene, patient safety and privacy, body mechanics, and documentation.

Procedure Steps

1. ✚ **Obtain the number of personnel needed** to make a safe transfer.

   For efficiency and patient and staff safety.

2. **Gather the patient's medications and label them** correctly for the new room.

   Ensures availability of medications when the patient arrives at the new unit; helps prevent medication administration errors.

3. **Notify the receiving unit** of the time to expect the transfer. Also notify other departments (e.g., dietary, pharmacy, admitting), primary care provider, and family of the transfer.

You need to schedule the transfer with the receiving nurse so he can plan his work and so you can arrange the transfer time to limit the number of interruptions during the handoff. Limiting interruptions minimizes the possibility of communication errors (e.g., forgetting information). Other departments must have the transfer data so that services such as meals and physical therapy treatments will not be interrupted. The primary care provider and family, of course, need to know where to find the patient.

4. **Gather the patient's personal belongings and supplies,** including treatment-related supplies and equipment (e.g., isolation supplies, clean dressings), and patient records. Place on a utility cart if necessary.
   Having the supplies and equipment "ready to go" makes the transfer more efficient for you and less stressful for the patient.

5. **Bring the wheelchair or transfer cart** to the bedside and assist the patient to the chair or cart. If using a wheelchair, the patient can hold personal belongings or supplies; if using a bed or cart, place supplies on the bed.

6. **Take the patient to the new room** and give the handoff report. Follow agency procedure for handoff reports. However, the method chosen should allow both the giver and receiver of patient information the opportunity for questioning.
   a. If you need to review content of an oral handoff report, see Chapter 18. In general, the report should include name, age, sex, physicians, surgical procedures, medical diagnoses, medications, allergies, laboratory data, special equipment (e.g., oxygen, suction), the patient's current health status, and whether there are advance directives and resuscitation status. Identify the nursing diagnoses and priorities for nursing care.
   b. Consistently use a structured framework or memory aid to guide the handoff process and the oral report.
      The objective of a handoff is to provide accurate information about the patient. The information communicated must be accurate in order to ensure patient safety.
   c. ✚ Be sure to point out to the nurse if the patient is taking corticosteroids, anticoagulants, diabetic medications, antibiotics, or narcotic analgesics.
      These medications can have serious side effects and need careful monitoring.

? What if . . .

■ **The patient has intravenous (IV) lines and other equipment that cannot be turned off?**

It is common to transfer patients with IV lines. Some wheelchairs are equipped with an IV pole; for others, you may need to obtain a rolling pole from the unit supply room. The patient may be able to maneuver the rolling pole. Most beds and transfer carts also have portable IV poles, sometimes stored along the underside. Portable oxygen and suction are also available for patients who must have them even during transfer. Be sure to obtain these, set them up, and check their functioning prior to moving the patient from his bed.

■ **The patient has too many personal belongings for one person to carry?**

If the patient's condition requires two staff members to transfer, one person can manage the utility cart while the other manages the patient. If only one person can make the actual move, load a utility cart and move all the supplies and belongings to the new room before transferring the patient.

■ **The patient is being transferred to the intensive care unit (ICU)?**

If this is an urgent transfer, you may need to notify the receiving nurse and move the patient with his records and medications. Later you can make the other notifications, finish the charting, and move belongings and other supplies. In some ICUs, the family may need to take the patient's personal belongings home.

Evaluation

With the receiving nurse, evaluate the patient's response to the move. The receiving nurse will take vital signs and make a preliminary admission assessment.

Documentation

■ Just before moving, document as much information as you can, including the patient's status at that time.
■ After handoff, document the information reported in the handoff, the name and title of the person who received the patient, and your report.
■ Sign the note. Some agencies have a standardized form for the transfer note.

Example documentation

3/13/18,   1615.   Client transferred to room 501 by stretcher, with both siderails up, with assistance of one.

Temperature 104.8°F, pulse 100 beats/min, BP 138/88, respirations 20 breaths/min and shallow. Drowsy upon arrival. Responds to verbal stimuli with moaning. Last pain medication given at 1515. Denies pain when asked. No urine noted since 12:00 pm; will encourage voiding by offering urinal every 2 hr. #22 IV in RAC and #18 IV in R hand flushed with 3 mL of normal saline; flushes without redness, edema, or induration. Receiving 3 L/min of oxygen during transfer. Placed on 3 L/min in room; will wean oxygen as tolerated. Handoff report given to Linda Hamm, RN. ————————————————— Sarah Fields, RN

Practice Resources

The Joint Commission (2016); Maxson, P. M., Derby, K. M., Wrobleski, D. M., et al. (2012); Riesenberg, L. A., Leisch, J., & Cunningham, J. M. (2010); Taylor, J. S. (2015).

Procedure 11-3 ■ Transferring a Patient to a Long-Term Care Facility

➤ For steps to follow in *all* procedures, refer to the Universal Steps for All Procedures found on the page facing the inside back cover.

Equipment

- Health record or chart
- Care plan
- Patient's medications
- Supplies for any ongoing treatments
- Patient's belongings, clothes, and personal care articles
- Standardized transfer form, if available
- A utility cart, if belongings are numerous
- Wheelchair or transfer cart

Delegation

If the patient's condition allows, you can delegate the physical transfer of the patient and have the NAP move the patient's supplies and belongings. However, as the nurse, you are responsible for obtaining and completing the necessary records, making the final assessment, and gathering and checking the medications. You must also give the handoff report to another nurse.

Pre-Procedure Assessment

- Make a final, brief focused physical assessment.
- Assess the patient's mobility and ability to assist.
- Assess for emotional and/or physical distress (administer medications, as needed).
- Assess the patient's ability to communicate and understand what is occurring.

➤ When performing the procedure, always identify your patient according to agency policy, using two identifiers, and be attentive to standard precautions, hand hygiene, patient safety and privacy, body mechanics, and documentation.

Procedure Steps

1. **Notify the patient and family well in advance** of the upcoming transfer to another facility. Include information about the reasons the patient is being transferred, as well as any alternatives to transfer. You will also need to determine which agency is to arrange transportation for the patient.
   Allows them time to adjust emotionally and to make any necessary plans.

2. **Prepare the patient's records.** You may need to send a copy of the patient's health record to the receiving facility. The original remains with the hospital. You will usually also send a copy of the comprehensive nursing assessment and a detailed nursing care plan, as well as prescriptions and cards for future appointments (e.g., with physicians or social workers).
   Ensures continuity of care, thus minimizing patient stress.

3. **Gather and pack the patient's personal** items and treatment supplies to send to the long-term care facility with the patient.
   Having the supplies and equipment "ready to go" makes the transfer more efficient for you.

4. ✚ **Be certain the medications are labeled correctly.**
   Ensures availability and correct administration of medications when the patient arrives at the new facility.

5. **Coordinate the transfer.** Notify the receiving facility of the time to expect the transfer and of any special equipment the patient will need (e.g., IV pole, portable oxygen); notify other hospital departments (e.g., dietary, pharmacy, admitting), primary care provider, and family of the transfer.
   You need to schedule the transfer with the receiving agency so they can plan their work and so you can arrange the transfer at a time that will limit the number of interruptions during the transfer. Other in-house departments must have the transfer data so that services such as meals and physical therapy treatments will be discontinued. The primary care provider and family, of course, need to know where to find the patient.

6. **Just before transfer, make your final quick assessment** and sign off your charting (usually there is a preprinted, standardized discharge form for this purpose).
   It is important to complete documentation in a timely manner, but it is also important to provide the most recent assessment data to the long-term care facility.

7. **Take the patient off the unit** and out of the hospital after you are notified that transportation has arrived (or delegate this task). Alternatively, a transporter may come to your unit to get the patient. (*Note:* Some agencies ask you to remove the patient's identification band at time of transfer.)
   Keeping the patient on the unit as long as practical helps to minimize his anxiety and fatigue that may occur from a long wait in the hospital lobby.

8. **Give an oral report** to the nurse at the long-term care facility. You will usually give a telephone report unless a nurse comes to your hospital to accompany the patient. The report should include, as appropriate for the care, treatment, and services provided, the following:
   a. The reason the patient is being transferred
   b. The patient's physical and psychosocial status
   c. A summary of care, treatment, and services provided and progress toward outcomes

d. Referrals, community resources provided to the patient

A report helps ensure continuity of care and provide a baseline for later changes in the patient's health status.

■ ✚ **It is best to consistently use a structured framework** or memory aid to guide the handoff process and the oral report.

The objective of a handoff report is to provide accurate information about the patient. The information communicated must be accurate in order to ensure patient safety.

■ ✚ **Notify the long-term care agency** if the patient is colonized or infected with methicillin-resistant *Staphylococcus aureus* (MRSA) or other contagious microorganisms.

The facility can arrange for and communicate any special isolation or care activities to their staff. MRSA is a serious problem for long-term care residents.

■ ✚ **Be sure to point out to the nurse if the patient is taking corticosteroids,** anticoagulants, diabetic medications, antibiotics, or narcotic analgesics.

These medications confer particularly high risk of adverse postdischarge drug events, and the long-term care nurses will need to continue careful monitoring.

? What if . . .

■ **The patient has IV lines and other equipment that cannot be turned off?**

It is common to transfer patients with IV lines. Some wheelchairs are equipped with an IV pole. If you need to hold the IV bag while taking the patient to the transporting vehicle, always hold the bag well above the patient's chest and arm so that blood does not back up in the tubing. Also, you should notify the long-term care

facility so they will have the necessary equipment in the transport vehicle. Portable oxygen and suction are also available for patients who must have them. Usually the receiving facility will bring these, but you need to coordinate that in advance.

■ ✚ **When you are ready to transfer the patient, her condition worsens and she becomes unstable?**

Perform interventions to stabilize the patient, call for help if needed, and notify the medical provider. Notify the transporter and the long-term care center of the change and postpone the transfer until further medical assessment is done.

Evaluation

The receiving nurse at the long-term care facility will evaluate the patient's response to the move.

Documentation

■ Just before the transfer, document your final assessment and complete the agency's discharge summary.

■ You will probably put your final nursing note on a transfer or discharge summary similar to those shown in Figures 11-5 and 11-6.

Practice Resources

The Joint Commission (2016); Maxson, P. M., Derby, K. M., Wrobleski, D. M., et al. (2012); Riesenberg, L. A., Leisch, J., & Cunningham, J. M. (2010).

Procedure 11-4 ■ Discharging a Patient From the Healthcare Facility

➤ For steps to follow in *all* procedures, refer to the Universal Steps for All Procedures found on the page facing the inside back cover.

Equipment

- Health record or chart
- Patient's medications
- Supplies for any ongoing treatments
- Patient's belongings, clothes, and personal care articles
- Standardized discharge form, if available, with instructions for patient
- A utility cart, if belongings are numerous
- Wheelchair

Delegation

If the patient's condition allows, you can delegate to the NAP such tasks as packing belongings, helping the patient dress, and

taking the patient out of the facility. However, as the nurse, you are responsible for obtaining and completing the necessary records, making the final assessment, gathering and checking the medications, and coordinating care.

Pre-Procedure Assessment

- Make a final, brief focused physical assessment.
- Assess the patient's mobility.
- Assess for emotional and/or physical distress.
- Assess the patient's ability to communicate and understand what is occurring.

➤ When performing the procedure, always identify your patient according to agency policy, using two identifiers, and be attentive to standard precautions, hand hygiene, patient safety and privacy, body mechanics, and documentation.

(continued on next page)

Procedure 11-4 ■ Discharging a Patient From the Healthcare Facility (continued)

Procedure Steps

1. **Notify the patient and family** as much in advance of the discharge as possible. This is often done early in the hospital stay.
   Allows them time to adjust emotionally and to make any necessary plans.

A Day or Two Before Discharge (Steps 2 and 3)

2. **Make or confirm necessary arrangements.**
   a. Arrange for or help the family arrange for services (e.g., home healthcare, physical therapy, intravenous therapy, social worker) that will be needed at home.

   NOTE: To reimburse for home care, insurers require a physician's order for all services, and the patient must meet certain eligibility criteria.

   b. Confirm or arrange for equipment needed in the home (e.g., portable oxygen).
   c. Confirm or arrange for transportation.
   d. Make necessary referrals (e.g., medical specialists, physical therapists); book appointments, if necessary and if in line with agency policy.
      Hospital stays are short, and many patients are still ill enough to require complex treatments and care by family members when they go home.

3. **Communicate and provide teaching** to the patient and caregivers.
   Patients who have a clear understanding of their after-hospital care (e.g., medications, follow-up visits) are less likely to visit the emergency department or be readmitted than patients who lack this information (Agency for Healthcare Research and Quality, 2014b).

   a. Discuss the patient's diagnosis, care needs, and functional abilities with the family/caregiver.
   b. Train the patient and caregiver in the use of equipment. Arrange for follow-up evaluation at home to check that equipment is working and being used correctly and that further training is given if needed.
      In the stress of illness and the disruption of transition home, patients may not retain what they are taught in the hospital. Therapies will be ineffective if equipment is used incorrectly, so follow-up is essential to help avoid further illness and hospital readmission.

   c. Educate about medication use and side effects.
      Medication errors at home are a frequent cause of adverse events and readmissions to the hospital.

   d. Ask relatives or the caregiver to bring clothing for the patient to wear home, if needed.
      If this was an unplanned admission, the patient may have come in nightwear and a robe.

Day of Discharge (Steps 4 Through 16)

4. **Make and document final assessments.**
   a. Assess that the patient's condition remains as expected.
   b. Confirm that the patient has house keys, heating is turned on, and food is available.
   c. Follow up on diagnostic and laboratory test results.

5. **Bring a wheelchair or other transport** device to the bedside.

6. **Make final notifications.**
   a. Contact the family or guardian; confirm transportation.
   b. Notify community service agencies and home health nursing of the discharge, as needed.

7. **Gather prescriptions and instruction sheets,** including a list of current medications and appointment cards; give to the patient along with the discharge instructions at discharge. **KEY POINT:** *Be certain that either the patient or caregiver can read the instructions. Inadequate literacy has been shown to be a risk factor for readmission.*

8. **Gather and pack the patient's personal items and treatment supplies.**
   Having the supplies and equipment ready to go makes the transfer more efficient for you and less stressful for the patient and family.

9. ✚ **Prepare the patient's medications.** Be certain the medications are labeled correctly; pack them and record which medications he is taking home.
   This ensures availability and correct administration of medications when the patient arrives home. It also provides a legal record that the patient left with the medications.

10. **Review the following discharge instructions** with patient and caregiver (and provide a written copy to take home):
    a. Medication instructions
    b. Symptom management and treatments
    c. Information about provider and location for the follow-up appointment(s)
    d. How to obtain further care, treatment, and services, as needed
    e. How and when to call the physician or primary care provider, including signs of a change in condition
    f. Emergency contact
    g. Diet restrictions
    h. Maintenance of hydration
    i. Activities of daily living, focusing on safety and mobility
       Teaching should occur throughout the hospital stay. However, it is important to reinforce with a last-minute summary and written instructions to take home. With the stress of illness and anticipation of discharge, patients may not retain what they are taught.

11. **Address any questions or concerns** of the patient and caregiver.
    Improves the ability to transition to home.

12. **Give new prescriptions to the patient,** as well as reminder cards for outpatient appointments (e.g., with social services, physicians) to the patient.
   Ensures continuity of care, thus minimizing patient stress.

13. **Document your final nursing note** and complete the discharge summary (the patient often receives a copy of the summary). The patient needs a copy of (1) his instructions for care at home, which may be called a discharge plan, and (2) his discharge summary, a summary of the progress of his illness and treatment from admission through discharge. Some agencies combine these into one form.
   It is important to document the patient's condition at the time he leaves the unit. This provides a baseline for comparison if his condition should deteriorate after discharge.

14. **Accompany the patient off the unit** and out of the hospital (or delegate this task) when you are notified that transportation has arrived.
   Keeping the patient on the unit as long as practical helps to minimize the anxiety and fatigue that may occur from a long wait in the hospital lobby while a family member brings a car to the door.

15. **Notify the admissions department** of the discharge. Depending on agency policy, notify the primary care or admitting physician.
   This will stop all scheduled services, such as meals, and notify the housekeeping department that the room needs to be cleaned.

16. **Ensure the patient's records are sent** to the medical records department.
   Whether paper or electronic, the health record is a legal document and remains permanently in storage in the healthcare institution.

? What if . . .

- ✚ **Near the time of discharge, the patient's condition worsens and he becomes unstable?**

   Perform interventions to stabilize the patient, call for help if needed, and notify the provider.

   Notify the family that discharge will be delayed.

   Communicate with other hospital departments and community agencies as necessary.

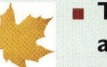

- ■ **The patient is an older adult?**

   Allow for more time to dress and leave the hospital.

   Allow for more time to communicate, teach, and answer questions.

   Obtain feedback to be certain the caregivers have heard and understood instructions.

   Consider having a geriatric nurse specialist make follow-up home visits.
   Hearing, visual, and mobility deficits become more common with advanced age.

- ✚ **The patient is taking "high-risk" drugs postdischarge?**

   Medications with a high risk of postdischarge adverse events include corticosteroids, anticoagulants, diabetic medications, antibiotics, anti-anxiety agents, sedatives, and narcotic analgesics.

   Provide teaching for patient, family, and other caregivers throughout the hospital stay. A day or two before discharge, review teaching with patient and family; evaluate their understanding.

   On discharge, summarize medication precautions and provide clear written instructions. Be sure the patient and family can read them.

Evaluation

A few weeks after discharge, the facility will contact the patient to evaluate the quality and appropriateness of the discharge process. This may be done by making a home visit, telephoning, or sending a questionnaire. As a nurse, you may or may not be involved in this evaluation. The best evaluation of the multidisciplinary care will be whether the patient must be readmitted to the acute care facility.

Documentation

- For the health record, the primary provider will write a discharge progress note that contains the following information:

   Reason for hospitalization

   Significant findings during the stay, including significant changes in status since admission

   Procedures performed; care, treatment, and services provided during the stay

   Status of goals for the stay

   Condition at discharge

- Agency policy determines the format and content of nursing documentation. This is often a combination of a structured discharge form or checklist and a narrative progress note. Regardless of format, you should document the following information:

   Your final assessment of the patient's health status

   Information and teaching provided to the patient and caregivers

   Referrals, medications

   How patient left the unit (e.g., in wheelchair) and who accompanied him (e.g., wife, name of staff member)
   The Joint Commission recommends standardized formats for documentation (2008, p. 367).

   To see examples of discharge summaries, see Figures 11-4 and 11-5.

Practice Resources

Agency for Healthcare Research and Quality (2013, 2014a, 2014b); Altfeld, S. J., Shier, G. E., Rooney, M., et al. (2013); Closson, B., Mattingly, L., Finne, K., et al. (2012); Greenwald, J. L., Denham, C. R., & Jack, B. W. (2007); Hunter, T., & Birmingham, J. (2013); The Joint Commission (2008, 2012, 2015); Lim, F., Foust, J., & VanCleave, J. (2016).

To explore learning resources for this chapter,

 Go to www.DavisAdvantage.com and find:

Answers and Suggested Responses for all questions in this chapter

Lists of NIC Interventions and NOC Outcomes

List of NANDA-I Diagnoses

Knowledge Map

References and Bibliography

Concept Map

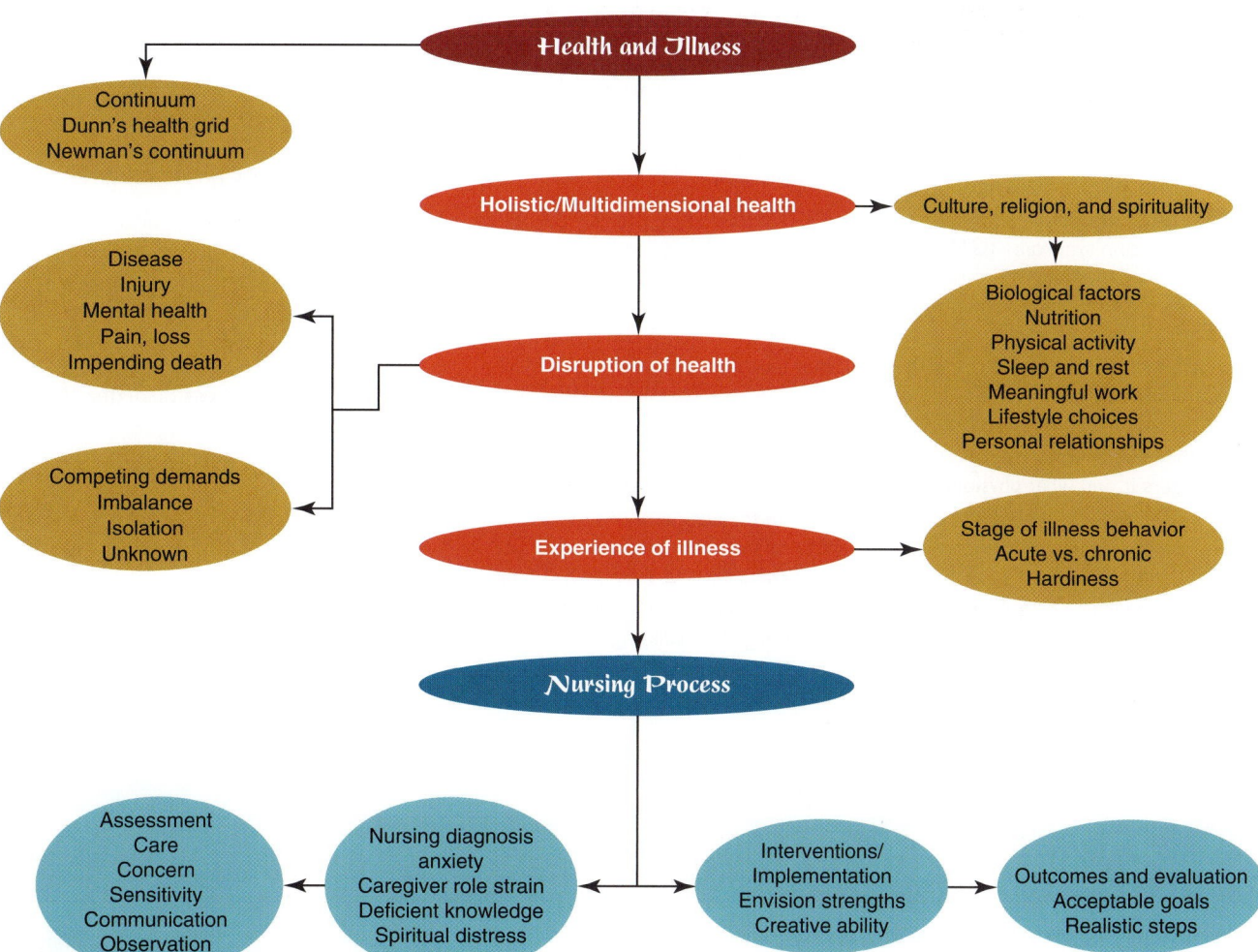

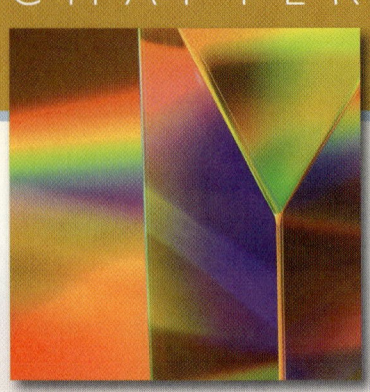

CHAPTER 12

Stress & Adaptation

Learning Outcomes

After completing this chapter, you should be able to:

➤ Define *stress*.

➤ Explain the difference between adaptive and maladaptive coping strategies.

➤ Explain the relationship between stressors, responses, and adaptation.

➤ Compare and contrast stages of Selye's general adaptation syndrome (GAS) with the local adaptation syndrome (LAS), including both physical and psychological changes that occur.

➤ Describe physical changes occurring during the three stages of Selye's general adaptation syndrome (GAS).

➤ Discuss the inflammatory response: What triggers it, and what physiological changes occur?

➤ Explain how anxiety, fear, and anger relate to stress.

➤ Describe the specific psychological responses to stress and discuss their relationships to the concept of stress.

➤ Provide examples and definitions of specific ego defense mechanisms.

➤ Compare and contrast hypochondriasis, somatization, somatoform pain disorder, and malingering.

➤ Describe the physiological effects of prolonged stress and unsuccessful adaptation on the various body systems.

➤ Compare and contrast crisis and burnout.

➤ State three ways in which you could assess for stressors and risk factors for stress.

➤ Discuss three ways to assess coping methods and adaptation to stress.

➤ Evaluate the adequacy of support systems and other personal attributes for successful or unsuccessful coping.

➤ Plan interventions or activities for preventing and managing stress.

Key Concepts

Adaptation

Coping

Stress

Related Concepts

Anxiety

Fear

See the Concept Map at the end of this chapter.

Example Problem

Post-traumatic stress disorder (PTSD)

Meet Your Patients

Gloria and her husband, John, live in a residential community from which John commutes to work in a nearby city. Gloria runs an accounting business from their home. They have two teenage boys who need transportation to many extracurricular activities. Gloria and John teach Sunday school and are Boy Scout leaders. Gloria's mother needs knee replacement surgery and cannot take care of Gloria's father, who has early-stage Alzheimer's disease. In addition to her own home responsibilities, Gloria must go to her parents' home to prepare meals and to provide care for them during the day. Gloria's sister sleeps in the parents' home during the night.

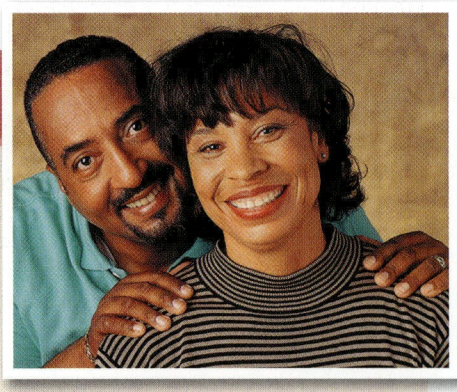

Theoretical Knowledge
knowing **why**

Everyone experiences stress as a part of daily life, but we each perceive and respond to stress in our own unique way. Failure to adapt to stress has been linked to several physical and mental illnesses. You will encounter many stressful situations in your career, so you must develop healthful ways of responding and of helping your clients to adapt to stressors.

ABOUT THE KEY CONCEPTS

The two overarching concepts for this chapter are **stress** and **adaptation.** To help you grasp those concepts, we present definitions and examples, as well as numerous subconcepts that relate to health and illness in various ways. Another important concept is **coping.** As a nurse, you need to understand stress to help your clients cope effectively and adapt to the stressors of illness and caregiving.

WHAT IS STRESS?

Stress is any disturbance in a person's normal balanced state. A **stressor** is a stimulus that the person perceives as a challenge or physical or emotional threat. Stress produces voluntary and involuntary **coping responses** aimed at reducing tension, pressure, or emotional strain. The changes that take place as a result of coping are called **adaptations.** We can also define *adaptation* as an ongoing effort to maintain external and internal equilibrium, or **homeostasis.**

Stress is not necessarily bad. It can keep you alert and motivate you to function at a higher performance level. However, if you become too anxious, you may not be able to think clearly or focus on the task.

Types of Stressors

The sources of stress are infinite; however, stressors are commonly categorized in the following ways:

Distress/Eustress **Distress** threatens health, and **eustress** (literally, "good stress") is protective. A passionate kiss can produce as strong a stress response as a slap in the face.

External/Internal Stressors may be **external** to the person, for example, death of a family member, a hurricane, or even something as simple as excessive heat in a room. Stressors may also be **internal,** for example, diseases, anxiety, nervous anticipation of an event, or negative self-talk.

Developmental stressors can be predicted to occur at various stages of a person's life. For example, school-age children may experience stress at school or among family or peers; and many middle-aged adults must adjust to aging parents and accepting their own physical changes. For theoretical knowledge about developmental stages, refer to the theories of Erikson and Havighurst in Chapter 9.

Situational stressors are unpredictable. You cannot predict if you will experience an automobile accident, a natural disaster, job conflict, or an illness. Situational stressors can occur at any life stage and can affect infants, children, and adults equally.

Time stressors can lead to angst over the lack of opportunity to tend to all the things that you have to do. Common examples of time stress include worrying about managing multiple demands or rushing to avoid being late for work or an appointment.

Anticipatory stressors are those that you experience concerning the future. Sometimes this stress can be focused on a specific event, such as an upcoming exam or clinical day. Anticipatory stress can also be undefined, such as a vague sense of concern about the future or a feeling that something will go wrong.

Physiological stressors are those that affect body structure or function. You can categorize them as follows; a few examples are given for each category:
Chemical—environmental toxins, medications, tobacco
Physical or mechanical—trauma, cold, joint overuse
Nutritional—vitamin deficiency, high-fat diet
Biological—viruses, bacteria
Genetic—inborn errors of metabolism
Lifestyle—obesity, sedentary lifestyle

Psychosocial stressors are external stressors that arise from work, family dynamics, living situation, social relationships, financial strain, and other aspects of our daily lives. The Holmes-Rahe Social Readjustment Scale contains examples of psychosocial stressors.

PICOT

Stress and Multiple Responsibilities

Situation: The nurse is preparing to meet with a mother who has two children: a 9-year-old with some behavior problems at school and a 5-year-old with Down syndrome (DS). The mother and her husband work alternate shifts, although she also has total responsibility for child care and household responsibilities.

PICOT Components:

P—Population/client	=	Siblings of Down syndrome children
I—Intervention/indicator	=	Parents with less satisfactory relationships
C—Comparator/control	=	Parents with psychosocial well-being
O—Outcome	=	Behavior problems
T—Time	=	During school

SEARCHABLE QUESTION: Do _____ (P) who receive/are exposed to _____ (I) demonstrate _____ (O) as compared with _____ (C) during _____ (T)?

Example of Evidence: While reports show there seems to be greater intimacy among siblings of children with DS, there are other factors that negatively influence sibling adaptation. One study associated the degree of adaptation in siblings to the level of parental distress. Parents who were depressed and had less satisfactory marital relationships tended to have less well-adapted children than those with psychosocial well-being. These children were more likely to show deviant behavior problems both at home and in school.

Reference: Choi, H., & Riper, M. (2013). Siblings of children with Down syndrome: An integrative review. *MCN, The American Journal of Maternal/Child Nursing, 38*(2), 72–78.

 Go to Davis Advantage, Resources, Chapter 12, **PICOT Box Suggested Responses.**

KnowledgeCheck 12-1

Refer to the Meet Your Patients scenario at the beginning of the chapter.

- What are Gloria's stressors? Classify each of them as follows: (1) Are they physiological or psychosocial? (2) Are they developmental or situational?
- What are John's stressors?

Models of Stress

Some theorists (Lazarus & Folkman, 1984) conceptualize stress as a complex, dynamic, and reciprocal exchange between person and environment. Other theorists (Holmes & Rahe, 1964) view stress solely as a stimulus that causes psychological or physiological responses that in turn increase vulnerability to disease. Hans Selye (1974, 1976) found that physical, emotional, psychological, and spiritual stressors, or the anticipation of a stressor (as in anxiety), can initiate nonspecific physiological *responses*. Selye defined these responses as stress.

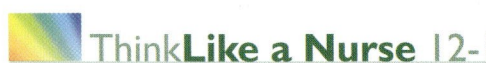

ThinkLike a Nurse 12-1

- Make a list of your own stressors in the following areas: work, school, family, and living situation.
- What physiological stressors do you have?

HOW DO COPING AND ADAPTATION RELATE TO STRESS?

Coping strategies are the thinking processes and behaviors a person uses to manage stressors. Coping strategies can be adaptive or maladaptive.

Adaptive (effective) coping consists of making healthy choices that reduce the negative effects of stress (e.g., exercising to relieve tension, hobbies, seeking support or advice). The difference between effective and ineffective coping may be in the degree to which a technique is used (for examples, see Ego Defense Mechanisms later in this chapter).

Maladaptive (ineffective) coping does not promote adaptation. Unhealthful coping choices include overeating, working too much, oversleeping, and substance abuse. Although a maladaptive behavior may temporarily relieve anxiety, it may have other harmful effects. For example, a person who smokes to relieve the tensions of a stressful work situation may experience an immediate decrease in anxiety, but with long-term risks to health.

Three Common Approaches to Coping

People use three approaches to cope with stress, at different times and in various combinations:

- **Altering the Stressor.** In some situations, a person takes actions to remove or change the stressor.
- **Adapting to the Stressor.** It is not always possible to remove or change a stressor. Adapting involves changing one's thoughts or behaviors related to the stressor. As Gloria (Meet Your Patients) gains experience as a caregiver, she may find more efficient, less stressful ways to care for her parents.
- **Avoiding the Stressor.** Sometimes it is healthful to avoid a stressor. In other situations, avoidance may be maladaptive. For example, a woman who discovers a lump in her breast fears that she may have cancer. She copes with her anxiety by putting it out of her mind and avoids seeking medical care, perhaps making eventual treatment less effective

The Outcome of Stress: Adaptation or Disease

Successful adaptation allows for normal growth and development and effective responses to changes and challenges in daily life. The outcome depends on the balance between the strength of the stressors and the effectiveness of the person's coping methods (Fig. 12-1). In the following equation, **E** is the event (stressor), **R** is the person's response (which is determined in part by past experiences, perception of the stressor, and coping methods used), and **O** is the outcome:

E	+	**R**	=	**O**
stressful event		response (experience, perception, coping methods)		outcome (adaptation or disease)

Some events produce more stress than others. However, a person with good coping skills can usually adapt to a single stressful event, even a demanding one. But suppose several stressors occur in a short period of time. As with Gloria, when there are many stressors or when stressors continue for a long period of time, adaptation is more likely to fail with fatigue, despair, and depleted resources for coping.

Personal Factors Influence Adaptation

Why do some people succumb to overwhelming stress, while others adapt and thrive? Successful adaptation does not depend entirely on being able to alter or avoid stressors. Various personal factors also influence the outcome:

Perception of the Stressor A person's perception may be realistic or exaggerated. Suppose two women with similar

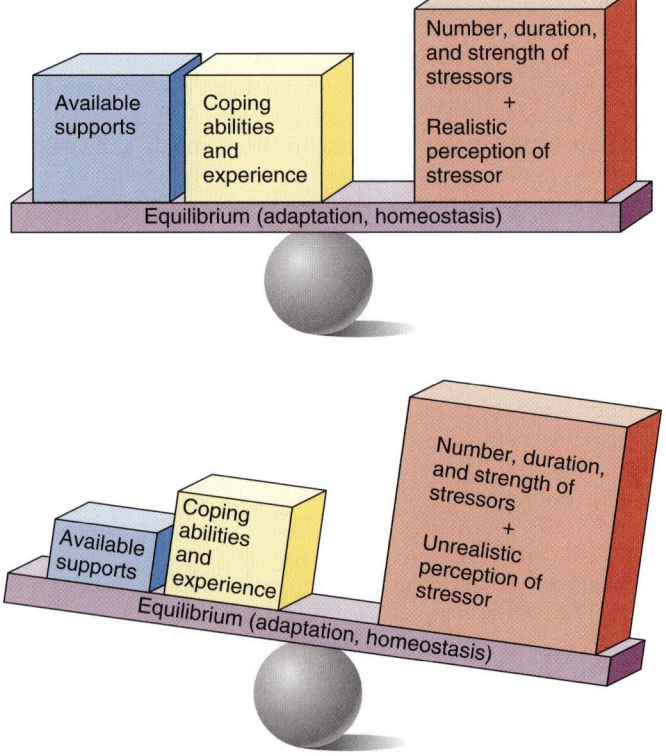

FIGURE 12-1 Adaptation occurs when a person has supports and coping abilities adequate to enable him to deal with the stressors. A realistic perception of the stressful event promotes adaptation, whereas an unrealistic perception makes adaptation more difficult.

coping skills and support systems both must have a mastectomy. One thinks, "Yes, I am losing a part of my body, but I am more than just my breasts. I am so grateful just to be alive." The other feels, "I will be so ugly. I feel less of a woman now." Which woman do you think is more likely to adapt successfully to this change in her body?

Overall Health Status Stressors may actually cause a healthy person to engage in constructive adaptive behaviors that improve health (e.g., by modifying his diet and exercising to control his blood pressure and prevent complications). However, a person who also has been coping for years with pain and immobility from arthritis may be too overwhelmed and exhausted to take any actions to lower his blood pressure.

Support System Friends, family, counseling and church groups, or people who share common interests often support each other in times of difficulty. A good support system can help a person adapt to stress and solve problems—for example, by providing emotional support, encouraging expression of feelings, and providing financial and other supports.

Hardiness People who thrive despite overwhelming stressors tend to have a quality that has been termed **hardiness.** They maintain three key attitudes that help them weather adversity: commitment, control, and challenge. *Commitment* lets them seek to be involved with ongoing events rather than feeling isolated. *Control* enables them to struggle and try to influence outcomes instead of becoming passive and feeling powerless. *Challenge* allows them to perceive stressful changes as opportunities for learning (Maddi, 2002; Maddi, Koshaba, Fazel, et al., 2009).

Other Personal Factors Age, developmental level, and life experiences all affect a person's response to stress. For example, infants and the very old may lack physiological reserves to adapt to physical stressors, such as temperature extremes, dehydration, or illness. Even with a positive attitude and good coping skills, excessive amounts of stress can lead to maladaptation and disease. **KEY POINT:** *Each person has a different ability to tolerate stress, but everyone has a breaking point at which stress becomes overwhelming.*

KnowledgeCheck 12-2

- True or false: The difference between adaptive and maladaptive coping is that maladaptive coping does not relieve stress.
- In addition to avoiding the stressor, what are two other approaches to coping?
- (Complete the sentence.) The outcome of stress (adaptation or disease) depends on the balance among the strength, number, and duration of the stressors and _____.

HOW DO PEOPLE RESPOND TO STRESSORS?

Although Selye's (1974, 1976) response-based model acknowledges physical, emotional, psychological, and spiritual *stressors,* his ideas about responses *(stress)* are primarily physiological. The body has various mechanisms for regulating its internal environment to maintain a balanced state, or homeostasis. Selye described the physiological responses to stress as either the general adaptation syndrome (GAS) or the local adaptation syndrome (LAS).

The General Adaptation Syndrome Includes Nonspecific, Systemic Responses

Would you be surprised to know that a near-miss automobile accident and kicking the winning field goal at a football game would both produce the same general body responses? Responses to stress involve the whole body, especially the autonomic nervous system and the endocrine system. The **general adaptation syndrome (GAS)** is Selye's name for the group of nonspecific responses that all people share in the face of stressors. The GAS has three stages: (1) the initial alarm stage, (2) resistance (adaptation), and (3) the final stage of either recovery or exhaustion (Fig. 12-2).

Alarm Stage—Fight or Flight

Has someone ever playfully grabbed you from behind and shouted, "Boo"? How did you feel? If you are not feeling a

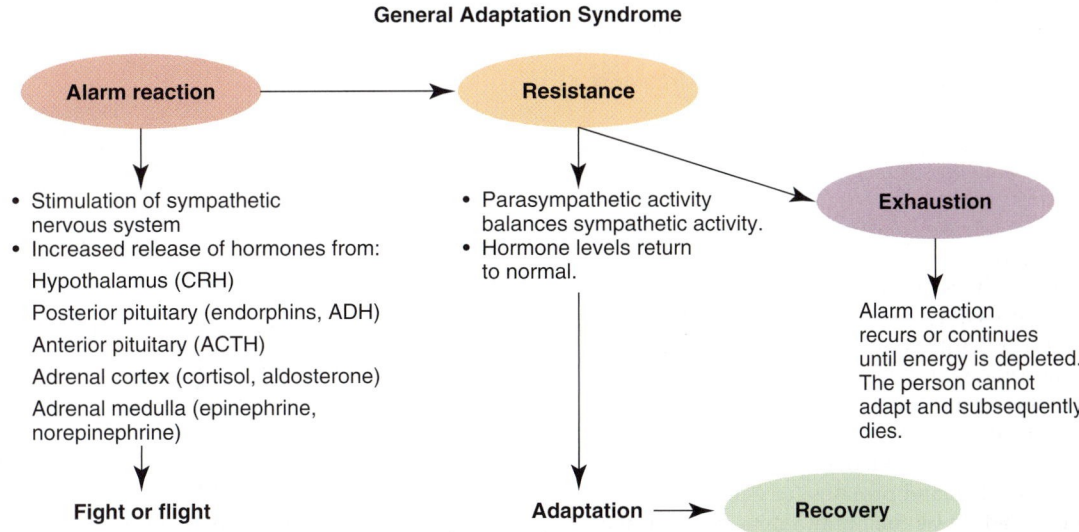

General Adaptation Syndrome

FIGURE 12-2 The stages of Selye's general adaptation syndrome (GAS) are (1) alarm (also called "fight or flight"); (2) resistance (or adaptation), in which the body enacts physical and psychological adaptive mechanisms to maintain homeostasis; and (3) either recovery or exhaustion (which usually ends in disease or death).

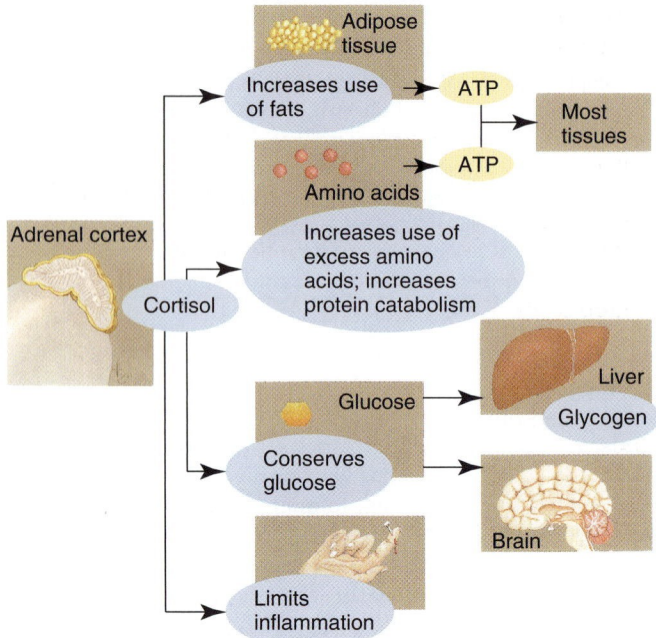

FIGURE 12-3 Functions of cortisol during the alarm stage of the GAS.

response to that, think back to a time when something else startled you. Did your heart pound? Did you breathe fast? Was there a flutter in your stomach? Did your muscles tighten? What were your emotions? Did you want to run away, or were you "frozen"? That exercise in imagination should help you to understand the experience of the alarm stage. The alarm stage has two phases: shock and countershock.

- The **shock phase** begins when the cerebral cortex first perceives a stressor and sends out messages to activate the endocrine and sympathetic nervous systems. A surge of epinephrine (adrenaline) and various other hormones prepare the body for *fight* or *flight*. The shock phase does usually last less than 24 hours, sometimes only a minute or two.
- In the **countershock phase,** all the changes produced in the shock phase are reversed, and the person becomes less able to deal with the immediate threat.

Various body systems produce responses when a stressor is perceived. See Figures 12-3, 12-4, and 12-5.

Endocrine System Responses

In response to a perceived stressor, the following endocrine responses occur:

1. The *hypothalamus* releases corticotropin-releasing hormone (CRH).
2. *CRH,* together with messages from the cerebral cortex, directs the pituitary gland to release adrenocorticotropic hormone (ACTH) and antidiuretic hormone (ADH).
3. *ACTH* stimulates the adrenal cortex to produce and secrete glucocorticoids (especially cortisol) and mineralocorticoids (especially aldosterone).
   Cortisol, in general, has a glucose-sparing effect. It increases the use of fats and proteins for energy and conserves glucose for use by the brain. Cortisol also has an anti-inflammatory effect. See Figure 12-3 for the effects of cortisol during the alarm reaction of the GAS.
   Aldosterone promotes fluid retention by causing the kidneys to reabsorb more sodium. In that way, it helps

to increase fluid volume and maintain or increase blood pressure.

4. *ADH* also promotes fluid retention by increasing the reabsorption of water by kidney tubules. See Figure 12-4 for the effects of aldosterone and ADH.
5. *Endorphins,* secreted by the hypothalamus and posterior pituitary, act like opiates to produce a sense of well-being and reduce pain.
6. *Thyroid-stimulating hormone (TSH)* is secreted by the pituitary gland to increase the efficiency of cellular metabolism and fat conversion to energy for cell and muscle needs.

Sympathetic Nervous System Responses

The cerebral cortex also sends messages via the hypothalamus to stimulate the sympathetic nervous system. The sympathetic nervous system then stimulates the adrenal glands to secrete adrenaline and norepinephrine, which increase mental alertness. This allows the person to assess the situation and aids in a decision to stand and fight or run away in flight. Adrenaline also increases the ability of the muscles to contract and causes the pupils to dilate, producing greater visual fields. See Figure 12-5 for the effects of adrenaline during the alarm reaction of the GAS.

Other Body System Responses in the Alarm Stage

The following are some body system responses that occur in the alarm stage as a result of endocrine and sympathetic nervous system activity. Refer to Figures 12-2 through 12-5 to see how these changes are produced.

- *Cardiovascular system.* The heart rate and contraction force increase. Peripheral and visceral vasoconstriction increase blood flow to vital organs (e.g., brain, lungs) and to muscles preparing for flight. Blood volume and blood pressure also increase, and the blood clots more readily.
- *Respiratory system.* The bronchioles dilate, thereby increasing the depth of respiration and tidal volume. This makes oxygen available for diffusion to muscle, brain, and cardiac cells.

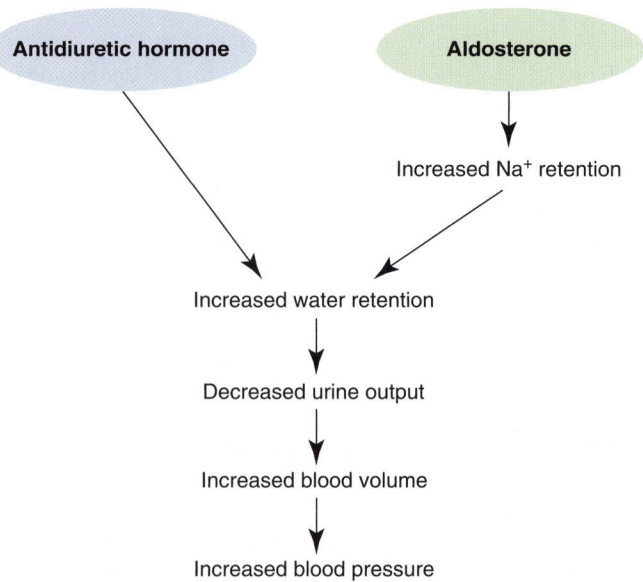

FIGURE 12-4 The release of ADH (from the posterior pituitary gland) and aldosterone (from the adrenal cortex) leads to sodium and water retention, increases blood volume, and increases blood pressure.

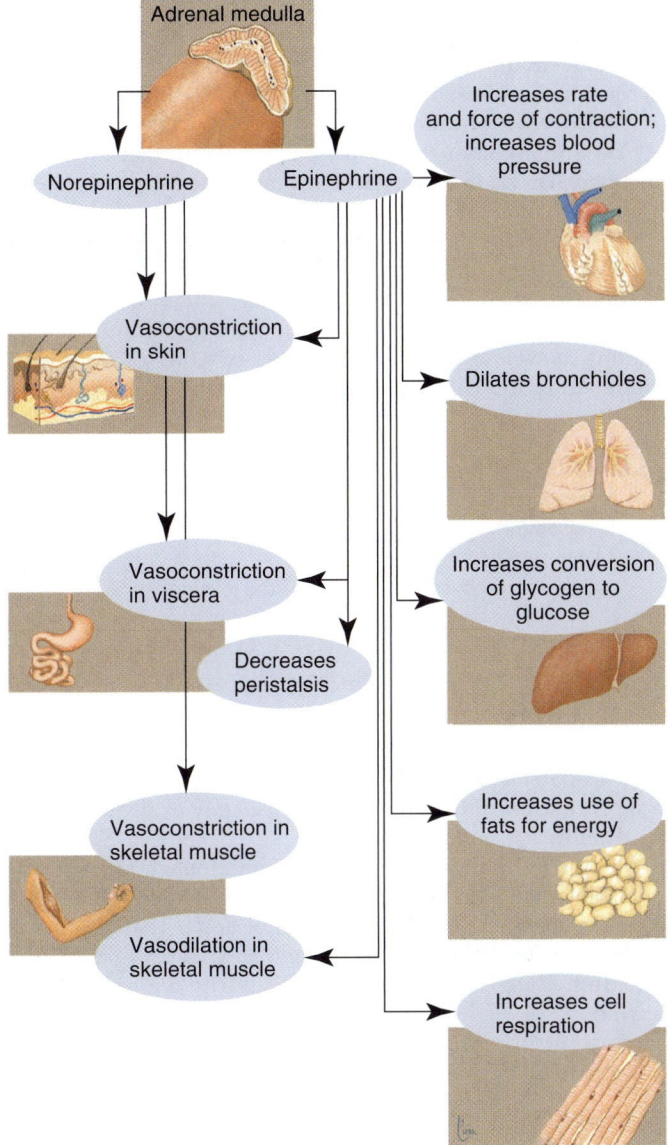

FIGURE 12-5 Functions of epinephrine and norepinephrine during the alarm stage of the GAS.

- *Metabolism.* The metabolic rate increases. The liver converts more glycogen to glucose *(glycogenolysis)*, making it available for energy. Except in the brain, the body uses less glucose for energy. The use of amino acids and the mobilization of fats for energy *(lipolysis)* increase.
- *Urinary system.* Blood flow to the kidneys decreases, and they retain more sodium and water. The kidneys secrete renin, which produces *angiotensin.* In turn, angiotensin constricts the arterioles and tends to increase blood pressure.
- *Gastrointestinal system.* Peristalsis and secretions of digestive enzymes decrease. The blood glucose level increases to fuel the energy needed for fight or flight.
- *Musculoskeletal system.* Blood vessels dilate, increasing flow of blood (and thus oxygen and energy) to skeletal muscles.

Resistance Stage—Coping With the Stressor

During the second stage of the GAS, **resistance** (or *adaptation*), the body tries to cope, protect itself against the stressor, and maintain homeostasis. Stabilization involves the use of

physiological and psychological coping mechanisms. Psychological defense mechanisms for coping are discussed in a subsequent section in this chapter. Physical adaptations help the heart rate, blood pressure, cardiac output, respiratory function, and hormone levels return to normal.

- *If the person adapts successfully* or if the stress can be confined to a small area (as in the inflammatory response), the body regains homeostasis.
- *If the stress is too great* (as in serious illness or severe blood loss), defense mechanisms fail, and the person enters the third phase of the GAS.

Exhaustion or Recovery Stage—Final Effort to Adapt

Exhaustion If stress continues and adaptive mechanisms become ineffective or are used up, a person enters the final stage, **exhaustion.** Physiological responses in this stage include vasodilation, decreased blood pressure, and increased pulse and respirations. Physical adaptive resources and energy are depleted. The body is unable to defend itself and cannot maintain resistance against the continuing stressors. Exhaustion usually ends in injury, illness, or death.

Recovery In contrast, if adaptation is successful, the final stage is **recovery.** For example, after a miscarriage, a couple participates in a support group and begins to focus more deeply on their relationship with each other. They are able gradually to resolve their grief.

KnowledgeCheck 12-3

- In general, what is the difference between the alarm stage and the resistance stage of the GAS?
- Name the gland that releases each of the following hormones in response to stress, and name each hormone's function: corticotropin-releasing hormone (CRH), antidiuretic hormone (ADH), adrenocorticotropic hormone (ACTH), aldosterone, cortisol, epinephrine, and norepinephrine.
- In the alarm stage of the GAS, what are the effects of the sympathetic nervous system on each of the following: heart, brain, glycogen stores, and skeletal muscle?
- What is the effect of Selye's resistance stage on the cardiovascular and respiratory systems? On hormone levels?

The Local Adaptation Syndrome Involves Specific Local Responses

Whereas the GAS is a whole-body response to a stressor, the **local adaptation syndrome (LAS)** is a localized body response; that is, it involves only a specific body part, tissue, or organ. It is a short-term attempt to restore homeostasis. The two most common LAS responses you will deal with as a nurse are the reflex pain response and the inflammatory response. Others include blood clotting and pupil constriction in response to light.

Reflex Pain Response

When you perceive a painful stimulus, especially in one of your limbs, you immediately and unconsciously withdraw from the source of pain. If you've ever accidentally touched a hot stove, you certainly didn't stop to ponder, "Hmmm, I think I will withdraw my hand"—you pulled your hand away before you could even think about it. This is a protective **reflex,** an involuntary, predictable response. Pain receptors send sensory impulses to the spinal cord, where they synapse with the spinal motor neurons. The motor impulses travel back to the site of stimulation, causing the flexor muscles in the limb to contract. This is a local, rather than a whole-body, response.

Inflammatory Response

The **inflammatory response** is a local reaction to cell injury, either by pathogens or by physical, chemical, or other agents (Box 12-1). **KEY POINT:** *Regardless of the injuring agent (stressor), its mechanisms are the same, and they produce the classic symptoms of inflammation: pain, heat, swelling, redness, and loss of function.* The inflammatory process includes a vascular response, a cellular response, formation of exudate, and healing.

Vascular Response   Immediately after injury, blood vessels at the site constrict (narrow) to control bleeding. The following also occur:

- *Response:* The injured cells release histamine.
  Effect: Local vessels dilate, increasing blood flow to the area **(hyperemia).**
- *Response:* The dying cells release kinin.
  Effect: Capillaries become more permeable, allowing fluid to move from capillaries into tissue spaces. This results in tissue **edema** (swelling).
- *Response:* **Leukocytes** (white blood cells) move into the area.
  Effect: Localized blood flow again decreases to keep WBCs in the area to fight infection.

Cellular Response   Specialized white blood cells **(phagocytes)** migrate to the site of injury and engulf bacteria, other foreign material, and damaged cells and destroy them. Sometimes they form a "wall" around an invading pathogen. The accumulation of dead white cells, digested bacteria, and other cell debris in the presence of infection is called *pus.*

Exudate Formation   The fluid and white blood cells that move from the circulation to the site of injury are called **exudate.** The nature and quantity of exudate depend on the severity of injury and the tissues involved. For example, a surgical incision may ooze serosanguineous (clear or pinkish) exudate for a day or two.

Healing   Healing is the replacement of tissue by regeneration or repair.

- **Regeneration** is replacement of the damaged cells with identical or similar cells. However, not all cells can regenerate

(e.g., some central nervous system neurons and cardiac muscle cells cannot regenerate).

- **Repair** occurs when scar tissue replaces the original tissue. Most injuries heal by repair. You will find a thorough discussion of wound healing in Chapter 36.

The inflammatory response is adaptive in that it protects the body from infection and promotes healing. However, chronic inflammation, as in arthritis, is itself a stressor.
KEY POINT: *Do not confuse inflammation with infection.* Inflammation is a mechanism for eliminating invading pathogens; therefore, you always see inflammation when there is infection. However, inflammation is stimulated by trauma as well as by pathogens (e.g., swelling of a sprained ankle); thus, it can occur when there is no infection.

KnowledgeCheck 12-4

- What are four characteristics of the local adaptation syndrome (LAS)?
- Name two LAS responses.
- What are the classic symptoms of the inflammatory process?

Psychological Responses to Stress Include Feelings, Thoughts, and Behaviors

Health professionals understand most human health disorders to be *biopsychosocial.* This means that we respond and adapt to stress physically, mentally, behaviorally, and even spiritually.

Psychological responses are both emotional and cognitive, and they include feelings, thoughts, and behaviors (Box 12-2). They may be fleeting, as in a flash of anger that is gone in seconds, or long term, as in the avoidance of relationships by an adult whose needs for love and security were not met as a child.

As with physical responses, psychological responses can be adaptive or harmful. Consider this example case:

> Both Mr. Laslow and Mr. Harvey have had heart attacks and are feeing anxious. To relieve his anxiety, Mr. Laslow uses problem-solving. He learns about diet, exercise, and lifestyle changes that he must make. Mr. Harvey uses denial, saying, "I feel fine. Even if I deny myself the burgers, beer, and cigarettes, I could still get hit by a truck and die tomorrow." Both of these men may experience some relief from anxiety. Which approach do you think is more adaptive in the long term?

Common emotional responses to stress include the concepts of anxiety, fear, anger, and depression.

Anxiety

Anxiety is diffuse and not easily defined. NANDA International (2015, p. 323) defines it as a "vague, uneasy feeling of discomfort or dread accompanied by an autonomic response (the source often nonspecific or unknown to the individual); a feeling of apprehension caused by anticipation of danger. . . ." Notice that the response is not to a danger but to the *anticipation* of danger—to imagining it. An anxious person worries; feels nervous, uneasy, and fearful; may be tearful; and often has physical symptoms, such as nausea, trembling, and sweating. However, he cannot say specifically what he is afraid of.

- *Mild to moderate anxiety*—may be adaptive because it motivates and mobilizes the person to action.

BOX 12-1 ■ Agents Causing Inflammatory Responses

The following agents stimulate the inflammatory response by causing cell injury:

- Autoimmune disorders
- Antigen–antibody responses
- Body substances (e.g., digestive enzymes leaking into the abdomen; accumulation of uric acid crystals in joints)
- Chemical injury (e.g., acid or alkali burns)
- Ischemia
- Neoplastic growth (i.e., cancer)
- Pathogens (e.g., bacteria, viruses)
- Physical agents:
  Heat or cold
  Radiation
  Electrothermal injury
  Mechanical trauma (e.g., abrasion, contusion, laceration, puncture, incision, fractures, sprains)

BOX 12-2 ■ Psychological Responses to Stressors

Cognitive Responses

Difficulty concentrating
Poor judgment
Decrease in accuracy (e.g., in counting money)
Forgetfulness
Decreased problem-solving ability
Decreased attention to detail
Difficulty learning
Narrowing of focus
Preoccupation, daydreaming

Emotional Responses

Adjustment disorders
Anger
Anxiety
Depression
Fear
Feelings of inadequacy
Low self-esteem
Irritability
Lack of motivation
Lethargy

Behavioral Responses

Academic difficulties
Aggressiveness
Crying, emotional outbursts
Dependence
Nightmares
Poor job performance
Substance use and abuse
Altered sleeping (too little or too much)
Change in eating habits (e.g., loss of appetite, overeating)
Decrease in quality of job performance
Preoccupation (i.e., daydreaming)
Illnesses
Increased absenteeism from work or school
Increased number of accidents
Strained family or social relationships
Avoiding social situations or relationships
Rebellion, acting out

■ *Severe anxiety*—consumes energy and interferes with the person's ability to focus on and respond to what is really happening.

See Chapter 13 for more information on theoretical knowledge of anxiety and fear, including levels of anxiety.

Fear

Fear is an emotion or feeling of apprehension (dread) from an identified danger, threat, or pain. The danger may be real or imagined. Anxiety and fear produce similar responses. However, some experts differentiate them as follows:

■ Fear is a cognitive response; anxiety is an emotional response.
■ Fear is related to a present event; anxiety is related to a future (or anticipated) event.
■ The source of fear is easily identifiable; the source of anxiety may not be identifiable.
■ Fear can result from either a physical or a psychological event; anxiety results from psychological conflict rather than physical threat.

ThinkLike a Nurse 12-2

Read the following two scenarios. In which situation are you most likely to feel fear rather than anxiety? Explain your reasoning.

1. You are a student assigned to a 6-hour day in the clinical area. Each time you have a clinical day coming up, you feel anticipation and look forward to working in the clinical area. However, you do not know what to expect. You think: "What will my patients be like? How will the day go? Do I know enough to handle it? Do I need to practice any procedures?" It is hard to answer these questions until you are actually on the unit and see your patients.
2. Given the same situation, suppose that when you begin your clinical day, your clinical instructor tells you that he will be in the agency asking questions, supervising, evaluating your performance, and, perhaps from your perspective, making your life miserable.

Ego Defense Mechanisms

When faced with a stressful situation, ego defenses may kick in to diminish inner tension. Just as the body responds physiologically to stressors, it has psychological responses that protect from anxiety and assist with adaptation (Table 12-1).

■ *When used sparingly,* and for mild to moderate anxiety, defense mechanisms can be helpful.
■ *When overused,* defense mechanisms become habits that give us the false illusion that we are coping.
■ *If psychological defense mechanisms are inadequate* to diminish the threat and restore equilibrium, the person may develop an anxiety disorder.

Anger and Depression

Anger is a strong, uncomfortable feeling of animosity, hostility, extreme indignation, or displeasure. When expressed appropriately and clearly (i.e., verbally), anger can be a healthy release of tension. When the conflict is in the open, those involved can deal with it.

A person who cannot control stressors may become apprehensive (anxious about what may happen) and respond with anger. Thus, anger is often a first protective response against anxiety. As anxiety increases and the person recognizes fear, he feels more threatened and may resort to bullying behavior to increase the personal feeling of power, control, and self-esteem.

Hostility is anger that involves destructive behaviors (e.g., physical or verbal abuse). Some people exhibit anger by shouting, throwing things, or hitting, or more subtly with sarcastic, caustic remarks. Others attempt to hide their emotions and soften their hurtful remarks, or make them more socially acceptable through the use of humor and joking. Even verbal expressions of anger can lead to resentment and alienation.

Depression is sometimes associated with unresolved anger and may result from stress. It is normal to feel depression in response to any loss or a traumatic event, but long-term depression is a reason for concern. See Chapter 13 for more information about anger and depression.

KnowledgeCheck 12-5

■ In addition to ego defense mechanisms, name four common emotional responses to stress.
■ Explain how mild to moderate anxiety can be adaptive.
■ True or false: One difference between anxiety and fear is that the danger in anxiety may be imagined, whereas in fear the danger is real.
■ What are ego defense mechanisms?

Table 12-1 ➤ Psychological Defense Mechanisms

DEFENSE MECHANISM	EXAMPLES	EXAMPLES AND CONSEQUENCES OF OVERUSE
Avoidance—Unconsciously staying away from events or situations that might open feelings of aggression or anxiety.	"I can't go to the class reunion tonight. I'm too tired; I have to sleep."	The person becomes socially isolated because of the tension he feels when around other people.
Compensation—Making up for a perceived inadequacy by developing or emphasizing some other desirable trait.	A small boy who wants to be on the football team instead becomes a great singer.	Use of drugs or alcohol to gain courage to enter a social situation.
Conversion—Emotional conflict is changed into physical symptoms that have no physical basis. The symptoms often disappear after the threat is over.	Feeling back pain when it is difficult to continue carrying the pressures of life; developing nausea that causes the person to miss a major exam.	Laryngitis, inability to speak on the anniversary of father's death. Continued anxiety can lead to actual physical disorders, such as gastric ulcers.
Denial—Transforming reality by refusing to acknowledge thoughts, feeling, desires, or impulses. This is unconscious; the person is *not* consciously lying. Denial is usually the first defense learned.	A student refuses to acknowledge that he is barely passing anatomy, does not withdraw from the class, and is now failing a nursing course. A person with alcohol dependence states, "I can quit any time I want to."	Overuse can lead to repression and dissociative disorders (e.g., dual personalities, selective amnesia).
Displacement—"Kick the dog." Transferring emotions, ideas, or wishes from one original object or situation to a substitute inappropriate person or object that is perceived to be less powerful or threatening.	Husband loses his job, goes home, and yells at his wife. (This mechanism is rarely adaptive.)	In extreme situations, this mechanism leads to verbal and physical abuse.
Dissociation—Painful events are separated or dissociated from the conscious mind.	A person who was sexually abused as a child describes the events as though they happened to a sibling.	May result in a dissociative disorder, such as multiple personality disorder.
Identification—A person takes on the ideas, personality, or characteristics of another person, especially someone whom the person fears or respects.	Children play cowboy, police, firefighter, or mommy.	Assumes mannerisms, wears clothing, and arranges hair and physical appearance to match those of the other person.
Intellectualization—Cognitive reasoning is used to block or avoid feelings about a painful incident.	When her husband dies, the wife relieves her pain by thinking, "It's better this way; he was in so much pain." A person says, "I think" rather than, "I feel."	"My husband loves me, but he doesn't like it when another man talks to me; that's why he loses his temper and releases his anger physically by hitting me."
Minimization—Not acknowledging or accepting the significance of one's own behavior, making it less important.	"It doesn't matter how much I drink. I never drive when I'm drinking."	Person engages in unhealthy or antisocial behavior; there is no motivation to change behavior.
Projection—Blaming others. Attributing one's own personality traits, mistakes, emotions, motives, and thoughts to another; "finger pointing."	"The clinical instructor makes me nervous, so I cannot do well." "I forgot to bake cookies because you did not tell me that cookies were due at school today."	Person cannot see his own responsibility for a situation, so he cannot make adaptive behaviors. Person criticizes habits in others that are the same as one's own bad habits.
Rationalization—Use of a logical-sounding excuse to cover up or justify true ideas, actions, or feelings. An attempt to preserve self-respect or approval or to conceal a motive for some action by giving a socially acceptable reason. Similar to intellectualization, but uses faulty logic.	"It was God's will that this happened to me." "If I didn't have to work, I would be a better wife."	This mechanism can lead to self-deception.

Table 12-1 ➤ Psychological Defense Mechanisms—cont'd

DEFENSE MECHANISM	EXAMPLES	EXAMPLES AND CONSEQUENCES OF OVERUSE
Reaction formation—Similar to compensation, except the person develops the opposite trait. The person is aware of her feelings but acts in ways opposite to what she is really feeling.	"It's okay that you forgot my birthday" (when it really is not okay).	Overuse can cause failure to resolve internal conflicts.
Regression—Using behavior appropriate in an earlier stage of development to overcome feeling of insecurity in a present situation.	Cooks and eats a comfort food (e.g., hot fudge sundae). A 60-year-old divorcee dresses and acts like a teenager.	Can interfere with perception of reality.
Repression—Unconscious "burying" or "forgetting" of painful thoughts, feelings, memories, ideas; pushing them from a conscious to an unconscious level. It is a step deeper than denial.	Having no memory of sexual abuse by sibling or father. An adolescent forgets to put out the trash because being "bossed" makes him angry, but he feels guilty if he consciously chooses not to do it.	Flashbacks, PTSD, and amnesia.
Restitution (undoing)—Making amends for a behavior one thinks is unacceptable to reduce guilt.	Giving a treat to a child who has been punished for wrongdoing.	May send double messages. Relieves the person of the responsibility for honesty about the situation.
Sublimation—Unacceptable drives, traits, or behaviors (often sexual or aggressive) are unconsciously diverted to socially accepted traits.	Anger is expressed by aggression when playing sports. A person who chooses not to have children runs a day-care center.	The "acceptable" behavior might reinforce the negative tendencies, and the person may still show signs of the undesirable trait or behavior. For example, a person indulges in child pornography to obtain sexual gratification.

Source: Adapted from Gorman, L. M., & Anwar, R. (Eds.). (2014). *Neeb's fundamentals of mental health nursing* (4th ed.). Philadelphia, PA: F.A. Davis.

Spiritual Responses to Stress

Spiritual responses vary among individuals—as do all human responses. Examples include the following:

- Depending on a higher power or religious community for support when coping with stress
- Searching for a larger meaning in the illness or other stressor
- Viewing stress as a test, a punishment, or a challenge.

Spiritual responses vary in different stages of stress.

- Alarm Stage—A common first response is to pray or ask for help (e.g., for healing, coping).
- Adaptation Stage—Prayer, meditation, and religious affiliation can also help during the second stage (adaptation).
- Exhaustion or Recovery—Spiritual resources may become exhausted, creating Spiritual Distress, leaving the person feeling abandoned, helpless, and hopeless.

WHAT PROBLEMS OCCUR WHEN ADAPTATION FAILS?

Living with continual stress strains adaptive mechanisms and can lead to exhaustion and disease—which in turn can lead to more stress. Once established, this type of feedback loop is difficult to break. When adaptation fails, three types of disorders that can develop are stress-induced organic responses, somatoform disorders, and psychological disorders.

Stress-Induced Organic Responses

As a result of repeated central nervous system stimulation and elevation of certain hormones, continual stress brings about long-term changes in various body systems. People who use maladaptive coping strategies (e.g., overeating, substance abuse) create additional stress on the body, further contributing to disease (Table 12-2).

Somatoform Disorders

Somatoform disorders are conditions characterized by the presence of physical symptoms with no known organic cause. They are believed to result from unconscious denial, repression, and displacement of anxiety. The physical symptoms allow the person to avoid a situation that, if confronted, would provoke extreme anxiety.

Certain people seem predisposed to somatoform disorders—for example, those who suffer from personality disorders and major psychiatric illness; those who do not handle anxiety well; and those who are dependent, emotionally needy, frustrated,

Table 12-2 ➤ Organic Responses Related to Failure of Adaptation

BODY SYSTEM	PHYSIOLOGICAL RESPONSE
Cardiovascular system	■ *Decreased cardiac output, oxygen depletion, and fatigue*—Continued secretion of epinephrine may cause angina, myocardial infarction, cardiomegaly, and congestive heart failure, all of which lead to decreased cardiac output. As cardiac output decreases, less oxygen circulates to meet cellular metabolic demands, and the body becomes fatigued. Stress has been directly linked to stroke (Richardson, Shaffer, Falzon, et al., 2012). ■ *Vasoconstriction causes hypertension*—Prolonged secretion of epinephrine and renin result in vasoconstriction, causing hypertension. ■ *Electrolyte imbalance and edema*—ADH, aldosterone, ACTH, and cortisol create electrolyte imbalance and retention of sodium and water, thus promoting peripheral edema.
Endocrine system	■ *Diabetes*—Consistent high levels of blood glucose and insulin can cause diabetes. ■ *Hyper- or hypothyroidism*—These metabolic disorders can result as persistent demands for thyroid hormone production cause a rebound failure of the gland. ■ *Prenatal effects*—Prenatal stress can increase the risk for preterm birth, low birth weight, and developmental delays and metabolic diseases later in life.
Immune system	■ *Autoimmune illness*—Stress reduces the ability of the body's immune cells to differentiate between self and non-self. Thus, the immune cells begin to attack body tissues, producing autoimmune illness (e.g., rheumatoid arthritis, allergies). ■ *Suppression of immunity*—Stress can weaken the immune system, leading to infection and illness. Indirectly, it is also linked to cancer (Ohio State University, 2013).
Gastrointestinal system	■ *Bowel inflammation and other disorders*—Stress can cause the bowel to react with constipation or diarrhea, gastroesophageal reflux, colitis, or irritable bowel syndrome. ■ *Gastric hyperacidity*—Continued secretion of hydrochloric acid produces gastric hyperacidity and erosion of the gastrointestinal tract, including the stomach, especially in the presence of *Helicobacter pylori*.
Musculoskeletal system	■ *Muscle tension and pain*—Constant readiness for fight or flight produces muscle tension and pain in various body sites. ■ *Tension headache and temporomandibular joint pain*—These can result from prolonged muscle tension in the head, neck, and spine.
Respiratory system	■ *Increased respiratory rate*—Epinephrine and circulating hormones dilate the bronchial tubes and increase the rate of respiration. ■ *Hyperventilation*—This can produce symptoms of alkalosis, including dizziness, tingling hands and feet, and anxiety. ■ *Exacerbation of existing asthma, hay fever, and allergies*—All of these can be provoked by distress in the respiratory system. In addition, stress aggravates chronic bronchitis and emphysema (Quick, Saleh, Sime, et al., 2006).

ACTH = adrenocorticotropic hormone; ADH = antidiuretic hormone; PTSD = post-traumatic stress disorder.

and resentful (Gorman & Anwar, 2014). The following are examples of somatoform disorders:

- **Hypochondriasis.** The person is preoccupied with the idea that he is or will become seriously ill. The person is abnormally concerned with his health and interprets his real or imagined symptoms unrealistically, fearing that they will get worse or become incurable. **KEY POINT:** *The person is not "faking it"; anxiety about his health may trigger the physical sensations.*
- **Somatization.** In this disorder, anxiety and emotional turmoil are expressed in physical symptoms, loss of physical function,

pain that changes location often, and depression. **KEY POINT:** *The patient is unable to control the symptoms and behaviors, and complaints are vague or exaggerated.*
- **Pain disorder.** Previously called *somatoform pain disorder*, this is emotional pain that manifests physically. Pain is the main focus of the person's life. The physical cause is either disproportionate to the pain level the patient reports or cannot be found at all. The pain does not change location.
- **Malingering.** Malingering is different from the other disorders because it is a *conscious* effort to use his symptoms to escape unpleasant situations or gain something

(e.g., calling in sick because the person does not want to go to work).

Stress-Induced Psychological Responses

Even if defense mechanisms are effective initially, with long-term stress exhaustion sets in and the mechanisms begin to fail. The person may then try maladaptive ways to cope. As work and personal relationships deteriorate, the person loses self-esteem. Prolonged stress can eventually result in crisis and burnout, which we discuss next (also see Fig. 12-6). More severe responses include psychiatric illnesses, such as anxiety disorders, clinical depression, and post-traumatic stress disorder (PTSD). Anxiety and depression are discussed in Chapter 13.

Crisis

A **crisis** exists when (1) an event in a person's life drastically changes the person's routine and he perceives it as a threat to self, and (2) the person's usual coping methods are ineffective, resulting in high levels of anxiety and inability to function adequately. Crisis events are usually sudden and unexpected (e.g., serious illness or death of a loved one, serious financial losses, an automobile accident, domestic violence, and natural disasters) (Fig. 12-6).

Each person has a different tolerance for stress; an event that creates a crisis for one may be just a minor nuisance for another. Nevertheless, most experts agree that people experiencing crisis go through five phases (Gorman & Anwar, 2014; Stuart, 2012).

1. *Precrisis.* In response to the event or anxiety, the person uses usual coping strategies; has no symptoms; denies feeling stress; and may even report a sense of well-being.
2. *Impact.* In this phase, anxiety and confusion increase. The person may have trouble organizing his or her personal life and may feel the stress but minimize its severity.
3. *Crisis.* The person experiences more anxiety and tries new ways of coping, such as withdrawal, rationalization, and projection (refer to Table 12-1). The person recognizes the problem but denies that it is out of control.
4. *Adaptive.* The person redefines the threat and perceives the crisis in a realistic way. Rational thinking and positive problem-solving help the person to regain some self-esteem and begin socializing again. Adaptation is more likely if the person can use effective coping strategies and if situational supports are available.
5. *Postcrisis.* In the aftermath of a crisis, a person may have developed better ways of coping with stress. Or, he or she may be critical, hostile, and depressed, and using maladaptive strategies (e.g., overeating or engaging in substance abuse) to deal with what has happened.

KEY POINT: *People in crisis are at risk for physical and emotional harm, so intervention is essential (see Crisis Intervention later in the chapter).*

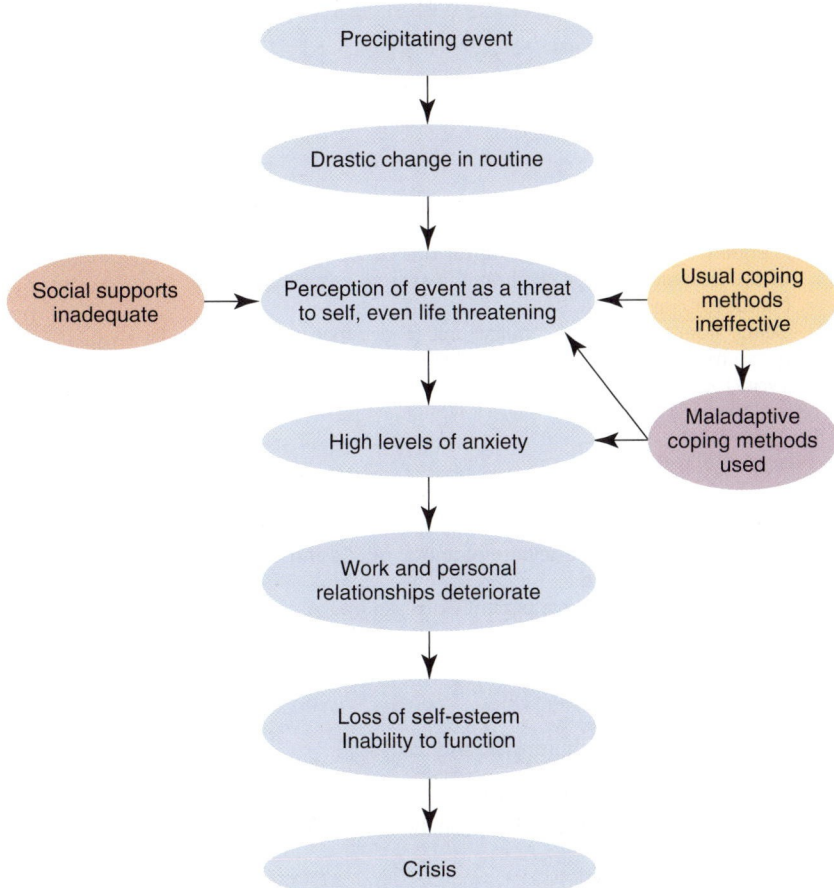

FIGURE 12-6 How a crisis develops.

ThinkLike a Nurse 12-3

Suppose you are the charge nurse on a 30-bed surgical unit. In addition, you must assume care of three more patients because another nurse called in sick. It is a normal, busy day with seven postoperative patients and eight discharges. In addition, a patient went into cardiac arrhythmia and was transferred to the coronary care unit. Because the sick nurse was supposed to work a 12-hour shift and no replacement has been found, you are told you must stay and work 4 hours of overtime. You had plans to have dinner with your spouse this evening because it is your anniversary. Now you will surely not be home before 8:00 p.m., and you will be exhausted.

- What would be the stressors for you in this situation?
- What thoughts and feelings would you have?
- What physical responses would you probably notice?
- What are some psychological responses that you would use to help you adapt and cope with this day?
- How would you probably react if the same thing happens on the following day?

Burnout

Burnout occurs when a person cannot cope effectively with the physical and emotional demands of the workplace. You will find examples of stressors specific to nursing in Box 12-3. Excessive demands, lack of respect, or little support from an employer or coworkers can serve as a catalyst for burnout.

BOX 12-3 ■ Stressors That Can Lead to Burnout

Relationship Stressors

- Dealing with difficult personalities (e.g., patients, supervisors, physicians)

Staffing Stressors

- Working 12-hour shifts with minimal breaks for food, water, or rest
- Frequent rotating shifts that upset the circadian rhythm of the body and lower the immune system response
- Mandatory overtime
- Being "floated" to an unfamiliar unit (e.g., a maternity nurse may be "floated" to an orthopedic unit)
- Workload: low staffing ratio (one nurse to many patients)

Nurse–Patient Stressors

- Frustration with patients (e.g., those who do not follow therapeutic routines)
- Need to constantly anticipate patients' needs and cope with the unexpected
- Feeling helpless against a patient's disease process or lack of healing
- Dealing with death and dying

Employer Issues

- Lack of rewards (both intrinsic and extrinsic)
- Lack of participation in decision making
- Inability to delegate responsibilities
- Organizational philosophy that conflicts with personal philosophy

---

In response, the nurse experiences anger or frustration, feels overwhelmed and helpless, or suffers low self-esteem and depression. Some nurses experience grief, moral distress, and guilt when the situation prevents them from performing as well as they believe they should. As a result, a nurse may develop a physical illness or a negative attitude, or may use maladaptive coping techniques such as smoking, engaging in substance abuse, or distancing from patients—"going through the motions" but not really interacting with patients in a meaningful way. Many nurses with these feelings may give up and leave nursing. You will find suggestions for preventing burnout later in the chapter.

Example Problem: Post-Traumatic Stress Disorder

Post-traumatic stress disorder (PTSD) is a severe form of anxiety following exposure to extreme psychological a violent trauma (e.g., natural disaster) or to physical or emotional abuse (e.g., rape, combat). For nursing care, see the accompanying Example Problem for PTSD.

KnowledgeCheck 12-7

Define *crisis, burnout,* and *post-traumatic stress disorder.*

PracticalKnowledge
knowing **how**

In the remainder of this chapter you will learn about planning and implementing care for patients experiencing stress. You will also have opportunities to practice clinical reasoning and critical thinking.

ASSESSMENT NP

People under stress may not think clearly or communicate effectively; therefore, you will need to demonstrate empathy, develop rapport, and relieve their immediate anxiety as much as possible before beginning an assessment. Focus the patient by asking short, direct questions and then proceeding to open-ended questions that will provide you with as much information as possible (see Chapter 20 for information on questioning techniques).

Assess Stressors, Risk Factors, and Coping and Adaptation

Data about the patient's stressors and risk factors should help you to:

- Determine whether the client has a realistic or an exaggerated perception of the stressors.
- Identify factors that increase risk for future stress.
- Identify interventions to reduce current stress and to provide anticipatory guidance to prevent future stress.

You might begin gathering these data by having the patient complete a stress inventory. Then follow up with observations such as those in the Focused Assessment box, Assessing for Stress: Questions to Ask.

Assess Responses to Stress

Stress responses are holistic. Therefore, you will need to assess physiological, emotional, behavioral, and cognitive indicators of stress. **KEY POINT:** *Be aware that if coping is*

EXAMPLE PROBLEM: Post-Traumatic Stress Disorder (PTSD)

General Definition: Anxiety following exposure to extreme psychological event or to physical or emotional abuse; feelings of harm and helplessness during a traumatic event.

Nursing Diagnosis (NANDA-I): Post-Trauma Syndrome: Sustained maladaptive response to a traumatic, overwhelming event
Other NANDA-I Diagnoses: Anxiety, Social Isolation, Situational Low Self-Esteem

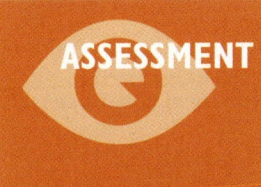
ASSESSMENT

Assess for these symptoms

Physical Increased BP and heart rate, rapid breathing, muscle tension, nausea, diarrhea, dizziness. See Box 12-4.

Cognition and Mood
Can begin or worsen after the traumatic event, but are not due to injury or substance use; may feel detached from friends or family
- Trouble remembering key features of the traumatic event
- Negative thoughts
- Distorted feelings (guilt or blame)
- Loss of interest in enjoyable activities
- Chemical abuse, dependence

Re-experiencing Words, objects, places, or situations that are reminders of the event and can trigger nightmares, fear, and **flashbacks** (reliving the trauma), including physical symptoms like racing heart or sweating

Avoidance—Reminders of the event may be the trigger to:
- Stay away from places, events, or objects that are reminders of the traumatic experience
- Feel emotionally numb
- Feel strong guilt, depression, or worry
- Lose interest in once enjoyable activities
- Difficulty remembering the event

Reactivity—Usually constant instead of being triggered by a reminder of the event
- Easily startled
- Agitation, irritability
- Difficulty sleeping
- Angry outbursts
- Excessive emotions
- Problems relating to others, including feeling or showing affection
- Difficulty concentrating

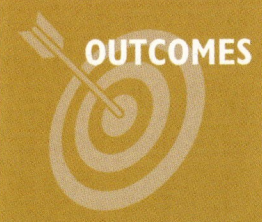
OUTCOMES

NOC Outcomes—Mood Equilibrium, Personal Resiliency, Personal Well-Being

Individualized goals/outcome statements
- Breaks up large tasks into small ones; sets priorities

- Breaks up large tasks into small ones; sets priorities
- Spends time with other people; confides in a trusted friend or relative.
- Expects symptoms to improve gradually, not immediately
- Is active in trying to reduce stress

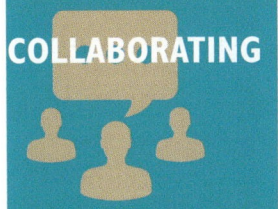
COLLABORATING

- Counseling or psychotherapy
- Exposure therapy
- Family therapy
- Group therapy

- Cognitive behavioral therapy
- Eye movement desensitization and reprocessing
- Medications (antidepressants)

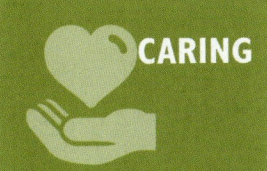
CARING

Encourage the client to seek out comforting situations, places, and people.

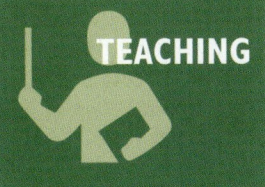
TEACHING

Help people to:
- Identify and deal with guilt, shame, and other feelings about the event.
- Change how they react to their PTSD symptoms (e.g., therapy helps people face reminders of the trauma).

Teach:
- Effects of trauma
- Relaxation and anger-control skills
- Tips for better sleep, diet, and exercise habits

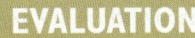
EVALUATION

Assess for the following indicators of improvement:
- Exhibits affect that fits situation
- Verbalizes positive outlook

- Removes self from abusive relationships.
- Expresses satisfaction with social relationships
- Demonstrates ability to control activities
- Performs usual roles

Assessing for Stress: Questions to Ask

1. **Assess stressors and risk factors.** Ask the client to complete a stress inventory, such as the Holmes-Rahe Social Readjustment Scale. Then ask the client the following questions:
   - ➤ What is causing the most stress in your life?
   - ➤ On a scale of 1 to 10 (1 being "not much" and 10 being "extreme"), rate the stress you are experiencing in each of these areas: work or school, finances, community responsibilities, your health, health of a family member, family relationships, family responsibilities, relationships with friends.
   - ➤ How long have you been dealing with the stressful situation(s)?
   - ➤ Can you track the accumulation of stress in your life?
   - ➤ How long have you been under this stress?
   - ➤ Note the client's developmental stage and determine whether he is functioning as expected for this stage. Review Chapter 9 if you need help in identifying developmental milestones. To help you assess for stressors that can be predicted to occur in each stage, you might ask questions such as the following:
     What challenges do you face as a result of your life and your age?
     Have you had recent life changes?
     Do you anticipate any life changes?

2. **Assess coping methods and adaptation.**
   - ➤ What coping strategies have you used previously? What was successful and what was not successful?
   - ➤ Tell me about previous experiences you have had with stressful situations in your life.
   - ➤ What do you usually do to handle stressful situations? (If the client needs prompting, you can ask, "Do you cry, get angry, avoid people, talk to family or friends, do physical exercise, pray? Some people laugh or joke, others meditate, others try to control everything, others just work hard and look for a solution. What is your usual response?")
   - ➤ How well do these methods usually work for you?
   - ➤ What have you been doing to cope with the present situation?
   - ➤ How well is that working?
   - ➤ During the interview, you should also observe for the use of psychological defense mechanisms. See Table 12-1.
     - ➤ If the patient has not exhibited any defense mechanisms, you could ask about the common ones. For example, "Do you ever cope with a situation by denying it exists or just by trying to put it out of your mind?"
   - ➤ Ask the client about physiological changes and diseases caused by ongoing stress. Check the client's records for a history of somatoform disorders. Ask the client:
     What physical illnesses do you have? How long have you had them?
     What, if any, physical changes have you noticed?
     Do you have other physical conditions, for example, hypertension, cardiac disease, diabetes, arthritis, joint pains, cancer?
     To review maladaptive responses to stress, see Table 12-2.

3. **Assess physiological responses to stress.**
   The following are examples of questions you should ask:
   - ➤ What do you do to stay healthy?
   - ➤ Tell me about your health habits.
   - ➤ How often do you have a checkup?
   - ➤ What are your health concerns?

4. **Observe for emotional and behavioral responses to stress.**
   Emotional Responses
   - ➤ Anger
   - ➤ Anxiety
   - ➤ Depression
   - ➤ Fear
   - ➤ Feelings of inadequacy
   - ➤ Low self-esteem
   - ➤ Lack of motivation
   - ➤ Lethargy

   Behavioral Responses
   - ➤ Crying, emotional outburst
   - ➤ Dependence
   - ➤ Poor job performance
   - ➤ Substance use and abuse
   - ➤ Sleeplessness or sleeping too much
   - ➤ Change in eating habits (e.g., diminished appetite or overeating)
   - ➤ Decrease in quality of job performance
   - ➤ Preoccupation or distraction
   - ➤ Listlessness
   - ➤ Increased absenteeism
   - ➤ Increased number of accidents
   - ➤ Reduced interest in social interactions or relationships
   - ➤ Rebellion, acting out

   Examples of Assessment Questions
   - ➤ Do you smoke?
   - ➤ How much alcohol do you drink every day?
   - ➤ What do you eat? What is your typical eating pattern?
   - ➤ How much fluid do you drink daily?
   - ➤ How many hours do you sleep at night? Do you feel rested when you wake up?
   - ➤ Do you often wake up very early in the morning and have difficulty getting back to sleep?
   - ➤ What prescribed medications, vitamins, over-the-counter medications, or herbs do you take?
   - ➤ What regular physical activity or exercise do you engage in?
   - ➤ How much time do you spend at work versus at leisure and play?
   - ➤ Do you constantly take work home with you? Do you think about work almost all the time?
   - ➤ How do you relax?
   - ➤ Have you given up activities and relationships you previously enjoyed because you "don't have enough time" or are too tired?
   - ➤ How do you express anger?
   - ➤ Do you try to be perfect?
   - ➤ Would you describe yourself as having the stress-filled lifestyle of a type A personality?
   - ➤ How often do you find yourself feeling hopeless? Sad?

Assessing for Stress: Questions to Ask—cont'd

5. **Assess cognitive responses to stress.**
   Observe for the following responses when you assess other functional areas:
   ➤ Difficulty concentrating
   ➤ Poor judgment
   ➤ Decrease in accuracy (e.g., in counting money)
   ➤ Forgetfulness
   ➤ Decreased problem-solving ability
   ➤ Decreased attention to detail
   ➤ Difficulty learning
   ➤ Narrowing of focus
   ➤ Preoccupation, daydreaming
6. **Assess support systems.**
   Ask the following questions:
   ➤ Tell me about your home. Describe your living environment. (Make a home visit if possible, or contact the case manager or social worker to arrange a home evaluation.)
   ➤ Who in your life provides the most support for you? In what ways do they support you?
   ➤ What support is available from family, friends, significant others, community agencies, and clergy that you may not have required until now?
   ➤ Do you have or do you seek spiritual support?
   ➤ How has your stress affected the family?
   ➤ What are your financial resources? What are your financial obligations?

---

successful, clinical signs and symptoms of stress may not be present.

- **Assessing Physiological Responses.** Because the GAS is nonspecific, you must obtain data from all body systems (for physical examination techniques, see Chapter 21).
  Vital signs—Elevations in pulse, respiration, and blood pressure will indicate whether the fight-or-flight response is present.
  General survey, or overview, of the patient—Note hygiene, grooming, facial expression, body language, posture, nonverbal expression, and ability to make eye contact.
  Box 12-4 summarizes physiological responses that indicate stress.
- **Assessing Emotional and Behavioral Responses.** Assess for the emotional and behavioral responses to stress that are described in Box 12-2 and in the Focused Assessment box. The client may or may not be aware that the feelings or behaviors are related to stress, so be sure to:
  Observe nonverbal behaviors and body language for cues to mood and affect.
  Check client records for evidence about destructive behaviors (e.g., drug abuse).
- **Assessing Cognitive Responses.** You can assess the client's cognitive functioning as you assess other functional areas. See Box 12-2 to review examples of cognitive responses. When you ask the client to describe and rate the intensity of the stressors, you can begin to assess whether he perceives the stressors realistically or in an exaggerated way.

Assess Support Systems

Recall that support systems, such as family, friends, and coworkers, are important to the success of a client's coping strategies. Conversely, these people may be affected by the same stressors or by the client's responses to them. For these reasons, you should determine the supports available and their ability to assist the client—that is, do the significant others have the sensitivity and skills to be supportive? (See the Focused Assessment box Assessing for Stress: Questions to Ask.)

ThinkLike a Nurse 12-4

Review the scenario of Gloria and John (Meet Your Patients). How much does it really tell you about the clients' situation?

- Which aspect of stress do you have the most information about: their stressors, their coping methods and adaptation, their responses to stress, or their support systems?
- What facts do you have about either Gloria's or John's physiological responses to their multiple stressors? What can you infer their responses might be?
- What facts do you have about the clients' emotional and behavioral responses to their stressors?
- What information do you have about how well they are adapting to stress?
- What data do you have about their support systems? What information do you need?

BOX 12-4 ■ Physiological Responses to Stressors

- Dilated pupils
- Muscle tension
- Stiff neck
- Headaches
- Nail biting
- Skin pallor
- Skin lesions (e.g., eczema)
- Diaphoresis, sweaty palms
- Dry mouth
- Nausea
- Weight or appetite changes
- Increased blood glucose
- Increased heart rate
- Cardiac dysrhythmias
- Hyperventilation
- Chest pain
- Water retention
- Increased urinary frequency or decreased urinary output
- Diarrhea or constipation
- Flatulence

ANALYSIS/NURSING DIAGNOSIS NP

Stress is nonspecific, so there is almost no limit to the number of nursing diagnoses that could be stress induced. Your theoretical knowledge of the holistic nature of stress should lead you to identify diagnoses in the physical, behavioral, cognitive, emotional, interpersonal, and spiritual domains. The following are some examples:

Physical	Constipation r/t decreased peristalsis secondary to stress
Behavioral	Ineffective Health Management r/t use of denial as an ego defense mechanism to relieve anxiety
Cognitive	Impaired Memory (short term) r/t overwhelming number and severity of stressors
Emotional	Anxiety r/t uncertainty about the future and ineffectiveness of usual coping mechanisms
Interpersonal	Impaired Parenting r/t maladaptive use of alcohol to cope with recent stress of divorce
Spiritual	Hopelessness r/t perceived lack of support and ability to change the present situation

It is important to identify the etiology of the diagnosis so that you can choose interventions to remove or modify the stressor. For example, if you believe a patient's diarrhea is being caused by stress, you would intervene by modifying the stressor, helping the patient to perceive the stressor differently, and so on. If, instead, a gastrointestinal virus is causing the diarrhea, your interventions would not have been helpful.

KnowledgeCheck 12-8

- How might you identify and assess Gloria and John's stressors (Meet Your Patients)?
- List three questions you could ask to find out how Gloria is coping and adapting to stress.
- List three questions you could ask to assess Gloria's physiological responses to stress. What observations might you also make?
- List three questions you could ask to assess Gloria's emotional and behavioral responses to stress.
- How might you determine whether stress is affecting Gloria's cognitive functioning?
- You know Gloria's sister is providing some support. How could you find out more about the extent of Gloria and John's support system?

PLANNING OUTCOMES/EVALUATION NP

NOC standardized outcomes, if achieved, demonstrate resolution of the problem stated in the nursing diagnosis. For example, if you make a diagnosis of Anxiety related to the client's perception that he will not be able to fulfill family responsibilities, you might use the NOC outcome Anxiety Control.

Individualized goal or outcome statements are also specific to each nursing diagnosis. Broad, general goals for clients experiencing stress are to (1) reduce the strength and duration of the stressor, (2) relieve or relieve responses to stress, and (3) use effective coping mechanisms. Examples of specific outcome statements you might write include the following:

- Reports (or physical exam reveals) reduction in physical symptoms of stress.
- Demonstrates less physical tension in facial expression and other muscle groups.
- Verbalizes increased feelings of control in the stressful situation.
- Uses problem-solving and anxiety-reducing techniques.
- Demonstrates relaxation and stress-reducing strategies.

PLANNING INTERVENTIONS/ IMPLEMENTATION NP

NIC standardized interventions for stress may be linked to both the problem and the etiology of the nursing diagnosis. Using the preceding example of Anxiety related to the client's perception that he will not be able to fulfill family responsibilities, some interventions may focus on supporting the client's ability to fulfill family roles (e.g., Caregiver Support); others may focus on general techniques for relieving anxiety, regardless of its cause (e.g., Anxiety Reduction, Calming Technique).

Specific nursing activities should be individualized on the basis of the patient's needs and the etiologies of the nursing diagnoses. Always consider the patient's ability and motivation to comply with the plan of care (Box 12-5).

Most stress-relieving interventions work by one or more of the following means:

- **Removing stressors,** or modifying them
- **Supporting coping abilities** (e.g., changing the person's perception of the stressor)
- **Treating responses** to stress (e.g., symptoms such as anxiety or diarrhea)

As you read through the following interventions, see whether you can identify which of the preceding provide a rationale for the actions.

Health Promotion Activities

People cannot always control the occurrence of a stressful event, and there are no high-tech treatments for coping with stress. However, a healthy lifestyle can prevent some stressors and improve the ability to cope with others. Chapter 27 provides an in-depth discussion of wellness promotion. The following suggestions are a brief guide to a healthy lifestyle:

Nutrition Nutrition is important for maintaining physical homeostasis and resisting stress. For example, adequate nutrition is essential to maintain the integrity of the immune system; proteins are needed for tissue building and healing. In addition, overweight and malnutrition are stressors that may lead to illness.

See Chapter 28 if you need detailed information about healthful nutrition.

BOX 12-5 ■ Will the Patient Comply?

- Does the person wish to use complementary or alternative care measures? How open is he to deviating from traditional biomedical therapies?
- Is the patient able to comply with the therapies?
- Is the patient willing to follow therapeutic suggestions?
- Confer and collaborate with patients to determine what will fit most comfortably into their lifestyle. Those are the interventions that will be most effective.

Healthy Nutrition for Coping With Stress

➤ Maintain a normal body weight.
➤ Limit the intake of fat (especially animal fat) to no more than 30% of daily calories.
➤ Limit the intake of sugar and salt.
➤ Eat more fish and poultry and less red meat.
➤ Eat smaller, more frequent meals to aid digestion.
➤ Consume 25 grams of fiber (fruits, vegetables, and whole grains) daily to promote bowel elimination.
➤ Consume no more than one or two alcoholic beverages per day but not every day.

Exercise Regular exercise promotes physical and emotional homeostasis. To achieve any health benefits, exercise of moderate to vigorous intensity for at least 150 minutes per week (U.S. Department of Health and Human Services, 2008). Additional health benefits occur with more activity. During exercise, the brain releases **endogenous opioids** (e.g., endorphins), which create a feeling of well-being. Exercise provides the following benefits:

▪ Improves muscle tone and helps to control weight
▪ Improves the functioning of the heart and lungs
▪ Reduces the risk of cardiovascular disease
▪ Promotes relaxation and reduces tension

Advise clients who are obese, chronically ill, or who have always been sedentary to consult a primary caregiver before beginning a new exercise program.

To promote adherence to the exercise routine, suggest that the client identify a variety of physical activities that he enjoys (e.g., swimming, bicycling, walking) and schedule regular sessions with one or more exercise "buddies," if possible.

See Chapter 33 for more specific physical activities to manage stress.

Sleep and Rest Sleep and rest restore energy levels, allow the body to repair itself, and promote mental relaxation. Most people need 7 or 8 hours of sleep a day; however, the amount of sleep varies among individuals. Stress, pain, and illness may interfere with the ability to sleep, so some clients may need help identifying and implementing techniques for relaxing and going to sleep (see Chapter 35 for more information on sleep, as needed).

Leisure Activities Compared with exercise, which not everyone enjoys, leisure activities are any activities that provide joy and satisfaction. They may involve physical activity, or they may be sedentary activities, such as reading, painting, or watching television. Leisure activities are a form of rest and, as such, are restorative.

Time Management People who manage their time efficiently and organize their life routines are likely to feel more in control and, therefore, less stressed. If clients feel overwhelmed, you can help them to prioritize tasks and make "to do" lists. Assist them to learn to do the following:

▪ *Delegate responsibilities and set boundaries on the use of time.* For example, a working couple with three children may need to reserve meals requiring time-consuming preparation for weekends.

▪ *Learn to say no.* People sometimes try to make everyone happy by agreeing to every request for assistance, from family and the community. Prompt clients to ask themselves:
How much can I realistically do?
What is essential to do?
What would be nice to do?

If you would like more information on time management, see Chapter 41, Leading and Managing.

Avoiding Maladaptive Behaviors Some people use maladaptive behaviors as a response to stress. For others, the behaviors themselves become stressors. Advise clients to avoid unhealthful behaviors, such as overuse of caffeine, alcohol, tobacco, recreational or prescription drugs, and even food. Counseling may be beneficial for those experiencing impaired social interactions, sexual dysfunction, poor sleep patterns, stress eating, and risk-taking behaviors.

Toward Evidence-Based Practice

Farrow, C. V., Haycraft, E., & Blissettt, J. M. (2015, May). Teaching our children when to eat: How parental feeding practices inform the development of emotional eating—a longitudinal experimental design. *American Journal of Clinical Nutrition, 101*(5), 908–913. doi:10.3945/ ajcn.114.103713

Researchers concluded that parents who exerted excess control on their children's food intake (e.g., by using food as a reward) may unintentionally teach children to rely on high-calorie foods to cope with stress and negative emotions.

Dewald, J. F., Meijer, A. M., Oort, F. J., et al. (2014). Adolescents' sleep in low-stress and high-stress (exam) times: A prospective quasi-experiment. *Behavioral Sleep Medicine, 12*(6), 493–506. doi:10.1080/15402002. 2012.670675

Researchers examining the influence of stress on the quality of adolescents' sleep compared 175 students during low-stress (regular school week) and high-stress (exam week) periods. They found their sleep more restless during stressful times, yet the onset of sleep and sleep duration were not changed under a stressful situation.

Torres, O. V., & O'Dell, L. E. (2016). Stress is a principal factor that promotes tobacco use in females. *Progress in Neuro-Psychopharmacology & Biological Psychiatry, 2016*(65), 260–268. doi:10.1016/j.pnpbp.2015.04.005.

Researchers studying the role of stress in tobacco use among women found that they are more likely to smoke in order to cope with stress than were men. During smoking abstinence, women experience more intense anxiety than do men and report that the calming effects of smoking are

(Continued)

Toward Evidence-Based Practice—cont'd

the main reason they continue to smoke and why they go back to it after abstaining.

1. Even children experience stress. How might you teach a child to cope with stress?

2. Hans Selye (1974, 1976) found that physical, emotional, psychological, and spiritual stressors or the anticipation of stressors can initiate a physiological stress response. What strategies might the adolescent use to improve sleep during times of stress?

3. These three studies examined the effect that stress can have on behaviors, such as eating, smoking, and sleeping. What other maladaptive behaviors might occur in people experiencing high levels of stress or chronic stress?

 Go to Davis Advantage, Resources, Chapter 12, **Toward Evidence-Based Practice Suggested Responses.**

KnowledgeCheck 12-9

Name and discuss at least four aspects of a healthful lifestyle that can help prevent or relieve stress.

Relieving Anxiety

Because anxiety is a common response to illness, medical tests, and treatments, you will use anxiety-relief interventions every day of your professional life. For example, when you tell patients what to expect before you perform a procedure or ask them to take deep breaths during a painful treatment, you lessen anxiety. If you have developed a therapeutic, trusting relationship, your very presence will help to ease the patient's anxiety. You will find specific interventions for anxiety in Chapter 13, and many of the interventions in the following sections provide anxiety relief as well. Also see the Complementary & Alternative Modalities (CAM) box, Using CAM for Stress Reduction.

Anger Management

Anger is a common response to stress. However, clients usually do not openly say, "I am angry." They may not even recognize that they are angry. Instead, they engage in angry behaviors (e.g., becoming hypercritical, verbally abusive, or demanding). You may have heard stories from nurses about the client who is "on the call light constantly." An angry response from the nurse blocks communication and may escalate the person's anger. For tips on managing anger, refer to Violence, in Chapter 23; and Clinical Insight 12-1, Dealing With Angry Patients.

Stress Management Techniques

Most stress management techniques focus on discharging tension or simplifying one's life to modify stressors or control stress responses. **Relaxation,** a state of reduced physical and mental arousal, is an important intervention because it reverses some stress responses. By elongating muscle fibers, relaxation reduces neural impulses sent to the brain and decreases the activity of the brain and other body systems. In a relaxed state, blood pressure, heart rate, respiratory rate, and oxygen consumption decrease, while peripheral skin temperature and brain alpha wave activity increase.

The techniques in this section are CAM therapies, and some require special training and licensing or credentialing. Many are discussed in detail in other chapters.

Complementary & Alternative Modalities (CAM)

Using CAM for Stress Reduction

van der Zwan, J. E., de Vente, W., Huizink, A. C., et al. (2015, June). Physical activity, mindfulness meditation, or heart rate variability biofeedback for stress reduction: A randomized controlled trial. *Applied Psychophysiology and Biofeedback, 2015.* doi: 10.1007/s10484-015-9293-x

Meditation and Exercise

In a study designed to evaluate the potential preventive effects of meditation or exercise, researchers found fewer episodes of stress, anxiety, and depressive symptoms, as well as more feelings of psychological well-being and sleep in those who meditated or exercised to relieve stress.

Altayar, O., Sharma, V., Prokop, L. J., et al. (2015). Psychological therapies in patients with irritable bowel syndrome: A systematic review and meta-analysis of randomized controlled trials. *Gastroenterology Research and Practice, 2015*(549308), 1–19. Retrieved from http://dx.doi.org/10.1155/2015/549308

Mindfulness Training

This article reports that psychological therapies, including cognitive-behavioral therapies, psychoeducational courses, mind-body therapy, psychodynamic interpersonal therapy, and contingency management, may improve the quality of life and symptom severity in irritable bowel syndrome.

Köhn, M., Lundholm, U. P., Bryngelsso, I-L., et al. (2013). Medical yoga for patients with stress-related symptoms and diagnoses in primary health care: A randomized controlled trial. *Evidence-Based Complementary and Alternative Medicine, 2013.* Retrieved from http://dx.doi.org/10.1155/2013/215348

Yoga

Yoga is effective in reducing levels of stress and anxiety in patients with stress-related symptoms in primary health care.

Exercise Exercise is used to treat, as well as prevent, stress. It releases tension held in muscles, improves muscle tone and posture, expresses emotions, and stimulates the secretion of endorphins, thus creating a feeling of well-being and relaxation.

Relaxation Techniques Relaxation techniques involve teaching the patient to relax individual muscle groups. **Progressive relaxation** in a quiet, meditative state or lying in bed, relaxing and contracting muscle groups, is much less traumatic and damaging to fragile joints and muscles than is active exercise. With **passive relaxation,** the person relaxes the muscle groups without first contracting them.

Meditation Managing stress through meditation involves heightening one's attention or awareness. Regular meditation facilitates harmony among mind, body, and spirit, thereby reducing anxiety and giving the person a sense of control.

Mindfulness is a type of mediation involving focus on the present and living each moment to the fullest. It promotes psychological well-being and decreases internal stress and feelings of nursing burnout (Heard, Hartman, & Buschardt, 2013)

Visualization or Imagery Visualization (imagery) techniques are often used to complement the effects of relaxation techniques. They are explained in Chapter 32 in this text and in Chapter 46 on DavisAdvantage.

Biofeedback Techniques of biofeedback use electronic instruments to measure neuromuscular and autonomic nervous system activity and provide information about those responses to the person. The immediate feedback helps the person become aware of and learn how to **voluntarily** control certain physiological responses, such as those produced by stress.

Acupuncture Acupuncture involves insertion of a needle into "meridian points" to regulate the flow of energy or life force throughout the body. It can modify pain perception and restore normal physiological functions (e.g., decrease the heart rate). If you want more information, see Chapter 32.

Chiropractic Adjustment Chiropractic adjustment involves manual realignment of the vertebrae. The theory is that misalignment of the vertebrae leads to pain, loss of function, and illness. Realignment is performed to free energy, release muscle tension, and improve body function and health. Chiropractors undergo special education and training before they are qualified to perform adjustments.

Reiki and Therapeutic Touch These touch therapies are focused on energy modulation. Healing energy is channeled through a practitioner's hands to improve well-being.

Massage Through manipulation of the soft tissues, massage relaxes muscles and releases body tension. This improves circulation and allows energy and blood to flow through muscles and soft tissues more readily. See Chapter 32 for more information. For instructions on how to give a back rub, also see Procedure 35-1.

Reflexology Reflexology is the application of pressure to specific points on the feet, hands, or ears; these points are thought to correspond with certain organs of the body. The goal is to relieve blockage, promote the flow of energy, and reduce tension—thus, reflexology may be helpful in treating stress-related illnesses (Korhan, Khorshid, & Uyar, 2014).

If you would like to have more information about CAM and stress management, see the accompanying CAM box, and

Go to **Bonus Chapter 46, Holistic Healing,** on Davis Advantage.

Other Activities The following are simpler activities you can recommend to most clients to aid in relaxation and stress reduction:

- **Humor.** Laughter releases endorphins and relieves feelings of stress. It enhances respiration and circulation, oxygenates the blood, suppresses the stress-related hormones in the brain, and activates the immune system. Some medical centers have begun implementing in-house humor programs (Bennett, Parsons, Ben-Moshe, et al., 2014; Cousins, 1979, 2005; du Pré, 1998; Tremayne, 2014). See the iCare box.
- **Listening to Music.** Listening to relaxing music reduces the stress response. A study comparing physiological and psychological effects of stress found those exposed to relaxing music produced higher levels of cortisol and salivary alpha-amylase (endocrine markers produced with exposure to stress) than rest alone or listening to soothing water. Music listening led to a lower perceived stress level and anxiety as well as quicker recovery after a stressful experience (Thoma, Thoma, Brönnimann, et al., 2013).
- **Engaging in Art Activities.** Painting, working with clay, and engaging in other art activities help to express emotions and release endorphins.
- **Dance and Sports.** Like other forms of exercise, dance and sports release pent-up physical tension and emotions. Steady-state exercises, such as running or swimming at a consistent pace, offer stress relief in a meditative manner through sustained deep breathing and movement. Physical activity can also enhance self-esteem and help people feel better by the simple act of accomplishing a personal goal.
- **Journal Writing.** Journal writing helps the person to reflect on experiences and express emotions. The venting of emotion that can occur in journal writing often provides insights into causes of stress and ways to modify stressors.

Changing Perception of Stressors or Self

Recall that altering one's perception is one way to improve adaptation to stress.

- **Cognitive restructuring** may be helpful for clients who have an unrealistic perception of the stressor and can imagine only negative outcomes. With this technique, you help clients to recognize their negative focus and to restructure their thinking in more positive and realistic ways. For example, you might encourage a working mother with demanding family members to take a single positive step, such as saying no to someone at least once a day.

♥ **iCare 12-1**

Using Humor

When using humor, the caring nurse considers the following:
- The nurse must be sensitive to patients' unique personalities, racial background, and other personal traits.
- Humor might not be appropriate when the patient is experiencing pain, is extremely ill, needs quiet time or privacy, needs to cry, or is overly stressed.
- When in doubt whether to use humor or not, remember that there is no substitute for compassion, care, and touch.

- **Identifying positive aspects of self and coping abilities** promotes self-esteem and helps clients to recognize and use the resources they have for coping with their stressors.
- **Self-affirmation** improves problem-solving under stress (Cresswell, Dutcher, Klien, et al., 2013).
- **Positive self-talk** is another method for increasing self-esteem. Each time you hear negative self-talk, stop the client and ask him to rephrase the statement so that it is positive.

Identifying and Using Support Systems

You can facilitate successful adaptation by helping clients to identify and contact people and groups who offer various supports (e.g., listening, encouragement, advice, problem-solving, help with household tasks, financial support). Be aware of the groups available in your community (e.g., Weight Watchers, Alcoholics Anonymous, Reach for Recovery). You may need to teach socialization skills to clients who are socially isolated so that they can begin to build a support system.

Reducing the Stress of Hospitalization

Illness and hospitalization are stressful for patients and their families. In addition to being sick, patients find themselves in unfamiliar surroundings, with little privacy, and a certain loss of control.

- *Promote patient-centered care* in the healthcare agency as much as you can.
- *Involve patients and families actively in their care.* This helps them adapt to the stressors of hospitalization.
- *Teach patients what to expect* from hospitalization and give them a few tips to help plan ahead to minimize the stress they experience (see the Self-Care box Teaching Clients How to Reduce the Stress of Hospitalization).

Providing Spiritual Support

In addition to helping clients obtain spiritual support from church groups and clergy, you can help to strengthen the client spiritually. You may wish to do the following:

- Pray for or with clients, if they desire, and if you are comfortable doing so. Prayer can help reduce their feelings of powerlessness and loneliness.
- Help clients to define their values and set boundaries that honor themselves and uphold their values.
- Teach clients to silently recite an affirming mantra (e.g., on inhalation, say, "I am free"; exhale and say, "Stress, leave me"). The client may prefer to use relevant spiritual passages.

  For other ways to provide spiritual support, see Chapter 16.

Crisis Intervention

As an entry-level nurse in acute and ambulatory care settings, you are more likely to see patients in the first three phases of crisis and not be present for the adaptive and postcrisis stages.

Crisis centers often rely on telephone counseling (hotlines). If telephone counseling is not adequate, or if observations of the home environment are needed, home visits may be necessary. See Clinical Insight 12-2 for a description of how to intervene at an entry level of practice when a patient is in crisis.

KnowledgeCheck 12-10

- Describe at least five specific interventions for dealing with an angry person.
- What is cognitive restructuring?
- What is the purpose of positive self-talk?

Self-Care

Teaching Clients How to Reduce the Stress of Hospitalization

Share the following tips with clients, preferably before hospitalization:

What to Bring

- ➤ Make a list of necessities and pack carefully before you leave home. For example, bring your own soap, toothpaste, lotion, pajamas, and slippers, or your favorite tea bags and sweetener. Having familiar things can make your stay more pleasant for you.
- ➤ Bring clothing that is washable, loose, and comfortable.
- ➤ If you will feel well enough, bring your computer, reading material, crossword puzzles, or whatever you like to do that can help prevent boredom and depression. You might want to bring a few family photos for your nightstand.
- ➤ Before your appointment jot down a few notes of what you want to remember to ask when your healthcare provider comes in the room.
- ➤ Do *not* bring jewelry, cash, credit cards, or other valuables.

Family and Friends

- ➤ Do not allow family or friends to visit if they are ill.
- ➤ Ask family or friends to stay at the bedside, particularly when the physician is "making rounds." They can advocate when you feel too ill to ask for what you need.
- ➤ Family or friends can also help you interpret and remember information and instructions that you will receive. There may be 30 care providers in your room each day, and when you don't feel well, it is hard to keep track of everything.
- ➤ Keep a bottle of hand sanitizer by your bed or insist visitors, including family members and care providers, use a hand hygiene product at the door when entering the room, just as you do.

Caregivers

- ➤ Know the name of your primary nurse (or nurses) on each shift, and ask as many questions as you need to.
- ➤ Even though some things seem to not make sense (e.g., taking your temperature at 3 a.m.), there is likely a medical reason for it. Try to be as patient and cheerful as possible.

- List the seven steps of crisis intervention.
- Why is relaxation an important stress intervention?

Stress Management in the Workplace

You will need to pay attention to your feelings, your body, and your personal responses to stress.

- Do you notice that you are eating more than usual or have lost your appetite?
- Are you feeling edgy or impatient with family or coworkers, or are you not sleeping well?
- Do you feel tired or often have headaches or gastrointestinal distress?
- Are the muscles in your face and shoulders tense?
- Do you often take work home with you?

- Are you unable to stop thinking about work, even when you are at home?
- Do concerns about finances or personal situations consume your thinking and create a sense of doom?

If you answered yes to many of those questions, you probably need to start managing your stress. When stressors arise from the workplace, the following actions are especially important:

- Set realistic expectations of yourself and others. Don't be overcritical; most people, including you, are doing the best they can.
- Ask for help. Seeking the support of others does not indicate weakness or incompetence. It can even make others feel good by giving them an opportunity to practice collegiality.
- Offer support to colleagues who need help with tasks or with their feelings. This adds to the overall good feeling on a unit and improves the efficiency of performing many tasks.
- Be proactive about the things you can change and accept the things that you cannot change. Get involved in constructive efforts to change a particular stressor. If you cannot effect the changes, and if you cannot accept things as they are, you may need to think about removing yourself from the situation.
- Be aware that complaining and negative talk add to your own stress and that of others.
- Join and support professional organizations that address workplace issues (e.g., the National Student Nurses Association and the American Nurses Association).

- Strive for balance in these seven key areas: family, financial responsibilities, health, social contributions, career, vocation or education, and spirituality or faith. Focus on the most important items and task; remember, work affects life, but your life also affects your work.
- Obtain counseling for stress that exceeds your ability to cope.

Making Referrals

This chapter has presented many assessments and interventions for reducing stress. Remember, though, you are not yet an expert nurse and no one, not even an experienced nurse, is an expert in all areas. It is important not to "get in over your head" and attempt to intervene beyond your abilities with clients who are showing maladaptive coping. You can help by recognizing your limitations and by referring the client to the appropriate professionals (e.g., a spiritual leader, a counselor, a social worker, a practitioner of complementary therapies, a physician, a psychologist, or a psychiatrist).

 ThinkLike a Nurse 12-5

Sally is a registered nurse seeking employment at a local nursing home. She left her previous employer because of stress and frustration with agency policy, for which the bottom line was financial gain rather than quality patient care. What can Sally do to help ensure that she will not experience the same problem in the new agency?

CLINICALREASONING

The questions and exercises in this section allow you to practice the kind of thinking you will use as a full-spectrum nurse. Critical-thinking questions usually have more than one correct answer, so we do not provide "correct answers" for these features. It is more important to develop your nursing judgment than to just cover content. You will learn by discussing the questions with your peers. If you are still unsure, see the Davis Advantage chapter resources for suggested responses.

Caring for the Nguyens

After having a comprehensive physical exam at the family health center, Yen Nguyen has been scheduled to have a mammogram and screening laboratory work. When she arrives at the clinic for her mammogram, she tells you she is very nervous. "I have a good friend who just found out she has breast cancer. She's very depressed now. Do I really have to do this test?"

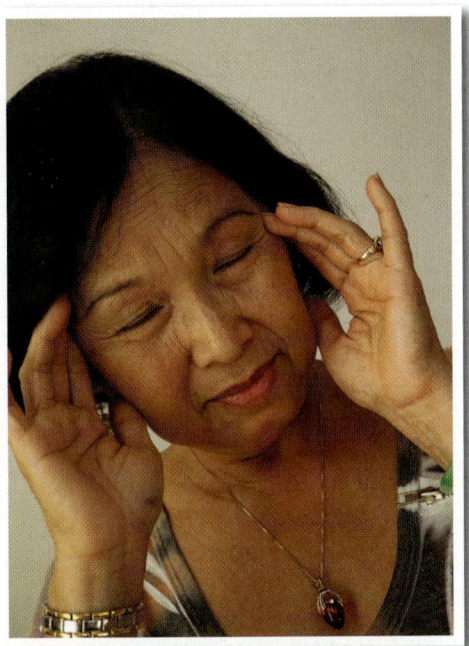

(Continued)

Caring for the Nguyens (continued)

A. What kind of stress is Yen experiencing?

B. Three days later, the radiologist contacts Yen, requesting that she return to the family health center for additional films of the upper outer quadrant of the right breast. "There are some calcifications I want to check out," explains the radiologist.
- What factors might affect Yen's adaptation to this stress?
- Evaluate what you know about Yen's perception of her stress, her overall health status, her support system, and her coping methods.

- What more do you need to know about these topics to fully answer this question?

C. Later, Yen calls the office, frantically explaining that she is very upset about this recent event. She says, "Not knowing is killing me. I'm so nervous I can't stand it! I can't sleep. I can't eat." She asks how she can handle the stress until she comes in for the additional tests next week. What strategies would you recommend to help Yen deal with the stress?

Applying the **Full-Spectrum Nursing Model**_____
PATIENT SITUATION

Mrs. Williams is a 76-year-old Indian American woman who was admitted yesterday after suffering a stroke that paralyzed her right side. She has had diabetes and high blood pressure for many years. Since the stroke, she has been unable to speak clearly and becomes frustrated as she attempts to communicate her needs. Her daughter says Mrs. Williams is a proud, independent, and tidy woman who has been living alone since her husband's death last year. Until her stroke, she had been driving her car, cleaning her house, doing her grocery shopping, and maintaining the yard and garden. She wears eyeglasses for reading and driving and has a hearing aid, although she rarely uses it.

THINKING

1. *Theoretical Knowledge:*
   a. What stroke risk factors probably functioned as stressors for Mrs. Williams? (*Hint:* Look up *stroke risk factors* in a medical–surgical nursing or pathophysiology text or online.)
   b. What are common stressors for patients who must be hospitalized?
2. *Critical Thinking (Contextual Awareness):* Now that Mrs. Williams is in the hospital, what new stressors might she have?

DOING

3. *Practical Knowledge:* What might you advise Mrs. Williams's daughter to do to help her mother adapt more comfortably to the stressors in the hospital?
4. *Nursing Process (Diagnosis):* Based on only the data in the scenario, write one actual nursing diagnosis for Mrs. Williams. Do not use potential diagnoses. Remember, the defining characteristics must be present in the scenario. State the data you would need in order to make the diagnosis more descriptive.

CARING

5. *Self-Knowledge:* Imagine yourself in Mrs. Williams's situation.
   a. What is the one thing that would cause you the most stress? Why would that be the most stressful thing?
   b. What is the single most important thing you would want your nurse to do for you?

PracticalKnowledge: clinical application

Clinical Insight 12-1 ➤ **Dealing With Angry Patients**

- **Be aware of how you are responding to angry patients.** Are you relieving your own stress, or are you relieving the client's stress? Responding angrily can provoke further anger in the patient and even escalate the situation to the point of violence.
- **Remind yourself not to take anger personally;** remind family members of this as well.
- **Recognize that anger and anxiety are normal feelings when facing adversity,** such as a debilitating illness.
- **Do not discount feelings** by saying something such as, "Please, don't be so angry," or "You shouldn't talk like that," or, "Everything will be okay. Don't worry."
- **Encourage the client and family to express feelings verbally and appropriately.**
- **Listen instead of defending.** If the patient yells, "Everything about this place stinks!":

  Don't defend. Don't respond with a comment such as, "We really are all trying to do the best we can for you."

  Do encourage the person to express his feelings or give you more information: "You seem really angry; what's going on?" or "Maybe I can help. Tell me a little more about what stinks."
- **Do not take responsibility for the patient's anger.** It is not your fault, so don't apologize—unless you really do have something to apologize for. In the preceding example, for instance, do *not* say, "I'm sorry we haven't been meeting your expectations."
- **Remain calm.** This reassures the patient.
- **Help the patient identify what is causing the anger and try to meet those needs.**
- **Be alert to your own and to the patient's safety needs.**

  Do not allow a patient to get between you and the door if he seems violent.

  Do not wear a stethoscope around your neck, dangling jewelry, or anything a patient might use to hurt you.

  Do not go into a room alone with a patient who seems to have a potential for violence.

  Do not turn your back on an angry patient.

  Remain at least an arm's length away from an angry and potentially violent patient.

  KEY POINT: *Be sure you know how to call for help from staff or security personnel if you think you or someone else is in danger.*
- **KEY POINT:** *If you believe the patient's anger may escalate to violence, your priority is your own safety and the safety of others in the area.*

  Also refer to the NIC intervention, Anger Control Assistance (Bulechek, Butcher, Dochterman, et al., 2013, pp. 81–82).

Clinical Insight 12-2 ➤ **Crisis Intervention Guidelines**

For nurses who are at an entry level of practice, crisis intervention includes the following (Brammer & MacDonald, 2003; Gorman & Anwar, 2014):

Assess the situation.

What is the nature of the patient's condition and the severity of the crisis?

Ensure safety.

- Call for help if you are or the patient is in physical danger.
- Do not leave the patient unless you think you are in imminent danger.
- First ensure your own safety; then provide for the patient's safety.

Defuse the situation.

- Keep in mind that a person in crisis may not be in control of his actions.
- Try to calm the person verbally.

- Attempt physical restraint only as a last resort and only when there is enough help to do it safely for both the staff and the patient.

Decrease the person's anxiety.

- Reassure the person that he is in a safe place and that you are concerned and want to help.
- Explain gently but firmly that you need his help and cooperation.
- Help the person to vent feelings of fear, guilt, and anger.
- Use physical contact very cautiously. The person in turmoil may interpret touch as aggression or a sexual approach.

Determine the problem.

- Find out what the patient believes to be the cause of the crisis.
- Remain calm and do not pressure the patient to give reasons. Any tension on your part will create further panic in the patient.

(Continued)

Clinical Insight 12-2 ➤ **Crisis Intervention Guidelines—cont'd**

Decide on the type of help needed.

- You may be able to calm the person enough for him to understand what just happened, or you may not. Evaluate your ability to calm the patient based on your assessment of his coping skills and resources.
- Put in place the help needed to restore the person to a minimal level of functioning. This may require long-term treatment. In that case, make the referrals.

Return the person to his precrisis level of functioning.

- *Crisis counseling.* The goal of crisis counseling is to provide immediate relief, solve the most urgent problems, and give long-term counseling if needed. Crisis centers often rely on telephone counseling (hotlines).
- *Home visits.* If telephone counseling is not adequate or if observations of the home environment are needed, home visits might be necessary.

To explore learning resources for this chapter,

Go to www.DavisAdvantage.com and find:

Answers and Suggested Responses for all questions in this chapter

List of **NIC/NOC Classifications**

List of **NANDA-I Diagnoses**

Knowledge Map

References and Bibliography

Concept Map

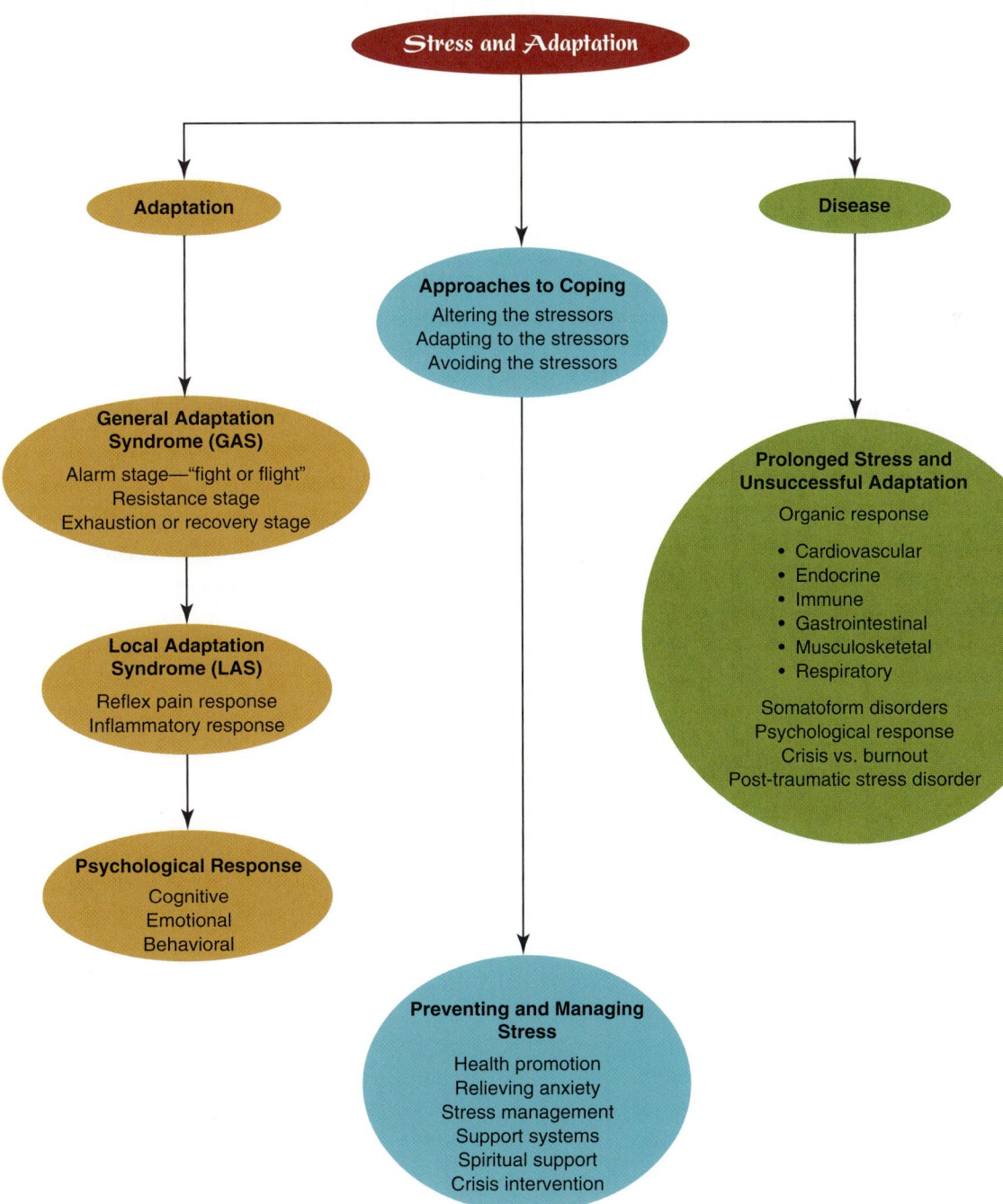

CHAPTER 13

Psychosocial Health & Illness

Learning Outcomes

After completing this chapter, you should be able to:

➤ Explain the relationship of psychosocial factors to overall health and development.

➤ Identify the factors that influence the development and stability of self-concept.

➤ List the four interrelated components of self-concept.

➤ Develop a nursing care plan for patients exhibiting disturbances in self-concept and self-esteem.

➤ Identify nursing diagnoses, outcomes, and interventions specific to body image disturbance.

➤ Describe interventions for preventing depersonalization.

➤ List the psychological and physiological effects of anxiety.

➤ Recognize the levels and symptoms of anxiety that are severe enough to merit referral to a mental health professional.

➤ Devise a nursing care plan for the nursing diagnosis of Anxiety.

➤ Differentiate between mild depression and that which should be referred to a mental health professional.

➤ Assess older adults for manifestations of depression.

➤ Plan outcomes and nursing interventions for patients who are depressed.

➤ Plan outcomes and nursing interventions for patients with a diagnosis of Risk for Suicide.

Key Concepts

Anxiety

Depression

Psychosocial health

Self-concept

Related Concepts

See the Concept Map at the end of this chapter.

Example Problems

Anxiety

Depression

Self-concept disturbance

Low self-esteem

Meet Your Patient

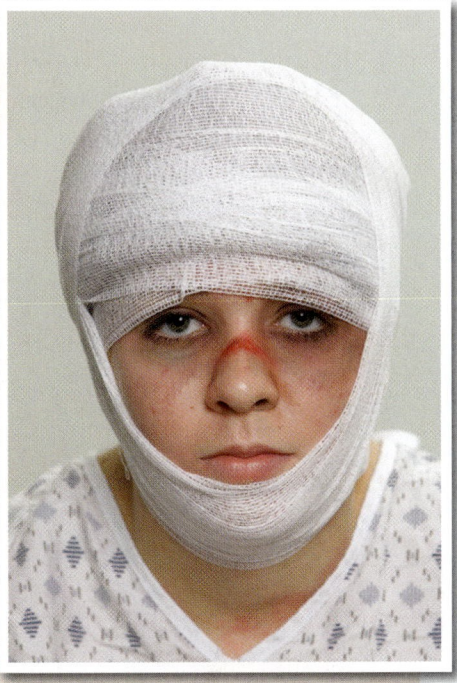

You are caring for a 16-year-old patient named Karli who is suffering from fractures to both arms and several ribs, as well as extensive first- and second-degree burns to 30% of her body, following a motor vehicle accident. Karli was driving her parents' car home from her part-time job when she lost control of the car and crashed into a wall. The car exploded in flames. A passerby quickly reported the accident, and fast action by the emergency response team saved Karli's life.

Karli is suffering from a moderate amount of shock and pain. She alternates between outbursts of anger, self-directed sarcasm, and despondence. She tells you that she cannot understand how the accident happened, that one moment she was adjusting the car radio, and the next moment she awoke in the hospital. Then suddenly she explodes. "It's not fair! I just took my eyes off the road for a second; that's all!" She bursts into tears. Picking at her bandages, she sobs, "No one will ever love me the way I'm going to look. My life is over. I hate myself!" You take her hand. "I used to be pretty," she says, "but now I'll look like a freak!

What did I do to deserve this? I know plenty of kids who drive drunk or high all the time. I wasn't doing anything wrong! Why did this happen to me?"

Before reading on, jot down a list of the multiple physical, psychological, and social issues that you would need to consider in developing a comprehensive care plan for Karli. You can revisit your list throughout this chapter to compare your answers.

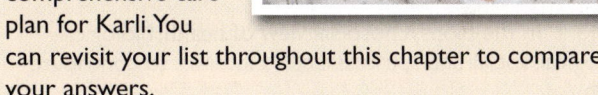

ThinkLike a Nurse 13-1

Review Chapter 9 as needed.

- What theoretical knowledge about Karli's developmental stage will assist you in determining nursing diagnoses, interventions, and outcomes?
- Considering that Karli will need a significant amount of assistance for activities of daily living (ADLs) because of her fractures and burns, how might you use the time to develop your therapeutic relationship?

ABOUT THE KEY CONCEPTS

This chapter introduces you to the key concepts of **psychosocial health, self-concept, anxiety,** and **depression.** As you study the related topics and terms in the chapter, you will gain a more complete understanding of the four key concepts. Conceptual thinking will help you organize the content in your mind so you can remember it longer.

PSYCHOSOCIAL HEALTH

This chapter is designed to help you provide basic psychosocial care for patients in general practice settings. **KEY POINT:** *Remember, the physical body is only one dimension of a person. What patients are thinking and feeling is equally important to their healing process.*

TheoreticalKnowledge
knowing **why**

The interactions of the mind and body are continuous and complex. One strength of nursing is that we can go beyond a

biomedical (disease-oriented) focus to care for the whole person. Nurses recognize that patient responses to illness are influenced not only by physical pathology but also by the person's psychosocial health and its relationship to her overall wellness.

The term *psychosocial* encompasses both psychological and social factors: A person's psychological state interacts with his social development and position within society to contribute to his overall—or biopsychosocial—well-being (Fig. 13-1). Figure 13-2 illustrates the interlocking psychosocial influences on health and personal development.

KEY POINT: *Any human dimension may dominate health needs at a given time.* For example, a patient suffering from a severe flare-up of psoriasis (a skin disease characterized by red, scaly patches) may require *physiological interventions* during the acute stage. He may not be ready to deal with body image issues *(psychological dimension)* until his skin lesions are better. Remember, though, that your patients' psychosocial needs are just as important as, for example, their dietary requirements or level of pain.

What Is Psychosocial Theory?

You can think of **psychosocial theory** as a method of understanding people as a combination of psychological and social events.

- **Erikson.** Of the many theories of psychosocial development, the works of the German psychologist Erik Erikson (1902–1994) are foremost. Using Erikson's theory, you can assess for successful completion of developmental tasks. Refer to Chapter 9 for more information about Erikson's theory.
- **Maslow.** Psychologist Abraham Maslow's theory of self-actualization and self-transcendence is another psychosocial theory that is relevant for healthcare providers (see Chapter 9). Maslow (1968) developed a widely accepted

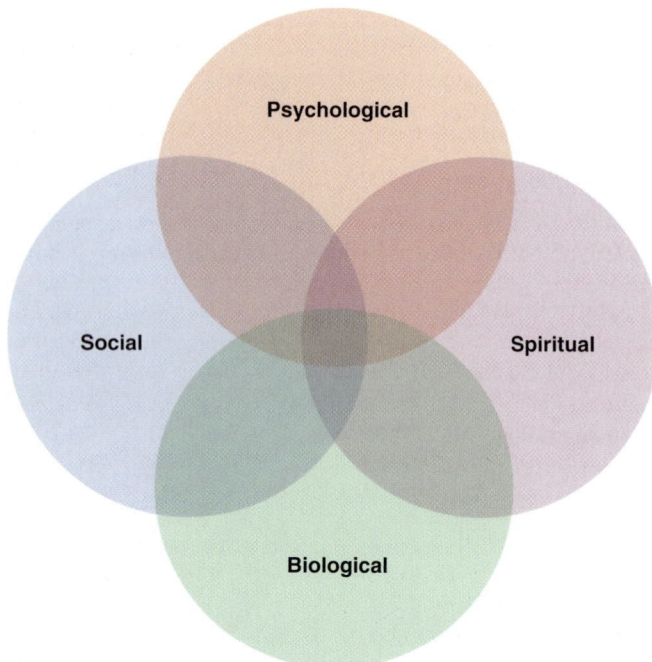

FIGURE 13-1 In the biopsychosocial view of health, biological, psychological, social, and spiritual factors interact to contribute to health.

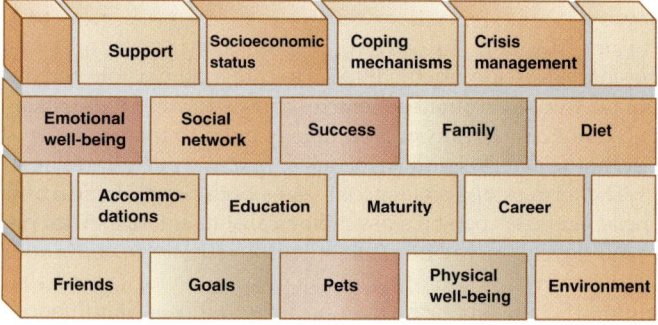

FIGURE 13-2 Interlocking psychosocial influences.

hierarchy of human needs and motivations in which essential needs (e.g., air, water, and food) must be met before higher needs (e.g., learning, creating, understanding, and self-fulfillment). Recall that, in order from most basic to highest need, Maslow's hierarchy includes physiological, safety and security, love and belonging, self-esteem, and self-actualization needs.

KnowledgeCheck 13-1

- Why is psychosocial theory relevant to healthcare?
- What does the term *biopsychosocial* mean?
- Explain the implication of Maslow's hierarchy of human needs for working with a homeless man with gangrene.

What Is Self-Concept?

Self-concept is one's overall view of oneself. It is your complete and unique answer to the question "Who do you think you are?" (e.g., "I am a student"; "I am successful and competent"). **KEY POINT:** *Self-concept forms out of a person's evaluation of*

his physical appearance, sexual performance, intellectual abilities, success in the workplace, friendship and approval from others, problem-solving and coping abilities, unique talents, and so on. A person with a healthy self-concept has a mostly positive perception of these evaluations of self.

- Self-concept influences social functioning.
  Example: Karli's self-concept is that she "looks like a freak." If this self-concept continues, she may withdraw from social interaction, and it will be difficult to form new relationships (social functioning).
- Self-concept is influenced by social functioning.
  Example: If others—for example, prospective employers—do see her as hideously ugly, she may have difficulty finding a place in society. This would reinforce her poor self-concept.

The "Dynamic Self" The self forms and changes in response to our environment. Margaret Mead (1934) states that we discover who we are through a lifelong process of differentiating from and comparing our self to others. As we experience life events, we continually develop our understanding of who we are. Dickstein (1977) called this idea the **dynamic self,** meaning that who we are (the self) is subject to change through social and environmental influence. But if our concept of self is changeable, what factors cause it to change? Can it be harmed? If so, how? How does it first develop? These questions are explored next.

How Is Self-Concept Formed?

Humans are not born with a concept of self; rather, it develops during infancy and childhood as the child interacts with family members, peers, and others. The broad steps of self-concept formation are as follows:

Infant—Learning that the physical self is different from the environment: "me; not me."

Child—Internalizing others' attitudes about the self, primarily parents and peers: "Who do *they* say that I am?"

Child and adult—Internalizing standards of society: "How do I compare to others?"

Adult—Self-actualization and self-adjustment: "This *is* who I am and who I will continue to be."

Change occurs gradually, and the steps overlap. Also, the age at which the stages occur varies widely among individuals.

 Think**Like a Nurse** 13-2

- Explain how each of Maslow's five basic needs is related to psychosocial development; that is, how might each of the needs affect psychosocial health if met or not met?
- To what extent do social relationships help or hinder a person in meeting each need?

What Factors Affect a Person's Self-Concept?

Some factors affecting a person's self-concept cannot be changed, for example, gender and developmental level. Others, such as socioeconomic status and family relationships, can be changed to a degree but are not fully under the person's control—and certainly not during childhood, when the self-concept is forming. Understanding that people may not be able to change such factors may help you provide more sensitive, compassionate care to patients experiencing impaired self-concept.

Gender

Certain aspects of self-concept differ by gender. Some of the differences appear to be related to the role expectations of boys and girls rather than any actual difference in ability. For example:

Girls typically rate teamwork and cooperation as important, whereas most boys place a higher value on individual achievement.

Physical appearance tends to seem more important to girls throughout life.

As role expectations and career choices for both men and women expand, these gender-based differences in self-concept may fade.

Developmental Level

As we mature, our self-concept becomes more inner guided. That is, others (e.g., friends, the media) have less influence on our ideas about who we are. We become less likely to view our failures and shortcomings as evidence of worthlessness and more likely to see them as challenges common to all humans.

Family and Peer Relationships

The family strongly influences a child's developing self-concept. As an infant's sense of self-permanence develops and becomes stable, categories of self begin to emerge. These include notions of gender, values, and a sense of having a distinct "place" among family members (Feiring & Taska, 1996). Social identity is first fostered by interactions between infants and their parents and broadens in toddlerhood through relationships with immediate and extended family members. For older children, peers become more important than family in this respect.

Locus of Control

Whereas the preceding external influences contribute to the *formation* of our self-concept, internal influences help us to *moderate* it. For example, biochemical brain processes influence perceptual acuity, interpretation abilities, and level of insight and judgment.

- **Internal Locus of Control.** People who allow their inner voice to influence their self-concept have what is called an **internal locus of control.** Such people feel they can exert control over their lives. They take appropriate responsibility for their life experiences and for their responses to them. This enables them to interpret unexpected adverse events (e.g., injuries and illnesses) in a more positive light.
- **External Locus of Control.** In contrast, people who have an **external locus of control** attribute control of their situation to external factors, including other people, institutions, and God. They may feel they lack the ability to change what happens to them.

KnowledgeCheck 13-2

- When does self-concept become stable?
- What factors have been determined to have an impact on our self-concept?

What Are the Components of Self-Concept?

Self-concept embraces four interrelated subconcepts: body image, role performance, personal identity, and self-esteem.

Body Image

How often do you hear someone say something like the following?

"Look at the muscles on that man. He looks good!"

"Look at her pigging out. She needs that candy like I need a hole in my head."

You probably grew up overhearing similar statements. Such preoccupations with food, weight, and appearance have led to prejudice against people who do not have perfect bodies. No wonder people engage in unhealthy behaviors in order to be thin or that patients such as Karli have difficulty coping with disfiguring accidents or with surgeries such as limb amputation and mastectomy.

Body image is your mental image of your physical self, including physical appearance and physical functioning. Both cognitive understanding and sensory input influence body image. Cognitive understanding is in turn influenced by family, social, ethnic, and cultural norms; education; and exposure to alternative values. The American media portray the ideal male as young, tall, and muscular; nevertheless, many older, short, slender men maintain a positive body image because they understand cognitively that they are in good health, are attractive to their partners, and so on.

Ideal, Perceived, and Actual Body Image People may not see their own bodies as objectively as others see them. Some psychological disorders interfere with the ability to interpret sensory data objectively.

Example: People with the eating disorder anorexia nervosa see themselves as fat even when their mirror reflects, and other people see, a normal or even an emaciated body.

The closer the match between a person's ideal body image and sensory input about his or her body (perceived body image), the more positive the person's body image is likely to be.

Appearance and Function A physical disability, such as blindness, deafness, or paraplegia, can interfere with the development of a positive body image. Children born with a physical disability are at risk for poor self-concept and depression, perhaps related to the person's perception that he has low social value. In contrast, an attractive appearance and superior functioning, whether in a career, sports, or academics, make it easier to develop a positive body image. Keep in mind, though, that cognitive understanding (e.g., of one's successes) can increase self-concept even in people who are average in appearance or achievement.

Gradual Versus Sudden Body Changes Gradual changes in physical appearance occur naturally as the body matures and grows old. Most people adapt to such changes relatively easily, especially because their friends and colleagues are aging, too. In contrast, when changes in appearance or functioning occur abruptly (e.g., following an acute illness or an accident, as happened to your patient, Karli), they are much more difficult to accept. Denial, anger, self-hatred, and despair are a few of many reactions that can follow such an abrupt change in body image.

Influence of Body Image on Health Body image influences health and health behaviors. A negative body image has been associated with the following health problems:

- Depression (Cargill, Clark, Pera, et al., 2012; McCabe & Ricciardelli, 2012; Muehlenkamp, & Brausch, 2012)
- Initiation of smoking among adolescents (Cargill, Clark, Pera, et al., 2012)
- Increased risk for unintended pregnancy and sexually transmitted infections, including HIV infection (Larson, Clark, Robinson, et al., 2012; Woertman & van den Brink, 2012)
- Increased incidence of being bullied (Brixval, Rayce, Rasmussen, et al., 2012)

In contrast, a positive body image was found to be a major contributor to overall life happiness in adult women (Walters-Brown & Hall, 2012).

Role Performance

Before you began your nursing program, what were your expectations? What activities did you imagine yourself engaged in, and what behaviors did you think would be expected of you? Together, these expectations make up your conception of the *role* of a nursing student. In addition to being a student, you probably play several other roles, such as parent, sibling, friend, breadwinner, caregiver, volunteer, and so on. These are your **role expectations.**

Role performance can be defined as the actions that a person takes and the behaviors that he demonstrates in fulfilling a role. Instead of being expectations, role performance is the reality.

- *Role strain.* If you expected that you would sail through your nursing program and instead you find yourself so overwhelmed that you have begun to skip classes, then you are experiencing **role strain,** a mismatch between role expectations and role performance.
- *Interpersonal role conflict.* In addition, your ideas about how to perform the nursing student role may be very different from those of your instructors. When that type of mismatch occurs, you are experiencing an **interpersonal role conflict.**
- *Interrole conflict.* Imagine you are a single parent and your child's illness causes you to miss a week of classes. When two roles make competing demands on an individual, **interrole conflict** occurs.

Personal Identity

Your **personal identity** is your view of yourself as a unique human being, different and separate from all others. Identity develops over time, beginning in childhood when you identified with your parents. Unlike body image, which is expected to change over time, personal identity is relatively constant and consistent.

- **Cultural identity is culturally determined and learned through socialization.**
  - *People with a strong sense of personal identity* are less likely to compare themselves to others or to be unduly influenced by them. They tend to appreciate the unique perspective and contributions of others, yet value their own perspectives and contributions.
  - *People with a weak sense of personal identity,* in contrast, have difficulty distinguishing their boundaries from those of others. They may interpret events in the environment personally, or interpret their personal experiences as belonging to everyone.
    Example: When the hospital's air-conditioning system fails, a patient with a weak personal identity may insist that it is a punishment for his complaint that his room was too cold.
- **Patients may experience an impaired sense of identity when they are challenged by a serious or chronic illness** (e.g., cancer, AIDS, or rheumatoid arthritis). They then place too many limitations on their activities or interpret the responses of others in light of their illness. For instance, a woman with osteoporosis (loss of bone density) might say, "I can't go bird watching anymore because I might trip and fall."

Think**Like a Nurse** 13-3

Think about Karli in the Meet Your Patient scenario. If you asked Karli to list 10 labels to identify herself, what do you think they would be? You may not have enough information to come up with 10, but think of as many as you can.

Self-Esteem

Self-esteem is, in the simplest terms, how well a person likes himself. It is the difference between the "ideal self" and "actual self," that is, between "what I think I ought (or want) to be" and "what I really am." The area of overlap in Figure 13-3 illustrates the extent of self-esteem. The more overlap there is, the higher the self-esteem.

When we succeed beyond our ambitions, we experience a high sense of self-esteem; but when we aim for an ideal self beyond our capabilities, we risk loss of self-esteem. Even mild illnesses and minor setbacks can cause some people to question their self-worth. It is not difficult to imagine how a sudden, disfiguring accident such as Karli's might provoke a crisis in self-esteem, because Karli's ideal self is currently out of her reach. This is especially true if the problem is interpreted as one incident in a continuing pattern—for example, a couple hoping to become parents who experience a third pregnancy loss.

As another example, if as a nursing student you find that you are more successful than you expected to be when you enrolled in your nursing program, that is a boost to your self-esteem. If, however, your expectations of being a skillful nurse outweigh your current abilities, then lower self-esteem is likely.

Think**Like a Nurse** 13-4

What if a person does not have any aspirations to success, but is content to meet each day as a learner, vitalized by her daily discoveries? How do you think a high score on an exam would affect her self-esteem? How do you think a poor score on a clinical skills test would affect her self-esteem?

Knowledge**Check** 13-3

- What four components contribute to an individual's self-concept?
- What is self-esteem?

Practical**Knowledge**
knowing **how**

Practical knowledge in this chapter consists of planning, implementing, and evaluating care to promote clients' mental health and provide support when they experience mental health problems. **KEY POINT:** *Remember, the physical body is*

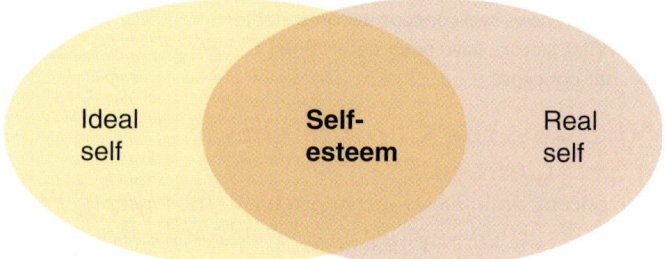

Ideal self: expectations and aspirations; "what I ought to be," "what I wish I were"

Real self: current skills, attributes, and successes; "what I really am"

FIGURE 13-3 Self-esteem is determined by the relationship between an individual's ideal self and real self.

only one dimension of a person. What patients are thinking and feeling is equally important to their healing process.

Communication and interpersonal skills are especially important in caring for patients' psychosocial needs. See Chapter 20. Physical illness may be particularly stressful when it occurs in combination with psychosocial issues. For example, think of Karli (Meet Your Patient). Might her condition have been less complicated if (1) her injuries were not disfiguring or (2) if she were an older adult at a developmental stage when appearance is generally less crucial?

ASSESSMENTS: PSYCHOSOCIAL NP

No matter what the patient's medical diagnosis, you need to perform accurate and ongoing psychosocial assessments to develop holistic nursing diagnoses and interventions. Most admission assessment forms have a few questions to screen psychosocial status. If any of the answers indicate risk for a problem, you may need to conduct a more comprehensive special needs (or system specific) assessment.

Psychosocial information is personal and sometimes sensitive. To encourage patients to share this information, you will need to use your developing communication skills. For example:

- Be aware of your own biases and discomforts that could influence your assessment.
- Use active listening through eye contact and verbal response. Be sensitive, though—eye contact is uncomfortable for some people.
- Proceed from general details ("How do you get along with your parents?") to the specific ("Does your mother ever hit you?").
- Use an open and positive voice tone, facial expression, and body language (e.g., avoid frowning, criticizing, or expressing shock).
- Keep the focus on the patient.
- Be respectful and sensitive to cultural and gender-specific details.
- Use open-ended questions (questions that cannot be answered with just a yes or no).
- Follow the patient's cues by using reflection and restating.
- Be flexible and use humor as appropriate.
- Provide empathetic feedback and touch as appropriate.

You will learn more about interviewing and communication skills in Chapters 3 and 21.

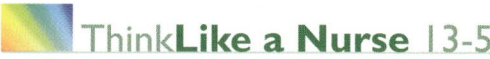 **Think**Like a Nurse 13-5

Psychologically, Karli is worried about the unfairness of her situation, and is probably struggling with body image issues. In addition, what do you think her *social* concerns might be?

ANALYSIS/NURSING DIAGNOSIS: PSYCHOSOCIAL NP

Psychosocial issues involve nearly all areas of patient functioning, so there is overlap between what we are calling *psychosocial* diagnoses and those used in the rest of the chapter to describe the more specific problems of self-concept, anxiety, and depression. That is, you may use some of these psychosocial diagnoses for clients who have problems of self-concept, anxiety, and depression. It would be impossible to list every possible psychosocial diagnosis; the following are but a few:

- *Family Coping [Compromised and/or Disabled].* Usual support (comfort and assistance) from a significant other is either compromised (insufficient or withdrawn) or disabled (competing or maladapted), causing a significant health challenge.
- *Parental Role Conflict.* A parent shows significant role confusion and/or conflict in response to crises.
- *Ineffective Coping.* The patient fails to comprehend and effectively judge stressors when he perceives incorrect or dangerous life choices as normal and when there is an inability to use available resources. Inability to identify strengths and resources may be secondary to low self-esteem.
- *Post-Trauma Syndrome.* There is a maladaptive learned response to a traumatic and distressing event.
- *Risk for Loneliness.* The person is separated from persons, culture, objects, or environments to which a person may have ongoing attachments.
- *Social Isolation.* The person experiences significant aloneness that has a negative impact on health, or perceives the isolation as a threat to health.
- *Risk for Other-Directed Violence.* Situations in which a person threatens or uses aggression or violence to harm others. The intention of harm may not be limited to physical harm.

Psychosocial issues can be a problem, a symptom of a problem, or the etiology of a problem. It is important to determine what is cause and what is effect, although this can be hard to unravel at times. What you identify significantly affects your choice of goals and nursing activities (Table 13-1).

PLANNING: PSYCHOSOCIAL OUTCOMES/ EVALUATION NP

Individualized goal/outcome statements will depend on the nursing diagnoses, client input, and expectations of what the client agrees to and can realistically achieve. For example:

- *For Compromised or Disabled Family Coping*—Examples of goal statements are "Involves family members in decision making" and "Expresses feelings and emotions freely."
- *For Impaired Social Interaction*—A goal statement might be for the client to develop the skills of "engagement, assertiveness, compromise, confrontation, and consideration."

The Psychosocial Health domain of the NOC taxonomy includes approximately 40 *NOC standardized outcomes* to describe psychological well-being, psychosocial adaptation, self-control, and social interaction. The following are a few examples:

Abusive Behavior Self-Restraint
Coping
Child Adaptation to Hospitalization
Psychosocial Adjustment: Life Change
Role Performance
Social Interaction Skills

Other NOC domains also include useful psychosocial outcomes. Examples include (Moorhead, Johnson, Maas, et al., 2013):

Family Coping
Family Functioning
Family Participation in Professional Care
Family Resiliency

PLANNING: PSYCHOSOCIAL INTERVENTIONS/IMPLEMENTATION NP

Psychosocial nursing interventions and activities will be determined by the nursing diagnoses you identify, especially by the etiologies.

NIC standardized interventions for psychosocial diagnoses are found primarily in the Behavioral and Family domains of the

Table 13-1 ➤ Implications of Identifying a Psychosocial Issue as Problem, Etiology, or Symptom

	AS PROBLEM	AS ETIOLOGY	AS SYMPTOM
Nursing Diagnosis	**Interrupted Family Processes** r/t tumult from parental divorce	Delayed Development r/t lack of stimulation **secondary to Interrupted Family Processes** (parental divorce)	Ineffective Individual Coping (Mother) r/t poor judgment and impaired reality perception, **as manifested by Interrupted Family Processes** and risk-taking behaviors
Sample Goals (based on problem)	**NOC Outcome** Family Functioning	**NOC Outcome** Child Development: 4 years	**NOC Outcomes** Coping, Decision Making, Role Performance, Social Support, Impulse Control
	Goals Members perform expected family roles. Family cares for dependent members.	**Goals** Child demonstrates age-appropriate motor activities. Child uses four- and five-word sentences.	**Goals** Identifies coping strategies that have been effective in the past. Discusses the implications of decision alternatives with family.
Sample Interventions and Activities (based on etiology)	**NIC Interventions** Family Integrity Promotion Family Process Maintenance Normalization Promotion	**NIC Interventions** Developmental Enhancement: Child Parent Education Health Screening	**NIC Interventions** Coping Enhancement Decision-Making Support Impulse Control Training Family Involvement Promotion Support Group Support System Enhancement
	Specific Activities Promote parental involvement in healthcare. Assist the family with skills and education of conflict resolution, coping skills, and problem-solving. Link the individual and family to the appropriate support and education services.	**Specific Activities** Establish time for one-on-one care. Provide for creative play (e.g., clay, blocks, painting). Teach parents appropriate stimulation. Teach parents about developmental milestones and expected behaviors. Assess changes in family processes.	**Specific Activities** Identify and discuss alternative behaviors. Encourage delaying decision making when under stress. Help the mother solve problems constructively. Assist her to evaluate her own behavior. Identify and discuss past successful coping behaviors that she has used.

NIC system. The following are some examples from the Behavioral domain:

Anger Control Assistance

Anxiety Reduction

Coping Enhancement

Decision-Making Support

Socialization Enhancement

Examples of interventions from the Family domain are:

Family Involvement Promotion

Family Support

Family Therapy

Parenting Promotion (Bulechek, Butcher, Dochterman, et al., 2013)

Specific, individualized nursing activities used to help patients maintain a sense of personhood are discussed in the following section, Preventing Depersonalization. The NIC taxonomy also has many nursing activities to achieve the nursing goal of enhancing socialization, providing conflict mediation, and strengthening and mobilizing the family.

Preventing Depersonalization

Illness, and especially hospitalization, can have a depersonalizing effect that alters the self-concept. The ill person may feel that she has become an object to be examined, poked, prodded, and discussed. ♥ **iCare** You can help patients maintain a sense of personhood by using a caring approach:

▪ Introduce yourself if the patient does not know you.

▪ Address the patient by her preferred name each time you enter the room and always speak respectfully.

- Listen actively when the patient speaks.
- Do not talk *about* the patient to others in the room (e.g., do not say, "He seems to be better today, don't you think?"); speak *to* the patient.
- Use eye contact and touch, keeping in mind that people vary in their desire to be touched.
- Always offer an explanation before beginning a procedure and warn the patient before you touch him ("I'm going to touch your leg now").
- Move, turn, and position the patient gently.
- Provide for privacy when performing procedures or discussing something personal or sensitive.

NURSING CARE FOR EXAMPLE PROBLEMS: SELF-CONCEPT DISTURBANCE AND LOW SELF-ESTEEM

As is true for psychosocial issues, self-concept and self-esteem issues are a part of the holistic care of well and ill patients in all settings. See the infographic, Example Problem: Self-Concept Disturbance and Low Self-Esteem.

PracticalKnowledge
knowing **how**

ASSESSMENT: SELF-CONCEPT AND SELF-ESTEEM NP

For an all-purpose assessment of self-concept you might use for screening in any setting, refer to the Focused Assessment box Assessing Self-Concept.

To assess self-esteem, see the Focused Assessment box Performing a Self-Esteem Inventory.

ANALYSIS/NURSING DIAGNOSIS: SELF-CONCEPT AND SELF-ESTEEM NP

Self-concept issues, like psychosocial issues, can be a problem, a symptom of a problem, or an etiology. As you can see in Table 13-1, your analysis significantly affects your choice of goals and nursing activities.

Self-Concept or Body Image as a Problem

Diagnose a body image or self-concept problem when it is the result of a particular condition and might not exist if not for the condition (e.g., a profoundly deaf adolescent develops self-worth problems). For diagnoses that may be useful for patients with either low overall self-concept or difficulties in specific domains of self-concept (e.g., self-esteem), see the Example Problem: Self-Concept Disturbance and Low Self-Esteem.

Self-Concept or Body Image as Etiology

Self-concept problems are an etiology when they precede and play a central role in a condition such as depression (e.g., low self-esteem causing and maintaining depression). The following are examples of nursing diagnoses with self-concept (e.g., self-esteem) as the etiology:

- *Ineffective Coping* should be used when a patient experiences difficulties in adapting perception and evaluation of self after changes in health status (e.g., loss of a limb).

Focused Assessment

Assessing Self-Concept

Assessment Category	Examples of Assessment Questions
Body image	➤ When you look in the mirror, what do you see? ➤ How do you think others see you? ➤ How does your current ability to engage in work and leisure activities compare with how you would like to be?
Role performance	➤ What are your three or four major roles (e.g., daughter, student)? ➤ How successful are you in each of these roles? ➤ How important is it to you to be successful in each of these roles? ➤ What is interfering with your ability to perform any of these roles? What can you do about it?
Personal identity	➤ How did you see yourself before your illness/injury/loss? ➤ How do you see yourself now? ➤ How would you describe yourself to others? ➤ What special abilities do you have? ➤ How do you think others see you?
Self-esteem (also refer to the Focused Assessment box Performing a Self-Esteem Inventory)	➤ How do you feel about yourself? ➤ What do you like about yourself? ➤ To what extent do you feel you are in control of your life? ➤ If you could change one thing about yourself, what would it be? ➤ Where would you like to be 5 years from now? ➤ How realistic are your expectations of yourself? ➤ How do you see your illness/injury/loss in relation to yourself?

- *Complicated Grieving* may develop in anticipation of or following body changes (e.g., hysterectomy) or loss of a key role (e.g., resulting from death of a spouse).
- *Deficient Knowledge* of a healthcare situation may occur because of low self-esteem and lack of confidence in ability to learn or to manage care. Low self-esteem diminishes the motivation to learn.
- *Impaired Social Interaction* may occur when the person's low self-esteem and external locus of control cause him to fear criticism or lack of acceptance from others.
- *Sexual Dysfunction* or *Ineffective Sexuality Pattern* may result from negative body image brought about by changes in body structure or function (e.g., pregnancy, diseases such as arthritis).

Focused Assessment

Performing a Self-Esteem Inventory

Place a check mark in the column that most closely describes the client's answer to each statement. Each check is worth the number of points listed.

	3 Often or a Great Deal	2 Some- times	1 Seldom or Occasionally	0 Never or Not At All
1. I become angry or hurt when criticized.				
2. I am afraid to try new things.				
3. I feel stupid when I make a mistake.				
4. I have difficulty looking people in the eye.				
5. I have difficulty making small talk.				
6. I feel uncomfortable in the presence of strangers.				
7. I am embarrassed when people compliment me.				
8. I am dissatisfied with the way I look.				
9. I am afraid to express my opinions in a group.				
10. I prefer staying home alone rather than participating in group social situations.				
11. I have trouble accepting teasing.				
12. I feel guilty when I say no to people.				
13. I am afraid to make a commitment to a relationship for fear of rejection.				
14. I believe that most people are more competent than I am.				
15. I feel resentment toward people who are attractive and successful.				
16. I have trouble thinking of any positive aspects about my life.				
17. I feel inadequate in the presence of authority figures.				
18. I have trouble making decisions.				
19. I fear the disapproval of others.				
20. I feel tense, stressed out, or "uptight."				

Problems with low self-esteem are indicated by items scored with a 3 or by a total score higher than 46.

Source: Townsend, M. C. (2015). *Psychiatric mental health nursing: Concepts of care in evidence-based practice* (8th ed., p. 250). Philadelphia: F.A. Davis.

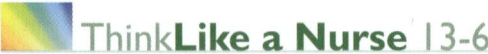

ThinkLike a Nurse 13-6

In the Meet Your Patient scenario, Karli perceives herself as unlovable "looking this way." You should not assume that you know exactly what Karli means by this. Also from the scenario: "Picking at her bandages, she sobs, 'No one will ever love me the

way I'm going to look. My life is over. I hate myself!' You take her hand. 'I used to be pretty,' she says, 'but now I'll look like a freak!'"

- Which of her words do you need to clarify with her?
- What might you say to her to get her to provide more information about the psychosocial meaning of her statement

EXAMPLE PROBLEM: Self-Concept Disturbance and Low Self-Esteem

Basic Definitions

Self-Concept
One's overall view of self
The answer to "Who am I?"

Self-Esteem
The difference between ideal self and real self
An important component of self-concept

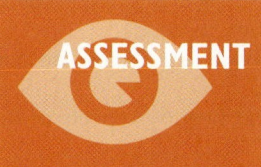
ASSESSMENT

Self-Concept

- Screen for problems, using the Focused Assessment box Assessing Self-Concept.
- **KEY POINT:** *If you suspect serious problems with self-concept, document the patient's responses in your nursing notes*

Self-Esteem

- To assess specifically for self-esteem, use the Focused Assessment box Performing a Self-Esteem Inventory.
- Observe for behaviors and comments associated with low self-esteem:

Avoids eye contact
Speaks hesitantly
Stooped posture
Overly critical
Moves slowly
Does not accept positive comments
Poor grooming
Apologizes frequently
Verbalizes feelings of powerlessness
Also see the Focused Assessment boxes on self-concept and self-esteem.

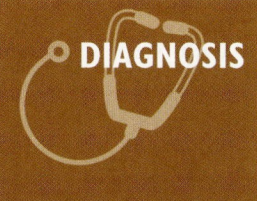
DIAGNOSIS

Analysis

- Avoid seeking simplistic cause-and-effect relationships.
- Avoid confusing low self-concept with clinical emotional and/or behavioral psychiatric diagnoses.

Diagnoses

- **Chronic Low Self-Esteem.** Expresses ongoing and long-standing overall self-dissatisfaction and negative self-appraisal (i.e., wide differences between "ideal" and "actual" or "perceived" self). *Etiology example: Depression*
- **Situational Low Self-Esteem.** Exhibits self-disapproval and negative self-evaluations as a specific reaction to loss or change. *Etiology example: Failure to adapt to a change in functioning*

- **Disturbed Personal Identity.** Exhibits negative and incorrect assessment of self-identity and inability to determine boundaries between self and others. *Etiology example: Mental illness*
- **Ineffective Role Performance.** Experiences or perceives difficulty in fulfilling a usual role, or there is a mismatch between role expectations and role performance (either perceived or societal expectations). *Etiology examples: Pain, Fatigue*
- **Disturbed Body Image.** Has a confused image of his physical self or negatively evaluates his body or an aspect of it. *Etiology example: eating disorder, gender conflict*

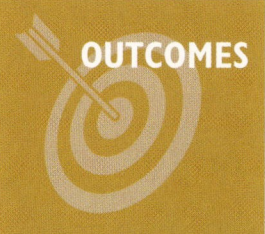
OUTCOMES

Nursing Diagnosis: Chronic Low Self-Esteem

NOC Outcome: Quality of Life
Individualized Outcome: Expresses pleasure in participating in activities

Nursing Diagnosis: Disturbed Body Image

NOC Outcome: Body Image
Individualized Outcome: Verbalizes positive aspects of body
Also refer to the NOC Outcomes list in the Chapter Resources on Davis Advantage.

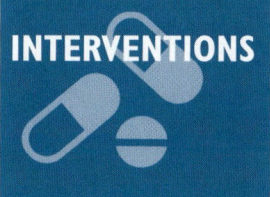
INTERVENTIONS

Common NIC Standardized interventions

Anticipatory Guidance
Decision-Making Support
Behavior Modification
Self-Esteem Enhancement

Also refer to the discussion on Planning Interventions: Self-Concept Disturbance and Low Self-Esteem in this chapter.

PLANNING OUTCOMES/EVALUATION: SELF-CONCEPT DISTURBANCE AND SELF-ESTEEM NP

You will choose outcomes based on the client's specific nursing diagnosis. For examples, refer to Example Problem: Self-Concept Disturbance and Low Self-Esteem.

When self-concept is the etiology of other problems (e.g., Sexual Dysfunction related to negative body image), choose outcomes based on the problem label (e.g., Sexual Functioning, Body Image). The overall goal, in all cases, is that the patient's self-concept (or some aspect of it) will improve.

PLANNING INTERVENTIONS/ IMPLEMENTATION: SELF-CONCEPT DISTURBANCE AND SELF-ESTEEM NP

Common *NIC standardized interventions* for self-concept and self-esteem diagnoses are found on in the Example Problem for self-concept and self-esteem. For more NIC self-concept and self-esteem interventions and activities, refer to the NIC list in the Chapter Resources on Davis Advantage.

Specific, individualized nursing activities for patients with self-esteem and self-concept problems are discussed in the following sections.

Promoting Self-Esteem and Self-Concept

The dependence that often accompanies illness and aging can bring about loss of self-esteem. Although the foundation for self-esteem is laid in childhood and affected by many sociocultural variables, your nursing approach can help preserve and enhance a patient's self-esteem.

Identifying Patient Strengths It is important to help the client identify past achievements and areas of strength. One way to do that is to point out areas of strength that you observe, such as the following:

Emotional strengths might include the ability to express emotions, to "feel" for others.

Relationship strengths include being sensitive to others' needs and being a good listener and making people feel comfortable.

Spiritual strengths may include faith in God and participation in church activities.

Evaluate the client's sense of humor, which can also be a strength, and be sure the client considers special aptitudes, such as cooking, arts and crafts, sports, work, and education.

Other Interventions The following are other nursing actions specific to self-esteem:

- Establish a therapeutic relationship emphasizing trust, consistency, honest communication, and unconditional positive regard.
- Encourage the client to be as independent as possible (e.g., by performing self-care).
- Monitor for and discourage self-criticism and negative self-talk.
- Teach the client to substitute positive self-talk for negative self-talk. For example, the client says, "I know my blood sugar is high, but I can't seem to stay on my diet. I ate way too much again today." You might remind the client that she exercised today and has been following her exercise program religiously. Eventually, she should learn to cue herself.

- Be supportive and accepting but do not invade the client's personal space.
- Help the client develop realistic goals that provide achievable challenges (no-fail situations).
- Encourage the client to take part in activities that offer opportunities for success.
- Role model communications skills that will help the person develop interpersonal relationships. Provide opportunities for practice.
- Refer to self-help and support groups, as needed.
- When possible, ask the client's advice (e.g., "How do you usually do this dressing change?").
- Point out good health practices and healthy aspects of the client's body functions.
- Refer to the Self-Care box for suggestions for teaching parents about promoting self-esteem in their children.

Promoting Positive Body Image

You can help parents promote a positive body image in their children, and you can help patients develop a different attitude toward their body. The following suggestions may be useful:

- Examine your own attitudes about what constitutes a healthy body and pay attention to the messages you convey to others.
- Encourage patients to discuss body changes resulting from their illness, surgery, or trauma.
- Provide the opportunity to interact with people who have had similar body changes.

Self-Care

Teaching Parents to Promote Self-Esteem in Children

Demonstrate love and acceptance by:
➤ Spending some one-on-one time with the child as often as possible: reading, playing, or just being together
➤ Being free with touches: a hug, a pat on the back
➤ Refraining from frequent negative criticism
➤ Providing nearly total acceptance of the child

Provide security by:
➤ Having clearly defined limits and consequences for breaking rules
➤ Being firm and consistent in applying the rules
➤ Being sure the rules are reasonable
➤ Allowing some latitude for individual actions within defined limits
➤ Treating the child with respect
➤ Establishing routines, such as bedtime activity, homework before play, dressing for school before breakfast in the morning, and so on
➤ Clearly defining every family member's role

Promote competence by:
➤ Setting realistic expectations about behaviors
➤ Assigning a few chores that are within the child's capability (e.g., picking up toys, making the bed)
➤ Modeling values, such as respect for others, honesty, and responsibility
➤ Providing positive feedback
➤ Helping the child accomplish goals
➤ Providing a stimulating and responsive environment
➤ Providing support in meeting challenges

Teach clients the following, some of which are the same as for developing self-concept and self-esteem. Provide feedback (e.g., about negative self-comments) as appropriate.

- **Healthy does not mean perfect.** Understand that healthy bodies come in a wide range of shapes and sizes. Fashion magazines portray an ideal body that is unrealistic and unhealthy for most people. If they make you feel bad by comparison, don't read them!
- **Focus on activity and healthy eating.** Be active and focus on healthy eating rather than starving and depriving yourself to lose weight.
- **Don't make negative comments about your body.** Be conscious of negative comments you make. Try not to talk negatively about body weight, size, or deformity; be kind to yourself. Ask support persons to point out when you are being unrealistically critical of you body.
- **Keep a list.** Keep a list of things you like about your body and refer to it when you are feeling down.
- **Accept compliments.** Practice accepting positive comments about your appearance. Ask support persons to coach your responses as needed (e.g., say, "Thank you" after a compliment).
- **Challenge critical comments.** Practice challenging critical comments from others about your appearance.
- **Surround yourself with positive people.** Surround yourself with positive people who support the changes you are trying to make in your image of your body. Avoid people who are critical.
- **Use a counter.** Buy a counter and click it each time you make a deliberate effort to accept positive feedback about your body or engage in positive body behaviors.

To see a care plan and care map for Body Image Disturbance,

 Go to Davis Advantage, Resources, Chapter 13, **Care Plan** and **Care Map.**

 Think**Like a Nurse** 13-7

- Refer to Karli in Meet Your Patient. Look at the preceding five NANDA-I labels for self-concept problems (Chronic Low Self-Esteem, Situational Low Self-Esteem, Disturbed Personal Identity, Ineffective Role Performance, Disturbed Body Image). Which one most clearly applies to Karli? Explain your thinking.
- For the interventions you did not choose, explain why.

Facilitating Role Enhancement

Sometimes the difficulty with self-concept centers on the inability to fulfill one's usual or desired role. Specific actions to enhance role satisfaction include the following:

- Help the client distinguish between ideal and actual role performance.
  - Help the person to identify her past, present, and future roles. For older adults, encourage reminiscence.
- Discuss boundaries, expectations, and management defined by lifestyle and family networks.
- Facilitate communication between client and significant other regarding the sharing of role responsibilities to accommodate role changes of the ill person.
- Help the client describe realistic roles and expectations tailored to specific health changes.

- Compare realistic roles with previous and less functional roles.
- Provide education about the difference between previous roles and current role.
- Provide a learning environment that focuses on positive and supportive change.
- Help the client identify and role-play behaviors needed in new roles.

KnowledgeCheck 13-4

Without looking back at the preceding material, see whether you can do the following:

- List three interventions for preserving self-worth.
- List three interventions for promoting self-esteem.
- List three interventions for fostering positive body image.
- List three interventions for promoting role enhancement.

Example Problem: Anxiety

I wake up in the middle of the night with a knot in my stomach and thinking about work. I go over and over my day and worry about my decisions and what I should have done instead. I replay the meetings in my head and think, "I know what that person said, but what did she mean by that?" I wonder whether I can handle the responsibility. My neck and shoulders are so tense that I get headaches. But when I try to relax and watch TV, I can feel my heart racing, and I feel shaky. I can't concentrate well enough to read.

TheoreticalKnowledge
knowing **why**

Anxiety is a common emotional response to a stressor—a "vague, uneasy feeling of discomfort or dread (the source often nonspecific or unknown to the individual) accompanied by an autonomic response; a feeling of apprehension caused by anticipation of danger" (NANDA International, 2018). An anxious person worries; feels nervous, uneasy, and fearful; may be tearful; and often has physical symptoms such as nausea, trembling, and sweating. Anxiety and fear produce similar responses; however, some experts differentiate them as follows:

Fear	*Response:* Cognitive
	Threat: Known; physical or psychological
	Event: Present;
Anxiety	*Response:* Emotional; psychological conflict (not physical threat)
	Threat: Known or unknown
	Event: Anticipated, not existing yet

Anxiety ranges from normal to abnormal, depending on its **intensity** and **duration**—how much anxiety is present and how long it has been present. See Table 13-2.

- **Normal anxiety** is an essential reaction to a realistic danger or threat to a person's physical or psychological integrity. It enables us to survive, and when the threat is no longer present to move on.
- **Abnormal anxiety** is out of proportion to the situation and lasts long after the threat is over, perhaps causing the person to alter her lifestyle.

Defense Mechanisms

To relieve anxiety, people use a variety of coping behaviors, such as exercising and talking with others (Bourne, 2011). Less adaptive behaviors include excessive sleeping, eating, smoking,

Table 13-2 ➤ Levels of Anxiety

DEFINITION OR DESCRIPTION	SYMPTOMS
Mild Anxiety	
This is normal anxiety, experienced in response to the events of day-to-day living. It heightens perception, sharpens the senses, enhances learning, and enables the person to function at his optimal level.	■ If present, symptoms may include muscle tension, restlessness, irritability, and a sense of unease. The person usually does not experience distress.
Moderate Anxiety	

As anxiety increases, the perceptual field narrows, and the person begins to focus on self and the need to relieve his discomfort.	■ Less alert to environmental events.
	■ Distracts easily.
	■ Shorter attention span.
	■ May need help with problem-solving but can attend to his needs with direction.
	■ Physical symptoms may include:
	  • Increased heart and respiratory rate
	  • Increased perspiration
	  • Gastric discomfort
	  • Increased muscle tension
	  • Rapid, loud, and higher pitched speech

Severe Anxiety	
Perceptual field is so narrow that the person can focus on only one particular detail or may shift focus to many extraneous details. Focus is totally on self and the need to relieve the anxiety.	■ Concentration and attention span are severely limited, so the person has difficulty completing simple tasks. ■ Anxiety prevents problem-solving and learning. ■ May report feelings of dread, confusion, and other unpleasant emotions. ■ Physical symptoms may include headaches, palpitations, tachycardia, insomnia, dizziness, nausea, trembling, hyperventilation, urinary frequency, and diarrhea.
Panic Anxiety	
The person becomes unreasonable and irrational and is unable to focus on even one detail in the environment. He may misperceive environmental cues or lose contact with reality (e.g., experience hallucinations or delusions).	■ May react wildly (e.g., shouting, screaming, running about, clinging to something) or withdraw completely. ■ Cannot function or communicate effectively (e.g., may speak incoherently or be unable to speak). ■ May feel terror and impending doom, believe he has a life-threatening illness, or that he is "going crazy." ■ Physical symptoms include dilated pupils, labored breathing, severe trembling, sleeplessness, palpitations, diaphoresis, pallor, and muscular incoordination (Townsend, 2014).

crying, pacing, fidgeting, drinking, laughing, cursing, nail biting, or finger tapping.

When anxiety is more severe, the person attempts to counteract the anxiety in some way. Each person develops unique patterns of coping with anxiety, called **defense mechanisms,** which are used consciously or unconsciously to relieve the anxiety. Examples of defense mechanisms are **denial** (refusing to acknowledge the existence of a real situation or associated feelings) and **displacement** (transferring feelings from one target to another that seems less threatening—for example,

kicking the dog when you are angry at your boss). See Chapter 12 for further discussion of defense mechanisms.

■ *When overused, defense mechanisms can be maladaptive* and can lead to psychological disorders such as obsessive–compulsive disorders and dissociative disorders (e.g., amnesia).

■ *Excessive or unrelieved anxiety may also contribute to **psychosis,*** which is a loss of ability to differentiate self from non-self. It may include impaired reality testing (e.g., knowing what is real and what exists only in one's mind). Examples of psychotic responses to anxiety include schizophrenia and delusional disorders. These disorders are beyond the scope of this book. If you need more information, refer to a mental health text.

KnowledgeCheck 13-5

- What is anxiety?
- When is anxiety a normal response to life?
- Identify at least three healthcare scenarios that might trigger anxiety in patients.

PracticalKnowledge
knowing **how**

As a nurse generalist, your independent role is to assess and document the patient's behavioral state as it relates to his medical–surgical condition rather than to diagnose and treat mental illnesses. An anxious client, for example, may not understand or recall instructions for self-care nor focus well enough to follow a medical regimen or keep appointments with healthcare providers. **KEY POINT:** *As a nurse, you should be prepared to recognize and provide care for anxious and depressed patients in all practice settings.*

For nursing care for Anxiety, see Example Problem: Anxiety.

ASSESSMENT: ANXIETY NP

In general practice, the focus of nursing care for clients with anxiety is (1) to differentiate between mild anxiety and that which is severe enough to require referral to a mental health professional (see Table 13-2) and (2) to provide interventions to relieve anxiety.

For a checklist to help you determine the patient's anxiety level, refer to the Focused Assessment box Anxiety Assessment Guide.

ANALYSIS NURSING DIAGNOSES: ANXIETY NP

Anxiety can be the etiology or a symptom of many other nursing diagnoses, such as Deficient Knowledge, Self-Mutilation, Ineffective Sexuality Pattern, or Insomnia. See the accompanying Example Problem.

KnowledgeCheck 13-6

- List five NANDA-I labels you could use to describe a problem of anxiety.
- List four observations that would alert you that anxiety is severe enough to merit referral to a mental health professional.

Focused Assessment

Anxiety Assessment Guide

Rating Scale: None = 0, Mild = 1, Moderate = 2, Severe = 3, Disabling (Panic) = 4

Physiological Effects	Rating	Psychological Effects	Rating
Shortness of breath (dyspnea)	____	Depersonalization (unreal)	____
Choking sensation	____	Feeling "on edge"	____
Dry mouth	____	Poor concentration	____
Pounding heart, increased heart rate	____	Poor memory	____
Chest pain	____	Depressed mood	____
Increased sweating and clammy	____	Loss of interest	____
Feeling faint, dizzy, unsteady	____	Restlessness	____
Nausea and abdominal upsets	____	Sense of panic	____
Numbness (pins and needles)	____	Worry, anticipation of the worst	____
Hot/cold flashes	____	Irritability	____
Trembling, shaking	____	Nightmares	____
Muscle tension and aches	____	Feeling of fear and foreboding	____
Exaggerated startle response	____	Excessive apprehension	____
Difficulties in falling asleep and staying asleep	____	Feeling lack of control	____

Assessing Overall Scores

0–28	Mild anxiety
29–56	Moderate anxiety
57–84	Severe anxiety
85–112	Disabling anxiety

Creating a total score from this table can help you assess whether overall anxiety is mild, moderate, severe, or disabling. However, individual physiological or psychological symptoms that are rated as severe (3) or disabling (4) may be more important and relevant to your nursing assessment. For example, your patient's overall or total assessment may be 26 (in the mild range, 0–27) but she has rated "Excessive apprehension" as 4 (disabling).

EXAMPLE PROBLEM: Anxiety

Defining Characteristics (Signs, Symptoms)
Behavioral—poor eye contact, restlessness, crying, trembling, rapid speech
Cognitive—confusion, difficulty concentrating, forgetfulness

Objective data—sweating, rapid pulse and respirations, dilated pupils
Subjective data—shortness of breath, nausea, insomnia, worry

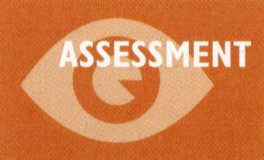

ASSESSMENT

- Consider a comprehensive physical assessment to rule out underlying disease or disorders.

- Identify the presence, level, and cause of anxiety. Each level requires different nursing actions.

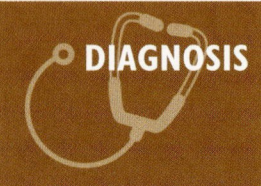

DIAGNOSIS

- Anxiety
- Death Anxiety

- Decisional Conflict.
- Fear

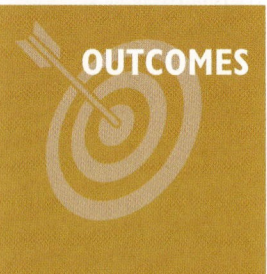

OUTCOMES

For Anxiety
- Plans coping strategies for anxious situations.
- Uses relaxation techniques as required.
- Reports absence of physical and psychological manifestations of anxiety.

For Death Anxiety
- Reports feeling less fearful.
- Discusses funeral arrangements with family.

For Fear
- Uses effective coping strategies.
- Maintains social relationships and control over life.

For Ineffective Denial
- Verbalizes understanding of the complications that may occur if the disease is not treated.
- Follows prescribed regimen for treatments and medications.

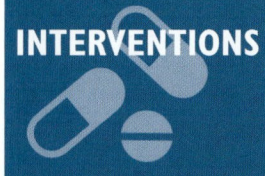

INTERVENTIONS

For Anxiety
- Recognize that the client is anxious.
- Identify the source of the client's anxiety.
- Deal with the symptoms of the client's anxiety.

Individualized Nursing Activities
- Provide a calm and safe environment to help patient stay focused.
- Establish a relationship of trust, caring, and unconditional positive regard.
- Be present; stay with the client to help allay fears, create trust, and promote safety.
- Use clear and factual knowledge tailored to the individual's circumstances.
- Explain and, if necessary, explore details of all healthcare procedures.
- Advise regular physical exercise unless contraindicated by a physical condition.
- Help identify triggers and situations that create anxiety.
- Administer and monitor anti-anxiety medication prn.
- Assist with relaxation methods. For information about such relaxation,

    Go to Bonus **Chapter 46, Holistic Healing,** on Davis Advantage.

Severe Anxiety

Individualized Activities

- ⊞ If you suspect severe or disabling anxiety, document the patient's responses.
- Involve a mental health professional immediately (same day) if you discover any of the following: suicidal thoughts, assaultive or homicidal thoughts and/or plans, loss of touch with reality (psychosis), or significant or prolonged inability to work and care for self or family.

Death Anxiety

Individualized Activities
- Stay physically close to the fearful patient.
- Obtain spiritual support for the patient and family.
- Honor specific patient/family requests for care.
- See Chapter 17 for more interventions.

For other NIC standardization interventions and activities for Anxiety, refer to the NIC list on Davis Advantage, chapter resources.

PLANNING OUTCOMES/EVALUATION AND INTERVENTIONS/IMPLEMENTATION FOR ANXIETY NP

Whether anxiety is a symptom, a problem, or the etiology (cause) of a problem, one of the desired outcomes is that the anxiety will be relieved. Interventions for anxious clients depend on the cause and level of anxiety. See the accompanying Example Problem for anxiety, as well as the NOC and NIC lists on Davis Advantage Chapter Resources.

EXAMPLE PROBLEM: DEPRESSION

Others imply that they know what it is like to be depressed because they have gone through a divorce, lost a job or broken up with someone. But these experiences carry with them feelings. Depression, instead, is flat, hollow, and unendurable.

— Kay Redfield Jamison (1997, p. 218), An Unquiet Mind

Theoretical Knowledge knowing **why**

The term *depression* is commonly used to describe a feeling of sadness or "the blues." But to healthcare professionals, it refers to a specific condition with characteristic symptoms and often devastating consequences if left untreated (Steptoe, 2007). For American Psychiatric Association (APA) criteria for depression, see Example Problem: Depression, later in the chapter.

Depression occurs in all age groups, even in very young children. It affects about 11% of the adult population in the United States and is one of the top three risks for functional decline. See Table 13-3 for common truths and myths about depression.

As a nurse generalist, your independent role is not to diagnose and treat mental illnesses. Rather, it is to assess and document the patient's behavioral state as it relates to his medical–surgical condition. A depressed patient, for example, may not have the energy or motivation to recall or follow a medical regimen or keep appointments with healthcare providers.

Unlike the feeling of true sadness, such as might accompany a divorce, death, or other loss, the depressed mood is typically marked by a sense of emptiness. This contributes to the depressed person's tendency to withdraw from social contacts and also explains the characteristically flat affect (Fig. 13-4).

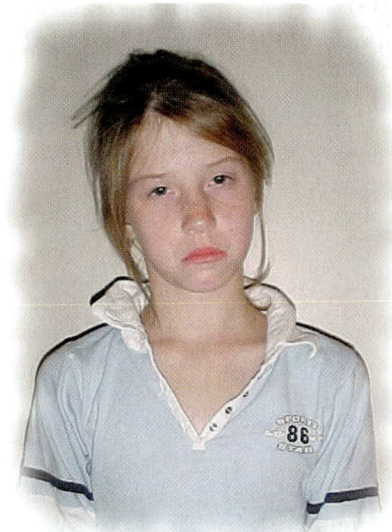

FIGURE 13-4 Depressed affect.

What Causes Depression?

Are our genes responsible for the development of depression? Is depression "anger turned inward"? Depression theories fall into the following four groupings:

- *Physiological theories* relate depression to biochemical imbalances stemming from hormonal, neurological, or genetic factors.
- *Psychodynamic theories* relate depression to loss, abandonment, and emotional detachment and to diurnal and seasonal mood variations.
- *Cognitive theory* relates depression to negative thinking.
- *Social/environmental theories* relate depression to poor family relationships, difficult interpersonal relationships, and socioeconomic and political factors.

Depression in Older and Middle Adults

Depressive symptoms are an important indicator of general well-being and mental health among older adults. People who report many depressive symptoms often experience higher rates of physical illness, greater functional disability, and higher healthcare resource utilization. While older adults were the demographic group with the highest suicide rates for decades, suicide rates for middle-aged adults (aged 24 to 62) have increased to comparable levels. In 2008, 16% of women aged 65 and over reported depressive symptoms compared with 11% of men (Federal Interagency Forum on Aging-Related Statistics, 2012).

Risk Factors Specific to Older Adults For older adults, risk factors for depression include disability, new medical illness, poor health status, prior depression, poor self-perceived health, sleep disturbance, bereavement, and female gender (Cole & Dendukuri, 2014).

Signs and Symptoms of Depression in Older Adults Depression is difficult to diagnose because in older adults and is, therefore, underdiagnosed and undertreated.

- Depression is more likely to be masked rather than exhibited by typical symptoms such as sadness.
- Symptoms are often physical or expressed as personality changes such as irritability.

Table 13-3 ➤ Depression: Truths and Myths	
TRUE	**FALSE**
Depressive disorders are more common among women than men (2:1) (Albert, 2015).	"Getting on with life" will cure depression.
Spiritual distress is associated with depression.	Everyone likes to talk about how they feel.
Depression can be defined as a maladaptive emotional response.	Medication is the answer to depression.
Low socioeconomic circumstances and social isolation correlate with depression.	Once depression has been cured, it does not return.

- **KEY POINT:** *Depression may occur along with, or be mistaken for, dementia and delirium. In older adults, all three conditions may include the symptoms of confusion, distractibility, and memory loss.*
- Some of the physical symptoms of depression (e.g., fatigue, anorexia, constipation, and psychomotor retardation) can be confused with physical illness, medication interactions, substance abuse, or "signs of old age."

KnowledgeCheck 13-7

- What distinguishes clinical depression from feelings of sadness?
- How might a child manifest depression?
- Why is the nurse–patient (therapeutic) relationship important when caring for depressed individuals?

Substance Abuse and Mental Illness

Substance abuse is a growing concern for the United States. It contributes to family crises, public health issues, and criminal justice concerns. Many people who regularly abuse drugs are also diagnosed with mental disorders and vice versa. By 2020, mental and substance use disorders will surpass all physical diseases as a major cause of disability worldwide.

- *Persons diagnosed with mood or anxiety disorders,* antisocial personality, or conduct disorders are about twice as likely to suffer also from a drug abuse or dependence (National Institute on Drug Abuse, 2010b).
- *Similarly, persons diagnosed with drug disorders* are roughly twice as likely to suffer from mood and anxiety disorders.

By far the most common issue connecting mental illness and substance abuse is the intention of patients to medicate the mental health symptoms that they find disruptive or uncomfortable by using alcohol and drugs. Some examples include the following:

- A depressed patient who uses marijuana to numb the pain
- A patient with low energy and lack of motivation who abuses Adderall, cocaine, or crystal meth to increase the drive to get things done

Treatment for Substance Abuse Treatment helps reduce the powerful effects of drugs on the body and brain, thereby helping people improve their physical health and everyday functioning and regain control of their lives. Depending on the substance(s) involved, treatment may include medications, behavioral treatments, or a combination. A physician, substance abuse counselor, or other health professionals play an important role in determining the right treatment for an individual.

Medications are available to treat addiction to opiates, nicotine, and alcohol, but none has yet been approved for treating addiction to marijuana, stimulants, or depressants. However, behavioral therapy can be helpful in these cases. Nursing care for these patients is complex and requires special training. A major role for the nurse is to help the patient understand and adapt to the various medications. To find out more about substance abuse, see Chapter 9 and,

 Go to Example Problem: Substance Abuse in Chapter 9.

PracticalKnowledge
knowing **how**

Of course, you will not be conducting psychotherapy in your general practice. However, you *will* care for patients who are taking antidepressant medications and who have situational or even clinical depression. There is much you can do to make their care more effective. See the accompanying Example Problem: Depression.

The nurse–patient relationship is vital when you work with a depressed person. A depressed person is likely to be apathetic, avoid your approach, or feel unworthy of your time and effort. Establishing a nurse–patient bond requires a specific, empathetic approach involving warmth, acceptance, and understanding (unconditional positive regard) even in the face of an unresponsive, even angry, patient response.

ASSESSMENT: DEPRESSION NP

You should be alert for risk factors and signs and symptoms of depression in all healthcare settings. If cues are present, you will need to perform a more thorough screening or comprehensive assessment, such as the Focused Assessment box Depression Assessment Guide: Patient Health Questionnaire (PHQ-9).

Assessing Older Adults: Depression, Delirium, or Dementia?

Unfortunately for older adults, cognitive difficulty and depression continue to be under-recognized and under-treated. Cognitive disorders, such as delirium and dementia, are sometimes confused with depression, because they share some symptoms. You can find more information about dementia in Chapter 10. Depression has been described on the preceding page.

Delirium, also called *acute confusion,* is an acute and potentially reversible disturbance of consciousness and cognition in response to underlying medical or mental illnesses, drug toxicity, and various other causes. An estimated 40% of cases of delirium are preventable (Kresevic, 2015). Delirium is an important consideration in quality of care and patient safety. Many aspects of nursing care, such as medication administration, evaluation of complications, and assessment of dehydration, nutrition, and sleep, are factors that can be modified to prevent the development of delirium.

Dementia is an irreversible decline in mental abilities. The APA (2013) defines dementia as part of **neurocognitive disorders (NCDs),** a group of disorders in which the primary clinical deficit is in cognitive function. Dementia can occur at any age, but is more common in older adults.

- NCDs are acquired rather than developmental.
- NCDs may be associated with Alzheimer's disease, vascular disease, Parkinson's disease, traumatic brain injury, HIV infection, or substance/medication-induced NCD.
- Dementia affects about 22% of adults aged 71 years and older.
- Prevalence increases with age: The rate is about 40% in those older than age 85.

KEY POINT: *Confusion may be present in patients with depression as well as those who have dementia or delirium.*

For a comparison of the symptoms of depression and dementia, see the Focused Assessment box Differentiating Depression and Dementia.

When Should I Refer the Patient to a Mental Health Specialist?

Figure 13-5 illustrates the continuum of mild to severe depression incorporating aspects of mood, behavior, thoughts, and physical symptoms.

Depression Assessment Guide: Patient Health Questionnaire (PHQ-9)

This is a valid and reliable measure of depression developed in 1999 by Pfizer, Inc. It can be self-administered (Kroenke, Spitzer, & Williams, 2001). It may be useful across cultures (Chen, Huang, Chang, et al., 2006).

Over the past 2 weeks, how often have you been bothered by any of the following problems? (Check or circle your answers.)

	Not At All	Several Days	More than Half the Days	Nearly Every Day
1. Little interest or pleasure in doing things	0	1	2	2
2. Feeling down, depressed, or hopeless	0	1	2	3
3. Trouble falling or staying asleep, or sleeping too much	0	1	2	3
4. Feeling tired or having little energy	0	1	2	3
5. Poor appetite or overeating	0	1	2	3
6. Feeling bad about yourself—or that you are a failure or have let yourself or your family down	0	1	2	3
7. Trouble concentrating on things, such as reading the newspaper or watching television	0	1	2	3
8. Moving or speaking so slowly that other people could have noticed. Or the opposite—being so fidgety or restless that you have been moving around a lot more than usual	0	1	2	3
9. Thoughts that you would be better off dead or of hurting yourself in some way	0	1	2	3

ADD COLUMNS   ☐ + ☐ + ☐

TOTAL: ☐

If you checked off any problems, how difficult have these problems made it for you to do your work, take care of things at home, or get along with other people?

Not difficult at all _____
Somewhat difficult _____
Very difficult _____
Extremely difficult _____

(Healthcare professional: For interpretation of TOTAL, please refer to the accompanying score card. [Note to students: Interpretation requires training. You should report the patient's score to your instructor or your immediate supervising nurse.])

Source: Pfizer, Inc. Retrieved from http://www.phqscreeners.com/

The presence of any of the following should alert you to document the patient's responses in your nursing notes make a referral to a mental health specialist:

- Personal or family history of recurrent depression or bipolar disorder
- Personal history of recurrence of depression within 1 year after stopping effective treatment
- Episode of major depression before age 20
- Severe, sudden, or life-threatening depressive episode (i.e., suicide attempt); if you believe there is a risk for suicide, make the referral immediately (Box 13-1)

For two alternative methods you can use to identify patients who should be referred to a mental health specialist for evaluation and/or treatment of depression, refer to the Focused Assessment box Identifying Depressed Patients Who Should Be Referred for Evaluation.

ANALYSIS/NURSING DIAGNOSIS: DEPRESSION NP

Depression is a psychiatric diagnosis, so you will not make that diagnosis. Nevertheless, you will need to describe associated problems that are appropriate for nursing intervention. The NANDA-I taxonomy does not have a diagnosis that uses the term *depression.* However, the nursing diagnoses on the accompanying Example Problem may be useful in describing the feelings and moods of patients who are depressed.

EXAMPLE PROBLEM: Depression

Criteria established by the American Psychiatric Association (APA) for major depressive disorder include the following:
- Depressed mood most of the day nearly every day for at least 2 weeks, typically accompanied by markedly diminished interest or pleasure in activities the person previously enjoyed
- Insomnia or hypersomnia
- Loss of energy
- Feelings of worthlessness
- Diminished ability to concentrate
- Feelings of emptiness
- Recurrent thoughts of death (APA, 2013)

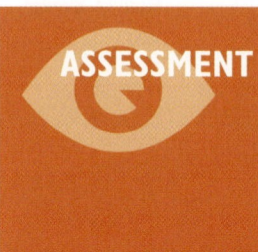
ASSESSMENT

Assess for Risk Factors
- Family history of depression, hormonal or nutritional imbalance, inability to externalize anger, low self-esteem, negative thinking, learned helplessness and hopelessness, prior success or failure in coping mechanisms, traumatic loss, catastrophic stressors (e.g., unemployment, disability, poor health, bereavement), chronic disease, female sex, sleep disturbance

- If present, perform focused assessment to determine whether depression is present.

Assess for Signs and Symptoms (APA Criteria)
- Feelings (Affect)
- Cognition (Thoughts)
- Behaviors
- Lifestyle Effects
- Physiological Effects

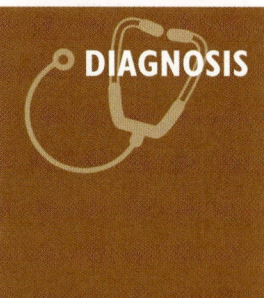
DIAGNOSIS

Hopelessness
Powerlessness

➕ **Risk for Suicide** must always be considered when a patient is depressed, especially when there is a history of prior attempts or the person is verbalizing the desire to die or the intent to kill himself.

Other Physical and Behavioral Diagnoses

Activity Intolerance
Ineffective Health Management

Constipation
Obesity
Overweight
Impaired Social Interaction
Self-Neglect
Insomnia
Risk for Overweight
Self-Care Deficit (Bathing, Feeding, Dressing, Toileting)

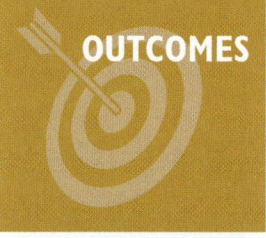
OUTCOMES

- Expresses positive belief in self, others, and meaning of life.

- Participates in healthcare decisions to extent possible.
- Sets realistic goals for self.

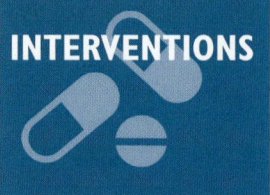
INTERVENTIONS

General Interventions for Depression
- Promote activity. Small group activities help build self-esteem.
- Promote and teach good nutrition and hydration.
- Use therapeutic communication.
- Assess use of, and provide information about, complementary and alternative therapies for depression.

- Assess suicide risk. Ask directly, "Have you thought about harming yourself? If so, what do you plan to do?"
- Institute measures to build self-esteem.
- Provide information on support groups.

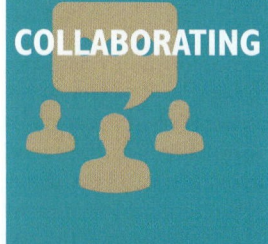
COLLABORATING

People who are clinically depressed cannot just "snap out of it." If untreated, the symptoms may continue for weeks or even years. The physiological theory of depression predominates in the medical community, and current evidence shows that biochemical processes determine moods, thought, cognition, and perception. Therefore, treatment of serious depression relies more heavily on antidepressant medication than on psychotherapy.

However, the medications have a number of unpleasant, and even serious, side effects, and some patients say that they do not effectively elevate their mood.

Psychotherapists acknowledge that individual tolerance of symptoms, coping resources, education, and social support networks all have an important effect on outcomes and treatment.

Differentiating Depression and Dementia

Use this tool to help identify older adults who should be referred for further evaluation to determine whether symptoms are related to depression or dementia.

➤ *To determine whether the patient should be referred to a mental health professional,* refer to the Focused Assessment box Identifying Depressed Patients Who Should Be Referred for Evaluation, later in this chapter.

Characteristic	Depression	Dementia
Cause/triggers	Loss (e.g., of spouse, of independence); stress	Physiological causes (e.g., Alzheimer's disease, brain infarcts)
Onset	Acute or chronic; can be related to specific events	Chronic, gradual, and insidious
Course	Varies, depending on cause	Progressive, over a long period of time
Alertness	Usually reduced	Usually normal
Memory	Memory loss and forgetfulness	Recent and remote memory impaired; loss of recent memory is first sign; some loss of common knowledge
Thinking	Inability to concentrate	Difficulty with abstraction and word finding, especially nouns; difficulty with calculations; decreased judgment
Response to questions	Often says, "I don't know"	Answers inappropriately or with "near misses"
Language	Speaks slowly; slow to respond to verbal stimuli	Disoriented, rambling, incoherent; difficulty using nouns
Sleep	Difficulty falling asleep, early morning awakening, much day sleeping	Sleep fragmented; awakens often during night
Reversibility	Potential	Irreversible, progressive

Source: Adapted from Edwards, N. (2003, December). Differentiating the three D's: Delirium, dementia, and depression. *MEDSURG Nursing, 12*(6), 347. Retrieved from http://nursing.advanceweb.com/Features/Articles/Delirium-Dementia-Depression.aspx

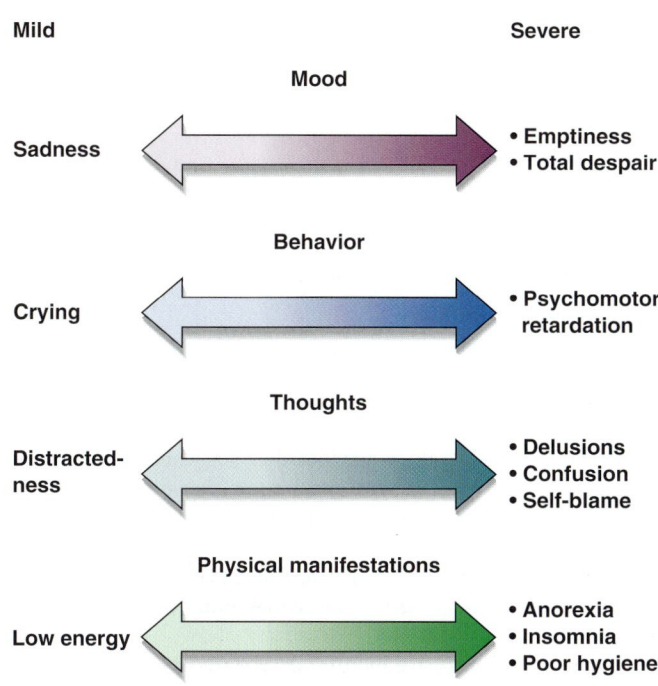

FIGURE 13-5 Depression assessment continuum incorporating mood, behavior, thoughts, and physical state.

PLANNING OUTCOMES/EVALUATION: DEPRESSION NP

Individualized goal/outcome statements should relate to the patient's specific nursing diagnosis, stating behaviors that will indicate that the problem is resolving. The following are a few examples:

For Depressed Mood:
Reports feeling less sadness and depression.
Interacts willingly and appropriately with others.

For Hopelessness:
Expresses positive belief in self, others, and meaning of life.
Demonstrates interest in life/activity.

For Powerlessness:
Participates in healthcare decisions to the extent possible.
Sets realistic goals for self.

For Risk for Suicide:
Verbalizes any suicidal ideas to staff.
Trusts staff enough to disclose any specific plans for suicide.

PLANNING INTERVENTIONS/ IMPLEMENTATION: DEPRESSION NP

Standardized interventions for Depression can be found on the NIC list in Davis Advantage, Chapter Resources. *Individualized interventions and activities* are discussed in the following pages.

BOX 13-1 ■ Cues Indicating a Possible Risk Factor for Suicide

Risk Factors

- Alcohol and other substance abuse
- Family history of mental disorders or substance abuse
- Family history of suicide
- Guns in the home
- Family violence, including physical or sexual abuse
- A significant medical illness, such as cancer or chronic pain
- Compulsive gambling
- Recent losses: physical, financial, personal
- Age, gender, race (elderly or young adult, unmarried, white, male, living alone)
- Recent discharge from an inpatient psychiatry unit

Warning Signs

➕ Patients with risk factors who exhibit any of the following warning signs clearly raise a red flag and merit immediate referral:

- Withdrawal from social contact
- Desire to be left alone

- Preoccupation with death and dying, or violence
- Risky or self-destructive behavior, such as drug use or unsafe driving
- Changes in routine, sleeping patterns
- Changes in eating habits
- Giving away belongings or getting affairs in order
- Personality changes, such as becoming very outgoing after being shy
- Saying goodbye to people as if they won't be seen again
- Talking about suicide (e.g., "I'm going to kill myself," I wish I were dead," or "I wish I hadn't been born")

Source: Maybury, B. C. (2008). Suicide prevention: Every nurse's responsibility. Nurse.com. Retrieved from http://news.nurse.com/article/20080310/NY02/80305017

Identifying Depressed Patients Who Should Be Referred for Evaluation

Focused Assessment

Two Yes/No Questions

One way to identify depression that is more than simple, situational depression is to ask the following two questions. A yes answer merits a referral.

1. "Over the past 2 weeks, have you felt down, depressed, or hopeless?"
2. "Over the past 2 weeks, have you felt little interest or pleasure in doing things?"

SIGECAPS

Another method is to use the mnemonic SIGECAPS, a concise version of the *DSM-IV-TR* diagnostic criteria. Ask the patient whether he has experienced, for 2 or more weeks:

Sleep increase/decrease
Interest in formerly compelling or pleasurable activities diminished
Guilt, low self-esteem
Energy poor
Concentration poor
Appetite increase/decrease
Psychomotor agitation or retardation
Suicidal ideation

Both of the following require referral for evaluation and treatment:

Major depression = depressed mood or interest *plus* 4 SIGECAPS for 2 or more weeks
Mild depression (mood disorder) = depressed mood or interest *plus* 3 SIGECAPS most days for 2 or more years

Source: U.S. Preventive Services Task Force. (2015a). Final update summary: Depression in adults: Screening. Retrieved from http://www.uspreventiveservicestaskforce.org/Page/Document/UpdateSummaryFinal/depression-in-adults-screening?ds=1&s=Depression

IN SAD CAGES

Some people prefer a mnemonic from an older source, IN SAD CAGES, which you would use in essentially the same way. Ask the patient whether he has experienced, for 2 or more weeks:

Interest reduced
Negative thoughts

Sleep disturbance
Appetite change
Decreased confidence or self-esteem

Concentration reduced
Affect blunt or flat
Guilt
Energy reduced
Suicidal ideas

The original reference does not include a suggested total that requires referral. However, you can assume that the more symptoms, the more severe the depression. We suggest the following:

IN (reduced interest and negative thoughts or depressed mood) plus 4 of the other **SAD CAGES** requires referral.

Do not try to differentiate mild and major depression with this method.

Adapted from: Leng, L. B. (2011). Overview of major depressive disorder. *The Singapore Family Physician, 37*(4), 18–21.

Complementary and Alternative Modalities (CAM) used for Depression

Many people use herbal therapies to relieve symptoms of anxiety and depression. Patients may self-treat with herbal remedies, or CAM practitioners may prescribe them. You should assess for CAM use to be sure that the method is not contraindicated and that the patient has informed the primary care provider about its use.

		DEPRESSION		
CAM	**Active Ingredients**	**Side Effects**	**Contraindications**	**Patient Teaching**
Ginkgo biloba	Ginkgetin, ginkgolic acid, ascorbic acid, flavonols, sterols	Nausea, vomiting, diarrhea (usually mild) Headache	Pregnant or breastfeeding Children Patients using anticoagulants (use with caution) Patients with peptic ulcer disease Cardiovascular disease	Can take 6–8 weeks for patient to feel any better. Mixing with some fruits and nuts could produce poison ivy–like reaction.
Ginseng	Ginsenosides, beta-elemene, sterols, flavonoids, peptides, vitamins B_1, B_2, B_{12}, nicotinic acid, fats, minerals, enzymes	(many) Nausea Vomiting Diarrhea Chest pain Headache Nosebleeds Palpitations Nervousness Insomnia	Hypertension Hypotension Diabetes Pregnancy or breastfeeding Patients with active bleeding Anticoagulants Antiplatelet medications	There are many kinds of ginseng; patient should research the specific type he is using. ✚ Discourage use by patients who are anticoagulated, or who have hypertension or diabetes.
Kava	Kava pyrones, pipermethystine	Visual disturbances Changes in reflexes and judgment Decreased platelet and lymphocyte counts Hepatotoxicity	Pregnancy Breastfeeding Use of alcohol, alprazolam, or central nervous system (CNS) depressants	May experience symptom relief within 1 week. Significant adverse reactions may occur. Kava enhances the effects of alcohol and CNS medications. Because of liver toxicity, the Centers for Disease Control and Prevention has cautioned consumers against using kava (CDC, 2002). Its use is severely limited and regulated in Australia (Therapeutic Goods Administration, updated 2015).
St. John's wort	Tannin, naphthodianthrones, flavonoids, bioflavonoids, phloroglucinols	Dry mouth Constipation GI upset Sleep disturbances Restlessness Photosensitivity Interferes with digoxin and indinavir	Pregnancy or lactation Children Use of monoamine oxidase inhibitors, selective serotonin reuptake inhibitors, alcohol, or over-the-counter cold and flu medications	Teach contraindications and side effects. Patients who are depressed should not take this herb without medical supervision.
S-Adenosyl methionine (SAMe)	Amino acid and adenosine triphosphate, which are produced naturally in the body and are now being reproduced artificially as well	Few side effects Gastric upset Hypomania (in patients with bipolar disorder) Anxiety (in patients with depression) Headache		Patients with bipolar disorder should not use this supplement unless under direct supervision of their physician. Use enteric-coated forms to decrease gastric irritation.

Anxiety

Kava	See Depression, preceding. Not recommended for use.

Source: Adapted from Beaubrun, G., & Gray, G. E. (2014). A review of herbal medicines for psychiatric disorders. *Psychiatric Services, 51*(9), retrieved from http://ps.psychiatryonline.org/doi/10.1176/appi.ps.51.9.1130; and Gorman, L. M., & Anwar, R. (2014). *Neeb's fundamentals of mental health nursing* (4th ed.). Philadelphia, PA: F. A. Davis.

Suicide Prevention Interventions

It is not only patients on psychiatric units who commit suicide. They may be the same patients you care for on a medical–surgical unit or in their homes. Illnesses such as advanced cancer and AIDS are often accompanied by uncontrolled pain and delirium. Because of the suffering and dependency these illnesses cause, they are associated with higher suicide rates.

KEY POINT: *Your most important nursing intervention is assessment. Be alert for risk factors and warning signs that may indicate the possibility of suicide (see Box 13-1).*

Remember that about 80% of those who attempt suicide give some prior verbal or indirect cues.

- Evaluate the patient's medications (e.g., certain antihypertensive agents, steroids, cancer chemotherapeutic agents, amphotericin-B can cause depression).
- If risk factors are present, put them prominently on the care plan and report them to other caregivers.
- Do not avoid the patient because you fear saying the wrong thing. Talking about suicide does not increase the risk.
- Be aware of your personal feelings and anxieties regarding suicide.
- If the patient mentions suicide specifically, be direct. Ask whether he is having thoughts of harming himself.
- If he answers yes, do not leave him. Have someone contact his primary care provider so that a psychiatric consult can be ordered, and possibly transfer the patient to a psychiatric unit if he is physically stable.
- Ask whether the patient has a plan for suicide, and if so, what it is.
- Remove items that might be used for self-harm, for example, razor blades and other sharp objects, shoelaces, belts, intravenous tubing, telephone cords, pills, and glasses. Search the room and the bathroom.
- Make sure the windows cannot be opened.
- Follow agency policy for continuous monitoring, moving to a room close to the nurses' station, and so on (Gorman & Anwar, 2014; Maybury, 2008).
- **KEY POINT:** *Most of all, never attempt to work with a suicidal patient by yourself. Involve other members of the team immediately.*

Nursing Interventions for Older Adults

KEY POINT: *Remember that (1) depression is not a normal part of aging, and (2) it is important to identify depression and not mistake it for dementia or "signs of old age."*

Team Communication If you identify signs of depression, be certain to communicate that to other members of the staff and to the primary care provider.

Medications Because metabolism changes with aging, the risk of adverse medication effects is high for older adults.

- Closely supervise patients being treated with antidepressants because severe side effects are possible.

- When a patient is admitted to a hospital, there is a risk that self-administered medications may be overlooked. Missed doses of an antidepressant combined with a physical illness may cause depression symptoms to worsen.

Reminiscence Encourage the patient to talk about significant positive and negative experiences that have occurred during her life.

Dementia Care The Progressively Lowered Stress Threshold (PLST) (Fletcher, 2012) provides a conceptual framework for the nursing care of patients with dementia:

- Monitor the effectiveness and side effects of medications given specifically to improve cognitive function or delay cognitive decline.
- Provide appropriate cognitive-enhancement techniques and social engagement.
- Ensure adequate rest, sleep, fluid, nutrition, elimination, pain control, and comfort measures.
- Avoid the use of physical and pharmacological restraints.
- Maximize functional capacity: Maintain mobility and encourage independence as long as possible.
- Address behavioral issues: Identify environmental triggers, medical conditions, or caregiver–patient conflict that may be causing the behavior.

- Ensure a therapeutic and safe environment.

- Encourage and support advance-care planning: Explain trajectory of progressive dementia, treatment options, and advance directives.
- Provide caregiver education and support.
- Integrate community resources into the plan of care to meet patient and caregiver needs.

Suicide Risk **KEY POINT:** *Keep in mind that depression is a significant predictor of suicide in older adults.* Rates of suicide for both men and women reach their highest peaks in the 85-and-older age group. Most elderly persons who attempt suicide or die by suicide suffer from depression. However, depression alone cannot adequately explain late-life suicidal behavior, given that only a minority of depressed elders actually attempts suicide. Other known risk factors for late-life suicide—such as loss of a significant other, disability, and prior suicide attempt—have limited explanatory power as well (Cheung, Merry, & Sundram, 2015).

Professional Help Encourage the patient to seek professional help. Older adults are likely to try to handle it themselves or even not think of depression as a health problem. Many think that it is normal to be depressed as they grow older.

♥ iCare 13-1

Relieving Anxiety for Patients With Confusion

People with dementia are often anxious and fearful. Find ways to reassure and help the person feel more comfortable as you converse, such as the following:

- Gently hold or pat the patient's hand.
- Realize that the person is probably distressed and is doing the best he can.
- Be affectionate, reassuring, and calm, even when things make no sense.
- Respond to the person's feelings instead of the content of his words. For example, if a woman is constantly searching for her husband, don't say, "Your husband is not here."

Rather, say, "You must miss your husband," or "Tell me about your husband."
- If the person has difficulty finding the right word, supply it for him unless doing so upsets him. This helps control his frustration.
- If you do not understand what the patient is trying to say, ask him to point to it or describe it (e.g., "What does a zishmer look like?").
- Consider using alternative therapy, such as music therapy, that may be soothing to the patient.

Toward Evidence-Based Practice

(Study A) Piderman, K., Lapid, M., Stevens, S., et al. (2011). Spiritual well-being and spiritual practices in elderly depressed psychiatric inpatients. *Journal of Pastoral Care & Counseling: JPCC, 65*(1–2), 3–31.

Researchers studied 45 elderly psychiatric inpatients to examine associations among spirituality, depression, and quality of life (QOL). They found that patients with spiritual well-being reported a higher QOL and those with poor spiritual well-being had a higher incidence of depression. During hospitalization, participants with increased spiritual well-being reported peacefulness and reduced hopelessness, worthlessness, and guilt.

(Study B) Judson, P., Dickson, E., Argenta, P., et al. (2011). A prospective, randomized trial of integrative medicine for women with ovarian cancer. *Gynecologic Oncology, 123*(2), 346–350.

This pilot trial evaluated the usefulness of complementary or integrative medicine (CM-IM) in women with newly diagnosed ovarian cancer, along with its effects on QOL, chemotherapy toxicity, and immunological profiles. The 43 women randomized to the experimental group received hypnosis, therapeutic massage, and healing touch with each cycle of chemotherapy; the control group received chemotherapy without complementary or integrative therapy. The researchers concluded that women who received CM-IM demonstrated no improvement in QOL or chemotherapy toxicity.

(Study C) Lin, P. C., Lin, M. L., Huang, L. C., et al. (2011). Music therapy for patients receiving spine surgery. *Journal of Clinical Nursing, 20*(7–8), 960–968.

This study compared the effects of music therapy with a quiet, uninterrupted rest period on pain intensity, anxiety, and physiological parameters after spinal surgery. A total of 60 patients receiving spinal surgery were randomly assigned to listen to selected music from the evening before surgery to the second day after surgery. The control group did not listen to music. Researchers found that patients who listened to music experienced a significant reduction in anxiety and pain, but that there was no effect on blood pressure, heart rate, or cortisol levels. They concluded that patients recovering from spinal surgery may benefit from music therapy.

1. To help you with your analysis for the following questions, complete the following table

	STUDY A	STUDY B	STUDY C
Intervention			
Type of patient			
Result/conclusion			

2. Which of the studies tested an intervention?

3. Which of the interventions was most successful in relieving anxiety? Explain your thinking.

4. Think about the study that did not test an intervention. What, if anything, is its value to nurses or patients?

 Go to Davis Advantage, Resources, Chapter 13, **Toward Evidence-Based Practice Suggested Responses**, on Davis*Plus*.

CLINICALREASONING

The questions and exercises in this section allow you to practice the kind of thinking you will use as a full-spectrum nurse. Critical thinking questions usually have more than one right answer, so we do not provide "correct answers" for these features. It is more important to develop your nursing judgment than to just cover content. You will learn by discussion the questions with your peers. If you are still unsure, see the Davis Advantage chapter resources for suggested responses.

Caring for the Nguyens

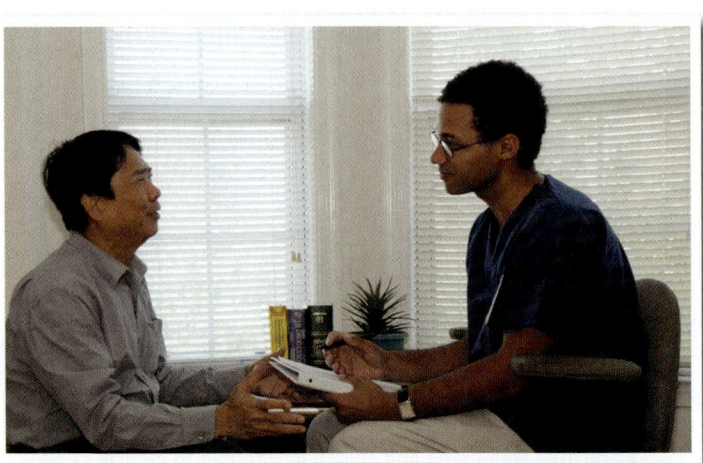

Recall the case of Nam Nguyen. Mr. Nguyen has been diagnosed with hypertension, obesity, and degenerative joint disease. At clinic visits he has made the following comments: "Every time I come in here, I get some new diagnosis. I guess it's amazing I'm not dead yet. I thought I had a lot more time left, but I'm not so sure anymore." When you ask him what his main concerns are, he tells you, "Just take a look at me! I'm a mess. Nothing is turning out the way I planned. I might as well just die now. It would save my family a lot of grief."

A. What information do you need in order to respond to Mr. Nguyen?

B. How should you respond to Mr. Nguyen?

C. What actions should you take?

D. What conclusions can you make about Mr. Nguyen's self-concept (body image, role performance, personal identity, and self-esteem)? What additional information do you need about his self-concept?

Applying the **Full Spectrum Nursing Model** _____

PATIENT SITUATION

Matthew has been admitted to the emergency department with extensive wounds to both forearms, including tendon and vascular damage, from a suicide attempt. Matthew seems very quiet, almost withdrawn, and answers most of your questions in monosyllables.

Matthew reports the following: He is the third child in a family of five. Matthew's middle-class parents are now retired, and his brothers and sisters are scattered across the country in various large cities. Although Matthew claims his schooling years were unremarkable, he recalls several occasions when he was bullied and physically beaten by gangs of older adolescents.

Matthew further states that he graduated from Harvard Law School and became vice president of an influential law firm. Despite his apparent success in life, he has continually questioned his self-worth since childhood. Plagued by worries and depression that have increased over the past few years, he says he wrote a note indicating that he now realizes what a failure he is and proceeded to slash both of his forearms with a sharp razor.

Matthew reports that he has not been eating much, feels tired all the time, and has no interest in going outside the house. He says, "I just don't feel like doing anything; I just want to sleep all the time."

THINKING

1. *Theoretical Knowledge:* Using just the information you have in the Patient Situation, use the SIGECAPS method to assess Matthew's level of depression (see the Focused Assessment box Identifying Depressed Patients Who Should Be Referred for Evaluation). You will need to assume that he is reporting what he has experienced in the past 2 weeks (unless he is obviously referring to the more distant past).
2. *Critical Thinking (Inquiry):* What items of the SIGECAPS cannot be completed with the information in the Patient Situation? What do you need to ask Matthew to complete them?

DOING

3. *Nursing Process (Interventions):* Based on your SIGECAPS data, what do you need to do right away (or be certain it was done in the emergency department)?

CARING

4. *Self-Knowledge:* What do you have in common with Matthew that might help you to empathize with him?
5. *Ethical Knowledge:* Try to put aside your own beliefs now, and answer the following questions from the perspective of (a) Matthew and (b) one of your nursing colleagues on the unit.
   a. Give one reason to support Matthew's claim that he has a right to commit suicide if his despair is too deep to bear.
   b. Give one reason to support a colleague's claim that he does not have a right to commit suicide, no matter how he feels.

To explore learning resources for this chapter,

Go to **www.DavisAdvantage.com** and find:

Answers and Suggested Responses for all questions in this chapter

Lists of NIC Interventions and NOC Outcomes

List of NANDA-I Diagnoses

Knowledge Map

References and Bibliography

Concept Map

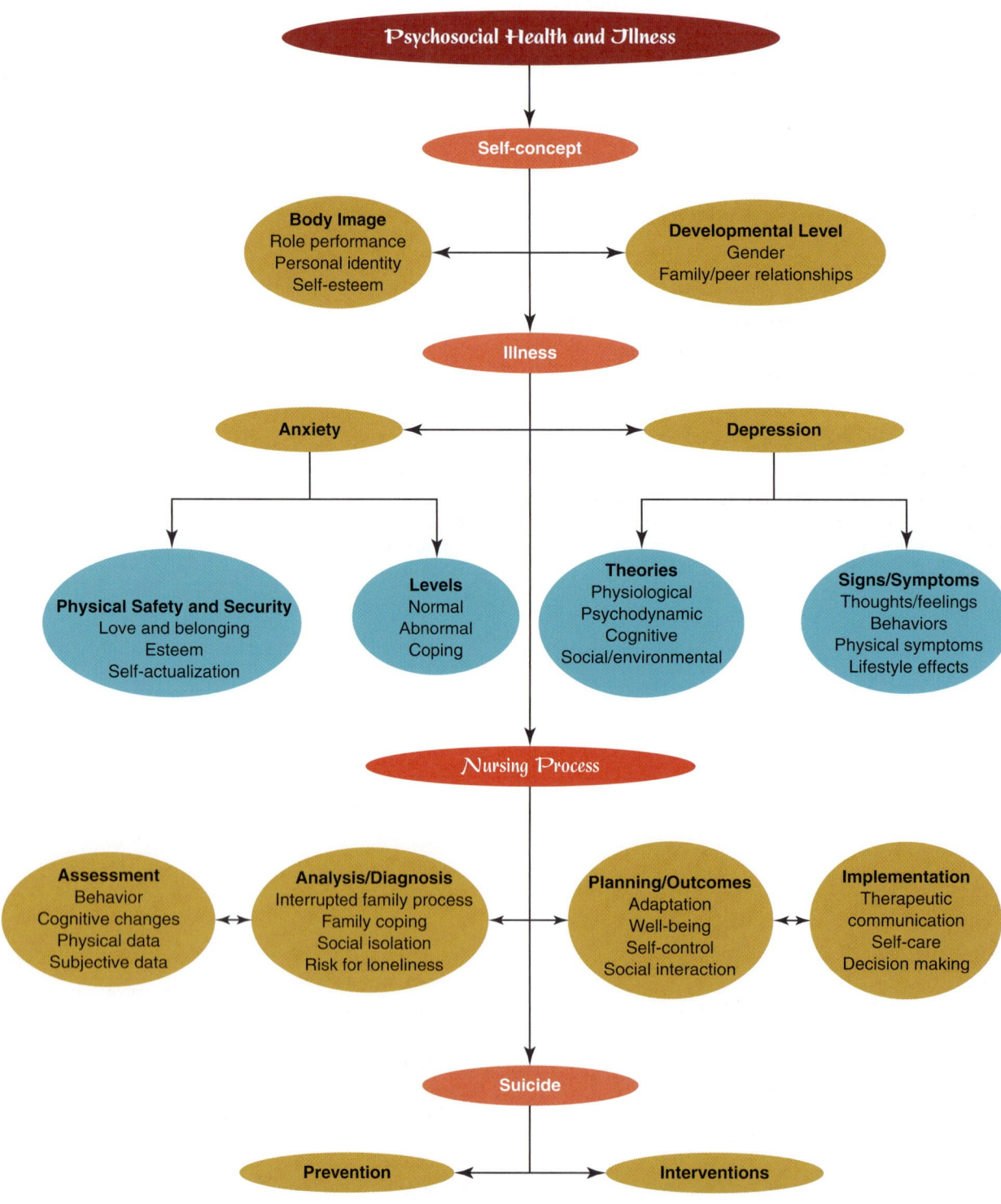

Psychosocial Health and Illness

Self-concept

Body Image
Role performance
Personal identity
Self-esteem

Developmental Level
Gender
Family/peer relationships

Illness

Anxiety

Depression

Physical Safety and Security
Love and belonging
Esteem
Self-actualization

Levels
Normal
Abnormal
Coping

Theories
Physiological
Psychodynamic
Cognitive
Social/environmental

Signs/Symptoms
Thoughts/feelings
Behaviors
Physical symptoms
Lifestyle effects

Nursing Process

Assessment
Behavior
Cognitive changes
Physical data
Subjective data

Analysis/Diagnosis
Interrupted family process
Family coping
Social isolation
Risk for loneliness

Planning/Outcomes
Adaptation
Well-being
Self-control
Social interaction

Implementation
Therapeutic
communication
Self-care
Decision making

Suicide

Prevention

Interventions

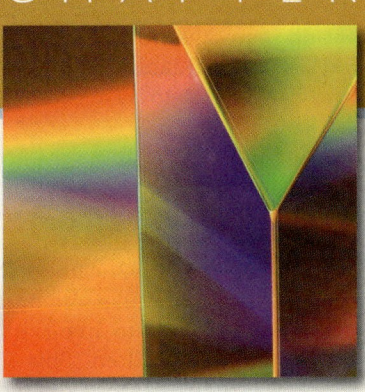

CHAPTER 14

Family

Learning Outcomes

After completing this chapter, you should be able to:

➤ Distinguish between different family structures.

➤ Describe approaches to working with various types of families to provide optimal care to both well and ill clients.

➤ Explain how family theories provide a framework to understand family functioning.

➤ Identify family risk factors across five different family stages.

➤ Discuss ways in which economic factors influence nursing practice, family care, and access to services.

➤ Discuss the effects of chronic and disabling illness on families.

➤ Identify populations most at risk for homelessness.

➤ Demonstrate an understanding of family violence.

➤ Conduct a family assessment.

➤ Identify common health beliefs and communication patterns in families.

➤ Identify appropriate nursing interventions when a family member is ill.

➤ Review how factors such as illness and death, substance abuse, violence, mental health disorders, financial hardship, unemployment, and other issues can change a family's structure, communication, and coping strategies.

➤ Discuss the sandwich generation and assessment and intervention strategies for caregiver burnout.

Key Concepts

Family
Family nursing

Related Concepts

See the Concept Map at the end of this chapter.

Example Problem

Caregiver role strain

Meet Your Patient

J. B. is an 80-year-old man who is hospitalized for end-stage renal disease. His wife died 4 years ago. His remaining family includes two married daughters and four grandchildren. J. B. has several siblings, but they live far away and rarely phone or visit.

J. B. has lived in the same neighborhood for more than 55 years. When he and his wife, Pamela, first moved into the neighborhood, they lived across the street from Mike and Lena. The two couples socialized, raised their children, and enjoyed many holidays and festivities together. After the children were grown, the two couples sold their homes and each moved into a townhouse near the center of town. They lived next door to each other and continued to spend time together. A year after Pamela died, Mike's wife, Lena, died of liver cancer.

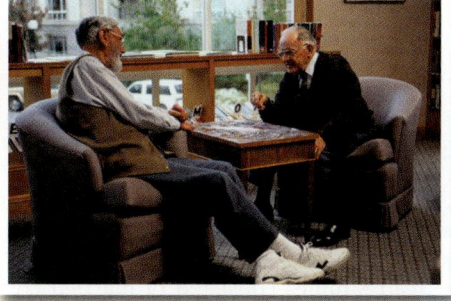

J. B. and Mike decided to share an apartment to reduce living expenses. They also wanted the security, support, and companionship that come with a roommate situation. Before starting their daily activities, they like to read the newspaper over breakfast—the local one for J. B. and the national one for Mike. They have season tickets to the baseball games and watch sports together on TV. "Thank goodness we have each other," says Mike. Mike comes to the hospital every morning. He brings both papers; he also brings breakfast muffins for the two of them and the nursing unit staff. He spends the day at the hospital and leaves shortly after dinner.

Theoretical Knowledge
knowing **why**

ABOUT THE KEY CONCEPTS

This chapter is about contemporary families and how they differ from those of the past. As you study the chapter, you will begin to see how **family, family nursing,** and other related concepts apply to J. B. and Mike (Meet Your Patient). The key concepts are the basis of the theoretical knowledge to which you will apply the nursing process and your nursing judgment. Integration of these concepts into your nursing care will help you meet the challenges of family health as a full-spectrum nurse.

WHAT IS A FAMILY?

Traditionally, people have thought of a family as consisting of a husband, wife, and children. However, with changes brought about by cultural diversity, less reliance on social traditions, and wider acceptance of differing lifestyles, the concept of family has become broader.

- **A family is formally defined** as two or more people related by birth, marriage, or adoption occupying the same household (Lofquist, Lugaila, O'Connell, et al., 2012).
- **A more holistic definition of family** is "two or more individuals who provide physical, emotional, economic, or spiritual support to each other." They may or may not be related by blood, but they maintain involvement in each other's lives.

Most often, people who consider themselves to be family live in the same household; however, adult children living apart from their parents continue to be part of a family unit, which may also include siblings, aunts, uncles, and cousins. **KEY POINT:** *In short, families come in many forms, living arrangements, and emotional connections.*

Changes in Family Structures

We continue to see significant changes in the living arrangements of families in the United States as a result of the following:

- Socioeconomic factors
- Aging population
- Increasing average age at first marriage
- High divorce rates
- Improvements in the health and financial status of the older population
- Changing residential preferences

In 2012, compared to 1970, we saw a 15% decrease in family households, a 20% decrease in households of married couples with their own children under age 18, and a 10% increase in the proportion of one-person households (Vespa, Lewis, & Kreider, 2013).

Traditional Families In the past, the majority of American families consisted of married couples with at least one child, a husband in the labor force, and a wife not employed outside the home. Trends in data show a consistent decline in married couples. Of all families, married couples with children under age 18 made up 52% of them in 1960 compared to 29% in 2015.

Similarly, the percentage of white married families with children under age 18 decreased from 83% in 1980 to 69% in 2015. A similar trend was seen for Hispanic parents, from 74% to 59%, and for black parents, from 48% to 35% (U.S. Census Bureau, 2015a).

Grandparent Families Grandparent households are a significant resource for single women with children and for families during economic distress. In 2012, the majority of grandparent households contained the mother and no father (40%), compared to the father and no mother (6%). Since the 2007 economic recession, multigenerational families (parents and grandparents) have slightly increased to 34% (Ellis & Simmons, 2014).

When parents are unable or unwilling to assume the parenting role, grandparents will raise their grandchildren to prevent them from going to foster care or an alternate placement. In 2012, the percentage of children under 18 raised by grandparents was 20% compared to 28% in 1992. Although the largest increase was seen for white non-Hispanic and Hispanic children, they were still less likely to live with grandparents compared to black or Asian children (Ellis & Simmons, 2014).

Adults Who Are Married but Do Not Have Children Once only a small number in American society, this group now accounts for 43% of family groups (U.S. Census Bureau, 2015a).

Dual-Earner Families A dual-earner family is one in which both parents are in the workforce.

- In 1960, 25% of households had dual family incomes compared to 60% in 2012.
- In 1960, the father was the main source of family income (70%), whereas in 2012 most families were dual earners (60%). The father was the only parent employed in 31% of households (Pew Research Center, 2015).

Single-Parent Families Single-parent families result from divorce or from the death of a partner, or result when partners choose not to marry or live together. In 2015:

- 11.4% of children under age 18 lived with only the mother; 2.2%, with the father (U.S. Census Bureau, 2015b).
- Black and Hispanic children had higher rates of living with one parent (Vespa, Lewis, & Kreider, 2013):
  - Black—55%
  - Hispanic 31%
  - Non-Hispanic white—21%
  - Asian—13%

Blended and Stepfamilies A **blended family** is established when single parents marry and either or both have children from a previous relationship. The nonbiological partner becomes the stepparent and a stepfamily is created. Commonly, biological parents who are not living together in the child's home alternate responsibilities for child care.

Extended Families It is not unusual for extended family members (e.g., grandparents, aunts, uncles, cousins) to be considered immediate family and live within a single dwelling or in proximity. Close friends may also be considered immediate family. In the Meet Your Patient scenario, what data allow you to infer that J. B.'s siblings are members of his extended family? What information allows you to infer that Mike is his immediate family?

Sandwich Generation The growing number of older adults has created **sandwich families** (Parker & Patten, 2013; Schumacher, MacNeil, Mobily, et al., 2012), in which middle-aged adults who still have children at home must care for and share their household with aging parents. Although competent in the caregiver role, they feel personally overwhelmed and emotionally conflicted, but overall reported being as happy as the nonsandwiched families.

Other Family Structures In addition to families bound by marriage and bloodlines, other family types exist, such as *unmarried heterosexual individuals who reside in a common* *household* or *unmarried gay and lesbian couples with or without children.* Although *individuals or couples who adopt children* or provide foster care are not biologically related, they are very much a family. They assume parenting roles in the child's life and share experiences that create an emotional attachment.

- **Cohabiting adults** may choose to live together but not marry or they may choose to live together as a "trial run" prior to marriage. Research indicated that couples who were over age 23 when they started living together had a higher probability of a successful marriage did than couples who began cohabiting before age 23 (Kuperberg, 2014).
- **Kith** refers to persons with a kinship bond. Recall that a family is a group of individuals who provide support and assistance to each other. Although J. B. and Mike (Meet Your Patient) are not blood relatives, they provide strong support for each other. For some, this bond is stronger than those created through bloodline.

Approaches to Family Nursing

Family nursing refers to nursing care that is holistically directed toward the whole family and to individual members (Fig. 14-1). Knowing the family unit is affected by acute or chronic illness, hospitalization, or healthcare interventions, the nurse best cares for the family by involving them in client care decisions.

With J. B.'s permission (Meet Your Patient), the nurses would support Mike's daily visits and involve Mike's and J. B.'s adult children in his care, discharge planning, and follow-up care at home. They would teach both Mike and J. B. about medications and treatments so that Mike can assist J. B. in his activities of daily living.

Three perspectives on family nursing include the family as (1) context for care, (2) unit of care, and (3) system. Family nursing is a specialty; to work with the family as a unit of care or as a system, you may need additional preparation.

Family as the Context for Care As a graduate nurse, you should be prepared to work, at the minimum, with the family as the context of care of an individual person. **KEY POINT:** *Your focus in this approach is on the ill individual.* From this perspective, you view the family as either a resource or a stressor to your client. Using this knowledge, you would recognize the importance of Mike (Meet Your Patient). Before discharge, you would ask J. B., "Will Mike or your daughters be able to help you when you go home?"

Family as the Unit of Care A slightly more complex approach views the family as the unit of care. You must assess

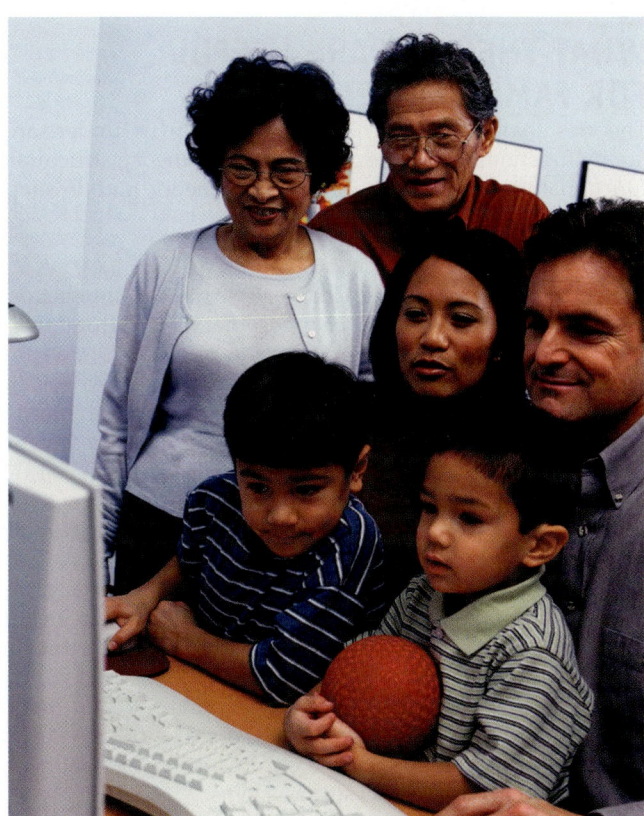

FIGURE 14-1 *Family nursing* refers to nursing care that is holistically directed toward the whole family as well as to individual members.

and provide care to each member because wellness is critical to promoting family health. **KEY POINT:** *Family health is viewed as the sum of all individual members; however, you might direct interventions to individual family members rather than the family as a whole.* For example, to use our previous example, you might check Mike's blood pressure when he visits J. B.

Family as a System **KEY POINT:** *In this approach, you focus on the family as a whole and as an interactional system.* Using this perspective, you direct your assessment and intervention to communications and interactions between family members.

The systems approach sees the family as embedded in and interacting with a larger community. You might ask, for example, "How has your family's relationship within the seniors' group at your townhouse complex changed since your illness?"

KnowledgeCheck 14-1

- Name at least three types of family structure.
- What are two topics that the nurse can discuss with the family as a unit?

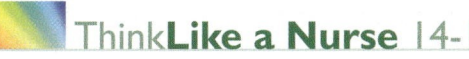 ThinkLike a Nurse 14-1

How can you promote family cohesion for a family whose members live great distances from one another?

♥ **iCare**

The Family

- "The family" will be slightly different for each and every patient you encounter.
- As a nurse, you must possess and exhibit a cultural awareness and competency for a broader definition of family as our society continues to change.
- Remember what defines "the family" is very different in today's changing society. There is no longer a traditional composition of whom and of what a family consists.
- Ask the following: *"Can you introduce me to your family?"* Doing so avoids assumptions and allows the patient to tell you about his or her family structure.

WHAT THEORIES ARE USEFUL FOR FAMILY CARE?

Theories that have been proposed to help us understand family functioning include general systems theory, structural–functional theories, family interactional theory, and developmental theory.

General Systems Theory

General systems theory (see Chapter 8) focuses on interactions between systems and the changes that result from these interactions.

- **Open system.** The family is considered an open system because the members function as individuals, are interdependent, and operate as a family unit (a whole, in systems language). Interactions can occur between members of the family or between multiple families.
- **Balance.** Healthy families strive to maintain a balance between external stress and internal relationships.
- **Interaction.** Changes in the behaviors or attitudes of an individual member affect the family unit, and changes in family structure and functioning affect individual members. Think of a system as a mobile; if one piece is moved, that movement sets the whole mobile in motion.
- **Suprasystems.** Broader systems that surround the family unit (e.g., the community, the city, the state, the healthcare system) are referred to as suprasystems.
- **Subsystems.** Smaller components that fit within the family system (e.g., the mother, the marital couple) are subsystems. Each subsystem has a particular function. For example, one family member might be viewed as the decision maker, another as the peacekeeper, and another as the disciplinarian for the children.

Structural–Functional Theories

Structural–functional family theories are based on the developmental theories of Freud, Erikson, and Havighurst (see Chapter 9) and include the concepts of family roles and interactions. The structural–functional approach includes the following assumptions (Parsons & Bales, 1955):

- A family is a social system with functional requirements.
- A family is a small group possessing certain features common to small groups.
- The family accomplishes functions that serve both the individual and society.
- Individuals act according to internalized norms that are learned through socialization.

KEY POINT: *Although they view the family as a social system, structural–functional theories, unlike systems theory, focus on* **outcome** *rather than* **process.** You would use this theory to assess how well the family functions internally (among family members) and externally (with outside systems). Examples of family functions include socialization of children; meeting the physical, financial, and emotional needs of family members; caring for older members; and being productive members of society.

Family Interactional Theory

Family interactional theory views the family as a unit of interacting personalities (Hill & Hansen, 1960). **KEY POINT:** *The major emphasis is on family roles. This approach to understanding families deemphasizes the influence of the external world on what occurs within the family.* Nurses working from an interactional perspective focus family healthcare on the interaction and communication between family members; their roles and power; family coping; and relationships with other people outside the direct family unit.

Developmental Theories

KEY POINT: *Developmental theories focus on the stage of family development.* Theorists typically identify eight stages in the family life cycle according to the ages of the children and parents: beginning family, childbearing family, family with preschool children, family with school-age children, family with teenagers and young adults, family launching young adults, postparental family, and aging family. Each stage is associated with developmental tasks the family needs to achieve. Most family development theories do not identify stages and tasks for families who remain childless throughout their lives. To learn about developmental tasks associated with family stages, including those without children, see Table 14-1.

Generally, the stages follow one another in a linear progression; however, some families may be in more than one stage at a time or may revert to previous stages. This overlap or reversion is most common in families that have children spaced far apart, in blended families, and in stepfamilies. See Chapter 9 for developmental theories applicable to individual family members.

KnowledgeCheck 14-2

- Which type of theory focuses on interactions among families, family members, and groups in the environment?
- What is the name of the theory that views families as a social system with a focus on outcomes?
- What are some examples of family functions as defined by structural–functional theories?

ThinkLike a Nurse 14-2

- Using systems theory, you could view J. B., his siblings, his children, and his grandchildren as a system. Refer to the section on family structures—how would you categorize this family structurally?
- Again using systems theory, what or who are the subsystems in the family system described in the preceding question?
- Considering J. B. alone, at what developmental stage is his "family"?

WHAT ARE SOME FAMILY HEALTH RISK FACTORS?

Many health risk factors are the same for families as they are for individuals, and they are similar across age-groups and family types.

For specific topics related to families, also see Chapters 9 and 10 covering the life span, Chapter 12 on stress and adaptation, Chapter 20 on communicating, and Chapter 26 on teaching.

Childless and Childbearing Couples

Adapting to new roles within the home creates stress for newly married couples; couples who are trying to become pregnant; and new parents who are inexperienced in the challenges and responsibilities of raising a healthy, happy, and safe child (Fig. 14-2). Use of maladaptive coping mechanisms can lead to health problems and deterioration in

Table 14-1 ➤ Family Developmental Tasks

STAGES	TASKS	CHILDREN'S AGES (IF ANY) (APPROXIMATE)
Beginning family	■ Relinquishing the family of origin as the major emotional and economic resource ■ Gaining a sense of autonomy and independence ■ Making the relationship/marriage work; investment in spouse as the major emotional resource ■ Finding a place in the kin network of each partner ■ Exploring options for career development ■ Deciding whether to have children	None
Childbearing family	■ Achieving pregnancy and birth ■ Adjusting to life changes after birth and to the infant's needs ■ Determining ways to meet all members' needs ■ Renegotiating marriage ■ Increasing contact with extended family	Newborn to 2 years
"No longer newlyweds" (with no children)	■ Establishing a sense of the permanence of the relationship ■ Establishing long-term residency ■ Being involved in the community/promoting the well-being of the community	*Not applicable*
Family with preschool children	■ Adjusting to increased costs associated with family life ■ Socializing the preschoolers ■ Coping with loss of parental energy and privacy	3–5 years
Mature family (with no children)	■ Renegotiating relationship on the basis of more maturity ■ Adjusting to changing levels of responsibility in work and community ■ If not done already, achieving financial security	Not applicable
Family with school-age children	■ Adjusting to the needs and demands of growing children ■ Promoting joint decision making among parents and children ■ Encouraging and supporting educational and school-related activities	6–12 years
Family with teenagers and young adults	■ Maintaining open communication among family members ■ Reinforcing ethical and moral values ■ For teens, balancing independence with parental rules	13–20 years
Family launching young adults	■ Maintaining support to young adults as they leave the security of family ■ Rediscovering marriage	18–30 years

(Continued)

Table 14-1 ▸ Family Developmental Tasks—cont'd

STAGES	TASKS	CHILDREN'S AGES (IF ANY) (APPROXIMATE)
Postparental family	▪ Preparing for retirement	Adult
	▪ Adjusting to children's moving into new phases of adulthood, marriage or other relationship, and childbearing and to becoming a grandparent	
Middle-aged couple (with no children)	▪ Accepting that it may be too late to reconsider childbearing or child rearing	None
	▪ Reaching the peak of a career or realizing that the peak may not occur	
	▪ Planning for retirement	
Aging family (applies to family with no children)	▪ Adjusting to retirement and changes associated with aging	Adult *(or none)*
	▪ Adjusting to the loss of a spouse and friendships	

Source: Adapted from Friedman, M. M., Bowden, V. R., & Jones, E. G. (2003). *Family nursing: Research, theory, and practice* (5th ed.). Upper Saddle River, NJ: Prentice Hall; Kaakinen, J., Coehlo, D., & Steele, R. (Eds.). (2015). *Family health care nursing: Theory, practice and research* (5th ed.). Philadelphia, PA: F.A. Davis.; McGoldrick, M., & Carter, E. (1985). The family life cycle: Its stages and dislocations. In J. Henslin (Ed.), *Marriage and family in a changing society* (4th ed., pp. 372–389). New York, NY: Free Press.

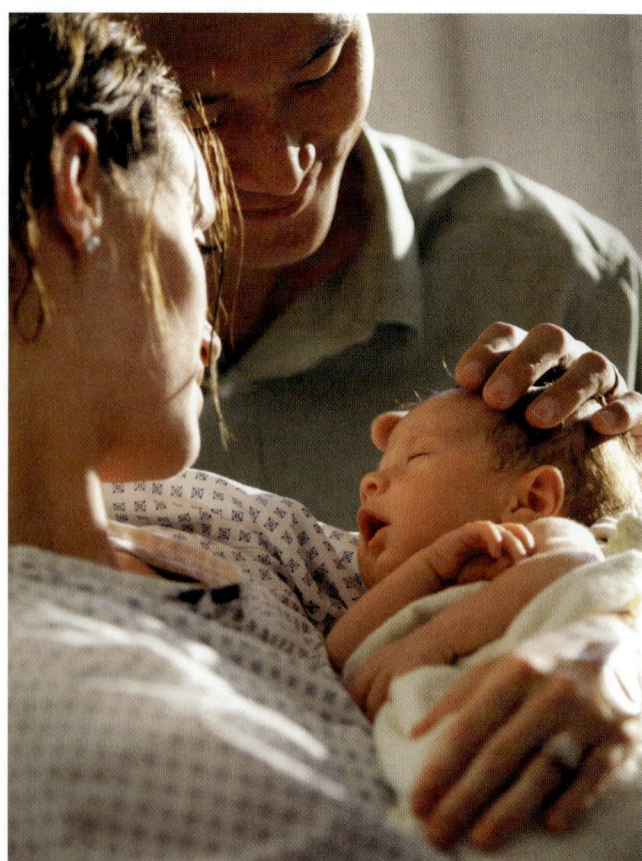

FIGURE 14-2 Newly married couples, couples who are trying to become pregnant, and new parents are vulnerable to stress as they adapt to new roles.

relationships. For example, when someone who uses alcohol to deal with stress:
▪ The individual is at risk for addiction, self-injury, and liver disease.
▪ The family can suffer the effects of neglect and family violence, as well as health risks related to pregnancy (e.g., miscarriage, congenital malformations, and genetic defects in the child).

Families With Young Children

Common parenting concerns center on the child's safety, development, socialization, education, discipline, nutrition, sleeping, and toileting.
▪ **Childcare.** Finding safe, nurturing, and affordable child care can be a major source of family stress for parents working outside the home.
▪ **Marital Relationship.** In addition, the demands of work and child rearing mean less time is available to nurture the couple's relationship, leaving them at increased risk for marital discord.
▪ **Contagious Diseases.** Injuries and illness create risks to family health. For example, children attending schools are exposed to contagious diseases that can spread to other family members. ✚ To reduce the risk for serious infectious diseases (e.g., polio or hepatitis B), parents need to adhere to the recommended childhood immunization schedule. You should teach the importance of vaccinations and provide accurate information to counter myths regarding vaccines.

Survey data revealed high levels of childhood vaccination coverage and low exemption rates. However, many states did not reach the national *Healthy People 2020* goal of ≥95% for kindergartners (Seither, Calhoun, Knighton, et al., 2015). Parents who refuse immunizations for their children cite various concerns, including personal perceptions and healthcare system issues (Luthy, Beckstrand, Callister, et al., 2012).

- **Disability or Chronic Illness.** For families who live with a chronic illness, (e.g., asthma or type 1 diabetes) or a developmental or learning disability (e.g., autism), the stress related to compromised health, falling behind in school, and financial burdens can become overwhelming.

Families With Adolescents

Families with adolescents are often concerned about teen risk-taking behaviors.

- **Social Pressure.** Adolescents may participate in risky behaviors to impress others, to feel cool or important, or to experience a feeling of power.
- **Risk Tolerance.** Research shows that when compared with their older peers, adolescents may be more likely to avoid clearly stated risks, but they have a higher tolerance for the unknown (Tymula, Belmaker, Roy, et al., 2012). Developmentally, adolescents typically do not feel or know the inherent dangers. Based on the formula "Risk taking = curiosity + challenge + excitement + denial," Pickhardt (2014) identified the parents' role as less control and lots of talking. You can educate parents to inform the adolescent of hidden risks and costs of these behaviors.
- **Specific Behaviors.** Specific risk-taking behaviors include using tobacco, alcohol, and other illicit drugs; engaging in extreme stunts; accepting dares; rebelling against authority; and being sexually promiscuous.
- **"Sandwich" Families.** Families with adolescents may also be dealing with aging parents or grandparents (Fig. 14-3). Parents may become "sandwiched" between the needs of the adolescents and the needs of their aging parents. Women are particularly at risk for stress in these situations because they are usually the caregivers for older relatives.

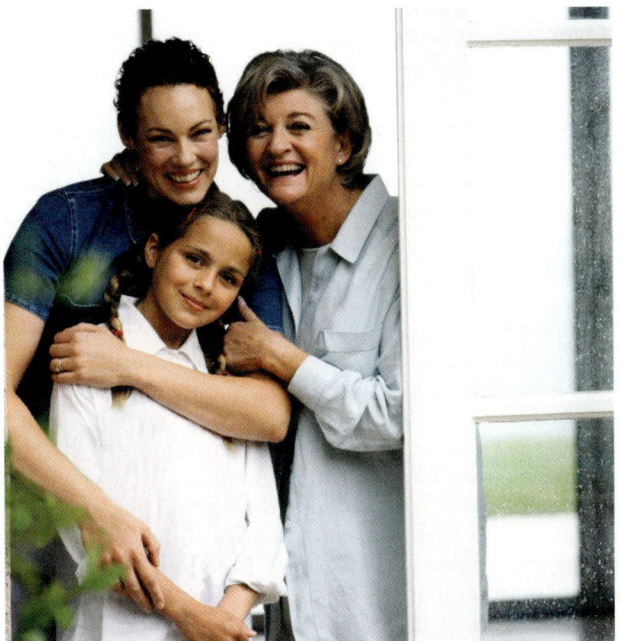

FIGURE 14-3 In families with adolescents or young adults, parents may become "sandwiched" between the needs of the growing adolescents and the needs of their own parents.

Families With Young Adults

Young adults commonly move out of the parental home as their school years end, taking on full-time jobs, many for the first time. This is a time when many marry and begin childbearing and rearing. Newly found autonomy and independence are both exhilarating and anxiety provoking. Some confront problems such as tight finances, inability to find meaningful work, nontherapeutic personal relationships, or other life challenges.

"Return to the Nest" Financial strain might cause a young adult, alone or with a newly formed family, to move back in with his parent(s) until he can "get back on his feet." This return to the nest, although sensible, can be a stress on the family. Although returning to the home of origin can represent a new opportunity for family attachment, the presence of young adults in the household commonly changes family dynamics. Role strain and poor communication are common. Roles within the family will evolve and families will need to find healthy ways to adapt.

Families With Middle-Aged Adults

The middle years are a time of examining life goals and coping with aging and the empty nest. This can be not only a satisfying time but also a time of self-doubt.

- **This can be a satisfying time** of role fulfillment, career success, financial security, and social comfort. Without the time demands of bringing up children, adults have more time available to pursue other personal interests or career paths. The quality of the spousal relationship might take on a new importance. The middle adult may experience a new sense of freedom and need for self-exploration and personal growth.
- **The middle years can also be a time of self-doubt** triggered by the changes caused by aging, menopause, an empty nest, care or death of parents, heightened career demands, or change in relationships, all of which can create emotional strain.
- **Some people suffer a midlife crisis,** which is a period of intense questioning about the meaning and direction in life and what brings personal fulfillment. Adults battling a midlife crisis might display signs of depression, anxiety, or rebellion from the status quo.
- **The effects of long-standing unhealthy behaviors** often become apparent in middle adulthood. For example, people who have used tobacco for many years may begin to notice an increase in cough and chest congestion or those who consumed high-fat diets may develop high blood pressure or elevated cholesterol levels.

Keep in mind that the health of the middle-aged person also affects family health.

Families With Older Adults

Falls and Trauma are a common health risk for families with older adults. For more information about falls, see Chapters 10 and 23.

Social Isolation and Loneliness are common in older adults and loneliness because of the loss of relationships that occurs with aging. Elderly adults have an increased risk for depression. Families should maintain frequent contact and communications to offset feelings of isolation and loneliness. Friends can also be a significant source of support (Fig. 14-4).

- *Family dynamics change* as the older person copes with the death of a spouse, sibling, friends, or other loved ones.
- *Loss and grief* can deeply affect an elderly person's quality of life, clarity of thinking, and physical and emotional well-being.

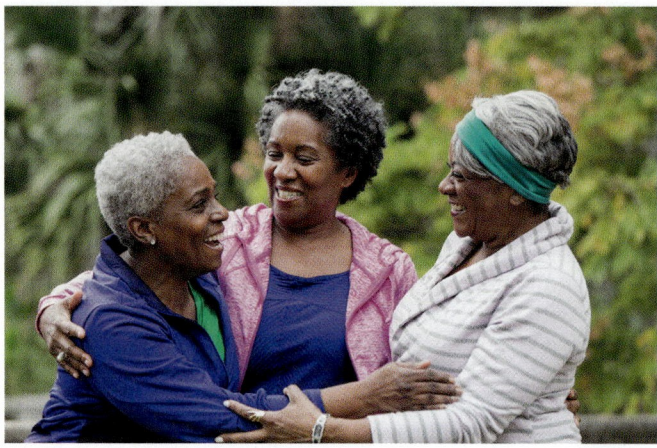

FIGURE 14-4 Friends play an important role in the support system of older people.

- *Retirement* can bring the simpler life that many people desire. However, retired individuals must deal with the loss of daily contact with colleagues in the workplace; some experience a reduced sense of responsibility or purpose.
- *Functional losses* may cause the person to limit physical activity, volunteer work, church attendance, and other social activities.

Nutrition and Hydration become more difficult to maintain as a person ages. The following are situations that may compromise the nutrition of older adults:

- Forgetting to eat (especially those who live alone)
- Inadequate or unreliable transportation to shop for food
- Lack of money to buy food
- Physical changes that alter taste (e.g., reduced sensitivity in the taste buds and less saliva for taste and swallowing)
- Loss of appetite
- Poorly fitting dentures

For more information about nutrition, see Chapter 27.

Memory and Problem-Solving abilities change with aging. Forgetfulness and confusion can pose safety risks for older adults, particularly for those living alone or those whose mental status is compromised. When older adults lose their ability to reason, they are vulnerable to physical harm. The demands of keeping the aging adult safe can lead to caregiver role strain and family stress.

It is easy to understand from the above scenarios the cascading effect that one deficit, such as lack of transportation, can have on the health of an older adult and her family—especially when it involves a frail elderly adult. Be sure to educate families about the availability of community resources, such as Meals on Wheels and home health aides, as many may not be aware that help is available.

ThinkLike a Nurse 14-3

- What developmental stage is your family in? How do you know?
- What basic attitudes, values, or beliefs influenced you in your childhood family?
- How were decisions made in your childhood family? Were people's feelings and individuals' needs considered?

- Can you remember good times and laughter that bonded you together as a family? In your present family life, how often do you laugh together?
- In the Meet Your Patient scenario, what health risks do J. B. and Mike face, considering their age and health?

WHAT ARE SOME CHALLENGES TO FAMILY HEALTH?

We have already mentioned the effect of some demographic changes, such as an aging population, on families. This section examines other regional and national trends that present challenges to family health.

Poverty and Unemployment

Poverty and unemployment involve interrelated social and economic factors.

Inadequate or No Health Insurance When families do not have adequate health insurance they (1) do not seek preventive medical care and (2) use the emergency room for their medical needs. The Affordable Care Act (ACA), passed in 2010, has provisions to provide healthcare coverage for people who cannot obtain private or employment-funded insurance.

- The percentage of uninsured persons decreased from 13.3 in 2013 to 10.4 in 2014 (U.S. Census Bureau, 2015b).
- For children under age 18, the uninsured rate decreased from 8.9% in 2008 to 5.5% in 2014 (Ward, Clarke, Freeman, et al., 2015).

Teenage Pregnancy Teen pregnancy is strongly associated with poverty, unemployment, and health risks. In 2013, the birth rate for U.S. teens aged 15 to 19 decreased by 10% from 2012. Although that was a record low, it remains higher than in other Western industrialized nations (Martin, Hamilton, Osterman, et al., 2015; Sedgh, Finer, Bankole, et al., 2015).

- Infants born to teen mothers are more likely to have health problems at birth.
- Teen mothers are more likely to have greater health disparities and high unemployment rates; their children have higher involvement in the juvenile justice system.

Overall Economic Climate When the economy takes a downturn, families may struggle to provide for basic needs such as food, shelter, and healthcare.

- *Single-parent and low-income families are hardest hit.* However, families in all socioeconomic levels can experience difficulties in an economic downturn. Most people living at or below the federal poverty level are minimum-wage or seasonal job workers. Jobs labeled nonessential may be eliminated in a sluggish economy. As a result, fewer workers are paying taxes in such an economy, so government programs supporting families in need may be underfunded. Although some families find creative solutions to family poverty (e.g., combining households), many experience extreme hardships.
- *Middle-income families are also affected by corporate downsizing or stock market fluctuations.* Even families who were prospering may not have sufficient funds to cover a period of unemployment or economic recession. They may find it impossible to keep up with credit card debt, home mortgages, car payments, insurance premiums, and perhaps school or other loans.

KnowledgeCheck 14-3

- Which socioeconomic group of families is hardest hit during poor economic periods?

- How are middle-income families affected by poor economic times?
- What concerns are associated with teenage pregnancies?

Infectious Diseases

Family health may be affected by infections caused by a variety of pathogens. For in-depth information about preventing infections, refer to Chapter 22.

New or Drug-Resistant Pathogens Any number of new or resistant pathogens, such as severe acute respiratory syndrome (SARS), methicillin-resistant *Staphylococcus aureus* (MRSA), the Zika virus, HIV, and H1N1, can cause illness. For example, influenza viruses cause illness especially among young children, pregnant women, people aged 65 years and older, and those with certain chronic diseases. Similarly, the Zika virus spreads to the fetus of pregnant women, causing serious birth defects.

HIV Infection HIV is a devastating disease that significantly impacts the family. In addition to the physical and financial stressors, women who infect their infants with HIV bear a tremendous burden of guilt, as do partners who infect the other partner. The populations at highest risk for contracting HIV are men who have sex with men, followed by heterosexual groups (CDC, 2012). When compared with white and Hispanic/Latino women, African American women have a disproportionately higher rate of HIV infections (CDC, 2016). Some families keep the diagnosis a secret and blame each other, whereas other families support each other and manage the illness as best they can.

Advances in treating HIV infection and preventing its spread have been made through public and patient education, vaccination, antiviral therapy, and other antimicrobial treatments for HIV-related complications. The nurse should emphasize the use of proper protective precautions to minimize the spread of the disease.

"Old" (Comeback) Diseases Even old diseases once thought to be eradicated can threaten family health. In recent years, diseases once controlled by immunization are making a comeback (e.g., pertussis [whooping cough], polio, mumps, and smallpox). Many families either refuse or fail to comply with immunization schedules. As a result, a reduction occurs in **herd immunity**, which is a group's protection from disease that occurs because a large proportion of the group is immune. You should educate parents that childhood immunizations save lives and prevent diseases.

KnowledgeCheck 14-4

- What populations are at highest risk of contracting HIV?
- Name two previously eradicated diseases that have become a threat again.

Chronic Illness and Disability

Individuals in the home with chronic illness and disability profoundly change the way families function.

- *Caregiving.* Family members' roles evolve over time, especially that of the caregiver, who often must assist with activities of daily living, such as getting around the home, feeding, bathing, dressing, toileting, and getting in and out of a chair or bed.
- *Financial strain.* Disability may mean inability to work or generate family income, creating financial strain or poverty.
- *Mental strain.* Long-term illness and disability cause mental, emotional, or physical limitations that affect family communication patterns.

- *Relationships.* Because of caregiver strain and issues related to dependency, relationships within the family may be difficult.
- *Abuse.* Long-term care of a family member may increase the risk for abuse and neglect, including maltreatment of frail, elderly family members.

The ADA (Americans With Disabilities) Amendments Act of 2008 defines one component of **disability** as a physical or mental impairment that substantially interferes with a person's ability to engage in major life activities (U.S. Equal Opportunity Commission, 2008). Individuals have a disability if they meet criteria involving limitations in mobility/ambulation, hearing, vision, learning, cognitive, self-care, or independent living, to name a few. In the United States (Department of Commerce, 2014, updated 2015):

- 57 million Americans had a disability, more people than the entire population of Canada.
- The prevalence of disability was lowest for children under age 15 (8%), and highest for adults 65 and older (50%).
- 6.5 million (32.6%) of noninstitutionalized people with disabilities were employed.
- About one-third of persons with a work disability or a broad disability were below the poverty level.
- In 2010, of individuals 21 to 64 years of age,
    11.7 million people had ambulatory disabilities and
    4.1 million had vision disabilities (Institute on Disability, 2015).

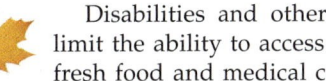

Disabilities and other mobility limitations can limit the ability to access needed resources such as fresh food and medical care. This can lead to poor health outcomes in older adults. In order to achieve better long-term health outcomes, it is essential that nurses collaborate with social work/case management to ensure that older adults have the resources needed to remain independent as long as possible.

Homelessness

Homelessness is a growing problem for individuals and families in many U.S. cities. Many homeless people sleep on the streets; others live temporarily with relatives or in mission shelters. Homelessness is far more complex than merely lack of housing. Several factors are involved, such as: financial crises, socially dysfunctional relationships, unemployment, lack of job skills, substance abuse, healthcare expenses, or the inability or lack of desire to live within the socially accepted norms of society. In the United States, deep poverty and homelessness often result from mental illness, disability, or other factors (e.g., economic recession, loss of a job).

Social Isolation Homeless families are often socially isolated. Many homeless children do not attend school, and those who do tend to perform poorly. Often, homeless families do not seek care for significant health problems because they do not know how to access the healthcare system and qualify for healthcare services. You should focus on helping the family meet basic needs of food and shelter, which according to Maslow's hierarchy of needs (see Chapters 4 and 8), must be met before the family can grow.

Groups at High Risk Those who are particularly vulnerable to homelessness and poverty are single women, members of minority groups, and single-parent families (Fig. 14-5).

- Divorced women commonly end up with less income than do their ex-husbands. In addition, some women also have sole custody of their children, which creates additional strain on their reduced income.

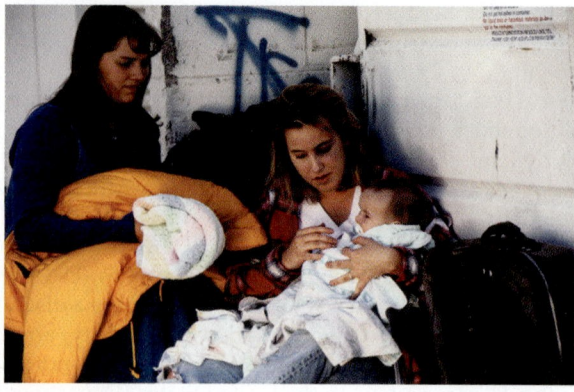

FIGURE 14-5 Many homeless people are single women and children.

- Some biological fathers struggle to pay child support while maintaining their own living expenses. Others may be incarcerated or not interested in being a father, or their whereabouts may be unknown.
- In many states, social services departments are underfunded and unable to enforce child support laws.

Violence and Neglect Within Families

Domestic violence—including physical, emotional, and sexual abuse—occurs throughout all strata of our society, among all racial, social, and economic groups.

- Approximately one in four women will be a victim of violence during her lifetime.
- More than 3 million children each year are reported to child protective services agencies as alleged abuse victims.
- Approximately 679,000 children were victims of child abuse and neglect in 2013. That represents one victim per 100 children (Children's Bureau, 2015).
- Race and ethnic data showed that nationwide, 44% of these child victims were white, 22.4% Hispanics, and 21.2% African Americans.

Victimization of Children   Children aged 3 and younger were the most frequent victims of fatalities (73.9%) resulting from abuse and neglect (Children's Bureau, 2015), with the highest rate occurring in children under 1 year of age (21.1/1000 children).

- Boys had a higher rate of fatalities than did girls.
- These children are the most vulnerable for many reasons, including their dependency, small size, and inability to defend themselves.

Long-Term Effects   Any type of violence is likely to have long-lasting effects on the victims and the family.

- **Loss of Family Integrity**—Disintegration of family relationships and structure may occur (e.g., sending the children to foster care, escaping to a battered women's shelter, living with others).
- **Health issues**—Effects of domestic violence include physical injury from the assault itself as well as chronic health problems that emerge as a complication of traumatic injury. Health problems may also result from the ongoing stress of violence or neglect:
  - *Families experiencing domestic violence have more unintended pregnancies, miscarriages, abortions, and low-birth-weight babies.*
  - *Victim's families have higher incidence of sexually transmitted infections (STIs) and higher rates of depression,*

post-traumatic stress syndrome, substance abuse, and suicide.
- *Often there are long-term effects involving emotional injury, marred self-esteem, or poor quality relationships, even though the emotional and physical pain may stop when the victim leaves the family environment.*
- *Victims of family violence learn patterns of ineffective coping that can be repeated in successive generations.*

KnowledgeCheck 14-5

- Name two causes of homelessness.
- Name two groups of individuals who are vulnerable to homelessness.
- Name two types of violence.
- Among children, which age-group is the most vulnerable to abuse and neglect?
- Describe the effects of family violence that generally endure after the physical injury has healed.

PracticalKnowledge
knowing **how**

A holistic view of family health integrates the biological, social, cultural, and spiritual aspects of life and refers to individual members as well as the whole family. Nurses play a vital role in promoting family wellness and encouraging them to take responsibility for their own family health. Your interactions with families can empower them to practice healing and health maintenance behaviors.

ASSESSMENT NP

Family health assessment is similar to that for individuals. Gather all essential information about each family member. Ensuring privacy is essential for obtaining an accurate and comprehensive assessment. (See Chapter 21 for additional information on physical assessment.) In addition to the individual's data, assess the health of the family unit.

For a description of a family assessment, refer to the Focused Assessment box Conducting a Family Assessment.

The following sections discuss in more detail the assessment of family health history, family health beliefs, communication patterns, coping processes, and caregiver role strain.

Assessing the Family's Health History

The family history can provide clues about a person's health and susceptibility for disease. Genetic linkages have been discovered for common, complex diseases, such as breast cancer, Alzheimer's disease, diabetes, macular degeneration, seizures, inflammatory bowel disease, lupus, and heart disease, to name a few.

What Is Genomics?   **Genomics** is the study of human genes and their function, including the interactions with other genes and the environment. Simply put, it is about the interplay between a person's genetic makeup and food and environmental factors (e.g., lifestyle, and stress).

How Can Genomics Be Useful?   Genomics can be used to personalized a patient's plan of care by:

- Identifying at risk individuals for certain conditions to provide more effective preventive care.
- More accurately detecting illness, even before symptoms appear.

Conducting a Family Assessment

In general, a family assessment should include the following:

Identifying data	Include information such as name, address, phone number, cultural/ethnic background, religious identification, and social affiliation.
Family composition	For each family member, include gender, age, relationship, date and place of birth, occupation, and education.
Family history and developmental stage	➤ This refers to the stages and developmental tasks in Table 14-1, Assessing Family Developmental Tasks. ➤ Include a genogram.
Environmental data	Include a description of the home, neighborhood, and larger community, as well as the family's social supports and transactions with the community.
Family structure	Identify the structural type of family (e.g., traditional nuclear, single-parent) Also assess: ➤ *Communication patterns:* Functional and dysfunctional patterns; the manner in which emotions are expressed and contextual variables that affect communication ➤ *Power and role structures* (e.g., How are family decisions made? What are the roles of each member? Have there been changes in these?) ➤ *Family values* (e.g., What are their values? What are their priorities? How do they compare with the values of their cultural group? Are there value conflicts in the family?)
Family functions	Assess the effectiveness of the family's: ➤ *Nurturing* (e.g., Are the members close? Are they separate or connected?) ➤ *Socialization and child rearing* (e.g., Who is[are] the socializing agent[s] for the children? What are their child-rearing practices? Are needs for play being met?)
Health beliefs, values, and behaviors	➤ How do they define health and illness? ➤ What are their dietary, sleep, physical, and drug habits? ➤ What are their dental and medical health practices, including physicals, eye examinations, immunizations, and exercise patterns? ➤ Do they have access to healthcare services?
Family stressors and coping	➤ What are their stressors (e.g., financial, family communication or relationships, neighbors, holidays, children's behavior?) ➤ What successful coping strategies have they used? ➤ What strategies are dysfunctional?
Family strengths	Assess what members view as their strengths. Identify the individual(s) who provide guidance and direction to the family. Who is the advocate to keep the family strong, connected, and healthy?
Abuse and violence within the family	Because of the prevalence of abuse and because families are likely to be ashamed to discuss it, you should assess every family to see whether any abuse or neglect is occurring. For detailed guidelines, go to Procedure 9-1, Assessing for Abuse.

- Tailoring healthcare to the individual while reducing a trial-and-error approach.
- Evaluating a person's response to the care, considering multiple factors.

Genomics helps us understand how people respond differently to particular drugs and medical treatments. For example, while one client with a genetic predisposition for high cholesterol can reduce its risk by a change in diet and active exercise regimen, another may require cholesterol-reducing drugs.

How Is a Genogram Constructed? When assessing the family history, you can use a pictorial tool, called a **genogram,** to display the relationship of family members with pertinent health-related information (Fig. 14-6). This type of family tree can provide a quick and useful context in which to evaluate an individual's health risks.

To construct a genogram, you will use a three-generation (or more) diagram, showing for each family member:
- Causes of death
- Important health problems

- Genetically linked diseases
- Environmental (e.g., toxin) issues
- Mental health issues (e.g., depression, alcohol abuse, suicide)
- Occupational diseases (e.g., asbestos)
- Infections (e.g., MRSA)
- Obesity

When developing a genogram, use symbols and abbreviations to denote family members, including a key for interpretation (Box 14-1).

Assessing the Family's Health Beliefs

Health beliefs can vary widely among families and among individuals within families, especially those of different generations. Generations may pass these beliefs to future generations. Some common health beliefs are expressed in such adages as "An apple a day keeps the doctor away" and "Feed a cold, starve a fever." Some families have an intense mistrust of medical care and hospitals; they may seek treatment only when absolutely necessary.

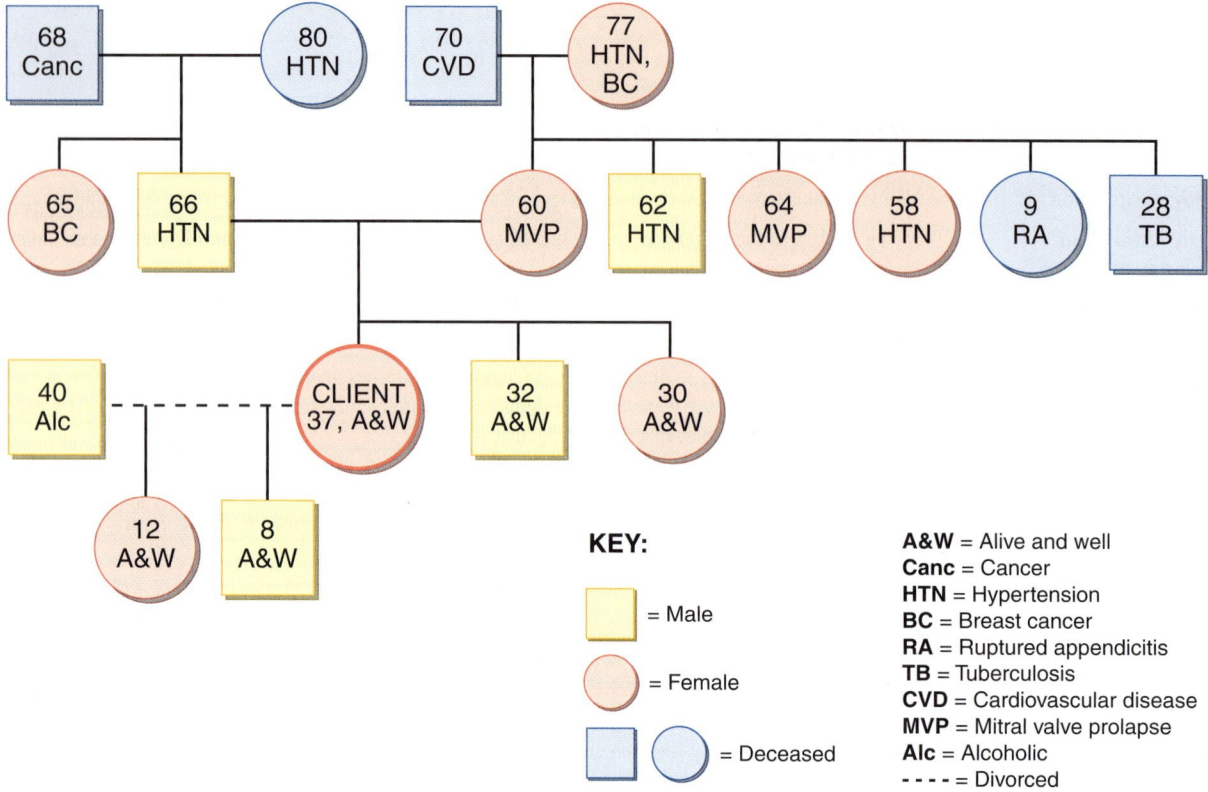

FIGURE 14-6 Family history by genogram.

The family's beliefs may influence individual decision making, even when a member shares only a few of the family's beliefs. Suppose a family is caring for a member who is elderly, frail, confused, and immobile. Imagine that one family member believes quality of life issues are more important than length of life. Yet another family member strongly disagrees with this belief and supports the right of the elderly adult to receive whatever care is needed for any length of time. In a situation like this, the family is at risk for interpersonal conflict, impaired communication, and caregiver strain. If you would like more information on health beliefs, see Chapter 27.

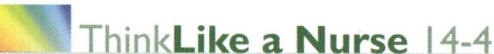

ThinkLike a Nurse 14-4

- As a nurse, how can you promote overall wellness in a family with a critically ill member?
- What health beliefs would you want to ask J. B.'s (Meet Your Patient) family about?

Assessing the Family's Communication Patterns

To assess family communication patterns, you will need to interview the family and carefully observe the interactions between family members. Try to uncover the following information:

- Who is the primary decision maker?
- How are family decisions made—by one person or by family conference?
- What is the most frequent type of communication among family members (e.g., visits to the home, telephone, texting, e-mail, social media)?

Family members who participate in dysfunctional communication patterns may not come to scheduled family meetings and may not be present during the initial interview. Additionally, when relationships among family members are strained or dysfunctional, they may distort the information about a home situation or another family member.

KEY POINT: *Do not rely solely on the information provided by the family members during the interview process.* Families usually want to "put on the best face" for healthcare providers, so they may be careful to give socially desirable responses.

BOX 14-1 ■ Family History by Listing Family Members

The following history is for a 37-year-old female patient:
Patient: Age 37, alive and well
Spouse: Age 40, divorced, alcoholism
Daughter: Age 12, alive and well
Son: Age 8, alive and well
Brother: Age 32, alive and well
Sister: Age 30, alive and well
Father: Age 66, hypertension (HTN)
Mother: Age 60, mitral valve prolapse (MVP)
Paternal aunt: Age 65, breast cancer
Maternal uncle: Age 62, HTN
Maternal uncle: Deceased age 28, tuberculosis (TB)
Maternal aunt: Age 64, MVP
Maternal aunt: Age 58, HTN
Maternal aunt: Deceased age 9, ruptured appendix
Paternal grandfather: Deceased age 68, cancer
Paternal grandmother: Age 80, HTN
Maternal grandmother: Age 77, HTN, breast cancer
Maternal grandfather: Deceased age 70, cardiovascular disease (CVD)

PICOT

Alcohol Treatment and Family Support

Situation:

The nurse is meeting with a family prior to the discharge of the husband/father from alcohol treatment. The teenage daughter asks the nurse whether her father will ever drink again.

PICOT Components:

P	Population/client	=	Alcoholic adults
I	Intervention/indicator	=	Family Support
C	Comparator/control	=	No family support
O	Outcome	=	Decreased risk of relapse; overall well-being
T	Time	=	Over time

Searchable Question:

Do _____(P) who receive/are exposed to _____(I) demonstrate _____(O) as compared to _____(C) during _____(T)?

Example of Evidence:

Alcohol abuse is a common social, family, and individual health problem. Research indicates that clients are less likely to relapse if they have spent more time in treatment and subsequent time in an abstinence-related treatment facility, and they also have overall family support. Family support did not need to be alcohol related; rather, support for the client in general was shown to have a positive effect on the client's sustained sobriety. In addition, family support was positively correlated to decreased stress and anxiety and overall well-being.

Practice Change:

The nurse made certain to assess family relationships and support for this and future clients.

References: Makilim, N., Valdir, A., Adriana, M., et al. (2013). Perception of family support in dependents of alcohol and others drugs: Relationship with mental disorders. *Adicciones, 25*(3), 220–225; Siddharth, D. (2015). Social support and treatment outcomes in alcohol dependence syndrome in armed forces. *Journal of Clinical and Diagnostic Research, 9*(11), VC01–VC05. doi:10.7860/JCDR/2015/14142.6739

Carefully observe the words people use and other cues such as body language, direct eye contact, and other nonverbal expressions, particularly among family members.

Assessing the Family's Coping Processes

The physiological manifestations of stress (e.g., anxiety, increased pulse rate) may decrease the effectiveness of interventions and negatively affect a client's health. Similarly, family members who are not coping effectively may cause the client to become tense or anxious or have problems sleeping. Assessing family coping is a first step to helping them develop more effective coping patterns.

Observe for physical indications of stress, anxiety, or loss of sleep in the ill person and for relationships and communication patterns among family members. As a nurse, you can assess whether family members are irritable and "snap at"

(speak harshly or curtly to) one another. Pay attention to who is visiting. Family members who are not coping well may avoid coming to visit the client, so this may be an indicator of who is coping and who is not.

KnowledgeCheck 14-6

- Why is it important for you to ask about family health beliefs?
- What factors may impede a family's ability to cope with an individual's illness?
- What is the significance of a genogram?

Assessing for Example Problem: Caregiver Role Strain

Conflicts between caregiving and other responsibilities can produce tremendous family stress. The physical, emotional, financial, and time demands involved in caring for family members who are chronically ill, disabled, or frail can add up, causing family caregivers to suffer from what NANDA-I terms Caregiver Role Strain. This is present when a person has difficulty in performing adequately in the family caregiver role. To learn more about this diagnosis and relevant nursing care, see the Example Problem: Caregiver Role Strain.

ANALYSIS/NURSING DIAGNOSIS NP

Recall that in the diagnostic process you must analyze the data for cues (data that deviate from norms). Therefore, you should be familiar with the characteristics of a healthy family so that you can use them as your basis for comparison (Box 14-2). For individual family members, any NANDA-I diagnosis may be appropriate for describing health status. **KEY POINT:** *Family diagnoses are meant to describe the health status of the family as a whole.* The following are examples:

Caregiver Role Strain (actual and risk for)
Family Coping: Compromised
Family Coping: Disabled
Dysfunctional Family Processes
Impaired Home Maintenance
Impaired Parenting (actual and risk for)
Ineffective Family Health Management
Ineffective Role Performance
Interrupted Family Processes
Readiness for Enhanced Family Coping
Readiness for Enhanced Parenting
Relocation Stress Syndrome
Risk for Impaired Attachment
Social Isolation

PLANNING OUTCOMES AND EVALUATION NP

NOC outcomes specifically for families as units are found in the NOC domain Family Health, which includes the classes Family Coping, Family Health Status, Family Integrity, and Parenting Performance. Outcomes from other domains may apply as well, depending on the nursing diagnosis you have made.

Individualized goals/outcome statements you might write for a family include the following examples, which represent some of the traits of healthy families in Box 14-2. The family:

Teaches respect for others within and outside the family.
Observes rituals and traditions (e.g., celebrates birthdays).
Respects the privacy of each member.
Communicates effectively and openly.

EXAMPLE PROBLEM: Caregiver Role Strain

Definition: Difficulty in performing family/significant other caregiver role (Herdman & Kamitsuru, 2014).
Defining Characteristics: Grouped into four main categories: caregiving activities, caregiver health status (physical, emotional, and socioeconomic), caregiver–care receiver relationship, and family processes.

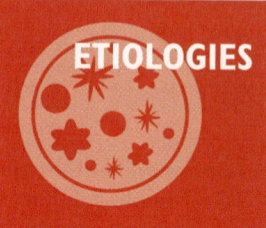

ETIOLOGIES

Causes & Risk Factors

- Poor communication
- Financial issues
- Client physical care demands (complex treatments, frailty)

- Conflicts between caregiving and other responsibilities
- Physical, emotional, and time demands involved in caring for family members who are chronically ill, disabled, or frail

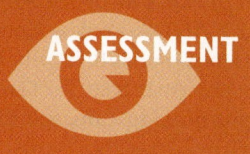

ASSESSMENT

Assess Caregiver Risk Factors & Symptoms

- Causes of role strain (see Etiologies)
- Dysfunctional communication, such as abusive language and aggression
- Apathy, withdrawal
- Emotional distress
- Caregiver depression, withdrawal, isolation, aggression, abusive communications

Assess Family Functioning

- Conflicts
- Avoidance
- Attachment
- Demanding
- Criticism of healthcare personnel or family

Assess Client

- Physical injuries
- Withdrawal, isolation
- Neglect
- Depression

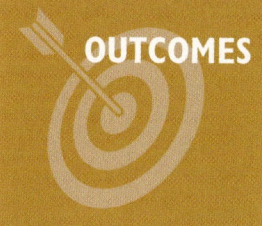

OUTCOMES

NOC Outcomes

- Caregiver Emotional Health
- Caregiver–Patient Relationship
- Caregiver Physical Health

- Caregiver Performance: Direct Care
- Caregiver Performance: Indirect Care

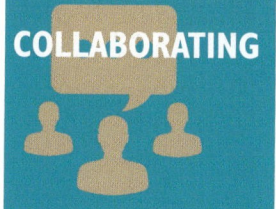

COLLABORATING

- Caregiver relief-respite
- Referral to family support groups

- Treatment of depression
- Symptomatic relief to client and caregiver

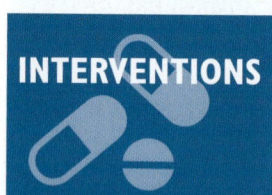

INTERVENTIONS

- Promote positive communications
- Promote family wellness
- Promote family cohesion during crisis (illness, hospitalization)
- Protect the client; assess for removal from environment
- Identify support systems to ensure caregiver support
- Refer for anger control assistance

- Promote expression of feelings, open communication of fears, anxiety, and concerns
- Praise positive relationships
- Praise/maintain family strengths
- Support family in problem-solving/decision making,
- Provide symptomatic treatment to client

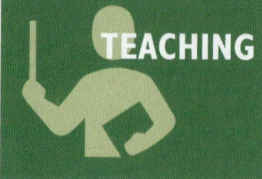

TEACHING

- Teach respect for others within and outside the family
- Teach caregiver skills and techniques for effective coping

- Teach how to address conflict
- Teach health promotion behaviors
- Teach relaxation methods

BOX 14-2 ■ Characteristics of a Healthy Family

A healthy family requires more than merely the absence of family dysfunction or disease in an individual member. Characteristics of a healthy family include the following:
- State of family well-being
- Sense of belonging and connectedness
- Clear boundaries between family members wherein the responsibilities of adults are clear and separate from responsibilities of growing children
- Sense of trust and respect
- Honesty and freedom of expression, including different opinions or viewpoints
- Spending time together, sharing rituals and traditions
- Relaxed body language, physical touch, and frequent eye contact
- Flexibility: adaptability and ability to deal with stress, openness to change
- Commitment: working together to maintain the family
- Spiritual well-being
- Respect for privacy of individual members
- Balance of giving and receiving
- Positive, effective communication
- Accountability, including acceptance when mistakes are made
- Appreciation and affection for each other
- Responding to the needs and interests of all members
- Health-promoting lifestyle of individual members

Remember the outcomes you develop for the care plan serve as the criteria for evaluating your client's responses to nursing interventions.

PLANNING INTERVENTIONS/ IMPLEMENTATION NP

NIC interventions for families as units are found in the NIC domain Family Integrity Promotion, which includes the classes for the Childbearing Family. Interventions from other domains also apply, depending on the nursing diagnosis you have made. The following are some examples:

> Caregiver Support, Family Integrity Promotion, Genetic Risk Identification, Home Maintenance Assistance, and Respite care.

Individualized nursing actions you might use with families include the following examples; other interventions are described in succeeding sections:
- Collaborate with family in problem-solving and decision making.

- Refer the family to support groups composed of other families dealing with similar problems.
- Monitor current family relationships.
- Assist family with conflict resolution.
- Encourage family to maintain positive relationships.
- Establish trusting relationship with family members.
- Counsel family members on additional effective coping skills for their own use.
- Refer for family therapy, as indicated.
- Tell family members it is acceptable to use their usual expression of affection when in a hospital setting.
- Encourage family members to verbalize their concerns, fears, and perceptions.

Promoting Family Wellness

Encourage families to value and incorporate health promotion into their lifestyles. This will also affect the health of individual members. Health promotion behaviors are typically learned within the family, so you can promote family wellness by addressing both individual and family needs. It is important to identify both strengths (see Box 14-2) and basic weaknesses of the family.

Involving the family in each phase of the nursing process promotes positive health outcomes and helps gain their trust. Wellness interventions may include contracting, health teaching, anticipatory guidance, and promoting family cohesion during a crisis (e.g., hospitalization of a family member). For specific health promotion activities, see Chapter 27.

Interventions When a Family Member Is Ill

When a family member is ill or hospitalized, other family members experience a range of emotions—especially when the illness is severe or of sudden onset. Family members may display signs of stress in a variety of ways, for example, by arguing with each other or with healthcare providers, insisting on immediate care for their loved one, avoiding the client's room, being critical of the care provided, or by frequently asking that information be repeated. These are normal reactions; do not take them personally.

The client and family need to understand the medical diagnosis, the plan of care, and the recovery process. In addition, often the nurse provides extensive discharge instructions to the client and family before they leave the hospital. To help family members manage stress when a family member is ill, see Box 14-3.

Interventions for Example Problem: Caregiver Role Strain

For nursing interventions specific to Caregiver Role Strain, see Example Problem: Caregiver Role Strain.

Toward Evidence-Based Practice

Doley, R., Bell, R., Watt, B., et al. (2015). Grandparents raising grandchildren: Investing factors associated with distress among custodial grandparent. *Journal of Family Studies, 21*(2), 101–119. Retrieved from https://dx.doi.org/10.1080/13229400.2015.1015215

This study measured the level of depression and life satisfaction of 100 grandparents who were the primary custodial parent for their grandchildren. Findings revealed that grandparents raising children with emotional and/or behavioral problems, who did not have a source of social support, reported more stress, anxiety, depression, and less overall life satisfaction did than their counterparts with adequate support systems.

Ivey, D. (2014). *Stressors and social support among African-American grandparents raising grandchildren* (Unpublished doctoral dissertation). University of Texas, Arlington.

Several themes emerged from focused group discussions with African American grandparents raising their grandchildren. Grandparents experienced social isolation because the high demands of parenting left little time to engage in leisurely activities. Church communities were the most common source of support. Despite the stressors, these grandparents did not want to release their grandchildren to social services or the parents.

Backhouse, J., & Graham, A. (2012). Grandparents raising grandchildren: Negotiating the complexities of role-identity conflict. *Child & Family Social Work, 17*(3), 306–315.

A qualitative study was conducted to identify common themes from the experiences of 27 grandmothers and 7 grandfathers who were raising their grandchildren, who ranged in age from 1 to 17 years. Some of the pain and challenges described by the subjects included feelings of grief and loss regarding their children's situations, emotional and financial costs of dealing with the legal and welfare systems, inability to meet the physical activity needs of their grandchildren, and the thought of dying before the grandchildren reached adulthood. Nevertheless, the positive experiences dominated the relationships. These included the emotional bond and attachment with the grandchildren, the satisfaction of providing them with security and stability, and having more tolerance and patience with child-rearing experiences.

1. Based on this research, if you were the nurse, what kinds of information would you want to gather from families in which grandparents provided custodial care to grandchildren?

2. What ways can you think of to support grandparents who assume major roles in rearing grandchildren?

 Go to Davis Advantage, Resources, Chapter 14, **Toward Evidence-Based Practice Suggested Responses**.

BOX 14-3 ■ Interventions to Help Family Cope With Hospitalization

- Provide written materials explaining the client's diagnosis or condition.
- Actively involve the family in team meetings.
- Promptly follow up with family concerns or questions.
- Encourage the family to go home and rest.
- Encourage the family to call for updates when they cannot be present.
- Suggest ideas for stress-reducing activities (e.g., walking, meditating).

- Inform the family about on-site availability of a clergy member or chapel.
- Encourage the family to participate in care activities as appropriate.
- Keep the family informed of the client's progress.
- Help the family to identify sources of stress and develop strategies to work through and dissolve the root cause.
- Provide anticipatory guidance regarding outcome and expectations for discharge.

CLINICALREASONING

The questions and exercises in this section allow you to practice the kind of thinking you will use as a full-spectrum nurse. Critical-thinking questions usually have more than one correct answer, so we do not provide "correct answers" for these features. It is more important to develop your nursing judgment than to just cover content. You will learn by discussing the questions with your peers. If you are still unsure, see the Davis Advantage chapter resources for suggested responses.

Caring for the Nguyens

Kim Phan, 3 years old, is the first grandchild for Nam and Yen Nguyen. Until recently, Kim lived with his mother, Trinh Phan, the Nguyens' daughter. Trinh was diagnosed with schizophrenia at age 18 and initially was functioning adequately on her medications. However, her condition has been worsening and for the past year she has not been taking her medications. When Trinh became unable to care for Kim, Nam and Yen assumed the child's care. Trinh rarely visits Kim. Nam and Yen convinced Trinh to obtain residential care at a mental health facility. Nam tells you at a clinic visit that he wishes his family were "normal."

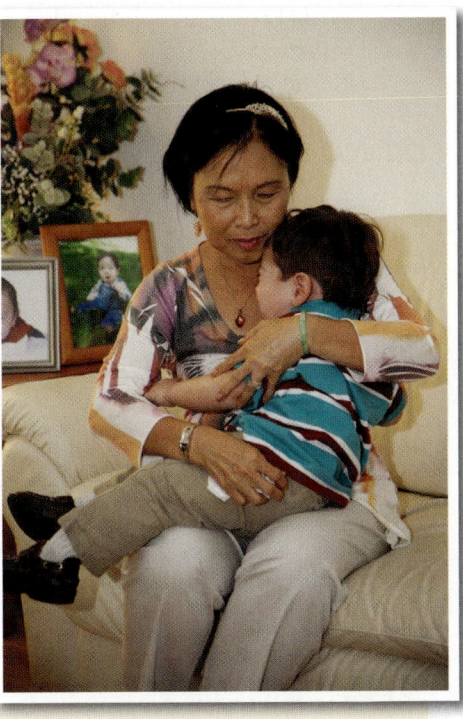

A. What do you need to clarify about Nam's statement regarding his family?

B. What do *you* think Nam means by a "normal" family?

C. How would you respond to Nam's comments?

D. What effect might this new family structure have on Nam's and Yen's health?

E. How might you promote family functioning for the Nguyens? What assessments should you make? What interventions should you consider?

F. What personal values or biases do you have that may affect your ability to care for the Nguyens?

Applying the **Full-Spectrum Nursing Model**

PATIENT SITUATION

Sandra Jackson is the 22-year-old single mother of an 18-month-old child. She has type 1 diabetes mellitus. Blood glucose control has been unstable, primarily during times of stress and illness. Sandra lives with her mother and three siblings. At times her boyfriend stays in the home, depending on the status of their relationship. Sandra works part-time at a retail chain, struggling to meet the financial responsibilities of rearing a child. She is showing physical signs of depression and distress (e.g., apathy, anorexia, excessive sleeping, and episodes of crying). During your home visit, Sandra says, "Something is really wrong with me. I can't snap out of this feeling of darkness. Life is too hard and it's nothing but pain. I can't take it anymore and want it to be over." You believe she needs immediate mental health support.

THINKING

1. *Theoretical Knowledge:*
   a. What facts and principles do you already know about stress and depression?
   b. How does the emotional well-being of one family member affect others living in the home and the family as a whole?
2. *Critical Thinking (Inquiry):*
   a. What factors in Sandra's life are possibly contributing to her feelings of hopelessness and thoughts of self-harm?
   b. Name at least three nursing diagnoses that would best suit Sandra's health needs.

DOING

3. *Practical Knowledge:* Based on the knowledge you have about stress and depression (see #1 above), how would you explain to the family about how best to support Sandra?
4. *Nursing Process (Evaluation):* What measures would you identify to determine whether your nursing plan of care was effective?

CARING

5. *Self-Knowledge:*
   a. How comfortable would you be in caring for a patient who is at risk for self-injury?
   b. What is one problem with Sandra and her family, not described in the scenario, that could possibly arise?
6. *Ethical Knowledge:* What ethical concerns might you have for a woman with a young child who is at risk for self-injury but has no financial resources to cover expenses of mental healthcare?

To explore learning resources for this chapter,

Go to **www.DavisAdvantage.com** and find:

Answers and Suggested Responses for all questions in this chapter

NIC/NOC Classifications

Alphabetical List of NANDA-I Diagnoses

Knowledge Map

References and Bibliography

Concept Map

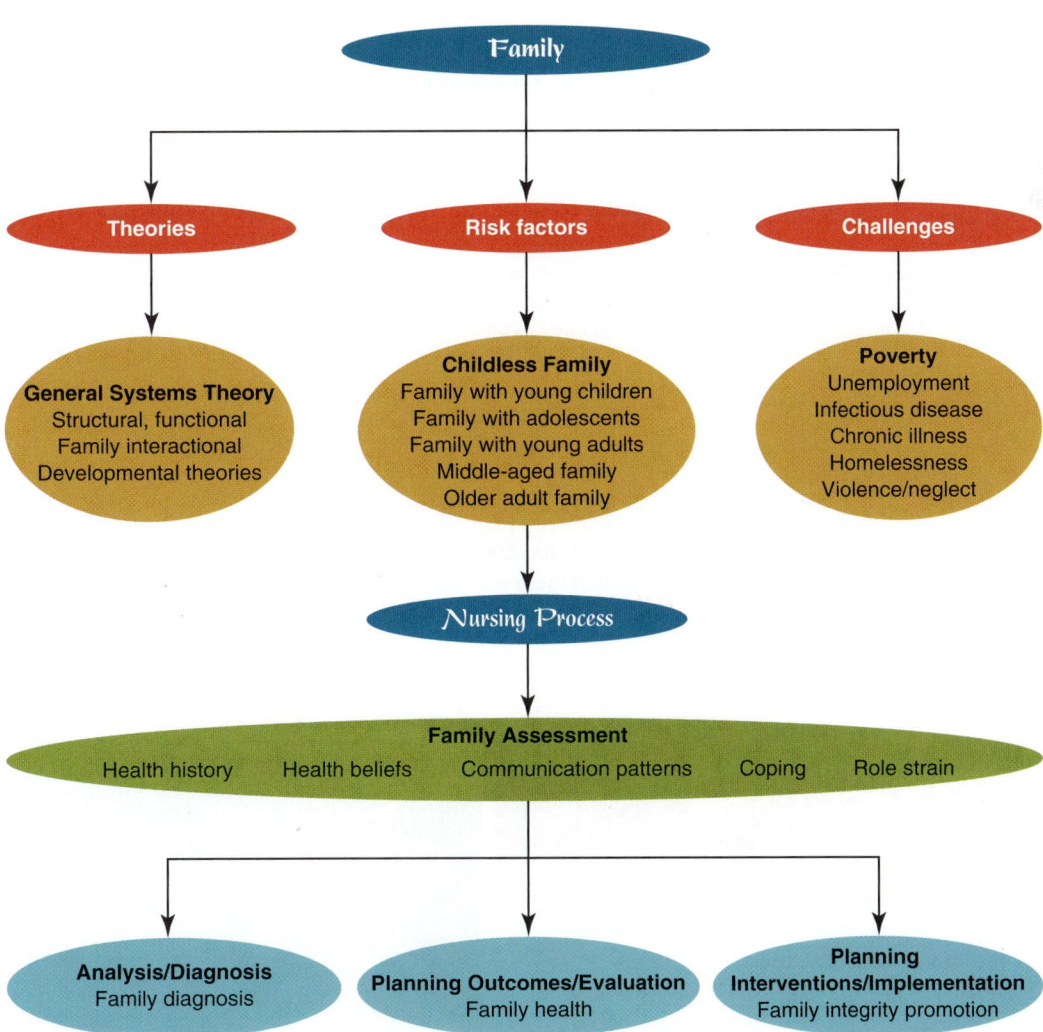

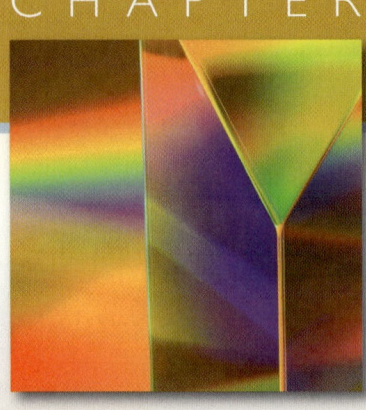
Culture & Ethnicity

Learning Outcomes

After completing this chapter, you should be able to:

➤ Explain why cultural competence is important for nurses.

➤ Explain what is meant by *culture* and *acculturation*.

➤ Discuss concepts pertaining to cultural diversity in nursing.

➤ Identify vulnerable populations in the United States.

➤ Define and give an example of culture universals and of culture specifics.

➤ Differentiate between cultural archetypes and cultural stereotypes.

➤ Describe the culture of the North American healthcare system, including professional subcultures.

➤ Identify the phenomena of culture, including how they can affect the nursing care needs of clients and families.

➤ Discuss the differing views of culturally diverse clients, including biomedical, holistic, and alternative health systems, such as folk medicine.

➤ Explain guidelines for performing a transcultural assessment, including a cultural assessment model.

➤ Recognize the cultural implications inherent in nursing diagnoses.

➤ Describe nursing strategies that promote delivery of culturally competent care to clients and their families.

➤ Identify techniques for communicating with clients when there is a language barrier.

Key Concepts

Cultural competence

Culture

Related Concepts

See the Concept Map at the end of this chapter.

Meet Your Patients

Your clinical assignment is to spend the day in a walk-in clinic with a primary care provider. Your assignment while there is to greet the clients and help them complete a health history form. These are the clients you see that day:

■ Romano Salvatore points to his head and moans. When you ask him what is wrong, he makes a gesture to convey to you that he does not understand what you are saying. He speaks a foreign language that sounds to you like Italian.

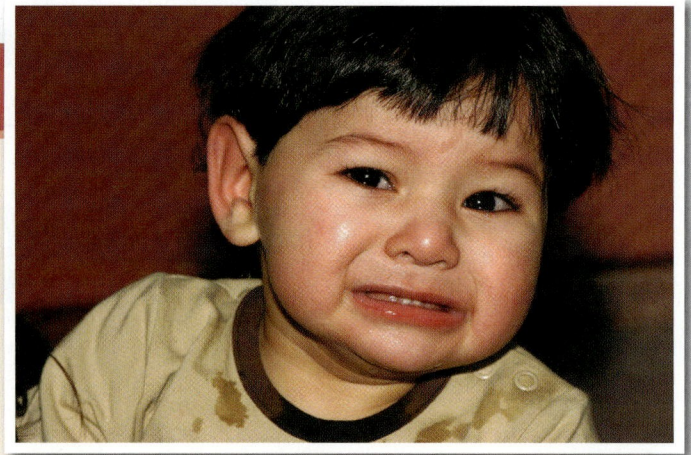

Meet Your Patients (continued)

- Rosanna is a frantic young mother, carrying her 4-year-old son, José, who is crying and coughing. Rosanna informs you that José complains of a sore throat and has a fever. She tells you she has been to her *curandero*, but José is not getting any better. You notice that José is wearing a heavy coat and knit hat although it is quite warm outside. When you question Rosanna about the child's clothing, she says that José is cold.

- Lee Chan, an elderly Chinese American man, is accompanied by eight family members. Because the waiting area is small, all except his daughter Kim are asked to wait outside. Mr. Chan is quiet and does not make eye contact with you. His daughter explains that her father has stomach cancer and is in a lot of pain because of disharmony. When you ask him to rate his pain, he just shakes his head and looks away. Would you wonder what disharmony means?

Theoretical Knowledge
knowing why

Try to answer the following questions about the clients you have just met. You may not have the theoretical knowledge to answer them all—you will acquire that in this chapter—but do your best based on the background you now have.

Think Like a Nurse 15-1

- Think about Romano Salvatore.
  If you could speak Italian, what would you ask him?
- Think about Rosanna and her child.
  One question that might spring immediately to your mind is, "What is a *curandero*?" How would you find out this information?
  Why do you think that the child is dressed more warmly than you would expect for the weather?
- Think about Mr. Chan and his family.
  How would you feel about so many of his family members coming with Mr. Chan to the clinic?
  Why do you think he is not looking at or speaking to you?
  How could you communicate with Mr. Chan? Would you assume that he does not speak your language? Explain your reasoning.

ABOUT THE KEY CONCEPTS

The overarching concepts for this chapter are **culture** and **cultural competence**. These and the concepts of *assimilation* and *culture universals* are important for nurses to understand and apply to the care of clients.

WHY LEARN ABOUT CULTURE?

You will care for clients from various cultures and likely work on a multicultural healthcare team (see Fig. 15-1). Having cultural knowledge can help you to provide culturally competent care.

The Population Is Diverse The United States is a multicultural society. We continue to see a trend of increasing immigration from other nations (e.g., Asia, Latin America, and the Middle East and North African region). Because of the growth in various population groups, the United States is expected to become a **majority-minority nation** by 2044 (Colby & Ortman, 2015). That is, no single group will have a majority share of the total population. Trend data from 2014 to 2060 show that the non-Hispanic whites will remain the largest single group.

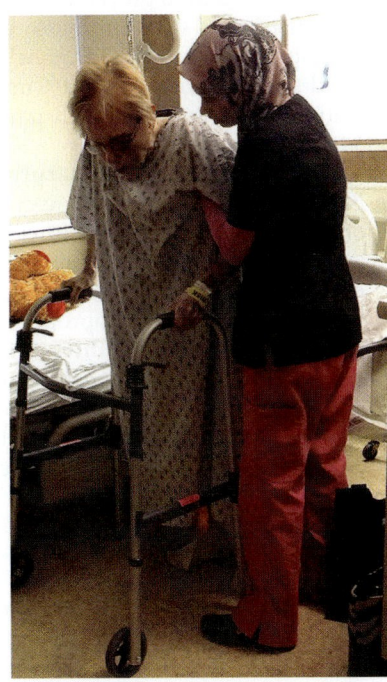

FIGURE 15-1 Nurses work with patients from many cultures.

Asians and Hispanics are the second and third fastest growing populations, respectively.

Think Like a Nurse 15-2

- With what cultural groups do you identify?
- In the neighborhood where you live, identify the cultural or ethnic groups that are different from your own. How many are there?
- In the school you are now attending, how many different cultural or ethnic groups are represented? What are they?

Health Disparities Exist Among Racial and Ethnic Groups A *Healthy People 2020* overarching goal is to eliminate disparities, achieve health equity, and improve the health of all groups (*Healthy People 2020*, n.d.).

- **Health Status.** One general disparity is that, except for Asians, minority groups experience higher rates of illness and death and, in general, poorer health status compared with the white, non-Hispanic population. For example:
  - When compared with those for whites, infant mortality rates are significantly higher for blacks and American

Indians and Alaska Natives (Kaiser Family Foundation, 2016a).

- Blacks and American Indians and Alaska Natives adults have a higher prevalence of asthma, diabetes, and cardiovascular disease (Artiga, 2016).
- Blacks are eight to 10 times more likely to have higher rates of HIV/AIDS diagnoses than are whites (Kaiser Family Foundation, 2016a).

- **Quality of care.** When compared by socioeconomic status, high-income households received better care than poor households. Disparities among racial groups are common, with whites receiving better care on 40% of quality measures than blacks, Hispanics, American Indians, and Alaska Natives (Agency for Healthcare Research and Quality, 2015).

- **Access to care.** Lack of access to preventive healthcare contributes to health disparities. The Affordable Care Act had decreased the number of uninsured. For nonelderly adults, the rate decreased from 17% in 2013 to 11% in 2015 (Kaiser Family Foundation, 2016a), although disparities remain among racial groups.

Nursing Is Challenged to Provide Culturally Competent Care   In North America the healthcare culture reflects the dominant, or European American, culture. However, as you know, nurses care for patients from many races and cultures. Nursing care that is appropriate for the dominant cultural group may be ineffective and inappropriate for people with a different cultural heritage. **KEY POINT:** *It is impossible to know about every culture, but it is important to learn about those you will encounter most often.* An understanding of culture and ethnicity will help you in providing direct care, teaching, supervising, and modeling culturally competent care to other care providers.

KnowledgeCheck 15-1

- What do recent demographic trends in North America indicate?
- Why should nurses know about the culture and ethnicity of clients?

WHAT IS MEANT BY CULTURE?

Culture is what people in a group have in common, but it changes over time. Purnell (2014) defined culture as "the totality of socially transmitted behavior patterns, arts, beliefs, values, customs, lifeways, and all other products of human work and thought characteristics of a population of people that guides their worldview and decision making" (p. 6). The following are some other definitions of culture:

- *Spector* (2017) explained culture in a unique way by asserting that we should view it by picturing the entire luggage each of us carries around on our lifetime journey. According to Spector, the luggage can be beliefs, habits, practices, likes and dislikes, and so on that we can learn from our families and can transmit to our children.
- *Leininger and McFarland* (2002, p. 47) view culture as "the learned, shared, and transmitted knowledge of values, beliefs, and lifeways of a particular group that are generally transmitted intergenerationally and influence thinking, decisions, and actions in patterned or in certain ways."
- *Purnell and Paulanka* (2008, p. 404) defined culture as "the totality of socially transmitted behavior patterns, arts, beliefs,

values, customs, lifeways, and all other products of human work and thought characteristic of a population of people that guide their worldview and decision making. Patterns may be explicit or implicit, are primarily learned and transmitted within the family, and are shared by the majority of the culture."

- The *Office of Minority Health* (2013, p. 10) defined culture as "the integrated pattern of thoughts, communications, actions, customs, beliefs, values, and institutions associated, wholly or partially, with racial, ethnic, or linguistic groups, as well as with religious, spiritual, biological, geographic, or sociological characteristics."

As you learn more about culture and cultural, recall the following characteristics:

- **Cultures consist of common beliefs and practices.** Most members of a culture share the same beliefs, traditions, customs, and practices as long as they continue to be adaptive and satisfy the members' needs. Culture can influence everything its members think and do.
- **Culture is both *universal*** (everyone has it) **and *dynamic*** (active). Cultural customs, beliefs, and practices are not static. They change over time and at different rates as members adapt and respond to their environment.
- **Cultural beliefs provide identity and a sense of belonging** if they continue to satisfy its members and do not conflict with the dominant culture.
- **Culture exists at many levels.** Culture exists in both the material (art, writings, dress, or artifacts) and the nonmaterial (customs, traditions, language, beliefs, and practices). See Figure 15-2.
- **Cultural values, beliefs, and traditions are passed down from generation to generation.** Learning occurs through life experiences shared with other members of the culture, either formally (e.g., in schools) or informally (e.g., in families). Some generations totally adopt the values, beliefs, and

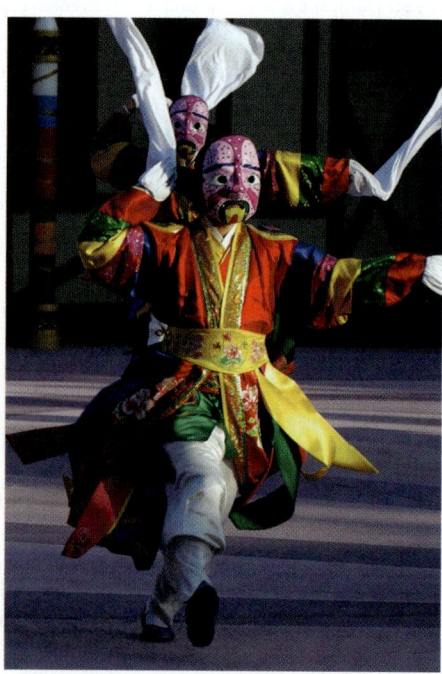

FIGURE 15-2 Traditional lunar New Year dancer in South Korea.

traditions of their elders; some partially accept them, while others reject them.

- **Cultural assumptions and habits are unconscious.** Thus, they may be difficult for members of the culture to explain to others or to identify as different from another culture.
- **Culture is diverse** and demonstrates the variety that exists among groups and among members of a particular group.

 Think**Like a Nurse** 15-3

Figure 15-2 depicts an example of ways in which members of particular cultural groups express their cultural uniqueness in dance. Can you think of other ways that people express their culture?

Ethnicity, Race, and Religion

You may hear the terms *culture, ethnicity,* and *race* used interchangeably, but in fact they have separate, specific meanings. Distinctions between culture, ethnicity, race, and religion might seem confusing, but think of it this way: You are a member of:

- The subculture of nursing
- An ethnic group (e.g., Portuguese Americans from the Azores)
- A racial group (e.g., white)
- A religion (e.g., Roman Catholicism)

Each of those groups has its own set of beliefs and values, so your culture is a blend of all of them.

Ethnicity

Examples of ethnic groups include French Canadians, Hmongs, and Latinos.

- **Ethnicity is similar to** *culture* in that it refers to groups whose members share a common social and cultural heritage that is passed down from generation to generation.
- **Ethnicity is also similar to** *subculture,* in that the members of an **ethnic group** have some characteristics in common (e.g., race, ancestry, physical characteristics, geographic region, lifestyle, religion) that are not shared or understood by outsiders
- **Ethnicity may include race, but it is not the same as race.** To demonstrate, the U.S. Census Bureau (2011) has numerous categories for *race* (see the next section). In addition, it identifies two categories for *ethnicity:* (1) Hispanic, Latino, or Spanish and (2) *Not* Hispanic, Latino, or Spanish.
  - **Hispanic** Americans are people who originally came from any Spanish-speaking country (e.g., Mexico, Spain).
  - **Latino,** strictly speaking, refers only to people from Central or South America.
  - **Spanish** implies origin in Spain.

If you know a client's country of origin, it is more accurate to use it when referring to the client's ethnicity (e.g., Mexican American, Colombian American) than to use the term *Hispanic, Latino,* or *Spanish.*

Race

Unlike ethnicity, race is strictly related to biology. **Race** refers to the grouping of people based on biological similarities, such as skin color, blood type, or bone structure (Purnell, 2013). The terms *race* and *ethnicity* overlap somewhat, because race can be a characteristic of a specific ethnic group. The U.S. Census Bureau (2011) asks people to choose the race with which they identify and divides the population into the following list of racial categories:

- White
- Black, African American, or Negro
- American Indian or Alaskan Native
- Asian Indian
- Chinese
- Filipino
- Japanese
- Korean
- Vietnamese
- Other Asian
- Native Hawaiian
- Guamanian or Chamorro
- Samoan
- Other Pacific Islanders

People of Hispanic, Latino, or Spanish origin may be of any race, because the U.S. Census Bureau includes Hispanic/Latino/Spanish as a sociocultural rather than a race category.

Race as a Social Construct   You usually cannot determine a person's race by his appearance. So, then, is race determined by heredity? What race is someone whose father is African American and whose mother is white? Historically, most North Americans would say that the person is African American. In some other countries (e.g., most of South America), that same person would be categorized as white. Many, including the U.S. Census Bureau, believe that race is socially (rather than biologically) determined. As a culturally sensitive nurse, ask people what race they identify with and what name they prefer to use for it. For more information on race as a social construct,

 Go to "Race Is a Social Construct, Scientists Argue," at http://www.scientificamerican.com/article/race-is-a-social-construct-scientists-argue/

KEY POINT: *We tend to group and categorize data to make them meaningful and useful, but we must be careful to avoid using these categories as the basis for interacting with people or providing care. When you need to designate a name for a group, be as specific as possible (e.g., Syrian American instead of white).*

Religion

Religion may be confused with ethnicity because people within an ethnic group may share the same religion. For example, the Jewish culture overlaps with the Jewish faith community. **Religion** refers to an ordered system of beliefs regarding the cause, nature, and purpose of the universe, especially the beliefs related to the worship of a God or gods (Andrews & Boyle, 2015). In many cultures, religion is a high priority (Figure 15-3).

Concepts Related to Culture

The concept **bicultural** describes a person who identifies with two cultures and integrates some of the values and lifestyles of each into his life. A child whose father is Jewish and mother is an Italian Catholic may choose to follow Jewish tradition while still holding some of the values and beliefs of her Italian heritage. A bicultural person may experience divided loyalties.

Multicultural refers to many cultures and is used to describe groups rather than individuals. Think of a hospital: Caregivers may be members of various ethnic, racial, and religious groups, and the nurses, providers, physical therapists, and students each make up a different subculture. A hospital is thus a multicultural setting.

Socialization, Acculturation, and Assimilation

Socialization is the process of learning to become a member of a society or a group. A person becomes socialized by

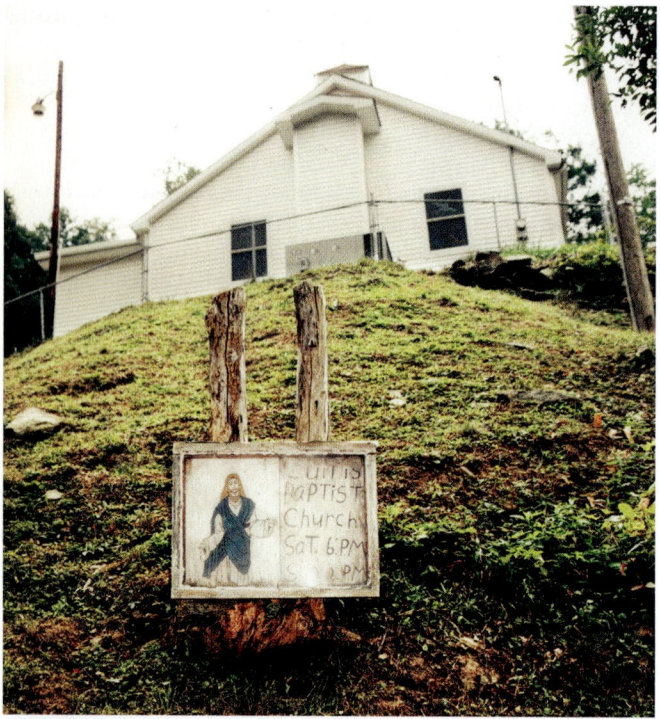

FIGURE 15-3 Even in this tiny community of rural Appalachia, people have built a place for worship.

learning social rules and roles; by learning behaviors, norms, values; and by perceptions of others in the same group or role. Your education program is socializing you into the role of a professional nurse. Families, schools, churches, peer groups, and the media are agents of socialization and foster their members' identification with the culture.

Acculturation is a learning process through which **immigrants** (new members of a group or country) assume the characteristics of that culture. A person who is acculturated accepts both his own and the new culture, adopting elements of each. Acculturation is the outgrowth of the minority group's need to survive and flourish in the new culture. It may take several years, perhaps three generations, for an immigrant group to become acculturated.

Assimilation occurs when the new members gradually learn and take on the essential values, beliefs, and behaviors of the dominant culture. Assimilation is complete when the newcomer is fully merged into the dominant cultural group. A person becomes assimilated by, for example, learning to speak the dominant language; marrying a member from the new (host) culture; and making close, personal relationships with members of the new group.

Dominant Cultures, Subcultures, and Minority Groups

Ethnocentrism is the tendency to think that your own group (cultural, professional, ethnic, or social) is superior to others and to view behaviors and beliefs that differ greatly from your own as somehow wrong, strange, or unenlightened. The tendency to ethnocentrism exists in all groups, not just in the dominant culture.

A Dominant Culture is the group that has the most authority or power to control values and reward or punish behaviors. It is usually, but not always, the largest group. The dominant group may assume their ways are the norm and that

everyone else is culturally different. What do you think is the current dominant culture of the United States? If you said white or Caucasian or European American, you would be only partially correct. The ancestors of most white Americans emigrated from Europe, and many were of Protestant or other Christian religions. Thus, the dominant culture in the United States and Canada is considered white Anglo-Saxon Christian of European descent.

Subcultures are groups within a larger culture or social system that have some characteristics that are different from those of the dominant culture (e.g., values, behaviors, ancestry, ways of living). People in subcultures have had different experiences from those in the dominant group because of status, residence, gender, sexual orientation, ethnic background, education, or other factors that unify the group (Purnell, 2013). You may be able to recognize subcultures by their speech patterns, dress, gestures, eating habits, lifestyles, and so on (e.g., street gangs, physicians, nurses, women, elderly adults, persons with disabilities, rural Midwesterners).

KEY POINT: *Nursing subcultures within hospitals can impact quality of care and thus patient outcomes. Nurses in specialty subcultures (e.g., critical care units, emergency rooms) had more autonomy, better quality of patient care, and fewer adverse events when compared with the medical–surgical nurse subculture (Mallidou, Cummings, Estabrook, et al., 2011).*

Minority Groups are also made up of individuals who share race, religion, or ethnic heritage. They usually have fewer members than the majority group. Depending on the type of group, they may or may not share beliefs, practices, or physical characteristics. The term *minority* is sometimes used to refer to a group of people who receive different and unequal treatment from others in society. You should consider that this term may be offensive to some because it suggests inferiority and marginalization.

KnowledgeCheck 15-2

- Define *culture*.
- Give an example of each: ethnic group, race, religion.
- How does culture provide identity for an individual?
- Give an example of *acculturation*.

Vulnerable Populations as Subcultures **Vulnerable populations** are groups that are more likely to develop health problems and experience poorer outcomes because of limited access to care, high-risk behaviors, and/or multiple and cumulative stressors (e.g., the homeless [Fig. 15-4], poor, or mentally ill; people with physical disabilities; the very young; and older adults). Some ethnic and racial minority groups are also vulnerable. For example, among American Indians and Native Alaskans, there is a higher incidence of type 2 diabetes in those under 20 years of age (Satterfield, DeBruyn, Santos, et al., 2016). **KEY POINT:** *Vulnerable populations are subcultures of all of the major cultural groups.*

One of the overarching goals of *Healthy People 2020* (n.d.) is to achieve health equity, eliminate disparities, and improve the health of all groups. Examples include the following:

Eliminating oral health disparities (Carrion, Castañeda, Martinez-Tyson, et al., 2011; Lester, Henderson, & Taylor, 2012)

Overweight/obesity among children of different ethnic groups (Long, Mareno, Shabo, et al., 2012)

Neighborhood disparities in access to health food (Hilmers, Hilmers, & Dave, 2012)

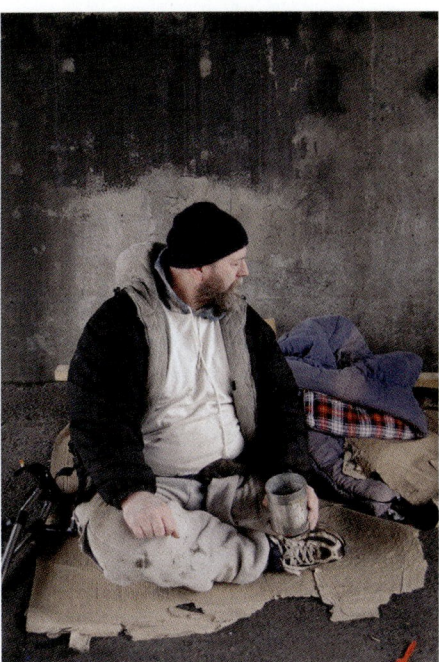

FIGURE 15-4 A homeless man sits on his cardboard, begging for spare change.

Gender as a Subculture It should come as no surprise that some behaviors are considered acceptable for men but not for women, and vice versa. There are values and responses considered more typical of one sex than of the other. For example, in the dominant culture it is more acceptable for women than it is for men to cry out in pain. Men are expected to be strong. Similarly, the U.S. culture tends to view caring and nurturing as the province of women; thus, men were historically excluded from the nursing profession. Today, however, the number of male nurses continues to increase. Research shows that they are well integrated and accepted by their peers and given fair, if not preferential, treatment in career advancement (McMurry, 2011).

🍁   **Old Age as a Subculture** Older adults, especially the very old, can be thought of as a vulnerable population in some respects. You should assess for elder abuse in *all* cultures and not assume that indicators of abuse are a result of cultural practice. For example, researchers used *promotores* (local Spanish-speaking Latinos) to assess for elder abuse among low-income Latino immigrants. Results reveal a variety of abuses, including psychological (25%), physical (11%), sexual (9%), financial (17%), and caregiver neglect (12%). Failure to report abuse may result from mistrust of the system, desire to protect the family, and/or language barriers (Deliema, Gassoumis, Homeier, et al., 2012).

HOW DO CULTURAL VALUES, BELIEFS, AND PRACTICES AFFECT HEALTH?

Values help to shape health-related beliefs and practices. Do you know what values are? What are the five ideals, principles, or things that are most important to you?

You may name, for example, learning, family, independence, faith, and cleanliness. Or you may have said something entirely different. Simply put:

■ A **personal value** is a principle or standard that has meaning or worth to an individual. (e.g., cleanliness).

■ A **belief**, in contrast, is something one accepts as true (e.g., "I believe that germs cause disease").

■ A **practice** is a set of behaviors that one follows (e.g., "I always wash my hands before preparing food").

Do you now see how values, beliefs, and practices are related?

■ Cultural values, beliefs, and practices are the principles, standards, ideas, and behaviors that members of a cultural group share. Some values of the dominant U.S. culture include cleanliness, youth, beauty, success, and independence.

■ You should not assume a client shares your values, beliefs, and practices—nor those of the dominant culture.

■ **KEY POINT:** *Remember, also, that individuals within an ethnocultural group vary widely and that learning commonalities is no substitute for careful assessment of each person.*

What Are Culture Universals and Specifics?

■ **Culture universals** are the values, beliefs, and practices that people from *all* cultures share. Leininger and McFarland (2002) call these *culture commonalities*.

■ **Culture specifics** (*culture diversities* in Leininger's theory) are those values, beliefs, and practices that are special or unique to a culture.

For example, all cultures celebrate the birth of a new baby in some way (a culture universal), but different cultures celebrate birth *rites* in different ways (a culture specific). Similarly, people from all cultures practice marriage rites in elaborate rituals that are culture specific (Fig. 15-5).

Archetype or Stereotype?

At this point in your efforts to be culturally sensitive, you might be thinking, "I went to a Chinese wedding, and it was no different from my own Italian wedding"; or "I know plenty of Greek people who don't put amulets on their babies." Of course, you are correct. However, acknowledging that there are commonalities within a group is not the same as saying that *all*

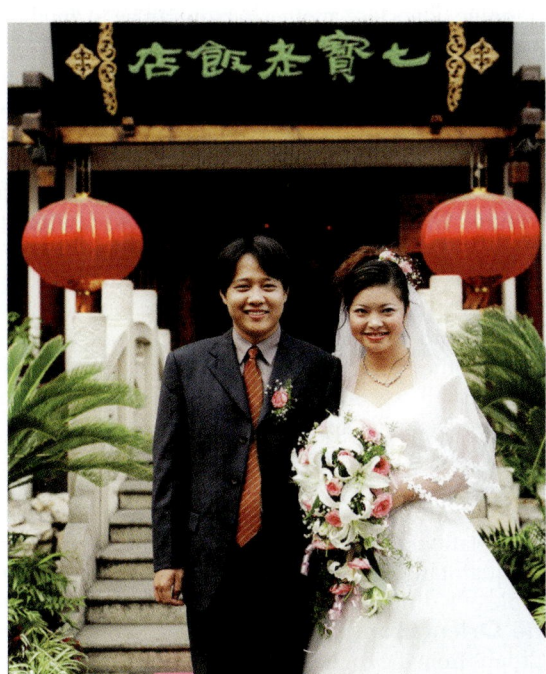

FIGURE 15-5 People of all cultures practice marriage rituals.

people in the group have those characteristics. You now understand the difference between an archetype and a stereotype.

- A **cultural stereotype** is an unsubstantiated belief that all people of a certain racial or ethnic group are alike in many respects. Stereotypes are often, but not always, negative. Someone may think, for example, that people of a particular heritage are "naturally intelligent" or "naturally athletic."
- A **cultural archetype** is a symbol for remembering some of the culture specifics and is usually not negative. For example, you might think of Mexican Americans as having brown skin or of European Americans as having blue eyes—these are not negatives.

Remember, there is probably more variation among people *within* an ethnic or cultural group than there is *between* the groups, and that variation stems from socioeconomic differences or regional origin as much as from race or ethnicity. **KEY POINT:** *The guiding principle for your practice is that each person must be seen as unique—as a member of an ethnic group, influenced by his heritage but not defined by it.*

How Do Culture Specifics Affect Health?

Culture specifics affect our health beliefs and behaviors. Thus, knowledge of the culture specifics of groups in your community will help explain why clients from different cultures have different expectations of healthcare. Ultimately, it will help you to provide culturally competent care. The following are six culture specifics that influence health as described by Giger (2016):

Communication is an exchange of information, ideas, and feelings. It includes verbal and nonverbal language (i.e., spoken language, gestures, eye contact, and even silences). Think how difficult it would be if you became ill in a foreign country whose language you did not know. How would you tell the caregivers your symptoms or understand the treatment plan? Language differences present one of the most difficult obstacles to providing care. Even when you and the client speak the same language, culture influences how feelings and thoughts are expressed and which verbal and nonverbal expressions are appropriate to use. See Chapter 20 for communication strategies, if you wish.

Space refers to a person's personal space, or the boundaries that determine how close another person can be to another person. A person's comfort level is related to space. If you are invading someone's personal space, a common reaction is for the person to move away from you. A similar concept, **territoriality**, means the geographic space a person views as owned or claimed, such as an area or room (Spector, 2017). When an individual's personal space is protected, he feels secure and safe, less anxious, and in control. The following are some examples of culturally influenced attitudes toward personal space (Purnell, 2013):

- Americans, Canadians of northern European ancestry, and the British typically keep at least 18 inches of space between themselves and the person with whom they are conversing.
- Arabs and others from the Middle East typically stand quite close when talking. They tend to keep steady eye contact, but not between men and women
- Germans usually require a great deal of space and consider even looking into a room an invasion of privacy.

Within all cultural groups, personal space varies depending on the relationship between the people speaking: intimates versus acquaintances, people of the same versus opposite sex, and people of a different position within the social hierarchy.

Time Orientation varies among people of different cultures. Groups from the Far East tend to be past oriented and value traditions and relationships over time and deadlines. In contrast, European Americans tend to be future oriented, and Latin Americans and Filipinos are more present oriented and enjoy living in the moment. Differences in time orientation can be important as you plan nursing interventions. For example, clients who are future oriented may be more focused on illness prevention; thus, you should provide teaching on health promotion.

ThinkLike a Nurse 15-4

- Suppose you say to a client, "You will need to exercise and follow a low-calorie diet to lose weight and control your diabetes." What kind of time orientation would a client most likely have in order to follow your directions?
- Suppose a client says, "I know I need to lose weight, but I work so much, and the children take so much time. I just don't have time to shop and cook for the right foods or to exercise." What time orientation does this illustrate?

Social Organization includes the family unit (e.g., nuclear, single parent, or extended family) and the wider organizations (e.g., community, religious, ethnic) with which the individual or family identifies (Spector, 2017).

- *A close social organization can be found in all cultures; however, the specifics vary.* For example, in Middle Eastern and Latino cultures, the man is likely to be the dominant family member. But many African American families are matriarchal—that is, the decision maker and family leader is a woman.
- *The social organization of your clients' cultures can provide clues about how they will act during life events,* such as birth, death, illness, and mourning. For example, a client who does not trust large institutions or government agencies is likely to use home remedies and delay seeing a conventional medical provider, even though Medicaid pays for her healthcare.
- *Kinship and social ties also determine who receives healthcare, and in what priority.* In the United States, for example, someone of high status (e.g., a celebrity or political figure) is likely to receive better care than an unknown poor person. In some cultures, men receive care before women and children.

Environmental Control refers to a person's perception of his ability to plan activities to control nature or direct environmental factors (Spector, 2017). A person's health and illness

---

♥ iCare 15-1

Culture and Ethnicity

Farik, an 84-year-old Middle Eastern Muslim male who does not speak English, has come to the ICU for multisystem failure. He arrives with multiple family members, all in a highly emotional state. It is expected in his culture that the male members collectively make decisions. They may elicit the guidance from an Imam, an experienced Muslim leader, regarding medical treatment decisions. The nurse's priority focus is Farik's immediate physical needs. However, it is equally important that she demonstrate caring by being respectful and sensitive to Muslim norms and practices. This is essential to providing appropriate, culturally sensitive, competent, and holistic care.

beliefs and practices are directly related to this concept. For example, if a person does not believe he has control over his health outcomes, he may not seek medical care, take his medications, or exercise. Consider most Asian Americans' perception and tolerance of pain. They do not view circumstances as something to be "controlled"; therefore, they tend to accept pain stoically and not demand relief. Think about why Mr. Chan (Meet Your Patients) just shook his head and looked away when asked to rate his pain.

Biological Variations include ways in which people are different genetically and physiologically. They include body build and structure, skin color, vital signs, enzymatic and genetic variations, and drug metabolism (Purnell, 2013; Spector, 2017). Biological variations create susceptibility to certain diseases and injuries and explain differences in responses to treatment. For example, studies have shown that African Americans have poorer responses to certain categories of antihypertensive drugs when compared with their white counterparts (Gupta, 2010; Wikoff, Frye, Zhu, et al., 2013). Consequently, clinical trials (drug studies) now recommend incorporating biological variations. For more information about biological variations and about biological susceptibility to diseases, see Clinical Insight 15-1.

Other Culture Specifics The following may also be culture specifics. The first two, religion/philosophy and education, vary among subcultures in the United States, whereas technology, politics/law, and the economy exert broader effects that can be seen among different countries, but less so among subcultures within a country.

- **Religion and Philosophy.** A person's religion may determine which healthcare treatments a person will permit. For example, some religions (e.g., Jehovah's Witnesses) do not accept blood transfusions.
- **Education.** Education influences perceptions of wellness and illness and the knowledge of options that are available for healthcare. These, in turn, affect the person's expectations for care.
- **Technology.** The availability of supplies and equipment in the healthcare setting becomes culturally expected. For example, nurses in most of North America assume they will have bed linens, water, electricity, prescribed medications, and diagnostic machines. In many parts of the world, however, these items are not available.
- **Politics and the Law.** Governmental policies (e.g., Affordable Care Act) affect healthcare by determining eligibility, allocation of funds, reimbursement for providers, and acceptable standards. Review Chapter 1 for an overview of governmental healthcare programs.
- **Economy.** The condition of the economy directly affects the availability of funds for publicly funded services. It also affects the individual's ability to pay for healthcare.

ThinkLike a Nurse 15-5

Consider this example: Mrs. Miyagi, a Japanese American, has been admitted to your care from the postanesthesia care unit after having undergone a major surgical procedure. She refuses pain medicine, although she appears to be in pain. As the hours pass, Mrs. Miyagi continues to refuse the pain medication, so eventually the nurses stop asking.

- Do you assume that she is experiencing no pain?
- Are you or the other nurses stereotyping her for her cultural response to pain?
- What would you do?

KnowledgeCheck 15-3

- Explain the difference between an archetype and a stereotype.
- Identify at least six culture specifics affecting health.
- How could you use this information about culture specifics to provide better care to your clients?

WHAT IS THE "CULTURE OF HEALTHCARE"?

The indigenous and professional healthcare systems can exist side by side in any culture (Leininger & McFarland, 2002; McFarland & Wehbe-Alamah, 2014). Each has its own culture.

The Indigenous Healthcare System consists of *folk medicine* and *traditional healing methods,* which may also include over-the-counter (OTC) and self-treatment remedies. Different groups have different folk practices, but all cultural groups probably use the professional healthcare system to at least some degree.

The Professional Healthcare System, in contrast, is run by professional healthcare providers who have been formally educated and trained for particular roles and responsibilities. In North America, professional healthcare is dominated by a biomedical healthcare system that combines Western biomedical beliefs with traditional North American values of self-reliance, individualism, and aggressive action. Table 15-1 summarizes the norms of this system, also called Western or allopathic medicine.

The professional healthcare system also includes practitioners formally trained in alternative healthcare, such as diet therapy, mind–body control methods, therapeutic touch, acupressure, reflexology, naturopathy, kinesiology, and chiropractic. If you would like more information about alternative healthcare,

 Go to **Bonus Chapter 46, Holistic Healing.**

Conflicts may occur when the professional provider does not understand the beliefs and practices of the indigenous healthcare systems and its traditional healers. The view that a practice is uncivilized and based on the supernatural creates distrust between the client and provider and benefits no one. As a nurse, you should become aware of and understand a variety of health beliefs and practices so that you can better meet the needs of your clients.

What Are Health and Illness Beliefs?

Generally speaking, people follow one of three major health belief systems: scientific/biomedical, magico-religious, or holistic (Andrews & Boyle, 2015).

- The **scientific/biomedical health system** is one with which you are already familiar.
- In the **magico-religious system,** belief in supernatural (mystical) forces dominates. This system is considered "alternative" or "indigenous" in the United States. One example is Voodoo, practiced in some developing nations in Africa, Latin America, and the Caribbean. The lion is a spiritual symbol (Fig. 15-6).
- The **holistic belief system** is similar to the magico-religious, but it focuses more on the need for harmony and balance of the body with nature.

Table 15-1 ➤ Summary of Cultural Norms of the North American Healthcare System	
NORM	**EXAMPLES**
Beliefs and Values	Standardized definitions of *health* and *illness*
	Significance of technology
	Reliance on the biomedical system
	Desire to conquer disease
	Defines *health* as absence or minimization of disease
Practices	Maintaining health through diet, exercise, adequate sleep
	Preventing disease through practices such as immunizations and avoidance of stress
	Annual physical examinations and diagnostic tests
Habits	Hand washing
	Use of jargon (e.g., "take your vitals")
	Use of problem-solving methods
Likes	Punctuality
	Neatness and organization
	Compliance (e.g., with medical "orders")
	Documentation
Dislikes	Tardiness
	Disorganization
	Messiness, lack of cleanliness
Customs	Use of procedures (e.g., circumcision, last rites) surrounding birth and death
	Professional respect and observance of hierarchy found in autocratic and bureaucratic systems
	Adherence to a set of ethical standards and codes of conduct
Rituals	Annual physical examination
	The surgical procedure

Sources: Adapted from Giger, J. (2016). *Transcultural nursing: Assessment and intervention* (7th ed.). St. Louis, MO: C.V. Mosby; Leppa, C. (2005). Transcultural communication within the health care subculture. In C. Munoz & J. Luckmann (Eds.), *Transcultural communication in health care* (2nd ed., pp. 74–83). Clifton Park, NY: Thomson Delmar Learning; Munoz, C., & Luckmann, J. (Eds.). (2005). *Transcultural communication in nursing* (2nd ed.). Clifton Park, NY: Thomson Delmar Learning; Purnell, L. (2014). *Guide to culturally competent health care* (3rd ed.). Philadelphia, PA: F.A. Davis; Spector, R. (2017). *Cultural diversity in health and illness* (9th ed.). Upper Saddle River, NJ: Pearson Education.

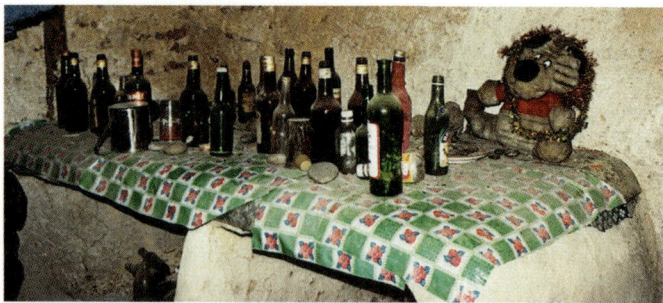

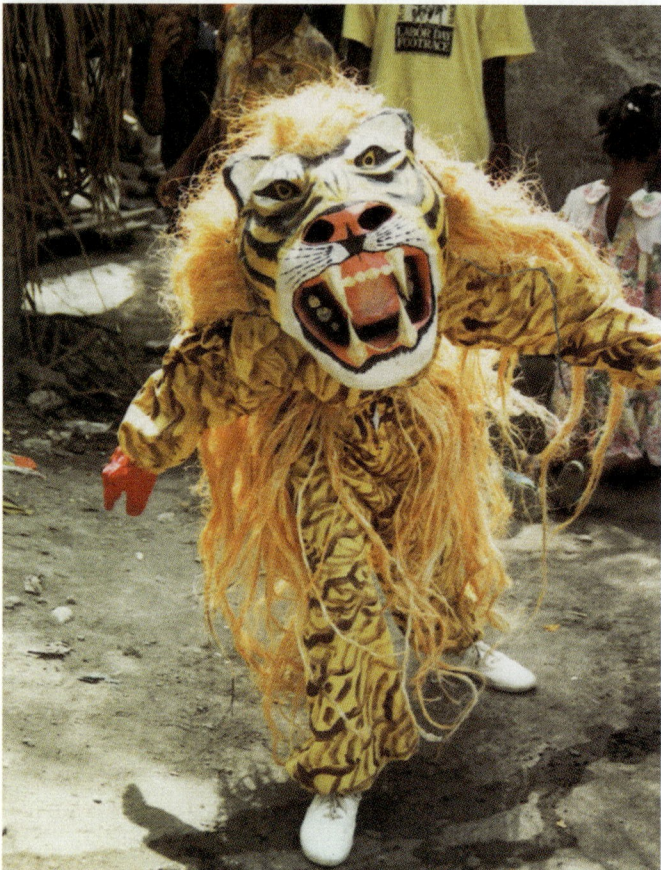

FIGURE 15-6 Voodoo is an example of a magico-religious belief system. *Top,* A Haitian voodoo shrine (notice the lion). *Bottom,* Here, a Haitian man is costumed for carnival as the spirit of the lion.

Think**Like a Nurse** 15-6

- What do you do to keep yourself healthy?
- What do you do to treat minor illnesses when you do not want to see a healthcare provider?

What Are Health and Illness Practices?

In addition to knowing their values and beliefs, you need to know health practices of people in various cultural groups to maintain wellness. Think about the patients in the Meet Your Patients scenarios. As you consider the following questions, keep in mind that cultural health practices can be efficacious (helpful), neutral (neither helpful nor harmful), or dysfunctional (harmful) (Giger, 2016):

- Would you support or discourage Mr. Chan's daughter's request for a Chinese priest to come to his room and perform a ceremony to restore his harmony?

- Would you support Rosanna's dressing her child in a heavy coat and knit hat although it is quite warm outside?
- Do you think the ceremony or dress is harmful or helpful?

You should encourage practices that could be helpful and discourage those that are harmful.

KnowledgeCheck 15-4

- List three types of alternative healthcare that are delivered by formally trained providers as a part of the professional healthcare system.
- What are magico-religious belief systems?
- As a nurse, in which of the following cultural health practices would you support your client: efficacious, neutral, dysfunctional, uncertain? Why?
- Refer to the Meet Your Patients feature. Identify an efficacious practice.

 ## ThinkLike a Nurse 15-7

- What aspects of the indigenous and professional systems have you used for yourself or your family? Give examples.

Nursing and Other Professional Subcultures

The biomedical healthcare system in the United States is a culture with its own set of norms. That culture can be further divided into subcultures, such as those of physicians, nurses, or therapists. Nursing is the largest subculture within the healthcare culture. Leininger (1978) defines the **culture of nursing** as the learned and transmitted lifeways, values, symbols, patterns, and normative practices of members of the nursing profession that are not the same as those of the mainstream culture. The nursing subculture's beliefs and values have been formed in part by the society at large, which historically has been dominated by white Anglo-Saxon Protestants.

Nursing Values include, in addition to those listed in Table 15-1, silent suffering in response to pain, caring, nursing autonomy, and use of the nursing process. In this book, we add knowledge and critical thinking to that list. Although these values may not be consistently rewarded in practice, we believe that a steadily increasing number of nurses realize that nursing is "knowledge work"—the nurse's knowledge and thinking are essential to the well-being of patients.

As you become more socialized into the nursing culture, you should continue to examine professional values to see how strongly you identify with them and how they affect your work with patients. For example, suppose you value silent suffering in response to pain. If your client, a woman in very early labor is screaming and crying even though her contractions are very mild on palpation, you might be tempted to view her as a whiner. Be careful not to lose your ability to understand health and illness from the patient's point of view.

Review the case of Rosanna and José (Meet Your Patients). After a positive strep test, the primary care provider prescribes an antibiotic for José's fever and sore throat. You observe that Rosanna does not seem to be happy with the medicine, so you stress to her that it is important for her to give the medication immediately to make José better. On her way out of the clinic, Rosanna throws the prescription in the trash. Why do you think she threw away the prescription? (See Table 15-2.)

Some people of Mexican heritage believe that illness is caused by the body's imbalance of "hot" and "cold" (not related to temperature). This problem might have been prevented if you or the primary care provider had assessed Rosanna's health beliefs and practices and discussed with her treatment options for José. For example, if she considered his ear infection to be "hot," then the provider might have been able to explain that the prescribed medication would get rid of the heat and pain that José is experiencing from the infection.

This is an example of what can happen when healthcare providers are so rigidly grounded in the beliefs of the professional healthcare culture that they fail to recognize and understand the health beliefs and practices of their clients. Such rigidity is a barrier to culturally competent care.

KnowledgeCheck 15-5

How do the cultural norms of the North American healthcare system differ from those of other cultural groups? Refer to Tables 15-1 and 15-2 in this chapter as needed.

Traditional and Alternative Healing

You need to know how healers from various cultures cure and care for members of their group. All cultures think of their healthcare system and beliefs as "traditional." We use *traditional* in this chapter to refer to alternative beliefs, those that are not of the Western, North American, biomedical, or professional healthcare system (previously discussed). You have already learned about different *healthcare beliefs and practices* that clients may have (e.g., biomedical or scientific, holistic, magico-religious). The following section focuses on the types of *healing systems* that you may find in all cultures throughout the world.

Folk Medicine

Folk medicine, defined as the beliefs and practices that the members of a cultural group follow when they are ill, includes both self-treatment and use of folk healers (Andrews & Boyle, 2015). When you feel as if you're getting a cold or the flu, what do you do? If you said that you take vitamin C or eat chicken soup, then you are practicing folk medicine. You most likely do what your mother or some other relative did for you in similar situations. Knowledge of these treatments is passed down from generation to generation by oral, and sometimes written, tradition.

- *Folk medicine* often involves natural medicines (e.g., herbs, plants, minerals, animal substances).
- *Magico-religious folk medicine* involves the use of charms, holy words, rituals, and holy actions to prevent and treat illnesses (Spector, 2017).

Why would someone want to see a folk healer rather than a professional healthcare provider? People of other cultures may seek out folk healers because they speak their native language, share their values and beliefs, charge less money, are readily available, and visit the sick at home, or, simply, people perceive that the professional healing system cannot meet their needs.

Many folk healing traditions are guided not only by cultural practices but also by religious beliefs and rituals. Religious rituals are often associated with births (e.g., circumcision) and deaths (e.g., who is allowed to wash the body and prepare it for burial). **KEY POINT:** *Although there is a strong association between culture and religious beliefs, you should never assume that because your patient is a member of a certain culture, he will also be of a certain religion. You should always ask as a part of your cultural assessment.*

Table 15-2 ➤ Values and Health and Illness Beliefs and Practices for Selected Ethnocultural Groups in North America

GROUP	DOMINANT VALUES	HEALTH AND ILLNESS BELIEFS	HEALTH AND ILLNESS PRACTICES
Native American	Bonding to family or group Acceptance of nature (Mother Earth) Tradition Sharing Belief in a spiritual power Respect of elders	Health means living in harmony with nature. Surviving under difficult circumstances Body treated with respect Illness is associated with disharmony or evil spirits. Illness is caused by an action that should not have been performed.	Rituals and ceremonies Chanting Purification Meditation Herbs
Asian and Pacific Islander	Extended family Respect for elders Group orientation Subordination to authority Conformity Self-respect and self-control Love of the land	Health is a state of physical and spiritual harmony. Illness is the disharmony of basic principles: *yin* and *yang*.	Acupuncture Amulets Moxibustion Meditation Herbs
Black or African American	Family bonding Matrifocal Spiritual orientation Present oriented	Health is harmony with nature (mind, body, and spirit). Illness is the result of disharmony or failure to eat proper foods.	Prayer Laying on of hands Magic rituals Voodoo Herbs
Hispanic or Latino	Extended family Group emphasis Fatalistic Faith and spirituality	Health is good luck or a reward for good behavior, a gift from God. Illness is body imbalance (hot or cold, wet or dry) or punishment.	Prayer Belief in miracles Wearing of religious medals or amulets Religious relics in home Herbs and spices Rituals "Hot" and "cold" therapy
White or European American	Independence Individuality Wealth Comfort Cleanliness Achievement Youth and beauty	Health is a state of physical and emotional well-being. Illness is contagion or contamination that is hereditary, psychosomatic, or supernatural.	Biomedical care Home remedies Religious traditions Diet and exercise

Note: Most people in North America use a combination of biomedical and traditional (specific to their culture) healthcare practices.

Sources: Adapted from Andrews, M., & Boyle, J. (2015). *Transcultural concepts in nursing care* (7th ed.). Philadelphia, PA: Lippincott Williams & Wilkins; Giger, J. (2016). *Transcultural nursing: Assessment and intervention* (7th ed.). St. Louis, MO: C.V. Mosby; Munoz, C., & Luckmann, J. (Eds.). (2005). *Transcultural communication in healthcare* (2nd ed.). Clifton Park, NY: Thomson Delmar Learning; Purnell, L. (2013). *Transcultural health care: A culturally competent approach* (4th ed.). Philadelphia, PA: F.A. Davis; Spector, R. (2017). *Cultural diversity in health and illness* (9th ed.). Upper Saddle River, NJ: Pearson Education.

Complementary and Alternative Medicine

- **Complementary medicine** is the use of rigorously tested therapies *to complement* those of conventional (i.e., biomedical) medicine (Andrews & Boyle, 2015).

    Examples include chiropractic care, biofeedback, and use of certain supplements.

- **Alternative medicine,** in contrast, is defined as therapies used *instead of* conventional medicine and whose reliability has not been validated through clinical testing in the United States.

    Examples include iridology, aromatherapy, and magnet therapy.

Some complementary and alternative modalities (CAMs) are derived from the ancient and indigenous healthcare systems of people of other countries, such as traditional Chinese medicine and **ayurveda,** the traditional healthcare system of India. Certain CAMs require a healer specially trained in their use (e.g., chiropractic, reflexology, massage therapy). For a more thorough discussion of CAMs,

 Go to **Bonus Chapter 46, Holistic Healing**.

KnowledgeCheck 15-6

- What is folk medicine?
- What are some common folk medicine practices?
- Why might members of some cultural groups seek out the local folk healer rather than the conventional healthcare provider?

WHAT IS CULTURALLY COMPETENT CARE?

The terms *cultural awareness, cultural sensitivity,* and *cultural competence* are often used interchangeably; however, they are not the same.

- **Cultural awareness** refers to an appreciation of the external signs of diversity.

- **Cultural sensitivity** has more to do with personal attitudes and being careful not to say or do something that might be offensive to someone from a different culture.
- **Cultural competence** is achieved on a continuum ranging from incompetent to competent (Purnell, 2014). You cannot achieve cultural competence overnight because it is a developmental process.

As you gain more knowledge and awareness of the needs of individuals from various ethnocultural groups, you will move forward on the journey toward cultural competence. The following are four descriptions of culturally competent nursing practice:

American Nurses Association

The American Nurses Association's *Nursing: Scope and Standards of Practice* (2015) devotes an entire standard to promoting cultural competency. Standard 8 highlights that registered nurses should practice in a manner that is congruent with cultural diversity and inclusion to ensure culturally congruent practice.

Safe, Effective Nursing Care (SENC)

Several of the SENC competencies ensure culturally competent care. For example, the client-centered care competency recognizes that nurses provide care that shows respect for client values, religious beliefs, needs, and preferences. Understanding cultural needs and preferences ensures the implementation of interventions to promote client comfort and safety.

Purnell Model

The Purnell model for cultural competence (Fig. 15-7) stresses teamwork in providing culturally sensitive and competent care to improve outcomes for individuals, families, and communities (Purnell, 2014; Purnell & Paulanka, 2013). In the context of nursing, Purnell's model defines **cultural competence** as "adapting care to be congruent with the patient's culture" (Purnell, 2014, p. 5).

Safe, Effective Nursing Care

How Cultural Competency Improves Patient Outcomes

Chapter Key Concepts: Cultural Competency

SENC Competency: Goal-Directed Client-Centered Care

Full-Spectrum Model: The full-spectrum nursing model concept that is most pertinent is "doing": *Show respect for client values, religious beliefs, needs, and preferences.*

Background. Every client is entitled to healthcare that is respectful of his cultural beliefs and practices. The SENC competency of providing goal-directed client-centered care protects and promotes the dignity of the client. Culturally competent healthcare empowers the client and facilitates participation in healthcare decisions. Research found that patients who rated their provider as highly culturally skilled also had high ratings for processes of care (trust, respect, communication) (Michalopoulou, Falzarano, Butkus, et al., 2014). The provider was able to establish a good interpersonal relationship with the patient, which is the foundation for mutual goal setting. Consistently Kersey-Matusiak (2012) reports that cultural competency promotes

better nurse–patient communication. This contributes to a cultural partnership and sensitivity, which results in the following:

- ➤ Both nurse and patient better understand the disease process and treatment management.
- ➤ The patient is more likely to adhere to the treatment protocols.
- ➤ Patient outcomes are improved (Kersey-Matusiak, 2012).

Think about it:
What is the relationship between cultural competence and healthcare disparities?

How can cultural competence by healthcare providers impact patient outcomes?

Sources: Kersey-Matusiak, G. (2012). Culturally competent care: Are we there yet? *Nursing Management, 43*(4), 35–39; Michalopoulou, G., Falzarano, P., Butkus, M., et al. (2014). Linking cultural competence to functional life outcomes in mental health care settings. *Journal of the National Medical Association, 106*(1), 42–49.

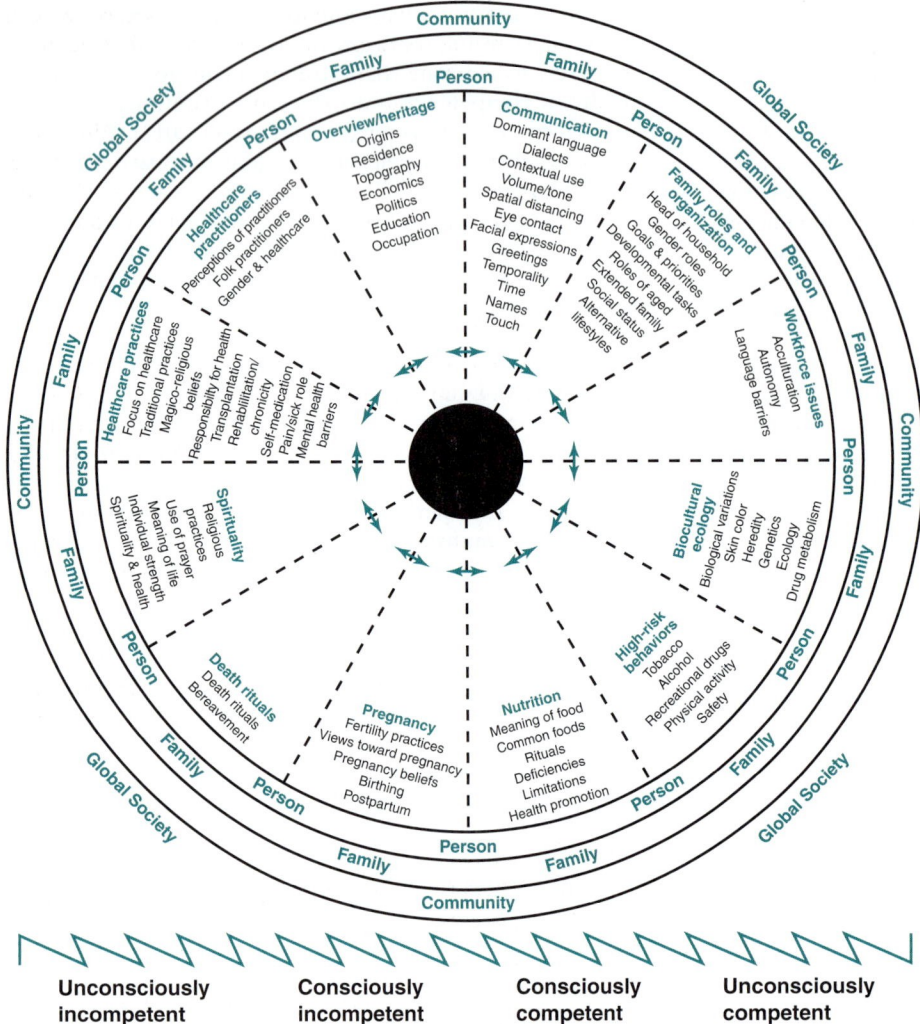

Unconsciously   Consciously   Consciously   Unconsciously
incompetent   incompetent   competent   competent

FIGURE 15-7 Purnell's model for cultural competence.

The model identifies levels of several levels of cultural competence. Think about the meaning of each level:

1. Unconscious incompetence—not being aware that you lack knowledge about another culture
2. Conscious incompetence—being aware that you lack knowledge about another culture
3. Conscious competence—learning about the client's culture, verifying generalizations about the culture (e.g., archetypes), and providing culture specific interventions
4. Unconscious competence—automatically providing culturally congruent care to clients of diverse cultures (Purnell, 2013)

Increasing one's consciousness of cultural diversity improves the possibilities for healthcare practitioners to provide culturally competent care.

Leininger

Although Madeline Leininger does not use the term *cultural competence,* her theory fits with that concept. The goal of her theory is to guide research that will assist nurses to provide *culturally congruent care* using her three modes of nursing care actions and decisions (to be explained later in the chapter). Nurses can achieve this goal by:

♥ **iCare** ▪ Discovering cultural care and caring beliefs, values, and practices
▪ Analyzing the similarities and differences of these beliefs among the different cultures

WHAT ARE SOME BARRIERS TO CULTURALLY COMPETENT CARE?

Your ability to provide culturally competent care may be hampered by various prejudices, attitudes, and language barriers. Self-knowledge and critical thinking are essential in helping you identify and manage them. You should avoid the following barriers in your practice:

- **Bias.** A lack of impartiality, one-sidedness; can be positive or negative.
- **Ethnocentrism.** The tendency of people to believe their own beliefs and values are right and that those of other cultures are wrong (or at least bizarre). This can cause your patient to feel that you disapprove of or don't understand or respect him.
- **Cultural stereotype.** The unsubstantiated belief that all people of a certain racial or ethnic group are alike in certain respects. A stereotype may be positive or negative.
  - **Prejudice.** Negative attitudes toward other people based on faulty and rigid stereotypes about race, gender, sexual orientation, status, and so on.
  - **Discrimination.** The behavioral manifestations of a prejudice (e.g., refusing to provide services or opportunities to certain racial or ethnic groups). Members of minority groups may still experience discrimination in housing, banking, and the job market.

Racism

Racism is a form of prejudice and discrimination based on the belief that (1) race is the principal determining factor of human traits and capabilities, and (2) racial differences produce an inherent superiority (or inferiority). The word *race* evokes powerful emotional responses for people who feel that they or their ancestors have been oppressed or exploited and equally for those who deny such a responsibility. In the United States, the history of discrimination against non-whites has created racial divisiveness. You must recognize that unconscious racism can play a major role in your ability to communicate with patients of other races.

Sexism

Sexism is the assumption that members of one sex are superior to those of the other sex. For example, assertiveness, a trait usually considered positive in men, is often viewed as aggressiveness and considered undesirable in women. Male nurses must also combat sexism, mainly the idea it is "unnatural" for men to engage in caring behaviors. Thus, male nurses may initially be rejected by their female peers and some patients.

Male chauvinism (assumption of male superiority) is common in many cultures and may be overt or subtle. When you have the opportunity to do so, observe a conversation between a male nurse and a male provider. You may note that the male nurse communicates more directly and uses more eye contact than female nurses do with this same provider. We are not assuming that all providers (or nurses) are chauvinistic; we are simply stating that you will probably be able to observe a different kind of interchange among some professionals between males and females. The assumption of equality (or inequality) changes the way people communicate.

Language Barriers

More than 60 million people in the United States speak a language other than English at home (Ryan, 2013). Language barriers, such as foreign languages, dialects, regionalisms (words or pronunciation particular to a specific region), street talk, and jargon, will obviously affect your ability to communicate with clients.

Recall Mr. Salvatore in the Meet Your Patients scenario. Suppose he has a brain tumor and you need his consent for immediate surgery even though he and his family do not speak English. You will need a certified interpreter. However, he may have difficulty understanding Mr. Salvatore completely if a different dialect or slang is used. In this case, you should review the policies of your healthcare facility to obtain additional resources. If there are no such policies, you would have

---

Toward Evidence-Based Practice

Govere, L., Fioravanti, M., & Tuite, P. (2016). Increasing the cultural competence levels of undergraduate nursing students. *Journal of Nursing Education, 55*(3), 155–159. Retrieved from http://dx.doi.org/10.3928/01484834-20160216-06

Researchers evaluated the effectiveness of several learning modules on improving the cultural competence level of undergraduate nursing students. The online modules were completed over a 2-week period. Students' competence level increased, from lowest to highest, as follows:

Before the modules: 89% culturally aware, 11% culturally competent, 0% culturally proficient
After the modules: 22% culturally aware, 67% culturally competent, 11% culturally proficient

Long, T. (2016). Influence of international service learning on nursing students' self-efficacy towards cultural competence. *Journal of Cultural Diversity, 23*(1), 28–33.

The researcher examined the effect of an international immersion learning experience on cultural competence of 16 associate degree nursing students. Results showed a significant improvement in self-efficacy, knowledge, and confidence of students toward working with a Hispanic ethnic group. Students without prior training in cultural competence had the highest improvement in cultural competence.

Witt, A. (2016). *The impact of cultural encounters on the cultural competence of baccalaureate nursing students.*

Retrieved from ProQuest Dissertations & Theses Global. (Order No. 1796375574).

In a study involving 453 baccalaureate nursing students, results revealed that students who had (1) a previous course in cultural competency, (2) a previous degree, (3) traveled internationally, or (4) lived abroad had higher levels of cultural competence. In addition, senior students scored higher on cultural awareness and knowledge. The researcher noted that cultural encounters had a significant impact on cultural competence.

Instructions: Staff nurses have expressed concerns that nursing students are not incorporating cultural differences in the patients' plans of care. They have asked that students receive more education on cultural care in their nursing program of study. Answer the following questions:

1. Which studies or results support the belief that education and learning activities on culture will improve cultural competence?

2. What is the importance of encounters with clients from various cultures on acquiring cultural competency?

3. Which study provides the best evidence for including cultural education in the nursing program of study?

 Go to Davis Advantage, Resources, Chapter 15, **Toward Evidence-Based Practice, Suggested Responses.**

Focused Assessment

Obtaining Minimum Cultural Information

You should obtain at least this much cultural information from every client. For some, you may need a more in-depth assessment.

➤ Begin the interview with open-ended questions, such as the following:

I would like to know more about your family.

Who will be able to help you when you go home?

What do you do to help keep yourself well?

➤ When you and the client are comfortable, be sure to ask a question such as, "What concerns you the most about your illness and treatment?" This allows you to focus on the individual rather than just on his culture.

➤ You will not need to perform an in-depth cultural assessment on every patient, but you will need to recognize situations in which this is needed. Lipson and Meleis (1985) suggest that the following minimum information is important:

Language(s) spoken; proficiency in the language of the host country	➤ What language(s) do you speak? ➤ Are you comfortable speaking [English], or would you like to have an interpreter?
Length of time client has been here; where client was raised	➤ Where were you raised? ➤ How long have you lived here?
Ethnic affiliation and identity	➤ With what racial and ethnic group(s) do you identify? ➤ How closely do you identify with the values of those groups?
Usual religious practices	➤ What religion do you practice, if any? ➤ Are there any special beliefs, rituals, or practices you want us to be aware of?
Nonverbal communication style	➤ You will need to observe the patient and draw on your theoretical knowledge of the patient's cultural group for this information.
Family roles, primary decision maker	➤ Who is in your family? ➤ What is your role in your family? ➤ Who makes most of the decisions? ➤ How are decisions made in your family? ➤ Whom should I talk to for decisions about your healthcare?
Social support in the new country	➤ Do you have family and friends here? ➤ Whom can you go to when you need help? ➤ Where do you work? ➤ Will you need any help with your healthcare expenses?

Sources: Giger, J. (2016). *Transcultural nursing: Assessment and intervention* (7th ed.). St. Louis, MO: C.V. Mosby; Spector, R. (2017). *Cultural diversity in health and illness* (9th ed.). Upper Saddle River, NJ: Pearson Education; Suzuki, L.A., & Ponterotto, J. G. (2007). *Handbook of multicultural assessment: Clinical, psychological, and educational applications* (3rd ed.). San Francisco, CA: Jossey-Bass.

---

to resort temporarily to nonverbal language and pictures to communicate.

KEY POINT: *If a consent issue is involved, the hospital must ensure adequate resources to comply with informed consent requirements.*

Street Talk, Slang, and Jargon These vocabularies can be as challenging as a foreign language. Their meanings change, and not everyone has the same interpretations of a word or a phrase. For example, the word *bad* can mean "bad" or "good," depending on context. African American Vernacular English (AAVE), also known as Ebonics, has in the past, been spoken primarily by African Americans, but many youths of other races now embrace AAVE as a way to connect with the street culture. Texting can be another form of jargon. Likewise, not everyone understands the abbreviations used in texting.

Healthcare Jargon Words or expressions used by a subculture, including nursing, are called jargon. In healthcare, we

often use our own peculiar terminology and abbreviations, which our clients do not understand. For example, many patients will not know what you mean if you ask, "Have you voided today?" Even worse, patients may hesitate to ask for clarification because they do not want to admit their lack of understanding of your words.

Other Barriers

- *Lack of knowledge* about the cultural and ethnic values, beliefs, and behaviors of people within their community is not unusual among healthcare providers. It can cause them to misinterpret a client's behaviors.
- *Emotional responses,* such as fear and distrust (both yours and the client's), can arise when members of different cultural groups meet.
- *Self-knowledge* is essential in removing barriers and helps you to effectively communicate with your clients.

Focused Assessment

Cultural Assessment Using the Transcultural Assessment Model

Assess information listed in the following categories:

Cultural Uniqueness

➤ Cultural and ethnic identification
➤ Place of birth
➤ Time in country

Communication

➤ Voice quality
➤ Pronunciation and enunciation
➤ Use of silence
➤ Use of nonverbal communication
➤ Touch
➤ Spoken language

Space

➤ Degree of comfort
➤ Distance in conversations
➤ Definition of space
➤ Body movement

Social Organization

➤ Normal state of health
➤ Marital status
➤ Number of children
➤ Parents living or deceased
➤ Friends
➤ Work
➤ Leisure

Time

➤ Orientation to time
➤ View of time
➤ Physiochemical reaction to time

Environmental Control

➤ Locus of control
➤ Value orientation
➤ Health and illness beliefs

Biological Variations

➤ Physical assessment (including body structure, skin color, skin discoloration, hair color and distribution, other visible physical characteristics, weight, height, lab variances)
➤ Susceptibility to illness
➤ Nutritional preferences
➤ Psychological characteristics

Other

In addition to the Giger and Davidhizar categories, obtain information about the following:
➤ Educational experiences (formal and informal)
➤ Family patterns of healthcare
➤ Family role and function
➤ Healthcare beliefs and practices (folk and professional)
➤ Religious practices and beliefs
➤ Social networks
➤ Values orientation

Source: Adapted from Giger, J. (2016). _Transcultural nursing: Assessment and intervention_ (7th ed.). St. Louis, MO: C.V. Mosby.

KnowledgeCheck 15-7

- Define _cultural competence._
- How do the barriers of ethnocentrism and language impede nursing care of diverse populations?

PracticalKnowledge
knowing **how**

Each phase of the nursing process presents an opportunity to provide culturally sensitive, congruent, and competent care. You must establish rapport before beginning data collection.

ASSESSMENT NP

Various regulating bodies (e.g., The Joint Commission and the Office of Minority Health) require healthcare organizations to integrate cultural data into a patient's health records. Cultural assessment consists of an interview and a physical assessment. When you perform a cultural assessment, you should gather data directly from your client, but if this is not possible you may ask for help from a friend or family member of the client. **KEY POINT:** _When an interpreter is needed, because of privacy concerns and legal guidelines you should not rely on a family member._

The Health History

Some information you obtain from a patient's health history may be sensitive or personal. Regardless of culture, to encourage patients to talk about themselves you must convey empathy, show respect, establish trust, listen actively, and provide appropriate feedback (Andrews, 2014; Cole & Bird, 2013). Ask open-ended questions when beginning a cultural assessment.

✚ Always ask clients about their use of alternative medicine and folk remedies so their effects on traditional biomedical medications and treatments can be evaluated. Some remedies may interfere with traditional treatments; others can be dangerous. Many people use folk remedies, but they may be reluctant to tell you because they fear ridicule or disapproval.

You will not need to perform an in-depth cultural assessment on every client, but you will need to recognize situations in which this is needed. The two accompanying Focused Assessment boxes will guide you in obtaining the information needed for a focused cultural assessment.

Physical Assessment

Physical assessment may reveal biocultural variations. To assess and evaluate clients accurately, you need to know the normal physiological variations among healthy members of selected populations (e.g., body proportions, vital signs, laboratory values, general appearance, skin, musculoskeletal system, and illness).

- ✚ **Assessing the Skin.** Knowledge of biocultural variations is essential in assessing for pallor, cyanosis, jaundice, erythema, rashes, and petechiae in dark-skinned clients. You must be more observant and detailed in your assessment. For helpful suggestions and for more information about assessing the skin, see Clinical Insight 15-1 and Chapter 35.

- **KEY POINT:** *Assessing for Pain. Culture influences the patient's responses to pain. Because pain and comfort are subjective, you need to quantify them as objectively as possible by using a pain measurement scale. It is essential to investigate the meaning of pain to each patient and his view of acceptable ways to express or cope with pain.*

  For descriptions of some cultural responses to pain, see Clinical Insight 15-2.

Cultural Assessment Models and Tools

Some agencies have special tools for in-depth cultural assessments. If yours does not, you can structure your assessments using any culture model. For example, you may want to search the Internet for the following models:

- Purnell's Domains of Culture
- Transcultural Nursing Assessment Guide (Andrews & Boyle, 2015)
- Leninger's Sunrise Model Depicting the Theory of Cultural Care, Diversity, and Universality
- Transcultural Assessment Model (Giger & Davidhizar, 2008)
- Spector's Heritage Assessment Tool. Unlike the preceding tools, which assess culture specifics, Spector's tool assesses heritage *consistency:* the degree to which a person's lifestyle reflects his traditional culture (country of origin, race, or ethnic group). This assessment tool also reveals the degree to which the client still identifies with his cultural origins.

ANALYSIS/NURSING DIAGNOSIS NP

There are no NANDA-I diagnoses that specifically address culture. However, cultural factors can be the etiology of various problems. Any of the NANDA-I diagnostic labels can be used for patients of any culture, provided that the defining characteristics are present. Some possible examples include the following:

- Risk for Imbalanced Nutrition: Less Than Body Requirements might apply to a patient who is hospitalized and cannot obtain foods prepared in the traditional manner of his ethnic group.
- Impaired Parenting could occur if the patient's traditional methods of discipline are not acceptable or appropriate in the dominant culture.
- Powerlessness might occur when the patient is unable to make healthcare personnel understand the importance of his cultural rituals or practices.
- Impaired Verbal Communication is sometimes used for patients who do not speak or understand the nurse's language.
- Ineffective Health Management might be used for clients and/or caregivers who do not follow an agreed on

health-promoting or therapeutic plan. The plan may be inconsistent with the patient's belief.

> *Example:* Suppose that a 60-year-old woman who works as a hotel housekeeper is repeatedly admitted to your hospital for uncontrolled hypertension. You diagnose Ineffective Health Management because she does not take her prescribed medication. But do you know that the cost of the antihypertensive medication does not fit into her budget? Or perhaps she believes that herbs, diet, and other practice will decrease her blood pressure.

Based on cultural norms or differences, you should know that nonadherence is a defining characteristic of *Ineffective Health Management*. This requires you to examine the cultural impact of care.

The preceding example illustrates the concern that standardized nursing diagnoses are not culturally sensitive—that is, they may not apply accurately to patients who are not from the dominant culture. Nursing diagnoses should describe responses that *patients* see as problematic. A nurse and patient who are from different cultures will likely have different perceptions of health and illness, which can lead to misdiagnosis. The nurse may either diagnose a problem that doesn't exist for the patient or diagnose a real problem but fail to describe it accurately (Wilkinson, 2012).

The following are a few NANDA-I nursing diagnoses that could be interpreted differently by people from different cultures. Undoubtedly there are others.

Acute Pain	Impaired Social Interaction
Anxiety	Ineffective Coping
Decisional Conflict	Ineffective Role Performance
Readiness for Enhanced Breastfeeding	Ineffective Health Management

KEY POINT: *The point is to use all labels carefully and to validate nursing diagnoses with the patient to be sure that the statement describes her health status as* **she** *sees it.*

PLANNING OUTCOMES/EVALUATION NP

The outcomes you choose, whether standardized or individualized, depend on the nursing diagnoses you have identified. If the diagnoses are culturally sensitive, the outcomes should be as well. However, you must involve the patient in order to be certain. For example, suppose you and a dying patient agree that her diagnosis is Acute Pain. Nevertheless, your goals will be different if you want her to be free from pain, whereas she wants to stay alert enough to interact with her family, even if it means enduring some pain. When your cultures differ, it is even more important to validate the goals with the patient. Some individualized goal/outcome statements associated with cultural differences might include the following:

- Agrees to take prescribed analgesic (pain medication) before bedtime and after family leaves for the evening.
- Talks to her spiritual adviser about conflicts between the treatment plan and her religious beliefs.
- Freely shares information about folk practices and OTC medications with the provider.

PLANNING INTERVENTIONS/ IMPLEMENTATION NP

To plan culturally appropriate care, you should become familiar with the cultural groups that are dominant in your area and that you will encounter in your nursing practice.

NIC standardized interventions related to culture and the provision of culturally competent care include the following examples:

Mutual Goal Setting (for Ineffective Health Management)

Self-Responsibility Facilitation (for Decision-making, Readiness for Enhanced)

Culture Brokerage (for Comfort, Impaired)

Culture Brokerage is defined as "the deliberate use of culturally competent strategies to bridge or mediate between the patient's culture and the biomedical healthcare system" (Bulechek, Butcher, Dochterman, et al., 2013, p. 136).

Individualized nursing activities and focused assessments are important for all patients. However, patients from different cultural and ethnic groups may have unique needs that require culturally competent care.

Nursing Strategies for Providing Culturally Competent Care

You will need information about clients' cultural values, beliefs, and practices to identify and implement the interventions that will support these practices (Wilkinson, 2011). For example:

- When you are teaching about a specific treatment regimen ordered by the provider, you should find out whether it conflicts with the patient's folk beliefs or alternative treatments. If so, suggest modifications.
- Remember to identify educational methods that are most appropriate for your client's needs (e.g., translated materials and/or diagrams) and to make community referrals as necessary.
- When caring for patients from vulnerable populations, it is important that you focus on their strengths and resources, not exclusively on their difficulties and risks.

KnowledgeCheck 15-8

- Describe, in general, how the nursing process can help you provide culturally competent care.
- How can nursing diagnoses cause bias in planning care for patients from different cultures?

How Should I Respond to a Client's Cultural Health Practices?

Theorists describe different situations in which nursing decisions and actions are needed regarding a client's cultural health practices (Giger, 2016; Leininger, 1991; McFarland & Wehbe-Alamah, 2014). See Table 15-3.

Negotiation The client's perspective may differ from yours about the effects of a particular practice. Negotiation acknowledges that gap. **KEY POINT:** *You must negotiate when folk or traditional practices might be harmful to the client.*

Example: The nurse negotiates with the client to continue seeing the *curandero* but also to come to the clinic every 6 weeks to have his blood pressure checked. If the client refuses all nursing or biomedical interventions, the avenue is still open to continue monitoring the client to identify changes in his health status. If a health crisis occurs, it may be possible to renegotiate the care.

Repatterning/Restructuring This occurs when you attempt to change your actions or the client's lifestyle (Leininger, 1991; McFarland & Wehbe-Alamah, 2014). You would support and encourage the client to greatly modify his behaviors and to adopt new, different, and beneficial health behaviors while still respecting his cultural values and beliefs.

Example 1: Change in nurse's actions. When the client refuses to take the prescribed pain medication, the nurse uses massage, distraction, and other nonpharmacological techniques to help relieve his pain.

Table 15-3 ➤ Possible Effects of a Patient's Cultural Health Practices

THE EFFECTS ARE:	EXAMPLE	NURSING APPROACH
Efficacious (helpful)	Family or friends bring ethnic foods that are appropriate for the client's prescribed diet.	Encourage practices that will likely improve client health and help her preserve cultural values related to health.
Neutral (neither helpful nor harmful)	Some people associate good health with eating properly and fasting to cure disease. Some may treat illness with prayers or simple foods such as dates, honey, salt, and olive oil (Purnell, 2013).	There should be no harm in allowing a patient to continue a neutral health practice. You would not want to interfere with these neutral practices.
Uncertain (unknown by you)	A client drinks a daily smoothie that consists of certain herbs and spices, such as ginger, cinnamon, and basil, for "good health."	You can neither encourage nor discourage these practices until you obtain more information about them. Do this as soon as possible.
Dysfunctional (harmful)	A client may refuse to give prescribed medication to her child.	Discourage folk practices that may cause harm. In such instances, you should support and enable the client to adapt to biomedical therapies (repatterning/restructuring) or negotiate with the client to achieve satisfying outcomes.

Example 2: Modification of the client's behaviors. A client refuses to see a biomedical doctor for her family's needs. However, when the folk healer is unsuccessful in treating her child's illness and the child becomes critically ill, the nurse convinces the client to bring the child to the emergency department.

How Do I Communicate With Clients Who Speak a Different Language?

Communicating with clients who do not speak your language can be especially challenging. The Internet and computer software allow patients to type information in their native language and translate it into English as a way to communicate with providers. However, the best way to provide culturally competent care to such clients is to use a professional medical interpreter or translator. Each must meet predetermined standards to participate in translation services.

You should review your facility's policies and procedures for translation resources. The Joint Commission views communication as an essential aspect of patient care (The Joint Commission, 2010). For guidelines additional guidelines, see Clinical Insight 15-3.

Culturally and Linguistically Appropriate Services (CLAS) Standards

CLAS standards promote culturally and linguistically appropriate services to ensure that care is respectful of and responsive to the person's cultural and linguistic needs. **KEY POINT:** *Healthcare facilities must provide language assistance services by, in order of preference, bilingual staff, face-to face interpretation by trained persons, or telephone interpreters. Healthcare interpreters should be used to obtain informed consent and to assist the patient to understand the treatment plan* (Office of Minority Health, 2013). For a complete listing of the CLAS standards,

 Go to the document published by the Office of Minority Health at http://minorityhealth.hhs.gov/assets/pdf/checked/finalreport.pdf

Developing Strategies

There are several strategies for you to consider and many resources to help you develop strategies specific to various cultural groups (Box 15-1). Consider the following as you move forward on your journey toward cultural competence:

Reflect and Know Yourself

- Understand your own cultural values and practices and appreciate how they may differ from those held by people of other cultures.
- Consider how your own biases about people and groups may affect the care you provide.
- Learn from your mistakes. Remember, a mistake twice is a decision!

Keep Learning

- Learn as much as you can about the cultural groups in your community and work area.
- Study nursing theories and principles pertaining to culture.
- Take advantage of every opportunity to interact with persons from different cultural groups.

Accommodate and Negotiate

- Make an effort to incorporate beliefs and practices from various cultures into your nursing care and teaching materials.
- Encourage helpful or neutral cultural practices, and discourage those that are dysfunctional (harmful).
- Suggest alternatives to harmful practices.
- Accommodate cultural dietary practices when possible. For inpatients, some dietary departments can make special foods, and you can encourage families to bring food from home. In all situations, help patients and families adapt cultural foods to therapeutic diets.

BOX 15-1 ■ Being Considerate of Cultural Specifics

Consider Verbal and Nonverbal Communication.

- Know, or find out, whether touch (e.g., a handshake) is expected or prohibited.
- Know, or find out, whether eye contact is expected or avoided. Avoiding eye contact, for some, is a sign of respect.
- Ask the client how he wishes to be addressed.
- Know, or find out, the ways people welcome each other.

Consider the Person's Need for Personal Space.

- Know the person's cultural and religious customs regarding touching and contact.
- Know the usual comfortable distance for conversing in the client's culture.

Consider Body Language.

- Gestures that are acceptable in one culture may be taboo in another. Know what is acceptable to the client.
- Be aware that smiling does not universally indicate friendliness.

Consider Time Orientation.

- Tell clients when you are coming and be on time.
- Avoid surprise visits.

- Share your own expectations about time.
- Ask clients what they expect regarding time, appointments, and so on.
- Be sure you know the times for and meanings of the client's religious and ethnic holidays.

Consider Social Organization.

- Know which person in the family is the leader or decision maker.
- Know what dates are important and whether gifts are expected or not.
- Know how special events, such as births and funerals, are celebrated, whether certain colors have meaning, and what the expected rituals are.

Consider the Person's Perspective on Environmental Control.

- Find out what the client's health traditions and practices are.
- Know whether the person believes she has any ability to "change things."
- Know the general influence of the culture on perception and tolerance of pain.
- Know what foods are forbidden, what foods may or may not be eaten together, and what and how utensils are used.

Collaborate

- Work with the folk medicine practitioner in the interest of the client.
- Advocate for all of your clients, but especially for those not from the dominant culture.
- Consider the cultural role of the family member who makes the primary decisions. To ignore this person is to doom your interventions to failure.

Respect

- Consider each client as a unique individual, influenced but not defined by his culture.
- Respect your clients regardless of cultural background and never force, pressure, manipulate, or coerce them to participate in care that conflicts with their values and beliefs.

This is by no means an exhaustive list. Most likely, you can think of other strategies. It may help you to "take a trip to BALI":

Be aware of your own cultural heritage.

Appreciate that the client is unique: influenced, but not defined by his culture.

Learn about the client's cultural group.

Incorporate the client's cultural values/behaviors into the care plan.

KnowledgeCheck 15-9

- List five factors to consider to help you develop strategies to become more culturally competent.
- What does the acronym "BALI" stand for?

How Can I Become Culturally Competent?

Of course you can't become culturally competent just by reading. Recall that people acquire cultural competence gradually, progressing through stages.

Theoretical knowledge can increase your awareness and appreciation of cultural differences, but you can achieve cultural competence only if you are motivated and even then only by interacting with people from different cultures (Musolino, Burkhalter, Crookston, et al., 2010). Carballeira (1997) sums up this process with the LIVE and LEARN model for culturally competent family services:

Like		Listen
Inquire		Evaluate
Visit	and	Acknowledge
Experience		Recommend
		Negotiate

KEY POINT: *If there were only one intervention you could use to improve your cultural competence, it should be to routinely ask patients what matters most to them in their illness and treatment.* No matter how busy you are, you can find time to do that. You can then use that information to incorporate cultural needs into the client plan of care.

ThinkLike a Nurse 15-8

What kind of knowledge do you need to become culturally competent (theoretical, practical, self, ethical)? Explain your answer. (Refer to Chapter 2 to review types of knowledge, if necessary.)

CLINICALREASONING

The questions and exercises in this section allow you to practice the kind of thinking you will use as a full-spectrum nurse. Critical-thinking questions usually have more than one correct answer, so we do not provide "correct answers" for these features. It is more important to develop your nursing judgment than to just cover content. You will learn by discussing the questions with your peers. If you are still unsure, see the Davis Advantage chapter resources for suggested responses.

Caring for the Nguyens

Review the initial assessment of Nam Nguyen in the front of the book, immediately preceding Chapter 1.

A. How might the Nguyens' cultural heritage affect their health beliefs?

B. What factors would you want to consider when performing a cultural assessment of the Nguyen family?

Applying the **Full-Spectrum Nursing Model**_____

PATIENT SITUATION

Mrs. Vasquez, a 70-year-old Mexican American woman, has diabetes mellitus and has come to the hospital because of a sore on her lower leg that will not heal. Mrs. Vasquez, a widow, cares for herself at home. She speaks only broken English and has some difficulty understanding your questions. After great effort on your part, you determine that she has missed the last appointment with her diabetes specialist because she has no transportation, so she has just been putting a dressing on the sore. Mrs. Vasquez tells you that she loves to see her grandchildren, who visit often, and that she enjoys cooking and eating Mexican food. She also says that she believes she is sick because she has not pleased God. However, God is a source of comfort and assurance to her. She prays and often has rosary beads in her hand.

THINKING

1. *Theoretical Knowledge (Recall of Facts and Principles):* List six important culture specifics.
2. *Critical Thinking (Application of Knowledge):* Based on your theoretical knowledge, what are your expectations about communicating with Mrs. Vasquez?
3. *Critical Thinking (Compare and Contrast):* Compare your expectations with the actual data you have about her ability to communicate.

DOING

4. *Nursing Process (Assessment):* What are some pertinent cultural data that you should assess for Mrs. Vasquez?
5. *Nursing Process (Analysis/Diagnosis):* Which nursing diagnosis do you think would be best for planning Mrs. Vasquez's care? (Recall that the etiology should suggest your nursing interventions, and the diagnostic label should suggest the expected patient outcome.) Explain your reasoning.
   - Ineffective Health Management (not adhering to clinic appointments) r/t lack of transportation
   - Impaired Skin Integrity r/t self-treatment of ulcer
   - Ineffective Health Management (not adhering to clinic appointments) r/t beliefs about God and illness

CARING

6. *Self-Knowledge:* What areas of commonality do you have with Mrs. Vasquez, around which you might form a caring relationship?
7. *Self-Knowledge:* Do you agree with Mrs. Vasquez that illness may be caused by displeasing God?
8. *Ethical Knowledge:* Suppose you do not agree with Mrs. Vasquez that she is ill because she has displeased God. Discuss whether you would explain to her that this is most likely not true and then teach her about the cause of diabetic ulcers.

 Go To Davis Advantage, Resources, Chapter 15, **Applying the Full-Spectrum Nursing Model Suggested Responses.**

PracticalKnowledge
clinical application

CLINICAL INSIGHTS

Clinical Insight 15-1 ➤ **Assessing for Biological Variations**

People differ genetically and physiologically. Some biological variations create susceptibility to certain diseases and injuries. The following are examples:

Body Build and Structure

- 12% of Native Americans have 25 vertebrae instead of 24, which relates to an increased number of back problems.
- Black and white men are on average about 3.5 inches taller than Asian American men and 2 inches taller than Mexican American men.
- Lower socioeconomic status increases the likelihood of obesity.

Skin Color

- Darker skin challenges you to be more observant when assessing skin color changes (e.g., when assessing oxygenation or skin rashes). Obtain a baseline skin color by asking a family member or someone who knows the patient well.
- To assess for oxygenation and cyanosis in dark-skinned people, examine the sclera, buccal mucosa, tongue, lips, nailbeds, palms of the hands, and soles of the feet.
- To assess for jaundice in Asians, examine the sclera.

Vital Signs

- The average systolic blood pressure of black men between the ages of 35 and 65 is 5 mm Hg higher than that of European American men of the same age.

Laboratory Tests

- Native Americans, Hispanic Americans, and Japanese Americans, on average, have higher blood glucose levels than do whites.
- Bone density is greater in whites than in Chinese, Japanese, and Eskimos.

Susceptibility to Disease

- Blacks have a higher incidence of hypertension and sickle cell anemia than do other groups.

- Asian Americans have a higher incidence of tuberculosis compared with the white population.
- Blacks, Native Americans, and Mexican Americans are more likely to have diabetes mellitus than their white counterparts.

Nutritional Variations

- All groups demonstrate food preferences.
- Soy sauce, used in many Asian foods, is high in sodium.
- There is a high incidence of diabetes mellitus in areas where sugar cane is a major crop.

Enzymatic and Genetic Variations and Body Secretions

- Lactose intolerance, caused by a deficiency of the enzyme lactase, is more commonly seen in blacks, Native Americans, and Asians.

Drug Metabolism

- Native Americans and Asians are more likely to experience facial flushing and palpitations after ingesting alcohol.
- Blacks metabolize alcohol, nicotine, antihypertensives, and beta blockers differently from European Americans; they are more susceptible to side effects of haloperidol and tricyclic antidepressants; and they respond better to diuretic therapy than do whites.
- Asian Americans tend to experience more gastrointestinal side effects from opiates, even though the analgesic effect is less pronounced.
- Chinese Americans are more sensitive to the cardiovascular effects of propranolol; they have increased absorption of antipsychotics, antihypertensives, and some narcotics.
- Recall that most drug studies in the past were normed on European Americans, so "variations" refer to differences from those norms.

Practice Resources

Andrews, M. M., & Boyle, J. S. (2015); Giger, J. (2016); Purnell, L. (2013); Purnell, L., & Paulanka, B. (2008); Spector, R. (2017); Suzuki, L., & Ponterotto, J. (2007).

Clinical Insight 15-2 ➤ Pain Perception in Selected Cultural Groups

The following are some general cultural beliefs about and responses to pain. Remember that these are only a starting point (archetypes) and that you must never stereotype a person on the basis of culture. Assess each person individually.

Cultural Group	Pain Perception and Responses
Black heritage	Depending on the religion, may believe that pain is inevitable and must be endured; therefore, may tolerate a great deal of pain. Depending on the religion, may seek prayers and the laying on of hands for pain relief. May see pain as a test of faith. May see pain as the only sign of illness or disease, so may not follow medical therapies (e.g., for hypertension) if pain is absent.
European American heritage, New England subculture	(These are chronic pain responses.) Copes by working and keeping busy. Stoicism; lack of expressiveness and behavioral pain response, including little wincing and groaning. Pain is viewed as a biological abnormality that can be treated and lived with; may be angry with care providers if treatment is ineffective. *Polish American subgroup*: Strong tendency for nonexpressiveness.
Arab heritage	View pain as unpleasant and something to be controlled. Expect medical science to be able to relieve their suffering. Express pain openly with family members, less so with health professionals. This may cause the nurse to evaluate pain relief as adequate even though the family may be demanding more medication for the patient.
Chinese heritage	Pain expression is similar to traditional U.S. culture, but description of pain may be different (i.e., described more often as "dull" and "diffuse"). Use external pain relief methods, such as massage, oils, warmth, and relaxation.
Filipino heritage	View pain as a part of living an honorable life or as an opportunity to atone for sins. Commonly tolerate severe pain, with stoic acceptance. May not complain of pain or ask for interventions.
Irish heritage	Value stoic response to pain. Ignore, deny, or minimize pain. Delay seeking treatment.
Italian heritage	Verbalization of pain is common and acceptable, even with chronic pain. Women are especially likely to report and express pain. Expect immediate treatment for pain.
Japanese heritage	It is a virtue and a matter of family honor to bear pain without expressing it. There may be taboos against use of narcotics for pain relief. May be more accepting of analgesics if reassured that pain control enhances healing.
Jewish heritage	Verbalization of pain is common and acceptable. Knowing the reason for pain is as important as obtaining relief.
Mexican heritage	View pain as the will of God or a part of life. May view pain as punishment for immoral behavior. May view enduring pain as a sign of strength. May endure pain longer and report it less frequently than other groups, or may express vocally with groaning and crying out. May delay seeking help for pain, hoping it will go away. May interpret pain as a loss of manhood or provider role.

Clinical Insight 15-2 ➤ Pain Perception in Selected Cultural Groups—cont'd

Navajo Indian heritage	View pain as a part of life. Do not express pain openly. May hide the intensity of pain. May not request pain medication. May prefer herbal medications for pain.
Puerto Rican heritage	Loud and outspoken expression of pain is not an exaggeration but a socially learned coping mechanism. May experience low self-esteem because of pain. Older or rural people may not be able to interpret pain-rating scales. Most prefer oral or intravenous analgesics to intramuscular or rectal routes. Many use herbal teas, heat, and prayer to manage pain.

Practice Resources

Andrews, M., & Boyle, J. (2015); Bates, M. S. (1996); Campbell, C., & Edwards, R. (2012); Giger, J. (2016); Giger, J., & Davidhizar, R. (2008); Purnell, L. (2013); Spector, R. (2017); Todd, K. (1996); Zborowski, M. (1952).

Clinical Insight 15-3 ➤ Communicating With Clients Who Speak a Different Language

When possible, use a qualified interpreter or a translator.

■ A **translator** merely restates into the targeted language.
■ An **interpreter** is specially trained to provide the meaning behind spoken words from one language to another. An interpreter can serve as a cultural broker by conveying the client's responses to questions, and by providing general information about the client's culture (Munoz & Luckmann, 2005; Purnell, 2014).
■ Because of confidentiality issues, do not use family or friends, especially a child or spouse, as interpreters except if requested by the patient.

Resources

■ Explore online translation services.
■ Download translation apps.
■ Use Communication Access Realtime Translation (CART).

When using any type of interpreter, it is important to do the following:

■ Avoid using an interpreter who is socially or politically incompatible with the client (e.g., you would not ask an Israeli to interpret for a Palestinian).
■ Be aware of gender and age differences. (It usually is preferable to have an interpreter of the same gender as the client.)
■ Have the interpreter spend some time alone with the patient.
■ Ask the interpreter to interpret the words used by the healthcare provider as closely as possible, except where literal translation might be offensive or misunderstood. In such cases, an interpreter (as compared with a translator)

would provide the meaning of your words in terms acceptable to the client.

■ Do not use metaphors ("happy as a clam") or medical jargon.
■ Observe nonverbal communication (e.g., body language) when the client is listening and talking to the interpreter.
■ Address your questions to the client, not the interpreter.
■ Maintain eye contact with both the client and interpreter.
■ Speak slowly and distinctly, facing the client; do not speak loudly.
■ Ask one question at a time; allow time for interpretation and response from the client before asking another question.
■ Use active rather than passive voice (e.g., say, "The doctor will see you tomorrow" rather than "You will be seen by the doctor tomorrow").
■ Be aware that many clients can understand more English words than they can express.
■ Have health education materials translated into the client's language or have an interpreter audiotape or videotape instructions.

If there is no one available to interpret for you:

In addition to the preceding strategies, you should do the following (Munoz & Luckmann, 2005; Purnell, 2014):

■ Greet the client with respect. Greet the person formally, using Mr., Ms., and so forth, until given permission to do otherwise. People in some groups consider it disrespectful to use a person's first name.
■ Identify the client's primary language, and use any words that you are familiar with in her language to show that you are trying to communicate.

(Continued)

Clinical Insight 15-3 ➤ **Communicating With Clients Who Speak a Different Language—cont'd**

- Use the Internet or computer software to translate words into the client's native language.
- If appropriate, use a third language that both of you speak. For example, some Vietnamese and some Cambodians speak French.
- Speak slowly and clearly, using simple sentences to talk about one question or need at a time.
- Use gestures to help convey meaning.

- Restate in different words, if needed.
- Use pictures or diagrams.
- Be aware that some clients may answer yes even if they don't understand what you have said.

Practice Resources
Munoz, C., & Luckmann, J. (2005); Purnell, (2014).

 To explore learning resources for this chapter,

 Go to www.DavisAdvantage.com and find:

Answers and Suggested Responses for all questions in this chapter

Lists of NIC Interventions and NOC Outcomes

List of NANDA-I Diagnoses

Knowledge Map

References and Bibliography

Concept Map

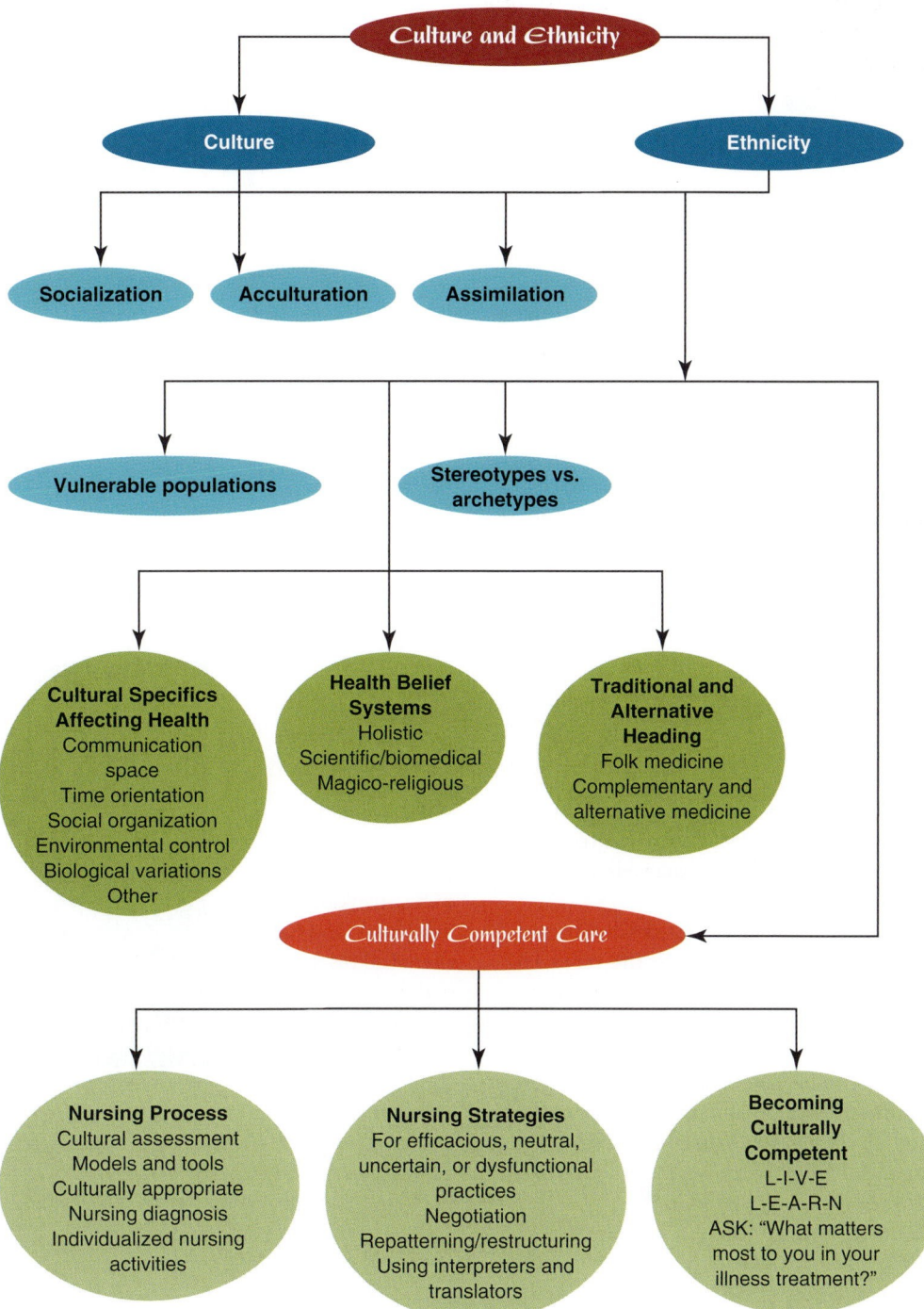

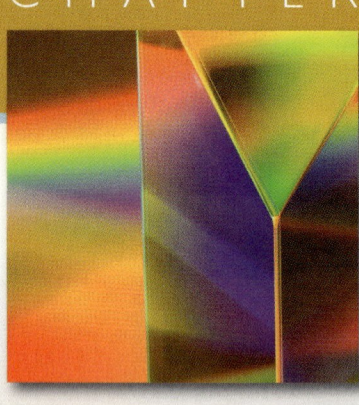
Spirituality

Learning Outcomes

After completing this chapter, you should be able to:

➤ Describe the differences and similarities between religion and spirituality.

➤ Discuss what is meant by *spirituality*.

➤ Describe the major beliefs and their implications for nursing care for each of the religions briefly covered in this chapter.

➤ Identify five barriers to spiritual care.

➤ Perform a spiritual assessment.

➤ Recognize the differences between spiritual care diagnoses and those that

may serve as etiologies of other nursing diagnoses.

➤ Plan nursing interventions based on the data obtained in a spiritual assessment.

➤ Examine your own level of comfort in terms of performing spiritual interventions.

➤ Describe collaborative efforts to ensure the spiritual care of the patient or family.

Key Concepts

Religion
Spiritual care
Spirituality

Related Concepts

See the Concept Map at the end of this chapter.

Meet Your Patient

Charles Johnson is a 75-year-old African American man with newly diagnosed lung cancer. His physicians want to start chemotherapy to try to increase his life span. He is unsure whether he wants to have chemotherapy.

Mr. Johnson was brought up in the Baptist Church, but has fallen away from practicing his faith over the years. He began smoking at age 15 and has been a heavy drinker all of his adult life. As a young man, he distanced himself from church. He explains: "Church folk are all a bunch of hypocrites. I choose not to be a part of any of that." Nevertheless, he says that he tries to be kind to and tolerant of others. "I've messed up my life, so I figure I don't have any business telling other people how to live. I just figure that how a person lives is between him and God."

Mr. Johnson has one surviving relative, a sister, who is concerned about him. His sister is a devout Jehovah's Witness, and she has tried several times to talk to Mr. Johnson about the importance of Jehovah in her life. She continually leaves religious pamphlets and materials in his mailbox to encourage him to think about religion again.

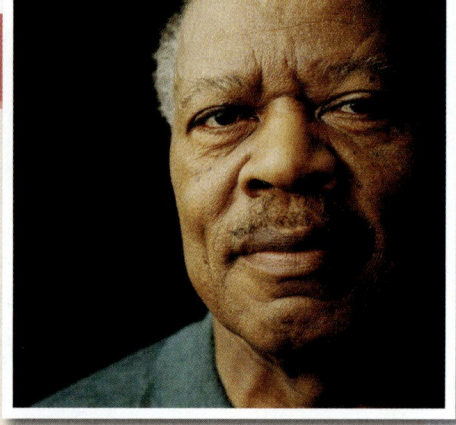

Mr. Johnson's wife divorced him 20 years ago because of his drinking behaviors, and he has alienated his two middle-aged children, so he rarely sees his grandchildren. He lives alone, is retired, and is having financial difficulties. He has one avid hobby: He loves to go out in a boat and fish all day with his buddy, Jim.

■ Mr. Johnson clearly has some physical and psychosocial difficulties. Can you identify them?

■ Assess Mr. Johnson's support system. Whom can he rely on for help?

■ How might you help Mr. Johnson to add some spiritual supports to his available resources?

This chapter presents a holistic interpretation of spirituality—one that views spirituality as a component of every person's life. It also encourages you to engage your own spirituality to improve your patients' health and wholeness. It should help you to answer some of the questions posed for Mr. Johnson.

TheoreticalKnowledge
knowing **why**

Spirituality in nursing has multiple layers. The following competing layers must be properly balanced to minimize your confusion, frustration, and avoidance of spiritual care:

- **Spirituality of the Nurse.** Each nurse's spirituality serves as part of the guiding framework for her practice.
- **Spirituality of the Patient and Family.** Spirituality will be understood in many different ways by patients and their families. It may or may not involve formal religion.
- **Effects of Nursing Education.** The emphasis placed on spiritual care differs among the nursing programs; however, many teach students to avoid imposing their spiritual beliefs on patients.
- **Demands of Nursing Practice.** Time constraints imposed by day-to-day patient care can negatively impact your ability to meet patients' spiritual needs. A therapeutic nurse–patient relationship is the foundation for meeting your patients' spiritual needs (Biro, 2012).

ABOUT THE KEY CONCEPTS

As you study this chapter, try to relate what you are reading to the key concepts of **spirituality** and **religion,** and try to understand the relationship between these two concepts. This will provide the foundation to understand the concept of **spiritual care** and its application to your patients.

HISTORY OF SPIRITUALITY IN NURSING

Through the ages, nurses and other caregivers have demonstrated deep concern for the spiritual as well as the physical and psychological needs of those who are sick and infirm.

- **In the pre-Christian era,** caring for the sick was an expression of the values of hospitality and charity. People prayed to the god(s) for healing and as an adjunct for primitive medical procedures.
- **In the early Christian era,** nursing the sick was honored and respected because it was one of Jesus Christ's primary teachings—a vital component of loving one's neighbor. Gradually, during the 4th through 12th centuries, religious communities combined the healing arts with religious care.
- **During the post-Reformation period** in Europe, nursing orders continued to flourish. For Florence Nightingale, spirituality was at the very heart of human nature and thus was fundamental to healing. She instilled this value in her nurses, particularly during their missions in the Crimea where "the lady with the lamp" brought comfort and relief to the sick and the dying (Dolarno, 2010; McDonald, 2013).
- **By the mid-20th century,** with advances in the sciences and as more nurses studied in university settings, the spiritual underpinnings of nursing were replaced by what could be seen and tested by the scientific method. Only recently has nursing (and the broader health community) reclaimed the spiritual dimension as a vital part of its identity and recognized its power to influence health.

KEY POINT: *Today, spiritual care cannot be the "overlooked" area of nursing practice. Professional standards of care make clear that meeting patients' spiritual needs is essential to provide holistic nursing care.* The Joint Commission (2014) has established standards for spiritual care. In addition, the American Nurses Association's *Code of Ethics for Nurses* (2015) instructs that nurses must incorporate factors such as culture and religious and spiritual beliefs in the plan of care for clients.

Safe, Effective Nursing Care

The Impact of Nurse Self-Awareness on Client Spiritual Care

Chapter Key Concepts: Spirituality; Goal-Directed, Client-Centered Care; Nurse Self-Awareness

Competencies: Provide goal-directed, client-centered care; show respect for client values, religious beliefs, needs, and preferences. (Thinking, Doing, Caring)

Background: Goal-directed, client-centered care includes addressing physical, psychosocial, and spiritual needs. Spirituality isn't always linked with religion. Rather, it is what the individual professes it to be (Schaefer, Stonecipher, & Kane, 2012). The SENC competency of goal-directed, client-centered care recognizes that the nurse must show respect for and incorporate the client's values, religious/spiritual beliefs, needs, and preferences into the plan of care. This implies holistic care.

➤ Establishing mutual goals with the client promotes holistic assessment and ensures that this vital aspect of client care is not overlooked.
➤ To provide holistic care, the nurse must understand the meaning of spirituality and have spiritual self-awareness.

Such self-awareness contributes to the ability to relate meaningfully to clients and to support their spiritual needs (Lee & Higgens, 2010; Pullen, McGuire, Farmer, et al., 2015).

Think about it:
Describe nursing interventions that would meet the spiritual needs of the client.
How does providing goal-directed, client-centered care attend to the spiritual needs of the client?
Discuss how spiritual self-awareness by the nurse might influence the spiritual care provided for the client.

Sources: Lee, D., & Higgens, P.A. (2010). Adjunctive therapies for the chronically critically ill. *AACN Advanced Critical Care, 21*(1), 92–106; Pullen, L., McGuire, S., Farmer, L., et al. (2015). The relevance of spirituality to nursing practice and education. *Mental Health Practice, 18*(5), 14–18; Schaefer, J., Stonecipher, S., & Kane, I. (2012). Finding room for spirituality in healthcare. *Nursing2012, 42*(9), 14–16.

WHAT ARE RELIGION AND SPIRITUALITY?

Spirituality and religion are related, yet they are two distinctly different concepts (Paloutzian & Park, 2014). One way to distinguish religion from spirituality is to think of religion as a map and spirituality as a journey, as shown in Table 16.1. For example, atheists and agnostics have no religious foundation but may have spiritual needs (Sessana, Finnell, Underhill, et al., 2011).

What Is Religion?

You may use a map to get to a certain location. The "map" of religion tells you what to believe and what values are essential. It provides codes of conduct that integrate beliefs and values into a way of living. The map itself may be in the form of a religious tradition (e.g., Christianity) or denomination (e.g., Baptist), which provides an identity and a "lens" for reading the world. The rituals, symbols, sacraments, and holy writings associated with religions serve as bases of authority and provide diverse ways to go beyond the physical and access the divine (e.g., God) (Fig. 16-1). Regardless of their differences, many of the world religions have the following in common:

- **Theology**—that is, discussions and theories related to God and God's relation to the world
- Sacred writings that are regarded as authoritative and/or reveal the nature of the divine in some way
- Notion of created order and purpose
- Definition of *human being* that includes important life events
- Notion of sin (primarily in Western religions)
- Explanation of the origin of evil and the nature of suffering
- Conception of either salvation (in Judeo-Christian religions) or enlightenment (in Eastern religions)
- **Eschatology,** or doctrines about the human soul and its relation to death, judgment, and eternal life (primarily a Western concept)

- Explanation of the nature of reality, the higher Self or soul, the relationship between humans and the divine, and the purpose of human existence

What Is Spirituality?

If religion is the map, spirituality is the day-to-day, moment-by-moment journey in life and living. Like a journey, spirituality involves personal, subjective experiences that take place over time. Many life events that prompt spiritual growth are fulfilling and joyful, but growth often results from painful life events that cause great internal upheaval, struggle, and challenge.

Like religion, spirituality allows various ways to experience the divine in our daily lives, to transcend the physical world, or simply to be still and introspective. You can also think of spirituality as the insight, value, purpose, and meaning of life derived from accumulated life experiences.

It is critical for you to recognize and respect the different ways that clients understand religion and spirituality. Most people are comfortable with their beliefs (or lack thereof); your primary goal is to support their healing, not convert them to a different view. You must also be able to recognize when a client may be experiencing spiritual distress and may need referral to professionals with more specialized training. These aspects of spiritual care are discussed later in this chapter.

KnowledgeCheck 16-1

- Regardless of their differences, what do many world religions have in common?
- Which can be compared to a journey: religion or spirituality?
- True or false: Both religion and spirituality allow a person various ways to access the divine.
- What is Mr. Johnson's religion (Meet Your Patient)?
- What is his sister's religion?

Table 16-1 ➤ Comparison of Religion and Spirituality

RELIGION (THE MAP)	SPIRITUALITY (THE JOURNEY)
A "roadmap" that defines: Beliefs Values Code(s) of conduct and ethics	One's journey through life; a personal quest to define meaning, fulfillment, and satisfaction in life; a will to live; a belief in self; an exploration of who you are
A tradition or system of worship that provides: Rituals Answers Norms Connection with God	A dynamic relationship with that which transcends; a capacity to know and be known (a sense of openness, expectation); connectedness with self, others, nature, and a higher power (Cavendish, Konecny, Mitzeliotis, et al., 2003); belief in a divine being or infinite source of energy (Beckman, Boxley-Harges, Bruick-Sorge, et al., 2007).
The roadmap and tradition define: What is to be believed How beliefs affect life Self-image and identity	A lifelong process of growth (which may involve joy and/or struggle); a constant process of taking in "truth" and then adding individual insight to arrive at a way of perceiving and acting in the world
Issues: Faith, belief, trust, the nature of good and evil, the meaning of suffering, judgment, or enlightenment	Issues: Faith, hope, love

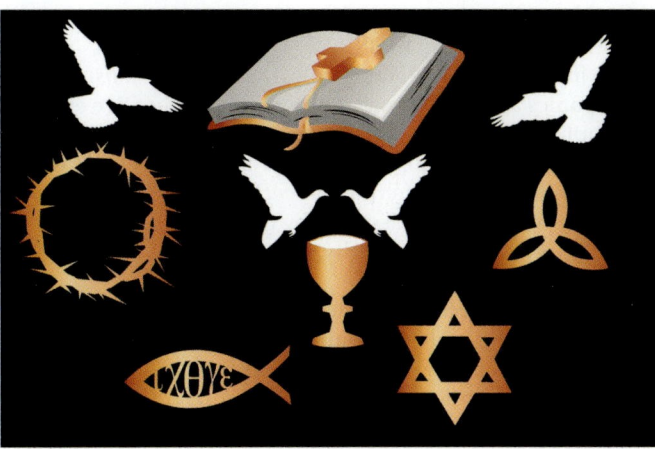

FIGURE 16-1 Associated with religion are various symbols and holy writings. For example, the Bible, cross, crown of thorns, trinity symbol, doves and chalice, and fish are all associated with Christianity, whereas the Star of David is associated with Judaism.

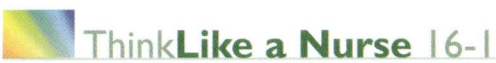

ThinkLike a Nurse 16-1

What do you know, or what can you speculate, about Mr. Johnson's (Meet Your Patient) spirituality?

What Are the Core Issues of Spirituality?

By now you know that spirituality has many dimensions. We limit discussion here to three core issues. In the New Testament of the Bible, the Apostle Paul identified "three things that last": faith, hope, and love. Following in this tradition, a manual for nursing care of the dying (Aspen Reference Group, 2002) identifies this same trio as the three core "issues" of spirituality.

Faith

Faith is an evolving pattern of believing that guides and grounds us and helps us make sense of the world and confront the challenges we face (Dyess, 2011; Rosmarin, Bigda-Peyton, Kertz, et al., 2013). Faith is expressed in terms of belief. It allows us to trust, to maintain an optimistic perspective on life events, and to find purpose in life. Like spirituality, faith represents a set of beliefs developed over time, through events that cause us to suffer and those that enable us to rejoice.

Faith struggles are common among people who experience illness and significant loss. People experiencing faith struggles might feel anger, guilt, self-judgment, and worthlessness. C. S. Lewis, a devout Christian, revealed that after the death of his wife, his grief caused him to doubt whether God exists at all, or if so, whether He is perhaps a "Cosmic Sadist" (1961, p. 35) who deliberately tortures us. Finally, Lewis came to understand that such shattering experiences are "one of the marks of His presence" (Lewis, 1961, p. 76).

Hope

Hope is a positive expectation and desire for future things to happen. It includes our basic human need to achieve, create, and to shape something of our life that will endure. Hope is rooted in purpose—who am I, what is my purpose, why have I been created? People who are confronting a debilitating or terminal illness often lose hope. Research shows that support systems, attitudes of healthcare providers, and skilled nursing care are important in fostering hope in patients who experienced traumatic injuries (Warwick, 2012). After suffering a near-fatal spinal cord injury, actor Christopher Reeve wrote in an essay, "Hope . . . is different from optimism or wishful thinking. When we have hope, we discover powers within ourselves we may have never known—the power to make sacrifices, to endure, to heal, and to love. Once we choose hope, everything is possible" (Reeve, 2002, p. 176).

Compassionate Love

Compassionate love, defined as "feelings of affection, compassion, caring, and tenderness for others," can be a source of reward and pain for patients, family members, and health care providers (Barsade & O'Neill, 2014). Many view love as a trade: We extend our love because we hope to find it returned in some way or to simply experience the emotional satisfaction of loving others.

Illness and sudden injury commonly prompt "struggles with love." For example, clients with debilitating illnesses who require increasing levels of care may view themselves as a burden to their loved ones. Family members are invaluable in showing their unconditional love to help restore the client's inner integrity and self-worth. Reeve stated that the most powerful words his wife spoke to him in the first days after his injury, "the words that saved my life," were, "You're still you. And I love you" (Reeve, 1998, p. 32). This support, combined with the compassionate love of healthcare providers, can help patients to overcome negative states, increase healing, and promote better quality outcomes (Barsade & O'Neill, 2014; Posadzki, 2010).

Cures, Miracles, and Spiritual Healing

A **miracle** is anything that allows for the presence of the transcendent (e.g., God, a higher being, or any brush with the divine). They may be spiritual phenomena, mysterious, and difficult to define or explain.

- **KEY POINT:** *We typically think of miracles as events that break with the natural order of things; however, miracles may proceed according to natural law.*
  Example: After the death of her client, a provider described the client's long-resisted acceptance of his impending death as the miracle, which prevented fruitless interventions and unnecessary suffering (La Madrid, 2012).
- **One aspect of miracle events is that they far exceed our expectations.** But as you can see, miracles do not always involve physical cures.
  Example: An elderly woman, bitter for decades over the death of her young daughter, "feels" her presence and dies in peace.
- **Miracles can be viewed as perfectly ordinary events or explained as the act of a "deity"** (McGrew, 2013). For example, a blind person suddenly can see, with no treatment or explanation.

Clients May Request a Prayer for Cure The client or family may request a prayer asking God for a cure when your expertise tells you that all curative measures have been exhausted. You should not say that a cure is impossible; however, you should avoid giving the patient and family to false hope. It may be possible for you to reframe the situation for them. Perhaps healing does not necessarily have to imply the elimination of suffering or of the disease. Instead, there may be various forms of healing. A transformation in a client's thinking or feeling or in acknowledging his belief in the spirit can be seen as a miracle.

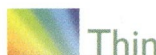

ThinkLike a Nurse 16-2

Faith is a constant search for comprehension and meaning. What are some of your struggles with faith, and what are some of the "joys" of your faith?

How Might Spiritual Beliefs Affect Health?

Religion and spirituality have been presented as two separate and distinct constructs; however, current research on their influence on health tends to combine them into one concept, namely, religion or religious involvement. Research findings are varied, as you will see in the following examples.

- One study found that religious involvement was instrumental in decreasing anxiety and depression and increasing overall quality of life (Huang, Hsu, & Chen, 2012).
- Another study found that African Americans and Hispanic Americans had a greater rate of religiosity; however, they did not experience greater mental health benefits. In addition, only white Americans experienced better mental health benefits from attending religious services (Sternthal, Williams, Musick, et al., 2012).
- The impact of the religious/cultural belief of *fatalism* among Hispanics and Asians was found to have a negative effect on compliance with preventive cancer screening. Both groups were highly pessimistic that preventive screening would lower their risk of getting cancer. (Fatalism and *fatalismo* view fatal diseases as destined by nature and acceptance as a sign of wisdom and maturity.) (Sternthal, Williams, Musick, et al., 2012).

Research on spirituality often involves self-reports of one's own religiousness, denominational affiliation, church attendance or membership (e.g. "On a scale of 1 to 5, how religious are you?" "How often do you attend church?'); thus, they do not allow for researchers to examine whether there might be potential harmful effects of religion.

There is growing awareness that religion and spirituality are complex variables involving cognitive, emotional, behavioral, interpersonal, and physiological dimensions. **KEY POINT:** *Research suggests that religion has a positive influence on health outcomes, but does not yet answer the how or why.*

Toward Evidence-Based Practice

Jim, H., Pustejovsky, J., Park, C., et al. (2015). Religion, spirituality, and physical health in cancer patients: A meta-analysis. *Cancer, 121*(21), 3760–3768. doi:10.1002/cncr.29353

The relationship between religion/spirituality and physical health (physical well-being, functional well-being, and physical symptoms) was studied in over 32,000 patients. Findings revealed that patients who reported greater overall religiousness/spirituality also reported better physical health, greater ability to perform their usual daily tasks, and fewer related physical symptoms of cancer and treatment. Although a strong cognitive aspect of religion/spirituality (ability to integrate the cancer into their religious or spiritual beliefs) was associated with self-reports of better physical health, there was not a relationship between physical health and the behavioral aspects of religion/spiritualty, such as church attendance, prayer, or meditation.

Sherman, A., Merluzzi, T., Pustejovsky, J., et al. (2015). A meta-analytic review of religious or spiritual involvement and social health among cancer patients. *Cancer, 121*(21), 3779–3788. doi:10.1002/cncr.29352

Social health was significantly associated with religion/spirituality in a study involving 14,277 patients. Findings revealed that patients who reported better social health had stronger spiritual well-being, perceptions of a benevolent God, or strong beliefs in their God. They also had the capacity to retain satisfying social roles and relationships in the face of cancer.

Salsman, J., Pustejovsky, J., Jim, H., et al. (2015). A meta-analytic approach to examining the correlation between religion/spirituality and mental health in cancer. *Cancer, 121*(21), 3769–3778. doi:10.1002/cncr.29350

Researchers found a positive correlation between religion/spirituality (e.g., coping, beliefs, experiences) and mental health (e.g., well-being, depression). The emotional dimension of religion/spirituality was more strongly associated with positive mental health than the behavior or cognitive dimensions. Patients who had a strong spiritual well-being experienced less distress, anxiety and depression.

Grudzen, C., Stone, S., Mohanty, S., et al. (2011). "I want to be taking my own last breath": Patients' reflections on illness when presenting to the emergency department at the end of life. *Journal of Palliative Medicine, 14*(3), 293–296.

Interviews conducted with 13 patients receiving palliative care treatment revealed that many were comforted by their faith in God but did not view themselves as controlling their fate. Many had not discussed their desire to die at home surrounded by their family with their provider.

1. Taken as a whole, what is the relationship between religion/spirituality and client experiences in the face of illness? Identify specific variables and explain the connections.

2. Suppose you are a hospital administrator in an institution where the focus is almost entirely on physical care. You are thinking about a program to teach and encourage your staff to integrate spiritual interventions into their client care. Evaluate the findings from each of the studies to see how useful it would be in supporting your idea. Explain your thinking.

 Go to Davis Advantage, Resources, Chapter 16, **Toward Evidence-Based Practice Suggested Responses.**

KnowledgeCheck 16-2

What are some of the ways that religion might positively influence health?

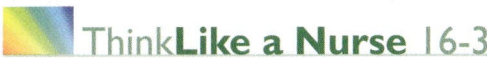

ThinkLike a Nurse 16-3

- How might religion negatively influence health?
- Recall a pivotal moment in your life, a moment of crisis or despair that eventually provided an opportunity for spiritual growth.

MAJOR RELIGIONS: WHAT SHOULD I KNOW?

Learning about other religions requires you to be open and nonjudgmental. When you care for a patient from a known religious background, you will need to think about how the person's beliefs affect her ideas of health, healing, hospitalization, and the experience of dying. To help you make these connections, the following brief descriptions of several of the world's major religious traditions provide you with several different "worldviews." To learn more about the effect of religions on dying, see Chapter 17.

- **KEY POINT:** *The more you know about the differences and similarities among the world's major religions, the more you will be able to offer comprehensive and compassionate care to patients.*
- **KEY POINT:** *There may be various beliefs and practices within a religious group, so always validate with your client to avoid stereotyping.*

Judaism

Judaism is one of the Western world's oldest religions and the foundation on which Christianity and Islam were built. The Jewish law is set down in the collective writings of the Torah. Judaism is based on the worship of one God (monotheism), obeying the Ten Commandments, and practicing charity and tolerance toward others. The degree to which Jews celebrate rituals and holy days depends on whether the person identifies with the Orthodox, Liberal, Conservative, or Reconstructionist beliefs (Oxtoby, Amore, Hussain, et al., 2015).

- **The Sabbath.** Jews celebrate the Sabbath from sunset on Friday to sunset Saturday evening. For Orthodox Jews, work is prohibited on the Sabbath. This includes writing, traveling, and switching on lights and appliances.
- **Holidays.** During Passover (in March or April), some Jewish patients may require special foods, dinnerware, and utensils. The Day of Atonement, or Yom Kippur (in September or October), is the holiest day of the Jewish calendar. It is a special day of fasting, but fasting is not required if it would be a danger to the patient. A Jewish patient will normally wish to keep that day to pray and rest. For Orthodox patients, you might offer alternatives to oral medication (e.g., injections or suppositories).
- **Dietary Practices.** Conservative Jews observe strict dietary laws: Only kosher foods are accepted. **Kosher foods** have been prepared under strict guidelines concerning how animals are slaughtered and do not contain pork, certain types of seafood, or combinations of dairy and meat. Meals are also double-packaged if kosher foods are heated in nonkosher heating units (Noble, Rom, Newsome-Wicks, et al., 2009). If possible, consult a rabbi or dietitian who is knowledgeable about Jewish dietary laws for assistance in planning dietary and activity modifications.
- **Clothing Practices.** Orthodox Jewish women prefer to have their bodies and limbs covered. They may also prefer to keep their hair covered with a scarf and often wear a wig. Orthodox men keep their head covered with a hat or skullcap (*kappel*).
- **Medical and Reproductive Practices.** Some Orthodox Jewish sects forbid contraception unless the woman's health is at risk. Nearly all Jewish boys are circumcised, usually 8 days after birth. Orthodox Judaism usually forbids organ transplants, but opinions vary and decisions may rest with the rabbinic authority.

Both Reconstructionist and Reform Judaism incorporate current societal values. Reconstructionists view Judaism not as a religion with rituals mandated by God but as a spiritual path with unity and connections developed among persons (Bronstein, 2012). Likewise, followers of Reform Judaism adhere to the traditional tenets, but practice inclusion, such as the acceptance of women as rabbis (Kaplan, 2013).

Christianity

Christianity is a major world religion. Christians worship Jesus Christ and believe that his death atoned for their sins by granting them forgiveness from God, which allows for eternal life. Their sacred text, the Bible, includes the Judaic Old Testament and the New Testament relating to the life of Christ. Rituals and practices vary among the Christian denominations, but the following are some similarities:

- **Baptism.** Many practice baptism, which is a sign of moral cleansing and correlates to being born again. The baptism of an infant, also known as "christening," indicates that the child will be raised with Christian values and influences, so when infants or children are very ill, baptism should be offered.
- **Dietary Practices.** Christians usually have no special dietary requirements, although some choose to abstain from eating meat on Fridays and/or during Lent and some abstain from alcohol. Others **fast** (abstain from food) to become closer to God, to pray for blessings, or before receiving Holy Communion.
- **Health and Reproductive Practices.** Most Christians do not object to blood transfusion or organ transplantation. Perspectives vary on using artificial birth control methods; however, natural family planning methods (e.g., rhythm) are widely accepted.

Christianity has many denominations, including Roman Catholicism (with allegiance to the pope in Rome), Orthodoxy (with allegiance to the patriarch of Constantinople), Protestant denominations (e.g., Lutheran, Baptist, United Methodist), and others (e.g., Jehovah's Witnesses, Mormons, Christian Scientists).

Roman Catholicism

In Roman Catholicism, the **sacraments** are a means to obtain grace.

- *Anointing the sick.* A Roman Catholic who is seriously ill might wish to receive the sacrament of *anointing the sick,* once known as the last rites. This sacrament can be repeated if the person recovers and then becomes ill at a later time.
- *Sacrament of reconciliation* (confession). Only a priest can hear the *sacrament of reconciliation,* during which God, through the priest, grants forgiveness for past sins.

- *The Eucharist* (communion bread). The *Eucharist* is consecrated at the *mass* (a religious service), and may be brought to hospitalized clients by a priest, deacon, or designated lay Eucharistic minister.

Other denominations within Christianity (e.g., Episcopalians and Lutherans) observe certain sacraments as well, although the meaning and details of the rituals may vary.

Christian Science

The Christian Science faith was established in 1879. Christian Scientists believe that illness is caused by faulty thinking, is evil, and is not part of God's plan, for God is good (Manca, 2013; Waldman, Perlman, & Chaudhry, 2010). Therefore, followers practice a reliance on God and prayer for healing. Although they may not believe in immunizations and vaccinations, they will follow the laws of the state (Christian Science, 2013).

- **Lifestyle and Nutrition.** Christian Scientists advocate proper nutrition, adequate sleep/rest, and avoidance of alcohol and tobacco. Strict believers may not drink tea or coffee.
- **Health Practices.** Parents usually consent to other medical care for their child if doctors consider it essential or the law so requires—but perhaps not for themselves. You will most likely encounter followers as patients only after accidents or because of family or legal pressures. While Christian Scientists do not oppose Western medicine, it is usually not their first choice to promote health and prevent illness.
- **Transfusions.** Adults will probably not accept a blood transfusion but will usually consent to transfusion for their child.

Jehovah's Witnesses

Many Jehovah's Witnesses adhere to the commands of God as written in both the Old and New Testaments of the Bible.

- **Blood Transfusions.** A practice that can create medical concerns is their refusal to accept blood transfusions or blood products, which they view as morally wrong. Patients who adhere to this faith would accept death rather than accept blood (Dyer, 2012; Hubbard, Waters, & Yazer, 2015). Autologous blood transfusions and donation or receipt of an organ through which blood flows are also not permitted. If blood is not involved (e.g., corneal transplants) then transplantations may be accepted
- **Dietary Practices.** Consistent with this practice, Jehovah's Witnesses will not eat raw meat, red meat, or meat that has not been bled properly.
- **Holidays.** Jehovah's Witnesses do not celebrate birthdays or holidays, except for the anniversary of the death of Christ. This date usually corresponds with the Christian Easter or Jewish Passover.
- **Lifestyle.** Although Jehovah's Witnesses abstain from tobacco and other recreational drugs, they may drink alcohol but do not condone drunkenness.

Mormonism

The Church of Jesus Christ of Latter-Day Saints (LDS) is commonly called the Mormon Church. Mormons believe in Jesus and one God and adhere to the sacred writing the Book of Mormon (which Joseph Smith translated from ancient records written on gold plates in 1830).

- **Clothing Practices.** Some Mormons (both men and women) wear a sacred undergarment (temple garments) that is "an outward expression of an inward commitment to follow the Savior" (The Church of Jesus Christ of Latter-Day Saints, 2013). The garments are only removed for purposes such as

hygiene, elimination, or being intimate in marriage. Nurses may also remove it before surgery, but it must at all times be considered intensely private and be treated with respect (Keddington, 2007).

- **Death and Dying.** Many believe in life before and after death; thus, death represents the passage to another life phase (Waldman, Perlman, & Chaudhry, 2012).
- **Nutrition and Lifestyle.** Mormons follow a strict health code, known as the Word of Wisdom, which advises healthful living and prohibits the use of tea, coffee, alcohol, and tobacco.

Seventh Day Adventism

The Seventh Day Adventist Church is distinguished mostly by observance of Saturday as the Sabbath, a day of rest and worship. To keep the Sabbath holy, Adventists do no secular work or unnecessary business on Saturday.

- **Sacraments.** Adventists usually practice communion, which begins with a foot-washing ceremony, four times a year.
- **Death and Dying.** Officially against active euthanasia, the church permits a passive form through withdrawal of medical support to allow the patient to die. Death is akin to sleep and the person is viewed as being in an unconscious state (Taylor & Carr, 2009).
- **Lifestyle and Adornment.** Most members avoid alcohol, tobacco, illegal drugs, and caffeinated beverages. The church also emphasizes culturally conservative principles and many Adventists refrain from body piercing, tattoos, and wearing jewelry.
- **Nutrition and Diet.** Some members believed that a healthy mind and body are essential elements of faith and worship and that both spiritual health and physical health are enhanced by good nutrition (Nath, 2010). Thus, the church recommends a vegetarian diet and avoidance of pork, shellfish, and "unclean" food in adherence to Old Testament kosher laws.
- **Reproductive Practices.** Although the church is generally antiabortion, in cases of serious dilemmas (e.g., threat to the woman's life or pregnancy resulting from rape or incest), women are counseled to make their own decisions. Birth control is permitted for married couples.

Islam

Islam was the third monotheistic religion to emerge, following Judaism and Christianity and is now the second largest (Abdel-Khalek, 2011). The word *Islam* means "submission." In particular, a Muslim is one who submits to Allah (God). Muhammad is the founder of Islam and a respected deity among the Muslims. The sacred book of authority in Islam, the Koran (Holy Qu'ran), is the result of messages from the angel Gabriel sent from God to the prophet Muhammad. It contains one message common to all faiths: There is a Supreme Being whose sovereignty is acknowledged in worship and whose teaching and commandments must be obeyed.

- **Blood Transfusion/Transplants.** There is no specific religious rule prohibiting blood transfusion or organ transplantation; however, strict Muslims will not usually agree to organ transplants.
- **Dietary Practices.** Muslims are forbidden to eat pork. They may eat other meat, but it has to be *halal* meat, that is, killed in a special manner stated in Islamic law. Fish and eggs are allowed, but not if they are cooked near pork or non-halal meat.

- **Holidays.** During the month of Ramadan, a Muslim fasts between sunrise and sunset; however, those who are sick are not expected to fast. Essential drugs and medicines are allowed at all hours during Ramadan.
- **Hygiene Practices.** Muslims always wash their hands before eating and it is customary to eat with the right hand (unless prevented by injury). Patients prefer to wash in free-flowing water, so if a shower is not available, provide a pitcher to use in the bath.
- **Modesty.** Women prefer to be treated by female staff. Some women may refuse vaginal examination by a male nurse or provider because they are forbidden to expose their bodies to or be touched by any man other than their husband.
- **Religious Symbols.** Women may wear a locket containing religious writing around the neck in a small leather bag. These are kept for protection and strength, so you should never remove them.
- **Reproductive Practices.** After the birth of a baby, prayers are whispered in the baby's ear so the first thing heard are words of prayer. Orthodox Muslims do not approve of contraception; however, individuals vary widely in their practices. Abortion is frowned on but may be tolerated for medical reasons.

Hinduism

Hinduism, seen as the oldest major religion, does not embrace a single body of beliefs and practices or the existence of one god. Hindus may worship several or even hundreds of gods and goddesses, including elements in the natural world such as rivers, fire, and so forth. Sacred Hindu texts include the *Vedas,* the *Bhagavad Gita* (Song of the Blessed One), and the *Ramayana,* the story of the life of the god Rama.

- **Dietary Practices.** Most Hindus are lactovegetarians, consuming milk but no eggs. Many will not eat beef and avoid bovine-derived medication because of the reincarnation of certain gods (Wilkins & Mailoo, 2010). Fasting, which may mean eating only "pure" foods, such as fruit or yogurt, is common during major festivals but is not expected of the sick.
- **Hygiene Practices.** Hindus prefer to wash in free-flowing water (e.g., a shower instead of a tub). If a shower is not available, provide a jug of water for the person to use in the bath.
- **Lifestyle and Health Practices.** Hindus practice **ayurvedic medicine,** which encompasses all aspects of life, including diet, sleep, elimination, and hygiene. Some believe in the medicinal properties of "hot" and "cold" foods (does not refer to temperature or spicy qualities). There is no religious objection to contraception, blood transfusion, or organ donation. The use of alcohol or tobacco may be accepted.
- **Modesty and Respect.** Women are modest and usually prefer to be treated by female medical staff. Some Hindus may consider touching a person's feet or on the head a sign of disrespect.
- **Religious Beliefs.** Hindus believe in the core concepts of karma, dharma, and reincarnation (Wilkins & Mailoo, 2010). Karma teaches that every action has or causes an effect. A person who does not fulfill his destiny or given purpose in life (dharma) will have bad karma. After death, persons begin a new life in a different body or spiritual form (reincarnation).
- **Religious Symbols.** Some Hindus wear "sacred thread" around the body or wrist. Do not remove or cut this thread without permission from the patient or next of kin. Jewelry often has a religious significance.

Buddhism

The Buddha, or the "Awakened One," is revered not as a god but as an example of a way of life (Fig. 16-2). Siddhartha Gautama was born into a royal family in 624 BCE in a part of northern India that is now in Nepal, gained enlightenment at the age of 35, and then began to teach others how to attain liberation from suffering for themselves and others.

One of the Buddha's core teachings is that suffering can be ended by following the eightfold path: right understanding, right intention, right speech, right action, right livelihood, right effort, right mindfulness, and right contemplation (Bodhi, 2007; Knierim, n.d.). **Nirvana,** similar to the Christian concept of heaven, can be attained only through an absence of desire, the achievement of perfection, and the lack of a unique identity. Buddhism is about finding spirituality within oneself. Like Hindus, Buddhists believe in karma and reincarnation.

- **Dietary Practices.** Food is an essential component of maintaining spiritual focus, meditation, and interactions with others (Nath, 2010). Many Buddhists follow a vegetarian diet; in some cases, the diet may include both milk and eggs. Fasting customs vary by tradition.
- **Reproductive Practices.** Buddhists accept contraception but typically condemn abortion and active euthanasia.
- **Transfusions and Transplants.** They will usually accept blood transfusion and organ transplantation.

Native American Religions

There are more than 400 federally recognized Native American nations or tribes in the United States. Although each has its own traditions and cultural heritage, some general beliefs underlie the more specific tribal idea. The Earth is considered to be a living organism, the body of a higher individual, and humankind has an intimate relation with this organism

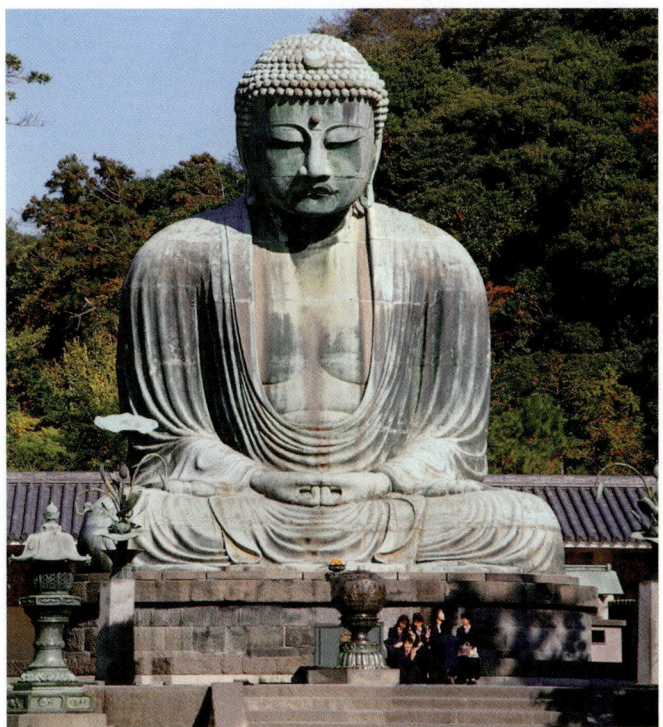

FIGURE 16-2 The Buddha is revered as an example of a way of life.

through nature. Thus, rather than having a designated sacred place to worship, Native American religions place value in the land, mountains, rivers, and meadows (Fowler, 2009; Minority Nurse Staff, 2013).

- **Communication.** Native Americans may converse in a low tone of voice and may maintain long periods of silence. Be sure the setting is quiet enough to allow you to hear the patient because it is impolite to indicate that you did not hear the communications. You should know that for some tribes, note taking by the professional is forbidden. Thus, when you take a history or perform an examination, you must rely on your memory and record findings later.
- **Health Practices.** Some Native Americans consider health as a state of harmony with nature. Whenever disharmony exists, disease or illness can occur. Because the traditional healer is wise in the interrelationships of land, humankind, and the universe, many Native Americans believe that the treatments they receive from medicine men and women are far better than those rendered by the dominant healthcare establishment, which often treats Native Americans with scorn or disrespect (Fig.16-3).

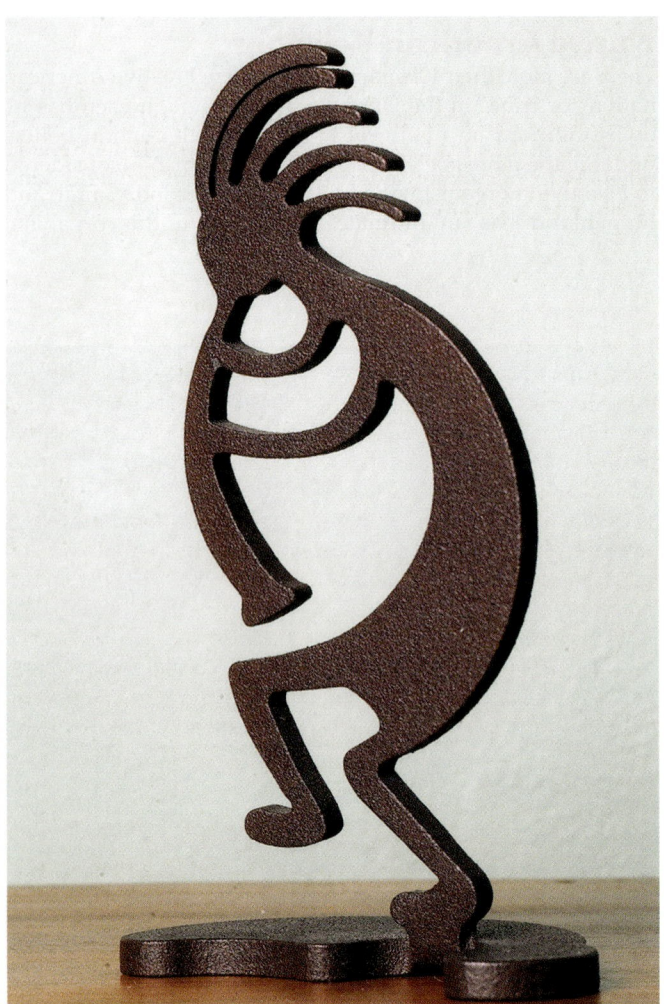

FIGURE 16-3 Kokopelli, the humpbacked flute player, has been a sacred figure to Native Americans of the Southwest for thousands of years. He is a legendary symbol of fertility who brought well-being to the people.

Rastafarianism

Rastafarianism is a personal religion that emphasizes dignity and a deep love of God. The authoritative writings include the Old and New Testaments of the Bible, but as a rule Rastafarians do not consider themselves to be Christian. There are no churches, services, or official clergy.

- **Clothing Practices.** The women dress modestly. Wearing secondhand clothing is taboo, so the patient may be unwilling to wear hospital gowns that have been worn by others. You may need to provide a disposable gown or allow the person to wear her own personal nightclothes.
- **Dietary Practices.** Rastafarians do not eat pork and shellfish, some are completely vegetarian, and some do not drink milk or coffee.
- **Health Practices.** Many prefer alternative therapies (e.g., herbalism, marijuana, or acupuncture), do not believe in contraception, and avoid any treatment that will contaminate the body.
- **Transfusions.** Many will accept blood transfusions but may require reassurance about its safety.

Atheism

Atheists do not believe in the presence of God or supernatural deities. Rather than receiving directives on living from external sources, atheists have their own personal moral code that is derived from their value systems, beliefs, and life experiences. They can be spiritual and even religious but focus on the humanistic, secular perspectives. A nurse recalls a patient's comment that he regretted putting "Atheist" on his admission paperwork because he would have welcomed the presence of a chaplain to discuss his spirituality (Mais, 2010). **KEY POINT:** *This comment does not imply that all atheists would react in the same way as this patient did. It does, however, reinforce that importance of a thorough assessment of patient needs instead of relying on categories and labels.*

KnowledgeCheck 16-3

- Which major religion believes in the anointing of the sick or dying?
- Which denomination or religion does not believe in blood transfusions?
- In terms of Native American beliefs and healthcare, who is the traditional healer or the person to be consulted in the event of "illness"?
- True or false: Most Hindus are vegetarian.

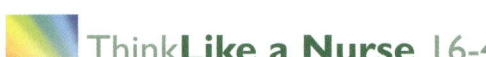

ThinkLike a Nurse 16-4

What are some of the ways that world religions might influence nursing care?

SELF-KNOWLEDGE: WHAT EVERY NURSE SHOULD KNOW

As you have seen, your patients' spiritual and religious backgrounds may be diverse and may involve ways of thinking and doing that seem strange to you or that you do not fully understand. Before trying to understand your patients' religious experience, you must give considerable thought to your own religious or spiritual journey. Attaining self-knowledge is an important aspect of becoming a full-spectrum nurse. This section will help to you in your reflections.

What Are Your Personal Biases?

We each carry our own perspectives with us at all times. We tend to view the world through lenses we acquired in childhood, adolescence, and early adulthood. In addition, our religious education is sometimes taught with a certain flavor of "upmanship"; that is, we are taught that our religious beliefs and practices are superior to all others. When you view your own experience as the norm or as the preferred way of organizing the world, you tend to limit the range of care you provide to the patient who believes differently. Spiritual care demands nonjudgmental attitudes and an open manner of thinking that invites rather than excludes.

 ThinkLike a Nurse 16-5

Consider the following examples. For each person, what moral/spiritual judgments should the nurse avoid?

■ A nurse is caring for a gay man who is hospitalized with end-stage AIDS.
■ A woman has come to the clinic to be treated for gonorrhea (a sexually transmitted infection). She says she has had at least six sexual partners this year.
■ A man comes to the emergency department (ED) at least once a month to ask for morphine to treat his back pain. He is known to abuse drugs and to visit other EDs for the same purpose.

If you are aware of your biases, it will be easier to avoid abuses of spiritual care.

What Are Some Barriers to Spiritual Care?

Although most nurses would acknowledge that clients have a spiritual dimension, few nurses actually identify spiritual problems or provide spiritual interventions. This may be a result of economic constraints, poor staffing, insufficient time, lack of privacy, and high-tech care, which force nurses to focus on physical needs to the exclusion of spiritual needs (Narayanasamy, 2014; Nardi & Rooda, 2011; Ronaldson, Hayes, Aggar, et al., 2012). You may judge these nurses less harshly after you understand more about the barriers to spiritual interventions by nurses.

Lack of General Awareness of Spirituality

A greater awareness of spirituality in general will help you tune into the spiritual needs of patients and improve your comfort in communicating about spiritual matters. Research consistently reveals that healthcare providers need more education on spiritual care to address commonly cited reasons for inadequately addressing the spiritual needs of patients. One study identified the barriers cited by nurses and providers as inadequate training, lack of time, lack of privacy, and not a component of their professional role (Balboni, Sullivan, Enzinger, et al., 2014). Another showed that patients at risk for spiritual distress are not identified (Blanchard, Dunlap, & Fitchett, 2012) or are inaccurately assessed (Highfield, 1992).

Lack of Awareness of Your Own Spiritual Belief System

To feel comfortable making spiritual interventions, you will need more than just theoretical knowledge. You will need introspection and an awareness of your own spiritual journey. Nurses who are aware of their own spirituality are better able to incorporate spiritual care in their practice (Pullen, McGuire, Farmer, et al., 2015). You can take steps to enhance your spiritual growth (Baldacchino, 2011; Koren & Papamiditriou, 2013),

gain a broader view of spirituality, and increase sensitivity to others' spiritual needs. You must:

1. Understand the differences between religion, spirituality, and spiritual care.
2. Develop an awareness of your own spirituality and how it is applied (or not) in meeting the patient's spiritual needs.
3. Open yourself by being totally present with the patient, including being an active listener. Allow the patient to share his feelings and emotions without reserve and reflect in your attitude and demeanor that you care and have the time to listen.
4. Develop your critical and reflective thinking abilities. Explore through reflection and discussions with others. Write your own epitaph: one or two lines summing up how you would like to be remembered.
5. Reflect on your thoughts and feelings about end-of-life issues. Imagine you have only a few weeks to live; think how you would feel.
6. Reflect on your personal experience with grief and loss. For example, what is the first death you can remember? What were your feelings at the time? How do you usually cope with loss? What actions by others comforted you?

These suggestions will help you find ways to take care of and nurture your own spiritual needs and to provide appropriate spiritual care to others.

Trying to Be All Things to All People

Acknowledge that you can't meet every patient's spiritual needs. Their backgrounds vary, as does the extent of spiritual care needed. Clearly, there are times when you should refer to others with more knowledge and experience in religion and spirituality (e.g., the agency's chaplain), with the patient's permission, of course.

Differences in Spirituality Between Nurse and Patient

When a patient's spiritual beliefs are different from your own, you must be careful not to impose your beliefs on the patient or discount the importance of the patient's beliefs and rituals. For example, if a client is near death, he and his family might be offended if their nurse inquires whether they are "saved" Christians. By remaining focused on the patient's need to talk about meaning, salvation, or other end-of-life issues, you provide full-spectrum spiritual care. In Meet Your Patient, do you think Mr. Johnson feels supported by his sister?

When the patient's views are similar to yours, take care not to make false assumptions about his spiritual needs. Although you share some commonalities, this does not mean that you will have the same perspectives or needs in all areas of spirituality or religion.

 ThinkLike a Nurse 16-6

■ How does your religion or spirituality differ from Mr. Johnson's (Meet Your Patient)?
■ How is it similar?
■ Can you think of problems these differences and similarities could cause you in caring for him?

Fear That Your Knowledge Base Is Insufficient

Nurses sometimes avoid giving spiritual care because they believe they lack knowledge of spirituality or of the patient's religion. This is a realistic concern. In several studies, nurses were found to be unsure of what constituted spiritual problems and spiritual interventions (Blanchard, Dunlap, & Fitchett, 2012; Smyth & Allen, 2011). In some cases, they did not identify the spiritual dimension of care, or they took religious aspects into account but did not place them into a broader spiritual perspective. Your ability to incorporate spiritual care into practice will increase with experience.

Fear of Where Spiritual Discussions May Lead

Many nurses fear that inquiring into the spiritual domain might cause harm to the patient. For example, what if a patient asks you, "Do you believe active euthanasia is morally wrong? Would it jeopardize my salvation?"

- You may not feel prepared to answer the questions.
- You might have an answer based on your personal religious beliefs but fear the patient may think you are imposing your beliefs on him.
- You might wonder whether communicating your own beliefs (e.g., in favor active of euthanasia) might jeopardize the client's spiritual life if your ideas turn out to be "wrong."

    The following thoughts may help counter your fears:

- The patient's addressing this concern with you indicates that you are open to the spiritual domain of care.
- The patient's questions about euthanasia could lead to discussions about his fears of pain, dependence, being a burden on family members, and dying alone.
- You should realize that being open to the spiritual realm and assessing the patient's need for spiritual intervention does not mean that you must be a chaplain or have the extraordinary ability to deal with all spiritual or religious questions or requests. You can collaborate with a chaplain, who is more prepared to deal with specific religious issues.

KnowledgeCheck 16-4

- What qualities can you demonstrate that may help you improve the quality of spiritual care you provide?
- What common barriers to spiritual interventions do nurses encounter?
- True or false: No matter how nonjudgmental and open we may think ourselves to be, we all carry our own unique biases and prejudices that have the potential to affect patient care.

ThinkLike a Nurse 16-7

- What are some of the possible errors made by nurses related to spiritual care?
- What are some ways that you can develop a greater awareness of the "spirit within the self"?
- Discuss ways that nurses and patients can nurture their own spiritual needs.

PracticalKnowledge
knowing how

Most hospital admission forms include a place to record the client's religious preferences. Unfortunately, some nurses believe that by completing such forms, they have addressed the client's spiritual needs. However, armed with your basic theoretical knowledge of spirituality and your growing spiritual

self-knowledge, you should be able to provide a level of support that extends beyond paperwork to compassion and caring. The good news is that spiritual care has never been more welcomed by patients. You now know the importance of and can provide care to meet your patient's spiritual needs. The Practical Knowledge section will provide a more detailed understanding of your role in spiritual care.

ASSESSMENT NP

You should always do a careful religious assessment (Wilkins & Mailoo, 2010). People of the same religion often vary greatly in the degree to which they follow religious practices. It is not enough to "fill in the religion blank" on an assessment form. You must assess each person individually to determine religious needs and practices, keeping in mind that this may be a sensitive area for some clients.

KEY POINT: *It may be difficult to obtain meaningful information on the initial admission assessment because of time constraints in completing the paperwork, collaboration with the healthcare team, and the stresses involved in getting the client introduced to the healthcare setting.* Obtain the essential data of the patient's church preference, name of clergy, whom to call in case of emergency, dietary requirements/restrictions, and any religious implications for medical care (e.g., refusal of blood transfusions). As you have further interactions with the client and family, trust will develop and you will be able to obtain more sensitive, complex, and meaningful spiritual/religious information.

Sources of Spiritual Data

You can acquire information about a patient's spirituality from a variety of sources other than interviews:

- **Client's environment.** Observe the client's environment for hints about her spirituality (e.g., pictures of family, the presence of sacred texts or reading materials, articles used in worship [a crucifix, rosary beads, statues], or copies of church bulletins).
- **Client's questions.** The client may ask questions that are indicative of spiritual comfort, longing, or distress. For example, the client may ask whether you attend church and, if so, whether it provides you with a sense of comfort and meaning.
- **Client's behaviors, moods, and feelings.** Emotional behavior gives a clear and certain indication that the client may be struggling with issues that have spiritual overtones. These warrant further assessment and nursing intervention. For example, a client may ask whether you have ever felt guilty about something you did as a child.
- **Nonverbal communication.** Body language may indicate hope or distress. For example, you may observe a client praying. Or when asking about spirituality, you may see the client roll his eyes, shake his head, and demonstrate muscle tension.

Spiritual Assessment Tools

Some healthcare agencies have focused spiritual assessment tools tailored to their particular setting. Several others have been developed, including the following:

    HOPE   The application of the HOPE questions is an easy-to-use screening method. Although not validated by research, they do allow for an open-ended exploration of spiritual resources and concerns (Gowri & Hight, 2001) (see the Focused Assessment box The HOPE Approach to Spiritual Assessment: Examples of Questions).

Focused Assessment

The HOPE Approach to Spiritual Assessment: Examples of Questions

Mnemonic	Examples of Questions
H—Sources of **hope**, meaning, comfort, strength, peace, love and connection	What are your sources of internal support? What do you hold on to to get you through difficult times? For some people, religious or spiritual beliefs are a source of comfort in dealing with life's ups and downs. Is this true for you?
O—Organized religion	Do you belong to a religious or spiritual community? Does it help you? How important is this to you? What aspects of your religion are helpful to you?
P—Personal spirituality/Practices	Do you believe in God? What is your relationship with God? Do you have personal spiritual beliefs that are not a part of organized religion? If so, what are they? What aspects of your spirituality are most helpful to you (e.g., meditation, prayer, reading scripture, listening to music, nature)?
E—Effects on medical care and end-of-life issues	Has your illness affected your relationship with God? Or to do the things that usually help you spiritually? Are you concerned about conflicts between your beliefs and your healthcare treatment plan? Do you have any dietary restrictions or other practices I should know about in planning your care? Would you like to speak to a clinical chaplain (or community spiritual leader)?

Source: Based on Gowri, A., & Hight, E. (2001). Spirituality and medical practice: Using the HOPE questions as a practical tool for spiritual assessment. *American Family Physician, 63,* 81–89.

JAREL The JAREL spiritual well-being scale was developed and is commonly used by nurses (Hungelmann, Kenkel-Rossi, Klassen, et al., 1996). Cutting across religious and atheistic belief systems, it assesses three key dimensions: (1) faith/belief, (2) life/self-responsibility, and (3) life-satisfaction/self-actualization.

SPIRIT The comprehensive spiritual assessment tool developed by Highfield (2000) involves an interview that is concerned with six key areas designated by the acronym SPIRIT. Refer to the Focused Assessment box S-P-I-R-I-T Assessment.

KnowledgeCheck 16-5

What are the six areas for spiritual assessment summarized in Highfield's (2000) acronym SPIRIT?

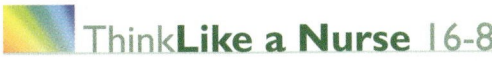 ThinkLike a Nurse 16-8

Complete the SPIRIT assessment on yourself. Discuss it with your classmates.

ANALYSIS/NURSING DIAGNOSIS NP

When analyzing spiritual assessment data, you must consider the person's developmental stage. People progress through stages of spiritual development in much the same way that they develop physically and cognitively. Spiritual behaviors that seem problematic in one stage may not be so in an earlier stage. To review developmental stages, refer to Chapters 9 and 10.

Spirituality Diagnoses

Box 16-1 contains NANDA-I diagnostic labels that specifically deal with religion and spirituality. The following are examples of full diagnostic statements you might write for spiritual problems:

- *Spiritual Distress* related to overwhelming anxiety associated with the need to have a surgical procedure that is not accepted by her religion
- *Risk for Spiritual Distress* related to unremitting pain and loss of hope for relief, as manifested by patient's question about the usefulness of prayer ("God has forgotten about me")

ThinkLike a Nurse 16-9

Which of these nursing diagnoses would you use for Mr. Johnson (Meet Your Patient): Spiritual Distress, Risk for Spiritual Distress, or Readiness for Enhanced Spiritual Well-Being? Why?

A Non–NANDA-I Diagnosis Millspaugh (2005) has suggested *Spiritual Pain* as a diagnosis. When a person experiences a combination of awareness of death, loss of relationships, loss of self, loss of purpose, and loss of control, Spiritual Pain may occur. However, this combination of negative experiences can be balanced by having a life-affirming and transcending purpose and an internal sense of control (Fig. 16-4). The presence and quality of Spiritual Pain is determined by the degree to which the person is experiencing each component, and by the relationship of the components to each other.

Spirituality as Etiology

In the spiritual realm, it is sometimes difficult to determine what is the problem and what is the etiology. Does the patient experience Spiritual Distress because of pain and hopelessness? Or did the patient first lose faith in God, which led to hopelessness and anxiety? Either way, spiritual support is needed.

S-P-I-R-I-T Assessment

➤ Obtain information from the patient when possible.
➤ In an emergency or if the patient cannot give information, consult the next of kin or a designated power of attorney for information as soon as possible.

S—Spiritual/religious belief system

Religion, tradition, sect, or denominational affiliation
Text/writing(s) that provide source of authority and codes for behavior
Name and phone number of church or other place of worship
Past experience with a belief system (positive or negative)
Beliefs about suffering, terminal or chronic illness, advance directives, autopsy, organ donation
Stigmas related to illness, if applicable

P—Personal spirituality

Individual beliefs and affiliation practices of the patient or family
Individual beliefs that may differ from affiliation beliefs
Whether spirituality is a part of personal experience of religion or a separate entity
Level of comfort discussing spirituality
Whether personal spirituality is viewed positively or negatively at the present time

I—Integration within a spiritual community

Name and title of religious or spiritual leader or authority figure(s)
Names and titles of religious groups that may need to be contacted: ministry, prayer group leader, prayer chain support person, shaman, medicine man or woman, men's or women's group within denomination
Role of patient in any of above-named groups

R—Ritualized practices and restrictions

Activities that the patient's or family's faith encourages or forbids
Needs for modesty and covering of body parts or appendages

Any special beliefs or needs in relation to drawing blood or to laboratory tests or procedures
Dietary needs and restrictions: food preferences, preparation of foods, and location of food preparation areas
Gender-specific roles and responsibilities of care providers
Prayer needs and restrictions: Who delivers and offers such practices?
Articles or other materials needed for worship, devotion, or prayer (rosaries, prayer beads, prayer books, religious tracts, Bibles, crosses, prayer shawls or cloths)

I—Implications for medical care

Beliefs and practices that healthcare providers should remember while providing care
Specific medications that may not be administered and withheld; implications for pain control
Specific medical procedures or products that may not be administered (abortion, blood products)
Communication patterns and needs for effective care delivery: Who makes decisions? What is the role of parents or guardians when children or other vulnerable populations are the recipients of care? Does the guardian reflect the beliefs of patient, if these are known?

T—Terminal events planning

Wishes for advance directives (cardiopulmonary resuscitation, intubation, ventilator assist, feeding tubes)
Wishes for transplantation or organ donation
Need for religious services (last rites, ministries of healing, baptism, initiation, confession, communion)
Clergy or ministry groups to be contacted and when
Ideas of an afterlife
Treatment of the body at the time of death
Funeral planning

Source: Adapted from Highfield, M. E. F. (2000). Providing spiritual care to patients with cancer. *Clinical Journal of Oncology Nursing, 4*(3), 115–120.

BOX 16-1 ■ NANDA-International Spirituality Diagnoses

Moral Distress	Experienced when the person makes an ethical or moral decision but then is unable to carry out the chosen action. Defining characteristics include an expression of anguish, powerlessness, anxiety, and fear over the inability to act on the moral choice.
Impaired Religiosity	Difficulty in exercising or impaired ability to exercise reliance on beliefs or to participate in rituals associated with one's faith (e.g., go to church, take communion).
Readiness for Enhanced Religiosity	The ability to increase reliance on religious beliefs and/or participate in rituals of a particular faith tradition. The client is not experiencing a problem but wishes to enhance his religious options, customs, or practices.
Readiness for Enhanced Spiritual Well-Being	Describes healthy spirituality. "A pattern of experiencing and integrating meaning and purpose in life through connectedness with self, others, art, music, literature, nature, and/or a power greater than oneself, which can be strengthened" (NANDA International, 2015, p. 213). It is the opposite of Spiritual Distress, so you will see positive expressions of hope, love, courage, acceptance, and purpose in life; healthy connections with others and with art, music, literature, and nature; and prayer and other expressions of a connection with a power higher than oneself.

BOX 16-1 ■ NANDA-International Spirituality Diagnoses—cont'd

Risk for Impaired Religiosity	Occurs when risk factors are present but symptoms are not. Risk factors may be categorized as developmental, environmental, physical, psychological, sociocultural, or spiritual. Specific examples include life transitions, lack of transportation, pain, depression, and inadequate social support/interactions.
Risk for Spiritual Distress	Difficulty in finding purpose in life; experiences unremitting pain and loss of hope for relief, as manifested by patient's question about the usefulness of prayer ("God has forgotten about me.")
Spiritual Distress	"A state of suffering related to the impaired ability to experience meaning in life through connections with self, others, the world, or a superior being" (NANDA International, 2015, p. 218). Defining characteristics (signs and symptoms) of this diagnosis include the following: Connections to self: Feelings of anger, guilt or being unloved; demonstrates ineffective coping Connections with others: Self-isolate from support system, spiritual leaders, family or friends; expressions of alienation Connections with art, music, literature, nature: No interest in nature; spiritual materials, or the creative arts. Connections with power greater than self: Inability to pray, inability or refusal to participate in religious activities, feelings of abandonment by God or other deity, expressions of anger toward God or other deity, requests to see a religious leader, sudden changes in spiritual practices (increased or decreased)

Source: Adapted from *Nursing Diagnoses—Definitions and Classification 2018–2020.* © 2010 NANDA International, ISBN 978-1-62623-929-6. Used by arrangement with the Thieme Group, Stuttgart/New York.

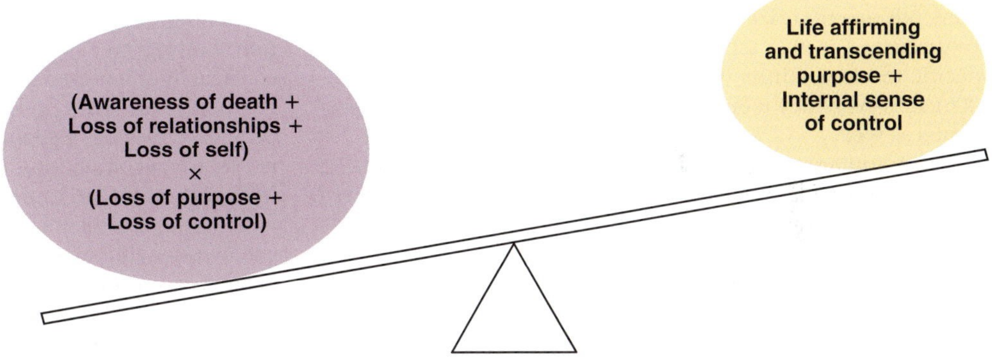

FIGURE 16-4 Components of spiritual pain.

Several of the NANDA-I diagnoses relate to spirituality as the etiology, or symptom, of other diagnoses. Examples include Anxiety, Chronic Sorrow, Death Anxiety, Decisional Conflict, Hopelessness, Interrupted Family Processes, Powerlessness, and Social Isolation. Non–NANDA-I etiologies include anger or resentment; feelings of guilt, shame, inadequacy, abandonment, or distrust; depression or sadness; and the inability to find meaning in life. The following are examples of diagnostic statements with spiritual etiologies:

Anxiety related to inability to reconcile decision to use birth control with religious proscriptions

Decisional Conflict related to confusion about the religious implications of the decision to forgo heroic treatment measures

Ineffective Health Management (nonadherence to treatment regimen) related to the belief that the illness is "God's will" and that healing will occur (without treatment) for the same reason.

KnowledgeCheck 16-6

Consider the following statement: A nursing diagnosis that reflects either an actual or a potential problem may reflect religious and/or spiritual dimensions of the human condition.

- Is this statement true?
- Would it be true for a *physical* diagnosis (e.g., Disturbed Sleep Pattern)? Explain your thinking.

PLANNING OUTCOMES/EVALUATION NP

The outcomes you establish in the planning stage of the nursing process serve as the criteria for evaluation of the patient's progress and the success of the nursing interventions.

NOC standardized outcomes associated with spirituality diagnoses include, but are not limited to, the following: Anxiety Level, Comfortable Death, Comfort Status: Psychospiritual, Dignified Life Closure, Hope, Loneliness Severity, Personal Resiliency, Personal Well-Being, Quality of Life, Spiritual Health, and Will to Live (Moorhead, Johnson, Maas, et al., 2013).

Individualized goals/outcome statements you might write for spiritual diagnoses include the following:

- **For Risk for Spiritual Distress**—Exhibits no signs or symptoms of spiritual distress (e.g., finds meaning in life, expresses hope and faith, follows usual religious practices).

- **For Spiritual Distress**—Returns to previous state of spiritual well-being and comfort (e.g., expresses a sense of peace, asks to see religious adviser).
- **For Readiness for Enhanced Spiritual Well-Being**—Experiences a higher level of connectedness with self, others, higher power, and/or nature.

To see a care plan and care map for a client with Spiritual Distress,

 Go to Davis Advantage, Resources, Chapter 16, **Nursing Care Plan: Spiritual Distress,** and **Care Map: Spiritual Distress**

PLANNING INTERVENTIONS/ IMPLEMENTATION NP

Spiritual interventions are those used to treat and prevent spiritual problems related to the patient's illness. You will direct some nursing activities to resolving the problem, others at removing the etiology, and still others at relieving symptoms. You will, of course, base your nursing activities on the patient's symptoms and the problem etiologies. However, there are some nursing interventions that are useful for all, or most, spiritual problems.

Standardized (NIC) Spirituality Interventions

A few NIC standardized interventions to promote spirituality are discussed in this section. The evidence base for these is specific to older adults (Gaskamp, Sutter, Meraviglia, et al., 2006); however, they would seem to be indicated for other age-groups as well.

When you are performing interventions of a spiritual nature, remember that you absolutely must follow the patient's lead and be caring and respectful without inserting your own beliefs into the conversation. Choose your language carefully—words such as *saved, repentance,* and so on, which may be a part of everyday conversation for people who follow some religions, may cause some patients to feel pressured or uncomfortable. Try to mirror, and not go beyond, the patient's religious terminology. It requires knowledge, skill, and practice to provide religious support without imposing your own beliefs. The safest course of action, of course, is to offer to contact a chaplain for the patient. However, patients cannot always—or may not always want to—wait for a chaplain.

Active Listening (NIC)

The Active Listening intervention allows the nurse to establish a trusting relationship and to hear, understand, and interpret what the client is saying. Listening actively involves four NIC interventions and one non-standardized activity.

Presence (NIC) Presence means to be with patient and family in meaningful ways. It requires:
- Your actual presence at the bedside
- Being open to issues and concerns of the patient
- Allowing the patient to lead discussions rather than setting the agenda or controlling the conversation
- Sincere communication
- Being fully available to the client
- Listening to the patient's "stories" about his illness

Touch (NIC) Caring touch, such as hand holding or touching an arm or shoulder, can facilitate communication. It conveys concern, comfort, and acceptance, especially during stressful experiences. At least one study has shown touch to improve life satisfaction and faith. Some people prefer not to be touched, so carefully observe the patient's responses.

Exploring Meaning (non-NIC) *Meaning* refers to a clear understanding of the illness or loss (e.g., loss of independence). It also refers to the concept of finding meaning and purpose in life or a sense of personal worthiness. You can facilitate the patient's search for meaning by asking probing questions, providing explanations, and reframing maladaptive interpretations of life events.

Reminiscence Therapy (NIC) **Reminiscence** is the recalling and sharing of past life events with another person. It promotes meaning-making by rethinking and clarifying previous experiences. As the patient reminisces, he may make spiritual links by expressing personal beliefs that helped him live through difficult life events. This intervention is more effective within a long-term relationship.

Spiritual Support (NIC)

NIC defines Spiritual Support as "assisting the patient to feel balance and connection with a greater power" (Bulechek, Butcher, Dochterman, et al., 2012, p. 353). Effective Spiritual Support is based on a focused spiritual assessment, including the person's belief system. It may include assisting with forgiveness, encouraging hope, praying, and reading scriptures or other texts the patient requests.

Forgiveness Facilitation (NIC) **Forgiveness** is the act of pardoning or being pardoned for an offense, debt, or obligation. Letting go of the resentment felt for another promotes constructive changes in a person's life; a sense of renewal; and reconciliation with God, church, and one's inner being. To provide this intervention, you must first assess the patient's needs for reconciliation with self, others, and God. If, like Mr. Johnson (Meet Your Patient), the person has lost contact with family members because of disagreements, you could collaborate with the social worker and chaplain about ways to facilitate a meeting.

Forgiveness is one aspect of love. People have a spiritual need to forgive others and to be forgiven.
- When a person cannot forgive others, it separates him from them and interferes with giving and receiving love.
- When a person cannot forgive himself, he may feel the pain of shame, guilt, and anger.
- The person may be hurting because he wants forgiveness from someone he has wronged or from God.
- Many people interpret their illness as punishment for sins.

You can help the patient achieve spiritual peace by listening when the person expresses self-doubt or guilt, providing guidance, praying with the patient if he requests it, inquiring whether he is ready to forgive someone else, or offering to contact his chosen spiritual leader if intensive spiritual support is needed.

Hope Inspiration (NIC) **Hope** is a subjective state of confidence in the possibility of a better future. It includes a positive orientation, faith, and will to live. **Hopelessness** is a state in which the person perceives limited or no alternatives or personal choices. To intervene effectively, it is important to know the source of the person's hope and the factors underlying the feelings of hopelessness. As a nurse, you can encourage spiritual growth, which is thought to facilitate hope, and you can refer your patient to a support group to help in stress reduction, coping, and hope.

Prayer (non-NIC) Prayer is an integral component of almost every religion. Research shows that the percentage of

Intercessory Prayer

Complementary & Alternative Modalities (CAM)

Many people pray when they are ill, and prayer seems to have positive effects. But what about the effects of *intercessory prayer*—the prayers of people for *others* who are ill? How useful is intercessory prayer? The following studies provide little support for the use of intercessory prayer as a CAM. However, this is not an exhaustive list of studies of intercessory prayer, and research is ongoing.

➤ **Struve, Lu, Hart, et al. (2015)**—Researchers studied the effect of intercessory prayer on disruptive behaviors in six late-stage clients with dementia over a 12-week period. Results showed a reduction in disruptive behaviors in 27 categories per week. The use of antipsychotic medication was reduced or discontinued in four clients. Researchers concluded that intercessory prayer improved the clients' quality of life by reducing their disruptive behaviors.

➤ **Schlitz, Hopf, Eskenazi, et al. (2012)**—Researchers explored the efforts of distant healing intention (DHI) (also known as intercessory prayer and spiritual healing) on wound healing of 72 postoperative women. The results showed that DHI did not affect wound healing or self-reported postoperative emotional or physical health. However, the women who knowingly received prayer had significantly longer surgeries. The groups that believed in and knowingly or unknowingly received DHI had worse physical and self-reported well-being outcomes.

➤ **Roberts, Ahmed, Hall, et al. (2011)**—Selecting 10 trials from the literature that randomized more than 7,800 participants, researchers concluded that there was not a significant difference in outcomes for those receiving intercessory prayer and those who did not. However, researchers noted that in a trial on high risk of death, people in the intercessory group who were at a high risk of death were significantly more likely to live. Another trial found that some complications were significantly more likely to occur in the nonintercessory prayer group, but the certainty of receiving prayer was associated with a lower incidence of postoperative complications.

---

adults who use prayer for health concerns increased from 42% to 49% over a 5-year period (Wachholtz & Sambamoorthi, 2011). Research found that clients who received intercessory prayer had a significant improvement in spiritual and emotional well-being (Olver & Dutney, 2012) and an improved quality of life (Struve, Lu, Hart, et al., 2015).

At least 49 million older adults pray for health. African Americans and Hispanic older adults are more likely to pray for health than whites. Women are considerably more likely (97%) to pray than men, and older adults at the lower income level who have chronic conditions are more likely to pray for health (Tait, Laditka, Laditka, et al., 2011). It is quite possible that a patient or a family member may ask you to pray for or with him. You must distinguish between *praying with* and *praying for*.

- If the patient asks you to pray *with* him, determine whether he simply wants you to be present while he or another person leads the prayer. You should ask whether he wants you to begin the prayer or whether he wants to begin the prayer.

- If a patient asks you to pray *for* him, assess what it is that he wants you to pray for. Often the patient is merely asking you to pray for him on your own time, as frequently as your schedule allows.

Regardless of the situation, if you feel comfortable doing so, then you should enter the experience of prayer with confidence. After all, the patient or family member has asked you to be present because he feels at ease with you and trusts in your abilities. However, if you feel at all uncomfortable about offering prayer, then you should state your feelings and offer to find someone who is comfortable with prayer. For example, you might say either of the following to the patient or family:

- "Thank you for asking me to pray with you; there is another nurse on the floor who is better at this than I am. May I have your permission to seek that person out for you?"

- "I am confident that the chaplain can help you in many ways with your request. May I make a referral to the chaplain for you?"

Prayer consists of those ways that we respond to and interact with the Supreme Being, whether by words, thoughts, or actions (e.g., the painting in Fig. 16-5). If you wish to pray with clients, understanding the different types of prayer may help. People tend to think of prayer in its narrowest sense as being requests for something (intercession), and this is an important and useful type of prayer. However, there are at least six other types of prayer, including adoration, praise, thanksgiving, penitence, offering, and petition (*Book of Common Prayer*, 1979).

The following is an excerpt from an aunt's e-mail to her family and friends. It movingly demonstrates a belief in the powerful nature of prayer and is an example that supports the research findings that many people rely on intercessory prayer during illness.

Example: I would really appreciate your prayers . . . for my nephew . . . who is newly diagnosed with Hodgkin's lymphoma. We go to the clinic at 10 a.m. to get his labs and then [to] the Children's Hospital to start his chemotherapy. . . . He is very sad and scared. His chest symptoms have increased . . . [and] we know the mass

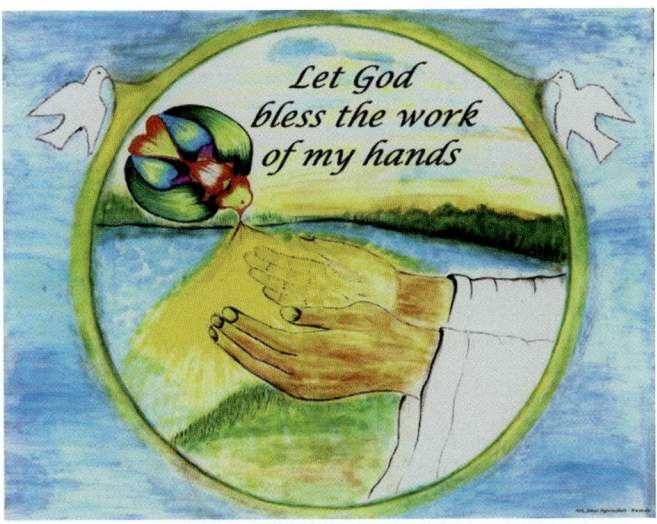

FIGURE 16-5 This painting may be an expression of prayer.

is still growing. Please pray . . . for wisdom and communication with the doctors and nurses. Pray all who come in contact with my nephew give peace, comfort, and soothing touch. Pray the side effects . . . are minimal. More than anything, . . . pray the chemo targets every cancerous cell . . . and specifically for greater than 70% shrinkage. [Pray also for] no more . . . fever, night sweats, weight loss, [and] chest pain. God truly can work miracles in times of trial and we are trusting fully in Him at this great time of need. (D. Wojcik, personal communication, March 1, 2013)

Prayer has a variety of purposes, expressions, and meanings to patients, families, and nurses. Prayer may provide for periods of intimacy with God, reveal the presence and love of God, and serve as a powerful source of comfort and hope.

Other Nursing Activities

Spiritual care involves you in relationships with people who have come face-to-face with a significant life event that creates a new sense of meaning and purpose. Specific nursing activities, to be individualized to each client's needs, are discussed, in the following list:

- **Make Referrals When Needed.** There are times when you should refer a client to others with more knowledge and experience in religion and spirituality. For example, a client may be experiencing Spiritual Distress because he believes he needs forgiveness for a past act, or a client may refuse medical treatment because she thinks her church would not approve. For hospitalized and hospice clients, you can usually ask the chaplain's office to refer the client and family to clergy or religious counselors in the community. For non-hospitalized clients, access a directory (Internet, telephone book) for local churches. Priests, ministers, rabbis, and other spiritual advisers are all resources for you and the client.

♥ iCare 16-1

Older adults have identified their spiritual needs in healthcare settings as understanding their spiritual practices; relationship with God; hope, meaning, and purpose of life; and interpersonal connections and therapeutic professional staff interactions (Hodge, Horvath, Larkin, et al., 2012).
- Taking those needs into account, what are some concrete things you might do to demonstrate caring with older adult patients?

♥ iCare 16-2

Spirituality
- Spirituality means different things to different people.
- Spirituality has a great impact on a person's well-being and outlook on healthcare situations.
- A caring nurse is respectful and open to different religious beliefs, recognizing that spirituality is an accumulation of life experiences and is very personal in nature.
- Exhibiting empathy and a nonjudgmental attitude can be supportive and helpful.
- Often, you will not need to say anything. Simply listening and "being present" in the moment is beneficial.

Complementary & Alternative Modalities (CAM)

Spiritual Care

Spiritual interventions, especially prayer, are a frequently used CAM:
- **Bekke-Hansen, Pedersen, Thygesen, et al. (2012)**—A recent study found that 76% of adult patients with acute coronary syndrome rated CAM treatments as having a positive influence on their quality of life. The most prevalent types of CAM used were dietary and exercise counseling and dietary and nutritional supplements.
- **Ben-Arye, Schiff, Vintal, et al. (2012)**—In this study, researchers found that oncology patients with a higher spiritual quest had an increased use of CAM and higher expectations that providers integrate CAM into their care.
- **Trinkaus, Burman, Barmala, et al. (2011)**—Of the 123 patients with advanced cancer on a palliative care unit, 85% had used CAM; 42% used it for curative intent. The use of CAM for cure was associated with increased spiritual faith but low existential well-being.
- **Matthews, A. (2013)**—A survey of 225 nurses identified their responses to a client's spiritual need request as providing prayer, referring a patient to the chaplain, showing respect for religious and cultural beliefs, providing comfort, encountering barriers, and sharing own faith beliefs. The study also found a positive link between religion/spirituality in the nursing curriculum, baccalaureate or higher education, and addressing client's spiritual needs.
- **Ellison, Bradshaw, & Roberts (2012)**—When compared with those who were only spiritual, participants who were both spiritual and religious were more likely to use body–mind therapies when it included the CAM of prayer, meditation, or spiritual healing and less likely (44%) when these CAMs were removed. Religious-only participants were not inclined to use CAM.

- **Encourage expression of feelings.** The best way to do this is simply to ask the client how he is feeling or what he thinks about a particular situation.
- **Help the client identify feelings of guilt.** You might ask the following after a patient has voiced a concern: "How do you feel about that?" or "You seem to feel bad about saying/doing that."
- **Help significant others understand the client's feelings and needs.** Encourage family members to talk with the patient or to just sit at the bedside. Periods of silence often lead into the most therapeutic of discussions.
- **Maximize the client's comfort.** This is one of the most important spiritual activities a nurse can perform. A client cannot think about spiritual issues when suffering physical pain or discomfort.
- **Listen to the client's "stories."** These tell the life history surrounding the person's illness and spiritual comfort or distress.
- **Assess the client's needs for reconciliation.** This may include reconciliation with self, others, and God. If the patient has lost contact with family members because of

disagreements related to past events, you could collaborate with the social worker and chaplain about ways to facilitate a meeting.

- **Explore with the client the possible meanings of** *healing,* *miracle,* **and** *cure.*
- **Collaborate with the dietary department.** Provide foods compatible with the client's religious needs. Encourage family members to bring foods from home, as appropriate.
- **Respect the client's dress (and other) requirements as determined by his religion.** This may include religious icons, jewelry, or special clothes.
- **Do not make assumptions about the client's and family's beliefs.** When a client dies, for example, a seemingly harmless statement such as "He's gone to a better place" assumes the family believes in an afterlife. If they ask, briefly share your beliefs, but reflect their questions back to them (e.g., "Tell me what *you* think happens after death").

KnowledgeCheck 16-7

- What is prayer?
- What are ways you can support a patient's prayer needs?
- When a patient asks you to pray for him, what might be your most effective first response?

ThinkLike a Nurse 16-10

A patient dying of lung cancer asks you to pray with him early one morning. You agree and ask him what he would like you to pray for. He responds, "That I may be cured of my cancer and go back home." He is on oxygen therapy, has pain medications given as prescribed, and is in a room by himself. Construct a prayer that might be meaningful and helpful.

Return to the scenario for Charles Johnson (Meet Your Patient). See whether you can answer the three questions more completely now than when you began reading the chapter.

Summary

In summary, the more you know about yourself, the more effectively you care for others. To work effectively with a diverse population, you must first obtain a great degree of self-knowledge. Try the following:

- Be open to the many possibilities for diverse thinking.
- Welcome challenging experiences that allow for personal growth.
- Take time to think about how your actions and biases might affect the care of others. As you know, communication and therapeutic relationships are important in supporting spirituality.

CLINICALREASONING

The questions and exercises in this section allow you to practice the kind of thinking you will use as a full-spectrum nurse. Critical-thinking questions usually have more than one correct answer, so we do not provide "correct answers" for these features. It is more important to develop your nursing judgment than to just cover content. You will learn by discussing the questions with your peers. If you are still unsure, see the Davis Advantage chapter resources for suggested responses.

Caring for the Nguyens

Kim Phan is the 3-year-old grandson of Nam and Yen Nguyen. The Nguyens are both practicing Catholics. Kim's mother, Trinh, is the Nguyens' daughter. Trinh feels that Catholicism is "a waste of time" and does not attend church. Kim has had no formal religious experiences or training.

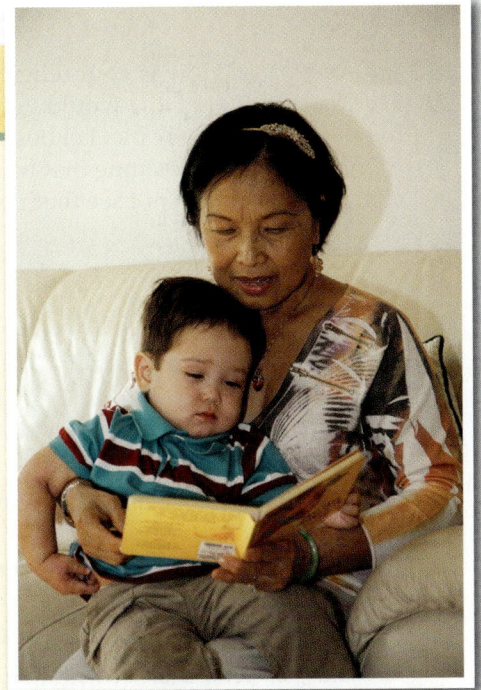

(Continued)

Caring for the Nguyens (continued)

A. At a clinic visit, Nam asks you what you think about keeping religion away from a child. How would you respond?

B. Mr. Nguyen explains his views on the situation: "If anything were to happen to him, he would go to hell. I think we should take him to church and get him baptized right away. I don't know how anyone can live like that. He has no connection to God." Do you agree with this statement? Explain your views.

C. Nam asks you to pray for Kim and his mother. How would you feel about this situation? What would you say to Nam?

Applying the **Full-Spectrum Nursing Model**_____

PATIENT SITUATION

Review the Meet Your Patient scenario to answer the questions below about Charles Johnson, a 75-year-old black man with newly diagnosed cancer of the lung. His physicians want to start chemotherapy to try to increase his life span. He is unsure whether he wants to have chemotherapy.

THINKING

1. *Theoretical Knowledge (Recall of Facts and Principles):* Define *forgiveness* and explain the benefits of forgiving self and others.
2. *Critical Thinking (Application of Knowledge):* Based on your theoretical knowledge about forgiveness, with whom might Mr. Johnson need to reconcile? Why do you think so?

DOING

3. *Practical Knowledge (HOPE Assessment):* Use the Focused Assessment box The HOPE Approach to Spiritual Assessment: Examples of Questions, and enter Mr. Johnson's data. Identify sections for which you need additional data.

CARING

4. *Self-Knowledge:* How is your religious background similar to or different from Mr. Johnson's?
5. *Self-Knowledge:* (a) How would you feel if Mr. Johnson said to you, "Church folk are all a bunch of hypocrites, if you ask me. I choose not to be a part of any of that"? (b) How would you respond?
6. *Ethical Knowledge:* Imagine that Mr. Johnson's sister comes to visit and leaves some religious pamphlets on a chair, where he will not see them before she leaves. What would you do?

 To explore learning resources for this chapter,

 Go to **www.DavisAdvantage.com** and find:

Answers and Suggested Responses for all questions in this chapter
Lists of NIC Interventions and NOC Outcomes
List of NANDA-I Diagnoses
Knowledge Map
References and Bibliography

Concept Map

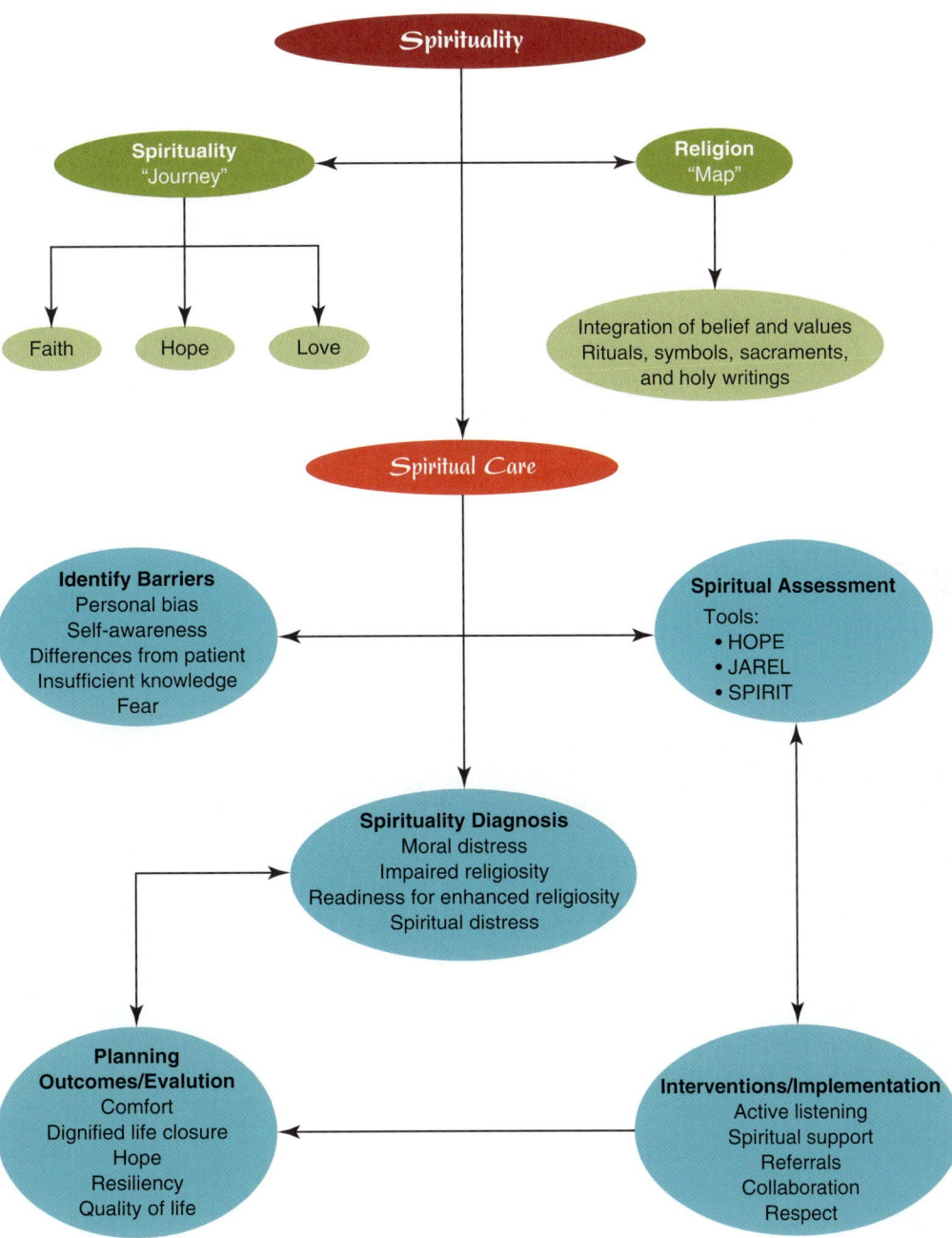

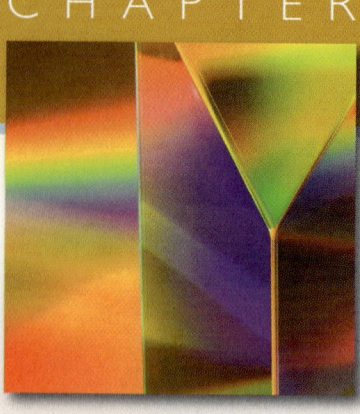

CHAPTER 17

Loss, Grief, & Dying

Learning Outcomes

After completing this chapter, you should be able to:

➤ Name and describe at least four types of loss.

➤ Identify the stages of grief as described by major theorists.

➤ Compare and contrast four types of grief.

➤ List and discuss at least five factors that affect grieving.

➤ Define *death* according to the Uniform Determination of Death Act.

➤ Give a definition of *higher-brain death.*

➤ Create a time line of the dying process, indicating the physiological signs and symptoms common to each stage.

➤ List and describe the models and theories of grief and bereavement.

➤ Define *end-of-life care, hospice care,* and *palliative care.*

➤ Identify the legal and ethical issues involved in death and dying.

➤ Apply the nursing process in the care of dying patients and their families.

➤ Describe the responsibilities of the nurse regarding postmortem care.

➤ Identify nursing interventions to help clients who are grieving.

Key Concepts

Death and dying

End-of-life care

Grief

Loss

Related Concepts

See the Concept Map at the end of this chapter.

Meet Your Patient

Thomas Manning is a 47-year-old man who is in the oncology unit with end-stage cancer of the pancreas. He is married and has three children, aged 18, 15, and 13. His oldest daughter has been away at college for only 6 months. Mr. Manning's father died 3 months ago of complications of alcoholism, and his mother has been withdrawn and grieving. His wife, Mary, tells you that Thomas "just wants to die" and does not want anyone trying to revive him or "jump on his chest" if he dies. Mary is distressed and wants him to "keep fighting."

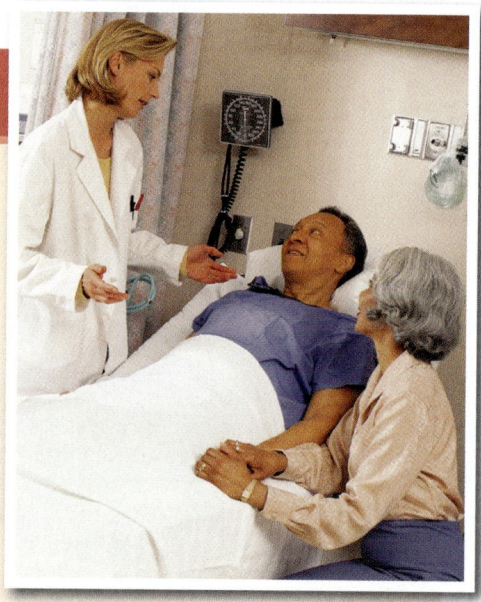

Theoretical Knowledge
knowing why

Throughout your nursing career, you will care for patients coping with loss—of youth, beauty, previous health, functioning, or quality of life. Some, like Thomas Manning, will be confronting their own approaching death, while family members will be facing loss of their loved one. You can use your theoretical and practical knowledge to help these people cope with their losses and grieve in a way that is healing, even transformative. As a foundation, you must understand your own feelings and attitudes about loss, grief, and dying.

ABOUT THE KEY CONCEPTS

In order to provide care for patients experiencing loss, you will need to understand the key concepts of **loss, grief, death and dying,** and **end-of-life care.** Related concepts, such as stages of death, depression, and grief education, will expand the way you think about the key concepts.

WHAT IS LOSS?

Do you associate *loss* with death? Many people think of loss as losing a loved one through death. Loss is a daily occurrence. **Loss** can be defined as the undesired change or removal of a valued object, person, or situation. It begins at birth when we lose the warmth and security of the womb and ends with the ultimate loss, the death of self. Examples of losses at each stage of development include the following:

- Infancy (birth through 12–18 months)—weaning from breast or bottle
- Toddler (18 months–3 years)—loss of the familiar setting; going to preschool
- Early childhood (3–6 years)—going to full-day school; moving and losing friends
- Middle childhood (6 years to puberty)—loss of the familiar; dealing with body changes
- Adolescence (puberty to 19 years)—loss of childhood; expectation to act grown up
- Young adulthood (20–45)—loss of single status/parents' home; changing relationships
- Middle adulthood (45–65 years)—children leaving home; job changes; medical issues
- Older adulthood (> 65 years)—loss of health, friends; retirement

Categories of Loss

Loss can be categorized in the following ways:

- **Actual loss** includes the death of a loved one (or relationship), theft, deterioration, destruction, and natural disaster. The loss can be identified by others, not just by the person experiencing it (e.g., hair loss during chemotherapy).
- **Perceived loss** is internal; it is identified only by the person experiencing it (e.g., a woman with a sexually transmitted infection may perceive loss of her purity).
- **Physical loss** includes (1) injuries (e.g., limb amputation), (2) organ removal (e.g., hysterectomy), and (3) loss of function (e.g., paralysis).
- **Psychological (internal) losses** are commonly seen in the areas of sexuality, control, fairness, meaning, and trust. Loss of youth, limbs, body disfigurement, or body functions can negatively impact one's perception of self. The effect is loss of hope, faith, or dreams.

- **External losses** are actual losses of objects that sentimental or monetary value (e.g., jewelry, a home).
- **Environmental loss** involves a change in the familiar, even if the change is perceived as positive (e.g., moving to a new home, getting a new job, and going to college).
- **Loss of significant relationships** includes, but is not limited to, actual loss of spouses, siblings, family members, or significant others through death, divorce, or separation.

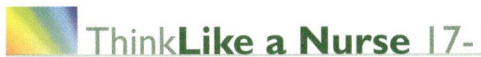

ThinkLike a Nurse 17-1

- Which kinds of loss do you think Thomas Manning (Meet Your Patient) is experiencing?
- Why is it important to recognize loss?

WHAT IS GRIEF?

Whenever there is significant loss, there is grieving. Although grieving requires energy and can interfere with health and delay healing, it is positive and essential to psychological healing after a loss. Consider the following losses and the different reactions of the women involved:

Both Mrs. Smith and Mrs. Jones have lost a dog. The dog that Mrs. Smith's son left with her when he went away to college last year has died of old age. Mrs. Jones's dog of 10 years and only companion since her husband died 5 years ago was killed by a car today. Which woman do you think will grieve her loss more? Why? Discuss this situation with a classmate. Do you both have the same opinion about this?

It is really impossible to decide who would feel "more" grief because the meaning of and attachment to the dog are different for each one. Both women probably felt sad. **KEY POINT:** *The intensity of the grief depends on the meaning the person attaches to the loss.*

You might have thought Mrs. Smith's loss was minor; however, her dog was owned by her son and may have represented him in her mind. Mrs. Jones's dog was a companion and a protector and may have represented security and friendship. Each woman must grieve what the loss represents to her. This is true for everyone who experiences grief.

- **Grief** is the physical, psychological, and spiritual responses to a loss.
- **Mourning** consists of actions associated with grief (e.g., wailing, wearing black clothing). These processes are normal and natural responses to a loss.
- **Bereavement** is the period of mourning and adjustment after a loss.

KEY POINT: *Although each person may express grief differently, some aspects of grief are shared by almost everyone.*

KnowledgeCheck 17-1

What types of losses commonly occur in our lives?

Theoretical Foundations of Grief

There is no single, correct way to grieve, nor do people move neatly from one stage or step of grief to the next. Rather, grieving is a fluid, ongoing process. Several theorists provide insight into the grieving process and its associated stages (see Table 17-1).

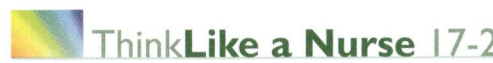

ThinkLike a Nurse 17-2

What are some of the similarities you see in the models/theories described?

Table 17-1 ➤ Theories and Models of Grief

STAGES	DESCRIPTION
George Engel (1961)—Three Stages of Grief.	
Uncomplicated grief is universal, has a clear onset and a predictable course (with modifications), and does not require treatment.	
Shock and disbelief	Initial phase. The sufferer denies the loss in an attempt to protect himself against the shock of reality.
Developing awareness of the loss	■ Painful feelings of sadness, guilt, shame, helplessness, hopelessness, loss, and emptiness
	■ Loss of interest in usual activities; impaired work performance
	■ Loss of appetite, sleep disturbances, physical symptoms of pain or other discomfort
Restitution and recovery	■ Final phase; prolonged and gradual
	■ Carries on the work of mourning and overcomes the trauma of the loss
	■ A state of health and well-being is reestablished.
John Bowlby (1982)—Phases of Grief.	
This attachment theory describes the reaction to strong emotional bonds that have been developed. The individual must work through each process to avoid complicated grief. Grief is a mature way of dealing with loss of attachment.	
Shock and numbness	■ Initial stage
	■ Disorientation
	■ Feelings of helplessness
Yearning and searching	■ The grieving person yearns to be reconnected with the deceased and searches for connections.
Disorganization and despair	■ Permanence of the loss now real
	■ Feelings of pain
	■ Emotions of grief to the fullest
	■ Feels there is no hope of reconnection
Reorganization	■ Adjusting to life without the deceased (or lost object)
	● Developing new coping skills
Theresa Rando (1984, 1986, 1993, 2000).	
Rando identified the three Processes of Grieving described below. In addition, she identified six tasks (6Rs) associated with grieving: (1) **R**ecognizing the loss, (2) **R**eacting to the separation, (3) **R**ecollecting memories of the deceased, (4) **R**elinquishing the old attachment, (5) **R**eadjusting to the new environment, and (6) **R**einvesting self.	
Avoidance	■ Shock, disbelief, denial, anger, bargaining
Confrontation	■ Begins to face the loss
	■ A very emotional and upsetting time when grief is felt most acutely
Accommodation	■ Begins to live with the loss
	■ Feels better
	■ Resumes some routine activities
William Worden (2002)—Four Tasks of Grieving.	
Accepting the reality of the loss	■ *Realizing that the loved one (or object) is gone.*
	■ In the hours and days after a significant loss, the grieving person typically feels numb and unable to accept the fact of the loss.

Table 17-1 ➤ Theories and Models of Grief—cont'd

STAGES	DESCRIPTION
	▪ Numbness is thought to be a helpful form of denial, which allows the person to "take in" only what the psyche is capable of handling.
	▪ The task of realizing the loved one or object is gone may take several days or, in the case of a sudden death, weeks.
Working through the pain and grief	▪ *Feelings and emotions that surface are intense and can change rapidly.*
	▪ Feels "out of control"
	▪ May say she feels as if "going crazy"
	▪ Usually the longest phase for two reasons:
	1. Because none of us likes to be in pain, we become expert at finding ways not to feel it. We overeat, overmedicate, overwork, and drink to excess to avoid feeling the pain, and we thereby prolong the process of grief.
	2. Caring people do not like to see their loved ones in pain, so they make attempts to remove the pain (e.g., by distraction) rather than letting the person experience it. Like avoidance, this well-meaning behavior also prolongs the process.
Adjusting to the environment in which the deceased is missing	▪ *Adjusting to the environment without the deceased.*
	▪ This may mean performing alone activities and tasks, such as going for walks or shopping, that were once shared.
	▪ It may include taking on roles and responsibilities that the deceased previously held.
	▪ Such experiences can be extremely sad, frustrating, and challenging, or very rewarding.
	▪ Once the person has established the new pattern, he or she typically feels satisfaction and increased self-esteem.
Emotionally relocating the deceased and moving on with life	▪ *Investing emotional energy.*
	▪ Initially all energy is focused on the deceased: thinking about the person, talking about him/her, reliving memories, and so on. It is nearly impossible to think of anything else.
	▪ Concentration is difficult, so the grieving person finds it hard to engage in activities such as reading.
	▪ When the person's energy begins to flow toward others or to different or former interests (e.g., working, socializing), the healing process is in progress.
Elisabeth Kübler-Ross (1969)—Five Stages of Grieving.	
Individuals may not experience every stage or go through the stages in a linear order. In addition, individuals may experience two or more stages simultaneously.	
Denial	▪ "Not me." "This cannot be happening." "I don't believe it."
	▪ The person is usually in a state of shock
	▪ Denial is not necessarily negative; it gives the person a chance to prepare psychologically for accepting the news.
Anger	▪ "Why me?" "Why is this happening?"
	▪ Anger can be obvious or subtle.
	▪ Anger is the person's response to the feeling that the situation is unfair.
	▪ The person may take his anger out on people who are "safe" (e.g., family, spouse) or from whom there will be no reprisals (e.g., nurses, provider).
Bargaining	▪ "If only I can live until . . ." "Yes me, but . . ." Usually this takes the form of a bargain with God or a Higher Power, in which the person asks to live to see a birth, graduation, wedding, and so forth.

(Continued)

Table 17-1 ➤ Theories and Models of Grief—cont'd

STAGES	DESCRIPTION
Depression	■ A withdrawn sadness, not to be confused with clinical depression. This is a response to the current loss as well as to any accumulated and/or future losses.
Acceptance	■ Not necessarily *wanting* death (or the loss), but coming to terms with it and ceasing to fight it. The person may seem almost devoid of feelings.

Margaret Stroebe and Henk Schut (1999)—Dual Process Model.

Mourning is cyclical. People oscillate between two dimensions in bereavement.

Loss-oriented response	■ Focuses on grief work
	■ Concentrates on appraising and processing the loss; searches for meaning
	■ Experiencing pain
Restoration-oriented response	■ Focuses on dealing with the consequences of the loss
	■ Establishes new routines and takes on new roles (paying bills, doing laundry)
	■ Reorients to the world without the decreased person

Dennis Klass, Phyllis R. Silverman, and Steven L. Nickman (1996)—Continuing Bond Model.

Bereavement, or grief, is never fully resolved.

■ The focus should not be on individuals' obtaining closure but instead on finding new ways to relate to the deceased.

■ The griever maintains a continuing bond with the deceased.

Negotiate and Renegotiate	■ The meaning of the loss is negotiated and renegotiated over time.
	■ However, the emphasis is not on achieving closure or forgetting.
	■ The emphasis is on establishing therapeutic expressions of continuing bonds to adapt to the loss (e.g., memorabilia, pictures).

Robert Neimeyer (1999)—Meaning-Making Model of Grief/Bereavement.

Grieving is a process of meaning reconstruction. The best predictor of a positive adaptation to loss is the ability to find meaning in the loss. The unsuccessful struggle to find meaning can result in complicated forms of grief.

Sources: Bowlby, J. (1982). *Attachment and loss* (Vols 1–3). New York, NY: Basic Books; Engel, G. L. (1961). Is grief a disease? A challenge for medical research. *Psychosomatic Medicine, 23*(1), 18–22; Kübler-Ross, E. (1969). *On death and dying.* New York, NY: Macmillan; Neimeyer, R. (1999). Narrative strategies in grieving therapy. *Journal of Constructivist Psychology, 12*(1), 65–68; Rando, T. (1984). *Grief, dying and death: Clinical interventions for caregivers.* Champaign, IL: Research Press; Smit, C. (2015). Theories and models of grief: Applications to professional practice. *Whitireia Nursing and Health Journal, 22*(1), 33–37; Stroebe, M., & Schut, H. (1999). The dual process model of coping with bereavement: Rational and description. *Death Studies, 23*(3), 197–224; Stroebe, M., & Schut, H. (2010). The dual process model of coping: A decade on. *Omega: Journal of Death and Dying, 61*(4), 273–289. doi:10.2190/OM.61.4.b; Worden, J. W. (2002). *Grief counseling and grief therapy: A handbook for the mental health practitioner* (3rd ed.). New York, NY: Springer.

Factors Affecting Grief

To begin thinking about factors affecting grieving, consider the exercise in Think Like a Nurse 17-3.

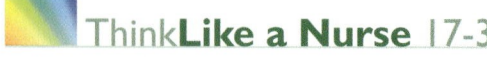

ThinkLike a Nurse 17-3

Mr. Klein is an 86-year-old man whose wife died of heart disease 2 months ago. He has two adult children, both of whom visit him regularly. He also has a very supportive pastor, Mr. Owens, who meets him in the park to share stories. Mr. Owens is 30 years old and has been raising his 5-year-old daughter alone for the past 6 months after the sudden death of his wife in an automobile accident. His parents and siblings live out of state. Each man misses his wife very much.

■ What factors do you think play a role in each man's grief?
■ Who do you think will "get over it" faster?
■ What are some issues that may make each man's grief uniquely difficult?

Many factors play a role in a person's grieving process. They include the following:

■ **Significance of the Loss.** The meaning the person has attached to the person or object lost will be different for each person. The greater the attachment, the more difficult the grieving will be.

- **Support System.** People with strong emotional and psychosocial support typically have less complicated grief.
- **Unresolved Conflicts.** Prolonged or complicated grief can occur with unresolved conflict. A conflict (e.g., an argument) left unresolved may cause prolonged grief.
- **Circumstances of the Loss.** The manner and circumstances of the death can leave the bereaved feeling guilty, responsible, or unprepared. Violent deaths (e.g., homicide, suicide, accident) can result in prolonged or complicated grief.
- **Previous Loss.** A person who has sustained several losses in a short period of time may experience complicated grief. In the hospital, you will frequently care for patients with multiple losses; for example, a patient suffering a stroke with paralysis has lost his mobility, independence, and familiar surroundings when moved to a skilled care facility.
- **Spiritual/Cultural Beliefs and Practices.** Spirituality and religious beliefs can help or hinder the grieving process. One person might believe that the deceased is in a place of contentment and happiness, where all suffering is over. Another may believe that the deceased person will be reborn into another form. Yet another may believe that death is final and there is no afterlife. Most cultures engage in rituals (e.g., funerals) that allow the bereaved to openly express their grief and pain (Fig. 17-1), whereas others may limit expressions of grief to private settings.
- **Timeliness of the Death.** The death of a child or a young person is almost universally more difficult to accept than the death of an older person. In addition to loss of the person, there is a sense of unfairness because of the loss of *potential*—of what the child might have become or achieved.

Developmental Stages and Grief

Based on Erik Erikson's stages of psychological growth, we all must achieve certain psychological milestones during a lifetime. Grief can affect the healthy development of life stages, and in turn, the person's stage of development affects the grieving process. If you need to review Erikson's theory, refer to Chapter 9.

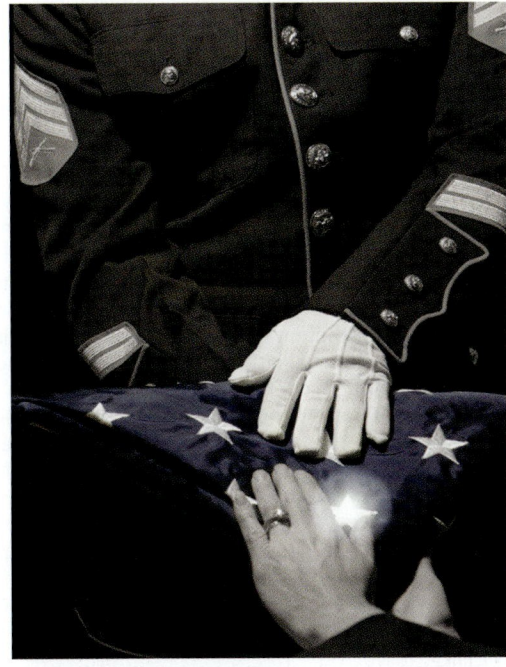

FIGURE 17-1 Rituals are used to facilitate grieving.

Childhood Because cognitive development is not yet complete, preschool children believe that death is temporary and reversible, as with cartoon characters that "die" and then "come to life" again. During early childhood, children begin to understand that death is permanent, but they believe it would never happen to them or anyone they know.

Young children believe they are the cause of what happens around them. This is known as *magical thinking*. Such thinking may cause them to feel guilt when there is a death of someone close to them. Other responses include regressing to a previous developmental stage: "acting like a baby," demanding food and attention, becoming incontinent, and talking "baby talk."

During the weeks after a death, a child may feel immediate grief, may or may not display sadness, or may continue to believe the person is still alive. These are normal reactions.

Adolescence The bereavement and emotions felt by adolescents along with confusion regarding their identity and role can create major uncertainty. The adolescent is struggling to learn who he is as a person as he breaks away from parental control. The loss of a parent while pushing the parent away may create a sense of guilt and unfinished business.

At the same time, the bereaved teen also faces psychological, physiological, social, and academic pressures. Although teens may look mature, they often lack emotional maturity but are often expected to be "grown up" and support a surviving parent or younger siblings. When they feel this responsibility, they do not have the opportunity, or the permission, to mourn and may turn to non-family members to discuss their feelings.

 Research shows that bereaved youths who have lost a parent have a higher frequency of engaging in health risk behaviors (Hamdan, Mazariegos, Melhem, et al., 2012). Adult caregivers must be alert to these behaviors and take appropriate interventions to meet the bereavement and safety needs of children and adolescents.

Adulthood Adults are cognitively able to understand the nature of death, and have usually experienced other types of loss. Over time, they perceive loss as a normal part of living. How they respond to loss depends on factors such as one's self-esteem and the availability of supports.

Older Adulthood A special difficulty for older adults is the cumulative effect of the many losses that they experience. Most deaths occur among older adults, so they are likely to lose friends and siblings in rapid succession, along with physical and functional losses and the loss of independence. In addition, they began the process of preparatory grief in anticipation of their own death (MacKenzie, 2011). The emotional effects may be devastating.

Research reveals that elderly adults who have suffered the loss of a child experience significant and sometimes irreparable mental and physical outcomes, accelerated disabilities, and loss of the ability to function independently. To minimize these negative outcomes, caregivers should use listening skills and metaphors and promote storytelling (Smith, Kerr, Galligan, et al. 2011).

KnowledgeCheck 17-2

- What are the main tasks of the grieving process?
- What factors affect the grieving process?

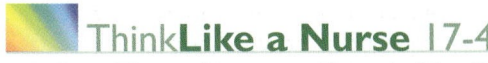 ThinkLike a Nurse 17-4

Refer to Thomas Manning and his wife (Meet Your Patient). Apply each of the preceding factors affecting grief to Thomas and to Mary (they may be different for each spouse). If the scenario does not provide enough information for you to comment, say so and then describe how you would obtain the data you need.

Types of Grief

Grief can be categorized in several ways, most of which have to do with timing and intensity.

Uncomplicated Grief (normal grief) is the natural response to the loss of a person or object. The bereaved person experiences the expected feelings, behaviors, and cognitions. Emotions are intense but gradually diminish over time (several months to several years). Some emotions will always be present, but the intensity will change.

Complicated Grief, also known as prolonged acute grief, is characterized by intensity of emotions and length of time. The person's responses are maladaptive, dysfunctional, unusually prolonged, or overwhelming (Germain, Shear, Walsh, et al., 2013). For example, the bereaved may become severely depressed, violent, or suicidal; become a "workaholic"; become socially isolated; or demonstrate addictive behavior. After several years the person may still be experiencing as much pain and disruption as in the first months after the loss. Chronic grief, masked grief, and delayed grief are all examples of complicated grief:

- **Chronic grief** begins as normal grief but continues long term, with little resolution of feelings and inability to rejoin normal life.
- **Masked grief** occurs when the person is grieving but expressing the grief through other types of behavior. For example, a man whose wife has died may begin drinking heavily, or a couple who lost a child start to argue more intensely with each other. They may not recognize this change in behavior as a part of their grief response.
- **Delayed grief** is grief that is put off until a later time (e.g., "I'll think about it later; right now, I'm busy trying to keep a roof over our heads and care for my children").

Disenfranchised Grief is experienced in connection with a loss that is not socially supported or acknowledged by the usual rites or ceremonies. Some examples include the unplanned termination of a child's foster placement or a mistress whose lover dies (Lang, Fleiszer, Duhamel, et al., 2011; Riggs & Willsmore, 2012). In each of these instances, the bereaved person lacks the familial or communal support that is helpful in grieving.

Anticipatory Grief is experienced before a loss occurs. A wife caring for her husband through a long illness may grieve as she sees the vibrant man she once knew change before her eyes as she anticipates his death. A potential negative outcome of anticipatory grief is that the survivor may detach from the person too early in the dying process, leaving the person without emotional support during that period. This does not always happen, of course.

ThinkLike a Nurse 17-5

Thomas Manning (Meet Your Patient) had a strained relationship with his father for most of his life. His father was an alcoholic and constantly fought with his mother while Thomas was growing up. A few months ago, his father was hospitalized for the third time for complications of alcoholism, and Thomas visited him. He confronted his father regarding his drinking and the problems and pain it had caused him and the family. The confrontation ended in an argument. That night, Thomas's father slipped into a coma and died a few days later without recovering consciousness.

- What issues does Thomas have to deal with?
- Why might this be a complicated grief process?

DEATH AND DYING

In mainstream North American culture, death is not seen as a natural part of life but rather as something to avoid at all costs. Dying is associated with the loss of physical control, function, independence, possibilities, and relationships. Death is viewed as the ultimate loss.

How Is Death Defined?

The definitions of death have evolved with considerations of technology.

- **Higher-brain death.** In the 1970s, many practitioners began using the term **higher-brain death,** which defines death as the irreversible cessation of all "higher" brain functions (e.g., cognitive functioning, consciousness, memory, reasoning). By this definition, a functioning brainstem could maintain both respiratory and cardiac activity, although the person does not make purposive responses to external stimuli; cephalic reflexes are absent; and the electroencephalogram shows no activity.
- **The Uniform Law Commission,** in 1978, redefined death broadly as the "irreversible cessation of all functioning of the brain, including the brainstem" as determined by reasonable medical standards. This definition did not provide clear guidance to states.
- **The Uniform Determination of Death Act** was adopted in 1981 to further clarify (see Box 17-1) and expand the previous definition to include the "irreversible cessation of circulation and respiratory functions" based on acceptable medical standards. Providers use several methods to assess for functioning of the brainstem (e.g., pupils fixed and unresponsive to light, no corneal reflex, absence of vestibulo-ocular reflexes).

What Are Coma and a Persistent Vegetative State?

A **coma** is a prolonged, deep state of unconsciousness lasting days or even years. The patient cannot be aroused and may or may not have decreased brainstem reflexes.

BOX 17-1 ■ Uniform Determination of Death Act

1. [Determination of Death] An individual who has sustained either (1) irreversible cessation of circulatory and respiratory functions, or (2) irreversible cessation of all functions of the entire brain, including the brain stem, is dead. A determination of death must be made in accordance with accepted medical standards.
2. [Uniformity of Construction and Application] This act shall be applied and construed to effectuate its general purpose to make uniform the law with respect to the subject of this Act among states enacting it.

Source: President's Commission for the Study of Ethical Problems in Medicine and Biomedical and Behavioral Research. (1981). *Defining death: A report on the medical, legal, and ethical issues in the determination of death* (p. 73). Washington, DC: Government Printing Office.

The loss of higher cerebral functions can result in a **persistent vegetative state (PVS).** The person does not purposefully respond to stimuli, is unaware of the environment, and has no cognition or affective mental functions. Thus, the person cannot speak or obey commands. Patients in a PVS may look somewhat normal and may occasionally grimace, cry, or laugh. They continue to have a sleep–wake cycle, may have some spontaneous movements, and may open their eyes in response to external stimuli. The family may believe that the patient is responding to the environment and thus not want to give up hope for recovery. Because they cannot work through the grieving process, they continue to grieve each day.

What Are the Stages of Dying?

To help dying patients and their families understand the dying process, your theoretical knowledge must include an understanding of both physiological and psychological processes.

Physiological Stages of Dying

The dying process is unique to each person. However, people experience many similar symptoms as they approach the end of life. Fewer than 10% of patients die suddenly and unexpectedly, as in an accident or massive heart attack. Ninety percent die after a long illness, progressively deteriorating until experiencing an active dying phase at the end (Emanuel, Ferris, von Gunten, et al., 2015; Knight & von Gunten, n.d.). The following time line describes the physiological responses of that group (Karnes, 1995; Scott, 2016):

One to Three Months Before Death The dying person begins to withdraw from the world and people. Sleep increases. It becomes difficult for the body to digest food, especially meats, and appetite and food intake decrease. Liquids are preferred. Anorexia and the resulting ketosis may be protective, as they can diminish pain and increase the person's sense of well-being.

One to Two Weeks Before Death A host of physical changes indicates the body is beginning to lose its ability to maintain itself. Cardiovascular deterioration brings reduced blood pressure, changes in pulse and skin color (e.g., a yellowish pallor), and extreme pallor of the extremities. Temperature fluctuates and perspiration increases. Respiratory rate may increase or decrease; during sleep, the dying person may experience brief periods of apnea. Congestion may cause a rattling sound and/or a nonproductive cough.

Days to Hours Before Death Often a surge of energy brings mental clarity and a desire to eat and talk with family members. However, as death approaches, patients tend to become dehydrated and have difficulty swallowing, which results in decreased blood volume. The tissues of the tongue and soft palate sag, and the gag reflex declines, so secretions accumulate in the oropharynx and/or bronchi. Often the mucous membranes become dry and tacky and lips become cracked. Dehydration during the last hours of dying is thought not to cause distress and perhaps acts to stimulate endorphin release (Emanuel, Ferris, von Gunten, et al., 2015; McGinley, 2014).

- **Respirations**—Breathing may be shallow, rapid, or irregular: Periods of apnea may lengthen to 10 to 30 seconds before breathing resumes.
  - Congestion causes a "death rattle" that can be quite loud.
  - **Cheyne-Stokes respirations** may occur. This is a cyclic pattern consisting of a 10- to 60-second period of apnea and then a gradual increase in depth and rate of respirations. Respirations gradually become slow and shallow, and then the cycle begins again with apnea.

- **Peripheral circulation** decreases, and the person perspires and feels "clammy."
  - Blood pressure decreases; pulse may be hard to detect.
  - Extremities become cool and mottled; the underside of the body may be much darker.
  - Decreased circulation also results in reduced kidney function and decreased urinary output.
- **Elimination**—As peristalsis slows, the patient may retain feces. Urine output decreases and urine often becomes more concentrated and foul smelling. Sphincters relax, and bowel and bladder incontinence can occur.
- **Muscles** throughout the body relax, causing the face to "droop."
- **Vision** blurs; the eyes may be open or partially open but unseeing. Instead, the patient may see things that are not visible to others.
- **Cognition**—In the final hours of life, many patients become restless and agitated. This response may be caused by medications, liver failure, cerebral hypoxia, renal failure, stool impaction, distended bladder, increased pain, or unresolved emotional or spiritual issues. Near to the time of death, some people unexpectedly become more coherent and energized for a time. Others become less communicative, quiet, and withdrawn (Pitorak, 2003; Scott, 2016). Fatigue is common.

Moments Before Death The dying person does not respond to touch or sound and cannot be awakened. Typically, there is a short series of long-spaced breaths before breathing ceases entirely and the heart stops beating (National Caregiver Library, n.d.; Scott, 2016).

Psychological Stages of Dying

Perhaps the best known author on the psychology of dying is Dr. Elisabeth Kübler-Ross (1969). She felt that if people understood what dying patients are experiencing, they would be more competent in caring for them. She found that people tend to experience one or more of five psychological stages during the period from the time of the terminal diagnosis to the actual death (see Table 17-1). When you study the Kübler-Ross stages, it is important to understand that dying people:

- May not go through *every* stage.
- May not go through the stages in a linear fashion, but rather in random order.
- Do not necessarily complete one stage and move on to the next.
- May experience two or three stages simultaneously.

KEY POINT: *Remember that it is not the nurse's responsibility to move people to the next stage so that dying patients accept death. It is our responsibility to accept and support people "where they are" and help them to verbalize their feelings. We need to understand patients, not change them.*

What Is End-of-Life Care?

When, precisely, is the end of life? There is no set, agreed-upon definition or set of criteria. A recent set of guidelines provides a working definition that includes the following three situations:

- The patient has a fatal condition.
- Death is likely with the next exacerbation of disease.
- The patient acknowledges the seriousness of the situation.

The goal is to ensure that end-of-life care is delivered with compassion, sensitivity, and competency. Some of these competencies include the following (Bednash & Ferrell, 2000; End-of-Life Nursing Education Consortium, 2012):

- Making a holistic assessment of patients and families (i.e., physical, psychological, social, and spiritual)

- Acknowledging diversity in patients' beliefs and customs
- Promoting the provision of comfort care to the patient by addressing symptoms (e.g., pain, dyspnea, constipation, anxiety, fatigue, nausea, vomiting, altered cognition)
- Evaluating the impact of traditional, complementary, and technological therapies on patient, families, and established outcomes
- Incorporating essential communication strategies that meet spiritual and cultural needs
- Applying legal and ethical principles to end-of-life care
- Demonstrating respect for the patients' views and wishes during end-of-life care
- Assessing patient, family, colleagues, and one's own success in coping with suffering, grief, loss, and bereavement at the end of life
- Recognizing one's own attitudes, feelings, values, and expectations about death and dying
- Providing quality postmortem care

End-of-life care includes palliative care and hospice care, which are similar in that both may involve caring for dying patients, and neither focuses on cure. Some people use the terms interchangeably; however, there are subtle differences.

Palliative Care

When patients reach a stage in their illness in which cure is no longer possible, or when they refuse further treatment, they may be eligible to receive "comfort care"—meaning that no further efforts will be made to stop the disease process or prevent the patient from dying. However, the patient will receive treatments to minimize unpleasant symptoms (e.g., pain, nausea). Although the correct interpretation of the term *comfort care* is

"Nothing more *can* be done to cure your loved one," members sometimes interpret it as "Nothing more *will* be done." In this situation, the term *palliative care,* which is provided by a holistic team of professionals, may be more acceptable. Some patients receive palliative care from their primary provider and even in acute care hospitals. These providers should be comfortable with and educated on end-of-life care (Emanuel, Ferris, von Gunten, et al., 2015; Higgins, Riet, Sneesby, et al., 2014).

Palliative care is actually aggressively planned comfort care. It addresses end-of-life care concerns that include supporting families and caregivers, promoting continuity of care, ensuring respect for persons, addressing emotional and spiritual concerns, managing symptoms (e.g., pain, dyspnea, depression), and ensuring informed decision making.

A patient does not necessarily have to be "actively dying" to receive palliative care. It can also be provided over a long period of time for those who have slowly progressive diseases. The overall goal of palliative care is increased patient/family satisfaction, improved symptom control, and cost savings for hospitals (Owens, Eby, Burson, et al., 2012).

Hospice Care

The hospice movement was set in motion in England by Dame Cicely Sanders, who founded the first modern-day hospice within a London hospital in 1968. Hospice care focuses on holistic care of patients who are dying or debilitated and not expected to improve. Unlike palliative care, for a patient to be eligible for hospice insurance benefits, a provider must certify that the patient is likely to die within 6 months.

Hospice care is based on two key premises: (1) The quality of life is as important as the length of life, and (2) those who are terminally ill should be allowed to face death with dignity and surrounded by the comfort of their homes and families. The purposes of admitting a patient are to:

- Provide a family with some respite for a period of time
- Stabilize a patient who requires symptom management
- Care for a patient who is in the end stage of a disease (e.g., AIDS or cancer) and needs a level of expert care that family members cannot provide at home

An interprofessional team plans holistic care with the patient and family. Family members are encouraged to be active in the team to the extent they are able. Nursing support is available 24 hours a day and families are taught what to expect as the disease progresses. As the patient nears death, hospice workers remain as long as necessary. After the patient dies, there is follow-up bereavement care for the families.

Complementary & Alternative Modalities (CAM)

End-of-Life Care

- **Hodgson (2013)** studied the effects of reflexology and Swedish massage on pain reduction and symptoms of agitation in 60 end-stage dementia patients. Results revealed that both CAMs promoted palliation of symptoms and pain reduction.
- **Heath, Oh, Clarke, et al. (2012)** interviewed parents of children who had died of cancer to determine the perceived efficacy of CAM and its effect on the overall end-of-life experience. The primary types of CAM used were organic foods, faith healing, and homeopathy, with 44% of respondents using more than one type. The majority (78%) reported a significant benefit from CAM use.
- **Kraft (2012)** reviewed research studies and reviews to determine the effect of CAM on depression, anxiety, grief, and other symptoms in advanced palliative care patients. Although short lived, yoga, acupuncture, aromatherapy, and some massage techniques had a positive effect on depression. These therapies also successfully treated anxiety, as did music therapy and mindfulness-based stress reduction. Acupuncture had a positive benefit on fatigue.
- **Rahim-Jamal, Sarte, Kozak, et al. (2011)** found that 81% of 49 hospice patients expressed an interest in CAM for pain relief, relaxation, and enhanced well-being. Of those, 79% had used CAM prior to entering the hospice setting.

♥ iCare 17-1

Rebecca

Rebecca is a 30-year-old woman who has end-stage colon cancer and been hospitalized for 21 days. You have gotten to know her very well and she shares with you that she always loved walking on the beach and feeling the sun on her face. After lunch, you inform Rebecca there is another important test that has been ordered. You have obtained administrative approval and surprise Rebecca by taking her outside for a little while and allowing her to feel the warmth of the sun on her face and to get a breath of fresh air.

Legal and Ethical Considerations at End of Life

The technology of life support makes it possible to prolong body functions almost indefinitely, leaving patients and families struggling with the appropriateness of prolonging life. More clients depend on nurses for education on patient rights and end-of-life care choices. Each situation is unique, and you should be able to explore with clients the various options available. See Chapters 43 and 44 for more information about the ethical and legal aspects of each of the following topics.

Advance Directives

An **advance directive** is a group of instructions (written or oral) stating a person's wishes regarding his healthcare if he were incapacitated or unable to make that decision. An ordinary power of attorney does not give another person the right to make healthcare decisions for the patient; only a durable power of attorney for healthcare can do that.

The **Patient Self-Determination Act (PSDA),** passed by Congress in 1990, requires that all healthcare providers who receive Medicare funds (e.g., hospitals, home care agencies, hospices, nursing homes) must educate staff and patients, provide patients with information on their rights to accept or refuse treatment, and provide an opportunity for all patients to complete an advance directive. The Joint Commission (2015) also requires institutions to address the wishes of the patient regarding end-of-life decisions. Laws in each state vary regarding advance directives. It is important for you to understand federal and state laws and the policies of your institution. The two types of advance directives serve different purposes.

- A **living will** is a document that provides specific instructions about the kinds of healthcare the person would wish (e.g., pain medication) or would wish *not* to have (e.g., ventilator support) in particular situations.
- A **durable power of attorney (DPOA)** for healthcare, or **healthcare proxy,** identifies another person to make decisions for the individual regarding healthcare choices when he is unable to do so based on circumstances (e.g., irreversible coma, dementia). The individual should provide specific instructions about his desires regarding hydration, feeding tubes, medication, resuscitation, and mechanical ventilation. Because this is a legal document, it should be properly prepared (executed) and can be changed or canceled at any time by the patient. Nurses should document whether the patient has an advance directive in the medical records.

Some people fear that once an advance directive is signed, no further care will be provided. Explain to families and patients that this is not true; instead, the directive is intended to make sure they will get however much or little care *they* wish. Remind them that they should formulate advance directives while they are healthy. Such explanations are independent nursing activities, for which you are responsible. To download a copy of your state's advance directives,

 Go to this URL: http://www.caringinfo.org/i4a/pages/index.cfm?pageid=3289

Prescriptions for DNR

A **do not resuscitate (DNR) prescription** is an order by a provider to *not* attempt resuscitation of the patient in the event of cardiac or respiratory failure. Some are recommending the acronym **AND** (allow natural death) to replace DNR (Breault, 2011), because the word *death* in the acronym makes clear the intent of the provider's prescription (American Nurses Association [ANA], 2012). Regardless, you must pay careful attention to these prescriptions, agency policies, and advance directives to be prepared if the patient suffers a cardiopulmonary arrest.

In many healthcare settings, cardiopulmonary resuscitation (CPR) is performed almost automatically. This practice may be slowly changing, as the American Heart Association now provides guidance on the appropriate use of CPR. For example, in considering whether DNR (AND) is appropriate, emphasis is placed on the efficacy of CPR attempts, balancing the benefits and burden and therapeutic goals (ANA, 2012).

You should carefully explain to patients and families what CPR involves and their available options. For example, the provider cannot write a DNR prescription without their permission, and they have the right to refuse CPR and may request a DNR (AND) prescription. The American Nurses Association (ANA, 2012) guides that DNR prescriptions must be clearly documented, reviewed, and updated to reflect changes in the patient's condition. Avoid language that is subject to interpretation or confusing (e.g., chemical code only, slow code, do nothing). Nurses have a duty to communicate with patients and the interprofessional team regarding the patient's wishes regarding end-of-life care and to clarify the treatment plan.

Interventions such as family meetings and interprofessional collaboration with the palliative care team improve decisions about end-of-life care (Lind, Nortvedt, Lorem, et al., 2013). See Box 17-2 for the additional recommendations by the ANA on DNR/AND.

Assisted Suicide

Assisted suicide means making available that which is needed for the patient to end his own life (e.g., pharmacological agents or weapons). The patient is physically capable of ending his own life, has expressed the intention to do so, and has turned to the healthcare provider merely to supply the means. Although physician-assisted suicide is legal in some states, the ANA opposes assisted suicide (2012). ANA "prohibits nurses' participation in assisted suicide and euthanasia because these are in direct violation of *Code of Ethics for Nurses With Interpretive Statements . . .* , the ethical traditions and goals of the profession, and its covenant with society" (ANA, 2013).

BOX 17-2 ■ Highlights of ANA Recommendations Concerning DNR/AND

- The competent patient's choices have highest priority when there is conflict.
- When the patient is not competent, give highest priority to advance directives or the surrogate decision makers.
- DNR orders should be discussed explicitly with the patient and significant others, preferably before a life-threatening illness.
- DNR orders must be documented, reviewed, and updated.
- Nurses should provide quality patient care regardless of DNR status.
- Nurses should be aware of and have an active role in developing DNR policies in the institutions where they work; they should participate in interdisciplinary mechanisms for resolving disputes among patients, families, and healthcare practitioners concerning DNR orders.
- Nurses should consider the acronym AND (allow natural death) because the word *death* makes the intent clear.
- Nurses have a responsibility to avoid participation in "slow codes" or "partial codes."
- Nurses have a duty to educate patients and families about technologies and termination of treatment decisions, and to encourage them to think about end-of-life preferences and make their wishes known in advance.
- Nurses have a duty to communicate relevant information and to advocate for a patient's end-of-life preferences to be honored.

Source: Adapted from American Nurses Association. (2012). Revised position statement: Nursing care and do not resuscitate (DNR) and allow natural death (AND) decisions. Retrieved from http://www.nursingworld.org/MainMenuCategories/EthicsStandards/Ethics-Position-Statements/Nursing-Care-and-Do-Not-Resuscitate-DNR-and-Allow-Natural-Death-Decisions.pdf

---

Assisted suicide violates the ethical principle of nonmaleficence (Friend, 2011).

Some advocate the use of continuous sedation until death as an alternative to assisted suicide (American Academy of Hospice and Palliative Medicine, 2014). The Hospice and Palliative Nurses Association promotes **palliative sedation** as the controlled and monitored use of sedatives and nonopioid medications to induce unconsciousness to relieve suffering from refractory and unendurable symptoms (Hospice and Palliative Nurses Association, 2016).

Euthanasia

The term **euthanasia** comes from the Greek word *euthanatos*, which means "good death." It refers to the deliberate ending of a life of someone suffering from a terminal or incurable illness.

Active euthanasia occurs as a result of a direct action (e.g., giving an overdose of medication). Active euthanasia can be *voluntary* (patient consents); *involuntary* (patient refuses); or *nonvoluntary* (patient is unable to consent, or someone else makes the decision and the patient is unaware of it).

Passive euthanasia occurs as a result of a *lack* of action (e.g., withholding medications or food necessary to sustain life). Honoring the refusal of treatments is not generally considered passive euthanasia and can be ethically and legally permissible.

For more information about the ethical and legal issues surrounding euthanasia, see Chapters 43 and 44, respectively.

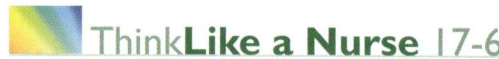

ThinkLike a Nurse 17-6

What are your feelings about assisted suicide, continuous sedation, and euthanasia? Focus on your feelings, not on principles, explanations, and rationales.

Autopsy

An **autopsy** is a medical examination of the body to determine the cause of death. Autopsies also provide relevant data about disease processes and causes. The pathologist performs a detailed internal and external evaluation of the body, removes body organs, and extracts sample tissues for further examination. The organs are then replaced in the body, and the body cavities are closed with sutures. An autopsy requires signed permission from the next of kin, except when required by law (e.g., suspicious or unwitnessed deaths).

Organ Donation

The Uniform Anatomical Gift Act (UAGA) provides guidance on tissue, eye, and organ donation (National Conference of Commissioners on Uniform State Laws, 2009). The act was amended to add language that would prevent others from overriding an individual's prior decision regarding organ donation. However, there remain ethical concerns that the UAGA might result in donors being maintained on life support against their family's wishes.

KEY POINT: *A conflict between a potential organ donor's advance directives and measures to ensure the viability of his organs (e.g., life support) must be resolved as soon as possible by one of the following, in this order: (1) the donor (if able), (2) the surrogate decision maker, or (3) another person as authorized under state law. Until resolution, maintaining the suitability of the organs has the highest priority. You should advocate that your patient's advance directives are clear on end-of-life care and organ donation.*

The UAGA has been adopted in all but four states (as of May 2016). In general, the UAGA states the following:

- As a rule, general donors must be at least 18 years of age or an emancipated minor.
- Next of kin can donate organs when a person dies, unless an objection is known.
- Relatives cannot revoke a person's donation, even after death.
- The person making the gift can amend or revoke it at any time.

Many states issue identification cards or allow driver's licenses to be amended to identify a person as an organ donor. However, even though donor cards are legal in all states, many institutions will not procure organs from the deceased if there is strong family objection Therefore, if a patient is planning to donate organs or tissues, be sure that he discusses these wishes with family members. If death is imminent, a healthcare team member (provider or nurse) should ask whether the patient has agreed to be an organ donor, has a donor card, or is registered with the state's donor database. In many institutions, a transplant coordinator contacts the family and makes the request for organ and tissue donation.

KnowledgeCheck 17-3

- What are advance directives?
- What is the ANA's position on assisted suicide?

PracticalKnowledge
knowing **how**

ASSESSMENT NP

When a patient is dying or has experienced a loss, you must carefully assess the patient and significant others for the common physical, emotional, behavioral, and cognitive grief reactions (see the Focused Assessment box). Also assess knowledge base, history of loss, coping patterns and abilities, meaning of the loss or illness, and support systems.

For dying patients, assess the following:

- Determine whether there are burial or cremation plans or other such tasks (e.g., calling family members) when the client and family are ready to discuss these topics.
- Determine whether the dying client has advance directives (e.g., living will, durable power of attorney for healthcare) and organ donation documents.

Is It Grief or Depression?

When you are performing a focused assessment for grief or loss, you will need to distinguish between grief and depression. Sadness and depression are an integral part of grief with several common symptoms (e.g., sadness, insomnia, poor appetite, and weight loss). However, lasting depression may be a sign that the stress of grieving has triggered a major depressive episode (Pies, Shear, & Zisook, 2014; Widera & Block, 2012). For help differentiating between them see the Focused Assessment box Assessing Grief and Loss.

KnowledgeCheck 17-4

What assessments should you make for your terminally ill patient and his or her family?

Focused Assessment

Assessing Grief and Loss

1. **Assess the patient and significant others for common grief reactions.**

Physical	Emotional	Behaviors	Cognition
Loss of appetite	Anger	Forgetfulness	Decreased concentration
Weight loss/gain	Sadness	Withdrawal	Forgetfulness
Fatigue	Guilt	Insomnia or too much sleep	Impaired judgment
Decreased libido	Relief	Dreaming of deceased	Obsessive thoughts of the deceased or lost object
Decrease in immune system	Shock	Verbalizing the loss	Preoccupation
Decreased energy	Numbness	Crying	Confusion
Possibly physical symptoms, such as headache or stomach pain	Loneliness	Loss of productivity at work or school	Questioning spiritual beliefs
	Fear		Searching to understand
	Anxiety		Searching for purpose and meaning
	Powerlessness		
	Helplessness		
	Depression		

2. **Assess knowledge base of patient and significant others.**
   a. Can they make informed decisions about healthcare choices? You might ask the following:
      ➤ "Tell me what you understand about your illness."
      ➤ "Are there any questions about your illness that you'd like me to answer?"
      ➤ "What are your options for treatment?"
      ➤ "Do you know how to reach your provider if you have questions about your care?"
   b. What and how much do the patient and family want to know? *Some people wish to have all the details of their condition and care. For others, the details cause anxiety.*

(Continued)

Assessing Grief and Loss—cont'd

3. **Assess the history of loss.** Determine whether the patient or family has sustained recent losses or major changes (e.g., death, moving, divorce, retirement). Ask the following:
   - "Have you had any recent changes in your life?"
   - "Tell me about your family."
   - "Are your parents still living?" (as appropriate)
   - "What previous experiences have you had with the loss of someone you loved (or with this condition)?"

4. **Assess coping abilities and support systems.** Ask the following:
   - "What do you do to reduce stress?"
   - "Which family/friends can you talk with?"
   - "What would you say is your greatest support when going through difficult times?"
   - "Tell me about a previous loss and what you did to cope with it."
   - "Are you using any community resources to help you get through this? Do you know what they are?"

   The way individuals have coped in the past will affect how they cope with dying or with their current loss. It may also be therapeutic for them to identify their resources and supports.

5. **Assess the meaning of the loss or illness.** Be alert for anything that may indicate the patient or family is struggling to find meaning, such as:
   - "I'm being punished."
   - "She doesn't deserve this."
   - "Why is this happening to me?"

   In trying to "make sense" of their loss or their dying, people try to attach a meaning to their suffering.

6. **Differentiate between grief and depressive disorder.**
   a. Symptoms common to both grief and depressive disorder: sadness, insomnia, poor appetite, and weight loss.

   Feelings of sadness and depression are a normal part of grief, provided the depression does not linger too long.

   b. Symptoms that indicate grief. For example, the person may feel relatively better in certain situations, such as when she is with friends and family. However, triggers, such as the deceased person's birthday, an anniversary, or holidays, cause the feelings to resurface more strongly.
   c. Symptoms that indicate depressive disorder:
      - The depression is more pervasive. That is, the person rarely gets any relief from the symptoms.
      - Feelings of guilt not related to the loved one's death
      - Thoughts about own death or of suicide (other than feelings the person would be better off dead now that the loved one is gone)
      - Preoccupation with own "worthlessness"
      - Sluggishness
      - Hesitant and confused speech
      - Prolonged and marked difficulty in carrying out activities of daily living
      - Hallucinations, other than thinking he hears the voice of or sees the deceased person

7. **Perform a physical assessment.** Look for signs of increased stress, such as tension, forgetfulness, distraction, increased or decreased appetite and sleep, weight gain or loss, fatigue, and decreased self-care (e.g., deficient hygiene). *A thorough physical examination adds data to help you determine how well the patient is coping with the loss or illness.*

8. **Perform a cultural and spiritual assessment.**
   a. Assess the patient's and family's religious beliefs, any spiritual needs they may have (e.g., forgiveness, hope, meaning, love), and cultural influences that may affect the way they cope.
   b. Do not assume that a person adheres closely to the dominant values of his religious or cultural group. Always assess. For example, ask, "To what religious and ethnic groups do you belong?" and "How closely do you identify with those groups?"

   See Chapters 15 and 16 for details of cultural and spiritual assessment, if you need them.

9. **Perform these specific assessments for dying patients. For dying patients, in addition to the other assessments in this guideline, you should also assess the following:**
   a. When the patient and family are ready, encourage them to talk about what the patient might want for burial or cremation or whether there are tasks that the person would like taken care of (e.g., giving away valuables, calling family members).
   b. Determine whether the dying person has a living will or advance directives.
   c. Discuss with the patient and family the possibility of organ donation if appropriate for the patient's circumstances.
   d. Observe for physical changes indicating the approach of death:

      1 to 3 months before death: Beginning withdrawal from others, increased sleep, decreased appetite, difficulty digesting food (especially meats), prefers liquids. *Anorexia may be protective, because the resulting ketosis can diminish pain and increase the person's sense of well-being.*

      1 to 2 weeks before death: Cardiovascular deterioration brings decreased blood pressure, pulse and respiration changes (decreased or increased), a yellowish pallor to the skin, extreme pallor of extremities. Observe for temperature fluctuations, increased perspiration, brief periods of apnea during sleep, rattling breathing sounds caused by congestion, nonproductive cough.

      Days to hours before death: A brief surge of energy and mental clarity, with a desire to eat and talk with family members.
      - Dehydration, difficulty swallowing, decreasing blood pressure, weak pulse
      - Mucous membranes dry and tacky; cracked lips. *Dehydration during the last hours of dying is thought not to cause distress and perhaps to stimulate endorphin release.*
      - Sagging of tongue and soft palate, diminished gag reflex, secretions accumulating in the oropharynx and/or bronchi

Focused Assessment

Assessing Grief and Loss—cont'd

➤ Shallow, rapid, or irregular breathing; respiratory congestion; Cheyne-Stokes respirations; apnea of 10 to 30 seconds; "death rattle." *Cheyne-Stokes breathing is a cyclic pattern consisting of a 10- to 60-second period of apnea and then a gradual increase in depth and rate of respirations. Respirations gradually become slow and shallow, and then the cycle begins again with apnea.*

➤ Decreased peripheral circulation, increased perspiration, "clammy" skin; extremities cool and mottled; dependent body parts darker than the rest of the body

➤ Decreased urinary output, concentrated and foul-smelling urine, secondary to decreased kidney function

➤ Slack facial muscles ("drooping")

➤ Retained feces; bowel and bladder incontinence. *Due to decreased peristalsis and relaxation of sphincters*

➤ Blurred vision; eyes open but unseeing

➤ Restlessness or agitation (check for impacted stool, distended bladder, pain, medications, cerebral hypoxia, unresolved emotional or spiritual issues)

➤ Decreased communication, quiet, withdrawal. Some become more coherent and energized for a time.

➤ Fatigue

Moments before death: Does not respond to touch or sound; cannot be awakened. There may be a short series of long-spaced breaths before breathing stops entirely and the heart stops beating. Auscultate to determine whether apical pulse and respirations are absent.

Sources: Blinderman, C., & Billings, A. (2015). Comfort care for patients dying in the hospital. *The New England Journal of Medicine, 373*(10), 2539–2561. doi:10.1056/NEJMra1411746; Carter, L. (2016). Understanding our role in bereavement. *International Journal of Childbirth Education, 31*(4), 28–30; Emanuel, L., Ferris, F., von Gunten, C., et al. (2015). The last hours of living: Practical advice for clinicians. *Medscape.* Retrieved from http://www.medscape.com/viewarticle/716463; Finocchiaro, D. (2016). Supporting the patient's spiritual needs at the end of life. *Nursing2016, 56*(5), 46–59; Pies, R., Shear, K., & Zisook, S. (2014). Distinguishing grief, complicated grief, and depression. *Medscape.* Retrieved from http://www.medscape.com/viewarticle/836977_2; Scott, P. (2016). 10 signs death is near. *Caring.Com.* Retrieved from https://www.caring.com/articles/signs-of-death; Widera, E., & Block, S. (2012). Death rattle: Prevalence, prevention and treatment. *Journal of Pain and Symptom Management, 23*(4), 310–317.

ANALYSIS/DIAGNOSIS NP

When you are analyzing patient data, keep in mind that most grief is normal, not complicated or dysfunctional. You must determine whether loss and grieving are the problem or the etiology, because the etiology influences your interventions. Also note that the same diagnoses can be used in the context of death, dying, grief, or loss.

Loss and Grieving as a Problem Various nursing diagnoses may be appropriate for a person who is dying or grieving. The most obvious are Grieving and Complicated Grieving. Complicated Grieving is disabling pain and grief, characterized by long-term grieving (perhaps years), functional impairment, and/or intense emotions. The person may deny or have difficulty expressing feelings of loss or may experience physical symptoms as a result of suppressing feelings.

Other diagnoses may include Ineffective Denial, Hopelessness, Powerlessness, Chronic Sorrow, Spiritual Distress, Self-Care Deficit, Constipation, and many other physiological diagnoses. Examples of defining characteristics of NANDA-I diagnoses, selected NOC outcomes, and selected NIC interventions for grief/grieving and complicated grief/grieving are presented in Table 17-2.

ThinkLike a Nurse 17-7

Refer to Table 17-2 mentioned in the preceding reference. Answer the questions in the table. Also refer to a nursing diagnosis handbook and NIC and NOC manuals.

Loss and Grieving as Etiology Loss, grief, and dying are an etiology when they create problems in other areas of patient or family function. The following are examples of such nursing diagnoses:

- Anxiety related to inability to cope with the loss; or related to unknown outcome of situation
- Death Anxiety (or Fear) related to impending death
- Decisional Conflict related to end-of-life treatment measures (e.g., knowledge that the treatment may lengthen life but decrease the quality of life)
- Fatigue related to demands of caring for a dying loved one
- Spiritual Distress related to loss of trust in a loving God

PLANNING OUTCOMES/EVALUATION NP

Encourage the patient and family to play an active role in planning care. Involving family members helps facilitate their acceptance of the diagnosis and may put the patient more at ease. Questions such as the following will help to elicit the patient's goals for end of life (Matzo & Sherman, 2014; Weissman, Quill, & Arnold, 2010):

- What do you still want to accomplish or do?
- What are the things you wish you could still do?
- Whom would you like to see?
- What would make you more medically comfortable?
- If you have pain, what would be an acceptable level for you on a 0 to 10 scale?
- Where do you want to spend the rest of your life? Where are you most comfortable?
- If spiritual peace is important to you, what would help you achieve it?"

Table 17-2 ➤ Examples of NOC Outcomes and NIC Interventions for Loss and Grieving Diagnoses

NURSING DIAGNOSES	SELECTED NOC OUTCOMES	SELECTED NIC INTERVENTIONS
Grieving ***Defining Characteristics:*** Anger; anticipatory loss of significant object (e.g., job, status, parts and processes of body); blame; pain; disturbed sleep pattern; making meaning of the loss; alterations in activity level, dream patterns, immune functions; anticipatory loss of significant other	Adaptation to Physical Disability Coping Dignified Life Closure Family Coping Grief Resolution Psychosocial Adjustment: Life Change Spiritual Health	Anticipatory Guidance Body Image Enhancement Coping Enhancement Counseling Emotional Support Family Integrity Promotion Family Support Grief Work Facilitation Grief Work Facilitation: Perinatal Death

Think about it.

■ Does Thomas Manning (Meet Your Patient) have any symptoms of Grieving?

Complicated Grieving ***Defining Characteristics:*** Grief Avoidance, decreased functioning in life roles, depression, persistent emotional distress, preoccupation with thoughts of the decreased, lack of acceptance of the death, persistent painful memories, anxiety	Anxiety Self Control Coping Family Coping Family Resiliency Fatigue Level Grief Resolution Psychosocial Adjustment: Life Change Role Performance Self-Care Status	Coping Enhancement Counseling Crisis Intervention Family Integrity Promotion Family Support Grief Work Facilitation Grief Work Facilitation: Perinatal Death Resiliency Promotion Role Enhancement Self-Awareness Enhancement

Think about it.

■ Most of the NOC outcomes are the same for Grieving and Complicated Grieving. How do the interventions differ? Do you understand why?
■ Notice that for both diagnoses, many of the defining characteristics include normal grief reactions. But for Grieving, the symptoms occur before the loss. For Complicated Grieving, they continue to occur for a long time after the loss, and/or they are more intense than normal.

Sources: Moorhead, S., Johnson, M., Mass, M., et al. (Eds.). (2013). *Nursing outcomes classification (NOC)* (5th ed.). St. Louis, MO: C.V. Mosby. Used with permission. Bulechek, G., Butcher, H., Dochterman, J. M., et al. (2013). *Nursing interventions classification (NIC)* (6th ed.). St. Louis, MO: C.V. Mosby. Used with permission; Herdman, T., & Kamitsuru, S. (Eds.). (2014). *Nursing Diagnoses—Definitions and Classification 2018–2020.* © 2010 NANDA International, ISBN 978-1-62623-929-6. Used by arrangement with the Thieme Group, Stuttgart/New York; Johnson, M., Moorhead, S., Bulechek, G., et al. (2012). *NOC and NIC linkages to NANDA-I and clinical conditions* (3rd ed.). St. Louis, MO: C.V. Mosby. Used with permission.

NOC standardized outcomes are determined by the diagnostic label you use (see Table 17-2)

Individualized goals/outcome statements you might write for a grieving or dying person include the following examples. The patient and/or family will:
1. Communicate openly among themselves and healthcare providers (e.g., express fear, concerns, pain).
2. Obtain satisfactory pain relief and symptom management.
3. Exercise control in the management of care to the extent possible.

As always, you will use the goals set in the planning stage as criteria for evaluating the patient's or family's health status.

KnowledgeCheck 17-5

- List three nursing diagnosis labels you might consider when dying or grieving is the primary problem.
- List three nursing diagnosis labels that might occur as a result of dying or grieving.

PLANNING INTERVENTIONS/ IMPLEMENTATION NP

NIC standardized interventions associated with death, dying, and bereavement are found Table 17-2.

Specific nursing activities are determined by the nursing diagnosis, especially by the etiology. A compassionate approach is essential but may be challenging. Watching patients struggle with pain, loss, grief, and death may stir our own deepest doubts and fears, and we may reject the challenge to respond from the heart. Employers usually reward nurses for what they *do* rather than who they *are* as people, so it is easy to rationalize that we have other tasks to accomplish that may be equally important. When we do that, we ignore the real gift we may have to offer the suffering patient: our willingness to "walk the walk" with them, if even for just a short time. **KEY POINT:** *Your ability to help someone who is grieving or dying is largely determined by your attitude. Full-spectrum nurses combine their psychomotor and thinking skills with compassion in ministering to those who are suffering.*

Some important nursing interventions involved in care of the dying person are discussed in the following sections. Also see the Nursing Care Plan and Care Map for Grieving.

Therapeutic Communication

Therapeutic communication is critical to building a trusting relationship with the dying or grieving patient and significant others. It is important to listen to the dying patient and to be alert for and respond to nonverbal cues. Encourage patients and family members to express their feelings and reassure them that their feelings are normal and not "wrong." In discussions about DNR (AND) or withholding or withdrawing treatments, it is important to find out why the patient is seeking that option: Does she wish to avoid suffering, or does she fear being a burden to loved ones?

Providers and nurses should always work to improve their communication skills because they are essential for achieving better outcomes at end of life (Galushko, Romotzky, & Voltz, 2012). See Box 17-3 for barriers to end-of-life communication.

♥ iCare 17-2

Loss, Grief, and Dying

Dealing with loss, grief, and dying is very difficult. As caregivers, we can display "caring" to patients, friends, and families by merely being present. Some people need space, while others may need acknowledgment and comfort.

When a death occurs, it is important to acknowledge the loss of life. How one does this can vary, depending on a patient's culture and beliefs. A moment of silence and/or spiritual reflection can exhibit "caring" to acknowledge the sacredness that a life has been lost for friends and family members as well as caregivers.

For tips on communicating with people who are dying or bereaved, see Clinical Insight 17-1.

If you need more information on communication and therapeutic relationships, refer to Chapter 20.

Facilitating Grief Work

Regardless of the source of grief (e.g., a loss of health, an impending death), you can help patients and families express their feelings, recall memories, and find meaning in their lives.

Expressing Feelings

It is the family, not just an individual patient, who grieves a death or loss. Grief is a normal process, and people must communicate their feelings to deal with it effectively. Sometimes people hold in their feelings, which interferes with their grief resolution. You may need to facilitate the process, using your therapeutic communication skills to help them feel comfortable (refer to Chapter 20 as needed). Several ways to facilitate expression of feelings include the following:

- Encourage questions and respond to them within a reasonable period of time.
- Sit beside the head of the bed; do not appear rushed.
- When you observe the patient or family member expressing feelings, either verbally or nonverbally, encourage him or her to continue.
- Expect and accept a wide range of feelings, including anger, fear, and loneliness.
- Ask, "How would you like me to help?" "What do you need?"
- Be sure that everyone on the healthcare team understands and follows the care plan.
- Ask yourself what you would do if this were your family member.
- Do not compare another person's loss with your own experience. Avoid comments such as "I know how you feel." Instead, say, "Tell me how you feel."

BOX 17-3 ■ Barriers to End-of-Life Communication

- Fear of one's own mortality
- Unresolved personal grief issues (e.g., the loss of one's own parent)
- Lack of experience with death and dying
- Fear of expressing emotion (i.e., crying)
- Fear of not knowing the answer to a question
- Not knowing whether to give an honest (and possibly unwelcome) answer to a question
- Not understanding the family's culture
- Keeping physical distance (e.g., standing away from the person or avoiding eye contact)
- Insensitivity: interrupting communication, patronizing, giving false reassurance

Sources: Malloy, P., Virani, R., Kelly, K., et al. (2008). End-of-life care: Improving communication skills to enhance palliative care. *Medscape.* Retrieved from http://www.medscape.org/viewarticle/574420; Sinuff, T., Dodek, P., You, J., et al. (2015). Improving end-of-life communication and decision making: The development of a conceptual framework and quality indicators. *Journal of Pain and Symptom Management, 49*(6), 1070–1080. doi:http://dx.doi.org/10.1016/j.jpainsymman.2014.12.007

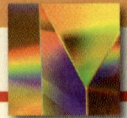

Nursing Care Plan

Client Data

You are participating in a special Caring for the Caregiver program set up by the public health nurse in your community. In this program, registered nurses visit primary caregivers to assess their needs and offer support services as needed. You are assigned to Wilma Peterson.

Wilma Peterson is caring for her son Henry who has AIDS. Henry is 20 years old; his older brother, William, died of AIDS-related pneumonia 2 years earlier at age 24. William had left home at 18 to live in Miami and returned to his home in rural Alabama when he became too ill to manage on his own. Henry stayed home to help his mother care for William and learned he was HIV-positive just before his brother died. Henry did not tell his mother of his diagnosis until he was hospitalized for the first time with cytomegalovirus infection. Since then, he has not followed nutritional and medical advice and has continued to stay out late and party when he feels well enough. His health has steadily declined.

Ms. Peterson is initially cordial when you visit but tells you, "This is my responsibility. I don't stop being his mother because he's grown up. I'm always his mama." As your discussion continues, Ms. Peterson wistfully talks about when William and Henry were boys. She says, "I didn't really understand this awful disease until William got so sick. Now, I look at Henry and I know what's waiting for him. I know we are going to lose him. Sad . . . just so sad. . . ." Her voice trails off as tears well in her eyes.

Nursing Diagnosis

Grieving related to the client's anticipating the loss of a second son, as evidenced by her previous experience caring for her other son who died at home of AIDS and by the client's stating, "I know what's waiting for him."

NOC Outcomes	Individualized Goals / Expected Outcomes
Family Coping (NOC 2600) Psychosocial Adjustment: Life Change (NOC 1305)	*(Short-term goals) At the end of the initial home visit, Ms. Peterson will:* 1. Identify community resources available to help her care for Henry at home during acute illnesses. 2. Begin to feel comfortable discussing her concerns with the nurse. *(Long-term goals) Within 6 weeks, Ms. Peterson will:* 1. Explore activities she would like to participate in once she is no longer caring for Henry. 2. Talk with Henry to learn what type of funeral he would like.

NIC Interventions*

Anticipatory Guidance (NIC 5210)
Coping Enhancement (NIC 5230)
Grief Work Facilitation (NIC 5290)

Nursing Activities	Rationales
1. Encourage Ms. Peterson to talk about her experiences caring for William before he died.	Grieving often occurs in the context of repeated caregiving (Somers, McLennan, & MacCourt, 2016) or in situations in which the caregiver has had previous experience with the same or a similar terminal illness. Supportive communication allows for asking questions, sharing information, and ultimately coming to terms with the loss (Ostler, 2010).

*Interventions are only a sample of those linked to this diagnosis by NIC. Activities should be individualized for each client.

Nursing Care Plan (continued)

Nursing Activities	Rationales
2. Ask her to relate similarities and differences between care for William and care for Henry.	Asking the client to discuss previous experiences allows the nurse to validate the nursing diagnosis (Mullen, Reynolds, & Larson, 2015) and provides an opportunity for the client to discuss her specific needs (Kelly, Malloy, Munevar, et al., 2010).
3. Ask Ms. Peterson to describe the elements of Henry's care and to identify which she considers to be the most important.	Clients are holistic and consider more than just medical treatment in the care of a family member. Their actions may be based on care needed, cultural and religious beliefs, and previous experiences instead of a medically based care plan. It is important that the client and healthcare provider are consistent in their identification of client needs (Mullen, Reynolds, & Larson, 2015). By asking for Ms. Peterson's priorities the nurse can learn from the client rather than making assumptions based on the healthcare perspective. By showing respect for her experience as a caregiver, the nurse can build a stronger relationship with Ms. Peterson, thereby facilitating future nursing interventions and anticipatory guidance (Reinhard, Given, Petlick, et al., 2008).
4. Talk with Ms. Peterson to find out what community resources she used when she cared for William and whether she has accessed them now in caring for Henry.	Isolation and loneliness are risk factors for sole caregivers at home. Assessing community resources helps the nurse determine whether Ms. Peterson is "connected" or isolating herself. Isolation and previous loss put her at risk for Complicated Grieving (Lobb, Kristjanson, Aoun, et al., 2010). Many community resources provide a sense of belonging and enhance and support coping strategies as well.
5. Promote shared decision making if this is acceptable to Henry Peterson.	Informing both Ms. Peterson and Henry about the disease, prognosis, treatment, and comfort options allows them to retain some control over their lives together, which is essential for effective palliative care (Lind, Nortvedt, Lorem, et al., 2013; Wilson, Gott, & Ingleton, 2013). Henry's permission must be obtained to preserve his autonomy.
6. Provide nonjudgmental emotional support to Ms. Peterson, and support healthy coping activities she is using.	Establishing a comfortable and emotionally safe environment will allow Ms. Peterson to share her concerns without fear of being judged because of her son's diagnosis (Milberg & Strang, 2011; Slatyer, Pienaar, Williams, et al., 2015).

Evaluation

Review the initial short-term outcomes and goals. Reassess your client to determine whether the goals are achieved in the stated time frame. In this case, long-term goals will fluctuate based on the progression of Henry's illness. The following occurred as the care plan was implemented:

- Ms. Peterson cried as she described the deterioration in William's health before he died. She worries that Henry will suffer and does not want him to lose his dignity the way she believes William did.

- Ms. Peterson's greatest concern is that Henry is not eating enough. Much of her self-value as a mother arises from her ability to prepare homemade meals to feed her family, and Henry doesn't have much of an appetite. This is very distressing to her.

- She has not contacted community agencies. She is holding off, hoping Henry will not be "so sick for so long. With these new drugs, he can get better."

- She remains involved in her church, which is the same one she attended as a little girl. However, she will not tell her church group that Henry has AIDS. "They talk too much," she says. Instead, she says he has leukemia.

Only one short-term goal is met at this visit—establishing a comfort level between the client and the nurse. Ms. Peterson has not identified community resources related to caring for Henry at this time.

(continued)

Nursing Care Plan (continued)

Plan for Further Evaluation

Additional supportive visits will be needed to help Ms. Peterson understand that contacting community agencies does not mean Henry will die sooner. An important coping mechanism for Ms. Peterson is denying the need for community help; however, it is not currently affecting her ability to care for her son. If his condition worsens, this issue will need to be promptly addressed.

References

Bulechek, G., Butcher, H., Dochterman, J. M., et al. (2013). *Nursing interventions classification (NIC)* (6th ed.). St. Louis, MO: C. V. Mosby.

Johnson, M., Moorhead, S., Bulechek, G., et al. (2013). *NOC and NIC Linkages to NANDA-I and clinical conditions* (3rd ed.). St. Louis, MO: C. V. Mosby.

Kelly, K., Malloy, P., Munevar, C., et al. (2010). Beyond bad news: Communication skills of nurses in palliative care. *Journal of Hospice and Palliative Nursing, 12*(3), 166–174.

Lind, R., Nortvedt, P., Lorem, G., et al. (2013). Family involvement in the end-of-life decision of competent intensive care patients. *Nursing Ethics, 20*(1), 61–71. doi:10.1177/0969733012448969

Lobb, E., Kristjanson, L., Aoun, S., et al. (2010). Predictors of complicated grief: A systematic review of empirical studies. *Death Studies, 34*(8), 673–698.

Milberg, A., & Strang, P. (2011). Protection against perceptions of powerlessness and helplessness during palliative care: The family members' perspective. *Palliative & Supportive Care, 9*(3), 251–262.

Moorhead, S., Johnson, M., Maas, M., et al. (2013). *Nursing outcomes classification (NOC)* (5th ed.). St. Louis, MO: C. V. Mosby

Mullen, J., Reynolds, M., & Larson, J. (2015). Caring for pediatric patients' families at the child's end of life. *Critical Care Nurse, 35*(6), 46–56. doi:10.4037/ccn2015614

Nursing Diagnoses—Definitions and Classification 2018–2020. © 2010 NANDA International, ISBN 978-1-62623-929-6. Used by arrangement with the Thieme Group, Stuttgart/New York.

Ostler, T. (2010). Grief and coping in early childhood: The role of communication in the mourning process. *Zero to Three, 31*(1), 29–35.

Reinhard, S., Given, B., Petlick, N., et al. (2008). Supporting family caregivers in providing support. In R. Hughes (Ed.), *Patient safety and quality: An evidence-based handbook for nurses* (Chapter 14). Rockville, MD: Agency for Healthcare Research and Quality. Retrieved from http://www.ncbi.nlm.nih.gov/books/NBK2665/

Slatyer, S., Pienaar, C., Williams, A., et al. (2015). Finding privacy from a public death: A qualitative exploration of how a dedicated space for end-of-life care in an acute hospital impacts on dying patients and their families. *Journal of Clinical Nursing, 24*(15/16), 2164–2174. doi:10.1111/jocn.12845

Somers, S., McLennan, M., & MacCourt, P. (2016). Education on grief, loss and dementia for family caregivers. *Canadian Nurse, 112*(7), 26–27.

Wilson, F., Gott, M., & Ingleton, C. (2013). Perceived risks around choice and decision making at end-of-life: A literature review. *Palliative Medicine, 27*(1), 38–53.

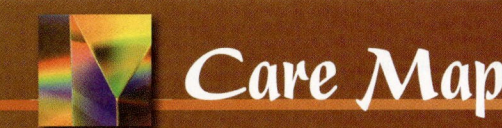

Care Map

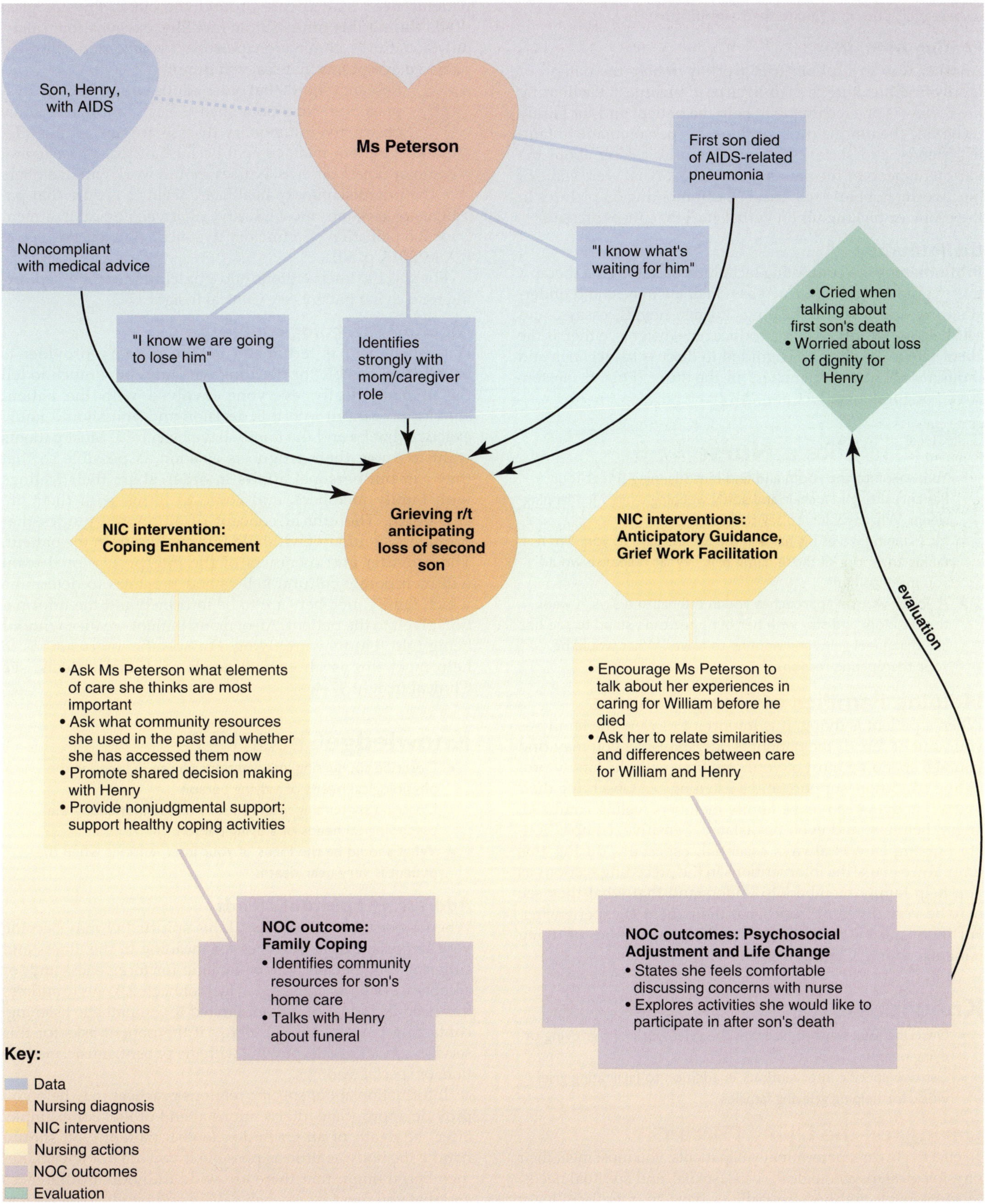

Son, Henry, with AIDS

Ms Peterson

First son died of AIDS-related pneumonia

Noncompliant with medical advice

"I know we are going to lose him"

Identifies strongly with mom/caregiver role

"I know what's waiting for him"

- Cried when talking about first son's death
- Worried about loss of dignity for Henry

Grieving r/t anticipating loss of second son

NIC intervention: Coping Enhancement

NIC interventions: Anticipatory Guidance, Grief Work Facilitation

evaluation

- Ask Ms Peterson what elements of care she thinks are most important
- Ask what community resources she used in the past and whether she has accessed them now
- Promote shared decision making with Henry
- Provide nonjudgmental support; support healthy coping activities

- Encourage Ms Peterson to talk about her experiences in caring for William before he died
- Ask her to relate similarities and differences between care for William and Henry

NOC outcome: Family Coping
- Identifies community resources for son's home care
- Talks with Henry about funeral

NOC outcomes: Psychosocial Adjustment and Life Change
- States she feels comfortable discussing concerns with nurse
- Explores activities she would like to participate in after son's death

Key:
- Data
- Nursing diagnosis
- NIC interventions
- Nursing actions
- NOC outcomes
- Evaluation

Recalling Memories

Grieving patients and family members may need to recall memories, both good and difficult. One way to encourage recall is to go through photo albums with them and ask questions about the people in the pictures. Also look for objects of sentiment (e.g., a family heirloom) in the environment and ask the dying or bereaved person to share their significance.

Finding Meaning

Another way to support grief work is to help the patient or family find meaning in their lives or in their past. Facilitating life review is one technique to help the patient and/or family recognize the unique contributions this person made to family, friends, and society. You can begin by asking about the various aspects of the patient's life (e.g., "What were some of his favorite hobbies/activities?"), commenting on pictures in the room, or picking up on verbal cues that are expressed.

Bibliotherapy

Bibliotherapy is a counseling technique used for grief therapy. It uses guided reading to increase client awareness and understanding and promote healing. Poems, novels, essays, and self-help literature can help produce new insights, either as the client retells the story or is guided to discuss his feelings and thoughts about the characters in the story (Pola & Nelson, 2014; Songprakun & McCann, 2012).

ThinkLike a Nurse 17-8

- You walk into the room and find Mrs. Manning (Meet Your Patient) sitting in a chair and softly weeping while Mr. Manning sleeps. What would you say to her?
- Mr. Manning waves his hand in the air and says to you, "I'm not taking any more of those damn pills." What response would you make to him?
- A young woman approaches you in the hall and says, "I want to visit Mom and stay with her, but I just can't stand to see her like that. I feel guilty for wanting to leave." What would be your therapeutic response?

Helping Families of Dying Patients

When a patient is dying, it is important to view the family as your unit of care. If the patient is unresponsive, you may find yourself spending most of your care time with the family providing education, support, and a listening ear. Observing their loved one dying can leave family members feeling confused, angry, helpless, and even devastated. Sensitive, compassionate nursing care is always essential, especially during this time. You can use the interventions in the preceding sections as you help family members to understand that what they see may be very different from what the patient is experiencing. For more specific interventions for helping families of dying patients, refer to Clinical Insight 17-2.

KnowledgeCheck 17-6

- Describe four ways to facilitate the grief work of a grieving or dying person.
- List two specific interventions, in addition to facilitating grief work, for helping grieving families.

Caring for the Dying Person

To effectively care for terminally ill patients, you must meet their physiological, psychological, social, sexual, and spiritual needs. Most hospitals and hospice facilities have an interdisciplinary team (e.g., provider, nurse, social worker, nutritionist, allied health therapists, clergy) to provide holistic care to dying patients and their families.

Meeting Physiological Needs

In the final 4 to 48 hours of life, as body systems fail, most patients need skilled care around the clock. Physiological needs during this time include mobility, oxygenation, safety, nutrition, fluids, elimination, personal hygiene, and control of pain and symptoms (nausea, vomiting).

 Research shows that older adults with refractory dyspnea from conditions such as heart failure or chronic obstructive pulmonary disease are not getting adequate symptom management because of fear of hastening death or other concerns. Nurses should work with members of the interdisciplinary healthcare team to ensure that patients receive the "most effective pharmacological treatment for the palliation of refractory dyspnea" (Lowey, Powers, & Xue, 2013, p. 50).

For specific interventions and guidelines to use when caring for a dying patient, see Clinical Insight 17-3.

Meeting Psychological Needs

When a patient is terminally ill, the primary provider is usually responsible for deciding what and how much to tell the person. Ideally, everyone involved with the patient should have input into this decision and you should know exactly what he and the family have been told. Most patients want to know their prognosis as soon as possible so that they can put personal affairs in order, share their feelings with family members, and come to terms with their life and death. The ethical concept of autonomy guides that providers should not withhold information from the patient. The provider and members of the interprofessional team will incorporate cultural beliefs and practices to determine which family members are to be informed and the information given to the patient. Also, many patients realize without being told that they are dying. For specific interventions to help meet the psychological needs of dying patients, see Clinical Insight 17-4.

KnowledgeCheck 17-7

- Describe six nursing interventions to use in meeting the physiological needs of a dying person.
- Describe six nursing interventions to use in meeting the psychological needs of a dying person.
- What should be the focus of your interventions when the patient is very near death?

Addressing Spiritual Needs

When a person is terminally ill, his spirituality may become very important as he searches for meaning in the illness and suffering. The person may be looking for forgiveness and/or acceptance or be reaching out to feel connected. Ways to address this need include (but are not limited to) empathetic listening, contacting pastoral care or clergy if the patient asks for this service, special rituals, praying with the patient, music, meditation, or special readings.

Information about specific religious practices may help you provide appropriate interventions at end of life. For example, after the death of an Orthodox Jewish patient, you should handle the body as little as possible if you are not Jewish. Remember, though, that there are wide individual differences and that you must assess each patient and family to determine

Toward Evidence-Based Practice

Fine, E., Reid, C., Shengelia, R., et al. (2010). Directly observed patient–physician discussions in palliative and end-of-life care: A systematic review of the literature. *Journal of Palliative Medicine, 13*(5), 595–603.

Researchers reviewed 20 studies that used direct observations in end-of-life/palliative communications. Several common themes emerged. Physicians tended to dominate the discussions and focused more on medical/technical aspects. Emphasis was not placed on emotional or quality-of-life issues. Patient satisfaction was associated with supportive behaviors by physicians.

Gramling, R., Norton, S., Ladwig, S., et al. (2013). Direct observation of prognosis communication in palliative care: A descriptive study. *Journal of Pain & Symptom Management, 45*(2), 202–212.

Researchers audio-recorded the initial visit of 71 seriously ill patients and their families who were referred for discussions of end-of-life decision making or goal clarification. Results identified these major themes: (1) Patient-focused quality-of-life discussions occurred more frequently than did survival discussions focused on the general population. (2) Pessimistic cues regarding prognosis occurred more often than did optimistic ones.

Periyakoil, V., Neri, E., & Kraemer, H. (2015). No easy talk: A mixed methods study of doctor reported barriers to conducting effective end-of-life conversations with diverse patients. *PLoS ONE, 10*(4), e0122321. doi:10.1371/journal.pone.0122321

A study of 1,040 physicians identified that 99.9% reported barriers in engaging in end-of-life discussions with their patients, especially with those of dissimilar ethnicity (87.5%). Some of the major barriers included the following: (1) language and medical interpretation issues, based on the technical jargon required in end-of-life discussions; (2) patient–family religious and spiritual beliefs about death and dying (e.g., will of God, taboo about withholding food/fluid); (3) lack of knowledge of cultural beliefs, practices, and values; and (4) cultural difference in truth handling and decision making, with some patients recusing themselves from conversations or family members who want the truth withheld to protect the patient. This research identified the importance of understanding religious/spiritual beliefs and cultural differences to effectively engage in end-of-life discussions with a diverse patient population.

1. Based on these research results, how do you think health professionals should inform patients when they have an advanced life-limiting (terminal) illness? What should be the focus of the communication? Explain your thinking.

2. What should be the goal of communications between health professionals and terminally ill patients related to end-of-life care?

 Go to Davis Advantage, Resources, Chapter 17, **Toward Evidence-Based Practice Suggested Responses**.

how closely they adhere to the rituals of their religion. Review Chapters 15 and 16, as needed.

Addressing Cultural Needs

Cultural values can influence a person's openness to discussions regarding death and his end-of-life healthcare preferences. Researchers found that regardless of ethnicity or gender, end-of-life concerns important to most people include comfort, physician communication, having responsibilities taken care of, support, hope and optimism, and honoring spiritual beliefs. Other concerns were being cared for, love and compassion, expressing feelings, fixing relationships, saying goodbye, having choices, making plans, not being in pain or unable to breathe, and being "ready to go" (ElGindy, 2013; Flanagan, 2015; Valente, 2010).

There is some overlap between religious and cultural practices. For example, most cultural groups engage in some type of religious ceremony that helps the bereaved begin the grieving process (Fig. 17-2). Nevertheless, some death rituals and expressions of grief may be culture based but not necessarily involve religion. For example, some cultures may emphasize keeping emotions subdued and limiting expressions of grief to private settings, whereas others gauge the value of the deceased by the amount of crying that occurs.

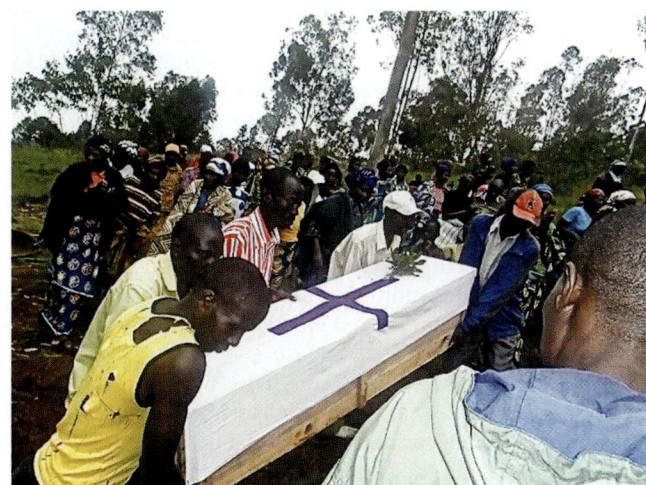

FIGURE 17-2 After death, rituals (e.g., the Rwandan burial shown here) are viewed as respect for the deceased and help friends and family bring closure.

Despite the commonalities among groups, there are some culture-specific differences. To provide culturally sensitive care at end of life, you will need some information about specific cultural practices surrounding death. For example, many Chinese families prefer to protect the patient from news that she has a terminal illness, or at least want to deliver the news themselves.

For general cultural information, see Chapter 15.

KEY POINT: *As with spiritual care, remember that you cannot assume that a person follows the practices of her cultural group; you must assess to be sure.*

ThinkLike a Nurse 17-9

Reflect on this passage by Theresa Rando from *The Gift of Presence:*

It is one of the most difficult things in the world to do to sit and listen while another's heart is breaking with grief, to hold the hand of a dying patient who cries silently while staring into space. The gift of presence, the gift of being with those in pain, is the only gift we can give. It is the sole armor patients have against the anguish. The very most we can do for dying patients is to make it better, with our presence and concern, than it would be if we were not there. . . . We cannot "do" anything that can get rid of the psychic pain of impending loss and death. (Rando, 1984, p. 272)

Close your eyes and visualize yourself sitting quietly beside a dying patient and holding her hand. Visualize the patient crying silently. Can you still your mind and remain silent, or do you feel you must say something to make the patient feel better?

Providing Postmortem Care

Postmortem care includes care of the patient's body after death and fulfilling any legal obligations, such as arranging transportation to the morgue or funeral home and determining the disposition of the patient's belongings. You will follow agency policies and respect cultural and spiritual preferences, along with the care that is commonly provided. In most states, the provider must pronounce death; in some areas, however, a coroner or a nurse may also perform this task. Changes in the body after death include the following:

- **Rigor mortis** (the stiffening of the body after death) is caused by contraction of the muscles from a lack of adenosine triphosphate. It occurs about 2 to 4 hours after death. Rigor mortis begins in the involuntary muscles (e.g., the heart). It appears next in the head, neck, and trunk, and finally in the extremities. It disappears about 96 hours after death.
- **Algor mortis** occurs when the blood stops circulating. The body temperature drops about 1.88°F (1°C) per hour until it reaches room temperature.
- **Livor mortis** occurs when the dependent parts of the body appear bluish and mottled. That happens when the blood stops circulating and the red blood cells break down, releasing hemoglobin.

If the family wishes to be alone with the body, straighten the bedcovers, remove all tubes (unless contraindicated), and make the patient look as natural as possible. Give family members whatever time they need before you prepare the body. Ideally, you will have already established a relationship with the family and will have begun to facilitate their grieving during the patient's dying period. And you will have prepared them as the death becomes imminent. For specific guidelines for care of the body and other immediate postmortem interventions to support family members, see Clinical Insight 17-5.

KnowledgeCheck 17-8

- Why is it important to position the body with a pillow under the head and shoulders soon after death?
- Why is it important to close the eyes and mouth of the deceased and position the body within at least 2 to 4 hours after death?

Providing Grief Education

At some point after the immediate postmortem period, explain the stages of grief and point out that it may take months or even years to resolve. Explain that grief may become more intense on the anniversary of the death (or other loss) and on significant dates (e.g., birthdays).

Recall that once the bereaved person accepts that the loss is real, his feelings may be so intense that he may wonder whether he is losing his sanity. The grieving person may be fatigued from not sleeping and disoriented or unable to concentrate and have numerous other symptoms. Reassure the person that such responses are expected and that there is no single right way to grieve (Holtslander & McMillan, 2011; Neimeyer, 2014; Pies, Shear, & Zisook, 2014). Inform him, too, that although the grief process takes time, the symptoms will not last forever.

Helping Children Deal With Loss

Some families may need information about helping children deal with grief, especially when there is a death in the family. You may need to explain that children perceive death differently from adults and the importance of addressing death and grief with children. See the Self-Care box for teaching surviving relatives how to help children deal with grief.

Self-Care

Helping Children Deal With Loss

Teach surviving relatives the following:

➤ If a child is frightened about attending a funeral, do not force him to go. It is important, however, to include the child in some service or observance, such as lighting a candle, saying a prayer, or visiting the gravesite, at a later time.

➤ Spend as much time as possible with the child, making it clear that the child has permission to show her feelings openly or freely.

➤ Let the child know that it is okay to want attachment items (e.g., picture, jewelry, special object).

➤ Be prepared for intermittent expressions of sadness and anger from the child over a long period of time.

➤ Be prepared for the possibility of regression to earlier developmental stages (e.g., talking "baby talk").

➤ Assure the child that he was in no way responsible for the death.

➤ Warning signs that may indicate the need for professional help, especially if they are prolonged, include an extended period in which the child loses interest in daily activities and events, inability to sleep, loss of appetite, fear of being alone, extended regression, repeated statements about wanting to join the dead person, withdrawal from friends, refusal to attend school, or a drop in academic performance.

Taking Care of Yourself

When caring for dying patients, you will confront your own feelings of mortality. It is important to understand your own attitudes, fears, and beliefs concerning death, so think about these before you encounter dying patients. This will enable you to deal in a healthier way with patients and their families. In addition, suppressing feelings associated with the death of patients can take a heavy toll on you emotionally.

When you become involved with dying persons and their families at such an intimate time in their lives, you become connected to them. There is nothing wrong with this emotional involvement; it helps you to be effective in your work. But just as you care for these families, you need also to care for yourself during these times.

- Recognize that feelings of grief and loss are normal, so do not be afraid to confront grief. If you deny your feelings and focus on caring for others, you will begin to wear down physically and emotionally.

- Talk with other colleagues about your feelings. Nurses are known for being able to take care of everyone but themselves! Don't be afraid to ask for what you need. Also recognize that your coworkers may need support. Form a nurses' support group that meets regularly to talk about the feelings of grief or loss and to remember those who have died. If you need or want a facilitator, pastoral care workers and social workers may be available for these services.

- When away from work, do some nice things for yourself on a regular basis (e.g., facial, quiet bubble bath, massage, a sports event). Set aside a special relaxation spot in your home; decorate it with items that help you focus on peaceful thoughts (e.g., candles, pictures, religious objects).

- If you wish, it is appropriate to attend calling hours and/or funeral services when one of your patients dies to help diffuse some of your feelings of loss. Also, it is meaningful to family members to know that you took the time to remember them and their loved one.

CLINICALREASONING

The questions and exercises in this section allow you to practice the kind of thinking you will use as a full-spectrum nurse. Critical-thinking questions usually have more than one correct answer, so we do not provide "correct answers" for these features. It is more important to develop your nursing judgment than to just cover content. You will learn by discussing the questions with your peers. If you are still unsure, see the Davis Advantage chapter resources for suggested responses.

Caring for the Nguyens

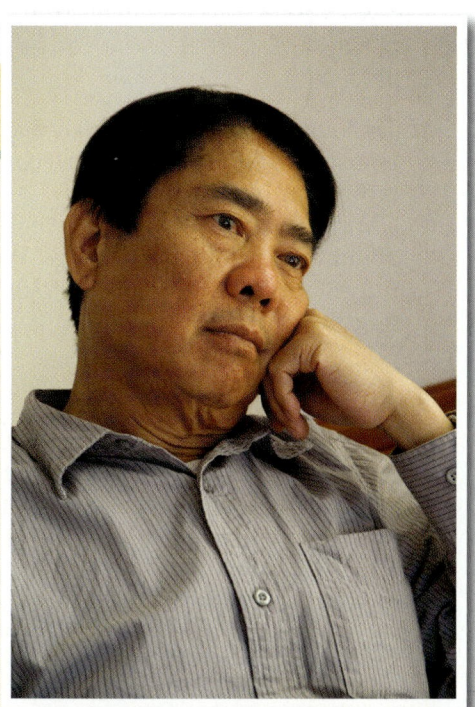

At a clinic visit, Nam Nguyen tells you that his father's health is declining rapidly: "I thought he was doing okay. I knew he had surgery for his prostate, so I thought it was all over. Lately he's been having lots of low back and hip pain. So my mom begged him to go to the doctor, and he told her he has cancer all over." Mr. Nguyen shakes his head and looks away from you. You notice tears in his eyes.

Mr. Nguyen tells you that his family has avoided discussions about serious illness and death. "It just never got discussed. The whole idea made my parents uncomfortable. When my father got sick the first time, he refused to discuss it. 'I'm going to get better. Don't even think about it,' he would say." Now Mr. Nguyen feels the need to discuss this situation with his parents but doesn't know how to bring up the topic. He asks for your advice.

(Continued)

Caring for the Nguyens (continued)

A. What would you think and feel when you see Nam's tears and when Mr. Nguyen asks for this advice?

B. What would you advise Mr. Nguyen?

C. What type of grief is Mr. Nguyen experiencing?

D. Examine the factors that affect grief. Apply these factors to Mr. Nguyen's situation. You will need to review the

family history included in the introduction to the Nguyens (in the front of this book) to fully answer this question. Indicate whether the information for any of the factors to be evaluated is insufficient.

 Go to Davis Advantage, Resources, Chapter 17, **Caring for the Nguyens—Suggested Responses.**

Applying the **Full-Spectrum Nursing Model**_____

PATIENT SITUATION

Marie is 84 years old and has had a right-sided cerebrovascular accident (CVA: stroke or brain attack). Doctors say she is unlikely to regain much physical function, if she even awakens from the coma. She was alert and active before her stroke and was able to maintain her independence with the help of a home health aide, who assisted her with activities of daily living and meal preparation three times a week. Kelly and Dan, her children, have met with the provider, who tells them that Marie's chance of survival is slim. He wants to put a feeding tube into Marie and has asked whether they want Marie to be resuscitated in case of cardiac or respiratory arrest. Kelly wants to do what is best for her mother, but she feels that Marie would not want to be kept alive in this condition. She is also concerned about putting her through uncomfortable procedures if there is no chance of recovery. Her brother, Dan, thinks Marie should have the feeding tube. Kelly asks to speak with you and wants to know the best thing to do for her mother.

THINKING

1. *Theoretical Knowledge (Recall of Facts and Principles):* If Kelly and Dan agree that they do not want Marie to be resuscitated, the provider will complete a DNR (AND) prescription. What do the letters *DNR* and *AND* represent?
2. *Critical Thinking (Problem-Solving):* At this stage of your education, you probably need more information about CVAs and tube feedings. Write a PICOT question you could use to search the literature for information about these two topics and how they are related. See Chapter 8 if you need to review PICOT questions.

DOING

3. *Practical Knowledge (Nursing Diagnosis):* Write a possible nursing diagnosis to describe Kelly's situation.
4. *Practical Knowledge (Basic Skills):* If Kelly and Dan agree to tube feedings for Marie, as her nurse what basic nursing skills will you need to perform? How will you learn to perform these skills if you do not already know how to do them?

CARING

5. *Ethical Knowledge:* How do you think the situation came to this point? What might Kelly, Dan, and Marie have done before the stroke to prevent this confusion and indecision?
6. *Self-Knowledge:* What are your responsibilities in this situation? What could you do to help Kelly and Dan?

 Go to Davis Advantage, Resources, Chapter 17, **Applying the Full-Spectrum Nursing Model—Suggested Responses.**

PracticalKnowledge: clinical application

CLINICAL INSIGHTS

Clinical Insight 17-1 ➤ **Communicating With People Who Are Grieving**

Perfect your listening skills. Listen for what is *not* said as well as what is said.

Be alert for and respond to nonverbal cues with appropriate touch and eye contact. A smile, a gentle touch, sitting with a patient, and eye contact all relay a message of genuine care and concern. You may not need to say very much at all.

Encourage and accept expressions of feelings.

- Receiving expressions of intense feelings (e.g., anger and guilt) may be painful for you. It may help to remember that it is therapeutic for people to express their feelings.
- You don't need to change the person's feelings or "make them better." As much as we would like to do this, it is not possible.
- You do need to validate the person's feelings (e.g., "It is normal to feel that way; it is okay").

Reassure the person that it is not "wrong" to feel anger, guilt, relief, or other feelings she may believe to be unacceptable. A dying patient might say, "I know it's awful, but I feel so angry with God for giving me this disease." Or a bereaved spouse might admit, "I shouldn't feel this way, but I'm relieved that it's finally over." Patients need to hear you say their feelings are not "wrong" or "bad" and that they are going through a normal process.

Increase your self-awareness. Become more conscious of your own attitudes and feelings regarding death and dying. *If you are comfortable with your perspective, you will be able to hear patients' expressions of anger, guilt, frustration, fear, and loneliness more comfortably.*

Continue to communicate with dying patients even if they are in a coma. Encourage family members to do so as well.

- Talk to the patient. Tell him what is going on around him, what care you are providing, and when you or others enter or are about to leave the room.
- Avoid discussing the dying person as though he were not present. *Research indicates that patients continue to hear even though they cannot respond, sometimes up to the moment of death.*

Practice Resources

Emanuel, L., Ferris, F., von Gunten, C., et al. (2015); Gibson, A., Hyde, Y., & Kautz, D. (2016); Holms, N., Milligan, S., & Kydd, A. (2014); The Joint Commission (2015); Wittenberg-Lyles, E., Goldsmith, J., Oliver, D., et al. (2012).

Clinical Insight 17-2 ➤ **Helping Families of Dying Patients**

- **View the family as your unit of care.** *Family members often rate communication with clinicians as one of their most important needs.*
- **Provide information, support, and a listening ear.** Include specific facts about the patient's condition and prognosis and whom to call about changes in condition.
- **Communicate medical updates daily.** *Information can relieve anxiety and is useful to the family when making decisions.*
- **Encourage family members to help with care if they are able.** Instruct and supervise as appropriate. If family members are not physically or emotionally able to provide care, accept that. *This helps meet their need to be useful, promotes family ties, and makes the patient more comfortable.*
- **Encourage family members to ask questions.** *They may hesitate to do so for various reasons (e.g., they may not want to interrupt busy care providers).*

- **Listen actively to the patient's and family's concerns.** Make eye content; clarify when you don't understand. *This helps you avoid misinterpreting the family's concerns and needs.*
- **Help the family to understand the goals of care and solve problems when needed.**
- **Follow up with other healthcare team members promptly** if the family has questions that are outside your scope of practice.
- **Arrange for a formal multidisciplinary meeting with the family** soon after the patient's admission, if possible. Discussions should cover personal, cultural, and religious traditions (e.g., how prayers are to be conducted, how the body is to be handled after death, and so on).
- **Encourage the family to visit the hospital chapel and to speak with a chaplain** or with their own spiritual adviser.

(Continued)

Clinical Insight 17-2 ▶ Helping Families of Dying Patients—cont'd

- **Provide anticipatory guidance regarding the stages of loss and grief** so that they will know what to expect after their loved one dies.
- **Acknowledge the family's feelings** and the loss they are experiencing. *Many times family members begin the grieving process before the loved one dies.*
- **Help the family members explore past coping mechanisms;** reinforce successful past coping mechanisms.
- **Refer for ethics consultation** if decision making may become a problem.
- **Remind family members and significant others to take care of themselves.** *Watching a loved one die is a very difficult experience. A sensitive, caring nurse can make it a little easier.*
  - Many times they need "permission" to go to eat or to go home and rest.
  - If the patient is near death and family and friends do not want to leave the patient's side, make them as comfortable as possible.
  - Provide comfortable chairs, coffee, and snacks (according to organizational policy) and be alert for other needs they may have.
- **Teach the family what to expect regarding medications, treatments, and signs of approaching death.** *If family members know what is normal, they will be less likely to panic or fear the inevitable.*

- **As physical signs of death become apparent, keep the family informed.** You may say something like, "Her blood pressure is becoming difficult to hear. That is one of the signs that she is closer to death." Help the family to understand what the patient is experiencing, as this may be very different from what they are seeing.
- **Reassure families of patients who become withdrawn near the time of death** that this does not mean the patient is rejecting them, but only that his body is conserving energy and that he has come to terms with dying and letting go of his connections with life.
- **When approaching death is apparent, ask family members directly, "Do you want to be present while he is dying?"** Tell them what to expect, if they do not know.
- **When an expected death occurs, shift the focus of your care** to the family and those who were caregivers. *Death does not end the relationship; family and caregivers need support during bereavement.*

Practice Resources

Emanuel, L., Ferris, F., von Gunten, C., et al. (2015); The Joint Commission (2014, 2015); Keely, M. (2016); Slatyer, S., Pienaar, C., Williams, A., et al. (2015); Stayer, D. (2016); Williams, B., Lewis, D., Burgio, K., et al. (2012); Yim, M., Vico, C., & Wai, C. (2013).

Clinical Insight 17-3 ▶ Caring for the Dying Person: Meeting Physiological Needs

Active dying usually occurs over a period of 10 to 14 days (although it can take as little as 24 hours). The "final hours" refer to the last 4 to 48 hours of life, in which failure of body systems results in death.

Encourage the patient to be as independent as possible. *This helps the patient maintain a sense of control.*

Provide adequate pain control. *This can be a major issue for patients and caregivers. In fact, dying patients are often more concerned about pain and loss of control than about dying itself. Pain is difficult to assess in semiconscious or unconscious patients. See Chapter 32 if you need more information about pain management.*

- Dispel the myths about pain medication (e.g., addiction, overdose). Effective pain control medications exist and can be administered by various routes. Assure the patient and family that analgesics will not be addictive in this situation.
- Respect the patient's informed decision to refuse pain medications. For example, a patient may prefer to endure

pain in order to be awake and alert when his family is at the bedside.
- Follow the prescribed pain protocols to ensure that pain is controlled.
- Administer pain medication on a regular schedule instead of waiting until the patient asks (prn) to ensure pain control.
- Teach and perform nonpharmacological pain-relief measures when you judge these may be helpful (e.g., meditation, heat/cold therapies, massage, distraction, imagery, deep breathing, and herbal-scented lotions). It may be soothing to play soft music, add "white noise," or turn off the television.
- Patients who are near death may moan or grunt as they breathe; this does not necessarily indicate pain. Be sure that families understand this. When accompanied by agitation and restlessness, these symptoms may indicate terminal delirium, which may require medications for control.

Clinical Insight 17-3 ➤ **Caring for the Dying Person: Meeting Physiological Needs—cont'd**

Monitor the patient's energy level. *Fatigue is a normal part of the dying process. Most dying patients sleep much of the time.*

- Perform hygiene and other care if the patient tires easily or lacks the energy for self-care (i.e., activities of daily living).
- Remove environmental stressors that interfere with sleep (e.g., noise, too much light, a room that is too hot or too cold).
- Identify psychosocial stressors (e.g., depression, anxiety, fear) that may keep the patient awake (see Clinical Insight 17-4).

Maintain skin integrity. *During the final hours of life, the goal changes from preserving skin integrity to providing comfort. Realize that during this time even excellent care may not prevent skin breakdown.*

- Turn the patient frequently unless contraindicated. Refer to the pain-control interventions in the preceding list.
- Assess for increased diaphoresis and/or incontinence.
- Maintain adequate nutrition.

If the patient is comatose or unconscious, provide special care for the eyes so they do not become too dry. Many agencies use a form of artificial tears for this purpose.

If the patient is not able to take fluids, wet the lips and mouth frequently with cool water or with a prepared product to prevent dryness and cracking of lips and mucous membranes of the nose, mouth, and eyes.

➤ *There is some evidence that glycerin swabs dry the mucous membranes and should not be used.*

Provide artificial hydration (unless the patient has an advance directive requesting no artificial hydration) per nasogastric (NG) or IV route. Monitor fluid balance. *IV fluids can cause edema, nausea, and even pain in a patient who is actively dying. Dehydration is thought not to cause distress during the last hours and may even be protective (Campbell, 2010; Emanuel, Ferris, von Gunten, et al., 2015).*

Take the vital signs often, unless contraindicated; observe for decreased level of consciousness and pallor.

Assess and provide interventions for constipation, urinary retention, and incontinence. *Constipation may be associated with decreased fluid intake, inactivity, weakness, hypercalcemia, hyperkalemia, and lack of privacy. It can contribute to pain, nausea, vomiting, and anorexia, so intervention is an important comfort measure. Incontinence may occur* because of fatigue and loss of sphincter control. It can be distressing to patients and family members.

- Administer laxatives, stool softeners, and lubricants for constipation.
- Catheterize the patient if he is unable to void and the bladder becomes distended.
- Use pads for incontinence, but change them frequently to prevent skin breakdown and, near the end, to promote comfort.
- Use a rectal tube if diarrhea is severe.

Intervene for "death rattle" if it occurs and if it is distressing to the family.

- Turn the patient on his side, and elevate the head of the bed.
- Administer antispasmodic and anticholinergic medications if necessary.

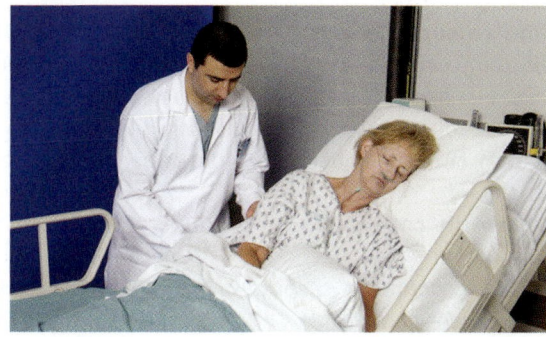

Provide medication for other symptoms, such as nausea and breathlessness.

Continue to speak to the patient as if he can hear.

Do not talk about the patient to others in his presence. *The patient is usually able to hear even after he can no longer respond to sounds and other stimuli. Assume the unconscious patient hears everything.*

Document changes in vital signs and level of consciousness. Record intake and output, noting changes. Document the times of cardiac arrest and cessation of respirations.

Practice Resources

Brennan, C., Prince-Paul, M., & Wiencek, C. (2011); Covington, M. (2013); Emanuel, L., Ferris, F., von Gunten, C., et al. (2015); Fahlberg, B. (2015a); Higgins, I., Riet, P., Sneesby, L., et al. (2013); The Joint Commission (2014, 2015); Kisvetrová, H., _koloudík, D., Joanovi_, E., et al. (2016); Steindal, S., Ranhoff, A., Bredal, I., et al. (2013).

Clinical Insight 17-4 ► Caring for the Dying Person: Meeting Psychological Needs

Patients experience many emotions at end of life, including anger, sadness, depression, fear, relief, loneliness, and grief. At this time, communication and support are most helpful. Discussing concerns and issues is a viable means of coping.

If there is an advance directive or living will, locate the documents. Review the documents to be certain you understand the patent's wishes. If you have not already done so, notify all relevant health professionals of the existence of these documents.

Answer all questions honestly.

Explain all care and treatments even if the patient is unconscious. *He may still be able to hear.*

Realize that the patient may feel he is losing control.

- Help the person recognize what he does have control over.
- Include the patient in care decisions as much as he is able.

Attend to social needs. *Relationships are a priority at this time. Some patients may simply need to keep the bonds with family members and friends intact. For other patients, this may be a time to reestablish or mend relationships.*

- Notify family members when the patient wishes to see them.
- Allow the patient and family to discuss death at their own pace.
- Offer to contact a chaplain or other spiritual leader if the patient chooses.
- Pray with the patient if he requests it and you are comfortable doing so.

Encourage the patient to express feelings. Be prepared to accept a wide range of feelings, including anger, hopelessness, loneliness, and depression.

Early in the dying process, assess the sources of financial support for the patient and family. *Finances may* be a concern and may place an additional burden on the family; the patient may feel his care is a burden to others.

Be aware of sexual needs. Provide realistic information about these issues. For example, suggest ways a couple can be close and affectionate at this time. Be aware that expressions of sexuality may change as a person becomes closer to death. *Some people may feel it is not right to have sexual feelings when the person they love is dying. Others may be afraid of harming the patient if they are sexually intimate.*

When the patient is very near death, focus on relieving symptoms (e.g., pain, nausea) and emotional distress.

If the person can communicate, ask about immediate concerns:

- "Are you in pain?" "Are you comfortable?"
- "What are you afraid of now?"
- "What can we do to help you go peacefully?"
- "Who do you want in the room with you right now?"

If the patient asks whether he is dying, be honest.

If the patient cannot communicate, ask a significant other what the patient would want. Ask the family member or person who is most likely to know.

When the patient is very near death, it may be helpful to say something like, "Your family will be fine" rather than, "It is okay for you to go now." *Be aware that some people seem to wait to die until after a significant date (birthday, anniversary, and so on) has passed. Others wait for family to gather, whereas others wait until loved ones leave so they will not upset the family by dying in their presence.*

Practice Resources

Brennan, C., Prince-Paul, M., & Wiencek, C. (2011); Coolen, P. (2012); Emanuel, L., Ferris, F., von Gunten, C., et al. (2015); Finocchiaro, D. (2016); Law, R. (2009); The Joint Commission (2015); Pola, A., & Nelson, R. (2014); Scogin, F., Fairchild, J., Yon, A., et al. (2014); Slatyer, S., Pienaar, C., Williams, A., et al. (2015).

Clinical Insight 17-5 ► Providing Postmortem Care

Supporting the Family

- **At the moment of death, do not interrupt or intrude on the family.** Wait quietly and observe, or if they would feel more comfortable being alone with the patient, leave the room. Give them as much time as they need. When they move away from the body or have expressed their last good-byes, then it is time to assess the patient and report the lack of vital signs.
- **Immediately after death, express sympathy to the family.** This is very important. Make a simple statement, such as, "I am sorry for your loss." Avoid statements that interpret the situation for the family, such as, "It's God's will." Also avoid attempts to mitigate the family member's grief, for example, "It will get better in time," or "You still have your son."

- **If the family wishes to be alone with the body,** straighten the bedcovers and make the patient look as natural as possible. Remove any tubes, IV lines, and so on, according to the institution's policy, and have the patient positioned in a way that appears comforting (e.g., bedcovers pulled up, hands at the side).
- **Be accepting of family members' behavior at this time,** no matter how strange it may seem to you. A family might want to take a picture, or the spouse may lie down beside the deceased person.
- **If no family members are present, identify the next of kin** and be sure the family is informed of the patient's death.
- **If family members arrive after the death, offer to take them to the bedside.**

Clinical Insight 17-5 ➤ Providing Postmortem Care—cont'd

- **If family members wish to be involved in postmortem care,** encourage them to do so. This can facilitate their grieving process.
- **Ask whether each family member wishes to spend time alone with the deceased person,** and arrange for them to do so. Never remove the body until the family is ready. Viewing the body is useful to many individuals.
- **Ask, "How can I help?" "What do you need?" "What would you like for me to do?"**
- **Locate personal effects and give them to the family/next of kin.** If you can't remove a ring, wrap it with gauze, tape it in place, and tie the gauze to the wrist to prevent subsequent loss.

Legal Responsibilities

- **Notify the primary provider of the death.** Usually the physician must pronounce death; however, in some areas a coroner or a nurse may also perform this task.
- **The person who pronounces death must sign the death certificate.** In some agencies, the nurse is responsible for checking to see that it has been signed.
- **If the patient is donating organs,** review and make any necessary arrangements.
- **If an autopsy is to be performed,** as a rule the physician (or other person designated by the institution) is responsible for obtaining signed permission from the next of kin.

Care of the Body

- **Follow agency policies and respect cultural and spiritual preferences.**
- **Wash the body if there has been any incontinence or drainage.** Place absorbent pads between the buttocks to absorb rectal drainage. Ask for the family's permission before washing the body. *In some cultures, the body is not washed, or family members arrange to have someone special do it.*
- **Dress the body in a clean gown, comb the hair, and straighten the bed linens.**
- **Place the body supine in a natural position.**
  Place the dentures in the mouth before rigor mortis occurs.
  Close the eyes and mouth before rigor mortis occurs. Close the eyes by gently pressing on the lids with your fingertips. If they do not stay closed, place a moist compress on the eyelids for a few minutes and then try to close them again.
  Tie a strip of soft gauze (e.g., Kling) under the chin and around the head if your institution requires it (not all do). Alternatively, you can place a folded towel under the chin to keep the jaw closed. *This keeps the mouth set in a natural position in case there is a viewing later.*

Place a pillow under the head and shoulders. *This prevents blood from settling there and causing discoloration.*
- **Be sure that dressings are clean and, unless an autopsy is to be done, remove all tubes and drains.** Be careful when removing tape or dressings. Apply small adhesive bandages to puncture sites. *After death, the skin loses its elasticity and can be torn easily.*
- **If the family asks about the coldness and color of the body, explain to them about algor mortis and livor mortis.**
- **After the family has spent time with the body, arrange to have it sent to the morgue,** where either an autopsy will be performed, or, if not, the funeral home in charge of arrangements will arrive to transport the body.
  Pad the wrists and ankles to prevent bruising; tie them together with gauze.
  Wrap the body in a shroud or body wrap for transfer to the morgue.
  If no relatives were present to receive patient belongings, bag them, label the bag, and send with the patient to the morgue.
  If possible, close doors to adjoining rooms before transport.
- **Make sure there are identification tags on the body, on the shroud or body bag, on the patient's possessions, and, if necessary, hazard labels.** Follow agency policy for number and location of tags. They will usually include the patient's name, room and bed numbers, date and time of death, and the physician's name. *Misidentification can create legal problems, for example, if the body is prepared incorrectly for a funeral.*
- **Follow institutional policy if the patient has died of a communicable disease.** By law, there are special preparations to perform in such cases.
- **Handle the body with dignity.**

Documentation

Documentation varies among healthcare facilities. However, you will almost always document the time that you noted absence of heartbeat and respirations, any auxiliary equipment still present (e.g., mechanical ventilator), the disposition of the patient's possessions (especially money and jewelry), and the date and time the body is transported to the morgue or funeral home.

Practice Resources

College of American Pathologists (2012, updated); The Joint Commission (2015); Olausson, J., & Ferrell, B. (2013); Smith-Stoner, M., & Hand, M. (2012).

To explore learning resources for this chapter,

Go to www.DavisAdvantage.com and find:

Answers and Suggested Responses for all questions in this chapter

Lists of NIC Interventions and NOC Outcomes

List of NANDA-I Diagnoses

Knowledge Map

Care Plan

Care Map

References and Bibliography

Concept Map

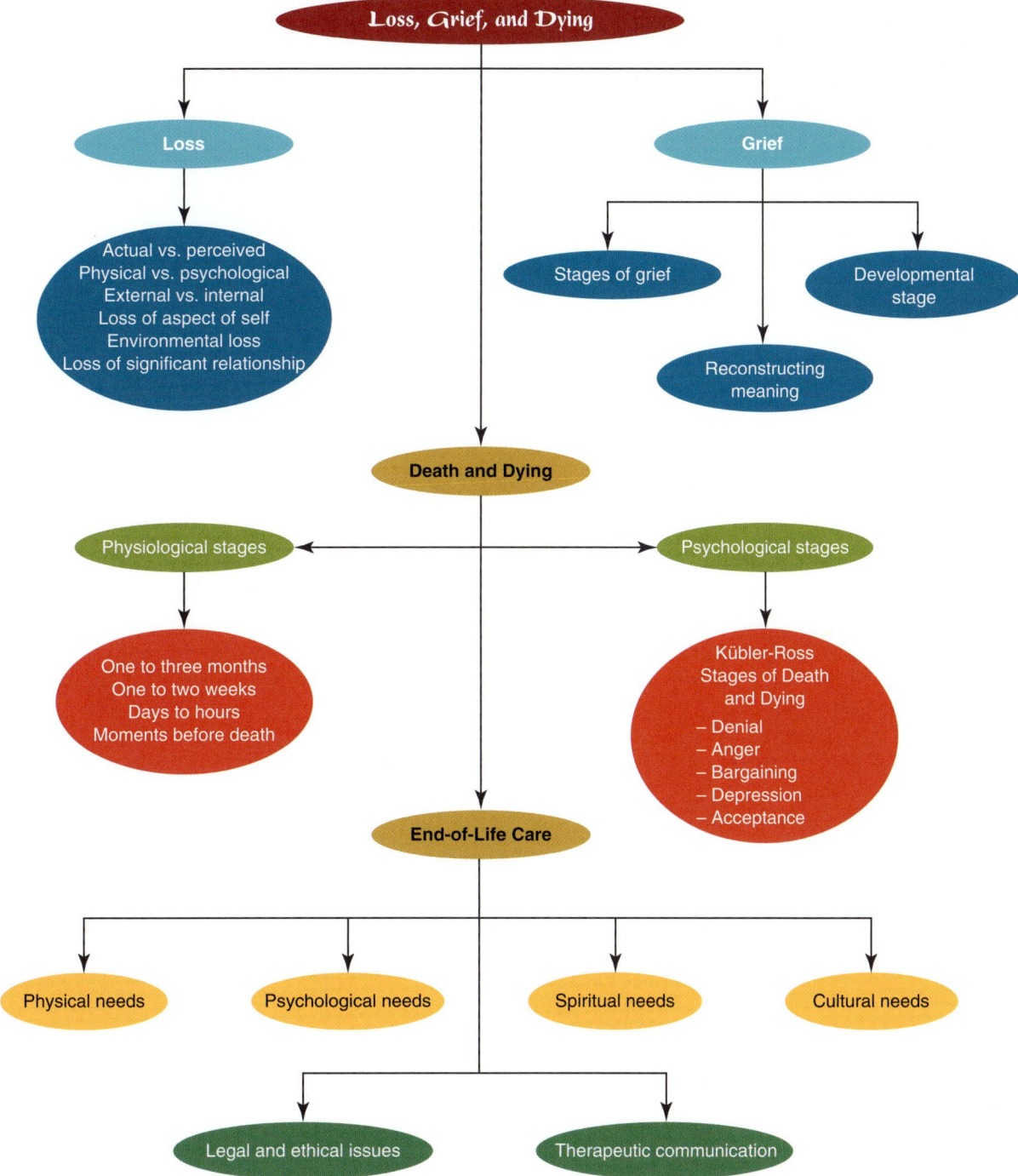

Essential Nursing Interventions

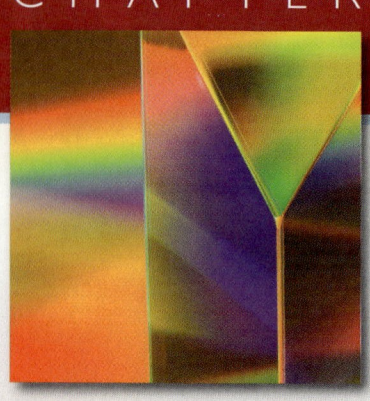

CHAPTER 18

Documenting & Reporting

Learning Outcomes

After completing this chapter, you should be able to:

- ➤ Explain the purposes of documentation.
- ➤ Compare and contrast electronic and written documentation.
- ➤ Identify a variety of charting formats and their purposes.
- ➤ Follow documentation guidelines to accurately record client health status, nursing interventions, and client outcomes in written and electronic formats.
- ➤ Identify approved abbreviations to use in documenting in clinical environments.
- ➤ Discuss the key elements of giving an oral client report.
- ➤ Explain the process for verifying or questioning a medical prescription.

Key Concepts

Documentation
Oral reporting

Related Concepts

See the Concept Map at the end of this chapter.

Meet Your Patient

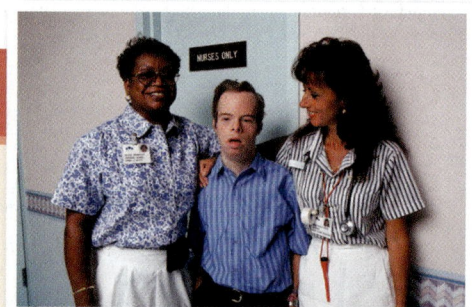

Steven Stellanski is a 16-year-old male who has just been released from the post-anesthesia care unit (PACU) after an emergency appendectomy. You are to admit him to your unit. Steven is groggy but moaning in pain. "Help me, help me," he whispers. He is holding his abdomen and grimacing. The PACU nurse tells you that Steven has Down syndrome and functions at an elementary school-age level.

Steven's vital signs are as follows: tympanic membrane temperature, 99.9°F (37.7°C); pulse, 104 beats/min; respirations, 24 breaths/min; and blood pressure, 104/68 mm Hg. An intravenous (IV) bag of lactated Ringer's solution is infusing at 125 mL/hr. The dressing on Steven's right lower abdomen is dry and intact. An indwelling catheter is draining pale yellow urine.

The provider has prescribed a patient-controlled analgesia (PCA) pump that will deliver morphine sulfate at 1 mg every 15 minutes, up to 4 mg per hour. Steven is to remain NPO (nothing by mouth) for now. His postoperative dressing is to be changed tomorrow morning and the nurses are to institute progressive ambulation as tolerated.

TheoreticalKnowledge
knowing **why**

When you imagine yourself working as a nurse, what do you think of? Most people picture themselves at the bedside working with clients. When you look at ads for nursing jobs, they often show a nurse performing interventions (e.g., hanging an IV bag or listening to heart sounds). The ads rarely show the nurse documenting or verbally reporting care. Yet healthcare professionals rely on these methods of communication to coordinate client care. In this chapter, we discuss paper, electronic, and oral communication.

ABOUT THE KEY CONCEPTS

Documentation and **oral reporting** are the two broad concepts to which all other concepts in this chapter are linked. As you read, think, "What does this have to do with documentation?" and "How does this relate to oral reporting?"

DOCUMENTATION

Documentation is the act of recording patient status and care. **KEY POINT:** *Documentation can be in written or electronic form or in a combination of the two forms.* Documentation is the act of making a written record. The terms *documenting, recording,* and *charting* are often used to mean the same thing. Oral communication about a patient's status is called **reporting**—that is discussed later in this chapter.

Historically, the collection of documentation, orders, and other care information for a patient had been called the **medical record** or **chart.** However, with the present emphasis on health promotion, it is now more often referred to as the **health record.** A patient's health record permanently documents:

- Care, in chronological order, provided by all healthcare providers
- The patient's responses to interventions and treatments
- Important facts about the patient's health history, including past and present illnesses, examinations, tests, treatments, and outcomes

As a nurse, you are responsible for managing and implementing the interprofessional plan of care, including the care provided and the progress made toward goals. Research shows that nurses routinely spend 15% to 25% of their workday documenting their care, and in some cases considerably more (Yee, Needleman, Pearson, et al., 2012).

How Do Healthcare Providers Use Documentation?

Clear, complete, concise, comprehensive, and correct documentation in a client health record serves a variety of purposes:

Communication Members of the interprofessional team use the health record to communicate about the client's status and care. For example, if it is not possible to speak directly to the respiratory therapist on your shift, you can at least review the progress notes. Communication enables healthcare professionals to plan and evaluate treatment and monitor health status over time.

Continuity of Care Communication promotes continuity of care. For example, if you are concerned that the client is at high risk for infection, you can include a nursing diagnosis of Risk for Infection on the written or electronic plan of care. You would then initiate nursing prescriptions for

other nurses to regularly observe for and document signs of infection.

Quality Improvement To improve overall quality of care, healthcare agencies must identify ways to decrease length of stay, control costs, and identify knowledge and practice gaps that can be addressed through inservice and continuing education. In an internal review, they

- Perform **manual chart audits** (directed reviews of client medical records) of written documentation.
- Run reports to analyze large amounts of data in electronic health record (EHR) systems.

External accrediting agencies, such as The Joint Commission, review written and electronic records to ensure delivery of quality care and public safety.

Planning and Evaluation of Client Outcomes Documentation enables providers, nurses, and other healthcare professionals to plan and evaluate treatment and monitor health status over time.

Legal Record The health record will be scrutinized by legal experts if a dispute about a client's care arises. In court, the health record is legal evidence of the care given to a client and is used to judge whether the interventions were timely and appropriate.

Professional Standards The American Nurses Association's (ANA) *Nursing: Scope and Standards of Practice* (2015) includes documentation in many of its standards. If you want to know which specific standards include documentation, see Box 18-1.

Reimbursement and Utilization Review Insurance companies, government and third-party payers, budget managers, and organization billing staff use client health records to determine the cost of care. They also use the health record for **utilization review** to determine whether the medical treatments and interventions were necessary and appropriate.

BOX 18-1 ■ ANA Standards of Practice Regarding Documentation

The ANA standards require nurses to:
- Document relevant data accurately and in a manner accessible to the interprofessional team (Standard 1—Assessment).
- Document diagnoses, problems, and issues in a manner that facilitates the determination of the expected outcomes and plan (Standard 2—Diagnosis).
- Document expected outcomes as measurable goals (Standard 3—Outcomes Identification).
- Document the plan using standardized language or recognized terminology (Standard 4—Planning).
- Document implementation and any modifications, including changes or omissions, of the identified plan (Standard—Implementation).
- Document the coordination of care (Standard 5A—Coordination of Care).
- Document the results of the evaluation (Standard 6—Evaluation).
- Document nursing practice in a manner that supports quality and performance improvement initiatives (Standard 14—Quality of Practice).

Source: American Nurses Association. (2015). *Nursing: Scope and standards of practice* (3rd ed.). Silver Spring, MD: Author.

Education and Research As a student, you are well aware that the health record provides a snapshot of what is going on with the client, enabling you to research unfamiliar diagnoses, orders, and treatments before beginning direct care. This helps you to deliver safe care.

The health record is also used to gather data for clinical research. The increasing use of EHRs enables rapid analysis of large numbers of health records. Use of large samples of health records and clinical data sets is an essential step toward better understanding the cause and progression of disease, treatment methods, and outcomes across varied populations and diseases.

Why Are Standardized Nursing Languages Important?

- **Make nursing visible.** As healthcare costs escalated, it became necessary to demonstrate the value of nursing—that is, to describe what nurses do and the outcomes that result. Standardized nursing terminology helps do that by making nursing care and its effect on patient outcomes more visible in patient records.
- **Support nursing research.** Documentation systems that use ANA recognized terminology (e.g., NANDA-I, NIC, and NOC) allow researchers to retrieve nursing data for aggregation and analysis and establish standards for the delivery of evidence-based nursing care. Such standards help close the gap between what research shows to be the best nursing practices and the interventions nurses actually use in practice.
- **Provide standardized terminology for use in EHR systems.** This is important in EHR systems because computers require standardized information that can be converted to numerical codes.

Several standardized nursing language models have been created and are used in nursing documentation, such as NANDA-I (for nursing diagnoses), NIC (for interventions), and NOC (for patient outcomes). To review using standardized nursing language in your own practice, see the standardized language sections in Chapters 4, 5, and 6. For lists of terms,

Go to Davis Advantage, Resources, Chapter 18, **List of: NANDA-I Diagnoses, List of NOC Outcomes, and List of NIC Interventions**

How Are Health Records Systems Organized?

A **health records system** is the overall process by which all client records are created, stored, and retrieved in an organization. In a sense, it consists of all the EHRs in an organization. Each healthcare agency determines the health record system that is used. Nursing leaders in each organization usually determine the documentation forms that nurses will use within the records system.

Source-Oriented Record Systems

Patients in hospitals and long-term care facilities commonly use **source-oriented records.** Members of each discipline record their findings in a separate section of the chart. A typical source-oriented record includes the following sections:

- *Admission data*—demographic information, insurance data, contact information
- *Advance directive*—information on client's wishes for the extent of care and medical support that should be given in the event of a life-threatening event

- *History and physical*—a detailed summary of the current health problem; past medical, surgical, and social history; medications taken; allergies; review of systems; and physical examination data
- *Provider's orders*—prescriptions for medications, treatments, and activities
- *Progress notes*—chronological charting by healthcare team members including client exams, problem identification, and response to therapy
- *Diagnostic studies*—reports detailing the findings of tests that have been performed, such as x-ray exam and ultrasound, or pulmonary function tests, such as complete blood count
- *Laboratory data*—results from diagnostic test results
- *Nurses' notes*—documentation of client care and response to treatment recorded by nurses (usually chronological)
- *Graphic data*—numerical data collected over time and displayed visually to allow analysis of trends. Examples include intake and output records; vital sign flow sheets; rating scales; and checklists regarding client activity, dietary intake, and activities of daily living (ADLs)
- *Rehabilitation and therapy notes*—chronological charting by therapists (e.g., physical, occupational, respiratory) about assessments, the treatment plan, and client response to therapy
- *Discharge planning*—includes data from utilization review, case managers, or discharge planners on anticipated client needs after discharge

Advantages In source-oriented records, you can easily locate the care provided by each discipline and the results of laboratory and diagnostic tests.

Disadvantages Data may be fragmented and scattered throughout the chart. That means you need to review all sections of the medical record to fully understand the client's condition and care. It is especially difficult with source-oriented records to track the treatments and client outcomes associated with a particular problem. For example, suppose a client with congestive heart failure is retaining fluids, causing her to be short of breath on exertion. To find the interventions that have been done for this problem, you would need to look in the:

1. Primary care providers' (PCP) prescriptions to see which drugs (e.g., cardiac or diuretics) were prescribed to help with the fluid retention
2. Respiratory therapist's notes for the client's response to breathing treatments
3. Nursing notes to determine positioning (head of the bed elevated to facilitate breathing)
4. Graphic section to evaluate urinary output in response to the medication

Problem-Oriented Record Systems

Problem-oriented records (PORs) are organized around the patient's problems. There are no separate sections for each discipline. The POR consists of four parts: database, problem list, plan of care, and progress notes.

- The **database** consists of many parts: demographic data, the history and physical, nursing assessment data, and family and social history. As the patient's condition changes, the database is updated to reflect his current status.
- The **problem list** is a concise listing of problems identified from the database. Once a problem is resolved, it is noted on the problem list. If a problem changes or is redefined, the problem list is updated to reflect the change. See Figure 18-1 for an example of a problem list.

Problem number	Date entered	Date resolved	Client problem
1	4/10/18	4/11/18	Abdominal pain (unknown etiology) Redefined 4/11/18
1A	4/11/18		Appendicitis resulting in emergency appendectomy
1B	4/11/18		Acute pain r/t abdominal incision 2 appendectomy
2	4/10/18		Down syndrome — functions at school-age level
3	4/11/18		Risk for constipation r/t opioid use for pain control and h/o appendicitis

FIGURE 18-1 A problem list for Steven Stellanski (Meet Your Patient). Note that Problem 1 was redefined after the cause of Steven's pain was determined. Note also that the list contains both medical and nursing diagnoses.

- The **plan of care** includes the PCP's prescription and the nursing care plan to address the identified problems. Other disciplines may also contribute to the plan.
- **Progress notes** are organized according to the problem list. Each discipline charts on shared notes. Charting is labeled according to problem number.

Advantages A common problem list allows for input from all disciplines, making it easy to monitor the patient's progress. Because each problem is readily identified in the notes, the findings of each discipline can easily be reviewed, which promotes greater collaboration.

Disadvantages To work well, the POR system requires a cooperative spirit among health providers as well as diligence in maintaining a current database and problem list.

Charting By Exception

Charting by exception (CBE) is a system of charting in which only significant findings or exceptions to standards and norms of care are documented. To use CBE effectively, you must know and adhere to professional, legal, and organizational guidelines for nursing assessments and interventions.

Preprinted flow sheets are used to document most aspects of care. Normal responses for various assessments are defined on either the front or back of the form. **KEY POINT:** *CBE assumes that all standards have been met and the client has responded normally, unless a separate entry is made (an exception).* Each flow sheet has entries for expected aspects of care and thus can vary by specialty or diagnosis.

Advantages CBE reduces the amount of time spent on documentation, reduces repetitive charting of routine care, provides a record that is easily read and understood, and clearly highlights any variations from the expected plan of care. EHRs can standardize common processes and list abnormal findings from the menu bar (Duffy, 2015).

Disadvantages The main problem associated with CBE is omissions of pertinent information. Omissions may result from disagreement over what constitutes a significant variation. Some define deviations based on the client's baseline

while others use normal physiological parameters (Kerr, 2013). Critics of CBE believe it:

- Requires nurses to be overly familiar with the organization's documentation standards and policies
- Makes it difficult to capture the skilled judgment of nurses
- Reduces care to such rote repetitions that the nurse may forget to chart an exception to the established standards

CBE can lead to errors because nurses may conclude that care has been completed when in fact it was not done. This system requires you to carefully assess and validate care provided.

Here is an example of what part of a CBE flow sheet for Steven Stellanski (Meet Your Patient) might look like. Notice in the first section that the day-shift nurse merely initials that she has made an assessment or taken one of the listed actions at each of the designated times:

DATE: 04/11/2018				
Hour	0800	0900	1000	1100
ACTIVITY				
Bedrest		LP		
Ambulate	LP*			
Sleeping				
BRP				
HOB elevated	LP	LP		

	DAY	EVENING	NIGHT	
Neurological		√		
Cardiovascular		√		
Pulmonary		√		
Gastrointestinal		*		Vomited 3×1, 100 mL clear yellow fluid at 0730. Given Promethazine 7 mg IV with relief.

Key: √ = normal findings, * = significant finding

Notice also the second table (with the checkmarks) is a summary for the day shift. This is where the nurse describes and discusses any of the significant findings noted at the individual assessment times.

Electronic Health Record (EHR) Systems

The EHR consists of records that are entered via computer. EHRs typically combine source-oriented and problem-oriented record styles, although the source-oriented system is most common. For example, a client's EHR often contains prescriptions, clinical documentation, and results of laboratory and other tests and procedures, as well as an integrated plan of care (IPOC), a problem and diagnosis list, and progress notes entered by providers, nurses, therapists, and other healthcare providers.

Figure 18-2 is a section of an electronic form for recording intake and output in source-oriented format. As you can see, the input and output (I&O) screen records numerical data. It also allows the nurse to add brief narrative comments in each field. Figure 18-3 is an electronic IPOC in problem-oriented format. The IPOC can be updated at the times specified by the organization and the I&O data can be entered at any time. Both exist within the same electronic records system.

Advantages

- **Enhanced communication and collaboration.** Communication is improved among healthcare providers.
- **Improved access to information.**
  - Multiple healthcare providers can access the same information at the same time.
  - Authorized persons can access information remotely (e.g., from a client's home).
  - EHRs integrate client information between multiple departments so that new information is immediately available to users in all areas. For example, when the laboratory enters a critical result, such as a clotting time, you do not need to wait for the lab to phone or e-mail to the nursing unit.
- **Time savings**
  - Nurses spend up to 25% less time documenting.
  - Stored information is quickly and easily retrieved.
  - Reports can be created quickly because of the computer's ability to aggregate data (e.g., a 24-hr graph of the client's vital signs).
  - Repetition and duplication are reduced.

- **Improved quality of care**
  - The system can use protocols to automatically enter prescriptions based on the client's condition. For example, some EHR systems will automatically enter a prescription to observe and document risk of falls when a client's "falls score" exceeds a certain level.
  - Embedded protocols enhance caregiver knowledge and the ability to follow clinical practice guidelines. For example, suppose there is a medical prescription to administer insulin based on a patient's blood glucose results. In some EHR systems, the nurse can activate an immediate link to the tables of information needed to decide how much insulin to administer to the client.
  - Medical errors are minimized by programmed alerts that are automatically displayed when a provider takes an action that could be harmful (e.g., when a provider prescribes a drug to which a patient is allergic).
  - Data can be analyzed at the time of collection, making immediate nursing decisions possible.
  - EHRs facilitate evidence-based practice by analyzing thousands of records in ways that cannot be done with paper forms. With aggregated data, nursing practice can be compared across populations and geographic locations to support nursing decisions and guide professional and organization quality improvement.
- **Information that is private and safe**
  - Information is permanently stored and not likely to be lost.
  - Confidentiality of client information is enhanced by restricting access, tracking everyone who accesses the healthcare record, and using proper security clearances, unique passwords, and front view screen protectors.

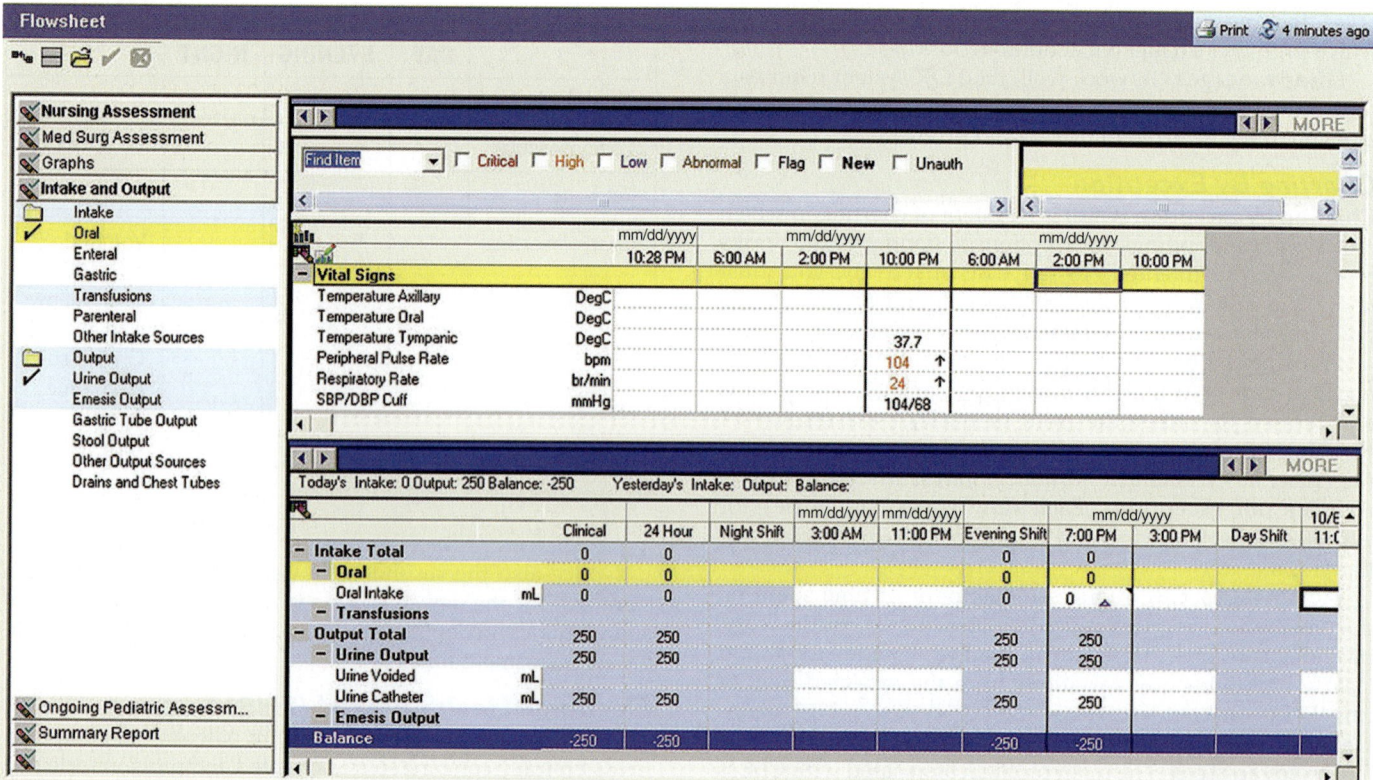

FIGURE 18-2 An electronic intake and output (I&O) entry form.

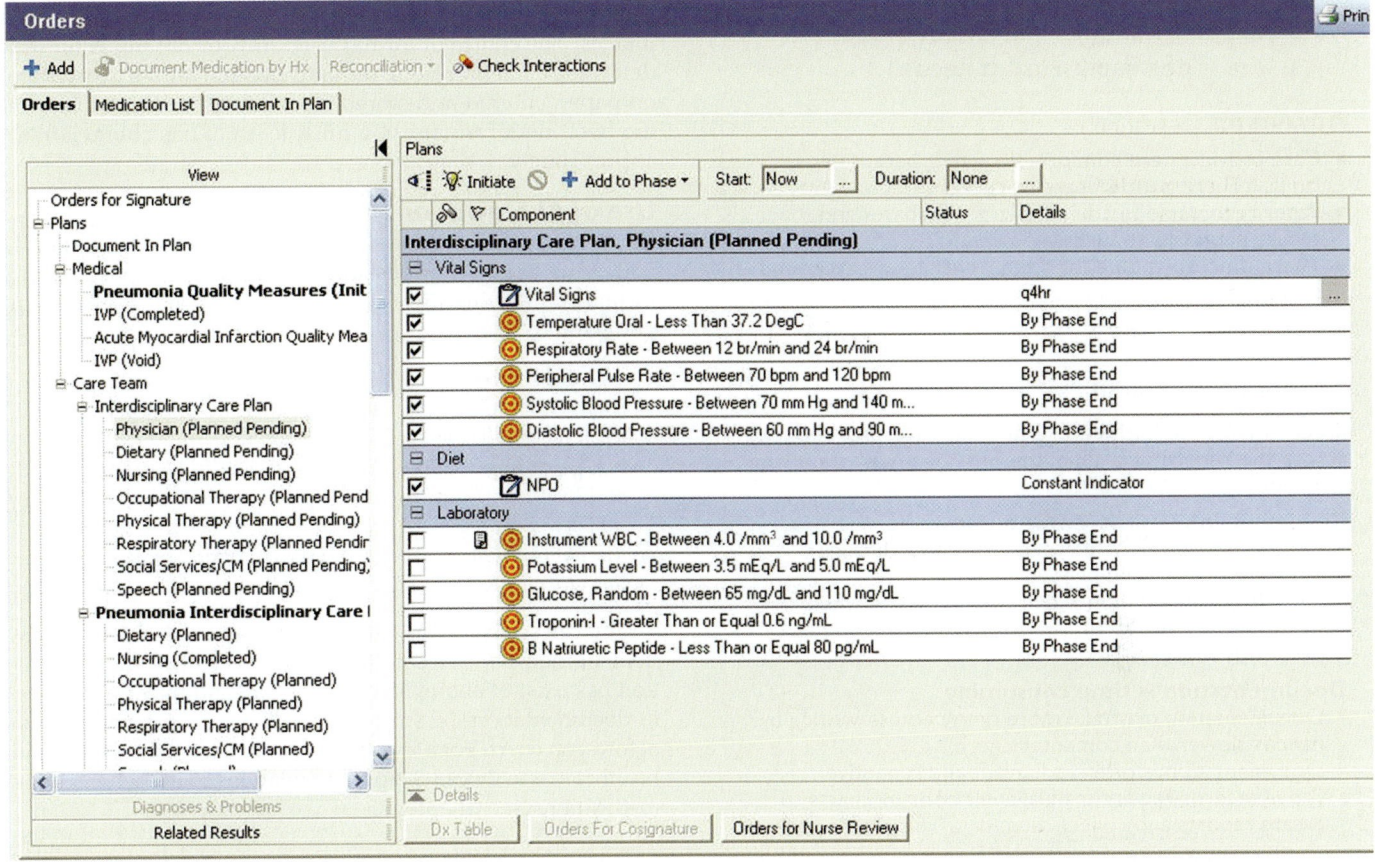

FIGURE 18-3 A portion of an electronic integrated plan of care (IPOC) form.

Disadvantages

- **Expense.** Electronic documentation systems are expensive.
- **Downtime.** Downtime processes must be in place for times when parts of the EHR are not available (e.g., because of power outages and system upgrades).
- **Difficulties associated with change.**
  - Learning to use some documentation systems can be challenging and time consuming.
  - Some healthcare providers resist the change to EHRs.
  - It is not easy to capture narrative nursing content from paper documentation into an electronic format.
  - Some EHRs are not user friendly (e.g., difficult to quickly find information needed to make care decisions).
  - Some systems do not control redundancy well, requiring caregivers to continuously ask the client for the same information.
- **Lack of integration.** Most EHRs are not integrated across the different departments: This means that sometimes a person with a legitimate reason to enter the record cannot see entries made by other departments and must then request verbal, e-mail, or paper reports (e.g., lab reports).

Paper Records

Healthcare environments are still transitioning from paper health records to electronic health records, so you may work in facilities that still use paper records. For a summary of the advantages and disadvantages of paper records, see Box 18-2.

KnowledgeCheck 18-1

- Identify the purposes of the client health record.
- What are the key differences in the organization of source-oriented records, problem-oriented records, electronic documentation systems, and charting by exception systems?
- What are three advantages of paper health records?
- What are three advantages of EHRs?

Documentation and the Nursing Process

The goal of nursing documentation is a clear, concise, comprehensive, and correct representation of the client's healthcare experience that is easily accessible and understood by all members of the healthcare team. Effective documentation allows you to help clients make sound health decisions. It also enables use of current and consistent data, problem statements, diagnoses, goals, and strategies to support continuity of care.

Research, however, continues to identify insufficient documentation of the steps in the nursing process (e.g., inadequate assessment information, lack of decisions based on a nursing diagnosis, inadequate evaluation and revisions in the plan of care) (Blair & Smith, 2012). Regardless of the type of documentation, you must ensure the nursing process is used and each client's problem is appropriately prioritized (Lavin, Harper, & Barr, 2015).

Assessment: Chart signs and symptoms that may indicate actual or potential client problems. At an initial assessment, document comprehensive data about all client systems.

BOX 18-2 ■ Advantages and Disadvantages of a Paper Health Record

Advantages

- Care providers are comfortable with it because it is familiar. There is little "learning curve."
- Paper records do not require large databases and secure networks to function.
- There is no downtime for system changes, weather, and so on.
- It is relatively inexpensive to create new forms and update old ones.

Disadvantages

Access may be delayed. Only one care provider can access the record at a time; the provider must be in the same location as the chart.

Retrieving information may be slow.
- Healthcare providers may need to search through multiple pages to find needed information.
- Specific documentation is difficult to retrieve when needed, especially when files are archived in another part of the building.

Documentation is time consuming.
- Documentation may take more time because writing by hand is slower than computer entry.
- Documentation is often redundant and repetitive.
- Paper records require manual audit of many charts to create reports and collect client data. This is time and resource intensive.

There is a relatively high risk for patient care error.
- Narrative documents are hard to read if the handwriting is illegible or messy. This means nurses have to take time from patient care to contact providers to clarify handwritten prescriptions.
- Papers can be lost from the chart or damaged, leading to duplicate assessments or medication errors.
- Paper records are often inconsistent in how the same client information is documented, even within the same organization. Often standardized terminology is not used.

Storage of paper records is expensive.

Confidentiality is difficult to protect. There is no way to know who may have access to the paper health record without proper authorization.

Diagnosis/Analysis: After analyzing assessment data, document your clinical nursing judgment about the client's response to actual or potential health conditions or needs.

Outcomes/Planning: Document measurable and achievable short-term and long-term plans of care with goals directed at preventing, minimizing, or resolving identified client problems or issues.

Implementation: After putting the plan of care into effect, record the specific interventions that were used.

Evaluation: Document client responses to nursing care; chart whether the plan of care was effective in preventing, minimizing, or resolving the identified problems; and then modify the plan as needed.

What Are Some Common Formats for Nursing Progress Notes?

Nursing documentation can take many forms, including paper charts, computerized electronic documents, audio or video files, e-mails, faxes, scanned paper documents, electronically stored photographs, x-ray findings, and other images. The choice of format used in your organization will determine whether your nursing documentation is written on paper, entered and stored electronically, or in a blend of the two. In all formats, you must learn to use abbreviations appropriately.

Use of Abbreviations

Recall the case of Steven Stellanski (Meet Your Patient). Following is a brief admission note using narrative charting format. Underline any words or entries that you do not understand.

> *4/11/2018 1600 Pt received on unit from PACU. VSS. TM temp 99.9°F (37.7°C), P 104, and BP 104/68. LOC unstable. Arouses when name called but quickly drifts off to sleep. PERRLA. Moaning, grimacing, holding abd, whispers "Help me. Help me." LR at 125 mL/hr infusing in R forearm. IV site patent. Urinary catheter draining pale yellow urine. Abd drsg dry & intact. Morphine sulfate PCA ordered. Will initiate. _____ Ray Allenby, RN. _____*

You can see from this entry that nurses use many abbreviations in their paper record charting. Every healthcare institution has a list of abbreviations that may and may not be used in documentation. Be sure to consult your organization's list before you chart. For a list of commonly used abbreviations in healthcare, see Box 18-3. For abbreviations to use when giving medications, see Chapter 25.

✚ The Joint Commission (2015) created a "do not use" list that directs medical personnel in healthcare organizations to write out the words rather than use the abbreviations (see Table 18-1).

Narrative Format

Narrative format is written in source-oriented and problem-oriented charts. The **narrative chart entry** tells the story of the client's experience in the order that it happens.

- It provides information on the details of the client's care—status, activities, nursing interventions, psychosocial context, and response to treatment.
- It tracks the client's changing health status and progress toward goals.
- Narrative charting is especially useful when attempting to construct a time line of events, such as a cardiac arrest or other emergency situations.
- A disadvantage is that the lack of standardization can result in lengthy notes, making it difficult to retrieve relevant data in a timely manner (Blair & Smith, 2012).

Problem–Intervention–Evaluation (PIE)

The **Problem–Intervention–Evaluation (PIE)** system organizes information according to the client's problems; it requires keeping a daily assessment record and progress notes. PIE eliminates the need for a separate care plan and provides a nursing-focused rather than medical-focused record.

Problem: Use data from your original assessment to identify appropriate nursing diagnoses.

Intervention: Document the nursing actions you take for each nursing diagnosis.

Evaluation: Document the client's response to interventions and treatments.

Problems are identified from the admission assessment. Subsequent entries begin with identification of the problem number. This type of charting establishes an ongoing care plan.

BOX 18-3 ■ Abbreviations Commonly Used in Healthcare

ABBREVIATION	MEANING
ADLs	Activities of daily living
ad lib	As desired, if the patient desires
AKA	Above-knee amputation
amb	Ambulation, ambulatory
amt	Amount
ASAP	As soon as possible
bid	Twice a day
BM	Bowel movement
BR	Bedrest
BRP	Bathroom privileges
BSC	Bedside commode
c̄	With
cal	Calories
Cath	Catheter
CBC	Complete blood count
CCU	Critical care unit or coronary care unit
c/o	Complaint of
CO₂	Carbon dioxide
CPR	Cardiopulmonary resuscitation
CVA	Cerebrovascular accident (stroke)
D&C	Dilation and curretage
DM	Diabetes mellitus
dsg or drsg	Dressing
DX or Dx	Diagnosis
EBL	Estimated blood loss
EKG/ECG	Electrocardiogram
ED/ER	Emergency department, emergency room
EEG	Electroencephalogram
EENT	Eyes, ears, nose, throat
ETOH	Alcohol
F	Female
FBS	Fasting blood sugar
Ft	Foot
Fx	Fracture
GI	Gastrointestinal
gtt(s)	Drop(s)
GU	Genitourinary
GYN	Gynecology
HA	Headache
HMO	Health maintenance organization
h/o	History of
hob or HOB	Head of bed
HOH	Hard of hearing
H&P	History and physical
hr	Hour
ht	Height

ABBREVIATION	MEANING
HTN	Hypertension
hyper	Above or high
hypo	Below or low
ICU	Intensive care unit
I&O	Intake and output
isol	Isolation
IV	Intravenous
IVP	Intravenous push (caution: do not use to mean "IV piggyback")
L	Liter
lb	Pound
LPN	Licensed practical nurse
LMP	Last menstrual period
LVN	Licensed vocational nurse
mcg	Microgram
MD	Medical doctor
med	Medication
mg	Milligram
mL	Milliliter
MN	Midnight
NAS	No added salt
N/V/D	Nausea, vomiting, diarrhea
NKA or NKDA	No known allergies or no known drug allergies
NG	Nasogastric
NGT	Nasogastric tube
noc	At night
NPO	Nothing by mouth
O₂	Oxygen
OB	Obstetrics
OOB	Out of bed
OPD	Outpatient department
ortho	Orthopedics
OR	Operating room
os	Mouth, opening
OT	Occupational therapy
oz	Ounce
pc	After meals
PCA	Patient-controlled analgesia
PO	By mouth
P, p̄	After
PPBS	Postprandial blood sugar
prn	As needed
Pt	Patient
PT	Physical therapy
q	Every

(Continued)

BOX 18-3 ■ Abbreviations Commonly Used in Healthcare—cont'd

ABBREVIATION	MEANING	ABBREVIATION	MEANING
qam	Every morning	STI or STD	Sexually transmitted infection or sexually transmitted disease
qh	Every hour	TB	Tuberculosis
qid	Four times a day	TO	Telephone order
RN	Registered nurse	TPR	Temperature, pulse, respirations
R/O	Rule out	tid	Three times a day
RX or Rx	Treatment or prescription	VO	Verbal order
$\bar{s}$	Without	VS	Vital signs
SCD	Sequential compression device	WBC	White blood count
SOB	Short of breath	w/c	Wheelchair
$\bar{ss}$	One-half	WNL	Within normal limits
SSE	Soapsuds enema	wt	Weight
Stat	Immediately		

KEY POINT: *Abbreviations vary among healthcare agencies. Furthermore, they change rather often because of regulating agency guidelines (e.g., The Joint Commission). Therefore, you will need to be familiar with the abbreviations in the agency in which you work.*

Table 18-1 ➤ Joint Commission "Do Not Use" List

DO NOT USE THIS ABBREVIATION	WRITE OUT THE WORD OR DOSE
"U" or "u"	Unit
"IU"	International Unit
Q.D., QD, q.d., qd	Daily
Q.O.D., QOD, q.o.d., qod	every other day
MS, MSO4, and MgSO4	either morphine sulfate or magnesium sulfate
The trailing zero for medications (X.0 mg)	X mg (e.g., 10 mg)
Lack of leading zero (.X mg)	0.X mg (e.g., 0.1 mg)

Other Recommendations

In consideration of furthering The Joint Commission's Patient Safety Goals, some institutions require the following to minimize common errors that occur in healthcare organizations:

- Write out "greater than" or "less than"—rather than using the symbols > or <.

- Write drug names in full—rather than using abbreviations.

- Use metric units—instead of apothecary units.

- Write "at" or "each"—rather than use the @ symbol.

- Write "mL" or "milliliters"—in place of the "cc" abbreviation.

- Write "mcg" or "micrograms"—instead of the "μg" abbreviation.

A PIE charting entry for Steven Stellanski (Meet Your Patient) might look like this:

> 4/11/18   1630
> *P:* 1B
> *I:* Pt c̄ 1 mg doses up to 4 mg morphine/hr. Groggy yet c/o pain. Has not triggered PCA independently. Rates pain as 8 on scale of 1–10. PCA use reviewed with Pt. Demonstrated use c̄ 1st dose at 1615.
> *E:* Still moaning & grimacing. Has not initiated another dose via PCA. 2nd dose given as additional demo. Will reevaluate in 1 hr. May need continuous infusion if unable to use to control pain. ——————————Ron Allen, RN

SOAP/SOAPIE/SOAPIER

The **SOAP format** is often used to write nursing and other progress notes. It can be used in source-oriented, problem-oriented, and electronic health records. The following list explains the acronyms SOAP, SOAPIE, and SOAP(IER):

- *Subjective data*—What the client or family members tell you about the client's signs and symptoms and the reason they are seeking healthcare. Typically, this is documented by quoting the actual words said.

- *Objective data*—Factual, measurable clinical findings such as vital signs, test results, and quality of breath sounds. Refer to Chapter 3 to review subjective and objective data.

- *Assessment*—Conclusions drawn from the subjective and objective data, usually client problems or nursing diagnoses. **KEY POINT:** *SOAP terminology is different from nursing process terminology. In the nursing process chapters, we referred to conclusions about data as inferences or problems and stated that assessment does **not** include conclusions about data. When using SOAP, you **should** chart your conclusions about the data under "A."*

- *Plan*—Short-term and long-term goals and strategies that will be used to relieve the client's problems.

- *Interventions*—Actions of the healthcare team that are performed to achieve expected outcomes.

- *Evaluation*—An analysis of the effectiveness of interventions.
- *Revision*—Changes made to the original care plan.

Components of a POR Recall that a POR is organized according to specific client problems and has five components: database, problem list, initial plan, progress notes, and a discharge summary. You will refer to and use the following four parts when charting in SOAP format:

- **Problem List.** A numbered list of the client's current problems in chronological order is compiled so that you can refer to the number when entering your notes.
- **Initial Plan.** This includes expected outcomes and plans for further care interventions and teaching. There is only one initial plan, so you update and change the plan in subsequent progress notes.
- **Progress Notes.** This is where you record the SOAP(IER) information. As a rule, you enter a note for each current problem every 24 hours or when the client's condition changes.
- **Discharge Summary.** At discharge, each problem on the list is addressed and a notation made about its status. Unresolved problems, with plans for each, are included when communicating with the client, other facilities, and home health agencies.

Following is an example of SOAP progress notes using the admission data of Steven Stellanski (Meet Your Patient). In the previous section, these same data were used to create a narrative note. Notice that the data are similar; however, the narrative note is organized by data source. Steven's SOAP(IER) charting entry related to his postoperative nausea and pain could look like this:

	0900	**A**—Postoperative pain **P**—Give analgesic as needed. _____ **I**—Morphine PCA initiated at 0835. Instructed on its use. 1st dose (1 mg) administered as demonstration. **E**—Still moaning & grimacing even after 2nd dose _____ given as additional demo. Still has _____ not initiated _____ additional _____ PCA dose. _____ ——Ron Allen, RN
	0930	**R**—Still no pain relief; still has not used PCA independently. Discussed w/Dr. Jadu. Continuous infusion begun at 2 mg/hr. Will supplement up to 4 mg/hr prn. _____ ——Ron Allen, RN

4/11/2018	0830	#1—Nausea related to anesthesia _____ **S**—States "I feel sick to my stomach. Help me." **O**—Vomited 100 mL clear, light yellow fluid. _____ **A**—Nauseated secondary to anesthesia. _____ **P**—Monitor nausea and give antiemetic as needed. **I**—Administer _____ Promethazine 7 mg IV at 0830. _____
	0900	**E**—States he feels less sick to his stomach. ———Ron Allen, RN
4/11/18	0830	#1B—Acute pain related to abdominal incision 2° appendectomy _____ **S**—States, "help me, help me." Moaning and grimacing. _____ **O**—Moaning and _____ grimacing; holding abd. Drsg dry & intact. BP 104/68 mm Hg, _____ P104 beats/min, _____ R24 breaths/min, and TM temp 99.9°F. PERRLA.

Disadvantages This type of charting can be inefficient and ineffective.

- You may find the same interventions and responses repeated in more than one section for patients with overlapping problems.
- You may also find that nurses write a complete narrative rather than a single problem entry.
- The use of SOAP has also been shown to shift the focus from the patient to the disease, thus promoting a medical model instead of the nursing process (Blair & Smith, 2012).

Focus Charting®

The term *focus* is used to encourage you to view the patient's status from a positive perspective rather than a problem-oriented, perspective. **Focus Charting®** uses assessment data to evaluate patient care concerns, problems, or strengths. It also identifies necessary revisions to the care plan as you record each entry. The focus is often:

- A nursing diagnosis (e.g., Ineffective Breathing Pattern)
- A sign or symptom (e.g., shortness of breath)
- Client behavior (e.g., inability to follow inhaler instructions)
- A special need (e.g., non-English-speaking)
- An acute change in condition (e.g., sudden appearance of chest pain)
- A significant event (e.g., surgery).

Focus Charting® works well in acute care settings, in areas with the same care, and where procedures are repeated frequently.

In focused charting, the first column contains the time and date, the second column identifies the focus or problem addressed in the note, and the third column contains charting in a DAR format. DAR is an acronym for *data, action,* and *response.*

- **Data.** Subjective and objective data (e.g., laboratory and diagnostic test results) that support the focus. This section reflects the assessment phase of the nursing process.
- **Action.** Describes interventions performed, such as administering medications or making calls to the primary provider. This section reflects the planning and implementation phases of the nursing process.
- **Response.** The client's response to your interventions. This section reflects the evaluation phase of the nursing process.

Advantages Focus Charting® is attractive because it addresses the client's concerns holistically.

Disadvantages The lack of a common problem list may lead to inconsistent labeling of the focus of notes, thus causing difficulty in tracking client progress. The following is an example of a Focus® note:

4/11/2018 1800	Focus: Developmental delay	**D:** 16 y.o. rec'd on unit at 1600 from PACU; post-appendectomy. Pt w/Down syndrome. Morphine PCA initiated. Pt unable to use PCA to control pain. Continuous infusion at 2 mg/hr begun at 1745. PERRLA. Alert, drifting in & out of sleep. PACU RN reports Pt functions at school-age level. **A:** Will discuss Pt status w/parents and adjust plan of care accordingly. —————— Ron Allen, RN
1830		**R:** Met w/parents, who report that Pt has significant developmental delays & needs supervision w/all ADLs. Pt comfortable on 2 mg/hr infusion of morphine. Use of PCA for supplementary pain control reviewed with parents. Parents demonstrated understanding; stated they will assist Pt w/PCA when meds are needed——————— ———Ron Allen, RN

FACT System

Noted for its individual elements, the **FACT documentation model** incorporates many charting-by-exceptions (CBE) principles and disadvantages. It includes four key elements:

- *Flow sheets* individualized to specific services
- *Assessment* features standardized with baseline parameters
- *Concise, integrated progress notes and flow sheets* documenting the client's condition and responses
- *Timely entries* documented when care is given

FACT documentation includes only exceptions to the norm or significant information about the patient. It eliminates the need to chart normal findings. The following is a FACT example for Steven Stellanski (Meet Your Patient).

DATE/TIME	04/12/2018 0900	04/12/2018 1330
Neurological Alert and oriented to time, place, and person. PERRLA. Symmetry of strength in extremities. No difficulty with coordination. Behavior appropriate to situation. Sensation intact without numbness or paresthesias.	√	√
Orient patient		
Refer to neurological flow sheet		
Pain No report of pain. If present, include pain scale intensity choice by patient (0–10) with location, description, duration, radiation, precipitating, and alleviating factors.	Abdominal incision pain— score 10	√
Location	RLQ	
Description	Dull, constant	
Relief measures	Percocet 1 tablet PO	
Pain relief: Y = yes / N = no	Y	
Cardiovascular Apical pulse 60 to 100. S1 and S2 present. Regular rhythm. Peripheral pulses (radial, pedal) present bilaterally. No edema or calf tenderness. Extremities pink, warm, moveable within patient's ROM.		
IV Solution and Rate	lactated Ringer's at 125 mL/hr	lactated Ringer's at 125 mL/hr

Electronic Entry

The Health Information Technology for Economic and Clinical Health Act has been instrumental in the widespread conversion from paper to electronic health records. Electronic clinical information systems streamline electronic processes, make them more accurate and efficient, and reduce the risk of human error. This frees you to do the expert work that only nurses can do. Electronic documentation requires changes in how you document your work:

- EHRs change documentation formats from paper to electronic.
- Documentation is done at the bedside instead of at the nurse's station.
- Decision-making processes change from gradual to immediate.

As a nurse, you will almost certainly need to have computer skills (Fig. 18-4). You will play a crucial role in the development and evaluation of effective EHR systems that make sense to nurses. You may even participate directly in the design–implementation–redesign cycle of the EHR system in your organization.

Electronic documentation forms and flow sheets (such as Fig. 18-2) include the information that your organization has decided is important to document. Reminders to document specific kinds of information, such as overdue medications and overdue nursing interventions, display automatically to help ensure your charting is accurate. The extensive use of clearly named data entry fields, drop-down menus, check boxes, and specially created templates allows you to enter your nursing documentation quickly and efficiently, usually with minimal keyboard typing.

Depending on the EHR system used and the associated charting form, progress notes may be documented electronically in prebuilt note formats. In some electronic systems, you may still need to write progress notes on lined paper, in narrative, SOAP, PIE, IPOC, Focus®, or FACT formats. Transitioning from paper to electronic documentation can be challenging. It usually takes a few days to know where to document your nursing care and feel confident that you haven't overlooked anything. EHR software is user friendly. Many organizations have printed information, classes, and Web-based tutorials that provide information about electronic documentation.

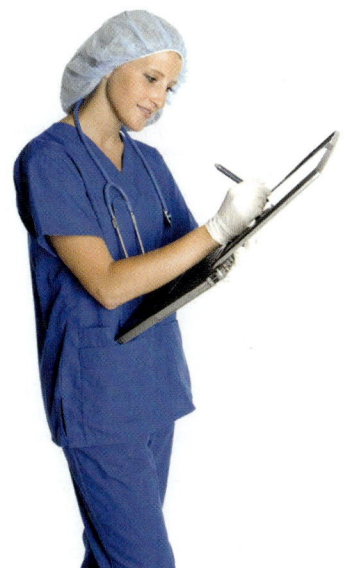

FIGURE 18-4 Many healthcare institutions are adopting computerized patient records.

Take advantage of opportunities to build your knowledge when they arise.

KnowledgeCheck 18-2

Summarize the characteristics of each of the different kinds of nursing documentation formats (narrative, PIE, SOAP, Focus®, CBE, FACT, and electronic entry).

ThinkLike a Nurse 18-1

Compare the documentation examples (narrative, PIE, SOAP, Focus®, CBE, FACT, and electronic documentation). If you have had experience with charting in the clinical setting, apply this experience as well. With which charting format do you feel most comfortable? Why?

What Forms Do Nurses Use to Document Nursing Care?

Documentation forms vary by purpose, institution, and unit. This section discusses the most commonly used paper and electronic documentation forms that are used in addition to the nursing progress notes discussed in the preceding sections.

Nursing Admission Data Forms

A separate nursing admission form or a combined interdisciplinary form is completed at the time the client enters the healthcare system. A baseline assessment is essential because it: (1) may be used as a benchmark to monitor change; (2) provides information about the client's support system and helps forecast future needs; (3) contains critical information (e.g., presenting illness or reason for admission, vital signs, allergy information, current medications, activities of daily living [ADL] status, physical assessment data, and discharge planning information).

You will use admission forms in all settings—for example, in ambulatory clinics, long-term care facilities, and hospitals. Long-term care admission forms are similar to hospital admission forms. Ambulatory care admission forms include demographic data, allergy information, current medications, family health data, social history, and the client's past medical history. The form completed by Nam Nguyen at his first clinic visit is an example (see Meet the Nguyens at the beginning of the book).

Discharge Summary

Discharge data are obtained with the admission assessment, but are often recorded on a separate form. **KEY POINT:** *A general principle in nursing is that discharge planning begins on admission. Therefore, discharge needs should be evaluated when the patient first enters a healthcare facility, especially in acute care facilities.* Ask yourself what this client would need if he were to go home in the next few days. For example, would he need help with food preparation? With his medicines?

A **discharge summary** is the last entry made in the paper chart. In the electronic chart, the discharge summary can begin any time after admission and revised throughout the hospitalization. A summary is completed when the client is transferred within the same organization, to another facility, or discharged to home. The discharge summary may be a multidisciplinary document or each discipline may write a separate summary.

The forms are different in each organization, but they contain similar data. For examples of an electronic discharge summary, see Figure 18-5. For a paper form, see Figure 11-5.

As you can see in Figure 18-5, there is a drop-down menu in which the Nursing Discharge Note is located. It is important to clearly document the client's condition on discharge because the discharge summary serves as baseline data for the healthcare professionals who provide follow-up care.

Flow Sheets and Graphic Records

Flow sheets and graphic records are used to do the following:

- *Document assessments and care that are performed frequently, on a recurring schedule, or as a part of unit routines* (e.g., I&O, weight, hygiene measures, ADLs, and medications).
- *Perform and document care activities.* How often you do so depends on your client's condition and the unit policy. In the first hour after surgery, for example, you would probably record vital signs every 15 minutes, then every 30 minutes for 1 hour, and then every 4 hours.
- *Allow you to see patterns of change* in client status. For instance, you may view a steady increase in the line representing a client's blood pressure compared to his pain score on an electronically generated graph. On a paper form, you may scan across a row to see that your client has not had a bowel movement for several days.

For examples of a paper graphic flow sheet, see Figure 3-3. For an electronic flow sheet, see Figure 18-2.

Checklists

Assessments and care may also be recorded on paper and electronic checklists. Common normal and abnormal findings are often organized according to body systems. Figure 18-6 is an example of a paper checklist.

Using a paper form, the nurse checks the box that reflects the current assessment findings. Some checklists include nursing actions, such as wound care, treatments, or IV fluid administration. Essentially, such forms are comprehensive charting documents. Client care activities, responses, and exceptions (deviations) are recorded in the narrative note section of the paper form.

Using an electronic field-based checklist, the nurse enters values or text in the appropriate fields and saves the documentation. Electronic flow sheets contain information similar to that on paper checklists but also include a greater range of potential documentation areas that can be opened as needed (e.g., treatments, IV fluid administration, and other parameters).

Intake and Output Records

You will enter data about the patient's fluid balance on a separate paper intake and output (I&O) form or an electronic flow sheet. Electronic systems have flow sheet sections to enter I&O and save it into the patient's EHR (see Fig. 18-2). I&O is usually totaled by shift and by 24-hour periods. Paper forms must be totaled manually, whereas electronic systems will automatically total I&O for you. See Figure 18-7 for a paper record. I&O paper graphics may be kept at the bedside. You might also input the I&O totals at the bedside using an electronic device (e.g., tablet, computer). Chapter 30 provides detailed information about monitoring intake and output.

Medication Administration Records

Medication administration records (MARs) contain information about the medications that have been prescribed for the client. The information and format vary by setting, with significant differences between outpatient and inpatient facilities.

- **Inpatient facilities:** Inpatient medication records not only contain a list of prescribed medications but also track medication administration and usage for the agency. For a comparison of the content of inpatient and outpatient MARs, see Table 18-2.

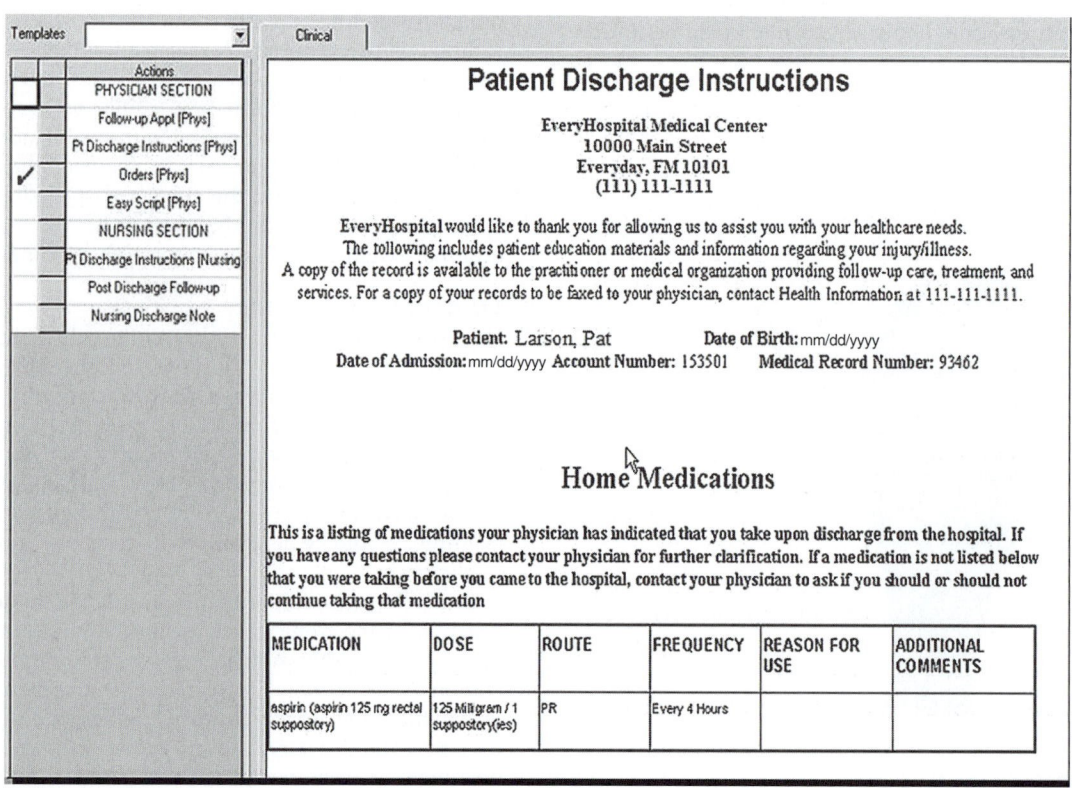

FIGURE 18-5 A portion of an electronic discharge planning form.

DATE / /

PHYSICAL ASSESSMENT - SHIFT _____

NEURO

LOC	ORIENTATION	SPEECH
❏ ALERT	❏ X3 ❏ FOR AGE	❏ APPROPRIATE
❏ SEDATED	❏ PERSON	❏ APHASIA
❏ LETHARGIC	❏ PLACE	❏ SLURRED
❏ UNRESPONSIVE	❏ TIME	❏ RAMBLING

SENSATION	FONTANELS	
❏ INTACT	❏ FLAT	❏ NA
❏ NUMBNESS	❏ SUNKEN	
❏ TINGLING	❏ BULGING	

CARDIOVASCULAR

RHYTHM	PULSE	EDEMA	CAP. REFILL
❏ REGULAR	❏ STRONG	❏ ABSENT	❏ < 3 SEC.
❏ IRREGULAR	❏ WEAK	❏ _____	❏ > 3 SEC.
❏ MURMUR	❏		

MONITOR RHYTHM

RESPIRATORY

EFFORT   BREATH
LU LL SOUNDS RU RL

❏ NORMAL	❏ DYSPNEA	❏❏	CLEAR	❏❏
❏ LABORED	❏ COUGH	❏❏	CRACKLES	❏❏
❏ NASAL FLARING	❏ SPUTUM	❏❏	RHONCHI	❏❏
❏ RETRACTIONS	❏ CRYING	❏❏	WHEEZING	❏❏
❏ IRREGULAR		❏❏	DIMINISHED	❏❏
		❏❏	ABSENT	❏❏

GASTROINTESTINAL

ABDOMEN

❏ FLAT	❏ FIRM	❏ NAUSEA
❏ ROUNDED	❏ TENDER	❏ VOMITING
❏ DISTENDED	❏ NON-TENDER	
❏ SOFT		
❏ GIRTH_____	CM	

BOWEL SOUNDS	STOOL	
❏ ACTIVE	❏ REGULAR	LAST BM
❏ ABSENT	❏ CONSTIPATED	
❏ HYPER	❏ DIARRHEA	_____
❏ HYPO	❏ INCONTINENT	

SUCTION
❏ INTERMITTANT   ❏ CONSTANT   ❏ CLAMPED
❏ FEEDING TUBE   ❏ PATENT
❏ NG   ❏ PLACEMENT ✔
DRNG COLOR:

GU

URINE		❏ CATHETER
❏ CLEAR, YELLOW / AMBER ❏ QS		❏ PAIN
❏ OTHER _____	❏ FREQUENT	
	❏ RETENTION	❏ INCONTINENT

MUSCULOSKELETAL

MOBILITY	MUSCLE TONE	ROM
❏ NORMAL	❏ GOOD	❏ FULL
❏ ASSIST X _____	❏ OTHER	❏ LIMITED
❏ AMBULATORY		
❏ BED REST		
❏ OTHER	❏ P.T. CONSULT	

SKIN

CONDITION	TURGOR	MUCOUS MEM
❏ WARM, DRY INTACT	❏ ADEQUATE	❏ MOIST
❏ BREAKDOWN	❏ DECREASED	❏ DRY

COLOR ❏ NORMAL
❏ PALE ❏ CYANOTIC ❏ FLUSHED ❏ _____

WOUND/INCISION/ DRESSING

LOCATION/CONDITION/DRAINAGE	HEALING NO S/S INFECTION
_____	❏
_____	❏
_____	❏

TUBES/DRAINS

LOCATION/CONDITION/DRAINAGE	GRAVITY	SUCTION
_____	❏	❏
_____	❏	❏
_____	❏	❏

IV'S

IV SITE / CONDITION	PATENT, NO REDNESS OR SWELLING	PUMP
_____	❏	❏
_____	❏	❏
_____	❏	❏

PAIN
❏ ABSENT   PAIN SCALE _____
❏ PRESENT   LOCATION _____
❏ CONTROLLED

PSYCHOSOCIAL

EYE CONTACT   ❏ YES ❏ NO

❏ APPROPRIATE	❏ RESTLESS	❏ COMBATIVE
❏ FLAT AFFECT	❏ AGITATED	❏ BELLIGERENT
❏ UNCOOPERATIVE	❏ CRYING	❏ ODOR
❏ ANXIOUS	❏ SUBSTANCE USE	

DISCHARGE

DISCHARGE PLAN

❏ NA	❏ ONGOING	❏ COMPLETED
❏ D.P. CONSULT	❏ O.T CONSULT	❏ H.H. CONSULT

EQUIPMENT

❏ BED ALARM	❏ CARDIAC MONITOR
❏ CPM	❏ FEEDING PUMP
❏ IV PUMP X_____	❏ K - PAD
❏ OXIMETER	❏ PCA PUMP
❏ PASSPORT	❏ POLAR ICE
❏ SUCTION	❏ TELEMETRY
❏ _____	❏ _____
❏ _____	❏ _____

SIGN

SIGNATURE X_____   TIME_____

REASSESSED BY X_____   TIME_____

OBSERVATION / INTERVENTION / EVALUATION
(TIME & INITIAL ENTRIES)

PHYSICAL ASSESSMENT - SHIFT _____

NEURO

LOC	ORIENTATION	SPEECH
❏ ALERT	❏ X3 ❏ FOR AGE	❏ APPROPRIATE
❏ SEDATED	❏ PERSON	❏ APHASIA
❏ LETHARGIC	❏ PLACE	❏ SLURRED
❏ UNRESPONSIVE	❏ TIME	❏ RAMBLING

SENSATION	FONTANELS	
❏ INTACT	❏ FLAT	❏ NA
❏ NUMBNESS	❏ SUNKEN	
❏ TINGLING	❏ BULGING	

CARDIOVASCULAR

RHYTHM	PULSE	EDEMA	CAP. REFILL
❏ REGULAR	❏ STRONG	❏ ABSENT	❏ < 3 SEC.
❏ IRREGULAR	❏ WEAK	❏ _____	❏ > 3 SEC.
❏ MURMUR	❏		

MONITOR RHYTHM

RESPIRATORY

EFFORT   BREATH
LU LL SOUNDS RU RL

❏ NORMAL	❏ DYSPNEA	❏❏	CLEAR	❏❏
❏ LABORED	❏ COUGH	❏❏	CRACKLES	❏❏
❏ NASAL FLARING	❏ SPUTUM	❏❏	RHONCHI	❏❏
❏ RETRACTIONS	❏ CRYING	❏❏	WHEEZING	❏❏
❏ IRREGULAR		❏❏	DIMINISHED	❏❏
		❏❏	ABSENT	❏❏

GASTROINTESTINAL

ABDOMEN

❏ FLAT	❏ FIRM	❏ NAUSEA
❏ ROUNDED	❏ TENDER	❏ VOMITING
❏ DISTENDED	❏ NON-TENDER	
❏ SOFT		
❏ GIRTH_____	CM	

BOWEL SOUNDS	STOOL	
❏ ACTIVE	❏ REGULAR	LAST BM
❏ ABSENT	❏ CONSTIPATED	
❏ HYPER	❏ DIARRHEA	_____
❏ HYPO	❏ INCONTINENT	

SUCTION
❏ INTERMITTANT   ❏ CONSTANT   ❏ CLAMPED
❏ FEEDING TUBE   ❏ PATENT
❏ NG   ❏ PLACEMENT
DRNG COLOR:

GU

URINE		❏ CATHETER
❏ CLEAR, YELLOW / AMBER ❏ QS		❏ PAIN
❏ OTHER _____	❏ FREQUENT	
	❏ RETENTION	❏ INCONTINENT

MUSCULOSKELETAL

MOBILITY	MUSCLE TONE	ROM
❏ NORMAL	❏ GOOD	❏ FULL
❏ ASSIST X _____	❏ OTHER	❏ LIMITED
❏ AMBULATORY		
❏ BED REST		
❏ OTHER	❏ P.T. CONSULT	

SKIN

CONDITION	TURGOR	MUCOUS MEM
❏ WARM, DRY INTACT	❏ ADEQUATE	❏ MOIST
❏ BREAKDOWN	❏ DECREASED	❏ DRY

COLOR ❏ NORMAL
❏ PALE ❏ CYANOTIC ❏ FLUSHED ❏ _____

WOUND/INCISION/ DRESSING

LOCATION/CONDITION/DRAINAGE	HEALING NO S/S INFECTION
_____	❏
_____	❏
_____	❏

TUBES/DRAINS

LOCATION/CONDITION/DRAINAGE	GRAVITY	SUCTION
_____	❏	❏
_____	❏	❏
_____	❏	❏

IV'S

IV SITE / CONDITION	PATENT, NO REDNESS OR SWELLING	PUMP
_____	❏	❏
_____	❏	❏
_____	❏	❏

NURSING ASSESSMENT   PATIENT NAME _____

FIGURE 18-6 A portion of a nursing assessment checklist.

INTAKE AND OUTPUT SHEET

DATE	Time	INTAKE						OUTPUT						SIGNATURE OF NURSE
		ORAL	IV	IV MED	BLOOD PRODUCT	OTHER	TOTAL	URINE	EMESIS	STOOL	SUCTION	OTHER	TOTAL	
	6 A.M.-2 P.M.													
	2 P.M.-10 P.M.													
	10 P.M.-6 A.M.													
	TOTAL													

FIGURE 18-7 Nurses use I&O records to record data about the patient's fluid status.

Table 18-2 ▶ Comparison of Content of MARs for Inpatient and Outpatient Facilities

INPATIENT MARS	OUTPATIENT MARS
▪ Drug name	▪ Drug name
▪ Dosage	▪ Dosage
▪ Route of administration	▪ Route of administration
▪ Frequency	▪ Number of pills, patches, and so on to be dispensed at each prescription refill
▪ Duration	
▪ Scheduled times of administration	▪ Number of refills ordered
▪ Charting of medication administration	▪ Directions for using the medication, including frequency and duration
▪ Signatures (written or electronic) of nurses administering medication	▪ Historical information about prescriptions, pharmacies used, and refills authorized

▪ **Outpatient facilities** (e.g., include clinics, primary care offices, and treatment facilities): Because patients do not stay at the facility, usually the MAR primarily contains information about how the patient is to use the medications prescribed. Patients retain responsibility for administering their own medications either independently or with the help of family or caregivers.

Some electronic MARs allow care providers to look up detailed information about the medication, including indications, contraindications, expected or adverse effects, and safe dosage ranged based on routes of administration. Figure 18-8 is a portion of an electronic medication record.

Terminology for Medication Administration Times
You will document medications according to the times they are given: scheduled, unscheduled, continuous, prn, STAT, and so on.

▪ **Scheduled medications** are medications that are to be given on a regularly scheduled basis.
▪ **Unscheduled medications** are medications that are to be given on call at the appropriate time. An example of an unscheduled medication is a preoperative medication to be administered immediately before the patient goes to the operating room.
▪ **Continuous infusions** are IV fluids that are infusing consistently unless stopped to administer an incompatible medication or blood transfusion.
▪ The letters **prn** mean "as needed." Medications administered prn are given only when the patient meets certain conditions that were established in the medication prescription. Typically, medications are prescribed prn for relief of pain, fever, nausea, and constipation. You should administer a prn medication when requested or your assessment of need is validated by the patient.
▪ A **STAT** medication is given immediately, only once, and documented immediately.
▪ A **single-order** medication is given once at a prescribed time but not necessarily immediately.

Charting Additional Information About Medications
For scheduled medications, you may only have to initial and make a checkmark in the column with times preprinted at the top. You will need to record additional information on the MAR and sometimes in the progress notes in the following circumstances:

▪ **Injections.** You must chart the type and site of the injection. This documentation protects the patient from repeated injections in the same location.
▪ **Assessment required before administration.** Some medications require you to make a specific assessment before giving the drug to ensure that it is safe to administer. You must document that assessment data on the MAR along with the time of administration and other required information (see Chapter 25). For example, you should not give digoxin (a cardiac medication) if the apical heart rate is below 60 beats/min, so you must auscultate the rate before giving

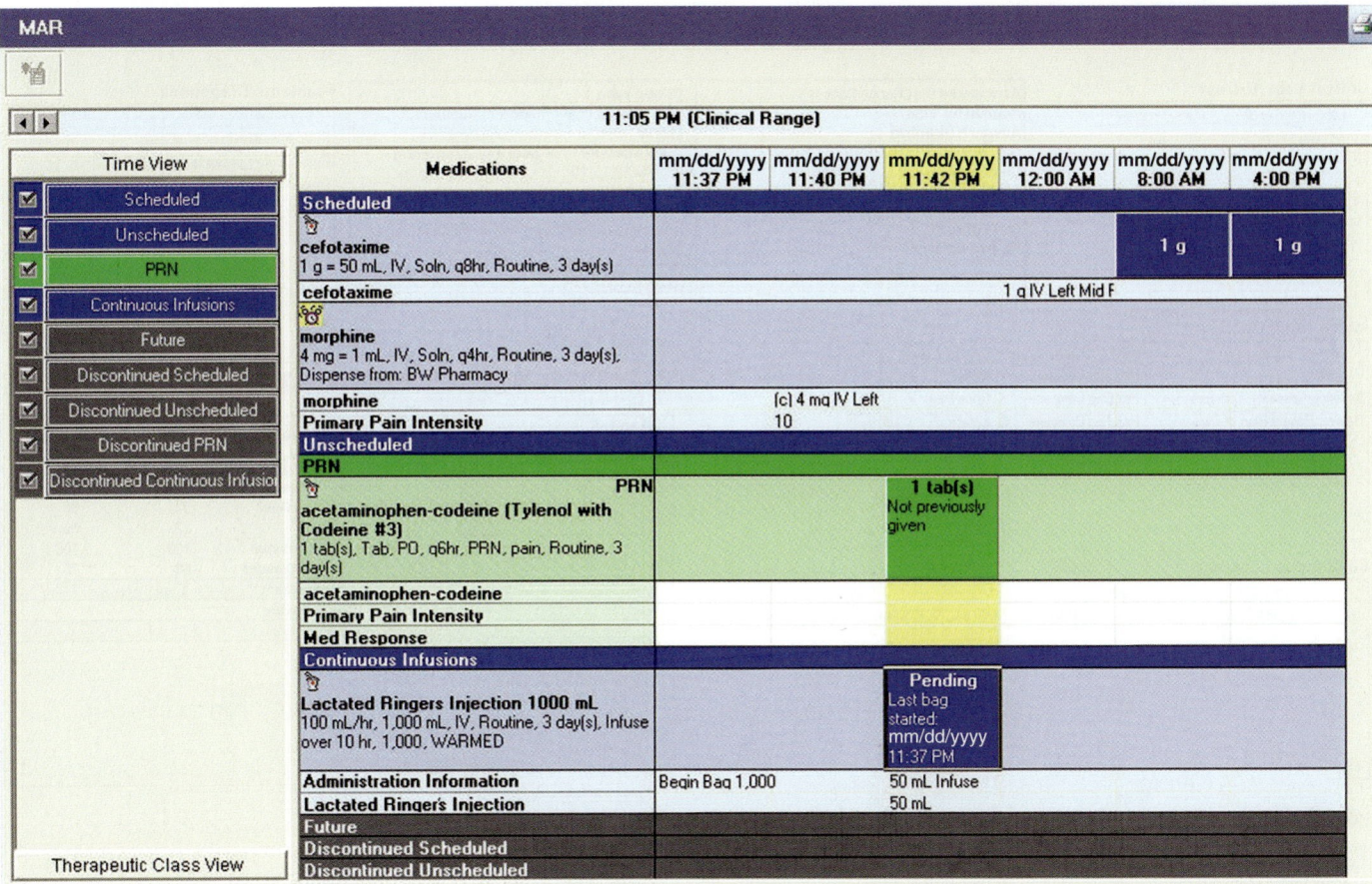

FIGURE 18-8 A portion of an electronic medication administration record.

the drug. Blood pressure, insulin, and anticoagulants medications also require assessments before administration.

- ◆ **Drug allergies.** Drug allergies are always noted on the MAR. This makes them easily visible for caregivers who are prescribing or administering medication. If the patient has an allergic reaction to a medicine, you must report this to the prescriber and record this response on the MAR and in the nurses' notes.

- **STAT, prn, unscheduled, and single-order medications.** Enter on the MAR the time the medication is given. Make a narrative note of your assessment findings and the patient's response to the medication in the appropriate location on the MAR. In an EHR, some documented data, such as the pain score before administration of an analgesic, may automatically migrate from other documentation sources to become visible on the MAR.

- **Dosage range orders.** You may occasionally see a prn order that provides a range of medication to be given based on your assessment of the patient. For example, "Titrate morphine 2–3 mg IV every 1–2 hours to achieve pain control."

  ◆ In the electronic MAR system, medication range orders (e.g., 1 to 2 mg) are difficult to order, so The Joint Commission and most agency protocols no longer allow dosage range orders.

- **Patient refusal.** If the patient refuses a medication, note the refusal on the MAR. Your organization's policy will determine how this is recorded. On paper, you might draw a circle around the scheduled time of administration. When documenting electronically, you can click on an option offered in the MAR, such as Not Given, and then select *Patient*

Refused from a drop-down field listing multiple reasons that a medication is not given.

- **Omitted medication or delayed administration.** It may be necessary to withhold a medication or delay its administration if the patient is not available or is experiencing health changes that require immediate interventions. On the paper MAR, you may find a boxed section at the bottom with a code to indicate why the medication was withheld or given at a different time. Circle the scheduled time and fill in the symbol. You will also have to document the omission or delay in your nurses' notes. However, in the electronic MAR, often it is possible to reschedule administration times for a single dose or permanently going forward. Many systems will require you enter the reason and the action taken.

Kardex® or Patient Care Summary

As discussed in Chapter 5, the Kardex is a special paper form or folding card that briefly summarizes a patient's status and plan of care. Paper Kardex and electronic patient care summaries typically pull patient data from multiple areas of the health record (medical and nursing diagnoses, prescriptions, treatments, results). Figure 18-9 is an example of an electronic patient care summary screen.

Paper Kardex are usually kept together in a portable file in a central location in the nurses' station to allow all team members access to patients' summary information. Each patient has a separate screen in an electronic summary. All authorized members of the care team can access the electronic care summary at the same time, even if they are away from the patient or even outside the organization in a remote location, depending on the

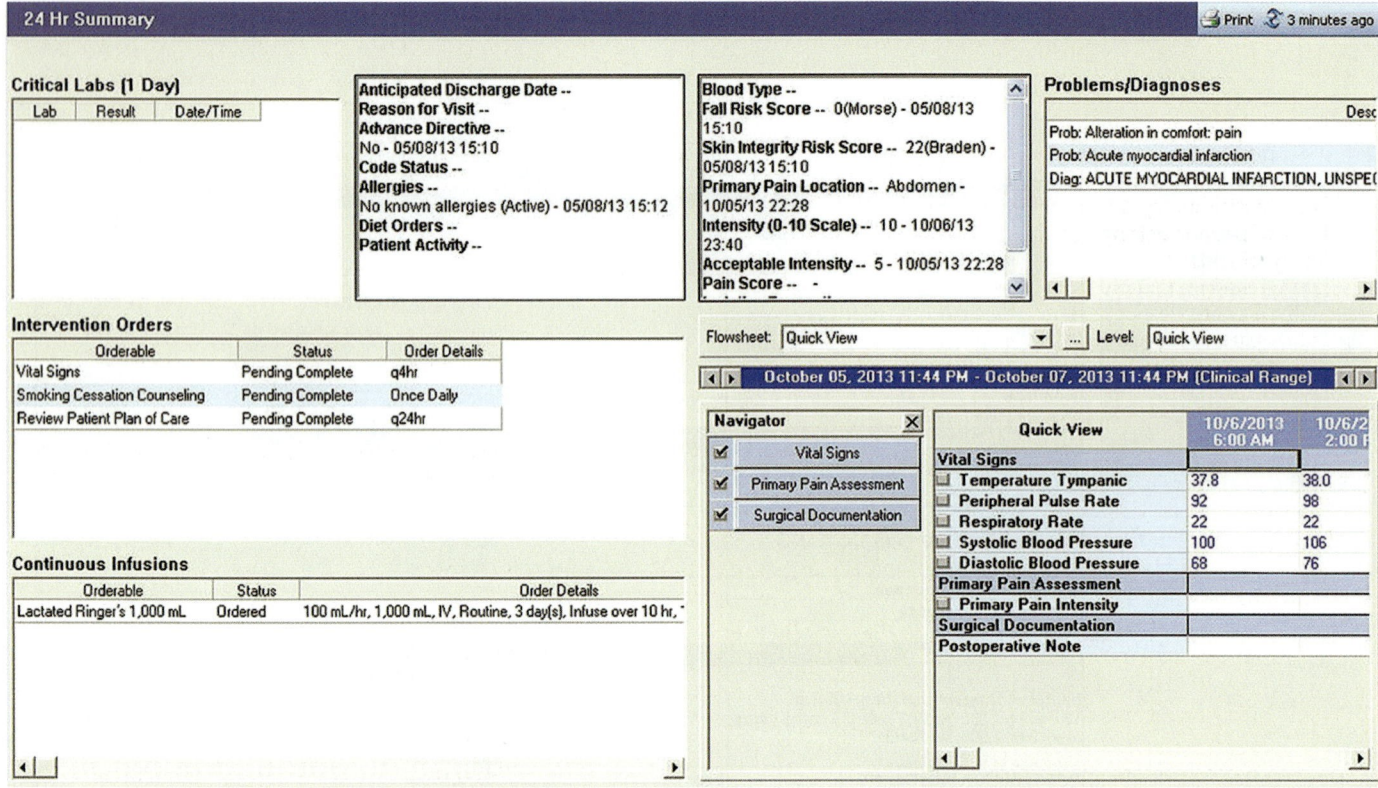

FIGURE 18-9 A portion of an electronic patient care summary screen.

institution's permission for access. Neither the paper Kardex nor the electronic care summary is a permanent part of the patient's health record.

Integrated Plan of Care (IPOC)

IPOCs are a combined charting and care plan form. An IPOC maps out, day by day, the patient goals, outcomes, interventions, and treatments for a specific diagnosis or condition from admission to discharge. Major aspects of the treatment plan are included (e.g., laboratory and diagnostic testing, medications, standardized interventions, therapies) are included in the pathway. IPOCs help administrators predict length of stay and monitor costs of care and can assist with staffing. They also eliminate duplicate charting, increase team effort, and enhance the nurse's teaching about what the patient can expect during the hospital stay. Figure 18-3 shows an example of an electronic IPOC.

Multiple patient diagnoses can be captured easily in an electronic IPOC. However, in special situations, you may need to individualize the paper IPOC by commenting on special issues in the space provided for narrative comments (e.g., developmental delay with patient Steven Stellanski).

Occurrence Reports

An **occurrence report,** or *incident report,* is a formal record of an unusual occurrence or accident. It is an organizational report used to analyze the event, identify areas for quality improvement, and formulate strategies to prevent future occurrences.

- The overall goal is to create safer processes and procedures for clients and staff.
- **KEY POINT:** *An occurrence report is not part of the client's health record and thus should never be referenced in the nurses' notes or in other sections of the health record.*

- The paper report is sent to risk management, according to agency protocol, whereas the electronic form is completed on the organization's secure internal network.
- You should report all errors, even if there was no adverse impact on the patient. This is important from a safety standpoint for improving your institution's quality of care and from a legal perspective to provide defensible information.
- When completing an occurrence form, be sure to:
  Clearly identify the client, date, time, and location.
  Briefly describe the incident in objective terms.
  Quote the client or persons involved if possible.
  Identify any witnesses to the event, equipment involved, and environmental conditions.
  Avoid drawing conclusions or placing blame.
  Document actions taken and the client response to the interventions.
- See Box 18-4 for examples of events that require the completion of an occurrence report. Chapter 45 provides additional information on occurrence reports.

KnowledgeCheck 18-3

- Identify at least five types of paper documentation forms.
- What should you document after administering a prn medication?
- What is the purpose of an occurrence report?
- Identify four events in which you will need to complete an occurrence report.
- Identify the following abbreviations:

abd	OOB	NKDA
BRP	pc	tid
DM	prn	q
fx	STD	LUQ

What Is Unique About Documentation in Home Healthcare?

Although you will perform many of the same assessments and interventions in home care that you do in other areas of healthcare, the documentation is unique. The Centers for Medicare & Medicaid Services (CMS) guidelines govern home healthcare documentation. Among the requirements for care are the following:

- Certification of homebound status
- A plan of care
- Ongoing assessment of the need for skilled care

The most commonly used paper home health documentation form is known as OASIS—the Outcome and Assessment Information Set. Because of the federal government emphasis on electronic health records, home health is moving toward electronic documentation. Home health nurses use electronic devices (e.g., tablets, laptop computers) to retrieve client data, record progress notes in the home, order supplies, and coordinate scheduling of follow-up visits.

In home care, a monthly summary describing the client's status and ongoing needs is required. The client's primary care provider signs this form, which is submitted for reimbursement. Chapter 41 provides further information about home care.

Home health documentation includes the following:

- Your assessment highlighting changes in the client's condition
- Interventions performed (e.g., wound care, dressing changes, teaching)
- The client's response to interventions
- Interaction or teaching that you conducted with caregivers
- Interaction with the client's primary care provider

If you would like to see an OASIS form,

 Go to http://www.oasisanswers.com/downloads/SAMPLE_FORMS_OAI_Manual_2008.pdf

 **Think**Like a Nurse 18-2

Why do you think it is essential to document homebound status and the ongoing need for skilled care?

What Is Unique About Documentation in Long-Term Care?

Documentation requirements for long-term care depend on the level of care the client requires.

- All clients in long-term care facilities must have a comprehensive assessment at admission.

- Federal law further requires that a resident be evaluated using the Minimum Data Set (MDS) for Resident Assessment and Care Screening within 14 days of admission.
- The MDS must be updated every 3 months and with any significant change in client condition.

For an example of an MDS Basic Tracking form,

 Go to the **CMS** Web site at www.cms.gov, and do a search for the form.

Legal requirements to protect older adults mandate that you report changes in a client's condition to the primary care provider as well as the client's family. You must also document your communications. If you are caring for a client receiving Medicare-reimbursed services, (e.g., IV therapy, wound care, rehabilitation services), documentation is required with each shift. In addition, a nurse must record a weekly summary that includes the following:

- A summary of the client's condition
- An evaluation of the client's ability to perform ADLs
- The client's level of consciousness and mood
- Hydration and nutrition status
- Response to medications
- Any treatments provided
- Safety measures (e.g., bed rails, bed alarm, wander guard)

Long-term care facilities also provide intermediate-care services for clients who need assistance with medications, nutrition, and ADLs. These clients require a nursing care summary every 2 weeks.

KnowledgeCheck 18-4

How do home care and long-term care documentation differ from hospital-based documentation?

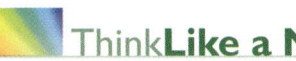 **Think**Like a Nurse 18-3

Why do long-term care clients require less frequent charting than clients in acute care settings?

ORAL REPORTING

The purpose of giving an oral report is to maintain continuity of care and engage in professional communications. Whether the source of the information shared is from a written report form, a paper Kardex®, or a summary view in the EHR, the quality of the report you give and receive influences how you and others plan the shift work. Restrict your oral reports to client-focused discussion and limit unimportant details and social conversation.

How Do I Give a Handoff Report?

The purpose of a **handoff report** (sometimes called *change-of-shift report* or *handover report*) is to promote continuity in care. The nurse is alerted to the client's status, recent status changes, planned activities, diagnostic testing, or concerns that require follow-up. A handoff report may be given at the bedside or in a conference room using paper notes or an EHR device.

As a student nurse, you will receive reports from either the off-going or on-coming shift nurse assigned to the client. Report any changes to the nurse assigned to the client during your shift and always give a report before leaving the unit.

- A **bedside report,** sometimes known as "walking rounds," allows you to observe important aspects of client care, such as appearance, IV pumps, and wounds. With a bedside report, the outgoing nurse introduces you to the client. If the client is alert, give her the opportunity to participate in the report and ask questions. Although this type of report is time consuming, it encourages continuity of care, team collaboration, and client/family communication. **KEY POINT:** *Ensure that the patient's privacy rights are protected when using bedside reports.*

- A **face-to-face oral report** may involve only the outgoing and oncoming nurse or may include the entire oncoming shift. When given in a conference room, an oral report does not let you directly observe the client, but it is time efficient and still allows interaction between nurses.

- An **audio-recorded report** is a convenient but sometimes time-consuming way to transmit information. The outgoing nurse audio-records a report on her clients. This method does not allow you to ask questions about the client; occasionally the audio quality is poor and the report is not clear. However, an advantage of this method is that the outgoing nurse continues to provide patient care while the incoming nurse receives report. ✚ To minimize communication errors, the outgoing and incoming nurses should speak directly to each other to update information or answer any questions about the client care.

✚ **Standardized Report Formats** Data indicate that "an estimated 80 percent of serious medical errors involve miscommunication between caregivers when patients are transferred or handed-off" (The Joint Commission, 2012a). No matter where or how the handoff report is given, nurses should use a consistent, structured (standardized) process that contains critical key items.

- The **PACE** format is an example of a specifically developed standardized approach to organize data for handoffs. The mnemonic stands for **P**atient/**P**roblem, **A**ssessment/**A**ctions, **C**ontinuing/**C**hanges, and **E**valuation (Schroeder, 2006).

- The **SBAR** (**S**ituation—**B**ackground—**A**ssessment—**R**ecommendation) is an easy-to-remember, concrete acronym useful for framing any conversation. Because nurses and providers communicate in very different ways, SBAR is useful for interprofessional communication, especially in critical situations requiring a clinician's immediate attention and action. SBAR allows for an easy and focused way to set expectations for how and what will be communicated among team members. The SBAR technique can be adapted for handoff reports. For additional information about communicating with SBAR and PACE, see Clinical Insight 18-1, Giving Oral Reports.

KnowledgeCheck 18-5

- What data should be included in a handoff report?
- What are the types of handoff reports?

What Is a Transfer Report?

Transfer reports are given when a patient is transferred from unit to unit or from facility to facility. If the client is being transported to another unit in the same facility, you will need to transport a paper chart, unless the receiving organization can electronically access the client record. Detailed information about the client's health history can be communicated between healthcare professionals or transmitted before transfer. You should review your facility's policy on what can be copied or electronically transmitted during client transfers.

Safe & Effective Nursing Care

Ensuring Safe, Effective Handoff Reports

Chapter Key Concepts: Documentation, Oral reporting

Competencies: Provide Safe, Quality Client Care; Embrace/Incorporate Technological Advances

Thinking: Consider the number of client handoffs per day among nurses and other providers. Factors that contribute to miscommunication and breakdowns in client care during handoff reports include the lack of a standardized protocol or form, lack of experience, and lack of dedicated time for reporting.

Caring: A primary role of the nurse is to ensure safe, quality client care. Caring influences the way you think and act and motivates the nurse to be attentive to safety. Because they care, nurses perform interventions to prevent harm to clients (e.g., report critical lab values, follow principles of documentation).

Doing: Collaborate with others in your facility to suggest the following strategies for improving quality of care, teamwork, and patient safety:

➤ Standardize the information (e.g., SBAR) to be conveyed.

➤ Include "if . . . , then . . ." statements for current problems (e.g., *if* the glucose level is still elevated, *then* call the provider for insulin orders).

➤ Develop an electronic form or other tool to reinforce and clarify the transfer of knowledge and responsibility.

➤ Conduct training sessions to lessen the chance of reporting errors.

Sources: Cloete, L. (2015). Reducing medication errors in nursing practice. *Nursing Standard, 29*(20), 50–59; Collins, S., Stein, D., Vawdrey, D., et al. (2011). Content overlap in nurse and physician handoff artifacts and the potential role of electronic health records: A systematic review. *Journal of Biomedical Informatics, 44*(4), 704–712; Riesenberg, L., Leisch, J., & Cunningham, J. (2010). Nursing handoffs: A systematic review of the literature. *American Journal of Nursing, 110*(4), 24–34.

Research shows that older adults are vulnerable to errors in care when transitioning from one healthcare facility to another. Medication errors were dominant, resulting in increased hospital readmissions, injuries, or death. MBAR (**M**edication—**B**ackground—**A**ssessment—**R**ecommendation) was developed to provide a structured handoff that promotes medication reconciliation during handoffs and transfers (Blank, Benyo, & Glover, 2012).

For a review of transfers and discharges, refer to

 Go to Chapter 11 and Procedures 11-2, 11-3, and 11-4.

How Do I Receive and Document Verbal and Telephone Orders?

✚ Although licensed nurses may find it necessary to accept verbal or telephone orders on occasion, they increase the risk of hearing or writing the order incorrectly. The Joint Commission recommends that you validate a verbal order or report of critical test results using a written and read-back process before taking any action (The Joint Commission, 2011).

Telephone Orders/Prescriptions

Telephone prescriptions can lead to errors because of differences in pronunciation, dialect, or accent; background noise; poor perception; and unfamiliar terminology. Taking a telephone or verbal prescription may be acceptable in the following situations:

- When there has been a sudden change in your client's condition and the provider is not in the hospital or cannot transmit prescriptions electronically.
- In a life-threatening emergency—but you must apply the "document and read-back" safeguard.

Faxes, text messages, and e-mail have reduced the need for telephone prescriptions; however, they may never entirely disappear. For guidelines to use when taking telephone prescriptions, refer to Clinical Insight 18-2.

Verbal Orders/Prescriptions

Verbal prescriptions are spoken directions for patient care given to you in person, usually during an emergency. Providers should never use verbal communications as a routine method of giving prescriptions. For guidelines to ensure safety see Clinical Insight 18-2, Receiving Telephone and Verbal Orders.

KnowledgeCheck 18-6

- What important factors should you document when receiving a telephone prescription?
- What is the purpose of a verbal prescription? When should it be used?

How Do I Question a Prescription?

✚ If you feel uncertain about a prescription, you must question it. As a student, you will first want to discuss your concerns with your clinical instructor or the nurse you are working with during your clinical time. Remember, the goal is to provide safe care. If you have concerns, do not remain quiet—act on them.

- Follow organization policy for clarifying prescriptions.
- If a prescription is written illegibly on paper or is entered into the EHR missing certain details or components, contact the provider directly for clarification. Generally, you should contact the provider who wrote the prescription.
- If, after contact, the provider leaves the prescription as-is and you still don't feel comfortable with it or believe there is an error, you may refuse to implement it.
  - Inform the chain of command at your organization about your refusal.
  - Usually you will speak with the charge nurse, who may then contact the nurse manager or nursing supervisor.
  - The nature of the prescription will determine how this situation is handled.
  - If you do refuse to follow a prescription, you must document your refusal and the actions you took to clarify the prescription.

As a new nurse, you may feel uncomfortable about questioning a prescription. Even experienced nurses sometimes feel uneasy with this challenge. If uncertain how to proceed, you can discuss your concerns with your colleagues, the charge nurse, or the supervisor before contacting the provider. **KEY POINT:** *If you believe an order is inappropriate or unsafe, you are legally and ethically required to question the order.*

PracticalKnowledge
knowing how

To document care effectively, you need to be familiar with the forms and requirements of your institution. Remember that the client's health record is permanent and that information contained inside is confidential. As a student, you are granted access to a client's charts for educational purposes. You have a duty to keep the information private and confidential. The Health Insurance Portability and Accountability Act (HIPAA) regulations govern access, storage, transfer, and discussion of client information. For more information about privacy, confidentiality, and HIPAA, refer to Chapters 42 and 43.

ThinkLike a Nurse 18-4

You note that your client with asthma is having increasing difficulty breathing. You call the provider, who gives you a telephone prescription for an asthma medication and then hangs up. When you enter the verbal prescription electronically, you find it is a nonformulary medication that your pharmacy does not carry.

- Was this an acceptable reason to take a verbal prescription?
- The provider gets irritated when you call back and says, "I prescribed what I wanted." How would you handle this situation?
- You entered the prescription electronically after the provider hung up. How could this situation have been avoided?

GUIDELINES FOR DOCUMENTING CARE

KEY POINT: *Your documentation should convey the care that you provided to the patient during your shift.* Thus, if you read your documentation 3 years later, as in the case of malpractice lawsuits, it should attest that the care you provided to the patient adhered to minimum standards of nursing practice. For a brief set of documentation tips, see Box 18-5. For detailed guidelines for documentation, see Clinical Insight 18-3. For ANA standards of practice referring to documentation, see Box 18-1.

Guidelines for Paper Health Records

To comply with HIPAA requirements, paper health records need to be stored in designated areas accessible only to healthcare providers. To ensure your written paper documentation is effective, the forms used must be efficient, comprehensive, and relevant to the client's healthcare needs. The forms should guide you to document appropriately according to your organization's policies and procedures. Use the following guidelines to documenting appropriately:

- **Maintain confidentiality.** Do not provide written or verbal information to anyone not involved in the direct care of the client without his consent.

BOX 18-5 ■ Documentation ABCs

Accurate	**E**asy to read
Bias-free	**F**actual
Complete	**G**rammatical
Detailed	**H**armless (legally)

- **Ensure you have the correct form (e.g., I&O sheet, graphic record) before you begin writing.**
- **Check that the chart and documentation forms are clearly marked with the client's name and identification number.**
- **Write legibly, neatly, and in an organized manner.** This enables others to read your entries and use them to make clinical decisions. Sloppy or illegible handwriting creates errors or at least leads to poor communication.
- **Always use black ink for handwritten notes (some agencies do permit blue ink).** Inks other than black or blue are not legible when a chart is photocopied. Do NOT use green or red pen. Remember that the medical records are legal documents.
- **Do not leave blank lines in the narrative notes.** If you need to leave space for clarity, draw a straight line through the area and begin on the next line. Open areas leave an opportunity for later tampering.
- **Draw a line through the incorrect documentation and initial it.** Never use a correction fluid, "ink over," or otherwise cover up written notes.
- **Sign all your paper charting entries with your first name, last name, and professional credentials, such as Judy Long, RN.**
- **Don't write in "shorthand" or your own abbreviated symbols. Use only abbreviations that are approved by your organization.**

Guidelines for Electronic Health Records

Well-designed nursing documentation forms and systems help you organize your work, manage your care plans, track client diagnoses and outcomes, and support decision making by healthcare providers.

How Can I Document Efficiently and Effectively in the EHR?

To ensure efficient and effective documentation in the EHR, keep the following in mind:

- **You must have basic computer, mouse, and software skills** to document effectively in the EHR.
- **If you are uneasy or more stressed using computers** or are unfamiliar with the software, it may take you longer to make the transition to documenting in the EHR.
- **Help keep client rooms clutter free** so that you have a place to use a portable computer in the room for direct charting.

What Is Unique About Entering the Data?

- **Before Charting.** Before opening charting forms, you must ensure that the client's name, identification number, and any other unique health record identifiers are correct.
- **Saving Documentation.** If your EHR allows you to save partially completed documentation before signing it, do complete the documentation and sign it as quickly as possible. In most EHR systems, saved documentation cannot be seen by others until it is signed.
- **Checklists.** Electronic forms and flow sheets are often built in a format similar to a checklist. This can make it more difficult to capture detailed client changes and findings.
- **Errors.** If you make an error (e.g., make entries on the wrong chart or enter and sign the wrong information), you can correct it. The entry can never be completely deleted, but only the corrected information will be visible to anyone viewing the records.

What Happens If the Computer Doesn't Work?

EHR systems can have periodic downtimes due to scheduled maintenance or network or interface problems. Client care does not stop, so you need to know the procedures to follow when the EHR is offline and inaccessible. Follow organization policies regarding the amount of time the EHR needs to be "down" before you begin documenting on paper form.

How Do I Maintain Confidentiality and Data Security?

Although the specific risks to and safeguards of confidentiality differ in detail between paper and electronic records, confidentiality is equally important in both. The following safeguards are specific to EHRs:

- *Ensure confidentiality and privacy*—Close the screen, lock the computer, or permanently log off of the EHR system when moving away from an open EHR. Most computer stations will automatically log off after a specified period of inactivity. This helps keep unauthorized viewers from having access to client information.
- *Use privacy filters*—Some computer screens are equipped with privacy filters to prevent unauthorized viewers from seeing the information.
- *Create a secure password*—not something obvious, such as your birth date, Social Security number, or family members' names. Instead, you might choose a password that is at least eight characters long and includes at least one capital letter (if the system is case sensitive), one number, and (if allowed by the system) one symbol. The system you are using will determine the specifications.
- *Change your password at regular intervals* even if your organization does not require it. Some systems will lock you out of the system if your password is not changed as required.
- *Do not share your personal username or password* with anyone. You are responsible for the data recorded using your electronic identity. If someone else enters data or accesses records under your identity, you may be held responsible if the client initiates legal action.
- *Do not leave client data displayed on the screen where others can see it.*
- *Do not leave the computer unattended after you have logged on.* This allows others access to confidential data and to document under your name.
- *Do not leave a portable device (e.g., a laptop or PDA) unattended in a public location,* such as on a countertop in the nurses' station. This increases the possibility of theft or unauthorized access to secured client information.
- *Never access client health records that you have no professional reason to view.* This is a severe breach of client privacy rules. Know your state and federal laws and the consequences for privacy violations.
- *Become familiar with your organization's policies* regarding network and client health record information security and confidentiality.

KnowledgeCheck 18-7

 Refer to Clinical Insight 18-3 to help you answer the following questions:

- What aspects of care should be documented?
- When should care be documented?
- How is documentation on paper different from documentation in an EHR or on an electronic digital form?

ThinkLike a Nurse 18-5

You are caring for two clients on a medical–surgical unit. One of your clients is short of breath and complaining of chest pain. Your other client is recovering from abdominal surgery. He is alert, stable, and free from pain at this time. After stabilizing your first client, you realize you are 45 minutes late administering a medication to the abdominal surgery client. You are not sure how to proceed.

- What theoretical knowledge do you need?
- You give the medicine as soon as you can (60 minutes late). How and where should you document the medication administered?
- If you had been aware that you were going to be late with the medication, what might you have done to be sure it was given on time?

Can I Delegate Charting?

In some facilities, each member of the team is responsible for documenting care provided to the client. Nursing assistants or other nursing assistive personnel (NAP) often chart ADLs, activity, and I&O on graphic records. You are responsible for documenting the nursing care you provide. Never chart the actions of others as though you performed them. If an action is crucial to a chain of events, you may document that action on paper or in the EHR, referring to the person who did the action clearly. For example, "Became dizzy; assisted to chair by Nora Roverdale, NAP."

KnowledgeCheck 18-8

- Can charting be delegated?
- You are a student nurse on a medical–surgical unit. You review your client's chart and notice that the provider entered prescriptions that do not appear to be appropriate for your client. The provider is still in the area. How would you handle this situation?

Toward Evidence-Based Practice

Burke, M., & Ellis, M. (2016). Electronic health records: Describing technological stressors of nurse educators. *Nurse Educator, 41*(1), 46–48. doi:10.1097/nne.0000000000000196

Research revealed the top three factors creating the highest levels of technostress for educators were lack of student access to training materials, the need of educators to learn new EHR systems, and the availability of technological support. Strategies to decrease technostress included more training, partnering with clinical facilities, and providing technological support resources.

Mitchell, J. (2015). Electronic documentation: Assessment of newly graduated nurses' competency and confidence levels. *Online Journal of Nursing Informatics, 19*(2). Retrieved from http://www.himss.org/ojni.

Research revealed new graduate nurses, even those with prior experiences, have difficulty learning the technological competencies/skills needed for EHR documentation. Providing more extensive training beyond the first week of orientation was recommended to ensure new graduates learn the functionality of the system and expectations of their roles.

Cherry, B., Ford, E., & Peterson, L. (2011). Experiences with electronic health records: Early adopters in long-term care facilities. *Health Care Management Review, 36*(3), 265–274.

Research revealed that administrators, nurses, and other system users in 10 long-term care facilities found that EHRs (1) were cost effective in improved quality of care, (2) increased documentation accuracy and implementation of evidence-based practices, (3) improved access to resident information, (4) reduced nursing overtime, and (5) resulted in an overall positive attitude among personnel.

Huryk, L. (2010). Factors influencing nurses' attitudes toward healthcare information technology. *Journal of Nursing Management, 18*(5), 606–612.

A systematic review of 13 articles of nurses' attitudes toward healthcare information technology revealed more positive attitudes were associated with (1) increased computer experience, (2) perceptions of enhanced patient care or safety, (3) positive attitude of administrators, and (4) user-friendly and well-integrated systems. Less positive attitudes were associated with (1) perceptions of dehumanizing patient care and (2) technological system issues/flaws.

1. What are factors that may contribute to the lack of competence of new graduates with EHR documentation? What factors may be derived from the findings of Burke and Ellis (2016)?

2. Which study identifies the importance of EHR? What does the study say about that?

3. What factors contribute to a positive attitude toward EHR by nurses?

 Go to Davis Advantage, Resources, Chapter 18, **Toward Evidence-Based Practice Suggested Responses.**

CLINICALREASONING

The questions and exercises in this section allow you to practice the kind of thinking you will use as a full-spectrum nurse. Critical-thinking questions usually have more than one correct answer, so we do not provide "correct answers" for these features. It is more important to develop your nursing judgment than to just cover content. You will learn by discussing the questions with your peers. If you are still unsure, see the Davis Advantage chapter resources for suggested responses.

Caring for the Nguyens

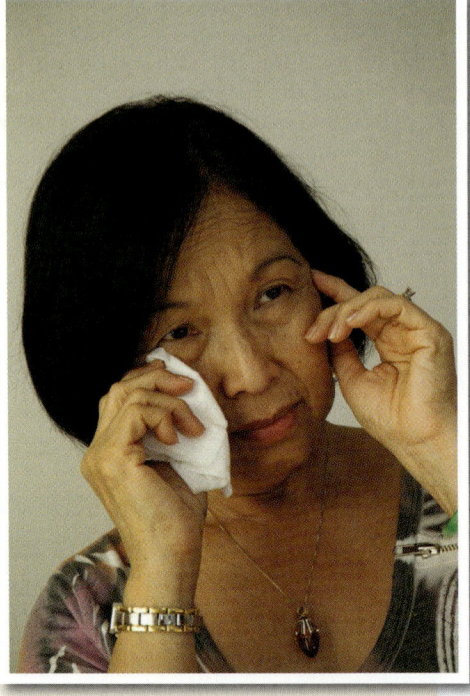

Yen Nguyen arrives at the Family Medicine Clinic complaining of pain and drainage from her right eye. She requests an appointment. As part of your clinical experience working as a triage nurse at the clinic, you must evaluate the client's status and determine whether she needs to be seen today. What follows is your conversation with Mrs. Nguyen:

Mrs. Nguyen: I don't have an appointment, but I need to see someone today. My husband is a patient here. I have an appointment in 2 weeks for a physical, but I've never been here before. I just can't wait 2 weeks.

You: What seems to be the problem?

Mrs. Nguyen: My eye is killing me. My right one. It burns and stings, and there's all this nasty gunk coming out. I think I need some medicine for it.

You: Tell me a little more about this problem. When did this start?

Mrs. Nguyen: I woke up yesterday with a painful, itchy eye. I used some saline drops, but the eye seems to be worse. I work at a preschool, and they won't let me work unless I take care of this. I also think I need to be checked for other things. I haven't had an appointment in a long time. I suppose I just need some tests. My husband just found out he has high blood pressure, but I don't think I do. I guess I'm not old enough. I'm 55, but

my mother got high blood pressure when she was 70.

As she is talking, you notice a large amount of thick, yellow-green drainage in the corner of her right eye and the eye is reddened. She is rubbing this eye vigorously and dabbing at it with a tissue. The skin is puffy around the eye as well. Her left eye is slightly red, but there is no drainage.

Her vital signs are as follows: blood pressure, 132/76 mm Hg; heart rate, 88 beats/min; respirations, 18 breaths/min; and temperature, 98.9°F (37.2°C). Based on your brief assessment, you ask the receptionist to give Mrs. Nguyen an urgent appointment.

A. Make two charting entries to describe the above events. First, make a brief narrative note.

B. Next, construct a SOAP(IER) note. Be sure to follow charting guidelines when you prepare your note

 Go to Davis Advantage, Resources, Chapter 18, **Caring for the Nguyens—Suggested Responses.**

Applying the **Full-Spectrum Nursing Model**

PATIENT SITUATION

Ellen is 85 years old and has sustained a right-sided cerebrovascular accident (CVA, or stroke or brain attack). Doctors say she is unlikely to regain much physical function, if she even awakens from the coma. Her children, Mary and Dale, have met with the provider, who tells them that Ellen is not likely to survive. The provider wants to insert a feeding tube and has asked whether they want Ellen to be resuscitated in case of cardiac or respiratory arrest. Mary tells you she wants to do what is best for her mother, but she feels that Ellen would not want to be kept alive in this condition. She is also concerned about putting her through uncomfortable procedures if there is no chance of recovery. Her brother, Dale, says, "Mom needs the feeding tube. I can't sit and watch her starve to death. As long as she's alive, there's hope."

THINKING

1. *Theoretical Knowledge (Recall of Facts and Principles):* You plan to use the Focus Charting® format to document this interaction.
   a. Write the focus for this note.
   b. What does the acronym *DAR* stand for?
2. *Critical Thinking (Contextual Awareness):*
   a. What aspects of this situation have you experienced or observed previously in your role as a caregiver?
   b. How might those past experiences affect your perception in this situation?

DOING

3. *Practical Knowledge (Handoff Report):* Ellen's last name is Smith; assume her children are also named Smith. Ellen is in room 820. Using the PACE format, what would you say to the oncoming nurse during handoff report? You will be able to address only a small amount of physiological information because the scenario does not provide it.

CARING

4. *Self-Knowledge:* In what way(s) can you identify with any of the people involved in this scenario?

 Go to Davis Advantage, Resources, Chapter 18, **Applying the Full-Spectrum Nursing Model—Suggested Responses.**

PracticalKnowledge: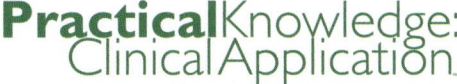
Clinical Application

CLINICAL INSIGHTS

Clinical Insight 18-1 ➤ **Giving Oral Reports**

For All Types of Report Formats:

Remember the acronym CUBAN (Currie, 2002):
Confidential, **U**ninterrupted, **B**rief, **A**ccurate, **N**amed nurse

Use a Standardized Format Such as the Following:

PACE

Patient/Problem—Include client's name, room number, diagnosis, reason for admission, and recent procedures. State the present problem. Briefly summarize medical history relevant to the current problem.

Assessment/Actions—Nursing assessments and interventions directed to the problem.

Continuing/Changes—Continuing needs and potential changes include:

- Client care and treatments that must be monitored on other shifts (e.g., dressing changes)
- Changes in the client's condition or the care plan, recent or anticipated (e.g., new orders, changes in discharge date)

Evaluation—Evaluation of responses to nursing and medical interventions, progress toward goals, and effectiveness of the plan

SBAR/SBAR-R

Identify yourself, the client, and the agency.
Situation—"Here's the situation . . ."
Background—"The supporting background information is . . ."
Assessment—"My assessment of the situation is that . . ."
Recommendation—"I recommend that you . . ."
[***Read back***—"To repeat the information and . . ."]
[***Questions***—Questions asked and answered]

(Continued)

Clinical Insight 18-1 ➤ **Giving Oral Reports—cont'd**

Include the Following Content:

In a handoff report:

- Client's name, age, and room number
- Client's admitting diagnosis—one or several may exist. Status of identified outcomes.
- Client's relevant past medical history
- Treatments the client has received during this admission, such as surgery, line placements, breathing treatments. Include consultations completed with other disciplines.
- Upcoming consultations, diagnostic tests, surgeries, or treatments

In a transfer report:

- Your name, facility, and phone number
- Client's name, age, gender, and admitting and current diagnoses
- Client's providers(s), if still following client
- Procedures or surgeries performed
- Current medications and last date/time each was taken/ time next dose is due
- Client status at present as well as progression since admission
- Last set of vital signs, plus any pertinent trends since admission

- Client restrictions, such as diet, bedrest, isolation, activity limits
- Plan of care, such as IV therapy, pain management, current medications, wound care, client or family concerns, discharge planning
- Significant assessment findings from the previous shifts
- Teaching conducted

- Tubes in place, such as IVs, catheters, drainage tubes, along with the intake and output of each tube or drain
- Presence of wounds or open areas of the skin plus current interventions for each
- Names and contact numbers for family and significant others
- Special directives, such as code status, presence of advance directives, preferred intensity of care, or isolation required
- Reason the client is being transferred
- Location of above information (on transfer form, in medical records, etc.)

When Your Report Is Finished:

- Ask the receiving nurse whether he has any questions.
- Get the nurse's full name and then record it plus the transfer date and time in your transfer documentation.

Practice Resources

Cornell, P., Gervis, M., Yates, L., et al. (2014); Gore, A., Leasure, A., Carithers, C., et al. (2015); Grbach, W., Vincent, L., & Struth, D. (2008); Haig, K., Sutton, S., & Whittington, J. (2006); Kaiser Permanente of Colorado (updated 2011); Schroeder, M. (2011); Schroeder, S. (2006).

Clinical Insight 18-2 ➤ **Receiving Telephone and Verbal Orders**

✚ You should accept verbal and telephone prescriptions only in specific situations when the primary provider is not able to electronically submit, write, or enter them personally.

- **Have a second nurse listen to the prescription,** if possible, to verify its accuracy.
- **Write or enter the prescription electronically only if you heard it yourself;** no third-party involvement is acceptable.
- **Repeat the written prescription** even if you believe you have clearly understood it. This validates that the prescription given is correct.
- **Spell unfamiliar names** aloud to be sure the spelling is correct.
- **Pronounce digits of numbers separately.** For example, instead of "seventeen," say "one, seven." Mishearing a number can lead to a serious error in medication dosage.
- **Make sure the prescription makes sense** given the client's current status.

- **Transcribe the prescription directly into the chart as quickly as possible.** Writing it on a piece of paper, then copying it again on a paper order sheet or into an EHR introduces an additional chance of error. If entering into an EHR, it's best to have the prescription entry area open and enter the prescription as the prescriber dictates it to you.
- **Write the prescription while the prescriber remains on the telephone or in the building** so that you can ask any necessary questions immediately without the need for a return call.
- **When writing on a paper prescription sheet, first document the date and time.** Next write the text of the prescription. Then, depending on how you received the prescription, write "TO" (telephone order) or "VO" (verbal order) next to the text of the prescription, followed by the ordering provider's name and then your name. The following is an example of a telephone prescription:

12/17/2018   0815 – Morphine 2 mg IV push ×1 for pain now. TO Dr. Clayton Kent/Sarah Hogan, RN; prescription read back for verification and validated.————

Clinical Insight 18-2 ➤ **Receiving Telephone and Verbal Orders—cont'd**

- **Sign electronically to activate the prescription.** If entering the prescription electronically, indicate during entry that it was given verbally or over the telephone, the date and time the prescription was given, and then search for and select the ordering provider's name. Click "sign" or whatever option in your EHR indicates the prescription is signed and is now active.
- **Be sure you have the provider's phone number** so that you can reach her if future questions arise.

- **All verbal and telephone prescription must be countersigned** by the provider within 24 hours.

Practice Resources

Buppert, C. (2012); National Coordinating Council on Medication Error Reporting and Prevention (2015).

Clinical Insight 18-3 ➤ **Guidelines for Documentation**

GUIDELINE	HOW TO APPLY	RATIONALE OR EXAMPLE
	When to Document	
Documentation begins at the start of your shift.	■ *Hospital or long-term care facility*—start of shift ■ *Home visit or outpatient facility*—when you first encounter the client ■ Document the condition of your patient when you first observed him. Was he awake? Was he in bed? Did he have any complaints? What did you do?	
Document immediately.	Discipline yourself to document as soon as possible after making an observation or providing care.	The longer you wait, the more likely you will forget important details.
Never chart ahead.	Never chart before performing an intervention.	It is impossible to see into the future and be sure that what you expect to happen will actually happen. To do this threatens the record's credibility.
Avoid "block" charting.	Each entry needs to be made individually; record the time each was done	Do not chart an entry time as "From 1300 to 1500."
Chart chronologically.	■ *On paper:* Document times in chronological order. ■ *EHRs:* Most automatically insert the current date and time when forms are opened. Follow the documentation system's guidelines for changing those dates and times before signing.	Chronological charting communicates the changing status of the client.
Designate late entries (paper).	■ If you forget to make an important entry while charting, you will later need to add "late entry" to the first available line. ■ Record the time and date you are making the addition; clearly designate it is a late entry. ■ If you know legal action is pending, do not place a late note in the health record without notifying the nurse manager or risk management officer first.	■ Late entry example: 5/11/2018, 1400; late entry for 5/11/2018, 1200 ■ It is a criminal offense to alter a client record after the organization's approved time limit for doing so has passed.
Designate late entries (EHR).	■ Open the appropriate form and change the automatically generated current date/time to the date/time your care was actually done; then sign. ■ Follow the agency policy regarding the time period for making a late entry.	

(Continued)

Clinical Insight 18-3 ➤ **Guidelines for Documentation—cont'd**

GUIDELINE	HOW TO APPLY	RATIONALE OR EXAMPLE
	What to Document	
Questions to aid your recall.	As your shift or visit progresses, you will perform assessments and nursing interventions. To remind yourself what to record, ask yourself the example questions in the right-hand column.	▪ What were your assessment findings? ▪ Did any abnormalities exist? ▪ What was the client's response to your intervention? Did any changes occur from the initial assessment?
Interventions, client responses, and evaluation of progress toward goals.	▪ These are often recorded on an IPOC. ▪ Clearly describe what your client is experiencing. ▪ **KEY POINT:** *Do not chart a symptom without also documenting what you did about it and how the client responded.*	(Symptom) Pt complained of pain, rated 6 on a 0–10 scale. (Intervention) Administered Tylenol 1,000 mg, by mouth, at 0900. At 1030, Pt rated pain as 3.
Significant events or changes in condition.	When possible, quote the client's interpretation of the event or change.	Quoting the client directly gives all health-care providers objective data.
Informed consent.	▪ If you are asked to obtain informed consent for a procedure, document your actions. ▪ In most states, your signature (paper or electronic) confirms only that the client signed the consent. ▪ For further discussion of informed consent, see Chapters 43 and 44.	The primary provider conducting the procedure is legally responsible for discussing the procedure and its risks and benefits.
Client teaching.	▪ Include instruction about medications and client diagnoses. ▪ Include discharge teaching. ▪ If the client's physical or cognitive condition prevents teaching, explain that in your documentation.	Documenting client teaching can positively affect insurance and other payments to the institution.
Spiritual or other concerns expressed by the client and/or family.	Document your interventions.	Addressing spiritual concerns ensures that the client receives holistic healthcare.
Attempts made to contact the primary care provider.	▪ Contacts may, for example, be to notify the provider of the client's condition, or to clarify orders. ▪ If you are unable to contact the primary provider, document your contacts with your charge nurse, nurse manager, supervisor, medical director, and hospital administrator.	You must indicate that you made every effort to communicate your concerns.
Client leaving the facility against medical advice (AMA).	▪ Chart the client's condition, any explanations of risks and consequences given to the client, the client's destination (if known), and your notification of the client's care providers. ▪ If your facility has specific forms for AMA departures, use the designated form. ▪ If the form is hard-copy paper, have the client sign the form before leaving. ▪ If the client refuses to sign, document this in your chart.	Your actions and responsibilities in the situation must be made clear in the record.
Client's refusal of treatment.	▪ Try to determine the reason for refusal. ▪ Quote the exact language the patient used in this situation whenever possible.	Doing so helps ensure charting facts instead of inferences.
Use of restraints.	▪ Most facilities have a separate form that allows you to document the reason for restraint use, the type of restraint, and frequent checks of the client.	▪ The primary care provider must place a signed order for restraints in the chart or in the EHR.

Clinical Insight 18-3 ➤ Guidelines for Documentation—cont'd

GUIDELINE	HOW TO APPLY	RATIONALE OR EXAMPLE
	■ You must have contacted the primary care provider.	■ Restraint orders must be reordered inside a specific time frame set by the organization or the restraints are discontinued (see Chapter 23).
"Occurrences."	■ Chart your findings accurately and objectively. ■ Fill out a separate occurrence form and send to the risk manager (paper forms). ■ Do not make reference to the occurrence form anywhere in your charting.	■ Examples of occurrences: falls and medication errors. ■ Occurrence forms are not part of the client's health record. See **Occurrence Reports,** earlier in the chapter.
Complete data about medications.	■ *Paper MAR*—Include the date, time, and medication given, and your initials. ■ *Electronic MAR*—Ensure your entry is accurate, then sign electronically that administration was accomplished successfully.	Accurate documentation is an essential component of the nurse's role.
prn, unscheduled, IV infusions, and STAT medications.	■ Record on the MAR. ■ Include comments regarding the medication in your narrative charting or insert a comment in your electronic charting. ■ Chart a timely evaluation of the client's response to the medication.	Certain prn medications require a follow-up response be documented within a specific period of time set by the organization, usually 15 to 30 minutes after the medication is given.
Medications not administered.	■ Document omission on the MAR. ■ If the client states a reason for refusing the medication: *Paper notes*—Quote the client in your narrative notes. *Electronic MAR*—Use pull-down or other menu.	■ *Examples:* Client refuses medication; dose accidentally omitted. ■ Most electronic MARs include an explanation with a selection from a drop-down list such as "Client refused" or "Patient not available." ■ Some MARs also contain a narrative section to type a comment about why a medication was not given.

How to Document

Know your organization's requirements for reimbursement.	■ Requirements typically specify frequency of charting and the type of data that must be recorded. ■ Fulfilling documentation requirements helps to ensure appropriate reimbursement. ■ Home care, hospitals, clinics, office settings, and long-term care facilities have specific guidelines for documentation necessary for payment.	
Date and time all your documentation.	Most organizations use a 24-hour clock or military time to avoid confusion between a.m. and p.m. In this system: ■ The day begins at 0001 (1 minute past midnight) and ends at 2400 (12 midnight). ■ *Morning hours*—Most people have little difficulty with early morning hours. Example: 9:00 a.m. is 0900. ■ *Hours after 12 noon*—To convert to military time after 12 noon, simply add 12 to the clock time. Example: 7:30 p.m. + 12 = 1930 in military time.	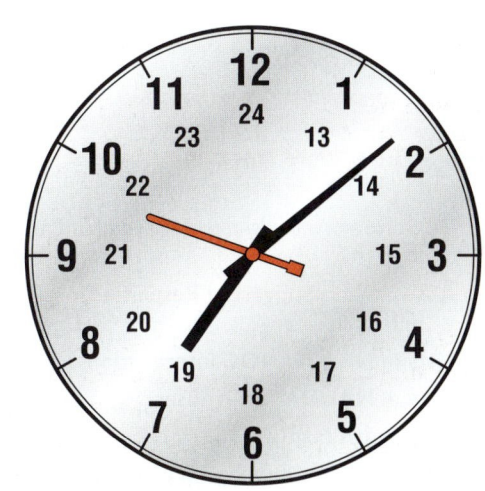 Many healthcare facilities use the 24-hour clock.

(Continued)

Clinical Insight 18-3 ➤ **Guidelines for Documentation—cont'd**

GUIDELINE	HOW TO APPLY	RATIONALE OR EXAMPLE
Document accurately and objectively, using nonjudgmental language.	■ Avoid labeling clients or team members. ■ Do not chart judgments about decisions made by members of the care team. ■ Document objective facts, so the reader can draw an informed conclusion. ■ Quote the client in his own words, when possible.	■ *Chart the client's words:* "I'm not taking that medicine. Take it away." ■ *Do not chart:* "Client obnoxious and refuses prescribed medication."
Avoid vague, subjective words.	■ When possible, give specific examples.	■ Terms such as *good, average,* or *normal* do not clearly define the status of the client. ■ Descriptive details allow caregivers to better understand your client's individual needs.
Use only the abbreviations authorized by your organization.	See Table 18-1 and Box 18-3.	
Use correct spelling and grammar.	Incorrect spelling may raise questions about what you are attempting to communicate. Incorrect grammar implies carelessness on your part and creates a question of your competence if your chart is reviewed.	
Chart your own nursing actions.	Do not allow anyone to chart for you. Do not document the actions of others as though you had performed them.	Each nurse is responsible for documenting his assessments, interventions, and evaluations. A deviation from this principle can imply cover-up, carelessness, or a blatant disregard of policy and standards of practice.
You may need to document the actions of someone else.	■ Try to avoid this, but if you must do it, be sure to designate clearly whose actions they are. ■ *EHRs*—You can indicate another person performed the action in an added comment or by searching for and selecting the other care provider in the appropriate field, then signing.	*Example:* If the NAP (nursing assistive personnel) helped the client ambulate: *Do not chart:* "Assisted to bathroom." *Do chart:* "J. Scott, NAP, assisted client to bathroom."
Avoid charting what someone else said, heard, felt, or smelled.	■ If the information is critical and you *must* chart it, use quotations, and attribute the remarks to the person who made them.	*Example:* "Wife stated, 'My husband told me that he is in a lot of pain, but does not want to bother the nurses.'"

To explore learning resources for this chapter,

Go to www.DavisAdvantage.com and find:

Answers and Suggested Responses for all questions in this chapter
Lists of **NIC** and **NOC** interventions
Lists of **NANDA-I Diagnoses**
Knowledge Map
References and Bibliography

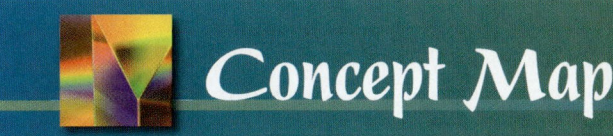

Concept Map

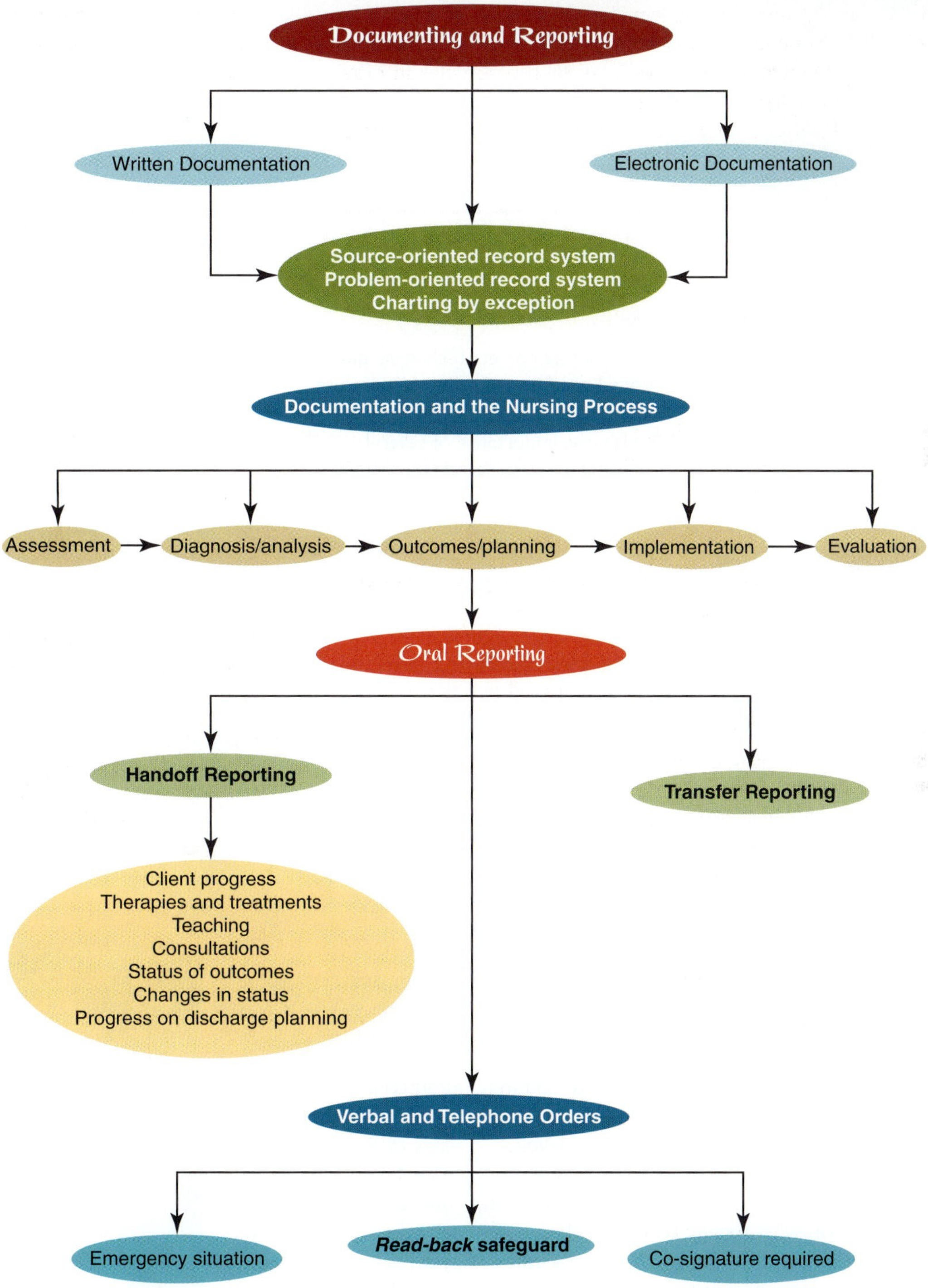

Documenting and Reporting

Written Documentation

Electronic Documentation

Source-oriented record system
Problem-oriented record system
Charting by exception

Documentation and the Nursing Process

Assessment → Diagnosis/analysis → Outcomes/planning → Implementation → Evaluation

Oral Reporting

Handoff Reporting

Transfer Reporting

Client progress
Therapies and treatments
Teaching
Consultations
Status of outcomes
Changes in status
Progress on discharge planning

Verbal and Telephone Orders

Emergency situation

Read-back **safeguard**

Co-signature required

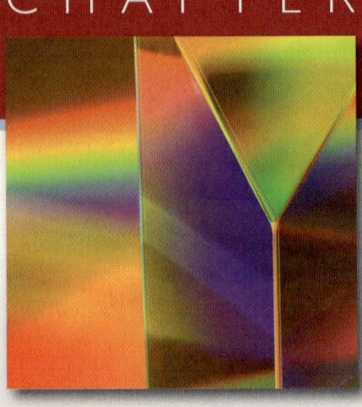

CHAPTER 19

Vital Signs

Learning Outcomes

After completing this chapter, you should be able to:

➤ Describe the physiological processes involved in regulating body temperature, pulse, respirations, and blood pressure.

➤ Convert between the Fahrenheit and centigrade temperature scales.

➤ Discuss expected normal vital signs findings for various age-groups.

➤ Recognize client vital signs readings that should be referred to the primary care provider.

➤ Define *arterial oxygen saturation, hypoxia, hyperventilation,* and *hypoventilation.*

➤ Define *hypotension, hypertension, essential hypertension,* and *secondary hypertension.*

➤ Select the correct site and equipment for measuring the temperature, pulse, respiration, and blood pressure of patients in various age-groups.

➤ Demonstrate correct technique and procedures for measuring temperature, pulse, respiration, and blood pressure.

➤ Explain the importance of several measurements to interpret a client's blood pressure.

➤ State at least one nursing diagnosis to describe a problem for each of the vital signs: temperature, pulse, respirations, and blood pressure.

➤ Describe nursing interventions for the client (1) with temperature alterations; (2) with impaired respiratory status; (3) diagnosed with high blood pressure (hypertension); and (4) with alterations in pulse parameters.

➤ Identify important tips to teach your clients in managing their hypertension.

Key Concepts

Oxygenation (respirations)

Perfusion (pulse, blood pressure)

Thermoregulation

Vital signs

Related Concepts

See the Concept Map at the end of this chapter.

Example Problems

Hyperthermia/Heat Stroke

Hypothermia

Hypertension

Hypotension

Meet Your Patients

Your instructor has scheduled a clinical day at a local community health fair for students to answer health-related questions, administer flu vaccines, check blood sugar levels, and take vital signs: temperature, pulse, respirations, and blood pressure (BP). You have been asked to check vital signs.

Jason. The first person who arrives at the booth is Rosemary, a young mother, with Jason, her 2-year-old son. She tells you he has been eating poorly and is very irritable. The child's skin is warm and dry and he is flushed. Rosemary explains that she does not have a thermometer, and she would like you to take her son's temperature. Jason's axillary temperature is 101.8°F (38.8°C).

Now it is time to think like a nurse! What could this temperature reading mean? What, if any, additional data should you collect? How will you explain your findings to Rosemary? What action would you advise Rosemary to take? You may not yet have all the theoretical knowledge you need to answer these questions, but try to do so anyway, based on your present knowledge base and your life experiences.

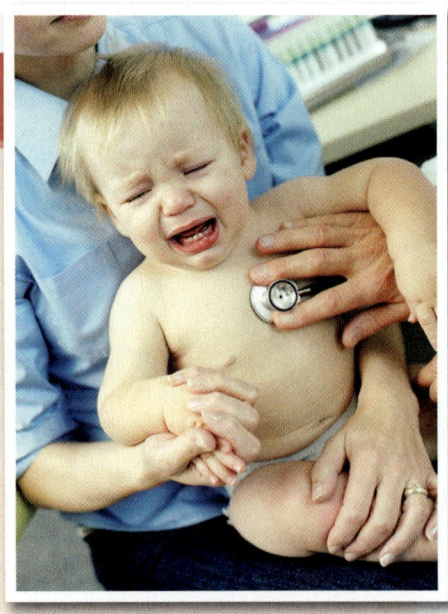

Meet Your Patients (continued)

Ms. Sharma. The next person to arrive at the booth is Ms. Sharma, an active 80-year-old woman who works part-time in a local literacy program and walks 3 miles four times per week. Ms. Sharma notes that she has "lost a little pep. I don't feel sick, but I'm tired lately." Her pulse is difficult to feel. The rhythm is irregular, and the strength of the pulse is uneven—some beats are strong, while others are weak. What might this finding mean? What questions do you have for Ms. Sharma? What, if any, additional data should you collect? How will you explain your findings to Ms. Sharma? What action would you advise her to take?

Mr. Jackson. As Mr. Jackson sits down next to you, you notice he is short of breath. His respiratory rate is 28 breaths/min, and he appears to be struggling to breathe. What do you think this respiratory rate means? What should be your next action? What would you say to Mr. Jackson?

Lucas. The next client to arrive is Lucas, a 35-year-old accountant who works for a firm in a nearby office building. Lucas tells you he has been under a lot of stress and is worried about his blood pressure. You measure his blood pressure as 150/98 mm Hg. Is this an acceptable blood pressure? What does this reading mean? What should you discuss with Lucas? What advice should you offer?

You will gain the theoretical knowledge you need to answer the preceding questions as you work through this chapter and learn more about vital signs.

ABOUT THE KEY CONCEPTS

The key concepts of **thermoregulation, perfusion,** and **oxygenation** pertain to specific **vital signs** you will learn about in this chapter (temperature, pulse, respirations, and blood pressure). A grasp of these underlying concepts will help you understand and remember the rationale for what you do when measuring and interpreting vital signs.

WHAT ARE VITAL SIGNS?

The concept of **vital signs (VS)** suggests assessment of vital or critical physiological functions. Variations in temperature, pulse, respirations, or blood pressure are indicators of a person's state of health and function of the body systems. These four assessments are among the most frequent you will make as a nurse. Because of their importance, accurate measurements and documentation of each vital sign is a top priority.

Do not become complacent when a patient's vital signs are within normal limits. Although stable vital signs may *indicate* physiological well-being, they do not *guarantee* it. Vital signs alone are limited in detecting some important physiological changes. For example, vital signs may sometimes remain stable even when there is a moderately large amount of blood loss. **KEY POINT:** *Evaluate the vital signs in the context of your overall assessment of the patient.*

Other Vital Signs Some experts have recommended adding other factors that affect client care and outcomes to the four traditional measures of physiological status:

- *Pain.* This is viewed by many as the fifth vital sign (The Joint Commission, 2011). See Chapter 32.
- *Oxygen saturation.* Pulse oximetry provides important information on arterial blood oxygen concentration.
- *Smoking status.* This is important to assess based on the impact of smoking on body functions and thus vital signs.
- *Emotional distress.* This can have an impact on overall physiological functioning.

Rather than being overly concerned about whether or not these parameters should be referred to as vital signs, we recommend that nurses include them in all of their ongoing assessments of clients.

♥ **iCare 19-1**

Measuring Vital Signs

Measuring vital signs seems pretty straightforward. How can you incorporate caring into this technical task?

Simple Solution: Approach every patient unhurriedly. Introduce yourself, make eye contact, and explain what you will be doing before you touch the person. "*Hello, Mr. Smith. My name is Annie Gates. I'm a student nurse. I need to take your vital signs, which includes taking your blood pressure and measuring your temperature, pulse, and breathing rate. Is it okay with you that I perform these tasks?*"

Introducing yourself and explaining your actions shows respect for the person's autonomy. In addition, you are informing and educating the patient about the plan of care and allowing him an opportunity to consent or refuse.

When Should I Measure a Patient's Client's Vital Signs?

In the Meet Your Patients scenario, patients asked you to take their vital signs. However, in many clinical settings, vital signs are measured and documented in the following commonly occurring circumstances:

- On admission to the hospital
- For inpatients, at the beginning of a shift
- At a visit to the healthcare provider's office or clinic
- Before, during, and after surgery or certain procedures
- To monitor the effects of certain medications or activities
- Whenever the patient's condition changes

The ideal frequency for assessing vital signs depends on the client's condition and the events taking place (Schulman & Staul, 2010). Agency policies also determine the frequency for monitoring and recording vital signs. The following list contains commonly used frequencies. However, one recent study suggests that low-risk clients might be allowed to rest instead of waking them up for routine vital signs during the night (Jordan, Yoder, Yuen, et al., 2013).

- In the hospital: once every 4 to 8 hours
- In the home health setting: at each visit

- In the clinic: at each visit
- In skilled nursing facilities, also known as convalescent hospitals: weekly to monthly

✚ It is up to the nurse to decide whether vital signs need to be monitored more frequently than prescribed by the primary care provider. You must always obtain an initial set of VS to establish the client's baseline. When a client's VS vary from their baseline, you should assess and document them more frequently to determine a trend in the degree and severity of the variation. As a beginning practitioner, you should validate your clinical assessments with a more experienced nurse and determine how often to reassess.

KEY POINT: *A baseline is important for evaluating a change in the client's physiological status. Such a change may be caused by a disease state, the effect of therapies, or changes in physical activity or environment.*

Table 19-1 shows average or normal findings for adults, but it is important to remember that each person has his or her own baseline for "normal." If a client's vital signs vary from established norms, compare the finding with that person's baseline.

Table 19-1 ➤	**Vital Signs: Average Normal Findings for Adults**
Mean Adult Temperature	
Oral	98°F (36.7°C)*
Rectal	98.6°F (37°C)*
Pulse	
Normal range	60–100 beats/min
Average	80 beats/min
Respirations	
Normal range	12–20 breaths/min
Blood Pressure	
Normal range	100–119 mm Hg systolic or 60–80 mm Hg diastolic
Prehypertensive	120–139 mm Hg systolic or 80–89 mm Hg diastolic
Average	110/70 mm Hg (the middle of the "normal" range) (Joint National Committee on Prevention, Detection, Evaluation, and Treatment of High Blood Pressure, 2003)

*This is revised downward from the traditional norms to reflect more recent research (Mackowiak, Wasserman, & Levine, 1992) and a systematic review of the literature (Sund-Levander, Forsberg, & Wahren, 2002).
- The systematic review reported the following mean normal temperatures: Oral 97.3°F (36.3°C), Rectal 98.3°F (36.9°C).
- The traditional Wunderlich (1871) average normal temperature is 98.6°F (37.0°C) to 99.5°F (37.5°C), depending on measurement site.

How Do I Document Vital Signs?

Most agencies have special flow sheets for documenting vital signs. If the VS are not within normal limits, you will also document them in the nurses' notes, along with any associated symptoms (e.g., cyanosis [blue-gray skin] with abnormal respirations). Because nurses are required to take appropriate actions based on their assessment finding, you must also document your interventions (e.g., elevating the head of the bed when the client has shortness of breath). For an example of a graphic flow sheet for documenting vital signs, see Figure 19-1.

BODY TEMPERATURE

Body temperature is the degree of heat maintained by the body. It is the difference between heat produced by the body and heat lost to the environment.

Theoretical Knowledge
Knowing Why

You must understand the concept of *thermoregulation* to assess and support regulation of body temperature at a professional level. You will learn the normal temperature range, how heat is produced by and lost from the body, and factors that influence body temperature.

What Is a Normal Temperature?

No single number can be considered "normal," because baseline body temperature varies among individuals as a result of differences in metabolism. Furthermore, each person's temperature fluctuates with age, exercise, and environmental conditions. However, the body does function optimally within a narrow temperature range.

"Average" Normal Temperature There is little definitive evidence about what, exactly, is a normal temperature. You may see different values in the many sources you read. We can at least conclude that the traditional belief of 98.6°F (37°C) for an average normal reading is too high, based on available research. A systematic review of the literature found a mean normal adult oral temperature of 97.3°F (36.3°C) (Sund-Levander, Forsberg, & Wahren, 2002). (See Table 19-1.) Research findings are inconsistent concerning whether older adults have lower body temperatures (Lu & Dai, 2009) and recommend that body temperature be evaluated based on individual variability (Sund-Levander, Grodzinsky, Loyd, et al., 2004). Table 19-2 shows age-related variations for all vital signs, including temperature.

Slight Variations in Temperature Temporary, slight variations of temperature above or below normal usually are not significant. Greater variations indicate a disturbance of function in some system or region of the body (Fig. 19-2). However, the degree of temperature elevation does not always indicate the seriousness of the underlying disease or condition. For example, some acute, even fatal, infections may cause only a mild temperature elevation. **KEY POINT:** *A continuous elevation, even if slight, is cause for concern and indicates a need for further evaluation.*

Core Temperature An adult's normal internal temperature, called the **core temperature,** ranges from about 97°F to 100.8°F (36.1°C to 38.2°C). The core temperature is typically 1°F to 2°F (0.6°C to 1.2°C) higher than surface (skin) temperature. Most research and clinical practice situations do not report core body temperature because it is not convenient to measure. Rectal and tympanic membrane measurements are

VITAL SIGNS
24 HOUR FLOW SHEET

ACCOUNT NO.	37681A
MED. REC. NO.	00005674321
NAME	Fred D Abbott
BIRTHDATE	1-25-39

DATE __mm/dd/yy__   WEIGHT __285 lb.__

ISOLATION __Standard Precautions__

TIME	04	05	08	12	14	15	16	17	18	19	21	23	24
PULSE RADIAL	78	80	80	90	102						78	76	74
APICAL					100	98	92	90	82	80			
RESP.	12	14	16	20	21	22	20	18	16	16	14	12	12
B/P	118 / 84		120 / 86	138 / 90	144 / 90	146 / 90	140 / 86	138 / 84	130 / 84	124 / 82	118 / 80		118 / 78
PAIN													
SAO₂	96%		96%	94%	94%		92%	96%	98%	99%	99%		98%

PAIN LEVEL
0–NONE
10–SEVERE

FIGURE 19-1 Graphic flow sheet for recording vital signs.

Table 19-2 ➤ Comparison of Normal Vital Signs for Various Ages**

AGE	TEMPERATURE AVERAGE °C (°F)	PULSE RANGE beats per min	RESPIRATIONS RANGE breaths per min	BLOOD PRESSURE AVERAGE mm Hg
Newborn	36.8 (98.2)* axillary	130 (80–180)	30–60	80/40
1–3 years	37.7 (99.9)* rectal	110 (80–150)	20–40	98/64
6–8 years	37.0 (98.6)* oral	95 (75–115)	20–25	102/56
10 years	37.0 (98.6)* oral	90 (70–100)	17–22	110/58
Teen	37.0 (98.6)* oral	80 (55–105)	15–20	110/70
Adult	36.7 (98) oral	80 (60–100)	12–20	<120/80
Adult older than 70 years	35 to 36.0 (95 to 96.8) oral	80 (60–100)	12–20	120/80, up to 160/95

*We speculate that based on recent literature for adult temperatures, these may all be slightly high. Definitive literature to support changes was not available.

**NOTE: Pulse and respirations are shown as ranges, not averages. This means that you might see either the low or high extreme for a short period of time without alarm. Ranges and averages should be used as guides, not absolutes.

Example 1: A normal newborn's respiratory rate may be as much as 60 when crying, or 30 when at rest.

Example 2: An older adult being treated for hypertension may regularly have a blood pressure reading of up to 160/95. Although this is not desirable or "normal," it may be normal for that patient, and would not in that case require special treatment.

 To interpret vital signs, you must know the patient's baseline and the activity at the time of the measurement.

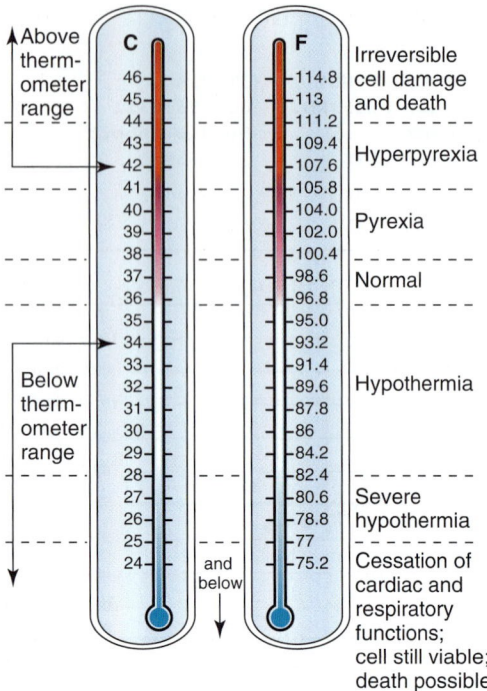

FIGURE 19-2 Ranges of normal and altered body temperatures.

used to represent core temperatures, whereas oral and axillary measurements reflect surface temperatures.

What Is Thermoregulation?

Thermoregulation is the process of maintaining a stable temperature. To keep body temperature constant, the body must balance heat production and heat loss. This balance is controlled by the hypothalamus, located between the cerebral hemispheres of the brain. Similar to a thermostat, the hypothalamus recognizes even small changes in body temperature that are sent to it by sensory receptors in the skin.

Decreasing the Body Temperature When heat sensors in the hypothalamus are stimulated, they send out impulses to reduce the body temperature.

- This activates compensatory mechanisms, such as peripheral vasodilation, sweating, and inhibition of heat production.
- **Vasodilation** (increase in the diameter of the blood vessels) diverts core-warmed blood to the body surface, where heat can be transferred to the surrounding environment.

Increasing the Body Temperature When sensors in the hypothalamus detect cold, they send out impulses to increase heat production and reduce heat loss.

- To produce heat, the body responds by shivering and releasing epinephrine, which increases metabolism.
- To reduce heat loss, the blood vessels constrict. **Vasoconstriction** (narrowing of the blood vessels) conserves heat by shunting blood away from the periphery (where heat is lost) to the core of the body, where the blood is warmed.
- **Piloerection** (hairs standing on end) also occurs, but it is not an important heat-conserving mechanism in humans.

Behavioral Control of Temperature People also engage in behaviors to maintain a comfortable body temperature. When people feel cool, they can turn up the thermostat, put on more clothing, or move to a warmer place. When they feel too warm, they can turn on an air conditioner, remove some clothing, or take a cool shower.

How Is Heat Produced in the Body?

The body produces heat through the interaction of three factors: metabolism, the movement of skeletal muscles, and nonshivering thermogenesis.

Metabolism is the sum of all physical and chemical processes and changes that take place in the body. Metabolism uses energy and generates heat. The **basal metabolic rate (BMR)** is the amount of energy required to maintain the body at rest. Body size, lean muscle mass, and numerous hormones influence BMR. For example:

- *Hyperthyroidism* (an increase in the thyroid hormone **thyroxine**) increases the BMR. Clients with *hyperthyroidism* often complain of feeling warm even when in a cool environment.
- By contrast, when the thyroxine level is low *(hypothyroidism)*, less heat is produced, and clients commonly report feeling cold. Epinephrine and norepinephrine also increase BMR and heat production.

Skeletal Muscle Movement Skeletal muscles are used in all body movements. Muscles need fuel to function.

- The breakdown (catabolism) of fats and carbohydrates in muscle produces energy and heat. While it requires very little muscle activity to sit and read this text, if you were to go for a run, you would use more skeletal muscles. After your run, your body temperature would be higher, perhaps as high as 101°F to 104°F (38.3°C to 40°C).
- In contrast, if you were to go outside without a coat when the temperature was 35°F (1.6°C), your hypothalamus would sense a drop in body temperature and you would begin to shiver to produce heat. This mechanism is so efficient that body heat production can rise to about four times the normal rate in just a few minutes.

Nonshivering Thermogenesis Nonshivering thermogenesis is the metabolism of brown fat to produce heat. It is used by infants because they cannot produce heat through shivering, as do adults and children. This mechanism disappears in the first few months after birth.

How Is Heat Exchanged Between the Body and the Environment?

Heat moves from an area of higher to an area of lower temperature; that is, cool air and objects "pick up" heat from warmer ones. The mechanisms that affect the exchange of heat between the body and the environment are radiation, convection, evaporation, and conduction (Fig. 19-3).

Radiation is the loss of heat through electromagnetic waves emitting from surfaces that are warmer than the surrounding air. If the uncovered skin is warmer than the air, the body loses heat through the skin. This is why a cool room warms by radiation when it is filled with many people. In contrast, a person can acquire heat by turning on a heat lamp or being in the sunlight. Radiation accounts for almost 50% of body heat loss.

Convection is the transfer of heat through currents of air or water. Nurses use this principle to intentionally effect changes in a patient's body temperature. Immersion in a warm bath may raise body temperature for a hypothermic client. In contrast, the currents of cool air produced by a fan can help reduce a fever. Together, the processes of convection and conduction account for approximately 15% to 20% of all heat loss to the environment.

Evaporation occurs when water is converted to vapor and lost from the skin (as perspiration) or the mucous membranes (through the breath). Evaporation causes cooling. Water loss by evaporation is called **insensible loss.** Evaporation is

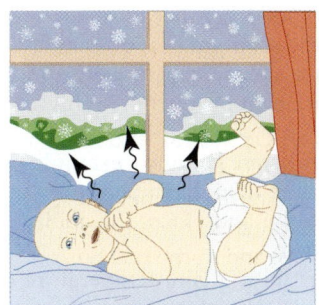
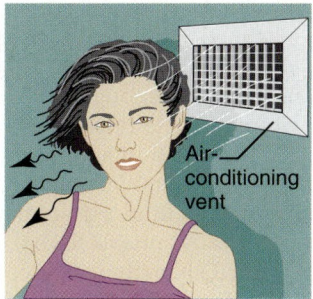
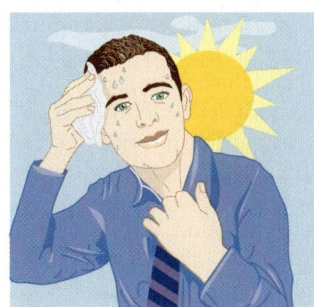
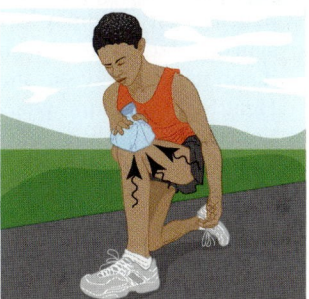

FIGURE 19-3 Mechanisms of heat exchange with the environment: radiation, convection, evaporation, and conduction.

affected by the relative **humidity** (moisture in the environment). If the air already contains much humidity, then less moisture evaporates from the skin and less cooling occurs.

Conduction is the process whereby heat is transferred from a warm to a cool surface by direct contact. Suppose that a patient's temperature is 98.6°F (37°C) while he is fully dressed in the examination room. If he puts on a thin hospital gown and lies on a cool metal radiology table, his temperature would drop, perhaps as much as a full degree Fahrenheit in the first hour.

What Factors Influence Body Temperature?

The following are examples of factors involved in the delicate balance of body temperature:

Developmental Level Infants and older adults are most susceptible to the effects of environmental temperature extremes.

■ **Infants** lose approximately 30% of their body heat through the head, which is proportionally larger than the rest of the body compared with adults. This places them at increased risk for decreased body temperature. Body temperature begins to stabilize during early childhood and remains relatively stable until older adulthood.

 ■ **Older adults** have difficulty maintaining body heat because of slower metabolism, decreased vasomotor control, and loss of subcutaneous tissue. Research revealed that older adults (aged 85 years and older) had mean body temperatures lower than 98.6°F (37°C) (Lu & Dai, 2009). Temperatures ranged from 94°F (34.4°C) to 99.6°F (37.6°C), but most were 98.6°F or lower (Gomolin, Aung, Wolf-Klein, et al., 2005). **KEY POINT:** *You can think of the average normal temperature for older adults as about 95°F to 96.8°F (35°C to 36°C).*

Environment While very high external temperatures can significantly increase internal temperatures, causing heat stroke, very cold environments can lower body temperatures and lead to hypothermia.

Gender A woman's body temperature varies (as much as 1°F, or 0.6°C) with her menstrual cycle and pregnancy. Body temperature is lower when progesterone levels are low and increases as progesterone levels increase. Hormonal fluctuations during menopause, when menses stop, often cause temperature fluctuations commonly known as *hot flashes,* which can produce episodes of intense body heat and sweating.

Exercise The increase in metabolism from strenuous exercise can increase body core temperature to 101°F to 104°F (38.3°C to 40°C). The sweat that is produced during exercise evaporates and helps to cool the body.

Emotions and Stress Emotional stress, excitement, anxiety, and nervousness stimulate the sympathetic nervous system, causing production of epinephrine and norepinephrine. These trigger an increase in the metabolic rate, which in turn increases body temperature.

Circadian Rhythm The body has an internal physiological 24-hour cycle called *circadian rhythms.* Certain physiological processes (e.g., changes in temperature and blood pressure) occur every 24 hours. Temperature can fluctuate 1°F to 2°F (0.6°C to 1.2°C) and is usually lowest in the early morning hours and highest in late afternoon or early evening.

ThinkLike a Nurse 19-1

■ You notice the following temperature readings in your client's chart:
0400: 97.4°F
0800: 97.9°F
1200: 98.4°F
1600: 99.6°F
2000: 100.9°F

■ When you assess the client's temperature at midnight, it is 101.2°F. What do you notice about the pattern of the temperature readings?
What is important in this scenario?
As a nursing student, what should you do?

KnowledgeCheck 19-1

■ Which age-groups are most susceptible to thermoregulation problems and why?
■ List five factors that affect body temperature.
■ What are the compensatory mechanisms for decreasing body temperature?
■ What are the compensatory mechanisms for increasing body temperature?

What Is a Fever (Pyrexia)?

■ **Fever,** or **pyrexia,** is an oral temperature higher than 100°F (37.8°C) or a rectal temperature of 101°F (38.3°C) in an adult. A person with a fever is said to be **febrile;** one without fever is **afebrile.**

■ A person's normal body temperature changes by as much as 1°F (0.6°C) throughout the day, so you need to take several readings at different times of the day.

■ A moderate fever is the body's natural defense against infection (up to 103°F, or 39.5°C) and although uncomfortable, it does not pose a threat to most clients. A fever is beneficial because it enhances the immune response. Specifically, it
1. Kills or inhibits the growth of many microorganisms
2. Enhances phagocytosis

3. Causes the breakdown of lysosomes and self-destruction of virally infected cells
4. Causes the release of interferon, a substance that protects cells from viral infection

- **KEY POINT:** *Hyperpyrexia, a fever above 105.8°F (41.0°C), is dangerous and requires intervention to prevent damage to body cells, especially in the brain, leading to confusion, delirium, seizures, or coma.* In addition, vascular collapse may follow, producing cerebral edema, shock, and death. Death usually results if body temperature becomes higher than 109°F to 112°F (43°C to 44°C) (McCance & Huether, 2014).

✚ Note that certain patients (e.g., those with epilepsy) are especially sensitive to even slight temperature elevations, so antipyretics might be used at the first sign of temperature elevation.

What Causes a Fever?
Fever occurs in response to **pyrogens** (fever-producing substances). When bacteria or other foreign substances invade the body, they stimulate **phagocytes** (specialized white blood cells), which ingest the invaders and secrete pyrogens (e.g., interleukin-1). Pyrogens induce secretion of **prostaglandins** (substances that reset the hypothalamic thermostat at a higher temperature). The reset value is called the **set point.** The body's heat-regulating mechanisms then act to bring the core temperature up to this new setting. When the stressor is removed, the set point resets at normal.

Fever occurs in three phases:

1. *Initial phase (febrile episode or onset):* The period during which body temperature is rising but has not yet reached the new set point. The onset of fever may be sudden or gradual, depending on the condition causing it. The person usually feels chilly and generally uncomfortable and may shiver.
2. *Second phase (course):* The period during which body temperature reaches its maximum (set point) and remains fairly constant at the new higher level. The person is flushed and feels warm and dry during this phase, which may last from a few days to a few weeks.
3. *Third phase (defervescence or crisis):* The period during which the temperature returns to normal. The person feels warm and appears flushed in response to vasodilation. Diaphoresis occurs, which assists with heat loss by evaporation. This phase is commonly referred to as the fever's "breaking."

Ways to Describe a Fever
The following are four important ways to describe a fever:

- **Intermittent fever:** Temperature alternates regularly between periods of fever and periods of normal or below-normal temperature without pharmacological intervention, or the temperature returns to normal at least once every 24 hours.
- **Remittent fever:** Fluctuations in temperature (greater than 3.6°F, or 2°C), all above normal, during a 24-hour period.
- **Constant (sustained) fever:** Temperature may fluctuate slightly (less than 1°F, or 0.55°C) but is always above normal.
- **Relapsing (or recurrent) fever:** Short periods of fever alternating with periods of normal temperatures, each lasting 1 to 2 days.

Example Problem: Hyperthermia/Heat Stroke

- **Hyperthermia,** like hyperpyrexia (fever), is a body temperature above normal. However, in hyperthermia, the elevated body temperature is higher than the set point. The hypothalamic regulation of body temperature is overwhelmed and does not reset the set point as it does in fever. Hyperthermia occurs because the body cannot promote heat loss fast enough to balance heat production or high environmental temperatures.
- **Heat exhaustion and heat stroke** are common examples of hyperthermia. With overexposure to high temperatures and inadequate fluid replacement, the body loses the ability to sweat and is unable to cool down.
  - **Heat Exhaustion** may occur with a core temperature of 98.6°F to 103°F (37°C to 39.4°C). Warning signs of heat exhaustion vary, but may include weakness, nausea, vomiting, syncope, tachycardia, tachypnea, muscle aches, headache, diaphoresis (heavy sweating), and flushed skin.
  - **Heat Stroke** occurs when the body's temperature regulation fails, usually when the hyperthermia progresses to a temperature above 103°F (39.4°C). Temperatures of 106°F (41.1°C) and higher may be reached.

For more information on heat exhaustion and heat stroke, see the Example Problem: Hyperthermia/Heat Stroke.

Example Problem: Hypothermia

The Centers for Disease Control and Prevention (CDC, 1988) defines *hypothermia* as an abnormally low core temperature, less than 95°F (less than 35°C). You must know the person's usual normal range of temperature because some people, especially older adults, have a normal temperature of less than 95°F. See the accompanying Example Problem: Hypothermia.

Practical Knowledge
knowing how

Now that you understand the concept of thermoregulation, you are ready to gain the practical knowledge of how to assess and support a client's body temperature.

ASSESSMENT NP

In our daily routines, we commonly assess temperature by touch. For example, you can use simple touch to detect fever, however, you cannot differentiate *degrees* of fever. Because vital signs are used as indicators of a client's health status, it is essential to have an accurate measure. To see the sequence of steps to take when measuring a patient's temperature, refer to Procedure 19-1.

Temperature Measurement Scales: Fahrenheit and Centigrade

Two scales are used for recording temperature: Fahrenheit and centigrade (or Celsius), a metric scale. Most people in the United States are familiar with the Fahrenheit scale; however, some healthcare agencies use centigrade.

- Electronic and tympanic membrane thermometers can usually measure temperature in either scale; often all you need to do is to flip a switch.
- Some types of thermometers only provide one scale (Fig. 19-4 shows both scales), so you may need to convert a reading from one scale to the other.
  - You may have a conversion app on your cell phone. If not, you can find conversion tools on the Internet.
- If you need to convert scales and do not have access to a conversion chart, you can use a mathematical formula.

EXAMPLE PROBLEM: Hyperthermia/Heat Stroke

Problem

Definition: The body temperature is dangerously high (103°F to 106°F, or 39.4°C to 41.1°C, or higher) and cannot promote heat loss fast enough to balance external temperatures or heat production. The body temperature is above normal and higher than the set point.

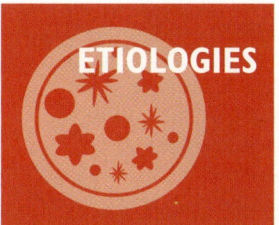

ETIOLOGIES

Prolonged exposure to hot environmental temperatures
Strenuous physical exertion in hot weather

Dehydration
Excessive alcohol intake in hot weather

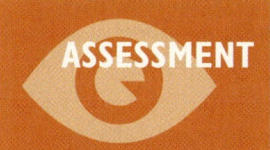

COMPLICATIONS

Untreated heat stroke can cause damage to the heart, brain, kidneys, and other vital organs, resulting in permanent disability and even death.

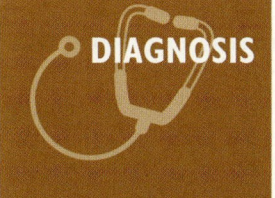

ASSESSMENT

Symptoms

The body is unable to sweat.
Rapid breathing; rapid, strong pulse; throbbing

Headache; delirium; confusion; slurred speech

Impaired judgment; lethargy; red, hot, dry skin; dizziness; seizures; coma

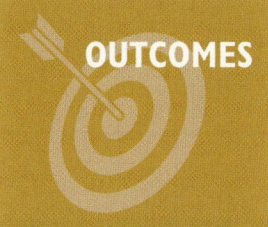

DIAGNOSIS

NANDA-I Nursing Diagnoses

- Deficient Fluid Volume—Decreased intravascular, interstitial, or intracellular fluid; refers to dehydration (water loss alone without change in sodium)
- Hyperthermia—Core body temperature above the normal range due to failure of thermoregulation

- Ineffective Thermoregulation—Temperature fluctuation between hypothermia and hyperthermia

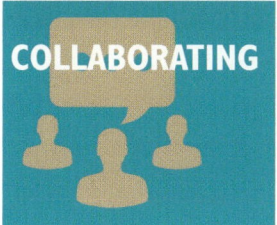

OUTCOMES

NOC Outcomes

Outcomes and goals will depend on the nursing diagnoses. Examples:
- Thermoregulation
- Vital Signs

Individualized Goals/Outcomes

- Body temperature 98.6°F (37°C)
- No damage to vital organs
- Good skin turgor
- No alterations in mental status (e.g., confusion)

COLLABORATING

- If treatments cause shivering, the provider may order a muscle relaxant.

- Administer antibiotics as prescribed if fever is caused by bacterial infections.

(Continued)

EXAMPLE PROBLEM: Hyperthermia/Heat Stroke—cont'd

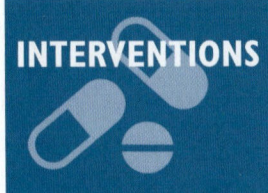

INTERVENTIONS

NIC Interventions

Outcomes and goals will depend on the nursing diagnoses. Examples are Fever Treatment, Temperature Regulation, and Vital Signs Monitoring.

Individualized Interventions

- Collect specimens (blood, sputum, urine) to determine the cause of the fever.
- Remove excess clothing.
- Provide cooling blankets that circulate water; cool at a controlled rate.
- Provide cool water mist on the skin with air fanned over the body.
- Provide cloth-covered ice packs or cool washcloths to the head, groin, neck, or axillae (arm pits).
- Instruct the client to use minimal bed covers. Keep clothing and bed linen dry to prevent chilling and shivering.
- Provide intravenous fluids to replace fluid loss and to prevent dehydration or hypovolemia.
- Provide appealing nutritional foods.
- Encourage good mouth care with a water-soluble lubricant to treat or prevent cracked lips, swollen tongue.
- Monitor temperature and vital signs at least every 2 hours.
- If outdoors, move person to a shady area.
- Provide cooling measures (e.g., place in cool bath tub, take cool shower, or sponge with cool water).

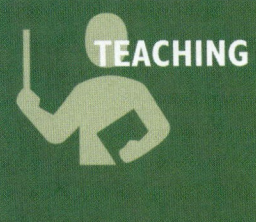

TEACHING

- Teach clients to:
  Wear loose-fitting, lightweight clothing.
  Drink plenty of fluids; avoid alcohol and caffeine.
  Avoid long periods of sun exposure in hot weather.
  Limit the amount of time working or exercising in hot weather.
- Teach signs of heat exhaustion (temperature up to 103°F [39.4°C], weakness, nausea, vomiting, syncope, tachycardia, tachypnea, muscle aches, headache, diaphoresis [heavy sweating], and flushed skin).
  - **Advise older adults to stay in air-conditioned buildings** when the outside temperature is extremely high; to take cool baths and showers; to limit physical activity; and to drink plenty of nonalcoholic and noncaffeinated fluids.
- **Advise family to check on elderly neighbors and family members** at least twice a day and make sure they have an electric fan.

 Although alcohol baths may be effective to reduce temperature, the topical application of large amounts of isopropyl alcohol can cause alcohol poisoning and toxicity in children and older adults (Smitherman, Janise, & Mathur, 2005; Thompson & Kagan, 2011)

EXAMPLE PROBLEM: Hypothermia

Definition

- A core body temperature of less than 95°F (< 35°C).
- As the body temperature drops, metabolic processes slow. Prolonged exposure to cold is no longer correctible by shivering and may prove fatal.

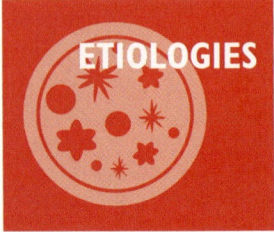

ETIOLOGIES

Caused by environmental exposure to extreme cold, drug intoxication, surgery, medically induced hypothermia, or metabolic or nervous system dysfunction (Meiman, Anderson, & Tomasallo, 2015)

EXAMPLE PROBLEM: Hypothermia—cont'd

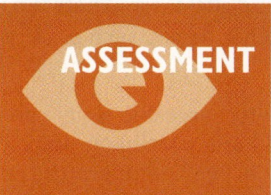

ASSESSMENT

- **Initial symptoms:** Cool skin, shivering, fatigue, confusion, loss of coordination, cyanosis of lips and fingers, decreased heart rate and respirations
- **Followed by:** Pain in the extremities, confusion, slowing of heart rate and respirations

- **Late symptoms:** Loss of ability to shiver; blue skin; dilated pupils; amnesia; hypotension; slow, impaired respirations; cardiac arrhythmias
- Death occurs when body temperature falls below 70°F to 75°F (21°C to 24°C). (Survival has been known to occur at a core temperature of 60.8°F [16°C], however.)

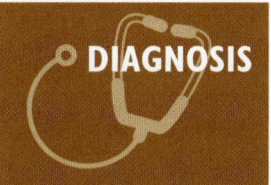

DIAGNOSIS

Hypothermia

Ineffective Thermoregulation

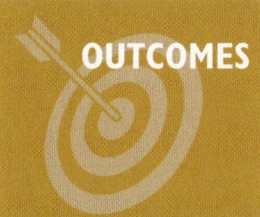

OUTCOMES

NOC Outcomes, Examples

- Thermoregulation
- Vital Signs
- Tissue Perfusion: Peripheral

Individualized Outcome Statements

- Oral temp > 97.6°F (or patient's baseline temp)
- Pulse and respiratory rates within normal limits.

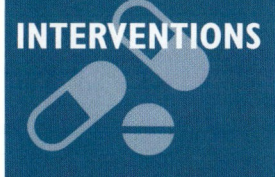

INTERVENTIONS

NIC Standardized Interventions and Activities

- Monitor vital signs
- Institute Warming Measures:
  - Move to a warm environment.
  - Remove cold, wet clothing.
  - Provide a warm bath or shower.
  - Apply head coverings, blanket, hot water bottle.
  - Warm the chest, neck, head, and groin areas first with external warming

  blankets or heating pads. Do not use electric blankets.
- Provide warm high carbohydrate beverages; avoid alcohol or caffeinated drinks.
- Monitor rate of rewarming. A severely hypothermic client should be rewarmed gradually.
- Monitor skin color and temperature.

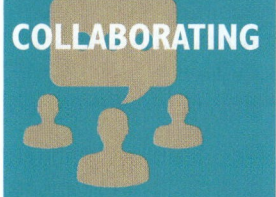

COLLABORATING

Administer warmed intravenous fluids as prescribed.

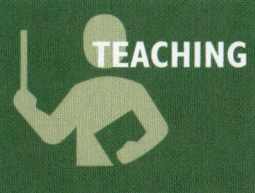

TEACHING

Teach Older Adults Ways to Prevent Hypothermia.

- Keep your home warm enough, at least 68°F to 70°F. Even mildly cool indoor temperatures of 60°F to 65°F can lead to hypothermia in older adults.
- Wear socks and slippers, long underwear under your clothes. Wear a hat or cap indoors.
- Cover your legs and shoulders with a blanket or afghan to keep warm.
- Wear a hat, scarf, and gloves or mittens when going outdoors in the cold. This

helps prevent loss of heat through your head and hands. A large portion of body heat can be lost through the head, so the cap is important.
- Dress in several layers of warm, loose clothing to trap warm air between the layers and keep in body heat. (National Institutes on Aging, 2010, updated 2016).

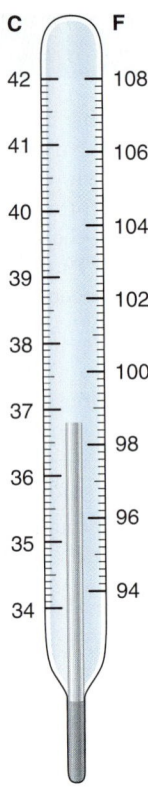

FIGURE 19-4 Some thermometers are available with degree markings in Fahrenheit or centigrade. *Left,* Centigrade scale. *Right,* Fahrenheit scale.

KEY POINT: *To convert from Fahrenheit to centigrade, subtract 32 from the Fahrenheit temperature and multiply by 5/9.*

  Example: A client has a temperature of 102°F. What is his temperature as measured in centigrade?

$$(102 - 32) \times 5/9 = (70 \times 5) \div 9 = 39°C$$

KEY POINT: *To convert a centigrade reading to Fahrenheit, multiply the centigrade temperature by 9/5, and add 32.*

  Example: A client has a temperature of 39°C

$$(39 \times 9/5) + 32 = (351 \div 5) + 32 = 102°F$$

What Equipment Do I Need?

Nurses measure temperature with various kinds of thermometers. Each type has advantages and disadvantages (see Table 19-3), so you need to think critically about the type of thermometer best suited for each client situation.

Glass Thermometers Historically, the thermometer was a mercury-filled glass tube marked in degrees and read visually. Researchers at Boston Children's Hospital found that children younger than 4 years of age suffered broken glass to the mouth or rectum, exposure to mercury, and/or required imaging to detect foreign objects in the body associated with the use of glass thermometers (Aprahamian, Lee, Shannon, et al., 2009). The U.S. Environmental Protection Agency and the American Hospital Association now advise against use of equipment containing mercury (U.S. Environmental Protection Agency [EPA], 2012). Most healthcare facilities have replaced glass-and-mercury thermometers with electronic digital thermometers or with glass thermometers containing other liquids, such as alcohol or gallium–indium–tin (galinstan).

Electronic Thermometers are rechargeable units consisting of an electronic probe attached to a portable unit by a thin wire. A beep sounds when the peak temperature is reached. The probe is covered with disposable plastic sheaths to prevent transmission of infection; the sheath is discarded after each use. Most units have a separate probe for rectal and oral temperatures, color-coded red and blue, respectively. Use the correct probe for each site.

Electronic Infrared Thermometers These rechargeable units contain a sensor that detects heat in the form of infrared energy given off by the body. The thermometer does not touch the actual sites (e.g., tympanic membrane, temporal artery). A beep sounds when the peak temperature is reached.

Disposable Chemical Thermometers A disposable chemical thermometer is a thin plastic strip, patch, or tape containing a matrix of chemicals that produces a color change at a designated body temperature. Most are used once for an oral or axillary reading and then discarded. Disposable thermometers are useful in the home and for patients in protective isolation. While measurements taken on children are as accurate as those done with electronic thermometers (Cincinnati Children's Hospital Medical Center, 2011), they may not be as accurate for adults (Barnason, Williams & Proehl, et al., 2012; Washington & Matney, 2008).

What Sites Should I Use?

You must choose the safest, most accurate, and most reliable site for each patient (Table 19-4). The sites for intermittent measurement are the mouth, rectum, axillae, tympanic membrane, and skin over the temporal artery. These sites allow the thermometer to contact body tissues that are well supplied with blood vessels, which is essential for accurate measurement.

Sites for Core Temperature Sites in the pulmonary artery, esophagus, and bladder accurately measure core temperature. These sites are used in surgery and intensive care, but they are invasive, expensive, and impractical for most clinical settings. Measurements from these sites require the use of specially designed thermometers and practitioners with advanced training. **KEY POINT:** *Pulmonary artery temperature is considered the gold standard with which other sites are compared.*

Temperature Variations at Different Sites Although research on site differences is conflicting, generally from lowest to highest readings, the sites are thought to be axillary, oral, tympanic membrane, rectal, and temporal artery. For axillary, oral, and rectal temperatures there is an approximately 0.8°F (0.4°C) difference between each site and the next higher one. For convenience, nurses tend to round the fraction up to a full 1°F (0.5°C). For example, an axillary temperature of 98.1°F is similar to an oral reading of 99.1°F or a rectal reading of 100.1°F.

Use this *only* to help you understand your patient's data. You cannot reliably convert temperatures mathematically between sites. When you measure a temperature, record the value you obtain and the site used.

Table 19-3 ➤ Advantages and Disadvantages of Various Thermometers

ADVANTAGES	DISADVANTAGES

Glass Thermometer

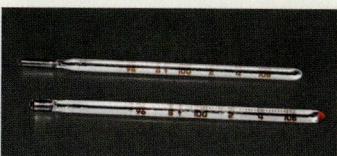

- Flexibility of use: Can be used for measuring oral, rectal, or axillary temperature.
- Inexpensive initial cost.
- Accuracy, as indicated by several studies.
- Easily disinfected.

➕ Do not use glass thermometers containing mercury. If you find one, recommend that it be replaced immediately.

- Easily broken, so there is ongoing cost of replacement and risk for injury. For this reason, glass is not recommended.
- Slow: It takes 3–8 min to obtain an accurate reading, depending on the site.
- Difficult for some people to read accurately.

Electronic Thermometer

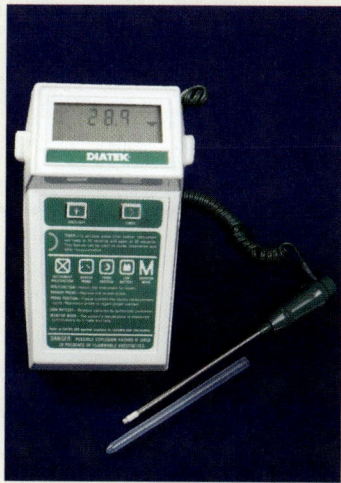

- Flexibility of use: Can be used for measuring oral, rectal, or axillary temperature.
- Ease of use.
- Rapid measurement: It takes 2–60 sec to obtain reading, depending on the unit.

- Expensive initial cost.
- Requires regular inspection and maintenance to ensure accuracy.
- Data are conflicting regarding their accuracy compared with other types of thermometers.
- Needs to be kept charged.

Electronic With Infrared Sensor

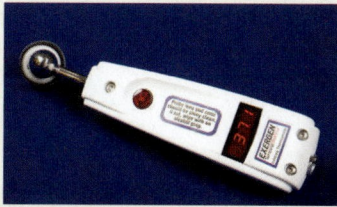

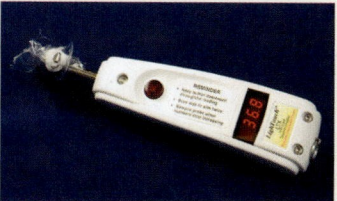

A, Temporal scanner   B, Otic thermometer

- Ease of use.
- Rapid measurement: It takes 2–5 sec to measure the temperature.

- Expensive initial cost.
- Less accurate than electronic or glass/plastic thermometers when used for tympanic membrane temperatures, as some studies indicate.

(Continued)

Table 19-3 ➤ Advantages and Disadvantages of Various Thermometers—cont'd

ADVANTAGES	DISADVANTAGES
■ May be the most cost-effective method because of time and labor savings from their rapid reading capabilities. ■ Low rate of operator error.	■ Requires regular inspection and maintenance to ensure accuracy. ■ Batteries require recharging.

Disposable Chemical Thermometer

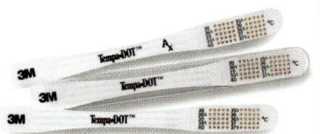 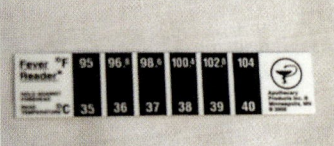

ADVANTAGES	DISADVANTAGES
■ Easy to use; requires no special training. ■ Equally as accurate as the electronic thermometer. ■ Less expensive than purchasing supplies for and maintaining an electronic thermometer. ■ Because it is disposable, it may prevent spread of infection among patients. ■ Recommended for measuring axillary temperature among pediatric patients over the age of 2 years (Cincinnati Children's Hospital Medical Center, 2011).	■ Less accurate/reliable than glass thermometers. ■ The skin must be dry. ■ Indicates only body surface temperature; does not reflect core. ■ Guidelines currently recommend only for pediatric patients.

Table 19-4 ➤ Disadvantages and Contraindications of Various Sites for Measuring Temperature

ADVANTAGES	DISADVANTAGES	CONTRAINDICATIONS
Temporal Artery		
■ Most accurate representation of core temperature. ■ Fast. Most scanners provide a reading in about 3 sec. ■ No discomfort is associated with the procedure. ■ Safe. Can be used even for those who cannot follow instructions (e.g., infants). ■ Less prone to error than tympanic thermometer.	■ Requires special scanning thermometer. ■ Any covering, hat, hair, etc., prevents heat from dissipating and causes the reading to be falsely high. This is also true for the side of the head lying on a pillow.	Not recommended for febrile adults and pediatric patients 0–3 months (National Guideline Clearinghouse, 2011).
Rectal		
■ Accurately represents core (internal) body temperature. ■ Use for clients who are unable to follow directions for oral temperature monitoring or in situations in which accuracy is crucial.	■ Most clients find this method objectionable or embarrassing. ■ ✚ Not recommended as the first choice of site because of the risk for injury to the rectal mucosa, especially infants. ■ Requires special positioning of the client.	■ ✚ Clients who may be injured by the method (e.g., clients who have a rectal disease, severe diarrhea, or rectal surgery; newborns, whose rectal mucosa is fragile).

Table 19-4 ➤ Disadvantages and Contraindications of Various Sites for Measuring Temperature—cont'd		
ADVANTAGES	**DISADVANTAGES**	**CONTRAINDICATIONS**
	■ Does not reflect changes in core temperature as soon as the oral method. ■ Presence of stool may cause inaccurate reading.	■ Clients with cardiac surgery and some heart conditions because this method can slow the heart rate by stimulating the vagus nerve. ■ Clients with hemorrhoids. ■ Immunosuppressed clients or those with clotting disorders.
Oral		
■ Simple, convenient. ■ Comfortable for most patients. ■ Safe for adults and children who are old enough to follow simple directions.	■ ✚ Glass thermometers can break if bitten. ■ Slow; requires up to 8 min to ensure an accurate reading (if glass thermometer used). ■ Patient must keep her mouth closed for several minutes (glass thermometers). ■ Eating, drinking (e.g., ice water, hot tea), and smoking in the 30 minutes before measurement affect the accuracy of the reading. ■ Bradypnea may create false temperature elevations.	■ ✚ Clients who cannot cooperate with the instructions or who might be injured (e.g., infants and small children; patients who have had oral surgery, breathe through the mouth, have chills, or are confused or unconscious).
Axillary		
■ Safe ■ Easy to use. ■ Can be used for children and for uncooperative or unconscious clients. ■ Recommended over rectal site for routine measurements.	■ Not reflective of core temperature. ■ Considered one of the least accurate sites. ■ Diaphoresis (sweating) can affect the reading. ■ Thermometer may need to be left in place for a long time (8 minutes if glass is used).	■ Clients who are perspiring heavily. ■ Does not accurately diagnose fever. If fever is suspected, confirm with measurement from another route.
Tympanic Membrane		
■ Fast (2–5 sec). ■ Can be used for children and for uncooperative or unconscious clients.	■ Requires a special thermometer, a relatively expensive initial purchase. ■ More variable than oral and rectal sites. ■ Must be carefully positioned to ensure accuracy; prone to caregiver measurement errors. ■ Presence of cerumen (earwax) may affect accuracy. ■ Significant differences have been found between readings in left and right ear of same patient. ■ Risk of injury to tympanic membrane if not positioned carefully to avoid touching it. ■ May be uncomfortable for the client. ■ Chemical thermometers (skin temperatures) have been found to be more accurate and reliable than tympanic membrane instruments. ■ Hearing aids must be removed.	■ ✚ Clients who have had recent ear surgery. ■ Contraindicated in the presence of ear infection.

(Continued)

ADVANTAGES	DISADVANTAGES	CONTRAINDICATIONS
Table 19-4 ▶ Disadvantages and Contraindications of Various Sites for Measuring Temperature—cont'd		
ADVANTAGES	DISADVANTAGES	CONTRAINDICATIONS
Skin (e.g., forehead)		
• Safe, convenient. • Easy to use for nonprofessionals. • Can be used when other sites are contraindicated. • Inexpensive (chemical paper or tape is used).	• Forehead skin temperature is generally 2°F–4°F (1°C–2°C) less than core temperature; if marked deviations in skin temperatures are detected, the readings must be confirmed via a more reliable route.	• Should not be used when accurate, reliable readings are required (e.g., in the presence of hypothermia or heatstroke). • Skin temperatures may be accurate and reliable when obtained with an infrared skin thermometer (DeCurtis, Calzolari, Marciano, et al., 2008).

ThinkLike a Nurse 19-2

- Convert the following temperatures and analyze the readings. What might they mean?
  a. 38.5°C _____ °F
  b. 96.5°F _____ °C
  c. 37.0°C _____ °F
- Rank the expected early evening temperatures of the following individuals from lowest to highest:
  a. A 22-year-old college athlete
  b. A 5-year-old kindergarten student
  c. An 88-year-old nursing home resident

ThinkLike a Nurse 19-3

Recall the clients in the Meet Your Patients scenario. Two-year-old Jason's axillary temperature was 101.8°F (38.8°C) and his skin was warm, dry, and flushed. His mother told you that he had been eating poorly and was very irritable.

- What changes in behavior alert you that something is wrong?
- Do you have enough theoretical knowledge or client information to know what is going on?
- What, if any, additional information about the client situation do you need?

PULSE

The concept of **perfusion** refers to the continuous supply of oxygenated blood through the blood vessels to all body cells. The **pulse** is the rhythmic expansion of an artery produced when a bolus of oxygenated blood is forced into it by contraction of the heart. How do you think the pulse affects perfusion? How might perfusion affect the pulse?

Theoretical Knowledge
knowing why

To assess and support regulation of a client's pulse, you will need to understand the concept of perfusion and know the normal pulse range, how the pulse is produced and regulated, and factors that influence pulse rate. An important reason to assess the pulse is to identify when more advanced monitoring is required.

What Is a Normal Pulse Rate?

Pulse rate is measured in beats per minute. The normal range for healthy young and middle-aged adults is 60 to 100 beats/min, with an average rate of 70 to 80 beats/min (see Table 19-1). Table 19-2 shows age-related variations for all vital signs, including pulse rate.

When the heart rate is of concern, you will most likely use a cardiac monitor to determine not only the rate but also the rhythm and intensity of the pulse.

How Does the Body Produce and Regulate the Pulse?

The pulse wave begins when the left heart ventricle contracts and ends when it relaxes. Each contraction forces blood into the already filled aorta, increasing pressure within the arterial system. The intermittent pressure and expansion of the arteries cause the blood to move along in a wave-like motion toward the capillaries. You can palpate a light tap at the peak of the wave, when the artery expands. The trough (low point) of a pulse wave occurs when the artery contracts to push the blood along its way.

- The **peak** of the wave corresponds to **systole,** or the contraction of the heart.
- The **trough** corresponds to **diastole,** or the resting phase of the heart.
- **Stroke volume** is the quantity of blood forced out by each contraction of the left ventricle. You will not usually know your patient's actual stroke volume, though it averages 70 mL in most healthy adults. If stroke volume decreases (as in a large blood loss, or *hemorrhage*), the body tries to maintain the same cardiac output by increasing the pulse rate.
- **Cardiac output** is the total quantity of blood pumped per minute. It is expressed in liters per minute and calculated as follows:

$$\text{Cardiac output} = \text{stroke volume} \times \text{pulse (heart) rate}$$

For a person with a pulse of 80 beats/min and an average stroke volume (70 mL), the cardiac output would be about 5,600 mL (or 5.6 L) per minute.

- **The autonomic nervous system** regulates the heart rate. Sympathetic stimulation increases the heart rate (and thus the cardiac output); parasympathetic stimulation decreases it. We discuss this in more detail in Chapter 38.

Toward Evidence Based Practice

Counts, D., Acosta, M., Holbrook, H., et al. (2014). Evaluation of temporal artery and disposable digital oral thermometers in acutely ill patients. *MEDSURG Nursing, 23*(4), 239–244, 250.

Research was conducted to evaluate the use of the disposable digital oral thermometer and the temporal artery thermometer as a replacement for the nondisposal digital oral thermometer. Forty-eight acutely ill patients were tracked over a 2-month period. Neither the digital disposable oral thermometer nor the temporal artery thermometer was an acceptable replacement based on the number of temperature differences, 21% and 44%, respectively.

Hamilton, P., Marcos, L., & Secic, M. (2013). Performance of infrared ear and forehead thermometer: A comparative study in 205 febrile and afebrile children. *Journal of Clinical Nursing, 22*, 2509–2518. doi:10.1111/jocn.12060

Researchers compared the precision and bias of the ear and temporal scan thermometers against the traditional and widely used "reference" thermistor-based contact thermometer. The ear thermometer had a lower rate of misclassifications when compared with the temporal artery thermometer. There was a threefold higher rate of false positives with the temporal scan thermometer. Researchers concluded that the ear thermometer was more consistent with measurements of the "reference" thermometer.

Wolfson, M., Granstrom, P., Pomarico, B., et al. (2013). Accuracy and precision of temporal artery thermometers in febrile patients. *MEDSURG Nursing, 22*(5), 297–302.

Researchers used an interrater reliability approach (two persons taking independent temperature measurements) to evaluate the accuracy of temporal artery thermometers on 34 postoperative patients over a 3-month period. The measurements were compared with the standard oral electronic thermometer. Both interrater reliability and the consistency between the temporal artery and oral thermometer were within the acceptable range. Researchers concluded that the temporal artery thermometer is an additional noninvasive method to accurately measure patients' temperatures.

Paes, B., Vermeulen, K., Brohet, R., et al. (2010). Accuracy of tympanic and infrared skin thermometer in children. *Archives of Disease in Childhood, 95*(12), 974–978.

Researchers evaluated the accuracy of the tympanic and infrared skin thermometers as alternatives to rectal temperature readings. In 100 hospitalized pediatric patients, the tympanic thermometer was less accurate than the rectal thermometer but was more accurate than the infrared skin thermometer.

1. Make a table containing the following:

   a. The name of the first researcher (e.g., Counts)

   b. The number and type of subjects in the study

   c. What each study found out about temperature measurements

2. Imagine that you are on a committee to make recommendations on the purchase of thermometers. Based on these studies, what recommendations would you make?

What Factors Influence the Pulse Rate?

In a healthy adult, the peripheral pulse rate is the same as the heart rate. Therefore, taking the pulse is a quick and simple way to assess the condition of the heart, blood vessels, and circulation. The pulse varies in response to:

- Changes in the volume of blood pumped through the heart
- Variations in heart rate
- Changes in the elasticity of the arterial walls
- Any condition that interferes with heart function.
- Impaired functioning of the nervous system. The heart and blood vessels are regulated by the nervous system, so conditions that interfere with normal functioning of the nervous system also affect the pulse.

Other factors that may cause variations in pulse rate, rhythm, or quality include the following:

- *Developmental level.* Newborns have a rapid pulse rate. The rate stabilizes in childhood and gradually slows through old age. The resting heart rate increases with age; however, variability decreases (Chester & Rudolph, 2011). Thus, you should not rely solely on changes in the pulse rate of older adults to detect their response to external stressors.

- *Gender.* Adult women have a slightly higher pulse rate than do adult men.
- *Exercise.* Muscle activity normally increases the pulse rate. After exercise, a well-conditioned heart returns to a normal rate more quickly. People who are well conditioned have lower heart rates, both before and during exercise, than those who are less conditioned.
- *Food intake.* Ingestion of a meal causes a slight increase in pulse rate for several hours.
- *Stress.* Stress triggers the fight-or-flight sympathetic nervous system response, which increases both pulse rate and strength of the heart contractions (stroke volume).
- *Fever.* The pulse rate tends to increase about 10 beats/min for each degree Fahrenheit of temperature elevation. The reasons are that (1) the metabolic rate increases and (2) in response to the fever, peripheral vasodilation occurs, causing a decrease in blood pressure. The body then causes the heart to beat faster to compensate for the decreased blood pressure.
- *Disease.* Diseases, such as heart disease, hyperthyroidism, respiratory diseases, and infections, are generally associated with increased pulse rates. Hypothyroidism is associated with decreased pulse rates.

- *Blood loss.* Small blood loss is generally well tolerated and produces only a temporary increase in pulse rate. Theoretically, a large blood loss stimulates the sympathetic nervous system, bringing about an increase in pulse rate to compensate for the decreased blood volume. However, research suggests that VS are limited in their ability to detect large blood losses; thus, a stable pulse and blood pressure are unreliable measures of the amount of loss.
- *Position changes.* Standing and sitting positions generally cause a temporary increase in pulse rate as a result of blood pooling in the veins of the feet and legs. This causes decreased blood return to the heart, decreasing blood pressure and subsequently increasing heart rate.
- *Medications.* Stimulant drugs (e.g., epinephrine) increase pulse rate. Cardiotonics (e.g., digitalis) and opioids (e.g., narcotic analgesics) or sedative drugs decrease pulse rate.

PracticalKnowledge
knowing **how**

Now that you understand some of the concepts and factors that produce the pulse, you are ready to learn the practical knowledge to assess and support this aspect of physical functioning.

ASSESSMENT NP

Assess the pulse by **palpation** (feeling) or **auscultation** (listening with a stethoscope). To palpate the pulse, select the pulse site and lightly compress the patient's artery against the underlying bone with your index and middle finger. When a patient's pulse is difficult to palpate, you may need to use a Doppler device, which has an ultrasound transducer that transmits the pulse sounds to an audio unit. For a summary of the steps for assessing a client's peripheral pulse, see Procedure 19-2.

What Equipment Do I Need?

To count the pulse, you need a watch or clock with a second hand or digital display. To auscultate the pulse, you will use a stethoscope. The stethoscope does not magnify sounds, but rather blocks out noise so that you can hear the heartbeat and other faint sounds.

- A **stethoscope** consists of a sound-transmitting device (bell and diaphragm), attached to earpieces by rubber tubing and hollow metal tubes (Fig. 19-5). Use the bell to hear low-frequency sounds (e.g., certain heart sounds); use the diaphragm to assess high-frequency sounds (e.g., lung sounds).
- **Stethoscopes can be either single lumen or double lumen.** A single-lumen stethoscope has one tube connected to the chestpiece; a double-lumen stethoscope has two tubes attached to the chestpiece. Double-lumen stethoscopes are more sensitive than single-lumen instruments.
- **Most stethoscopes come with soft earpieces** that help seal your ear canal to block room noise from interfering with the sound.
- **Stethoscopes have varying lengths of tubing.** Short tubing requires you to be close to the patient and to bend more, but the sound may be a bit better than with longer tubing, which is more likely to rub against the body or clothing. Some stethoscopes are made to work effectively through clothing; however, you should place the instrument directly on the skin unless you know you are using that type.

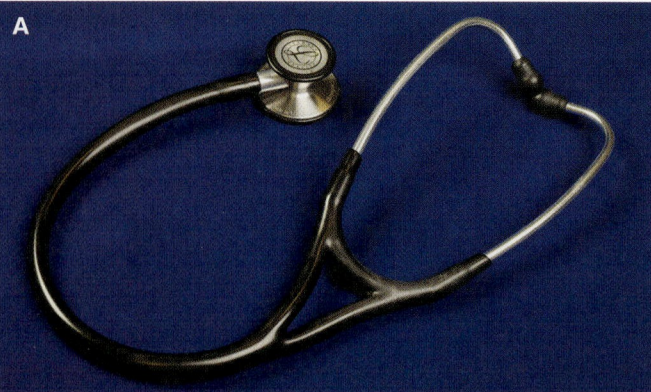

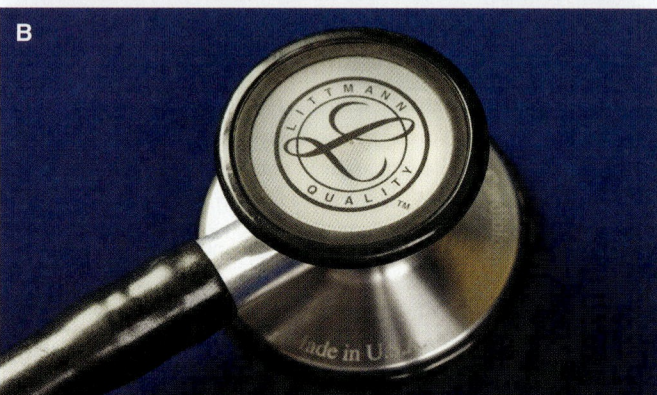

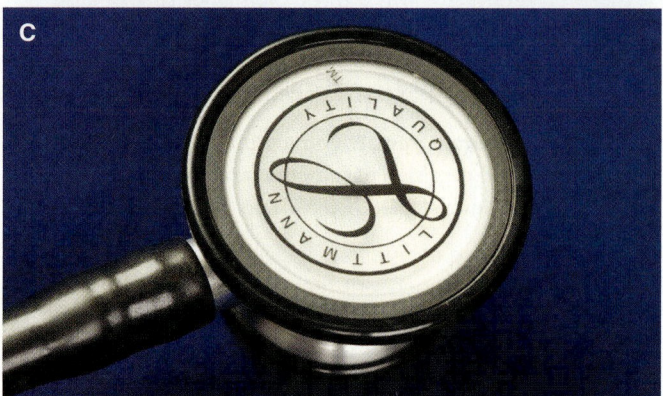

FIGURE 19-5 (A) A stethoscope. (B) The bell, for low-frequency sounds. (C) The diaphragm, for high-frequency sounds.

- **Digital stethoscopes** are also available to provide sound clarity in noisy environments, for obese patients, and for care providers who have impaired hearing.
- **To prevent injury,** do not wear a stethoscope around your neck.
- **To prevent cross-contamination,** always clean your stethoscope before and after using it to examine a patient. Use a 70% alcohol or benzalkonium chloride wipe. Bacteria colonize most stethoscopes, although not many are pathogenic. Cleaning can reduce the bacterial count by 94% to 100% (CDC, 2008; Rutala & Weber, 2004). Researchers found that the mean skin flora colony–forming unit on stethoscopes decreased from 27 prior to cleaning to 1 after cleaning (Mitchell, DeAlwis, Collins, et al., 2010). Similarly, subjects in the pre-cleaning group had bacterial growth on their stethoscopes compared with no bacterial growth in the post-cleaning group (Russell, Secrest, &

Schreeder, 2012). Antimicrobial stethoscope covers have been developed to prevent surface contamination; however, research has associated them with higher colony counts (Wood, Lund, & Stevenson, 2007).

What Sites Should I Use?

Nurses assess the pulse at the apex of the heart **(apical pulse)** or at a place where an artery can be pressed by the fingers against a bone **(peripheral pulses).** Peripheral sites are shown in Figure 19-6.

The choice of pulse site depends on the reason for assessing the pulse and/or the accessibility of a site. You would, for example, use the:

- *Radial artery* for routine assessment of vital signs. This is the most commonly used site because it is easily found and readily accessible.
- *Brachial artery* when performing cardiopulmonary resuscitation (CPR) of infants.
- *Carotid artery* during CPR of adults and for assessing circulation to the brain.
- *Temporal artery* when assessing circulation to the head or when other sites are not easily accessible.
- *Dorsalis pedis* (also called *pedal pulse*) and *posterior tibial arteries* for assessing peripheral circulation to the feet and legs.
- *Femoral artery* to determine circulation to the legs and for children.
- *Popliteal artery* for assessing circulation to the lower leg.

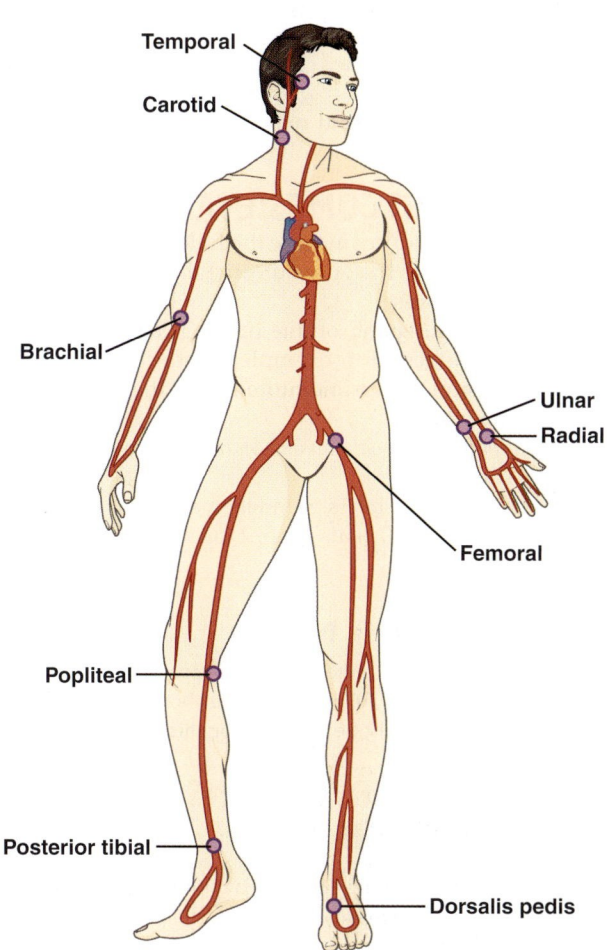

Temporal
Carotid
Brachial
Ulnar
Radial
Femoral
Popliteal
Posterior tibial
Dorsalis pedis

FIGURE 19-6 Sites commonly used for assessing a pulse.

ThinkLike a Nurse 19-4

- If you obtain a very slow radial pulse, how might you check to be sure your count is accurate?
- What kind of nursing knowledge does this require (i.e., theoretical, practical, self, or ethical)?

When Should I Take an Apical Pulse? The apical pulse reading is the most accurate of the pulses. In a healthy person, the apical and peripheral pulses should be about the same rate. However, in some cardiovascular diseases, they can differ. If the heartbeat is weak, for example, some beats may be too weak to feel in a peripheral site. In this case, you would obtain a lower count for the radial than for the apical pulse. Use the apical site when:

- The radial pulse is weak or irregular.
- The rate is less than 60 beats/min or greater than 100 beats/min.
- The patient is taking cardiac medications (e.g., digitalis).
- The patient is an infant or is a child up to age 3 (because peripheral pulses may be difficult to palpate).

For step-by-step instructions for assessing the apical pulse, refer to Procedure 19-3. For children, the location is different, depending on age (Fig. 19-7).

When Should I Take an Apical-Radial Pulse? You will sometimes need to obtain a radial and apical pulse reading at the same time to assess for heart function or the presence of heart irregularities. A difference between the two counts **(pulse deficit)** indicates that not all apex beats are being transmitted or felt at the radial artery. As you are listening at the apical site, you will hear a beat without feeling a pulse at the radial artery. You may detect a pulse deficit in conditions that interfere with peripheral perfusion, such as atrial fibrillation. You should promptly report pulse deficits to the primary care provider. See Procedure 19-4.

KnowledgeCheck 19-2

For each of the following, would you expect the pulse rate to be greater or less than the normal adult rate of 80 beats/min?

- A healthy, professional tennis player
- A newborn infant
- An adolescent who has just finished running track
- A client who has just undergone a painful procedure
- A client with a fever
- An accident victim who is hemorrhaging
- A 90-year-old man

What Data Should I Collect?

You will need data about three characteristics of the patient's pulse: rate, rhythm, and quality.

Pulse Rate

To assess the pulse **rate,** count the number of beats per minute while palpating or auscultating. Begin the count with one rather than zero (Hwu, Coates, & Lin, 2000). For normal healthy adults, you can determine the rate of a regular heart rhythm by counting the pulse for 15 seconds and multiplying the result by 4 or 30 seconds and then multiply by 2. If the pulse is irregular or slow, always count for 1 full minute. Table 19-1 identifies average pulse rates for adults, while Table 19-2 provides pulse rates for other age-groups.

Rates below 60 beats/min are known as **bradycardia** (*brady* = slow, *cardia* = heart). Rates over 100 beats/min are known as **tachycardia** (*tachy* = rapid, *cardia* = heart).

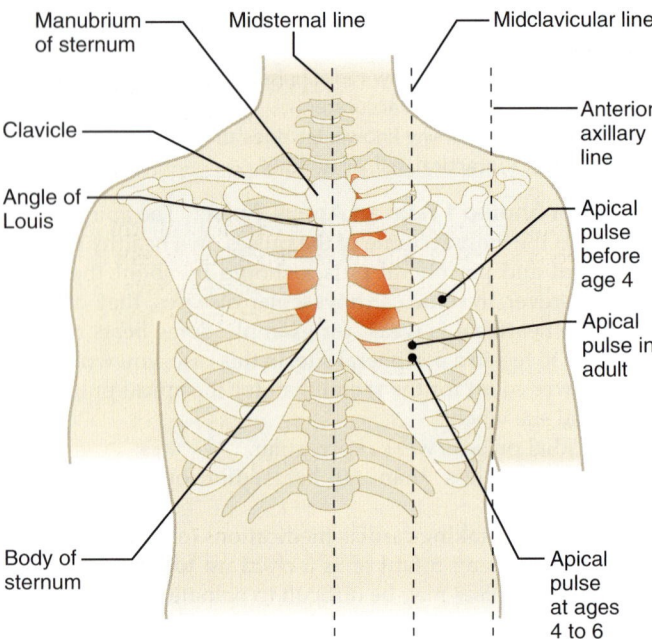

FIGURE 19-7 Location of apical pulse for adults and children.

Pulse Rhythm

The intervals between heartbeats establish a pattern known as the **rhythm.** Normally, the heart beats at regular intervals, much like a metronome. When the intervals between beats vary enough to be noticeable, the rhythm is abnormal **(dysrhythmia).** Abnormal rhythms may be single beats that occur too early or too late or a group of irregular beats that form a pattern.

When assessing an irregular pulse, it is important to determine whether the beat is *regularly irregular* (an irregular rhythm that forms a pattern) or *irregularly irregular* (an unpredictable rhythm). To make this distinction, you must count the rate for a full minute. An irregular heart rhythm can be very serious and may require additional assessment by **electrocardiogram (ECG),** a procedure that traces the electrical pattern of the heart.

Pulse Quality

The **quality** of the pulse is assessed by determining the pulse volume and bilateral (both sides) equality of pulses.

Pulse Volume refers to the amount of force produced by the blood pulsing through the arteries. Normally, the pulse volume for each beat is the same. The following terminology refers to pulse volume; the numbers are assigned on a scale of 0 to 3:

0—Absent: Pulse cannot be felt.
1—Weak (thready): Pulse is barely felt and can be easily obliterated by pressing with the fingers.
2—Normal quality: Pulse is easily palpated, not weak or bounding, obliterated by finger pressure.
3—Full: Pulse is easily felt with little pressure; not easily obliterated.
4—Bounding: Forceful, obliterated only by strong finger pressure.

Bilateral Equality is useful in determining whether the blood flow to a body part is adequate. Assess bilateral equality by comparing the pulses on both sides of the body for equal volume. For example, if you are concerned about the circulation to the left hand, assess both the right and left radial arteries to determine whether the volume is the same. If the pulses feel the same, they are said to be *equal in strength bilaterally.* If one pulse is stronger than the other, then the pulses are *unequal*

bilaterally. You would record, "Radial pulses unequal in strength bilaterally; weaker in left arm." Or you might use a pulse volume scale. For example, you could record, "Radial pulses unequal in strength bilaterally; Right 2, Left 1."

Absent or Weak Pulse If a peripheral pulse is absent or weak, it may be because the circulation is compromised in that extremity. Assess for pallor or cyanosis to confirm this.

- **Cyanosis** is a bluish or grayish discoloration of the skin resulting from deficient oxygen in the blood.
- **Pallor** refers to the paleness of skin in one area when compared with another part of the body. For example, when circulation to the lower extremities is compromised, the feet often appear pale in comparison with the trunk or arms, the dorsalis pedis and/or posterior tibial pulses may be weak or absent, and the feet may feel cool to the touch.

ANALYSIS/NURSING DIAGNOSIS NP

Pulse changes are symptoms, not problems. Therefore, nursing diagnoses are useful for describing the condition that is *causing* the pulse changes. By itself, a change in pulse (e.g., weak and thready) is not adequate to support the following diagnoses. Other symptoms must also be present.

- **Ineffective Tissue Perfusion (Peripheral)** can be used when a pulse is absent or weak and cool, pale skin is present.
- **Risk for Impaired Skin Integrity** and **Risk for Impaired Tissue Integrity** may be used as secondary diagnoses when Ineffective Tissue Perfusion is present. If tissue is not adequately perfused, tissue ischemia and *necrosis* (death of tissue) may occur.
- **Deficient Fluid Volume** may cause the pulse to be weak and thready.
- **Excess Fluid Volume** may cause the pulse to be bounding and full.
- **Decreased Cardiac Output** may cause tachycardia, bradycardia, or changes in pulse volume.

PLANNING OUTCOMES/EVALUATION NP

NOC standardized outcomes include the following:
- Vital Signs Status is the only outcome that directly pertains to assessing the pulse.
- Other outcomes depend on the nursing diagnosis causing the pulse changes. For example, Ineffective Peripheral Tissue Perfusion can be monitored with the NOC label of Circulation Status.

Some *individualized goal/outcome statements* you might write for pulse status follow:
- Apical pulse 60 to 80 beats/min when at rest.
- Pedal pulses 80 to 100 beats/min, 2 (on a scale of 0 to 3), and equal bilaterally.

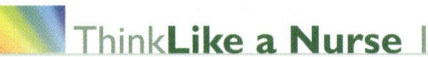

ThinkLike a Nurse 19-5

Did you notice that the pulse rates in the preceding two goals are not the same as the full normal range shown in Table 19-1? What do you think might be a reason for this?

PLANNING INTERVENTIONS/ IMPLEMENTATION NP

NIC standardized interventions include the following:
- Dysrhythmia Management—applies to monitoring an abnormal pulse
- Vital Signs Monitoring—may be used for general evaluation of clients who do not have an identified problem with the pulse

Specific nursing activities and focused assessments for a patient with a dysrhythmia depend on the cause of the problem and on specific orders from the physician. For example, a client with a pulse rate of 50 beats/min is usually considered to have bradycardia. However, such a slow resting heart rate would be perfectly normal for a well-trained athlete. Some dysrhythmias are *benign*; that is, they are not dangerous to the client, and they require no interventions. Nursing strategies that address dysrhythmias, regardless of cause, include the following:

- *Closely monitor the client's VS.* A reduced heart rate may alter blood pressure and tissue perfusion. The extent of intervention depends on the effect of the dysrhythmia on the client's other vital signs.
- *Monitor the client's activity tolerance.* Degree of activity, orientation, and level of fatigue while the dysrhythmia is present are indicators of the patient's ability to tolerate the dysrhythmia.
- *Collect and assess laboratory data as prescribed.* Cardiac function depends on normal electrolyte balance, particularly potassium, calcium, and magnesium levels. If a client is receiving medications that affect cardiac rhythm, serum levels of these medications must be checked periodically.
- *Help determine the cause of the dysrhythmia.* Determine when the client experiences the dysrhythmia. Are there precipitating or alleviating factors?
- *Administer antidysrhythmic medications* (if prescribed) at regular intervals to control the heart rhythm.
- ♥ **iCare** • *Provide emotional support.* The client experiencing a dysrhythmia may be frightened by the experience. Explain all procedures to the client, and maintain a calm presence. Family members may also be frightened. Be sure to include them in your explanations and teaching.

Think**Like a Nurse 19-6**

- Which of the following findings should be referred to the primary healthcare provider so that an ECG can be prescribed? Why?
  Patient A, who has a radial pulse of 100 beats/min, regular, and equal bilaterally
  Patient B, who has a regular apical pulse of 100 beats/min
  Patient C, who has a very irregular apical pulse of 78 beats/min
- Recall the clients in the Meet Your Patients scenario. Ms. Sharma is an active 80-year-old woman who works part-time and exercises four times per week. She is complaining of feeling tired. You find that her pulse is irregular and uneven.
  What other client data do you need to know? How would you go about getting this additional information?
  What actions should you consider taking while meeting with Ms. Sharma?
  What theoretical knowledge (rationale) supports your beliefs and actions?

RESPIRATION

Respiration is the exchange of oxygen and carbon dioxide in the body. The process of respiration has two aspects: mechanical and chemical.

- **Mechanical.** The mechanical aspects of respirations involve the active movement of air into and out of the respiratory system. This is known as **pulmonary ventilation** or, more commonly, *breathing.*

- **Chemical.** The chemical aspects of respiration include the following:
  External respiration—The exchange of oxygen and carbon dioxide between the alveoli and the pulmonary blood supply
  Gas transport—The transport of these gases throughout the body
  Internal respiration—The exchange of these gases between the capillaries and body tissue cells
  This chapter focuses on the mechanical aspects of respiration. Chapters 37 and 38 explore gas exchange and transport throughout the body.

Theoretical Knowledge
knowing **why**

To assess and support clients' respirations, you will need to know the normal range of respiratory rates, how respiration is regulated, the mechanics of breathing, and factors that affect respiration.

What Is a Normal Respiratory Rate?

Respiratory rate normally varies with age, exertion, emotions, and other factors. Normal adult respirations are identified in Table 19-1; Table 19-2 provides normal respiratory rates at other developmental stages.

How Does the Body Regulate Respiration?

Special respiratory centers in the medulla oblongata and pons of the brain, along with nerve fibers of the autonomic nervous system, regulate breathing in response to minute changes in the concentrations of oxygen (O_2) and carbon dioxide (CO_2) in the arterial blood. **KEY POINT:** *The primary stimulus for breathing is the level of CO_2 tension in the blood.*

- **Central chemoreceptors,** located in the respiratory centers, are sensitive to CO_2 and hydrogen ion (pH) concentrations. Minor increases in either stimulate respirations.
- **Peripheral chemoreceptors** are located in the carotid and aortic bodies. The partial pressure of oxygen in arterial blood (Pa_{O_2}) is normally between 80 and 100. When the Pa_{O_2} falls below normal, peripheral chemoreceptors stimulate respirations.

  Usually breathing is an involuntary action that requires little effort. However, it is possible to exert conscious control over respiration (e.g., a young child holding his breath during a temper tantrum; a person holding her breath when swimming).

What Are the Mechanics of Breathing?

Pulmonary ventilation depends on changes in the capacity of the chest cavity (Fig. 19-8).

Inspiration In response to impulses sent from the respiratory center along the phrenic nerve, the thoracic muscles and the diaphragm contract. The ribs move upward from midline ½ to 1 inch (1.2 to 2.5 cm), the diaphragm moves downward and out about 0.4 inch (1 cm), and the abdominal organs move downward and forward, expanding the thorax in all directions. As expansion causes airway pressure to decrease below atmospheric pressure, air moves into and expands the lungs. This stage of respiration (drawing air into the lungs) is termed **inspiration.**

Expiration When the diaphragm and thoracic muscles relax, the chest cavity decreases in size, and the lungs recoil,

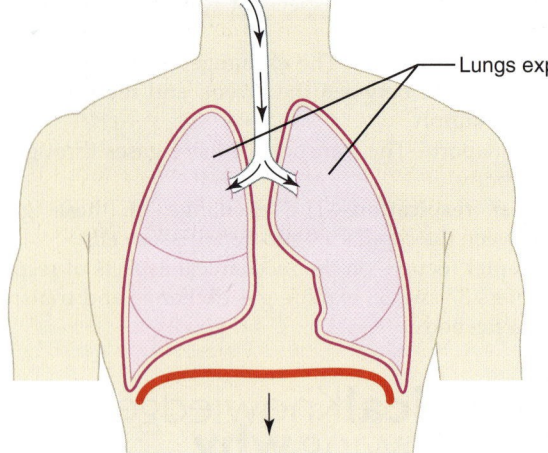

A   During inspiration (diaphragm contracting)

Lungs expand

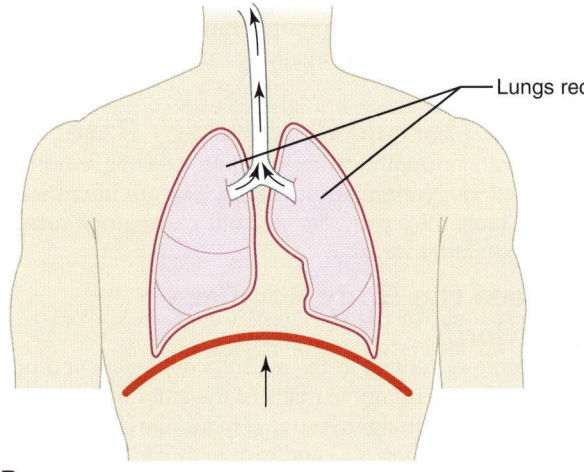

B   During expiration (diaphragm relaxing)

Lungs recoil

FIGURE 19-8 Changes in thoracic cavity during inspiration and expiration. (A) During inspiration. (B) During expiration.

forcing air from the lungs until the pressure within the lungs again reaches atmospheric pressure. This stage, which involves the expulsion of air from the lungs, is called **expiration.** Expiration is passive and normally takes 2 to 3 seconds, compared with 1 to 1.5 seconds for inspiration. During normal breathing, the chest wall and abdomen gently rise and fall.

KnowledgeCheck 19-3
- Which two gases are exchanged through respiration?
- Which respiratory process involves the movement of air into and out of the lungs?
- What is external respiration?
- What is the primary stimulus for breathing?
- What mechanical forces allow the lungs to expand?

What Factors Influence Respiration?
To interpret the meaning of your clients' respiratory data, you need to be aware of factors that influence breathing.
- *Developmental level.* A newborn's respiratory rate usually ranges from 40 to 60 breaths/min. However, some references give an upper limit of 90 breaths/min so long as it is for a short period of time (transient tachypnea). The rate gradually decreases until it reaches the normal adult rate

of 12 to 20 breaths per minute. The respiratory rate decreases slightly in older adults.

Respiration is often thought of as the forgotten vital sign (Parkes, 2011). However, research has shown that respiratory rates greater than 27 beats/min are highly predictive of adverse events in older adults (Chester & Rudolph, 2011). You must remember that an accurate measurement of respiratory rate is an essential component of the assessment of older adults.
- *Exercise.* Muscular activity causes a temporary increase in respiratory rate and depth to increase oxygen availability to the tissues and to rid the body of excess carbon dioxide.
- *Pain.* Acute pain causes an increase in respiratory rate but a decrease in depth.
- *Stress.* Psychological stress, such as anxiety or fear, may markedly influence respiration as a result of sympathetic stimulation. The most common change is an increase in rate.
- *Smoking.* Chronic smoking increases resting respiratory rate as a result of changes in airway compliance (elasticity).
- *Fever.* When heart rate increases because of fever, respiratory rate also increases. For every 1°F (0.6°C) the temperature rises, the respiratory rate may increase up to 4 breaths/min.
- *Hemoglobin.* Respiratory rate and depth increase as a result of anemia (reduced hemoglobin), sickle cell anemia (abnormally shaped red blood cells), and high altitudes. When hemoglobin is decreased or abnormal, the rate and depth of respirations, as well as the heart rate, may increase to maintain adequate tissue oxygenation. High altitudes inhibit the binding of oxygen to hemoglobin and trigger similar compensation efforts.
- *Disease.* The rate of breathing may be increased or decreased by various diseases. For example, brainstem injuries and increased intracranial pressure may interfere with the respiratory center, inhibiting respirations or altering respiratory rhythm.
- *Medications.* Central nervous system depressants, such as morphine or general anesthetics, cause slower, deeper respirations. Caffeine and atropine can cause shallow, fast breathing.
- *Position.* Standing up maximizes respiratory depth; lying flat reduces respiratory depth. Slumping (sitting with shoulders forward and the back curved in a C shape) prevents chest expansion, which impedes breathing.

ThinkLike a Nurse 19-7
Consider the following client situations. What effect would they have on respirations?
- A client with four fractured ribs
- A woman who is 9 months pregnant
- A young child excited at her birthday party
- An adult who has consumed alcoholic beverages

PracticalKnowledge knowing how

Although the adequacy of external and internal respiration is assessed in various ways, it is pulmonary ventilation (breathing) that you assess as a vital sign. Accurate assessment of respirations depends on your ability to recognize normal breathing, abnormal breathing, and factors that affect breathing. This chapter discusses only assessment of respirations.

For nursing diagnoses, outcomes, and interventions for respiratory problems, see Chapter 37.

ASSESSMENT NP

Because people can control their breathing rate, it is best to count respirations when the client is unaware of what you are doing. One way to do this is to palpate and count the radial pulse, and then count the respirations before removing your fingers from the client's wrist. To learn this skill, see Procedure 19-5.

What Equipment Do I Need?
- For measuring respiratory rate—a watch with a second hand or digital display
- For auscultating respirations—a stethoscope
- Many electronic thermometers have counter displays and signals that indicate 15-, 30-, and 60-second time intervals for counting respirations.

What Data Should I Obtain?

In addition to measuring the respiratory rate, you will also observe indicators of overall respiratory function, including depth, rhythm, and effort, among others. For additional information on respiratory assessment, see Chapter 21 and Procedure 21-12.

Respiratory Rate

The **respiratory rate** is the number of times a person breathes (or completes a cycle of inhalation and exhalation) within 1 full minute. You can easily count and observe respirations by:
- Placing your hand on the client's chest (palpating) or observing (inspecting) the number of times the client's chest or abdomen rises (inspiration) and falls (expiration)

- Placing your stethoscope on the client's chest (auscultation) and counting the number of inhalation and exhalation cycles

KEY POINT: *For a new patient or when you need to ensure accuracy, you must count for 60 seconds (Morton & Rempher, 2012; Vital Signs, 1999).* In some situations, for example, for a patient you know well and for whom respiratory rate is not directly relevant to the assessment, you may count for only 30 seconds and multiply by 2. If respirations vary from normal, you should count for 1 minute by auscultation. Normal adult respirations are identified in Table 19-1. Table 19-2 includes normal rates for other developmental stages.

A person can tolerate **apnea,** cessation of breathing, for only a few minutes. If apnea continues for more than 4 to 6 minutes, brain damage and even death can occur. See Table 19-5 for terminology to describe respiratory rhythms.

Respiratory rate is a measure of the client's general condition, but rate alone is not a good indicator of the adequacy of respiration. You must also assess other characteristics of the respirations.

Respiratory Depth

Tidal volume is the amount of air taken in on inspiration—about 300 to 500 mL for a healthy adult. Specialized equipment is required to measure tidal volume. However, you can estimate the adequacy of tidal volume by observing the depth of a client's respirations. This is a subjective evaluation of how much or how little the chest or abdomen rises during breathing. Respiratory depth is described as *deep* (taking in a very large volume of air and fully expanding one's chest or abdomen), *shallow* (when the chest barely rises and is difficult to observe), or *normal* (between shallow and deep).

Table 19-5 ▶ Respiratory Rates and Rhythm		
TYPE	**DESCRIPTION**	**ILLUSTRATION**
Eupnea	Normal respirations, with equal rate and depth, 12–20 breaths/min	
Bradypnea	Slow respirations, < 10 breaths/min	
Tachypnea	Fast respirations, > 24 breaths/min, usually shallow	
Kussmaul's Respirations	Respirations that are regular but abnormally deep and increased in rate	
Biot's Respirations	Irregular respirations of variable depth (usually shallow), alternating with periods of apnea (absence of breathing)	
Cheyne-Stokes Respirations	Gradual increase in depth of respirations, followed by gradual decrease and then a period of apnea	
Apnea	Absence of breathing	

Respiratory Rhythm

Rhythm is assessed simply as *regular* or *irregular*. Generally, the period between each respiratory cycle is the same, and there is a regular breathing pattern (see Eupnea in Table 19-5). Infant breathing rhythms are more likely to be irregular than adult rhythms. An abnormal breathing pattern may indicate other healthcare problems and deserves further assessment. Two abnormal breathing patterns, Cheyne–Stokes and Biot's breathing, are discussed in Chapter 37.

Respiratory Effort

Respiratory effort refers to the degree of work required to breathe. Normal breathing is effortless. When diseases such as asthma or pneumonia are present, the person must work harder to breathe.

- **Dyspnea** is increased effort with breathing or labored breathing. It is uncomfortable for the client and frequently produces fatigue and fear.
- **Orthopnea** is difficulty or inability to breathe when in a horizontal position. You will observe this in some clients with respiratory or cardiac conditions.

Breath Sounds

You will use a stethoscope to listen for breath sounds. Normal respirations are quiet. Abnormal (adventitious) sounds include the following:

- **Wheezes** are high-pitched, continuous musical sounds, usually heard on expiration. They are caused by narrowing of the airways and can often be heard without a stethoscope.
- **Rhonchi** are low-pitched, continuous gurgling sounds caused by secretions in the large airways. They often clear with coughing.
- **Crackles** are caused by fluid in the alveoli. They are discontinuous sounds usually heard on inspiration, but they may be heard throughout the respiratory cycle. They may be high-pitched, popping sounds or low-pitched, bubbling sounds, and they have been described as being similar to the sound made by rubbing strands of hair together with the fingertips.
- **Stridor** is a piercing, high-pitched sound that is heard without a stethoscope, primarily during inspiration in infants who are experiencing respiratory distress or in someone with an obstructed airway.
- **Stertor** refers to labored breathing that produces a snoring sound. It is common with mouth breathing due to nasal congestion. The "death rattle" is a type of stertorous breathing.

  See Chapter 21 for further discussion of abnormal breath sounds.

Chest and Abdomen Movement

The chest or abdomen normally rises with inspiration and falls with expiration in a gentle and rhythmic pattern. When a person is having difficulty moving air into or out of the lungs, respiratory patterns change.

- **Intercostal retraction** refers to the visible sinking of tissues around and between the ribs that occurs when the person must use additional effort to breathe.
- **Substernal retraction** exists when tissues are drawn in beneath the sternum (breastbone).
- **Suprasternal retraction** exists when tissues are drawn in above the clavicle (shoulder girdle).

Associated Clinical Signs

When you assess respiration, it is important to assess for clinical signs of oxygenation and perfusion.

- **Hypoxia**—Signs of **hypoxia** (inadequate cellular oxygenation) include pallor or cyanosis, restlessness, apprehension, confusion, dizziness, fatigue, decreased level of consciousness, tachycardia, tachypnea, and changes in blood pressure.
  - When evaluating cyanosis, the tongue and oral mucosa are the best indicators of hypoxia.
  - Cyanosis of the nails, lips, and skin may be caused by hypoxia but may also be related to cold or reduced circulation in that area.
  - Chronic hypoxia causes **clubbing** (loss of the nail angle) of the fingers.
- **Cough**—A **cough** is a forceful or violent expulsion of air during expiration. Coughs may be symptoms of allergic reactions, lung disease, respiratory infection, or heart conditions
  - Coughs may be *constant* (occurring frequently and consistently) or *intermittent* (occurring occasionally).
  - The cough is **productive** if secretions are expectorated (coughed up). The cough is **nonproductive** or **dry** if no secretions are produced,
  - A **hacking cough** is a series of dry coughs that occur together, whereas a **whooping cough** is a sudden, periodic cough that ends with a whooping sound on inspiration.

KnowledgeCheck 19-4

- How can you estimate a client's tidal volume?
- What is the range of normal for an adult's respiratory rate?
- Besides the rate, what other characteristics of a client's respirations should you observe?
- What are some common clinical signs associated with poor oxygenation?

Arterial Oxygen Saturation

The rate, quality, and depth of the respirations are indicators of the general health of the respiratory system. However, they do not measure the amounts of oxygen and carbon dioxide present in the blood—information that is essential for evaluating the effectiveness of respiratory effort. Two methods exist to measure O_2 and CO_2 blood levels. One method is invasive; the other is not.

- **Arterial blood gas (ABG) sampling** directly measures the partial pressures of oxygen and carbon dioxide and blood pH, the gases in the arterial blood. This method requires the puncture of an artery followed by laboratory testing of the sample. It provides comprehensive data, but it is invasive, painful, time consuming, and relatively expensive. If you need more information about this diagnostic test, consult a medical–surgical nursing or laboratory tests text.
- **Pulse oximetry** is a noninvasive method of monitoring oxygenation with a device that measures **oxygen saturation** (an indication of the oxygen being carried by hemoglobin in the arterial blood). The oximeter emits light, and a photosensor placed on the client's finger or earlobe measures the light passing through the site and calculates a pulse saturation (SpO_2) that is a good estimate of arterial oxygen saturation. The only risk in pulse oximetry is that clinicians may become too dependent on it or trust erroneous readings. Do not neglect the other aspects of holistic respiratory assessment. In many situations oxygen

saturation is monitored routinely along with the other vital signs. To learn how to apply a pulse oximeter, see Procedure 37-2.

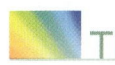

ThinkLike a Nurse 19-8

- Mrs. Dowell has smoked two packs of cigarettes per day for 45 years. She has recently been diagnosed with pneumonia—an infection of the lungs. What VS assessments would be important for Mrs. Dowell, and why?
- Recall the clients in the Meet Your Patients scenario. Mr. Jackson is short of breath and struggling to breathe. His respiratory rate is 28 breaths/min. What else do you need to know about the client situation? What is important and what is not important in this scenario? What is probably least important?

ANALYSIS/NURSING DIAGNOSIS NP

As noted earlier, *hypoxia* refers to inadequate cellular oxygenation. It results from decreased oxygen intake, decreased ability of tissues to remove oxygen from blood, impaired ventilation or perfusion, impaired gas exchange between the blood and alveoli, or inadequate levels of hemoglobin. The following are two common alterations in respiration:

- **Hyperventilation** occurs when rapid and deep breathing result in excess loss of CO_2 **(hypocapnia).** A client who is hyperventilating may complain of feeling lightheaded and tingly. Causes of hyperventilation include anxiety, infection, shock, hypoxia, drugs (e.g., aspirin, amphetamines), diabetes mellitus, or acid–base imbalance.
- **Hypoventilation** occurs when the rate and depth of respirations are decreased and CO_2 is retained or alveolar ventilation is compromised. Hypoventilation may be related to chronic obstructive pulmonary disease, general anesthesia, impending respiratory failure, or other conditions that result in decreased respirations.

Two nursing diagnoses commonly used to describe various respiratory problems are Impaired Gas Exchange and Ineffective Breathing Patterns. For a more complete list, see Chapter 37.

BLOOD PRESSURE

Blood pressure (BP) is the pressure of the blood as it is forced against arterial walls during cardiac contraction.

- **Systolic pressure** is the peak pressure exerted against arterial walls as the ventricles contract and eject blood.
- **Diastolic pressure** is the minimum pressure exerted against arterial walls, between cardiac contractions when the heart is at rest.

Adequate blood pressure is essential for healthy tissue perfusion and is an important indicator of overall cardiovascular health. Blood pressure is measured in millimeters of mercury (mm Hg) and is recorded as systolic pressure over diastolic pressure (e.g., 110/74 mm Hg).

Pulse Pressure is the difference between the systolic and diastolic. For a BP of 120/80 mm Hg, the pulse pressure is 40 mm Hg. It is an indication of the volume output of the left ventricle. Generally, the pulse pressure should be no greater than one-third of the systolic pressure, as in the example of a BP of 120/80 mm Hg, with a pulse pressure of 40 ($1/3 \times 120 = 40$).

KnowledgeCheck 19-5

- For a client whose BP is 150/80 mm Hg, what is the pulse pressure?
- Is that normal? If so, explain. If not, what should the pulse pressure be?

TheoreticalKnowledge knowing **why**

To assess and support clients' blood pressure, you will need to understand how the concepts of systolic and diastolic blood pressure contribute to **tissue perfusion.**

1. Contraction of the heart (systolic pressure) forces a bolus of oxygenated blood into the arterial circulation to provide a continuous supply of oxygen to all body cells *(perfusion).*
2. The heart then rests and refills with blood (diastolic pressure), which is pumped out to the tissues.
3. Any factor that interferes with this cycle can cause impaired tissue perfusion.

You will also need to know that an expert panel has classified as "normal" a systolic BP below 120 and a diastolic BP below 80 (Table 19-6) (Joint National Committee on Prevention, Detection, Evaluation, and Treatment of High Blood Pressure, 2004). You will learn in this section how to classify BP readings, how the body regulates blood pressure, and what factors affect the blood pressure.

How Does the Body Regulate Blood Pressure?

Blood pressure regulation is a highly complex process. It is influenced by three factors: cardiac function, peripheral vascular resistance, and blood volume. The body constantly regulates and adjusts arterial pressure to supply blood to body tissues via perfusion of the capillary beds. For in-depth discussion, see Chapter 38.

Cardiac Function

Recall that *cardiac output* is the volume of blood pumped by the heart per minute, and that it reflects the functioning of the heart. An increase in cardiac output causes an increase in BP; a decrease in cardiac output causes a decrease in BP (if all other factors remain the same). A change in either stroke volume or heart rate alters cardiac output.

Increased Stroke Volume Conditions that increase cardiac output by increasing stroke volume include the following:

- Increased blood volume (e.g., as occurs during pregnancy)
- More forceful contraction of the ventricles (e.g., as occurs during exercise)

Decreased Stroke Volume Conditions that decrease cardiac output by decreasing stroke volume include the following:

- Dehydration
- Active bleeding
- Damage to the heart (as seen after myocardial infarction, or heart attack)
- A very rapid heart rate (up to a point). While an increase in heart rate increases cardiac output, a very rapid heart rate limits the time allotted for the ventricles to fill, resulting in decreased stroke volume and, ultimately, decreased cardiac output.

Table 19-6 ➤ Classification of Adult Blood Pressure*

CATEGORY	SYSTOLIC (mm Hg)		DIASTOLIC (mm Hg)	FOLLOW-UP
Normal	< 120	and	< 80	Encourage lifestyle modification if there are risk factors. Recheck in 1–2 years or sooner if there are risk factors.
Elevated	120–129	or	< 80	Encourage lifestyle changes. Recheck in 3-6 months of nonpharmacologic therapy.
Stage I Hypertension	130–139	or	80–89	Low atherosclerotic cardiovascular disease (ASCVD): Encourage lifestyle changes. Recheck in 3-6 months of nonpharmacologic therapy. **High ASCVD**: Manage with both nonpharmacologic and antihypertensive drug therapy with repeat BP in 1 month.
Stage II Hypertension	≥ 140	or	≥ 90	Evaluation by a primary care provider within 1 month of diagnosis; treat with nonpharmacologic therapy and two different classes of antihypertensive drugs. Recheck BP in one month.

Note: If SBP and Diastolic fall within two categories, classify based on the higher category.
Source: Data from the 2017 Guideline for the Prevention, Detection, Evaluation, and Treatment of High Blood Pressure in Adults, an update of the 2003 Seventh Report of the Joint national Committee on Prevention, Detection, Evaluation and Treatment of High Blood Pressure. (2017). Whelton, P., Carey, R., Arownow, W., et al., (2018). 2017 ACC/AHA/AAPA/ABC/ACPM/AGS/APhA/ASH/ASPC/NMA/PCNA Guideline for the Prevention, Detection, Evaluation, and Management of High Blood Pressure in Adults. *Journal of the American College of Cardiology*, 71(19), e127-e248. DOI: 10.1016/j.jacc.2017.11.006. Retrieved on September 23, 2018 from, http://www.onlinejacc.org/content/71/19/e127?_ga=2.117871433.119615486.1537818239-291529677.1537536713 Ühobanian, A., Bakris, G., Black, H., et al. (2003). Seventh Report of the Joint National Committee on Prevention, Detection, Evaluation, and Treatment of High Blood Pressure. *Hypertension*, 42(6), 1206–1252.
*For adults aged 18 and older, based on the average of two or more readings taken at each of two or more visits after an initial screening.

Peripheral Resistance

Peripheral resistance refers to arterial and capillary resistance to blood flow as a result of friction between blood and the vessel walls. Increased peripheral resistance creates a temporary increase in BP. The amount of friction or resistance depends on blood **viscosity** (thickness), arterial size, and arterial **compliance** (elasticity). The walls of the veins are thin and very distensible, so they have little influence on peripheral resistance and BP.

- **Blood Viscosity.** Blood viscosity influences the ease with which blood flows through the vessels. Viscosity is determined by the **hematocrit** (the percentage of red blood cells in plasma). Any disorder that increases hematocrit (e.g., dehydration) increases blood viscosity and, therefore, BP. Conversely, a low hematocrit, as seen in anemia, lowers viscosity and may reduce BP.
- **Arterial Size.** The smaller the radius of a blood vessel, the more resistance it offers to blood flow. Constricted arteries prevent the free flow of blood and, subsequently, increase BP. Dilated arteries allow unrestricted flow of blood, thereby reducing blood pressure. The sympathetic nervous system controls vasoconstriction and vasodilation.
- **Arterial Compliance.** Arteries with good elasticity can distend and recoil easily and adequately. When age- or disease-related changes in arterial structure cause a loss of elasticity, peripheral resistance, and possibly BP, increase. **Arteriosclerosis** (hardening of the arteries) is a common contributor to increased BP in middle-aged and older adults.

Blood Volume

The normal volume of blood in the body is about 5 liters (5,000 mL). A significant loss of blood, as occurs with hemorrhage, reduces vascular volume, and BP falls. When vascular volume is increased above the norm, as occurs with renal (kidney) failure and fluid retention, BP increases.

What Factors Influence Blood Pressure?

KEY POINT: *Blood pressure normally changes from minute to minute with changes in activity or changes in body position. Therefore, you must establish BP patterns rather than relying on individual BP readings when determining whether a client's BP is normal or abnormal.* This is even more important for older adults because their BP tends to fluctuate even more. The following are some factors that affect the BP:

- **Developmental Stage.** An average newborn has a systolic BP of about 60 to 80 mm Hg and a diastolic BP of 40 to 50 mm Hg (Lowdermilk, Perry, Cashion, et al., 2016). It increases gradually throughout childhood. A child's or adolescent's BP depends on body size; therefore, a smaller child or adolescent has a lower blood pressure than does a larger child or adolescent. Both systolic and diastolic BP continue to increase with age as a result of decreased arterial compliance and changes in the left ventricular wall. These normal aging process changes can lead to cardiovascular instability (Lange, 2012).
- **Gender.** The average BP for men is slightly higher than that for women of comparable age. After menopause, a woman's BP tends to increase, possibly due to a decrease in estrogen.
- **Family History.** A family history of hypertension markedly increases the likelihood of an individual's developing hypertension.
- **Lifestyle.** Increased sodium consumption, smoking, and consumption of three or more alcoholic drinks per day have been shown to elevate BP. Caffeine may raise BP for a short while after ingestion, but it has no long-term effect on the BP.
- **Exercise.** Physical fitness has been shown to reduce BP in many individuals. However, muscular exertion temporarily increases BP as a result of increased heart rate and cardiac output. You should, therefore, wait about 30 minutes before you assess the BP of someone who has been physically active.

- **Body Position.** BP is higher when a person is standing than when she is sitting or lying down. Readings are higher if taken with the client's arm above heart level or if the arm is unsupported at the client's side. Seated readings are higher if the client's feet are dangling rather than resting on the floor or if the legs are crossed at the knees.
- **Stress.** Fear, worry, excitement, and other stressors cause BP to rise sharply because of sympathetic nervous system stimulation (fight-or-flight response). For example "white-coat hypertension" occurs when a patient's BP is elevated in the provider's office or clinic—a situation in which he is likely to experience stress—but not at other times. However, if BP is consistently elevated with stress, treatment may be indicated.
- **Pain.** Pain often causes an increase in BP. However, severe or prolonged pain can significantly decrease BP.
- **Race.** African Americans have a higher rate of hypertension and related complications than do European Americans (McCance & Heuther, 2014).
- **Obesity.** As a rule, obesity increases BP due to (1) the additional vascular supply required to perfuse the large body mass and (2) the resultant increase in peripheral resistance.
- **Diurnal Variations.** Generally, BP varies according to the person's daily schedules and routines. BP is lower while the person is sleeping and upon wakening, rising during the day and dropping again toward bedtime.
- **Medications.** Many medications alter BP. This effect may be intended, as with antihypertensive medications, or unintended, such as the drop in BP that often results when a client receives pain medication. Many over-the-counter preparations, herbal products, and illicit drugs can affect BP.

➕ Teach your client to consult with a pharmacist to identify the effect these products can have when taken with regularly prescribed medications.

- **Diseases.** BP may be affected by diseases that affect the circulatory system or any of the major organs of the body (e.g., the kidneys).
- **Genetic Variations/Genes.** Researchers used the recognized 29 genetic variants known to influence systolic and diastolic blood pressure to develop a genetic risk score. Twenty-nine percent of people with the top 10% of genetic risks had hypertension compared with 16% in the lowest risk groups (National Institutes of Health, 2011).

Think**Like a Nurse** 19-9

- Evaluate the following adult blood pressures. Are they high, low, or normal?
  116/90 mm Hg
  80/50 mm Hg
  184/102 mm Hg
  140/90 mm Hg
  40/0 mm Hg
- What theoretical knowledge did you use to evaluate the blood pressures?

PracticalKnowledge
knowing **how**

Now that you understand the concept of perfusion and how blood pressure is maintained and regulated, you are ready to gain practical knowledge of how to assess and support this aspect of physical functioning.

ASSESSMENT NP

Blood pressure may be assessed directly or indirectly.

Direct Method In the *direct method*, a catheter is threaded into an artery under sterile conditions and attached to tubing that is connected to an electronic monitoring system. The pressure is constantly displayed as a waveform on the monitor screen. This method is very accurate and is mostly used in critical care and surgery because of the risk of sudden arterial blood loss.

Indirect Method Usually, you will measure BP via the *indirect*, or *noninvasive, method*. This provides an accurate estimate of arterial BP that can be performed in any setting. For a procedure for noninvasive blood pressure monitoring, see Procedure 19-6.

What Equipment Do I Need?

You will need a stethoscope, a blood pressure cuff and sphygmomanometer, or an electronic blood pressure monitor. Electronic monitoring is gradually replacing the stethoscope and sphygmomanometer in client care settings. However, a common stethoscope and sphygmomanometer are sufficient to hear most clients' blood pressures. When blood pressure is weak, ultrasonic stethoscopes are useful for magnifying sound waves occurring during systole.

Evidence-based guidelines suggest that using the bell of the stethoscope enables you to hear blood pressure sounds more accurately, especially at diastolic pressures (Perloff, Grim, Flack, et al., 1993; Vital Signs, 1999). However, most people use the diaphragm because it is easily placed and because some stethoscopes do not have a bell (see Fig. 19-5). The key to clarity of sound is to use a high-quality stethoscope with short tubing.

Sphygmomanometers A **sphygmomanometer** consists of a vinyl or cloth cuff, a pressure bulb with a regulating valve, and a manometer (Fig. 19-9). Blood pressure cuffs contain an inflatable rubber bladder.

The cuff is attached to a gauge or manometer and a valved pressure bulb that inflates the bladder (Fig. 19-10). Cuffs can be placed on either the upper arm or midthigh and are supplied in various sizes.

Sphygmomanometers are either aneroid or mercury.

- **Aneroid** manometers have dials that register BP by pointers attached to a spring. They require frequent calibration to ensure accuracy.
- **Mercury** manometers measure BP using a calibrated upright tube containing mercury (see Fig. 19-9, top). As the bladder of the cuff is inflated, the pressure pushes the column of mercury up the tube. The column of mercury falls as the cuff is deflated. Although they are easier to maintain and more accurate than aneroid manometers, mercury manometers pose a health hazard if the mercury tube is broken. Based on the 1998 recommendation of the American Hospital Association and the EPA (EPA, 2012), many healthcare agencies have eliminated mercury-containing equipment (Mercury-Free Health Care, n.d.).

Electronic Blood Pressure Monitors use either microphones to sense sounds or sensors that detect pressure waves as blood flows through arteries (Fig. 19-9, bottom). They can be set to monitor and record BP at timed intervals and do not require the use of a stethoscope. They measure systolic, diastolic, and mean arterial pressures. Electronic monitors are useful when you must monitor BP frequently (e.g., during surgery, in critical care units). ➕ To ensure accuracy, you should auscultate a baseline BP before initiating automatic monitoring.

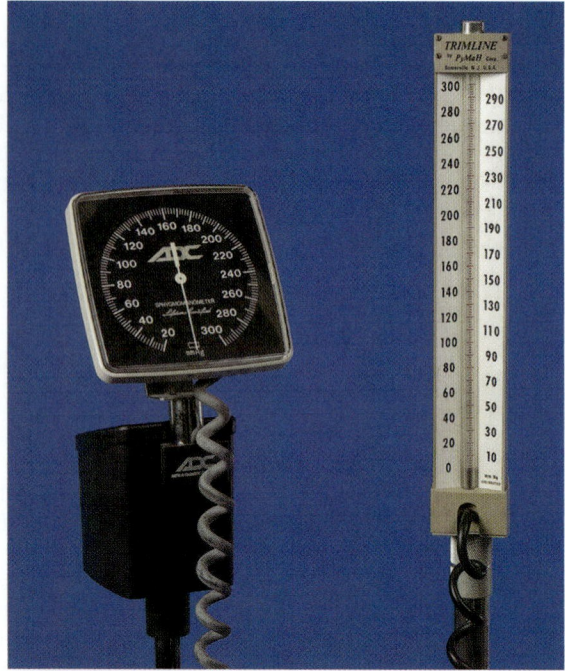

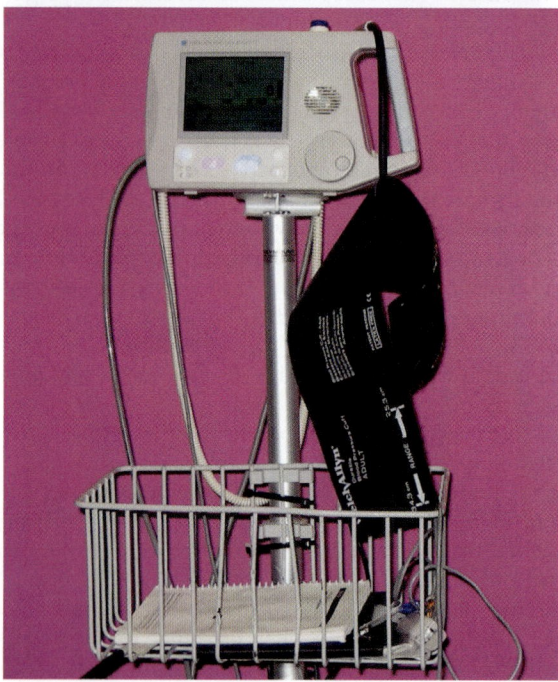

FIGURE 19-9 Types of manometers. *Top left,* aneroid. *Top right,* mercury. *Bottom,* electronic.

Electronic monitors may be less accurate than those with an aneroid monitor, or they may malfunction.

Numerous models of the electronic BP monitor can be purchased for client home use. Teach clients to know their baseline and seek follow-up care when readings are not within their normal range. See the accompanying Home Care box for further topics to teach clients about using electronic BP monitors.

What Cuff Size Should I Use?

The *width* of the bladder of a properly fitting cuff will cover approximately two-thirds of the *length* of the upper arm (or other extremity) for an adult and the entire upper arm for a child

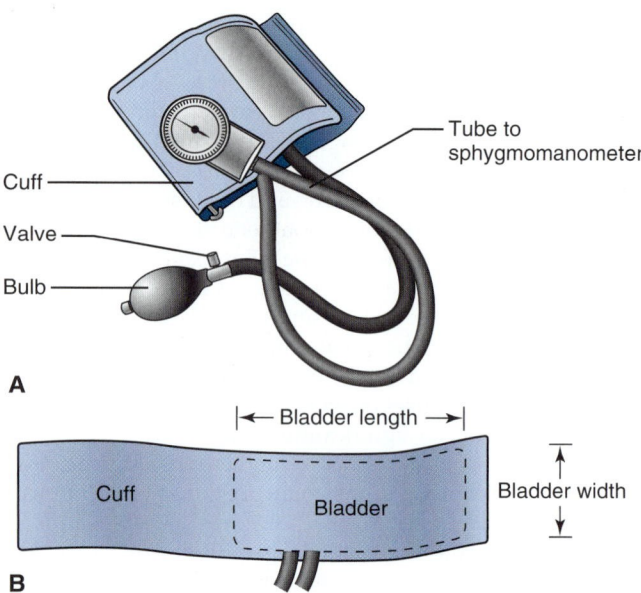

FIGURE 19-10 (A) Parts of the blood pressure cuff. (B) Placement of bladder within the cuff.

(Fig. 19-11) (National Heart, Lung, and Blood Institute, 1996, revised 2005). Alternatively, you can check that (1) the *cuff width* is 40% of the arm circumference and (2) the *length* of the bladder encircles 80% of the arm in adults (Tomlinson, 2010).

Using a cuff or bladder of the incorrect size can result in a measurement error of as much as 30 mm Hg. If the cuff is too narrow, your reading will be too high; if it is too wide, the reading will be too low. Although cuffs are manufactured in various sizes, in practice you will probably have access to only two or three different adult sizes. If you must use a cuff of the improper size, (1) it is better to use one that is too large than one that is too small, and (2) be sure to document the cuff size along with the BP reading. Refer to Figure 19-11 and Table 19-7 for information about cuff sizes in centimeters. Also see Clinical Insight 19-1.

Which Site Should I Use?

You usually use the *brachial artery* for assessing BP. However, the condition of the client's arm as well as other factors can interfere with accurate BP measurement.

- Avoid assessing blood pressure in an arm that has an intravenous access device, renal dialysis fistula, skin graft, extensive trauma, a cast, or a dressing.
- Do not use the arm that is paralyzed or on the same side of previous breast or shoulder surgery.
- You can use the forearm, thigh, or calf in these situations; however, remember that systolic pressure may be 20 to 30 mm Hg higher in the lower extremities than in the arms, but diastolic pressures are similar. Also, forearm and upper arm readings may not be interchangeable.
- Always document the site used. See Procedure 19-6 for techniques for measure blood pressure.

Auscultating Blood Pressure

Blood pressure can be measured indirectly by auscultation or palpation. The preferred, and most commonly used, method is auscultation; however, palpation is useful in certain situations. When auscultating BP, place your stethoscope over an artery, inflate the cuff, and listen for sounds as you deflate the cuff.

The sounds you listen for when you assess BP are called **Korotkoff sounds.** These sounds, described by Russian

Home Care

Teaching Your Client Self-Monitoring of Blood Pressure

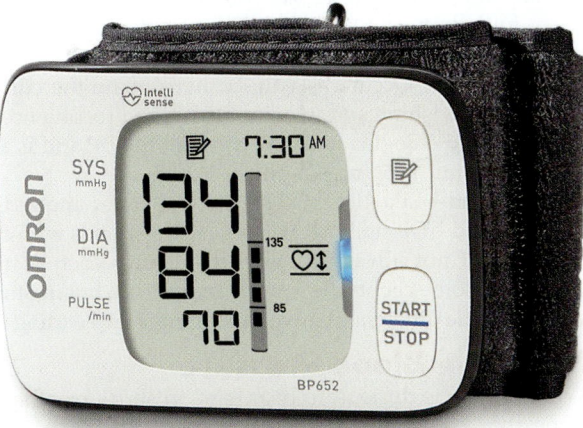

➤ With a portable home device, the client simply pushes a button, and the cuff inflates and deflates automatically. The device provides an electronic digital readout of the BP. Because these devices are sensitive, arm movement or improper cuff placement can cause inaccurate readings.

➤ Some grocery stores, fitness clubs, and other public places have stationary automatic BP devices for public use. The machine gives a visual display of the BP reading. The accuracy of these machines varies.

Benefits of Self-Monitoring

➤ May detect high BP in those who have not previously had a problem (screening).

➤ Allows for observation of the BP *pattern* over time, rather than a one-time office reading. The results can be analyzed to distinguish "white-coat hypertension" from actual hypertension.

➤ For clients with hypertension, self-monitoring increases participation in treatment and may improve compliance with treatment.

Disadvantages of Self-Monitoring

➤ Possible incorrect use of the BP device.

➤ May cause needless anxiety over a single elevated reading.

■ Clients with hypertension may make adjustments to their medications based on the BP readings without consulting their care provider.

Nursing Implications

■ Teach proper use of the self-measurement devices.

■ Periodically evaluate the client's technique.

■ Teach the meaning of BP readings and the need to look for patterns from multiple readings, not just a single reading.

■ Explain the need for calibration of the home-monitoring device at least once a year or according to the manufacturer's instructions.

■ Have the client bring the home-monitoring device to clinical visits so that readings can be compared with simultaneously recorded auscultatory readings.

■ Teach the client to have abnormally high or low readings (occurring on more than one occasion) rechecked by a healthcare provider. Home readings of 135/85 or higher should be considered elevated.

■ Advise the client to keep a written record of BP readings, including the date and time for each, and bring it to each clinic or office visit.

Safe, Effective Nursing Care

Using Evidence to Support Clinical Practice

Chapter Key Concept: Perfusion (blood pressure)

Competency: Evidence-Based Practice (Thinking, Doing)

Background: It is essential to measure blood pressure accurately for appropriate treatment and management (Elliott & Coventry, 2012). Accuracy and reliability of blood pressure measurement are improved by proper patient position, arm position, and timing. Research shows a correlation between increased readings and timing of the measurement, positioning of the patient (standing versus sitting in a chair versus sitting on an examining table) and positioning of the arm at the level of the heart (Jahangir, 2015; Mayo Clinic, 2015; Tomlinson, 2010; Turner, Burns, Chaney, et al., 2008).

Scenario: A 70-year-old obese patient with a history of hypertension and peripheral vascular disease is seen at the ambulatory care setting. You are assessing her vital signs to provide data for medication management. Prior to taking the patient's blood pressure, you obtain an aneroid sphygmomanometer and then request she sit in a chair and extend one arm while supporting the arm at level of the heart. Another nurse states, "You don't need to do all that."

Think about it:

■ What factors could influence the accuracy of the blood pressure assessment in this patient?

■ What evidence will you give the other nurse for your actions, and how will you locate best evidence to support your response?

■ What other actions should you institute to maintain accuracy in blood pressure measurement?

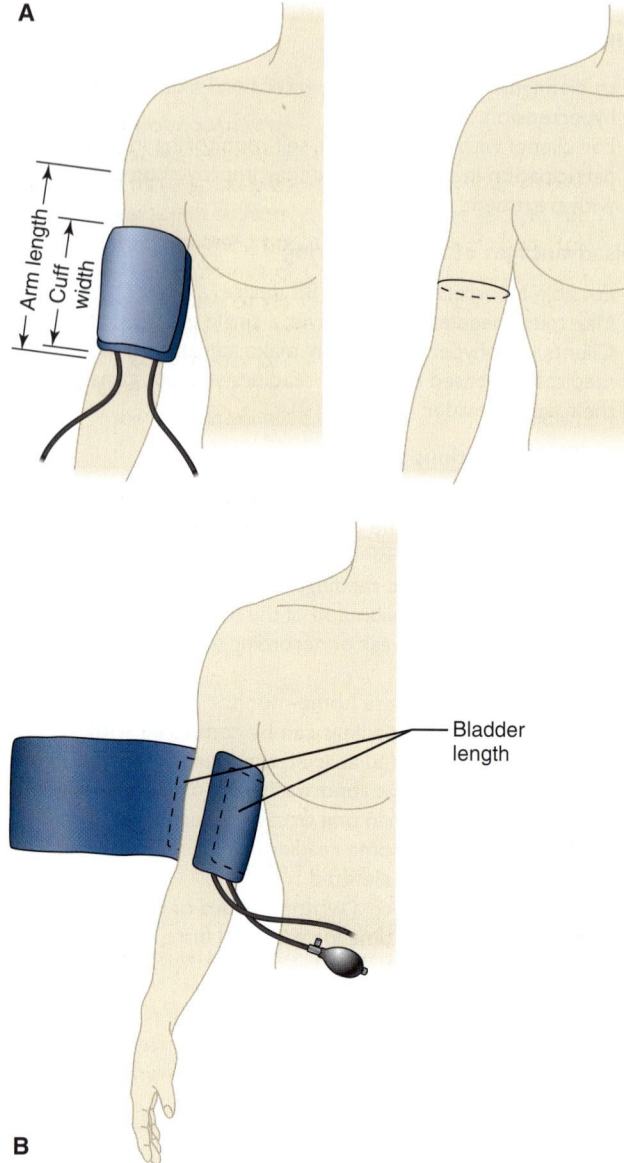

A

B

FIGURE 19-11 Determining correct BP cuff size. (A) The cuff width should be two-thirds of the length of the upper arm or should encircle 40% of the arm. (B) The length of the bladder should encircle 80% of the upper arm.

neurologist Nicolai Korotkoff in 1906, are used to describe the sounds of blood pulsating through arteries (Fig. 19-12).

1st sound—Systolic BP. As you deflate the BP cuff, you will initially hear a sound that occurs during systole. It is a tapping sound that corresponds to the pulse.

2nd sound—Occurs as you further deflate the cuff. It is a soft, swishing sound caused by blood turbulence.

3rd sound—Begins midway through the BP and is a sharp, rhythmic tapping sound.

4th sound—Like the third sound, but softer and fading.

5th sound—Diastolic BP. Silence; it corresponds with diastole.

You will not always be able to identify each of the five sounds. In some clients the sounds are distinct, but in others you will note little difference between beginning and ending sounds.

Palpating Blood Pressure

When the BP is difficult to hear (e.g., in shock or other conditions that compromise circulation) you can use palpation alone. You can usually palpate only the systolic BP, because diastolic pressure is difficult to feel. To learn this technique, see Procedure 19-6, Variation D, Palpating the Blood Pressure.

Using Palpation With Auscultation

You should use palpation with auscultation for calculating the proper cuff inflation pressure before auscultating the BP and for detecting an auscultatory gap, discussed below.

Calculating Proper Inflation Pressure The first time you measure a client's BP, you will not know what the systolic BP is. Should you pump the cuff to 200 mm Hg just to be sure you don't miss the first sound? The answer is NO. If you overinflate the cuff, the patient will feel discomfort. However, if you underinflate it (e.g., stop inflating at 110 mm Hg), you may miss the first sound and obtain an incorrect reading. You can use palpation with auscultation to estimate the systolic BP. This helps ensure that you inflate the cuff to the proper level to obtain an accurate reading. To learn how to perform this method, see Procedure 19-6, Measuring Blood Pressure.

Recognizing an Auscultatory Gap If the client has hypertension, as you auscultate the BP during deflation of the cuff you may note the loss of sounds for as much as 30 mm Hg, followed by the return of sound. This loss and later return of sound is referred to as an *auscultatory gap*. Palpating first and then auscultating (as described in the preceding paragraph and Procedure 19-6) ensures that you

CUFF TYPE—>	NEWBORN	INFANT	CHILD	SMALL ADULT	ADULT	LARGE ADULT	ADULT THIGH
Arm circumference at midpoint (cm)**	< 6	6–15	16–21	22–26	27–34	35–44	45–52
Bladder width (cm)	3	5	8	12	16	16	16
Bladder length (cm)	6	15	21	22	30	36	42

Table 19-7 ▶ Blood Pressure Cuffs: Acceptable Bladder Sizes*

Sources: Perloff, D., Grim, C., Flack, J., et al. (1993). *Human blood pressure determination by sphygmomanometry* (AHA Medical/Scientific Statement, Product Code: 88:2460–2467). Dallas, TX: American Heart Association; Pickering, T., Hall, J., Appel, L., et al. (2005). Recommendations for blood pressure measurement in humans and experimental animals: Part 1: Blood pressure measurement in humans: A statement for professionals from the subcommittee of Professional and Public Education of the American Heart Association Council on High Blood Pressure Research. *Hypertension, 45*(1), 142–161.

*The National Heart, Lung, and Blood Institute states that practically speaking, "correct cuff size equals the largest cuff that will fit on the upper arm with room below for the stethoscope head" (2007).

**Arm circumference is half the distance from the acromion to the olecranon process. If correct size not available, use next larger (rather than smaller) size.

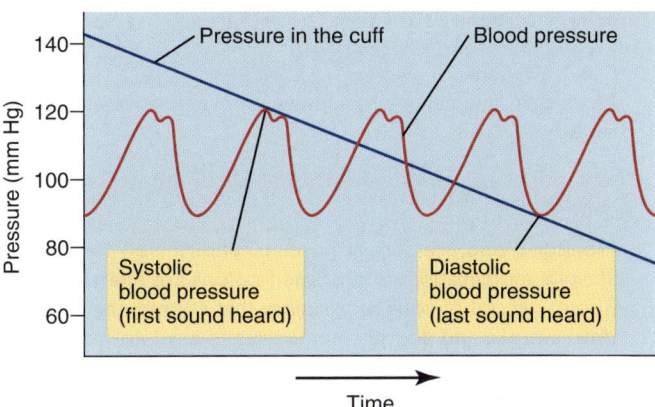

FIGURE 19-12 Relationship of blood pressure to changes in cuff pressure and the 1st and 5th Korotkoff sounds (BP 120/80).

will not miss the isolated first sound. You should record the range of pressures in which the gap occurs (e.g., BP left arm, sitting, 170/90 with an auscultatory gap from 170 to 140). Failure to recognize an auscultatory gap can result in a serious misreading of the systolic BP. For tips that will help ensure the validity of your BP measurements, see Clinical Insight 19-2.

KnowledgeCheck 19-6

- Which of the Korotkoff sounds would you record as the systolic pressure?
- Which of the Korotkoff sounds would you record as the diastolic pressure?
- A nurse is auscultating a BP. He hears the first sound at 170 mm Hg. The sound disappears immediately. At 150 mm Hg, the sound appears again and continues until there is silence at 80 mm Hg. The pressures were taken in the client's right arm with the client supine.
  How should the nurse record these pressures?
  How do you explain what happened?

ANALYSIS/NURSING DIAGNOSIS NP

Hypotension and hypertension are medical diagnoses or, more commonly, symptoms rather than nursing diagnoses. However, they may be the etiology of nursing diagnoses—for example, Risk for Falls related to orthostatic hypotension. For more information about hypotension and hypertension, and for goals and interventions, see the Example Problems for Hypotension and Hypertension.

You may use the new NANDA-I diagnosis, Unstable Blood Pressure, when the patient is "susceptible to fluctuating forces of blood flowing through arterial vessels which may compromise health" (NANDA-I, 2018).

PLANNING OUTCOMES/EVALUATION NP

Because hypotension and hypertension are collaborative problems, you may need goals for overall blood pressure monitoring. However, you will more likely use goals for problems related to hypotension and hypertension (e.g., Risk for Falls).

PLANNING INTERVENTIONS/ IMPLEMENTATION NP

NIC standardized interventions planning client care. Refer to the Example Problem. Also see CAM Box: Alternative Therapies for Lowering Blood Pressure.

Complementary & Alternative Modalities (CAM)

Alternative Therapies for Lowering Blood Pressure

According to an American Heart Association's Scientific Statement, some alternative methods—particularly aerobic exercise and resistance training—can be considered adjunctive to the medical therapies of diet and medication to reduce blood pressure. Biofeedback techniques (isometric handgrip exercise and device-guided slow breathing) are likely to reduce blood pressure by a small amount, but the evidence is not as strong. Evidence is insufficient to support use of the following as adjunctive treatments for hypertension: meditation, yoga, relaxation therapy, stress-reduction techniques, and acupuncture.

Source: Brook, R., Appel, L., Rubenfire, M., et al. (2013). AHA Scientific Statement. Beyond medications and diet: Alternative approaches to lowering blood pressure. *Hypertension, 61*(6), 1360–1383. Retrieved from http://hyper.ahajournals.org/content/61/6/1360.long

KnowledgeCheck 19-7

- Which of the clients with the following BP has hypertension? One with a BP of:
  150/80 mm Hg on two separate occasions
  180/100 mm Hg on one occasion
  138/88 mm Hg on two occasions
- Which of the following client(s) has/have *primary* hypertension?
  Client A, who is obese and has a high sodium intake
  Client B, who is in renal failure
  Client C, who has hypertension induced by pregnancy
  Client D, who has a family history of hypertension

ThinkLike a Nurse 19-10

Recall the clients in the Meet Your Patients scenario. Lucas is 35 years old. He has been under a lot of stress. His blood pressure is 150/98 mm Hg.

- To evaluate his BP, what else do you need to know about Lucas's situation (the context)?
- What possible actions should you consider while meeting with Lucas?
- What is the theoretical knowledge (rationale) to support your decisions?

PUTTING IT ALL TOGETHER

Regardless of clinical setting, you will need to use clinical judgment about which VS to measure and how often to measure them.

Evaluating Vital Signs

You should evaluate the client's VS on the basis of known norms as well as the particular client's trends. When you note a deviation in the client's VS, evaluate it in the context of his medication, diagnosis, procedures, environment, activity, and so on to understand the theoretical basis for the change. Assess your client for other clinical signs to determine your course of action.

KEY POINT: *A sudden change in the client's condition requires a thorough assessment. You must report your findings to the primary care provider.*

Self-Care

Teaching Your Client About Hypertension

Teach the client and family about lifestyle changes for preventing and managing hypertension.

➤ Limit salt intake to 1 teaspoon per day (2,400 mg of sodium).

➤ Consume a diet high in potassium (e.g., fresh fruits and vegetables such as bananas, potatoes, and acorn squash).

➤ Consume a diet high in calcium (e.g., milk and milk products [yogurt], sardines, molasses, tofu).

➤ Limit alcohol intake to 1 or 2 drinks per day for men; 1 for women. (One drink is a can of beer, one jigger of liquor, or a glass of wine. Wine is preferred.)

➤ Maintain ideal body weight; lose weight if overweight.

➤ For overall cardiovascular health, reduce saturated fat and cholesterol intake.

➤ Eliminate smoking.

➤ Engage in aerobic exercise (30 to 45 minutes several days a week, or a total of 150 minutes per week).

➤ Try to reduce stress and stressful situations.

➤ Teach the client that even one lifestyle change has effects similar to treatment with a single antihypertensive drug.

Teach the need for follow-up assessments.

More than one change has an even more positive effect on BP.

Teach the client about monitoring his blood pressure at home.

➤ Monitor blood pressure at home to determine whether lifestyle modifications and/or medications are effective.

➤ Keep a record of your BP readings that contain the date, time, systolic and diastolic numbers, and any information that you want your provider to know.

➤ Take your BP whenever you experience symptoms such as headaches or dizziness.

➤ Use an upper arm or wrist BP monitor that has been validated.

➤ Take your BP equipment when you visit your healthcare provider to check your monitor for accuracy.

➤ Follow the researchers' and manufacturer's guidelines for arm position and recalibration. This is especially true for wrist monitors (Dourmap, Girerd, Marquand, et al., 2010; Zheng, Huang, Sheng, et al., 2012).

For BP of:			Teaching Points
Systolic		**Diastolic**	**Analysis and Client Action**
< 120 mm Hg	and	< 80 mm Hg	Normal Blood Pressure Recheck at each healthcare encounter or at least every 2 years.
120–139 mm Hg	Or	80–89 mm Hg	Prehypertension Review lifestyle modifications and make follow-up visits as your primary healthcare provider advises. If you have not seen a provider, consult one within 1 to 2 months.
140–159 mm Hg	Or	90–99 mm Hg	High Blood Pressure—Stage 1 Review lifestyle modifications and schedule follow-up with a healthcare provider within 1 to 2 months.
160 or higher mm Hg	Or	100 or higher mm Hg	High Blood Pressure—Stage 2 Consult the primary care provider within 1 week, or immediately if the clinical situation warrants.

Source: Joint National Committee on Prevention, Detection, Evaluation, and Treatment of High Blood Pressure. (2004). *JNC 7 complete report. The seventh report of the Joint National Committee on Prevention, Detection, Evaluation, and Treatment of High Blood Pressure.* Bethesda, MD: National Institutes of Health. Retrieved from http://www.nhlbi.nih.gov/guidelines/hypertension/index.htm

Delegating Vital Signs

VS may usually be obtained by nursing assistive personnel (NAP). ✚ When working with complex or critical patients, you should carefully consider whether to delegate VS to a NAP. The significance of the VS results must be analyzed in relation to other assessment data.

■ **If you are the registered nurse (RN)** working in a team nursing model, you are responsible for reviewing and interpreting the findings of all NAPs. This includes evaluating their

technique and the accuracy of their measurements. The professional nurse is *always* responsible for interpreting VS trends and making decisions based on abnormal VS findings.

■ **As a student nurse,** you are responsible for functioning within your scope of knowledge. If unsure how to interpret the meaning of a patient's VS, discuss the findings with your instructor and/or the nurse assigned to care for your client. Even though you are participating in the client's care, the assigned nurse maintains responsibility for client oversight.

EXAMPLE PROBLEM: Hypotension

Problem

Low blood pressure: Systolic blood pressure less than 100 mm Hg. Not usually a problem unless the decrease from baseline BP causes dizziness, fatigue, concentration problems, activity intolerance, or shortness of breath. Very low BP (hypovolemic shock) is a medical emergency.

Risk Factors for Orthostatic Hypotension: Older adults, pregnant women, prolonged bedrest, decreased blood volume (e.g., from dehydration or recent blood loss)

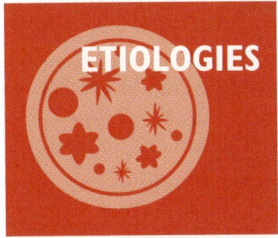

ETIOLOGIES

- Position changes
- Medications: Side effects of numerous medications (e.g., antihypertensives, diuretics)
- Medical conditions: Hypothyroidism, diabetes, heart failure, dehydration, hemorrhage

- **Orthostatic or Postural hypotension**— Sudden drop of 10 mm Hg on moving from a lying position to a sitting or standing position, causing dizziness and/or fainting

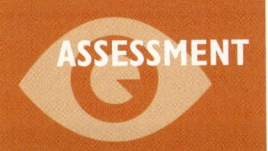

ASSESSMENT

Assess for:
- Changes in BP
- Orthostatic hypotension
- Pale skin

- Complaints of dizziness, fatigue, concentration problems, activity intolerance, or shortness of breath

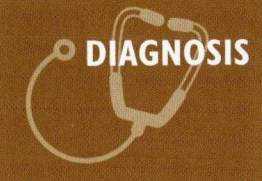

DIAGNOSIS

- Hypotension is a medical diagnosis, not a nursing diagnosis.
- Examples of nursing diagnoses associated with hypotension are:
  - Risk for Falls related to dizziness secondary to postural hypotension

- Fear of falling related to fainting secondary to postural hypotension
- Unstable Blood Pressure related to cardiac arrhythmias and decreased cardiac output

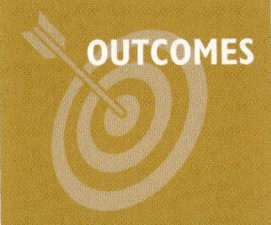

OUTCOMES

- NOC outcomes and goals will depend on the nursing diagnosis; however the outcome Hypotension Outcome is likely to be useful.

- Examples of individualized outcomes:
  - BP > 110/70
  - Increase in circulatory volume
  - No falls while walking

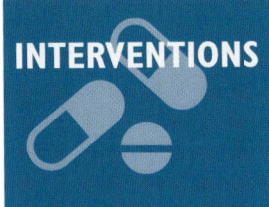

INTERVENTIONS

- NIC standardized interventions will depend on the nursing diagnoses.
- Examples of individualized interventions:
  - Monitor I&O; volume depletion can cause hypotension.
  - Monitor VS as client condition requires.
  - Assess for orthostatic or postural hypotension.
  - Assist the client to lie down, if dizzy.
- Surveillance: Safety for older adults, pregnant women, clients on prolonged bedrest, and clients with decreased blood volume.
- Increase fluid intake.
- Eat small, low carbohydrate meals to minimize the drop in blood pressure that occurs after meals.

Interventions for Orthostatic Hypotension

- Help the client lie down.
- Obtain orthostatic vital signs—take the pulse and BP with client supine, sitting, and standing. Take each reading 1 to 3 minutes after each change of position. Notify the provider of change in measurements.
- When documenting orthostatic VS, record the client's position in addition to the pulse and BP (e.g., supine P = 80, BP = 150/90; sitting P = 84, BP = 140/84; standing P = 90, BP = 104/60).

(Continued)

EXAMPLE PROBLEM: Hypotension—cont'd

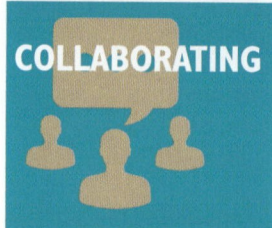
COLLABORATING

- Hemodynamic regulation
- Administer intravenous fluids.

- Administer prescribed medications.
- Treat underlying cause.

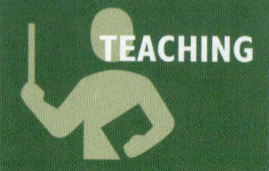
TEACHING

- Teach client to change position slowly.

- Counsel on safety activities (avoid driving, sports, etc.).

EXAMPLE PROBLEM: Hypertension

Problem
Prehypertension: Systolic BP of 120 to 139 mm Hg; or Diastolic BP of 80 to 89 mm Hg; based on 2–3 readings (taken 6 minutes apart, with the patient sitting).
Hypertension: Systolic BP > 140 mm Hg or diastolic BP > 90 mm Hg, based on two or more readings on separate occasions.

Risk Factors
Family history, age, race, obesity, diet, heavy alcohol consumption, smoking history, high cholesterol levels, and stress

Complications
Hypertension increases the stress on the heart and blood vessels. If untreated, it may lead to heart attack, heart failure, peripheral vascular disease, kidney damage, or stroke (American Heart Association, n.d.a).

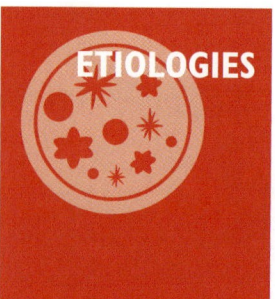
ETIOLOGIES

- Physiologically, hypertension is related to thickening of arterial walls and decreased elasticity of the arteries.
- As blood pressure rises, peripheral resistance increases. Over time, the heart is unable to compensate, and cardiac output declines.

Essential Hypertension:

No known cause

Secondary Hypertension:

- Renal and endocrine disorders
- Prescription and nonprescription drugs (e.g., NSAIDs)
- Oral contraceptives, some decongestants
- Adrenal steroid hormones
- Nicotine
- Illicit drug use (e.g., cocaine, amphetamines)
- Stressful lifestyle

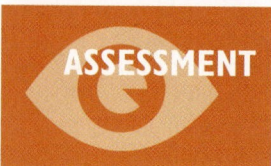
ASSESSMENT

Client may not have symptoms.

Assess for complaints of early morning suboccipital headaches, fatigue, and visual changes.

EXAMPLE PROBLEM: Hypertension—cont'd

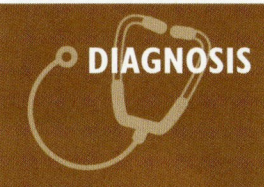
DIAGNOSIS

Risk for Decreased Cardiac Output
Risk for Unstable Blood Pressure

Hypertension may be the etiology of other diagnoses.

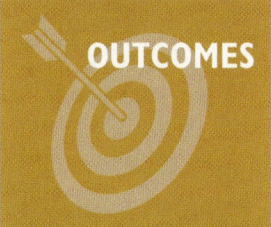
OUTCOMES

NOC Outcomes:

Cardiac Pump Effectiveness
Vital Signs

Individualized Outcome:

Will have systolic and diastolic BP of nor more than 15 mm/Hg over his baseline

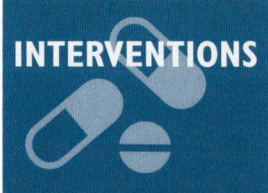
INTERVENTIONS

NIC Standardized Interventions

Will depend on the nursing diagnoses. Examples: Smoking Cessation Assistance, Cardiac Risk Management

Individualized Interventions:

- Monitor VS.
- Monitor the patient's activity tolerance to determine activity tolerance (level of fatigue).

- Monitor I&O; fluid retention can increase blood volume and pressure.
- Observe for edema—sign of fluid retention.
- Monitor weight gain—can indicate fluid retention or poor dietary/activity compliance.
- Assess the client's attitude and beliefs about taking antihypertensive medications and making lifestyle changes.

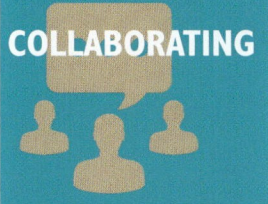
COLLABORATING

- Hemodynamic regulation
- Laboratory tests to identify cause(s): Blood urea nitrogen (BUN), creatinine, electrolytes, hemoglobin, hematocrit, and lipid levels. The American College of Physicians and the American Academy of Physicians recommend initiation of

pharmacologic treatment in adults 60 years and older to achieve a target systolic B/P of < 150 mm/Hg.
- Treat underlying cause.
- Administer prescribed antihypertensive medication.

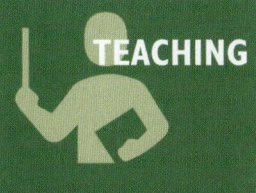
TEACHING

- Teach client the needed lifestyle changes: balanced weight loss diet, increased activity, decreased alcohol intake, stress management and relaxation techniques.
- Encourage self-management: self-monitoring of BP, compliance with medication and therapeutic regimen.
- Refer to the Self-Care box, Teaching Your Client About Hypertension.
- Teach regarding the timing of taking medications (e.g., avoid diuretics at night).
- Educate about medications that can be taken at night. Research shows that taking

at least one antihypertensive medication at night decreases the risk of cardiovascular disease (Keller, 2011).

 • Help the client understand and gain realistic expectations regarding the medication therapy. Research shows that older adults with negative beliefs about their medication are more likely to be noncompliant in maintaining the medication regime (Ruppar, Dobbels, & Geest, 2012).

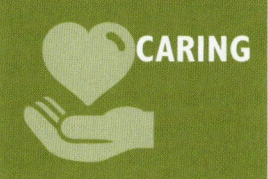
CARING

♥ **iCare** • Praise the client for indicators that show compliance.

- Continue to provide encouragement and realistic expectations.

CLINICALREASONING

The questions and exercises in this section allow you to practice the kind of thinking you will use as a full-spectrum nurse. Critical-thinking questions usually have more than one correct answer, so we do not provide "correct answers" for these features. It is more important to develop your nursing judgment than to just cover content. You will learn by discussing the questions with your peers. If you are still unsure, see the Davis Advantage chapter resources for suggested responses.

Caring for the Nguyens

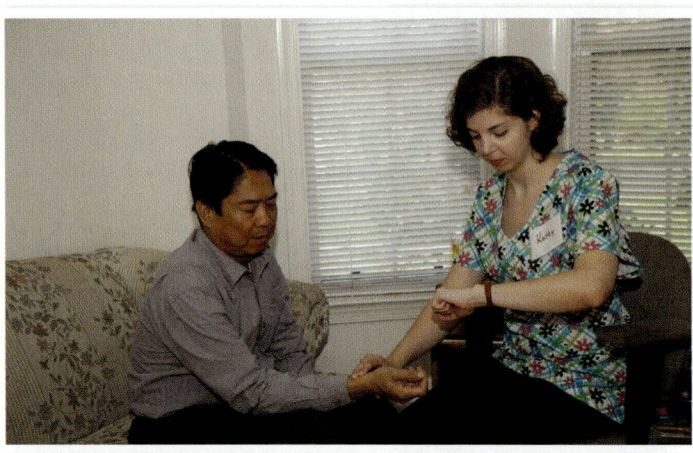

Recall that on Nam Nguyen's preliminary visit to the Family Medicine Center, his blood pressure (BP) was 162/94 mm Hg. On subsequent visits, his BP was 168/100 and 174/96 mm Hg, and he was continuing to gain weight. Mr. Nguyen was diagnosed with hypertension and prescribed an antihypertension medication to be taken each morning. This morning Mr. Nguyen has come to the clinic for follow-up. The following information is gathered as he checks in for his visit.

VS: BP, 168/92 mm Hg; pulse, 80 beats/min; respirations, 20 breaths/min; temperature, 98.4°F (36.9°C)
Weight: 180 lb (82 kg)

Review the preliminary data and the preceding information to answer the following questions:

A. What patterns do you see in the data?

B. Do you have enough information to draw any conclusions? If not, what other information should you gather?

C. Identify three alternatives that may explain what is happening with Mr. Nguyen's vital signs.

D. How could you determine which of these alternatives provides the best explanation of what is happening?

E. Why is it important to intervene in this situation?

Applying the **Full-Spectrum Nursing Model**

PATIENT SITUATION

A patient in the critical care unit had a stable pulse and BP for the first few days. He has become more ill and now his pulse and BP are weak and difficult to palpate. His last BP reading was abnormally low, so it must be monitored frequently. He is receiving intravenous fluids in both arms.

THINKING

1. *Critical Thinking (Reflecting and Deciding What to Do):* Which of the patient's vital signs (temperature, pulse, respiration, and BP) might you be able to delegate to a NAP?

DOING

2. *Practical Knowledge:* How would you take the patient's blood pressure? Be specific:
  a. What site would you use?
  b. What equipment would you use?
3. *Nursing Process (Assessment):*
  a. Will you need to validate any of the vital signs you obtain? If so, why?
  b. How could you validate those vital signs?

CARING

4. Assume that you are very busy. How would you demonstrate caring to this patient while you are assessing his vital signs (the ones you did not delegate to a NAP)?

PracticalKnowledge:
clinical application

CLINICAL INSIGHTS

Clinical Insight 19-1 ➤ **Choosing a Blood Pressure Cuff Size**

- The *width* of the bladder should cover approximately two-thirds of the *length* of the upper arm (or other extremity) for an adult and the entire upper arm for a child.
- Another method for sizing: (1) The cuff width should be 40% of the arm circumference, and (2) the *length* of the bladder should encircle 80% of the arm.
- Perhaps the easiest sizing method is to measure *arm circumference* and follow these guidelines:

For arm circumference	**Cuff should be**
22–26 cm (8½ × 10¼ in.)	"small adult" size: 12 × 22 cm (4¾ × 8¾ in.)
27–34 cm (10½ × 13½ in.)	"adult" size: 16 × 30 cm (6¼ × 11¾ in.)
35–44 cm (13¾ × 17¼ in.)	"large adult" size: 16 × 36 cm (6¼ × 14¼ in.)
45–52 cm (17¾ × 10½ in.)	"adult thigh" size: 16 × 42 cm (6¼ × 16⅝ in.)

Practice Resources

Pickering, T., Hall, J., Appel, L., et al. (2005).

Clinical Insight 19-2 ➤ **Taking an Accurate Blood Pressure**

To improve your technique and accuracy of measurement, use the following tips in addition to Procedure 19-6:

- Explain the procedure, particularly on admission or when changing the routine.
  Reduces patient anxiety.
- Wait 30 minutes before assessing BP after client has ingested caffeine or smoked.
- Do not assess BP while the client is in pain.
- Apply the cuff over bare skin, if possible. Controversy surrounds this issue, so follow the manufacturer's instructions and agency policy. Advise clients who are home monitoring to apply the cuff over bare skin.
- Instruct the client not to talk during BP measurement. You should not talk either.
- Keep environmental noise and client movement to a minimum.
- Hold the stethoscope lightly but completely against the skin; do not put your thumb on top of the bell or diaphragm. Try not to allow the tubing to brush against your clothing or the bed.

- Do not be influenced by the client's previous BP measurements.
- Use the same limb for each measurement, unless you are comparing arms or averaging readings from both arms.
- For the initial reading, measure the BP in both arms and use the arm with the higher reading for subsequent measurements.
- If you obtain an elevated reading, confirm in the other arm.
- Do not draw conclusions based on one reading. Take two or more readings, at least 2 to 5 minutes apart, and average them. If the readings differ by more than 5 mm Hg, obtain and average additional readings.

Practice Resources

Bunker, J. (2014); Handler, J. (2009); Joint National Committee on Prevention, Detection, Evaluation, and Treatment of High Blood Pressure (2004); Ma, G., Sabin, N., & Dawes, M. (2008); McKay, D. (2008); Tomlinson, B. (2010).

PROCEDURES

Procedure 19-1 ■ Assessing Body Temperature

➤ For steps to follow in *all* procedures, refer to the Universal Steps for All Procedures found on the page facing the inside back cover.

Equipment

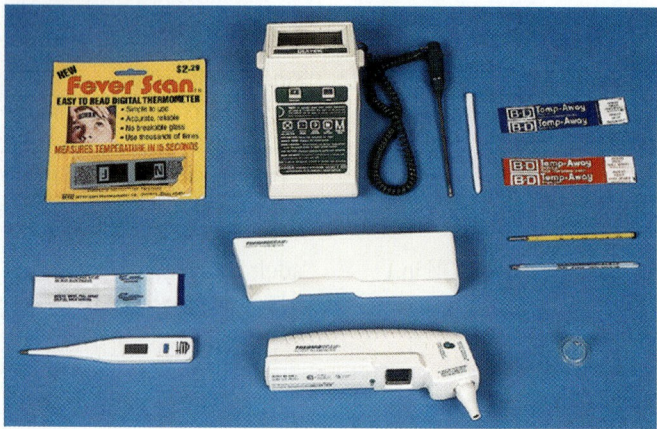

- Thermometer (An oral thermometer generally has a blue tip. A rectal thermometer generally has a red tip.)

- ✚ Glass-and-mercury thermometers should not be used in any healthcare setting. However, because some people still use them at home, we include them in this procedure. They should be used with disposable covers and cleaned and sterilized regularly according to the manufacturer's instructions.

- Thermometer cover, if needed
- Procedure gloves, if taking a rectal temperature or if there is risk of contact with body fluids (e.g., saliva)
- Water-soluble lubricant, if taking a rectal temperature
- Towel, if needed, for taking an axillary temperature (to dry the axillae)
- Tissues

Delegation

You can delegate temperature measurement to a nursing assistive personnel (NAP) if you conclude that the condition and the NAP's skills allow. Perform the pre-procedure assessments and inform the NAP of the route and type of thermometer used. Explain any special considerations (e.g., tell the NAP if the patient had food or oral fluids in the last 20 to 30 minutes; inform the NAP if the patient is confused). Ask the NAP to record and report the temperature to you, and to report immediately if the temperature is elevated (e.g., greater than 100°F [37.8°C]).

Pre-Procedure Assessments

- Determine the most appropriate site. Consider comfort, safety, and accurate measurements. For example, do not use the oral route for a patient who is unable to hold the thermometer properly, for children, or for others who cannot follow instructions (e.g., unconscious), or for those who are "mouth breathing."

- For an oral temperature: Determine how long it has been since the patient smoked, had anything to eat or drink, or chewed gum. If so, wait 20 to 30 minutes before taking the temperature.
  Smoking, eating, drinking, and chewing gum can all affect an oral reading.

- Assess for any contraindications to using the site you have chosen. For example:
  Tympanic: Assess for impacted earwax or hearing aid.
  Rectal: Check the client record for diarrhea or impacted stool.
  Axillary: Check the client record for presence of fever or hypothermia.
  Skin: Assess for conditions that require a very precise, reliable reading (e.g., fever, hypothermia).
  Some conditions increase the risk for client injury; others contribute to inaccurate, unreliable temperature measurement.

- What were the previous recordings, if any?
  Noting changes over time is important in all client assessments.

- Assess for clinical signs and symptoms of temperature alterations.

Procedure 19-1A ■ Taking an Axillary Temperature

➤ When performing the procedure, always identify your according to agency policy, using two identifiers, and be attentive to standard precautions, hand hygiene, patient safety and privacy, body mechanics, and documentation.

Procedure Steps

1. **Position the client supine or sitting.**

2. **Dry the client's axilla,** as needed.
   Moisture from perspiration alters the temperature reading.

3. **Slide the thermometer into a protective sheath** (depending on type of thermometer).
   A protective sheath provides a barrier to prevent transmission of organisms.

4. **Place the thermometer tip** in the middle of the axilla.

5. **Position the client's upper arm down,** with the lower arm across the chest.

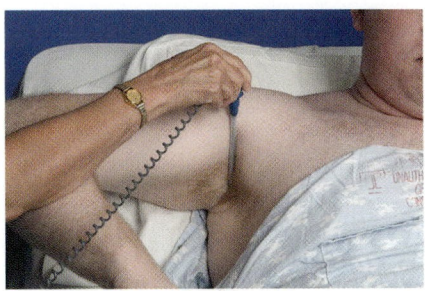

Puts the thermometer in close proximity to the axillary blood vessels, allowing it to better reflect the core temperature. ▼

6. **Hold the thermometer in place** for the recommended time.
   a. Leave an electronic probe in place until it beeps.

b. Leave a plastic, or glass if you must use it, thermometer in place for 8 minutes or according to agency policy (usually 5 minutes for children).
   Study findings differ for accuracy of temperature measurements at the axillary site. Follow agency policy.

7. **Read the temperature.**
   a. **Electronic thermometer:** Read the digital display; remove the thermometer.
   b. **Glass thermometer:** Remove the thermometer; hold at eye level, and rotate it until the markings are clear. Avoid using glass, if possible.

8. **After removing the thermometer,** discard the cover. If there is no cover, wipe the thermometer with a tissue.
   Removes any moisture that may have accumulated in 8 minutes' time.

9. **Clean and replace the thermometer** in the storage base, following agency policy.
   Prevents microbial growth on thermometers and recharges the battery.

Procedure 19-1B ■ Taking an Oral Temperature

> ➤ When performing the procedure, always identify your patient according to agency policy, using two identifiers, and be attentive to standard precautions, hand hygiene, patient safety and privacy, body mechanics, and documentation.

Procedure Steps

1. **If you must use a glass thermometer,** shake down the liquid if necessary.
   a. Stand in an open area away from tables and other objects.
      Prevents thermometer breakage.
   b. Hold the end opposite the bulb between your thumb and forefinger, and snap your wrist downward.
   c. Shake the thermometer until the reading is less than 96°F (36°C).
      The reading must be lower than the anticipated temperature measurement.

2. **Slide the thermometer into** a protective sheath.
   Provides a barrier to prevent transmission of microorganisms.

3. **Place the thermometer tip** under the tongue in the posterior sublingual pocket (right or left of frenulum).
   Puts the tip in close proximity to the major blood vessels under the tongue, allowing the thermometer to reflect the core temperature. ➤

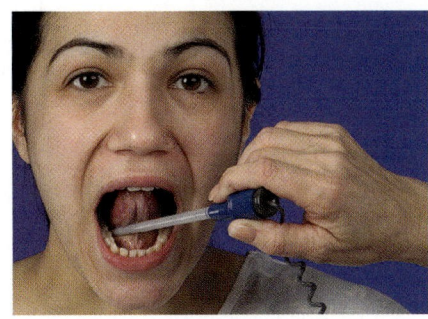

4. **Have the patient close her lips** around the thermometer, cautioning her not to bite down on it.
   Protects the thermometer from exposure to the air, which could alter the reading. Biting may break a glass thermometer, injuring the mouth.

5. **Leave the thermometer in place** for the recommended time.
   a. Glass thermometer: 5 to 8 minutes
   b. Electronic (digital) thermometer: Until it beeps
   c. According to agency policy
      Research findings differ on the optimal time for measuring an oral temperature, so follow agency policy.

6. **Read the temperature.**
   a. **Glass thermometer:** Remove the thermometer, position it at eye level, and rotate it until the markings are clear. ▼

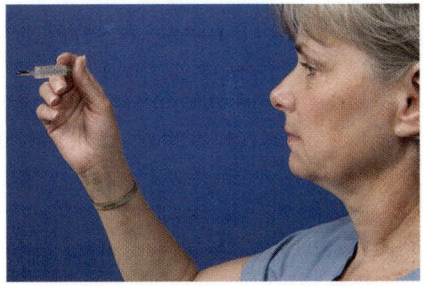

   b. **Electronic thermometer:** Read the digital display, then remove the thermometer.

7. **After removing the thermometer,** discard the cover. If there is no cover, wipe the thermometer with an antimicrobial or alcohol-based wipe.
   Wiping removes mucus that can make the markings on a glass thermometer difficult to read.

8. **Clean and replace the thermometer.** Follow agency policy.
   Prevents microbial growth on thermometers and recharges battery of electronic thermometers.

(continued on next page)

Procedure 19–1 ■ Assessing Body Temperature (continued)

Procedure 19–1C ■ Taking a Rectal Temperature

➤ When performing the procedure, always identify your patient according to agency policy, using two identifiers, and be attentive to standard precautions, hand hygiene, patient safety and privacy, body mechanics, and documentation.

➤ *Note:* This procedure primarily describes use of an electronic (digital) thermometer.

Procedure Steps

1. **Slide the thermometer into** a protective sheath.
   A protective sheath provides a barrier to prevent transmission of microorganisms.

2. **Position an adult patient** in Sims' position (on the side with the knees flexed). Drape the patient so that only the anal area is exposed. ▼

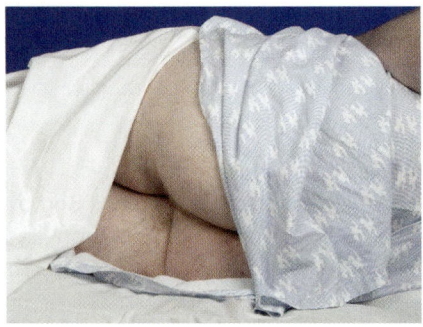

Step Variation Taking a Rectal Temperature for a Small Child
Place a child in the prone position. You can lay the child face down across your lap or a parent's lap.
Flexing the knees helps relax the muscles to ease insertion and aid in visualization. Draping provides privacy and decreases embarrassment.

3. **Lubricate the tip** of the thermometer by squeezing water-soluble lubricant onto a tissue and then applying it to the thermometer.
   Prevents injury to the rectal mucosa and eases insertion. Inserting the thermometer into the lubricant container would contaminate contents of the container.

4. **Don a procedure glove** on your dominant hand or on both hands if necessary.

5. **With your nondominant hand,** separate the patient's buttocks to visualize the anus.

6. **Gently insert** the thermometer approximately:
   Adult: 1 to 1.5 in. (2.5 to 3.7 cm)
   Child: 0.9 in. (2.5 cm)
   Infant: 0.5 in. (1.5 cm)
   The thermometer must be placed past the rectal sphincter.

   a. Have the patient take a deep breath. Insert the thermometer as he exhales.
      Taking a deep breath helps relax the anal sphincter.

   b. If you feel resistance, do not use force.
      Inserting the thermometer too far or forcing against resistance may injure the rectal mucosa. ➤

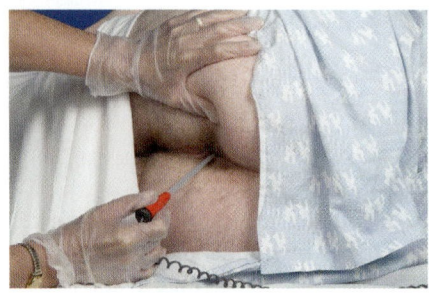

7. **Hold the thermometer in place** until it beeps. (For a plastic or glass if you must use it, thermometer, hold the thermometer 3 to 5 minutes.)
   The thermometer must be held in place to prevent inadvertent injury to the patient. An electronic thermometer will beep when a constant temperature is reached. Research differs on the optimal time for measuring a rectal temperature, so follow agency policy.

8. **Remove the thermometer,** discard the cover, and read the digital display.

9. **Remove the procedure glove(s)** and discard in a biohazards container.

10. **Follow agency policy** for cleaning and storing thermometers.
    Prevents microbial growth on thermometers and recharges electronic thermometer battery.

Procedure 19–1D ■ Taking a Temporal Artery Temperature

➤ When performing the procedure, always identify your patient according to agency policy, using two identifiers, and be attentive to standard precautions, hand hygiene, patient safety and privacy, body mechanics, and documentation.

Procedure Steps

NOTE: *If the patient has been lying down, do not measure the temperature on the side that was lying on the pillow. Do not measure if a cap or hair has been covering the area over the temporal artery.*

These can prevent heat dissipation and produce a falsely high reading.

1. **Remove the protective cap** from the instrument; clean the lens/probe according to the manufacturer's instructions.

2. **Place the probe flat** on the center of the forehead, midway between the eyebrow and the hairline. ➤

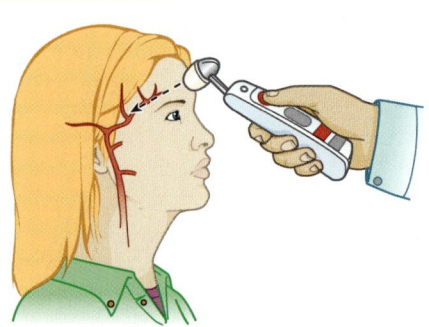

3. Press and hold the button while you stroke the thermometer medially to laterally across the forehead; keep the lens/probe flat and in contact with the skin and slide in a reasonably straight line until you reach the hairline. ▼

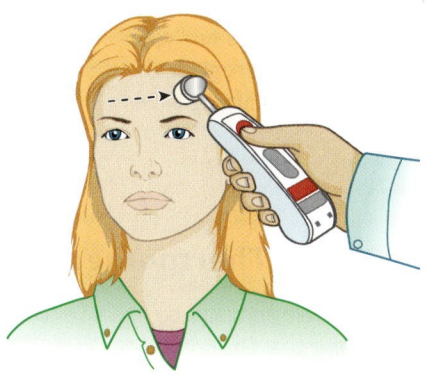

4. Still holding the button, touch the thermometer lens/probe behind the ear lobe, in the soft depression below the mastoid.
This step is necessary for an accurate reading if there is any moisture at all on the patient's forehead. ▼

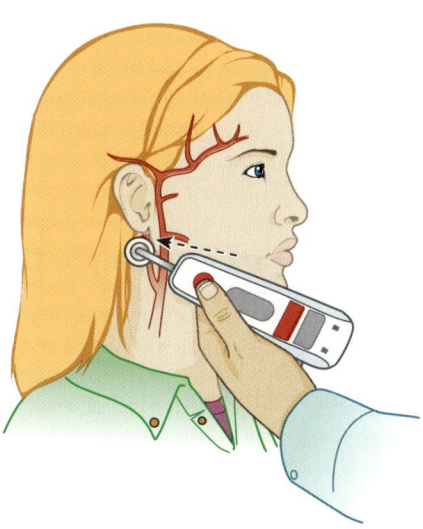

5. Release the button for the temperature reading. ▼

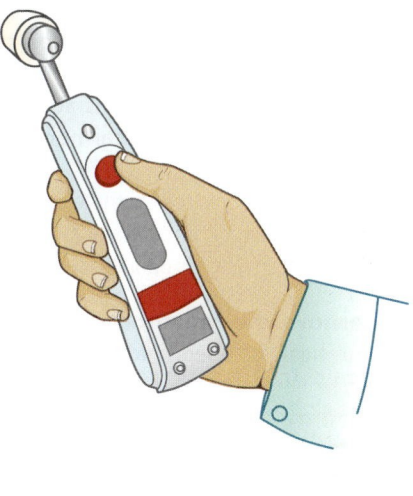

Procedure 19-1€ ■ Taking a Tympanic Membrane Temperature

➤ When performing the procedure, always identify your patient according to agency policy, using two identifiers, and be attentive to standard precautions, hand hygiene, patient safety and privacy, body mechanics, and documentation.

Procedure Steps

1. Make sure the thermometer lens is intact and clean.
Ensures an accurate reading.

2. Place a disposable cover tightly over the lens, making sure the clear film is smooth across the lens.
Ensures an accurate reading and prevents cross-contamination.

3. Position the patient's head to one side. If you are right-handed, try to use the right ear; if you are left-handed, use the left ear.
This allows you to better visualize the ear canal.

4. Straighten the ear canal or follow the manufacturer's instructions. As a rule: ▼

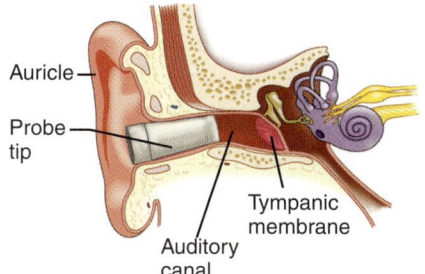

Auricle

Probe tip

Tympanic membrane

Auditory canal

a. For an adult, pull the pinna up and back. ▼

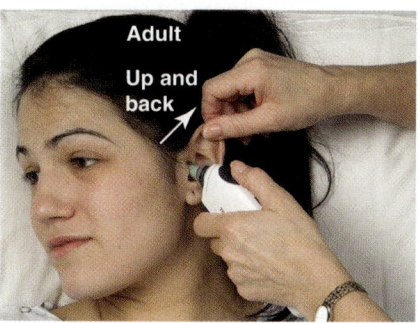

b. For a child, pull the pinna down and back. ▼

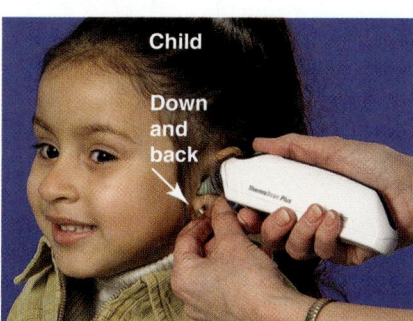

Some tympanic thermometers require you to straighten the ear canal; others do not. Some instruct, for adults, to pull the ear up, backward, and slightly away from the head. Some models instruct, for a child, to pull the pinna straight back instead of down and back. The external auditory canal is curved upward in children younger than 3 years of age. In an adult, it is a slightly S-shaped structure.

5. Insert the probe into the ear canal gently and firmly, directing it toward the tympanic membrane and inserting far enough to seal the opening.
Creates a seal to obtain an accurate reading without causing trauma to the ear canal.

6. Rotate the probe handle toward the jaw (for some thermometer models). Follow the manufacturer's instructions; not all models require this.
Aims the lens toward the tympanic membrane.

(continued on next page)

Procedure 19–1 ■ Assessing Body Temperature (continued)

7. Take the measurement.
   a. Press and release the button to obtain the reading.
   b. Follow the instructions for the specific tympanic thermometer being used.
   Some tympanic thermometers record the reading immediately; for some you must wait for about 3 seconds.

8. Remove the thermometer when you hear a beep and the display flashes. Note the reading in the display window.

9. Repeat the measurement in the other ear.
   A study of 132 adults found significant differences in temperature in the left compared with the right ear. In addition, the left ear tended to register a lower temperature than the right ear at temperatures below 36.7°C (98.1°F) and a higher temperature above 36.7°C (Heusch & McCarthy, 2005) or when taken by a female (Helton & Carter, 2011).

10. Discard the probe cover (usually you will press an "eject" button to do this) and replace the thermometer in its charging base.
   Recharges the battery and protects the instrument.

Procedure 19–1F ■ Taking a Skin Temperature Using a Chemical Strip Thermometer

> ➤ When performing the procedure, always identify your patient according to agency policy, using two identifiers, and be attentive to standard precautions, hand hygiene, patient safety and privacy, body mechanics, and documentation.

Procedure Steps

1. Place the thermometer strip (paper or tape) on the patient's skin, generally on the forehead or abdomen.
The thermometer strip must be in contact with the skin to work properly. ▼

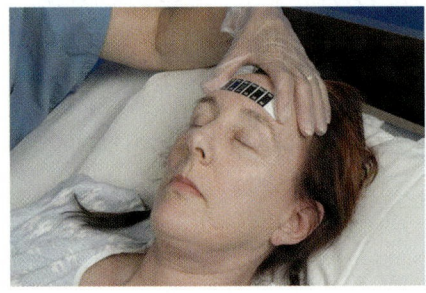

2. Leave the thermometer strip in place 15 to 60 seconds (or as the manufacturer directs).

3. Observe for color changes.
Chemical strips have indicators that change colors to indicate temperature changes.

4. Read the temperature before removing the strip from the patient's skin.
Ensures the most accurate reading.

5. Remove and discard the thermometer strip.

? What if . . .

■ **The patient's temperature is not within normal range?**

Identify whether the temperature reading indicates hypothermia, fever, or hyperthermia (e.g., heat stroke).
Perform other assessments to determine the cause or severity of the findings.
Assess for clinical signs to confirm an abnormal temperature reading.

Institute interventions to raise or lower temperature, as appropriate.
Provide comfort measures (e.g., change linens if they are wet from diaphoresis).

■ **You are using a glass thermometer?**

✚ Be sure the thermometer does not contain mercury.

Before and after using, shake down the thermometer as needed.
Clean the thermometer before and after using with soap and water or approved solution; rinse.
Use disposable covers, if available.
When reading the thermometer, hold it at eye level and rotate it until the markings are clear and easy to read.
Handle carefully and store in an appropriate container to avoid breakage.

Evaluation

- Compare with normal range for developmental stage, site used, and client's baseline data.
- Look for trends to identify potential concerns.
- Notify the appropriate healthcare provider of abnormal findings.

Patient Teaching

- Inform the patient of the temperature reading.
- Explain the significance of the temperature reading and any interventions that may be needed.

Home Care

- Clients commonly use chemical strip (disposable), glass, or tympanic membrane thermometers at home. Teach the following points:

  - Do not use an oral thermometer to take a rectal temperature. Use a specially shaped, more rounded, rectal thermometer *to avoid injury to the rectum.*

  - Do not use glass-and-mercury thermometers. If you discover a glass-and-mercury thermometer, urge the client to replace it with a safer instrument. Arrange for an exchange if there is a procedure for this in your agency or community.

Glass-and-mercury thermometers carry the risk of breakage, cuts, and exposure to toxic mercury.

- If you obtain a high or low reading using a chemical strip or a tympanic thermometer, retake the temperature using a glass or digital thermometer.
- Teach the same procedures you have learned for measuring temperature. Observe as the client takes a temperature to ensure correct technique.
- Clients often use the oral site. Remind them not to drink, eat, or smoke for 30 minutes before taking the temperature.
- Reinforce the following points about care of reusable thermometers:
  - If you use the same thermometer for more than one person, use disposable covers, if possible; clean the thermometer well between uses.

- If the person has an infection or communicable illness, soak the thermometer in 70% isopropyl alcohol between uses.
- Clean the thermometer after each use, even if it is used for only one person. Wash with soap and water, rinse with cold water, dry well, and store in a clean, dry container.
- If you store a thermometer in alcohol, rinse it with cold water before taking the temperature.
- Do not use the same thermometer for both oral and rectal temperatures.

Documentation

You will usually record temperature on a graphic flow sheet (see "Flowsheets and Graphic Records" in Chapter 18). In some situations (e.g., a fever), you may need to write a nurse's note. If so, follow these suggestions:

- Document the temperature, indicating the route of measurement, according to agency policy.
- Notify the appropriate provider of abnormal findings.
- Document supporting findings, such as "Skin is hot and dry" and state whether the temperature reading is consistent with the client's condition.

Sample documentation

mm/dd/yyyy   1230   Oral temperature 105°F: it has risen steadily since the first elevation at 0630, when it was 100°F. Skin hot and dry. Patient is voiding only small amounts, but states no burning. Urine dark but clear. No chills. I&O begun. Gave Tylenol 650 mg by mouth and notified Dr. Anderson of patient's condition and medication ——————————— Mary Clinton, RN

Practice Resources

Amoore, D. (2010); Lockwood, C., Conroy-Hiller, T., & Page, T. (2004); Morrow-Barnes, A. (2014). Rabinowitz, R., Cookson, S., Wasserman, S., et al. (1996); Vital Signs (1999).
Insert:

The video, **Assessing Body Temperature,** along with questions and suggested responses, is available on the *Davis's Nursing Skills Videos* Web site on *DavisPlus.*

Procedure 19-2 ■ Assessing Peripheral Pulses

➤ For steps to follow in *all* procedures, refer to the Universal Steps for All Procedures found on the page facing the inside back cover.

Equipment

- Watch with a second hand or digital readout
- Pen, pencil, and flow sheet or personal digital assistant (PDA)

Delegation

- You can delegate measurement of pulses to the nursing assistive personnel (NAP) if you conclude that the patient's condition and the NAP's skills allow. For example, if pedal circulation is critical and you suspect it may be difficult to palpate, you should not delegate assessment of the pedal pulse.
- If you do delegate, perform the pre-procedure assessments and tell the NAP which site (e.g., radial, brachial) to use. Inform the NAP of any special considerations (e.g., to note what the patient's activity has been just before taking the pulse).

- Ask the NAP to record and report the pulse to you and to report immediately if it is outside normal limits (you must specify what is "normal" for each patient).

Pre-Procedure Assessments

- Determine why assessment of pulses is indicated.
  Conditions requiring an assessment of pulses include blood loss, cardiac or respiratory disease, diabetes mellitus, and other conditions that affect oxygenation.
- Assess factors that may alter the pulse, such as activity and medications. If the patient has been active recently, wait 5 to 10 minutes before measuring.
  Activity increases the pulse rate; increased intracranial pressure decreases the rate; medications such as digoxin decrease the rate; other medications, such as albuterol, increase the pulse rate.

Procedure 19-2A ■ Assessing the Radial Pulse

➤ When performing the procedure, always identify your patient according to agency policy, using two identifiers, and be attentive to standard precautions, hand hygiene, patient safety and privacy, body mechanics, and documentation.

Procedure Steps

1. **With the patient sitting or supine,** flex the patient's arm and place the patient's forearm across his chest.

2. **Palpate the radial artery.**
   The radial site is the most frequently used to calculate the patient's heart rate because it is generally the easiest site to use.

   a. Place the pads of your index or middle fingers (or both) in the groove on the thumb side of the patient's wrist, over the radial artery.
   b. Press lightly but firmly until you are able to feel the radial pulse. Start with light pressure to prevent occluding the pulse and gradually increase the pressure until you feel the pulse.
   The fingertips are the most sensitive parts of the hand to palpate arterial pulsations. Avoid using the thumb, because it has its own pulsation and may interfere with the accuracy of your count. ➤

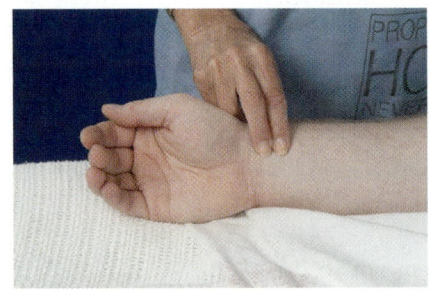

3. **Note the rhythm and quality** of the pulse. Note whether the thrust of the pulse against your fingertips is bounding, strong, weak, or thready.
   The rhythm and quality of the pulse are a reflection of the patient's cardiac output. The strength of the pulse reflects the volume of the blood that is ejected against the arterial wall with each contraction of the heart. An irregular or weak pulse indicates decreased cardiac output. A bounding pulse indicates increased cardiac output.

4. **Count the pulse:**
   a. Count for 60 seconds the first time you take a patient's pulse. After that, you can count a pulse with a regular rhythm for 15 seconds and

   multiply by 4, or count for 30 seconds and multiply by 2 to get the beats per minute. If you do not know the patient well, count for a full minute to be certain to detect irregularities. See Step 4c rationale.
   b. Begin timing with the count of 1—starting with the first beat that you feel.
   c. Count an irregular pulse for 1 full minute (60 seconds).
   Research is conflicting. Some studies indicate that a 60-second count is most accurate; others say that accuracy is not affected by a 30-second, or even a 15-second, count if the pulse is regular. You must count an irregular pulse for 1 full minute to be accurate.

5. **For an admission assessment** or peripheral vascular check, palpate the radial pulses on both wrists simultaneously. Note any difference in the quality of the pulse between arms. Is the pulse on one side weaker than that on the other?
   Palpating simultaneously enables the recognition of small differences in the peripheral circulation.

Procedure 19-2B ■ Assessing the Brachial Pulse

➤ When performing the procedure, always identify your patient according to agency policy, using two identifiers, and be attentive to standard precautions, hand hygiene, patient safety and privacy, body mechanics, and documentation.

Procedure Steps

1. **Palpate the brachial artery.**
   a. Using firm pressure, press in the inner aspect of the antecubital fossa until you palpate the brachial artery.
   b. If you have difficulty palpating the pulse, ask the patient to pronate the forearm (i.e., turn the palm of the hand downward).

This brings the brachial artery over a bony prominence and makes the pulse easier to feel. ▼

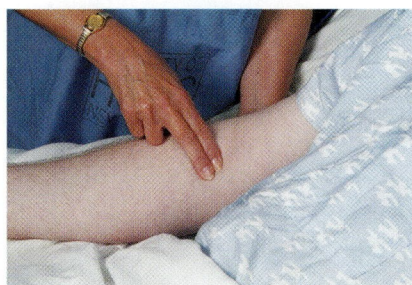

2. **Assess pulse rate, rhythm,** and **quality,** and assess bilaterally (see Procedure 19-2A).
   The brachial pulse is used most frequently to assess blood pressure and to identify the presence of a pulse during cardiopulmonary resuscitation (CPR) in an infant.

Procedure 19-2C ■ Assessing the Carotid Pulse

➤ When performing the procedure, always identify your patient according to agency policy, using two identifiers, and be attentive to standard precautions, hand hygiene, patient safety and privacy, body mechanics, and documentation.

✚ **Caution!** Do not palpate the carotid pulse except during cardiopulmonary resuscitation in an adult, and in certain situations to assess for circulation to the head. Persons not trained in CPR should not assess the carotid pulse.

Pressure on the carotid (especially in older adults) can stimulate the vagus nerve, causing the pulse and blood pressure to drop suddenly and perhaps fainting or circulatory arrest. It can also decrease circulation to the brain.

Procedure Steps

1. **Palpate the carotid artery lightly.** Place your fingers on the patient's trachea and slide them to the side into the groove between the trachea and the sternocleidomastoid muscle.
   Compressing or massaging the carotid arteries can stimulate the carotid bodies and significantly decrease the patient's heart rate and blood pressure. ➤

✚ NEVER compress the carotid artery on both sides of the neck at the same time.

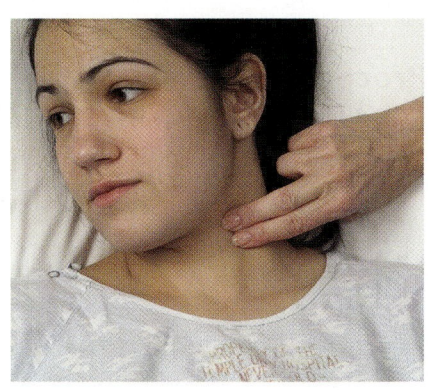

2. **Assess the rate, rhythm,** and quality, and compare bilaterally.

Procedure 19-2D ■ Assessing the Dorsalis Pedis Pulse

➤ When performing the procedure, always identify your patient according to agency policy, using two identifiers, and be attentive to standard precautions, hand hygiene, patient safety and privacy, body mechanics, and documentation.

Procedure Steps

1. **Palpate the dorsalis pedis pulse.**
   a. Run your fingers up the groove between the great and first toes to the top of the foot.
   b. Palpate very lightly.
      The dorsalis pedis pulse is easily obliterated, so use very light pressure. The dorsalis pedis pulse is used to access circulation of the foot.

 Owing to atherosclerosis or hardening of the arteries, the dorsalis pedis may be difficult to palpate in older adults.

2. **Assess pulse rate, rhythm,** and quality, and assess bilaterally. ▼

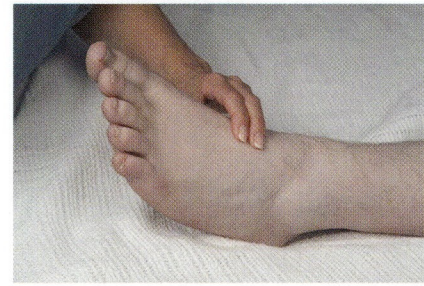

3. **If you are unable to palpate the dorsalis pedis pulse,** use a Doppler ultrasound device to assess the pulse and circulation to the lower extremity.

(continued on next page)

Procedure 19-2 ■ Assessing Peripheral Pulses (continued)

Procedure 19-2E ■ Assessing the Femoral Pulse

➤ When performing the procedure, always identify your patient according to agency policy, using two identifiers, and be attentive to standard precautions, hand hygiene, patient safety and privacy, body mechanics, and documentation.

Procedure Steps

1. **Palpate the femoral pulse** by pressing deeply in the groin midway between the anterosuperior iliac spine and the symphysis pubis.

   The femoral artery lies very deep and requires significant pressure to palpate. You may need to use both hands to feel the pulse on an adult. ➤

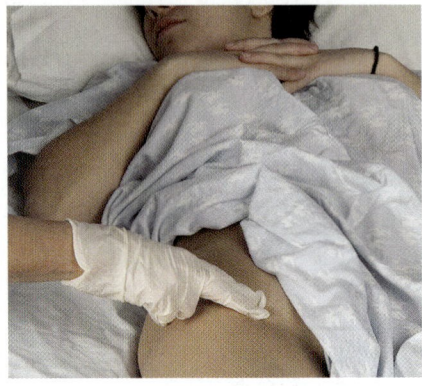

2. **Assess pulse rate, rhythm, and quality, and assess bilaterally.**

   The femoral pulse is used to determine the presence of a pulse during CPR and to assess circulation to the leg.

Procedure 19-2F ■ Assessing the Posterior Tibial Pulse

➤ When performing the procedure, always identify your patient according to agency policy, using two identifiers, and be attentive to standard precautions, hand hygiene, patient safety and privacy, body mechanics, and documentation.

Procedure Steps

1. **Palpate the posterior tibial pulse** by pressing on the inner (medial) side of the ankle below the medial malleolus.

   The posterior tibial pulse is usually palpated easily, but it may be deeper in some people. So, press down moderately and then increase pressure until you feel the pulse. It is relatively easy to obliterate. ➤

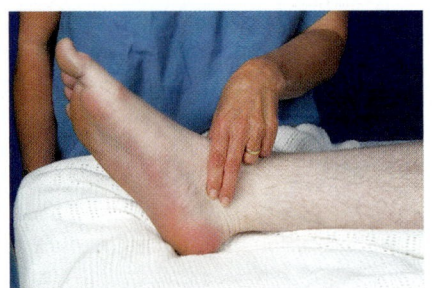

2. **Assess pulse rate, rhythm, and quality, and assess bilaterally.**

   The posterior tibial pulse is used to assess circulation to the lower extremity; it is assessed along with the dorsalis pedis pulse.

Procedure 19-2G ■ Assessing the Popliteal Pulse

➤ When performing the procedure, always identify your patient according to agency policy, using two identifiers, and be attentive to standard precautions, hand hygiene, patient safety and privacy, body mechanics, and documentation.

Procedure Steps

1. **Palpate the popliteal pulse** by pressing behind the knee in the middle of the popliteal fossa.

   The popliteal pulse can be difficult to feel. It is used only when specifically indicated because of absence of pedal pulses or for taking a thigh blood pressure. ➤

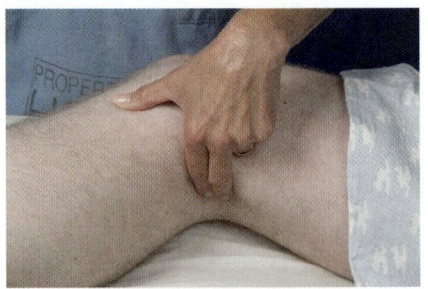

2. **Assess pulse rate, rhythm, and quality, and assess bilaterally.**

   The popliteal pulse is used to assess circulation of the lower leg and auscultate a thigh blood pressure.

Procedure 19-2H ■ **Assessing the Temporal Pulse**

➤ When performing the procedure, always identify your patient according to agency policy, using two identifiers, and be attentive to standard precautions, hand hygiene, patient safety and privacy, body mechanics, and documentation.

Procedure Steps

1. **Palpate the temporal pulse** by pressing lightly lateral (outside area) and superior to (above) the eye. ▼

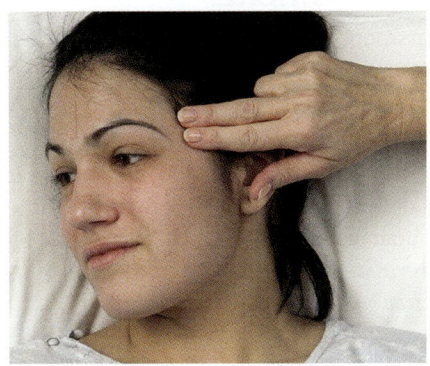

2. **Assess pulse rate, rhythm,** and quality, and assess bilaterally as for the radial pulse (see Procedure 19-2A).
   The temporal pulse is easily accessible and is used frequently in infants.

? What if . . .

- **The patient is an infant or a child younger than age 3 years?**

   Auscultate an apical pulse rate. Rates are faster and small arteries more difficult to feel in a child or infant.

If a parent is present, encourage the parent to hold the child to reduce anxiety.
Fear increases the pulse rate.

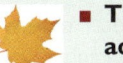

   ■ **The patient is an older adult?**

   Have the patient at rest for 15 to 20 minutes after activity and before assessing the pulse.
   The pulse tends to return to baseline more slowly in older adults.

   If the pulse is fast, take repeated measures; if a pattern of fast rate emerges, note this for the primary care provider for further evaluation.
   An elevated heart rate is related to increased mortality in older adult women, so it is a simple index of general health status.

- **The pulse is faint or weak?**

   Use a Doppler ultrasound device to detect blood flow.
   Lack of pulses indicates inadequate circulation to the lower extremities. If you cannot feel the pulse, you must determine whether the pulse is absent or whether you are having difficulty feeling. To draw

the conclusion that the pulse is "absent," you must use a Doppler.

Apply transmission gel to the end of the probe. Do not use water-soluble lubricant as a substitute for transmission gel.

Place the probe lightly on the skin over the artery you are using.

Turn on the instrument and set the volume control to the lowest setting.

Tilting the probe to a 45° angle to the artery, move the probe slowly in a circular motion to locate the signal (a rhythmic hissing noise). Count for 60 seconds.
Move the probe slowly to avoid distorting the signal.

When you are finished, wipe the gel off the patient's skin. Clean the probe with soapy water or an antiseptic solution. Do not immerse the probe or bump it against anything hard.
Clean the probe to prevent cross-contamination to other patients. Probes are fragile and may malfunction if bumped against a hard surface.

Evaluation

Especially if pedal pulses are decreased, observe for other indications of inadequate circulation, such as cool skin, decreased capillary refill, and bluish or ashen skin tone. You must provide supporting evidence if you chart that pedal pulses are decreased or absent. The complete absence of a pulse requires immediate intervention.

Patient Teaching

- Teach the patient about the significance of any abnormalities in pulse rate or rhythm.
- Explain any interventions that may be needed.

Home Care

Assess the skill level of the person who will be assessing the client's peripheral pulses in the home and provide instruction if necessary.

Documentation

Usually you will document routine vital signs (VS), including pulse, on a flow sheet or graphic. If you record it in a nurse's note, document the pulse rate, rhythm, quality, and site (e.g., "radial pulse 64 beats/min, regular, and strong bilaterally").

Practice Resources

Alexis, O. (2010); Lewis, R. (2013); Lockwood, C., Conroy-Hiller, T., & Page, T. (2004); Nicholson, C. (2014); Vital Signs (1999).

 The video, **Assessing Peripheral Pulses,** along with questions and suggested responses, is available on the **Davis's Nursing Skills Videos** Web site on DavisPlus.

Procedure 19-3 ■ Assessing the Apical Pulse

➤ For steps to follow in *all* procedures, refer to the Universal Steps for All Procedures found on the page facing the inside back cover.

Equipment
- Watch with a second hand or second readout
- Stethoscope
- Alcohol wipes (to clean stethoscope)

Delegation
You can delegate measurement of the apical pulse to the nursing assistive personnel (NAP) if you conclude that the patient's condition and the NAP's skills allow.
- First perform the pre-procedure assessments.
- Then inform the NAP of any special considerations (e.g., to note what the patient's activity has been just before taking the pulse or to mark the time exactly so you can compare it with the patient's ECG).

- Ask the NAP to record and report the pulse to you, and to report immediately if it is outside normal limits (you must specify what is "normal" for each patient).

Pre-Procedure Assessments
- Determine why assessment of the apical pulse is indicated.
  Conditions that require assessment of the apical pulse include digitalis therapy, blood loss, cardiac or respiratory disease, or other conditions that affect oxygenation status.

- Assess factors that may alter the pulse, such as activity and medications. If the client has been recently active, wait 10 to 15 minutes before obtaining a measurement.
  Activity can increase the pulse rate. Relate above factors to baseline pulse rate to determine their effect.

➤ When performing the procedure, always identify your patient according to agency policy, using two identifiers, and be attentive to standard precautions, hand hygiene, patient safety and privacy, body mechanics, and documentation.

Procedure Steps

1. **With the client supine or sitting,** expose the left side of the chest, but only as much as necessary.
   Prevents distortion of sound from the patient's gown rubbing on the stethoscope, while also protecting the patient's privacy. ▼

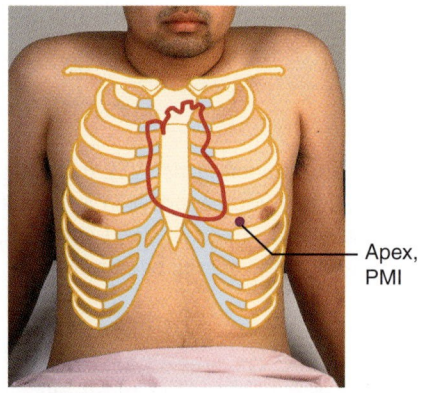

— Apex, PMI

2. ✚ **Wipe the stethoscope with** a 70% alcohol or benzalkonium chloride wipe before and after examining the patient.
   Cleaning can reduce the bacterial count by up to 100%.

3. **Palpate the 5th intercostal space** at the midclavicular line for the apical pulse.

The left ventricle of the heart and the point of maximum impulse lie in this area. The apical pulse is generally best heard at the point of maximum impulse (PMI), over the apex of the heart.

a. To locate the 5th intercostal space, slide your finger down from the sternal notch to the angle of Louis (the bump where the manubrium and sternum meet).
b. Slide your finger over to the left sternal border to the 2nd intercostal space.
c. Now place your index or ring finger (depending on which hand you use) in the 2nd intercostal space, and count down to the 5th intercostal space by placing a finger in each of the spaces.
d. Slide over to the midclavicular line, keeping your finger in the 5th intercostal space.

The apical pulse is generally best heard at the PMI in the 5th intercostal space at the midclavicular line. The PMI is located over the apex of the heart. For an adult, this site is on the anterior chest at 3 inches (8 cm) or less to the left of the sternum, at the 4th, 5th, or 6th intercostal space at the midclavicular line.

4. **Palpate the apical pulse** (also called the point of maximal impulse [PMI]).
   The pulse area should be about the size of a quarter, without lifts or heaves.
   A larger than normal pulsation may indicate ventricular hypertrophy.

5. **Warm the stethoscope** in your hand for 10 seconds. Then place the diaphragm over the PMI, and listen to the normal S_1 and S_2 heart sounds ("lub dub"). Count each pair of sounds ("lub-dub") as one heartbeat.
   A cold stethoscope placed on the skin may startle the patient and increase the heart rate. Heart sounds result when blood moves through the valves of the heart. The first heart sound is louder at the apical area and should be audible when the pulse is auscultated.

6. **Count the apical heart rate** for 1 full minute.
   Ensures accuracy. Because the apical heart rate is needed as an assessment measure for the administration of some medications (e.g., digoxin), accuracy is essential. Some cardiac conditions cause either slow or irregular rates, both of

which must be counted for a full minute to ensure accuracy.

? What if . . .

- **The apical rate is less than 60 beats/min?**
  - ➤ (*Note:* You may also see "bpm" as an abbreviation for "beats per minute" or for "beats/min.")

If the patient is taking cardiac medications, withhold them and consult with a physician about whether to adjust dosage.

Certain cardiac medications (e.g., digoxin) are given to slow the heart rate; bradycardia may indicate that blood levels are too high.

Assess for chest pain, dizziness, dyspnea.

May indicate decreased cardiac output.

- **The apical rate is greater than 100 beats/min?**

Obtain a complete set of vital signs. Assess for pain, anxiety, fever, dehydration, decreased oxygenation, hypotension, and decreased exercise.

These factors may increase pulse rate.

Evaluation

- Are the findings within normal limits?
- Are there other factors supporting the findings?
- What are the trends over time?
- Is the skin pink, warm, and dry?
- Is there any cyanosis?

Patient Teaching

- Teach the patient about the significance of any abnormalities in the pulse rate or rhythm.
- Explain any interventions that may be necessary.

Home Care

- Assess the skill level of the person who will be assessing the client's apical pulse in the home and provide instruction if necessary.
- Teach the home caregiver when to hold medications and/or to call primary care provider (e.g., to hold the digitalis if the rate is < 60).
- Before leaving the home, clean the stethoscope with detergent or disinfectant when possible, or place it in a plastic bag for transporting to the reprocessing location.

- ▪ ✚ If the patient has a multidrug-resistant organism infection, reusable equipment such as stethoscopes should remain in the home. If the stethoscope cannot remain in the home, clean and disinfect it before leaving the home, using a low to intermediate level disinfectant. If this is not practical, place the stethoscope in a plastic bag and transport it to another site for cleaning and disinfection.

Documentation

Document the pulse rate, rhythm, and site.

Sample documentation

mm/dd/yyyy —— 0800 —— Apical pulse regular rhythm, and strong, rate of 64. —— Janice Jonas, RN

Practice Resources

Alexis, O. (2010); Best Practices (2007); CDC (2008); Lockwood, C., Conroy-Hiller, T., & Page, T. (2004); Vital Signs (1999).

The video, **Assessing Apical Pulse,** along with questions and suggested responses, is available on the **Davis's Nursing Skills Videos** Web site on DavisPlus.

Procedure 19–4 ▪ Assessing for an Apical-Radial Pulse Deficit

> ➤ For steps to follow in *all* procedures, refer to the Universal Steps for All Procedures found on the page facing the inside back cover.

Equipment

- Watch or clock with a second hand or second readout
- Procedure gloves, if indicated
- Stethoscope
- Alcohol or other antiseptic wipes to clean the stethoscope

Delegation

Instead of delegating measurement of an apical-radial pulse to a NAP, you would most likely ask the NAP to assist you in this procedure because it is best performed by two persons working together.

Pre-Procedure Assessments

- Determine why assessment of pulse deficit is indicated.
  Conditions that require assessment of pulse deficit include digitalis therapy, blood loss, cardiac or respiratory disease, and other conditions that affect oxygenation status.
- Assess factors that may alter the pulse, such as activity and medications.
- Obtain another nurse to assist with the procedure.

(continued on next page)

Procedure 19-4 ■ **Assessing for an Apical-Radial Pulse Deficit** (continued)

➤ When performing the procedure, always identify your patient according to agency policy, using two identifiers, and be attentive to standard precautions, hand hygiene, patient safety and privacy, body mechanics, and documentation.

Procedure Steps

1. ✚ **Wipe the stethoscope with** a 70% alcohol or benzalkonium chloride wipe before and after examining the patient.
   Cleaning can reduce the bacterial count by up to 100% and prevent the transmission of microbes.

2. **Expose the left side** of the patient's chest, minimizing patient exposure.
   Prevents distortion of sound from the patient's gown rubbing on the stethoscope and protects privacy.

3. **Place the watch so that the** second hand is visible to both nurses (if two nurses are performing the procedure).
   Using one watch increases accuracy of counts.

4. **Nurse 1 prepares to auscultate** the radial pulse. She palpates the 5th intercostal space at the midclavicular line, then places and holds the stethoscope in that spot, using firm pressure until Nurse 2 says "Start."
   Aids in hearing high-pitched sounds and ensures good contact between the

diaphragm of the stethoscope and the skin. ▼

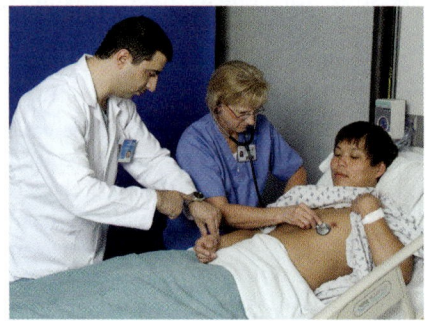

5. **Nurse 2 palpates to locate** the radial pulse, preparing to assessing rate, rhythm and quality.

6. **Nurse 2 says "Start"** when ready to begin and "Stop" when finished. Both nurses count the pulses simultaneously for 1 full minute.
   Count simultaneously to ensure accuracy. Counting for 1 full minute is necessary for an accurate assessment of any discrepancies that may exist between the two sites.

7. **To obtain pulse deficit, subtract** the radial rate from the apical rate.

   Apical Rate – Radial Rate =
   Pulse Deficit

Atrial and ventricular dysrhythmias may cause beats that do not perfuse, so although you hear an apical heartbeat, you do not feel a peripheral pulse. The pulse deficit is the number of heartbeats that do not perfuse.

? **What if . . .**

■ **There is not another nurse available to assist?**

Hold the stethoscope in place with the one hand while palpating the radial pulse with the hand wearing the watch.
Even if you cannot manage to count both rates, you should be able to feel any differences between the apical and radial pulses.

■ **There has been an increase in pulse deficit since the last measurement?**

An increase in pulse deficit means that the patient's cardiac output has decreased.

Evaluation

- Identify the presence of an apical-radial pulse deficit, and compare to previous findings.
- Assess other measures of cardiopulmonary status to identify a decline in the patient's condition.
- Look for trends.
  The presence of any apical-radial pulse deficit is abnormal.

Patient Teaching

- Teach the patient about the significance of an apical-radial pulse deficit.
- Explain any necessary interventions.

Home Care

- Assess the skill level of the person(s) who will be measuring the client's apical-radial pulse deficit in the home and provide instruction if necessary.
- Before leaving the home, clean the stethoscope as described in the Home Care section of Procedure 19-3.

Documentation

Document the apical-radial pulse deficit.

Sample documentation

MM/DD/YYYY   0900   *Apical-radial pulse deficit is 4 beats/min.* ——————— *Jon Albertson, RN*

Practice Resources

Alexis, O. (2010); Best Practices (2007); CDC (2008); Lockwood, C., Conroy-Hiller, T., & Page, T. (2004); National Guideline Clearinghouse (2003, revised 2014); Vital Signs (1999).

 The video, **Assessing for an Apical Radial Pulse Deficit,** along with questions and suggested responses, is available on the **Davis's Nursing Skills Videos** Web site on Davis*Plus.*

Procedure 19–5 ■ Assessing Respirations

➤ For steps to follow in *all* procedures, refer to the Universal Steps for All Procedures found on the page facing the inside back cover.

Equipment
- A watch with a second hand (or a wall clock)

Delegation
You can delegate the counting of respirations to the nursing assistive personnel (NAP) if you conclude that the patient's condition and the NAP's skills allow.
- Perform the pre-procedure assessments.
- Inform the NAP of any special considerations (e.g., the need to keep the patient in a certain position).
- Ask the NAP to record and report the respirations to you and to report immediately if they are not within the normal range for this patient (specify the range).

Pre-Procedure Assessments
- Observe for signs of respiratory distress—breathing faster or slower than normal, gasping breaths, confusion, circumoral (around the month) cyanosis.
  Signs of hypoxemia may indicate that the patient is not adequately oxygenated.
- Determine the baseline respiratory rate and character of respirations.
- Assess for factors that may affect the respiratory rate (e.g., pain, activity, fever, respiratory disorders).

➤ When performing the procedure, always identify your patient according to agency policy, using two identifiers, and be attentive to standard precautions, hand hygiene, patient safety and privacy, body mechanics, and documentation.

Procedure Steps

1. **Position the patient.** With the patient in a sitting position (preferably), flex the patient's arm and place her forearm across her chest.
   Aids in counting the patient's pulse rate by making the rise and fall of the chest more discernible and by making the patient less aware that you are measuring the respiratory rate. The patient's awareness might alter the respiratory rate and/or pattern because respirations are partially under voluntary control. ▼

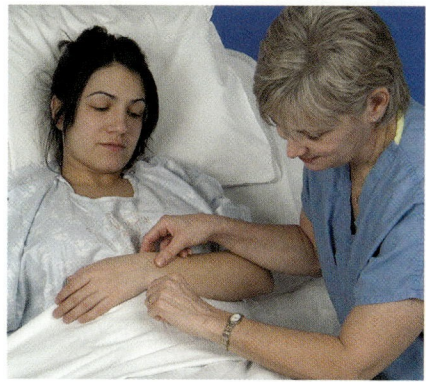

2. **Palpate and count the radial** pulse; remember that number.

3. **Then, keeping your hand** on the patient's wrist, count the respirations.
   Allows you to count the respirations unobtrusively.

4. **Observe the respiratory rate,** rhythm, and depth.
   - *Rate:* Normal for patient's age, fast (tachypnea), or slow (bradypnea)
   - *Rhythm:* Regular or irregular
   - *Depth:* Normal, shallow, or deep (e.g., Kussmaul's)
   All of these characteristics are necessary to evaluate respiratory status. Different pathologies affect each of these characteristics differently.

5. **Count the number of breaths** per minute. Begin timing the respirations with a count of 1, not 0 (the same as with pulse measurement).
   a. If the respiratory rhythm is regular, count the rate (one inhalation and one exhalation is one respiration) for 30 seconds, and multiply by 2.
   b. If the rhythm is irregular, count the rate for 1 full minute (60 seconds).
   Variations in rhythm may cause an inaccurate rate when counted for less than 1 minute.

? What if . . .

- **The patient is an infant?**
  Place your hand on the abdomen to assess the respiratory rate. Auscultate breath sounds with a stethoscope.

Infants and young children breathe rapidly and are abdominal breathers, so it is difficult to see each and every rise and fall of the abdomen. Using a stethoscope increases the accuracy of the count as well as providing information about the breath sounds.

For infants and very young children, count for 1 full minute.
Infants and young children have irregular respirations. Counting for a full minute provides a more accurate rate for irregular respirations.

- **The patient is receiving oxygen therapy, or requires careful assessment of respiratory status?**

  Apply a pulse oximeter (see Procedure 37-2, Monitoring Pulse Oximetry).
  Evidence suggests that pulse oximetry is useful for detecting deterioration of physiological function that might otherwise be missed (e.g., during the perioperative period or in seriously ill patients).

(continued on next page)

Procedure 19-5 ■ Assessing Respirations (continued)

Evaluation

- Compare the respiratory rate and rhythm with previous readings.
- Note other vital signs, especially temperature.
- Look for trends and note whether the respiratory rate and rhythm are changing in conjunction with changes in the other vital signs.

  If the patient has an elevated temperature, the respiratory rate will increase. Corresponding elevation in pulse with respiratory rate may indicate hypoxemia. If respirations are not within normal parameters, assess oxygenation with a pulse oximeter.

Patient Teaching

Teach the patient about factors that affect respiratory status, such as smoking and activity.

Home Care

Assess the skill level of the person(s) who will be measuring the client's respiratory rate in the home and provide instruction as needed.

Documentation

You will document routine VS (including respirations) on a graphic or flow sheet. When a nurse's note is needed, follow the following guidelines:

- Document the respiratory rate, depth, and rhythm.

  Document that respirations are either labored or unlabored.

If labored, describe in what way (e.g., intercostal retractions, use of accessory muscles, nasal flaring).

Example of Electronic Health Record

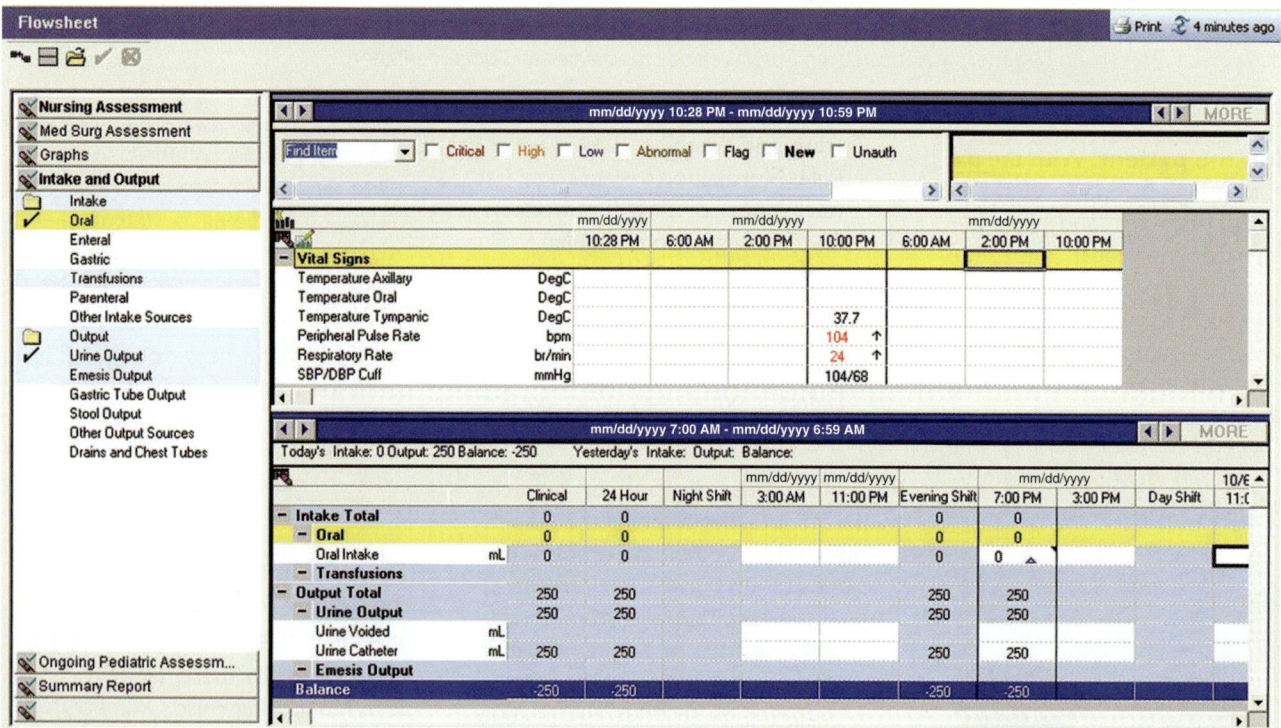

Practice Resources

CDC (2008); Hunter, J., & Rawlings-Anderson, K. (2008); Lockwood, C., Conroy-Hiller, T., & Page, T. (2004); Parkes, R. (2011); Vital Signs (1999).

 The video, **Assessing Respirations,** along with questions and suggested responses, is available on the *Davis's Nursing Skills Videos* Web site on DavisPlus.

Procedure 19-6 ■ Measuring Blood Pressure

➤ For steps to follow in *all* procedures, refer to the Universal Steps for All Procedures found on the page facing the inside back cover.

Equipment

■ Stethoscope

■ ✚ *NOTE: Do not wear a stethoscope around your neck. There is a slight risk that you can entangle it in intravenous and other lines. There is also a risk that a psychotic or delirious patient could use it to harm you. Also, wearing a stethoscope can be a source of cross-contamination.*

■ Use 70% alcohol or benzalkonium chloride wipes.
For cleaning stethoscope before and after use. Clean all parts.

■ Sphygmomanometer with a cuff of the appropriate size. Refer to Clinical Insight 19-1.
A cuff that is too small will produce a false-high reading; a cuff that is too large will produce a false-low reading.

NOTE: This procedure describes the use of an aneroid manometer or an electronic measuring device.

Delegation

You can delegate measurement of BP to the NAP if you conclude that the patient's condition and the NAP's skills allow.
■ Perform the pre-procedure assessments.
■ Inform the NAP of the site (e.g., radial, brachial) to use.

■ Inform the NAP of any special considerations (e.g., not to place a BP cuff on the same side as the site of a mastectomy).
■ Ask the NAP to record and report the BP to you, and to report immediately if it is outside normal limits (you must specify what is "normal" for each patient).
■ Tell the NAP that if BP is elevated to note which arm, the patient's position during measurement, and activity immediately preceding the measurement.

Pre-Procedure Assessments

■ Check for factors or activities that may alter the readings.
Caffeine, smoking, exercise, and stress can all elevate the BP. Be certain the patient has been lying or sitting for at least 5 minutes (30 minutes after strenuous exercise) and is relaxed.

■ Check the previous recording, if any.
Noting changes over time is important with all patient assessments. Because BP changes constantly and because so many factors affect it, you cannot draw conclusions from a single measurement.

➤ When performing the procedure, always identify your patient according to agency policy, using two identifiers, and be attentive to standard precautions, hand hygiene, patient safety and privacy, body mechanics, and documentation.

➤ Note: To improve the accuracy of your readings, also refer to Clinical Insights 19-1 and 19-2.

Procedure Steps

1. **Clean the stethoscope before** and after the procedure.
Although only a small percentage of microorganisms are pathogenic, cleaning can reduce the bacterial count by 94% to 100%.

2. **Position the patient** comfortably, ensuring that:
a. The legs are uncrossed, the back is supported, and the feet are resting on the floor (if the patient is sitting in a chair); or that the patient is supine.
This position allows for the most accurate reading. Crossing the legs may elevate the BP reading.

b. The measurement arm is supported at heart level, slightly flexed, with the palm facing upward.

The blood pressure will decrease if the arm is above the heart and increase if the arm is below the heart or not supported.

3. **Fully expose the arm,** being careful that clothing is not tight. Remove clothing rather than rolling up a sleeve. *Note:* There is some evidence to suggest that readings taken over sleeves do not affect blood pressure results, and that it may actually be preferable because of concerns about hygiene, privacy and religious beliefs (Pinar, Ataalkin, & Watson, 2010). While you are learning, and until there is more evidence, we advise that you will find it easier to hear the BP sounds on a bare arm.
Clothing that is tight enough to restrict blood flow will alter the reading.

4. **Place the cuff** on the upper arm. ▼

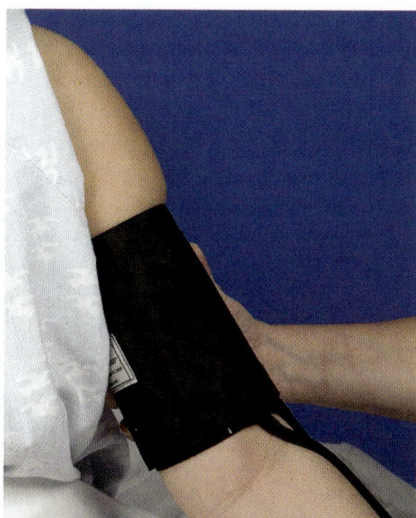

a. Wrap the cuff snugly.
b. Ensure that the cuff is totally deflated and palpate the brachial artery.

(continued on next page)

Procedure 19-6 ■ **Measuring Blood Pressure** (continued)

c. Place the bottom edge of the cuff approximately 1 in. (2.5 cm) above the antecubital space.

d. Place the center of the cuff bladder directly over the brachial artery (the center is often indicated with an arrow on the BP cuff).
The center of the cuff bladder needs to be directly over the brachial artery to obtain an accurate reading. Loose application of the cuff results in overestimation of the pressure.

5. **Place the stethoscope ear pieces** in your ears, pointing slightly forward.
When the earpieces point slightly forward, they direct sound into the ear canal, making the sounds more audible.

6. **Palpate the brachial artery** on the arm with the cuff. (Use the radial artery for this step if you prefer.)
For correct stethoscope placement.

7. **Inflate the cuff, as follows:**
a. Close the sphygmomanometer valve and inflate the cuff rapidly to about 80 mm Hg.

b. Then palpate the pulse while you continue inflating in 10 mm Hg increments until you no longer feel the pulse.

c. As you *inflate* the cuff, the artery is occluded as the pressure of the cuff exceeds the pressure in the artery. At that point, blood flow through the artery is halted, and no sound can be heard. Note the pressure at which the pulse disappears.

d. Go to step 8 or the variation, as you prefer.
Palpating the artery while inflating the cuff ensures that the cuff is inflated higher than the systolic BP. If the patient has an auscultatory gap, the systolic pressure can be mistakenly identified as lower than it actually is. Palpation is particularly important if the baseline systolic BP is unknown or if the patient is hypertensive.

8. **Continue inflating the cuff** to a pressure that is 20 to 30 mm Hg above the level at which the pulse disappeared. Move to Step 9.
Helps ensure you will not miss an auscultatory gap or a faint first sound.

Step Variation in Cuff Inflation Technique

■ Do not continue palpating after the pulse disappears; instead, deflate the cuff rapidly.

■ Wait 2 minutes, then place the stethoscope over the brachial artery and inflate the cuff to a pressure that is 20 to 30 mm Hg above the palpated level.

■ Continue with steps 9 and 10.

9. **Place the stethoscope over** the brachial artery as follows: ▼

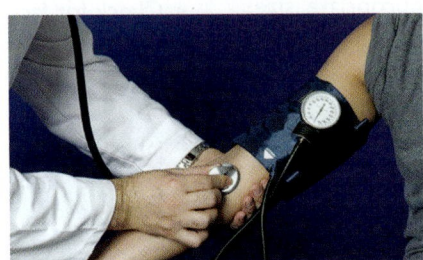

a. Be certain that the stethoscope tubing is not touching anything and that the diaphragm is not tucked under the edge of the cuff.
When the tubing rubs against clothing, for example, it produces artifact sounds that make it difficult to hear the BP sounds. Placing the bell or diaphragm under the cuff can partially occlude the brachial artery, delaying the appearance of the Korotkoff sounds.

b. Using the bell will enable you to hear BP sounds more accurately, especially at diastolic pressures. However, most people use the diaphragm because it is easily placed and because some stethoscopes do not have a bell.

10. **Deflate the cuff slowly** (2 to 3 mm Hg per second or per beat), listening for the Korotkoff sounds as you deflate.
Deflating the cuff slowly increases patient discomfort and may alter the reading. Deflating the cuff faster may cause errors in hearing the Korotkoff sounds.

a. As you *deflate* the cuff, blood begins to flow rapidly through the partially open artery, producing turbulence that you will hear through the stethoscope as a tapping sound. Note the point

on the manometer at which you hear the first sound. This is the *systolic BP.* (If you are using an electronic BP device, read the digital screen when the numbers appear. Follow the manufacturer's instructions.)
The 1st Korotkoff sound is the systolic pressure.

b. Continue deflating the cuff and note the level at which the sounds become muffled and disappear. The artery is no longer compressed and sound will disappear. Record the point at which the sound disappears as the *diastolic pressure.*
The 5th Korotkoff sound (the disappearance of sound) is the diastolic BP in adults. The 4th Korotkoff sound (the muffling of sounds) is the diastolic BP in children. The American Heart Association recommends recording the first sound, muffling, and last sound in children younger than 13 years, pregnant women, and people with high cardiac output or peripheral vasoconstriction.

11. **If you need to repeat** the measurement, deflate the cuff completely, and wait 2 minutes before reinflating it.
Prevents venous congestion and false high readings.

? **What if . . .**

■ **You cannot feel the brachial pulse?**
While supporting the arm at the elbow, have the patient pronate her forearm.
This moves the brachial artery more over a bony prominence, making the pulsation easier to feel.

■ **You have difficulty hearing BP sounds for many patients?**
You may need a stethoscope with a built-in amplifier.

■ **You are not certain of the systolic reading when you begin to deflate the cuff?**
Do not stop cuff deflation to recheck the systolic reading. Deflate the cuff

completely and wait 1 to 3 minutes before taking another measurement. *Stopping deflation and retaking the BP too soon can lead to a muffling of the Korotkoff sounds and inaccurate results.*

- **You must use a mercury manometer?**

  ✚ Because mercury is a health hazard, mercury manometers should not be found in healthcare agencies. Use an aneroid manometer or an electronic BP device if one is available. If you must use a mercury manometer, be certain the meniscus of the mercury is at eye level when taking the reading. Take care not to bump equipment against the glass cover over the column of mercury.

- **You are using an automatic blood pressure device?**

  Follow the same guidelines as for a manual BP (e.g., cuff size and placement, patient position):
  Turn on the machine; be sure the cuff is deflated.
  Apply the cuff.
  Press the button to start the measurement.
  At the tone, read the digital measurement.

- **You do not have a cuff size to fit the upper arm?**

  Use the forearm, thigh, or calf. See Procedure Variations A, B, and C, below, respectively.

- **The patient requires contact or isolation precautions?**

  Follow agency guidelines for equipment (e.g., stethoscope, BP cuff). Generally the equipment remains in the room with the patient; otherwise, it must be disinfected before leaving the room. For information about contact precautions and protective isolation, see Chapter 23, Clinical Insights.

Procedure Variation A: Measuring Blood Pressure in the Forearm

- Place a properly sized cuff on the forearm, midway between the elbow and the wrist. Auscultate over the radial artery.
- Note that a forearm reading is not interchangeable with an upper arm reading.

Procedure Variation B: Measuring Blood Pressure in the Thigh

- Use the thigh or the calf if the cuff will not fit either the upper or lower arm.

  NOTE: The thigh systolic measure may be 20 to 30 mm Hg higher than an arm BP reading. The diastolic reading is generally comparable.

- Place the patient in a prone position. If patient cannot be prone, place supine with knee slightly bent.
- Choose the correct cuff size. Wrap the cuff snugly around the thigh so that the lower edge of the cuff is approximately 1 in. (2.5 cm) above the popliteal fossa and the center of the cuff bladder is positioned directly over the popliteal artery (often indicated with an arrow on the blood pressure cuff).
- Palpate and auscultate over the popliteal artery. ▼

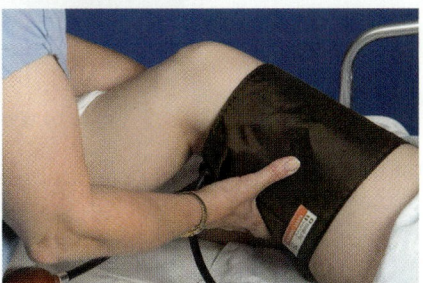

Procedure Variation C: Measuring Blood Pressure in the Calf

- Use the thigh or the calf if the cuff will not fit either the upper or lower arm.
- Place the patient supine.
- Choose the correct size cuff. Wrap the cuff snugly around the calf so that the lower edge of the cuff is approximately 2.5 cm above the malleoli or ankle.
- Place the stethoscope over either the dorsalis pedis or the posterior tibial artery.

NOTE: Calf BP measurements are not equivalent to upper arm measurements in adults; they tend to produce a higher systolic BP.

Procedure Variation D: Palpating the Blood Pressure

- Apply the cuff and palpate for the radial or brachial pulse.
- Begin to inflate the cuff. When you can no longer feel the pulse, inflate the cuff about 30 mm Hg more.
- As you release the valve and slowly deflate the cuff, note the reading on the manometer at which you once again feel the pulse.
- Record the palpated blood pressure according to the way it was assessed (e.g., "Palpated, low Fowler's, left arm 86/——" [or "86 systolic"]).

(continued on next page)

Procedure 19-6 ■ **Measuring Blood Pressure** (continued)

Evaluation

- Compare the BP reading with previous readings.
- Look for trends. Is the BP slowly decreasing (e.g., impending shock) or slowly increasing (e.g., hypervolemia)?
- Look for a corresponding change in pulse rate, indicating potential hypoxemia.
- If this is the first BP measurement for the client, check readings in both arms.
  A difference of 10 mm Hg or less is normal.
- Report any significant changes in the BP reading.

Patient Teaching

Teach the patient about:

- Normal BP values (keep in mind that prehypertension is diagnosed at a lower level when using self-monitored readings).
- Significance of the BP reading.
- Further follow-up that may be necessary.

Home Care

- The American Heart Association and other guidelines recommend self-monitoring of BP at home. It is thought that self-measurement of BP provides more reliable data than office BP because of the availability of multiple readings. It is also thought to improve adherence to treatment regimens.
- If possible, use the same equipment each time to prevent false changes in measurement.
- Explain the need for frequent recalibration of the home-monitoring device.
- Assess the skill level of the person(s) who will be measuring the patient's BP in the home and provide instruction if necessary.
- Assess whether self-monitoring is causing the client to be anxious.
  Some clients do become overly anxious when they know they must monitor their BP or when they obtain a high reading. Self-monitoring should not be used if it produces too much anxiety; this raises the BP even more.
- Teach clients not to change their medication dosage without consulting their primary provider when their BP goes up or down.
- Before leaving the home, clean the stethoscope and sphygmomanometer with detergent or disinfectant, when possible, or place them in a plastic bag for transporting to the reprocessing location.

- If the client has an infection with a multidrug-resistant organism, reusable equipment such as stethoscopes should remain in the home. If the stethoscope and sphygmomanometer cannot remain in the home, clean and disinfect them before leaving the home, using a low to intermediate level disinfectant. If this is not practical, place them in a plastic bag and transport them to another site for cleaning and disinfection.

Documentation

- You will usually document BP on a flow sheet (such as in Procedure 20-5, Documentation).
- Document the blood pressure systolic/diastolic readings (e.g., 130/80).
- If you hear the 4th Korotkoff sound or muffling, document systolic/muffling/diastolic (e.g., 130/80/70). If you hear an auscultatory gap, document "systolic/diastolic with an auscultatory gap from…" For example, "170/90 with an auscultatory gap from 170 to 140."
- Follow agency policy regarding the recording of muffled sounds.
- If you chose an alternate site, document the site used and the reason for not using the upper arm.

Practice Resources

Alexis, O. (2010); American Association of Critical-Care Nurses (2010); American Heart Association (n.d.a, 2016b); CDC (2011); Joint National Committee on Prevention, Detection, Evaluation, and Treatment of High Blood Pressure (2004); Pinar, R., Ataalkin, S., & Watson, R. (2010); Vital Signs (1999).

 The video, **Measuring Blood Pressure,** along with questions and suggested responses, is available on the **Davis's Nursing Skills Videos** Web site on DavisPlus.

To explore learning resources for this chapter,

Go to **www.DavisAdvantage.com** and find:

Answers and Suggested Responses for all questions in this chapter

Lists of NIC interventions and NOC outcomes

List of NANDA-I Diagnoses

Knowledge Map

References and Bibliography

Concept Map

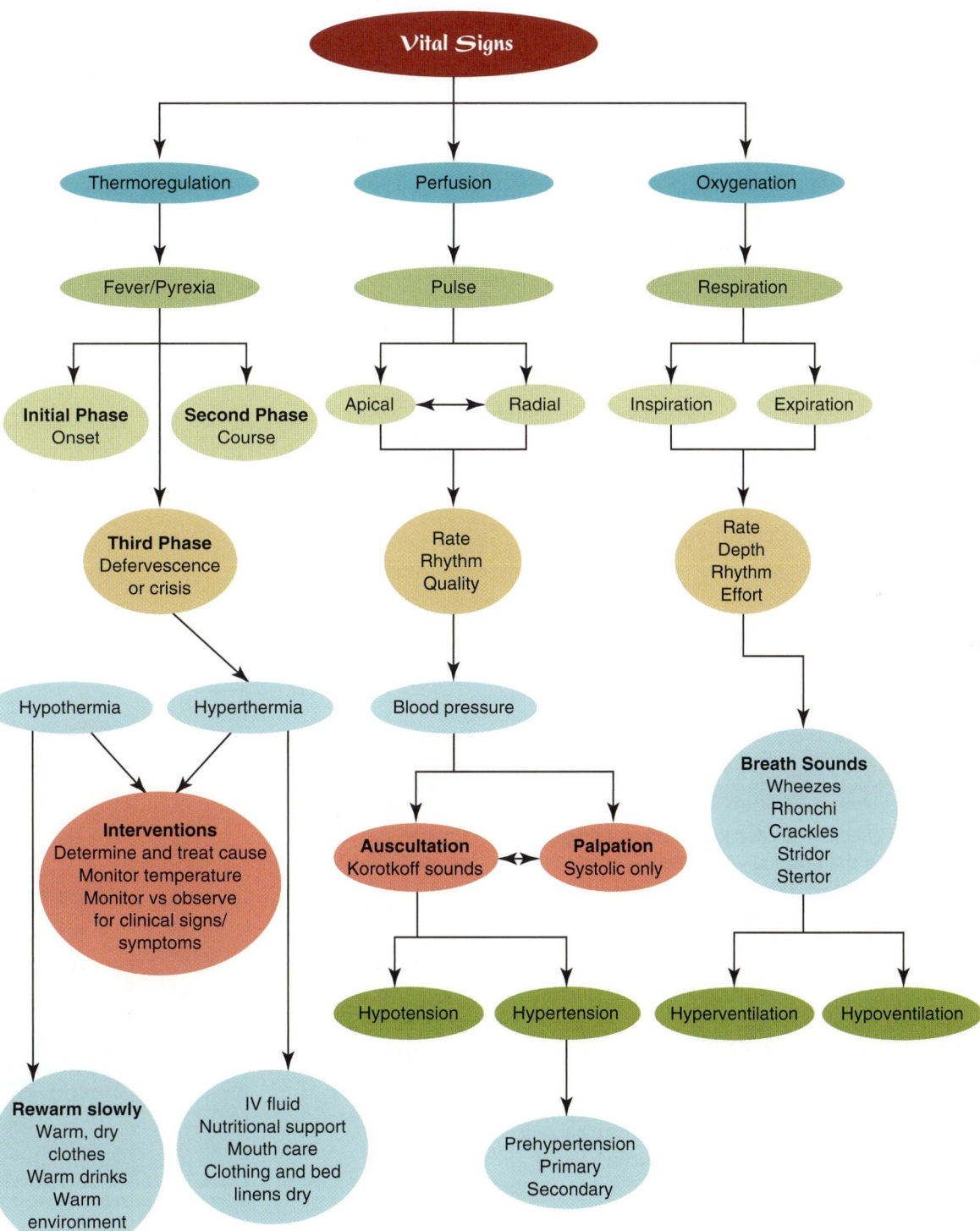

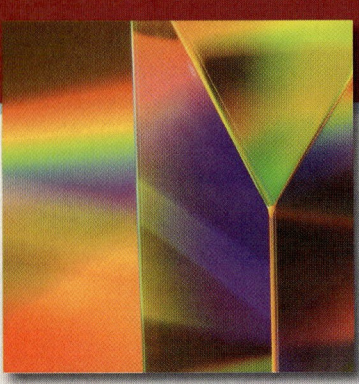

CHAPTER 20

Communicating & Therapeutic Relationships

Learning Outcomes

After completing this chapter, you should be able to:

- Discuss the three basic levels of communication.
- Describe the process of communication between sender and receiver; include all five elements.
- List the characteristics of verbal and nonverbal communication.
- Analyze factors that influence the communication process.
- Describe some characteristics of collaborative professional communication.
- Explain how relationships and roles influence communication.
- Describe the role of communication in each of the four phases of the therapeutic relationship.
- Compare and contrast techniques that enhance communication with those that hinder communication.
- Communicate with clients with impaired hearing, speech, or cognition.
- Communicate with clients whose culture or language is different from yours.
- Plan nursing care for a client experiencing impaired communication.

Key Concepts

Communication techniques

Therapeutic relationships

Related Concepts

See the Concept Map on at the end of this chapter.

Meet Your Patient

You have been assigned to care for John Barker, a 56-year-old man admitted to the hospital with bleeding in the lower gastrointestinal tract. When you enter the room to introduce yourself, his wife is at the bedside. They are holding hands, and clearly both have been crying. You begin by saying, "Good afternoon, Mr. Barker, I am a nursing student from the university. I've been assigned to care for you tomorrow." Mr. Barker swallows hard and says, "I don't think you'll be able to do anything for me!" His wife says, "Don't take it personally. It's not a good time right now. Please just leave us alone."

You leave the room, unsure how to respond. At the unit station when you review the chart, the charge nurse says,

"Oh my! You've been assigned to him? I hope you've got a lot of experience." As you read the chart, you realize that Mr. Barker was just informed that he has advanced stage colon cancer.

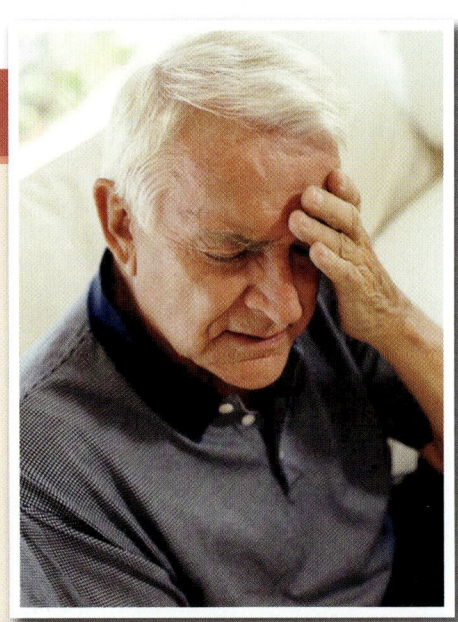

Theoretical Knowledge
knowing why

As a resource to you while you are learning what it means to care for patients in difficult situations such as Mr. Barker's, you might look to the following professional and regulatory agencies that stress the importance of good communication:

- **The Joint Commission National Patient Safety Goal 2, effective 2015,** aims to improve patient safety by improving communication among caregivers.
- **The Joint Commission** states that patients have the right to receive effective, understandable information and the right to have a language interpreter. This is an essential component of quality care and patient safety (The Joint Commission, 2010).
- **Quality and Safety Education for Nurses (QSEN).** To provide for patient safety, nurses need to effectively communicate their concerns about hazards and errors to patients, families, and the healthcare team (Cronenwett, Sherwood, Barnsteiner, et al., 2007).

ABOUT THE KEY CONCEPTS

In this chapter you will learn how **communication techniques** link to the concept of **communication** and how they both help you to form **therapeutic relationships** with patients, families, and members of the healthcare team.

WHAT IS COMMUNICATION?

Communication is a dynamic, reciprocal process of sending and receiving messages using words, sounds, expressions, body movements, written symbols, and behaviors. Communication forms the basis for sharing meaning, expressing needs, and building effective working relationships among individuals, families, and the healthcare team. Communication is more than the act of talking and listening (Box 20-1).

Communication Occurs on Many Levels

Communication is not just an exchange of words between two individuals. It occurs in inner dialogue, between people, and among groups.

Intrapersonal Communication is conscious internal dialogue, sometimes known as self-talk. For example, if you discover your patient is pale, diaphoretic (perspiring profusely), and moaning, you may ask yourself, "What's happened? This patient appears to be in a lot of pain."

- *Constructive affirmations, or positive self-talk* (e.g., "This will work! I can do it"), promotes success in a task.
- *Negative self-talk* (e.g., "I can't do this, it is too difficult") may adversely affect a person's ability to complete a task.

BOX 20-1 ■ What Is Communication?

Communication is . . .
- Bidirectional exchange of thoughts or feelings
- A way to meet physical, psychosocial, emotional, and spiritual needs
- A process—the act of sending, receiving, interpreting, and responding to a message
- Content—the actual subject matter, words, gestures, and substance of the message

---

Interpersonal Communication occurs between two or more people. Nurses use interpersonal communication to gather information during assessment, to teach about health issues, to explain care, and to provide comfort and support. In addition, professional nurses communicate with other nurses and healthcare team members to provide comprehensive care for clients. In order to appropriately delegate activities, they must also communicate effectively with nursing assistive personnel (NAP).

Group Communication is interaction occurring between more than two people. *Group communication* occurs when you engage in an exchange of ideas with two or more individuals at the same time. Examples of small-group communication include staff meetings, committee meetings, educational groups, self-help groups, and family teaching sessions. Working with groups requires effective communication skills and a basic understanding of group processes—discussed later in the chapter.

Public Speaking is a unique form of group communication. Generally, the speaker addresses a group with varying degrees of interaction. Nurses engage in public speaking to educate various-sized groups of people about health issues, to lobby for health legislation, and to address colleagues at professional conferences.

KnowledgeCheck 20-1

- What is the purpose of communication?
- Describe the three levels of communication.
- What level of communication was used in the Meet Your Patient scenario?

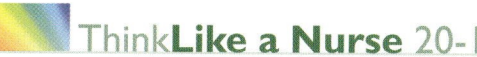 ThinkLike a Nurse 20-1

Evaluate your own skills with the three levels of communication.

Communication Involves Content

The **content** of communication is the actual subject matter, words, gestures, and substance of the message. It is the message that everyone can hear or see. For example, suppose your client said, "I slept through lunch." The content of that statement is open to interpretation. It does not tell you whether he thinks this is a good thing because he needed rest or a bad thing because he is so exhausted. As you can see, the words are just a part of communication. You must also consider the process.

Communication Is a Process

Process refers to the act of sending, receiving, interpreting, and reacting to a message. Figure 20-1 illustrates the relationship between the following five elements of the communication process.

- The **sender** (source or encoder) uses verbal and nonverbal methods to deliver a message (content) to another person.
- **Encoding** refers to the process of selecting the words, gestures, tone of voice, signs, and symbols used to transmit the message. For example, as a beginning nursing student, you might feel anxious about caring for Mr. Barker (Meet Your Patient). To communicate your concerns to your instructor, you might say directly, "It makes me nervous to be assigned to him." Or you might avoid eye contact and tell your instructor, "I'm going to need some help today." Both styles communicate your anxiety, but they are encoded differently.
- The **message** is the verbal and nonverbal information the sender communicates. It might be content of a conversation, a speech, a gesture, a letter, and so forth. Effective messages are complete, clear, concise, organized, timely, and expressed

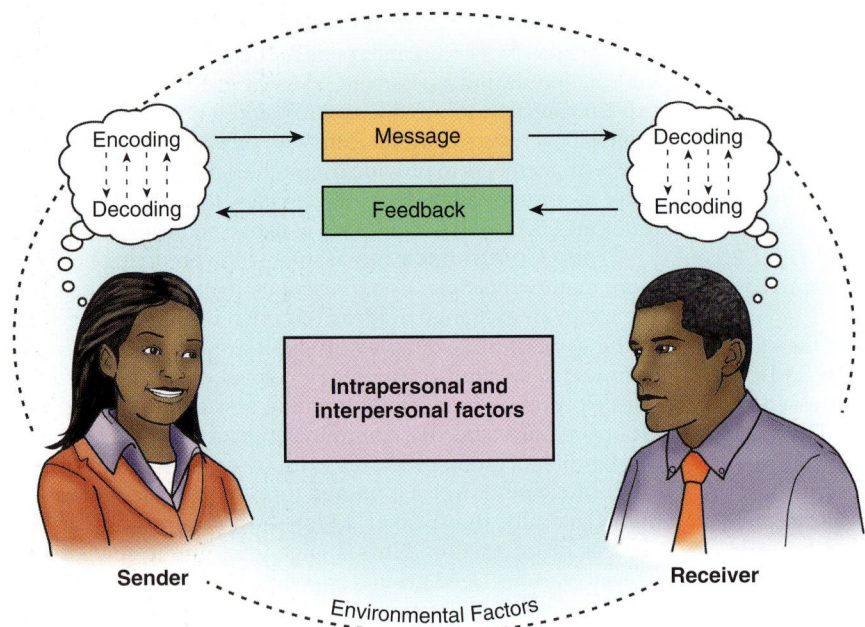

FIGURE 20-1 Communication: A sender encodes and transmits a message to a receiver, who decodes it and transmits feedback.

in a manner that the receiver can understand. The message must be appropriate for the situation and for the developmental level of the person receiving the message.

- The **channel** is the method in which the message is conveyed. Face-to-face communication is a commonly used channel. Nurses frequently use touch as a nonverbal way to communicate caring and concern. Other channels include written pamphlets, audiovisual aids, recordings, telephone and text messages, and the Internet. When choosing the best channel for communicating, consider the type of message, its purpose, and the size of the audience.

- The **receiver** is the observer, listener, and interpreter of the message. The receiver interprets, **(decodes)** by relating the message to past experiences to determine the sender's meaning. The receiver uses visual, auditory, and tactile senses to decode the message. If the sender's intended meaning matches what the receiver thinks it means, then the message was effective. Messages are sometimes misinterpreted, especially when the receiver is not physically or emotionally ready to receive the message.

    For example, if you approached your instructor to discuss your concerns about your patient when she was assisting with an emergency, she might be unable to receive your message.

- **Feedback** may be verbal, nonverbal, or both. Once the receiver has received and interpreted the message, he may be stimulated to respond by providing feedback to the sender. Feedback validates that the receiver received the message and understood it as the sender intended.

KnowledgeCheck 20-2

Using the Meet Your Patient scenario, identify at least one sender, one message, one receiver, one channel, and one example of feedback.

Verbal Communication

People send and receive messages both verbally and nonverbally. The two forms of communication occur spontaneously and simultaneously. **Verbal communication** is the use of spoken and written words to send a message. It is influenced by

educational background, culture, language, age, and past experiences. Verbal communication is generally a conscious act in which the sender chooses the most effective words to communicate a message. The goal of a verbal message is for the receiver to understand both your words and your meaning. The following factors affect how a message is received:

Vocabulary

Healthcare workers have a large vocabulary of technical terms and jargon. However, laypersons are often unfamiliar with the language of healthcare and find its use intimidating or at best, puzzling. Consider the following example, in which a nurse says:

> *You need to be NPO after 2400. I'll be in to prep the op site at about 8. You'll need to void before your pre-med. Then we'll transfer you to a gurney and take you to the holding area.*

Do you think most patients would understand this message? Do *you* understand all the words? How much better it would be if the nurse had said:

> *You will not be able to eat or drink anything after midnight. I'll come in about 8 in the morning to clean your hip and get it ready for your surgery. You'll need to urinate before I give you some medicine to relax you. Then, we'll put you on a cart and take you to the operating area.*

KEY POINT: *Use medical terms only when you are certain that the listener will understand them.*

Denotative and Connotative Meaning

Denotation is the literal (dictionary) meaning of a word. **Connotation** is the implied or emotional meaning of the word. Consider the following examples:

A mother says to her infant, "Don't cry, Baby."
A 40-year-old man says to his nurse, "Would you rub my back, Baby?"
A 10-year-old boy says to another boy, "You're a baby!"

The denotative meaning of *baby* is a very young child who is not yet able to walk. However, the connotative meaning is different in each example. In the first example, the connotative meaning is the same as the denotative meaning. The nurse might interpret the second example as a sexist remark; and in the last example, the 10-year-old boy undoubtedly meant *baby* as an insult. As you can see, words are often value laden or biased. **KEY POINT:** *Use terms that provide clear, objective data and are not open for misinterpretation.*

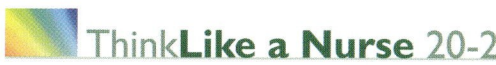

ThinkLike a Nurse 20-2

Think of two other examples in which the connotative meaning of a word may be different from its denotative meaning.

Pacing

The pace and rhythm of the delivery can alter the receiver's interpretation of the message. The pace must be slow enough for the receiver to interpret one thought before the sender moves on to the next thought, but must also be fast enough to maintain the listener's interest. When a lecturer talks too slowly, does your mind wander (e.g., "I need to get milk on the way home.")?

Intonation

"Tone of voice," or **intonation,** reflects the feeling behind the words. We listen for:
- *Pitch* (high or low)
- *Cadence* (rising and falling of the pitch)
- *Volume* (soft or loud).

For example, experiment with different ways you might say, "Your test results are in."

Pitch, cadence, and volume can reinforce or contradict the message while conveying various emotions. People tend to tune out when someone speaks in a **monotone** (does not vary the pitch, cadence, and volume). Before presenting lengthy information, whether to an individual or to a group, experiment with pitch, cadence, and volume to ensure that the listener remains engaged with your topic.

In an electronic message (e.g., text, e-mail), the receiver does not have the advantage of intonation or body language. This may lead to miscommunication. People sometimes insert *emojis* and *emoticons* (symbols such as "smiley faces") or use upper-case text to provide cues to the emotional tone of a message.

Clarity and Brevity

A conversation that is clear and brief holds the interest of all parties and effectively conveys the intended messages.
- **Clarity**—requires (1) that you select words that convey the intended meaning and (2) that you make sure your spoken words and the nonverbal language send the same message.
- **Brevity**—You can achieve brevity by using the fewest words possible.

Timing and Relevance

Timing is crucial. Before starting a conversation, assess your client. A person who is unable to concentrate (e.g., pain, hunger) will not receive the message as you intended it. Similarly, a client attempting to cope with stressors (e.g., limited finances, an upcoming surgery) may be too distracted to listen effectively. Consider the following principles:
- *Timing:* **Consider the presence of others.** If you ask a client about a personal issue in the presence of others, you may receive a different response than if you ask the question privately. In contrast, if you are instructing a client about a recommended diet, be sure that the person who does the shopping and cooking is also present.
- *Timing:* **Interaction must allow ample time for response.** A rapid flow of questions or one-sided conversations inhibits interaction.

- *Relevance:* **Communication is effective when those involved find the discussion to be important.** When teaching your client about his medication, begin by reminding him of the purpose of the discussion: "Let's talk about how you can take this medication to get the best control of your pain."

Credibility

Patients judge the **credibility** (or believability) of the message by the trustworthiness of the sender. Your credibility depends on a pattern of honest, factual, and timely responses to patient concerns, as well as congruence between your verbal and nonverbal communication.
- **Always be open and honest with patients.** Deceiving patients can take many forms, including false reassurance, but it always destroys trust.
- **Give information only if you are certain of the facts.** A response such as, "I don't know, but I will find out for you," is far better than an incorrect answer, guess, or opinion.
- **If a situation makes you uncomfortable, it is better to acknowledge your discomfort than to risk loss of credibility.** For instance, you may feel uncomfortable talking to Mr. Barker (Meet Your Patient) about his recent diagnosis. You may be tempted to say, "Maybe the test results are wrong," or "You can beat this." However, a more honest approach would be to tell Mr. Barker that you would like him to talk with a counselor or hospital chaplain.
- **To be credible, your body language must be consistent with your spoken words.**

Humor

Laughter can create physiological changes that contribute to well-being and provide an emotional release in a tense situation, thus positively influencing the patient's attitude and healing. Humor is highly subjective and personal, and it also depends on cultural norms. Use humor cautiously, and never direct humor at the client, disease process, or treatment team. Misused humor can have a negative effect on self-esteem, self-confidence, or the client's confidence in care providers.

Nonverbal Communication

Nonverbal communication (or body language) is the exchange of messages without the use of words. Because it emerges from feelings on a more unconscious level, your patient's body language, including posture, gesture, movement, facial expression, and eye gaze, can tell you how he is coping with what he is hearing and how he is processing the information.

♥ **iCare**   Your body language is equally important. When speaking to your patient who is sitting or lying in bed, it is helpful to crouch or kneel down to be at eye level, rather than speaking from an elevated, standing position. This can put him at ease and help form a genuine connection. Eye contact and face-to-face interactions are certainly important; however, genuine empathy and warmth are the most powerful in making a connection with your patient and fostering good communication.

Facial Expression

Expressions of the face and especially the eyes are the most obvious forms of nonverbal communication. Facial expressions communicate joy, anger, sadness, concern, or fear. Raised eyebrows, staring, squinting, or darting eyes all convey meaning. A mismatch between your verbal message and facial expression may be confusing or cause the client to doubt your credibility (Fig. 20-2).

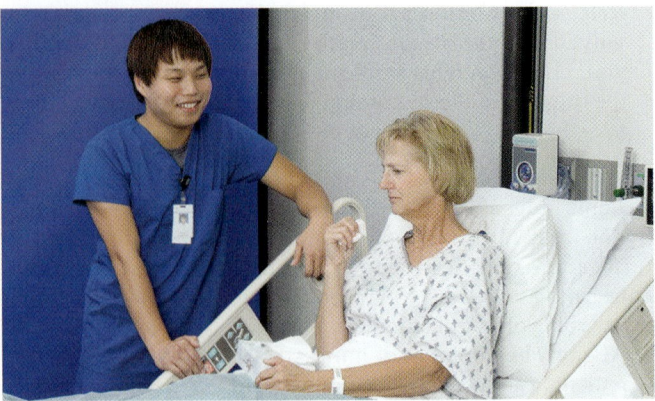

FIGURE 20-2 The nurse's facial expression is not appropriate because the patient appears to be in distress.

KEY POINT: *The interpretation of facial expressions is culturally dependent. For example, downcast eyes may indicate sadness, poor self-esteem, desire to avoid the conversation, respect, powerlessness, or submissive behavior. In Western cultures, eye contact usually indicates an interest in the conversation and a willingness to communicate; however, in Eastern cultures, the amount of eye contact considered acceptable varies.* Chapter 15 discusses cultural variations.

Posture and Gait

Body position, gait, and posture offer clues to a person's attitudes, emotions, physical well-being, and self-concept. When you see someone with an erect posture, head held high, and a quick gait, what do you think? In Western culture, these are nonverbal indicators of health and a sense of self-assuredness. In contrast, a slow, shuffling gait may signify someone who is ill, depressed, or has poor self-esteem.

Personal Appearance

Personal appearance provides clues to a person's feelings, socioeconomic status, culture, and religion. A person who is ill, tired, or depressed may lack energy for hygiene and grooming. That would be especially significant in a person who typically engages in meticulous grooming. As with all nonverbal data, you need to investigate the meaning of personal appearance to avoid drawing erroneous conclusions.

Dress and accessories are powerful cultural clues. Does the patient dress in a style that differs from local custom? Are pieces of jewelry or religious medallions visible? These are clues to the patient's values, socioeconomic status, livelihood, and religion, for example. Pay attention to these clues, but do not make assumptions about them. Religious jewelry or tattoos may not actually represent the patient's religious beliefs.

KEY POINT: *Have you thought about what your own personal appearance conveys to your patients and colleagues?*

Most people express their individuality through their clothing, hairstyle, and so on. Nurses, however, must also consider how patients perceive them and whether their appearance helps or hinders patient relationships. Issues of safety and cleanliness are also essential when choosing clothing, hairstyles, and body adornment (e.g., jewelry, nail polish, body piercings).

Gestures

Hand and body gestures emphasize and clarify the spoken word.

- Gestures are good indicators of the feeling tone behind the words. Imagine that your patient says, "I'm okay." What might it mean if he accompanies his statement with raised arms? What might it mean if, instead, he lowers his head to his hands?
- Gestures vary among individuals and cultures, so use them with caution. Suppose someone makes a V with the second and third fingers of the hand. To some people, this is a peace sign; to others, it could be a victory sign, the number two, or have no meaning to it at all.
- Gestures can help you communicate with individuals with impaired verbal communication.

Touch

♥ **iCare** Touch can convey affection, caring, concern, and encouragement (Fig. 20-3). Avoid using touch when dealing with someone who is angry or mentally disturbed because the touch may be misinterpreted (e.g., as a sign of aggression or sexual attraction). Although touch can be highly effective, use it with sensitivity to the situation, environment, culture, and receptivity of the patient.

For examples of therapeutic nonverbal behaviors and how patients may interpret them, see Clinical Insight 20-1.

KEY POINT: *In summary, eye contact, common language, face-to-face interactions, and other techniques are certainly important. However, genuine empathy and warmth are the most powerful in making a connection with your patient and fostering good communication.*

KnowledgeCheck 20-3

- Identify the components of verbal and nonverbal communication.
- What action should you take when there is a discrepancy between the client's spoken word and nonverbal body language?

ThinkLike a Nurse 20-3

- Observe an interaction between family members or your fellow students. Look for congruence between verbal and nonverbal communication. Strategize what you would say to validate the intended meaning when the two modes of communication are not in agreement.
- Recall the brief interaction with the charge nurse in the Meet Your Patient scenario. What might you say or do in response?

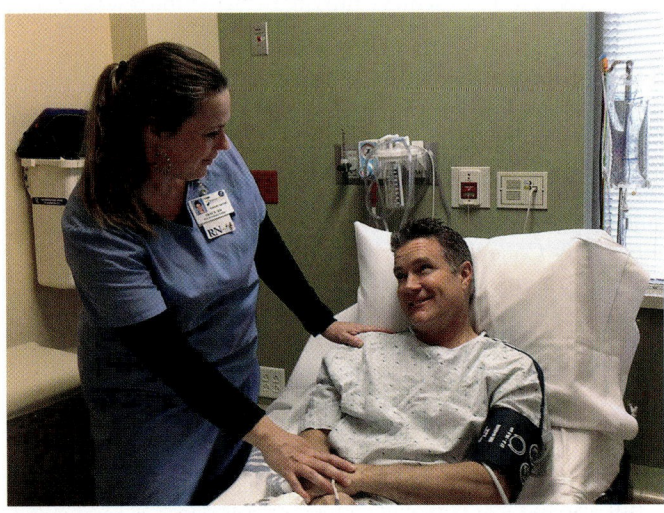

FIGURE 20-3 The nurse conveys genuine caring using touch.

WHAT FACTORS AFFECT COMMUNICATION?

The following sections contain a discussion of the major factors other than verbal and nonverbal language that affect communication.

Environment

Communication is most successful in an environment that is quiet, private, free of unpleasant smells, and at a comfortable temperature. You may not even notice the noise and distractions in the healthcare setting, but you need to be sensitive to how the environment is affecting your client. Background noise is distracting, interferes with hearing, and can create confusion. Being around others in pain or distress creates anxiety and fear; lack of privacy may cause embarrassment. All of those feelings may prevent your patient from sharing personal information or understanding your message.

You may be able to find a comfortable location for conversation in hospital chapels, foyers, and activity rooms. To discuss private matters, consider talking with the patient in a conference room rather than a shared room. If none of these is possible, at least close privacy curtains and turn off the radio or television.

Developmental Variations

Physical and cognitive development, language skills, level of education, and maturity influence communication. Therefore, you will need to modify your strategies to communicate effectively, respectfully, and compassionately with patients at all developmental stages. For detailed information for each developmental stage, see Chapters 9 and 10.

- *Infants* require attachment to a parent or caregiver, nurturing, social interaction, and physical stimulation, such as soothing talk and gentle touch, in order to achieve normal neurological development (National Institutes of Health, 2015).
- *Young toddlers* with limited language skills communicate nonverbally. Your response may combine verbal and nonverbal communication. For example, if a hospitalized 1-year-old cries out for his mother, you might cuddle the child with his favorite toy and reassure him by saying, "Mama will be back very soon."
- *Older toddlers and preschoolers* have more verbal ability. Although they may prefer to have a parent present, they are likely to talk with you and answer questions.
- *School-age children* are usually comfortable interacting verbally. Pay attention to their vocabulary as they speak and match it as closely as possible, using words and phrasing that the child will understand.
- By the time children reach *adolescence*, most can process abstract concepts. As a result, they are usually able to understand disease processes, treatments, and other health issues. Bear in mind that children with chronic health problems, who have required frequent interventions, are often more knowledgeable than would be expected for their age.
  - *Older adults* may be affected by sensory alterations, such as hearing loss or vision changes, or any of a variety of healthcare problems that affect cognition and expression, such as dementia.

Gender

Males and females communicate differently and may interpret the same communication differently.

- Women tend to communicate not only to convey a message but also to form personal connections and establish relationships (Tannen, 2001).

- Male communication is more purpose driven. It typically focuses on goals, tasks, information, and maintaining independence, as well as achieving favorable positions in a hierarchy.

Gender differences are important because male and female patients may communicate their needs very differently. Similarly, the gender of the nurse may affect the response to the patient's requests. For example, a female patient might state, "I feel so lousy today." A female nurse may interpret this as a desire to talk. In contrast, a male nurse may discuss pain control.

Personal Space

People vary in the amount of physical space they prefer when communicating. The distance they maintain is influenced by the relationship of the individuals, the nature of the conversation, the setting, and culture (Fig. 20-4). Also see Chapter 15 for cultural preferences for personal space. Hall (1992) describes four distinct distances for communication: intimate, personal, social, and public:

Intimate Distance is the area immediately surrounding a person that is defined as her private space. People prefer to maintain intimate distance between themselves and others during conversations. In Western cultures, intimate distance is typically about 18 inches. Within this distance, people can easily interpret facial expression, maintain eye contact, hear each other speaking at a low volume, and even sense each other's smell and body heat.

It is also at this distance that body contact occurs. As a nurse, you invade a client's personal space to perform assessments and procedures, or even while using touch to offer support. This may make some clients uncomfortable.

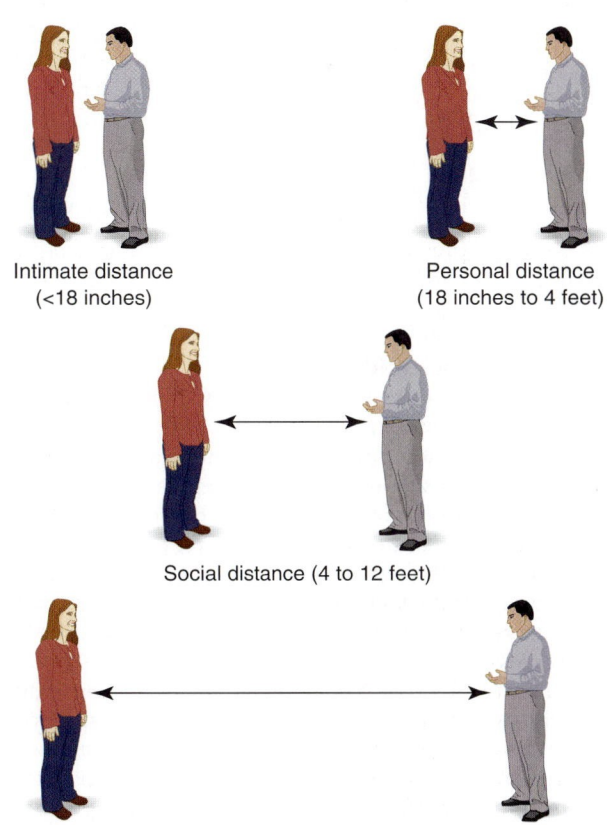

Intimate distance
(<18 inches)

Personal distance
(18 inches to 4 feet)

Social distance (4 to 12 feet)

Public distance (12 feet)

FIGURE 20-4 The distance that individuals engaged in communication maintain between one another is influenced by their relationship, the nature of the conversation, the setting, and cultural background(s).

♥ **iCare** Before providing nursing interventions in the client's intimate distance, discuss what you are about to do. It is best to ask the client's permission, even for gentle touch, if you are in the slightest doubt about his receptivity. If the touch is not optional, say, "I'm going to touch you now."

Personal Distance is from 18 inches up to 4 feet. Interactions with clients and healthcare team members will commonly occur in this range. This distance facilitates sharing of feelings or personal thoughts and is appropriate when communicating caring or concern.

Social Distance is generally between 4 to 12 feet; and is common for formal interaction or when communicating with a group. At this distance, individuals are not within range to be physically touched. The volume of the spoken words may be loud enough for others to overhear, so people share personal feelings and thoughts less often at this distance. For example, if you stand at the client's bedside and ask how she is feeling, you will likely receive a more personal response than if you were to ask the same question while standing at the door.

Public Distance is considered to be beyond 12 feet. This distance requires loud and clear enunciation for communication. This distance is characterized by a lack of individuality and a greater focus on the group or community, as in a lecture.

Territoriality

Territoriality refers to the space and things that an individual identifies as his own. In a hospital setting, many patients consider the hospital room and their personal belongings to be their territory. ♥ **iCare** Patients may be offended if you change, rearrange, or interfere with this personal space by moving furniture, discarding objects, or borrowing items from the room, even if they are institutional property. To establish trust, you must request permission to rearrange the patient's territory. Also recognize that hospitalized patients are not in their "home" territory. They are therefore likely to be less at ease during interactions.

Sociocultural Factors

Culture and socioeconomic status strongly influence communication, affecting facial expressions, nonverbal communication, and even selecting with whom and how to interact. For example, in some cultures it would be unacceptable for a male nurse to address and provide personal care to a female patient.

Roles and Relationships

Social roles and status (or hierarchy) affect the sender's and receiver's choice of vocabulary, tone of voice, use of gestures, and distance associated with the communication. Have you ever been present while a physician explained a treatment plan to a patient? Often the patient asks no questions or nods approval and waits until the physician leaves to ask you questions or express concerns. This may be because many patients perceive more comfortable social distance between themselves and the nurse. Social distance can also play a role in how health professionals view patients.

Patients are often unclear about the nurse's responsibilities within the healthcare team. Some might be confused by the fact that many healthcare workers, all of whom may be wearing "scrub clothes," call themselves nurses even though they are not legally qualified to use the title. If you are working with NAPs, medical assistants, or other team members, be sure to clarify their roles with the patient so he can communicate his questions and concerns to the appropriate healthcare provider. For easier identification, some agencies are assigning colors for various workers' scrubs (e.g., blue for physicians, purple for nurses).

KnowledgeCheck 20-4

- What are the major factors that affect communication?
- In what distance(s) do most nurse–client interactions occur?

WHAT IS COLLABORATIVE PROFESSIONAL COMMUNICATION?

Communication is essential to collaborative practice among nurses, physicians, and health professionals from other disciplines. You might recognize collaborative professional communication by the following characteristics:

- Uses an assertive style
- Ideally, makes use of standard communication tools
- The patient rounds approach is one example

Each discipline shares the common goal of providing optimal patient care. This goal should guide the way you communicate—at the bedside, at the nurse's station, in care conferences, or via the patient record.

Nurses also communicate with peers and colleagues to contribute to their professional development. See Box 20-2 for statements from professional organizations about collaborative communication.

Communication Styles

Think of communication styles as a continuum from passive through assertive to aggressive.

- A **passive approach** avoids conflict and allows others to take the lead. It tends to be submissive, helpless, indecisive, apologetic, or whining. For example, "Whatever you want. I'll just sit here and wait for you to decide what you're going to do."
- An **aggressive approach,** in contrast, forces others to lose. The goal is to win and be in control (for example, you might say, "My way is the correct way. You don't know what you're talking about."). Aggressive communication can be bossy, arrogant, opinionated, sarcastic, manipulative, intolerant, or overbearing.

Why might you adopt a **nonassertive style** of communication? When speaking to physicians, some nurses still communicate their needs in a style that assures physicians that they are not telling them what to do (e.g., "Do you think Mrs. King's heart rate is a little fast today?" instead of "Mrs. King's heart rate was 120 beats per minute at 0800"). This has been referred to as the *doctor–nurse game* (Stein, Watts, & Howell, 1990). Such unclear, indirect communication contributes to frustration, reduced nurse role satisfaction, errors, and poor patient outcomes. The following section will help you to learn to communicate assertively, thereby improving outcomes.

Communicating Assertively

Assertive communication is the expression of a wide range of positive and negative thoughts and feelings in a style that is direct, open, honest, spontaneous, responsible, and nonjudgmental. Assertiveness recognizes your rights while still respecting the rights of others. It allows you to take responsibility for your own thoughts and actions without blaming others, encourages feedback, and enables you to find mutually satisfying solutions to conflict by confronting people constructively.

✚ Effective communication and teamwork are essential for high-quality, safe patient care. To avoid communication failures that can lead to adverse events in patients, you must speak up when you have concerns and take the necessary steps to communicate assertively and collaboratively with the healthcare team. You must question care decisions that don't seem right to you and assertively discuss errors or poor clinical judgment with coworkers.

BOX 20-2 ■ Collaborative Professional Communication

American Nurses Association (2015)

Standards of professional performance stress the importance of communication to collegiality and collaboration. The following are some of the competencies for these three standards:

Standard 9. Communication

The registered nurse:

- Communicates effectively in all areas of practice.
- Assesses one's own communication skills and effectiveness.
- Demonstrates cultural empathy when communicating.
- Assesses communication ability, health literacy, resources, and preferences of healthcare consumers to inform the interprofessional team and others.
- Uses language translation resources to ensure effective communication.
- Incorporates appropriate alternative strategies to communicate effectively with healthcare consumers who have visual, speech, language, or communication difficulties.
- Uses communication styles and methods that demonstrate caring, respect, deep listening, authenticity, and trust.
- Conveys accurate information.
- Maintains communication with the interprofessional team and others to facilitate safe transitions and continuity in care delivery.
- Contributes the nursing perspective in interactions with others and discussions with the interprofessional team.
- Exposes care processes and decisions when they do not appear to be in the best interest of the healthcare consumer.
- Discloses concerns related to potential or actual hazards and errors in care or the practice environment to the appropriate level.
- Demonstrates continuous improvement of communication skills (American Nurses Association, 2015, p. 71).

Standard 10. Collaboration

The registered nurse:

- Communicates effectively with the healthcare consumer, the family, and healthcare providers regarding healthcare consumer care and the nurse's role in the provision of care (American Nurses Association, 2015, p. 73).

Standard 11. Leadership

The registered nurse:

- Communicates to manage change and address conflict (American Nurses Association, 2015, p. 73).

Standard 14. Quality of Practice

The registered nurse:

- Collaborates with the interprofessional team to implement quality improvement plans and interventions (American Nurses Association, 2015, p. 79).

Standard 15. Professional Practice Evaluation

The registered nurse:

- Provides peers with formal or informal constructive feedback regarding their practice or role performance (American Nurses Association, 2015, p. 81).

American Association of Critical-Care Nurses (2015)

Standard 4: Communication

Competencies for skilled communication for nurses caring for acutely and critically ill patients include the following:

- Assessing the preferred and most effective style for communicating with acutely and critically ill patients, families, and the interprofessional team
- Seeking to protect and advance collaborative relationships among colleagues while exhibiting respect for the perspectives of others
- Contributing professional perspective and seeking the rationale and relevant perspectives supporting patient care decisions
- Continually improving professional communication and conflict-resolution skills
- Reporting observations or expressing concerns related to the safety of patients, hazards in the healthcare environment, or possible errors in care
- Communicating clearly with other providers to minimize risks associated with patient handoffs, transfers, and transitions in care

The Joint Commission, 2015 National Patient Safety Goals

Goal 2: Improve the effectiveness of communication among caregivers.

The Joint Commission added NPSG.02.03.01 to improve staff communication by reporting important test results to the right staff person on time.

Source: American Nurses Association. (2015). *Nursing: Scope and standards of practice* (3rd ed., pp. 71, 73, 79, 81). Silver Spring, MD: Author; The Joint Commission. (2015). *The Joint Commission hospital accreditation program: National patient safety goals effective January 1, 2015.* Retrieved from http://www.jointcommission.org/assets/1/6/2015_NPSG_HAP.pdf

---

A study by Garon (2012) found that open communication, in which nurses feel free to speak up, leads to better patient care, improved safety, and better staff satisfaction (Garon, 2012).

So how can you communicate assertively?

- *Speak clearly and firmly in a positive manner; convey a "can do" attitude.*
- *Maintain professional composure.*
- *Question care decisions openly and honestly.* Do not begin your statements with timid or self-effacing statements that fail to take credit for your contributions (e.g., "You may disagree with this, but . . ."). Be frank, but be flexible and open-minded.

- *Use "I" statements.* An "I" statement should include the elements of behavior (or facts), feeling, and effect (on you). For example, instead of saying, "Why haven't you ordered Mrs. Nobu's pain medications yet?" you might say, "I telephoned you this morning about Mrs. Nobu's pain, but I don't see a change in her analgesic order. I am concerned about her discomfort and the effect it may have on her willingness to ambulate."
- *Focus on the issue, not the participants.* For example, say, "I think this approach might be the best, but I'd like to hear your thoughts."

- *Use effective nonverbal language.* Your body and verbal language should be congruent. Eye contact demonstrates interest and shows sincerity. Use a calm, well-modulated voice tone and add appropriate gestures for emphasis. Posture also communicates your attention and interest in the dialogue.
- *Don't invite negative responses.* For example, say, "I would really appreciate it if you could help me weigh Mr. Kudari on the bed scale," rather than, "Would you want to help me weigh him?"
- *Learn to accept criticism without becoming anxious or defensive.* Acknowledge that you might not have had experience with a particular patient situation or have depth of knowledge in an area. Suppose Mrs. Nobu's prescriber says, "Are you playing pharmacist today?" You might respond, "It's true I am not an expert on analgesics. However, Mrs. Nobu needs pain relief and I need your help prescribing pain medication." Take responsibility for your imperfections (e.g., knowledge, experience) and take action later to remedy them. You will earn more respect from your healthcare team and patients than by acting defensive, insecure, or sarcastic.
- *Use negative inquiry.* You might choose, in the preceding situation, to use negative inquiry. You would reply, "So you believe that I do not have adequate knowledge to discuss Mrs. Nobu's pain control?"
- *Strive for a workable compromise,* but not if it affects patient well-being or your feelings of self-respect. Suppose an administrator comes to a patient's room while you are inserting a nasogastric tube and says, "I need to see you right now. Come to the desk immediately." An example of a workable compromise would be to say, "I understand that you need to talk to me right away, and I need to finish what I am doing. So what about meeting you at the desk as soon as I finish, in about 10 minutes?"
- **KEY POINT:** Use "critical language (CUS)." *Remember the words* C*oncerned,* U*ncomfortable, and* S*afety—as in, "I'm concerned; I'm uncomfortable; this is unsafe; or I'm scared"* (*Agency for Healthcare Research and Quality, 2013 revised; Leonard, Graham, & Bonacum, 2004*).

 Some organizations identify a code phrase for themselves, for example, "I need clarity." When anyone there says, "I need clarity," the receiver of the request must stop and listen attentively while the sender asserts the issues that need to be clarified (Amer, 2013).

It may help to practice ahead of time how you want to look and sound before attempting assertive communication. Assertiveness is a learned skill. Role-playing with a colleague can build your confidence.

Using Standardized Communication Tools

Nurses are taught to be more descriptive of clinical situations and patient responses, whereas physicians learn to be concise and precise. Standardized communication tools are effective in overcoming differences in nurse–physician communication styles and conveying key information clearly and concisely. Structured communication tools ensure accuracy and also create an environment in which individuals can express concerns that facilitates the exchange of information for healthcare professionals involved in the patient's care.

A well-known and highly effective method for team communication and collaboration is the **SBARQ** model. The acronym represents **S**ituation, **B**ackground, **A**ssessment, **R**ecommendation, **Q**uestions. See Clinical Insight 20-2.

If you need other information about giving a verbal report, also see Chapter 18.

Using the Patient Rounds Approach

Patient rounding is a collaborative approach in which physicians and nurses gather at the patient's bedside to discuss goals for care and/or changes in the plan of care and to answer any questions the patient, family, and healthcare staff may have. Meeting for rounds allows the nurse to provide input, which results in improved nurse and physician working relationships and professional satisfaction (Chapman, 2009).

WHAT IS THE ROLE OF COMMUNICATION IN THERAPEUTIC RELATIONSHIPS?

♥ **iCare** Caring is integral to a therapeutic nurse–patient relationship, which according to Benner (1984) is the hallmark of nursing practice. She uses the terms *connectedness* and *involvement* to describe nursing. These terms are also the foundation of meaningful communication (Alpers, Jarrell, & Roxena, 2013). In their demanding environments, nurses multitask and function with many competing priorities. Because of this, they run the risk of conveying a rushed, noncaring attitude to patients. This can be frustrating to patients and exhausting for nurses.

A **therapeutic relationship** focuses on improving the health of the client, whether an individual or community. **Therapeutic communication** is client-centered communication directed at achieving client goals. It is used to establish the therapeutic relationship, provide and obtain healthcare information, and express interest in and concern for the client and family.

Communication Is Essential to All Phases of the Therapeutic Relationship

The therapeutic relationship consists of four phases. As you read about each phase, notice the fundamental role of client-focused communication.

Pre-interaction Phase **Pre-interaction** occurs before you meet the client. You lay the groundwork for communication by gathering information about the client, but you do not communicate directly with the client. As a student, you initiate this phase as you prepare for clinical days. The client also experiences a pre-interaction phase, which begins when she identifies the need for healthcare.

Orientation Phase The **orientation** phase begins when you meet the client and introduce yourself and your role in the relationship. You then address him by his preferred name and/or title. Before collecting personal or health data, inform the client that pertinent information will be shared with the healthcare team.

The goal of the orientation phase is to establish rapport and trust by using verbal and nonverbal communication. When rapport is established, patients are more likely to express their concerns openly and seek emotional support (Joanna Briggs Institute, 2011). Assess the patient's readiness to communicate; be sensitive to the patient's mood, past experiences, and overall physical and psychological state. Try to understand the cause of the client behaviors, comments, and attitudes, and respond with patience and wisdom. Orientation ends when the relationship has been defined.

Working Phase Most therapeutic communication occurs in the **working phase,** the active part of the relationship. During this phase, the nurse communicates caring, the patient expresses thoughts and feelings, mutual respect is maintained, and honest verbal and nonverbal expression occurs. Key communication goals are to assist the client to clarify feelings and concerns. A professional relationship is courteous, trustworthy, and confidential, and accomplished by active listening.

Termination Phase The conclusion of the relationship marks the **termination phase,** whether at the end of the nurse's shift or on the client's discharge from the unit, facility, or service. Reviewing and summarizing help to bring the relationship to a comfortable closure. If communication has been effective, the termination phase prepares the nurse and client for future interactions. Unsuccessful communication may affect the client's health outcomes or understanding of his disease process, as well as affect the nurse's job satisfaction.

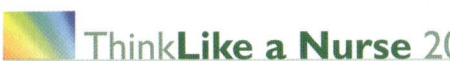

ThinkLike a Nurse 20-4

Recall the scenario of Mr. Barker (Meet Your Patient).

- What phase of the therapeutic relationship is illustrated in the scenario?
- How might the interaction between you and Mr. Barker change if it occurred in a different phase of the therapeutic relationship?
- What could you have done differently?

Therapeutic Communication Has Five Key Characteristics

The therapeutic relationship requires *therapeutic use of self:* conscious use of your knowledge and skills to effect change in the patient. Therapeutic use of self requires practice so that you will be able to recognize boundaries and focus on the patient rather than on your own feelings and experiences.

Five qualities characterize communication in the therapeutic relationship: empathy, respect, genuineness, concreteness, and confrontation. Later in the chapter you'll learn specific strategies for enhancing communication, as well as barriers to therapeutic communication. Look for these techniques and barriers in any conversation you analyze.

Empathy The desire to understand and be sensitive to the feelings, beliefs, and situation of another person is called **empathy.** It requires you to be willing to adapt your style, tone, vocabulary, and behavior to create the best approach for each client situation. It is relatively easy to have empathy for people who are like you and who are likeable. It is more difficult to connect with people you see as difficult or different. To empathize with a client, you must look beyond outward appearance or behavior and put yourself, mentally and emotionally, in the client's place. The empathy with which you care for your patient, deliver difficult news, or guide him through complex decisions can make an enormous difference to that patient's and family's experience and adaptation to illness.

Respect ♥ iCare In the therapeutic relationship, you communicate respect by valuing the client and being flexible to meet the client's needs in the way you address him and the words and intonation you choose. Making even minor adjustments, such as delaying breakfast for an hour to allow the client to sleep, communicates that you respect the client's wishes. When a relationship is grounded in respect, both parties maintain power and self-esteem.

Genuineness When interviewing clients, we expect them to respond truthfully. Similarly, clients have a right to expect truthful responses from healthcare providers.
- **Genuineness requires honesty.** If you are unable to answer a client's question, do not offer guesses. Make a response such as "I don't know, but I'll find out and let you know."
- **Genuineness also involves willingness to self-evaluate.** How well did I communicate? Did I handle that situation appropriately? How could I improve my communication?

Concreteness In a therapeutic relationship, you must offer understandable responses to a client's questions and concerns. To do so requires you to express in concrete, specific terms what you mean. The message must be constructed and delivered in a manner that is suitable for the client.

Confrontation If your client is unable to express his thoughts clearly, you must be willing to ask him directly to say it another way or clarify his point further. Similarly, you must be willing to be challenged if you are unclear.

Communication Is Important in Group Helping Relationships

Nurses frequently communicate with groups—for example, when you interact with a family, a community, or a committee. Groups can enhance problem-solving and creativity, generate understanding and support, enhance morale, and provide affiliation. However, *groupthink,* a pattern of communication in which consensus overrides creativity in problem-solving, can emerge, particularly in cohesive groups or those with unbalanced power structure.

Task Groups are formed to address a task or fulfill a need. Typically, members are chosen based on ability to complete the task. Other times members are selected for reasons of convenience, such as availability, interest, or agenda, rather than for the skills needed to accomplish the goal of the group.

Short-term groups disband once the task is completed (e.g., a task force to address holiday scheduling or a panel to critique response to a disaster drill). Because the group members' time together is limited, the focus of communication is on the task at hand. Therefore, time to develop rapport or relationships is limited.

Ongoing Groups address recurrent issues. Committees are a form of an ongoing task group. Ongoing committees in healthcare organizations include quality improvement, infection control, and discharge planning. Members have designated roles within the group (e.g., recorder, time keeper). A leader or chairperson is usually appointed or elected.

In small groups, members have an opportunity to communicate their opinions. In larger groups, patterns of communication form; some members voice their opinion regularly, whereas others are often silent. When not all members speak, it is essential to examine nonverbal behavior to determine whether the non-speaking members agree with those who participate verbally.

Self-Help Groups are voluntary organizations composed of individuals with a common need. Alcoholics Anonymous may be the most widely recognized self-help group. Other well-known self-help groups include Weight Watchers, Narcotics Anonymous, and Reach to Recovery (for women with breast cancer).

Members are encouraged to share experiences and seek support from other members of the group. Members who have met the goals of the group often serve as the group facilitator by leading the interactions or simply arranging meeting logistics. Nurses or experts in the field may be consulted to offer guidance or education to the group. Self-help groups most often have face-to-face meetings, but they may also participate online.

Therapy Groups are organized to help individual members cope with challenging personal issues or stressful life events, such as divorce, death of a spouse, or new motherhood. Therapy groups may also address ways improve relationships and improve communication. Also called self-awareness or growth groups, they may be ongoing or have a designated length of operation.

Work-Related Social Support Groups help members of a profession cope with the stress associated with their work. The helping professions can be emotionally draining. Members have an opportunity to share concerns and offer mutual support through facilitated formal meetings or informal drop-in events. Formation of a group does not guarantee its success. To be successful, a group must have characteristics that allow the group to function and achieve its goals (Box 20-3).

KnowledgeCheck 20-5

- Identify and describe the phases of the therapeutic relationship.
- What are the five characteristics of therapeutic communication?
- Describe the difference between a task group and a self-help group.
- Compare and contrast the role of a therapy group with that of a work-related support group.

ThinkLike a Nurse 20-5

Review the local newspaper, hospital bulletin board, the Internet, and the school intranet. Identify at least three group helping experiences available. How might you learn more about these organizations? How would you determine whether they are resources that you might make available to your patients?

PracticalKnowledge
knowing how

Therapeutic communication is used throughout the nursing process. In the next few sections we explore communication problems as well as therapeutic interventions.

BOX 20-3 ■ Characteristics of a Successful Group

A successful group includes the following:
- Clearly defined purpose
- Shared set of guidelines under which the group functions
- Sense of shared responsibility
- Shared leadership
- Mutual trust
- Comfort among members
- Climate that is cohesive but does not stifle individuality
- Members who are willing to share feelings, concerns, or beliefs
- Flexibility to change what is not working

ASSESSMENT NP

Assessment is essential to effective communication. You should assess for factors that alter a client's ability to receive, process, or transmit information, such as developmental delays, physical and cognitive impairment, substance abuse, and so forth. See the Focused Assessment box, Communication.

ANALYSIS/NURSING DIAGNOSIS NP

Communication can be the problem or the etiology of a nursing diagnosis. The following NANDA-I diagnosis labels describe communication problems. Note that communication problems may involve the inability to receive, interpret, or express spoken, written, and nonverbal messages.

- *Readiness for Enhanced Communication* is appropriate when the client expresses willingness to improve communication that is already effective.
- *Impaired Verbal Communication* is useful if the client has (1) expressive aphasia or a physiological problem such as dyspnea, stuttering, or laryngeal cancer that impairs the ability to speak; or (2) receptive aphasia or sensory deficits that impair the ability to receive messages.
- *Impaired Communication* is the preferred diagnosis if the client is unfamiliar with the dominant language or has some other difficulty receiving and sending messages. *Note:* This is not a NANDA-I label.

Etiologies of Communication Diagnoses

Your assessment data will help you determine whether communication impairment is the primary problem or whether it is a result of other health problems. Some nursing diagnoses may cause or contribute to communication problems. For example:

- Acute or chronic confusion may cause difficulty expressing or receiving verbal and nonverbal messages. Confusion may be related to physical or mental health problems, a side effect of medications, or sleep deprivation.
- Mental health problems can also lead to communication problems. For example:
  Anxiety impairs the ability to deliver and receive messages.
  Chronic or Situational Low Self-Esteem often results in limited interaction with others.

Communication as Etiology of Other Nursing Diagnoses

Impaired Verbal Communication may be the etiology of other nursing diagnoses, for example:

- Anxiety r/t inability to communicate needs
- Impaired Social Interaction r/t inability to carry on conversation
- Chronic Low Self-Esteem r/t fear of conversing with others secondary to stuttering

PLANNING OUTCOMES/EVALUATION NP

Individualized client outcomes and goals depend on the nursing diagnosis you identify. For example, for Impaired Verbal Communication, you might write the following desired outcomes for a client:

- Uses alternative methods of communication (e.g., writing, picture board, gestures) effectively.
- Demonstrates minimal frustration with communication difficulties.
- Communicates effectively using a translator or interpreter.

Focused Assessment

Communication

A focused assessment should identify factors that alter a patient's ability to receive, understand, and transmit verbal and nonverbal messages.

Medications

➤ Is the patient taking medications that might interfere with speech, cognition, or level of consciousness?
➤ Does the patient use alcohol or other substances? Is he intoxicated?

Language, Vocabulary, Literacy

➤ What is the patient's primary language?
➤ Does the patient have sufficient command of the dominant language?
➤ Is an interpreter (foreign language or sign language) required?
➤ Can the patient read and write? At what level and in what language?

Cognitive Function

Communication difficulties may signal cognitive impairment. Look for history of developmental delays and pathology or injury of the central nervous system.
➤ What is the patient's level of consciousness?
➤ Is there short-term or long-term memory loss, or both?
➤ Is intellectual function at, below, or above expectations for age?
➤ Can the patient read simple instructions?
➤ Can the patient follow simple spoken instructions?
➤ Can the patient understand a yes or no choice?
➤ Are there symptoms or a diagnosis of mental illness or dementia?
➤ If the patient is unconscious, are there nonverbal responses that indicate that he can hear you (e.g., blinking, moving the head, squeezing your hand)?

Hearing

➤ Ask the patient, and observe, whether there are hearing problems.
➤ Is the patient wearing a hearing aid? If so, is it working properly? Does the patient appear to be reading your lips?

➤ Is the patient trying to use sign language to communicate?
➤ Refer to Chapter 21 for tests of hearing (e.g., ticking watch).

Vision

➤ Is the patient wearing glasses or contact lenses?
➤ Is the patient able to see adequately?
➤ Refer to Chapter 21 for vision tests.

 Also see the Davis's Nursing Skills Video, **Brief Bedside Assessment.**

Aphasia

➤ Is there a history of stroke or a diagnosis of aphasia?
➤ Is there receptive aphasia (inability to receive or interpret verbal or nonverbal messages)?
➤ Is there expressive aphasia (inability to express verbal or nonverbal messages)?

Physiological Barriers

Does the patient have conditions that cause difficulty speaking, such as
➤ Dyspnea?
➤ Artificial airway?
➤ Oral problems, such as poorly fitted dentures?
➤ Cleft palate or other structural problems?

Communication Style

➤ Is it difficult to understand what the patient says (e.g., slurring words, stuttering, inability to pronounce certain sounds)?
➤ Does the patient speak readily or refuse to speak?
➤ Does the patient speak slowly or rapidly, spontaneously, or hesitantly?
➤ Is the vocabulary adequate for the purpose needed?
➤ Has the vocabulary changed from the person's normal vocabulary?

Other

➤ Are verbal and nonverbal communication congruent?

▪ Interprets messages accurately, as evidenced by appropriate verbal or nonverbal feedback.

NOC standardized outcomes associated with Impaired Verbal Communication are: Communication, Expressive Communication, and Receptive Communication. Using NOC indicators with those outcomes, you can develop goals for clients' communication problems.

PLANNING INTERVENTIONS/ IMPLEMENTATION NP

Specific nursing activities for communication problems depend on the etiology of the problem and on the goals selected. The focus of nursing interventions is to facilitate communication and to resolve or reduce the factors interfering with it.

NIC standardized interventions for Impaired Verbal Communication are: Active listening, Assertiveness Training, Communication Enhancement (Hearing or Visual Deficit), Presence, and Touch.

Enhancing Therapeutic Communication

The following sections contain techniques and activities you can implement immediately to improve your communication with patients and others.

Addressing the Patient

KEY POINT: *When you first meet your client, use a formal title—Mr., Ms., Dr., and so on. In the orientation phase of the relationship, ask your patient how he would prefer to be addressed.* If the patient is unable to respond, ask family members

Limits and Boundaries of Therapeutic Relationships

Chapter Key Concept: Therapeutic Relationships

SENC Competency: Patient-Centered Care

What are boundaries? Boundaries define personal space and allow people to communicate comfortably. Professional relationships have stricter boundaries than do personal relationships: Questions and comments made to friends may be inappropriate with clients. Moreover, boundaries between patients and nursing students, and even nurses, are not equal and are not always clear. Patients are asked intimate details about their lives, are physically exposed, and are often dependent on the care provider. Behaviors that suggest you might have boundary issues include the following:

➤ Thinking about or socializing with the patient while away from work
➤ Disclosing personal information
➤ Sharing patients' private information publicly
➤ Engaging in physical contact, flirting, or discussing sexual attraction, including texting or online messaging

Think about it: How do those factors make patients vulnerable? What thinking and doing and caring do you need to develop trust-based therapeutic relationships with patients and families? What can you do to help them maintain their dignity?

For example, most healthcare experiences strip the client of power—personal clothing is swapped for hospital-issued garments; roles are changed; people are separated from loved ones and familiar surroundings; and schedules are altered.

Actions: In developing therapeutic boundaries, try to achieve the "zone of helpfulness." That is, find a balance between underinvolvement (distancing, disinterest, neglect) on one end and overinvolvement (boundary violations, professional sexual misconduct) on the other (National Council of State Boards of Nursing [NCSBN], 2014). The NCSBN calls for nurses to:

➤ Show respect for human dignity.
➤ Avoid personal gratification at the patient's expense.
➤ Never interfere in the patient's personal relationships.
➤ Promote patient autonomy and self-determination.
➤ Understand that the nurse–patient relationship is based on trust.

KEY POINT: *Nurses have a moral duty to protect patients from inappropriate relationships. Patient-centered care is only possible when boundaries are respected and patients and their families feel safe to communicate freely and truthfully.*

Sources: Hall, K. (2011). Professional boundaries: Building a trusting relationship with patients. *Home Healthcare Nurse, 29*(4), 210–217; Hanna, A., & Suplee, P. (2012). Don't cross the line. Respecting professional boundaries. *Nursing2012, 42*(9), 40–48. doi:10.1097/01. NURSE.0000419445.29116.e1; Holder, K., & Schenthal, S. (2007). Watch your step: Nursing and professional boundaries. *Nursing Management, 38*(2), 24–29; National Council of State Boards of Nursing. (2014). *A nurse's guide to professional boundaries.* Chicago, IL: Author. Retrieved from https://www.ncsbn.org/ProfessionalBoundaries_Complete.pdf

---

♥ iCare 20-1

Caring Using Active Listening

Active listening behaviors convey caring, signal a willingness to listen, and provide a comfortable environment for the client to share his concerns. To listen actively:

- Keep your attention in the moment and on the patient. Do not multitask.
- Do not look at your smartphone or watch; never text while the patient is talking.
- Do not interrupt the patient.
- Pay attention to verbal and nonverbal communication and look for congruence.
- If a message is unclear, seek clarification through use of probing questions or reflective comments, such as "Tell me more," or "When you say . . . what do you mean?"
- Face your client, lean in, and make eye contact.
- Focus the conversation on issues of importance to the client (see Fig. 20-5).
- Using a mobile device during a conversation distracts you from active listening. If you must take notes, record only key words to stimulate your memory at another time.
- Do not casually talk with coworkers while the patient is waiting.

how to address her. This conveys respect, which is essential to a therapeutic relationship.

Active Listening

At first glance, the term *active listening* appears to be an oxymoron. People often think of listening as a passive activity. If you have ever been in a one-sided conversation, you know that listening can be passive. In contrast, an *active listener* uses all senses to focus on the sender's message and allows the sender the opportunity to complete comments without interruption (Fig. 20-5).

Failure to listen to your client will result in missed messages or misinterpretation. Consider the following example:

Patient:	I guess I'm going to have surgery tomorrow.
Nurse:	*[Checking the IV fluids and hanging a medication.]* Uh-huh.
Patient:	The surgeon says I'll be in intensive care for a few days.
Nurse:	*[Looking at the drainage in the urine collection bag.]* Okay. Your urine looks good.
Patient:	I guess this is pretty risky surgery.
Nurse:	*[Recording on the flow sheet.]* Yep.

How do you think the patient must feel in this situation? The patient is clearly expressing concern about his upcoming surgery and seems to want to talk about it with the nurse.

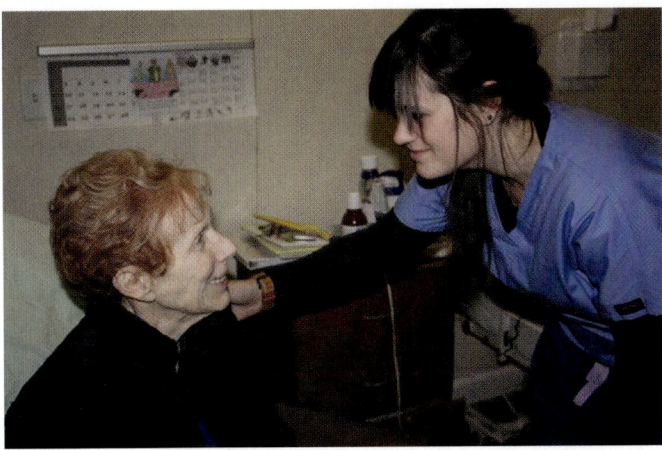

FIGURE 20-5 Active listening using full attention, direct eye contact, and caring touch.

However, the nurse is busy with a variety of tasks and is not paying attention to the conversation. Undoubtedly the patient will continue to feel anxious. In fact, his unsuccessful attempts to communicate may even increase his anxiety. If the nurse were listening, this would be an excellent opportunity to discuss the patient's concerns, provide preoperative teaching, and help the patient ease his anxiety.

Establishing Trust

Honesty and disclosure cannot exist without trust. That is why mutual trust is an essential component of professional and therapeutic communication. As trust grows, the client can more easily relay information and share feelings. To establish trust, always greet the client by name, listen actively, respond honestly to the client's concerns, and provide competent, consistent care.

Being Assertive

An assertive person is able to express himself effectively and directly communicate his point of view while still respecting the viewpoint and beliefs of others. Because assertive communication is based on mutual respect and freedom to confront difficult issues, the therapeutic relationship is a safe place for clients to convey their needs and concerns without feeling judged.

Restating, Clarifying, and Validating Messages

These three techniques help to identify client concerns and focus communication. They are especially helpful if the client is unclear or vague about a message.

- **Restating** means using your own words to summarize the message you received from the client. This demonstrates concern, active listening, and understanding of what the patient has said. The following is an example:

  Client: I'm so worried about my diabetes. I have young kids. I want to see them grow up. Every diabetic I've known has died young.

  Nurse: Diabetes is a serious disease. I understand your worry about its effects on you. That's why we want to focus on becoming well controlled so that you can avoid complications.

- **Clarifying** messages helps ensure that you have accurately interpreted the information. For instance, you might state, "I'm not sure what you mean when you say you're so worried about your diabetes." Or, "When you say you're worried, what do you mean?"

- **Validate** the message, by asking the client whether you are making a correct interpretation: "When you say you're worried about your diabetes, do you mean you are afraid you will die soon?"

Interpreting Body Language and Sharing Observations

Be attentive to what the patient says and how she says it. Note the tone of voice, rate of speech, distance, eye movement, facial expressions, and gestures. If the spoken and the nonverbal messages are inconsistent, you can share your observations by describing the patient's body language or tone of voice. For example, you might say, "I know you said you feel well, but your voice and hands are trembling. How can I help you?" Or more simply, "You're frowning. Has something upset you?"

Exploring Issues

Ask open-ended questions to obtain a clear understanding of an issue and follow your client's thoughts (see Chapter 3). Probing comments such as "Tell me more" encourage your client to share information.

Using Silence

Learn to be comfortable with silence, especially when your client is emotionally upset. When you remain attentive, silence demonstrates acceptance and allows the client to organize his thoughts and so provide further information.

Summarizing the Conversation

At the end of the conversation, summarize what you have heard. For example, you might say, "Today we talked about diet, exercise, and medications for high blood pressure. Your job now is to review the handouts and start taking your medication every morning. I'll see you in 2 weeks at your follow-up visit." Summarizing demonstrates active listening and allows the client to clarify any misunderstandings.

Using Process Recordings

A strategy commonly used to improve therapeutic communication skills is called **process recording.** In process recording, ideally two people converse while a third records the conversation. Sometimes two people converse while one of them takes notes or records from memory after the conversation.

- Audio recording effectively captures the words and intonation of the conversation, but it must be supplemented by notes describing the nonverbal communication.
- Video recording allows participants to examine both verbal and nonverbal communication.

  Afterward, the participants analyze the interaction. As you examine an interaction, evaluate how well you showed empathy, respect, and genuineness. Identify techniques you used to enhance the communication (e.g., active listening, restating). Be alert for barriers to therapeutic communication.

Barriers to Therapeutic Communication

As you learn to communicate therapeutically, you may find yourself thinking, doing, or saying things that seem to shut down your conversation. If so, acknowledge your error and return to therapeutic patterns. The following sections describe the most common barriers to therapeutic communication.

Asking Too Many Questions

Asking questions at the appropriate time is important. However, asking too many questions, especially closed questions (requiring only a yes or no answer), can make clients feel that they are being interrogated. It may also suggest insensitivity or lack of respect for the client's issues, as in the following dialogue:

Patient:	I feel lousy today.
Nurse:	Didn't you sleep well?
Patient:	No, hardly at all.
Nurse:	Did you take anything to help you sleep?
Patient:	No.
Nurse:	Do you think you should have taken something?
Patient:	I guess.
Nurse:	Why didn't you tell the night nurse you needed something?
Patient:	I don't know.

As you can see, this approach controls the range and nature of client responses. In contrast, open-ended questions stimulate conversation and exploration. Consider the preceding conversation in comparison with the following conversation:

Patient:	I feel lousy today.
Nurse:	Lousy? Tell me more.
Patient:	Well, my back and neck hurt, and I hardly slept at all. I thought it would go away, but I just lay in bed last night worrying.
Nurse:	What kind of things are you worrying about?
Patient:	I'm worried about . . .

Notice that the nurse's open-ended questions encouraged the patient to discuss his concerns.

Fire-Hosing Information

Sometimes a healthcare provider might meet with a patient or family and deliver an overwhelming amount of information in a short time. Those involved might understand what the provider said, but afterward remember only a fraction of it. Or they might feel stunned, confused, intimidated, or helpless. It is better to engage your patient in a *dialogue* in which you give important information and prompt your patient to share his own concerns and questions. You can then ask him for his understanding of what has been shared and clarify when needed.

Asking Why

Sometimes we need to learn why a patient acted or responded as he did. However, directly asking for reasons suggests criticism to some people. If you ask, "Why did you stop taking your medication?" the patient may become defensive and stop talking. A subtle approach is more comfortable for the patient. You might ask, "What concerns do you have about your medicines?" or "Tell me more about your experience with the medication." Both approaches will help you obtain more information about the client's concerns without suggesting criticism.

Changing the Subject Inappropriately

Try not to abruptly change the topic of discussion, because you will seem uninterested. This often occurs when the nurse is intent on one issue and the patient is focused on another, or if the topic is difficult to discuss (e.g., abnormal test results, poor prognosis).

Notice when the patient changes the subject, as in the following example:

Nurse:	Your wife is very sick. Do you think she will get better?
Patient's spouse:	It's tough, I know. Her condition reminds me of a movie I saw last night. She even looks like the leading actress.

Toward Evidence-Based Practice

Milic, M. M., Puntillo, K., Turner, K., et al. (2015, July). **Communicating with patients' families and physicians about prognosis and goals of care.** *American Journal of Critical Care,* 24(4), e56–e64. doi:10.4037/ajcc2015855

At the request of nurses providing care to acutely and critically ill patients in the intensive care unit, researchers designed an interactive workshop to improve communication and coping skills. Nurses used role playing to practice communication methods, such as reflection statements, "Tell me more," hope/worry statements, and ask-tell-ask. After the workshop nurses reported greater confidence discussing difficult topics with patients, families, and the healthcare team. Those participating in the workshop reported increased confidence in their communication skills with the healthcare team. They also described improved coping with stress, moral distress, and compassion fatigue.

Hammer, M., Fox, S., & Hampton, M. D. (2014). **Use of a therapeutic communication simulation model in pre-licensure psychiatric mental health nursing: Enhancing strengths and transforming challenge.** *Nursing and Health,* 2(1), 1–8. doi:10.13189/nh.2014.020101

Researchers implemented a simulation model for nursing students in a pre-licensure psychiatric mental health course to practice therapeutic communication techniques. Using unscripted, videotaped simulation, students were evaluated for effectiveness of verbal and nonverbal responses. Active listening behaviors included clarifying, imparting information, self-disclosure, silence, and focusing. The therapeutic communication simulation experience provided a safe, challenging, and experiential learning environment.

After participating in an educational activity to improve your communication skills, suppose you are the nurse providing care for a patient suffering with a bipolar mood disorder.

1. What nonverbal cues might you use to convey caring?

2. What nonverbal behaviors communicate a noncaring attitude or poor listening?

3. What verbal skills might you use to establish a therapeutic relationship with the client?

4. What nonverbal behaviors interfere in the therapeutic relationship between the nurse and the client?

 Go to Davis Advantage, Resources, Chapter 20, **Toward Evidence-Based Practice Suggested Responses.**

Your relationship with your patient's husband and the facts of the situation determine whether you would redirect this conversation back to the original subject or allow him to digress. You may choose to give the husband more time to be comfortable with you before approaching this topic again.

Failing to Probe

Failing to ask relevant questions can convey a lack of caring. It can also result in incomplete assessment and affect the quality of your care. When assessing, you should explore issues in detail. Review the following conversations:

Patient:	I'm having a lot of discomfort in my back.
Nurse:	How much does it hurt?
Patient:	Quite a bit. I had trouble sleeping last night.
Nurse:	I'll get you something for pain.

Compare that conversation with the next example, in which the nurse gathers additional data:

Patient:	I'm having a lot of discomfort in my back.
Nurse:	Tell me about the discomfort.
Patient:	It hurts a lot. I had trouble sleeping last night.
Nurse:	When did you first notice this pain?
Patient:	It started in the middle of the night.
Nurse:	What does it feel like?
Patient:	I feel sore. I'd like to turn over to my side, but I can't because of this heavy cast.
Nurse:	Let me help you turn. [*Assists patient to turn and uses pillows to hold the patient on her side.*]
Patient:	Oh, that feels better!
Nurse:	I'm glad you're feeling better. Would you like something for pain as well?
Patient:	I think I'm okay now.

In the second example, the nurse followed her original question with additional probing questions. A few additional questions helped clarify what the patient needed and led to immediate comfort.

Expressing Approval or Disapproval

Nurses need to be sensitive about expressing both approval and disapproval to a patient. Although it may seem supportive, expressing approval can inhibit further sharing—it puts you in the position of being the judge of what is "right." This often prompts the patient to continue to seek approval. He thinks, "I'd better be careful; she may not approve of the next thing I was going to tell her. She expects me to be *this* way." Consider instead offering recommendations and allowing the patient to choose. Read the following exchange:

Patient:	I've decided I'm going to have the surgery.
Nurse:	That's great. I think you made the right choice.

Compare that conversation with the following example:

Patient:	I've decided I'm going to have the surgery.
Nurse:	Tell me about your decision.
Patient:	Well, my shoulder has been bothering me for several months now. I know I said I wanted to put off surgery, but I think I'll have a faster recovery if I just get the surgery done now.
Nurse:	So your choices are to do a trial of physical therapy and anti-inflammatory medicines, to try a steroid injection, or to have surgery.
Patient:	Right. But there's a good chance I'll still need surgery even if I try the therapy or medicines. The only thing that will actually fix the problem is surgery. The others don't guarantee improvement.

Can you see how the conversation changes if the nurse does not express approval? By encouraging the patient to discuss the choices, the nurse empowers the patient to make his own healthcare decisions.

Offering Advice

Avoid statements such as "If I were you . . ." or "You should . . ." These statements impose your opinion on your clients. In effect, your statements function as approval if they agree with the client's thoughts or disapproval if they do not. As with other forms of approval or disapproval, conversation halts. If the client asks, "What should I do?" help clarify the options and provide her with information about the choices. Giving the client your solution deprives the client of opportunity to participate as a partner in the decision-making process.

Providing False Reassurance

- **Providing realistic reassurance helps to ease concern, offers comfort, and communicates empathy.** Therefore, it is an appropriate and therapeutic action—if the reassurance is warranted. For example, suppose a patient presents to the emergency department (ED) for treatment of an acute episode of asthma. Because anxiety exacerbates asthma, it is certainly therapeutic to reassure the client that he will be cared for promptly and effectively.
- **In contrast, false reassurance is a barrier to therapeutic communication.** When patients or family members ask for information or tell you that they are worried, it is easy to reassure them that everything will be fine. However, such responses are uninformed and inaccurate and may feel dismissive—even condescending.
  - *Example:* You are a nurse working at the triage station in the local ED. Your role is to evaluate the condition and prioritize the care of all clients presenting for treatment. An ambulance arrives with a man experiencing severe chest pain. He is ashen and short of breath. He tells you his pain is "crushing." Suspecting a heart attack, you immediately move him to the critical care bay of the ED and request urgent evaluation. Several minutes later his wife arrives. She anxiously asks you, "How is my husband?" How would you respond?

Your first instinct may be to respond: "Don't worry, everything will be all right." But do you really know that will be the case? A better approach is to provide accurate information: "I had him immediately taken in for treatment. I'll get you in to see him as soon as I can. Please have a seat, and I'll check on him." This comment is accurate and calming and avoids misleading the person.

Stereotyping

As discussed in Chapter 15, racial, cultural, religious, age-related, or gender stereotypes distort assessment and prevent you from recognizing the patient's uniqueness. Examples of statements reflecting a stereotype include the following: "He's old; he won't remember anything you tell him," and "Men are always the biggest wimps about pain." Such comments may block communication and escalate tension.

Stereotypes and generalizations may be blatant or subtle. Some are easily recognized and may create an intense reaction. Others are harder to identify but may be equally disruptive to care, for example:

- Assuming patients will understand their healthcare because of their educational level or work experience (e.g., expecting that a physician who has suffered a heart attack needs little or no explanation of her care)

- Believing a patient will be calm and know what to expect because he has had previous hospitalizations for the same diagnosis, has had previous surgeries or other procedures, or was given information about his condition
- Expecting all patients with the same surgery or diagnosis to experience similar responses

Using Patronizing Language

Patronizing language communicates superiority or disapproval. Statements such as "You ought to know . . ." are patronizing and offensive to the client. Condescending approaches, such as "You should have used the call button before you got up; you're lucky you didn't hurt yourself" do not communicate respect for the client.

Elderspeak, another form of patronizing, describes ways that healthcare workers may unintentionally show disrespect to elderly patients by speaking to them in a high-pitched, slow, repetitive, childlike voice and calling patients "Sweetie," "Dearie," or "Mama." Staff may also alter pronouns, saying, for example, "Are we ready for our bath?" Although the intent is to communicate caring, many patients are offended because it sounds as though you are speaking to a child. Research indicates that mentally competent nursing home residents are irritated by elderspeak, and that people with moderate Alzheimer's disease become more agitated and resistant to care if they are addressed in this manner (Williams, Herman, Gajewski, et al., 2009).

KnowledgeCheck 20-6

Identify at least five barriers to communication.

Enhancing Communication With Clients From Another Culture

The way you address your patient will vary according to culture. In the United States and many other countries, people use a formal salutation (Mr., Mrs., Ms., Dr.). The given name (personal name) precedes the surname. Other countries, such as Korea and China, go by surname, followed by first name. Some people from another culture adapt their name to fit within the culture in which they are living. **KEY POINT:** *Be sensitive to the practices of your patient and ask his preference.*

Healthcare facilities should provide interpretation (including translation) services as necessary (The Joint Commission, 2010).

- Many health facilities have in-house translation services for non-English-speaking patients. Translators may also be available through telephone contact; a few are linked via computer to a healthcare interpreter network to enable video teleconferencing.
- Internet and mobile technologies offer applications for translating English into various other languages. Try learning

♥ iCare 20-2

Communicating With Caring Presence

Lisa is admitting Ana, a 30-year-old-female. Ana is visiting from Brazil and speaks only Portuguese. While shopping, she experienced severe right lower quadrant abdominal pain and was rushed to the hospital by ambulance. She is alone and scared. Although medical interpreters have been provided, none of her family or friends has arrived yet. Lisa, recognizing Ana's fear, takes the time to sit with her, reassuring her through nonverbal communication such as smiling, making eye contact, and gently touching her shoulder. She sits quietly, holding her hand. Her presence seems to reassure Ana, who stops crying and remains calm until her friends arrive.

a few key words in your patients' primary language to communicate basic care and understand their basic needs. For a list of a few useful Spanish terms and for guidelines for communicating with clients from other cultures, see Clinical Insight 20-3.

- Use relatives as translators only if there are no other options. It is often culturally unacceptable to have family members ask personal questions. As a result, translations may be altered or questions remain unasked.
- See Chapter 15 for additional information on the use of translators.

Enhancing Communication With Clients Who Have Impaired Speech

For guidelines to help you communicate with clients who have speech deficits, see Clinical Insight 20-4.

Enhancing Communication With Clients Who Have Impaired Cognition or Reduced Level of Consciousness

Communicating with cognitively impaired clients can be difficult, time consuming, and frustrating for even the most experienced nurse. This might be a patient with acute illness or neurological injury, a patient with congenital abnormality, a person with sensory or language deficits, or an older adult with dementia. In the hospital setting, impairments are heightened because of illness, changed routines and environment, and medication. As a result, the patient may be unable to understand explanations, follow directions, ask for help, or report symptoms (Zembrzuski, 2013, revised).

♥ iCare *It is critical that you make every effort to communicate regardless of whether the client can understand you.*

For guidelines to help you communicate with clients with impaired cognition or consciousness, see Clinical Insight 20-5.

CLINICALREASONING

The questions and exercises in this section allow you to practice the kind of thinking you will use as a full-spectrum nurse. Critical-thinking questions usually have more than one right answer, so we do not provide "correct answers" for these features. It is more important to develop your nursing judgment than to just cover content. You will learn by discussing the questions with your peers. If you are still unsure, see the Davis Advantage chapter resources for suggested responses.

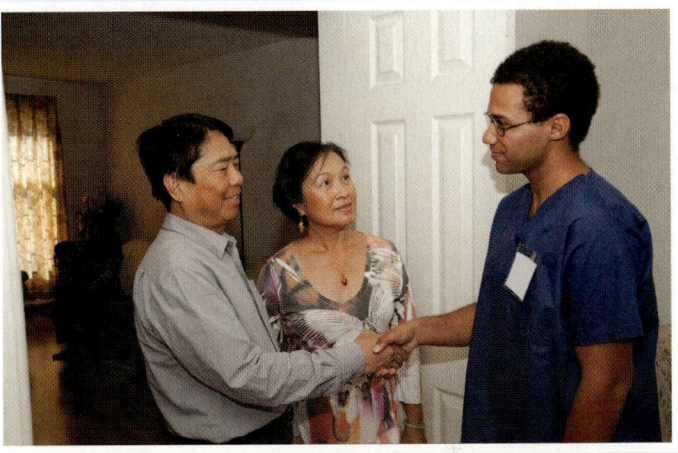

Caring for the Nguyens

Below is a transcript of an interaction that occurred during Nam Nguyen's first visit to the family healthcare clinic. As you may recall, Zach Miller is a family nurse practitioner who is examining Nam Nguyen. Analyze the interaction. Identify open-ended and closed questions and therapeutic communication techniques. Comment on responses that Zach might have improved on.

Zach: Are your parents still living?

Nam: Yes, they're both alive. My father is 80 years old and my mother is 76.

Zach: I'd like to hear a little more about your family history. Tell me about your father's cancer. How old was he when he was first diagnosed? Has he had treatment?

Nam: He was probably about 60 when he first found out about it. I know he had some kind of surgery and takes medicines, but I don't know the details. He seems all right though.

Zach: Your father also has high blood pressure and heart disease. Please tell me a little more about that.

Nam: My father and mother both have high blood pressure and heart disease. They both take medication for their blood pressure. My father had a small heart attack about 10 years ago. My mother has never had a heart attack that I know of, but she sometimes has chest pain.

Zach: Your mother also has diabetes?

Nam: She's had that for a long time. A lot of people in my family, especially on my father's side, have diabetes but nobody in my mother's family. Yet my mother is the one with the diabetes!

Yen: A lot of people in my family have diabetes, too. But so far I'm okay, I think.

Zach: Have you had a health exam lately, Mrs. Nguyen?

Yen: Not in about a year, but I'm going to schedule an appointment here.

Applying the **Full-Spectrum Nursing Model**_____

Choose two of the following communication techniques and plan to consciously use them with your next patient. Use the following thinking, doing, and caring questions to reflect on your interaction.

Active listening
Communicating assertively using "I" statements
Restating a message
Clarifying messages
Validating messages
Sharing observations about body language
Asking open-ended questions
Using silence
Summarizing the conversation

THINKING

1. *Critical Thinking (Contextual Awareness):* Before you have the conversation, make a note of what is going on in the situation (e.g., values, environment, culture) that might influence the effectiveness of the two techniques you will be using.

DOING

2. *Nursing Process (Assessment):* Before using the two techniques, assess for factors that might affect the patient's ability to communicate. Make a note of them.
3. *Nursing Process (Implementation):* As soon as possible after using the techniques, record the conversations. Try to remember the exact words.
4. *Nursing Process (Evaluation):* Evaluate your ability to use the two techniques you chose.
   a. Did you use them at an appropriate time in the conversation—for example, as an appropriate response to something the patient said?
   b. What effect did your communication have on the interaction? How did the patient respond to what you said?
   c. Do you think your communication was therapeutic for the patient?

CARING

5. *Self-Knowledge:*
   a. What were your thoughts and feelings before, during, and after the interaction?
   b. In what way has your comfort level with these two techniques changed?
   c. Describe the type of patient or situation in which you would be the least confident in your ability to communicate therapeutically.

PracticalKnowledge:
clinical application

This section provides clinical insights and focused assessments for communication.

CLINICAL INSIGHTS

Clinical Insight 20-1 ▶ **Enhancing Communication Through Nonverbal Behaviors**	
Nonverbal Behaviors	**Interpretation**
Direct eye contact	Demonstrates interest and attention. Consider the client's cultural heritage when determining how much eye contact is appropriate.
Concerned facial expression **Leaning forward** **Personal space**	Lends credibility, if congruent with conversation. Shows interest in the conversation. A distance of 18 inches to 4 feet allows most clients to feel comfortable during the interaction. Adjust the distance within that range based on the client's preference.
Professional appearance	Gives people an impression of how you may act in your role as a healthcare provider.
Sitting down to talk	Communicates willingness to listen and a sense of not wanting to rush the interaction with the client.
Touch	Conveys caring and concern when used appropriately.

Clinical Insight 20-2 ➤ Communicating With SBARQ*

Situation	In 10 seconds, identify yourself and the patient and describe the present situation that prompted you to call. State ■ Your name ■ Your unit ■ The patient's name and room number ■ The problem
Background	Give other information pertinent to the situation—not the patient's entire history since admission, but circumstances leading up to the situation (e.g., medications, lab results, current symptoms).
Assessment	State the problem and what you think is causing it. This is an inference rather than traditional data collection.
Recommendation	State what you think will correct the problem, or what you need from the physician.
Question	■ Allow an opportunity to ask or answer any questions. ■ Review specific concerns.

*If you need other information about SBARQ, see Chapter 18.

Practice Resources

De Meester , K., Verspuy, M., Monsiers, K. G., et al. (2013); Institute for Healthcare Improvement (2011a, updated 2013); Military Health System, U.S. Department of Defense. (n.d.); Potter, Mostek, Sobeski, et al. (2013).

Clinical Insight 20-3 ➤ Communicating With Clients From Another Culture

General Guidelines

■ Most important: Be aware of your own cultural beliefs and attitudes.
■ Learn about other cultures, especially those in your area.
■ Convey empathy and show respect.
■ Be certain the communication strategies you usually use are culturally appropriate for the individual.
   Is direct eye contact viewed as aggressive or impolite? Or is it perceived as engaged and caring?
   How much space should you keep between yourself and the patient?
■ Use touch cautiously. In some cultures, it is inappropriate to touch certain parts of the body.
■ Proceed slowly. Rushing may cause the patient to be more anxious and is offensive to some.

■ Smile and be polite, but not overfriendly or casual. Use the patient's title and last name when introducing yourself.
■ Use short words and sentences. Don't give too much information in one sentence.
■ Present one idea at a time.
■ Provide written teaching materials.

If There Is a Language Barrier

■ Written information provided must be appropriate to the population served and the language of the patient (The Joint Commission, 2010).
■ Use a trained medical interpreter, if possible.
■ To review guidelines for communicating with clients who speak a different language, refer to How Do I Communicate With Clients Who Speak a Different Language? in Chapter 15 of this book.

Some medical dictionaries or Web-based resources have a comprehensive list of English–Spanish phrases, for example:

English	Spanish	English	Spanish
How do you feel?	¿Como se siente?	Cough	Tosa
Good	Bien	Open your mouth	Abra la boca
Bad	Mal	Take a deep breath	Respire profundamente
Have you any difficulty breathing?	¿Tiene dificultad al respirar?	You may eat	Puede comer
Are you thirsty?	¿Tiene sed?	Tea	Té
Have you any pain?	¿Tiene dolor?	Coffee	Café
Show me where	Enséñeme dónde	I will give you something for	Le dare algo para eso
Is it worse now?	¿Está peor ahora?	A pill	Una píldora

Clinical Insight 20-4 ➤ **Communicating With Clients Who Have Impaired Speech**

Healthcare agencies should address the communication needs of those with vision, speech, hearing, language, and cognitive impairments.

- Nonverbal communication is the key to communication with clients with impaired speech.
- Ask the client to use hand gestures and a picture board, as appropriate.
- Solicit family assistance in understanding the client's speech.

- Provide a comfortable environment for the client to practice speaking.
- Be positive and patient.
- Although the client may have difficulty speaking, you should continue to speak and explain all procedures.
- A referral to a speech pathologist may be necessary.

Practice Resources

The Joint Commission (2010).

Clinical Insight 20-5 ➤ **Communicating With Patients Who Have Impaired Cognition or Consciousness**

Patients Who Are Cognitively or Developmentally Impaired or With Dementia

Always try to communicate.	Make every effort to communicate, even if you think that the client cannot understand you.
Address the patient slowly and from the front.	Convey nonthreatening approach with a friendly demeanor and direct eye contact.
Don't rush the patient.	Provide adequate time to allow the patient to communicate. He needs time to respond to your questions or commands.
Use multiple communication modalities.	Provide verbal and written discharge instructions. Review the instructions several times with the patient before discharge and include family members in the teaching.
Provide reminders.	Use memory aids, schedules, and reminder notices to reinforce information.
Orient the client.	Verbally orient to time, person, and place, and provide visual orientation materials, such as a calendar or schedule.
Eliminate distractions.	Background noise, such as TV or smartphone, can interfere with the patient's ability to concentrate and follow communication.
Stimulate memory.	If the patient loses his place in the conversation, stimulate his memory by repeating his last expressed thought. For instance, you might say, "We were talking about your back pain. Tell me more about your back pain." Or if the patient cannot "find" the word, encourage her instead to describe that word. This will reduce frustration.
Use short sentences.	Use short sentences, containing a single thought, such as "Are you hungry?" Avoid complex statements. You could say, "You look hungry. Would you like a sandwich or a milk shake, or can you hold off until dinner?"
Ask "yes/no" questions.	Ask direct questions that require only a yes or no answer. ("Are you hungry?")
Ask one question at a time.	Likewise, when giving instructions, be sure to take a step at a time.
Limit choices.	Limit choices to avoid confusing or frustrating the patient.
Be concrete and specific.	Do not use vague comments to indicate that you are listening. The patient may be unable to interpret comments, such as "I see." Instead, repeat the patient's words and directly state your response. "You are cold. I will bring you a blanket."

Clinical Insight 20-5 ➤ **Communicating With Patients Who Have Impaired Cognition or Consciousness—cont'd**

Avoid slang and jargon.	The patient may not understand. For instance, if you say to your patient, "Are you cool?" she might think you mean body temperature when you might actually mean, "Are you feeling okay?"
Use gestures.	Model desired behaviors. You might say, "Brush your teeth now," and then enact brushing your teeth.
Don't assume.	Bear in mind that the patient cannot behave differently and that he may be confused about reality. When the person is talking about superficial, routine matters, he may seem more competent than he is.

Clients with expressive difficulties

- If you are sure of the word the person is trying to say, repeat it. Don't guess, though.
- Pay close attention to nonverbal communication.
- Assess for and anticipate unmet needs, such as hunger, thirst, and pain.
- Respond to the emotion, not the words.
- Do not reprimand the patient if she curses or is aggressive.

Patients Who Are Unconscious

- Touch and speak to unconscious or sedated patients; advise them of the care that you are providing. Although the patient may not be able to respond, she may be able to hear your comments.
- Consult with previous caregivers or the family to determine what the patient responds to.
- Begin each interaction by identifying yourself and calling the patient by name.
- Speak calmly and slowly, even if the patient doesn't seem to be alert and oriented.
- Explain all healthcare procedures as you are doing them.
- Provide soothing music and periods of rest.

Patients Who Have Suffered a Stroke

- Remember that many stroke survivors may have trouble communicating their thoughts. They also commonly experience emotional ups and downs. Do not take these moods personally.
- With aphasia, speak more slowly, not louder. Be careful not to use a patronizing tone.
- Be a good listener and allow time for the patient to express his thoughts.
- **Augmentative and alternative communication (AAC)** might be helpful to patients experiencing expressive aphasia. AAC includes all forms of communication other than speech to express thoughts, needs, wants, and ideas, such as communication boards and electronic devices.

Practice Resources

Alzheimer's Society (2015); American Heart Association (2012); American Speech-Language-Hearing Association (n.d.); deVries, K. (2013); Simoes, J., Jesus, L. M. T., & Voegeli, D. (2009); Zembrzuski, C. (2013, revised).

To explore learning resources for this chapter,

Go to **www.DavisAdvantage.com** and find:

Answers and Suggested Responses for all Questions in this Chapter

Lists of NIC Interventions and NOC Outcomes

List of NANDA-I Diagnoses

Knowledge Map

References and Bibliography

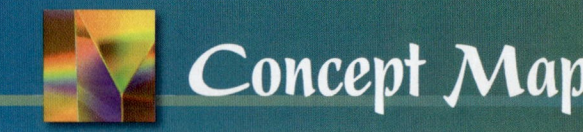
Concept Map

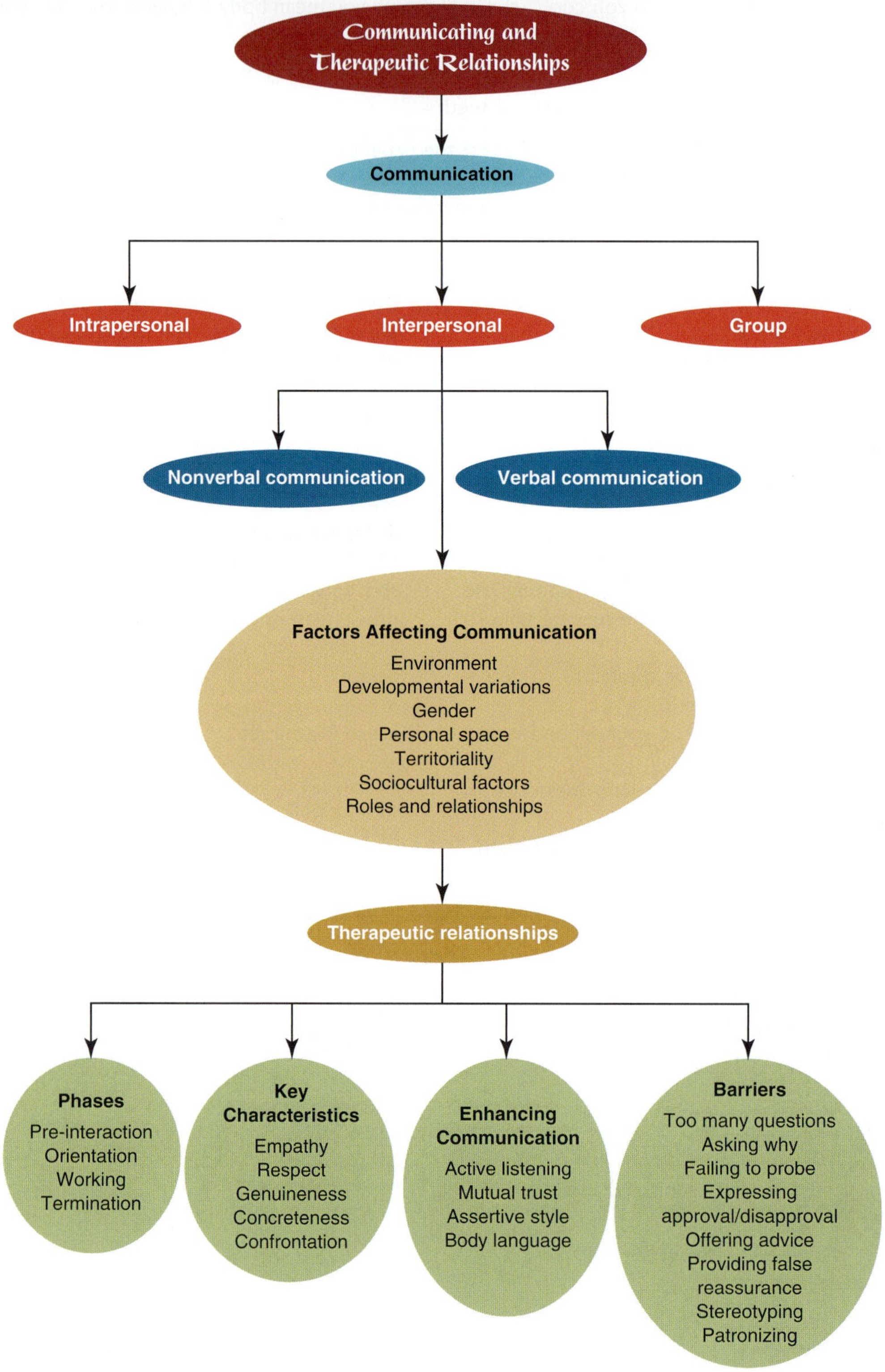

Communicating and Therapeutic Relationships

↓

Communication

Intrapersonal   **Interpersonal**   **Group**

Nonverbal communication   **Verbal communication**

Factors Affecting Communication

Environment
Developmental variations
Gender
Personal space
Territoriality
Sociocultural factors
Roles and relationships

↓

Therapeutic relationships

Phases

Pre-interaction
Orientation
Working
Termination

Key Characteristics

Empathy
Respect
Genuineness
Concreteness
Confrontation

Enhancing Communication

Active listening
Mutual trust
Assertive style
Body language

Barriers

Too many questions
Asking why
Failing to probe
Expressing approval/disapproval
Offering advice
Providing false reassurance
Stereotyping
Patronizing

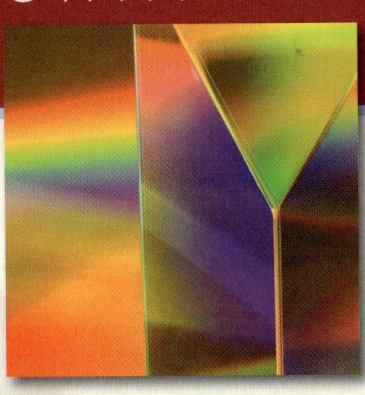

CHAPTER 21

Physical Assessment

Learning Outcomes

After completing this chapter, you should be able to:

➤ Identify the purposes and components of a physical examination.

➤ Discuss the differences between comprehensive, focused, and ongoing physical examinations.

➤ Describe how to prepare for a physical examination.

➤ Demonstrate the skills used in physical examination.

➤ Explain adaptations that may be required when you examine clients of various ages.

➤ Identify the components of the general survey.

➤ Conduct a full physical examination of a client.

➤ Discuss the expected findings of a physical examination.

➤ Document the findings of a physical examination.

➤ Perform a brief bedside physical examination.

Key Concepts

Health assessment

Nursing assessment

Physical examination

Related Concepts

See the Concept Map at the end of this chapter.

Meet Your Patient

Nam Nguyen is scheduled for a comprehensive physical examination at the family health center at 1400 today. As you recall, he has previously been seen and evaluated by Zach Miller, RN, FNP. Mr. Nguyen has medical diagnoses of hypertension, degenerative joint disease, obesity, and heavy tobacco use. During his earlier visit, Zach instructed Mr. Nguyen about a low-salt, low-fat diet and advised him to lose weight and quit smoking. Zach also ordered laboratory work to establish a baseline for wellness and detect abnormalities that might indicate illness.

At today's visit, Zach will perform a comprehensive physical exam of Mr. Nguyen and review his lab results. You will find the results following the Caring for the Nguyens

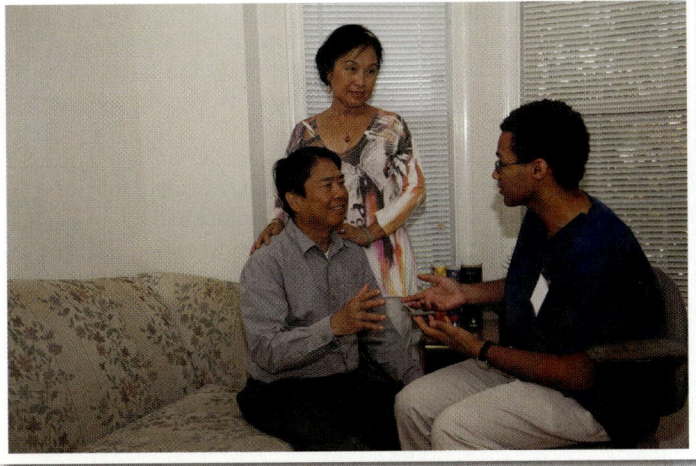

feature later in this chapter. After Nam's appointment, Yen Nguyen will also have a comprehensive exam.

Theoretical Knowledge
knowing why

In this chapter, theoretical knowledge consists mostly of information about the key concepts. You will see how an understanding of the key concepts will prepare you and the client for the examination and help you to modify your assessments for different age-groups.

ABOUT THE KEY CONCEPTS

A **health assessment** is a comprehensive assessment of the physical, mental, spiritual, socioeconomic, and cultural status of an individual, group, or community. **Nursing assessments** focus on the client's functional abilities and physical responses to illness and other stressors. In contrast, medical assessments focus on disease and pathology. As a nurse practitioner, Zach Miller combines the nursing and medical approaches.

A **physical examination** consists of the techniques used in a health or nursing assessment to gather objective data about the body.

PHYSICAL EXAMINATION

A complete health assessment includes both a nursing history and a physical examination. In addition to the physical examination, you will also ask questions to obtain subjective data about each body system or area. Questioning may be done in a separate nursing interview or as you perform the physical examination. Both the interview and the exam require tact and sensitivity.

Purposes of a Physical Examination

A physical examination is performed for any of several reasons:

- *To obtain baseline data.* Data about the patient's physical status and functional abilities to serve as a comparison as the patient's health status changes.
- *To identify nursing diagnoses, collaborative problems, and wellness diagnoses.* Problem statements form the basis for the plan of care and help you to address the patient's nursing care needs.
- *To monitor the status of a previously identified problem.* For example, Mr. Nguyen has already begun treatment for hypertension. Today's examination will be linked to the lab results to further explore the status of his hypertension.
- *To screen for health problems.* Regular checkups can help to identify health problems at early stages. Because Mr. Nguyen has an enlarged prostate, a prostate-specific antigen test was done to screen for prostate cancer.

Types of Physical Examination

The type of physical examination you perform will depend on the client's health status, the nature of the client encounter, and the setting.

- **Comprehensive physical examination** (also called physical assessment) includes a health history interview and a complete head-to-toe examination of all body systems. For example, you would perform a comprehensive physical exam at an outpatient appointment for an annual physical, a client's admission to an inpatient setting, and at the initial home health visit.
- A **focused physical assessment** (or examination) pertains to a particular topic, body part, or functional ability rather than overall health status, and it adds to the database created by the comprehensive assessment. For example, in an emergency situation, your assessment will be rapid and focused on the presenting problem

- A **system-specific assessment** is a focused assessment limited to one body system (e.g., the lungs, the peripheral circulation). The following are examples of focused and system-specific physical assessments, respectively:

    Assessing bowel sounds when a client has abdominal pain

    Listening to breath sounds, counting respirations, and obtaining pulse oximetry readings to assess a patient's respiratory status

- **Ongoing assessment** is performed as needed after the initial database is completed and, ideally, at every interaction with the patient. For example, on a medical–surgical unit, each nurse who provides care to a client conducts a brief ongoing assessment to determine changes in the client's status. For more details on the types of assessment, see Chapter 3. To learn how to perform a brief bedside assessment, see Procedure 21-20.

Preparing for a Physical Examination

Develop a systematic approach and follow the same order each time you perform a physical exam. This will help you recall the steps and include all the important data.

- A **head-to-toe approach** starts at the head and neck and progresses down the body, examining the feet last.
- A **body systems approach** examines each system in a predetermined order (e.g., musculoskeletal, cardiovascular, neurological).

    Whatever the approach, prepare yourself, the environment, and the client before you begin.

Prepare Yourself

- Preparing for a physical examination requires *theoretical knowledge* of:

    Anatomy and physiology

    Examination equipment and techniques

    Therapeutic communication, and documentation

- *Self-knowledge* is also important:

    How comfortable are you when performing an examination?

    What skills do you need to review or practice?

    Will you need assistance to perform some aspects of the exam?

    Will you need help documenting your findings?

    Honestly evaluate your strengths as well as areas that need improvement.

    Be sure to seek help from your instructor, an experienced nurse, fellow students, or other healthcare providers as needed.

- *Before approaching the patient, familiarize yourself with his situation.*

    What are the patient's main health concerns?

    What is the purpose of your exam? For instance, if you are doing a focused assessment of a client's wound, you will need to learn about the wound being examined.

    Is there a dressing over the wound? What supplies will you need to remove and replace the dressing?

    Has the patient required pain medication before exams in the past?

- *Finally, unless this is an initial assessment, review the nursing plan of care* and keep it in mind as you examine the patient. Reviewing previous findings helps you to work efficiently and formulate questions you might want to ask the patient. Furthermore, your assessment data may lead to modification or updating of the care plan.

Prepare the Environment

- **Privacy. KEY POINT:** *Physical examination requires you to observe and touch the client's body, so privacy is essential.*
  - You will need a room with curtains or a door to shield the client from view.
  - For additional privacy, drape your client and uncover only the area you are examining.
  - For convenience you may use bed linens and/or a gown to drape. Disposable paper drapes are also available.

- **Noise.** Because you will need to hear the patient and listen to a variety of sounds during the exam, turn off the television, radio, or other media.
- **Lighting.** You will need good lighting to observe subtle changes in skin and body contours.
- **Temperature.** Adjust the temperature of the room according to patient comfort.
- **Equipment.** Determine the instruments and equipment you will need (see Box 21-1). Take everything you need so that you will not have to leave the client to obtain supplies.

BOX 21-1 ■ Equipment Needed for Physical Examination: Usual Equipment for Ongoing Assessment

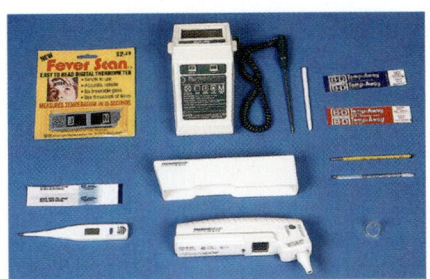

Thermometer (for measuring temperature)

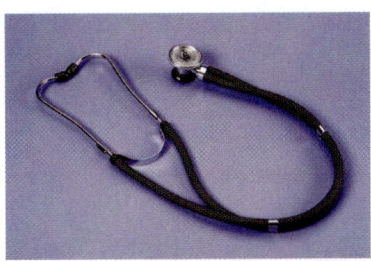

Stethoscope (for measuring blood pressure and listening to heart, lung, and bowel sounds)

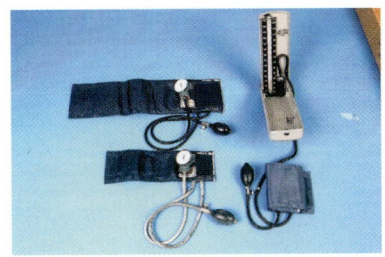

Sphygmomanometer (for measuring blood pressure)

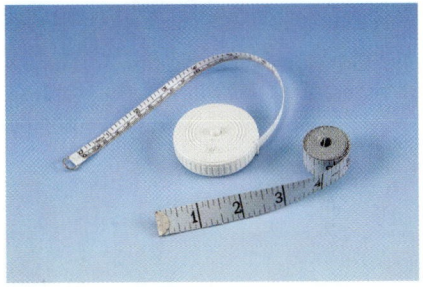

Tape measure (to measure circumference and length)

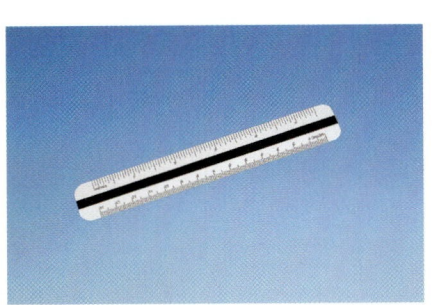

Pocket ruler (to measure size or distance)

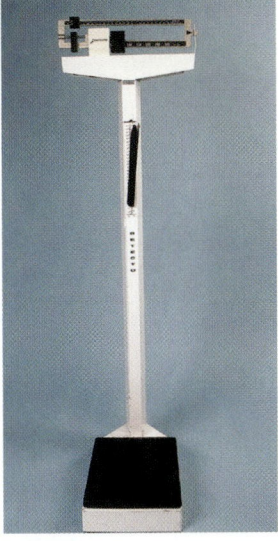

Scale (to measure weight and height)

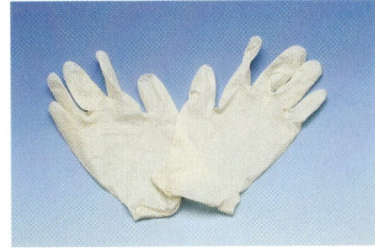

Gloves (to wear if there is any possible exposure to blood or body fluids)

(Continued)

BOX 21-1 ■ Equipment Needed for Physical Examination: Usual Equipment for Ongoing Assessment—cont'd

Additional Equipment for a Comprehensive Assessment

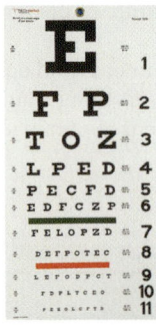

Snellen acuity chart (for screening vision)

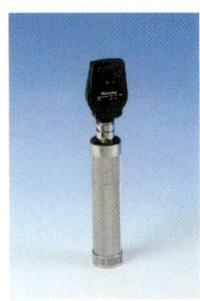

Ophthalmoscope (for inspection of the internal structures of the eye)

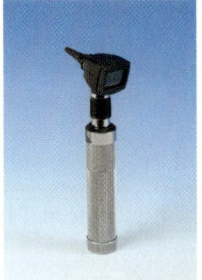

Otoscope (for examining the external auditory canal and tympanic membrane)

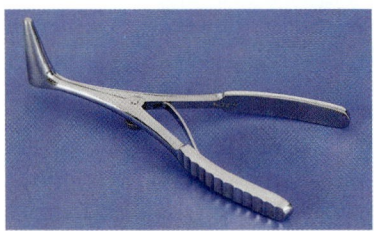

Nasal speculum (for examining the nasal turbinates)

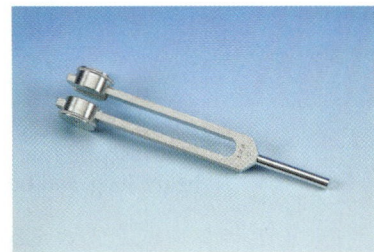

Tuning fork (for auditory screening and assessment of vibratory sensation during the neurological exam)

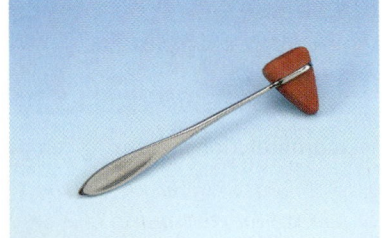

Percussion hammer (for eliciting deep tendon reflexes)

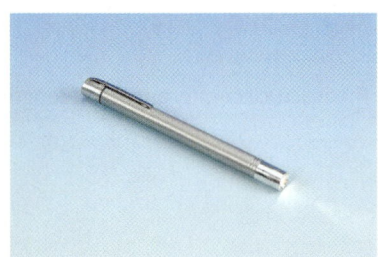

Penlight (for visualizing the eyes and inside of mouth, or highlighting a skin lesion)

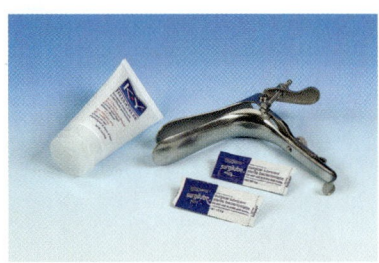

Vaginal speculum and lubricant (for examining the female pelvis; lubricant is also used for rectal exams)

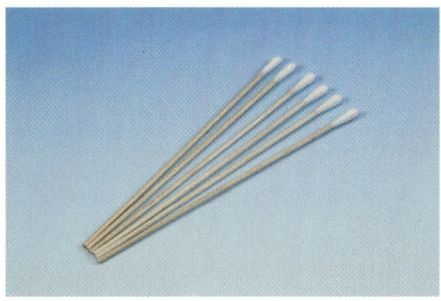

Cotton-tipped applicators (for obtaining specimens)

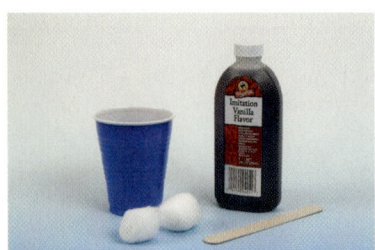

Cotton balls, tongue depressor, strong-smelling substance, a glass of water (for testing various cranial nerves)

Prepare the Client

In most clinical settings, you must examine a client often to evaluate a changing status, and timing will be decided by the client's condition rather than by convenience. However, when possible, select a time when the client is comfortable and receptive to the exam. Avoid conducting the exam when the client is in pain or is hungry, tired, anxious, or unwilling to cooperate in the assessment.

♥ **iCare**   Take the time to establish rapport with the client; this will help him relax and cooperate fully in the assessment.

- Introduce yourself, ask the client how he wishes to be addressed, and explain what you will be doing.
- Ask the client to void before the examination; this promotes relaxation and also makes it easier to palpate the abdomen.
- Always alert the client before touching him. For example, before you start to palpate the neck for lymph nodes, say, "I'm going to feel your neck now."
- Proper positioning during the exam also promotes comfort (see the following section).
- Pay attention to the pace of your exam, being careful not to prolong it and tire the client.

KEY POINT: *Consider developmental and cultural differences. For example, some clients may wish to have a family member present during an exam; some may require a same-sex clinician. If you and the client do not speak the same language, arrange to have an interpreter present.*

KnowledgeCheck 21-1

- What are the purposes of a physical examination?
- Describe how you would prepare for a physical exam.

ThinkLike a Nurse 21-1

- The nurse conducts a physical examination for Nam and Yen Nguyen (see Meet Your Patient) at an outpatient clinic. Discuss the differences between their planned experience and a focused physical exam of a hospital inpatient.
- Identify a plan to practice and improve your assessment skills.

Positioning the Client for the Examination

The client will need to assume a variety of positions during a comprehensive physical examination. As you place your client in positions that allow you to best observe each body system, be alert to special needs that call for you to modify the position. For example, a patient with a cervical spine problem would need a neck roll when lying supine.

- Table 21-1 illustrates and describes the major positions you will need to use.

KnowledgeCheck 21-2

Identify the best positions for examining the lungs, heart, pulses, and abdomen.

Physical Examination Techniques

You will use the physical examination techniques in the following order, with one exception: inspection, palpation, percussion, auscultation, and sometimes olfaction. *Exception:* When performing an abdominal assessment, perform auscultation

---

Safe, Effective Nursing Care

Health Assessment and Cultural Adaptation

Related Concepts: Developmental Stages

SENC Competencies: Goal-directed, client-centered care (Thinking, Doing, Caring)

Background: When performing a health assessment, adaptation for the developmental age of the client is a widely accepted nursing practice. It is also important to adapt for the client's culture. In order to engage diverse clients and respond to their preferences and values, culturally competent communication must be an integral component when initiating the health assessment according to Chircop, Edgecombe, Hayward, et al. (2013). The Thinking, Doing, Caring dimensions of goal-directed, client-centered care promotes the same principle. Four areas that demonstrate cultural adaptation in the health assessment are eliciting client preferences regarding: (1) comfort with touch, (2) comfort with exposure (modesty), (3) need for personal space, (4) and need for the presence of a support person.

Scenario: A client who speaks Portuguese requires an interpreter while hospitalized. You are assigned to complete the initial health assessment.

Think about it: The following items are for your own reflection or discussion with peers.

1. The nurse directs questions and makes eye contact with which of the following when obtaining the history: the interpreter or the client? Discuss how your response supports cultural adaptation.
2. Formulate questions for the nursing history to elicit client preferences regarding comfort with touch, comfort with exposure, personal space, and the presence of a support person.

Source: Chircop, A., Edgecombe, N., Hayward, K., et al. (2013). Evaluating the integration of cultural competence skills into health and physical assessment tools: A survey of Canadian schools of nursing. *Journal of Transcultural Nursing*, 24(2), 195–203. doi:10.1177/1043659612472202

---

before percussion and palpation to avoid disturbing the abdominal sounds.

Inspection is the use of sight to gather data. You begin to use inspection the moment you meet the client and continue as you observe the person's gait, personal hygiene, affect, and behavior during the general survey, and as you evaluate each body system.

- Adequate lighting and proper positioning aid inspection.
- The otoscope, ophthalmoscope, and penlight also enhance your inspection abilities.

Palpation is the use of touch to gather data. Use palpation to assess temperature; skin texture; moisture; anatomical landmarks; and such abnormalities as edema, masses, or areas of tenderness. As you move through the assessment of each body system, always inform the client when you are about to touch him. Use a gentle approach and be certain your hands are warm. Begin with light pressure to detect surface characteristics. Then move to deep palpation to assess the underlying structures. Examine last any areas of discomfort or sensitivity. (Palpation section continues on page 506.)

Table 21-1 ➤ Positioning the Client

POSITION AND DESCRIPTION	COMMENTS
Standing	
Upright posture with both feet flat on the floor.	Use to examine the musculoskeletal and neurological systems and to assess gait and cerebellar function. Clients who are weak or who have poor balance may not be able to assume this position.
Sitting	
Sitting upright at side of bed or exam table 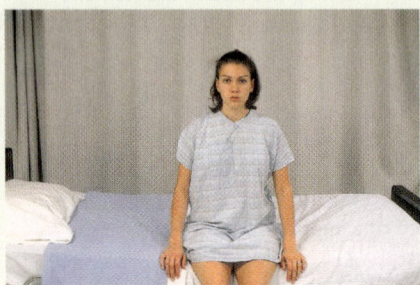	Use to assess vital signs, head and neck, chest, cardiovascular system, and breasts. If your client is weak, he may need assistance to maintain this position.
Supine	
(Including Fowler's and semi-Fowler's positions). Lying flat on the back with arms and legs fully extended 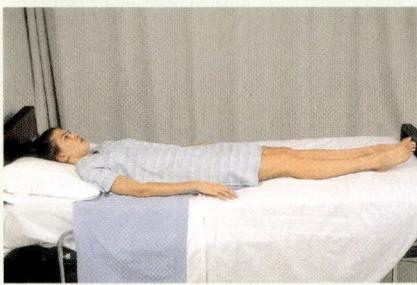	Use to assess the abdomen, breasts, extremities, and pulses. If your client becomes short of breath, raise the head of the bed (HOB). In **Fowler's position,** the head is elevated 60°. In **semi-Fowler's position,** the head is elevated only 30°–45°.
Dorsal Recumbent	
Supine with knees flexed 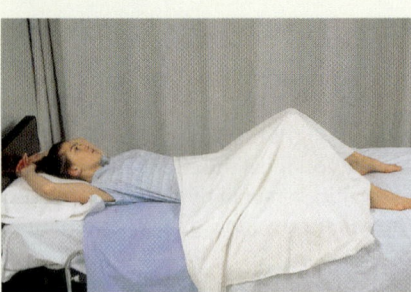	Use for abdominal assessment if your client has abdominal or pelvic pain. Flexing the knees promotes relaxation of the abdominal muscles.

Table 21-1 ➤ Positioning the Client—cont'd

POSITION AND DESCRIPTION	COMMENTS
Lithotomy	
Dorsal recumbent position at end of table with feet in stirrups, legs flexed, and widely open 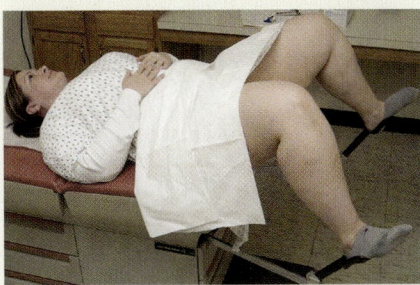	Use for a female pelvic exam; provides maximum exposure of genitals. Older patients may need support to assume and maintain this position. The patient's legs are exposed here to illustrate position. To see a privacy drape, refer to Procedure 24-4.
Sims'	
Flexion of the hip and knees in a side-lying position 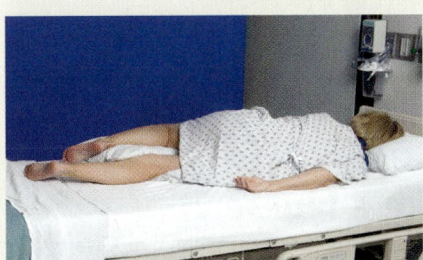	Use to examine the rectal area. Use for a female pelvic exam if the patient is unable to assume the lithotomy position. Do not use if the client has had total hip replacement.
Prone	
Lying on stomach (A small pillow under the abdomen makes this position more comfortable.) 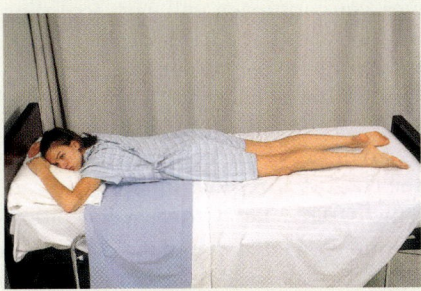	Use to examine the musculoskeletal system, especially hip extension; may also be used to examine the back and buttocks. May be difficult to assume by clients with respiratory problems.
Lateral Recumbent	
Lying on the side in a straight line 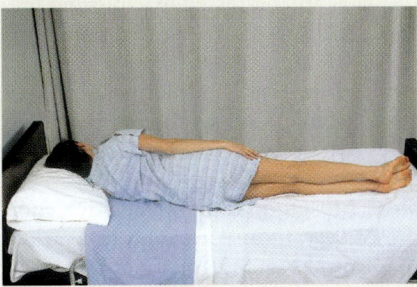	Left lateral recumbent is used to evaluate heart murmur or during a thorough cardiovascular assessment. This position brings the heart closer to the chest wall. If the client cannot assume this position, listen to the heart with the client seated and bending forward.

(Continued)

Table 21-1 ▸ Positioning the Client—cont'd	
POSITION AND DESCRIPTION	**COMMENTS**
Knee–Chest	
On hands and knees with head down and buttocks elevated 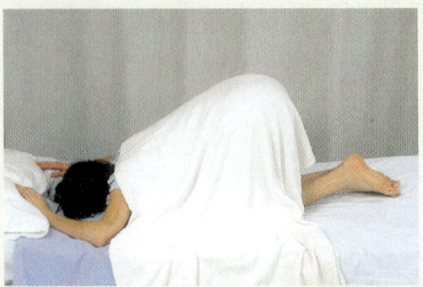	Provides good visualization for examining the rectal area. However, it is not used often because it is embarrassing and uncomfortable for the client.

Following is a list of the most common palpation techniques, using different parts of the hand:

- *Fingertips:* Use for fine tactile discrimination, including assessment of skin texture, swelling, and specific locations of pulsations and masses.
- *Dorsum of hand:* Use for temperature determination.
- *Palmar surface of hand:* Use for locating general area of pulsations.
- *Grasping with fingers and thumb:* Use to detect the position, shape, and consistency of a mass.

Percussion is tapping your fingers on the skin using short strokes. Tapping (percussing) produces vibrations, and the resulting sound allows you to determine location, size, and density of underlying structures. Percussion is especially useful when assessing the abdomen and lungs (Procedures 21-12 and 21-14). A quiet environment allows you to perceive the subtle differences in percussion notes.

Percussion takes practice. To learn more about percussion, see Clinical Insight 21-1.

Auscultation is the use of hearing to gather data.

- **Direct auscultation** is listening without using an instrument. If you have heard wheezing or chest congestion without the use of a stethoscope, you have already performed direct auscultation.
- **Indirect auscultation** is listening with the help of a stethoscope.

To improve your skill in indirect auscultation, see Clinical Insight 21-2.

Olfaction is the use of the sense of smell to gather data. Some clinicians may not consider this a formal assessment skill; however, you will certainly use this skill in the clinical setting. Olfaction adds information to the data you collect through the other techniques. Consider these examples:

- If a client is slurring his words, you will want to look for data that reveal the cause of the problem. Slurred speech might be caused by a stroke or by sedative medications. However, if the client smells of alcohol, you would first investigate recent alcohol use as a probable cause for the slurred words.
- If an older client smells of urine, you would want to assess for problems with leakage of urine or inability to perform self-care.
- If the client's breath has a "fruity" or "acetone" odor, you would suspect ketoacidosis, which may accompany diabetes.

You would know to assess the urine for ketones and contact the primary care provider if necessary.

KnowledgeCheck 21-3

- Identify five physical assessment skills.
- In what order are these skills performed?

ThinkLike a Nurse 21-2

Think about olfaction as an assessment technique. Give two or three additional examples of data you might collect through the use of smell.

Modifications for Different Age-Groups

The basic techniques of physical examination remain the same for everyone. However, your approach will vary according to the developmental stage of your patient. As a rule, encourage parents of infants and children to be present for the exam.

Infants Use the assessment as an opportunity to teach the parent about normal growth and development. Infants usually feel most secure if a parent holds them during the examination, either against the chest or, for older infants who can sit without support, on the parent's lap. Otherwise, position an infant on a padded examination table. If there are siderails, raise them to prevent falls. Do not leave the infant's side or turn your back on the infant.

Toddlers The following list includes some tips for examining toddlers:

- **Include parents.** Toddlers are interested in exploring the environment, but they also like to stay close to a parent, often in the parent's lap.
- **Perform invasive procedures last.** Toddlers may be fearful of invasive procedures, such as examination of the oral cavity or inner ear. If they are upset, it will be more difficult to examine other body areas.
- **Give the child choices.** Most toddlers enjoy making choices, so this will promote cooperation. For example, you might say, "Should I listen to your chest first, or should we see how much you weigh?"
- **Allow the child to show you his developmental skills.** If he needs assistance to remove clothing, have the parent help and observe how the parent and child interact.

- **Use praise freely.** Praise the toddler for his abilities and co-operation. This sets the stage for positive feelings about healthcare.

Preschoolers Preschool children are developing initiative and, as a result, usually cooperate with an examination. However, children of this age have fantasies and fears that may arise during the examination. For example, they may object to a noninvasive procedure because they believe it will cause pain or injury, or they may refuse to step on the scale because to them it resembles a monster.

- **Combat fears** by demonstrating the procedure on a doll or having the parent step on the scale before you approach the child.
- **Allow the preschool child to sit on a parent's lap** if she wishes. By age 5, most children will be comfortable enough to lie on the examination table if a parent is present.
- **Let the child help with the exam.** For example, have her hold equipment or remember her height and weight.
- **Give reassurance** as you go through the examination, for example, "Your lungs sound very healthy."
- **Always compliment the child on her cooperation.**

School-Age Children The school-age child has a rapidly expanding vocabulary and usually seeks approval of parents, teachers, and healthcare providers.

- **Develop rapport** by asking the child about his favorite school or play activities.
- **Support independence.** Allow the child to undress himself and get up on and down from the exam table.
- **Demonstrate your equipment** and let the child touch it before you use it. This makes the equipment seem less threatening.
- **Allow time for teaching.** The school-age child will be interested in how his body works, so use this opportunity for teaching.

Adolescents The adolescent is self-conscious and introspective and may wish to be examined without parents or siblings present, at least during the more personal aspects of the exam. Offer the adolescent this choice.

- **Provide privacy.** Adolescents often worry about the "normalcy" of their changing bodies and appreciate respect for their privacy.
- **Be certain to discuss the normal physiological changes** that accompany puberty. If you need to review those changes, see the section on adolescence in Chapter 9.
- **Be aware that adolescent behavior is strongly influenced by peer values.**
- **Emphasize lifestyle habits that promote wellness,** including a healthful diet, adequate rest and exercise, and avoidance of tobacco, alcohol, and other drugs.
- **Discuss sexually transmitted infections and cancer,** particularly testicular cancer and human papillomavirus.
- **Prepare the adolescent, if necessary, for a pelvic examination and breast examination,** which usually begin in the teen years.
- **Screen for depression and suicide risk.** Suicide is the third leading cause of death among adolescents (see Chapter 13 for a review of depression and suicide).

Young and Middle Adults Most young and middle adults are able to cooperate during a physical examination and do not require a modified approach. Modifications may be required if the client has acute or chronic illness or cannot understand or follow instructions.

 Older Adults Allow extra time to interview and examine older adults. They are adjusting to changes in physical abilities and health. As part of a comprehensive exam:

- Assess the client's support system and ability to perform activities of daily living. Observe your client's energy level during the physical examination and provide rest periods if needed.
- If the client tires easily, arrange the exam sequence to limit position changes.
- Be aware that stiff muscles and arthritic joints may make it impossible for the client to assume certain positions.
- Adapt your techniques when examining older adults with impaired vision or hearing. Obtain feedback to be sure the patient is seeing and hearing you adequately.

The acronym SPICES will help you to remember common problems of older adults that require nursing intervention (Fulmer, 1991, 2007) and to focus your assessment as you perform a comprehensive physical examination:

S—Sleep disorders
P—Problems with eating or feeding
I—Incontinence
C—Confusion
E—Evidence of falls
S—Skin breakdown

KnowledgeCheck 21-4

What exam modifications, based on developmental stage, should you consider for the following clients (Meet Your Patient):

- Nam Nguyen?
- Nam's 3-year-old grandson, Kim Phan?
- Nam's elderly mother, Mai Nguyen?

PracticalKnowledge
knowing **how**

The remainder of the chapter discusses each of the components of a comprehensive physical examination. For a step-by-step approach to perform each assessment, see the Procedures later in the chapter. To understand your patient's overall health status, you will need to be aware of the results of various diagnostic tests associated with each of the body systems you assess. Refer to the agencies' lab "norms" and to diagnostic studies handbooks, as needed, to interpret the tests.

THE GENERAL SURVEY

The general survey is your overall impression of the client. It begins at first contact and continues throughout the exam. **KEY POINT:** *Be sure to consider cultural background because this may influence your findings and interpretation.*

When you discover a deviation from normal in the general survey, you will explore it further during focused assessment of that body system. For example, if on meeting the patient you notice a drooping eyelid **(ptosis)** on one side of her face, you will keep that in mind as you perform the neurological assessment. Ptosis may be caused by a stroke or neurological injury.

Once you have completed your general survey of the client, you can begin to focus on each body system. Whether you are doing a complete or focused physical examination, remember that all body systems are interrelated. A problem in one system may affect or be affected by other systems. The following are aspects of the general survey. For a step-by-step approach for assessing them, see Procedure 21-1.

Appearance and Behavior   Refer to Procedure 21-1, Performing the general survey, steps 1, 2, and 3, for details about assessing appearance and behavior.

Body Type and Posture   Posture is a clue about overall health status. Focused assessments in the remainder of the general survey will help to reveal the exact meaning of such cues.

Speech   As you speak with the client and ask health-related questions, look for clues offered by his speech.

- **Inappropriate or illogical responses** may be associated with psychiatric disorders.
- **Difficulty speaking or changes in voice quality** may indicate a neurological problem.
- **Rapid speech** may be a sign of anxiety, hyperactivity, or use of stimulants.
- **Hoarseness** could indicate inflammation in the throat from infection, overuse, a foreign body, or perhaps a tumor or other obstructive material.
- **Slow speech** may be due to depression, sedation from medications, or neurological disorders.
- **Vocabulary and sentence structure** provide information about the client's educational level and comfort with the language.
- **A foreign accent with hesitancy and/or sparse verbalization** may signal a language barrier and a need for an interpreter.

Mental State   Mental state includes level of consciousness and capacity to interact. If the client has an altered mental status, ask a family member about the onset of the change.

 Keep in mind that many medications, especially in older adults, may contribute to confusion or other changes in mental status.

Dress, Grooming, and Hygiene   A client's ability to dress and perform personal hygiene is affected by physical and emotional well-being. It is often a cue to mental or physical self-care deficits.

Vital Signs   You should assess vital signs as a part of the general survey and with subsequent assessments. Analyze for trends. See Chapter 19 for a complete discussion of vital signs, if needed.

Height and Weight   Height and weight provide valuable information about your client's growth and development, nutritional status, overall general health, and risk for various diseases such as diabetes and heart disease (Fig. 21-1). These data are important for proper dosing of medication. When possible, the client should wear minimal clothing (gown) and no shoes. Because children have frequent changes in growth, their measurements are documented on growth charts for easy monitoring and comparison to age- and gender-related standards.

Body mass index (BMI) evaluates the relationship between height and weight. You can calculate the BMI for adults using a BMI calculator or table (see Procedure 21-1, step 10). **KEY POINT:** *Because the proportion of fat to muscle affects BMI calculation, the BMI is* **not** *useful for the following:*

- *Athletes (who have a larger proportion of muscle, which is denser than fat mass)*
- *Pregnant and lactating women (who have a larger blood and tissue volume)*
- *Growing children*
- *Frail and sedentary older adults*

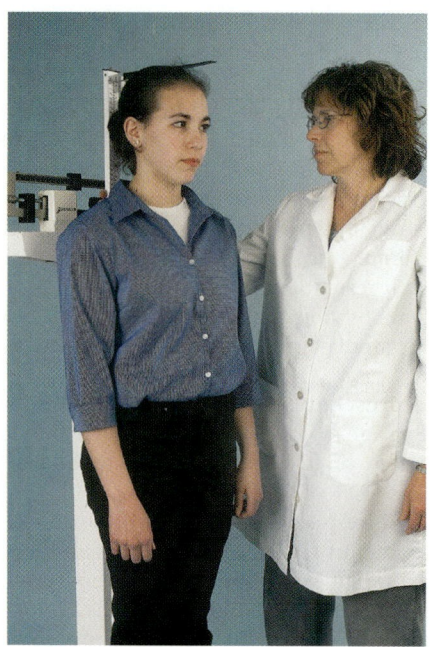

FIGURE 21-1 For adults, measure height with the client's back to the platform scale.

THE INTEGUMENTARY SYSTEM

The integumentary system consists of the skin, hair, and nails. In a comprehensive exam, you assess this system briefly in the general survey and then in greater detail as you move to examine other areas of the body. This allows the client to remain draped as long as possible. Also refer to Procedure 21-2.

The Skin

To perform a skin assessment, observe skin color, lesions, and other characteristics. Also notice unusual odors.

- An unpleasant body odor may be a sign of poor hygiene, the presence of a wound, or underlying disease.
- Excessive sweating may be related to activity (e.g., if the client has just finished exercising), thyroid problems, or overactive sweat glands.
- An odor of urine or stool may indicate a nursing diagnosis of Self-Care Deficit or Bowel or Urinary Incontinence.

Skin Color

Skin color variations commonly seen in neonates and infants include the following:

- **Mongolian spots** are benign, blue-black birthmarks that occur on the lower back and buttocks of African American, Hispanic, Native American, and Asian babies. They are due to pigmented cells in the deeper areas of skin. Most fade by age 2 but can persist until early adolescence.
- **Capillary hemangiomas,** sometimes known as "stork bites," are small, irregular pink-red areas that are often seen around the face and nape of the neck in newborns. They typically disappear in infancy, although they can persist until age 5.
- **Café-au-lait spots** are light brown birthmarks that can occur anywhere on the body. The name of these birthmarks is French for "coffee with milk" because of their light-brown color. Most often café-au-lait spots are not associated with medical problems, although they can sometimes signal a genetic disorder.

Table 21-2 discusses the significance of other skin color variations that may be seen in clients of any age.

Table 21-2 ➤ Common Skin Color Variations

Pallor	
In light-skinned clients: extreme paleness; skin appears white; loss of pink or yellow tones. In dark-skinned clients: a loss of red tones	May be related to poor circulation or a low hemoglobin level (anemia). Best sites to assess for pallor include the oral mucous membranes, conjunctiva, nailbeds, palms, and soles of feet.
Cyanosis	
A blue-gray coloration of the skin, often described as ashen	■ If seen in the lips, tongue, mucous membranes, and facial features, it is known as *central cyanosis* and is associated with hypoxia. **Acrocyanosis,** which is bluish discoloration of palms and soles in the first few hours to days of life, is normal in newborns. ■ Cold causes the lips to turn blue but the tongue is not affected. Cyanosis may also be seen in the extremities, especially hands and feet, after exposure to extreme cold.
Jaundice	
A yellow-orange cast to the skin	■ Often associated with liver disorders. ■ Best sites to assess for jaundice include the sclera, mucous membranes, hard palate of the mouth, palms, and soles of feet. ■ Jaundice in the newborn is a normal finding in the first few weeks of life unless there is blood incompatibility or a congenital disorder.
Flushing	
A widespread, diffuse area of redness	Generalized redness of the face and body may occur as a result of fever, excessive room temperature, sunburn, polycythemia (an abnormal increase in red blood cells), vigorous exercise, or certain skin conditions, such as rosacea.
Erythema	
A reddened area	Associated with rashes, skin infections, prolonged pressure on the skin, or application of heat or cold.
Ecchymosis	
Bruised (blue-green-yellow) area	■ May be seen anywhere on the body. ■ The color will vary based on the age of the injury. ■ May indicate physical abuse, internal bleeding, side effect to medication, or bleeding disorder. ■ Refer to Chapter 9 to review assessing for abuse.
Petechiae	
Tiny, pinpoint red or reddish-purple spots	■ Visible in the skin due to extravasation (leakage from vessels) of blood into the skin. ■ May be associated with a variety of disorders and medications.
Mottling	
Bluish marbling	■ Occurs in light-skinned clients, especially when cold. ■ In newborns mottling indicates overstimulation of the autonomic nervous system.

Skin Characteristics

As does color, the temperature, texture, and turgor of the skin offer clues to the client's health status. Although it is not technically a skin characteristic, you should also check for edema while you are assessing the skin.

Skin Temperature The skin should feel warm, but keep in mind that the temperature should be consistent with the room temperature and the patient's activity level.

Skin Moisture Excessive moisture may result from hyperthermia, thyroid hyperactivity, anxiety, or **hyperhidrosis** (excessive sweating). Dry skin may result from dehydration, chronic renal failure, hypothyroidism, excessive exposure, or overzealous hygiene.

Skin Texture The following factors affect skin texture:
■ *Exposure.* Exposed areas tend to be drier and coarser in texture, as do the elbows and knees.

- *Age.* The skin of infants and young children is very smooth because of lack of exposure to the environment.
- *Hyperthyroidism and other endocrine disorders.* These may cause the skin to become coarse, thick, and dry.
- *Impaired circulation.* Peripheral arterial insufficiency is associated with smooth, thin, shiny skin with little to no hair. In contrast, venous insufficiency leads to thick, rough skin that is often hyperpigmented.

Skin Turgor refers to the elasticity of the skin, which provides data about hydration status. **Edema,** which is an excessive amount of fluid in the tissues, is an abnormal finding. It is common in clients with congestive heart failure, kidney disease, peripheral vascular disease, or low albumin levels. A client with edema may tell you his skin feels "tight" or say, "My shoes don't fit anymore." Swollen tissue may feel tender to touch. Edema is not actually a condition of the skin, but it is convenient to assess for it while assessing the skin.

Skin Lesions

Any lesion, variation in pigment, or break in continuous tissue requires assessment.

Normal Lesions Lesions considered to be normal variations and not harmful include:

- *Milia.* White raised areas on the nose, chin, and forehead of newborns. These lesions, which resemble "whiteheads," are due to retention of sebum in the maturing sebaceous glands. They disappear during infancy.
- *Nevi (moles), freckles, birthmarks*
- *Skin tags.* Tiny tags or fleshy buds of skin usually around skin creases in middle-aged and older adults
- *Striae.* Silver-to-pink "stretch marks" in pregnant women, women who have had children, and anyone who has experienced significant weight fluctuations.

Abnormal Lesions Abnormal lesions are classified as primary or secondary.

- *Primary skin lesions* develop as a result of disease or irritation. The pustules of acne are an example.
- *Secondary skin lesions* develop from primary lesions as a result of continued illness, exposure, injury, or infection, such as the crusts that form from ruptured pustules.
- *Evaluate all skin lesions for the possibility of malignancy,* especially those located in a site exposed to chronic rubbing or other trauma. You can remember the warning signs of malignant lesions by thinking of the letters ABCDE (**A**symmetry, **B**order irregularity, **C**olor variation, **D**iameter greater than 0.5 cm, and **E**levation above skin surface).
- *To help you categorize and describe lesions,* see the table Describing Skin Lesions at the end of Procedure 21-2.

KnowledgeCheck 21-5

- What aspects of the skin should you assess?
- What assessments should you perform if you find a lesion?
- What warning signs lead you to suspect a malignant lesion?

The Hair

When assessing the hair, use inspection and palpation to obtain data about color, texture, distribution, and condition of the scalp. A client who does not properly groom her hair may need help with other self-care tasks.

- **Color.** There is a wide range of naturally occurring hair color. Age-related graying of the hair varies among individuals according to their genetic background.

- **Texture.** Normal hair texture varies from fine to coarse.
- **Distribution.** Generally, the hair is evenly distributed on the scalp, and fine body hair is present over the body. Alterations in hair distribution may be an indication of disease.
- **Alopecia.** Hair loss along the temples and in the center of the scalp is considered a normal balding pattern in men and is largely genetically based.
    - *Diffuse alopecia* can be caused by chemotherapy for the treatment of cancer, by nutritional deficiencies, or by endocrine disorders.
    - *Thinning hair* can also occur in the perimenopausal period when hormone levels are fluctuating.
    - *Patchy hair loss* may be the result of fungal infections of the scalp, hair pulling, constant wearing of caps, or **alopecia areata,** a benign autoimmune disorder.
- **Hirsutism.** Excess facial or trunk hair may be due to endocrine disorders or steroid use.
- **Scalp.** Normally the scalp is smooth, firm, symmetrical, nontender, and without lesions.
- **Pediculosis.** The hair should be free of **pediculosis** (head lice infestation). Head lice are tiny, very mobile, and difficult to see. You may find it easier to see the eggs, or **nits,** that are deposited on the hair shaft close to the scalp.

For a step-by-step description of assessing the hair, see Procedure 21-3.

The Nails

Variations in color, shape, or texture of the nails may indicate health problems. For illustrations of nail variations and a step-by-step description of nail assessment, see Procedure 21-4.

Nail Color Pink nails with rapid capillary refill indicate circulation to the extremities. Other color abnormalities that you may encounter include the following:

- *Half-and-half nails,* in which a distal band of reddish-pink covers 20% to 60% of the nail. These occur in clients with low albumin levels or renal disease.
- *Mees' lines,* which are transverse white lines in the nailbed. They are seen in clients who have experienced severe illnesses or nutritional deficiencies.
- *Splinter hemorrhages,* small hemorrhages under the nailbed, are associated with bacterial endocarditis or trauma.

Nail Shape A change in nail shape may indicate underlying disease. Clubbing, in which the nail plate angle is 180° or more, is associated with long-term hypoxic states, such as occurs with chronic lung disease.

Nail Texture Nails and surrounding epidermis are normally smooth. Chronic nail-picking results in callus formation around the nail. Occasionally, the surrounding skin becomes inflamed. This condition, known as paronychia, is painful and may require drainage if infection is present.

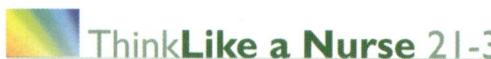

ThinkLike a Nurse 21-3

You are caring for a woman who has no hair on her head. How might you determine the cause of her hair loss? What other assessments should you perform?

THE HEAD

Assessment of the head is often referred to by the acronym HEENT: **H**ead, **E**yes, **E**ars, **N**ose, and **T**hroat. You will use all the assessment techniques—inspection, palpation, percussion, and auscultation—in the HEENT exam.

The Skull and Face

Taking individual variation into account, on inspection the skull should be rounded and the face symmetrical in appearance and movement. Head size is familial.

- A large head in an adolescent or adult may be associated with **acromegaly,** a disorder associated with excess growth hormone.
- **Microcephaly,** an abnormally small head size, is seen in clients with certain types of mental disorders.
- Asymmetry may be the result of trauma, surgery, neuromuscular disorder, paralysis, or congenital deformity.
- In infants and children, a head that is growing disproportionally faster than the body may be a sign of **hydrocephalus** (an accumulation of excessive cerebrospinal fluid).
- Facial appearance that is inconsistent with gender, age, or racial/ethnic group may indicate an inherited or chronic disorder, such as Graves' disease, hypothyroidism with myxedema, or Cushing's syndrome.

To learn how to assess the skull and face and to view some facial abnormalities, see Procedure 21-5.

The Eyes

In examining the eyes, you will inspect and palpate the external eye structures, assess vision, and examine the internal eye structures. For step-by-step instructions, see Procedure 21-6. For convenience, you may wish to perform some cranial nerve testing along with the eye exam (e.g., corneal reflex, pupillary reaction, accommodation, and extraocular movements). For instructions on performing a cranial nerve examination, see Procedure 21-16.

Visual Acuity

Visual acuity is a measure of the eye's ability to detect the details of an image. When testing visual acuity, you will assess distant, near, peripheral, and color vision, usually with a Snellen chart. Nurses commonly perform screening tests of visual acuity. Other testing is performed by nurses in advanced or specialty practice or by an optometrist or ophthalmologist as needed. To test visual acuity, see Procedure 21-6.

Distance Vision **Normal vision** is clear vision at 20 feet (20/20) in the right eye, left eye, and both eyes. **Myopia,** or diminished distant vision, is associated with a smaller fraction. For example, 20/100 vision means that to see text a person with normal vision can read at 100 feet, the client has to stand just 20 feet from the Snellen chart

Near Vision A client with normal near vision will be able to read the newsprint from a distance of 35.5 cm (14 in.) without hesitation with either eye and with both eyes.

Color Vision **Color vision** is the ability to detect color. Color blindness may be genetically inherited (usually seen in males), or it may result from macular degeneration or other diseases that affect the cones of the eye. Use the color bars at the base of the Snellen chart to test color vision. **Ishihara cards** are specialized cards that enable thorough testing for color blindness. They contain embedded figures within a field of color (see Procedure 21-6).

Visual Field Visual field is the area the eye is able to observe. It is related to peripheral vision and extraocular muscle (EOM) function. Visual field abnormalities may be caused by problems with cranial nerves III, IV, and VI or with the retina. Poorly controlled diabetes, cataracts, macular degeneration,

and advanced glaucoma are other disorders that limit the visual field.

- **Peripheral vision** describes the boundaries of the visual field while the eye is in a fixed position. The common phrase "I see you out of the corner of my eye" refers to peripheral vision.
- **The EOMs** control the movement of the eye and eyelids and allow you to track movement. Three cranial nerves (CN) innervate the EOM. They are CN III (oculomotor), CN IV (trochlear), and CN VI (abducens). CN III also works together with CN II (optic) to control the pupillary reaction to light. Figure 21-2 illustrates the eye positions affected by the EOM and the corresponding cranial nerves.

External Structures of the Eye

To review the structure of the external eye, see Figure 21-3. There should be no pallor, dryness, or edema.

Eyelids and Lashes The following are common abnormal findings on the eyelids and lashes:

- A **pterygium** is a growth or thickening of conjunctiva from the inner canthus toward the iris.
- **Ectropion,** an everted eyelid, is commonly seen in older adults secondary to loss of skin tone. It can lead to excessive dryness of the eyes.
- **Entropion,** an inverted eyelid, can lead to corneal damage.
- **Ptosis,** or drooping of the lid, may be seen in clients who have experienced a stroke (cerebrovascular accident [CVA]) or Bell's palsy (paralysis of the facial nerve, see Procedure 21-5). For ptosis and other eye abnormalities, refer to Procedure 21-6.

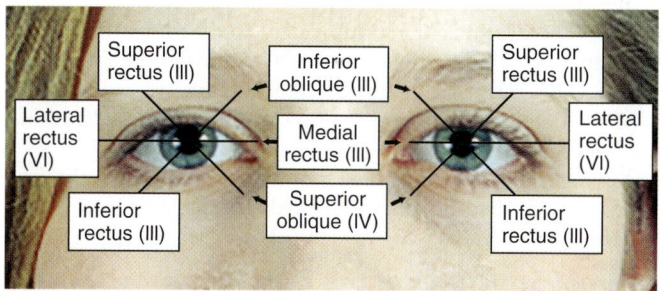

FIGURE 21-2 Cranial nerves and the extraocular muscles.

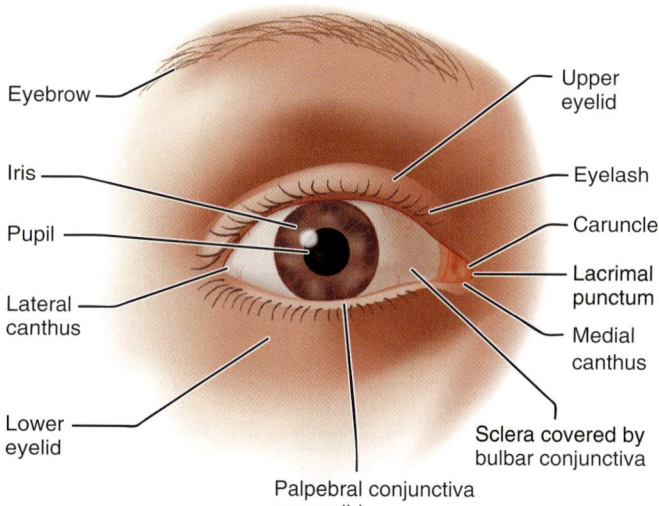

FIGURE 21-3 The external eye and eyelid.

Sclera and Conjunctiva Associated disorders may include infection, allergies, injuries, and liver disorders. For example, yellow (**icteric**) sclera may be seen with an elevated bilirubin. Blood visible in the sclera is known as a **subconjunctival hemorrhage** and may be related to trauma or hypertension.

Lens and Cornea The lens and the **cornea** or outermost layer of the eyeball, are transparent, smooth, and moist. Roughness or irregularity of the cornea is seen with trauma or a corneal abrasion.

Pupils The **pupils** should be uniform in color, equal in size, and round. They should **accommodate** equally, that is, the pupils constrict and the eyes converge (cross) as a person attempts to focus on an object moving toward him. This is typically charted as PERRLA: **P**upils **E**qual, **R**ound, **R**eactive to **L**ight and **A**ccommodation. The following are common pupillary abnormalities:

- Sluggish accommodation may be caused by anticholinergic drugs or advanced age.
- Failure of one or both pupils to accommodate may reflect a cranial nerve III problem or **exophthalmos** (associated with hyperthyroidism).
- Congenital cataracts, although rare, may be seen in infants and are checked during an eye exam using the "red reflex." Congenital cataracts cause "lazy eye" or amblyopi and can lead to other eye problems such as nystagmus, strabismus and inability to fix a gaze upon objects.

  - Cloudy pupils, a finding related to cataracts, are commonly seen in older adults.

- **Mydriasis** (enlarged pupils) may be seen with glaucoma, an increase in intraocular pressure.
- Many medications affect pupil size. Medications called **mydriatics** are used to dilate the pupil to allow better visualization of the internal eye during examination.
- **Miosis** (constricted pupils) often results from medications to treat glaucoma.
- **Anisocoria** (unequal pupils) may be seen with central nervous system disorders. In some individuals, anisocoria may be normal.

Internal Structures of the Eye

Use an ophthalmoscope to visualize the internal structures of the eye (the optic disc, physiological cup, retinal vessels, retinal background, and macula). This is an advanced assessment technique; however, advanced practice nurses and registered nurses (RNs) on specialty units do perform it with training. This technique provides information about certain diseases that affect the eye, such as hypertension and diabetes.

KnowledgeCheck 21-6

- What are the major components of an eye assessment?
- Identify the cranial nerves involved with eye movement and function.

The Ears and Hearing

The ears are involved in both hearing and equilibrium.

- The **external ear** collects and conveys sound waves to the middle ear. It protects the middle ear from environmental factors such as humidity and temperature and prevents entry of foreign matter.
- The **middle ear** contains the tympanic membrane and cavity, the eustachian tube, and the **ossicles** (the small bones of the middle ear: the malleus, incus, and stapes). The middle ear conducts sound waves to the inner ear.
- The **inner ear** is responsible for hearing and equilibrium. Figure 21-4 illustrates the structures of the ear.

For procedure steps and guidelines for using the otoscope and tuning fork to examine the ears, see Procedure 21-7. As with the eyes, nurses are usually responsible only for screening and making referrals. However, in some settings nurses perform advanced assessments.

Examining the External and Middle Ear

- **On inspection,** the ears should be of equal size and similar appearance. Normally the pinna is level with the corner of the eye and within a 10° angle of vertical position (shown in Procedure 21-7).
- **On palpation,** the external structure of the ear is smooth, nontender, pliable, and without nodules. A painful auricle or tragus may be associated with **otitis externa** (an outer ear infection), whereas tenderness behind the ear is seen with **otitis media** (a middle ear infection).

Otoscopic Examination As you begin the otoscopic examination, you may notice that the external auditory canal contains **cerumen** (wax), which protects the middle ear from

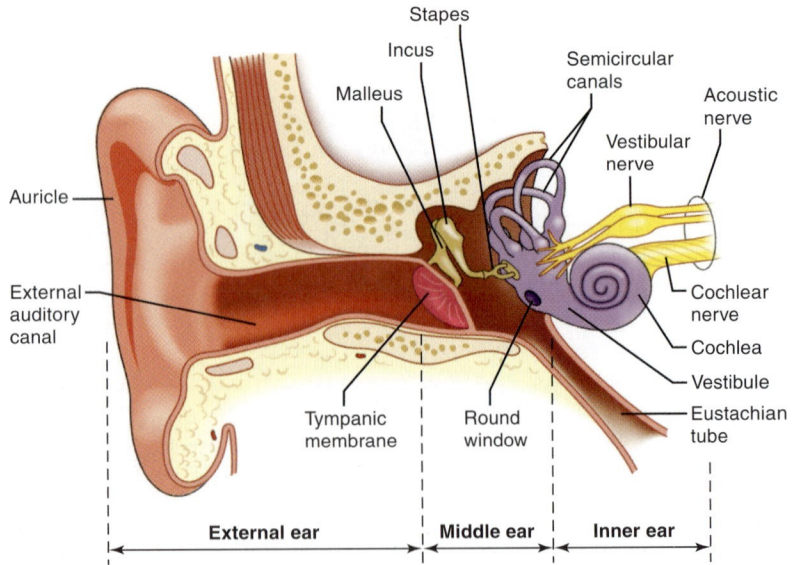

FIGURE 21-4 Cross section of the ear.

excessive drying. However, it should not completely obstruct the ear canal. Cerumen may be black, dark red, yellowish, or brown in color and waxy, flaky, soft, or hard, with no odor; all are normal variations. Be careful as you manipulate the otoscope, because the inner two-thirds of the canal can be tender from the pressure and manipulation of the otoscope head.

Normally the **tympanic membrane (TM)** is pearly gray, shiny, and translucent. Changes in its appearance arise from abnormalities such as otitis media (which causes a red, bulging TM) and the presence of pressure equalization tubes in young clients with chronic ear infections.

Assessing Hearing

To assess hearing, you will need a quiet room and a tuning fork. Gross hearing ability includes the ability to hear both high- and low-pitched tones. See Procedure 21-7.

The Weber and Rinne Tests Hearing involves transmission of sound vibrations and generation of nerve impulses along CN VIII.

- The **Weber test** assesses both aspects. When you place a vibrating tuning fork on the center of the client's head, he should be able to sense the vibration equally in both ears. Record a positive Weber test if the vibration is louder in one ear. If the Weber test is positive, you will need to perform the Rinne test to assess the type of hearing problem.
- The **Rinne test** also uses a tuning fork to compare air conduction (AC) and bone conduction (BC). Normally AC is twice as long as BC. For step-by-step instructions for performing the Weber, Rinne, and Romberg tests, see Procedure 21-7.

The Romberg Test Along with the cerebellum and midbrain, *vestibular cells* in the ear are responsible for maintaining equilibrium. To assess equilibrium, perform the Romberg test. You may prefer to perform the Romberg test with examination of the neurological system instead of with the ears

KnowledgeCheck 21-7

Your client has a negative Weber test. What further testing is required?

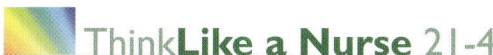

ThinkLike a Nurse 21-4

What type of symptoms would you expect a client to be experiencing if he had a positive Romberg test?

The Nose

The nose and sinuses are the organs of smell and are a part of the respiratory system. Vaporized molecules sniffed into the upper nasal cavities trigger receptors that generate impulses along the olfactory nerve (CN I) that travel to olfactory centers in the temporal lobes. To identify the paranasal sinuses and for a procedure for assessing the nose and sinuses, see Procedure 21-8.

The Mouth and Oropharynx

The structures of the mouth include the lips, tongue, teeth, **gingiva** (gums), uvula, hard and soft palate, and salivary glands and ducts. For an illustration of structures of the mouth and for instructions on examining the mouth and oropharynx, see Procedure 21-9.

- **The Lips, Buccal Mucosa, and Gingiva.** The lips, buccal mucosa (mucous membrane of the cheeks), and gums should be smooth, moist, and pink in color. Increased pigmentation

(e.g., bluish or dark patches) occurs in dark-skinned clients. When inspecting the mouth, be sure to ask your client about use of tobacco, either smoked or chewed. Both forms are associated with increased risk for oral cancer.

- **The Teeth.** Tooth decay and periodontal (gum) disease are common. Poor oral hygiene is a major contributing factor for both. As you examine the mouth and teeth, talk to the patient about his oral care. Recommend toothbrushing after each meal, daily flossing, and dental checkups every 6 months. See Chapter 24 for a more complete discussion of oral hygiene and prevention of periodontal disease.
- **The Tongue and Oropharynx.** When inspecting the mouth, carefully examine the oropharynx and all aspects of the tongue: dorsal, ventral, and lateral. Procedure 21-9 for illustrations of abnormalities.

THE NECK

The neck has components of the musculoskeletal, neurological, vascular, respiratory, endocrine, and lymphatic systems. The sternocleidomastoid and trapezius muscles form the landmarks of the neck, known as the **anterior and posterior triangles.** The symmetrical neck muscles center and coordinate movement of the head.

The trachea, thyroid gland, anterior cervical nodes, and carotid arteries are positioned in the anterior triangle; the posterior cervical nodes are in the posterior triangle. You will palpate the tracheal rings and the cricoid and thyroid cartilage in the midline of the anterior neck. To see instructions for assessing the neck and illustrations of structures of the neck consult Procedure 21-10.

The Cervical Lymph Nodes The cervical lymph nodes occur in three chains (see Procedure 21-10, step 2). The lymph nodes are generally not palpable, although occasionally they can be felt, especially in young children. Normal nodes are small in size (less than 1 cm), mobile, soft, and nontender.

The Thyroid Gland Normally the thyroid is smooth, firm, nontender, and often nonpalpable. However, thyroid abnormalities are common. An enlarged thyroid may be associated with either hypothyroidism or hyperthyroidism. Thyroid masses may be malignant but are usually benign.

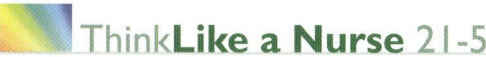

ThinkLike a Nurse 21-5

A client complains of sore throat, fever, chills, and runny nose. What assessments should you perform?

THE BREASTS AND AXILLAE

The breasts consist of glandular, adipose, and connective tissue; smooth muscle; and nerves. The functions of the female breast are sexual stimulation and milk production for nourishing offspring. Breast size and shape vary among women, and commonly one breast is slightly larger than the other. At puberty, the ovaries produce estrogen and progesterone, which stimulate the breasts to develop. The menstrual cycle, pregnancy, and breastfeeding also enlarge breast tissue. Although breasts are thought of as female organs, men also have breasts. However, because of limited estrogen and progesterone levels, normal male breasts develop only minimally.

Breast tissue and lymph drainage for the breast extend up into the axilla. The majority of breast tumors are found in the tail of Spence, in the axilla. A breast exam, therefore, always includes an exam of the axillae. Many women have breast reconstruction, either after breast removal due to cancer or breast augmentation for cosmetic reasons. These women should not omit breast examination, and it is performed in exactly the same way as for natural breasts.

Clinical Breast Exam You should perform a breast exam for the woman if she cannot do it herself and demonstrate the procedure as part of client teaching for self-care. Clinical breast exams are not recommended for average-risk women at any age (American Cancer Society, n.d.b, last revised 2015).

Breast Self-Exam KEY POINT: *Researchers agree that patients who perform a breast self-exam (BSE) should be trained in proper technique in order to avoid falsely negative findings (American Congress of Obstetricians and Gynecologists, 2012, reaffirmed 2014; Smith, Cokkinides, Brooks, et al., 2011; Smith, Duffy, & Tabár, 2012).* For a step-by-step guide to examining the breasts and axillae, see Procedure 21-11.

Mammography and Thermography The American Cancer Society (n.d.b, last revised 2015) recommends that women with average risk of breast cancer undergo regular screening mammography or breast thermography starting at age 45 years. Women aged 45 to 54 years should be screened; women 55 years and older should transition to bi-ennial screening or have the opportunity to continue screening annually. Women should have the opportunity to begin annual screening between the ages of 40 and 44 years if history warrants and should continue as long as a woman is in good health and is expected to live 10 more years or longer (Oeffinger, Fontham, Etzioni, et al., 2015).

 Think**Like a Nurse** 21-6

What strategies might encourage more women to regularly perform breast self-examination?

THE CHEST AND LUNGS

The chest, or thorax, is the bony cage that protects the heart, lungs, and great vessels. The ribs, sternum, and vertebrae form the chest. **KEY POINT:** *Be systematic in your assessment: Always assess the areas of the chest and lungs in the same order.* To learn how to assess the chest and lungs, see Procedure 21-12.

Chest Landmarks

Before beginning the thoracic exam, review the following important landmarks that will help you visualize the underlying structures and perform an accurate assessment:

- *Anterior chest*—Identify positions vertically on the anterior chest in relation to the ribs. For example, the space between the 5th and 6th ribs is known as the 5th intercostal space (5th ICS). You can easily palpate the ribs and count the spaces if you remember that the 1st rib is tucked up next to the clavicle (Fig. 21-5A).

    Use a series of imaginary vertical lines (Fig. 21-5B) to further aid in identifying locations on the anterior chest. For instance, the apex of the heart is usually located in the 5th intercostal space at left midclavicular line (5th ICS MCL).
- *Posterior Chest*—Identify positions vertically in relation to the vertebra (Fig. 21-6B). The prominent vertebra at the base of the neck is the 7th cervical vertebra (C7). The next one down is T1 (1st thoracic). Counting down to about T9 should be adequate.
- *Lateral and Posterior Chest*—Use imaginary lines on the lateral and posterior chest as well. Figure 21-6, parts A and C, illustrates the location of these lines. Notice that the anterior

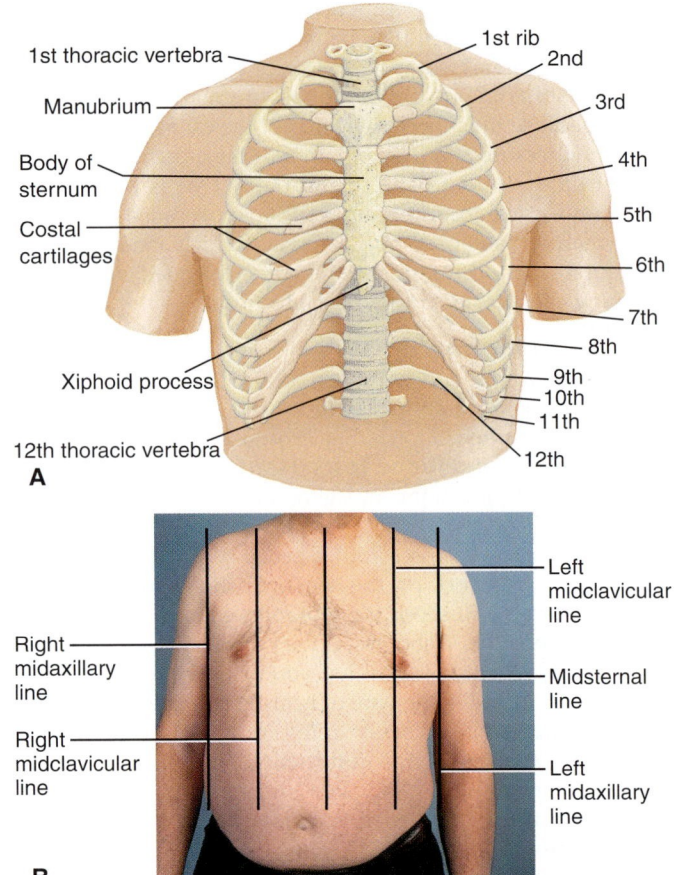

FIGURE 21-5 (A) The anterior thoracic cage and the bony landmarks. (B) A series of imaginary vertical lines is used to describe locations on the chest.

axillary line can be used to locate sounds on both the anterior and lateral chest.

Chest Shape and Size

The chest diameter expands up to 3 in. (7.6 cm) with deep inspiration. The anteroposterior diameter of the chest is half the size of the lateral diameter (written as AP:Lateral = 1:2).

 Musculoskeletal changes associated with aging result in a gradual increase in the anteroposterior diameter. This change is also seen, regardless of age, in clients who have chronic obstructive pulmonary disease (COPD), a disorder associated with long-term smoking. Figure 21-7 illustrates normal and "barrel" chest shapes.

Osteoporosis, a common disorder accompanying aging, is associated with increased porosity of the vertebrae. As a result, vertebrae may compress or collapse, shortening the length of the spine and pushing the ribs forward and downward.

Breath Sounds

Listen to breath sounds in a quiet room by auscultating one full respiratory cycle at each site. Directly apply the stethoscope to the client's skin. Compare breath sounds bilaterally. See Figure 21-8.

- **Normal Sounds.** Three types of normal breath sounds are heard: bronchial, bronchovesicular, and vesicular. To find a description of normal lung sounds, see the table Normal Lung Sounds at the end of Procedure 21-12.

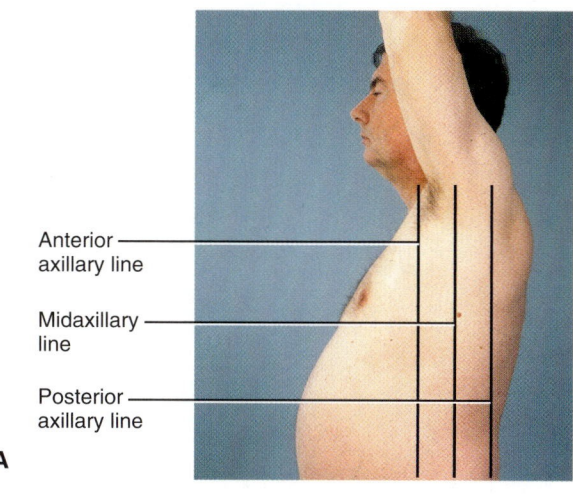

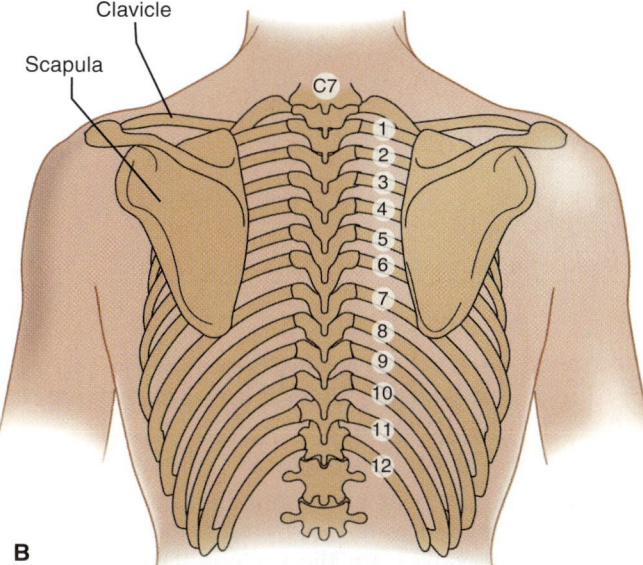

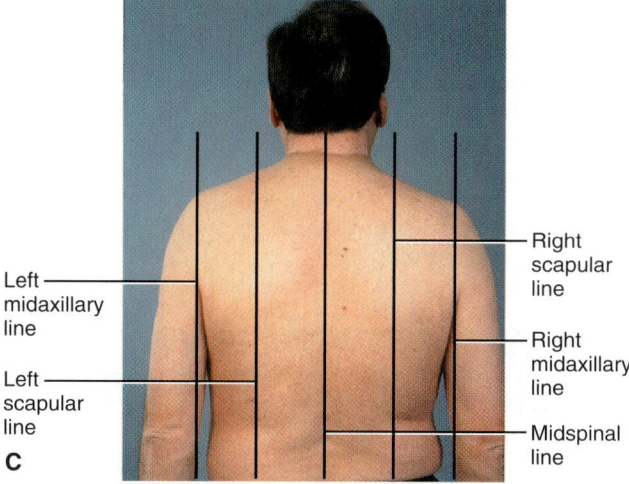

FIGURE 21-6 (A) Lateral chest landmarks. (B) The vertebrae are the landmarks on the posterior chest. (C) Landmark lines on the posterior chest.

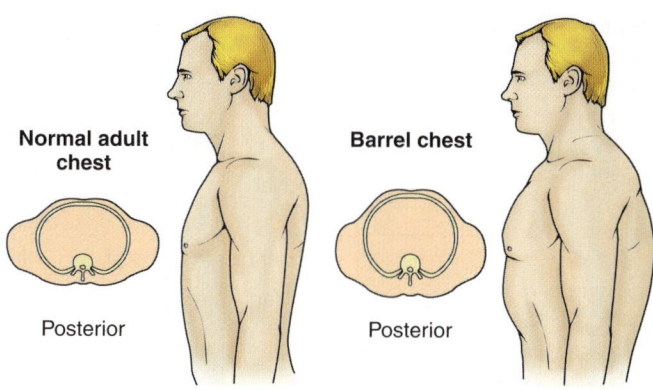

FIGURE 21-7 The normal anteroposterior to lateral ratio is 1:2. The lateral aspect of the chest increases dramatically with COPD, leading to a barrel chest appearance.

- **Abnormal Sounds.** Breath sounds that differ from those three are abnormal. To find a description of abnormal breath sounds refer to the table Abnormal Lung Sounds at the end of Procedure 21-12.

KnowledgeCheck 21-8

- List and describe the location of the horizontal and vertical landmarks of the anterior chest.
- List and describe the location of the horizontal and vertical landmarks of the posterior chest.
- List and describe the location of the vertical landmarks of the lateral chest.

THE CARDIOVASCULAR SYSTEM

The cardiovascular system consists of the heart and the blood vessels. The heart is a muscle that pumps blood throughout the body. In a healthy adult, it is about the size of a clenched fist. The blood vessels, which make up the vascular system, have two main networks: the pulmonary circulation and the systemic circulation. See Chapter 38 if you need to review the anatomy of the cardiovascular system.

- **Pulmonary circulation.** Oxygen-depleted blood circulates from the heart into the lungs, where it is oxygenated, then back to the heart. This system is known as the **pulmonary circulation.**
- **Systemic circulation.** The left ventricle pumps blood from the heart into the **systemic circulation** via the arterial system.
- **Capillaries.** The arteries subdivide many times, becoming smaller and smaller until they separate in the tissues and organs into **capillaries.** It is at the capillary level that oxygen is delivered to the tissues.
- **The venous system** collects the oxygen-depleted blood and returns it to the right atrium of the heart to begin the circuit again.
- **Coronary circulation,** which circulates blood through the heart itself, is a part of the systemic circulation.

For further discussion on pulmonary circulation and oxygenation, see Chapter 37. For a complete step-by-step procedure for assessing the heart and vascular system, refer to Procedure 21-13.

The Heart

The heart is positioned at an angle on the left side of the chest in the 3rd, 4th, and 5th intercostal spaces (ICS). To facilitate auscultation of specific heart sounds, perform the cardiac

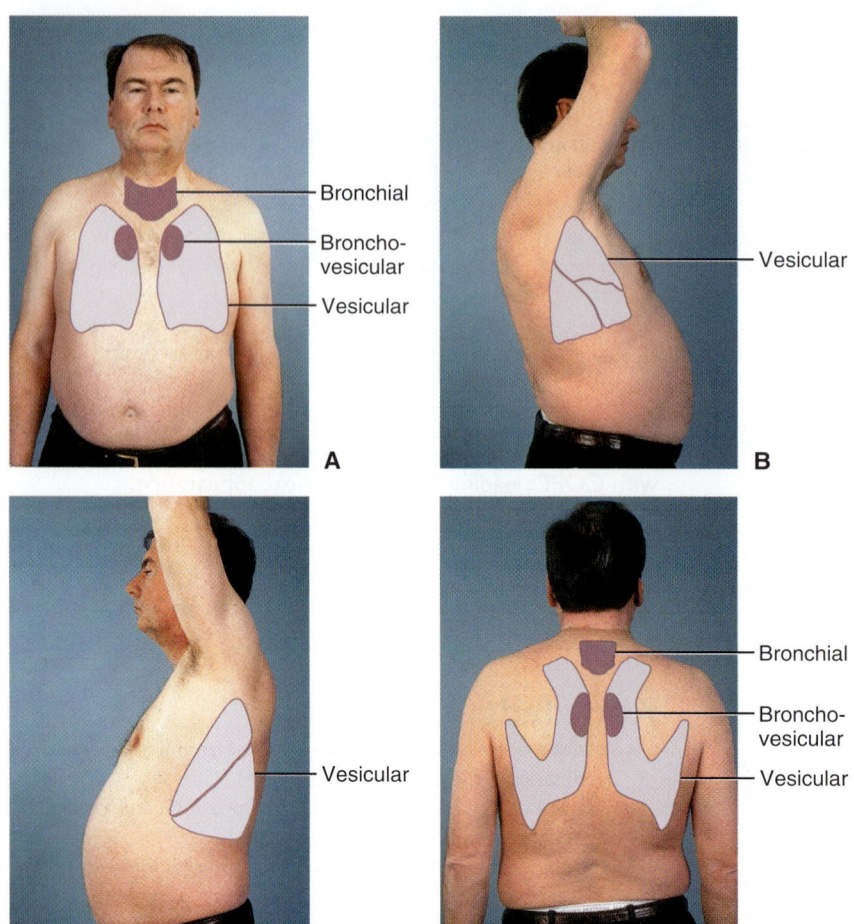

Bronchial
Broncho-
vesicular
Vesicular

A

Vesicular

B

Vesicular

C

Bronchial
Broncho-
vesicular
Vesicular

D

FIGURE 21-8 Normal breath sounds. (A) Anterior. (B) Right lateral. (C) Left lateral. (D) Posterior.

assessment with the client in three positions: sitting, supine, and left lateral recumbent. ✚ Clients with chronic heart or lung problems may have little cardiac reserve, so minimize position changes to conserve your client's energy.

♥ **iCare** To help minimize your client's anxiety, explain that it always takes time to examine the heart and circulatory system.

The Cardiac Cycle

During a cardiac cycle, the atria and ventricles alternately contract and relax to fill and empty; while the atria are contracting (emptying), the ventricles are relaxing (filling) and vice versa. **Systole** refers to the contraction, or emptying, of the ventricles. **Diastole** refers to the relaxation, or filling, phase of the ventricles.

Inspecting and Palpating the Heart

Begin your assessment of the heart with the client sitting. Observe the **precordium**, the area of the chest over the heart, for visible pulsations. A small pulsation at the 5th ICS midclavicular line, also known as the **point of maximal impulse (PMI)**, is normal.

Also palpate for vibrations. A **thrill** is a vibration or pulsation palpated in any area except the PMI. A thrill is associated with abnormal blood flow and usually has an accompanying **murmur** (additional heart sound).

Auscultating the Heart

Auscultate to establish cardiac rate and rhythm and to identify normal and abnormal heart sounds. A quiet room is

essential. You can hear heart sounds from any location on the anterior chest wall. However, the four sites located over the heart valves are the preferred listening areas. Table 21-3 describes these locations; they are also shown in Procedure 21-13, step 8.

Auscultate in an orderly fashion. Start at the aortic area and move gradually through each landmark. The following is a mnemonic you may use to recall the order of the heart sound landmarks:

*A*unt	Aortic
*P*olly	Pulmonic
*T*akes	Tricuspid
*M*eds	Mitral

Table 21-3 ➤ Locations for Assessing the Heart

STRUCTURE TITLE	VALVE ASSESSED	LOCATION
Base Right	Aortic valve	2nd ICS right sternal border
Base Left	Pulmonic valve	2nd ICS left sternal border
Left Lateral	Tricuspid valve	4th ICS left sternal border
Apex	Mitral valve	5th ICS MCL

Listen carefully at each site to each component of the heart sounds. You will find information about abnormal heart sounds in step 8 of Procedure 21-13.

First Heart Sound S_1 (or "lub") results from the closure of the valves between the atria and ventricles. "Lub" is a dull, low-pitched sound, louder over the mitral and tricuspid areas. S_1 marks the beginning of systole.

Second Heart Sound S_2 (or "dub") corresponds to closure of the semilunar valves (between the ventricles and the great arteries exiting the heart). "Dub" is higher in pitch and shorter than the S_1 "lub." The S_2 is loudest at the aortic and pulmonic areas. S_2 marks the beginning of diastole. Normally the mitral and tricuspid valves and the aortic and pulmonic valves close within a fraction of a second from each other. This near-simultaneous closure results in a singular S_1 and S_2 sound. However, a split sound may occur, at either S_1 or S_2, if there is a delay in closure of one of the valves.

Third Heart Sound A third heart sound (S_3), heard immediately after S_2, has a gallop cadence that follows the rhythm of the word "KenTUCKy." It is best heard at the apical site with the client lying on his left side.

Fourth Heart Sound A fourth heart sound (S_4), heard immediately before S_1, has a rhythm that follows the word "FLOrida." S_4 is best heard at the apical site, using the bell of the stethoscope, with the client lying on his left side.

Murmurs Murmurs are additional sounds produced by turbulent flow through the heart. Some murmurs are "innocent," but others represent pathology such as alteration in valve structure. Identifying and classifying a murmur are advanced skills that require practice. To learn more about assessing murmurs, see Procedure 21-13.

ThinkLike a Nurse 21-7

What findings would you anticipate when assessing Mr. Nguyen's (Meet Your Patient) thorax?

THE VASCULAR SYSTEM

The vascular system is a network of arteries and veins that transport oxygen, carbon dioxide, and nutrients to the cells of the body.

- **Arteries carry blood away from the heart.**
  - *The pulmonary arteries* carry oxygen-depleted blood from the right ventricle to the lungs.
  - *The systemic arteries* carry oxygenated blood from the left ventricle to the body periphery.
- **Veins carry blood toward the heart.**
  - The *pulmonary veins* transport oxygenated blood from the lungs to the left atrium.
  - The *systemic veins* return oxygen-depleted blood from the periphery to the right atrium of the heart.

The Central Vessels

The carotid arteries and internal jugular veins run alongside the sternocleidomastoid muscle on both sides of the neck (see Procedure 21-13 for illustrations). These central vessels provide circulation to the brain.

The Carotid Arteries Because the carotid arteries are large and close to the heart, you can easily feel a pulse over the carotid artery even when it is difficult to palpate a peripheral pulse.

- Never palpate both carotid arteries at the same time because bilateral pressure may impair cerebral blood flow.

- As a general rule, avoid palpating the carotids except during cardiopulmonary resuscitation or when it is necessary to assess them for a specific reason (such as in a comprehensive physical exam or when an underlying pathology makes it necessary to establish that circulation to the head is adequate).

- Turbulent blood flow through the carotid artery produces a whooshing sound known as a **bruit,** which you can auscultate using a stethoscope. Bruits are common among older adults.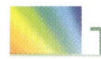

The Jugular Veins return blood from the brain to the superior vena cava. The *external jugular veins* are superficial; the internal *jugular veins* are deep. Normally the jugular veins are flat when the client is in an upright position and distend when the client lies flat. Jugular venous distention (JVD) is seen when the right side of the heart is congested because of inadequate pump function. The best position for assessment of JVD is semi-Fowler's (30° to 45° angle).

The Peripheral Vessels

The peripheral vessels supply blood to all the body cells. The **arteries** are a high-pressure system with several palpable pulse sites. The **veins** are a low-pressure system with valves to prevent backflow due to gravity. The veins return blood to the heart via the continuing pressure from the arterial system and pumping action of the adjacent skeletal muscles.

You will assess the peripheral vascular system by:
- *Measuring the blood pressure* (see Chapter 19). Usually you will measure the blood pressure at the start of the exam as part of the general survey.
- *Palpating the peripheral pulses* (see Chapter 19). In a healthy individual, pulses will be regular, strong, and equal bilaterally. Weak, absent, or asymmetrical pulses may indicate partial or complete occlusion of the artery. Other signs of arterial occlusion include pain, pallor, cool temperature, paresthesia, or paralysis.
- *Inspecting and performing tests for adequate perfusion.* The data you obtain when inspecting and palpating the integumentary system provide some information about peripheral tissue perfusion. Recall that when an area is not adequately oxygenated, the skin may be pale, cyanotic, cool, and shiny; hair growth may be sparse; and there may be clubbing of the nails. Inadequate tissue oxygenation may be a result of chronic pulmonary problems; however, it can also result from impaired central or peripheral circulation.

Refer to Procedure 21-13 for assessment of the peripheral vessels.

KnowledgeCheck 21-9

Identify the precautions to take when evaluating the carotid arteries.

THE ABDOMEN

The method most commonly used to identify the location of assessment findings is the four-quadrant method, which divides the abdomen into four sections by "drawing" a line vertically from the xiphoid process to the symphysis pubis and a horizontal line at the level of the umbilicus (see Procedure 21-14, step 4).

- To promote comfort during the assessment, ask the client to empty his bladder before the examination.

■ **KEY POINT:** *When examining the abdomen, inspect and auscultate first, before percussing and palpating. Percussion and palpation stimulate the bowel and may alter bowel sounds; therefore, the examination sequence differs from other body systems.*

■ If the client has a painful area, examine that area last to minimize discomfort during the rest of the exam.

Inspecting the Abdomen The skin over the abdomen is usually paler than that over other parts of the body. In clients with abdominal distention, the skin will appear taut. Distention may be normal, as with pregnancy, or it may be due to gas or fluid retention or to bowel obstruction. See Figure 21-9 for normal variations in abdominal shape.

Auscultating the Abdomen Proceed in an organized manner, listening in several areas in all four quadrants (Procedure 24-14, step 4c). Use the same pattern for every examination so that it becomes a habit.

■ **First, Auscultate Bowel Sounds.** Bowel sounds are high-pitched, irregular gurgles or clicks lasting one to several seconds and occurring every 5 to 15 seconds (or 5 to 30 times per min) in the average adult. Abnormal bowel sounds are described in Procedure 21-14.

■ **Next, Auscultate the Major Arteries.** Major arterial vessels lie in the abdomen below the intestines. Listen over the aorta and the renal iliac and femoral arteries for the presence of bruits.

Percussing the Abdomen Use indirect percussion to assess for fluid, air, organs, or masses. Some practitioners include percussion of the kidney with the abdominal examination.

Palpating the Abdomen Begin with light palpation to put the patient at ease. Palpate for tenderness and guarding in all four quadrants (see Procedure 21-14). Palpation of the liver and spleen is an advanced technique not usually performed by staff nurses, except perhaps in some specialty areas.

KnowledgeCheck 21-10

■ What strategies can you use to make the client more comfortable during an abdominal assessment?
■ Identify the sequence of assessment for the abdominal exam.

THE MUSCULOSKELETAL SYSTEM

The musculoskeletal system consists of bones, muscles, and joints. Bone is complex living tissue that responds to nutrition, stress, and illness.

■ **The bones** include:
  Long bones, such as the humerus and tibia
  Flat bones, such as the sternum and ribs
  Irregular bones, such as the vertebrae and pelvis

■ **Tendons, ligaments, and cartilage** serve as connecting structures.
■ **Bursae,** small disc-shaped, fluid-filled sacs, act as cushions to reduce friction between the joint and the tendons that cross over the joint (Fig. 21-10).

The musculoskeletal system provides shape and support to the body, allows movement, protects internal organs, produces red blood cells in the bone marrow, and stores calcium and phosphorus. Assessment of the musculoskeletal system includes evaluation of the client's posture, gait, bone structure, muscle function, and joint mobility. See Procedure 21-15.

Body Shape and Symmetry

To assess bone structure, examine body shape and symmetry. Major deformities in bone structure affect posture and gait. The client should be able to stand upright with the neck and head midline. There are four normal curvatures of the spine (see Procedure 21-15). The cervical and lumbar curves are concave, and the thoracic and sacral are convex.

Commonly seen abnormalities include:
■ **Kyphosis**—accentuated thoracic curve
■ **Scoliosis**—lateral S deviation of the spine
■ **Lordosis**—accentuated lumbar curve

Balance, Coordination, and Movement

Walking is a complex task involving balance, coordination, and movement. Pay attention to the *base of support* and *stride* as the client walks. If the client has an altered gait, try to identify the specific portion of the gait that is abnormal. If you need additional information on gait, see Chapter 33 and the illustrations in Procedure 21-15. Tests for *balance, movement,* and *coordination* are also explained in Procedure 21-15.

♥ **iCare**   As you perform each assessment, pay attention to the client's stability and level of comfort. Do not attempt movements that may produce pain or cause the client to fall. For example, recall that Mr. Nguyen (Meet Your Patient) has bilateral knee pain. Before asking him to perform deep knee bends or hop in place, you would want to assess his pain and its triggers.

Joint Mobility and Muscle Function

Any joint deformity requires investigation. Color changes in a joint indicate inflammation or infection. If you see erythema or swelling, investigate further by feeling for warmth. Determine any effect the deformity has on function. To assess function, test range of motion (ROM) and muscle strength.

■ **Active ROM** requires the client to move the joint through its full ROM.
■ **Passive ROM** is used when the client is unable to exercise each joint independently. Instead, you support the body and move each joint through its ROM.

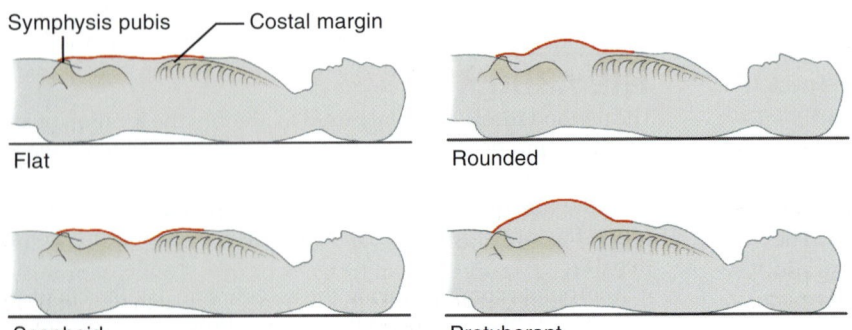

FIGURE 21-9 Normal variations in abdominal contour.

Flat   Rounded

Scaphoid   Protuberant

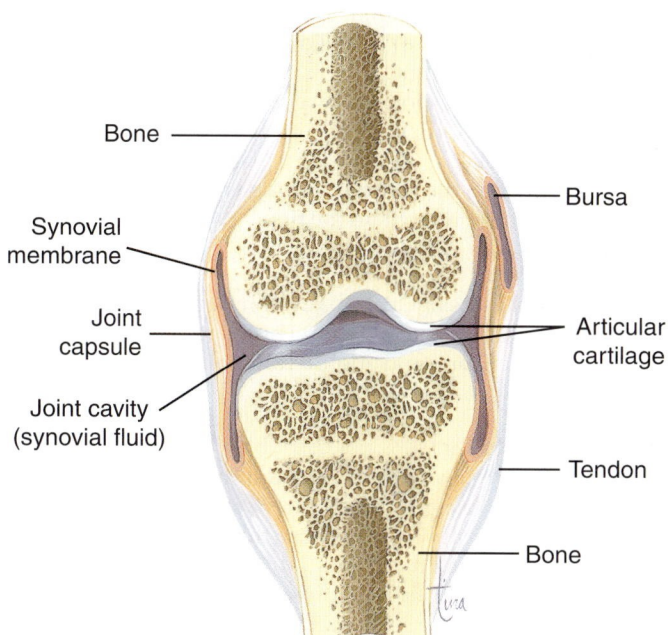

Bone

Bursa

Synovial membrane

Joint capsule

Articular cartilage

Joint cavity (synovial fluid)

Tendon

Bone

FIGURE 21-10 Many synovial joints have bursae that act as cushions against friction.

Assess **muscle strength** along with movement by asking the patient to perform ROM while you apply resistance to the part being moved. For more information about the musculoskeletal system, see Chapter 33.

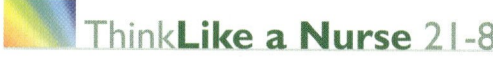

ThinkLike a Nurse 21-8

As you recall, Mr. Nguyen (Meet Your Patient) is moderately obese and has been having pain in both of his knees.

- What history questions would you ask him to assess his knee pain?
- What would you do to examine his knees?

THE NEUROLOGICAL SYSTEM

The neurological system controls or affects the function of all body systems and allows interaction with the external world. Its work is carried out through the transmission of chemical and electrical signals between the brain and the rest of the body. The basic functions of the nervous system are cognition, emotion, memory, sensation and perception, and regulation of homeostasis.

A comprehensive neurological assessment takes hours to complete and is usually reserved for clients with symptoms of neurological problems. As a staff nurse in general practice, you usually perform only portions of a neurological exam. In the next few sections and in Procedure 21-16 we look at the components of a focused neurological exam.

Developmental Considerations

When interpreting a neurological exam, consider the following developmental changes and modifications:

Infants Reflexes present at birth include rooting, sucking, palmar grasp, tonic neck reflex (fencing), and Moro. These reflexes disappear during infancy. With neurological injury, as may occur with stroke or trauma, these reflexes may return, indicating severe problems (see Chapter 9).

Young Children Because language skills and motor development are age-dependent, the Denver Developmental Screening Test (Denver II, 1990) is used as a neurological screening test for young children. The Denver II examines motor, language, and coordination skills. It requires specialized training to administer and evaluate. For toddlers and older children, you can usually perform a comprehensive neurological exam with age-appropriate modifications. For example, when testing for smell, use materials that a young child knows, such as bananas or apples.

Older Adults With advanced age, changes commonly observed are slower reaction time, a decreased ability for rapid problem-solving, and slower voluntary movement. The number of functioning neurons decreases. However, intelligence, memory, and discrimination do not change with normal aging.

Neurological deficits in older adults are usually the result of adverse effects of medications, nutritional deficits, dehydration, cardiovascular changes that alter cerebral blood flow, diabetes, degenerative neurological conditions (e.g., Parkinson's disease or Alzheimer's disease), alcohol or drug use, depression, or abuse.

Cerebral Function

Cerebral function refers to the client's intellectual and behavioral functioning. It includes level of consciousness, mental status, cognitive function, and communication.

Level of Consciousness

Level of consciousness (LOC) includes arousal and orientation.

Arousal may range from alert to deeply comatose. Arousal is classified based on the type of stimuli (auditory, tactile, or painful) required to produce a response from the client. An alert client responds to *auditory stimuli* (e.g., verbal communication or noise). **KEY POINT:** *Remember, if your client does not speak your language he may not respond to questions or commands.*

Orientation refers to the client's awareness of time, place, and person.

- **Orientation to time** includes awareness of the year, date, and time of day. Hospitalized patients are subjected to lights and noise around the clock; are roused in the middle of night for medications or time-sensitive treatments; and are given anesthesia and pain medications that alter their sense of awareness, so they easily become disoriented to time.
- **Orientation to place** involves awareness of surroundings. The patient should know that he is, for example, in the hospital and not in church. Patients who have been moved (e.g., from the emergency department to a ward bed) may not recall their room number but are easily reoriented.
- **Orientation to person** involves recognition of familiar persons and self-identity. The client should be able to state her name or identify people in photographs at the bedside. Because a client may meet many health professionals during a hospitalization, she may not be able to recall your name unless you have had repeated encounters with her.

Mental Status and Cognitive Function

Mental status and cognitive function include behavior, appearance, response to stimuli, speech, memory, communication, and judgment. By this point in the exam, you would have already interviewed the client and talked with him while performing the exam, so you would have a good deal of information about his mental status and cognitive function. You would have already assessed posture, gait, motor movements, dress, and hygiene through the general survey and the musculoskeletal exam; you would be aware of the client's mood based on his tone of voice, actions, and statements.

Many clinicians choose to screen for mental status and cognitive function by working questions into the interaction with the client as they assess other body systems. This type of informal assessment is not only more natural for the client but it is also more accurate. If you choose this method, observe for clarity of thought, appropriate content, concentration, memory, and ability to perform abstract reasoning.

Documenting Cerebral Function

Document LOC by describing the client's response or using the Glasgow Coma Scale (GCS) to grade eye, motor, and verbal responses. The GCS evaluates eye opening, motor responses, and verbal responses. Its limitations are that it relies heavily on vision and verbal interaction, and does not evaluate brainstem reflexes.

A systematic review of evidence suggests that best practice should include use of the GCS plus other evaluation of brainstem reflexes, eye examination, vital signs, and respiratory assessment. A new tool, the **Full Outline of UnResponsiveness (FOUR)**, provides additional information beyond that of the GCS. Both scales are included at the end of Procedure 21-16.

If you are not using the GCS, use the following terms to describe arousal:

- **Alert**—Follows commands in a timely fashion.
- **Lethargic**—Appears drowsy; easily drifts off to sleep.
- **Stuporous**—Requires vigorous stimulation before responding.
- **Comatose**—Does not respond to verbal or painful stimuli.

Although these terms are widely used, a thorough description is preferable. Look at the following two chart entries:

Example 1: Pt. lethargic.
Example 2: Pt. responds to repeated tactile and verbal stimulation. Quickly drifts off to sleep if stimulation is discontinued.

As you can see, the second charting entry provides significantly more information than the first.

Cranial Nerve Function

Cranial nerve assessment is a key component of the neurological exam (Procedure 21-16). The cranial nerves control a variety of sensory and motor functions (Table 21-4 and Fig. 21-11).

Reflex Function

Deep tendon reflexes (DTRs) are automatic responses that do not require conscious thought from the brain. A reflex produces a rapid, involuntary response that occurs at the level of the spinal cord (see Procedure 21-16, step 24, for an illustration). Because the brain is not involved, muscle response is instantaneous. Intact sensory and motor systems are required for a normal reflex response. Each DTR corresponds to a certain level of the cord and is graded on a 0 to 4+ scale (see Procedure 21-16, step 24).

You can elicit **superficial reflexes** by swiftly and lightly stroking a body part (e.g., with the reflex hammer). Superficial reflexes are graded as positive or negative.

Sensory Function

To assess sensory function, ask the client to keep his eyes closed as you apply various stimuli. Ask him to indicate when he feels a sensation. Vary your location and approach so that you test sensation, not pattern recognition. If you notice an area of altered sensation, systematically assess the

Table 21-4 ➤ Cranial Nerves

CRANIAL NERVE NUMBER & NAME	TYPE OF NERVE	FUNCTION OF NERVE
I. Olfactory	Sensory	Smell
II. Optic	Sensory	Visual acuity, visual fields, and ocular fundi
III. Oculomotor	Motor	EOM, pupil constriction
IV. Trochlear	Motor	EOM
V. Trigeminal: 3 branches	Sensory and motor	Corneal reflex; scalp, teeth, and facial sensation; and jaw movement
VI. Abducens	Motor	EOM
VII. Facial	Motor and sensory	Facial movement, sense of taste
VIII. Auditory	Sensory	Hearing and equilibrium
IX. Glossopharyngeal	Motor and sensory	Swallowing, gag response, tongue movement, taste, secretion of saliva
X. Vagus	Motor and sensory	Sensation of pharynx and larynx; motor activity of swallowing and vocal cords; sensory in cardiac, respiratory, and blood pressure reflexes; peristalsis; digestive secretions
XI. Spinal accessory	Motor	Head movement and shoulder elevation; motor to larynx (speaking)
XII. Hypoglossal	Motor	Tongue movement

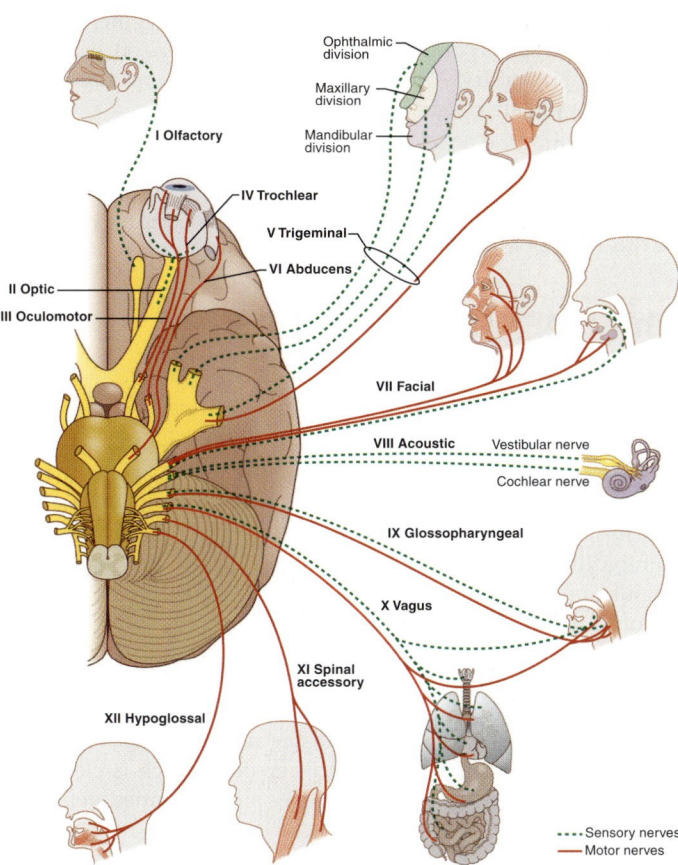

FIGURE 21-11 Origin of cranial nerves.

area to define the border of the change. Usually you will limit your testing to the upper and lower extremities and the trunk. If the client has known or suspected deficits, you should test at numerous other sites. For techniques for assessing reflexes and sensory function, see Procedure 21-16.

Motor and Cerebellar Function

The neurological system coordinates the function of the skeleton and muscles. Motor pathways transmit information between the brain and muscles and the muscles control movement of the skeleton. The cerebellum helps coordinate muscle movement, regulate muscle tone, and maintain posture and equilibrium. The cerebellum is also largely responsible for **proprioception,** or body positioning. Disorders of motor and cerebellar function result in pain or problems with movement, gait, or posture. Thus, when you assess the musculoskeletal system, you also assess the motor functions of the neurological system.

KnowledgeCheck 21-11

- Identify and describe the components assessed in the neurological exam.
- What approach to assessment should you take if:
  Your client has no neurological problems but you are performing a comprehensive exam?
  Your client is hospitalized for a documented cerebrovascular accident?
  Your client has been admitted with an acute head injury and the extent of neurological injury is unknown?

THE GENITOURINARY SYSTEM

In most practice settings, nurses assess only the patient's external genitalia and inguinal lymph nodes. Nurse practitioners and physicians perform comprehensive examinations of the female and male reproductive and urinary systems, as do nurses working in specialty areas. However, even as a novice nurse you may assist with exams or just be present as a witness or to provide emotional support to the client.

♥ **iCare** The genitourinary system includes both the reproductive system and the urinary system. Because a genitourinary (GU) assessment focuses on sexual and reproductive function, it might be embarrassing or uncomfortable for many people. A competent, professional approach is needed. Your confidence and ease with these topics will help the client to feel more relaxed.

The Male Genitourinary System

A complete examination includes assessment of the external genitalia, evaluation for hernias, and a rectal exam for prostate screening. The penis and scrotum are examined by inspection and palpation. You will assess some of the urinary system organs when examining the back (kidneys, ureters) and the abdomen (bladder); the prostate gland is palpated during the exam of the rectum and anus (discussed later in this chapter). For illustrations and steps to follow in examining the male genitourinary system, see Procedure 21-17.

As a result of the scarcity of clear, scientific evidence, the American Academy of Pediatrics (2012) no longer recommends **circumcision** (excision of the foreskin of the penis) as a routine practice. Nevertheless, they do acknowledge the benefits of infant circumcision (Baskin, Lockwood, Bartlett, et al., 2015). Also, circumcision is tied to some religious and cultural beliefs (e.g., among Jews and Muslims), so it is still common.

A **hernia** is a protrusion of the intestine (or other organ) through the wall that contains it. A hernia may be a small protrusion or it may cause pain and distention. In men, a hernia is most likely to be a protrusion of the intestine either through the abdominal wall **(direct hernia)** or into the inguinal canal and possibly into the scrotum **(indirect hernia).** An **umbilical hernia** (fairly common in infants) is an outward bulging due to delayed closure around a small muscle around the umbilicus (belly button). For an illustration of an umbilical hernia, see Procedure 21-14.

KnowledgeCheck 21-12

- What assessment techniques are used when examining the male genitourinary system?
- What is the most common hernia occurring in men?

The Female Genitourinary System

You may be called upon to assist with a comprehensive examination. For a procedure for inspecting external female genitalia and palpating inguinal lymph nodes, see Procedure 21-18.

External Examination

For adolescents and young women who are not sexually active, an external GU examination includes the inspection of the amount and distribution of pubic hair, the skin of the pubic area, and the external genitalia and palpation of the inguinal lymph nodes.

Internal Examination

Women who have abnormal findings on external examination; who have abdominal, pelvic, or genitourinary complaints; or who are on hormone therapy require an internal genital examination (Qaseem, Humphrey, Harris., et al., 2014). The exam includes the following:

- Palpation of Bartholin's glands and Skene's ducts (see Procedure 21-18)
- Assessment of vaginal muscle tone and pelvic musculature
- Speculum examination
- Bimanual examination, wherein the examiner palpates the cervix, uterus, and adnexal tissues with the use of one or two fingers within the vagina and the other hand on the outside to help bring the inner structures toward the two hands

Pap Smear   Recent changes to major guidelines recommend, in general, less frequent routine Papanicolaou tests (Pap smears) to screen for cervical and uterine cancer. They recommend the following for women:

- Younger than age 21: Not screened, regardless of whether they are sexually active or have other risk-taking behaviors.
- Ages 21 through 29: Screen every 3 years.
- Ages 30 to 65: Screen every 3 to 5 years (and follow the advice of their provider).

- Older than age 65: Do not routinely screen unless they are at high risk. However, a recent study states that the cancer incidence rates used for guidelines do not account for the high rates of hysterectomy in the United States. This has the largest impact on older black women. Authors recommend that the risk and screening guidelines be reconsidered (Rositch, Nowak, & Gravitt, 2014).

- Those with certain vulnerabilities (e.g., weakened immune system, HIV positive) should have a Pap test every year (American Cancer Society, n.d.b, revised 2015; National Guideline Clearinghouse, 2005, revised 2016).

KEY POINT: *National screening guidelines vary and they change frequently.*

Additional cultures or screens may be done if there is unusual discharge or risk of sexually transmitted infection. A **speculum examination** is performed to collect specimens and assess the cervix. To learn about assisting with a speculum exam, see Clinical Insight 21-3.

KnowledgeCheck 21-13

What are the responsibilities of the nurse during an internal exam of the female genitourinary system?

The Anus, Rectum, and Prostate

Examining the rectum and anus is the last aspect of a comprehensive examination. For the female client, this exam is usually performed at the end of a bimanual pelvic examination while the client is still in the lithotomy position. For a male client you will usually perform the exam after completing your examination of the genitals. For a step-by-step procedure, see Procedure 21-19.

Inspect the anus and rectum for skin condition and hemorrhoids and palpate for muscle tone, masses, and tenderness. Skin irritation and erythema are common in clients who have diarrhea and in infants and toddlers who wear diapers. **Hemorrhoids** (dilated, usually painful, anal vessels) may be seen in clients with a history of constipation. Many women develop hemorrhoids with pregnancy and childbirth.

A comprehensive examination for a man should include a digital rectal examination to assess for prostate enlargement.

An enlarged prostate may indicate benign enlargement of the prostate, which is common in men older than age 50, or it may indicate prostatitis. A hard nodule or multiple nodules may indicate prostate cancer.

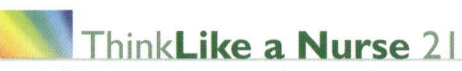

ThinkLike a Nurse 21-9

How will examination of the rectum and anus differ for Nam and Yen Nguyen (Meet Your Patient)?

DOCUMENTING PHYSICAL EXAMINATION FINDINGS (NAM NGUYEN)

Zach Miller has completed his physical examination of Nam Nguyen (Meet Your Patient). What follows is his charting entry. Recall that Zach is an advanced practice nurse and has performed a comprehensive physical exam. Therefore, this examination and charting entry are more extensive than what would be expected of a staff nurse. Keep in mind that you should use only abbreviations that are on your clinical agency's approved list.

General Survey   56-year-old moderately obese man presents to the clinic for a physical exam in no apparent distress. Pt. appears stated age; is well dressed and groomed; and alert and oriented to time, place, and person. Speech is clear, response and affect appropriate. Moves all extremities well, gait steady and balanced. Smells of cigarettes.

Height	5 ft 4 in.
Weight	185 lb (84 kg)
BP	166/100 mm Hg
Pulse	88 beats/min
RR	22 breaths/min
Temp	98.5°F (36.9°C), oral
BMI	33

Integumentary   Skin even in color, warm & dry, good turgor, no suspicious lesions. Well healed scar in right inguinal area. Hair clean, coarse, evenly distributed. Some graying. Nails pink, brisk capillary refill, no clubbing.

Head & Neck   Normocephalic, erect, midline. Scalp mobile, no lesions, tenderness, or masses. Facial features symmetrical. Thyroid gland symmetrical and not enlarged; cervical lymph nodes not palpable or tender.

Eyes   Snellen = right eye 20/100, left eye 20/100, both eyes 20/100. Color vision intact. Difficulty noted with near vision. Visual fields normal by confrontation. Extraocular movements intact. PERRLA at 3 mm by direct and consensual. Eyes clear and bright, + blink, no lid lag or abnormalities. Anterior chamber clear. Cornea & iris intact. Sclera white, conjunctiva clear. Lacrimal glands and ducts nontender. + red reflex bilateral, discs flat with sharp margins, vessels intact, retina & macula even in color.

Ears, Nose, & Throat   Skin intact, no masses, lesions, or discharge. Position WNL. External ears nontender to palpation. + whisper test. Weber—no lateralization. External canals clear without redness, swelling, lesions, or discharge. Tympanic membranes intact, light reflex and bony landmarks visible; frontal and maxillary sinuses nontender. Nares patent, able to distinguish familiar odors, mucosa pink, no discharge, septum intact with no deviation.

Mouth   Lips, oral mucosa, gingivae pink with no lesions. All teeth present and in good repair. Pharynx pink, tonsils absent, palate intact. Symmetrical rise of the uvula, + gag and swallow reflex. Tongue smooth, pink, symmetrical, mobile, without lesions, taste intact (correctly identified sweet, salty, and sour).

Respiratory Respirations 22 breaths/min and unlabored. Trachea midline, AP less than transverse chest diameter. Chest expansion symmetrical. No tenderness, scars, masses, or lesions. Diaphragmatic excursion 5 cm. Lungs clear to auscultation.

Cardiovascular PMI @ MCL at 5th ICS, P 85, regular, no murmurs, gallops, or thrills present; pulses +2, no bruits or thrills, no varicosities; jugular venous pulsation 2 cm at 45°. Carotids without bruits.

Breasts Symmetrical. No masses, lymphadenopathy, or discharge.

Abdomen Abdomen soft, rounded; no masses or pulsations. Surgical scar right inguinal area. +bowel sounds, +tympany throughout.

Musculoskeletal Normal spinal curvature. Joints and muscles symmetrical, no deformity. +Bilateral knee pain (right more than left). Full ROM in upper and lower extremities; +5 muscle strength; moderate crepitus right knee.

Neurological Awake; alert; and oriented to time, place, and person. CN I–XII intact. Gait steady and coordinated; negative Romberg; unable to do deep knee bends due to pain. Point-point localization; superficial and deep sensation intact; +2 deep tendon reflexes.

Genitourinary Circumcised male; penis nontender, no masses, urethral meatus midline, no discharge; testicles descended bilaterally, nontender, inguinal and femoral canals free of masses, prostate small, smooth, mobile, nontender. Rectal wall smooth, no masses, stool hemoccult negative.

CLINICALREASONING

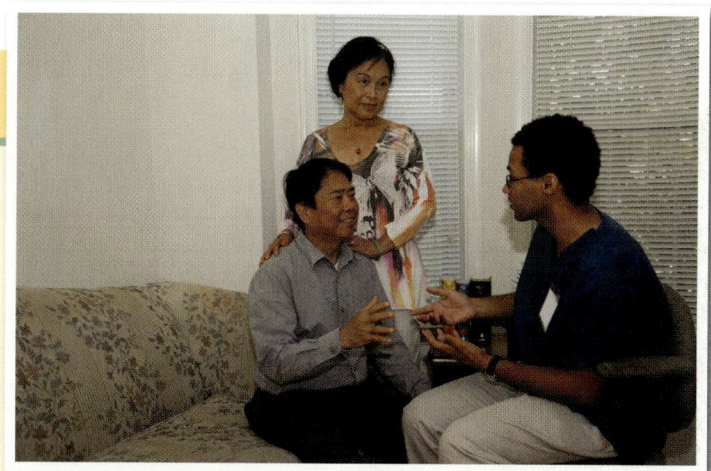

Caring for the Nguyens

Nam Nguyen has had a comprehensive physical examination with Zach Miller, the nurse practitioner. Review the note written by Zach, preceding; and also the Laboratory Data for Nam Nguyen, below.

A. Discuss how each of the following would differ from the examination Zach Miller conducted and what would be expected if:
- A registered nurse conducted the exam.
- A nursing student performed the exam.

B. Review Zach's documentation of the exam. Identify the abnormal findings.

C. Review the laboratory work. Identify the abnormal findings.

D. What conclusions, if any, can you draw from these findings? What actions should you consider based on these conclusions?

E. Identify at least two nursing diagnoses based on these findings.

F. Zach Miller has identified a problem of Obesity for Mr. Nguyen.
- What information do you need to determine the etiology of this problem?

- Because you do not have that information, write a two-part diagnostic statement describing Mr. Nguyen's nutritional status.

G. Now rewrite the nutrition statement as a three-part statement, using "as evidenced by."

H. Zach Miller has identified the diagnosis Acute Pain (knees) for Mr. Nguyen. If the pain is caused by a medical condition, osteoarthritis, how would you write a two-part diagnostic statement to describe this health status?

I. How would the examination of Yen Nguyen differ from the exam Nam experienced?

J. How would the examination of Kim Phan, Nam's 3-year-old grandson, differ?

K. If you were responsible for examining Nam Nguyen, what aspects of the exam would you find most challenging? Explain why.

(Continued)

Caring for the Nguyens (continued)

Name: Nam Nguyen   **Age:** 56
Acct#: K00205412   Family Medicine Center, Z. Miller

Test	Result	Reference Range*
CBC/Differential		
WBC	5.6 x 10³/mm³	5–10 x 10³/mm³
Hemoglobin	14.8 g/dL	M: 14–18 g/dL F: 12–16 g/dL
Hematocrit	45.1%	M: 42–52% F: 37–47%
RBC count	5.1 million/mm³	M: 4.7–5.14 million/mm³ F: 4.2–4.87 million/mm³
MCV	84 mm³	85–95 mm³
MCH	29 pg	28–32 pg
MCHC	34%	33–35%
Neutrophils	57%	59%
Lymphocytes	30%	34%
Monocytes	5%	4%
Eosinophils	2.5%	2.7%
Basophils	0.7%	0.5%
Platelet count	197,000/mm³	150,000–400,000/mm³

Test	Result	Reference Range*
Comprehensive Metabolic Panel		
Sodium	138 mEq/L	135–145 mEq/L
Potassium	4.3 mEq/L	3.5–5.0 mEq/L
Chloride	101 mEq/L	97–107 mEq/L
Carbon dioxide	27 mEq/L	23–29 mEq/L
BUN	16 mg/dL	10–31 mg/dL
Creatinine	0.8 mg/dL	M: 0.6–1.2 mg/dL F: 0.5–1.1 mg/dL
Glucose	156 mg/dL	75–110 mg/dL
Albumin	4.0 g/dL	19–60 years: 3.2–4.8 g/dL
Total protein	7.2 g/dL	6.8–8.0 g/dL
ALT (alanine aminotransferase, also called SGPT)	18 units/L	M: 10–40 units/L F: 7–35 units/L
ALP (alkaline phosphatase)	43 units/L	M: 35–142 units/L F: 25–125 units/L
AST (aspartate aminotranspeptidase, also called SGOT)	26 units/L	M: 19–48 units/L F: 9–36 units/L
Bilirubin, total	0.7 mg/dL	0.3–1.2 mg/dL
Calcium	8.5 mg/dL	8.2–10.2 mg/dL

Test	Result	Reference Range*	
Lipid Panel**			
Total cholesterol	201 mg/dL	<200 200–239 >240	-Desirable -Borderline high -High
LDL cholesterol (Primary target of therapy)	140 mg/dL	<100 mg/dL 100–129 mg/dL 130–159 160–189 >190	-Optimal -Near optimal/ above optimal -Borderline high -High -Very high
HDL cholesterol	34 mg/dL	<40	-Low
Triglycerides	196 mg/dL		

**To interpret lipid panel results, follow the most recent guidelines of the National Cholesterol Education Program (NCEP) Expert Panel on Detection, Evaluation, and Blood Cholesterol in Adults available at www.nhlbi.nih.gov/guidelines/cholesterol/atglance.pdf. The reference range figures in this table will undoubtedly be revised (and lowered) by NCEP in the near future.

Also, the norms for an individual patient's lipid panel depend on the calculation of risk factors. Nam is hypertensive, is obese, and has an elevated blood sugar. His norms reflect high risk for coronary heart disease; they would be about <160 for total cholesterol, <100 for triglycerides, <100 for LDL, and >45 for HDL.

Test	Result	Reference Range*
Urinalysis		
Appearance	Clear	Clear
Color	Amber	Light yellow to amber
Odor	Aromatic	None–aromatic
pH	6.0	5.0–9.0
Specific gravity	1.012	1.001–1.035
Leukocyte esterase	Negative	Negative
Nitrites	Negative	Negative
Ketones	Negative	Negative
Protein	5 mg/dL	<20 mg/dL
Crystals	None	In acid urine: uric acid, calcium oxalate, amorphous urates In alkaline urine: triple phosphate, calcium phosphate, ammonium biurate, calcium carbonate, amorphous phosphates
Casts	None	None, except rare hyaline
Glucose	Negative	Negative
WBC	1/hpf	<5/hpf
RBC	1/hpf	<5/hpf

PSA (prostate-specific antigen)	2.8 ng/mL	<4 ng/mL
Fecal occult blood screen		
Sample #1 — negative		
Sample #2 — negative		
Sample #3 — negative		

*For most studies, each laboratory establishes its own reference range.

PracticalKnowledge
clinical application

CLINICAL INSIGHTS

Clinical Insight 21-1 ➤ **Performing Percussion**

Direct Percussion

Tap lightly with the pads of the fingers directly on the skin.

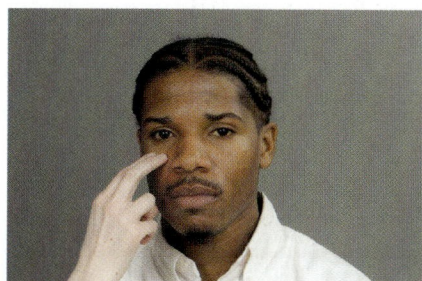

Direct percussion over the sinuses

Indirect Percussion

- Keep your fingernails short.
- Strive for a quiet environment: Turn off all entertainment media and music, shut the door, and so on. *This allows you to better perceive the subtle differences in percussion notes.*
- One hand is considered the stationary hand; the other is the striking hand.
- Hyperextend the middle finger of your stationary hand and place its distal portion firmly against the client's skin over the area you wish to percuss.
- Lift the rest of your fingers off the patient's skin. *Prevents dampening the sounds produced.*
- Be sure both of your hands are relaxed to best perform the technique. *Stiff hands will not effectively produce the percussion sounds for assessment.*

- Use the middle finger of your dominant hand as the striking finger **(plexor)** and tap the distal portion of the middle finger of the stationary hand using a quick motion from your wrist.

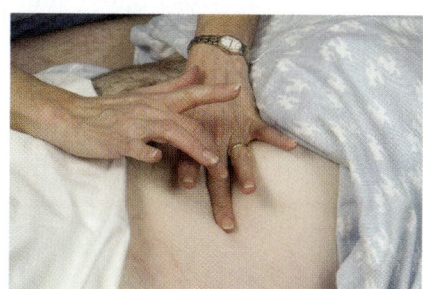

Indirect percussion

- Use enough force to elicit a clear sound.
- Percuss two times over each location, then move to a new body location and repeat.

Describing Sounds

Use the terms in the following list to describe the sounds you hear. The terms are based on the components of the sounds produced by percussion.
- *Amplitude*—The loudness or softness of a sound
- *Pitch*—The number of vibrations per second; can be either high or low in nature
- *Quality*—A distinctiveness about the sound produced
- *Duration*—How long the sound lingers

Percussion Notes					
SOUND	**AMPLITUDE**	**PITCH**	**QUALITY**	**DURATION**	**EXAMPLE**
Resonant	Medium-loud	Low	Hollow	Medium	Normal lung
Hyperresonant	Louder	Lower	Booming	Longer	Hyperinflated lung (as in emphysema)
Dull	Soft	High	Muffled thud	Short	Liver/spleen
Flat	Very soft	High	Absolute dullness	Very short	Thigh or tumor
Tympany	Loud	High	Musical	Longest	Gastric air bubble, intestinal air

Clinical Insight 21-2 ➤ Performing Auscultation

- Provide a quiet environment to facilitate auscultation.

- ✚ Clean your stethoscope with a 70% alcohol or benzalkonium chloride wipe before and after using it to examine a patient. Most stethoscopes are colonized by bacteria, although only a small percentage are pathogenic. Cleaning can reduce the bacterial count by 94% to 100%.

- **Use the diaphragm to listen to high-pitched sounds** that normally occur in the heart, lungs, and abdomen. Press the diaphragm hard enough to produce an obvious ring on the patient's skin.
- **Use the bell to hear low-pitched sounds,** such as extra heart sounds (murmurs) or turbulent blood flow (bruits). Apply the bell lightly with just enough pressure to produce an air seal with its full rim.
- Place the earpieces facing forward. *Seals the ear canal and improves detection of sounds.*

- Warm the stethoscope before you place it on the client's skin.
- Place the stethoscope directly on the client's skin. Do not listen through clothing. *Clothing can create artifact or reduce the quality of auscultation.*
- If body hair prevents good contact with the skin, dampen the hair before you listen.
- Close your eyes as you listen through the stethoscope to improve your focus.
- Concentrate on one sound at a time. Do not try to evaluate breath and heart sounds at the same time.

Practice Resources

Centers for Disease Control and Prevention (2009); Muniz, J., Sethi, R. K., Zaghi, J., et al. (2012); Russell, A., Secrest, J., & Schreeder, C. (2012).

Clinical Insight 21-3 ➤ Assisting With a Speculum Exam

Equipment

- Patient drape
- Nonsterile gloves
- Vaginal speculum (see accompanying figure)
  The speculum may be plastic or metal.
  The size of the speculum depends on the patient's history. Use a small speculum for a woman who has never been sexually active or an older woman who is not sexually active.
  If a culture or a Pap smear is to be obtained, lubricate the speculum with warm water. Otherwise, use a water-soluble lubricant.
- Lubricant
- Pap smear slide, spatula, brush, or specimen broom and container with solution
- Fixative, if the smear technique is used
- Genital culture supplies
- Additional light source

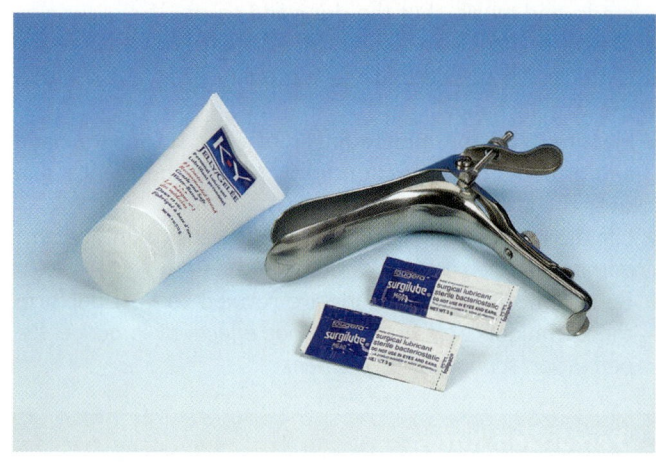

Equipment. A vaginal speculum.

Clinical Insight 21-3 ➤ Assisting With a Speculum Exam—cont'd

Preparing the Patient

- Explain to the patient that an internal examination of her vagina and pelvic organs will be performed. The examination usually takes only a few minutes, and although it might not be comfortable it should not be painful.
- Have the woman urinate before the examination if needed. *Emptying the bladder helps the patient to feel more comfortable during the exam.*
- Provide privacy and keep the patient warm during the procedure.
- Assist the woman to the lithotomy position and cover her with a drape.

Inserting the Speculum

The speculum is inserted into the vagina to visualize the cervix (see accompanying figure). Once the speculum is inserted, you may need to adjust the light source for the examiner.

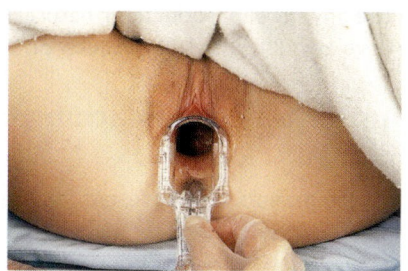

(A) A vaginal speculum examination. Placement of the speculum in the vagina.

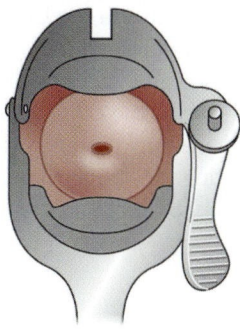

(B) View through the speculum.

Collecting Specimens

If a routine screening for cervical and uterine cancer is being done, a specimen will be collected. Additional cultures or screens may be required if there is unusual discharge or risk of sexually transmitted infection. Genital cultures are endocervical smears.

Pap Smear Procedure

Most commonly, the examiner inserts a small brush through the cervical os and rotates it to obtain cells from within the cervical canal (endocervical smear). The brush is then rolled onto the slide.

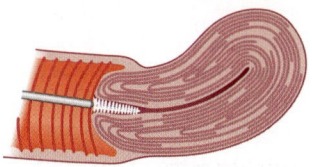

Using a specimen broom to obtain endocervical cells.

A second specimen may be obtained by lightly scraping the cervix with a wooden spatula to obtain cells from the ectocervix (the lowest portion of the cervix that protrudes into the vagina).

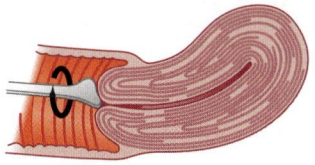

Using a spatula to obtain ectocervical cells.

The spatula is then smeared on the slide. Some examiners use both specimen sources and then apply a fixative, usually a spray or liquid, on top of the specimen to preserve it for examination. After the samples are obtained, the speculum is removed.

Pap Smear, Alternative Method

- The examiner inserts a specimen broom into the cervical os and rotates it. The broom is then inserted into a fixative solution and rotated to disperse cells into the solution. After the samples are obtained, the speculum is removed. This technique is gaining popularity because it is considered more sensitive for detection of cervical changes.

Bimanual Exam

After removing the speculum, the examiner inserts lubricated gloved fingers into the vagina while pressing down on the lower abdomen and suprapubic area. This is known as a **bimanual exam.** It is used to assess the consistency of the cervix; the size of the uterus; and to detect tenderness over the ovaries, fallopian tubes, or with movement of the cervix.

Post-Procedure

- Assist the woman to a sitting position at the end of the exam.
- You may need to assist the woman with perineal care.
- If there is any bleeding or discharge, provide a perineal pad.
- Document the date and time of the procedure, the name of the examiner, the patient's tolerance of the procedure, and any nursing assessments or interventions performed.

Practice Resources

American Congress of Obstetricians and Gynecologists (2014); U.S. Preventive Services Task Force (2012).

PROCEDURES

KEY POINT: *As the RN, you are responsible for (1) performing the initial assessment to establish a baseline and for (2) follow-up assessments for any changes.* You can instruct nursing assistive personnel (NAP) to report any changes to you. You can delegate measurement of height, weight, and vital signs to the NAP. However, you may want to obtain the first set of vital signs yourself, because they will serve as a baseline.

Together, the procedures in this section represent a comprehensive physical examination you can use for initial and ongoing physical assessments. Procedure 21-20 provides a brief bedside assessment. The following procedures are described mainly for adult patients. To review ways in which to modify your examination to people of different ages, see the earlier section Modifications for Different Age-Groups. Also note the following:

- *Developmental Modifications* for various age-groups are given just before the procedure steps. Use these to help you adapt your examination techniques to the specific patient.
- *Developmental Variations* are provided in the procedure in column 2, under Expected and Abnormal findings. Use these when you are analyzing assessment findings.

Procedure 21-1 ■ Performing the General Survey

➤ For steps to follow in *all* procedures, refer to the Universal Steps for All Procedures found on the page facing the inside back cover.

Equipment
See Box 21-1.

Positioning

- Have the client seated as you begin the examination (on an exam table or on the side of the bed). Face the client and make eye contact.
  Helps build rapport and put the client at ease.

- If the client is unable to sit, use Fowler's or semi-Fowler's position.
  An upright position allows the client to expand his lungs fully and is useful for assessing vital signs, the head and neck, the heart and lungs, the back, and the upper extremities.

Focused History Questions

- How are you feeling today?
- (If the client is an outpatient) What brings you to the clinic today?
- Are you in any discomfort or pain?
- Have you had any hospitalizations or surgeries?
- What medicines do you take? That includes prescribed as well as over-the-counter drugs.
- How much alcohol do you drink per day? Do you smoke cigarettes? If so, how many per day and for how long? Do you use drugs for non-medical purposes?
- Do you use any herbal products or natural remedies?
- Do you have any difficulty falling asleep or staying asleep?

Developmental Modifications for Infants and Children

- Encourage the parents to be present for the examination.
  Infants and toddlers usually feel most secure if a parent is present.

- Adolescents should be examined without parents or siblings present unless they request otherwise. Provide privacy.

- *Older adults*—Assess the older adult's functional status. You can use the Lawton Instrumental Activities of Daily Living (IADL) found in the Assessment Guidelines and Tools in Chapter 3.

- *Older adults*—Work the SPICES assessment into the examination of various body systems: **S**leep disorders, **P**roblems eating or feeding, **I**ncontinence, **C**onfusion, **E**vidence of falls, **S**kin breakdown.

➤ When performing the procedure, always identify your patient according to agency policy, using two identifiers, and be attentive to standard precautions, hand hygiene, patient safety and privacy, body mechanics, and documentation.

Procedure Steps

Observe the client's general characteristics.

1. **Identify signs of physical or emotional distress** (e.g., pain, fear, or anxiety). If signs of distress are present, perform a focused assessment, and address the immediate problem.

Findings

Expected findings: The client is in no apparent distress. The client appears relaxed, with no evidence of pain, fear, or anxiety.

Abnormal findings: Pain, grimacing, breathing problems, skin color changes

2. **Observe apparent age, sex, and race.** Ask the patient, "What racial or ethnic group do you identify with?" Ask yourself,
   - Is apparent age consistent with biological age?
   - Are there cultural or gender-related factors that influence the exam or findings?

Expected findings: Client appears his stated age. Makes eye contact consistent with his cultural norms. Is reasonably comfortable with being examined.

3. **Note facial characteristics,** including facial expression, symmetry of facial features, and the condition and color of the skin. Ask yourself,
   - What is the client's face telling me?
   - Is the facial expression appropriate to the situation?
   - Are facial features symmetrical (palpebral fissure and nasolabial folds)?
   - Are there any changes in condition or color of skin?
   - Does the client maintain eye contact?
   - Does the client appear older than his stated age?

Expected findings: Face is symmetrical; visible skin is intact without excessive wrinkling, discoloration, or deformity.

Abnormal findings: Excessive wrinkling may be from sun exposure, tobacco use, or illness.

4. **Note body type and posture.** Greet the client with a handshake. Be aware that shaking hands is not acceptable in all cultures.
   Allows you to assess muscle strength and surface skin characteristics while at the same time conveying that you care.

   Ask yourself:
   - Is the body build stocky, slender, average, obese, or **cachectic** (very thin, wasted appearance)?
   - Are the body parts proportional to the client's overall size?
   - Is body fat distributed normally?
   - Does the client assume a specific position for comfort (e.g., sitting versus supine)?

Expected findings: Posture is upright, and body appears proportionate. Grip is strong.

5. **Observe gait, and note any abnormal movements.** If the client has Impaired Bed Mobility, determine ability to move and amount of assistance needed. Ask yourself,
   - Does the client move in a coordinated manner?
   - Are there any obvious gait problems?
   - Does the client walk with a wide base of support or short stride length?
   - Does the client use assistive devices, such as a cane?
   - Are there any abnormal or spastic movements?

Expected findings: Movements are smooth and coordinated; gait is steady; does not use assistive devices.

Abnormal findings: Unstable or shuffling gait, spastic movements, stiff movements may be associated with joint, muscle, or neurological disorders. A slumped position may indicate fatigue, depression, osteoporosis, or pain

6. Listen to your client's speech pattern, pace, quality, tone, vocabulary, and sentence structure while you are examining the body systems. Ask yourself,
   - Are the responses appropriate (a) to the situation, and (b) for developmental stage?
   - Is there any difficulty with speech?
   - Does the client's tone of voice match her statements
   - Is the voice hoarse?
   - Does the client have a foreign accent; is there hesitancy and/or little verbalization?

Expected findings: Client responds appropriately to questions. Tone of voice matches responses. Speech is clear, evenly paced, and rises and falls based on content.

Abnormal findings: Rapid speech, slow speech, slurred speech, illogical responses, language barrier

(continued on next page)

Procedure 21-1 ■ Performing the General Survey (continued)

7. Assess mental state and affect.
  a. Determine level of consciousness.
  b. Determine orientation to time, place, and person.
  Ask yourself,
  - If the client is disoriented, does he reorient easily?
  - What is the client's mood? Is it appropriate for the situation?

  NOTE: If you note any abnormal findings, be sure to focus on them when you assess mental status during the sensori–neurological examination.

Expected findings: Awake, alert, and oriented to time, place, person, and self. Mood is appropriate for the situation.

Abnormal findings:
- Confusion and irritability may indicate hypoxia or medication side effects.
- Inability to recall information or provide history may indicate a neurological disorder.
- Lethargy and somnolence may be due to medications; depression; or a neurological, thyroid, liver, kidney, or cardiovascular disorder.
- Bizarre responses may signal a psychiatric problem.

8. Observe dress, grooming, and hygiene. Ask yourself,
  - Is the client appropriately and neatly dressed?
  - Is the client well groomed?
  - Are there any unusual odors?

Expected findings: Client is dressed appropriately for the climate. Skin is clean, and clothing is in good repair. No noticeable odor.

Abnormal findings: Poor hygiene, dirty skin or nails, uncombed hair, visible soiling of clothing, mismatched or wrinkled clothing, objectionable odor; may indicate a self-care deficit, chronic pain, fatigue, depression, or low self-esteem.

9. Measure vital signs: blood pressure, temperature, radial pulse, respiratory rate. If your initial observations and interview indicate that the client is in pain, perform a pain assessment, as well (see Chapter 32.)

Expected findings:

BP: < 120/80 mm Hg

Temperature: 97.3°F–98.6°F (36.3°C–37°C) oral

Pulse: 60–100 beats/min, regular, and easily palpated

Respiratory rate: 12–20 breaths/min, regular and even

Abnormal findings: See Chapter 19.

10. Measure height and weight.
  a. For adults: Calculate BMI, or use the accompanying table.

$$\frac{Wt \ (lb) \times 703}{Ht \ (in.)^2} = BMI$$

  b. For children: Plot height and weight on growth chart.

Developmental Modifications

Adults

- Use a platform scale with a sliding ruler (see Fig. 21-1), or a bed scale if the client cannot stand safely.

Infants and children

- Weigh infants without clothing; weigh older children in their underwear.
- For infants and children younger than age 2 yr, use a stationary measure (e.g., infant scale) if available. Position supine to measure height; be sure knees are extended.
- For infants and children younger than age 2 yr, also measure head circumference.

Expected findings: For adults: BMI is 18.5–24.9.

For children: Height and weight are consistent with previous trend on growth chart.

Abnormal findings:

BMI < 18.5 = underweight

BMI 25–29.9 = overweight

BMI ≥ 30 = obese

BMI 30–34.9 Level I Moderate obesity

BMI 35–39.9 Level II Severe obesity

BMI > 40 Level III Morbid obesity

NOTE: For growth charts for males and females from birth to 20 years of age,

 go to the CDC, National Center for Health Statistics Web site at www.cdc.gov/growthcharts/clinical_charts.htm

? What if . . .

- **There is an apparent language barrier?**

Obtain an interpreter; and refer **to Clinical Insight 20-3 in Chapter 20** of this book.

Use this table to find body mass index, based on height and weight, or use a BMI calculator such as the ones found at

http://www.nhlbi.nih.gov/health/educational/lose_wt/B MI/bmicalc.htm and http://www.cdc.gov/healthyweight/ assessing/bmi/adult_bmi/english_bmi_calculator/ bmi_calculator.html ▼

Weight (lb)

Height (ft/in)	120	130	140	150	160	170	180	190	200	210	220	230	240	250	260	270	280	290	300	310	320	330
4'5"	30	33	35	38	40	43	45	48	50	53	55	58	60	63	65	68	70	73	75	78	80	83
4'6"	29	31	34	36	39	41	43	46	48	51	53	56	58	60	63	65	68	70	72	75	77	80
4'7"	28	30	33	35	37	40	42	44	47	49	51	54	56	58	61	63	65	68	70	72	75	77
4'8"	27	29	31	34	36	38	40	43	45	47	49	52	54	56	58	61	63	65	67	70	72	74
4'9"	26	28	30	33	35	37	39	41	43	46	48	50	52	54	56	59	61	63	65	67	69	72
4'10"	25	27	29	31	34	36	38	40	42	44	46	48	50	52	54	57	59	61	63	65	67	69
4'11"	24	26	28	30	32	34	36	38	40	43	45	47	49	51	53	55	57	59	61	63	65	67
5'0"	23	25	27	29	31	33	35	37	39	41	43	45	47	49	51	53	55	57	59	61	63	65
5'1"	23	25	27	28	30	32	34	36	38	40	42	44	45	47	49	51	53	55	57	59	61	62
5'2"	22	24	26	27	29	31	33	35	37	38	40	42	44	46	48	49	51	53	55	57	59	60
5'3"	21	23	25	27	28	30	32	34	36	37	39	41	43	44	46	48	50	51	53	55	57	59
5'4"	21	22	24	26	28	29	31	33	34	36	38	40	41	43	45	46	48	50	52	53	55	57
5'5"	20	22	23	25	27	28	30	32	33	35	38	38	40	42	43	45	47	48	50	52	53	55
5'6"	19	21	23	24	26	27	29	31	32	34	36	37	39	40	42	44	45	47	49	50	52	53
5'7"	19	20	22	24	25	27	28	30	31	33	35	36	38	39	41	42	44	46	47	49	50	52
5'8"	18	20	21	23	24	26	27	29	30	32	34	35	37	38	40	41	43	44	46	47	49	50
5'9"	18	19	21	22	24	25	27	28	30	31	33	34	36	37	38	40	41	43	44	46	47	49
5'10"	17	19	20	22	23	24	26	27	29	30	32	33	35	36	37	39	40	42	43	45	46	47
5'11"	17	18	20	21	22	24	25	27	28	29	31	32	34	35	36	38	39	41	42	43	45	46
6'	16	18	19	20	22	23	24	26	27	29	30	31	33	34	35	37	38	39	41	42	43	45
6'1"	16	17	19	20	21	22	24	25	26	28	29	30	32	33	34	36	37	38	40	41	42	44
6'2"	15	17	18	19	21	22	23	24	26	27	28	30	31	32	33	35	36	37	39	40	41	42
6'3"	15	16	18	19	20	21	23	24	25	26	28	29	30	31	33	34	35	36	38	39	40	41
6'4"	15	16	17	18	20	21	22	23	24	26	27	28	29	30	32	33	34	35	37	38	39	40
6'5"	14	15	17	18	19	20	21	23	24	25	26	27	29	30	31	32	33	34	36	37	38	39
6'6"	14	15	16	17	19	20	21	22	23	24	25	27	28	29	30	31	32	34	35	36	37	38
6'7"	14	15	16	17	18	19	20	21	23	24	25	26	27	28	29	30	32	33	34	35	36	37
6'8"	13	14	15	17	18	19	20	21	22	23	24	25	26	28	29	30	31	32	33	34	35	36
6'9"	13	14	15	16	17	18	19	20	21	23	24	25	26	27	28	29	30	31	32	33	34	35
6'10"	13	14	15	16	17	18	19	20	21	22	23	24	25	26	27	28	29	30	31	32	34	35

Less risk   **More risk**

Documentation

- Document BP as right or left arm, and note the patient's position: sitting, standing, or lying.
- Document temperature measurement route: oral, rectal, or tympanic membrane.
- If you need more information about documenting, see Documenting Physical Examination Findings (Nam Nguyen), immediately preceding the Clinical Reasoning section of this chapter.

- For a graphic flow sheet for recording vital signs, see Figure 19-1.

Practice Resources

Centers for Disease Control and Prevention (2015, last updated); CDC (2012, last updated); National Guideline Clearinghouse (2013); National Heart, Lung, and Blood Institute (n.d.).

Procedure 21-2 ■ **Assessing the Skin**

➤ For steps to follow in *all* procedures, refer to the Universal Steps for All Procedures found on the page facing the inside back cover.

Equipment

- Nonlatex gloves (if exposure to body fluids is a possibility)
- Flexible transparent ruler
- Penlight
- Magnifier
- Pen and record form

Focused History Questions

Ask the patient about the history or presence of any:
- Rashes
- History of allergies
- Areas of skin that have changed color
- Skin lesions
- Skin with rough or unusual texture

- Skin that is always warm or cool, regardless of room temperature

 ### Developmental Modifications for Older Adults

- Assess the level of risk for pressure ulcers. For assessment tools (Braden scale, Norton scale), go to Chapter 36 in this textbook.

  As adults age, the subcutaneous tissue layer thins. The dermal layer loses elasticity as a result of changes in collagen fibers, and the strong bond between the epidermal and dermal layers decreases. These changes make the skin prone to breakdown.

➤ When performing the procedure, always identify your patient according to agency policy, using two identifiers, and be attentive to standard precautions, hand hygiene, patient safety and privacy, body mechanics, and documentation.

Procedure Steps

1. **Inspect skin color, including mucous membranes, tongue, and conjunctiva.**

   To assess color changes of exposed and unexposed areas. Color changes and odors may indicate underlying disease and should be fully investigated.

   a. Provide good lighting.
   b. In dark-skinned clients, look for color changes in the conjunctiva or oral mucosa, tongue, lips, nailbeds, palms of the hands, and soles of the feet.

   Skin color varies widely among individuals by age and ethnicity, but in each individual, skin color is fairly uniform over his body. ▼

   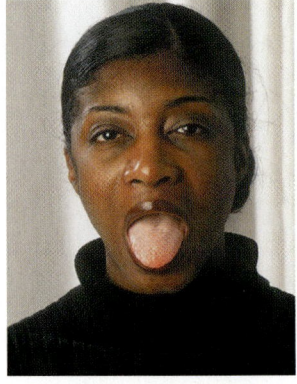 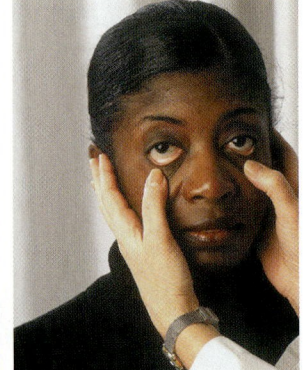

   c. Note any unusual odors.
   d. To assess for cyanosis, be sure to examine the tongue.

   Exposure to cold causes the lips to turn blue, but not the tongue. Cyanosis affects the color of the skin, mucous membrane, and tongue.

Findings

Expected findings: Skin color is uniform, with darker exposed areas. Mucous membranes and conjunctiva are pink and moist. No unusual odors.

Developmental Variations

Newborns—May be jaundiced for a few weeks. Blue-black mongolian spots and pink-red capillary hemangiomas are common and fade with time.

 Older adults—May have thin, translucent skin and wrinkles due to loss of elasticity. Fragile skin is not uncommon among lighter skinned, older adults.

Abnormal findings: Pallor, jaundice (may require further investigation), cyanosis, erythema, hyperpigmentation, hypopigmentation

- Café-au-lait spots, although usually normal, may sometimes signal a genetic disorder.
- If there are abnormal findings, ask the patient (or someone who knows him well) about the baseline skin color.

For more information about skin color and lesions, see Table 21-2.

2. Palpate skin for temperature.
   a. Wear procedure gloves and discard after examining any open areas of the skin.
   b. Use dorsal aspect of hand or fingers.
   c. Compare bilaterally, and compare to the feet.
      The dorsa of the hands and the fingers are most sensitive to temperature variations.
   d. Check the skin temperature over any area of erythema.
   e. If skin feels excessively warm, validate your data: assess for fever.

Expected findings: Skin is warm; temperature is the same bilaterally.

Abnormal findings: Local area(s) that are warmer or cooler than the rest of the skin; generalized temperature increase or decrease.
- Localized warmth with erythema can indicate an infection.
- Cool skin might be a sign of compromised circulation, shock, exposure to cold, hypothyroidism, or dehydration, particularly in the older adult.

---

3. Palpate skin for turgor. Test an unexposed area, such as the area below the clavicle, inner thigh, sternum, or forehead, by gently pinching up the skin, noting its return when you release it.

Developmental Modifications

Infants—Check skin turgor on the abdomen.

 Older adults—Check skin turgor over the sternum or clavicle.* ▼

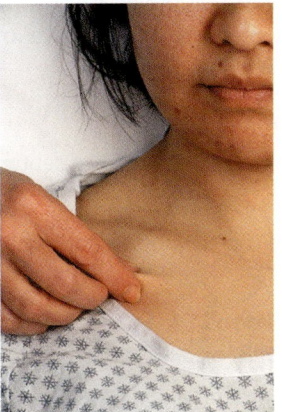

Expected findings: Skin returns immediately to its original position.

Developmental Variation

 Older adults—Decreased skin turgor due to decreased elasticity.

Abnormal findings: Decreased or increased turgor.
- *Tenting (decreased turgor):* Skin takes several seconds to return to original position.
- *Decreased turgor (tenting)* is seen with dehydration or normal aging. It predisposes the patient to skin breakdown.
- *Increased turgor:* Skin tension does not allow the skin to be pinched up; may be due to edema or scleroderma.

---

4. Palpate the skin for texture.
   Texture varies, depending on the area being assessed and the age of the client.

Expected findings: Skin is smooth and soft. Exposed areas and extensor surfaces (e.g., elbows and knees) are drier and coarser than other areas.

Developmental Variations

Infants and young children—Have smooth skin.

Abnormal findings: Coarse, thick, rough, or dry skin; very smooth, thin, fine-textured, shiny skin

---

5. Palpate skin for moisture/hydration. Use the dorsum of your hand.

Expected findings: Skin is warm and dry.

Developmental Variations

 Older adults—Skin may be dry and flaky because of decreased activity of sebaceous and sweat glands.

Adolescents—May have skin that is oilier than normal.

Abnormal findings: Increased moisture (skin feels damp, visible diaphoresis); decreased moisture (skin feels dry)

(continued on next page)

Procedure 21-2 ■ **Assessing the Skin** (continued)

6. Inspect for edema.
a. Press firmly with your fingertip for 5 sec over a bony area, such as the tibia.
b. Release your finger, and observe the skin for the reaction.
c. If edema is present, note the location, degree, and type of swelling. For example, if you observe edema in the lower leg, how far up the leg does it extend?

Expected findings: No edema. Normally there will be no evidence of the pressure once you release your finger. If pitting edema is present, you will see a depression in the skin.

Grading System

Trace: Minimal depression with pressure.

+1: 2-mm depression; rapid return of skin to position.

+2: 4-mm depression that disappears in 10–15 sec.

+3: 6-mm depression that lasts 1–2 min. Area appears swollen.

+4: 8-mm depression that persists for 2–3 min. Area is grossly edematous.

Abnormal findings: Edema is an abnormal finding.

7. Identify any skin lesions.
a. Inspect and palpate lesions.
b. When you notice bruises, be alert for signs of abuse (see Chapter 9).
c. Ask the client: "Do you have any new moles or other lesions? Has there been any change in existing moles/lesions?"
d. Assess for malignant lesions using ABCDE:
   A. (asymmetry)
   B. (irregular borders)
   C. (color variations)
   D. (diameter > 0.5 cm)
   E. (elevation).

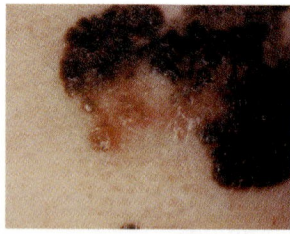

Malignant melanoma

Expected findings: No lesions are present.

Normal variations include moles, freckles, birthmarks, striae (in pregnant women or clients who have lost much weight), and wrinkles.

Developmental Variations

Newborns—**Milia** (tiny collections of sebum, usually on the face) are common.

Adolescents—Acne is a common, abnormal finding among adolescents.

Adults—**Acrochordons** (skin tags) may be seen around the neck, axillae, skinfolds, or areas where clothing rubs.

Older adults—Flat beige or brown macules are common on exposed skin areas.

Abnormal findings: See Describing Skin Lesions, following, and the table Describing Skin Lesions following this procedure.

Describing Skin Lesions

When you observe a lesion, evaluate and describe the following:
■ **Size.** Measure the length, width, and depth of the lesion.
■ **Shape and pattern.** Describe the *shape* of individual lesions. If there are clusters or groups, describe the *pattern*. Is it linear or circular? Are the *borders* distinct, or do they run together? Is the border smooth or irregular?
■ **Color.** Describe the color of the lesion, and determine whether there is any variation of color within the lesion.
■ **Distribution.** Are the lesions distributed over the entire body? Are they confined to a specific region? What parts of the body are affected?

■ **Texture.** The texture (e.g., smooth, rough, scaly) of a lesion helps with classification.
■ **Surface relationship.** To assess surface relationship, you will need to palpate the lesion. Is it flat, raised, or depressed? Is it firmly attached to the surrounding skin or mobile?
■ **Exudate.** Examine the lesion(s) for signs of drainage. Describe the color, appearance, amount, and odor of drainage, if present.
■ **Tenderness, pain, or itching.** Press on the lesion, and determine the patient's reaction. Does touching the lesion cause pain or discomfort?

Patient Teaching

Teach the patient the signs and symptoms of skin cancer, the importance of the skin exam, and preventive measures.

Home Care

- Assess the skill level of the caregiver. Instruct the caregiver in the importance of skin assessment and measures to prevent skin breakdown.

- ✚ Be alert for lesions (e.g., burns, bruises) that may signal physical abuse. For more signs of abuse, refer to Procedure 9-1.

Documentation

- If lesions are present, describe the history: onset, duration, associated or aggravating factors (e.g., itching), factors that relieve symptoms, treatments that have been used, and responses to treatment.
- Sketch the location of skin lesions on body diagrams, if available (see example); or sketch a body if necessary.

If you need more information about documenting, review Documenting Physical Examination Findings (Nam Nguyen) earlier in the Theoretical Knowledge section of this chapter. ▼

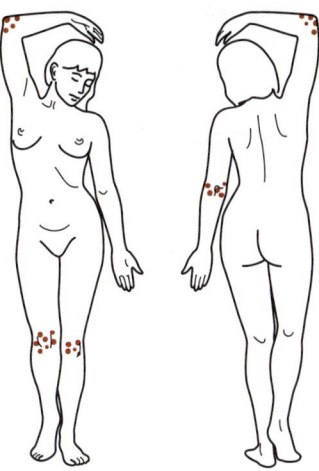

Practice Resources

Kottner, J., & Surber, C. (2016); Linton, C. P. (2011), Reddy, M. (2008).

Describing Skin Lesions		
PRIMARY LESIONS		
Types		**Description**
Macule (nonpalpable, < 1 cm)	Macule (nonpalpable, < 1 cm)	Flat and colored. Examples: freckle, petechiae, birthmark, mongolian spot
Papule (palpable), < 1 cm; plaque, > 1 cm 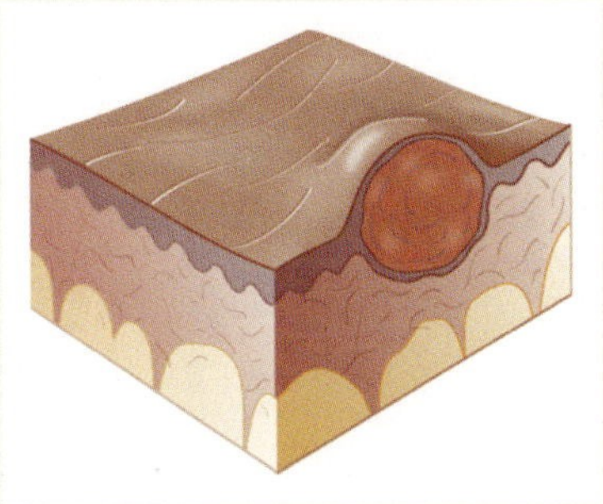	Papules (seborrheic keratosis) 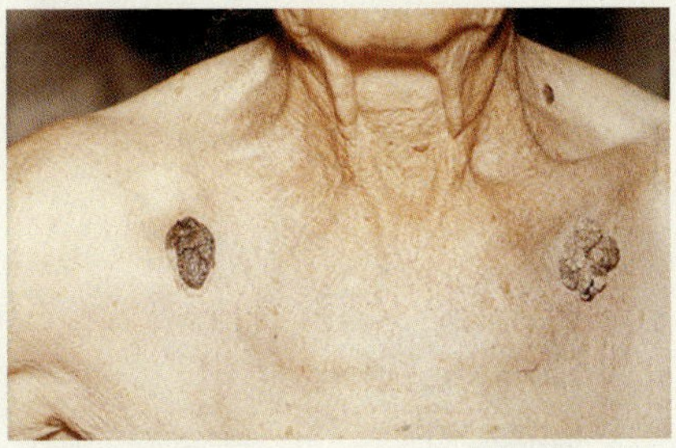	Elevated and raised, but superficial. Examples: mole, psoriasis

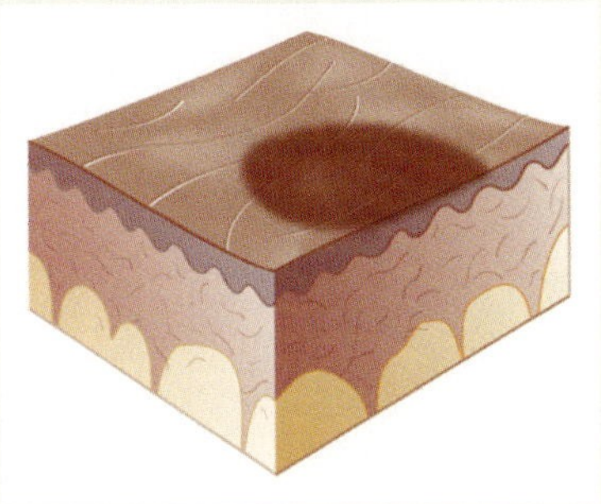

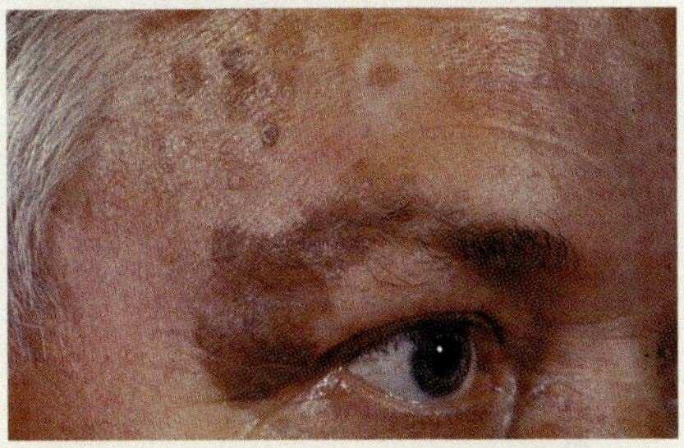

(continued on next page)

Procedure 21-2 ■ Assessing the Skin (continued)

Describing Skin Lesions—cont'd

PRIMARY LESIONS

Types		Description
Vesicle (palpable), < 1 cm; bulla, > 1 cm 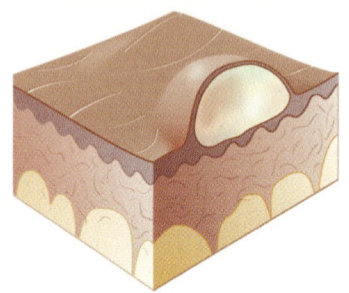	Vesicles (blisters) 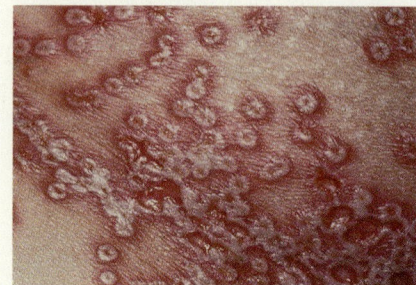 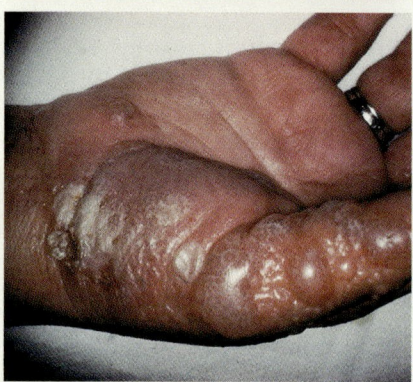	Elevated and filled with serous fluid. Examples: blister, herpes simplex
Cyst (palpable), < 2 cm 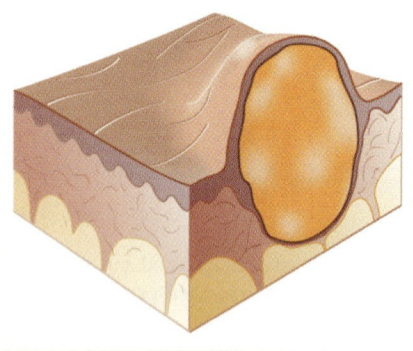	Keratogenous cyst 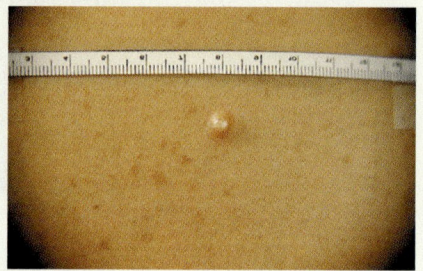	Palpable, fluid filled, and encapsulated. If not fluid filled, called a *nodule*
Pustule (palpable). 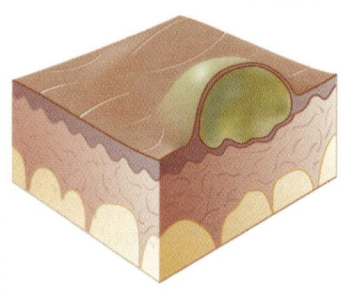	Pustules (acne) 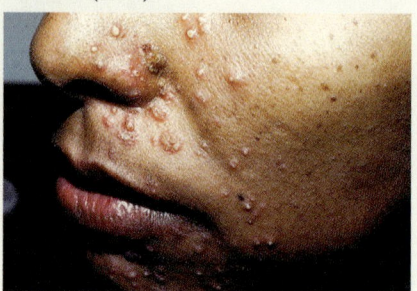	Elevated and filled with pus. Examples: acne, folliculitis, impetigo

Describing Skin Lesions—cont'd

PRIMARY LESIONS

Types		Description
	Nodule (palpable) 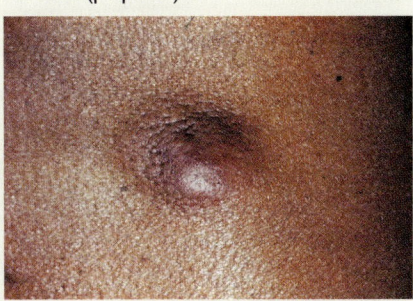	Elevated, solid, and firm, with depth into dermis. Examples: wart, lipoma (fatty cyst)
Wheal 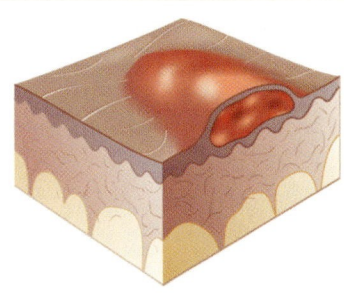	Hive 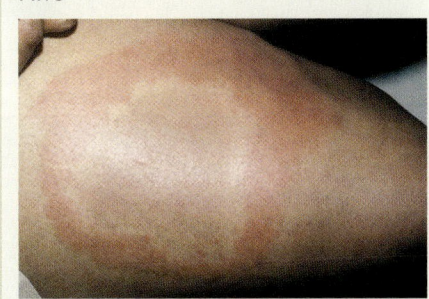	Elevated, superficial, with localized edema. Examples: insect bites, hives

SECONDARY LESIONS

Excoriation 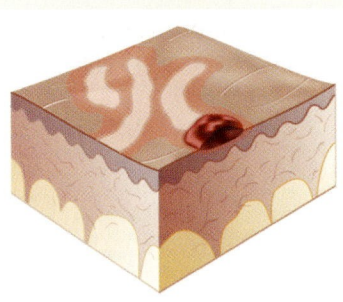	Excoriation from pruritus 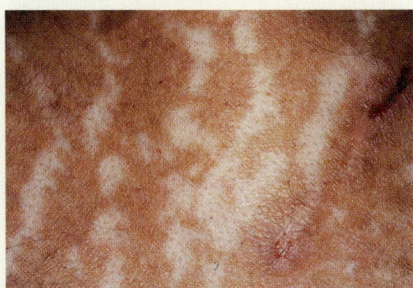	Abrasion or loss of skin that does not extend beyond the superficial epidermis. Examples: scratches, stasis dermatitis, atopic dermatitis
Erosion 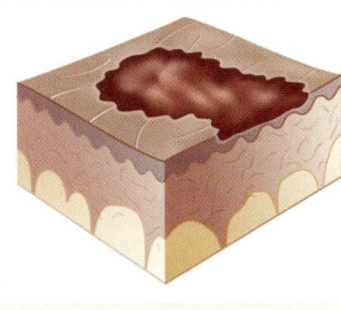	Erosions 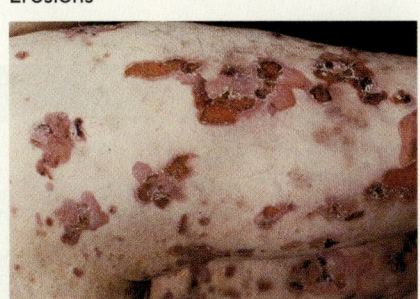	Loss of superficial epidermis, usually secondary to rupture of a blister. Examples: abrasions and impetigo

(continued on next page)

Procedure 21-2 ■ Assessing the Skin (continued)

Describing Skin Lesions—cont'd
SECONDARY LESIONS

Types		Description
Fissure 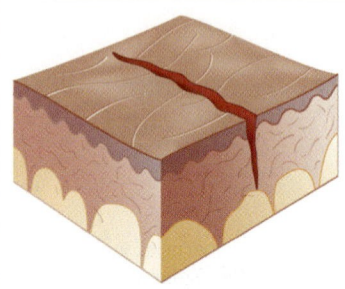	Cheilitis 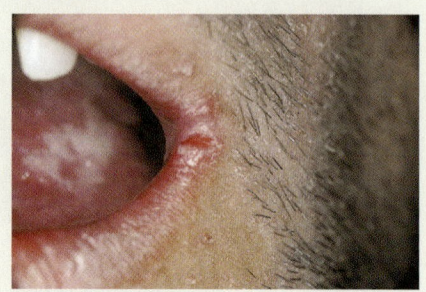	Linear break in the skin ("crack"); may extend to the dermis. Examples: athlete's foot, cheilitis
Ulcer 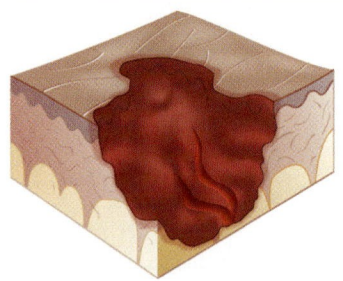	Stasis ulcer 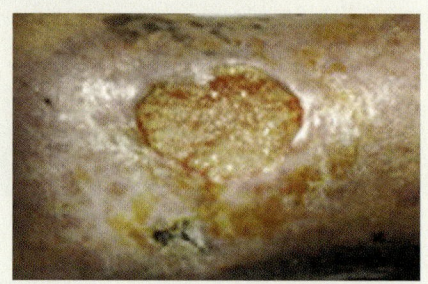	Irregularly shaped with loss of tissue. Graded based on depth and tissue involvement. Examples: pressure ulcers, stasis ulcers
Crust 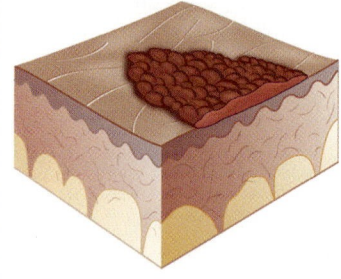	Crust 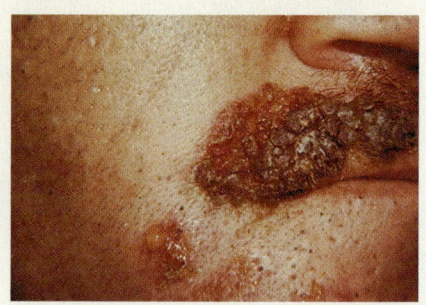	Elevated, rough texture with dried exudate. Examples: impetigo, herpes simplex
Scales 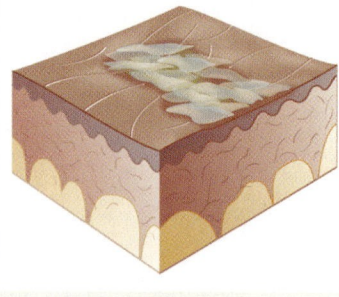	Psoriasis 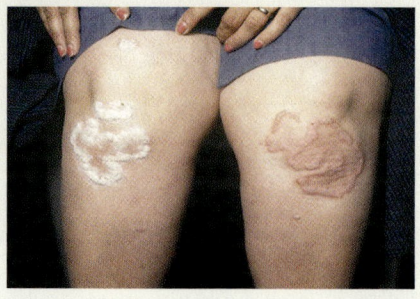	White to tan flaking, dead skin cells; may be adherent or loose. Examples: psoriasis and dandruff

Describing Skin Lesions—cont'd

SECONDARY LESIONS

Types		Description
Scar		Fibrous tissue at site of injury, trauma, or surgery. Examples: surgical site, trauma site
Keloid	Keloids	Raised and irregular scar due to excess collagen formation. Examples: surgical scars, ear piercing

Sources: Linton, C. P. (2011). Describing the configuration of skin lesions. *Journal of the Dermatology Nurses' Association, 3*(6), 379; Reddy, M. (2008). Skin and wound care: Important considerations in the older adult. *Advances in Skin & Wound Care, 21*(9), 424–436..

Procedure 21-3 ■ Assessing the Hair

➤ For steps to follow in *all* procedures, refer to the Universal Steps for All Procedures found on the page facing the inside back cover.

Equipment

- Nonlatex procedure gloves (if exposure to body fluids is a possibility)
- Pen and record form

Focused History Questions

- Have you had any changes in hair texture?
- Have you had any hair loss?
- Do you use dyes or chemical treatments for curling or straightening?

(continued on next page)

Procedure 21-3 ■ **Assessing the Hair** (continued)

➤ When performing the procedure, always identify your patient according to agency policy, using two identifiers, and be attentive to standard precautions, hand hygiene, patient safety and privacy, body mechanics, and documentation.

Procedure Steps

1. **Inspect the hair and scalp.** Check the color, quantity, and distribution of the hair and the condition of the scalp. Note the presence of lesions or pediculosis.

   Sex, genetics, and age affect hair distribution on the head, legs extremities, pubis, and axillae. With aging, melanocyte function declines and sebaceous gland function decreases.

Findings

Expected findings: The hair is evenly distributed on the scalp, and fine body hair is present over the body (men often have more hair on face, chest, and back; alopecia is considered normal in men). The hair is clean and free of debris or pediculosis.

Developmental Variations

Infants—May have very little scalp hair.

   Adolescents—May have oily hair. Puberty marks the onset of pubic hair growth and increased hair growth.

      Older adults—Scalp, axillary, leg, and pubic hair may be dry and thin; hair of the ears, nostrils, and eyebrows may become coarse.

Abnormal findings:
- Generalized hair loss not attributed to genetics or aging; patchy hair loss.
- **Hirsutism** (excess facial or trunk hair).
- White hair accompanied by very pale skin is seen in a condition known as **albinism** (lack of pigment).
- Alterations in hair distribution may be signs of disease.

2. **Palpate the texture of the hair.**

Expected findings: Hair texture varies (fine, medium, coarse) depending on genetics and treatments.

Abnormal findings: Very coarse, dry hair may indicate hypothyroidism; thinning and very fine hair may indicate hyperthyroidism.

3. **Palpate the scalp for mobility and tenderness.**

Expected findings: Scalp is smooth, firm, symmetrical, nontender, and without lesions.

Abnormal findings: Common deviations include an asymmetrical or bumpy scalp due to trauma or lesions and scaly flakes or patches due to fungal infection (e.g., dandruff), dermatitis, or psoriasis. Tenderness, lesions.

Developmental Variation

Infants: In newborns **cradle cap**—scaly white patches over the scalp due to secretion of sebum—is common. It can be removed with washing and gentle scrubbing.

Patient Teaching

If indicated, teach the patient to check for head lice, and provide preventive measures.

Documentation

If you need more information about documenting, review Caring for the Nguyens and Documenting Physical Examination Findings (Nam Nguyen).

Procedure 21-4 ■ Assessing the Nails

➤ For steps to follow in *all* procedures, refer to the Universal Steps for All Procedures found on the page facing the inside back cover.

Equipment

- Nonlatex gloves (if exposure to body fluids is a possibility)
- Pen and record form

Focused History Questions

- Have you had any recent changes in the way your nails grow or look?
- Have you had any recent trauma to your nails?
- Do you use acrylic nails?
- Do you have any medical problems, such as peripheral vascular disease or diabetes?

➤ When performing the procedure, always identify your patient according to agency policy, using two identifiers, and be attentive to standard precautions, hand hygiene, patient safety and privacy, body mechanics, and documentation.

Procedure Steps

1. **Inspect nails.**
   - Check nails for color, condition, texture, and shape.
   - Examine nails on both hands and feet. However, for efficiency you may defer examination of the toenails until the assessment of peripheral circulation. ▼

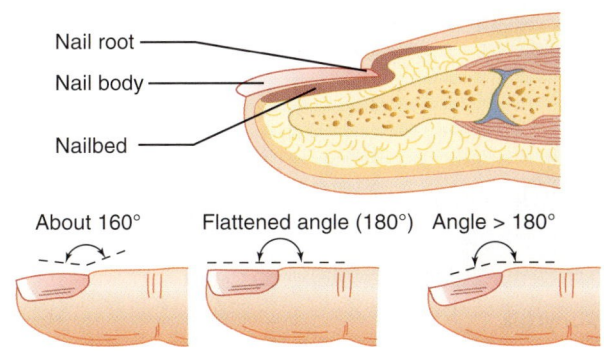

Nail root
Nail body
Nailbed

About 160°   Flattened angle (180°)   Angle > 180°

Findings

Expected findings: Healthy nailbeds are level, firm, and similar to the color of the skin. The shape is convex, with a nail plate angle of about 160°.

Developmental Variations

Newborns—Have very thin nails.

Children—May bite their nails. Most children outgrow this habit.

Older adults—Nails grow more slowly, become thicker, and tend to split.

Abnormal findings:

- Black discoloration resulting from blood under the nail is seen after local trauma.
- Pale or cyanotic nailbeds are seen in circulatory or respiratory disorders that result in anemia or hypoxia.
- White spots may indicate zinc deficiency.
- Spoon-shaped (concave) nails are associated with iron deficiency.

2. **Inspect and palpate for texture.**
   Grooves or lines in the nails provide information about nutrition and health problems.

Expected findings: Nails are smooth and uniform in texture; surrounding tissue is smooth.

Abnormal findings: Thickened nails with yellowing may indicate fungal infection, known as *onychomycosis*.

- Brittle nails are seen with hyperthyroidism, malnutrition, calcium and iron deficiencies, and repeated use of harsh nail products.
- Soft boggy nails are seen with poor oxygenation.
- Paronychia.

(continued on next page)

Procedure 21-4 ■ Assessing the Nails (continued)

3. **Assess capillary refill:** Briefly press the tip of the nail with firm, steady pressure; then release and observe for changes in color.

This test assesses circulatory adequacy rather than the nails themselves. However, circulatory insufficiency affects the nails and nailbeds. It is convenient to perform the assessment at this point in the exam. ▼

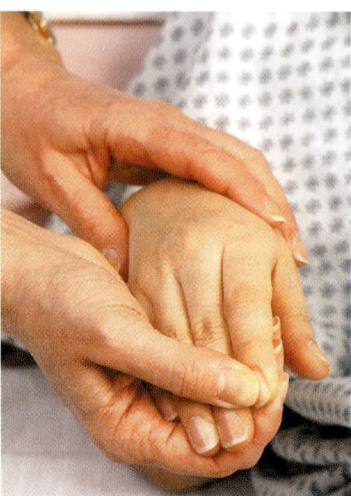

Expected findings: Normal capillary refill is < 2 to 3 sec.

Developmental Variations

 Older adults—Capillary refill time (CRT) is slower.

Males—CRT faster than in women

Environment—CRT is slower in a cool environment.

Abnormal findings: Delayed capillary refill.

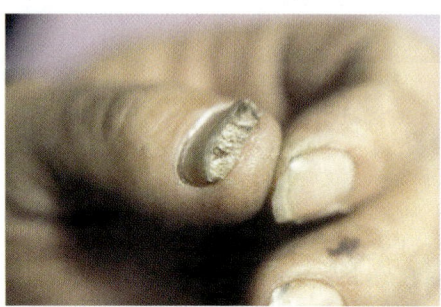

Fungal infection

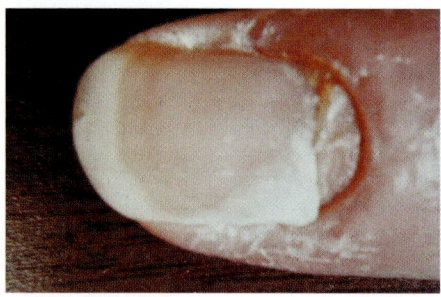

Paronychia

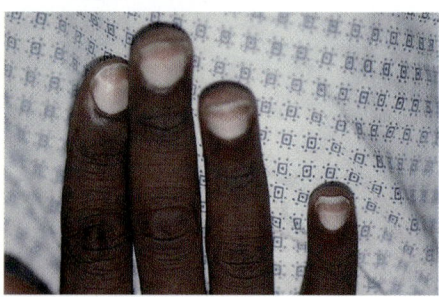

Half-and-half nails

Documentation

- If you need more information about documenting, review Caring for the Nguyens, including Documenting Physical Examination Findings (Nam Nguyen).

Practice Resources

Lima, A., & Bakker, J. (2015), Linton, C. P. (2012).

Procedure 21-5 ■ Assessing the Head and Face

➤ For steps to follow in *all* procedures, refer to the Universal Steps for All Procedures found on the page facing the inside back cover.

Equipment

- Nonlatex gloves (if exposure to body fluids is a possibility)
- Penlight (to transilluminate the sinuses)
- Pen and record form

Positioning

The client should be sitting, if possible.

Focused History Questions

- Have you had any recent headaches?
- Have you ever had a head injury or loss of consciousness?
- Have you ever had a seizure?
- Do you have jaw or facial pain?

➤ When performing the procedure, always identify your patient according to agency policy, using two identifiers, and be attentive to standard precautions, hand hygiene, patient safety and privacy, body mechanics, and documentation.

Procedure Steps

1. **Inspect the head: Check for size, shape, symmetry, and position.**
   If size seems unusual, measure it.

Developmental Modifications

Newborns and infants—Assess and transilluminate fontanels, and measure head circumference.

Findings

Expected findings: There is wide variation in head size and shape, although the shape should be symmetrical and rounded. The head should be erect, midline, and proportional to the body size based on age.

Developmental Variations

Newborns and infants—Cranial bones are not fused at birth, and head shape may reflect normal pressure or trauma during vaginal birth for several weeks. The anterior fontanel ("soft spot") fuses at about 18 mo; the posterior, at about 8 wk. Infants normally cannot hold their head up until about 6 mo.

Abnormal findings: Larger or smaller than expected size for age; asymmetry of skull.

2. **Inspect the face.** Note the client's facial expression. Ask yourself:
   - Are the facial features symmetrical?
   - Are there any abnormal facial movements?
   - Are there any visible lesions or abnormal hair distribution?

   Helpful hint: Look for symmetry in the palpebral fissures and the nasolabial folds. ▼

Expected findings: Facial expression is appropriate for the situation. No visible lesions. Facial features and movement are symmetrical.

Abnormal findings: Facial appearance inconsistent with sex, age, or racial/ethnic group; asymmetry of facial features or facial movement. ▼

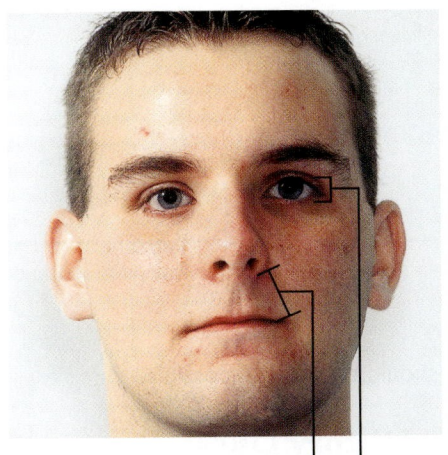

Nasolabial fold
Palpebral fissure

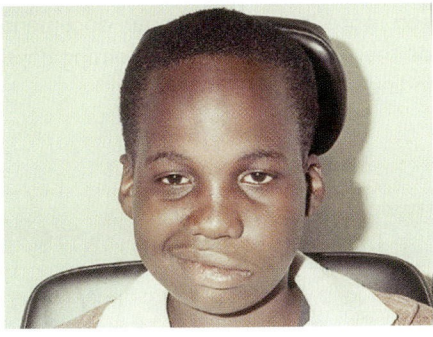

Bell's palsy

(continued on next page)

Procedure 21-5 ■ Assessing the Head and Face (continued)

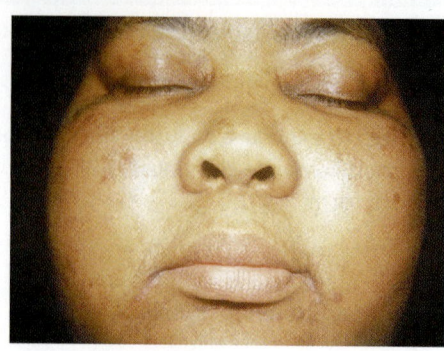

Cushing's syndrome

3. Palpate the head. Check for masses, tenderness, and scalp mobility.

Developmental Modifications

Newborns and infants—Palpate anterior and posterior fontanels.

Expected findings: The head should be nontender, relatively smooth and symmetrical; and with unusual contours, bulges, or lesions.

Abnormal findings: Contour abnormalities (e.g., indentations, "bumps") or tenderness can result from trauma, congenital anomalies, or surgery.

4. Palpate the face for symmetry, tenderness, muscle tone, and temporomandibular joint (TMJ) function. ▼

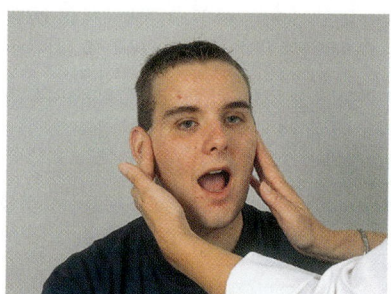

Palpating the TMJ

Expected findings: Smooth, symmetrical movement with no pain, crepitus, or clicking of the jaw

Abnormal findings: Irregular or uneven movement of the jaw; pain or popping/cracking with movement may indicate TMJ syndrome.

Documentation

- If you need more information about documenting, review Caring for the Nguyens and Documenting Physical Examination Findings (Nam Nguyen).

Procedure 21-6 ■ Assessing the Eyes

➤ For steps to follow in *all* procedures, refer to the Universal Steps for All Procedures found on the page facing the inside back cover.

Equipment

- Nonlatex gloves—if exposure to body fluids is a possibility
- Visual acuity chart with color bars (Snellen)
- A card—to cover one eye during the acuity exam
- Penlight
- Cotton ball and cotton-tipped applicator
- Ophthalmoscope
- Pen and form

Position

The client should be sitting, if possible.

Focused History Questions

- Have you noticed any changes in your vision?
- Do you wear glasses or contact lenses?
- Have you ever had an eye injury?
- Have you ever had an eye infection or stye?

- Do you have problems with excessive tearing or dry eyes?
- Have you ever had eye surgery?
- Have you ever experienced blurred vision?
- Do you have difficulty with nighttime vision?
- Do you ever see halos of light, spots or floaters, or flashes of light?

- Do you have a history of eye problems, such as glaucoma, or medical problems, such as diabetes or hypertension?
- When was your last eye exam?
- Do you use any prescription or over-the-counter eye medications?

➤ When performing the procedure, always identify your patient according to agency policy, using two identifiers, and be attentive to standard precautions, hand hygiene, patient safety and privacy, body mechanics, and documentation.

Procedure Steps

1. **Test distance vision.**
   - Depending on patient's age and literacy level, use the Snellen standard eye chart or Snellen E chart (for those who cannot read). Picture charts are available for preschoolers.
   - If the client wears corrective lenses, they should be worn during a test.
   a. Have the patient sit or stand 6 m (20 ft) from the chart. With a card, cover the eye not being tested; ask the patient to read the smallest line of print that he can distinguish. Consider a line to be read correctly if the client makes no more than two mistakes in that line. If he hesitates when reporting the letters or symbols, document "with hesitation."
   b. Test the opposite eye.
   c. Test both eyes together.
   d. At the end of each line of the Snellen chart is a fraction—the top line is 20/200. After each test, record the resulting fraction: the number at the end of the smallest line the patient could read with no more than two errors. If there were more than 2 errors in a line, record the number of items missed. ▼

Findings

Expected findings: 20/20 vision in the right eye, left eye, and both eyes. The top number of the fraction indicates the distance the person was standing from the chart; the bottom number is the distance from which a person with normal vision would be able to read the chart.

Developmental Variations

Children—Distance vision does not reach 20/20 until around age 6 or 7 yr.

Middle adults—At about middle age, the lens of the eye begins to lose some ability to accommodate to near objects.

Abnormal findings: A smaller fraction (e.g., 20/100) indicates diminished distant vision or *myopia*. A larger fraction (e.g., 20/15) indicates diminished near vision, called *hyperopia*.

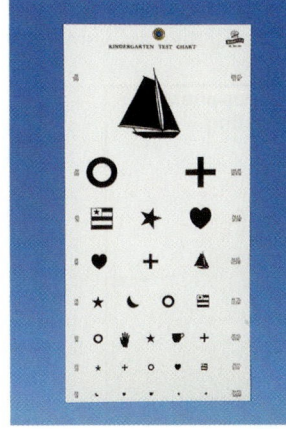
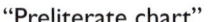

"Preliterate chart"

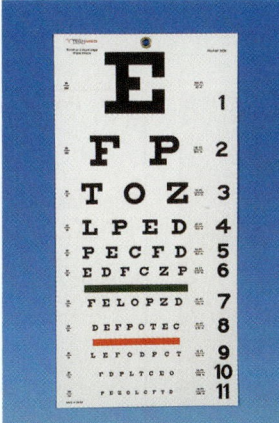

"Snellen Standard"

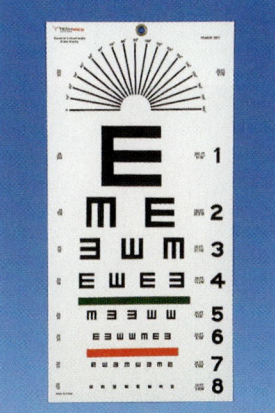

"Snellen E chart"

2. **Test near vision.** Test the client's ability to read newsprint at a distance of 35.5 cm (14 in.) from the eyes. Use print-sized pictures if the patient is unable to read.

Expected findings: The client reads newsprint at a distance of 35.5 cm (14 in.).

Developmental Variation

Adults: The lens of the eye naturally loses some ability to accommodate to near objects. In clients older than 45 years of age, diminished near vision is known as presbyopia.

(continued on next page)

Procedure 21-6 ■ **Assessing the Eyes** (continued)

3. Test color vision.

  a. Have the patient differentiate patterns of colors on color cards or identify the color bars on the Snellen eye chart.

  b. Inability to distinguish colors requires a thorough evaluation using the Ishihara cards to determine the scope of the color deficit. ▼

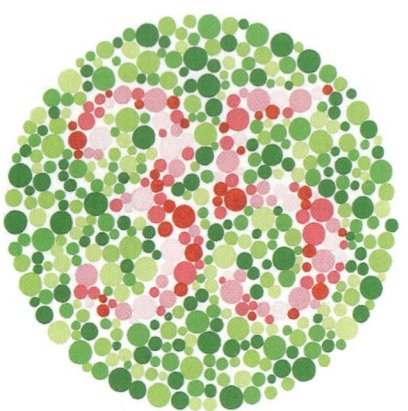

Ishihara card

Abnormal findings: The need to hold the print at a greater distance indicates **hyperopia** or **presbyopia.**

Expected findings: Color vision is intact.

🍁 *Developmental Variations*

Older adults—Experience some decline in color vision, especially in the ability to see purples and pastels.

Abnormal findings: Inability to distinguish colors.

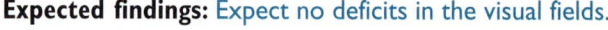

4. Test peripheral vision.

  a. Seat the client 60–90 cm (2–3 ft) from you.

  b. Have client cover one eye and fix the gaze straight ahead while you bring an object in from the periphery to the center of the visual fields. Be sure to begin by holding the object well outside the range of normal peripheral vision. Instruct the client to identify when the object becomes visible.

  c. Repeat this in each of the four visual fields, moving clockwise.

Expected findings: Expect no deficits in the visual fields.

Abnormal findings:

■ **Strabismus** (crossed eye) is a condition in which one or both eyes deviate from the object they are looking at. Constant strabismus of one eye may result in **amblyopia** ("lazy eye"), in which the brain does not fully acknowledge the images seen by the amblyopic eye. This creates reduced vision in that eye, not correctable by glasses or contact lenses

■ Loss of peripheral vision. Report gross deficits to an ophthalmologist for further assessment. ▼

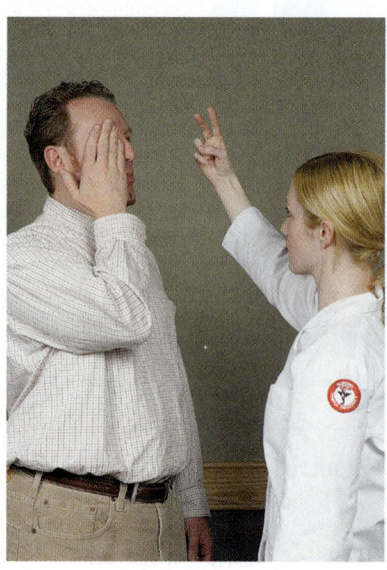

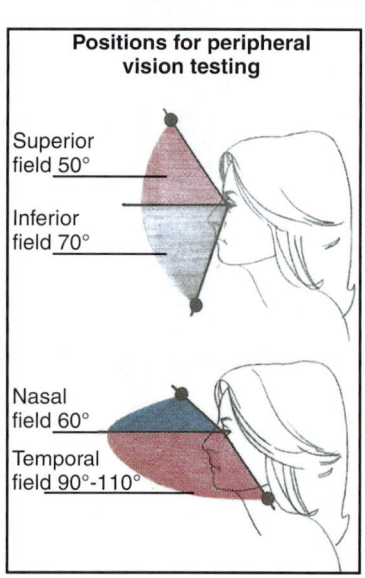

Positions for peripheral vision testing

Superior field 50°

Inferior field 70°

Nasal field 60°

Temporal field 90°-110°

Developmental Variation

Infants: Strabismus is normal during the first 1 or 2 months of life. After that, it may be caused by weak intraocular muscles or a lesion on the oculomotor nerve.

5. Assess extraocular movements.

  a. **Inspect the eyes for parallel alignment.**

  b. **Test the corneal light reflex** by shining a penlight at the bridge of the nose. Note where the light reflects on the cornea of each eye.

  c. **Test the six cardinal fields of gaze.** Stand in front of the patient, and have the patient follow an object through the six cardinal fields without moving his head. ▼

  a. **Expected findings:** The eyes should be in parallel alignment.

  b. **Expected findings:** Corneal light reflex appears at the same position in each eye.

Abnormal findings: An asymmetrical corneal light reflex may indicate weak extraocular muscles or strabismus.

  c. **Expected findings:** The eyes move through all six gaze positions.

Abnormal findings: Inability to move through all gaze positions.

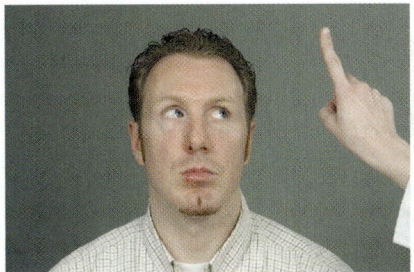

Up Left

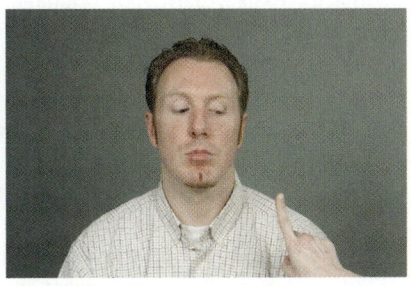

Side Left

Down Left

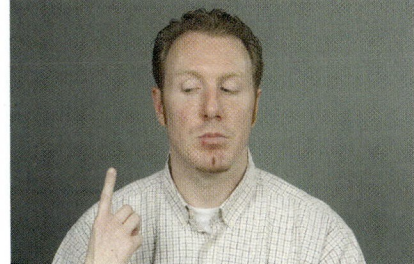

Down right

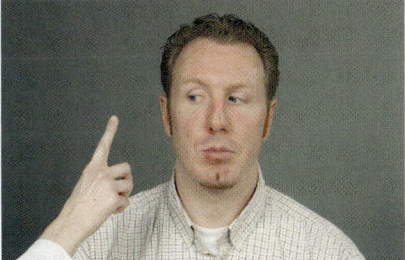

Side right

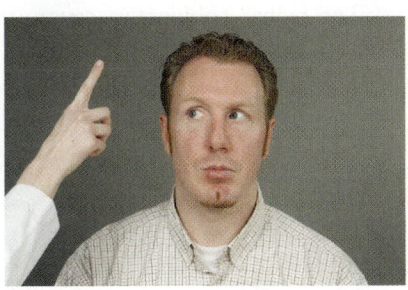

Up right

  d. **Perform the cover/uncover test.** Cover one eye and have the patient gaze at a distant object. Uncover the eye. Repeat on the opposite side.

  d. **Expected findings:** The gaze should be steady when the eye is covered and uncovered.

Abnormal findings: A shift in gaze indicates weak eye muscles.

6. Inspect the external structures.

  a. **General appearance:** Check the color and alignment of the eyes.

  a. **Expected findings:** Eyes clear, bright, and in parallel alignment.

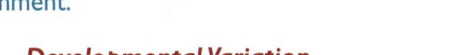 ***Developmental Variation***

Older adults—A decrease in periorbital fat may give the eyeballs a sunken appearance.

Abnormal findings: Glazed eyes may indicate a febrile state.

  b. **Inspect eyelids.** Note the presence of any lesions, edema, or lid lag (ptosis).

  b. **Expected findings:** Eyelid margins moist and pink. No crusting, scales, or lesions present; lids move freely. Upper eyelid covers half of the upper iris; lower eyelid appears at bottom edge of iris.

Developmental Variation

Older adults—The lower lids may sag; skinfolds are prominent in the upper lids.

Abnormal findings: Asymmetry of lids may result from CN III damage or from a stroke. Lesions may be benign (e.g., a stye) or pathological (e.g., basal cell carcinoma).

(continued on next page)

Procedure 21-6 ■ Assessing the Eyes (continued)

c. **Inspect the eyelashes.** Note symmetry and distribution.

c. **Expected findings:** Eyelashes are evenly distributed and curve outward. No crustations or infestations are present.

Abnormal findings: Inflammation of the eyelids, which may be caused by infection; inverted eyelashes (entropion); everted eyelashes (ectropion); visible sclera between the iris and upper lid.

d. **Inspect the lacrimal ducts and glands.** Note any edema, excessive tearing, or drainage.

d. **Expected findings:** No periorbital edema or lesions are present. No drainage.

Abnormal findings: Swelling, redness, drainage, or tenderness.

e. **Inspect the conjunctivae.** Note the color, moisture, and contour of the conjunctivae.
   (1) The palpebral conjunctivae cover the lids. To assess, have the patient look up as you place a cotton-tipped applicator on the upper lid, gently grasp the upper lid and lashes, and evert the lid over the cotton-tipped applicator.
   (2) The bulbar conjunctiva covers the eyeball. To assess, pull the lower lid down. ▼

e. **Expected findings:** The *palpebral conjunctivae* are smooth, glistening, and peach in color. Minimal blood vessels are present. The *bulbar conjunctivae* are clear with few underlying blood vessels and white sclera visible.

    Developmental Variation

Older adults—The conjunctivae may be pale or have a slightly yellow tint due to fat deposits.

Abnormal findings: Pallor, dryness, edema; pterygium; subconjunctival hemorrhage.

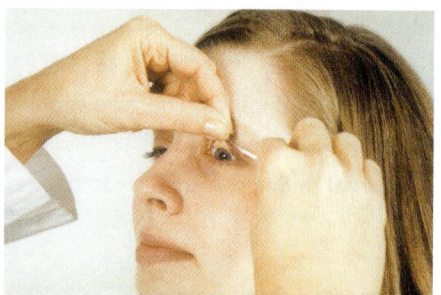

Examining the palpebral conjunctiva

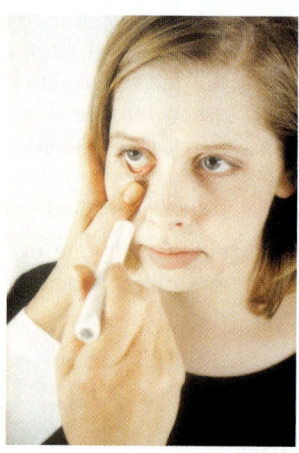

Examining the bulbar conjunctiva

f. **Inspect the sclera.** Note the color of the sclera and whether lesions are present.

f. **Expected findings:** The sclera should be smooth, white, and glistening. Dark-skinned patients may have a yellowish cast to the peripheral sclera or small brown spots more centrally.

Abnormal findings: Yellow (icteric) sclera.

g. **Inspect the cornea and lens.** As the client looks straight ahead, shine a penlight at an angle to the eye, and move it across the corneal surface. Note the color and whether any lesions are present.

g. **Expected findings:** The cornea and lens are clear, smooth, and glistening.

Older adults—Arcus senilis (white, gray, or blue opaque ring in the corneal margin) is a normal variant.

Abnormal findings: Lens opacities (cataracts); roughness or irregularity of the cornea.

h. **Test the corneal reflex.** Touch the cornea with a wisp of sterile cotton, or use a needleless syringe to shoot a small amount of air over the cornea.

> ✚ *NOTE:* This is not routinely performed on conscious patients. A conscious person can blink intentionally, so there is no need. In addition, there is a slight risk of corneal abrasion from cotton.

i. **Inspect the iris and pupils.** Note the color, size, shape, and symmetry.

j. **Test pupillary reaction.** In a dimly lighted room, have the patient look straight ahead. Bring a penlight in from the side, and shine the light onto one eye. Note the reaction, equality, and speed of response of both eyes. (For example, when you shine a light onto the right eye, the right pupil reaction is direct; the left eye is consensual.) Repeat the test on the opposite eye. ▼

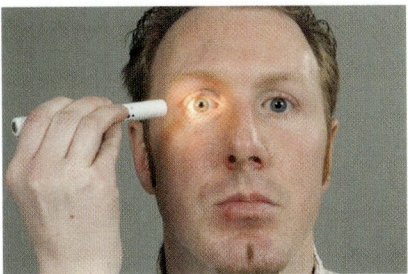

Testing pupillary reaction to light

k. **Test pupil accommodation.** Have the patient look straight ahead and focus on an object about 30 cm (12 in.) from his face. Slowly bring the object in toward the patient's eyes. Note pupil size and location.

h. **Expected findings:** Blink reflex is prompt.

Abnormal findings: Failure to blink may result from neurosensory deficits.

i. **Expected findings:**
- The iris is blue, green, brown, or a combination of these colors; its shape is circular.
- The pupils are round and of equal size. Unequal pupils **(anisocoria)** can be a normal variation if the difference is less than 0.5 mm.

🍁 *Developmental Variation*

Older adults—Pigment degeneration may cause the iris to be pale with brownish discolorations.

Abnormal findings:
- Damage to one eye may cause the iris to be a different color.
- Absence of part or all of the iris is a congenital problem.
- Unequal pupils (anisocoria) may result from CN III damage, stroke, brain herniation, or increased intracranial pressure.
- Enlarged pupils (mydriasis); constricted pupils (myosis).
- Cloudy pupils.

j. **Expected findings:** Normal direct and consensual response to light is brisk, with equal constriction of both pupils.

🍁 *Developmental Variation*

Older adults—Pupil reaction may be slower but should be symmetrical.

Abnormal findings: Sluggish or fixed pupils may result from CN III damage or brain injury. Absence of consensual response may result from nerve compression or anoxia.

k. **Expected findings:** The pupils constrict and the eyes cross as a person attempts to focus on a near object.

🍁 *Development Variation*

Older adults—Accommodation may be slow.

Abnormal findings: One or both pupils fail to accommodate, or they accommodate slowly.

(continued on next page)

Procedure 21-6 ■ Assessing the Eyes (continued)

l. **Inspect the anterior chamber.** Shine a penlight across the eye from the side as the patient looks straight ahead. Observe color, size, shape, and symmetry. ▼

l. **Expected findings:** The chamber should be clear and symmetrically curved.

Abnormal findings: Blood or pus in the chamber.

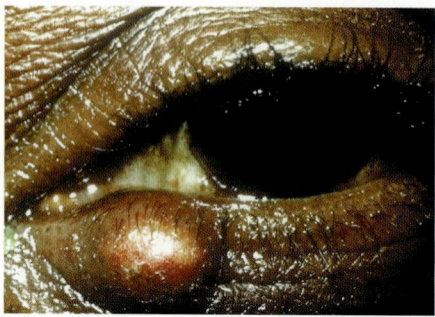

Hordeoleum

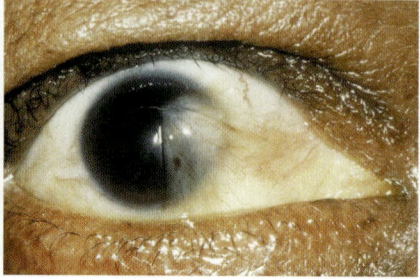

Pterygium

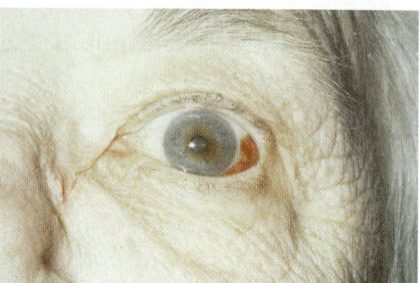

Subconjunctival hemorrhage

7. **Palpate the external structures.**
   a. Gently palpate the globe (eyeball) with your fingertips on the upper lids over the sclera. Note the consistency and any tenderness. ▼

Expected findings: The globe is firm and nontender. Lacrimal glands are nonpalpable; no tenderness is present.

Abnormal findings: Firm or tender globe; swelling and tenderness over the lacrimal glands.

   b. Palpate the lacrimal glands and ducts by palpating below the eyebrow and below the inner canthus of the eye. Note tenderness and excessive tearing or discharge.

8. **Assess the internal structures via ophthalmoscopy.** This is an advanced physical assessment technique.
   a. Darken the room.
   b. Stand about 1 ft from the patient at a 15° lateral angle.
   c. Dial the lens wheel to zero with your index finger. Hold the ophthalmoscope to your brow.

Expected findings: A positive red light reflex. On internal examination, the optic disk is round with sharp margins. There are no opacities and the cup:disk ratio is 1:2. The disk is yellow with a white cup.

Abnormal findings: Any findings not consistent with the above should be reported promptly.

d. Have the patient look straight ahead while you shine the light on one pupil and identify the red light reflex. ▼

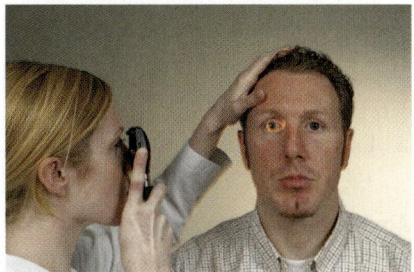

Checking red reflex

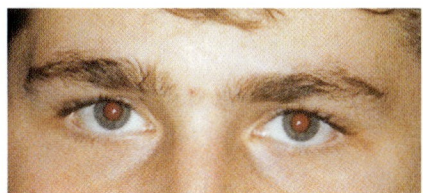

Red reflex over pupil area

e. Once you identify the red light reflex, move in closer to within a few inches of the eye and observe the internal structures of the eye. Adjust the lens wheel to focus as needed. Use your right eye to examine the patient's right eye, and your left eye to examine the patient's left eye. ▼

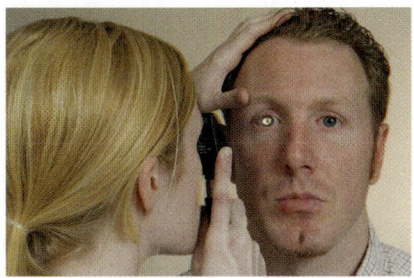

Examining internal structures of the eye

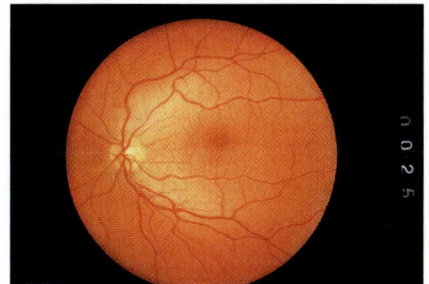

Normal fundus

f. **Repeat for the opposite eye.**

Patient Teaching

Teach the patient the importance of routine eye examinations.

Documentation

- If you need more information about documenting, review Caring for the Nguyens and Documenting Physical Examination Findings (Nam Nguyen).

Procedure 21-7 ■ Assessing the Ears and Hearing

➤ For steps to follow in *all* procedures, refer to the Universal Steps for All Procedures found on the page facing the inside back cover.

Equipment

- Nonlatex gloves (if exposure to body fluids is a possibility)
- Tuning fork
- Watch that ticks (or a similar device)
- Otoscope with pneumatic tube
- Pen and record form

Position

Have the patient seated, if possible.

Focused History Questions

- Do you have any hearing problems?
- Have you ever had ringing in your ears?
- Have you had any changes in your hearing?
- Do you have any ear drainage? If yes, how much and what color?
- Do you have any ear pain?
- Do you have any balance problems, dizziness, or vertigo?
- Do you have a history of head trauma?
- Are you exposed to noise pollution at work or in your home environment?

(continued on next page)

Procedure 21-7 ■ Assessing the Ears and Hearing (continued)

➤ When performing the procedure, always identify your patient according to agency policy, using two identifiers, and be attentive to standard precautions, hand hygiene, patient safety and privacy, body mechanics, and documentation.

Procedure Steps

1. Inspect the external ear.

a. Check the placement and angle of attachment of the ear. ▼

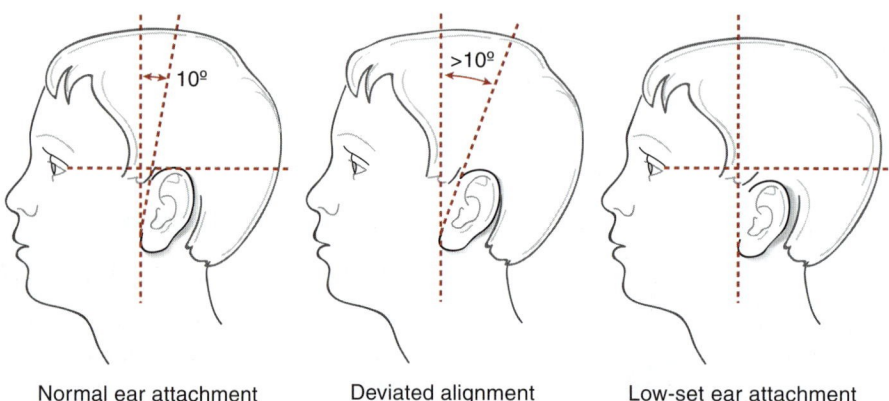

Normal ear attachment   Deviated alignment   Low-set ear attachment

b. Note the shape, size, and symmetry of the ears. ▼

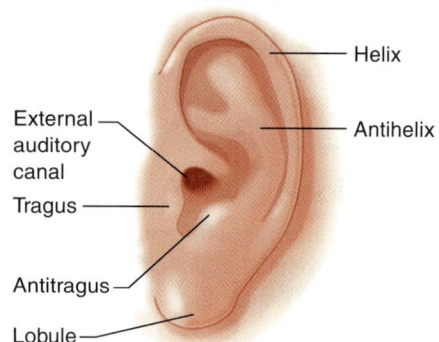

- Helix
- External auditory canal
- Antihelix
- Tragus
- Antitragus
- Lobule

c. Observe the color of the ear.

d. Observe the condition of the skin; observe for drainage and visible lesions.

Findings

a. **Expected findings:** The normal angle of attachment is 10° of vertical position.

Abnormal findings: High or low placement of the ear may be a sign of hearing deficit or genetic problems, for example Down syndrome.

b. **Expected findings:** The helix, antihelix, antitragus, tragus, and lobule are present. The ears are 4–10 cm in length and symmetrical in size and shape.

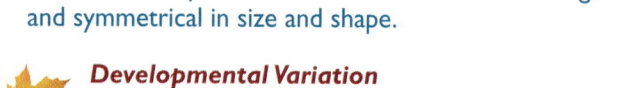 **Developmental Variation**

Older adults—The ear changes shape as the lobe elongates.

Abnormal findings: Absence of any of the landmarks may indicate a hearing deficit. Ears that are less than 4 cm long or greater 10 cm long may indicate a genetic disorder.

c. **Expected findings:** Color is consistent with skin color.

Abnormal findings: Redness may indicate inflammation or infection.

d. **Expected findings:** Skin is intact with no drainage or lesions. Piercings may be present.

Developmental Variations

Older adults—May have coarse hair on the helix, antihelix, and tragus; skin may be dry.

Abnormal findings: Bloody drainage may result from trauma. Purulent drainage may be seen with infection. The ears are a common location for skin cancer.

2. **Palpate the external structures of the ear.** Note the consistency of the skin, the presence of lesions, and any signs of tenderness.

Expected findings: Skin is soft, pliable, and nontender. No nodules or lesions are present.

Abnormal findings: Tenderness is often associated with infection (e.g., otitis externa, otitis media).

3. **Perform an otoscopic exam.**
   This is an advanced physical assessment technique.
   a. Use a speculum with the largest diameter and shortest length that the ear canal can accommodate. 4 mm is a common size for adults.
   b. Have the patient tilt his head to the side not being examined.
   c. For adults, grasp the pinna and gently pull upward and back. For a child, position the pinna down and back.
      Positions the ear canal with more direct alignment, allowing for improved visualization.
   d. Insert the speculum no further than halfway into the ear canal. As you advance the speculum, examine the canal for redness, open areas, drainage, foreign objects, and so on. ▼

Expected findings: The ear canal is light in color and patent, with a small amount of yellow cerumen (color may vary). Tympanic membrane (TM) is shiny, pearly gray, and translucent with a cone of reflective light on the nasal aspect (this would be 7 o'clock in the left ear and 5 o'clock in the right ear). Bony landmarks are visible through the TM. The TM is mobile. No bulging or retraction of the TM. ▼

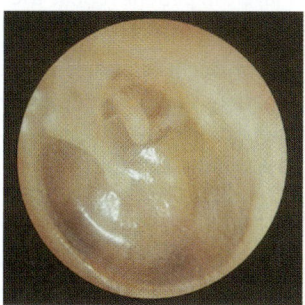

Normal TM left ear

Developmental Variations

Older adults—May have dry earwax. The TM is translucent, and the light reflex may be diminished.

Abnormal findings: Excessive wax may occlude the canal. TM that is red, with a distorted light reflex, suggests otitis media. A change in the position or shape of the cone of light reflex indicates an imbalance in middle ear pressure. ▼

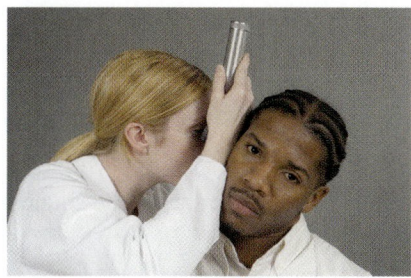

Otoscope insertion with handle up

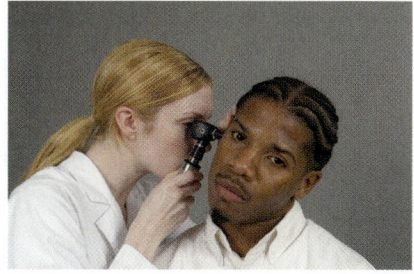

Otoscope insertion with handle down

   e. Look through the magnifying lens.
      (1) Observe the ear canal.
      (2) Observe the tympanic membrane.
   f. Test the mobility of the tympanic membrane by using the otoscope's pneumatic tube to gently "puff" air into the external ear canal while observing movement of the cone of light.

NOTE: The ears are mirror images, with the cone of light at 7 o'clock in the left ear and 5 o'clock in the right ear.

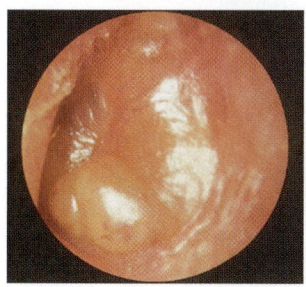

Otitis media

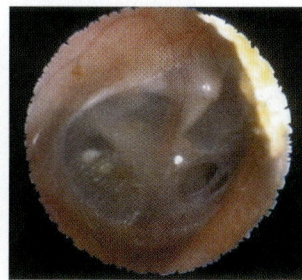

Perforated TM

(continued on next page)

Procedure 21-7 ■ **Assessing the Ears and Hearing** (continued)

Developmental Modifications

Children—Many young children fear the otoscopic examination. Demonstrating the procedure on a parent or a doll may relieve their anxiety.

    g. Carefully remove the otoscope from the ear canal, being careful not to traumatize the delicate tissue.

---

4. **Test gross hearing.**

    a. Stand 1–2 ft behind the patient. Have the patient cover one ear as you whisper some words. Repeat on the other side. Have the patient repeat the words she heard.
   A test of hearing also indicates cranial nerve XIII is intact.

    b. Have the patient occlude one ear. Hold a ticking watch next to the patient's unobstructed ear. Slowly move it away until the patient says she can no longer hear the sound. Repeat for the opposite ear.

Developmental Modifications

Infants—For infants younger than age 3 months of age, loudly clap your hands behind the infant and observe whether he startles. After age 3 months of age, the infant should turn his head or eyes toward a sound, for example, when the parent stands behind the infant and calls his name.

Expected findings: The patient is able to hear you whisper on both sides. The patient hears the watch at a distance of about 12 to 13 cm (5 in.).

🍁 Developmental Variation

Older adults—Often have a generalized loss of hearing. It first occurs in the high-frequency sounds (*f, s, sh,* and *ph*) and then progresses to include all frequencies.

Abnormal findings: Problems with the whisper test indicate low-tone hearing loss. Problems with the watch-tick test indicate a high-pitch deficit.

---

5. **Perform the Weber test:** Place a vibrating tuning fork on top of the patient's head. Ask the patient whether the sound is the same in both ears or louder in one ear. ▼

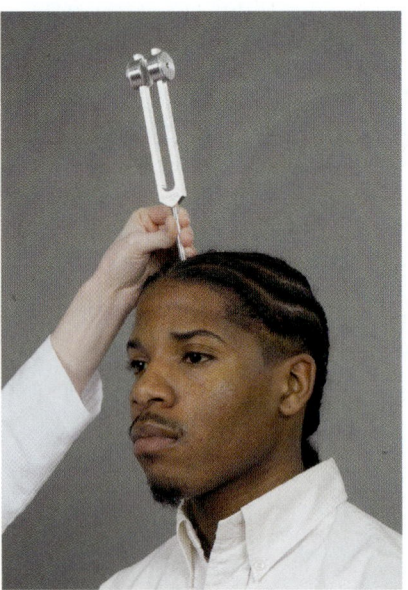

Weber test

Expected findings: The patient hears the sound equally in both ears.

Abnormal findings: Sound is louder in one ear.

  ■ If there is a *conductive hearing loss,* the vibration will be louder in the impaired ear. Conductive hearing loss may be caused by external or middle ear problems, such as infection, blockage of the canal by cerumen, or trauma to the TM.

  ■ If there is a *sensorineural hearing loss,* the sound will be louder in the unaffected ear. Sensorineural loss may result from inner ear problems or from some medications.

6. **If the Weber test is positive: Perform the Rinne test.**

   a. Strike a tuning fork on the table. While it is still vibrating, place it on the patient's mastoid process.
   Tests bone conduction of sound.

   b. Measure the elapsed time in seconds that the patient hears the vibration.

   c. Move the tuning fork to 2.5 cm (I in.) in front of the ear, and measure the elapsed time until the patient can no longer hear the vibration.
   Tests air conduction of sound.

   Repeat for the opposite ear. ▼

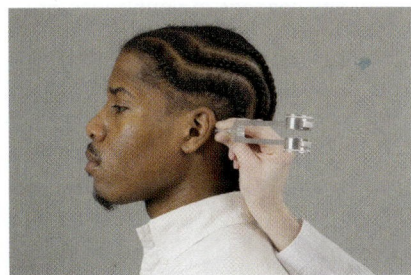

Rinne test

Expected findings: Normally, sound transmission through air (step 6c) is twice as long as transmission through bone (step 6b); that is,

$$AC = 2 \times BC.$$

The ratio of air conduction (AC) to bone conduction (BC) is similar in both ears.

Abnormal findings:
- *Conductive loss:* AC < 2 × BC.
- *Sensorineural loss:* AC is > BC but not 2 × longer; or the patient is unable to hear the tuning fork through BC.
- A difference between ears indicates unilateral hearing loss.
- Inability to hear the tuning fork through BC indicates sensorineural hearing loss.

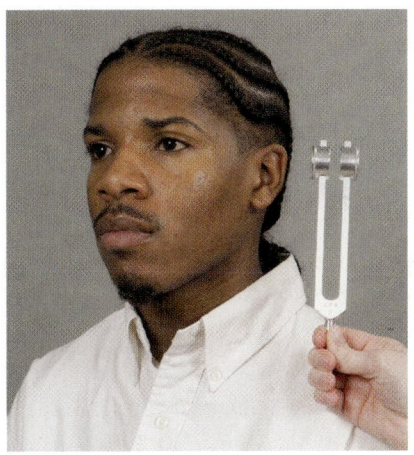

Step 6c

7. **Perform the Romberg test:** Have the patient stand with feet together, hands at side, with eyes opened and then with eyes closed. Note the patient's ability to maintain balance. Stand nearby in case the client loses his balance.

    Stand nearby in case the client loses his balance.

   Tests for balance. Strictly speaking, it does not assess the ears but rather the vestibular nerve and other parts of the central nervous system. Therefore, you may prefer to perform the test during the neurological exam.

Expected findings: The patient maintains balance with minimal sway.

Abnormal findings: Positive Romberg (swaying) is seen with vestibular and cerebellar disorders.

Patient Teaching

Teach the patient the importance of routine hearing examinations.

Documentation

- If you need more information about documenting, review Caring for the Nguyens and Documenting Physical Examination Findings (Nam Nguyen).

Procedure 21-8 ■ Assessing the Nose and Sinuses

> ➤ For steps to follow in *all* procedures, refer to the Universal Steps for All Procedures found on the page facing the inside back cover.

Equipment

- Nonlatex procedure gloves (if exposure to body fluids is a possibility)
- Penlight
- Nasal speculum or otoscope with a wide-tipped speculum
- Pen and record form

Positioning

Have the patient seated, if possible.

Focused History Questions

- Do you have any nasal congestion?
- Do you have a history of nose or sinus problems?
- Do you have problems with seasonal or environmental allergies?
- Do you have a history of sinus headaches?
- Do you experience nosebleeds *(epistaxis)*?
- Have you ever broken your nose?
- Have you had any changes in your sense of smell?
- Do you use nasal sprays or allergy medications?

> ➤ When performing the procedure, always identify your patient according to agency policy, using two identifiers, and be attentive to standard precautions, hand hygiene, patient safety and privacy, body mechanics, and documentation.

Procedure Steps

1. **Position the client for the exam.**

2. **Inspect the external nose.** Note the position, shape, and size. Observe for discharge and flaring.

3. **Check for patency of the nasal passages.** Ask the patient to close his mouth, hold one naris closed, and breathe through the other naris. Repeat with the opposite naris.

4. **Inspect the internal structures.**
   a. Use a nasal speculum or an otoscope with a large speculum (or a penlight with a speculum) to assess the internal structures.
   b. Tilt the patient's head back to facilitate speculum insertion and visualization.
   c. Brace your index finger against the patient's nose as you insert the speculum.

Findings

Expected findings: The nose is midline and symmetrical. No discharge or flaring.

Abnormal findings:
- Asymmetry suggests congenital deformity or trauma.
- Flaring suggests respiratory distress (especially in infants, who cannot breathe through the mouth).
- Clear drainage suggests allergy; yellow or green drainage suggests upper respiratory infection; bloody drainage may result from trauma, hypertension, or a bleeding disorder.

Expected findings: The client breathes freely through both nares.

Expected findings: Nasal mucosa is pink and moist. Septum is intact and midline. No lesions.

Developmental Variation

Older adults—The sense of smell diminishes in older adults because of a gradual decrease in and atrophy of the olfactory nerve fibers.

Abnormal findings: Deviated septum; polyps.
- Pale boggy mucosa is seen with allergies; bright red mucosa is associated with rhinitis, sinusitis, and cocaine use.
- Clustered vesicles suggest herpes infection.
- Erosion of nasal mucosa should signal you to investigate further for other signs or history of crack/cocaine use.

d. Insert the speculum about 1 cm into the nares. Use the other hand to position the client's head and to hold the penlight if you do not have a lighted scope. ▼

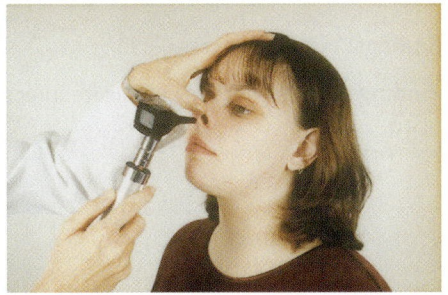

Step 4d

e. Observe the nasal mucosa for color, edema, lesions, erosion or ulceration, blood, and discharge. Inspect the septum for position and intactness.

f. Check for sense of smell using commonly recognized objects, such as a lemon or vanilla. Do not use a noxious odor. You can defer this test until the sensorineurological part of the exam if you choose, but keep the same order for every exam.

Cranial nerve I is intact when the patient shows an ability to detect odor.

Developmental Modifications

Infants and children—You will not need a speculum to examine internal structures. Push the tip of the nose upward with your thumb, and direct a penlight into the nares.

5. **Transilluminate the frontal and maxillary sinuses.**
First, darken the room.
a. *Frontal sinuses:* Shine a penlight or the otoscope with speculum below the eyebrow on each side. ▼

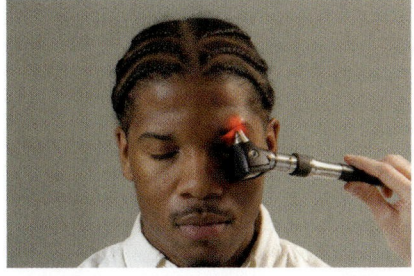

b. *Maxillary sinuses:* Place the light source below the eyes and above the cheeks. Look for a glow of red light at the roof of the mouth through the client's open mouth. ▼

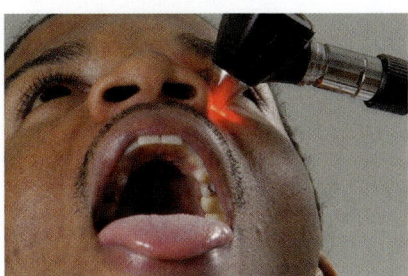

Step 5b

■ Blood in the nasal passage indicates trauma, nosebleeds, or polyps. ▼

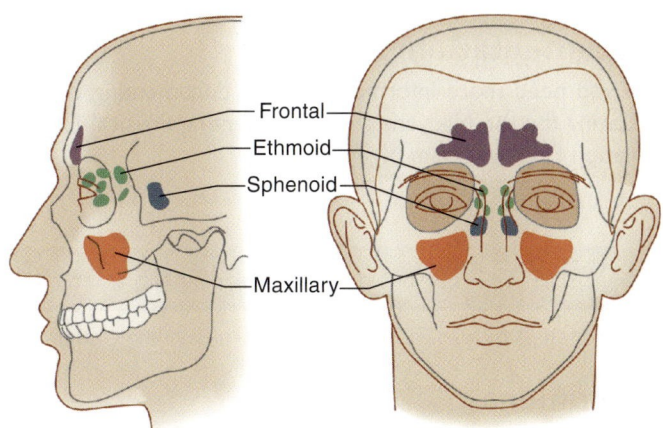

Paranasal sinuses: frontal, ethmoid, sphenoid, and maxillary

a. **Expected findings:** A red glow is seen above the eyebrow, indicating that the frontal sinus is patent.

b. **Expected findings:** A red glow may be (but is not always) seen in the roof of the mouth, indicating that the maxillary sinus is patent.

Abnormal findings: Absence of transillumination may result from mucosal thickening or sinusitis.

(continued on next page)

Procedure 21-8 ■ Assessing the Nose and Sinuses (continued)

6. Palpate the external structures.

Expected findings: No tenderness, lesions, or deformity.

7. Palpate the frontal and maxillary sinuses.

Expected findings: No tenderness.

Abnormal findings: Tenderness may indicate infectious or allergic sinusitis.

Documentation

- If you need more information about documenting, review Caring for the Nguyens and Documenting Physical Examination Findings (Nam Nguyen).

Procedure 21-9 ■ Assessing the Mouth and Oropharynx

➤ For steps to follow in *all* procedures, refer to the Universal Steps for All Procedures found on the page facing the inside back cover.

Equipment

- Nonlatex procedure gloves
- Penlight
- Tongue blade
- Small gauze pad
- Pen and record form

Positioning

Have the patient seated, if possible.

Focused History Questions

- Do you have any problems with your mouth or teeth?
- When was your last dental exam?
- Do you have any discomfort in your mouth or throat?
- Have you had any recent changes in your mouth or teeth?
- How often do you brush your teeth? Floss?
- Do you smoke or chew tobacco?
- Do you have any sores or irritation in your mouth? If so, when did you first notice this?

➤ When performing the procedure, always identify your patient according to agency policy, using two identifiers, and be attentive to standard precautions, hand hygiene, patient safety and privacy, body mechanics, and documentation.

Procedure Steps

I. Inspect the mouth externally. Locate the placement of the lips and their color and condition. Ask the client to purse his lips.

Findings

Expected findings: The lips are midline, symmetrical, moist, and intact with no lesions. Coloring is consistent with ethnic group/race. The client can purse his lips.

Abnormal findings:
- Asymmetry—may be due to congenital deformity, trauma, paralysis, or surgical alteration
- Pallor, cyanosis, redness
- Inability to purse lips—may indicate facial nerve damage
- Lesions—may be caused by bacteria, viruses, or trauma

2. **Note the color and condition of the oral mucosa and gums.**
   a. Don procedure gloves.
   b. **Inspect and palpate the lower lip.** Pull the lower lip away from the teeth, and inspect the inner side of the lip. Palpate any lesions for size, mobility, and tenderness. ▼

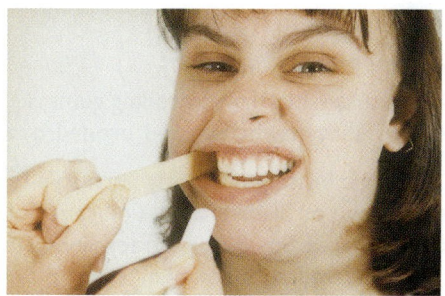

Step 2b

   c. **Inspect the buccal mucosa,** top to bottom and back to front.
   ▪ Ask the client to open his mouth. Use a tongue depressor to retract the cheek, then shine a penlight onto the mucosa.
   ▪ Using a tongue blade and penlight, inspect the Stensen's duct openings to the parotid glands.
   ▪ Finally, palpate inside each cheek by placing a finger inside and thumb outside. Grasping the cheek between them, move the finger about. Repeat on both sides.
   d. Also **examine the gums** as you are inspecting the buccal mucosa. Check for color, bleeding, edema, retraction, and lesions. Press gum tissue gently with gloved finger or tongue blade to assess firmness. ▼

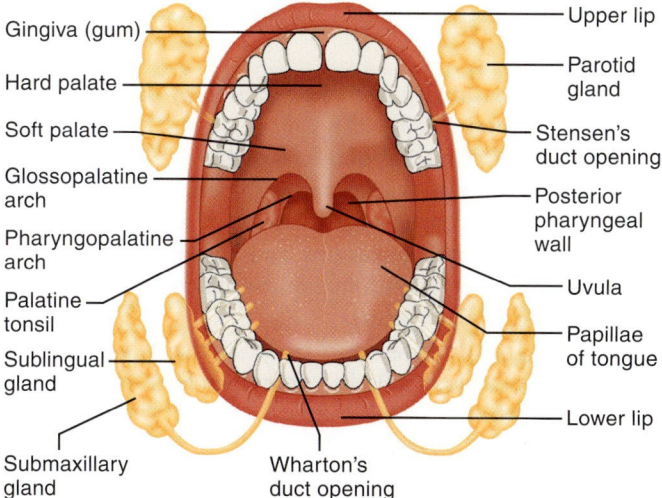

Structures of the mouth and oropharynx

Labels (left side, top to bottom): Gingiva (gum), Hard palate, Soft palate, Glossopalatine arch, Pharyngopalatine arch, Palatine tonsil, Sublingual gland, Submaxillary gland, Wharton's duct opening

Labels (right side, top to bottom): Upper lip, Parotid gland, Stensen's duct opening, Posterior pharyngeal wall, Uvula, Papillae of tongue, Lower lip

Expected findings: *Oral mucosa* is pink, moist, and intact; no lesions. *Gingiva* is consistent in color with the other mucosae and is intact, with no bleeding. *Buccal mucosa* is pink and moist, with no lesions. Mucosa is darker in dark-skinned clients. ▼

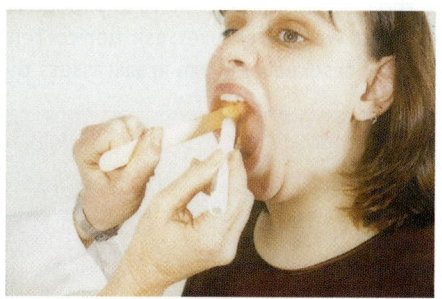

Step 2b

🍁 *Development Variations*

Older adults—Mucosa is drier than in young adults because of decreased salivary gland activity; brownish pigmentation of gums may be seen, especially in dark-skinned people.

Abnormal findings: Pallor may indicate anemia or inadequate oxygenation. The following are types of abnormal lesions.
▪ **Gingivitis** is a sign of periodontal disease. You will see red, swollen, or spongy, bleeding gingiva and receding gumlines. The gums may be tender.
▪ **Parotitis** is an inflammation of the parotid salivary gland.
▪ **Stomatitis** is inflammation of the oral mucosa.
▪ **Leukoplakia** (thick, elevated white patches) that do not scrape off may be precancerous lesions; white, curdy patches that scrape off and bleed indicate **thrush** (a fungal infection).
▪ **Redness or abrasions** of the gingiva may be caused by poorly fitted dentures.
▪ **Aphthous ulcers** are small, painful vesicles with a reddened periphery and a white or pale-yellow base. **Canker sores** are a benign type of aphthous ulcer believed to be caused by viral infection, allergies, stress, or trauma. So-called *major* aphthous ulcers may be caused by herpes simplex virus, HIV, and bacterial infections.

(continued on next page)

Procedure 21-9 ■ Assessing the Mouth and Oropharynx (continued)

3. **Inspect the teeth.** You can do this while you are inspecting the oral mucosa and gums, in step 2.
   a. Observe the number, color, and condition of the teeth. Note the occlusion ("bite") and any loose teeth.
   b. If the client wears dentures, ask her to remove them. Inspect for cracked or worn areas; assess the fit. ▼

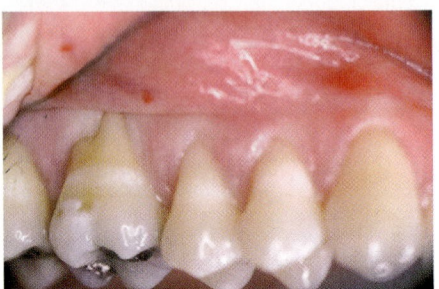

Gingival recession

Expected findings: Most adults have 28 teeth, or 32 if the wisdom teeth have erupted. Children have 20 teeth. The teeth should be white, in good repair, with no caries and good occlusion. The top front teeth should slightly override the lower ones.

> 🍁 ***Developmental Variations***
>
> *Older adults*—May have receding gums, so teeth appear longer. Teeth may be chipped, eroded, or stained.

Abnormal findings: Missing or poorly anchored teeth; misalignment; brown or black enamel (indicative of dental caries or staining, e.g., from taking tetracycline). White spots may indicate excessive fluoride intake.

4. **Inspect the tongue and the floor of the mouth.**
   a. Ask the client to "stick out" his tongue. Examine the upper surface for its color, texture, position, and mobility.
   b. Ask the client to roll his tongue upward and move it side to side.
   c. Have the client place the tip of his tongue on the roof of his mouth, as far back as possible. Using the penlight, inspect the underside of the tongue, the frenulum (which fastens the tongue to the floor of the mouth, in the center), and the floor of the mouth.
   d. Inspect the two Wharton's duct openings to the submaxillary glands, on either side of the frenulum.
   e. Use a tongue blade or gloved finger to move the tongue aside and examine the lateral aspects of the tongue and the floor of the mouth bilaterally. Use caution when placing your finger into the mouth of a non-compliant client. ▼

Expected findings: Tongue is moist with a rough surface; coloring is consistent with the client's race. Mucosa has no lesions or discoloration. Papillae are intact. Tongue is symmetrical, midline, with full mobility. The base of the tongue is smooth with prominent veins. There is no tenderness, no palpable nodules. A geographic tongue is a common normal variant.

> 🍁 ***Developmental Variation***
>
> *Older adults*—May have varicosities under the tongue.

Abnormal findings:
- Limited mobility
- Deviation from midline—may be caused by damage to the hypoglossal nerve (CN XII)
- **Glossitis** (inflammation of the tongue)
- A dry, furry tongue—associated with dehydration
- A black, "hairy" tongue—associated with fungal infections
- Reddened mucosa, ulcerations, and absence of papillae—may indicate allergy, inflammation, or infection
- Swelling, nodules, or ulcers
- A smooth, red tongue—may occur in clients who have a deficiency of iron, vitamin B_{12}, or vitamin B_3

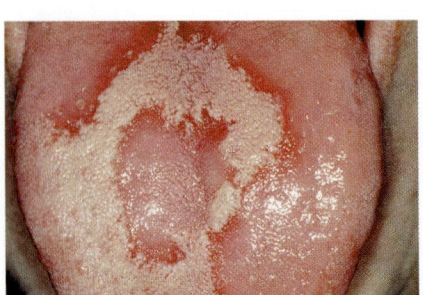

Geographic tongue

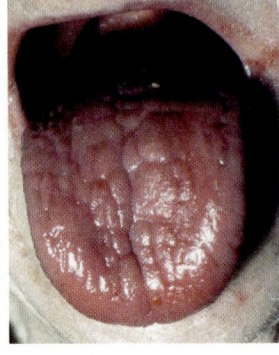

Red, beefy tongue

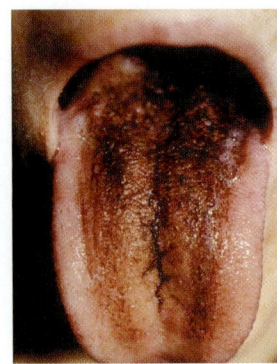

Black, hairy tongue

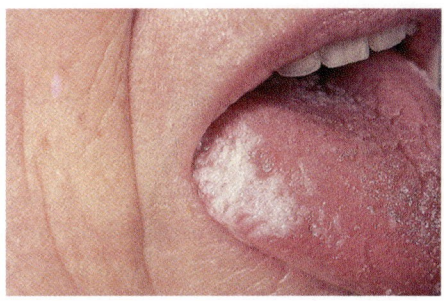

Leukoplakia

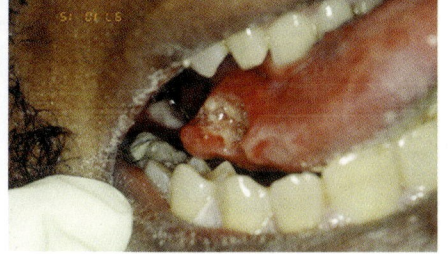

Cancer of the tongue

---

5. **Palpate the tongue and floor of the mouth.** Stabilize the tongue by grasping it with a gauze pad. Palpate top, bottom, and sides with your other index finger.

---

6. **Inspect the oropharynx (hard/soft palate, tonsils, and uvula).** Note the color, shape, texture, and condition.
   a. Have the client tilt his head back and open his mouth as widely as possible. Depress the tongue with a tongue blade, and shine a penlight on the areas to be inspected.
   b. To inspect the uvula, ask the client to say, "Ah," and watch the uvula as the soft palate rises.
   c. Inspect the oropharynx by depressing one side of the tongue at a time, about halfway back on the tongue.
   d. Note the size and color of the tonsils; note any discharge, redness, swelling, or lesions.
   e. Look and palpate for cleft palate, especially in infants.

Expected findings: Hard and soft palate are pink, smooth, moist, and intact. Uvula is midline and rises symmetrically on vocalization. Tonsils, if present, are small, pink, symmetrical, and without lesions or exudate

Developmental Variation

Children—Until about age 12, the tonsils may extend beyond the palatine arch.

Abnormal findings:
- Redness, edema, lesions, plaques, drainage; yellow or greenish streaks on the posterior wall of pharynx (indicate postnasal drainage).
- Tonsils that are red, edematous, or enlarged or have white or pale patches of exudates.
- Asymmetrical rise of the uvula—may indicate a problem with CN IX or X.

---

7. **Test the gag reflex** by touching the back of the soft palate with a tongue blade.

Expected findings: Positive gag reflex is present.

 Developmental Variation

Older adults—May have a slightly slower gag response.

Abnormal findings:
- Absence of a gag reflex is seen with extreme sedation, head injury, or damage to CN IX and X.
- Inability to articulate the specified words indicates CN XII is not intact.

---

8. Ask the client to repeat the following words: *Light, tight, dynamite.* Again, you may defer this test to the sensorineurological portion of the exam if you choose.

Patient Teaching

Instruct the patient in the importance of dental care and the need for regular checkups.

Documentation

- If you need information about documenting your findings, review Caring for the Nguyens and Documenting Physical Examination Findings (Nam Nguyen).

Procedure 21-10 ■ Assessing the Neck

➤ For steps to follow in *all* procedures, refer to the Universal Steps for All Procedures found on the page facing the inside back cover.

Equipment
- Stethoscope and antiseptic wipe
- Pen and record form

Positioning
- Have the client seated, if possible.
- For infants and children, use a supine position.

Focused History Questions
- Do you have any difficulty swallowing?
- Do you have any neck pain or stiffness?
- Do you have any neck masses or lumps?
- Do you have any history of thyroid disease?
- Do you have any difficulty swallowing?

➤ When performing the procedure, always identify your patient according to agency policy, using two identifiers, and be attentive to standard precautions, hand hygiene, patient safety and privacy, body mechanics, and documentation.

Procedure Steps

1. **Inspect the neck.** Note symmetry, ROM, and the condition of the skin.
   a. Inspect the neck in a neutral position.
   b. Inspect the neck when it is hyperextended.
   c. Inspect the neck when the patient swallows water.

2. **Palpate the cervical lymph nodes.** Note the size, shape, symmetry, consistency, mobility, tenderness, and temperature of any palpable nodes.
   a. Use light palpation with one or two fingerpads in a circular movement.
   b. Palpate the cervical nodes in the following order:
      (1) *Preauricular*—in front of the ear
      (2) *Posterior auricular*—behind the ear
      (3) *Tonsilar*—at the angle of the jaw
      (4) *Submandibular*—halfway up the lower jaw
      (5) *Submental*—under the tip of the chin
      (6) *Occipital*—at the base of the skull in the occipital area
      (7) *Superficial cervical*—below the tonsilar node over the sternocleidomastoid muscle
      (8) *Deep cervical*—under the sternocleidomastoid muscle
      (9) *Posterior cervical*—in posterior triangle along trapezius muscle
      (10) *Supraclavicular*—above the clavicle

   NOTE: Use the same sequence every time so that the steps will become automatic and you will not omit any area.

Findings

Expected findings: Neck is erect, midline, and symmetrical with full ROM. No masses are present; skin is intact. Larynx and trachea rise with swallowing. Thyroid is not visible.

Abnormal findings:
- Asymmetrical head position may result from damage to the muscles, swelling, or masses.
- Painful or erratic movement may be due to a benign condition, such as muscle spasm, or to significant problems, including meningitis, neurological injuries, or chronic arthritis.
- Swollen lymph nodes may be visible.
- An enlarged thyroid may be visible in the lower half of the neck.

Expected findings: Lymph nodes are supple and nontender; no palpable masses. ▼

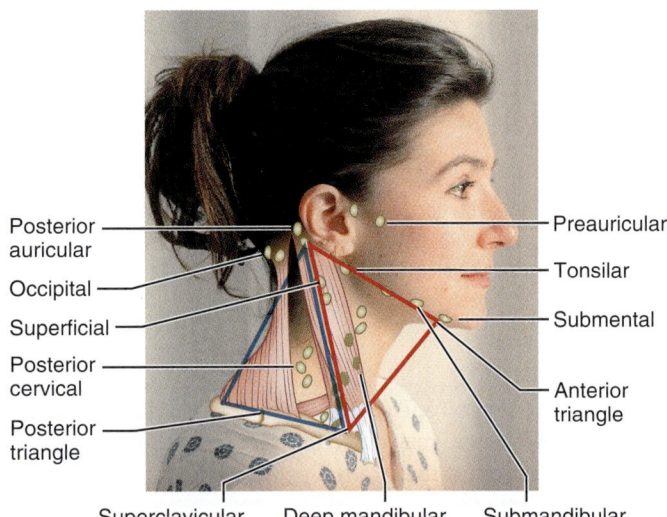

Abnormal findings: Lymphadenopathy (palpable nodes 1 cm or greater). Enlarged, immobile, or tender nodes may indicate malignancy, inflammation, or infection in the area they drain.

3. Palpate the thyroid.

To use the posterior approach:

a. Stand behind the client, and ask her to flex her neck slightly forward and to the left.

b. Position your thumbs on the nape of the client's neck.

c. Using the fingers of your left hand, locate the cricoid cartilage, which is located below the thyroid cartilage. Push the trachea slightly to the left with your right hand as you palpate just below the cricoid cartilage and between the trachea and sternocleidomastoid muscle.

d. Ask your client to swallow (give her small sips of water if necessary), and feel for the thyroid gland as it rises up.

e. Reverse and repeat the same steps to palpate the right thyroid lobe (use the fingers of your left hand to displace the trachea to the right, while using the fingers of your right hand to palpate the thyroid to the right of the trachea).

To use the anterior approach:

f. Stand in front of the client, and ask her to flex her neck slightly forward and in the direction you intend to palpate.

g. Place your hands on the neck, and apply gentle pressure to one side of the trachea while palpating the opposite side of the neck for the thyroid as the client swallows.

h. Reverse and repeat the same steps on the opposite side.

Expected findings: The thyroid is generally nonpalpable. If some tissue is palpable, the consistency is firm and smooth. There is no nodularity, enlargement, or tenderness.

Abnormal findings: An enlarged thyroid may signify a tumor or goiter (hypo- or hyperthyroidism). A tender thyroid is associated with inflammation. ▼

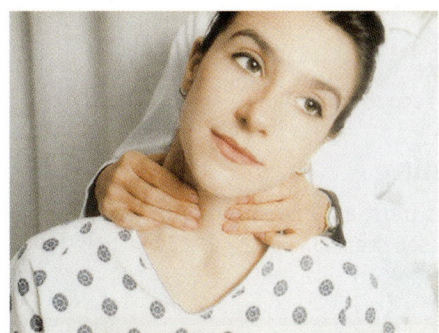

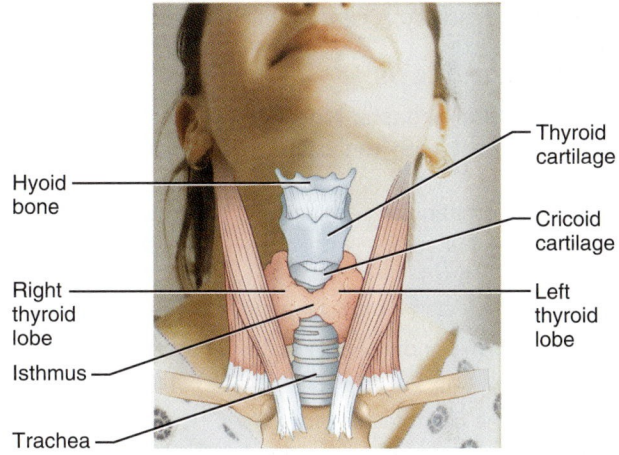

Hyoid bone

Thyroid cartilage

Cricoid cartilage

Right thyroid lobe

Left thyroid lobe

Isthmus

Trachea

Steps 3a–d

? What if . . .

■ **The thyroid gland is enlarged or there is a mass?**

Auscultate the thyroid for bruits using the bell portion of the stethoscope. Ask the client to hold her breath as you auscultate. There should be no bruits.

Patient Teaching

Teach the patient how to perform a "neck check"—self-check the thyroid with a glass of water and a handheld mirror. Tell the patient, "Hold the mirror in your hand and focus on your neck just below the Adam's apple and above your collarbone. Tip your head back, take a drink of water, and swallow. As you swallow look at your neck. Check for any bulges in this area as you swallow." To download neck check instructions, and for more information about thyroid health,

 Go to https://www.verywell.com/how-to-do-a-neck-check-for-thyroid-disease-3232914 or http://www.thyroidawareness.com/neck-check

Documentation

■ Describe enlarged nodes (greater than 1 cm in diameter) according to their location, size, shape, consistency, mobility, and tenderness.

■ If you need more information about documenting your findings, review Caring for the Nguyens and Documenting Physical Examination Findings (Nam Nguyen).

Procedure 21–11 ■ Assessing the Breasts and Axillae

➤ For steps to follow in *all* procedures, refer to the Universal Steps for All Procedures found on the page facing the inside back cover.

Equipment

- Nonlatex procedure gloves, if exposure to body fluids is possible
- Glass slide
- Culturette
- Pen and record form

Positioning

The patient must assume several positions during breast examination (see step 1).

Focused History Questions

- Do you have a lump or thickening in your underarm or breasts that persists throughout your menstrual cycle?
- Do you have any breast pain or discharge?
- Have you noticed any changes in the skin on your breasts, nipples, or underarms?
- Have you had any changes in your nipples?
- Have your breasts changed in size, shape, or contour?
- Do you perform breast self-examination (BSE)?
- Are you taking any medications or hormones?
- If you are premenopausal, when was your last period?

➤ When performing the procedure, always identify your patient according to agency policy, using two identifiers, and be attentive to standard precautions, hand hygiene, patient safety and privacy, body mechanics, and documentation.

Procedure Steps

1. **Inspect the breasts.** Note size, shape, symmetry, and color. Inspect with the client in each of the following positions:

   a. Sitting or standing with arms at her side

   b. Sitting or standing with arms raised slightly but not over her head
      Aids in detecting dimpling or retraction of breast tissue

   c. Seated or standing with her hands pressed on her hips
      Aids in detecting dimpling or retraction of breast tissue

   d. With the client leaning forward
      Helpful when examining large, pendulous breasts

   e. With the client supine with a pillow under the shoulder of the breast being examined
      Helps spread the breast tissue over the chest wall

Findings

Expected findings: The breasts are symmetrical; however, the dominant side may be more developed, resulting in a slightly asymmetrical appearance. Skin color is lighter than exposed areas, and there are no lesions, redness, or edema. Texture is smooth, with no dimpling or retraction. Striae are a normal variation.

Developmental Variations

Newborns—You may see breast enlargement and watery, white discharge from the nipples during the first 2 wk of life.

Children—Breasts typically begin to develop at about age 13 yr; the breasts may not develop at equal rates.

Pregnancy—Breast size increases; areolae and nipples darken; superficial veins become prominent; stretch marks may be present; colostrum (a thick, yellow precursor to breast milk) can sometimes be expressed as early as the second trimester.

 Older adults—Breasts lose firmness and become flaccid and pendulous.

Abnormal findings:

- Asymmetry warrants further investigation.
- Swelling or erythema may be seen in infection (mastitis).
- **Peau d'orange** (dimpled skin texture) skin changes may be seen with lymphatic obstruction that is present in some forms of breast cancer.
- Puckering, lesions, and retraction may also be seen with breast cancer.
- **Gynecomastia** (enlargement of breasts in males) may indicate hormone imbalance.

2. Inspect the nipples and **areolae.** Note color, shape, and symmetry. Observe for any discharge.

Expected findings: The areolae and nipples are darker in color than breast tissue. Nipples are everted and point in the same direction. No discharge present, except in newborns and during pregnancy and lactation. No lesions or erosion present.

Abnormal findings:
- Nipple discoloration that is not associated with pregnancy
- Nipples pointing in different directions. Such findings warrant follow-up as a potential sign of an underlying mass.
- Flat or inverted nipples, which are caused by shortening of the mammary ducts. May make breastfeeding difficult.
- Any nipple discharge not associated with newborns, pregnancy, or breastfeeding requires a thorough evaluation
- Cracks and nipple redness, which may occur with breastfeeding

3. Inspect the axillae. Note the color, condition of the skin, and hair distribution.

Expected findings: Skin is intact with no lesions or rashes. Presence of hair depends on the age of the client and personal preference. Axillary hair develops with puberty. Some women shave the hair, whereas others allow it to grow.

Abnormal findings:
- Rashes, redness, or unusual pigmentation may indicate infection or allergy to deodorants.
- Dark-pigmented, velvety skin may be seen with acanthosis nigricans, a condition associated with obesity and type 2 diabetes mellitus.

4. Palpate the breasts, wearing procedure gloves if necessary. Using the fingerpads of your three middle fingers, make small circles with light, medium, and deep pressure.

Begin at an imaginary line drawn straight down the side from the underarm; move across the breast to the middle of the sternum. Check the entire breast area, moving down until you feel only ribs and up to the clavicle.

Follow one of the following three patterns (evidence suggests the vertical strip method is best).

a. *Vertical strip method:* Start at the sternal edge, and palpate the breast in parallel lines until you reach the midaxillary line. Go up one area and down the adjacent strip (like "mowing the grass"). ▼

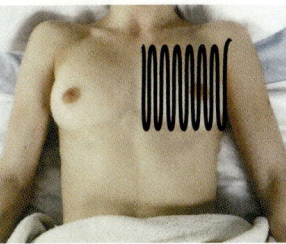

Vertical strip method

Expected findings: Breasts are soft and nontender with no lesions or masses.

Developmental Variations

Consistency depends on age: Premenopausal women have firm and elastic tissue, whereas postmenopausal women have softer tissue that may be stringy or cordlike.

Abnormal findings: Breast lumps or masses may be benign or malignant and require follow-up.

Technique Hints
- Do not remove your fingers from the skin surface once you have begun palpating. Move from area to area by sliding the fingers along the skin.
- Most breast lesions in women are found in the upper outer quadrant.
- Most breast cancer in men occurs in the areola.

(continued on next page)

Procedure 21–11 ■ **Assessing the Breasts and Axillae** (continued)

b. *Pie wedge method:* This method examines the breast in wedges. Move from one wedge to the next. ➤

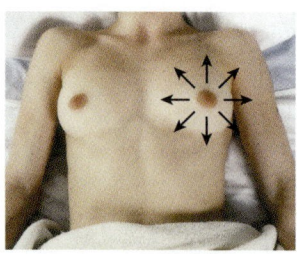

Pie Wedge Method

c. *Concentric circles method:* Start at the outermost area of the breast at the 12 o'clock position. Move clockwise in concentric, ever smaller, circles. ➤

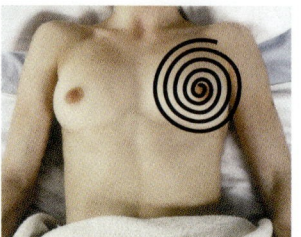

Concentric circles method

5. **Palpate the nipples and areolae.**
   a. If the woman is supine, place a small pillow or folded towel under the shoulder of the breast you are examining.
   b. Squeeze the nipple gently between your thumb and finger to check for discharge.
   c. Note tissue elasticity and tenderness.

Expected findings: Nipples are elastic and nontender. No discharge is present.

Developmental Variations

Nipple tenderness is normal when establishing breastfeeding.

Abnormal findings:
- Loss of elasticity may indicate underlying malignancy.
- Bloody, purulent discharge may indicate infection. Other forms of drainage may indicate malignancy.

6. **Palpate the axillae and clavicular lymph nodes.**
   a. Have the woman sitting with her arms at her sides or supine.
   b. Using your fingerpads, move your fingers in circular fashion.
      - *Central nodes:* located high in the midaxillary region
      - *Anterior pectoral nodes:* located on the lower border of the pectoralis major in the anterior axillary fold
      - *Lateral brachial nodes:* located high in the axilla on the inner aspect of the humerus
      - *Posterior subscapular nodes:* located high in the axilla on the lateral scapular border
      - *Epitrochlear nodes:* located above the elbow
      - *Infraclavicular nodes:* located below the clavicle
      - *Supraclavicular nodes:* located above the clavicle

Expected findings: Nodes are nonpalpable.

Abnormal findings: Palpable nodes may be seen with infection or malignancy. Enlarged lymph nodes caused by infection are tender. ▼

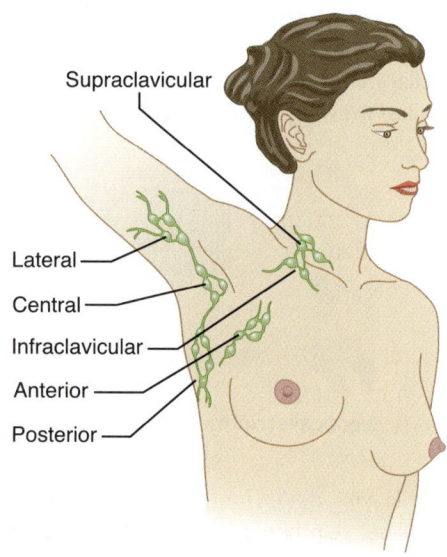

Location of normal lymph nodes

? What if . . .

■ **There is a nipple discharge?**

If there is nipple discharge in a woman who is not pregnant or breastfeeding, obtain a specimen by placing a glass slide up to the breast to capture a drop of discharge. Transport the slide to the laboratory as soon as possible. If there is ample discharge, obtain a swab of the discharge with a culturette.

Patient Teaching

You should demonstrate BSE procedure as part of client teaching for self-care if the patient chooses to perform BSE. Instruct clients that clinical breast exams should be done annually for women aged 40 and older and every 1 to 3 years for women aged 20 to 39 (American Congress of Obstetricians and Gynecologists, 2012, reaffirmed 2014). Guidelines vary as to the age at which women should start having clinical breast exams (CBE) and mammograms to screen for breast cancer. Annual or biennial mammograms or breast thermography most commonly begin after age 40, or at a younger age and more often for those at high risk. (American Cancer Society, n.d.b, revised 2015, n.d.c, revised 2016). Evidence at present does not support the need for a CBE if a mammogram is done (Agency for Healthcare Research and Quality, 2014).

Documentation

■ If you palpate a mass or lump, document its size, shape, symmetry, mobility, tenderness, and skin color changes. To document the location, divide the breast into four quadrants by intersecting vertical and horizontal lines. With the nipple as the center, locate the mass or lump as though the breast were a clock; state the distance in centimeters from the nipple (e.g., 4 o'clock, 2.5 cm from nipple).

■ If you need more information about documenting your findings, review Caring for the Nguyens, including Documenting Physical Examination Findings (Nam Nguyen). ➤

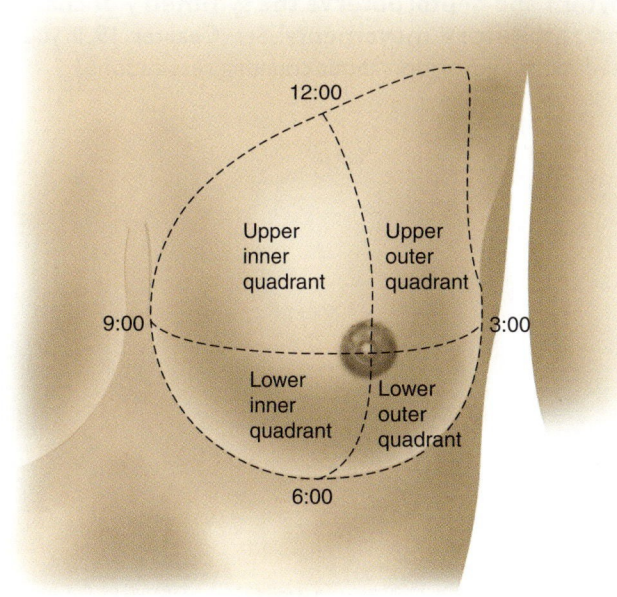

Practice Resources

Agency for Healthcare Research and Quality (2014); American Congress of Obstetricians and Gynecologists (2012, reaffirmed 2014); American Cancer Society (n.d.b, revised 2015, n.d.c, revised 2016); Maurice, A., Evans, D. G., Affen, J., et al. (2012); Smith, R. A., Duffy, S. W., & Tabár, L. (2012).

Procedure 21-12 ■ Assessing the Chest and Lungs

> ➤ For steps to follow in *all* procedures, refer to the Universal Steps for All Procedures found on the page facing the inside back cover.

Equipment

■ Stethoscope and antiseptic wipe
■ Felt-tipped marker and ruler
■ Pen and record form

Positioning

■ Have the client sitting, if possible, and leaning forward for the posterior approach.
  If the client is unable to sit up, findings will be distorted.

■ If the client is lying down, findings are more evident on the dependent side; help her change positions so that you can assess with each side dependent.

Focused History Questions

■ Do you have fatigue or activity intolerance?
■ Do you have any current respiratory problems?
■ Have you had any recent respiratory problems?
■ Do you have a cough?
■ Do you have any difficulty breathing?
■ What, if anything, causes you to be short of breath?
■ Have you had any chest pain?
■ Do you have a history of allergies or asthma?
■ Do you smoke? If so, how much and for how long?
■ If you smoke, have you tried to quit? Would you like to quit?
■ Are you exposed to air pollutants at home or at work?

(continued on next page)

Procedure 21-12 ■ Assessing the Chest and Lungs (continued)

➤ When performing the procedure, always identify your patient according to agency policy, using two identifiers, and be attentive to standard precautions, hand hygiene, patient safety and privacy, body mechanics, and documentation.

Procedure Steps

1. **Count the respiratory rate, and observe the rhythm and depth; observe the symmetry of chest and respiratory movements.** See Chapter 19 if you need more information about counting respirations.)

Findings

Expected findings:

- Respirations are quiet with a regular rhythm and depth. Respiratory rate is 12–20 breaths/min for adults. Chest movement is symmetrical, rising and falling with respirations.

Developmental Variations

Infants and children—The normal respiratory rate varies by age. A newborn may have a respiratory rate of 40–90 breaths/min. The rate gradually declines as the child matures. Newborns breathe abdominally, so you will see little chest movement. The chest in young children is apple shaped.

 Older adults—Rate changes very little; however, respirations decrease in depth as muscles become weakened.

Abnormal findings:

- Chest asymmetry may be seen with musculoskeletal disorders of the spine, such as kyphosis or scoliosis.
- Asymmetrical chest movement during breathing is seen in rib fractures, pneumothorax, and atelectasis; affected chest area may not move at all with respiration.
- Sternal and intercostal retractions are seen with hypoxia, respiratory distress, and airway obstruction.
- Respiratory rate may be increased with activity, smoking, fever, pain, or anemia.

2. **Inspect the chest.**
   a. Inspect the anteroposterior (AP): lateral ratio.

   a. **Expected findings:** Normal adult AP: lateral ratio is 1:2.

   Developmental Variations

   Infants—AP is equal to the lateral diameter.

    Older adults—Kyphosis (excessive curvature of the thoracic spine), scoliosis (lateral curvature of the spine), and osteoporosis alter the shape of the thoracic cage; weakening thoracic and diaphragm muscles allow the chest to widen and become more barrel-shaped, as does COPD.

   Abnormal findings: AP:lateral ratio is increased in COPD (barrel chest).

b. Inspect the costal angle. ▼

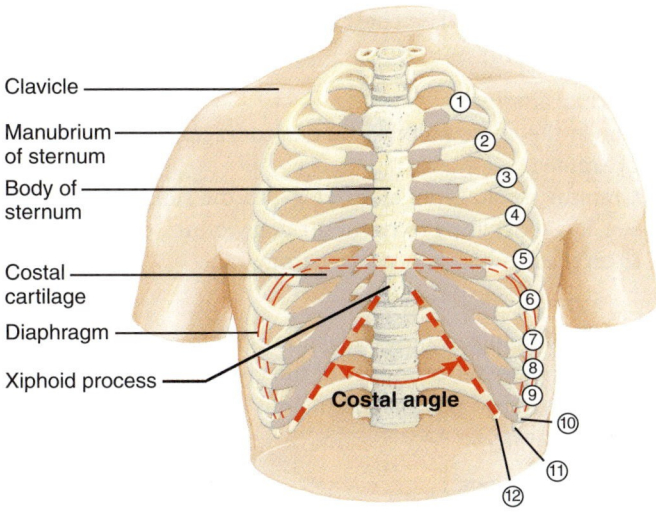

Clavicle

Manubrium of sternum

Body of sternum

Costal cartilage

Diaphragm

Xiphoid process

Costal angle

① ② ③ ④ ⑤ ⑥ ⑦ ⑧ ⑨ ⑩ ⑪ ⑫

b. **Expected findings:** The costal angle is < 90°.

Abnormal findings: Costal angle is > 90° in COPD.

c. Identify any spinal deformities. ▼

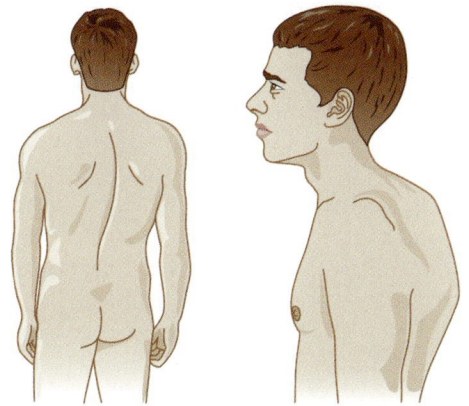

Scoliosis and Kyphosis

c. **Expected findings:** The spine is straight without lateral curvature or deformity.

Abnormal findings: Scoliosis is a lateral curvature of the spine. Kyphosis is excessive thoracic curvature.

d. Observe the effort required to breathe.

d. **Expected findings:** Respirations appear effortless. No retraction or use of accessory muscles.

Abnormal findings: Sternal and intercostal retractions are seen in severe hypoxia or respiratory distress.

e. Note the color and condition of skin.

e. **Expected findings:** Skin color and hair distribution are consistent with the client's gender, ethnicity, and exposure to the sun. The skin is intact with no scars.

Abnormal findings: Cyanosis of the chest wall (due to extreme hypoxia or cold temperature).

3. **Palpate the trachea.** Place your fingers and thumb on either side of the trachea and note its position. (In a comprehensive exam, you may have already done this with the neck examination.)

Expected findings: Trachea is in the midline.

Abnormal findings: Tracheal deviation may occur from a mass in the neck (e.g., thyroid enlargement) or from excess pressure in the lungs (e.g., **tension pneumothorax).**

Developmental Modifications

Infants—Neck is short, so it may not be possible to palpate the trachea.

(continued on next page)

Procedure 21-12 ■ Assessing the Chest and Lungs (continued)

4. Palpate the chest.

- Observe for tenderness, masses, or **crepitus** (crackling skin due to air in the subcutaneous tissue).
- Palpate the anterior, posterior, and lateral chest by placing your hands on the chest wall.

Expected findings: The chest is nontender. No masses or crepitus present.

Abnormal findings:

- Pain in the chest wall may be due to fracture, inflammation, or trauma.
- Crepitus results from air leaking into the subcutaneous tissue. It is most likely to occur around wounds, central IV line sites, chest tubes, or a tracheostomy.

5. Palpate chest excursion (expandability).

a. Place your hands at the base of the client's chest with fingers spread and thumbs about 5 cm (2 in.) apart (at the costal margin anteriorly and at the 8th to 10th rib posteriorly).

b. Press your thumbs toward the client's spine to create a small skinfold between them.

c. Have the client take a deep breath, and feel for chest expansion. This may be performed on the anterior or posterior portion of the chest, or both. ▼

Expected findings: Chest excursion is symmetrical on the anterior and posterior aspect of the chest (you should feel equal pressure on your hands; thumbs should move apart equal distances).

Abnormal findings:

- Limited chest excursion may occur with shallow breathing, restrictive clothing, or restrictive airway disease.
- Asymmetrical excursion may result from airway obstruction, pleural effusion, or pneumothorax.

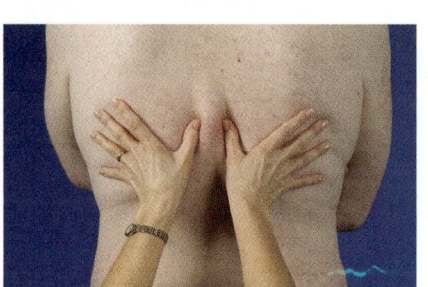

6. Follow the same pattern and sequence for palpating fremitus, percussing, and auscultating the chest. See the accompanying diagrams. ▼

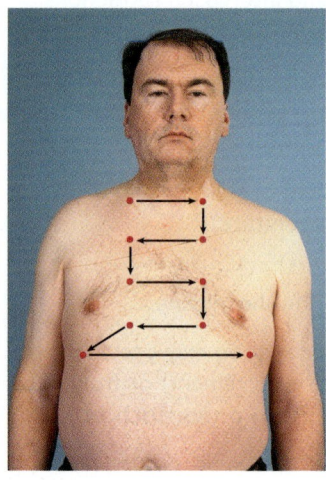 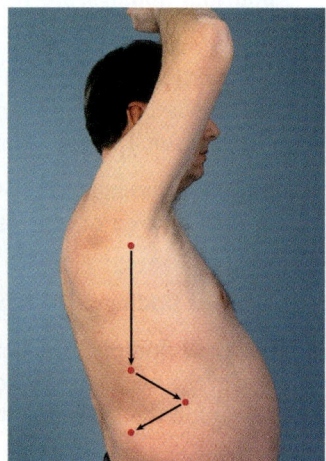 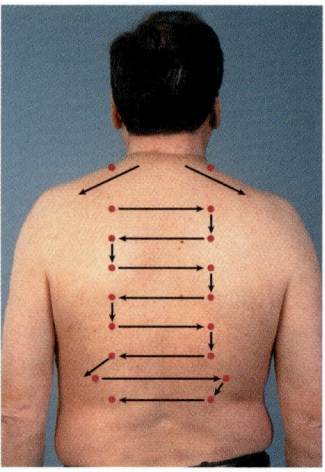

7. Palpate the chest for tactile fremitus.

a. Use the palmar surface of your hands, but raise the fingers off the client's chest so that you palpate with the bony metacarpophalangeal joints of your hands.
Bony prominences are best for detecting vibrations.

b. Palpate for vibrations as the client says, "99" ▼

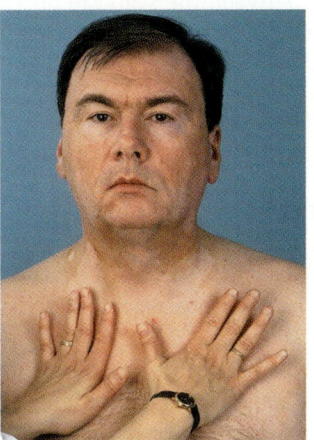

Expected findings: Tactile fremitus is equal bilaterally on the anterior and posterior chest; it is diminished at midthorax. Fremitus is normally diminished if the chest wall is very thick or the voice very soft.

Developmental Variations

Children and thin adults—May have increased fremitus.

Abnormal findings: Increased fremitus occurs with conditions that cause fluid in the lungs (e.g., pulmonary edema). Decreased or absent fremitus occurs when there is decreased air movement or tissue consolidation (e.g., emphysema, asthma).

Developmental Modifications

Infants—Place your hand over the chest while the infant is crying.

8. Percuss the chest. Compare the right side to the left side.

a. Percuss over the intercostal spaces rather than over the ribs.
Percussion over bone produces less resonance.

b. Use the indirect percussion method on the anterior, posterior, and lateral chest, following the pattern in the diagram in step 6.

Expected findings:

- The anterior chest is resonant to the 2nd ICS on the left and to the 4th ICS on the right.
- The lateral chest is resonant to the 8th ICS.
- The posterior chest is resonant to T12.

Abnormal findings: Dullness is heard with fluid or masses in the lungs. Hyperresonance is heard with air trapping that occurs with emphysema.

9. Percuss the posterior chest for diaphragmatic excursion.

a. Percuss the level of the diaphragm on full expiration. Have the client exhale completely and hold his breath while you percuss (beginning just below the scapula) from resonance over the lung downward toward the diaphragm. The sound will become dull at the diaphragm. Mark the area with a pen.

b. Percuss the diaphragm level on full inspiration. Have the client take a deep breath and hold it as you percuss again. Mark the location.

c. Measure the distance between the two marks.

Expected findings: Diaphragmatic excursion (the distance between the two marks) is normally 3–6 cm.

Abnormal findings: Decreased excursion may indicate paralysis, atelectasis, or COPD with overinflated lungs. ▼

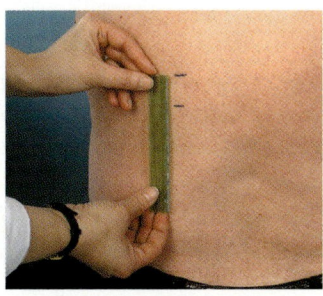

(continued on next page)

Procedure 21-12 ■ **Assessing the Chest and Lungs** (continued)

10. Auscultate the chest.
  a. **Routine daily assessment:** Follow the *pattern* in step 6, using fewer locations, when making a routine daily bedside assessment.
  b. **For a focused assessment**, auscultate more areas while still following the pattern in step 6.
    Following a "pattern" allows you to compare findings side-to-side.
  b. Use the diaphragm of the stethoscope.
  c. Have the client take slow, deep breaths through his mouth as you listen at each site through one full respiratory cycle.
To review lungs sounds, see the tables at the end of this procedure.

Expected findings: No abnormal or adventitious sounds are heard. Lung fields are clear to auscultation.
  ■ *Bronchial* breath sounds are heard over the trachea. *Bronchovesicular* breath sounds are heard over the sternum anteriorly and between the scapulae posteriorly.
  ■ *Vesicular* breath sounds are heard over most of the lung fields.

Developmental Variations

Infants—Breath sounds are louder than in adults.

Abnormal findings: Crackles or rales, rhonchi, wheezing, stridor, friction rub, grunting.
  ■ **Diminished breath sounds** are heard with poor inspiratory effort, in the very muscular or obese, or with restricted airflow.
  ■ **Misplaced breath sounds** (e.g., bronchial breath sounds heard over the lung fields) indicate constriction of flow.
  ■ **Adventitious breath sounds,** such as wheezes, rhonchi, and rales, are sounds heard over normal breath sounds. **KEY POINT:** *If an abnormal sound is heard, have the client cough and listen again.*

11. Auscultate for abnormal voice sounds if there is evidence of lung congestion. Follow the pattern in step 6.
  a. Assess for *bronchophony* by having the client say, "1, 2, 3" as you listen over the lung fields.
  b. Assess for *egophony* by having your client say "eee" as you listen over the lung fields.
  c. Assess for whispered *pectoriloquy* by having your client whisper, "1, 2, 3" as you listen over the lung fields.

Expected findings: No abnormal voice sounds are heard.

Abnormal findings:

  a. **Bronchophony** is present if the words are clearly heard over the lungs.
  b. **Egophony** is present if the sound you hear is "ay."

  c. **Whispered pectoriloquy** is present if you hear "One, two, three" clearly.

Patient Teaching

Instruct the patient about the dangers of tobacco use, especially smoking; exposure to air pollutants and environmental pollutants, such as radon or asbestos; and the signs and symptoms of lung cancer.

Home Care

■ Instruct clients or caregivers to identify any pollutant within the home that may cause respiratory problems, such as radon, dirty heating/air-conditioning systems, or mold.

■ Instruct caregivers or patients with allergies and/or asthma to eliminate potential allergens, such as cigarette smoke, dust, feathers, and pet dander.

Documentation

If you need information about documenting your findings, review Caring for the Nguyens, including Documenting Physical Examination Findings (Nam Nguyen).

Normal Lung Sounds			
NORMAL SOUNDS	**LOCATION**	**DESCRIPTION**	**ILLUSTRATION**
Bronchial or Tubular: Produced by air moving through the trachea	Heard best: *Anteriorly:* Over the trachea *Posteriorly:* Below the nape of the neck	Blowing, hollow sounds; inspiration is shorter than expiration and lower pitched	Inspiration / Expiration

Normal Lung Sounds—cont'd

NORMAL SOUNDS	LOCATION	DESCRIPTION	ILLUSTRATION
Bronchovesicular: Produced by air moving through the bronchial airways	Heard best: *Anteriorly:* Over the 1st and 2nd ICS adjacent to the sternum anteriorly *Posteriorly:* Over the scapula posteriorly	Medium-pitched, medium intensity, blowing sounds; inspiration and expiration are equal length and similar pitch	Inspiration Expiration
Vesicular: Produced by air moving through the smaller airways	Heard over the lung fields	Soft, low-pitched, breezy sounds; inspiration is longer, louder, and higher-pitched than expiration	Expiration Inspiration

Abnormal Lung Sounds

ABNORMAL LUNG SOUNDS	CAUSE	CHARACTERISTICS	EXAMPLES
Crackles (sometimes called rales)	Air bubbling through moisture in the alveoli	Bubbling, crackling, popping. Soft, high-pitched, and very brief sounds, usually heard during inspiration	Pneumonia Congestive heart failure (CHF) Bronchitis Emphysema
Rhonchi	Mucus secretions in the large airways	Course, snoring, continuous low-pitched sounds heard during inspiration and expiration. May clear with coughing.	Bronchitis Emphysema Narrowed airways Fibrotic lungs
Wheezes	Narrowing of small airways by spasm, inflammation, mucus, or tumor	High-pitched musical or squeaking sounds heard during inspiration or expiration	Acute asthma Emphysema
Stridor*	Partial upper airway obstruction or tracheal or laryngeal spasm	High-pitched, continuous honking sounds heard throughout the respiratory cycle but most prominent on inspiration	Acute respiratory distress Foreign body in airway Epiglottitis
Friction rub	Rubbing together of inflamed pleural layers	A high-pitched grating or rubbing sound that may be heard throughout the respiratory cycle. Loudest over lower lateral anterior surface.	Pleuritis
Grunting	Retention of air in the lungs	A high-pitched tubular sound heard on expiration	Emphysema

*Patients with stridor need immediate medical evaluation.

Procedure 21-13 ■ Assessing the Heart and Vascular System

➤ For steps to follow in *all* procedures, refer to the Universal Steps for All Procedures found on the page facing the inside back cover.

Equipment

- Combination stethoscope with bell and diaphragm
- Alcohol or other antiseptic wipe
- Two rulers
- Pen and record form

✚ Clean stethoscope and rulers before and after using unless they are only used for one patient.

Positioning

Place the client in three positions: sitting, supine, and left lateral (to facilitate hearing specific sounds).

Focused History Questions

- Have you experienced any fatigue or activity intolerance?
- Do you have a history of high blood pressure or stroke?
- Have you ever passed out or felt light-headed?
- Do you have any problems with your heart or circulation?
- Do you ever experience chest pain? If so, describe the circumstances that triggered the pain.
- What was the pain like? What did you do to relieve it?
- Do you ever experience palpitations or a rapid heart beat?
- Do you ever feel short of breath?
- Do you ever get swelling in your feet?
- What medications are you taking?

➤ When performing the procedure, always identify your patient according to agency policy, using two identifiers, and be attentive to standard precautions, hand hygiene, patient safety and privacy, body mechanics, and documentation.

Procedure Steps

1. **Inspect the neck.**
   a. With the patient supine, inspect the carotid and jugular venous system in the neck for pulsations.
   b. *Assess jugular flow:* Compress the jugular vein below the jaw. The vein collapses, and the jugular wave is more prominent at the supraclavicular area.
   The jugular venous pulse is easily obliterated with gentle pressure.
   c. *Assess jugular filling:* Compress the jugular above the clavicle. The vein distends and the jugular wave disappears.

Findings

Expected findings: Carotid pulsation is easily visible. A slight pulsation in the supraclavicular area or suprasternal notch indicates jugular venous pressure. The pulsation should be easily obliterated when you apply pressure to the area.

Abnormal findings: Significant jugular vein distention suggests right-sided heart failure. ▼

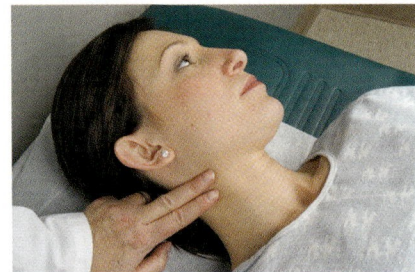

Assessing jugular flow

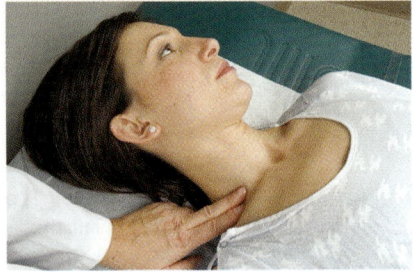

Assessing jugular filling

2. **Measure jugular venous pressure (JVP).**
   a. Elevate the head of the bed to a 45° angle.
   b. Identify the highest point of visible internal jugular filling.
   c. Place a ruler vertically at the sternal angle (where the clavicles meet).

Expected findings: Normal jugular venous pressure is < 3 cm.

Abnormal findings: Elevated JVP (in CHF or constricted flow into the right side of the heart); low JVP (in hypovolemia).

d. Place another ruler horizontally at the highest point of the venous wave.
e. Measure the distance in centimeters vertically from the chest wall. ▼

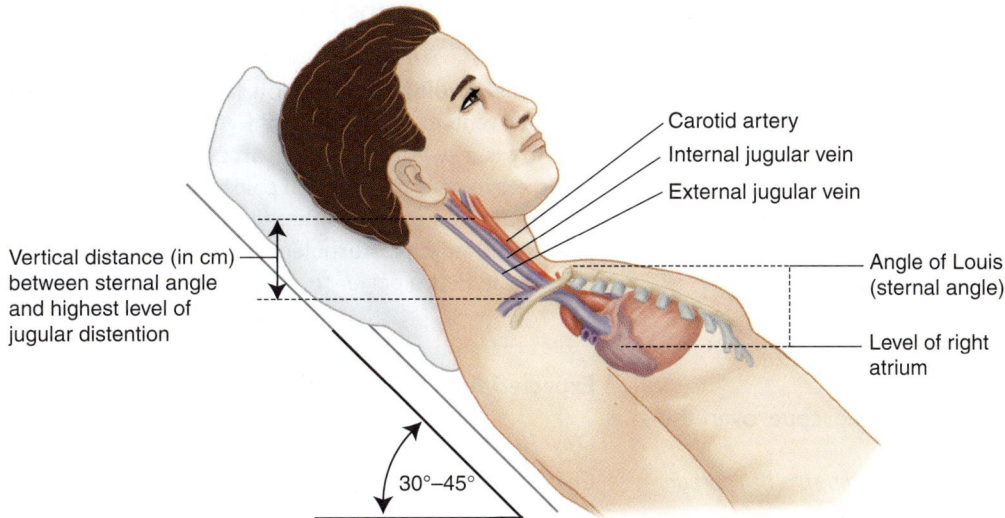

Measuring jugular venous pressure

---

3. **Inspect the precordium for pulsations**. (Position the patient supine with tangential lighting.)

Developmental Modifications

Children—Look for the PMI more medially and at about the 4th ICS in children younger than age 8.

Expected findings: Visible pulsation at the point of maximal impulse (PMI, the 5th ICS in the midclavicular line)

Developmental Variations

In thin adults and children, a pulsation may also be visible over the base of the heart.

Abnormal findings:
- A pulsation (a heave or lift) displaced toward the axillary line indicates left ventricular hypertrophy.
- Pulsations to the right of the sternum may indicate an aortic aneurysm.

---

4. **Very gently palpate the carotid arteries.**

✚ NOTE: that this step is not done for all patients. It is a part of a thorough cardiovascular assessment and is done only when indicated.

a. ✚ Palpate each side separately; never at the same time.

Bilateral pressure may impair cerebral blood flow.

b. Avoid massaging the carotid artery as you palpate.
Increased pressure on the carotid will lead to a drop in the heart rate and blood pressure and can lead to cardiac arrest.

c. Note the rate, rhythm, amplitude, and symmetry of the pulse.
d. Note the contour, symmetry, and elasticity of the arteries.
e. Note any thrills.

Expected findings:
- Rhythm is regular with +2 amplitude.
- *Contour:* There should be a smooth upstroke with less acute descent.
- *Symmetry:* Pulses are equal bilaterally.
- *Elasticity:* Carotids are soft and pliable.

Developmental Variation

Pulse rate is age dependent.

 Older adults—The carotids may be stiff and cordlike.

Abnormal findings: A thrill indicates turbulent flow.

(continued on next page)

Procedure 21-13 ■ Assessing the Heart and Vascular System (continued)

5. Palpate the precordium.
   a. For this part of the examination, have the patient sit up and lean forward. If lying down, have him turn to the left side.
   Brings the apex of the heart closer to the chest wall.
   b. Palpate in all five areas: apex, left lateral sternal border, epigastric area, base left, and base right.
   c. Feel for pulsations, lifts, heaves, and thrills.
Helpful hint: *Perform cardiac palpation and ausculta-tion from the patient's right side, whenever possible.*
This allows you to stretch the stethoscope during auscultation so that you minimize interference and "static."

Expected findings: PMI is palpable at the apex over a 1-cm to 2-cm area. Slight pulsation from the abdominal aorta may be felt at the epigastric area. No pulsations, lifts, heaves, or thrills are palpable.

Abnormal findings: A pulsation, lift, or heave may be seen with left ventricular hypertrophy.
   - A **lift** is a pulsation that is forceful enough to seem to lift the examiners fingers with palpation.
   - A **heave** is a pulsation that feels rolling under your fingers.
   - A **thrill** indicates turbulent flow and feels like a vibration over the PMI.

6. Auscultate the carotids.
   a. Place the bell portion of the stethoscope over the carotid artery to listen for bruits.
   Bruits are low-pitched sounds, best heard by the bell portion.
   b. Have the patient hold his breath as you listen.
   Breath sounds over the trachea are loud and could interfere with the ability to hear a bruit.

   NOTE: If you hear a bruit, lightly palpate the neck for thrills (pulsations or vibrations), which further confirm turbulent flow.

Expected findings: No audible bruit is present.

Developmental Variations

Children—Bruit may be heard because of a high-output state.

Abnormal findings: In adults, a bruit suggests carotid stenosis, increased cardiac output secondary to fluid overload, use of stimulants, or hyperthyroidism.

7. Auscultate the jugular veins.
   a. Place the bell portion of the stethoscope lightly over the jugular veins to listen for a low-pitched venous hum.
   b. Have the patient hold his breath as you listen.

Expected findings: No venous hum is audible.

Developmental Variations

Children—A venous hum may be heard. This is a benign condition whereby blood travels to the brain and back down again to the heart, causing the vein walls to vibrate.

8. Auscultate the precordium. To review heart sounds, **KEY POINT:** *Be systematic. To keep from missing impor-tant parts of the exam, always auscultate in the same order to all the areas.*
   - Ask the patient to sit upright and lean forward a bit.
   This will position the heart closer to the chest wall for clearer auscultation.
   - Listen for the S_1, S_2, S_3, and S_4 sounds.
   - Listen for murmurs.
   - Listen with both the bell and the diaphragm at the sites in the accompanying figure:
   These sites are located along the pathway the blood takes as it flows through the atria, ventricles, and valves of the heart.

Expected findings: No extra sounds are heard. No murmurs, clicks, or rubs are present.
An S_4 sound is normal in athletes.

Developmental Variations

Infants—You may hear a split S_2 when the child takes a deep breath.

Children—The chest wall is thinner, so heart sounds are louder than in adults. An S_3 is normal in young children and adolescents when they are sitting or lying, but it disappears when they stand or sit up.

Pregnancy—An S_3 is a normal variant in the third trimester of pregnancy.

Older adults—An S$_4$ sound is considered normal; extra systoles per minute are considered normal. ▼

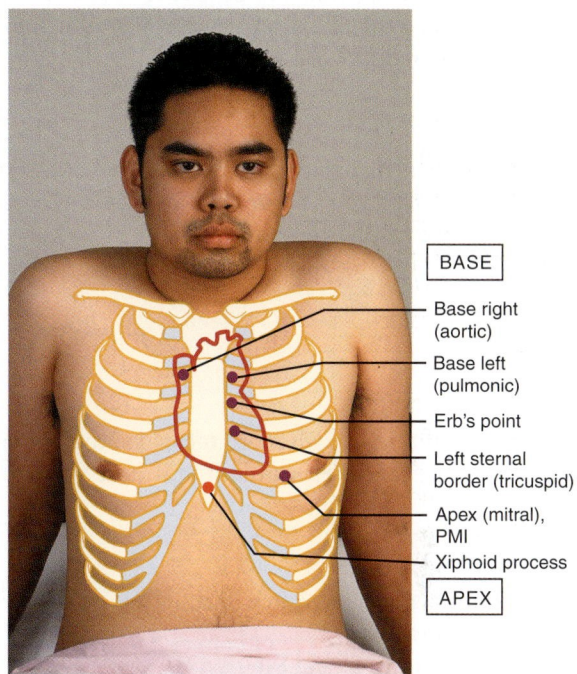

BASE
- Base right (aortic)
- Base left (pulmonic)
- Erb's point
- Left sternal border (tricuspid)
- Apex (mitral), PMI
- Xiphoid process

APEX

Cardiac auscultation sites

Abnormal findings:
- A split sound at either S$_1$ or S$_2$ may occur if there is a delay in closure of one of the valves.
- An S$_3$ that does not disappear with position change is abnormal and represents heart failure or volume overload.
- An S$_4$ may be heard in adults with coronary artery disease, hypertension, and pulmonic stenosis.

a. *Base right (aortic valve).* Locate the angle of Louis (the prominence on the sternum, two to three fingerbreadths below the suprasternal notch). Slide your fingers laterally until you feel the 2nd ICS.
The right 2nd ICS is the best place to auscultate the aortic valve.

a. **Expected findings:** S$_1$ < S$_2$

b. *Base left (pulmonic valve).* Locate the angle of Louis (the prominence on the sternum, two to three fingerbreadths below the clavicular notch). Slide your fingers laterally until you feel the 2nd ICS.
The left 2nd ICS is the best place to auscultate the pulmonic valve.

b. **Expected findings:** S$_1$ < S$_2$

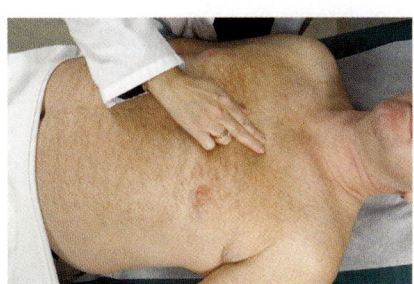

(continued on next page)

Procedure 21-13 ■ Assessing the Heart and Vascular System (continued)

c. *Apex (mitral valve).* You may be able to locate the apex by observing the pulsation at the PMI. It is at the 5th ICS in the midclavicular line.

d. *Left lateral sternal border (LLSB) (tricuspid valve).* From the apex, *slide* your finger up to the 4th ICS, then move close to the sternum.

Assessing Murmurs

Auscultating murmurs is an advanced technique that requires practice and experience. However, if you hear a murmur, assess its:
- Location
- Quality
- Frequency (high, medium, or low pitch)
- Intensity (loudness)
- Timing (in relation to S_1 and S_2)
- Duration
- Configuration (constant or crescendo/decrescendo)
- Radiation (can you hear this in other locations?)
- Respiratory variation (does it change with breathing?)

c. **Expected findings:** $S_1 > S_2$

Developmental Variation

Children—You will hear S_3 at the apex in about 30% of children.

d. **Expected findings:** $S_1 \geq S_2$. You may hear a split S_1.

Abnormal findings: Extra sounds (S_3 or S_4), murmurs, clicks, or rubs. *NOTE:* A diastolic murmur or a murmur greater than grade 3/6 is never innocent. Also, *in infants,* a split S_2 sound during normal respirations may indicate an atrial–septal defect.

Classifying Murmurs

Grade
- $1/6$ Very faint, comes and goes
- $2/6$ Quiet, but heard immediately
- $3/6$ Moderately loud
- $4/6$ Loud, associated with a thrill
- $5/6$ Heard with stethoscope half off the chest wall; thrill present
- $6/6$ Heard with stethoscope entirely off the chest wall; thrill present

---

9. **Inspect the periphery for color, temperature, and edema.** (You will probably already have done this when examining the integumentary system.)

Expected findings: Skin is warm. No edema is present. Color is appropriate for race.

Abnormal findings: Pallor, cyanosis, coolness, shininess, sparse hair growth, and clubbing of the nails (may indicate pulmonary oxygenation problems or impaired central or peripheral circulation).

---

10. **Palpate the peripheral pulses:** radial, brachial, femoral, popliteal, dorsalis pedis, and posterior tibial.
    a. Using the distal pads of your second and third fingers, firmly palpate pulses.
    b. Palpate firmly but not so hard that you occlude the artery.
    c. If you have trouble finding a pulse, vary your pressure, feeling carefully at the correct anatomical location.
    d. Assess pulses for rate, rhythm, equality, amplitude, and elasticity.
    e. Describe pulse amplitude on a scale of 0–4:
       0—Absent: Pulse cannot be felt.
       1—Weak (thready): Pulse is barely palpable and can be easily obliterated by pressing with the fingers.
       2—Normal quality: Pulse is easily palpated, not weak or bounding, obliterated by finger pressure.
       3—Full: Pulse is easily felt with little pressure; not easily obliterated.
       4—Bounding, forceful, obliterated only by strong finger pressure.

Expected findings: All pulses are regular, strong, and equal bilaterally. Pulse amplitude is +2.

Developmental Variation

Older adults—Arterial pulses may be difficult to palpate because of decreased arterial perfusion.

Abnormal findings: Weak, absent, or asymmetrical pulses may indicate partial or complete occlusion of the artery. Other signs of arterial occlusion include pain, pallor, cool temperature, paresthesia, or paralysis.

11. Inspect the venous system. If a client has varicosities, assess for valve competence with the manual compression test, following.
  a. With the client standing, compress the distal portion of the vein.
  b. Still holding the distal portion, compress the proximal portion.
  c. Feel for a pulsation with your lower (distal) hand.
    ■ **If the valves are competent,** you will not feel backflow when you compress the vein.
    ■ **If the valves are incompetent,** you will feel a wave pulsation with your lower hand as a result of backflow when you press on the proximal segment.

Expected findings:
Veins are not distended. Superficial spiderlike veins, especially on the lower extremities, may occur with normal aging.

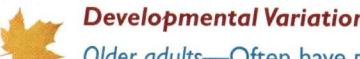
  Developmental Variation
  Older adults—Often have peripheral edema as a result of chronic venous insufficiency.

Abnormal findings: Ropelike, distended, tortuous, or painful veins **(varicosities).**

? What if . . .

■ **The patient is obese and heart sounds are difficult to hear?**

The larger the body mass over the heart, the more difficult it is to hear heart sounds clearly. However, it may help to have the patient sit upright and lean forward as you auscultate.

■ **Findings from inspecting and palpating peripheral pulses are abnormal?**

If inspection or palpation findings are abnormal, perform tests in the table More Extensive Tests for Abnormal Findings at the end of this procedure.

Patient Teaching

Instruct the patient in the risk factors of heart disease and stroke and in the signs and symptoms of heart disease.

Documentation

■ If you need information about documenting your findings, review Caring for the Nguyens and Documenting Physical Examination Findings (Nam Nguyen).

■ If you need more information about assessing apical pulse and peripheral pulses and measuring blood pressure,

 Go to **Davis's** *Nursing Skills Videos,* **Vital Signs,** on the **Davis's** *Nursing Skills Videos* Web site on Davis*Plus.*

More Extensive Tests for Abnormal Findings	
TESTS	**EXPECTED FINDINGS**

1. ***Perform the capillary refill test*** anywhere you note signs of diminished blood flow.
  a. Press the skin with sufficient pressure to produce blanching.
  b. Release the pressure and observe the return of color.
	1. Color returns in less than 3 sec.

2. ***Perform Allen's test*** to assess abnormal pulse findings and arterial flow in the hands.
  a. Have the client form a tight fist with one hand.
  b. With her fist still clenched, compress her radial and ulnar arteries.
  c. Ask the client to open her hand; observe for pallor.
  d. Release the ulnar artery and watch for natural color to return.
  e. Then repeat the process, but release the radial artery
	2. In a healthy individual skin color returns rapidly with each maneuver. Failure to return to normal color indicates impaired flow through the open artery. Normally pallor resolves in 3–5 sec.

(continued on next page)

Procedure 21-13 ■ Assessing the Heart and Vascular System (continued)

More Extensive Tests for Abnormal Findings—cont'd

TESTS	EXPECTED FINDINGS
3. ***Check the ankle–brachial index (ABI)*** to assess circulatory impairment of the feet. a. Use a Doppler (handheld ultrasonic device) to measure blood pressure at the posterior tibialis or dorsalis pedis pulse sites. b. Compare that pressure with blood pressure obtained over the brachial artery. c. To calculate the ABI, divide the systolic pressure at the ankle by the systolic pressure at the brachial site.	3. Normally ankle pressure is higher than brachial pressure. The following is a summary of ABI findings: Normal: 1 or greater Minimal disease: 0.8–0.95 Moderate disease: 0.79–0.4 Severe disease: 0.39–0 *Example:* If the systolic pressure at the ankle is 75 and at the brachial artery is 100, the ABI is 75/100, or 0.75. This indicates moderate peripheral vascular disease.
4. ***Perform the color change test*** to assess arterial circulation in the legs. a. While the client is lying supine, elevate the legs to increase venous return. b. Have the client quickly move to a sitting position with the feet dangling.	4. Normal color should return to the feet in less than 10 seconds. Pallor with the legs elevated and dependent **rubor** (reddish-purple color) are signs of arterial insufficiency.

Procedure 21-14 ■ Assessing the Abdomen

➤ For steps to follow in *all* procedures, refer to the Universal Steps for All Procedures found on the page facing the inside back cover.

Equipment

- Stethoscope and antiseptic wipe
- Felt-tipped marker
- Tape measure and ruler
- Penlight or examination light
- Pen and record form

✚ Clean stethoscope and other equipment before and after using unless they are only used for one patient.

Positioning

Begin with the client supine, arms at sides, with small pillows under the head and knees.
Relaxes the abdominal muscles, allowing for more effective palpation.

Focused History Questions

- What types of foods do you typically eat?
- Are there any foods that you cannot eat? If so, why?
- How many cups of coffee, tea, cola, or caffeinated beverages do you drink per day?
- Do you smoke? If so, how much and at what age did you start?
- Do you drink alcohol? If so, how many drinks per day? Per week?
- Do you use any drug for non-medical purposes?
- Do you have any abdominal pain?
- How often do you have a bowel movement (BM)?
- Have you noticed any changes in your BMs?

- Are you having any problems with constipation, diarrhea, or getting to the bathroom in time to use the toilet?
- Have you ever seen blood in your stool or noticed blood when you wipe after a BM?
- Have you ever had black, tarry stools?
- How often do you use antacids, laxatives, enemas, aspirin, or anti-inflammatory medicines, such as Anaprox or Motrin?
- What home remedy, herbal, or over-the-counter medicines do you use?
- What prescription medicines do you use?
- Have you ever been immunized for hepatitis?
- Have you ever had a blood transfusion?
- What is your occupation?
- Have you ever been diagnosed with an ulcer, hemorrhoids, hernia, bowel problem, cancer, hepatitis, liver problems, cirrhosis, or appendicitis?
- Have you ever had abdominal surgery? If so, when, what type, and what if any follow-up was done for the problem?
- Do you have any family history of abdominal problems, such as ulcers, gallbladder disease, bowel disease, or cancer?
- Do you ever have trouble with: swallowing, heartburn, nausea, vomiting, diarrhea, bloating, excess gas, yellowing of the skin?

🍁 ***Developmental Modifications***

Older adults—Recall that "Problems with eating" is a part of the SPICES assessment. Ask clients, for example:

- Do you have difficulty chewing or swallowing your food?
- How is your appetite?
- Are you able to shop for and prepare your food?

➤ When performing the procedure, always identify your patient according to agency policy, using two identifiers, and be attentive to standard precautions, hand hygiene, patient safety and privacy, body mechanics, and documentation.

Procedure Steps

1. Have the client void before the exam.
Empties the bladder so that you do not mistake a full bladder for a mass.

2. Position the client supine with the knees slightly flexed.
Relaxes the abdominal muscles for more effective palpation.

3. Inspect the abdomen.
  a. Observe the size, symmetry, and contour of the abdomen.
    (1) Stand at the client's side and view across the abdomen.
    (2) If distention is present, use a tape measure to measure girth at the level of the umbilicus.
    (3) Have the client raise his head and check for bulges.
    Accentuates hernia, if present.

  b. Observe the condition of skin and skin color. Look for lesions, scars, striae, superficial veins, and hair distribution (if you have not already done this in your examination of the integumentary system).

  c. Note abdominal movements.

Findings

Expected findings:
Abdomen is flat, slightly rounded, scaphoid (concave), or slightly protuberant; sides are symmetrical. No visible masses or distention present.

Developmental Variations

Infants and toddlers—Protuberant abdomen is normal.

Abnormal findings:
- *Asymmetry* may be caused by tumors, cysts, or scoliosis.
- *Distention* may be due to gas, fluid retention, or bowel obstruction.

Expected findings: Skin color is consistent with ethnicity but is usually lighter in color than exposed areas. No lesions are present. Hair distribution is appropriate for age and gender. Striae, superficial veins, and scars are common variations.

Abnormal findings:
- Skin color changes may be associated with bruising, internal bleeding, or jaundice.
- Striae occur after periods of rapid growth or weight gain. Pink striae are new. Older striae are silver-white in color.
- Dilated veins are associated with liver disease and obstruction of the vena cava.

Expected findings: On a thin client, peristalsis and aortic pulsations may be visible. Men tend to use their abdominal muscles for breathing.

Developmental Variations

Infants and children—Peristaltic waves are often visible. Abdominal breathing is common in infants and young children.

 Older adults—Abdomen may be more rounded because of decreased muscle tone.

Abnormal findings:
- Peristaltic waves may be seen if there is intestinal obstruction.
- Abnormal respiratory movements may be seen with respiratory distress.
- Pulsations (in other than a thin client) may indicate an aortic aneurysm.

(continued on next page)

Procedure 21-14 ■ Assessing the Abdomen (continued)

d. Note the position, contour, and color of the umbilicus. ▼

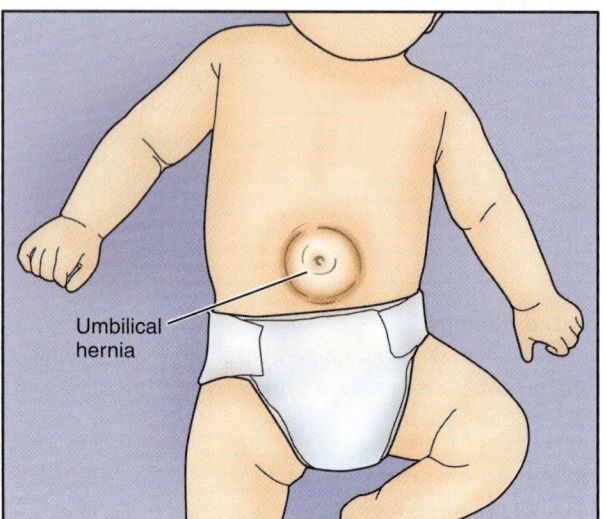

Umbilical hernia

Expected findings: Umbilicus is inverted and in the midline. No discoloration or discharge is present. ▼

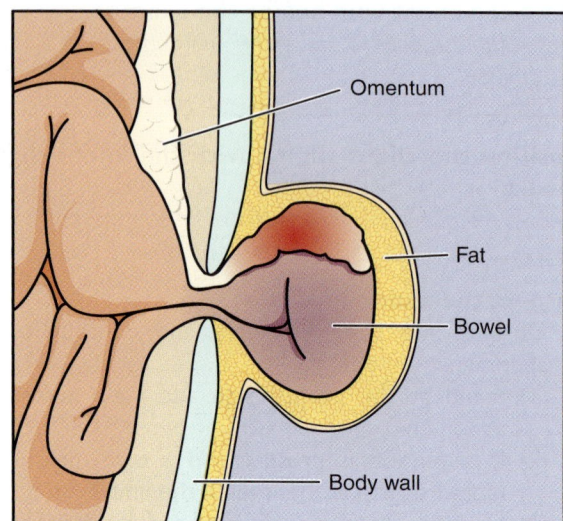

Omentum

Fat

Bowel

Body wall

Abnormal findings: Protrusion of the umbilicus may result from a hernia or underlying mass.

4. **Auscultate the abdomen.**

   a. Ask the client when he last ate.

   Bowel sounds are loudest 5 or 6 hr after the person eats, when the small intestine contents empty through the ileocecal valve into the large intestine. They also increase immediately after eating.

   b. Listen for bowel sounds.

   (1) Using the stethoscope diaphragm, listen in several areas in all four quadrants (see the figure).

   The diaphragm of the stethoscope is used because bowel sounds are high-pitched.

   (2) If bowel sounds are infrequent or difficult to hear, listen to the right of the umbilicus over the ileocecal valve.

   (3) Listen for 5 min before concluding that bowel sounds are absent.

Expected findings: Audible bowel sounds, occurring every 5–15 sec or 5–30 times per min in a healthy adult.

Abnormal findings:

■ Hyperperistalis (hyperactive): > 2 or 3 sounds per sec or > 30 sounds per min.

■ Hypoperistalsis (hypoactive) < 5 sounds per min; faint sounds.

■ Absent bowel sounds: none after listening for 5 min.

c. Use the stethoscope bell to listen for bruits over the aorta and the renal, femoral, and iliac arteries. ▼

Expected findings: No audible bruits are present.

Abnormal findings: A bruit is abnormal and may indicate an aneurysm or altered blood flow. ▼

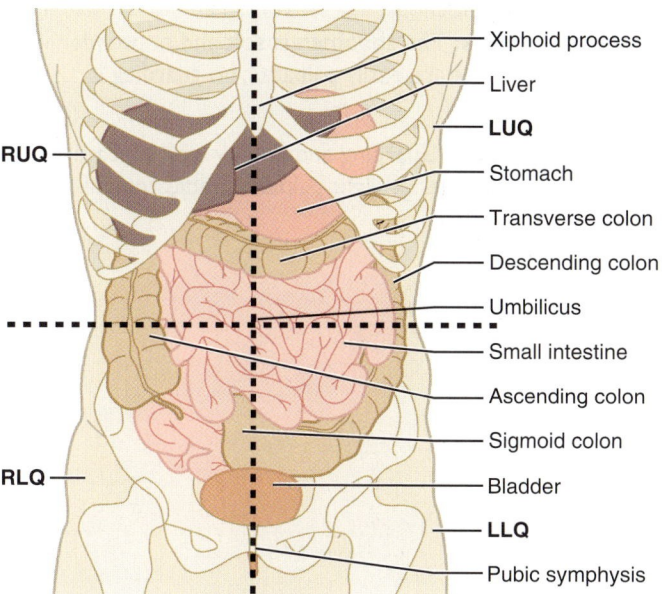

The four abdominal quadrants

Labels: Xiphoid process, Liver, **LUQ**, Stomach, Transverse colon, Descending colon, Umbilicus, Small intestine, Ascending colon, Sigmoid colon, Bladder, **LLQ**, Pubic symphysis, **RUQ**, **RLQ**

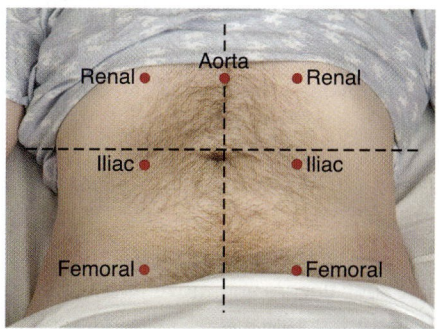

Locating abdominal arteries

Labels: Renal, Aorta, Renal, Iliac, Iliac, Femoral, Femoral

5. Percuss the abdomen. (See Clinical Insight 21-1.)
   a. Use indirect percussion to assess at multiple sites in all four quadrants.
   b. Estimate organ size by noting the change in sounds as you percuss over the liver, spleen, and bladder. ▼

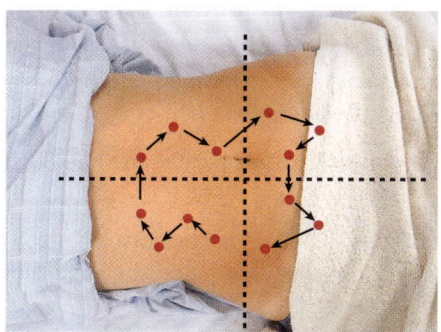

Expected findings: Tympany, with dullness over organs or fluid, is present (due to presence of gas). No tenderness; no masses.

Abnormal findings: Extremely high-pitched tympanic sounds are heard with distention. Extensive dullness indicates organ enlargement or underlying mass.

6. Using fist or blunt percussion, percuss the costovertebral angle (where the end of the rib cage meets the spine) bilaterally to assess for kidney tenderness. ▼

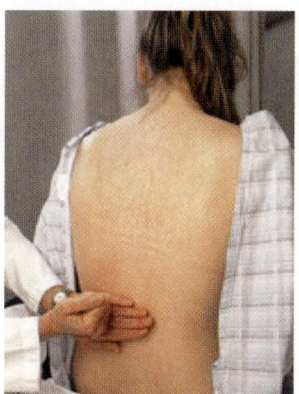

Expected findings: No costovertebral angle tenderness is present.

Abnormal findings: Pain or tenderness is associated with kidney infection or musculoskeletal problems.

(continued on next page)

Procedure 21–14 ■ Assessing the Abdomen (continued)

7. Palpate the abdomen.

a. **Begin with light palpation** throughout the abdomen. Identify surface characteristics, tenderness, muscular resistance, and turgor.

(1) If the client is having pain in one area of the abdomen, palpate that area last.

A guarding response to pain from palpation can interfere with your assessment of the other areas.

(2) Using your fingertips, press down 1–2 cm in a rotating motion.

(3) Lift your fingers and move to the next site.

(4) Palpate the entire abdomen if possible.

(5) Proceed in an organized fashion through all quadrants, using the same sequence in every examination.

(6) Observe for grimacing, guarding, or verbal statements of tenderness or pain.

Expected findings: The abdomen is soft and nontender, with no masses. Muscles are easily palpated; no guarding is present.

Abnormal findings: Guarding and rigidity may indicate peritonitis. Tenderness on light palpation indicates the need for further evaluation.

Developmental Modifications

Encourage a child to place her hand lightly over yours as you palpate.

✚ Caution: Do not palpate the abdomen if the client has a Wilms' tumor, a large diffuse pulsation, or a history of organ transplant.

b. **Use deep palpation** to palpate organs and masses. See the table Deep Palpation Techniques at the end of this procedure.

a. Tenderness may be noted in a normal adult near the xiphoid process and over the cecum and sigmoid colon.

🍁 ***Developmental Variation***

Older adults—May have a higher pain threshold, so they may not react to palpation even if there is an abnormality in the abdomen.

Abnormal findings: A mass indicates the need for further evaluation.

Expected findings: The liver is not normally palpable unless the client is very thin. If it is palpable, the edge should be smooth and nontender.

Developmental Variation

Children—Liver is relatively large and can be palpated 1–2 cm (0.5–1 in.) below the right costal margin.

Abnormal findings: Palpation below the costal margin indicates liver enlargement.

c. **Palpate the liver.**

(1) Stand at the client's right side.

(2) Place your right hand at the client's right midclavicular line under the costal margin, parallel to the right costal.

(3) Place your left hand under the client's back at the lower (11th to 12th) ribs, and press upward. This elevates the liver toward the abdominal wall.

(4) Ask the client to inhale and deeply exhale while you press in and up, gently but deeply, with your right fingers.

Alternative approach: Hooking technique. Place your hands over the right costal margin, and hook your fingers over the edge. Have the client take a deep breath, and feel for the liver's edge as the liver drops down on inspiration and then rises up over your fingers during expiration. ➤

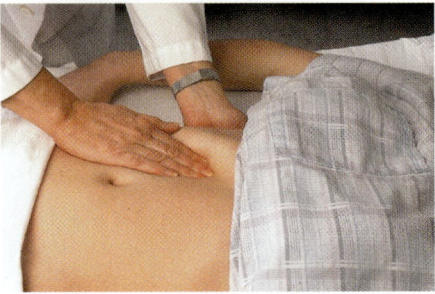

d. **Palpate the Spleen**
(1) Stand at the client's right side.
(2) Reach across the client to place your left hand under the costovertebral angle, and pull upward to move the spleen anteriorly.
(3) Place your right hand under the left anterior costal margin, and have the client take a deep breath.
(4) During exhalation, press your hands together (inward) to try to palpate the spleen. ➤

Expected findings: The spleen is not normally palpable.

Abnormal findings: Splenic enlargement or tenderness may result from infection, enlargement, trauma, or cancer.

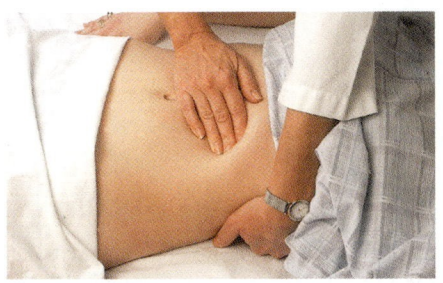

? What if . . .

■ **The patient has a nasogastric (NG) tube attached to suction?**

Discontinue suction or clamp the tube while auscultating so that you will not mistake the sound of suction for bowel sounds.

■ **The patient is ticklish or guarding when you palpate the abdomen?**

Distract the person by giving her a task, such as "Count aloud to 10" or "Count backward from 100." Alternatively, have the client place her hand on her abdomen; place your hand on hers and begin light palpation. When she begins to feel more relaxed, slip your hand underneath hers and continue.

■ **The patient complains of abdominal pain?**

Check for rebound tenderness: Place your hand perpendicular to the abdomen. Press firmly and slowly then release quickly.
If pain increases when you remove your hand, this indicates peritoneal irritation. Rebound tenderness in the right lower quadrant may be a sign of appendicitis.

Patient Teaching

Instruct the patient in the importance of proper diet, the signs and symptoms of colorectal cancer, and the importance of screening colonoscopy.

Documentation

■ If you need more information about documenting your findings, review Caring for the Nguyens and Documenting Physical Examination Findings (Nam Nguyen).

Deep Palpation Techniques

DEEP PALPATION: ONE-HANDED TECHNIQUE	DEEP PALPATION: BIMANUAL TECHNIQUE
■ Using your fingertips, press down 4 to 6 cm in a dipping motion. ■ Proceed in an organized fashion through all four quadrants.	■ This technique is useful when palpating a large abdomen. ■ Place your nondominant hand on your dominant hand. ■ Depress your hands 4 to 6 cm (1.5 to 2 in.) in a dipping motion. ■ Proceed in an organized fashion through all four quadrants.

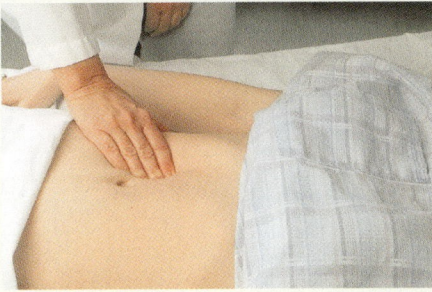

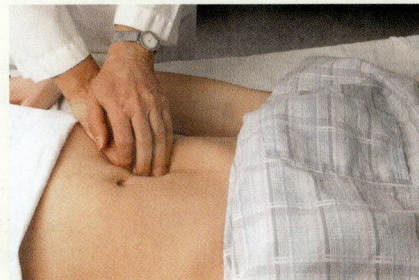

? What if . . .

■ **You palpate a mass?**

Have the client tighten her abdominal muscles.
If the mass is in the abdominal wall, it will become easier to palpate. If it is deep in the abdomen, it will be difficult to palpate.

Procedure 21-15 ■ Assessing the Musculoskeletal System

➤ For steps to follow in *all* procedures, refer to the Universal Steps for All Procedures found on the page facing the inside back cover.

Equipment

- Tape measure
- Goniometer
- Pen and record form

Developmental Modifications

Older adults—recall that "Problems with falls" is a part of the SPICES assessment. If your facility has a falls assessment tool, perform that focused assessment.

Focused History Questions

- Do you have any difficulty with coordination (e.g., folding clothes, brushing your teeth)?
- Do you now have, or have you ever had, musculoskeletal problems, pain, or disease? If so, what medications or treatments are you using?
- Have you ever injured your bones or joints?
- Do your joints, muscles, or bones limit your activities?
- Do you lose your balance or fall?
- Do you have any occupational hazards that could affect your muscles and joints?

➤ When performing the procedure, always identify your patient according to agency policy, using two identifiers, and be attentive to standard precautions, hand hygiene, patient safety and privacy, body mechanics, and documentation.

Procedure Steps

1. **Assess posture.**
   a. Note the body and head position.

   b. Check the alignment and symmetry of the shoulders, scapula, and iliac crests. Inspect from the front, back, and side.

Developmental Modifications

Newborns—Palpate clavicles for fractures that may have occurred at birth. Check for congenital hip dysplasia (dislocation) by examining for asymmetry of the gluteal folds or shortening of the femur.

   c. Assess the spinal curvature by:
   (1) Observing the client's profile while he is standing erect.
   (2) Having the client bend forward at the waist with arms hanging free at the sides. ▼

Findings

Expected findings: Posture is erect, with the head in the midline.

Expected findings: The shoulders, scapula, and iliac crests are symmetrical.

Expected findings: Cervical and lumbar curves are concave; thoracic and sacral curves are convex.

Developmental Variation

Children—**Lordosis** (exaggerated lumbar curve) is normal before age 5.

Abnormal findings: Kyphosis, scoliosis, lordosis.

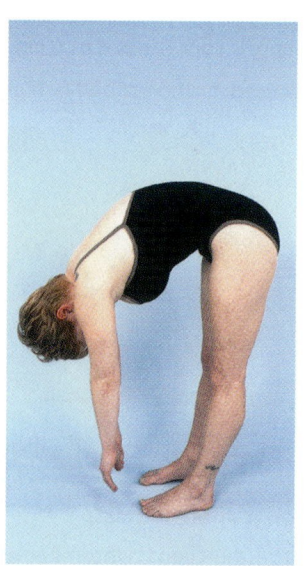

Cervical
(concave)
Thoracic
(convex)
Lumbar
(concave)
Sacral
(convex)

Assessing for normal curves   Assessing for kyphosis and scoliosis

d. Have the client stand upright with the feet together. Note the position of the knees. ▼

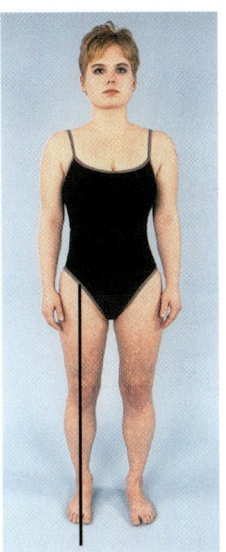

Expected findings: Patella is in the midline on an imaginary line drawn from the anterior superior iliac crest to the feet.

Developmental Variation

Children—**Genu varum** (bowlegs) is normal for 1 year after a child begins to walk.

---

2. Assess gait by observing the client walking.

Developmental Modifications

Children—Observe them at play.
  a. Pay attention to the *base of support* (distance between the feet) and *stride length* (distance between each step).

  b. Observe the phases of the gait.

a. **Expected findings:**
Average base of support for an adult —5–10 cm (2–4 in.)
Average stride length is 30–35 cm (12–14 in.)
The longer the legs, the longer the stride length.

Abnormal findings:
- *Abnormal gait* can be caused by muscle weakness, joint stiffness, pain, deformities, lumbar disc problems, central nervous system dysfunction, muscle atrophy or hypertonicity (e.g., from stroke or brain tumor), Parkinson's disease, cerebral palsy, multiple sclerosis, and spinal tumors.
- *A wide base of support and shortened stride length* reflect a balance problem, placing the client at risk for falls.

b. **Expected findings:** Movements are smooth and coordinated, weight is evenly distributed, arms swing in opposition, and toes point forward.

Abnormal findings: Toeing in or out, jerky or shuffling movements, touching the floor first with the toe rather than the heel, arms held out to the side or front.

Stance Phase ▼

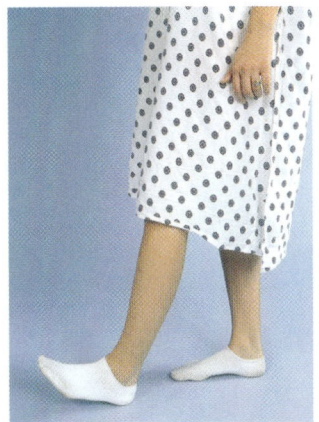

Heel strike

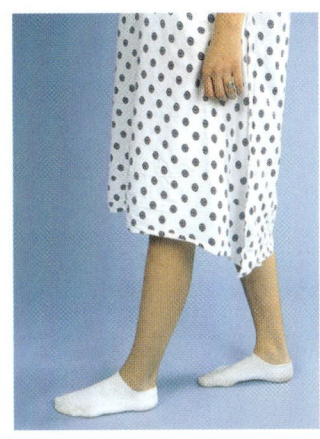

Foot flat

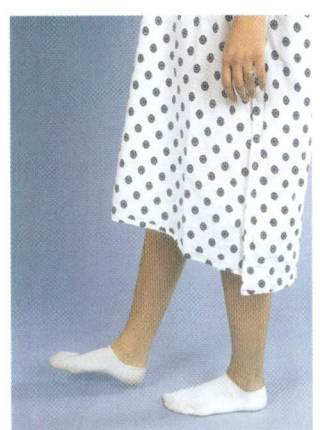

Midstance

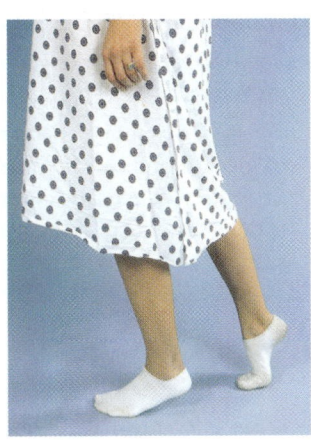

Push-off

(continued on next page)

Procedure 21-15 ■ Assessing the Musculoskeletal System (continued)

Swing Phase ▼

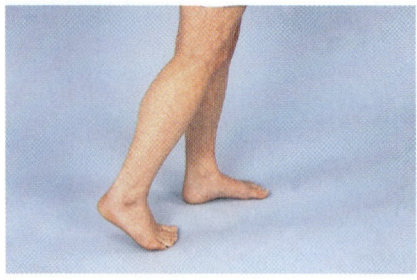
Accelerate

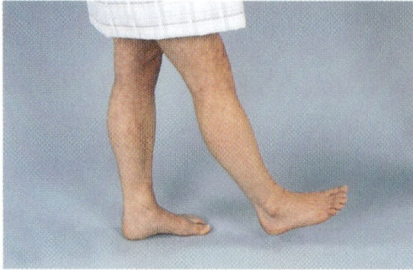
Swing-thru

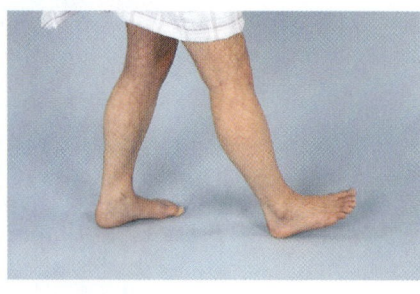
Decelerate

3. Assess balance.

KEY POINT: *If the client was unsteady when walking, do not complete this portion of the exam. Proceed only if the gait is steady; stand nearby in case the client loses his balance.*

   a. Have the client tandem walk heel-to-toe.

   b. Have the client walk alternately on heels and toes.

   c. Ask the client to do a deep knee bend.

   d. Ask the client to hop in place on each foot several times.

   e. Perform the Romberg test (if you did not already do so when examining the ears): Have the client stand with feet together and eyes open. Then have him close his eyes and stand still. ▼

Expected findings:

■ The client is able to perform each of these maneuvers smoothly.

■ The Romberg test (see Procedure 21-7) is negative—the client is able to maintain balance with minimal sway with eyes open and closed.

Developmental Variation

Infants—Should be able to sit alone by age 8 mo.

Abnormal findings: Balance problems may indicate a cerebellar disorder, an inner ear problem, or muscle weakness.

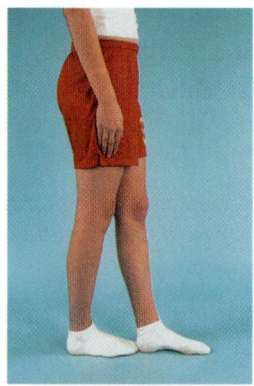
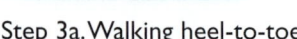
Step 3a. Walking heel-to-toe

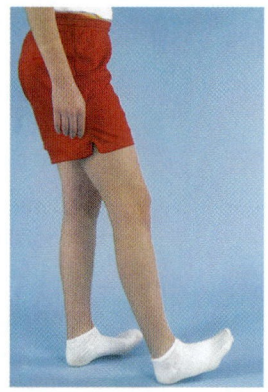
Step 3b. Walking on heels

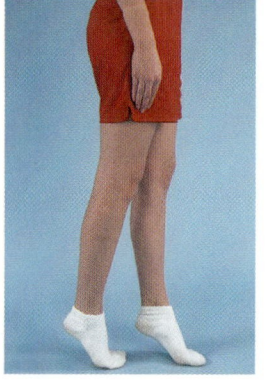
Step 3b. Walking on toes

Developmental Modifications

Infants—Observe sucking, swallowing, and kicking movements.

Children—To assess a child's movement, coordination, range of motion, and so on, watch the child at normal play. Cerebellar function cannot be tested on infants and toddlers because of their immature neuromuscular system.

4. **Assess coordination while the client is seated.**
   a. Test upper extremity coordination by having the client perform finger–thumb opposition. Test one side and then the other.

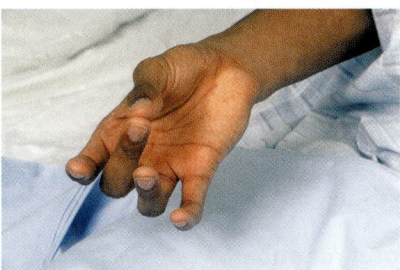

   b. Test rapid alternating movements by having the client alternate between supinating and pronating her hands.
   c. Assess lower extremity coordination by having the client perform rhythmic toe-tapping, one side at a time.
   d. Have the client run the heel of one foot down the shin of the other leg. Repeat on the opposite side.

Expected findings: The client is able to perform these movements smoothly and in a coordinated fashion. The dominant side (usually the right) may be slightly more coordinated.

Developmental Variations

> *Older adults*—Decreased coordination and reaction time may result from slower nerve conduction and loss of muscle tone.

Abnormal findings: Slowness or awkwardness with movement may indicate a cerebellar disorder or muscle weakness.

---

5. **Test accuracy of movements.** Have the client touch his finger to his nose with his eyes open. Repeat with his eyes closed.

Expected findings: The movement is accurate with eyes open and closed.

Abnormal findings: Inaccurate movements indicate cerebellar dysfunction.

---

6. **Measure the limbs.**
   a. Measure arm length from the acromion process to the tip of the middle finger.
   b. *Apparent leg length*—Measure from the umbilicus (a nonfixed point) to the medial malleolus.
   c. *True leg length*—Measure from the anterior superior iliac crest, crossing over the knee to the medial malleolus ▼

Expected findings: The differences in length between the right and left arm and leg are 1 cm or less.

Abnormal findings: Leg length discrepancies may cause back and hip pain and gait problems. An *apparent leg length* discrepancy may result from a pelvic tilt or flexion deformity of the hip; a *true leg length* discrepancy results from unequal bone length.

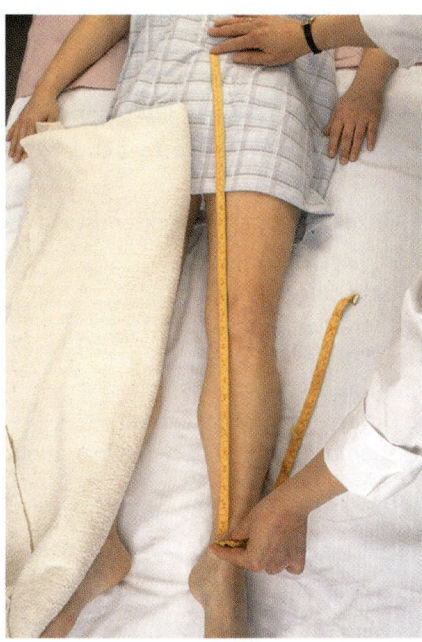

Apparent leg length

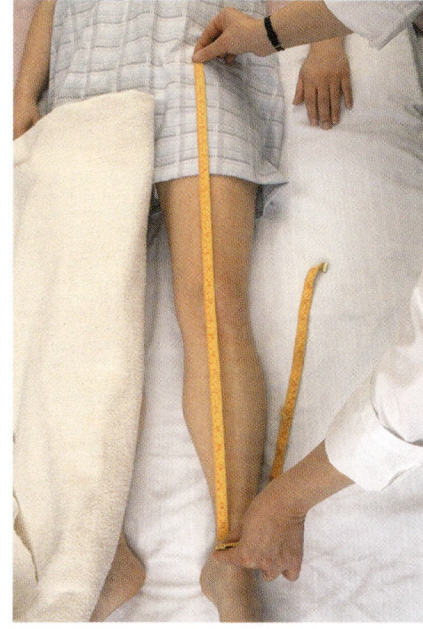

True leg length

(continued on next page)

Procedure 21-15 ■ Assessing the Musculoskeletal System (continued)

d. Measure the circumference of the forearms, upper arms, thighs, and calves.

Expected findings: The differences in circumference between the right and left extremity are 1 cm or less.

Abnormal findings: Circumference differences > 1 cm may reflect atrophy or hypertrophy.

---

7. Inspect muscles and joints bilaterally for symmetry and shape.

Expected findings: Size and shape are symmetrical. Muscles and joints are smooth, nontender, and similar in color and temperature to surrounding tissue.

Developmental Modifications

Older adults—Observe for surgical scars indicating joint replacement or joint surgeries.

Developmental Variation

Older adults—Muscle mass and tone decrease.

Abnormal findings:

- Hot, red, swollen, stiff, or painful joints may indicate injuries, arthritis, gout, bursitis, or other inflammatory diseases.
- **Heberden's nodes** are hard, painless nodules over the distal interphalangeal joints—usually seen with degenerative joint disease (DJD), but they may be seen with rheumatoid arthritis (RA).
- Severe misalignment and deformity are more often a result of DJD than of RA.
- Crepitus may be heard in DJD.

---

8. Test active ROM by asking the client to move the following joints through ROM
  a. Temporomandibular joint (TMJ)

  b. Neck

  c. Thoracic and lumbar spine

  d. Shoulder

  e. Upper arm and elbow

  f. Wrist
  g. Hands and fingers

Expected findings:

TMJ—Able to flex, extend, move side to side, protrude, and retract the jaw.

Neck—Flexes, extends, hyperextends, bends laterally, and rotates side to side.

Spine—Able to bend at the waist, stand upright, hyperextend (bend backward), bend laterally, and rotate side to side.

Shoulder—Able to move the arm forward and backward, abduct, adduct, and rotate internally and externally.

Upper arm and elbow—Able to bend, extend, supinate, and pronate the elbow.

Wrist—Flexes, extends, hyperextends, and moves side to side.

Hands and fingers—Able to:
  Spread the fingers (abduct)
  Bring them together (adduct)
  Make a fist (flex)
  Extend the hand (extend)
  Bend fingers back (hyperextend)
  Bring thumb to index finger (palmar adduction).

h. Hip

i. Knee

j. Ankles and feet

Hip—Able to:
   Extend the leg straight
   Flex the knee to the chest
   Abduct and adduct the leg
   Rotate the hip internally and externally
   Hyperextend the leg.

Knee—Able to flex and extend the knee.

Ankles and feet—able to dorsiflex, plantar flex, evert, invert, abduct, and adduct the feet and ankles.

KEY POINT: *If a patient cannot move the limb, put the joint through passive ROM. Never force a joint against resistance or if it causes discomfort.*

Joint Movements ▼

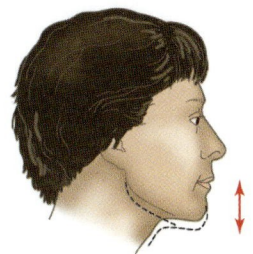

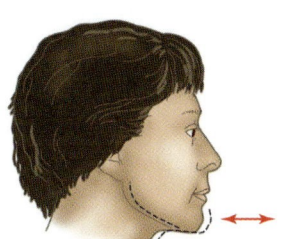

Depression: lowering a body part
Elevation: raising a body part

Retraction: moving backward
Protraction: moving forward

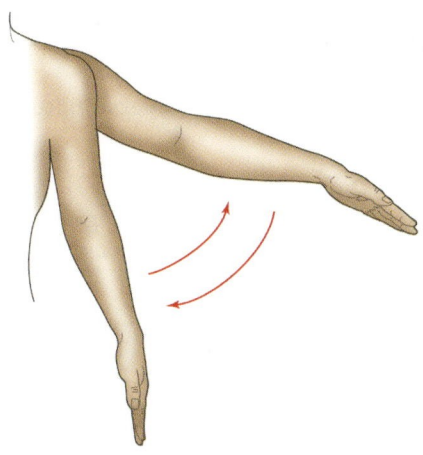

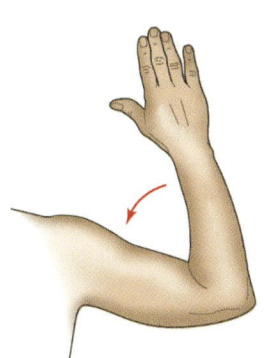

Abduction: moving away from midline
Adduction: moving toward midline

Flexion: bending, decreasing joint angle

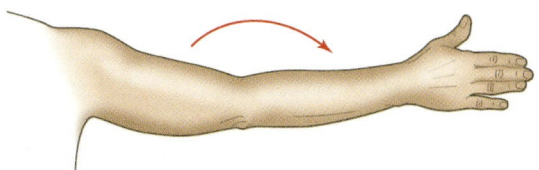

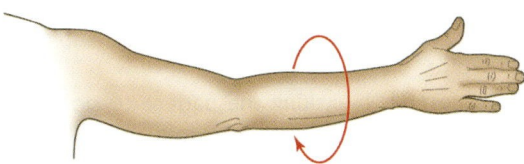

Extension: straightening, increasing joint angle

Circumduction: moving in a circular fashion

(continued on next page)

Procedure 21-15 ■ Assessing the Musculoskeletal System (continued)

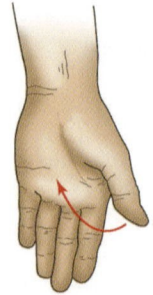
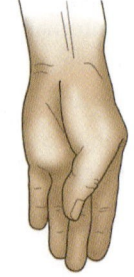

Resposition   Opposition

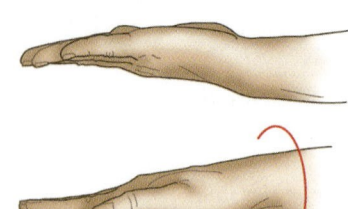

Supination: turning upward

Pronation: turning downward

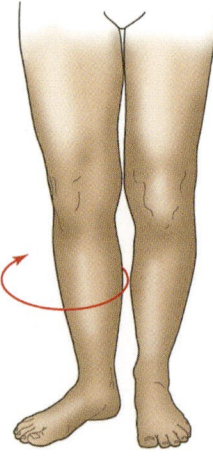
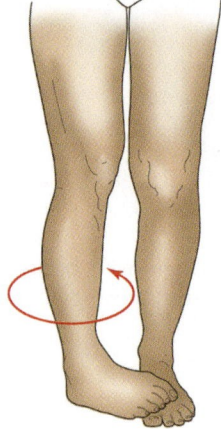
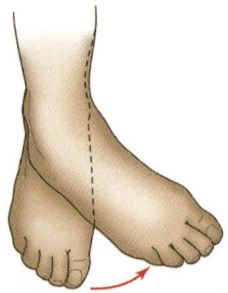
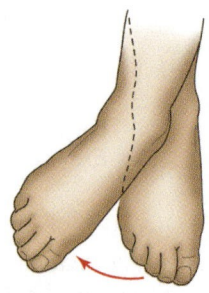

External rotation: turning away from midline

Internal rotation: turning toward midline

Inversion: turning inward

Eversion: turning outward

---

9. **Test muscle strength by repeating ROM against resistance.** Use the rating scale at the end of this step.
   a. **Test handgrip** by crossing your middle and index fingers and asking the patient to squeeze. (*Tip: If you are wearing rings, a strong handgrip on those fingers can be painful.*)
   b. **Test biceps strength.** Place one hand on the client's biceps and have the patient raise the forearm (flex the elbow) as you apply resistance at the wrist.
   c. **Test triceps strength** by having the client straighten the arm at the elbow (extend the elbow) as you apply resistance at the wrist.
   d. **Test leg strength** by having patient raise leg (straighten the knee) against your hand as you apply resistance.
   e. **Test ankle strength** by asking the patient to point the toes downward (plantar flexion). Hold the ankle while you apply resistance to the plantar surface of the foot.
   f. **Test ankle strength** by having the client point the toes toward the knee (dorsiflexion) as you apply resistance to the top of the foot.

Expected findings: Active motion against full resistance. There should be no crepitus (clicking) or pain with joint movement. ▼

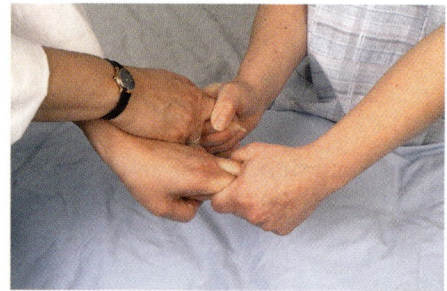

Muscle Strength Rating Scale		
RATING	CRITERIA	CLASSIFICATION
5	Active motion against full resistance	Normal
4	Active motion against some resistance	Slight weakness
3	Active motion against gravity	Weakness
2	Passive ROM	Poor ROM
1	Slight flicker of contraction	Severe weakness
0	No muscular contraction	Paralysis

? What if . . .

- **There is limited ROM in a joint?**

  Use a goniometer to measure the limited motion in degrees. Place the goniometer over the joint, matching the angle of the joint.

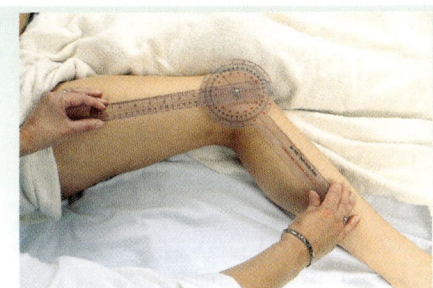

Using a goniometer

Documentation

- If you need information about documenting your findings, review Caring for the Nguyens, including Documenting Physical Examination Findings (Nam Nguyen).

Procedure 21-16 ■ Assessing the Sensory–Neurological System

➤ For steps to follow in *all* procedures, refer to the Universal Steps for All Procedures found on the page facing the inside back cover.

➤ *NOTE:* This procedure provides guidelines for performing a comprehensive neurological exam. Steps 1–10 assess cognitive status, and the box at the end of the procedure contains questions that are useful for screening cognitive status.

Equipment

- Pen and record form
- Wisp of cotton
- Sharp object, such as a toothpick or sterile needle
- Objects to touch, such as a coin, button, or key
- Something fragrant, such as coffee or rubbing alcohol
- Something to taste, such as sugar, salt, or lemon
- Tongue blade
- Two test tubes
- Reflex hammer
- Ophthalmoscope

Developmental Modifications for Children

- For children younger than age 5 years, use the Denver Developmental Screening Test II to assess neurological and motor function.

- Check the child's ability to understand and follow instructions.

Developmental Modifications for Older Adults

- You may need to perform the sensory–neurological exam over several sessions. The full exam is lengthy, and older adults fatigue easily. If the client seems to be getting tired, stop the test and finish at a later time.

Focused History Questions

- Do you have any neurological ("nerve") problems?
- Have you ever had head trauma, loss of consciousness, dizziness, headaches, or seizures?
- Do you have memory problems, forgetfulness, or inability to concentrate?

(continued on next page)

Procedure 21-16 ■ Assessing the Sensory–Neurological System (continued)

- Have you noticed any changes in your ability to see, smell, taste, hear, feel, or maintain balance?
- Do you have any weakness, numbness, or paralysis?
- Do you have any problems performing activities of daily living (ADLs)?
- Do you have any problems walking?
- Do you have mood problems or depression?

- Do you use alcohol or drugs for non-medical purposes? If so, how much and how often?
- Have you ever been treated for neurological or psychiatric problems?
- Do you have a history of hypertension, diabetes, stroke, or circulation problems?

➤ When performing the procedure, always identify your patient according to agency policy, using two identifiers, and be attentive to standard precautions, hand hygiene, patient safety and privacy, body mechanics, and documentation.

Procedure Steps

1. **Assess behavior.** Note the client's facial expression, posture, affect, and grooming.

2. **Determine level of arousal (LOA):**
   a. Note the client's response to verbal stimuli.
   b. If the client does not respond to verbal stimuli, try **tactile stimulation:** Gently shake the client's shoulder. **KEY POINT:** *Clients who have hearing deficits lip-read to compensate. Catch the client's attention by combined auditory and visual stimuli (e.g., touch her hand).*
   c. If the client does not respond to tactile stimuli, try **painful stimuli:** Squeeze the trapezius muscle, rub the sternum, apply pressure on the mandible at the angle of the jaw, or apply pressure over the "moon" of the nail.

   NOTE: *Clients who respond to painful stimuli withdraw when pressure is applied.*

   The Glasgow Coma Scale and the FOUR Scale at the end of this procedure provide standard references for assessing LOA for a patient with head injury.

3. **Determine the level of orientation.**

   a. *Orientation to time:* Ask the client to state the year, date, and time of day.

   b. *Orientation to place:* Ask the client to state where he is (i.e., city, state, where he lives).

Findings

Expected findings: The client is well groomed, with an erect posture, pleasant facial expression, and appropriate affect.

Abnormal findings: Inappropriate behavior may result from neurological or psychological problems, as well as from a variety of medications, alcohol, and street drugs.

Expected findings: The patient is awake and alert and readily responds to verbal stimuli.

Abnormal findings: Lethargy, stupor, or coma may result from trauma, neurological disorder, hypoxia, or chemical substances.

✚ A changing level of arousal (along with forgetfulness, restlessness, or sudden quietness) is one of the earliest indicators of increased intracranial pressure, which can be life threatening.

Expected findings: The client is awake, alert (see step 2), and oriented to time, place, and person (AAO × 3).

a. **Expected findings:** Hospitalized patients commonly lose track of date and time of day, but they easily reorient. As a rule, they should at least know the year.

Abnormal findings: Older adults who become disoriented to time usually think it is an earlier date. If a client offers a bizarre time or futuristic date, consider psychiatric concerns as the cause of disorientation.

b. **Expected findings:** Interpret data carefully. In some situations (e.g., after an automobile accident away from home), the patient may know he is in the hospital but not know which hospital or which city.

c. *Orientation to person:* Ask the names of family members. Ask, "Do you know who I am?" If the client cannot answer these questions, ask him to state his name. *Self-identity remains intact the longest.*

c. Patient should know you are a healthcare worker, but not necessarily your name.

Developmental Variations

 Older adults—The stress of an unfamiliar situation can create confusion in an older adult.

Abnormal findings: Disorientation may result from physical or psychological problems. Bizarre responses are usually associated with psychiatric problems.

4. **Assess memory.**
   a. *Assess immediate memory* by asking the client to repeat a series of three numbers that you speak slowly (e.g., 1, 5, 8). Gradually increase the length of the series until the client cannot repeat the series correctly. Record the length of the last correct series (e.g., "Successfully repeats a series of 7 numbers correctly.")
   b. *Repeat the test,* beginning with a series of three numbers, but ask the client to repeat them back to you in reverse order.
   c. *Assess recent memory* by naming three items (e.g., "mirror, truck," and "the letter X") and asking the client to recall them later during the exam. Alternatively, you can ask questions such as, "How did you get to the hospital? What did you have for breakfast?" However, you will need to verify the patient's answers.
   d. *Assess remote* memory by asking the client his birth date or the date of a major historical event.

Developmental Modifications

Children—Assess memory by using names of toys (e.g., truck, ball, puzzle), names of people in his family, or names of familiar cartoon characters.

Expected findings: Immediate, recent, and remote memories are intact. Average series recall is 5–8 numbers in sequence and 4–6 numbers in reverse order.

Developmental Variations

Children—Number of objects recalled is usually fewer than the child's age in years.

 Older adults—Loss of immediate and recent memory is common; long-term memory is usually not impaired.

Abnormal findings: Memory problems may be benign or may signal underlying neurological problems. Temporary memory loss may occur after trauma.

5. **Assess mathematical and** calculation **skills.**
   a. Have the client solve a simple mathematical problem, such as 3 + 3.
   b. If he is able to solve that problem, present a more complex example, yet simple enough that regardless of math skills the client could still determine the appropriate response, such as, "If you have $3 and you buy an item for $2, how much money will you have left?"
   c. To assess both calculation skills and attention span, ask the client to count backward from 100.
   d. A more difficult test is to have the client perform serial threes or serial sevens. Ask him to begin at 100 and keep subtracting 3 (or 7).

Consider the person's language, education, and culture in deciding whether this test is appropriate for him.

Expected findings: Mathematical and calculation ability is appropriate for the patient's age, education level, and language ability. The average adult can solve simple mathematical problems and can complete serial sevens in about 90 seconds with 3 or fewer errors.

Abnormal findings: Inability to calculate at a level appropriate for age and educational level may indicate neurological impairment or developmental delay.

6. **Assess general knowledge.**
   You can ask questions directly or work this into the overall interaction with the client.

   NOTE: Ask the client how many days in the week or months in the year.

Expected findings: Vocabulary and general knowledge are intact.

(continued on next page)

Procedure 21-16 ■ Assessing the Sensory–Neurological System (continued)

7. Evaluate thought processes. Assess throughout the exam. Notice attention span, logic of speech, ability to stay focused, and appropriateness of responses.

Expected findings: Thought processes are clear, client responds appropriately, and speech is coherent and logical.

Abnormal findings: Alteration in thought processes may be due to physical disorders, such as dementia; psychiatric disorders, such as psychosis; or alcohol and drugs.

8. Assess abstract thinking. Ask the client to interpret a maxim (or saying), such as "A penny saved is a penny earned" or "A rolling stone gathers no moss."

Expected findings: Abstract thinking is intact.

Abnormal findings: Inability to think abstractly is associated with dementia, delirium, mental retardation, and psychoses.

Developmental Modifications

Children—The ability to think abstractly does not develop until the late school-age years or adolescence. To assess a child younger than age 12 years, ask her to describe things that are like and unlike a named object (e.g., "Tell me something that is like a cup.")

9. Assess judgment. Ask the client to respond to a hypothetical situation, such as, "If you were walking down the street and saw smoke and flame coming from a house, what would you do?"

Expected findings: Judgment is intact.

Abnormal findings: Impaired judgment may be associated with dementia, psychosis, or substance abuse.

10. Assess communication ability.

   a. **Listen to the client's speech.** Note the rate, flow, choice of vocabulary, and enunciation.

Expected findings: Speech flows easily, and patient enunciates clearly. Vocabulary is consistent with the client's age, education, and language fluency.

Abnormal findings: Problems with flow (e.g., halting speech, stuttering, very rapid speech, slurred words) may be due to language problems, nervousness, anxiety, or neurological problems.

   b. **Test spontaneous speech**: Show the client a picture, and have him describe it.

Expected findings: Spontaneous speech is intact.

Abnormal findings: Impaired spontaneous speech is associated with cognitive impairment.

   c. **Test motor speech** by having the client say "Do, re, mi, fa, so, la, ti, do." Assess ability to swallow. Observe for clarity of speech, facial mobility, drooling, and oral hypotonia. Ask the client to repeat a short phrase 2 or 3 times and observe for lack of coordination.

Expected findings: Motor speech is intact.

Abnormal findings: Impaired motor speech is associated with problems with CN XII or with coordination of speech muscles.

   d. **Test automatic speech** by having the client recite the days of the week.

Expected findings: Automatic speech is intact.

Abnormal findings: Cognitive impairment or memory problems cause difficulty with automatic speech.

   e. **Test sound recognition** by having the client identify a familiar sound, such as clapping hands.

Expected findings: Sound recognition is intact

Abnormal findings: Temporal lobe problems may be the cause of impaired sound recognition.

   f. **Test auditory–verbal comprehension** by asking the client to follow simple directions (e.g., "Point to your nose; rub your left elbow").

Expected findings: Auditory–verbal comprehension is intact.

Abnormal findings: Temporal lobe problems affect reception. Frontal lobe problems affect expression.

g. **Test visual recognition** by pointing to objects and asking the client to identify them.

Expected findings: Visual recognition is intact.

Abnormal findings: Impaired visual recognition indicates parieto-occipital lobe problems.

h. **Test visual–verbal comprehension** by having the client read a sentence and explain its meaning.

Expected findings: Visual–verbal comprehension is intact.

Abnormal findings: Impaired visual-verbal comprehension indicates cognitive impairment.

i. **Test writing** by having the client write her name and address.

Expected findings: Writing ability is intact.

j. **Test ability to copy figures** by having the client copy a circle, letter X, square, triangle, and star.

Expected findings: The client is able to copy figures.

---

11. Test cranial nerve I—olfactory nerve

NOTE: You can assess CN I with your examination of the nose and sinuses (see Procedure 21-8).

a. Before testing, check the patency of the nostrils by gently occluding each nostril and having the client sniff.

b. Have the client occlude one nostril and hold an aromatic substance (e.g., lemon, coffee, vanilla, alcohol) under the nostril.

c. Repeat with a different substance under the other nostril.

Expected findings: The client can identify the substances.

Developmental Variation

Older adults—May have a decreased sense of smell.

Abnormal findings: Anosmia is the loss of the sense of smell. It may be genetic, related to chronic nose or sinus problems, heavy tobacco use, snorting cocaine, or zinc deficiency.

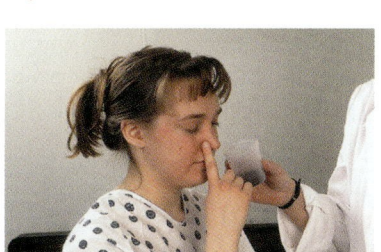

Developmental Modifications

Children—Select a substance that you are certain the child is familiar with (e.g., bananas or apples).

---

12. Test cranial nerve II—optic nerve.

NOTE: You can assess CN II with your examination of the eyes (see Procedure 21-6).

a. Test visual acuity by asking the client to identify the smallest print readable on the Snellen chart.

Expected findings: Visual acuity is 20/20 in the right eye, left eye, and both eyes.

Abnormal findings: Many visual deficits are correctable with eyeglasses or contact lenses. They are not necessarily caused by optic nerve damage.

Developmental Modifications

Use picture chart for small children, Snellen E for school-age children.

b. Identify visual field by having the client describe the boundaries of the visual field while her eye is in a fixed position.

Expected findings: Peripheral vision range is approximately 50° in the superior field, 70° in the inferior field, 60° in the nasal field, and 90°–110° in the temporal field.

c. Perform a fundoscopic exam (see Procedure 21-6).

Expected findings: Disc margins are sharply demarcated. The cup is half the size of the disc or less.

Abnormal findings: CN II deficits may be due to tumor or CVA.

(continued on next page)

Procedure 21–16 ■ Assessing the Sensory–Neurological System (continued)

13. Test cranial nerves III, IV, and VI—oculomotor, trochlear, and abducens nerves.
   a. Test EOMs by having the client move the eyes through the six cardinal fields of gaze while holding her head steady. ▼

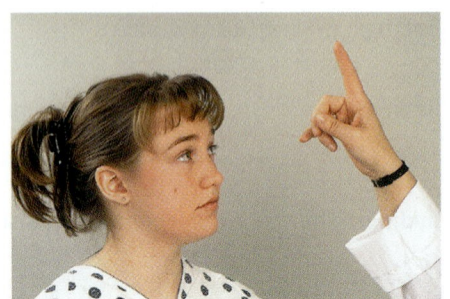

   b. Test pupillary reaction to light and accommodation.

   NOTE: See Procedure 21-6 for further details on each of these tests.

Expected findings: Client can move her eyes through the six cardinal fields of gaze. Pupils are equal in size and react to light and accommodation.

Abnormal findings: Changes in intracranial pressure (ICP) may affect EOMs and pupillary reaction.

---

14. Test cranial nerve V—trigeminal nerve.
   a. **Test motor function** by having the client move his jaw from side to side, clenching his jaw, and biting down on a tongue blade.

   NOTE: You can assess this function in your examination of the mouth and oropharynx (see Procedure 21-9).

   b. **Test sensory function** by having the client close her eyes and identify when you are touching her face at the forehead, cheeks, and chin bilaterally—first with your finger and then repeat with a toothpick.
   c. **Test the corneal reflex** by touching the cornea with a wisp of cotton or puffing air from a syringe over the cornea.

   ✚ The corneal reflex is not usually tested on a conscious person because the procedure is unpleasant and a corneal abrasion can occur. A conscious person can blink intentionally, so there is no need to stimulate the blink.

   NOTE: You can assess the corneal reflex in your examination of the eyes (see Procedure 21-6).

Expected findings: The client is able to perform all motor functions and can perceive light touch and superficial pain bilaterally; corneal reflex is intact.

Abnormal findings: Inability to perceive light touch and superficial pain may indicate peripheral nerve damage. An absent corneal reflex is an ominous neurological sign.

---

15. Test cranial nerve VII—facial nerve.
   a. Test motor function by having the client make faces, such as smile, frown, or whistle.

   NOTE: You can assess this function in your examination of the head and face (see Procedure 21-5).

   b. Test taste on the anterior portion of the tongue by placing sweet (sugar), salty (salt), or sour (lemon) substance on the tip of the tongue. Do not test taste by using pungent, bitter, or markedly unpleasant flavors.

   NOTE: You can assess this function in your examination of the mouth and oropharynx (see Procedure 21-9).

Expected findings: The client is able to perform all movements and can distinguish sweet, salty, and sour tastes.

Developmental Variations

 Older adults—Have decreased taste sensation, especially sweet and salty, due to taste bud atrophy and diminished sense of smell.

Abnormal findings: Asymmetrical movement may be seen with nerve damage from a CVA or Bell's palsy. Impaired taste may be associated with nerve damage, chemotherapy, or radiation to the face or neck.

16. Test cranial nerve VIII—acoustic nerve.

NOTE: *You can assess this function in your examination of the ears (see Procedure 21-7).*

a. Perform watch-tick test for hearing by holding a watch close to the client's ear.
b. Perform Weber and Rinne tests to assess air and bone conduction.
c. Test balance with the Romberg test, if it has not already been performed.

See Procedures 21-7 and 21-15 for further details on these tests.

Developmental Modifications

Children—Romberg test is appropriate only after age 3.

Expected findings: Hearing is intact. Romberg test is negative.

Abnormal findings: Hearing loss, loss of balance, or vertigo may result from acoustic nerve damage.

---

17. Test cranial nerves IX and X—glossopharyngeal and vagus nerves.

a. Observe ability to talk, swallow, and cough.
b. Test motor function by asking the client to say, "Ah" while you depress a tongue blade and observe the soft palate and uvula.
c. Test sensory function by taking a tongue blade and gently touching the back of the pharynx to induce a gag reflex.
d. Test taste (sweet, salty, and sour) on the posterior portion of the tongue. Avoid bitter or repulsive tasting substances.

Expected findings: Swallow and cough reflex are intact. Speech is clear. The uvula and soft palate rise symmetrically, and the gag reflex is intact. Taste on the posterior tongue is intact.

Developmental Variations

 Older adults—Have decreased taste sensation, especially sweet and salty, due to atrophy of the taste buds and a diminished sense of smell.

Abnormal findings: Damage to CN IX and X impairs swallowing. Damage to CN X changes voice quality.

---

18. Test cranial nerve XI—accessory nerve.

NOTE: *You can assess this motor nerve function with your examination of the musculoskeletal system (see Procedure 21-15).*

a. Place your hands on the client's shoulder, and have the client shrug his shoulders against resistance.
b. Have the client turn his head from side to side against resistance. ▼

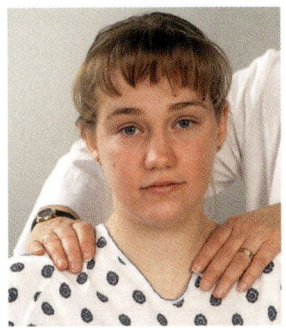

Expected findings: Movement is symmetrical and pain free. Full ROM of the neck with +5 strength.

Abnormal findings: Asymmetrical movement, pain, or absent movement indicates CN XI disorders.

---

19. Test cranial nerve XII—hypoglossal nerve.
a. Ask the client to say, "d, l, n, t."
b. Have the client protrude the tongue and move it from side to side.

Expected findings: The client can articulate the sounds and move the tongue easily.

Abnormal findings: Tongue paralysis

(continued on next page)

Procedure 21-16 ■ Assessing the Sensory–Neurological System (continued)

20. Test superficial sensations.

a. Begin with the most peripheral part when testing the limbs (e.g., test the foot before the leg). ➤
If the client can feel sensation in the most peripheral part, you can assume the sensory nerve is intact to that point.

b. If the client does not perceive the touch in an area, determine the boundaries of the dysfunction by testing at about every inch (2.5 cm). Sketch the area of sensory loss.

c. Wait about 2 sec before moving to each site.
Wait so that you can be sure that the patient is perceiving each stimulus separately.

d. *Light touch:* With the patient's eyes closed, brush a cotton wisp on various areas of the body, comparing sides. Ask the client to say, "Now," when he feels your touch and to point to the spot you are touching.

e. *Pain:* With the patient's eyes closed, use a toothpick (or sterile needle) with dull and sharp ends. Touch various areas of the body (except the face), and have the patient identify whether the sensation is dull or sharp. Alternate the dull and sharp ends as you move from spot to spot. Compare sides of the body.

f. *Temperature sensation:* Test only if the patient's perception of pain is abnormal. Use test tubes filled with hot and cold water. Touch the tube to various areas of the body, comparing sides; have the client say "Hot," "Cold," or "Don't know."
If pain sensation is intact, temperature will be, too, because sensations for pain and temperature are transmitted along the same tracts.

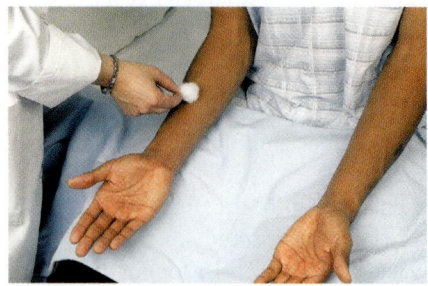

Testing light touch

Expected findings: Able to identify areas of light touch.

Abnormal findings: Diminished sensation or areas of absent perception

Expected findings: The client is able to identify the areas stimulated and the type of sensation.

Abnormal findings:
- **Hyperalgia:** increased pain sensation
- **Analgesia:** no pain sensation
- **Paresthesia:** numbness and tingling

Developmental Variations

Older adults—May have a decreased perception of temperature and deep pain.

21. Test deep sensations.

a. *Assess vibratory sensation* by placing a vibrating tuning fork on a metatarsal joint and distal interphalangeal joint. Have the patient identify when she feels the vibration and when it stops. ▼

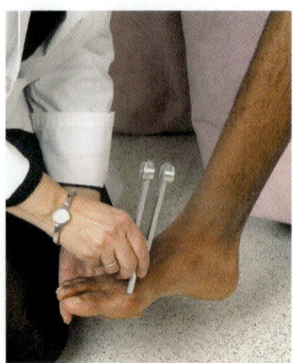

Expected findings: Vibratory sense is intact bilaterally in the upper and lower extremities.

Abnormal findings: Diminished or absent vibration sense is seen with peripheral nerve damage from vascular disease, diabetes, alcoholism, or damage to the posterior column of the spinal cord.

22. **Test kinesthetic sensation (position sense)** by holding the client's finger or toe on the sides and moving it up or down. Keeping her eyes closed, have the client identify the direction of the movement. ▼

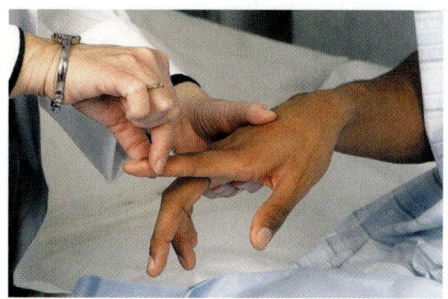

Expected findings: Position sense is intact bilaterally in the upper and lower extremities.

Developmental Variation

 Older adults—May lose position sense in the great toes.

Abnormal findings: Diminished or absent position sense indicates nerve or spinal cord damage.

23. **Test discriminatory sensations.**
   a. *Assess stereognosis* by placing a familiar object (e.g., a coin or a button) in the palm of the client's hand and having her identify it.
   b. *Assess graphesthesia* by drawing a number or letter in the palm of your patient's hand and having the patient identify what was drawn.
   c. *Test two-point discrimination* with toothpicks. Have the patient close her eyes. Touch her on the finger with two toothpicks simultaneously. Gradually move the points together, and have the patient say, "One," or "Two," each time you move the toothpicks. Document distance and location at which she can no longer feel two separate points. ➤

Expected findings: **Stereognosis** (the ability to recognize the form of solid objects by touch) is intact bilaterally.

Expected findings: **Graphesthesia** (the ability to recognize outlines, numbers, or symbols written on the skin) is intact bilaterally.

Expected findings: **Point discrimination** (recognizing whether 1 or 2 areas of the skin are being touched). Discriminates between two points on fingertips no more than 0.5 cm apart.

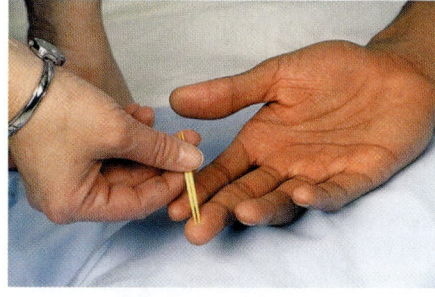

   d. *Test point localization* by having the patient close her eyes while you touch her. Have her point to the area you touched. Repeat on both sides and the upper and lower extremities.
   e. *Test sensory extinction* by simultaneously touching the patient on both sides (e.g., on both hands, both knees, both arms). Have the patient identify where he was touched. ▼

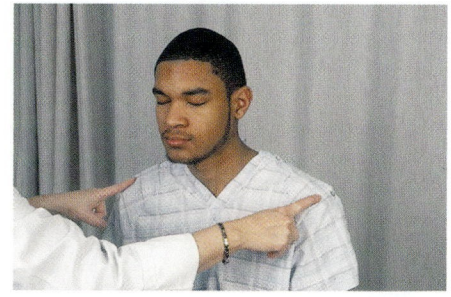

Expected findings: **Point localization** (the ability to identify where one is being touched) is intact bilaterally in the upper and lower extremities.

Expected findings: Extinction is intact: Client should feel the sensation on both sides of his body.

Abnormal findings: Abnormalities in any of the discriminatory sensation tests may indicate a lesion or disorder of the sensory cortex or disorder of the posterior column of the spinal cord.

Developmental Modifications

 Older adults—May need more time to respond to a stimulus, as reaction time may be slower.

(continued on next page)

Procedure 21-16 ■ Assessing the Sensory–Neurological System (continued)

24. Test deep tendon reflexes.
Use the accompanying scale to grade responses.

Deep Tendon Reflex Grading Scale

0 No response detected

+1 Diminished response

+2 Response normal

+3 Response somewhat stronger than normal

+4 Response hyperactive with **clonus** (involuntary contractions that continue after the first contraction is elicited by the hammer)

   a. **Biceps reflex** (spinal cord level C5 and C6). Rest the patient's elbow in your nondominant hand, with your thumb over the biceps tendon. Strike the percussion hammer to your thumb. ▼

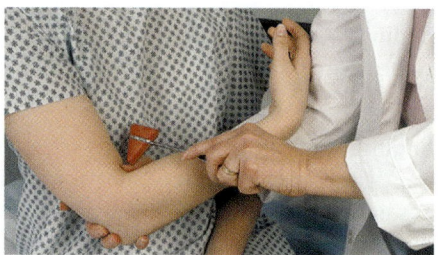

   b. **Triceps reflex** (spinal cord level C7 and C8). Abduct the patient's arm at the shoulder, and flex it at the elbow. Support the upper arm with your nondominant hand, letting the forearm hang loosely. Strike the triceps tendon about 2.5–5 cm (1–2 in.) above the olecranon process. ▼

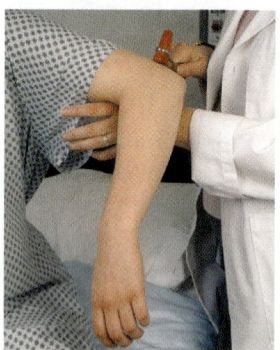

Developmental Variations

   Older adults—Reflex responses may not be as strong as in young adults. Reaction time is slower as well.

Expected findings: +2 response: You can feel the biceps contract with your thumb; slight flexion of the elbow.

Expected findings: +2 response: Contraction of triceps with slight extension at elbow

c. **Brachioradialis reflex** (spinal cord level C3 and C6). Rest the client's arm on her leg. Strike with the percussion hammer 2.5–5 cm (1–2 in.) above the bony prominence of the wrist on the thumb side. ▼

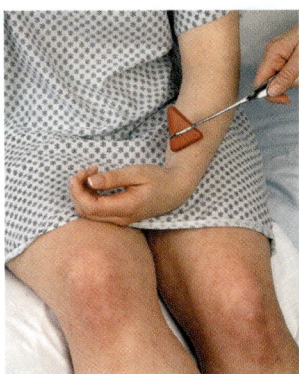

Expected findings: +2 response: Flexion at elbow and supination of forearm

d. **Patellar reflex** (spinal cord level L2, L3, and L4). Have the client sit with her legs dangling. Strike the tendon directly below the patella. ▼

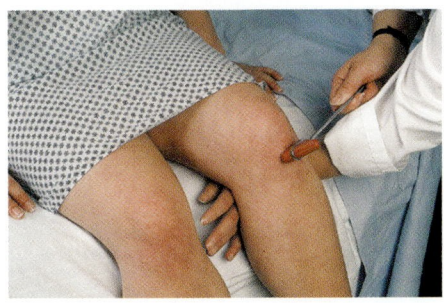

Expected findings: +2 response: Contraction of quadriceps with extension of leg

e. **Achilles reflex** (spinal cord level S₁, S₂). Have the patient lie supine or sit with her legs dangling. Hold the patient's foot slightly dorsiflexed, and strike the Achilles tendon about 5 cm (2 in.) above the heel with the percussion hammer. ▼

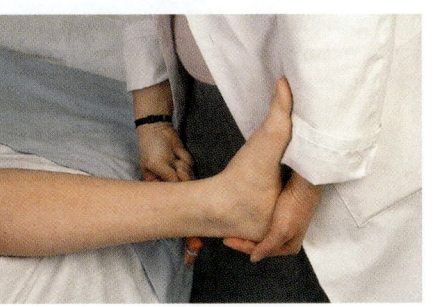

Expected findings: +2 response: Plantar flexion of foot.

Developmental Modifications

Newborns—test the following reflexes:

- **Rooting reflex**—Stroke the cheek; the head should turn to the side you touched.
- **Palmar grasp**—Place one finger in the baby's hand; his fingers should curl around your finger.
- **Tonic neck reflex**—Position the baby supine; turn his head to one side. The arm and leg on that side should extend, and those on the other side will flex.

Developmental Variation

 Older adults—May lose this reflex.

Abnormal findings:

- Absent or diminished responses are seen with degenerative disease, nerve damage, or lower motor neuron disease.
- Hyperactive reflexes are seen with spinal cord injuries and upper motor neuron disease.
- Rooting, palmar grasp, and tonic neck reflexes present after age 6 mo.

(continued on next page)

Procedure 21-16 ■ Assessing the Sensory–Neurological System (continued)

25. Test superficial reflexes:
Plantar reflex (Babinski's response): With your thumbnail or pointed object, stroke the sole of the client's foot in an arc from the lateral heel to medially across the ball of the foot. Record response as negative (normal) or positive (abnormal). ▼

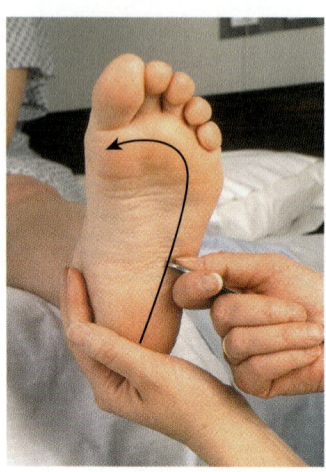

Expected findings: Babinski's response is negative: All the toes curl downward or there is no response.

Infants and children—Positive Babinski's is normal until age 2 yr or until the child begins walking.

Abnormal findings: A positive Babinski's response: dorsiflexion of the great toe and fanning of the other toes. Seen with drug or alcohol intoxication or upper motor neuron disease

Developmental Modifications

Older adults—This reflex may be difficult to elicit.

26. Mental status screening.
The following questions may be used for a rapid evaluation of cognitive status. You may have already assessed for some aspects of mental status (e.g., orientation to time).

Questions for Evaluating Cognitive Status

This complete set of questions is included so that you can use them for a mental status exam that is not part of a comprehensive assessment. In a comprehensive assessment, do not repeat questions you have already covered in other portions of the assessment.

QUESTION	FUNCTION ASSESSED
What is today's date?	Orientation to time
What time is it?	Orientation to time
Where are you?	Orientation to place
What is the reason for your visit? (If the patient is hospitalized, modify the question: Why are you in the hospital?)	Communication, vocabulary, thought processes, recent memory
Ask the patient to count backward from 100.	Word comprehension, abstract reasoning
Ask the patient to name several objects that you point to. Be sure to use common objects such as a pen, shoe, or window.	Vocabulary, general knowledge, and word comprehension
Write a brief command, such as "Clap your hands," on a slip of paper. Hand the paper to the patient and ask him to follow the instructions.	Reading comprehension
Ask the patient to write the names of his family members, along with their relationship to him.	Writing, thought processes, memory, sound recognition

Questions for Evaluating Cognitive Status—cont'd

QUESTION	FUNCTION ASSESSED
Ask the patient to name three things that begin with the letter D.	Auditory comprehension, thought processes
Ask the patient to draw a circle, square, and triangle next to each other on a sheet of paper.	Word comprehension, mathematical and calculation skills, communication (naming)
Difficulty with any of these questions requires further evaluation.	

? What if . . .

- **The patient is an older adult?**

For a mental-status exam for older adults, you may wish to use tools from the following Web sites:

The Mini-Cog (mental status assessment of older adults)

http://www.alz.org/documents_custom/minicog.pdf

Mini-Mental Status Exam

http://infotechsoft.com/products/aspect_forms.aspx?formID=MMSE

You should also assess older adults for dementia, which is characterized by these four features:

- Mental status change of sudden onset or fluctuating course

- Difficulty focusing attention, distractible
- Disorganized, illogical thinking
- Increased or decreased level of consciousness (e.g., hyperalert, lethargic)

Delirium occurs in 15% to 60% of older hospitalized patients. You should assess them frequently to facilitate prompt identification and management of delirium.

For a reliable tool for assessing confusion and dementia in older adults, go to the following Web site or search in your browser for The Confusion Assessment Method Instrument: **http://www.hospitalelderlifeprogram.org/delirium-instruments/short-cam/**

Home Care

Instruct caregivers in home safety if the client has cerebral function deficits or sensory or motor deficits.

Documentation

If you need information about documenting your findings, review Caring for the Nguyens and Documenting Physical Examination Findings (Nam Nguyen).

Glasgow Coma Scale

EYE RESPONSE	SCORE	MOTOR RESPONSE	SCORE	VERBAL RESPONSE	SCORE
Opens spontaneously	4	Obeys verbal commands for movement	6	Oriented and converses	5
Opens to verbal commands	3	Reacts purposefully to localized pain	5	Disoriented but converses	4
Opens to pain	2	Withdraws in response to pain (generalized body response)	4	Uses inappropriate words	3
No response	1	Assumes flexor posture (decorticate posturing—arms flexed to chest, hands clenched and internally rotated) in response to pain. *Indicates problem is at or above the brainstem*	3	Makes incomprehensible sounds	2
		Assumes extensor posture (decerebrate posturing—arms extended, hands clenched and hyperpronated); Indicates problem at the brainstem level	2	No response	1
		No response	1		
Totals	____		____		____

(continued on next page)

Procedure 21-16 ■ **Assessing the Sensory–Neurological System** (continued)

Full Outline of UnResponsiveness (FOUR)

Eye Response

4—Eyelids open or opened, tracking, or blinking on command
3—Eyelids open but not tracking
2—Eyelids closed but open to loud voice
1—Eyelids closed but open to pain
0—Eyelids remain closed with pain

Motor Response

4—Thumbs-up, fist, or peace sign
3—Localizing to pain
2—Flexion response to pain
1—Extension response to pain
0—No response to pain or generalized myoclonus status

Brainstem Reflexes

4—Pupil and corneal reflexes present
3—One pupil wide and fixed
2—Pupil or corneal reflexes absent
1—Pupil and corneal reflexes absent
0—Absent pupil, corneal, and cough reflexes

Respirations

4—Not intubated, regular breathing pattern
3—Not intubated, Cheyne-Stokes breathing pattern
2—Not intubated, irregular breathing
1—Respirations greater than ventilator rate
0—respirations at ventilator rate or apnea

NOTE: Education is necessary to use this scale properly. To see how to use it,

Go to Mayo Clinic Proceedings, Wolf, Wijdicks, Bamlet, et al., 2007. Further validation of the FOUR Score Coma Scale by intensive care nurses, figure 1, is found at http://www.ncbi.nlm.nih.gov/pmc/articles/PMC2719522/

Sources: Okasha, A. S., Fayed, A. M., & Saleh, A. S. (2014). The FOUR Score predicts mortality, endotracheal intubation and ICU length of stay after traumatic brain injury. *Neurocritical Care, 21*(3), 496–504; Rauen, C., Chulay, M., Bridges, E., et al. (2008). Seven evidence-based practice habits: Putting some sacred cows out to pasture. *Critical Care Nurse, 28*(2), 98–124; Wijdicks, E. F., Kramer, A.A., Rohs, T., Jr., et al. (2015). Comparison of the Full Outline of UnResponsiveness Score and the Glasgow Coma Scale in predicting mortality in critically ill patients. *Critical Care Medicine, 43*(2), 439–444.

Procedure 21-17 ■ **Assessing the Male Genitourinary System**

➤ For steps to follow in *all* procedures, refer to the Universal Steps for All Procedures found on the page facing the inside back cover.

Equipment

- Nonlatex procedure gloves
- Penlight
- Pen and record form

Developmental Modifications for Children

- Obtain the parent's permission to perform this assessment.
- Explain to the child what you are going to do, and expect some resistance or embarrassment.

  Children are taught not to let strangers touch their genitals, and many children are modest.

Developmental Modifications for Older Adults

- Assess for incontinence.

  Incontinence is one of the elements of the SPICES assessment model for older adults.

Focused History Questions

- Have you noticed any redness, swelling, discharge, or odor in your genital area?
- Have you noticed asymmetry, lumps, or masses in your genitals? If so, describe them, and show me where they are.

- Have you ever been told you have a hernia?
- Have you ever had trauma to your genitals?
- Are you having any problems urinating?
- Are you sexually active? If not, have you ever been?
- Do you have sex with men, women, or both?
- What types of sexual activity do you engage in? Oral, anal, genital?
- Do you have more than one partner? How many partners have you had in the past 6 months?
- Do you use birth control? If so, what type and how often?
- Have you ever been treated for a sexually transmitted infection (STI)? If so, what type?
- Are you concerned about STIs or HIV?
- Do you take any precautions to avoid infections?
- Do you have any concerns about your sexual function?
- Do you have any difficulty achieving or maintaining an erection?
- Have you been taught to examine your testicles?

  In spite of the low prevalence of testicular cancer, men should be aware that a lump in the testicle, feeling of heaviness or swelling in the scrotum could be a sign of testicular cancer and should report these findings to his healthcare provider immediately (American Cancer Society, n.d.a).

- How often do you do testicular self-examination?
- Have you had any surgery of your reproductive tract?

➤ When performing the procedure, always identify your patient according to agency policy, using two identifiers, and be attentive to standard precautions, hand hygiene, patient safety and privacy, body mechanics, and documentation.

Procedure Steps

1. **Instruct the client to empty his bladder and undress** to expose the groin area.

2. **Have the patient stand while you sit at eye level to the genitalia;** alternatively, the patient can lie supine on the exam table with his legs slightly apart.

3. **Inspect the external genitalia.**
   a. *Hair.* Note the hair distribution pattern and condition of pubic hair. See the table discussing Tanner staging at the end of this procedure.
   The appearance of the external genitalia depends on the client's developmental stage.

   b. *Skin.* Inspect the condition of the skin of the penis. Observe for the presence or absence of the foreskin. Note the position of the urethral meatus and any lesions or discharge.

   c. **Scrotum.** Observe the condition, size, position, and symmetry of the scrotal sacs.

   d. **Inguinal area.** Note the condition of the inguinal areas. Look for swelling or bulges. The best way to do this is to have the client bear down while you palpate the inguinal canal.

4. **Palpate the penis.**
   a. With a gloved hand, use your thumb and fingers to palpate the shaft of the penis. Note consistency, tenderness, masses, or nodules.
   b. Retract the foreskin if present.

Findings

Expected findings: Hair distribution is triangular and appropriate for age. No pediculosis is present.

Abnormal findings: Sparse or absent hair may result from genetic factors, aging, or local or systemic disease.

Expected findings: Skin is intact with no lesions or discharge. Color is consistent with ethnicity. The urethral meatus is midline. The foreskin may be absent (circumcised); if present, it covers the glans and easily retracts.

Developmental Variations

Infants—Foreskin is difficult to retract in the uncircumcised male until about age 3 mo.

 Older adults—Penis and testes decrease in size.

Abnormal findings: Ulcerations or lesions (may be seen with a number of STIs, such as genital warts and genital herpes); **phimosis** (foreskin cannot be retracted and becomes swollen)

Expected findings: The skin should be free of lesions, nodules, swelling, rash, and erythema. The skin is rugated and deeper in color than the rest of the body.

Size and shape vary greatly. The left scrotal sac is usually lower than the right.

Abnormal findings:
- A rash may be caused by **tinea cruris,** a fungal infection often called "jock itch."
- Swelling may indicate hernia, tumor, or infection.

Expected findings: The inguinal area should be free of swelling or bulges.

Abnormal findings: A bulge may indicate a hernia or enlarged lymph node.

Expected findings: The penis is nontender with no masses or nodules. Pulsations are present on the dorsal side. The foreskin, if present, easily retracts.

Abnormal findings:
- Inability to palpate a pulse may indicate vascular insufficiency.
- Difficulty retracting the foreskin or problems with its return to position need further evaluation.

(continued on next page)

Procedure 21-17 ■ **Assessing the Male Genitourinary System** (continued)

5. Palpate the scrotum, testes, and epididymis.

a. Don a procedure glove and use your thumb and fingers to palpate. ▼

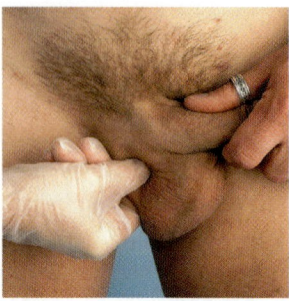

b. Note size, shape, consistency, mobility, masses, nodules, or tenderness.

c. Transilluminate any lumps, nodules, or edematous areas by shining a penlight over the area in a darkened room. ▼

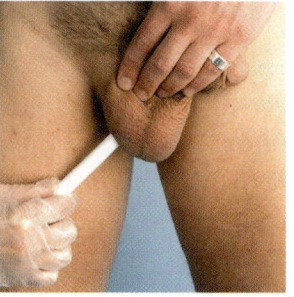

Expected findings:

- The scrotal skin is rough but without lesions.
- Each testicular sac contains a testicle and epididymis.
- The testes are rubbery, round, movable, and smooth. They are sensitive to pressure but nontender.
- The epididymis is comma shaped.
- The spermatic cord is smooth and round.
- There is no swelling or nodules.
- The left scrotal sac is usually lower than the right.

Abnormal findings:

- A unilateral mass
- Painless intratesticular masses may represent testicular cancer.
- A testicle that is swollen or tender may indicate infection or torsion.

6. Palpate the inguinal and femoral area for hernias. ▼

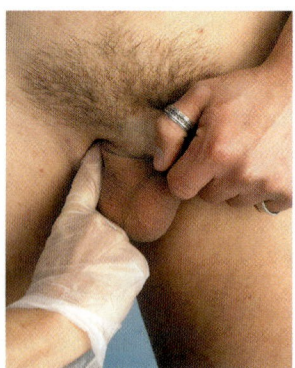

a. Assess for inguinal hernias with a gloved hand. Have the patient hold his penis to one side. Place your index finger in the client's scrotal sac above the testicle, and invaginate the skin. Follow the spermatic cord until you reach a slit-like opening (Hesselbach's triangle). Ask the client to cough or bear down as you feel for bulges.

b. Palpate for femoral hernias by palpating below the femoral artery while having the client cough or bear down.

Expected findings: No bulges or palpable masses are present in the inguinal or femoral area.

Abnormal findings: A bulge or mass often represents a hernia.

Direct hernia: protrusion through the abdominal wall.

Indirect hernia: protrusion into the inguinal canal or into the scrotum.

7. **Palpate the lymph nodes** in the groin area and the vertical chain over the inner aspect of the thigh.

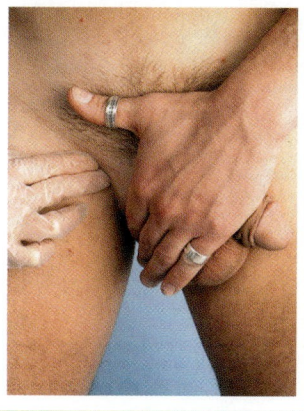 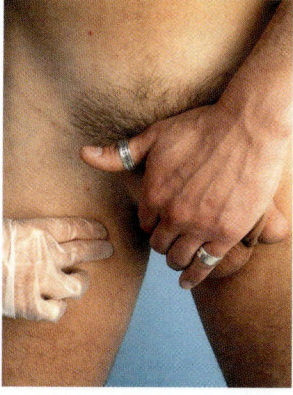

Expected findings: Nodes should be < 1 cm in size and freely mobile.

Abnormal findings: Enlarged or tender lymph nodes may indicate local or systemic disease.

Documentation

If you need more information about documenting your findings, review Caring for the Nguyens and Documenting Physical Examination Findings (Nam Nguyen).

Tanner Staging			
STAGE	**PUBIC HAIR**	**PENIS**	**TESTES AND SCROTUM**
Stage 1: Preadolescent	No pubic hair except for fine body hair similar to that on abdomen	Same size and proportions as in childhood	Same size and proportions as in childhood
Stage 2	Sparse growth of long, slightly pigmented, downy hair, straight or only slightly curled, chiefly at base of penis	Slight or no enlargement	Testes larger, scrotum larger, somewhat reddened and altered in texture
Stage 3	Darker, coarser, curlier hair spreading sparsely over pubic symphysis	Larger, especially in length	Further enlarged
Stage 4	Coarse and curly hair, as in adult; area covered greater than in stage 3 but not as great as in adult	Further enlarged in length and breadth, with development of glans	Further enlarged; scrotal skin darkened

(continued on next page)

Procedure 21-17 ■ Assessing the Male Genitourinary System (continued)

Tanner Staging—cont'd			
STAGE	**PUBIC HAIR**	**PENIS**	**TESTES AND SCROTUM**
Stage 5: Adult	Hair same as adult in quantity and quality, spreading to medial surfaces of thighs but not up over abdomen	Adult in size and shape	Adult in size and shape

Source: Adapted from Tanner, J. (1962). *Growth at adolescence* (2nd ed.). Oxford, England: Blackwell Scientific.

Procedure 21-18 ■ Assessing the Female Genitourinary System

➤ For steps to follow in *all* procedures, refer to the Universal Steps for All Procedures found on the page facing the inside back cover.

Equipment

- Patient drape
- Additional light source
- Nonlatex procedure gloves (if exposure to body fluids is a possibility)
- Pen and record form

Positioning

Lithotomy position, if possible.

🍁 Developmental Modifications for Older Adults

- Assess for incontinence.
Incontinence is one of the elements of the SPICES assessment model for older adults.
- Older women may have arthritis, which, along with muscle weakness, may make it difficult for them to assume the lithotomy position. You may need to use Sims' position and/or provide support for them to maintain a position.

Developmental Modifications for Children

- Obtain parental permission for this examination.
- Explain to the child what you are going to do, and expect some resistance or embarrassment.
Children are taught to not let strangers touch their genitals, and many children are modest.
- **KEY POINT:** *Do not perform internal assessment of an adolescent unless the girl is sexually active.*

Focused History Questions

- Are you having any problems urinating?
- Have you noticed any redness, swelling, discharge, or odor in your genital area?
- Have you ever been told you have a hernia?
- Have you ever had trauma to your genitals?
- Are you sexually active? If not, have you ever been?
- Do you have sex with men, women, or both?
- What types of sexual activity do you engage in? Oral, anal, or genital?
- How many partners do you currently have?
- How many partners have you had in the past 6 months?
- Do you use birth control? If so, what kind and how often?
- Have you ever been treated for a sexually transmitted infection (STI)? If so, what type?
- Are you concerned about STIs or HIV?
- Do you take any precautions to avoid infection?
- Do you have any concerns about your sexual function?
- Have you had any surgery of your reproductive tract?
- When was your last menstrual period?
- How often are your periods?
- Do you have any problems with your periods, such as cramping, breast pain, or heavy flow?
- How often do you have a gynecological health exam?
- When was your last Pap smear?
- Have you ever had an abnormal Pap smear? If so, how was it treated?
- How many times have you been pregnant?
- How many children do you have?
- Have you ever had a miscarriage? An abortion?

➤ When performing the procedure, always identify your patient according to agency policy, using two identifiers, and be attentive to standard precautions, hand hygiene, patient safety and privacy, body mechanics, and documentation.

Procedure Steps

1. Inspect the external genitalia.

a. Note the hair distribution pattern and the condition of pubic hair. See the table Maturation Status in Females at the end of this procedure.

The appearance of the external genitalia depends on the developmental stage of the client.

b. **Inspect the condition of the skin of the mons pubis and labia.** Observe for color, condition, lesions, and discharge.

Findings

Expected findings: Hair distribution in the pubic region is inverse triangular. Some hair may extend onto her abdomen and upper thighs. Hair distribution is appropriate for age.

Abnormal findings: Sparse or absent hair (may result from genetic factors, aging, or local or systemic disease).

Pediculosis pubis (lice), **nits** (white lice eggs), or flecks of dried blood on the skin.

Expected findings: Skin is intact with no lesions or discharge. Labia majora and minora are symmetrical with smooth to moderate wrinkling. Skin color is consistent with ethnicity. No ecchymosis, excoriation, nodules, edema, rash, or lesions are present.

Developmental Variations

 Older adults—Labia and vulva are atrophied.

Abnormal findings: Ulcerations or lesions may occur with a number of STIs.

---

2. Inspect the clitoris, urethral meatus, and vaginal introitus.

a. Wearing gloves, use your thumb and index finger to separate the labia and expose the clitoris. Observe the clitoris for size and position. ▼

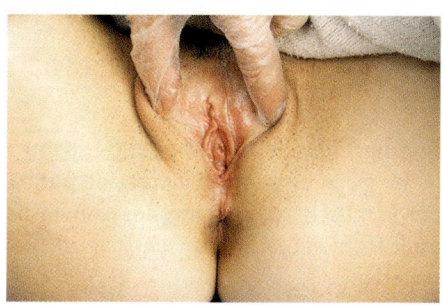

b. With the labia separated, observe the urethral meatus and vaginal introitus. Observe for color, size, and presence of discharge or lesions.

c. Have the client bear down while you observe the introitus.

Expected findings: The clitoris is about 2 cm long and 0.5 cm in diameter. No redness or lesions are present.

Abnormal findings: Enlargement of the clitoris may result from androgen excess or swelling related to trauma.

Absence of the clitoris, along with parts of the labia, is seen with female circumcision.

Expected findings: The urethral meatus is slit-like; midline; and free of discharge, lesions, swelling, or erythema. The mucosa of the introitus is pink and moist. Some clear to white discharge may be present and is odor free.

Expected findings: The introitus is patent, and there is no bulging or discomfort with bearing down.

Abnormal findings:
- Discharge, redness, or swelling may result from infection.
- Pale and dry mucosa may result from aging or use of topical steroids.
- Bulging may indicate prolapse of the uterus, bladder, or rectum.

(continued on next page)

Procedure 21-18 ■ Assessing the Female Genitourinary System (continued)

3. Palpate Bartholin's glands, the urethral glands, and Skene's ducts.
   a. Lubricate the index and middle fingers of your dominant hand with water-soluble lubricant.
   b. To palpate Bartholin's glands, insert your lubricated fingers into the vaginal introitus, and palpate the lower portion of the labia bilaterally between your thumb and fingers. ▼

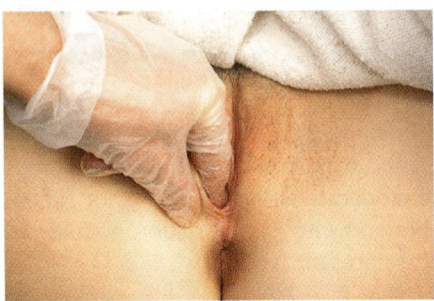

   c. To palpate Skene's ducts, rotate your internal fingers upward, and palpate the labium bilaterally.
   d. To milk the urethra, apply pressure with your index finger on the anterior vaginal wall, and observe for urethral discharge. Culture any discharge you see. ▼

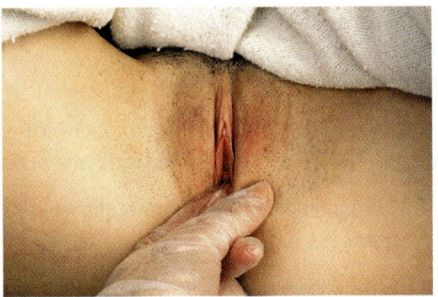

Expected findings:
- No swelling, masses, or tenderness of the glands.
- No urethral discharge.
- Labia uniform in texture; no discharge or pain with palpation.
- Perineum is smooth and firm in **nulliparous** women (women who have had no children), thinner in **parous** women (women who have had children).

Abnormal findings:
- Pain or discharge from the glands may indicate infection.
- Fissures or tears in the perineum are painful and require treatment.

---

4. Assess vaginal muscle tone and pelvic musculature.
   a. Insert two gloved fingers into the vagina.
   b. Ask the woman to constrict her vaginal muscles and then to bear down as though she were having a bowel movement.

Expected findings: Muscle tone should be strong in women who have never given birth. With increasing **parity** (number of births), pelvic muscle tone diminishes. Diminished tone may also result from injury, age, or medication. No bulges should be noted.

---

5. Palpate the inguinal and femoral area for hernias.

Expected findings: No bulges or palpable masses are present in the inguinal or femoral area.

---

6. Palpate the lymph nodes in the groin area and the vertical chain over the inner aspect of the thigh.

Expected findings: Nodes should be < 1 cm in size and freely mobile.

Abnormal findings: Enlarged or tender lymph nodes may indicate local or systemic disease.

Documentation
- If you need more information about documenting your findings, review Caring for the Nguyens and Documenting Physical Examination Findings (Nam Nguyen).

Maturation Status in Females

STAGE OF DEVELOPMENT	BREASTS	PUBIC HAIR
Stage 1: Prepuberty	Elevation of papilla.	No pubic hair except for fine body hair similar to hair on abdomen.
Stage 2	Breast bud. Elevation of breast and nipple and increased diameter of areola.	Sparse growth of long, slightly pigmented, downy hair, straight or only slightly curled, mostly along labia.
Stage 3	Areola deepens in color and enlarges further. Glandular tissue begins to develop beneath areola.	Hair becomes darker, coarser, and curlier and spreads sparsely over pubic symphysis.
Stage 4	Areola appears as a mound; breast appears as a mound; papilla and areola form a secondary mound.	Pubic hair is coarse and curly as in adults. It covers more area than in stage 3, but does not extend to the medial thighs.

(continued on next page)

Procedure 21-18 ■ **Assessing the Female Genitourinary System** (continued)

Maturation Status in Females—cont'd

STAGE OF DEVELOPMENT	BREASTS	PUBIC HAIR
Stage 5: Adult	Mature breast. Areola recesses to general contour of breast; nipple projects forward.	Quality and quantity are consistent with adult pubic hair distribution and spread over medial surfaces of thighs but not over abdomen.

Source: Adapted from Tanner, J. (1962). *Growth at adolescence* (2nd ed.). Oxford, England: Blackwell Scientific.

Procedure 21-19 ■ **Assessing the Anus and Rectum**

➤ For steps to follow in *all* procedures, refer to the Universal Steps for All Procedures found on the page facing the inside back cover.

Equipment

- Water-soluble lubricant
- Hemoccult test
- Nonlatex procedure gloves
- Pen and record form

Developmental Modification for Infants and Children

You will not usually perform a rectal exam on infants and children.

Focused History Questions

- Do you have any pain or discomfort around your anus?
- Do you ever have difficulty passing stool?
- Have you ever noticed blood on your stool or when you wipe?
- Do you have or have you ever been told you have hemorrhoids?
- For men: Have you ever had a prostate exam or a prostate-specific antigen blood test? If so, what were the results?

➤ When performing the procedure, always identify your patient according to agency policy, using two identifiers, and be attentive to standard precautions, hand hygiene, patient safety and privacy, and body mechanics.

Procedure Steps

1. **Inspect the anus.** Note the condition of the skin and the presence of any lesions.

Findings

Expected findings: Anal area is intact, with no inflammation or lesions. Anus is a darker color than surrounding tissue.

Abnormal findings:

- A fissure or tear may be due to trauma, severe constipation, or an abscess.
- External hemorrhoids or skin tags may be visible.

2. **Palpate the anus and rectum.**
   a. **For women,** change gloves to prevent cross-contamination. Insert a lubricated index finger gently into the rectum. Palpate the rectal wall, noting masses or tenderness.
   b. **For males,** have the client bend over the exam table or turn on his left side if recumbent. Insert a lubricated index finger gently into the rectum. Palpate the rectal wall, noting, masses or evidence of tenderness. ▼

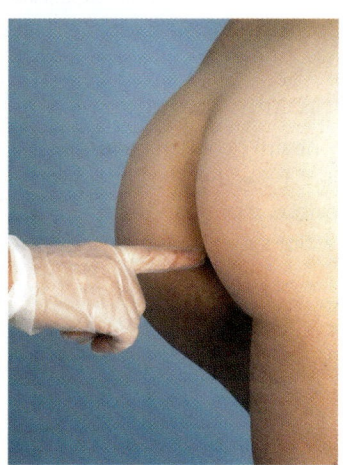

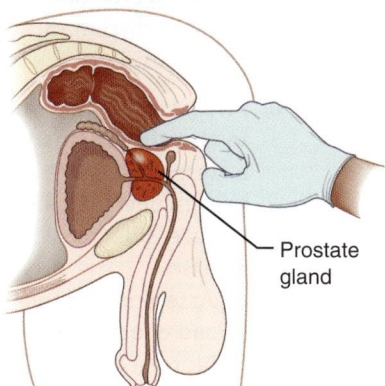

— Prostate gland

   c. Test any stool on the gloved finger for occult blood. See Procedure 29-1.

Expected findings: Good sphincter tone. Rectum is nontender. No palpable masses or hard stool. The stool is brown and negative for occult blood.

Abnormal findings:
- Hard stool in the rectum indicates impaction.
- Positive occult blood indicates bleeding in the GI tract.
- A palpable mass or enlarged prostate gland requires further evaluation.
- Internal hemorrhoids may be present.

Patient Teaching

Instruct the client in the importance of colonoscopy and prostate exam.

Documentation

If you need more information about documenting your findings, review Caring for the Nguyens, including Documenting Physical Examination Findings (Nam Nguyen).

Procedure 21-20 ■ Brief Bedside Assessment

➤ *NOTE:* This assessment is not as detailed as in Procedures 21-1 through 21-19. You might perform a brief bedside assessment to determine changes in the client's status. For daily patient assessments, you will modify the procedure to fit the patient's health status. You may be able to omit some portions, and you may need to add in-depth, focused assessments of some body systems. The entire brief assessment should take no more than 15 minutes after you become skilled.

➤ For steps to follow in *all* procedures, refer to the Universal Steps for All Procedures found on the page facing the inside back cover.

Equipment
- Thermometer, stethoscope, sphygmomanometer
- Procedure gloves

Focused History Questions
- Ask about any health problems, allergies, or medications.
- Ask your patient how she feels currently and how she felt during the previous month and year.
- Ask other questions as you assess each body system.

➤ When performing the procedure, always identify your patient according to agency policy, using two identifiers, and be attentive to standard precautions, hand hygiene, patient safety and privacy, body mechanics, and documentation.

Procedure Steps

1. **Greet the patient and explain what you need to do.** Ask the patient her name and confirm by checking her identity band.
   Assures that you have the correct patient and also allows you to assess mental status and communication.

2. **Observe the environment** (e.g., IV lines, oxygen, urinary catheter) and patient's general appearance (including signs of distress).
   This allows you to identify any immediate actions you may need to take before performing the assessment.

3. **Begin by measuring the vital signs** (patient supine or sitting):
   a. Temperature, pulse, respirations, blood pressure
   b. Pain status
   c. Pulse oximetry

4. **Now assess each body system.**
   a. Use a systematic approach such as head-to-toe.
   b. As you assess each system, observe for mobility, ROM, balance, and coordination.
   c. As you talk with the patient, observe her thought processes and level of consciousness.

5. **Assess the integument.**
   a. Ask about any hair, nail, or skin changes, including rashes.
   b. With each body system, inspect skin color, rashes, and lesions and palpate for temperature, turgor, and texture. Also inspect the hair and nails in that area (e.g., when assessing the legs and feet).
   c. Assess wounds: appearance, size, drainage, dressings, drains.
   d. Inspect and palpate the hair and scalp.

6. **Assess the head and neck.**
   a. Ask the patient about any problems with the head and neck.
   b. **KEY POINT:** *Remember to continue assessing mental status and orientation to time, place, and person.*
   c. Inspect the external ears; observe for apparent hearing deficit.
   d. Check the eyes for pupil reaction and cardinal fields of gaze. Ask about and observe for any problems with vision.
   e. Inspect the color of the lips, mucous membranes, and conjunctiva.
   f. Inspect the tongue and oropharynx.
   g. Inspect for hydration, color, and lesions of the mucous membranes.
   h. Lightly palpate the carotid pulse (only if indicated by patient's condition) and listen for carotid bruits.

   ➕ Do not palpate both carotid arteries at the same time. See Procedure 21-13.

7. **Assess the heart.**
   a. Have the patient sit up and lean forward a bit.
   b. Ask about any cardiovascular problems.
   c. Auscultate heart sounds. Note rate, rhythm, S_1, S_2, and extra sounds.

8. **Assess the back while patient is in the sitting position.**
   a. Inspect skin.
   b. Auscultate breath sounds; compare side to side and apex to base.
   c. Assess respiratory rate, rhythm, and effort.
   d. Note cough, secretions, how many pillows used to sleep on, and whether head of bed is elevated for breathing.
   e. Check oxygen order, SaO_2, ability to use incentive spirometer.

9. **Assess the anterior chest.**
   a. Ask about any respiratory or cardiovascular problems.
   b. Palpate skin turgor, temperature, and PMI.
   c. Auscultate breath sounds.

10. **Assess the abdomen, with the patient supine.**
    a. Inspect the size, shape, symmetry, and condition of the abdominal skin.
    b. Observe abdominal movements including respirations, pulsations, and peristalsis.

c. Auscultate bowel sounds in all four quadrants, and the aorta for bruits.

d. Palpate all four quadrants for tenderness, guarding, and masses; and inspect for rebound tenderness.

e. Ask the patient about any weight changes, GI complaints, a change in appetite or diet.

f. Review the pattern for bowel movements and when examining a woman, ask her the date of last menstrual period.

11. **Assess urinary status.**
   a. Review voiding pattern with the patient (including frequency and dysuria).
   b. If there is an indwelling catheter, observe for patency, kinks in the tubing, and color of urine; monitor intake and output.
   c. Palpate for bladder distention.

12. **Assess the upper extremities.**
   a. Ask about any problems with the hands and arms, such as weakness; arthritis; change in sensation, temperature, or color.

b. Inspect the condition of the skin and nails.

c. Palpate skin temperature and bilateral brachial and radial pulses.

d. Check capillary refill.

e. Note any stiffness or limited ROM of the hands and arms.

f. Test muscle strength by having the patient grip your hands or two fingers.

g. Note whether the patient has any casts, traction, splints, or slings.

h. Observe for edema.

13. **Assess the lower extremities.**
   a. Ask about any problems with the legs, such as weakness; numbness; tingling; arthritis; edema; and change in sensation, temperature, or color.
   b. Observe ROM and ability to ambulate or move about in bed.
   c. Inspect the condition of the skin and nails.
   d. Palpate skin temperature and pedal pulses; check capillary refill.

e. Test for leg strength by asking the patient to raise the leg against your counterpressure. (This is more easily done with the patient sitting.)

d. Check sensation through light touch, proceeding to pain as needed.

e. Observe for problems such as paralysis.

f. Observe for edema.

14. **Ask the patient to stand, and inspect for:**
   a. Gross spinal deformities
   b. Balance and coordination of movements
   c. ROM and gait

15. **With the patient seated in bed, legs extended, check for:**
   a. Babinski's reflex
   b. Homans' sign

Documentation

- Document your findings and report any significant changes or findings to the primary care provider. As a student, report your findings to the instructor and the patient's assigned RN for validation and action.
- If you need more information about documenting your findings, review Caring for the Nguyens, including Documenting Physical Examination Findings (Nam Nguyen).

Thinking About the Procedure

To practice applying clinical reasoning to this procedure,

 The video **Brief Physical Assessment,** along with questions and suggested responses, is available on the **Davis's *Nursing Skills Videos*** Web site on DavisAdvantage.

 To explore learning resources for this chapter,

 Go to **www.DavisAdvantage.com** and find:

Answers and Suggested Responses for all questions in this chapter

Lists NIC and NOC terms

List of NANDA-I Diagnoses

Knowledge Map

References and Bibliography

Concept Map

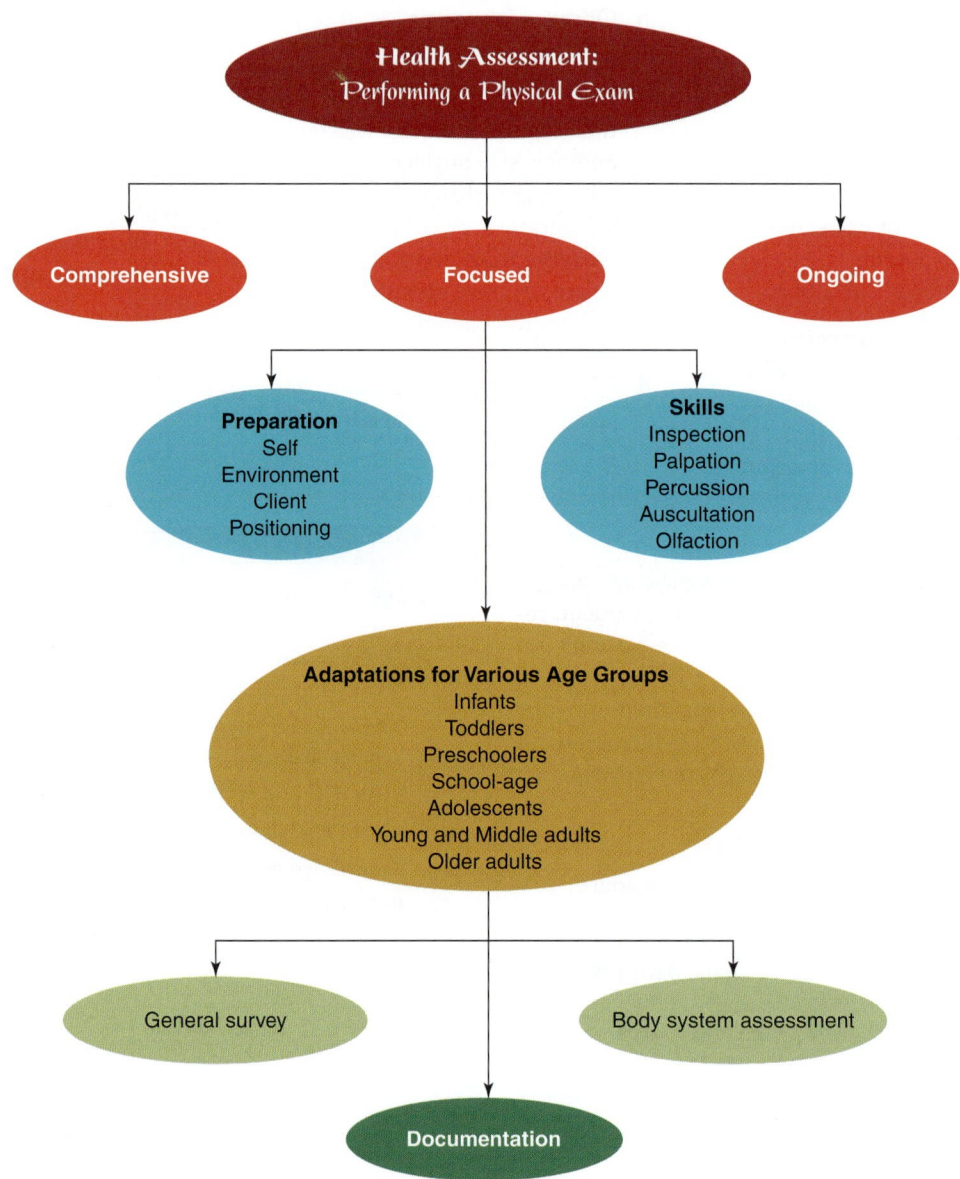

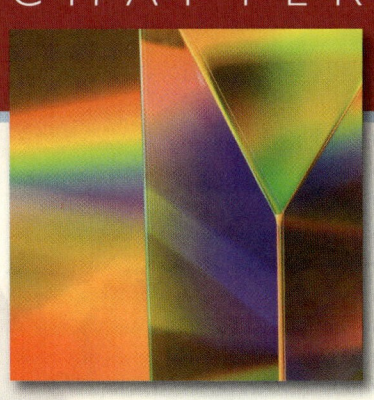

CHAPTER 22

Infection Prevention & Control

Learning Outcomes

After completing this chapter, you should be able to:

- ➤ Discuss the six links in the chain of infection.
- ➤ Describe the stages of a typical infectious process.
- ➤ Describe processes involved in the body's primary, secondary, and tertiary defenses.
- ➤ Identify activities that promote immune function.
- ➤ Discuss the factors that increase the risk for infection.
- ➤ Explain why it is important to be aware of emerging infectious diseases.
- ➤ Explain why multidrug-resistant organisms are of special concern in healthcare.

- ➤ Use standard precautions to prevent transmission of infection through blood and body fluids.
- ➤ Describe additional precautions that must be taken when there is concern about contact, droplet, or airborne disease transmission.
- ➤ Compare and contrast methods of breaking the chain of infection.
- ➤ Use medical asepsis and sterile technique, when appropriate.
- ➤ Discuss infection prevention and control measures in the home and community.
- ➤ Discuss the nurse's role in recognizing, preventing, and helping to contain a biological epidemic.

Key Concepts

Body defenses

Infection

Infection prevention and control

Medical asepsis

Surgical asepsis

Related Concepts

See the Concept Map at the end of this chapter.

Example Problem

Multidrug-Resistant Organism (MDRO) Infections—Prevention

Meet Your Nursing Role Model

Jason Sergei works as a nurse on a busy labor and delivery unit in a major medical center. One night at the dinner table, his 7-year-old daughter, Stephanie, asks, "Daddy, what was the most important thing you did at work today?" Jason considers his reply. Finally, he answers, "I washed my hands—a lot."

Jason says that he also assisted in the birth of five infants, resuscitated one of the infants who was struggling for breath, and identified several problems that prevented complications for mothers in labor. "Daddy, I don't understand why washing your hands was so important," Stephanie protested. "Look at all the *really* important things you did today!"

As you read this chapter, think back to Jason's discussion with his daughter. Perhaps you will someday say the same thing to your child or anyone who asks about your day.

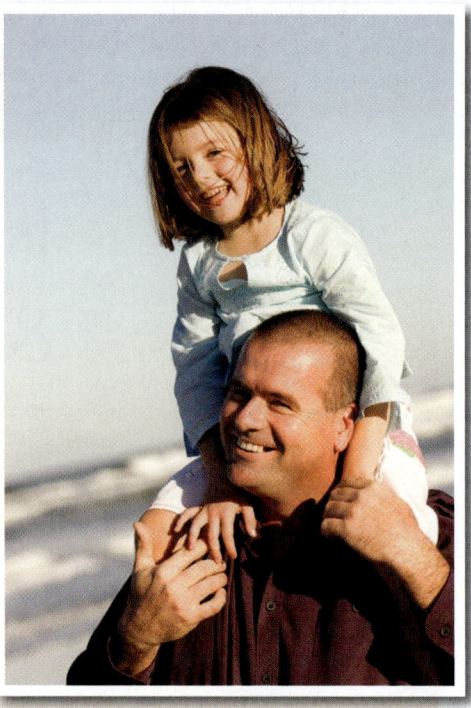

Theoretical Knowledge
knowing **why**

In the theoretical knowledge section, you will learn how infections occur and about measures to prevent them. We will discuss healthcare-associated infections and related professional standards and guidelines.

ABOUT THE KEY CONCEPTS

Infection is invasion of and multiplication in the body by a pathogen (a microorganism capable of causing disease). A grasp of the broad concept of infection will enable you to use **infection prevention and control** measures to promote biological safety for your clients. Those activities include **medical and surgical asepsis** and interventions to support patients' **body defenses.**

WHY SHOULD NURSES KNOW ABOUT INFECTION PROCESSES?

The goals of infection prevention and control for nurses are to:
- Protect patients from infections.
- Meet professional standards and guidelines.
- Protect yourself from diseases (e.g., how to avoid contact with infectious material and microorganisms, especially MDROs).
- Help lower the cost of healthcare.

Healthcare-Associated Infections

The term **healthcare-associated infection (HAI)** refers to infections associated with healthcare given in any setting (e.g., hospitals, home care, long-term care, and ambulatory settings). **Nosocomial infection** refers more specifically to hospital-acquired infections. HAIs aggravate existing illness and lengthen hospital stay and recovery time.
- HAIs are the leading complication of hospital care and one of the 10 leading causes of death in the United States (Agency for Healthcare Research and Quality, 2011; Siegel, Rhinehart,

Jackson, et al., 2007); however, they are preventable (Cardo, Dennehy, Halverson, et al., 2010).
- Approximately 1 out of every 25 hospitalized patients will contract an HAI (Centers for Disease Control and Prevention, 2016b).
- *Clostridium difficile* was the most commonly reported pathogen (causing 12.1% of HAIs) (Magill, Edwards, Star, et al., 2014).

The following are some reasons for the high incidence of healthcare-related infections:
- In hospitals and other facilities, patients encounter many care providers who can transmit pathogens to them.
- Ill patients are vulnerable to infection due to lowered resistance, and they are a source of infection for others.
- Inpatients undergo many invasive procedures (e.g., injections), which can be a source for microbes to enter.

Professional Standards and Guidelines

Various government, professional, and accrediting organizations have published quality-control guidelines for healthcare agencies and professionals. The following are important examples:

The Centers for Disease Control and Prevention (CDC) The mission of this federal agency is to protect Americans from health, safety, and security threats through education, research, and action. To access this site and retrieve Infection Control Guidelines,

 Go to the CDC Web site at http://www.cdc.gov/hai/

The primary goal of the U.S. Department of Health and Human Services (2013, updated 2015) for the healthcare setting is to keep patients from becoming injured or sicker during their care. Specific aims are to reduce:
- Central line–associated bloodstream infections (CLABSI)
- Surgical site infections (SSI)

- Catheter-associated urinary tract infections (CAUTI)
- Ventilator-associated pneumonia (VAP)
- Multidrug-resistant organisms (MDROs)

The Agency for Healthcare Research and Quality (AHRQ) The AHRQ Web site features links to information, tools, and resources on HAIs for both healthcare providers and consumers. To access this site,

 Go to http://www.ahrq.gov.

The Joint Commission This is a quality oversight agency. Its standards of performance include extensive criteria describing what healthcare organizations must do to minimize the risks of infection. In addition, Goal 7 of the National Patient Safety Goals for 2016 is to "reduce the risk of health care associated-infections" (The Joint Commission, 2016). They include strategies for healthcare providers to prevent infection in inpatient and community-based settings. To read these initiatives,

 Go to http://www.jointcommission.org/assets/1/6/2016_NPSG_HAP.pdf

Quality and Safety Education for Nurses (QSEN) This is a group of educators that was formed to identify the competencies necessary to improve the quality and safety of nurses' places of work. Some nursing schools have adopted these as standards. Safety is one of the competencies you should have on completing your nursing education. Although QSEN does not specifically say so, you should assume that safety includes being safe from infection (Cronenwett, Sherwood, Barnsteiner, et al., 2007).

To access the QSEN Web site,

 Go to http://www.qsen.org/

American Nurses Association (ANA) Standard 5 of the ANA *Nursing: Scope and Standards of Practice* (2015) applies to infection prevention and control:
- "Partners with the healthcare consumer to implement the plan in a safe and timely manner.
- Implements the plan in a timely manner in accordance with the patient safety goals" (ANA, 2015, p. 61).

Limiting the Spread of Infectious Diseases

Cooperative efforts among many disciplines and organizations worldwide are required to limit the spread of infectious diseases. The World Health Organization (WHO) is committed to reducing healthcare-associated complications, prevent surgical site infection, combat antimicrobial resistance (also called MDROs), prevent sepsis and catheter-associated bloodstream infections, prevent catheter-associated urinary tract infections, and improve Ebola response and recovery (WHO, n.d.). The Joint Commission (Soule, Memish, & Malani, 2012) requires hospitals to have an emergency management plan for responding to large numbers of infectious patients who might need to be treated as a result of an epidemic or pandemic event.

HOW DOES INFECTION OCCUR?

Imagine that your clinical instructor alerts you to an outbreak of infectious disease in the hospital where you have your assignment. So far, only 14 people have become infected, and one has died. Would that prompt you to wonder how the infection was spread and why it seems to affect some people more than others?

Infections Develop in Response to a Chain of Factors

Infections spread through a **chain of infection.** It is made up of six links (described below), all of which must be present for the infection to be transmitted from one individual to another (Fig. 22-1). Later in the chapter we discuss how to interrupt the chain to limit the spread of infection.

Infectious Agent

Some microorganisms are harmful. Others live on or in the human body without causing harm (e.g., the *Staphylococcus* bacteria that grow on human skin). Other microorganisms are beneficial or even essential for human health and well-being. They are referred to as **normal flora.**

Normal Flora Normal flora in the intestine aid in digestion; synthesize vitamin K; and release vitamin B_{12}, thiamine, and riboflavin when they die. In addition, they limit the growth of harmful bacteria by competing with them for available nutrients. There are two types of normal flora: transient and resident.
- **Transient flora** are normal microbes you acquire by coming in contact with objects or another person (e.g., when you touch a soiled dressing). Hand washing can remove these.
- **Resident flora** are permanent inhabitants of the skin and cannot usually be removed with routine hand washing. They live and multiply harmlessly deep in skin layers.

Pathogens are microorganisms capable of causing disease.
- *The largest groups of pathogenic microorganisms* are bacteria, viruses, and fungi (which include yeasts and molds).
- *Less common pathogens* are protozoa, **helminths** (commonly called worms), and **prions,** which are infectious protein particles that cause certain neurological diseases.

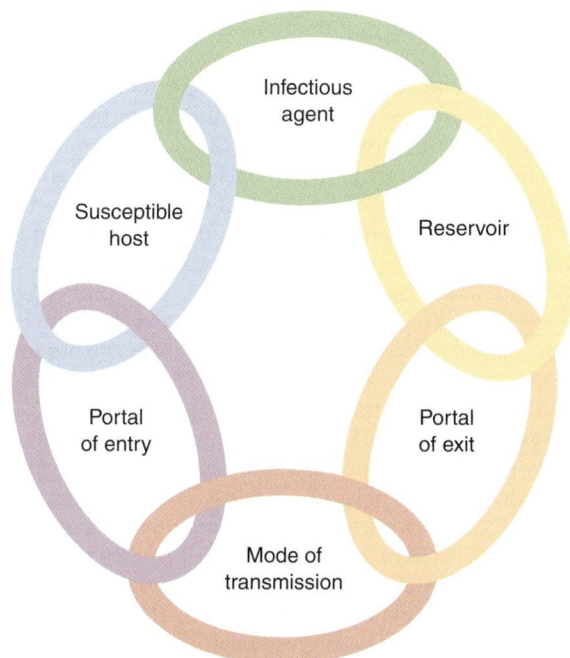

FIGURE 22-1 All six links in the chain of infection must be present for infection to be transmitted from one person to another.

■ *Normal flora may become pathogenic* when a patient is especially vulnerable to disease, or if they enter regions of the body they do not normally inhabit (*Escherichia coli,* harmless in the bowel, cause infection when they multiply in the urinary tract).

Once a pathogen enters a host, four factors determine whether the person develops infection:

■ **Virulence** of the organism (its power to cause disease)
■ Ability of the organism to survive in the host environment
■ Number of organisms (the greater their number, the more likely they are to cause disease)
■ Ability of the host's defenses to prevent infection

Reservoir

A **reservoir** is a source of infection: a place where pathogens survive and multiply. **KEY POINT:** *Most pathogens flourish in a warm, moist, dark environment. This is why the human body is the most common reservoir for pathogens.* Animals and insects are other living reservoirs. Nonliving reservoirs include soil, water, food, and environmental surfaces (e.g., contaminated water, soiled diapers, wet equipment or medical fabrics, and wound dressings).

In healthcare facilities, many surfaces act as reservoirs, such as sinks, toilets, bed rails, and bed linens, because of their proximity to patients, family members, and healthcare providers harboring pathogens.

Some people, called **carriers,** are capable of defending themselves from active disease but harbor the pathogenic organisms within their bodies. They have no symptoms, yet they serve as reservoirs and can pass the disease to others.

Nutrients To live and thrive in humans, microbes must be able to use the body's precise balance of nutrients, electrolytes, pH, and temperature. Bacteria can rapidly multiply in food left at room temperature. For example, the bacteria *Salmonella enteritidis,* which causes salmonellosis ("food poisoning"), can multiply in raw and undercooked meat and eggs.

Moisture Pathogens require moisture for survival, for example, the moist environment of wounds, the genitourinary tract, and the throat and airways. However, bacteria form spores that allow them to live without water (e.g., the *Bacillus* and *Clostridium* species, both of which cause food-borne disease).

Temperature For most pathogens, the ideal temperature is 95°F (35°C). Environments that are too hot or too cold for a species will slow its growth or even kill the entire population. In part, the microbes that are pathogenic to humans are so because they thrive at about the same temperature as the human body. Thus, the body produces a fever in response to infection to inhibit and even kill invading pathogens.

Oxygen Many bacteria and most protozoa and fungi are **aerobic.** That is, they must have oxygen to live and grow (e.g., the yeast *Candida albicans*). **Anaerobic** organisms do not require oxygen for growth and may even be killed in its presence. One example is *Clostridium tetani,* which can cause tetanus.

pH and Electrolytes To live in humans, pathogens need the body's precise balance of sugars, pH (acidity), and electrolytes. Most prefer a pH range of 5 to 8. Therefore, they cannot survive in the highly acidic environment of the stomach. When patients take antacids, stomach pH increases (acidity decreases) and removes this defense, allowing the pathogens to multiply and cause infection in other organs, such as the lungs.

Light Microbes These grow best in dark environments (e.g., inside the body, deep in wounds, and under dressings). Ultraviolet light is sometimes used to remove pathogens such as *Staphylococcus, Salmonella,* and viruses from surgical instruments and other objects. It is also used to disinfect contaminated drinking water.

KnowledgeCheck 22-1

■ What is a pathogen?
■ What is the role of normal flora?
■ Identify at least five reservoirs of infection.

Portal of Exit

A contained reservoir is only a potential source of infection. For infection to spread, a pathogen must exit the reservoir. In the case of human or animal reservoirs, the most frequent **portal of exit** is through body fluids.

■ *Expelling foreign materials.* The body's natural response to foreign materials, including pathogens, is to try to expel them. For example, if you have a pathogen in the respiratory system, they exit when you cough and sneeze. If it is in the gastrointestinal system, they exit when you vomit or experience diarrhea.
■ *Non-intact skin.* Wounds, bites, and abrasions also provide an exit for body fluid. Blood and pus seeping from a wound help transport pathogens away from the broken skin. In healthcare-related infections, puncture sites, drainage tubes, feeding tubes, and intravenous lines serve as exit routes for pathogens.

Mode of Transmission

Contact, either direct or indirect, is the most frequent **mode of transmission** of infection.

■ **Direct contact** usually involves physical contact, sexual intercourse, and contact with wound drainage, but it can involve scratching and biting.
■ **Indirect contact** involves contact with a **fomite,** a contaminated object that transfers a pathogen. For example, suppose while you are entering data into the patient record, you sneeze or cough. If you cover your nose and mouth with your hand and then resume using the keyboard, you may transmit pathogens to the next person who touches that surface. Shoes, eyeglasses, stethoscopes, and other commonly worn items also serve as fomites. Some microbes can live only a few seconds on fomites; others can live for years, depending on the environment.
■ **Droplet transmission** occurs when a pathogen travels in water droplets expelled as an infected person exhales, coughs, sneezes, or talks, or during suctioning and oral care. The droplet usually enters the eye of or is inhaled by a susceptible host. Although droplets can travel only a few feet, within that distance they readily contaminate fomites that then transmit the organism by contact.
■ **Airborne transmission** occurs when microorganisms float considerable distances on air currents to infect large numbers of people. Airborne pathogens can travel through heating and air-conditioning systems. Sweeping a floor or shaking out contaminated bed linens can also launch microorganisms into the air. Common airborne pathogens are the agents of measles, tuberculosis, and many fungal infections.
■ A **vector** is an organism that carries a pathogen to a susceptible. The mosquito is a common vector for diseases, including malaria, yellow fever, and the West Nile virus. Ticks, fleas, and some animals can also be vectors.

Portal of Entry

Pathogens can enter the body through various **portals of entry.** Normal body openings, such as the conjunctiva of the eye, the nares (nostrils), mouth, urethra, vagina, and anus are potential portals of entry, as are abnormal openings, such as minor wounds and abrasions. Vectors, such as mosquitoes, create portals of entry when they bite or sting through the skin. In healthcare settings, common portals of entry include more severe wounds, surgical sites, and insertion sites for tubes or needles.

Susceptible Host

A **susceptible** (or compromised) **host** is a person who is at risk for infection because of inadequate defenses against the invading pathogen. Among the factors that increase susceptibility are:

Age (very young, very old)

Compromised immune system (immune suppression for organ transplantation or treatment of cancer)

Chronic illness

Immune deficiency (e.g., HIV, leukemia, malnutrition)

KnowledgeCheck 22-2

- Identify the six links in the chain of infection.
- What kinds of microbes favor the human body as a reservoir of infection?

 ThinkLike a Nurse 22-1

You are working as a nurse on a medical–surgical unit. What roles might you play in the chain of infection?

Infections Can Be Classified by Location and Duration

Infections are classified according to their location in the body, whether it is the patient's first infection, where it was acquired, and how long it lasts.

Local or Systemic

- **Local infections** are those that cause harm in a limited region of the body, such as the upper respiratory tract, the urethra, or a single bone or joint.
- **Systemic infections** occur when pathogens invade the blood or lymph and spread throughout the body.

   Bacteremia is the clinical presence of bacteria in the blood.

   Septicemia is symptomatic systemic infection spread via the blood.

Primary or Secondary

- **A primary infection** is the first infection that occurs in a patient.
- **A secondary infection** is one that follows a primary infection, especially in immunocompromised patients.

   Example: A frail client is infected with pneumonia. Under the stress of illness, she may develop herpes zoster (shingles), a viral infection related to past infection with varicella.

Exogenous or Endogenous
Healthcare providers need to determine the source of pathogens in a patient infected while he is in the facility.

- In **exogenous** healthcare-related infections, the pathogen is acquired from the healthcare environment.
- In **endogenous** healthcare-related infections, the pathogen arises from the patient's normal flora, when some form of treatment (e.g., chemotherapy or antibiotics) causes the normally harmless microbe to multiply and cause infection.

   Example: Candidal vaginitis (yeast infection) may develop in a client after frequent use of antibiotics.

Acute or Chronic

- **Acute infections** have a rapid onset but last only a short time (e.g., the common cold).
- **Chronic infections** (e.g., an abscess) develop slowly and last for weeks, months, or even years. Some chronic infections (e.g., relapsing fever caused by an infection from a tick bite) recur after periods of remission.
- **Latent infections** cause no symptoms for long periods of time, even decades. Tuberculosis and HIV are examples.

Infections Follow Predictable Stages

Infections usually follow a predictable course, although the precise duration and intensity of symptoms in each stage vary from one individual to another:

- **Incubation.** Infection begins in this stage between successful invasion of the pathogen into the body and the first appearance of symptoms. In this stage, the person does not suspect that he has been infected but may be capable of infecting others. This stage may last only a day, as with the influenza virus, or as long as several months or even years, as with tuberculosis.
- **Prodrome.** The prodromal stage is characterized by the first appearance of vague symptoms at the onset of illness. For example, a person infected with a cold virus may experience a mild throat irritation. Not all infections have a prodromal stage.
- **Illness.** The patient becomes ill when the first signs and symptoms of the disease occur. If the patient's immune defenses and medical treatments (if any) are ineffective, this stage can end in death.
- **Decline.** When the patient's immune defenses, along with medical therapies, successfully reduce the number of pathogenic microbes, the infection begins to decline. As a result, the clinical manifestations of the infection begin to fade.
- **Convalescence.** Healing begins as the remaining number of microorganisms approaches zero. Convalescence may require only a day or two or, for severe infections, as long as a year or more.

Why Should Nurses Be Aware of Emerging Pathogens and Diseases?

Continental and intercontinental travel allow for many ways of spreading emerging diseases. Infected travelers serve as reservoirs for pathogens. The closed spaces and recirculated air systems in airplanes provide an ideal environment for the transmission of airborne pathogens and for both direct and indirect contact contamination between passengers. Air travel also enables a person to infect many people headed for widespread locations, often even before the reservoir person shows symptoms of the disease.

An **epidemic** is an outbreak of a disease that suddenly affects a large group of people in a geographic region (e.g., a city or state) or in a defined population group (e.g., children, healthcare workers). A **pandemic** is an exceptionally widespread epidemic—that is, one that affects many people in an entire country or worldwide. Examples of pandemics are Ebola, H1N1 influenza ("swine flu"), and malaria.

You should also know the term **emerging infectious disease.** Although there are various definitions, you can think of emerging infectious diseases as:

- *Newly identified diseases* caused either by an unrecognized microorganism (e.g., the virus causing AIDS was unknown before 1981) or by a known organism (e.g., *Streptococcus* infection causing toxic shock syndrome).

- *Diseases occurring in new geographic areas* (e.g., Ebola virus in western Africa) or settings (e.g., *C. difficile* was primarily a hospital-acquired infection and now occurs in the community).
- *Microorganisms in animals or insects that extend their host range to begin infecting humans* (e.g., H1N1 virus from swine, or Zika virus, which is carried by mosquitos and can cause birth defects when acquired during pregnancy).
- *Microbes that evolve to become more virulent* (e.g., a strain of *E. coli,* which now causes severe illness).
- *Known diseases that dramatically increase in incidence* as a result of failed or poor compliance with public health measures to control outbreaks, such as immunization (mumps) and water treatment (cholera) (e.g., mumps and pertussis, also known as whooping cough).
- *Many viruses show a high mutation rate* and can rapidly yield new strains. For example, the influenza virus is difficult to eradicate and immunize against because of its adaptability.
- *Organisms that are deliberately altered for bioterrorism* (e.g., the contamination of U.S. government mail with *Bacillus anthracis* [anthrax]).
- *Many emerging pathogens are viruses.* In 2015 the World Health Organization prioritized the following emerging pathogens for which few or no medical countermeasures exist: ebola virus, Zika virus, SARS, MERS, Crimean Congo haemorrhagic fever, and others.

Multidrug-Resistant Organisms

Antibiotic resistance is one of the most significant challenges in treating patients with severe infectious diseases. During the past several decades, the prevalence of multidrug-resistant organisms (MDROs) in U.S. hospitals and medical centers has increased steadily. MDROs are a serious problem because options for treating MDRO infections are limited. Furthermore, they are associated with serious illness, increased mortality, and increased hospital lengths of stay and costs. See the Example Problem: Multidrug-Resistant Organism (MDRO) Infections—Prevention.

ThinkLike a Nurse 22-2

- Why are emerging infections of special concern in healthcare?
- Why are multidrug-resistant organisms (MDROs) of special concern in healthcare?

WHAT ARE THE BODY'S DEFENSES AGAINST INFECTION?

The human body has three "lines of defense" against infectious disease:

- Certain anatomical features limit the entry of pathogens.
- Protective biochemical processes fight pathogens that do enter.
- The presence of pathogens activates immune responses against specific, recognized invaders.

The first two (primary and secondary) lines of defense are nonspecific; that is, they have no means of adapting their response to each specific invader. Instead, they act in precisely the same way against all intruders, from a simple cold virus to deadly fungal spores.

Primary Defenses

The "soldiers" in the first line of defense are the structural barriers of the human body. These **primary defenses** prevent organisms from entering the body.

- **Normal flora of the body**. Any treatment that disturbs the balance between the normal flora and other microorganisms can increase the risk of developing disease. For example,

when broad-spectrum antibiotics are used to treat infection, they may eliminate normal flora in addition to those causing the infection. This allows other kinds of pathogens to multiply, producing a **superinfection** or another opportunistic infection.
- **Skin.** Intact, healthy skin prevents entry of many pathogens. Normal skin flora inhibit multiplication of other organisms that land on the skin.
- **Respiratory tree.** The nares, trachea, and bronchi are covered with mucous membranes that trap pathogens. The nose contains hairs that filter the upper airway; the nasal passages, sinuses, trachea, and larger bronchi are lined with **cilia,** tiny hair-like cells that sweep microorganisms upward from the lower airways. Coughing and sneezing forcefully expel organisms from the respiratory tract.
- **Eyes.** The lacrimal glands produce tears that contain lysozyme, an antimicrobial enzyme. The tears help wash infective organisms from the eyes.
- **Mouth.** The mouth normally has many pathogenic microorganisms, but saliva, like tears, contains lysozyme and continually washes microbes from the teeth and gums. The rich blood supply of the mouth swiftly transports defensive blood cells, and the normal flora of the mouth compete with invading organisms for nutrition, thus keeping the microorganisms in check.
- **Gastrointestinal tract.** Many pathogens are destroyed in the acidic environment of the stomach. Those that enter the small intestine face the antimicrobial action of bile. Normal peristalsis as well as diarrhea and vomiting remove pathogens that invade the gastrointestinal tract. In addition, normal flora in the intestine secrete antibacterial substances.
- **Genitourinary tract and the anus.** The epithelial cells lining the mucous membranes of the urethra, vagina, and anus secrete mucus, which adheres to pathogens to promote their excretion through urine and stool. Urine itself is highly acidic and contains lysozyme (an antibacterial enzyme). In addition, the high acidity and normal flora of the vagina keep pathogens in check.

Secondary Defenses

Pathogens that dodge the primary defenses and enter the body begin to release wastes and secretions and to cause the breakdown of cells and tissues. The presence of such chemicals activates a set of **secondary defenses.**

Phagocytosis is the process by which **phagocytes** (specialized white blood cells [WBCs]) engulf and destroy pathogens directly. Table 22-1 summarizes the types of WBCs and their roles in defending against infection.

Complement cascade is a process by which a set of blood proteins, called *complement,* triggers the release of chemicals that attack the cell membranes of pathogens, causing them to rupture. Complement also signals basophils (WBCs) to release histamine, which prompts inflammation.

Inflammation is the process that begins when histamine and other chemicals are released either from damaged cells or from basophils being activated by complement. With inflammation, blood vessels dilate and become more permeable, which increases the flow of phagocytes, antimicrobial chemicals, oxygen, and nutrients to the affected area. The classic signs and symptoms of inflammation are localized warmth and erythema (redness), which develop as blood flow is increased. In addition, fluid leaking from the more permeable blood vessels accumulates in the surrounding tissue, causing edema, which in turn exerts pressure on nerve endings, causing prompts pain.

Fever is a rise in core body temperature that increases metabolism, inhibits multiplication of pathogens, and triggers

EXAMPLE PROBLEM: Multidrug-Resistant Organism (MDRO) Infections—Prevention

Definition: Microbes that have mutated to develop resistance to one or more classes of antimicrobial drugs; associated with serious illness, increased hospitalization, higher death rates

Transmission: From: (1) one person to another via the hands of healthcare personnel and visitors; (2) bed linens, bed rails, medical equipment, personal items, other . . . contaminated . . . inanimate objects

Types
- **Methicillin-resistant *Staphylococcus aureus* (MRSA).** Spread by skin-to-skin contact, especially in crowded living conditions. Most are skin and soft tissue infections. May cause bloodstream infections **(sepsis),** pneumonia, and surgical site infections.

- **Vancomycin-resistant enterococci (VRE).** Most occur in hospitals. Spread by failure to follow infection control measures.
- ***Clostridium difficile* (*C. diff.*).** Elderly, immunocompromised, and people who have had prolonged treatment with antibiotics are at greater risk. *C. diff.* are found in the feces. Spores can survive for days on doorknobs and toilet seats.
- **Other significant MDROs** include multidrug-resistant tuberculosis (MDR-TB), penicillin-resistant *Streptococcus pneumoniae*, multidrug-resistant *E. coli*, and *Klebsiella pneumoniae*.
- **Antibiotic-resistant superbug.** Mutant strains that are resistant to conventional antibiotic therapy (e.g., a strain of drug-resistant *E. coli* that can pass its resistance to other species of bacteria).

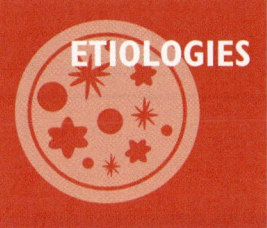

ETIOLOGIES

Risk Factors
- Previous exposure to antibiotics
- Impaired body defenses caused by underlying disease or immune deficiency

- Severe illness
- Invasive procedures and devices
- Repeated hospitalization, especially ICUs
- Advanced age

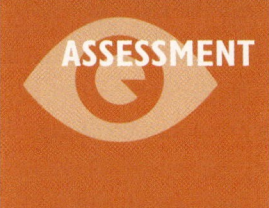

ASSESSMENT

Symptoms
- Observe for symptoms of infections: fever, swelling, redness, excessive warmth, pain, or drainage.
- Wounds that are slow or fail to heal with antibiotics

Diagnostic Tests
- Cultures and sensitivities of wound and skin, blood, sputum, urine, cerebral spinal fluid (CSF), CBC with differential
- Complete blood count (CBC) with differential
- Some institutions require screening cultures at admission or on specialty units (ICU).

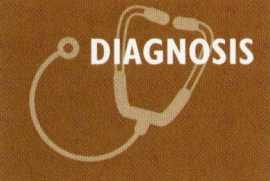

DIAGNOSIS

Risk for Infection (MDRO) r/t open skin lesions and long-term antibiotic use

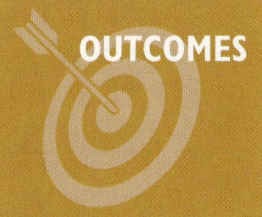

OUTCOMES

Patient
- No signs of localized infection
- Verbalizes improved comfort
- Effective coping behaviors while isolated

Nurse
- Practices MDRO prevention
- Recognizes the signs of MDRO infection

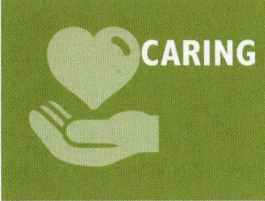

CARING

- Be sensitive to the patient's emotional needs, as many feel "dirty." Some may be embarrassed by the odor of wound infection. Others may feel anger or experience depression during extended isolation.

- Provide measures to relieve boredom (Isolation reduces sensory input)
- Patients may be socially isolated because other people fear they will be infected.
- Encourage visitors to spread out visits and be mindful of patient's feelings of loneliness.

(Continued)

EXAMPLE PROBLEM: Multidrug-Resistant Organism (MDRO) Infections—Prevention—cont'd

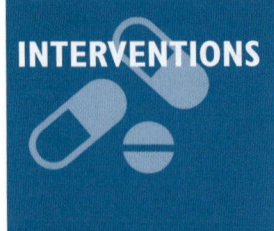

INTERVENTIONS

- Adhere strictly to guidelines for hand hygiene, glove use, and isolation precautions for all patient contact until cultures are negative.
- Ensure patient areas are cleaned well and often.
- Disinfect high-touch surfaces (bed rails, door handles, sink).

- Wear gowns and gloves for all contact patient and contaminated items.
- Dedicate noncritical equipment (stethoscope, thermometer) to use for individuals with MDRO infection.
- Use masks and eye protection, especially when splashes are possible.
- Use private rooms as needed.

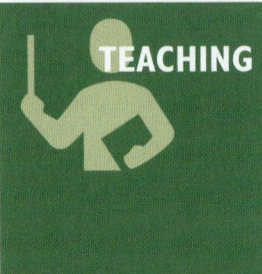

TEACHING

Teach patient and caregiver:

- Ways to limit further spread of infection to close contacts
- Difference between bacterial and viral infection
- Importance of avoiding overuse of antibiotics
- Those unable to keep infected wounds covered and practice strict hand washing

should be excluded from activities involving close contact with others (e.g., day care, contact sports).
- Also see the Self-Care box Teaching Your Patient About Preventing Spread of CA-MRSA, and the Home Care box Preventing Infection in the Home and Community.

Table 22-1 ➤ Types and Functions of White Blood Cells	
TYPE	**FUNCTION**
Granular WBCs	
Basophils: 0.5%–1% of total WBCs	Release histamine and heparin granules as part of the inflammatory response. Percentage normal during infections.
Eosinophils: 1%–3% of total WBCs	Bind to helminthes and release toxins to destroy them; mediate allergic reactions; have limited role in phagocytosis. Percentage increases in parasitic infections.
Neutrophils: 55%–70% of total WBCs	Phagocytize pathogens
Agranular WBCs	
Lymphocytes: 20%–35% of total WBCs	T cells—responsible for cell-mediated immunity; recognize, attack, and destroy antigens.
	B cells—responsible for humoral immunity; produce immunoglobulins to attack and destroy antigens. Percentage of total lymphocytes increases in viral infection and chronic bacterial infection; decreases in sepsis.
Monocytes: 3%–8% of total WBCs	Able to phagocytize directly as well as to differentiate into macrophages, which help clean up damaged tissue, infection, and cellular debris. Percentage increases in tuberculosis, protozoal, and rickettsial infections.

Note: Laboratory values alone are not adequate for diagnosing infection. Presence of clinical signs (e.g., fever, pus, swelling) must be assessed.

specific immune responses. Believing that low-grade fevers are a necessary natural defense mechanism, many clinicians do not treat a fever unless it's greater than 102°F (38.9°C).

Tertiary Defenses

Immunity against an infection is achieved through the presence of antibodies that neutralize or destroy toxins or disease-producing organisms. **Active immunity** occurs when the body makes its own antibodies or T cells to protect the body against a pathogen. Immunity can also be achieved when a person is given antibodies to a pathogen rather than producing them through her own immune system, called **passive immunity** (Box 22-1).

Why is it that most people who recover from an infectious disease such as measles or chickenpox never get the disease again, even if they are repeatedly exposed to the virus? The answer lies in **specific immunity:** the process by which the body's immune cells "learn" to recognize and destroy pathogens they have encountered before. The cells involved in specific immunity are the **lymphocytes,** WBCs produced from stem cells in

BOX 22-1 ■ Four Types of Immunity

Natural active immunity—After a person acquires an infection, the body produces its own antibodies to fight the disease-causing organism and protect from infection by this organism in the future (e.g., influenza).

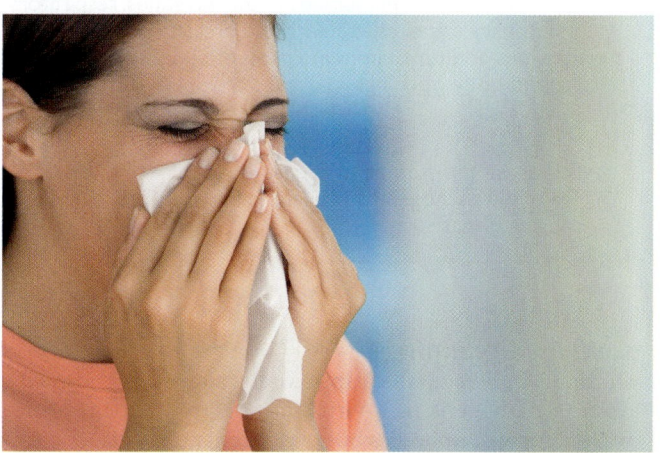

Natural passive immunity—Immunity results when natural antibodies are passed from one body to another, such as from mother to baby through the placenta or through breastfeeding.

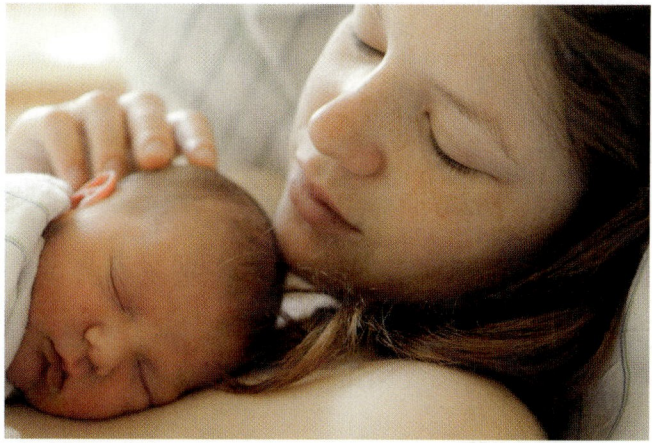

Artificial active immunity—An immune response occurs when the body is exposed to weakened or dead pathogens in a vaccine. The body then makes T cells or antibodies to keep from developing the illness (e.g., tetanus, measles). This type of immunity offers long-lasting or even lifetime protection.

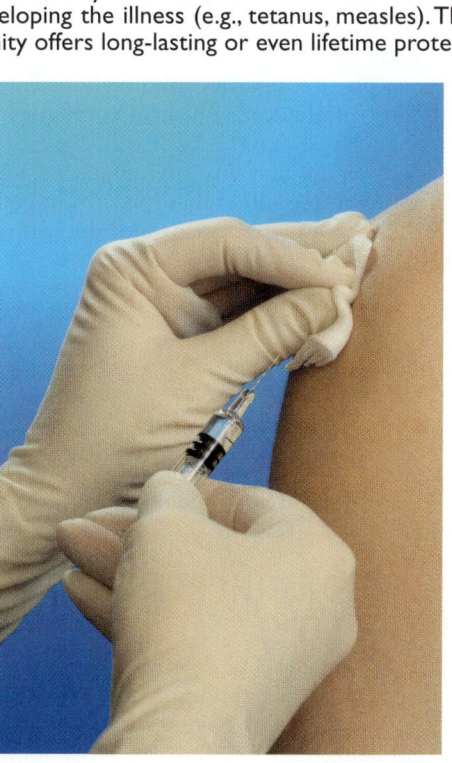

Artificial passive immunity—Protection from infection is achieved when a person receives serum from another person or animal that has already produced antibodies against the pathogen (e.g., serum for treatment of rabies or botulism).

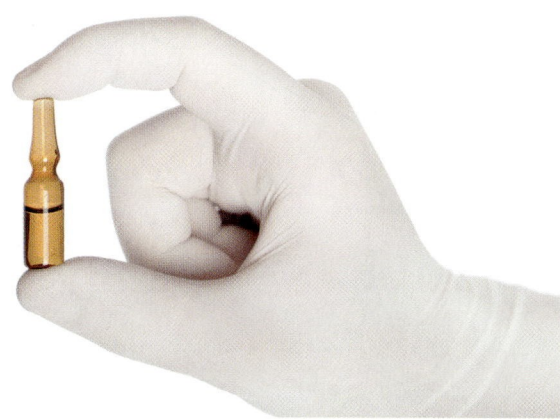

the red bone marrow. Refer to the heading, Cellular Immunity, following.

KEY POINT: *Remember that* **T** *cells mature in the* **T***hymus, and* **B** *cells mature in* **B***one marrow.*

Humoral Immunity

The humoral immune response (or antibody-mediated response) protects the body by circulating antibodies to fight against pathogens (e.g., bacteria). The body's defense system acts by producing specialized white blood cells (leukocytes) to seek out and destroy invaders by any of the following methods (Fig. 22-2):

- *Phagocytosis.* Immunoglobulins, which are the specialized proteins in the body's immune system that function as antibodies. Antibodies (see Box 22-2) signal leukocytes (macrophages and neutrophils) to phagocytize the pathogens to which the antibodies are bound.
- *Neutralization.* By binding to a pathogen's attachment sites, antibodies disable the pathogens' machinery for adhering to and invading body cells. Thus, although they are not destroyed, the pathogens become ineffective.
- *Agglutination.* Antibodies have two attachment sites; therefore, each antibody can attach to two pathogenic cells in a population. This characteristic causes the pathogens to clump together (agglutinate), reducing their activity and increasing the likelihood that the group will be detected and phagocytized by leukocytes.
- *Activation of complement and inflammation.* Antibodies trigger the complement cascade and stimulate the release of inflammatory chemicals to destroy the antigen.

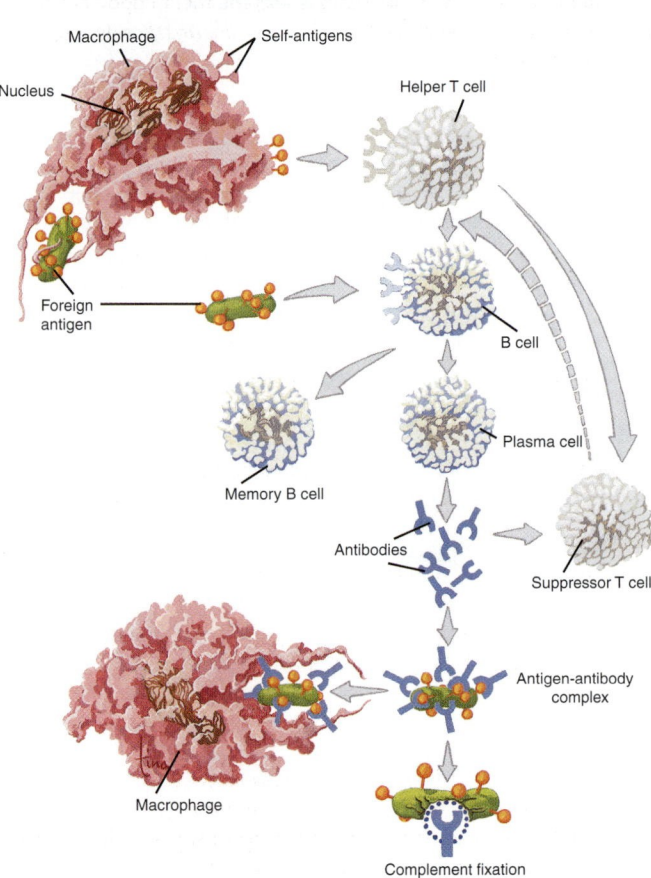

Macrophage · Self-antigens · Nucleus · Helper T cell · Foreign antigen · B cell · Memory B cell · Plasma cell · Antibodies · Suppressor T cell · Antigen-antibody complex · Macrophage · Complement fixation lysis of cellular antigen

FIGURE 22-2 The humoral immune response produces antibodies to destroy antigens.

Cellular Immunity

Cellular (cell-mediated) immune response acts directly to destroy pathogens (i.e., viruses, fungi, protozoans, cancers) without using antibodies but rather activating phagocytes and T and B cells (lymphocytes). After maturing, most T cells and B cells travel to the lymph nodes, spleen, and other sites of lymphatic tissue. Some circulate in blood and lymph. Four types of T cells play a role in fighting infection:

- *Cytotoxic (killer) T cells* directly attack and kill pathogens and infected body cells.
- *Helper T cells* play a supportive role in cell-mediated responses by secreting **interleukin,** which attracts infection-fighting white blood cells.
- *Memory T cells.* The first time an antigen invades the body, T cells form that respond to that specific antigen. The memory T cells increase the speed and amount of the T-cell response.
- *Suppressor T cells* are thought to stop the immune response when the infection has been contained.

KnowledgeCheck 22-3

- Identify and describe the purpose of the body's three major lines of defense against infection.
- If a patient's lab work reveals that IgM, but not IgG, is present in the blood, what could you conclude about this infection?

WHAT FACTORS INCREASE HOST SUSCEPTIBILITY?

Anything that weakens the defenses makes a person more susceptible to infection. In addition, any factors that increase the person's exposure to pathogens, such as working at a day-care center or being a nurse, increase the risk for infection.

Developmental Stage Young children are vulnerable because their immune systems are immature and they have had limited exposure to pathogens. Children frequently begin to have more infections when they start interacting with people outside of their family (e.g., when they begin day care or start school). Acquiring active immunity is a part of the developmental process.

Older adults are also susceptible hosts because the immune response declines with aging. Skin, a primary defense, becomes less elastic and more prone to breakdown with aging. Elders also tend to be less active, and their nutrition may be inadequate.

Breaks in the First Line of Defense A break in the skin, whether caused by a surgical procedure, skin breakdown, an insect bite, or insertion of an intravenous device, creates a portal of entry for infectious microorganisms.

Illness or Injury Recuperation from infection or injury limits the physical resources available to combat a new pathogen.

Tobacco Use

- Tobacco interferes with the ability to move the chest, cough, sneeze, or have full air exchange.
- Chemicals in tobacco paralyze cilia, so secretions pool in the lower airways, creating a hospitable environment for bacteria.
- Smoking adversely affects the immune system, so along with chronic exposure to secondhand smoke (e.g., bartenders, children of smokers) are at risk for a wide range of infections.

Substance Abuse This includes alcohol as well as other substances.

- Alcohol curbs hunger. As a result, many chronic alcohol users do not consume an adequate diet, leading to vitamin, mineral, and protein deficiency. Alcohol is also toxic to the liver and to the cells lining the intestinal mucosa.
- Inhaled substances, such as marijuana and cocaine, affect respiratory cilia in a manner similar to tobacco.
- Any substances that affect orientation and energy level (e.g., heroin, cocaine) will diminish food intake, activity, rest, and hygiene—factors that support host defenses.
- Injecting substances leads to breaks in skin integrity, further increasing the risk of infection.

Multiple Sexual Partners The more sexual partners a person has, the higher his risk of acquiring a sexually transmitted infection.

Environmental Factors Environmental factors can increase exposure to pathogens, irritate respiratory airways, or cause breaks in the skin that increase risk for infection. Increased exposure to pathogens occurs in some work situations (e.g., kindergarten teacher, healthcare worker) and living situations (e.g., nursing home, parents with young children who are in preschool).

Chronic Disease Poor circulation prevents antibodies and T cells from reaching the pathogens and damages tissue, making it easier for pathogens to enter and thrive.

- Diseases that impair peripheral circulation, such as uncontrolled hypertension (high blood pressure) and diabetes mellitus, make the patient prone to infection in the extremities.
- Leukemia, a form of cancer of the blood, increases the production of abnormal white blood cells, but these cells are ineffective in combating infection.
- Because HIV infects T cells, patients with AIDS have a reduced ability to fight off secondary infections.

Medications Some medications are given to intentionally reduce the immune response, for example, to patients receiving organ or tissue transplants. For most patients, though, decreased immunity is an unwanted side effect of treatment.

- Even common medications, such as NSAIDs (e.g., ibuprofen), decrease the immune response.
- As a side effect, some medications, such as chemotherapeutic agents, decrease the production of white blood cells or cause the cells produced to be abnormal.
- Antibiotics can also increase the risk for infection. For example, an antibiotic given for a respiratory infection may cause a vaginal yeast infection because it destroys colonies of normal vaginal flora, allowing the harmful microbes to thrive. Such **superinfections** (opportunistic growth of harmful transient pathogens that are normally kept in check) can be extremely challenging to treat.

Nursing and Medical Procedures Several procedures are associated with an increased risk of infection. For example, urinary catheterization may injure the fragile urethral mucosa, provide a direct pathway for pathogens into the bladder, and prevent the normal flushing of the urethra.

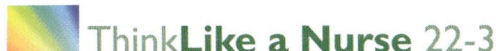

KnowledgeCheck 22-4

What factors increase a client's risk for infection?

ThinkLike a Nurse 22-3

- Consider your current lifestyle. How would you evaluate your ability to support your body's defenses?
- Recall the scenario of Jason Sergei, the labor and delivery nurse, and his daughter (Meet Your Nursing Role Model). Why did Jason say that hand washing was the most important thing he did at work that day? Explain your answer by referring to all of the links in the chain of infection.

PracticalKnowledge knowing **how**

As a nurse you will have direct contact with patients who are infected with a variety of pathogens or who are at increased risk for infection. The remainder of this chapter provides practical information for preventing infection in your clients and for caring for clients with infection.

ASSESSMENT NP

Some elements of the nursing history and physical assessment focus specifically on the risk factors and symptoms of infection.

Nursing History

To elicit information related to infection, ask the client about the following:

- Any exposure to pathogens in the environment, including at work, recent or international travel, contact with people who are ill, and unprotected sexual behavior
- If the patient is febrile, ask, "Have you recently traveled outside the country?"
- Any unusual foods or products ingested
- Past and present disease or injury history
- Medications, over-the-counter preparations, herbal products, alcohol intake, and any substances currently in use
- Current level of stress
- Immunization history
- Symptoms of illness

♥ iCare 22-1

About Protecting Patients From the Spread of Infection

Care enough to:
- Be knowledgeable about your organization's policy and procedures.
- Spend the time with thorough hand washing and strict aseptic technique when needed.
- Never use shortcuts when it comes to hand hygiene and asepsis.
- Remind others about diligent hand hygiene and use of personal protective equipment and sterile techniques.
- Be bold and call people out on breaks in aseptic technique when violated.
- Caring is being an advocate for infection prevention.

Physical Assessment

The following observations focus specifically on infection.

- **General appearance.** Does he seem fatigued? Is he diaphoretic (perspiring profusely)? Is he wrapped in blankets or complaining of feeling chilled? Does the patient appear well nourished? Are the mucous membranes dry?
- **Skin.** Examine the skin thoroughly for:
  - Normal elasticity (turgor)
  - Signs of local infection evidenced by pain, redness, swelling, and warmth
  - Presence or absence of any rashes, skin breaks, or reddened areas
  - *Note:* Patients with poor peripheral circulation often have skin discoloration, rather than signs of inflammation, when experiencing an infection.

- **Lymph nodes.** Swollen lymph nodes may indicate the presence of an infection in the area that drains into the nodes.
- **Temperature and pulse.** Elevated temperature and pulse rate are classic signs of an infection.

The presence of one infection does not eliminate the risk for an additional infection. For example, a patient being treated with IV medications for a wound infection is at risk for infection at the IV site, as well as for a superinfection or an infection related to insufficient immunizations.

For a list of tests commonly used to evaluate evidence of or risk for infection, see the accompanying Diagnostic Testing box. Each specific test should be evaluated based on the patient's condition, age, and coexisting conditions.

ANALYSIS/NURSING DIAGNOSIS NP

Only one NANDA-I diagnosis directly pertains to infection: Risk for Infection.

Infection, Risk for Virtually all patients in a healthcare setting are at risk for becoming infected because of exposure to pathogens in the environment. **KEY POINT:** *Use this diagnosis only for patients who are at higher than usual risk (e.g., those with poor nutritional status) and who need nursing interventions to help prevent infection. Do not use it for the generic assessments you do routinely for all patients (e.g., assessing temperature, routine examination of surgical incision).* Examples of appropriate use of this diagnosis include the following:

- Risk for Infection r/t altered immune response secondary to corticosteroid therapy
- Risk for Infection r/t impaired skin integrity and poor nutritional status.
- Risk for surgical site infection r/t transverse abdominal incision.

Actual Infection There is no NANDA-I diagnosis of "actual infection" because once an infection develops, it is

Diagnostic Testing

Common Tests for Evaluating the Presence of or Risk for Infection

Test	Description
White blood cell (WBC) count with differential	A breakdown of the number and types of WBCs; normal WBC count is 5,000–10,000/mm³.
Blood cultures	A sample of blood placed on culture media and evaluated for growth of pathogens. Normally, should show no growth of infectious microorganisms.
Urine cultures	Urine is normally sterile with no microorganism growth.
Throat cultures, wound cultures	Presence of microorganisms is normal, but there should be no growth of infectious microorganisms. To yield the most reliable results, blood cultures should be obtained from peripheral sites, using venipuncture by trained phlebotomists, unless a culture is specifically ordered from a central catheter or peripherally inserted central catheter.
Disease titers	Blood tests for specific disease immunity (e.g., to rubella)
Panels to evaluate specific disease exposure	Blood tests to evaluate exposure to specific diseases (e.g., HIV, hepatitis)
Immunoglobulin (IgG, IgM) levels	Blood tests to evaluate humoral immunity status
C-reactive protein (CRP)	A blood test to measure inflammatory change or bacterial infection
Agglutinins, warm or cold	Used to diagnose atypical infections by detecting antigens in the blood
Erythrocyte (red blood cell) sedimentation rate (ESR or sed rate)	A measure of inflammatory changes. Sed rate increases with inflammation. Normally it is at 15 mm/hr for men and < 20 mm/hr for women.
Iron level	Normally 60–90 g/100 mg. Lower in chronic infection.

managed collaboratively with the healthcare team. Infection is a medical diagnosis.

- *Infection may be the etiology of other nursing diagnoses,* such as Fatigue, Risk for Imbalanced Body Temperature, or Pain.
- *Patients with infection may have other nursing diagnoses* due to their infected status. For example:

Social Isolation r/t communicable disease (e.g., tuberculosis [TB])

Decreased Diversional Activity r/t inability to leave room secondary to protective isolation

- Other diagnostic statements may apply, depending upon the patient's condition, treatment ordered, and the patient's response to illness.

For a care plan and care map for Risk for Infection,

 Go to Davis Advantage, Resources, Chapter 22, **Care Plan** and **Care Map.**

PLANNING OUTCOMES/EVALUATION NP

NOC standardized outcomes for a diagnosis of Risk for Infection are:

Community Risk Control	Infection Severity
Communicable Disease	Risk Control: STDs
Immune Status	Wound Healing: Primary Intention
Immunization Behavior	Wound Healing: Secondary Intention

Individualized goals/outcomes statements depend on the specific nursing diagnosis and etiology. For example, for an undernourished woman, if the nursing diagnosis is Risk for Infection r/t indwelling central line and inadequate nutrition, an appropriate goal would be the following:

Patient will show no signs of localized infection at the infusion site, as evidenced by the absence of swelling, redness, excessive warmth, pain, or drainage.

You will evaluate the nursing care plan by examining the extent to which such goals have been met.

PLANNING INTERVENTIONS/ IMPLEMENTATION NP

When caring for a patient at risk for infection, nursing activities are aimed at breaking the chain of infection at every possible link. Some of the most common reasons that patients are diagnosed with Risk for Infection are exposure to pathogens, bypass of their normal defense mechanisms, increased physiological stress, or inadequate immune response. Direct nursing care toward these concerns and provide the following broad interventions:

- Reduce exposure to pathogens by using aseptic technique.
- Maintain skin integrity and support natural defenses against infection.
- Reduce stress.
- Promote immune function through immunization, healthy diet and activity, sleep, and lifestyle.
- Provide supportive measures to decrease the length of time that a patient needs invasive devices, such as intravenous lines and urinary catheters.

NIC standardized interventions for patients with infections include:

Communicable Disease Management	Infection Protection
Immunization/Vaccination Management	Surveillance
Incision Site Care	Teaching: Safe Sex
Infection Control	Wound Care

For more information about NIC interventions, refer to a standardized language handbook. Also,

 Go to Davis Advantage, Resources, Chapter 22, **Alphabetical List of NIC Outcomes.**

Specific nursing activities will be based on the unique situation of the client, as described in the etiology of the diagnostic statement. For example:

- **For clients who have had surgery and general anesthesia or who are at risk for pneumonia**—Promote coughing and deep breathing on a regular basis.
- **For clients being mechanically ventilated**—Provide special oral care designed to prevent ventilator-associated pneumonia.

 For older adults, especially those who are frail or in a debilitated state and those living in a group residence—Encourage immunizations that can help them to acquire immunity from some communicable diseases, such as influenza.

- **Community health nurses can limit disease transmission**—Through surveillance of the community, tracking of disease patterns, and initiation of prompt treatment.
- **For clients who have surgical incisions or breaks in the skin**—Provide regular assessment for infection status and follow appropriate medical or surgical asepsis guidelines.
- **For all clients at risk for infection**—Provide care that is based on principles of medical asepsis.

Teaching Infection Prevention

Clients and caregivers are usually at less risk for infection in their homes than they are in the hospital because:

- They share the same potential pathogens and antibodies.
- There is limited exposure to others with illness.

Nevertheless, to protect their own health and the health of others, clients need to understand basic principles of medical asepsis, personal hygiene, and infection control. You should also teach them to recognize signs and symptoms of infection; and for those who have an infection, help them to understand their specific organism and disease process. See the following boxes:

- Home Care: Preventing Infection in the Home and Community—For information about teaching infection control in the home and community
- Self-Care: Teaching Your Patient About Preventing the Spread of Community-Acquired MRSA—To help clients avoid acquiring or spreading community-acquired MRSA (CA-MRSA)

Wellness Promotion to Support Host Defenses

Lifestyle factors that strengthen host defenses and help break the chain of infection are healthful nutrition, good hydration, adequate hygiene, rest and exercise, stress reduction, and immunizations.

Nutrition It is important to monitor and support client nutrition, including protein, vitamins, minerals, and water. An acute infection depletes the body's nutritional stores. Nutrients are required to replace lost stores, to maintain production of white blood cells, and to repair damaged tissues. Common defenses against infection are increased mucus secretions and fever (which increases the metabolic rate). These common defenses against infection increase water loss. Chapter 28 further discusses the importance of adequate nutrition.

Safe, Effective Nursing Care

Preventing Ventilator-Associated Pneumonia (VAP)

Key Concepts: Infection Prevention and Control

SENC Competencies: Provide safe, quality client care; Collaborate with the interdisciplinary healthcare team

You and your colleagues can help improve the quality of patient care. Think about the following project and consider what Thinking, Doing, and Caring skills are required for its success.

Scenario: Nurses and physicians at the Mercy Medical Center wanted to reduce the rate of ventilator-associated pneumonia (VAP) in the intensive care unit.

1. **They collected data** to establish the current VAP rate of 12.6 cases per 1,000 ventilator days.
2. **Then they developed and implemented an intervention.** Nurses provided oral care with cetylpyridinium chloride (Oral-B) using a suction toothbrush every 4 hours. After that, they cleaned the patient's mouth with a hydrogen peroxide–treated suction swab, performed deep oropharyngeal suctioning, and applied mouth moisturizer.

3. **The result.** Incidence of VAP declined 72%, and after changing the tooth cleanser to chlorhexidine gluconate, VAP declined by 90% (Hutchins, Karras, Erwin, et al., 2009).

Otherwise, researchers interested in preventing VAP reviewed 28 clinical trials in the scientific literature. They found chlorhexidine rinses, gels, and swabs also lower the risk for HAIs for patients receiving mechanical ventilation (El-Rabbany, Zaghlol, Bhandari, et al., 2015).

Think About It.

Reflect on the following and discuss the questions with your peers:

➤ What information did nurses and team members need before changing the care of patients on ventilators?
➤ How does the intervention improve patient comfort?
➤ How significant do you think the team's work was? How will their efforts affect patients?
➤ What do you think the team should measure to determine whether the intervention worked?

Home Care

Preventing Infection in the Home and Community

Levels of disinfection and sterilization may differ in home care because clients and caregivers share the same potential pathogens and antibodies, and there is limited exposure to others who are ill and to care providers carrying unusual pathogens.

➤ To disinfect the home environment, mix a solution of 1 part regular-strength bleach to 50 parts water. The mixture may be stored for a month in an opaque container. **KEY POINT:** *NEVER mix the solution with other household cleaners.*
➤ Procedures performed using sterile technique in the hospital (e.g., urinary catheterization) are often performed by clean procedure in the home.
➤ Healthcare workers can carry pathogens into the home and must use good hand hygiene to avoid infecting the client.
➤ If the client or family member is capable and willing to perform the required treatment, provide the necessary teaching.
➤ Assess for signs of infection: temperature increase, fatigue, lymph gland enlargement, delayed healing of wounds, fever, chills, or drainage.
➤ Teach clients and family members the signs and symptoms of infection and how and when to report these findings to their care provider.
➤ Advise those planning international travel to get vaccinations before departing, especially for travel to sub-Saharan Africa, South-Central Asia, or Latin America, where they may contract malaria, dengue, rickettsiosis, and hepatitis.

Basic Infection Prevention Measures in the Home

Teach clients and family members the following basic hygiene and infection prevention measures:

➤ Always wash hands before preparing food, before eating, and before putting the hands near the face, and after going to the bathroom or blowing the nose.
➤ Keep the home environment clean.
➤ Prepare and store food safely. Growth of pathogens in foods can be prevented by:
   Cooking at high temperatures and storing in a cool place.
   Using highly concentrated solutes (e.g., salting meat and preserving fruit jellies, jams, and preserves).
➤ Do not share personal care items (e.g., towels, washcloths, toothbrushes, combs).
➤ Washing dishware and eating utensils in a dishwasher with hot water and detergents is sufficient decontamination

Avoiding Infection Outside the Home

Teach clients and family members actions to help prevent infection when they are outside the home, for example:

➤ Wash hands and do not touch surfaces in a public bathroom.
➤ Carry and use antibacterial hand gel as needed while in public places.
➤ Wash hands upon returning home (e.g., from shopping).
➤ Ask healthcare providers to wash their hands before touching you, if they have not done so.
➤ Use tongs, not fingers, to get food from serving trays in grocery stores.

Self-Care

Teaching Your Patient About Preventing the Spread of Community-Acquired MRSA

Everyone should take the following measures to prevent CA-MRSA:

➤ Take antibiotics as prescribed. Take *all* the medication, or as recommended.
➤ Contact your healthcare provider if the infection doesn't improve after a few days of taking an antibiotic.
➤ Never use antibiotics prescribed for someone else; do not give your medication to others.
➤ Follow your healthcare provider's recommendations for influenza and pneumonia vaccinations. Preventing respiratory infections decreases antibiotic use.
➤ Make sure your healthcare providers clean their hands before they touch you. This is one of the most important infection prevention and control measures.
➤ Wash your hands often with soap and water. Wash for 15 to 30 seconds or as long as it takes to sing the "Happy Birthday" song.
➤ Use alcohol-based hand sanitizer if soap and water are not available or hands are not visibly soiled. Sanitizer should contain at least 60% alcohol.
➤ Avoid sharing personal items (e.g., towels, makeup, combs, clothing).
➤ Pay attention to symptoms that may indicate an infection (e.g., drainage or inflammation of a wound) and contact your healthcare provider immediately.
➤ Cough and sneeze into your elbow and wash your hands after using a tissue.

Clients who have MRSA on their skin or who are infected with MRSA should be taught to:

➤ Keep all wounds clean and covered with bandages.
➤ When changing a bandage:
   Don't touch the sore with your bare hands. Wear gloves. Immediately discard the soiled bandage and gloves in a plastic bag where no one else can touch them.
   Wash your hands after removing the gloves.
➤ Avoid touching other people's wounds or bandages.
➤ Avoid close-contact activities until your skin infection is healed, unless you can ensure that your sore will not come in contact with another person (e.g., if your sore can be well covered by a bandage and clothing).
➤ Shower daily, using antibacterial soap if your healthcare provider advises it.
➤ Wash your clothing, towels, and bedding separately from other family members' items. Use warm or hot water and bleach, if possible. Use warm or hot setting on the dryer.
➤ Wash exercise clothes after each use.

Sources: Adapted from CDC. (2015a, April 17, updated). Antibiotic resistance questions & answers. Retrieved from http://www.cdc.gov/getsmart/community/about/antibiotic-resistance-faqs.html; CDC. (2016e, March 24, updated). General information about MRSA in healthcare settings. Retrieved from http://www.cdc.gov/mrsa/community/index.html

---

Hygiene Encourage frequent hand washing and regular showering or bathing. Good hygiene is crucial to decrease the bacterial count on the skin and maintain intact skin, a primary host defense. However, overzealous cleanliness diminishes the skin's natural oils and may lead to cracking of the skin.

Chapter 24 focuses on the importance of hygiene for health. Also see the Home Care box Preventing Infection in the Home and Community.

For the immunocompromised or bed-bound hospitalized patient, provide daily bedside baths using filtered tap water, disposable basins, and prepackaged bathing products. Nurses should use disposable cloths with 2% chlorhexidine gluconate (CHG) to reduce colonization of specific bacteria and infections with MDROs (Petlin, Schallom, Prentice, et al., 2014; Power, Peed, Burns, et al., 2012).

Rest and Sleep Sleep of 6 to 9 hours per night is considered fully restorative for most people. However, sleep needs and patterns vary. Rest and sleep conserve energy needed for healing.

Exercise and Activity Exercise is just as important as rest and sleep. Too little activity causes circulation to slow and the lungs to supply less oxygen. Too much exercise leads to fatigue and joint injury. Chapters 33 and 35 provide in-depth discussion on activity, exercise, rest, and sleep.

Stress Reduction Laughing increases immune responses, improves oxygenation, and promotes body movement. In contrast, physical or mental stress decreases the body's immune defenses. Studies demonstrate a correlation between stress and disease (Cousins, 1979; Franco, de Barros, Nogueira-Martins, et al., 2003; Tegethoff, Greene, Olsen, et al., 2011). See Chapter 12 if you want further details on the effects of stress.

Immunizations Encourage clients to follow recommendations for immunizations (e.g., via vaccination). Encourage clients to follow recommendations for immunizations to protect against several common infectious diseases (e.g., measles, mumps, pertussis, polio, pneumonia, influenza, smallpox, and shingles). Unfortunately, some pathogens, such as the common cold virus, mutate too rapidly for an immunization to be developed. **KEY POINT:** *For most diseases, at least 85% of the population must be immunized in order to protect the entire population from the disease.* If you need specific recommended immunizations throughout the life span and their role in health promotion, see Chapters 9 and 10 for various age-groups, and

 Go to the links on the CDC page, Immunizations for Health Professionals, at http://www.cdc.gov/vaccines/schedules/hcp/index.html

Knowledge Check 22-5

What actions improve host ability to prevent infection?

The remainder of the chapter will discuss the infection prevention measures of medical asepsis and surgical asepsis.

PRACTICING MEDICAL ASEPSIS

Asepsis is a term that means absence of contamination by disease-causing microorganisms. **Medical asepsis** ("clean technique") refers to procedures that decrease the potential for the spread of infections. You probably already practice medical asepsis in other settings without realizing it. For example, at home you wash your hands before and after handling foods. In the healthcare setting, medical asepsis includes hand hygiene, environmental cleanliness, standard precautions, and protective isolation.

✚ Infection prevention, including the patient's safety, depend on nurses' rigorously and consistently following the principles of asepsis. When you are hurrying, you may be tempted to take shortcuts or forget to follow a guideline. Remember: Cutting corners can put your patient, and possibly yourself, at risk for a serious infection.

Maintaining Clean Hands

KEY POINT: *Hand hygiene is the single most important activity for preventing and controlling infection.*

The WHO (2009) chose as the first Global Patient Safety Challenge the reduction of HAIs, with the theme, *clean care is safer care.* Hand hygiene is the cornerstone strategy because it is simple, standardized, low-cost, and based on solid scientific evidence.

Although you may think you already know how to wash your hands, decisions about the type of hand hygiene to use, how long to wash, when to wash, and so on based on the amount of contact you have with patients or contaminated objects, as well as the patient's infection status and susceptibility to infection. Hand washing involves five key factors: time, water, soap, friction, and drying.

- **Time.** In a nonsurgical setting, wash the hands vigorously for at least 15 seconds, longer if hands are visibly soiled. In a surgical setting wash for 2 to 6 minutes, depending on the soap or other product used.
- **Water.** Use warm water and rinse off soap completely.
- **Soap.** Use agency-approved soap; or The CDC recommends (2002) use a 60% alcohol-based solution (rubs, sprays, gels) for routine hand cleansing and plain or antimicrobial soap and water when hands are visibly dirty. Iodine compounds are also effective, but usually too irritating for regular hand hygiene.

✚ **If there is a potential for contact with bacterial spores** (e.g., when caring for a client with a *C. difficile* infection), you must wash your hands with soap and water; alcohol-based solutions are not effective against spores.

For more specific details and guidelines for hand hygiene, see Clinical Insight 22-1 and Procedure 22-1, Hand Hygiene.

- **Friction.** Rub all surfaces of the hands and wrists vigorously, including the backs of the hands and between the fingers. Remove jewelry and clean areas underneath. Clean underneath the fingernails using an orangewood stick.
- **Drying.** Use single-use towels or hand dryers to remove all moisture after washing the hands. If using antimicrobial hand gels, apply and rub hands until dry.

Failure to perform standards of care constitutes medical negligence and can result in harm to the patient. In addition, Medicare does not reimburse for patient complications arising from certain HAIs, many of which result from poor hand washing. Despite the importance of clean hands, research demonstrates that clinical staff do not consistently observe hand hygiene guidelines (Pratt, Pellowe, Wilson, et al., 2007). You can help improve clinical practice by serving as a role model for good hand hygiene.

Maintaining a Clean Environment

A clean environment includes the surfaces in a patient's room, as well as supplies, equipment, and other objects brought into the room. The floor, soiled dressings, used tissues, sinks, commodes, and bedpans are examples of contaminated items. An object becomes contaminated or unclean if it comes in contact with a contaminated surface—or if you suspect, for whatever reason, that it may contain pathogens. Agency policies determine whether a reusable item is cleaned, disinfected, or sterilized, based on how the item is used.

Cleaning

Cleaning is the removal of visible soil (organic and inorganic) from objects and surfaces. In healthcare agencies, it is usually accomplished manually or mechanically using water with detergents or enzymatic products formulated to inhibit microbial growth. A goal of medical asepsis is to keep all public and patient care areas within the facility clean and free from dust, debris, and contamination. Any spilled liquids, dirty surfaces, or potentially contaminated areas should be cleaned immediately. Items must be cleaned thoroughly before they can be disinfected or sterilized.

Disinfecting

Disinfection removes pathogens on inanimate objects by physical or chemical means, including steam, gas, chemicals, and ultraviolet light. Chemical germicides can achieve three levels of disinfection (Box 22-3).

Disinfection is used for semicritical and noncritical items:

- **Semicritical items** are those that contact mucous membranes or nonintact skin. They must be free of all microorganisms except bacterial spores, so they must at least be disinfected and sometimes sterilized.
  Examples: Reusable devices, such as flexible endoscopes, and respiratory therapy and anesthesia equipment
- **Noncritical items** are supplies and equipment that come in contact with intact skin but not mucous membranes. They do not carry a high risk of infection transmission, and they can be decontaminated where they are used. Disinfection is adequate for noncritical items.
  Examples: Bedpans, stethoscopes, and blood pressure cuffs
  Examples of noncritical environmental surfaces: Floors, food utensils, bed linens, and bed rails (CDC, 2009a).

Sterilizing

Sterilization is the elimination of all microorganisms (except prions) in or on an object. The major sterilizing methods used in hospitals are (1) autoclaving with moist heat, also called immediate use steam sterilization, (2) gas or vapor (e.g., ethylene oxide or hydrogen peroxide), (3) dry heat, (4) ozone, and (5) liquid chemicals (e.g., peracetic acid) (Spry & Connor, 2012).

- **Critical items** are those that pose a high risk for infection if they are contaminated with any microorganism—that is,

---

BOX 22-3 ■ Level of Disinfection

High-level disinfection kills all organisms except high levels of bacterial spores.
Intermediate-level disinfection kills bacteria, mycobacteria, and most viruses.
Low-level disinfection kills some viruses and bacteria.

those that enter the vascular system or sterile tissue or those items through which blood flows.

Examples: Intravenous catheters, needles for injections, urinary catheters, surgical instruments, some wound dressings, and chest tubes

As a nurse, you must be familiar with the agency's policies and procedures for cleaning, handling, and transporting items to be disinfected and sterilized, and for working collaboratively with other departments and specially trained personnel (e.g., Environmental Services) to keep the patient care area as clean and free of clutter as possible.

For more specific information about maintaining a clean environment in institutional and home care, see Clinical Insight 22-2.

CDC Guidelines for Preventing Transmission of Pathogens

In addition to hand washing and maintaining a clean environment, you should follow other precautions to protect yourself and your patients. CDC guidelines provide for two tiers of protection (Siegel, Rhinehart, Jackson, et al., 2007):

- **Standard precautions,** the first tier of protection, apply to care of all patients. You must assume that every patient is potentially colonized or infected with an organism that could be passed to others in the healthcare setting.
- **Transmission-based precautions,** the second tier of protection, are for patients with known or suspected infection or colonization with pathogens. Recall from the discussion on the chain of infection that pathogens may be transmitted by contact, droplet, or air. Each mode of transmission requires

a different approach to prevent infection. ♥ **iCare** For all transmission-based precautions, institute measures to counteract negative effects of isolation on patients (i.e., anxiety, depression, perceptions of stigma, reduced contact with staff, and increases in preventable adverse events).

- Table 22-2 provides a comparison of standard and transmission-based precautions. For detailed guidelines to aid you in following both types of precautions, refer to Clinical Insights 22-3 and 22-4.

KnowledgeCheck 22-6

Under what circumstances are standard precautions used?

Personal Protective Equipment The CDC recommends and the U.S. Occupational Safety and Health Administration requires employers to provide personal protective equipment (PPE) for healthcare workers (e.g., gloves, gowns, face masks, and eye protection [Fig. 22-3]) (U.S. Department of Labor, n.d.a). This equipment is to be used in standard precautions as well as transmission-based precautions. To learn how to don and remove PPE, refer to Procedures 22-2 and 22-3.

Protective Environment in Special Situations

Patients who are immunosuppressed (e.g., receiving chemotherapy) are sometimes placed in a special form of isolation, called *protective isolation* or *reverse isolation*. However, the CDC states that standard and transmission-based precautions are adequate protection for most of those patients. They recommend a "protective environment" only for a special class of

---

Table 22-2 ▶ Comparison of CDC Standard and Transmission-Based Precautions

STANDARD PRECAUTIONS	TRANSMISSION-BASED PRECAUTIONS
"Tier One" Precautions	**"Tier Two" Precautions**
Use with all clients, in all settings, regardless of suspected or confirmed presence of infection.	Use for patients known or suspected to be infected or colonized with infectious agents.
Principle: All blood, body fluids, secretions, excretions except sweat, nonintact skin, and mucous membranes may contain pathogens.	*Principle:* Routes of transmission for some microorganisms are not completely interrupted using standard precautions alone. Used *in addition to* standard precautions.
Include: Hand hygiene; use of gloves, gown, mask, eye protection, or face shield (depending on expected exposure) and safe injection practices.	**Three categories of precautions:** *Contact Precautions*—For organisms spread by direct contact with the patient or his environment. This is the most common form of transmission.
Added for protection of patients more than of healthcare personnel: Safe injection practices, respiratory hygiene and cough etiquette, and wearing a mask when performing special lumbar puncture procedures.	*Droplet Precautions*—For pathogens spread through close respiratory or mucous membrane contact with respiratory secretions (e.g., sneezing, coughing, talking); pathogens that do not remain infectious over long distances.
Standard precautions do not completely protect against microorganisms spread by contact, droplets, or through the air.	*Airborne Precautions*—For pathogens that are very small and remain infectious over long distances when suspended in the air and are easily transmitted through air currents (e.g., fanning linens, ventilating systems).

Source: Siegel, J. D., Rhinehart, E., Jackson, M., et al. (2007). *2007 guideline for isolation precautions: Preventing transmission of infectious agents in the healthcare setting.* Retrieved from http://www.cdc.gov/hicpac/2007IP/2007isolationPrecautions.html

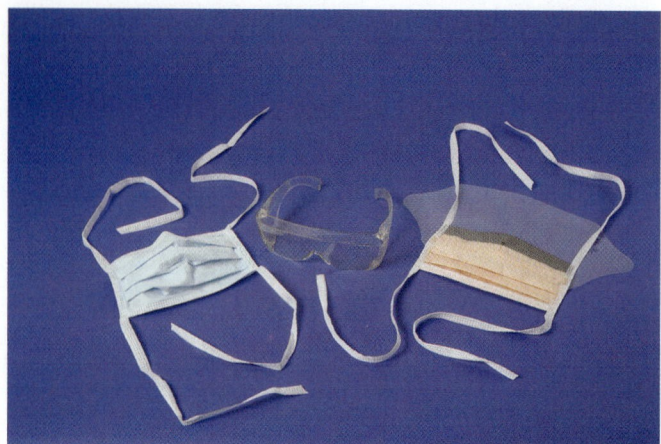

FIGURE 22-3 Several types of face masks and eye shields are available.

stem cell–transplant patients who have neutropenia (low white blood cell count) secondary to chemotherapy. Most of the recommendations are engineering and environmental services rather than nursing measures. Refer to Clinical Insight 22-5 as a guide to providing a protective environment.

Patients with compromised immunity are more likely to become infected by pathogens harbored in their own bodies than from pathogens transmitted by other people (Siegel, Rhinehart, Jackson, et al., 2007). Therefore, except for the special situations described above, standard and transmission-based precautions should protect nearly all vulnerable patients from organisms brought in by healthcare workers and visitors.

Nevertheless, in practice you may see what has been called **protective isolation** being used for clients with low WBC counts, clients undergoing chemotherapy, or clients with large open wounds or weak immune systems. Protective isolation usually includes following standard precautions; placing the patient in a private room; restricting visitors; wearing a mask, gown, and gloves for patient care; and special cleaning or disposal of the patient's equipment and supplies. Some units, such as neonatal intensive care units, burn units, and labor and delivery suites, may follow some aspects of protective isolation all the time.

Control of Potentially Contaminated Equipment and Supplies

Whenever possible, use disposable equipment in an isolation room. Nondisposable equipment and supplies require special handling.

- **Protective Isolation.** If a client is in protective isolation, be sure that equipment has been disinfected *before* it is taken into the room. Take linen and dishes directly to the protective isolation room, and hand them to someone wearing the required protective clothing.
- **Transmission-Based Isolation.** If the client is in transmission-based isolation, disinfect the equipment *on removal* from the room. When removing linen or nondisposable items from a room with contact, droplet, or airborne isolation, place them in special isolation bags.

Disposing of Used Isolation Supplies Place contaminated disposable equipment and materials containing body fluids in special isolation bags; use the bags *only* for contaminated materials. This process requires two healthcare workers. The worker inside the room wears protective clothing and

handles only contaminated items. The second worker stands at the door and holds the isolation bag open. The first worker places items inside the bag without touching the outside of the bag. If the bag contains linens, the isolation bag is closed and placed in a laundry hamper. Securely close the isolation trash bag and place it in a special isolation trash container. Special disposal methods are used to prevent these objects from going into a landfill, where they could become a reservoir of infection.

Sharps Disposal Always place disposable needles, syringes, and other sharp items and glass in special disposable sharps containers immediately after use. Never recap a contaminated needle. Refer to Chapters 23 and 25 if you need further information on preventing needlestick injuries.

Laboratory Specimens Laboratory specimens contain blood and body fluids and are always considered contaminated. Label the specimen container in a clean area before taking it to the patient. Have the specimen collected by a healthcare worker wearing appropriate protective clothing. Once the specimen is collected, place it in a special transport bag. Do not allow the outside of the bag to touch any contaminated item, especially your gloves.

For more guidelines on care of contaminated equipment and supplies, refer to Clinical Insights 22-2, 22-3, and 22-4, as needed.

KnowledgeCheck 22-7

- If you needed to disinfect a sink in a client's home, what would you use?
- List at least three actions clients can take to help avoid infection when they are out in the community.

PRACTICING SURGICAL ASEPSIS

If an object is sterile, it contains no life and therefore no infectious organisms. Inanimate objects, such as surgical equipment, gauze dressings, or wound irrigation fluid may be sterilized. However, it is impossible to rid the human body of all microorganisms, either in or on it.

♥ iCare 22-2

About Supporting the Psychological Needs of Patients in Isolation

Keep in mind that it is the disease that is being isolated, *not* the person who has the disease. Patients in isolation continue to have a need for human contact. In fact, isolation may produce anxiety and increase the desire for human contact. Search for ways to reassure and maintain contact with the patient in protective isolation.

- Use touch as much as possible (when wearing required protective equipment).
- Set aside time to ask about how the client is coping with isolation.
- If the patient is in droplet isolation, remember that the danger area is 3 feet from the patient. You can go to the door of the room and speak to the patient without a mask.
- Reassure the patient that precautions are temporary.
- Explain that the precautions and the PPE protect you and the patient, as well as family members and other patients.

Toward Evidence-Based Practice

Scott, E., Goodyear, N., Nicoloro, J. M., et al. (2015). Laundering habits of student nurses and correlation with the presence of *Staphylococcus aureus* on nursing scrub tops pre- and postlaundering. *American Journal of Infection Control,* 43(9), 106–108. doi:http://dx.doi.org/10.1016/j.ajic.2015.05.007

Researchers studied the effect of laundering on microbial colonization of scrubs. Students were asked to swab their scrub tops after their clinical shifts and after laundering. After work in the clinical setting, 17% of swabs tested positive for *Staphylococcus aureus.* Yet after laundering, only 64.3% of the bacteria were eliminated from contaminated scrubs.

Cassir, N., Guillemette, T., Hraiech, S., et al. (2015). Chlorhexidine daily bathing: Impact on health care–associated infections caused by gram-negative bacteria. *American Journal of Infection Control,* 43(6), 640–643. Retrieved from http://dx.doi.org/10.1016/j.ajic.2015.02.010

Healthcare-associated infections (HAIs) are a major cause of illness in intensive care unit (ICU) patients. Research was conducted to evaluate the effectiveness of bathing patients daily using chlorhexidine gluconate (CHG) on HAIs, specifically ventilator-associated pneumonia, bloodstream infections, and urinary tract infections. Patients who received daily skin cleansing with 2% CHG–impregnated cloths were found to have a lower incidence of clinical cultures positive for gram-negative bacteria than those who were bathed daily with soap and water.

1. From these studies, what can you conclude about the transmission of HAIs?

2. What measures do these two studies suggest for reducing microbial colonization that could lead to the spread of HAIs? What else could nurses do to further lessen the risk for spreading microbes in the clinical setting?

 Go to Davis Advantage, Resources, Chapter 22, **Toward Evidence-Based Practice—Suggested Responses.**

Surgical asepsis, or **sterile technique,** requires creation of a sterile environment and use of sterile equipment. It differs from medical asepsis in that it is more complex and it is not necessary to use it with all patients. Sterilization can be accomplished through the use of special gases or high heat. Surgical equipment and implanted devices are examples of materials that must be sterilized.

To create a sterile area, environmental services personnel perform thorough cleaning using special solutions and procedures. All personnel working in the area must wear appropriate surgical attire and perform a surgical hand scrub.

Levels of Asepsis   Recent guidelines suggest using modified sterile technique for many bedside procedures that have traditionally used sterile technique (e.g., tracheostomy care and wound care). The following summarizes the practical differences in sterile, modified sterile, and clean techniques:

- **Sterile technique** is the use of sterile gloves and sterile supplies (e.g., drapes, bandages, instruments, water).
- **Modified sterile technique** is use of nonsterile procedure gloves with sterile supplies.
- **Clean technique** is use of clean hands or nonsterile gloves and clean, rather than sterile, supplies (e.g., tap water).

Performing a Surgical Scrub

A **surgical scrub** is a modification of the hand-washing procedure described earlier (see Table 22-3 for a comparison). It traditionally involves an extended scrub of the hands using a sponge, nail cleaner, and a bactericidal scrubbing agent. A newer method uses a brushless scrub, using a bactericidal scrubbing agent. All methods require a prewash before the surgical scrub. For the steps, refer to Procedures 22-4 and 22-5.

Donning Surgical Attire

Burn units; labor and birth units; and some surgical suites, intensive care units, newborn nurseries, and oncology floors require surgical attire for aspects of patient caregiving. In each of these units, nurses care for clients who are at increased risk for infection or are undergoing an invasive procedure that places them at increased risk. The goal is to protect patients from infection transmitted by healthcare workers.

Clean Surgical Attire   Staff working in these areas don *clean,* not sterile, surgical attire, or scrub suits, when they arrive on the unit. These scrub suits should not be worn outside the unit. If you must transport a patient to another area or leave the unit to gather supplies, wear a covering over the scrub suit. Remove the covering on your return to the unit. Additional precautions may include a disposable head cover, shoe coverings, and face masks.

Sterile Surgical Attire   Personnel involved in surgery or certain invasive procedures must dress in *sterile* surgical attire. As a beginning student, you will soon find yourself in such a situation. Initially your role will be limited to observation, but you will need to be prepared for these experiences.

First you will change into scrub apparel, apply shoe coverings, and put on a disposable hat; wash your hands; and apply a facemask. If there is potential for spray of fluids, wear a face mask with an eye shield. Be sure to fit the mask so that it is comfortable to breathe through. Then perform the surgical scrub. If a surgical gown is required, don it after the hand scrub.

- **Closed Gloving.** If you are applying full surgical attire, you will need to don gloves using a closed method, after you have put on your gown. Once you are wearing sterile gloves, you may touch only sterile items. To learn how to don sterile gloves and gown using the closed method, see Procedure 22-6.
- **Open Gloving.** You will often wear sterile gloves for procedures that do not require full surgical attire. For this, you will use the open method of gloving. For complete instructions for open-method sterile gloving, refer to Procedure 22-7.

KEY POINT: *Be sure to open the glove packaging slowly, avoid fanning the wrapping or touching the gloves, and put the first glove on your dominant hand. (See Figure 22-4.)*

KEY POINT: *A general rule to consider when applying the second glove is to touch glove-to-glove and skin-to-skin. The already-gloved hand may touch any of the sterile surfaces of the second glove. The second hand may touch only the inside of the glove—the portion that will have contact with the skin. (See Figure 22-5.)*

Using Sterile Technique in Nursing Care

Healthcare providers use sterile technique to perform a variety of procedures. Some of the procedures require full surgical PPE; others do not. Examples of procedures that use both sterile technique and principles of medical asepsis are administering an injection, starting an IV line, and performing a sterile dressing

Table 22-3 ▶ Different Types of Hand Hygiene				
METHODS	**AGENT**	**PURPOSE**	**AREA**	**DURATION (MINIMUM)**
Routine handwash	Water and non-antimicrobial soap (i.e., plain soap)	Remove soil and transient microorganisms	All surfaces of the hands and fingers	15 seconds
Antiseptic handwash	Water and antimicrobial soap (e.g., chlorhexidine, iodine, and iodophors)	Remove or destroy transient micro-organisms and reduce resident flora (persistent activity)	All surfaces of the hands and fingers	15 seconds
Antiseptic handrub	Alcohol-based handrub	Remove or destroy transient micro-organisms and reduce resident flora (persistent activity)	All surfaces of the hands and fingers	Until the hands are dry
Surgical antisepsis	1. Water and anti-microbial soap (e.g., chlorhexidine, iodine, and iodophors) 2. Water and non-antimicrobial soap (i.e., plain soap) followed by long-acting, alcohol-based surgical hand scrub product	Remove or destroy transient microorganisms and reduce resident flora (persistent activity)	Hands and forearms	1. 2–6 minutes 2. Follow manufacturer instructions for surgical hand scrub product with persistent activity

Source: Centers for Disease Control and Prevention. (2013). Infection control: Frequently asked questions—hand hygiene. Retrieved from http://www.cdc.gov/oralhealth/infectioncontrol/faq/hand.htm

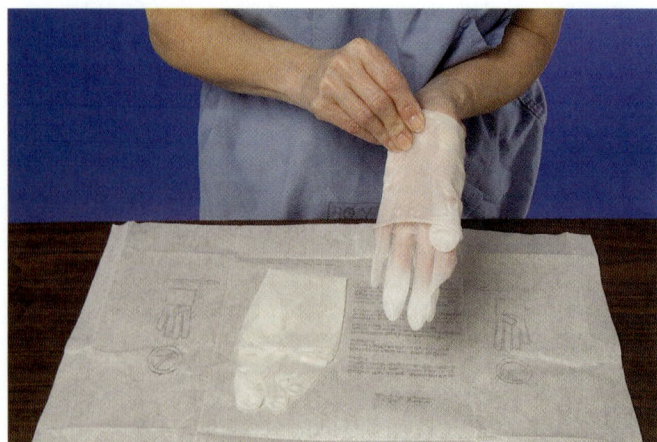

FIGURE 22-4 When applying the first glove, touch only the inside cuff of the glove.

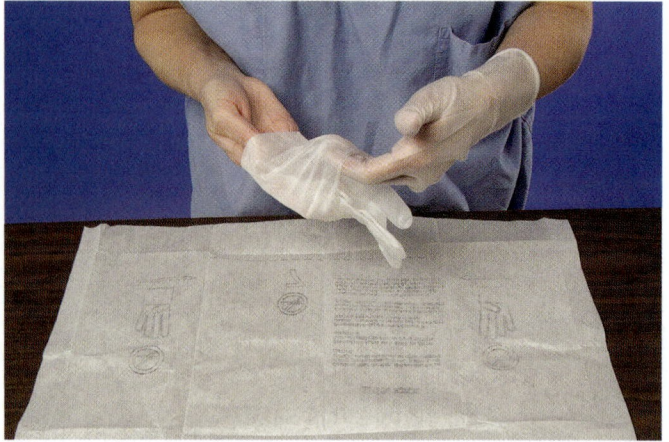

FIGURE 22-5 When applying the second glove, consider this general rule: glove-to-glove, skin-to-skin.

change. To clarify, when administering an injection, you prepare the patient; cleanse the injection site; and remove the needle cap using standard precautions. You do not don sterile gloves, but for the rest of the procedure you observe sterile technique by taking care not to touch or otherwise contaminate the exposed needle.

Before performing a sterile procedure, determine what supplies you will need and whether you will need assistance. If the patient is unable to maintain a position required for the procedure, you will need a helper to hold the patient during the procedure.

Preparing and Maintaining Sterile Fields There are some variations in how you might set up sterile fields. Sometimes it is as simple as opening a package of supplies wrapped in a sterile disposable cover. At other times, you may work with a larger, reusable or disposable sterile drape (wrapped in an outer wrapping). To learn a procedure for maintaining a sterile field, as well as adding supplies and sterile liquids to it, see Procedure 22-8A.

Adding Supplies to a Sterile Field Some supplies (e.g., urinary catheter kits) are packaged in a wrapper that can serve as a sterile field. The outside of these packages is considered clean, and the inside is sterile. You must open these packages in a way that does not contaminate the inside of the wrapping. Be cautious when adding supplies to a sterile field. If any object falls only partly on the field, it is no longer sterile. For detailed instructions on how to add supplies to a sterile field, see Procedure 22-8B.

Adding Sterile Solutions to a Sterile Field Add sterile liquids to a sterile field by slowly pouring them into a container on the field. Some sterile drapes contain an impermeable membrane between layers that serves as a barrier to moisture and prevents wicking. With this type of drape, you may pour sterile liquid directly on gauze pads on the field. Pour only an amount of liquid that is sufficient to make the gauze pads damp. Excess fluid may run off the field, causing the field to become contaminated—a wet field is not sterile because it does not provide a barrier to microorganisms on the unsterile surface under the drape (see Box 22-4 about common breaks in sterility). For step-by-step instruction in how to add sterile solutions to a sterile field, refer to Procedure 22-8C.

KnowledgeCheck 22-8

- When will you need to don sterile gloves using the closed method?
- True or False: Some procedures require both standard precautions and sterile technique.
- What part(s) of a sterile field are considered to be unsterile?

BOX 22-4 ■ Avoiding Common Breaks in Sterility

What Areas Are Considered Sterile?

- A sterile field is sterile only on the horizontal plane (e.g., the draped table top). *Material that drapes over the horizontal plane may easily be contacted by nonsterile clothing or equipment.*
- Consider a 1-inch margin along the borders of a sterile drape unsterile even if it remains on a horizontal surface. *Because it is in contact with contaminated surfaces.*
- If you are wearing sterile attire, consider only the front of your body from the chest to the level of the sterile field to be sterile, nothing else.
- Sleeve cuffs are considered unsterile when your hands pass beyond the cuff (cuffs are sterile if you don gloves using the closed method).

Protecting the Equipment on the Sterile Field

- **KEY POINT:** *Sterile touches sterile. Unsterile touches unsterile. Only sterile items can be placed on a sterile field.*
- Wash your hands before gathering materials from the sterile supply area and then gather the other required supplies and equipment.
- Handle sterile equipment only if you are wearing sterile gloves.
- Sterile liquids must be contained in sterile containers on the field or the sterile drape must be nonpermeable to avoid wicking. *If the drape is permeable, liquid can seep through to the underlying surface and act as a wick for contaminants to travel upward to the sterile field.*
- Make sure you are opening equipment packaged with labels indicating it has been sterilized properly, packaging intact and dry, and not expired.
- If packages are light and small, gently add them to the sterile field by separating the package flaps and allowing them to fall onto the field.

- If the object is large (e.g., an irrigation bowl), slowly unwrap the packaging and, grasping it through the outside wrapper, place the bowl on the field.

Protecting the Sterile Field

- Move slowly and deliberately.
- Never reach across a sterile field.
- If you see someone else contaminate a sterile field or object, identify the break and cover the area with sterile drapes or replace with a new sterile setup, gown, or gloves.
- Remain at least 1 foot away from nonsterile areas if you are wearing sterile garb.
- Never turn your back to a sterile field. A sterile field and open sterile items must be kept above waist level and in constant view. *You are responsible for monitoring and maintaining the sterility. If you cannot see the field, you do not know whether it has become contaminated.*
- Make sure your clothing or lab coat never touches any part of the sterile field.
- Keep your fingernails short and clean. Avoid nail polish and artificial nails.
- Avoid wearing jewelry that dangles or can fall into the sterile field.
- Keep long hair pulled back or covered by a head covering designed for sterility.
- Change your gown or reinforce with additional sterile drapes if it is soaked through.
- Avoid splashing any kind of solution onto the sterile field.
- Keep doors closed so turbulent airflow does not contaminate a sterile area with airborne microbes.
- Clean wounds and prep sterile sites from clean to dirty.

Source: Adapted from Simko, L. (2012). Breaking sterility: Procedural violations in healthcare. *Nursing2012, 42*(8), 22–26. doi:10.1097/01. NURSE.0000415839.66736.4c

INFECTION CONTROL AND PREVENTION FOR HEALTHCARE WORKERS

It is critical that you learn how to protect yourself from infections—not only to avoid personal illness but also to avoid becoming a reservoir for infection. Nurses and other patient care workers are at increased risk of acquiring infections because they come in contact with a variety of pathogens. Skin and mucous membrane contact and puncture wounds often serve as portals of entry.

As a nurse, you need to monitor other healthcare workers, patients, and visitors for adherence to infection control measures. As well, nursing assistive personnel (NAP), hospital personnel, and volunteers are often present on nursing units. You need to protect them and yourself from potential hazardous exposure as well as from microorganisms brought into the unit.

What Role Does the Infection Preventionist Nurse Play?

The task of the infection prevention nurse is to minimize the number of infections in the healthcare facility. Infection preventionists must keep current with information about pathogens, antibiotic resistance, and infection control. The infection prevention nurse also functions as an epidemiologist, tracking down the source of HAIs and strengthening measures to prevent their recurrence. Finally, all members of the infection prevention team enforce compliance with federal, state, and local regulations related to infection control and prevention.

What Should I Do If I Am Exposed to Bloodborne Pathogens?

Exposure to blood, body secretions, or body tissues containing blood or secretions requires immediate action. See Box 22-5 for complete instructions. The first step is to minimize the exposure by washing the area thoroughly. Then notify the appropriate people, complete an injury report, and seek medical attention.

BOX 22-5 ■ If You Are Exposed to Blood or Other Body Fluids

✚ If you are stuck by a needle or other sharp or get blood or other potentially infectious materials in your eyes, nose, mouth, or on broken skin:

1. Immediately flood the exposed area with water and clean any wound with soap and water or a skin disinfectant if available.
2. Report the exposure immediately to the appropriate person in the agency. If you are a student, also report immediately to your instructor.
3. Seek immediate medical attention. Consent to testing and follow-up treatment as advised.
4. Complete an incident or injury report.
5. Attend counseling sessions provided by the agency.

Source: Bloodborne pathogens and needlestick prevention. Evaluating and controlling exposure. (n.d.). Occupational Safety & Health Administration. U.S. Department of Labor. Retrieved from https://www.osha.gov/SLTC/bloodbornepathogens/evaluation.htm

---

Anyone exposed to bloodborne pathogens should have baseline lab work done to check for hepatitis and HIV. If the patient source is known, the infection preventionist will arrange to have the patient tested. Subsequent testing and possible preventive treatment are based on the type of exposure and what is known about the source and the injured person. To limit risks from the exposure, the infection prevention team will provide counseling and recommendations as soon as possible after the event. Chapters 23 and 25 present information on preventing needlestick injuries.

How Can I Minimize the Effects of Bioterrorism and Epidemics?

Bioterrorism is the intentional release, or threatened release, of disease-producing organisms or substances intended to cause death, illness, harm, economic damage, or fear. Diseases with recognized bioterrorism potential are anthrax, botulism, pneumonic plague, smallpox, viral hemorrhagic fevers, and tularemia.

Recognize an Outbreak Should a biological event occur, either as a result of bioterrorism or a naturally occurring epidemic, a major factor in minimizing its effects is the ability to quickly recognize unusual disease patterns and detect the presence of infectious diseases. Some electronic health record systems include special features to identify the pattern of infectious diseases. However, there is no substitute for direct, clinical observation skills.

Nurses need to assess not only the individual patient's condition but also clusters of symptoms. Hospital, emergency department, and clinic nurses are in key positions to recognize outbreaks because they see patients from multiple primary care providers. Nurses must keep the following questions in mind:

- Am I seeing an unexpected number of infectious diseases or diseases possibly caused by infectious organisms?
- Am I seeing similar cases that are not responding to medical treatment?
- Are healthcare workers who provide care to infectious patients becoming ill?

Notify the Safety Officer After identifying a suspicious pattern, you should notify the institution's interventionist or safety officer as soon as possible. Appropriate cultures will be needed, and the federal and state health departments should be notified. If the infectious organism is unknown, samples must be preserved for future analysis.

Institute Appropriate Level of Standard Precautions
KEY POINT: *In the event of an epidemic, the essential principles of hand hygiene and standard precautions will be the core of your infection prevention and control measures.* Patients with similar symptoms should be cared for by a minimum number of healthcare personnel, and those personnel must use appropriate isolation precautions. If the etiology and transmission route of the causative organism are unknown, standard, contact, and airborne precautions should be implemented as needed. The U.S. Department of Labor (n.d.a) defines types of personal protective equipment and situations in which you are required to wear it.

Prepare Clients for a Pandemic Disease Outbreak
Isolation and personal protective equipment (PPE) are important in preventing the spread of most pandemic infections. Preparing for pandemic disease is similar to preparing for other general kinds of emergency preparedness, such as natural disasters.

SUMMARY

After studying this chapter, you should be armed with the basic concepts and skills you need to protect yourself and your clients from infection. However, knowledge and skill are not enough. **KEY POINT:** *Research continues to show that healthcare professionals too often fail to comply with guidelines for infection prevention, even the simple measures such as hand hygiene and standard precautions.* Although healthcare workers must wash their hands, patients do not necessarily feel comfortable asking them to do so (Ottum, Sethi, Jacobs, et al., 2012). Your role as a nurse is to integrate the best current evidence with your clinical expertise and to minimize harm to patients and others with your own performance. This includes using technology and standardized practices that support patient safety and quality.

 Wash your hands! Follow standard precautions!

CLINICALREASONING

The questions and exercises in this section allow you to practice the kind of thinking you will use as a full-spectrum nurse. Critical-thinking questions usually have more than one correct answer, so we do not provide "correct answers" for these features. It is more important to develop your nursing judgment than to just cover content. You will learn by discussing the questions with your peers. If you are still unsure, see the Davis Advantage chapter resources for suggested responses.

Caring for the Nguyens

Mrs. Nguyen works as a preschool teacher in her community. Kim, her grandchild, has been attending the preschool since he came to live with his grandparents. Mrs. Nguyen tells you at a recent visit to the clinic that Kim has had "a lot of problems with colds and a runny nose since he started preschool."

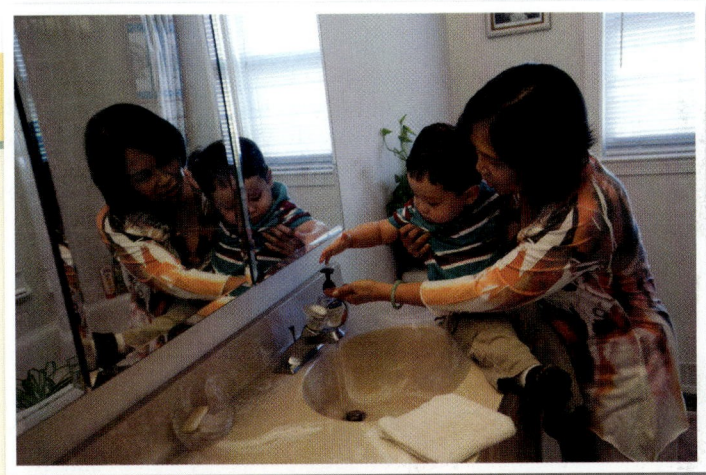

A. Based on your theoretical knowledge of asepsis and immunity, what is the most likely explanation for Kim's symptoms?

B. Do you have enough patient data to make any conclusions? If not, what other information should you gather?

C. Identify three alternatives that may explain what is happening.

D. What strategies could you recommend that Mrs. Nguyen implement at the preschool to help limit the number of infections? Identify at least two strategies.

 Go to Davis Advantage, Resources, Chapter 22, **Caring for the Nguyens—Suggested Responses.**

Applying the **Full-Spectrum Nursing Model**

PATIENT SITUATION

Mr. Long, a frail elderly man, is in the hospital because he has become dehydrated and needs supportive care. The nurse administered intravenous fluids. Mr. Long also has a fairly large pressure injury, which was cultured recently and found to be infected with *Staphylococcus aureus*. The nurse wore gloves to treat the ulcer. While doing so, she noticed that the IV was infusing too fast and, without thinking, regulated the IV without removing her contaminated gloves. The next nurse to regulate the IV did so with her bare hands, and then, without realizing it, rubbed her neck. Later, the nurse developed a boil on her neck, which was infected with *S. aureus*.

THINKING

1. *Theoretical Knowledge:*
   a. What are the six links in the chain of infection?
   b. Why do you think the *S. aureus* was able to thrive in Mr. Long's decubitus ulcer?
   c. What are the three modes of transmission of microorganisms? Which one is the most frequent mode of transmission?
2. *Critical Thinking (Reflecting):*
   a. What was the reservoir for the *S. aureus*?
   b. What was the exit from Mr. Long?
   c. What was (were) the fomite(s) for transmission to the nurse?
   d. What was the portal of entry into the nurse?

DOING

3. *Nursing Process (Implementation):* In addition to wearing gloves, what other PPE (if any) does the nurse need if she is performing decubitus care and changing Mr. Long's bed linens?

CARING

4. *Self-Knowledge and Ethical Knowledge:* Think of one instance in the clinical setting in which you did *not* follow standard precautions. Why do you think that happened?

Go to Davis Advantage, Resources, Chapter 22, **Applying the Full-Spectrum Nursing Model—Suggested Responses**.

PracticalKnowledge
clinical application

As a nurse, you play a vital role in preventing transmission of infection. Most infection control measures are independent nursing activities that do not require a medical prescription. You do need theoretical knowledge and scrupulous medical and surgical asepsis technique. The Clinical Insights and procedures in this section provide the guidance you will need to give safe, effective nursing care.

CLINICAL INSIGHTS

Clinical Insight 22-1 ➤ **Guidelines for Hand Hygiene**

Hand Washing

When to Wash

- When hands are visibly dirty or soiled with blood or body fluids
- When arriving on and leaving the patient care unit
- Before direct contact with a patient, even if you intend to wear procedure gloves
- Before donning and after removing gloves (either procedure or sterile)
- When gloves are changed during a procedure
- After removing gloves
- After contact with a patient's intact skin (e.g., when taking a blood pressure)
- After contact with body fluids, mucous membranes, non-intact skin, and wound dressings even if hands are not visibly soiled
- When moving from a contaminated body site to a clean body site during patient care

- Before and after contact with objects and equipment in the patient's immediate vicinity
- Before and after touching any area on your face and hair

What to Use

- Use alcohol-based handrub (at least 60% alcohol) for routine hand hygiene and if hands are not visibly soiled. *Note:* Iodine compounds are also effective, but usually too irritating for regular hand hygiene.
- Use soap and water:
  When hands are dirty or visibly soiled.
  After using a restroom.

➕ **If there is potential for exposure to *Bacillus anthracis* (or other spore-producing bacteria such a *C. difficile*).** *Alcohol-based solutions are not effective against spores.*

- Use warm, not hot, water.
- Use disposable paper towels.

Clinical Insight 22-1 ▶ Guidelines for Hand Hygiene—cont'd

■ Apply non-petroleum-based, fragrance-free lotions. *Drying, chafing, and chapping commonly occur with frequent hand washing and application of petroleum-based skin products. Breaks in the skin can harbor microbes.*

How to Wash

Refer to Procedure 22-1, Hand Hygiene.

Fingernails

■ Keep natural fingernails short (1/4 inch or less) and avoid wearing fingernail polish or artificial nails in the perioperative setting (AORN, 2013a; WHO, 2009). *Chipped nail polish can contaminate a sterile environment when gloves are not worn or are punctured or torn. Artificial nails, including gels, acrylics, and resins harbor microorganisms and impede proper hand hygiene.*

■ Scrub the undersides of fingernail with soap and water and nail brush every time you wash your hands.

■ Clean nail grooming tools before use.

■ Avoid biting or chewing nails or cuticles. Never rip a hangnail; instead, trim with a sanitized nail trimmer (CDC, 2009b).

Jewelry

■ Remove all jewelry before beginning hand hygiene, or surgical hand scrub. CDC (2013). *Hand jewelry may make donning gloves more difficult and cause gloves to tear more readily.*

■ The WHO (2009) prohibits any jewelry or watches on the hands of the surgical team. *Skin underneath rings is more heavily colonized than comparable areas of skin on bare fingers.*

■ We recommend that you not wear a watch or rings in the clinical setting, especially rings with stones. If your agency permits you to wear jewelry, clean it thoroughly and often.

Practice Resources

AORN (2013b, 2016); Boyce, J., & Pittet, D. (2002); CDC (2009b); Conner, R., Spruce, L., Burlingame, B., et al. (2013); Pratt, R. J., Pellowe, C. M., Wilson, J. A., et al. (2007); Rupp, M. E., Fitzgerald, T., Puumala, S., et al. (2008); Siegel, J. D. Rhinehart, E., Jackson, M., et al. (2007); WHO (2009).

Clinical Insight 22-2 ▶ Providing a Clean Patient Environment

Use the following guidelines along with standard precautions for all patients:

Supplies and Equipment

■ Do not stock rooms with unnecessary supplies.

■ Consider supplies brought into a patient's room contaminated. Do not return them to the linen or supply cart; handle them according to agency policy.

■ Items brought from the patient's home, gifts from visitors are considered unclean.

■ Mobile computing devices should be cleaned (e.g., pagers, smartphones, point-of-care keyboards, and medication administration devices). Be sure to wash your hands after using such a device.

■ Wipe stethoscopes with alcohol before use on a patient. *Stethoscopes are often contaminated with S. aureus.*

■ Disinfect reusable equipment that is soiled with blood or body fluids according to agency policy—typically, cleaning then autoclaving or using ethylene oxide gas or dry heat.

■ Do not reuse equipment for the care of another patient until it has been cleaned and reprocessed appropriately.

■ Dispose of single-use equipment soiled with blood or body fluids in biohazard containers.

■ Wear gloves when handling visibly contaminated equipment. Perform hand hygiene.

Linens

■ While wearing gloves, carefully handle contaminated linens. *To prevent skin and mucous membrane exposure, contamination of clothing, and transfer of microorganisms to other patients or the environment.*

■ Bag and remove soiled linens from the room immediately. *Linens may harbor microorganisms that may transfer to your clothing, open skin, or mucous membranes, which could then be carried to other clients or environment.*

Uniforms and Lab Coats

■ Do not wear a uniform (e.g., scrubs) or a lab coat for more than 1 day without laundering. *Care provider clothing is often contaminated when moving from patient to patient. The traditional white lab coats are considered vehicles for the transfer of pathogens (Association for Surgical Technologists, 2008b; CDC, 2009a).*

■ Visibly soiled, wet, and/or contaminated scrub attire must be changed as soon as possible. (Scott, Goodyear, Nicoloro, et al., 2015).

■ If you wash your clinical uniforms at home, use warm or hot water and detergent (except in the case of possible exposure to multidrug-resistant organisms, for which you should add bleach).

■ Home laundering of surgical attire is not recommended.

(Continued)

Clinical Insight 22-2 ▶ Providing a Clean Patient Environment—cont'd

Spills and Waste

- Empty and clean bedpans, urinals, and emesis basins immediately after use.
- Place soiled dressings, drains, and so forth in appropriate waterproof bags for disposal; never in an open trashcan.
- Wipe up small spills from tabletops and floors. Notify the housekeeping or environmental services department for large spills.

Needles and Sharps

✚ Do not recap, bend, break, or hand-manipulate used needles. If recapping is necessary, use a one-handed "scoop" technique. Place used sharps in puncture-resistant containers.

Practice Resources

Association for Surgical Technologists (2008b); AORN (2016); Carling, P. C., Parry, M. F., & Von Beheren, S. M., for the Healthcare Environmental Hygiene Study Group (2008); CDC (2009a); Siegel, J. D., Rhinehart, E., Jackson, M., et al. (2007).

Clinical Insight 22-3 ▶ Following CDC Standard Precautions

Standard precautions (Tier 1) apply to all clients and should be used whenever there is a possibility of coming in contact with blood, body fluids (except sweat), excretions and secretions, mucous membranes, and breaks in the skin. *These precautions are designed to protect you from exposure to potential pathogens, to decrease the likelihood that you will transmit pathogens among patients, and to protect the patient from microorganisms that you may carry.*

✚ Assume that every person may be infected or colonized with an organism that could be transmitted to others.

STANDARD PRECAUTIONS	RECOMMENDATIONS
Hand Hygiene	■ Perform hand hygiene after touching blood, body fluids, secretions, excretions, contaminated items; immediately after removing gloves; between patient contacts. Refer to Clinical Insight 22-1 for details.
Respiratory Hygiene/Cough Etiquette for Patients	■ Instruct symptomatic persons to cover mouth/nose when sneezing/coughing. ■ Provide and use tissues and dispose in a no-touch receptacle. ■ Perform hand hygiene after soiling hands with respiratory secretions or after using a tissue or covering the mouth/nose. ■ Wear a surgical mask if tolerated or do not come within 3 feet of another person if possible. Some patients may not be able to tolerate the decreased oxygen that is available when breathing room air through a mask.
Masks and Eye Protection (for the Nurse)	■ Wear a mask and eye protection or a face shield to protect mucous membranes of the eyes, nose, and mouth during patient care activities that are likely to generate splashes or sprays of blood, body fluids, secretions, and excretions. *Barrier protection helps keep microorganisms from accidentally entering your mucous membranes, eyes, nose, or mouth.*
Patient Placement	■ Place in a single-patient room if: 1) the patient is at increased risk of transmitting or acquiring infection, 2) does not maintain appropriate hygiene, 3) is likely to contaminate the environment, or 4) is at increased risk of developing adverse outcome following infection.
Gowns	■ Wear a clean, nonsterile, nonpermeable gown during procedures and activities when you anticipate contact of clothing or exposed skin with blood or body fluids, secretions, and excretions (e.g., when there is a risk of spray or splash onto clothing).

Clinical Insight 22-3 ➤ **Following CDC Standard Precautions—cont'd**

STANDARD PRECAUTIONS	RECOMMENDATIONS
	■ Promptly remove the gown once it is soiled. Avoid contaminating clothing when removing the gown.
	■ Wash hands after removing the gown.
	■ See Procedures 22-2 and 22-3, Donning and Removing PPE.
✚ *Needles and Sharps*	■ Never recap, bend, or break used needles; otherwise manipulate them using both hands; or use any other technique that involves directing the point of a needle toward any part of the body. Instead, use either a one-handed "scoop" technique or a mechanical device designed for holding the needle sheath (see Procedure 25-10, Recapping Needles . . .).
	■ Use safety features when available.
	■ Place "sharps" (e.g., scalpels, needles) in puncture-resistant containers for disposal.
Patient Resuscitation	■ Use one-way valve mouthpieces, resuscitation bags, or other ventilation devices as an alternative to mouth-to-mouth resuscitation methods in situations when the need for resuscitation is predictable.
	To prevent contact between rescuer's and client's mucous membranes and airflow, preventing transmission of microorganisms.
Soiled Patient-care Equipment, Environment, Textiles, & Laundry	■ See Clinical Insight 22-2 for details.
	■ Wear gloves if the equipment or laundry is visibly contaminated.
	■ Handle equipment, textiles, and laundry in a manner to prevent transfer of microorganisms to others and the environment.
	■ Perform hand hygiene.
	■ Develop procedures for routine care, cleaning, and disinfection of environmental surfaces, especially frequently touched surfaces in patient care areas.
Gloves	**When to Wear**
	■ If you have an area of irritation or a break in the skin, wear gloves or apply an occlusive dressing during patient contact.
	■ Wear gloves when contact with blood or other potentially infectious materials, mucous membranes, and nonintact skin could occur.
	When to Remove or Change
	■ Remove gloves immediately after caring for a patient. Avoid touching clean items, environmental surfaces, or another patient.
	■ Do not wear the same gloves for care of more than one patient; do not wash gloves and reuse gloves between patient contact.
	■ Change gloves during patient care if moving from a contaminated body site to a clean.
	■ Change gloves between tasks or procedures on the same patient if you have made contact with material that may contain a high concentration of microorganisms.
	Use and Storage
	■ When preparing for a procedure, first collect equipment and place at the bedside ready for use; then wash your hands and put on gloves just before performing the procedure. Donning gloves ahead of time allows them to become contaminated before the procedure.
	■ Do not carry gloves in your pocket. Keep them in their original box and remove them when and where required.
	■ Do not store gloves on top of trash containers or on windowsills.
	✚ ■ Hand washing or disinfection is required regardless of whether gloves are used or changed. Gloves are not completely impermeable to microorganisms; furthermore, they may leak or tear. Hands can be easily contaminated when removing gloves.

Practice Resources

Boyce, J., & Pittet, D. (2002); Pratt, R. J., Pellowe, C. M., Wilson, J. A., et al. (2007); Siegel, J. D., Rhinehart, E., Jackson, M. et al. (2007); U.S. Department of Labor (n.d.a, n.d.b).

Clinical Insight 22-4 ➤ Following Transmission-Based Precautions

Refer to Clinical Insight 22-3 if you need to review standard precautions.

When to Use: Pathogens may be transmitted by contact, droplet, or air. Each mode of transmission requires a different approach to prevent infection and has a different set of precautions. Use transmission-based (Tier 2) precautions when the routes of transmission are not completely interrupted using standard precautions alone.

Contact Precautions

When to Use: Use contact precautions when direct contact with the patient or the patient's environment can lead to spread of the pathogen. Indirect contact, or contact with fomites, can also transmit pathogens that spread by this method.

Patient Placement and Transport

- Ideally, consult with an infection preventionist for patient placement.
- Place in a private room, if available.
- If no private room is available, place patient in a room with a patient with an active infection caused by the same organism and no other infections.
- When transporting the patient, ensure that infected or colonized areas of the body are contained and covered.
- *Ambulatory care:* Place the patient in an exam room or cubicle as soon as possible.

Personal Protective Equipment (PPE)

- Don clean, nonsterile gloves when touching the patient's intact skin. Put them on when entering the patient's room.
- Wear a clean gown if you anticipate your clothing may contact the patient or any contaminated items in the room.
- Remove PPE and observe hand hygiene before leaving the room. Be careful that your skin and clothing do not contact environmental surfaces on your way out of the room.

Equipment, Supplies, and Environment

- Keep contact precaution supplies just outside the patient's room on a cart.
- Double bag all linen and trash (or use a single waterproof bag) and clearly mark them contaminated.
- Use disposable equipment (e.g., blood pressure cuffs) if possible; otherwise, clean and disinfect the equipment per institutional policy before removing it from the room and before use on another patient.
- Ensure that the patient room is cleaned and disinfected at least daily.
- *Home care:* Limit nondisposable equipment brought into the home. If possible, leave the equipment in the home until discharge from home care. If not, clean and disinfect items before taking them from the home or place them in a plastic bag for transport to a reprocessing area.

Other

- Follow additional precautions specific to the microorganism.
- Discontinue contact precautions according to pathogen-specific recommendations.

Droplet Precautions

When to Use: Droplets can spread infection by direct contact with mucous membranes or through indirect contact—for example, suctioning or touching a bedside table that was contaminated with droplets and then rubbing your eyes. Use droplet precautions when the pathogen can be spread via large droplets (e.g., sneezing, coughing, talking).

Patient Placement and Transport

- If no private room is available, ensure patients are physically separated by more than 3 feet. Keep the privacy curtain closed. *Consult with an infection preventionist for patient placement. A private room provides the most effective protection.*
- Limit transport outside the room to medically necessary purposes; if transport is necessary, the patient should wear a mask.

Personal Protective Equipment

- Keep droplet precaution supplies near the patient's room on a cart.
- Wear a mask when working within 3 feet of the patient. Don the mask on entry into the room. Whether to wear goggles is an unresolved issue. Follow agency policy.
- Change PPE and perform hand hygiene between contact with patients in the same room, regardless of whether one or both patients are on droplet precautions.

Other

- Instruct patients to observe respiratory hygiene/cough etiquette.
- Discontinue droplet precautions according to pathogen-specific recommendations.

Airborne Precautions

When to Use: Use airborne precautions to control the spread of infections that are transmitted person-to-person on air currents.

Patient Placement and Transport

- Place the patient in an airborne infection isolation room (AIIR)—one with negative pressure that discharges and exchanges the air outside or through a high-efficiency particulate air (HEPA) filtration system. Monitor air pressure daily (usually this is via an electronic device with an alarm).
- If such a room is not available, transfer the patient to a facility where one is available.

Clinical Insight 22-4 ➤ **Following Transmission-Based Precautions—cont'd**

- Keep the room door closed when not required for entry and exit. To maintain the negative pressure and contain the airborne organisms.
- In the event of an outbreak involving large numbers of patients who require airborne precautions, consult with infection preventionists for patient placement.
- Limit moving the patient outside the room to medically necessary purposes. If transport is necessary, cover any infectious skin lesions and have the patient wear a mask. Notify the receiving department. The receiving department can take airborne precautions if notified.
- *Ambulatory or emergency care:* Triage and identify patients with suspected airborne precautions upon entry to the agency. Place the patient in an AIIR as soon as possible. If one is not available, place a mask on the patient and place him in an exam room. Do not reuse the room for at least an hour after the infected patient leaves it.

Personal Protective Equipment

- Keep airborne isolation supplies just outside the patient's room on a cart.
- Don a mask on entering the room. Wear a special fit-tested and approved mask (e.g., N-95 respirator) if the patient is suspected of having pulmonary tuberculosis or smallpox.

- Remove your respirator/mask outside the room after closing the door. If the respirator is not disposable, clean and store according to the manufacturer's instructions.
- When using a respirator mask, check the seal. Hold your hands over the respirator and exhale. If you feel air around your nose, adjust the nosepiece; if you feel air at the edges, adjust the straps.
- When the patient has rubeola, varicella (chickenpox), or disseminated zoster, the CDC makes no recommendation about use of PPE if, based on your history of vaccination or disease, you think you are presumed immune to the disease. If the hospitalized patient has or is suspected of having rubeola or varicella, only immune caregivers should provide care.

Other

- Discontinue airborne precautions according to pathogen-specific recommendations of the CDC.
- Tape a waterproof bag to the bedside. *To facilitate proper disposal of tissues.*

Practice Resources

Pratt, R. J., Pellowe, C. M., Wilson, J. A., et al. (2007); Siegel, J. D., Rhinehart, E., Jackson, M., et al. (2007); U.S. Department of Labor (n.d.a).

Clinical Insight 22-5 ➤ **Maintaining a Protective Environment in Special Situations**

The CDC recommends a protective environment (isolation) for a special class of stem cell transplant patients, who are neutropenic (and therefore immunocompromised) secondary to chemotherapy.

Some facilities may use protective isolation for other types of patients, as well. However, in most instances, standard and transmission-based precautions are adequate protection for those patients.

In special situations:

- **Follow standard precautions** meticulously, including hand hygiene before and after patient contact.
- **Follow transmission-based precautions** as indicated by a suspected or proven infection.

Patient Room

- Maintain a protective environment (PE) room.
- Avoid a standing collection of water in the room (e.g., vases containing fresh flowers or humidifier containing water). To prevent fungi and bacteria typically found in this water.

Personal Protective Equipment

- PPE is not required for care providers or visitors for routine entry into the room, unless approaching the patient.

- If the patient must be taken out of the PE room for diagnostic or other procedures, provide respiratory protection (e.g., an N-95 respirator, minimal contact with others).
- Visitors and care providers should don gown, gloves, and mask according to standard precautions and as indicated for suspected or proven infections for which they are recommended.
- Refer to Procedures 22-2 and 22-3 to review donning and removing PPE.

Care Providers, Visitors

- Only healthy caregivers should provide care. Also restrict visitors who have a cold or contagious illness.
- Healthcare workers caring for patients in protective isolation should not also be providing care for other patients with active infections.

Housekeeping/Environmental Services

- Carpeting in patient rooms or halls traps soil and can wick moisture, facilitating growth of microbes.
- Upholstered furniture and furnishings tend to harbor microbes.
- Avoid dusting methods that scatter particles in the air.

(Continued)

Clinical Insight 22-5 ► Maintaining a Protective Environment in Special Situations—cont'd

- If vacuum cleaning is necessary, use a vacuum cleaner equipped with a HEPA filter.
- Wet-dust horizontal surfaces daily with EPA-registered disinfectant or detergent.

Engineering

- Use of 99.7% efficiency particulate air (HEPA) filters to remove particles for incoming air at a specified flow rate of air
- Well-sealed rooms—no air leaks

- Ventilation as for airborne precautions
- Directed air flow within the room
- Positive room air pressure in relation to the corridor
- Backup ventilation equipment (e.g., portable fans or filters)
- For patients who require both protected environment and airborne isolation, use an anteroom to control air in and out of the room.

Practice Resources

AORN (2013a); Siegel, J. M., Rhinehart, E., Jackson, M., et al. (2007).

PROCEDURES

Procedure 22-1 ■ Hand Hygiene

> ► For steps to follow in *all* procedures, refer to the Universal Steps for All Procedures found on the page facing the inside back cover. For this procedure, also refer to Clinical Insight 22-1 as needed.

Equipment

- Liquid soap (antimicrobial) or alcohol-based handrub
- Paper towels
- Warm, running water
- Hand moisturizer (optional)

Pre-Procedure Assessments

- Check your hands for breaks in the skin.
  Breaks in the skin provide a route for microbial entry.

- Inspect the condition of your nails.
  Nails should be no longer than $1/4$ inch from the fingertips.
  Do not wear artificial nails or extensions.
  Nail polish should not be chipped.
  Preferably, do not use polish.
  Research indicates the area under the nails, artificial nails/extensions, and chipped polish act as reservoirs for microorganisms. Additionally, if your glove were to tear or perforate, chipped nail polish could potentially go into the surgical wound.

Procedure 22-1A ■ Using Soap and Water

> ► When performing the procedure, always identify your patient according to agency policy, using two identifiers, and be attentive to standard precautions, hand hygiene, patient safety and privacy, body mechanics, and documentation.

Procedure Steps

1. **Bare your hands and forearms.** Push your sleeves above your wrists, and remove your wristwatch and rings.
   Moist clothing facilitates transfer of microorganisms; jewelry harbors bacteria and creates a moist area on the skin, which facilitates bacterial growth.

2. **Turn on water. Use electronic faucet when possible.** Adjust water to warm, not hot.
   Hands-free electronic faucets lessen risk of recontamination of hands after washing as there is no need to manually turn

off the water. Warm water opens pores and helps remove microorganisms without removing skin oils. It also reduces chapping. Hot water increases the risk for skin breakdown.

3. **Wet your hands and wrists.** Keep your hands below your wrists and forearms.
   Prevents water from running from hands to the wrists and forearms. Hands are considered more contaminated than the wrists and arms.

   a. Avoid splashing water onto clothing.

   b. **Avoid touching the inside of the sink.**
      Microorganisms travel in moisture. The inside of the sink is considered contaminated. ▼

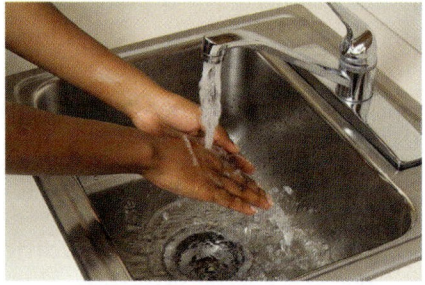

4. **Apply enough liquid soap to cover all hand surfaces** (typically 3 to 4 pumps from a dispenser).
From 3 to 5 mL of liquid soap provides enough to completely cover the hands for maximum removal of transient microorganisms.

5. **Vigorously rub your hands together** for at least 15 seconds
Lather all surfaces, interlacing fingers, rubbing around each finger and thumb, rubbing the backs and palms of the hands in a circular motion.
It takes at least 15 seconds for mechanical removal of microorganisms and for antimicrobial products to be effective. Research indicates areas of the hands

most often missed are the thumb, the wrist, and areas between the fingers. ▼

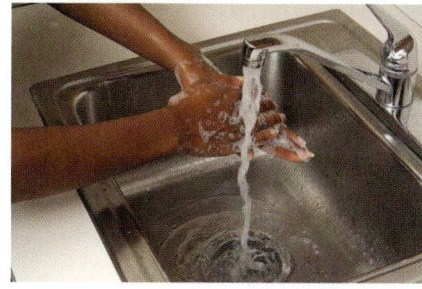

6. **Clean under your fingernails,** if needed, using a disposable nail cleaner.
Areas under the nails harbor high concentrations of microorganisms.

7. **Rinse your hands thoroughly.** Keep your hands below your wrists and forearms.

8. **Dry your hands thoroughly,** moving from your fingers up to your forearms and blotting with paper towel.
Move from the area you wish to keep cleanest (hands). Blotting decreases skin irritation.

9. **Turn off the faucet.**
If faucet is not hands-free, hold a dry paper towel in your hand to turn it off. Do not handle the paper towel with the opposite hand.
A paper towel acts as a barrier to prevent contamination of hands from the faucet. After the towel has contacted the contaminated faucet, it can transfer microorganisms to your clean hand. Many pathogens can live on faucets and countertops.

10. **Apply a hand moisturizer** at least twice daily; use hand care products recommended by infection preventionists. (Many agencies use soaps that contain moisturizers.)
Hand moisturizer helps prevent drying and chafing, which may lead to skin damage and increase the risk for transmission of infection. Petroleum-based products cause latex gloves to become permeable.

Procedure 22-1B ■ Using Alcohol-Based Handrubs

➤ When performing the procedure, always identify your patient according to agency policy, using two identifiers, and be attentive to standard precautions, hand hygiene, patient safety and privacy, body mechanics, and documentation.

Procedure Steps

1. **Use alcohol-based handrubs when** hands are not visibly soiled and when certain pathogens are suspected.
Antiseptic solutions are not effective when organic material or dirt is present. Alcohol handrubs cannot remove spores, and therefore should not be used for hand hygiene when Clostridium difficile or Bacillus anthracis is suspected of being present.

2. **Bare your hands and forearms.** Push your sleeves above your wrists. Remove jewelry and wristwatch.

3. **Apply antiseptic solution** in a quantity sufficient (at least 3 mL) to cover the hands and wrists.

4. **Vigorously rub antiseptic solution into your hands,** covering all surfaces, for at least 20 seconds (or if no clock is available, as long as it takes to sing "Happy Birthday").
Cover all surfaces of the hands: interlacing fingers, rubbing around each finger and thumb, and rubbing the backs and palms of the hands in a circular motion, including under

the nails, until the solution is completely dry.
A period of 15 to 30 seconds is required for effective disinfection by alcohol handrubs (CDC, 2009b). All surfaces must be thoroughly covered with product to effectively remove microorganisms. ▼

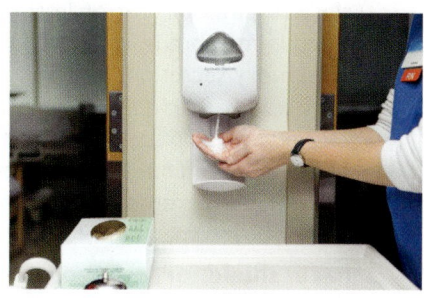

Evaluation
Hands are free of handrub and dry.

Documentation
Hand hygiene is a responsibility of all healthcare providers. It usually does not require documentation.

Thinking About the Procedure
To practice applying clinical reasoning to this procedure,

➤ The videos **Hand Hygiene: Using Soap and Water** and **Hand Hygiene: Using Alcohol-Based Handrubs,** along with questions and suggested responses, are available on the **Davis's** *Nursing Skills Videos* Web site on DavisPlus.

Practice Resources
AORN (2016); Boyce, J., & Pittet, D. (2002); CDC (2009b); Siegel, J. D., Rhinehart, E., Jackson, M., et al. (2007).

Procedure 22-2 ■ Donning Personal Protective Equipment (PPE)

➤ For steps to follow in *all* procedures, refer to the Universal Steps for All Procedures found on the page facing the inside back cover. For this procedure, also refer to Clinical Insights 22-3 and 22-4 if you need more information.

Equipment

Following CDC recommendations, you will usually use some combination of gloves, gown, mask, and eye protection; depending on the organism and level of precaution. In certain situations, you may need hair covers and shoe covers (e.g., when full barrier precautions are needed). Determine the availability of appropriate PPE.

- Disposable gloves of the proper size
- Disposable isolation gown

- Face mask (or N-95 respirator mask, as indicated)
- Face shield or goggles
- Hair cover (if needed)
- Shoe covers (if needed)

➤ When performing the procedure, always identify your patient according to agency policy, using two identifiers, and be attentive to standard precautions, hand hygiene, patient safety and privacy, body mechanics, and documentation.

Procedure Steps

1. **Assess the need for and gather PPE**.

   a. **Gloves:** When you may be exposed to body secretions directly or indirectly

   Gloves provide a barrier against body fluids. All patients are considered potentially infected per standard precautions.

   b. **Gowns:** When your uniform (e.g., scrubs) may become exposed to potentially infective secretions.

   Examples include excessive wound drainage, fecal incontinence, or other discharges from the body, or when fluids may be splashed (as in eye irrigation).

   c. **Face mask:** To prevent transmission of pathogens spread through close respiratory (3 ft or less) or mucous membrane contact with respiratory secretions.

   Surgical masks provide a barrier to large-particle droplets (> 5 microns in diameter), helping prevent transmission of pathogens to the nurse's mucous membranes.

   d. **Face shield or eye goggles:** When splashing might occur and fluids enter your eyes (e.g., blood splashes, respiratory droplets, wound débridement).

   To protect the entire facial area, wear a face shield. It should protect the crown and chin and wrap around the face to the ear.

   Helps prevent pathogens from entering the conjunctiva directly or indirectly.

   e. **N-95 respirator mask:** When caring for clients infected with airborne organisms (< 5 microns) such as the tuberculosis bacillus.

   This device prevents airborne transmission of the tuberculosis bacterium. The respirator mask is disposable; others are reusable. ▼

   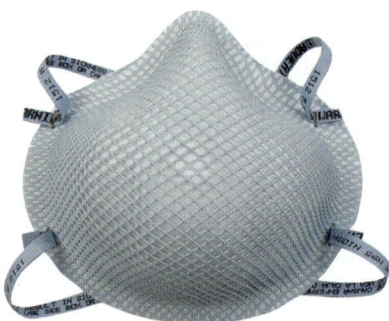

   f. **Hair covers:** When there is a potential for spraying or splashing body fluids.

   Although not included in the CDC report (Siegel, Rhinehart, Jackson, et al., 2007), agency policy may advise hair covers in certain situations.

   g. **Shoe covers:** When there is a potential for contamination of shoes with body fluids.

   The floor (and anything in contact with it) is considered contaminated. However, certain categories of pathogens require full protective gear, and in those circumstances shoe covers are necessary.

2. **Don the isolation gown. KEY POINT:** *Do not substitute a patient gown for a disposable isolation or protective gown.*

   Isolation gowns must be made of moisture-repelling materials to prevent contamination of underlying clothing and skin.

   a. Pick up the gown by the shoulders, allowing it to fall open without touching the floor or other surfaces.

   Touching the floor or other surfaces will contaminate the gown with environmental pathogens. ▼

   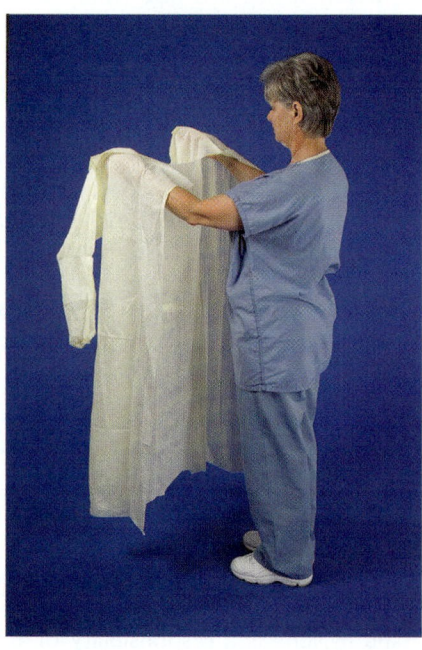

b. Slip your arms into the sleeves. ▼

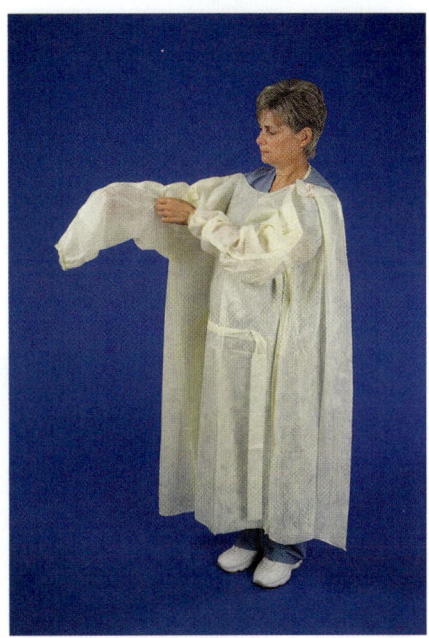

c. Fasten ties at the neck.
d. Position the gown so that it covers the back, and fasten the ties at the waist. Do not bring ties around to the front of the gown.
The front of the gown is considered contaminated after you enter the patient's room. If the ties are at the front of the gown, they will be contaminated, making it difficult to remove the gown safely.
e. If the gown does not completely cover your clothing in the back, wear two gowns.
- Put on the first gown so that the opening is in the front.

- Then place the second gown over the first, so that the opening is in the back.

3. **Don the face mask or N-95 respirator.**
   a. Determine how the mask is secured. Identify the top edge of the mask by locating the thin metal strip (nosepiece) that goes over the bridge of the nose.
   Surgical masks may be secured by ties at the back of the head and neck, loops around the ears, or elastic bands.
   b. Pick up the mask with the top ties or ear loops. Place the mask over your nose, mouth, and chin. Press the flexible metal strip so that it conforms to the bridge of your nose.
   The mask must fit snugly to your face for maximum barrier protection. Correct positioning will also keep your glasses or goggles from fogging. ▼

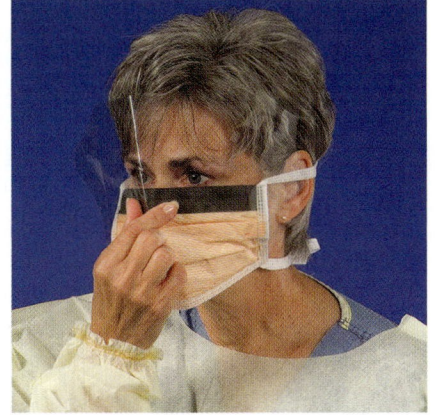

c. Tie the upper ties to the back of your head and the lower ties to the back of your neck or slip the loops around your ears or place the elastic bands as with the ties.
d. Place the lower edge of the mask below your chin and tie the lower ties.
Covering the nose and mouth creates a barrier to prevent droplet pathogens from entering through the nasal and oral mucous membranes or the respiratory system.

4. **Don the face shield or goggles.**
   a. *Face shield:* Place the shield over your eyes, adjust the metal strip over the bridge of your nose, and tuck the lower edge below your chin. Secure the straps behind your head.
   b. *Safety glasses or goggles:* Set them over the top edge of the mask.

5. **Don hair cover, if indicated.**

6. **Don shoe covers, if indicated.**

7. **Don gloves.**
   a. Select nonsterile disposable gloves of the appropriate size.
   The correct size will prevent gloves from falling off or ripping while you are working with the client.
   b. If you are wearing a gown, make sure that the glove cuff extends over the cuff of the gown. If skin is visible between the gown and the glove, tape the glove cuff to the gown cuff, covering all visible skin.

Patient Teaching

Answer questions the patient may have and educate about the need for PPE, his disease process, and the purpose of isolation.

Home Care

- Identify the type of PPE needed and ensure that the necessary supplies are available.
- Develop a plan with the client and family for using and disposing of personal protective equipment and contaminated items.
- Teach family members to don PPE as needed.
- Obtain referral for a home health agency to provide support.

Documentation

The use of personal protective equipment is generally assumed and usually does not require documentation.

Practice Resources

AORN (2013a); Minnesota Dept. of Health (n.d.); Siegel, J. D., Rhinehart, E., Jackson, M., et al. (2007).

Thinking About the Procedure

To practice applying clinical reasoning to this procedure,

 The video **Donning Personal Protective Equipment (PPE),** along with questions and suggested responses, is available on the **Davis's** *Nursing Skills Videos* Web site on Davis*Plus.*

Procedure 22-3 ■ Removing Personal Protective Equipment (PPE)

➤ For steps to follow in *all* procedures, refer to the Universal Steps for All Procedures found on the page facing inside back cover. For this procedure, also refer to Clinical Insights 22-3 and 22-4 if you need more information.

KEY POINT: *Considered contaminated: front areas, sleeves, mask, and gloves of the PPE (as well as head and shoe covers if you are wearing them).*

KEY POINT: *Considered clean: the inside of the gown, gloves, the ties on the mask, and ties at the back of the gown (as well as the inside of the head and shoe covers if you are wearing them).*

➤ When performing the procedure, always identify your patient according to agency policy, using two identifiers, and be attentive to standard precautions, hand hygiene, patient safety and privacy, body mechanics, and documentation.

Procedure Steps

1. **Remove gloves first** (unless the gown ties in front; in that case, see "What if . . .").

   Gloves are the most contaminated PPE and must be removed first to avoid contamination of clean areas of the PPE during removal.

   a. **Remove the first glove by grasping** the outside cuff of the glove with the opposite gloved hand and pulling downward so that the glove turns inside out. Do not touch the skin of your wrist or hand with your gloved hand.

   The outside of both gloves are contaminated. To prevent contamination of your skin, touch only the outside (contaminated) surface of first glove to outside (contaminated) surface of second glove. "Dirty touches dirty" and "clean touches clean." ▼

   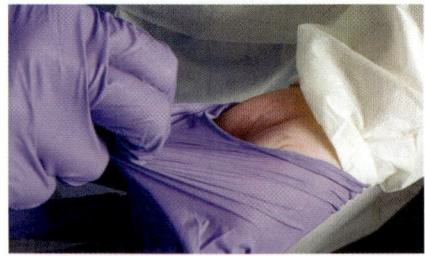

   b. **To remove the second glove:**
   - Hold the removed glove in the palm of your gloved hand.
   - Slip two ungloved fingers inside the cuff of the remaining glove.
   - Pull the glove off, inside out, over the glove that hand is holding.

     The insides of the gloves are considered "clean" because they have not been in contact with client or contaminated surfaces. Therefore,

   you can touch the insides with your bare hands. ▼

   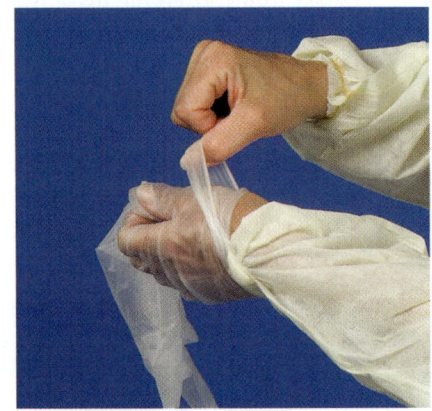

   c. **Dispose of gloves** in a designated waste receptacle. Keep them away from your body.

2. **Remove the gown:**
   a. **Release the waist ties and** the neck ties of the gown, bending slightly forward to allow the gown to fall forward.

   Allowing the gown to fall forward exposes the clean area for the hands to grasp more readily.

   b. **Slip your hands inside the neck** and peel the gown away from the shoulders.
   - Reach inside to pull off the cuff and remove your arm from the sleeve.
   - Repeat the maneuver to remove the second sleeve.
   - Do not touch the front of the gown, even if it is not visibly soiled. ➤

   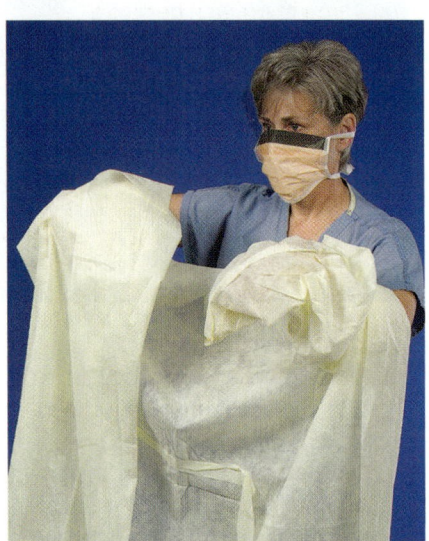

3. **Fold the gown so the inside** of the gown is to the outside. Holding the gown away from your uniform, roll it up with the contaminated front and sleeves in the center, and place in the *designated waste receptacle.*

   Folding the gown prevents contamination of your hands, the clothing, and the environment. ▼

   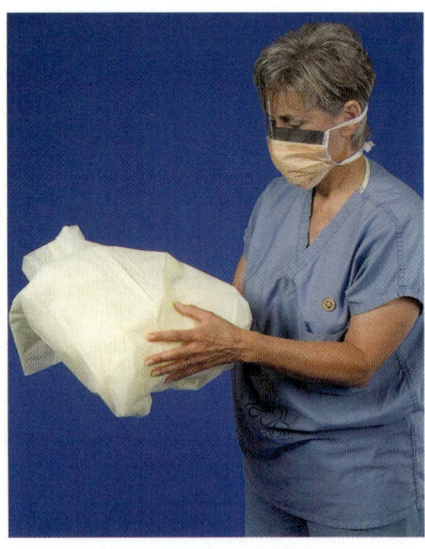

4. Remove goggles.
   a. Grasp only the earpieces or head band of the goggles and pull off the face.
   b. If the goggles are not disposable, place in the receptacle provided for disinfection.
   Earpieces are considered clean. Some goggles are cleaned and reused.

5. Remove your mask or face shield.
   a. Untie the lower ties first.
   b. Untie the upper ties next, being careful not to let go of the ties.
   c. Touch only the ties; do not touch the front of the mask.
   d. Dispose of the mask, placing it in a designated waste receptacle.
   Touching it would contaminate your bare hands.

6. Remove your hair covering.
   a. Slip your bare fingers under the edge of the hair cover—do not touch the outside of it.
   b. Lift it up and away from your hair.
   c. Touching only the inside, place the mask in a designated waste receptacle.
   The inside of the hair covering is considered clean, so you may touch it with your bare hands.

7. Remove shoe covers. Be careful to touch only the insides of the covers.

8. Perform hand hygiene before leaving the room.
   Even if wearing gloves, hands may become contaminated.

9. **Close the door.**
   Keeping the door closed contains contaminants and makes signage more visible.

? What if . . .

- **The gown is tied in front?**

Untie the front gown ties before removing your gloves; then remove the gloves and untie any back ties (e.g., at the neck). (This would be an unusual circumstance.) *Because the front of the gown (including a front tie) is considered contaminated, once you remove your gloves, you could not use your bare hands to untie a front tie.*

- **You are wearing two gowns (top one tied in back, inner one tied in front)?**

Remove gloves; untie waist ties of outer gown, remove the gown and fold it inside out. Remove the inner gown by untying it in front. Fold inner gown inside out. Take off goggles and face mask or shield.

Patient Teaching

See Procedure 22-2.

Home Care

See Procedure 22-2.

Documentation

The removal of personal protective equipment is generally assumed and does not require documentation.

Practice Resources

AORN (2013a); Conner, R., Spruce, L., Burlingame, B., et al. (2013); Siegel, J., Rhinehart, E., Jackson, M., et al. (2007); U.S. Department of Labor (n.d.a, n.d.b).

Thinking About the Procedure

To practice applying clinical reasoning to this procedure,

The video **Removing Personal Protective Equipment (PPE),** along with questions and suggested responses, is available on the **Davis's** *Nursing Skills Videos* Web site on Davis*Plus*.

Procedure 22-4 ■ Surgical Hand Washing: Traditional Method

➤ For steps to follow in *all* procedures, refer to the Universal Steps for All Procedures found on the page facing the inside back cover. For this procedure, also refer to Clinical Insights 22-3 and 22-4 if you need more information.

Equipment

- Antimicrobial soap (60% to 95% alcohol, or other FDA-approved for surgical hand asepsis)
- Soft, nonabrasive scrub sponge
- Disposable single-use nail cleaner
- Deep sink with foot or knee controls
- Surgical shoe covers, cap, and face mask
- Sterile gloves of the correct size
- Surgical pack containing a sterile towel

(continued on next page)

Procedure 22-4 ■ **Surgical Hand Washing: Traditional Method** (continued)

➤ When performing the procedure, always identify your patient according to agency policy, using two identifiers, and be attentive to standard precautions, hand hygiene, patient safety and privacy, body mechanics, and documentation.

Procedure Steps

1. Determine that sterile gloves, gown, and towel are set up for use after the scrub.

To maintain sterility, the sterile towel, gown, and gloves must be ready for use immediately after you scrub. If you need to gather supplies after the scrub, you must start the scrub procedure over again.

2. Determine the agency policy for the duration of the surgical scrub and the type of cleansing agent used.

The type of cleansing agent determines how long to scrub. Typically, an alcohol-based antimicrobial soap requires 2 to 6 minutes.

3. Avoid nail polish or artificial nails. Trim so nails do not extend beyond fingertips. Remove rings, watches, and bracelets.

Rings are a substantial risk factor for harboring moisture and gram-negative bacilli and S. aureus; and artificial nails and polish are more likely to carry gram-negative pathogens, including Pseudomonas, because water collects between the artificial and real nails.

4. Don surgical shoe covers, cap, and face mask before the surgical scrub.

5. Perform a prewash before the surgical scrub (see Procedure 22-1).

The prewash removes visible soil, reduces the number of microorganisms on your skin, and allows you to begin the surgical scrub with clean hands.

6. Remove debris from underneath your nails using a single-use nail file under running water.

Decreases the number of microorganisms ➤.

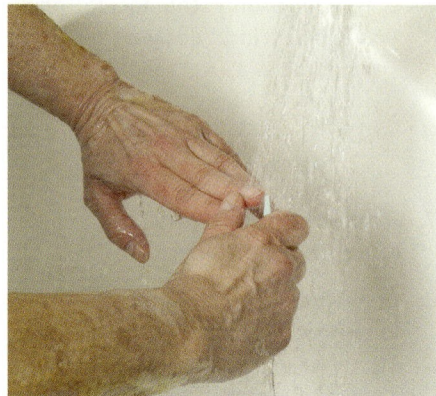

7. To begin the surgical scrub, turn on the water, using the knee or foot controls or motion sensors. Adjust the temperature so that the water is warm.

Hot water removes the skin's protective oils. Knee and foot controls help to prevent contamination of the hands. You cannot touch any unsterile surfaces once you begin the surgical hand wash. ▼

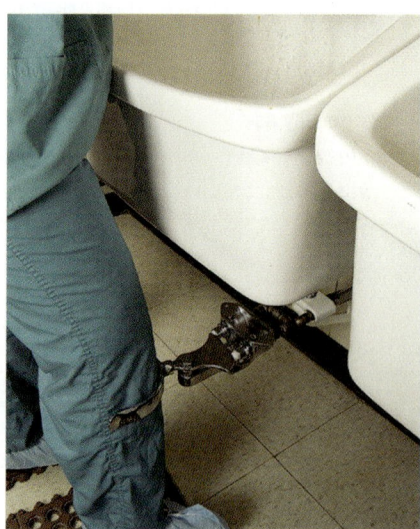

8. Wet your hands and **forearms** from elbows to fingertips, keeping hands above elbows and away from your body. If using a scrub sponge, wet the sponge.

Prevents water running down from your "dirty" elbows and forearm over "clean" rinsed hands.

9. Apply antimicrobial soap, a liberal amount, on to your hands and the sponge.

- Lather well to 2 inches above the elbow.
- Do not touch the inside of the sink with your fingers, hands, or elbows.
- Avoid splashing your surgical attire.

Scrub brushes are harsh on the skin. Soft, nonabrasive sponges are recommended instead. Antimicrobial soap reduces the number of microorganisms.

10. Scrub one hand and arm, all surfaces, using a circular motion.

- Start at the fingers. Scrub at least 10 strokes each on nail, all four sides of each finger, hands, and arms.
- When scrubbing the arm, use 10 strokes each for the lower, middle, and upper areas of the forearm.
- Keep hands higher than elbows.

Cover all surfaces to remove maximum number of microorganisms from the skin. Keep hands higher than elbows so that water from the area nearest the unscrubbed skin does not run downward and contaminate the hands. ▼

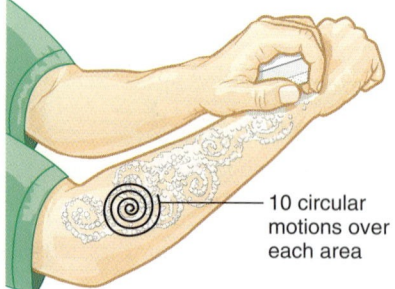

10 circular motions over each area

11. Rinse the brush and reapply antimicrobial soap. Repeat the scrub on the second hand and arm. Normally the scrub takes at least 2 to 6 minutes.

The length of the scrub depends on the time needed for the particular scrub agent to be effective in removing microorganisms on the hands.

12. **Rinse your hands and arms,** keeping fingertips higher than elbows. ▼

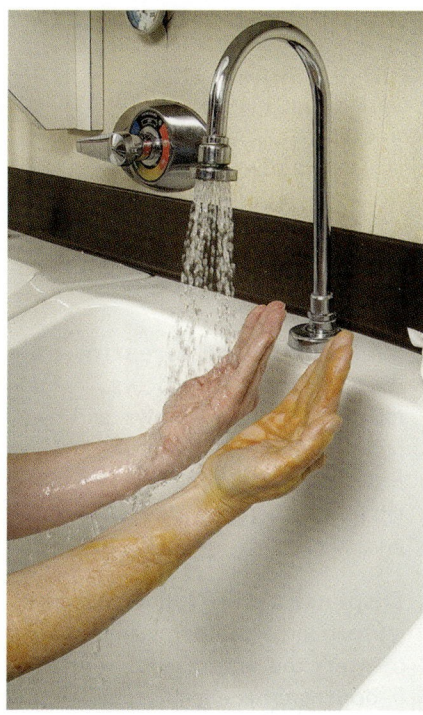

13. **Repeat steps 8 through 12** if directed to do so by the soap manufacturer or agency policy.

14. **With arms flexed and your hands** held higher than your elbows and away from your body, turn and move toward the sterile towel and gown.
    Avoids contamination of hands from water runoff.

15. **Grasp the sterile towel** and step back while not turning your back or your eyes from the sterile field.
    Backing away keeps the sterile field dry and prevents you from inadvertently brushing against the table, which would contaminate the field. ▼

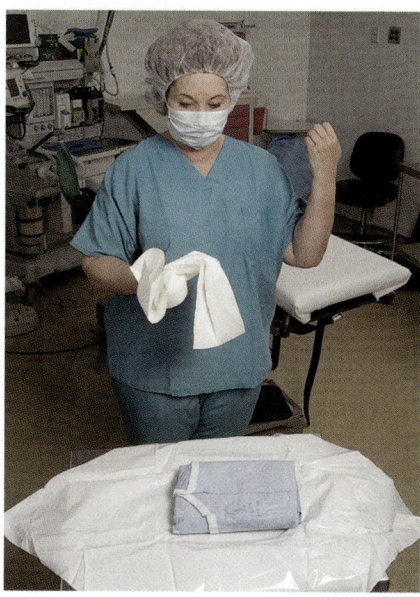

16. **Lean forward slightly,** and allow the towel to fall open, being careful not to let it touch your clothing.
    The towel would be contaminated if it brushed against your uniform.

17. **Use one end of the towel** to dry one hand and arm. Use the opposite end to dry the other hand and

arm. Be certain your skin is thoroughly dry before donning sterile gloves.
Drying skin prevents maceration and enables gloves to go on more easily. Use a separate section of the towel to prevent rewetting the skin or contaminating an already clean area.

? What if . . .

- **The agency uses an alcohol-based surgical hand-scrub product?**
  a. Perform steps 1 through 6. Omit steps 7 through 17.
  b. Using the indicated amount of handrub, rub all surfaces of the hands, including the nails and up the arm to 2 inches above the elbow, according to the manufacturer's recommendations and agency policy.
     Many different products are on the market. Be careful to follow the manufacturer's guidelines for use for maximum effectiveness.
  c. Allow the handrub to dry completely before you don sterile gloves.

Patient Teaching

If the patient is able to observe the procedure, explain the purpose of the surgical scrub and sterility.

Documentation

A surgical hand scrub does not require documentation. Instead, chart the procedure (or surgery) and how the patient tolerated it.

Practice Resources
AORN (2016); Boyce, J., & Pittet, D. (2002); Siegel, J., Rhinehart, E., Jackson, M., et al. (2007).

Procedure 22–5 ■ **Surgical Hand Washing: Brushless System**

➤ For steps to follow in *all* procedures, refer to the Universal Steps for All Procedures found on the page facing the inside back cover. For this procedure, also refer to Clinical Insights 22-3, 22-4 if you need more information.

Equipment

- Antimicrobial soap (60% to 95% alcohol or other FDA-approved for surgical hand asepsis)
- Disposable single-use nail cleaner
- Deep sink with foot or knee controls
- Surgical shoe covers, cap, and face mask
- Sterile gloves of the correct size
- Surgical pack containing a sterile towel

➤ When performing the procedure, always identify your patient according to agency policy, using two identifiers, and be attentive to standard precautions, hand hygiene, patient safety and privacy, body mechanics, and documentation.

Procedure Steps

1. **Determine agency policy** for the type of cleansing product to be used and for duration of the surgical scrub (typically 2 to 6 minutes).
   Policies vary from institution to institution, although all should be based on sound principles for infection control in accordance with guidelines from CDC and the Association of periOperative Registered Nurses (AORN), as well as manufacturer's directions for product use. The type of cleansing agent determines how long to scrub. Typically, alcohol-based handrub is rubbed on to hands and arms until dry.

2. **Before starting the surgical scrub,** gather supplies and set up sterile gloves, gown, and towel for use after the scrub.
   To maintain sterility of the hands after the scrub, the sterile gloves, gown, and towel must be ready before washing.

3. **Observe recommended hygiene.**
   a. Avoid wearing artificial nails and extenders; nails should be free of polish and not extend beyond the end of the fingers.
   The AORN and CDC recommend this when in direct contact with patients, in high-risk situations such as the perioperative setting, or among those receiving immunosuppressant therapy. Artificial nails have been shown to harbor more pathogenic organisms in the subungual area than natural nails, particularly gram-negative bacilli (especially Pseudomonas) and various strains of yeast. Long and poorly groomed nails can tear gloves.

   b. Remove rings, watches, and bracelets before starting the surgical scrub.
   Hand jewelry can prevent the handrub from reaching all skin areas, leaving potential pathogens on the skin. Risk of infection from microorganisms increases exponentially in relation to the number of rings worn.

4. **Don shoe covers, a cap, and a mask.** Tuck hair completely under the cap.
   Masks filter out possible airborne pathogens carried in the nose or mouth, preventing contamination of sterile areas. Covering the hair reduces the transmission of pathogenic organisms that adhere to the hair shaft or scalp.

5. **Perform a prewash before the surgical scrub.** Use a pick and running water to remove dirt and debris from under the nails; discard.
   Prewash removes any visible soil, reduces the number of microorganisms on your skin, and allows you to begin the surgical scrub with clean hands. The area under the nails harbors dirt, debris, and microorganisms.

6. **Turn on the water,** using the knee or foot controls or motion controls. The temperature usually adjusts automatically in a surgical scrub sink. If it does not, adjust to warm.
   Water temperature that is too hot can cause injury to the skin, making it prone to drying, chafing, and cracks. It can also remove normal flora and natural oil, which have a protective effect on the skin.

7. **Wet hands and forearms** from the fingertips to elbows, keeping hands above the elbows and away from the body at all times.
   Prevents water running down from your elbows and forearm over washed and rinsed hands.

8. **Dispense a palm full of** antibacterial soap into your dominant hand.
   a. Insert the fingertips of your nondominant hand into the soap using a twisting motion to apply the product to the fingertips and nails.
   b. Then rub the hands together to distribute the soap over the hands. ▼

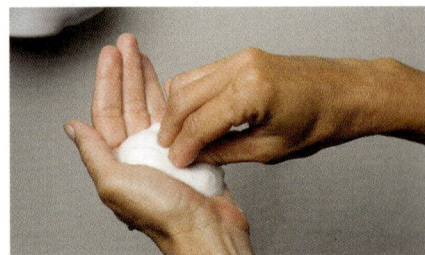

9. **Vigorously rub all surfaces** of your nondominant hand and fingers, adding water as needed.
   - Be sure to rub each finger on all sides.
   - Do not touch the inside of the sink during the cleansing procedure.
   Complete contact and friction are necessary for removal of microorganisms adherent to the skin's surface. The inside of the sink is considered contaminated with microbes. Incidental contact necessitates repeating the cleansing procedure.

   a. Rub the hands together palm to palm.
   b. Using your dominant palm, clean the back of your nondominant hand.

c. Then rub your nondominant palm over your dominant hand.

d. Then rub your palms together with your fingers interlaced.

e. Rub the back of your fingers on your closed right hand back and forth across your nondominant palm, with your curved fingers interlaced. Do the same with your other hand. ▼

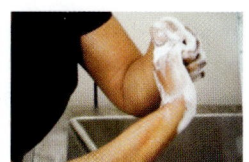

f. With your nondominant hand, clasp your dominant thumb and make rotational movements to cleanse the thumb. Repeat on the other hand.

g. Hold your fingers together on the dominant hand and move them back and forth and in a circular pattern against your other palm, and vice versa.

Although the palmar surface carries more organisms than the back side of the hands and arms, this area nonetheless should be cleansed thoroughly to reduce microbial count.

10. **Rinse, using deep basin sink** with knee-, foot-, or motion-operated controls.

Improved adherence to sterile technique commonly results from use of motion- or foot/knee-operated controls for faucets.

11. **Next cleanse the remaining** ⅔ of the arms, beginning at the wrist, to 2 inches above the elbow. Cover every aspect of the middle and upper third of the forearm.

12. **Dispense cleansing solution** into the hands each time you cleanse a new area. Be sure the dispenser is not blocked

A blocked dispenser can interfere with obtaining the amount of product needed for reducing bacterial colonization.

13. **First, scrub the nondominant arm** wrist-to-elbow. Then repeat the wrist-to-elbow scrub on the dominant arm. Rinse each arm thoroughly and independently.

14. **This completes one washing cycle**.

a. Using the same motions, beginning with step 8, perform a second cycle.

b. Then finish with a third cycle in which you scrub only the hands (steps 8–11).

c. The scrub is complete after cleansing every aspect of the hands and forearms for 3 full minutes.

AORN promotes a 2- to 3-minute scrub time using an antiseptic detergent to achieve maximal microbicidal activity while avoiding irritant contact dermatitis. Reduced time required to perform the surgical scrub often results in increased compliance with the prescribed technique.

15. **With arms flexed and hands** held higher than the elbows away from the body, move to the area with the sterile towel and gown.

This position prevents water running down from your elbows and forearm over rinsed hands.

16. **Grasp the sterile towel,** and back away from the sterile field. Lean forward slightly and allow the towel to fall open, being careful not to let it touch clothing or gown.

This motion is performed to maintain a dry sterile field and prevent inadvertent brushing against the table and contaminating the field. Do not turn your back on any sterile field.

17. **Use one end of the towel** to dry one hand and arm.

Dry the other hand and arm with the opposite end of the towel.

Use of a separate section of the towel guards against inadvertently rewetting the skin or contaminating an already clean area.

18. **Allow time for the skin to dry** thoroughly before donning sterile gloves.

Dry skin prevents maceration and allows the gloves to go on more easily. Moisture left on the skin can be a source of further microbial contamination.

19. **Once the brushless scrub is complete,** keep your hands in front of your body and above the waist. It may be necessary to enter backward through the door of the surgical suite.

These actions help prevent contamination of the hands and forearms when moving from the scrub sink.

Documentation

A brushless surgical hand scrub does not require documentation in the patient's medical record, although there may be a checklist. However, you must adhere to the institution's policy for performing the technique.

Patient Teaching

If the patient is able to observe the procedure, explain the purpose of a diligent approach to surgical scrub for promoting a low-risk environment for infection.

Home Care

Sinks in the home environment typically do not have knee- or foot-operated controls or motion-sensor on/off devices.

Therefore, when scrubbing for a sterile procedure in the home, contact with the faucet handles is performed with barrier objects (e.g., a paper towel or a sterile towel for a sterile scrub) between the clean hands and the environmental surface.

Practice Resources

AORN (2013a, 2013b); Association for Surgical Technologists (2008a); CDC (2002); George, D., & Bhabra, M. A. (2010).

Thinking About the Procedure

 The video **Surgical Hand Washing: Brushless System,** along with questions and suggested responses, is available on the **Davis's *Nursing Skills Videos* Web** site on DavisPlus.

Procedure 22-6 ■ Sterile Gown and Gloves (Closed Method)

➤ For steps to follow in *all* procedures, refer to the Universal Steps for All Procedures found on the page facing the inside back cover. For this procedure, also refer to Clinical Insights 22-3 and 22-4, if you need more information.

Equipment
- Sterile gloves of the correct size
- Sterile gown

You should find these lying on a sterile field. If they are not, you will need to create a sterile field to place them on.

➤ When performing the procedure, always identify your patient according to agency policy, using two identifiers, and be attentive to standard precautions, hand hygiene, patient safety and privacy, body mechanics, and documentation.

Procedure Steps

1. **Grasp the gown at the neckline.**
   - Hold the gown up and allow it to fall open as you step back from the table.
   - Be careful not to allow the gown to come into contact with non-sterile areas while you are lifting it off the table and opening it.
   The gown will be contaminated if it touches unsterile objects. ▼

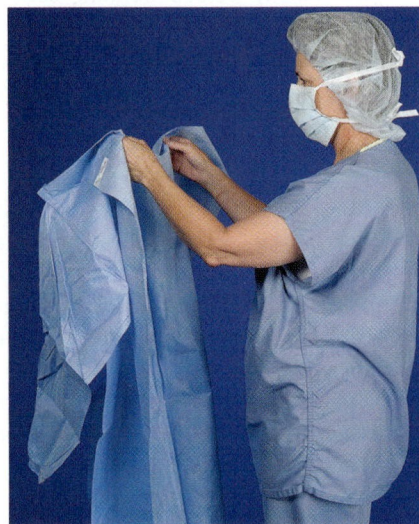

2. **Slide both arms into the sleeves,** but do not extend your hands through the cuffs. ▼

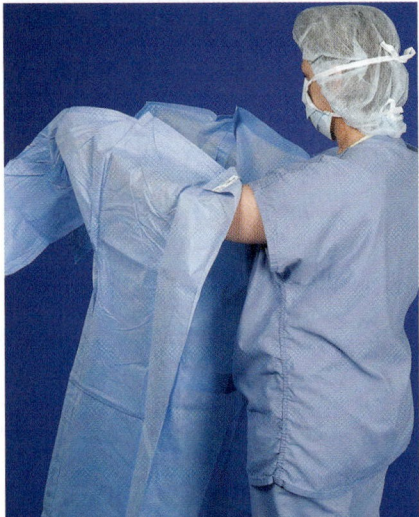

3. **Keep the sleeves of the gown** above waist level.
   Hands will contaminate the sleeve edge if allowed to pass through the cuff.

4. **Have a coworker (or the circulating nurse,** if you are in the operating room) stand behind you and pull the shoulders of the gown up and tie the neck tie. The coworker touches only the inside of the gown while pulling it up.
   Touching only the inside prevents contamination of the gown with the nurse's hands.

5. **Don sterile gloves** using the closed method.
   Open the sterile glove wrapper, keeping your fingers inside the sleeve of the gown. (The outer wrapper has already been discarded.)

   Glove the dominant hand first:

   a. With your nondominant hand, keeping your hands inside the gown sleeves, grasp the cuff of the glove for your dominant hand. Turn your dominant hand palm up.
   Keeping the hand inside the cuff ensures that you are making contact with the sterile gown; sterile is touching sterile.

   b. Lay the glove on the dominant gown cuff, thumb side down with the glove opening pointed toward the fingers, and thumb of glove positioned over the thumb side of the hand. ▼

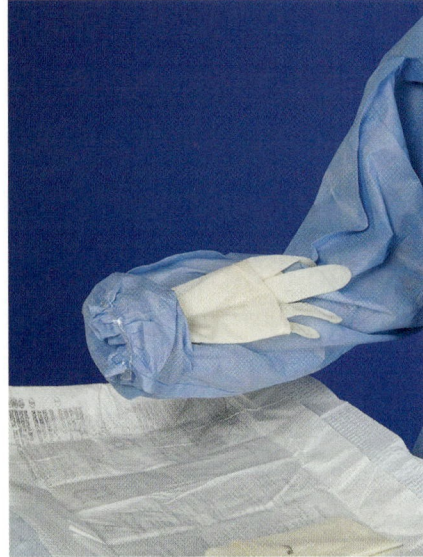

c. Keeping your dominant hand inside the sleeve, grasp the inside of the glove cuff. ▼

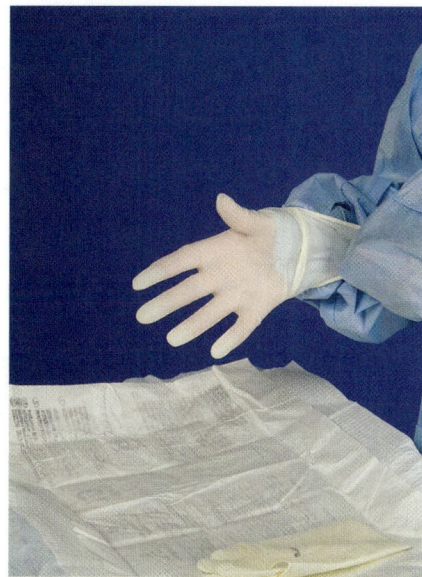

d. With your other hand (inside its sleeve), grasp the upper side of the glove cuff and stretch it over the gown cuff.

e. Pull the sleeve of your gown up to pull the glove cuff over your wrist as you move your fingers into the glove fingers.

Glove the nondominant hand.

a. Place the fingers of your gloved hand under the cuff of the second glove.
   ▪ Lay the glove on the forearm of your nondominant hand.

▪ Grasp and anchor the inside glove cuff with your nondominant (ungloved) hand through the gown, being careful to keep fingers inside the gown.

b. With your dominant (gloved) hand, pull the glove cuff over the cuff of the gown as you move your fingers into the glove. ▼

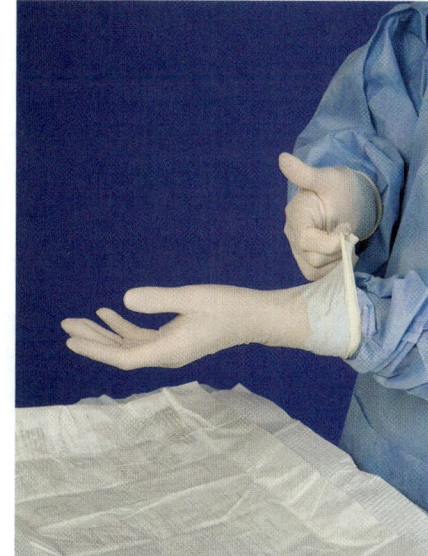

c. **Adjust the fingers in both** gloves so the excess glove is pulled over the fingertips.
   Maintains sterility of the gown and gloves by maintaining a closed system. The final adjustment of the gloves is done when both gloves are in place to prevent contaminating the gloves. Taut gloves, especially over the fingertips, allow better feel and dexterity.

6. **Grasp the waist tie on the gown,** and hand the tie to the circulating nurse or a coworker who is wearing a hair cover and mask. Your coworker will grab the tie with sterile forceps.
   The tie is considered sterile. You will need help pulling it around you. A coworker can help you. Using sterile forceps keeps the tie sterile. ▼

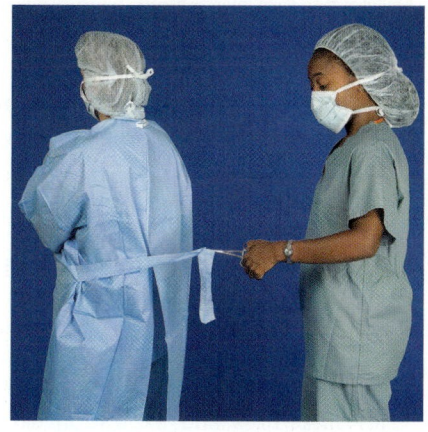

7. **Make a three-quarter turn** and receive the tie from your coworker.
   Because only areas within your field of vision are considered sterile, a coworker must pull the waist tie around you.

8. **Secure the waist tie.**
   Ensures that the gown is secured and will not expose clothing to a sterile field.

Patient Teaching

If the patient is alert during the procedure, explain:
▪ The need for the sterile procedure
▪ Why he must not touch the drapes
▪ Why he must not move or talk once the drapes are in place
▪ Any special precautions during the procedure

Documentation

▪ Donning sterile gown and gloves does not require documentation.
▪ You will need to chart the procedure performed and how the patient tolerated it.
▪ In the operating room, the circulating nurse charts about the surgery and the patient's response.

? What if . . .

▪ **Your hand inadvertently comes through the cuff opening when putting on the gown?**

   Change gowns. The cuff would have been contaminated and would then contaminate your glove.

Practice Resources
AORN (2013a, 2013b, 2016); CDC (2002).

Thinking About the Procedure

To practice applying clinical reasoning to this procedure,

 The video **Sterile Gowns and Gloves (Closed Method),** along with questions and suggested responses, is available on the **Davis's *Nursing Skills Videos*** Web site on Davis*Plus.*

Procedure 22-7 ■ Sterile Gloves (Open Method)

> ➤ For steps to follow in *all* procedures, refer to the Universal Steps for All Procedures found on the page facing the inside back cover. For this procedure, also refer to Clinical Insights 22-3 and 22-4 if you need more information.

Equipment
- Sterile gloves of the correct size

> ➤ When performing the procedure, always identify your patient according to agency policy, using two identifiers, and be attentive to standard precautions, hand hygiene, patient safety and privacy, body mechanics, and documentation.

Procedure Steps

1. Determine the correct size of sterile gloves. The gloves should be snug but not tight.

Gloves that are too loose are more easily contaminated and make handling equipment or supplies difficult. Gloves that are too tight are uncomfortable and may tear during use.

2. ✚ Assess the glove package for intactness and expiration date. Do not use the gloves if the package is torn, has become moist, or is past the expiration date.

Torn packaging may allow the gloves to become contaminated. Moisture allows wicking and may cause contamination. Expired gloves are not considered sterile. ▼

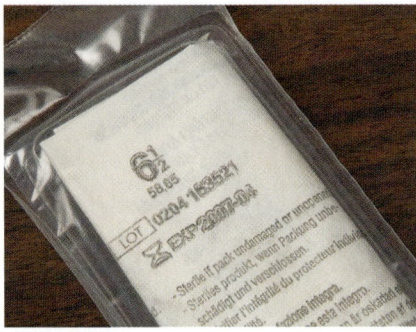

3. Assess the patient's environment for a space that is clean and has adequate space to allow you to open the glove package. Don the gloves without touching a nonsterile item.

4. Open the outer wrapper and place the inner glove package on a clean, dry surface.

Prevents contamination of the gloves inside the package.

5. Open the inner glove package so that the glove cuffs are closest to you. Be careful to fully open the package flaps so that they do not fold back over and contaminate the gloves.

The outer 1-inch border of the glove package is considered contaminated. ▼

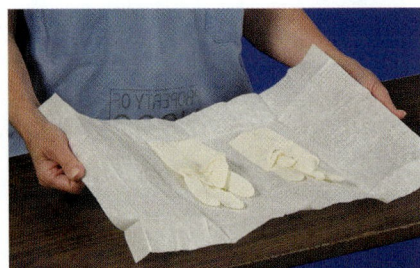

6. With your nondominant hand, grasp the inner surface of the glove for the dominant hand.
- Lift the glove up and away from the table, keeping it away from your body.
- Take care to not touch anything else on the sterile field.

  The inside of the glove is not sterile because it is in contact with your skin. Lifting the glove up and away from the table prevents you from contaminating the glove by accidentally touching the table or your clothing while donning it.

7. Slide your dominant hand into the glove, keeping your hand and fingers above your waist and away from your body.

The area below the waistline is considered contaminated. Keeping gloves away

from your body prevents accidental contamination. ▼

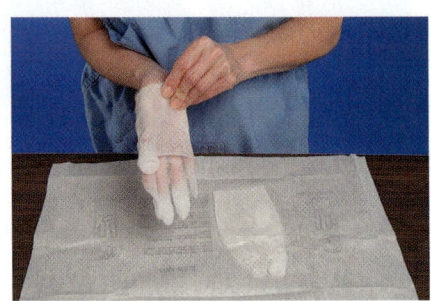

8. Slide your gloved fingers under the cuff of the remaining glove, keeping your gloved thumb well away from your ungloved hand. Lift the glove up and away from the table and away from your body.

The outside of the glove is sterile and may be touched with your sterile gloved hand. ▼

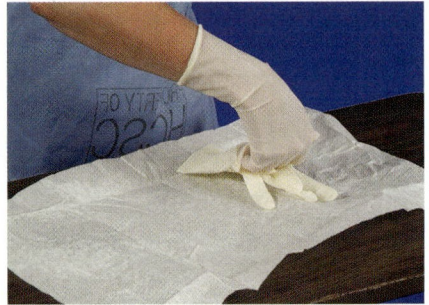

9. **With gloved fingers still under the cuff,** slide your nondominant hand into the glove and pull it on, being careful to avoid contact with your gloved hand, especially the thumb. ▼

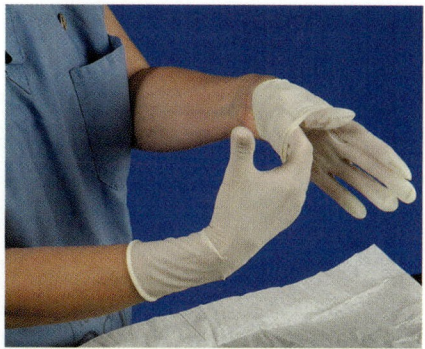

10. **Adjust both gloves to fit your fingers.** If necessary, pull the fingers of the gloves down so that no excess is at the fingertips.
Adjusting your gloves after both have been donned decreases the risk of contamination and allows for greater dexterity during the procedure.

11. **Keep your hands between shoulder** and waist level in front of you.
Keeps the gloves within your field of vision to avoid contamination.

To remove soiled gloves after the procedure, refer to Procedure 22-3.

Patient Teaching

Explain why sterile gloves are needed for the procedure.

Home Care

- Many home care procedures are clean rather than sterile. The client is in his own environment and not surrounded by other patients, who may serve as hosts for infection.
- You may need to teach caregivers how to apply sterile gloves for some procedures. No modifications are required. Demonstrate the procedure, and have the caregiver do a return demonstration.

Documentation

- No special documentation is needed for sterile gloving.
- Chart the procedure you performed and the patient's response to the procedure.

Practice Resources
AORN (2013a, 2013b, 2016).

Thinking About the Procedure

To practice applying clinical reasoning to this procedure,

 The video **Sterile Gloves (Open Method),** along with questions and suggested responses, is available on the **Davis's** *Nursing Skills Videos* Web site on Davis*Plus.*

Procedure 22-8 ■ Sterile Fields

➤ For steps to follow in *all* procedures, refer to the Universal Steps for All Procedures found on the inside back cover. For this procedure, also refer to Clinical Insights 22-3, 22-4, and 22-5. If you need more information, review the section Using Sterile Technique in Nursing Care and Box 22-4, earlier in this chapter.

Equipment

- Package of sterile supplies required for the procedure
- Sterile gloves of the correct size

(continued on next page)

Procedure 22-8 ■ Sterile Fields (continued)

Procedure 22-8A ■ Setting Up a Sterile Field

➤ When performing the procedure, always identify your patient according to agency policy, using two identifiers, and be attentive to standard precautions, hand hygiene, patient safety and privacy, body mechanics, and documentation.

Procedure Steps

- Close doors and limit the number of people in the area.
  Air currents can carry dust and microorganisms.

- Prepare a sterile field as close as possible to the time of use.
  To minimize the opportunity for contamination via air currents.

1. **Assess the sterility of all packages and equipment.** Check to make sure the packaging is intact and the expiration dates have not passed.
   Only sterile items should enter a sterile field. Any compromise in packaging means that the item is assumed not to be sterile.

2. **Arrange the environment** for performing the sterile procedure.
   a. Remove all items from the surface you will use to set up the sterile field.
   Inadequate space causes inadvertent contamination during sterile procedures.
   b. Position the patient as needed for the procedure.
   Allows you to immediately proceed with the planned procedure. Once the sterile field is established, air movement can create contamination of the sterile items.

Procedure Variation Using Sterile Packaged Equipment

3. **Place the sterile package** on a clean, dry surface.
   Prevents contamination of the sterile item. If a surface is damp, strike through of moisture may occur, making the item unsterile. ▼

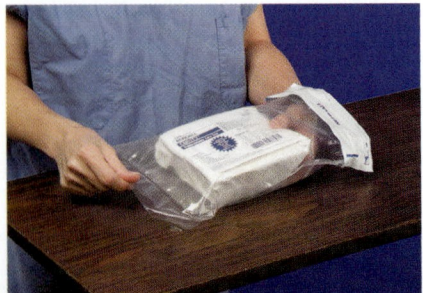

4. **Open the flap away from you first.**
   To prevent passing an unsterile arm over the sterile items. If you move an unsterile item over a sterile field, the field is no longer considered to be sterile. ▼

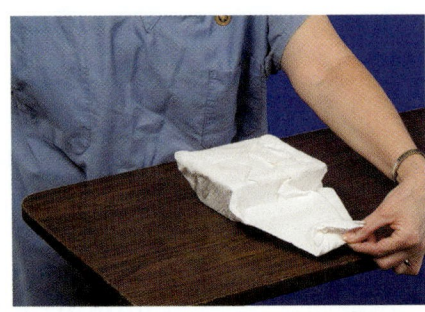

5. **Open the side flaps.** ▼

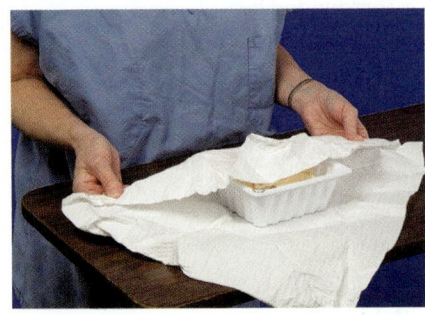

6. **Pull the final flap toward you.** The wrapper is now the sterile field. Touch the inside of the wrapper only after you don sterile gloves.
   - The area 1 inch from the edge of the wrapper and 1 inch from the table edge is considered unsterile.
   - Do not readjust the sterile area after the package has been opened.
   Only the horizontal surface of the draped area is considered sterile. Any part of the sterile wrapper that falls below the level of the sterile area (e.g., top of the table) is considered unsterile. If you move the field after opening, the field shifts and places

unsterile areas of the wrapper on the surface. ▼

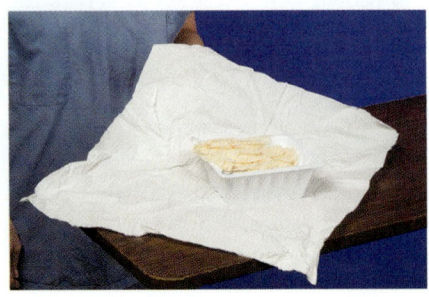

Procedure Variation Opening a Fabric- or Paper-Wrapped Sterile Package

7. **Check and remove** the chemical indicator strip.
   The indicator tape per manufacturer or institution confirms that the package was sterilized. The pack usually is also dated.

8. **Remove the outer wrapper** and place the inner wrapped package on a clean, dry surface.
   The outer wrapper is not considered sterile and is discarded.

9. **Open the inner wrapper** following the same technique described in steps 3 through 6.

Procedure Variation Placing a Sterile Drape
Omit steps 3 through 9.

10. **To place the package on a clean, dry surface:**
    a. With the outer wrapper still on the package, hold the edge of the package flap down toward the table.
    b. Grasp the top edge of the package, and peel back.
    The sterile drape is inside the outer wrapper. This maneuver opens the

package without contaminating the sterile drape. ▼

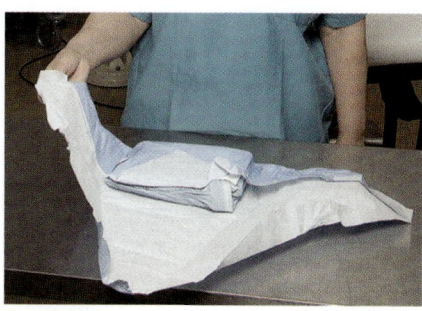

11. Pick up the sterile drape by the corner.
  - Allow the drape to fall open, away from your body and away from

unsterile surface, touching only the outside (unsterile side) and edge of the drape.
  - Avoid fanning the sterile drape as you unfold it to cover the table surface.
  - Drape musts extend over the edge of the table, but not touch the floor.

A 1-inch border around the sterile drape is considered unsterile.

12. In some situations, when placing a sterile drape (e.g., under a patient) you may need to protect your gloved hands by cuffing the drape over your hands. ▼

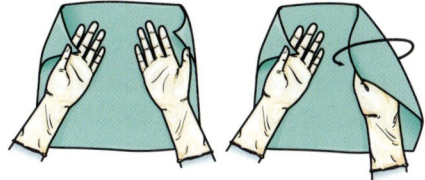

Protecting gloved hands

Procedure 22-8B ■ Adding Supplies to a Sterile Field

➤ When performing the procedure, always identify your patient according to agency policy, using two identifiers, and be attentive to standard precautions, hand hygiene, patient safety and privacy, body mechanics, and documentation.

Procedure Steps.

1. ✚ **Before adding items to a sterile field,** inspect them for proper packaging, integrity, and inclusion of a sterilization indicator. Never assume an item is sterile. If there is any doubt about its sterility, consider it contaminated.

2. Hold the sterile package in your dominant hand. Grasping the corner of the wrapper, peel each corner back with your nondominant hand.
The inside of the wrapper is sterile and will be used as a barrier when placing the sterile item onto a sterile field.

3. Holding the contents several inches above the field, allow the supplies to drop onto the field inside the 1-inch border of the sterile field. Do not let your arms pass over the sterile field.
By holding the package upside down, you ensure that the sterile part of the package is facing the sterile field and that you deposit the item onto the sterile field. ▼

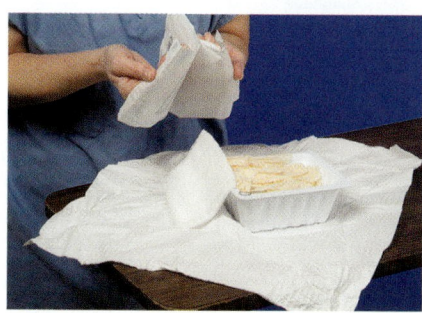

4. Dispose of the wrapper and continue opening any needed supplies for the procedure.
KEY POINT: *Once sterile gloves are on, you will not be able to add items without contaminating the gloves.*

(continued on next page)

Procedure 22-8 ■ Sterile Fields (continued)

Procedure 22-8C ■ Adding Sterile Solutions to a Sterile Field

➤ When performing the procedure, always identify your patient according to agency policy, using two identifiers, and be attentive to standard precautions, hand hygiene, patient safety and privacy, body mechanics, and documentation.

Procedure Steps

1. **Use a sterile bowl or receptacle.** Place it on the side of the sterile field closest to you.
Prevents you from reaching over and thereby contaminating the field.

2. **Check that the sterile solution is correct** and confirm that the expiration date has not passed and that the solution and concentration are correct and have not expired. ▼

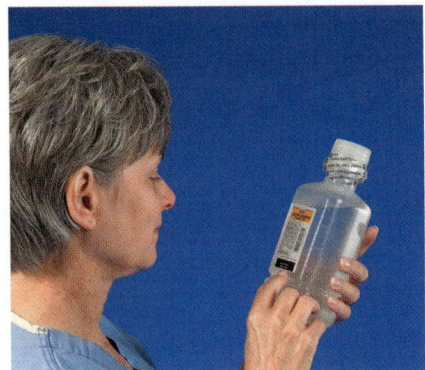

3. **Remove the cap from the solution bottle** by lifting it directly up. Throw it away.
The edge of the container is considered contaminated after the contents have been poured and the sterility of the contents cannot be ensured if the cap is replaced.

4. **Hold the bottle 4 to 6 inches** above the bowl and pour the needed amount of the solution into the bowl.
Prevents you from inadvertently touching the sterile bowl with the bottle and thereby contaminating the bowl. Limited height reduces the risk of splashing, with strike through of a permeable sterile field. A disposable sterile drape generally has a plastic membrane in the middle to prevent strike through. ▼

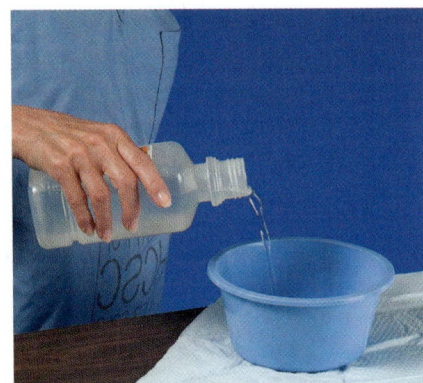

5. **Discard the remaining solution.**
Reusing open containers may cause contamination because of drops contacting the unsterile areas and running back over the container opening.

6. **Before donning sterile gloves** to perform the procedure, double-check that all supplies have been added to the field.
   - Do not leave the sterile field unattended.
   - Do not turn your back to the sterile field.
   If a sterile item is out of your field of vision, it is no longer considered sterile because airborne particles, insects, or liquids could contaminate the field.

Home Care

- Most sterile procedures in the home are done by visiting nurses.
- Procedures performed by clients or family members are usually clean rather than sterile.

Documentation

- You will not usually document the actual setting up of the sterile field.
- Document the procedure, your assessment of the patient's tolerance for the procedure, and your assessment of the area being treated by the procedure.

? What if . . .

- **The nurse observes a breach in sterility by the surgeon?**

The nurse's duty is to protect the patient above all else, even when fearing an uncomfortable confrontation with the healthcare provider. The nurse is obligated to follow the institution's policy and advocate for patient safety.

Practice Resources

AORN (2013b, 2016); Association for Surgical Technologists (2008a); Siegel, J. D., Rhinehart, E., Jackson, M., et al. (2006); Simko, L. (2012).

Thinking About the Procedure

To practice applying clinical reasoning to this procedure,

 The videos **Setting Up a Sterile Field—Sterile Packaged Equipment; Setting Up a Sterile Field—Sterile Fabric- or Paper-Wrapped Sterile Package; Setting Up a Sterile Field—Sterile Drape; Adding Supplies to a Sterile Field— Sterile Packaged Equipment; Adding Supplies to a Sterile Field—Fabric- or Paper-Wrapped Sterile Package; Adding Supplies to a Sterile Field—Sterile Drape; Adding Sterile Solutions to a Sterile Field—Sterile Packaged Equipment; Adding Sterile Solutions to a Sterile Field—Fabric- or Paper-Wrapped Sterile Package;** and **Adding Sterile Solutions to a Sterile Field—Sterile Drape,** along with questions and suggested responses, are available on the Davis's **Nursing Skills Videos** Web site on DavisPlus.

To explore learning resources for this chapter,

 Go to www.DavisAdvantage.com and find:

Answers and Suggested Responses for all questions in this chapter

Lists NIC and NOC

List of NANDA-I Diagnoses

Knowledge Map

Care Plan

Care Map

References and Bibliography

Concept Map

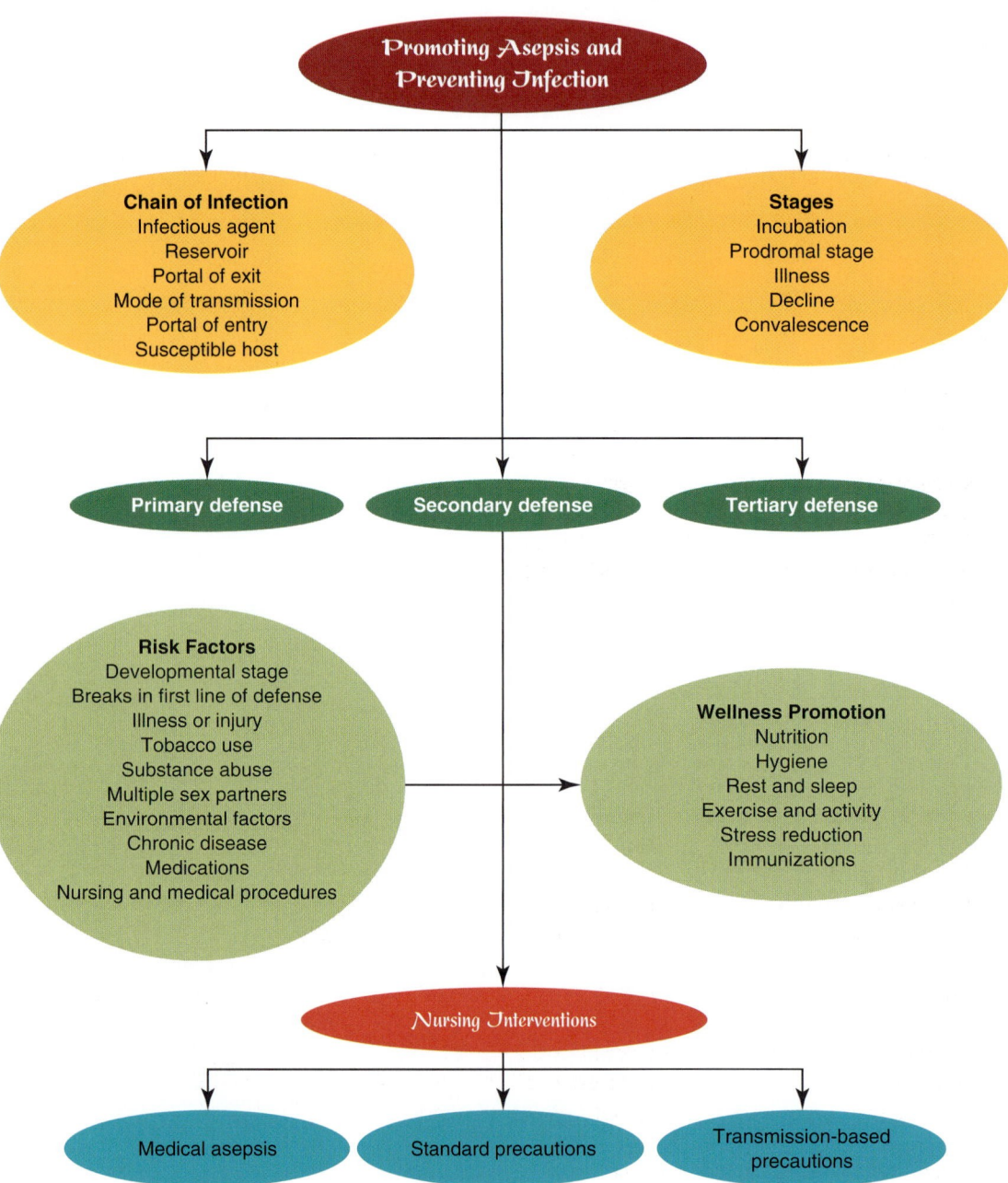

Promoting Asepsis and Preventing Infection

Chain of Infection
Infectious agent
Reservoir
Portal of exit
Mode of transmission
Portal of entry
Susceptible host

Stages
Incubation
Prodromal stage
Illness
Decline
Convalescence

Primary defense

Secondary defense

Tertiary defense

Risk Factors
Developmental stage
Breaks in first line of defense
Illness or injury
Tobacco use
Substance abuse
Multiple sex partners
Environmental factors
Chronic disease
Medications
Nursing and medical procedures

Wellness Promotion
Nutrition
Hygiene
Rest and sleep
Exercise and activity
Stress reduction
Immunizations

Nursing Interventions

Medical asepsis

Standard precautions

Transmission-based precautions

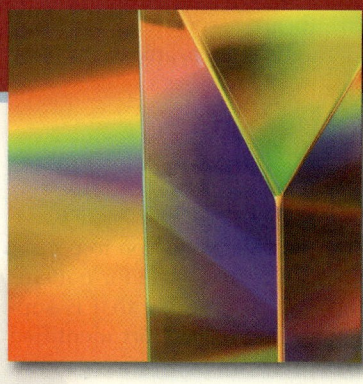

CHAPTER 23

Safety

Learning Outcomes

After completing this chapter, you should be able to:

➤ List the three leading causes of accidental death in the United States.

➤ Discuss developmental and individual factors that create safety risks.

➤ Identify at least five safety hazards in the home environment and interventions to prevent injury from them.

➤ Discuss the steps to follow when you suspect that a client has ingested a poisonous substance.

➤ Describe the choking rescue maneuver and identify instances when it is appropriate to use it.

➤ Describe the four main physical hazards that are found in the community and interventions to prevent injury from them.

➤ Describe and give examples of hazards encountered in the healthcare agency.

➤ Identify four interventions to prevent falls in the healthcare agency.

➤ Discuss the appropriate use of siderails in the healthcare agency.

➤ Properly apply restraints and discuss measures to prevent injury in clients who are restrained.

➤ Discuss at least one data collection instrument that is used to assess the client who is at risk for falls.

➤ Plan and implement nursing care to promote safety and prevent injury in clients who are at risk.

Key Concepts

Patient Safety

Safety

Related Concepts

See the Concept Map at the end of this chapter.

Example Problem

Falls

Meet Your Patients

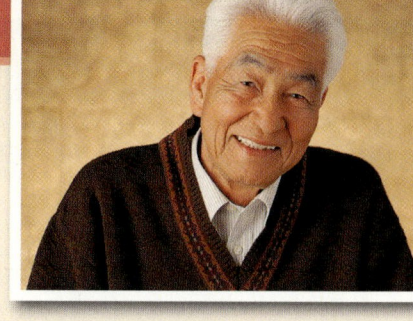

■ **Alvin Lin.** Alvin Lin is a 79-year-old man who was just transferred from a long-term care facility to your medical unit. His admitting diagnosis is dehydration and pneumonia. The night nurse reported that he had rested well during the night and was alert and oriented. When you enter his room, he is confused and does not know where he is. He becomes combative and tries to get out of bed. How should you respond to the situation?

■ **Teresa.** Suppose you are a nurse making a home visit to Teresa, who lives in a rural area. Teresa is 20 years old and has a 2-year-old daughter. She is also responsible for caring for her elderly grandmother, who is recovering

from a hip fracture. Teresa says that it is getting more difficult to keep up with her toddler, who is "into everything," and to care for the needs of her grandmother. Her grandmother has a fear of falling and is reluctant to do anything for herself.

Theoretical Knowledge
knowing **why**

This chapter will increase your ability to recognize safety hazards in the home, community, and healthcare facility and to plan interventions that promote safety for clients of all ages, such as the two in the Meet Your Patients scenario. Many accidental injuries can be prevented by being aware of hazards and taking reasonable precautions.

ABOUT THE KEY CONCEPTS

Safety is a basic human need, second only to survival needs such as oxygen, nutrition, and fluids. As a nurse, the concept of **safety** is fundamental to providing safe, effective, high-quality care to your clients. Nurses contribute to **patient safety,** in any setting, by coordinating and integrating the multiple aspects of quality into the nursing care, and across the care delivered by others. You must also be concerned with your own safety and the safety of other care providers. Many accidental injuries can be prevented by being aware of hazards and taking reasonable precautions.

IMPORTANCE OF SAFETY

According to the Centers for Disease Control and Prevention (CDC, 2015b), accidents, or unintentional injuries, are the fourth leading cause of deaths in the United States. An estimated 130,000 people die each year as a result of accidents. Expressed another way, one person dies from an accident every 5 minutes. Poisoning is now listed as the number one cause of unintentional death, followed by motor vehicle accidents, firearms, falls, drowning, and fires (see Table 23-1).

Of course, the death rate was not the only noteworthy number in the CDC report: Millions of people received injuries that disabled them beyond the day of injury. Many healthcare organizations are campaigning for safer patient care in an effort to reduce the cost of healthcare and the burden of suffering. The following are examples:

- **The Joint Commission,** the accrediting body for healthcare facilities, each year publishes National Patient Safety Goals.

For example, the 2016 goals include improving the accuracy of patient identification, improving the safety of medication use, reducing the risk of healthcare-associated infections, and preventing mistakes in surgery. For a link to the 2016 National Patient Safety Goals,

 Go to the Web site of The Joint Commission at https://www.jointcommission.org/standards_information/npsgs.aspx.

- **Institute of Medicine's (IOM)** report *To Err Is Human: Building a Safer Health System* brought public attention to patient safety. It stated that it is simply not acceptable for patients to be harmed by the same healthcare system that is supposed to offer healing and comfort. The report identified five critical principles to ensure safe healthcare systems: Provide leadership, recognize human limits in process design, promote effective team functioning, anticipate the unexpected, and create a learning environment (IOM, 2001). To learn what is meant by the "culture of safety" in the healthcare setting, read the accompanying Safe, Effective Nursing Care box.
- The **American Nurses Association's (ANA)** *ANA's Health System Reform* agenda (2010) recommends six major public policy changes that can raise the quality of healthcare. Quality Aim 1 is safe healthcare.
- **Quality and Safety Education for Nurses (QSEN),** a task force to improve nursing education, identified and described six competencies that all nursing students should have by graduation. Safety is one of those competencies (Cronenwett, Sherwood, Barnsteiner, et al., 2007; Cronenwett, Sherwood, & Gelmon, 2009).
- **Medicare** is a federal agency that has identified **"never events"** or hospital-acquired conditions (HAC): costly errors that cause serious injury or death, and that are mostly preventable (falls, injuries from restraints). Medicare will no longer pay institutions for care required to treat the effects of such errors (Centers for Medicare & Medicaid Services, 2006a, modified 2015).

WHAT FACTORS AFFECT SAFETY?

To promote client safety, you will need theoretical knowledge about developmental stages and individual risk factors that affect clients' ability to avoid accidental injury. This chapter discusses specific risk factors and describes hazards the home, the community, and the healthcare agency.

Developmental Factors

The type and incidence of accidents vary among age-groups. You will find interventions for all age-groups integrated into the topics throughout this chapter. The descriptions given for each age-group are characteristics common to most people in that group. However, individuals progress through developmental stages at their own pace, so there will always be people who do not fit the group description closely. For supplemental discussion of safety needs during different developmental stages, review Chapters 9 and 10.

Infant/Toddler Infants and toddlers are completely dependent on others for their care. They are able to walk and manipulate objects before they have the judgment to recognize dangers. Infants and toddlers are curious and tend to explore the environment by putting objects in their mouth. This is why the incidence of choking is highest between 6 months and 3 years of age. As mobility continues to improve, toddlers gain more freedom, and their curiosity leads them to explore

Table 23-1 ▶ Leading Causes of Unintentional Deaths in the United	
MECHANISM OF INJURY	**TOTAL ANNUAL DEATHS, ALL AGE-GROUPS**
Poisoning and exposure to noxious substances	42,917
Motor vehicles	33,687
Firearms	31,672
Falls	26,852
Drowning	3,782
Fires, flames, and smoke	2,845

Source: Murphy, S. L., Xu, J. Q., & Kochanek, K. D. (2013). Deaths: Final data for 2010. *National Vital Statistics Reports, 61*(4).

Creating a Culture of Safety

Chapter Key Concept: Safety (Thinking, Doing, Caring)

Competency: Collaborate with the interdisciplinary healthcare team; Provide safe, quality client care

Background: Until recently the healthcare industry took patient safety more or less for granted. It assumed that all dedicated practitioners would perform correct actions and that people who made mistakes were "bad apples" to be fired. Mistakes were hushed up. Certainly the patient or family was never told an error had occurred. This culture of secrecy and blame still exists.

In the past 20 years, advisory bodies have reported the cost to society and the huge impact of medical mistakes on patients and their families. The Institute of Medicine (IOM) has called for (1) healthcare organizations to work to dismantle the culture of secrecy and blame and create a culture of safety and (2) that nurses be leaders in these efforts.

Safe, Effective Nursing Care (SENC) activities were created specifically to help prepare nurses for these roles. SENC describes the skills you need to become part of the new culture of safety. Baseline knowledge and skills you will need to acquire include:

> Thinking in terms of systems.
> Understanding how systems create a mistake-prone environment.
> Understanding the types of errors that occur in your facility

KEY POINT: *People make the mistakes. Systems set the stage for them.*

Think About It: It is equally important to determine what systems need to be in place to build the culture of safety.

Some critical system features include the following, along with questions for your reflection or discussion:

> All levels of leadership make safety a visible priority and take actions that promote safety.
Why is leadership important in changing culture?
> All staff members providing care are formally encouraged to communicate their concerns to the team.
Why do you think nurses or junior doctors might not communicate concerns?
> All information needed to appropriately manage the patient across shifts, units, facilities, or after other handoffs is available at all times.
What types of errors can occur during handoffs?
> Facility adopts a nonpunitive response to errors and uses strategies such as root cause analysis to identify system issues.
What effect might a punitive culture have on error reporting?
> Facility recognizes both individual and system causes of errors but emphasizes a systems approach to error reduction.
Describe one system that can break down and make errors more likely.
> Each person providing care acknowledges own potential for error and values own role in preventing errors.
What can you do to help prevent errors?

Sources: Institute of Medicine. (2001). *Crossing the quality chasm: A new health system for the 21st century.* Washington, DC: The National Academies Press. Retrieved from http://www.nap.edu/openbook.php?record_id=10027&page=R1; Institute of Medicine. (2011). *The future of nursing: Leading change, advancing health.* Washington, DC: The National Academies Press. Retrieved from http://books.nap.edu/openbook.php?record_id=12956

---

cupboards, stairs, open windows, swimming pools, and other hazards (CDC, 2012).

- Drowning is the leading cause of death for children aged 1 to 4, followed by motor vehicle accidents ("Vital Signs," 2012).
- Falls, choking, sudden infant death and ingesting poisons are other critical safety concerns.

Preschooler After age 3 years, children are a little less prone to falls because their gross and fine motor skills, coordination, and balance have improved. However, as they begin to play outside more often (e.g., playgrounds, pools, front yards) there are additional safety concerns.

- *Accidental deaths*—Motor vehicle injuries are a major cause, along with drowning, fires, and poisoning.
- *Nonfatal injuries*—Falls are the primary cause of nonfatal injuries.

Although preschoolers become more aware of dangers and limitations, adult supervision is essential.

School-Age Child School-age children have developed more refined muscle coordination and control, and improved decision-making skills. However, because they become more involved in activities outside the home, bone and muscle injuries are common. Injuries are often related to sports, skateboarding, bicycle riding, and playground injuries. Most school-age children are less fearful than are toddlers and are ready to try any new skill with or without practice or training. Exposure to the wider school and neighborhood environment also increases the safety risks for children from people outside the home (e.g., abduction).

- *Accidental deaths*—Motor vehicles continue to be the leading cause in this age-group.
- *Nonfatal injuries*—Falls are the leading cause of nonfatal injuries.

Adolescent Peak physical, sensory, and psychomotor abilities give teenagers a feeling of strength and confidence, yet they lack the wisdom and judgment of adults. This, along with feelings of being indestructible, makes them more likely to participate in risk-taking behavior, and, in turn, more prone to injury.

- *Accidental death*—Motor vehicle accidents are the leading cause, followed by homicide. Both are frequently associated with alcohol and drug use.
- *Accidental injuries*—Sports and recreational injuries, including diving and drowning incidents, are also common, especially when drinking and drug use are involved.

Adult Workplace injury may be a significant concern. Other injuries to adults are related to lifestyle (e.g., excessive alcohol use), stress, carelessness, abuse, and decline in strength and stamina.

- *Accidental death*—Unintentional poisoning causes more deaths than do motor vehicle accidents (CDC, 2015a).

- *Accidental injuries*—For many, work and family responsibilities leave little time for regular physical activity, increasing the risk of musculoskeletal injury in the so-called weekend athlete.

Older Adult Although many older adults have intact senses and continue to enjoy life as they age, physiological changes do occur (e.g., reduced muscle strength and joint mobility; slowing of reflexes; decreased ability to respond to multiple stimuli; and sensory losses, particularly hearing and vision). These changes increase the older adult's risk for falls, burns, car accidents, and other injury.

Accidental death—Falls are the most common cause of accidental death for adults aged 65 and older (CDC, 2015b).

Individual Risk Factors

In addition to developmental stage, individual factors also influence a person's risk for unintentional injury. These include lifestyle, cognitive awareness, sensoriperceptual status, ability to communicate, mobility status, physical and emotional health, and awareness of safety measures. Table 23-2 summarizes individual risk factors.

KnowledgeCheck 23-1

- What are some important developmental considerations when providing a safe environment for a preschool child?
- What is the main cause of injuries during the adolescent period?
- What are some ways that the aging process makes the older adult more prone to injury?
- Based on your theoretical knowledge and the scant patient data you have, why do you think Teresa's toddler (Meet Your Patients) is at risk for accidents? What about Teresa's grandmother?

Table 23-2 ▶ Individual Risk Factors for Injury

RISK FACTORS	BEHAVIOR MANIFESTATION
Lifestyle	Smoking, alcohol abuse, risk-taking behaviors
Cognitive awareness	Confusion due to stress and loss of short-term memory
Sensory and perceptual status	Loss of senses (e.g., vision, hearing, pain) that provide first line of defense
Impaired communication	Language barriers and hearing and speech impairment related to disease processes
Impaired mobility	Impaired strength with accompanying problems in mobility, balance, and endurance
Physical and emotional well-being	Reduced physical stamina and depression, with feelings of loss of control and helplessness
Safety awareness	Reduced cognitive awareness (e.g., of older adult) and immature development of the child

SAFETY HAZARDS IN THE HOME

What safety issues in the home environment would you need to assess with regard to Teresa's toddler and grandmother (Meet Your Patients)? The overview of home safety hazards in this section should help you answer this question.

Except for motor vehicle accidents, most fatal accidents occur in the home. The leading causes of death in the home are poisonings, falls, fires and burns, and choking. For children, maternal mental health problems and having older siblings are associated with less safe homes (Myhre, Thoresen, Grøgaard, et al., 2012).

Poisoning

Poisoning death rates have more than quadrupled in the past 20 years. Although young children are frequent victims, the increase has been mainly adults. In many poisoning cases, the person does not die but becomes ill or suffers other effects. Poisoning exposure accounts for about 7,000 emergency department visits per day (CDC, 2010a, updated 2015).

- *Young children* are poisoned most often by improper storage of household chemicals, medicines and vitamins, and cosmetics (see Box 23-1). The use of lead in paint was banned in 1978, but lead-based paint can still be found in older homes and in toys produced in some foreign countries. Some soil (which young children often put in their mouth) contains high levels of lead. In the United States, poor, urban, and immigrant populations are at higher risk for lead exposure than are other groups.
- *Older children and adolescents* may attempt suicide by overdosing with medicines or being poisoned accidentally when experimenting with recreational or prescription drugs intended for adults.
- *Adults* experience poisonings as a result of illegal drug use or misuse or abuse of prescription drugs, especially narcotic medications, tranquilizers, and antidepressants.
- *Prescription analgesics,* or prescription painkillers, have caused deaths related to their use to reach epidemic levels in the past decade, greater than deaths from heroin and cocaine combined. A big part of the problem is nonmedical use—using pain medications without a prescription or using them just for the high they cause. A 2014 survey found

BOX 23-1 ■ Poisonous Agents Commonly Ingested by Children

- Household cleansers, including oven cleaner, drain cleaner, toilet bowl cleaner, and furniture polish
- Medicines, including cough and cold preparations, vitamins, pain medications, antidepressants, anticonvulsants, and iron tablets, which to children may look like candies
- Indoor houseplants, including poinsettia, dieffenbachia, philodendron, and many others
- Cosmetics, hair relaxer, nail products, mouthwash
- Pesticides
- Kerosene, gasoline, lighter fluid, paint thinner, lamp oil, antifreeze, windshield washer fluid, lighter fluid, and other chemicals
- Alcoholic beverages
- Wild plants and mushrooms
- Pesticides, rodent poisons

that there were 4.3 million current nonmedical users of painkillers (National Safety Council, 2016).

- *Treatment choice* depends on the poison ingested. For most poisonings, the most effective intervention is professional administration of activated charcoal orally or via gastric tube. However, charcoal is not effective for ethanol, alkali, iron, boric acid, lithium, methanol, or cyanide. Depending on the situation, other options for medical treatment include gastric lavage, dialysis, administration of antidotes, and forced diuresis.

Carbon Monoxide Exposure

Carbon monoxide (CO) is a colorless, tasteless, odorless toxic gas. Exposure can cause headaches, weakness, nausea, and vomiting; prolonged exposure leads to seizures, dysrhythmias, unconsciousness, brain damage, and death. Each year in the United States, CO poisoning causes approximately 500 unintentional deaths (Sircar, Clower, Shin, et al., 2015).

- Most CO exposures occur at home.
- Most CO exposures involve females, children under the age of 17 years, and adults aged 18 to 44 years.
- CO poisoning accounts for the majority of deaths at the scene of fires and is also a relatively common method of suicide.
- Many CO deaths occur during cold weather among older adults and the poor who seek nonconventional heat sources (e.g., gas ranges and ovens) to stay warm.

Scalds and Burns

The following are common causes of scalds and burns:

- *Scald injuries* (e.g., from hot water, steam, or grease) are the most common cause of burns in children younger than age 3. Scalding burns (especially on both feet or both hands) and cigarette burns in children and vulnerable older adults should always prompt you to assess for abuse (see Procedure 9-1).
- *Warming food or formula in the microwave* may cause the food to become hotter than intended, leading to burns in infants and young children.
- *Sunburn* can cause a first- or second-degree burn.
- *Contact burns* may occur from contact with metal surfaces and vinyl seats when cars are parked in the sun. The risk of contact burns in all age-groups is greater in the presence of heating devices such as kerosene heaters, wood-burning stoves, and home sauna heating elements. People may use these as heat sources when they cannot afford the cost of traditional furnace fuels.
- *Chemical agents,* such as acid, alkali, or other organic compounds, can also cause localized burns.

Fires

Home fires are a major cause of death and injury. Older adults and children under age 5 have the greatest risk of fire death. *Cooking fires* are the number one cause of home fires and home fire injuries. Most *fatal home fires* occur while people are asleep, and most fire-related deaths occur from smoke inhalation. The following are other common causes of fire in the home:

- *Smoking* (e.g., cigarettes) is the leading cause of fatal home fires.
- *Heating equipment* is equally responsible during the winter.
- *Home oxygen administration equipment*—in 75% of the home fires involving oxygen, smoking materials are the ignition source.
- *Other causes of fire* include unsupervised children playing with matches, improper use of candles, and faulty wiring.

Example Problem: Falls

Falls are the third leading cause of injury-related deaths—the leading cause for older adults. An average of 4 in 100 people experience a nonfatal fall for which they seek medical advice. More than half of all falls occur in the home, and about 80% of home falls involve people aged 65 years and older. The rate triples for adults older than 75 years (Adams, Barnes, & Vickerie, 2008). See the Example Problem: Falls, later in the chapter, for more information.

Firearm Injuries

Gun ownership is a controversial issue, so keep that in mind when you address patients. Some people keep guns in the home for protection and/or recreation (e.g., hunting, target shooting). However, guns are a source of unintentional injury and death. Gun safety and security are especially important when there are children or someone in the home who abuses substances. Household access to firearms has been implicated as a risk factor for youth and domestic homicide, as well as unintentional injury (Fowler, Dahlberg, Haileyesus, et al., 2015; Weinberger, Hoyt, Lawrence, et al., 2015). Because of the frequency and severity of unintentional firearm injuries involving children, the American Academy of Pediatrics and other groups have mounted efforts to educate parents about firearm safety.

ThinkLike a Nurse 23-1

- What are some initial questions you might ask Teresa (Meet Your Patients) regarding the home environment?
- What are some basic interventions you might suggest to Teresa to help childproof her home? To answer this question, you will need to recall information about:
  Safety hazards that we encounter in the home
  Developmental and lifestyle factors that affect safety
  Specific nursing activities that can be used to prevent accidents or injuries related to the environmental hazards (e.g., firearms)

Suffocation/Asphyxiation

Suffocation by smothering is the leading cause of death for infants younger than 1 year. Suffocation may be caused by drowning, choking on a foreign object, or inhaling gas or smoke.

- *Infants*—Suffocation of infants is often related to bed or crib hazards, such as excess bedding or pillows, or toys hung from long ribbons inside the infant's crib. Infants can become entangled in cords from window blinds or in the ribbon or string used to hang a pacifier around an infant's neck.
- *Ages 1 to 18 years*—Drowning is an important cause of accidental death in children age 1 to 18 years. **KEY POINT:** *Children up to age 4 years are especially at risk for drowning.*
- *Nonfatal incidents*—Food items (e.g., hot dogs, raw vegetables, popcorn, hard candies, nuts, and grapes) are responsible for most nonfatal choking.
- *Fatal incidents*—Nonfood items (e.g., latex balloons and plastic bags) cause the majority of suffocation deaths in young children.

KnowledgeCheck 23-2

- What are the most common poisonous agents ingested by children?
- Name one source of CO (carbon monoxide) poisoning.

Take-Home Toxins

Take-home toxins are hazardous substances transported from the workplace to the home. The National Institute for Occupational Safety and Health (NIOSH) reports that pathogenic microorganisms, asbestos, lead, mercury, arsenic, pesticides, caustic farm products, and dozens of other agents cause significant morbidity and mortality in workers' homes (NIOSH, 2003, updated 2014). These toxins are most likely transported on the workers themselves, on their clothing, or on objects brought from the workplace. In the home, contamination occurs via any of three sources:

- Direct skin-to-skin contact or direct contact with contaminated clothing
- Arthropod vectors, such as ticks
- On dust particles that are inhaled (e.g., anthrax spores, arsenic in mine and smelter dust)

SAFETY HAZARDS IN THE COMMUNITY

This section discusses four hazardous agents: motor vehicle accidents, pathogens, pollution, and weather hazards. These are a major contributor to illness, disability, and death worldwide.

Motor Vehicle Accidents

Motor vehicle accidents (MVAs) are a leading cause of accidental death in the United States. Teens and young adults aged 15 to 29 years accounted for 38% of the Emergency Room visits for treatment of injuries following an accident (Bergen, Peterson, Ederer, et al., 2014). Older drivers are at higher risk of being injured or killed in a car crash. Every day, on average 500 people over age 65 are injured in an automobile accident.

- *Failure to use seat belts* and proper child car seats are the major contributing factors.
- *Air bag deployment* when young children are improperly placed in the front passenger seat also causes severe injuries and death.
- *Driver distraction*, especially due to cell phone use is a major concern. In most states, laws curtail or ban cell phone use while driving. However, a survey of drivers revealed at that 21% of respondents in the UK and 69% in the United States had done so at least once in the previous 30 days. Drivers who had read or sent emails at least once in the past 30 days ranged from 15% in Spain to 31% in Portugal and the United States ("Mobile Device Use," 2013).
- *Other risk factors* for MVAs and related injuries and deaths include speed, alcohol, and nonuse of motorcycle helmets.

Pathogens

A **pathogen** is any microorganism capable of causing an illness. Pathogens can enter the body through several sources in the environment: food, mosquitoes, and other insects; rodents and other animals; and unclean water.

Food-Borne Pathogens

Food poisoning is a nonspecific term that describes illness caused by ingesting bacteria and other microorganisms, or their toxins, in food.

- Improper food storage and preparation are a major cause of food poisoning.
- Raw foods are commonly associated with food-borne illness, for example raw meat, poultry, eggs, shellfish, raw fruits and vegetables, and unpasteurized milk and fruit juice.
- Poisonous chemicals in the environment, such as mercury, arsenic, zinc, and potassium chlorate, may also contaminate foods.

Vector-Borne Pathogens

Vectors are organisms that transmit pathogenic bacteria, viruses, and protozoa from one host to another. The following are examples:

Mosquitoes The severity of the reaction to a mosquito bite depends on the degree of allergy to the mosquito's saliva. In addition to the discomfort caused by bites, infected mosquitoes can transmit diseases such as West Nile virus and malaria. They can also transmit parasites to domestic animals (e.g., canine heartworm, equine encephalitis).

Other Insects Other insects, such as roaches, fleas, sand flies, lice, and ticks (which are, technically, arachnids and not insects) can also transmit serious diseases and produce a wide variety of allergens. Allergic sensitivity to cockroaches, for example, is a predictive factor for asthma severity (Salo, Jaramillo, Rose, et al., 2015).

Animals Structural defects in a building (e.g., roofs and walls) permit entry of birds, rodents, and other small animals, and dead spaces in walls permit their circulation among apartments in multiunit dwellings. Rodents and other animals can also act as vectors and allergens. Examples include the following:

- Rabies can be spread through the bite of a rabid animal.
- Some fungal diseases can spread via the inhalation of bird droppings.
- Mouse proteins have been implicated in the occurrence of asthma.

Water-Borne Pathogens

Sanitation refers to measures to promote and establish favorable health conditions, especially those related to the community's water supply. People who live in substandard housing may not have safe drinking water, hot water for washing, or adequate methods of waste disposal. People in rural areas often depend on private wells, which may not be adequately maintained and tested for pathogens such as *Giardia lamblia*, *Cryptosporidium*, and *Escherichia coli*. These are primarily community health problems.

Pollution

Pollution is any harmful chemical or waste material discharged into the air, water, or soil. Examples of pollutants are gaseous fumes, asbestos, carbon monoxide, and cigarette smoke. Each year Americans generate 254 million tons of trash. Of this, they recycle or compost about 87 million tons (U.S. Environmental Protection Agency [EPA], 2015).

Air Pollution occurs indoors as well as outside.

- *Outdoor air pollution*—Motor vehicle emissions are a major cause in the United States. Other toxic outdoor air pollutants include asbestos, toluene; metals such as mercury and lead compounds, and emissions from sources such as factories and power plants.
- *Indoor pollutants* include radon, carbon monoxide, and allergens from dust mites, cockroaches, mold, rodents, and pets.

  Passive exposure to tobacco smoke is associated with respiratory disease and cancer, and environmental air pollution is linked to cardiovascular disease and respiratory viral infection (Kit, Simon, Brody, et al., 2013; U.S. Department of Health and Human Services, 2014).

Water Contamination Contamination in lakes, rivers, and streams affects both recreation and food production. Pollution occurs when inadequately treated or inappropriate quantities of human, industrial, or agricultural wastes are released into the water systems. If the pollution is severe enough, the water may become unsafe for human consumption.

Noise Substantial exposure to noise is associated with various adverse health effects, including hearing loss, stress, elevated blood pressure, and loss of sleep. Noise is pervasive in our society, caused by, among other sources, road traffic, airplanes, garbage trucks, construction equipment, lawn mowers, and loud music. People who live or work near major roads, bus depots, airports, and trucking routes are at greater risk, as are those in certain work environments (e.g., railroad workers).

Soil Improper waste disposal and excessive use of pesticides can contaminate soil. Agricultural, industrial, and manufacturing processes create solid and toxic waste. Animal, radioactive, and medical wastes pose special problems. Household products (e.g., paints, cleaners, oils, batteries, and pesticides) contain corrosive or toxic ingredients that contaminate the environment when disposed of improperly.

Weather Hazards

More than 1,000 people die each year in the United States as a result of weather hazards. The most likely killer is heat. The number of deaths caused by lightning, tornadoes, and hurricanes has fallen steadily during the 21st century, and deaths related to floods have declined because of advances in technology and warning systems (National Weather Service, 2015). For additional information about weather hazards,

 Go to the Web site of the Surgeon General and view National Hazard Statistics at http://www.surgeongeneral.gov/library/reports/50-years-of-progress/consumer-guide.pdf

KnowledgeCheck 23-3

- What are the major causes of injuries from MVAs?
- List at least three tips for preventing food poisoning.
- List three sources of noise pollution.

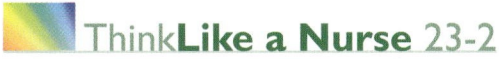 **ThinkLike a Nurse** 23-2

Identify an environmental problem in your neighborhood. What are some possible solutions?

SAFETY HAZARDS IN THE HEALTHCARE FACILITY

The Institute of Medicine (IOM) (1999) estimated that as many as 98,000 people die as a result of medical injuries each year in U.S. hospitals. The estimated number of deaths has grown over time to more 400,000 people each year as a result of medical errors, which are the third leading cause of death in the United States (Leap Frog Group, 2015). This increase may be due in part to better reporting and measuring of outcomes.

Healthcare facilities embody several safety hazards for residents and workers. We have already discussed the hazard of infection in Chapter 22. Box 23-2 lists The Joint Commission's National Patient Safety Goals for 2016, which should give you an idea of the types of accidents that occur in healthcare agencies. If you would like to see a full explanation of the patient safety goals,

 Go to the Web site of The Joint Commission at https://www.jointcommission.org/standards_information/npsgs.aspx

BOX 23-2 ■ The Joint Commission 2016 Patient Safety Goals

For a full understanding of TJC Patient Safety Goals,

 Go to http://www.jointcommission.org/

Goal 1. Identify patients correctly.
Goal 2. Improve staff communication.
Goal 3. Use medicines safely.
Goal 6. Use alarms safely.
Goal 7. Prevent infection.
Goal 15. Identify patient safety risks (specifically, suicide risk).
***UP 1.** Prevent mistakes in surgery.

***Universal Protocol (UP 1):** "Prevent mistakes in surgery" is a preprocedure verification process to make sure that all documents, information, and equipment are available, and that the correct procedure is performed on the correct person and site.

Source: Adapted from The Joint Commission. (2015). The Joint Commission: Accreditation program, Hospital. National patient safety goals (effective January 1, 2016). Retrieved from http://www.jointcommission.org/assets/1/6/2016_NPSG_HAP_ER.pdf

Organizational factors contribute to errors and to safety problems in healthcare, including the following:
- Poor design
- Maintenance failures
- Unworkable procedures
- Shortfalls in training
- Less than adequate tools and equipment
- Inadequate staffing
- Disruptive behavior and intimidation in the workplace
- Culture of disrespect among healthcare professionals

Healthcare Culture Healthcare has traditionally been a hierarchy with the physician at the top. However, healthcare professionals, including nurses, have been taught to practice with autonomy. This combination of factors sets the stage for a culture that does not respond well to questions about possible problems with patient care, particularly from subordinates. It is clear that such a culture needs to be repaired, and many healthcare organizations are working to address disrespectful behavior, staff reluctance to speak up about risks and errors, and blatant disregard of expressed concerns.

Quality Nursing Care **KEY POINT:** *Because nurses are the healthcare professionals who spend the greatest amount of time with patients, research documents what physicians, patients, and nurses themselves have long known: The quality of nursing care affects patient health and outcomes and sometimes can be a matter of life and death.* In providing quality care and patient safety, nurses are indispensable. Studies have shown that:
- Greater numbers of patient deaths are associated with fewer nurses to provide care (Aiken, Clarke, Sloane, et al., 2001; Brennan, Daly, & Jones, 2013; Kutney-Lee & Aiken, 2015).
- Less nursing time provided to patients is associated with higher rates of infection, gastrointestinal bleeding, pneumonia, cardiac arrest, and death from these and other causes (Kalisch, Tschannen, & Lee, 2012; Stimpfel & Aiken, 2013; Unruh & Zhang, 2012).

What Are Never Events?

Never events, also known as **Serious Reportable Events (SREs),** are healthcare-acquired complications that (1) can cause serious injury or death to a patient and (2) should *never* happen in a hospital. The list of never events has been expanded over time to mean events that are (1) clearly identifiable and measurable, (2) serious, and (3) usually are prevented. You can gain insight into healthcare facility hazards by examining the following list of never events (National Quality Forum, 2011). Be aware that this list may grow and change more over time.

- Foreign object (such as a sponge) left in patients after surgery
- Air embolism
- Administering the wrong type of blood
- Severe pressure injuries
- Falls and trauma
- Infections associated with urinary catheters
- Infections associated with intravenous catheters
- Symptoms resulting from poorly controlled blood sugar levels
- Surgical site infections following certain elective procedures (e.g., certain orthopedic surgeries, bariatric surgery for obesity)
- Deep vein thrombosis or pulmonary embolism following total knee and total hip replacement procedures.

The Institute for Healthcare Improvement (IHI) (n.d.b), an independent, not-for-profit organization, recently completed the 5 Million Lives Campaign as a follow-up to its 100,000 Lives Campaign. The IHI Campaign recommended healthcare changes to reduce morbidity and death in American healthcare. At least three of the 5 Million Lives goals supported the list of never events: Prevent adverse drug events, prevent central line infections, and prevent surgical site infections. To read the entire list of recommendations and the results of the campaign,

 Go to the IHI Web site at http://www.ihi.org/engage/initiatives/completed/5MillionLivesCampaign/Pages/default.aspx

 Think**Like a Nurse** 23-3

Many never events can be reduced by good nursing care. By preventing complications and maximizing reimbursement, nurses can prove their value to an organization and make the case for better staffing. Over which of the never events do you think nurses have the most control? Explain your thinking.

Understanding Errors in Healthcare: Root Cause Analysis

Root cause analysis (RCA) tries to solve problems by identifying and correcting the underlying causes of events as opposed to simply addressing their symptoms. The goal is to decrease the likelihood that the problem will recur. A root cause is typically a finding related not to individual error but to a process or system that has a potential for redesign to reduce risk. Therefore, a root cause finding is usually used for the purpose of redesigning a process or system, rather than preventing an individual error. RCA provides an organized structure for analysis of errors and is designed to answer three basic questions:

1. What happened?
2. Why did it happen?
3. What can be done to prevent it from happening again?

Toward Evidence-Based Practice

Compton, J., Copeland, K., Flanders, S., et al. (2012). **Implementing SBAR across a large multihospital health system.** *Joint Commission Journal on Quality and Patient Safety,* 38(6), 261–268.

Researchers assessed by survey (1) nurses' use of SBAR (Situation, Background, Assessment, and Recommendations) standardized communication tool and (2) physician perception of communication quality after SBAR implementation. More than half of nurses who participated in the study already used SBAR for critical communication. Findings indicated that:

- 72.6% of nurses demonstrated good or high proficiency with SBAR.
- Of 155 physicians, 78.1% said that the last report they received was adequate to make clinical decisions.
- Of the 27 physicians who indicated that the last report was not adequate, 25 had not received the report in SBAR format.

Vardaman, J., Cornell, P., Gondo, M., et al. (2012). **Beyond communication: The role of standardized protocols in a changing health care environment.** *Health Care Management Review,* 37(1), 88.

A qualitative case study of two hospitals collected data from 80 interviews with nurses, nurse managers, and physicians. Results indicated that in addition to standardizing communication among nurses and physicians, SBAR may:

- Aid in rapid decision making by nurses, leading to better patient outcomes.
- Provide a tool for less-tenured nurses to feel confident in communication.

1. Identify a recent interaction you have had in which communication was difficult. What issues specific to the healthcare setting may encourage communication difficulties?

2. Communication problems among healthcare personnel can jeopardize patient safety. SBAR, a structured-communication technique, has been adapted from aviation and the military as a strategy for clear communication based on a statement of the Situation, Background, Assessment, and Recommendations related to a clinical issue. Based on the findings from each of the studies, identify specific ways that the use SBAR can impact patient safety.

 Go to Davis Advantage, Resources, Chapter 23, **Toward Evidence-Based Practice—Suggested Responses.**

The Joint Commission requires healthcare agencies to perform RCA for all unexpected occurrences involving death or serious physical or psychological injury, also known as **sentinel events.**

Culture of Safety

A positive nursing unit culture helps improve patient outcomes. Culture is a way of thinking, behaving, or working in a place or organization. **KEY POINT:** *In a culture of safety, nurses practice in an environment where all staff work together to create a safe unit, disclose errors without fear, and address any safety concerns.* Key components of a culture of safety include (Helbling & Huwe, 2015):

- *Team empowerment.* Every individual has the opportunity to be heard, feel important, and be a valued team member for the contribution offered.
- *Communication.* Open and honest lines of communication are needed between the team members and from the team to other hospital units.
- *Transparency.* Team members are united in their efforts to eliminate rumors and operate with only the facts, contributing to mutual team goals.
- *Accountability.* Staff claim ownership for human error and are willing to disclose the error and help prevent similar errors

Also refer to the accompanying iCare box.

High Reliability Organizations High reliability industries are everywhere; most people just don't realize it—they range from amusement parks and zoos to oil drilling rigs, air

traffic control, and nuclear submarines. **High reliability** is the ongoing safe operation of an organization without a mishap or adverse event (Chassin & Loeb, 2013). The concept has been slow to catch on in the healthcare industry. In healthcare, being a high reliability organization means having *no preventable harm incidents and causing no harm to patients* (The Joint Commission Center for Transforming Health Care, n.d.). High reliability is an ongoing journey, not a one-time achievement. It is a commitment to a culture of patient safety and quality healthcare.

Example Problem: Falls

Although most falls occur in the home, they are a major concern in healthcare facilities as well. Falls are by far the most common incident reported in hospitals and long-term care facilities. As a result, most agencies have established procedures and safety features to prevent falls.

Infants and older adults are especially at risk for injury from falls. Many cases involve falling from a bed, and falls occur more frequently at night and on weekends and holidays. For risk factors, see the Example Problem: Falls, later in the chapter.

Equipment-Related Accidents

Equipment-related accidents usually occur because of equipment malfunction or improper use—for example, when suction devices and infusion pumps are not working properly, oxygen cylinders are transported incorrectly, or wheelchairs and beds are not locked during transfer activities.

Alarm Fatigue

"Failure to recognize and respond to actionable clinical alarms. . . in a timely manner" is second highest-ranked patient safety risk (ECRI Institute, 2016). Missed alarms cause harm most commonly when (1) the medical device does not detect the alarm condition, (2) the alarm is not communicated to a medical practitioner, or (3) it is communicated but not adequately addressed.

Thousands of alarms go off every day in hospitals. **Alarm fatigue** occurs when nurses become overwhelmed by the number of alarm signals and begin to ignore, delay response to alarms, or even deactivate them. Missed alarms or delayed responses have resulted in sentinel events, including patient deaths. The Joint Commission has named alarm desensitization a National Patient Safety Goal and requires that healthcare facilities provide the following:

- A comprehensive alarm management program that includes input from nurses, other healthcare workers, and management
- Education for staff about the purpose and proper operation of alarms systems for which they are responsible (The Joint Commission, 2015)

Fires and Electrical Hazards

Fire in a healthcare agency is more often related to anesthesia or improperly grounded or malfunctioning electrical equipment than to smoking. Most healthcare agencies have policies for preventing electrical hazards. Nevertheless, patients and visitors do break the rules, so smoking cannot be discounted as a hazard.

When a fire occurs, an announcement is made over the communication system. Often, words such as "Code Red" or "Code Yellow" are used in an effort to prevent panic among patients and visitors. The announcement may ask visitors to leave the building.

♥ iCare 23-1

Caring Is Creating a Culture of Safety

Safety is a basic need for all persons. Your commitment to safety is one way for you to show caring. As the person closest to and most constantly with the patient, you can facilitate a culture of safety by:

- Speaking up for Safety. Use CUS words:
  - C—state your concern
  - U—say why you are uncomfortable
  - S—state "this is a safety issue"; explain how and why
- Stopping the line (e.g. calling for a pre-procedure "time-out" when there is a concern)
- Escalating the safety issue when needed, communicating through the appropriate chain of command
- Being open and transparent with patients/families/colleagues
- Participating in *safety huddles* (quick conversations with a focus on safety)
- Opening all meetings with the topic of Safety, allowing time for stories/concerns
- Using SBAR (Situation, Background, Assessment, Recommendation) communication
- Validating and Verifying when unsure (have second nurse check)
- *200% accountability* (calling other nurses or healthcare disciplines on hand washing or use of personal protective equipment)
- Reporting both actual and "near miss" medication errors, policy deviations, treatment and outcome variations and adverse events
- Participating in your organizations Patient and Caregiver Safety committee

Restraints

A **restraint** is a device or method used for the purpose of restricting a patient's freedom of movement or access to his body, with or without his permission. The most obvious form of restraint is the use of physical force by another person. A restraint may also be (1) a mechanical device, material, or equipment, such as a cloth vest or siderails; or (2) a chemical restraint (e.g., sedatives and psychotropic medications) given to control disruptive behavior.

- **Devices such as casts and traction are not considered restraints** (Centers for Medicare & Medicaid Services, 2008; The Joint Commission, 2009).
- **Physical holding of a patient is not always considered restraint.** Sometimes it is necessary to use devices or methods that involve the physical holding of a patient for routine physical examinations or tests.
- **Restraints are classified according to the reason for their use:** medical–surgical restraints or behavior management restraints. Medicare has specific guidelines for each circumstance. Guidelines are more restrictive when restraints are used for behavior management.

Nurses traditionally restrained highly dependent older adults, patients with poor mobility, and impaired cognition, and others they judged to be at risk for falls. However, it has been found that restraints make care more time consuming and do not reduce falls. Restraints are themselves a safety hazard, and actually increase the likelihood of injury.

✚ A restrained person has a natural tendency to struggle and try to remove the restraint. As a result, the person can become entangled, suffer nerve damage or circulatory impairment, and even suffocate.

- *Potential Physical Effects.* Restraint-imposed immobility can cause pressure injuries, contractures, and loss of strength and affect nearly every body system.
- *Potential Emotional Effects.* The person may suffer anger, fear, humiliation, and diminished self-esteem.

Restraint Free Environments

Research indicates that less restraint use saves time and money and reduces patient injuries (Chan, LeBel, & Webber, 2012; Cleary & Prescott, 2015). The American Nurses Association and other healthcare organizations have established evidence-based guidelines. These show that a restraint-free environment is the standard of care. When the decision is made to avoid restraints, alternatives must be provided for keeping the patient safe.

    KEY POINT: *Restraints never resolve the underlying problem; addressing the reason behind the patient's behavior is key to calming the patient (Said & Kautz, 2013).*

To provide the safest possible care environment, The Joint Commission encourages healthcare facilities to do the following:

- Promote a commitment to reduce the use of restraints and seclusion among all direct-care staff.
- Educate caregivers before they take part in any restraint-related activity.
- Document restraint episodes specifically, in detail.
- Maintain one-to-one viewing of patients in restraint and seclusion.
- Include staff members when deciding whether to explore new technology that is considered a safe alternative to traditional restraint devices.
- Budget for an adequate number of qualified staff to attend to patients.

Restraint Is Sometimes Necessary

Organization guidelines differ slightly, depending on whether restraints are used to support medical healing or for a behavioral health reason (e.g., when a patient is irrational and pulling out his intravenous [IV] lines). Use restraints only as a last resort. Better anticipation of patient needs and the use of technology (such as bed alarms) should be used instead of restraints.

✚ If you must use restraints, Medicare, The Joint Commission, and other regulators require both of the following:

- Restraints must be medically prescribed.
- You must first try all less restrictive interventions.

Do Not Depend on Siderails

Based on Medicare standards, siderails can be viewed as a restraint.

- *A full-length siderail* is a restraint when it is used to prevent the patient from getting out of bed regardless of whether he is able to do so safely.
- *A half- or quarter-length upper siderail* can be an aid to independence if it is used by the patient for the purpose of getting into and out of bed.
- *Split rails* are not considered restraints if a client requests them in order to feel more secure.

Remember that older or cognitively impaired adults may regard siderails as a barrier rather than as a reminder that they need assistance. **KEY POINT:** *Several studies have shown that siderails may lead to serious falls and injuries.* These findings have led healthcare providers to recommend that siderails not be used routinely (Cleary & Prescott, 2015; Kirk, McGlinsey, Beckett, et al., 2015).

KnowledgeCheck 23-4

- What is a typical cause of fire in healthcare facilities?
- What measures should you take, and in what order, if a fire occurs in the hospital?

Mercury Exposure

Mercury is a heavy, odorless, silver-white liquid metal. Mercury is toxic in both acute and chronic exposure. It can be inhaled, ingested, or absorbed through the skin. It accumulates in muscle tissue and can cause renal and neurological disorders, especially in fetuses and neonates. Because of its shiny color and ability to form beads or balls, mercury is appealing to curious children. See Table 23-3 for potential health effects.

Products containing mercury include thermometers, thermostats, batteries, fluorescent light bulbs, blood pressure devices, and electrical equipment and switches.

Since 1998, the American Hospital Association and the EPA have sponsored a program to eliminate mercury-containing waste in the healthcare industry and prevent it from entering the environment via incinerators, landfills, and wastewater.

- *Thermometers and Sphygmomanometers.* Mercury thermometers are no longer being made in the United States. However, some people may still have them in their homes. Most, but not all, healthcare facilities have eliminated mercury thermometers and sphygmomanometers. Some hospitals conduct thermometer exchanges, providing free or low-cost nonmercury thermometers to anyone who brings in a mercury thermometer.
- *Mercury Spills.* Healthcare facilities must have policies and procedures for hazardous waste spills, as required by

Table 23-3 ➤ Potential Health Effects of Mercury

PRIMARY ROUTE	POTENTIAL HEALTH EFFECTS
Acute Effects	
Toxicity	Symptoms of chills, nausea, malaise, chest tightness and pain, dyspnea, coughing, stomatitis, gingivitis, excess salivation, and diarrhea. High levels can cause severe respiratory irritation, digestive disturbances, and severe renal damage.
Inhalation	Respiratory damage, wakefulness, muscle weakness, anorexia, headache, ringing in the ears, chest pain, inflammation of the mouth, and pneumonitis
Eye	Irritation and corrosion
Skin	Irritation and allergic dermatitis
Ingestion	Intestinal obstruction
Chronic Effects	
Primarily central nervous system	Numbness or tingling of the hands, lips, and feet; behavior and personality changes
Other	Fatigue, weakness, anorexia, weight loss, and gastrointestinal disturbances

The Joint Commission, the EPA, the Occupational Safety and Health Administration (OSHA). You are not likely to encounter mercury exposure in acute care and ambulatory agencies.

Biological Hazards

As a nurse, you will place a high priority on the biological safety of patients. Institutionalized patients are at especially high risk from infectious microorganisms, some of which are highly resistant to antibiotics. To learn about or review healthcare-related infections, asepsis, and infection control, refer to Chapter 22.

Hazards to Healthcare Workers

Nursing is an active profession, and workplace injuries are all too common. Common accidents include back injuries, needlestick injuries, radiation injury, and violence.

Nurses sometimes hesitate to report an injury because they fear consequences such as being labeled a complainer or troublemaker or being denied opportunities for promotion. However, OSHA (1) requires that employers show employees how to report a workplace injury and (2) prohibits discrimination against employees who make such reports.

➕ You should always report an injury. By doing so, you help (1) pinpoint trends and areas of need in safety and (2) ensure you will receive necessary treatment and follow-up.

Back Injury

Nursing personnel are consistently listed in the top 10 occupations for work-related musculoskeletal disorders (MSDs). Most often the MSD involves the shoulders and back (Bureau of Labor Statistics, 2012). The ANA reports that 52% of nurses report chronic back pain (ANA, 2013), likely because many nursing tasks require bending and twisting of the torso, activities that can cause injury when the nurse does not use correct body mechanics. Among the most stressful activities are transferring patients (e.g., from toilet to chair),

weighing patients, lifting a patient in bed, repositioning patients in beds or chairs, and changing bed linens.

Healthcare facilities have not consistently implemented safe patient handling guidelines and laws. In response, the ANA (2013) developed national standards to guide healthcare agencies in this regard. The ANA aims to:

- Create a culture of safety by requiring employers to develop a safe handling and moving program with policies, appropriate equipment, training and accommodations for injured employees.
- Empower nurses to (1) actively participate in creating and implementing safe handling measures and (2) promptly report hazards, incidents, and injuries in a "blame free" environment.

Refer to Chapter 33 for information about body mechanics and how to safely lift and move patients. For more information about ANA's campaign to prevent musculoskeletal injuries,

 Go to the ANA's Safe Patient Handling Web site at http://nursingworld.org/MainMenuCategories/WorkplaceSafety/Healthy-Work-Environment/SafePatient

Needlestick Injury

Healthcare workers, mostly nurses and housekeeping staff, suffer up to 1 million injuries per year from needles and other sharps, putting them at risk for infectious diseases, such as hepatitis B and AIDS. The operating room is a high-risk area; surgeons experience about a quarter of all "sharps" injuries (Waljee, Sunitha, & Chung, 2013).

The federal Needlestick Safety and Prevention Act and OSHA standards require employers to maintain a log of sharps injuries and to purchase needleless systems and safer medical and needle devices. Needlestick injuries declined by more than 36% during the 3-year period following passage of that law. Nevertheless, OSHA (2013) estimates that each year 385,000 needlestick injuries and other sharps-related injuries occur. This is an average of approximately 1,000 sharps injuries per day in U.S. hospitals. The risk of needlestick injury increases for nurses who:

- Work in stressful environments
- Work varying or long shifts (12 consecutive hours or longer)
- Have low skill level, based on education or experience

Other risk factors include a lack of protective equipment, recapping needles and working in an area that requires higher than average use of needles.

Although OSHA has fined hospitals for noncompliance, some employers still have not complied completely with the regulations. For suggestions about how you can prevent needlestick injuries, see Clinical Insight 23-1.

Radiation Injury

Radiation is the process of emitting radiant energy in the form of waves or particles. Ionizing radiation is used in computerized tomography (CT scans) in diagnostic radiology, linear accelerators in radiotherapy, and positron emission tomography (PET scans) in nuclear medicine. Patients are deliberately exposed to radiation during diagnostic tests and certain medical treatments. Healthcare workers who care for these patients are unavoidably exposed to small doses of radiation.

Take precautions to avoid excessive radiation exposure for the patient and yourself during x-ray procedures. **KEY POINT:** *Follow the principles of time, distance, and shielding when caring for a patient who is being treated with an internal radioactive implant:*

- **Time:** Organize nursing care to limit the amount of time with the patient.
- **Distance:** Perform near the patient only the nursing care that is absolutely necessary.
- **Shielding:** Wear protective shielding (e.g., a lead apron), if available. If you deliver care that regularly exposes you to radiation, wear a film badge to indicate any radiation exposure.

Violence

The impact of violent acts on healthcare workers is widespread and results in injuries, higher-than-average staff turnover, increased requests for medical leaves, unusually high levels of time-off and attendance issues, and stress-related illnesses (Papa & Venella, 2013). Hospital security may not be sufficient to protect you from injury if violence breaks out among patients, visitors, and/or staff. This is especially true in the following situations:

- **A crowded or chaotic environment**—For example, the emergency department (ED), which has 24-hour accessibility, is often both crowded and chaotic.
- **Anxiety and anger**—Under the stress of an acute illness, patients and family members may become anxious and angry and act out in unpredictable ways. **KEY POINT:** *Violence typically begins with anxiety and escalates in stages through verbal aggression and then physical aggression. If you can relieve a patient's anxiety, you may be able to halt the progression to physical violence.*
- **Certain emotional and physical conditions**—These often increase the risk for patient aggression (refer to Assessing the Risk for Violence).
- **Gang activity**—Now widespread in many U.S. cities, gang activity is another potential source of violence. As gangs increase, so does the likelihood that gang members will be treated in the ED or admitted to the hospital (Gillespie, Gates, & Berry, 2013; Taylor & Rew, 2011).

PracticalKnowledge
knowing how

This section provides focused safety assessments, general interventions for addressing patient safety, and specific nursing interventions for safety hazards discussed in the preceding Theoretical Knowledge section.

ASSESSMENT NP

It is important to assess the client's immediate environment, developmental stage, and individual risk factors. The following will help you to perform focused assessments for falls risk, home safety, and risk for violence:

Assessing for Example Problem: Falls

Use of a standardized falls prevention tool has been shown to decrease fall rates (Coppedge, Conner, & Sin Fan, 2016). You will find more information in the Example Problem: Falls.

- Assess all inpatients for falls risk when they are admitted to the healthcare setting.
- For patients at risk for falls, repeat the risk assessment every 8 hours and increase the frequency of monitoring.
- Be sure to identify medications that increase the risk for falling.

Most institutions have policies and guidelines for assessing risk for falls. The following are methods you might use:

Morse Fall Scale   The Morse scale is a rapid and simple method of assessing a patient's likelihood of falling. Ideally, the scale should be calibrated specifically for each nursing unit so that fall prevention strategies are targeted to those most at risk. Institutions implementing the Morse scale should train personnel in the proper use of the scale (Morse, 1997, 2008, 2009).

The Morse Fall Scale uses the following questions to assess a person's risk for falls:

1. Does the patient have a history of falling?
2. Does the person have more than one medical diagnosis?
3. Does the person use ambulatory aids such as crutches or a walker?
4. Does the person have an IV line or a saline lock?
5. Is the person's gait normal or stooped or otherwise impaired?
6. What is the person's mental status (e.g., disoriented, forgetful)?

You can easily score, tally, and record those six variables on the patient's chart. The risk of falling varies greatly with different patient populations, different times of day, and different stages of the patient's illness. Age alone is not a predictor of falls, but the items scored by the scale are more common in older adults (Morse, 2001).

Assessing Older Adults for Falls

 As a part of the routine assessment of all older adults, ask the patient (or caregivers) about falls. For a flowchart summarizing falls assessment for older adults, refer to Figure 23-1.

EXAMPLE PROBLEM: Falls

Complications of Falls

Falls may cause serious injuries, disability, loss of independence, and even death.

Risk Factors

- History of falls
- Age > 80 years
- Impaired vision
- Weakness/dizziness
- Gait or balance problems
- Pain
- Hypotension

- Cognitive impairment
- Chronic conditions (e.g. arthritis)
- Medication side effects
- Polypharmacy
- Home hazards
- Unfamiliar environment
- Alcohol use

KEY POINT: *Clients usually have multiple risk factors.*

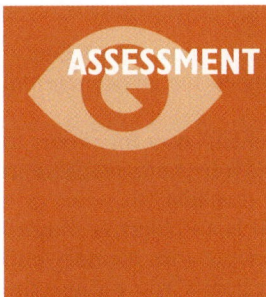

ASSESSMENT

- Identify modifiable risk factors—Different conditions require different nursing interventions.
- Ask older adult (or caregivers) about falls at least once a year.
- Use standardized tools, such as the Get Up and Go test, the Timed Up and Go test, or the Morse Fall Scale for fall risk assessment.

Get Up and Go Test Have the patient:
- Move from sitting to standing without using arms to help them rise.
- Walk several paces, turn, and return to the chair.
- Sit back in the chair without using arms for support
- If patient has difficulty, refer for a comprehensive falls assessment (see column 2).

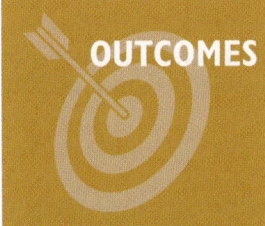

OUTCOMES

NOC Outcomes
- Balance
- Fall Prevention Behavior

Other
- Injury-free
- Maintains independence

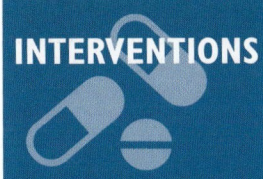

INTERVENTIONS

Nursing Care In the Home

Prevention is key!
- Teach to get up slowly to prevent a drop in BP with position change; teach what to do if dizziness occurs.
- Review medications; identify drugs that increase fall risk; explore alternatives.
- Avoid excessive alcohol.
- Review home environment for safety (remove throw rugs, cords, etc.).
- Provide gait training and advice on the safe use of assistive devices.

Teach what to do if a fall occurs!
- Don't panic.
- Stay still for a few minutes to get over the shock.
- If you think you are okay, slide over to a sturdy piece of furniture, assume a kneeling position, and push yourself up; then sit down until you recover. If you cannot move, try to cover yourself to keep warm until help arrives. Also see the Home Care box, Interventions for Example Problem: Preventing Falls in the Home.

Nursing Care in the Healthcare Facility

- Review medications, especially psychotropic medications. Modify as needed.
- Place call light within reach. Have patient demonstrate ability to call for the nurse.
- Orient patient to surroundings (e.g., bathroom, chairs); you may need to label items.
- Place disoriented patients in rooms near the nurse's station.
- Keep water, urinal, bedpan, and tissues within easy reach of patient.
- Provide a night-light.
- Keep floors dry and free of clutter.
- Teach fall prevention strategies to patient and family.
- For patients at risk for falls, place a warning sticker on the chart or door. See Box 23-3.

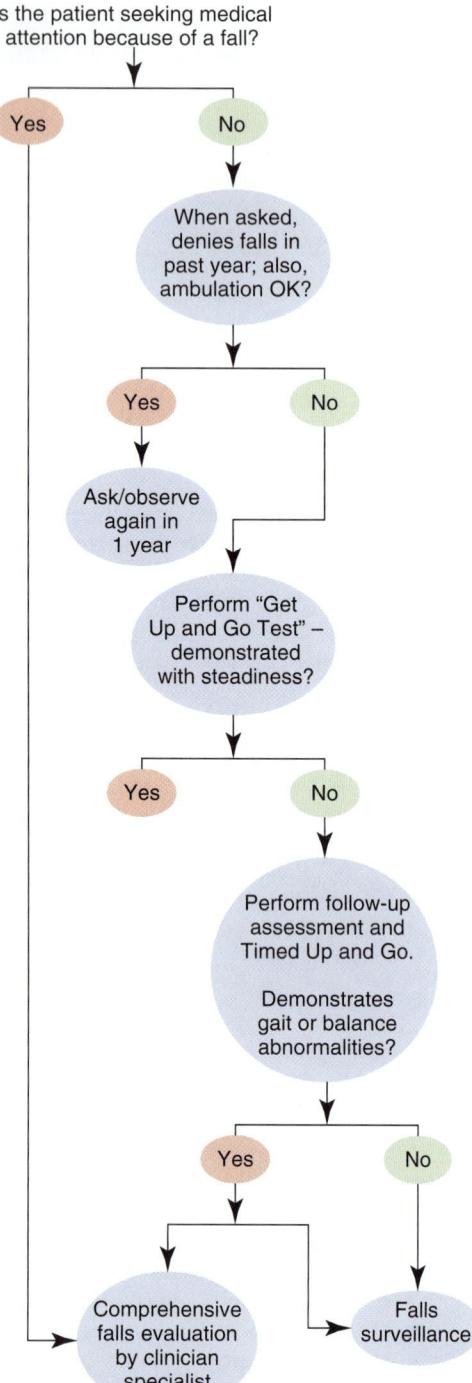

Is the patient seeking medical attention because of a fall?

Yes → No

No → When asked, denies falls in past year; also, ambulation OK?

Yes → Ask/observe again in 1 year

No → Perform "Get Up and Go Test" – demonstrated with steadiness?

Yes → (Ask/observe again in 1 year)

No → Perform follow-up assessment and Timed Up and Go.

Demonstrates gait or balance abnormalities?

Yes → Comprehensive falls evaluation by clinician specialist

No → Falls surveillance

FIGURE 23-1 Falls assessment flowchart.

Get Up and Go Test Use if there is a history of falls. If patient or caregiver reports a single fall or risk factors, conduct the Get Up and Go test to identify whether the patient needs further evaluation. Have the patient do the following:

- Move from a sitting position and stand without using his arms to help him rise and stand.
- Walk several paces, turn, and return to the chair.
- Sit back in the chair without using his arms for support.

  Those who have difficulty or demonstrate unsteadiness performing this test require a focused, comprehensive falls assessment.

Timed Up and Go Test If the patient is seeking care because of a fall or if you observe any difficulty with ambulation, refer him to a practitioner with advanced skills and experience for a Timed Up and Go test and a comprehensive fall evaluation. This is a version of the Get Up and Go test, in which the patient is asked to get up and walk 8 feet in 8.5 seconds or less. Primary care providers should annually perform a Timed Up and Go test for fall risk assessment for all patients over age 65 (American Academy of Neurology, n.d.a, n.d.b; Kenny, Rubenstein, Martin, et al., 2011; Podsiadlo & Richardson, 1991). To see the Timed Up and Go test,

 Go to the CDC Web site at http://www.cdc.gov/steadi/pdf/ tug_test-a.pdf

Assessing for Home Safety

Many accidents occur in the home (e.g., fire, poisoning). Everyone should take a few minutes to check for environmental safety hazards.

- **A home safety checklist** is a convenient way for clients to identify potential hazards. Many such lists are available in an Internet search for "home safety checklist."
- **The safety assessment scale (SAS)** is an objective way to evaluate the dangers incurred by people with memory and cognitive deficits who live alone at home. You can use the short version of the SAS (Fig. 23-2) to assess risk status and decide whether the person should have an in-depth evaluation. In addition to assessing risk for injury, this scale evaluates whether the cognitively impaired person is capable of taking medications and performing other activities of daily living (ADLs) independently.

Assessing the Risk for Violence

You can be prepared to intervene and perhaps even prevent violence if you recognize risk factors and early warning signs (Arnetz, Hamblin, Essenmacher, et al., 2015; Woodrow & Guest, 2012).

1. **Assess for factors that increase the risk for aggression:**
   - Mental disorders, such as dementia, delirium, schizophrenia, and bipolar disorder
   - Being under the influence of alcohol or other drugs
   - Withdrawal from alcohol or other drugs
   - History of violence
   - Clinical conditions such as high fever, epilepsy, head trauma, and hypoglycemia
2. **Assess for signs of anxiety:**
   - Agitation and restlessness
   - Pacing
   - Talking loudly, speaking rapidly
   - Gesturing widely
   - Verbal aggression, such as threats, sarcasm, and swearing

KnowledgeCheck 23-6

- Which assessment tool would you use for a slightly confused home care client to assess her ability to safely live alone and perform activities of daily living?
- List the six risk factors that are assessed on the Morse Fall Scale.
- How should you screen older adults to see whether they need a comprehensive falls evaluation?

Name
_____

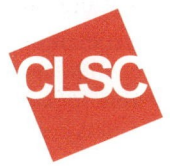 **CÔTE-DES-NEIGES**

S.A.S. **SAFETY ASSESSMENT SCALE**

CAREGIVER AND LIVING ENVIRONMENT ①

a) This person lives on her own.   Yes [1]   No [0]   _____

b) This person is alone at home.
Always [4]   Most of the time [3]   Occasionally [2]   Never [1]   _____

SMOKING ②

This person leaves cigarette bum marks on the floor, furniture or clothing.
Yes [1]   No [0]   _____

FIRE AND BURNS ③

a) The stove on/off buttons are located...
on the front of the stove [1]   on the top of the stove [2]
behind the hotplates [3]   _____

b) This person is capable of turning on the stove him/herself
Yes [1]   No [0]   Doesn't know [1]   _____

c) This person cooks his/her own food.
Always [4]   Most of the time [3]   Occasionally [2]   Never [1]   _____

d) This person forgets a pan on the stove.
Very often [4]   Often [3]   Sometimes [2]   Never [1]   _____

e) The heating system uses...
electricity [1]   natural gas [2]   wood [3]   _____

NUTRITION ④

a) This person receives meals-on-wheels or other prepared meals.
More than once a day [1]   Once a day [2]
A few times a week (2 to 6 times a week) [3]   Once a week or less [4]   _____

b) This person's meals contain foods from different food groups
(dairy products, meat or fish, cereals, fruit and vegetables).
Always [1]   Most of the time [2]   Occasionally [3]   Never [4]   _____

FOOD POISONING AND TOXIC SUBSTANCES ⑤

This person can tell the difference between food that is fresh and food
that is spoiled.   Yes [0]   No [1]   _____

MEDICATION AND HEALTH PROBLEMS ⑥

a) This person takes, on a regular basis...*
1 to 3 medications [2]   4 to 6 medications [3]
7 medications or more [4]   Does not take any medication [1]
*prescribed medications only   _____

b) This person takes medication to help him/her sleep or relax.
Yes [1]   No [0]   _____

c) Does this person suffer from any physical health problem?
None [1]   Minor [2]   Moderate [3]   Severe [4]   _____

d) This person accepts treatment for his/her physical health problems.
Yes [0]   No [1]   Does not apply [0]   _____

WANDERING AND ADAPTATION TO CHANGING TEMPERATURE ⑦

a) This person gets lost in familiar surroundings.
Very often [4]   Often [3]   Sometimes [2]   Never [1]   _____

b) Has this person ever gotten lost?   Yes [1]   No [0]   _____

c) Can this person find his/her way home?   Yes [0]   No [1]   _____

d) Does this person dress appropriately according
to the changing temperature, both indoors and outdoors?
Yes [0]   No [1]   _____

An Affiliated University Centre
Affiliated with McGill University

Assessed by _____

SCORE

47

Source: Dr. Louise Poulin de Courval ©CLSC Côte-des-Neiges. Used with permission.

FIGURE 23-2 Safety assessment scale (SAS).

ANALYSIS/NURSING DIAGNOSIS NP

A few examples of NANDA-I labels to use in describing safety problems include the following:

Hyperthermia   Risk for Injury
Hypothermia   Risk for Poisoning
Risk for Aspiration   Risk for Suffocation
Risk for Contamination Risk for Physical Trauma
Risk for Falls

KEY POINT: *Use the diagnosis Risk for Injury only when the risk cannot be described by one of the more specific nursing diagnoses.*

Etiologies How would your interventions differ for each the following two nursing diagnoses?

Risk for Falls r/t poor vision secondary to cataracts
Risk for Falls r/t to muscle weakness, joint instability, and poor sense of balance

The nursing diagnoses listed above illustrate that problem etiologies are important because they affect your choice of interventions. Etiologies may include environmental hazards as well as the developmental and individual risk factors discussed in the preceding sections. Keep in mind that you must state *specific* etiologies for each individual—not just general ones such as "environmental hazards." For example:

Correct: Risk for Falls r/t cluttered home environment and joint instability
Incorrect: Risk for Falls r/t environmental and physical factors

PLANNING OUTCOMES/EVALUATION NP

The *NOC standardized outcomes* you use will depend on the nursing diagnosis. The following are some examples:

Aspiration Prevention   Personal Safety Behavior
Community Disaster   Physical Injury Severity
   Response   Respiratory Status: Airway
Fall Prevention Behavior   Patency
Parenting: Infant/Toddler   Safe Home Environment
   Physical Safety   Thermoregulation

Individualized goals/outcome statements you might write for a client's safety diagnoses include the following examples:

- The child will be free of injury.
- (Client) will experience no physical injury due to environmental hazards.
- Family members will describe their planned escape routes in case of fire.

PLANNING INTERVENTIONS/IMPLEMENTATION NP

NIC standardized interventions will be determined by the nursing diagnosis you use. A few examples of NIC interventions include the following:

Aspiration Precautions   First Aid
Dementia Management   Home Maintenance
Emergency Care   Assistance
Environmental   Sports-Injury Prevention:
   Management: Safety   Youth
Fall Prevention   Surveillance: Safety

To see the more than 50 interventions in the NIC Safety domain (category),

 Go to Davis Advantage, Resources, Chapter 23, **Alphabetical List of NIC Interventions.**

General Interventions Related to Safety

Specific nursing activities are designed to monitor and manipulate the physical environment to promote safety. The following general activities provide an overview of your role in safe, effective nursing care (Thinking, Doing, Caring) in all types of settings and circumstances:

- Assess and continually monitor the safety needs of patients, based on their level of physical and cognitive function and past history of behavior.
- Provide client education to foster informed decisions, to promote involvement in care, and to facilitate post-discharge health.
- Evaluate and use techniques/processes to avoid medical/nursing errors in the delivery of client care.
- Remove hazards from the environment or modify the environment to minimize hazards and risk.
- Use technology to deliver safe effective care
- Establish mutual goals with clients and teach clients about specific safety measures.
- If an accident or injury occurs in the healthcare setting, file an incident report according to agency policy. See Chapters 18 and 44 for more information on this topic.
- Urge patients to be active members of the healthcare team

For more information to help patients participate in their care,

 Go to The Joint Commission (TJC), Speak Up: Know Your Rights Web site at http://www.jointcommission.org/multimedia/speak-up-know-your-rights/

Home Care Safety Interventions

The following specific interventions address particular hazards in home care. After a brief discussion, you will find a series of boxes containing specific home safety interventions.

Prevent Poisoning in the Home

✚ In all cases of suspected poisoning, call 911 or the local emergency number right away. Even if the person is having no symptoms, call the poison control center (PCC) as soon as possible. **The National PCC number is (800) 222-1222; they will connect you to a local PCC.**

✚ Never induce vomiting when the ingested material is acidic or caustic to the esophagus. Although the American Academy of Pediatrics no longer recommends inducing emesis (e.g., with syrup of ipecac), some practitioners may still do so. The National Poison Control Center does not support routinely stocking ipecac in households with young children. It should be given only on specific recommendation from a poison center or qualified medical personnel (American Academy of Pediatrics, 2003).

For Children Nursing interventions focus on teaching parents how to childproof the home and what to do if someone ingests a poisonous substance. All homes should be equipped to handle an emergency if poisoning occurs. Teach parents:

- To keep the telephone number for the nearest PCC easily accessible.
- If they suspect a child has ingested a poisonous substance, it is crucial to obtain help immediately so there is less time for the substance to enter the child's system.

For Adults Unintentional poisoning can affect people at all ages and from all walks of life. However, it may surprise you that middle-aged adults have the highest unintentional poisoning death rates. Advise clients of the following:

- Take only medications prescribed by a healthcare professional.
- Never take larger or more frequent doses of medications to try to get faster or better relief, particularly prescription pain medications.
- Never share or sell your prescription drugs.
- Be sure to follow directions on the medications and read all warning labels.

 Advise families with older adults to prevent accidental overdose or misuse of prescribed medications by using a medication organizer with compartments for the days/times the pills are to be taken. The patient or a family member may fill the organizer once a week.

For steps to prevent poisoning, see the Home Care box Preventing Poisoning in the Home. For actions to take if poisoning occurs at home,

 Go to the Mayo Clinic Web site, Poisoning First Aid, at http://www.mayoclinic.org/first-aid/first-aid-poisoning/basics/art-20056657

Home Care

Preventing Poisoning in the Home

Young children will eat and drink almost anything. Most victims of accidental poisoning are children younger than the age of 5. Tips to prevent poisoning include the following:

Careful Words and Actions

➤ Never leave a small child unattended near household cleaning supplies or medicines. If you must answer the phone or doorbell, take the child with you. *Children act fast; it takes only a moment for them to swallow something.*
➤ Avoid taking medicines in front of children. *Children tend to imitate adults.*
➤ Never call medicines or vitamins "candy." Instead, use the correct name (e.g., "cough medicine").

Careful Storage

➤ Store medicines or household chemicals on high shelves or in locked cabinets and drawers. Never leave them on kitchen or bathroom counters.
➤ Store all household chemicals away from food.
➤ Keep medicines and household chemicals in their original containers. Leave the original labels on them. Do NOT store chemicals in containers that normally hold food.
➤ Use child-resistant packaging for medicines and household chemicals. Close the container securely after each use.
➤ Do not assume your child is safe around substances in child-resistant containers. *Research has shown that many toddlers and preschoolers can open them.*

Careful Disposal

➤ Teach clients to take advantage of community programs that take back medications for safe disposal (e.g., call the local trash service or a local pharmacy for options in your area).
➤ Teach clients how to safely dispose of outdated prescription medications:
  Crush the medication or add water to dissolve it.
  Mix the drugs with an undesirable substance such as kitty litter or used cooking grease *To make it less desirable for pets and children to eat.*

Place the mixture in an empty can or resealable bag and put it in the trash.
Remove all identifying information from prescription labels before throwing containers in the trash or recycling them.
If disposal options are not available, medicines can be flushed down the sink or toilet when they are no longer needed (Food and Drug Administration, 2015). For a list of medicines recommended for disposal by flushing,

 Go to The FDA Web site at http://www.fda.gov/Drugs/ResourcesForYou/Consumers/BuyingUsingMedicineSafely/EnsuringSafeUseofMedicine/SafeDisposalofMedicines/ucm186187.htm#Flush_List.

Careful Environment Checks

➤ Verify that house plants are nontoxic. Examples of toxic plants are rhododendron, philodendron, English ivy, holly, mistletoe, and lily of the valley.
➤ Find out whether any plants growing in your yard are poisonous, and, if so, remove them.
➤ Teach children that they must never eat berries, wild mushrooms, or other edible-looking plants in yards, fields, and forests. *A wide variety of plants can cause illness and even death in young children.*
➤ Warn parents to keep children from chewing on windowsills and to carefully clean up flakes of paint. Advocate for clients who need to have lead-based paint replaced in their homes. *Lead-based paint can still be found in older homes, and some soil contains a high lead content. Young children often put dirt in their mouths and chew on furniture and windowsills, especially when they are teething.*

Prevent Carbon Monoxide Poisoning

If carbon monoxide (CO) intoxication is suspected, the person should be treated with 100% humidified oxygen. A simple blood test may be done to confirm CO levels in the blood. Teach prevention measures, such as the following:

- Buy, install, and maintain a home CO detector.
- Ensure that gas or wood-burning appliances are adequately vented to the outside.
- Repair rust holes or defects in vehicles that could allow exhaust fumes to enter the passenger compartment.
- Do not use a kerosene heater, gas oven, or gas range to heat a house, even for a short time.
- Never operate gasoline-powered engines such as automobiles, generators, or lawn mowers near open doors or windows or in confined spaces, such as garages or basements.
- Never burn charcoal inside a home, cabin, recreational vehicle, or tent—not even in a fireplace.

Prevent Home Fires

Nursing interventions include teaching families how to prevent fires and measures to take should a fire occur. Stress the following:

- **Have a warning system.** Have working smoke alarms and change batteries at least every six months. Keep a phone near the bed or chair for people who have limited mobility.
- **Have an escape plan.** Develop a fire escape plan and practice it at least twice a year. Keep a rope or other type of ladder for escape from rooms above ground level. Have a fire extinguisher in the home and know where it is located and how to use it. Check fire extinguishers regularly and replace them when they become outdated.
- **Have a preventive frame of mind.** When decorating Christmas trees and the exterior of your home, always use fire-safe lights. Do not leave old light sets hung on the outside of your home year after year. Always unplug Christmas tree lights before leaving home and remove the Christmas tree from the home when it becomes dry. Other cautions include the following:

  Never leave burning candles unattended. Do not use candles near curtains or other flammable materials.

  For charcoal grills, use only charcoal starter fluids designed for barbecue grills.

  For gas grills, be sure that the hose connection is tight and check hoses for leaks.

  Store flammable materials (e.g., oil-soaked rags) in appropriate containers (e.g., metal container with a tight lid).

  Do not smoke, especially in bed—and especially in a home where oxygen is in use.

  Never use an open flame when oxygen is in use.

- **Promote electrical safety in the home.** Make sure electrical outlets have covers. Routinely inspect electrical appliances for damaged cords; replace frayed cords. Do not place electrical cords under carpets and make sure cords do not hang off tables and countertops.
- **Know what to do if a fire occurs.** The actions you take to extinguish a small fire depend on the source of the fire. For example, never pour water on a grease fire and never discharge a fire extinguisher into a pan fire. If there is an oven fire, turn off the heat and keep the door closed. If there is a microwave fire, keep the door closed and unplug the microwave. **KEY POINT:** *If the house is on fire, follow your escape plan. Crawl or stay low to the floor as much as possible to avoid the smoke.*

Prevent Scalds and Burns in the Home

Fire is not the only cause of thermal injuries. Teach clients how to avoid scalds and burns from other causes:

- Turn pot handles toward the back of the stove so that children cannot grab and tip them over.
- Never wear loose-fitting clothing (e.g., wide sleeves) when cooking.
- **KEY POINT:** *Avoid warming infant formula and food in the microwave. Many parents ignore this advice; therefore, tell them to always check the temperature of formula and food carefully before giving it to the child.*
- Remove coverings from microwaved food carefully.
- Do not smoke, use matches, or drink hot liquids while holding an infant. Do not leave burning cigarettes unattended.
- Always check bath water temperature for children and older adults and set water heater temperature low enough to prevent scalds.
- Place guardrails in front of radiators and fireplaces.
- Wear protective clothing and sunscreen when outside.

Intervention for Example Problem: Prevent Falls at Home

Teach clients, especially older adults, measures for increasing the safety of their home environment. Use the material in the Home Care box Preventing Falls in the Home and also the material found in Example Problem: Falls.

KnowledgeCheck 23-7

- Identify four safety measures that decrease the risk of burns in the child.
- What are some specific activities that reduce the possibility of fires in the home?

Prevent Firearm Injuries

Education is an essential intervention to prevent unintentional firearm injuries involving children. The American Academy of Pediatrics and other groups have mounted efforts to educate parents so that they will be able to make smart choices related to gun safety. You can help by teaching gun owners that it is important to store firearms unloaded and in a secure, locked container when not in use, and to store ammunition in a different location from the firearm. Suggest that they participate in gun safety courses and know the following rules for safe gun handling (National Rifle Association Headquarters, n.d.a):

- Always keep the gun pointed in a safe direction so that even if it were to go off it would not cause injury or damage.
- Never put your finger on the trigger until you are ready to shoot.
- Always keep the gun unloaded until ready to use it.
- Before cleaning a gun, make absolutely sure that it is unloaded. If you do not know how to open the gun and inspect the chamber(s), leave it alone and get help from someone who does.

✚ **Teaching Children** Even if parents do not have guns in their own home, it is possible that children will encounter them in other places. Urge parents to teach children safe behavior around firearms and to be sure children know what to do if they see a gun (e.g., at a friend's house or in school):

1. Stop.
2. Don't touch it.
3. Leave the area.
4. Tell an adult (National Rifle Association Headquarters, n.d.b).

Home Care

Interventions for Example Problem: Preventing Falls in the Home

Exercise Regularly

➤ Exercise at least 30 minutes every day. Any activity is better than none; the amount depends on age, physical condition, and the intensity of the exercise. See Chapter 33 for more specific information. Tai chi, yoga, and weight training are ways to improve balance, coordination, flexibility, and strength.

➤ Learn to use assistive devices, such as walkers and canes, safely. Be sure rubber tips are not worn. Keep the walking aid by the bed at night.

Take Your Time

➤ You are more likely to fall when you are tired, sick, rushed, or emotionally upset.

➤ Walk carefully without hurrying; be careful not to be distracted while walking about.

➤ Do one thing at a time; complete it before going on to the next task.

➤ Get out of bed or a chair slowly and check your balance before standing or walking. Postural hypotension and dizziness on rising may be caused by medications for high blood pressure and other conditions.

Lighten Loads—Brighten Paths

➤ Carry things in small loads so that you are able to see over them, especially on stairs. Carry several small loads rather than one very large load.

➤ Use bags with handles instead of large boxes or laundry baskets to carry items.

➤ Have your eyes checked at least once a year.

➤ Clean eyeglasses frequently.

➤ Make sure rooms are adequately lighted, use dim light (e.g., a night-light) at night, and turn on the lights before entering a room.

Don't Trip Yourself Up

➤ Ensure that shoes fit properly and wear slippers with nonskid soles. Do not go barefoot.

➤ Avoid loose, trailing clothes. Keep hems of clothing at a length to prevent tripping.

➤ Older adults with leg or hip stiffness and pain may shuffle when walking; use of a cane or walker may help.

➤ Tips of assistive devices, such as canes, walkers, and crutches, should have intact nonskid covers.

➤ Use a ladder or step stool; do not stand on the top step of a stepladder; never climb on a chair.

Clear the Floor

➤ Tape or otherwise fasten phone and electrical equipment cords to the baseboard.

➤ Arrange furniture to provide wide walking areas.

➤ Keep clutter (e.g., toys, magazines, clothing) out of the walkways.

➤ Remove all scatter or throw rugs (or at least be sure they have nonskid padding under them).

➤ Wipe up all foods and fluids from the floor immediately.

➤ Apply an ice-melt product, salt, or sand to icy sidewalks, steps, and porches.

Use Caution on Stairs

➤ Keep stairs well lit.

➤ Keep stairs free of clutter.

➤ Install sturdy handrails and slip-resistant floor coverings on staircases.

 ➤ For older adults and those with vision problems, paint the top and bottom steps white or put white stripes on the front edges of steps.

Minimize Bathroom Hazards

➤ Use shower chairs and raised toilet seats.

➤ Install grab bars and use a nonskid mat in the shower and tub.

➤ Install handheld shower attachments to make it easier to sit while showering and minimize the need to move and turn.

Childproof the Home

➤ Install window guards; never leave a window wide open.

➤ Use gates at the top and bottom of stairways for small children.

➤ Never leave a child alone on a changing table, even for a moment. Supervise young walkers to protect from falls.

➤ Remove chairs near counters or other areas where young children would be likely to climb. Push chairs all the way under dining table tops.

➤ Teach children to pick up their toys.

➤ Be sure that children wear helmets and other appropriate protective gear for bicycling, skateboarding, and other active sports.

 For Older Adults or Those With Limited Mobility:

➤ Use beds that are low to the floor.

➤ Keep a cordless phone in each room and by the bedside to make it easier to call for help if needed.

➤ Ask your doctor or pharmacist to review your medicines—both prescription and over the counter—to reduce side effects and interactions that might interfere with balance and coordination. This is especially important for psychotropic medications.

➤ Get treatment for postural hypotension and cardiovascular disorders, including dysrhythmias.

Prevent Suffocation

Clients should recognize and teach children the universal sign for choking: grasping the neck between the thumb and index finger or clutching the neck with both hands (Fig. 23-3). It is also important to teach clients the following measures to prevent suffocation or asphyxiation:

- Inspect toys for small, removable parts.
- Do not attach pacifiers, rattles, or other infant toys to ribbons or strings.
- Do not use sweatshirts or jackets with necktie strings.
- Position mobiles well above the crib, and remove once the baby begins to push up on his hands and knees or by age 5 months, whichever comes first.
- Keep window blind cords out of a child's reach.
- Store plastic bags away from young children in a secure place.
- Ensure that the crib is designed to meet federal regulations: Crib slats must be less than $2\frac{3}{8}$ in. (6 cm) apart, and the mattress must fit snugly.
- When feeding children meat, cheese, or other firm foods, cut the food into very tiny pieces.
- Do not give a young child hard candy, chewing gum, nuts, popcorn, grapes, or marshmallows.
- Supervise children's balloon play and dispose of burst balloons promptly.

Choking Rescue

Teach adults the universal sign for choking (Fig. 23-3) and basic first aid for choking, but explain that choking rescue is a skill that is best taught using supervised practice with a mannequin. Recommend that clients attend classes presented by organizations such as the Red Cross or the American Heart Association. **KEY POINT:** *The most important thing to remember when someone is choking is to have someone call 911 immediately.*

The Choking Rescue Maneuver is an emergency procedure for removing a foreign object lodged in the airway. It lifts the diaphragm and forces enough air from the lungs to create an artificial cough. The cough should move and expel the obstruction from the airway. The **Heimlich maneuver** makes use of abdominal thrusts only. The American Red Cross (2011) alternates five back blows with five abdominal thrusts until the blockage is dislodged.

- **For adults**-If you suspect airway obstruction in an adult, do the following:
  1. Determine whether the victim is able to speak or cough forcefully (other signs include noisy breathing, loss of consciousness, and dusky skin, lips, and nailbeds).
  2. Ask, "Are you choking?"
  3. If the person cannot speak or indicates he is choking, perform the Heimlich or choking rescue maneuver. You can obtain an summary and illustration of the Heimlich from the U.S. National Library of Medicine, MedlinePlus, at **https://medlineplus.gov/ency/image pages/18152.htm**
     There is also a YouTube video at **https://www.youtube.com/watch?v=XOTbjDGZ7wg&feature=youtu.be**
- **Infants under 1 year**—Management of choking is different for adults and children. Do not use the Heimlich maneuver for infants under 1 year of age. For a summary and illustration of choking first aid for an infant under one year, go to MedlinePlus, at **https://medlineplus.gov/ency/presentations/100221_1.htm**

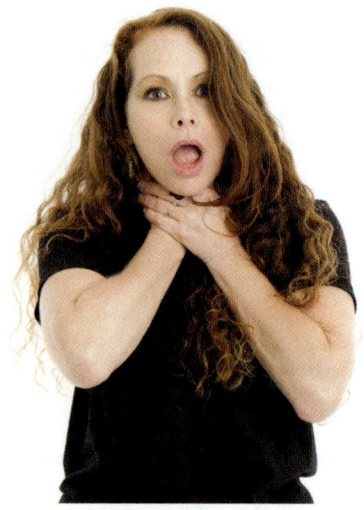

FIGURE 23-3 The universal sign for choking.

Prevent Drowning

Drowning is a form of suffocation but is discussed separately here for convenience. Teach clients the following water safety measures:

- Supervise activity when the child is near any source of water.
- Children up to age 4 should never be left unattended in or near a bathtub, hot tub, swimming pool, or other source of water. Even wading pools, toilets, and mop buckets hold enough water to drown a small child.
- Do not allow children to run around a pool or to dive in shallow areas.
- If you have a pool, be sure it has a barrier (e.g., tall fence) to prevent children from gaining access.
- Insist that children use personal flotation devices (e.g., lifejackets, not float toys). This is controversial, however. Some authorities regard flotation devices as toys that provide false security; others say anything that reduces a child's fear of the water is positive, because it is the fear reaction that leads to drowning.

Prevent Take-Home Toxins

Most preventive measures for toxins apply to the workplace. However, you can teach clients who are at risk to remove work clothing and to shower, preferably in an open-air shower, before leaving work. If shower facilities are not available, patient advocacy may be appropriate. (To learn about advocacy, see Chapters 41 and 43.) If exposed workers have not showered at work, they should remove their clothing and shower immediately before entering their home. When handling contaminated clothes or objects, they should wear gloves to reduce the risk of skin transmission. Laundering may not be effective in removing certain toxins in clothes.

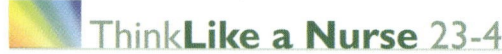

ThinkLike a Nurse 23-4

You are having dinner in a restaurant and notice that the guest at the table beside you seems to be choking.

- What is the universal sign for choking?
- What is the first action you should take?

KnowledgeCheck 23-8

- List two things a person who works around workplace toxins can do to prevent bringing them into the home.
- What specific safety measures would you discuss with a mother to prevent choking in her 9-month-old child?s

Community Intervention: Teaching for Safety Self-Care

In addition to teaching home safety to clients, you should also promote safety self-care related to particular hazards in the community and environment.

Motor Vehicle Safety

Anticipatory guidance and educational programs are important measures for improving motor vehicle safety for all age-groups. You may also wish to become politically active on the issue of motor vehicle safety. For instance, you might petition your city council for a stop sign at a dangerous intersection or a reduced speed limit on a highway.

Also teach clients the following measures for avoiding motor vehicle injuries:

- Be cautious when walking or bicycling on the roadway and observe the laws.
- Do not drink alcohol or take unprescribed or recreational drugs and drive. Have a designated driver.
- Do not engage in distracting activities while driving (e.g., using cell phones, texting, changing the music, applying cosmetics).
- Observe the speed limits.

- Always wear seat belts and periodically check them to ensure safe operation.
- Buckle children properly in age-appropriate safety seats in the back seat of the car. If in doubt about how to use safety seats, ask the local police department to check the installation. See Table 23-4.

 Older Adults Age-related changes increase the risk for injury or death in a car crash, especially after age 70. But driving helps older adults maintain mobility and independence. Urge them to have regular vision checks and to leave a large distance between themselves and the car in front of them.

Food Safety

Teach clients safe food handling and other preventive measures, such as the 4 **C**s of food safety: **C**lean, **C**ook, **C**ombat cross contamination, **C**hill. For further explanation of the 4 **C**s, refer to the Self-Care box Food Safety.

Fighting Vector-Borne Pathogens

The following are points you can use to teach clients about strategies to combat the vectors, mosquitoes, ticks, and rodents (CDC, 2015c; U.S. Environmental Protection Agency, 2016).

Mosquitoes

Public strategies to control mosquitoes include spraying programs and digging ditches to promote drainage from stagnant areas. Individuals can help by taking the following actions:

Table 23-4 ➤ Types of Car Safety Seats

AGE		TYPE OF SEAT	GUIDELINES
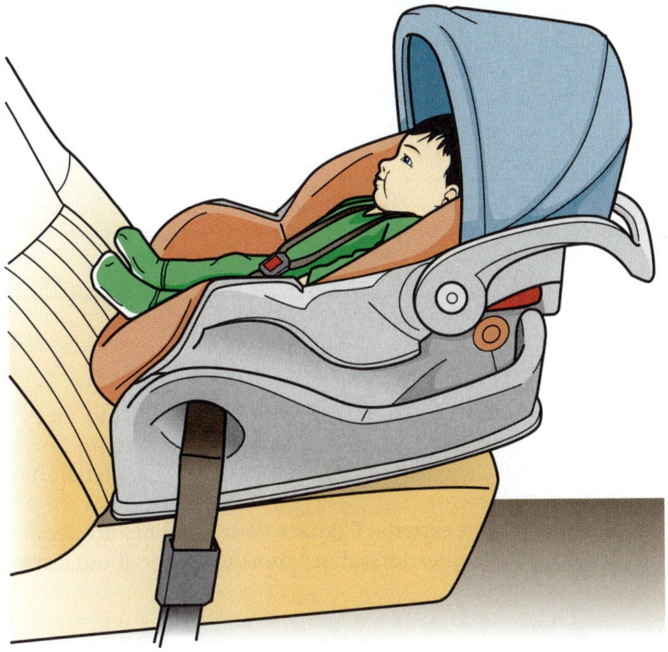 Infant car seat with infant in rear-facing position in the middle of the back seat. Infants younger than age 1 yr		"Infant-only" (These are small and may have carrying handles or be part of a stroller system.)	Use rear-facing seats until the infant is age 1 yr and weighs at least 20 lb (see figure).

(Continued)

Table 23-4 ▸ Types of Car Safety Seats—cont'd

AGE	TYPE OF SEAT	GUIDELINES
Toddlers and preschoolers	"Convertible" (can be used rear facing, then converted to forward facing) or "forward facing"	Rear-facing seats are safer for toddlers until they are age 2 yr. It is best to ride rear facing as long as possible (until they reach the height and weight maximum specified by the seat manufacturer).
School-age children	Booster seats	After outgrowing their car safety seat, children should stay in a booster seat until the car seat belts fit properly (usually at about 4 ft 9 in. tall and ages 8 to 12 yr). Booster seats are safer than a seat belt alone.
Older children	Car lap and shoulder belts	Children who have outgrown their booster seats should ride in the back seat until age 13 yr. Some experts recommend that anyone weighing less than 110 lb, regardless of age, ride in the back seat. Riding in the back seat is associated with a 40% reduction in the risk of fatal injury, and up to 46% in cars with airbags.

Note: These are guidelines, not legal requirements. Some states may also have laws governing types and use of car safety seats. You should be familiar with the laws in your area.

For in-depth information about child safety seats,

 Go to the American Academy of Pediatrics Web site at https://healthychildren.org/English/safety-prevention/on-the-go/Pages/Car-Safety-Seats-Information-for-Families.aspx

Sources: American Academy of Pediatrics. (2015). *Car seats safety: A guide for families 2015.* Retrieved from https://healthychildren.org/English/safety-prevention/on-the-go/Pages/Car-Safety-Seats-Information-for-Families.aspx; CDC (2010b, updated 2015). Child passenger safety. Retrieved from http://www.cdc.gov/features/passengersafety/

- **Remove sources of stagnant water.** Empty standing water in old tires, buckets, toys, or other outdoor containers. Change water in birdbaths, fountains, wading pools, and potted plant trays at least once a week to destroy mosquito habitats. Keep rain gutters unclogged. Treat swimming pools with the proper chemicals and keep the water circulating.
- **Kill or repel mosquitoes.** Use "bug zappers" or citronella candles for evening outdoor activities. Use EPA-registered mosquito repellents when necessary and follow label directions carefully. All repellents and pesticides should have the name and amount of active ingredient on the label. No pesticide is 100% safe, so use them cautiously.
- **Avoid mosquitoes, if you can.** Repair holes in window and door screens. Replace outdoor lights with yellow "bug" lights. They will attract fewer mosquitoes, but they are not repellents. In areas with high mosquito populations (e.g., salt marshes, deep woods), use head nets, long sleeves, and long pants. If there is a mosquito-borne disease alert, stay indoors during the evening, when mosquitoes are active.
- **Consult the experts.** Contact your local health department if you have questions about mosquitoes or about a spraying program.

Ticks

When walking in tick-infested areas:

- Use DEET-containing insect repellant. Reapply it every few hours (or according to the label). Formulations as high as 50% are recommended for adults and children over age 2 months. Use with caution for children. Wash off repellent at night before going to bed.
- When wearing sunscreen, apply sunscreen first and then repellent.

Food Safety

Clean

➤ Wash hands and surfaces often. Always wash your hands with soap and water before handling or preparing food and before eating.
➤ Don't be a source of food-borne illness yourself:
  ➤ Avoid preparing food for others if you yourself have a diarrheal illness.
  ➤ Avoid changing a baby's diaper while preparing food.
➤ Wash produce. Rinse fresh fruits and vegetables in running tap water to remove visible dirt.
➤ Remove and discard the outermost leaves of a head of lettuce or cabbage.
➤ Never use a cutting board, knife, or other object that was used to prepare meat, poultry, or fish for any other purpose until it has been thoroughly washed in hot, soapy water.
➤ Be careful not to contaminate foods while slicing them up on the cutting board. Bacteria grow well on the cut surface of fruits or vegetables.
➤ Wash hands with soap after handling reptiles, birds, or baby chicks and after contact with pet feces.

Cook

➤ Use a thermometer to measure the internal temperature of meat.
➤ Cook to temperatures sufficient to kill bacteria.
  Ground beef to an internal temperature of 160°F (71°C)
  Leftovers and casseroles, 165°F (74°C)
  Beef, lamb, and veal, 145°F (63°C)
  Pork and ground beef, 160°F (71°C)
  Whole poultry and thighs, 180°F (82°C)
  Poultry breasts, 170°F (77°C)
  Ground chicken or ground beef, 165°F (74°C)
  Stuffed fish, 165°F (74°C)
  Roast meats at an oven temperature of 300°F (149°C) or above
➤ Cook eggs until the yolk is firm. Do not eat raw or partially cooked eggs.
➤ Hold hot food above 140°F (60°C) and do so for no more than 2 hours.

Combat Cross Contamination (Separate)

➤ Avoid cross contaminating foods by washing hands, utensils, and cutting boards after they have been in contact with raw meat or poultry and before they touch another food.
➤ Put cooked meat on a clean platter, rather than back on one that held the raw meat.

Chill

➤ Refrigerate leftovers within 4 hours. Bacteria multiply quickly at room temperature.

➤ Avoid leaving cut produce (e.g., fruits, vegetables) at room temperature for a prolonged time.
➤ Chill cooked foods rapidly in a shallow (2 in. in depth) container. Large volumes of food will cool more quickly if they are divided into several shallow containers for refrigeration.
➤ Do not buy partially thawed items. Be sure they are frozen solid.
➤ Use a cooler to transport foods when the temperature is above 80°F (27°C).
➤ Store deli meat for only 1 or 2 days.
➤ Use thermometers in the refrigerator and freezer. Keep freezer temperature at 0°F (−18°C) or below. Keep refrigerator temperature at 40°F (4°C) or below.
➤ Thaw foods in the refrigerator or under cold running water. Use the microwave to thaw foods only if you are going to continue cooking them at that time.
➤ Pack lunches in insulated containers. You can refrigerate or sometimes freeze sandwiches before packing to keep them cold.

Store

➤ Cover and date food.
➤ Store vegetables and fruit separately from uncooked meats.
➤ Do not store food in decorative containers unless they are labeled safe for food. Some crystal and pottery, for example, have high lead content.
➤ Store cleaning supplies away from food.

Report

Report suspected food-borne illnesses to your local health department, which is an important part of the food safety system. Often calls from concerned citizens are how outbreaks are first detected.

Other

➤ Never eat any food that has an odor or that might be spoiled.
➤ Be aware that some imported folk remedies, such as *greta* (which is used by some Hispanic patients for colic), may be contaminated with lead.
➤ Observe sanitation reports for selecting eating establishments in the community.

Sources: CDC. (2015e). Food safety. Information for consumers. Retrieved from http://www.cdc.gov/foodsafety/groups/consumers.html; FoodSafety.gov. (n.d.). Keep food safe. Retrieved from http://www.foodsafety.gov/keep/index.html; U.S. Food and Drug Administration. (2016). Food. Retrieved from http://www.fda.gov/Food/default.htm

■ Treat clothing with permethrin-containing or other insect repellent.
■ Wear light-colored clothing. Ticks are attracted to dark colors; also, it is easier to see a tick on light-colored clothing.
■ Wear long-sleeved shirts, tucked in. Pull socks up over pant legs.

■ After walking in wooded areas, inspect your body, especially in the hair and skinfolds. Use a mirror to view all parts of your body.
■ Remove ticks right away. This can prevent some infections, such as Lyme disease or Rocky Mountain spotted fever. For instructions on how to remove attached ticks,

Go to the CDC Web site at http://www.cdc.gov/ticks/removing_a_tick.html

Rodents and Other Animals

To control rodents, raccoons, and other small animals, remove as many food and water sources as possible. Advise clients to do the following:

- Cover food and clean up immediately after meals.
- Do not leave unwashed dishes on counters and in sinks.
- Keep garbage in closed containers that cannot be overturned.
- Repair holes and cracks in the exterior structure of the home, as well as in walls, closets, attic, around sinks and cabinets, and so on.
- Use commercial traps or hire professional exterminators.
- Participate in neighborhood cleanup projects.

- ✚ Keep in mind that rat and mice poisons and baits can be fatal to humans and should not be used in areas accessible to children and pets.

Reducing Pollution

Teach families they can help to reduce solid pollution and hazardous wastes as well as air and noise pollution of the environment. Refer to the following tips:

Air Pollution To help reduce air pollution, pay attention to air quality warnings, and restrict time spent in high-traffic areas. You might also participate in car pools or use public transportation whenever possible.

Noise Pollution Two specific interventions you can teach clients to help prevent irreversible hearing loss are to (1) avoid exposure to high noise levels and (2) wear protective devices (e.g., ear plugs) in environments with a high noise level.

Hazardous Waste The following are tips for safe disposal:

- **Information.** Contact the local refuse disposal company for instructions about proper disposal of hazardous waste (e.g., paints, solvents, pesticides, cleaners, rechargeable batteries).
- **Product.** Use nonhazardous or less hazardous products; use only the amount necessary for a project. Share leftover materials with neighbors.
- **Motor Oil.** Never dump motor oil into storm drains. Instead, call your local waste management company, a local quick-lube, or tire dealer for recommendations regarding disposal. You can also,

 Go to http://www.valvoline.com/auto-resources/motor-oil-faq-recycled

- **Batteries.** Talk to an automotive dealer or repair service about recycling or trading in car and other batteries.

Solid Waste Proper disposal and recycling of solid wastes helps to prevent pollution. Remember the 4 **R**s: **R**educe, **R**euse, **R**ecycle, and **R**espond.

   Reduce the amount of trash discarded (e.g., don't buy products that have unnecessary packaging).
   Reuse containers, bags, and products; sell or donate instead of throwing items out.
   Recycle by using and buying recyclable and recycled products; compost yard trimmings.
   Respond by educating others, expressing preferences for less waste (e.g., to manufacturers, merchants).

Weather Hazard Safety Measures

Teach clients that if they are aware of what weather event is about to impact their area, they are more likely to survive it. Before severe weather strikes, suggest that clients:

1. **Develop a disaster plan** at home, work, school, and when outdoors. The American Red Cross offers planning tips and information on a putting together a disaster supplies kit at:

    the American Red Cross Web site, http://www.redcross.org/

2. **Identify a safe place to take shelter.** For information on how to build a Safe Room in your home or school,

    Go to the Federal Emergency Management Agency Web site at https://www.fema.gov/safe-rooms

3. **Know the county/parish in which you live or visit** and in what part of that county you are located. The National Weather Service issues severe weather warnings on a county/parish basis or for a portion of a county/parish.
4. **Keep a highway map nearby** to follow storm movement from weather bulletins.
5. **Have a Weather Radio receiver unit with a warning alarm** tone and battery backup to receive warning bulletins.
6. **Check the weather forecast before leaving for extended periods outdoors.** Watch for signs of approaching storms.
9. **If severe weather threatens, check on people** who are elderly, very young, or physically or mentally disabled. Don't forget about pets and farm animals.

Intervention: Promoting Safety in the Healthcare Facility

The following interventions will help you to prevent common accidents in healthcare settings. Also see Box 23-3.

Example Problem Interventions: Preventing Falls

Perhaps the most important thing you can do to prevent falls is to identify those who are at risk for them. Nursing interventions to prevent falls are based on the risk factors identified at the initial assessment. You will find other interventions in Box 23-3. For a summary of interventions, review the Example Problem: Falls.

To see a care plan and care map for Risk for Falls,

 Go to Davis Advantage, Resources, Chapter 23, **Care Plan** and **Care Map.**

Reducing Electrical Hazards

Electrical hazards are a major cause of fires in healthcare agencies. The following interventions help reduce electrical hazards:

- Before use, have all electrically powered equipment and accessory equipment evaluated by facilities management.
- The Joint Commission standards mandate that all employees participate in education and training programs for electrical safety.
- If you suspect an electrical safety hazard, clearly label the malfunctioning equipment and send it for inspection.
- Use three-pronged electrical plugs whenever possible.
- Observe for breaks or frays in electrical cords.

BOX 23-3 ■ Intervention for Example Problem: Preventing Falls in Healthcare Facilities

Provide a Safe Environment

- Determine the appropriate use of siderails based on the patient's cognitive and functional status. Recent research suggests that removing or lowering siderails may help to prevent falls that occur when patients climb over them (Capezuti, Wagner, Brush, et al., 2007).
- Keep the bed in a lowered position, except when giving care; lock wheels.

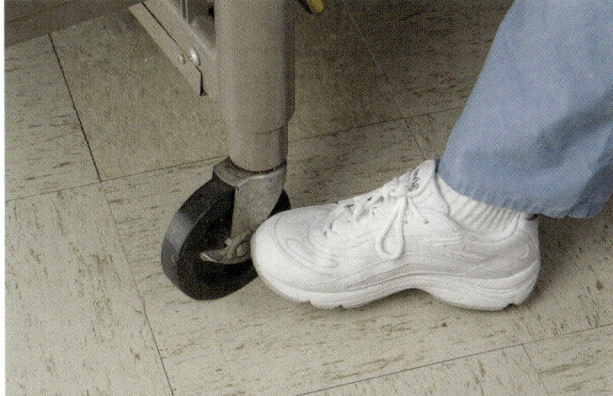

Locking bed.

- Make sure to lock wheels of wheelchairs, especially during patient transfer.

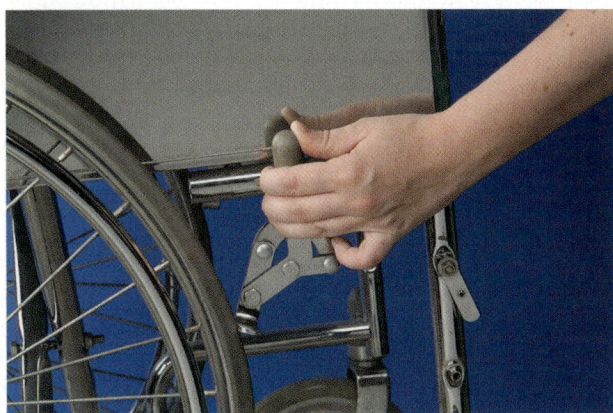

Safety locks on wheelchairs.

- Provide nonskid slippers.

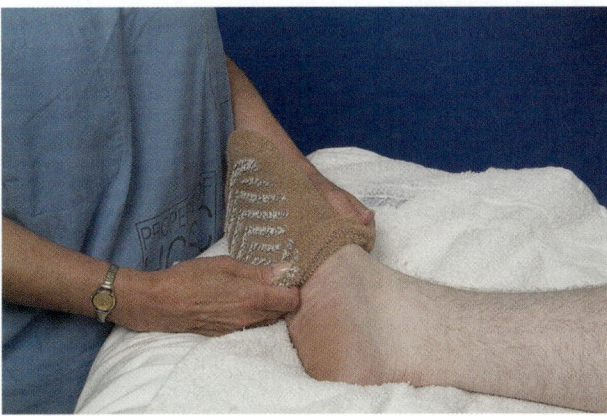

Applying nonskid slippers.

- Keep water, urinal, bedpan, and tissues within easy reach of the patient.
- Place the call light within reach. Have the patient demonstrate the ability to call for the nurse.
- Provide a night-light.
- Keep floors dry and free of clutter.
- For patients at risk for falls, place a warning sticker on the chart or door.

Assess, Teach, and Support

- Review and suggest needed modification of medications, especially psychotropic medications.
- Provide gait training and advice on the appropriate use of assistive devices.
- Orient the person to the surroundings (e.g., bathroom, chairs; you may need to label items).
- Offer to assist with toileting and transfer activities.
- Educate the patient and family regarding fall prevention strategies.

Policies, Procedures, Routines

- Consider instituting hourly rounds on your unit. This has proved effective in reducing the number of falls.
- Place disoriented patients in rooms near the nurses' station.
- Provide regular nursing surveillance of hospitalized older adults. Research suggests that this can significantly reduce patient falls rate (Pappas, Davidson, Woodard, et al., 2015).
- Ask patients at risk for falling to wear red or brightly colored socks to alert caregivers.
- Communicate falls risk status during handover and transfer reports.
- Document changes in the patient's condition in the patient record.

Sources: Adapted from CDC. (2013). National Center for Injury Prevention and Control. Preventing falls: How to develop community-based fall prevention programs for older adults. Retrieved from http://www.cdc.gov/ncipc/preventingfalls/CDC_Guide.pdfh; Centers for Disease Control and Prevention.(2015d). Take a stand on falls. Retrieved from http://www.cdc.gov/features/older-adult-falls/index.html; Joanna Briggs Institute. (2010). Interventions to reduce the incidence of falls in older adult patients in acute care hospitals. *Best Practice, 14*(1); Kenny, R., Rubenstein, L. Martin, F., et al. (2011). Summary of the updated American Geriatrics Society/British Geriatrics Society clinical practice guideline for prevention of falls in older persons. *Journal of the American Geriatrics Society, 59*(1), 148–157; National Guideline Clearinghouse. (2012). Fall prevention. In *Evidence-based geriatric nursing protocols for best practice.* Rockville, MD: Agency for Healthcare Research and Quality. Retrieved from http://www.guideline.gov/content.aspx?id=43933

Responding to Fires

You must know your agency's procedures for responding to a fire, including how to evacuate patients from the building. Remember: **R-A-C-E.**

- **Rescue the patient.** Remove the patient from immediate danger. Move patient(s) into the corridor and close doors to the affected area.
- **Activate the alarm.** Report the location and kind of fire and identify yourself. Activate the nearest alarm.
- **Confine the fire.** Close all doors and windows. Turn off all oxygen valves after coordinating with the charge nurse.
- **Extinguish the fire.** Use the proper extinguisher. Stay between the fire and the path to safety. Keep low.

KEY POINT: *If you discover a fire, your first instinct may be to contain or put out the fire. Fight that instinct! Your first action is to rescue the patient. You should try to extinguish (the E step) the fire only* **after** *the R-A-C steps are completed, and only if it is a* **small** *fire that is contained to one area, such as a trash can. If the fire gets out of control, leave the area immediately.*

Extinguisher Classifications   You should know where the extinguishers are located in your facility and know how to use them. Most agencies use multipurpose (Class ABC) extinguishers.

Class A	Wood, paper, rubber, textiles, plastics
Class B	Flammable liquids, gases, oils, solvents, paints, or greases
Class C	Live electrical wires or equipment
Class D	Combustible metals (e.g., potassium, magnesium, titanium)
Class K	Kitchen fires involving cooking oils and fats

Preventing the Need for Restraints

KEY POINT: *Restraints are a last resort. The current standard of care is restraint free.* The following nursing interventions provide less restrictive alternatives to using restraints for patients who are confused or otherwise cognitively impaired.

Provide Consistency   Keep the environment and the caregivers as consistent as possible. To help relieve anxiety, encourage family and friends to:

- Remain with the patient around the clock for a few days after admission.
- Help with the patient's care.
- Bring familiar objects from home.

Review the Patient's Medications   Determine whether they may affect mental status or balance.

Provide Relaxation and Relieve Anxiety   Relieving anxiety helps to prevent wandering. You may wish to try some of the following measures:

- Orient patients and families to their surroundings; reorient as often as necessary.
- Provide consistency of caregivers and environment, as discussed above.
- Use therapeutic touch and relaxation techniques, such as massage.
- Use the least invasive and most comfortable method to deliver care. For example, use a toileting schedule or provide a bedpan instead of inserting a urinary catheter, or encourage and provide oral fluids to avoid inserting an IV for hydration.
- Discontinue treatments that cause discomfort or agitation as soon as possible. For example, some patients become agitated and pull at or try to escape sensations from indwelling catheters, intravenous catheters, and nasogastric tubes.

Provide Frequent Assessment and Surveillance   Use one-to-one supervision as needed and encourage family members and friends to stay or to hire sitters for clients who need supervision. Place near the nursing station those patients with cognitive deficits or who need supervision for other reasons. Check on them frequently. Assess all patients regularly for cognitive changes.

Find Ways to Communicate   This is essential, even though it may be difficult to communicate with patients who have cognitive deficits. Assess the patient's communication abilities to determine whether he can let you know what he needs and wants. You will need to be especially alert for body language, such as gestures, nods, and eye contact, as these may be the patient's only way of communicating.

- Speak clearly, calmly, and slowly.
- Smile and face the patient.
- Ask the patient directly what he needs, for example, "Do you need the bathroom?"
- Word questions so the patient can answer with a yes or no.

Modify the Environment   Some simple ways to prevent agitation and confusion are to:

- Reduce noise on the unit and provide adequate light.
- Use music therapy for a calming effect.
- Use wedge cushions and body props for patients sitting in chairs to help them maintain good posture in the chair. These help keep them from slumping and falling out of the chair.
- Use low beds for patients who are likely to fall or wander.
- It may be best to remove bed rails in some situations.
- Keep doors to the unit locked if this is feasible and acceptable.
- In long-term care facilities, also lock outside doors. Have a staff member at main entrances and exits.

For types of alarms and specific instructions about using bed alarms, see Procedure 23-1.

Anticipate Unmet Needs   Often patients try to get out of bed because they have a need they cannot express. The best way to achieve restraint-free care is to individualize care to avoid the risky behavior. Look for the meaning of disruptive behaviors (e.g., is the wandering patient thirsty or in pain)? The following are examples of actions to anticipate patient needs:

- Plan an elimination routine based on the patient's history. Patients often try to get out of bed because they need to go to the toilet.
- Provide pain relief and other comfort measures to decrease agitation.
- Provide diversional activities.

KEY POINT: *Sometimes restraints are necessary to ensure the immediate physical safety of the patient or others.* When that occurs, follow organization policies and always use the least restrictive restraint that ensures safety. To learn more about applying and using restraints, see Clinical Insight 23-2, What You Should Know About Using Restraints, and Procedure 23-2, Using Restraints, later in the chapter.

Responding to Mercury Spills

If a mercury spill is not properly cleaned, the mercury can remain in cracks and crevices for long periods of time and cause continuous exposure to mercury vapors. Large spills usually must be cleaned by a pollution control agency and can be very costly. It is especially difficult to remove mercury spills from carpets, so they usually have to be disposed of as hazardous waste. If you must clean mercury spills of 25 mL or less, consult Box 23-4.

BOX 23-4 ■ What to Do If There Is a Mercury Spill

⬥ Do not touch mercury droplets. Mercury vaporizes; the toxic vapors can be inhaled or absorbed through the skin.

In the Healthcare Agency

⬥ If you are not trained in the procedure, do not attempt to clean up a mercury spill. Notify the environmental services department.

- Keep people and animals away from the area.
- Clean the spill promptly.
- If you are trained, use a commercially made mercury spill kit. All healthcare facilities should have them. Spill kits should contain gloves, protective glasses, mercury-absorbing powder, special mercury sponges, and a disposal bag. Some kits have filtered vacuum equipment.
- Follow agency guidelines and instructions in the kit.
- Clean beads off skin, clothing, and disposable items. Place cleaning materials and disposable items in the disposal bag and seal. Follow agency policy for laundering clothing.
- On hard surfaces, use a flashlight to search for beads.
- Change clothing that has been contaminated.
- Wash well. Shower and wash your hair as soon as possible so you do not unknowingly carry mercury home.
- Ventilate the area well to reduce the concentration of mercury vapors. Promote exhaust ventilation if possible.
- Complete an occurrence report.

In the Home and Community

- If you do not have a spill kit, wear rubber gloves and eye protection; use paper towels for cleanup and a plastic bag for disposal.
- Keep people and pets away from the area.
- Wipe beads off skin, clothing, and disposable items. Place disposable items in the plastic bag and seal with tape.
- On hard surfaces, use cardboard to scrape up the beads and pour them into a can or jar with a lid. Then wash the area.
- Shower or wash well.
- Keep the area well ventilated for several days.
- Do not use a broom or vacuum cleaner. These will just spread the mercury around and they will become contaminated by it.
- Do not flush mercury or cleaning materials down a toilet or drain.
- Do not wash and reuse contaminated materials.

Keeping Equipment Safe

The following interventions help ensure safe use of equipment:
- Seek advice if you are unsure how to operate the equipment.
- Make sure medical equipment has been properly inspected.
- Be alert to signs that the equipment is not functioning properly.
- Make sure that rooms are not cluttered with equipment.

- Follow agency policies regarding equipment brought from the patient's home (e.g., hair dryers, electric shavers, radios); usually these should be inspected for proper grounding and safe cords.

Reducing Alarm Fatigue

The American Association of Critical-Care Nurses suggests the following nursing actions:
- Provide proper skin preparation for ECG electrodes.
- Change ECG electrodes at least daily.
- Set alarm parameters and levels on ECG monitors to meet individual needs.
- Collaborate with the interprofessional team to customize delay and threshold settings on oxygen saturation via pulse oximetry (SpO$_2$) monitors.
- Provide education about devices with alarms.
- Establish interprofessional teams to address issues such as the development of policies and procedures related to alarms.
- Monitor only those patients with clinical indications for monitoring, as determined by the interprofessional team.

For more explanation about the AACN strategies to reduce alarm fatigue and improve patient safety,

 Go to the *AACN Practice Alert: Alarm Management* at http://www.aacn.org/wd/practice/docs/practicealerts/alarm-management-practice-alert.pdf

Coping With Violence

Some agencies have a "public safety room." Patients who have been arrested and brought to the hospital for blood and urine testing for alcohol and drug levels, or any hostile patient who has risk factors for violence, should receive care in the public safety room. The following are other interventions for preventing and protecting yourself from violence (Ackley & Ladwig, 2010; Bulechek, Butcher, Dochterman, et al., 2012; Doenges, Moorhouse, & Geissler-Murr, 2010; Flores, 2008; Wilkinson & Barcus, 2017).
- Intervene to relieve anxiety. Anxiety often precedes violent behavior.
- Treat underlying medical conditions. For example, give medications or check blood glucose levels.
- Administer sedatives such as diazepam or lorazepam. There may be standing prescriptions for these.
- Use a calm, reassuring approach.
- Avoid using threatening, aggressive body language.
- Don't respond to anger with anger.
- Don't defend when the patient is verbally aggressive.
- Don't wear a stethoscope around your neck, dangling jewelry, or anything a patient might use to hurt you.
- If you know you will be receiving an angry patient, remove objects from the room that could be used as a weapon.
- Don't go into a room alone with an angry patient.
- Keep the room door open; do not let the patient get between you and the door.
- Remain at least an arm's length away from the angry patient.
- Do not turn your back on an angry patient.
- Do not touch the patient without permission, unless you intend to physically restrain him.
- Protect others in the environment. Follow the department's safety guidelines.
- As a last resort, use mechanical restraints if ordered and as necessary.
- Your priority must be your own safety and the safety of others in the area.

Which Safety Interventions Can I Delegate?

As nurse manager or a primary care nurse, you may need to delegate safety promotion interventions to nursing assistive personnel (NAP). For all delegation decisions, refer to the discussion and guidelines in Chapter 7.

- **Restraints.** One safety activity you might delegate is applying restraints. You must first be sure that the NAP is competent to perform the skill. Although you may delegate the application of the restraints, you may *not* delegate the assessment of the patient's status nor the evaluation of her response to the restraints. You may assign the NAP to (1) remove and reapply restraints to provide skin care and allow for supervised movement and (2) observe for skin excoriation under or around restraint location and report it to you.
- **Other Measures.** You should be sure assistive personnel are aware of and follow all safety measures and institutional procedures. For example, you can expect the NAPs to remove clutter and spills in patient rooms, to provide patients with nonskid slippers, and to lock beds and wheelchairs.

CLINICALREASONING

The questions and exercises in this section allow you to practice the kind of thinking you will use as a full-spectrum nurse. Critical-thinking questions usually have more than one correct answer, so we do not provide "correct answers" for these features. It is more important to develop your nursing judgment than to just cover content. You will learn by discussing the questions with your peers. If you are still unsure, see the Davis Advantage chapter resources for suggested responses.

Caring for the Nguyens

Refer to the assessment data for Nam Nguyen in the front of this book. Use full-spectrum thinking to identify safety hazards for Mr. Nguyen, his 3-year-old grandchild (Kim Phan, who lives with him), and his widowed mother, Mai Nguyen, who lives alone.

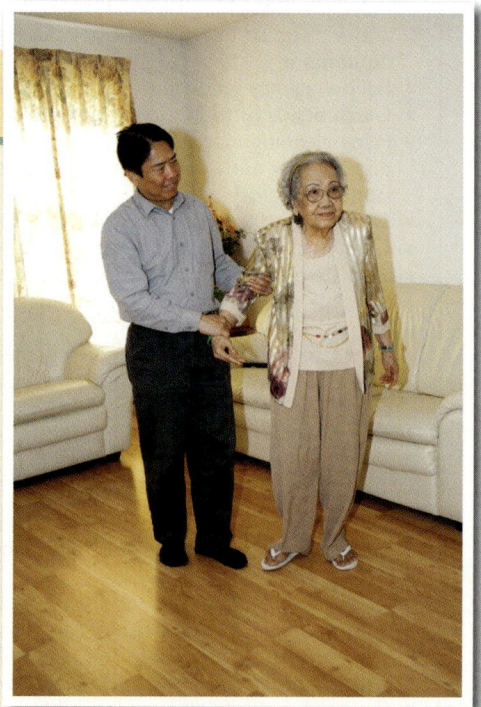

A. Without using any of Nam's patient assessment data (except ages), what theoretical knowledge do you have that will help you to identify risks that commonly occur in the developmental stages represented by these three clients?
Mr. Nguyen
Mr. Nguyen's 3-year-old grandchild, Kim
Mr. Nguyen's widowed mother, Mai

B. From Mr. Nguyen's assessment, what data can you put with your theoretical knowledge to identify the most likely safety risks for him? What are those risks?

C. From the risks and possible risks you have identified, for which one do you definitely need more data before deciding whether it increases his risk for accidents? That is, which piece of data is especially vague? What do you need to find out?

D. You know the theoretical (or possible) risks for Mr. Nguyen's mother. What data do you need in order to determine her *actual* safety risks?

E. What, if any, data do you have that would help you to identify any *actual* safety risks for Mr. Nguyen's grandchild? What, if any, are those risks?

F. What would you want to assess at the child's preschool to be sure that safety measures exist for preventing falls?

Applying the **Full-Spectrum Nursing Model**_____

PATIENT SITUATION

Recall your patient, Alvin Lin, from the Meet Your Patients scenario. Mr. Lin is a 79-year-old man who was just transferred from a long-term care facility to your medical unit. His admitting diagnoses are dehydration and pneumonia. In the handoff report you were told he had rested well during the night and was alert and oriented. When you enter his room, he is confused and does not know where he is. He is becoming combative and is trying to get out of bed.

THINKING

1. *Theoretical Knowledge:*
   a. What is the pathophysiology of pneumonia?
   b. When the oxygen level of the blood falls, what is the effect on the central nervous system? If you do not know the answer to this question, consult a reliable reference.
   c. What are the defining characteristics for the NANDA-I diagnosis, Deficient Fluid Volume?
2. *Critical Thinking (Considering Alternatives):*
   a. Which of the three defining characteristics (in 1c) may increase Mr. Lin's risk for falls? Why?
   b. What else may be increasing his confusion and his risk for falls?

DOING

3. *Practical Knowledge:* Suppose you have tried all the less restrictive restraints, but Mr. Lin still attempts to get out of bed. He has even pulled out his intravenous line. You decide you must apply restraints to keep him safely in bed. You have called the physician, but he has not returned your call. You cannot wait any longer because you have other patients who need you, and yet you must stay with Mr. Lin to keep him from falling. What should you do right now?
4. *Nursing Process (Diagnosis):* Which nursing diagnosis seems more useful to you in planning care for Mr. Lin?
   a. Confusion related to disease process
   b. Risk for Falls related to confusion and possibly r/t weakness

CARING

5. *Self-Knowledge:*
   a. Do you think having a restraint-free facility is a valuable goal or not? Explain your thinking.
   b. How did you come to believe that?
6. *Ethical Knowledge:* Suppose Mr. Lin is too confused to give consent for restraints, and you cannot reach his family by telephone. How can you justify applying restraints, and what must you do later to follow up?

Practical Knowledge:
clinical application

CLINICAL INSIGHTS

Clinical Insight 23-1 ➤ Preventing Needlestick Injury

✚ Use needleless systems (e.g., retractable needles) when possible. More than 80% of needlestick injuries can be prevented with the use of safe needle devices (ANA, 2002).

Before beginning a procedure:

- Provide adequate lighting and space to perform the procedure.
- Place the sharps container near the work area, if it is moveable.
- Obtain assistance if there is a risk that the patient may be uncooperative, combative, or confused.
- Inform the patient about the procedure and explain the importance of avoiding any sudden movement.

During the procedure:

- Be sure you can see the sharps container at all times.
- When handling a sharp, be aware of other persons in the immediate area.
- Do not hand-pass exposed sharps from one person to another.
- When using a safety needle, observe for audio or visual cues that the feature has engaged.

Handling needles:

- Do not shear or break contaminated needles.
- Avoid recapping, bending, or removing contaminated needles and other sharps unless there is no feasible alternative.
- When you must recap a sterile needle, use a mechanical recapping device or a modified "scoop" technique (see Procedure 25-10).
- Never carry syringes in your uniform pocket.

Sharps containers:

- Keep puncture-proof needle disposal containers in every room.
- Place sharps containers at eye level; do not overfill the container.
- Make sure the container is large enough to hold the entire sharp device.

- Dispose of sharps immediately. Do not wait until you have finished the procedure.
- Inspect sharps and waste containers for protruding sharps. If found, notify safety personnel for removal of the hazard.

If your agency does not use needleless systems or protective devices, you should do the following:

- Explain the OSHA Bloodborne Pathogens Standard (BPS) to your employer, including the need to provide needleless systems or protective devices for blood products and parenteral medication administration.

 Refer your employer to the OSHA Web site at www.osha.gov/needlesticks/needlefaq.html

- OSHA requires worker involvement in evaluating, selecting, and implementing the use of safer needle products; volunteer to serve on that committee.
- Ask your agency for a copy of their exposure control plan, which is required by the BPS for monitoring compliance with the new law.
- Keep a record of needlestick injuries on your unit and of "near-misses" (e.g., overfilled sharps containers, sharps left on bed or overbed table).
- Submit written concerns to your employer.
- If your employer refuses to purchase safety devices, you may want to file an OSHA complaint. If you do, refer to whistleblowing in Chapter 43. Complaints can be filed anonymously.
- For complaint filing,

 Go to http://www.osha.gov/as/opa/worker/complain.html

Practice Resources

Adapted from ANA (2002); Centers for Disease Control and Prevention (2011); National Institute for Occupational Safety and Health (n.d., reviewed 2012); U.S. Department of Labor, U.S. Department of Labor, Occupational Safety and Health Administration (2001).

Clinical Insight 23-2 ➤ What You Should Know About Using Restraints

- **Agency policy,** professional guidelines, and state laws should guide restraints use.
- **Use restraints only for safety** to ensure the immediate physical safety of the patient or others.
- **You must obtain a medical prescription** from a physician or other licensed care provider.
- **No standing orders** or "as needed" orders for physical restraint are allowed.
- **You must renew restraint prescriptions every 24 hours** (more often for behavioral restraints).
- **You must modify the plan of care** to reflect the application of restraints and the plan for monitoring.
- **Explain the need for the restraints** if you must use them.
- **Obtain consent** from the patient and family when feasible.
- **Medications are considered a restraint** when they are used to restrict the patient's freedom of movement or to manage behavior.

- **Physical holding of a patient is not always considered restraint.** Sometimes it is necessary to use devices or methods that involve the physical holding of a patient for routine physical examinations or tests.
- **Monitor and reassess.** These are critical components of caring for patients in physical restraints. Assess restraints every 30 minutes (more frequently for patients with behavioral restraints, who may need continuous monitoring).
- **Remove restraints for assessment, feeding, toileting, and skin care every 2 hours.** Patients in medical-surgical restraints should be evaluated by an RN at least every 2 hours. Those in behavioral restraints require more frequent monitoring.
- **Always use the least restrictive restraint that ensures safety.**
- **Remove the restraint as soon as possible.**

PROCEDURES

Nursing activities to promote safety in the home focus mainly on patient teaching. In inpatient facilities, however, you will take a more active role in preventing injury to patients. You will need skills and techniques to prevent falls and to apply and manage restraints safely.

Procedure 23-1 ■ Using Bed and Chair Monitoring Devices

➤ For steps to follow in *all* procedures, refer to the Universal Steps for All Procedures found on the page facing the inside back cover.

Equipment

Bed or chair exit monitoring device
At least four types of notification systems are used to warn caregivers that a patient is leaving a bed or chair: (1) pressure sensitive, (2) posture indicators, (3) motion sensors, and (4) pull-cord and combination alarms.

Delegation

As the nurse, you must determine whether a monitoring device is needed. You must also select the appropriate device and provide ongoing evaluation of its effectiveness. You may delegate to a nursing assistive personnel (NAP) the installation of the device, after verifying the NAP has the necessary knowledge and skill.

Pre-Procedure Assessments

Assess for intrinsic factors that increase the risk for falls.
- Older than age 75
- History falling
- Bowel or bladder incontinence (particularly urge bladder incontinence)
- Cognitive impairment

- Mood changes, lability
- Dizziness
- Functional impairment
- Medications (especially new medications or changes)
- Comorbidities (e.g., dementia, hip fracture, Parkinson's disease, arthritis, and depression)
- Assess for factors that increase risk for more severe injury in the case of a fall. These include use of anticoagulants (e.g., Coumadin, Plavix or aspirin) and osteoporosis.

Assess for extrinsic (environmental) factors that increase the risk of falling.
- Use of an assistive device
- Equipment in the room
- Wet or uneven floors
- Use of physical restraints
- Poorly fitting footwear
- Poor lighting
- Lack of grab rails and bars in the bathroom
- Furniture and adaptive aids that are in disrepair or unstable (e.g., bed rails, IV poles)
- Clothing that may cause tripping
- Check the alarm on the monitoring device to ensure that it is working properly.

(continued on next page)

Procedure 23-1 ■ Using Bed and Chair Monitoring Devices (continued)

➤ When performing the procedure, always identify your patient according to agency policy, using two identifiers, and be attentive to standard precautions, hand hygiene, patient safety and privacy, body mechanics, and documentation.

Procedure Steps

1. Apply the device.

Variation: Bed or Chair Monitor

Place sensor pads under the patient's buttocks.

The sensor will alarm when the patient attempts to get out of the bed or chair; it alarms when there is no weight on it for more than a few seconds. For some devices, you may need to set alarm sensitivity. For example, you may set the system to alarm when the patient exits the bed, when the patient attempts to exit the bed, or even when the patient moves in the bed. ▼

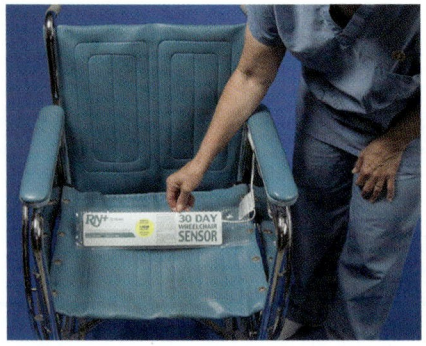

Variation: Leg Sensors

Place sensors on the patient's thigh.

The alarm will sound when the leg assumes a near-vertical position. ▼

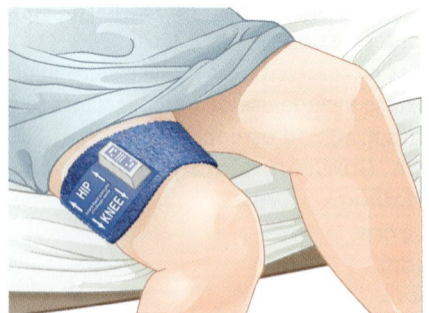

Variation: Infrared Beam Detector

Attach next to the bed or on the wall. ▼

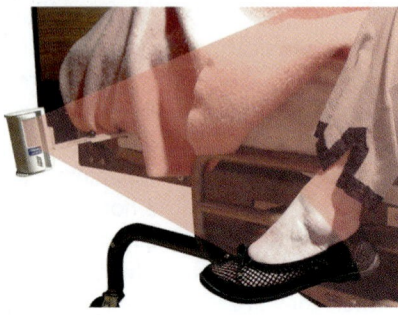

Variation: Cord-Activated Sensor

Attach one end of the cord (clip) to the patient's garment. Attach the other end to the control unit. The cord should be long enough to allow moderate movements but short enough to prevent false alarms. Be sure the cord is free to pull straight out from the monitor and is not blocked by pillows, bedding, or bedrails.

The alarm is activated when the patient's movement causes the cord to be detached from the control unit. Some patients will deactivate the alarms, including removing the alarms clipped to their garments. ▼

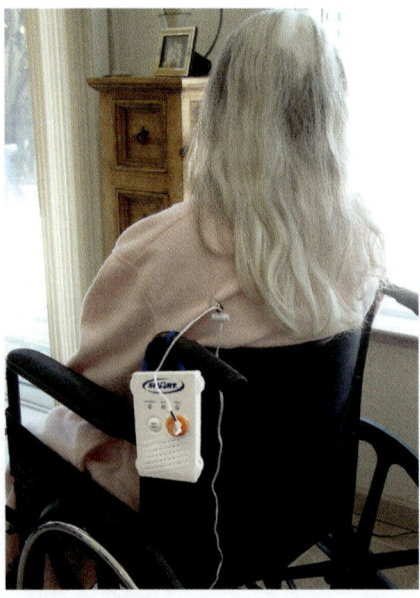

2. Connect the control unit to the sensor pad.

Variation: Bed or Chair Monitor

Mount the control unit on the bed or chair.

Variation: Leg Sensor

Mount the control unit directly on the leg sensor.

Variation: Infrared System

Mount the control unit next to the bed or on the wall.

Variation: Cord-Activated System

Mount the control unit next to the bed or on the wall.

3. Connect the control unit to the nurse call system, if possible.

Allows for a quicker response; however, not all call systems will accommodate this.

4. Before assisting the patient out of the bed or chair, disconnect or turn off the alarm.

Prevents false alarms. Some systems have a standby setting to allow the alarm to be temporarily suspended.

5. Reactivate the alarm after assisting the patient back to the bed or chair.

Helps improve the timeliness of staff response, which may prevent patient falls.

6. Be sure the patient can access the nurse call light easily.

Evaluation

- Assess the sensitivity of the monitoring device, and adjust as needed to ensure that the alarm is activated if the patient tries to get out of the bed or chair.
- Continue to assess fall risk per agency policy and as indicated by the patient's physical and/or mental status.
- In the event of a fall, perform a post-fall assessment to identify possible causes. Monitor patients closely for 48 hours after a fall.

Patient Teaching

- Explain to the patient and family that a bed or chair exit monitoring device alerts the staff when the patient tries to get out of the chair or bed.
- Explain that the purpose of the device is to help prevent falls using the least restrictive method possible to reassure the patient and family.
- Explain to the patient that she will need to call for assistance when she wants to get up.
  Calling for assistance will prevent the alarm from sounding. Summoning for help can prevent the patient from falling.

Documentation

- Document the initial sensor placement, including type of sensor used and the location of placement.

- After documenting initial placement, follow agency policy for documenting the use of bed exit monitor. Usually, the minimum documentation for exit monitors is every 8 hours.
- Place the patient on fall risk precautions according to agency policy.
- Document on the fall risk assessment sheet, restraint flow sheet, and nursing notes according to agency policy.

Sample documentation:

9/06/18, 1230. Continues to be confused and to stand up without assistance. Wheelchair exit alarm placed on wheelchair and monitoring clip attached to back of client's gown. Notified client's daughter, June Kennedy, via telephone. Daughter agreed the exit alarm would help keep her father from falling. ———————————— Mary Clinton, RN

Practice Resources

Gray-Micelli, D., & Quigley, P. (2011); National Guideline Clearinghouse (2012); Park, M., & Tang, J. (2007).

Thinking About the Procedure

 The video **Using Bed and Chair Monitoring Devices,** along with questions and suggested responses, is available on the **Davis's *Nursing Skills Videos*** Web site on Davis*Plus.*

Procedure 23-2 ■ Using Restraints

➤ For steps to follow in *all* procedures, refer to the Universal Steps for All Procedures found on the page facing the inside back cover.

➤ *Caution:* This procedure describes Medicare standards, but state and agency policies may be more restrictive.

Equipment

- Restraint of the appropriate size: belt, vest, wrist or ankle, or mitt
- Soft gauze or cotton padding for bony prominences

Delegation

As the nurse, you must determine whether restraints are needed in each specific situation. You must also select the least restrictive type of restraints, evaluate their effectiveness, and continue to assess for complications that may occur. You may delegate to the NAP the application and periodic removal of ordered restraints, after verifying that the NAP has the knowledge and skill to do so.

Pre-Procedure Assessments

- Assess the patient's risk for falls, including mobility status and level of awareness.

- Assess for need for restraints: The immediate physical safety of the patient, a staff member, or others is threatened.
  If a patient must be temporarily restrained so that a procedure may be performed, this is not considered "restraint."
- Determine that all less restrictive interventions have been tried unsuccessfully.
- Identify the appropriate restraint:
  - The least restrictive possible
  - Does not interfere with care or exacerbate patient's medical condition
  - Does not pose a safety risk to the patient
  - Can be changed easily to keep it clean

(continued on next page)

Procedure 23-2 ■ **Using Restraints** (continued)

➤ When performing the procedure, always identify your patient according to agency policy, using two identifiers, and be attentive to standard precautions, hand hygiene, patient safety and privacy, body mechanics, and documentation.

Procedure Steps

1. **Determine whether dangerous** behaviors continue despite attempts to eliminate causal factors using less restrictive interventions.

2. **Obtain a prescription** for restraint, including type of restraint, indications for use, site of restraint application, and duration. Determine if the restraint is being used for medical–surgical or behavioral reasons.
   Federal and state regulations and laws permit healthcare facilities to use restraints only when they are medically needed. Restraints can be used only with a physician's or advanced practice nurse's order for a specified and limited time. When you apply restraint in an emergency, obtain the order as the restraint is being applied or as quickly as possible afterward. When the restraint prescription expires (maximum 24 hr), physician assessment and a new prescription are needed.

3. **Notify the family of the change** in patient status and the need for restraints. Obtain patient and family consent when clinically feasible.
   Patients have the right to refuse treatment. Consent may not be necessary if there is an immediate threat to patient safety; however, as a rule, the family must be notified of the use of restraints if the patient has cognitive impairment. Many times family members prefer to sit with the patient as an alternative to restraint.

4. ✚ **Pad bony prominences** and apply the appropriately sized restraint, using appropriate knotting techniques.
   - Use a quick-release knot, such as the half-bow, when tying restraints to the bed frame or wheelchair.

Do not tie restraints to the siderails. ▼

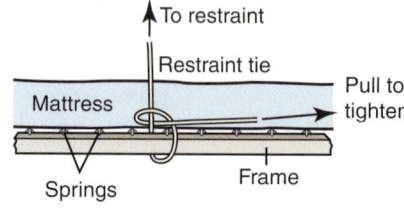
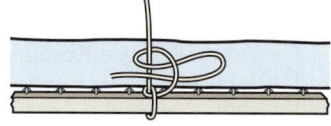
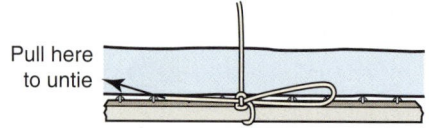

A quick-release knot is used to prevent patient injury and for ease in caring for the patient. Tie the knot on an immovable part of the bed to prevent injuring the patient if the siderails or head of bed are lowered. A quick-release knot will not tighten or slip when the patient moves about, but it will untie quickly when you pull on the loose end.

Variation: Belt Restraint

a. Place the belt restraint at the patient's waist, removing any wrinkles.
b. Make sure that the belt is snug but does not constrict the patient's waist.
c. Some belts have a key-locked buckle to prevent slipping.
   A belt restraint is used mainly to prevent a patient from falling when getting up from a chair or wheelchair

and may be used to remind a patient not to get out of bed unassisted. ▼

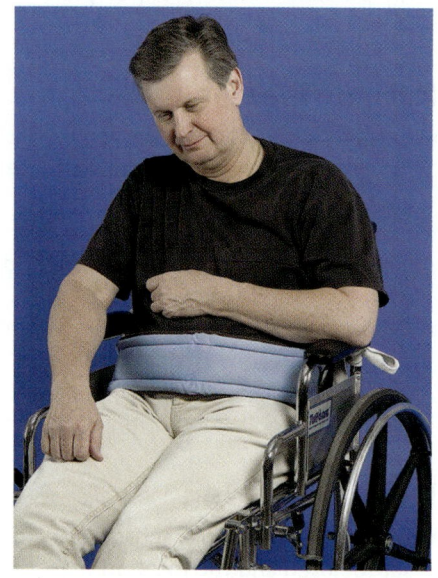

Variation: Vest or Jacket Restraint

a. Place the patient in the vest restraint. A zipper-style vest is preferred.
   A vest restraint with a rear zipper is less likely to accidentally strangle the patient.

b. Attach the vest straps to the bed or wheelchair.
   A vest restraint is used mainly to prevent a patient from falling out of a chair or wheelchair and sometimes to prevent a patient from getting out of bed unassisted. ▼

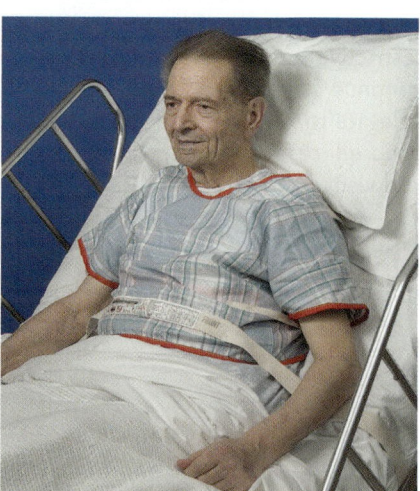

Variation: Wrist or Ankle Restraint

a. Apply the padded portion of the wrist or ankle restraint around the patient's wrist or ankle.

b. Make the restraint snug enough to prevent the patient from being able to slip it off but not tight enough to impair circulation.

c. Attach the restraint strap to the bed frame. Do not attach to bed rails.

A wrist restraint is used mainly to prevent an agitated patient from pulling at tubes, such as IV sites and nasogastric tubes. ▼

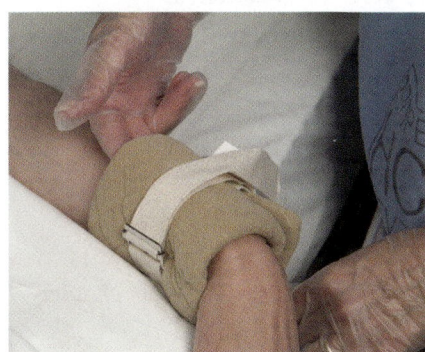

Variation: Mitt Restraint

a. Place patient's hand in the mitt restraint, ensuring that fingers are slightly flexed in the mitt.

b. Attach restraint strap to the bed frame if necessary.

A mitt restraint is used mainly to prevent a patient from pulling at tubes, such as IV sites and nasogastric tubes. Mitt restraints limit the use of the fingers, which may be enough to prevent the patient from grasping the tube. If this is the case, mitts that are

not tied to the bed frame are the least restrictive restraint. ▼

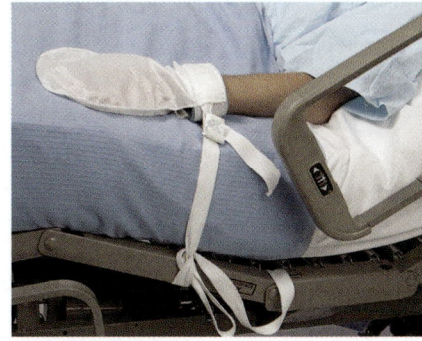

Variation: Enclosed Bed

a. Place patient in the bed and zip all sides. Be sure zippers are completely closed and zipper tabs are positioned in the upper aspects of the net panels out of the patient's reach.

b. Adhere to the manufacturer's minimum height and weight recommendations.

c. Never leave the bed in the high position with the patient unattended.

An enclosed bed is a canopy-like padded bed that is used mainly to keep a patient from wandering or from falling out of bed. The bed has nylon netting on all four sides, with zippered panels that can be opened to provide care. The patient has full freedom of movement and access to all parts of his body. Patients in enclosed beds have a higher risk of becoming entrapped between the bed rails and the mattress, risking suffocation. The dangers are greater for smaller patients and when the bed is left in a high position.

5. **Adjust the restraint** to maintain good body alignment, comfort, and safety. You should be able to slide two fingers under a wrist or ankle restraint.
The restraint should be snug enough to prevent it from slipping off, but not tight enough to impair circulation.

6. ✚ **Release restraints at least** every 2 hours to provide skin care, passive and active range of motion (ROM), ambulation, toileting, hydration, and nutrition. Assess for the continued need for restraint.

Prevents impaired circulation and injury. Medicare- and Medicaid-certified healthcare agencies must ensure that a patient's abilities do not decline unless the decline cannot be avoided because of the patient's medical condition. Patients often lose the ability to bathe, dress, walk, toilet, eat, and communicate when they are regularly restrained. If restraints are necessary, they must be used in a way that does not cause these losses.

7. **Place the patient on fall risk** precautions according to agency policy.
Patients who are restrained have a higher incidence of falls.

? What if . . .

■ **I must apply a restraint in an emergency, for the safety of the patient or others?**

In such an emergency, an RN may initiate a restraint. When you apply restraint in an emergency, obtain the order as the restraint is being applied or as quickly as possible afterward.

Evaluation

■ Assess the initial restraint placement, circulation, and skin integrity. Observe for pallor, cyanosis, and coolness of extremities when extremities are restrained.

■ Check the restraint every 30 minutes (more often for a behavioral restraint).

■ Release the restraint to assess circulation, the patient's response to the intervention, and the need for continuing the use of the restraint every 2 hours; remove it when it is no longer needed.

KEY POINT: *Patients in behavioral restraints require more frequent monitoring and in some circumstances require continual observation.*

Ensures that the restraint is still functioning as intended. Monitoring and reassessment are critical components of caring for patients in physical restraints. Frequency of monitoring is determined by the type of restraint (behavioral vs. medical–surgical).

(continued on next page)

Procedure 23-2 ■ Using Restraints (continued)

- Check every 24 hours to see that the restraint prescription has been renewed.
- Remove the restraint as soon as possible.
- Modify the plan of care to reflect the application of restraints and the plan for monitoring.

Patient Teaching

- Explain to the patient and family the need for the restraints.
- Explain that the restraints will be removed as soon as possible.

Home Care

- The same guidelines apply to clients in the home.
- Evaluate caregivers' knowledge and skill in using restraints and provide teaching as needed (e.g., regarding padding bony prominences and the need to periodically release restraints).
- If an enclosed bed is used in the home, instruct the caregiver in safe use.

Documentation

Document the following:

- All nursing interventions that were done to eliminate the need for the restraint (e.g., moving patient closer to the nurses' station, asking a family member to remain with the patient, reorienting the patient)
- Reasons for placing the restraint (e.g., patient behaviors)
- The initial restraint placement, location, circulation, and skin integrity
- The teaching session with the patient and family members
- Circulation checks, range of motion, and restraint removal per agency protocol
- Entries on fall risk assessment sheet, restraint flow sheet, and nursing notes according to agency policy

Sample Documentation

1/24/18 1230.   Continues to be confused, pulling at IV lines. Physician notified and evaluated patient. Mitt restraints ordered and placed on bilateral hands. Fall risk precautions initiated. Mitt restraints explained to patient and wife. Wife agreed that mitt restraints would help keep her husband from removing IV lines . —— Mary Clinton, RN

Practice Resources

American Nurses Association (2012); Centers for Medicare & Medicaid Services (2006b, revised 2015).

Thinking About the Procedure

To practice applying clinical reasoning to this procedure:

 The video, **Using Restraints,** along with questions and suggested responses, is available on the **Davis's** *Nursing Skills Videos* Web site on Davis*Plus*

 To explore learning resources for this chapter,

 Go to **www.DavisAdvantage.com** and find:

Answers and Suggested Responses for all questions in this chapter

Lists NIC interventions and NOC Outcomes

List of NANDA-I Diagnoses

Knowledge Map

Care Plan

Care Map

References and Bibliography

Concept Map

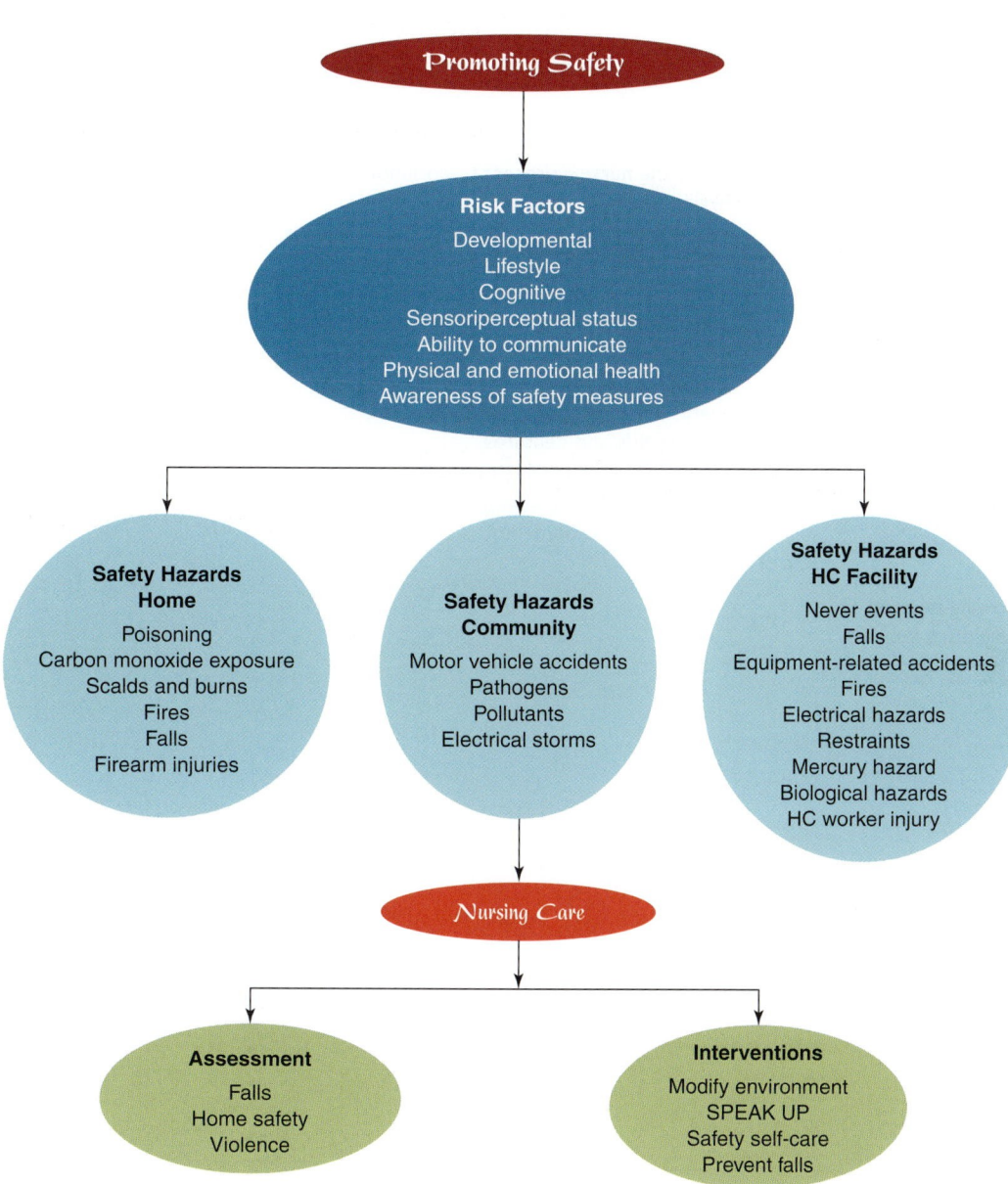

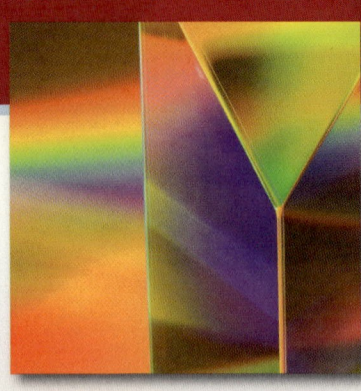

CHAPTER 24

Hygiene

Learning Outcomes

After completing this chapter, you should be able to:

➤ Explain how personal hygiene relates to health and well-being.

➤ Identify factors influencing personal hygiene practices.

➤ Discuss delegation of hygiene activities to nursing assistive personnel (NAP).

➤ Discuss the nurse's role in determining a client's self-care ability.

➤ Identify nursing diagnoses related to self-care ability and hygiene practices.

➤ Describe routine assessments to make when providing hygiene care of the skin, feet, nails, mouth, hair, eyes, ears, and nose.

➤ Describe the following types of baths: complete, assist, partial, towel, bag, shower, tub, and therapeutic.

➤ Apply the nursing process to common hygiene-related problems of the skin, feet, nails, mouth, hair, eyes, ears, and nose.

➤ Demonstrate nursing skills to promote patient hygiene (such as bathing, foot care, and bed making).

➤ Demonstrate care of the eyes, ears, and teeth, including glasses, contact lenses, hearing aids, and dentures.

➤ Discuss the relationship between a patient's overall well-being and the immediate environment.

Key Concepts

Activities of daily living

Hygiene

Self-care ability

Related Concepts

See the Concept Map at the end of this chapter.

Example Problem

Hygiene Self-Care Deficit

Meet Your Patients

You and a NAP (nursing assistive personnel) are to assist the following patients with their hygiene:

- Mrs. Williams, a 76-year-old woman of Indian heritage who was admitted yesterday after suffering a stroke that paralyzed her right side. She is now unable to speak clearly and becomes frustrated as she attempts to communicate her needs. Her daughter says Mrs. Williams is a proud and tidy woman who has been living alone and caring for herself independently since her husband's death last year, even maintaining the yard and garden. She wears eyeglasses for reading and driving and has a hearing aid.
- Mr. Gold, a 68-year-old Orthodox Jewish man admitted last week after a massive heart attack. Although his eyes are open, he does not respond to external stimuli. Because of Impaired Swallowing, Mr. Gold is unable to take food or fluid orally. A feeding tube was placed to ensure adequate nutrition and hydration. His oral mucous membranes and lips are dry and crusty. He is incontinent

of urine and stool. Mr. Gold's son, Ira, tells you that Mr. Gold adheres to Orthodox Jewish law and requests that you respect this in his care.

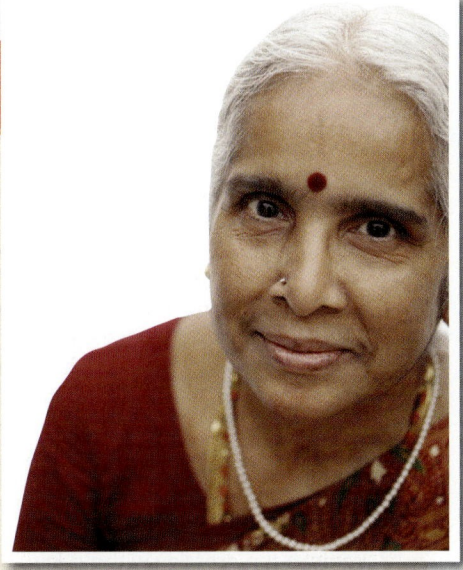

Think about the following questions now, then again after you have read the chapter: What immediate concerns come to your mind about each of these patients? How will you ensure that their hygiene needs are met? Are there any safety issues? Which parts of their hygiene care can you delegate, if any?

Theoretical Knowledge
knowing why

This chapter provides the theoretical knowledge you need to answer the preceding questions, as well as others that will arise as you care for patients. It begins first with an explanation of the concepts of hygiene, activities of daily living, and self-care.

ABOUT THE KEY CONCEPTS

Hygiene is the broadest of the key concepts because everything in the chapter is related to hygiene. However, every aspect of hygiene includes consideration of the key concepts of **activities of daily living** and **self-care ability**. That is, you need to know the patient's ability to perform an activity of daily living in order to know how to give appropriate hygiene care (e.g., can he wash his entire body, or just his hands and face?).

HYGIENE AND SELF-CARE

Hygiene describes activities involved in maintaining personal cleanliness and grooming. **Activities of daily living (ADLs)** (e.g., taking a bath or shower, washing hair, or brushing and flossing teeth) promote comfort, improve self-image, and decrease infection and disease. Healthy people perform their own personal hygiene; however, some patients need assistance because of illness or injury. **KEY POINT:** *As a nurse, you are responsible for providing the necessary assistance and, at the same time, encouraging as much self-care as possible to promote activity, independence, and self-esteem.*

What Factors Influence Hygiene Practices?

♥ **iCare** Every patient is unique, so as you would expect, personal hygiene practices vary greatly. To reflect caring, expand your understanding of the concepts of hygiene to respect and accommodate each person's preferences and differences whenever possible.

Personal Preferences Some people prefer a shower, others a bath. One person may shower in the morning to wake up, whereas another bathes in the evening to relax before going to sleep. Choice of soaps and shampoos varies as well.

Culture and Religion or Spirituality Cultural and spiritual values and beliefs about hygiene form the foundation for our beliefs as adults. Generally, people in North America consider daily bathing, use of deodorant, and brushing the teeth necessary to eliminate body odors, whereas people in some cultures may find a weekly bath sufficient. Some religious or spiritual beliefs also influence hygiene practices. For example, Orthodox Judaism prohibits receiving personal care from a member of the opposite sex.

Economic Status or Living Environment Inadequate bathing facilities or lack of money for hygiene supplies (e.g., lack of access to running water) can influence how often a person bathes. People living in poverty must focus on meeting basic needs for food and shelter before they can spend money and energy on hygiene.

Developmental Level Parents and other caregivers provide hygiene care for infants and young children. Older children learn practices that become habits, such as brushing and flossing the teeth. As children begin to perform their own hygiene independently, they are influenced by the media and societal norms.

Chapter Key Concepts: Hygiene, Self-Care Ability (Thinking, Doing, Caring)

Competency: Provide goal-directed, client-centered care

Background. Promotion of health and safety requires patient engagement and patient-provider partnership. An active partnership establishes trust and encourages self-care. **KEY POINT:** *Hand hygiene is considered the most significant action in breaking the chain of infection.* Best practice regarding hand hygiene has infrequently considered the role of the patient in the chain of infection (Landers, Abusalem, Coty et al., 2012). Salcido (2012) reported an increase in hand hygiene compliance in healthcare workers (HCW) when patients were reminded to ask the HCW, "Did you wash/sanitize your hands?" (p. 342).

Scenario: The student is caring for a patient with a surgical incision. A nurse enters the room and begins to remove the dressing without initiating hand hygiene.

Think about it: Reflect on the following questions or discuss them with your peers:

1. In this situation what are the implications for the student nurse in maintaining safe and effective care and preventing infection?
2. Identify specific strategies to engage the patient in self-care management to reduce the risk of infection.
3. Debate the value of utilizing the patient-engagement strategy of asking, "Did you wash/sanitize your hands?" as reported by Salcido (2012).

Resources: Landers, T., Abusalem, S., Coty, M. B., et al. (2012). Patient-centered hand hygiene: The next step in infection prevention. American Journal of Infection Control, 40(4), Supplement 1, S11–S17; Salcido, R. (2012). Patient safety: It is in our hands. Advances in Skin and Wound Care, 25(8), 342.

For example, some preteens may bathe only under parental duress, but teenagers, who are typically very self-conscious, may take several showers a day. Many teenagers have oily skin and can tolerate frequent bathing, but as we age, the oil-producing sebaceous glands become less active. For adults, frequent bathing and the use of deodorant soap further dries the skin. Older adults may find it necessary to bathe only every 2 or 3 days, use less soap, and increase the use of skin moisturizers.

Knowledge and Cognitive Levels Not everyone has the knowledge needed to make appropriate decisions. Patient teaching is an important part of your hygiene care because most people will, eventually, take care of their own personal hygiene. For example:

- Some people may not know the importance of flossing.
- Some women may not be aware of the importance of cleansing the perineum from front to back after using the toilet.

 Think**Like a Nurse** 24-1

Think about Mrs. Williams and Mr. Gold (Meet Your Patients). After reviewing each of the preceding factors, determine the following for each patient:

- Which factor(s) will have the most influence on the hygiene practices of this patient?

- Why do you think so?
- How will this factor affect the individual plan of care?

How Does Health Status Affect Self-Care Ability?

Both physiological and emotional factors can interfere with a person's ability or willingness to perform hygiene measures.

Pain Pain limits the person's ability and motivation to perform ADLs. The pain itself, limited mobility caused by the pain, and drowsiness from analgesics used to manage the pain may all contribute to a self-care deficit.

Limited Mobility Limited mobility (e.g., from joint and muscle problems, injury, weakness, fatigue, surgery, prescribed bedrest, or pain) makes it difficult to perform hygiene activities. For example, a patient may be unable to bend over to wash her lower legs and feet, cut her toenails, or even raise her arms to wash and dry her hair. A patient who is weak or "light headed" may be afraid of falling and be reluctant to move about. Such a person needs help, especially getting into the bathtub or shower. Obstacles such as IV lines, oxygen tubing, nasogastric tubes, indwelling urinary catheters, or casts may also interfere with the patient's ability to perform self-care.

Sensory Deficits Sensory deficits diminish a person's ability to perform hygiene measures safely and independently. Safety is a priority for patients with sensory deficits. Consider these examples:

- A patient with macular degeneration (a visual deficit) is admitted to the hospital. Because he is unfamiliar with the new surroundings, he is unable to gather necessary supplies for grooming. You would need to provide direction, assistance, and understanding.
- A patient with a hearing loss is taking an anticoagulant (a medication to delay blood clotting). You may need to provide written instructions about the importance of using an electric razor instead of his preferred double-edged razor.

Cognitive Impairment Patients with conditions such as dementia, delirium, psychosis, stroke, Alzheimer's disease, or traumatic brain injury may find it impossible to initiate their own grooming. The patient may be unable to recognize the need for hygiene, much less know how to accomplish related tasks.

- *Example:* A patient with advanced Alzheimer's disease may actually forget how to care for himself and will need step-by-step direction. Because the person may have difficulty interpreting stimuli in the environment, he may be fearful and resistant to hygiene measures performed by the nurse. Such cognitive deficits require new or modified hygiene plans.

Emotional or Other Mental Health Disturbances A depressed patient may neglect his grooming and hygiene because of a profound lack of energy or motivation. Patients experiencing altered reality states, such as psychoses, delusions, or hallucinations, may:

- Dress inappropriately for the weather or the situation
- Have poor hygiene practices
- Be unable to make decisions about "what to do next" when bathing, dressing, and so on

Knowledge Check 24-1

- What are the benefits of personal hygiene?
- Why should you respect and accommodate your patient's hygiene preferences?

- Identify two economic or living environmental factors that may influence how frequently a person bathes.
- Identify one example of a cognitive impairment that may make independent initiation of grooming impossible.
- Why may people experiencing depression neglect their grooming and hygiene?

Practical Knowledge
knowing **how**

This section of the chapter will assist you to assess for and promote self-care abilities and to plan care for patients with Self-Care Deficits. **KEY POINT:** *Plan hygiene care around the patient's needs, not facility routines or staff convenience.*

For guidelines for assessing, diagnosing and planning and evaluating deficits in hygiene self-care, see the box Example Problem: Hygiene Self-Care Deficit.

ASSESSMENT (Self-Care) NP

Focus on the patient's *ability* to perform hygiene measures and the need for assistance, not necessarily on the *quality* of these measures. To learn what to include in an assessment of self-care and hygiene, see the Focused Assessment box Guidelines for Assessing Hygiene.

ANALYSIS/NURSING DIAGNOSIS (Self-Care) NP

Following are NANDA-I diagnoses specific to self-care abilities, except for the diagnosis Self-Neglect. Self-Neglect occurs when the person is capable of performing self-care but fails to maintain a socially accepted standard of health and well-being (which might include hygiene).

Readiness for Enhanced Self-Care	Feeding Self-Care Deficit
Bathing Self-Care Deficit	Toileting Self-Care Deficit
Dressing Self-Care Deficit	Self-Neglect

ThinkLike a Nurse 24-2

Answer the following questions for Mrs. Williams (Meet Your Patients):

- What factor(s) may interfere with Mrs. Williams's self-care ability?
- How can you ensure maximum independence with hygiene for her?
- How might you encourage her to strive toward optimal functioning?

PLANNING OUTCOMES/EVALUATION (Self-Care) NP

NOC standardized outcomes for Self-Care Deficit diagnoses are determined by the specific diagnosis. Useful outcomes might be:

- For patients who have more than one activity deficit—Use Self-Care: Activities of Daily Living (ADLs).
- For patients who have a single self-care deficit—Choose from these outcomes: Self-Care: Bathing; Self-Care: Oral Hygiene; Self-Care: Dressing; Self-Care: Eating; and Self-Care: Toileting.

When using NOC outcomes to write goals, rank the patient's abilities by using the NOC scale for self-care indicators: (1) dependent, does not participate, (2) requires assistive person and device, (3) requires assistive person, (4) independent with assistive device, and (5) completely independent. For example:
- Chooses clothing (5)
- Buttons clothing (4)

PLANNING INTERVENTIONS/ IMPLEMENTATION (Self-Care) NP

NIC outcomes for self-care deficits include the following examples:

Energy Management	Perineal Care
Bathing	Oral Health Maintenance
Environmental Management	Self-Care Assistance: Bathing
Foot Care	Self-Assistance: Dressing
	Self-Assistance: Toileting

Individualized interventions depend on the extent of the client's Self-Care Deficit, as well as the etiology of the problem. Refer to the accompanying Example Problem, Hygiene Self-Care Deficit. The following are some examples for Dressing Self-Care Deficit:
- Demonstrate the use of assistive devices (e.g., to help patient grasp and pull on socks).
- Use Velcro fasteners instead of buttons and zippers.

You will find a thorough discussion of specific hygiene-care activities (e.g., care of the skin, oral hygiene) in the remainder of this chapter. To access a bathing and hygiene plan of care and care map,

 Go to Davis Advantage, Resources, Chapter 24, **Care Plan** and **Care Map.**

ThinkLike a Nurse 24-3

- Which NANDA-I self-care diagnoses apply to Mrs. Williams and Mr. Gold (Meet Your Patients)?
- Explain the reasoning for your choices.
- For each patient, what are the related factors for his or her Self-Care Deficit?
- Write a self-care diagnostic statement for Mrs. Williams and one for Mr. Gold.

Types of Scheduled Hygiene Care

The following types of scheduled hygiene care are provided in most inpatient facilities (e.g., hospitals and long-term care settings).
- **Hourly rounds (comfort rounds or safety rounds)** consist of seeing the patient every hour, on schedule, to offer help with self-care needs (e.g., pain relief, positioning, and toileting). Hourly rounding improves patient safety and greatly reduces call light use.
- **Early morning care** is provided soon after the patient awakens to prepare the patient for breakfast or other activities, such as diagnostic tests. As needed, assist with toileting, washing the face and hands, giving mouth care, and providing comfort measures.
- **A.M. (morning) care** occurs after breakfast. Depending on the patient's self-care ability, assist with toileting, bathing, oral hygiene, skin care, hair care (including shaving if needed), dressing, and positioning or helping the patient transfer to a chair. Change or straighten bed linens, according to agency policy, and tidy the room.

EXAMPLE PROBLEM: Hygiene Self-Care Deficit

PROBLEM

Definition
- A **self-care deficit** exists when a person is unable to perform one or more ADLs (e.g., bathing).
- A **hygiene self-care deficit** occurs when the person lacks ability to bathe himself, including washing the whole body, combing hair, brushing teeth, doing skin care and nails, and applying makeup.

Adverse Effects (of hygiene care)
Although cleanliness can contribute to well-being, comfort, and health, it can also be stressful—for example, to critically ill patients, the frail elderly, and those with dementia. Adverse events include:
- Decreased oxygenation or ventilation
- Hypertension
- Hypotension
- Intracranial hypertension
- Cardiorespiratory arrest

ETIOLOGIES
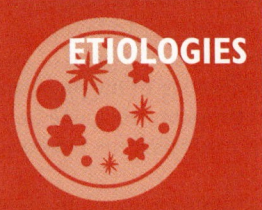

- Pain
- Fatigue
- Impaired cognitive ability
- Impaired physical functioning
- Sensory disturbances
- Impaired mobility
- Emotional or mental health disturbances
- Environmental barriers

ASSESSMENT
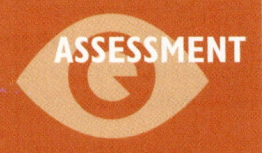

Assess Self-Care Ability

Use a standardized functional status rating to assign a score to each response. For the commonly used Katz ADL,

 Go to the Clinical Nursing Web site at https://consultgeri.org/try-this/general-assessment/issue-2.pdf

You can also create your own scale, such as the following:
1. Completely independent; needs no assistance.
2. Needs device or special equipment (e.g., walker).
3. Requires assistance or teaching from another person.
4. Requires assistance from a person, as well as special equipment.
5. Totally dependent; does not participate in the activity

Obtain a Health History

- Identify underlying illness, injury, or disease.
- Identify cognitive impairment.
- Assess for depression, psychoses, or delusions.
- Assess for other factors (see list of etiologies).
- Determine preferences and practices.

DIAGNOSIS
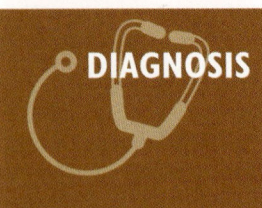

- NANDA-I self-care diagnoses related to hygiene are Self-Care Deficit: Bathing, Dressing, Toileting, and Feeding; and sometimes Self-Neglect (2014).
- Classify the patient's functional level (see preceding scale).
- Use descriptive terms such as *mild, moderate, severe,* and *total.*
- Example diagnostic statement, using a scale: Bathing Self-Care Deficit **(2)** related to severe knee pain secondary to degenerative joint disease

OUTCOMES
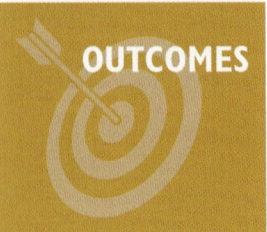

- *The NOC standardized outcome* **Self-Care: Activities of Daily Living (ADLs)** *is appropriate for all of the Self-Care Deficit diagnoses.*
- *Individualized goals/outcome statements you might write include the following:*
  Verbalizes satisfaction with body cleanliness and oral hygiene after A.M. care.
  Accepts assistance with ADLs or total care, if needed.
  By May 4, will complete bath independently, except for back and feet, after nurse provides equipment and assists patient to the bathroom.

EXAMPLE PROBLEM: Hygiene Self-Care Deficit—cont'd

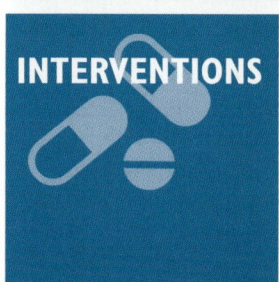

INTERVENTIONS

- Offer pain medication before ADLs.
- Allow sufficient time for all ADLs to prevent fatigue and frustration.
- Modify care to meet individual needs.
- Evaluate patient responses continually as you work.
- Provide care in small segments, allowing the patient to rest after brushing his teeth.
- Promote eventual self-care.
- Critically ill patients need rest, so you will not push them to perform at their highest level of function.
- If the patient is able to perform self-care, allow him to rest while you perform part of the care—for example, washing his feet and legs.

Focused Assessment

Guidelines for Assessing Hygiene

Assessment of Functional Abilities

The Katz Index of Independence in Activities of Daily Living (ADL) is used extensively to assess functional abilities in activities of daily living (bathing/hygiene, dressing/grooming, feeding, toileting). To use the Katz ADL,

 Go to the Clinical Nursing Web site at https://consultgeri.org/try-this/general-assessment/issue-2.pdf

Observe Self-Care Abilities

When bathing, dressing, eating, and toileting, which of the following best describes the patient's ability?

➤ Is completely independent; requires no assistance.
➤ Requires a device or special equipment (e.g., a walker, a large-handled spoon).
➤ Requires help, supervision, or teaching from another person.
➤ Requires help from another person, as well as a device or special equipment.
➤ Is totally dependent; does not participate in the activity (e.g., total bed bath).

The Environment

➤ Is the room temperature comfortable?
➤ Are the siderails up, when indicated? Is the bed in low position?
➤ Are bed wheels locked?
➤ Are bed linens clean and wrinkle free?
➤ Is the patient's call device within reach?
➤ Is the overbed table clean and uncluttered?
➤ Is the walking space uncluttered?
➤ Are there unpleasant odors?

Skin

Subjective Data

Patients may be sensitive about skin problems or poor hygiene practices, so direct your questions to the patient in a nonjudgmental, respectful manner. General questions to ask include the following:

➤ How often do you prefer to bathe?
➤ How do you usually care for your skin?

➤ What soaps, lotions, or other skin care products do you use?
➤ Do you have difficulty controlling body odor?
➤ Have you ever had an allergic skin reaction to food, medications, plants, skin care products, or other materials?
➤ What problems have you had with your skin in the past?
➤ What problems are you having with your skin now?
➤ For each problem identified, ask:
What symptoms are you having (e.g., any rash or itching)? Where is the problem located?
➤ How long have you had this problem?
➤ What have you done to provide relief from the symptoms?
➤ Do you use any prescription, over-the-counter (OTC), or herbal remedies to treat this problem?
➤ Have you seen a healthcare provider about this problem?
➤ Was a diagnosis made? If so, what was it?
➤ How has this problem affected your life?
➤ How can I best help you with your skin care?
➤ Also ask about the presence of diseases or other factors that are known to cause skin problems—for example, decreased mobility, decreased circulation, incontinence, inadequate nutrition, or deficient knowledge.

Objective Data

➤ Note the skin's overall cleanliness, condition, color, texture, turgor, hydration, and temperature.
➤ Observe for rashes, lumps, lesions, and cracking.
➤ Look for drainage from wounds or around tubes.
➤ Observe for four significant color changes: pallor, erythema, jaundice, and cyanosis.

Feet

Subjective Data

Ask the patient the following questions or obtain the data from his records:

➤ What is your normal foot care routine?
➤ What type of footwear do you usually wear? Observe what the patient is wearing.
➤ Have you had any foot problems; what treatments have you had for them?
➤ Do you examine your feet on a regular basis?
➤ Do you have diabetes mellitus or peripheral vascular disease?

(Continued)

Focused Assessment

Guidelines for Assessing Hygiene—cont'd

Objective Data

Compare findings for both feet:

➤ Observe for cleanliness and skin integrity. Note open areas, drainage, or redness.

➤ Inspect for swelling, inflammation, or infection.

➤ Palpate for edema.

➤ Check the skin between the toes for cracks or signs of a fungal infection.

➤ Notice the color and temperature of the feet; are they the same bilaterally? The color and temperature provide data about circulation and oxygenation. For example, cold, dusky feet may indicate impaired circulation or tissue perfusion secondary to a peripheral vascular disease.

➤ Check capillary refill. How many seconds does it take for the color to return after you apply pressure?

➤ Note the presence of foot odors, if any.

Nails

Subjective Data

Ask about the patient's usual nail care practices and history of nail problems and their treatments.

Objective Data

Inspect the nails for the following:

➤ Shape, contour, and cleanliness

➤ Presence of broken nails, hangnails, or cracked cuticles

➤ Hands: Do the fingernails appear neatly manicured, or does the patient bite the nails?

➤ Feet: Are the toenails trimmed appropriately, straight across?

➤ Presence of redness or swelling at the nail base or sides

Oral Cavity

Subjective Data

➤ Usual hygiene practices

➤ History of periodontal disease or other oral problems

➤ Financial or insurance problems that limit access to dental care

➤ Nutritional status and dietary habits (e.g., intake of refined sugars)

➤ Medications, such as anticonvulsants or diuretics

➤ Medical treatments, such as radiation therapy, oxygen therapy, and nasogastric tubes

➤ Other factors known to cause oral problems (smoking, alcohol use, NPO status, dehydration, mouth breathing)

➤ Self-care deficits (e.g., cognitive impairment, activity intolerance, impaired mobility, depression, lack of knowledge, lack of motivation)

Objective Data

➤ Observe the lips, which should be pink and moist without lesions.

➤ Inspect the oral mucosa and gums, which should also be pink, moist, smooth, and free of lesions.

➤ Healthy gums should have a well-defined margin at each tooth. There should be no visible bleeding.

➤ Instruct the patient to stick out his tongue and to move it around. It should move freely. The tongue should be symmetrical and pink, with a slightly rough surface.

➤ Assess the teeth for the presence of any loose, missing, or decaying teeth.

➤ Examine the hard and soft palates for color, lesions, patches, or petechiae.

➤ Note any unusual mouth odors or halitosis.

Hair

Subjective Data

➤ Use of special products or medicated shampoos

➤ History of hair problems or current conditions needing treatment (e.g., pediculosis)

➤ History or presence of disease or therapy that affects the hair (e.g., chemotherapy)

➤ Factors influencing the patient's ability to manage hair and scalp care (e.g., Impaired Mobility)

➤ Personal or cultural preferences for styling of the hair

Objective Data

➤ Note the condition, cleanliness, texture, and oiliness of the hair.

➤ Inspect the scalp for dandruff, pediculosis (head lice), alopecia (hair loss), secretions, or lesions.

Eyes

Subjective Data

➤ If the patient wears glasses, ask when he uses them (e.g., for reading, for driving) and ask how well he sees without them.

➤ If the patient wears contact lenses, determine:

  ➤ The type of lens (hard, soft, long-wearing, disposable).

  ➤ How often he wears them (daily, occasionally) and for how long at a time. Are they worn during sleep?

  ➤ History of, or present, problems with lens usage (e.g., cleaning, removal).

  ➤ Usual practices for cleaning and storage.

➤ History of or current problems with the eyes (e.g., redness, tearing, irritation, dryness, or "scratchy feeling").

Objective Data

➤ Inspect the eyes for redness, lesions, swelling, crusting, excessive tearing, or discharge.

➤ Check the color of the conjunctivae.

▪ **P.M. (afternoon) care** consists of preparing patients for afternoon rest or to receive visitors. As needed, assist non-ambulatory patients with toileting, hand washing, and oral care; straighten bed linens; reposition the patient; and offer other comfort measures (e.g., pain medications).

▪ **H.S. (hour of sleep) care** is given before the patient goes to sleep. Offer the same care as given in the afternoon, adding a back massage to help relax the patient. Also place within easy reach the call light, water glass, urinal, or anything else the patient may need during the night.

Hygiene Routines

When performing morning hygiene for your patient, ask how she would prefer her routine. This can be as simple as asking:

- What part of your care are you able to participate in?
- What soap do you prefer?
- How would you like your hair styled?
- What clothes do you like to wear?

These questions show caring, compassion, and respect for each patient.

Turn off lights and TV and close the door before leaving the room (according to patient needs and preferences). For a back-massage procedure, see Procedure 35-1.

Delegating Hygiene Care

In many institutions, NAPs perform most of the hygiene care. However, you will need to carefully assess patients to ensure that it is safe to delegate their care. If the patient is unstable or the NAP is inexperienced or unfamiliar with the patient's limitations, you must assist or perform the care yourself. Read the section "What Should I Know About Delegation and Supervision?" in Chapter 7 for a review of making delegation decisions. Also see Figure 24-1.

Before assigning a NAP to assist with a bath, shower, or toileting, give instructions about the following:

- Patient's limitations and restrictions, and amount of assistance necessary
- Use of assistive devices (e.g., cane, walker, or gait belt)
- Specific safety precautions (e.g., use of gait belt or shower chair)
- Presence of obstacles (e.g., drainage tubes, catheters, IV tubing, or bandages) and how to maintain them during bathing and toileting

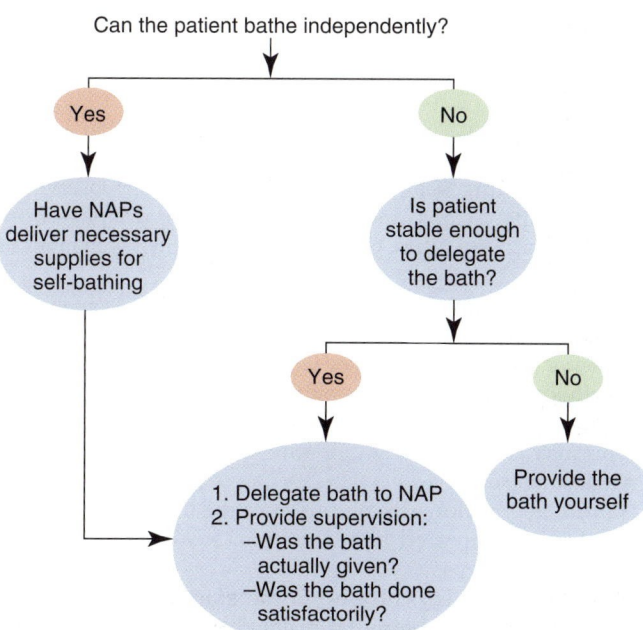

FIGURE 24-1 The RN should assess the patient, delegate bathing as appropriate, and provide supervision.

- Observations to make during the procedure and why they are important. Examples include the following:

    Skin condition: presence of lesions; areas of special concern over bony prominences and under abdominal folds and breasts

    Presence, appearance, and amount of urine or stool, or the need to collect a specimen

Remember, as the professional nurse, you are responsible for making assessments and determining the meaning of the data reported to you by the NAP. Assisting with or supervising hygiene care is an excellent opportunity for you to assess the patient's level of consciousness, short- and long-term memory, ability to follow instructions, range of motion, skin condition, activity tolerance, and overall self-care ability.

ThinkLike a Nurse 24-4

Think about Mrs. Williams (Meet Your Patients). You have delegated her bathing and oral hygiene to a NAP.

- What information do you need to share with the NAP about this patient's needs, limitations, or preferences?
- What, if any, specific observations will you ask the NAP to make for Mrs. Williams?
- What, if any, specific observations will *you* need to make for Mrs. Williams?
- What action will you take if you determine that the patient's needs and preferences were not met by the NAP?

CARE OF THE SKIN

The preceding sections introduced you to the broad topic of hygiene, self-care, and activities of daily living. The rest of the chapter will deal with specific topics, such as care of the skin.

Theoretical Knowledge
knowing why

To assist patients with skin care, you must have theoretical knowledge about personal hygiene measures and the structure and function of the **integument** (skin).

Anatomy and Physiology of the Skin

The **integumentary system** consists of the skin, the subcutaneous layer directly under the skin, the hair, the nails, and the sweat and sebaceous glands. The skin has two distinct layers (see Fig. 36-1):

1. The **epidermis** (the thicker, outer layer) consists of stratified squamous epithelial tissue composed of keratinized (dead) cells, which make the skin waterproof.
    - The epidermis continually sheds (**desquamates**) and is completely replaced every 3 to 4 weeks.
    - The epidermis contains melanin, a pigment that provides protection against the ultraviolet rays of the sun and that, together with circulating blood, gives skin its color.
2. The **dermis** (the thinner, second layer) contains blood and lymphatic vessels, nerves, bases of hair follicles, and sebaceous and sweat glands.

Functions of the Skin

The skin has the following five main functions:

1. *Protection.* Intact skin is the body's first line of defense against bacteria and other microorganisms that can enter the body. Skin protects underlying tissues from thermal, chemical, and mechanical injury. **Sebaceous glands** secrete

an oily substance called *sebum,* which helps to waterproof and lubricate the skin and decrease bacterial growth.

2. *Sensation.* The skin contains sensory organs or receptors for heat, cold, pressure, touch, and pain.

3. *Regulation.* The skin helps maintain fluid and electrolyte balance by preventing the escape of excess water and electrolytes from the body. It helps to regulate body temperature by dilating and constricting blood vessels and activating or inactivating sweat glands. **Sweat glands,** concentrated in the axillae and external genitalia, excrete water in the form of perspiration; evaporation produces a cooling effect on the skin.

4. *Secretion/excretion.* The sweat glands secrete fatty acids and proteins and excrete nitrogenous wastes *(urea),* sodium chloride, and water in perspiration.

5. *Vitamin D formation.* The skin contains a form of cholesterol that is changed to vitamin D on exposure to ultraviolet light from the sun.

See Chapter 36 for more information about the structure and functions of the skin.

Factors Affecting the Skin

In addition to a person's hygiene practices, health status and developmental stage also affect skin condition.

Health Status

Anything that interferes with the hydration, circulation, and nutrition of the skin creates a risk to skin integrity. As you read each of the following factors, think about whether it would be present for Mr. Gold (Meet Your Patients):

- **Dampness.** Excessive perspiration (e.g., in fever) and incontinence of urine or bowel cause the skin to become damp. The skin then breaks down more easily, especially in the skinfolds. This is called **maceration.**
- **Dehydration.** Fluid loss (e.g., from vomiting, diarrhea, or fever) and insufficient fluid intake can cause dehydration, causing the skin to become dry and to crack easily.
- **Nutritional Status.** Very thin or very obese people are at increased risk for skin irritation and injury. *Morbid obesity* makes it physically difficult to reach and clean all areas of the body and can lead to development of odor and fungal conditions.
- **Insufficient Circulation.** Immobility, vascular disease, and inadequate nutritional status compromise circulation. This predisposes the patient to local tissue death and ulceration when skin cells do not receive enough oxygen.
- **Skin Diseases.** Skin diseases such as impetigo (a bacterial infection of the skin) and systemic diseases such as measles and chickenpox cause lesions that create discomfort and require special hygiene care.
- **Jaundice.** Certain diseases cause a yellow skin discoloration brought about by accumulation of bile pigments in the skin. Jaundice causes the skin to be itchy and dry.
- **Lifestyle and Personal Choices.** Some people damage their skin by exposure to ultraviolet rays because they want to be tan. Some use sunscreen; some do not. As another example, many people have skin tattoos or piercings, creating the risk for systemic and local infection and scarring.

Developmental Stage

- Infants have fragile, easily injured skin.
- As a child matures, the skin becomes more resistant to injury and infection, but children need adults to provide or supervise the cleanliness of their skin.

- In adolescence, the sebaceous glands enlarge, and secretions increase. The skin becomes oily and susceptible to acne.
- With aging, numerous skin changes increase the older adult's risk for skin problems such as pressure ulcers and reduced ability to heal. Refer to Table 24-1 for a description of normal skin changes in older adults.

KnowledgeCheck 24-2

- What are five functions of the skin?
- How does the skin help regulate body temperature?
- What changes take place in the skin as a person ages?

PracticalKnowledge
knowing **how**

ASSESSMENT (SKIN) NP

For a thorough discussion of skin assessment, including how to describe and document your observations, see Chapter 21. However, as you provide skin hygiene you should routinely make the following observations.

♥ **iCare** Patients may be sensitive about skin problems or poor hygiene practices, so as you interview and examine the patient, do so in a nonjudgmental, respectful manner. Protect the patient's privacy by closing the curtain and exposing only the area being bathed or examined. Be mindful of the room temperature and try to reduce drafts to avoid chilling the patient.

Subjective Data Ask the patient about his usual bathing and skin care practices and preferences, as well as the following:
- Past and current skin problems, including their effects on the patient's life
- Prescription and over-the-counter (OTC) or herbal skin remedies being used
- Allergic skin reactions to food, medications, plants, skin care products, and so on
- History of diseases or other factors known to cause skin problems, including decreased mobility, decreased circulation, incontinence, inadequate nutrition, or deficient knowledge

Objective Data Inspect each area of the skin in an orderly, head-to-toe manner, noting overall cleanliness, condition, color, texture, turgor, hydration, and temperature. Observe for rashes, lumps, lesions, and cracking. Look for drainage from wounds or around tubes. Observe for the following changes in skin color:
- **Pallor** in a light-skinned person may appear as pale skin without underlying pink tones. In a dark-skinned person, observe for an ashen gray or yellow color.
- **Erythema** is redness of the skin related to vasodilation and inflammation. It is difficult to see in dark-skinned people, so you may discover it by palpating the skin for areas of increased warmth.
- **Jaundice,** a yellow discoloration of the skin, occurs in patients with impaired liver function. It is best seen in the sclerae of the eyes.
- **Cyanosis,** a bluish coloring of the skin, is caused by decreased peripheral circulation or decreased oxygenation of the blood. It may be related to cardiac, pulmonary, or peripheral vascular problems. In dark-skinned patients,

Table 24-1 ▶ Normal Skin Changes in Older Adults

STRUCTURE	CHANGE IN STRUCTURE AND ACTIVITY	CLINICAL EFFECTS
Epidermis	Thinner; decreased rate of cell turnover	Skin appears pale and somewhat translucent; slower healing.
Subcutaneous tissues	Thinner and more fragile, less fat	Decreased protection of bony prominences and thermoregulation
Collagen and elastin fibers in the dermis	Weaken and become less elastic	Skin becomes wrinkled.
Sebaceous and sweat glands	Activity decreases.	Skin becomes dry, scaly, and itchy. Temperature regulation in hot weather becomes more difficult.
Hormones (estrogen and progesterone)	Production decreases.	Contributes to drying and thinning of the skin.
Skin	Vascularity decreases.	Skin becomes cool and pale.
Hair follicles	Diminish in number and activity.	Hair becomes thin, grows more slowly.
Melanocytes (pigment cells)	Numbers decrease.	Hair turns gray or white; skin may become unevenly pigmented.
Nails	Thicken; become softer; growth rate diminishes.	Nails tear easily.
Skin growths	Become more common (e.g., warts, "liver spots," "age spots").	Most are caused by years of sun exposure; most are harmless (except for skin cancers, which are fairly common but not normal changes).

you can best see cyanosis by examining the conjunctivae, tongue, buccal mucosa, and palms and soles for a dull dark color.

KnowledgeCheck 24-3

- True or False: The professional nurse is responsible for making assessments.
- True or False: Assisting with the bath is an excellent time to assess the patient.
- To inspect for pallor in a dark-skinned person, which areas would you assess for an ashen gray or yellow color?
- What is the term that means "a bluish color of the skin"?
- Name two physiological causes of erythema.
- Where can you best see jaundice?

ANALYSIS/NURSING DIAGNOSIS (Skin) NP

You should be familiar with the following common skin problems and observe for them as you provide skin care:

- **Pruritus** (itching) may lead to scratching and breaks in the skin.
- **Dry skin** tends to crack, burn, or itch.
- **Maceration** is softening of the skin from prolonged moisture (e.g., urinary incontinence). It makes the epidermis more susceptible to injury.
- **Excoriation** is a loss of the superficial layers of the skin caused, for example, by scratching and by the digestive enzymes in feces.

- **Abrasion,** a rubbing away of the epidermal layer of the skin, especially over bony areas or prominences, is often caused by friction or shearing forces that occur when a patient moves or is moved in bed.
- **Pressure injuries** are lesions caused by tissue compression and inadequate perfusion. See Chapter 36.
- **Acne** is an inflammation of the sebaceous glands that is common among adolescents and young adults.
- **Burns** are a type of traumatic injury caused by thermal, electrical, chemical, or radioactive agents.

To see illustrations of most of those skin problems, see Procedure 21-2.

Impaired Skin Integrity as the Problem

When you wish to focus on prevention or treatment of the skin condition, use the following NANDA-I diagnostic labels (2014):

- **Risk for Impaired Skin Integrity.** *Definition:* At risk for alteration in epidermis and/or dermis.
  Risk factors: The general conditions that affect the skin are dampness, dehydration, inadequate circulation, immobility, nutritional status (thin or obese), skin diseases, systemic diseases, and jaundice.
  Example: Risk for Impaired Skin Integrity related to immobility secondary to casts and traction
- **Impaired Skin Integrity.** *Definition:* Altered epidermis or dermis.
  Defining characteristics: Invasion of body structures, destruction of skin layers (dermis) or of skin surface (epidermis).

Example: Impaired Skin Integrity related to decreased peripheral circulation secondary to arteriosclerosis

Impaired Skin Integrity as the Etiology

Impaired Skin Integrity may be the etiology of other nursing diagnoses. Certain skin problems create a risk for infection by causing cracks or breaks in the skin. Others may contribute to discomfort and low self-esteem. The following are examples:

Risk for Infection related to skin lacerations and abrasions
Situational Low Self-Esteem related to appearance and self-consciousness about skin lesions secondary to severe eczema

ThinkLike a Nurse 24-5

- Why are Mrs. Williams and Mr. Gold (Meet Your Patients) at risk for Impaired Skin Integrity?
- What are the specific kinds of skin integrity problems that pose an increased risk to both patients?

PLANNING OUTCOMES/EVALUATION (Skin) NP

NOC standardized outcomes for problems of the skin, feet, nails, mouth, teeth, hair, eyes, ears, and nose, include the following:

Oral Hygiene (and Self-Care: Oral Hygiene)	Wound Healing: Primary Intention
Tissue Integrity: Skin and Mucous Membranes	Wound Healing: Secondary Intention
Self-Esteem	Immobility Consequences: Physiological

Individualized goals/outcome statements you might write for a patient with skin problems include the following:

- Skin will remain intact and free of secretions.
- Skin will remain free of lesions.
- Patient will follow a regimen to improve skin dryness.

PLANNING INTERVENTIONS/ IMPLEMENTATION (Skin) NP

Examples of NIC standardized interventions for skin integrity and skin care include the following:

- **For Impaired Skin (or Tissue) Integrity**—Bathing, Cutaneous Stimulation, Perineal Care, Pressure Management, Skin Surveillance, and Wound Care
- **For Risk for Impaired Skin Integrity**—Add to the above: Bed Rest Care, Circulatory Precautions, Pressure Ulcer Prevention, and Positioning

Individualized nursing activities for patients with Impaired Skin Integrity include bathing and massage, which are presented in this section. You will usually delegate patient bathing to NAPs (see Fig. 24-1). However, you must make certain that the patient actually gets a bath.

Bathing   Bathing serves three purposes: health promotion, social interaction, and pleasure or relaxation.

- Bathing removes perspiration and bacteria from the skin surface, helping to prevent body odor.
- The warmth from the bath solution and the friction of bathing dilate the blood vessels near the surface of the skin, increasing the circulation.
- Bathing stimulates depth of respirations and provides sensory input.
- Bathing can be a time to strengthen the nurse–patient relationship.

- Bathing promotes relaxation and comfort, enhances well-being, and improves self-image.

Back Massage   Regardless of the type of bath used, when possible end the bath with a back massage to provide relaxation and stimulate circulation. As with all procedures, be sure there are no contraindications to massage (e.g., fractured ribs, burns, recent heart surgery). To learn a procedure for giving a back massage, see Procedure 35-1.

Choosing the Type of Bath to Meet Patient Needs

The type of bath you give depends on your nursing judgment; the patient's preference, self-care ability, and endurance; and the medical plan of care.

- **Assist bath**—the nurse helps the patient with areas that may be difficult to reach, such as the back, feet, and legs.
- **Complete bath**—the nurse washes the patient's entire body without assistance from the patient. For complete instructions see Procedures 24-1 through 24-3.
- **Partial bath**—the nurse cleanses only the areas that may cause odor or discomfort, such as the axillae and perineum. If a complete bath would be stressful to the patient, you may choose to give a partial bath.

The following sections discuss types of baths in detail.

Bed Baths and Modified Bed Baths

A **bed bath** is for patients who must remain in bed but who are able to bathe themselves. You will assist by placing the bath supplies on the bedside stand or overbed table. The following are four types of bed bath:

Prepackaged Bathing Products   Recent guidelines and evidence support the now widespread use of **prepackaged bathing products** (Nøddeskou, Hemmingsen, & Hørdam, 2015; Ritz, Pashnik, Padula, et al., 2012). These are a set of commercially prepared and packaged premoistened, disposable washcloths. Studies suggest the following benefits:

- Helps assure consistency of bathing technique among caregivers
- Prevents inconsistent applications of emollients (moisturizers)
- Decreases the skin damage due to rough washcloths

- ✚ Decreases the potential for colonization of the skin and the spread of microorganisms with the use of tap water and basins. This is especially true of products containing chlorhexadine (Ritz, Pashnik, Padula, et al., 2012; Rubin, Louthan, Wessels, et al., 2013; Sievert, Armola, & Halm, 2011).

Towel Bath   When giving a **towel bath,** you will place a large towel and a bath blanket in a plastic bag, saturate them with a warmed, commercially prepared mixture, and use them to bathe the patient. The solution dries rapidly, so there is no need to towel-dry the patient. Patients find towel baths satisfactory, and they require less nursing time than a traditional bed bath. **KEY POINT:** *This is a preferred method for patients who have mild to moderate Impaired Skin Integrity or Activity Intolerance and for patients with dementia (e.g., Alzheimer's disease).* See Procedure 24-2.

Bag Bath   A **bag bath** uses 8 to 10 washcloths instead of a towel and bath blanket. They are moistened with water (preferably sterile, filtered or distilled) or a pH balanced no-rinse soap. They are warmed, and each section of the patient's body is cleansed with a fresh cloth.

Basin and Water Bath   This is a type of bed bath in which you use a disposable basin with water, washcloths, lotion, and pH-balanced no-rinse soap or a chlorhexidine-and-water solution. This may be done, for instance, if a patient refuses the prepackaged bath or if the patient is grossly soiled (e.g., large amounts of blood or feces). When you use a basin and water bath, you must be aware of the potential for healthcare-acquired infections (HAIs) related to (1) reusable basins becoming a reservoir for microorganisms and (2) the presence of biofilm in hospital waterlines and plumbing.

- **Bath water.** Depending on the patient's condition, it may be safer to use distilled, sterile, or filtered water in place of tap water to prevent skin contamination with bacteria biofilm. Some agencies have a serious problem with biofilm, whereas others do not; and some agencies have filtering systems that make the water safe to use. When using tap water, it is a good idea to bathe the patient with a solution of chlorhexadine and water to combat any bacteria that may be present (Rubin, Louthan, Wessels, et al., 2013; Rutala & Weber; HICPAC, 2008).
- **KEY POINT:** *One size does not fit all! The more vulnerable the patient, the more caution you must exercise regarding basin and water bathing.*
- For guidelines for bathing adults, see Box 24-1. **KEY POINT:** *Guidelines change frequently; be alert for practice changes.*

Shower

Most ambulatory patients prefer a shower. It is a time-saver and refreshing as well as cleansing. In a hospital or long-term care facility, some clients can manage a shower mostly on their own. For complete information, refer to Clinical Insight 24-1.

Tub Bath

If a client is ambulatory but requires assistance with bathing (e.g., because of pain and stiffness in the hands and arms) you may prefer a tub bath (see Clinical Insight 24-1). It will be easier for you to wash and rinse the patient, and you will not get as wet as when you help with a shower. Immersion in water also helps to soak areas that are crusty, scaly, or soiled and relaxes stiff, sore muscles and joints. Overall, tub baths are thought to be of greater benefit than sponge or bed baths.

The tub should have handrails and a nonskid surface to prevent falls. Some patients need assistance getting into and out of a tub. Some kneel or squat first and then sit in the tub. For completely dependent patients, specially designed tubs reduce the need to lift patients into and out of the tub. You can also use a hydraulic lift and a regular tub (Fig. 24-2).

Therapeutic Bath

The primary care provider may prescribe **therapeutic baths** for some patients. These are baths given for a specific purpose (e.g., to relax muscles, to remove scales and crust from the skin). Given that current research suggests that hospital water supplies may serve as a reservoir for pathogens and play a role in the spread of HAIs, use of distilled or sterile water would seem preferable, if in accord with provider prescription and facility policy.

It is your responsibility to add the medically ordered substance, ensure prescribed water temperature, and assist the patient into the tub. Use a disposable sitz tub if one is available. If not, clean the tub thoroughly at the end of the bath, preferably with a chlorhexidine-based product. Examples of therapeutic baths include the following:

- Oatmeal or coal tar baths, used to treat specific skin conditions, such as psoriasis

---

BOX 24-1 ■ Guidelines for Bathing the Adult Patient

Bathing Frequency

For patients who are unable to provide self-care, assist with or provide a bath:

- Daily or more frequently for comfort purposes (on patient request)
- To respond to diaphoresis
- To address a significant incontinence episode

Privacy and Timing of the Bath

Maintain patient privacy throughout the procedure.

Bath time should be determined based on:

- Patient preference
- Clinical stability
- Patient's physiological tolerance to activity
- Sleep pattern (uninterrupted sleep is essential to the healing process)

Bath Supplies and Products

Prepackaged bath products should be used in place of basin and tap water for regular bathing:

- Remove reusable basins from the environment to encourage use of prepackaged bathing products.
- If using a basin, use sterile or distilled water in place of tap water.
- No-rinse pH-balanced cleansers with emollients help to protect the barrier function of the skin and reduce the risk of dry skin.

Chlorhexidine gluconate (CHG) 2% prepackaged cloths are recommended to decrease the colonization of bacteria on the skin.

- Do not rinse; retain 2% CHG on the skin at all times.
- Do not use on mucous membranes (face or perineal area).

Source: Veje, P. L., & Larsen, P. (2014). The effectiveness of bed bathing practices on skin integrity and hospital-acquired infections among adult patients: A systematic review protocol. *The JBI Database of Systematic Reviews and Implementation Reports,* 12(2), 71–81. Retrieved from http://joannabriggslibrary.org/jbilibrary/index.php/jbisrir/article/view/1422/1848

- A warm sitz bath, to help to cleanse the perineum and soothe inflammation of perineal, vaginal, or rectal tissues.

Perineal Care

The **perineum** (the area between the anus and vulva in a female, or the anus and scrotum in a male) is a dark, warm, moist area that supports bacterial growth. Perineal care promotes comfort and prevents odor, skin excoriation, and infection. You will usually give perineal care (including the external genitalia) along with a complete bed bath, but it may be needed at other times as well. Give perineal care more frequently if the patient is incontinent of urine or feces or has drainage from the area.

Whether you and the patient are of the same or opposite sex, perineal care may at first be embarrassing for you both. Perform care in a professional manner and provide privacy (e.g., shut the door, pull bed curtains, drape properly). A matter-of-fact, sensitive approach puts most patients at ease.

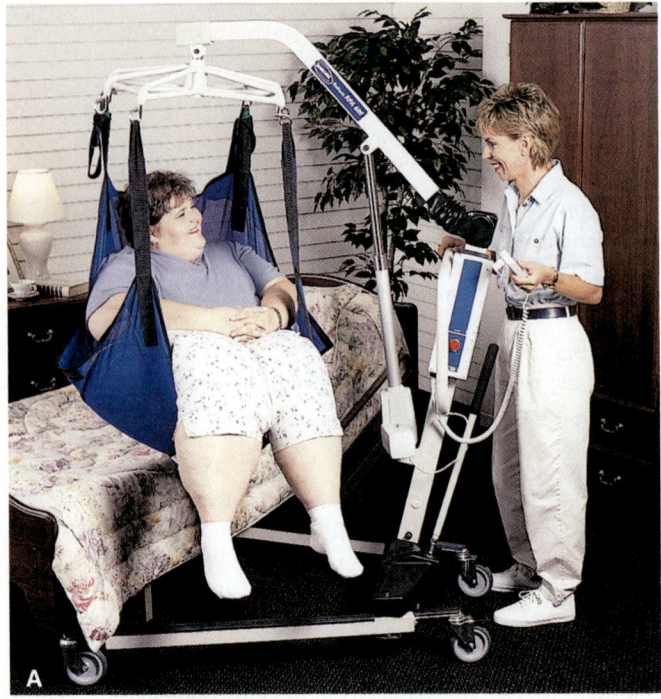

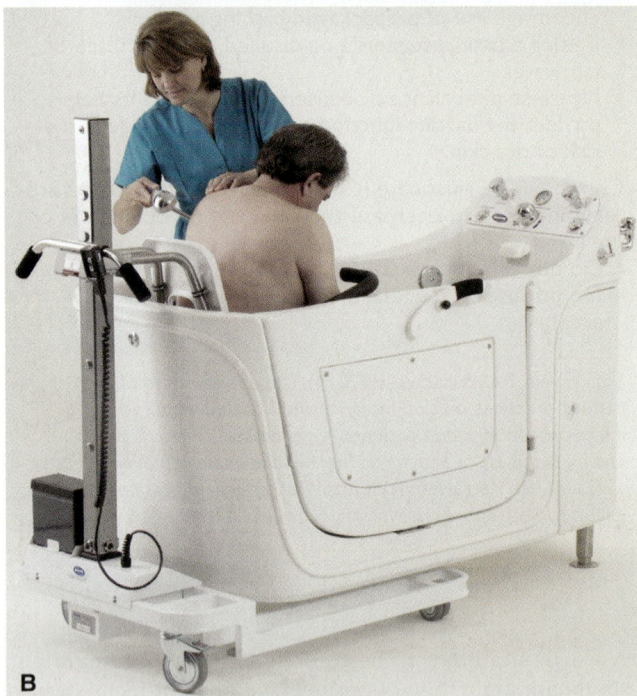

FIGURE 24-2 A. A hydraulic lift allows you to transport a patient to a bath or shower. B. A tub with a side-opening door enables patients to safely and easily enter the tub. (Courtesy of Carroll Health Care, London, Ontario, Canada.)

For complete information about providing perineal care, refer to Procedure 24-4.

KnowledgeCheck 24-4

- What causes body odor?
- What is the best intervention to rid the skin of body odor?
- What is the rationale for providing perineal care?
- How can you protect patient privacy during perineal care?

ThinkLike a Nurse 24-6

- Which of your patients (Meet Your Patients) will require nurse-assisted perineal care? Explain your reasoning.
- Which patient, if you are a woman, is most likely to be embarrassed by perineal care? Explain your reasoning.
- If you need more theoretical knowledge to answer these questions, what is it? Where could you find the information?

Bathing Patients With Dementia

Bathing should be a pleasant experience, not a stressful one. But patients with dementia tend to become agitated when told it is time to bathe, and they often yell or scream at their caregivers or pinch or hit them (Konno, Stern, & Gibbs, 2013; Wolf & Czekanski, 2015). The reason for agitation is usually that they experience pain, cold, fear, and loss of control. When you meet the patient's comfort needs (e.g., by adjusting the water temperature or taking special care when washing arthritic joints), the patient becomes less agitated and aggressive behavior declines significantly. You can significantly reduce aggressive behaviors by giving a towel bath or bag bath instead (Konno, Stern, & Gibbs, 2013). Despite the common myths about bathing, keep in mind that:

- The patient does not always need to have a daily tub bath or shower. It does not take a large amount of water to get a person clean. Using prepackaged bathing products can help you finish the bath more quickly, possibly reducing the patient's agitation.
- The patient will not be at more risk for skin problems or infections if a towel bath is used.
- It is not necessary to bathe a person who is resisting. You can adapt the approach, method, and time.
- Patients who are forced to bathe do not "just forget about it"; many stay upset and agitated for hours.

For more discussion of bathing myths and for instructions about providing a bath for a person with dementia, see iCare 24-2.

ThinkLike a Nurse 24-7

Suppose you have been providing towel baths to a patient who has mild dementia. One day a visiting family member says, "My father tells me he has not had a bath all week. What's going on here?" What would you do? How could you help to prevent this misunderstanding in the future?

Bathing Morbidly Obese Patients

Obesity is traditionally defined as a body mass index (BMI) of 30 or higher (about 20% to 40% above ones ideal weight). **Severe,** or **morbid, obesity** exists when BMI is 40 or higher (or body weight is 50% more than ideal weight).

For the morbidly obese person, thorough skin assessment is essential, but it is difficult. Be sure to obtain adequate assistance to reposition the patient during the bath and skin exam, so that you do not miss any areas. Pay special attention to skinfolds. The following are preventive interventions for problems related to hygiene, moisture, pressure, shear and friction, and nutrition (Rose & Drake, 2008):

Hygiene Morbidly obese clients find it physically difficult to reach all areas of the body. In addition, they may have limited mobility. Inability to maintain good hygiene may lead to odor and fungal infections.

- Ask how the patient handles skin care at home. Use the same adaptations, if possible.

Caring Tips for Bathing a Patient With Dementia

- **Focus on the patient,** not the task; provide choices.
- **Distract** with food or by playing relaxing music.
- **Use a gentle type of showerhead** for rinsing. A strong spray may frighten the patient.
- **Be creative:** Try bathing one part of the body each day.
- **Bathe at a regular time,** preferably the same time that the patient bathed at home.
- **Ensure continuity of care,** so the patient can build a relationship with the caregiver and be less fearful.
- **Provide privacy.** Patients with dementia do not necessarily lose their modesty and sense of privacy.
- **Avoid sensory overload:** Turn down lights, warm the room, play soft music, speak calmly. People with dementia have difficulty processing information. Sensory overload may trigger aggression.
- **Foster independence.** Encourage the patient to wash her own face if able, so that she may feel like an active participant.
- **Explain the procedure simply,** using short sentences.
- **Let the patient know before you touch her or spray her** with any fluids. Sudden actions are often frightening.
- **Do not rush.** The patient will feel the tension and may become agitated.
- **Teach techniques to caregivers at home** (e.g., being flexible with time, using a towel bath)
- Also refer to the "What if . . ." section of Procedure 24-1.

- Provide a trapeze to assist the patient to lift and reach difficult areas.
- Provide a handheld shower and long-handled brushes.
- Experts vary on the use of soap. Certainly the skin should be rinsed and dried well.

Moisture Skin in skinfolds stays damp because perspiration cannot evaporate.

Moisture contributes to the development of fungal and other skin infections.

- Use moisture barrier creams, particularly in skinfolds and the perineal area.
- Use fans, if permitted.
- Change linens often.
- Manage incontinence.
- If fungal infections occur, you may need a medical prescription for antifungal powders, sprays, cream, or ointment.

Pressure Pressure can be caused by limited mobility, by skinfolds where skin rubs on skin, by tight clothing, catheters, and so on.

- Reposition the patient frequently to redistribute the pressure of the skinfolds.
- Reposition catheters and tubes often; use tube holders to prevent rubbing.
- Separate the skinfolds with towels.

Shear and Friction The patient is at risk for friction and shearing injury from pulling skin across the linens when moving in the bed and chair.

- Provide a trapeze.
- Do not use sheepskins.

- Use a waterproof and breathable mattress cover.
- Keep linens wrinkle free.

The American Nurses Association's position is that you should use specialized lifts and other equipment to move patients safely and avoid injury to yourself (de Castro, 2004). If in an emergency you must move the patient, obtain sufficient help to avoid pulling the skin across the sheet or other surfaces.

Bathing Older Adults

KEY POINT: *For older adults, especially the bedbound and frail elderly, goals are to prevent drying of and injury to the skin.* At the same time, you should promote comfort and encourage independence in ADLs. This requires proper skin care and bathing techniques.

- Bag baths adequately address the problems of skin itching and irritation, improve skin integrity, and are far less distressing to frail older adults (Kottner, Lichterfeld, & Blume-Peytavi, 2013).
- Use a no-rinse pH-balanced cleanser to further protect the barrier function of the skin.
- Other interventions include avoiding use of soap, cleaning the skin immediately after soiling, and applying skin moisturizer.
- Also see "What if . . . Your Patient Is an Older Adult?" in Procedure 24-1.

KnowledgeCheck 24-5

- A nurse has given a bath in which he washed a bedridden patient's entire body without assistance from the patient. What is the term for this bath?
- What are the advantages of a towel or bag bath?
- For which type of bath will you most likely have a medical prescription?

ThinkLike a Nurse 24-8

Which type of bath would be most app\\ropriate for each of your patients (Meet Your Patients)? Provide rationales for your choices.

CARE OF THE FEET

Foot care is a necessary part of hygiene and essential at any age for tissue health, proper posture, and ambulation.

TheoreticalKnowledge knowing why

When providing foot care, you will need theoretical knowledge about the structure of the feet, life span variations, and common foot problems. The feet provide support for the weight of the entire body and absorb a significant amount of shock during walking. Their structure is complex, consisting of 26 bones and many muscles, tendons, and ligaments.

Foot problems tend to increase with aging. Because of diseases such as arteriosclerosis and peripheral vascular insufficiency, older adults often have decreased circulation to the lower extremities. This increases their risk for foot ulcers and infection. The incidence of diabetes is high among older adults, further increasing the risk for infection secondary to delayed healing. In addition, the skin becomes dry, predisposing the skin to cracking.

Common Foot Problems

In a recent survey in the United States, 83% of adults aged 21 and older reported their foot health to be good to excellent. However, 78% reported that they had had at least one foot problem (e.g., pain, blisters, athlete's foot) (Institute for Preventive Foot Health, 2012). Many foot problems are the result of improperly fitting shoes.

- A **corn** is a cone-shaped thickening of the epidermis caused by continuous pressure (e.g., from improperly fitting shoes) over bony prominences (e.g., toe joints).
- **Calluses** are usually found over the weight-bearing part of the foot: the heels, soles, or plantar surfaces. They are similar to corns but cover a wider area and are not painful.
- **Tinea pedis,** or athlete's foot, is a fungal infection of the skin, aggravated by moisture accumulation in unventilated shoes. Symptoms include itching and burning skin with blisters, scaling, and cracking, especially between the toes. Athlete's foot may be contracted by walking barefoot in public showers.
- An **ingrown toenail** grows inward into the soft tissues around it and the tissue at the nail border becomes swollen, inflamed, and painful. It may result from improperly trimming the toenails and wearing poorly fitting shoes. The nail may need to be surgically removed.
- **Foot odor** is produced when microorganisms growing on the feet interact with perspiration. The warm, moist environment created by shoes encourages both perspiration and bacterial growth.
- **Plantar warts** are painful growths caused by a virus. They may occur on any part of the sole of the foot but often develop under pressure points, such as the heel or ball of the foot.
- **Pressure injuries** are lesions caused by unrelieved pressure that impairs the circulation; this usually occurs over a bony prominence. In patients who are immobile, the back of the heels, the ankles, and the great toes are common locations; pressure ulcers do, of course, occur over other bony prominences.
- A **bunion** (hallux valgus) is a progressive disorder that begins with the enlargement of the first metatarsal joint at the base of the great toe and then progresses to leaning of the big toe, gradually changing the angle of the bones. A characteristic bump occurs slowly and continues to become increasingly prominent with aging. Tight-fitting shoes (particularly with high heels) are thought to be the cause of bunions in most patients. Genetics also play a role, as do some diseases, such as arthritis. For optional illustrations and more information about bunions,

 Go to the Web site of the American College of Foot and Ankle Surgeons, at http://www.acfas.org/

PracticalKnowledge
knowing **how**

The nursing focus for foot care is on prevention and early identification of problems.

ASSESSMENT (Feet) NP

This chapter describes routine observations that you can make when giving foot care. The color and temperature of the feet provide data about circulation and oxygenation. For example, cold, dusky, or pale feet may indicate impaired circulation or tissue perfusion secondary to peripheral vascular disease. For a thorough discussion of foot assessment, see Chapter 21 and the Pre-Procedure Assessments in Procedure 24-5. For specific questions to ask, see the Focused Assessment box Guidelines for Assessing Hygiene.

ANALYSIS/NURSING DIAGNOSIS (FEET) NP

The feet can be affected by congenital malformations, injuries, improper footwear, and medical conditions. The following are examples of nursing diagnoses associated with the feet:

- Impaired Skin (or Tissue) Integrity (feet) r/t mechanical pressure from wearing shoes that do not fit properly
- Risk for Impaired Skin Integrity (feet) r/t (1) altered sensation secondary to diabetes mellitus and (2) impaired circulation to the feet secondary to arteriosclerosis
- Impaired Walking r/t foot pain secondary to arthritis

PLANNING OUTCOMES/EVALUATION (FEET) NP

NOC outcomes for foot care are the same as for other areas of the body, as they relate to circulation, infection, tissue integrity, wound healing. For example, Tissue Integrity: Skin and Mucous Membranes is useful for any area of the body.

Individualized goals/outcome statements you might write for a patient with foot problems include the following:

- Avoids trimming calluses.
- Wears shoes that fit properly.
- Inspects feet regularly.

PLANNING INTERVENTIONS/ IMPLEMENTATION (FEET) NP

Examples of *NIC standardized interventions* include Foot Care; Circulatory Care: Arterial Insufficiency (or Venous Insufficiency); Skin Surveillance; and Teaching: Individual.

Individualized nursing activities related to care of the feet are those that prevent infection, odor, and trauma to the soft tissues of the feet. To learn how to administer foot care, see Procedure 24-5.

Teaching Your Client About Foot Care

While performing foot care, use the opportunity to teach the patient self-care for the feet. This is especially important for clients who have diabetes. Include the information in the accompanying Self-Care box in your patient teaching.

Diabetic Foot Care The following self-care measures are especially important for people who have diabetes or poor peripheral circulation. Those who have diabetes should have their feet checked regularly by a professional. People who have diabetes are at high risk for problems with their feet because they often have impaired circulation and delayed healing, as well as an increased risk for infection. Furthermore, if they have neuropathy, they may not experience pain with a foot injury, so treatment may be delayed. If untreated, a seemingly minor foot lesion can progress to gangrene and require amputation.

KnowledgeCheck 24-6

- What are some causes of ingrown toenails?
- What is the cause of foot odor?
- Why should you not apply lotion between the toes?

Self-Care

Teaching Your Client About Foot Care

While performing foot care, use the opportunity to teach the patient self-care for the feet. This is especially important for clients who have diabetes. Include the following in your patient teaching.

Daily Foot Inspection

➤ Inspect the feet daily, using a mirror to view all surfaces. Check between the toes for cracks or redness. Look for calluses, blisters, wounds and lesions, or dry areas.
➤ If you cannot check your own feet, have someone else do it.

Hygiene for Feet and Nails

➤ Wash, rinse, and dry the feet well.
➤ Avoid soaking the feet if you are diabetic, or if there is decreased circulation to the feet.
➤ Apply a water-soluble lotion to feet but not between the toes, because it may cause maceration.
➤ Use an antifungal powder, if needed, for athlete's foot.
➤ Do not cut or file callused areas.
➤ Cut and file toenails straight across. Do not use a razor blade on the nails or feet.

Shoes and Stockings

➤ Wear cotton or wool socks, which absorb perspiration.
➤ Wear well-fitted, sturdy shoes with nonskid soles and arch support. Natural materials, such as canvas and leather, are best because they allow air to circulate and perspiration to evaporate. Shoes should allow ½ to ¾ inch of toe room.
➤ Avoid open-toed shoes, sandals, high heels, and thongs or flip-flops. They do not protect the feet.
➤ Before putting on shoes, check for foreign objects; check that the inside of the shoe is smooth.

Protecting the Feet

➤ Avoid measures that impair circulation to the feet, such as wearing tight garters or knee stockings or crossing the legs.
➤ Do not go barefoot, even when getting out of bed at night. Wear slippers.
➤ Do not put tape or OTC corn medicines or pads or other medications (e.g., hydrogen peroxide) on the feet.
➤ Do not smoke. This constricts arterioles and decreases circulation to the feet.

When to Seek Medical Attention

➤ Pain in the feet or legs. This may be a sign of loss of circulation, serious infection, or nerve damage (neuropathy)
➤ Wounds or ulcers on the feet, especially if they don't seem to be healing
➤ Cut to the feet or lower legs that extends deep into the skin and bleeds significantly
➤ Cuts or cracks in the feet
➤ Generalized redness or red streaks surrounding a wound or ulcer on the feet or lower legs. This might be a sign of infection of the tissue (cellulitis).
➤ Fever greater than 101°F (38.5°C)
➤ Confusion. This can be a sign that a wound infection has entered the bloodstream (septicemia). A change in mental status might indicate low blood sugar, which occurs with serious infection or if the patient is diabetic.
➤ Numbness or tingling, decrease in sensation, cold skin temperature, corns, ingrown toenails, and for trimming very thick nails—especially if you have diabetes

CARE OF THE NAILS

The nails are part of the integumentary system. Like the hair and skin, they are composed of epithelial tissue. Healthy nailbeds are usually clean, pink, smooth, convex, and evenly curved. Present at birth, the nails change very little throughout life; however, as one ages, nails thicken, become ridged, and may yellow or become concave in shape. Other changes are caused by certain pathological conditions. For example:

- Trauma to the nail can lead to nail bruising or falling out.
- Inadequate diet or metabolic changes can cause the nails to become brittle.
- Patients with diabetes mellitus are much more prone to infection.

ASSESSMENT (Nails) NP

When assessing the nails, obtain subjective data about the patient's usual nail care practices, any history of nail problems, and their treatments. To obtain objective data, inspect the nails for shape, contour, and cleanliness and observe whether they are neatly manicured and trimmed appropriately, straight across. Unclean or rough fingernails may scratch or abrade the skin and create a risk for infection. Other nail changes may reflect an underlying disease process. In addition, the area under the nail can harbor dirt and bacteria, which can be another source for transmitting microbes.

ANALYSIS/NURSING DIAGNOSIS (Nails) NP

There are no NANDA-I labels to describe nail problems. However, the following are examples of nursing diagnoses related to nail care:

- Risk for Impaired Tissue Integrity related to ingrown nails secondary to trimming too close to the cuticle
- Risk for Infection related to loss of skin integrity secondary to hangnails, cracked cuticles, or trauma from using sharp scissors or nail clippers

PLANNING OUTCOMES/EVALUATION (Nails) NP

There are no NOC outcomes that relate specifically to nail care, but you can use outcomes that relate more generally to circulation, infection, tissue integrity, or wound healing.

Individualized goals/outcome statements you might write for a patient with problems associated with nail care may include the following:

- Demonstrates proper care of the nails.
- Seeks care of a **podiatrist** (physician who specializes in foot care) for toenail care.

PLANNING INTERVENTIONS/ IMPLEMENTATION (Nails) NP

Examples of *NOC standardized interventions* for nail care include Nail Care and Self-Care Assistance.

Individualized nursing activities related to proper care of the nails include providing nail care for dependent patients. The procedure for care of the fingernails is the same as for care of the toenails. Also see Procedure 24-5.

Teaching Your Client About Nail Care Teach clients the following self-care measures:

- Inspect the nails daily.
- Trim nails with a nail clipper. People with diabetes or circulatory problems should file only, because cutting poses a risk for injury to the slow-healing tissues.
- File the nails straight across, rounding the corners slightly to prevent scratching. Do not cut deeply into the lateral corners because this may cause ingrown nails.
- Remove hangnails by carefully removing them with cuticle clipper.
- Clean under the nails with an orangewood stick or other blunt instrument.
- Push back the cuticles gently.
- Use a moisturizing lotion to soften cuticles.
- Avoid biting nails.
- Consult a podiatrist for ingrown toenails or other nail problems.
- Recommend to patients with diabetes, circulatory insufficiency, or nail problems that they seek nail care from a podiatrist.

KnowledgeCheck 24-7

- True or False: Healthy nails are usually clean, smooth, and convexly curved.
- List at least three nail changes that occur with aging.
- List at least four things you should teach clients about self-care of their nails.

ORAL HYGIENE

To maintain the integrity of the mucous membranes, teeth, and gums and to prevent tooth loss and gum disease, it is important to have (1) routine dental checkups, (2) adequate nutrition, and (3) daily mouth care (oral hygiene). The following are benefits of mouth care:

- It removes food particles and secretions.
- A clean mouth helps to promote a better appetite.
- It reduces the incidence of healthcare-acquired pneumonia in older adults and critically ill patients in acute care settings.

TheoreticalKnowledge knowing **why**

Digestion of food begins in the mouth (oral cavity). The tongue and teeth begin digestion by breaking up food and mixing it with saliva.

- **Incisors** (front teeth) are for biting and tearing.
- **Molars** (in the back of the mouth) are used for chewing.

- **Wisdom teeth** are the very back molars on either side of each jawbone.

Saliva, produced by three pairs of salivary glands in the mouth, also acts as a mechanical cleaner of the mouth. The structures of the mouth pertinent to oral hygiene include the tongue, **gingiva** (gums), and teeth.

Developmental Variations

The first set of teeth (**deciduous teeth**) erupts between ages 6 months and 2 years. By age 2, a child usually has 20 teeth (Fig. 24-3). Between ages 6 and 12 years, the deciduous teeth loosen and fall out and are eventually replaced with 32 permanent teeth (Fig. 24-4).

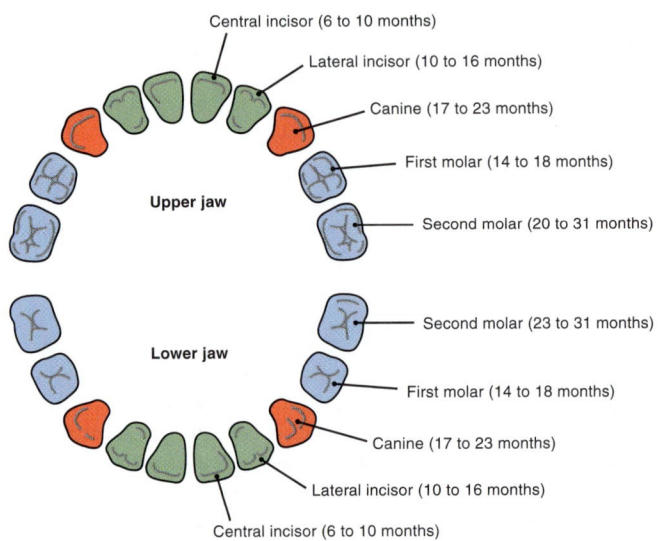

FIGURE 24-3 The 20 deciduous teeth. (Courtesy of P. Dillon. [2015]. *Nursing health assessment* [3rd ed.]. Philadelphia, PA: F.A. Davis.)

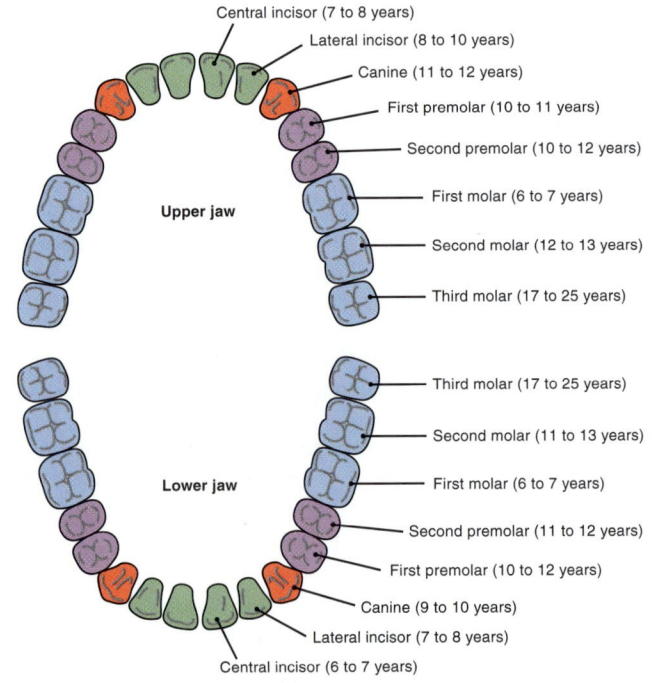

FIGURE 24-4 Most adults have 32 permanent teeth. (Courtesy of P. Dillon. [2015]. *Nursing health assessment* [3rd ed.]. Philadelphia, PA: F.A. Davis.)

The tooth surface wears away with aging and the gums may begin to recede, resulting in bone and tooth loss, possibly necessitating the use of dentures (false teeth). Other changes common in aging are a brownish pigmentation of the gums and dryness of the oral mucosa, which is caused by decreased saliva production.

Risk Factors for Oral Problems

Oral health is influenced by heredity, nutrition, and oral hygiene. Therefore, any condition that prevents good oral hygiene can lead to oral problems. Risk factors include the following:

- **History of periodontal disease**
- **Lack of money or insurance** for dental care
- **Pregnancy.** The gums may bleed easily and become puffy and tender during pregnancy because of increased estrogen, which increases the vascularity of the gingiva. Good hygiene is needed to prevent infection.
- **Poor nutrition or eating habits.** Adequate intake of calcium, phosphorus, and vitamin D is essential for healthy teeth and gums. Excessive intake of refined sugars leads to dental decay. One example of this is **baby-bottle tooth decay,** which occurs when parents put an infant or toddler to bed with a bottle or sippy cup of milk, fruit juice, or other sugary beverage. Carbohydrates in the fluid cause demineralization of the tooth enamel, leading to major decay of the teeth.
- **Medications.** The anticonvulsant phenytoin (Dilantin) causes gingival hyperplasia (excessive growth of cells). Other medications cause dryness of the mouth (e.g., diuretics, medications used to treat cancer, numerous calcium channel blocker agents [especially nifedipine], and tranquilizers such as chlorpromazine [Thorazine] and diazepam [Valium]).
- **Medical treatments.** Medical treatments affecting the oral cavity include the following:
  Jaw surgery, which requires scrupulous oral hygiene to prevent infection
  Radiation treatments of the head and neck, which can permanently damage the salivary glands
  Oxygen therapy, which dries the oral mucosa
- **Any situation that causes dry mouth** predisposes to cracking of the mucosa, including heavy cigarette smoking, excessive alcohol use, inadequate fluid intake (e.g., being NPO), dehydration, and mouth breathing
- **Compromised self-care abilities** may be caused by:
  Decreased level of consciousness (e.g., a person who is comatose or heavily sedated), serious illness or injury, weakness, activity intolerance, or paralysis
  Cognitive impairment (e.g., developmental delay, dementia)
  Depression
  Lack of knowledge or motivation to perform self-care

KnowledgeCheck 24-8

- How do the teeth aid in digesting food?
- How many deciduous teeth does a child usually have?
- List at least three factors that cause dry mouth.
- List at least two medications or medical treatments that can cause oral problems.
- Name four situations that can compromise self-care ability for oral hygiene.

ThinkLike a Nurse 24-9

- For which of your patients, Mrs. Williams or Mr. Gold, does the scenario indicate that the patient is at risk for oral problems? What are the data?

- Why is the patient's nursing diagnosis Risk for Impaired Oral Mucous Membrane Integrity instead of Impaired Oral Mucous Membrane Integrity?

Common Problems of the Mouth

Dental **caries** (cavities) and periodontal disease are the two most frequent problems affecting the teeth. They are discussed here along with other common mouth problems:

- **Dental caries** are primarily caused by the failure to remove plaque. **Plaque** is an invisible bacterial film that builds up on the teeth and eventually leads to destruction of the tooth enamel. The plaque builds up with dead bacteria and forms hard deposits at the gumlines (**tartar**). The tartar causes deterioration of the supporting structures that hold the teeth in the gums and also attacks the bone tissue, causing the teeth to become loose. Other causes of cavities include excessive intake of refined sugars, a lack of brushing and flossing, and infrequent visits to the dentist.
- **Periodontal disease (pyorrhea)** is the major cause of tooth loss in adults 35 years and older. It is an inflammation characterized by bleeding and receding gums and destruction of the surrounding bone structure. The patient experiences halitosis and complains of a bad taste in the mouth. When pyorrhea is advanced, the gums become infected, and the teeth loosen and may fall out or need to be removed.
- **Gingivitis** is inflammation of the gum tissue surrounding the teeth. If untreated, it may progress to periodontal disease.
- **Halitosis,** also known as bad breath, results from poor oral hygiene, eating certain foods (e.g., garlic, onions), tobacco use, dental caries, infections, or even systemic diseases, such as uncontrolled diabetes or liver disease.
- **Stomatitis,** an inflammation of the oral mucosa, has numerous causes, including bacteria, mechanical trauma, irritants, nutritional deficiencies, and systemic infection. Symptoms may include pain, halitosis, and increased salivation.
- **Glossitis,** an inflammation of the tongue, is caused by deficiencies of vitamin B_{12}, folic acid, and iron.
- **Cheilosis** is a cracking and/or ulceration of the lips, in the form of reddened fissures at the angles of the mouth. It is usually caused by vitamin B–complex deficiencies.
- **Oral malignancies** must be detected as early as possible. Teach patients to see a dentist immediately if any of the following are present in the mouth: lumps, ulcers, white or red patches, bleeding, pain, persistent sores, or numbness.

KnowledgeCheck 24-9

- Identify and define several causes of halitosis.
- What are the two most common problems affecting the teeth?
- What is the end result of severe periodontal disease?

PracticalKnowledge
knowing **how**

You should assess the patient's oral cavity when performing or assisting with oral hygiene. This is particularly important for older adults because of the association between oral health and systemic disease.

ASSESSMENT (Oral Cavity) NP

You might begin your subjective assessment by asking the patient about his usual hygiene practices. You should also interview the patient or examine his records for the risk factors for oral problems discussed in the preceding section. Ask about tobacco and alcohol use.

As part of your objective assessment, inspect the lips, oral mucosa, gums, and tongue. Mucosa and gums should be pink and moist without lesions or bleeding. Look for loose, missing, or decaying teeth; tartar; and stomatitis; and note any unusual odors or halitosis. Check to be sure the tongue is normal in color and without lesions.

 The Kayser-Jones Brief Oral Health Status Examination (BOHSE) is used to assess the oral cavity of older adults. It was specifically designed for nursing home residents with both normal and impaired cognitive functioning, and it can be used by a variety of nursing personnel. The tool assigns a numerical rating to findings for items such as lips, tongue, tissue inside the mouth, gums, saliva, condition of natural teeth, condition of artificial teeth, pairs of teeth in chewing position, and oral cleanliness. To learn more about the BOHSE, and see a copy of the tool, you can search the Web or,

 Go to the Clinical Nursing Web site at https://consultgeri. org/try-this/general-assessment/issue-18.pdf

To learn more about physical assessment of the oral cavity, refer to Chapter 21. Also refer to the Focused Assessment box Guidelines for Assessing Hygiene.

ANALYSIS/NURSING DIAGNOSIS (Oral Cavity) NP

In addition to Self-Care Deficit, discussed in the first part of the chapter, the following are examples of nursing diagnoses that may be useful in describing problems of the mouth:

- Risk for Infection related to mouth lesions
- Impaired Dentition (caries) related to inability to afford dental care
- Impaired Oral Mucous Membrane Integrity related to inability to manage mouth care secondary to impaired mobility
  Oral and dental problems can be the etiology of other nursing diagnoses, for example:
- Imbalanced Nutrition related to lack of teeth for mastication
- Pain related to mouth lesions

PLANNING OUTCOMES/EVALUATION (Oral Cavity) NP

NOC standardized outcomes for oral problems include Oral Hygiene; Self-Care: Oral Hygiene; and Knowledge: Health Behavior.

Individualized goals/outcome statements you might write for mouth problems include the following examples:

- Oral mucous membranes will remain pink, moist, and intact.
- Demonstrates correct technique for brushing and flossing.
- Makes preventive dental visits every 6 months.

PLANNING INTERVENTIONS/ IMPLEMENTATION (Oral Cavity) NP

For some clients, you may need only to provide the necessary supplies for mouth care. For others, you will need to assist with or provide complete care as often as necessary to keep the mouth clean and moist. Rinsing with mouthwash is not a substitute for a thorough cleaning of the teeth and mouth.

NIC standardized interventions for mouth care include Oral Health Maintenance; Self-Care Assistance; and Teaching: Individual.

Individualized nursing activities related to oral hygiene include teaching for self-care (and assisting with and providing oral hygiene for dependent patients), which is discussed in the following section.

Teaching Your Client About Oral Self-Care

Teach the following self-care measures to promote oral health and prevent periodontal disease:

Preventing Caries and Periodontal Disease

- Eliminate between-meal snacks with high sugar content (ice cream, soft drinks, candy, gum, jams and jellies).
- Include in the diet cleansing, fibrous foods, such as raw fruits and vegetables.
- Include an adequate intake of calcium, phosphorus, and vitamins A, C, and D.
- Have regular dental checkups every 6 months.
- Brush teeth with a soft brush and toothpaste after each meal and at bedtime (some dentists say twice a day). Bacteria do the most damage to the teeth in the first 24 hours after eating.
- Floss between the teeth daily to remove food debris and stimulate the blood flow to the gingiva.
- Use a fluoride toothpaste to strengthen tooth enamel.
- You can make your own cleanser by combining one part baking soda with two parts salt.
- Follow the dentist's recommendations for topical applications of fluoride.

Brushing and Flossing

- Make sure the brush is small enough to reach all teeth. If it is too firm, it can injure enamel and gum tissue.
- Electric toothbrushes are effective; however, you should consult your dentist about using water-spray units, because they can force debris into pockets of the gums.
- Brush at a 45° angle, from the gum to the tooth crown, using small circular or vibrating motions.
- When flossing (1) wrap one end of the floss around each of your middle fingers. (2) Hold about 1 to 2 inches of floss tightly between the fingers. (3) Insert floss between the teeth by gently moving it back and forth; do not force it. (4) Floss adjacent sides of both teeth to the gum tissue, but not into the gum, because you may injure the tissue. (5) Use a fresh section of floss when it becomes soiled or frayed. (6) Rinse your mouth well when you are finished. A variety of convenient flossing devices are available as an alternative to this method (Fig. 24-5).

Oral Hygiene for Children

- Begin oral hygiene when the first tooth erupts. Use a washcloth, cotton ball, or gauze pad moistened with water.
- Do not put a child to bed with a bottle or sippy cup. Milk, juice, or any other liquid with sugar can lead to dental caries in the young child when the liquid sits on the teeth at night or during naps.
- Begin brushing the child's teeth with a soft toothbrush when she is about 18 months old. Start first using water only. Later, switch to a fluoride-containing toothpaste.
- Follow your dentist's instructions for giving a fluoride supplement.

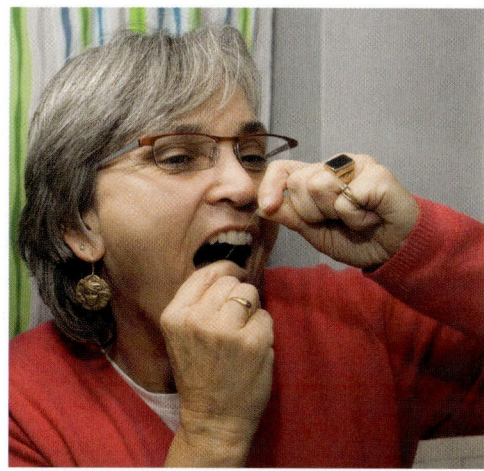

FIGURE 24-5 Flossing between the teeth is an essential part of oral hygiene.

- Schedule a visit to the dentist when all 20 deciduous teeth have erupted.
- See your dentist if you notice any problems, such as chipping, redness or swelling, caries, or misalignment.
- For school-age children, parents may need to supervise mouth care to be sure it is done adequately.

Denture Self-Care

- If you have dentures or other removable prostheses ("bridges"), wear them. If you do not, the gums are likely to shrink, and you will have further gum loss.
- Clean dentures and bridges at least once a day, preferably after each meal.
- Remove dentures from the mouth to clean them.
- Use regular toothpaste or special denture-cleaning compounds.
- Do not use hot water on dentures; it may damage them.
- If the dentures have metal parts, do not soak them overnight in cleaning solutions.
- Store dentures in a denture cup, in water, to prevent drying. Do not wrap them in tissues because they may accidentally be thrown away.
- Clean dentures over a plastic pan or towel in the sink (Fig. 24-6). They are fragile and may break if dropped.

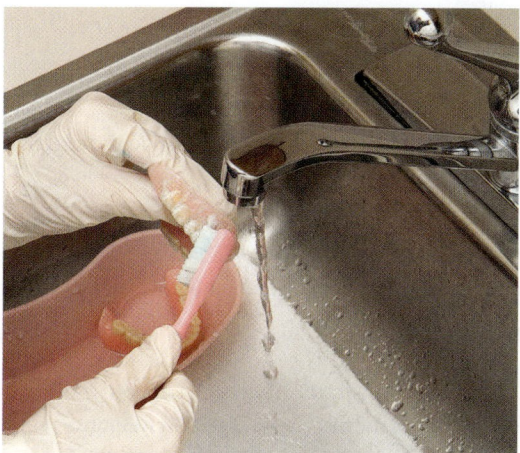

FIGURE 24-6 Dentures must be cleaned thoroughly as a part of daily oral hygiene.

- Flossing between the teeth is an essential part of oral hygiene.
- Dentures must be cleaned thoroughly as a part of daily oral hygiene.

Assisting With Denture Care

A patient may have a complete set of removable dentures or just an upper or lower plate. A **bridge,** or partial plate, consists of one or more artificial teeth. A bridge may be permanently fastened to other teeth, or it may be removable. Artificial teeth are fitted to the individual and should not be used by anyone else. If the person leaves the prosthesis out of his mouth for long periods, the shape of the gums will change, and the prosthesis will no longer fit properly. Poorly fitted or loose dentures can lead to chewing difficulties and even nutritional deficiencies. Recent research suggests that elderly persons should remove dentures at bedtime to prevent problems such as tongue and denture plaque and gum inflammation. In addition, elderly persons who wore dentures during sleep were more likely to develop pneumonia (Iinuma, Arai, Abe, et al., 2015).

The nurse's role is to ensure cleanliness by teaching for self-care (above) or to provide denture care for dependent clients. For further information, refer to Procedure 24-7.

Oral Care for Critically Ill Patients

Patients in long-term care settings and critically ill patients in acute care settings are at high risk for healthcare-associated pneumonia. This is especially true for those dependent on a ventilator. Ventilator-associated pneumonia (VAP) is the most common healthcare-acquired infection in critically ill patients. A simple and inexpensive way to reduce the risk of pneumonia for these patients is to keep their teeth clean, thus reducing the number of bacteria that cause pneumonia (American Association of Critical-Care Nurses, 2010, El-Rabbany, Zaghlol, Bhandari, et al., 2015; Lin, Xu, Huang, et al., 2015). The regimen includes the following:

- Brush the teeth twice a day.
- Use a soft toothbrush.
- Moisturize oral mucosa and lips every 2 to 4 hours.
- Use a chlorhexidine gluconate (0.12%) rinse twice a day during the perioperative period for adult patients who undergo cardiac surgery.
- Use mouthwash inside the mouth twice a day for adult patients who are on a ventilator.

Oral Care for Unconscious Patients

Oral care for unconscious patients is particularly important because they often breathe through the mouth. If the patient is receiving oxygen per cannula or has a nasogastric or feeding tube inserted, the mucous membranes become even drier. To learn more about how to provide oral care for unconscious patients, see Procedure 24-8.

An unconscious patient often responds to oral stimulation by biting down, so use a padded tongue blade instead of your fingers to hold the mouth open. Also use a padded tongue blade when providing oral care for a patient with seizures to avoid the patient biting you.

Follow agency practices for the type and frequency of special mouth care. Some patients may need it every hour or two. You may use commercially packaged applicators or foam swabs to clean the mouth.

- **Do not use** lemon-glycerine swabs because they are drying to the mucosa and may causes changes in tooth enamel.
- **Do not use** hydrogen peroxide because it is irritating to oral mucosa and may alter the balance of normal flora of the mouth.

Oral Care for Patients With Dementia

Poor oral health and dental pain impact on general well-being—specifically, on the ability to eat, type of diet, weight, speech, hydration, appearance, and social interactions. Dental disease and pain may be the source of some of the behavior problems of older adults with dementia. Because it is a challenge to provide oral hygiene for patients with dementia, staff sometimes neglect care. Residents may be uncooperative: refusing care, refusing to open the mouth, biting the toothbrush, and so on. Research is needed to identify the best interventions (Bedi, 2015). Meanwhile, for experts' suggestions for ways to provide oral care to patients with dementia, see the "What if . . ." section in Procedure 24-6.

KnowledgeCheck 24-10

How would you position Mr. Gold (Meet Your Patients) to perform his oral hygiene?

CARE OF THE HAIR

Hair is an accessory structure of the skin.
- **Vellus hair** is the short, fine hair present over much of the body.
- **Terminal hair,** which is coarser, darker, and longer, is found on the scalp, eyebrows, axillae, perineum, and legs

The hair helps to maintain body temperature, serves as a receptor for tactile sensation, and influences a person's self-image. Sebaceous glands at the base of the hair follicle secrete sebum, or oil, to lubricate hair and scalp. See Chapter 21 for more information about changes in hair that occur through the life span and as a result of illness.

ASSESSMENT (Hair) NP

For the purposes of hygiene, you will need information about the patient's history of hair problems or current conditions needing treatment (e.g., pediculosis), diseases or therapy that affect the hair (e.g., chemotherapy), and factors influencing the patient's ability to manage her hair and scalp care (e.g., Impaired Mobility). Ask the patient about special products she uses and about her preference for styling her hair. Inspect the condition and cleanliness of the hair, and inspect the scalp for dandruff, lesions, and so forth. For more complete information

---

Toward Evidence-Based Practice

American Association of Critical-Care Nurses. (2007, revised 2010). AACN practice alert. Oral care in the critically ill. Retrieved from http://classic.aacn.org/AACN/practiceAlert.nsf/Files/OC/$file/Oral%20Care%20in%20the%20Critically%20Ill%20.pdf

This evidence report reviewed 14 references and graded the evidence for the conclusions they drew. They used a scale of I to VI, with Level VI being the strongest support and Level I being the weakest (manufacturer's recommendations only). The following are two AACN recommendations for oral care in the critically ill:

- Use oral chlorhexidine gluconate (0.12%) rinse twice a day for adult patients undergoing cardiac surgery; not routinely for all patients. (Level V)
- Brush teeth, gums, and tongue at least twice a day. (Level II)

Ames, N., Sulima, P., Yates, J., et al. (2011). Effects of systematic oral care in critically ill patients: A multicenter study. American Journal of Critical Care, 20(5), 103–114.

Researchers examined the effects of an oral care protocol on oral health for critically ill patients in an intensive care unit. The intervention included toothbrushing that was performed at least every 12 hours and in a systematic way to prevent missing any areas. After oral care, chlorhexidine, delivered as a spray, was applied to teeth and mucosa. Researchers concluded that the evidence-based oral healthcare program effectively and statistically improved oral health in the critically ill patient.

Lin, Y. J., Xu, L., Huang, X. Z., et al. (2015). Reduced occurrence of ventilator-associated pneumonia after cardiac surgery using preoperative 0.2% chlorhexidine oral rinse: Results from a single-centre single-blinded randomized trial. Journal of Hospital Infection, 91(4), 362–366.

These researchers explored the effects of a chlorhexidine rinse compared with a saline rinse in preventing ventilator-associated pneumonia (VAP) in patients scheduled for heart surgery. Patients gargled three times with 0.2% chlorhexidine or saline 30 min after each meal and 5 min after toothbrushing at bedtime. VAP occurred in 8.5% of the chlorhexidine group compared with 24% of the saline group.

1. Suppose you are a critical-care nurse using the AACN Practice Alert guidelines. For which of the two AACN recommendations would you most want to have further research evidence?

2. Which of the latter two studies provide additional support for that guideline? Explain your thinking. (*Note:* This question does not include the AACN Practice Alert.)

3. How are the patients in the Ames et al. and Lin et al. studies alike or different from the patients for whom the AACN Practice Alert was designed?

 Go to Davis Advantage, Resources, Chapter 24, **Toward Evidence-Based Practice—Suggested Responses.**

about assessing the hair, see Chapter 21. Also see the Focused Assessment box Guidelines for Assessing Hygiene, earlier in the chapter.

ANALYSIS/NURSING DIAGNOSIS (HAIR) NP

Common problems associated with the hair and scalp include the following (also see Chapter 21):

- **Dandruff** is a condition in which there is excessive shedding of the epidermal layer of the scalp. Primary symptoms include itching and flaking of the scalp, which may be caused by fungal infection.
- **Pediculosis** is an infestation of head lice. Though frequently associated with poor hygiene practices, it knows no socioeconomic boundaries. Head lice spread through sharing of combs, brushes, hair ornaments, hats, and caps.
- **Alopecia,** or hair loss, can be very stressful and affect self-image. Abnormal hair loss, which may be gradual or sudden, can be caused by an autoimmune disorder, hormonal imbalance, thyroid disease, stress, fever, certain medications, or chemotherapy.

There are no NANDA-I labels that apply specifically to the hair. When the difficulty lies with self-care ability, you can use Dressing Self-Care Deficit and Bathing Self-Care Deficit. Examples of other nursing diagnoses that may apply include the following:

- Risk for Impaired Skin Integrity related to secretions on the scalp
- Situational Low Self-Esteem related to alopecia secondary to chemotherapy

KnowledgeCheck 24-11

- List at least four assessments you should make of a patient's hair.
- What is pediculosis?
- What is alopecia?

PLANNING OUTCOMES/EVALUATION (HAIR) NP

As always, select outcomes based on the client's nursing diagnoses. *Individualized goals/outcome statements* you might write for a patient with problems related to the hair include the following:

- Scalp and hair are clean.
- By 9/18, brushes own hair.
- Hair and scalp are free from infestation, infection, irritation, or dryness.
- Verbalizes improved comfort and self-esteem.

PLANNING INTERVENTIONS/ IMPLEMENTATION (Hair) NP

NIC standardized interventions specific to hair care are: Hair Care, Skin Surveillance, and Infection Protection.

Individualized nursing activities related to the care of the hair include daily brushing and combing, shampooing, and, for men, shaving and beard care.

Providing Hair Care

- Brush the hair daily to remove tangles, massage the scalp, stimulate the circulation, and distribute oil down the hair shaft.

- Use a stiff-bristled brush, but be sure the bristles are not sharp enough to injure the patient's scalp. Likewise, a comb with broken or uneven teeth or one that is too fine can break or snarl the hair and scrape the scalp.
- Comb tightly curled hair with a wide-toothed comb or pick.
- Encourage patients to brush and comb their own hair, if they are able to do so.
- Encourage family members to assist with hair care. This promotes their participation and reduces feelings of helplessness.
- Do not cut a patient's hair unless he consents to the haircut.

Shampooing the Hair Shampooing cleans the hair and scalp. It is soothing and relaxing to many patients. Hair can be shampooed while the person is in the shower, standing or sitting over a sink, or in bed. Protect the patient's eyes with a dry washcloth and make sure the water temperature is appropriate for the patient. For patients who are unable to tolerate a standard shampoo procedure, you can use a dry shampoo as an alternative. However, it is not as effective as shampooing with water. Commercially prepared shampoo caps are available and have, in most institutions, replaced the dry shampoo method. See Procedure 24-9.

Hair Care for African Americans Hair care is equally important for all patients, so if a patient's hair requires special care, you must learn how to do it. The hair of African Americans varies in texture from some other ethnicities—it may be long or short, straight or kinky, thick or thin. Worn naturally, very curly hair can easily become entangled or matted, and it tends to be fragile and easily broken.

Shampoo and groom the hair according to the person's preference. In general, though, you should comb and brush the hair daily and apply a light oil to the scalp. Ask a family member to bring from home the product the patient prefers to use. Do not apply chemical relaxers to a patient's hair. Only a licensed beautician should do this. See Procedure 24-9 for shampooing.

Beard and Mustache Care

Beards and mustaches tend to collect food particles. They should be washed daily during a bath or shower and combed and trimmed as necessary. Use agency-approved (e.g., filtered) water. Do not shave a patient's mustache or beard without permission to do so. For details of beard and mustache care, see Procedure 24-10.

Shaving

Depending on the culture, shaving is an important part of grooming and helps patients feel better about their appearance. Many men shave their facial hair every day. Women may shave to remove axillary and leg hair. ✚ If the patient has a bleeding disorder or is taking anticoagulant medication, you should use an electric razor. For important points about shaving, see Procedure 24-11.

Some dark-haired men (e.g., African Americans and Italians) have tightly curled facial hair, which curls back into the skin when shaved. An inflammatory reaction may occur, resulting in the formation of papules and pustules ("razor bumps"). If the man wishes to use a **depilatory** (hair-removing agent) instead of shaving, be sure to keep the chemical from contacting his eyes, nose, mouth, and ears. Do not use a straight or safety razor to remove the depilatory, because it will irritate the skin. Some men with this condition prefer to grow a beard, especially when they are ill and unable to care for themselves.

CARE OF THE EYES

Usually you will not need to provide special hygiene care for the eyes. The eyelids and lashes keep dust and debris from entering the eyes, and tears continually cleanse and lubricate them. When necessary, you may gently cleanse the eyes, from the inner to the outer canthus, with a moistened washcloth, with no soap. If there is drainage or crusting, use a different cloth for each eye to prevent cross-contamination.

ASSESSMENT (Eyes) NP

When performing hygiene care, inspect the eyes for redness, lesions, swelling, crusting, excessive tearing, or discharge. Also check the color of the conjunctivae. You should also ask the patient or check his records to see whether he wears glasses or contact lenses. If the patient wears glasses, ask when he uses them (e.g., for reading, for driving), and ask how well he sees without them. If the patient wears contact lenses, determine the following:

- The type of lens (hard, soft, long wearing, disposable)
- How often he wears them (daily, occasionally) and for how long at a time
- Whether they are worn during sleep
- History of or current problems with lens usage (e.g., cleaning, removal)
- Usual practices for cleaning and storage
- History of or current problems with the eyes (e.g., redness, tearing, irritation, dryness, or "scratchy feeling")

These should be adequate data for hygiene care. However, it is not a complete eye assessment. For detailed information about assessing the eyes, see Chapter 21.

ANALYSIS/NURSING DIAGNOSIS (Eyes) NP

Other than Bathing Self-Care Deficit, there are no NANDA-I labels specific to the eyes. Other diagnoses that might occur include the following:

- Risk for Infection related to improper hand washing and improper lens cleaning
- Risk for Injury (to eyes) related to wearing lenses longer than recommended

PLANNING OUTCOMES/EVALUATION (Eyes) NP

The only *NOC standardized outcome* specific to the eyes is Sensory Function: Vision.

Individualized goals you might write for eye care include these examples:

- Demonstrates proper cleaning and storage of contact lenses.
- Eyes appear clean and without redness or drainage.

PLANNING INTERVENTIONS/ IMPLEMENTATION (Eyes) NP

There are no *NIC standardized interventions* specific for eye care. However, for a Risk for Infection and Risk for Injury diagnosis, Infection Protection, Self-Care Assistance, and Individual Teaching might be useful.

Individualized nursing activities related to the care of the eyes include providing eye care to unconscious clients, caring for eyeglasses and contact lenses, and caring for artificial eyes.

Eye Care for the Unconscious Client

✚ Having lost the blink (corneal) reflex, comatose or critically ill patients need more frequent eye care (every 2 to 4 hr). Keep their eyes lubricated with saline or artificial tears to protect them from corneal abrasions and drying. You may also need to use a protective eye shield to keep the patient's eyes closed. Instill eye ointment or drops in the lower lids as prescribed.

To review a procedure for administering ophthalmic medications, refer to Procedure 25-2.

Caring for Eyeglasses and Contact Lenses

Eyeglasses need to be cleaned at least once a day. Using warm water and a soft cloth, clean gently to prevent scratching of the lens. Ask the patient whether the lenses require a special cleaning solution; some patients bring their own. **KEY POINT:** *Label each patient's glasses and store them in a safe place within the patient's reach, preferably in a glasses case in the drawer of the bedside table. They are expensive, so take care that they are not lost or damaged.*

An alternative to glasses, contact lenses are plastic discs worn on the cornea over the pupil. They float on the tears of the eye and stay in place because of surface tension. The cornea is nourished mainly by oxygen from the atmosphere and from tears, so in order to ensure an optimal supply of oxygen, contact lenses must be removed periodically. Wearing time varies from daily wear to about 30 days, depending on the type of lens.

People usually care for their own contact lenses. Contact lens users must be careful to keep them free of infectious microorganisms and to be careful to avoid eye irritation.

✚ The Centers for Disease Control and Prevention (n.d., updated 2014) recommends that lenses should be kept away from all water.

1. Water can cause soft lenses to swell and stick to the eye, possible scratching the cornea.
2. Water is not germ free, and serious eye infections can result. The Centers for Disease Control and Prevention recommends contact lens removal before showering, swimming, or using a hot tub.
3. Users should not store lenses in water.
4. If water touches the lenses, the wearer should remove and discard them.

Teach cleaning and disinfecting measures to clients as needed (see the Self-Care box Teaching Clients About Cleaning and Storing Contact Lenses), and follow those measures when you must care for a client's lenses.

If you need to remove a patient's lenses during an emergency, follow universal precautions and handle the lenses as you would any other valuable patient property. ✚ Never use your fingernails to remove a lens, as you may scratch the eye or damage the lens. For more detailed instructions, see Procedure 24-12.

Caring for Artificial Eyes

An artificial eye is made to look like a natural eye. It can be made of glass or plastic. Some artificial eyes are permanently implanted in the socket, but others must be removed daily for cleaning of the prosthesis and the eye socket. If the patient is not able to perform his own eye care, follow his usual routines

Teaching Clients About Cleaning and Storing Contact Lenses

➤ Cleaning and disinfecting procedures and solutions vary among manufacturers. Depending on the type of lens, use saline solutions or special rinsing and soaking solutions.

➤ Use a special container for the lenses, with a cup labeled for the left and right lens. Some lenses are stored in a solution; others are stored dry. Follow manufacturer's instructions.

➤ Always wash your hands before touching the eyes or the lenses.

➤ Be careful not to allow the lenses to come in contact with soaps, hair sprays, or cosmetics.

➤ Do not wear soft lenses while using eye drops or ointment (wait 1 hr after using drops and at least 4 hr for ointment).

➤ Be aware of the risk for eye irritation when in the presence of smoke or chemical vapors.

when possible. For details about removing, cleaning, and replacing an artificial eye, see Procedure 24-13.

KnowledgeCheck 24-12

- True or False: Eyes should be cleansed from the outer to the inner canthus.
- How can a contact lens wearer help prevent eye infections?
- After you have cleaned a prosthetic eye, should you dry it before reinserting it, or leave it wet?

CARE OF THE EARS

Healthy ears require minimal care. However, you will need to help patients who have limited self-care abilities and teach others about self-care. For example, **cerumen** (wax) impaction is a common cause of functional hearing loss, especially in older adults. People sometimes believe that hearing loss is a normal part of aging and fail to seek treatment. Encourage them to see their primary care provider whenever hearing loss occurs.

✚ Teach patients to avoid using rigid objects such as bobby pins or toothpicks to clean their ears. Such instruments can traumatize the ear canal and may rupture the **tympanic membrane** (eardrum). Likewise, never use cotton-tipped applicators; they will push the cerumen farther into the ear, causing a blockage.

For dependent patients, assess for drainage, excess cerumen, and hearing loss during the bath. Clean the auricle and remove wax from the canal with the tip of the moistened washcloth or disposable wipe. If cleansing does not effectively remove excess wax buildup, obtain a prescription for **cerumenolytic** drops and water irrigation. You can delegate ear cleaning and hearing aid care to the NAP if you are sure that the NAP knows how to perform these tasks. See Chapter 31 for information about ear irrigations.

Care of Hearing Aids A hearing aid is a battery-powered device that amplifies sound. Three types of hearing aids are shown in Figure 24-7. Some patients wear a hearing aid in the temple pieces of their eyeglasses. People with severe hearing

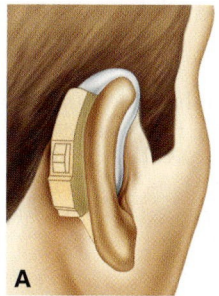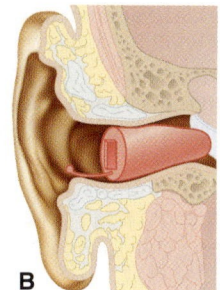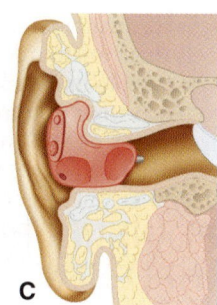

FIGURE 24-7 Hearing aids. A. The postaural (behind-the-ear) aid is the most widely used. A plastic tube connects it to an earmold. B. An in-the-canal aid is the least visible. C. The in-the-ear aid is made in one piece; all components are in the earmold.

loss may wear a body hearing aid that clips onto the clothing or a harness-type carrier that connects by a cord to the earpiece. Digital hearing aids are rapidly replacing the analog models.

Hearing aids are expensive and often essential to the patient, so handle and store them properly. They require regular cleaning and replacement of batteries. Even with good care, they usually need to be replaced every 5 to 10 years, and earmolds usually need adjustment more often than that. **KEY POINT:** *Never place a hearing aid in water.* Additionally, humidity can reduce their effectiveness. To learn how to remove, clean, and replace a hearing aid, refer to Procedure 24-16.

CARE OF THE NOSE

Usually the nose requires no special care. Have the patient remove excess secretions by gently blowing into a tissue with both nostrils open. Holding one nostril shut can force secretions into the eustachian tubes.

- **In debilitated or unconscious patients,** dried secretions can interfere with respirations. Remove secretions by gently inserting a moistened cotton-tipped applicator into the nostrils. Occasionally you may need to instill saline into the nares and suction secretions to keep the airway patent.
- **If the patient has an NG tube,** the constant pressure on the skin may cause breakdown. Provide special skin care and a lubricant at the point where the tube touches the nares.

THE CLIENT'S ENVIRONMENT

♥ **iCare** A comfortable environment contributes to the client's well-being. It is your responsibility to see that the bedside unit and surroundings are clean, safe, and comfortable.

ASSESSMENT (Scanning the Environment) NP

Each time you enter a patient's room, you should scan the environment to see whether you need to make adjustments to ensure patient safety and comfort:

- Is the room temperature comfortable?
- Are the siderails up, when indicated?
- Is the bed in low position, and the wheels locked?
- Are bed linens clean and free of wrinkles?
- Is the patient's call device within reach?

- Is the overbed table clean and uncluttered?
- Is there uncluttered walking space?
- Are there unpleasant odors?

Each time you leave the room, ask, "What else can I do for you?" This ensures that you have not overlooked anything.

PLANNING INTERVENTIONS/ IMPLEMENTATION (The Environment) NP

♥ **iCare** Adequate ventilation, proper room temperature, low noise level, and neat, clean surroundings are important to ensure patient comfort. A caring nurse provides for patient well-being by attention to the environmental details following.

Prevent and Eliminate Odors

Body secretions such as urine, feces, vomitus, or draining wounds cause odors in both inpatient facilities and the home. Odors can be offensive, and patients often feel embarrassed by them, so work quickly to free the environment of any sources of odors.

- Cleanliness is the best way to prevent odors.
- Provide good ventilation, if this is under your control. For example, open a window or use a fan.
- Empty urinals, bedpans, or emesis basins promptly.
- Dispose of soiled dressings or other malodorous items in appropriate containers and immediately remove them from the room.
- Unless use of a room deodorizer is contraindicated by the patient's illness, you can use one to help eliminate odors.
- Most institutions ban smoking in patient rooms, in part because of the odor.

Control Room Temperature

Although preferences may vary, a room temperature between 68°F and 74°F (20°C and 23°C) is usually comfortable for most patients. Those who are very ill, very young, or very old may need a warmer room. If there is no thermostat in the room, you may need to provide blankets, open a window, provide a fan, and so on to adjust the room temperature.

Limit Noise

People who are ill are often sensitive to environmental noises, such as an ice machine, suction equipment, paging systems, loud talking, and laughter. Make it a priority to control noise. Keep unnecessary conversations to a minimum and speak quietly. Some hospitals have instituted a "quiet hour" each day to promote better rest. Others have installed decibel meters to help nurses be mindful of noise escalation during activity in the nurses' station.

Standard Bedside Equipment

In a hospital, standard bedside equipment usually includes a bed, bedside stand (end table), overbed table, and one or two chairs. The wall unit may consist of a call light, oxygen, suction and electrical outlets, and light fixtures and switches. The patient's personal items are usually kept in the bedside stand. Therefore, you should request permission from the patient before opening the stand. Personal hygiene items, bedpan, and urinal may also be kept in the lower cabinet of this stand.

Hospital Beds   Hospitalized patients spend a significant amount of time in bed. Hospital beds can be uncomfortable and may contribute to restlessness and poor sleep.

- Memory foam and moisture control mattresses are available and provide more comfort. However, they are expensive and not used routinely.
- Hospital beds are higher and narrower than a home bed. This allows you to reach the patient more easily and safely.
- Hospital beds are usually electronically controlled, so the patient and nurse can raise and lower the head and foot separately by the push of a button (see Fig. 24-8 for bed positions).

Safety Concerns for Beds   To help prevent falls, a common cause of injury, be aware of and use bed safety features.

- ⊕ **Bed height.** Patient safety is your priority, so although you should raise the entire bed to a comfortable working level, be sure to place the bed in the lowest position before leaving the bedside. Long-term care settings usually have low beds to make it easier for ambulatory patients to transfer into and out of bed. As a part of the admission process, teach patients how to use the bed controls.

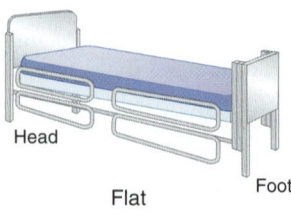
Head   Foot
Flat

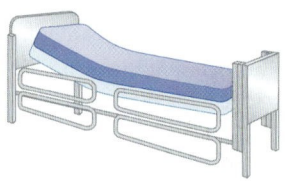
Semi-Fowler position (30° angle)

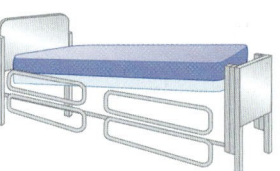
Trendelenburg position

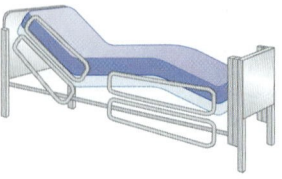
Fowler position (45° angle)

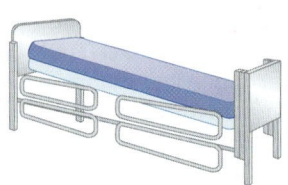
Reverse Trendelenburg position

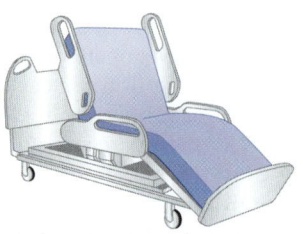
Sitting position (special wound-care beds; also adjust to standing position)

FIGURE 24-8 Hospital beds adjust to several positions.

- **Siderails.** Patients may use siderails when moving into and out of bed. Siderails may help to prevent falls for patients with decreased consciousness. However, they are considered a passive restraint and may pose risk to a patient with a cognitive impairment. See Chapter 23 for additional information about the safe use of siderails and other equipment.

- 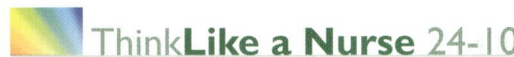 **Wheel locks.** To help prevent falls, always be sure to lock the wheels on a hospital bed when it is stationary, when you are helping the patient to a sitting position on the side of the bed, and when you are assisting with a transfer to a chair or stretcher. An unlocked bed could roll out from under an ambulatory patient or one you are assisting to get out of bed.

Mattresses and Linens Mattresses are usually firm and covered in a water-repellant material that resists staining and soiling and may be easily wiped down with a germicidal cleaner. A variety of therapeutic mattresses are available to help reduce the effects of pressure over the bony prominences (e.g., sacrum, heels). See Chapter 36 for further discussion of special mattresses.

- **Mattress Covers.** A mattress cover and/or pad promotes patient comfort and prevents soiling of the mattress. Mattress covers may lose their effectiveness over time, allowing moisture, blood, or bacteria to penetrate the mattress. Regularly check each medical bed mattress cover. If you find any visible signs of damage or wear (e.g., cuts, tears, cracks, pinholes, snags, or stains), the cover should be immediately replaced to reduce the risk of infection (U.S. Food and Drug Administration, 2013).

- **Linens.** Sheets may be fitted or flat. Other linens include drawsheets, washable incontinence pads, pillowcases, blankets, bedspreads, and gowns. If a plastic surface lies directly under the sheet, you should place a cloth or other absorbent pad between the patient and the sheet. Because plastic mattress covers or pads do not allow moisture to escape, they contribute to skin maceration for patients who are incontinent or diaphoretic.

Bed Making Clean, wrinkle-free bed linens help promote a sense of well-being. In contrast, wrinkled and soiled linens can contribute to skin breakdown and pressure areas. Linens are generally changed daily after the bath and when soiled. If patients are up and about during the day, such as on a rehabilitation unit, beds are made daily, but bed linens may be changed weekly or when soiled. If the patient is immobile or on bedrest, you or the NAP can make the bed while the patient occupies it. For more information about bed making, see Procedures 24-15 and 24-16.

ThinkLike a Nurse 24-10

For which of your patients (Meet Your Patients) will you most surely need to make an occupied bed? Why?

CLINICALREASONING

The questions and exercises in this section allow you to practice the kind of thinking you will use as a full-spectrum nurse. Critical-thinking questions usually have more than one correct answer, so we do not provide "correct answers" for these features. It is more important to develop your nursing judgment than to just cover content. You will learn by discussing the questions with your peers. If you are still unsure, see the Davis Advantage chapter resources for suggested responses.

Caring for the Nguyens

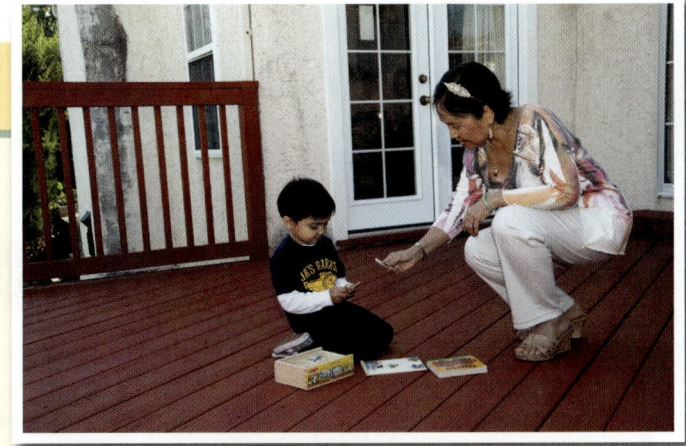

Yen Nguyen works as a preschool teacher. She schedules a clinic visit to discuss a variety of concerns. For each of the concerns she mentions, answer the following four questions:

1. What theoretical knowledge do you need?
2. Where could you find it?
3. What, if any, additional patient information do you need?
4. How would you respond to Mrs. Nguyen's concerns?

A. Yen tells you that her skin is very dry and irritated.

B. Yen tells you that several of the children at the preschool have recently been diagnosed with head lice. She would like to know how to assess for pediculosis.

C. Yen tells you that her 3-year-old grandson, Kim, frequently refuses to bathe. She asks for advice on how to handle this.

 Go to Davis Advantage, Resources, Chapter 24, **Caring for the Nguyens—Suggested Response**

Applying the **Full-Spectrum Nursing Model**＿＿＿＿＿＿＿

PATIENT SITUATION

Alice Baker is a frail elderly woman, 93 years old, who lives in a nursing home. She has almost total Self-Care Deficit related to her weakness, painful joints, and dementia. Her mental and physical conditions are not likely to improve. Imagine that your charge nurse has instructed you to provide a complete bed bath and other hygiene care for Ms. Baker. When you enter her room with bath supplies and say, "Good morning, Ms. Baker, it's time for your bath," she screams, "Go away from me. I just had a bath. I don't want a bath." You discuss this with the charge nurse, who says, "She has not had a bath, and she needs one today. You will need to do it whether she likes it or not." You tend to agree that Ms. Baker needs a bath because her clothing and linens have food stains, and she smells of urine and perspiration.

THINKING

1. *Theoretical Knowledge:*
   a. What benefits does a bath have for Ms. Baker?
   b. What are the disadvantages of bathing a patient with dementia who is resisting the bath?
2. *Critical Thinking (Considering Alternatives, Deciding What to Do):*
   a. What do you think Ms. Baker is feeling and experiencing, and how does that help you know what to do?
   b. What are some alternatives to a complete bed bath that would achieve the same purposes?

DOING

3. *Practical Knowledge:* Imagine that you have, indeed, decided that Ms. Baker needs a bath. Which type of bath you will give her? What supplies will you need, and where will you find them in the clinical agency you have attended most recently?

CARING

4. *Self-Knowledge:* What is your greatest concern about bathing Ms. Baker; what is the cause of your concern?

 Go to Davis Advantage, Resources, Chapter 24, **Applying the Full-Spectrum Nursing Model—Suggested Responses.**

PracticalKnowledge:
clinical application＿＿＿＿＿＿＿＿＿＿＿＿＿

The following Clinical Insights and procedures provide the practical knowledge you will need to assist patients with personal cleanliness and grooming. Patient Teaching and Home Care content in the procedures help you to promote increased activity and independence for patients.

CLINICAL INSIGHTS

Clinical Insight 24-1 ➤ **Assisting With a Shower or Tub Bath**

Inpatient Care

■ Assess the patient's self-care abilities: sensorimotor, musculoskeletal, and cognitive function; activity tolerance; level of knowledge.
■ Ensure that the patient has the necessary supplies (e.g., soap, washcloth, towel, clean gown).
■ If using prepackaged bath product, be sure to warm bathing products before use.
■ Hang a sign on the door to ensure privacy and place the call device within reach.

■ Help wash and dry any areas that the patient cannot reach (e.g., feet, back).

Preventing Nosocomial Infections

■ If using tap water for bath, check agency policy regarding the safety of the tap water for general use in bathing patients, including the following:
   ■ The hot water temperature is maintained above 55°C (131°F).
   ■ Routine sampling for bacteria is done.

Clinical Insight 24-1 ➤ **Assisting With a Shower or Tub Bath—cont'd**

- ✚ Avoid showering and exposure to faucet water for in-patients who are immunocompromised, the frail elderly, newborns, the critically ill, those having recent surgery or other loss of skin integrity, and patients requiring mechanical ventilation. Use prepackaged wipes instead.

- ✚ Verify water temperature for clients with impaired cognition or decreased sensory perception. Bath water should be 110°F to 115°F (43°C to 46°C) to avoid burns.

- ✚ Tubs should be stringently maintained and cleaned, preferably with a chlorhexidine gluconate (CHG)-based product, to prevent nosocomial infections related to the use of tubs (e.g., biofilm).

Preventing Falls

- ✚ Assist the patient to the shower or bathroom as needed.
- Ensure that there is a nonskid surface or mat in the shower or tub.
- Use a shower chair in the shower or tub for patients who have impaired mobility or activity intolerance.
- Be sure that the shower or tub is safe (e.g., with grab bars and handrails).
- Provide a call device for the patient to obtain help if needed; point out the emergency call device if there is one in the bathroom (usually it is a red button or cord on the wall).

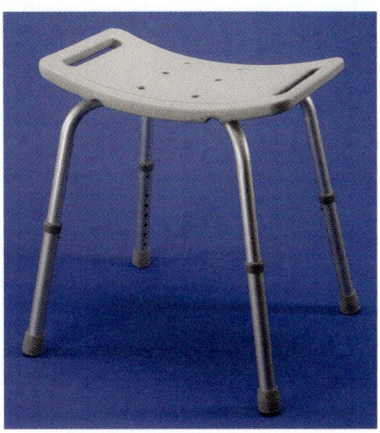

Shower chair

Home Care

- ✚ Encourage clients and families to install hand bars on the sides of the bathtub and on the wall next to the tub.
- Advise parents never to leave a child alone in the tub or shower and to have a way to unlock the bathroom door from outside the room.
- Advise older adults or those who are ill not to lock the bathroom door while bathing so that help can be summoned if needed (e.g., if they fall).
- Help families to obtain benches for transferring into the bathtub, or use a plastic chair in the shower.
- Ensure that there is a nonskid surface or mat in the shower or tub.

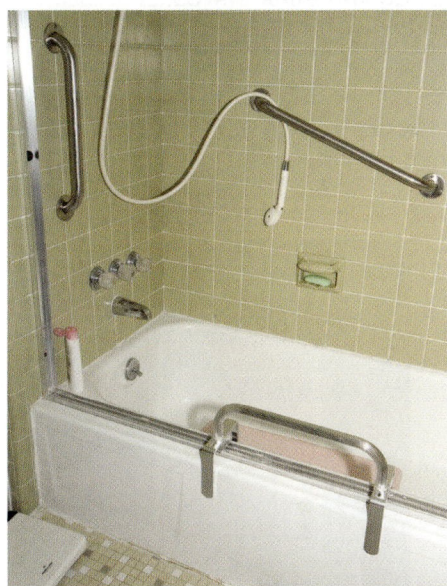

Bathtub with handrail and grab bars

PROCEDURES

Procedure 24-1 ■ Bathing: Providing a Complete Bed Bath Using a Prepackaged Bathing Product

➤ For steps to follow in *all* procedures, refer to the Universal Steps for All Procedures found on the page facing the inside back cover.

Equipment

- Prepackaged bathing product with disposable wipes (e.g., Comfort Bath)
- Bath blanket
- Clean patient gown (with shoulder snaps or Velcro closures if the patient has an IV line)
- Clean bed linen
- Orangewood stick
- Deodorant, lotion, and/or powder as needed
- Emollient (if not included in prepackaged bathing product)
- Procedure gloves (for anal and perineal care)
- Bedpan or urinal
- Laundry bag
- Plastic trash bag for used wipes and other disposable soiled items ▼

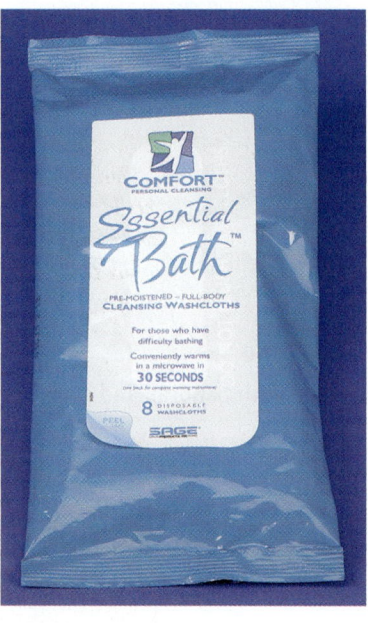

Delegation

You can delegate this procedure to the NAP if you conclude that the patient's condition and the NAP's skills allow. Perform the following assessments, and inform the NAP of the specific type of bath (e.g., packaged bath, towel bath); the amount of help the patient needs; and any special considerations, such as IV lines, drains, and so on. Ask the NAP to report the condition of the patient's skin, level of self-care, and ability to tolerate the procedure.

Pre-Procedure Assessments

- Assess mobility, activity tolerance, type of bath needed, and ability to perform bathing self-care.
  Decreased activity tolerance or mobility (e.g., chest pain or shortness of breath with exertion) may limit the bathing self-care ability. Having the patient assist as much as possible increases mobility and sense of control and comfort.

- Check for positioning or activity restrictions (e.g., maintaining hip abduction following a total hip replacement).
  Prevents injuring the patient during the procedure.

- Determine the number of people you need to safely bathe and reposition the patient.
  Helps prevent injury to the patient or the nurse.

- Assess for personal and cultural issues that may be of concern to the patient regarding the bath.
  Bathing may conflict with the patient's sense of privacy or modesty. Cultural norms and individual preferences must be considered.

- Assess for specific patient needs and preferences during a bath, such as lotions and extra wipes or towels.
  Advanced age, certain skin conditions, or skin breakdown may require special soaps and/or lotions. Incontinence or drainage may require additional wipes, towels, and precautions. Meeting patient preferences helps prevent depersonalization and promotes patient cooperation with the procedure.

➤ When performing the procedure, always identify your patient according to agency policy, using two identifiers, and be attentive to standard precautions, hand hygiene, patient safety and privacy, body mechanics, and documentation.

➤ Note: You may find that you need to adapt the bathing order and other steps to meet individual needs.

Procedure Steps

1. **Provide for patient privacy** and comfort.
   a. Close the door or privacy curtains, adjust room temperature, and assist the patient with elimination as needed.

   b. Ask the patient and family whether they wish family members to assist with the bath.
   Assisting the patient with elimination before beginning helps prevent interruptions during the procedure. Bathing practices and privacy needs differ among cultures and individuals. The patient or family may wish to
   have a family member assist with the bath, or the patient may prefer that they leave the room.

2. **Peel open the label on the commercial bath** without completely removing it.
   Allows for steam to escape as contents .heat without spilling the contents.

3. ✚ **Heat the package** in the microwave for no longer than 1 minute. The temperature of the contents should be approximately 105°F (41°C). Some references suggest instead, for safety, using the commercial bag bath at room temperature.
Heating to 105°F (41°C) brings contents to a safe and comfortable temperature. This must be done with caution to prevent burning, especially in patients who have fragile skin.

If Using a Warmer Unit

You do not need step 3 because the bags are always warm.

4. **Adjust the bed** to working height, lower the siderail nearest you, and position the patient supine close to the side of bed you will be working on.
   ✚ Raise the siderail before you leave that side of the bed.
   Prevents falls and keeps you from having to lean over the patient or reach across the siderail, which can cause back strain or injury.

5. **Remove the bedspread** and spread the bath blanket over the top sheet; then ask the patient to hold the bath blanket in place while you remove the top sheet.
   Protects modesty and prevents chilling. If no bath blanket is available, you can use the top sheet in its place. However, if the sheet becomes damp, it may chill the patient. ▼

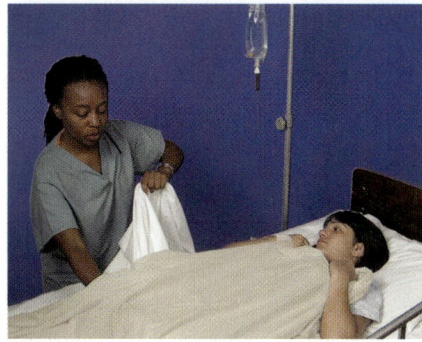

NOTE: *Before proceeding, assist the patient with oral hygiene as needed. See Procedures 24-6 and 24-7.*

6. **Remove the patient's gown,** keeping the patient covered with the bath blanket. During the bath, expose just the part of the body you are bathing.
Maintains the patient's modesty and prevents chilling.

Patient With an IV Line

If the patient has an IV line and is wearing a gown that does not have snap-open sleeves:

If there is a 2-way, needlefree connector on the IV tubing:

Some systems include a needlefree 2-way connector that allows you to disconnect the tubing while still maintaining a closed line. In that case, you simply open the connection, remove the gown, and then reconnect the tubing. After the bath, follow the same procedure to place the clean gown on the patient.

If there is no 2-way, needlefree connector on the IV tubing,

   a. Remove the gown first from the arm without the IV.
   b. Lower the IV container and pass the gown over the tubing and the container, taking care to keep the container above the level of the patient's arm. ▼

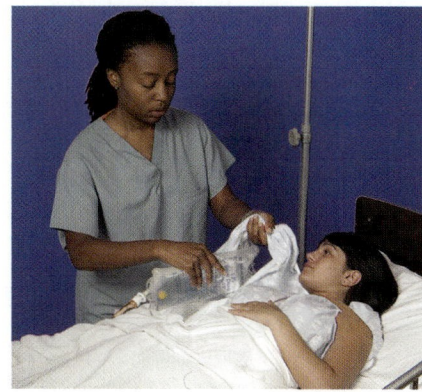

   c. ✚ Never disconnect this type of IV connection; this breaks the sterile system and provides a portal of entry for pathogens.
   d. Rehang the container; check the flow rate.
   Manipulating the IV equipment may change the flow rate; flow rate must be maintained as prescribed.
   e. After the bath, replace the gown by threading the IV equipment from inside the arm of the gown and onto the affected arm. Then

place the unaffected arm through the other gown sleeve.

7. **Don clean procedure gloves** if exposure to body fluids is likely or if either you or the patient has any breaks in the skin.
Follows universal precautions; helps prevent transfer of microorganisms.

8. **Wash the patient's face, neck, and ears.**
   a. Fold the wipe around the hand to make a mitt, tucking in loose corners.
   Keeps loose ends from dragging across the skin. This is uncomfortable because loose ends cool quickly.
   b. Wash the face using one wipe.
   c. Use a different corner of the wipe to gently wipe each eyelid outward from the inner canthus.
   Some wipes contain chlorhexidine gluconate (CHG), an antimicrobial, which can be irritating to the eyes and mucous membranes. Use pH-balanced prepackaged wipes for the face, or use gauze squares moistened with sterile or filtered water or normal saline. **KEY POINT:** *A major principle is cleaning from "clean to dirty" to prevent contamination of a cleaner area. The inner canthus is considered the cleanest area. Prevents moving debris toward the nasolacrimal duct, which is located near the inner canthus.* ▼

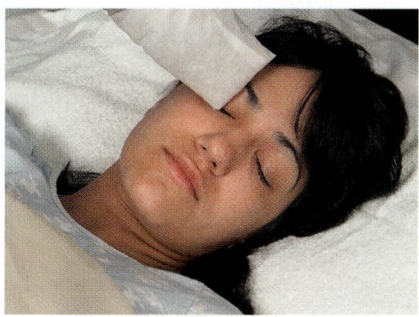

   d. Wash the rest of the patient's face, neck, and ears.
   Move sequentially through the bath to make it less tiring for the patient and more efficient for the nurse.
   e. Allow areas to air dry. Do not rinse.
   Prevents the emollient and surfactant skin protectants from being removed.

(continued on next page)

Procedure 24-1 ■ Bathing: Providing a Complete Bed Bath Using a Prepackaged Bathing Product (continued)

9. **Discard each wipe after use.**
   Ensures following the "clean to dirty" principle.

10. **Wash the patient's arms** using a new, clean wipe.
    a. Fold the bath blanket off one arm at a time and place a folded bath towel under the arm. Beginning with the patient's far arm, support the arm, and wash the arm from the hands upward using long strokes.
    Long strokes increase circulation in the extremity. Washing from distal to proximal increases venous return from the periphery. Lifting the arm provides range of motion (ROM) to preserve joint mobility.

    b. Continue to support the arm while washing the axilla.
    Prevents potential injury to the joints. A sprain, subluxation, or dislocation of the joint can occur when an extremity is not properly supported, especially in older adults.

    c. Allow the areas to air dry; do not rinse.
    Prevents the emollient and surfactant skin protectants from being removed.

    d. Apply deodorant and/or powder if desired.
    Follow patient preferences whenever possible to increase comfort.

    e. Clean under the nails with an orangewood stick as needed.

    f. Repeat the preceding steps 9a–d for the arm nearest you.

11. **Wash the patient's chest,** using a new clean wipe.
    a. Cover the patient's chest with a bath towel and lower the bath blanket to the patient's waist.
    Maintains patient comfort and modesty.

    b. For women, gently lift each breast to wash the skinfold if needed. Keep the chest covered between the wash and rinse.
    Skinfolds are a source of odor and can become irritated because of skin-to-skin friction and dampness from perspiration.

    c. Cover to maintain privacy and warmth.

    d. Allow the areas to air dry; do not rinse.
    Prevents the emollient and surfactant skin protectants from being removed.

12. **Wash the abdomen,** using a new, clean wipe.
    a. Fold the bath blanket down to the perineal area and cover the chest with a bath towel.

    b. Wash the abdomen, including the umbilical area; allow to air dry. Pay special attention to skinfolds.
    Perspiration and moisture do not evaporate well from skinfolds, predisposing them to maceration.

    c. Cover the abdomen and chest with the bath blanket.
    Prevents chilling, maintains privacy.

13. **Wash the legs and feet,** using a new, clean wipe for each leg.
    a. Uncover one leg at a time, beginning with the leg farthest from you. Place the bath towel under the leg.
    Keeps the sheet dry; prevents chilling.

    b. Wash the leg from distal to proximal with long, gentle strokes. Allow the leg to air dry.

    ➕ **Do not massage the calves of the legs.**
    Washing from distal to proximal may help to promote venous return. If a venous thrombus is present, massaging might dislodge the clot and cause an embolus. ▼

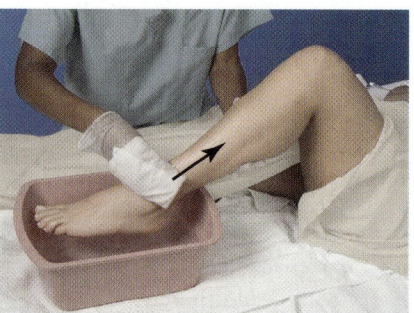

    c. Thoroughly wash the foot and toes. Allow the foot to air dry. Apply lotion if the prepackaged bath product does not include emollient and as needed, but not between the toes.
    Disease processes frequently decrease circulation to the feet and lower legs, increasing the likelihood that minor skin irritations may become more severe. Applying emollient between the toes can lead to skin breakdown.

    d. Repeat the procedure on the other leg and foot.

14. **Wash the back and buttocks,** using a new, clean wipe.
    a. Position the patient on his side with his back facing you or in the prone position. Make sure the siderail on the far side of the bed, facing the patient, is still up.
    Provides for clear visualization of back and access to the area.

    b. Exposing only the back and buttocks, place the bath towel under the back and buttocks. Wash the back first and then the buttocks. Observe for redness and skin breakdown in the sacral area.
    Maintains the principle of "clean to dirty." The sacral area is a common site of pressure sores. ▼

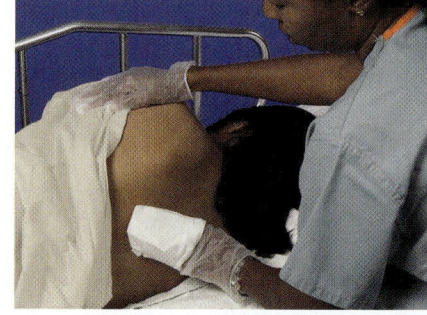

    c. Unless contraindicated, give the patient a back rub, applying lotion to the back and buttocks (see Chapter 35, Procedure 35-1: Giving a Back Rub).
    Stimulates circulation and maintains the health of the skin. Because the patient is in bed, he is at risk for

skin irritation and breakdown from immobility and friction. A back rub may be contraindicated for patients with musculoskeletal injuries or cardiovascular disease.

d. **Don procedure gloves if you have not already done so, and wash the rectal area**, removing any fecal matter with tissues before washing with the wipe. Wash from front to back.
Washing the rectal area at this time removes the need for the patient to turn to his side again and helps prevent soiling clean linen when changing the linen in an occupied bed. Fecal matter usually contains microorganisms. Washing from front to back helps prevent transferring bacteria from the rectum to the vagina and urethra. ▼

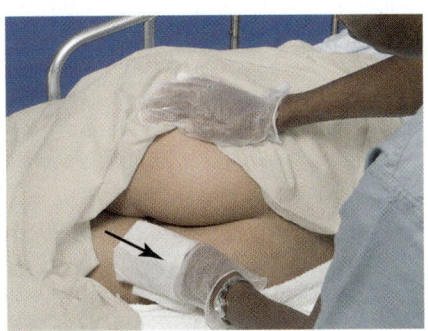

e. Discard the soiled wipe. If linens are soiled, cover them with a clean sheet before repositioning the patient.

f. Remove soiled gloves and wash hands or use an alcohol-based handrub. Don new procedure gloves before providing perineal care.
Prevents transferring microorganisms from anal to genital area—cleansing the gluteal and anal areas contaminates the wipe. Maintains standard precautions during the bath and prevents soiling of clean linens during bed change and cross-contamination to other body sites.

15. **Cleanse the perineal area.** See Procedure 24-4: Providing Perineal Care.

16. **After providing perineal care,** reposition and cover the patient with the bath blanket. Remove soiled gloves and wash hands or use alcohol-based handrub. Help the patient put on a clean gown, and attend to other hygiene needs (e.g., hair grooming).
Prevents contaminating clean linen with soiled gloves. Ensures proper body position and warmth.

17. **Change the bed linen** as needed, including soiled linen or linen that became damp during the bath. Properly dispose of soiled items by placing it in a linen bag. See Procedure 24-15: Making an Occupied Bed.
Ensures patient safety, comfort, and privacy.

? What if . . .

■ **You are bathing the patient without assistance, or you are not tall enough to comfortably reach across the patient?**

These situations put you at risk for back strain. Thus, you may want to bathe one side of the body—that is, the right arm, trunk, right leg—and then move to the other side of the bed to bathe the opposite side of the body (instead of the order given in steps 8 and 9). Move the patient close to you before beginning the bath.

■ **You are bathing a patient in leg traction?**

You may decide to bathe the arms and trunk first. Then have the patient sit forward so that you can cleanse his back. Then have the patient lift up slightly so that you can wash his buttocks. Finally, wash the lower extremities.

■ **You are bathing a patient with dementia?**

Use your knowledge of the person's bathing practices and preferences to determine a time of day and a routine the person will accept. Keep stimulation to a minimum. Turn on some calming music, speak softly and reassuringly, and don't rush. Keep the patient warm. If the patient becomes agitated and you cannot calm him, do not force him to bathe. You may wish to consider a towel bath as an alternative (Procedure 24-2). Also refer to iCare 24-2, Caring Tips for Bathing a Patient With Dementia.
Many steps in the bathing process may be misinterpreted or stressful for the patient, who may become disruptive or agitated. If forced to bathe, the patient may be upset for hours. Towel baths are effective hygiene measures.

■ **Your patient becomes agitated and uncooperative during the bath?**

Speak calmly and softly. Give the patient a few minutes to calm down. Discontinue the bath if the patient remains upset.

■ **Your patient is an older adult?**

a. Some clinicians recommend bathing older adults every other day instead of daily, and it is generally agreed that they should not bathe more than once a day unless soiling occurs.
Helps prevent skin dryness.

b. Assure that the wipes are warm prior to use, but not hot.
Prevents burns (older adults may have decreased sensation in their extremities).

c. If you are not using a commercial packaged bath, use antibacterial soap or a mild soap substitute. If you must use soap, it should not be perfumed and should be rich in moisture. If you use soap, rinse the skin well.
To avoid skin irritation.

d. Pat the skin dry or air dry; do not rub.

e. Immediately after drying, wash your hands and apply moisturizer while there is still moisture in the skin.

f. Cleanse the skin immediately after every incident of soiling (e.g., when the patient has a bowel movement).
Prevents maceration and irritation from enzyme activity.

(continued on next page)

Procedure 24-1 ▪ Bathing: Providing a Complete Bed Bath Using a Prepackaged Bathing Product (continued)

Evaluation

- Assess how well the patient tolerated the procedure. Was there any discomfort, shortness of breath, and so on?
- Observe the patient's mobility, both ROM and ease of movement.
- Note the condition of the patient's skin, including redness and other abnormal findings, especially in skinfolds.
- Ask the patient whether he is comfortable and satisfied.
- If you delegate the procedure, you must still evaluate the care to be certain that it was done and performed satisfactorily.

Patient Teaching

- Discuss the need for activity (e.g., moving about in bed) and the hazards of immobility.
- Discuss usual skin care and how to increase the health of the skin.
- Demonstrate bathing procedure to family or other caregivers.

Home Care

NOTE: *(1) Many of the following apply to older adults and others with self-care deficits. (2) The following include all types of home bathing, not just to Procedure 24-1:*

- ✚ Evaluate the home for bathing safety considerations (not limited to bed bath), such as the following:
  Safety bars in the bathroom?
  To facilitate transfers and provide support while washing.

  A safe water supply for bathing?
  Bathing supplies that are available and accessible?
  Nonskid mat or abrasive strips for shower or tub?
  Stool for shower; transfer bench or stool for getting into the tub?
  Handheld shower spray?
  Long-handled brush or sponge?

- Assess the client's ability to help with the bath or to bathe independently.
- Ask how the client usually bathes (e.g., shower, at the sink). Follow the client's preference as much as possible.
- Ask what supplies the client usually uses for the bath, and ask where they are stored. You will need to adapt the

procedure depending on the available equipment and supplies.
- Suggest the use of large plastic trash bags or a shower curtain to protect the mattress during a bed bath.
- Instruct caregivers to wear gloves when handling linens that are soiled with blood or other body fluids. Such linens should be washed in cold water, separately from other household laundry, and then washed again, using hot water, detergent, and bleach.
  Hot water coagulates proteins in the blood and makes it more difficult to remove. Detergent and bleach are used to destroy pathogens.

Documentation

Chart the type of bath given, how much patient was able to help with the bath, how well the patient tolerated the procedure, the patient's mobility, and any abnormal findings. Hygiene care is charted on checklists and flow sheets in most agencies.

Sample documentation

0630   *complete bed bath given, pt. unable to assist in care. Patient tolerated procedure well, VSS, denied pain. Patient turned side to side with assist of one. Skin warm, dry and intact. Emollient applied to dry areas. Encouraged patient to shift weight while in bed to prevent injury to skin ———————— K. Barnett, RN*

Practice Resources

D'Hondt, A., Kaasalainen, S., Prentice, D., et al. (2012); Konno, R., Stern, C., & Gibbs, H. (2013); Nøddeskou, L. H., Hemmingsen, L. E., & Hørdam, B. (2015); Powers, J., & Fortney, S. (2014); Powers, J., Peed, J., Burns, L., et al. (2012); Sievert, D., Armola, R., & Halm, M. (2011).

Thinking About the Procedure

To practice applying clinical reasoning to this procedure,

 The video, **Bathing: Providing a Complete Bed Bath Using a Prepackaged Bathing Product,** along with questions and suggested responses, is available on the **Davis's** *Nursing Skills Videos* Web site on Davis*Plus*.

Procedure 24-2 ▪ Bathing: Providing a Towel Bath

➤ For steps to follow in *all* procedures, refer to the Universal Steps for All Procedures found on the page facing the inside back cover.

➤ Note: Because the towel bath is a variation of the bed bath, only the steps differing from a bed bath are listed.

Equipment

- Large plastic bag containing a bath blanket (or a very large towel, about 3 ft (6 ft), one standard bath towel, and two or three washcloths
- Dry bath blankets (two or more) and dry bath towels
- Pitcher and approximately 2 qt (2,000 mL) of warm distilled, sterile, or filtered water (105°F [41°C]), according to agency policy

- 30 mL of no-rinse liquid soap or commercial solution of soap, moisturizer, and disinfectant (preferably a CHG and water solution)
- Other supplies for a bed bath; see Procedure 24-1.

Delegation

You can delegate this procedure to the NAP if you conclude that the patient's condition and the NAP's skills allow. Perform the pre-procedure assessments and inform the NAP of the amount of help the patient needs and any special considerations, such as IV lines and drains. Ask the NAP to report the condition of the patient's skin, level of self-care, and ability to tolerate the procedure.

Pre-Procedure Assessments

- Assess the patient's mobility and activity tolerance to determine whether she will be able to assist with the bath, whether a towel bath is appropriate, and the amount of help you will need.

  Decreased activity tolerance or mobility (e.g., because of chest pain or shortness of breath) may limit the patient's ability to assist with the bath, making a towel bath the most appropriate choice. For severely compromised patients, having two nurses give the bath will make the procedure much quicker and less demanding on the patient.

➤ When performing the procedure, always identify your patient according to agency policy, using two identifiers, and be attentive to standard precautions, hand hygiene, patient safety and privacy, body mechanics, and documentation.

Procedure Steps

1. **Prepare the towel bag.**
   a. Fold the bath blanket.
   Allows for organized application and ease of handling the blanket.

   b. Fill a large pitcher with 2,000 mL warm water (approximately 105°F [41°C]). Distilled, sterile, or filtered water is recommended; follow agency policy.
   - Tap water exposes patients to pathogens if biofilm is present in the water lines or faucets. This differs among agencies.
   - The amount of water varies depending on the size of the bath blanket and bath towel. Use enough water to saturate them.
   - Hot water can injure the patient and removes more of the skin's protective oils, but if the water is too cool, the patient may become chilled.

   c. Add 30 mL of no-rinse soap or commercial solution to the water according to the manufacturer's instructions.
   Adding a prescribed amount of soap to the water before pouring into the bag prevents excessive sudsing.

   d. Pour about 2,000 mL of the solution into the bag, over the bath blanket, bath towel, and wash cloths. Ensure even distribution.

2. **If you do not plan to change** the linen, work one dry bath blanket under the patient.
   Protects the linen and provides warmth.

3. **Spread a dry bath blanket** over the patient; remove the patient's clothing, working underneath the blanket.
   Protects privacy and prevents chilling.

4. **Replace the dry blanket with** the wet blanket:
   a. Take the wet bath blanket or towel out of the bag, squeezing out excess water so that it does not drip.
   b. Push the dry bath blanket down to the patient's waist, and place the wet bath blanket on the patient's chest.
   c. Continue to unfold the wet bath blanket until it covers the patient, pushing the dry bath blanket out of the way as you do so.
   The wet bath blanket will feel warm and relaxing. You will use the dry bath blanket to dry the patient.

   d. If necessary, place yet another dry blanket on top of the wet one.
   This helps hold in the warmth if the patient is chilling or the room is cool.

5. **Bathe the patient,** beginning at the feet and working toward the head.
   a. Keeping the patient covered, use the wet bath blanket to wash the legs, abdomen, and chest.
   b. As you work, replace the wet bath blanket with the dry one.
   Keeps the patient from chilling. ➤

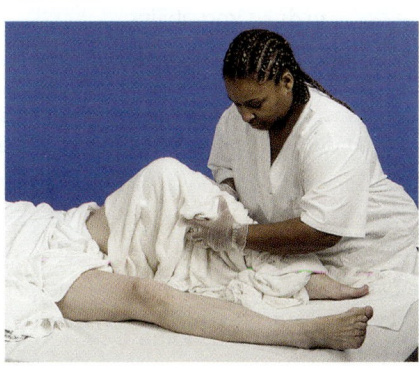

   c. Fold the wet bath blanket as each area is bathed, allowing only clean surfaces to contact clean surfaces.
   Prevents contamination of the clean side of the wet bath blanket.

   d. Use one of the wet washcloths to wash the patient's face, neck, and ears.
   Notice that this varies from the order of most baths, which proceed from head to toe. However, this is the most efficient way to accomplish a towel bath. It does not really compromise the "clean to dirty" principle because the legs, abdomen, and chest are usually equally "clean," and you are washing those before the back, buttocks, and perineum.

6. **Don procedure gloves.** Roll the client to one side, unfold the wet bath towel so the clean surface covers the patient, and use the wet bath towel to wash the back and then the buttocks.

(continued on next page)

Procedure 24-2 ■ Bathing: Providing a Towel Bath (continued)

7. **Remove procedure gloves;** wash your hands. Wash the perineal area with a washcloth. See Procedure 24-4: Providing Perineal Care.

8. **Finish the bath** as in Procedure 24-1. Follow patient preferences whenever possible to increase feelings of comfort.

9. **Change linen as needed,** including soiled linen or linen that became damp during the bath. You will almost certainly need to change the linen if

you have not padded the bottom sheet well before the bath.
Ensures patient safety and comfort. Because the bath is finished rapidly, there is no real need to pad the bottom sheet if you know that you will have time to change the linens after the bath.

? What if . . .

■ **Your patient becomes agitated and uncooperative during the bath?**

Speak calmly and softly. Give the patient a few minutes to calm down. Discontinue the bath if the patient remains upset.

Practice Resources
Konno, R., Stern, C., & Gibbs, H. (2013); Larkin, C. (2011); Warchol, K. (2010); Wolf, Z. R., & Czekanski, K. E. (2015).

Procedure 24-3 ■ Bathing: Using a Basin and Water

KEY POINT: *Evidence indicates that (1) bath basins can become a reservoir for microorganisms and for cross-contamination of the immediate environment and healthcare personnel; and (2) biofilm is commonly present in hospital water lines and faucets. Use this method only when a patient is grossly contaminated or a patient refuses other types of bath.*

➤ For steps to follow in *all* procedures, refer to the Universal Steps for All Procedures found on the page facing the inside back cover.

Equipment

■ Disposable, water basin for single-patient use
■ Tap, distilled, filtered, or sterile water (depending on facility policy)
■ CHG and water solution (for bathing the patient and cleaning the basin)
■ Lotion, deodorant, and/or powder as needed
■ Bath blanket
■ Clean patient gown (gown with shoulder snaps or Velcro closures if the patient has an IV line)
■ Clean linen
■ Procedure gloves

Delegation

You can delegate this procedure to the NAP if you conclude that the patient's condition and the NAP's skills allow. Perform

the pre-procedure assessments, and inform the NAP of the amount of help the patient needs and of any special considerations, such as IV lines and drains, Ask the NAP to report the condition of the patient's skin, level of self-care, and ability to tolerate the procedure.

Pre-Procedure Assessments

Assessments are the same as in Procedure 24-1: Bathing: Providing a Complete Bed Bath Using a Prepackaged Bathing Product.

➤ When performing the procedure, always identify your patient according to agency policy, using two identifiers, and be attentive to standard precautions, hand hygiene, patient safety and privacy, body mechanics, and documentation.

Procedure Steps

✚ **Fill the disposable basin** with warm water (approximately 105°F [41°C]). Check the temperature with a thermometer or your hand. If possible, ask the patient to test the water temperature.

Using tap water for bathing exposes patients to waterborne pathogens; use distilled, filtered, or sterile water if available. This differs among institutions, so follow

agency requirements. Use water that is comfortable for the patient. Hot water removes protective skin oils and can injure the patient. If the water is too cool, the patient may become chilled.

1. **Prepare a solution** of 60 mL CHG solution diluted in 3 qt (2.85 L) of water for bathing the patient (Powers, Peed, Burns, et al., 2012).
Evidence indicates that use of CHG is effective in preventing the bath basin

from becoming a reservoir for microorganisms, thus helping to prevent HAIs.

2. **Prepare the patient for the bath** by doing the following (refer to Procedure 24-1 for rationales):
   a. Adjust the bed to working height.
   b. Remove the bedspread and spread bath blanket over top sheet.
   c. Remove the patient's gown, keeping the patient covered with the bath blanket.

d. If the patient has an IV:
  - For a needle free 2-way connector, open the connection, remove the gown and reconnect the tubing.
  - If there is no 2-way, needlefree connector, remove the gown first from the arm without the IV, lower the container, and pass gown over the container and tubing, taking care to keep the container above the level of the patient's arm. Rehang the container and check the flow rate.
  - After the bath, replace the gown by threading the container from inside the arm of the gown and onto the affected arm. Then place the unaffected arm through the other gown sleeve.

e. Don clean procedure gloves if exposure to body fluids is likely or if either you or the patient has any breaks in the skin.

3. **Using a clean, rinsed washcloth,** wash the patient following the following sequence:
Face, neck, ears
Eyes
Chest and arms
Abdomen
Legs and feet
Back and buttocks and rectum and perineal

Rinse and wring water from the washcloth as you move from each body area. Change water and use a clean washcloth to wash the perineal area. *Rinsing keeps washcloth warm and clean. Changing water prevents cross-contamination and contamination of wounds with dirty bath water.*

4. **Rinse body area as needed** (e.g., if you use soap) and pat dry. *Preserves skin integrity by preventing the drying effect of the soap.*

5. **Apply deodorant, lotion, and/or powder as desired or as needed.**

6. **Put used washcloths in the laundry** for future use.

7. **Help patient don a clean gown.**

8. **Provide a back rub,** if not contraindicated.

9. **Reposition patient,** as needed.

10. **Change linens,** as needed, and bag soiled linen for laundering.

11. **Clean and dry the basin** according to agency policy.

✚ *Evidence supports single-patient use of a disposable basin, cleaning it with chlorhexidine solution, drying the basin after each use, storing it upside down, not storing anything (e.g., bathing supplies) in it, and not reusing it (Powers, Peed, Burns, et al., 2012).*

For Evaluation, Documentation, and Patient Teaching, see Procedure 24-1: Bathing: Providing a Complete Bed Bath Using a Prepackaged Bathing Product.

Practice Resources

Doughty, D., Junkin, J., Kurz, P., et al. (2012); Powers, J., Peed, J., Burns, L., et al. (2012); Ritz, J., Pashnik, B., Padula, C., et al. (2012); Rönner, A. C., Berland, C. R., Runeman, B., et al. (2010); Wolf, Z. R., & Czekanski, K. E. (2015).

Procedure 24-4 ■ Providing Perineal Care

➤ For steps to follow in *all* procedures, refer to the Universal Steps for All Procedures found on the page facing the inside back cover.

Equipment

- Procedure gloves
- Prepackaged bathing wipes (i.e., Comfort Care)
- Bedpan or portable sitz tub (optional)
- Bath towel
- Toilet paper
- Plastic trash bag for used wipes and other disposable soiled items
- Perineal ointment or lotion if needed

If prepackaged bathing product is not available:

- Sterile, filtered, distilled, or tap water, according to agency policy
- Disposable basin or perineal wash bottle, if needed
- Perineal cleansing solution or no-rinse soap
- Wash cloths

Delegation

You can delegate perineal care to the NAP if the patient's condition and the NAP's skills allow. Perform the pre-procedure assessments, and inform the NAP of the amount of help the patient needs and any special considerations (e.g., presence of a urinary catheter, vaginal drainage). Ask the NAP to report the condition of the patient's perineum, level of self-care, and ability to tolerate the procedure.

Pre-Procedure Assessments

- Assess the patient's mobility and activity tolerance.
  Determine whether the patient will be able to assist with the perineal care. Doing as much self-care as possible increases the patient's sense of independence and maintains modesty.

- Check for positioning or activity restrictions, such as maintaining hip abduction following a total hip replacement. *Prevents injuring the patient during the procedure.*

- Assess for psychosocial issues related to perineal care. *Consider personal and cultural norms to ensure that the perineal care is appropriate for the patient. For example, in some cultures a woman would find it completely unacceptable for a male nurse to perform her perineal care (pericare).*

- Assess for the specific patient needs, such as presence of a urinary catheter, perineal surgery, lesions, incontinence, or skin breakdown. *You may need to adapt the procedure (e.g., clean around an indwelling urinary catheter or surgical incision, use special soaps). Incontinence requires assessment and follow-up to prevent Impaired Skin Integrity.*

(continued on next page)

Procedure 24-4 ■ **Providing Perineal Care** (continued)

➤ When performing the procedure, always identify your patient according to agency policy, using two identifiers, and be attentive to standard precautions, hand hygiene, patient safety and privacy, body mechanics, and documentation.

Procedure Steps

1. **Adjust the room temperature** and assist with elimination as needed. *Assisting the patient with elimination before perineal care helps prevent interruptions during the procedure and allows for thorough cleansing. Adjusting room temperature prevents chilling.*

2. Warm the perineal bathing product with disposable wipes.

If Using a Microwave

✚ Heat the package of disposable wipes in the microwave for no longer than 1 minute. The temperature of the contents should be approximately 105°F (41°C). This step is controversial. Some references suggest, for safety, using the commercial wipes at room temperature.

If Using a Warmer Unit

You do not need step 2 because the package of disposable wipes is always warm.

3. **Prepare the patient.**
   a. Position the patient on her back (supine). Place waterproof pads under the patient if they are not already in place. You may wish to place the patient on a bedpan or portable sitz tub, especially if the perineum is grossly soiled. Place a waterproof bag within reach to discard wipes.
   Placing the patient on a bedpan raises the hips to increase visualization and allows for more thorough cleansing. A bedpan also allows for using water when needed.

   b. Wear procedure gloves (and other protective wear as needed) when providing perineal care. If you are using a basin and water, wear a procedure gown and goggles if you are concerned about splashing (e.g., if the patient is confused and may be unable to follow instructions).
   When providing perineal care there is a possibility of coming in contact with urine, vaginal secretions, or fecal material.

   c. Drape the patient to protect privacy.

For Female Patients

- Drape the bath blanket so that one point faces the patient's head (drape it in the shape of a diamond).
- Take one of the side points of the diamond, and wrap it around the patient's leg. Anchor the end of the blanket under the patient's foot.
- Repeat on the other leg with other point of the diamond. ▼

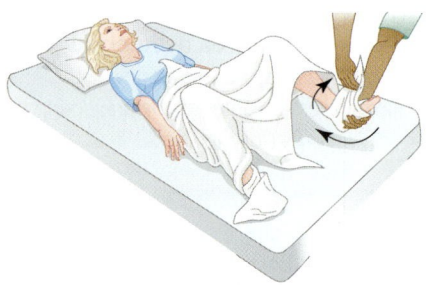

- Fold the center lower point of the diamond up to expose the patient's perineum. ▼

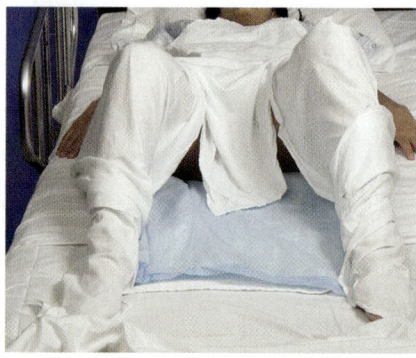

This draping technique covers the patient as much as possible, which helps maintain privacy and prevents chilling during the procedure. The patient can also relax her legs against the bath blanket.

For Male Patients

- Place the bath blanket over the patient's chest.
- Fold the bed linens down to expose only the patient's groin.
   d. Remove any fecal material with toilet paper.
   Prevents contamination of the perineum with feces, which can lead to

bladder or incisional infections. If you are providing perineal care as part of giving a bed bath, you will have cleaned the anal area when the patient was in the lateral position.*

4. **Wash the perineum,** using a warm disposable wipe. In both males and females, cleanse the skinfolds of the groin area thoroughly. Examine the skin creases for redness or excoriation.

For Female Patients

Wash the perineum from front to back, using a clean portion of the wipe for each stroke. Cleanse the labial folds and around the urinary catheter, if one is in place.
Prevents contaminating the urethra with fecal material. Any fecal particles that are left can cause skin breakdown due to enzyme activity and may increase the risk of a urinary tract infection because of the presence of Escherichia coli in the feces. ▼

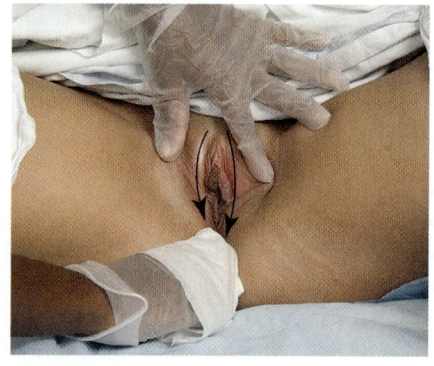

Male Patient

Retract the foreskin, if present, and gently cleanse the head of the penis using a circular motion. Replace the foreskin and finish washing the shaft of the penis, using firm strokes. Then wash the scrotum, using a clean portion of the wipe with each stroke. Handle the scrotum with care, because the area is sensitive.
To adequately clean the head of the penis in an uncircumcised male, you must retract the foreskin. After cleaning, replace the foreskin to prevent constriction and edema of the penis. Firm strokes may help to prevent an erection. Using a clean portion of the wipe

for each stroke prevents fecal contamination of the urethra and perineum. ▼

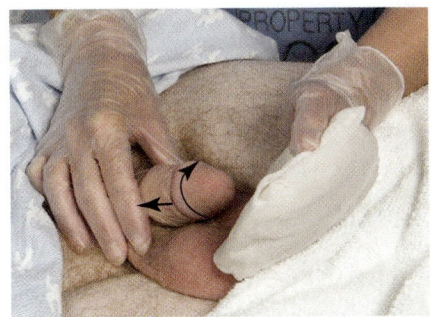

Detects and prevents excoriation in skinfold areas, where moisture accumulates.

5. **Allow body areas to air dry;** do not rinse.
   Prevents the emollient and surfactant skin protectants from being removed.

6. **Discard each wipe after use,** or place on the waterproof pad to discard when finished.
   Ensures following the "clean to dirty" principle.

7. **If perineal care is not being** done as part of the bath, also clean the anal area. Ask the patient to turn to the side and then wipe the buttocks and anal area as needed.
   Fecal contamination of the perineum can lead to urinary tract infections and skin irritation. Therefore, the anal area is cleansed last.

8. **Apply skin protectants** as needed. Powder only if the patient requests it.
   If urinary or fecal incontinence is present, skin barriers may be used to

prevent urine, feces, or other drainage from contacting the skin. This helps prevent skin breakdown. For female patients, powder is a medium for bacterial growth. In the presence of moisture, it also creates a paste, which irritates the skin.

9. **If the patient has an indwelling** catheter and if agency policy requires special catheter care, you will usually provide the care at this point. Don clean gloves before providing catheter care, and follow the agency's procedure. For more information about catheter care, see Clinical Insight 30-1: Caring for a Patient With an Indwelling Catheter.

10. **Reposition and cover the patient** with the bath blanket. Remove soiled gloves, discarding in a waterproof bag.
    Prevents contaminating clean linen with soiled gloves.

11. **Change linen as needed,** including soiled linen or linen that became damp during perineal care.
    Ensures patient safety, comfort, and privacy.

? What if . . .

- **The patient is unable to control bowel and/or bladder?**

Gently cleanse the perineal/perigenital area after each incontinence/soiling

and apply a moisture barrier according to agency protocols.
Minimizing contact with irritants such as moisture, urine, and stool can decrease the development of incontinence-associated dermatitis.

Use a spray, no-rinse cleanser, and soft wipes.
These aid in preventing irritation from friction and reduce drying effects on the skin.

Follow agency policy and use skin assessment tools (some geared particularly to perineal skin).

Assess for signs of secondary infection in addition to irritation and report as needed.

Consider bowel and bladder retraining and scheduling to reduce frequency of incontinence.

- **Your patient is postpartum?**

Educate the patient about perineal care. Include the importance of hand washing before and after cleansing the perineum, measures to keep the perineum clean, frequent changing of sanitary pads, and checking for signs and symptoms of abnormal lochia. If the patient had an episiotomy, laceration, or tear, teaching should also include management of discomfort and signs of wound infection.

Evaluation

- Assess the patient's responses to the procedure (e.g., any discomfort?).
- Observe for difficulty with movement or ROM during the procedure.
- Note the condition of the skin, including redness and other abnormal findings.
- Ask the patient whether she feels comfortable now.

Patient Teaching

- Discuss adaptations to perineal care. For example, if the area is tender, (1) wash the area with warm moistened wipe after going to the bathroom, instead of using toilet paper, or (2) use a skin protectant on the area.
- Review the importance of hand washing after elimination.

- If appropriate, teach the caregiver how to provide perineal care, including the major concept of cleaning front to back ("clean to dirty"). Stress the importance of wearing gloves and washing hands.
- Advise women not to douche because it disturbs the balance of normal vaginal flora and can irritate or injure mucosal cells.
- Explain that scented and deodorant feminine hygiene products are not necessary for cleanliness and may even be harmful. Daily cleansing is the most effective means of odor control.

Home Care

- Evaluate the ability of the client or caregiver to provide perineal care.

(continued on next page)

Procedure 24-4 ■ **Providing Perineal Care** (continued)

- Determine the availability of supplies needed for perineal care.
- You will need to adapt the procedure depending on the available equipment and supplies. Major issues involved in perineal care in the home are the lack of clean water and/or linens. In some instances, you may need to use bottled water or boil water for the procedure. One option is to use prepackaged moistened towelettes to provide the care (e.g., Comfort Bath towelettes).

Documentation

Usually perineal care is part of routine hygiene care and is charted on a flow sheet. If you need to write a narrative note, chart that perineal care was given, any patient responses to the procedure, and the condition of the perineal area.

Sample documentation

8/16/18   1430   *Perineal care given. Patient had no complaint of discomfort. No redness or discharge noted.* ──────────── *Nora Noyes, RN*

Practice Resources

National Guideline Clearinghouse (2013a); Powers, J., Peed, J., Burns, L., et al. (2012).

Thinking About the Procedure

To practice applying clinical reasoning to this procedure,

 The video, **Providing Perineal Care,** along with questions and suggested responses, is available on the **Davis's *Nursing Skills Videos*** Web site on Davis*Plus.*

Procedure 24-5 ■ **Providing Foot Care**

➤ For steps to follow in *all* procedures, refer to the Universal Steps for All Procedures found on the page facing the inside back cover.

➤ *Note:* This procedure describes foot care using a basin and water. It may also be done with prepackaged wipes, along with the bath.

Equipment

- Procedure gloves (if there are open lesions)
- Pillow (if procedure is done with the patient in bed)
- Disposable basin for water (distilled, sterile, or filtered tap water, per agency requirements)
- Liquid no-rinse soap
- Bath towel and washcloth
- Waterproof pad
- Orangewood stick
- Toenail clippers and nail file
- Lotion or prescribed ointment or cream

Delegation

You can delegate foot care to the NAP if the patient's condition and the NAP's skills allow. For example, as a rule you should not delegate care if the patient has impaired peripheral circulation or foot ulcers. Perform the following pre-procedure assessments, and inform the NAP of the amount of help the patient needs and any special considerations (e.g., ability to sit in a chair). Ask the NAP to report the condition of the patient's skin and nails, level of self-care, and ability to tolerate the procedure.

Pre-Procedure Assessments

- As you assess the feet and toenails, compare findings for both feet.
- Assess bilateral dorsalis pedis pulses, capillary refill, skin color, and warmth. Compare right and left feet. Palpate pulses at the same time bilaterally to determine whether one side is weaker than the other.

Decreased circulation to the feet increases the risk for tissue injury and infection. A variety of diseases can cause poor circulation. For example, cardiac or renal disease may cause pedal edema, which impairs circulation to the skin, and diabetes causes vascular changes leading to poor circulation to the lower extremities.

- Assess for diseases (e.g., diabetes mellitus and peripheral vascular disease) that create risks for foot problems.
- Thoroughly assess all areas of the feet for skin integrity, edema, condition of toenails, and any abnormalities. Check carefully between the toes.

Decreased circulation in the feet commonly causes problems such as thickened toenails, dry skin, and increased risk of infection. Changes in vision and mobility can increase the risk for injuries to the feet. Patients with diabetes also may have neuropathy, which prevents them from knowing when they have injured their feet. Identifying abnormalities enables you to provide interventions to help prevent potential problems. ▼

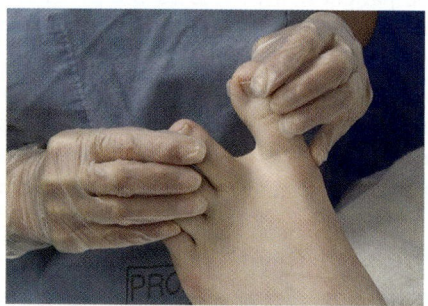

- Check institutional policy to verify whether a nurse is allowed to trim nails. Obtain a primary provider's prescription, if necessary.

Patients who have diabetes or impaired circulation to the lower extremities require a prescription for trimming their nails. Refer the patient to a podiatrist if the circulation is severely compromised or if edema would make the procedure difficult.

- **Assess the patient's usual footwear.**
Improperly fitting shoes, especially if they are too tight, are a common cause of foot problems (e.g., bunions, ingrown toenails).

- **Assess the patient's self-care ability to provide foot care.** Evaluate the need for a referral. Determine whether the patient has the necessary vision and mobility to be able provide his own foot care.

- Assess the patient's knowledge about foot care, including usual foot care practices.

➕ Identify potential deficits in understanding that may require additional teaching or referral to a podiatrist, general practice physician, or advanced practice nurse.

Many home remedies for foot problems can damage the tissue. For example, corn pads can increase pressure on the tissue, compromising circulation and causing local tissue ischemia. Cutting the sides of the toenails can lead to ingrown toenails.

➤ When performing the procedure, always identify your patient according to agency policy, using two identifiers, and be attentive to standard precautions, hand hygiene, patient safety and privacy, body mechanics, and documentation.

Procedure Steps

1. **Wear procedure gloves** and other protective wear as needed when providing foot care.
Follows standard precautions. The heel is a common place for skin breakdown, so use gloves if you are unable to see the area without lifting the foot. If the patient has significant drainage to the area, such as a draining wound, you may need to wear a protective gown.

2. **Ask the patient to sit in a chair** with a waterproof pad or bath towel under the feet, if possible. If the patient is unable to sit in a chair, place him in semi-Fowler's position in bed; place a pillow under his knees.
It is easier to perform the procedure with the patient in a chair. The pillow supports the knee joints and prevents muscle fatigue.

3. ➕ **Fill the basin halfway** with warm water (approximately 105°F to 110°F [40°C to 43°C]).
Recent research recommends the use of filtered, distilled, or sterile water. Using tap water for bathing exposes patients to waterborne pathogens that may be contained in biofilm in water lines and faucets. Hot water can injure the skin. Warm water promotes circulation. Filling the basin halfway prevents spilling when the patient places his foot in the water.

4. **Help the patient place one foot** in the water, first checking with the patient that the temperature is comfortable.
   a. If the patient is in a chair, place the basin on the floor (on the waterproof pad).

   b. If the patient is in bed, place the basin near the foot of the bed on the waterproof pad; pad the basin with a towel.
   The waterproof pad keeps the bed dry. Padding the basin prevents pressure on the back of the leg, which could cause discomfort and interfere with circulation.

5. **Allow the foot to soak** for 5 to 20 minutes, depending on the patient's tolerance and the condition of his feet.

   ➕ Soaking is not recommended for patients with diabetes or peripheral vascular disease (PVD).

   Soaking softens the skin and helps relax the patient. For patients who have diabetes or PVD, soaking is not recommended because it may remove natural oils, cause cracking of the skin, and may cause burns even if the water is at the recommended temperature.

6. **Cleanse the foot** with mild or no-rinse soap.
Removes loose debris. No-rinse soaps do not dry the skin. ▼

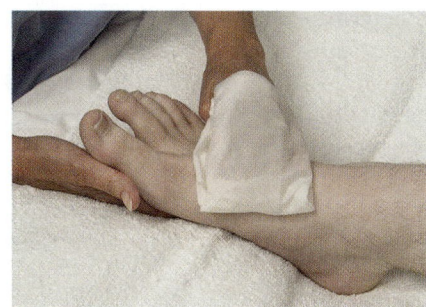

7. **Clean under the nails** with the orangewood stick while the foot is still in the water.
Water softens the nails and makes cleaning easier.

8. **Remove the foot from** the water, and dry it gently and thoroughly.
Remaining moisture, especially between the toes, can cause maceration and promotes development of fungal infections.

9. **Change the water.**
Ensures proper temperature and prevents cross-contamination.

10. **Soak the opposite foot** while performing steps 11 through 14 for the first (clean) foot.
Efficient use of time.

11. **Gently push the cuticles back** with the orangewood stick or towel.
Increases cuticle health. Do not damage the cuticle; doing so can increase the risk of infection.

12. **Trim the nails straight across** with toenail clippers, if not contraindicated by the patient's condition and if permitted by agency policy. Note whether the nail has cut into the skin of the toe being trimmed or the adjacent toes. If the nails are brittle or thick, allow the foot to soak for 10 to 20 minutes before trimming.
Trimming straight across prevents ingrown toenails. Early recognition and

(continued on next page)

Procedure 24-5 ■ **Providing Foot Care** (continued)

treatment of problems will prevent further complications, such as infection. ▼

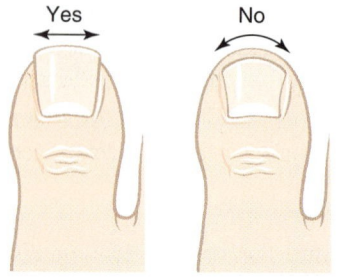

Yes   No

13. File the nails with an emery board.
Smooths the edges to prevent scratching the skin with the toenails.

14. Apply cream, lotion, or foot powder lightly to the feet and toes.
Cream hydrates the skin; however, excess cream can cause maceration. Foot powder absorbs moisture and functions as a nonirritating deodorant for patients whose feet perspire heavily.

15. Repeat steps 11 through 14 with the second foot.

16. Check the patient's footwear for rough edges that may injure feet.

? What if . . .

■ **My patient has Impaired Bed Mobility?**

Apply protective devices (e.g., lamb's wool) as needed.

■ **My patient has an injury, lesions, or pain?**

You may need to use a bed cradle to keep the pressure of the bedding off the patient's feet. Refer to Chapter 36 for other measures to preserve skin integrity.

■ **My patient has diabetes mellitus?**

In addition to controlling blood glucose levels, adhering to a specific foot care plan is essential for people with diabetes. Include the following in your teaching:

■ The importance of inspecting the feet daily

■ Ways to protect the feet (e.g., by wearing shoes when out of bed)
■ Potential complications involving the feet
■ Management of symptoms
■ When to seek advice from a healthcare professional
■ What to include in the foot care regimen (apply moisturizing lotion on tops and bottoms of feet but not between toes)—and what not to do (cut corns and calluses, use topical corn removers, or soak the feet)

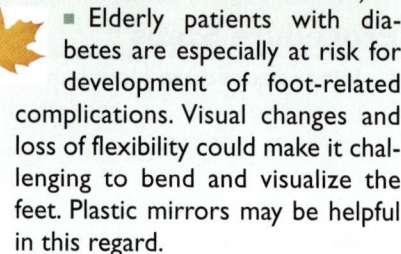

■ Elderly patients with diabetes are especially at risk for development of foot-related complications. Visual changes and loss of flexibility could make it challenging to bend and visualize the feet. Plastic mirrors may be helpful in this regard.
Early detection and treatment of problems can minimize foot-related complications.

Evaluation

■ Observe that feet are clean, smooth, and intact; nails are trimmed and smooth; skin is pink and warm.
■ Be sure that foot problems are identified and interventions provided.
■ Ask the patient to demonstrate or describe correct foot care.

Patient Teaching

For patient teaching, refer to the Self-Care box Teaching Your Client About Foot Care in this chapter.

Home Care

The procedure does not vary in the home. The nurse must:
■ Work with the client and care provider to determine the availability of supplies needed for foot care (clean water and so on).
■ Identify home care practices and teach the client and/or caregiver proper foot care techniques. Influencing older adults can be especially difficult if they have usual routines, such as walking barefoot, that put them at risk for injury. For clients with diabetes, the biggest risk to foot health is inadequate regulation of their blood glucose levels.

Documentation

In most agencies you will not document routine foot care (except, perhaps, on a checklist) unless there are problems. If you do document, chart that foot care was given and chart assessment findings.

Sample documentation

09/25/18   0900.   Foot care given. 2 cm circular reddened area on right heel. Skin abrasion outer lateral aspect of 5th toe, left foot— bio-occlusive dressing applied. ————————— Ann Hopkins, RN

Practice Resources
Bonner, T., Foster, M., & Spears-Lanoix, E. (2016); National Guideline Clearinghouse (2015); Powers, J., Peed, J., Burns, L., et al. (2012); Siegel, J., Rhinehart, E., Jackson, M., et al. (2007).

Thinking About the Procedure

To practice applying clinical reasoning to this procedure,

 The video, **Providing Foot Care,** along with questions and suggested responses, is available on the **Davis's *Nursing Skills Videos*** Web site on Davis*Plus*.

Procedure 24-6 ■ Brushing and Flossing the Teeth

➤ For steps to follow in *all* procedures, refer to the Universal Steps for All Procedures found on the page facing the inside back cover.

Equipment

- Toothbrush or sponge toothettes
- Toothpaste
- Dental floss (two pieces, each about 10 in. long) and floss holder (optional)
- Tonsil-tip suction connected to suction source (if aspiration is a concern)
- Emesis basin
- Towel
- Glass of water (distilled, sterile, or filtered water, according to agency requirements)
  KEY POINT: *Recent studies recommend that hospitalized patients at high risk for infection avoid exposure to hospital water. Follow agency policy.*
- Mouthwash and/or lip moisturizer, if desired
- Procedure gloves; mask and goggles if splashing may occur

Delegation

You can delegate oral hygiene to the NAP if the patient's condition and the NAP's skills allow. Perform the following assessments, and inform the NAP of the specific type of oral care and the amount of help the patient needs. Ask the NAP to report the condition of the patient's mouth, level of self-care, and ability to tolerate the procedure.

Pre-Procedure Assessments

- Assess the patient's ability to assist with oral care.
  Having the patient assist whenever possible promotes independence and supports a positive self-image.
- Determine whether the patient has dentures, bridgework, or partial plates.
  Determines how you will provide oral care.
- Assess general oral health, including gag reflex and the condition of the teeth, gums, and mucous membranes. If a patient has dentures, examine the mouth with and without the dentures.
  (a) If the patient has a hypoactive or absent gag reflex, you will need a suction setup to prevent aspiration. (b) Inflammation or lesions in the mouth increase the patient's risk of infection and may make eating difficult or painful, leading to malnutrition. (c) Poorly fitting dentures can cause irritation of the gums.
- Assess the patient's usual oral care, including cultural practices.
  Helps determine the type of oral care you will provide and identifies areas of patient teaching needed.

➤ When performing the procedure, always identify your patient according to agency policy, using two identifiers, and be attentive to standard precautions, hand hygiene, patient safety and privacy, body mechanics, and documentation.

Procedure Steps

1. **Position the patient** in a high-Fowler's position or in a chair, if possible. Position the patient on her side if the head of the bed cannot be elevated.
   Prevents aspiration and makes the procedure easier.

2. **Set up suction,** if needed. Attach suction tubing and tonsil-tip suction; check suction.
   Suctioning equipment may be needed to prevent aspiration of secretions during the procedure, especially if the gag reflex is decreased.

3. **If the patient is able to perform self-care:**
   a. Arrange supplies within the patient's reach.

   Promotes the patient's ability to do self-care and therefore independence.

   b. Assist the patient with brushing and flossing as needed.
   Ensures that the teeth are thoroughly cleaned.

Procedure Variation for Nurse-Administered Brushing and Flossing

4. **Place the towel across** the patient's chest.
   Prevents getting the patient's gown or linen wet during the procedure.

5. **Don procedure gloves** as needed. Wear gown and goggles if splashing might occur, such as with a confused patient.
   Follows standard precautions.

6. **Adjust the bed to working** height; lower the siderail nearest you.
   Prevents you from having to lean over the patient or reach across the siderail, possibly causing back strain or injury.

7. **Moisten a small, soft toothbrush** and apply a small amount of toothpaste. See Equipment for type of water to use.
   A small toothbrush fits more easily into the mouth and reaches more areas. The soft bristles can be used to brush the tongue and also the gums if the patient is edentulous. Excessive toothpaste does not increase the cleaning, and toothpaste residue has a drying effect on the mucosa. Moistening the toothbrush increases patient comfort because patients frequently have a dry mouth.

(continued on next page)

Procedure 24-6 ■ Brushing and Flossing the Teeth (continued)

8. **Place, hold, or ask the patient** to hold the emesis basin under the chin.
   Collects oral secretions and protects clothing and linens.

9. **Brush the teeth,** holding the bristles at a 45° angle to the gumline.
   a. Using short circular motions, gently brush the inner and outer surfaces of the teeth, from the gumline to the crown of each tooth.
   b. Brush the biting surface of the back teeth by holding the brush bristles straight up and down to the teeth and brushing back and forth.
      This is the most effective technique for removing all food particles and plaque from the teeth and gums. Removing debris and subsequent plaque helps to decrease microbial colonization.
   c. If the patient is frail, perform oral suctioning when fluid accumulates in the mouth.
      Prevents choking and aspiration. ▼

Brush teeth, holding bristles at a 45° angle to the gumline. Using short circular motions, gently brush the inner and outer surfaces of the teeth, including the gumline.

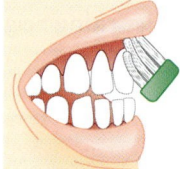

Clean front teeth.

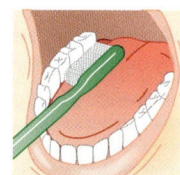

Clean both inner and outer surfaces of the teeth.

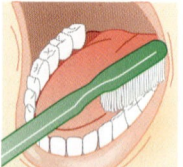

Brush the biting surfaces of the back teeth with the brush bristles straight up and down.

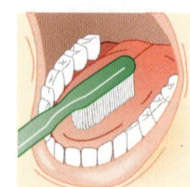

Brush the surface of the tongue.

10. **Gently brush the patient's tongue.**
    Removes coating and accumulated debris that can be a reservoir for bacteria. Brush gently to prevent gagging or vomiting.

11. **Floss the teeth.** Grasp dental floss in both hands, or use a floss holder. ▼

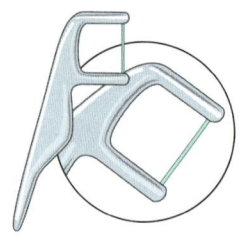

If you are not using a floss holder
a. Wrap one end of the floss around the middle finger of each hand. ▼

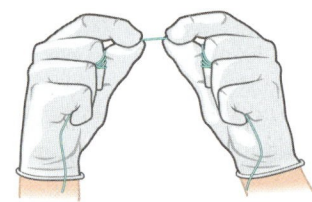

b. Stretch the floss between your thumbs and index fingers, and move the floss up and down against each tooth. ▼

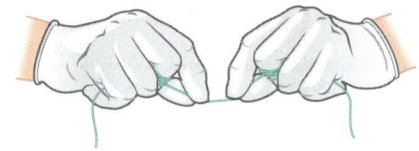

c. Floss between and around all teeth.
   Moving the floss up and down instead of back and forth prevents damaging the gums. ▼

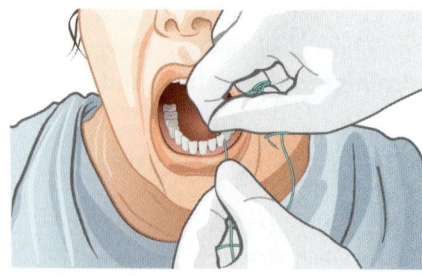

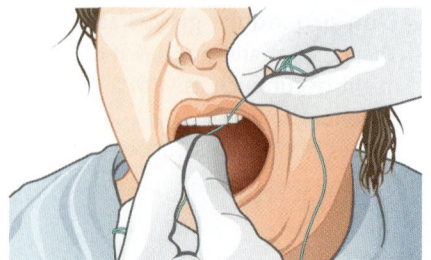

12. **Assist the patient in rinsing** his mouth, suctioning as needed. Or, ask the patient to rinse vigorously and spit the water into the emesis basin.
    Removes food particles from mouth. Suction if the patient has a decreased or absent gag reflex.

13. **Offer a mild or dilute** mouthwash, and apply lip moisturizer, if desired.
    Prevents irritation of the mucous membranes. Apply lip moisturizer for dry lips, for unconscious patients, or those on a ventilator, or per patient preference.

14. **Reposition the patient** as needed and return the bed to the low position.
    Ensures patient comfort and safety.

? What if . . .

- **My patient has an excessively dry oral cavity?**

  You may need to use a saliva substitute. *Aging, adverse medication effects, and illness often lead to decreased salivary production.*

- **My patient has viscous (thick) mucus?**

  Use appropriately diluted sodium bicarbonate to dissolve viscous mucus.

- ✚ **My patient has a high risk of gum bleeding (e.g., such as associated with thrombocytopenia), has painful mouth lesions, or toothbrushing is otherwise contraindicated?**

  You may use foam or cotton mouth swabs instead of a toothbrush. Do not use glycerin swabs, lemon glycerin swabs, or gauze squares. Use normal saline mouthwash.
  Foam swabs are less effective in removing debris and plaque, so it is best to brush when not contraindicated. Lemon glycerin swabs are drying to the mucosa and may cause decalcification of tooth enamel. Mouthwashes may be painful.

- **My patient has dementia or is uncooperative and agitated for other reasons?**

Use dementia-focused behavior management strategies:

Older adults with dementia frequently accumulate greater amounts of plaque and calculus, exhibit a higher incidence of periodontal gingival bleeding, and demonstrate a greater prevalence of denture-related oral mucosal lesions, yet they often resist oral care.

- Provide oral hygiene at the same time every day, not necessarily at bathing time.
- Use as many staff members as necessary.
- Give care in a quiet, distraction-free environment. Keep stimulation to a minimum, turn on some calming music.
- Speak softly; give one-step directions in short, simple sentences.
- Use a relaxed, slow approach; be sure your facial expression does not reflect tension.
- Give reassuring body contact and use gentle touch.
  Promotes trust. Quick or forceful touch may frighten the patient.
- Provide diversion.
  Occupies the patient's hands and prevents "grabbing."
- ✚ Never place your fingers between the teeth.
- Try placing a spare toothbrush or a rolled facecloth in the patient's hands while you provide oral care.
  Minimizes "grabbing."

- Use the "hand over hand" technique to gently guide the patient's own hand.
- Try starting the task (e.g., brushing), then having the resident help finish it.
- If the procedure is not going well, find another caregiver to come in and attempt the task.
- Use modified equipment and aids, if available (e.g., mouth props, backward-bent and suction toothbrushes).

■ **My patient is on a ventilator, is a frail older adult, or has undergone cardiac surgery?**

Be certain the teeth are brushed twice a day.

In addition to brushing, use moisturizer on lips and oral mucosa every 2 to 4 hours.

Apply a 0.12% chlorhexidine gluconate solution twice daily to complement oral care.

■ **My patient is receiving chemotherapy?**

Stress the importance of good oral hygiene, including brushing the teeth after meals and before going to bed.

Chemotherapy can cause neutropenia (reduced white blood cell count), predisposing the patient to infections. The oral cavity is a common site for infections in patients with neutropenia.

Routine rinses of mouthwashes with chlorhexidine are not recommended. Instead, use a bland rinse of diluted salt and/or sodium bicarbonate. Patients should swish for a minimum of 30 seconds and then expectorate the residue.

Chlorhexidine products have not proved superior to bland rinses in preventing or reducing either chemotherapy/radiation-induced mucositis or yeast colonization. In addition, chlorhexidine products may contain alcohol, may cause discomfort, may alter taste sensations, and may stain teeth. Bland rinses containing 1 teaspoon of salt or sodium bicarbonate per pint of water reduce the acidity of oral secretions, lessen mucus accumulation, and discourage yeast colonization.

An antifungal agent or a multiagent rinse (sometimes labeled "magic" or "miracle" rinse) may be used, followed by a short NPO period of 30 to 60 minutes. If other mouthwashes or rinses are also being used, allow 30 minutes to pass between their use and the use of an antifungal agent.

✚ *Multiagent rinses typically contain lidocaine. The resulting numbing effect may pose risks for a biting injury or aspiration. These rinses can neutralize antifungal agents.*

Evaluation

- Inspect the teeth, gums, and mucous membranes to verify that they are free of food particles.
- Inspect for abnormalities, such as bleeding, that may have been stimulated by the brushing or flossing.
- Observe for patient discomfort or gagging during the procedure.
- If the procedure was performed by the NAP, the nurse should still perform an evaluation of the care. This includes a physical assessment of the oral cavity as well as objective and subjective findings related to the patient's tolerance of and satisfaction with the care.

Patient Teaching

- Discuss the importance of daily oral care.
- Review any areas of brushing or flossing that the patient has not been performing adequately.

- Discuss any problems that need further follow-up, such as inflammation, bleeding, dryness, caries, missing teeth, or broken or missing dentures.

Home Care

The procedure does not vary in the home. The nurse must:

- Work with the client and care provider to determine supplies needed for the home.
- Determine whether suction is needed (e.g., if the client is unconscious or has a decreased gag reflex). Explain to the client and/or caregiver how to obtain a portable suction unit.
- Demonstrate how to position the client and perform the procedure if the height of the bed is not adjustable or if both sides of the bed are not accessible.

(continued on next page)

Procedure 24-6 ■ Brushing and Flossing the Teeth (continued)

Documentation

Document that oral care was given, the patient's response, any abnormal findings, and nursing interventions. Oral care is usually charted on a flow sheet.

Sample documentation

Mm/dd/yyyy   0815   Oral care given. Mucous membranes intact, pink and dry. No choking or complaints of discomfort. Patient encouraged to increase fluid intake. ———————————— Nancy Botha, RN

Practice Resources

American Association of Critical-Care Nurses (2007, revised 2010); Berry, A., Davidson, P., Nicholson, L., et al. (2012); Cuccio, L., Cerullo, E., Paradis, H., et al.

(2012); Philip, P., Rogers, C., Kruger, E., et al. (2012); Weening-Verbree, L., Huisman-de Waal, G., van Dusseldorp, L., et al. (2013).

Thinking About the Procedure

To practice applying clinical reasoning to this procedure,

 The video, **Brushing and Flossing the Teeth,** along with questions and suggested responses, is available on the **Davis's *Nursing Skills Videos*** Web site on Davis*Plus.*

Procedure 24-7 ■ Providing Denture Care

➤ For steps to follow in *all* procedures, refer to the Universal Steps for All Procedures found on the page facing the inside back cover.

Equipment

- See Procedure 24-6: Brushing and Flossing the Teeth.
- Denture cup

Delegation

You can delegate denture care to the NAP if the patient's condition and the NAP's skills allow. Perform the pre-procedure

assessments, and inform the NAP of the specific care and the amount of help the patient needs. Ask the NAP to report the condition of the patient's mouth and dentures, level of self-care, and ability to tolerate the procedure.

Pre-Procedure Assessments

See Procedure 24-6: Brushing and Flossing the Teeth.

➤ When performing the procedure, always identify your patient according to agency policy, using two identifiers, and be attentive to standard precautions, hand hygiene, patient safety and privacy, body mechanics, and documentation.

Procedure Steps

1. **Don gloves and remove** dentures (if the patient cannot do so).

   a. *Upper denture:* With a gauze pad, grasp the denture with your thumb and forefinger and move it gently up and down. Tilt the denture slightly to one side to remove it, without stretching the lips. Place the denture in the denture cup.

   The gauze gives you a better grip. Breaking the seal on the top dentures can be difficult; movement breaks the suction. Always place dentures in a denture cup as soon as you remove them to prevent accidental breakage. ➤

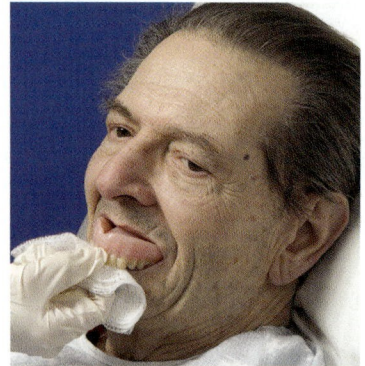

   b. *Lower denture:* Use your thumbs to push up gently on the denture at the gumline to release from the lower jaw. Grasp the denture with your thumb and forefinger and tilt it to remove it from the patient's mouth. Place the denture in the denture cup.

A gauze pad is not usually needed to grasp the lower dentures; however, you can use one if the dentures are difficult to grasp. Pushing up on the dentures breaks the seal. Rotating the dentures is necessary to remove the dentures from the patient's mouth. ▼

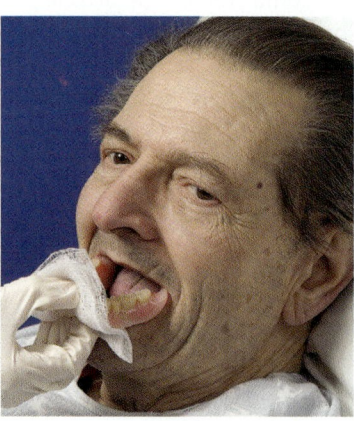

2. **Place the towel in the sink** and pour cool water (in accordance with agency policy) over the dentures to cleanse them.

Heat can damage some dentures. It's best to cleanse in the sink, under running water and over a plastic pan or towel. Running water facilitates cleansing; the towel/pan helps keep dentures from breaking. Dentures are expensive and usually not reimbursed by insurance. Institutions vary with regard to the existence of biofilm in the water lines

a. Apply a small amount of special denture paste to a soft-bristled toothbrush.

Denture paste assists in cleaning. Toothpaste and stiff-bristled brushes may be too abrasive for dentures. However, follow the patient's preference in use of denture cleaner. Some patients prefer to soak their dentures in a cleanser overnight. If dentures have been soaking, rinse them well before placing them in the patient's mouth.

b. Brush all surfaces of each denture.
Loosens all food particles and any old denture adhesive.

c. Rinse thoroughly with cool water.
Removes loosened particles and the cleaning agent. Do not use hot water with dentures, because hot water can react to make the denture material sticky. Patients at high risk for infection should avoid exposure to hospital water, so use distilled, sterile, or filtered water instead.

NOTE: *You can soak stained dentures in a commercial cleaner, following the manufacturer's instructions. Do not soak the denture overnight if the appliance has metal parts.*

Soaking can cause corrosion of the metal parts.

3. **Inspect dentures** for rough, worn, or sharp edges.
These can irritate the tongue, gums, or mucous membranes of the mouth.

4. **Inspect the patient's mouth** under the dentures for redness, irritation, lesions, or infection.
If present, refer to a dentist to check the fit of the dentures or to make needed repairs.

5. **Apply denture adhesive** as needed (ask the patient whether he uses denture adhesive).
Adhesives are needed to "seal" some dentures and prevent slipping and irritation of the gums.

6. **Moisten the top denture,** if it is dry. Then insert the top denture, at a slight tilt, and press it up against the roof of the mouth.
Moistening the dentures eases insertion. You can tell when you have securely seated the dentures by checking to feel for any slippage or to confirm that the dentures stay in place. Because the top denture is larger, it is removed first and inserted first for ease of insertion.

7. **Moisten the bottom denture,** if it is dry. Then insert bottom denture, rotating it as you put it in the patient's mouth.
Because it is smaller, the bottom denture is inserted after the top one. ▼

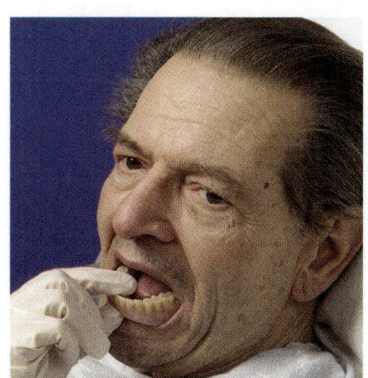

8. **Ask the patient whether** the dentures are comfortable.
Ensures that the dentures are properly placed.

9. **If the patient does not wish to** wear the dentures, cover them with water in a clean denture container with a lid. Label the container with the patient's name and the agency identifying number. Place denture container in bedside drawer rather than on top of bedside table for safekeeping.
Drying can cause dentures to warp. Hospitalized patients at high risk for infection avoid exposure to hospital water and use sterile water instead. Having the denture out of the mouth for several hours a day relieves pressure on the oral tissues, allows saliva to clean the tissues, and helps to minimize gingival irritation.

10. **Offer mouthwash.**

? What if . . .

■ **My patient develops *Candida*-related denture stomatitis?**

Follow agency protocols. Microwave disinfection of complete dentures has been documented as an effective treatment of *Candida*-related denture stomatitis and can reduce the recurrence of infections.

Denture stomatitis ranges in severity. Treatment includes good oral and denture hygiene and administration of antifungal agents. Recurrence of infection after treatment can be due to colonization of Candida on the dentures.

Evaluation

■ See Procedure 24-6: Brushing and Flossing the Teeth.
■ Check to see that dentures are comfortable and fit properly.

Other

For Documentation, Patient Teaching, and Home Care, see Procedure 24-6: Brushing and Flossing the Teeth.

Practice Resources

National Guideline Clearinghouse (2012); Siegel, J., Rhinehart, E., Jackson, M., et al. (2007); Silva, M., Mima, E., Colombo, A., et al. (2012).

Thinking About the Procedure

To practice applying clinical reasoning to this procedure,

The video, **Providing Denture Care,** along with questions and suggested responses, is available on the **Davis's *Nursing Skills Videos*** Web site on Davis*Plus*.

Procedure 24-8 ■ Providing Oral Care for an Unconscious Patient

➤ For steps to follow in *all* procedures, refer to the Universal Steps for All Procedures found on the page facing the inside back cover.

Equipment

- Toothbrush with soft bristles or sponge oral swabs
- Toothpaste
- Denture cup, if the patient has dentures
- 4 in × 4 in. gauze pad to remove dentures if present
- Tonsil-tip suction connected to suction source (you may use a product that combines the toothbrush or oral swab with the suction device)
- Tongue blade (padded) or bite-block
- Towel
- Waterproof linen protector
- Disposable emesis basin
- Water-soluble lip moisturizer
- Procedure gloves and goggles ▼

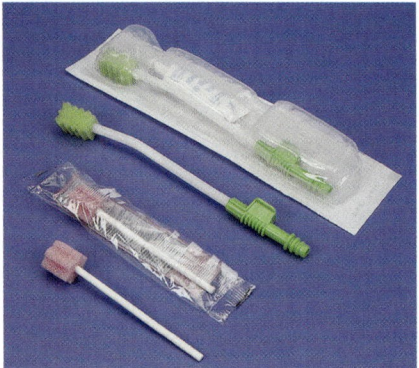

Source: Courtesy of Sage Products, Inc., Cary, IL.

Delegation

As a rule, you probably should not delegate oral hygiene for an unconscious patient to a NAP. However, in some situations it may be acceptable—for example, when agency policy permits, when the NAP has a great deal of experience caring for unconscious patients, and when the NAP's ability to perform oral hygiene safely for them is documented. Perform the preprocedure assessments, and inform the NAP of any special considerations for care (e.g., if the patient must have the head of the bed elevated to facilitate breathing). Ask the NAP to report the condition of the patient's mouth and the patient's ability to tolerate the procedure (e.g., ask the NAP to take vital signs before and after the procedure, or to note the oxygen saturation if it is being monitored).

Pre-Procedure Assessments

- **Determine whether the patient has dentures or partial plates.**
  The presence of these appliances determines how you will provide oral care. You may leave dentures out for an unconscious patient to decrease the risk that the dentures will be damaged or block the airway. However, when possible keep the dentures in place to help ensure they will fit adequately later. Remove partial plates in an unconscious patient to prevent the plate from causing aspiration or damage to the mouth if it becomes loosened.

- **Assess the patient's gag reflex.**
  If the patient has an intact gag reflex, the risk of aspiration is lower.

- **Assess the patient's general oral health, including the condition of the teeth and gums and hydration of the mucous membranes. If the patient has dentures, examine the mouth with and without the dentures.**
  Unconscious patients tend to breathe through the mouth, so oral mucosa are often dry. Because the oral mucosa acts as a barrier against microorganisms, inflammation or lesions in the mouth increase the risk for infection. The lips, gums, and mucous membranes should be pink, moist, and intact. The teeth should be intact and clean. The condition of the mouth determines what you will use to provide oral care. Assess the fit of dentures and the condition of the skin under the dentures to determine whether the fit is proper and whether any irritation is present.

➤ When performing the procedure, always identify your patient according to agency policy, using two identifiers, and be attentive to standard precautions, hand hygiene, patient safety and privacy, body mechanics, and documentation.

Procedure Steps

1. ✚ **Position the patient side-lying** with head turned to the side and, if possible, with the head of the bed down.
   Secretions will pool in the dependent side of the mouth. This position helps prevent aspiration and facilitates the removal of secretions by gravity.

2. **Don procedure gloves and eye goggles.**
   Follows standard precautions. Eye protection is needed when suctioning because of the risk of splashing.

3. **Place a waterproof pad** and then a towel under the patient's cheek and chin.
   The towel and pad will absorb water and keep the bed linens dry.

4. **Set up suction.** Attach suction tubing and tonsil-tip suction; check suction.
   Suctioning helps ensure that the patient does not aspirate oral secretions during mouth care.

5. **Brush the patient's teeth.**
   a. Use a padded tongue blade or bite-block, as needed, to hold the patient's mouth open.
   A padded tongue blade or bite-block is used to hold the mouth open so

you can visualize and reach the different areas of the mouth without injuring the oral mucosa. It also keeps the patient from biting the nurse's fingers. ▼

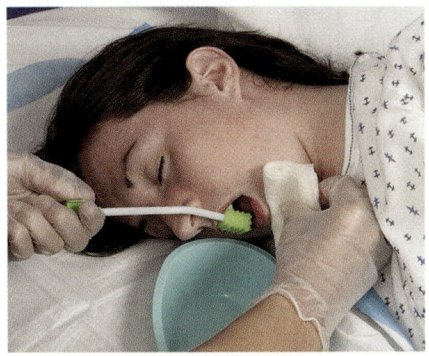

b. Place an emesis basin under the patient's cheek.
Catches the secretions draining from the patient's mouth.

c. Moisten the toothbrush and apply a small amount of toothpaste. Use hospital-approved water (e.g., sterile, distilled, or filtered tap water).
Excessive toothpaste does not increase the cleaning. Brushing the teeth with a soft-bristled brush stimulates the mucosa, which increases the health of the gums.

d. Brush the teeth, holding the bristles at a 45° angle to the gumline.
(1) Using short, circular motions, gently brush the inner and outer surfaces of the teeth, including the gumline.
(2) Brush the biting surface of the back teeth by holding the brush bristles vertical to the teeth and brushing back and forth.
(3) Brush the patient's tongue.
This is the most effective technique for removing plaque and debris from the teeth and gums. The tongue can be a reservoir for bacteria.

e. ✚ Perform oral suctioning when fluid accumulates in the mouth.
Removing fluid prevents choking and aspiration.

f. Draw about 10 mL of distilled, sterile, or filtered water, or mouthwash (e.g., dilute hydrogen peroxide) into a syringe; eject it gently into the side of the mouth. Allow the fluid to drain out into the basin, or suction as needed.
Removes any toothpaste residue, which may have a drying effect. Remove all fluid from the mouth to prevent aspiration into the lungs. Use a minimal amount of solution to prevent aspiration.

6. **Provide denture care,** if necessary. See Procedure 24-7: Providing Denture Care.

7. **Clean the tissues in the oral cavity** according to agency policy. Use foam swabs or a moistened gauze square wrapped around a tongue blade. Use a clean swab for each area of the mouth: cheeks, tongue, roof of the mouth, and so on.
Oral tissues may be dry and sticky from mouth breathing. Using separate swabs prevents transfer of microorganisms from one area to another.

8. **Remove and dispose of the basin,** dry the patient's face and mouth, and apply water-soluble lip moisturizer.

✚ *Petroleum-based lip moisturizers (e.g., mineral oil, petroleum jelly) are not recommended because of the possibility of aspiration, which might cause pneumonia. Never use petroleum-based jelly for patients receiving oxygen therapy; it can cause burns.*

9. **Remove the waterproof pad** and towel; turn off suction equipment; discard gloves and used supplies.

10. **Reposition the patient** as needed.
Maintains good body alignment.

11. **Cleanse and store reusable** oral hygiene tools in clean containers, separate from other articles of personal hygiene.
Prevents possible contamination from the environment and other personal hygiene tools.

? What if . . .

■ **You are providing oral care to a patient receiving mechanical ventilation?**

Provide oral cleansing, including subglottic suctioning, at least every 2 hours and prn. Brush the teeth at least twice a day.
Keeping the oral cavity clean and clear of secretions has been proved to decrease the incidence of ventilator-associated pneumonia (VAP). Pooled oral secretions become rapidly colonized with pathogens that contribute to VAP.

Avoid tap water. Use normal saline or a half-strength solution of saline for oral rinses.
Studies show hospital plumbing and tap water are often colonized with microbial organisms.

Apply a 0.12% chlorhexidine gluconate solution twice daily to complement oral care.

■ **It is difficult to floss the patient's teeth, or the patient doesn't tolerate flossing?**

Handheld interdental tools may be used instead of floss. These devices are special small brushes, picks, or sticks.
Toothbrush bristles can't reach between teeth to dislodge food particles and bacteria. Interdental cleaners can be as effective as floss in keeping these areas clean.

■ **Oral tissues are dry and sticky?**

Use appropriately diluted sodium bicarbonate to dissolve viscous mucus.

(continued on next page)

Procedure 24-8 ■ Providing Oral Care for an Unconscious Patient (continued)

Evaluation

- Inspect the teeth, gums, and mucous membranes for cleanliness.
- Observe the oral mucosa and gums for hydration, inflammation, bleeding, or infection.
- Observe the patient's overall responses to the procedure (e.g., gagging, coughing, vital signs, skin color).

Patient Teaching

- Discuss with family members any problems that need further follow-up.
- Teach oral hygiene measures, as needed.

Home Care

The procedure steps do not vary in the home.

- Work with the client and caregiver to determine supplies needed for the home.
- Determine whether suction is needed and explain to caregivers how to obtain a portable suction unit.
- Demonstrate how to position the client and perform the procedure if the height of the bed is not adjustable or if both sides of the bed are not accessible.

Documentation

Document that oral care was given, any abnormal findings, and nursing interventions. Typically, though, oral care is documented on a checklist or flow sheet.

Sample documentation

> 11/22/18   0730   Oral care given. Mucous membranes pink and moist. White coating on tongue—physician notified. Patient had no coughing during procedure. Gag reflex intact. Respiratory rate 18. ————————————Susan Hiam, RN

Thinking About the Procedure

To practice applying clinical reasoning to this procedure,

 The video, **Providing Oral Care for an Unconscious Patient**, along with questions and suggested responses, is available on the **Davis's *Nursing Skills Videos*** Web site on DavisPlus.

Practice Resources

American Association of Critical-Care Nurses (2007); American Dental Association (n.d.); Ames, N., Sulima, P., Yates, J., et al. (2011); Berry, A., Davidson, P., Nicholson, L., et al. (2012); Karki, S., & Cheng, A. C. (2012); National Guideline Clearinghouse (2012).

Procedure 24-9 ■ Shampooing the Hair

➤ For steps to follow in *all* procedures, refer to the Universal Steps for All Procedures found on the page facing the inside back cover.

Delegation

You can delegate this procedure to the NAP if the patient's condition and the NAP's skills allow. Perform the pre-procedure assessments, and inform the NAP of the specific type of procedure needed (e.g., in bed, at sink, disposable shampoo equipment) and the amount of help the patient needs. Inform the NAP of any special considerations, such as scalp lesions or positions the patient cannot assume. Ask the NAP to report the condition of the patient's scalp and hair, level of self-care, and ability to tolerate the procedure.

Pre-Procedure Assessments

- Assess for contraindications to a shampoo (e.g., scalp sutures or limited head or neck movement). A rinse-free shampoo would be more appropriate in these cases.

- Determine the patient's ability to assist with the procedure. *Promotes independence and provides active ROM.*

- Assess the condition of the patient's hair and scalp. Note any dryness or irritation. *Dry and brittle hair may indicate hypothyroidism or malnutrition and may require special shampoos or conditioners.*

- Determine the need for special hair care products. *Dandruff, lice, and dry hair are examples of conditions that require medicated shampoos or conditioners.*

- Ask the patient how she normally cares for her hair.

Procedure 24-9A ■ Shampooing the Hair for a Patient on Bedrest—Using Rinse-Free Shampoo

➤ When performing the procedure, always identify your patient according to agency policy, using two identifiers, and be attentive to standard precautions, hand hygiene, patient safety and privacy, body mechanics, and documentation.

Equipment

- Rinse-free shampoo (no water is needed); conditioner is optional
- Bath towel
- Brush or hair pick and comb
- Procedure gloves (if scalp lesion or infestation present)

Procedure Steps

1. **Elevate the head** of the bed, if possible.
   Makes it easier to maintain good body mechanics during the procedure.

2. **Place a protective pad** or bath towel under the patient's shoulders.
   Prevents the linen from getting wet.

3. **Don procedure gloves** if lesions or infestations are present.
   Helps prevent transmission of disease.

4. **Work your fingers through the hair,** or comb the hair to remove tangles before washing. If the patient has her hair in small braids, do not take out the braids to wash the hair.

5. **Apply rinse-free shampoo.** Apply enough shampoo to thoroughly wet the hair. One application is usually sufficient to clean the hair.

6. **Work the shampoo through the hair** from scalp down to ends.
   Helps prevent pulling on and damaging the hair.

7. **Dry the hair** with a bath towel.
   Removes the shampoo. Leaves the hair feeling clean and soft.

8. **Comb or brush hair** to remove tangles, starting at the ends and working toward the scalp.
   Prevents excessive pulling on the patient's hair, which may cause breakage.

9. **Dry the hair** with a hair dryer at a medium temperature, if desired.
   Use a medium temperature to prevent burning the patient.

10. **When you are finished,** be sure that the patient's clothing and bed linens are dry. Wash and store brushes and combs.

Procedure 24-9B ■ Shampooing the Hair Using Rinse-Free Shampoo Cap

> ➤ When performing the procedure, always identify your patient according to agency policy, using two identifiers, and be attentive to standard precautions, hand hygiene, patient safety and privacy, body mechanics, and documentation.

Procedure Steps

1. **Warm the shampoo cap** using a water bath or microwave according to package instructions. Be careful to not overheat. Check the temperature before placing on the patient's head to prevent burns.

A commercial no-rinse shampoo cap is a microwavable cap that contains a no-rinse shampoo and conditioner. Different products are available. Be sure to follow the directions on the package.

2. **Place the cap on the patient's hair** and gently massage.

3. **Remove the cap** and towel-dry the patient's hair.
   Removes the shampoo and excess water.

4. **Complete hair care** according to the patient's needs (see Procedure 24-9A, steps 7 through 10, preceding).

Procedure 24-9C ■ Shampooing the Hair Using a Basin and Water

KEY POINT: *The use of prepackaged shampoo products is recommended. However, some patients prefer the traditional shampooing technique or may have excessive soiling of the hair and scalp, requiring the use of water and basin. The traditional method of hair hygiene can result in significant variation from caregiver to caregiver and increase the risk of healthcare-associated infection from contaminated basins and/or tap water. Such techniques also require more nursing time and may be more tiring for the patient.*

Equipment

- Shampoo; conditioner is optional
- Disposable shampoo tray or commercial system, if available
- Disposable washbasin, plastic pail, small easy-to-handle plastic container
- Towels (2), washcloth, bath blanket
- Waterproof pads or plastic trash bag
- Brush and comb
- Procedure gloves, if indicated by the presence of lesions or infestation
- Hair dryer
- For inpatients, filtered tap water, distilled, or sterile water (see Key Point, above). Follow agency policy, as conditions vary among institutions.

> ➤ When performing the procedure, always identify your patient according to agency policy, using two identifiers, and be attentive to standard precautions, hand hygiene, patient safety and privacy, body mechanics, and documentation.

Procedure Steps

1. **If lesions or infestation is** present, don procedure gloves.
   Observes standard precautions.

2. **Unless contraindicated** (e.g., by a neck condition), lower the head of the bed, take the pillow from under the patient's neck, and place it under her shoulders.
   Hyperextends the neck and helps keep water from the eyes.

3. **Place the waterproof pad or plastic trash bag** under patient's shoulders, and cover with towels. A commercial system will have a drain hose to use.
   Protects the bed from getting wet.

4. **Collect warm, not hot, water** (see Equipment) in a container and bring to the bedside.

5. **Place the shampoo tray under the patient's shoulders** (or head, depending on the type of tray). If you are using a hard plastic tray, pad the neck area with a towel. An inflatable shampoo tray needs minimal padding,

(continued on next page)

Procedure 24-9 ■ Shampooing the Hair (continued)

but you will need to inflate it before beginning the procedure, either by mouth or with an air pump.
Protects the patient from lying on a hard surface and prevents water from leaking out onto the bed.

6. **Ensure that the tray will drain** into the washbasin or plastic pail.
Prevents water draining onto the bed or floor.

7. **Fold the top linens down** to the patient's waist, and cover her upper body with a bath blanket.
Keeps the linen dry; keeps the patient warm.

8. **Work your fingers through the patient's hair,** or comb the hair to remove tangles prior to washing.
It is easier to remove tangles from dry hair. Note that very tangled or matted hair may sometimes indicate a lice infestation.

9. **Wash the hair.**
   a. Wet the hair, pouring warm water from the pitcher. Do not get water in the person's eyes or ears.
   b. Next, apply shampoo and lather well, working from the scalp out and from the front to the back of the head.
   c. Gently lift the patient's head to rub the back of the head.

10. **Rinse thoroughly.**
Shampoo is drying if left in the hair. ▼

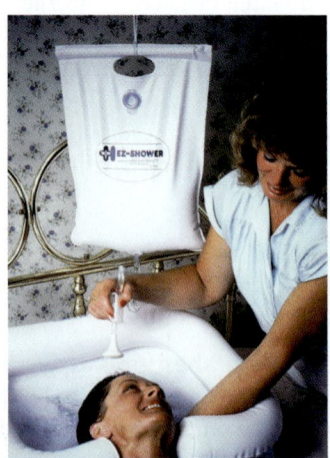

11. **Apply conditioner to the hair,** if desired, especially for patients with hair that tangles easily, such as dry, long, curly, or kinky hair. Rinse if needed. Leave-in conditioner can be used and is recommended for curly hair.

12. **Remove the tray** and blot-dry the hair with the towel. Do not use circular motions to dry the hair.
Circular motions will increase tangles.

13. **Comb or brush hair** to remove tangles, starting at the ends and working toward the scalp.
Prevents excessive pulling on the patient's hair, which may cause breakage.

14. **Dry the hair** with a hair dryer at a medium temperature, if desired.
Use a medium temperature to prevent burning the patient.

15. **When you are finished,** be sure that the patient's clothing and bed linens are dry. Wash the shampoo tray and the brushes and combs.

Procedure Variation Shampooing the Hair of African American Patients

16. **If the hair is in cornrows or braids,** do not take out the braids to wash the hair. You may need to apply a cloth or net cap to the head prior to shampooing.

17. **Handle the patient's hair very gently,** being careful not to pull on the hair.
Many African Americans have fragile hair that breaks easily. Apply moisturizer, if needed, to untangle the hair.

18. **When shampooing,** thread your fingers through the hair from the scalp out to the ends. Do not massage the hair in circular motions.

19. **Rinse thoroughly,** then apply a conditioner on the hair if the hair is dry and fragile.
A leave-in conditioner helps minimize tangles and breakage.

20. **Comb through the hair.**
   a. Use a wide-toothed comb or hair pick. Do not use a brush or fine-toothed comb.
   b. Part the hair into four sections and begin combing near the ends of the hair, working through each section.
   c. Use additional moisturizer to help soften and ease combing.
   Never pull on the hair, because it will break easily.

21. **Apply a natural oil to the hair,** if desired. Examples of natural oils are coconut, sweet almond, shea butter, and avocado. Many commercial products use these oils.
Mineral oil and petroleum jelly tend to clog pores and damage the hair, so use them only if the patient still prefers them after receiving this information.

22. **Let the hair air-dry** if possible.
Prevents the hair from becoming frizzy. A high temperature, such as from a hair dryer, will also damage the hair.

? What if . . .

■ **You discover head lice or nits as you begin the shampoo?**

Stop the procedure. Discuss your findings with the patient and offer reassurance. Leave the patient in a position of comfort and safety. Perform hand hygiene. Report the findings and obtain an order for a prescriptive shampoo.

■ **You do not have a shampoo tray?**

Improvise by using a new bedpan, and reserve it only for washing the hair. Pad it liberally with towels.

Evaluation

- Observe that the hair is clean, dry, and free of tangles.
- Observe for patient discomfort or fatigue during the procedure.
- Ask the patient how the hair and scalp feel.

Patient Teaching

- Educate patients and their families about how bathing technology has changed to improve patient care and reduce risk of infection. Products such as rinse-free shampoos or a shampoo cap can make shampooing easier to accomplish for a bedridden patient.
- Advise patients with coarse hair to wash it less frequently (every 3 to 7 days, depending on dryness). Leave-in conditioners are often recommended for dry, curly, or kinky hair.

Home Care

- In the home care setting, determine how the client usually washes her hair.
- If the client is confined to bed, work with the caregiver to develop an effective plan for washing the client's hair. For example, if a shampoo tray is not available, you can make one by using a plastic garbage bag and pillows or rolled towels.
- The newer rinse-free products or the inflatable shampoo tray may be good choices for the client.

- If the client cannot afford the adaptive equipment needed, refer the caregiver to the local resources, such as senior services.
- If the client is ambulatory, recommend a shower stool. The stool needs to fit into the shower or bathtub securely, without wobbling, to prevent the client from falling.
- If the client has only a bathtub, an adaptor for the faucet can be used to attach a handheld showerhead. Using a shower stool will make the procedure easier.

Documentation

Chart that hair was shampooed, the condition of the hair and scalp, and the patient's responses to the procedure.

Sample documentation

mm/dd/yyyy   2045   Hair shampooed, Scalp without signs of irritation. Hair dry. Conditioner applied. No c/o discomfort. Pt states "My hair feels wonderful now, and my head doesn't itch anymore." ———————— Alicia Nelson, RN

Practice Resources

"EZ-Shampoo Hair Washing Tray Instructions" (2015); Thompson Healthcare, Inc. (2012). [Caveat: These are not research articles; they are manufacturers' recommendations.]

Procedure 24-10 ■ Providing Beard and Mustache Care

> For steps to follow in *all* procedures, refer to the Universal Steps for All Procedures found on the page facing the inside back cover.

Equipment

- Scissors or beard trimmer
- Wide-toothed comb
- Mild shampoo; conditioner for coarse and/or dry hair
- Basin (single-patient use, disposable)
- Bath towel
- Procedure gloves (if skin nicks occur, contact with blood may occur)

Delegation

You can delegate beard and mustache care to the NAP if the patient's condition and the NAP's skills allow. Perform the pre-procedure assessments, and inform the NAP of the specific type of care needed (e.g., in bed, at sink, safety razor, electric razor). Inform the NAP of any special considerations, such

as skin irritation or activity intolerance. Ask the NAP to report the condition of the patient's skin and beard, level of self-care, and ability to tolerate the procedure

Pre-Procedure Assessments

- Ask the patient or family about preferences for beard and mustache care.
  Beards and mustaches may have personal and/or cultural meaning. Men in some cultures never cut or trim their beards. Some patients use a comb and scissors to do a slight trim of their beard and/or mustache, whereas others use a beard trimmer for a closer trim.

- Assess the patient's skin and hair condition.
  Determine whether the skin has any reddened or dry areas and whether skin treatments are needed.

> When performing the procedure, always identify your patient according to agency policy, using two identifiers, and be attentive to standard precautions, hand hygiene, patient safety and privacy, body mechanics, and documentation.

Procedure Steps

1. **Drape the towel around** the patient's shoulders.
   Protects the patient's clothing from falling pieces of hair and water from shampooing the beard or mustache.

2. **Trim the beard and mustache** when they are dry.
   The beard and mustache are often shorter when dry. If they are cut when wet, they may be shorter than desired after they dry.

If Using a Comb and Scissors

   a. Comb through the beard, and cut the hair on the outside of the comb. Be conservative; cutting too little is better than cutting too much.

(continued on next page)

Procedure 24-10 ▪ Providing Beard and Mustache Care (continued)

Trimming too much off the beard can be upsetting for the patient, whereas if you cut too little, you can always trim off more.

b. Trim from the front of the ear to the chin on one side, and repeat on the other.
Keeps the beard equal on both sides of the face.

If Using a Beard Trimmer

c. Select the trimming guide to the correct length. Adjust the guide to a longer length rather than a shorter length.
Ensures that you do not cut the beard too short.

d. Trim from the front of the ear to the chin on one side, and repeat on the other.

3. **Trim the mustache.**
   a. Comb the mustache straight down.
   Cuts the length equally so that the mustache is just above the upper lip. ▼

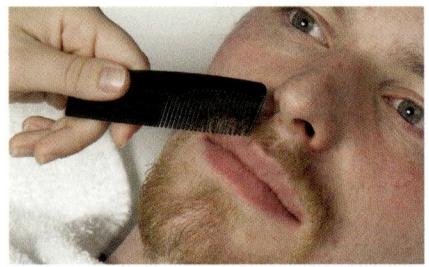

b. Using either scissors or a beard trimmer, start in the middle, and trim toward one side of the mouth and then toward the other. Do not trim the top of the mustache.
Trimming from the center out toward each side helps you cut both sides equally.

4. **Define the beard line** by one of the following methods:
   a. Using either the scissors or a beard trimmer, trim the line of the beard so that it is well defined. Trim very little to ensure that you only define the beard and do not change the length. ▼

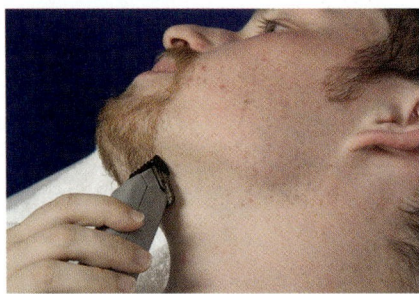

b. Shave the neck to define the beard line, particularly for short beards.

5. **Apply procedure gloves,** if needed, and shampoo the beard and mustache using warm sterile, distilled, or tap water and a mild shampoo.
The skin under a beard or mustache can be tender, so treat it gently with a mild shampoo. Follow standard precautions, because it is possible to nick the skin and cause bleeding. Policies about use of tap water vary among institutions.

6. **Rinse well, and pat and wipe** the beard and mustache dry with the towel.
Any shampoo left can irritate the skin, as can rubbing motions with the towel.

7. **Apply conditioner,** if desired.

8. **Comb the beard and mustache** with a wide-toothed comb or a brush.
Do not use a fine-toothed comb, because it will pull the hair.

Evaluation

- Make sure that the beard and mustache are trimmed to the desired length and are clean.
- Verify that skin problems are identified and treatment initiated.

Home Care

No adaptations are required in the home. The patient's usual supplies are sufficient, as a rule.

Documentation

Chart that beard and mustache were trimmed and shampooed; chart the condition of the skin.

Practice Resource

Procter & Gamble (n.d.). [*Caveat:* This is not an evidence-based practice article. It is a manufacturer's recommendation.]

Procedure 24-11 ■ Shaving a Patient

➤ For steps to follow in *all* procedures, refer to the Universal Steps for All Procedures found on the page facing the inside back cover.

Equipment

- Safety razor or electric razor
- Shaving cream or soap; after-shave lotion, if desired
- Shaving brush, if desired
- Warm water (sterile, distilled, or tap water per agency policy)
- Face towel and bath towel
- Procedure gloves

Delegation

You can delegate shaving to the NAP if the patient's condition and the NAP's skills allow. Perform the pre-procedure assessments, and inform the NAP of the amount of help and specific type of care (e.g., safety or electric razor, in bed, or at the sink) the patient needs. Inform the NAP of any special considerations, such as skin irritation or activity intolerance. Ask the NAP to report the condition of the patient's skin, level of self-care, and his ability to tolerate the procedure.

Pre-Procedure Assessments

- Determine how much assistance the patient needs.
  Helps you promote as much independence as possible.

- ✚ Assess the patient's skin and hair condition for redness, skin lesions, or moles.
  Identifies skin problems and determines whether skin treatments are needed or the procedure must be modified. To prevent abrading the skin, do not shave any areas that have skin lesions or moles.

- Assess the patient's usual shaving method, including use of electric razor or safety razor.
  When possible, follow the patient's routine. The patient may or may not use shaving cream or shaving soap, shaving brush, and after-shave lotion.

- ✚ Check for any contraindications to shaving, such as an increased risk of infection or bleeding (e.g., because of neutropenia, thrombocytopenia, or the administration of anticoagulants, such as warfarin or heparin).

➤ When performing the procedure, always identify your patient according to agency policy, using two identifiers, and be attentive to standard precautions, hand hygiene, patient safety and privacy, body mechanics, and documentation.

Procedure Steps

1. **Don procedure gloves.**
   To prevent exposure to blood if skin is nicked or scratched.

2. **Place a warm, damp face towel** on the patient's face for 1 to 3 minutes.
   Opens the pores and softens the beard to prevent pulling. Do not use hot water, because it will dehydrate the skin and can burn sensitive skin.

3. **Apply shaving lotion** to the face with your fingers or a shaving brush. Lather well for 1 to 2 minutes.
   Lathering well helps to further soften the beard. Do not use shaving creams that contain numbing agents, because they close the pores and stiffen the beard.

4. **Shave the patient.**
   a. Pull skin taut with your nondominant hand, and gently pull the razor across the skin. If you are using a safety razor, hold the blade at a 45° angle to the skin.
   b. Shave the face and neck in the same direction of hair growth (the direction is not the same for all people). Using short strokes, start shaving at the sideburns, and work down to the chin on each side and then the neck.
   c. Last, shave the chin and upper lip. *Usually the hair on the face will grow down toward the chin and on the neck up toward the chin. The hair is generally thickest on the chin and upper lip, so shaving them last allows more time for the shaving cream to soften the hair. Shave in the same direction as the hair is growing to prevent skin irritation.* ▼

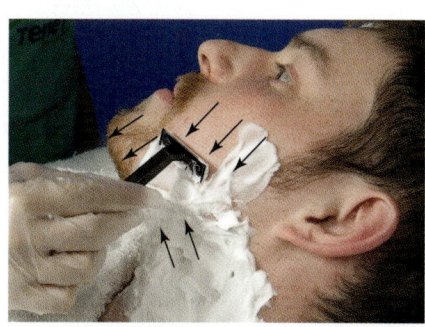

5. **Rinse the razor** frequently while you are shaving.
   Avoids clogging the blade.

6. **When you are finished shaving,** rinse the patient's face with cool water (see Equipment), and gently pat it dry.
   Cool water helps close the pores. Pat dry, do not rub, to prevent irritating the skin.

7. **Apply after-shave lotion,** if desired.
   After-shave lotions that contain alcohol are not recommended, because alcohol stings and dries out the skin. A moisturizer is recommended.

8. **Dispose of the single-use razor** in the sharps container.
   Prevents cutting injury to others.

If Using a Multiuse Razor

Shake the razor to remove excess moisture. Do not bang the razor against objects or dry with a towel. Store the razor in a covered container.
Banging or wiping the razor edge will dull the razor and may damage the holding mechanism. A covered container protects others from a cutting injury.

Procedure 24-11 ■ Shaving a Patient (continued)

? What if . . .

- Your patient has a condition that predisposes him to bleeding (e.g., thrombocytopenia) or infection (e.g., neutropenia)?

✚ **Such patients must be shaved carefully using an electric razor, if at all.**
A razor scratch or cut causes a break in skin integrity, providing a portal of entry for pathogens. This could be especially serious for a patient whose defenses against infection are compromised. For a patient with a delayed clotting time, a cut could cause excessive blood loss.

Evaluation

- Inspect the patient's face and closeness of the shave, and inspect for nicks or cuts.
- If the procedure was performed by the NAP, ask the patient about his satisfaction with and tolerance of the care.

Patient Teaching

Teach patients about changes that need to be made in their shaving technique as a result of changes in health status. For example, a patient who has begun taking anticoagulants may need to change from a blade to an electric razor because of an increased risk of bleeding.

Home Care

The procedure does not vary in the home. The nurse must:
- Determine the availability of supplies
- Assess the client's or caregiver's ability to perform the procedure.

Documentation

Chart that the patient was shaved and the condition of the skin. There will probably be a flow sheet or checklist for this information.

Practice Resources

Dunkley, S., & McLeod, A. (2015); Procter & Gamble (n.d.); *Men's Health* (2016). [*Caveat:* The *Men's Health* reference is not an evidence-based resource. It is information from manufacturers.]

Procedure 24-12 ■ Removing and Caring for Contact Lenses

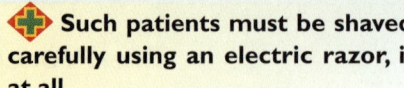

➤ For steps to follow in *all* procedures, refer to the Universal Steps for All Procedures found on the page facing the inside back cover.

Equipment

- Contact lens wetting solution
- Contact lens soaking solution
- Sterile saline (optional)
- Contact lens case
- Contact lens remover (optional)
- Procedure gloves

Delegation

You can delegate this procedure if the patient's condition and the NAP's skills permit. For example, if the patient is unconscious, you must determine whether contact lenses are present, and you should not delegate their removal.

Pre-Procedure Assessments

- Determine whether the patient is wearing contact lenses. If the patient is unconscious, examine the eyes for the presence of contact lenses by shining a penlight across the eye. You should be able to see the edge of the lens.
- Determine the type of contact lenses in place.
  Hard lenses are smaller than soft lenses. Each type of contact lens has different care requirements. Hard lenses can be worn for only up to 18 hours. Rigid gas-permeable lenses may be worn overnight or for about 7 days, depending on the kind. Soft contacts are used for either short or longer periods.
- Ask the patient whether he is able to remove his contact lenses.

➤ When performing the procedure, always identify your patient according to agency policy, using two identifiers, and be attentive to standard precautions, hand hygiene, patient safety and privacy, body mechanics, and documentation.

➤ *Note:* It is difficult to remove a contact lens when wearing procedure gloves. For hard lenses, you can use a suction cup device if one is available. ✚ If you must use ungloved hands (e.g., in an emergency situation), it is extremely important to wash your hands thoroughly before and after the procedure. *Do not* use your fingernails.

➤ *Note:* Lens cases are marked "L" and "R" to indicate left and right lenses. Clean, rinse, and place the lens you remove first into its designated cup before removing the second lens.

Procedure Steps

1. **Perform hand hygiene** and don gloves.

2. **Instill one to two drops** of contact lens wetting solution to moisten the lenses.
   Aids in lens removal.

3. **Remove the lenses.**

For Hard or Gas-Permeable Contact Lens

■ *Alternative 1:* If the lens is not centered over the cornea, place your finger on the patient's lower eyelid, and apply gentle pressure to move it into position. Place your index finger at the outer corner of the eye, and gently pull sideways toward the ear; position your other hand below the eye to "catch" the lens. Ask the patient to blink. As the skin tightens, the palpebral fissure narrows and the lids catch on the edge of the lens and pop it out. ▼

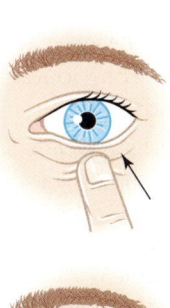

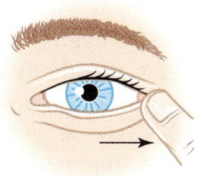

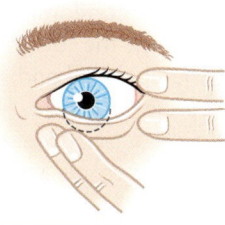

■ *Alternative 2:* Use a small suction cup contact lens remover. Gently press the suction cup end of the remover on to the contact lens, and lift straight up off the eye.

■ *Alternative 3:* Gently pull the top eyelid up and the lower lid down beyond the top and bottom edges of the lens. Then gently press the lower eyelid up against the bottom of the lens. When the lens is slightly tipped, move the eyelids together. This should cause the lens to slide out. ▼

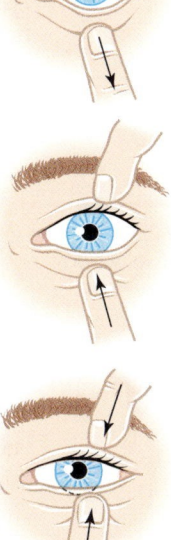

For Soft Contact Lens

a. Hold the eye open with your non-dominant hand.
   Allows you to visualize the contact lens.

b. Gently place the tip of your index finger on the contact lens and slide it down off the pupil to the white area of the eye.

To prevent potential damage to the eye, do not pinch a lens directly over the pupil. ▼

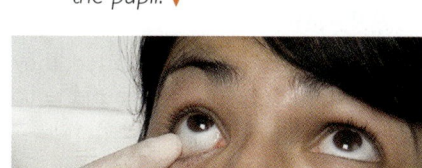

c. Using your thumb and index finger pads, gently pinch the lens and lift it straight up off the eye. If the edges stick together, moisten with a few drops of wetting solution. Rub gently until edges separate.
   A soft contact lens is very flexible and pinches easily. ▼

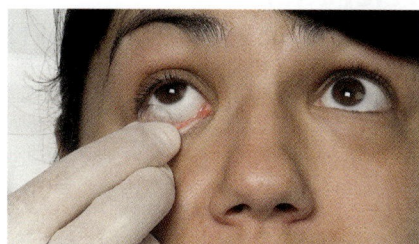

4. **Clean the lens** according to the instructions on the cleaning solution bottle. If there is no lens cleaner, use sterile saline. Be careful not to tear soft lenses.

5. **Rinse the lenses** with contact lens solution or sterile saline.
   Removes any particles from the lenses.

6. **Place the lenses in a contact** lens case containing soaking solution or sterile saline (see note above regarding lens cases). ✚ **Never use water.**
   Prevents bacterial growth on the contacts and keeps the lenses from drying out.

(continued on next page)

Procedure 24-12 ■ Removing and Caring for Contact Lenses (continued)

Evaluation

Examine the eyes for redness or irritation.

Patient Teaching

- Review with the patient and/or family the importance of keeping the contact lenses clean and moist.

- ✚ Teach the patient that contact lenses should not be worn or stored in water. If water touches the lens, remove and discard the lens.

- If hard contact lenses are used, they must be removed at bedtime to prevent hypoxia of the cornea.

Documentation

Chart that contacts were removed, what type of lenses they are, what solution they are stored in, and the condition of patient's eyes.

Practice Resources

American Academy of Ophthalmology (2015); Bausch & Lomb (2015, 2016); Massachusetts Eye and Ear Infirmary (2016).

Procedure 24-13 ■ Caring for Artificial Eyes

➤ For steps to follow in *all* procedures, refer to the Universal Steps for All Procedures found on the page facing the inside back cover.

Equipment

- Procedure gloves
- Normal saline solution
- Labeled container filled with saline or sterile, distilled, or filtered water
- Cotton balls

Delegation

You can delegate this procedure to the NAP if the patient's condition and the NAP's skills allow. Perform the pre-procedure assessments, and inform the NAP of any special considerations. Ask the NAP to report the patient's ability to tolerate the procedure.

Pre-Procedure Assessments

- Assess the patient's activity tolerance and whether you will need another caregiver to assist.

➤ When performing the procedure, always identify your patient according to agency policy, using two identifiers, and be attentive to standard precautions, hand hygiene, patient safety and privacy, body mechanics, and documentation.

Procedure Steps

1. **Wash hands and don gloves.**

2. **Position the patient lying down.**
   If you drop the eye when removing it, it will fall onto the bed instead of the floor.

3. **To remove the artificial eye:**
   a. Raise the upper eyelid with your nondominant hand, and depress the lower lid with your dominant hand.
   b. Apply slight pressure below the eye to release the suction holding it in place.
   c. Catch the eye in the palm of your dominant hand.
   d. Alternatively, you can use a small bulb syringe, place it directly on the eye, and squeeze to create suction and lift the eye straight up from the socket. ➤

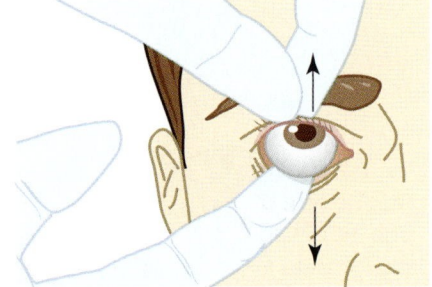

4. **Clean the eye with saline,** and store it in a labeled container filled with saline or sterile, distilled, or filtered water. ✚ Do not use solvents, disinfectants, or alcohol. These chemicals may irritate the socket or damage the artificial eye.

5. **Wipe the edge of the patient's** eye socket with a moistened cotton ball, wiping from outer canthus toward the nose.

6. **Inspect the socket** for redness, swelling, or drainage.
   Irritation or infection can occur if debris has entered the socket.

7. **To reinsert the eye:**
   a. Remove the prosthetic eye from the container, but do not dry it.
   b. Hold the eye between your thumb and the index finger of your dominant hand.
   c. With your nondominant hand, pull down on the lower lid while lifting the upper lid and guide the eye into the socket.
   The prosthesis will slide into place more easily when it is wet.

Evaluation

- Observe that the eye has been placed correctly in the socket.
- Ask the patient how the eye area feels.
- Observe the eye area for redness or irritation.

Patient Teaching

- Advise the patient to periodically inspect the eye area.
- Review the importance of hand hygiene and proper handling of the eye.
- If the eye wearer experiences dryness or irritation, a lubricant made for ocular prosthetics can be used.
- If the eye needs to be wiped but not removed, wipe from outer canthus toward the nose.
  Wiping outward may dislodge the prosthesis.
- Encourage the patient to sleep in the prosthesis at night and remove it every 1 to 3 weeks for cleaning (follow prosthesis specialist's advice). Some patients do find that it is necessary to remove and clean the prosthesis every day.
  Frequent removal irritates the lining of the socket and increases the amount of discharge produced by the eye socket.

- The eye should be professionally polished every 6 to 12 months. Symptoms that may indicate the need for a polish are irritated or itchy lids, increased drainage or discomfort, or changes in the appearance of the artificial eye.

Home Care

- In the home care setting, determine how the client usually performs eye care.
- Discuss ways to promote the safety of the artificial eye.
- Work with the client or caregiver to develop a plan of care for cleaning the eye and care of the area associated with the socket.

Documentation

Chart that the artificial eye was cleansed, the condition of the socket, care given to the area around the socket, and the patient's responses to the procedure.

Practice Resources

"Artificial Eye Service" (2010); Erikson Labs Northwest (n.d.); Peters, R. (2010).

Procedure 24–14 ■ Caring for Hearing Aids

➤ For steps to follow in *all* procedures, refer to the Universal Steps for All Procedures found on the page facing the inside back cover.

Equipment

- Face cloth, dry towel
- Damp cloth
- Cotton applicators
- Wax-loop and wax brush, if available
- Pipe cleaner or toothpick, if wax-loop and wax brush unavailable
- Procedure gloves (to prevent contact with earwax or ear drainage)

Delegation

You can delegate hearing aid care to the NAP if the patient's condition and the NAP's skills allow. Perform the pre-procedure assessments, and inform the NAP of the specific type of care needed (e.g., type of hearing aid) and the amount of help the patient needs. Inform the NAP of any special considerations, such as skin irritation or usual volume setting. Ask the NAP to report the condition of the patient's ears, level of self-care, his ability to tolerate the procedure, and his ability to hear in a normal conversation.

Pre-Procedure Assessments

- Determine how much assistance the patient needs.
  Aids you in promoting independence as much as possible.
- Determine the type of hearing aid in use. The three common types of hearing aids are (1) postaural hearing aid, (2) in-the-canal hearing aid, and (3) in-the-ear hearing aid.
  The cleaning procedure varies according to the type of hearing aid.

To review the types of hearing aids,

 Go to **Figure 24-7.**

- Assess the patient's ear and outer canal for redness, skin lesions, earwax buildup, or drainage.
  Identify skin problems and determine whether any symptoms of infection exist. Earwax buildup increases with age and doesn't necessarily indicate a health problem.

➤ When performing the procedure, always identify your patient according to agency policy, using two identifiers, and be attentive to standard precautions, hand hygiene, patient safety and privacy, body mechanics, and documentation.

Procedure Steps

1. **Don procedure gloves.**
   The hearing aid may contain earwax buildup or drainage.

2. **Place a towel on a nearby table or flat surface.**
   The towel helps prevent the hearing aid from breaking if it is accidentally dropped. Hearing aids are expensive.

3. **To remove the hearing aid:**
   a. Turn the hearing aid off by applying slight pressure against the volume control wheel and turning it backward (away from the nose).
      Stops the hearing aid from whistling.

(continued on next page)

Procedure 24-14 ■ Caring for Hearing Aids (continued)

b. Rotate the earmold slightly forward (toward the nose) and gently pull it out. Do not pull on the battery door or the volume wheel.

Pulling on the battery door or the volume wheel may damage the faceplate.

c. Place the hearing aid on the towel.

The towel will prevent the hearing aid from rolling off the table or banging against the table.

4. Clean the hearing aid.

a. Wipe all external surfaces with a damp cloth.

b. Clean the canal portion of the hearing aid using the wax-loop and wax brush, cotton-tipped applicator, pipe cleaner, or toothpick. Clean the top portion only. Do not insert anything into the hearing aid itself.

Poking utensils into any part of the hearing aid except for the canal portion may damage the hearing aid.

Detachable Earmold

c. Disconnect the earmold, and soak it in soapy water. Rinse and dry well, and then reattach it. Do not use alcohol. Never immerse a hearing aid in water, only the earmold.

Detaching an earmold that is glued or fastened by a small metal ring will break the hearing aid. Alcohol will damage the earmold material.

d. Check the hearing aid and any tubings for cracks and loose connections.

A damaged hearing aid will be less effective and may cause injury to the ear. Early detection of hearing aid damage may allow for repair rather than replacement of the device.

5. Cleanse the outer ear using the corner of a washcloth or a cotton-tipped applicator. Inspect these areas for redness, abrasions, swelling, drainage, or other irregularities.

Poorly fitting or improperly positioned hearing aids may cause trauma to the ear.

6. Insert the hearing aid.

a. Check that the battery is functioning. Hold the hearing aid in your hand. Close the battery compartment door if open. Turn the power on, turn the volume high, and listen for a whistling sound.

Whistling indicates proper power level and functioning of the battery.

b. Set the volume control to "Off."

Prevents whistling during insertion and a sudden loud noise.

c. Handle the hearing aid by the edges using your thumb and forefinger.

Prevents whistling during insertion.

d. Holding the hearing aid in your dominant hand, use your nondominant hand to gently pull the ear up and back.

Opens the ear canal slightly for an easier insertion and better fit.

e. Insert the canal portion of the hearing aid into the ear. Apply slight pressure and gently rotate the hearing aid back and forth until the canal portion rests flat in the ear.

Allows a better fit and prevents hearing aid from falling out.

When Inserting a Postaural Hearing Aid

Insert the earmold first and then place the earmold over the ear.

When Inserting an In-the-Canal Hearing Aid

Insert with the volume control at the top. The canal should be facing away from your hand.

When Inserting an In-the-Ear Hearing Aid

Insert with the volume control at the bottom.

7. Turn the hearing aid on and adjust the volume by turning the volume control wheel toward the nose. Set the volume control as low as possible.

Normal setting requires a one-third to two-thirds turn of the volume control wheel. A noisier environment requires less volume, or one-fourth turn.

8. Protect the hearing aid from curling irons, hair dryers, and hair spray and other hair products.

Heat and moist aerosols will damage the hearing aid.

Procedure Variation Storing the Hearing Aid

9. Open the battery compartment and place the hearing aid in a closed container labeled with the patient's name.

Saves battery power and allows any moisture to evaporate. Protects the hearing aid from accidental damage or loss.

10. If the hearing aid is to be kept stored and not worn for a week or more, remove the battery completely.

Prevents battery acid from leaking and damaging the hearing aid.

11. Store the hearing aid in a cool, dry place, preferably in the bedside drawer. Keep the hearing aid away from children and pets.

Moisture and heat will damage the hearing aid. Hearing aids and containers are easily lost. A child may choke on the hearing aid. Dogs and cats are attracted to the whistling noise and odor of the hearing aid and sometimes attempt to eat the device.

Procedure Variation Replacing the Battery

12. Use your finger to swing the battery door open. Never force the door.

13. Peel the tab off the new battery.

14. Hold the battery with the positive (+) side up and slide it into the door, not into the hearing aid itself.

15. Gently close the battery door. Never force the door.

16. Dispose of the old mercury-free battery in the regular trash.

NOTE: If the battery contains mercury, refer to the package for disposal instructions.

Guidelines for Care of the Batteries

- Always dispose of old batteries. Do not throw into a fire.
  Minimizes damage from leaking battery acid and prevents mistaking fresh battery from used battery. Heat and fire may cause the battery to explode.

- Store batteries in a cool, dry place. Do not place zinc-air batteries in the refrigerator.
  Heat shortens the life of the battery. Cold batteries warming to room temperature are exposed to condensation and subsequent corrosion.

- Do not store batteries near coins or other metals.
  Contact with other metals can short-circuit the batteries.

- Do not remove the tab from the battery until the battery is ready for use.
  The tab keeps air out of the battery. Once the tab is removed, the battery is activated. Early removal decreases the life of the battery.

- ✚ Keep batteries away from children, confused adults, and pets.
  Minimizes accidental swallowing.

? What if . . .

- **The hearing aid becomes wet?**

  If the hearing aid becomes exposed to moisture, dry it as thoroughly as possible. Remove the battery and throw it away. Keep the battery door open. Place the hearing aid in its container and allow it to dry overnight. Do not place a new battery in the hearing aid until the next morning.
  Moisture will cause the battery to corrode.

- **The patient wears bilateral hearing aids?**

  Be sure to identify which hearing aid is for the left ear and which hearing aid is for the right ear. Most hearing aids have a color marking for easy identification: red = right ear and blue = left ear.
  Attempting to force a hearing aid into the wrong ear may cause trauma to the ear.

- **The patient continues to have hearing difficulties despite hearing aids?**

  Hearing aids will not restore full hearing. General tips when communicating with a person with a hearing deficit are listed in Clinical Insight 31-3: Communicating With Hearing-Impaired Clients.
  Hearing aids will not block out background noise. A clear, distinct, low-pitched voice helps the client to understand what is being said.

Evaluation

- Assess how well the patient tolerated the procedure. Was there any discomfort, difficulty with insertion, and so on?
- Note the condition of the patient's skin, including pain, redness, and abnormal discharge.
- Note the condition of the hearing aid itself.
- Assess the patient's ability to hear normal speaking voices.
- Ask the patient whether he feels comfortable and hears satisfactorily.

Patient Teaching

- Discuss the importance of daily hearing aid care.
- Review any areas of care that the patient has not been performing adequately.
- Discuss any problems that need further follow-up, such as earwax build up, faulty or broken hearing aid, or ill-fitting hearing aid.

Home Care

The procedure does not vary in the home. The issues are that the nurse must:

- Work with the patient and care provider to determine supplies needed for the home.

- Determine whether further knowledge is required (e.g., if the patient must expose hearing aids to prevailing weather conditions, uses a telephone extensively, must make several adaptations from quiet to noisy environments throughout the day).
- Provide a list of available resources (e.g., AARP, National Institutes of Health, Better Hearing Institute).

Documentation

Chart that the patient is wearing a hearing aid, the condition of the ear, and the ability to hear. There will probably be a flow sheet or checklist for this information.

Practice Resources

Department of Veterans Affairs (n.d.); National Institute on Deafness and Other Communication Disorders (2015); U.S. Food and Drug Administration (2009).

Procedure 24-15 ■ Making an Unoccupied Bed

➤ For steps to follow in *all* procedures, refer to the Universal Steps for All Procedures found on the page facing the inside back cover.

Equipment

- Bottom and top sheets, possibly drawsheet
- Pillowcase for each of the pillows
- Linen bag or hamper
- Procedure gloves (if exposure to body fluids is possible)
- Moisture-proof gown (if heavy soiling of linens with body fluids is possible).

Delegation

You can delegate this procedure to the NAP. You are responsible for supervising to ensure that the procedure is performed correctly.

Pre-Procedure Assessments

- Check to see whether the linen (including the mattress pad, blanket, and bedspread) needs to be changed, and what linens are needed.
- Assess whether the patient is able to be out of bed during the linen change.
- Assess for drainage or incontinence to determine whether personal protective equipment, such as procedure gloves and gown, is needed.

NOTE: This procedure describes bed making by one person. It is more efficient for two people to work together on opposite sides of the bed.

➤ When performing the procedure, always identify your patient according to agency policy, using two identifiers, and be attentive to standard precautions, hand hygiene, patient safety and privacy, body mechanics, and documentation.

Procedure Steps

1. **Assist the patient to a chair.** Provide a robe and/or blanket if needed.
   Ensures that the patient is comfortable and will be warm enough during the bed change.

2. **Prepare the environment:** Position the bed flat, raise to appropriate working height, put on the brakes, and lower the siderails. Move the overbed table and other furniture, as needed. Place the linen bag or hamper conveniently near the bed.
   Maintains good body mechanics and prevents back strain during the procedure. Remove obstacles to allow easy access to the bed. Place all items so you can work efficiently, saving time and energy.

3. **Don protective gloves** and other gear if necessary. Loosen all the bedding.
   This observes standard precautions and reduces the risk of contaminating your clothing.

4. **If the blanket or bedspread is** clean, fold it and place it on a clean area (e.g., on the back of a chair). Do *not* place on another patient's bed or furniture.
   Reuse the blanket and/or bedspread if it is not soiled. Placing the item on a clean area prevents cross-contamination.

5. **Remove the bottom and top sheet,** draw sheet, and pillowcases.
   a. Do not shake the linens.
      Minimizes dispersal of dust, skin cells, and microorganisms into the environment.
   b. Holding the items away from your body, place them in a laundry bag or hamper. Never place linen on the floor. Place the pillows on a clean area (e.g., on a chair).
      Hold dirty linen away from your uniform to prevent contamination. Cross-contamination can occur if you place linens on the floor. ▼

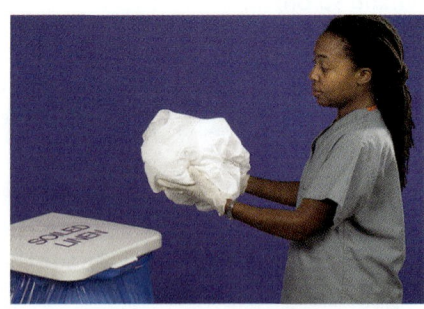

6. **Working from one side of bed,** to save steps:

   For a Contour-Bottom Sheet
   a. Fit the contour-bottom sheet on one side of the bed, and smooth it out over half the mattress.

   For a Flat-Bottom Sheet
   b. Fold the flat-bottom lengthwise with the center crease in the middle of bed and unfold with the rough side facing down.
   c. Position the bottom sheet so that approximately 10 inches hang over at the top and sides. The hem of the bottom sheet should be just even with the bottom edge of the mattress.
   d. Tuck in the sheet, mitering the sheet at the top corner (see step 11).
      When using a flat bottom sheet, having extra sheet at the top helps keep it in place when the head of the bed is raised and lowered. Unfold the sheet rather than shake or fan to reduce dispersing microorganisms into the air. The sheet will not be long enough to tuck in at the bottom.

7. **Place the drawsheet** with the center fold in the middle of the mattress and unfold. Tuck the side in under the mattress, and smooth out over half of the mattress.
   Ensures that all wrinkles are out of the bottom sheet and drawsheet. ▼

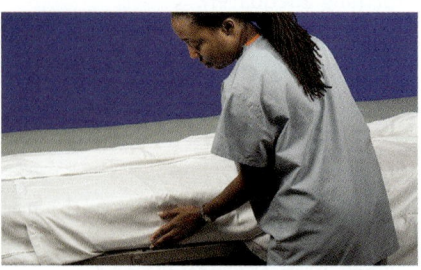

8. **Go to the other side** of the bed, straighten the linen, and finish tucking in the bottom sheet and drawsheet.
   a. Make the drawsheet tight, and smooth any wrinkles in the bottom sheet and drawsheet.
   b. If desired, place a waterproof pad on or under the drawsheet.
      Pulling the drawsheet tight helps prevent wrinkles from developing under the patient when she moves around in bed. ▼

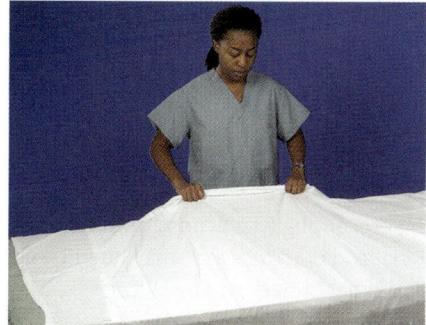

9. **Place the top sheet and** bedspread along one side of the mattress. Center the top sheet and bedspread, so that when you straighten them from the other side of the bed, they fall equally over each side of the bed.
   Putting the linen on one side of the bed saves steps.

10. **At the foot of the bed** make a small pleat in the top sheet and bedspread.
    Prevents the top covers from placing pressure on the patient's toes. ▼

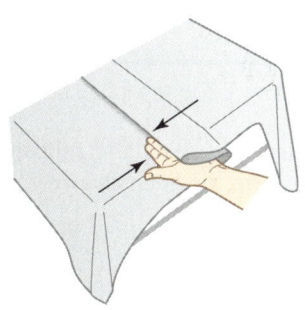

11. **Tuck in the top sheet** and bedspread at the same time, mitering the corners.
    Tuck in the sheet and bedspread at the bottom of the mattress. ▼

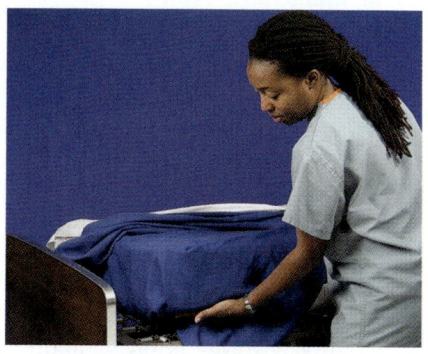

   a. Bring the edge of sheet and the bedspread up to make a right angle. ▼

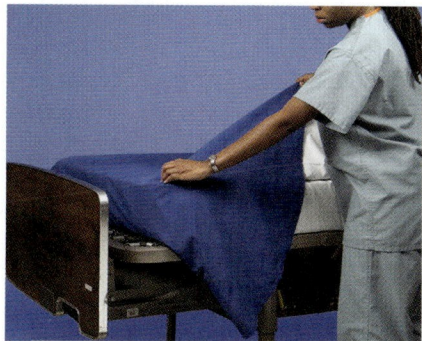

   b. Tuck the lower edge of sheet and bedspread under the mattress.
      Mitered corners help secure the linen at the foot of the bed. ▼

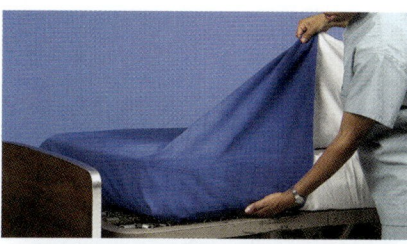

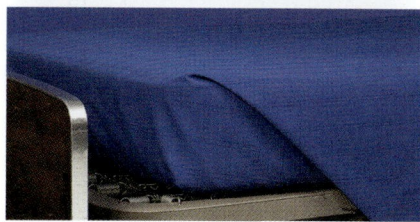

12. **Move to the other side** of the bed, smooth top linens, and repeat step 11. At the head of the bed, fold the edge of sheet down over the bedspread.
    Prevents the bedspread from rubbing against the patient's skin. ▼

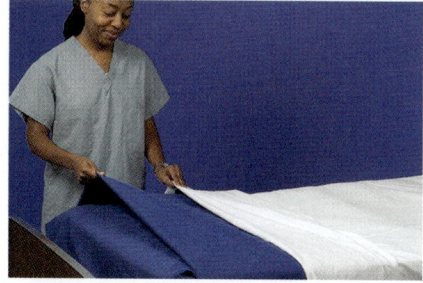

13. **Fanfold the top sheet** and bedspread back to the foot of the bed.
    Makes it easier for the patient to get into bed. ▼

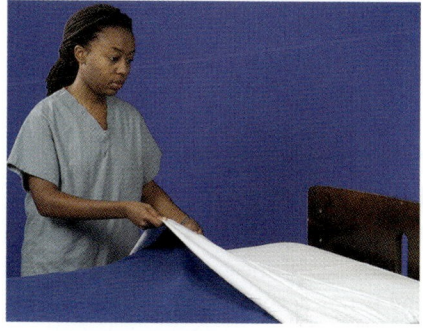

14. **Change pillowcases.**
    a. Turn the pillowcase wrong side out.
    b. Grasp the middle of the closed end of the pillowcase.
    c. Reaching through the pillowcase, grasp the end of the pillow. ▼

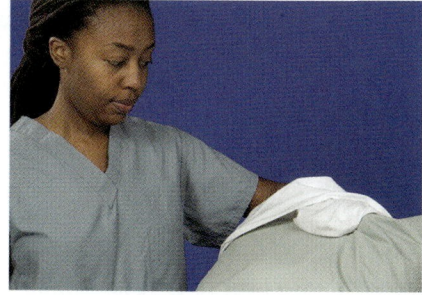

(continued on next page)

Procedure 24-15 ■ Making an Unoccupied Bed (continued)

d. Continuing to grasp the end of the pillow, pull the pillowcase down over the pillow.

Do not hold the pillow under your arm or chin to put on pillowcase because contamination can occur. ▼

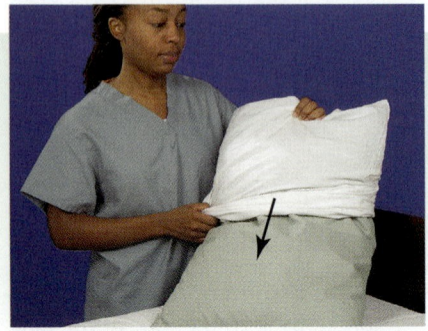

15. **Assist the patient back to bed,** return the bed to the low position, place the call signal within reach, and place the bedside table and overbed table so that they are accessible to the patient.

Provides for patient comfort and safety.

? What if . . .

■ **The linens have been contaminated by body fluids?**

Follow recommended infection control procedures for laundering of linens (e.g., wear procedure gloves, place linens in moisture-proof bags).

■ **The mattress has become contaminated by body fluids?**

Follow agency policies for cleaning the mattress before putting on clean linens. This often involves notifying another department, such as housekeeping or environmental services, whose members are trained in this procedure.

■ **The mattress cover is damaged or worn?**

If routine assessments review that the mattress cover is stained, damaged, or worn, remove from use, according to

the healthcare facility's procedures, and immediately replace any damaged mattress cover to reduce the risk of infection to patients.

■ **The patient has a specialty bed or specialty mattress?**

Several products are available with specific criteria to match patients' needs in terms of comfort, prevention, or treatment of pressure injuries, and movement (e.g., specialty beds designed for bariatric patients). Follow the manufacturer's directions (e.g., a recommendation for a specific mattress may be to use only one layer of sheet over the mattress for maximum benefit). If you find the sheets are not large enough to accommodate a specialized mattress, you may need to use two flat sheets to cover it.

Home Care

The only adaptations at home depend on the type of bed the patient has. If the height of the bed is not adjustable or the bed is not accessible from both sides, the procedure may be more difficult.

Documentation

Linen changes are generally recorded on a checklist, if at all. Additional charting would need to be done only if something

abnormal occurred—for example, "The drawsheet had a 20-cm circular area of serosanguineous drainage."

Practice Resources

Mitchell, B., Wilson, F., McGregor, A., et al. (2012); Sergent, A. P., Slekovec, C., Pauchot, J., et al. (2012); Siegel, J., Rhinehart, E., Jackson, M., et al. (2007); U.S. Food and Drug Administration (2013).

Procedure 24-16 ■ Making an Occupied Bed

➤ For steps to follow in *all* procedures, refer to the Universal Steps for All Procedures found on the page facing the inside back cover.

Equipment

- Bottom and top sheets; drawsheet
- Pillowcase for each of the pillows
- Bath blanket (as needed)
- Linen bag or hamper
- Procedure gloves (if exposure to body fluids is possible)
- Moisture-proof gown (if heavy soiling of linens with body fluids is possible).

Delegation

You can delegate this procedure if the patient's condition and the NAP's skills permit. For example, if the patient is very ill, in

pain, or requires two people for turning and repositioning, you should assist with or perform the linen change yourself.

Pre-Procedure Assessments

- Determine the patient's ability to assist with the procedure and whether additional help or assistive devices are needed.
- Make other assessments listed in Procedure 24-15.

➤ When performing the procedure, always identify your patient according to agency policy, using two identifiers, and be attentive to standard precautions, hand hygiene, patient safety and privacy, body mechanics, and documentation.

➤ *Note:* If linen change is done at the same time as the bed bath, some of these steps will vary.

Procedure Steps

1. **Prepare the environment:** Move the overbed table and other furniture, as needed, to allow access to the bed. Place the linen bag or hamper conveniently near the bed.
To allow easy access to the bed and enable you to work efficiently, saving time and energy.

2. **Don protective gloves** and other gear if necessary.
This observes standard precautions and reduces the risk of contaminating your clothing.

3. **Position the bed flat** if possible, and raise it to working height. Lower the siderail nearest you.
Maintains good body mechanics and prevents back strain during the procedure. Having the head of the bed flat makes it easier to smooth the bottom sheet. To prevent the patient from falling out of bed, lower the siderails only on the side where you are standing.

4. **Disconnect the call device** and remove the patient's personal items from the bed.
Prevents items from getting lost.

5. **Check that no tubes** (e.g., IV, nasogastric) are entangled in the bed linens.
Prevents dislodging tubes accidentally.

6. **If the blanket or bedspread** is clean, fold it and place it on a clean area (e.g., the back of a chair); do not place it on another patient's bed or furniture.
Reusing the blanket and/or bedspread if it is not soiled conserves resources.

7. **Cover the patient** with a bath blanket, if available, or leave the top sheet over the patient.
Covering the patient prevents chilling and preserves modesty.

8. **Slide the patient to the far side** of the bed and place him in a side-lying position, facing the siderail. Place a pillow under his head. If needed for support, place a pillow between the patient and the siderail.
Placing the patient close to the siderail will allow you to place the clean linen over a larger area, making it easier to roll the patient back onto the clean linen. Patients who cannot maintain the side-lying position should have a pillow placed between their chest and the siderail to prevent them from accidentally rolling into the siderail.

9. **Roll or tightly fanfold** the soiled linens toward the patient's back. Tuck the roll slightly under the patient. Cover any moist areas with a waterproof pad.
Cover any moist areas to prevent contact with the clean linen or patient. ▼

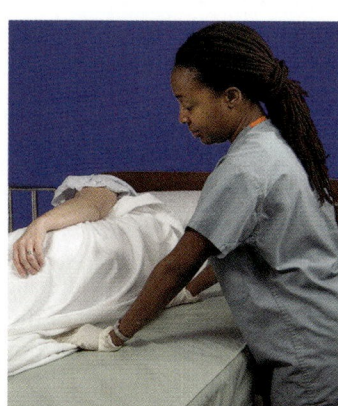

10. **Remove soiled gloves,** perform hand hygiene, and don clean gloves.

11. **Place the clean bottom sheet** and drawsheet (or pad) on the near side of the mattress, with the center vertical fold at the center of the bed. Fanfold the half of the clean linen that is to be used on the far side, folding it as close to the patient as possible and tucking it under the dirty linen. Tuck the lower edges of clean linen under the mattress. Smooth out all wrinkles.

Wrinkles under the patient can cause skin irritation. ▼

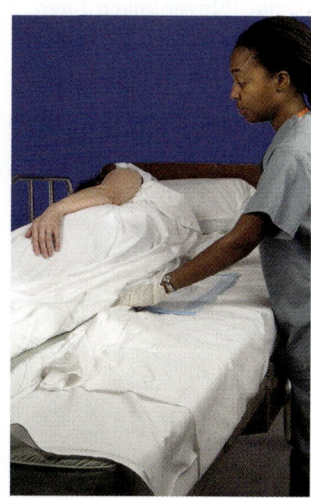

12. **Roll the patient over the clean and dirty linen,** turning him toward you. Explain to him that he will be rolling over a "lump," and then gently pull the patient toward you so that he rolls onto the clean linen. ▼

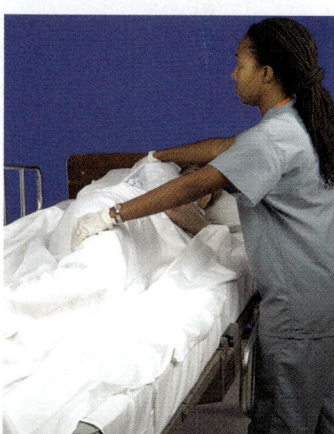

13. **Raise the siderail** on the clean side of the bed.
Prevents the patient from falling.

14. **Move the pillows** to the clean side. Position the patient comfortably on his side, near the siderail.
Always ensure patient comfort and safety before going to the other side of the bed.

(continued on next page)

Procedure 24-16 ■ Making an Occupied Bed (continued)

15. **Go to the opposite side of bed** and lower the rail. Pull the soiled linen from under the clean linen, and then place it in laundry bag or hamper. Never place linen on the floor.
Prevents cross-contamination. ▼

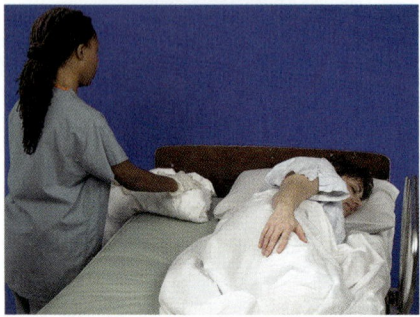

16. **Remove soiled gloves and** don clean gloves. Pull clean linens through and tuck them in. Pull taut, starting with the middle section.
Ensures that no wrinkles will be under the patient. ▼

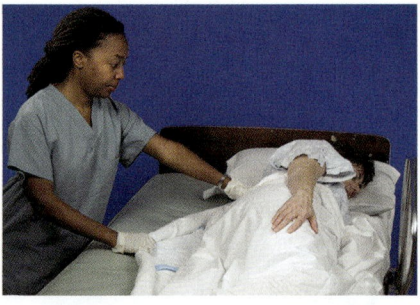

17. **Assist the patient to a supine** position close to center of the mattress

18. **Place the top sheet** and bedspread along one side of the mattress, and continue making the bed as in Procedure 24-15, steps 9 through 14, *except* remove the bath blanket from under the top linens before tucking them in. ▼

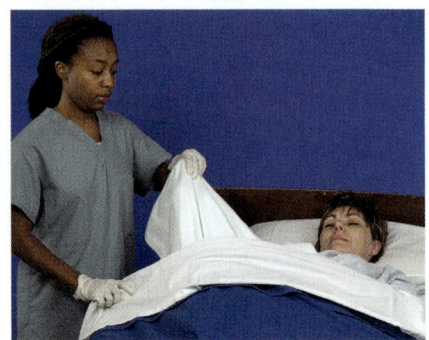

19. **Return the bed to the low** position, raise the siderails, and attach the call light within patient's reach. Position the bedside table and overbed table within patient's reach.
Ensures patient safety and comfort.

? What if . . .

■ **You are making the bed with a patient in leg traction?**

It may be easier to make the bed from top to bottom, as follows:
- Loosen all bed linens and bring the dirty linens from the top of the bed to hip area. Put the clean bottom sheet on the top corners of the mattress, bring down to hip level,

and tuck under the dirty linen. Cover any moist areas with a waterproof pad.
- Ask the patient to grasp the trapeze and raise his buttocks. If the patient is unable to raise his buttocks, use an assistive device per agency policy.
- Bring the dirty bottom sheet along with the clean bottom sheet toward the foot of the bed. Remove dirty linen and place in the laundry bag.
- Tuck the clean sheet under the mattress. Cover with the top sheet. To accommodate traction equipment, do not tuck in the top sheet.

■ **You need to move or reposition a patient in bed who is not able to assist or is obese?**

 Before making the occupied bed, assess the patient's ability to move. Use assistive equipment such as friction-reducing devices, mechanical lifts, air-powered mattresses, and lateral-transfer devices.
These are essential tools in preventing work-related injuries. Limit the need to use your own strength while lifting, turning, or repositioning the patient in bed because of the stress placed on the weaker muscles in the arms and shoulders.

Follow agency policies and use of patient moving devices appropriately.
Many healthcare facilities have adopted safe lifting and patient-handling policies as a means to protect both the patient and the healthcare worker.

Evaluation

- Assess how well the patient tolerated the procedure. Was there any discomfort, shortness of breath, and so on?
- Ask the patient whether he feels comfortable.

Home Care

The only adaptations at home depend on the type of bed the client has. If the height of the bed is not adjustable or the bed is not accessible from both sides, the procedure may be more difficult.

Documentation

Linen changes are usually recorded on a checklist. Additional charting needs to be done only if something abnormal occurred.

Practice Resources

Centers for Disease Control and Prevention (2009); Pegram, A., & Bloomfield, J. (2015). Siegel, J., Rhinehart, E., Jackson, M., et al. (2007).

Thinking About the Procedure

To practice applying clinical reasoning to this procedure,

The video, **Making an Occupied Bed**, along with questions and suggested responses, is available on the **Davis's *Nursing Skills Videos*** Web site on Davis*Plus*.

To explore learning resources for this chapter,

 Go to www.DavisAdvantage.com and find:

Answers and suggested responses for all questions in this chapter

Lists of NIC Interventions and NOC Outcomes

List of NANDA-I Diagnoses

Knowledge Map

Care Plan

Care Map

References and Bibliography

Concept Map

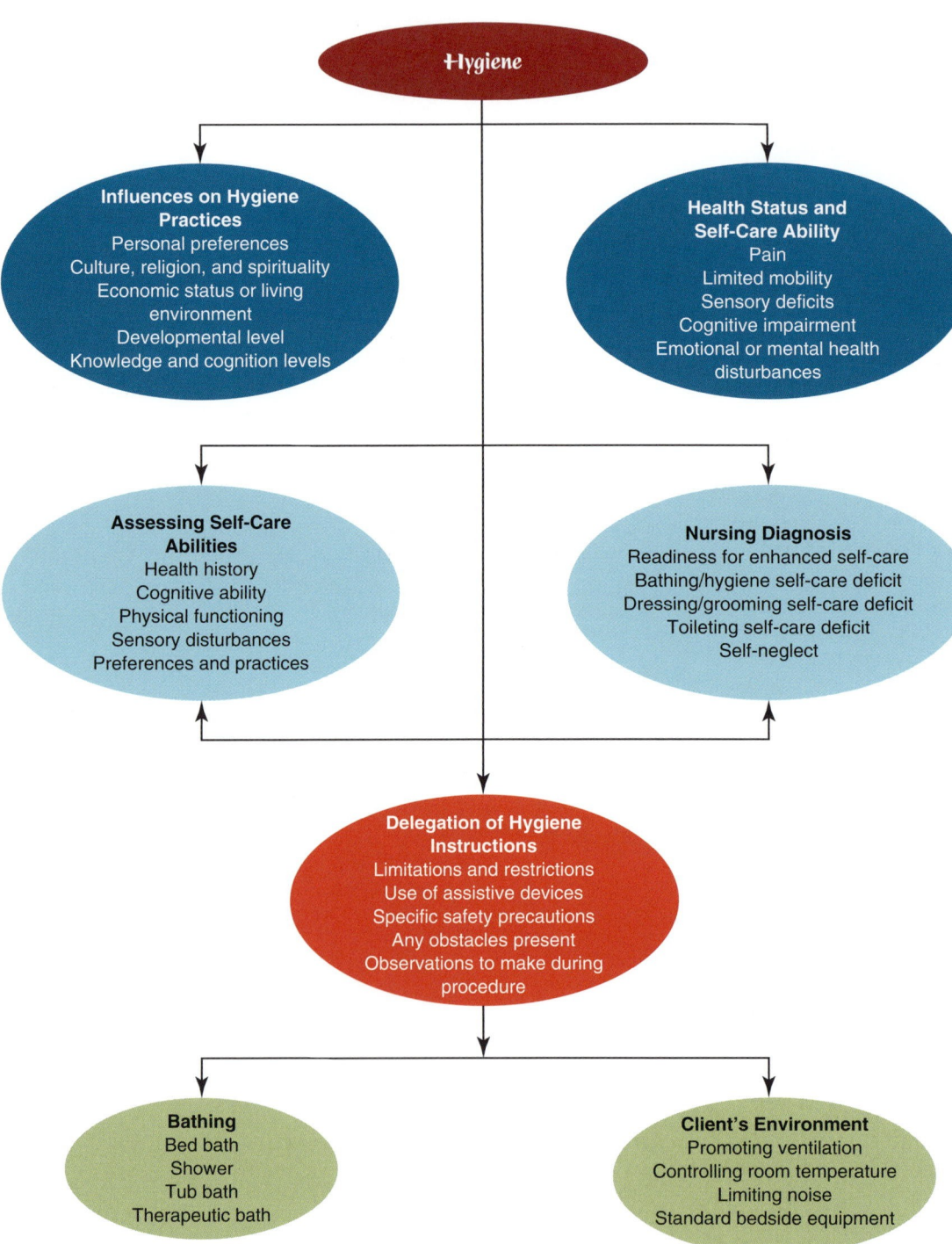

Hygiene

Influences on Hygiene Practices
Personal preferences
Culture, religion, and spirituality
Economic status or living environment
Developmental level
Knowledge and cognition levels

Health Status and Self-Care Ability
Pain
Limited mobility
Sensory deficits
Cognitive impairment
Emotional or mental health disturbances

Assessing Self-Care Abilities
Health history
Cognitive ability
Physical functioning
Sensory disturbances
Preferences and practices

Nursing Diagnosis
Readiness for enhanced self-care
Bathing/hygiene self-care deficit
Dressing/grooming self-care deficit
Toileting self-care deficit
Self-neglect

Delegation of Hygiene Instructions
Limitations and restrictions
Use of assistive devices
Specific safety precautions
Any obstacles present
Observations to make during procedure

Bathing
Bed bath
Shower
Tub bath
Therapeutic bath

Client's Environment
Promoting ventilation
Controlling room temperature
Limiting noise
Standard bedside equipment

CHAPTER 25

Administering Medications

Learning Outcomes

After completing this chapter, you should be able to:

- ➤ Name at least five sources of medication information.
- ➤ Distinguish between various nomenclature systems for naming and classifying drugs.
- ➤ Discuss the concepts and processes of pharmacokinetics, including drug absorption, distribution, metabolism, and excretion.
- ➤ Define onset, peak, and duration of drug action; therapeutic level, peak level, and trough level; and biological half-life.
- ➤ Compare and contrast primary, secondary, cumulative, and side effects and adverse, toxic, allergic, anaphylactic, and idiosyncratic reactions.
- ➤ Define drug-drug interaction, antagonistic drug relationship, synergistic drug relationship, drug incompatibility, and medication contraindications.
- ➤ Correctly calculate drug dosages, including (1) conversion among the metric, apothecary, and household measurement systems and (2) working with units and milliequivalents (mEq).
- ➤ List the types of and methods for communicating medication prescriptions.

- ➤ Discuss the agencies and legislation that help to ensure drug quality and safety.
- ➤ Describe nursing assessment before, during, and following the administration of a drug.
- ➤ Plan care for clients with diagnoses of Risk for Injury and Ineffective Health Management related to medications.
- ➤ Administer medications using the "three checks" and "rights of medication."
- ➤ Describe appropriate steps to take when communicating a medication error.
- ➤ Demonstrate the correct procedure for administering medications by the oral, enteral, inhalant, and parenteral routes.
- ➤ Demonstrate the intramuscular injection procedure at the following sites: ventrogluteal, deltoid, and vastus lateralis.
- ➤ Explain why the dorsogluteal site is not recommended for intramuscular injections.
- ➤ List five steps to incorporate in your practice to ensure safe medication administration and prevent a medication error.

Key Concepts

Medication administration
Medication safety
Pharmacology

Related Concepts

See the Concept Map at the end of this chapter.

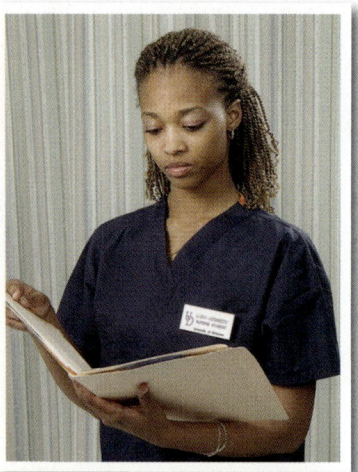

Meet Your Patients

As a new nurse, you are scheduled to administer medications to five patients on the medical–surgical unit today for the first time. Your preceptor will be available as a resource. Your patients are:

- Margaret Marks, an 82-year-old woman who has a fractured hip and experiences periods of confusion
- Cary Pearson, a 70-year-old man with feeding and swallowing difficulties who receives his medications through a gastrostomy tube
- Cyndi Early, a 32-year-old woman with diabetes who is scheduled for surgery at 1000 today
- James Bigler, a 44-year-old man who had a repair of a compound fracture of the right arm and is receiving intravenous fluids and medications
- Rebecca Jones, an 84-year-old woman with compression fractures of two lumbar vertebrae resulting from a fall

You have reviewed your assignment but are unsure of where to begin. Should you visit your patients first and perform an assessment? Should you review the charts first? What should you do with the medication administration records (MARs)? There are so many questions running through your head, and you are a little nervous being on

your own. Perhaps you could use the model of full-spectrum nursing (Chapter 2) to focus your thinking. In general, any time you give a medication, you will need to incorporate the following:

1. *Theoretical Knowledge:* Find out about the actions and expected effects of the medications you are to give.
2. *Patient Situation:* Assess the health status (e.g., disease process) of each patient as it relates to his medications.
3. *Critical Thinking:* Why is the drug being given? Is there anything about the patient's physiology that may alter his responses to the drug? Do you need to modify the administration procedure in any way?
4. *Practical Knowledge:* Be sure that you know the procedures for administering each medication safely.

By the time you complete this chapter, you will have the information you need to make those kinds of judgments. Your instructor and the staff nurses will be there for support.

Theoretical Knowledge
knowing **why**

Pharmacology is the science of drug effects. It deals with all drugs used in society, legal and illegal, prescription and nonprescription, and "street" drugs. You should thoroughly understand the benefits of the medications you administer, as well as their potential to cause harm.

ABOUT THE KEY CONCEPTS

The broadest concepts identified in this chapter are **medication administration** and **medication safety.** An understanding of the theoretical knowledge of **pharmacology** (another key concept) and practical knowledge about safe procedures will help you safely administer medications. As you learn other concepts (e.g., pharmacodynamics, pharmacokinetics), relate them to the three key concepts. This helps to organize information so you can remember it better.

HOW ARE DRUGS NAMED AND CLASSIFIED?

A **drug** is a chemical that interacts with a living organism and alters its activity. In healthcare, drugs are used in diagnosing, treating, or preventing a disease or other medical condition. The term *drug* is used interchangeably with *medication,* although some people may think the term *drug* refers to an illegal substance.

Drug Names

A drug may have multiple names.

- **Chemical name** is the exact description of the drug's chemical composition and molecular structure. For example, *2-(p-isobutylphenyl) propionic acid* is the chemical name of the anti-inflammatory drug ibuprofen. The chemical name is rarely used in nursing practice.
- **Generic (nonproprietary) name** is assigned by the United States Adopted Names Council (USAN Council) when the developing manufacturer is ready to market the drug. This is usually similar to the chemical name, but in a simpler form.
- **Official name** is also the generic name that is listed in publications such as the *United States Pharmacopeia (USP)* and *National Formulary (NF).* For example, *ibuprofen* is both a generic and an official name.
- **Brand (trade** or **proprietary) name** is what the drug is sold as in stores. The brand name is easily recognized because it begins with a capital letter and sometimes has a registration mark (®) at the upper right of the name. Different manufacturers of the same medication may give it different brand names. For example, Advil, Nuprin, and Motrin are all brand names for ibuprofen.

Prescription drugs require a written prescription from a healthcare provider (e.g., physician or advanced practice nurse) who is licensed by the state to prescribe or dispense drugs. **Nonprescription,** or **over-the-counter (OTC),** drugs may be purchased without a prescription and are assumed to be safe for the general population if consumers follow the manufacturer's directions. Ibuprofen and acetaminophen are examples.

Drug Classifications

It is not realistic to know everything about every drug, so "looking it up" must become second nature. If you learn the common characteristics for a drug classification, then when you encounter a new drug, you will be able to associate it with its classification and make inferences about its basic characteristics.

- By usage—why the drug is used
- By body system—where the drug works
- By chemical or pharmacological class

A drug can be placed in more than one category in a classification system. Classified by usage, for example, ibuprofen (Motrin) can be an analgesic, anti-inflammatory, and an antipyretic agent. A drug can act on more than one body system, as well; in fact, most do. For example, diazepam (Valium) is used for its anti-anxiety effects, but it also decreases the activity of the intestinal system and other smooth muscles.

KnowledgeCheck 25-1

- Name three ways a drug may be classified.
- List at least four ways a drug could be named.

WHAT MECHANISMS PROMOTE DRUG QUALITY AND SAFETY?

Before the 20th century, the United States did not have mechanisms for publishing drug ingredients, regulations to govern the contents of drugs, or limitations regarding drug sales. Now, reliable sources of drug information, state and federal regulations and standards controlling drug administration, and a variety of systems for storing and distributing medications in healthcare agencies all work together to protect consumers.

Drug Listings and Directories

KEYPOINT: *When in doubt, look it up!* As a nurse, you are professionally, ethically, legally, and personally responsible for every dose of medication you administer. Always use current information when researching a medication. The following have become relied upon references for the healthcare industry:

- **Pharmacopoeia and formularies.** The United States Pharmacopeia and National Formulary (USP-NF) is the official recognized directory for drugs approved to be marketed in the United States. It contains information such as drug substances, composition, dosages forms, therapeutic values, and compounded preparations. Any drug included in this book has met rigorous standards of quality, strength, and purity and the manufacturer is permitted to use the letters USP-NF after the drug name.
- **Nursing drug handbooks.** These are a quick resource for drug dosage, side effects, and associated nursing interventions.
- *Physician's Desk Reference (PDR).* The *PDR* is commercially compiled by the pharmaceutical companies. It lists manufacturers' prescribing information and is a standard resource for professionals prescribing and administering medication. The *PDR* contains information on dosing, routes of administration, and side effects, but does not include nursing interventions.
- **Pharmacology texts.** A textbook provides more information about physiology, pathophysiology, mechanism of action, and drug classifications than the drug formulary or a handbook. However, it may or may not have detailed information about the specific drug you are administering.
- **Electronic and Internet-based formularies.** The Internet, computer software, PDAs, and other handheld devices offer convenient access to formulary databases.
- A **clinical pharmacist** can assist you with medication-related concerns (e.g., dosage calculations, compatibility).
- **Medication package inserts** are packaged in most medications. The insert provides information identical to that found in the drug formulary and specific for that particular drug.
- **Institutional medication policies and procedures.** You should know the policies and protocols for medication administration for each institution in which you practice.

ThinkLike a Nurse 25-1

Mr. Pearson (Meet Your Patients) has a medication, metoprolol (Lopressor), due at 0800. You are not familiar with this medication.

- What do you need to know before giving the drug?
- What resources might you use to learn about this medication?
- Which is the generic and which is the brand name of this medication?
- Select a nursing drug handbook and research this medication. What kinds of information are available to you in the book?
- Now look up the drug in a pharmacology text. How is that information similar to and different from the information in the handbook?

Legal Considerations

Federal, state, and local laws control drug administration. Standards of nursing practice, state nurse practice acts, and organizational policies and procedures define your role and responsibilities in administering medications. You must be familiar with them to know what you can and cannot do, as well as limitations based on your own experience, skills, and knowledge.

The Food and Drug Administration (FDA) of the U.S. Department of Health and Human Services regulates the testing, manufacture, and sale of all medications. This agency also monitors the safety and effectiveness of medications available to consumers. This process helps to ensure that ineffective or unsafe drugs are not marketed or are recalled, if later found unsafe. However, some medicinal products (e.g., herbal remedies, naturopathic supplements) are *not* regulated by the FDA. Considered "food products," they are advertised as providing health benefits.

Nurse Practice Acts

In most states, a nurse cannot prescribe or administer medications without an authorized provider's (e.g., physician, advanced practice nurse) prescription. The Board of Nursing also regulates the types and routes of medications that can be administered by the various levels of nurses. For example, a licensed practical nurse (LPN) in some states cannot administer intravenous medications, whereas other states require additional education and experiences before LPNs can perform this skill. You should refer to your state's nurse practice act for your scope of practice. If you violate the nurse practice act (e.g., by giving medications without a prescription), your state's nursing board could revoke your license to practice nursing.

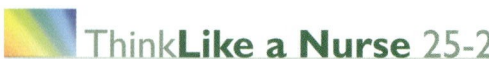

ThinkLike a Nurse 25-2

Obtain a copy of the nurse practice act for the state in which you work. To find a copy,

 Go to the National Council of State Boards of Nursing Web site at **https://www.ncsbn.org/index.htm**

What does your state's nurse practice act tell you about administering medications?

U.S. Drug Legislation

Each state must conform to the regulations of the various federal agencies that regulate the manufacture and sale of medications to protect consumers. Examples:

- Harrison Narcotics Act—regulated the manufacture, sale, and use of drugs that caused dependence (e.g., opium, cocaine, marijuana)
- Durham-Humphrey Amendment—specified which drugs required a prescription and mandated the appropriate labeling
- Comprehensive Drug Abuse Prevention and Control Act—regulated the manufacture, distribution, and sale of controlled substances.

In addition, states may institute additional controls. Local governments may enact regulations for the use of alcohol and tobacco.

Regulation of Controlled Substances

Controlled substances are drugs considered to have either limited medical use or high potential for abuse or addiction. Under the Controlled Substances Act (CSA) of the Comprehensive Drug Abuse Prevention and Control Act of 1970, it is illegal to possess a controlled substance without a valid prescription. Controlled substances are classified by schedules:

- Schedule I identifies drugs that have a high potential for abuse and no acceptable medical use (e.g., heroin, LSD, Ecstasy, peyote, mescaline).
- Schedule II identifies drugs that have an acceptable medical use, but a high potential for abuse (e.g., opium, morphine, cocaine, oxycodone [OxyContin]).
- Schedule III identifies medically acceptable drugs that may cause dependency (e.g., paregoric, Codeine < 90 mg [Tylenol with Codeine]; Hydrocodone < 15 mg [Vicodin]).
- Schedule IV identifies medically acceptable drugs that may cause mild physical or psychological dependence (e.g., diazepam [Valium], alprazolam [Xantax], triazolam [Halcion]).
- Schedule V identifies medically acceptable drugs with limited potential to cause dependence (e.g., Robitussin AC, hydrochloride with atropine sulfate).

Controlled substances must be stored, handled, disposed of, and administered according to regulations established by the U.S. Drug Enforcement Administratrion (DEA):

- Only prescribers with a *national provider identification number* have the authority to prescribe controlled substances.
- Controlled substances must be **double locked**—stored in locked drawers within a second locked area.
- The facility must keep a record of every dose administered. A count of all controlled substances is performed at specified times, usually at change of shift.

- To facilitate counting and tracking inventory, drug manufacturers package many narcotics in sectioned containers, with each tablet separately and consecutively numbered (Fig. 25-1).

ThinkLike a Nurse 25-3

Locate the controlled substance area on your nursing unit.

- Is a double-locking system in place?
- Who is responsible for "carrying" the narcotics keys?
- What is the process if there is a discrepancy between a narcotics sign-out sheet and the actual number of narcotics doses present?

Systems for Storing and Distributing Medications

Most inpatient healthcare facilities have specific areas designed for preparation of medications. Usually this is a central room ("medication room") or mobile cart. Some nursing units store drugs and supplies in a locked cabinet in or near patient rooms. Whatever the method, all drugs are secured in designated areas accessible only to nurses.

Stock Supply

Medications used most frequently may be kept in **stock supply** (bulk quantity), labeled, and in a central location. For example, acetaminophen elixir and cough syrups may be kept in large multidose bottles. Stock supplies require you to measure the dose each time a patient needs it, so the potential for measurement error occurs more frequently. However, a bulk supply of medication is often very cost-effective.

Unit-Dose System

A locked mobile cart is used, with drawers containing separate compartments for each patient's medications (Fig. 25-2). Extra drawers contain supplies, such as medication cups, syringes, and alcohol swabs. The pharmacy staff refills the drawers each shift or every 24 hours. Limited amounts of **prn** ("give according to patient need") medications and stock medications are also kept in the mobile cart.

A **unit dose** is the prescribed amount of drug the patient receives at a single time. For example, if 800 mg of ibuprofen (Motrin) is prescribed to be given every 8 hours, the unit dose is 800 mg. Each unit dose (usually one tablet) is individually

FIGURE 25-1 To facilitate counting, many narcotics are packaged in sectioned containers with each tablet numbered consecutively.

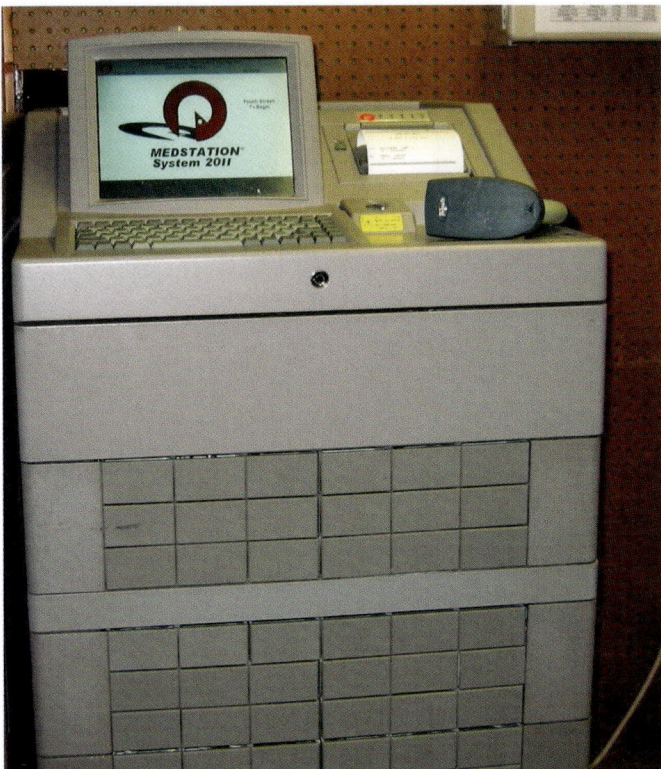

FIGURE 25-2 Medications may be kept in locked, mobile carts, with a drawer for each patient. Mobile (portable) medication carts are linked to the automated dispensing unit.

packaged and labeled with drug name, dose, and expiration date. The pharmacist checks each unit dose before sending the drug to the nursing unit. **KEY POINT:** *Nevertheless, you must recheck the drug and dose when preparing it for administration.* The unit-dose system not only saves nursing time but also is the safest method because of the double-check system.

Automated Dispensing System

An automated dispensing system is a computerized system similar to a unit-dose system. The locked cart contains all the medications frequently used on a particular nursing unit. The computer database contains prescriptions, records, and counts of the medications for each patient on the unit. Each nurse uses a password to access the machine and enters the data about the needed drug, after which the machine dispenses the medication. The medications are usually packaged in unit doses, but some bulk medications may also be kept on the cart. This method allows for immediate availability and administration of newly prescribed and prn medications.

Self-Administration

At times while in the hospital, patients may self-administer medications (SAM). For example, some patients self-administer sublingual nitroglycerin (used for chest pain) at home, and some can continue SAM of the drug while in the hospital. Drugs prescribed for SAM are supplied in individual containers and stored at the bedside. Remind the patient to tell you when he takes the dose. This method promotes independence and allows you to evaluate the patient's ability to manage medications safely and accurately before discharged. Check the policy in your institution to determine whether self-administration is allowed.

KnowledgeCheck 25-2

- What legislation defines controlled substances in the United States?
- How is medication quality managed?

WHAT IS PHARMACOKINETICS?

Pharmacokinetics refers to the absorption, distribution, metabolism, and excretion of a drug (Fig. 25-3). These four processes determine the intensity and duration of a drug's actions. Each drug has unique pharmacokinetic characteristics. As you study these concepts, relate them to each other and to the key concepts of pharmacology and medication administration and safety.

What Factors Affect Drug Absorption?

Absorption refers to the movement of the drug from the site of administration into the bloodstream. The rate of absorption determines when a drug becomes available to exert its action; thus, absorption also influences metabolism and excretion. Absorption depends on the route of administration, form of the drug, drug solubility, effects of pH, blood flow to the area, and body surface area. **Bioavailability** is a subcategory of absorption. It refers to the proportion of a drug that enters the circulation and is able to have an active effect.

Route of Administration

Drugs are manufactured for a specific route of administration and are absorbed at different rates depending on the route. The form (preparation) of a drug usually determines its route of administration. Table 25-1 summarizes the preparations and the advantages and disadvantages of the various routes of administration.

Drugs are given for either local or systemic effect.
- **Local effects** of a drug occur at the site of application (e.g., certain topical applications of drugs to the skin), so little if any absorption occurs.
- For a **systemic effect,** the drug must be absorbed into the bloodstream before it can be distributed to a distant location. A drug may enter the circulation either by injection into a vein or by absorption from other areas (e.g., muscle, stomach lining, mucous membranes).

The choice of route is crucial in determining the suitability of the drug for a particular patient. For example, if your patient is vomiting, an oral drug will not be absorbed effectively in the stomach and would likely be expelled during vomiting. If the patient has diarrhea, rapid motility of the gastrointestinal (GI) tract would decrease absorption. If your patient Cary Pearson (Meet Your Patients) has a prescription for an oral medication, would you question the route? Why or why not?

Solubility of the Drug

Solubility refers to the ability of a medication to be transformed into a liquid form that can be absorbed into the bloodstream. Typically, absorption occurs more rapidly with highly soluble drugs. *Oral medications* must be water soluble and at least partially lipid soluble to be absorbed in the GI tract. Liquids (e.g., suspensions or solutions) are absorbed faster than tablets or capsules because the liquids are already dissolved.
- *Water-soluble drugs.* Drugs must be water-soluble in order to dissolve in the *aqueous* (watery) contents of the GI tract. Therefore, these drugs are more rapidly absorbed from the GI tract and take effect faster.
- *Lipid-soluble drugs.* Lipid-soluble drugs can penetrate lipid-rich cell membranes and enter the cells, whereas

(Text continued on page 780)

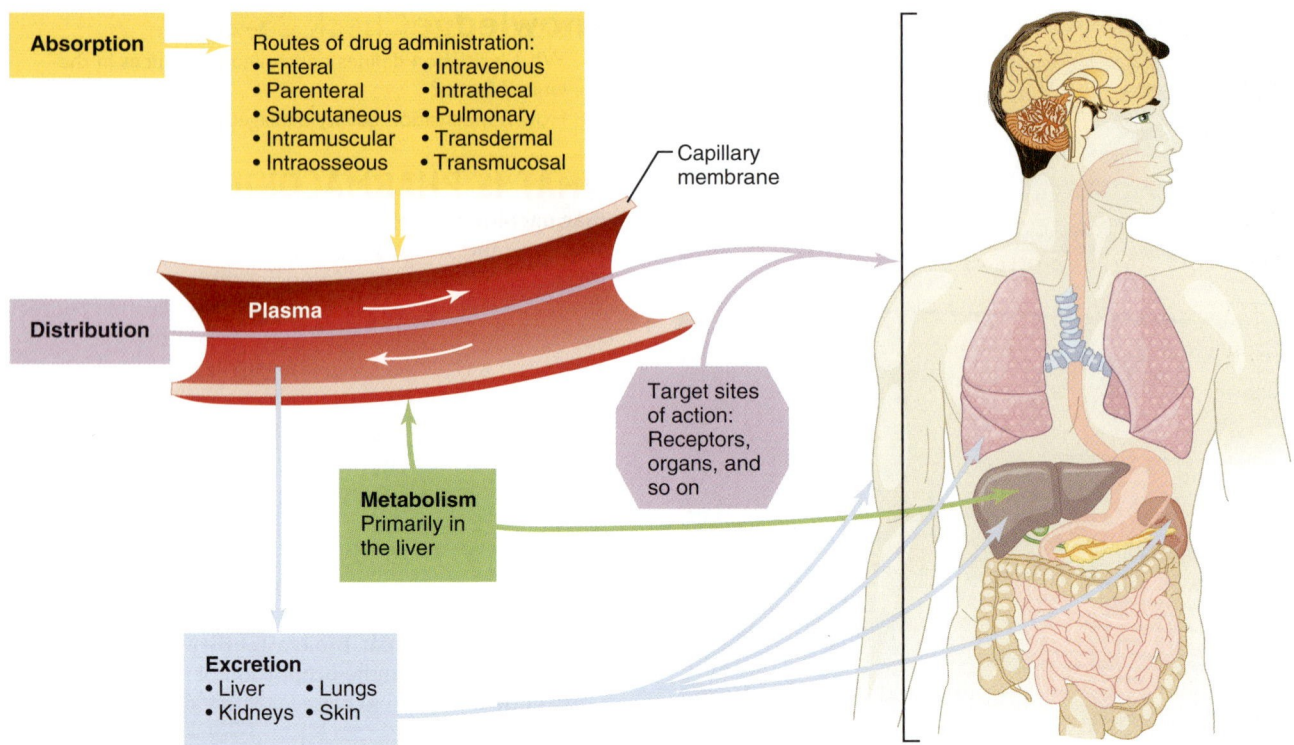

FIGURE 25-3 Pharmacokinetics is the study of drug absorption, distribution, metabolism, and excretion, which determine the intensity and duration of a drug's actions in the body.

Table 25-1 ➤ Advantages and Disadvantages of Routes of Administration

ROUTE: ORAL The drug is swallowed and absorbed from the stomach or small intestine.

Preparation Types

- **Capsule**—A gelatinous container that holds the liquid, powder, or oil form of the drug. When swallowed, the gelatin container dissolves in the gastric juices.

- **Pill**—This term is rarely used now. *Tablet* is the preferred term.

- **Tablet**—A powdered drug is compressed into a hard, compact form (e.g., round, oval) that is easy to swallow and then breaks up into a fine powder in the stomach. The tablet is the most common oral preparation. *Enteric-coated tablets* have an acid-insoluble coating to keep them from dissolving in the stomach; they disintegrate in the alkaline secretions of the small intestine.

- **Time-released tablet or capsule**—A tablet or capsule formulated so that it does not dissolve all at once, but gradually releases medication over a few hours.

- **Elixir**—A liquid containing water and about 25% alcohol that is sweetened with volatile oils (e.g., aromatic elixir); not as sticky or as sweet as syrups.

- **Extract**—A very concentrated form of a drug made from animals or vegetables; may be a syrupy liquid or a powder.

- **Fluid extract**—An alcohol-based solution of a drug from a vegetable source (e.g., belladonna); the most concentrated of the fluid preparations.

- **Spirits**—A concentrated alcohol-based solution of a volatile (easily evaporated) substance or oil (e.g., ammonia, peppermint oil, orange oil); contains larger amounts of the substance than can be dissolved in water.

- **Syrup**—An aqueous solution of sugar; used to disguise unpleasant taste of drugs.

- **Tincture**—An alcohol or water-and-alcohol (with a high percentage of alcohol) solution made by extracting potent plants; may also be used externally (e.g., tincture of iodine).

- **Powder**—Finely ground drug(s), usually mixed with a liquid before ingesting; some are used internally, others externally. (Some are mixed with diluents for parenteral injection.)

- **Solution**—Drug(s) dissolved in a liquid carrier. *Aqueous solutions* are medications dissolved in water. (May be used orally, externally, and parenterally.)

- **Suspension**—Drug(s) that are suspended (not completely dissolved) in a liquid. *Aqueous suspensions* are suspended in water. *Never* used for IV or intra-arterial routes.

Table 25-1 ➤ Advantages and Disadvantages of Routes of Administration—cont'd

ADVANTAGES	DISADVANTAGES
■ Convenient	■ Unpleasant taste may cause noncompliance.
■ Sterility is not needed for oral use.	■ May irritate gastric mucosa.
■ Economical	■ Patient must be conscious.
■ Noninvasive, low-risk procedure	■ Digestive juices may destroy drug.
■ Easy to administer, good for self-administration	■ Cannot use if patient has nausea and vomiting or decreased gastric motility.
■ Capsule can mask unpleasant taste of a drug.	■ Cannot use if patient has difficulty swallowing.
■ Capsule can be time-release	■ Potential for aspiration
	■ May be harmful to teeth.
	■ Onset of action is slow.

ROUTE: ENTERAL The drug is given directly into the stomach or intestine (e.g., through a nasogastric [NG] or gastrostomy tube).

Preparation Types

Same as for oral medications

ADVANTAGES	DISADVANTAGES
■ Can be used for patients with Impaired Swallowing, as an alternative to parenteral administration.	■ Not all tablets or capsules can be crushed; medications can clog the NG tube.
	■ NG tube itself presents some risk of aspiration.

ROUTE: SUBLINGUAL (a variation of transmucosal administration)—The drug is held under the tongue and absorbed across the sublingual mucous membrane.

Preparation Types

Lipid-soluble lozenge (troche)—A flat, round preparation that dissolves when held in the mouth. May act locally or be absorbed through mucosa for systemic effect.

Tablet (See oral route.)

ADVANTAGES	DISADVANTAGES
■ Used for local or systemic effects	■ May inadvertently be swallowed in the saliva.
■ Convenient	■ Not useful for drugs with unpleasant taste
■ Sterility not needed	■ May irritate the oral mucosa.
■ Quick delivery to general circulation	■ Patient must be conscious.
■ Bypasses stomach and intestines; absorbed directly into bloodstream.	■ Useful only for highly lipid-soluble drugs
	■ Patient must hold the drug in place until it is dissolved, which may take a few minutes.
	■ Limited period of effectiveness, requiring frequent redosing

ROUTE: BUCCAL/TRANSMUCOSAL ADMINISTRATION Medication is held against the mucous membrane of cheek until it dissolves.

Preparation Types

Lipid-soluble lozenge or tablet (See oral and sublingual routes.)

Spray—Can be dispersed to the nasal or pharyngeal mucosa for rapid absorption.

ADVANTAGES	DISADVANTAGES
■ Same as sublingual	■ Same as sublingual
■ Rapid, convenient, portable	

(Continued)

Table 25-1 ➤ Advantages and Disadvantages of Routes of Administration—cont'd

ROUTE: TOPICAL (SKIN) The drug acts locally or is absorbed directly through skin (transdermal or percutaneous absorption).

Preparation Types

Gel or **jelly**—A clear or translucent semisolid substance that liquefies when applied to the skin.

Liniment—An oily liquid to rub into the skin.

Lotion—An *emollient* (softening or soothing agent) for use on the skin; may be a clear solution, suspension, or emulsion.

Ointment—A semisolid, fatty (usually petroleum jelly or lanolin based) substance for skin or mucous membranes; usually not water soluble.

Paste—Similar to an ointment, but thicker and stiffer.

Tincture (See oral route.)

Transdermal patch—Releases constant, controlled amounts of medication, for systemic effect.

Aerosol spray or **foam**—A liquid or foam that is sprayed by air pressure onto the skin.

Cream—A non-oily, semisolid substance applied to the skin.

ADVANTAGES	DISADVANTAGES
■ Continuous dosing	■ Effective only for lipid-soluble drugs and must be specially formulated.
■ Sterility is not needed.	
■ For local or systemic effects	■ May cause local irritation, especially if the patient is allergic to latex or tape.
■ Long-acting systemic effect	■ Discarded patches may pose danger of poisoning.
■ Useful if patient is unable to take oral medications	■ Leaves residue on skin.
■ Acceptable to most patients	■ Accurate doses can be difficult to obtain when the drug is in a tube or jar.

ROUTE: TOPICAL: INSTILLATIONS The drug is placed into a body cavity (e.g., urinary bladder, rectum, vagina, ears, nose, eye).

Preparation Types

Solutions (for nose, ears, eyes; enemas per rectum)—Drug(s) dissolved in a liquid carrier.

Suppositories (for bladder, vagina, rectum)—Drug(s) mixed with a glycerin-gelatin or cocoa butter base and shaped for insertion into the body. They dissolve gradually at body temperature.

Jellies, creams (for vagina and rectum)—See skin route.

ADVANTAGES	DISADVANTAGES
■ Continuous dosing	■ May be embarrassing for the patient.
■ Sterility is not needed.	■ Absorption from the rectum is slow and if stool is present, there is local irritation, or if the patient defecates before the suppository melts.
■ Useful if patient is unable to take oral medications, when the oral drug has an unacceptable taste or odor.	
■ Preferred when the patient is vomiting or unconscious.	■ Pain, if the patient has hemorrhoids.
■ May be used for local or systemic effects.	■ As a rule, contraindicated when there is active rectal bleeding.

ROUTE: TOPICAL: INHALATION A device (e.g., nebulizer, face mask) breaks the drug into finely dispersed particles, which are breathed into the respiratory passages. Some drugs are intended for local effects in the respiratory passages; others (e.g., anesthetic gases) are for systemic effects, especially in the brain.

Preparation Types

Aerosols—Aerosols are liquids in very fine particles that can be inhaled into the lungs; they are sprayed under air pressure.

Gases—Gas is a basic form of matter (i.e., solid, liquid, and gas). A gas must be kept in a closed container; otherwise, the fast-moving molecules escape into the air. Examples are oxygen, nitrogen, carbon dioxide, and anesthetic gases.

Table 25-1 ➤ Advantages and Disadvantages of Routes of Administration—cont'd

ADVANTAGES	DISADVANTAGES
■ Quick and efficient local and systemic route through the lungs ■ May be given to unconscious patient. ■ Allows continuous dosing, and dosage can be easily modified.	■ Requires special equipment. ■ May irritate lung mucosa. ■ Useful only for drugs that are gases at room temperature. ■ May have unexpected systemic effect when only local effect is desired.

ROUTE: ALL PARENTERAL ROUTES Drug taken into the body other than through the digestive system.

Preparation Types

Depends on route.

ADVANTAGES	DISADVANTAGES
Patient may be conscious or unconscious.	■ Requires sterile procedures. ■ Poses risk for infection because skin is broken. ■ Requires skill. ■ May cause some pain. ■ Produces anxiety. ■ More expensive than oral administration.

ROUTE: PARENTERAL: INTRAVENOUS The drug is injected directly into the vein, either by bolus or slow infusion.

Preparation Types

Aqueous solutions—Drug(s) dissolved in water.

ADVANTAGES	DISADVANTAGES
■ Rapid effect because absorption is bypassed; therefore, good for emergency situations ■ Patient needs only one needlestick, even for multiple doses.	■ Poses risk of transient drug concentrations if drug is injected too rapidly. ■ Limited to highly soluble medications. ■ Poses risk for sepsis because pathogens may be introduced directly into the bloodstream. ■ The patient must have usable veins. ■ Cost of supplies and medications.

ROUTE: PARENTERAL: INTRAMUSCULAR The drug is injected into the muscle mass.

Preparation Types

Primarily aqueous solutions (see intravenous route), although some preparations (e.g., penicillin) are suspensions.

ADVANTAGES	DISADVANTAGES
■ Rapid absorption, except for oily preparations or suspensions ■ Allows use of drugs that are not stable in solution. ■ Causes less pain (than do subcutaneous injections) from irritating drugs because they are deep in the muscle. ■ Allows administration of a larger volume than does subcutaneous administration. ■ Allows more rapid absorption than does subcutaneous or oral administration.	■ May cause irritation and local reactions. ■ Poses risk for tissue and nerve damage if site is improperly located. ■ Cannot be used where tissue is damaged (e.g., bruised) or peripheral circulation is decreased.

(Continued)

Table 25-1 ➤ Advantages and Disadvantages of Routes of Administration—cont'd

ROUTE: PARENTERAL: SUBCUTANEOUS   The drug is injected into the subcutaneous tissue under the skin.

Preparation Types

Primarily solutions—Drugs dissolved in a liquid carrier.

ADVANTAGES	DISADVANTAGES
■ Allows faster action than does oral administration. ■ Allows better absorption of lipid-soluble drugs than does intramuscular administration.	■ Only very small amounts can be given. ■ Absorption is relatively slow and often confined to the injected area.

ROUTE: PARENTERAL: INTRADERMAL   The drug is injected under the skin, into the dermis. Most commonly used for diagnostic testing or screening or for injecting local anesthetic.

ROUTE: PARENTERAL: OTHER

Preparation Types

Intraspinal—Injection of drug into the spinal canal.

Intrathecal—Injection of drug into the subarachnoid space around the spinal cord.

Epidural—Injection of drug between the vertebral spines into the extradural space. Most commonly used for regional anesthesia and pain control.

ADVANTAGES	DISADVANTAGES
■ Most rapid absorption ■ Highly effective	■ Some patients may be anxious about administration method. ■ Spinal route can produce hypotension, nausea, urinary retention, or headache.

water-soluble drugs (e.g., penicillin) cannot. That is why a highly fat-soluble drug (e.g., nitrous oxide) can easily pass through the blood–brain barrier and cause sedation. Lipid-soluble drugs are preferred when a much longer acting effect is desired, because they are more slowly released into the circulatory system. Lipid solubility depends partly on the drug's chemical structure and the environment at the site of absorption. Some lipid-soluble drugs are prepared as a *lozenge (troche)*, a flat, round preparation that dissolves when held in the mouth. Some act locally and some are absorbed through mucosa for systemic effect.

- **Enteric-coated** drugs cannot be broken down by gastric acids because the coating prevents the medication from being diluted before it reaches the intestines. In this way, the coating delays the action of the drug, which decreases the irritating effects on the stomach.
- **Timed-release (sustained-release)** medications are formulated to dissolve slowly, releasing small amounts for absorption over several hours. ✚ You should never crush or break enteric-coated and time-released medications; to do so would destroy their protective coatings.

Which of your patients (Meet Your Patients) is most likely to receive a water-soluble medication?

Effects of pH and Ionization

The **pH** (relative acidity or alkalinity) of the local environment also affects the absorption of a drug. The acid content of the stomach aids in transporting the medication across the mucous membranes, so *acidic* medications, such as aspirin, are more readily absorbed in the stomach than are *basic* (alkaline) medications, such as sodium bicarbonate, which are readily absorbed in the more alkaline small intestine. For best absorption, should Mr. Pearson's (Meet Your Patients) medications be acidic or alkaline preparations?

In solution, some of a drug's molecules are in **ionized** (electrically charged) form, and others are **nonionized** (neutral or noncharged). The ionized molecules are lipid insoluble and thus cannot pass easily through the phospholipid layer of cell membranes. Drug molecules can be converted easily from one form to the other, depending primarily on the pH of the environment. For example, when aspirin is dissolved in the stomach acid, most of its molecules remain nonionized because of the low pH, so they easily pass through the membranes of the gastric mucosa and enter the bloodstream. If the person ingests an antacid before taking aspirin, the pH will increase and the aspirin will become more ionized, thus reducing the absorption and effect of the aspirin.

Blood Flow to the Area

Medications are absorbed rapidly in areas where blood flow to the tissue is greatest (e.g., oral mucous membranes). Areas with poor vascular supply (e.g., the skin, scarred areas) experience delayed absorption. Consider the following examples:

- Excessive exercise draws blood away from the stomach and intestines to the muscles. Which route would promote absorption for a person who has just exercised heavily: oral or intramuscular (IM)? Why?

■ A person in shock has poor peripheral circulation. Which route would promote faster absorption: intramuscular or intravenous (IV)? Why?

For the first question, the IM route would be better for the person who has recently engaged in heavy activity. This is because medication injected deep into the muscle where there is a rich blood supply would be absorbed more readily, whereas medication administered orally must first dissolve and be absorbed in the GI tract.

For the second question, the IV route is more efficient for the person with poor circulation because drugs act more rapidly, even in healthy people, when they are injected directly into the bloodstream and do not have to be absorbed.

KnowledgeCheck 25-3

■ Define *absorption*.
■ How are drugs absorbed?
■ What factors affect absorption?

How Are Drugs Distributed Throughout the Body?

Distribution is the transportation of a drug in body fluids (usually the bloodstream) to the various tissues and organs of the body. Because blood goes to all parts of the body, theoretically a drug can produce effects (intended or unintended) anywhere. The rate of distribution is influenced by:

■ Adequate local blood flow in the **target area** (the site where the drug effects occur)
■ The permeability of capillaries to the drug's molecules
■ The protein-binding capacity of the drug.

Local Blood Flow The blood supply of the target site affects distribution of a drug. For example, it is difficult to deliver a systemic medication to the skin and toes, where the blood vessels are very small.

■ Factors that cause vasodilation in an area increase circulation to area tissues (e.g., application of warmth to an injection site).
■ Factors that cause vasoconstriction decrease circulation to the target tissue (e.g., shock, chilling of the body).

Membrane Permeability Drug molecules must leave the blood and cross capillary membranes to reach their sites of action. The capillary networks in some organs consist of tightly packed endothelial cells that prevent some drugs from crossing them. For example, the blood–brain barrier allows distribution into the brain and cerebrospinal fluid of only those drugs that are (1) lipid soluble (e.g., anesthetics and barbiturates) and (2) not tightly bound to plasma proteins. This barrier can be bypassed by injecting medications intrathecally (via the spinal canal) into the cerebrospinal fluid.

Protein-Binding Capacity For a given amount of a drug, some molecules bind to plasma proteins, and the remainder will be "free." Only free (unbound) drug molecules can produce pharmacological effects because only free molecules can be metabolized or excreted. For example, nearly all acetaminophen (Tylenol) molecules are free in the bloodstream and are therefore pharmacologically active. By contrast, about 99% of the anticoagulant warfarin (Coumadin) is bound in the blood; its effects are produced by only the 1% of warfarin molecules that are free.

A drug's tendency to bind to plasma proteins depends mostly on its chemical structure. Some medical conditions also affect protein binding. For example, malnourishment and liver disease reduce the amount of protein (serum albumin) available for binding.

KnowledgeCheck 25-4

■ Define *distribution*.
■ What factors affect distribution of drugs in the body?

How Are Drugs Metabolized in the Body?

Metabolism (or **biotransformation**) is the chemical inactivation of a drug through its conversion into a more water-soluble compound or into metabolites that can be excreted from the body. Once a medication reaches its site of action, it is metabolized (changed into the inactive form) in preparation for excretion. Metabolism takes place mainly in the liver, but medications can be detoxified also in the kidneys, blood plasma, intestinal mucosa, and lungs.

If liver function is impaired (e.g., liver disease or aging), the drug will be eliminated more slowly, and toxic levels may accumulate. Disease states also affect drug metabolism. For example, patients with diabetes do not metabolize sugar effectively, so they should not take elixirs, which are high in sugar content.

First-Pass Effect Oral medications are absorbed from the GI tract and circulate through the liver before they reach the systemic circulation. This inactivation is known as the **first-pass effect.** For this reason, oral medications are formulated with a higher concentration of the drug than are parenteral medications. Some medications can be given parenterally, allowing the drug to be distributed directly to target sites before it passes through the liver. For example, nitroglycerin undergoes this first-pass effect when taken orally; therefore, it is given sublingually or intravenously so that it bypasses the stomach and liver and reaches therapeutic levels in the blood.

KnowledgeCheck 25-5

■ Define *drug metabolism*.
■ Where are drugs metabolized?
■ What factors affect drug metabolism?

How Are Drugs Excreted From the Body?

A drug continues to act in the body until it is excreted. For **excretion** to occur, drug molecules must be removed from their sites of action and eliminated from the body. Drugs may be metabolized completely, partially, or not at all when they are excreted. The following are common organs of excretion:

Kidneys The kidneys are the primary site of excretion. Adequate fluid intake facilitates renal excretion. If your patient has decreased renal function (e.g., as indicated by an elevated creatinine level), you should monitor for medication toxicity. Obtain a prescription for adjusted dosing if signs of toxicity are present.

Liver and GI Tract Some drugs broken down by the liver are excreted into the GI tract and eliminated in the feces. Others (e.g., fat-soluble agents) are reabsorbed by the bloodstream, distributed to the target site, and returned to the liver. This is called **enterohepatic recirculation.** The kidneys later excrete these compounds. Anything that increases peristalsis (e.g., diarrhea, laxatives, enemas, chronic bowel disease) accelerates drug excretion via feces. Inactivity, poor diet, and decreased peristalsis delay excretion, increasing the effects of a drug.

Lungs Most drugs removed by the lungs are not metabolized first. Gases and volatile liquids (e.g., general anesthetics) administered by inhalation usually are removed through exhalation. Other volatile substances, such as ethyl alcohol and paraldehyde, are highly soluble in blood and are excreted in limited amounts by the lungs. Examples include the following:

- Strenuous exercise and deep breathing increase pulmonary blood flow and thereby promote excretion.
- Decreased cardiac output (as in shock) and hypoventilation prolong the period of time for drug elimination.

Exocrine Glands Drug excretion through the **exocrine** (sweat and salivary) **glands** is limited. The elimination of metabolites in sweat is frequently responsible for such side effects as dermatitis. Drugs excreted in the saliva are usually swallowed and absorbed as other orally administered agents.

 ThinkLike a Nurse 25-4

You are notified of a patient being transferred from the intensive care unit (ICU) to your unit. The patient is 79-year-old Hattie Banks, admitted 2 days ago to the ICU for digoxin toxicity.

- What theoretical knowledge do you have about the metabolism and excretion of digoxin (Lanoxin)?
- What assessments are important to make for Ms. Banks?

Other Concepts Relevant to Drug Effectiveness

In addition to the processes of absorption, distribution, metabolism, and excretion, you need to understand four other concepts related to a drug's effectiveness: (1) onset, peak, and duration of drug action; (2) therapeutic range; (3) bioavailability of the drug; and (4) concentration of the drug at target sites. As you read about them, try to relate these concepts to the key concepts of medication administration and medication safety.

Onset, Peak, and Duration of Drug Action

- **Onset of action**—The time needed for drug concentration to reach a high enough blood level for its effects to appear. This is the **minimum effective concentration.**
- **Peak action**—When the concentration of medication is highest in the blood.
- **Duration of action**—That period of time in which the medication has a pharmacological effect (before it is metabolized and excreted) (Fig. 25-4).

If the serum level of a medication falls below the minimum effective concentration, then the drug is not effective during that time. If the drug level exceeds the peak level, toxicity occurs.

 ThinkLike a Nurse 25-5

Refer to Table 25-1. James Bigler (Meet Your Patients) is having right arm pain and needs relief quickly.

- Would it be better to give him oral acetaminophen with codeine or an IM injection of a similar-strength medication? Why?
- Do you have enough information to be completely sure your choice of route will bring the quickest onset of action? Explain.

Therapeutic Range

Even after absorption stops, distribution, metabolism, and excretion continue. When giving multidose medication (e.g., an

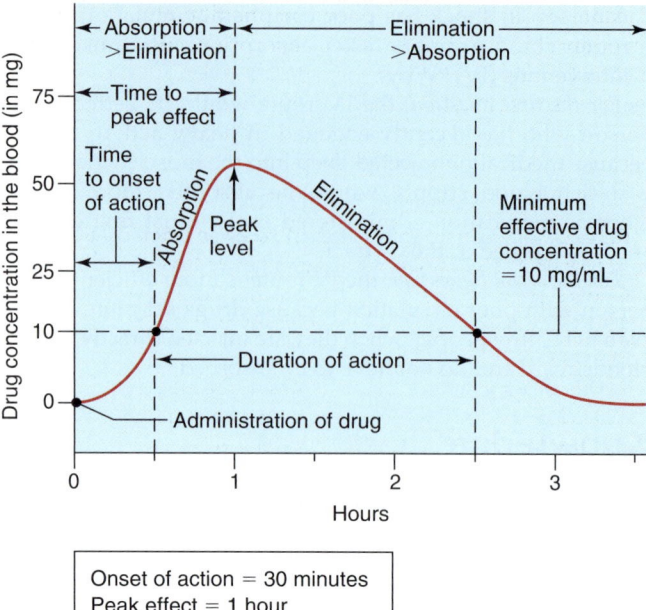

Onset of action = 30 minutes
Peak effect = 1 hour
Duration of action = 2.0 hours

FIGURE 25-4 Once the drug is administered and absorption begins, blood levels begin to rise. When the *minimum effective concentration* is reached, drug effects begin *(onset of action)*. *Maximum effect* occurs at peak blood level.

antibiotic), the goal is to achieve a constant, therapeutic blood level. Because a fraction of the drug is constantly being excreted, repeated doses of the medication are given to achieve and maintain a constant therapeutic concentration.

Therapeutic range of a drug is a range of therapeutic concentrations. At onset of action, serum drug level is minimal.

Therapeutic level is the concentration of a drug in the blood serum that produces the desired effect without toxicity.

Peak level occurs when the drug is at its highest concentration (when the rate of absorption is equal to the rate of elimination). After that, metabolic and excretory processes begin to remove the drug from the tissues and blood.

Trough level occurs when the drug is at its lowest concentration, right before the next dose is due.

A test called a *peak and trough* helps to ensure the safety and effectiveness of certain drugs. The peak level occurs when the drug is at its highest level in the patient's bloodstream and thus must be measured when absorption is complete. This, of course, depends on all the factors that affect absorption. The trough level is the lowest level in the patient's blood and thus is typically measured about 30 minutes before the next dose of the drug is due. The drug's *half-life* (below) and the time between doses affect the trough level. You will sometimes need to monitor serum drug levels so the primary care provider can adjust the dose and timing of a medication as needed.

Biological Half-Life

A medication's **biological half-life** is the amount of time it takes for half of the drug to be eliminated.

Example: Tramadol has a half-life of approximately 6 hours. This means if you take a 50-mg dose at 0800, by 1400 half of that dose (25 mg) will still be left in your body. In 12 hours, one-fourth of the initial dose (12.5 mg) will be left in your body.

Half-life is affected by drug composition and distribution. Liver and kidney disease, aging, absence of food, and slowed metabolic rate all prolong half-life because of their effects on metabolism and excretion.

 Think**Like a Nurse** 25-6

Rebecca Jones (Meet Your Patients) received tramadol 50 mg for pain at 0800. The prescription allows her to have the drug every 6 hours. So at 1400, you give her another dose of tramadol 50 mg. The drug is metabolized in the liver and excreted mainly in the urine.

- When this medication reaches onset of action, about how much tramadol does Ms. Jones now have in her body?
- If the "normal" half-life of tramadol is 6 hours, you would expect that Ms. Jones would still have about 25 mg of her first dose left in her body at the time of the second dose. Given her age, though, do you think she probably has more or less than 25 mg left at 6 hours? Why?

Concentration of Active Drug at Target Sites

The effectiveness of a medication depends ultimately on its concentration at the intended site. For example, a medication such as nitrofurantoin may be prescribed to treat a urinary tract infection. This drug is used because it is highly soluble in urine and therefore tends to accumulate and concentrate in the bladder and kidneys, where the infection exists.

What Factors Affect Pharmacokinetics?

A drug's pharmacokinetics and therefore its effectiveness and safety are affected by the following factors:

- **Age.** Infants and young children need smaller doses because of their smaller body mass and immature body systems. Older adults may have declining liver and kidney function and are therefore at higher risk for drug toxicity.

  Table 25-2 summarizes life span variations in pharmacokinetics.

- **Body Mass (Weight).** The average adult dose is based on the drug quantity that will produce a particular effect in 50% of

PHARMACOKINETIC PROCESS	CHILDREN		OLDER ADULTS
Table 25-2 ➤ **Drug Therapy Across the Life Span**			
Absorption	■ Exaggerated in infants as a result of lack of gastric acidity and shorter intestines		■ Delayed but more complete
	■ More complete topical absorption results from a larger body surface and thinner epidermis.		■ Gastric pH is less acidic because of decreased acid production in the stomach.
	■ Enteral route is unpredictable.		■ Decreased gastric pH delays absorption of medications absorbed in acid environments.
	■ Decreased muscle tone makes absorption of parenteral drugs unpredictable.		■ Because of decreased intestinal motility, drugs remain in the system longer, allowing for more absorption.
	■ Gastric pH is higher, so that medications absorbed in acid environments are absorbed much more slowly.		
Distribution	■ Protein binding may be a problem.		■ Low albumin level could create a problem with plasma protein binding.
	■ Greater chance of toxicity because of low albumin levels.		■ Increased risk of toxicity due to multiorgan slowdown.
	■ Water content in the child's body is higher than in adults, so water-soluble drugs are less concentrated in the child and fat-soluble drugs are more highly concentrated.		■ Altered because of less lean mass.
			■ Less body water, greater body fat.
			■ Dehydration, poor nutrition, and electrolyte imbalances decrease absorption.
Metabolism	■ Metabolism may be altered because of immature liver.		■ Presence of diseases may decrease metabolism of the drug.
	■ Best to base dosage on body weight to avoid toxicity.		■ Changes from age, higher blood concentration, and less excretion cause greater chances of toxicity.
			■ Some drugs interfere with the liver's ability to metabolize another drug.
Excretion	■ Excretion is delayed as the result of immature kidneys.		■ Decreased glomerular filtration rate inhibits excretion from the kidneys.
	■ Repeat dosing may cause problems.		■ Diminished renal function inhibits excretion, thereby increasing the risk of toxicity.

people 18 to 65 years of age and weighing 150 lb. Obviously, a person who is much larger or smaller than this "average" requires an adjusted dose.

- **Gender.** Men and women absorb drugs differently because women usually have lower muscle mass than men, a different hormone profile, and different fat and water distribution.
- **Pregnancy.** Most drugs are contraindicated during pregnancy because of their possible adverse effects on the embryo or fetus. Drugs known to cause developmental defects are called **teratogenic** drugs (e.g., alcohol, the anticonvulsant phenytoin [Dilantin]).
- **Environment.** Heat and cold affect peripheral circulation. A noisy environment may interfere with a person's response to antianxiety, sedative, or pain medications.
- **Route of Administration.** The route of administration influences the amount of a drug absorbed into the circulatory system and the distribution to the sites of action.
- **Timing of Administration.** The presence or absence of food in the GI tract affects an oral drug's pharmacokinetics. Biorhythms and cycles (e.g., drug-metabolizing enzyme rhythms, blood pressure cycles) also influence drug action.
- **Fluids.** Insufficient fluid intake affects the absorption of solid dosage forms.
- **Pathological States.** Intense pain decreases the effect of opioids; diseases causing circulatory, hepatic, or renal dysfunction interfere with pharmacokinetic processes.
- **Genetic Factors.** Abnormal susceptibility to certain chemicals is genetically determined. Enzyme deficiencies and altered metabolism change a patient's responses to a drug. For example, African Americans usually respond better to diuretics for blood pressure control than do other racial groups; people of Asian descent metabolize some opioids at a slower rate. Use your critical thinking now. What important nursing intervention should you perform after you administer an opiate to an Asian patient? (If you said you would need to observe closely for unexpected side effects, good thinking!)
- **Psychological Factors.** Some patients have the same response to a placebo—a pharmacologically inactive substance—as they do to the active drug. If a person has faith that a drug will help him, a *placebo effect* similar to the effect of an active drug may occur. Emotional states, such as anxiety, may cause may cause resistance to tranquilizing drugs.

WHAT IS PHARMACODYNAMICS?

Pharmacodynamics, another subconcept of pharmacology, is the study of *how* medications achieve their effects at various sites in the body—how specific drug molecules interact with target cells and how biological responses occur. You will use pharmacodynamics concepts to help you administer medications safely and to evaluate patient outcomes.

What Are Primary Effects?

Primary or **therapeutic effects** of medications are effects that are predicted, intended, and desired. They are, in short, the reason the drug was prescribed.

- **Palliative effects** relieve the signs and symptoms of a disease but have no effect on the disease itself. For example, morphine sulfate may be given to a patient with cancer to manage pain, but it does not destroy cancer cells. The goal of palliative therapy is to make the patient as comfortable as possible when treatment options have been exhausted.
- **Supportive effects** support the integrity of body functions until other medications or treatments can become effective. For a patient with a bacterial infection, you may give acetaminophen to control fever until blood levels of the prescribed antibiotic are effective in combating the infection causing the fever.
- **Substitutive effects** replace either body fluids or a chemical required by the body for improved functioning. You may, for example, administer insulin to a diabetic patient to replace the insulin no longer produced by the pancreas.
- **Chemotherapeutic effects** destroy disease-producing microorganisms or body cells. Two examples are (1) antibiotics, used to treat infections by killing or limiting the reproduction of certain bacteria, and (2) antineoplastic drugs, used to treat cancer by limiting cell reproduction and destroying malignant cells.
- **Restorative effects** return the body to or maintain the body at optimal levels of health. For example, vitamin and mineral supplements are administered to many patients recovering from surgery.

KnowledgeCheck 25-6

- Name and define the four pharmacokinetic processes.
- How does absorption differ in children and older adults?
- What factors affect excretion?
- You are to administer the following drugs to Cyndi Early (Meet Your Patients): (1) insulin subcutaneously for her diabetes and (2) morphine intravenously to relieve her pain. For which primary effect is each of these drugs being given?

What Are Secondary Effects?

All medications can cause secondary effects (e.g., side effects, adverse reactions, allergic reactions), which can either be harmless or cause injury that may sometimes be predicted.

Side Effects

Side effects are unintended, often predictable, physiological effects of the medication to which patients usually adapt. They occur at the usual prescribed dose and may be immediate (e.g., dizziness) or delayed (e.g., constipation). For hospitalized patients, you will most often see side effects caused by analgesics, antibiotics, antipsychotics, and sedatives. The most common side effects are nausea, vomiting, diarrhea, dizziness, drowsiness, dry mouth, abdominal distention or distress, and constipation.
KEY POINT: *Your role as a primary nurse includes teaching the patient what side effects to anticipate and how to manage them.*

♥ iCare 25-1

Medicating Patients

- Medicating patients is routine for nurses but remember that receiving medications can be anxiety producing for patients.
- Listen to the message the patient is giving you with his questions, observations, knowledge, or fears.
- **STOP** if there is any uncertainty.
- Verify and validate all aspects of the medication process prior to administration. This helps ensure safe medication practices. Being safe is one aspect of caring.

Adverse Reactions

Adverse reactions are harmful, unintended, usually unpredicted reactions to a drug administered at the normal dosage. They are more severe than side effects and often require discontinuation of the drug.

- *Dose-related* adverse reactions result from known pharmacological effects of the medication. For example, a diabetic patient treated with insulin may develop very low blood sugar if too much insulin is administered.
- *Patient sensitivity* adverse reactions occur because the patient is unusually susceptible to the effects of the drug. Box 25-1 lists patients at high risk for adverse reactions.

The FDA defines **severe adverse reactions** as those that (1) are life threatening; (2) require intervention to prevent permanent impairment or death; or (3) lead to congenital anomaly, disability, hospitalization, or death. Health professionals must document serious adverse reactions according to agency policy and report them to the FDA MedWatch program. To make a report, contact the FDA by calling 1-888-INFO-FDA (1-888-463-6332), or

 Go to the FDA Medwatch Web site at http://www.fda.gov/medwatch/

You can also contact the Institute for Safe Medication Practices (ISMP) to report errors, close calls, or hazardous conditions, using this URL: https://www.ismp.org/reporterrors.asp. ISMP guarantees the confidentiality and security of the information received.

Toxic Reactions

Toxic reactions are dangerous, damaging effects to an organ or tissue. They are more severe than adverse reactions, sometimes even causing permanent damage or death. It may help to think of toxicity as poisoning. Antidotes are available for some medications—for example, naloxone is given for opiate toxicity. Toxicity may be caused by any of the following:

- *Overdosing* (administrating a dose that exceeds the prescribed amount). Examples are respiratory depression from excessive morphine and hypoglycemia from too much insulin.

- *Accumulation* of the drug in the tissues (related to long-term use or incomplete metabolism/excretion)
- *Abnormal sensitivity* or allergic response to the drug
  Toxic reactions can be:
- Localized to a particular tissue or organ or can affect several organ systems.
- Reversible (e.g., tinnitus caused by aspirin) or permanent (e.g., hearing loss caused by aminoglycoside antibiotics).
- Immediate and evident soon after administration, or they can develop months or even years after administration (e.g., drug-induced cancers).

ThinkLike a Nurse 25-7

- You have just looked up the antihypertensive drug lisinopril (Zestril) and found the following side effects:

  Neutropenia, dizziness, headache, fatigue, depression, somnolence, paresthesia, hypotension, chest pain, nasal congestion, diarrhea, nausea, dyspepsia, impotence, rash, cough, muscle cramps, angioedema, lethargy, hypokalemia, decreased libido

What strategy could you use to help you remember all the above side effects?

- You have checked the MAR for Margaret Marks (Meet Your Patients) and prepared her next dose of antibiotic for intravenous administration. The MAR also indicates that she is receiving morphine for pain and that her last dose was given 1 hour ago. When you enter the room, you find her apparently sleeping. You are not able to awaken her to verify her identity. What do you suspect is happening and how should you respond? (If you need information about antibiotics and morphine, look it up in an appropriate reference.)

Allergic Reactions

In an **allergic reaction,** the immune system identifies a medication as a foreign substance that should be neutralized or destroyed. The patient experiences no problems with the first dose of the medication, but it acts as an antigen, activating the formation of antibodies against the drug. When the drug is again administered, the antigen–antibody-binding complex prompts an allergic reaction.

Allergic reactions range from minor to serious; however, even a small amount of a medication can cause a severe reaction. Urticaria (hives), pruritus (itching), edema of soft tissue and mucosa, and rhinitis (inflammation of the nasal mucosa) usually occur within minutes to 2 weeks after exposure and are considered mild. Such reactions often disappear after the medication is discontinued and the blood level of the drug falls. Medications most frequently implicated in allergic reactions are antibiotics, biological agents, and diagnostic agents. See Table 25-3.

An Anaphylactic Reaction is a life-threatening allergic reaction that occurs immediately after administration.

- Anaphylaxis produces sudden constriction of bronchioles, edema of the larynx and pharynx, severe shortness of breath, wheezing, and severe hypotension (low blood pressure).
- Immediate treatment includes discontinuing the medication and giving epinephrine, IV fluids, steroids, and antihistamines. Respiratory support (e.g., oxygen, intubation, ventilation) may also be required.

- ✚ A patient who is allergic to one drug may also be allergic to other medications in the same class. For example, many patients who are allergic to penicillin are also allergic to cephalexin (Keflex), a synthetic penicillin.

BOX 25-1 ■ Risk Factors for Adverse Drug Reactions

Behavioral and Situational Factors

- History of allergies or previous adverse drug reactions
- Receiving treatment from two or more providers at the same time
- Taking multiple prescription drugs in addition to over-the-counter preparations and herbal remedies and supplements. This is also called polypharmacy.
- Taking a drug inconsistently
- Long-term use of a drug (may promote accumulation, leading to toxicity)

Physical Factors

- Concurrent illnesses (e.g., diabetes and renal failure)
- A change in the ability to absorb, metabolize, or excrete the drug (e.g., impaired hepatic or renal function)
- Confusion/cognitive impairment
- Very old or very young age
- Obesity or extreme thinness
- Dehydration or rapid change in hydration status

Table 25-3 ➤ Medications Frequently Triggering Allergic Reactions

DRUG CLASSIFICATION	EXAMPLE DRUGS	
Analgesics, Anesthetics, and Anti-inflammatory Agents	Codeine Morphine NSAIDs (ibuprofen, acetaminophen, naproxen) Indomethacin	Aspirin Tranquilizers Local anesthetic agents, such as tetracaine, phenylbutazone, procaine, lidocaine, cocaine, benzocaine, general anesthetics
Antiseizure Drugs	Phenytoin Carbamazepine	
Antibiotics	Cephalosporins Erythromycin Neomycin Penicillin	Streptomycin Sulfonamides Tetracycline Vancomycin
Biological Agents	Allopurinol Antitoxins Corticotropin (ACTH) Enzymes	Gamma globulin Insulin Vaccines
Diagnostic Agents	Iodinated media contrasts Intravenous pyelogram (IVP) dye	
Other Drugs	Dextran Histamines Iodines	Iron Phenothiazides Quinidine

- Always ask the patient about allergies and his reaction to the medications.
- People with severe allergic reactions should wear a MedicAlert bracelet (Fig. 25-5) that identifies the person and the allergen and carry epinephrine for emergency injection.

ThinkLike a Nurse 25-8

You are administering medications to your assigned patients (Meet Your Patients). What should you do in each of the following situations? Which patient should you attend to first? Explain your thinking.

- Ms. Jones has ibuprofen prescribed for her back pain. She tells you she cannot take this medication because it makes her feel nauseated.

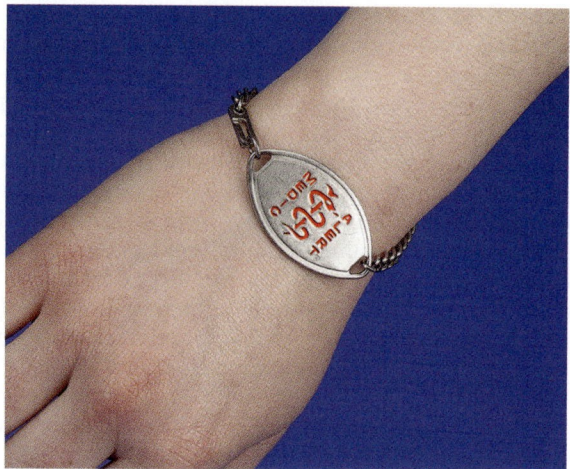

FIGURE 25-5 People with severe allergies to a medication should wear a MedicAlert bracelet.

- Mr. Bigler had an open reduction internal fixation of his arm performed yesterday and is receiving an antibiotic, cefazolin, 500 mg IV every 8 hours. He has already received three doses of this medication, and you initiated his 0800 dose about 10 minutes ago. He tells you that he thinks his throat is closing shut.

Idiosyncratic Reactions

An **idiosyncratic** reaction is an unexpected, abnormal, or peculiar response to a medication. It may take the form of extreme sensitivity to a medication, lack of response, or a paradoxical (opposite of expected) response, such as agitation in response to a sedative.

Cumulative Effect

A **cumulative effect** is the increased response to repeated doses of a drug that occurs when the rate of administration is greater than the rate of metabolism and excretion (e.g., liver or kidney disorders). Unless the dose is changed, the medication accumulates in the system until a toxic level is reached. Opiates and barbiturates are known for their cumulative effects.

KnowledgeCheck 25-7

- Differentiate between primary and secondary effects of medications.
- List one adverse reaction for each of the following systems: blood, gastrointestinal, neurological, cardiovascular, hepatic, and renal.
- What are some of the symptoms you will see in an anaphylactic reaction?
- What type of patient is most likely to experience an allergic reaction?

How Do Medications Interact?

The more drugs a patient takes, the higher the risk of a drug interaction. Drugs may also interact with certain foods. There are several types of medication interactions:

- **Drug interaction** occurs when one drug alters or modifies the action of another.
- **Antagonistic drug relationship** happens when one drug interferes with the actions of another and decreases the resultant drug effect.
- **Synergistic drug relationship** is an additive effect; the effect of both drugs together is greater than the individual effects.

- **Drug incompatibilities** occur when multiple drugs are mixed together, causing a chemical deterioration of one or both drugs. ✚ You can usually recognize an incompatibility when the mixed solution takes on a changed appearance. However, you should always consult medication resources and compatibility charts *before* mixing medications. Then, after mixing, double-check the medication for changes in appearance. If an incompatibility occurs, do not administer the drug.

KnowledgeCheck 25-8

- What type of interaction occurs when one drug interferes with the action of another?
- What interactions occur when one drug has an additive effect on another drug?
- What is drug incompatibility?

What Should I Know About Drug Abuse or Misuse?

You should be able to differentiate between concepts that describe nontherapeutic use or effects of drugs:

- **Tolerance** is a decreasing response to repeated doses of a medication. The person then requires more of the drug to achieve the desired effect.
- **Dependence** is a person's reliance on, or need for, a drug. It leads to compulsive patterns of drug use wherein the user's lifestyle centers on procuring and taking the drug.
- **Drug misuse** is the nonspecific, indiscriminate, or improper use of drugs, including alcohol, OTC medications, and prescription drugs. Older adults are especially prone to misuse of laxatives in the self-treatment of constipation. Continued use of laxatives can lead to dependence and other medical problems.
- **Drug abuse** is the inappropriate intake of a substance by amount, type, or situation, continuously or periodically. For example, consuming alcohol at work is considered abuse, but having a glass of wine with dinner is not. Drug abuse may or may not lead to drug dependence.
- **Illicit drugs,** also known as street drugs, are drugs sold illegally. Many are prescription drugs (e.g., hydrocodone) sought for their mood-altering effects. Prescription drugs can be abused when taken for purposes other than medically intended.

HOW DO I MEASURE AND CALCULATE DOSAGE?

Medications are not always available in the exact dosage the patient needs. Therefore, you must be proficient in calculating drug dosages to be sure your patients receive the correct amount of medication.

Medication Measurement Systems

Medications are usually prescribed and measured using the metric system; however, a few are still dispensed using the apothecary and household systems. You will sometimes need to make conversions from one measurement system to another.

- **Metric System.** The metric system is the preferred system to measure drug dosages because it promotes accuracy by allowing for calculation of small drug dosages. A disadvantage of this system in the United States is that many people outside the healthcare system are not familiar with it.
- **Apothecary System.** The British apothecary system of measurement (Roman or Arabic numerals) has been in use in the United States since colonial times. Only a few medications

(e.g., aspirin) are measured using this system because it is less convenient and less precise. For example, *5 grains* might be written as *grains V* or *gr V.* ✚ To avoid a dosage error, write out the intended unit of measurement. For example, write grains so gr (grains) is not mistaken for gm (grams) (The Joint Commission, 2016a).

- **Household System.** Although it is easier to teach a patient about home medications using this system (e.g., teaspoons, ounces, cups), nurses do not often use it because drug dosages are less precise and can lead to medication dosing errors.

Special Measurements: Units and Milliequivalents

Units Insulin, a drug used by diabetics to help control blood sugar, is measured in **units,** with 100 international units (U100) being the standard strength preparation. In this strength, 1 mL of the fluid medication contains 100 units of insulin. The following is a prescription using units: "NPH insulin 14 units subcutaneously every morning." Heparin (an anticoagulant) and penicillin are also prescribed in units.

✚ Be aware that not all units are the same. For example, 1 mL of heparin does not contain 100 units of heparin. You must always read the container label to know the number of units per milliliter.

Milliequivalents (mEq) indicate the strength of the ion concentration in a drug. A milliequivalent is the number of grams of a solid contained in 1 mL of a solution. Electrolytes, such as potassium chloride (KCl), are measured in mEq. The following is a medication prescriptions using mEq: "D_5W 1000 mL with KCl 40 mEq every 8 hours."

KEY POINT: *Note that units and mEq cannot be directly converted to the apothecary, metric, or household system.*

Calculating Dosages

You should be able to calculate accurately using several different methods and formulas. Inaccurate calculations result in incorrect dosages and could harm the patient.

One easy formula to remember is the following:

$$\frac{\text{Dose on hand}}{\text{Quantity (or volume) on hand}} = \frac{\text{Desired dose}}{\text{Quantity (or volume) desired}}$$

Or

$$\frac{\text{DH}}{\text{QH}} = \frac{\text{DD}}{\text{X}}$$

Remember: You must pay attention to *both* the milligrams (weight of the drug) marked on the medication container *and* the milliliters (amount of liquid in which the medication is dissolved). For example, the provider prescribes meperidine (Demerol) 25 mg IM now. You have a prefilled syringe containing Demerol 50 mg in 1 mL volume. How much of the liquid (how many mL) would you administer to the patient?

$$\frac{\text{DH}}{\text{QH}} = \frac{\text{DD}}{\text{X}} \quad \text{or} \quad \frac{50 \text{ mg}}{1 \text{ mL}} = \frac{25 \text{ mg}}{\text{X}}$$

Therefore (recalling your algebra),

$$50X = 25 \text{ mL,}$$
$$\text{so } X = 25 \text{ divided by } 50,$$
$$\text{so } X = 0.5 \text{ mL}$$

Here is an alternative formula you can use for calculating dosages:

$$\frac{\text{Dose desired (DD)}}{\text{Dose on hand (DH)}} \times \text{quantity on hand (QH)} = \text{desired quantity}$$

How Should I Calculate Dosage for a Child?

You must be very careful when calculating medication dosages for children and infants.

✚ Confusion between pounds and kilograms is a source of dosing error in pediatrics. Most drug references list normal pediatric ranges, which can serve as additional verification.

KEY POINT: *The standard measurement for pediatric patients is kilograms, and prescriptions for pediatric dosages are usually either calculated by the prescriber or stated in terms of "milligrams per kilogram of body weight."* For example, you might have a prescription for "Erythromycin 30 mg/kg of body weight." You know that 1 kg equals 2.2 lb. and that the child weighs 44 lb.

- Convert the weight to kilograms by dividing 44 by 2.2: the child thus weighs 20 kg.
- Multiply the prescribed dose (30 mg) by body weight (20 kg): 30 mg × 20 = 600 mg
- 600 mg is the dosage for a 20-kg child.

You should rarely need to calculate a child's dosage on the basis of an adult dose, because medication prescriptions should specify the exact dosage for the individual child, and the medication is dispensed using pediatric-specific medication formulations and concentrations. However, if you must calculate a child's dosage, use either the Body Surface Area (BSA) Formula by using a Nomogram for Children, or Clark's Rule for Children to verify the safety of pediatric orders.

Nomograms To find a child's BSA using the nomogram, you must know the child's height and weight. To use a nomogram, you draw a straight line between the child's height (on the left scale) and weight (on the right scale) and note where the lines cross midline. To see a nomogram example,

 Go to http://www.manuelsweb.com/images/nomogram.png

Clark's Rule Another formula used in pediatrics to determine safe dosage range is Clark's Rule; this rule is mostly used for children aged 2 and younger. A good example of how to employ this rule is with the drug erythromycin, which has a *usual adult dose* for erythromycin of 250 to 500 mg. To determine the safe dosage range of erythromycin for a child 2 years and younger, use Clark's Rule.

1. Using this formula, you assume that an average adult weighs 150 lb (68 kg) (this is the standard for the rule).

$$\text{Adult dose} \times \frac{\text{child's weight in lb}}{150} = \text{child's dose}$$

2. According to Clark's Rule, if the maximum adult dose of erythromycin is 500 mg, then the maximum dose for an infant weighing 15 lb is:

$$500 \times 0.1 = 50 \text{ mg}$$

If you need a Web-based dosage calculator,

 Go to http://www.manuelsweb.com/nrs_calculators.htm

WHAT MUST I KNOW ABOUT MEDICATION PRESCRIPTIONS?

Before administering any medication, you must obtain a **prescription** from the primary care provider and verify that it is complete and legible.

- *For inpatients*, prescriptions for medications are either entered into an electronic health record for automated dispensing or printed in the medical orders section of the paper chart. This was traditionally referred to as an *order*.
- For *outpatients* and for medications that will be filled by the patient (instead of the agency pharmacy), a prescription is written and given to the patient or family. See Figure 25-6 for an example of a *prescription*.

A written or printed outpatient medication prescription should contain the following essential elements:

- Patient's full name (some agencies and some states require the address of the patient)
- Name, address, and telephone number of the prescriber, including relevant credentials and legal registration number, such as the National Provider Identification (NPI) in the United States. Providers who are prescribing controlled substances must register with the federal Drug Enforcement Administration (DEA). The prescriber's DEA number must be included on the prescription.
- Date and time prescription was written
- Name of medication
- Dosage (including size, frequency, and number of doses)
- Route of administration
- Signature of prescriber

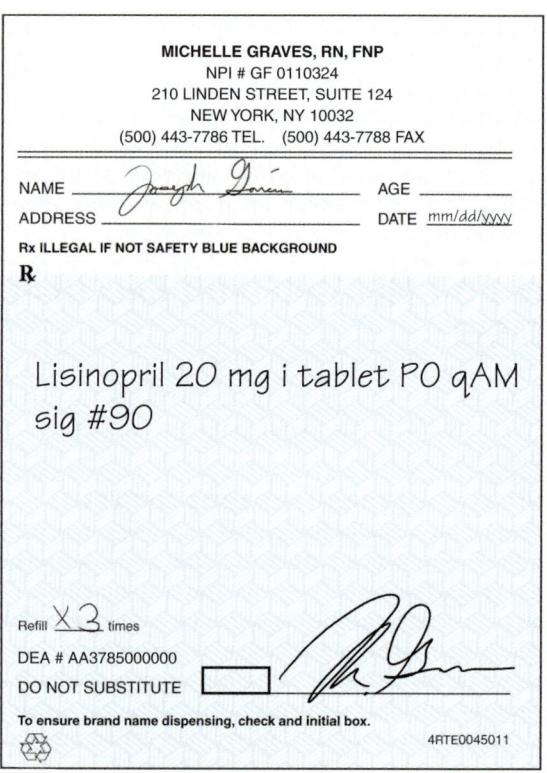

FIGURE 25-6 Example of a prescription.

KnowledgeCheck 25-9

- What are the essential parts of a medication prescription?
- How does an inpatient prescription (order) differ from an outpatient prescription?

What Abbreviations Are Used in Medication Prescriptions?

For a list of medication-related abbreviations you may see when reviewing and documenting medications, see Table 25-4. Because abbreviations can be easily misread, you should write out drug names in full. However, some are used in medication administration (e.g., mL, mEq), so you should be familiar with them and your facility's approved list of abbreviations.

Consult The Joint Commission's official Do Not Use list (Table 18-1). Also be familiar with the Institute for Safe Medication Practices (ISMP) List of Error-Prone Abbreviations, Symbols, and Dose Designations in Table 25-5.

Types of Medication Prescriptions

Common types of medication prescriptions are based on the duration, frequency, and/or urgency of the prescription.

- **Standard written prescriptions** apply without a renewal date until the prescriber writes a prescription to alter or discontinue the medication or indicates a specific stop date on the original prescription. For example, "Give furosemide 20 mg IVP twice a day for 5 days." After 5 days, the prescription is discontinued, unless the provider renews it.
- **Automatic stop dates** are protocols that hospitals use for discontinuing medications after a certain length of time. Most narcotics prescriptions are in effect for only 7 days. If the medication is needed after the automatic stop date, the provider must write another prescription.
- **STAT** prescription means that a single dose of medication is to be given immediately and only once. For example, "Give furosemide 20 mg IV push STAT," or "Give lorazepam 1 mg IV push now."

Table 25-4 ▶ Common Medication-Related Abbreviations

ABBREVIATION	EXPLANATION	ABBREVIATION	EXPLANATION
ac	before meals	pc	after meals: Example: 0900, 1300, 1900 hours
ad lib	as desired	PM	Evening
a.m.	Morning	po or PO	by mouth
bid	twice a day	prn	as needed
c̄	With	qh, qr (q1h, q1hr)	Every hour
fl oz	fluid ounce	q2h, q2hr	every 2 hours: Example: 0800, 1000, 1200 hours, etc.
g, gm, or GM	Gram	q3h, q3hr	every 3 hours: Example: 0900, 1200, 1500 hours, etc.
gtt	Drop	q4h, q4hr	every 4 hours: Example: 0200, 0600, 1000, 1400, 1800, 2200 hours
h, hr	Hour	q6h, q6hr	every 6 hours: Example 0600, 1200, 1800 hours, 2400.
IM	intramuscular	qid or QID	four times a day: Example 1000, 1400, 1800, 2200
IV	Intravenous	qs	sufficient quantity
IVPB	intravenous piggyback	s̄	Wthout
Kg or kg	Kilogram	Stat or STAT	at once
KVO	keep vein open	sup or supp	Suppository
L or l	Liter	susp	Suspension
mEq	Milliequivalent	tab	Tablet
mL or ml	Milliliter	Tbsp	Tablespoon
OTC	over-the-counter	tid or TID	three times a day: 1000, 1400, 1800 hours
oz	Ounce	T or tsp	Teaspoon

Table 25-5 ▶ Institute for Safe Medication Practices (ISMP) List of Error-Prone Abbreviations, Symbols, and Dose Designations

ABBREVIATIONS	INTENDED MEANING	MISINTERPRETATION	CORRECTION
μg	Microgram	Mistaken as "mg"	Use "mcg."
AD, AS, AU	Right ear, left ear, each ear	Mistaken as OD, OS, OU (right eye, left eye, each eye)	Use "right ear," "left ear," or "each ear."
OD, OS, OU	Right eye, left eye, each eye	Mistaken as AD, AS, AU (right ear, left ear, each ear)	Use "right eye," "left eye," or "each eye."
BT	Bedtime	Mistaken as "bid" (twice daily)	Use "bedtime."
cc	Cubic centimeters	Mistaken as "u" (units)	Use "mL."
D/C	Discharge or discontinue	Premature discontinuation of medications if D/C (intended to mean: "discharge") has been misinterpreted as "discontinued" when followed by a list of discharge medications	Use "discharge" and "discontinue."
ij	Injection	Mistaken as "IV" or "intrajugular"	Use "injection."
IN	Intranasal	Mistaken as "IM" or "IV"	Use "intranasal" or "NAS."
HS	Half-strength	Mistaken as bedtime	Use "half-strength."
hs	At bedtime, hours of sleep	Mistaken as half-strength	Use "bedtime."
*IU	International units	Mistaken as IV (intravenous) or 10 (ten)	Use "International units."
o.d. or OD	Once daily	Mistaken as "right eye" (OD-oculus dexter), leading to oral liquid medications administered in the eye	Use "daily."
OJ	Orange juice	Mistaken as OD or OS (right or left eye); drugs meant to be diluted in orange juice may be given in the eye	Use "orange juice."
per os	By mouth, orally	The "os" can be mistaken as "left eye" (OS-oculus sinister)	Use "PO," "by mouth," or "orally."
*q.d. or QD	Every day	Mistaken as q.i.d., especially if the period after the "q" or the tail of the "q" is misunderstood as an "i"	Use "daily."
qhs	Nightly at bedtime	Mistaken as "qhr" or every hour	Use "nightly."
qn	Nightly or at bedtime	Mistaken as "qh" (every hour)	Use "nightly" or "at bedtime."
*q.o.d. or QOD	Every other day	Mistaken as "q.d." (daily) or "q.i.d." (four times daily) if the "o" is poorly written	Use "every other day."
qld	Daily	Mistaken as q.i.d. (four times daily)	Use "daily."
q6PM, etc.	Every evening at 6 PM	Mistaken as every 6 hours	Use "6 PM nightly" or "6 PM daily."
SC, SQ, subQ or subq	Subcutaneous	SC mistaken as SL (sublingual); SQ mistaken as "5 every"; the "q" in "sub q" has been mistaken as "every (e.g., a heparin dose ordered sub q 2 hours before hours before surgery) surgery" misunderstood as every 2	Spell out "subcutaneous."
ss	Sliding scale (insulin)	Mistaken as "55"	Spell out "sliding scale"; use "one-half."
SSRI, SSI	Sliding scale regular insulin	Mistaken as selective-serotonin reuptake inhibitor; mistaken as Strong Solution of Iodine (Lugol's)	Spell out "sliding scale (insulin)."

Table 25-5 ➤ **Institute for Safe Medication Practices (ISMP) List of Error-Prone Abbreviations, Symbols, and Dose Designations—cont'd**

ABBREVIATIONS	INTENDED MEANING	MISINTERPRETATION	CORRECTION
i/d	One daily	Mistaken as "tid"	Use "1 daily."
TIW or tiw	3 times a week	Mistaken as "3 times a day" or "twice in a week"	Use "3 times weekly."
*U or u	Unit	Mistaken as the number 0 or 4, causing a 10-fold overdose or greater (e.g., 4U seen as "40" or 4u seen as "44"); mistaken as "cc" so dose given in volume instead of units (e.g., 4u seen as 4cc)	Use "unit."

DOSE DESIGNATIONS OR OTHER INFORMATION	INTENDED MEANING	MISINTERPRETATION	CORRECTION
*Trailing zero after decimal point (e.g., 1.0 mg)	1 mg	Mistaken as 10 mg if the decimal point is not seen expressed in whole numbers	Do not use trailing zeros for doses.
*No leading zero before a decimal dose (e.g., .5 mg)	0.5 mg	Mistaken as 5 mg if the decimal point is not seen	Use zero before a decimal point when the dose is less than a whole unit.
Drug name and drug dose run together (e.g., Inderal 40 mg)	Inderal 40 mg	Mistaken as Inderal 140 mg	Place adequate space between the drug name, dose, and unit of measurement.
Numeric dose and unit of measurement run together (e.g., 10 mg)	10 mg	The "m" can be mistaken for a zero, leading to a 10-fold dosing error	Place adequate space between the drug name, dose, and unit of measurement.
Abbreviations such as mg. or mL. with a period following the abbreviation	mg or mL	The period is unnecessary and could be mistaken as the number 1 if written poorly	Use mg, mL, etc., without a period.
Large doses without properly placed commas (e.g., 100000 units or 1000000 units)	100,000 or 1,000,000 units	100000 has been mistaken for 10,000 or 1,000,000; 1,000,000 has been mistaken for 100,000	Use commas for dosing units at or above 1,000 or use such words as 100 "thousand" or 1 "million" to improve readability.

DRUG NAME ABBREVIATIONS	INTENDED MEANING	MISINTERPRETATION	CORRECTION
Note: Pharmacies do not accept orders for abbreviated medications.			
ARA A	vidarabine	Mistaken as cytarabine (ARA C)	Use the complete drug name.
AZR	zidovudine (Retrovir)	Mistaken as azathioprine or aztreonam	Use the complete drug name.
CPZ	prochlorperazine (Compazine)	Mistaken as chlorpromazine	Use complete drug name.
DPT	Demerol-Phenergan-Thorazine	Mistaken as diphtheria-pertussis-tetanus	Use complete drug name.

(Continued)

Table 25-5 ➤ Institute for Safe Medication Practices (ISMP) List of Error-Prone Abbreviations, Symbols, and Dose Designations—cont'd

DRUG NAME ABBREVIATIONS	INTENDED MEANING	MISINTERPRETATION	CORRECTION
DTO	Diluted tincture of opium, or deodorized tincture of opium (Paregoric)	Mistaken as tincture of opium	Use complete drug name.
HCl	hydrochloric acid or hydrochloride	Mistaken as potassium chloride (The "H" is misinterpreted as "K.")	Use complete drug name unless expressed as a salt of a drug.
HCT	hydrocortisone	Mistaken as hydrochlorothiazide	Use complete drug name.
HCTZ	hydrochlorothiazide	Mistaken as hydrocortisone (seen as HCT 250 mg)	Use complete drug name.
*MgSO$_4$	magnesium sulfate	Mistaken as morphine sulfate	Use complete drug name.
*MS, MSO$_4$	morphine sulfate	Mistaken as magnesium sulfate	Use complete drug name.
MTX	methotrexate	Mistaken as mitoxantrone	Use complete drug name.
PCA	procainamide	Mistaken as patient-controlled analgesia	Use complete drug name.
PTU	propylthiouracil	Mistaken as mercaptopurine	Use complete drug name.
T3	Tylenol with codeine No. 3	Mistaken as liothyronine	Use complete drug name.
TAC	triamcinolone	Mistaken as tetracaine, adrenaline, cocaine	Use complete drug name.
TNK	TNKase	Mistaken as "TPA"	Use complete drug name.
ZnSO$_4$	zinc sulfate	Mistaken as morphine sulfate	Use complete drug name.

STEMMED DRUG NAMES	INTENDED MEANING	MISINTERPRETATION	CORRECTION
"nitro drip"	nitroglycerine infusion	Mistaken as sodium nitroprusside infusion	Use complete drug name.
"Norflox"	norfloxacin	Mistaken as Norflex	Use complete drug name.
"IV Vanc"	intravenous vancomycin	Mistaken as Invanz	Use complete drug name.

SYMBOLS	INTENDED MEANING	MISINTERPRETATION	CORRECTION
ʒ	dram	Symbol for dram mistaken as "3"	Use the metric system.
♏	Minim	Mistaken as "mL"	Use the metric system.
×3d	for 3 days	Mistaken as "3 doses"	Use "for 3 days."
< and >	greater than and less than	Mistaken as opposite of intended; mistakenly using incorrect symbols	Use "greater than" or "less than."
/ (slash mark)	separates two doses or indicates "per"	Mistaken as the number 1 (e.g., "25 units/ 10 units" misread as "25 units and 110" units)	Use "per" rather than a slash mark to separate doses.
@	at	Mistaken as "2"	Use "at."
&	and	Mistaken as "2"	Use "and."
+	plus or and	Mistaken as "4"	Use "and" or "plus."
°	hour	mistaken as zero (e.g., q2° seen as q 20)	Use "hr", "h", or "hour."

Source: Used with permission from the Institute for Safe Medication Practices. Report medication errors or near misses to the ISMP Medication Errors Reporting Program (MERP) at 1-800-FAIL-SAF(E) or online at www.ismp.org.
*These abbreviations are included on The Joint Commission's "minimum list" of dangerous abbreviations, acronyms, and symbols that must be included on an organization's "Do Not Use" list, effective January 1, 2004. Visit www.jointcommission.org for more information about this Joint Commission requirement.
From: https://www.ismp.org/Tools/errorproneabbreviations.pdf

- **Single** (or *one-time*) prescription indicates that the medication is to be given only once at a specified time usually before surgery or diagnostic procedures. For example: "Give Versed 25 mg intramuscularly on call for when surgical staff requests premedication to be administered."
- **Standing prescriptions (orders)** occur when a unit has a standard population of patients and the primary care provider develops a set of *standing prescriptions* for treating a particular disease or set of symptoms. (e.g., coronary care, postpartum patients). These are officially accepted sets of prescriptions to be applied routinely by nurses for the care of patients. For example: "Give nitroglycerin 0.4 mg sublingually q3–5 min for chest pain, to a maximum of 3 doses in 15 min" may be a standing order in coronary care units.
- **prn prescription** means the provider may prescribe a medication to be given whenever the patient requires (prn). A prn prescription requires the nurse to determine, within the established parameters and in collaboration with the patient, when the medication is to be given. The prescription specifies (1) the condition for which the medication is to be given and (2) the minimum time intervals between doses—for example, "Morphine sulfate 10 mg intramuscularly q3–4hr prn incisional pain." **KEY POINT:** *The medication cannot be given more frequently than prescribed, even if symptoms persist.* Pain medications, antiemetics (antinausea medications), antipyretics, and laxatives are usually given prn.

How Are Medication Prescriptions Communicated?

Providers communicate medications prescriptions in writing (including electronically) and verbally. The nursing implications are slightly different for each.

Written Prescriptions You will find written prescriptions either hand written on a prescription form or on preprinted standard medication order sheets and protocols. Some agencies accept medication prescriptions transmitted electronically or via facsimile from the prescriber to the nurse, with the original copy provided later.

Verbal Prescriptions A prescriber may sometimes give a verbal prescription, which is an oral order spoken to the nurse. The registered nurse (RN) then writes the prescription and signs it with the provider's name followed by the nurse's name and credentials. Medication names that sound the same can be confusing and lead to administering the wrong drug (Box 25-2). Repeat the prescription to the provider and spell the medication name to ensure accuracy. Verbal prescriptions increase the risk for miscommunication and errors and should only be used in urgent situations.

A provider may give you a verbal prescription via telephone **(telephone prescription)** usually in response to a call you have placed to report a change in the patient's condition or the results of laboratory or other tests. The provider usually must cosign oral and telephone prescriptions within 24 hours.

What Should I Do If I Think a Prescription Is Incorrect?

KEY POINT: *As a nurse, you are legally responsible for medications you administer.* If you believe a prescription is incorrect, do the following:

- Look up the medication in a reliable resource (e.g., drug formulary) to verify spelling, usage, dosages, and routes.
- Ask another nurse or provider to check the prescription and compare it with your resource data.

BOX 25-2 ■ Medications With Similar-Sounding Names

Alprazolam—lorazepam	Morphine—meperidine
Baclofen—Bactroban	NovoLog—Humalog
Cefzil, Keflin—Keflex	NovoLog—Novalin R
Celebrex—Celexa, Cerebyx	Ophthalgan—Auralgan
Cytoxan—Ciloxan	Percocet—Percodan
Demerol—dicumarol	Phenergan—Phenaphen
Digoxin—digitoxin	Procardia—Procardia XL
Glyburide—glipizide	Quinine—quinidine
Humalog—Humulin R	Ranitidine—amantadine
Keflex—Kantrex	Serzone—Seroquel
Lamictal—Lamisil—Ludiomil—Lomotil	Taxotere—Taxol
	Zantac—Xanax
Lodine—iodine	Zantac—Zyrtec—Zyprexa
	Zostrix—Zestril

- Contact the prescriber for clarifications, concerns, or questions.

Do not assume you are correctly interpreting the prescription if you have any question at all. Use your knowledge, common sense, and intuition when administering medications. To avoid errors, you must know and understand the procedures at your facility, be familiar with the medications you give, and always check the prescription. Each agency will have a policy specifying the procedure for checking medication prescriptions. For example, a unit secretary may transcribe the original prescription into a medication administration record (MAR), but the nurse must check to ensure the transcription is correct.

✚ Most medication errors occur during the prescribing process; however, 50% are detected before these errors reach the patient (Mckay, 2012). Thus, this double-check system is imperative.

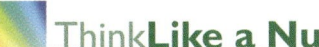

ThinkLike a Nurse 25-9

Find the errors in the following list of medication prescriptions. Use a drug formulary or nursing drug handbook to check dosages, spellings, and so on.

- Ancef 10 g q6hr IV
- Capatril 25 mg orally twice a day
- Digoxin 0.125 mg daily
- Lasix 400 mg by mouth
- NTG gr 1/150 prn chest pain
- Tylenol orally prn fever

MEDICATION ERRORS

A **medication error** is any preventable event that may cause or lead to inappropriate medication use or harm to a patient. Medication errors affect nearly 5% of inpatients, making them the most common adverse events that occur in hospitalized patients (Agency for Healthcare Research and Quality, 2015b). The National Coordinating Council for Medication Error Reporting and Prevention (2012) estimated that 98,000 hospitalized patients die annually as a result of medication errors.

The most common medication errors made by nurses are related to confusion caused by similar drug names, lack of knowledge of the drug, and lack of information about the patient. Box 25-3 describes several causes of medication errors by nurses. For a list of drugs that can have devastating consequences when erroneously administered,

 Go to the ISMP Web site at http://www.ismp.org

BOX 25-3 ▪ Why Do Medication Errors Occur?

The following are several factors associated with medication errors:

Lack of Knowledge or Information

- Lack of knowledge of the drug (e.g., incorrect dosages, incorrect mixing, overly rapid infusion, drug interaction, adverse effects) is the most common factor contributing to medication errors.
- Lack of information about the patient (e.g., allergies, other medications, lab results, medical condition for which the medication is contraindicated) is the second most frequent cause of errors.
- A drug is given by the wrong route.

Faulty Communication

- The written prescription is unclear, illegible, or transcribed incorrectly, resulting in administering the wrong drug or dosage (e.g., confusion between drugs with similar names).
- The telephone prescription is taken incorrectly.
- Protocol is not understood or is violated.
- A drug prescription is written on the wrong patient's chart.
- The wrong dosage is prescribed (e.g., by misplacing a zero or decimal point).
- Abbreviations are misunderstood.
- Poor, or no, documentation can result in error. For example, a nurse administers a medication yet fails to record it immediately afterward. A second nurse checking the patient's chart thinks the drug has not been given so administers a dose. The patient receives a double dose.

Equipment Errors

- Wrong equipment is used to administer the drug.
- Equipment malfunctions or is not used properly.

Calculation and Measurement Errors

- An error in calculating the dosage is made, so the patient receives the wrong dose.
- There is confusion in the unit of measurement; for example, a drug is prescribed based on kilograms and dispensed or administered based on pounds (and vice versa).

Other

- Medication is improperly handled or stored.
- The patient's identity is not checked, and the wrong patient receives the medication.
- Lighting is inadequate.
- The nurse is fatigued, distracted, or interrupted.

Sources: Durham, M., Suhayda, R., Normand, P., et al. (2016); Hayes, B., Klein-Schwartz, W., & Gonzales, L. (2009); Mckay, M. (2012); Pretorius, R., Gataric, G., Swedlund, S., et al. (2013).

How Can I Avoid Errors?

To ensure patient safety, begin by following the "three checks" and the six-plus "rights" found in the section Ensuring Safe Medication Administration, later in this chapter. You must also be familiar with and follow the variety of systemwide measures designed to prevent medication errors in your agency. For example, The Joint Commission recommends standardizing protocols for prescribing, administering, and documenting medication.

Medication Safety

PICOT

Situation: The student is preparing to administer medications to two clients in the subacute nursing setting. There are several medications to be administered to each client. The student has researched the medications and knows that there are oral, subcutaneous, and intravenous medications to administer. Prior to preparing the medication, the student reviews the medications and calculates the doses to ensure accuracy.

PICOT Components:

P Population/client	=	Nursing students
I Intervention/indicator	=	Medication administration simulation
C Comparator/control	=	Math testing only
O Outcome	=	Safe medication administration skills
T Time	=	Initial practice after graduation

Searchable Question: Do _____ (P) who receive _____ (I) demonstrate _____(O) as compared to _____(C) during _____ (T)?

Example of Evidence: Medication errors have been identified as a cause of 5% of all sentinel events in 2015 (The Joint Commission, 2016b). They result in increases in hospitalization, but can cost up to $8,700 per injury (Anderson & Townsend, 2015). Nursing students are often tested on medication calculation skills separately from the skill of administering medications. Research showed that simulation in medication administration fostered critical thinking and increased student success on the medication administration exam (Harris, Pittiglio, Newton, et al., 2014). Shanks (2011) noted that psychomotor and cognitive skills needed to be integrated. Simulations that included calculating a pediatric dosage (mg/kg/day), administration of the medication, documentation, and evaluation of the efficacy allow the skills to be practiced in an environment that does not expose clients to harm. During the debriefing or reflection session that follows the simulation, the factors that contributed to an error or near miss can be identified, and further remediation can be utilized.

Practice Change. Simulation allows students and new graduates to gain the knowledge and confidence to work through medication problems and arrive at accurate results (Harris, Pittiglio, Newton, et al., 2014; Shanks, 2011).

References: Harris, M., Pittiglio, L., Newton, S., et al. (2014). Using simulation to improve the medication administration skills of undergraduate nursing students. *Nursing Education Perspectives, 35*(1), 26–29; The Joint Commission (2016b). Sentinel events summary data. Retrieved from https://www.jointcommission.org/sentinel_event_statistics_quarterly/; Shanks, L. (2011). Medication calculation competency. *American Journal of Nursing, 111*(10), 67–69.

Critical thinking may be your best way to avoid errors and improve patient care and safety. Ask "are we," "what if," and "why" questions:

- Are we following standardized protocols for prescribing, administering, and documenting medication?
- What will happen if I don't do something or if I do something wrong?
- What assessments are required before and after I give this medication?
- Why am I hanging this IV or giving this medication?

Error-Prevention Technology

Technology has been integrated throughout the medication management process to decrease errors by improving access to information and communication among health professionals. Some healthcare agencies provide nurses with laptops and handheld mobile devices, allowing them to tap into detailed information about diseases, similar-sounding drugs, interactions, and side effects.

- **Computerized Prescriber Order Entry (CPOE)** helps prevent errors in transcription due to illegible handwritten prescriptions. Electronic prescribing systems are safer when combined with decision-support tools that automatically alert prescribers to possible interactions, allergies, and other potential problems.
- **Barcode medication administration,** especially when combined with CPOE, provides a highly effective system for identifying the right patient. It transfers data electronically, eliminating the error-prone paper transcription process. When used correctly, barcoding at the unit-dose level prevents nurses from selecting an incorrect medication.
- **Smart pumps** (IV infusion technologies used at the point of care) can help you avoid programming the wrong dose into the pump to ensure the correct dose is delivered. Once programmed, the delivery rate does not change. An alarm will sound or the pump will stop if a nurse attempts to program outside dosing limits or the flow is interrupted (e.g., blocked line). For more information on smart pump technologies, cases involving medication errors, and risk management strategies,

 Go to the FDA Web site at http://www.fda.gov/Safety/MedWatch/default.htm

- **Automated dispensing cabinets** minimize human handling of drugs in the pharmacy and are known to reduce medication errors when the built-in safety features are used. See the Safe, Effective Nursing Care box for examples of errors that can occur when technologies for administering medication are misused.

✚ Technology complements other safety regimes and cannot substitute for the need to adhere to all guidelines in medication administration. Rubin, Nash, and Safran (2012) presented a case scenario that resulted in the death of a premature infant and a pretrial settlement of $8.25 million. The numerous systems in place failed to detect human error that caused the infant to receive an IV that contained 60 times the normal dose of sodium.

What Should I Do If I Commit a Medication Error?

As a nurse, you have a duty to do no harm. If you make a medication error, even though you might be anxious about having put your patient at risk, be embarrassed to admit that you

Safe, Effective Nursing Care

Understanding the Limitations of Technologies for Medication Safety

Chapter Key Concept: Medication Safety

Competencies: Safety (Knowledge); Informatics (Knowledge, Skills, Attitudes)

It is important to understand the limitations of safety-enhancing technologies so that you can apply them correctly (Incorporate Technological Advances) and reduce the risk of patient harm (Safety).

Computerized provider order entry (CPOE). CPOE was hailed as the answer to prescribing errors and it has had many positive effects. However, several studies have reported mixed results: One documented 22 new types of errors, and one reported an *increase* in mortality after CPOE implementation. Factors contributing CPOE errors include:

➤ "Alert fatigue": the tendency for users to ignore frequent interruptions from warning messages
➤ Rigid programs that take users through multiple unnecessary screens or force unnecessary decisions. These encourage users to bypass decision points.
➤ The origin of the system—commercial versus designed in-house
➤ False sense of security generated by the belief that automated systems prevent errors

Bar-code-assisted medication administration (BCMA). A high rate of false-positive alerts has led to practitioner overrides and work-around actions. Of particular concern is the practice of "back scanning" in which the patient's bar code is scanned *after* medication administration. This greatly increases the risk of error and constitutes negligence.

Smart pump problems. These include software limitations and practitioner misuse (e.g., turning off the pump's dose-checking feature and bypassing alerts). Such actions are ethically and legally indefensible, and do not meet standards of care.

➤ How does Incorporate Technological Advances competency relate to the Provide Safe Quality Care competency?
➤ How can you avoid risky behaviors, contribute to the redesign of safety technologies, and put safe quality patient first when administering medications?

Sources: Agrawal, A. (2009); Ehteshami, A., Rezaei, P., Tavakoli, N., et al. (2013); Elias, B., & Moss, J. (2011); Goedert, J. (2010); Poon, E., Keohane, C., Yoon, C., et al (2010); Radley, D., Wasserman, M., Olsho, L., et al. (2013); Sittig, D., & Singh, H. (2011); Trbovich, P., Pinkney, S., Cafazzo, J., et al. (2010).

made a mistake, or fear you could lose your job, you must immediately assess the patient's vital signs and physical status and then report your findings to the patient's primary care provider. For detailed guidelines about actions to take if you commit a medication error, see Clinical Insight 25-1: Taking

Action After a Medication Error. Follow your institution's policy regarding incident reporting and other actions. Although an error does not actually occur until the patient has *taken* a medication, you may be required to file a report for a "near miss." These are errors detected during the checking procedure before drug administration (e.g., the pharmacy sent the wrong medication for a patient).

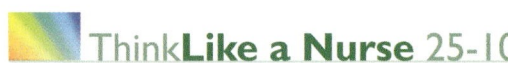

PracticalKnowledge
knowing **how**

Regardless of the type of medication or the route of administration, when administering a medication you should perform a medication-focused assessment, follow procedures for safe administration, and perform related interventions (e.g., explaining that a certain drug should be taken with food). The rest of this chapter explains these activities to you. You should become familiar with the **Medication Guidelines: Steps to Follow for All Medications (Regardless of Type or Route)** in the Practical Knowledge: Procedures section of this chapter.

ThinkLike a Nurse 25-10

Mr. Pearson (Meet Your Patients) refuses to take his 1400 dose of antibiotic, stating that he had just taken it. What actions should you take to ensure sound decision making and maintain patient safety?

ASSESSMENT NP

During your initial patient assessment, you will gather data that you need to administer medications safely. The following are highlights of medication-related assessments:

Before medicating patients:
- Measure vital signs.
- Assess whether the patient's general condition is appropriate for the medication.
- Evaluate your knowledge of the medication.
- Identify biological factors that affect drug metabolism.

While administering medications, assess:
- Mental status
- Coordination
- Ability to self-administer the drug
- Swallowing (for oral medications)

After medicating patients, assess:
- Effectiveness of the drug
- Side effects
- Signs of adverse reactions or toxicity

When Taking a Medication History explore the patient's allergy history (e.g., medication and food allergies), type of reactions, and treatment required. You should also ask about the patient's history of illness, attitudes toward medications, learning needs, and whether the patient (if a woman) is pregnant or breastfeeding. Also check relevant laboratory test results and obtain a list of current medications (prescribed and OTC) and prescribing providers. Ask the patient about his ability to have his prescriptions filled. Some patients are non-compliant because they cannot afford the medications.

Physical Examination helps you to identify potential problems and the need for adapting medication administration procedures. For example, laboratory tests results are used to monitor serum drug levels and evaluate proper dosages for the patient. You will also assess relevant body systems and vital signs to confirm the need for the drug (e.g., apical pulse before administering digoxin) and to provide a baseline for evaluating the patient's responses to it. For oral medications, assess the patient's ability to swallow; for intramuscular medications, assess muscle mass.

ANALYSIS/NURSING DIAGNOSIS NP

The following are some NANDA-I nursing diagnosis labels that might be useful when medicating patients:
    Deficient knowledge
    Risk for Allergic Reaction
    Ineffective health management
    Ineffective family health management
    Risk for Poisoning
    Risk for Aspiration
    Constipation
    Diarrhea
The following are some examples of nursing diagnoses you might write for patients receiving medications:
    Deficient Knowledge related to lack of motivation to learn
        about medications
    Ineffective Family Health Management related to anxiety
        over child's health status
    Risk for Aspiration related to Impaired Swallowing
    A few nursing diagnoses represent medication side effects; however, because a wide range of adverse effects is possible, no attempt was made to include them all. The following sections discuss Risk for Injury and Ineffective Health Management (nonadherence).

Risk for Injury

Risk for Injury may be related to polypharmacy and misuse, overuse, or underuse of medications.

Polypharmacy is the ingestion of numerous medications in an attempt to treat many conditions simultaneously. Many people self-prescribe or rely on OTC medications for symptom relief (e.g., insomnia, headaches, joint pains, indigestion). They may continue taking them in combination with prescribed medications. Polypharmacy increases the potential for adverse reactions and dangerous drug and food interactions.

   In older older adults, the likelihood of increased sensitivity to medications, drug interactions, and adverse drug effects increases as the number of medications taken increases (Perry, 2011). You should conduct an in-depth medication history to identify combinations that can be especially dangerous to them.

Misuse, Overuse, Underuse Some patients misuse, overuse, underuse, or use drugs inconsistently. They may even use them when contraindicated. For example, a person takes an antibiotic, "feels better" after a few days of the medication, and then stops taking it when symptoms are gone. The inconsistent dosage schedule hinders the body's ability to achieve a therapeutic blood level of the medication to treat the infection. Some drugs, such as beta blockers, can be dangerous or even life threatening when taken inconsistently.

Nonadherence

Nonadherence is failure to follow the treatment plan (e.g., not taking a prescribed medication or skipping doses). As you assess the patient's reasons for nonadherence, be prepared to address the numerous reasons, such as lack of symptoms, intolerable side effects, forgetfulness, inability to afford the medication, disagreement with the treatment plan, or lack of knowledge. Some patients, particularly older adults, have visual and motor deficits that limit their ability to read labels and manipulate access (e.g., bottle caps, syringes).

KnowledgeCheck 25-10

- What are the risks involved for patients who engage in polypharmacy?
- List at least three reasons for nonadherence to a medication regimen.

PLANNING OUTCOMES/EVALUATION NP

NOC standard outcomes depend on the specific nursing diagnoses you choose. The following are examples of NOC outcomes.

Knowledge: Medication, Treatment Regimen
Adherence Behavior
Bowel Elimination
Compliance Behavior
Comfort Status
Medication Response
Motivation
Risk Control: Drug Use
Self-Care: Non-Parenteral Medication, Parenteral Medication
Swallowing Status

Individualized goals/outcome statement you might write for a client should be stated so their achievement reflects resolution of the problem (NANDA-I label). The following are examples:

After explanation, and within 1 week, describes the expected actions and side effects of his medications.

Self-administers his medications in the correct amounts and on the prescribed schedule.

PLANNING INTERVENTIONS/ IMPLEMENTATION NP

NIC standardized interventions depend on the patient's nursing diagnoses, especially on the etiologies. Examples include:

Aspiration Precautions
Teaching: Psychomotor Skill, Prescribed Medication
Diarrhea Management
Discharge Planning
Health Education
Health System Guidance
Behavior Modification
Medication Management
Mutual Goal Setting
Self-Responsibility Facilitation
Surveillance

Specific individualized nursing activities include preparing and administering medications and teaching clients to self-administer their medications. You will use specific, step-by-step procedures for these activities. However, only the general principles are presented in this chapter.

TEACHING PATIENTS ABOUT MEDICATION SELF-ADMINISTRATION

Teach the following information to patients to help them safely administer their own medications.

Know and Understand What You Are Taking in order to take your drugs safely and effectively.

- **When you are prescribed a new medication, ask why you are taking it,** how long you should take it, what side effects to expect, whether you should take it with food, and about any special precautions.

- **Keep a list of your medications,** including doses and times taken. Take this list with you when you visit any healthcare provider or emergency department.

Take Your Drugs as Prescribed

- **Take the drug in its prescribed dose for the entire length of time** to receive its full benefit (e.g., some patients may take only part of an expensive antibiotic, hoping to "save it for later"). This can lead to infection or an antibiotic resistance may develop, leading to "superinfection," such as methicillin-resistant *Staphylococcus aureus* (MRSA).

- **Older adults may forget to take their medications.** A simple plan you can follow at home, such as a written schedule or a meds calendar, might help, especially if the drugs are taken other than at mealtimes and bedtime.

- **If you cannot see well,** ask a family member to write the schedule in large, black letters. Display it in a highly visible place.

- **Some older adults may take the medication, only to forget shortly thereafter that they did so.** Use a divided pill container or a small glass filled with the medications for each dosage time during the day. If the a.m. container is empty, you will know you have taken the morning drugs and won't accidentally repeat them.

Communicate With Your Prescriber Notify your prescriber if you have side effects, adverse reactions, or questions. If you become pregnant, notify your primary care provider as soon as possible so your medications can be discontinued or adjusted.

Think About Safety Be aware of your safety and the safety of others.

- **Wear a MedicAlert bracelet** or necklace if you are a diabetic, take anticoagulants, or have allergies to any medication.

- **Do not take medications prescribed to others** and do not share your medications with others.

- **If you take a variety of medications,** post a list of them in a prominent place that is easy to see in the event of an emergency.

- **Use childproof caps** if children have access to your medications. If no children are in the home, replace with simple closure cap for elderly patients who might have difficulty opening the containers. ✚ Families with young children visiting the homes of older adults need to be alert to the risk of accidental ingestion of medication.

- **Dispose of expired medications safely.** Do not place them in the trash. Disposing of drugs in the sink or toilet is not environmentally sound (e.g., they can appear in the community water supply). Your community may sponsor a "discard medications day" or provide a place to discard drugs. Check with your local pharmacy.

Administer Your Drugs Correctly as follows:

- **Read the label carefully on the bottle each time** you take the medication so that you take the correct medication in the prescribed dose. Many tablets look alike.

- **To measure liquids, use kitchen measuring spoons** rather than tableware, which can vary in volume.

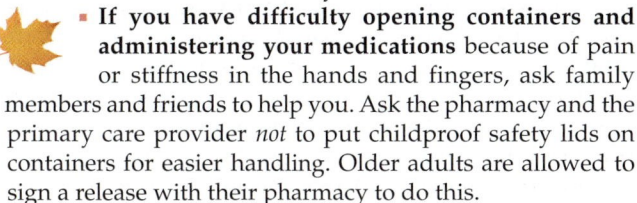

- **If you have difficulty opening containers and administering your medications** because of pain or stiffness in the hands and fingers, ask family members and friends to help you. Ask the pharmacy and the primary care provider *not* to put childproof safety lids on containers for easier handling. Older adults are allowed to sign a release with their pharmacy to do this.

Store Your Drugs Safely Do not store a drug in a different container from the one it came in. The medication may lose its strength, or you may take the wrong medication. Store all your medications in a dry place out of sunlight and away from heat. If a medication requires a cold storage, be sure you return it to the refrigerator immediately after use.

Maintain Your Supply Your drugs need to be up to date and available when you need them.

- **Monitor your prescription amounts and get refills before you run out.** If you get medications by mail, be sure you order them in plenty of time.
- **Check expiration dates** and properly discard any outdated medications.
- **Do not take expired medications;** they may have lost their strength.

ENSURING SAFE MEDICATION ADMINISTRATION

Medication errors are the most common type of healthcare adverse events. One such error is giving the dose to the wrong patient. Many other errors occur as a result of interruption or distraction. It is best not to stop what you are doing when preparing or giving medication. One recommendation is to create a "quiet zone" when preparing your medications. You can do this by putting up "do not disturb" signs, using the medication room, or wearing a bright yellow apron.

To help prevent errors, perform "three checks" and the "rights of medication" when giving medication. Also see **Medication Guidelines: Steps to Follow for All Medications (Regardless of Type or Route)** in the Practical Knowledge: Procedures section.

Three Checks

Check each medication three times:
1. *BEFORE you pour, mix, or draw up a medication,* check its label against the entry on the MAR. Be sure that the name, route, dose, and time match the MAR entry.
2. *AFTER you prepare the medication,* and before returning the container to the medication cart or discarding anything, check the label against the MAR entry again.
3. *AT THE BEDSIDE, check the medication again* before actually administering it.

Observing the "three checks" rule will help you to practice the "rights of medication."

Rights of Medication

Following the **rights of medication** means that you will give the (1) right medication to the (2) right patient in the (3) right dose using the (4) right route at the (5) right time with the (6) right documentation of the medication administration. This system helps you to prevent medication errors.

Right Drug

Obviously, you must always administer the correct medication. That is one reason for reading each label three times (see the "three checks"). Other ways to ensure giving the correct drug are to:
1. *Think Critically.*
   - Strictly adhere to the guidelines for taking verbal prescriptions.
   - Always check the MAR to ensure it is the right drug, dose, time, and route.

- Know the drugs you administer. If unsure or you don't know, look it up.
- Ask yourself whether the medication prescription is suitable for the patient's condition. If not, question the prescriber.
- Participate in daily patient rounds so you will be better informed about your patient's plan of care and why the medications are prescribed.

2. *Be aware of the pitfalls in abbreviations, units of measurement, and handwriting.*
   - Double-check all prescriptions transcribed by hand to the MAR.
   - Do not attempt to decipher illegible handwriting or confusing abbreviations. When in doubt, ask the prescriber to clarify.
   - Be alert for names that look very similar (e.g., Keflex and Keflin). It may be impossible to differentiate them when they are handwritten. Do not administer a drug prescribed by a nickname; be sure it is written out in full.

3. *Perform the "three checks" of the label against the MAR.* Include all of the following as part of the process:
   - Read the label before and after you prepare the medication, and again at the bedside to verify that you selected the correct product name and strength.
   - Select the prescribed medication from the patient's drug drawer (unless it is a stock drug). Do not "borrow" from another patient's drawer.
   - Do not substitute one medication for another.
   - Even when using a unit dose, read the label. Avoid selecting medications based on size and color because many medications are the same size, shape, and color as others.
   - Be alert for similar-looking labels. If you are accustomed to withdrawing oxytocin (given IV to stimulate uterine contractions) from a small vial with a green label, you might be surprised to find that the small green-label vial in your hand is actually hydroxyzine, which is harmful if given IV.
   - If a label is hard to read or comes off the container, return the container to the pharmacy. Never give a medication from such a container. Also, do not transfer medications from one pharmacy container to another.

4. *Take Special Care With Heparin.* Physically separate the highly concentrated heparin sodium (10,000 units/mL in 1-mL vials) from the more diluted 1-mL vials for flushing heparin locks. There is a risk for fatal hemorrhage if the highly concentrated heparin solution is mistakenly used to flush an IV line. Note the FDA-approved labeling that includes new color and design to distinguish the various heparin concentrations in the vials.

Right Dose

The right dose is the dose prescribed for a particular patient. Be sure the dose is within the recommended range for the patient's age, weight, and condition. The following are suggestions for avoiding dose errors:

- **Perform the "three checks" of the container against the MAR.** If the pharmacist has sent a dose different from the one prescribed, calculate how much of it to give. It is a good idea to have another nurse check your calculations. You should also know the drug's dosage range.
- **For IV medications, use smart infusion pumps** to help ensure that the correct dose is delivered.
- **Prepare the medications with precision** because *how* you prepare it can affect the dose the patient receives. When you must break a tablet, use a knife or a cutting device. If the

tablet does not break evenly, you should discard and account for it. When crushing a tablet to mix with liquid or food, clean the crushing device completely before and after using to remove any pieces of a previously crushed drug.

- **Read and write measurements carefully.** It is easy to misread "mg" instead of "mL." There is a significant difference between 1 mg and 1 mL of IV morphine.
- **Write out "international units"** instead of abbreviating as "IU." IU can be confused with IV.
- **Know how and when to use a zero.** Always write a zero *before* a decimal point. It is easy to mistake .15 for 115 if the decimal point is written large or the 1 is written small (e.g., write "Lanoxin 0.125 mg," not "Lanoxin .125 mg"). Conversely, never write a decimal point and a zero *after* a whole number. The decimal point may be mistaken for a 1 (e.g., write "5 mg," not "5.0 mg").
- **Question prescriptions for multiple tablets or vials** as a single dose; most doses are one or two tablets or one single-dose vial.
- **Question abrupt and excessive increases in dosage;** most dosages increase gradually.
- **Question prescriptions that are not consistent with the standard (protocol) dosage range** for the patient's age, weight, and condition.
- **Examine the standards of care and practice in your institution** to see whether they comply with The Joint Commission's National Patient Safety Goal for high-risk medications.

Right Time

- Check the prescription against the time to give the drug, and document the exact time of administration on the MAR.

   ✚ If the drug is not charted, never assume the patient received it as scheduled. If you do, the patient may not receive an essential medication; if you assume it has not been given and give it, the patient may receive an overdose.

- As a rule, you can give scheduled medications within a "window" of one-half hour before and one-half hour after the scheduled time.
- Time oral medications in relation to food. Give drugs that are irritating to the stomach (e.g., potassium, aspirin) with food; give drugs that absorb better on an empty stomach (e.g., tetracycline, iron supplement) before meals.
- Determine whether your patient is scheduled for any diagnostic or surgical procedures that require him to remain NPO. If so, you may need to hold oral or enteral medications, or have them changed to another route or time to maintain a therapeutic blood level.

Right Route

Recall that drug absorption is highly dependent on the route of administration. The following are suggestions for ensuring the right route:

- **Do not guess.** If the prescription does not specify a route, clarify with the prescriber. Many medications are available in multiple forms; others are made for one specific route. For example, cephalexin, an antibiotic, comes in capsules, suspensions for oral use, and injectable forms for IM and IV administration. By contrast, the antibiotic penicillin G procaine is prepared for IM injection and is *not* to be given intravenously.
- **The right route also includes right site.** If an intramuscular injection is prescribed, be sure the site is appropriate considering the age of the patient and the medical condition.
- **Use an oral syringe to draw up oral liquids** to avoid inadvertent IV administration.

Right Patient

- **Always double-check the patient's identification (ID) bracelet** just before giving the medication. This helps ensure that you have the correct patient. Always use two methods of patient identification; thus you should also ask the patient to state his name. It is best to say, "Please tell me your name," because patients with hearing impairment or confusion might respond "yes" incorrectly when asked, for example, "Are you Mary Smith?" Never skip this step, even if you are familiar with the patient. If you are busy and distracted, it is possible to enter the wrong room. Also, patients, especially when they are confused or emotionally disturbed, may enter the wrong room.
- **Do not leave medications at the bedside.** Suppose you are taking an oral tablet to a patient's room and find him in the bathroom. If you leave it on the table, how would you know whether he really took it? Someone else could come in and take or discard the medication.
- **Be alert for patients with the same last names.** It is common to have two patients with same or similar last names (e.g., Williamson, Wilkinson, Wilson, Wilkerson). Look for and place special alerts on charts and MARs to call attention to names that look or sound similar.
- **Ensure that order entry is made in the correct patient record** with the use of technological systems (e.g., CPOE, bar coding).

Right Documentation

Most nurses consider documentation the sixth right. After administering a medication, document it immediately on the patient's MAR, as in Figure 25-7. To see an electronic MAR, refer to Chapter 18. Be sure to document the following information:

- Name of medication given
- Dose of medication given
- Route of administration and injection site for parenteral medications
- Date and time administered
- Your name or initials as administering nurse

Most MARs are preprinted with the patient's name, name of the medication, dosage, and route administered (e.g., intramuscular, oral, or intravenous). If so, you need only to write the time you actually gave the medication, initial each medication, and sign the form one time. As for all charting, write legibly in ink.

If for some reason you do not administer a prescribed medication (e.g., patient refusal, NPO for tests or procedures), document that information on the MAR and write a nurse's note explaining why it was not given. For example:

mm/dd/yyyy 0800—Pt NPO for surgery this a.m. 0800 meds held as prescribed.————————————Janet King, RN.

When giving a prn medication, in addition to recording on the MAR, write a nursing note documenting your assessment and the time the drug was given. Then, after allowing time for the medication to be absorbed and take effect, evaluate and document the patient's responses. For example:

mm/dd/yyyy 0800—Pt reports abdominal pain at incision site rated as a #6 on a scale of 1–10. Active bowel sounds auscultated. Resp 16 breaths/min, HR 88 beats/min, BP 130/84. Denies N/V. Morphine 10 mg given intramuscularly in right vastus lateralis. No injection-related complaints (see MAR). ————Janet King, RN mm/dd/yyyy 0900—States pain relieved; "about 3" (scale of 1–10). Resp 14 breaths/min, HR 68 beats/min. BP 126/80. ————J. King, RN

HOSPITAL MEDICATION ADMINISTRATION RECORD

Codes For Injection Sites

A - Left Anterior Thigh	H - Right Anterior Thigh
B - Left Deltoid	I - Right Deltoid
C - Left Gluteus Medius	J - Right Gluteus Medius
D - Left Lateral Thigh	K - Right Lateral Thigh
E - Left Ventral Gluteus	L - Right Ventral Gluteus
F - Left Lower Quadrant	M - Right Lower Quadrant
G - Left Upper Quadrant	N - Right Upper Quadrant

Mary Smith 086432

age 46   John Miller, M.D.

ALLERGIES: *PCN, Sulfa*

				mm/dd/yyyy	mm/dd/yyyy	mm/dd/yyyy
mm/dd/yyyy		Lanoxin 0.25mg po Q D	0900	09 JW		
mm/dd/yyyy		Rocephin ÷1 gm IV Q D	1200	1200 JW		
mm/dd/yyyy		Zinacef ÷1 gm IV Q 8 hr	0800 ⎫	08 JW		
			1600 ⎬			
			2400 ⎭			

SIGNATURE / SHIFT INDICATES	7-3	JW	
NURSE ADMINISTERING MEDICATIONS	3-11		
J Wilson, RN	11-7		

FIGURE 25-7 After administering a medication, immediately document the date, time, dose, route, and person administering the medication on the MAR.

KEY POINT: *You are responsible for documenting the client's responses to all medications, including therapeutic effects, side effects, and unexpected or adverse reactions.* ✚ Never document a drug before you give it; never document a medication given by someone else; and do not ask someone else to document medications you administer.

Other Rights

In addition to the rights already discussed, patients also have the following rights about medications they receive:

- **Right Reason.** This includes the right not to receive unnecessary medications. For example, a tranquilizer or sleeping pill should be given because the patient is very anxious or cannot sleep, not for the convenience of caregivers who are weary of his incessant demands.
- **Right to Know.** You should tell the patient the name of the medication, why it is being given, its actions, and potential side effects.
- **Right to Refuse.** The patient has the right to refuse a medication regardless of her reasons and regardless of the consequences, except under certain circumstances (e.g., incompetency).

KnowledgeCheck 25-11

- What are the rights of medication?
- Give an example of each one.
- How many times, and when, should you check the medication against the MAR?

ADMINISTERING ORAL MEDICATIONS

The oral route is the one most commonly used for medications. Recall what you already know about oral medications: Where are they absorbed? What are their advantages and disadvantages? What assessments should you make? For procedural steps for administering various the following types of oral medications, see Procedure 25-1.

Pouring Liquid Medications

Liquid medications are frequently used for children and older adults. They usually come in multidose bottles, so you will need to pour individual doses into a disposable, calibrated cup.

✚ Numerous safety organizations recommend the removal of the dram scale on the oral liquid dosing cup because of adverse medication errors. These cups should only contain the measurement in mL (Agency for Healthcare Research and Quality, 2015a).

When pouring, hold the bottle so the liquid does not run over the label, making it difficult to read. Hold the cup at eye level when measuring (Fig. 25-8).

Buccal and Sublingual Medications

Although placed in the mouth, these medications are rapidly absorbed in the mucous membranes rather than in the GI tract. **Buccal medications** are held in the cheek; **sublingual medications** are held under the tongue (see Procedure 25-1). Some soluble forms of medications and enzyme preparations are administered by this route and absorbed within seconds.

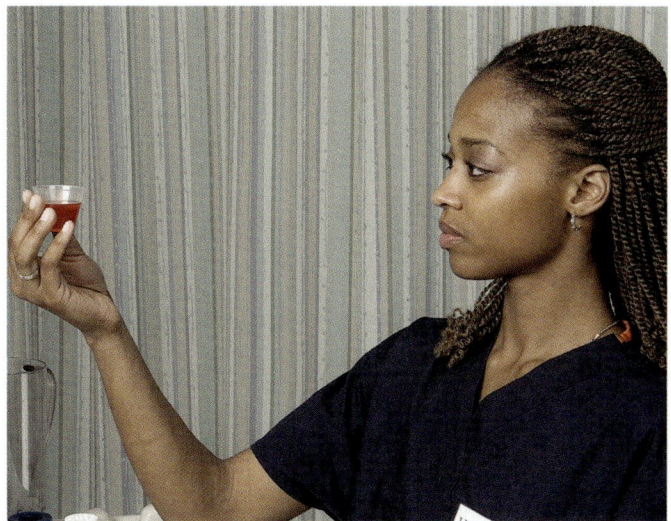

FIGURE 25-8 When pouring a liquid medication, measure the dose while holding the calibrated cup at eye level.

Enteral (Nasogastric and Gastrostomy) Medications

For patients who cannot swallow or who have feeding tubes, you can give oral medications through nasogastric (NG), gastrostomy, or jejunal tubes. Observe the following special considerations when administering enteral medications:

- *Hydrophilic medications,* such as psyllium (Metamucil)—Do not administer these through feeding tubes because they attract water and will solidify in the tube.
- *Crushing tablets*—Some tablets (e.g., enteric-coated or extended-release medications) should not be crushed, because crushing can change their action. Always check.
- *Continuous tube feedings*—Disconnect before giving medications.
- *Enteral tube suction*—Discontinue the suction for 30 minutes after administration and keep the tube clamped to allow time for the drug to be absorbed, if applicable.

For other procedures related to gastric and enteral tubes, see Procedures 27-2, 27-3, and 27-4.

Special Situations

For oral medications that discolor or damage tooth enamel, have an objectionable taste, are difficult to swallow, or cause the patient to gag, offer immediate oral hygiene. Also, follow these tips:

- **Medications that discolor the teeth.** Mix such drugs with liquid, have the patient drink the solution through a straw, and drink a liberal amount of flavored liquid (e.g., juice) or water afterward to dilute the medication, unless contraindicated.
- **Medications with an objectionable taste.** Have the patient suck on ice chips for several minutes before taking the medication to numb the taste buds. Unless contraindicated, you can store the medication in the refrigerator. The smell and taste are less objectionable when chilled, especially for oily liquids. When administering, place the medication on the back of the patient's tongue because there are fewer taste buds.
- **Contraindications to oral medications.** Do not give the drug to patients who are NPO, comatose, at risk for aspiration, or experiencing nausea or vomiting. Obtain a prescription for an alternative route or request permission to give the medication with small sips of water.

- **Patients who have difficulty swallowing medications.** Crush soluble tablets and place them in liquids or in a small amount of applesauce or pudding, unless contraindicated (e.g., time-released tablets).

KnowledgeCheck 25-12

- Describe two ways to ensure an accurate dosage when pouring liquid medications.
- What instructions should you give to a patient who is taking a sublingual medication?
- Explain the special step required when administering enteral medications to a patient who is receiving continuous tube feedings.
- Describe three methods for disguising the taste of objectionable tasting drugs.
- For which patients are oral medications contraindicated?

Administering Oral Medication to Children

Children are not motivated by logic. They do not grasp the cause and effect of "Take this; it will make you feel better." If they do not like the taste, they simply will not swallow the medication. Be aware that young children may not be able to swallow tablets and capsules. Therefore, most oral medications for children are prepared as sweetened and flavored liquids or chewable tablets. Always take special care to prevent choking and aspiration. Ask parents how they get their child to take medicines. You may also need to teach techniques for administering medications at home (see the Self-Care box Teaching Parents About Medicating Children).

Administering Oral Medications to Older Adults

Many interventions for older adults (e.g., facilitating swallowing) are the same as those discussed in the preceding section on Teaching Patients About Medication Self-Administration and in Procedure 25-1: Administering Oral Medication.

However, because of physiological changes associated with aging (see Table 25-2), older adults usually require smaller dosages of drugs, and physical responses to some medications are unpredictable. Therefore, you must carefully observe for both therapeutic and undesired effects. *Note:* The following interventions are for nurse-administered drugs (also see Box 25-4) and are not described in the self-administration discussion:

- **Address swallowing difficulties.** As the desire to drink decreases with age, the mouth often becomes drier, making it difficult to take large tablets. Crush tablets (if acceptable) or give drugs in liquid form. Try gently massaging the area just below the chin to initiate swallowing. For other strategies, collaborate with an occupational or speech therapist.
- **Accommodate slower reflexes and reasoning ability.** Allow more time to explain and administer medications. When teaching, keep instructions simple and repeat them often. Also reinforce the need to take the medication as prescribed. Some patients may think, "I don't feel any better when I take all this stuff." In the hospital, they may refuse to take medications, or they may put the tablets in their mouths and spit them out when you leave the room. Stay with the patient until you see that he has swallowed the medications.

Self-Care

Teaching Parents About Medicating Children

1. Mark each bottle or syringe containing medication with a different color of tape or adhesive label. This makes each clearly distinguishable because many medication bottles look alike.

2. You can reuse syringes for oral medications until the markings or tape begins to wear off or the plunger becomes difficult to move. Wash syringes with warm, soapy water, rinse well, and allow to air dry.

3. Take your time when giving medication, and find a quiet environment. Don't rush the process. It can be frustrating to struggle with a young child who is resisting taking a medication, especially if your time is limited.

4. Give the medication at the same time each day so it becomes a matter of routine. It is easier to remember when a pattern is established.

5. If the child is old enough to understand, warn him when a medication has an unpleasant taste (e.g., "John, this doesn't taste very good, but you can have a big drink of juice as soon as you swallow it"). You may lose his trust if you surprise him with a bad taste.

6. Give the child a frozen fruit bar or frozen flavored ice pop just before the medication. This helps to numb the taste buds to weaken the taste of the medication.

7. To mask bad-tasting medicines, you can crush tablets or empty the contents of a capsule and mix with soft foods, such as applesauce, hot cereal, or pudding. This is helpful for children who might aspirate liquids. (**Caution:** Check a drug reference book or with the prescriber before crushing a tablet or emptying a capsule. Some medications should not be crushed.)

8. Do not use essential foods in the child's diet (e.g., milk or orange juice) to mask the taste of medications. The child may later refuse a food he associates with the medicine.

9. To prevent choking or aspiration when giving liquids to infants and toddlers, hold the child in a sitting or semi-sitting position. Use a medicine dropper or syringe to place the medication between the gum and cheek. Instill the medication; avoid giving too much, too fast.

10. Always praise the child after she swallows the medication.

BOX 25-4 ■ Reducing Risk for Medication Errors for Older Adults

- **Be alert to unnecessary drug therapy.** It is not unusual for prescribers to be reluctant to stop a medication or simply forget to do so. The likelihood of a poor outcome increases as the number of drugs prescribed increases.
- **Request the indication for use** on all medication prescriptions.
- **Suggest nonpharmacological interventions** (e.g., warm massage, guided imagery) before prescribing medication for new symptoms.
- **Consider the "snowball effect."** This occurs when the provider prescribes a drug to counter the side effects of the initial treatment drug. A third drug is then prescribed to counter the side effect of the second drug and so on. To interrupt this phenomenon, the prescriber can discontinue the medication, reduce the dose, or substitute one that the patient tolerates better.
- **Verify that a newly prescribed medication** does not have a documented drug-drug interaction. Check that the prescribed dosage is correct within the desired range.
- **When titrating drug doses, start low and go slow.** It's best to start with the lowest possible dose when starting a medication because adverse drug effects are dose related and older adults tend to be more sensitive.
- **Assess urinary status.** Many drugs are cleared through the renal system. Some have toxic effects on the kidneys, particularly for older adults.
- **Recommend safer drugs** if the prescriber initiates medication associated with adverse outcomes for older adults. The benefit must exceed the risk to the patient (Zwicker & Fulmer, updated 2012).

KnowledgeCheck 25-13

- What is the chief danger when administering oral medications to children?
- How can you help a person who has some difficulty swallowing oral medications?
- How can you be sure that patients are not spitting out their medications after you leave the room?

ADMINISTERING TOPICAL MEDICATIONS

Topical medications are applied directly to a body site or placed in body cavities by irrigation or instillation. Their action depends on how the drug is prepared:

- *Local effects*—Examples are zinc oxide ointment to protect the skin against irritation associated with bowel and bladder incontinence and corticosteroid creams for itching.
- *Systemic effects*—These are absorbed through the skin and mucous membrane (e.g., estrogen patches; also see Transdermal Medications, following).

Lotions, Creams, and Ointments

Before applying medications to the skin, assess for contraindications (e.g., skin irritation, open lesions). Use a cotton swab, tongue blade, or gloved finger to apply these types of medications so your skin does not absorb them. For step-by-step instructions, see Procedure 25-7A.

Transdermal Medications

Designed to be absorbed through the skin, transdermal medications are prepared as patches made of a special membrane. Patches allow constant, controlled amounts of medications to be released over 24 hours or more, giving a prolonged systemic effect (e.g., nitroglycerin, used to control angina or chest pain; scopolamine, used to treat motion sickness; nicotine, used to control smoking urges). Most patches are prepared with the correct dose already applied and should not be cut; however, some can be cut and are self-adherent (e.g., lidocaine). Check the package insert or ask a pharmacist about proper handling, application, and disposal of patches. Always wear gloves to prevent absorption of the drug (see Procedure 25-7D).

PERFORMING IRRIGATIONS AND INSTILLATIONS

Washing out a body cavity with a steady stream of fluid or water is called **irrigation.** Sterile water, saline, or antiseptic solutions are flushed into the eyes, ears, throat, vagina, rectum, or urinary tract to wash out the cavity. **Instillation** is the insertion into a body cavity (e.g., eye drops) of medication for retention or absorption. Some medications need to remain in the body cavity for a period of time to achieve their maximum effect. Irrigations and instillations are performed to:

- Remove discharge or foreign bodies (e.g., from the eye or ear).
- Apply heat and cold to an area.
- Apply medications (e.g., antiseptics).
- Prepare an area for surgery (e.g., an enema for cleansing the bowels).

You will usually not use sterile technique unless there are breaks in the skin. Specific types of syringes are used for irrigating and instilling medications and fluids. Each is calibrated to allow you to control the amount and speed of solution delivered into the cavity (Fig. 25-9).

Ophthalmic Medications

Ophthalmic ointments or solutions are used for their local effects to treat eye infections and glaucoma, to lubricate to counter dryness, or to irrigate the eye to remove foreign bodies, secretions, or harmful chemicals. During an eye examination, medications may also be used to anesthetize the eye, dilate the pupil, or temporarily stain the cornea to identify abraded areas.

✚ Ophthalmic medications are packaged in small bottles or tubes with a label that states, "*For ophthalmic use only.*" Do not place any medication in the eye unless that statement appears on the container. Damage to the eye can result in permanent blindness.

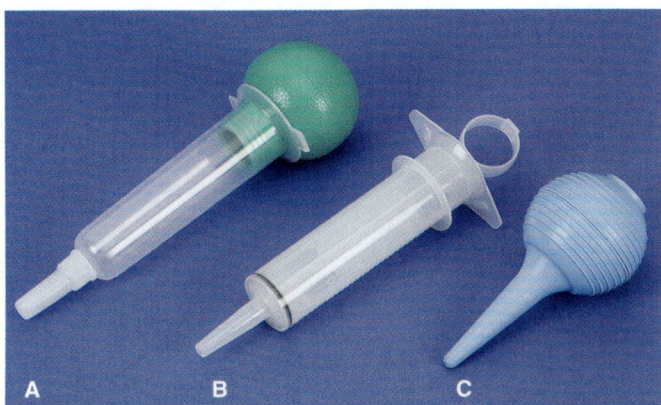

FIGURE 25-9 Syringes for administering enteral medications and performing irrigations and instillations. A. Asepto syringe: Plastic syringe with rubber bulb. B. Toomey (piston) syringe: Calibrated plastic syringe with removable tip that fits into the end of a tube (e.g., urinary catheter or enteral tube). For deep wound and bladder irrigations and administration of enteral medications. C. Rubber bulb syringe, for ear irrigations.

The **cornea** (the transparent part of the sclera in front of the iris and pupil) is easily injured, so you should not place medications directly on the eyeball. Do not touch the tip of the dropper or tube to the eye or conjunctiva; this may lead to bacterial growth on the container or damage the eye. For the step-by-step procedure, see Procedure 25-2. See Chapters 21 and 31 for information about the structure and function of the eyes.

Otic Medications

Medications or solutions may be dropped into the ear to treat internal and external ear infections, to apply heat to the area, and to soften and remove earwax. Use solutions at room temperature because a solution that is too hot or too cold may cause vertigo, nausea, and pain. You will use clean technique when administering otic medications. ✚ To prevent infection, use sterile technique if the tympanic membrane (eardrum) has been ruptured or a surgical procedure has been done.

See Chapters 21 and 31 for information about the structure and function of the ear. To learn the skill, see Procedure 25-3.

Nasal Medications

Clients usually self-administer nasal drops and sprays, many of which are available without a prescription. The most common nasal medications are used in the treatment of nasal congestion from colds and sinus infections. Nasal decongestants are used to shrink swollen mucous membranes and allow for better airflow and drainage of mucus. Caution your patient that long-term use of decongestants may cause a **rebound effect** that requires continual use of the drug to achieve nasal decongestion. The nasal congestion is relieved immediately after use, but recurs and even increases when the effects of the drug wear off. See Chapters 21 and 31 for information about the structure and function of the nose. For complete procedure steps, see Procedure 25-4.

Vaginal Medications

Vaginal medications come in various forms, including foams, jellies, liquids (douches), creams, tablets, and suppositories. They are used for several purposes: contraception, to destroy bacteria before gynecological surgery, to reduce dryness, to treat itching or infection, or to induce labor. To keep suppositories firm, store them in the refrigerator before use. Foams and jellies are inserted using an applicator or inserter. Provide a clean perineal pad to absorb drainage. For the complete procedure, see Procedure 25-5.

A **douche** is a vaginal irrigation using low pressure. Douches are used to administer antimicrobial solutions, remove irritating discharge, or apply heat or cold to reduce inflammation.

KEY POINT: *Teach women that douching may be harmful because it disturbs the normal pH and healthy balance of microorganisms in the vagina. Research has shown a connection between douching and ovarian cancer (Gonzalez, O'Brien, Aloisio, et al., 2016).*

Rectal Medications

Rectal suppositories and liquid instillations **(enemas)** are used to encourage bowel movements or to treat systemic complaints such as nausea (antiemetic medication). The rectal route may provide for higher blood levels of the medication than does the oral route because venous blood from the rectum does not pass through the liver before entering the general circulation. They can also be given in a colostomy stoma in certain patients. For a procedure for inserting a rectal suppository, see Procedure 25-6; for administering an enema, see Procedure 29-3.

ADMINISTERING RESPIRATORY INHALATIONS

Nebulization is the production of a fine spray, fog, powder, or mist from a liquid drug. The patient inhales the medication mixture by breathing deeply through a mouthpiece attached to the nebulizer. Absorption is rapid owing to the vascularity of the airways and alveoli.

Types of Nebulizers

The following are four types of devices for achieving nebulization:

1. *Atomizers* disperse the medication in the form of large droplets.
2. *Aerosol sprayers* suspend the droplets of medication in a gas (e.g., oxygen).
3. *An ultrasonic (handheld) nebulizer* mixes a small volume of medication, usually less than 1 mL, with 3 mL of normal saline. The device forces air through the nebulizer and delivers medication and humidity as a fine mist that can be inhaled deep into the lungs.
4. *A metered-dose inhaler (MDI)* (Fig. 25-10) is a type of nebulizer that delivers measured doses of a nebulized drug.

No matter which device is used, the smaller the droplets, the farther the medication can be inhaled into the respiratory tract.

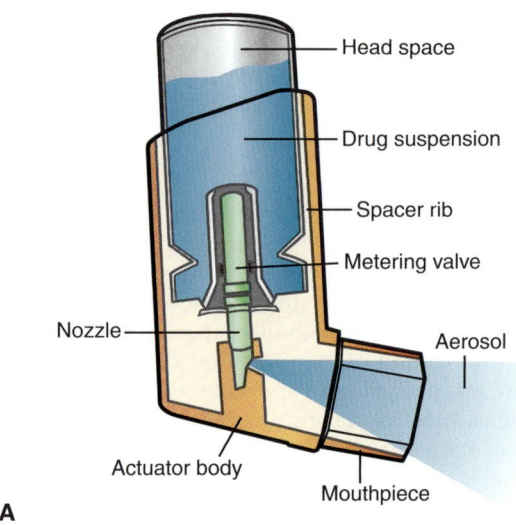

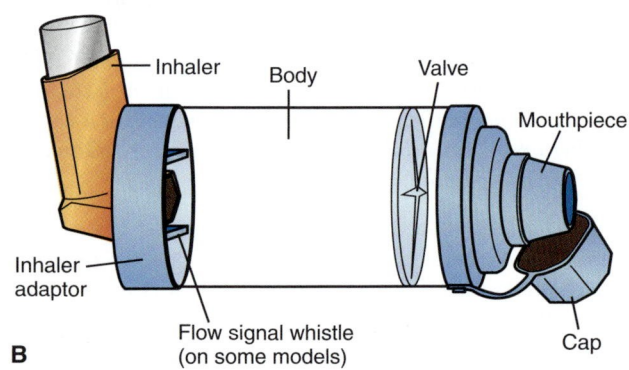

FIGURE 25-10 Inhalers. A. Metered-dose inhaler. B. Inhaler with a spacer.

Metered-Dose Inhalers and Dry Powder Inhalers

A **metered-dose inhaler (MDI)** is a pressurized container prefilled with several doses of a drug and an ecofriendly substance, hydrofluoroalkane, to propel the medication forward. The advantage of MDIs is that high doses of medication can be rapidly instilled in the lungs, producing local effects directly in the airway while avoiding systemic side effects. The patient inhales while pushing the canister's pump to release a measured dose of medication through a mouthpiece (see Fig. 25-10A). Sometimes an extender (spacer) is attached to the mouthpiece to enhance the delivery of medication into the respiratory tract (see Fig. 25-10B). Medication is pumped into the extender instead of directly into the patient's mouth. The patient inhales the drug from the chamber.

A **dry powder inhaler (DPI)** is activated by a pump rather than by inhalation. Once the dose is loaded, the patient simply takes a deep breath. DPIs are not designed to be used with a spacer. Patients frequently self-administer inhalations (most often bronchodilators or steroids) using an MDI. Teach your patient how to coordinate the inhalation of the medication and the pushing of the canister, to inhale and exhale deeply to correctly administer the dose (Fig. 25-11), and to track the number of puffs used to avoid the canister being unexpectedly empty when needed. See Procedure 25-8 to learn how to administer a metered-dose inhaler and keep track of the remaining doses.

KnowledgeCheck 25-14

- Why should you use a cotton swab, tongue blade, or gloved finger to apply corticosteroid creams and other topical medications?
- Most of the following routes are used for both local and systemic effects. Which one is used *only* for medications intended for systemic absorption (i.e., which one is *not* used for local effects): lotions, creams, ointments, transdermal patches, or irrigations?
- When administering eye drops, how can you prevent injury to the cornea?
- When should you use sterile technique when performing otic instillations?
- What are two of the undesired effects of self-administered nasal decongestants?
- What possible harm can result from vaginal douching?

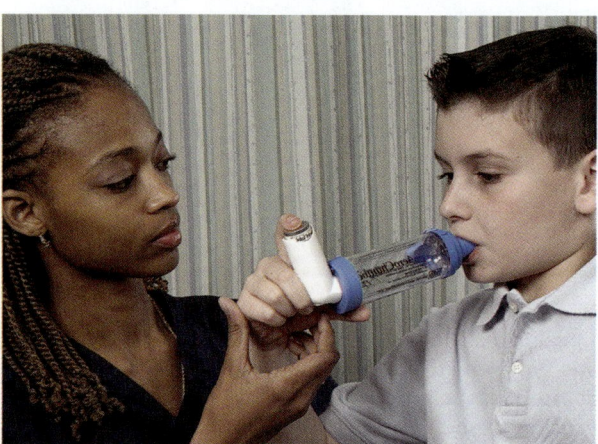

FIGURE 25-11 Child using a metered-dose inhaler with an extender.

- When is rectal instillation of a drug preferred over oral administration?
- When, as a rule, are rectal medications contraindicated?
- Define *nebulization*.
- What is the best way to determine whether a metered-dose inhaler is empty?

ADMINISTERING PARENTERAL MEDICATIONS

Parenteral medications include those that are injected or infused into body tissues or into the bloodstream via the intradermal, subcutaneous, intramuscular, or intravenous routes. Parenteral injections are absorbed faster and more completely than drugs given by other routes; therefore, the results are more predictable and the dosage can be measured more accurately. You must prepare and administer parenteral medications accurately, because the medications, once given, cannot be retrieved. Tissue damage may result if the pH, osmotic pressure, or solubility of the medication is not appropriate to the tissue where the medication is given. For example, medications intended for injection into muscle may damage subcutaneous tissue.

Equipment for Parenteral Medications

When administering injectable (parenteral) medications, you must know about various kinds of needles and syringes. You will need to decide, based on each situation, what size and type of needle and syringe to use. For a summary of the sites and equipment used for parenteral administration, refer to Table 25-6.

Reusing Equipment at Home Many people (e.g., those who have diabetes) must give themselves repeated injections, perhaps several each day. Supplies for home use are expensive. Insurance may or may not cover the cost, or the person may not have insurance. Therefore, although health professionals and manufacturers recommend that disposable syringes and needles be used only once, some people find it practical to reuse them. If they do, you can help them to do it more safely by teaching them the content in Clinical Insight 25-2: Reusing Needles and Syringes: Home Care

Table 25-6 ▶ Parenteral Injections: Comparison of Sites and Equipment

ROUTE	SITE	MAX VOLUME (mL)	NEEDLE GAUGE	NEEDLE LENGTH (inch)	SYRINGE SIZE (mL)	ANGLE OF INJECTION (degree)
Intradermal	Inner aspect of forearm	0.1	26–28	⅜	1.0	5°–15°
Subcutaneous Insulin	Fatty area over triceps, abdomen, anterior thigh	0.3, 0.5, and 1.0	28–31	3⁄16–1 (max ⅝ for upper arm)	0.3, 0.5, 1 (0.3–0.5 for upper arm)	45°–90°
Subcutaneous Other	Fatty area over triceps, abdomen, anterior thigh	0.5–1	25–27	⅜–⅝	1.0–3.0	45°–90°
Intramuscular	Deltoid	0.5–1	22–25	⅝–1 (infants and children) 1–1½ (adults)	1.0	90°
	Rectus femoris (*not recommended*)	2	22–25	1½–3	1.0	90°
	Vastus lateralis	1.0 (infants < 12 months) 1–2 (infants and children 1–12 years) 3–5 (adults, depending on muscle size)	22–25	1 (infants < 12 months) 1–1¼ (infants 12–24 months) 1½–3 (adults, depending on if obese)	1.0–3.0	45°–90°
	Ventrogluteal	2.5–3	20–25	1½–3	3.0	90°
Intravenous	Cephalic veins	Continuous infusion	18–25	1–1½		N/A
	Basilic veins	Continuous infusion	18–25	1–1½		N/A

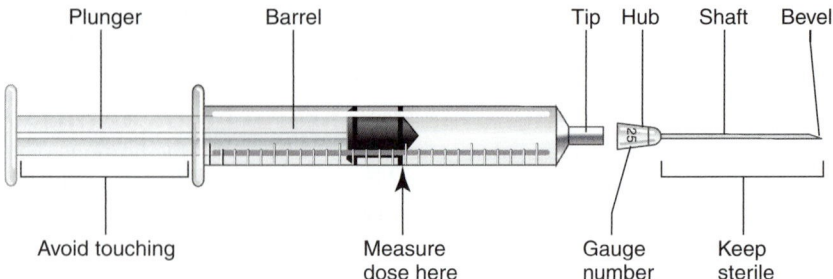

Plunger   Barrel   Tip Hub   Shaft   Bevel

Avoid touching   Measure   Gauge   Keep
                      dose here   number   sterile

FIGURE 25-12 Parts of a needle and syringe.

Needles

Needles are disposable stainless steel sheaths that attach to a syringe. Figure 25-12 shows the parts of a needle. Needles are made in various lengths and gauges and with different bevel sizes.

Gauge refers to the inside diameter of the needle lumen. Needle gauges are numbered 14 through 30: the smaller the gauge, the larger the diameter (i.e., a 16-gauge needle has a larger diameter than does a 20-gauge needle). Choose the gauge based on the patient's size and skin condition, the viscosity of medication used, and the speed of administration desired. Smaller needles (25- to 30-gauge) cause less pain and trauma to the tissue, so they are useful for patients who must have frequent or long-term injections (e.g., insulin and heparin). Larger needles (14- to 18-gauge) are used for blood and more viscous medications, to mix intravenous (IV) medications, or for rapid infusion of IV medications.

Bevel is the slanted tip with a narrow slit. The slant of the tip creates an opening that will close quickly to prevent leakage of medication, blood, and serum. A long bevel tip is sharper and narrower and therefore causes less discomfort during injection. Long bevels are usually used for subcutaneous and intramuscular (IM) injections. Short bevels are used for intradermal or IV injections. To see bevel types, refer to the Equipment list in Procedure 25-11.

Needle Length is the distance from the tip to the hub (bottom) of the needle. They usually range from ⅜ inch to 3 inches. Choose the length according to the thickness of the patient's muscle and adipose tissue and the site in which the drug is to be injected. For example, use a longer needle for intramuscular injections and a shorter one for intradermal injections. A 1 ½-inch needle is common for intramuscular injections, but you would use a shorter one for a child or a very thin person.

Filter Needles and Filter Straws are used to trap rubber or glass fragments when drawing up a medication from a vial or an ampule. You must replace the filter needle with a regular needle before injecting the medication into the patient or into the IV solution.

Safety Needles Many safety needle devices are available. Examples include a resheathing system with a sliding barrel that shields the needle, syringes with retractable needles, and needles with attached covers that reduce the risk of accidental puncture with contaminated needles (Fig. 25-13).

ThinkLike a Nurse 25-11

- You are to give an intramuscular injection of 1 mL of a thin, watery medication to a frail patient with very little muscle mass (5 ft 5 in. tall, weighs 96 lb). You have these needle sizes available: 16 gauge, 20 gauge, 25 gauge. Which would you use and why?
- For the same patient, you have needles available in 1-inch and 1½-inch lengths. Which would you use and why?

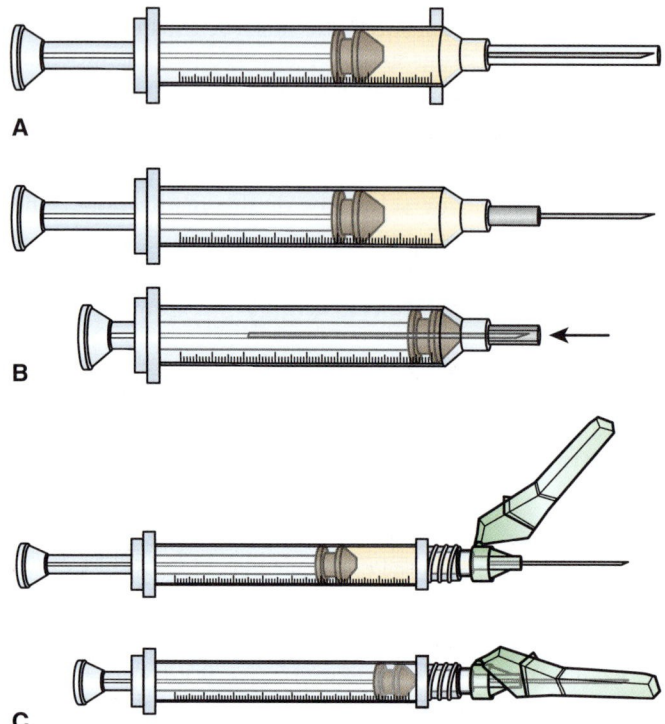

A

B

C

FIGURE 25-13 Needle safety features. A. Self-sheathing safety feature: Sliding needle shields attached to disposable syringes and vacuum tube holders. B. Syringe with retractable needle. C. Needles with covers.

Syringes

A syringe consists of a barrel, plunger, and syringe tip (Fig. 25-14). Because injections require strict sterile technique, you may touch the outside of the barrel and end of the plunger but not the inside of the barrel, hub, shaft of the plunger, or needle.

Syringes are usually made of plastic and are disposable. Some have the needle attached; others do not. The syringe tip, either **luer-lock** (twist on) or **non-luer-lock** (slip on), fits into the needle hub (Fig. 25-14). Syringes are made in various sizes, from 0.5 mL to 60 mL. The larger sizes are used for instillations and irrigations. You will usually use a 2-mL or 3-mL syringe for intramuscular injections (Fig. 25-15).

- **Standard syringes** are supplied in 3-, 5-, and 10-mL sizes. They are commonly supplied without needles or with 18-, 21-, 23-, or 25-gauge needles that are 0.5 to 3 inches long. To ensure accurate measurement of drugs, syringes are calibrated and marked in 0.1-mL and 1- or 2-mL increments.
- **Tuberculin syringes** have a 1-mL capacity and are calibrated in 0.01-mL increments; they come with a small (usually 25- to 28-) gauge, short (½- to ⅝-in.) needle. Use tuberculin syringes to administer small, precise doses of

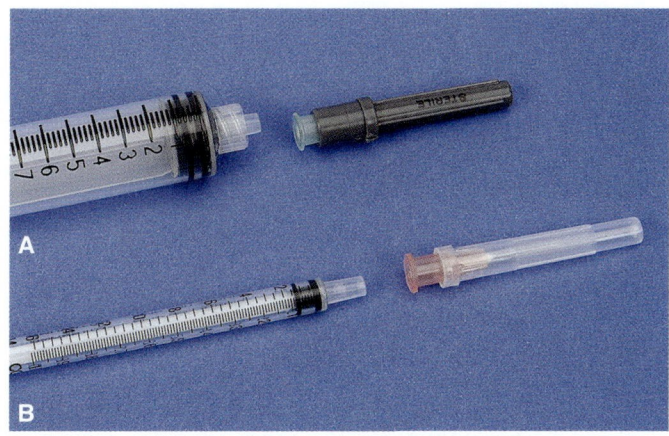

FIGURE 25-14 Syringe tips. A. Luer-lock (twist-on) tip.
B. Non-luer-lock (slip-on) tip.

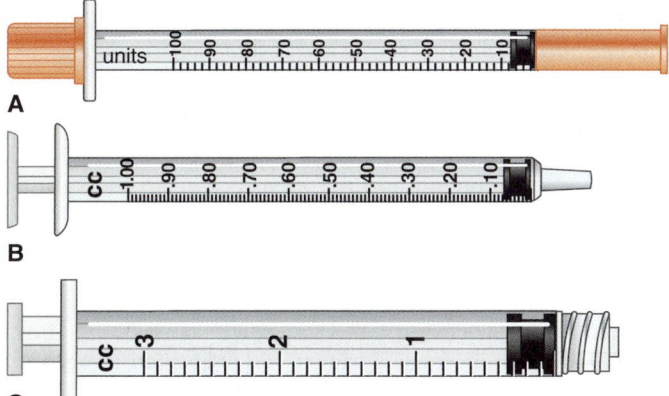

FIGURE 25-15 Syringe types. A. 100-unit insulin syringe
marked in units. B. 1-mL tuberculin syringe marked in
increments of 0.01 mL. C. 3-mL standard syringe marked
in increments of 0.1 mL.

medication (e.g., infants or children); for allergy tests; or
when administering potentially dangerous medications,
such as heparin.
- **Insulin syringes** are calibrated in units and are used to administer insulin. Insulin syringes are marked in 100 units
per milliliter. They are made in 0.3-, 0.5-, or 1-mL sizes with
very small-gauge needles (26- to 30-gauge).
- **Prefilled unit-dose systems** are reusable syringe holders
that hold disposable, single-dose, prefilled medication cartridges. No medication preparation is necessary, but you
must check each cartridge and dose carefully because all of
the cartridges look alike. You simply insert the cartridge into
the holder and lock it in place. After administering the medication, dispose of the cartridge; keep the holder for reuse.
- **Disposable prefilled, self-contained systems** are available for hospitals, office practices, nursing homes, and
self-administration. The injection plunger is attached to
the medication barrel and twists in directly. This ready-to-
use syringe reduces the risk of constituting or dosing
errors. Because you do not need to remove the cartridge
from the holder after using it, the risk of a needlestick
injury is reduced (Fig. 25-16). For guidelines for using
prefilled syringes, see Clinical Insight 25-3.
- **Safety needles.** Several devices are available, including devices featuring a resheathing system with a sliding barrel

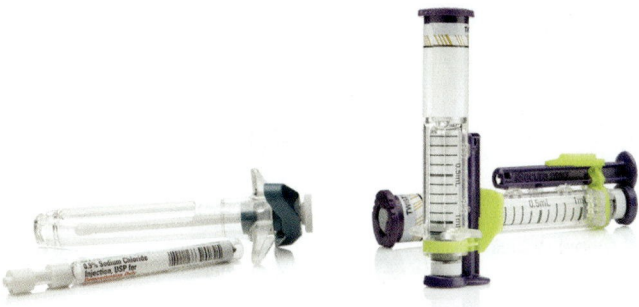

FIGURE 25-16 *(Left)* Prefilled unit-dose system. *(Right)*
Disposable, prefilled, self-contained system.

that shields the needle (Fig. 25-17); syringes with retractable
needles that spring back into the barrel of the syringe; and
needles with attached covers that reduce the risk of accidental puncture with contaminated needles.

KnowledgeCheck 25-15

- What does the term *parenteral* mean?
- What are two disadvantages of the parenteral route?
- To maintain sterile technique, which part of a syringe must you
  not touch?
- You need to irrigate a wound. Which syringe size do you need:
  0.5 mL, 3 mL, 5 mL, or 50 mL?
- Which syringe would you use for an intramuscular injection,
  as a rule: tuberculin, 50-mL, 5-mL, or 3-mL syringe?

Drawing Up and Mixing Medications

Most injectable medications are packaged in single-dose or
multidose ampules and vials.

Drawing Up Medications From an Ampule

An **ampule** is a thin-walled, disposable glass container with a
narrow neck that you must snap off to access the medication.
To prevent injuries, use an ampule opener to snap the glass
(Fig. 25-18). Each ampule holds a single dose of a liquid medication, usually 1 mL to 10 mL, but some hold 50 mL. To learn
how to use ampules, see Procedure 25-9A.

Drawing Up Medications From a Vial

A **vial** is a single-dose or multidose plastic or glass container
with a rubber stopper that reseals the top after each needle
introduction. A plastic or metal cap covers the rubber stopper to protect it until it is used (Fig. 25-19). Because the vial
is a closed system, you must inject air into it to withdraw the
solution. Otherwise, a vacuum is created in the vial that

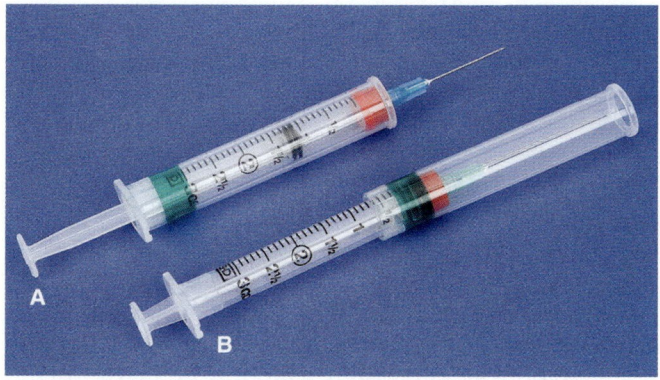

FIGURE 25-17 Safety syringe. A. Needle guard position before
injection. B. Needle guard position after injection.

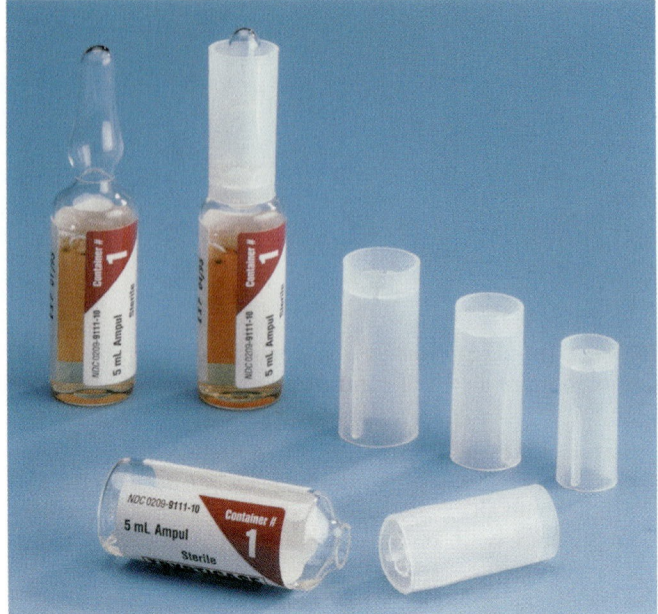

FIGURE 25-18 Safety device for opening glass ampules.

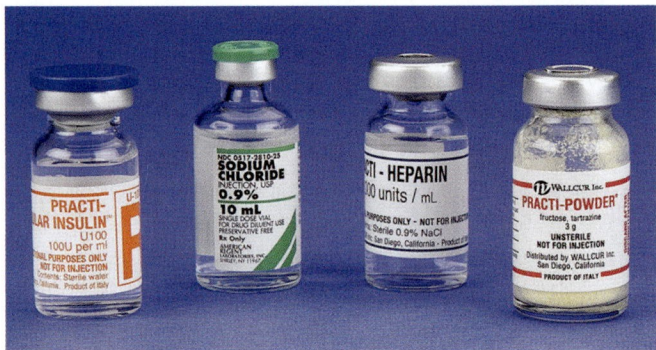

FIGURE 25-19 Vials containing medications.

makes withdrawal difficult. To learn how to use vials, see Procedure 25-9B.

Nurses traditionally wipe the rubber stopper with alcohol after removing the cap, even on a single-dose vial. The practice removes dust and rubber particles from the top of the vial as does using a filter needle or straw. Always follow your institution's policy.

Reconstituting Medications

Medications that are not stable in solution are dispensed as powders in vials. You must add a diluent or solvent to the powder to create a solution for injection. The diluent is usually sterile water or saline; however, each packaged vial includes the manufacturer's instructions for the amount and kind of solvent to add. For safety, use a plastic vial access cannula instead of a needle when possible. For guidelines, refer to Clinical Insight 25-4.

Mixing Medications in the Same Syringe

You can mix two medications in the same syringe (1) if they are compatible, (2) if the total dose is within accepted limits, and (3) if they are both prescribed by the same route. This technique allows for efficient use of supplies and fewer patient injections.

Medications are **compatible** if they can be mixed without affecting their constituents or actions. Package inserts

and medication references usually include compatibility information.

➕ Always check the compatibility before mixing medications together. If the contents of the syringe become discolored, there are visible particles in the solution, or there is a change in consistency, do not administer the medications.

When mixing medications in one syringe, you must follow these principles:

- Maintain sterile technique (as with all parenteral medications).
- Do not contaminate one container with medication from the other container. In most cases, you must use a separate needle to withdraw from each vial.
- A single-use vial contains only one dose of medication. Even if you do not administer the entire dose, the remaining amount must be discarded.
- Ensure the total, final dosage is correct by adding the volumes of the two medicines together before administering (see Procedure 25-9C).

KEY POINT: *A single-dose vial should only be used one time for one patient, using a sterile needle and sterile syringe.*

Accounting for Needle "Dead Space"

Some nurses believe a small amount of the patient's medication remains in the needle when an injection is given. Therefore, they recommend adding 0.2 mL of air to the syringe after measuring a medication for IM injection. Nurses are not in agreement regarding this practice and, unfortunately, there is scant research to provide evidenced-based guidance. Theoretically, on injection the air clears the needle of medication, ensuring that the patient receives the entire dose. However, because syringes are calibrated to account for medication left in the needle, and because the medication left in the needle after injection is the same amount as before the injection, many believe that air should not be added. We recommend that you add air only in the following situations:

1. *When the medication is irritating to subcutaneous tissues,* add 0.2 mL of air after measuring the proper dose. The air drives the medication deep into the subcutaneous tissue and creates an air lock above the medication, preventing it from tracking through subcutaneous tissue.
2. *When you change needles after drawing up the medication (e.g., replace a filter needle).* The new needle has air in it instead of medication. If you push the plunger until you see a drop of medication at the tip of the needle, you will see that you no longer have a complete dose in the syringe. Pulling in 0.2 mL of air before changing the needle and then pushing the plunger until you see a drop of medication at the tip of the new needle will prevent the loss of medication with the needle change.

Also refer to Clinical Insight 25-5 for technique.

Preventing Needlestick Injuries

Workplace injuries occur from needles and other sharps, putting healthcare workers at risk for bloodborne diseases (e.g., hepatitis B, hepatitis C, HIV) (see Chapter 23). Needleless systems reduce the risk of needlestick. Figure 25-20 shows three such devices. Also see Clinical Insight 23-1 in Chapter 23, and Procedure 25-10: Recapping Needles Using a One-Handed Technique.

The Centers for Disease Control and Prevention (CDC) and the Occupational Safety and Health Administration (OSHA) recommend the use of "needleless" systems. Most systems

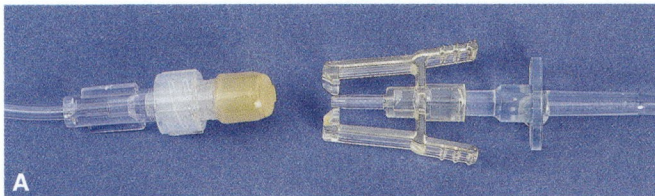
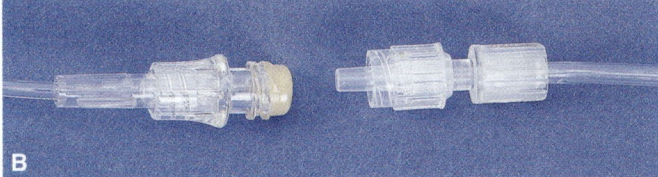
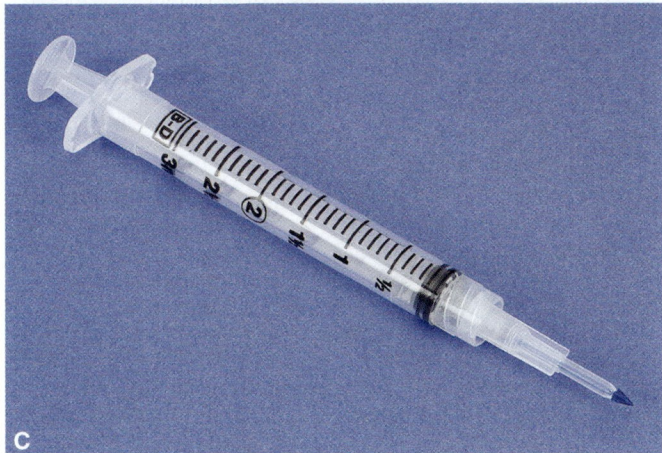

FIGURE 25-20 Needleless systems. A. Lever-lock cannula. B. Threaded lock cannula. C. Blunt-tipped syringe for drawing up medication.

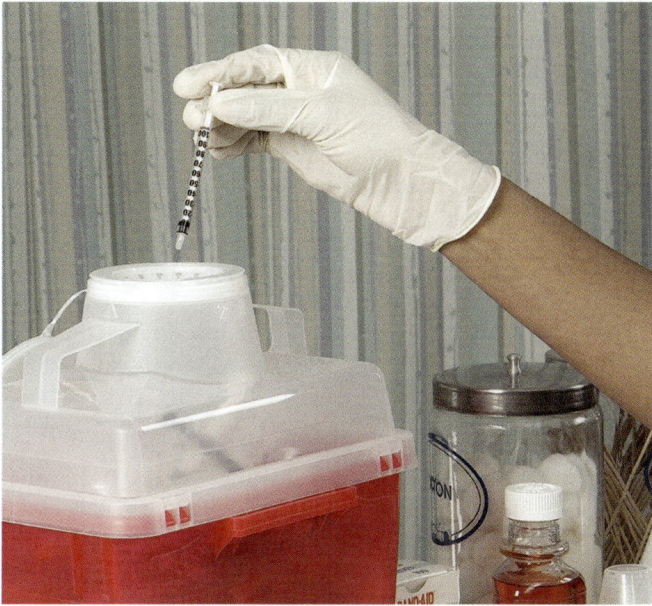

FIGURE 25-21 Disposal system for sharp objects, such as needles and glass. The container must be clearly marked, usually in red, and puncture-proof.

involve adapters that can be used with regular intravenous tubing and medication vials, permitting access through a valve system without a needle.

Another needle-free system is the jet injection most often used for immunizations. The jet injectors drive liquid medication into the intradermal, subcutaneous, or intramuscular tissues by creating a narrow stream under high pressure that penetrates the skin. However, local reactions or injury, such as redness, bruising, and pain, occur more often with jet injectors than by use of a needle.

✚ Always dispose of needles, glass, and other "sharps" in clearly marked, usually red, puncture-proof containers (Fig. 25-21). Never force a needle into an already full container; you may be injured by sharps protruding from the top. Never put a needle or other sharp in a wastebasket or in your pocket or leave it at the patient's bedside.

For tips to prevent needlestick injury, see Clinical Insight 23-1: Preventing Needlestick Injuries.

Recapping Contaminated Needles You should never recap a contaminated needle (e.g., after giving an injection); place it uncapped, needle pointing downward, directly into a sharps disposal container. However, you may occasionally find that you must recap a contaminated needle. The OSHA Fact Sheet (2011) requires bending, recapping, or needle removal using a mechanical device or a one-handed technique. For step-by-step instructions, refer to Procedure 25-10: Recapping Needles Using a One-Handed Technique.

Recapping Sterile Needles OSHA and the National Institute of Occupational Safety and Health (updated 2016) do not advise against recapping sterile needles (e.g., after drawing up a medication), except to recommend needleless systems and safety systems. We suggest that you not use the one-handed "scoop" technique to recap a sterile needle because the risk of contaminating it is high. Consider one of the other methods described in Procedure 25-10.

Comfort and Safety Considerations

Parenteral techniques are invasive. They carry the potential for tissue trauma and provide a portal of entry for pathogens through the skin. You must maintain strict aseptic (sterile) technique to minimize the risk of infection. Moreover, your injection technique and choice of injection site are critical to patient comfort and safety. When choosing a site, consider:

Type, viscosity, and volume of the medication to be administered

The anatomical landmarks underlying injection sites

Patient's situation (e.g., the condition of the tissues at the injection site, the accessibility of certain sites)

The following are examples of judgment and technique errors and their consequences:

- Injecting a large volume of medication into a small muscle causes pain and may damage the tissues.
- Injecting into the wrong tissue (e.g., giving an intramuscular medication too shallowly into the subcutaneous tissue) may (1) accelerate or delay the rate of absorption and (2) cause tissue injury and pain.
- Incorrectly locating an injection site may result in bone or nerve injury when you insert the needle.
- An unsteady needle and syringe while injecting the drug could lead to pain and tissue trauma.
- Forgetting to aspirate before injecting risks administration of medication into an artery or vein instead of the muscle. This could result in an adverse, even fatal, effect.

Minimizing Discomfort

The discomfort associated with an injection comes from three sources: (1) the prick of the needle, (2) the pressure of the volume of the drug in the tissues, and (3) chemical irritation caused by certain drugs. Fear and anxiety magnify discomfort. Use the following techniques to reduce discomfort:

- **Use the smallest needle suited** for the site and medication.
- **Use two needles when drawing up medications:** one to withdraw the medication from the container, and the second one for the injection. If the needle is not free of medication, it may irritate tissues as it is inserted.
- **Do not administer too much solution into an injection site.** If the total volume is more than the recommended amount, give it in two injections and at two sites.
- For intramuscular injections, **help the patient assume a position that reduces muscle tension.**
- For intramuscular injections, **use the Z-track technique,** discussed later in this chapter, to minimize pain and tissue irritation.
- **Pull the skin taut and insert the needle quickly** to avoid pulling the tissues. Remove the needle quickly and at the same angle you inserted it.
- **Steady the syringe** with one hand while injecting the medication.
- **Inject the medication slowly.**
- **Distract the patient** from the procedure by talking to her.
- **Apply gentle pressure** (not massage) after injection unless contraindicated.
- **Especially with children, acknowledge that they will feel some pain** (e.g., "This may hurt a little bit"). If you deny or minimize the pain, the patient might lose trust in you and be even more anxious about future injections.
- **After injecting a child, pat or hug him,** speak softly to him, and perhaps play with him, so that he does not associate you only with pain.
- **Other methods** for decreasing pain can be cooling the skin (e.g., applying ice) or flicking or tapping over the injection area before injecting. Both send distracting signals to the brain so that when the needle comes, it can't process the stimulus as easily.

Intradermal Injections

Intradermal injections are given into the **dermis,** which is the layer of the skin located beneath the skin surface. The intradermal route is commonly used for allergy or tuberculosis (TB) testing. Most nurses use the patient's nondominant arm for TB screening and the dominant arm, chest, or upper back

for all other tests (Fig. 25-22). Give only small amounts of medication by this route—about 0.1 mL. Use a 1-mL syringe and a short, small (26- to 28-gauge) needle, and insert at an angle of 5° to 15° (see Fig. 25-23). ✚ Do not apply pressure or massage the injection site, because the capillaries in the dermal tissue will quickly absorb the medication. For procedure steps, see Procedure 25-11.

Subcutaneous Injections

Subcutaneous (subQ) injections are given into the subcutaneous tissue, the layer of fat located below the dermis and above the muscle tissue. Absorption is slower than it is through the intramuscular route because subcutaneous tissue does not have as rich a blood supply as does muscle. However, speed of absorption varies with the subcutaneous site selected. Absorption is fastest in sites on the abdomen and arms; it is slower on the thigh and upper buttocks. Medication is absorbed more evenly from the abdomen than from the thighs and buttocks because it is affected less by activity.

You do not need to aspirate for blood return when giving a subcutaneous injection because of the shallow depth of the needle into the subcutaneous layer under the skin. For a full procedure, see Procedure 25-12.

Choosing a Subcutaneous Site

Avoid sites in which the subcutaneous tissue lies beneath burns, birthmarks, inflamed tissue, or scars. Do not use sites with lesions or sites over bony prominences, large underlying vessels, or nerves. When using the abdominal site, do not

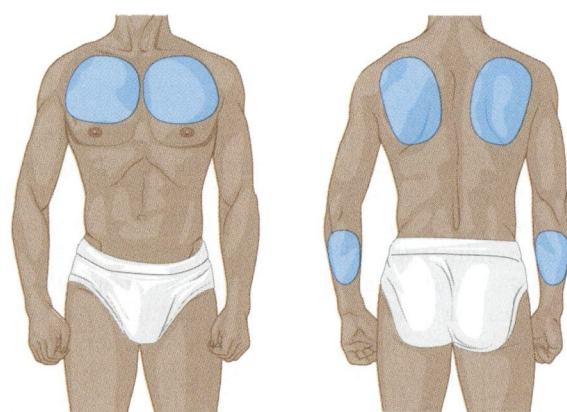

FIGURE 25-22 Sites commonly used for intradermal injection.

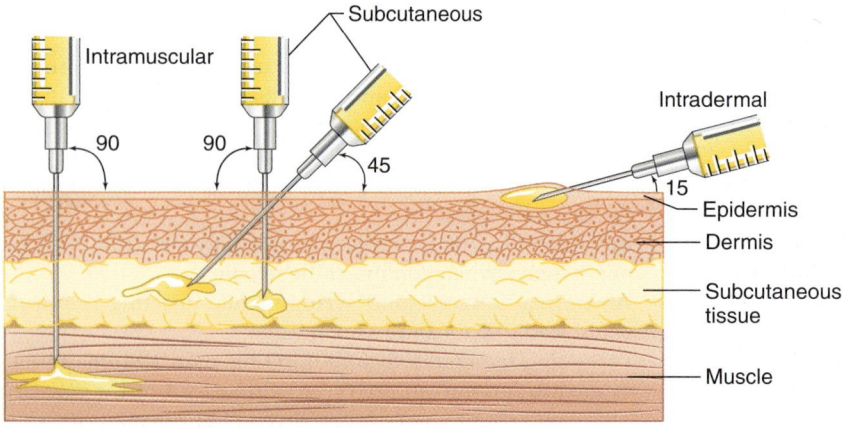

FIGURE 25-23 Standard angles of insertion for intramuscular, subcutaneous, and intradermal injections.

Toward Evidence-Based Practice

Benjamin, A., Hendrix, T., & Woody, J. (2016). Effects of vibration therapy in pediatric immunizations. *Pediatric Nursing, 42*(3), 124–129.

Researchers investigated the effect of vibration therapy without cold analgesia on 100 children, aged 2 months to 7 years, who received immunizations. Results revealed that the vibration therapy alone did not reduce the pain experienced by children aged 2 months to 4 years. However, pain was heightened in children aged 4 to 7 years. Researchers concluded that increased cognition of anticipating the immunizations overrode the effectiveness of the physical intervention in this age-group.

Pourghaznein, T., Azimi, A. V., & Jafarabadi, M. A. (2014). The effect of injection duration and injection site on pain and bruising of subcutaneous injection of heparin. *Journal of Clinical Nursing, 23*(7/8), 1105–1113. doi:10.1111/jocn.12291

Researchers measured the effects of various injection and withdrawal times on pain and bruising in 90 patients receiving heparin injections in the thighs and abdomen. Bruising was significantly lower when injections were administered over 15 seconds and waiting 5 seconds before withdrawing the needle. Injections in the abdomen were associated with lower pain when compared with those in the thighs.

Tuğrul, E., & Khorshıd, L. (2014). Effect on pain intensity of injection sites and speed of injection associated with intramuscular penicillin. *International Journal of Nursing Practice, 20*(5), 468–474.

Researchers investigated the effect of injection site (dorsogluteal, ventrogluteal) and injection duration (5 seconds/mL, 10 seconds/mL) on pain intensity from an intramuscular penicillin injection. Results revealed no significant difference in pain between the two injection durations at either injection site.

1. You are providing care to an adult patient who is receiving heparin therapy via subcutaneous and IM penicillin injections. Based on the Pourghaznein et al. study, would you give subcutaneous doses over 5, 10, or 15 seconds? What factors should be considered when administering IM penicillin injections?

2. You are working in a pediatric clinic. You want to administer IM immunizations to children in as pain-free a way as possible. What factors would you consider in administering these immunizations?

 Go to Davis Advantage, Resources, Chapter 25, **Toward Evidence-Based Practice Suggested Responses.**

---

inject any closer than 5 cm (2 in. horizontally and vertically) from the umbilicus. For repeated injections, each injection should be at least an inch apart. It is important to rotate sites for repeated injections to minimize scarring and hardening of fatty tissue that will interfere with the absorption of medication. See Figure 25-24 for sites to use for subcutaneous injections.

Choosing a Subcutaneous Needle

As a general rule, use a syringe with a small-gauge, short needle that is long enough to penetrate into the fatty subcutaneous layer but not into the muscle.

- **Needle length** will vary depending on the amount of adipose the patient has and the type of injection that is needed (e.g., insulin, immunization). For most subcutaneous injections, a ⅜- to ⅝-inch needle is preferred. However, shorter needles (e.g., ³⁄₁₆ to ⁵⁄₁₆ in.) are more comfortable for some insulin users.
- **Needle gauge** for subcutaneous injection is typically 25 to 27 gauge.
  - Insulin users often prefer finer needles (e.g., 28 to 31 gauge)
  - For children and persons with little or average subcutaneous fat, insert a standard length needle (⅝ in.) at a 45° angle; however, when using a shorter needle, inject at a 90° angle.
  - Obese patients will need a longer needle (e.g., 1 in.) and a 90° angle for injection (Fig. 25-24), and the nurse needs to spread the skin taut rather than pinching.

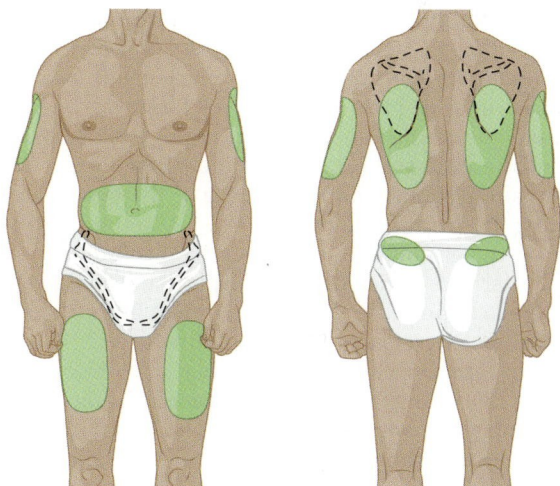

FIGURE 25-24 Sites used for subcutaneous injections.

➕ Inject only small amounts (0.5 to 1 mL) of water-soluble medication subcutaneously to avoid creating sterile abscesses (hardened, painful lumps under the skin).

Administering Insulin

Insulin must be administered subcutaneously or intravenously because it is a protein and would be destroyed in the gastrointestinal tract. Insulin is administered using a special insulin syringe. Insulin vials contain 100 units/mL. The prescriber will specify the number of units (not milliliters or milligrams) to administer. Insulin may be routinely prescribed in specific dosages at specific times or on a **sliding scale,** in which the dosage prescribed is based on the patient's blood glucose level.

However, some view the sliding scale as a reactionary, potentially dangerous practice (DeYoung, Bauer, Brady, et al., 2011), whereas others view it as effective, if it is timed appropriately (Trotter, Conaway, & Burns, 2013). Although basal insulin and insulin pumps are commonly used, the sliding scale is beneficial when initiating insulin therapy and during times of physical stress (e.g., illness, surgery). Follow your institution's policy and prescriber guidance.

Categories of Insulin   To correctly mix and safely administer insulin, you need to understanding the categories of insulin and how they are used to control blood sugar.

- **Basal insulin** is given to cover the body's energy needs without taking the diet into account. Common basal insulins are NPH, insulin glargine (Lantus), and insulin detemir (Levemir).
- **Prandial** (mealtime) and **preprandial insulins** such as regular insulin (e.g., Humulin R, Novolin R), are given to prevent high blood sugar after eating a meal. However, analogs with a more rapid acting onset than regular insulin (e.g., insulin lispro [Humalog], insulin aspart [NovoLog/NovoRapid], and insulin glulisine [Apidra]) are being prescribed (Magaji & Johnston, 2011).
- **Combination insulins** are manufactured mixtures of a fast-acting and long-lasting insulin. These types of insulins result in fewer injections but require careful monitoring. Similarly, you can mix insulins in the same syringe (see Clinical Insight 25-6).

Insulin Equipment   Insulin can be administered in a variety of ways.

- **Disposable syringes** for subcutaneous injection are the most common.
- **Automatic injectors** are used by some patients for subcutaneous dosing. By pressing a button on the device, the injector releases the needle into the skin, releasing the insulin dose.
- **Insulin pumps** are becoming more common as a way to maintain glycemic control because of the benefit of fine-tuning the dosing. The pump consists of a tube with a needle on the end of it that is taped to the abdomen and a computerized device that is worn at the waist. Insulin is received continuously from the pump. A button is pressed at mealtime to release an extra insulin dose.
- **Insulin pen devices** contain a cartridge and disposable needles to deliver certain doses with each injection. They are convenient and may help patients to avoid medication errors. Incorporating best practices with insulin pens can counter its known risk of cross-contamination in inpatient settings (Haines, Miklich & Rochester-Eyeguokan, 2016; Institute for Safe Medication Practices, 2013)
- **Nondisposable syringes** (glass syringe and metal needle) may be used repeatedly if they are sterilized after each use.
- **Spray injectors** forcefully spray the insulin dose into the skin. This involves a wider area of skin than would a regular injection.

KnowledgeCheck 25-16

- List three errors in technique that can occur when giving parenteral injections. State their possible consequences.

- Describe at least four ways to minimize the discomfort of an injection.
- Name two reasons for giving an intradermal injection.
- As a rule, what gauge and length of needle would you use for a subcutaneous injection?
- Why should people rotate injection sites when they must have repeated injections over a long period of time?

ThinkLike a Nurse 25-12

- What do intradermal and subcutaneous injections have in common?
- How are they different?

Administering Heparin

Heparin is a fast-acting medication that interrupts the blood-clotting process. It may be used for patients at risk for harmful clot formation (e.g., immobile after major surgery; post-vascular surgery; cerebrovascular accident [stroke, brain attack]; myocardial infarction [heart attack]). Because heparin is absorbed poorly from the gastrointestinal tract, it is given intravenously or subcutaneously. If mistakenly given intramuscularly, it will cause hematoma and pain.

Give the injection deep into the subcutaneous tissue of the abdomen, at least 5 cm (2 in.) away from the umbilicus and rotate sites. Because of the anticoagulant properties of heparin, you will need to modify your injection technique. For guidelines to use when injecting anticoagulants subcutaneously, refer to Clinical Insight 25-7.

Heparin dosage is based on the patient's weight and results of blood coagulation studies, so always check laboratory values for coagulation studies before administering.

Intramuscular Injections

Intramuscular (IM) injections (injections into muscle tissue) are absorbed faster than subcutaneous medications because of the rich blood supply in the muscles. Large muscles (e.g., vastus lateralis, ventrogluteal) can tolerate 3 or up to 5 mL of liquid. The smaller the muscle is, the less fluid it can tolerate. For example, 0.5 to 1 mL can be injected into the average deltoid muscle.

Conventional practice requires you to aspirate (pull back on the plunger of the syringe) before injecting medication intramuscularly to be sure the needle tip is not in a blood vessel. However, there are insufficient evidence-based studies to support this conclusion. *Aspiration is not recommended for:*

- The vastus lateralis and deltoid muscles because there are no large blood vessels at these sites (Centers for Disease Control and Prevention, n.d.a; 2016)
- Children, because the idea is to give the injection quickly in order to minimize pain (Walden & Vangilder, 2013).

Others would limit the practice of aspiration to IM injections of large molecule medications such as penicillin (Crawford & Johnson, 2012). You should follow your institution's policies and procedures for IM injections.

Choosing an Intramuscular Site

When selecting an IM site, you should look for a site that is:

- A safe distance from nerves, large blood vessels, and bones
- Free from injury, abscesses, tenderness, necrosis, abrasion, or other pathology
- Large enough to accommodate the volume of medication to be given

Muscles commonly used are the vastus lateralis, ventrogluteal, and deltoid. **KEY POINT:** *Because of their proximity to major nerves and vessels, the rectus femoris and dorsogluteal are no longer recommended sites (Walsh & Brophy, 2011).* See Procedure 25-13.

Ventrogluteal Muscle—Site of Choice

This is the preferred site for intramuscular injections for adults and young children who are walking because it is located away from major blood vessels and nerves. However, some medications (e.g., vaccines) may recommend the deltoid. The ventrogluteal site, located on the lateral hip, involves the gluteus medius and gluteus minimus muscles (see first figure in Procedure 25-13A).

When learning to locate this site, many students notice that it feels "hard" when they palpate it. They worry the needle will hit the bone. In part, the muscle feels hard because there is little subcutaneous tissue over it. To reassure yourself it is safe, examine a skeleton model with the muscles attached. Notice the ilium is concave (curves in) and the muscle lies deep down in the "cup" it forms. If you are sure you have located the anterosuperior iliac spine and if you follow the procedure steps, you will not hit a bone. In fact, you are less likely to do so than if you use other sites. For guidelines in locating the ventrogluteal site, refer to Procedure 25-13A.

Dorsogluteal Site—Site to Avoid

The dorsogluteal site consists of the gluteal muscles of the buttocks. ✚ Avoid using this site for IM injections because its proximity to the sciatic nerve and superior gluteal artery increases the risk of (1) injection into a major blood vessel and (2) damage to the sciatic nerve. Furthermore, the site is difficult to identify accurately in older adults and in people with flabby skin.

You may observe some nurses continuing to use the dorsogluteal site because of tradition, ease of use, or lack of knowledge. Your avoidance of the dorsogluteal site gives you the opportunity to role model patient safety by demonstrating correct technique for locating the preferred site.

Deltoid Site

The deltoid site is located in the middle third of the upper arm. It is small and lies close to the radial nerve and brachial artery (see second figure in Procedure 25-13B). The area has a small muscle mass with little subcutaneous tissue, so medications are absorbed rapidly. This muscle is easily accessible but is not well developed in many older adults. You should use it only for small amounts of up to 1 mL or when other sites are inaccessible. Avoid using the deltoid site in infants and assess children for adequate muscle mass before use. Some medications (e.g., vaccines, flu shot) may specify the deltoid muscle.

When locating the deltoid, do not merely roll up the sleeve. You must fully expose the entire upper arm and shoulder. Otherwise, you may miss the muscle mass and injure a nerve or blood vessel. For a guide to locating the deltoid site, see Procedure 25-13B.

Vastus Lateralis Site

The vastus lateralis muscle, located in the anterolateral thigh (see second figure in Procedure 25-13C), is the preferred site for young infants, particularly before walking age (Bartley, 2012a; Jackson, Peterson, Nelson, et al., 2013). It is usually the best developed and contains no large nerves or blood vessels, minimizing the risk for injury. Other advantages include the following: (1) Drugs are rapidly absorbed from this area, (2) it can accommodate a larger volume of medication than can the deltoid, and (3) it is a convenient location for those who self-administer injections.

A disadvantage is that the patient can see you administer the injection, and the psychological effect may create some discomfort. An ambulatory patient may notice more residual soreness because the muscle is used in walking.

For children and adult patients with small muscle mass, you should grasp ("pinch up") the body of the muscle during injection to be sure that the medication reaches muscle tissue and the needle does not penetrate to the underlying bone. For a guide to locating the vastus lateralis site, refer to Procedure 25-13C.

Rectus Femoris Site—For Adults Only

✚ The rectus femoris site, located in the anterior thigh, is no longer recommended for infants and children. You will only use this site for adults when other sites are inaccessible and the medication needs to be administered intramuscularly. It is often used by patients who self-administer their intramuscular injections because it is easy for them to reach. A disadvantage is that it is usually painful. A shorter needle can be used when injecting this site. For a guide to locating the rectus femoris site, refer to Procedure 25-13D.

Choosing an Intramuscular Needle

Although a 1½-inch needle is considered "standard" for IM injections, you should choose the needle gauge and length based on the site, the size of the muscle, the amount of medication to be given, and the amount of adipose tissue over the muscle. In the deltoid muscle, for example, you might use a 23- or 25-gauge, 1-inch needle. But if the solution is viscous, you would need a larger-bore needle (e.g., 20 gauge). For a very thin person, you could use a 1-inch needle, even when injecting into the larger muscles. For an obese person, you might need a needle as long as 3 inches to penetrate adipose tissue and reach the muscle (unfortunately, long needles may not be available in some settings). As a rule, the angle of insertion for an intramuscular injection is 90° (see Fig. 25-23). See Table 25-7 for needle length recommendations for immunizations.

Z-Track Technique

The Z-track technique seals the needle track and prevents medication from leaking out of the muscle up through the needle track and into the subcutaneous tissues after the needle is withdrawn. The Z-track method is recommended for all IM injections because it is less painful and helps to prevent irritation of subcutaneous tissues. It is also useful for irritating medications (e.g., iron preparations) that irritate or discolor subcutaneous tissue and for older adults who have reduced muscle mass. ✚ For this technique, it is best to use the larger muscles: the ventrogluteal and vastus lateralis.

Knowledge Check 25-17

- Name three sites for giving intramuscular (IM) injections.
- What is the preferred IM injection site for adults? Why?
- From which route is medication absorbed more rapidly: subcutaneous or IM? Why?
- For an "average" adult, what is the standard needle length for IM injections?
- Why is the dorsogluteal site *not* recommended?
- What are the disadvantages of the deltoid site?
- When using the vastus lateralis to give an intramuscular medication to a person with small muscle mass, how can you ensure the medication reaches muscle tissue and the needle does not penetrate to the underlying bone?

Table 25-7 ➤ Appropriate Needle Size Based on Age and Site for Vaccinations and Immunizations

AGE		NEEDLE LENGTH	SITE
Newborns (first 28 days)		⅝"*	Anterolateral thigh
Infants (1–12 months)		1"	Anterolateral thigh
Toddlers (1–2 years)		1–1¼"	Anterolateral thigh
		⅝–1"*	Deltoid
Children and Teens (3–18 years)		⅝–1"*	Deltoid
		1–1¼"	Anterolateral thigh
Adults (19 years and older)			
Male or Female	Less than 130 lb	⅝–1*"	Deltoid
Male	130–260 lb	1–1½"	Deltoid
Female	130–200 lb	1–1½"	Deltoid
Male	260+ lb	1½"	Deltoid
Female	200+ lb	1½"	Deltoid

*A ⅝" needle may be used with the skin stretched tight and injection given at a 90° angle.

Source: Adapted from: Centers for Disease Control and Prevention (n.d.b, updated 2016). Administering vaccines: Dose, route, site, and needle size. Retrieved from http://www.immunize.org/catg.d/p3085.pdf

Intravenous Medications

Intravenous (IV) medications are given through a catheter, or cannula, inserted into a vein. The onset of medication action takes place within seconds, so IV administration is especially useful in emergencies. Without a known antidote, there is no way for you to stop its action if an adverse reaction occurs. Review Table 25-1 for advantages and disadvantages of using the IV route. The following sections explain various methods for administering IV medications. You should see Chapter 39 for procedures for initiating and maintaining IV fluids.

IV Push Medications

IV push (bolus) medications are injected directly into a vein and enter the systemic circulation immediately (see Procedure 25-16). Many IV push medications are irritating to vein walls and can cause damage (sloughing, pain, abscesses) if accidentally injected into the tissues (Fig. 25-25). To prevent these complications, you should:

- Assess the patient before, during, and after giving the medication.
- Determine the compatibility of the drug with the IV fluid that is infusing and the plastic IV bag and tubing. Consult a pharmacist as needed.
- Use sterile technique.
- Administer the medication slowly.
- Observe the patient carefully for signs of adverse reactions.
- Have an antidote on hand if the drug has potentially serious side effects. Be aware, though, that many drugs do not have an antidote.
- If your patient shows signs of serious allergic reaction, you will need to prepare to support the patient's airway, deliver oxygen, and administer medication to reduce the reaction.
  Read the package insert or consult with the pharmacist or prescriber for specific guidelines on how fast the drug can be

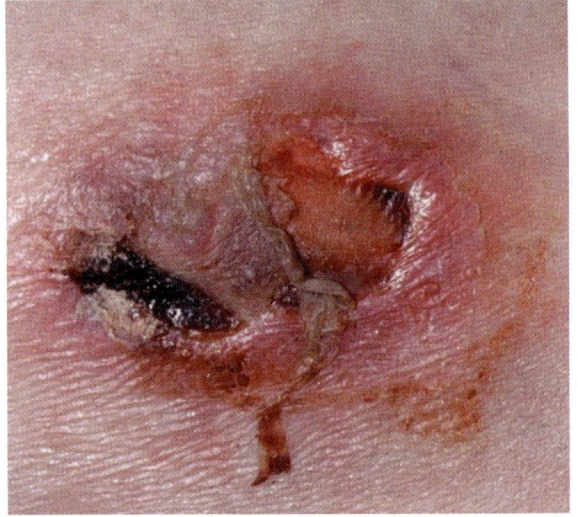

FIGURE 25-25 Tissue and skin injury after intravenous medication leaks into an infiltrated site.

pushed (usually incrementally over 1 to 3 minutes, or longer). One minute can seem like a very long time when you are pushing a medication, so don't guess—look at your watch!

✚ Take note that "IV push" does not mean the same thing as "give rapidly." If given too rapidly, IV drugs—particularly potassium—can be quite dangerous. Because you cannot retrieve the medication once it is injected, there is no margin for error. Safety is essential.

Adding Medications to IV Bags

One way to administer a drug intravenously is to mix it into a bag of IV fluid and administer it through a port on the primary IV line. Vitamins, potassium chloride, oxytocin, and several blood pressure and cardiovascular drugs are commonly administered this way. The drug is usually premixed with the fluid in the pharmacy. In some facilities, the nurse may need to add the drug to a small IV bag of fluid, though. This method is useful when the drug can be infused continuously to achieve the desired effect. The main disadvantage is the danger of infusing too much fluid, especially for children, older adults, and people with cardiac or renal disease.

- ✚ **Adding medications from multidose vials**—One safe method for adding medication to IV fluids when using multidose vials, while providing sterile air filtration, is to use a reconstitution device. **A reconstitution device** is designed with a sharp, thin, piercing spike to minimize coring and permit easy penetration of the rubber top of a vial (Fig. 25-26). The luer-lock port maintains a secure closure between the device and the syringe. The hinged cap and the sheath over the spike help maintain sterility before use, minimize "touch" contamination, and ensure a closed system for disposal.
- **Transfer needle**—Another safe method for adding medications to an IV container is to use a **transfer needle** or **cannula**: a blunted plastic needle with a double beveled tip (Fig. 25-27). One end is inserted into the powdered or liquid medication and the other end is inserted into a port of the IV bag. Solution is transferred from the IV bag into the medication vial, which you shake lightly to mix the medication. Then the medication is transferred back into the IV bag for administration.

Intermittent Infusion

Many medications, such as antibiotics, are administered intravenously by intermittent infusion. Intermittent infusions may be given through the port of an infusing IV line or, if the patient does not need the IV fluids, through an intermittent injection port, also called a saline or heparin lock (Fig. 25-28).

Infusion Setup Most intermittent infusion medications are supplied in bags containing 50 to 250 mL of 5% dextrose in water (D_5W) or normal saline. The drug is given over a period of time, usually 30 to 60 minutes, and at regular intervals (e.g., every 6 hours). The small bag of diluted medication (the "secondary" bag) is attached to the primary IV infusion line for administration, usually with a **piggyback setup** (Fig. 25-29). The smaller (secondary) container is connected to the primary (continuous) infusion line at the upper primary port. This setup allows for intermittent use only and the infusion of one solution at a time (see Procedures 25-17A and B).

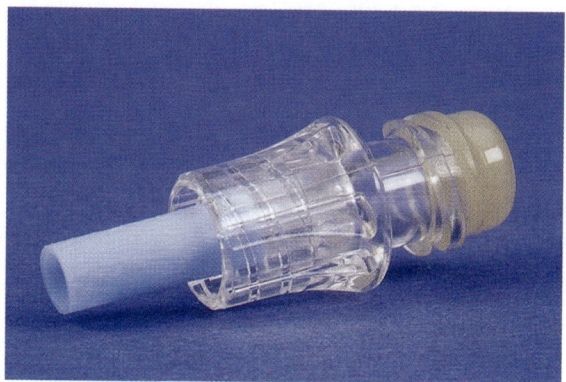

FIGURE 25-28 Intermittent injection port.

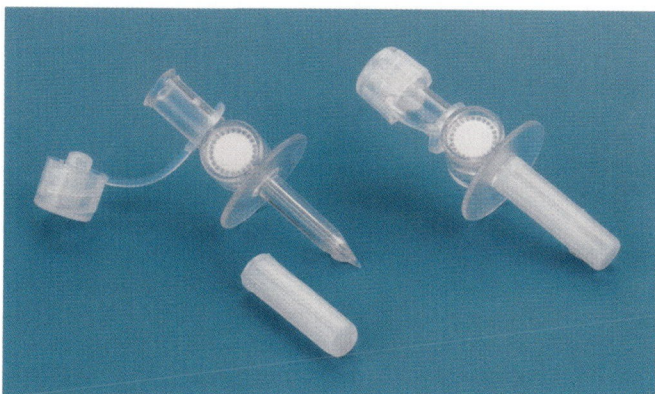

FIGURE 25-26 A reconstitution device is used to add medication from multidose IV vials while providing sterile air filtration.

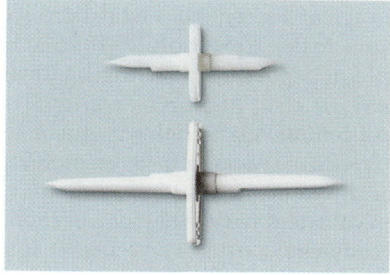

FIGURE 25-27 Transfer needles.

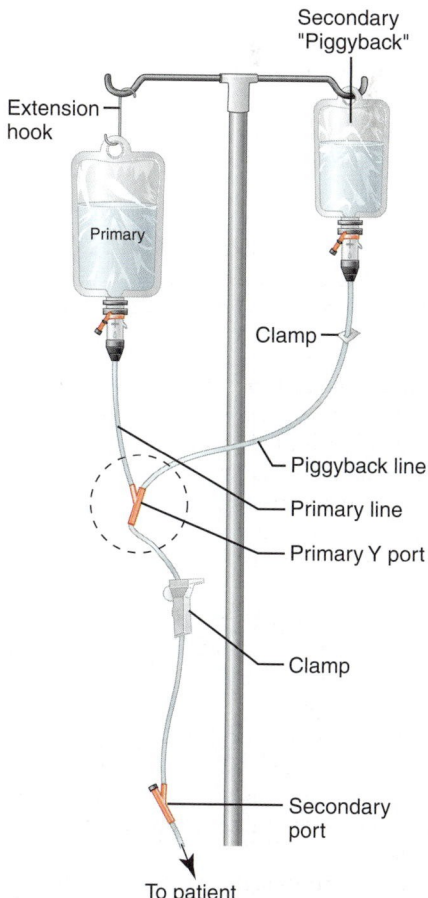

FIGURE 25-29 Piggyback setup is attached to the primary (continuous infusion) IV line at the upper port, allowing for intermittent infusion only.

A **tandem setup** allows for the simultaneous infusion of two IV bags, but is less commonly used than is a piggyback setup. ✚ For safety, most healthcare facilities require tandem infusions to be regulated via an IV pump.

Needleless Connections Traditionally, the secondary tubing was attached to the primary set tubing by inserting a needle into the port and taping it in place. However, most agencies now use needleless systems (see Fig. 25-20), which use a threaded or lever-type lock to make the connection. In addition to decreasing needlestick injuries, a needleless system prevents contact contamination at the IV connection site. **KEY POINT:** *You can help prevent catheter-related bloodstream infections by scrubbing the needleless IV connector for 15 seconds. Remember: "Scrub the Hub."* When the secondary tubing is no longer needed, a disinfection cap containing either alcohol or chlorhexidine/alcohol solution is placed over the port (Fig. 25-30).

Volume-Control Infusion Sets

To effectively control the infusion of smaller amounts of solutions, particularly with pediatric patients, a volume-control infusion set (e.g., Buretrol, Soluset, Volutrol, or Pediatrol) may be used (Fig. 25-31). These are small fluid containers (100 to 150 mL) that are attached directly below the primary fluid container. The medication and the desired amount of IV fluid are added to the volume-control container and administered through the primary line (see Procedure 25-17C). This system decreases the risk of overhydration because the amount of fluid that can infuse into the patient is limited to the amount that you place in the small container.

Central Venous Access Devices

Intravenous medication can be delivered through a central or peripheral vein. The most common reasons for a patient to have a central venous access device (CVAD) are to:

- Give long-term IV therapy
- Provide total parenteral nutrition when the patient cannot eat normally

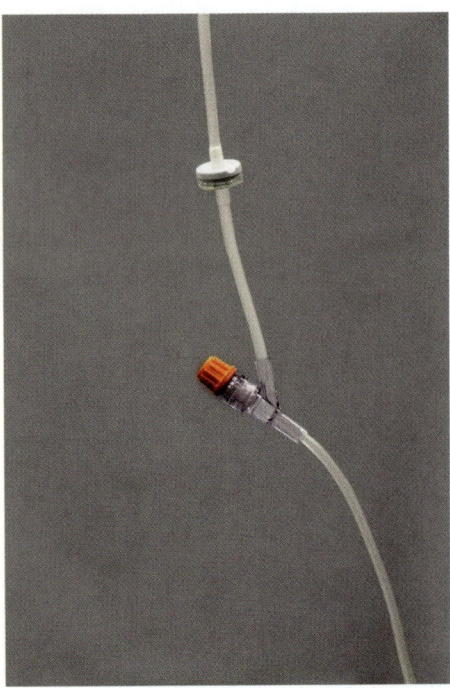

FIGURE 25-30 Disinfection cap for luer-lock needleless hubs.

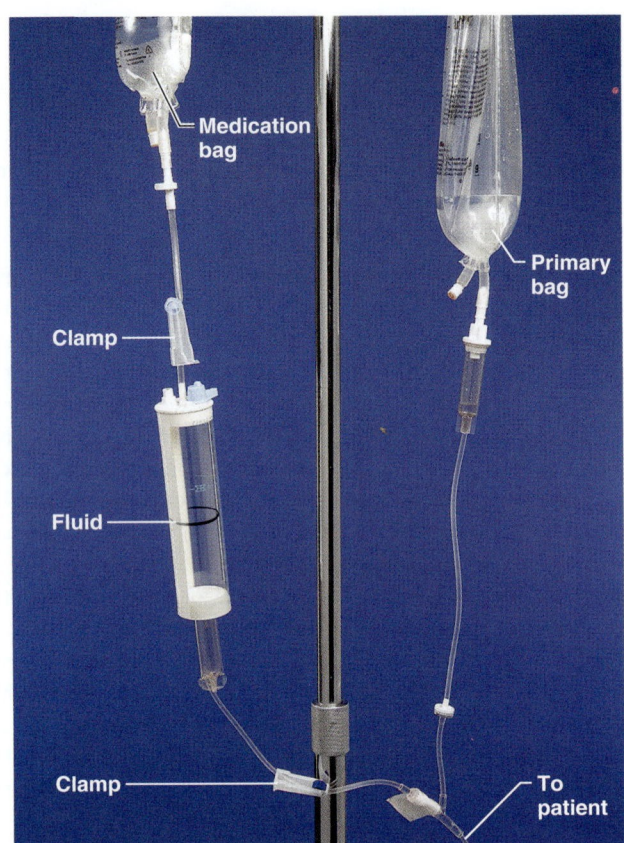

FIGURE 25-31 Volume-control infusion set for intermittent infusion administration; used when the fluid volume is critical and must be carefully monitored.

- Have blood drawn without the trauma and complications of repeated venipuncture
- Provide vascular access when peripheral IV placement is difficult

External CVADs can be either tunneled or nontunneled. The *tunneled devices* are surgically implanted peripherally and tunneled to a central vein, typically the superior vena cava. *Nontunneled catheters* are inserted near the destination site. These catheters can be single or multilumen. This category includes peripherally inserted central catheters (PICCs), which are inserted into the central circulation via a peripheral vein and can remain in place for months. For short-term use, the nontunneled central catheter can be inserted into the jugular, subclavian, or femoral veins.

An **internal**, or **implantable**, **port** is a CVAD that can remain in place and be functional for years. Access is gained through the skin via a hollow port with a self-sealing silicone cap. These devices are inserted when long-term IV medication is needed or the medication is too irritating for a peripheral site (see Procedure 25-18). See Figure 25-32A for an example of a port for injecting medication into the subclavian vein.

Catheters for central venous delivery can be single- or multilumen (Fig. 25-32B). Although they are more convenient for administering different medications and fluid, some types of multilumen catheters have a higher infection rate than do single-lumen catheters.

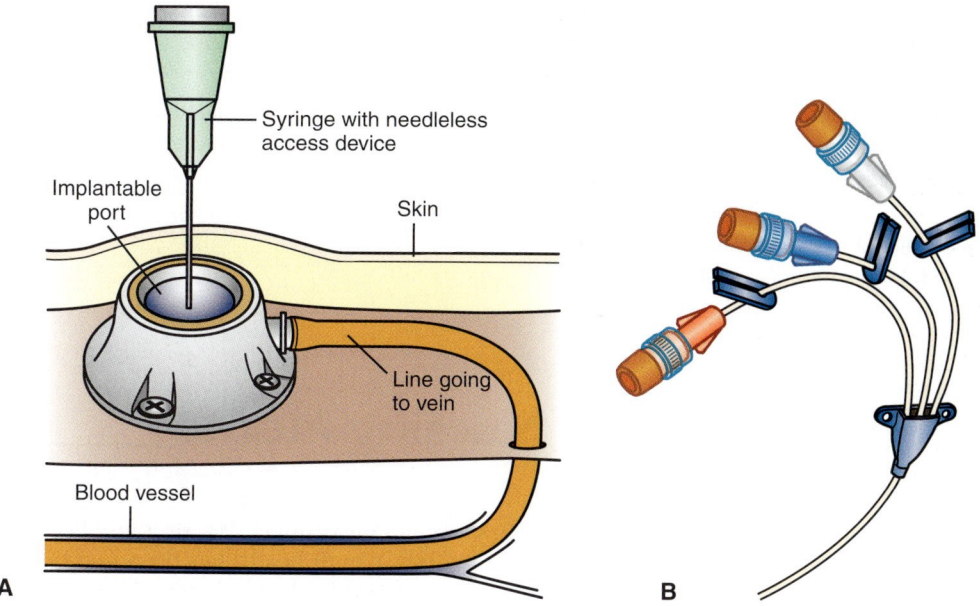

FIGURE 25-32 Central vascular access device. A. Implantable device. B. Multilumen catheter with blunt cannula, split septum, needleless access device.

CLINICALREASONING

The questions and exercises in this section allow you to practice the kind of thinking you will use as a full-spectrum nurse. Critical-thinking questions usually have more than one correct answer, so we do not provide "correct answers" for these features. It is more important to develop your nursing judgment than to just cover content. You will learn by discussing the questions with your peers. If you are still unsure, see the Davis Advantage chapter resources for suggested responses.

Caring for the Nguyens

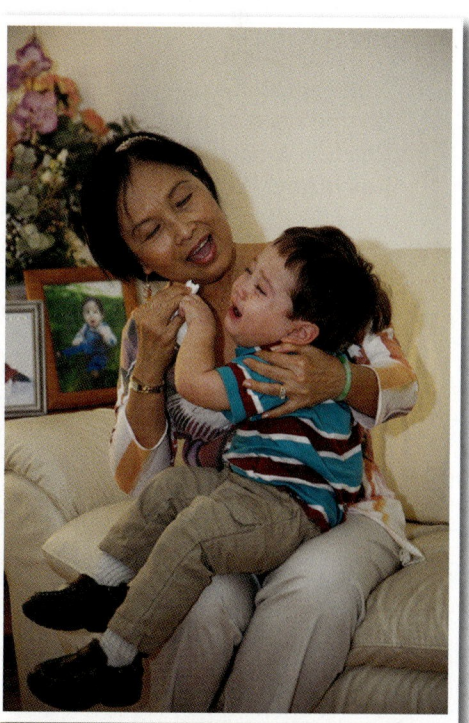

Kim Phan, the 3-year-old grandson of Nam and Yen Nguyen, has been tired and observed to be sitting down a great deal at preschool. Last week, he developed coughing, wheezing, shortness of breath, nasal congestion, and extreme fatigue. The pediatrician at the Family Medicine Center diagnosed asthma. He prescribed a 5-day tapering course of prednisone, a leukotriene inhibitor (Singulair) 4 mg orally daily at bedtime, and periodic treatments with albuterol through a home nebulizer system.

Nam's mother, Mai Nguyen, became very upset when she saw the bottle of prednisone elixir. She was even more upset when she learned that Kim received an injection of the medicine in the office. She advised Yen not to give Kim the medicine because she said it causes weak bones and stunts growth. Yen has called the clinic, asking for advice on how to handle this problem. (Look up the medications and use your knowledge of different routes of administration.)

A. What theoretical knowledge do you need to answer these concerns?

B. What are some reliable sources where you might find this information?

(Continued)

Caring for the Nguyens (continued)

C. What rationale could you offer to Yen to explain the safety of the prednisone prescription? You will need to use a variety of references to answer this question.

D. Yen asks you to explain why Kim received both a shot and pills. How would you respond?

E. Why is Kim receiving a leukotriene inhibitor (Singulair) orally and albuterol by nebulizer?

Applying the **Full-Spectrum Nursing Model**_____

PATIENT SITUATION

Leonard LeMonte is a 57-year-old African American man who has come to his primary care provider because of persistent headaches that increase in intensity over the course of the day. His overall health has been good, although he is approximately 50 to 60 pounds overweight. Past medical history is significant for borderline primary hypertension and non-insulin-dependent diabetes, type 2 (diet controlled). Leonard tells you he works in a high-stress environment. He shares great concern with you that he fears losing his job and not being able to pay his bills and meet other financial commitments for his family. He also states that he has little time for hobbies or recreational outlets because he works so many hours.

THINKING

1. *Theoretical Knowledge (Facts and Principles):* You see in the chart that the provider prescribed repaglinide (Prandin) to treat Mr. LeMonte's diabetes. By what route is this medication given?
2. *Critical Thinking (Inquiry):* If you did not know the answer to the first question, specifically how did you get that information? State your source.

DOING

3. *Nursing Process (Assessment):* To evaluate Mr. LeMonte's response to his diabetes medication, what questions do you need to ask him?
4. *Practical Knowledge (Skills):* Mr. LeMonte tells you that he forgot to take his Prandin this morning and also at lunchtime. What should you do?

CARING

5. *Self-Knowledge:* In what areas do you feel compassion for Mr. LeMonte, on which you might build a caring relationship?
6. *Self-Knowledge:* What do you identify as your strength in dealing with Mr. LeMonte's healthcare needs?
7. *Ethical Knowledge:* Mr. LeMonte tells you that he frequently skips doses of his Prandin because he can't afford the expense. He asks you not to tell his wife about this because he doesn't want her to worry. What will you do?

 Go to Davis Advantage, Resources, Chapter 25, **Applying the Full-Spectrum Nursing Mode—Suggested Responses.**

PracticalKnowledge: clinical application_____

Clinical Insights and Procedures in this section will assist you to prepare, measure, and administer various types of medications, locate injection sites, and handle needles safely.

CLINICAL INSIGHTS

Clinical Insight 25-1 ▶ Taking Action After a Medication Error

✚ First, check the patient. Take his vital signs and perform assessments related to the medication that was given.

- If you are unfamiliar with the side effects of the medication, consult a drug reference source.
- Verify that you have made a medication error and identify the type of error.
- Consult the charge nurse for guidance if this is your first error.
- Notify the prescriber and follow her prescriptions for intervention.
- Document on the chart that the medication was given, but do not indicate that it was given in error. This alerts anyone reviewing the chart that an error was made.

- Complete an incident report according to the facility's policies. Ask for assistance if you are unfamiliar with the format or requirement of this form. It is important that the information you provide is factual and accurate.
- **KEY POINT:** *Do not document in the patient's chart that an incident report was filed. This alerts anyone reviewing the chart that an error was made and makes the incident report available for legal review in the event of a lawsuit.*
- When you are calmer and can think clearly, critically reflect on the error. Identify the influences that led to your making the error. Were you rushed? Did you check the prescription? Did you follow the rights of medication? Whatever the reason, use this situation as a learning experience to improve your practice.

Clinical Insight 25-2 ▶ Reusing Needles and Syringes: Home Care

Assess for the Following:

- Is the patient is capable of safely recapping a syringe: adequate vision, manual dexterity, and no obvious tremor?
- Are there contraindications to needle reuse (e.g., poor personal hygiene, an acute illness, open wounds on the hands, or decreased resistance to infection)?

Teach How to Use Needles Safely:

- Consult your healthcare provider before beginning this practice.
- Examine the needle carefully before reusing it. The new 30- and 31-gauge needles can easily be bent at the tip to form a hook, which can lacerate tissue or break off within the skin. Never reuse a needle that is deformed in any way.
- Recap the needle immediately after use if you plan to use it again.
- To recap a needle, hold the syringe in one hand, rest that arm or hand on a solid surface, and with the other, replace the cap with a straight motion of the thumb. Do *not* guide both the needle and cap to meet in midair, because this frequently results in needlestick injury.
- Do not mix insulin types if you reuse needles and syringes. Use one syringe for each insulin type. That means more injections, but certain insulins cannot be mixed without reducing their effectiveness.
- Dispose of needles safely. Do not bend or break a needle; doing so increases the chance of injury. Use a coffee can or other puncture-proof container with a lid to dispose of needles.

Teach Your Patient When to Discard a Needle:

- Discard needles when they become dull. Usually they cannot be used more than 10 times.
- When a needle hurts too much, it's time to discard it. Increased pain means that the silicone coating is wearing off.
- Do not reuse a needle if it has come in contact with anything other than the injection site.

Teach How to Clean and Store Needles:

- Do not use alcohol to cleanse the needle. Alcohol may remove the silicone coating that makes for less painful skin puncture. It is best not to clean the needle after use; just carefully recap it.
- You may store the syringe and needle at room temperature. The potential benefits or risks of refrigerating the syringe are unknown.

✚ Teach How to Recognize and Avoid Infection:

- Be aware that reusing needles and syringes increases the risk of infection, although most insulin preparations have bacteriostatic additives that inhibit growth of bacteria commonly found on the skin.
- Inspect injection sites for redness or swelling. If these signs are present, do not reuse a needle; consult your healthcare provider.
- Never share syringes or needles with another person. This poses a risk of acquiring a bloodborne viral infection (e.g., hepatitis).

Clinical Insight 25-3 ➤ Using Prefilled Unit-Dose Systems

Prefilled systems are commonly used in a variety of health-care settings and in self-administration.

Technique

1. Check each medication cartridge and dose carefully, because all of the cartridges look alike.
2. No medication preparation is necessary.
3. Insert the cartridge into the holder.
4. Swing or twist the plunger into place, depending on the type of syringe you use. Lock it securely at the needle end.
5. Attach the plunger, if necessary. (The system may come with plunger attached.)

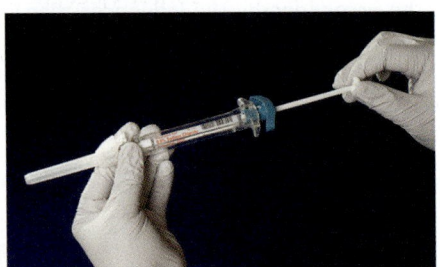

6. Expel air and excess medication.
7. Don gloves.
8. Administer the medication.
9. Dispose of the empty cartridge. Some types are available for reuse.

Technique Variations

The Needle Gauge or Length is Not Correct for the Patient.

You can transfer the medication into a regular disposable syringe, maintaining sterile technique. There are two ways you can do this:

Cartridge without removable needle:

1. Pull back on the plunger of the regular disposable syringe and keep a capped, sterile needle ready.
2. Insert the cartridge needle through the open tip of the disposable syringe.

3. Eject the medication into the regular syringe.
4. Replace the capped needle onto the regular syringe.
5. Eject the air and check for the correct dosage.

Cartridge with removable needle:

The capped needle can be removed from some prefilled cartridges, allowing the cartridge to be used as a vial. This allows you to safely draw the medications into a different (disposable) syringe, using a vial access device or safety needle. Do not inject air into a cartridge, because the excess pressure may eject the movable bottom.

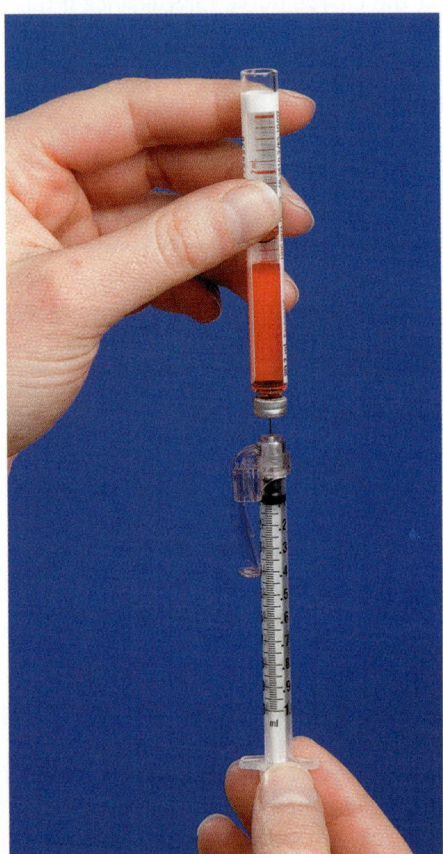

Clinical Insight 25-4 ➤ Reconstituting Medication

1. **Remove the caps of both the medication and diluent vials.**
2. **If a multidose vial is used, scrub the tops of both vials** with alcohol or other antiseptic wipe.
   To clean the cap of dust and reduce the number of microorganisms.
3. **Use a VAD or, if agency policy allows, attach a filter needle to the syringe.**
   To prevent withdrawing glass and rubber particles, which have been found in medications withdrawn from vials and ampules.

4. **Draw up the diluent into the syringe.**
   a. Draw air into the syringe in a volume equal to the amount of diluent you will be withdrawing.
   b. Insert the filter needle (or VAD) carefully through the center of the rubber cap and, keeping the bevel of the needle (or cannula) above the diluent, inject the air.
      The air prevents negative pressure inside the vial when you withdraw the diluent, allowing you to withdraw the diluent easily. Keeping bevel above diluent helps prevent bubbles.
   c. Withdraw the diluent in the specified amount.

Clinical Insight 25-4 ➤ **Reconstituting Medication—cont'd**

5. **Inject diluent into the medication vial** by inserting the VAD carefully through the center of the rubber cap and then injecting the diluent.

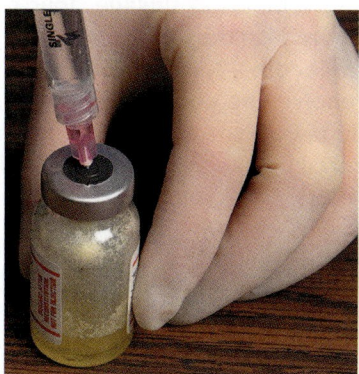

6. **Mix the medication, taking care not to create bubbles** (e.g., roll, do not shake, the vial). If medication does not mix easily, remove the needle or cannula from the vial, and place the syringe and needle on a sterile field (e.g., the wrapper the syringe came in) while you mix more. Alternatively, recap the sterile needle (see Procedure 25-10A).

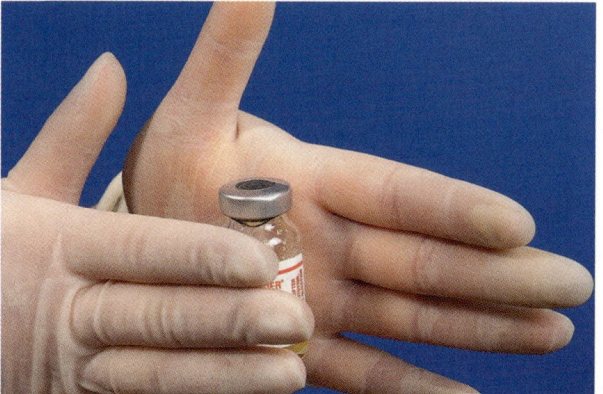

7. **Reinsert filter needle or VAD if it was removed** and withdraw the reconstituted medication into the syringe.

8. **Remove the filter needle or the cannula from the syringe** and replace it with a sterile needle before measuring the medication.
   This ensures that the dose is correct and minimizes discomfort. It also prevents tracking of medication through the tissues; filter needles are usually larger than you need for an injection. In addition, you should not eject fluid through a filter needle.

9. **Hold the syringe vertically, and carefully eject all air** from the syringe, but do not eject the medication. Read the dosage.

10. **If necessary, hold the syringe horizontally to eject unneeded medication** from the syringe to reach the prescribed dose.

Clinical Insight 25-5 ➤ **Measuring Dosage When Changing Needles**

Note: These are not the old "air lock" techniques.

Using a Nonfilter Needle

When drawing medication from a multidose vial, you may sometimes need to use two regular needles. Alternately, you may use a needleless reconstitution device that is designed with a dispensing spike instead of a needle on one end and a luer-lock port on the other end that attaches to the syringe.

Equipment

One needle (or needless reconstitution device) for drawing up the medication, and one needle for injecting the medication into the patient.

1. **Using Needle #1, draw up the prescribed amount of medication.** When using a vial, inject air into the air pocket within the vial. Then withdraw the correct amount of medication from the vial. Be sure to keep the tip of the

(Continued)

Clinical Insight 25-5 ➤ Measuring Dosage When Changing Needles—cont'd

needle in the fluid in order to avoid aspirating air bubbles into the syringe.

2. **Remove bubbles; eject the air.** After drawing up the medication, tap on the barrel of the syringe to remove air bubbles, if necessary. Then eject the air from the syringe (keeping the syringe vertical) while retaining the correct amount of medication in the syringe. Check the volume closely at eye level.

3. **Remove the Needle #1 and discard it** into a needle-safe container. Put on a fresh needle (Needle #2) for injection.

4. **Using Needle #2, pull back on the plunger** and draw an extra 0.2 mL of air to account for the air within the needle.

5. **Check the medication dosage.** Your plunger should be 0.2 mL more than the ordered dose.

6. **Still using Needle #2, when you inject the patient, she will receive the correct dose.** The air will drive the medication from the needle into the patient's tissues. This is important when giving irritating medications, such as iron. (This is called an air lock.)

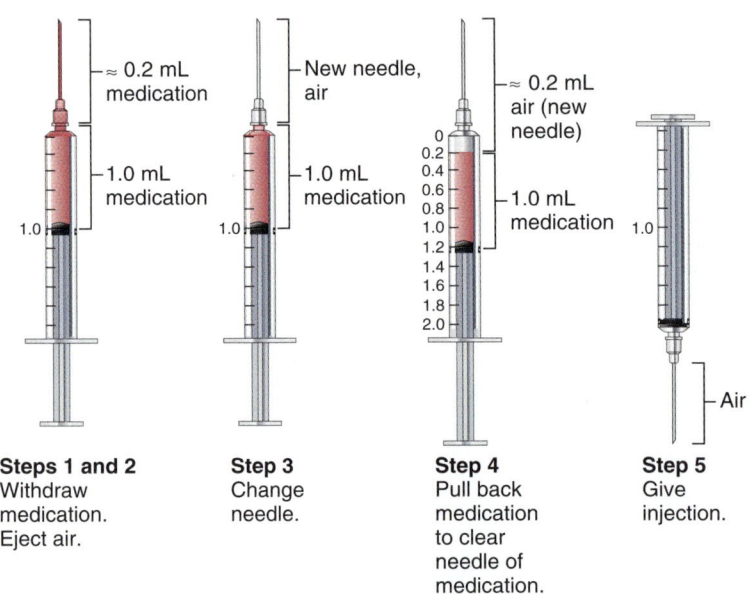

Steps 1 and 2 Withdraw medication. Eject air.	**Step 3** Change needle.	**Step 4** Pull back medication to clear needle of medication.	**Step 5** Give injection.

Nonfilter needles.

Using a Filter Needle

Always use a filter needle to withdraw medications, if one is available. You must change needles to give the injection because:

■ Filter needles are too large. To give the injection, you must use a needle of the correct gauge and length.

■ You should not push medication out of the syringe through the filter needle because it can break the filter and release glass (and other) fragments; however, you cannot measure dosage accurately with air in the syringe.

In the following method, pulling air into the syringe allows for exact dosage when the medication is injected. When ejected, the air will clear the needle so that the patient receives all the medication that is in the syringe.

Equipment

One filter needle (or filter cannula) and one regular needle.

1. **With the filter needle (or cannula), withdraw** the exact amount of medication, keeping the syringe vertical

as needed to obtain correct dose. Remember, you must not eject fluid through the filter needle.

2. **Pull back on the plunger to withdraw all the medication from the filter needle (or filter cannula) into the syringe.** Depending on the size of the access cannula, this may be as much as 0.2 mL. It will now appear that you have more than the ordered dose in the syringe (but you do not; the air is taking up some of the space).

3. **Change to the needle you are going to use for injection.** Needle #2 has air in it instead of medication.

4. **Hold the syringe vertically and eject air until you see a drop** of medication at the tip of the needle ("drop to the top").

5. **Measure the medication.** It should be at the correct syringe marking. If it is not, then tip the syringe horizontally and eject the medication until the dose is correct.

Clinical Insight 25-5 ➤ Measuring Dosage When Changing Needles—cont'd

6. **When you inject the patient, she will receive the correct dose** even though some medication will remain in the needle.

7. **If you are giving an irritating medication** (e.g., iron), draw 0.2 mL of air into the syringe before giving the injection. (This is called an air lock.)

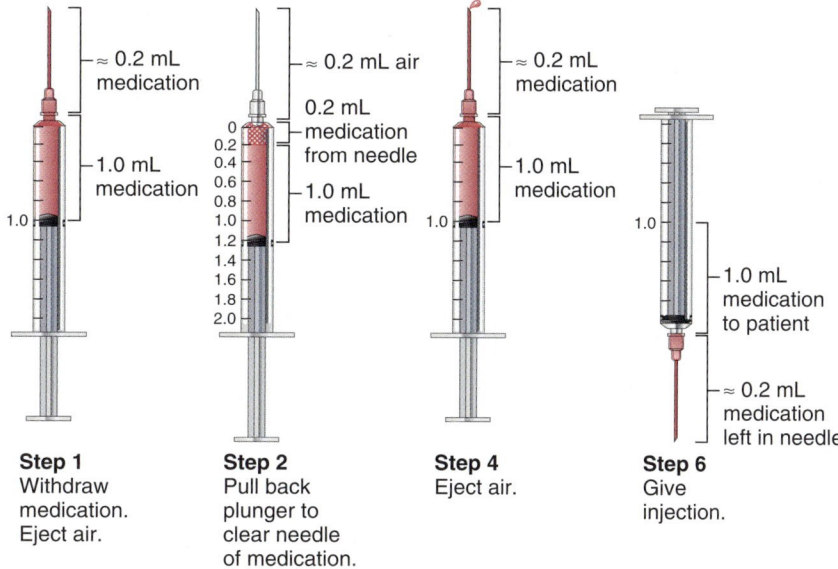

Step 1
Withdraw medication. Eject air.

Step 2
Pull back plunger to clear needle of medication.

Step 4
Eject air.

Step 6
Give injection.

Filter needles.

Clinical Insight 25-6 ➤ Mixing Two Kinds of Insulin in One Syringe

What You Should Know

Various combinations of rapid-acting, intermediate-acting, and long-acting insulin may be prescribed. Some can be mixed; some cannot.

- Lente insulins (Lente and Lantus) can be mixed with each other but not with neutral protamine Hagedorn (NPH).
- Even though they are compatible, do not mix Lente with regular insulin, except for patients who are already controlled on this mixture. Lente will bind with regular insulin, delaying the onset of action.
- A general rule is "clear before cloudy." Regular insulin is clear; all other types are cloudy because of the addition of proteins, which slow the absorption of the drug, giving it an intermediate to long duration of action. Therefore, you would draw up regular insulin into the syringe before Lente or NPH insulin, which are modified. If you draw up a modified type first, the needle may transfer it into the unmodified (regular) vial.

What You Should Do

Follow these steps when drawing up insulin from two vials into one syringe. The procedure assumes you are mixing regular (unmodified) insulin with a modified (e.g., NPH) insulin. *Note:* If regular insulin is cloudy, do not use it. Return it to the pharmacy.

1. **Maintain sterile technique throughout.**
2. **Before preparing the insulin**—Rotate the vials between the palms of your hands for at least 1 minute and invert them to ensure an adequate concentration. Do not shake the vials because this can create bubbles, which take up space and make it difficult to measure the dose precisely.
3. **Scrub vial stoppers** with alcohol or other antiseptic (they are usually multidose vials).
4. **Inject air into "cloudy" vial**—Using an insulin syringe and needle, inject an amount of air equal to the amount of insulin to be withdrawn from the vial of modified insulin (cloudy vial). Do not allow the needle tip to touch the insulin.
5. **Inject air into "clear" vial**—Using the same syringe, inject the appropriate amount of air into the vial of regular insulin (clear vial).
6. **Withdraw insulin from "clear" vial**—Do not withdraw the needle; withdraw the correct dose of regular insulin.

(Continued)

Clinical Insight 25-6 ➤ **Mixing Two Kinds of Insulin in One Syringe—cont'd**

7. **Measure the dose of "clear"**—Remove the syringe from the regular insulin. Eject air, and remove all air bubbles to measure the correct dose.
8. **Calculate combined dose**—Calculate the total amount on the syringe that the combined types of insulin should measure.
9. **Withdraw insulin from "cloudy" vial.**
   a. Return to the (first) vial of modified insulin (cloudy) ⅝ and draw the correct dose into the syringe. (For example, if you have 5 units of regular insulin in the syringe and you need 10 units of NPH, the plunger should be at the 15-unit mark when you have drawn up the NPH.)
   b. Recall that you have already added air to this vial in a previous step. Draw up the medication slowly and exactly to the total dose, being very careful not to create bubbles and to withdraw only the amount needed. You cannot return any excess to the vial because it is now a mixture of two medications.
10. **Administer the insulin mixture** within 5 minutes after preparation. Even NPH insulin will bind with regular insulin and delay the onset of its action.

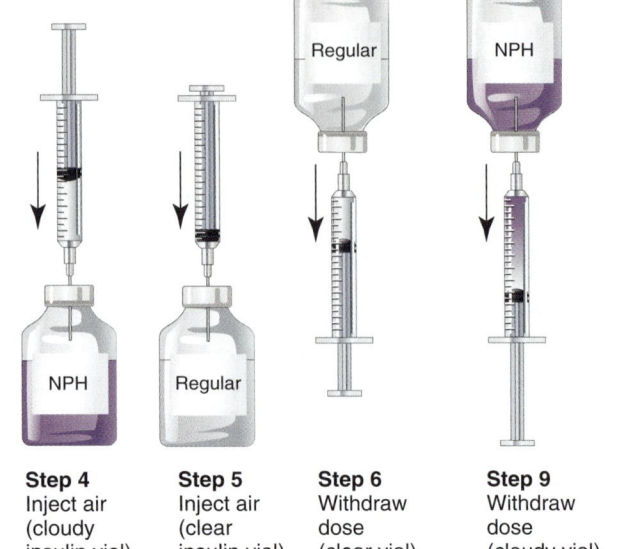

Step 4
Inject air (cloudy insulin vial).

Step 5
Inject air (clear insulin vial).

Step 6
Withdraw dose (clear vial).

Step 9
Withdraw dose (cloudy vial).

Total dose is mixture of clear and cloudy insulins.

Clinical Insight 25-7 ➤ **Administering Anticoagulant Medication Subcutaneously**

Because of the anticoagulant properties of heparin and enoxaparin (Lovenox), you will need to adapt your technique for subcutaneous injections in the following ways:

- Enoxaparin-prefilled syringes and graduated prefilled syringes are available with a system that shields the needle after injection.
- Use a ⅜-inch, 25- or 26-gauge needle.
- After drawing up the correct dose, add 0.2 mL of air to the syringe.
  To ensure that all of the medication is injected into the subcutaneous tissue and is not tracked into the superficial tissue.
- Do not expel the air bubble from the syringe before the injection.
  To avoid the loss of drug when using prefilled syringes.
- With your nondominant hand, pinch or spread the skin; insert the needle at a 90° angle, using your dominant hand.
  - If the patient has very little subcutaneous tissue, use a ⅝-inch needle and insert it at a 45° angle.
  - Introduce the whole length of the needle into a skinfold held between the thumb and forefinger; hold the skinfold throughout the injection.

- Alternate administration among sites on the abdomen. Give the injection subcutaneously deep on the abdomen, at least 2 inches away from the umbilicus.
- Do not aspirate before injecting.
  This can traumatize tissue and cause bruising.
- Do not massage the site after injecting.
  This can cause bleeding and bruising. It may also cause the heparin to be absorbed more rapidly than desired.
- Keep a record of the sites used. Most agencies have a chart of the body on which to record the sites injected.

✚ Several mix-ups between heparin and insulin have been reported. To help avoid this, in addition to observing the "3 checks and 6 rights":

1. Do not store heparin and insulin vials beside each other.
2. Have another RN check your preparation before administering IV heparin or insulin.
3. Think critically (e.g., ask yourself whether giving heparin—or insulin—makes sense given the patient's diagnosis) (Mattox, 2012).

PROCEDURES

Use the following Medication Guidelines for all medication administration.

Medication Guidelines: ■ Steps to Follow for All Medications (Regardless of Type or Route)

➤ For steps to follow in *all* procedures, refer to the Universal Steps for All Procedures found on the page facing the inside back cover.

KEY POINT: *Regardless of the type or route of the medication you are giving, you should always follow the steps below.*

Equipment

- Medication administration record (MAR)
- Medication drawer or portable cart with, as needed, keys to the medication drawer
- Gloves for the procedure, as needed
- Other supplies and equipment needed for the specific procedure (e.g., water, antiseptic wipes)

Delegation

As a registered nurse (RN), you can usually delegate administration of medications (except for intravenous [IV]) to a licensed practical nurse/licensed vocational nurse (LPN/LVN). You cannot delegate this task to nursing assistive personnel (NAP). You can instruct a NAP in the therapeutic and side effects of medications and to report any effects observed.

Nurse practice acts (NPAs) governing medication administration vary from state to state, as do policies in healthcare agencies. In some states, with additional education and training LPN/LVNs can administer IV medications and NAPs can administer some medications. You must know the scope of practice described in your state's NPA. The RN is always responsible for evaluating client responses, which include both therapeutic effects and side effects.

Pre-Procedure Assessments

- Assess your knowledge of the medication (e.g., drug action, purpose, recommended dosage, time of onset and peak action, common side effects, contraindications, drug interactions, and nursing implications).

- Determine whether the prescribed dosage is appropriate for the patient's age and weight.
  Dosages are generally decreased for children because of both age and weight. Usually dosing for elderly patients is not based on weight but on renal function. Both groups have less efficient liver and renal function, increasing the length of time a drug stays in the body before being excreted.

- Check for any history of allergies to medications or food.
  Some medications (e.g., penicillin and cephalosporin) have cross-sensitivity, that is, a patient with a penicillin allergy is at high risk for also being allergic to cephalosporin. Medications can also have cross-sensitivity with certain foods.

- At least the first time you administer medications to a patient, assess his knowledge of the medications being given.
  The patient will be more likely to take the medication correctly if she understands why she is taking the medication.

- Assess for factors that could interfere with drug absorption (e.g., diarrhea, inadequate circulation, foods, impaired liver function, edema, inflammation, age-related changes, and other medications).

- Assess vital signs and check lab studies specific to the medication to determine whether the medication can be safely administered.
  Medications are metabolized more slowly in a person with decreased liver function.

- Assess for situations in which it would not be reasonable to administer the medication (e.g., oral medications prescribed for a patient who is NPO, vomiting, or sedated or has swallowing difficulties).
  If the medication does not seem reasonable, question the prescriber.

➤ When performing the procedure, always identify your patient according to agency policy, using two identifiers, and be attentive to standard precautions, hand hygiene, patient safety and privacy, body mechanics, and documentation.

Procedure Steps

1. **Check the MAR** for the patient's name and identification number, medication, dose, route, time, and drug allergies. The rights of medication administration are the right patient, right drug, right dose, right route, right time, and right documentation. At the beginning of your shift, check the MAR to determine when medications are due **(first check).**
   Medication prescriptions may change even during your shift; checking the MAR helps ensure that you do not miss medication changes.

2. **Verify the prescription.** It should include the patient's name, patient identifier, medication name, dose, route, time, and patient allergies.
   You must note whether it has changed (e.g., since the last time you gave the drug). Clarify any discrepancies before giving the medication.

3. **Follow agency policies** for medication administration, including the time frame. Most agencies allow medications to be given 30 minutes before or 30 minutes after the time indicated on the MAR. Do not prepour medications.
   The time of administration is important for some medications. For example, if an anti-infective agent is given early or late, a therapeutic blood level may not be maintained.

4. **Perform hand hygiene.**
   Hand hygiene minimizes transmission of microorganisms.

(continued on next page)

Medication Guidelines: ■ Steps to Follow for All Medications (Regardless of Type or Route) (continued)

5. **Access the patient's medication** drawer, unlock the medication cart, or log on to the medication dispensing computer.

6. **Obtain the narcotics cabinet key** (or code) when administering a narcotic or barbiturate and sign out the medication, including the patient's name, drug, dose, and other pertinent information per agency policy. Note the drug count when removing a narcotic.
Federal law governs administration of controlled substances. All narcotics and barbiturates are counted and signed by an outgoing and oncoming nurse every shift.

7. **Select the prescribed** medication. Read the label and compare medication with the MAR for the first five rights (patient, drug, dose, route, time); check for drug allergies:
   - An inpatient should be wearing an identification band with the drug allergies identified.
   - Allergies should be clearly marked in the chart and on the MAR or in the electronic health record (EHR).
   - Ask the patient about allergies the first time you administer a medication and before giving a newly prescribed medication.
   These actions ensure that the correct drug is being given to the correct patient at the correct time in the correct dose by the correct route.

   KEY POINT: *Correct drug includes the correct form of the drug (e.g., oral, IV).*

8. **Calculate the medication dosage.** Double-check it. If you are unable to measure the dose exactly, contact the pharmacist.

9. **Check the expiration date** (on the label or on the box) of all medications.
A medication that has expired is no longer guaranteed to be effective.

10. **Do a second check** after preparing the medications to verify the correct patient medication, dose, route, and time **(second check).**
Verifies the first five rights of medication administration.

11. **Lock the medication cart.** Never leave an unlocked medication cart unattended.
This guards against pilferage and protects children, older adults with dementia, or anyone wanting to open the cart.

12. **Administer the medications.**
   a. Take the medication and MAR or a handheld portable device with the EHR into the patient's room.
   You must be able to do the final check in the patient's room and verify that you are administering the correct medication to the correct patient.

   b. Identify the patient using two forms of identification, according to agency policy: Check the identification bracelet, have the patient state her name, compare the patient with a posted picture of her, and check the patient's date of birth against the MAR.
   Agencies have different means of identifying patients. The Joint Commission requires two forms of identification. ▼

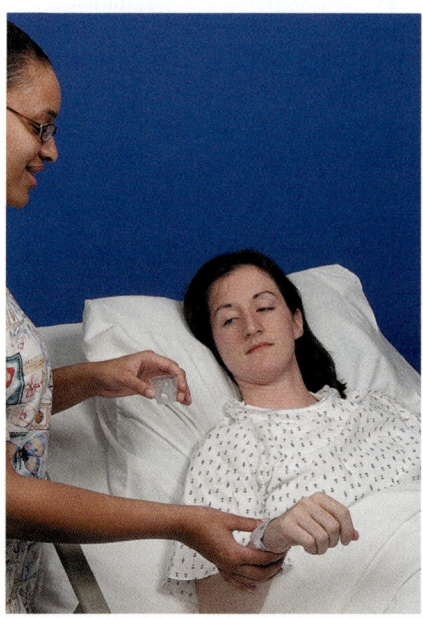

   c. Do a check of the rights of medication: right patient, right medication, right dose, right route, and right time **(third check).**
   Checks for the rights of medication are always required to prevent medication errors. Although it is not actually an "error" until the patient has taken a medication, you may be required to file a report for a "near miss" that was detected during the pre-administration checking process.

   d. Perform any necessary assessments, such as checking the pulse or blood pressure.
   Some medications can be given only if physical findings or vital signs are within certain parameters. For example, antihypertensive medications may need to be held if the blood pressure is lower than the patient's normal baseline.

   e. Explain to the patient that you are there to administer the medication; teach her about the medication.
   Patient teaching increases the patient's understanding of and compliance with treatment. The patient may then be able to identify potential errors in medication administration.

   ✚ *If the patient questions a medication, double-check the medication to be sure you are giving the correct drug and dosage.*

   f. Administer the medication using appropriate technique (see the procedures for administering medications by the specified route).

   g. Remain with the patient until you are sure that she has taken the medication.
   If you leave a medication at the bedside, someone else (e.g., another patient or a child) might take it, or the patient might discard it.

   h. Document the medication given in the patient's medication record (date, dose, route, and your name).
   Your initials on the MAR means that you administered the medication to

the patient. If the documentation is not in the patient's record, there is a risk that another nurse will assume the medication was not given and administer it again.

? What if . . .

- **The patient tells you the tablet you are ready to give him is a different color from what he normally takes of a certain prescribed medication?**

Determine why the tablet is different from what the patient is used to taking to be sure you are giving the correct drug and dose. Always verify the identity of the drug, especially when it is called into question by the patient who is familiar with the medication he normally takes.

Double-checking whenever you are uncertain about a medication you are about to administer helps prevent medication errors—it is possible you have the wrong drug or dosage.

- **The label on the medication shows an expiration date that has passed?**

Do not give the medication. Send it back to the pharmacy for replacement. *Expired medication can lose its potency.*

- **The patient refuses to take the prescribed medication?**

Discuss with the patient his concerns about the medication. Hold the dose and notify the prescriber of the patient's refusal and explain the patient's concerns.
The patient has a right to refuse medication.

- **You cannot decipher the prescriber's handwritten medication prescription?**

Hold the dose and contact the prescriber for clarification. Never administer medication if you are unable to read the entire prescription.

Handwriting that is hard to read is a common cause of preventable error. Electronic prescribing can help to avoid this.

- **Your patient's medication is not available from the pharmacy at the time the dose is due?**

Do not borrow the medication from another patient's supply. Administer only medication prescribed for that particular patient. Notify the pharmacy of the need to immediately dispense the medication.
Using another patient's medication increases the risk for error because drug dilution or dosage might vary among patients; or the drug names might sound similar, but they might be different medications. Also the safety system for charges and refills is bypassed when doses are borrowed from other patients, resulting in missing doses or erroneous charges.

Evaluation

- Evaluate the therapeutic effects of the medication (e.g., check blood pressure after administering an antihypertensive medication, or check pain level after an analgesic).
- Be alert for any adverse reactions, side effects, or allergic reactions. If present, notify the appropriate care provider.

Patient Teaching

- Describe how the drug is prescribed and when the patient should take the medication.
- Discuss the importance of taking the medication as prescribed.
- Explain the need for any laboratory tests for monitoring the medication, such as tests to measure drug level in the blood, if appropriate.
- Explain the purpose, common side effects, and drug interactions of the medications the patient is taking.
- Teach the patient to observe for side effects that signal the need to contact the prescriber.
- Discuss ways to minimize the side effects of a medication, such as avoiding the sun when taking a medication that causes photosensitivity or rising slowly when taking a medication that causes orthostatic hypotension.
- Discuss potential cultural issues related to taking the medication (e.g., in some Hispanic/Latino cultures, a patient may refuse a medication that is considered "hot" if he believes a "cold" treatment is needed).

- Teach the patient to self-administer medications (e.g., ear drops), as appropriate.

Home Care

- Assess the client's ability to safely self-administer medications.
- Determine the client's financial ability to obtain medications.
- Instruct the client about safe storage of medications.
- Provide instructions for use of each medication.
- Determine whether the client or caregiver has had past problems or present concerns about taking the medications as prescribed.
- If problems have occurred in the past or there are present concerns, discuss possible remedies. For example, you might teach the client or caregiver to use a medication storage container with compartments for the times and days of the week the medication(s) need to be taken.

Documentation

- Chart the medication; time, dose, and route given; preadministration assessments; and your signature.
- Do not document before giving the drug; do not document for anyone else; do not ask another nurse to document a drug you have given. Document only *after* administering the medication.
- Document all therapeutic and any adverse effects of the medication. Also document your nursing interventions and patient teaching regarding potential adverse effects.

(continued on next page)

Medication Guidelines: ■ **Steps to Follow for All Medications (Regardless of Type or Route)** (continued)

■ Record the scheduled medications on the MAR. Record prn medications in the nursing notes and on the MAR, including the reason the medication was given and the patient's response to the medication.

■ If the patient is unable or refuses to take the medication, document on the MAR that the medication was not administered and the reason, and inform the provider.

■ For parenteral medications, chart the site of injection.

Practice Resources

Institute for Safe Medication Practices (2015b); National Coordinating Council for Medication Error Reporting and Prevention (2015); U.S. Food and Drug Administration (2012, updated 2016).

 The video **Medication Guidelines: Steps to Follow for All Medications (Regardless of Route),** along with questions and suggested responses, is available on the **Davis's *Nursing Skills Videos*** Web site on Davis*Plus*.

Sample EHR documentation

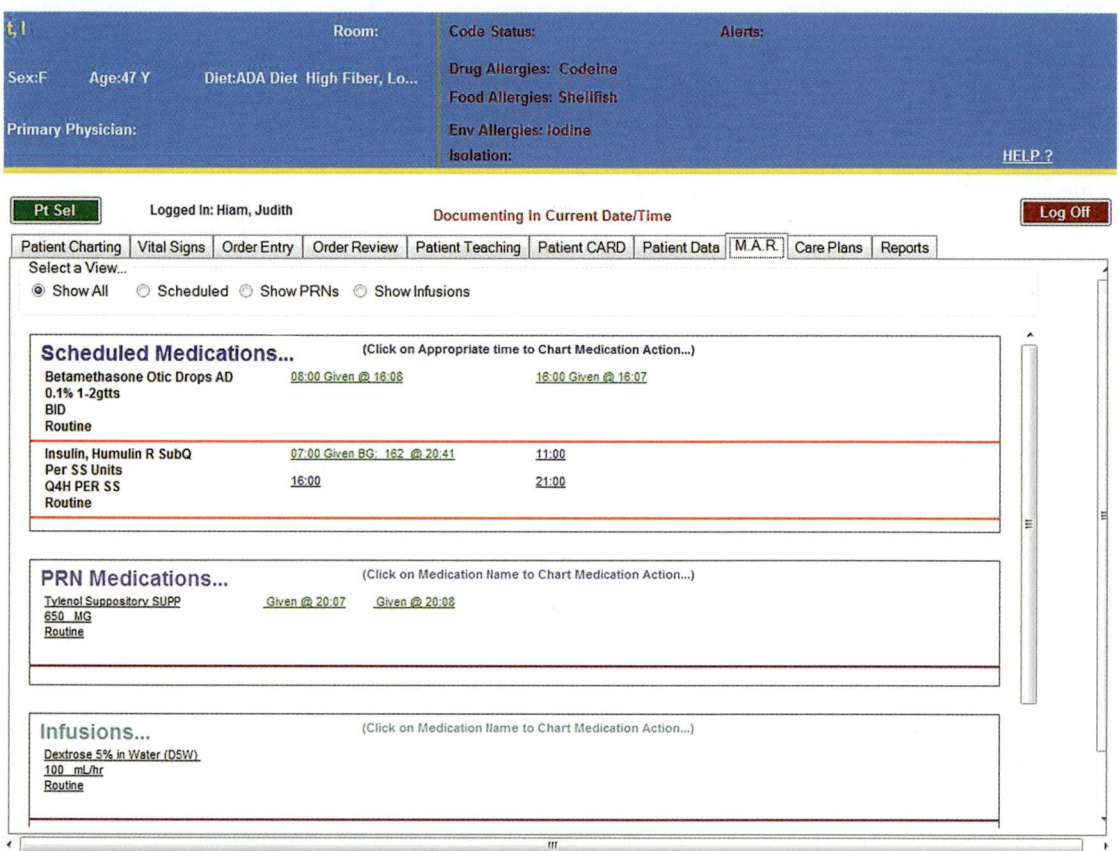

Procedure 25-1 ■ **Administering Oral Medication**

➤ For steps to follow in *all* procedures, refer to the Universal Steps for All Procedures found on the page facing the inside back cover. Also refer to **Medication Guidelines: Steps to Follow for All Medications (Regardless of Type or Route).**

Equipment

■ Desired liquid for swallowing medications
■ Disposable medication cup
■ Drinking straw, if needed
■ Procedure gloves, if you will need to place a tablet in the patient's mouth
■ For enteral medication:
  Water (for diluting and flushing the feeding tube)
  60-mL catheter-tip syringe
  Clean gloves

■ Stethoscope (*e.g., to check the apical pulse before administering some cardiac medications*)

Delegation

■ As a rule, you can delegate this skill to an LPN/LVN, depending on the medication, but not to a NAP, except under special policies and situations.

Pre-Procedure Assessments

- Assess the patient's condition to determine whether there are contraindications to oral medications or to the specific medication, for example, the patient's ability to swallow. *Impaired swallowing increases the risk for aspiration.*

- Check fluid needs and restrictions. If the patient is NPO (nothing by mouth), check with the prescriber to determine whether the medication should be given by another route or can be given with small sips of water.

A prescriber may decide it is medically necessary to administer oral medication to a patient who is NPO. If there is a fluid restriction, you need to consider how much fluid you can give with medication. Give additional fluid to a patient with dehydration; offer only sips for the patient with a fluid restriction.

- For enteral medications, check that the NG tube is in the stomach and is patent.

➤ When performing the procedure, always identify your patient according to agency policy, using two identifiers, and be attentive to standard precautions, hand hygiene, patient safety and privacy, body mechanics, and documentation.

Procedure Steps

1. **Prepare the medication** for administration.

For Tablet or Capsule

a. If you are pouring from a multi-dose container, do not touch the medication. Pour the tablet into the cap of the container, then into the medication cup.

b. If the medication is unit-dose, do not open the package. Place the entire unit-dose package into the cup.

c. Many institutions allow combining all tablets or oral caplets scheduled for the same time for the same patient into the same cup. However, even if the agency protocol permits dispensing from a single container, you will need separate cups for medications that require pre-administration assessment (e.g., checking the apical pulse rate prior to administering digoxin).
If a medication is held because of a pre-administration assessment finding, you can identify it more readily when it has been poured into a separate cup.

d. You may break scored tablets with a knife or a tablet cutter if necessary.
Only scored tablets may be broken. Breaking an unscored tablet would deliver an imprecise dose.

e. If a patient has difficulty swallowing, check to see whether the medication can be crushed. If so, use a mortar and pestle to grind it. If the medication is in a unit-dose package, grind it while it is still inside the package. Mix the ground medication with a small amount of soft food such as applesauce or pudding.
Crushing some medications (e.g., capsules, enteric-coated tablets, and sustained-release formulas) may alter their effectiveness or result in an overdose due to rapid absorption.

For Liquid Medications

f. Check to see whether you must shake the liquid before opening the container.
Some liquids, such as suspensions, will precipitate and need to be shaken to mix the active ingredient with the suspension liquid.

g. Remove the bottle cap and place it flat side down on the cart or counter.

h. Hold the bottle cap with the label in the palm of your hand.
Keeping the label on the upward side of the bottle prevents the liquid from dripping down onto the label and obscuring it. ▼

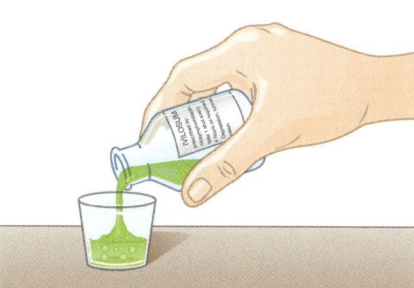

i. Hold or place the plastic medication cup at eye level, and pour the desired amount of medication. Read the dosage where the lowest part of the concave surface (meniscus) of the fluid is on the line. You can, instead, place the cup on a level surface, pour the medication, then hold the cup at eye level to read the amount.
Measuring liquids above or below eye level will cause you to read the dose incorrectly and pour too much or too little medication.

j. As you finish pouring medication, slightly twist the bottle to prevent the medication from dripping down the lip of the bottle. If medication does drip down over the lip, wipe the outside of the lip with a tissue or paper towel.
Wiping the outside of the bottle helps prevent contamination, particularly for thicker solutions such as elixirs or syrups containing sugar.

2. **Administer the medication.**

a. Assist the patient to a high Fowler's position, if possible.
An upright position facilitates swallowing and prevents choking.

b. **Powder:** Mix with liquid at the bedside and give the mixture to the patient to drink.
Some powders thicken very quickly and must be mixed immediately before administration.

c. **Lozenge:** Instruct the patient not to chew or swallow it whole.
Medication is absorbed through the oral mucosa and is generally inactivated by the acidity in the stomach.

d. **Tablet or capsule:**
1) If the patient is able to hold the medication in her hand, place the tablet or medication cup in her hand.
Promotes independence and is easier for the patient.

(continued on next page)

Procedure 25-1 ■ Administering Oral Medication (continued)

2) Give the patient water or other liquid.

Giving the medication with liquid moistens the mouth and helps the patient swallow the tablet or capsule.

3) If the patient is unable to hold the tablet, don procedure gloves, place the medication cup up to her lips, and tip the tablet or capsule into her mouth.

Encourage the patient to do as much as possible. Getting the tablet or capsule to the back of the mouth will assist in swallowing.

e. **Sublingual medications:** Have the patient place the tablet under the tongue and hold it there until it is completely dissolved.

Sublingual medications are made to be rapidly absorbed through the oral mucosa. The area under the tongue is

very vascular, so sublingual medications act very rapidly. Sublingual medications are inactivated by gastric acid if swallowed. ▼

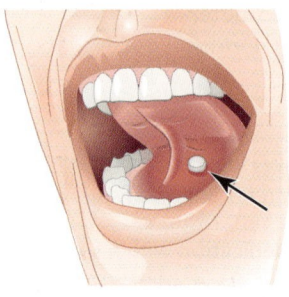

f. **Buccal medications:** Have the patient place the tablet between the cheek and teeth or tongue.

Buccal medications act by being absorbed through the oral mucosa or by being dissolved and swallowed in the saliva. ➤

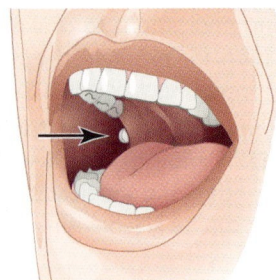

3. **Stay with the patient until** all medications have been swallowed or dissolved.

Some patients will "chipmunk" the medication in the side of the mouth without swallowing it or spit it out. Staying at the bedside until the patient swallows the oral medication ensures that the patient receives the dose.

Procedure 25-1A ■ Administering Medication Through an Enteral Tube

➤ For steps to follow in *all* procedures, refer to the Universal Steps for All Procedures found on the page facing the inside back cover. Also refer to **Medication Guidelines: Steps to Follow for All Medications (Regardless of Type or Route).**

Preparation

■ If the patient is receiving a continuous tube feeding, disconnect it before giving the medications. Leave the tube clamped for a few minutes after administering the medication, according to agency protocol.

■ If the enteral tube is connected to suction, you will usually discontinue the suction for 20 to 30 minutes after administration and keep the tube clamped to allow time for the drug to be absorbed.

➤ When performing the procedure, always identify your patient according to agency policy and be attentive to standard precautions, hand hygiene, patient safety and privacy, body mechanics, and documentation.

➤ *Note:* Follow steps 1a through 1j of Procedure 25-1: Administering Oral Medication. Also follow precautions for administering enteral medications.

Procedure Steps

1. **Prepare the medication.**

a. Give the liquid form of medication, if possible. If the solution is hypertonic, be sure to dilute with 10 to 30 mL of sterile water before instilling through a feeding tube.

Hyperosmolar substances administered too rapidly into the gut can cause bloating, nausea, and osmotic diarrhea.

b. If tablets must be given, verify that the medication can be crushed and given through an enteral tube.

Some tablets (e.g., sustained-release or enteric-coated tablets) should not

be crushed because doing so changes their action.

c. Crush the tablet and mix it with approximately 20 mL of water or obtain a liquid medication. If you are giving several medications, mix and administer each one separately.

If you are using a small-bore tube, such as a PEG tube, Keofeed NG feeding tube, or jejunostomy tube, always obtain the liquid form of the medication, because the small-bore tubes clog easily. Ensure that the medication is diluted enough to pass easily through the tube. Instilling

drugs one at a time allows you to identify each medication.

2. **Don nonsterile procedure gloves.**

Gloving maintains standard precautions.

3. **Place patient in a sitting (high Fowler's)** position, if possible.

An upright position reduces the risk for choking and aspiration.

4. **For NG tubes, check tube placement** (see Chapter 28, Clinical Insights 28-4 and 28-5) by aspirating stomach contents or measuring the pH of the aspirate, if possible. Other, less accurate, methods are injecting

air into the feeding tube and auscultating or asking the patient to speak; however, these are not confirmatory methods (DiMatteo, 2012).

➕ Never rely on only one bedside method for checking tube placement; use a combination of methods.

NG tubes can become displaced or positioned in the lungs. If medications are given through a misplaced NG tube, the patient may develop aspiration pneumonia.

5. **Check for residual volume** (see Chapter 28, Procedure 28-3).

6. **Flush the tube.** Based on the type of tube, use a piston tip or luer-lock syringe (usually a 30- to 60-mL syringe). Remove the bulb or plunger; attach the barrel to the tube; and pour in 20 to 30 mL of water.
   Flushing ensures patency of the tube and also clears the tube of feeding solution that could clump with medication.

7. **Instill the medication by depressing** the syringe plunger or using the barrel of the syringe as a funnel and pouring in the medication. A smaller tube or thicker medication will require instilling the medication with a 30- to 60-mL syringe, but when larger tubes are used, the medication can be poured. ▼

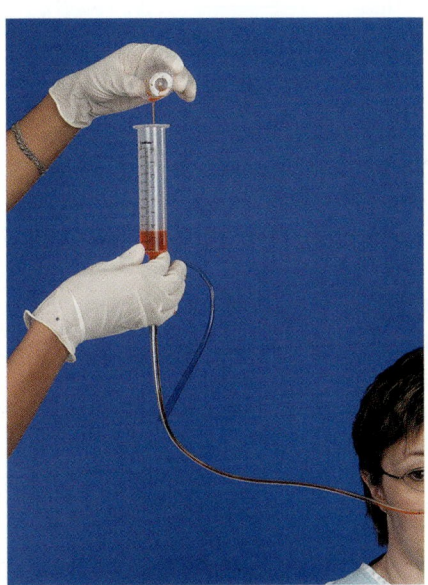

For Viscous Medication
Instill the medication by depressing the syringe plunger.

8. **Flush the medication through** the tube by instilling an additional 20 to 30 mL of water.
   Flushing ensures that all the medication has been administered and prevents the tube from clogging.

9. **If there is more than one medication,** give each separately, flushing after each.
   Some medications are less effective when given in combination, or there may be an additive effect if they have similar actions.

10. **Have the patient maintain a sitting position** for at least 30 minutes after you administer the medication.
    Minimizes the risk of aspiration.

❓ What if . . .

■ **My patient vomits shortly after taking oral medication?**

Notify the prescriber for instructions about whether or not to repeat the dose.

■ **My patient is unable to sit upright to take oral medication?**

Assist the patient into a side-lying position and offer a straw to take water with capsules or tablets.

■ **My patient has difficulty drinking from a cup?**

Use a syringe without a needle to place the medication in his mouth. Place the patient in a side-lying or upright position. Place the syringe between the gum and cheek in the back corner of the mouth, and slowly push the plunger to administer the liquid.

■ **My patient is NPO (nothing by mouth)?**

Check with the prescriber to determine whether the medication should be given by another route or can be given with small sips of water.

■ **My patient is on fluid restriction?**

Use the smallest amount of water needed to swallow or dissolve tablets and to flush enteral tubes.

■ **My patient is cognitively impaired?**

Request the patient open his mouth to see whether he has swallowed the medication; look under the tongue or side pocket near the inside of the cheek.

 My patient is an older adult who is to receive medication through an enteral tube?

Check level of consciousness, mentation, or alertness. Check for potential aspiration risk by checking the patient's swallow and gag reflexes.

■ **My patient is a child who is to receive medication through an enteral tube?**

Use only medications that are prepared in liquid form.
Prevent occlusion of the tube.

Position an infant in a prone, side-lying, sitting, or reverse Trendelenburg position for 30 minutes to 1 hour following medication administration.
These positions facilitate peristalsis and transport of medication through the intestine.

■ **The prescribed medication should be given on an empty stomach?**

Stop the feeding 30 minutes before giving the drug. Resume 30 minutes later.
These times allow for the stomach to empty and for drug absorption to occur before the feedings resume.

(continued on next page)

Procedure 25-1 ■ **Administering Oral Medication** (continued)

Evaluation

For medications administered orally:

- Note whether the patient has difficulty swallowing, gags, or coughs while swallowing oral medication.
- Evaluate for gastric discomfort, nausea, vomiting, or diarrhea.
- Assess for any signs of drug allergy or intolerance to the medication.

  For medications administered through a feeding tube:

- In addition to the preceding assessments, assess that the NG tube is correctly placed and patent before and after administering the medication.

Patient Teaching

- Refer to **Medication Guidelines: Steps to Follow for All Medications (Regardless of Type or Route).**
- Discuss drug safety measures with the patient, including use of child-safety caps (or using an easy-open cap for an elderly population or with those likely to have difficulty opening containers of this type); keeping the medication in its original container; discarding expired medications; avoiding transferring medication to another container; and carefully reading the label and directions for each medication.
- Discuss the relationship between food and the medication, if needed. For example, is the medication to be taken with food or not? Does taking the medication on an empty stomach contribute to nausea or gastric irritation? Does the medication interact with any foods?

For enteral medications:

Cover the preceding topics for patient teaching about oral medications, plus the following:

- Discuss the importance of upright positioning for 20 to 30 minutes after taking medication through an enteral tube.
- Instruct the patient to immediately notify his healthcare provider if he chokes or has difficulty breathing during or shortly after medication is given by enteral tube. He should stop the medication immediately, and emergency care might be necessary.

Home Care

Advise clients who are receiving enteral medication at home to do the following:

- Notify the healthcare provider: (1) if any of the following lasts for more than a day: diarrhea, constipation, nausea, dark urine, bad-smelling urine, or dry mouth; (2) if the tube becomes clogged or seems to be moving farther out or in; (3) if the feeding tube falls out; or (4) if you cannot confirm that the end of the tube is in the stomach.
- To prevent a clogged feeding tube, flush the tube with water each time after giving a medication or feeding.
- Brush your teeth at least twice daily if an NG tube remains in place continuously.
- Clean daily the area where the NG tube goes into the nostrils. Use a cotton-tip applicator moistened with warm

water. If your nose becomes sore, you might apply water-soluble lubricant.

- Change the nasal tape every other day or when it is loose or soiled.

Documentation

- Scheduled medications are often recorded only on the MAR.
- Document the drug, dosage, time, route, and your name as the healthcare provider administering the medication.
- Document any suspected drug reaction, intolerance, or patient response to the medication.
- For patients whose intake and output are being measured, document the amount of liquid medication and the water given. Some patients may be on fluid restrictions, so all intake. Follow your clinical facility protocol.

For enteral medications:

Document the following:

- Patency, residual volume, and verification of tube placement.
- Any difficulty with administering the medications through the feeding tube.
- On the intake and output form, record the amount of liquid medication and the water used for flushing. Some providers prescribe a specific amount of water to flush with each medication administration or feeding. Some healthcare facilities use a protocol amount of water to flush gastrostomy tubes. Follow the protocol in your clinical facility.

Sample documentation for a prn oral medication

mm/dd/yyyy   1800   Placed client in Fowler's position. Administered Lasix 20 mg. PO tablet with 30 mL water. Patient tolerated medication with no swallowing difficulties. ———— S. Smith, RN

Sample documentation for an enteral medication

mm/dd/yyyy   1400   Placed client in Fowler's position. GT placement confirmed with pH of 4.5 gastric aspirate. Administered 10 mL of liquid medication and flushed with 20 mL of water. Tolerated medication with no complaints. ———— S. Smith, RN

Thinking About the Procedure

 The videos **Administering Oral Medications: Tablet or Capsule, Administering Oral Medications: Sublingual, Administering Oral Medications: Buccal,** and **Administering Oral Medications: Liquid Medications,** along with questions and suggested responses, are available on the **Davis's Nursing Skills Videos** Web site on DavisPlus.

Practice Resources

Emami, S., Hamishehkar, H., Mahmoodpoor, A., et al. (2012); Kelly, J., Eggleton, A., & Wright, D. (2011); Morris, H. (2012).

Procedure 25-2 ■ Administering Ophthalmic Medication

➤ For steps to follow in *all* procedures, refer to the Universal Steps for All Procedures found on the page facing the inside back cover. Also refer to the **Medication Guidelines: Steps to Follow for All Medications (Regardless of Type or Route).**

Equipment

- Eye drops or ointment
- Tissue

For irrigation, add:

- Prescribed eye irrigation solution (e.g., 500 to 1,000 mL of normal saline or lactated Ringer's solution are commonly used)
- IV tubing or eye irrigation insert, such as the Morgan lens (Follow manufacturer's directions for this specialized equipment.)
- Ocular anesthetic, according to protocol or provider's orders
- pH paper
- Basin and towel

Delegation

An RN can usually delegate eye instillations to an LPN/LVN. You usually cannot delegate this task to a NAP, unless the NAP has special training for a specific, defined situation (e.g., "medication aides" in some long-term-care settings). **See Delegation, in Medication Guidelines: Steps to Follow for All Medications (Regardless of Type or Route).**

Pre-Procedure Assessments

- Assess the patient's eyes for redness, discharge, or other signs of irritation.
- Determine whether the eyes need to be cleansed before administration of the medication.
  Excess tearing, debris, or excess mucus in the eye could interfere with the absorption, and thus effectiveness, of the medication.

✚ Check the prescription for place to instill medication. (*NOTE:* **We do not advise using these abbreviations**—they have been disallowed by The Joint Commission—but you may still see them written in prescriptions.) *Clarify with the provider the correct site.*

OD = **right eye**   **OS** = **left eye**   **OU** = **both eyes**

For irrigations also assess the following:

- Determine the cause of the eye problem—acid, alkaline, or other chemical burn or body fluid splash, or nonembedded foreign body.
  Irrigations are generally used to remove chemical or physical irritants, but they may be done following surgery or to treat a severe infection. Normal saline (NS) or lactated Ringer's is the solution generally recommended for high-volume eye irrigations because the pH of 6 to 7.5 is closest to the normal tear pH of 7.1. Volumes of 500 to 1,000 mL are generally used.

- Assess the patient's eyes for swelling, redness, drainage, or complaints of pain.
  A baseline assessment is useful for determining the need for and effectiveness of irrigation. Sclera should be smooth, white, and glistening.

- Determine the patient's level of discomfort and ability to cooperate with the procedure.
  Combative or otherwise uncooperative patients refusing instillation of medication can interfere with the efficiency of the procedure. If the patient cannot hold still for the procedure, he may need to be sedated.

- Assess the pain level.
  Debris, chemicals, and some liquids in the eye can be extremely painful. The eye may need to be anesthetized before irrigation or a general systemic pain medication given.

➤ When performing the procedure, always identify your patient according to agency policy, using two identifiers, and be attentive to standard precautions, hand hygiene, patient safety and privacy, body mechanics, and documentation.

Procedure Steps

1. **Assist the patient to a high Fowler's position** with head slightly tilted back, if possible.

   ✚ Do not tilt the head back if the patient has a neck injury or other contraindication. The medication can be given with the patient supine.

   An upright position keeps eye drops in the eye and helps prevent eye drops from draining into lacrimal duct.

2. **Don procedure gloves.**
   Gloving complies with standard precautions.

3. **Cleanse the edges of the eyelid** from the inner to outer canthus, if needed.
   By following the principle of "clean to dirty," you avoid transferring debris into the nasolacrimal duct.

Procedure Variation A Instilling Eye Drops

(Follow steps 1–3. Note, however, that some sources recommend that the patient lie supine for eye drops.)

4. **Gently rest your dominant** hand (the one with the eyedropper) on the patient's forehead.
   Stabilizes the hand in the event the patient moves—prevents accidental injury to the eye.

(continued on next page)

Procedure 25-2 ■ Administering Ophthalmic Medication (continued)

5. With your nondominant hand, pull the lower lid down to expose the conjunctival sac.
Allows visualization of the area where you will administer the medication.

6. Position the eyedropper about 1.5 to 2.0 cm (½ to ¾ in.) above the patient's eye. Ask the patient to look up, and drop the prescribed number of drops into the conjunctival sac. Do not let the dropper touch the eye.
Keeping the dropper away from the globe of the eye reduces the risk of accidental injury to the eye and avoids contamination of the dropper. Having the patient look up helps to decrease the blink reflex. ▼

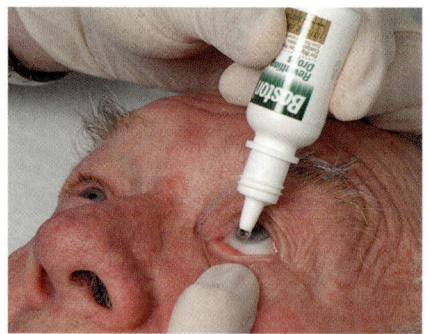

7. Ask the patient to gently close his eyes.
Closing the eyes helps to distribute the medication.

8. If the medication has systemic effects, press gently against the same side of the nose for 1 to 2 minutes to close the lacrimal ducts.
Reduces systemic absorption through the lacrimal duct. ➤

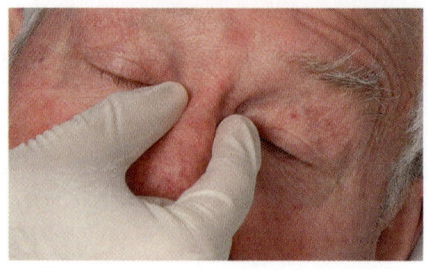

Procedure Variation B
Administering Eye Ointment
(Follow steps 1–3, then move to step 9.)

9. Gently rest your dominant hand, the one with the eye ointment, on the patient's forehead.
Stabilizing your hand helps to prevent accidental injury to the eye.

10. With your nondominant hand, pull the lower lid down to expose the conjunctival sac.
Allows visualization of area where you will administer the medication.

11. Ask the patient to look up as you apply a thin strip of ointment—usually about 2 to 2.5 cm (1 in.)—in the conjunctival sac; twist your wrist to break off the strip of ointment. Do not let the tube touch the eye.
If the medication ribbon is not broken off, lifting the tube will pull the medication out of the conjunctival sac. ▼

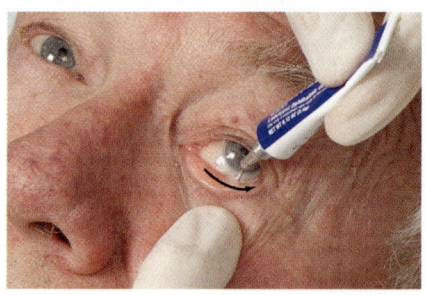

a. Ask the patient to gently close his eyes for 2 to 3 minutes. Alternatively, release the eyelids and have the client blink several times.
Helps to distribute the medication.

b. Explain to the patient that his vision will be blurred for a short amount of time after administration of the ointment.
The viscosity of the ointment can cause blurring.

? What if . . .

■ **My patient is a child who won't open his eye for the application?**

Try distracting the child by turning on the television or offering an age-appropriate toy in view.
Distraction and bribery are effective techniques for coaxing a child when cooperation is essential.

Ask a family member to help you gain cooperation of the child.
It might be fear or mistrust that is causing him to be unwilling to open his eyes.

■ **My patient wears soft contact lenses?**

Have the patient remove contact lenses before administering the medication and wait at least 15 minutes after instilling eye drops before reinserting the lenses.

Procedure 25-2A ■ Irrigating the Eyes

➤ When performing the procedure, always identify your patient according to agency policy, using two identifiers, and be attentive to standard precautions, hand hygiene, patient safety and privacy, body mechanics, and documentation.

Procedure Steps

1. Assist the patient to a low-Fowler's position, with the head tilted toward the affected eye, if possible.
This position helps to drain the irrigating solution from the eye and prevents contamination of the unaffected eye.

2. Place the towel and basin under the patient's cheek to absorb the drainage.
The patient will be more comfortable when he is clean and dry.

3. Check the pH by gently touching the pH paper to secretions in the conjunctival sac.
A litmus test determines the correct irrigating solution and whether the irritant is alkaline or acidic. The normal pH of tears is approximately 7.1.

4. Follow the agency protocol or prescriber's order regarding use of ocular anesthetic drops.
The ocular anesthetic will be washed out by the irrigation fluid, so it needs to be reinstilled every 2 to 3 minutes, or it can be added to the irrigation solution.

5. Connect the solution and tubing, and prime the tubing.
Priming the tubing prevents blowing air across the cornea, which would be uncomfortable.

6. Irrigate the eye.
a. Hold the tubing about 2.5 cm (1 in.) from eye.
A safe distance helps prevent accidental trauma to the eye.

b. Separate the eyelids with your thumb and index finger.
It is easier to irrigate the cornea when the eyelids are separated.

c. Direct the flow of solution over the eye from the inner canthus to the outer canthus.
The inner canthus is considered clean, primarily because of the open duct in this area. Flowing irrigation solution in this manner follows the principle of "clean to dirty." ▼

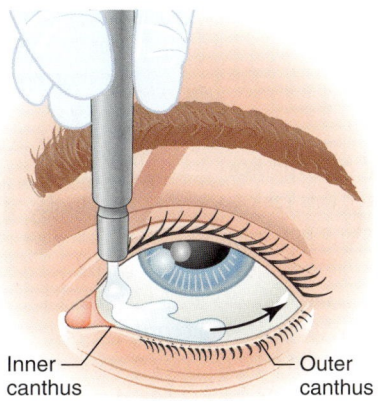

Inner canthus — Outer canthus

7. Recheck pH and continue to irrigate the eye as needed.
With alkaline or acidic chemical injuries, the pH of the eye needs to be returned to normal as soon as possible to prevent further eye injury.

Evaluation

- Examine the eyes for redness or drainage.
- Observe the patient's ability to follow instructions during the procedure.
- Observe the pain level during the procedure.
- After an irrigation, check for decrease in eye pain.

Patient Teaching

- Discuss how to prevent contaminating eye drops or ointment.
- Teach the best technique for instilling eye drops or ointment.
- Discuss the use of an eye drop guide if the patient needs assistance with instilling drops.
- Discuss the signs and symptoms to report to the provider, including eye pain and increased redness or drainage.

For irrigations:

- Discuss the cause and prevention of eye injuries, including use of protective goggles.
- Discuss the need for follow-up treatment. If the patient will be instilling eye medications or applying eye patches, ensure that he demonstrates the correct technique.

Home Care

If a splash occurs to the eyes in the home, teach the client to immediately flood his eyes with cool water (as follows):
- Hold your eyelids open and put your head under a faucet or pour water from a clean container.
- Roll your eyes as much as possible while running water across your eyes.
- Flood your eyes for at least 20 minutes.
- Get medical help immediately after rinsing your eyes.

Documentation

- *For instillations:* Chart assessment data before, during, and after instillation. Record on the MAR, as for all medications.
- *For irrigations:* Chart the condition of the patient's eyes before the irrigation, including complaints of pain or burning. Document the eye pH, instillation of anesthetic drops, the type and amount of irrigation fluid used, the eye pH following irrigation, and the patient's response. Also record other treatment (e.g., instillation of lubricating and/or antibiotic ointment; application of eye patches).

Sample documentation

mm/dd/yyyy   1200   In preparation for discharge and after teaching, patient correctly self-administered Garamycin eye drops 1 gtt in right eye as prescribed. Patient closed her eyes and gently pressed against the right side of the nose for 1 minute after instillation. Stated, "I will not have a problem doing this at home. Thank you for teaching me the right way." No redness, discharge, or complaints of pain. ——————————— S. Smith, RN

Thinking About the Procedure

 The video **Administering Ophthalmic Medication,** along with questions and suggested responses, is available on the **Davis's *Nursing Skills Videos*** Web site on Davis*Plus*.

Practice Resources

Centers for Disease Control and Prevention (2011a); Glaucoma Research Foundation (n.d., reviewed 2016); Heller, J. L. (2011, updated); Mason, I., & Stevens, S. (2010); Terrie, Y. (2012).

Procedure 25-3 ■ Administering Otic Medication

> For steps to follow in *all* procedures, refer to the Universal Steps for All Procedures found on the page facing the inside back cover. Also refer to the **Medication Guidelines: Steps to Follow for All Medications (Regardless of Type or Route).**

Equipment

- Ear drops
- Dropper with flexible rubber tip
- Cotton-tipped applicators
- Cotton ball

Delegation

The RN can usually delegate administration of otic medications to an LPN/LVN. You usually cannot delegate this task to a NAP, unless allowed by the state's nurse practice act.

Pre-Procedure Assessments

- Assess the external ear and canal for erythema, drainage, and cerumen.
  You may need to clean the external ear to remove obstructions so that the medication can be distributed throughout the ear canal. Use the otoscope to evaluate the tympanic membrane if the drainage is bloody or the patient complains of pain or decreased hearing acuity. Use sterile technique if the tympanic membrane is ruptured.
- Assess for any ear pain or hearing impairment.
  Establishes a baseline that can be used to evaluate the effects of treatment.

> When performing the procedure, always identify your patient according to agency policy, using two identifiers, and be attentive to standard precautions, hand hygiene, patient safety and privacy, body mechanics, and documentation.

Procedure Steps

1. **Hold the ear drop bottle** in your hand to warm it, or place it in warm water (not hot). Gently shake the bottle before using the drops.
   Warm solution is more comfortable than cool. Placing cool solutions in the ear can cause dizziness. Gently shaking the bottle disperses the medication throughout the solution.

2. **Assist patient to a side-lying** position, with the appropriate ear facing up.
   Facilitates administering the drops and prevents drops escaping from the ear.

3. **Clean the external ear** with a cotton-tipped applicator, if necessary.
   Cleaning the ear allows ear drops to reach all areas of the ear canal without trauma. Be careful not to push cerumen further into the ear canal.

4. **Fill the dropper** with the correct amount of medication.

5. **For infants and young children,** ask a parent or another caregiver to immobilize the child while you administer the medication.
   Mobilization and restraint reduce the risk for injury for the child who struggles during the procedure.

6. **Straighten the ear canal.**
   a. For a child younger than 3 years old, pull the pinna down and back. ▶

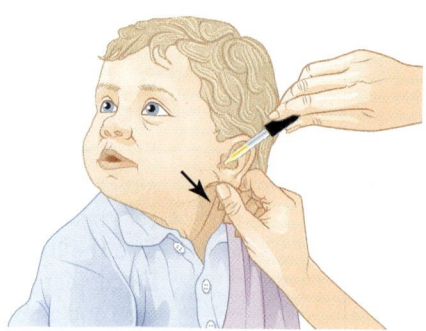

b. For children 3 years and older and adults, pull the pinna up and back. ▼

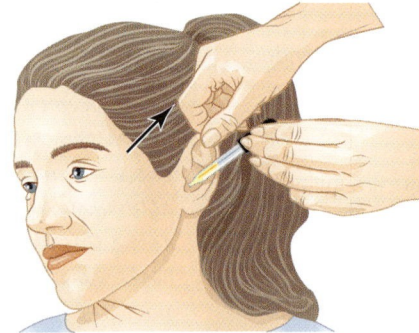

These positions straighten the ear canal for proper channeling of the medication.

7. **Instill the ordered number** of drops along the side of the ear canal, being careful not to touch the end of the dropper to any part of the ear.
   Reduces the risk of contaminating the dropper.

8. **Gently tug on the external** ear after drops are instilled.
   Facilitates flow of medication into the auditory canal.

9. **Instruct the patient** to remain on her side for 5 to 10 minutes.
   Assists in distributing the medication and prevents drops from escaping the ear canal.

10. **Place a cotton ball,** or a piece of it, loosely at the opening of the auditory canal for 15 minutes.

    A cotton ball will absorb excess fluid and keep the medication from flowing out.

    ✚ *Keep in mind that cotton left near an infant can be a choking hazard and must be carefully supervised.*

? What if . . .

- **My patient is a child and rolls over so most of the otic medication flows back out of the ear?**

  Estimate the amount of the dosage that was lost. Replace it by repeating the procedure for instillation of the medication, except next time position the child securely until you are confident the medication has had time to penetrate the ear canal.

- **There is too much cerumen (ear wax) in the canal to instill otic drops?**

   You can use special drops for softening the cerumen and allow for easier removal. Gentle irrigation with warm saline is effective, unless the patient has a perforated tympanic membrane or myringotomy tubes.

You should not use a metal syringe (Pomeroy syringe) for the removal of cerumen because (1) this type of syringe is heavy and difficult to control and (2) because of the pressure exerted, it may be associated with a higher risk of perforations of the tympanic membrane.

Oral jet irrigators have also been associated with some trauma, including tympanic membrane perforation.

You should not attempt to remove impaction by "ear candling," which is the application of hot candle wax.

Evaluation

- Assess for discomfort or pain during the procedure and for relief afterward.
- Evaluate for wax buildup, redness, swelling, or drainage.

Documentation

- Assess the amount, color, character, and odor of drainage, if present.

- Note any swelling or redness in the ear canal.
- Document pain or discomfort and hearing loss.

Thinking About the Procedure

The video **Administering Otic Medication,** along with questions and suggested responses, is available on the **Davis's** *Nursing Skills Videos* Web site on Davis*Plus.*

Procedure 25-4 ■ Administering Nasal Medication

➤ For steps to follow in *all* procedures, refer to the Universal Steps for All Procedures found on the page facing the inside back cover. Also refer to the **Medication Guidelines: Steps to Follow for All Medications (Regardless of Type or Route).**

Equipment

- Medication drops, spray, or aerosol
- Tissues

Delegation

As an RN, you can usually delegate administration of nasal instillations to an LPN/LVN. You usually cannot delegate this task to a NAP.

Pre-Procedure Assessments

- Check for nasal obstruction and congestion.
  Nasal obstruction or congestion can prevent the medication from reaching the nasal mucosa.

- Assess nasal discharge for color, consistency, and odor.
  The appearance of drainage is not always diagnostic of infection, especially for people with chronic sinus problems or polyps. Color can be indicative of the body's response to viral, bacterial, and allergic sources.

- Assess nasal mucous membranes for redness, color, moisture, excoriation, or trauma.

   Check the dropper tip to be sure it is not cracked or chipped.
  A cracked or chipped tip might interfere with drawing up the medication and scratch the nasal mucosa.

➤ When performing the procedure, always identify your patient according to agency policy, using two identifiers, and be attentive to standard precautions, hand hygiene, patient safety and privacy, body mechanics, and documentation.

Procedure Steps

1. **Explain to the patient** that the medication may cause some burning, tingling, or unusual taste.
   The taste of nasal medications can cause nausea and vomiting. The medication is more likely to cause burning or tingling if the nasal mucosa is inflamed.

2. **Ask the patient to gently blow** his nose and wash his hands afterward.
   Removing nasal discharge allows the medication to contact the mucous membranes without traumatizing already inflamed mucosa.

3. **Don procedure gloves.**
   Prevents transmission of microorganisms.

4. **Position the patient.**

   When Medicating the Frontal Sinuses With Spray
   "Head down and forward." Remember: "To spray your nose, look at your toes!" If the patient can comfortably assume this position, ask him to lean forward or kneel on the bed with his head

(continued on next page)

Procedure 25-4 ■ Administering Nasal Medication (continued)

down. Administer the medication, and then ask the patient to tilt his head back to medicate the nasal passages.

Radionuclide studies have demonstrated that using nasal drops or sprays with the patient sitting and leaning the head back causes poor distribution of the medications into the nasal complex and sinuses. ▼

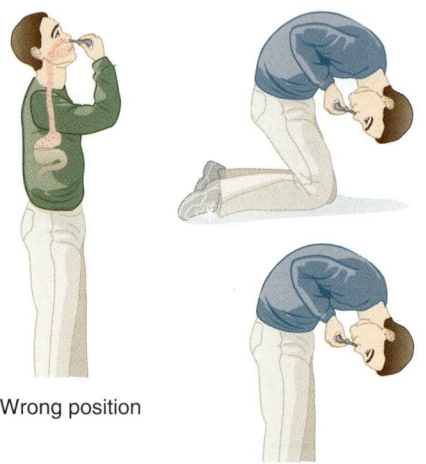

Wrong position

Correct positions

When Medicating the Ethmoid and Sphenoid Sinuses

Assist the patient into a supine position, tilt head back with his head over the edge of the bed. Support the patient's head. Alternatively, place a towel roll behind the patient's shoulders, and allow the head to drop back.

These positions help to prevent straining of the neck muscles and facilitate distribution of the medication to the ethmoid and sphenoid sinuses. ▼

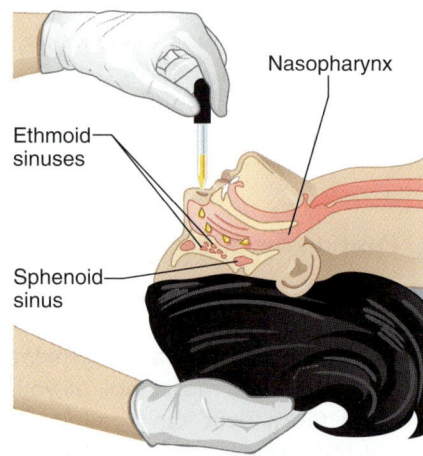

When Medicating the Frontal and Maxillary Sinuses With Drops

With patient supine, tilt the head back over the edge of the bed or place a pillow under the head and turn toward the affected side.

Titling the head promotes gravity to distribute the medication to the frontal sinuses. ▼

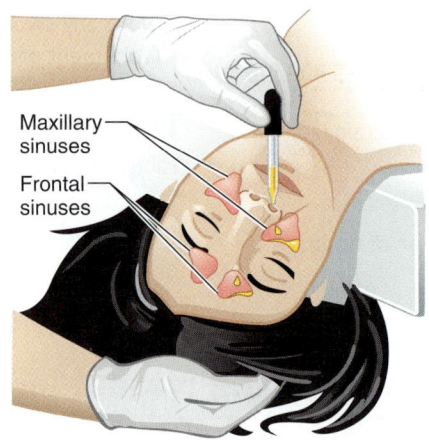

5. **Ask the patient to exhale** and then close one nostril.

   Blocking one nostril provides for deeper inhalation.

6. **Then ask the patient to breathe in** deeply through the nose and while he is breathing in, press down firmly and quickly once on the applicator. Ask patient to breathe out through the mouth. After spray, lean head backward for a few seconds. If a dropper is used, do not touch the sides of the nostril.

   Inhaling through the mouth prevents aspiration of the drops into the trachea and bronchi. Touching the dropper to the nostril will contaminate the dropper.

7. **Repeat for the other nostril.**

8. **If nose drops are used,** ask the patient to stay in the same position for 1 to 5 minutes (depending on the manufacturer's guidelines).

   Maintaining this position promotes better absorption by using gravity to disperse the medication throughout the

nasal passages and sinuses instead of draining out the nose.

9. **Instruct the patient** not to blow his nose for several minutes.

   To prevent expelling the medication.

? What if . . .

- **My patient cannot assume the "head down and forward" position?**

  Help him to hold his head upright to administer the drops or spray.

- **My patient can taste the medicine after it is administered?**

  That means his head was not down enough or he did not inhale long enough. Instruct him to put his head back down and sniff again without the medicine.

- **My patient has an excoriated area on the inside septum?**

  Assess further, examining other areas of the nasal mucosa. Determine whether the patient has a history of substance abuse or frequent nasal inhalations. Report the findings to the prescriber before administering nasal medication.

- **My patient begins to have nosebleeds after using nasal medication?**

  First, control the nosebleed. Then hold the medication and notify the prescriber. Assess for other signs of bleeding, bruising, or other petechiae.

Evaluation

Assess for a reduction of symptoms 15 to 20 minutes after administration.

Patient Teaching

- Teach the procedure for administering nasal drops or sprays, including proper positioning.
- Discuss the correct use of the medication and the adverse effects of overusing nasal decongestants.
- Explain the implications of the color of nasal secretions.

Documentation

Chart according to Medication Guidelines: Steps to Follow for All Medications (Regardless of Type or Route). For example, record the administration of the medication on the MAR.

For nasal instillation, document:

- Pre-medication assessment
- Type and amount of solution administered

- Discomfort the patient experienced during the procedure
- Patient's report of response to nasal administrations, such as nasal discharge, obstruction of nasal passage, bleeding, or other complication following the procedure

Sample documentation

mm/dd/yyyyy   1340   Client complained of nasal stuffiness. Administered mometasone furoate (Nasonex) 2 sprays per nostril as ordered. Client noted nasal tingling following administration of this medication. Client left resting in recliner chair. —————— H. Peratta, RN.

 The video **Administering Nasal Medication,** along with questions and suggested responses, is available on the **Davis's *Nursing Skills Videos*** Web site on Davis*Plus*.

Practice Resource

Mundlia, J., Kumar, M., & Amardeep, A. (2015).

Procedure 25-5 ■ Administering Vaginal Medication

➤ For steps to follow in *all* procedures, refer to the Universal Steps for All Procedures found on the page facing the inside back cover. Also refer to the **Medication Guidelines: Steps to Follow for All Medications (Regardless of Type or Route).**

Equipment

- Medication: foam, jelly, cream, suppository, douche, or irrigating solution
- Applicator (if indicated)
- Perineal wash solution or wipes for perineal care as needed
- Water-soluble lubricant
- Toilet tissue
- Perineal pad
- Bath blanket
- **For irrigation:** you will also need a waterproof pad, bedpan, vaginal irrigation set (consists of a solution container, nozzle, tubing, and clamp; may be disposable), and IV pole.

Delegation

An RN can usually delegate the administration of vaginal medications to an LPN/LVN. Delegation of this task to a NAP will

vary depending on the state's nurse practice acts and the healthcare facility policies. However, the RN is always responsible for evaluating patient responses, both therapeutic and side effects. You can instruct a NAP on the expected therapeutic effects and the side effects she should report.

Pre-Procedure Assessments

- Assess for vaginal burning, pruritus, and pain.
  A baseline assessment helps to determine the patient's level of comfort and later the effectiveness of treatment. Infections can cause vaginal burning, itching, and pain.
- Inspect the labia and vaginal orifice for redness and lesions.
  This is a good time to assess the perineal area for signs of sexually transmitted infection or other findings requiring healthcare.
- Check for vaginal discharge, including color, amount, consistency, and odor.

➤ When performing the procedure, always identify your patient according to agency policy, using two identifiers, and be attentive to standard precautions, hand hygiene, patient safety and privacy, body mechanics, and documentation.

Procedure Steps

1. **Ask the patient to void** before you insert the vaginal medication.
   A full bladder could cause discomfort during the instillation of vaginal medications.

2. **Position the patient** in a dorsal recumbent or Sims' position; drape with a bath blanket so that only the perineum is exposed.
   a. **Dorsal recumbent position**—supine with knees flexed and legs rotated outward.

   b. **Sims' position**—semiprone on the left side with the right hip and knee flexed.
   These positions allow for visualization during administration and promote retention of the medication following administration. Draping protects the patient's modesty.

(continued on next page)

Procedure 25-5 ■ Administering Vaginal Medication (continued)

3. Prepare the medication.

- Suppository: Remove the wrapper and place the suppository on the wrapper or in a medication cup.
- Applicator: Fill the applicator according to the manufacturer's instructions.
- For irrigation: Use a warm solution of approximately 105°F (40.5°C).
  Some suppositories come with applicators. Using a warm irrigation solution promotes patient comfort and prevents injury to the vaginal tissue. ▼

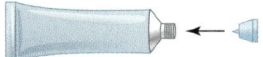

Invert cap and pierce end of medication tube

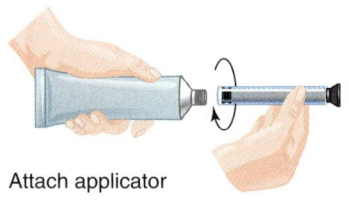

Attach applicator

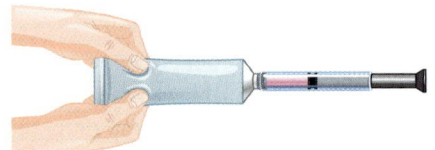

Squeeze medication into applicator

4. Don procedure gloves.
Prevents contaminating your hands and spreading microorganisms.

5. Inspect and clean around vaginal orifice.
Prevents the introduction of microorganisms into the vagina during medication administration.

6. Administer the medication.

For a Suppository

a. Apply water-soluble lubricant to the rounded end of the suppository and to your gloved index finger on your dominant hand.
   Eases insertion and prevents injury to the vaginal tissue.

b. Separate the labia with your non-dominant hand.
   Allows visualization of the vaginal orifice.

c. Insert the suppository along the posterior vaginal wall (about 8 cm, or 3 in.) or as far as it will go. If using an applicator, place the suppository in the end of the applicator, insert the applicator into the vagina, and press the plunger.
   The posterior vaginal wall is about 2.5 cm (1 in.) longer than the anterior wall. ▼

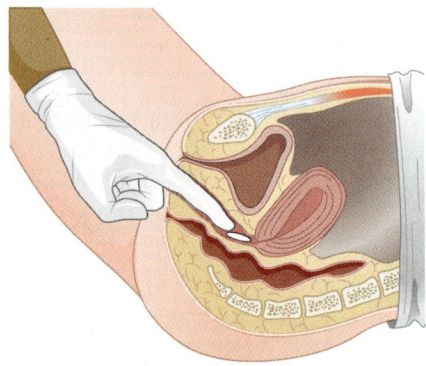

d. Ask the patient to remain in a supine position for 5 to 15 minutes. You may wish to elevate her hips on a pillow.
   Lifting the hips promotes retention and absorption of the medication.

For Applicator Insertion of Cream, Foam, or Jelly

e. Separate the labia with your non-dominant hand.

f. Insert the applicator approximately 8 cm (3 in.) into the vagina along the posterior vaginal wall.

g. Depress the plunger on the applicator, inserting the medication into the vagina.

h. Dispose of the applicator, or place it on a paper towel if the applicator is reusable. You will later wash it in the appropriate solution.

i. Instruct the patient to remain in a supine position for 5 to 15 minutes.
   A flat position promotes retention and absorption of the medication.

For Irrigations

j. Hang the irrigation solution approximately 30 to 60 cm (1 to 2 ft) above the level of the patient's vagina.

Uses gravity to create enough pressure for continuous irrigation without increasing the pressure so much that it causes the patient discomfort and possibly damages the vaginal tissue. ▼

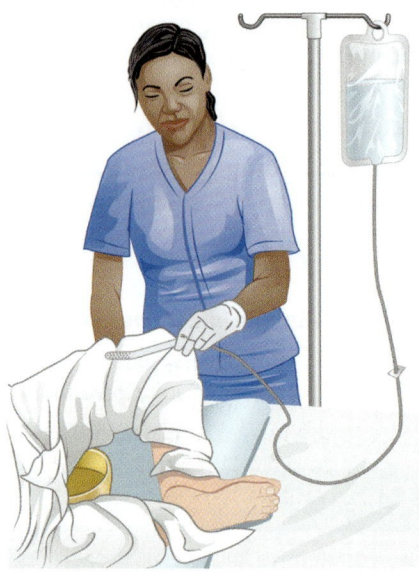

k. Assist the patient into a dorsal recumbent position, and position a waterproof pad and bedpan under the patient.
   This position is the easiest for performing a vaginal irrigation. Positioning the patient on the bedpan and using a waterproof pad protects the bedding.

l. If using a vaginal irrigation set with tubing, open the clamp to allow the solution to completely fill the tubing.
   Flushing the tubing prevents introducing air into the vagina, which can cause discomfort.

m. Lubricate the end of the irrigation nozzle.
   Lubrication reduces discomfort and irritation to the vaginal mucosa.

n. Insert the nozzle approximately 8 cm (3 in.) into the vagina, directing it toward the sacrum.

o. Start the flow of the irrigation solution, and rotate the nozzle intermittently as solution flows.
The rotation ensures even distribution of the solution throughout the vagina.

p. After all irrigating solution has been used, remove the nozzle.

q. Assist the patient to a sitting position on the bedpan.
Promotes removal of all the irrigating solution by gravity.

7. **Remove the bedpan and clean** the perineum with perineal wash solution and a washcloth or wipes. Dry the perineum.
Drainage could cause skin irritation.

8. **Apply a perineal pad** if necessary to absorb drainage.

? What if . . .

■ **The labia are reddened?**
Pour warm water (bottled or specially filtered tap water) over the labia with an irrigation bottle to soothe irritation and cleanse the area.

Evaluation

■ Assess for complaints of vaginal burning, pruritis, or pain.
■ Assess for purulent vaginal discharge.

Patient Teaching

■ Discuss with the patient personal hygiene and pericare.

■ ✚ Teach women that douching may be harmful because it disturbs the normal pH and healthy balance of microorganisms in the vagina. Research has revealed a relationship between douching and ovarian cancer (Gonzalez, O'Brien, Aloisio, et al., 2016).

Documentation

■ **For vaginal medications,** chart according to **Medication Guidelines: Steps to Follow for All Medications (Regardless of Type or Route).**

■ **For vaginal irrigations,** chart assessment; the type and amount of solution administered; discomfort the patient experienced during the procedure; and the patient's report of decreased vaginal pain, itching, and/or burning following the procedure.

Sample documentation

mm/dd/yyyy   1500   Explained medication and procedure. Client place in dorsal recumbent position with knees flexed at 90° angle. Vaginal suppository lubricated with water-soluble lubricant and inserted using two fingers. Instructed client to retain suppository as long as possible. Tolerated procedure well with no voiced complaints of pain or discomfort. ———— S. Snider, RN

Procedure 25-6 ■ Inserting a Rectal Suppository

➤ For steps to follow in *all* procedures, refer to the Universal Steps for All Procedures found on the page facing the inside back cover. Also refer to the **Medication Guidelines: Steps to Follow for All Medications (Regardless of Type or Route).**

Equipment

■ Suppository
■ Water-soluble lubricant
■ Toilet tissue

Delegation

An RN can usually delegate administration of rectal medications to an LPN/LVN. Although in some institutions you can delegate the administration of a glycerine suppository

(nonmedicated) to a NAP, you generally cannot delegate administration of rectal medications to a NAP.

Pre-Procedure Assessments

■ Determine the presence of contraindications for rectal administration, such as recent rectal surgery, rectal bleeding, or cardiac disease.
■ Assess the rectal area for hemorrhoids or irritation.

➤ When performing the procedure, always identify your patient according to agency policy, using two identifiers, and be attentive to standard precautions, hand hygiene, patient safety and privacy, body mechanics, and documentation.

Procedure Steps

1. **Ask whether the patient needs** to defecate before the suppository insertion.
Stool in the rectum interferes with insertion of medication against the rectal wall

and therefore with retention of the medication.

2. **Assist patient to Sims' position**— lying on the left side with the right hip and knee flexed. Drape the

patient, keeping her covered as much as possible.
Sims' position allows visualization of the anus and promotes retention of the medication because the descending colon is on the left side. It also helps

(continued on next page)

Procedure 25-6 ■ Inserting a Rectal Suppository (continued)

relax the external anal sphincter. Keeping the patient covered prevents chilling and maintains privacy.

3. Don procedure gloves.
Gloving prevents exposure to feces and spread of microorganisms; maintains standard precautions.

4. For an uncooperative patient, such as a confused patient or a young child, ask someone to help immobilize the patient while you insert the suppository.
Help with holding the patient allows proper instillation of medication and prevents injury to the rectal mucosa.

5. Prepare the suppository: Remove the wrapper. Using a water-soluble lubricant, lubricate the smooth end of the suppository and the tip of glove on the index finger. If no lubricant is available, apply cool tap water to the rectal opening.
Lubrication eases insertion and prevents friction damage to the rectal mucosa during insertion.

6. Explain that there will be a cool feeling from the lubricant and a feeling of pressure during insertion.
The patient should not experience severe pain with the insertion of a suppository, but will feel the coolness of the lubricant and pressure as the suppository is inserted past the rectal sphincter.

7. Using your nondominant hand, separate the buttocks.
Separation of the buttocks allows you to visualize the anus.

8. Ask the adult patient to take deep breaths in and out through the mouth.
Deep breathing helps relax the rectal sphincter. Pushing a suppository through a constricted sphincter produces discomfort.

9. Insert the suppository:
a. Using the index finger of your dominant hand, gently insert the lubricated smooth end first, or follow the manufacturer's instructions.
Lubrication eases insertion. ▼

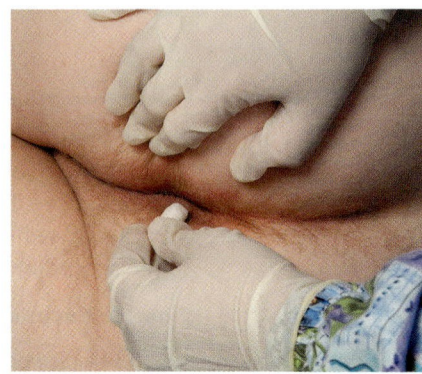

b. **Never force the suppository during insertion.**
Forcing the insertion of the suppository into a fecal mass would affect absorption. Forcing anything into the rectum may cause rectal irritation.

c. Push the suppository past the internal sphincter and along the rectal wall (½ to 1 in. in infants and 1 to 3 in. in adults).
The suppository must be in contact with the rectal wall for the medication to be absorbed. Inserting past the internal sphincter promotes retention. For a child, inserting the suppository too far could damage the rectal mucosa. ▼

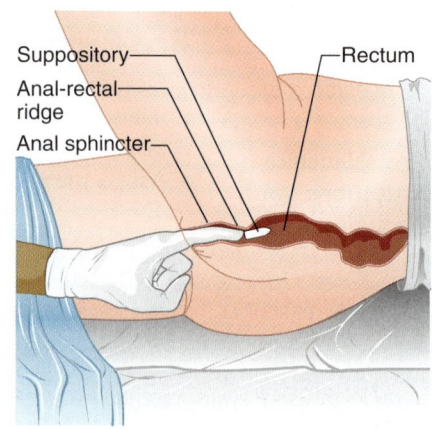

Suppository — Rectum
Anal-rectal ridge
Anal sphincter —

10. Ask the patient to try to retain the suppository if he is able. If he has difficulty retaining the suppository, hold his buttocks together for a short time.

11. Wipe the patient's anus with toilet tissue.
Wiping maintains hygiene and comfort.

12. Explain to the patient the need to remain in the side-lying position for 5 to 10 minutes.
Sims' position promotes retention and absorption of the medication. Explanation promotes compliance.

13. Discard used materials into a biohazard receptacle and wash hands thoroughly.

14. Leave the call device within reach and bedpan handy, if the suppository was a laxative.
In case the patient has a sudden urge to defecate or cannot retain the suppository for the recommended time.

? What if . . .

■ **The prescribed dose is only half of the suppository?**
Cut the suppository lengthwise with a clean, single-edge razor blade.

■ **My patient is a child? What is the best way to give a rectal suppository so the child doesn't expel it?**
For pediatric patients, it may be necessary to gently hold the buttocks together for 5 to 10 minutes.

■ **My patient is an older adult? Is there anything special I should know?**
Older adults may have difficulty retaining a suppository because of poor sphincter control. You may need to put the bedpan under the patient while you are inserting the suppository.

Evaluation

- Assess for pain or burning during and after insertion of the medication.
- Determine that the patient retained the suppository for the desired length of time after insertion (reinsertion may be required).

Patient Teaching

Explain that suppositories may take up to 30 minutes to be absorbed, depending on the medication.

Documentation

- Refer to **Medication Guidelines: Steps to Follow for All Medications (Regardless of Type or Route).**
- Chart the condition of anal tissue if abnormalities are present, any complaints of discomfort that are outside of the expected feelings and experience, and the length of time that the suppository was retained.
- Chart responses to medication (e.g., symptom relief, side effects).

Sample documentation

mm/dd/yyyy   2015   Patient temperature
103.2°F and complains of nausea. Tylenol grain
X suppository given per rectum with patient in Sims'
position. Instructed to remain in this position for
15 minutes. Voiced understanding. No rectal abnormalities
observed. Tolerated procedure well with no complaints
of pain or discomfort. ———————— J. Kinsley, RN

Practice Resources
Bartley, N. (2012b); Lowry, M. (2016).

Thinking About the Procedure

 The video **Inserting a Rectal Suppository,** along with questions and suggested responses, is available on the **Davis's *Nursing Skills Videos*** Web site on Davis*Plus*.

Procedure 25-7 ■ Applying Medication to Skin

➤ For steps to follow in *all* procedures, refer to the Universal Steps for All Procedures found on the page facing the inside back cover. Also refer to the **Medication Guidelines: Steps to Follow for All Medications (Regardless of Type or Route).**

➤ *Note:* Follow agency policy or provider's prescription regarding whether to use prepackaged wipes or soap and water to cleanse the skin.

Delegation

An RN can usually delegate administration of most topical medications to an LPN/LVN. In some institutions you can delegate the administration of an over-the-counter medication to a NAP. Refer to agency policy regarding administration of topical medication.

Pre-Procedure Assessments

- Assess for skin irritation, open lesions, area of hypersensitivity, or other skin abnormality.
- Determine the presence of contraindications for dermal application. Document and report these before administering medication.

Procedure 25-7A ■ Applying Topical Lotion, Creams, and Ointment

➤ When performing the procedure, always identify your patient according to agency policy, using two identifiers, and be attentive to standard precautions, hand hygiene, patient safety and privacy, body mechanics, and documentation.

Procedure Steps

1. **Don clean procedure gloves.**
   Complies with universal precautions and protects your skin from the topical medication.

2. **Cleanse the skin** with cleansing wipes or soap and water (according to agency policy) and pat dry before applying.
   Clean skin enhances absorption. Moisture on the skin can interfere with

   adherence of topical ointment, depending on the product used to suspend the medication.

3. **Warm the medication** in your gloved hands.
   This will be more comfortable for the patient and make the preparation easier to apply.

4. **Use gloved hands or an applicator** to apply and spread the medication evenly, following the direction

   of hair growth when coating the area.
   Excessive application may irritate the skin. Gloves prevent absorption of the medication through your own skin. ▼

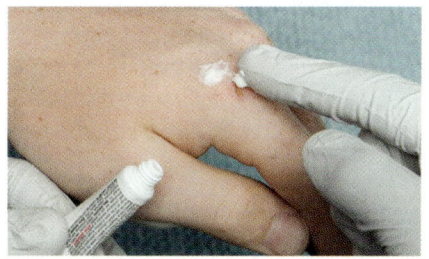

(continued on next page)

Procedure 25-7 ■ Applying Medication to Skin (continued)

Procedure 25-7B ■ Applying Topical Aerosol Spray

➤ When performing the procedure, always identify your patient according to agency policy, using two identifiers, and be attentive to standard precautions, hand hygiene, patient safety and privacy, body mechanics, and documentation.

Procedure Steps

1. **Don clean procedure gloves.**

2. **Cleanse the skin** with cleansing wipe or soap and water (according to agency policy) and pat dry before applying to enhance absorption.

3. **Shake the container to mix** the contents.

To ensure that active ingredients are be evenly distributed throughout the aerosolized suspension.

4. **Hold the container** at the distance specified on the label (usually 6 to 12 in.) and spray over the prescribed area.
Prevents excess application to a local area.

5. **Hold most containers upright** when spraying. If you are spraying near the patient's head, cover his face with a towel.
Prevents him from inhaling the spray.

Procedure 25-7C ■ Applying Prescribed Powder

➤ When performing the procedure, always identify your patient according to agency policy, using two identifiers, and be attentive to standard precautions, hand hygiene, patient safety and privacy, body mechanics, and documentation.

Procedure Steps

1. **Don clean procedure gloves.**

2. **Cleanse the skin** with a cleansing wipe or soap and water and pat dry before applying to enhance absorption.

Powder applied to a moist surface creates a pasty solution, which may irritate the skin.

3. **Spread apart skinfolds** and apply a very thin layer.

4. **Be careful that the patient does not inhale the powder.**
Particulate matter, such as powder, can irritate lung tissue and lead to pneumonitis or other inflammatory processes.

Procedure 25-7D ■ Applying Transdermal Medication

➤ When performing the procedure, always identify your patient according to agency policy, using two identifiers, and be attentive to standard precautions, hand hygiene, patient safety and privacy, body mechanics, and documentation.

Procedure Steps

1. **Don clean procedure gloves.**
Complies with universal precautions and protects your skin from the topical medication.

2. **Remove the previous patch,** folding the medicated side to the inside.
This helps to prevent unintentional contact of the medication on a different area of the patient's skin.

3. **Dispose of the old patch** carefully in an appropriate receptacle, keeping it away from children and pets.
Even a used patch has some active medication on it. Proper disposal is important to prevent medication exposure to others.

4. **Cleanse the skin of traces** of remaining medication. Allow the skin to dry.
A clean, dry surface optimizes the effectiveness of adherence and absorption of the medication.

5. **Remove the new patch from** its protective covering, and then remove the clear, protective covering without touching the adhesive or the inside surface that contains the medication. ▼

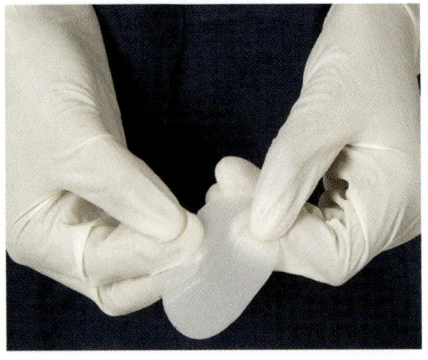

6. **Apply the patch to** a clean, dry, hairless (or little hair), intact skin area, pressing it down for about 10 seconds with your palm. Be sure the area is free of scars, lesions, and irritation.
A smooth surface maximizes the contact between medication and the skin. Skin that is disrupted can become irritated by topical mediation. Lesions involving thickened layers of skin can compromise absorption.

7. **Rotate application sites** with each new application. Common sites are the trunk, lower abdomen, lower back, and buttocks.
Rotating sites prevents irritation to local areas of the skin.

8. **Advise the patient *not*** to use a heating pad over the area.
Heat can cause some ointments to irritate or even burn the skin.

9. **Write the date, the time,** and your initials on the new patch.
Complete documentation helps to reduce medication errors.

10. **Remove your gloves and** perform hand hygiene.

11. **Observe for local side effects,** such as skin irritation, itching, and allergic contact dermatitis.
If an adverse response occurs at the local site, remove the patch, wipe the skin clean, and notify the prescriber.

? What if . . .

- **The medication is packaged as an ointment form with calibrated paper?**
Wear gloves; apply the ointment in a continuous motion along those marks to measure the required dose. Fold the paper in half to distribute the ointment evenly on the patch.

- **My patient is a child who does not want the medication to be applied?**

Hold the child securely while medication is applied. Then cover the site with a dressing to keep the child from disrupting the application of medication.

- **My patient is an older adult and has fragile skin?**
Avoid areas where penetration of the cream or ointment is likely to be reduced or cause irritation. Be gentle with the application and diligent with your assessment of the skin response to medication. Avoid using tape; use tape alternatives.

Evaluation

- Assess for rash, excoriation, hives, redness, swelling, or signs of allergy or skin sensitivity to topical medication.
- Ask the patient whether he feels burning, itching, pain, tenderness, or other sensation to skin where medication was applied.
- Assess for improvement in the patient's condition.

Patient Teaching

- Explain that topical medication may take up to 30 minutes to be absorbed, depending on the medication.
- Tell the patient never to ingest or inhale topical medication.
- Advise the patient to avoid touching his eyes after handling topical medication.
- Inform the patient not to use more medicine than prescribed or directed.

Documentation

- Refer to **Medication Guidelines: Steps to Follow for All Medications (Regardless of Type or Route).**
- Record the skin condition if abnormalities are present and complaints of discomfort during or after administration.
- Document responses to medication (e.g., symptom relief, side effects).

Sample documentation

mm/dd/yyyy   0835   Transdermal nitroglycerine 74.6 mg patch applied to upper chest. Pt instructed to leave patch intact for 12 hours. Patient reported mild, transient headache approximately 45 minutes after application of patch. No evidence of flushing, faintness, or dizziness. Patient denies chest pain.. ————————— M. Finegold RN

mm/dd/yyyy   0830   Fentanyl patch dated mm/dd/yyyy   removed from upper left arm. Skin intact, no irritation noted. Fentanyl patch applied to the left anterior chest wall below the clavicle. Patient stated, "This patch really helps my back feel better.". ————————— M. Finegold, RN

Thinking About the Procedure

The video **Applying Transdermal Medication,** along with questions and suggested responses, is available on the **Davis's *Nursing Skills Videos*** Web site on Davis*Plus*.

Procedure 25-8 ■ Administering Metered-Dose Inhaler (MDI) Medication

➤ For steps to follow in *all* procedures, refer to the Universal Steps for All Procedures found on the page facing the inside back cover. Also refer to the **Medication Guidelines: Steps to Follow for All Medications (Regardless of Type or Route).**

Equipment
- Metered-dose inhaler
- Spacer
- Tissues

Pre-Procedure Assessments

Assess the respiratory status before administration of medication to establish a baseline for evaluating the effects of treatment.

Delegation

An RN can usually delegate administration of MDI medications to an LPN/LVN. You usually cannot delegate this task to a NAP, unless the NAP has special training for a specific defined situation (e.g., "medication aides" in some long-term care settings in some states). If the patient is having respiratory distress, you should not delegate this task. Refer to **Medication Guidelines: Steps to Follow for All Medications (Regardless of Type or Route).**

➤ When performing the procedure, always identify your patient according to agency policy, using two identifiers, and be attentive to standard precautions, hand hygiene, patient safety and privacy, body mechanics, and documentation.

Procedure Steps

1. **Determine the number of** remaining inhalations of medication in the canister based on the start date and instructions for use. **KEY POINT:** *Do not use the old method of floating the canister in water, as it is not an accurate estimate.* Replace the canister promptly when it is nearly empty.

   ✚ Historically, patients have been instructed to float the canister in water to determine how much medication remains. However, propellants affect the weight of the canister and may lead to false reassurance that there is medication in an empty container.

   ✚ Some MDI medications are used as rescue agents during asthma attacks or periods of dyspnea. It is important always to have medication available for use.

2. **Assist the patient to a seated** or high Fowler's position if in bed.
   Facilitates the ability to take a deep inhalation when medication is administered.

3. **Ask the patient to rinse** out his mouth and spit the fluid out (not to swallow it).
   Helps prevent transfer of bacteria from the mouth to the inhaler.

4. **Shake the inhaler.** Then remove the mouthpiece cap of the inhaler and insert the mouthpiece into the spacer while holding the canister upright.
   A spacer is the most efficient method to deliver inhaled medications. It should be used if the patient has difficulty coordinating the use of the inhaler, is using a corticosteroid, or if it is prescribed.

5. **Remove the cap from the spacer.**

6. **Ask the patient to breathe out** slowly and completely. If a patient is unable to use the MDI independently, time the use of the device with the patient's own respirations.
   Deep breathing helps the patient to time the dose with his natural breathing.

7. **Place the spacer mouthpiece** into the patient's mouth and have him seal his lips around the mouthpiece (see Fig. 25-11). Sharply press down on the inhaler canister to discharge one puff of medication into the spacer.

If No Spacer Is Used

If a spacer is not used, place the canister 1 to 2 inches (2.5 to 5.0 cm) from or directly into the mouth.
A good seal allows proper delivery of medication.

8. **Ask the patient to inhale slowly** and then hold his breath for as long as possible. Encourage the patient to hold his breath for 10 seconds if possible.
   When the patient holds his breath, the medication can be delivered deep into the more distal bronchioles of the lungs.

9. **If a second puff is needed,** wait at least 1 minute before repeating steps 6 through 8.
   Allows the medication to be absorbed and the canister to recharge.

10. **If a corticosteroid inhaler** was used, assist the patient to rinse out his mouth with water and spit out the rinse.
    Prolonged exposure of this medication to the oral mucosa is irritating and can lead to thrush in some patients.

11. **Wipe the mouthpiece** with a tissue or moist cloth and replace the cap. Periodically rinse the spacer, mouthpiece, and cap with water.
    Proper cleaning of the MDI keeps the dispenser from clogging.

The following illustrations summarize the steps for using an MDI: ▼

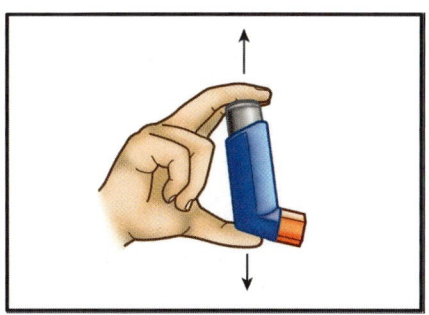

Shake canister.

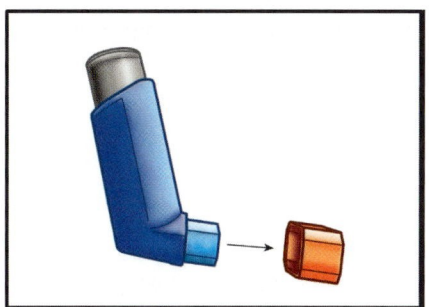

Remove cap. Discharge 2 puffs.

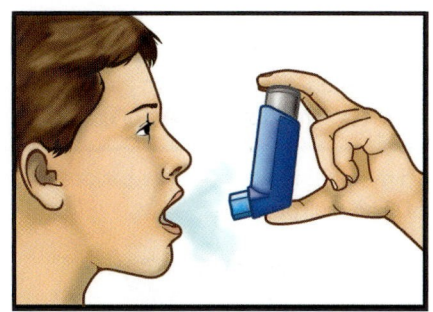

Deep breath out.

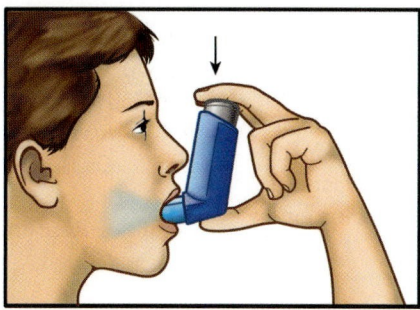

Press top. Inhale med slowly.

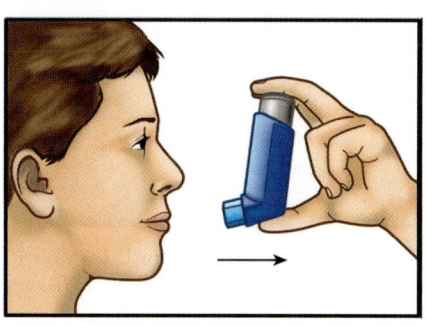

Hold breath. Exhale slowly.

Remove inhaler from mouth.
Wait 1 minute before next puff.

? What if . . .

- **My patient is a small child or frail older adult who is unable to assist with taking medication from the inhaler?**

  You will need to time discharge of the medication with the client's inspiration if the patient is unable to administer the medication with his own deep breaths.

Evaluation

Assess for change in respiratory status after medication administration.

Patient Teaching

- Explain when to use the inhaler and what side effects to anticipate.
- Teach and demonstrate how to correctly use a spacer and MDI.
- Explain how to determine whether the MDI canister is nearly empty.
- Explain that some inhalers are used in combination with others and must be used in correct order to receive the desired effect.
- Be aware that many patients who have not been taught to use dry powder inhalers do not get any medication into their lungs.

- Errors in using dry powder inhalers increase with age and illness severity. Carefully supervise older adults and seriously ill patients.

Home Care

General Information to Tell Patients

- Show your healthcare provider how you are using your MDI. If you are having trouble, ask for tips or to recommend another device.
- Never puncture or break the canister.
- Do not immerse the MDI in water.
- Keep the MDI where you can get it quickly when needed, but out of children's reach.
- Store the MDI at room temperature. If it gets cold, warm it by rubbing the canister between your palms. Never use anything else to warm it.

(continued on next page)

Procedure 25-8 ■ Administering Metered-Dose Inhaler (MDI) Medication (continued)

Determining the Number of Remaining Doses

- When you begin using a new MDI, write the start date on the canister.
- The only reliable method for determining the number of doses remaining in a canister is to subtract the number of doses used from the number available. Some devices are equipped with counters. Floating MDIs in water is not accurate for assessing remaining doses and often will clog the valve.

Cleaning the MDI

- Clean your apparatus regularly to avoid drug buildup that might keep the medication from reaching the lungs. Specific maintenance procedures may vary with the manufacturer.
- Remove the metal canister that contains the medication by pulling it out.

Documentation

- Refer to **Medication Guidelines: Steps to Follow for All Medications (Regardless of Type or Route).**
- Document the response to medications.

Sample documentation

mm/dd/yyyy   0800   pt. c/o shortness of breath. RR 26 and labored. Combivent MDI 2 puffs administered with spacer. ——————— S. Smythe, RN

0815   RR 20   regular, even comfortable. ——————— S. Smythe, RN

Thinking About the Procedure

 The video **Administering Metered Dose Inhaler (MDI) Medication,** along with questions and suggested responses, is available on the **Davis's *Nursing Skills Videos*** Web site on Davis*Plus*.

Practice Resources
Gandhi, K., Dahiya, A., Taruna-Kalra, A., et al. (2012); Lareau, S., & Hodder, R. (2012).

Procedure 25-9 ■ Preparing, Drawing Up, and Mixing Medication

➤ For steps to follow in *all* procedures, refer to the Universal Steps for All Procedures found on the page facing the inside back cover. Also refer to the **Medication Guidelines: Steps to Follow for All Medications (Regardless of Type or Route).**

Equipment

- Medication vials, ampules, and/or prefilled syringe
- Alcohol prep pad (70% alcohol) or chlorhexidine gluconate (CHG)–alcohol product
- Syringe of the appropriate size for medication volume and viscosity
- Needle of the appropriate size for the site and viscosity to be aspirated through the vial access device (VAD)
- VAD, filter needle, or safety needle.
- Gauze pad or ampule snapper, if you are using ampules ▼

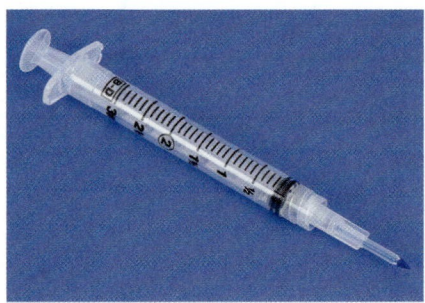

Vial access device.

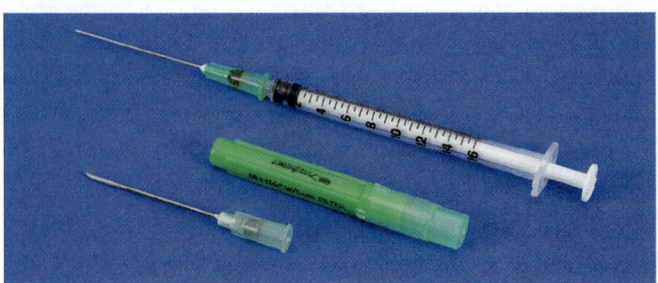

Top: Syringe with a regular needle. *Bottom:* Filter needle.

Delegation

An RN can delegate administration of some parenteral medications to an LPN/LVN. You usually cannot delegate this task to a NAP. Nurse practice acts governing medication administration vary from state to state, and policies vary further among healthcare agencies. Nevertheless, the RN is always responsible for supervising and evaluating delegated care. You can instruct a NAP in the therapeutic effects expected from the medication.

Pre-Procedure Assessments

- Check the ampule or vial for intactness, cloudiness, particles, and color.
  A change in color, cloudiness, particles, or cracks indicate the medication is altered or contaminated and should not be used.

- Check the compatibility of the medications to be mixed.
  Some medications are either chemically or physically incompatible and cannot be mixed. Other medications may be compatible for only 20 to 30 minutes, so they must be given promptly after

they are mixed. Although physically incompatible medications can frequently be identified by a change in appearance, such as precipitation, no such indication exists for chemically incompatible medications.

- Determine the total volume of medications and whether the total volume is appropriate for the administration site.
  Although the reason for mixing medications is to limit the number of injections a patient receives, the total volume of the injections must not be greater than what is appropriate for the site.

Procedure 25-9A ■ Drawing Up Medication From Ampules

➤ When performing the procedure, always identify your patient according to agency policy, using two identifiers, and be attentive to standard precautions, hand hygiene, patient safety and privacy, body mechanics, and documentation.

Procedure Steps

1. **Gently flick or tap the top** of the ampule with your index finger to remove medication trapped in the top of the ampule. Alternate method: Shake the ampule by quickly turning and snapping your wrist, like shaking down a mercury thermometer.
   Medication left in the top of the ampule may lead to administering an inadequate dose. All the medication must be in the bottom of the ampule before you open it.

2. ✚ **Use an ampule snapper,** if available. Alternatively, wrap a 2 in. × 2 in. gauze pad (or an unopened alcohol wipe) around the neck of the ampule. Snap the top off, breaking it away from you.

   Prevents you from cutting your fingers or spraying glass fragments toward you. Do not use an opened alcohol wipe to break the ampule, because it is not thick enough to prevent injury. ▼

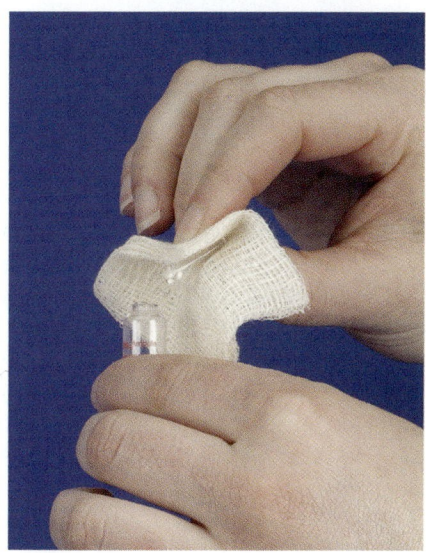

3. **Attach a filter needle** or filter straw to the syringe. If the syringe has a needle in place, remove both the needle and the cap and place them on a sterile surface (e.g., a newly unwrapped alcohol pad still in the open wrapper), then attach the filter needle or straw.
   Opening a glass ampule produces a spray of tiny fractured glass particles, which can enter the ampule and contaminate the contents. The filter needle or straw filters the solution drawn up from glass ampules to remove glass particles.

4. **Withdraw the medication** from the ampule with a filter needle by using one of the following techniques. Be careful not to touch the neck of the ampule with the filter straw or needle while withdrawing medication.
   Touching the neck of the ampule with the needle or straw increases the risk of contamination.

   a. *Invert the ampule,* place the filter needle or straw tip in the liquid, and withdraw the prescribed amount of medication. Be careful not to insert needle through the medication into the air at the top of the inverted ampule.
   This method is particularly useful with small ampules. The medication's surface tension prevents the liquid from leaking from the inverted ampule. However, if you insert the needle too far (into the air pocket above the medication), the medication will run out. ▼

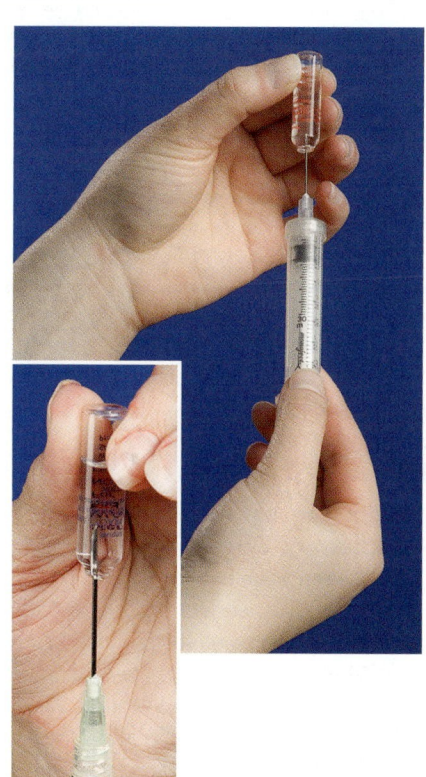

b. *Alternatively, tip the ampule,* place a filter needle or straw in the liquid, and withdraw all medication. Reposition the ampule so that the needle or straw tip remains in the liquid.
   This method allows for easier stabilization of the ampule while you withdraw the medication, and may help keep you from contaminating the needle on the edge of the vial opening. ▼

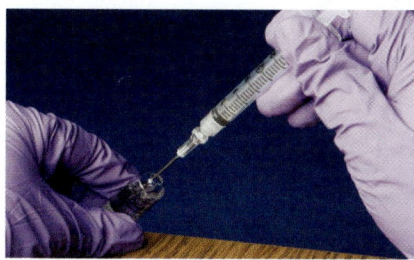

(continued on next page)

Procedure 25-9 ■ Preparing, Drawing Up, and Mixing Medication (continued)

5. **Holding the syringe vertically,** draw 0.2 mL of air into the syringe (see Clinical Insight 25-4). Draw up and measure the exact medication dose, plus 0.2 mL of air (the syringe plunger should be at 0.2 mL more than the prescribed dose).

6. **Remove the filter needle** or straw, and reattach the "saved" needle for administering the injection.

7. **Eject the 0.2 mL of air, and read** the dose. After all of the air is removed, if you need to eject some medication to make the dose correct, tip the syringe until it is horizontal to push out the medication.
   - Pulling air into the syringe allows for an exact dose when the medication

is injected; the air will clear the needle (after the medication) so that the patient receives all the medication that is in the syringe.
The syringe must be vertical to eject air. However, if you eject the medication while holding the syringe vertically, the drug will run down the needle and then track through the patient's tissue during the injection.

For a filter needle
Use a filter needle only to withdraw, not to measure, medication. Do not eject medication from it.
Pushing the medication out through the filter needle could cause the filter to break and release the glass fragments.

KEY POINT: *This is not the old "air lock" technique; you will eject the air before administering the medication to the patient.*

For medications that are irritating to tissues (e.g., parenteral iron)
You can leave the 0.2 mL of air in the syringe for injection. But be sure to account for the air when you read the dose markings on the syringe.

8. **Dispose of the top and bottom** of the ampule and the filter needle in a sharps container.
   Disposal into a puncture-proof container prevents accidental needlestick injury.

Procedure 25-9B ■ Drawing Up Medication From Vials

➤ When performing the procedure, always identify your patient according to agency policy, using two identifiers, and be attentive to standard precautions, hand hygiene, patient safety and privacy, body mechanics, and documentation.
  This procedure assumes you are using a vial access device (VAD), because that is preferred. Use a needle only when a filter needle is required.

Procedure Steps

1. **Mix the solution in the vial,** if necessary, by gently rolling the vial between your hands.
   Aqueous suspensions will settle to the bottom of the vial, so they need to be mixed. Rolling the vial between your hands will mix the medication without forming air bubbles. Shaking the vial traps air in the medication.

2. **Place the vial on a flat** work surface and thoroughly scrub the rubber top of the vial with an alcohol prep pad or CHG-alcohol product.
   The alcohol prep pad removes dust, grease, and microorganisms.

3. **Uncap the VAD** without touching the tip or shaft. If you are using a VAD, attach the device to the syringe, and remove the cap.
   VADs can be used only with single-use vials, unless the vial is designed for use with access pins, such as a LifeShield vial.

4. **Place the VAD cap** on a clean surface, or hold the cap open-side out

between two fingers of your non-dominant hand.
This method prevents contamination of the cap and the needle during recapping.

5. **Draw air into the syringe** equal to the amount of medication to be withdrawn from the vial.
   Injection of air into the vial makes withdrawing the medication easier. For small unit-dose vials, you may not have to instill air prior to withdrawing the medication, but you will need to maintain backward pressure on the plunger until the needle is completely withdrawn. If you release the plunger, the negative pressure in the vial will pull the medication back into the vial.

6. **Insert the VAD** into the vial without coring and while maintaining sterile technique. Use a needle *only* if for some reason (e.g., the type of medication) a filter needle is required.
   a. Place the tip of the VAD or filter needle in the middle of the rubber

top of the vial, with the bevel up at a 45° to 60° angle. ▼

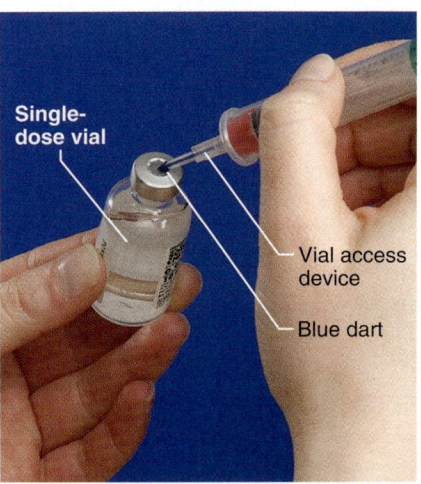

Single-dose vial

Vial access device

Blue dart

b. While pushing the VAD into the rubber top, gradually bring the syringe (and VAD) upright to a 90° angle.
   This method helps prevent coring, which occurs when a small piece of the rubber top is trapped inside the VAD during insertion. Coring is more

likely to occur with large-gauge needles and VADs. ▼

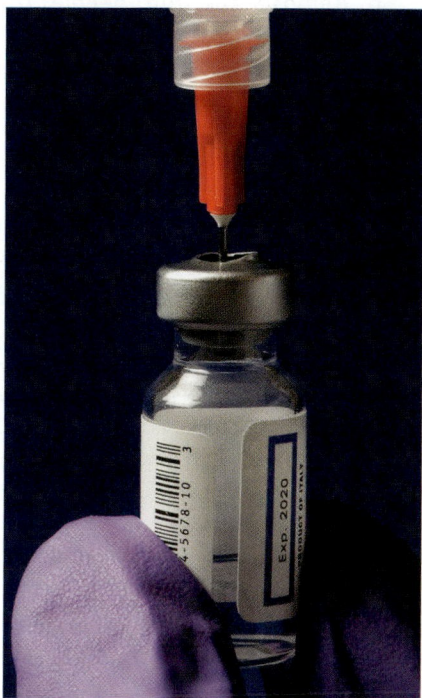

7. With the tip of the VAD above the fluid line, inject the air in the syringe into the air in the vial.
The air creates positive pressure in the vial, making the medication easier to withdraw. Injecting air into the medication would create air bubbles, which interfere with dosage measurement. ▼

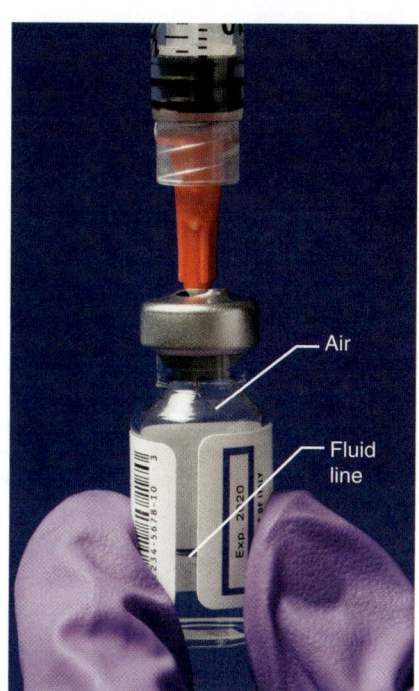

"Air to air."

8. Invert the vial, keep the VAD vertical in the medication, and slowly withdraw the medication.
The vial needs to be inverted so that all the medication can be withdrawn. Keeping the VAD in the medication and slowly drawing the medication will help prevent you from drawing excess air into the syringe. ▼

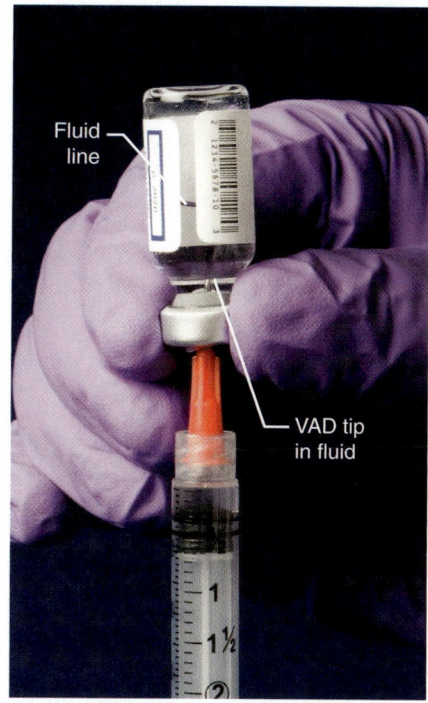

9. Keeping the VAD in the vial, remove any air from the syringe:
When the VAD is connecting the vial and syringe, a sterile unit is formed. The volume of air in the hub of the syringe and inside the needle/VAD, dead space, will be drawn back into the syringe. Air bubbles alter the dose of medication being administered, so they must be expelled. You can use a pen to tap the syringe if extra force is needed. ▶

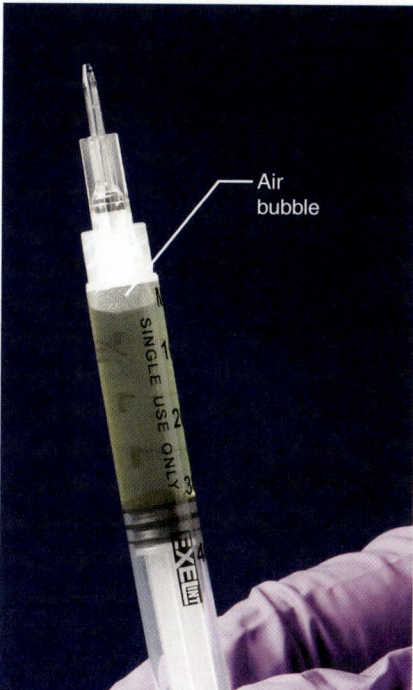

A. **Incorrect**—If syringe is not vertical, air is trapped near the hub.

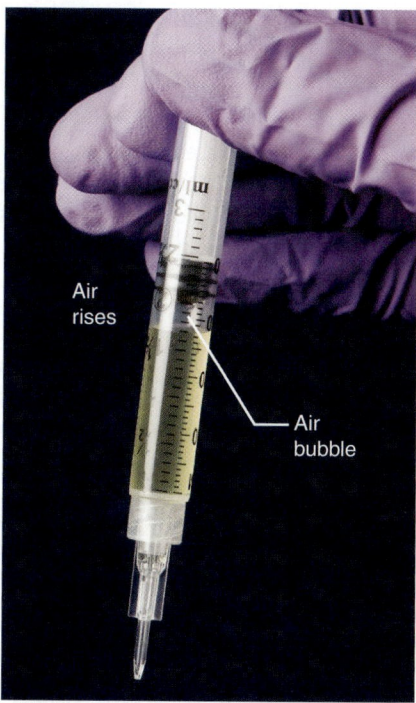

B. **Incorrect**—If tip is down, air is trapped at the plunger.

(continued on next page)

Procedure 25-9 ■ Preparing, Drawing Up, and Mixing Medication (continued)

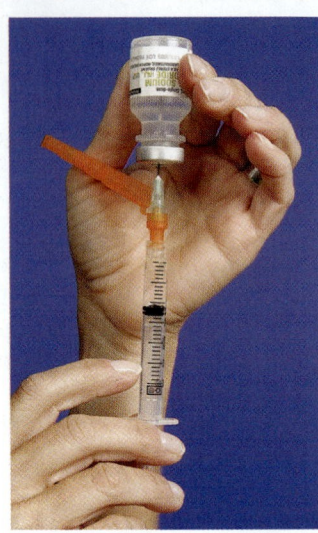

C. Correct—Syringe is vertical.

a. Carefully stabilize the vial and syringe, and firmly tap the syringe below the air bubbles. When air bubbles are at the hub of the syringe, make sure the syringe is vertical (straight up and down) and push the air back into the vial.
Remember that air rises, so if the syringe is tilted, air will be trapped in it.

b. If additional medication is necessary to obtain the correct dose, withdraw it before removing the VAD from the inverted vial.
When working with only one vial, you can withdraw and eject medication

into the vial as many times as needed to expel bubbles from the syringe and obtain the correct dose.

10. **When the dose is correct,** withdraw the needle or VAD from the vial at a 90° angle.
A vertical angle prevents accidental contamination or bending of the needle.

11. **Hold the syringe upright** at eye level to recheck the medication dose.
Reading the syringe at an angle can result in inaccurate measurement.

12. **Recap the VAD** or vial access needle using a recapping device or the one-handed method. See Procedure 25-10.
Although recapping a sterile needle does not present a threat of bloodborne pathogen exposure, using a mechanical recapping device or the one-handed method helps develop safe habits.

13. **Change the VAD or filter needle** before you inject the medication:
a. Before changing the VAD or filter needle, draw back on the syringe plunger to remove all medication from dead space in the old needle (or VAD).

b. Remove the old needle (or VAD), and reattach a new needle for injection (see Clinical Insight 25-5).
You should not eject medication through a filter needle; you cannot inject a patient with a VAD.

c. Hold the syringe vertically and expel the air. If it is necessary to expel some medication, hold the syringe horizontally to do so.
The difficulty with changing the needles is that you may slightly alter the dose. If you are planning to change the needles, draw slightly more than the ordered dose unless you are combining in one syringe. After changing the needle, re-measure the dose. Holding the syringe horizontally prevents medication from running down the needle and tracking into the patient's skin.

14. **Dispose of the vial, VAD,** or any needles in a sharps container.
This prevents sharps injury to healthcare workers or others in the vicinity. Proper disposal also reduces the risk of transmitting infectious organisms.

Procedure 25-9C ■ Mixing Medication From Two Vials

➤ First review the **Medication Guidelines: Steps to Follow for All Medications (Regardless of Type or Route)**; Procedure 25-9B: Drawing Up Medication From Vials; and Procedure 25-10A: Recapping Contaminated Needles.

➤ ✚ Always use a VAD instead of a needle whenever possible. If you must use a needle, use a safety needle.

➤ When performing the procedure, always identify your patient according to agency policy, using two identifiers, and be attentive to standard precautions, hand hygiene, patient safety and privacy, body mechanics, and documentation.

Procedure Steps

1. **Scrub the tops of both vials** with an alcohol pad or CHG-alcohol product.

   NOTE: Some experts omit this step for single-dose vials.

Not all pharmaceutical companies ensure the sterility of the rubber top on vials, even when they are first opened. However, be aware that once your fingers touch the alcohol pad, it is no longer sterile; therefore, you are not sterilizing but rather cleaning the vial top.

2. **Draw air into the syringe** in the same amount as the total medication doses for both vials (e.g., if the order is for 0.5 mL for vial A and 1 mL for vial B, then draw up 1.5 mL of air). ➤

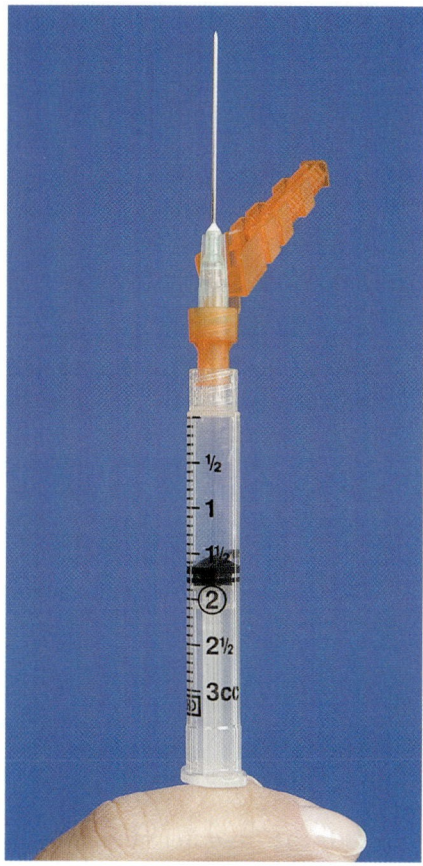

Vial A

3. Inject air into the vials.

a. Maintaining sterility, insert the vial access device or safety needle into the vial in the middle of the rubber top of the vial with the bevel up at a 45° to 60° angle. While pushing the VAD (or needle) into the rubber top, gradually bring the needle upright to a 90° angle. ▼

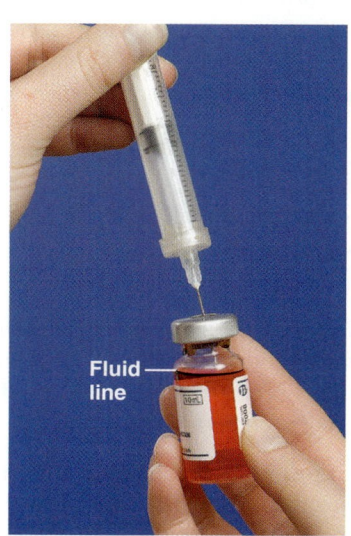

Fluid line

Vial A

This method helps prevent coring of the rubber top.

b. Keeping the tip of the VAD (or safety needle) above the medication, inject an amount of air equal to the volume of drug to be withdrawn from the first vial (e.g., 0.5 mL for vial A in step 2); then inject the rest of the air into the second vial (1.0 mL for vial B). Take care to prevent coring. ▼

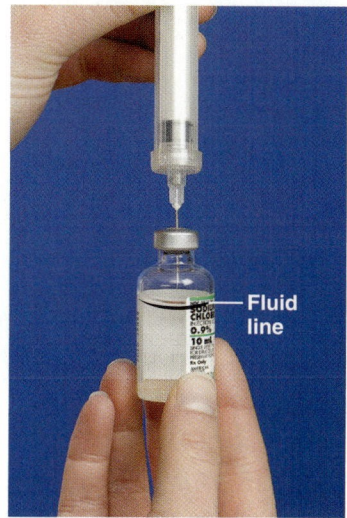

Fluid line

Vial B

Medication is easier to withdraw from a vial with positive pressure. For small unit-dose vials, it may be possible to withdraw the medication without instilling air, but you will need to maintain a slight backward pressure on the plunger until the needle is completely withdrawn. If you release the plunger, the negative pressure in the vial will pull the medication back in. Therefore, it is always safer to instill air.

Using One Multidose Vial and One Single-Dose Vial
You must withdraw medication from the multidose vial before withdrawing from the single-dose vial. However, the needle tip should stay above the medication at all times in steps 2 and 3.
This is an extra precaution to prevent contamination of the multidose vial with medication from the single-dose vial.

When Mixing Two Types of Insulin
If you are mixing two types of insulin at step 3, put air into the regular insulin last (see Clinical Insight 25-6 for mixing two types of insulin).

4. Without removing the VAD, or needle, from the second vial (B), invert it and withdraw the ordered amount of medication. Expel any air bubbles and measure the dose. Remove the VAD from the vial, then pull back on the plunger enough to pull all medication out of the VAD into the syringe (see Clinical Insight 25-5). Read the dose at eye level. Tip the syringe horizontally if you need to eject any medication.

Allows you to withdraw all the medication. Keeping the needle in the medication and withdrawing the medication slowly helps prevent drawing excess air into the syringe and prevents bubbles. ▼

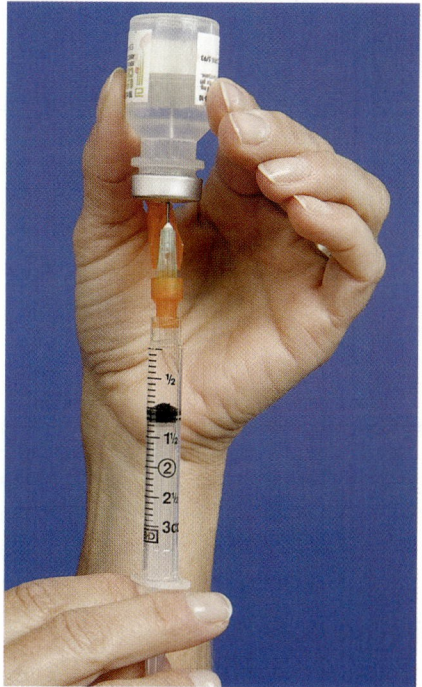

Vial B (step 4)

5. Insert the VAD or needle into the first vial (A), invert, and withdraw the exact ordered amount of medication, holding the syringe vertical.

■ When finished, the plunger should be at the line for the total/combined dose for vials A and B.

(continued on next page)

Procedure 25-9 ■ **Preparing, Drawing Up, and Mixing Medication** (continued)

(Using the example in step 2, you would have 1.5 mL of the mixed medications in the syringe.)

■ Be very careful not to withdraw excess medication; keep your index finger or thumb on the flange of the syringe to prevent medication from being forced back by pressure. If this occurs, you must discard the medication in the syringe and start over.

✚ *Because the medications are mixed, withdrawing extra from the second vial makes the entire mixture incorrect. If you draw up too much of the second drug or if your final measurement of the total for both drugs is incorrect, you cannot eject medication, because you cannot know how much of that is medication A and how much of it is medication B you are ejecting. You must discard the syringe and medication and begin again.*

You do not need to change the needle before step 5 because even if one vial is a multidose vial, you would have withdrawn the medication from it first (in step 4). It will not matter if you track medication into the single-dose vial. ➤

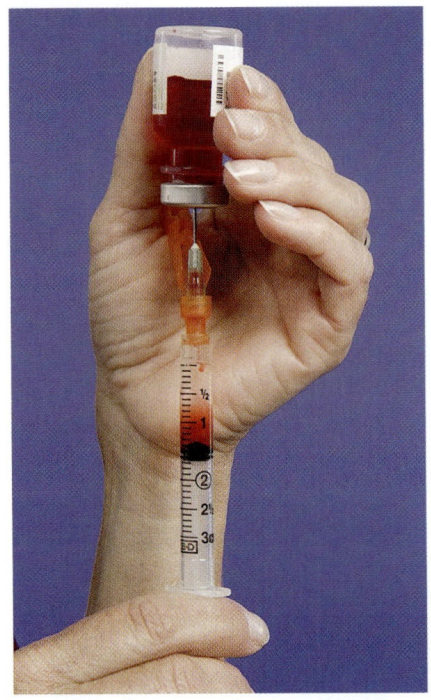

Vial A (step 5)

6. **Recap the VAD or access needle** using a needle-capping device or the one-handed scoop method (see Procedure 25-10: Recapping Needles Using One-Handed Technique).
Although recapping a sterile needle does not present a threat of bloodborne pathogen exposure, using a mechanical

recapping device or the one-handed method helps develop safe habits. As a rule, we do not recommend using the one-handed scoop for sterile needles; however, this needle will be discarded anyway, so if it is accidentally contaminated with a one-handed scoop, it will not be a major error.

7. **Remove the VAD (or access needle)** and attach a new sterile needle on the syringe for the injection.
Obviously, you must replace a VAD with a needle for injection. In addition, if you used a needle instead of a VAD, by the time you are finished withdrawing both medications you will have put it through a rubber vial top at least three times. This dulls the needle. A sharp needle causes less trauma to the patient on injection. A new needle also prevents tracking of the medication through the skin and subcutaneous tissues.

8. **Hold the needle vertically** to expel all air and recheck the dosage (the total for both medications).
Allows for more accurate accounting of the dose.

9. **If you have used a VAD or filter needle,** refer to Clinical Insight 25-5.

Procedure 25-9D ■ **Mixing Medications From One Ampule and One Vial**

➤ First review the **Medication Guidelines Steps to Follow for All Medications (Regardless of Type or Route)**; Procedure 25-9A: Drawing up Medications from Ampules; Procedure 25-9B: Drawing Up Medications From Vials; and Procedure 25-10A: Recapping Contaminated Needles.

➤ When performing the procedure, always identify your patient according to agency policy, using two identifiers, and be attentive to standard precautions, hand hygiene, patient safety and privacy, body mechanics, and documentation.

Procedure Steps

1. **Begin with the vial.** Scrub the stopper of the vial using an alcohol wipe or CHG-alcohol combination product.
Protects against microbial contamination.

2. **Attach a VAD and draw the same** volume of air into the syringe as the dose prescribed for the medication in the vial.

3. **Keeping the tip of the VAD** (or safety needle) above the medication, inject the amount of air equal to the volume of drug to be withdrawn

from the vial. The needle should be injecting air-to-air within the vial.
Draw from the vial first because you do not need to add air to ampules before drawing up the medication. In addition, if it is a multidose vial, you would contaminate it with the medicine if you withdrew from the ampule first.

Injecting air into the vial makes withdrawing the medication easier. For small unit-dose vials, it may be possible to withdraw the medication without instilling air, but you will need to maintain a slight backward pressure on the plunger until the needle is completely withdrawn.

If you release the plunger, the negative pressure in the vial will pull the medication back into the vial. Therefore, it is safer always to instill air.

4. **Invert the vial.** Withdraw the prescribed volume (dosage) of medication, keeping the VAD tip in the fluid. See Procedure 25-9B.

5. **Expel any air bubbles** and measure the dose at eye level. Recheck the dosage, and withdraw more or eject the drug as needed.
This prevents air from entering into the needle or VAD.

6. **After safely recapping** the VAD, remove it from the syringe. You may place it on an opened, sterile alcohol pad if you need your hands to open the filter needle packaging.

Keeps the needle sterile, if you are using one; you will reuse it. **KEY POINT:** *You would not reuse a VAD from this step on.*

7. **Attach a filter needle** or filter straw to the syringe.

The use of a 5-micrometer (μm) filter minimizes the possibility of withdrawing small glass fragments.

8. **Flick or tap the top** of the ampule (or snap your wrist) to remove medication from the neck of the ampule.

Flicking the neck of the ampule will help the fluid to drain down into the main part of the ampule, thus, reducing waste.

9. **Open the ampule** by wrapping the neck with a folded gauze pad or an unopened alcohol wipe or use an ampule snapper. Snap open away from you.

Snapping outward prevents you from cutting your fingers or spraying glass fragments toward your face. Do not use an opened alcohol wipe to break the ampule; the wipe is not thick enough to prevent injury.

10. **Withdraw the exact** prescribed amount of medication from the ampule into the syringe (see Procedure 25-9A). **KEY POINT:** *Be very careful in drawing up the second medication; if the total amount of the two medications is incorrect, you must discard the syringe contents and start over.*

11. **Draw 0.2 mL of air into the syringe.**

The extra bit of air clears the filter needle (see Clinical Insight 25-5).

12. **Confirm the dose is correct** by holding the syringe vertically and checking the dose at eye level.

Ensures the total volume in the syringe equals the ordered amount of both medications plus 0.2 mL of air from the needle.

13. **Recap the filter needle** using a needle-capping device or the one-handed technique recommended in Procedure 25-10B.

Although recapping a sterile needle does not present a threat of bloodborne pathogen exposure, using a mechanical recapping device or the one-handed method helps develop safe habits. Nevertheless, some scoop techniques pose a significant risk of contaminating the needle, so you must watch carefully that you maintain sterile technique.

14. **Remove the filter needle** or straw and discard it in a sharps container. Replace with a fresh safety needle for administering the medication to the patient.

This needle-recapping method prevents accidental needlestick injury. You cannot measure the dose accurately with a filter needle. You should not eject medication through the filter needle because of risk of breaking the filter. See Clinical Insight 25-5.

15. **After placing the administration needle** on the syringe, eject the 0.2 mL of air and check for the correct dose. If there is excess medication in the syringe, you must discard it and start over.

16. **Discard used needles and ampules** in a puncture-proof sharps container.

Procedure 25-9E ■ Using a Prefilled Cartridge and Single-Dose Vial—For Intravenous Administration

➤ *Note:* It is best not to use this technique with multidose vials because there is a risk of contaminating the multidose vial with the cartridge medication.

➤ First review the **Medication Guidelines: Steps to Follow for All Medications (Regardless of Type or Route).** Review Procedures 25-9 and 25-10, as needed.

➤ When performing the procedure, always identify your patient according to agency policy, using two identifiers, and be attentive to standard precautions, hand hygiene, patient safety and privacy, body mechanics, and documentation.

Procedure Steps

1. **Scrub the rubber stopper** of the vial thoroughly with an alcohol prep pad or CHG-alcohol-based product.

2. **Assemble the prefilled cartridge** and holder (see Clinical Insight 25-3).

3. **Remove the needle cap** from the prefilled cartridge, expel the air, and measure the correct dose of medication.

You must confirm that the dose of the first medication is correct before you mix it with the second medication.

4. **Holding the cartridge with** the needle up, draw in an amount of air equal to the volume of medication you need from the vial.

5. **While continuing to hold** the syringe with needle straight up (vertically), invert the vial and insert the needle into it until the tip of the needle shows in the air above the medication. Then inject the air into the vial. Maintain counterpressure on the plunger so that air and/or medication do not flow back into the syringe.

(continued on next page)

Procedure 25-9 ■ Preparing, Drawing Up, and Mixing Medication (continued)

Injecting air into the vial creates pressure, making the medication easier to withdraw. ▼

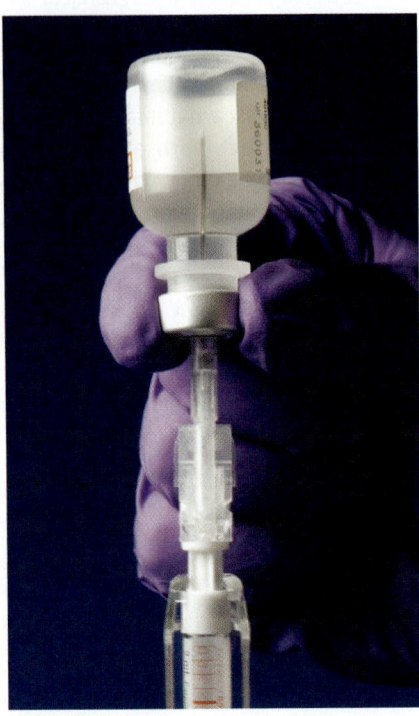

6. **While maintaining counterpressure** on the plunger, pull the needle down into the fluid and allow the pressure in the vial to push the medication into the syringe. Withdraw the prescribed amount of vial medication, being careful not to withdraw any excess.

7. **The pressure will generally push** a little less than you need, so carefully withdraw the amount you need for a correct dose—again, do not withdraw any excess.

   Withdrawing excess medication will result in an altered mixed dose, so you would need to discard the syringe and start over.

8. **Recap the needle** (use a one-handed method) and if possible remove the needle from the prefilled syringe and replace it with a sterile injection cannula for IV administration.

   For an intramuscular (IM) injection, if the prefilled cartridge does not have a safety needle, you would need to transfer the medication to a new syringe with a sterile safety needle for injection.

   VADs and injection cannulas prevent needlestick injury. Unless there is a needle safety device for the prefilled syringe, it is not recommended for IM injections.

? What if . . .

■ **I note particulate matter in the ampule or vial?**

Discard the medication and order a new one.

Documentation

Document on the MAR.

Thinking About the Procedures

 The videos **Drawing Up Medication From Ampules, Drawing Up Medication From Vials, Mixing Medication From Two Vials,** and **Mixing Medications From One Ampule and One Vial,** along with questions and suggested responses, are available on the **Davis's *Nursing Skills Videos*** Web site on Davis*Plus.*

Practice Resources

Centers for Disease Control and Prevention (n.d.a, updated 2016); Denholm, B. (2013); Manchikanti, L., Falco, F., Benyamin, R., et al. (2012).

Procedure 25-10 ■ Recapping Needles Using a One-Handed Technique

➤ For steps to follow in *all* procedures, refer to the Universal Steps for All Procedures found on the page facing the inside back cover. Also refer to **Medication Guidelines: Steps to Follow for All Medications (Regardless of Type or Route).**

Equipment

- Mechanical recapping device, if available
- Needle cover
- Safety syringe, if available
- Other supplies depending on the method used. ▼

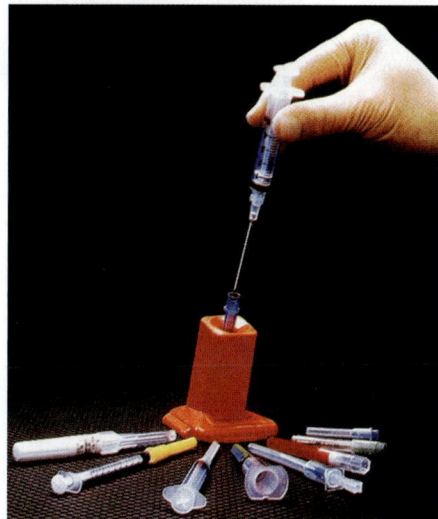

Needle-recapping device.

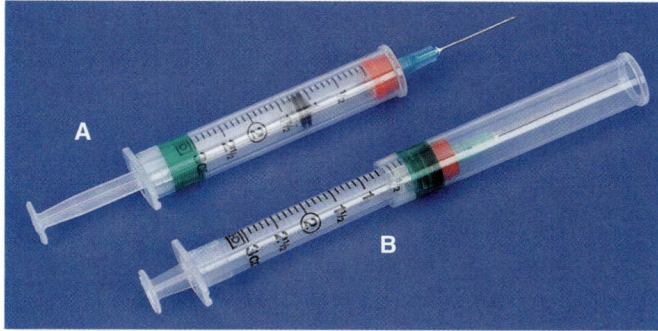

Safety syringe. A. Before injection. B. Cover slides up after injection.

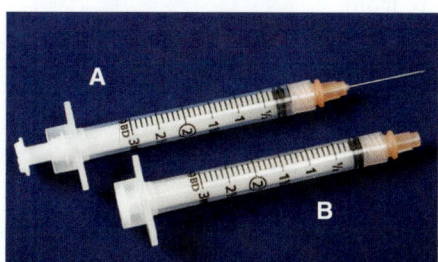

Safety syringe. A. Before injection. B. Needle retracted after injection.

Delegation

Delegation is not usually an issue because recapping needles is done in conjunction with administering parenteral medications, which you will usually not delegate. If you do delegate administration of parenteral medications to an LPN/LVN, you must supervise and evaluate recapping to ensure that the nurse uses proper technique.

Preparation

- **Assess the need to recap the needle.**

  Recap a contaminated needle only if doing so is absolutely unavoidable, according to Occupational Safety and Health Administration (OSHA) standards. As a rule, place a contaminated syringe and needle directly into a puncture-proof sharps container without capping, bending, or breaking the needle.

- **Identify whether the needle is sterile or contaminated.**

  Although a one-handed technique is used to recap both sterile and contaminated needles, different considerations exist.

  Sterile needle—*When you use the one-handed method for recapping a sterile needle, it is easy to contaminate the needle without realizing it. You should modify the technique to help prevent that—the main consideration is to "protect" the needle.*

  Contaminated needle—*The danger in recapping a dirty needle is that you will stick yourself with it, exposing yourself to pathogens. The main consideration is to protect yourself.*

- **Determine the availability of mechanical recapping device or safety syringe.**

  KEY POINT: *Always use a mechanical recapping device or safety syringe, if one is available.*

(continued on next page)

Procedure 25-10 ■ Recapping Needles Using a One-Handed Technique (continued)

Procedure 25-10A ■ Recapping Contaminated Needles

➤ When performing the procedure, always identify your patient according to agency policy, using two identifiers, and be attentive to standard precautions, hand hygiene, patient safety and privacy, body mechanics, and documentation.

Procedure Steps

1. **If you are using a safety needle,** engage the safety mechanism to cover the needle. (See Equipment.)
   OSHA regulations require the use of safety syringes to prevent needlestick injuries. You must engage the safety mechanism before placing the needle and syringe into the sharps container.

2. **Alternatively, place the needle** cap in a mechanical recapping device, if one is available. (See Equipment.)

3. **If a mechanical recapping device** is not available, use the one-handed scoop method to recap the needle.
   a. Place the needle cover on a flat surface.
      Keeps the needle cover from rolling during the needle-capping procedure. ➤

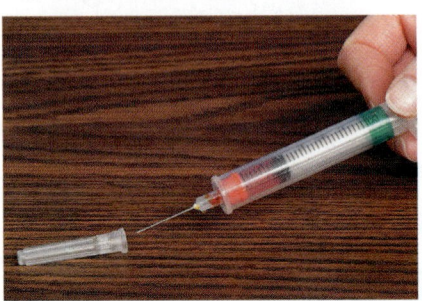

b. Then, holding syringe in your dominant hand, scoop the needle cap onto the needle. Tip the syringe vertically to slip the cover over the needle. Do not hold on to the needle cap with your non-dominant hand while scooping.
   A mechanical recapping device protects against needlestick injury. If it is unavailable, the one-handed method of recapping will prevent injuries when your own or the patient's safety is a concern. ▼

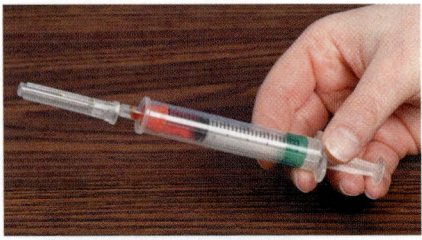

c. Secure the needle cap by grasping it near the hub.
   Prevents an accidental stick if the needle goes through the needle cap. Needles are sharp enough to go through the needle cap if inserted at an angle. ▼

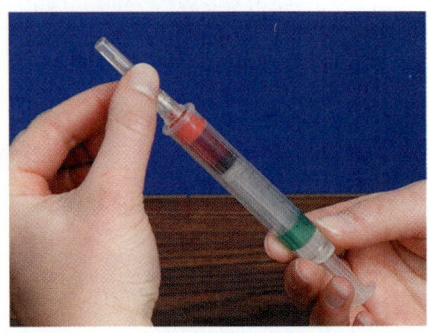

Procedure 25-10B ■ Recapping Sterile Needles

➤ When performing the procedure, always identify your patient according to agency policy, using two identifiers, and be attentive to standard precautions, hand hygiene, patient safety and privacy, body mechanics, and documentation.

Use one of the following techniques to ensure that you do not contaminate a sterile needle. If you contaminate the needle, microorganisms will be introduced with the injection.

Procedure Steps

1. **Place the needle cap** in a mechanical recapping device, if one is available.
   The device is specially developed to provide safe recapping.

2. **Alternative method: Medication cup.** Place the cap into a small liquid medication cup with the open end facing up. You can then insert the sterile needle into the cap, keeping your free hand well away from the cup.
   This step performs the same function as a mechanical recapping device. The needle and cover need to be taller than the cup you are using, so that the open end of the cap protrudes above the cup. ➤

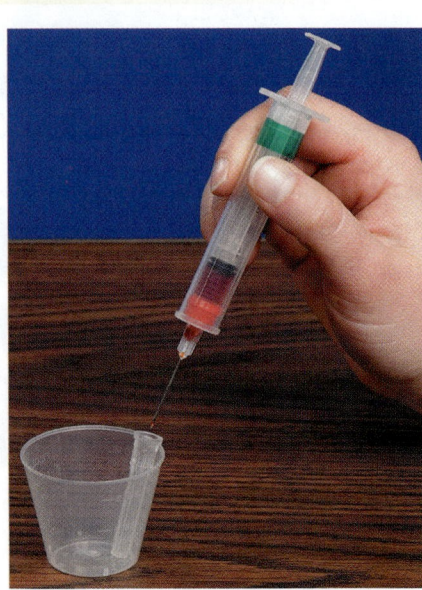

3. **Alternative method: Scoop technique.** Place the cap on a clean surface so that the end of the needle cap protrudes over the edge of the counter or shelf, and scoop with the needle; keep your free hand well away from the needle and cap as you are recapping.

This method prevents you from inadvertently hitting an unsterile surface with the needle. ▼

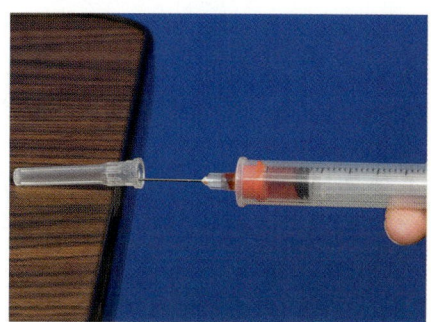

stand the container on its large end, invert the needle cap, and place it in the top of the hard container. Insert the needle downward into the cap. ▼

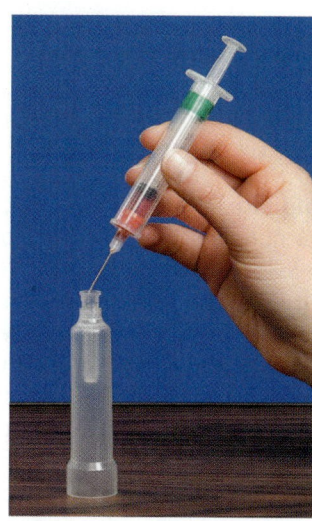

surface, such as on an open alcohol prep pad, and use the one-handed scoop technique. Be very careful not to touch anything with the needle other than the inside of the needle cap.

The alcohol prep pad provides a sterile barrier. Because you must bring the needle parallel to the flat surface, and because the alcohol pad is so small, it is easy to contaminate the needle using this method. ▼

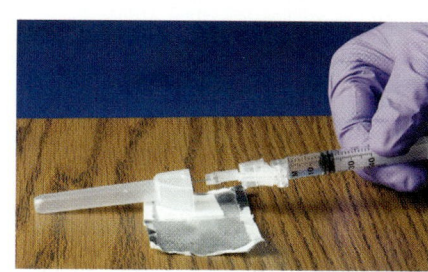

4. **Alternative method: Tubular container.** If the syringe is packaged in a hard plastic tubular container,

5. **Alternative method: Alcohol wipe.** Place the needle cap on a sterile

Documentation

No documentation needed for recapping needles.

Practice Resources

National Institute for Occupational Safety and Health (updated 2016); Waqar, S., Siraj, M., Razzaq, Z., et al. (2011).

Procedure 25-11 ■ Administering Intradermal Medication

➤ For steps to follow in *all* procedures, refer to the Universal Steps for All Procedures found on the page facing the inside back cover. Also refer to **Medication Guidelines: Steps to Follow for All Medications (Regardless of Type or Route).**

Equipment

- Alcohol prep pad or CHG-alcohol product
- 2 in. × 2 in. gauze pad
- Pen (ink or felt)
- 1-mL syringe (tuberculin) with intradermal needle (25- to 28-gauge, ¼- to ⅝-inch with short bevel) ▼

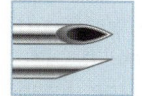 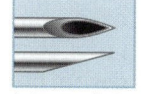 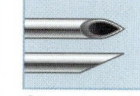

Regular bevel | Intermediate bevel | Short bevel

Delegation

As an RN, you can usually delegate administration of parenteral medications to an LPN/LVN. You usually cannot delegate this task to a NAP.

Pre-Procedure Assessments

- Assess for allergies, previous reaction to skin testing, and the skin for signs of irritation (e.g., bruising, swelling, tenderness).

  Some skin tests, such as the tuberculin test, should not be repeated after positive test results. Do not give intradermal skin tests if skin abnormalities are present. Also avoid giving them in areas where reading the results may be difficult, such as areas of heavy hair growth.

Preparation

- Have appropriate antidotes (usually epinephrine hydrochloride, a bronchodilator, and an antihistamine) readily available before the start of the procedure.

  Because many intradermal injections are used for allergy testing, this is an important consideration.

- Know the location of resuscitation equipment (artificial airway, Ambu bag, and code cart).

  Allergic reactions can be fatal.

(continued on next page)

Procedure 25-11 ■ Administering Intradermal Medication (continued)

> ➤ When performing the procedure, always identify your patient according to agency policy, using two identifiers, and be attentive to standard precautions, hand hygiene, patient safety and privacy, body mechanics, and documentation.

Procedure Steps

1. **Draw up the medication** from the vial (see Procedure 25-9B). The usual dose is 0.01 to 0.1 mL.
Intradermal sites can accommodate only small volumes of medication.

2. **Select the site for injection.** Usual sites are the ventral surface of the forearm and upper back. The upper chest may also be used. If you need to review site locations, see Figure 25-22.
Use areas where subcutaneous fat is less likely to interfere with administration and absorption. The forearm is the standard initial starting point because it has the least amount of subcutaneous tissue. The forearm and upper back usually have little hair, permitting easier visualization to interpret results accurately.

3. **Assist the patient to a** comfortable position. If you are using the forearm, instruct her to extend and supinate her arm on a flat surface. If you are using the upper back, ask the patient to lie prone or lean forward over a table or the back of a chair.
This method stabilizes the injection site. The procedure will be more comfortable if the patient is able to relax his muscles. Tension, in general, increases pain perception.

4. **Don procedure gloves.**
Procedure gloves are not required by OSHA for intradermal injections, but they are recommended by the CDC to prevent accidental exposure to bloodborne pathogens.

   ✚ *Remember, gloves cannot prevent needlestick injuries.*

5. **Scrub the injection site** with an alcohol prep pad or CHG-alcohol product pad. Allow the site to dry before administering the injection.
Cleansing to remove microorganisms follows the principle of "clean to dirty." Alcohol can interfere with the test results if a small amount is introduced during the injection. If the alcohol has not evaporated, it may cause the skin to sting during the injection.

6. **Grasp the syringe between** the thumb and index finger of your dominant hand.
Enables you to administer the solution at the correct angle.

7. **Hold the client's skin taut** with your nondominant hand using one of the following methods:
   a. If using the forearm, you may be able to place your hand under the client's arm and pull the skin tight with your thumb and fingers.
   b. Stretch the client's skin between your thumb and index finger.
   c. Pull the client's skin toward the wrist or down with one finger.
   A downward motion while stretching the skin eases needle insertion. Holding the skin tight can be difficult because of the low angle of administration.

8. **Continuing to hold the skin** taut with your nondominant hand, hold the syringe in your dominant hand with the needle bevel up and parallel to the client's skin at a 5° to 15° angle. Slowly insert the needle. There is some controversy about whether it is better to have the bevel down or up; however, the CDC recommends bevel up.
The low angle of insertion is necessary to place the needle tip in the intradermal layer instead of the subcutaneous tissue. Having the bevel up likely decreases the chance of injecting the medication deeper into the subcutaneous tissue. Patients receiving intradermal injections report bevel up as more comfortable. ▼

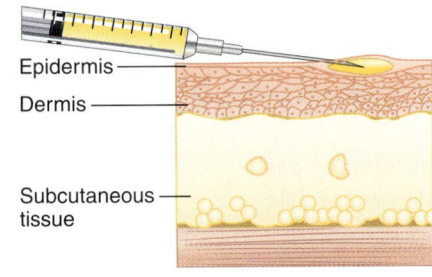

Epidermis
Dermis
Subcutaneous tissue

9. **Advance the needle** approximately 3 mm (⅛ in.) so that the entire bevel is covered. The bevel

should be visible just under the skin.
If the entire bevel is not inserted, the solution will leak out of the tissue. If you can see the bevel under the surface of the skin, you can be sure that the bevel is not in the subcutaneous tissue.

10. **Do not aspirate.** Hold the syringe stable with your nondominant hand and release the tightened skin.

11. **Release the taut skin and lowly inject the solution.** You should feel firm resistance. A pale wheal, about 6 to 10 mm (¼ in.) in diameter, will appear over the needle bevel.
The dermis does not have room to absorb the solution, so a wheal forms, stretching the skin. Slow administration gives you time to terminate the injection should a systemic reaction occur. If a bleb (wheal) forms, you have administered the drug properly. The size of the bleb depends on the amount of medication you injected. ▼

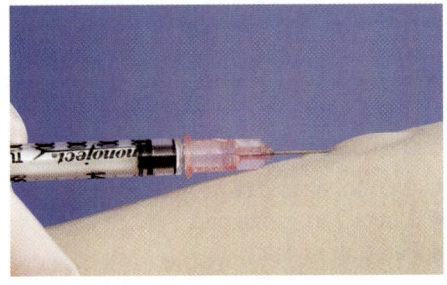

12. **Remove the needle,** engage the safety device, and dispose of the needle in a biohazard, puncture-proof container. If there is no safety device, place the uncapped syringe and needle directly in a biohazard, puncture-proof container.
Prevents needlestick injuries.

13. **Gently blot any blood** with a dry gauze pad. Do not rub the skin or cover it with an adhesive bandage.
Rubbing may cause the drug to leak out and alter absorption. An adhesive bandage can cause irritation and interfere with the skin test.

14. With a pen, draw a 1-inch circle around the bleb/wheal.

Marking the site helps you to identify any change in the size of the wheal at a later time.

? What if . . .

- **My patient has a history of a skin reaction to PPD testing?**

Obtain details about the type and severity of the reaction. If the previous reaction involved ulceration at the site, further Mantoux testing is contraindicated. Report this to the prescriber.

- **My patient is pregnant, is receiving chemotherapy, or has severe eczema?**

Before administering the tuberculosis skin test, engage in discussions with the prescriber to fully explore any contraindications.

- **My patient received a live vaccine at the time of tuberculosis skin testing?**

Tuberculosis skin testing should be deferred for one month after live viral vaccines or other major viral infection.

- **My patient has topical anesthetic cream on the skin?**

Use a site where the topical anesthetic cream was not applied or reschedule tuberculosis skin testing for another date.

Evaluation

- Reassess the client at 5 and 15 minutes after administration for allergic reactions that may subsequently occur.
- Read the site within 48 to 72 hours of injection, depending on the test.
- Observe that a wheal (about 6 to 8 mm in diameter) forms at the site and that it gradually disappears.
- Observe for minimal bruising that may develop at the site of injection.

Patient Teaching

- Explain when the patient needs to have the intradermal injection read to determine whether the result is positive or negative.
- Explain that mild itching, swelling, or irritation may occur at the injection site and is normal.

  If the patient has antigens to the injected solution, a histamine response occurs, causing itching, swelling, or irritation. This response generally subsides within a week.

- Discuss the significance of a positive or negative skin test result. Explain that some signs of irritation may occur that do not mean a positive test result.
- Instruct the patient not to scratch, apply lotions or creams, cover the site with a bandage, or scrub the site.

  This might cause irritation and interfere with the test, which may produce false-positive results.

Documentation

- See the information in **Medication Guidelines: Steps to Follow for All Medications (Regardless of Type or Route).**
- Some medications require documentation of lot numbers (check agency policy).
- Chart when the test is to be read.

Sample documentation

mm/dd/yyyy   0800   Explained purpose and procedure for Mantoux skin test. Client stated, "I need a PPD so that I can go to the long-term care facility." 0.2 mL of tuberculin purified protein placed in left forearm per physician order. No reaction noted 5 minutes after procedure. Will read test at 0800 on mm/dd/yyyy. ———————————— M. Saleh, RN

Thinking About the Procedure

 The video **Administering Intradermal Medication,** along with questions and suggested responses, is available on the **Davis's *Nursing Skills Videos* Web** site on Davis*Plus.*

Practice Resources

Centers for Disease Control and Prevention (n.d.a, n.d.b, 2011a); Diggle, J. (2014); Felicilda-Reynaldo, R. (2014); Garner, S. (2013).

Procedure 25-12 ■ Administering Subcutaneous Medication

➤ For steps to follow in *all* procedures, refer to the Universal Steps for All Procedures found on the page facing the inside back cover. Also refer to **Medication Guidelines: Steps to Follow for All Medications (Regardless of Type or Route).**

Equipment

- Syringe and needle appropriate for volume and site
- Alcohol prep pad or CHG-alcohol product
- Gauze pad (optional)

Delegation

As an RN, you can usually delegate administration of parenteral medications to an LPN/LVN. You usually cannot delegate this task to a NAP.

Pre-Procedure Assessments

- Check the selected site for inflammation, bruising, lumps, or other abnormalities that may contraindicate use of the site.
- Check the area for previous injection sites.
  Alternating among the arms, thighs, abdomen, and back changes the absorption rate of the medication. Absorption is fastest from the abdomen, then the arms, and lastly the thighs and back. Rotate sites within the same extremity or location, approximately 1 inch from the previous injection. Rotating the site helps prevent fat deposits and skin lumps.

- Do focused assessments for the specific medication being administered.
  Insulin—Check capillary blood sugar level and determine when the patient will be having the next meal; check for signs of hypoglycemia or hyperglycemia.
  Insulin must be balanced with food intake to prevent the patient from developing hypoglycemia or hyperglycemia. Different insulins have specific rates of absorption, peak action, and duration. Some insulins, such as Humalog and regular insulin, are rapid acting. Before you administer rapid-acting insulin, the capillary blood sugar must be within the normal range or above, and the patient must be ready to eat. With Humalog, the patient's food tray should be in front of him before you administer the insulin.

  Heparin—Check activated partial thromboplastin time (aPTT) and for signs of overt bleeding (e.g., bleeding from gums, IV injection sites) and covert bleeding (e.g., blood in urine and stool).
  Heparin is an anticoagulant, so the major side effect is bleeding.

  NOTE: The aPTT will not be monitored as frequently with the low-molecular-weight heparins (LMWHs) because bleeding is less likely to occur.

➤ When performing the procedure, always identify your patient according to agency policy, using two identifiers, and be attentive to standard precautions, hand hygiene, patient safety and privacy, body mechanics, and documentation.

Procedure Steps

1. **Select an appropriate syringe** and needle.
   a. For insulin administration, you must use an insulin syringe—typically 0.3, 0.5, or 1.0 mL. Most insulin needles are 28 to 31 gauge. Needle length is often ³⁄₁₆ to 1 inch. For more information about giving insulin, see Clinical Insight 25-6.

   ➕ Although both insulin and tuberculin (TB) syringes come in a 1-mL size, they are not interchangeable. Insulin syringes are calibrated in units; they have a permanent (nonremovable) needle and a very small amount of dead space.

   b. For other medications, for volumes less than 1 mL, use a tuberculin (TB) syringe with a 25- to 27-gauge, ³⁄₈- to ⁵⁄₈-inch needle.
   Because of the small increments on the TB syringe, small doses can be measured more accurately. ➤

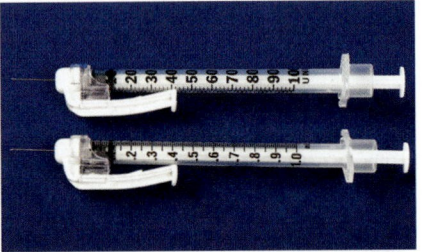

Top: Insulin syringe. *Bottom:* TB syringe.

   c. For administering a volume of 1 mL, you may use a 3-mL syringe with a 25- to 27-gauge, ³⁄₈- to ⁵⁄₈-inch needle.
   Although you can measure 1 mL with a TB syringe, it will be difficult to handle the syringe because the plunger will be pulled back as far as it can go. It is easy to pull it inadvertently out of the end of the syringe. Some medications are supplied in prefilled syringes. Examples are enoxaparin sodium (Lovenox) and the other LMWHs.

2. **Draw up the medication.** See Procedure 25-9.

3. **Select an injection site** with adequate subcutaneous tissue. If you need to review site locations, see **Figure 25-24.**
   Helps you avoid accidentally injecting into the muscle.

   a. The usual sites are the outer aspect of the upper arms, abdomen (at least 2 inches away from the umbilicus), anterior aspects of the thighs, and high on the buttocks near waist level.
   These areas usually have good circulation and are easily accessible. The buttocks are more convenient when someone other than the patient is giving the injection.

   b. The anterolateral and posterolateral abdomen ("love handles") sites are the only subcutaneous site used for administering heparin or LMWHs. For more information about giving heparin, see Clinical Insight 25-7.

The tissue 2 inches away from the umbilicus poses less risk of bleeding when an anticoagulant is administered.

4. **Position the patient** so that the injection site is accessible and the patient is able to relax the appropriate area. Check the site for inflammation, bruising, lumps, or other abnormalities.

Avoid areas with skin abnormalities, which may alter the absorption rates or increase patient discomfort during the injection.

5. **Don procedure gloves.**

To prevent exposure to bloodborne pathogens. You may prefer to don gloves before step 4.

6. **Scrub the injection site** with an alcohol prep pad or CHG-alcohol product. Allow the site to dry before administering the injection. For alcohol, circle from the site outward; for CHG, use a back-and-forth motion. Do not go back over already cleaned area.

7. **Remove the needle cap.**

The needle cap is more difficult to remove when using a one-handed technique.

8. **With your nondominant hand,** pinch the tissue at the injection site and determine the angle at which to inject the needle. Insert the needle using a 45° to 90° angle, depending

on the amount of adipose tissue (the less adipose tissue, the lower the angle). If the adipose tissue pinches 2 inches or more (client is obese), use a longer needle and spread the skin taut instead of pinching.

Grasping and lifting the tissue prevents you from accidentally injecting into the muscle. The subcutaneous injection must be given in the fatty tissue and not into intradermal layer. Traditionally, injections had been given using a 45° angle to ensure medication is deposited into the subcutaneous layer. ▼

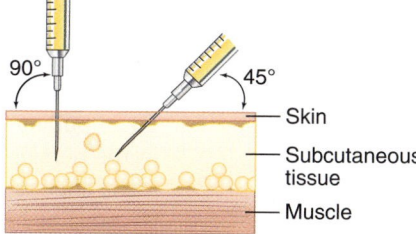

9. **Holding the syringe between** thumb and index finger of your dominant hand like a pencil or dart, insert the needle at the appropriate angle into the skinfold.

Quickly inserting the needle through the skin minimizes discomfort.

10. **Using the thumb or index finger** of your dominant hand, press the plunger slowly to inject the medication while stabilizing the syringe with your other hand. Alternatively, after inserting the needle, you can continue to hold the barrel with

your dominant hand and use your nondominant hand to depress the plunger.

Slow administration allows the medication to disperse and decreases discomfort. Subcutaneous injections do not need to be aspirated beforehand, because accidental entry into a blood vessel is rare. Stabilize the syringe to avoid discomfort and tissue damage from the needle.

11. **Remove the needle** smoothly along the line of insertion.

Prevents pulling against the skin and tissue and thus minimizes discomfort.

12. **Gently blot the site with gauze** if needed. Do not massage the site unless directed to do so by prescription or policy.

Occasionally there will be blood at the site after the needle is removed. You might have nicked a surface blood vessel when you injected, and blood is following the needle track out to the surface. Massaging or rubbing the site will alter the rate of absorption of the medication.

13. **Engage the needle safety device** and dispose of the needle in a biohazard container. If there is no safety device, place the uncapped syringe and needle directly into a biohazard, puncture-proof container.

A sharps container prevents needlestick injuries.

Evaluation

- Observe for minimal bruising that may develop at the site of injection.
- Reassess the patient for anticipated response and adverse reaction to medication.

  For insulin, observe for signs that the patient's blood sugar level has returned to normal and for signs of hypoglycemia.

  For heparin, observe that the patient has no signs of bleeding.

  For other medications, observe for known side effects.

Patient Teaching

- Discuss possible lifestyle adaptations that the patient may need to undertake while receiving the medication (e.g., diet and exercise recommendations for managing diabetes mellitus).

Home Care

- Discuss with the client or caregiver the options for insulin administration to determine the most appropriate choice for the person administering the injections.

  Many options are available, including specially designed syringes that are easier to handle and read, pen injectors, and prefilled syringes.

- In the home environment, the client might not routinely use an alcohol wipe to cleanse the site. This is acceptable as long as the skin is clean.

  In the home environment, there is less risk for superinfection with resistant strain organisms and other healthcare-acquired infections.

- Do not encourage reusing needles and syringes. However, if the client or caregiver believes he needs to reuse syringes and needles in the home, teach him how to do so safely (Clinical Insight 25-2).

(continued on next page)

Procedure 25-12 ■ **Administering Subcutaneous Medication** (continued)

■ 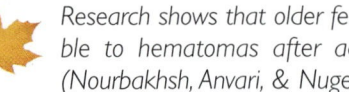 The very small insulin needles (30 gauge) bend very easily and are not recommended for reuse.

Determine whether reusing syringes is appropriate for the patient. Contraindications include inadequate hygiene, immunocompromised status, and difficulty handling equipment to prevent contamination of the needle.

■ 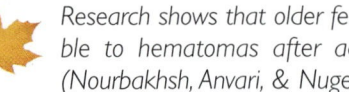 Discuss safety concerns regarding subcutaneous medication administration in the home, such as how to dispose of biohazardous wastes correctly and where to obtain a puncture-proof biohazard container.

The patient or caregiver may use a large plastic bottle or a coffee can. Local regulations regarding disposal must be followed.

■ Discuss with the patient the need to rotate sites and reasons for doing so. Recommend that he give injections at the same time of the day in the same body location about 1 inch from the previous injection site.

Repeatedly giving the medication in the same site can cause abnormalities in the tissue and alter absorption rates.

■ Remind the patient that when changing sites (thigh, arm, abdomen), the absorption rate may be altered.

■ If the patient is receiving heparin or LMWHs, discuss the need to avoid NSAID medications such as acetylsalicylic acid (aspirin) and ibuprofen (Motrin, Advil).

These drugs increase the risk of bleeding.

■ For patients receiving heparin or LMWHs, discuss home safety and the need to avoid falls.

The patient is at risk for bleeding and needs to follow safety guidelines to prevent injury.

Research shows that older females are more susceptible to hematomas after administration of LMWH (Nourbakhsh, Anvari, & Nugent, 2011). Nurses should carefully assess for abdominal bruising and complaints of abdominal pain.

Documentation

■ Chart according to **Medication Guidelines: Steps to Follow for All Medications (Regardless of Type or Route).**

■ Some agencies have a specific code for documenting subcutaneous injections, which allows exact site documentation on an outline of the body.

■ In the nursing notes, document any related patient assessment findings, such as capillary blood sugar, signs of hypoglycemia or hyperglycemia, bruising, and so on.

■ Document in the nursing notes as well as MAR any medication that was given prn.

Sample EHR documentation

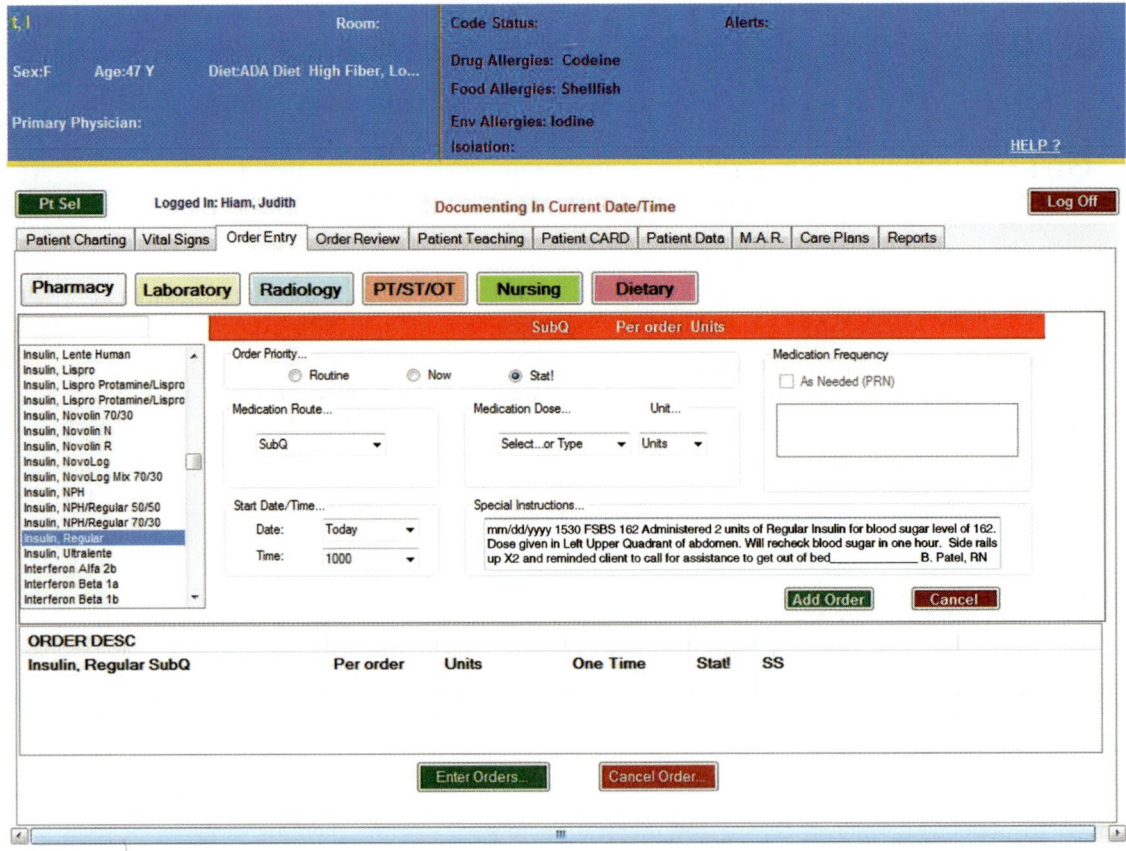

Thinking About the Procedure

 The video **Administering Subcutaneous Medication,** along with questions and suggested responses, is available on the **Davis's *Nursing Skills Videos*** Web site on DavisPlus.

Practice Resources

Bartley, N. (2012a); Nourbakhsh, E., Anvari, R., & Nugent, K. (2011); Ogston-Tuck, S. (2014b); Pledger, J., Hicks, D., Kirkland, F., et al. (2012); Pourghaznein, T., Azimi, A. V., & Jafarabadi, M. A. (2014).

Procedure 25-13 ■ Locating Intramuscular Injection Sites

➤ For steps to follow in *all* procedures, refer to the Universal Steps for All Procedures found on the page facing the inside back cover. Also refer to **Medication Guidelines: Steps to Follow for All Medications (Regardless of Type or Route).**

Delegation

As an RN, you can usually delegate administration of parenteral medications (including locating injection sites) to an LPN/LVN. You usually cannot delegate this task to a NAP. If you delegate the skill, you are responsible for evaluating the LPN/LVN's ability to locate injection sites correctly.

Pre-Procedure Assessment

Always palpate the landmarks and the muscle mass to ensure correct placement of the needle. Because patients' body shapes differ, the site locations will vary slightly.

Procedure 25-13A ■ Locating the Ventrogluteal Site

➤ When performing the procedure, always identify your patient according to agency policy, using two identifiers, and be attentive to standard precautions, hand hygiene, patient safety and privacy, body mechanics, and documentation.

Procedure Steps

1. **Ask the patient to assume a** side-lying position with the legs straight, if possible.
   This position makes the site easier to locate.

2. **Locate the greater trochanter,** anterior superior iliac spine, and the iliac crest.

3. **Place the palm of your hand** on the greater trochanter, your index finger on the anterior superior iliac spine, and your middle finger pointing toward the iliac crest. (Use your right hand on the patient's left hip; use your left hand on the patient's right hip.) Note that if your hands are very large or very small, the location of the "triangle" will be higher or

lower on the hip. Be sure you locate it well in the muscle mass. ▼

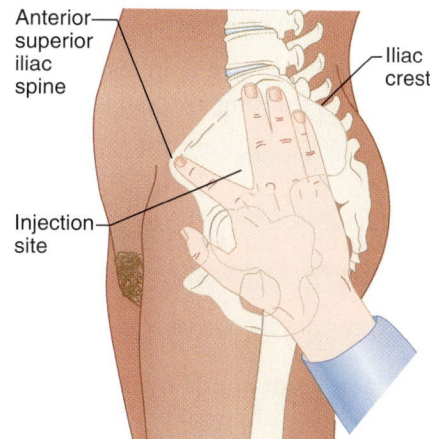
Anterior superior iliac spine — Iliac crest — Injection site

4. **The middle of the triangle** between your middle and index fingers is the injection site.
   This is a safe site for IM administration because it is not in proximity to any

major blood vessels or nerves. The landmarks are easy to find. This large muscle can take volumes up to 5 mL in the average adult. It is safe for patients of all ages and the preferred site for adults and children older than 7 to 12 months (there is some disagreement over the age; always palpate to assess adequacy of muscle mass, regardless of age). ▼

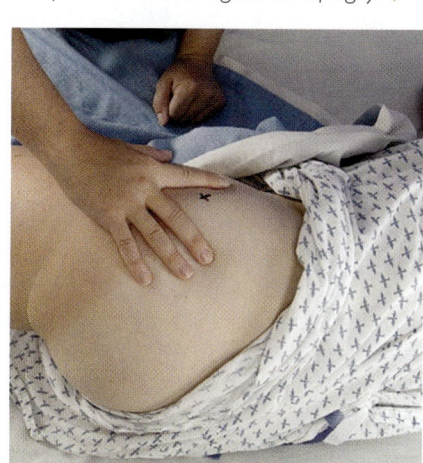

(continued on next page)

Procedure 25-13 ■ Locating Intramuscular Injection Sites (continued)

Procedure 25-13B ■ Locating the Deltoid Site

➤ When performing the procedure, always identify your patient according to agency policy, using two identifiers, and be attentive to standard precautions, hand hygiene, patient safety and privacy, body mechanics, and documentation.

Procedure Steps

1. Completely expose the patient's upper arm. Remove the garment; do not roll up the sleeve.
Incomplete exposure of site and landmarks creates a risk of injecting into other than muscle tissue. This is a small site, and it is easy to make an error in location.

2. Locate the lower edge of the acromion process (knobby part of shoulder), and go two to three fingerbreadths down (3 to 5 cm) to locate the midpoint of the lateral arm. ▼

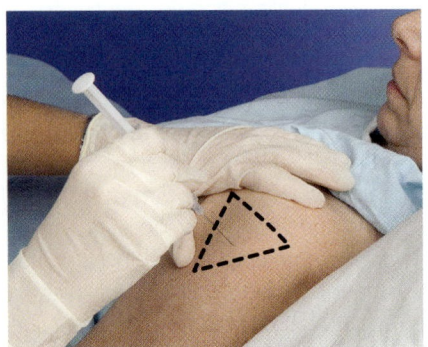

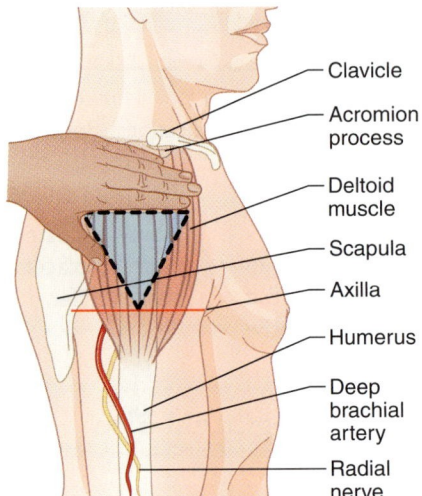

Clavicle
Acromion process
Deltoid muscle
Scapula
Axilla
Humerus
Deep brachial artery
Radial nerve

3. Draw an imaginary line from each end of the triangle base downward 1 to 2 in (3 to 5 cm) to the midpoint of the lateral arm.

4. The deltoid site is in the center of the resulting inverted triangle.

5. An alternative approach is to place four fingerbreadths across the deltoid muscle, with your top finger on the acromion process. The injection goes three fingerbreadths below the process in the midline of the upper arm.
Locates the appropriate site while avoiding the radial nerve and deep brachial artery. Because it is a fairly small muscle, only 0.5 to 1 mL of medication can be administered.

Procedure 25-13C ■ Locating the Vastus Lateralis Site

➤ When performing the procedure, always identify your patient according to agency policy, using two identifiers, and be attentive to standard precautions, hand hygiene, patient safety and privacy, body mechanics, and documentation.

Procedure Steps

1. Position the patient lying supine or sitting.
The patient may perceive the injection as less painful if supine because he cannot see the needle enter his leg. For some people this provokes anxiety and intensifies pain.

2. Locate the greater trochanter and the lateral femoral condyle.

3. Place your hands on the thigh, with one hand against the greater trochanter and the other edge of the hand against the lateral femoral condyle.

4. Visualize a rectangle between your hands across the anterolateral thigh.
  ■ The index fingers of your hands form the smaller ends of the rectangle.

  ■ The long sides of the rectangle are formed by (a) drawing an imaginary line down the center of the anterior thigh and (b) drawing another line along the side of the leg, halfway between the bed and the front of the thigh.
  ■ This box marks the middle third of the anterolateral thigh, which is the injection site.
  The rectus femoris lies on the top (or anterior) portion of the thigh and

partially covers the edge of the vastus lateralis. Therefore, do not inject too near the midline of the anterior thigh. Because it is not near any major blood vessels or nerves, the vastus lateralis site is safe for patients of all ages and is the recommended site for children younger than 7 months. ➤

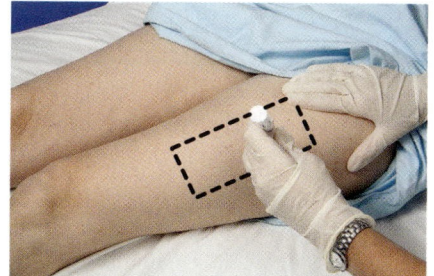

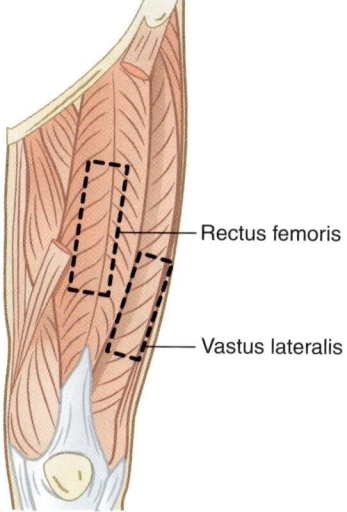

—Rectus femoris

—Vastus lateralis

Procedure 25-13D ■ Locating the Rectus Femoris Site

➤ When performing the procedure, always identify your patient according to agency policy, using two identifiers, and be attentive to standard precautions, hand hygiene, patient safety and privacy, body mechanics, and documentation.

Procedure Steps

✚ **Use this site only if no other sites are accessible** and no other medication routes are feasible.

1. **Position the patient** lying supine or sitting.

2. **Divide the top of the thigh** from the groin to the knee into thirds and identify the middle third.

3. **Visualize a rectangle** in the middle of the anterior surface of the thigh. This is the location of the injection site. Also refer to the drawing of the adult thigh in Procedure 25-13C. ➤

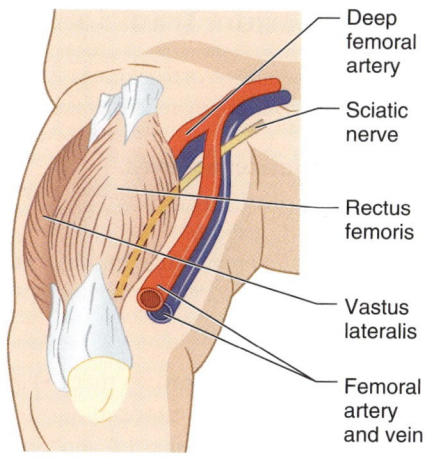

— Deep femoral artery

— Sciatic nerve

— Rectus femoris

— Vastus lateralis

— Femoral artery and vein

? What if . . .

- **My patient is a child? What is the best site to give an IM injection?**

  Because an infant's muscles are not fully developed, site selection is limited.

  For children who are walking, use the ventrogluteal site.

  For children who are not yet walking, use the vastus lateralis. Once the gluteal muscles are further developed, which occurs with walking, the ventrogluteal site can be used.

Thinking About the Procedure

The videos **Locating the Ventrogluteal Site, Locating the Deltoid Site,** and **Locating the Vastus Lateralis Site,** along with questions and suggested responses, are available on the **Davis's** *Nursing Skills Videos* Web site on Davis*Plus.*

Procedure 25-14 ■ Administering an Intramuscular Injection

> ➤ For steps to follow in *all* procedures, refer to the Universal Steps for All Procedures found on the page facing the inside back cover. Also refer to **Medication Guidelines: Steps to Follow for All Medications (Regardless of Type or Route).**
>
> ➤ The Z-track method is preferred for all IM injections, except in a rare instance in which it is contraindicated.

Equipment

- Syringe and needle appropriate for volume and site
- Alcohol prep pad or CHG-alcohol product
- Gauze pad or adhesive bandage
- Medication
- Procedure gloves
- Biohazard (sharps) container
- Small piece of gauze or cotton ball
- Small adhesive bandage

Delegation

As an RN, you can usually delegate administration of parenteral medications to an LPN/LVN. You cannot delegate this task to a NAP.

Pre-Procedure Assessments

- Identify the site of the previous injection.
- Assess the site for adequate muscle mass, bruises, edema, tenderness, redness, or other abnormalities.
  Muscle mass must be large enough to absorb the amount of medication prescribed. Abnormalities at the site increase patient discomfort and alter the absorption rate of the medication.
- Assess for factors that might affect absorption of the medication, such as decreased intramuscular blood flow, as found in shock or muscle atrophy.
  Decreased peripheral circulation or muscle atrophy decreases the absorption of the medication.

Procedure 25-14A ■ Intramuscular Injection: Traditional Method

> ➤ When performing the procedure, always identify your patient according to agency policy, using two identifiers, and be attentive to standard precautions, hand hygiene, patient safety and privacy, body mechanics, and documentation.

Procedure Steps

1. **Select the appropriate syringe and needle.**
   a. The usual syringe size is 1 to 3 mL, depending on volume of medication to be given. For doses less than 1 mL, you can use a tuberculin syringe with an intramuscular needle.
   b. The needle size is usually 21 to 25 gauge, 1½ in. in length for adults (or 1 in. for deltoid site), but a longer needle (3 in.) might be necessary to penetrate the muscle if the patient is obese.
   For IM administration, the needle gauge must be appropriate for the viscosity of the medication, and the needle must be long enough to deliver the medication into the muscle.
   c. Some medications are supplied in prefilled syringes, which are used for administration.

2. **Draw up the medication** (see Procedure 25-9A) or obtain prescribed unit dose and verify medication. If the volume for injection is more than 3 to 5 milliliters, divide the dose for separate injections.

3. **Don procedure gloves.**
   Procedure gloves are required by OSHA to prevent exposure to bloodborne pathogens. You may prefer to don gloves at step 6, while waiting for the antiseptic to dry.

4. **Position the patient** so that the injection site is well exposed and the patient is able to relax the appropriate muscles. Be sure the lighting is adequate.
   When the patient's muscles are relaxed (and not tense), it is easier to perform the injection and it reduces patient discomfort during injection. You must be able to fully visualize and safely access the site.

   a. *Deltoid site:* Position the patient with the arm relaxed at the side or resting on a firm surface, and completely expose the upper arm.
   b. *Ventrogluteal site:* Position the patient on the opposite side, with the upper hip and knee slightly flexed.
   This position may cause the trochanter to become more prominent, making it easier to locate the site.

   c. *Vastus lateralis:* Position the patient supine or sitting, if the patient prefers.
   d. *Rectus femoris:* Position patient supine. Because this site often causes more discomfort than others, use it only if all other sites are inaccessible and no other route is feasible.

   > ✚ *Dorsogluteal:* Do not use this site because of the muscle's proximity to the sciatic nerve and major blood vessels.

5. Using appropriate landmarks, identify the injection site (see Procedure 25-13). If the client is to receive more than one injection, rotate sites.
   Volumes of 1 to 5 mL may be given, depending on the muscle size (for adults, 0.5 to 1 mL in the deltoid, and typically 1 to 3 mL but up to 5 mL in the vastus lateralis site). If the volume for injection is more than 3 to 5 mL, then divide the dose for a separate injection. Rotating sites reduces discomfort and tissue trauma.

6. Gently but thoroughly scrub the injection site. Do not "go back over" already cleansed areas.

   a. If using an alcohol prep pad, thoroughly clean the site by circling from the center of the site outward.

   b. If using a CHG-based antiseptic, you may use a back-and-forth motion.

   Cleanse to remove microorganisms; follow the principle of "clean to dirty."

7. Place the wipe on the patient's skin outside the injection site, with a corner pointing to the site. Allow the site to dry before administering the injection. Do not fan the site.

Leaving the antiseptic prep pad on the skin with a corner pointing to the injection site helps identify the location for the injection. If the antiseptic has not evaporated, it may cause the skin to sting during injection.

8. Remove the needle cap.

9. With your nondominant hand, spread the skin taut between your thumb and index finger.

It is quicker, easier, and less painful to insert a needle through the skin that is taut.

10. Tell the patient what you are going to do and that he will feel a prick as you insert the needle. Then hold the syringe between thumb and fingers of your dominant hand like a pencil or dart and insert the needle at a 90° angle to the skin surface. Insert fully.

Quickly inserting the needle through the skin minimizes discomfort. A 90° angle is needed for the needle to penetrate through the subcutaneous and adipose tissue to the muscle.

11. Stabilize the syringe with your nondominant hand.

This prevents the needle from moving around in the tissue, thereby causing discomfort and possible tissue trauma.

12. Aspirate by pulling back on the plunger and waiting for 5 to 10 seconds. If you obtain a blood return, remove the needle, discard the syringe, and prepare the medication again. If there is no blood return, continue with step 12.

Aspirating blood indicates that the needle is in a blood vessel. Injecting would result in administering the medication intravenously instead of intramuscularly. If the needle is in a small vessel, it may take a few seconds for the blood to appear in the syringe. **KEY POINT:** *There are variations in practice regarding the requirement to aspirate for blood.*

Be sure to check with your instructor or the institution's protocol for the recommended method.

13. Using the thumb or index finger of your dominant hand, press the plunger slowly to inject the medication (5 to 10 sec/mL).

Slow administration allows the medication to disperse and decreases discomfort.

14. Remove the needle smoothly along the line of insertion.

Removing the needle in this way prevents pulling against the skin and tissue and minimizes discomfort.

15. Engage the safety needle device and dispose of the entire syringe in a biohazard container. If there is no safety device, place the uncapped syringe and needle directly into a biohazard puncture-proof container.

The biohazard sharps container prevents needlestick injuries.

16. Gently blot the site with a gauze pad, and apply an adhesive bandage as needed.

Apply pressure to stop the bleeding but do not massage or rub the site after IM injection. This can cause medication to disperse into the subcutaneous tissue where the needle was injected, which might be irritating to the tissue.

Procedure 25-14B ■ Intramuscular Injection: Z-Track Method

➤ When performing the procedure, always identify your patient according to agency policy, using two identifiers, and be attentive to standard precautions, hand hygiene, patient safety and privacy, body mechanics, and documentation.

Procedure Steps

1–8. Follow Procedure 25-14A, traditional method, preceding, except for this variation:

For Z-Track Method, use the larger muscles:

   a. *Ventrogluteal site:* Position patient on the side with upper hip and knee slightly flexed.

   b. *Vastus lateralis:* Position patient supine or sitting.

9. With the side of your nondominant hand, displace the skin away from the injection site, about 2.5 to 3.5 cm (1 to 1.5 in.).

This displaces the skin and subcutaneous tissue over the muscle, so that when it is released after the injection, the medication is sealed in the muscle. ▼

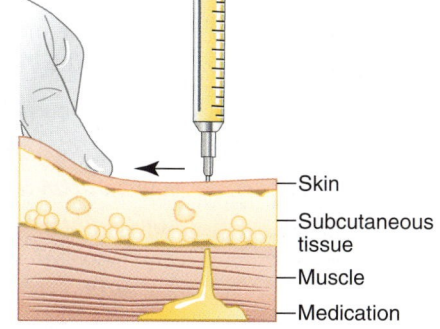

— Skin
— Subcutaneous tissue
— Muscle
— Medication

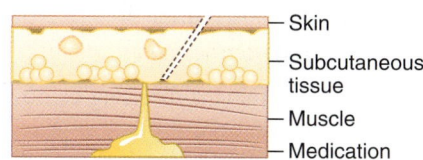

— Skin
— Subcutaneous tissue
— Muscle
— Medication

10. Holding the syringe between the thumb and fingers of your dominant hand like a pencil or dart, insert the needle at a 90° angle to the skin surface. Insert smoothly, quickly, and fully.

Quickly inserting the needle through the skin minimizes discomfort. A 90° angle is needed for the needle to penetrate through the subcutaneous and adipose tissue to the muscle.

(continued on next page)

Procedure 25-14 ■ Administering an Intramuscular Injection (continued)

11. **Stabilize the syringe** with the thumb and forefinger of your non-dominant hand while continuing to displace the skin with your other three fingers. Do not release the skin to stabilize the syringe.
Stabilizing the needle reduces discomfort and possible tissue injury. You must keep the skin retracted to create a seal after the medication is injected and the skin released.

12. **Aspirate by pulling back slightly** on the plunger for 5 to 10 seconds. If you obtain a blood return, remove the needle, discard the syringe, and prepare the medication again. You should follow your institution's policy regarding aspiration with parenteral injections.
Aspirating blood indicates that the needle has penetrated a vein. Continuing could result in administering the medication intravenously instead of intramuscularly. ▼

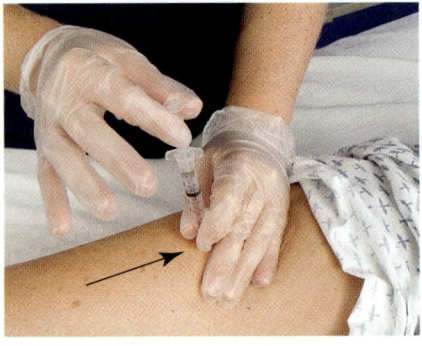

13. **Using the thumb or index finger** of your dominant hand, press the plunger slowly to inject the medication (5 to 10 sec/mL).
Slow administration allows the medication to disperse and decreases discomfort.

14. **Wait for 10 seconds,** then withdraw the needle smoothly along the line of insertion, then immediately release the skin.
Waiting before withdrawing the needle leaves a zigzag needle track that traps the medication in the muscle, preventing it from leaking up into the subcutaneous tissue.

15. **Engage the safety needle device,** and dispose of it in a biohazard container. If there is no safety device, place the uncapped syringe and needle directly in a biohazard puncture-proof container.

16. **Hold a cotton ball** or gauze pad with light pressure over the injection site. Do not massage the site. Apply an adhesive bandage if necessary.
Light pressure will stop superficial bleeding at the injection site. Massaging and rubbing can force medication into the subcutaneous tissues.

? What if . . .

■ **My patient is unable to cooperate during the procedure?**

Ask another healthcare provider or family member to help keep the patient from moving during the injection or to help position the patient.

■ **My patient is a child? Is there anything different about giving an IM injection to a child?**

Adapt the procedure to decrease pain: Apply topical anesthetic cream (e.g., EMLA) or a topical cooling spray if time permits. If not, distract the child with conversation, give him something to do, such as squeeze a hand, or apply a cold compress over the site.

Adapt the way you spread the skin to inject: In infants and small children, grasp the muscle with your thumb and index finger; in obese children, spread the skin and then grasp the muscle.

Adapt the medication volume: Inject no more than 1 mL in a single injection, 0.5 mL in a small infant.

The CDC recommends 1- and 1¼-inch needles for children 1-year-old or younger. Follow agency procedures.

■ **My patient is an older adult?**

Many older adults have decreased muscle mass, so use a shorter needle; spread the skin and grasp the muscle to localize and stabilize the site for injection.

Older adults tend to bleed from the site after injection because of reduced tissue elasticity. Apply a small pressure bandage if needed.

Evaluation

■ Observe for minimal bruising or oozing that may occur at the site of injection.
■ Observe for local reactions at site (e.g., pain, swelling, redness).

Home Care

■ Discuss safety concerns with administering medication intramuscularly in the home, such as correct disposal of biohazardous wastes and where to obtain a puncture-proof biohazard container.
The caregiver or patient can use a large plastic bottle. The local regulations must be followed for disposal.
■ Discuss with the client the need to rotate sites.
Repeatedly giving the medication in the same site can cause abnormalities in the tissue and alter absorption rates.

Documentation

■ Refer to **Medication Guidelines: Steps to Follow for All Medications (Regardless of Type or Route).**
■ Document related assessment findings, such as pain level or presence of nausea.
■ Unless the medication is prn you will typically document it only on the MAR.

Sample documentation for prn medication:

mm/dd/yyyy   1600   Client reports of nausea after ambulating 150 feet with assistive device. Phenergan 25 mg administered IM in right ventrogluteal site. No complaints of pain or discomfort. See MAR. —————————— M. Santos, RN.
Mm/dd/yyyy   1700   Client reports "I don't feel like I'm going to vomit anymore." ——————
—————————— M. Santos, RN.

Practice Resources

Advisory Committee on Immunization Practices (n.d.); Centers for Disease Control and Prevention (n.d.a); Bartley, N. (2012a); Ogston-Tuck, S. (2014a); Walden, A., & Vangilder, M. (2013); Walsh, L., & Brophy, K. (2011).

Thinking About the Procedure

 The videos **Intramuscular Injection: Traditional Method** and **Intramuscular Injection: Z-Track Method,** along with questions and suggested responses, are available on the **Davis's *Nursing Skills Videos*** Web site on Davis*Plus*.

Procedure 25-15 ■ Adding Medications to Intravenous Fluids

➤ For steps to follow in *all* procedures, refer to the Universal Steps for All Procedures found on the page facing the inside back cover. Also refer to **Medication Guidelines: Steps to Follow for All Medications (Regardless of Type or Route).**

Equipment

- Prescribed IV solution
- Syringe for measuring medication
- Needleless access device or safety needle (if a VAD is not available)
- Antimicrobial swab
- Label with medication, dose, date, time, and your initials

Delegation

As an RN, you would not usually delegate adding medications to IV fluids to LPN/LVNs. Nurse practice acts governing IV medication administration vary from state to state, and policies can further vary among healthcare agencies regarding which additives may be added by LPN/LVNs. Even if you delegate the skill, you are always responsible for evaluating the patient's responses, both therapeutic effects and adverse effects.

Pre-Procedure Assessments

- Assess the patency of the IV site.
- Assess the appearance of the IV site.
- Check the medication insert or *PDR* for appropriate time or rate for infusion and for compatibility.

➤ When performing the procedure, always identify your patient according to agency policy, using two identifiers, and be attentive to standard precautions, hand hygiene, patient safety and privacy, body mechanics, and documentation.

Procedure Steps

1. **Determine whether** the medication(s) are compatible with the IV solution and with each other.

 Not all medications or other additives can be mixed with the glucose or saline normally found in the primary IV bag. Multiple additives increase the possibility of incompatibility.

2. **Calculate or verify the amount** of medication to be instilled into the IV solution, and the rate of administration.

 Verifying the dose and the rate of infusion prevents medication errors.

3. **Remove any protective covers,** and inspect the bag or bottle for leaks, tears, or cracks. Inspect the fluid for clarity, color, and presence of any particulate matter. Check the expiration date.

 Double-checking the IV solution reduces the risk of infusing contaminated or expired solutions.

4. **Using the appropriate technique,** draw up the prescribed medication (see Procedures 25-9, as needed). Alternatively, insert a VAD transfer device into the medication vial.

 Medications can come in vials, ampules, or bags, within differences in techniques.

5. **Scrub all surfaces of the IV** additive port with an alcohol or CHG-alcohol combination product.

 Diligent scrubbing with antimicrobial products reduces the transmission of microorganisms and helps maintain sterility of the solution.

6. **Remove the cap from the syringe,** insert the needle or the needleless access device into the injection port, and inject the medication into the bag, maintaining aseptic technique. ▼

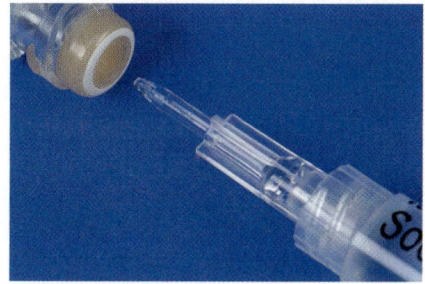

7. **Mix the IV solution and medication** by gently turning the bag from end to end.

 Ensures even distribution of the medication or additive into the solution.

(continued on next page)

Procedure 25-15 ■ Adding Medications to Intravenous Fluids (continued)

8. **Place a label on the bag** so that it can be read when the bag is hung; include the medication name, dose, route, and your name. Be sure the label does not cover the solution label or volume marks.

   A label informs you and others of additives to IV solutions. ➤

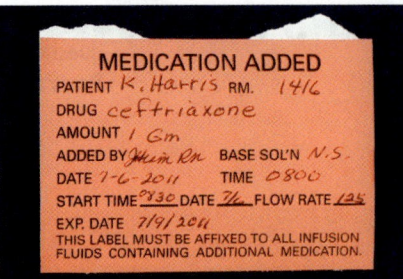

MEDICATION ADDED
PATIENT K. Harris RM. 1416
DRUG ceftriaxone
AMOUNT 1 Gm
ADDED BY Hum Rn BASE SOL'N N.S.
DATE 7-6-2011   TIME 0800
START TIME 0830 DATE 7/6 FLOW RATE 125
EXP. DATE 7/9/2011
THIS LABEL MUST BE AFFIXED TO ALL INFUSION
FLUIDS CONTAINING ADDITIONAL MEDICATION.

9. **Dispose of used equipment,** syringe, or VAD appropriately.

Evaluation

- Check the IV line at least once every hour to ensure that the ordered or calculated rate is maintained.
- Assess the patient for complaints of pain or signs of infiltration at the infusion site (e.g., redness, swelling).

Patient Teaching

- Discuss reasons the medication is being given intravenously.
- Explain whether it is a continuous or intermittent infusion.
- Explain the need to report immediately any reactions to the medication, such as breathing problems, rashes, or pain at the IV insertion site.

Documentation

- Document information according to **Medication Guidelines: Steps to Follow for All Medications (Regardless of Type or Route).**
- Document any findings on an IV flow record rather than in the nursing notes. Chart a nursing note only if there is something outside of the expected findings (e.g., if the IV has infiltrated).

Practice Resources

Infusion Nurses Society (2011a); Lavery, I. (2011).

Procedure 25-16 ■ Administering IV Push Medication

> ➤ For steps to follow in *all* procedures, refer to the Universal Steps for All Procedures found on the page facing the inside back cover.
> Also refer to **Medication Guidelines: Steps to Follow for All Medications (Regardless of Type or Route).**

Equipment

- Syringe appropriate for medication volume and the type of line (e.g., peripheral IV, PICC)
- If you are administering through an intermittent device:
  - Two 5- to 10-mL syringes, or one 10-mL syringe with 2 to 10 mL of normal saline or heparin for flushing the line. Heparin 100 units/mL rather than with saline solution is recommended (Bertolino, Pitassi, Tinelli, et al., 2012).

    Although either is acceptable, separate syringes pose less risk of contamination.

  - Depending on site and facility policy, one 5- to 10-mL syringe containing 2 to 5 mL of heparin flush (or saline) solution

    Evidence-based support and agency procedures differ: Some use saline to flush; others use heparin. New evidence recommends using heparin 100 units/mL (Bertolino, Pitassi, Tinelli, et al., 2012).

- Alcohol prep pad or CHG-alcohol combination product and gauze pad
- Procedure gloves

Pre-Procedure Assessments

- Check the compatibility of the medication with the existing IV solution, if it is infusing.

  Medications can be physically or chemically incompatible with the IV solution. Physical incompatibility is often obvious because precipitation may occur. Chemical incompatibility is not obvious and may result in the medication's having a weaker or a stronger effect than anticipated.

- Assess the patency of the IV line.

  If the line is occluded, you will not be able to instill the medication.

- Check the site for redness, swelling, tenderness, and other signs of infiltration or phlebitis.

  Some medications are irritating and may be toxic to the tissue. If the IV line is infiltrated, the medication may leak into the tissue and cause injury. IV medications can also irritate the veins and cause phlebitis. Do not infuse a medication into a compromised site.

Delegation

As an RN, you may, in some situations, be able to delegate administration of parenteral medications to an LPN/LVN. However, this is not a common practice.

Procedure 25-16A ■ **Administering IV Push Medications Through a Primary IV Line**

➤ When performing the procedure, always identify your patient according to agency policy, using two identifiers, and be attentive to standard precautions, hand hygiene, patient safety and privacy, body mechanics, and documentation.

Procedure Steps

1. **Determine how fast the medication** may be administered and whether the medication needs to be diluted for administration. Also check to be sure the medication is compatible with the solution infusing.

   IV push medications are frequently injected over 1 minute. Some must infuse over a longer time period, and some require diluting before administration. Giving an IV push medication too fast and/or undiluted can result in local or systemic adverse reactions.

2. **Prepare the medication** from a vial or ampule or obtain the prescribed unit dose and verify medication with the prescription (refer to Procedure 25-9). Dilute as needed. Temporarily pause the infusion pump to administer the medication. If the primary bag is infusing by gravity, simply clamp the tubing.

3. **Don procedure gloves** and thoroughly scrub all surfaces of the injection port closest to the patient with an alcohol prep pad or CHG-alcohol combination product.

   (1) Scrub time: Follow agency policy. Some facilities require nurses to cleanse the port for 1 minute when accessing venous access devices. (2) The port: Using the port closest to the patient minimizes the distance the medication must travel and gets it into the patient's circulation faster. You must use an injection port, which is self-sealing because if you puncture the plastic IV tubing, it will leak. (3) Scrub agent: Use povidone-iodine solution (Betadine) only if the patient is sensitive to alcohol or CHG-alcohol combination.

4. **Insert the medication syringe** into the injection port. If a needleless system is not available, use a syringe with a safety needle.

   Using a needleless system prevents needlestick injuries.

5. **Pinch or clamp the IV tubing** between the IV bag and the port.

   Occluding the tubing upline of the port prevents the medication from being injected back toward the IV bag. ▼

   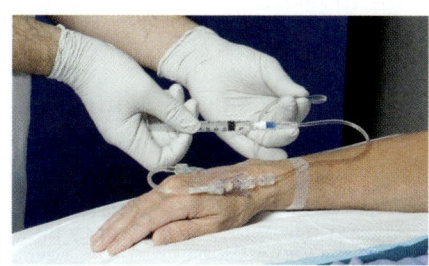

6. **Gently aspirate** by slowly pulling back on the plunger to check for a blood return.

   NOTE: Some newer connectors do not require or allow for aspiration. Follow institutional policy.

   (a) A blood return is one indication that the IV catheter is in the vein. An IV site may still be patent if no blood is returned, and an infiltrated IV line may have a blood return. Use the blood return as one indication of patency. (b) Injecting an IV medication into an IV site that is not patent administers the medication into the local tissue at the IV site. Some medications will cause tissue irritation and even necrosis if infused into the subcutaneous tissue. In addition, the patient would not receive the immediate therapeutic benefit from the drug.

7. **If you have aspirated and blood is returned,** administer a small increment of the medication while observing for reactions to the medication.

   Slow injection allows you to observe adverse reactions to the medication before all the medication has been injected. Administering IV push medications carries the highest potential risk to the patient because immediate, life-threatening reactions can occur.

8. **Administer another increment** of the medication (you may pinch the tubing while injecting medication and release it when not injecting; this is optional).

9. **Repeat steps 7 and 8 until** the full dose of medication has been administered over the prescribed amount of time.

   Medications require different administration times. Follow agency guidelines, provider prescriptions, and pharmaceutical information regarding whether the medication needs to be diluted and the rate of administration.

10. **If you clamped the IV tubing** during the infusion, open it now and reset the pump at the correct infusion rate, if necessary.

11. **Dispose of used supplies safely** and according to agency procedures.

(continued on next page)

Procedure 25–16 ■ Administering IV Push Medication (continued)

Procedure 25-16B ■ Administering IV Push Medications Through an Intermittent Device (IV Lock) When No Extension Tubing Is Attached to the Venous Access Device

➤ When performing the procedure, always identify your patient according to agency policy, using two identifiers, and be attentive to standard precautions, hand hygiene, patient safety and privacy, body mechanics, and documentation.

Procedure Steps

1. **Determine how fast the medication** may be administered and whether it needs to be diluted for administration.

   IV push medications are frequently injected over 1 minute. Some medications must be administered over a longer time period, and some medications must be diluted before administration. Giving an IV push medication too fast and/or undiluted can result in an adverse local or systemic reaction.

2. **Prepare the medication** from a vial or ampule. Dilute as needed. Refer to Procedure 25-9.

3. **Select the appropriate size** of syringe for flush solution.

   Smaller syringes exert more pressure against the wall of the IV catheter than do larger syringes. Check with the IV catheter manufacturer for specific recommendations, and follow agency policy.

4. **Don procedure gloves.**

5. **Thoroughly scrub all surfaces** of the injection port closest to the patient with an alcohol prep pad or CHG-alcohol combination product.

   Follow agency policy. Some facilities require nurses to scrub all surfaces of the port with an alcohol-based antimicrobial product for 1 minute when accessing venous access devices. Using the port closest to the patient minimizes the amount of medication in the IV line. Scrub: Use povidone-iodine solution (Betadine) only when the patient cannot tolerate an alcohol-based disinfectant.

6. **Insert the flush syringe** into the injection port and gently aspirate by pulling back on the plunger to check for a blood return.

NOTE: Some newer connectors do not require or allow for aspiration. Follow institutional policy.

A blood return is an indication that the IV catheter is in the vein. An IV site may still be patent if no blood is returned; conversely, an infiltrated IV may have a blood return. Use the blood return as only one indication of patency.

7. **Administer a flush solution** (usually 1 to 3 mL) to clear the line if you aspirated and blood was returned. Use a forward pushing motion on the syringe, with a slow, steady injection technique. If blood is not returned, see the "What if . . ." section at the end of Procedure 25-16.

   (a) Flush syringes may be prefilled; in some cases, the amount to inject may be a part of agency policy. (b) Rapid flushing causes a jet effect that can cause the catheter tip to migrate to other venous locations; this should be avoided. (c) Injecting an IV medication into an IV site that is not patent administers the medication into the local tissue at the IV site. Some medications will cause tissue irritation and even necrosis if infused into the subcutaneous tissue.

8. **Continue to hold the injection** port, remove the flush syringe, and again scrub the port with the alcohol prep pad or CHG-alcohol combination product.

   Cleansing the port reduces the risk of introducing microorganisms into the bloodstream. Scrub: Use povidone-iodine only when the patient is sensitive to alcohol-based disinfectants.

9. **Attach the medication** syringe and inject the medication in small

increments over the correct time interval. Use a slow, steady injection technique until the correct dose is instilled over the prescribed amount of time.

For example, if 1 mL of the medication is to be given over 1 minute, inject approximately 0.25 mL every 15 seconds. ▼

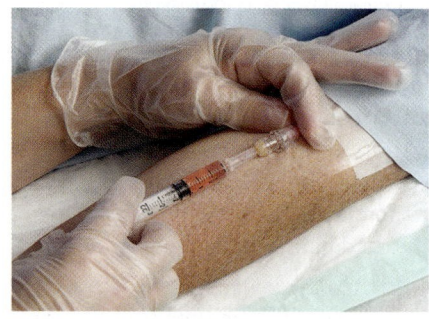

10. **Continuing to hold the injection** port, remove the medication syringe, and vigorously scrub all surfaces of the port with alcohol prep pad or CHG-alcohol–based product for at least 15 seconds. Attach the flush syringe.

    Vigorous scrubbing reduces the chance of contamination of the port.

11. **Administer the flush solution** usually 1 to 3 mL, or according to prescription or agency policy.

    Flushing ensures that all the medication has been administered and prevents occlusion of the IV catheter.

12. **Use a slow, steady injection** pressure technique when removing the syringe by placing your thumb or index finger to avoid movement of the plunger. (Follow equipment guidelines; you may not always need to do this.) Continue to administer

the flush solution while withdrawing the syringe cannula from the injection port.

This positive-pressure technique prevents blood backflow into the IV catheter, which might cause an occlusion. Follow equipment guidelines because some injection ports maintain positive pressure by removing the syringe and then closing the clamp. ➤

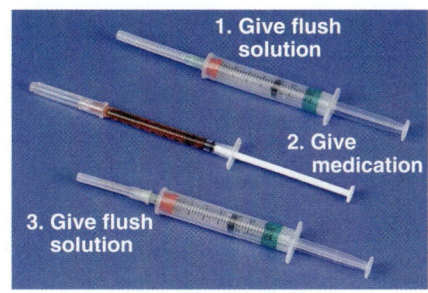

1. Give flush solution
2. Give medication
3. Give flush solution

13. Discard the flushing syringe from the needleless connector into a safety disposal container.

Procedure 25-16C ■ Administering IV Push Medications Through an Intermittent Device With IV Extension Tubing

➤ When performing the procedure, always identify your patient according to agency policy, using two identifiers, and be attentive to standard precautions, hand hygiene, patient safety and privacy, body mechanics, and documentation.

Procedure Steps

1. Determine how fast the medication may be administered and whether the medication needs to be diluted for administration.

IV push medications are frequently injected over 1 minute. Some must be administered over a longer time period, and some require diluting prior to administration. Giving an IV push medication too fast and/or undiluted can result in a local or systemic adverse reaction.

2. Prepare the medication from a vial or ampule. Dilute as needed. Refer to Procedure 25-9.

3. Determine the volume of any extension tubing attached to the access port.

The volume of extension sets can be greater than the IV push medication being given. If not accounted for, all the medication may be injected into the patient's bloodstream at once when the second flush solution is given.

4. Don procedure gloves.

5. Scrub all surfaces of the injection port with an antiseptic wipe.

6. Insert the flush syringe into the injection port. If a needleless system is not available, use a syringe with a safety needle. Depending on the equipment, you may then need to aspirate for a blood return as one sign

of vein patency. Some equipment does not require or allow for aspiration.

(a) In tubing that allows for or requires aspiration, a blood return is one sign that the IV catheter is in the vein. However, an IV site may still be patent even if no blood is returned. (b) Using a needleless system prevents needlestick injuries.

7. Administer the flush (commonly 1 to 3 mL): If blood appears in the tubing, during aspiration administer the rest of the flush. If blood is not returned, assess patency by administering a small amount of the flush solution and monitoring for ease of administration, swelling at the IV site, or patient complaint of discomfort at the site.

8. Again scrub the port. Attach the medication syringe and inject a volume of medication equal to the volume of the extension set at the same rate as the flush solution.

- When using a 5-mL syringe for peripheral lines and a 10-mL syringe for central lines, administer the flush solution briskly.
- When you use a smaller syringe, use a slower rate to prevent excess pressure damaging the vein or shearing of the IV cannula.

The medication clears the line of saline solution and fills it with medication; it also flushes the IV catheter with

saline as the medication pushes the saline through the catheter. ▼

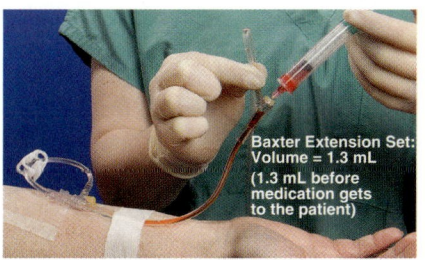

Baxter Extension Set: Volume = 1.3 mL (1.3 mL before medication gets to the patient)

9. Using a slow, steady injection technique, administer the remainder of the medication over the prescribed time interval for the specific medication.

Rapid flushing can create a jet effect that can cause the catheter tip to migrate to an unintended venous location.

10. Continuing to hold the injection port connector, remove the medication syringe, vigorously scrub all surfaces of the connector for at least 15 seconds, and then attach the flush syringe. **KEY POINT:** *The only time you should open the catheter hub is when the needleless connector or primary continuous IV set must be changed, usually at 96-hour intervals or as otherwise prescribed.*

11. Administer the same amount of flush solution at the same rate as the medication, using a slow, steady injection technique. For example, if the extension tubing has a

(continued on next page)

Procedure 25–16 ■ **Administering IV Push Medication** (continued)

volume of 1.3 mL, give the first 1.3 mL of the flush solution at the same rate as the medication. Then administer the remainder of the flush solution.

(a) At this step, the extension tubing contains all the medication. Administering the flush solution all at once pushes the medication too fast (it will enter the vein all at once). (b) Once you have incrementally cleared the medication from the extension tubing and all the medication is already in the vein, then the rate no longer matters as far as the medication is concerned.

12. **Use a slow, steady injection** pressure technique when removing the syringe. Continue to administer the flush solution while withdrawing the syringe cannula from the injection port. Follow equipment instructions regarding the method and order of removing the syringe, closing the clamp, and maintaining positive pressure.

13. **Discard the flushing syringe** from the needleless connector into a safety disposal container.

? What if . . .

■ **No blood is returned when I aspirate?**

Do not give IV push medication until you can verify the patency of the IV site. If the patency of the IV site is questionable, restart the IV at another site.

Further assess the patency of the IV line by administering a small amount of the saline flush and monitoring for ease of administration, swelling at the IV site, or patient complaint of discomfort at the site.

Another technique to determine patency is to lower the IV bag below the level of the IV site—a blood return should occur.

If the IV catheter is a small gauge, a blood return may not always be aspirated.

■ **There is resistance when flushing the line?**

Never force the flush solution into the VAD; look for a closed clamp on the catheter or tubing. Or you may check to see whether an inline filter is clogged. Do not proceed with the medication infusion until you are sure the catheter is still correctly positioned and that the fluid pathway is unobstructed.

■ **The IV infusing a dextrose solution infiltrates into the surrounding tissue of a peripheral catheter?**

Immediately stop the running fluid and remove the catheter. Initially apply a cool, moist compress to the site and later use heat to promote comfort. *Infiltration can cause tissue injury, inflammation, and edema and may even lead to tissue necrosis and sloughing.*

Some medications, such as vasopressors (e.g., dopamine), might need intradermal injection of an antidote, such as phentolamine (Regitine), to reverse the effects of extravasation. *If the IV fluid contains dextrose at greater than 10% concentration, calcium salts, potassium salts, sodium bicarbonate, blood, and parenteral nutrition, contact the primary care provider, who will likely prescribe injection of hyaluronidase (Amphadase) into the surrounding tissue.*

Evaluation

■ Assess the patient for complaints of pain or discomfort at the site.

Patient Teaching

■ Discuss why the medication is being administered intravenously.
■ Explain the need to report immediately any reaction to the medication.

Home Care

■ Discuss with the client and/or caregiver how to care for the IV site, including flushing. Many IV push medications need to be administered by a nurse. However, cost-cutting efforts have led to short hospital stays, and some clients are now being taught to administer their own IV antibiotics at home.
■ Explain how to identify problems with the IV site, such as infiltration and phlebitis.
■ Determine whether the client has adequate facilities for storing the medication, such as refrigeration if needed.
■ Discuss safety issues, such as keeping medications and needles and syringes secure and away from children and pets.

Documentation

In addition to charting according to **Medication Guidelines: Steps to Follow for All Medications (Regardless of Type or Route)**, document related patient assessment findings, such as the appearance of the IV site and patient complaints of pain or discomfort during IV administration. You will usually document on an IV flow record and/or MAR rather than in the nursing notes. Chart a nursing note only if there is a problem (e.g., if the patient experiences pain when you administer the medication).

Practice Resources

Centers for Disease Control and Prevention (2011a); Infusion Nurses Society (2011a, 2011b); Phillips, L. (2015).

Thinking About the Procedure

 The videos **Administering IV Push Medications Through a Primary IV Line, Administering IV Push Medications Through an Intermittent Device (IV Lock) When No Extension Tubing Is Attached to the Venous Access Device,** and **Administering IV Push Medications Through an Intermittent Device With IV Extension Tubing,** along with questions and suggested responses, are available on the **Davis's *Nursing Skills Videos*** Web site on Davis*Plus*.

Procedure 25-17 ■ Administering Medication by Intermittent Infusion

➤ For steps to follow in *all* procedures, refer to the Universal Steps for All Procedures found on the page facing the inside back cover. Also refer to **Medication Guidelines: Steps to Follow for All Medications (Regardless of Type or Route).** For step-by-step instructions in using volume-control devices (pumps), see Procedure 39-3, Setting Up and Using Volume Control Pumps.

Equipment

- Correct size syringe for measuring medication
- Needleless access cannula or safety needle
- Volume-control IV set (e.g., Buretrol, Volutrol, Soluset) or small bag of diluted medication with piggyback tubing
- Primary IV solution and tubing (unless one is already infusing)
- Antimicrobial swabs
- Labels for the IV tubing and medication administration system

Delegation

Nurse practice acts governing IV medication administration vary from state to state, and policies can further vary among healthcare agencies regarding which medications or methods of administration the LPN/LVN may perform. You cannot delegate this procedure to a NAP.

Pre-Procedure Assessments

- ✚ Check the compatibility of the medication with the IV solution.
  Medications can be physically or chemically incompatible with the IV solution. Physical incompatibility will be obvious if precipitation occurs. Chemical incompatibility is not obvious and may result in the medication having a weaker or a stronger effect than anticipated.

- Assess the patency of the IV line.
  If the line is occluded or if the fluid has infiltrated the medication will not infuse.

- ✚ Check the site for redness, swelling, tenderness, and other signs of infiltration or phlebitis.
  Some medications are irritating to the tissue. If the IV fluid has infiltrated, medication would leak into the tissue and cause injury. IV medications can also irritate the veins and cause phlebitis. Do not infuse a medication into a compromised site.

- **Determine the amount of IV solution needed to administer the specific medication.**
  Most medications specify (on the order or on the label) specific dilution to prevent potential harm to the patient.

- **Determine the time period over which the solution needs to be infused.**
  Infusing a medication too slowly may result in an inadequate blood level to achieve therapeutic levels, and infusing a medication too rapidly can cause harm.

- **Perform assessments that will provide a basis for evaluating the drug's effectiveness,** such as checking blood pressure after administering an antihypertensive agent.

Procedure 25-17A ■ Using a Piggyback Administration Set With a Gravity Infusion

➤ When performing the procedure, always identify your patient according to agency policy, using two identifiers, and be attentive to standard precautions, hand hygiene, patient safety and privacy, body mechanics, and documentation.

Procedure Steps

1. **Obtain the medication.** IV medications usually are premixed in small bags by the pharmacy. Rarely, you may need to draw up the medication and inject it into the piggyback solution (see Procedure 25-15). Date and label the medication bag label. Verify that it has the patient's name, amount of medication, date, and time given.

2. **Obtain and attach** the piggyback tubing to the medication bag. Do not touch the spike.
   Tubing connects the piggyback to the primary line. The piggyback tubing is

short. *Prevents contamination of tubing and solution.*

3. **Be sure the slide clamp is closed.** Squeeze the drip chamber, filling it one-third to one-half full.
   Clamping prevents excess air coming into the line when you are priming the tubing.

4. **Open the clamp and prime** the tubing, holding the end of the tubing lower than the bag of fluid. Do not let more than one drop of fluid escape from the end of the tubing. Close the clamp.

Alternative: "Backflushing" the Piggyback Line

a. Clamp the piggyback tubing.
b. Scrub all surfaces of the primary "Y" port, and attach the piggyback setup with the needleless connector.
c. Open the clamp on the piggyback tubing, and lower the bag below the primary bag to prime the piggyback line.
d. Once all the air is expelled from the piggyback tubing, clamp the tubing and finish the procedure.
Priming removes air from the tubing and maintains sterility of the system.

(continued on next page)

Procedure 25-17 ■ **Administering Medication by Intermittent Infusion** (continued)

Medications are diluted in small amounts of fluid (usually 50 to 100 mL), so you cannot waste any medication. The backflush method ensures you will not do so.

5. **Label the piggyback tubing** with the time, the date, and your initials.
   Tubing used for intermittent infusions can be used for 48 to 72 hours, depending on facility policy; labeling allows the nurse to know when it must be changed.

6. **Hang the piggyback container** on the IV pole. Lower the primary IV container to hang below the level of the medication bag.
   Gravity causes the higher bag (the piggyback IV setup) to flow instead of the primary IV setup. When the piggyback IV solution has infused, the primary IV line will resume infusing.

7. **Open the clamp** of the piggyback line, and regulate the drip rate with the roller clamp on the primary line.

Regulate to the prescribed infusion rate for the medication. ▼

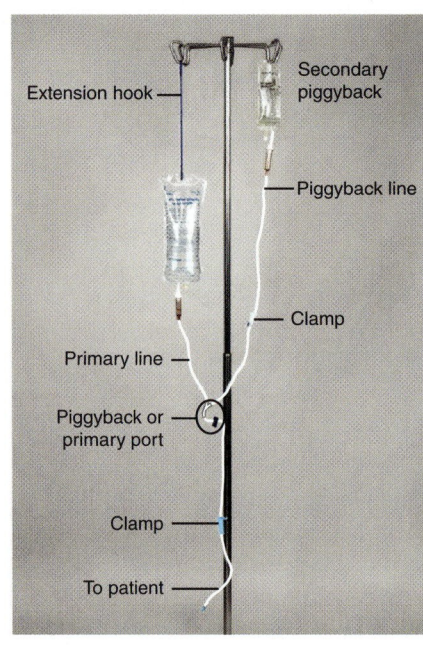

Because the piggyback is the only bag running, the primary roller clamp regulates the speed of the piggyback bag.

8. **When the medication is all infused,** clamp the piggyback tubing and move the primary bag back to its original height. Use the roller clamp to reset the primary bag to its correct infusion rate.
   This ensures that the primary fluids infuse at their ordered rate rather than flowing at the rate the piggyback medication was flowing—which would probably be either faster or slower than the prescribed primary fluid rate.

Procedure 25-17B ■ **Using a Piggyback Administration Set With an Infusion Pump**

➤ For step-by-step instructions in using intermittent infusion devices (pumps), also see Procedure 39-3.

➤ *Note:* This procedure describes the use of a one-piston infusion pump. The steps for using a two-piston pump vary slightly.

➤ When performing the procedure, always identify your patient according to agency policy, using two identifiers, and be attentive to standard precautions, hand hygiene, patient safety and privacy, body mechanics, and documentation.

Procedure Steps

1. **Obtain the medication.** IV medications usually are premixed in small bags and labeled by the pharmacy. If this is not the case, inject the medication into the prescribed piggyback solution (see Procedure 25-15). Date and initial the medication bag label. Verify that it has the patient's name, amount of medication, date, and time given.

2. **Be sure you have the correct secondary infusion tubing.** Hang the piggyback container on the IV pole. Attach the piggyback tubing to the medication bag. Do not touch the spike.
   Piggyback tubing is short; tandem tubing is much longer. Secondary tubing connects

the piggyback to the primary line. Touching the spike would contaminate the tubing and solution.

3. **Be sure the slide clamp** is closed. Squeeze the drip chamber, filling it one-third to one-half full.
   Clamping prevents excess air coming into the line when you are priming the tubing.

4. **Open the clamp and prime** the tubing, holding the end of the tubing lower than the bag of fluid. Do not let more than one drop of fluid escape from the end of the tubing. Close the clamp.

Alternative: "Backflushing" the Piggyback Line

a. With the drip chamber one-third filled, air will be in the secondary tubing.
b. Pause the infusion pump.
c. Scrub all surfaces of the "Y" port on the primary line and attach the piggyback setup with a needleless connector.
d. Open the clamp on the piggyback tubing and lower the bag below the primary bag to prime the piggyback line. The fluid from the primary line will flow up through the secondary tubing until all air is removed from the tubing. Restart the pump.

e. Once the line is primed, clamp the tubing and finish the procedure.

Priming removes air from the tubing and maintains sterility of the system. Medications are diluted in small amounts of fluid (usually 50 to 100 mL), so you cannot waste any medication. The backflush method ensures you will not do so.

5. **Label the piggyback tubing** with the time, the date, and your initials.

Tubing used for intermittent infusions can be used for 48 to 72 hours, depending on facility policy; labeling allows the nurse to know when it must be changed.

6. **Hang the piggyback container** on the IV pole. Lower the primary IV container to hang below the level of the piggyback medication bag.

The tubing system works such that the higher bag (the piggyback IV setup) flows instead of the primary IV setup.

7. **Program the pump** by selecting the secondary infusion button.

This converts the fluid infusing from the primary line to the secondary line.

8. **Program the rate and total volume** to be infused. (Some pumps allow you to select the medication and dose.)

Ensures accurate infusion amount and restart of primary fluids.

9. **Scrub the port** of the primary line.

Minimizes the introduction of microorganisms.

10. **Remove the cover from** the secondary tubing and connect it to the connection port of the primary line. (This was done at step 4 if the blackflush priming method was used.)

11. **Open the clamp** on the secondary tubing.

12. **Press "start"** on infusion pump.

13. **Check drip chambers** to ensure that the secondary solution is infusing and the primary solution is not.

This ensures that medication is infusing and patient does not receive an overload of fluids.

14. **Check the pump information** again to ensure the correct rate and volume.

15. **At the end of the infusion,** the primary IV line will resume infusing. Once the secondary infusion is complete, the pump programming will re-set to the previously programmed primary rate.

This ensures that the primary fluids infuse at their ordered rate rather than flowing at the rate the piggyback medication was flowing—which would probably be either faster or slower than the prescribed primary fluid rate.

Procedure 25-17C ■ Using a Volume-Control Administration Set

➤ For step-by-step instructions in using volume-control devices (pumps), see Procedure 39-3. If you have not already done so, affix a label to the secondary bag indicating the name and amount of medication, date and time given, and your name or initials.

➤ When performing the procedure, always identify your patient according to agency policy, using two identifiers, and be attentive to standard precautions, hand hygiene, patient safety and privacy, body mechanics, and documentation.

Procedure Steps

1. **Prepare the volume-control set.**
   a. Close both the upper and lower clamps on the tubing, if they are not already closed.

   Clamping prevents air bubbles from forming in the tubing.

   b. Open the clamp of the air vent on the volume-control chamber.

   Venting allows air to escape, which lets the IV solution enter the chamber.

   c. Maintaining sterile procedure, attach administration spike of the volume-control set to the primary IV bag.

   d. Fill the volume-control chamber with the desired amount of IV solution by opening the clamp between the bag and the volume-control chamber. When the correct amount of solution is in the chamber, close the clamp.

   The drip chamber provides solution for priming the tubing and diluting the IV medication.

   e. Prime the rest of the tubing by opening the clamp below the chamber and running the IV fluid until all the air has been expelled.

   Priming clears the IV tubing of air.

   f. Recheck the amount of fluid in the volume-control chamber, and add more fluid to the desired amount, if needed.

   Priming the tubing alters the volume in the chamber. You must fill to the desired amount.

2. **With an alcohol or CHG-alcohol swab,** vigorously scrub all surfaces of the injection port closest to the patient.

   Vigorous cleansing is necessary to remove microorganisms and particles from the IV port, which could potentially enter the patient's bloodstream.

(continued on next page)

Procedure 25-17 ■ **Administering Medication by Intermittent Infusion** (continued)

3. **Connect the end of the volume-control IV line** to the patient's IV site (e.g., directly to the IV catheter, to the extension tubing, or to the injection port closest to patient).

4. **Vigorously scrub the injection port** on the volume-control chamber, attach the medication syringe (preferably with a blunt, needleless device), and inject the medication into the solution in the chamber.

5. **Gently rotate the chamber** to mix the medication in the IV solution. *Distributes the medication within the IV solution.*

6. **Open the lower clamp** and start the infusion at the correct flow rate. *Unclamping allows the infusion of the medication. A correct flow rate infuses the* medication over the correct amount of time and prevents a toxic reaction to it.

7. **Label the volume-control chamber** with the date, time, medication and doses added, and your initials, according to agency policy.

8. **When the medication has finished infusing,** add a small amount of the primary IV fluid to the chamber and flush the tubing. For the flush volume, use two times the volume in the dead space of the tubing; check the tubing package for the amount. *Flushing the line ensures all the medication is given to the patient and does not adhere to the tubing.*

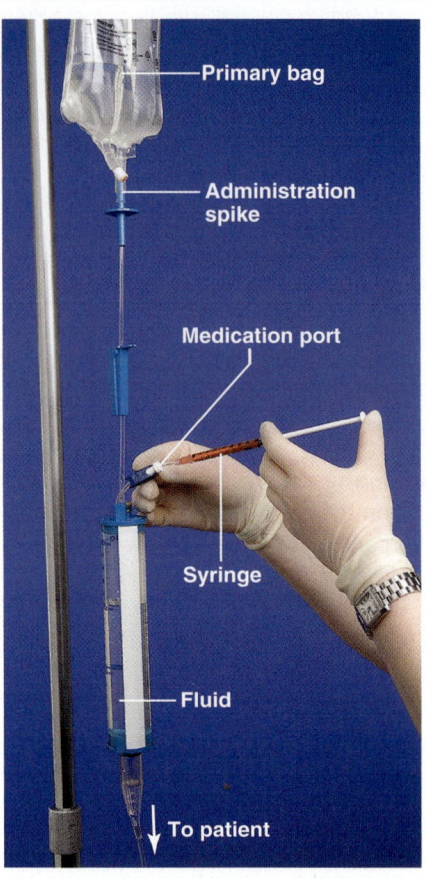

Primary bag

Administration spike

Medication port

Syringe

Fluid

↓ To patient

Evaluation

■ Assess for pain or discomfort at the site.
■ Intermittent infusions via a pump are generally infused over 30 to 60 minutes; therefore, you need to assess the patient as soon as the medication begins infusing and every 15 to 20 minutes until it is absorbed.

Patient Teaching

■ Discuss why the medication is being administered intravenously.
■ Explain the need to report immediately any reaction to the medication.
■ Ask the patient to activate the call device if the infusion pump starts to alarm. Explain common reasons for the alarm to minimize anxiety.

Home Care

■ Discuss with the client and/or caregiver how to care for the IV site. Only a nurse should add medications to the IV.
■ Explain how to identify problems with the IV site, such as infiltration and phlebitis.
■ Assess whether the client has adequate facilities for storing the medication, such as refrigeration if needed.

■ Discuss safety issues, such as keeping medications, needles, and syringes secure and away from children and pets.

Documentation

■ Chart information according to **Medication Guidelines: Steps to Follow for All Medications (Regardless of Type or Route).**
■ Document related patient assessment findings, such as the appearance of the IV site and patient complaints of pain or discomfort during the administration.

Thinking About the Procedure

The videos **Using a Volume-Control Administration Set, Using a Piggyback Administration Set With a Gravity Infusion,** and **Using a Piggyback Administration Set With an Infusion Pump,** along with questions and suggested responses, are available on the **Davis's** *Nursing Skills Videos* Web site on DavisPlus.

Practice Resources
Infusion Nurses Society (2011a, 2011b); Hamilton, S. (2014).

Procedure 25-18 ■ Administering Medication Through a Central Venous Access Device (CVAD)

➤ For steps to follow in *all* procedures, refer to the Universal Steps for All Procedures found on the page facing the inside back cover. Also refer to **Medication Guidelines: Steps to Follow for All Medications (Regardless of Type or Route).**

Equipment

See Figures 25-32A (Implantable device) and 25-32B (Multilumen catheter with blunt cannula, split septum, needleless access device).

- Syringe appropriate for medication volume (10 mL or larger)

  ✚ *Use of syringes smaller than 10 mL when flushing a CVAD can cause increase pressure and may rupture the CVAD.*

- Needleless device or safety syringe with a filter needle for drawing up the medication (you would also need a sterile needle for injection)
- Two syringes for the flush solution
- Saline or heparin flush solution, as prescribed. New evidence supports flushing peripheral venous catheters with heparin 100 units/mL rather than with saline solution (Bertolino, Pitassi, Tinelli, et al., 2012).
- Prep pad: CHG-alcohol combination product or appropriate antiseptic solution and gauze pad
- One pair nonsterile procedure gloves

Pre-Procedure Assessment

- Carefully palpate the area around the insertion site through the dressing. If the patient has tenderness, assess further for other signs of infection. Check the surrounding catheter insertion site for intact sutures, redness, swelling, warmth, or drainage.
  This can indicate catheter-related infection.

- Assess the patient's external chest wall for engorged veins at the surface of the skin. If the jugular's site is used, also assess for difficulty moving the neck or jaw, headache, or ear pain.
  This can indicate vein thrombosis.

- PICC line sites should be observed daily for swelling, tenderness, drainage, or streaking. Take site measurements at regular intervals during dressing changes and compare to pre-insertion arm circumference.
  May indicate problems with phlebitis and/or catheter sepsis.

- Conduct a comprehensive pain assessment, looking for unusual pain or discomfort.
  Pain can be associated with the catheter's position in the vein, especially if the line is not in an optimal position.

➤ When performing the procedure, always identify your patient according to agency policy, using two identifiers, and be attentive to standard precautions, hand hygiene, patient safety and privacy, body mechanics, and documentation.

Procedure Steps

1. **Prepare the medication.**
   a. Check compatibility of the medication with the existing IV infusion.
   b. ✚ Verify the medication that can safely be administered through a central site. Double-check the infusion rate as well.

   Some medication might be incompatible with infusion solution or additives. Because dosage may be different for medications given centrally versus peripherally, and because the medication enters the heart almost instantly, any error is potentially life threatening.

   c. Draw up the medication using a needleless device or needle with a filter. Then change to a sterile safety needle or needleless device for administering the medication.
   Filter needles prevent small particles from entering into the line.

   d. Recap any needles throughout, using a needle-capping device or approved one-handed technique that has a low risk of contaminating the sterile needle (see Procedure 25-10B: Recapping Sterile Needles).
   Recapping prevents needlestick injury and, performed correctly, maintains the sterility of the needle.

   e. Dilute the medication, if needed. Fill the medication syringe to the exact volume to be infused; expel excess volume.

   f. Label the syringe with the contents, including medication name, dilution, time to be administered, route, and name of person constituting the medication.
   Excess volume of medication in the syringe is a risk for inadvertent overdosing.

2. **Flush the line.**
   a. Obtain heparinized or saline solution for flushing the CVAD,

   following the institution's protocol or the prescription.
   The usual concentration for heparin is 10 to 100 units/mL of solution for adults. The recommended volume of flush varies by institution. Most facilities recommend 3 to 5 mL of solution to flush the catheter, although some are flushed with 10 mL to flush the line. Some medication might be incompatible with infusion solution or additives.

   ✚ *Dosage for centrally administered drugs is critical because the medication enters the heart almost instantly, so any error is potentially life threatening*

   ✚ *Using heparin flush in venous access devices is becoming more controversial because of the potential for heparin-induced thrombocytopenia. Be sure to follow the manufacturer's guidelines, prescriber's prescription and the policy of your institution.*

(continued on next page)

Procedure 25-18 ■ **Administering Medication Through a Central Venous Access Device (CVAD)** (continued)

b. Before flushing the CVAD, examine the syringe for bubbles. Remove them by flicking the syringe. Eject the air and bubbles, but be sure you have enough flush solution remaining in the syringe.

Flicking causes the bubbles to rise to the top. Remove bubbles from the syringe before giving medication through the CVAD port to avoid injecting air into the patient's vein and causing an embolus.

c. With clean procedure gloves, using pressure and friction, vigorously scrub all surfaces of the CVAD connectors as well as the luer-locking threads, and the luer-lock, including the extension "tail," with an alcohol wipe, CHG-alcohol combination product, or other antimicrobial product for at least 15 seconds. Then let it dry for 15 seconds. Do not touch this connector after cleansing.

Antimicrobial swabs reduce the risk of line-related infection by decreasing colonization of the port and tubing.

d. Insert the flush syringe at a vertical (90°) angle into the port using a needleless system or safety syringe.

A 90° angle reduces stress on the access port, which may cause shearing or mechanical trauma to the material.

e. Open the clamp between the syringe and the patient.

The clamp between the access port and the tubing that goes to the patient must be patent for medication to be injected through the CVAD.

f. Check for blood return, if necessary. Equipment differs regarding the need to aspirate, so follow agency protocols.

In some administration systems, aspiration is one indication that catheter placement is in the vein.

g. Inject saline or heparinized flush solution into the line, per agency protocol or provider's prescriptions and type of catheter. Some

catheter types (e.g., Groshong) do not require heparin in the flush solution. Close the clamp.

Saline or heparin flush is used, depending on the type of CVAD, institutional protocol, and manufacturer recommendations.

■ Saline is generally indicated when simple clearing of the line is needed.
■ If blood is likely to backflow into the line, then heparin might be used in the flush solution in order to reduce the risk of clot formation.
■ Most often heparin is used for implanted CVADs to reduce the risk of occlusion from a clot forming on the device.
■ Different catheters require different volume of flush solutions. Some are more prone to clot formation, depending on whether they are open or closed system devices. The initial flush maintains patency of the line and removes any heparin that was left if the catheter was used previously.

h. ➕ Never force the flush solution into the venous access device if you feel resistance. Look for a closed clamp on the catheter or tubing. Check to see whether an inline filter is clogged.

Forcing fluid creates a risk of rupturing the catheter.

i. Disconnect the flush syringe. **CAUTION:** Techniques of flushing and clamping may vary depending on the type of connector you are using. Consult agency protocols and manufacturer's instructions.

If using a needleless connector, do one of the following:

If Using Negative Fluid Displacement Device

Use a positive-pressure technique:
■ For a blunt cannula with split septum, or mechanical valve, withdraw the cannula before the syringe is completely empty, keeping your thumb on the syringe plunger.
■ For a mechanical valve device with negative displacement, maintain pressure

on the syringe plunger, close the clamp on the IV line between the needleless connector and the patient, and then disconnect the syringe.

If Using a Positive Fluid Displacement Device

Do not use a positive-pressure technique. Flush using a push-pause technique. Wait 10 seconds (or per manufacture guidelines) to allow fluid displacement to occur. Remove syringe, and only then may you clamp the catheter.

The positive-pressure technique would keep the internal mechanism from functioning properly.

For Neutral Fluid Displacement Devices

Any flushing technique can be used. The clamping and disconnecting sequence does not matter.

The clamping sequence is directly dependent upon the needleless connector being used and is critical for the final locking solution.

j. After removing the flush syringe from the port, discard it into a safety disposal container.

3. **Administer medication** through the CVAD.

a. Scrub all surfaces of the external ports, tubing, and connectors with a CHG-alcohol combination product for at least 15 seconds. Allow the port to dry for 15 more seconds or follow manufacturer's guidelines.

Antimicrobial swabs reduce the risk of line-related infection by decreasing colonization of the port and tubing.

b. Close the clamp to the infusion if a primary IV is running.

The medication could travel back up the line rather than infuse into the patient if the clamp is open.

c. Inject medication into the port, according to the medication order (infusion time).

Some medication is infused as a bolus; other medication is given over a period of time.

4. **After scrubbing all surfaces** of the port again with a CHG-alcohol product or other approved antiseptic, administer the second syringe of flush solution.

   The flush prevents incompatible medication or fluid from mixing at later administrations and ensures that all of the medication clears the catheter and enters the bloodstream.

5. **Clamp the tubing** between the syringe and the CVAD port. If there is an infusing primary IV, make sure the tubing is open between the IV fluid and the patient.

? What if . . .

- **My patient is a child? How should I secure the line?**

  Dress infants and younger children in a one-piece undershirt that fastens between the legs and tape the line to the shirt, leaving a little bit of slack to allow for movement.

- **The line does not flush easily?**

  - Make sure all clamps are unclamped.
  - Check to see whether the central line is kinked or twisted.
  - After straightening lines, attempt to flush the central line again. If the flush solution cannot be injected easily from the syringe into the CVAD, do not force the flush.

    Too much flush pressure may dislodge a clot that has formed in the central line.

  - Check to see whether an inline filter is clogged.
  - Assess the insertion site to see whether the stabilization device or dressing may be causing the occlusion.
  - Try to reposition the patient to lying down and turn to one side.
  - You might also have the patient lift his arms above his head and then attempt to flush the central line.
  - If it is still difficult to flush after repositioning, notify the provider.

- **The central line inadvertently comes out?**

  Hold firm, constant pressure on the site to control bleeding. Have a colleague notify the provider immediately.

- **The central line is cracked or leaking?**

  Close the clamp between the break or leakage in the line and the patient's line insertion site. Wrap an alcohol wipe and gauze around the broken part of the line. Immediately change the tubing.

- **The clamp on the line is broken?**

  Change the tubing. Assure the clamp works properly on the new tubing. This is essential for patient safety.

- **The central line gets caught on or pulled by the patient's clothing?**

  Loop the tubing over the dressing and secure with tape.

- **My patient is short of breath or complains of chest pain?**

  Notify the provider immediately.
  These symptoms could be a sign of fluid overload or other complications, such as a dislodged clot or embolism.

- **My patient feels pain in the neck or ear on the side where an implantable CVAD is located? Or the patient hears swishing noises or has palpitations?**

  Notify the provider immediately.
  In this case, the implanted device might be dislodged. Placement must be confirmed by x-ray.

Patient Evaluation

- Monitor for signs of catheter complications (e.g., shortness of breath, chest pain, palpitations).
- Monitor for signs of catheter dislodgement (e.g., neck swelling or pain, bleeding at the site or within the line, palpitations, gurgling noise).
- Assess for signs of catheter-related infection (e.g., fever, increased WBC count, redness, warmth at the site).
- Observe for leaking or blood backup at the injection ports, tubing connections, and the site.
- Observe for bleeding at the CVAD site.
- Assess for signs of allergic response or adverse effects to medication.

Patient Teaching

- Teach patients, families, and caregivers that the overall goal is to maintain a patent CVAD or PICC line that is free of infection, occlusion, or dislodgement.
- Avoid obtaining blood pressure readings in the arm where a PICC line is inserted.
- If a PICC line is in place, do not immerse the arm in water. The patient may shower if the site is covered by an occlusive dressing.
- Follow prescribed activity restrictions.
- Teach signs of catheter complications including line-related infection, thrombosis, and accidental dislodgement.
- Teach signs of catheter dislodgement to include pain or swelling in the neck or area near the ear of the affected side of the CVAD. Gurgling sounds might also indicate a problem with the placement of the CVAD.

Home Care

- The goals of home care for clients receiving medication through a CVAD or PICC line are medication safety and maintaining an infection-free line.
- Candidates for home IV therapy through a CVAD or PICC line are those who:
  - Have a family member or other caregiver who can competently provide or assist with care of the line.
  - Have telephone access—either via landline or cell phone.

(continued on next page)

Procedure 25-18 ■ Administering Medication Through a Central Venous Access Device (CVAD) (continued)

- Have access to reliable transportation in case of a line-related emergency.
  - Ideally, caregivers should be able to read instructions for home care.
- Procedures in the home environment are similar to the hospital setting, except clean technique is used instead of sterile.
- Home health supplies may be different than the ones used in the hospital.
- After discharge, follow-up care in the home environment is important to ensure safety.

Documentation

- Document any signs of allergic response to or adverse effects of medication.
- Note any signs of catheter complications or dislodgement.
- Document signs of catheter-related infection.
- Record the date and time tubing and port cap are changed.
- Document all medications infused through the CVAD.

Sample Documentation

mm/dd/yyyy   1200   PICC line insertion site clean and dry. No redness, swelling, or drainage. Arm circumference 16 inches; same as pre-insertion measurement. Pt reports no pain at site. Flushed with 10 ml of NS, no resistance noted. ———— Sue Creas, RN

Thinking About the Procedure

 The video **Administering Medication Through a Central Venous Access Device,** along with questions and suggested responses, is available on the **Davis's *Nursing Skills Videos*** Web site on Davis*Plus*.

Practice Resources

Bertolino, G., Pitassi, A., Tinelli, C., et al. (2012); Centers for Disease Control and Prevention (2011b); Infusion Nurses Society (2011a, 2011b).

Concept Map

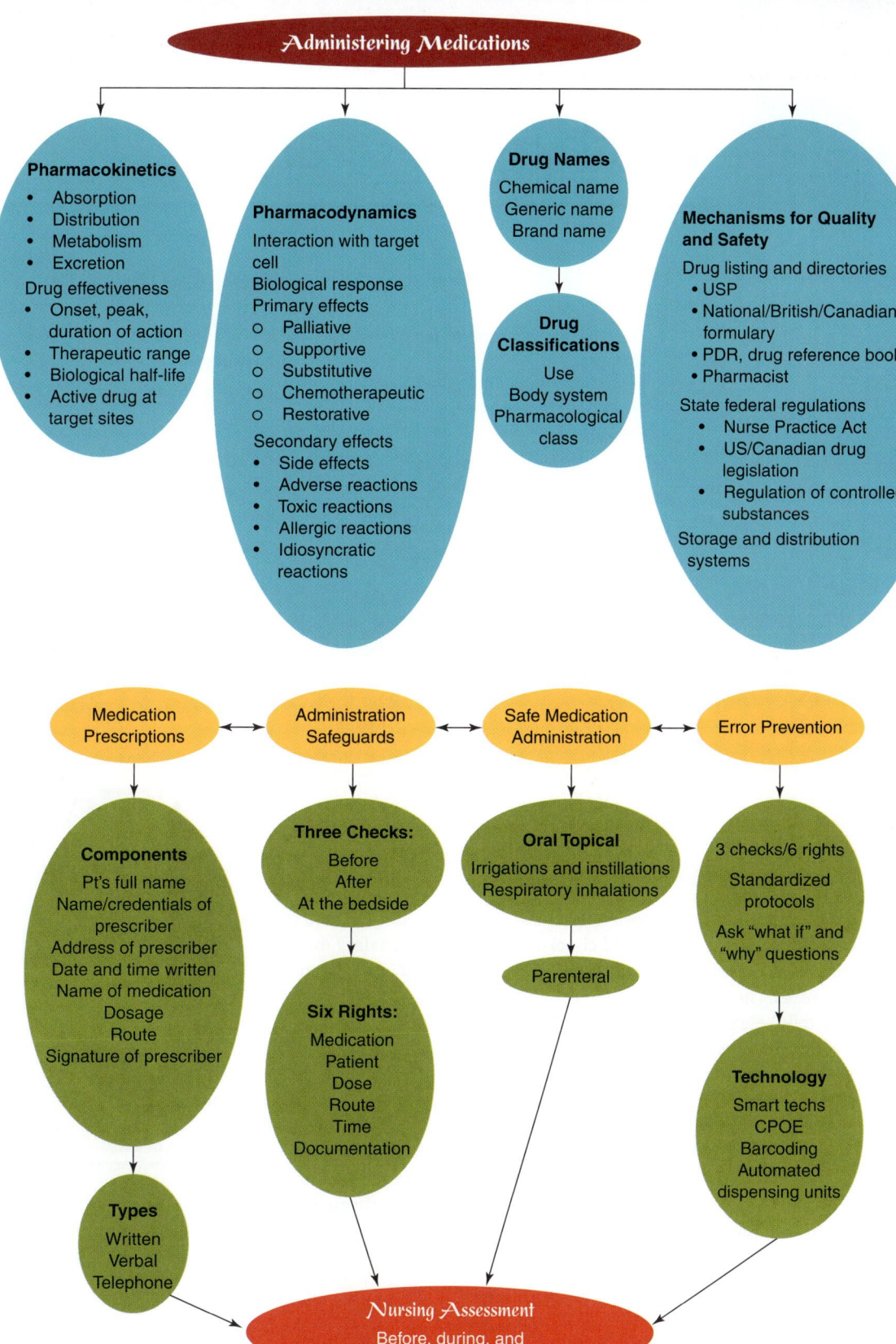

Administering Medications

Pharmacokinetics
- Absorption
- Distribution
- Metabolism
- Excretion

Drug effectiveness
- Onset, peak, duration of action
- Therapeutic range
- Biological half-life
- Active drug at target sites

Pharmacodynamics
Interaction with target cell
Biological response
Primary effects
- ○ Palliative
- ○ Supportive
- ○ Substitutive
- ○ Chemotherapeutic
- ○ Restorative

Secondary effects
- Side effects
- Adverse reactions
- Toxic reactions
- Allergic reactions
- Idiosyncratic reactions

Drug Names
Chemical name
Generic name
Brand name

Drug Classifications
Use
Body system
Pharmacological class

Mechanisms for Quality and Safety
Drug listing and directories
- USP
- National/British/Canadian formulary
- PDR, drug reference book
- Pharmacist

State federal regulations
- Nurse Practice Act
- US/Canadian drug legislation
- Regulation of controlled substances

Storage and distribution systems

Medication Prescriptions ↔ **Administration Safeguards** ↔ **Safe Medication Administration** ↔ **Error Prevention**

Components
Pt's full name
Name/credentials of prescriber
Address of prescriber
Date and time written
Name of medication
Dosage
Route
Signature of prescriber

Types
Written
Verbal
Telephone

Three Checks:
Before
After
At the bedside

Six Rights:
Medication
Patient
Dose
Route
Time
Documentation

Oral Topical
Irrigations and instillations
Respiratory inhalations

Parenteral

3 checks/6 rights

Standardized protocols

Ask "what if" and "why" questions

Technology
Smart techs
CPOE
Barcoding
Automated dispensing units

Nursing Assessment
Before, during, and after administration

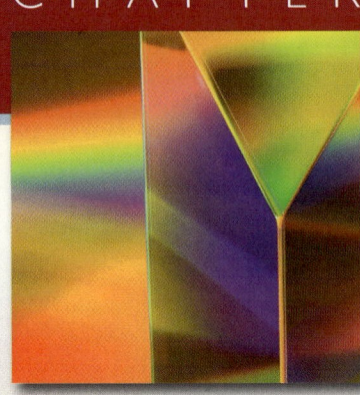

CHAPTER 26

Teaching & Learning

Learning Outcomes

After completing this chapter, you should be able to:

▶ Present three factors contributing to the expanding role of teaching in professional nursing.

▶ Describe the concepts of teaching and learning.

▶ Name, define, and give one example of each of Bloom's three, updated domains of learning.

▶ Describe the six levels of cognitive thinking in the modified (Krathwohl) Bloom's classification.

▶ Discuss the factors that can affect learning.

▶ List at least six barriers to teaching and learning.

▶ Describe some strategies for motivating learners.

▶ Develop strategies for working with clients with cultural or learning differences.

▶ Perform learning assessments.

▶ Apply the nursing diagnosis Deficient Knowledge appropriately to various patient situations.

▶ Develop teaching plans for clients.

▶ List four methods for evaluating the outcomes of teaching and learning.

▶ Document teaching content, methods, and patient responses to learning.

Key Concepts

Health literacy

Learning

Learning environment

Teaching

Related Concepts

See the Concept Map at the end of this chapter.

Meet Your Patient

Heather, a 20-year-old mother, and her 4-year-old preschooler come to the clinic for a well-child checkup. During the visit, you notice that the child speaks only in one- or two-word phrases. The mother's tone is impatient. "Stop using that baby talk." Heather says, "All her friends are taller and talking more. She was even small when she was born, so I suppose it's my fault."

Your assessment shows the child is below the fifth percentile for height and weight. You assess for teaching needs and provide anticipatory guidance to the mother. How would you begin to address Heather's learning needs without reinforcing her feelings of self-blame? What health teaching could you provide that might help resolve this problem?

Your guidance should include safety measures, immunizations, and nutrition for a 4-year-old, as well as expected growth and development. How can you evaluate whether the teaching has been effective and further promote Heather's retention of this new information?

By the time you finish working through this chapter, you should be able to answer these questions and provide teaching to meet the unique needs of other patients you encounter.

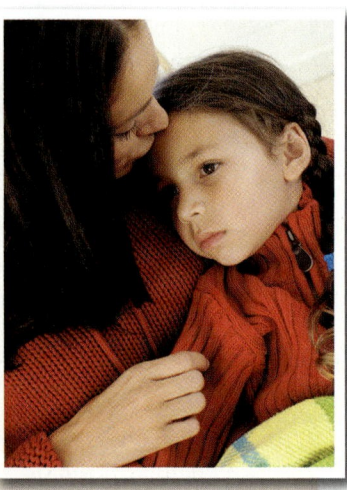

ABOUT THE KEY CONCEPTS

This chapter covers concepts that underlie how people take in and offer information within the healthcare setting. A firm grasp of **teaching, learning, health literacy,** and the **learning environment** will allow you to call to mind the information that you will need when teaching patients in a variety of settings.

Theoretical Knowledge knowing **why**

Nurses have been teaching patients since Florence Nightingale taught about the value of good nutrition, fresh air, exercise, and personal hygiene (Nightingale, 1860/1992). Since that time, teaching has become progressively more important, owing in part to the following:

Patients Participate in Healthcare Decisions Primary care providers expect patients to share the responsibility for their own health. Patients and families require accurate, clear, and complete information so that they can make *informed* decisions. You can help patients find answers to their questions, identify reliable resources, and develop self-care and health promotion behaviors.

Hospital Stays Are Brief A great deal of complex care is provided in patients' homes and the community. Patients are often sent home still requiring medication, dressing changes, and skilled procedures such as urinary catheterization. Nurses have a responsibility to instruct family members how to provide care and to teach patients to care for themselves as they are able.

Healthcare Is Expensive Patient education can help to decrease the overall cost of healthcare. It does so by helping to increase patient understanding and compliance with medical and nursing regimens, which can shorten hospital stays and reduce readmissions (Bastable, 2014; Peter, Robinson, Jordan, et al., 2015).

The basic purpose of teaching and learning is to provide information that will empower clients and families to (1) perform self-care and (2) make informed decisions about their healthcare options. Like other interventions, you can use teaching to promote wellness, prevent or limit illness, restore health, adapt to changes in body function, and facilitate coping with stress, illness, and loss.

WHO ARE THE LEARNERS?

As a nurse, your learners are clients, families, and others who care for the client. You will often provide informal, one-to-one teaching while performing other nursing interventions. For example, as you give a medication, you will teach about its therapeutic and side effects. Or you may do more formal teaching to groups of people in a variety of healthcare settings (e.g., demonstrating a baby bath to a class of expectant parents).

As a nurse, you will also be responsible for teaching healthcare workers whom you supervise. For example, you may instruct nursing assistive personnel (NAP) when you observe an error in technique. Or you may help a new nurse learn to how to use new equipment on the unit. Nurses in practice are also involved in clinical instruction of nursing students, new graduates, and other members of the healthcare team. Most of this teaching may be informal, although you might also present specific topics at unit meetings and conferences. For example, if there is a change in the agency's documentation system, you might teach a group of the nurses on your shift to learn the new system.

WHAT ARE MY TEACHING RESPONSIBILITIES?

Teaching is a major component of clinical practice skills and is an independent nursing function. In many states, nurses' teaching role and responsibility are defined in the nurse practice act. The organizations discussed in this section provide standards for nurses and patients/healthcare consumers, as outlined.

The American Nurses Association (ANA) The ANA's *Code of Ethics for Nurses With Interpretive Statements* (2015a) holds that nurses are responsible for promoting and protecting health, safety, and rights of patients. Patient teaching is essential in fulfilling that responsibility.

Nursing: Scope and Standards of Practice Standard 12 states, "The registered nurse seeks knowledge and competence that reflects current nursing practice and promotes futuristic thinking" (American Nurses Association, 2015b, p. 76). Registered nurses' teaching activities include the following:

- Providing health teaching that addresses topics such as healthy lifestyles, risk-reducing behaviors, developmental needs, activities of daily living, and preventive self-care.
- Using health promotion and health teaching methods appropriate to the situation and the healthcare consumer's values, beliefs, health practices, developmental level, learning needs, readiness and ability to learn, language preference, spirituality, culture, and socioeconomic status.
- Seeking opportunities for feedback and evaluation of the effectiveness of the strategies used.
- Using information technologies to communicate health promotion and disease prevention information to the healthcare consumer in a variety of settings.
- Providing healthcare consumers with information about intended effects and potential adverse effects of proposed therapies.

The Joint Commission These standards require educators in healthcare organizations to provide education based on patients' assessed needs and to consider the literacy, desire and motivation to learn, developmental and physical limitations, barriers to communication, culture, and religious beliefs of every patient (The Joint Commission, 2015).

Advisory Commission on Consumer Protection and Quality in the Health Care Industry (1997) The American Hospital Association's (2003) Patient Care Partnership (previously the Patient's Bill of Rights) describes in simple language the right of consumers to accurate and easily understood information about health plans, healthcare professionals, and healthcare facilities. If patients speak another language, have a physical or mental disability, or just do not understand something, they have the right to receive help so they can make informed healthcare decisions.

WHAT ARE SOME BASIC LEARNING CONCEPTS AND PRINCIPLES?

The educational process consists of both teaching and learning. **Teaching** is an interactive process that involves planning and implementing instructional activities to meet intended learner outcomes or providing activities that allow the learner to learn

(Bastable, 2014). Teachers must have effective communication skills to (1) adequately convey information, (2) assess verbal and nonverbal feedback, and (3) accommodate various learning styles. In patient education, nurses can use teaching, counseling, and behavioral modification together to achieve effective client learning.

Learning is a change in behavior, knowledge, skills, or attitudes. Information alone will not change behaviors. Change occurs as a result of motivation to learn and with planned or spontaneously occurring situations, events, or exposures. The "five rights" in Box 26-1 describe how some basic principles of learning help with planning patient education.

Learning Theories

Social learning theory explains the characteristics of the learner. *Self-efficacy* is a major concept in social learning theory. It refers to a person's *perceived* ability to successfully perform a task.

- *Behavioral learning theory* is characterized by explicit identification of information to be taught and immediate reward for correct responses. It has its roots in psychology and the belief that the environment influences behavior and, in fact, is the essential factor in determining human action. I. Pavlov (1927), B. F. Skinner (1953), and Albert Bandura (1971) are behavioral theorists.
- *Cognitive theory* sees learning as a complex cognitive (mental) activity. Learning is an intellectual or thinking process in which the learner structures and processes information. Cognitive theory also recognizes the importance of developmental stage and social, emotional, and affective influences on learning. Bloom (1956) is one of the major cognitive theorists.
- *Humanism* focuses equally on the learner's affective (emotional), cognitive (intellectual), and attitudinal qualities. It emphasizes the learner's active participation and responsibility in the learning process. Learning is thought of as self-motivated, self-initiated, and self-evaluated, and its purpose is self-development and achievement of the learner's full potential.

KnowledgeCheck 26-1

- Identify at least three reasons nurses have a responsibility to teach clients.
- Define *teaching*.
- Define *learning*.

Learning Occurs in Three Domains

People learn in three ways, or *domains:* cognitive, psychomotor, and affective (Bloom & Krathwohl, 1956). You should include each of these domains, involving thinking, doing, and caring/feeling, when writing objectives and planning teaching and evaluation strategies. Table 26-1 provides examples of client learning in each of the domains.

Krathwohl (2002) adapted Bloom's model describing learning using a more outcomes-based approach: Remember, understand, apply, analyze, evaluate, and create (Fig. 26-1).

Cognitive Learning

Cognitive skills are the mental activities for processing incoming information. Learning is not about how many facts you can recall but rather how meaningful the information is and how effectively you can use it when needed. After capturing your patients' attention and getting them to perceive the need to learn the information you are trying to teach, your goal is then to expand their learning beyond simple *remembering* and *understanding.* You will promote their thinking to a higher level that involves *applying, evaluating,* and *creating* ways to meet their own healthcare needs. Strategies and tools for promoting cognitive learning include lectures, one-to-one instruction, print and online reading materials, panel discussions and webinars, digital applications, and problem-based learning (e.g., case studies and care plans).

Psychomotor Learning

Psychomotor learning involves performing skills that require both mental and physical activity. It requires the learner to value learning the skill (the affective domain) as well as understand and implement the skill (the cognitive domain). Strategies and

---

BOX 26-1 ■ Five Rights of Teaching

When you are making a teaching plan, you can use this list to ensure that you consider each of the five "rights" of teaching.

Right Time

- Is the learner ready, free of pain and anxiety, and motivated?
- Have you and the learner developed a trusting relationship?
- Have you set aside sufficient time for the teaching session?

Right Context

- Is the environment quiet, free of distractions, and private?
- Is the environment soothing or stimulating, depending on the desired effect?

Right Goal

- Is the learner actively involved in planning the learning objectives?
- Are you and your client both committed to reaching mutually set goals of learning that achieve the desired behavioral changes?

- Are family or friends included in planning so that they can help follow through on behavioral changes?
- Are the learning objectives realistic and valued by the client; do they reflect the client's lifestyle?

Right Content

- Is the content appropriate for the client's needs?
- Is it new information or reinforcement of information that has already been provided?
- Is the content presented at the learner's level?
- Does the content relate to the learner's life experiences or is it otherwise relevant to the learner?

Right Method

- Do the teaching strategies fit the learning style of the learner?
- Do the strategies fit the client's learning ability?
- Are the teaching strategies varied?

Table 26-1 ➤ Bloom's Domains of Learning

DOMAIN AND LEVELS OF BEHAVIOR	EXAMPLES OF CLIENT BEHAVIORS
Cognitive (thinking)	
Includes memorization, recall, comprehension, and the ability to analyze, synthesize, apply, and evaluate ideas.	Reports the names and doses of the three medications he is taking.
	Explains the expected effect of the medication she has been prescribed.
	Designs a planned schedule for dressing changes for a wound on her leg.
	Describes how to distinguish between normal inflammation and signs of infection in a wound.
	Recognizes the need for behavioral changes to decrease the chance of recurrence of infection.
Psychomotor (skills)	
Includes sensory awareness of cues involved in learning, as well as imitation and performance of skills and creation of new skills.	Identifies that he needs to read directions before starting a project.
	Brings personal equipment to a teaching session.
	Follows the instructor who is demonstrating diapering of her newborn, imitating her movements.
	Diapers a newborn after observing a demonstration.
	Independently changes her complex dressing; the wound heals with no signs of infection.
	Creates a new approach to giving his daily injections.
Affective (feelings)	
Includes receiving and responding to new ideas, demonstrating commitment to or preference for new ideas, and integrating new ideas into a value system.	Makes eye contact with the nurse as she explains the admission process.
	Asks questions about what to expect during a procedure he is to undergo.
	A parent of a child who has just been admitted to the hospital expresses commitment to staying with her child after the nurse explains the impact of hospitalization.
	A client who has overcome drug addiction chooses to present his story to high school groups.

Source: Adapted from Bloom, B. S., & Krathwohl, D. R. (1956). Taxonomy of educational objectives: The classification of educational goals. In *Handbook I: Cognitive domain.* New York, NY: Longmans, Green; and Bloom, B. S., Mesia, B. B., & Krathwohl, D. R. (1964). *Taxonomy of educational objectives: Vol. 1. The affective domain. Vol. 2. The cognitive domain.* New York, NY: David McKay.

tools used to teach psychomotor skills include demonstration and return demonstration, simulation models, streaming video, journaling and self-reflection, and printed materials, especially those containing photographs and illustrations.

Affective Learning

Affective learning involves changes in feelings, beliefs, attitudes, and values. It is considered the "feeling domain." Strategies and tools for promoting affective learning include role modeling, group work, digital storytelling, panel discussion, role playing, mentoring, one-to-one counseling and discussion, interactive applications, and digital and printed materials.

KnowledgeCheck 26-2

- What are the three domains of learning?
- What strategies and tools are used to promote learning within each of the three domains of learning?
- Give an example of each of the domains of learning.

ThinkLike a Nurse 26-1

By now, you have probably already learned how to assess a patient's blood pressure (BP).

- Think about how you were taught to perform that *skill.* What would have been the best way for *you* to learn to take a BP? To read a book and look at the photos closely? To watch a YouTube video? To have someone tell you how to do it? To have someone demonstrate the skill? Perform the blood pressure measurement yourself? Some other way?
- Now think about the *principles* involved with BP (e.g., normal ranges, the physiological regulation of the BP). What, for you, would have been the best way to learn the principles? Read a book? Listen to a lecture? Physically obtain a BP reading for a patient? Work a case involving BP? Some other way?
- From your answers to the two preceding questions, what (if anything) can you conclude about different domains of learning and the kinds of activities to use in teaching and learning in each domain?

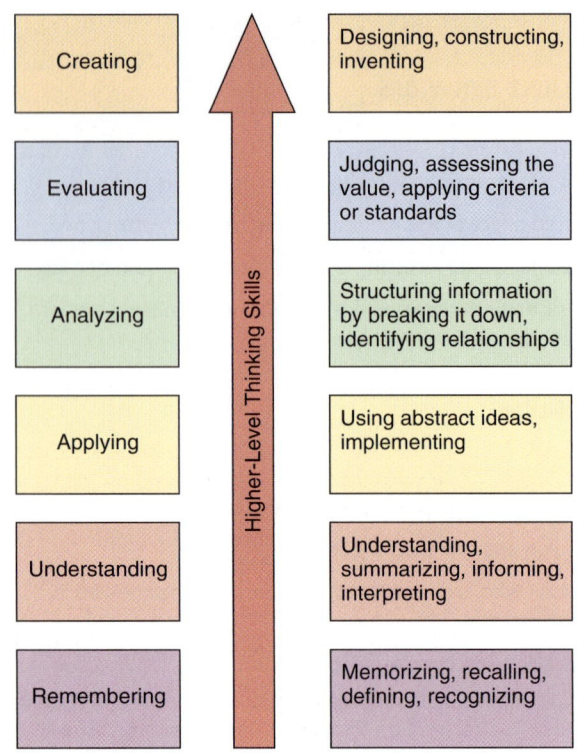

FIGURE 26-1 Bloom's revised taxonomy for higher order thinking skills.

Many Factors Affect Patient Learning

Learning is complex. Many factors can either enhance or interfere.

Motivation

Motivation is desire from within. Little learning can occur without it. Motivation is greatest when clients:

- Recognize the need for learning,
- Believe it is possible to improve their health, and
- Are interested in the information they are being given.

Think about classes you have taken. Have you studied harder in some than in others? What motivated you? Was it because you were intrigued by the information, wanted to earn a good grade, or had other incentives?

Motivation may be based on physical, emotional, and social needs; the need for task mastery or success; and health beliefs. In your teaching, try to apply the following principles for motivating learners:

- Convey your interest in and respect for the learner and the learning process to help motivate the learner.
- Create a warm, friendly environment. This can enhance social needs motivation, as can your enthusiasm.
- Helping clients identify a practical need can be motivating. For example, Heather (Meet Your Patient) may not be aware that her child is at risk for injury from home hazards. Helping her to understand the normal behavior of a 4-year-old may motivate her to childproof her home.
- Use rewards and incentives. The need for achievement and competence is related to task mastery and self-efficacy. When a person succeeds at a task, he is usually motivated to continue learning.
- The patient will be motivated to learn only if she believes that health is important. For example, Heather may understand

that a 4-year-old likes to explore and may recognize there are safety hazards in the home; however, she will not be motivated to learn safety measures if her attitude is that "it is no big deal."

Readiness

Readiness is the demonstration of behaviors that indicate the learner is both *motivated* and *able* to learn *at a specific time*. You must consider readiness in your planning. For instance, a client may not be "ready" for teaching right before scheduled diagnostic tests or treatments because anxiety makes it difficult to concentrate.

Physical Condition   Physical factors (e.g., pain, strength, coordination, energy, senses, mobility) and attention contribute to a patient's readiness to learn. For example:

- Pain interferes with the ability to concentrate on the teaching.
- The patient needs adequate strength, coordination, energy, and mobility to demonstrate psychomotor learning.
- Patients with impaired hearing or vision require adaptations in your teaching and evaluation strategies.

Emotions   Severe anxiety, stress, or emotional pain interferes with the ability to learn. In addition, the learning itself, and the idea that behaviors must be changed, can create anxiety. However, a mild level of anxiety can enhance learning by providing motivation. For example, a patient newly diagnosed with diabetes may not be experiencing physical complications related to the disease, so he may not be interested in learning about diabetes. You may be able to motivate him (i.e., create some anxiety) by pointing out the potential and serious complications (e.g., blindness, kidney damage) of uncontrolled diabetes. But do so carefully so that the client does not interpret your words as a threat, excessive negativity, or preaching.

Timing

You must present information at a time when the learner is open to learning. Timing is therefore everything.

- People retain information better when they have an opportunity to use it soon after it is presented. For example, one student reads about insulin; another reads the same information and also administers different types of insulin to several patients. At the test 2 weeks later, the second student will have an advantage at test time.
- For some concepts, the learner might need more time to absorb and apply information, especially when complex thinking is required.

Active Involvement

Learning is more meaningful when the patient is actively involved in the planning and in the learning activities. **KEY POINT:** *Learners retain 10% of what they read, but they retain 90% of what they speak and do (London, 1999).* Passive listening is not typically as effective for processing and retaining information as are activities involving more than one style of learning, especially hands-on learning. For instance, a demonstration with a return demonstration and a patient education brochure is an effective way to teach patients how to perform a new skill.

Feedback

Feedback is information about the learner's performance. For example, a test grade is feedback for students, conveying the message, "You need to work on that content some more," or "You have successfully mastered the lesson." Feedback in the

Teaching Clients Through Collaborative Relationships to Reduce Rehospitalization

Chapter Key Concepts: Teaching, Learning, Learning Environment

SENC Competencies: Client-Centered Care, Interdisciplinary Collaboration

Background

Patients with chronic illnesses or multiple health problems have learning needs to understand their health conditions and care after discharge. When nurses engage patients in the teaching/learning process, they are better equipped to make informed health decisions, prevent complications, and reduce hospital readmission.

Think about it:

➤ Using a patient-centered, collaborative approach, what should be your first step in order to teach effectively?

➤ Discuss what you might do to involve the patient in the teaching/learning process.

➤ Reflect on how patient partnership and empowerment have the potential to change patient health behaviors.

_____

Reference: Peter, D., Robinson, P., Jordan, M, et al. (2015). Reducing readmissions using teach-back: Enhancing patient and family education, *Journal of Nursing Administration*, 45(1), 35–42. doi:10.1097/NNA.0000000000000155

---

clinical setting or skills lab might be, "You consistently maintained sterile technique."

KEY POINT: *Positive feedback encourages learners who are tackling difficult content or devoting the time and effort needed to get the most out of the learning process. This is especially critical when significant behavioral changes are required.*

When teaching or coaching, you may sometimes need to suggest alternatives or point out errors. Do so in a positive way when you can. Be careful not to seem judgmental when clients are learning a new skill or are giving home care. Fear of failure or judgment can be a barrier to learning at what could be the client's most teachable moment.

Repetition

The patient is more likely to retain information and incorporate it into his life if the content is repeated. For example, often patients forget what medication is prescribed for certain conditions. Repeating the name of the drug can help patients remember it. This is especially true for learning psychomotor skills. Do you remember the first time you counted a radial pulse? Even that simple skill may have been difficult at first. By now it is probably very easy for you.

ThinkLike a Nurse 26-2

Use examples from your own experience, if you can. Do not use examples you have read in the preceding sections.

■ Give an example to illustrate the importance of relevance in learning.

■ Give an example to illustrate the importance of repetition in learning.

■ Give an example to illustrate the importance of timing in learning.

Learning Environment

For most people, an ideal learning environment is private, quiet, physically and psychologically comfortable, and free from distractions. If a separate space is not available, you can at least try to find a quiet corner, pull the bed curtain shut, close the door, or sit close to the patient so that you can talk softly (Fig. 26-2). Make the best of what you have to work with. However, some learners are best motivated and engaged when teaching occurs in a group.

When you are planning a teaching session, provide good lighting and comfortable seating that are conducive for conversations. Have your teaching materials at hand to avoid long pauses in the teaching session. If you have an area that is set aside for teaching, try to use inspirational or motivational accessories (e.g., photographs, posters).

Scheduling the Session

Plan for uninterrupted time to allow you to adequately assess and understand the patient. The teaching time doesn't need to be long, just uninterrupted (e.g., by procedures, physical therapy). Based on the patient's condition (e.g., activity intolerance, attention span, fatigue, pain), shorter teaching sessions may be best for comprehension and retention. Finding suitable time to teach can be a challenge, but a moment can be a teaching session, as shown in Box 26-2.

Amount and Complexity of Content

The more complex or detailed the content is, the more difficult it is for most people to learn and retain, as you probably know from your own learning experiences. For example, imagine teaching parents about the need for isolation precautions for their newborn who has just been diagnosed with a complex immune disorder. In comparison, teaching parents how to diaper their healthy newborn would be far less challenging.

The greater the change, the greater will be the challenge for both teacher and patient. For example, a patient rehabilitating after a stroke who has to relearn using eating utensils, swallowing, and other basic tasks for daily hygiene and

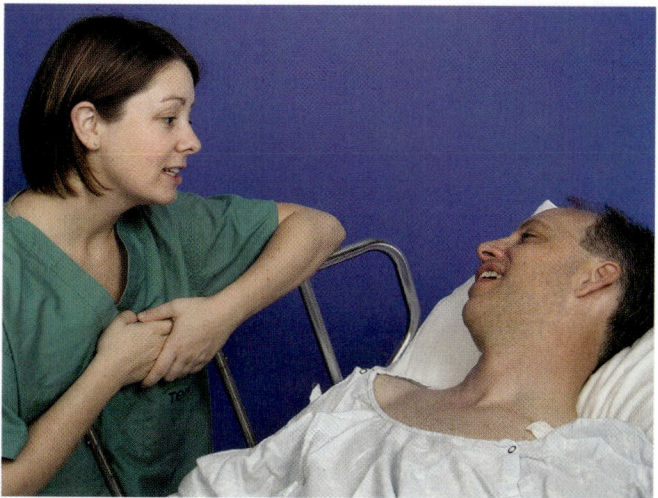

FIGURE 26-2 Sit or stand close to the patient so that you can talk privately.

BOX 26-2 ■ Teachable Moments

A student nurse walks into her patient's room. This week in class she has been studying patient teaching. Her instructor has informed the students that she expects them to incorporate teaching into each clinical day. But the student ponders, "I am way too busy to find time to teach. What am I going to do?" Later in the day, she asks the nurse who is co-assigned to her client for suggestions. The nurse asks, "Did you take the patient's blood pressure?" When the student answers that she did, the nurse says, "Did you explain why you were doing that and what the BP readings mean?" Again the student says, "Yes." The nurse asks, "When you gave your patient his medications, did you explain why you were giving each one?" The student says, "Yes, and the side effects, too." A light goes on! The student begins to understand that almost every patient contact presents an opportunity for teaching, even when the contact lasts for only a short time.

self-care will experience a more demanding learning challenge than one who has to learn only a daily schedule for taking medications.

Communication

Communication is central to the teaching and learning process in which teachers and learners exchange information, perceptions, and feelings. Attend carefully to verbal and nonverbal feedback that the client gives; it can tell you whether or not the learner is attentive and focusing on the learning activities. For more information about communication, see Chapter 20.

Special Populations

For patients who have special needs (e.g., those with learning disabilities, attention deficit-hyperactivity disorder [ADHD], mental illness, affective or communication disorders, mental illness, or brain injury), you must plan carefully to ensure that you maximize learning by adapting teaching strategies to the patient's special learning needs. Consider a variety of approaches—one size does not fit all. For example, you may need to do one or more of the following:

- Use brief, frequent learning sessions.
- Pay special attention to minimizing distracting stimuli in the environment.
- Present information slowly.
- Use repetition.
- Be satisfied with slower progress.

If you are not familiar with the patient's condition, you must acquire theoretical knowledge of it. Include a family member, caregiver, or other significant person in the teaching to reinforce the learning and act as a safety net for implementing the information.

Developmental Stage

An understanding of intellectual development will help you to gear your teaching strategies and content to the level of the learner. For example, when teaching psychomotor skills, you will need to assess the person's fine and gross motor development. A young child may not have adequate fine motor skills to complete a task. If you would like to review an extensive discussion of intellectual development, including Piaget's theory (1966), refer to Chapter 9.

ThinkLike a Nurse 26-3

A client who has a brain injury needs to learn how to administer insulin. Another learner, who must learn to change a wound dressing, has ADHD.

- How do you think these clients' health status might affect:
  1. Their motivation to learn?
  2. Their ability to be actively involved in the learning?
- What approaches or changes might you need to make in:
  1. The learning environment?
  2. The timing of the teaching session?
  3. The use of repetition?
  4. Your communication?
  5. The amount and complexity of content presented in a session?
  6. Your use of feedback?
  7. The amount of teacher support?

Stages of Cognitive Development

Piaget identified three stages of cognitive development that are especially important in client teaching in the cognitive domain:

- **Preoperational Stage** (2 to 7 years old), in which the child begins to acquire language skills and find meaning through use of symbols and pictures.
- **Stage of Concrete Operations** (7 to 11 years old), in which the child learns best by manipulating concrete, tangible objects and can classify objects in two or more ways (e.g., identify a shape as a triangle and also as green). Logical thinking begins, and the child can understand the relationship between numbers and the idea of reversibility. He also can begin to recognize and adapt to the perspective of others. Before reaching the stage of formal operations, clients learn best from examples instead of definitions and they understand concrete terms rather than abstract terms.
- **Formal Operational Stage** (age 11 years or older), in which the person can use abstract thinking and deductive reasoning. The person can relate general concepts to specific situations, consider alternatives, begin to establish values, and try to find meaning in life. Not everyone reaches this stage, including some adults.

Teaching Older Adults

When teaching older adults, consider the many factors that can adversely affect the teaching (e.g., vision and hearing impairments, illness, pain, reduced social interaction, reduced mobility, medication effects, sensory deficit, sociocultural factors, and a noisy or chaotic environment). Assess for these barriers so you can adapt your style according to any restrictions. Allow extra time for teaching and stop occasionally for rest periods. Refer to Table 26-2 for some principles that apply specifically to adult learners as well as tips for effectively teaching older adults.

Teaching Children

When you work with children, use strategies to gain trust, reduce their anxiety, promote cooperation, and enhance their emotional readiness to learn. For instance, for a child who needs surgery, schedule a tour of the hospital at least 1 week before the admission date and introduce the child to staff members and other patients of the same age (if possible). Teach the child breathing exercises to practice before

Table 26-2 ➤ Incorporating Principles of Adult Learning Into the Teaching of Older Adults

ASSUMED CHARACTERISTICS OF ADULT AND OLDER ADULT LEARNERS	TIPS FOR TEACHING ADULTS
Attitudes	
Adults are independent and self-directed.	Help them to identify their own learning needs.
Adults must recognize the need to learn before they become willing to learn.	Explain why the information or new skill is important. Include materials with practical tips and realistic goals for learning.
Some adults may be uneasy about the learning process because of (1) anxiety, (2) past unsatisfactory experiences with educational processes, (3) having received their formal education many years ago, (4) feeling that "being taught" is for those who don't know, or (5) fear of failure.	■ Present content in a nonthreatening environment where there is no risk of judgment or embarrassment in front of peers. Privacy is often necessary. ■ Offer feedback simply to improve important skills and not for the sake of a grade. ■ Remember, the intent of patient education is to improve clinical outcome. ■ Respect learners for what they already know.
As adults are goal-directed learners, they are more motivated to learn if they think they will be able to use the information or skills immediately.	Plan the teaching session close to the time the patient will need the information or need to perform a new skill. Relevancy and practicality are key.
Adults prefer to be partners in the learning process—to have some control over what they learn and how they learn it.	■ Encourage learners to tell you first what they intend to gain from the educational session. ■ Spell out the goals of your session in advance and allow the learner to customize it.
Some adults are resistant to the need to learn new information. They may feel, "I've been just fine all these years without needing to know that; why should I learn it now?" Or they may believe that they are "too old to learn." These may be defenses to avoid failure or to resist change.	■ Work with the learner to establish the "need to know" at the onset of the program. ■ Involve the learner in defining what he or she intends to gain from the educational session. ■ Reassure the learner about the importance of the information. ■ Encourage the learner to tackle a little at a time.
Older adults tend to be socially less connected and might perceive bias, ageism, or isolation.	As for any group of people, you must honor cultural backgrounds, local customs and practices, and personal preferences.
Experience	
Adults have previous life experiences that can enhance learning.	■ Assess what they already know. Then build teaching based on what they need to know. ■ Relate new content to learners' past experiences and knowledge; have them use their experiences to solve problems. ■ Encourage older adults to share life experiences.
Messages are best received when they are part of the real-life experience.	Model the message you are conveying to your audience: "Walk the walk" and not just "talk the talk."
Learning Environment	
Many adult learners do well when a hands-**on approach is used.** Older adults must practice a new skill, or rehearse new information, in order to learn it.	■ Offer active participation and opportunities for interaction with instructor and other learners. ■ Demonstrations and practical tips are useful for adult learners, particularly older adults.
Many older adult learners need to review new information away from the initial learning environment in order to retain it. The information might not sink in until later.	Use take-home materials, such as colorful posters, table tents, tip sheets, and patient-friendly brochures, to reinforce information.

(Continued)

Table 26-2 ➤ Incorporating Principles of Adult Learning Into the Teaching of Older Adults—cont'd

ASSUMED CHARACTERISTICS OF ADULT AND OLDER ADULT LEARNERS	TIPS FOR TEACHING ADULTS
Older adult learners can be distracted and annoyed by cellular phones and other electronic devices.	Request phones, radios, or other electronic devices be turned off for the educational session. Silence your own phone as well.
Most older adults were raised during a time when technology was not as prevalent as it is today. Learning occurred primarily through the reading, discussion, and retelling of stories.	■ Use informal teaching sessions that include storytelling. Keep your stories short. ■ Convey your genuine interest in your learners before sharing personal stories. ■ To elicit stories, you must be a patient and empathetic listener. ■ Allow more time for older adults, especially those with chronic illness, to tell their own stories. ■ Tie the patient's past experiences to the lesson. ■ Ask open-ended questions and be willing to wait for the answer.
Older people may bring family members or other caregivers to the teaching session to help interpret or remember information presented. Sometimes the extra people in the room can be noisy and distracting to the patient's learning situation.	If others in the room are distracting, it may be helpful to ask them to minimize their conversations or in some circumstances to leave the room for a time.
Older adults usually learn better when they are not overwhelmed with multiple needs, topics, or skills at one time.	■ Introduce only a few topics at a time. Usually tackling one to three new topics or skills is enough. ■ Identify what is the most important information for your learner to walk away with. Define those topics and cover them well. ■ Remember, slow and steady wins the race, especially when it comes to learning information that is essential to the patient's health.

Sensory and Physical

Changes in visual distance, depth, acuity, and light perception occur with aging, diminishing the ability to take in information. **Older adults experience increased sensitivity to glare and reduced color perception.** **Processing of sensory information is slower in the later decades of life.**	■ Avoid colors such as blue, green, and lavender because they are difficult for older adults to differentiate. ■ Remove physical barriers that could compromise the field of vision (e.g., projector position, tables). ■ In teaching materials, choose fonts that are bold, black, and a minimum size of 18-point. Fancy lettering is harder to decipher. ■ A nonglare background without a stylized pattern is easier to see and process than are complex designs. ■ For those who cannot read or who have severe visual impairment, consider recording instructional material.
Older adults may have experienced changes in hearing. Older adults may have reduced: ■ Hearing acuity ■ Perception for various tones ■ Filtration of extraneous	■ Speak slowly, using a normal tone of voice. ■ If you must speak more loudly than normal, be careful not to sound condescending, as though speaking to a child. Learners should not perceive annoyance in your tone. ■ Many older adults do some lip-reading, although they may be unaware of it. You can facilitate lip-reading by not distorting your facial features with exaggerated pronunciation. ■ Provide a quiet setting and decrease background noise. Close the door or windows if outside noise interferes.

Table 26-2 ▶ Incorporating Principles of Adult Learning Into the Teaching of Older Adults—cont'd

ASSUMED CHARACTERISTICS OF ADULT AND OLDER ADULT LEARNERS	TIPS FOR TEACHING ADULTS
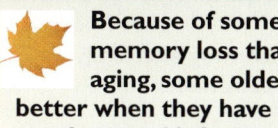 Because of some short-term memory loss that occurs with aging, some older adults learn better when they have a source of supplemental information or support.	▪ Reinforce your teaching with follow-up opportunities and connections to the community for information and support in grasping new information or acquiring a new skill.
Older adult learners can be particularly affected by fatigue, illness, medication, pain, stress, and other personal factors.	Plan the teaching session when the patient is well rested, as pain free as possible, and comfortable.

admission. Give the child (or parent) a coloring book explaining the upcoming surgery.

If the child is in the preoperational stage, simplify the information and use pictures or video and concrete examples. Preschoolers will not understand detailed rationale for taking medication. Instead, tell him that the medicine will make him feel better, use pictures of a child drinking from a medicine cup, or give the child a calendar to mark each time she takes a dose.

Cultural Factors

Awareness of norms, values communication, social structure, time orientation, and cultural identification are important in planning teaching (Chapter 15). If the client is not fluent in the prevailing language, you may need to use an interpreter.

♥ **iCare**   Nurses care by being culturally sensitive. This involves respect for clients' identity and needs, regardless of who they are, where they're from, how they speak, how old they are, their religious and spiritual practices, whether they are disabled, their financial status, how much they weigh, how socially popular they are, or any other aspect that can lead to unfair treatment. Box 26-3 highlights key concepts of teaching with a culturally competent approach.

Health Literacy

The Patient Protection and Affordable Care Act of 2010, Title V, defines **health literacy** as "the degree to which an individual has the capacity to obtain, communicate, process, and understand basic health information and services to make appropriate health decisions" (Centers for Disease Control and Prevention, 2016, updated). It does not refer simply to a person's ability to read and write but rather how a person can effectively:

▪ Find information and services to meet health needs for self and others.
▪ Communicate health needs to others.
▪ Understand and apply information and services to meet health needs.

Health illiteracy exists when the person is unable to apply language skills to understanding information about his healthcare. This occurs, for example, when the language spoken is not the patient's preferred language, or perhaps the format through which the information is communicated is not suited to the patient. Learning gaps can occur in the following examples:

▪ The patient has a hearing impairment, discharge teaching is done verbally, so the client misunderstands the words.

▪ A healthcare provider uses medical terminology that is unfamiliar or misinterpreted by the patient, thus resulting in an unintended message or lack of meaningful information.
▪ Limited health literacy is more common among the medically underserved community, minority populations, and older adults.

Patients with low health literacy are not as likely to understand the connection between risky behavior and health. They encounter problems such as difficulty taking medications as prescribed, difficulty managing complex or chronic health problems, and higher rates of emergency department (ED) visits, hospitalization, rehospitalization, and death.

Promoting Health Literacy   In the United States, one in five people does not speak English at home (Sarkar, Karter, Liu, et al., 2010). To enhance understanding between you and your patients, refer to the following tips for promoting health literacy:

▪ Ask questions that involve "how" and "what" rather than "yes" and "no."
▪ Assist patients in completing forms and/or health histories as needed.
▪ Organize information so the most important material stands out and is repeated for emphasis and clarity.
▪ Present information in three to five "chunks" at a time.
▪ Speak using simple words and short sentences and by structuring sentences with active rather than passive voice. For example, instead of saying, "The pill should be taken every 8 hours," say, "Take the pill every 8 hours."
▪ Write out instructions and appointments using simple language, avoiding medical jargon and technical terms.
▪ For those with low health literacy, provide printed materials with words of three or fewer syllables and sentences with fewer than 15 words. Be aware, though, that paragraphs made of short, simple sentences can make information too basic and therefore may not accurately communicate complex information (Badarudeen & Sabharwal, 2010).
▪ Use as many drawings and photographs as possible to illustrate your statements.

For those with limited English proficiency, provide information in their primary language, use online or software translation tools, or seek an interpreter to translate.

Barriers to Teaching and Learning

As you gain teaching experience, you will begin to recognize the factors we have just discussed (e.g., timing, the environment) and to manipulate those that can be changed to enhance teaching and learning. The most common barriers are identified in the sections that follow.

BOX 26-3 ■ Culturally Competent Teaching

Assessments

- Inquire about or observe interactions between family members so you can identify the decision maker and how decisions are made.
- Assess for customs or taboos that may conflict with the information you plan to present.
- Observe verbal and nonverbal communication patterns.
- Assess whether the family is past, present, or future oriented.
- Determine whether the patient and/or family prefers a same-sex nurse to teach a client about personal topics, such as birth control and sexually transmitted infections. Different cultures vary in their ideas about what is appropriate for discussion between men and women.
- Determine whether the client's values and wishes are in congruence or conflict with the family.
- Find sources of information that can help you learn about the culture and its healthcare practices.

Self-Knowledge

- Admit unfamiliarity with the culture, but express willingness to learn.

Caring

- Respect, accept, and validate the client's beliefs.
- Find ways to incorporate the client's current healthcare practices and beliefs into the plan.
- Respect, accept, and validate the client's health beliefs unless there is potential for harm.

Interventions

- Include the family in the planning and teaching.
- Allow the patient to include cultural practices in the plan of care.
- Speak slowly and clearly; avoid slurring syllables.
- Do not use slang expressions.
- Use short sentences and concrete rather than abstract words. Present only one idea in each sentence.
- Use pictures and other visual aids to help communicate your meaning, as needed.
- Provide teaching materials in the client's language. If you cannot read it, have it translated so that you can judge its appropriateness.
- Avoid using humor; jokes often do not translate well because of connotations, jargon, and culture-specific context.

Feedback

- Obtain feedback carefully. Do not assume that a client who smiles, nods, and says yes really understands what you are teaching. The client may be embarrassed to ask questions or may feel that it will embarrass you.
- Encourage the client to ask questions; stop often to evaluate client understanding.

Barriers for the Teacher

The following are barriers to effective teaching:

- Competing demands on the nurse's time (e.g., to prepare for teaching)
- Conflicting schedules between the nurse's available time for teaching and the patient's available time to learn
- Ineffective coordination of class lecture with clinical experience

- Lack of space and privacy
- Teaching not seen as a priority (by the nurse or the organization)
- No third-party reimbursement for teaching
- Frustration with the amount of documentation needed

Barriers for the Learner

The following are barriers to learning effectively:

- Illness, fatigue, other physical conditions
- Anxiety, personal stress
- Low literacy; low health literacy
- Environmental not conducive to learning
- Lack of time to learn
- Overwhelming amount of behavioral change needed
- Overwhelming complexity of the condition or treatment to be learned
- Lack of support and ongoing positive reinforcement
- Lack of motivation, willingness to take responsibility
- Language barrier
- Teaching not suited to learning preferences and style
- Provider uses jargon and technical terms
- Does not perceive need for the information taught

Barriers to Technology-Based Learning

Although technology is an asset to learning, it may also create some barriers. Some of the barriers are the same as in the classroom; others are unique, including the following:

- Lack of social interaction
- Poor learner motivation
- Diverse learning styles
- Time issues
- Technical problems (software or devices)
- Access to the Internet, for some learners

KnowledgeCheck 26-3

- List and define six factors that affect the learning process.
- What is one strategy you could use to motivate a client who seems uninterested in learning?
- What are some aspects of the environment that can enhance or interfere with learning?
- What two strategies might you use with a learner functioning with low cognitive ability?

ThinkLike a Nurse 26-4

- List some actions you can take to avoid each of the teaching barriers.
- Give an example of each of the barriers to the learner. For "anxiety, personal stress," here is one example: A patient is frightened after having a heart attack, worried about the cost of the medical treatment, and worried about not being able to go to work, so he cannot concentrate on the material being presented to him.

Note: These questions may be difficult, depending on your knowledge and experience. Work with others to answer the questions, as necessary.

PracticalKnowledge
knowing **how**

The teaching process parallels the nursing process. You will assess learning needs and readiness, make educational diagnoses, write learning objectives, plan and implement teaching strategies, and evaluate client learning.

ASSESSMENT NP

A learning assessment will help you to determine the right setting for the teaching, the content to cover, learning goals, and teaching strategies. Your initial assessment consists of general information about the amount of time and resources available for your teaching. Also be clear about your intended audience. You can assess the learner in several ways: through informal conversations, structured interviews, focus groups, questionnaires, tests, observations, and information obtained from the client's chart. You will pick up many cues in your initial comprehensive assessment of the client. For questions to ask when assessing learning, see the accompanying Focused Assessment box.

ANALYSIS/NURSING DIAGNOSIS NP

Deficient Knowledge is the most frequently used (and perhaps misused) nursing diagnosis for a teaching plan. It may be either a problem or the etiology of a diagnosis.

Deficient Knowledge as the Primary Problem

KEY POINT: *You should use Deficient Knowledge only if you believe that the lack of knowledge is the **primary problem**. Use it to describe conditions in which the patient needs new, additional, or extensive knowledge.*

Identify the specific knowledge deficit as the problem and follow with the etiology and related signs and symptoms, for example: *Deficient Knowledge (diabetic foot care) related to lack of prior experience, as manifested by anxiety and many questions about foot care.*

Incorrect Uses of Deficient Knowledge

KEY POINT: *Always look beyond the knowledge deficit to see what problematic responses it produces.*

- **Beware of routine or premature diagnosing.** It is easy to see that a patient lacks information, label it as a Deficient Knowledge problem, and try to solve the problem by giving

---

Learning Assessment

Pre-Assessment

Before assessing the learner, think about the following:
- Time constraints. How much information do you need to present? How much time do you have to do it?
- Available resources. What equipment and supplies do you have to work with? Do you have audiovisual equipment? A dry erase board? A copy machine? Books?

Assessing the Learner

A teaching/learning assessment should include the following:
- **Intended audience.**
  Who are you teaching?
  What is the person's age, occupation, developmental level, and cultural affiliation?
  Will you be teaching a person or a group?
- **Learning needs.**
  What is the client's medical (or other) problem?
  What behavioral changes are needed?
  What self-care knowledge and skills does the client need?
- **Knowledge level.** Determine what the client already knows so that you can reinforce knowledge or adapt the teaching plan to the client's learning needs. Ask questions such as:
  What do you think caused your health problem?
  What are your concerns about it?
  How has the problem affected your usual activities?
  What are your concerns about treatment [tests, surgery, etc.]?
- **Health beliefs and practices.**
  Ask the client to give a general description of her health. Ask:
  What do you usually do to stay healthy?
  What problems do you think you are at risk for?
  What lifestyle changes would you be willing to make in order to improve your health?"

- **Physical readiness.** Check ability to concentrate, manual dexterity skills, and pain level.
- **Emotional readiness.**
  Find out whether the client is experiencing anxiety or emotional distress that will interfere with the learning process.
  Ask the client whether she would like a family member or friend to be present during the learning.
- **Ability to learn.**
  What are the learner's cognitive and psychomotor developmental abilities?
  How does the client learn best (e.g., by memorization or recall, or by problem-solving or applying information)?
  How well does the client recall previously presented material?
- **Health literacy level.**
  Does the patient have the ability to understand basic health information and services needed to make appropriate healthcare decisions?
  Can the person read and write?
  Do the patient and healthcare provider speak the same language?
- **Neurosensory factors.**
  What is the client's ability to feel, see, hear, and grasp?
  Does the client have a medical condition that causes neurosensory compromise?
- **Learning styles.** Ask the person:
  How do you prefer to learn new things? For example, do you prefer to read about them, talk about them, watch a DVD, be shown how to do it, listen to the teacher, or use a computer?
  Do you like to read?
  Where do you get information about your health—from the Internet, books, magazines, your family, your healthcare provider?
  Do you learn best alone or with other people?

information—but information may not be what the patient needs at all.

- **Do not use Deficient Knowledge routinely as a problem label for all patients** (Jarrell, Alpers, & Wotring, 2011). There are information needs associated with almost every medical and nursing diagnosis. However, you cannot assume a particular patient needs to be taught that information. For example, a person with a foot ulcer secondary to long-standing diabetes may already know more than you do about foot care. **KEY POINT:** *For most nursing diagnoses (e.g., Anxiety, Imbalanced Nutrition), you can merely write a nursing order to provide the informal teaching needed instead of writing a Deficient Knowledge diagnosis.*
- **Do not use Deficient Knowledge for problems involving the client's** *ability to learn.* To accurately describe such situations, use non-NANDA-I diagnoses such as:

  Impaired Ability to Learn r/t fear and anxiety
  Impaired Ability to Learn r/t delayed cognitive development
  Lack of Motivation to Learn r/t feelings of powerlessness

Deficient Knowledge as the Etiology

Deficient Knowledge is usually most effective as the etiology of other nursing diagnoses, such as the following:

- Ineffective Health Maintenance related to (r/t) Deficient Knowledge of immunizations
- Risk for Impaired Parenting r/t Deficient Knowledge of child's developmental need for stimulation
- Ineffective Family Health Management r/t Deficient Knowledge of the procedure for drawing up and injecting insulin
- Risk for Imbalanced Nutrition: Less Than Body Requirements r/t Deficient Knowledge about additional calories and nutrients needed during pregnancy and fear of "getting fat"

Wellness Diagnoses

Teaching is the primary intervention for wellness diagnoses such as Effective Breastfeeding, Readiness for Enhanced Communication, and the more than 25 other NANDA-I labels beginning with the phrase "Readiness for Enhanced."

PLANNING OUTCOMES NP

Before making a teaching plan, educators contract with the learner for what they want to accomplish together. A **learning contract** is a statement of understanding between teacher and learner about how to achieve mutually set goals. The contract usually describes the responsibilities for both teacher and learner, time frame for the teaching, content to be included, and expectations of all participants. Learning contracts increase the learner's commitment to reaching the teaching and behavioral goals. They are usually informal.

Teaching goals are broad in scope and set down what is expected as the final outcome of the teaching and learning process. They should address all three domains of learning. In contrast, **learning objectives** are single, specific behaviors that must be completed to accomplish the goal. They are short term and ideally are accomplished in one or two sessions. Similar to patient outcomes in the nursing process, learning objectives/goals should include an action verb, an activity that can be measured or observed, the circumstances of the learner's performance, and how learning will be measured. For example:

Goal: Demonstrate ability to perform newborn care in 3 days.

Learning Objectives: (1) Changes infant's diaper, making sure that umbilical cord remains outside the diaper. (2) Demonstrates bathing baby while maintaining newborn's axillary temperature of greater than 98.5°F (36.9°C).

See Table 26-3 for examples of active verbs for each domain of learning. See Chapter 5 for a review of goals and outcomes.

NOC standardized outcomes for Deficient Knowledge depend on the content that needs to be taught. *Nursing Outcomes Classification (NOC)* (Moorhead, Johnson, Maas, et al., 2013) has identified more than 60 Health Knowledge outcomes for specific topics, for example, Knowledge: Diabetes Management and Knowledge: Infant Care.

If you use Deficient Knowledge as the etiology of another diagnosis (e.g., Imbalanced Nutrition) then you would use NOC outcomes linked to that diagnosis (e.g., Knowledge: Diet, or Nutritional Status).

Individualized goals/outcome statements you might write for a client with a diagnosis of Deficient Knowledge include examples such as the following:

- Deficient Knowledge (Child Physical Safety)—After demonstration and explanation, parents will fasten preschooler safely and securely in a car seat.
- Deficient Knowledge (Diabetes Management)—After reading pamphlets, client will explain the relationship of carbohydrate intake and exercise to blood sugar.

As you can see, the outcome is directly related to the area in which the client lacks knowledge or information. The outcomes you choose depend on whether you have used Deficient Knowledge in the problem clause or the etiology clause of the nursing diagnosis.

Table 26-3 ➤ Examples of Active Verbs for Domains of Learning		
COGNITIVE DOMAIN	**AFFECTIVE DOMAIN**	**PSYCHOMOTOR DOMAIN**
Compare	Cry	Apply
Define	Choose	Arrange
Describe	Defend	Assemble
Differentiate	Discuss	Change
Explain	Display	Construct
Give examples	Express	Create
Identify	Initiate	Demonstrate
List	Justify	Inject (e.g., medication)
Name	Relate	Manipulate
Plan	Revise	Move
State	Select	Organize
Summarize	Share	Start
	Smile	Work

ThinkLike a Nurse 26-5

A client has just been diagnosed with diabetes mellitus. He must monitor and record his blood glucose three times a day. The two of you establish as a goal that he will be able to perform glucose testing independently within 1 week. What objectives would you need to write to achieve this goal?

PLANNING INTERVENTIONS/ IMPLEMENTATION NP

In Chapters 5 and 6, you learned about creating a nursing care plan. For clients and families with special learning needs, you will create individualized teaching plans. The teaching plan is often a part of the client's complete nursing care plan.

Creating Teaching Plans

The process of creating a teaching plan differs from that of creating a nursing care plan in two key ways:

1. In a teaching plan, the interventions are actually teaching strategies.
2. When planning teaching, you will plan content, sequencing, and the types of instructional materials to be used.

Let's apply these aspects of a teaching plan, using Heather (Meet Your Patient) as an example. You have assessed the need for anticipatory guidance regarding safety for her 4-year-old. Your nursing diagnosis is Deficient Knowledge (safety for a 4-year-old) related to the mother's inexperience.

Teaching Strategies are the method used to present content. For Heather, they might include one-to-one instruction and printed information. You must use plain language always. The Joint Commission recommends "teach-back" and "show-back" techniques to assess and ensure patient understanding

(N.A., 2016, *Teach-back. . .*; The SHARE approach. . ., 2014). You may use drawings, models, technology, or devices to demonstrate your teaching message (Fig. 26-3). Always encourage your patients to ask questions to avoid misunderstanding.

Content of your teaching includes the information your learner must understand to reach the desired goal. It can include facts, skills, or emotions. For Heather (Meet Your Patient), the content of your informal teaching might include the following:

- *Poison control and prevention*—Curiosity and lack of ability to understand danger puts the preschooler at greater risk.

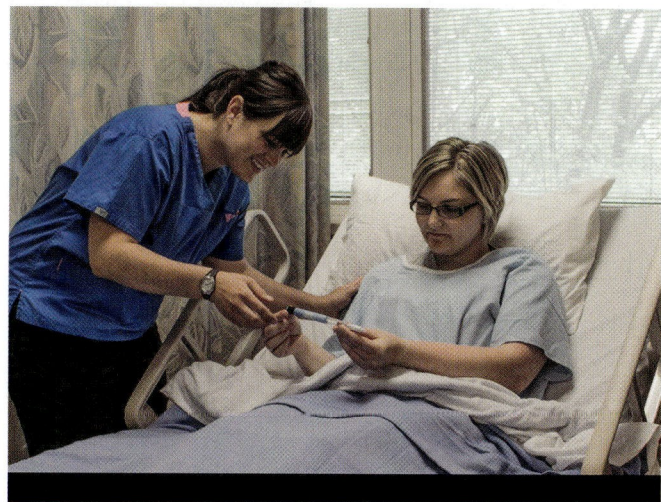

FIGURE 26-3 The nurse uses demonstration and return demonstration to teach a patient how to give herself an insulin injection.

General Tips for Effective Patient Teaching

Create a Conducive Learning Environment.

➤ **Provide private space to talk** with your patient and other designated family members. Be sure the setting allows for privacy and is free of distractions and interruptions.

➤ **Time the session to be held when the patient is in the best state of mind to concentrate** on what you are saying. For example, you will want to be sure the patient has pain under control but is not drowsy from pain relievers. Anxiety, depression, and fatigue also interfere with learning.

➤ **Help your patient decide who should be involved in the teaching session.** On the one hand, caregivers assisting in the care after discharge would benefit from the learning process. On the other hand, some patients may not want others to be present because of modesty or cultural practices.

Plan and Communicate Information According to Your Patient's Needs.

➤ **Be considerate of cultural, religious, or other issues** that might influence the way your patient receives information.

➤ **Developmental delays or cognitive impairment can also hamper learning.** Adjust learning style and level of complexity accordingly. Likewise, modify teaching approach for patients with visual or hearing deficits. Consider limited English proficiency, mental health, and emotional stress when communicating with patients.

➤ **Find out what your patient needs to know before making a teaching plan.** Involve him in the learning process. This not only improves your patient's motivation to learn but also helps your patient to get more out of the education.

➤ **Be sure you provide the vital information needed for home care.** As time, staffing, and resources are limited in the healthcare setting, decide what is most important and set that as priority teaching.

- *Accident prevention*—This would include the need for car seats, increased supervision when exploring, and the use of a helmet when the child rides a tricycle.
- *Risk of choking*—Foods that are hard to swallow or chunky (e.g., hot dogs) are a concern for a 4-year-old.
- *Need for immunizations and physical checkup*—These are important and should be scheduled during the next year.

Scheduling and Sequencing refer to both the information and the timing of the teaching session.

- *Sequencing—how you organize the information.* This refers to the order in which you present content. As a rule, you should begin with simple and nonthreatening topics, and then present complex and difficult ones. To enhance patients' understanding, limit the information you present to two or three important points at a time.
- *Timing—when the teaching session(s) are to be scheduled.* This should be based on the client's and teacher's needs. When extensive content is involved, it is best to schedule a teaching session in advance; the teacher and learner are then committed and prepared for the session. Meeting for short periods of time can be most effective if teaching is succinct and organized.

In the example at the beginning of this chapter, you could teach Heather about poison control and accident prevention in the lobby while she and her preschooler are waiting for the child to be examined. During the child's examination, you could review immunizations and the need for an annual checkup. At the end of the examination, when discussing the child's nutrition, you might include a discussion of foods that are a choking hazard, such as a hot dog.

Instructional Materials refer to what you will use to introduce information and reinforce learning. You might give Heather printed handouts with number for the Poison Control Center hotline or a link to a YouTube video demonstrating how to properly install a child car seat. To involve the child, you might include a coloring book and stickers about one of the topics.

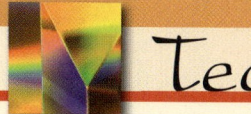

Teaching Plan

Client Data

Emily O'Connor is the advanced practice nurse in charge of the student health center on campus at State University. A research project revealed that 60% of students surveyed on campus reported they spent 300 minutes per week of moderate intensity exercise, which was consistent with a study examining compliance with the Physical Activity Guidelines for Americans (Tucker, Welk, & Beyler, 2011). However, researchers found 62% adherence by self-report but only 10% when measured via accelerometer. Thus, Emily decides to teach students and interested campus staff members about the importance of physical activity for physical and emotional well-being. To reinforce the content, Ms. O'Connor develops colorful brochures with photos and charts to make the information more visually appealing and an interactive teaching session to capture learners' attention. She also provides food, so people will have additional motivation to attend.

Nursing Diagnosis

Potential Deficient Knowledge (health behaviors) about physical activity as evidenced by campus-wide survey results showing that less than two-thirds of students comply with the U.S. Department of Health and Human Services recommendation for physical activity.

NOC Outcome

Knowledge: Health Behavior (1805)

NIC Intervention

Teaching: Group (5604)

Teaching Environment

1. Provide an environment conducive to learning. Promote comfort by making personal introductions and offering refreshments during break time.

   Rationale: When adult learners are in an environment in which they feel comfortable, they are less distracted and more able to learn. Participants' physical and emotional comfort is important for creating a positive atmosphere for adult learning. The environment influences a learner's interest level and actual motivation to acquire new knowledge (Edutopia, 2011).

Overall Strategy / Approach

1. Focus on real-world problems.
2. Emphasize application of content to everyday life.
3. Relate content to life experience.
4. Explain how the education will solve a problem.
5. Involve learners in the educational process.
6. Use a variety of methodologies.

   Rationale: Utilizes principles of adult learning. Using a variety of methodologies is important because different people learn in different ways.

Instructional Materials

1. Printed materials (brochures, fact sheets)

   Rationale: Print materials at an appropriate reading level (usually 6th grade) for the target audience allow participants to review information when it is convenient for them (Choudhry, Baghdadi, Wagie, et al., 2015; U.S. Department of Health and Human Services, National Institutes of Health, 2016, updated). In a study looking at the effectiveness of five different types of media (print materials, online PDF, audio files, audio with text Web page, and streaming video demonstration) for improving patient's learning, findings show that although participants preferred multimedia presentations, patients retained information using supplementary materials regardless of the form in which the content was presented (Wilson, Makoul, Bojarski, et al., 2012).

2. YouTube, DVDs, texting, wearable technologies, or other interactive applications on the computer to accompany PowerPoint slides

   Rationale: In a study examining the effectiveness of streaming video on medical student learning, researchers found a positive effect on learning when it was used to complement other in-class methods and multimedia sources (Bridge, Jackson, & Robinson, 2009; Wilson, Makoul, Bojarski, et al., 2012). In another study investigating the effectiveness of video for patient education, findings indicate patients using streaming video reported video as better than text for presenting health information (Hoffman, Salzman, Garbaccio, et al., 2011).

(Continued)

Teaching Plan (continued)

Learning Objective	Schedule/Sequence	Content	Teaching Strategy
By the end of the first educational session, participants will be able to explain why physical activity is important.	April 1–8	1. Determine date, time, and content of class to be held.	Advertise the educational session by using posters on campus, the campus newspaper, newsletter, social networking sites, and text and e-mail blasts.
	April 9 6:30–7:00 p.m.	2. Social hour. Healthy snacks and beverages. Get acquainted.	
	7:00–7:30 p.m.	3. Identify barriers to engaging in at least 300 minutes of moderate intensity or 150 minutes of vigorous intensity physical activity per week.	Lecture with PowerPoint slides, including photos
	7:30–7:50 p.m.	4. Describe how physical activity helps to promote health, prevent illness, control weight, and enhance overall quality of life.	Projected information (e.g., PowerPoint, YouTube)
	7:50–8:00 p.m.	5. Provide thorough instruction for proper technique for exercises to build strength, improve balance, and increase flexibility.	Video demonstration of various types of exercises with playback of class participants' technique
	8:00–9:00 p.m.	6. Promote awareness and track activity recorded in fitness logs in follow-up contact with participants.	Questions and answers
		7. Provide access to group fitness classes at the local community center.	Hand out printed passes or shareURL for downloading them from the community center's Web site, if available.

Rationale: Content is based on the Health Belief Model, designed by the U.S. Public Health Service. It identifies four key factors that promote health-seeking behavior (adapted for this setting): (1) Person perceives she is at risk for disease (low activity level). (2) Person perceives poor fitness is harmful and has serious consequences. (3) Person believes the suggested intervention (300 min/week of physical activity) will improve health and. (4) Person believes treatment (physical activity) effectiveness is worth overcoming barriers (Hochbaum, 1958).

Evaluation

Eighteen women and 20 men attended the session. When Emily O'Connor began the educational session, the participants were seated in chairs facing the front of the room, where the screen was set up for a YouTube video presentation. She distributed the printed handout materials and provided a short introduction. Before she began teaching, two women began talking about their battle with obesity and difficulty getting out to exercise. Three women shared stories about friends and family members who had suffered poor health and immobility. One had a question about sports-related injuries. During this discussion, the participants turned their chairs to face each other and talked among themselves.

Teaching Plan (continued)

Ms. O'Connor realized that learning takes place when participants share stories with facilitation by the group leader. Teaching does not have to be led exclusively by the facilitator. Even though she had a teaching plan, she was flexible enough to modify the plan to meet participants' needs. She turned off the PowerPoint, turned on the lights, and, instead of lecturing or showing videos from the CDC Web site, she shared information by answering questions and guiding the discussion.

During this process, Ms. O'Connor realized she had made assumptions about the participants' goals for this educational program and their educational needs. She learned that the women who attended came to the program with an understanding of the benefits of exercise and consequences of low levels of physical activity; they knew that exercise is important for health and fitness. They wanted to talk about their obstacles, concerns, and questions; they wanted to separate myths from facts; and they wanted to learn proper technique and how they could maintain motivation to perform at least 300 minutes per week of moderate intensity physical activity

After the session, Ms. O'Connor realized that she needed to revise her plan and offer a second session in a week or two. Her assumption that a lack of knowledge was responsible for the low number of people adhering to the Physical Activity Guidelines for Americans was not confirmed by discussion with the participants. She developed the following new goals for the second session:

1. By the end of the educational intervention, participants will:
   a. State that questions pertaining to weekly physical fitness have been addressed.
   b. Identify the factors that act as a barrier to engaging in physical activity.
   c. Share strategies for overcoming barriers to engaging in physical activity.
   d. Suggest at least five ways to perform at least 300 minutes of moderate intensity physical activity per week.
   e. List steps to follow if an injury occurs while engaging in physical activity.

2. At the 1-year follow-up visit, participants will report that they increased physical activity by 60 minutes per week during the past 12 months.

References

Choudhry, Baghdadi, Wagie, et al. (2015); Edutopia (2011); Hochbaum (1958); Tucker, Welk, & Beyler (2011); U.S. Department of Health and Human Services, National Institutes of Health (2016, updated); Wilson, Makoul, Bojarski, et al. (2012).

Selecting NIC Interventions

NIC standardized interventions related to patient learning depend on the nursing diagnoses you identify. The *Nursing Interventions Classification (NIC)* (Bulechek, Butcher, Dochterman, et al., 2013) lists 30 patient education interventions from which to choose, depending on the content being taught. An example is Health Education and Teaching: Disease Process.

 Go to the Lists of NIC Interventions and NOC Outcomes on DavisAdvantage.

Selecting Specific Teaching Strategies

Before selecting one of the many teaching strategies, consider the learner's needs and learning style and advantages and disadvantages of each method. For a comparison of advantages and disadvantages of each of the teaching formats discussed following, see Table 26-4.

The nurse may reinforce material taught by various methods by asking, "What questions do you have?" Avoid asking, "Do you understand?" as some patients are likely to answer "yes" out of embarrassment or a need to cooperate.

Table 26-4 ➤ Formats for Patient Teaching: Advantages and Disadvantages

Lecture

Advantages
- Efficient and cost-effective way to impart information, especially to large groups.
- Useful for conveying basic concepts and information that serve as the foundation for higher-level, critical thinking later.
- Presenter can use media-rich formats within the lecture to reach learners with auditory and visual learning styles.
- Lectures can be recorded for future use.

Limitations
- Does not allow for individualization of teaching.
- Passive-learning technique, usually not suited for optimal retention of information.
- May not be geared to the level of the learner.
- Not effective for teaching in the psychomotor or affective domains.
- Can lead to oversaturation if too much information is presented in too short a time.
- Boredom is common.
- Not a good strategy for promoting critical thinking.
- Little opportunity for assessing learner comprehension.

Group Discussion

Advantages
- A learner-centered and effective method for teaching in the affective and cognitive domains.
- Many students enjoy a learning environment with opportunities for interaction with peers.
- Social involvement can enhance content.

Limitations
- Less effective with large groups.
- The teacher must be comfortable with less structure and with unpredictable learner responses.
- Managing group discussion requires that the instructor have good leadership skills.
- Not well suited for teaching in the psychomotor domain.
- Quality of group work can be negatively affected by "groupthink"— a force that stifles creativity by succumbing to the subtle pressure of agreeing with the group even though affirmation doesn't reflect the learner's individual opinion.
- Brainstorming fails when participants are distracted or fail to contribute ideas because of fears of rejection or ridicule by peers. Some might even hold back with brainstorming when anticipating the ideas to be unpopular with the instructor.
- Individuals who dominate can be equally problematic when crowding out less confident participants.
- Those who are disruptive or intentionally sabotage the activity can interfere in successful group discussion.

Demonstration and Return Demonstration

Advantages
- Is most effective in teaching psychomotor skills (e.g., use of equipment, self-injection, dressing changes).
- Can be used in small groups if enough equipment is available.
- When the task or skill is performed correctly, return demonstration can increase self-confidence.

Limitation
- Does not work well with large groups or for those who do not learn best by observing others.
- May not be well suited for participants who learn at different rates; some might need repeated demonstration or slow enactment of steps, while others do not.
- Time consuming and labor intensive.

Table 26-4 ▶ Formats for Patient Teaching: Advantages and Disadvantages—cont'd

- Allows for targeted questions and answers and discussion of practical matters, rather than theory.

- Involves preparation time to set up equipment.

- Space must be suitable for the demonstration format.

- Demonstrator must have specialized expertise if technical skills are involved.

One-to-One Instruction and Mentoring

Advantages

- Gives the teacher the opportunity to establish a relationship with a learner; convey interest in his learning needs; and tailor the teaching to the learner's needs as the session proceeds.

- Mentoring allows reluctant learners to more readily ask questions.

- Enables the teacher to obtain frequent feedback so that material can be repeated and clarified as needed.

- Useful for teaching in all three domains: affective, psychomotor, and cognitive.

- Provides an opportunity for learners to build skills and problem-solve in situations with expert supervision, guidance, and feedback.

Limitations

- Can be labor intensive and reaches the fewest numbers of learners.

- May be overwhelming to learners if a large quantity of information is given in a short period of time, and therefore may not promote retention.

- Tends to isolate the learner from peers who may share the same learning needs and who could provide support.

- Can be hampered by personality conflicts.

- Relies heavily on the instructor, preceptor, or nurse being a good role model and having effective teaching skills.

Printed Materials

Advantages

- Allows for standardized information to be presented to each client but with some room for individualization.

- Hard-copy documents are a good way to reinforce material taught in lecture, demonstration and return demonstration, or one-to-one instruction.

- Handouts allow the teacher to cover just the main ideas while using the time more efficiently for face-to-face instruction.

- Printed materials are portable, so people can read the information when it most convenient.

Limitations

- Assumes literacy, proficiency in the dominant language, motivation to read the content, organization to keep track of materials, and visual acuity to decipher the print.

- Materials must be written at a 6th grade reading level with words that most people understand.

Role Modeling

Advantages

- Allows the learner to identify with the teacher.

- Can be a subtle but powerful method to increase motivation and ability to perform a desired behavior.

- Tends to generate high learner interest, and doesn't usually require additional preparation on the part of the role model.

Limitations

- Learners need to be aware of and receptive to this type of teaching.

- A role model who does not effectively represent desired behaviors can send the wrong message.

Online Sources of Information

Advantages

- The Internet makes a vast amount of health-related information readily available. This makes it possible for consumers to participate in self-care and make informed decisions.

- Patients feel empowered when they have access to relevant and understandable information.

- Patients often cope better and experience less uncertainty when health information is available.

- Using audiovisual materials engages both sight and hearing and can accommodate large groups.

Limitations

- The teacher has little control over the quality of information learners access via the Internet.

- Before recommending particular Web sites to a patient, you need to read it yourself to be sure the information is accurate and the format and reading level are best suited to your patient.

- See Chapter 45 for information about evaluating materials you obtain from a Web site.

- Audiovisual hardware and software can be expensive and must be replaced, upgraded, or updated.

KEY POINT: *A patient's lack of questions does not necessarily mean that she understands what's been taught; it could in fact mean the opposite (Dickens & Piano, 2013).*

Lecture Lecture is a traditional method of teaching in which one or more presenters orally share information while learners listen. Teachers can engage learners with an attention-getting opening and by supporting teaching points with stories, quotes, images, analogies or metaphors, and humor. Lectures can be further enhanced by including discussion and question-and-answer periods for clarifying content and by audiovisuals such as specialized applications, computer-projected slides, streaming video, flip charts, posters, brochures, and models.

Group Discussion In a group discussion, several participants discuss topics, exchange information, and present their points of view. The teacher acts as a facilitator to achieve objectives shared with the group at the beginning of the session. Effective group discussion requires: an atmosphere of trust that encourages everyone to participate, openness to new ideas, and confidentiality of the content expressed.

One type of group discussion is **brainstorming,** which is a process for generating multiple ideas for solving a problem. Participants suggest a maximum number of ideas in a short period of time, consider and analyze the various options, identify a best solution, and develop a plan of action.

Demonstration and Return Demonstration In this method, the teacher explains and demonstrates a skill or task. The learner then demonstrates comprehension by returning the demonstration. Return demonstrations should be scheduled close to the initial teaching of the skill. Mannequins are being used more and more in clinical teaching (Fig. 26-4).

One-to-One Instruction and Mentoring One-to-one instruction generally involves one teacher and one learner. They mutually formulate objectives at the beginning of the session. Frequently the learner receives printed or audiovisual materials to reinforce the information presented. You will often use this method for patient teaching.

Mentoring involves a more personal interaction between teacher and learner, involving not only the exchange of information but also role modeling and problem-solving. It offers an opportunity to directly observe and offer feedback on the learner's performance. Mentoring often involves learners in an authentic clinical setting.

Printed Materials Printed materials may be available in the form of fact sheets, discharge instructions, printed pamphlets, or detailed booklets. When you are creating your own teaching materials, remember the tips for ensuring readability in the Health Literacy section of this chapter:

- Include specific step-by-step actions you want learners to take.
- Avoid abstract words in the instructions. Action words are clearer.
- Be sure the materials do not contain jargon, abbreviations, or acronyms that readers might not be familiar with.
- Create patient materials geared to a general reading level of grade 6 (Fig. 26-5).
- Create printed materials in an easy-to-read font.
- Phrase directions positively to reinforce what you want patients to remember (e.g., say "do" rather than "don't" or "never").
- Use active verbs (e.g., "Take the pill" rather than "The pill should be taken").
- Provide a take-home summary of the main points they need to remember. Having something to refer to at a later time can be useful for reinforcing important information.
- To be sure clients understand the information, provide an opportunity for them to ask questions after they have read the materials.
- For children, use age-appropriate printed books, apps, coloring books, and electronic applications.

Digital Sources of Information Learners can obtain extensive information through applications (apps) for smartphones, tablets, and computers, as well as authority source, scientific, and credible Web sites (e.g., Centers for Disease Control and Prevention [CDC]). Learners can connect with

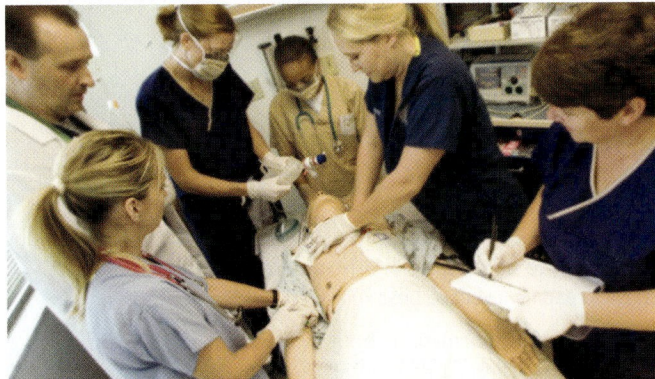

FIGURE 26-4 Simulation mannequins can offer realism and relevance to the educational experience.

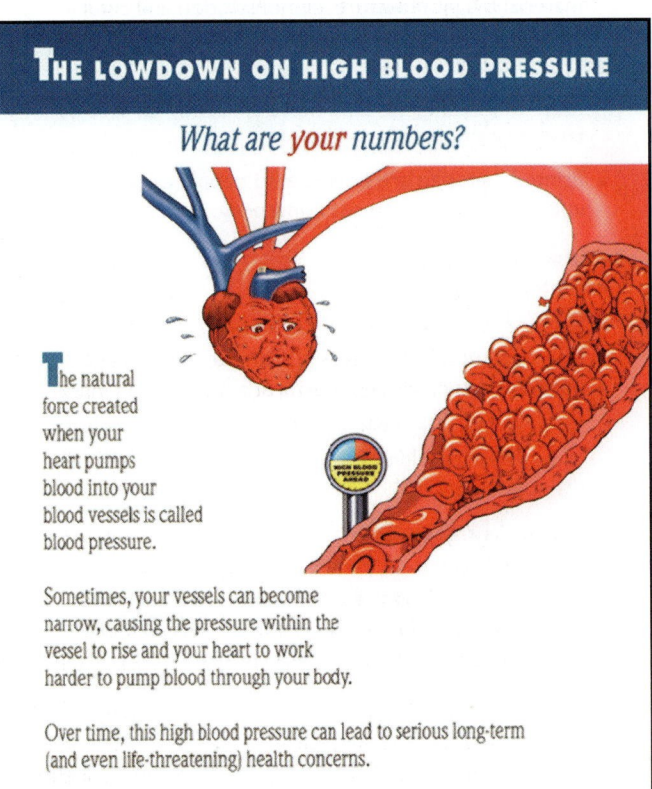

FIGURE 26-5 Reading level of this patient teaching aid is grade 6.

THE LOWDOWN ON HIGH BLOOD PRESSURE

What are your numbers?

The natural force created when your heart pumps blood into your blood vessels is called blood pressure.

Sometimes, your vessels can become narrow, causing the pressure within the vessel to rise and your heart to work harder to pump blood through your body.

Over time, this high blood pressure can lead to serious long-term (and even life-threatening) health concerns.

others and share a common interest through blogs, chats, threaded discussions, and social media special interest groups. They can exchange information, express opinions, offer support, promote interests and activities, and network for personal or professional reasons.

Mobile technology offers convenient access to a variety of learning tools. For example, smartphone and tablet apps include customizable medication reminders, rewards systems for healthy behaviors, and educational components. Health tracking devices and apps offer data regarding activity, diet, and other healthy lifestyle behavior, which can be the basis for a customized health teaching plan.

Role Modeling In role modeling, the nurse teaches by example, demonstrating the behaviors and attitudes that learners should adopt.

- Role modeling is more effective when the teaching point is congruent with the role model's action.
- Learning occurs unconsciously as well as intentionally. Therefore, you must consider what you are communicating both verbally and nonverbally.
- For children, role modeling using a puppet, stuffed animal, or a child's own doll can be helpful in reducing anxiety and enhancing the child's learning. For instance, you can suggest that the child be "the nurse" and "feel Miss Bunny's

pulse," or have a puppet "suggest" to a child, "When I get a shot, I say, 'Ouch!' real loud, and then it's all over!"

KnowledgeCheck 26-4

- True or false: When a patient has a learning disability, you should use a non-NANDA-I diagnosis (e.g., impaired ability to learn) to describe the problem.
- True or false: Learning objectives are short-term and, ideally, should be accomplished in one or two teaching sessions.
- List and state the advantages and disadvantages of at least six teaching strategies.

EVALUATION OF LEARNING

Patient learning is an outcome that is achieved or not. Evaluation of the effectiveness of the teaching plan is essential to improving the quality of instruction. You should evaluate the entire nursing process (as you may recall from Chapter 7). Was your assessment adequate, or did you fail to notice that the patient was physically uncomfortable and therefore not ready to learn? Was your nursing diagnosis accurate? Were your learning objectives realistic? When evaluating the teaching, consider the type of strategy you used, the timing of the teaching, the content, the amount of information, and the

---

Toward Evidence-Based Practice

Free, C., Phillips, G., Galli, L., et al. (2013). The effectiveness of mobile-health technology-based health behavior change or disease management interventions for health care consumers: A systematic review. *PLoS, 10*, e1001363. Retrieved from http://www.ncbi.nlm.nih.gov/pmc/articles/PMC3548655/

A rigorous scientific review of 75 controlled trials examined the effectiveness of mobile technology for healthcare consumers.

- Text messaging improved educational adherence for (a) low-income patients receiving antiretroviral therapy and (b) a smoking cessation group in a high-income setting. It showed short-term benefit in glucose management, physical activity, and psychological support for patients with diabetes. Attendance for vaccination was increased with text reminders and information.
- PDA-based education increased scores for confidence in self-care for patients with lung transplantation.

Deniard-Thompson, N. R., Steven, S. S., & Wofford, J. L. (2012). iPod technology for teaching patients about anticoagulation: A pilot study of mobile computer-assisted patient education. *Primary Health Care Research and Development, 13*(1), 42–47. doi:10.1017/S146342361100034X

Education modules using mobile tablet technology (iPod) were a practical and sustainable strategy for office-based patient education. More patients preferred the educational experience using the mobile technology as compared with print materials. This method also standardized the

educational content, improved clinic efficiency, and contributed to higher numbers of patients receiving patient education.

Niegarandeh, R., Mamoodi, M., Noktehdan, H., et al. (2013, July). Teach back and pictorial image educational strategies on knowledge about diabetes and medication/dietary adherence among low health literate patients with type 2 diabetes. *Primary Care Diabetes, 7*(2), 111–118. doi:10.1016/j.pcd.2012.11.001

This study found that nurses using pictorial images and teach-back educational strategies improved the adherence to medication and diet regimens among patients with type 2 diabetes and low health literacy.

---

1. In the first article discussing mobile technology for patient education and compliance, why was text messaging for conveying health information and reminders more effective for patient teaching than traditional methods?

2. Based on the results of the second study, why might mobile devices be an effective method of instruction for office- or clinic-based healthcare or even inpatient care?

In addition to patients with low health literacy, what other patients might benefit from nurses using pictures and teach-back methods for learning about complex healthcare after discharge?

 Go to Davis Advantage, Resources, Chapter 26, **Toward Evidence-Based Practice Suggested Responses.**

teaching materials. The client is your best source for feedback. He can tell you whether the materials and methods were helpful, uninteresting, and so on.

The following methods are commonly used for outcomes evaluation (client learning):

- *Oral questions/interviews/questionnaires/checklists* allow clients to evaluate their own progress. You may obtain more information by talking with the client; however, you may obtain more honest responses from anonymous written evaluations.
- *Direct observations of client performance* are descriptive notes that you make of the learner's performance. They will help you in providing feedback either to reinforce accurate learning or to correct misinformation.
- *Client's reports and client records* of performance and results. You can evaluate the data and give feedback. Provide criteria and clear expectations to help the client document.
- *Tests and written exercises* can be used in a formal learning setting to measure retention and progress toward meeting cognitive objectives. This method requires the learner to have adequate literacy skills.

Clients will not remember everything you teach them. That is normal. If you start to question your effectiveness as a teacher, think about one of the courses you took last semester. Did you score 100% on every test? How much of the material presented in that course do you remember now? Repetition, reinforcement, and practice are necessary for retention, and so is information made memorable, relevant, and interesting.

Documentation of Teaching and Learning

As is true for all nursing interventions (as you learned in Chapter 7), it is important to record the responses of the client and family to teaching. Documentation also is legal evidence that teaching was done and communicates the information to other health professionals. Write objective statements about what was taught and the client skills and behaviors that demonstrate learning. For informal teaching that occurs during other care activities, you may simply record in the nursing notes or use agency-provided documentation forms.

CLINICALREASONING

The questions and exercises in this section allow you to practice the kind of thinking you will use as a full-spectrum nurse. Critical-thinking questions usually have more than one right answer, so we do not provide "correct answers" for these features. It is more important to develop your nursing judgment than to just cover content. You will learn by discussing the questions with your peers. If you are still unsure, see the Davis Advantage chapter resources for suggested responses.

Caring for the Nguyens

Nam Nguyen has medical diagnoses including hypertension, type 2 diabetes mellitus, obesity, and osteoarthritis. There is a positive history of tobacco abuse. Based on the information you know about Nam and his family, consider the following questions:

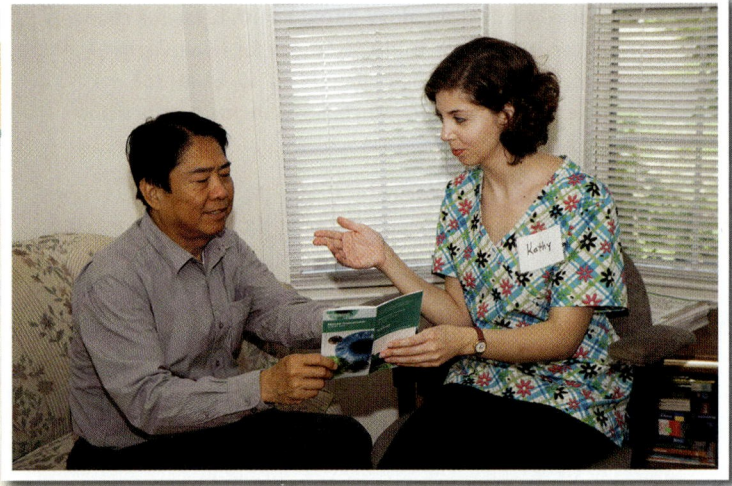

A. What kinds of information does Nam probably need?

B. What would be the best approach to teach Nam about his healthcare conditions?

C. You have been asked to teach Nam about weight loss. What theoretical knowledge must you have and where can you obtain it?

D. What patient information do you need to know before planning your teaching?

E. Nam tells you that he feels overwhelmed with his recent diagnoses. He does not believe he can begin a weight-loss program or attend any teaching sessions. How might you handle this concern?

F. Nam has been prescribed the following medications. Devise one or more teaching sessions focused on these drugs. You will need to use your pharmacology reference books to devise this plan. As you plan your teaching, recall that Nam is overwhelmed by his recent diagnoses.
Lisinopril 20 mg PO daily
Hydrochlorothiazide 25 mg PO daily
Metformin 500 mg PO bid

Applying the **Full-Spectrum Nursing Model** _____

PATIENT SITUATION

Katrina Peplowski, a 22-year-old college student from Ukraine, is transported to the emergency department after passing out in her dorm room. Before this episode, Katrina had a viral illness for 5 days, with fever, nausea, vomiting, and diarrhea. She had been drinking large amounts of Gatorade because of her insatiable thirst, thought to be related to the fever and vomiting. Even before the illness, Katrina's friends and family had commented about her remarkable weight loss since she started school 2 months earlier, especially in light of her increased appetite. On arrival to the ED, Katrina's blood sugar is 585 mg/dL. She is diagnosed with type 1 diabetes mellitus (DM). After stabilization of her blood sugar with fluid therapy and insulin infusion, Katrina regains consciousness. Although Katrina speaks some English, her proficiency is limited.

THINKING

1. *Theoretical Knowledge (Recall of Facts and Principles):* As your patient is newly diagnosed with type 1 DM, there are many areas in which Katrina will need healthcare education. List at least six important topics that are relevant to her care.
2. *Critical Thinking (Application of Knowledge):* What will you consider as you are devising a teaching plan for Katrina?
3. *Critical Thinking (Synthesis of Knowledge):* What factors are important for customizing her teaching plan, considering the communication limitations?

DOING

4. *Nursing Process (Assessment):* What are some pertinent personal factors that you should assess for Katrina when adapting a teaching plan to suit her learning needs?
5. *Nursing Process (Planning):* As you think about involving other members of the healthcare team in her care, how would you plan to optimize Katrina's motivation to learn about managing her diabetes after discharge?

CARING

♥ **iCare** 6. *Self-Knowledge:* What areas of commonality do you have with Katrina around which you might form a caring relationship?

7. *Ethical Knowledge:* Suppose Katrina refuses to receive information from you about DM. She states she is not interested in knowing how to give herself insulin because she doesn't want to give herself injections at home. How should you respond to Katrina's requests?

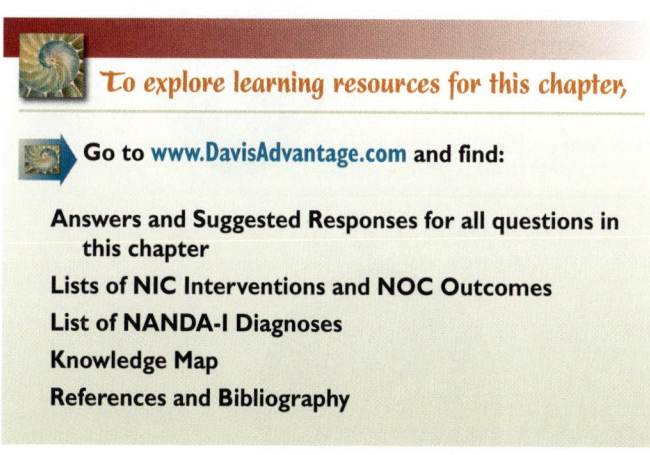

To explore learning resources for this chapter,

Go to **www.DavisAdvantage.com** and find:

Answers and Suggested Responses for all questions in this chapter
Lists of NIC Interventions and **NOC Outcomes**
List of NANDA-I Diagnoses
Knowledge Map
References and Bibliography

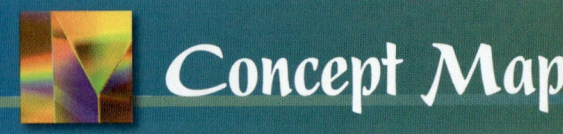

Concept Map

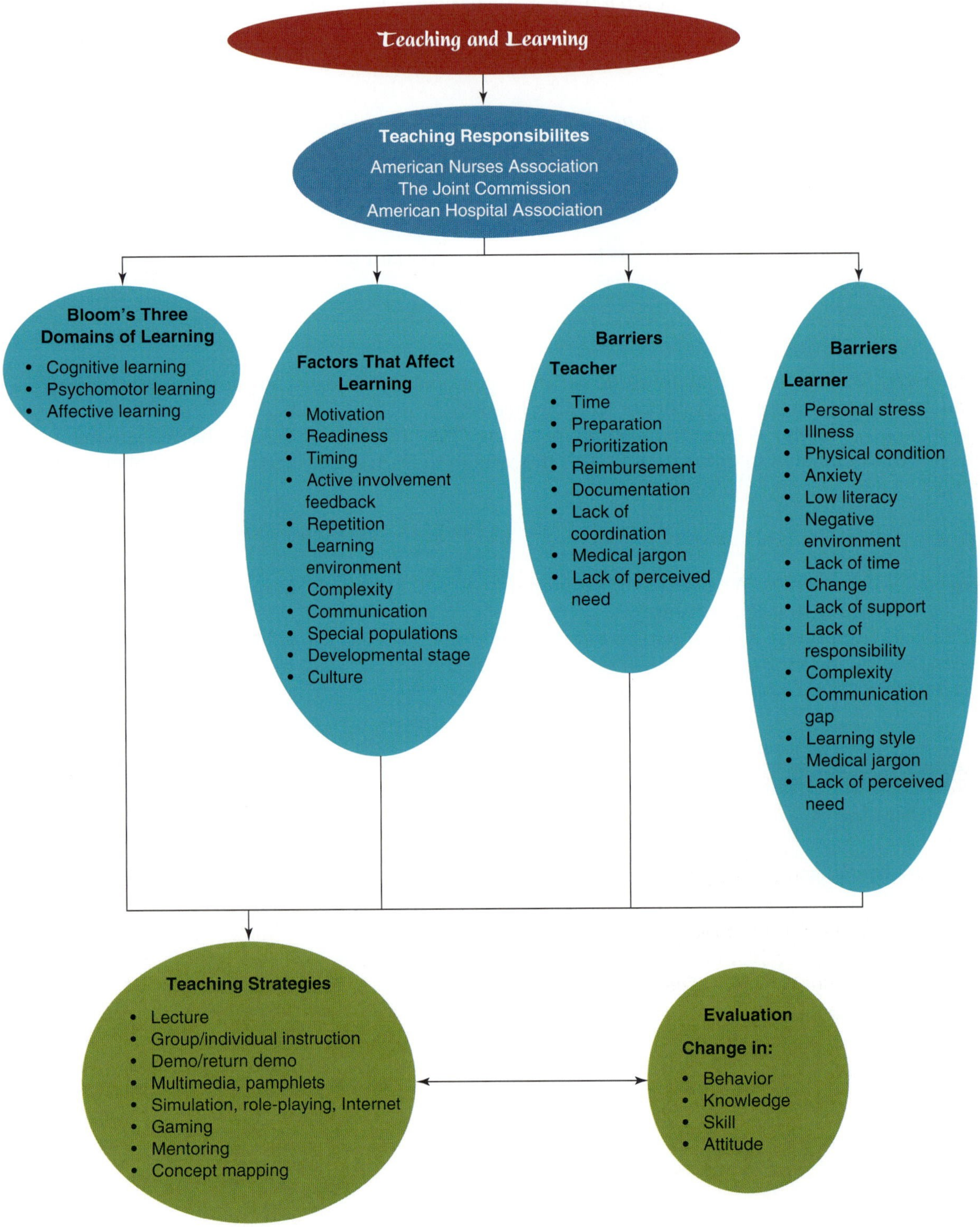

Teaching and Learning

Teaching Responsibilites

American Nurses Association
The Joint Commission
American Hospital Association

Bloom's Three Domains of Learning

- Cognitive learning
- Psychomotor learning
- Affective learning

Factors That Affect Learning

- Motivation
- Readiness
- Timing
- Active involvement feedback
- Repetition
- Learning environment
- Complexity
- Communication
- Special populations
- Developmental stage
- Culture

Barriers

Teacher

- Time
- Preparation
- Prioritization
- Reimbursement
- Documentation
- Lack of coordination
- Medical jargon
- Lack of perceived need

Barriers

Learner

- Personal stress
- Illness
- Physical condition
- Anxiety
- Low literacy
- Negative environment
- Lack of time
- Change
- Lack of support
- Lack of responsibility
- Complexity
- Communication gap
- Learning style
- Medical jargon
- Lack of perceived need

Teaching Strategies

- Lecture
- Group/individual instruction
- Demo/return demo
- Multimedia, pamphlets
- Simulation, role-playing, Internet
- Gaming
- Mentoring
- Concept mapping

Evaluation

Change in:

- Behavior
- Knowledge
- Skill
- Attitude

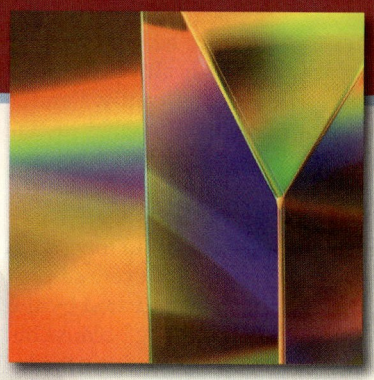

CHAPTER 27

Health Promotion

Learning Outcomes

After completing this chapter, you should be able to:

- ➤ Define *health, health promotion,* and *health protection.*
- ➤ Identify health prevention activities and categorize them as primary, secondary, or tertiary levels of prevention.
- ➤ Discuss the *Healthy People 2020* report in relation to leading causes of death and to health promotion strategies: nutrition, exercise, lifestyle, and environment.
- ➤ Apply Pender's Health Promotion Model to plan activities designed to change unhealthy behavior.
- ➤ Identify Prochaska and DiClemente's four stages of change.

- ➤ Identify specific health promotion strategies (including immunizations and screenings) across the life span.
- ➤ Discuss nurses' roles in health promotion and list health promotion activities that a nurse may conduct in acute care facilities, the workplace, local communities, and schools.
- ➤ Identify the areas of assessment in relation to developing a health promotion plan.
- ➤ Construct a health promotion plan of care using the nursing process, NANDA-I taxonomy, Nursing Outcomes Classifications, and Nursing Interventions Classifications.

Key Concepts

Health promotion
Health protection
Illness prevention
Wellness

Related Concepts

See the Concept Map at the end of this chapter.

Meet Your Peer

You are now enrolled in your first nursing course. In addition to classroom work, you spend a lot of time studying, preparing for clinical work, writing care plans, and completing follow-up assignments from clinical. You have other non-nursing course work and family responsibilities, as well. You usually get about 4 to 6 hours of sleep at night. By the end of the week, you're exhausted. You don't have time to cook so you pick up fast food several times a week. Even though it is not the healthiest choice, at least this way you can get something to eat. You have little time to exercise, and when you do have time, you feel too tired and uninterested. You use cigarettes to relax you and help you cope with stress. On the weekends, you let loose with friends,

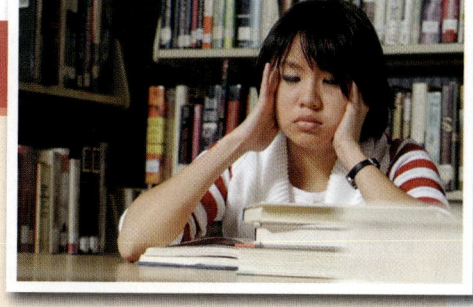

drinking beer and having a good time.

You spend most of your time learning about health and illness. Given your current lifestyle, do you consider yourself healthy? How did you make that decision? Your answer is based on your personal beliefs about health and what you have learned in your nursing course work. In this chapter, we explore health promotion. As you learn more about this topic, you may develop a plan to promote your own health as well as the health of clients.

Theoretical Knowledge
knowing **why**

To begin, we explore what others have written about the concepts. Various descriptions and definitions use the concepts health and wellness interchangeably, and we do the same in this chapter.

ABOUT THE KEY CONCEPTS

In Chapter 11, we considered the concepts of health, wellness, and illness. In this chapter, the emphasis is on strategies to support those concepts: **health promotion, health protection, illness prevention,** and **wellness.** As you study various concepts, such as health screening, role modeling, and health behaviors (to name a few examples), try to understand how they relate to the key concepts.

WHAT IS HEALTH PROMOTION?

To promote health, we must first identify what we mean by *health* and *wellness.* The following are some common descriptions of health:

World Health Organization The World Health Organization (WHO) defines health as "a state of complete physical, mental and social well-being and not merely the absence of disease or infirmity" (WHO, 1948). At the first conference for health promotion, WHO defined **health promotion** as the process of equipping people to have control over, and to improve, physical, emotional, and social health (WHO, 1986).

Jean Watson This nursing theorist proposed that health consists of three elements: (1) a high level of overall physical, mental, and social functioning; (2) a general adaptive-maintenance level of daily functioning; and (3) the absence of illness (or the presence of efforts that lead to its absence). She also refers to health as being a state of mind, the perception of the individual. A person may have a terminal illness and yet consider himself healthy (Watson, 1979).

Betty Neuman This nurse theorist describes health as an expression of living energy available to an individual. The energy is displayed as a continuum, with high energy (wellness) at one end and low energy (illness) at the opposite end. Individuals have varying levels of energy at various stages of life. When more energy is generated than expended, there is wellness. When more energy is expended than is generated, there is illness, possibly death (Neuman, 1995).

Myers, Sweeney, and Witmer In 2000, these theorists defined wellness as "a way of life oriented toward optimal health and well-being in which body, mind, and spirit are integrated by the individual to live more fully within the human and natural community" (p. 252). This definition includes lifestyles and habits as components of health and permits people who have been diagnosed with disease to be considered healthy.

Synthesis Applying aspects of these reflections on health, **health promotion** means finding ways to help individuals develop a state of physical, spiritual, and mental well-being. Health promotion activities are useful to all individuals, whether well or sick, because they encourage optimal function. How does this compare to the WHO definition of health promotion you read earlier?

Health Promotion Versus Health Protection

For the most part, the activities that promote health also protect health. Nevertheless, the ideas behind health promotion and health protection differ subtly but significantly. Pender and Murdaugh (2014) explain that motivation is what distinguishes the two activities.

- *Health promotion* is motivated by the desire to increase well-being.
- *Health protection* is motivated by a desire to avoid illness.

For instance, the 40-year-old who begins an exercise program to improve strength and endurance is motivated by the benefits of health promotion. If he starts exercising because his father died of a heart attack at age 50, he may be motivated by the need to protect his health.

Levels of Prevention

Leavell and Clark (1965) identified three levels of activities for health protection (illness prevention): primary, secondary, and tertiary. Interventions are classified according to where they occur in the disease process. This timing directs the types of interventions needed.

- **Primary prevention** activities are designed to prevent or slow the onset of disease. Examples include eating healthy foods, exercising, wearing sunscreen, obeying seat belt laws, and keeping up with immunizations.
- **Secondary prevention** involves screening activities and education for detecting illnesses in the early stages. Examples are breast self-examination, testicular exams, regular physical examinations, blood pressure and diabetes screenings, and tuberculosis skin tests.
- **Tertiary prevention** focuses on stopping the disease from progressing and returning the individual to the pre-illness phase. Rehabilitation is the main intervention during this level.

Patients and health providers move among these levels of prevention. For example, a patient hospitalized for a total hip replacement would receive the following:

- *Tertiary prevention* strategies focus on helping her recover from surgery, preventing complications of surgery, and, later on, helping her regain her strength and learn to walk again.
- *Secondary prevention* strategies may have been used previously, for example, to screen for osteoporosis that leads to bone fragility and fractures.
- *Primary prevention* strategies help her after she returns home, for example, limiting her salt intake and eating a balanced diet that is low in fat and refined sugar.

Health Behaviors

For the overall population, life expectancy (at birth) is 78.8 years, up from 75.4 years in 1990. The gap between men and women has narrowed from 7.0 years in 1990 to 4.8 years in 2013 (Centers for Disease Control and Prevention [CDC], 2016a). Health status is affected by health behavior.

Teen Pregnancy

Pregnant teenagers are less likely to receive early prenatal care. They are more likely to drop out of school and to live in poverty than are older pregnant women. The birth rate for teenagers aged 15 to 19 years dropped 9% from 2013, to 24.2%, a historic low for the United States (CDC, 2016b).

Abuse of Alcohol and Illicit Drugs

The risk of disease, injuries, and intentional death (suicide and homicide) increases with substance abuse.

- *Excessive alcohol use* increases the risk of harmful health conditions, such as injuries (motor vehicle crashes, falls, drowning), violence, alcohol poisoning, and risky sexual behavior. Over time, excessive alcohol use can lead to the development of chronic diseases. More than 88,000 deaths per year are attributable to alcohol misuse, which is the estimated third leading cause of preventable deaths in the United States. The U.S. Preventive Services Task Force (USPSTF) (2012) recommends that clinicians screen adults aged 18 years or older for alcohol misuse and provide persons engaged in risky or hazardous drinking with brief behavioral counseling interventions to reduce alcohol misuse. (Note: This guideline is under revision. Be sure you are using the latest version.)
- *Marijuana (cannabis)* is the most commonly used illicit drug in the United States. In 2013, an estimated 2.4 million persons aged 12 years and older had used marijuana for the first time. (Azofeifa, Mattson, Schauer, et al., 2016). Medical use of marijuana is now legal in several states. ✚ Substance abuse in adolescents is associated with a greater frequency of suicide attempts, more lethal (successful) attempts, an increased seriousness of intent, and greater suicidal ideation.

Tobacco Use

Cigarette smoking increases the risk of lung cancer, tuberculosis, heart disease, emphysema, and other diseases.

- The percentage of middle and high school students who reported smoking cigarettes in the past month was 7.4% and 25.3%, respectively (CDC, 2016c).
- Electronic cigarettes are the most commonly used products among middle (5.3%) and high school (16%) students
- Overall, the percentage of high school students and adults who reported using tobacco products remained stable at 20% to 23%, after declining from 36% in the previous decade.
- Men were more likely to be current cigarette smokers than women (24% compared with 18%) (CDC, 2010, updated 2013).
- The southern United States contains the highest percentage of tobacco users (CDC, 2010, updated 2013).
- Smoking as few as three cigarettes/day can increase the risk for cardiovascular disease and increase the risk of infections (pneumonia, active tuberculosis).

Obesity

The risk of heart disease, diabetes, and stroke increases with obesity.

- In 2011 to 2014, more than 17% of U.S. children and adolescents were obese. The prevalence of obesity was higher among adolescents than among preschool-age children. The same pattern was seen in both males and females (CDC, 2015).
- More than 36.5% of U.S. men and women were obese in 2011 to 2014. The prevalence of obesity among women (38.3%) was higher than among men (34.3%). Adults aged 60 years and over were more likely to be obese than were younger adults (CDC, 2015).

Sedentary Lifestyle

Exercise reduces the risk of disease and enhances mental and physical health. American adults have made little progress toward achieving recommended levels of physical activity or strength training. Between 2006 and 2015, the percentage of adults 18 years of age and over engaged in regular leisure-time physical activity or strength training activities increased from 41.4% to only 49.5%.

KnowledgeCheck 27-1

- How does health promotion differ from health protection?
- Which level of prevention is represented by the following activities?
  Mumps, measles, rubella (MMR) vaccination
  Tuberculosis (TB) skin test
  Physical therapy after repair of a hip fracture

Health Promotion Models

A model illustrates a system or framework to help explain what you see in clinical practice. The most common frameworks used for designing health promotion programs are described next.

Pender's Health Promotion Model

Pender's Health Promotion Model (HPM) (Fig. 27-1) identifies three groups of variables that affect health promotion: (1) individual characteristics and experiences, (2) behavior-specific cognitions and affect, and (3) behavioral outcome. The HPM is based on seven assumptions that reflect both nursing and behavioral science perspectives (Pender & Murdaugh, 2014). The first two general assumptions concern the interpersonal environment:

1. Health professionals constitute a part of the interpersonal environment, which exerts influence on persons throughout their life span.
2. Self-initiated reconfiguration of person–environment interactive patterns is essential to behavior change.

The next five assumptions are characteristics of people, whom the theorist assumes:

3. Seek to create conditions of living through which they can express their unique human health potential.
4. Have the capacity for reflective self-awareness, including assessment of their own competencies.
5. Value growth in directions viewed as positive and attempt to achieve a personally acceptable balance between change and stability.
6. Seek to actively regulate their own behavior.
7. Interact with the environment in all their biopsychosocial complexity, progressively transforming the environment and being transformed over time.

Pender's model has been used extensively in several disciplines in research and professional practice focused on health promotion. As a nurse, you should find Pender's focus applicable to your work.

ThinkLike a Nurse 27-1

- How might peers influence health behaviors? At what age might peers have more influence?
- Apply Pender's model to a person trying to lose weight. What might be some perceived barriers (see Fig. 27-1)?

Wheel of Wellness

Several authors have likened the different facets of health to the spokes of a wheel (Hettler, 1984; Myers, Sweeney, & Witmer, 2000; Witmer & Sweeney, 1992). If one of the spokes is weak, the whole wheel is weak. The "spokes" of the health

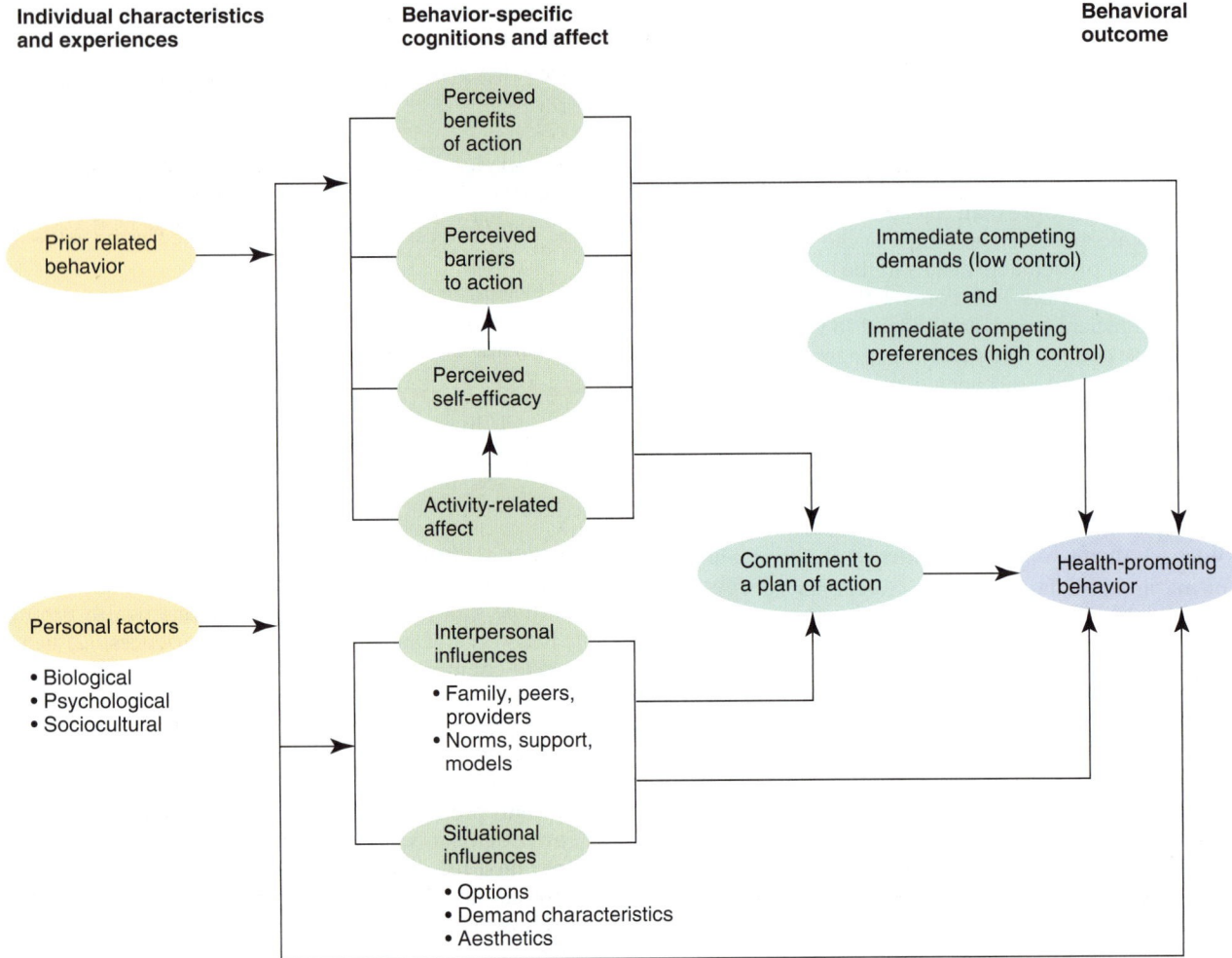

FIGURE 27-1 Pender's Health Promotion Model.

wheel represent the dimensions of health: emotional, intellectual, physical, spiritual, social/family, and occupational (Fig. 27-2). The level of wellness progresses from the center to the outer part of the wheel. The center represents the least amount of wellness, and the outer part represents optimal wellness. If one area of an individual's life is not functioning at optimal level, life will not be as fulfilling as it could be. As a nurse, you should assess each dimension for strengths and weaknesses.

Transtheoretical Model of Change

The Transtheoretical Model of Change (Prochaska & DiClemente, 1982) may serve to alter unhealthy behaviors. Health promotion and protection involve either changing the individual's response to the illness-producing stimuli or changing the environment so that the person will be less likely to encounter illness-producing stimuli. Either idea involves change. The Prochaska and DiClemente model identified four stages of change: Stages 2 through 5, in which change is occurring and Stages 1 and 6 that preceded and followed the stages of change.

Stage 1   In the **precontemplation** stage there is no intention to change behavior in the foreseeable future, because patients are unaware or underaware of their problems. They do not yet contemplate change.

Stage 2   **Contemplation**—Patients are seriously thinking about overcoming a problem but have not yet made a commitment to take action.

Stage 3   **Preparation**—Individuals are intending to take action in the next month and are reporting some small behavioral changes ("baby steps").

Stage 4   **Action**—The plan is implemented; this requires considerable **commitment** of time and energy.

Stage 5   **Maintenance**—Individuals are working to prevent relapse and they grow increasingly more confident that the change can be sustained.

Stage 6   The **termination** stage completes the maintenance. Persons who enter into the termination stage have changed the behavior and are not in danger of relapse.

Ideally, the stages would progress in this order. Realistically, a person may progress and regress in any of the stages. The change process in persons with some unhealthy habits (e.g., cigarette smoking, substance abuse, excessive eating) may best be described as a revolving door. An individual may exit at any point as the door goes around. If the exit occurs during or at the end of the maintenance period, the behavioral change is successful. If the exit occurs before the end of the

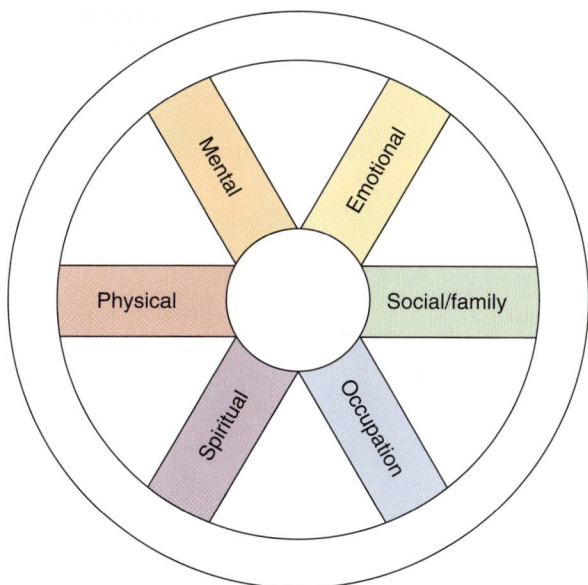

FIGURE 27-2 Wheel of Wellness.

maintenance period, relapse will occur, and the individual will return to the previous lifestyle.

Health Promotion Programs

Health promotion programs help a person advance toward optimal health. In the sections that follow we discuss several program types.

Disseminating Information To recognize a problem and understand the options for change, people need information. Information may be disseminated at three levels, as illustrated in the following examples:

- Individual level—Teaching a client how to modify his personal dietary intake
- Group level—Classes offered at the local hospital, prenatal education programs, and worksite programs
- Community level—A billboard that presents the dangers of smoking, health blogs on the Internet, and health fairs

Changing Lifestyle and Behavior These are group-level programs that provide information and offer support for activities such as weight loss, smoking cessation, exercise, nutrition, and stress management. Some include a maintenance program to help sustain the change.

Protecting the Environment Environmental control programs promote health by focusing on air and water quality, toxic waste, healthy homes and communities, infrastructure and surveillance, and global environmental health.

Assessing Wellness and Appraising Health Risk A **wellness assessment** tends to focus on the healthy behaviors. It supports positive change to improve health. A **health risk appraisal** identifies risky behaviors that promote disease. These tools are available on the Internet, in magazines, and at fitness centers.

KnowledgeCheck 27-2

- What are the six dimensions of health represented by the spokes on the wellness wheel?
- Identify the stages of change identified by Prochaska and DiClemente.
- Describe the four main types of health promotion programs.

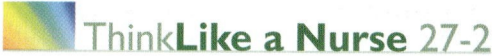

ThinkLike a Nurse 27-2

J.T. drinks a vodka and tonic while eating lunch with his coworkers. He keeps a bottle of vodka in his office desk for use during the day. Later, he stops at a local bar for a drink on the way home. At home, he drinks a six-pack of beer while watching the game. What information do you need to determine which of Prochaska and DiClemente's stages of change he is experiencing? How would you find this information?

Settings for Health Promotion Programs The most common sites for health promotion programs are health facilities, worksites, and schools.

- In *healthcare settings,* each interaction between patient and healthcare provider is an opportunity for health promotion. Unfortunately, most interactions focus on the disease process and compliance with treatments. You will need to make a conscious effort to help clients focus on behaviors that prevent illness and promote health.
- Nurses work in *health clinics within large companies* may be contracted to provide specific health promotion programs, such as smoking cessation, stress management, weight reduction, and fitness training. Employers have found that health programs decrease work-related injuries and sick leave.
- *Local school districts* are another setting for health promotion. Health learning can begin at an early age, and nurses and teachers can regularly reinforce healthy behaviors and redirect unhealthy behaviors. Schools provide a setting that allows for continued exposure to information. Interventions may be directed at general health promotion issues, such as physical activity, or they may focus on specific health risks, such as tobacco and alcohol use. School nurses work closely with teachers and parents to provide health promotion services in the schools.

Health Promotion Throughout the Life Span

Health promotion is a lifelong process that begins at conception. Table 27-1 describes the focus of health promotion programs at each developmental stage as well the types of screenings recommended for each age-group.

♥ iCare 27-1

Health Promotion

An effective way for you to promote health and wellness to your patients is to be a role model and engage in healthy behaviors yourself.

- Strive to maintain a healthy BMI. Patients are more apt to listen to your counseling about the importance of a normal BMI if you are a good role model.
- Do not smoke.
- Limit alcohol consumption.
- Exercise or engage in other stress-relieving activities such as yoga/meditation.
- Eat a well-balanced diet.
- Get enough sleep/rest.
- Maintain a healthy work/life balance.
- Practice preventive medicine (e.g., keep current with health appointments and screenings, annual physicals, dental appointments, and eye exams).

Table 27-1 ➤ Health Promotion Throughout the Life Span

Conception to Birth

Health Promotion Focus	**Health Screening**
Education about pregnancy	Alpha-fetoprotein level screening for gestational diabetes
Abstinence from alcohol, cigarettes, and illicit drugs	Prenatal care
Nutrition, including folic acid and iron requirements	Abuse
Exercise to maintain strength and muscle tone and to control weight gain	Additional screenings that may be offered:
Parenting education	• Ultrasound
	• Amniocentesis
	• Chorionic villus sampling

Infancy

Health Promotion Focus	**Health Screening**
Nutrition (breast vs. bottle)	Hearing evaluation
Introduction of solid foods	Screening for birth defects
Placing the infant on her back for sleep without a pillow to reduce the risk of sudden infant death	Blood work to rule out certain metabolic conditions
Sensory stimulation	Monthly examinations until at least 6 mo of age
Safety	After age 6 mo, visits every 2 or 3 mo
Motor vehicle safety	Growth and development
Oral health	Abuse

Toddler and Preschooler

Health Promotion Focus	**Health Screening**
Adequate supervision	Annual examinations
Safety, including storage of poisons	Growth and development
Toilet training	Cognitive skills
Motor vehicle safety	Abuse
Nutrition	Kindergarten readiness
Immunizations	
Oral health	
Sleep and rest	

School Age

Health Promotion Focus	**Health Screening**
Nutrition	Annual examinations
Physical activity	Growth and development
Safety	Cognitive skills
Sexuality	Abuse
Stranger danger	
Oral health	

Adolescence

Health Promotion Focus	**Health Screening**
Peer pressure	Growth and development
Motor vehicle safety	Sexually transmitted infection (STI) screening
Safety	Breast self-exam (BSE) (optional)

Table 27-1 ▶ Health Promotion Throughout the Life Span—cont'd

Self-esteem	Testicular self-exam (TSE) (optional)
Physical activity	Mental health
Suicide and depression	Stress
Firearm safety	Alcohol and drug use
Violence	Abuse
Sexuality	
Substance use and abuse	
Limiting sun exposure	
Update of immunizations	
Oral health	

Young Adult

Health Promotion Focus	**Health Screening**
Physical activity	Comprehensive exam at least every 3 yr
Motor vehicle safety	Lifestyle
Safety	Pap smear
Violence	STI screening
Sexuality	BSE
Substance use and abuse	TSE
Limiting sun exposure	Mental health
Update immunizations	Stress
Oral health	Alcohol and drug use
	Abuse

Middle Adult

Health Promotion Focus	**Health Screening**
Physical activity	Comprehensive exam at least every 3 yr to age 40, yearly after age 40
Safety	Blood pressure (BP) screening
Obesity	Lipid panel
Sexuality	Blood glucose
Lifestyle	Stress
Update of immunizations	Mammograms or thermography
Oral health	Digital rectal exam (DRE) for rectal polyps or prostate evaluation in men
Substance use and abuse	Prostate-specific antigen (PSA) for men
	Annual eye exam
	Sigmoidoscopy or colonoscopy
	Stool for occult blood with comprehensive exam
	Bone density
	Abuse

(Continued)

Table 27-1 ➤ Health Promotion Throughout the Life Span—cont'd	
Older Adult	
Health Promotion Focus	*Health Screening*
	Functional skills (activities of daily living [ADLs] and instrumental activities of daily living [IADLs])
Physical activity	
Nutrition	Hearing
Safety	Falls risk
Obesity	Stress
Sexuality	Eye exam and glaucoma screen
Lifestyle	BP screening
Update of immunizations	Lipid panel
Oral health	Blood glucose
	Mammograms
	DRE for prostate evaluation in men
	PSA for men who have a life expectancy of at least 10 yr
	Stool for occult blood
	Bone density
	Follow-up sigmoidoscopy or colonoscopy
	Mental health
	Abuse

Practical Knowledge
knowing **how**

Pender and Murdaugh (2014) summarized the health promotion process as a series of nine steps that involve the client and the nurse. Notice that many steps of this process are similar to the nursing process:

1. Review and summarize data from assessment.
2. Reinforce the client's strengths and abilities.
3. Identify health goals and related behavioral change options.
4. Identify behavioral or health outcomes that will indicate that the plan has been successful from the client's perspective.
5. Develop a behavior change plan based on the client's preferences, on the stages of change, and on "state-of-the-science" knowledge about effective interventions.
6. Reiterate benefits of change and identify incentives for change from the client's perspective.
7. Address environmental and interpersonal facilitators and barriers to behavior change.
8. Determine a time frame for implementation.
9. Commit to behavior-change goals, and structure the support needed to accomplish them.

ASSESSMENT NP

A health promotion assessment involves obtaining a health history, physical examination, fitness assessment, lifestyle and risk appraisal, life stress review, analysis of health beliefs, nutritional assessment, and screening activities.

History and Physical Examination

Assessment should begin with a thorough health history, review of body systems, and a physical examination.

- **Health History.** Ask the client about family history of health disorders and cause of death of family members. Keep in mind that the accuracy of reporting is higher for relatives without, rather than those affected by, a given disease (Qureshi, Wilson, Santaguida, et al., 2009). Gather the history directly from the client. As always, provide privacy and comfort while conducting the history and exam.
- **Physical Examination.** The level of detail of the physical examination depends on the health history. At a minimum, the exam should include vital signs, weight, body mass index (BMI) or waist circumference, auscultation and palpation of the chest and abdomen, inspection of the skin, and palpation of peripheral pulses.
- **Laboratory Studies.** Recommended lab work depends on the history and exam findings. For most adult clients, a screening lab consists of a complete blood count, comprehensive metabolic panel (also known as a chem 20 panel), lipid panel, thyroid function panel, and urinalysis (American College of Sports Medicine [ACSM], 2013).
- **Disease-Specific Studies.** In clients with known cardiac or pulmonary disease, additional disease-specific studies may be performed (e.g., electrocardiogram, carotid ultrasound, or pulmonary function tests).

Physical Fitness Assessment

A physical fitness assessment includes the following:

- *Cardiorespiratory fitness* is reflected in the ability to perform large-muscle, moderate- to high-intensity exercise for prolonged periods of time (ACSM, 2013). There are many different modes of testing, such as field tests (walking or running), treadmills, stationary bicycles, and step testing. Results depend on age and gender.

- *Muscular fitness* refers to both muscle strength and endurance. Muscle strength is a measure of the amount of weight a muscle (or group of muscles) can move at one time. Muscle endurance refers to the ability of a muscle to perform repeated movements.

- *Flexibility* is the ability to move a joint through its range of motion. The most common assessment is to evaluate low back and hip (trunk) flexion.

  For information and guidelines for assessing physical fitness (cardiorespiratory, muscular, and flexibility), see the Focused Assessment box Health Promotion: Physical Fitness Assessment.

Health Promotion: Physical Fitness Assessment

Cardiorespiratory Fitness

There are many modes of testing, such as field tests (walking or running), motor-driven treadmills, stationary bicycles, and step testing.

➤ **Field tests** for running are good for children. A 9-year-old child should be able to complete a 1-mile run in approximately 10 minutes, and a 17-year-old boy should be able to complete a 1-mile run in approximately 7½ minutes (http://www.presidentschallenge.org).

➤ The **step test** is appropriate for most adults. Using a 12-inch bench, instruct the participant to step up and down at a rate of 24 steps per minute for 3 minutes. At the end of 3 minutes, he should check his heart rate. Stop testing immediately if the participant experiences any chest pain, shortness of breath, or light-headedness. Results depend on age and gender and are available below.

Step Test Evaluation Charts

3-Minute Step Heart Rate Test (Men)

Physical Condition	18–25 yr	26–35 yr	36–45 yr	46–55 yr	56–65 yr	65+ yr
Excellent	< 79	< 81	< 83	< 87	< 86	< 88
Good	79–89	81–89	83–96	87–97	86–97	88–96
Above average	90–99	90–99	97–103	98–105	98–103	97–103
Average	100–105	100–107	104–112	106–116	104–112	104–113
Below average	106–116	108–117	113–119	117–122	113–120	114–120
Poor	117–128	118–128	120–130	123–132	121–129	121–130
Very poor	> 128	> 128	> 130	> 132	> 129	> 130

3-Minute Step Heart Rate Test (Women)

Physical Condition	18–25 yr	26–35 yr	36–45 yr	46–55 yr	56–65 yr	65+ yr
Excellent	< 85	< 88	< 90	< 94	< 95	< 90
Good	85–98	88–99	90–102	94–104	95–104	90–102
Above average	99–108	100–111	103–110	105–115	105–112	103–115
Average	109–117	112–119	111–118	116–120	113–118	116–122
Below average	118–126	120–126	119–128	121–129	119–128	123–128
Poor	127–140	127–138	129–140	130–135	129–139	129–134
Very poor	> 140	> 138	> 140	> 135	> 139	> 134

Muscular Fitness

➤ **Muscle strength** is recorded as a ratio of weight pushed (or lifted) divided by body weight. For example, a woman weighing 150 pounds who is able to lift 86 pounds will have a ratio of 86 divided by 150, or 0.57.
  ➤ Instruct the participant warm up and stretch before the test. Weight benches are ideal sites for testing upper body and leg strength.

➤ Compare the ratio obtained to normative standards or to previous personal scores to evaluate improvement.

➤ **Muscle endurance** is evaluated by the push-up or curl-up (crunch) test. Ask the participant to perform as many push-ups or curl-ups as possible without pausing.
  ➤ The number of repetitions is the score. Once again, compare scores to norms or previous performance.

(Continued)

Health Promotion: Physical Fitness Assessment—cont'd

Flexibility

The **sit-and-reach test** evaluates low back and hip (trunk) flexion.

➤ Ask the participant sit on a floor mat with legs fully extended and feet flat against a box. Have her extend her arms and hands forward as far as possible and hold for a count of 3.

➤ Using a ruler, measure the distance in inches that the client can reach beyond the proximal edge of the box. If the

client cannot reach the edge, measure the distance of the fingertips from the edge, and report it as a negative number.

➤ Norms for trunk flexion vary among men and women. The desired range for men is +1 to +5 inches and for women it is +2 to +6 inches (Pender & Murdaugh, 2014).

Lifestyle and Risk Appraisal

Lifestyle refers to the manner in which a person conducts his life: physically, emotionally, spiritually, and mentally. Lifestyle includes all of the activities that promote optimal living, such as taking responsibility for one's health, physical activity, nutrition, interpersonal relations, spiritual growth, and stress

management. You can gather this information by interview or by using a variety of questionnaires. A **health risk appraisal (HRA)** is a questionnaire that evaluates risk for disease based on current demographic data, lifestyle, and health behaviors. There are many HRA tools available; many are online. See the Focused Assessment box Lifestyle and Risk Assessment.

Lifestyle and Risk Assessment

The following is an example of an HRA.

Name _____   Age _____   Gender _____

Health View

In general, would you say your present health is?
☐ Excellent   ☐ Good   ☐ Fair
☐ Very good   ☐ Poor

General Practices

1. **Physical activity.** How many days each week do you get at least 30 minutes of physical activity, such as brisk walking, cycling, active gardening, active dance, swimming, jogging, or active sports? _____
2. **Strength exercises.** How many days each week do you do strength-building exercises, such as weight lifting or isometric exercises? _____
3. **Smoking status.** Indicate your present smoking status.
   ☐ Current smoker   ☐ Ex-smoker
   ☐ Nonsmoker, never smoked regularly.
   Environmental smoke. Do you live with or work with smokers and breathe second-hand smoke regularly?
   ☐ Yes   ☐ No
4. **Alcohol.** How many drinks do you typically have on a day you drink? *One drink is a bottle or can of beer (12 oz), a glass of wine or wine cooler (3.5 oz), or a shot glass of liquor (1.5 oz).*
   ☐ Never drink.
   ☐ Have no more than one drink in a day.
   ☐ Have no more than two drinks in a day.
   ☐ Sometimes have three or four drinks in a day.
   ☐ Sometimes have five or more drinks in a day.
5. **Sleep.** How many hours of sleep do you usually get each night? _____

Eating Practices

6. **Breakfast.** How many days each week do you usually eat breakfast (more than just coffee and a roll)? _____
7. **Bread/grains.** How many servings of whole-grain breads and cereals do you eat daily? *One serving =1 slice bread, $^1/_2$ cup dry cereal, $^1/_2$ cup cooked oatmeal or other whole-grain cereal or brown rice.* _____
8. **Fruits and vegetables.** How many servings of fruits and vegetables do you eat daily? *One serving =1 medium fruit, 6 oz fruit or vegetable juice, 1 cup raw fruit or vegetables, $^1/_2$ cup cooked fruit or vegetables.* _____
9. **High-fat and high-cholesterol foods.** How often do you eat foods high in saturated fat and cholesterol (e.g., steak, hamburger, hot dog, sausage, bacon, cheese, fried chicken, French fries, ice cream, cheesecake, or other desserts)?
   ☐ Daily
   ☐ Eat these foods three or more times a week.
   ☐ Seldom or never eat these foods.
10. **Nuts/seeds.** How many servings of nuts do you usually eat each week? *One serving = 1 oz or a small handful, or 2 tablespoons of natural nut butter.* _____
11. **Legumes.** How many times a week do you eat legumes (peas, beans, lentils, garbanzos)? *One serving = $^1/_2$ cup cooked.* _____
12. **Refined foods.** How often do you eat highly refined foods (soda pop, snack foods, chips, refined cereals, pastry, candy)?
    ☐ Daily
    ☐ Eat these foods three or more times a week.
    ☐ Seldom or never eat refined foods.
13. **Weight.** How many pounds have you gained since you were 21 to 24? (Enter 0 if you weigh the same, weigh less, or are younger than 21 years.) _____

Lifestyle and Risk Assessment—cont'd

14. **Water intake.** How many glasses (8 oz) of water do you typically drink each day? _____

Mental/Social Health

15. **Happiness.** How happy have you been during the last month?
    - ☐ Very happy
    - ☐ Pretty happy
    - ☐ Not too happy
    - ☐ Very unhappy
16. **Mood/feelings**
    (a) During the past month, have you often been bothered by feeling down, depressed, or hopeless?
    - ☐ Yes   ☐ No
    (b) During the past month, have you often been bothered by having little interest or pleasure in doing things?
    - ☐ Yes   ☐ No
    (c) Have your feelings in the past month caused you significant distress or impaired your ability to function socially or at work (or school)?
    - ☐ Yes   ☐ No
17. **Stress and coping.** How much of the time do you feel stressed out and unable to cope with life?
    - ☐ Seldom or never
    - ☐ Occasionally
    - ☐ Much of the time
    - ☐ Most of the time

Social Support

18. **Support.** Do you have family or friends you can get help from if needed?
    - ☐ Yes   ☐ No
19. **Social Interaction.** Do you have frequent social contact with family or friends?
    - ☐ Yes   ☐ No

Community

20. **Community support.** Do you meet regularly with a faith community or other group that gives you support, comfort, meaning, and direction in your life?
    - ☐ Yes   ☐ No

Safety

21. **Seat belts.** What percentage of the time do you wear seat belts when riding in a car? _____
22. **Smoke alarm.** Do you have a working smoke alarm on each floor of your home, including the area in which you sleep?
    - ☐ Yes   ☐ No   ☐ Don't know for sure.
23. **Helmet.** When biking or rollerblading, do you always wear a helmet and protective gear?
    - ☐ Yes   ☐ No
24. **Substance use and driving.** Do you ever drive soon after drinking alcohol or taking drugs or ride with someone who has been using illicit substances or alcohol?
    - ☐ Yes   ☐ No

Safer Sex

25. **Practice safer sex.**
    (a) Are you in a monogamous relationship?
    - ☐ Yes   ☐ No
    (b) Do you always use condoms, or abstain from sexual relations?
    - ☐ Always   ☐ Don't always practice safer sex.

Preventive Exams

26. Do you keep current on recommended preventive exams (see list below) and immunizations?
    - ☐ Yes   ☐ No   ☐ Don't know for sure.

Recommended Preventive Exams
- ➤ Periodic checkup, including blood pressure, height and weight, and cholesterol check as recommended by your doctor.
- ➤ Pap tests within last years, for women 21 or older.
- ➤ Mammogram within last 2 years, for women 45 or older.
- ➤ Colorectal cancer screening for all persons 50 or older.
- ➤ Prostate exam, for men 50 or older.
- ➤ Flu immunization, for everyone 6 months and older.
- ➤ Pneumonia immunizations, for everyone 65 or olde.r

Height _____
Weight _____
Blood pressure _____
Blood cholesterol _____ (mg/dL)

(Continued)

Lifestyle and Risk Assessment—cont'd

——————————————————————— Scoring ———————————————————————

Your score is the number of good health indicators you meet out of the 17 possible listed (below) in this assessment. The higher your score, the healthier your lifestyle. The Average Health Style Score is 9.4

Health Indicator	Guidelines for Good Health
1. Physical activity	Get 30 or more minutes of physical activity most days of the week.
2. Strength training	Do strength-building exercises at least twice per week.
3. Not smoking	Avoid all tobacco use and frequent exposure to secondhand smoke.
4. Alcohol use	Alcohol is not recommended, but if you drink alcohol, limit to one to two drinks in a day.
5. Adequate rest	Get adequate rest, at least 7 to 8 hours of sleep daily for best health.
6. Breakfast daily	Eat a nutritious breakfast daily for optimal physical and mental performance.
7. Whole grains	Choose whole-grain breads and cereals, at least three or more servings/per day.
8. Fruits and vegetables	Eat at least five servings of fruits and vegetables daily.
9. Fats, cholesterol	Limit high-fat meats, whole milk, and butter. Vegetable oils are healthier than oils from animals.
10. Nuts and legumes	Nuts, such as almonds, contain healthy fats and protect against heart disease. Legumes prevent carbohydrate cravings, prevent metabolic syndrome, provide protein and energy, protect against cancer, and are a source of calcium and other vitamins and minerals.
11. Healthy weight	Maintain a healthy weight by eating well and participating in regular, moderate-intensity physical activity.
12. Mental health	Develop effective coping skills and maintain a happy, hopeful outlook.
13. Social support	Maintain good social support and frequent contact with family and friends.
14. Community	Participate regularly in a faith community or other group that provides meaning, direction, and support in your life.
15. Safety	Be safety conscious; wear safety belts in the car and helmets when biking.
16. Safer sex	Remain in a monogamous relationship, or always use condoms, or abstain.
17. Regular exams	Get regular exams, including age/gender-recommended preventive exams.

Source: Adapted from Hall, D. R. (2004). *Lifestyle check assessment.* Vanderbilt University Health and Wellness. Retrieved from http://www.vanderbilt.edu/nursing/kwallston/mhlcforma.htm

 ## ThinkLike a Nurse 27-3

- Evaluate your own compliance with recommended health screenings for your age-group. What activities should you incorporate into your own health promotion plan?
- Answer the questions in the Lifestyle and Risk Assessment. How did you score? What additional activities should be added to your health promotion plan?

Life Stress Review

In 1976, Hans Selye proposed that stress triggers physiological responses that may, over time, induce illness.

Stressful Life Change Events Likewise, Richard Rahe (1974) identified some stress-inducing life change events and researched their possible effects on health. Rahe discovered that a high score on a life-change event scale is associated with a greater likelihood of a negative health change—that is, the more stressful life change events a person has, the more likely he is to experience a disruption in health. To see and use a life-change event scale,

 Go to the American Institute of Stress Web site at http://www.stress.org/holmes-rahe-stress-inventory/.

Alternatively, you might want to interview your patient to assess the following:
- His belief in his ability to control the experience (e.g., an impending decision, an illness)
- How deeply involved he is in the activity that is producing stress (i.e., is it something he can change, or wants to change?)

- Whether he is able to view such a change as a challenge to grow

Daily Stresses Other researchers have focused on daily stresses and their effects on actual health or on one's perception of health. Daily stresses involve travel to and from work, taking children to activities, daily chores, waiting in lines at shops, raising teenagers, and traffic jams. Researchers have found these stresses may gradually erode one's coping mechanisms, producing an inability to cope with daily events and an increased likelihood of illness.

Hardiness Research has also demonstrated that in the face of life events, some people develop hardiness rather than vulnerability (Abdollahi, Talib, Carlbring, et al., 2016; Steptoe, Deaton, & Stone, 2015). Kobasa (1979) identified **hardiness** as a quality in which an individual experiences high levels of stress yet does not fall ill. There are three general characteristics of the hardy person:
- **Control**—belief in the ability to control the experience
- **Commitment**—feeling deeply involved in the activity producing stress
- **Challenge**—ability to view the change as a challenge to grow

If you need additional information on hardiness, review Chapter 11.

ThinkLike a Nurse 27-4

- Undoubtedly you are experiencing stress as a student in a nursing program. How would you rate your level of hardiness?
- What statements would demonstrate a hardy personality in each area (commitment, control, challenge)?

Health Beliefs

A health promotion assessment would not be complete without investigating an individual's health beliefs. Health beliefs are embedded in one's culture and personal experiences. Culture influences beliefs and practices affecting wellness and disease prevention. For example, some people may use certain foods (e.g., garlic to prevent heart disease, orange juice to prevent a cold) or herbs to protect or restore health. Why do you think it is important for you to respect cultural and religious views while working with clients to adopt personal health goals?

Locus of Control It will be helpful to know whether health outcomes are a result of actions the person takes, actions of powerful others, or chance. The Multidimensional Health Locus of Control scale (MHLC) helps you obtain this information (Wallston, Wallston, & DeVellis, 1978, modified 2007). The MHLC measures the person's perception of the extent of control from each source. The person rates her level of agreement with statements such as "I am in control of my health," "No matter what I do, if I am going to get sick, I will get sick," and "Regarding my health, I can only do what my doctor tells me to do."

Identifying a patient's locus of control is of practical importance for several reasons:

- People who feel powerless about preventing illness are least likely to engage in health promotion activities.
- People who respond to direction from respected authorities often prefer a health promotion program that is supervised by a healthcare provider.
- Clients who feel in charge of their own health are the easiest to motivate toward positive change.

You can find a copy of the MHLC to print out and use with your patients if you

 Go to the Vanderbilt University Web site at http://www.vanderbilt.edu/nursing/kwallston/mhlcforma.htm

or do a Web search for "Multidimensional Health Locus of Control scale."

Nutritional Assessment

A nutritional assessment is a key component of an overall wellness assessment. Unhealthy eating habits occur across all ages, ethnicities, and socioeconomic classes. Assessment involves an evaluation of typical eating patterns correlated with physical examination findings and BMI. Body composition is important in identifying health risks. The usual methods for determining body fat composition clinically are by measuring height, weight, circumferences, and skinfolds (Chapter 28).

The pattern of body fat distribution is an important predictor of health risks. People with fat stored around the trunk and abdominal area have a higher incidence of metabolic syndrome, hypertension, hyperlipidemia, heart disease, type 2 diabetes, and premature death than do those who have the fat stored in the extremities (Ashwell & Gibson, 2016).

Health Screening Activities

Health screening activities are secondary prevention activities designed to diagnose specific diseases at an early stage so that treatment can begin before the disease can spread or become debilitating. Many of these screening activities are part of your usual care. For example, each time you check a client's blood pressure, you are performing a screen for hypertension. Table 27-1 identifies the typical health screening activities with each developmental stage. With regard to health screening guidelines, clinicians must take all of the following into consideration when they decide which screening tests to offer to their patients:

1. Different agencies and groups generate different guidelines for type and frequency of screening. For example, the American Cancer Society has different Pap screening recommendations than does the U.S. Preventive Services Task Force; the American Congress of Obstetricians and Gynecologists may have yet another recommendation.

2. Most evidence-based guidelines make use of cost-benefit analysis to arrive at their recommendations.

3. Various third-party payors have different policies regarding the type and frequency of screening for which they will reimburse.

4. Guidelines and recommendations change often.

Lipid Screening Guidelines

- Adults aged 20 years or older—Have a fasting lipid panel at least once every 5 years. If total cholesterol is 200 mg/dL or greater—or high-density lipoprotein is less than 40 mg/dL—then frequent monitoring is required.
- Children aged 9 to 11 years—Universal screening is recommended, regardless of risk factors for cardiovascular disease (National Guideline Clearinghouse [NGC], 2011).
- Children aged 2 to 8 years—Screening is recommended if a parent, grandparent, aunt/uncle, or sibling has a history of myocardial infarction, angina, stroke, coronary artery bypass graft/stent/angioplasty, or hyperlipidemia (NGC, 2011).

Dental Health Screening Clients should have regular dental checkups to detect early signs of oral health problems such as tooth decay, gingivitis (gum disease), and oral cancers.

Colon Cancer Screening Both men and women should have a fecal occult blood test using a multiple stool take-home test every year beginning at age 50 and a screening colonoscopy based on risk factors. If there is a strong family history of colorectal cancer or polyps, screening should begin at an earlier age and be conducted more frequently (American Cancer Society, 2013a).

Breast Cancer Screening All women should be familiar with how their breasts normally look and feel and report any changes to a healthcare provider right away. Although research does not show a clear benefit for physical breast exams done by either a health professional or by patients for breast cancer screening (ACS, 2016; American Academy of Family Physicians, 2016b), women should be encouraged to discuss the risks and benefits of breast self-examination (BSE) and clinical breast exam with their healthcare provider. **KEY POINT:** *Beginning at age 45 years, women at average risk for breast cancer should have the choice to start annual breast cancer screening with mammograms (American Cancer Society, 2016; Nelson, 2015; NGC, 2016).*

Cervical Cancer Screening A Papanicolaou (Pap) smear is used to detect cellular changes in the cervix.

- *All women* should begin cervical cancer screening at age 21.
- *Women between the ages of 21 and 29* should have a Pap test every 3 years. They should not be tested for human papillomavirus (HPV) unless it is needed after an abnormal Pap test result.
- *Women between the ages of 30 and 65* should have both a Pap test and an HPV test every 5 years. This is the preferred approach, but it is also okay to have a Pap test alone every 3 years.
- *Women older than age 65* who have had regular screenings with normal results should not be screened for cervical cancer. Women who have been diagnosed with cervical pre-cancer should continue to be screened (American Cancer Society, 2013a; NGC, 2005; Smith, Manassaram-Baptiste, Brooks, et al., 2015).

Testicular Cancer Screening In spite of the low prevalence of testicular cancer, men should be aware that a lump in the testicle or a feeling of heaviness or swelling in the scrotum could be a sign of testicular cancer and should report these findings to their healthcare provider immediately (American Cancer Society, 2012).

Prostate Cancer Screening The U.S. Preventive Services Task Force (USPSTF) recommends against routine prostate-specific antigen (PSA)-based screening for prostate cancer but understands that some patients may request testing. PSA screening should be done only if it includes shared decision making that enables an informed choice by patients. However, healthcare professionals may consider offering the PSA and digital rectal exam (DRE) yearly to men age 50 years and older at risk for prostate cancer and with at least a 10-year life expectancy. If there are risk factors, testing should begin at age 40 to 45 years (American Cancer Society, 2013a).

Skin Cancer Screening Screen during any health assessment or a specialized dermatological exam.

- A general survey of the skin using the ABCD criteria is a useful approach for assessing for skin malignancy: **A**symmetry, **B**order irregularity, **C**olor variability, **D**iameter greater than 6 mm.
- Rapidly changing lesions are also associated with an increased risk for cancer.

- Any suspicious lesions should be biopsied (Agency for Healthcare Research and Quality, 2014; National Cancer Institute, 2016).

KnowledgeCheck 27-3

- Identify at least three common sites for health promotion activities.
- What assessments are part of a health promotion assessment?
- What role does stress play in health promotion?

 ThinkLike a Nurse 27-5

Your 55-year-old aunt tells you she hasn't had a physical examination in 20 years. She is a registered nurse. "I don't need one because I feel fine and I can take care of myself." How would you respond?

ANALYSIS/NURSING DIAGNOSIS NP

A **health promotion diagnosis** is a clinical judgment about a individual's, family's, group's, or community's motivation and desire to increase well being and to actualize health potential. Such motivation and desire are expressed by readiness to enhance specific health behaviors. The diagnosis can be used

---

Toward Evidence-Based Practice

Cooley, M. E., Finn, K. T., Wang, Q., et al. (2013). **Health behaviors, readiness to change, and interest in health promotion programs among smokers with lung cancer and their family members: A pilot study.** *Cancer Nursing, 36*(2), 145–154.

Data were collected once from 37 lung cancer patient–family member dyads. Lung cancer patients and their family members had high rates of continued smoking, low intake of fruits and vegetables, and high rates of physical inactivity. Patients and family members indicated readiness to change behaviors within the next 6 months and interest in participating in a behavioral risk reduction program.

Hoffman, A. J., Brintnall, R. A., Brown, J. K., et al. (2013). **Too sick not to exercise: Using a 6-week, home-based exercise intervention for cancer-related fatigue self-management for postsurgical non-small cell lung cancer patients.** *Cancer Nursing, 36*(3), 175–188.

Seven participants with early-stage lung cancer performed light-intensity walking and balance exercises using the Nintendo Wii Fit Plus. Exercise started the first week after hospitalization for surgical removal of the tumor and continued for 6 weeks thereafter. The intervention positively impacted cancer-related fatigue severity; fatigue self-management, walking, and balance; fatigue self-management behaviors; and functional performance (number of steps taken per day). Researchers concluded that a home-based, light-intensity exercise intervention for patients after surgery for lung cancer is feasible, safe, well

tolerated, and highly acceptable, showing positive changes in cancer-related fatigue self-management.

Cooley, M. E., Emmons, K. M., Haddad, R., et al. (2011). **Patient-reported receipt of and interest in smoking cessation interventions after a diagnosis of cancer.** *Cancer, 117*(13), 2961–2969.

Data were collected from questionnaires and medical records from 160 smokers or recent quitters with lung or head and neck cancer. Eighty-six percent of smokers and 75% of recent quitters reported that healthcare providers gave advice to quit smoking. Fifty-one percent of smokers and 20% of recent quitters expressed an interest in a smoking-cessation program. An individualized smoking-cessation program was the preferred type of program. Among smokers, younger patients with early stage disease and those with partners who were smokers were more interested in programs.

1. Based on these studies, why is it important to assess a patient's interest in smoking-cessation programs?

2. Why do you think a patient's diagnosis of lung cancer might influence his willingness to participate in healthy activities?

3. In light of the research, what might you do to facilitate health promotion in your patient with a lung cancer diagnosis?

 Go to Davis Advantage, Resources, Chapter 27, **Toward Evidence-Based Practice—Suggested Responses.**

in any health state along the wellness-illness continuum. When the patient is unable to express his readiness, the nurse may make the health promotion diagnosis and act on the patient's behalf (NANDA-I, 2018). NANDA-I health promotion labels are preceded by the phrase "Readiness for Enhanced" and are now one-part statements with no etiology. Following are some examples of health-promotion diagnoses: Readiness for Enhanced Breastfeeding, Readiness for Enhanced Nutrition, and Readiness for Enhanced Self-Concept. For other examples, see the accompanying Standardized Language box.

PLANNING OUTCOMES/EVALUATION NP

NOC standardized outcomes related to health promotion vary depending on the focus area. For example, if the nursing diagnosis is Readiness for Enhanced Nutrition, a NOC outcome might be Nutritional Status. For examples of other NOC health promotion outcomes, see the accompanying Standardized Language box.

Individualized goals and outcomes might include losing 20 pounds or exercising for 30 minutes five times per week.

KEY POINT: *The nurse's role in health promotion primarily is to motivate clients and facilitate change. Clients are independently responsible for most of their health promotion activities.* You may need to help them identify goals, but it is essential that the goals be the clients', not yours.

Healthy People 2020 Goals. You may need aggregate wellness goals for groups as well as individualized goals. The following are four broad goals for the U.S. population set by the *Healthy People 2020* initiative (U.S. Department of Health and Human Services [USDHHS], 2009):

- Attain high-quality, longer lives free of preventable disease, disability, injury, and premature death.
- Achieve health equity, eliminate disparities, and improve the health of all groups.
- Create social and physical environments that promote good health for all.
- Promote healthy development and healthy behaviors across every stage of life.

Interventions to achieve these goals are targeted at the 37 topic areas shown in Box 27-1. Public health agencies at

---

Standardized Language

Examples of NIC & NOC Standardized Language for Health Promotion Diagnoses

Nursing Diagnosis/Definition	Selected NOC Outcomes and Goals Using NOC Indicators	Selected NIC Interventions and Nursing Activities
Sedentary Lifestyle Life that is characterized by low physical activity.	**NOC Outcomes** Exercise Participation Physical Fitness **Goals** Meets mutually defined goals of increased mobility. Verbalizes feeling of increased strength and ability to move.	**NIC Interventions** Exercise Promotion Self-Modification Assistance **Nursing Activities** Screen for mobility skills: ➤ Bed mobility ➤ Supported and unsupported sitting ➤ Transition movements standing and walking Prior to activity, treat pain. Obtain any assistive devices needed. Encourage independence in activities of daily living. Develop mutually agreed-on goals of increased activity.
Risk for Frail Elderly Syndrome Vulnerable to deterioration in physical, psychological, functional, or social health leading to increased risk for adverse health effects.	**NOC Outcomes** Self-Care Status Nutritional Status: Food and Fluid Intake **Goals** Maintains ability to perform basic tasks and personal care independently with or without assistive device.	**NIC Interventions** Hope Inspiration Health Education Self-Care Assistance **Nursing Activities** Assess home environment for safety. Evaluate depression or cognitive impairment. Provide suggestions for managing energy use. Encourage participation in low-intensity aerobic chair exercise. Provide opportunities for socialization and sensory stimulation.

(Continued)

Standardized Language

Examples of NIC & NOC Standardized Language for Health Promotion Diagnoses—cont'd

Nursing Diagnosis/Definition	Selected NOC Outcomes and Goals Using NOC Indicators	Selected NIC Interventions and Nursing Activities
Deficient Community Health One or more health problems that deter wellness or increase the risk of health problems experienced by groups.	**NOC Outcomes** Community Health Status Community Immune Status Community Risk Control: Communicable Disease **Goals** Community actions reduce the spread of infectious agents that threaten public health.	**NIC Interventions** Communicable Disease Management Health Screening Program Development Surveillance: Community **Nursing Activities** Monitor immunization status of community. Facilitate access to immunizations. Provide immunizations to prevent communicable disease. Provide health education. Teach hand washing. Participate in community surveillance.
Readiness for enhanced health management A pattern of integrating into daily life a regimen for the treatment of illness and its sequelae, which can be strengthened.	**NOC Outcomes** Compliance Behavior Health Promoting Behavior Participation in Healthcare Decisions **Goals** Participates in activities to enhance management of therapeutic regimen.	**NIC Interventions** Decision-Making Support Health Education Health System Guidance Mutual Goal Setting Risk Identification Self-Modification Enhancement Teaching: Individual **Nursing Activities** Create an accepting, nonjudgmental atmosphere. Encourage consideration of values underlying choices and consequences of the choice. Determine ability and motivation of patient and partner to correctly participate in therapeutic regimen. Include family/support person in instruction. Provide financial resource assistance if needed.

Sources:

Bulechek, G. M., Butcher, H. K., Dochterman, J. M., et al. (Eds.). (2012). *Nursing interventions classification (NIC)* (6th ed.). St. Louis, MO: C.V. Mosby. Used with permission;

Moorhead, S., Johnson, M., Maas, M., et al. (Eds.). (2012). *Nursing outcomes classification (NOC)* (5th ed.). St. Louis, MO: C.V. Mosby. Used with permission; *Nursing Diagnoses—Definitions and Classification 2018–2020.* © 2010 NANDA International, ISBN 978-1-62623-929-6. Used by arrangement with the Thieme Group, Stuttgart/New York.

the local, state, and federal levels use these focus areas as a blueprint to design programs aimed at improving the health status of the community (USDHHS, 2009). To view those objectives,

 Go to the *Healthy People 2020* Web site at https://www. healthypeople.gov/2020/topics-objectives

Whether standardized or individualized, expected outcomes for wellness diagnoses describe behaviors or responses that demonstrate health maintenance or achievement of an even higher level of health.

> *Example:* During the next year, Mr. Needham will continue to eat a balanced diet, with more emphasis on including whole grains and fiber.

By using the highest number (5) on the rating scale, you can use the NOC to write wellness outcomes.

> *Example:*
> *Nursing diagnosis:* Readiness for Enhanced Nutrition
> *Expected outcome:* Nutritional Status: (5) Not compromised

BOX 27-1 ■ Topics Areas of *Healthy People 2020*

1. Access to health services
2. Adolescent health
3. Arthritis, osteoporosis, and chronic back conditions
4. Blood disorders and blood safety
5. Cancer
6. Chronic kidney disease
7. Diabetes
8. Disability and secondary conditions
9. Early and middle childhood
10. Educational and community-based programs
11. Environmental health
12. Family planning
13. Food safety
14. Genomics
15. Global health
16. Health communication and health information technology (IT)
17. Healthcare-associated infections
18. Hearing and other sensory or communication disorders
19. Heart disease and stroke
20. HIV
21. Immunization and infectious diseases
22. Injury and violence prevention
23. Maternal, infant, and child health
24. Medical product safety
25. Mental health and mental disorders
26. Nutrition and overweight
27. Occupational safety and health
28. Older adults
29. Oral health
30. Physical activity and fitness
31. Public health infrastructure
32. Respiratory diseases
33. Sexually transmitted diseases
34. Social determinants of health
35. Substance abuse
36. Tobacco use
37. Vision

Source: U.S. Department of Health and Human Services, Office of Disease Prevention & Health Promotion and Human Services. (2009). *Healthy People 2020* topics and objectives. Retrieved from https://www.healthypeople.gov/2020/topics-objectives

PLANNING INTERVENTIONS/ IMPLEMENTATION NP

Community and public health nurses focus on the problems contributing to disease, such as poor housing conditions, sanitation, and nutrition; poverty; and substance abuse. The wellness focus in acute care is to educate patients about both health and disease.

Once the client identifies his goals, help him to identify the steps that he must take to reach the goals. Change occurs in stages. To create positive change, the client will need to understand the benefits of change, overcome the barriers to change, and make a commitment to follow through on the plan.

For *NIC standardized interventions* for health promotion, see the accompanying Standardized Language box. NIC does not have a special domain, or grouping, for wellness interventions. Instead, they are found throughout all areas of the taxonomy, particularly in the Behavioral, Safety, Family, Health System, and Community domains. Specific NIC nursing activities for health promotion include those in following subsections: Nutrition, Exercise, and Lifestyle Changes. The remainder of the chapter provides some strategies to promote their use.

Nutrition To guide people in making nutritional choices that promote health and prevent disease, the U.S. Department of Agriculture and the USDHHS revised the *Dietary Guidelines for Americans* (you will find these in Chapter 28) to include "MyPlate," a picture of a plate that is divided into four sections—fruits, vegetables, grains, and protein. MyPlate is a quick, simple reminder to people to be more mindful of the foods they eat. The symbol is part of a healthy eating initiative that conveys seven key messages:

- Enjoy food but eat less.
- Avoid oversized portions.
- Make half of the plate fruits and vegetables.
- Drink water instead of sugary drinks.
- Switch to fat-free or low-fat (1%) milk.
- Compare sodium in foods.
- Make at least half your grains whole grains.

Exercise Regular physical activity each week, sustained for months and years, can produce long-term health benefits including a lower risk for heart disease, stroke, type 2 diabetes, hypertension, high cholesterol, metabolic syndrome, certain types of cancer, and depression. Regular physical activity also prevents weight gain; improves cardiorespiratory and muscular fitness; prevents falls by increasing muscle tone, strength and balance, and promotes better memory and cognition in older adults (ACSM, 2013). Encourage physical fitness lifestyle habits in people of all ages and abilities. The most health benefits occur with at least 150 minutes (2 hours and 30 minutes) a week of moderate-intensity physical activity, such as brisk walking. Additional benefits occur with more physical activity (USDHHS, 2008). Children and teens should engage in at least 1 hour of age-appropriate physical activity daily. Activity should be vigorous in intensity and varied in type, not only to prevent boredom but also to promote muscle and bone strengthening as well as flexibility (Fig. 27-3).

For more information, do a Web search or,

 Go to the President's Challenge Web site at http://www. presidentschallenge.org

Lifestyle Changes For healthy living, adults and teens must choose a lifestyle without tobacco and recreational drugs and with little alcohol. Getting enough sleep and managing stress are also important. In general, adults need 6 to 9 hours of sleep a night. Children need more sleep (see Chapter 35). Inadequate sleep is linked to weight gain and obesity.

Role Modeling

A **role model** teaches by example, demonstrating the behaviors and/or attitudes to be learned. Models provide inspiration and strategies for health promotion behavior.

Example: A morbidly obese female joins a weight loss group led by a woman who has lost nearly 100 pounds. She admires the leader for her determination and success and selects her as a role model.

It may be helpful for you to guide the client in choosing a role model and to keep the following in mind:

- Consider the client's age, culture, values, and preferred activities.

Health Promotion

Situation: The student has noticed that many of his classmates have gained significant amounts of weight as the school year has advanced. In addition, it seems as though there is always someone who is sick in class. Students are complaining about the cost of co-payments and over-the-counter medications. The student wonders whether there are practical ways to improve this situation at his school.

PICOT Components

P	Population/client	=	Young adult students
I	Intervention/indicator	=	Health promotion information
C	Comparator/control	=	None
O	Outcome	=	Decreased risk of health problems
T	Time	=	None

Searchable Question

Do _____ (P) who receive/are exposed to _____ (I) demonstrate _____ (O) as compared to _____ (C) during _____ (T)?

Example of Evidence: The World Health Organization defined *health promotion* as the process that enables people to improve their own health by improving control over the determinants of health. Healthcare spending in the United States exceeded $3.5 trillion in 2015. America's worsening health habits, particularly obesity, are contributing to this massive growth in spending. Cost-effective health promotion measures include educating people about preventable health problems such as obesity, diabetes, hypertension, and other chronic diseases. Nursing educators will be at the forefront in evaluating nursing programs and teaching future nurses according to the needs of global health.

Practice Changes: The student talks to his professor about organizing a wellness group to share health promotion ideas.

_____
Reference: Jadelhack, R. (2012). Health promotion in nursing and cost-effectiveness, *Journal of Cultural Diversity, 19*(2), 65–68.

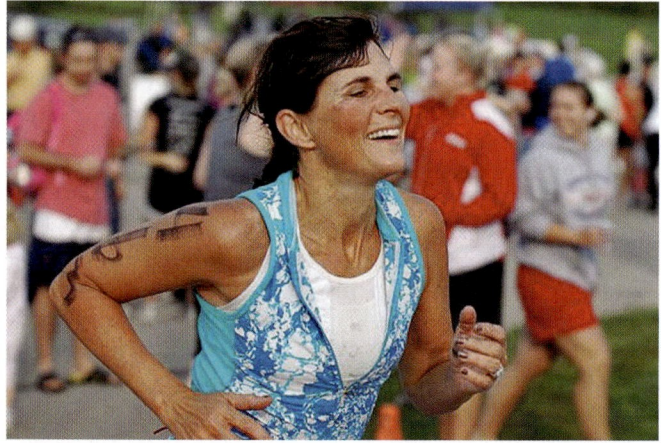

FIGURE 27-3 Vigorous-intensity exercise promotes muscle and bone strength and improves cardiovascular health.

- The model should be someone with whom the client identifies.
- Ideally, the role model should be accessible to the client during the early stages of change.
    Example: During the next year, Mr. Needham will continue to eat a balanced diet. This allows for interacting and for exchanging information.

Nurses also serve as role models. Therefore, we should provide an example of healthy behaviors. It is difficult to advocate for healthy behavior if you do not follow the behavior that you recommend to clients. Imagine the trust a client loses when he finds out that the nurse who tells him not to smoke cigarettes has a two-pack per day habit. To what extent do you role model healthy behaviors?

Providing Counseling

Counseling is an interpersonal communication process that helps a client to identify problems and make changes. In the context of health promotion, counseling promotes personal growth and helps clients change their lifestyle. Counseling may be formal or informal, one-to-one or a small-group discussion, face-to-face or offered via telephone or online. Each meeting with a client is a potential counseling session.

Individual Counseling

Face-to-face interaction may be helpful when clients are attempting major lifestyle change. In an individual session, you can customize and map out the steps required to meet the client's goals.
- **Contracting.** Counseling may include writing a contract detailing the client's expected behaviors. Print out the contract and have the client sign it to reinforce his commitment. Suggest that the client post the plan in a location where he will see it often so that it serves as a frequent reminder.
- **Reinforcing.** During counseling sessions, remember to reinforce health-promoting behaviors that have already been established. For example, the client who uses tobacco may eat a balanced diet; reinforce the healthy habit to boost self-esteem. Stress to the client that you believe the client can succeed in making the desired behavior change.

Telephone Counseling

Telephone counseling may be used as a primary counseling approach or as follow-up. Clients with hectic schedules may find it easier to arrange telephone counseling than to schedule a face-to-face interaction. The disadvantage is that telephone counseling does not allow you to detect nonverbal communication.

- When using telephone counseling, set goals and map out the strategy for change just as you would in face-to-face counseling.
- Let the client know how and when you can be reached if questions arise.
- If you are using the telephone for follow-up counseling, it is best to schedule a time to speak. Having an appointment helps keep the patient accountable to the expected behavior and to reinforce the information.

Providing Health Education

- Health education may focus on self-care strategies, caregiver concerns, or how to be an effective healthcare consumer.
  - **Self-care programs** typically cover nutrition, exercise, stress management, or disease prevention.
  - **Caregiver education programs** may teach caregivers how to perform nursing tasks or prevent injuries, or they may provide a list of community resources for respite care.
- Programs may consist of lectures, printed material, billboards, or posters. For example, the accompanying Self-Care box, Teaching Clients How to Prevent Upper Respiratory Infections, might be reproduced and posted in the lounge, restrooms, or locker areas of a worksite during cold and flu season to decrease absenteeism.
- Nurses can teach clients how to be effective healthcare consumers, how to interact with healthcare providers, and how to maneuver through the healthcare system.
- For a review of teaching and learning, see Chapter 26.

Providing and Facilitating Support for Lifestyle Change

Changing one's lifestyle is difficult and most clients need support to do so. You can provide support during interactions and counseling sessions. You can also help the client to identify available resources within the community and from family, friends, and coworkers.

Group support exists for a variety of lifestyle changes. For example,

- Weight Watchers®—for clients who want to lose weight.
- Alcoholics Anonymous—for clients who want to become and stay sober.

Group support provides opportunity to meet people experiencing the same difficulties and perhaps to find a role model. As a nurse, you should be familiar with various programs available in your community and refer clients to them.

KnowledgeCheck 27-4

Identify four strategies to help a client engage in positive lifestyle changes.

Self-Care

Teaching Clients How to Prevent Upper Respiratory Infections

- ➤ **Maintain a healthy lifestyle.** That means adequate sleep, good nutrition, and physical exercise. A balanced diet and physical fitness can boost your immune system to fight infection if it occurs.
- ➤ **Wash your hands often and teach children to do so.** This helps prevent spread of infection.
- ➤ **When using public restrooms, wash your hands.** Turn off the faucet with a paper towel and use a paper towel to open the door as you leave the room.
- ➤ **Avoid touching your eyes, nose, and mouth** because doing so spreads any virus your hands have contacted (e.g., on doorknobs).
- ➤ **Avoid crowds when there is a cold or influenza epidemic.**
- ➤ **Throw away tissues as soon as you use them.**
- ➤ **When someone in the family has a cold,** keep bathrooms and the kitchen very clean and do not drink from the same glass or use the same utensils.
- ➤ **When someone at home or at work has a cold,** wipe telephone receivers with soap and water or an antibacterial solution.
- ➤ **If a child has a cold,** wash his toys and commonly used items well.
- ➤ **When choosing child care, look for a clean environment;** ask what rules are in place concerning keeping the children clean (e.g., washing hands before snack time).
- ➤ **Don't smoke.** Cigarette smoke can irritate the respiratory tract, making you more susceptible to colds and illness.
- ➤ **Control stress.** People experiencing emotional stress tend to have weakened immunity to fight infection.
- ➤ **Consider taking echinacea or zinc lozenges,** although there is no conclusive evidence of their effectiveness (Singh & Das, 2011). Consult your primary healthcare provider.

CLINICALREASONING

The questions and exercises in this section allow you to practice the kind of thinking you will use as a full-spectrum nurse. Critical-thinking questions usually have more than one correct answer, so we do not provide "correct answers" for these features. It is more important to develop your nursing judgment than to just cover content. You will learn by discussing the questions with your peers. If you are still unsure, see the Davis Advantage chapter resources for suggested responses.

Caring for the Nguyens

Nam and Yen Nguyen, their 3-year-old grandson, Kim Phan, and Mai Nguyen, Nam's 76-year-old mother, are all patients at the Family Medicine Center. Zach Miller, the family nurse practitioner at the center, asks you to devise a health promotion program for each member of the family.

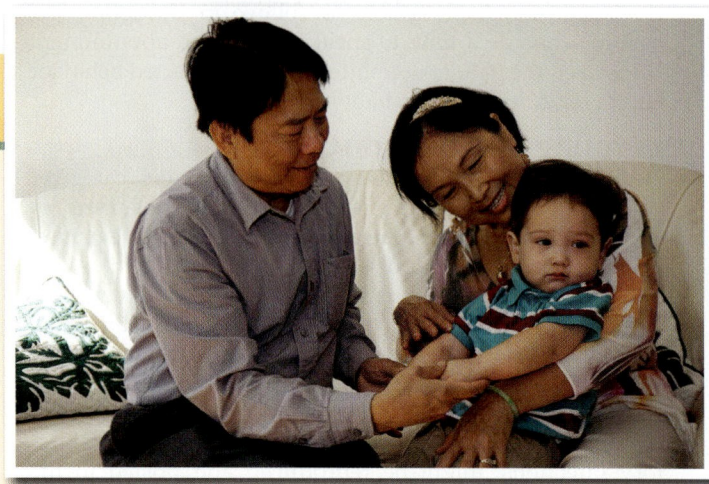

A. What information should you gather before you begin?

B. How might you obtain this information?

C. How will the plans differ for each?

D. Review Meet the Nguyens in the front of this textbook; also review Nam's physical exam findings in Chapter 21. What health promotion strategies and health screenings should you recommend to Nam Nguyen?

E. How would you begin to organize and prioritize a health promotion program for Nam?

F. Using therapeutic communication, give examples of appropriate questions to ask Nam about his health beliefs.

Go to Davis Advantage, Resources, Chapter 27, **Caring for the Nguyens—Suggested Responses.**

Applying the **Full-Spectrum Nursing Model**_____

PATIENT SITUATION

Shandra Shane is a single 37-year-old woman with three children ages 12, 15, and 17. She is raising the children on her own, although her sister occasionally helps with transportation or gives advice about disciplining her teenage daughters. Ms. Shane is a night-shift worker at the hospital. Her typical schedule is 3 to 4 hours of sleep in the morning soon after she gets home and then a short nap in the early evening before going back to work. She smokes 1 to 1½ packs of cigarettes per day but tells you she has been trying to smoke less around her children. Her job stress level is high, as the hospital is cutting back on the number of staff. Ms. Shane also takes care of her aging mother, who has Alzheimer's and lives with her. Ms. Shane's outlet for stress is going out with friends and drinking beer on the weekend. She is seeking your professional guidance to lose some weight (about 60 pounds) and to feel more energetic.

THINKING

1. *Theoretical Knowledge:*
   List health behaviors that negatively influence health status.
2. *Critical Thinking (Contextual Awareness):*
   What factors in this situation would you consider threatening Ms. Shane's health and could lead to disease later in life?

DOING

3. *Nursing Process (Planning/Intervention):*
What suggestions might you make about Ms. Shane's diet that could help her to lose weight? Why might these actions be effective for weight loss?

4. *Practical Knowledge:*
What areas of her daily living other than her diet might you explore further and offer recommendations for improving to promote better health and prevent illness?

CARING

5. *Self-Knowledge:*
Have you ever been in a situation in which you felt stressed and tired and wanted the gratification offered by food, nicotine, or alcohol? Describe your experience.

6. *Ethical:*
In what ways could you demonstrate genuine caring for Ms. Shane?

 Go to Davis Advantage, Resources, Chapter 27, **Applying the Full-Spectrum Nursing Model Suggested Responses.**

 To explore learning resources for this chapter,

 Go to www.DavisAdvantage.com and find:

Answers and Suggested Responses for all questions in this chapter

Lists of NIC Interventions and NOC Outcomes

List of NANDA-I Diagnoses

Knowledge Map

References and Bibliography

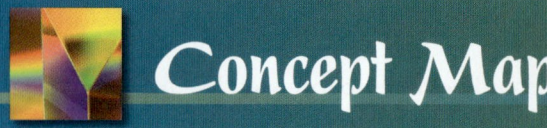

Concept Map

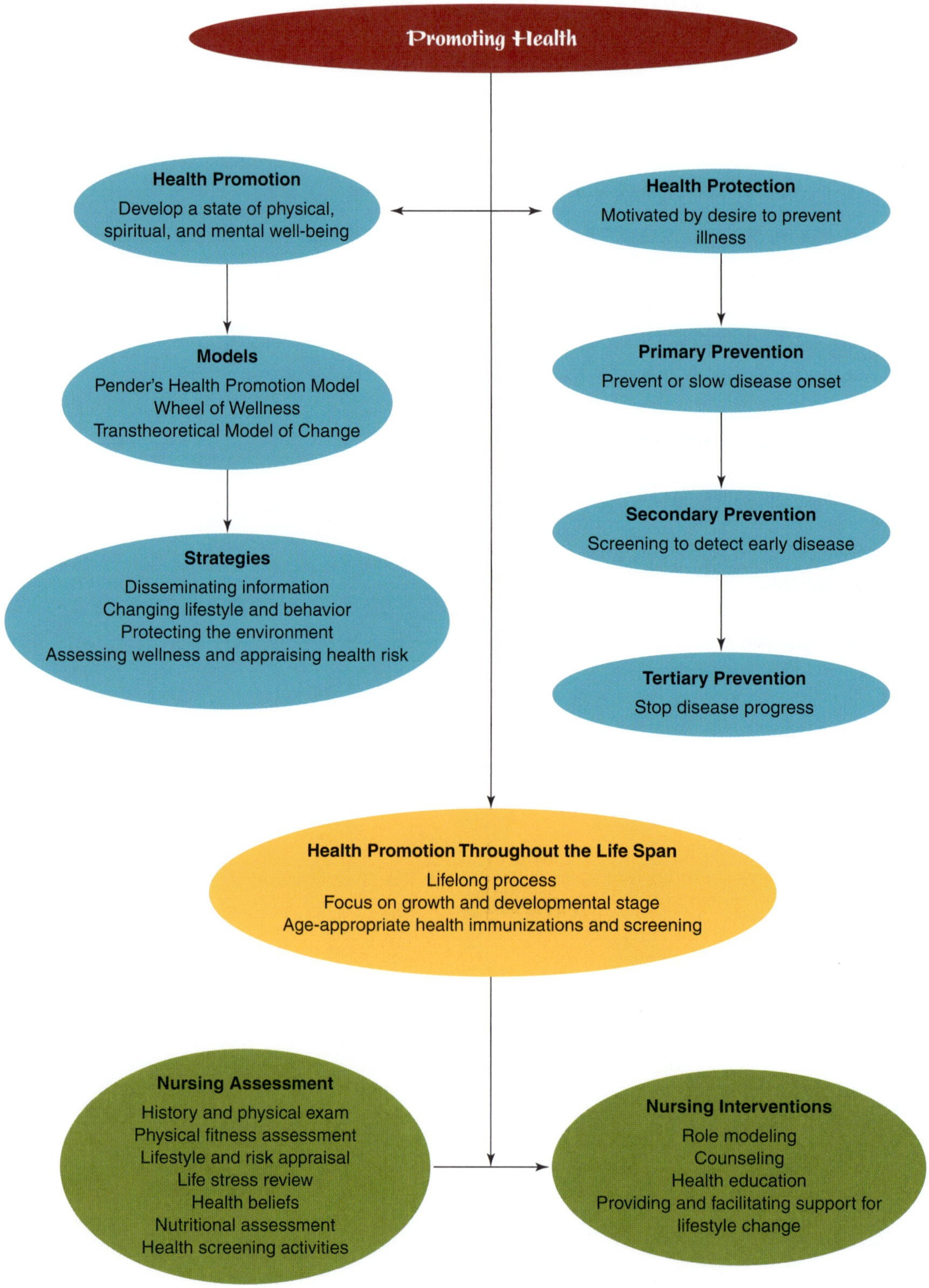

Promoting Health

Health Promotion
Develop a state of physical, spiritual, and mental well-being

Health Protection
Motivated by desire to prevent illness

Models
Pender's Health Promotion Model
Wheel of Wellness
Transtheoretical Model of Change

Primary Prevention
Prevent or slow disease onset

Strategies
Disseminating information
Changing lifestyle and behavior
Protecting the environment
Assessing wellness and appraising health risk

Secondary Prevention
Screening to detect early disease

Tertiary Prevention
Stop disease progress

Health Promotion Throughout the Life Span
Lifelong process
Focus on growth and developmental stage
Age-appropriate health immunizations and screening

Nursing Assessment
History and physical exam
Physical fitness assessment
Lifestyle and risk appraisal
Life stress review
Health beliefs
Nutritional assessment
Health screening activities

Nursing Interventions
Role modeling
Counseling
Health education
Providing and facilitating support for lifestyle change

Supporting Physiological Function

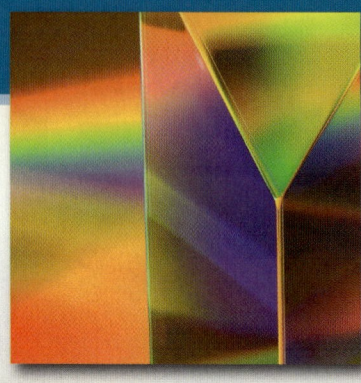

CHAPTER 28

Nutrition

Learning Outcomes

After completing this chapter, you should be able to:

➤ Identify the types, functions, metabolism, and major food sources of (1) energy nutrients, (2) vitamins, (3) minerals, and (4) water.

➤ Differentiate among the various sources of nutritional information (e.g., USDA dietary guidelines, ChooseMyPlate, DRIs, Nutrition Facts labels).

➤ Identify the primary nutritional considerations for various developmental stages.

➤ Discuss the effects of each of the following: nutritional status; also explain how each is affected by nutritional status: lifestyle choices, vegetarianism, dieting for weight loss, culture and religion, disease processes, functional limitations, and special diets.

➤ Describe tools and techniques for gathering subjective data about nutritional status.

➤ Perform various anthropometric measurements.

➤ Calculate a client's basal metabolic rate.

➤ Calculate the body mass index for a client and explain its significance.

➤ List at least five physical assessment findings that indicate nutritional imbalance.

➤ Identify laboratory values that are indicators of nutritional status.

➤ Discuss the need for and advisability of vitamin and mineral supplementation.

➤ Describe nursing interventions for patients with special nutritional needs: Impaired Swallowing, NPO, older adults, and Nausea.

➤ Identify and discuss at least six nursing interventions for each of the following diagnoses:

Imbalanced Nutrition: Less than Body Requirements

Obesity

Overweight

➤ Safely provide enteral and parenteral nutrition for patients.

Key Concepts

Energy
Metabolism
Nutrition

Related Concepts

See the Concept Map at the end of this chapter.

Example Problems

Overweight/Obesity

Underweight/Malnourished

Meet Your Patients

As part of a class assignment, you are to assist a local business with its wellness program. You will complete health risk appraisals and gather the following data on the employees: height, weight, medical and nutritional history, and lifestyle practices. Today you will screen two employees, and then each will have blood drawn for a complete blood count (CBC), comprehensive metabolic panel, and lipid panel:

- **Isaac Schwartz**, a 65-year-old accountant, works long hours. He describes a sedentary lifestyle, no tobacco use, infrequent alcohol use, no medical problems, and a nutritional history of skipping meals and daily consumption of restaurant food. You measure his height as 69 in. and weight as 245 lb.
- **Sujing Lee**, a 29-year-old project manager, regularly works 65 hours per week. Sujing is 30 weeks pregnant. She does not smoke or drink and has never been hospitalized or had surgery. She has gained a total of 25 lb since becoming pregnant. Her diet consists mainly of traditional Chinese food. She eats three meals a day

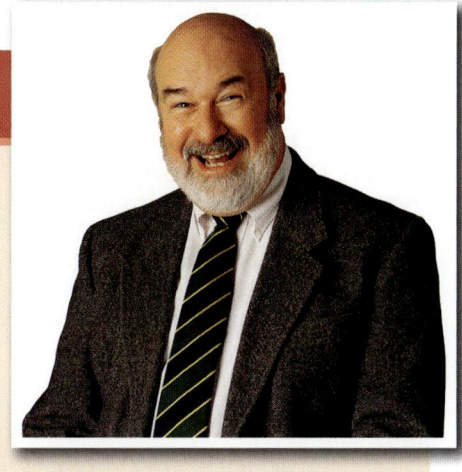

and always brings lunch from home. Lately she has felt "tired all the time." At the screening, she weighs 126 lb and measures 63 in. tall.

At the end of your clinical day, you need to compile a report on the clients you have seen. How would you interpret the data on height, weight, and nutrition? What, if any, additional information do you need to help you evaluate their nutritional status? In this chapter, you will read about dietary recommendations, energy balance, and nutritional concerns across the life span. You will gain the theoretical knowledge to answer these questions, as well as practical knowledge about managing nutritional problems.

Theoretical Knowledge
knowing why

Organic, natural, gluten-free, low-fat, sugar-free, reduced-calorie, low-sodium, calcium-enriched . . . these are just a few of the hundreds of claims that you find on packaged foods. Multimedia ads hype nutritional supplements, weight-loss pills, and new diets, while the health news carries conflicting reports on the benefits and dangers of phytochemicals, antioxidants, and *trans*-fatty acids. With so many options and different recommendations about what's healthy or not, it's no wonder that many people are confused about what to eat.

ABOUT THE KEY CONCEPTS

Nutrition is the study of food: how it affects the human body and influences health. **Metabolism** is the process by which the body converts food into energy. Good nutrition is essential to wellness, and poor nutrition contributes to disease; so clients need accurate, current, and appropriate nutritional information. Before you can give effective individualized advice, you need to know about the nutrients found in foods. In this chapter you will learn about concepts related to **energy**—for example, energy balance, macronutrients, micronutrients, and factors that influence nutritional status.

WHAT ARE SOME RELIABLE SOURCES OF NUTRITION INFORMATION?

Standards and guides provide credible nutrition information.

- **Standards** are a reference for nutrient intake thought to meet the nutritional needs of most healthy population groups. They list nutrient amounts in measurements, such

as grams and milligrams, and are not intended to indicate individual requirements or therapeutic needs.

- **Food guides** are more practical tools that you can use to educate patients and families. They specify the number of servings of foods needed daily so nonprofessionals can use them in making healthful meal choices.
- **KEY POINT:** *In general, standards and guides provide recommendations to healthy individuals but they are not specific to the needs of people with metabolic or other medical problems.*

Dietary Reference Intakes

The National Academy of Sciences, in collaboration with Health Canada, established nutrition standards to promote health consumption of micronutrients (vitamins, minerals, and trace elements) and macronutrients (carbohydrates, proteins, fats) and other substances (fiber) to prevent deficiencies and lower the risk of chronic disease. The DRIs are used for planning and assessing diets for healthy individuals.

The DRIs encompass four types of nutrient reference values for males and females in different age groups:

- Estimated Average Requirement (EAR)—the amount of a nutrient that is estimated to meet the requirement of half of all healthy individuals within a given age and gender group.
- Recommended Dietary Allowance (RDA)—the average daily dietary intake of a nutrient that is sufficient to meet the nutritional requirements of approximately 98% of healthy people.
- Adequate Intake (AI)—the amount of a nutrient consumed by a group of healthy people.
- Tolerable Upper Intake Level (UL)—the maximum daily intake of a nutrient that is likely to be without adverse health effects for almost all individuals.
- Acceptable Macronutrient Distribution Range (AMDR)—the percentage of protein, fat, and carbohydrate associated

with reduced risk of chronic disease, provided there is an intake of other essential nutrients (U.S. Department of Agriculture [USDA] and U.S. Department of Health and Human Services [USDHHS], 2015).

USDA Dietary Guidelines

The U.S. Department of Agriculture (USDA) developed the *Dietary Guidelines for Americans 2015–2020* to help people improve their nutritional habits. The guidelines do not specify daily amounts of food and nutrients (Box 28-1).

These USDA dietary guidelines are intended as a primary source of health information for nutrition educators, policy makers, and healthcare providers. They are based on scientific evidence and provide information about choosing a nutritious diet, maintaining healthy weight, achieving adequate exercise, and food safety. The dietary guidelines are updated every 5 years.

MyPlate

MyPlate (Fig. 28-1) is a five-color food guide that visually illustrates a healthy meal—red for fruits, green for vegetables, orange for grains, and purple for protein, as well as a separate blue section for dairy on the side.

The MyPlate Web site promotes healthy nutrition based on the USDA *Dietary Guidelines for Americans 2015–2020* in food choices and variety, portion size, activity, and tools for successful nutritional lifestyle.

Adapted Versions of MyPlate

- **MyPlate in Spanish.** The Spanish version is available on the ChooseMyPlate Web site.

 - **MyPlate for Older Adults.** This visual good guide illustrates healthy food choices and portions specific for the nutrition and hydration needs of older adults. It is consistent with the *Dietary Guidelines for Americans 2015–2020*. Both recommend limiting foods high in *trans-* and saturated fats, salt, and added sugars; and emphasize whole grains. It also stresses the importance of fluids and promotes physical activity. To see MyPlate for Older Adults,

 Go to https://www.choosemyplate.gov/older-adults

Food Guides Developed by Other Groups

- **Traditional Asian, Latin American, Mediterranean, and African heritage and vegetarian/vegan diets.** Although recipes are seasoned with culturally specific ingredients, these different diets similarly emphasize eating fresh local and seasonal foods. This back-to-earth style of eating is typically home-cooked and avoids excess sugar, salt, and solid fats. For healthy living, portion sizes are moderate (Oldways, n.d). You can find specific diets at the Oldways Preservation and Exchange Trust Web site.

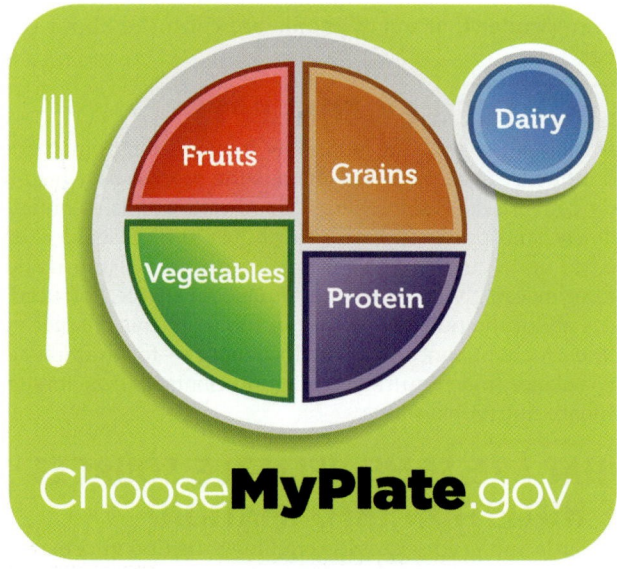

FIGURE 28-1 Build a healthy eating style using the USDA ChooseMyPlate.gov.

■ **Diabetes Food Plate.** The American Diabetes Association offers an online interactive tool called Create Your Plate to help diabetics manage blood glucose and lose weight. The diabetes food plate emphasizes a diet higher in nonstarchy carbohydrates and proteins.

Nutrition Facts Label

You are likely familiar with the **Nutrition Facts label** shown in Figure 28-2, because the U.S. Food and Drug Administration (USFDA) requires this label on all packaged foods sold in the United States. The Nutrition Facts panel contains important information about serving size, number of servings per package, total calories and calories from fat per serving, a list and amounts of the key nutrients in the food, and the *percent daily values* (% DV) for the nutrients listed on the panel. The % DV identifies the percentage that a serving of the food contributes to a consumer's daily intake of the nutrient listed. Teaching your patients how to use these labels will help them to make wiser dietary choices.

KnowledgeCheck 28-1

■ What are the DRIs?
■ List the current USDA dietary guidelines for Americans.

ThinkLike a Nurse 28-1

How might you use the various sources of nutritional information to evaluate the nutritional status of the clients introduced in the Meet Your Patients scenario?

WHAT ARE THE ENERGY NUTRIENTS?

The cells and tissues of the body depend on **nutrients** for growth, maintenance, and functioning. Any one food may contain a variety of nutrients; for instance, cheese contains carbohydrates, protein, fats, sodium, vitamins, and minerals.

■ **Macronutrients** supply the body with energy (kilocalories). Table 28-1 lists the sources of and requirements for macronutrients.

■ **Micronutrients** help manufacture, repair, and maintain cells.

Through the process of **metabolism,** the body converts food into complex forms of chemical energy and then into usable energy, which is then carried to individual cells. Metabolism encompasses all the ways in which the body changes and uses nutrients for vital processes and bodily functions. Most metabolic reactions are triggered by enzymes; each is specific and catalyzes only one type of reaction. Two types of

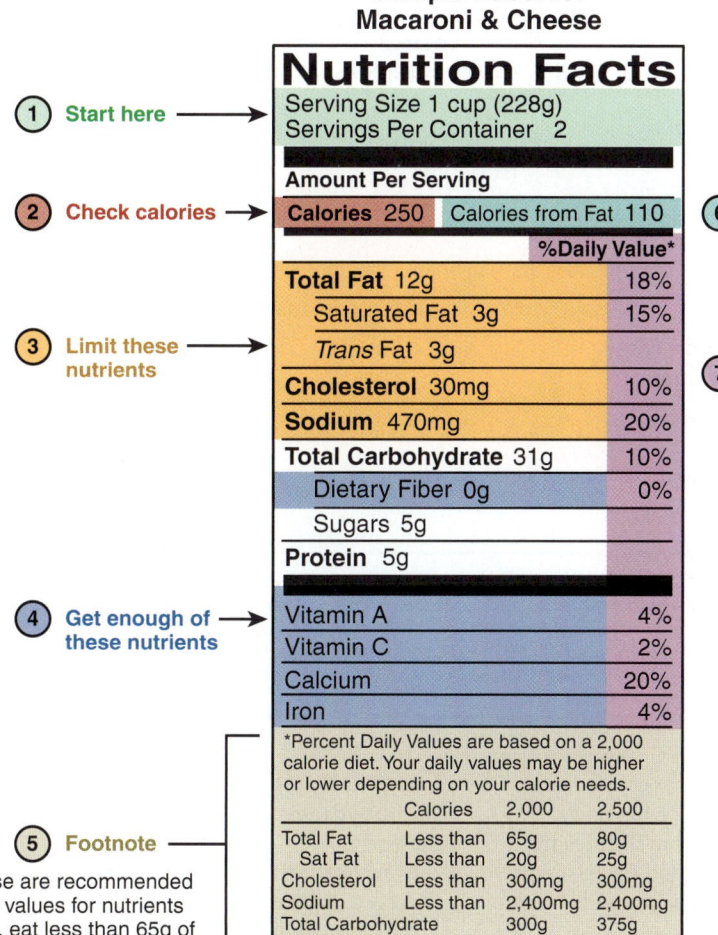

Sample Label for Macaroni & Cheese

① Start here

② Check calories

③ Limit these nutrients

④ Get enough of these nutrients

⑤ Footnote
These are recommended daily values for nutrients (e.g., eat less than 65g of fat per day; eat at least 25g of dietary fiber).

Nutrition Facts

Serving Size 1 cup (228g)
Servings Per Container 2

Amount Per Serving

Calories 250   Calories from Fat 110

%Daily Value*

Total Fat 12g	18%
Saturated Fat 3g	15%
Trans Fat 3g	
Cholesterol 30mg	10%
Sodium 470mg	20%
Total Carbohydrate 31g	10%
Dietary Fiber 0g	0%
Sugars 5g	
Protein 5g	

Vitamin A	4%
Vitamin C	2%
Calcium	20%
Iron	4%

*Percent Daily Values are based on a 2,000 calorie diet. Your daily values may be higher or lower depending on your calorie needs.

	Calories	2,000	2,500
Total Fat	Less than	65g	80g
Sat Fat	Less than	20g	25g
Cholesterol	Less than	300mg	300mg
Sodium	Less than	2,400mg	2,400mg
Total Carbohydrate		300g	375g
Dietary Fiber		25g	30g

⑥ Calories from fat help people to keep fat intake to less than 30% of total calories

⑦ Quick guide to % DV

Shows how the food fits into the overall daily diet

• 5% or less is low

• 20% or more is high

% is based on a 2,000 calorie diet

FIGURE 28-2 A Nutrition Facts label.

Table 28-1 ➤ Energy Nutrients

NUTRIENTS	SOURCES	ENZYMES INVOLVED IN DIGESTION	REQUIREMENTS
Carbohydrates	*Simple sugars* occur mainly in corn syrup, honey, milk, table sugar, molasses, sugar cane, sugar beets, and fruits. *Complex carbohydrates* occur in vegetables, breads, cereals, pasta, grains, and legumes.	Salivary amylase (mouth) Ptyalin (mouth and stomach) Pancreatic amylopsin Intestinal: Sucrase, lactase, maltase	DRI requirements for healthy adults are 45%–65% of calories from CHOs, or 130 grams per day (g/day). Body size and activity level affect the amount of carbohydrate used by the body. There is debate about the amount of dietary carbohydrate needed. Many popular diet plans alter carbohydrate intake. Some focus on low carbohydrate intake; others recommend a high intake of complex CHOs.
Proteins	*Complete proteins* come mostly from animal sources: meat, poultry, fish, eggs, and milk products. *Incomplete proteins* are supplied by plant sources (e.g., grains, nuts, legumes, seeds, vegetables). They can be combined to make complete proteins.	Stomach: Pepsin Pancreas: Trypsin, chymotrypsin, carboxypeptidase Intestine: Aminopeptidase, dipeptidase	10%–35% of the adult diet should be calories from protein, or 0.8 g/kg of body weight (46–56 g/day for an "average" person). Protein needs depend on age, body size, and physical state. Needs are increased during growth periods such as childhood and pregnancy.
Lipids	*Saturated fats* occur in pork, beef, poultry, seafood, egg yolk, and dairy; coconut oil and palm oil. *Unsaturated fats (from plants)* occur in olives, olive oil, vegetable oils (peanut, soybean, cottonseed, corn, safflower), nuts, and avocados. *Essential fatty acids (linoleic acid [omega-6] and alpha-linolenic acid [omega-3])* occur in polyunsaturated vegetable oils and in fatty fish (e.g., salmon). *Trans-fats* occur in hydrogenated oils, some margarines, packaged baked goods, and many processed foods.	Lingual: Lipase Gastric: Lipase, tributyrinase, bile salts Pancreatic lipase (steapsin)	Healthy adults should get 20%–35% of their calories from fat; children, 25%–40%. The American Heart Association recommends that people obtain < 30% of their calories from fat; < 7% of calories should come from saturated fats and < 1% from *trans*-fat. People with increased risk for heart disease may need stricter control.

Sources: Adapted from American Heart Association. (2015). Fats and oils: AHA recommendation. Retrieved from http://www.heart.org/HEARTORG/ GettingHealthy/FatsAndOils/Fats101/Fats-and-Oils-AHA-Recommendation_UCM_316375_Article.jsp; Institute of Medicine, Food and Nutrition Board, and the Panel on Macronutrients, Subcommittees on Upper Reference Levels of Nutrients and Interpretation and Uses of Dietary Reference Intakes, and the Standing Committee on the Scientific Evaluation of Dietary Reference Intakes. (2002/2005). *Dietary reference intakes for energy, carbohydrate, fiber, fat, fatty acid, cholesterol, protein, and amino acids.* Washington, DC: The National Academies Press. Retrieved from http://books.nap.edu/openbook.php?record_id=10490&page=R1

metabolic reaction, anabolism and catabolism, occur continually and are adjusted according to the needs of the body.

- **Anabolism** involves the formation of larger molecules from smaller ones. For example, if protein is needed for tissue repair, amino acids are recombined to form proteins. This process requires energy.
- **Catabolism** involves the breakdown of larger molecules into smaller components. This process releases energy.

Carbohydrates

Carbohydrates (CHOs) are the primary energy source for the body.

- **Simple carbohydrates,** commonly called *sugars,* are named according to the number of sugar (or *saccharide*) units making up their chemical structure.

  Monosaccharides (simple sugars) consist of a single unit.

  Disaccharides are molecules made up of two saccharides.

- **Complex carbohydrates** consist of long chains of saccharides, called **polysaccharides. Dietary fiber,** a polysaccharide, is the indigestible "fibrous skeleton" of plant foods. Humans do not have the enzymes to digest fiber; thus, it provides no usable glucose.

Functions of CHOs Carbohydrates perform several functions:

1. *Supply energy for muscle and organ function.* Carbohydrates are more easily and quickly digested than proteins and lipids. They fuel strenuous, short-term skeleton muscle activity and provide nearly all the energy for the brain. Humans store glucose in liver and skeletal muscle tissue as **glycogen.** Glycogen is converted back into glucose to meet energy needs. This process is called **glycogenolysis.**

2. *Spare protein.* If glycogen stores are low (e.g., in an undernourished person), physical activity causes the body to catabolize stores of protein **(gluconeogenesis)** and lipids (fats) to use for energy. However, when proteins are used for energy, they are not available for their primary functions of tissue growth, maintenance, and repair. Fats are then converted directly into an alternative fuel called **ketones,** which raise the acidity of the blood and can lead to acid–base imbalance.

3. *Other physiological functions* included the following;
   - Increase satiety (feeling of fullness and satisfaction).
   - Improve absorption of sodium and excretion of calcium.
   - Enhance insulin secretion. **Insulin** is a pancreatic hormone that promotes the movement of glucose into the cells for use.

Proteins

- **Proteins** are complex molecules made up of *amino acids.* Every amino acid consists of a central carbon atom connected to a hydrogen atom, an acid, an *amine* (a region of the molecule containing nitrogen), and a side chain. Just 20 different amino acids are the building blocks of most of the proteins in the human body.

- **Essential amino acids** are significant in our diets because the body cannot manufacture them. They must be supplied by food or nutritional supplements.

  Examples: Arginine, histidine, isoleucine, leucine, lysine, methoionine, phenylalanine, threonine, tryptophan, and valine

  Some consider arginine to be nonessential because it cannot be synthesized at a rate that will support growth; it is essential for children, but not for adults.

- **Nonessential amino acids** can be synthesized in the body, so we do not need to obtain them from food.

  Examples: Alanine, asparagine, aspartic acid, cysteine, glutamic acid, glutamine, glycine, proline, serine, and tyrosine

- Cysteine is considered essential in some situations, such as in immaturity or severe stress.

  For protein synthesis to occur, every amino acid necessary to build that protein must be available.

- **Complete proteins** contain all of the essential amino acids necessary for protein synthesis. These usually come from animal sources.

- **Incomplete proteins** (e.g., nuts, grains) do not provide all of the essential amino acids. However, by combining two incomplete proteins, a complete protein can be made. For instance, peanut butter on whole-grain bread constitutes a complete protein.

Protein Metabolism and Storage

Although protein digestion begins in the stomach, it occurs mostly in the small intestine, where enzymes break it down into amino acids (Table 28-1).

- The body continually breaks down and rebuilds protein into tissues, adjusting as needed to maintain overall protein balance.

- The body also maintains a balance between tissue protein and plasma protein.

Nitrogen Balance When amino acids are catabolized, the nitrogen-containing part is converted to ammonia and excreted in the urine as urea. Therefore, nitrogen level reflects how well body tissues are being maintained.

- **Nitrogen balance** occurs when intake and output of nitrogen are equal.

- **Positive nitrogen balance** exists when nitrogen intake exceeds output, making a pool of amino acids available for growth, pregnancy, and tissue maintenance and repair.

- **Negative nitrogen balance** exists when nitrogen loss exceeds nitrogen intake. This occurs in illness, injury (e.g., burns), and malnutrition.

Functions of Protein

Dietary proteins perform the following functions:

- *Tissue building.* Protein is essential for growth, maintenance, and repair of body cells and tissues. Except for water, protein makes up the biggest portion of the body.

- *Metabolism.* **Enzymes** facilitate cellular reactions throughout the body. Proteins are precursors to digestive enzymes and hormones (e.g., thyroxine). In addition, proteins combine with iron to form hemoglobin, the oxygen carrier in red blood cells.

- *Immune system function.* **Lymphocytes** (specialized white blood cells [WBCs]) and **antibodies** (components of our immune system that defend against foreign invaders) are proteins.

- *Fluid balance.* Because they attract water, proteins in cells and the bloodstream help regulate fluid balance.

- *Acid–base balance.* Blood proteins function as buffers, helping to regulate acid–base balance.

- *Secondary energy source.* As noted earlier, proteins can be broken down to provide energy when stores of the fats and CHOs are inadequate (Thompson & Manore, 2014).

  Lean meat is nourishing and healthy as long as it is consumed in modest amounts, is low in saturated fat, and is not processed. Many North Americans eat more protein than they need, especially in the form of red meat. Animal proteins high in saturated fat increase the risk for certain cancers and coronary artery disease.

Lipids

Lipids are organic (carbon-containing) substances that are insoluble in water. They are made up of carbon, hydrogen, and oxygen—the same basic elements that make up carbohydrates.

- **Fats** are solid at room temperature.
- **Oils** are liquid at room temperature.

For example, butter is a fat even when it is melted, because it would be solid at room temperature. You will hear the terms *lipids* and *fats* used interchangeably.

Fat is an essential nutrient for brain and nerve function, but certain types, when consumed in excess, can also be a health hazard. Lipid metabolism occurs in the small intestine. Because lipids are insoluble in water and because blood is primarily water, lipid absorption requires a solvent carrier.

Types of Lipids

The three types of lipids found in foods are glycerides, sterols, and phospholipids.

Glycerides   Also called **true fats,** glycerides consist of one molecule of glycerol attached to one, two, or three fatty acid chains.

- *Glycerol* is an alcohol composed of three carbon atoms.
- *Fatty acids* are long chains of carbon and hydrogen atoms ending in an acid.
- *Triglycerides* are the main glycerides found in foods. They are compounds consisting of a glycerol molecule attached to three fatty acids.

Sterols   are lipids, but are not made of fatty acids. The most important sterol in the body is **cholesterol,** a wax-like substance needed for the formation of cell membranes, vitamin D, estrogen, and testosterone. Cholesterol is synthesized in the liver, and it is also found in animal foods.

Phospholipids are a key component of **lipoproteins,** which consist of phospholipids and a protein. Because they are water soluble, lipoproteins are the major transport vehicles for lipids in the bloodstream. By "wrapping" triglycerides with water-soluble phosphates and proteins, lipoproteins deliver these substances to body cells.

- **Low-density lipoproteins (LDLs)** transport cholesterol to body cells. Diets high in saturated fats increase LDLs circulating in the bloodstream and may result in fatty deposits on vessel walls, causing cardiovascular disease. As a result, LDL is often known as the "bad cholesterol."
- **High-density lipoproteins (HDLs)** remove cholesterol from the bloodstream, returning it to the liver, where it is used to produce bile. Thus, a high blood level of HDL is considered protective against cardiovascular disease. It is often known as the "good cholesterol."

Saturated and Unsaturated Fatty Acids   Fatty acids are classified as saturated, unsaturated, or *trans*-fats (Table 28-2). Saturation means that a substance is holding all that it is capable of holding.

- An **unsaturated fatty acid** is not filled with all the hydrogen it can hold. Therefore, it is lighter and less dense
- **Monounsaturated fat** molecules have one unfilled spot where hydrogen is not attached.
- **Polyunsaturated fatty acids** contain two or more unfilled spots for hydrogen. At the spot(s) where no hydrogen is attached, the molecule becomes kinked and does not pack together. This is why these fats are liquid at room temperature. Dietary fat should mainly be polyunsaturated and unsaturated, to reduce the risk of heart disease and stroke.
- **Saturated fatty acids** are those in which every carbon atom is fully bound to (or "saturated" with) hydrogen. The molecules pack tightly together at room temperature and are dense, solid, and heavy.

Table 28-2 ▶ Dietary Fats

TYPE OF FAT	SOURCES	EFFECT ON BLOOD CHOLESTEROL
Monounsaturated	Olives; olive oil, canola oil, and peanut oil; cashews, almonds, peanuts, and most other nuts; avocados	Lowers LDL and raises HDL.
Polyunsaturated	Corn, soybean, safflower, sesame, sunflower, and cottonseed oils; fish, nuts, and seeds	Lowers LDL and raises HDL.
Saturated	Whole milk, butter, cheese, and ice cream; red meat; chocolate; coconuts, coconut milk, and coconut oil; palm oils; cocoa butter; processed foods	Raises LDL and HDL.
Trans-fats	Most margarines; vegetable shortening; partially hydrogenated vegetable oil; deep-fried chips; many fast foods (e.g., French fries, donuts); most commercial baked goods	Raises LDL.
Dietary Cholesterol	Foods from animals: meats, egg yolks, dairy products, organ meats (e.g., heart, liver), fish, and poultry	Raises cholesterol.

American Heart Association Recommendations

Limit foods high in saturated fat, *trans*-fat, and/or cholesterol. Instead, choose foods low in saturated fat, *trans*-fat, and cholesterol. Here are some helpful tips (AHA, 2015):

- Limit intake of whole-milk dairy products, fatty meats, tropical oils, partially hydrogenated vegetable oils, and egg yolks.
- Include a variety of fruits and vegetables in the diet.
- Eat a variety of grain products; include whole grains.
- Eat fish, particularly fatty fish, at least twice a week.
- Include fat-free and low-fat milk products and legumes.
- Choose skinless poultry and lean meats.
- Choose fats and oils with 2 g or less saturated fat per tablespoon (e.g., liquid and tub margarines, canola oil).

Trans-fatty acids are saturated fats created when food manufacturers add hydrogen to polyunsaturated plant oils, such as corn oil, to break the double carbon bonds and straighten out the molecules. This process solidifies the fat and extends the shelf life of the food. *Trans*-fats are found in processed foods containing *hydrogenated vegetable oils.*

Saturated fats and *trans*-fats are the main dietary factors in increasing blood cholesterol levels. They raise LDL cholesterol levels. The FDA mandates that *trans*-fat content be listed on all food labels.

Essential and Nonessential Fatty Acids A fatty acid is considered essential if (1) the body cannot manufacture it and (2) its absence creates a deficiency disease. The essential fatty acids, linoleic acid (omega-6) and alpha-linolenic acid (omega-3), help protect against heart disease.

Functions of Lipids

Lipids perform the following functions:

1. *Supply essential nutrients.* Food fats supply the essential fatty acids and aid in the absorption of fat-soluble vitamins.
2. *Energy source.* The body burns fat for energy when engaging in sustained light activity, when glycogen stores are exhausted, and when at rest. During strenuous physical activity, carbohydrates are the primary energy source.
3. *Flavor and satiety.* Lipids give food its creamy taste and texture and promote satiety (the feeling of being "full"). Fats are digested more slowly than carbohydrates, so stomach emptying time slows.
4. *Other functions.* Body fat provides insulation, protects vital organs, aids in thermoregulation, and enables accurate nerve-impulse transmission. In addition, lipids are a component of every cell membrane and are essential to cell metabolism.
5. *Cholesterol functions.* Cholesterol is a component of every cell in the body, where it lends suppleness and support. It is also an ingredient of bile, which helps digest fats, and serves as a precursor to all steroid hormones, including sex hormones. When lipid metabolism is "disordered," cholesterol contributes to atherosclerosis.

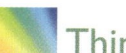

ThinkLike a Nurse 28-2

Review the information you collected on the two employees (Meet Your Patients).

- What conclusions, if any, can you make about their intake of carbohydrates, protein, and fats?
- How might you gather additional data on their intake of the energy nutrients?

WHAT ARE THE MICRONUTRIENTS?

Vitamins and minerals are called **micronutrients** because they are required by the body in only very small amounts. Although they provide no energy, they are critical in regulating a variety of body functions.

Vitamins

Vitamins are organic substances that are necessary for metabolism or preventing a particular deficiency disease. They are critical in building and maintaining body tissues, supporting the immune system to fight disease, and ensure healthy vision. Vitamins are especially critical during periods of rapid growth, pregnancy, lactation, and healing. Because the body cannot make vitamins, they must be supplied in food or supplements.

Table 28-3 summarizes specific functions of vitamins and Dietary Reference Intakes (DRIs). Although The Joint Commission includes the abbreviation *IU* on its "do not use" list, the abbreviation is used in other settings (e.g., on vitamin labels). Allowances (RDAs) represent the daily

Table 28-3 ▶ Vitamins: Adult Dietary Reference Intakes (DRIs)					
VITAMIN	FUNCTION	RDA/AI*	SOURCES	EFFECTS OF DEFICIENCY	SYMPTOMS OF EXCESS
Fat-Soluble Vitamins					
A	Night and color vision Cellular growth and maturity Maintaining healthy skin and mucous membranes Growth of skeletal and soft tissues Reproduction	*Females:* 600 mcg/day, 9–13 yr; 700 mcg/day, 14 yr and older *Males:* 600 mcg/day, 9–13 yr; 900 mcg/day, 14 yr and older	Fish liver oil, liver, butter, cream, egg yolk, yellow fruit, green leafy vegetables, fortified milk	Night blindness, xerosis, xerophthalmia, keratomalacia, skin lesions	GI upset, headache, blurred vision, poor muscle coordination, fetal defects
D°	Regulates blood calcium levels Regulates rate of deposit and resorption of calcium in bone	600 IU/day aged 1 to 70 800 IU/day after age 71	Fish liver oil, fish, fortified milk, sunlight exposure	Bone and muscle pain, weakness, softening of bone, fractures, rickets	Fatigue, weakness, loss of appetite, headache, mental confusion, mental retardation in infants

(Continued)

Table 28-3 ➤ Vitamins: Adult Dietary Reference Intakes (DRIs)—cont'd

VITAMIN	FUNCTION	RDA/AI*	SOURCES	EFFECTS OF DEFICIENCY	SYMPTOMS OF EXCESS
Fat-Soluble Vitamins					
E	Antioxidant Protects red blood cells and muscle tissue cells	15 mg/day, aged 14+	Vegetable oils, nuts, milk, eggs, muscle meats, fish, wheat and rice germ, green leafy vegetables	Hyporeflexia, ataxia, hemolytic anemia, myopathy	Insufficient blood clotting, impaired immune system
K	Synthesis of clotting factors Bone development	*Females:* 90 mcg/day (AI), aged 19+ *Males:* 120 mcg/day (AI), aged 19+	Green leafy vegetables, liver (Intestinal bacteria synthesize a form of vitamin K, so deficiency is unlikely.)	Increased bleeding	Jaundice and hemolytic anemia in infants
Water-Soluble Vitamins					
Thiamin	Cellular metabolism (producing energy from glucose and storing energy as fat) Nervous system function Gastrointestinal system function Cardiovascular system function	*Females:* 1.1 mg/day, aged 19+ *Males:* 1.2 mg/day, aged 14+	Whole grain enriched cereal, beef, pork, liver, peas, beans, nuts	Peripheral neuritis, loss of muscle strength, depression, memory loss, anorexia, constipation, dyspnea, decreased alertness and reflexes, fatigue, irritability, beriberi	Unlikely; readily excreted
Riboflavin	Cellular metabolism Antioxidant Tissue health and growth	*Females:* 1.1 mg/day *Males:* 1.3 mg/day	Milk, cheese, eggs, green vegetables, whole grain enriched cereals, bread, organ meats, poultry, fish	Tissue inflammation and breakdown: Sore throat, stomatitis, swollen tongue, facial dermatitis, anemia; poor wound healing	Unlikely; readily excreted
Niacin	Cellular metabolism to produce energy	*Females:* 14 mg/day *Males:* 16 mg/day	Enriched breads and cereals, chicken, tuna, liver, peanuts, dairy products	Weakness, poor appetite, indigestion, dermatitis, diarrhea, headache, dizziness, insomnia. *Chronic:* CNS damage (confusion, neuritis, dementia), pellagra	Facial flushing, itching, nausea, liver damage

Table 28-3 ➤ Vitamins: Adult Dietary Reference Intakes (DRIs)—cont'd

VITAMIN	FUNCTION	RDA/AI*	SOURCES	EFFECTS OF DEFICIENCY	SYMPTOMS OF EXCESS
Water-Soluble Vitamins					
B₆ (pyridoxine)	Protein (and some carbohydrate) metabolism RBC production Neurotransmitter synthesis	*Females:* 1.3 mg/day, younger than 50 yr 1.5 mg/day, aged 50+ *Males:* < 50 yr: 0.3 mg/day, ≥ 50 yr: 1.7 mg/day	Meats, poultry, fish, beans, nuts, seeds, dairy products, enriched cereals	Rash, stomatitis, seizure, peripheral neuritis, depression	Irreversible nerve damage (i.e., extremity numbness, walking difficulties)
Pantothenic Acid	Cell metabolism of fat and cholesterol Amino acid activation Heme formation	*All adults:* 5 mg/day (AI); 6 mg/day during pregnancy; 7 mg/day while lactating	Occurs widely in most foods. Best sources: Meats, whole grain cereals, legumes	Deficiency is unknown.	Unlikely; readily excreted
Folacin (folate, folic acid)	Cellular metabolism Neurotransmitter synthesis Cell division DNA synthesis Hemoglobin formation	400 mcg/day (folic acid); 600 mcg/day when pregnant Females capable of becoming pregnant should take a daily supplement of 400–800 mcg	Green leafy vegetables, asparagus, liver, yeast, eggs, beans, fruits, enriched cereals	Megaloblastic anemia, neural tube defects	Increased seizure activity, hives, respiratory distress, itching, rash
B₁₂ (cyanocobal-amin)	Metabolic reactions Maintain myelin sheath Hemoglobin synthesis	2.4 mcg/day	Dairy products, meat, poultry, fish, liver, milk, cheese, eggs	Pernicious anemia, irreversible nerve damage, memory loss, dementia	Unlikely; readily excreted
C	Collagen synthesis "Cementing" substance for capillary walls Antioxidant Iron absorption Immune function	*Females:* 75 mg/day *Males* (aged 19+): 90 mg/day Additional 35 mg/day for those who smoke	Citrus fruits, tomatoes, potatoes, green vegetables, cauliflower	Anemia, tissue bleeding, easy bone fracture, gingivitis, petechiae, poor wound healing, joint pain, scurvy	Stomach inflammation, diarrhea, oxalate kidney stones

Note: 1 mcg = 40 International Units (IU).
• **Recommended Dietary Allowances (RDAs)**—Intake sufficient to meet the needs of 97%–98% of individuals in a group.
• **Adequate Intakes (AIs)**—Recommended intake believed to cover the needs of all individuals in the group. These are used when RDAs can't be determined.
• **Upper Intake Levels (UIs)**—The maximum daily intake likely to pose no risk of adverse effects.
*RDAs are usually less than adult values for infants and children, more for pregnant women, and highest for lactating women. RDAs for some vitamins (e.g., vitamin A) are higher for older adults and higher for men than for women.
†The American Academy of Pediatrics recommends 10 mcg/day of vitamin D for infancy through adolescence (Wagner, & Greer; Section on Breastfeeding and Committee on Nutrition, 2008). Other clinicians and researchers have suggested that the RDA for adults should be dramatically increased as well, to 20–25 mcg (800–1000 IU) for adults aged 50 and older (Jockers, 2007).
Sources: Lutz, C., Mazur, E., & Litch, N. (2015); National Institutes of Health, Office of Dietary Supplements (n.d); U.S. Department of Agriculture and U.S. Department of Health and Human Services (2015).

dietary intake that is adequate to meet the needs of men, women, infants, and older adults.

Fat-Soluble Vitamins   The fat-soluble vitamins are A, D, E, and K. They are stored primarily in the liver and adipose tissues, although vitamin E is deposited in all body tissue.

- *Stored in the body.* Because the body can store these vitamins, we do not need to consume them every day if we are consuming them in adequate amounts. However, diets extremely low in fat and disorders affecting fat digestion and absorption can lead to deficiency of fat-soluble vitamins.
- *Not readily excreted.* Because they are not readily excreted, excessive supplementation with the fat-soluble vitamins can lead to toxicity.
- *Some need more vitamin D.* The Institute of Medicine and other guidelines recommend that those with little sun exposure, oseteoporosis, dark skin, or taking medication interfering with vitamin D absorption may require more than the daily recommendation (Ross, Taylor, Yaktine, et al., 2011).

Water-Soluble Vitamins   The water-soluble vitamins include vitamin C and the B-complex vitamins (Table 28-3). Because these vitamins are soluble in water, excess amounts are regularly excreted in the urine. Thus:

- Toxicity is rare except in people with renal disease.
- The body cannot store these vitamins, so they need to be consumed every day.

Minerals

Minerals are inorganic elements found in nature. They occur in naturally in foods, as food additives, and in supplements.

- **Major minerals (macrominerals)** are minerals that the body needs in amounts of 100 mg/day or greater.
- **Trace minerals** are essential, but in a lower concentration.

Functions   Minerals assist in fluid regulation, nerve impulse transmission, and energy production; they are essential to the health of bones and blood and help rid the body of by-products of metabolism. Evidence also shows that minerals play key roles in disease prevention and treatment. For example:

1. Adequate *calcium* intake throughout the life span decreases the likelihood of osteoporosis (a condition marked by porous bones). The recommended daily intake is difficult to achieve by diet alone. In the United States, calcium deficiency is one of the most common mineral deficiencies (Table 28-4).
2. *Iron* deficiency causes anemia, the most common nutritional problem worldwide.
3. *Magnesium* deficiency increases the risk of hypertension and coronary artery disease in women.
4. *Sodium,* consumed in high amounts (> 2,500 mg/day), increases the risk for high blood pressure, heart attacks, and stroke.

If the body is deficient in a mineral, it absorbs more; if the body has enough, it absorbs less and excretes more in the feces. Minerals interact with other minerals, vitamins, and other substances to accomplish absorption and metabolism and perform their functions. For example, iron absorption is enhanced in the presence of vitamin C, and vitamin D deficiency inhibits calcium absorption.

WHY IS WATER AN ESSENTIAL NUTRIENT?

Water is made up of hydrogen and oxygen and makes up about half of total body weight (55% to 65% in men and 50% to 55% in women). This is because men have greater muscle

Table 28-4 ➤ Minerals: Adult Dietary Reference Intakes*					
MINERAL	**FUNCTION**	**RDA†**	**SOURCES**	**EFFECTS OF DEFICIENCY**	**SYMPTOMS OF EXCESS**
Macrominerals					
Calcium (Ca)	Bone and teeth formation, blood clotting, nerve conduction, muscle contraction, cellular metabolism, heart action	700 mg/day (AI), aged 1–3; 1,000 mg/day (AI) aged 4–8; 1,300 mg/day (AI), aged 9–18; 1,000 mg/day, aged 19–70 (although females aged 51–70 years need 1,200 mg/day); 1,200 mg/day, aged 70 and older.	Dairy products, sardines, green leafy vegetables, broccoli, whole grains, egg yolks, legumes, nuts, fortified products	Bone loss, tetany, rickets, osteoporosis	Kidney stones, constipation, intestinal gas
Magnesium (Mg)	Aids thyroid hormone secretion, maintains normal basal metabolic rate, activates enzymes for carbohydrate and protein metabolism, nerve and muscle function, cardiac function	Females: 310 mg/day (AI), aged 19–30 Males: 400 mg/day (AI), aged 19–30; 420 mg/day, aged 31+	Whole grains, nuts, legumes, green leafy vegetables, lima beans, broccoli, squash, potatoes	Tremor, spasm, convulsions, weakness, muscle pain, poor cardiac function	Weakness, nausea, malaise

Table 28-4 ▶ Minerals: Adult Dietary Reference Intakes*—cont'd

MINERAL	FUNCTION	RDA†	SOURCES	EFFECTS OF DEFICIENCY	SYMPTOMS OF EXCESS
Phosphorus (P)	Bone and tooth strength, overall metabolism, formation of enzymes, acid–base balance	700 mg/day (AI), aged 19+	Dairy products, beef, pork, beans, sardines, eggs, chicken, wheat bran, chocolate	Bone loss, poor growth	Tetany, convulsions
Potassium (K)	Intracellular fluid control, acid–base balance, nerve transmission, muscle contraction, glycogen formation, protein synthesis, energy metabolism, blood pressure regulation	4.7 g/day (AI)	Unprocessed foods, especially fruits, any vegetables, meats, potatoes, avocados, legumes, milk, molasses, shellfish, dates, figs	Muscle weakness (including weakness of heart and respiratory muscles), weak pulse, fatigue, abdominal distention. (Rarely occurs as a result of inadequate dietary intake. More likely due to losses from prolonged vomiting, diarrhea, or some diuretic drugs.)	Cardiac dysrhythmias, cardiac arrest, weakness, abdominal cramps, diarrhea, anxiety, paresthesia
Sodium (Na)	Water balance, acid–base balance, muscle action, nerve transmission, convulsions	1.5 g/day (AI), aged 19–50; 1.3 g/day, aged 51–70; 1.2 g/day, aged 70+	Table salt (NaCl), milk, meat, eggs, baking soda, baking powder, celery, spinach, carrots, beets	Dizziness, abdominal cramping, nausea, vomiting, diarrhea, tachycardia, convulsions, coma	Thirst, fever, dry and sticky tongue and mucous membranes, restlessness, irritability, convulsion
Trace Minerals					
Copper	Aids in iron metabolism, works with many enzymes in protein metabolism and hormone synthesis	900 mcg/day (AI), aged 19+	Liver, seafood, cocoa, legumes, nuts, whole grains	Rarely occurs: anemia, low WBC count, poor growth	Vomiting, nervous system disorders
Fluoride	Increases resistance to dental caries	Females: 3 mg/day (AI), aged 14+ Males: 4 mg/day (AI), aged 19+	Fluorinated water, toothpaste, dental treatment, seaweed, fish, tea	Increased dental caries	Stomach upset, staining of teeth, bone pain

(Continued)

Table 28-4 ▶ Minerals: Adult Dietary Reference Intakes*—cont'd

MINERAL	FUNCTION	RDA†	SOURCES	EFFECTS OF DEFICIENCY	SYMPTOMS OF EXCESS
Iodine	Synthesis of the thyroid hormone, thyroxine	150 mcg/day, aged 14+	Iodized salt, salt water fish, dairy products, enriched white bread	Goiter, poor infancy growth, cretinism, hypothyroidism	Skin lesions, thyroid malfunction
Iron	Synthesis of hemoglobin, general metabolism (e.g., of glucose), antibody production, drug detoxification in the liver	*Females:* 18 mg/day, aged 19–50; 8 mg/day, aged 50+ *Males:* 8 mg/day, aged 19+	Meats, eggs, spinach, seafood, broccoli, peas, bran, enriched breads, fortified cereals	Small, pale RBCs, anemia	Hemochro-matosis
Zinc	Cofactor for many enzymes involved in growth, insulin storage immunity, alcohol metabolism, sexual development and reproduction	*Females:* 8 mg/day *Males:* 11 mg/day	Primarily red meats and poultry; oysters; also legumes, peas, and whole grains	Skin rash, diarrhea, decreased appetite, hair loss, poor growth and development, poor wound healing, taste abnormalities, mental lethargy	Reduced copper absorption, altered iron function, diarrhea, cramps, depressed immune function

*Dietary Reference Intakes (DRIs) represent:
• Recommended Dietary Allowances (RDAs)—Intake set to meet the needs of 97%–98% of individuals in a group.
• Adequate Intakes (AIs)—Believed to cover the needs of all individuals in the group.
• Upper Intake Levels (UIs)—The maximum daily intake likely to pose no risk of adverse effects.
• Values in table are RDAs unless marked (AI).
†RDAs are usually less than adult values for infants and children, more for pregnant women, and highest for lactating women. RDAs for some minerals are higher for older adults and different for men and women.
Sources: Institute of Medicine, Food and Nutrition Board (2005); Lutz, C., & Przytulski, K. (2015); National Institutes of Health, Office of Dietary Supplements (n.d., 2016); U.S. Department of Agriculture and U.S. Department of Health and Human Services (2015).

mass, and muscle contains a relatively large amount of water. Water is distributed in two body compartments.

- **Intracellular fluid** is the water contained within each living cell. It makes up about 40% of the total body weight.
- **Extracellular fluid** is external to the cell membrane (e.g., in the fluid portion of blood and lymph and in the gastrointestinal [GI] tract); it accounts for 20% of body weight.

Water is critical to the body because its functions are essential to life:

- **Solvent.** Water is the basic solvent for the body's chemical processes.
- **Transport.** As a component of blood, water serves as a medium for transporting oxygen, nutrients, and metabolic wastes.
- **Body structure and form.** Water "fills in the spaces" in body tissues (e.g., in blood, lymphatic material, and muscle) and by way of diffusion and osmosis transports ions into and out of cells.

- **Temperature.** Water helps maintain body temperature. When body temperature rises, evaporation of sweat helps cool the body.
- **Lubricant.** Fluid reduces friction between moving surfaces, such as in joints, and in thoracic and abdominal cavities where organs need to move freely.
- **Catalyst.** Water is a part of many biochemical reactions, such as the conversion of carbohydrates and proteins into energy during the digestive process.

The amount of water a person requires varies according to the environmental humidity and temperature, activity level, age, and metabolic needs. The average AI is about 2.7 liters of water per day for adult women and 3.7 liters for men (Lutz, Mazur, & Litch, 2015; Sawka, Cheuvront, & Carter, 2005). Eighty percent of those amounts should come from fluids. We also obtain water in the foods we eat.

Overall fluid balance is maintained when fluid intake (in liquids, foods, and metabolic reactions) matches fluid output (through urine, feces, respiration, and sweat.) Fluid and electrolyte balance is discussed in Chapter 39.

PICOT

Fluid Balance

Situation: The nurse working in the emergency department is reviewing an elderly client's intake and output (I&O) with him. The I&O are out of balance. The nurse begins to question the client further about other potential consequences of dehydration. How might she phrase a question to design a personalized patient teaching plan prior to discharge to home?

Searchable Question: Do _____ (P) who are _____ (I) demonstrate _____ (O) as compared to _____ (C) during _____ (T)?

PICOT Components

P	Population/patient	=	Elderly inpatients
I	Intervention/indicator	=	Dehydration
C	Comparator/control	=	Elderly community dwellers
O	Outcome	=	Complications of dehydration
T	Time	=	During hospitalization

Searching for the Evidence: Overall fluid balance is affected by diet, exercise, temperature, illness, and medication. Older people are also more susceptible to dehydration because of cognitive, sensory, and motor impairments, which affect their activities of daily living. They tend to take more medications and have more illness that can increase the risk for fluid imbalance. For example, the frail older person with exercise intolerance related to chronic pain may become easily dehydrated. If that person becomes ill, it is even more likely that the client will be unable independently to take in sufficient amounts of fluid. It is important to encourage all elderly people, inpatient and in the community, to consume small amounts of fluids throughout the day in order to maintain adequate fluid balance. Assessment questions that might point to a fluid imbalance would include those regarding intake, activity, and elimination patterns.

_____

Boltz, M., Capezuti, E., Fulmer, T., et al. (2016). *Evidence-based geriatric nursing protocols for best practice* (5th ed.). New York, NY: Springer.

KnowledgeCheck 28-2

- What is the body's most usable energy source?
- Which nutrient's primary function is growth and repair of tissue?
- Identify five functions of adipose tissue (body fat).
- Which type of vitamin requires daily consumption to maintain appropriate levels?
- What distinguishes a major mineral from a trace mineral?
- Identify at least four functions of water.

WHAT MUST I KNOW ABOUT ENERGY BALANCE?

The energy in carbohydrates, proteins, and lipids is measured in terms of **calories,** or, more precisely, **kilocalories (kcal).** A kcal is the amount of heat required to raise the temperature of 1 kg of water 1° centigrade. To maintain a stable weight, the number of kcal consumed must equal the number of kcal burned.

- **Too few dietary kcal** results in weight loss and is likely to lack essential nutrients, causing weakened immunity, stunted growth, and hormonal disruption.
- **Too many dietary kcal** can cause weight gain and obesity, which increases the risk for chronic diseases.

Below is the amount of energy liberated from the metabolism of 1 gram of energy nutrients:

Carbohydrates = 4 kcal/g
Protein = 4 kcal/g
Fat = 9 kcal/g

KEY POINT: *In determining total energy (kilocalorie) needs, consider the client's basal metabolic rate and the duration and intensity of daily physical activity.*

KnowledgeCheck 28-3

Imagine that you have just eaten a food consisting of 4 grams of protein, 18 grams of carbohydrate, and 1 gram of fat.

- What would your total kcal intake be?
- What percentage of your kcal is from carbohydrates? Protein? Fat?

What Is Basal Metabolic Rate?

The **basal metabolic rate (BMR)** is a measure of the energy used while at rest in a neutral temperature environment—the energy required for vital organs such as the heart, liver, and brain to function.

Direct measurement of BMR requires use of a **calorimeter**: an insulated unit that measures temperature changes of water that are produced by exposure to a fasting individual at rest. Although it is very accurate, it is rarely used because most institutions do not have calorimeters and because the test requires a controlled environment and a 12-hour fast. Direct measurement of BMR is used primarily by researchers.

Indirect calculation of BMR, sometimes called the resting energy expenditure, includes the following:

- Measuring oxygen uptake per unit of time. This can be done in an exercise lab or with portable machines at the bedside. It is most often done for patients in intensive care units. Not all facilities have this capability.
- Serum thyroxine levels (a blood test).
- A formula for calculating BMR when precise measurement is not required (Box 28-2).

What Factors Affect Basal Metabolic Rate?

When interpreting test results, consider the following factors that influence BMR:

- *Body composition.* Lean body tissue has greater metabolic activity than fat and bones. This explains why women, who have on average more adipose tissue than men, also have lower BMRs.
- *Growth periods.* BMR increases during periods of growth, such as the first 5 years of life, adolescence, pregnancy, and lactation.
- *Body temperature.* The BMR increases 7% for each 1°F (0.83°C) rise in body temperature.
- *Environmental temperature.* Cold weather, especially temperatures below freezing, causes a slight rise in the BMR to generate body heat and maintain normal body temperature.

BOX 28-2 ■ Calculating Basal Metabolic Rate (BMR)

Females:	0.9 kcal/kg of body weight per hour
Males:	1.0 kcal/kg body weight per hour
Example:	Isaac Schwartz (Meet Your Patients) weighs 245 lb.

1 kilogram = 2.2 pounds.

Divide 245 by 2.2 to convert pounds to kilograms:

$$245 \div 2.2 = 111.3$$

Now complete the calculation:

$$1.0 \times 111.3 \times 24 \text{ hours} = 2671.2$$

■ *Disease processes.* Diseases and injuries involving increased cellular activity result in BMR elevation (e.g., cancer, anemia, cardiac failure, hypertension, asthma, severe burns, traumatic injury).
■ *Prolonged physical exertion.* Examples: chopping wood, running.

How Do I Calculate a Client's Total Energy Needs?

A person's total daily energy requirement is the number of kcal necessary to replace those used for basic metabolism plus those used in physical activities. The following are simple, general estimates based on activity level and age:
■ Sedentary women and older adults need 1,600 kcal/day.
■ Children, teenage girls, active women, and most men need 2,200 kcal/day.
■ Teenage boys, active men, and very active women need 2,800 kcal/day.

To calculate energy use more precisely, you need to know the person's age, weight, and physical activity, including the intensity and duration of the activity (Table 28-5).

Heightened emotional states may also increase energy needs because they increase muscular activity in the form of muscle tension, restlessness, and agitated movements.

KnowledgeCheck 28-4

You have already calculated the expected BMR for Mr. Schwartz (Meet Your Patients) for a 24-hour period.

■ If Mr. Schwartz describes himself as working at a desk 8 to 10 hours per day, lawn mowing manually every other week during the summer, and playing an occasional game of golf, how would you classify his general activity level?

■ After interviewing Mr. Schwartz, you estimate his average caloric intake to be approximately 3,000 kcal per day. Determine whether his kcal intake is sufficient or insufficient to maintain his present activity level.

What Are Some Body Weight Standards?

Weight standards have been established to correlate weight with good health and longevity and to help determine a client's ideal body weight. The **general ideal weight guide** uses a formula to determine a reasonable weight based on height:

Men: 106 lb (47.7 kg) for the first 5 ft (150 cm), then add 6 lb/in. (2.7 kg/2.5 cm)
Women: 100 lb (45 kg) for the first 5 ft (150 cm), then add 5 lb/in. (2.25 kg/2.5 cm)
Add 10% for large body frame; subtract 10% for small body frame.

Various **height and weight tables** have been developed over the years. World Health Organization (WHO) child growth standards are based on statistical estimates and often include variations for age, sex, and body frame. Type **who.int/childgrowth** into your browser and follow the links if you want to see the World Health Organization (WHO) child growth standards.

Body composition analysis attempts to quantify lean body mass versus percentage body fat. Lean body mass includes muscle, bone, and connective tissue. Lean tissue weighs more than fat; thus, a person who engages in regular weight-bearing exercise and is physically fit may actually weigh more than an individual of similar appearance who is sedentary and unfit. Various methods to assess body composition, known as *anthropometric measurements,* are provided in the Assessment section later in the chapter.

ThinkLike a Nurse 28-3

Examine your dietary intake for the next 3 days to determine how balanced your diet is.

■ How does your diet compare with the USDA MyPlate in terms of:
   a. Servings of bread, cereal, rice, and pasta? _____
   b. Servings of vegetables? _____
   c. Servings of fruits? _____
   d. Servings of milk, yogurt, and cheese? _____
   e. Servings of meat, poultry, fish, dry beans, eggs, and nuts? _____
   f. Servings of fats, oils, and sweets? _____
■ From what you have learned from this activity, what habits could you change in patterns of eating in order to achieve optimal nutrition?

Table 28-5 ➤ Energy Needs Based on Weight and Activity

For *each pound of body weight,* a person needs the following per day:

ACTIVITY LEVEL	UNDERWEIGHT	NORMAL WEIGHT	OVERWEIGHT
Sedentary	13 kcal	13 kcal	9–11 kcal
Moderately active	18 kcal	16 kcal	13 kcal
Active	18–23 kcal	18 kcal	16 cal

EXAMPLE PROBLEM: Overweight/Obesity

Definition

- **Overweight or Obesity:** Weight higher than considered healthy for a given height
- **Body measurements:** Body weight 20% > ideal for height and frame

- **Body mass index (BMI)** 25–29.9 = overweight
  BMI ≥ 30 = obesity
- **Percentage of body fat:**
Obesity:	Men – > 25%	Women – > 33%
Overweight:	Men – 21%–25%	Women – 31%–33%

COMPLICATIONS

Physical

- Type 2 diabetes
- Heart disease, hypertension, hyperlipidemia, stroke
- Metabolic syndrome
- Cancer
- Breathing problems, increased asthma, shortness of breath
- Sleeping problems, sleep apnea
- Gallbladder disease
- Joint pain & injuries, osteoarthritis

- Erectile dysfunction, infertility, irregular menstruation
- Skin ulcers, heat rash, fungal infection, acne

Emotional

- Reduced self-esteem, shame, guilt
- Loneliness and social isolation
- Depression, anxiety, obsessive compulsive disorder (binge eating)

ETIOLOGIES

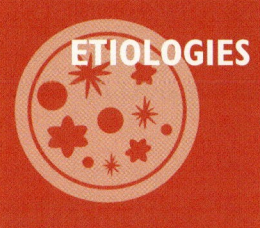

Risk Factors

- *Genetic factors/family predisposition*
- *Dietary intake*—poor quality, high-calorie, high-fat, high-salt, sugary, and processed foods; larger portions; habit of overeating and binging; snacking
- *Sedentary lifestyle*—high screen time, low physical activity
- *Medical condition*—Prader-Willi syndrome, endocrine and neurological disorders

- *Hormonal changes, slowing metabolism, menopause*
- *Medication*—steroids, some psychiatric drugs
- *Learned behaviors / emotional eating*—conflict, depression, reward for good behaviors; comfort when feeling sad or lonely; expression of love

---

DIAGNOSIS

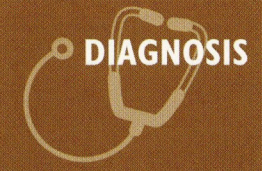

Obesity
Overweight
Overweight, Risk for

Examples:

- Overweight r/t insufficient physical activity, high-fat and high-sugar diet
- Obesity r/t metabolic disorder

OUTCOMES

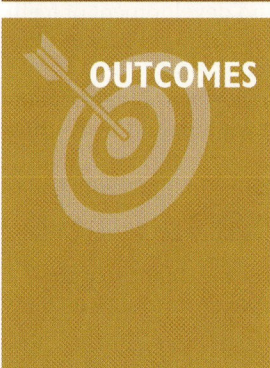

NOC Outcomes

Weight
Body Mass
Weight Loss Behavior
Weight Maintenance Behavior
Nutritional Status: Food and Fluid Intake
Nutritional Status: Nutrient Intake

Individualized goals/outcome statements

- Progressively gains weight toward desired goal.
- States factors contributing to weight gain.
- Designs dietary plan for long-term weight control.
- Reaches desired weight loss in an achievable time frame.
- Incorporates physical activities into daily life.

(Continued)

EXAMPLE PROBLEM: Overweight/Obesity—cont'd

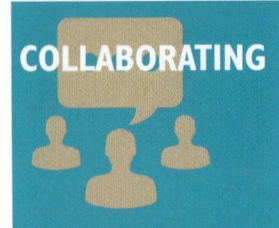

COLLABORATING

Weight-loss options for BMI > 40

- Appetite suppressant on an individual basis
- Consult with a dietitian for weight management.
- Refer for appropriate counseling as needed.

- Gastric bypass, laparoscopic adjustable gastric banding, gastric sleeve, biliopancreatic diversion with duodenal switch, vagal nerve blockade

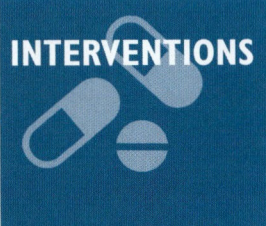

INTERVENTIONS

Weight control

- Set realistic expectations for weight loss and exercise goals.
- Encourage regular exercise, beginning gradually with low-impact activities. Minimum 300 min/week.
- Suggest the client keeps a food diary, uses a diet tracker mobile application, or blogs.
- Weigh the client weekly at the same time.

- See Self-Care box Teaching Weight-Loss Tips
- For children, recommend:
  5 – Servings of fruits and vegetables each day
  2 – Hours or less of "screen" time per day
  1 – Hour of physical activity per day
  0 – Servings of sweetened beverages

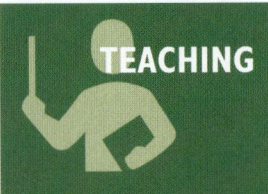

TEACHING

- Teach MyPlate dietary plan: more whole grains, fruits and vegetables, and lean protein.
- Teach client to reduce portion sizes; restrict high-carbohydrate, high-fat, sweetened foods and beverages.

- Warn clients to be wary of quick weight-loss plans and fad diets.
- Suggest weight-loss support group.
- **KEY POINT:** *Exercise and diet are both essential to weight control.*

CARING

Be encouraging and nonjudgmental, especially when there are setbacks.

WHAT FACTORS AFFECT NUTRITION?

Several factors influence nutritional needs and choices. Some can be modified; some cannot. The most influential factors are development, knowledge, lifestyle, culture, disease processes, and functional limitations. Parents and caregivers are the most important influences on the eating habits of children.

Developmental Stage

At specific developmental stages, nutritional needs and eating patterns vary according to physiological growth, activity level, metabolic processes, disease prevention, and other factors.

Infants to 1 Year

Humans grow most rapidly during the first year of life. Nutritional needs per unit of body weight are greater than at any other time.

Calories and Protein The infant needs adequate protein for tissue building and enough carbohydrates to furnish energy and "spare" the protein. **KEY POINT:** *The period from conception into the second year of life is most critical to brain development; therefore, the baby needs optimal nutrition.* Severe protein-calorie deficiency in the last trimester of pregnancy or the first 6 months of life may decrease the number of brain cells by 20%.

Vitamins and Minerals Fetal iron stores are depleted at 4 to 6 months, so intake of iron becomes important. The infant also needs calcium for bone growth and development of teeth, calcium and vitamin C for iron absorption, and vitamin D for calcium regulation.

Fluids Compared with adults, infants have a higher metabolic rate. Infants need proportionately more fluid than adults because infants:
- Have greater water loss through the skin, and skin makes up a greater proportion of the infant body.
- Have immature kidneys.

To meet nutritional and fluid needs, the infant requires 1.5 to 2 ounces of breast milk or formula per pound of body weight per day.

Infant Feedings KEY POINT: *The only safe choices for meeting fluid and nutrient needs in the first months of life are breast milk and commercially prepared formulas.* Breast milk is the ideal nutrition for infants and is sufficient to support healthy growth and development in infancy (American Heart Association, 2016). Breastfeeding has the following benefits:
- Enhances maturation of the infant's immune system and provides passive immunity against a number of infections, including pneumonia, acute otitis media, and gastroenteritis.

- Lower risk of sudden infant death syndrome (SIDS) (American Academy of Pediatrics, Task Force on Sudden Infant Death Syndrome, 2016).
- For infants receiving breast milk in the first 6 months of life it may also decrease the risk of developing diabetes mellitus later in life, obesity, asthma, and childhood leukemia (American Academy of Pediatrics, 2012; Crume, Ogden, Maligie, et al., 2011; Yamakawa, Yorifuji, Inoue, et al., 2013).

The American Heart Association recommends breastfeeding for 12 months with the addition of solid foods for micronutrients, beginning 4 to 6 months of life (2016). When breastfeeding is contraindicated or the mother chooses not to breastfeed, numerous commercial formulas are available. The most commonly used formula is iron-fortified, cow's milk protein available in powder, liquid concentrate, or ready-to-use liquid. Other types include iron-fortified, soy, and protein hydrolysate formulas.

✚ Infants younger than 1 year should not receive fresh cow's milk because it may cause gastrointestinal bleeding and may stress the infant's kidneys. It also can contribute to iron-deficiency anemia.

✚ Honey and corn syrup should not be used as a source of carbohydrates in preparing infant formula. They are potential sources of botulism toxin, which can be fatal in children younger than 1 year old (Centers for Disease Control and Prevention, 2014).

Whether to boil water prior to constituting infant formula depends on the water quality of the tap supply. When in doubt, consult the local health department. If unsure, the FDA recommends boiling rapidly for a minimum of 1 full minute and cooling completely before adding it to infant formula.*

Healthy infants born at term have sufficient iron for their first 4 months. Iron supplements are usually given beginning at 4 to 6 months (depending on whether breast- or formula-fed), and they may continue after 12 months if iron needs are not being met (Baker & Greer; Committee on Nutrition, 2010). Solids foods are generally introduced beginning with cereal at four to 6 months of age.

Toddlers

Toddlers grow more slowly in comparison with infants and have fewer energy demands. Toddlers generally require about 1,000 kcal and 1,250 mL of fluid per day, depending on body weight. As the GI system matures, they are able to eat most foods and adjust to the adult pattern of three meals a day. By age 3, most children have all of their deciduous teeth and can chew adult food.

- ✚ **Food should be cut into small pieces** to avoid choking in toddlers who sometimes are "too busy" to chew food sufficiently.
- **Sometimes young children "chipmunk" their food** and can later choke on it.
- **Do not give food when the child is in a car seat or bouncy chair,** where choking is more likely and can occur without a parent's noticing.

---

*Water that is purified or bottled for use in infant formulas does not contain fluoride. Fluoride might be prescribed in this situation and for infants without a fluoridated water supply.

- **Toddlers' diets are often deficient in nutrients,** commonly iron, calcium, and vitamins A and C. One- and 2-year-old children should drink reduced-fat (2%) milk or, in some cases, whole milk to provide adequate essential fatty acids for the still-growing brain.
- **Parents need to offer a variety of foods to provide essential nutrients.** Each meal should contain at least one fruit or vegetable; juice intake should be limited. This can be a challenge, because toddlers refuse foods to assert their autonomy or manipulate their parents. They may take a long time to eat or refuse to eat at all.
- **Parents should not turn mealtime into a battle of wills or use foods to punish or reward;** such reactions may affect the child's attitude toward food or magnify problem feeding behaviors. To encourage the child to eat, you may offer parents the suggestions in the accompanying Home Care box.

Preschoolers

Between ages 4 and 6, caloric need is typically 1,200 to 1,400 kcal/day. Dietary fat should provide only 25% to 30% of the child's intake (American Heart Association, 2015). Children's appetites naturally regulate food intake, depending on physical needs for energy and nutrition. It is important that parents and caregivers do not overfeed. Preschoolers are similar to toddlers in their growth and nutritional needs; however, their eating patterns typically improve.

- They begin to form responses to specific foods, such as refusing green vegetables or drinking less milk.
- They often refuse casseroles and foods with sauces.
- They might also eat only one particular food for several days.
- Because they are active, preschoolers require nutritious between-meal snacks.

Home Care

Tips for Encouraging Toddlers to Eat

➤ Be a good food role model. Children don't learn as much by listening to what you say but rather more by watching what you do.

➤ Keep only nutritious foods in the house to avoid battles over nutrient-poor snacks.

➤ Offer healthy foods that are easy to eat (e.g., "finger foods" or those easily chewed).

➤ Serve foods in a child-friendly way; for example, arrange tortillas, cheese, tomato slices, and beans in a smiling face.

➤ Allow the child to "graze" throughout the day on healthful foods rather than insisting that she sit for formal meals at the table.

➤ Avoid "combined" foods, such as casseroles and stews.

➤ Limit consumption of sweets and snack foods.

➤ Do not use dessert as a reward for eating other foods (e.g., "You can't have cookies until you eat your meat"). Reward with attention (hugs, kind words) instead of food.

➤ Include your child in food shopping. Let your child help select nutritious foods and serve them at home.

➤ Commit to family mealtimes to connect with each other. Turn off TV and cell phones. Get everyone involved.

- Lifelong food habits are developed during this stage, so encourage families to widen the variety of foods offered to preschoolers and to investigate the diet provided by their child's day care or preschool. A variety of foods is essential for children to get enough carbohydrates, protein and other nutrients.

School-Age Children

In the school-age period, growth and body changes occur gradually. Permanent teeth erupt, and the digestive system matures. Sedentary school-age children need about 1,600 to 1,800 kcal/day; active children typically require and additional 200 to 400 more kcal per day (American Heart Association, 2016).

- **Nutrients.** An adequate supply of vitamins and minerals is critical because the body is still growing and preparing for the demands of adolescence. Foods should be low in saturated fat, *trans*-fat, cholesterol, salt (sodium), and added sugars.
- **Eating behaviors.** Parental control over food intake declines because advertising influences the child's food choices. The child eats away from home and may buy junk food with his lunch money or choose less nutritious foods in the school cafeteria. Even if the child brings lunch from home, he may trade his food or not eat lunch at all. Parents should encourage their children to eat breakfast to provide nutrients and energy to fuel problem-solving skills, memory, and sports and playground activities.

Adolescents

Adolescence is a time of rapid growth and development of the reproductive system. Boys experience an increase in muscle tissue and bone length and density. At menstruation, girls experience fat deposition. The needs of the adolescent body for energy, vitamins, and minerals approach those of the infant. In particular, adolescents need protein, calcium, iron, and B and D vitamins.

Adolescents have active lifestyles and snack often, preferring convenience foods such as chips and cookies, and fast foods. Unfortunately, most such foods have little nutrient value. Adolescents are responsible for their own food decisions, so the best approach for parents is to keep only healthful snack foods (e.g., cheese, fruit, raw vegetables) in the home and role model a positive attitude toward healthy eating.

Eating disorders are a concern in this group. Most people with eating disorders exhibit their first symptoms before age 20, some as early as age 10. The majority of those with eating disorders are female (National Association of Anorexia Nervosa and Associated Disorders, n.d.).

Adults

Note: Underweight adults have a higher risk of early death 1.8 times greater than people of a healthy weight. Overweight people face a risk 1.2 times greater, and obese people 1.3 times greater (Cao, Moineddin, Urquia, et al., 2014).

- **Young adults** continue to require adequate amounts of protein, vitamins, and minerals, but not at the same levels as in adolescence. If adults continue unhealthful behaviors developed in earlier stages, repercussions will begin to show up in adulthood. Calcium, vitamin D, folic acid, and iron continue to be critical, especially in women, for bone and reproductive health.
- **Middle adults.** The BMR decreases in middle-age, potentially causing weight gain if dietary intake and activity level are unchanged. Individuals may begin to experience

chronic illnesses such as diabetes, hypertension, obesity, hyperlipidemia, and certain types of cancer. Often these are a result of heredity or poor lifestyle choices; however, dietary modification and exercise are essential to control these diseases.

Pregnant and Lactating Women

Nutritional requirements increase dramatically during pregnancy as the mother provides for the nutritional needs of the fetus.

- *Folic acid* intake is critical in the first trimester of pregnancy (the first 13 weeks) to prevent neural tube defects; a daily supplement of 600 to 800 mcg is recommended during pregnancy (American Academy of Pediatrics, 1999; Centers for Disease Control and Prevention, 2016, January, updated; U.S. Preventive Services Task Force, 2014).
- *Adequate protein and calcium* are important for growing muscle, brain, and bone tissues; iron is essential to maintain maternal and fetal blood supplies and stores during pregnancy.
- *Supplements*—It is almost impossible to consume the recommended amount of dietary *iron,* so supplements are commonly prescribed, as are supplements of *folic acid* and *calcium.*
- *Calories*—Pregnant women need about 300 additional kcal/day in the second and third trimesters of pregnancy.
- *Women who are breastfeeding* need 500 additional kcal per day. They continue to need additional protein and calcium, as well as increased fluid intake to make adequate amounts of breast milk. The nutritional quality of the milk remains the same even if dietary intake is not adequate.
- *Pregnant women also need to be screened for gestational diabetes.* Complications include increased childhood obesity, fetal macrosomia, and primary cesarean section (Hartling, Dryden, Guthrie, 2012).

Older Adults

Nutritional needs of older adults vary only slightly from those in middle adulthood (Table 28-6). Lean body mass, physical activity, and BMR decrease, so older adults tend to need fewer kcal; however, they still need the same or higher levels of nutrients.

Factors Affecting Nutrition Changes of aging often make it difficult for the older adult to achieve good nutrition.

- It is not unusual for older adults to lose interest in eating and to experience a decreased sensation of thirst.
- Older adults with chronic diseases may need to adjust to therapeutic diets low in salt, simple sugars, or fat. Unfortunately, the ability to taste and smell diminishes with age, and many clients find these diets unappealing.
- Other sensory changes, such as diminished vision or hearing, limit mobility and interaction, making it more difficult to purchase and prepare food.
- Tooth loss and gum disease limit chewing ability, forcing many older adults to eat only soft food.
- Arthritic hands may create difficulty preparing and eating food, and when they are no longer able to drive, many older adults must rely on local markets, where food choices may be limited and expensive.
- Other physical problems that may affect nutrition include gastroesophageal reflux, decreased gastric secretions, decreased intestinal peristalsis, and glucose intolerance.

Dietary Supplements Many older adults may need supplements of calcium, vitamin D, and vitamin B_{12}. For

EXAMPLE PROBLEM: Underweight/Malnourished

Definition of Underweight/Undernourished: Intake of nutrients insufficient to meet metabolic needs, based on activity, sex, height, and weight. BMI < 18.5; involuntary weight loss of more than 5% in 30 days or 10% in 180 days. For patients with serious illness, increased mortality is associated with a BMI < 21.

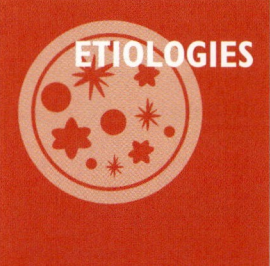

ETIOLOGIES

Risk Factors

Most common in

Underdeveloped nations; children, older adults

People with chronic illnesses (cancer, HIV, COPD)

Others at risk:

Serum albumin level < 3.5 g/dL

Clear liquid diet or NPO for > 3 days

Increased nutritional requirements (wound healing, burns)

Unplanned loss of 10% or > of Pt's usual weight

Etiologies

Eating Disorders

Anorexia nervosa—psychiatric disorder characterized by self-starvation.

Bulimia nervosa—binge eating with self-induced vomiting or laxative abuse to purge food; more common in women; onset before the age of 20.

Malnutrition—Long-term deficiency in energy &/or nutrient intake

- **Kwashiorkor**—severe deficiency of dietary protein
- **Marasmus**—severe protein and overall caloric deficit

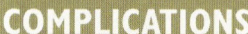

COMPLICATIONS

Emotional

Reduced self-esteem, shame, guilt

Loneliness and social isolation

Depression, anxiety

Physical

Osteoporosis, increased risk for fractures

Reduced resistance to infection

Metabolic disorders

Cardiac dysrhythmia

Organ failure

Death

Other diseases develop as a result of specific vitamin and mineral deficiencies:

- Beriberi (neurological deficits)
- Scurvy (delayed wound healing, poor bone growth)
- Pellagra (diarrhea and dementia)

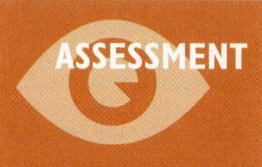

ASSESSMENT

Malnutrition

Physical Signs—Reduced physical activity, weight loss, reduced height, abdominal enlargement, hair loss

Eating Disorders

Physical Signs—Hair loss, abnormal weight loss, cold intolerance, absent or irregular menstruation, low blood pressure, weakness, atrophy of breasts

Emotional Behaviors—Intense fear of gaining weight, often overachieving or type A personality

Body Image Behaviors—Wears baggy clothes; perceives self as fat

Food Behaviors—Takes only tiny portions; skips meals. Will not eat in front of others. Always has an excuse not to eat. Often has a diet soda or coffee in hand. Eats only food that is low in fat or sugar. Deliberate self-starvation.

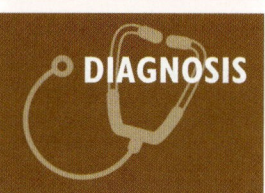

DIAGNOSIS

NANDA-I Nursing Diagnosis

- Imbalanced Nutrition, Less than Body Requirements

(Continued)

EXAMPLE PROBLEM: Underweight/Malnourished—cont'd

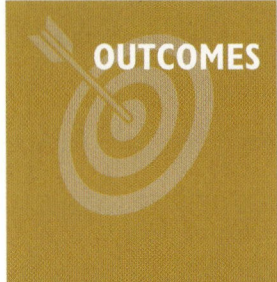

OUTCOMES

NOC Outcomes

Weight
Body Mass
Weight Gain Behavior
Weight Maintenance Behavior
Nutritional Status: Food & Fluid Intake

Individualized goals/outcome statements

Progressively gains weight toward goal.
Verbalizes willingness to take action for weight gain.
Lab values, body mass, and weight within normal limits (WNL).
Recognizes factors contributing to underweight.

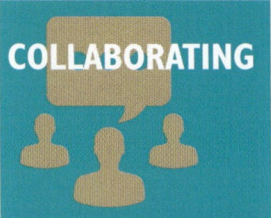

COLLABORATING

- Appetite stimulants on an individual basis.
- Consult with a dietitian about strategies to increase the nutritional content of foods.
- For eating disorders, refer for appropriate counseling.

- Suggest community resources for access to food.

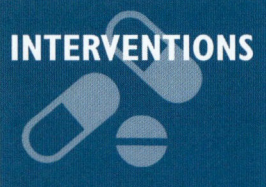

INTERVENTIONS

Stimulating Appetite

- Assess underlying cause (pain, fatigue, illness).
- Offer frequent, small, nutrient-dense meals when the person is most likely to be hungry.
- Offer high-protein supplements between meals.
- Restrict liquids with meals to prevent feeling full before Pt eats sufficient nutrients.
- Control pain; avoid painful treatments before meal.
- Provide or assist with frequent oral hygiene.

- Keep Pt environment neat, clean, and free of unpleasant sights, odors, and medical equipment.
- Order a late food tray or warm the food if Pt is not in his room during mealtime.
- Suggest smokers refrain for 1 hour before a meal.
- Position Pt comfortably for mealtime; arrange the tray within easy reach.
- Determine need for tube feedings or IV fluids.
- Teach caregiver how to promote healthy eating.

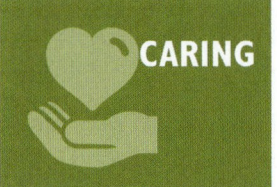

CARING

- Encourage others to bring foods the Pt likes to eat.
- Vary food textures, colors, flavor; serve attractively.

- For those who live alone, encourage meals with family or friends or meals at a senior center.

---

example, (1) as bone density decreases, calcium requirements increase, especially in women at risk for *osteoporosis;* and (2) low concentrations of vitamin B$_{12}$ and vitamin D have been linked to cognitive decline in older adults (Health Quality Ontario, 2013; Toffanello, Coin, Perisinotto, et al., 2014).

Frail Elderly Syndrome With advancing age, older adults face many losses (e.g., institutionalization). As a result, depression and social isolation are common. Both negatively affect appetite. **Frail Elderly Syndrome** is a complex disorder characterized by weight loss, decreased activity and interaction, and increasing frailty.

KnowledgeCheck 28-5

- Why is breast milk an ideal food source for infants?
- Why are an infant's nutritional needs per unit of body weight greater than at any other period of development?
- Why is it sometimes a challenge to meet the nutritional needs of toddlers?
- What is the challenge in meeting the nutritional needs of school-age children?
- Which age-group experiences a growth spurt second only to that of infants?
- Why are energy (kcal) requirements less for older adults?

Table 28-6 ▶ Daily Food Requirements for Adults Older Than Age 70

FOOD GROUP	ADULTS > 70 YEARS
Supplement of calcium, vitamin D, vitamin B_{12}, minerals, and fiber	As prescribed. Not everyone needs supplements. People should consult their healthcare providers.
Fats, oils, sweets, and salt (sodium)	Use sparingly
Milk, yogurt, and cheese group	3 servings
Meat, poultry, fish, dry beans, eggs, and nuts	2 or more servings
Fruit and vegetable group	Half a plate
Bread, fortified cereals, rice, and pasta group (whole grains and refined grains)	Half a plate
Water equivalents	8 or more servings

Notice that compared with adult requirements, the main difference is that older adults require smaller quantities of most foods. Older adults need fiber and plenty of fluid to prevent constipation and dehydration, unless their medical condition contraindicates.

Source: U.S. Department of Agriculture and U.S. Department of Health and Human Services (2015).

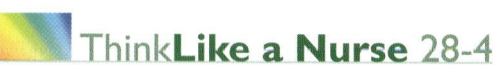

ThinkLike a Nurse 28-4

Make a list of all the food products you have seen advertised on television and in magazines. What are the implications for the nutritional status of the public?

Lifestyle Choices

Nutrition-related lifestyle choices include the following:

- **Dietary Patterns.** The type of food consumed is equally important as the amount of food to a person's overall health.
- **Work Environment.** Physically demanding work can cause fatigue and affect the quantity and quality of food consumed. When time pressure makes it difficult to prepare and eat healthy food during a short lunch break, some workers may rely on convenience foods to save time.
- **Cooking Methods.** Up to half of the water-soluble vitamin content (vitamins B and C) is lost in the cooking water of boiled vegetables. Keeping foods hot longer than 2 hours results in even further loss.
- **Oral Contraceptive Use.** This method of family planning lowers the serum level of vitamin C and several B vitamins. Women with marginal nutrient intake may need vitamin supplements.
- **Food to Relieve Stress.** Food is commonly used to cope with stress, depression, loneliness, or boredom. Skipping meals, binge eating, or consuming too much of a single food (e.g., snack foods, chocolate) can result in poor nutrition, obesity, and low self-esteem.
- **Tobacco Use.** Smokers use vitamin C, an antioxidant, faster than nonsmokers. The more a person smokes, the more vitamin is lost, and the more the body needs vitamin C to counteract the damage smoking causes to cells. Low levels of vitamin C also are linked to iron deficiency. If the person cannot quit smoking, a vitamin C supplement (2,000 mg/day) may help to compensate (Aghdassi, Royall, & Allard, 1999).

- **Alcohol.** Alcohol contributes to obesity. A 12-oz beer contains 150 calories; a juice-based cocktail contains about 160 calories. In addition, alcohol significantly decreases the rate of fat metabolism. Excessive alcohol use interferes with adequate nutrition by (1) replacing the food in the person's diet, (2) depressing the appetite, (3) decreasing the absorption of nutrients by its toxic effects on intestinal mucosa, and (4) impairing the storage of nutrients. People who use alcohol heavily need multivitamin supplements, especially B vitamins and folic acid.
- **Caffeine.** Many of our accepted beliefs about the danger and benefits of coffee are myths. Coffee does not create risk for dehydration, heart disease, or cancer and has little role in hypertension. Caffeine may be associated with bone loss; however, its negative effect can be offset by a small amount of milk. In high doses, it can sometimes cause anxiety and stomach upset. Caffeine can boost mood and mental and physical performance. It aids the ability to burn fat for fuel instead of carbohydrates and has been linked to a lower risk of Parkinson's disease, type 2 diabetes, stroke, and dementia (Ding, Bhupathiraju, Satija, et al., 2014).

Vegetarianism

All vegetarian diets exclude red meat and poultry, but beyond this distinction is a wide spectrum of diets.

- **Semi-vegetarians** are the most inclusive, allowing fish, eggs, and dairy products as well as plant-based foods.
- **Ovo-lacto vegetarians** are less inclusive in that they do not eat fish.
- **Lacto-vegetarians** consume only dairy and plant-based foods.
- **Vegans** eat only foods of plant origin.
- A **fruitarian** diet includes only fruits, nuts, honey, and vegetable oils.

Obtaining Nutrients Soybeans, soymilk, tofu, and processed protein products can be used by all but fruitarians to enhance the nutritional value of the diet. Although ovo-lacto vegetarians have no higher rate of nutrient deficiencies than the meat-eating population, they must choose foods carefully to include enough of the following nutrients:

- **Vitamin B$_{12}$** is found only in animal products, such as eggs and milk. Vegans must eat foods fortified with B$_{12}$ or take B$_{12}$ supplements. Long-standing B$_{12}$ deficiency can result in severe and irreversible neurological impairment.
- **Vitamin D** may be inadequately supplied by vegetarian diets, so vitamin D-fortified foods or supplements should be included. Soymilk and dairy milk are usually vitamin D fortified. Adequate sun exposure also helps to compensate for lack of dietary intake.
- **Iron.** The iron from plant foods is not absorbed as well as that from animal sources. However, iron is easier to absorb when it is eaten with foods containing vitamin C, so eating fruit or vegetables containing vitamin C with meals helps to compensate.
- **Calcium.** Vegans especially may find it difficult to obtain enough dietary calcium. It is important to include fortified soymilk and calcium-rich vegetables (e.g., kale, broccoli). Calcium-fortified cereals are also available. This is especially important for growth of vegan children and women who are pregnant or lactating.
- **Zinc** that is normally found in beef and chicken is also readily available from various seed and bean sources, such as pumpkin, sesame, squash, and watermelon seeds; wheat; chickpeas (hummus); wheat germ; dark chocolate; and garlic.
- **Protein** may be inadequate, especially in vegan children who do not care for the taste of soymilk, tofu, and other soy-based meat substitutes. For adults, a varied diet that meets normal nutrient and energy needs is also likely to supply adequate amounts of essential amino acids. Complementary proteins should be eaten throughout the day, but careful meal-by-meal balance of amino acids is usually not necessary. Review Table 28-1 and the discussion of complete and incomplete proteins earlier in the chapter.

Client Resources To ensure adequate nutrients it may be wise for vegetarians to consult a qualified nutrition professional, especially during periods of growth, breastfeeding, pregnancy, or recovery from illness. For recommended servings of vegetarian food groups, see MyVeganPlate (Fig. 28-3). This is presented in a similar manner to the ChooseMyPlate.gov nutritional guidelines. MyVeganPlate includes recommendations for food from each food group for those following a vegetarian diet.

Eating for Health

In recent decades the consumption of processed foods, grains, and beverages—which include *trans*-fats, preservatives, and chemical additives—is cited as a cause of diseases (e.g., type 2 diabetes and obesity, heart disease, and cancer). A diet high in meats and fish, fresh fruits and vegetables, nuts and seeds, eggs, and other natural whole foods is biologically healthier than the modern diet. Proponents of the Paleolithic (paleo) diet advocate returning to a "caveman" diet for improved health, nutrition, and athletic performance. Foods to avoid in the paleo diet are all processed foods, grains containing gluten, diary, refined sugar, legumes, potatoes, processed oils, and caffeine.

Eating for Weight Loss

Many diets, including the *Dietary Approaches to Stop Hypertension* (DASH) diet, the American Heart Association diet, and others, are nutritionally sound, but many others are fad

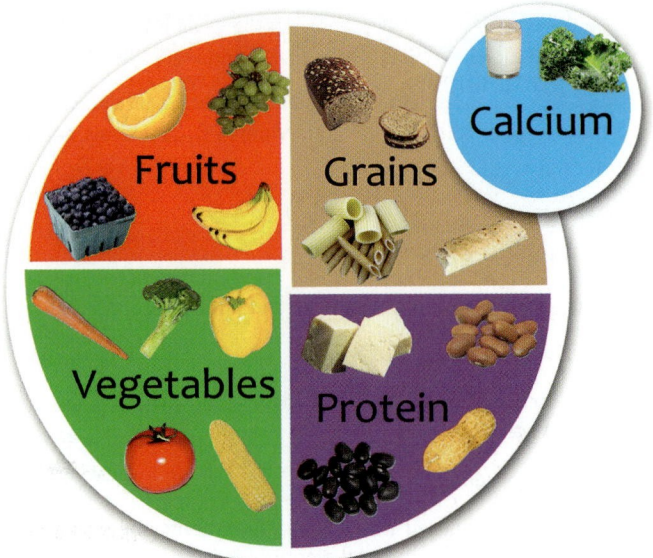

FIGURE 28-3 MyVeganPlate. Nutrition guide for vegatarians.

diets, claiming to produce rapid, effortless, almost miraculous weight loss. You can recognize fad diets by the following characteristics. They:

- Promise quick and dramatic weight loss, which is usually only temporary because it results from loss of body fluids.
- Limit the range of foods from which the dieter can select (e.g., only fruits and vegetables for the first week), leading to an imbalance in nutrients.
- Often recommend purchase of supplements and/or special packaged meals; in many cases, these are brands that they endorse or produce.
- Fail to include practical strategies that help dieters permanently change eating and activity patterns.
- Revert to former eating habits and regain the weight soon after achieving their weight-loss goal.

In contrast, more moderate calorie-restriction diets such as the American Heart Association diet:

- Describe food selection and preparation tips and other behavior modifications that can lead to slow, sustained weight loss.
- Promote a diet that includes a variety of food choices and a balance of nutrients.
- Encourage healthy habits (e.g., physical activity, sleep, reduced stress) as a cornerstone of weight loss.
- Emphasize self-monitoring, cognitive strategies, and behavior modification.

Ethnic, Cultural, and Religious Practices

Religion and culture can have a major impact on diet and lifestyle (see Chapters 15 and 16)

- Language barriers may make it difficult for a client to understand nutritional information. For those patients, simple visual aids may be useful.
- Ethnic/cultural food choices often reflect the foods that are plentiful in the region of origin (e.g., fish in coastal communities), as well as foods that are readily grown in the native soil.
- Other diet choices reflect a concern for food preservation; for instance, people from various geographic regions eat salted meats and dried fruits and cook with spices to combat microbes.

- Certain religions may require fasting or abstaining from certain foods. For example, some Roman Catholics don't eat meat on certain days of the religious calendar; kosher dietary laws prohibit eating pork.
- The prevalence of obesity is lower among non-Hispanic Asians than other ethnic groups (U.S. Department of Health and Human Services, Centers for Disease Control and Prevention, & National Center for Health Statistics, 2015, updated).
- Cultural beliefs, perceptions, and attitudes about weight issues may often not match those of health providers. For example, some parents may perceive their children as cute and healthy, even though their body mass index (BMI) indicates they are obese. A slim body is not the ideal in all cultures.

Traditional Diets of many cultures are healthful and should not be discouraged; in fact, contemporary adaptations made to these diets may compromise their nutritional quality.

- **Mediterranean Diet**—Rich in olive oil, fish, fruits, vegetables, and nuts and low in dairy foods, processed foods and saturated fats, and red meat; includes a glass of red wine per day. Linked to weight loss, a reduced risk of deaths due to cancer, coronary artery disease, hypertension and high blood cholesterol (Estruch, Ros, Salas-Salvado, et al., 2013; Mitrou, Kipnis, Thiébaut, et al., 2007; Panagiotakos, 2014).
- **Asian Diet**—A plant-based diet with a low amount of animal products. Consists of rice, fresh fruits, and vegetables, such as melons, bananas, tangerines, cabbage, and green leafy vegetables. Protein intake primarily consists of beans, nuts, and seeds, and occasional poultry, shellfish, and eggs. Health benefits of this diet include lower incidence of cardiovascular disease, diabetes, colon cancer, and obesity. Green and black teas contain antioxidants that may lower the risk of cancer.
- **Indian Diet**—The traditional diet contains fresh, home-cooked foods containing a wide array of spices. Meat selection is based on religious preference (e.g., traditionally, Muslims don't eat pork, Hindus aren't permitted to eat beef, and Buddhists are vegetarian). People who eat a traditional Indian diet (high in fruits, vegetables, legumes, and nuts, and low in processed foods) reap the benefit of low incidence of diabetes, heart disease, and other chronic diseases.
- **Hispanic Diet**—Relies heavily on grains, especially rice, and legumes (e.g., beans), and corn-based products. Beans as a staple are rich in fiber, B vitamins, calcium, phosphorus, and iron; however, when prepared with lard (refried), the health benefits diminish. The traditional Hispanic fare includes few fresh vegetables, except for tomatoes, which are rich in vitamins A and C, as well as potassium and iron. Diabetes type 2 is more prevalent among nonwhite Hispanics because of a high rate of obesity. Sugary fruit beverages and soda are a common part of the contemporary Hispanic diet.

Disease Processes and Functional Limitations

Chronic diseases (e.g., diabetes mellitus, GI disorders) can alter nutrient intake, digestion, absorption, use, and excretion. Any illness, especially when accompanied by fever, increases the need for protein, water, and kcal to meet the demands of increased metabolism. A variety of other physical and psychological disorders and/or their treatments can adversely affect a client's nutrition:

- **Traumatic Injury** (e.g., burns, surgery) requires extra protein and vitamin C for wound healing and tissue rebuilding.

- **Long-term Insufficient Calorie Intake** (e.g., patients with cancer) causes *protein-calorie malnutrition,* which is characterized by weight loss and muscle and fat wasting.
- **Alcoholism.** Poor appetite, common in alcoholism, results in decreased intake of food and therefore of nutrients. Alcohol can also interfere with the function of some vitamins.
- **Cognitive Function.** A person with a developmental delay, severe mental illness, head trauma, confusion, or memory loss may be unable to remember what, when, or whether she has eaten.
- **Ability to Obtain and Prepare Food.**
  - *Paralysis or hemiplegia* (e.g., from a stroke and other medical and physical conditions) can cause functional limitations and impaired mobility, limiting the ability to shop for and prepare food.
  - *Social factors* also limit the ability to purchase food. People with limited income may be forced to choose between buying food or paying for medication or household utilities.
  - A person with *severe dyspnea* or *fatigue* may not have the stamina or time to prepare a nutritious meal. Instead, she may eat prepared foods that are high in sodium content. Dyspnea and fatigue are associated with chronic obstructive pulmonary disease (COPD) advanced chronic disease, severe anemia, pregnancy, depression, and excess work.
- **Chewing and Swallowing.** Decayed or missing teeth and ill-fitting dentures make chewing difficult. The person often resorts to eating only soft foods or liquids, many of which lack fiber. Acute disorders affecting the throat, such as pharyngitis, make swallowing painful. Oral cancer and esophageal strictures also make swallowing painful or difficult, and frequently lead to avoiding food.
- **Stomach Function.** Heartburn, indigestion, and other stomach disorders are common. People may eat only bland foods or avoid certain foods to prevent the pain or burning that follow eating.
- **Peristalsis.** The wave-like action that propels food through the intestinal tract is called **peristalsis.** Bowel inflammation or infection, diverticula (outpouchings of the intestine), or tumors may increase peristalsis, thereby decreasing absorption of nutrients. In addition, high stress levels may either speed or slow transit time. If peristalsis is slow, the stomach may not empty properly (gastroparesis). This could lead to early satiety, nausea, or vomiting and affect nutrient intake.
- **Intestinal Surface Area.** When the amount of intestinal surface area is diminished by surgery or disease, absorption of nutrients is decreased. This may result in malnutrition despite the fact that the patient is consuming adequate calories and protein.
- **Enzyme Secretion.** Liver, gallbladder, or pancreas problems affect the secretion of digestive enzymes. Lactose intolerance is prevalent in the United States and worldwide, primarily among blacks, Native Americans, and Asian people (National Institute of Diabetes and Digestive and Kidney Diseases, 2014).
- **Bariatric surgery** alters digestion to achieve rapid weight loss. Restrictive procedures limit the stomach's capacity to hold food and reduce the passage through the GI tract (e.g., adjustable gastric banding). Malabsorption surgeries are done to impair the uptake of food nutrients and fats (intestinal bypass). A combined approach uses stomach restriction and a partial bypass of the small intestine. Bariatric weight-loss procedures increase the risk of nutrient deficiency, especially

iron, copper, zinc, selenium, thiamine, folate, and vitamins B_{12} and D (Choban, Dickerson, Malone, et al.; American Society for Parenteral and Enteral Nutrition, 2013).

Medications

In addition to the direct effects of diseases and disorders, nutrition may be affected by the drugs and therapies used to treat them, as in the following examples:

- *Some medications directly decrease appetite,* for example, dextroamphetamine (Adderall), aspirin, diphenhydramine (e.g., Benadryl), and lithium carbonate (e.g., Lithobid).
- *Chemotherapy and radiation therapy* may cause oral ulcers, intestinal bleeding, or diarrhea—which interfere with eating and absorbing nutrients from food.
- *Certain drugs alter nutrient metabolism;* some increase or decrease nutrient excretion; others may also alter taste, changing overall nutrient intake.
- *A drug may affect specific nutrients.* For example, acetylsalicylic acid (aspirin) decreases folate levels and increases excretion of vitamin C; laxatives may cause calcium and potassium depletion; and thiazide diuretics decrease the absorption of vitamin B_{12}.
- *Almost all oral medications have the potential to cause nausea or vomiting,* thereby decreasing appetite.

KnowledgeCheck 28-6

- List at least three nutrients that may be more difficult to supply through a vegetarian diet.
- When selecting a program for weight loss, what factors should a person consider?
- Why should you encourage clients from various cultures to follow their traditional diets?
- Describe the effects on nutrition of (1) smoking and (2) heavy alcohol use.

Special Diets

Many people must follow a modified diet to assist in managing their illness. In addition, all inpatients at healthcare facilities must have a diet prescribed by their primary care provider. The following are the most commonly prescribed diets:

Regular Diet A regular diet, also called the "house diet," is appropriate for clients without special nutritional needs. This diet is a balanced meal plan that supplies 2,000 kcal per day. Many facilities provide vegetarian and ethnic variations (e.g., Asian menu, kosher). Typically, inpatients choose each meal from a list of menu choices.

Have you ever heard someone complain that "hospital food is bland and unimaginative"? There is some justification for that complaint. House diets must accommodate the varied tastes of all patients, so they are usually lightly seasoned. Selections are limited to avoid unpopular items (e.g., Brussels sprouts) and restrict fatty, fried, or gas-producing foods, which many patients tolerate poorly. However, you should refrain from making negative comments to patients about the food.

NPO means no food or fluid (including water) by mouth. This may be ordered before surgery or an invasive procedure to limit the risk of aspiration. A common example is "NPO after midnight." Most well-nourished, well-hydrated patients easily tolerate short-term NPO status. However, no one can tolerate prolonged periods of NPO. Intravenous fluids may be given to provide hydration, and clients who must remain NPO for a lengthy period need enteral (through a stomach tube) or parenteral (IV) nutrition to prevent malnutrition.

Diets Modified by Consistency Patients undergoing surgery, bowel procedures, or acute illness may, for a short period of time, need a diet modified by consistency (see Table 28-7). Patients with chronic health concerns that affect their ability to chew or swallow (e.g., Impaired Dentition and Impaired Swallowing) may need long-term changes in the consistency of their diet.

Table 28-7 ▶ Diets Modified by Consistency

DIET DESCRIPTION AND FOODS INCLUDED	COMMENTS
Clear Liquids. Provides fluids to prevent dehydration and supplies some simple carbohydrates to help meet energy needs. *Foods:* Water, tea, coffee, broth, clear juice (usually apple, grape, or cranberry juice), popsicles, carbonated beverages, and gelatin.	▪ Does not supply adequate calories, protein, and other nutrients, so timely progression to more nutritious diets is recommended. ▪ If clear liquids are required for more than 3 days, commercial clear liquid supplements are usually prescribed.
Full Liquids. Contains all the liquids included in the clear liquid diet plus any food items that are liquid at room temperature. *Foods:* Add to clear liquid diet: soups, milk, milk shakes, puddings, custards, juices, some hot cereals, and yogurt.	▪ Difficult to obtain a balanced diet on a full liquid plan; use for a short time only. ▪ If needed for a longer time, a professional dietitian should be involved in planning of the diet. ▪ High-calorie, high-protein supplements are often added.
Mechanical Soft Diet. The diet of choice for people with chewing difficulties resulting from missing teeth, jaw problems, or extensive fatigue. *Foods:* Add to the full liquid diet: soft vegetables and fruits; chopped, ground, or shredded meat; and breads, pastries, eggs, and cheese.	▪ This diet can supply a full range of nutrients but is quite low in fiber. As a result, constipation is a risk. ▪ Many food items can be added to this diet by cooking them extensively or blending or grinding to alter their texture.
Pureed Diet. A pureed diet is a blended diet. Some foods may or may not be excluded.	Often liquids are added to the food to create a texture that may be scooped onto serving plates.

Diets Modified for Disease Some health conditions require modification of dietary intake. The following are the most common diets:

- *Calorie-restricted.* For clients requiring weight reduction
- *Sodium-restricted.* For clients with hypertension, Ménière's disease (inner ear problem), or fluid balance problems
- *Fat-restricted.* For clients with elevated cholesterol or triglyceride levels; may also be prescribed for general weight loss
- *Diabetic.* To manage calories and carbohydrate intake for clients with diabetes mellitus
- *Renal diet.* To manage electrolytes and fluid for clients with renal insufficiency
- *Protein-controlled diet.* To manage liver and kidney disease
- *Ketogenic diet.* To treat difficult-to-control epileptic seizures in children
- *Antigen-avoidance diets.* For clients allergic to or intolerant of certain foods, such as a gluten-free diet for clients with celiac disease
- *Calorie-protein push.* Used when there is a need to heal wounds, maintain or increase weight, or promote growth. If the person cannot consume enough kcal by adding fats and proteins to his regular diet, high-calorie, high-protein supplements may be used.

ThinkLike a Nurse 28-5

Analyze the following diets. Which nutrients are missing or difficult to obtain from these diets?

- Clear liquid
- Full liquid

PracticalKnowledge
knowing **how**

Good nutrition is essential for health and also is a key aspect of disease management. In the rest of this chapter, you will learn about assessing nutritional status and diagnosing and planning care for common nutrition problems (e.g., swallowing).

Nutrition is a basic human need. But more than a physical necessity, it also has emotional associations. We eat when we are hungry, but we also eat for pleasure because the food tastes good! Food has become a part of most social events and activities. A certain food may symbolize one's cultural or religious affiliation or even be a political statement. When supporting patients' nutritional needs, it is wise to keep in mind that personal beliefs, habits, and preferences are as important as nutritional knowledge in determining what a person eats.

ASSESSMENT NP

There are two kinds of nutritional assessment: (1) screening assessments and (2) thorough, focused nutritional assessments. Usually you will perform a screening exam. If you identify nutritional risk factors, you then perform a focused nutritional assessment.

HOW DO I SCREEN CLIENTS FOR NUTRITIONAL PROBLEMS?

KEY POINT: *All hospitalized patients, especially those with obesity and patients at risk for nutritional deficiency, should receive a nutritional screening support plan within 48 hours of inpatient admission* (Choban, Dickerson, Malone, et al.;

American Society for Parenteral and Enteral Nutrition, 2013). **Cursory screening** consists of evaluation of height, weight, and body mass index (BMI) coupled with a brief dietary history.

Clients who are found to have risk factors should be evaluated more fully (e.g., with the SGA, NSI, or MNA):

- *The subjective global assessment (SGA)* is a commonly used screening method that makes use of information from the overall medical history and physical examination to evaluate a client's nutritional status. See the Focused Assessment box Subjective Global Assessment.
- *The Nutrition Screening Initiative (NSI),* developed for older adults, identifies indicators of impaired nutritional status. Refer to the Focused Assessment box Nutrition Screening Initiative (NSI) for Older Adults: Indications of Impaired Nutritional Status.
- *The Mini Nutritional Assessment (MNA),* developed for older adults, can be used with clients of all ages (DiMaria-Ghalili & Guenter, 2008). It is a quick and easy method for identifying clients with nutritional risks or malnutrition. The first part screens for nutritional risk. The second part is completed only if the person is found to be at risk. The total of both parts, determines whether malnutrition exists and requires multidisciplinary follow-up. To see and use the MNA,

 Go to the Web site www.mna-elderly.com

FOCUSED NUTRITIONAL ASSESSMENT

If screening reveals nutritional problems, perform a more thorough focused nutritional assessment to evaluate the client.

 It is especially important to assess nutritional status in elderly clients carefully to ensure that you detect marginal deficiencies before major problems occur. The nutrition component of a focused nutritional assessment

---

Subjective Global Assessment

Focused Assessment

In this method, an experienced clinician examines the general medical history and physical examination to evaluate a client's nutritional status. There are six components pertinent to nutritional status:

➤ *Weight history*—over previous 6 months
➤ *Dietary history*—including a comparison of usual, recommended, and current intake, as well as changes in eating patterns over the past weeks or months
➤ *Gastrointestinal symptoms history*—anorexia, nausea, vomiting, and diarrhea
➤ *Energy level*—including activity level and functional abilities
➤ *Existing disease*—evaluation of the metabolic demands of any disease states along with acute stressors that may alter those demands
➤ *Physical examination data*—regarding loss of fat stores, muscle wasting, and the presence of edema and ascites

The effectiveness of this method depends largely on the experience of the clinician (Detsky, McLaughlin, Baker, et al., 1987).

Focused Assessment

Nutrition Screening Initiative (NSI) for Older Adults: Indications of Impaired Nutritional Status

This portion of the NSI identifies indicators of impaired nutritional status:

Major Indicators	Minor Indicators	Symptoms	Physical Signs	Lab Values
➤ Significant weight loss over time ➤ Significant high or low weight for height ➤ Significant change in functional status ➤ Significant and inappropriate food intake ➤ Significant reduction in midarm circumference ➤ Significant decrease in skinfold ➤ Osteoporosis or osteomalacia ➤ Folate or vitamin B deficiency	➤ Concurrent syndromes ➤ Alcoholism ➤ Cognitive impairment ➤ Chronic renal insufficiency ➤ Multiple concurrent medications ➤ Malabsorption syndromes	➤ Anorexia, nausea, or dysphagia ➤ Early satiety ➤ Changed bowel habits ➤ Fatigue or apathy ➤ Memory loss	➤ Poor oral or dental status ➤ Dehydration ➤ Poorly healing wounds ➤ Loss of subcutaneous fat or muscle mass ➤ Fluid retention	➤ Reduced levels of serum albumin, transferrin, or prealbumin ➤ Folate deficiency ➤ Iron deficiency ➤ Zinc deficiency ➤ Reduced levels of ascorbic acid

includes both subjective (history) and objective (physical examination) data.

Dietary History

You can obtain a dietary history during any routine assessment. Whether you use a self-administered form or an interview, you will collect general knowledge of the client's basic eating habits, food attitudes and preferences, cultural factors, and use of dietary supplements. A dietary history creates a picture of the client's food habits and eating behaviors. To collect detailed data on what the client is actually eating, ask him to keep a food diary. The following are three types of food diaries:

24-Hour Recall A 24-hour recall requires the client to name all foods eaten within a day. Simply ask questions such as "Yesterday, what did you eat for breakfast/lunch/dinner/snacks?" A 24-hour recall is simple; however, accuracy of the data may be questionable because some people have difficulty remembering everything they ate the previous day, and any single day may be atypical. Sometimes, a family member can help the client recall intake more accurately, particularly when the client is ill.

Food Frequency Questionnaire A food frequency questionnaire asks the client to identify the number of times per day, week, or month a particular food group is eaten (e.g., fruits, red meats). You can modify the questions according to the client's specific issues. Food frequency questionnaires provide a broader view of the client's nutritional intake than the 24-hour recall; however, accuracy is still a problem.

Food Record A food record is the most accurate food diary. It provides information on the quantity as well as the types of foods eaten. You ask the client in advance to keep a record of measured and weighed amounts of all foods he eats in a 3-day period. From the detailed information collected, you can analyze the total kcal and nutrient content for the recorded period. Although the food record provides meaningful results, it requires cognitive and psychomotor skills that not all clients have. It also requires commitment to the process for 3 days, which may be difficult for some people. You might remind some patients there are Web sites and apps that can help with journaling their diet and tracking nutritional intake, goals, weight management, and so on.

Physical Examination

You should correlate physical examination findings with other assessments, such as nutritional and medical history, dietary intake, anthropometric measurements, and laboratory results. Refer to Chapter 21 as needed for a review of physical examination techniques. For guidelines in performing a nutrition-focused physical examination, see the Focused Assessment box Nutritional Assessment.

Assessing Body Composition

You will use **anthropometric measurements** when assessing body composition (the proportion of fat in the body). These are noninvasive physical examination techniques to determine body dimensions such as height and weight. Anthropometric measurements are used to:

- Assess growth rate in children
- Indirectly assess adults' protein and fat stores
- Assess overweight, obesity, and underweight

To obtain accurate data, you must use standardized equipment and procedures and compare the data with existing reference standards for men and women. Keep in mind that body weight measurement alone is insufficient for assessing body composition.

Skinfold Measurements

Approximately half of body fat is located subcutaneously. Therefore, skinfold thickness provides an estimate of a person's body fat content. It reveals information about current nutritional status as well as long-term changes in fat stores.

- Use a caliper to obtain the most accurate measurement.
- The most reliable location is the triceps for children and women and the subscapular area in men.
- The combined measurements of triceps skinfold and mid-upper arm circumference yield a better estimate of muscle and fat areas than does a single measurement.
- Accurate reading can be difficult for those who are obese.
- See Clinical Insight 28-1

Circumferences

Another method of estimating the percentage of body fat is to use girth, or circumference, measurements.

- *Mid-upper arm circumference* is routinely measured as part of screening.

Focused Assessment

Nutritional Assessment

If you identify nutritional problems or risks using the screening tools, you should perform a more in-depth nutritional assessment, such as the following:

Nutritional History

Item	Components
Demographic data	Name, date, age, sex, date of birth, address, occupation, workplace
Chief complaint	Client's subjective statement of health problem, including onset and duration
Present illness and current health	Detailed data about chief complaint as it relates to nutrition status Recent diet changes and reasons Recent weight loss or gain and over what period of time Usual body weight: 20% above or below desirable weight? Change in appetite Unusual stress/trauma (surgery, job, family) Medications, prescriptions Alcohol, nicotine, caffeine consumption
Health history	Previous illnesses, trauma, major dental problems, or issues that could interfere with ability to shop, prepare food, chew, or swallow Allergies (i.e., environmental, foods, drugs) Eating disorders Chronic disease or surgery that affects gastrointestinal tract Substance abuse Nutritional programs Depression
Family health history	Genetic/familial disorders that could affect nutritional status: cardiovascular or gastrointestinal disorders, Crohn's disease, diabetes, cancer, sickle cell anemia, allergies, celiac disease, other food intolerances, obesity
Dietary history	Current food intake pattern using one of the following methods: 24-hour, 7-day recall, as appropriate; food frequency questionnaire; food record; and comparison with dietary guidelines and DRIs Special dietary considerations, restrictions Fad diets Vitamin and mineral supplements Commercial dietary supplements Nonconventional dietary supplements Food preferences, dislikes Dietary influences from ethnic, cultural, or religious practices Counseling needs (based on food knowledge)
Medication history	Recent use of steroids, immunosuppressants, chemotherapy, anticonvulsants, or oral contraceptives

Item	Components
Socioeconomic factors	Adequate food storage, refrigeration, food preparation, payments: Supplemental Security Income (SSI), SNAP, USDA WIC (Women, Infants, and Children) program Who shops for, prepares, and cooks food?
Personal factors	Stress/coping mechanisms, self-concept, social supports Daily activity level and exercise regimen

Nutrition-Focused Physical Examination

Correlate the following physical examination findings with the dietary history, screening methods, anthropometric measurements, and laboratory results:

I. The General Survey
Assess vital signs, height, weight, and overall impressions.
- **Overall appearance.** Does the client look ill? Does he appear adequately nourished? You will want to investigate any hunches as you move through the physical exam.
- **Temperature.** An increase in temperature raises the client's metabolic rate and need for fluid, is a sign of infection, and may decrease the client's appetite.
- **Blood pressure (BP) and heart rate** are affected by fluid status. An elevated BP may be related to fluid volume excess; a low BP may be a sign of dehydration. Heart rate usually increases when fluid volume is low.
- **Height and weight.** Calculate the body mass index (BMI) on the basis of these measures:

$$\text{BMI} = \text{weight in kilograms} \div (\text{height in meters})^2$$

II. Integumentary System
- **Skin turgor** is an indicator of fluid status. Poor skin turgor may result from dehydration. Swelling may result from overhydration.
- **Skin integrity** reflects overall nutritional status. Poor wound healing may suggest inadequate intake of protein, vitamin C, or zinc. Patients with uncontrolled diabetes often experience slow-healing wounds, especially in the feet and legs.
- **Areas of warmth or erythema.** These are signs of inflammation or infection.
- **Other nutrition-related skin changes** include red, swollen skin lesions (due to niacin deficiency); excessive bleeding seen as petechiae or ecchymosis (due to vitamin K or C deficiency); and xerosis (dry skin).
- **Abnormal nail findings** include spoon-shaped, brittle nails (due to iron deficiency); dull nails with transverse ridge (due to protein deficiency); pale, mottled nails (due to vitamin A or C deficiency); bruising or bleeding beneath nails (due to protein or caloric deficiency); and splinter hemorrhages (due to vitamin C deficiency).
- **Hair** will grow slowly, thin, or break easily if protein is deficient.

(Continued)

Nutritional Assessment—cont'd

III. The Head and Neck

The condition of the mouth, teeth, and gums has a major effect on a client's choice of food, ability to chew, and ability to swallow.

➤ *Facial paralysis or drooping* of one side of the face may be a result of stroke, injury, or nerve irritation, which also affects the ability to chew and swallow (dysphagia).

➤ *Enlarged thyroid gland.* Look for swelling of the thyroid, which may be related to hypothyroid or hyperthyroid states. Both disorders affect metabolic rate and energy requirements.

➤ *Eyes.* Nutritional deficits may cause the eyes to be red and dry and the conjunctiva pale.

➤ *Lips and tongue.* The lips may be chapped, red, or swollen. The tongue may be bright red, purple, or swollen or may have longitudinal furrows.

➤ *Teeth and gums.* Look for cavities, mottled or missing teeth, and spongy, bleeding, or receding gums.

➤ *Lymph nodes.* Palpate for enlarged or tender lymph nodes under the chin and along the neck. Nodes that are swollen can signal infection, such as a sore throat.

IV. Cardiovascular System

You will have gained initial information about the cardiovascular system by taking the vital signs. As you follow up and listen to the heart and check pulses, you should explore any abnormal vital signs.

➤ *Bounding pulses* are associated with fluid overload, fever, and hypertension.

➤ *Weak, thready pulse* may indicate dehydration, shock, or hypotension.

➤ *Edema in the extremities* may be a sign of fluid overload, inadequate protein stores, or electrolyte imbalance.

V. Abdominal Exam

➤ *Scaphoid or concave abdomen* indicates loss of subcutaneous fat, possibly caused by malnutrition.

➤ *Round or protuberant abdomen* points to obesity caused by excess caloric and/or high-fat intake.

➤ *Generalized enlarged abdomen* may signify **ascites** (fluid in the abdominal cavity) resulting from liver malfunction. Ascites results from three mechanisms: abnormal movement of protein and water into the abdomen; sodium and fluid retention; and decreased albumin production in the liver.

➤ *Hyperactive bowel sounds* are heard with gastrointestinal infection, laxative use, and malabsorption disorders.

➤ *Hypoactive bowel sounds* suggest sluggish motility in the GI tract.

VI. Musculoskeletal System

➤ *Thin extremities with excess skinfolds* may indicate muscle atrophy and fat loss related to malnutrition, especially protein and calories. This may also occur as a result of prolonged bedrest and inadequate food intake. Skinfold measurement is also useful in assessing muscle and fat stores.

➤ *Swelling, deformities, or limitation in range of motion* of the joints.

➤ *Kyphosis* of the spine may indicate osteoporosis and possible insufficient calcium intake.

➤ *Joint pain* on palpation or with movement is a sign of arthritis or gout. Arthritis may affect ability to shop for groceries, prepare food to eat, and use utensils for eating and drinking. Gout is often induced by diets high in purines (food substances that break down into uric acid), obesity, and excess alcohol intake.

VII. Neurological System

The neurological examination will give you insight into the client's ability to perform independent tasks.

➤ *Altered level of consciousness or signs of behavioral disturbances and dementia* through general conversation and appropriateness of answers to specific questions.

➤ *Coordination and reflexes.*

➤ *Cognitive deficits or severe psychiatric disorders.* A client with cognitive deficits or severe psychiatric disorders may have difficulty preparing food or judging appropriate nutrient choices.

➤ *Motor or sensory deficits.* Clients with motor or sensory deficits may be unable to purchase, prepare, or eat a variety of foods.

➤ *Confusion, weakness, diminished reflexes, paresthesia, and sensory loss* may be cues to vitamin B deficiencies.

➤ *Tetany or severe and generalized muscle spasm* may indicate calcium or magnesium deficits.

VIII. Signs of Severe Malnutrition

➤ Symptoms of undernutrition due to insufficient food include reduced physical activity, weight loss, and reduced height

➤ Children, older adults, and people with chronic illnesses such as cancer, HIV infection, and chronic obstructive pulmonary disease (COPD) are most likely to experience malnutrition.

➤ To assess for malnutrition in children, compare weight, height, and head circumference with the standards (norms) for the child's age. In cases of severe malnutrition, abdominal circumference can signal worsening disease. Other indicators in children include the presence of iron deficiency anemia.

➤ In adolescents, look for a delay of stages of sexual maturation.

- The *abdominal circumference*, measured at the iliac crest, is a simple and inexpensive method to assess body fat distribution. This method is highly accurate and should accompany the BMI measurement for assessing adiposity.
- *The waist-to-hip ratio (WHR)* evaluates obesity by assessing abdominal fat. Ideally, women should have a WHR ratio of 0.8 or less; men should have a WHR ration of 0.95 or less.

For specific instructions on measuring mid-upper arm circumference and WHR, see Clinical Insight 28-2.

KnowledgeCheck 28-7

- What are the most reliable locations for skinfold measurement?
- What are the implications of an increased WHR?

Body Mass Index

Body mass index (BMI) is another method of assessing body composition. It can be precisely measured using scanning devices that measure *bioelectrical impedance*—the conduction of a harmless electrical charge through the client's body. Lean tissue readily conducts the charge, whereas adipose tissue does not. However, you will usually roughly estimate BMI by using the calculation formula in Box 28-3. You may also consult tables with precalculated values based on height and weight (National Heart, Lung, and Blood Institute, n.d.). For an example of a height and weight BMI table, see Procedure 21-1: Performing the General Survey. You can also find BMI calculators on the **Centers for Disease Control and Prevention** and **National Heart Lung and Blood Institute** Web sites.

BOX 28-3 ■ Calculating Body Mass Index (BMI)

BMI = weight in kilograms ÷ (height in meters)^2

Example:
Robert weighs 165 lb. Convert his weight to kilograms:
$$165 \div 2.2 = 75 \text{ kg}$$
He is 71 inches tall. Convert his height to meters.
$$1 \text{ meter} = 39.37 \text{ inches}$$
Divide 71 inches by 39.37 inches; he is 1.8 meters tall (rounded off)
$$\text{His BMI is } 75 \text{ kg} \div (1.8)^2 = 23$$

The normal BMI for adults ranges from 18.5 to 24.9.

Classification of Body Mass Index Values

Classification	BMI (kg/m^2)
Severely underweight	< 16
Moderately underweight	16–16.99
Severe thinness	< 16
Moderate thinness	16–16.99
Mild thinness	17–18.49
Underweight	< 18.5
Healthy weight	18.5–24.9
Pre-obese	25.0–29.9
Obese class I	30.0–34.9
Obese class II	35.0–39.9
Obese class III	> 40.0

Source: Adapted from World Health Organization (2006a).

The normal BMI for adults ranges from 18.5 to 24.9 (although this may vary slightly among professional organizations). Limitations of the usefulness of BMI values are limited for:

- Athletes—because of their larger muscle mass.
- Pregnant and postpartum women—because they have a higher fluid composition.
- Older adults—values are often inaccurate because with age, adults lose height. Also older adults are typically less active and lose muscle mass. Because BMI is calculated based on height and weight, the index can be a less sensitive measure of weight status.

Despite these limitations, BMI is generally useful in identifying underweight and obese individuals.

KnowledgeCheck 28-8

- What is the most accurate type of food diary?
- Compare and contrast four nutritional screening approaches: cursory screening, subjective global assessment, Mini Nutritional Assessment, and Nutrition Screening Initiative.
- Identify three nutritional risk factors.

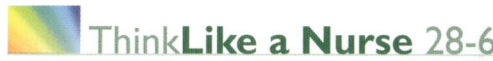

ThinkLike a Nurse 28-6

1. Calculate your waist-to-hip ratio (WHR).
2. Use Box 28-3 to calculate your BMI. Evaluate the result.
   - How useful are these data?
   - Do you feel you need to pursue a program of weight loss? Why or why not?

Underwater Weighing

Hydrodensitometry, or underwater weighing, is another method of determining body composition. It requires total submersion of the patient in a tank of water. Because fat readily floats, the person's buoyancy will vary depending on his percentage of body fat. This method is considered the gold standard for body composition measures. However, clinical use of this method is limited because it is impractical to use with children, the elderly, or individuals who are severely ill.

KnowledgeCheck 28-9

- Identify at least 10 physical examination findings that would lead you to suspect nutritional problems.
- What factors would lead to poor wound healing?

What Laboratory Values Reflect Nutritional Status?

The following laboratory or biochemical indicators provide information about nutritional status. Norms are given in the Diagnostic Testing box Tests Reflecting Nutritional Status: Norms.

Blood Glucose

The blood glucose level indicates the amount of fuel available for cellular energy. Levels above normal trigger the release of insulin, which causes the glucose to move into body cells and to be stored in the liver and muscles. A level below normal triggers the release of glucagon, leading to the release of glucose from storage.

Hypoglycemia limits the fuel supply to the body, resulting in symptoms ranging from weakness to coma. Hypoglycemia is usually defined as blood glucose of less than 50 mg/dL, but some people may feel symptoms at higher levels. Often the cause is insufficient food intake, excessive physical exertion, or a disproportionate amount of hypoglycemic agents.

Tests Reflecting Nutritional Status: Norms

Note: Norms are for adults (aged 19 to 65) unless otherwise noted.

Blood Glucose	Less than 70 mg/dL to 100 mg/dL. ➤ Capillary blood sugar is frequently assessed at the bedside with a simple fingerstick. ➤ Serum blood glucose is assessed by drawing a venous blood sample. The level is measured in the laboratory. The American Diabetes Association (2016, last edited) recommends for diabetic patients a preprandial plasma glucose level of 80 to 130 mg/dL.
Serum Albumin	3.4–4.8 g/dL
Prealbumin	12–42 mg/dL (aged 6 yr–adult)
Globulin	2.3–3.4 g/dL
Blood Urea Nitrogen (BUN)	5–18 mg/dL (children) 8–21 mg/dL (aged 14–adult); 10–31 mg/dL (adult older than 90)
Creatinine	0.5–1 mg/dL (female) 0.6–1.2 mg/dL (male)
Hemoglobin	13.2–17.3 g/dL (male) 11.7–15.5 g/dL (female) 12.6–17.4 g/dL (male, older adult) 11.7–16.1 g/dL (female, older adult)

BOX 28-4 ■ When to Assess for Diabetes

- Adults with BMI > 25
- Physical inactivity
- High-risk ethnicity for obesity (e.g., American Indians, Alaskan Natives)
- First-degree relative with diabetes
- Women diagnosed with gestational diabetes during pregnancy or who have delivered a baby weighing more than 9 lb
- Hemoglobin A_{1c} > 5.7% (test for glucose control over a 2- to 3-month period)
- HDL cholesterol < 35 mg/dL and/or triglyceride > 250 mg/dL
- History of cardiovascular disease and/or hypertension
- Physical signs indicating low blood sugar (sweating, shakiness, anxiety, confusion, irritability, dizziness, difficulty speaking, lethargy, or loss of consciousness)
- Physical signs indicating high blood sugar (flushed skin, confusion, weakness, labored breathing, sweet or fruity breath, nausea, loss of consciousness)
- Clinical conditions associated with insulin resistance (e.g., foot ulcers that are slow to heal)

If diabetes testing is normal, the American Diabetes Association (2014) recommends repeat evaluation every 3 years or more frequently, depending on risk factors.

Hyperglycemia (blood glucose greater than 109 mg/dL fasting or greater than 126 mg/dL at random) may be a sign of diabetes mellitus, an endocrine problem, which may develop as a result of either insufficient insulin production or resistance to the existing supply of insulin (Box 28-4). A high blood glucose level does not mean that there is more fuel available for cellular energy. A characteristic of diabetes is that although there is more than enough glucose in the blood, it cannot enter and be used by the cells. Repeated blood glucose measures are required before diagnosing diabetes mellitus, because glucose levels may be temporarily elevated as a result of excessive carbohydrate intake or emotional and physical stressors.

- **Symptoms and sequelae.** A rise in blood sugar may produce weakness or fatigue. Prolonged elevations lead to weight loss, blurred vision, **ketosis** (metabolism of fat due to inability to use carbohydrates as fuel), renal failure, and **peripheral neuropathy** (damage to nerves due to prolonged exposure to high glucose levels).
- **Monitoring.** Patients with diabetes usually monitor their own blood sugar levels, but you may need to do it for some. Usually this is done by a fingerstick to obtain capillary blood

for testing. Some glucometers can use blood from alternative sites such as upper arm, forearm, base of thumb, or thigh. Other types of monitors include:

A disposable sensor, placed just under the skin. The sensor communicates with a receiver that reads the levels.

A skin-testing device, worn like a watch, pulls tiny amounts of fluid from the skin without puncturing it.

For complete fingerstick steps, see Procedure 28-1.

Serum Protein Levels and Indices

Protein molecules dissolve in blood to form plasma proteins. Tissue proteins are a combination of albumin and globulin, so serum protein levels are indicators of protein stores.

- **Albumin** is synthesized in the liver and constitutes 60% of total body protein. Low levels of albumin are associated with malnutrition; malabsorption; acute and chronic liver disease; and repeated loss of protein through burns, wounds, or other sources. The half-life of albumin is 18 to 21 days. As a result, there is a lag in detecting nutritional problems based on serum albumin. Albumin is also affected by fluid status and, therefore, is not an accurate measure in the patient with fluid imbalance.
- **Prealbumin** level fluctuates daily and is considered a better marker of acute change than albumin.
- **Transferrin** is a protein that binds with iron. Because it has a half-life of only 8 to 9 days, it allows for faster detection of protein depletion than does measuring albumin. Transferrin can be measured directly or indirectly (by a total iron-binding capacity test [TIBC]). It also reflects iron status. In a person with iron deficiency, the TIBC will be increased; in a person with anemia, the TIBC will be decreased.

Other markers are used to monitor protein metabolism:

- **Urea** is formed in the liver as an end product of protein metabolism and is excreted through the kidneys. As such, the serum blood urea nitrogen (BUN) level is an indicator of liver and kidney function. An elevated BUN level is seen with

Toward Evidence-Based Practice

Panagiotakos, D. (2014, March). *Mediterranean diet and diabetes development: A meta-analysis of 12 studies and 140,001 individuals* (Abstract 139). Presented at the American College of Cardiology 2014 Scientific Sessions, Washington, DC.

Findings from a meta-analysis of 19 studies involving more than 162,000 low- and high-risk people in multiple countries showed that following the Mediterranean diet may prevent the development of diabetes. Earlier research has shown this diet is also associated with weight loss, lower blood pressure and blood cholesterol levels, and a reduced risk of heart disease with related death.

Siu, A. L, on behalf of the U.S. Preventive Services Task Force. (2015). *Screening for abnormal blood glucose and type 2 diabetes mellitus: U.S. Preventive Services Task Force recommendation statement. Annals of Internal Medicine,* 15(163), 861–868. doi:10.7326/M15-2345

The USPSTF recommends that overweight or obese adults aged 40 to 70 years should be screened for abnormal blood glucose as part of cardiovascular risk. Those with abnormal blood glucose should receive intensive behavioral counseling interventions to promote a healthful diet and physical activity.

Suez, J., Korem, T., Zeevi, D., et al. (2014). *Artificial sweeteners induce glucose intolerance by altering the gut microbiota. Nature,* 514(7521), 181–186. doi:10.1038/nature13793

Clinical research with nondiabetic participants showed that long-term consumption of artificial sweeteners (e.g., aspartame, sucralose, saccharin) was associated with measures of obesity and glucose intolerance, even when adjusted for body mass index.

1. You are the nurse providing health education and screening for a middle-aged, overweight man. His total cholesterol level is 230 mg/dL (high), LDL (bad cholesterol) is also elevated, and HDL (good cholesterol) is within normal limits. Your patient's fasting blood sugar (FBS) is 120 (prediabetes), and hemoglobin A_{1c} (Hb A_{1c}) is 6.5 (prediabetes). Based on these evidence-based resources, what dietary counseling would you offer to this patient?

2. In counseling this patient, what other recommendations might you make to reduce his risk for developing metabolic syndrome (diabetes, obesity, hypertension, and hyperlipidemia)?

---

impaired kidney function, dehydration, excessive protein breakdown (often seen with diabetes mellitus, hyperthyroidism, or starvation), or excessive dietary protein intake. Low levels are seen with impaired liver function, fluid overload, and low protein intake.

- **Creatinine,** an end product of skeletal muscle metabolism, is excreted through the kidneys and is an excellent indicator of renal function. Increased levels may indicate impaired kidney function or loss of muscle mass.

May I Delegate Nutritional Assessments?

You may safely delegate to nursing assistive personnel (NAP) the measurement of weight, height, and intake and output; other nursing staff (e.g., licensed practical/vocational nurses) can collect a nutritional history. However, the registered nurse (RN) is responsible for reviewing and interpreting these findings. When delegating these tasks, you must also tell the NAP or licensed practical nuse (LPN) how often the measurements are to be made. Review Chapter 7 for making delegation decisions.

KnowledgeCheck 28-10

- What are the likely causes of hyperglycemia?
- Why is it important to identify the serum albumin level?

ThinkLike a Nurse 28-7

The Nutrition Screening Initiative (NSI) is completed for a 70-year-old.

- What major indicator on the NSI would indicate impaired nutritional status?
- What minor indicator would you likely see?

- What would malnourishment look like in the adult?
- What type of anthropometric findings would be typical of an older adult with poor nutrition patterns?
- What type of laboratory values would support impaired nutritional status?

ANALYSIS/NURSING DIAGNOSIS NP

For clients who have no symptoms of or risk factors for nutrition problems, use the diagnostic label Readiness for Enhanced Nutrition. NANDA International (NANDA-I) defines this as "a pattern of nutrient intake, which can be strengthened" (2014, p. 162).

Nutrition as the Problem

You can use the following NANDA-I labels to describe general nutrition problems:

- Frail Elderly Syndrome (and Risk for Frail Elderly Syndrome)
- Imbalanced Nutrition: Less than Body Requirements
- Nutrition, Readiness for Enhanced
- Obesity
- Overweight
- Overweight, Risk for
- Self-Care Deficit, Feeding
- Ineffective adolescent eating dynamics
- Ineffective child eating dynamics
- Ineffective infant eating dynamics

  Etiologies of Nutrition Problems Nutrition problems have many contributing factors:

- **Etiologies for undernutrition** include eating disorders, difficulties with chewing and swallowing, vomiting, alcoholism, food intolerances, metabolic disorders, digestive disorders, and absorption disorders.
- **Etiologies for Overweight and Obesity** include overeating, insufficient of exercise, and metabolic or endocrine disorders.

- **Other nursing diagnoses may contribute to nutrition problems,** for example, Diarrhea, Impaired Swallowing, Nausea, and Deficient Knowledge (nutrition).

Nutrition as the Etiology

Nutritional problems can also be the etiology of problems in other functional areas, for example:

- Ineffective Breastfeeding r/t insufficient breast milk production 2° insufficient intake of calories and fluids
- Constipation r/t insufficient intake of fluids and fiber
- Impaired (or Risk for Impaired) Skin Integrity r/t inadequate intake of protein and/or vitamin A
- Disturbed Sleep Pattern r/t excessive caffeine intake or to eating fatty and spicy foods near bedtime
- Impaired Social Interaction r/t low self-esteem 2° Obesity

PLANNING OUTCOMES/EVALUATION NP

The overall *Healthy People 2020* nutrition goal for the United States population is to "promote health and reduce chronic disease associated with diet and weight" (U.S. Department of Health and Human Services, 2010, updated 2016).

NOC Standardized Outcomes directly linked to nutritional problems include the following:

Applicable to most nutrition problems:

Appetite	Nutritional Status:
Nutritional Status	Nutrient Intake
Nutritional Status: Food	Self-Care: Eating
and Fluid Intake	

In addition to the above, the following are outcomes for more specific diagnoses:

For Frail Elderly Syndrome:

Knowledge: Health	Self-Care Status
Behavior	Will to Live
Nutritional Status: Food	
and Fluid Intake	

For Obesity and **Overweight:**

Adherence Behavior:	Knowledge: Healthy Diet
Healthy Diet	Weight: Body Mass
Eating Disorder	Weight Loss Behavior
Self-Control	

For Underweight/Malnutrition:

Same as for Obesity/Overweight, except for Weight Loss Behavior.

You could choose other NOC outcomes based on the patient's nursing diagnosis. For example:

For Situational Low Self-Esteem related to obesity—you might use Self-Esteem.

Individualized Goals/Outcome Statements you might write for a patient with nutrition-related problems include the following:

Loses 1 lb per week until ideal weight is attained.

Follows the prescribed modified diet that, at a minimum, meets the DRIs.

PLANNING INTERVENTIONS/ IMPLEMENTATION NP

NIC Standardized Interventions directly linked to nutrition problems include the broad interventions that could probably be used for most nutrition problems, regardless of the etiologies. Examples are:

Nutrition Management	Nutritional Monitoring
Nutrition Therapy	Teaching: Individual
Nutritional Counseling	

For other nutrition-related nursing diagnoses, the following NIC interventions are appropriate:

For Frail Elderly Syndrome:

Cognitive Stimulation	Nutrition Therapy
Hope Inspiration	Self-Care Assistance

For Overweight/Obesity:

Behavior Modification	Nutritional Monitoring
Exercise Promotion	Weight Management
Nutrition Management	Weight Reduction Assistance
Nutritional Counseling	

For Underweight/Malnutrition:

Eating Disorders	Self-Care Assistance:
Management	Feeding
Enteral Tube Feeding	Swallowing Therapy
Fluid/Electrolyte Management	Weight Gain Assistance
Nutrition Management	Weight Management

To see the entire alphabetical list of NIC interventions,

Go to Davis Advantage, Resources, Chapter 28, **List of NIC Interventions.**

Individualized Nursing Actions are determined by the patient's nursing diagnosis. Examples are discussed in the following sections:

Vitamin and Mineral Supplementation

Noncredentialed nutrition "experts" recommend, and sell, many kinds of vitamin and mineral supplements to prevent cancer and heart attacks, improve your sex life, prevent aging, and offer more energy. Conservative health professionals may disregard the need for supplements, insisting that a nutritious diet supplies all the micronutrients you need. Somewhere in the middle, most likely, lies the truth. A growing body of research suggests that certain supplements provide health benefits. Remember, too, that RDAs are for "average" needs; individual needs for micronutrients vary. Given the modern diet of processed foods, it may be difficult to get enough nutrients from diet alone during periods of increased nutrient demands.

NIC Intervention—Nutritional Counseling

Supplements of specific vitamins and minerals may be needed during growth periods (i.e., pregnancy, lactation, and adolescence). **KEY POINT:** *However, as a rule healthy adults eating balanced diets do not need supplements.* When teaching clients about supplements, keep the following principles in mind:

1. **Dietary supplements may be appropriate** for people whose diet does not provide the recommended intake of specific vitamins or minerals. With a few exceptions, taking nutritional supplements in appropriate amounts is not harmful.

2. **Individual needs vary,** and those needs should determine the specific nutrients and amounts used. For example:
   - Newborn infants are given a *vitamin K* injection to prevent hemorrhaging because they do not yet have bacterial flora in the gut to synthesize enough vitamin K.
   - *Folic acid* supplementation is recommended for people taking methotrexate (a drug used to treat certain types of cancer).
   - Women of childbearing age should take supplemental *folic acid.*
   - People who do not eat dairy products need supplemental *calcium and vitamin D.*

- Most adults older than 50 years should obtain vitamin B_{12} from fortified foods or supplements. Woman aged 50 and older should take calcium supplements to prevent osteoporosis; men may need to do so as well.

3. **Supplements do not replace the need to eat a nutritious diet.** Specific supplements are more effective if the person also has an adequate diet.
4. **Read supplement labels carefully.** They provide information about toxicity levels, dosage, and side effects.
5. **Encourage patients to ask their primary care provider's advice** before taking vitamins.
6. **Advise patients to follow the DRIs or RDAs dosages.**
7. **Be certain that any health claims made for a supplement** are based on sound research.
8. **The long-term effects of most nutritional supplements** have yet to be fully researched.

Nutritious Foods on a Limited Budget

When your clients cannot afford to buy food, you should teach them about available assistance and make appropriate referrals to programs such as the following:

- **The Supplemental Nutrition Assistance Program (SNAP)** is the current name for the federal Food Stamp Program. For low-income households, this program issues a SNAP card that can be used to buy food to cover the household's needs.
- **Commodity Supplemental Food Program.** The federal government buys surplus food to support certain agricultural products. These include both perishable and nonperishable commodities (e.g., peanut butter, cheese, green beans). The foods are made available to low-income pregnant and breastfeeding women, infants, children younger than age 6 years, and older adults at least age 60 years.
- **Women, Infants, and Children (WIC).** This federal program provides free food to low-income women who are pregnant or breastfeeding and to children younger than age 5 years. Typical available foods are milk, eggs, cheese, cereals, juice, and infant formulas. They are not meant to supply all necessary food for the household, but are intended to supplement the diet with protein, iron, and vitamins.
- **National School Lunch and Breakfast Programs.** These federally assisted programs subsidize schools that provide free or reduced-rate breakfasts and/or lunches to qualifying children.

NIC Intervention—Teaching: Individual

You can help your clients to use their food dollars creatively by teaching them to follow the suggestions in the Self-Care box Teaching Your Patients on a Limited Budget to Buy Nutritious Foods.

Supporting Special Nutritional Needs

Patients with special needs (e.g., patients with impaired dietary intake and those who have difficulty with swallowing or digestion) require specific nutrition interventions.

Impaired Dietary Intake

Nutritional health is related to the type and amount of food patients consume. Physical illnesses that alter appetite, taste, and smell impair dietary intake. Medical restriction in intake, such as NPO, also affects nutritional status. Other factors leading to poor nutritional health include impaired ability to purchase and prepare nutritious food, and feed self.

♥ iCare 28-1

Nutrition

In order to promote health and healing, you need to perform a keen assessment of a person's physical status, food and fluid intake, weight changes, and response to treatment. How do you do this?

- Document daily weights, I/O, food preferences, consumption, tolerances, and intolerances at every meal.
- Be supportive of a patient's/family's wishes regarding artificial hydration and nutrition.
- Realize that different cultures have different beliefs.
- Put your own beliefs aside.

Self-Care

Teaching Your Patients on a Limited Budget to Buy Nutritious Foods

Plan Ahead

- Advance planning will help you to control impulse buying and extra trips to the store.
- Avoid eating at fast-food restaurants. Meals are more expensive and less nutritious than those you can prepare at home.
- Try planting a garden; you can use pots if you live in the city.

Buy Wisely

- Buy generic instead of more expensive and widely advertised brands.
- Watch for sales of nutrient-dense items. Stock up on and freeze them for later use if you do not need them right away.
- Buy in quantity—if it results in real savings and if you can use that amount of food before it spoils.
- Limit convenience foods (e.g., frozen dinners), breads, canned goods, chips, and many cheeses; they are often high in fat and sodium.

- Buy foods when they are in season; for example, fresh tomatoes are less expensive, and better tasting, in the summer than in the winter.
- Purchase oatmeal and cream of wheat instead of cold, sugared cereals. Buy in bulk rather than single-serving packages, but not so much that food spoils.
- Avoid shopping at convenience stores. Items are usually more expensive than in supermarkets.
- Buy inexpensive cuts of meat but not high-fat grades; avoid processed lunchmeats and hot dogs.
- Buy frozen concentrated of fresh-squeezed fruit juices instead of juice in plastic jugs and cardboard boxes.
- Substitute dairy products, beans and lentils, and peanut butter for more expensive meat. Substitute powdered milk for whole milk.
- Read the Nutrition Facts panels on prepared foods to be sure you obtain the most nutrition for the money.

Patients Who Have Nausea

Nausea can cause vomiting and loss of appetite, leading to Impaired Nutrition. After assessing for the cause of the nausea (e.g., anxiety, pain, constipation, dehydration, post-anesthesia, chemotherapy, pancreatitis). Nursing interventions include assessing for the cause of the nausea, and providing comfort and prevention measures, and stimulating the appetite. Glare, Miller, Nikolova, et al. (2011) suggest the following:

- Determine the cause of the nausea.
- Assess for dehydration (you may need to administer parenteral fluid and electrolytes).
- Keep tissues and cool water to rinse the mouth at the bedside.
- Maintain a calm environment.
- Provide cool, fresh air.
- Instruct the patient to wear loose clothing.
- Avoid wearing perfumes.
- Immediately remove any food that the patient cannot or will not eat. The sight and smell of food can induce nausea.
- Provide or assist with frequent oral hygiene.
- Ask the patient to sit in an upright position for 30 to 45 minutes after eating, unless contraindicated.
- If vomiting, limit all food and drink until vomiting stops; wait 30 to 60 minutes and then start sips of clear liquid. Once tolerated, offer dry, starchy food (e.g., crackers, dry toast). Then progress to protein-rich food. Dairy is the last food to add back into the diet.
- Provide small, frequent, bland meals and snacks; avoid greasy, warm, spicy, excessively salty, or aromatic foods. For some, cold food is better tolerated. Allow the patient to eat what she finds appetizing and tolerates well.
- Provide cool (not cold or iced) cola to drink.
- Have the patient suck on an ice cube, sorbet, or a piece of frozen fruit (pineapple, kiwi, or apple). Lemon or peppermint may be helpful.
- Encourage sips of fluid in between meals, even if the patient doesn't feel thirsty.
- Recommend a dietary consultation if nausea and vomiting persist.
- For malnourished patients, consult a dietitian. Consider dietary supplements; however, these are often poorly tolerated and may sometimes cause even more nausea.
- When the nausea is related to anxiety, stress, or anticipation of nausea, try certain psychological techniques, such as distraction, relaxation techniques, guided imagery, systematic desensitization, self-hypnosis, biofeedback, and music therapy.
- Administer antiemetics as prescribed or per protocol.

Other Factors Affecting Intake

- **Loss of Appetite; Diminished Sense of Smell and Taste.** Refer to the Intervention Stimulating Appetite in the Example Problem: Underweight/Malnourished.
- **Nothing by Mouth (NPO).** Patients who are NPO for prolonged periods must receive glucose and electrolytes through either intravenous (IV) fluids or total parenteral nutrition and IV lipid infusion meet the body's fluid and nutritional needs. Provide comfort measures for patients who cannot take food and fluids orally:
  - Assist the patient with or provide oral hygiene.
  - If allowed, provide ice chips, hard candy, chewing gum, or sips of water for rinsing the mouth.
  - Advise family or visitors not to eat or drink around the patient, and try to schedule other activities for the patient at mealtimes.

 Remember that remaining NPO for more than 3 days puts the patient at risk for malnutrition.

When older adults must be NPO for tests or procedures, schedule them early in the day to decrease the length of time the patient must be NPO. If testing must be late in the day, ask the primary care provider whether the patient can have an early breakfast.

- **Unwise Food Choices.** Advise clients to eat nutrient-dense foods and to eat essential foods first. Because the sense of taste is decreased, older adults may prefer concentrated sweets; and because they may also have a poor appetite, once they eat sweets they may not be hungry enough to eat other foods.

- **Limited Income.** Adults and children living in impoverished situations may qualify for government entitlement (e.g., SNAP, National School Lunch Program) to supplement nutritional needs. Additionally, private, religious, and other charitable agencies (e.g., Harvesters) offer meals to those in need. Refer to the Self-Care box Teaching Your Patients on a Limited Budget to Buy Nutritious Foods.

For older adults in the United States, regardless of income, can eat hot noon meals at a community center. Those who are ill or disabled can receive Meals on Wheels at home. Socially or medically needy and impoverished people are given priority.

Impaired Swallowing

The NANDA-I diagnosis Impaired Swallowing may be caused by a host of anatomical or physiological defects, for example: mechanical obstruction (e.g., tumor), neuromuscular impairment (e.g., facial paralysis), stroke, and cerebral palsy. Patients with impaired swallowing, or **dysphagia,** are at risk for choking and aspiration. Nutritional support should focus on helping your patient feel more comfortable while swallowing, and making mealtime safer and more enjoyable. Consider the activities from the NIC intervention, Swallowing Therapy (Bulechek, Butcher, Dochterman, et al., 2013, pp. 369–370):

- Provide/use assistive devices, as appropriate.
- Avoid use of drinking straws.
- Assist the patient to position [her] head in forward flexion in preparation for swallowing (chin tuck).
- Assist patient to place food at the back of the mouth and on the unaffected side.
- Monitor the patient's tongue movements while she is eating.
- Check mouth for pocketing of food after eating.
- Monitor body weight.
- Monitor body hydration (e.g., intake, output, skin turgor, mucous membranes).

In addition, you must also take the following Aspiration Precautions (Bulechek, Butcher, Dochterman, et al., 2013, p. 87):

- Monitor level of consciousness, cough reflex, gag reflex, and swallowing ability.
- Position the patient upright 90° or as far as possible.
- Keep suction setup available.
- Feed in small amounts.
- Cut food into small pieces.
- Inspect oral cavity for retained food or medications.
- Keep head of bed elevated for 30 to 45 minutes after feeding.

You will sometimes also offer a special dysphagia diet, depending on the degree of difficulty the patient has with swallowing: dysphagia puree, dysphagia mechanically altered, dysphagia advanced, and regular. Liquid diets vary in *viscosity,* or thickness, based on degree of swallowing impairment. Clinicians are encouraged to prescribe the minimal level of thickness needed for swallowing safety (Chichero, 2013).

Impaired Digestive Function

Nutritional health is due in part to digestive function from mastication (chewing) all the way through passing stool. Dysfunction of the GI tract can reduce the transport, absorption, and elimination of food nutrients.

- **Gastroesophageal Reflux.** Advise clients not to eat just before bedtime, and advise them to elevate the head of the bed 30° to 40°. It is also important for them to avoid overeating, to avoid bending over, and to take their prescribed medications. They should also avoid fruit juices, fatty foods, chocolate, alcohol, and smoking; all of these stimulate reflux. If overweight, the client with reflux should lose weight.
- **Decreased Gastric Secretions.** People with this problem should eat regularly scheduled meals, chew their food thoroughly, and take prescribed medications. They should be certain to eat foods rich in vitamin D to ensure calcium absorption.
- **Dry Mouth.** This is most often an age-associated change. Advise clients to avoid caffeine, alcohol, tobacco, and dry, bulky, spicy, salty, or highly acidic foods. Offer hard candy or chewing gum to stimulate salivation (unless the patient has dementia). Use lip moisturizer and encourage frequent sips of water.
- **Glucose Intolerance.** Obviously, patients with glucose intolerance should avoid concentrated, refined sugars (e.g., candy, ice cream, desserts), unless they have been told to use it to treat hypoglycemia. Complex carbohydrates (e.g., whole-grain cereals, vegetables) are better tolerated. Smaller, more frequent meals may also be necessary.
- **Decreased Intestinal Peristalsis.** To prevent constipation, advise patients to eat a diet high in fiber, including a minimum of five servings of fresh fruits and vegetables every day (prunes and prune juice are often effective); exercise or at least walk regularly; drink at least eight glasses of water or other fluids per day; and eat meals on a regular schedule.

Older Adults

Evidence suggests that dementia, especially Alzheimer's disease, is less common among people who eat fruits and vegetables daily, eat fish once a week, and use fats rich in omega-3 fatty acids (e.g., walnut and soy oil) (Barberger-Gateau, Raffaitin, Letenneur, et al., 2007). Of course, this doesn't suggest that diet alone can prevent dementia; it merely suggests there may be a connection.

Assisting Patients With Meals

Some patients are at risk for nutritional deficits as a result of a Self-Care Deficit (Feeding), which may be caused by loss of cognitive, musculoskeletal, or neuromuscular function; weakness; pain; or environmental barriers. Elderly patients especially are at risk for undernutrition or malnourishment in inpatient settings. You should institute special nutrition interventions in patients who have one of the following:

- An involuntary weight loss of more than 5% in 30 days or 10% in 180 days.
- Leaving more than one-fourth of their food in the past 7 days or two-thirds of meals (based on a 2,000-kcal diet).
- A BMI of 18.5 or less.

NIC Interventions for this situation are Feeding and Self-Care Assistance: Feeding. Important nursing actions include

assisting patients with meals. Other nursing activities include the following:

- Assess for functional deficits that contribute to Feeding Self-Care Deficit or Imbalanced Nutrition.
- Monitor intake for nutritional adequacy. Some patients may need liquid oral supplements of protein and calories.
- Collaborate with occupational and physical therapists in planning care.
- See that the patient has protein- and energy-enriched meals.
- Provide midafternoon snacks.
- Ensure the nutrition prescribed is implemented. Assign someone to be responsible for assisting the patient with meals as necessary. Include this in your instructions to NAPs and other assistive personnel.
- Fix food on a tray; for example, cut meat into smaller pieces, peel an egg, open packages.
- Provide a cup with a large handle or a straw, if necessary and if not at risk for choking.
- Refer the patient and family to an agency that can help them obtain a home health aide (Bulechek, Butcher, Dochterman, et al., 2013, pp. 195, 336).

For guidelines more specific to assisting with meals, including care of patients with dementia, see Clinical Insight 28-3.

Interventions for Example Problem: Overweight/Obesity

- Refer to the Example Problem: Overweight/Obesity.
- See the Self-Care box Teaching Weight-Loss Tips.
- To see a sample care plan and care map for Overweight/Obesity,

 Go to Davis Advantage, Resources, Chapter 28, **Care Plan** and **Care Map.**

Providing Enteral Nutrition

If a patient cannot meet his nutritional needs through an enhanced diet and measures to stimulate the appetite, you may need to use an alternative feeding method. Feeding can occur through the intestinal tract as enteral nutrition or intravenously as parenteral nutrition. **Enteral nutrition** (*tube feeding*) refers to the delivery of liquid nutrition into the upper intestinal tract via a tube. Tube feeding may be used in addition to or instead of oral intake. It is the preferred method of feeding for a patient who has a functioning intestinal tract but needs nutritional support (e.g., patients with swallowing disorders, certain bowel diseases).

Enteral feedings are preferred to parenteral (i.e., intravenous) nutrition because they have a lower incidence of sepsis and maintain intestinal structure and function. However, there are several risks associated with enteral feedings:

- If enteral formula is aspirated into the lungs, it can lead to infection, pneumonia, abscess formation, adult respiratory distress syndrome, and in some cases death.
- The high glucose content of enteral formulas provides a medium for bacterial growth.
- Other complications include diarrhea, nausea and vomiting, nasopharyngeal trauma, alterations in drug absorption and metabolism, and various metabolic disturbances.

For more about safe use of parental nutrition, see the Safe, Effective Nursing Care box. For complete instructions on tube feedings, see Procedure 28-3.

Preventing Tubing Misconnections There have been some instances in which enteral feedings have been mistakenly

Self-Care

Teaching Weight-Loss Tips

Getting Ready

Make a commitment.
- ➤ Promise yourself; promise others. "I will do this."

Set realistic goals.
- ➤ Aim to lose 1 to 2 lb/wk. To do this you need to burn 500 to 1,000 calories more than you consume. Losing weight faster usually means losing water weight or muscle tissue rather than fat.
- ➤ Set "process" rather than "outcome" goals. For example, "I will exercise for at least 30 minutes every day" instead of "I will lose 10 pounds this month." Changing your habits (your "processes") is the key to weight loss.
- ➤ Write your goals, your plan for achieving them, and your start date. This makes it reality, not just a thought.
- ➤ Review your goals each week. Readjust them as needed. If you are exercising more than you thought, adjust your goal upward, for example.

Plan for setbacks.
- ➤ Identify situations that might trigger eating or interfere with exercise; plan specific actions you will take to overcome them.

Beginning New Behaviors

Eat healthier foods.
- ➤ Eat more fruits and vegetables.
- ➤ Limit fatty foods and sugar-sweetened beverages.

Get active and stay active.
- ➤ If you have not been exercising, start to do so slowly.
- ➤ Work up to at least 300 min per week to lose weight and maintain the loss.

Get adequate sleep.
- ➤ For most people, this is 7 to 8 hr a night.
- ➤ Sleep deprivation can affect levels of the appetite-regulating hormones leptin and ghrelin (Knutson, Spiegel, Penev, et al., 2007).
- ➤ Sleep loss can affect the type of food you crave. When you are tired you are less able to cope with stress and emotional triggers for eating, and more likely to crave comfort foods such as chocolate and ice cream.

"Sticking With It"

Keep a food diary.
- ➤ This can double your weight loss.

Decide what and when to eat.
- ➤ Decide what foods you will eat as well as when you will eat. For example, "I will eat only at the table, three meals and two snacks daily."
- ➤ Make a conscious effort to take small bites and eat slowly.
- ➤ Serve your food on small plates.

Shop wisely.
- ➤ Shop for food on a full stomach.
- ➤ Read food labels when purchasing food (for information about calorie and fat content).

Find ways to exercise.
- ➤ Lay out your work-out clothing ahead of time (e.g., at night if you exercise in the morning).
- ➤ Use the stairs instead of the elevator; park in the back of the parking lot, as far from the door as possible.
- ➤ Walk or bike to work when possible.

Get emotional support.
- ➤ Family members can help by not offering you desserts. Weight-loss support groups let you know you are not alone. An exercise partner can help keep you motivated.

Recognize that lifestyle changes must be permanent.

Remember: Healthy eating, physical activity, and sleep are necessities, not options!

---

connected to intravascular (IV) lines and feeding solutions have been infused into veins. These events, termed "tubing misconnections," are potentially fatal to the patient (Institute for Safe Medication Practices, 2010; The Joint Commission, 2007, 2014; U.S. Food and Drug Administration, n.d.b, updated 2016). An enteral device manufacturer and a professional organization dedicated to advancing the science and practice of nutrition support therapy cooperated to develop the "Be A. L. E. R. T." Safety Campaign° (along with Be A. W. A. R. E. [see Boxes 28-5 and 28-7]) to increase the safety of patients on enteral nutrition.

Patients may receive enteral or parenteral nutrition in the home as well as in inpatient settings. The Home Care box Home Nutritional Support reviews teaching related to alternative feeding methods in the home. You should review these topics with the patient or caregiver.

Types of Enteric Tubes

Enteric tubes are available in various materials, lengths, diameters, and types. Choose the type of tube you need based on the intended use and the length of time you anticipate it will be left in place. This chapter focuses on the use of enteral tubes

Safe, Effective Nursing Care

Safe Use of Parenteral Nutrition

Chapter Key Concept: Nutrition

Competency: Collaborate with the interdisciplinary healthcare team; Validate evidence-based research to incorporate in practice; Provide safe, quality client care

Clinicians at Scripps Memorial Hospital (SMH) in La Jolla, California, theorized that their poor processes and variation in methods in use of parenteral nutrition (PN) were producing inconsistent patient outcomes, thus increasing patient risk. The following is a description of how they set out to correct this by identifying the root causes of the problems and standardizing care:

➤ **Problems Identified:** Clinicians first organized a multidisciplinary team to collect and analyze data, develop better practices, and evaluate outcomes. They found several problems: inappropriate use of PN, poor glycemic control in patients on PN, inconsistent and confusing ordering practices, insufficient calorie replacement, and insufficient laboratory monitoring.

➤ **Corrective Interventions:** Implementing the American Society for Parenteral and Enteral Nutrition's (A.S.P.E.N.) guideline for PN, revising the PN order form, educating physicians and other clinicians, and establishing twice weekly PN rounds. The group measured specific quality indicators before and after implementing the new

procedures. Changes in the top four measures over a 2-year period included the following:
1. Compliance with 10 Mandatory Components of an A.S.P.E.N. PN Order Form
2. Appropriate use of parenteral nutrition
3. Baseline labs ordered before initiating PN
4. Calories delivered within 10% of estimated need

Results/Conclusions: In addition to improving compliance, the new procedures resulted in significant costs savings.

➤ **Think About It:** Parenteral nutrition is a high-risk treatment associated with serious complications, including death.

➤ Do the above measures mean that patient outcomes are improved?

➤ In what specific ways does this QI project demonstrate the QSEN competencies of Quality Improvement, Safety, and Evidenced-Based and Practice?

➤ Which specific knowledge, skills, and attitudes does it address?

Source: Boitano, M., Bojak, S., McCloskey, S., et al. (2010). Improving the safety and effectiveness of parenteral nutrition. *Nutrition in Clinical Practice, 25*(6), 663–671.

Home Care

Home Nutritional Support

To assist the client or caregiver with the management of home nutritional therapy, teach the following aspects:
1. ***Formula.*** Review the type of formula the patient should receive. Enteral or IV solutions are clearly marked with their contents. Emphasize that the caregiver double-check that the correct solution is being used and that the expiration date and time have not been reached before administering any feeding.
2. ***Administration.*** Carefully review how to administer the feeding. Emphasize the need for hand washing before hanging the infusion. After a period of time, the client may be able to tolerate delivering 1 to 3 L of enteral feeding at night. The rate must be increased at the beginning and decreased when ending the delivery. If parenteral nutrition is administered at home, be sure that the client or caregiver is aware of proper technique.

3. ***Access device.*** Review the care required for the access device, including site care, dressing changes, and flushing.
4. ***Storage.*** Stored enteral and parenteral nutrition must be refrigerated to prevent bacterial contamination.
5. ***Monitoring.*** Instruct the client or caregiver to report a rise in temperature, weight loss, change in bowel movements, decrease in urine output, or change in condition.
6. ***Follow-up.*** Arrange for the client to be weighed and assessed regularly to monitor the adequacy of the feedings. Often clients weigh at home and report to the primary care provider's office or the nutrition support team for ongoing monitoring of progress and review of lab work.

These are complicated therapies to manage at home. These patients will typically go home with a referral for a home care nurse to assist in the transition from hospital to home and follow-up with nutritional support service.

---

as a route for feeding; however, they are inserted for other reasons as well:

- Lavage of the stomach (e.g., when there is disease, surgery, or bleeding in the GI tract, and in cases of poisoning or medication overdose)
- Collecting a specimen of stomach contents for laboratory tests
- To prevent nausea, vomiting, and gastric distention postoperatively

When a nasogastric (or orogastric) tube is placed to empty the stomach (lavage), larger bore, tubes made of polyvinyl chloride (PVC), are used. These are called **Salem sump tubes** (Fig. 28-4). A Salem sump tube has a lumen for drainage and one to allow air to enter the stomach. The air port (pigtail) is usually blue. A **Levin tube,** also used for drainage, has a single lumen, with holes in the tip and along the sides.

Selecting a Feeding Tube

Short-term (less than 6 wk) enteral feedings are usually delivered through a nasogastric (NG) or a nasoenteric (NE) tube. The **lumen** (inside diameter) of a feeding tube is measured using the **French (Fr) scale:** the larger the lumen, the larger the

BOX 28-5 ■ Be A.L.E.R.T.©

To reduce errors and help ensure safe enteral nutrition, use the following mnemonic:

A   **Aseptic** technique.....................................   When preparing and delivering enteral formula, practice good hand hygiene; wear gloves when handling feeding tube; avoid touching can tops, container openings, spike, and spike port.

L   **Label** enteral equipment...........................   with patient name and room number, formula name and rate, date and time of initiation, and nurse initials.

E   **Elevate** the head of the bed.....................   a minimum of 30° for feedings whenever clinically possible; may mitigate risk of reflux and aspiration of gastric content.

R   **Right** patient, **Right** formula, **Right** tube....   Match formula to patient's feeding order; verify **enteral** tubing set connects formula container to feeding tube.

T   **Trace** all lines and tubing back to patient......   Avoid misconnections—trace all lines from origin to patient; only enteral-to-enteral connections.

Sources: © 2009 Nestlé HealthCare Nutrition, Inc. The BE A. L. E. R.T. © Poster is a joint effort of the American Society for Parenteral and Enteral Nutrition (A.S.P.E.N.) and Nestlé HealthCare Nutrition, Inc. Retrieved from http://www.nutritioncare.org/guidelines_and_clinical_resources/toolkits/enteral_nutrition_toolkit/related_publications_and_tools/; Bankhead, R., Boullata, J., Brantley, S., et al.; American Society for Parenteral and Enteral Nutrition (A.S.P.E.N.) Board of Directors. (2009). Special report: Enteral nutrition practice recommendations. *Journal of Parenteral and Enteral Nutrition, 20*(10). doi:10.1177/0148607108330314

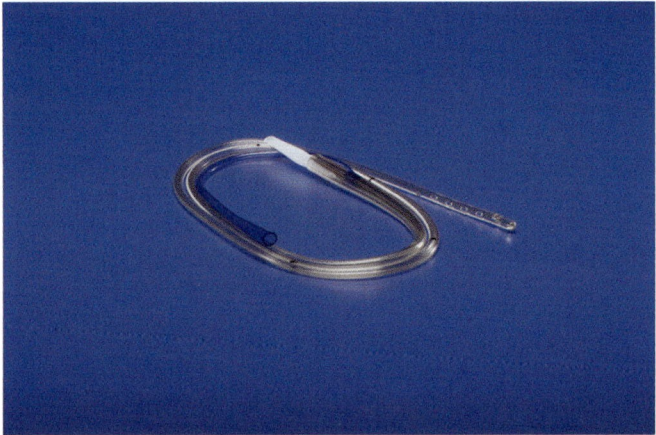

FIGURE 28-4 A large-bore, PVC Salem sump tube used for gastric lavage.

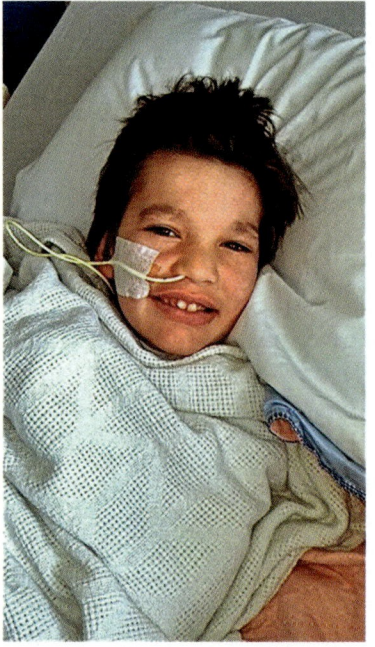

FIGURE 28-5 A small lumen, flexible nasoenteric feeding tube provides continuous nutrition to patients with impaired swallowing.

diameter. Most feeding tubes for adults are 8 to 12 Fr and 90 to 108 cm (36 to 43 in.) long. Each Fr unit is about 0.33 mm, so a 12 Fr tube is about 4 mm in diameter.

- **Small-bore NG tubes.** As a nurse, you may be asked to place a small-bore **NG feeding tube.** The tube is inserted through one naris, passed through the nasopharynx into the esophagus, and finally into the stomach. See Procedure 28-2.
- **An NE tube** is longer than an NG tube, extending through the nose down into the duodenum or jejunum (if it extends into the jejunum, it is called an NJ tube). A small, flexible tube is preferred for feeding (see Fig. 28-5). An NE tube may be used instead of an NG tube for patients at risk for aspiration (e.g., decreased level of consciousness, absent or diminished gag reflex, or severe gastroesophageal reflux).
- **Large-bore (larger than 12 Fr) NG tubes,** such as the Salem sump (Fig. 28-4), are occasionally used for feeding, but are converted to a smaller tube within the first 2 days. They are less flexible, less comfortable, and more commonly used if it is necessary to empty (lavage) the stomach. Figures 28-5 and 28-6 show three types of feeding tubes.

- **Tubes for long-term feedings.** A **gastrostomy tube (G-tube), percutaneous endoscopic gastrostomy tube (PEG)** (Figs. 28-7, 28-8), **jejunostomy tube (J-tube, PEJ),** or **gastrostomy button (G-button)** (Fig. 28-9) is preferred for long-term feedings. These are placed surgically or laparoscopically through the skin and the abdominal wall into the stomach or jejunum. The surgical incision is sometimes sutured tightly around the tube to hold it in place and prevent leakage. A gastrostomy tube can be converted to a **G-button** once healing has taken place. The G-tubes and G-buttons, which can be capped off flush with the abdominal wall when not in use, are the most comfortable of all for long-term use. Patient comfort

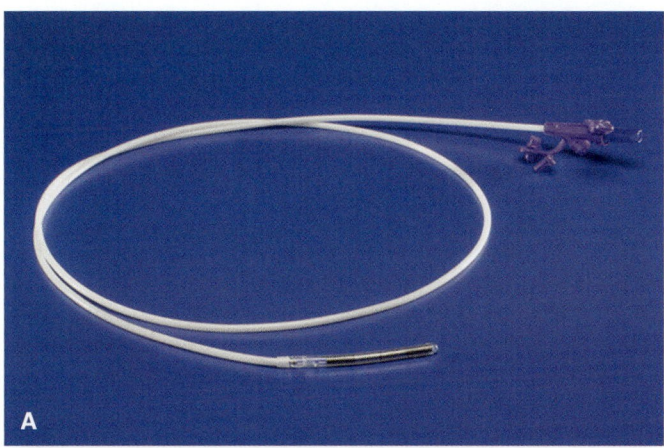

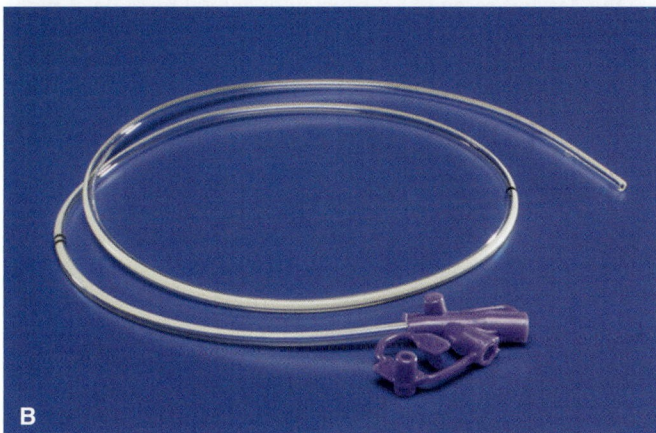

FIGURE 28-6 A. A double-lumen, weighted (Dobhoff) feeding tube. B. A nonweighted (kangaroo) feeding tube.

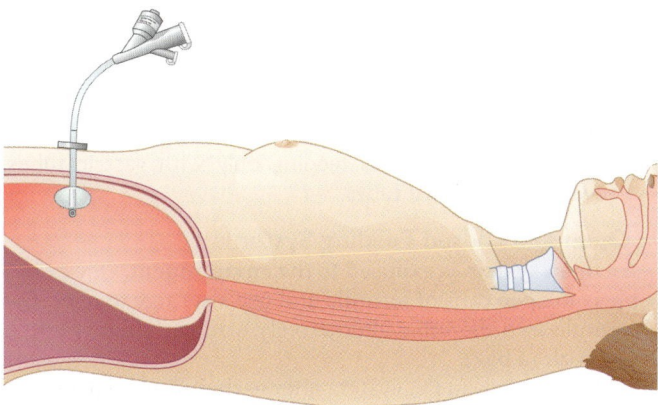

FIGURE 28-7 A percutaneous gastrostomy (PEG) tube for feeding.

and improved technology leading to ease of insertion have made PEG or PEJ an option even for short-term use.

Checking Feeding Tube Placement

✚ NG and NE feeding tubes are placed without direct visualization. As a result, there is risk of placing the tube into the respiratory tract. Therefore, you must check the location of the tip of the feeding tube before each enteral feeding or once per shift for continuous feedings. Failure to verify placement could be disastrous because it may result in infusion of formula into the lungs.

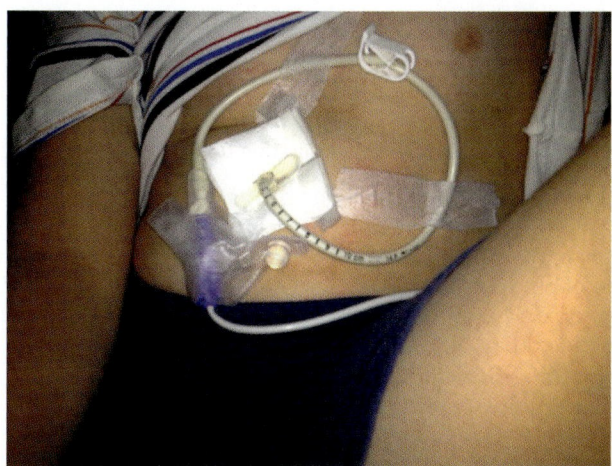

FIGURE 27-8 A PEG feeding tube is more convenient and comfortable than a nasogastric tube.

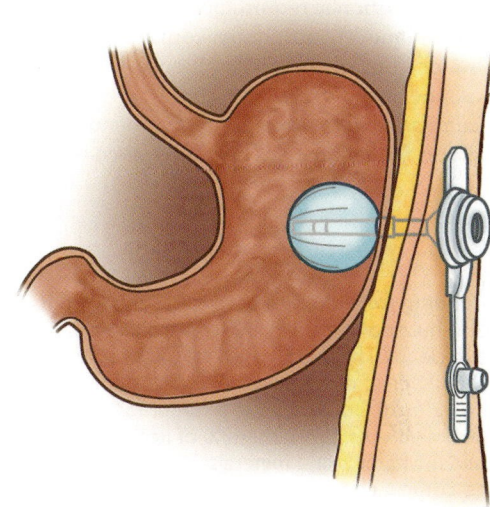

FIGURE 28-9 A gastrostomy button (G-button) in place for feeding.

KEY POINT: *Radiographic verification is the most reliable method for confirming tube placement and must be performed before the first feeding is administered.* However, x-ray is not practical for ongoing verification of placement. Reliable bedside assessment is necessary because even when the tube is initially placed correctly in the stomach (or intestine), it may later move upward.

No bedside method alone reliably verifies tube placement, so you must use the pH of the aspirate in combination with other methods for bedside verification (see Clinical Insight 28-4). If at any time after the initial x-ray you are in doubt about tube placement, obtain another one to verify the tube location.

✚ **No longer recommended:** Adding dye to enteral feedings as a method for identifying aspiration of gastric contents is not recommended. This is because dye has been associated with several adverse effects, including gastric bacterial colonization, diarrhea, systemic dye absorption, and death, and it is not effective in detecting aspiration (Metheny & the American Association of Critical-Care Nurses, 2005, updated 2016).

KnowledgeCheck 28-11

- When is enteral nutrition the preferred alternative feeding method?
- Identify and describe the types of enteral nutrition tubes.
- List four tube placement verification techniques.

Administering Enteral Feedings

In a few institutions, enteral feeding formulas are blended in the kitchen, but most use a commercially prepared product. The type of product selected depends on the patient's health condition. Products vary in nutritional components and caloric concentration (Box 28-6).

Feeding Schedules

- **Continuous feedings** provide a constant flow of formula and an even distribution of nutrition over 24 hours. Continuous infusions are usually administered into NG, NJ, PEG, or PEJ tubes, or G-buttons, to patients who require intensive nutritional support. Feedings may be interrupted for periodic instillation of medications or flushing with water. Continuous feedings allow the lowest possible hourly feeding rate to meet nutritional requirements, which can be better tolerated for some. Additionally, continuous infusion can lead to better control of blood glucose levels (American Diabetes Association, 2011).
  - *Pump-controlled infusions* are recommended for jejunal feedings and for gastrostomy feedings given by continuous

infusion to decrease gastroesophageal reflux (American Diabetes Association, 2011; American Gastrointestinal Association, 1995). A feeding pump ensures a steady flow rate.
  - *Gravity feedings* can also be used for continuous infusions, but the rate of delivery is not precise and they increase the risk of gastroesophageal reflux, diarrhea, and aspiration. You regulate the drip rate by adjusting a clamp on the tubing, much the same as adjusting an IV rate.
- **Cyclic feedings** are administered regularly; however, the infusion time less than 24 hours per day. The cyclic feeding schedule is more physiological, which is useful in the transition from continuous feedings to eventual oral intake
  - *Nocturnal feedings* are a form of cyclic feedings. The patient is able to eat meals and participate in activities throughout the day but receives an infusion of enteral formula at night while at rest.
  - A *20-hour infusion* is another variant, during which a 4-hour break allows time for the feeding pump to be disconnected for hygiene and other activities.
- **Intermittent feedings** are given to supplement oral intake or for patients who want greater mobility to take part in activities such as physical therapy. Feedings are given on a regular or periodic basis several times a day, usually over 30 to 60 minutes. An example of a prescription for a regular feeding is "Give 250 to 500 mL of enteral nutrition every 4 to 6 hours." Periodic feedings are often based on oral intake and are considered to be more physiologically similar to normal eating patterns. For example, if a patient consumes 90% or more of the ordered diet, no additional feeding is given. The less he consumes, the more formula is given after the meal.
  - The **bolus method** is sometimes used for intermittent feedings. In this method, you use a syringe to deliver 300 to 400 mL of formula through the tube over a 5- to 10-minute period. This is the easiest method to teach family members for home care, and it frees the patient from mechanical devices that limit activity. But because the fluid is given more rapidly by this method, it increases the risk for respiratory aspiration and for stomach distention.

    ✚ You can use bolus feeding only with gastric tubes, never with intestinal tubes.

Open and Closed Feeding Systems

- **An open system is exposed to the environment.** One example is to open cans of formula and use a syringe to inject the formula into the tube; alternatively, you can pour it into a reservoir (a bag).

    Flush and clean the system after each delivery.

    Most agencies require that an open-system feeding not hang for more than 4 hours.
- **A closed system is a prefilled system** (bag or bottle) that functions much like IV fluid. The nurse spikes the container with tubing that is attached to the feeding pump or run through a manually controlled drip chamber.

    Closed systems decrease the risk of contamination.

    A prefilled closed-system container can safely hang for 24 to 48 hours if you use sterile technique.

    You can measure out the specified amount in the drip chamber, allowing the remainder of the container to be used later in the day.

Monitoring Patients Receiving Enteral Nutrition

For patients receiving enteral nutrition, you will need to monitor tube placement, skin condition, laboratory values

---

BOX 28-6 ■ Types of Enteral Feeding Solutions

- ***Basic feeding formulas*** are used for clients who have no significant nutritional deficits but are unable to eat or drink sufficiently. They provide 1 kcal/mL of solution and meet the needs of most clients. A standard formula contains 12%–20% of kcal from protein, 45%–60% of kcal from carbohydrates, and 30%–40% of kcal from fats. They also contain vitamins and minerals. They are usually lactose free and contain complex forms of carbohydrates, fats, and proteins. Therefore, they require digestion and absorption.
- ***High-protein formulas*** are for clients who have a substantial need for protein, such as those with burns, open wounds, or malnutrition.
- ***Elemental formulas*** do not contain complex proteins; instead, they contain amino acids or peptides. They are reserved for patients with severe small bowel absorptive dysfunction. These formulas are fiber free and highly osmotic. Their use is controversial.
- ***Diabetic formulas*** are for clients who require tube feedings to meet nutritional needs but have type 1 or type 2 diabetes mellitus. These formulas control carbohydrate intake.
- ***Renal formulas*** are for clients who require tube feedings to meet nutritional needs but have renal failure or renal insufficiency as comorbidity. These formulas limit potassium, sodium, and nitrogen intake.
- ***Pulmonary formulas*** provide 55% of the calories as fat so that less CO_2 is produced per unit of oxygen consumed. They are used, for example, for patients with lung disease.
- ***Fiber-containing formulas.*** Because fiber has a potential protective effect for multiple disease states, including diverticulosis, colon cancer, diabetes, and heart disease, fiber-containing formulas may be used for patients in long-term care facilities or patients who require enteral feedings for a prolonged period of time.

(especially blood glucose, BUN, and electrolytes), feeding residual, and gastrointestinal status (Clinical Insight 28-5). This will allow you to detect complications that affect metabolism or fluid and electrolyte balance and to assess responses to enteral feeding. Feedings may need to be increased or decreased depending on the patient's changing clinical condition.

Preventing Contamination of Enteral Feedings

Enteral feeding solutions provide an ideal medium for bacterial growth. To prevent infection in patients receiving enteral feedings, be sure to:

- Check dates on feeding solutions and supplies. Do not use any that are expired.
- When hanging, label feeding containers with the patient's name and the date and time hung; document the time in the patient record.
- Use meticulous hand hygiene; wear nonsterile gloves.
- Use sterile equipment and supplies; once you have opened them, handle them as little as possible.
- Disposable feeding equipment is meant for one-time use. Do not wash and reuse.
- Replace feeding equipment after 24 hours.
- Replace the feeding tube according to the manufacturer's recommendations, or agency policy if that is sooner (Dietitians Association of Australia, 2011).
- Store opened feeding solutions in the refrigerator in covered and labeled containers. Allow the solution to return to room temperature before giving it to the patient. Discard after 24 hours.
- Keep unopened solutions at room temperature.
- Never allow a feeding to hang below the level of the patient's stomach.

- Follow agency policy regarding how long a solution may be left hanging. Usually sterile feedings may be hung for up to 24 hours (or unit policy).
- Nonsterile feedings (i.e., reconstituted powder feedings) may hang for up to 4 hours or unit policy.
- Do not transfer sterile feedings into a second container.
- Use sterile water for (1) flushing the tube after medication, (2) unclogging the tubing or to check for leakage at a hub, (3) patients who are immunocompromised, (4) patients receiving jejunal feeds, or (5) initially following a gastrostomy insertion.
- See Box 28-7 for guidelines.

Removing Feeding Tubes

When a patient's condition has stabilized and she no longer requires enteral nutrition, the feeding tube may be removed. A PEG tube is usually clamped if feedings are no longer required. For steps to follow when removing feeding tubes, see Procedure 28-4.

ThinkLike a Nurse 28-8

Your client has dementia and is frequently agitated. She has been progressively losing weight. An interprofessional team recommended enteral nutrition because of poor oral intake; however, the client has repeatedly pulled out her NG tube and had an episode of aspiration pneumonia last month. What recommendations might you consider at the next meeting?

Providing Parenteral Nutrition

Parenteral nutrition (PN) is the delivery of nutrition intravenously into a large, central vein. This is the preferred

---

BOX 28-7 ■ Be A.W.A.R.E.©: Practice Safe Enteral Medication Delivery

To reduce errors and optimize safe enteral nutrition, use the following mnemonic:

A	**Ask** the pharmacist about:	<ul><li>Drug-nutrient interactions</li><li>Drug-drug interactions</li><li>Adverse drug reactions</li><li>Appropriate dosage form</li><li>Risk of a drug clogging the tube</li><li>Whether location of the feeding tube's distal end allows safe and adequate drug delivery</li></ul>
W	**Water** only.	<ul><li>To dilute medications (including liquid meds)</li><li>To routinely flush the tube</li><li>Flush before/after each medication administered, using an amount appropriate for the patient's age and condition</li><li>Use water ONLY (no carbonated beverages, juices, coffee, other liquids.)</li></ul>
A	**Administer** medications.	<ul><li>Identify whether tube location (distal end) allows for safe and adequate drug delivery.</li><li>I medication at a time—do not mix drugs together.</li><li>Do not add medication directly to formula.</li><li>Identify medications that must be separated.</li></ul>
R	**Remember** the **Rights.**	<ul><li>Right patient, drug, time, dose, route</li><li>Right syringe, drug formulation, dilution, tube, and medication port</li></ul>
E	**Establish** evidence-based protocols.	<ul><li>Follow your facility's medication protocols.</li><li>Establish specific enteral medication protocols based on: National Guidelines Practice Recommendations http://www.nutritioncare.org/</li></ul>

method of feeding for clients who cannot be nourished through the gastrointestinal tract. Some clients (e.g., those with shortened small bowel secondary to injury or disease) who are able to partially meet their nutritional needs orally may supplement with PN to add calories and nutrients. Others (e.g., clients who are severely malnourished, have extensive burns or trauma, or have conditions that require resting the gastrointestinal system) are nourished entirely by PN.

Parenteral Nutrition Solutions usually contain a 10% to 70% concentration of dextrose in water (but usually not more than 20%), along with amino acids. They can provide 20 to 30 kcal per kilogram per day, depending on the patient's calculated energy need. **KEY POINT:** *Note, though, that the most common concentrations of glucose provide only 200 kcal per liter.* PN also contains vitamins, minerals, and trace elements. Standard PN can be modified to meet individual needs.

The type of venous access device used to administer PN will depend on the components of the PN and the anticipated duration of PN.

- **Large, high-flow vein.** Because PN solutions are hypertonic, they should be administered in a large, high-flow vein through a central venous access catheter. The subclavian vein has been the site of choice; however, the jugular vein is preferred for tunneled catheters and implanted ports.
- **PICC lines.** Peripherally inserted central catheter (PICC) lines are also used for PN.
- **Peripheral vein.** Some types of PN solutions may be infused via a peripheral vein, but this is not usual.

➕ **Confirming placement.** Whatever the insertion site, all PN catheters must have chest x-ray confirmation that the tip is in the lower portion of the superior vena cava adjacent to the right atrium (see Fig. 28-10) before beginning the first infusion. High blood flow through that vessel causes rapid dilution of the concentrated PN and thereby prevents vessel damage.

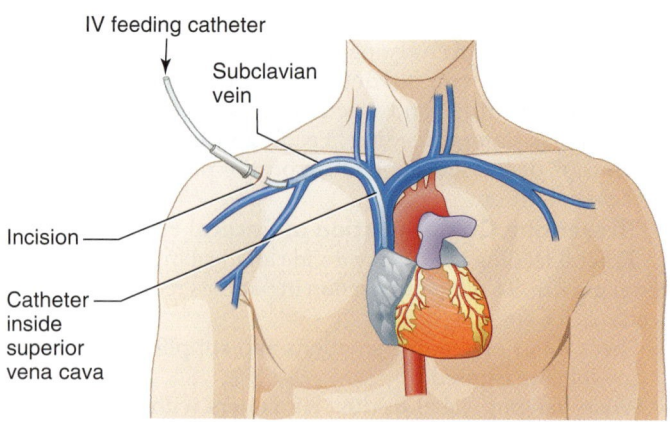

FIGURE 28-10 The subclavian vein is the site of choice for parenteral nutrition.

Lipid Emulsions contain essential fatty acids, triglycerides, and supplemental kcal. They are administered weekly for patients who rely on PN to prevent essential fatty acid deficiency. Lipids also add calories to the PN mixture so that lower glucose concentrations can be used, thus reducing the risk of glucose fluctuations. Most IV fats are supplied by safflower or soybean oil and provide 1.1 to 3 kcal/mL.

- You may administer lipids at the same time as the PN, through a peripheral line or by Y-connector tubing through a central line.
- Lipids are also sometimes added to the PN solution (this is called a 3-in-1 admixture), and administered over a 24-hour period.

To learn about monitoring and maintenance for patients receiving parenteral nutrition, see Clinical Insight 28-6.

CLINICALREASONING

The questions and exercises in this section allow you to practice the kind of thinking you will use as a full-spectrum nurse. Critical-thinking questions usually have more than one correct answer, so we do not provide "correct answers" for these features. It is more important to develop your nursing judgment than to just cover content. You will learn by discussing the questions with your peers. If you are still unsure, see the Davis Advantage chapter resources for suggested responses.

Caring for the Nguyens

Nam Nguyen has been diagnosed with hypertension, type 2 diabetes mellitus, obesity, osteoarthritis, and tobacco abuse. Zach Miller has advised an 1,800-kcal diabetic diet with no added salt and a brisk daily 30-minute walk. Mr. Nguyen discusses these challenges with his daughter, Trinh.

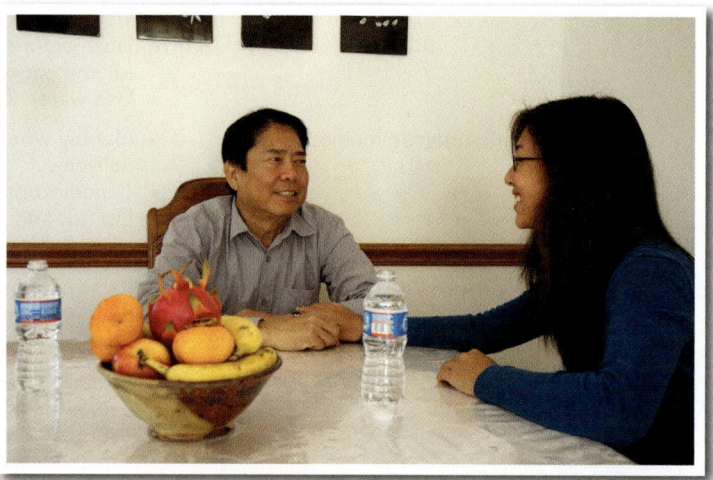

Caring for the Nguyens (continued)

A. Why might Zach have selected this diet plan? Discuss the rationale for each component (i.e., 1,800 kcal, diabetic diet, no added salt).

B. Mr. Nguyen's diet is complex. He tells you he is overwhelmed by the many changes asked of him. How might Zach streamline his instructions about his diet?

C. Nam asks what the best way is for him to monitor his weight-loss progress at home and how Zach Jackson will monitor his progress. How would you respond?

D. Identify teaching tools that might help Nam understand his diet.

Applying the **Full-Spectrum Nursing Model**_____

PATIENT SITUATION

Mrs. Ong is a 75-year-old retired schoolteacher who suffered a stroke 8 months ago. Since leaving the hospital, she has been living in a nursing home. Mrs. Ong has residual weakness on the right side—her dominant side—and has not mastered the use of tableware with her left hand. On admission to the nursing home 7 months ago, she weighed 150 pounds. Today she weighs only 125 pounds. Mrs. Ong refuses to go to the dining room for meals. The NAPs report that she eats a few bites of most foods, but never eats more than half of anything.

THINKING

1. *Theoretical Knowledge:*
   a. Based on Mrs. Ong's gender, age, and activity level, make a rough estimate of the number of kcal/day she needs.
   b. What are two other more precise ways you could determine Mrs. Ong's ideal body weight?
2. *Critical Thinking (Considering Alternatives):* What are some possible explanations for why Mrs. Ong is not eating all her food?

DOING

3. *Practical Knowledge:*
   a. Suppose you have decided to use the general ideal weight guide to determine Mrs. Ong's ideal weight. What, specifically, would you need to do? You do not need to actually calculate; just list the action steps.
   b. Suppose you have decided to determine Mrs. Ong's body mass index (BMI). What equipment would you need?
   c. What is the formula for calculating BMI from the height and weight?
4. *Nursing Process (Diagnosis):* Write a nursing diagnosis for Mrs. Ong. Use just the data provided in the situation. Assume her BMI is 20.

CARING

5. *Self-Knowledge:* What would you be feeling if you were in Mrs. Ong's situation?
6. *Ethical Knowledge:* What are one or two things you would do to help Mrs. Ong feel cared for and cared about?

PracticalKnowledge:
clinical application_____

To apply concepts that support patient nutrition, you will need to master techniques for assessing nutritional status, feeding patients, administering supplemental feedings, and working with nasogastric and nasoenteric tubes.

CLINICAL INSIGHTS

Clinical Insight 28-1 ➤ **Skinfold Measurement**

- Take measurements directly on the skin, not through clothing.
- Take each reading as soon as the jaws of the caliper come into contact with the skin and the reading has stabilized.
- In each site, take three readings in quick succession and average the results to the nearest 0.1 mm. *Accuracy of this method varies with the technique.*
- Add the averages of all skinfold sites to arrive at a total skinfold measurement.
- To determine the percentage body fat, compare the final calculated measurement with the values in the appropriate body fat and skinfolds table for the age and gender of the patient.

Measuring Triceps Skinfold

- Locate the midpoint on the posterior side of the dominant upper arm.
- With the client's arm hanging loosely at the side, palpate the measurement site at the midpoint to become familiar with distinguishing muscle from adipose soft tissue.
- From 1 cm above the midpoint, grasp a vertical pinch of skin and only the subcutaneous fat layer between the thumb and index finger. Gently pull the skinfold away from the underlying muscle.
- Place the skinfold caliper at the midpoint, and slowly release the jaw of the caliper while maintaining a grasp of the skinfold (see the figure).

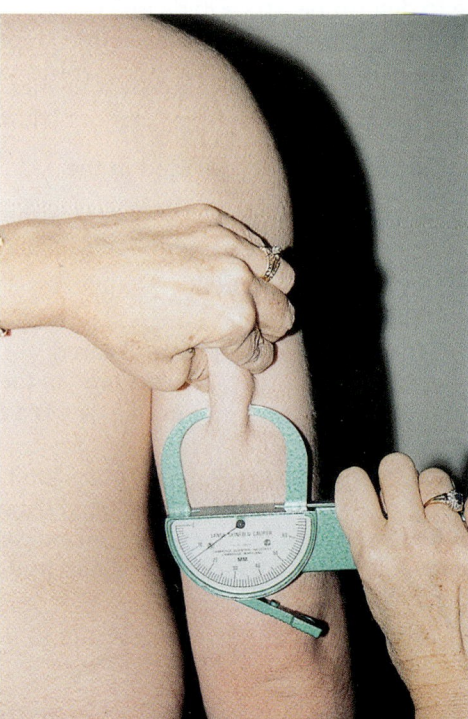

Triceps skinfold.

Measuring Subscapular Skinfold

- Follow the same procedure, except measure on the back, just under the shoulder blade. Grasp below the tip of the inferior angle of the scapula 45° to vertical.

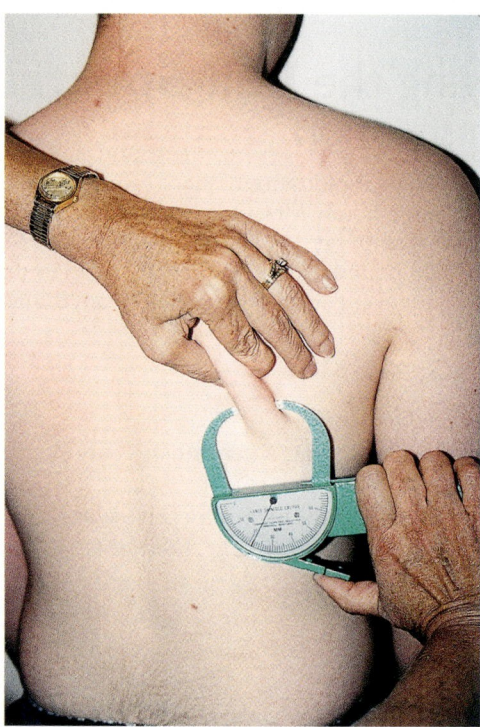

Subscapular skinfold.

Measuring Biceps Skinfold

- Follow the same procedure, except measure the muscle belly of the biceps. With the patient's arm hanging loosely at the side, grasp the skin and subcutaneous fat layer on the front of the upper arm, over the biceps, about level with the nipple.

Measuring Suprailiac Skinfold

- Follow the same procedure, except measure approximately 1 inch above the hipbone, above the iliac crest in the mid-axillary line.

Clinical Insight 28-2 ➤ Measuring Circumferences to Evaluate Body Composition

Measuring Mid-Upper Arm Circumference

- Keeping the client's dominant arm parallel to the body, bend the elbow 90°.
- Using a tape measure, measure the distance between the **acromion** (the bony protrusion of the back of the upper shoulder) and the **olecranon process** (tip of the elbow).
- Mark the midpoint between these two landmarks.
- Ask the client to relax the arm, so that it hangs loose and parallel to the body.
- Position the tape around the upper arm at the marked midpoint. Make sure the tape is snug but not so tight as to indent or pinch the skin.
- Record the circumference to the nearest 0.1 cm.

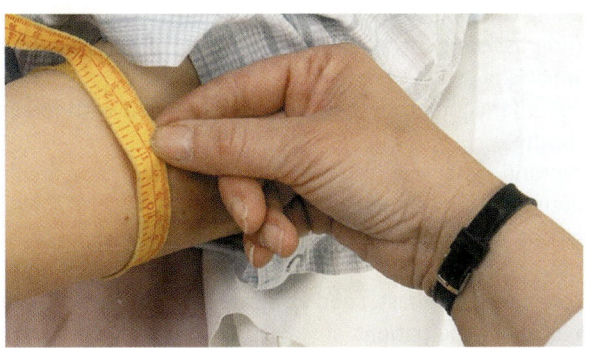

Calculating Waist-to-Hip Ratio (WHR)

- Use a tape measure to measure the circumference of the waist (at the umbilicus with stomach muscles relaxed).
- Use a tape measure to measure the circumference of the hips at their widest point.
- Calculate the waist-to-hip ratio using the following formula:

  waist circumference (in.) ÷ hip circumference (in.)

  Example: Robert's waist measurement is 32 inches, and his hip measurement is 34 inches. His WHR is 32 ÷ 34 = 0.94.

  (Obesity = > 1.0 in males and > 0.8 in females)

Clinical Insight 28-3 ➤ Assisting Patients With Meals

General Guidelines

- Recommend having one staff person for every two or three patients who need assistance, allowing about 20 to 30 minutes to feed a patient. Prolonged mealtimes do not promote appetite, nor does hurrying.
- Feeding assistants should be supervised by an RN or LPN.
- Do not interrupt meals with medications.
- Encourage family members to share mealtimes.
- If the patient's condition allows, encourage him to get out of bed for meals.
- Position upright for meals. Correct positioning and helping patients with their meal improves total food intake (Young, Allia, Jolliffe, et al., 2016).
- Encourage residents in long-term care settings to eat meals in the dining room instead of in the bedroom.

Preparation

- Assess for rituals used before meals (blessings of food, etc.).
- Implement a fixed mealtime schedule.
- Provide an opportunity for toileting, oral hygiene, and hand washing before meals.

- Assist the patient to eat and drink only as necessary; encourage independence.
- Provide privacy during meals if the patient is embarrassed; to further maintain dignity, use a napkin, not a bib, over the patient's clothes.
- Check for proper fit of dentures.
- Provide music during the meal if the patient wishes.
- Demonstrate the use of assistive devices and alternative methods for eating and drinking.

Assisting the Patient

- If the patient must eat in bed, place the head of the bed at the highest tolerable level and adjust the overbed table to be in easy reach.
- If the patient can feed himself, prepare the food on the tray for him (e.g., open food containers, cut the meat, peel an orange, open the milk and butter containers, mash food if needed).
- If the client is visually impaired, identify the locations of the meal on the tray based on a clock face (e.g., "The coffee is at 1 o'clock above the plate on the right").

(Continued)

Clinical Insight 28-3 ➤ Assisting Patients With Meals—cont'd

Feeding the Patient

- Feed the patient if she is unable to feed herself.
- Sit down while feeding the patient; do not rush.
- Position yourself so that you can make eye contact.
- Be sure to provide adequate time for her to chew and swallow.
- If possible, ask her what food she would like next.
- Serve one food at a time; serve small amounts.
- Serve finger foods (e.g., fruit, bread) to promote independence.
- Cue older adults whenever possible with words or gestures.
- Have casual conversation with the patient while feeding her to make mealtime more pleasant and relaxed.

After the Meal

- Help the patient to wash hands or use the rest room after the meal.
- Record the amount of food and fluid the patient consumed.
- Document feeding behaviors.
- Document changes in nutritional status.
- Document staffing and staff education, and availability of a supportive interdisciplinary team.

Assisting Older Adults With Dementia

As do all people, older adults with dementia differ in their abilities to eat and communicate. The following are general tips, but you should tailor interventions to each person's specific abilities to achieve the best results. In addition to many of the preceding interventions, try some of the following measures:

- Assess the patient's self-feeding abilities.
- Assess the patient's cognitive limitations and communication abilities.

- Assess for and treat pain.
- Minimize distractions: Turn off the TV; discourage people from entering the room.
- Help the patient to a comfortable chair if possible.
- Assist with oral hygiene and hand hygiene.
- Remove any unnecessary eating utensils; serve only one food at a time.
- Remove items that should not be eaten (e.g., packets of salt or pepper) and hot items that could be spilled.
- Cue the patient verbally to help with self-feeding (e.g., "take a bite," "chew," "swallow").
- Pantomime eating motions if necessary, so the patient can learn by imitating them.
- Place your hand over the patient's to begin and guide self-feeding (hand-over-hand).
- When assisting, sit at eye level and interact socially with the patient.
- Involve family members if they have assisted with feeding at home.
- Train and supervise NAPs in interacting with and feeding patients with dementia.
- Do not assist too soon—give the patient time to eat independently.
- Do not feed too fast. Feed at a rate that is safe and comfortable for the patient.

Practice Resources

Amella, E. (2008, updated 2012); Amella, E., & Lawrence, J. F. (2007a, 2007b); Chan, C., & Kwan, Y. K. (2014); Ebersole, P., Hess, P., Touhy, T., et al. (2013); Joanna Briggs Institute (2011).

Clinical Insight 28-4 ➤ Checking Feeding Tube Placement

✚ Tube placement must be verified by x-ray before the initial feeding is given. Because none of the bedside methods is foolproof, always use pH measurement in combination with one of the other methods for subsequent feedings.

Aspirating Stomach Contents

- Don procedure gloves. This is a clean, not sterile, technique.
- Just before feeding, draw up 10 to 30 mL of air in a 30- to 60-mL syringe, insert the syringe in the distal end of the feeding tube, and inject air.
  To flush out formula, medications, and other substances. This also helps keep a small-bore tube from collapsing when you aspirate.

- With the same syringe, aspirate the air and 20 to 30 mL of stomach or intestinal contents. Use slow, gentle suction—over 3 to 5 minutes if necessary.
  It can take a long time to obtain enough fluid, especially from a small-bore tube.
- If you could not aspirate any fluid, inject another 20 mL of air and use a smaller syringe to aspirate again.
  Using a small (< 10 mL) syringe for very small tubes creates less negative pressure and makes it less likely the tube will collapse.
- If you still do not aspirate fluid, repeat the procedure with this variation: Insert air with the large syringe; insert the small syringe into the end of the tubing, and leave it for 15 minutes to allow fluid to accumulate before aspirating.

Clinical Insight 28-4 ➤ Checking Feeding Tube Placement—cont'd

- If you are still unsuccessful, reposition the patient and try again after 20 minutes.

  Repositioning may move the tube into a place where fluid has pooled.

Inspecting the Aspirate

- Aspirate stomach contents, as described above. Gastric contents are normally greenish brown and liquid. If the patient is receiving enteral feedings, gastric contents should be curdled and white or a greenish color; intestinal contents will be a more yellow (bile) color with no curdling.

  ✚ Intestinal contents are usually yellow-green because of the influence of bile. The colors of gastric and pulmonary secretions are altered by a variety of conditions, so observation of the visual characteristics of feeding tube aspirates is of little value in differentiating between respiratory and GI placement (Joanna Briggs Institute, 2010a, 2010c).

Measuring the Volume and pH of the Aspirate

- Aspirate stomach contents, as described above. Then measure the residual volume of the aspirate.

  Unexpected changes in volume of the aspirate can indicate poor GI motility. Gastric volumes will generally be larger than intestinal or esophageal volumes.

- Measure the pH of the aspirated fluid using nitrazine paper.

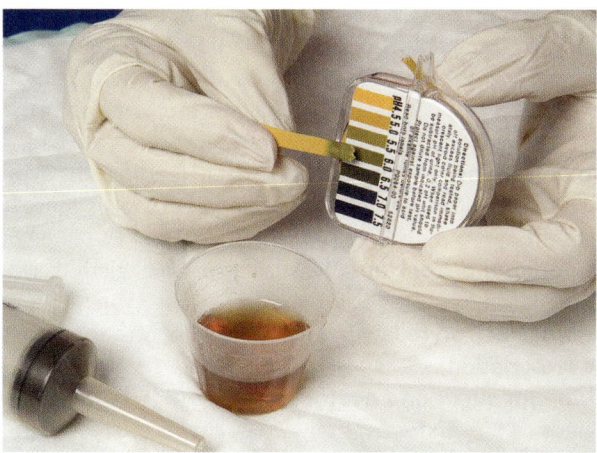

- The lower the pH, the more likely that the tube is in the stomach. The pH of gastric contents is typically 1 to 5.5.

Measuring the pH is useful only if the fluid you aspirate is acidic, indicating gastric placement.

- Intestinal contents usually have a pH of 6 or greater.
- The pH of respiratory secretions is 7 or higher; however, respiratory secretions may occasionally have a pH as low as 6.

- Remember that many variables can make the gastric pH results unreliable (e.g., blood in the stomach, antacid medications).

- Measuring bilirubin, trypsin, and pepsin in the aspirate can also be used to diagnose placement of a feeding tube in the respiratory tract (Cirgin Ellet, Cohen, Croffie, et al., 2014; Joanna Briggs Institute, 2010a).

Measuring and Observing the Length of the Tube That Extends From the Body

When the tube was inserted, it should have been marked with indelible marker where it exits the body (e.g., the naris), and the external length recorded. Compare the external length with previous measurements and with the mark made on the tube when it was inserted. If tube placement does not change, the external length should remain the same.

Injecting Air Into the Feeding Tube

KEY POINT: *This method is no longer recommended, although some professionals still do inject air into the feeding tube. It is the least accurate of the bedside methods and should never be used alone.*

- Draw 5 to 30 mL of air into a syringe; place the tip of the syringe in the end of the feeding tube.
- Place a stethoscope over the stomach.
- Listen with the stethoscope as you inject the air through the tube. If you hear a gurgling or whooshing sound in the left upper quadrant, the tube may be in the stomach. *Note:* You cannot be sure of this because the lungs and stomach lie close together, and the sounds created by sending air through the tube can cause you to err in determining placement.

Ongoing Patient Assessments

The following require repeated assessments over time to be useful for confirming other methods of tube placement:

- ***Observe for respiratory distress.*** Note cyanosis or difficulty breathing, coughing, choking. These symptoms are indicators that the tube is in the respiratory tract, but keep in mind that the tube could instead be in the stomach and the symptoms caused by something else. Absence

(Continued)

Clinical Insight 28-4 ➤ Checking Feeding Tube Placement—cont'd

of symptoms does not necessarily indicate correct placement in the stomach. The tube might be in the airway and not be causing any respiratory symptoms.

■ **Assess whether the patient can speak.** Keep in mind that some clients can speak even when the tube is in a lung.

Other Bedside Verification Methods

Capnometry measures of carbon dioxide concentration in expired gases. Capnometry and additional tests of gastric juices may also serve as measures to help verify that the tube is correctly placed.

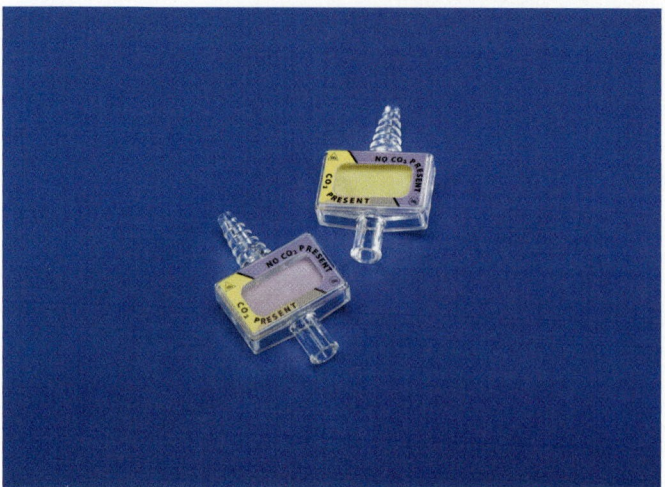

A carbon dioxide detector for checking feeding tube placement.

Clinical Insight 28-5 ➤ Monitoring Patients Receiving Enteral Nutrition

For patients receiving enteral nutrition, monitor the following:

■ **Position of the feeding tube.** Periodically check the placement of the tube. As a rule, check on each shift or at each intermittent feeding. For double-lumen tubes, keep the air vent above the level of the patient's stomach so it will not act as a siphon and leak stomach contents.

■ **NG or NE tube insertion site.** An NG or NE tube is secured by adhesive to the nose. Regularly check the skin, gently cleanse the area (with soap and water, as for normal washing; avoid harsh skin cleansers), and retape the tube as needed. Report tissue breakdown, epistaxis (nosebleed), or sinusitis.
These findings may signal a need for insertion of a percutaneous endoscopy gastrostomy (PEG) tube.

■ **Gastrostomy tube, PEG/PEJ insertion site.** Inspect the insertion site for erythema or drainage, which are signs of infection. Clean it daily with soap and water.

■ **Fluid balance.** Measure all intake and output.

■ **Weight.** To assess the adequacy of the feeding, regularly weigh patients receiving enteral nutrition. There is usually a medical prescription for frequency of weighing. Frequent weight checks allow adjustment of the feeding orders to achieve the desired goal.

■ **Tube feeding residual volume.** To assess residual volume, aspirate the feeding tube to determine the amount of feeding remaining in the stomach.
If you are able to aspirate a quantity equal to or greater than the formula flow rate for 1 hour (or alternatively, a

total of 150 mL), the patient may be receiving too much fluid or may have delayed gastric emptying. However, you should not automatically stop the feeding; if you obtain a single sample of an increased residual volume, recheck it in 1 hour. See Clinical Insight 28-4.

■ **Frequency of bowel movements.** Bowel movements should occur regularly.
Constipation is usually due to inadequate water or fiber. Some commercial feedings contain fiber. To alleviate constipation, you may add free water and perhaps fiber to the formula. Diarrhea may indicate intolerance of the formula, excessive feeding, or gastrointestinal disease.

■ **Bowel sounds.** Check before each feeding, or every 4 to 8 hours for continuous feedings. Peristalsis must be present.

■ **Abdominal distention.** Measure abdominal girth daily, at the umbilicus.

■ **Serum electrolyte levels.** Monitor regularly (per protocol or prescription).

■ **Urine for sugar and acetone.** This is sometimes done as a bedside screen for hyperglycemia. However, treatment is based on blood sugar levels.

■ **Skin turgor, hematocrit, and urine specific gravity.** These are indicators of dehydration and overhydration.

■ **Serum blood urea nitrogen (BUN) and sodium levels.** This is especially important for high-protein formulas.
Insufficient fluid intake combined with high protein intake may overload the kidneys so that nitrogenous wastes are not excreted adequately.

Clinical Insight 28-6 ➤ Monitoring and Maintenance for Patients Receiving Parenteral Nutrition

Monitoring

For patients receiving PN, you will need to monitor the following:

Catheter insertion site

- Assess catheter insertion site for swelling, redness, drainage, or tenderness.
  These are signs of infection (and/or phlebitis in PICC lines). The hypertonic PN creates a risk for phlebitis.
- Observe for swelling in the extremity on the same side of catheter insertion.
  This is a sign of infiltration or phlebitis.
- Observe for catheter retraction from the vein; observe the length of the catheter from the insertion site to the hub at insertion and periodically.

Supplies and equipment

- Monitor tubing connections to see that they are secure.
- Monitor to see that the dressing is secure and dry.
- Check the rate and amount infused at least hourly.
  To ensure the line is patent, the PN is flowing freely, and the pump is functioning properly.

Weight

Regularly weigh the patient (according to medical order or agency policy, but commonly daily or 3 times per wk).
(1) Frequent weight checks allow for assessing the adequacy of the formula and making adjustments as needed to achieve the desired goal. (2) Because of the hypertonicity of the solutions, fluid overload can occur. Rapid weight increase is an indicator.

Glucose

- Check blood glucose every 4 to 6 hours until stable, and then at least daily.
  The high proportion of glucose in the formulas can cause hyperglycemia, the most common complication of PN. The risk for hyperglycemia is less with 3:1 PN solutions.
- You may need to administer regular insulin according to a sliding scale (or the pharmacist may add it directly to the PN solution).

Diuresis and dehydration

These can occur if hypertonic dextrose is infused too rapidly.

Intake and output

Evaluate nutrient intake, fluid balance, and renal function.

Lab values

Patients receiving PN require regular lab studies (the following are examples and not a comprehensive list). The frequency of the studies depends on the patient's condition.

- Electrolytes, blood sugar, albumin, BUN, and creatinine
  These values are used for formula adjustment and to evaluate electrolyte balance and glucose metabolism.
- Albumin, transferrin, transthyretin (prealbumin), or retinol-binding protein
  May be used to assess visceral protein status.
- 24-hour urine for urine urea nitrogen (weekly)
  To assess for nitrogen balance.
- CBC and differential.
  To monitor changes in immune function.
- Liver function studies
- Serum zinc
- Plasma urea
- Plasma and urine osmolality
- Blood gases

Symptoms of complications

- *Electrolyte imbalances:* Symptoms depend on the electrolytes affected. Monitor lab values.
- *Sepsis:* Temperature greater than 100°F (37.8°C) orally, rapid pulse from baseline, chills, hypothermia, edema or erythema of skin, exudate from catheter insertion site, malaise, leukocytosis (increased WBC count), altered level of consciousness.
- *Air embolus:* Cyanosis, tachypnea, hypotension, heart murmur
- *Catheter dislodgement or thrombosis:* Swelling of arm or neck, pain, difficulty flushing catheter, difficulty infusing PN

Nutritional status

- Calculate the daily calorie intake.
- Perform nutritional assessment at 2-week intervals.
- Possibly measure arm circumference and triceps skinfold thickness.
- Most agencies have specialized nutrition teams who will monitor these parameters.

Maintenance

- Change the dressing over the catheter every 24 hours or according to agency policy, or when it becomes wet, soiled, or nonocclusive. Use sterile technique.
- Secure connections with luer-lock connectors; do not use tape.

(Continued)

Clinical Insight 28-6 ➤ Monitoring and Maintenance for Patients Receiving Parenteral Nutrition—cont'd

- Change the filter every 24 hours.
- Do not hang PN bottles for more than 12 hours (some guidelines and agency policies specify 24 hr).
  PN solutions are prepared in batches under strict aseptic conditions. Its high nutrient concentration makes PN an excellent feeding alternative; however, it also makes the solution ideal for bacterial growth.
- Use sterile aseptic technique when changing the dressing for a central line, as well as when changing the solution and tubing.
- Do not use the PN infusion line for administering any other medicines or solutions.
  To decrease the risk of contamination and infection.

- Infuse PN by pump with a reliable, audible alarm.
  To protect against "free flow."
- If an infusion falls behind schedule, do not increase the rate in an attempt to catch up.
  This can cause osmotic diuresis and dehydration.
- When PN is discontinued, it may be done gradually (perhaps over as many as 48 hr).
  To prevent a sudden drop in blood sugar.

PROCEDURES

Procedure 28-1 ■ Checking Fingerstick (Capillary) Blood Glucose Levels

➤ For steps to follow in *all* procedures, refer to the Universal Steps for All Procedures found on the page facing the inside back cover.

Equipment

- Blood glucose meter
- Test strip
- Sterile lancet (and injector, if available)
- Alcohol (or other antiseptic) pad, if required by policy
- 2 in. × 2 in. gauze pad or cotton ball
- Procedure gloves

✚ Glucometers should be assigned to individual patients. If this is not possible, you must clean and disinfect the device between patients. Do not use insulin pens for more than one person. Injectors, too, should be assigned to individual patients; if possible, use single-use lancets that permanently retract upon puncture. Keep trays or carts with these supplies outside patient rooms. If there are unused supplies, do not use them for another patient. Do not carry supplies in your pocket. Change gloves and perform hand hygiene between fingerstick procedures.

These measures help prevent needlestick injury and transmission of bloodborne pathogens (Centers for Disease Control and Prevention, 2013a).

Delegation

You can delegate this procedure to a licensed practical nurse (LPN) or nursing assistive personnel (NAP) who have been adequately trained in performing the skill if the patient's condition allows. Most patients perform this procedure independently at home.

Pre-Procedure Assessments

- Assess the patient's comprehension of the procedure.
  Understanding reduces anxiety and promotes cooperation.
- Assess potential puncture sites for bruising, inflammation, open lesions, poor circulation, or edema.
  Avoid such sites because of risk for infection and inaccurate results.
- Check for factors such as anticoagulant therapy, bleeding disorders, or low platelet count.
  These place the patient at risk for bleeding after skin puncture.

➤ When performing the procedure, always identify your patient according to agency policy, using two identifiers, and be attentive to standard precautions, hand hygiene, patient safety and privacy, body mechanics, and documentation.

➤ *Note:* The steps of this procedure will vary depending on the type of glucose meter used.

Procedure Steps

1. Verify the medical prescription for frequency and timing of testing.
A prescription is necessary for testing. Timing and frequency of testing are crucial for accurate insulin dosing.

2. Ask the patient to wash her hands with soap and warm water, if able, and to dry completely using a clean towel.
Reduces the risk for infection and dilates capillaries at the puncture site. Also ensures that the testing site is free of any sugar residue.

3. Turn on the blood glucose meter. Calibrate it according to the manufacturer's instructions.
Calibration readies the meter for testing and checks it for accuracy of the machine.

4. Check that the strip is the correct type for the monitor. Check the expiration date on the container of reagent strips. If the strips are expired, replace them.
Expired strips may alter test results. Different brands of monitors use different kinds of reagent strips.

5. Don procedure gloves.
Gloving protects against exposure to blood.

6. Remove the reagent strip from the container and place it into the blood glucose meter. Then tightly seal the container.
A tight seal protects reagent strips from exposure to air and light.

7. Select and clean a fingerstick site with an alcohol (or other antiseptic) pad, according to facility policy. Let it dry thoroughly.
Helps protect the patient from infection by removing some surface microorganisms. Allowing the alcohol to dry thoroughly will decrease pain of the skin puncture. Using alcohol is controversial, however, because it may interfere with the reagent on the strip, giving a false low reading; it also dries the skin. Follow agency policy and consult practice guidelines periodically.

8. Use a different site each time you check the glucose.
Adult and child: the lateral aspect of a finger (palmar surface, distal phalanx)
Infant: heel or great toe
The lateral aspect of the finger contains fewer nerve endings than does the central fingertip, so it hurts less.

9. Position the finger (or heel or great toe for an infant) in a dependent position, and massage from the base toward the tip of the finger.
A dependent position promotes blood flow to the site via gravity and pressure, ensuring an adequate specimen. The massaging action increases blood flow to the tip of the finger, which may prevent the need for repuncture.

10. Prick the finger (or other site) with the lancet:

Exposed-Blade Disposable Lancet
a. Remove the cover from the lancet, if there is a cover.
b. Place the back of the patient's hand on the table, or otherwise secure the finger (e.g., hold the finger and hand firmly).
c. Use a darting motion to puncture the site, at a 90° angle to the skin.

Semiautomatic Injector
d. Engage the sterile injector and remove the cover.
e. Place the disposable lancet firmly in the end of the injector.
f. Place the back of the patient's hand on the table, or otherwise secure the finger (e.g., hold the finger and hand firmly).

g. Position the end of the injector firmly against the skin, perpendicular (at a 90° angle) to the chosen puncture site.
h. Push the release switch, allowing the needle to pierce the skin.
Proper positioning and stabilization of the site ensure that the lancet pierces to the correct depth. This prevents patient injury and allows for adequate blood sampling. Patients tend to pull away as you perform the puncture. ▼

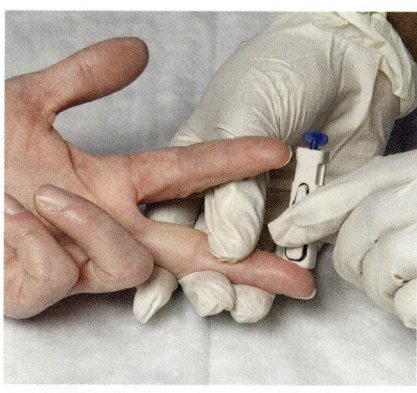

11. Lightly squeeze the patient's finger above the puncture site until a drop of blood has collected.
Squeezing promotes a better blood sample for testing without causing injury to the puncture site.

12. Place the reagent strip test patch close to the drop of blood. Allow contact between the drop of blood and the test strip. Do not "smear" the blood over the reagent strip.
This ensures adequate blood sample for testing. ▼

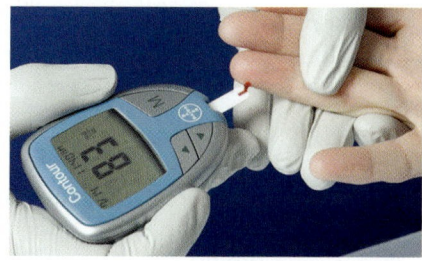

(continued on next page)

Procedure 28-1 ■ **Checking Fingerstick (Capillary) Blood Glucose Levels** (continued)

13. **Insert the strip into the glucometer meter,** if it is not already inserted (follow the manufacturer's instructions); allow the blood sample to remain in contact with the test strip for the amount of time specified by the manufacturer.
For some glucometers you insert the test strip before pricking the finger; with others you put the blood on the reagent strip and then insert the strip into the meter. The blood sample must be on the reagent strip for the specified amount of time to ensure accurate test results.

14. **Using a gauze pad,** gently apply pressure to the puncture site.
Pressure stops the bleeding by promoting coagulation.

15. **After the glucometer signals, read** the blood glucose level indicated on the digital display. ▼

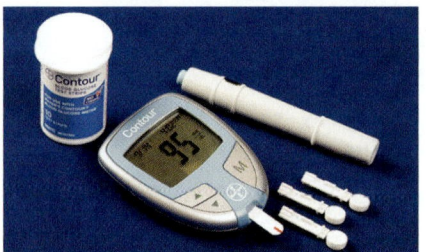

16. **Turn off the meter** and dispose of the reagent strip, gauze pad, alcohol pad, and lancet in the safe collection containers (e.g., a sharps container for the lancet).
Proper disposal prevents sharps injury and the spread of infection via bloodborne pathogens.

17. **Remove the procedure gloves** and dispose of them in the proper container. Perform hand hygiene.
Hand hygiene and gloving reduce the transmission of microbes.

? **What if . . .**

■ **The patient has poor circulation or is a child or older adult?**

Place a heel warmer or warm cloth on the site for about 10 minutes before obtaining the blood sample. Alternatively, position the patient's hand below the waist for 1 minute.
Capillaries in infants are very small; older adults may have poor peripheral circulation. The warmth may dilate the capillaries, helping you obtain an adequate amount of blood; the dangling of extremities allows blood to pool in the extremity, making it easier for you to obtain the quantity of blood needed.

■ **The patient is taking an anticoagulant such as warfarin sodium (Coumadin)?**

After the procedure, hold pressure for 2 minutes and then apply a pressure bandage if needed. Recheck the site after 5 minutes to make sure bleeding has stopped.

■ **The monitor shows an extremely unusual result or an error message?**

Repeat the process using a different finger or site.

■ **The patient uses a noninvasive method to measure blood glucose?**

A continuous glucose monitor (CGM) is used to more closely track blood sugar. One type of CGM is worn like a wristwatch. Using an electrical current, it pulls fluid from the skin to give a blood glucose reading. Another style uses a small sensor just below the skin of the abdomen and measures glucose in the interstitial fluid.
  - The CGM will take readings automatically every 5 to 30 minutes and will download data to a computer, tablet, or smartphone.
  - Advise the patient to shave his arm if it is very hairy, or the reading may not be accurate.
  - The patient should wear the device for a 3-hour warm-up before taking a reading, and should not bathe or swim during that time.
    This does not replace the patient's fingerstick method. Its purpose is to track trends in blood glucose. It also benefits patients whose blood sugar go dangerously low overnight, which could go undetected.

Evaluation

■ Assess the puncture site for bleeding or bruising.
■ Evaluate the patient's understanding of the procedure and the test results.
■ Promptly notify the provider of abnormal test results, or administer insulin based on test results, if prescribed.

Patient Teaching

■ Explain the procedure, test results, and treatment to the patient.
Information allows the patient to participate in his plan of care and typically increases adherence to the therapeutic regimen.

■ If the patient will be performing fingerstick blood glucose testing at home, teach the patient how to perform the procedure. Ask the patient to perform a return demonstration.
■ Discuss the importance of maintaining glycemic control.
■ If the patient will be performing fingerstick blood glucose testing at home, teach the patient to do the following:
Read the manufacturer's instructions carefully and contact the company if you have any questions.
Always use the test strips that are recommended for the meter.
Take your meter to your health provider's office so she can make sure you are measuring your blood sugar correctly.

Perform quality control checks (read the instructions) to make sure the glucometer is measuring accurately.

Clean the meter according to the manufacturer's directions. Some meters will give you an electronic alert telling you when to clean them.

Home Care

- Assess the client's ability to perform fingerstick blood glucose monitoring independently.

  A change in the patient's condition may not allow the patient to perform testing. Certain conditions, such as arthritis and limited vision, may limit dexterity.

- Advise the patient about purchasing home glucose monitoring equipment.

- Explain how to dispose of lancets in a labeled, puncture-proof container, such as an empty bleach container.

- Instruct caregivers to wear gloves when obtaining a blood sample for glucose monitoring.

- At home, patients do not need to cleanse their fingers with an alcohol wipe before puncturing it. However, they should wash their hands with soap and water and dry well.

Documentation

- Record the fingerstick blood glucose result in the progress notes or special flow sheet, including the date and time the test was performed.

- Note whether the provider was notified and record any treatment given.

- Document patient teaching.

- If the fingerstick is performed in response to patient symptoms, you may need to write a narrative note.

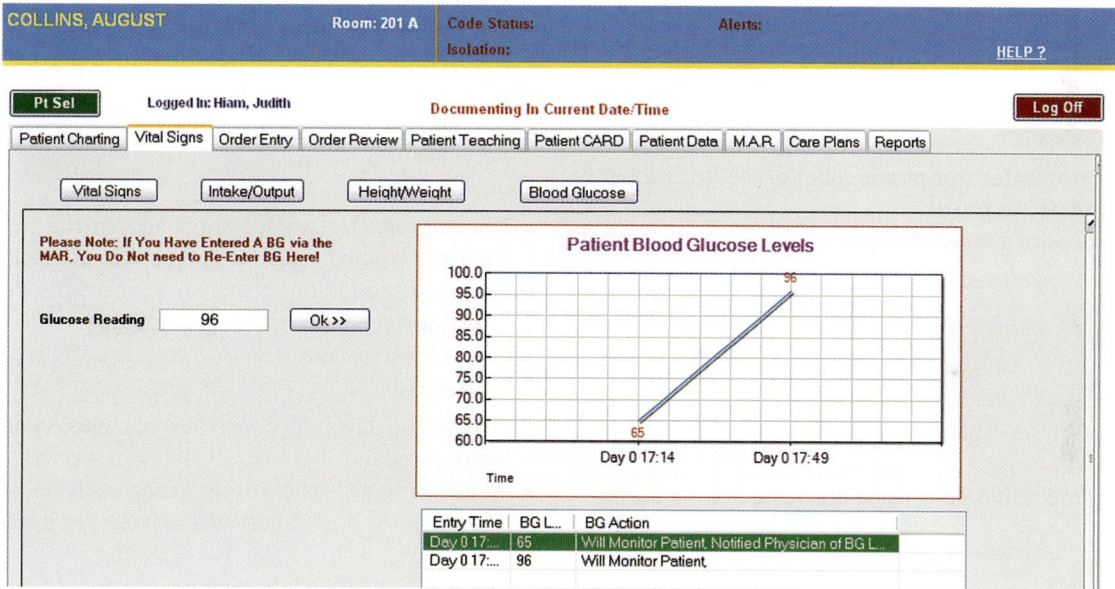

Practice Resources

American Diabetes Association (2016, last edited); CDC (2005); Hortensius, J., Slingerland, R. J., Kleefstra, N., et al. (2011); USFDA (2009, updated 2015, n.d.a, updated 2014).

Thinking About the Procedure

 The video **Checking Fingerstick (Capillary) Blood Glucose Levels,** along with questions and suggested responses, is available on the ***Davis's Nursing Skills Videos*** Web site on *DavisPlus.*

Procedure 28-2 ■ Inserting Nasogastric and Nasoenteric Tubes

➤ For steps to follow in *all* procedures, refer to the Universal Steps for All Procedures found on the page facing the inside back cover.

Equipment

- Nasogastric tube (commonly 16 or 18 Fr for adults, but sometimes smaller) or nasoenteric (small bowel) tube (8 Fr, 10 Fr, or 12 Fr)
- Stylet or guidewire (for small-bore tubes), according to agency policy
- Procedure gloves
- Linen-saver pad or towel
- Water-soluble lubricant
- 50- to 60-mL catheter-tip syringe or bulb syringe for Salem sump tubes; 30-mL luer-lock syringe for small-bore feeding tubes
- Hypoallergenic tape (about 2.5 cm [1 in.] wide) or tube fixation device
- Indelible marker
- Skin adhesive
- Stethoscope
- Emesis basin
- Basin with warm water (for plastic tube) or ice (for rubber tube). Most tubes are plastic.
- Glass of water with a straw
- Penlight
- Tongue blade
- pH test strip
- Tissues
- Safety pin
- Gauze square or small plastic bag
- Rubber band
- Suction equipment (if tube is being connected to suction)

Delegation

This procedure should not be delegated because it requires knowledge of anatomy and physiology and the ability to adapt the procedure based on patient responses. You can, however, delegate associated oral hygiene needs.

Pre-Procedure Assessment

- Verify the medical prescription for type of tube to be placed and whether it is to be attached to suction or drainage.
- Verify the patient's need for NG or NE intubation (e.g., surgery involving the gastrointestinal [GI] tract, impaired swallowing, or decreased level of consciousness).

  NG or NE intubation decreases the risk for aspiration in these patients. In many institutions, only specially trained nurses are allowed to place small bowel feeding tubes.

- Assess each naris for patency, deviated septum, and skin breakdown. Ask the patient to close each nostril alternately and breathe. Select the nostril with the greatest air flow. Ask the patient to blow her nose, if not contraindicated.

  A septal defect or facial fracture may cause obstruction, placing the patient at risk for nasal membrane trauma if insertion is attempted through the affected naris.

- Check health history for anticoagulant therapy, coagulopathy, nasal trauma, nasal surgery, epistaxis, deviated septum, and other conditions that may indicate the need for tube insertion via endoscope or fluoroscope.

  The medical provider should be notified if patient history or status places the patient at risk for injury during NG or NE insertion.

- Assess the level of consciousness and ability to follow instructions.
- Assess for a gag reflex, using a tongue blade.

  Diminished or absent gag reflex places the patient at risk for aspiration.

➤ When performing the procedure, always identify your patient according to agency policy, using two identifiers, and be attentive to standard precautions, hand hygiene, patient safety and privacy, body mechanics, and documentation.

Procedure Steps

1. Prepare the tube.

Plastic Tube

Wrap the tube around your index finger and then unwrap it and proceed or place in a basin of warm water for 10 minutes and proceed.

Rubber Tube

Place in a basin of ice for 10 minutes.

Small-Bore Tube

Insert a stylet or guidewire and secure into position, according to agency policy. (Small-bore tubes may come with the guidewire in them. If so, flush the tube with sterile water to lubricate the wire for easy removal. Leave the wire in place until the tube is positioned and its placement has been checked on x-ray film. Once the guidewire is removed, do not reinsert it.) Agency policy determines which nurses are authorized to place small-bore tubes.

Warm water softens a plastic tube, and ice stiffens the rubber tube to make it easier to insert. (Most tubes are polyurethane or silicone based.) Wrapping a plastic tube around your index finger helps the tube flex into a curve and aids in insertion. A guidewire facilitates passage of small-bore tube but can cause trauma if not secured in a proper position.

2. **Assist the patient into a high Fowler's position** with pillow behind the head and shoulders. Raise the bed to a comfortable working level.

   This position facilitates tube insertion and prevents aspiration should the patient vomit during tube insertion. Gravity facilitates passage of the tube. Raising the bed reduces strain on the nurse's back.

3. Measure the tube for placement.

Nasogastric Tube

Measure the length of the tube to be inserted by measuring from the tip of the nose to the earlobe, and from the earlobe to the xiphoid process. Mark the length with tape or indelible ink.

This measurement indicates the distance the tube must be inserted to reach the stomach. ▼

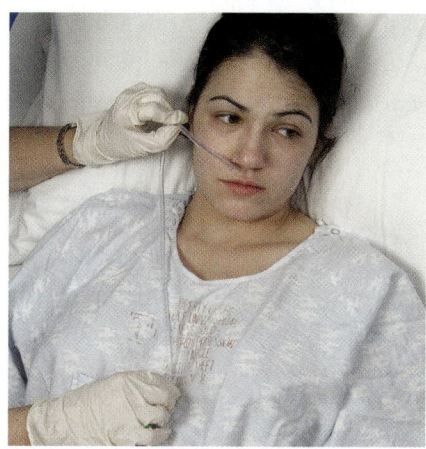

Nasoenteric Tube

Add 8 to 10 cm (3 to 4 in.) to the NG tube measurement, as directed, and mark the tube.

4. If you are right-handed, stand on the patient's right side; if you are left-handed, stand on the patient's left side. **Drape** a linen saver pad over the patient's chest, and hand her an emesis basin and facial tissues.

Draping protects the patient's gown from becoming soiled during tube insertion.

5. Prepare the fixation device. Cut a 10-cm (4-in.) piece of hypoallergenic tape if securing tube with tape; split the bottom end lengthwise 2.5 cm (2 in.). If using a commercial feeding tube attachment device, have it ready at this time.

To secure the tube after insertion.

6. Arrange a signal by which the patient can communicate if she wants to stop (e.g., raising her hand).

Relieves anxiety by giving the patient some control over the procedure.

7. Don procedure gloves if you have not already done so.

Reduces the spread of microorganisms.

8. Wrap 10 to 15 cm (5 to 6 in.) of the end of the tube tightly around your index finger, then release.

Forms the tube into a curve that helps it conform more easily to the shape of the nasopharynx.

9. Lubricate the distal 10 cm (4 in.) of the tube with a water-soluble jelly.

Lubrication eases the passage of the tube and prevents injury to the nasal mucosa. Water-soluble lubricant will dissolve if it is aspirated, whereas oil-based lubricants do not dissolve in the respiratory tract and would cause inflammation and blockage of airways if they enter the lungs. Some nurses prefer water as a lubricant because aqueous jelly dries and can block nasal passages, which is irritating to the patient. Some tubes have a surface lubricant and require only that you dip them in room-temperature water.

10. Hand the patient a glass of water with a straw, if she is awake, alert, and able to swallow.

Instructing the client to swallow water during insertion eases passage.

11. Instruct the patient to hold her head straight up and extend her neck back against the pillow (slightly hyperextended).
a. Grasp the end of the tube above the lubricant with the curved end pointing downward.
b. Carefully insert the tube along the floor of the nasal passage, on the lateral side, aiming toward the ear.
c. You will feel slight resistance when the tube reaches the nasopharynx; use gentle pressure, but do not force the tube to advance. The patient's eyes may tear; if so, provide tissues.
d. Continue inserting the tube until just past the nasopharynx by

gently rotating the tube toward the client's opposite naris.

Hyperextending the neck straightens the curve where the nasal passage meets the pharynx (nasopharyngeal junction). Gentle insertion prevents trauma to the nasal mucosa. Forcing against resistance can traumatize the mucosa. Tears are normal. ▼

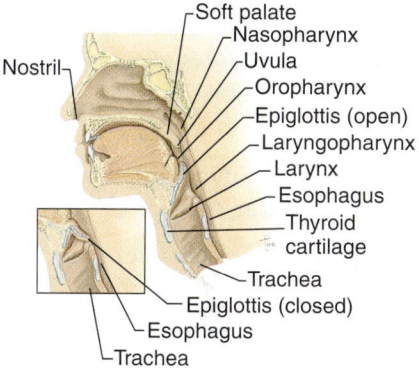

12. Pause for a moment to allow the patient to relax and perhaps use tissues. Explain that the next step requires her to swallow.

Stopping to relax can give the patient a feeling of control. The rest can also reduce gagging.

13. Instruct the patient to flex her head toward the chest, take a small sip of water, and swallow.

This maneuver closes the trachea and opens the esophagus. ▼

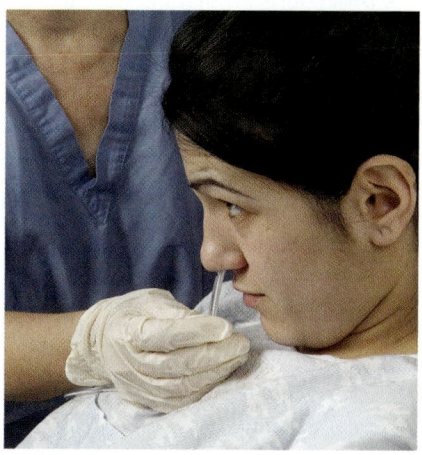

14. Rotate the tube 180°.

Rotation helps to redirect the tube so that it will not enter the patient's mouth.

(continued on next page)

Procedure 28-2 ■ Inserting Nasogastric and Nasoenteric Tubes (continued)

15. Direct the patient to sip and swallow the water as you slowly advance the tube. (If the patient is not allowed water, instruct her to dry swallow or suck air through the straw.) Advance the tube 5 to 10 cm (2 to 4 in.) with each swallow.
Moving the tube with each swallow uses normal peristaltic movement to help advance the tube into the stomach. Swallowing closes the epiglottis so that the tube cannot advance into the trachea.

16. Continue advancing the tube to the desired distance.

17. ✚ Temporarily secure the tube with one piece of tape. Then verify tube placement (see Clinical Insight 28-4). Never rely on a single bedside method. You can use a combination of the following methods to verify placement at the bedside; however, radiographic verification is the only reliable method and should be done before medications or fluids are given through the tube for the first time (Joanna Briggs Institute, 2012).

If you do not secure the tube, at least temporarily, it may move out of position—especially if you are waiting for placement to be confirmed by x-ray film.

a. Inspect the posterior pharynx for presence of coiled tube.
Visualization confirms that the tube has gone beyond the oropharynx.

b. Aspirate gently to withdraw stomach contents and measure aspirate pH. Aspirate gently over a period of up to 5 minutes, if necessary, to obtain gastric fluid.
The pH of stomach contents is normally 1 to 5.5; however, many situations commonly alter the pH of gastric contents, so the usefulness of this method is limited. pH testing is helpful only if the fluid is acidic; if it is alkaline, the gastric contents may have been altered (e.g., by enteral feedings or antacids and other medications), or the tube may be in the

lung. *This procedure does not reliably confirm gastric placement and should be used in combination with other methods.*

c. Take note of the amount, color, and consistency of the aspirate.
Gastric aspirates are often white or greenish and may be curdled. Intestinal aspirates will be smaller in quantity, yellowish due to the presence of bile, and not curdled.

d. Inject air into the NG tube and listen with a stethoscope over the stomach. Use this only to confirm other methods; do not use as the primary method of verification because it is the least reliable method.
If the tube is in the stomach, injecting 5 to 30 mL of air with the syringe should produce a gurgling sound. However, because the lungs and stomach are so close together, a tube inadvertently placed in the respiratory tract or esophagus can transmit a sound similar to that of air in the stomach.

e. Ask the patient to speak.
If she can do so, the tube is probably in the stomach. Use this only to confirm other methods; it is not reliable enough to use as the primary method of verification.

18. If the tube is not in the stomach, advance it another 2.5 to 5 cm (2 to 4 in.) and repeat steps 17a through 17e.

19. After you confirm proper placement, clamp the end of the tube or connect it to the drainage bag, feeding, or suction machine.

20. Secure the tube using one of the following methods:

Securing the Tube With 1-Inch (2.5-cm) Tape

a. Apply skin adhesive to the patient's nose, and allow it to dry.
A skin adhesive helps the tape to adhere and protects skin from breakdown.

b. Use the 5-cm (2-in.) piece of hypoallergenic tape, split lengthwise for 2.5 cm (1 in.) at one end.
A split tape can be wrapped around the tube in opposite directions to hold the tube in place more securely.

c. Apply the intact end of tape to the patient's nose.

d. Wrap the split strips around the tube where it exits the nose.

Securing the Tube With ½-Inch Tape

e. Use ½-inch (1.3-cm) tape, 4 inches (10 cm) long. Apply one end of tape to the patient's nose and wrap the other end downward around the tube and then back up to secure on the opposite side of the nose. ▼

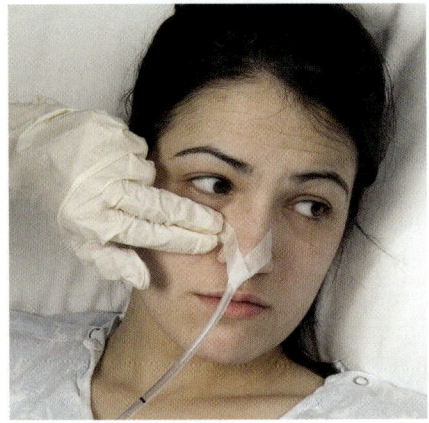

Securing the Tube With a Tube Fixation Device

f. Peel the backing off the pad and place the wide end of the pad over the bridge of the nose.

g. Position the connector around the NG or NE tube where it exits the nose. ▼

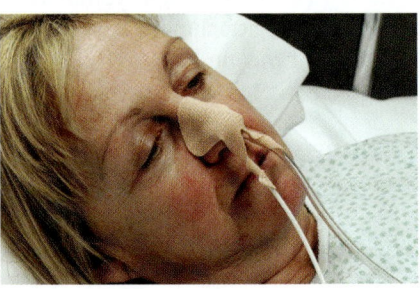

21. **Curve and tape the tube to the patient's cheek** (not necessary with some commercial tube fixation devices).

    Securing the tube to the cheek reduces the tension on the naris.

22. **Fasten the tube to the patient's gown:** Tie a slipknot around the tube with a rubber band. Loop a rubber band in a slipknot near the connection. (Alternatively, wrap a short piece of tape around the tube to form a tab.) Then fasten the rubber band or the tab to the gown with a safety pin (or tape).

    Reduces discomfort produced by the weight of the tube and prevents movement that may cause dislocation of the tube and irritation of the nose.

23. **Elevate the head of the bed** 30° unless contraindicated.

24. **Mark the tube** where it enters the naris with tape, or measure the length from the naris to the connector.

    A marked tube allows you to easily notice whether tube placement has changed.

? What if . . .

- **The patient is confused, combative, or comatose?**

  a. If the patient is comatose, place him into a semi-Fowler's position. Have a coworker use a pillow to help position the patient's head forward for insertion.

  b. If the patient is confused and combative, ask a coworker to assist you with insertion.

- **The patient gags, coughs, or chokes (at steps 11 and 15)?**

  a. Stop advancing the tube. Ask the patient to take deep breaths and drink a few sips of water.

  Helps suppress the gag reflex.

  b. Instruct the patient to breathe easily and take some sips of water.

  c. If coughing continues, pull the tube back slightly.

  d. If gagging continues, use a tongue blade and penlight to check the tube position in the back of the throat.

  The tube may be coiled in the back of the throat.

  e. Continue to advance the tube to the desired distance.

  f. If the tube is coiled in the back of the throat, the patient coughs excessively during insertion, the tube does not advance with each swallow, or the patient develops respiratory distress (e.g., gasping, coughing, or cyanosis), withdraw the tube completely and allow the patient to rest before reinserting.

  The tube may be in the patient's trachea.

- **You are unable to obtain an aspirate (at step 17b) when confirming tube placement?**

  a. Use a 50-mL syringe and aspirate very slowly over at least 5 minutes.

  b. Flush the tube with air, then aspirate.

  c. Turn the patient to the left side, wait 20 minutes, then aspirate again.

- **The prescription states the tube needs to be in the jejunum?**

  a. To advance the tube into the jejunum after the tube has been placed in the stomach, position the patient on the right side.

  Positioning on the right side allows gravity to assist tube passage through the pyloric sphincter.

  b. Advance the tube 5 to 7.5 cm (2 to 3 in.) hourly, over several hours (up to 24 hr) until x-ray confirms placement.

  Weighted tubes will advance by gravity and peristalsis if a loop of the designated length is made at the entrance to the naris. After reading the initial x-ray, the radiologist or primary physician can provide the measurement needed to advance the tube to the desired position. Note that specially trained nurses usually place these tubes at the bedside.

- **The procedure is anticipated to cause pain or discomfort?**

  Commercial viscous lidocaine is sometimes used to aid in patient comfort. Some practitioners use them for all NG insertions.

  a. You may insert 2% viscous lidocaine into the nasal passage with a syringe before tube placement.

  b. Alternatively, you can apply an anesthetic spray to the nasal and oropharyngeal mucosa.

- **The patient is a child?**

  a. Children usually require a tube of a smaller diameter.

  b. Encourage parents to comfort infants and children and participate in their care.

  c. You may need to apply restraints during insertion.

  To prevent dislodging of the tube.

  d. Monitor more frequently for complications.

  Small children are not able to communicate problems with the tube.

(continued on next page)

Procedure 28-2 ■ Inserting Nasogastric and Nasoenteric Tubes (continued)

Evaluation

- Assess how well the patient tolerated the procedure (e.g., discomfort, gagging, coughing?)
- Note the color, consistency, and pH of NG or NE aspirate.
- Ask the patient whether she feels comfortable.
- Assess respiratory status.

Patient Teaching

- Explain that the sensation of the tube should decrease with time.
- Explain the importance of immediately reporting tension on the tube or displacement of the tape or fixation device.
- Discuss the need for frequent mouth care while the tube is in place.

Home Care

- Assess the client or caregiver's ability to maintain an NG or NE tube at home.
- Assess the home environment to determine the client's risk for infection.
- Instruct the client or caregiver about aspirating stomach contents and measuring pH.
- Teach the client or caregiver how to verify tube placement.
- Explain to the client or caregiver how to properly secure the NG or NE tube.
- Reinforce the need for frequent mouth care.

Documentation

- Chart the date and time of insertion, size and type of the NG or NE tube and insertion site (which naris), length of tube from tip of the nose to the end of the tube, tolerance of the procedure, any abnormal findings, and methods for confirming NG or NE tube placement.
- Document the volume and description of gastric contents.
- Document respiratory status, including any sign of distress.
- NG or NE tube insertion is documented in the progress notes and flow sheets in most agencies.

Practice Resources

American Association of Critical-Care Nurses (n.d., revised 2009); Emergency Nurses Association (2010, revised 2015); Institute for Safe Medication Practices (2010); Joanna Briggs Institute (2010a, 2010c, 2012); The Joint Commission (2007); Metheny, N., & American Association of Critical-Care Nurses (2005, revised 2016); Metheny, N. A., Stewart, B. J., & Mills, A. C. (2012); National Institutes of Health (n.d., updated 2014); Shlamovitz, G. Z. (n.d., updated 2015); Simons, S. R., & Abdallah, L. M. (2012); Wiegand, D. (2011).

Thinking About the Procedure

 The video **Inserting Nasogastric and Nasoenteric Tubes,** along with questions and suggested responses, is available on the **Davis's Nursing Skills Videos** Web site on DavisPlus.

Procedure 28-3 ■ Administering Feedings Through Gastric and Enteric Tubes

➤ For steps to follow in *all* procedures, refer to the Universal Steps for All Procedures found on the page facing the inside back cover.

Equipment

- Prescribed feeding formula at room temperature
- Filtered water or prescribed diluent, if ordered
- Tube feeding administration set and bag
- 60-mL luer-lock or catheter-tip syringe (two needed for syringe feeding)
- Connector to connect administration set to the feeding tube
- Stethoscope
- Enteral feeding infusion pump, recommended for continuous and cyclic feedings
- IV pole
- Linen-saver pad
- Graduated container
- pH strip
- For gastrostomy and jejunostomy tubes: a small precut gauze dressing

Delegation

You can delegate the procedure to the NAP or LPN if the patient's condition is stable and the NAP's skills allow. You must verify peristalsis, tube placement, and feeding tube patency before the feeding is started. Remind the NAP to position the patient upright and to report patient discomfort and any difficulty with the infusion.

Pre-Procedure Assessment

- **Verify the feeding tube is in proper placement** prior to starting the procedure. See Clinical Insight 28-4 for methods you might use.

➕ Tube placement after insertion must be verified by radiography before the first feeding. For subsequent feedings, use more than one bedside method for verifying correct tube placement. One method is to aspirate and measure gastric residual volume. *(NOTE: For patients with a jejunostomy tube, do not measure the residual volume.)*

- You can also estimate tube placement by checking the length of the exposed tube: (1) Compare the length from the naris with the connector recorded after x-ray confirmation of placement; or (2) observe the mark that was made on it where it entered the nostril after insertion.
  These methods help confirm that the tube has not become displaced since radiography. If there is significant change in length, tube position must again be confirmed by radiography.

- Assess fluid status by checking breath sounds, mucous membranes, skin turgor, edema, and intake and output.
  These signs indicate fluid volume excess or insufficiency.

- Obtain baseline weight and laboratory studies.
  Weight change is a sensitive measure reflecting fluid and nutritional status.

- Monitor vital signs before and after feedings.
  Vital signs may vary from baseline because of pain, impaction, or dehydration.

- Auscultate for bowel sounds before each feeding or every 4 to 8 hours for continuous feedings. Also check for distention, nausea, vomiting, and diarrhea.
  These symptoms may indicate intolerance of tube feedings. If GI motility is impaired, feedings accumulate in the stomach along with gastric secretions, predisposing the patient to reflux and aspiration. Some medications (e.g., opioids) also slow gastric emptying.

- Assess frequency of bowel movements.
  Diarrhea may indicate intolerance of the formula, excessive feeding, or gastrointestinal disease.

- Check patient history for food allergies.
  Helps prevent allergic reaction to ingredients in the feeding formula.

- ***For gastrostomy and jejunostomy tubes:*** Assess the exit site at every shift. Report redness or drainage to the physician.
  Leaking of gastric or intestinal contents may cause skin breakdown.

Procedure 28-3A ■ Administering Feedings Through Gastric and Enteric Tubes Using a Closed System

➤ When performing the procedure, always identify your patient according to agency policy, using two identifiers, and be attentive to standard precautions, hand hygiene, patient safety and privacy, body mechanics, and documentation.

Procedure Steps

1. **Check the medical prescription** for the type of feeding, rate of infusion, and frequency of feeding.
   A medical prescription is required for enteral feedings. Rate and frequency of feeding are crucial for providing adequate nutrition.

2. **Elevate the head of the bed** at least 30 to 45-degrees, unless contraindicated.

3. **Check the expiration date** of the tube feeding formula.
   Expired formula should be discarded.

4. **Prepare the formula.**

   a. ✚ Inspect the container of feeding solution. If the bag, bottle, or can has been opened or damaged in any way, don't use it.

   b. ✚ Shake the feeding formula thoroughly. Examine the solution. It should be uniform in color and consistency. Most often the formula is room temperature. Follow the manufacturer's instructions for safe storage.

   Because the formula goes directly into the stomach and is not warmed
   by the mouth and esophagus, cold formula may cause abdominal cramping and increase the risk for diarrhea.

5. **Prepare the equipment for** administration.

   a. Don procedure gloves. Fill a disposable tube feeding container with a 4- to 6-hour supply of feeding formula. Or use a prefilled bottle with feeding formula. Follow similar procedure for flush bag if using a two-bag system.
   Limit hang-time to help prevent bacterial growth and prevent air from entering the GI tract.

   b. Label the container with the patient's name, room number, date, start time, formula type, feeding rate, and your initials. ✚ Write a warning using large, bold letters—for instance, "WARNING! For Enteral Use Only—NOT for IV Use."

   Labeling identifies the formula and prevents misconnection of the feeding tube into an IV line. Labeling also helps avoid administering formula past the expiration date.

   c. ✚ Be sure adapters and connectors used in the enteral system are incompatible with female luer-lock rigid connectors used for IV infusion.
   Prevents tube feeding misconnection with an IV line.

   d. Hang the tube-feeding container on an IV pole with the label facing forward. A prefilled container can safely hang for 24 to 36 hours (some agencies allow for 48 hours).
   Closed systems decrease the risk of contamination and prevent air from entering the GI tract.

   e. Open the administration set package. Make sure the tubing does not touch the floor.

   f. Close the clamp on the tubing before attaching the set to the container.

   g. Remove the cap from the end of safety connector.

   ✚ This adaptor must *not* be compatible with IV tubing. Do not touch the end of the connector or let it touch another surface.

(continued on next page)

Procedure 28-3 ■ Administering Feedings Through Gastric and Enteric Tubes (continued)

h. Insert the proximal end of the tubing (with the safety adaptor) into the cross-shaped opening of the port on the feeding tube bag. Twist the collar in a clockwise direction until it is securely fastened. ▼

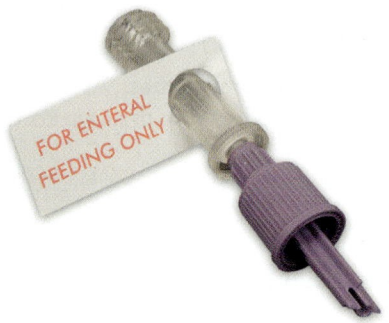

6. **Prime the tubing with the feeding solution.**

7. **Thread the administration set** tubing through the infusion pump according to the manufacturer's instructions. Be sure to close the roller clamp.
    Clamping the tube prevents air from entering the stomach or gastric contents from leaking out. ▼

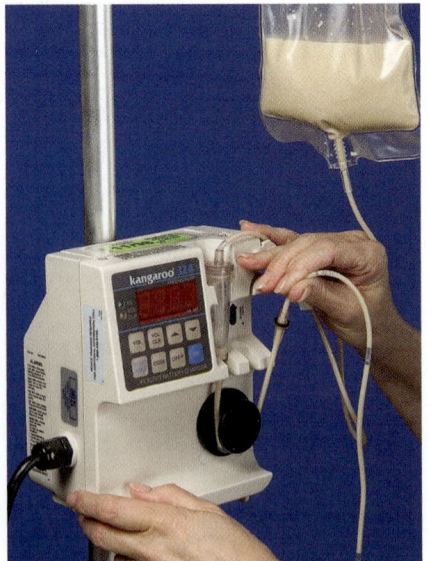

8. **Connect the distal end of the tubing** primed with feeding solution to the connector or directly to the NG or NE tube.

9. **Turn on the infusion pump.** Set the correct infusion rate and volume to be infused. Follow the pump manufacturer's instructions.

    ✚ Trace the tubing from the bag back to the patient before starting the feeding to ensure that you have not inadvertently hooked the feeding bag or bottle to the IV line.

10. **Unclamp the tube** and begin the infusion.

11. **When the feeding volume is complete,** stop the flow, flush the tube, and disconnect the feeding by turning off the pump and closing the roller clamp.

12. **Disconnect the feeding tube** from the administration tubing.

13. **Flush feeding tube** with the prescribed amount of water—typically 15 to 50 mL, if there is no fluid restriction.

14. **Cap the proximal end of the feeding tube.**
    Prevents leaking of gastric contents and stops air from entering the stomach.

15. **Keep the head of the bed elevated** at least 30° to 45° for 1 hour after administering the tube feeding.
    Reduces the risk for aspiration of gastric contents

16. **Provide or assist with regular oral hygiene** and encourage frequent gargling.
    Reduces oropharyngeal discomfort from the tube

17. **When you finish the procedure,** remember the Universal Steps that apply after all procedures. For example, leave the patient in a safe, comfortable position with the call device in easy reach.

Procedure 28-3B ■ Administering Feedings Through Gastric and Enteric Tubes Using an Open System: Syringe

Procedure Steps

First follow steps 1 through 4, above. Then proceed as follows:

1. **Prepare the equipment** for administration.
   a. Don procedure gloves.
   b. Label the syringe with the patient's name, room number, date, time, formula type, feeding rate, start time, and your initials. ✚ Write a warning using large, bold letters— for instance, "WARNING! For Enteral Use Only—NOT for IV Use."

   Labeling: identifies the formula, prevents misconnection of the feeding tube into an IV line, and helps avoid administering formula past the expiration date.

2. **Remove the plunger from the syringe.**

3. **Clamp or pinch off** the end of the feeding tube to begin the feeding.
   Prevents air from entering the feeding tube.

4. **Attach the syringe to** the proximal end of the feeding tube.

5. **Fill the syringe** with the prescribed amount of formula.

6. **Unclamp the feeding tube**, and elevate the syringe. Do not elevate the syringe more than 18 inches (45 cm) above the insertion site. Allow the feeding to flow slowly.
   Gravity facilitates the flow of formula through the feeding tube. Rate of flow is determined by the height of the syringe. Feeding slowly prevents sudden stomach distention, which can lead to diarrhea, cramping, nausea, and vomiting. ➤

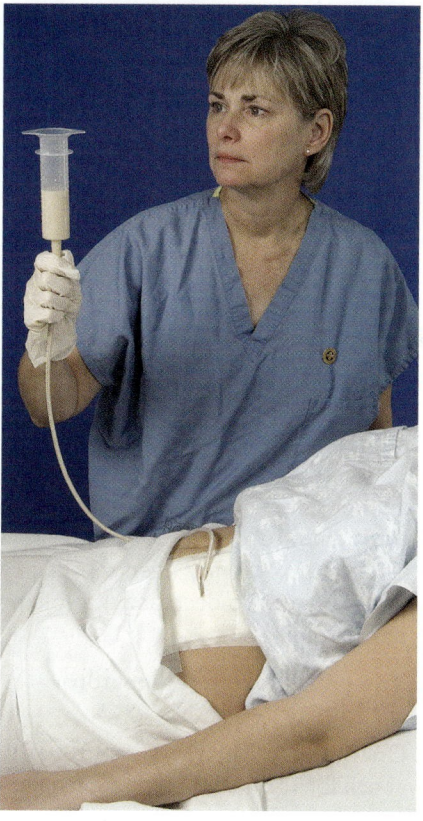

7. **When the syringe is nearly empty**, refill the syringe until the prescribed amount of feeding has been administered.
   If the tubing runs dry, air may enter the stomach and cause discomfort associated with gas.

8. **When the feeding volume** is infused, clamp or pinch the end of the feeding tube.

9. **Disconnect the syringe** from the feeding tube.

10. **Flush feeding tube** with the prescribed amount of water—typically 15 to 50 mL, if there is no feeding restriction.

11. **Cap the proximal end** of the feeding tube.
    Prevents spillage of gastric contents and stops air from entering the stomach.

12. **Keep the head of the bed elevated** at least 30° to 45° for 1 hour after administering the tube feeding.
    Elevation reduces the risk for aspiration of gastric contents.

13. **Provide or assist with** regular oral hygiene and encourage frequent gargling.
    Oral care reduces oropharyngeal discomfort from the tube.

? What if . . .

- **When checking for residual, the volume is more than the formula flow rate for 1 hour?**

  Reinstill the gastric residual volume. Residual gastric contents should be reinfused in the absence of pain or abdominal distension.

  If the residual is > 250 mL and if there is no abdominal pain or distension, continue the infusion. Recheck in 1 hour. If the residual is still > 250 mL, stop the infusion for 4 hours and recheck. If still > 250 mL, call healthcare provider (Bankhead, Boullata, Brantley, et al., 2009).

  If residual is < 250 mL, restart the infusion at 50% original rate and monitor (Kenny & Goodman, 2010).

  If the gastric residual volume is ≥ 250 mL after a second gastric residual check, a promotility agent may be considered in adult clients (American Society for Parenteral and Enteral Nutrition (A.S.P.E.N.) Board of Directors, 2009a; Bankhead, Boullata, Brantley, et al., 2009).
  High residual volumes indicate delayed gastric emptying.

- **When checking for residual, none is obtained?**

  Use a large syringe (e.g., 60 mL) and inflate 20 mL of air into the tube, if agency policy permits; this may move the tube away from the gastric wall or clear the tube of any residual formula, medication, or water.

(continued on next page)

Procedure 28-3 ■ Administering Feedings Through Gastric and Enteric Tubes (continued)

- **When irrigating the feeding tube (at step 10), resistance is met? Or when instilling the feeding, the fluid does not flow?**

- Do not force the solution.
- Do not use any fluid other than water for flushing.
- Check for kinks in tubing and that the pump is working correctly.
- Turn the client onto his left side.
- Remove any enteral feeding solution remaining in the tube. Try instilling 5 mL of warm water into the tube and clamping the tube for 5 minutes. Then apply gentle negative pressure to the tube with a syringe.
- Try flushing with a smaller (e.g., 10 or 20 mL) syringe.
- If these measures fail, the tube may need to be removed and a new one inserted; contact the primary care provider. (*Note:* There are other methods, such as the alkalinized enzyme method; they require a medical prescription.)
Forcing the solution may damage the tube. However, you can use a smaller syringe to exert slightly more pressure.

- **The patient has a cuffed tracheostomy tube?**

Inflate the cuff before administering the feeding, and keep the cuff inflated for at least 15 minutes afterward.
Cuffing helps to prevent aspiration.

- **During the feeding, the patient vomits or complains of nausea or feeling too full?**

Stop the feeding and assess the patient's condition. Flush the tube, wait an hour, then measure gastric contents and restart the feeding at a slower rate. You may need to obtain a medical order to decrease the volume of the feedings.

- **The patient has a jejunostomy tube?**

Do not instill air into the tube or check for residual before feeding.
The tube is in the jejunum rather than the stomach, and the jejunum isn't normally a reservoir; therefore, no residual volume is present in the jejunum. Gastrostomy and jejunostomy tubes are often placed through the upper abdominal wall; such tubes, of course, cannot inadvertently migrate into the airway. Injecting air into the tube is not necessary and introduces air into the GI tract, causing the patient discomfort from gas.

Clean the insertion site daily with soap and water. You may apply a small, precut gauze dressing to the site.
Helps prevent bacterial growth; prevents infection.

Be aware that the delivery rate will likely be slower for jejunostomy tubes because of the unavailability of the stomach as a reservoir.

Evaluation

- Evaluate the patient's tolerance to the tube feeding; did the patient have any abdominal discomfort, nausea, vomiting, or diarrhea?
- Auscultate bowel sounds and vital signs every 4 hours.
- Check gastric residual volume every 4 hours.
- Monitor intake and output every 8 hours.
- Weigh patient at least 3 times per week.
- Assess the exit site for signs of skin breakdown.
- Assess frequency of bowel movements.
- Check laboratory values to evaluate nutritional status.

Patient Teaching

- Demonstrate the procedure to the patient and caregiver if the patient will be continuing tube feedings at home.
- Explain the importance of flushing the feeding tube with sterile water every 4 hours while the patient is awake to maintain tube patency and fluid and electrolyte balance.
- Discuss the importance of remaining upright for at least 1 hour after the feeding.

Home Care

- Provide written instructions.
- Be sure the client has a 7-day supply of enteral feedings.
- Identify with the client the person who will be responsible for care of the enteral tube and administration of feedings at home.
- Explain to the client and caregiver how to measure the prescribed amount of tube feeding formula and water for flushes by using household measuring equipment.
- Explain the importance of washing reusable equipment thoroughly with soap and water to prevent the spread of infection.
- Discuss how and where to purchase and store the formula.
- If home feedings are to be delivered by pump:
  Facilitate a home care visit to provide training about the feeding pump.
  Arrange for delivery of the feeding pump before discharge (or refer to the appropriate professional for this).
  Ensure that the client has a 7-day supply of disposable feeding sets and 50-mL syringes upon discharge.

Documentation

- Chart the type of tube feeding, rate and volume of infusion, amount of gastric residual volume (if any), and tolerance of procedure.
- Tube feeding intake is documented on the intake and output portion of the flow sheet in most agencies.
- Record all flushes as intake. Subtract any liquids that you aspirate and do not reinstill (e.g., when gastric residual is too high).

Practice Resources

American Society for Parenteral and Enteral Nutrition (A.S.P.E.N.) (2009a, b); Bankhead, Boullata, Brantley, et al., & A.S.P.E.N. (2009); Dietitians Association of Australia (2011); Cincinnati Children's Hospital Medical Center (updated 2012);

Durfee, S. M., Adams, S. C., Arthur, E., et al.; Home and Alternate Site Task Force; American Society for Parenteral and Enteral Nutrition (2014); The Joint Commission (2014); McClave, S. A., Taylor, B. E., Martindale, R. G., et al. (2016); Metheny, N., & American Association of Critical-Care Nurses (2005, revised 2016); U.S. Food and Drug Administration (n.d.b, updated 2016).

Thinking About the Procedure

 The videos **Administering Feedings Through Gastric and Enteric Tubes With Infusion Pump** and **Administering Feedings Through Gastric and Enteric Tubes Using an Open-System Syringe,** along with questions and suggested responses, are available on the ***Davis's Nursing Skills Videos*** Web site on Davis*Plus*.

Procedure 28-4 ■ Removing a Nasogastric or Nasoenteric Tube

➤ For steps to follow in *all* procedures, refer to the Universal Steps for All Procedures found on the page facing the inside back cover.

Equipment

- Linen-saver pad
- 60-mL luer-lock or catheter-tip syringe
- Procedure gloves
- Stethoscope
- Disposable plastic bag
- Emesis basin
- Gauze square

Delegation

This procedure should not be delegated to the LPN or NAP.

Pre-Procedure Assessments

- Auscultate the abdomen for the presence of bowel sounds.
  Bowel sounds and flatus confirm peristalsis, which indicates bowel function is present.
- Assess the patient's ability to consume an oral diet.
  Confirms readiness for discontinuing the NG or NE tube.
- Determine how long it has been since the patient's last enteral feeding.

➤ When performing the procedure, always identify your patient according to agency policy, using two identifiers, and be attentive to standard precautions, hand hygiene, patient safety and privacy, body mechanics, and documentation.

Procedure Steps

1. **Check the patient's health record** to confirm removal of the tube. For feeding tubes, make sure tube feeding has been stopped at least 30 minutes before removal.

2. **Assist the patient to a sitting** or high Fowler's position.
   Proper body alignment facilitates tube removal.

3. **Place the plastic bag and emesis basin** on the bed or within reach. Hand the patient facial tissue. Explain that the procedure may cause some

gagging or nasal discomfort, but it will be brief.
Patients often need to blow their nose after this procedure.

4. **Drape a linen-saver pad or towel** across the patient's chest, and don procedure gloves.
   Draping protects the gown and linens from soiling. Maintains universal precautions.

5. **If you have not already done so,** wash your hands and put on gloves.

6. **If the NG tube is connected** to suction, turn off suction and disconnect the tube.

7. **Stand on the patient's right side** if you are right-handed and left side if left-handed.

8. **Attach the syringe** to the proximal end of the NG or NE tube and flush the tube with 15 mL of water, normal saline, or air.
   Flushing clears the tube of feeding formula or gastric secretions that could cause irritation or be aspirated during tube removal.

9. **Unfasten the tube** from the patient's gown and then remove the tape from the patient's nose. Use an adhesive-remover pad to help loosen the tape as necessary.

(continued on next page)

Procedure 28-4 ■ Removing a Nasogastric or Nasoenteric Tube (continued)

10. Clamp or pinch the end of the tube in your hand. Hold gauze up to the patient's nose and be ready to grab the tube with the towel in the opposite hand upon removal.
Prevents gastric fluids from leaking out the end of the tube onto the nurse or patient.

11. Ask the patient to take a deep breath and hold it.
Breath holding closes the epiglottis to prevent aspiration.

12. Quickly, steadily, and smoothly withdraw the tube and place it in the plastic bag.
Rapid removal in one steady motion prevents tissue trauma. The plastic

bag acts as a barrier to gastric fluids until the tube can be placed in the trash. Seeing and smelling the tube may cause the patient to become nauseated.

13. If the patient cannot do so, clean her nares and provide mouth care. Remove the tape residue from her nose with adhesive remover.
Promotes patient comfort and prevents infection.

14. If the NG tube was connected to suction, measure the drainage and note the character of the content. Dispose of the tube and

drainage equipment according to facility policy.
For patients receiving enteral feedings or gastric suction, record their intake and output. Proper equipment disposal prevents the spread of infection.

15. Remove and dispose of gloves in the nearest receptacle.

Evaluation

- Assess the nares for signs of skin breakdown or bleeding.
- Monitor the patient for signs of GI dysfunction, such as food intolerance, nausea, vomiting, and abdominal distention. Auscultate for bowel sounds.
  GI dysfunction could necessitate reinsertion of the tube.
- Monitor intake and output every 8 hours.
- Weigh the patient regularly.
- Check laboratory values to evaluate nutritional status.

Patient Teaching

- Instruct the patient or caregiver on how to remove the feeding tube.
- Explain the importance of reporting nausea, vomiting, food intolerance, or abdominal distention to the physician.
- Explain the importance of and procedure for drinking fluids, if not contraindicated.

Home Care

The procedure does not require special adaptation for home care, except that you might want to place the tube in

a plastic zippered storage bag before discarding it in the trash receptacle.

Documentation

- Chart the date and time of removal as well as the patient's tolerance of the procedure.
- Document the amount of drainage if the tube was connected to suction.
- Note any complications following NG or NE tube removal, such as food intolerance, nausea, vomiting, and abdominal distention.

Practice Resource

National Institutes of Health (n.d., updated 2014).

Thinking About the Procedure

 The video **Removing Nasogastric or Nasoenteric Tube,** along with questions and suggested responses, is available on the ***Davis's Nursing Skills Videos*** Web site on Davis*Plus*.

Procedure 28-5 ■ Administering Parenteral Nutrition

➤ For steps to follow in *all* procedures, refer to the Universal Steps for All Procedures found on the page facing the inside back cover.

Equipment

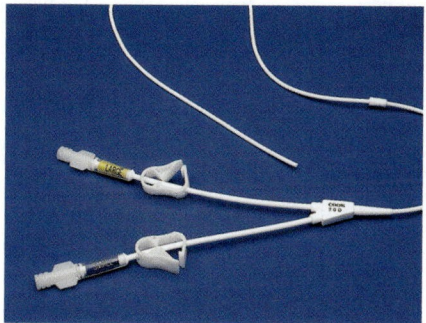

- Parenteral nutrition solution
  - Keep the PN refrigerated until 60 minutes before use; do not give cold. Do not hasten warming by placing in a microwave oven or hot water bath.
    Cold solution can cause pain, hypothermia, and venous spasm. Nutrients in PN solution are stable only for this short period of time. Nutrients could precipitate, causing catheter blockage or emboli.
  - Some pharmacies deliver the solution before infusion. Be sure the PN has not been mixed more than 24 hours beforehand. However, in home care you may find that solutions are mixed and delivered weekly.
- Procedure gloves
- Sterile gloves
- Intravenous administration set, extension set if indicated (free of plasticizers, such as DEHP, when fat emulsion is to be infused)
- 0.22-micron filter (1.2-micron filter if solution contains albumin or lipids)
  A 0.22-micron filter will remove most particulates and microorganisms that might have been introduced during mixing, but it is too fine for larger-molecule lipids to infuse properly.
- Time tape
  Even though the PN is delivered by infusion pump, there have been numerous recalls of infusion pumps because of malfunction. This simple tape provides valuable information quickly and is an additional safety measure.
- 70% alcohol pads or chlorhexidine gluconate (CHG)-based pads (e.g., 2% CHG in 70% isopropyl alcohol)
- Infusion pump
- 10-mL syringe and saline
  To check for catheter patency

- Blood glucose testing monitor
- Intake and output record
- Transparent dressing or sterile gauze and tape (if dressing is to be changed)
- Catheter stabilization device (e.g., StatLock)
  These are recommended for all catheters and must be changed with each dressing change.
- If the dressing is to be changed, you also need a transparent dressing or sterile gauze, tape, and a mask.

Delegation

Do not delegate this skill to the LPN or NAP because administration of parenteral nutrition requires advanced assessment and critical-thinking skills. The LPN or NAP can assist by monitoring vital signs and verifying patient identity with you. Instruct them about complications associated with PN and ask them to inform you of any signs or symptoms or change in the patient's condition.

Pre-Procedure Assessments

- Assess nutrition status and nutritional needs (e.g., daily weights, intake and output [I&O], lab results). Patients requiring PN have complex nutritional needs, and actual nutritional status is assessed by a nurse or dietician specializing in nutritional support.
- Check the prescriber's orders for type and concentration of additives in each container and for rate of infusion. (Standardized order forms are recommended by the American Society for Parenteral and Enteral Nutrition [A.S.P.E.N.].)
- Check the patient's record to confirm that proper CVC tip placement has been established before the initial PN administration.
- Check agency policy.
  Some agencies may require tubing and filter change with every bottle or bag. The CDC recommends changing the PN set every 72 hours and a fat emulsion set at least every 24 hours.
- Check the blood glucose level.
- Assess for apparent patency of the IV site.
  If PN is being administered continuously by pump, the infusion is running, and there is no leakage from the insertion, you can begin the first few steps of the procedure. Actual patency is confirmed at step 14.

(continued on next page)

Procedure 28-5 ■ Administering Parenteral Nutrition (continued)

➤ When performing the procedure, always identify your patient according to agency policy, using two identifiers, and be attentive to standard precautions, hand hygiene, patient safety and privacy, body mechanics, and documentation.

Procedure Steps

1. **Gather equipment and place** at the bedside.
   Promotes efficient use of time.

2. ✚ **Identify the patient,** using two identifiers, according to agency policy. Some institutions require, as an extra precaution, that two people identify the patient.
   Multiple patient identifiers help to avoid "wrong-patient" errors. PN solutions are mixed to meet individual needs.

3. **Explain to the patient** the procedure and the rationale for it.
   Respects the patient's right to be informed.

4. **Perform hand hygiene** and don procedure gloves.
   Reduces transmission of infectious microorganisms.

5. **Position the patient supine** in bed.

6. **Obtain and examine the PN** container. Check for leaks, cloudiness, or floating particles. Do not use if any of these are present. Some agencies require that two people examine the solution.

Solutions Containing Lipids (3-in-1 Admixture)

✚ Do not administer the admixture if it has a brown layer, oil droplets, or oil on the surface. This indicates that the emulsion has "broken," and the large lipid droplets can cause fat emboli if administered.

KEY POINT: *Note that this solution requires a 1.2-micron filter.*
To reduce the risk of adverse events such as fat emboli.

7. **Compare the bag with the patient's identification band;** check for correct bag number, expiration date, and additives and their concentration. Compare with the original prescription. Have a coworker verify with you.
   Ensures that the correct solution is administered. Check the expiration date to ensure that the solution will be discarded after that date and time. PN solutions are carefully calculated and prepared using the latest recommendations for sterile compounding of solutions. Therefore, the nurse should not add anything to the bag, either before it is hung or while it is infusing.

8. **Connect the IV tubing to the PN** solution; prime the tubing. Note that priming may be done manually now or later (on the pump after the tubing is loaded into the pump), depending on the design of the pump.
   ✚ Be sure to identify the correct port and IV line. Trace the PN tubing from the bag to the patient.
   Priming tubing removes air bubbles and prevents air from entering the patient's bloodstream, possibly causing air embolism. If there is PN already infusing, the old tubing must be removed from the pump and the rate regulated manually for the short period it takes to prime the new administration set.

When Using IV Tubing Without an Inline Filter

If the IV tubing does not have an inline filter, attach the filter and the extension tubing before priming. Attach the filter as close to the catheter site as possible.

9. **Place the IV tubing in the infusion pump.** (Prime the tubing if not previously done). Set the pump to the prescribed rate.
   Administration via pump (preferably volumetric) helps prevent complications associated with too-rapid infusion. PN solutions must be administered by infusion pump with reliable, audible alarms. Catheter tip placement must be confirmed before initial PN administration.

10. ✚ **Identify the correct IV catheter** and lumen for the PN. This is usually a peripherally inserted central catheter (PICC line) or a centrally inserted venous line designated solely for PN.
    PN must be administered via a central venous catheter (e.g., subclavian catheter, internal jugular, or PICC), the tip of which is positioned in the superior vena cava/right atrial juncture. Most guidelines state that a specific intravenous line be reserved for parenteral nutrition and not used for any other purpose. If a single-lumen catheter is used, it is used only for PN. If a multilumen catheter is used, one lumen will be dedicated for the PN, and blood and other fluids should not be given through that lumen.

11. **Clamp the catheter and the old PN administration set,** if still connected, before disconnecting the tubing.
    a. A clamp should be present on the central line catheters with valves built into the catheter itself.
       The central line for the PN should already be clamped if no PN is running. If a previous bag is running, always clamp the PN line near the patient before disconnecting. Clamping prevents air from entering the catheter when you open the connection.
    b. As an additional safety measure, instruct the patient to perform the Valsalva maneuver just as you change the tubing.
    c. If Valsalva is contraindicated for a patient, instruct the patient to exhale at a specific time when the lumen is open.
       The Valsalva maneuver increases intrathoracic pressure and creates positive pressure in the central vessels, also helping prevent air embolism.

12. **Remove and discard gloves.** Perform hand hygiene.

In steps 1 through 11, you were observing Universal Precautions. From this step forward, the emphasis is on preventing the introduction of microorganisms into the catheter lumen or the catheter insertion site.

13. **Don clean gloves (or sterile gloves,** if your agency policy requires them). Disconnect the old administration set. Using a chlorhexidine gluconate (CHG)–alcohol pad or a 70% alcohol pad, thoroughly scrub all surfaces of the central line injection cap and extension leg (in a needleless system) or the luer-lock, including threads.

Because PN solutions are a good medium for growth of pathogens, and because the IV line enters the central circulation, the risk for sepsis is relatively high.

14. **Determine patency of the line.** Use a 10-mL syringe to aspirate for blood, looking for a brisk return; then flush with saline. If the PN is running continuously on a pump, there are no occlusion alarms, and the dressing is dry and intact, these are also signs—but not proof—of patency.

When PN is running continuously on a pump, the pump creates a constant fluid flow through the lumen to help keep it patent. There is some controversy about this step. Some experts prefer to aspirate for blood only for the first bag of a continuous infusion, and thereafter to flush without aspirating. As always, follow agency policy.

15. **Attach the infusion tubing** to the designated PN port and then turn the luer-lock to secure the connection. ✚ "Luer-slip" connections should not be used. Do not use tape.

Securing the connection with a luer-lock connection prevents separation of the connection and decreases the risk for sepsis or embolism. Tape, even sterile tape, has been found to be a medium for bacterial colonization.

If the Previous Infusion Is Still Connected

Be sure the access line and the line to the "old" infusion bag are clamped (step 11). Quickly disconnect from the central line, thoroughly cleanse the port, and connect the new infusion.

16. ✚ **Trace the tubing from the patient back to the bag.** Then start the infusion. Check again to make sure the catheter-tubing connection is secure. Infuse at the rate prescribed (depending on the patient's tolerance). PN is usually started at a rate of 40 to 50 mL/hr and then advanced 25 mL/hr every 6 hours.

PN solutions may contain as much as 70% dextrose. A gradual rate increase allows the patient's pancreatic beta cells time to increase their insulin output to handle the increased glucose load. For lower concentrations of dextrose, you can usually run the same rate for the complete 24-hour volume. Tracing the tubing back to the bag is a double-check against misconnections.

17. **Label the tubing** with the date and time of change (if it is new tubing or if you have changed the tubing).

Labeling allows other nurses to know when tubing is due to be changed and a new solution must be hung.

18. **Remove and discard gloves.** Perform hand hygiene.

❓ What if . . .

- ✚ **When you flush the catheter (at step 14), you meet resistance?**

Examine the insertion site for leaking fluid or inflammation. Aspirate and try again to flush *gently*. Never forcibly flush against resistance. Reposition the patient and ask him to cough. Roll the patient's shoulder or raise the arm on the same side the catheter is on. If these measures fail, notify the primary care provider.

Occlusion may be caused by a clot, drug precipitation, or catheter migration, kinking, or compression. Forceful flushing may

discharge a clot into circulation. Other measures to clear a catheter require a medical order.

- ✚ **The rate falls behind or the pump gives occlusion alarms?**

First check to be sure the pump is turned on, the bag is not empty, and all clamps are fully open. Change the filter if it is clogged. Perform the steps in the preceding item. If those measures do not work, change the pump and send it to biomedical engineering to be checked. ✚ Do not attempt to catch up by increasing the rate.

A slow rate may indicate a clogged filter or injection cap, a kinked catheter, or a malfunctioning pump. A clogged filter must be changed; you cannot run the PN without a filter.

- ✚ **The 24-hour total deviates from the prescribed infusion rate by 10% or more?**

Notify the primary provider or nutrition support team.

- ✚ **A PN solution must be discontinued abruptly for any reason?**

Notify the primary provider or nutrition support team. Another solution of 5% or 10% dextrose may be started.

The dextrose solution is started to prevent rebound hypoglycemia. Note that if it is a catheter complication that requires this discontinuation, 10% dextrose is the highest concentration that can be infused through a peripheral vein because infiltrated hyperosmolar fluid causes tissue injury.

- ✚ **The patient no longer needs parenteral nutrition?**

You may need to decrease the rate gradually, perhaps over 48 hours, before discontinuing the infusion completely. Be sure the patient either receives enteral nutrition or consumes food during the next few hours after stopping PN.

To prevent rebound hypoglycemia.

(continued on next page)

Procedure 28-5 ■ Administering Parenteral Nutrition (continued)

Evaluation

These are post-procedure evaluations. For ongoing monitoring, see Clinical Insight 28-6.

- Assess vital signs, I&O, and weight.
- Observe that the solution is infusing at the prescribed rate.
- Assess patient's tolerance to the infusion (e.g., observe for pulmonary edema; check lab results).
- Observe for skin rashes, flushing, color changes, or other signs of allergic reactions; notify the primary provider. *NOTE: These are not common.*
- Monitor blood glucose and do not increase the infusion rate until glycemic control is established.

Patient Teaching

- Inform the patient and family of the purpose and duration of the nutritional support.
- Teach them to recognize and report to the nurse symptoms of complications associated with PN.
- Teach the patient that the dressing must remain occlusive, and to notify nurse if it comes loose or gets wet.
- Teach the patient the importance of measures to prevent blood infections.

Home Care

- The home environment must provide dry storage space for supplies, a refrigerator for storing admixtures, a clean low-traffic area for procedure preparation, and electronic outlets for any electronic equipment.
- Teach safe disposal of supplies.
- Provide verbal and written instructions of the procedures; demonstrate and ask for a return demonstration. Role play "what would you do if . . . ?" situations with the patient.
- Clients at home often administer their daily 24-hour total over 12 to 16 hours during the night. This allows them to disconnect from the infusion in the morning, flush the central line, and be free to pursue their usual activities during the day.
- Instruct about solution hang time and management of the access device.
  Depending on the anticipated length of therapy, patients may be sent home with a permanent venous access device.
- Provide 24-hour phone numbers for the primary care provider and home care agency.
- Home PN is less expensive than treatment in the hospital and in many cases is associated with a lower risk of infection.
- Home nutritional support is usually under the direction of specialized nutrition support teams.

Documentation

- A special form may be used for documenting PN administration.
- Bag number, date and time hung, volume, type of fluid, rate of delivery, additives
- Date and time of dressing or tubing change (if performed)
- Patient's tolerance of procedure
- Pre- and post-administration assessment data, including complications and response to therapy
- Results of fingerstick blood glucose checks
- If insulin is required, type, amount, and route/site administered
- Weight
- I&O

Practice Resources

American Society for Parenteral and Enteral Nutrition (A.S.P.E.N.) Board of Directors (2009a); A.S.P.E.N. Board of Directors and Task Force on Parenteral Nutrition Standardization; Kochevar, M., Guenter, P., Holcombe, B., et al. (2007); Ayers, P., Boullata, J., Gervasio, J., et al. (2014); Boitano, M., Bojak, S., McCloskey, S., et al. (2010); Infusion Nurses Society (2016); McClave, S. A., Taylor, B. E., Martindale, R. G., et al. (2016).

Procedure 28-6 ■ Administering Lipids

➤ For steps to follow in *all* procedures, refer to the Universal Steps for All Procedures found on the page facing the inside back cover.

➤ *Note:* If administering through a central line, refer to Procedure 28-5 for precautions associated with central lines.

➤ *Note:* This procedure is for administering fat emulsions. If you are administering an admixture with the parenteral nutrition solution, use Procedure 28-5.

Equipment

- Intravenous lipid solution (not refrigerated)
- Special tubing (infusion set) for lipids
  Must be without plasticizers (DEHP). Set should be labeled to that effect.
- Needleless cannula (if using a split septum needleless connector that requires it)
- 70% isopropyl alcohol pads or chlorhexidine gluconate
- Procedure gloves
- Time tape
- Infusion pump
- Intake and output record
- If a filter is used, it must be a 1.2-micron filter
  Lipid particles are large and will clog a smaller size.

Delegation

Do not delegate this skill to the LPN or NAP because administration of lipids requires advanced assessment and critical-thinking skills. The LPN or NAP can assist by monitoring vital signs and verifying patient identity with you. Instruct them about complications associated with lipids and ask them to inform you of any signs or symptoms or change in the patient's condition.

Pre-Procedure Assessments

- Assess for rash, eczema, dry, scaly skin, poor wound healing, and sparse hair.
  These are signs of essential fatty acid deficits.

- Check the history for anemia, coagulation disorders, and abnormal liver, pancreatic, or respiratory function.
  These factors predispose to fat emboli. Your role as a staff nurse is to be certain the PN prescriber is aware of these factors; they do not necessarily contraindicate giving the PN.

- Check peripheral IV site for erythema, infiltration, and patency. Check the central venous access site for erythema or other signs of infection.

- Take baseline vital signs just before infusing the lipids.
  An immediate reaction can occur upon starting the infusion. Note that not all guidelines require this action.

- Check patient's blood glucose level before infusing.
  Lipid infusion can raise the patient's blood glucose.

➤ When performing the procedure, always identify your patient according to agency policy, using two identifiers, and be attentive to standard precautions, hand hygiene, patient safety and privacy, body mechanics, and documentation.

Procedure Steps

1. **Review the prescriber's orders,** including rate of infusion; identify the patient; and explain the purpose of the procedure.
   Verifying helps to prevent dosage and wrong-patient errors. Explaining respects the patient's right to be informed and encourages cooperation.

2. **Gather supplies** and place at bedside. Adjust lighting as needed.
   Organization promotes efficient use of time.

3. **Perform hand hygiene** and don procedure gloves.
   To reduce transmission of infectious microorganisms.

4. **Position the patient supine** in bed.

5. **Be certain lipids are not cold.**
   Cold infusion can cause discomfort.

6. **Examine the bottle** for a layer of froth (indicates leakage) or for separation into fat globules or layers, or cloudiness.
   Do not use the lipids if these occur.

7. **Label the bottle** with the patient's name and identifier, room number, date, time, rate, and start and stop times. Label the tubing with date and time. *Note:* When lipids are infused with parenteral nutrition, the lipid infusion must be completed within 12 hours.
   Labeling helps ensure that the patient receives the correct infusion.

8. **Compare the lipids bottle** with the patient's wrist band; compare with the prescription (bag number, expiration date). Have a colleague verify.

9. **Determine patency of the IV line** (see Procedure 28-5).

10. **Cleanse the stopper** on the IV bottle with an antiseptic swab; allow to dry.

11. **Connect the special DEHP-free** lipids-infusion tubing to the bottle, twisting the spike as you insert it. **KEY POINT:** *You must use new tubing for each bottle.*
    Twisting the spike helps ensure that particles from the stopper do not fall into the bottle. New tubing reduces the growth of microorganisms (the feeding provides a medium for fungal growth).

12. **Place the primed tubing** in the pump and attach the tubing to the IV catheter lumen.

    ✚ Identify the correct IV line and port for the infusion. Trace the tubing from the bag back to the patient.

    a. Thoroughly scrub the catheter injection port or hub and the luer-lock threads with an antiseptic wipe.
    b. If you are infusing lipids simultaneously with PN, attach the primed lipid tubing to the injection port/hub closest to the patient, below the tubing filter, or through a Y-connection at the catheter hub.
    c. Turn the luer-lock to secure the connection.
    d. ✚ NOTE: *If a previous infusion has been running, clamp the catheter lumen and the old administration set tubing before disconnecting and changing the tubing.*
       Prevents blood backup in the line.

13. **Begin the infusion.** Ideally, infuse slowly at first: 1.0 mL/min for adults and 0.1 mL/min for children (or as prescribed by the physician). Check again to be sure the catheter-tubing connection is secure.
    Slow infusion allows time to assess if the patient will have an adverse reaction to the lipids. Nausea, vomiting, and elevated temperature have been reported when lipids are infused quickly.

14. **Take the vital signs now,** then every 10 minutes for 30 minutes, and according to agency protocol. Observe for side effects (e.g., chills, fever, flushing, dyspnea, nausea, vomiting, headache, back pain).

15. **If no reactions occur,** adjust to the prescribed infusion rate and continue monitoring according to your agency's protocol.

(continued on next page)

Procedure 28-6 ■ Administering Lipids (continued)

16. **Remove gloves and perform hand hygiene.**

17. **When the infusion is finished,** discard the bottle or bag and IV administration set.
    Formula contains sugars that are a medium for growth of pathogens.

 What if . . .

- **The entire bottle of lipids is not used?**

Discard partially used bottles.
Prevents contamination.

Evaluation

- If ordered, monitor serum lipids 4 hours after discontinuing the infusion.
- Monitor the IV site for infection, inflammation, and infiltration.
- Monitor for symptoms of fat emboli.
- Monitor the IV line for patency.
- Monitor for allergic reactions (nausea, vomiting, headache, chest pain, back pain, fever).
- Monitor for lipid intolerance (triglyceride levels, liver function tests, hepatosplenomegaly, decreased coagulation, cyanosis, dyspnea).

Patient Teaching

- Inform the patient and family of the purpose and duration of the nutritional support.
- Teach the patient to recognize and report symptoms of complications associated with lipids infusion.

Home Care

- The home environment must provide dry storage space for supplies, a refrigerator for storing solutions, a clean low-traffic area for procedure preparation, and electronic outlets for any electronic equipment.
- Teach safe disposal of supplies.
- Provide verbal and written instructions for the procedures; demonstrate and ask for a return demonstration.
- Instruct about solution hang time and management of the access device.
- Provide 24-hour phone numbers for the primary care provider and home care agency.

Documentation

- A special form may be used for documenting lipids and PN administration.
- Bottle number, date and time hung, volume, type of fluid, and rate of delivery
- Status of dressing, and date and time of dressing or tubing change (if performed)
- Patient's tolerance of the procedure and any problems encountered
- Pre- and post-administration assessment data and blood tests, if any
- Condition of the IV site
- Weight
- I&O

Practice Resources

Infusion Nurses Society (2016, revised); McClave, S. A., Taylor, B. E., Martindale, R. G., et al. (2016).

 To explore learning resources for this chapter,

Go to **www.DavisAdvantage.com** and find:

Answers and Suggested Responses for all questions in this chapter

Knowledge Map

References and Bibliography

Lists of NIC Interventions and NOC Outcomes

List of NANDA-I Diagnoses

Concept Map

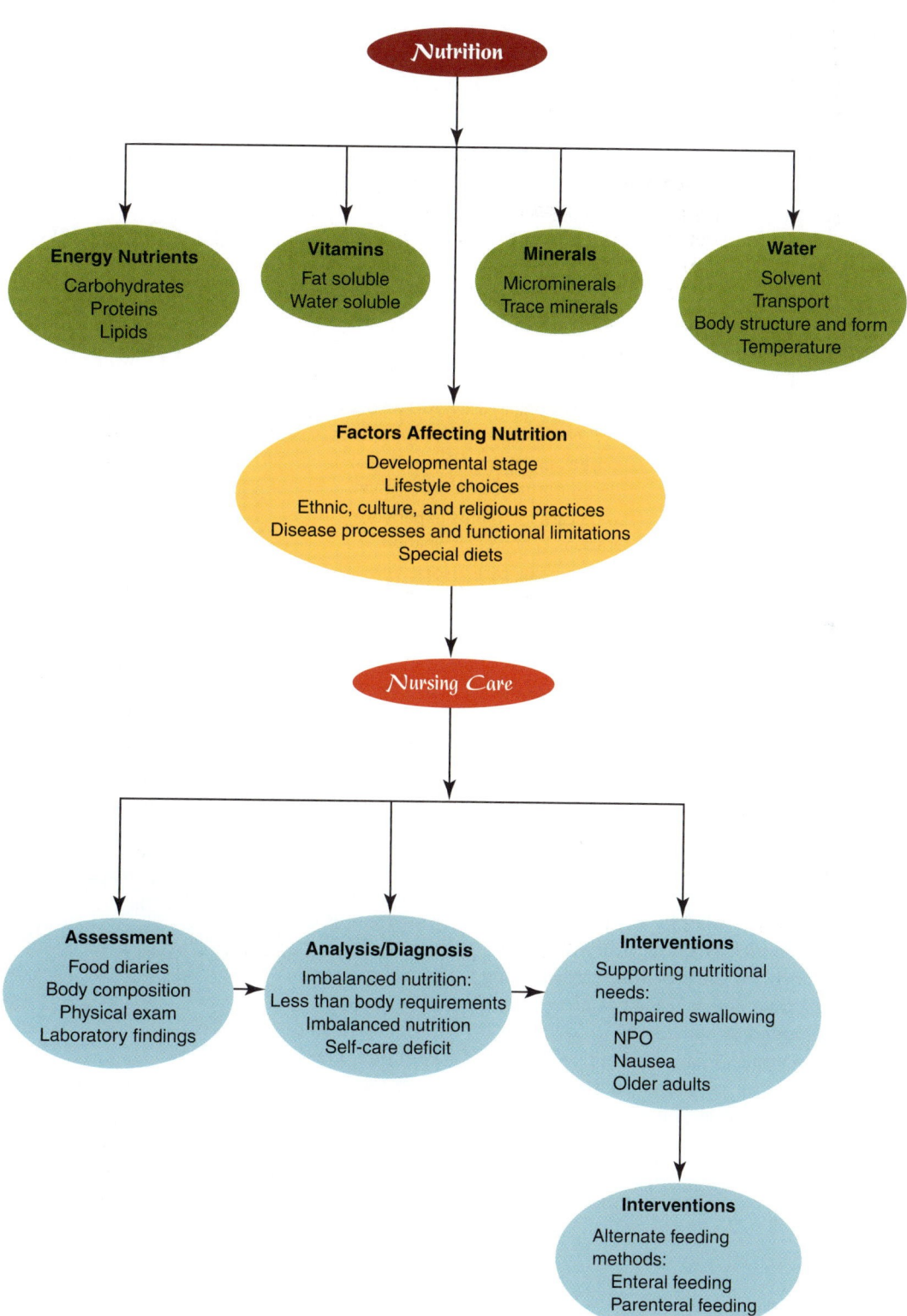

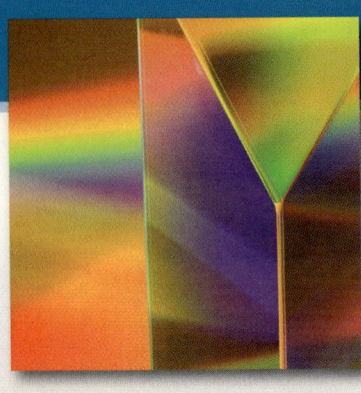

CHAPTER 29

Bowel Elimination

Learning Outcomes

After completing this chapter, you should be able to:

- ➤ Identify the basic structures and functions of the gastrointestinal system.
- ➤ Discuss factors that affect bowel elimination.
- ➤ Describe normal bowel elimination.
- ➤ Differentiate between the various types of bowel diversions.
- ➤ Discuss common bowel elimination problems.
- ➤ Identify appropriate nursing history questions to assess bowel elimination problems.
- ➤ Perform a physical examination focused on bowel elimination.
- ➤ List and describe diagnostic tests used to identify bowel elimination problems.
- ➤ Formulate nursing diagnoses associated with altered bowel elimination.
- ➤ Describe nursing interventions that promote normal bowel elimination.
- ➤ Provide care for clients experiencing alterations in bowel elimination.
- ➤ Discuss nursing care associated with the use of bowel diversions.

Key Concepts

Bowel elimination

Motility

Related Concepts

See the Concept Map at the end of this chapter.

Example Problems

Diarrhea

Constipation

Bowel incontinence

Meet Your Patient

You are assigned to care for Mrs. Zeno, a frail 96-year-old woman who broke her hip last month after a fall at home. Mrs. Zeno was hospitalized for surgical repair of her hip and is now in a skilled nursing facility for rehabilitation. The nursing assistive personnel (NAP) informs you that Mrs. Zeno has eaten poorly for the past week, only picking at the food on her meal trays and refusing the protein supplements that were added to her diet. Mrs. Zeno tells you she would like to go home: "I have my routine and the foods I like. I think I'd be better off there." As you review the chart in preparation for clinical, you note that she has not had a bowel movement (BM) for 3 days. Her last BM was small and very hard.

What additional assessments should you perform? What, if anything, is of concern about her bowel pattern? What actions should you take with Mrs. Zeno?

In this chapter, you will gain theoretical and practical knowledge to help you answer those questions and provide care for clients with bowel elimination concerns.

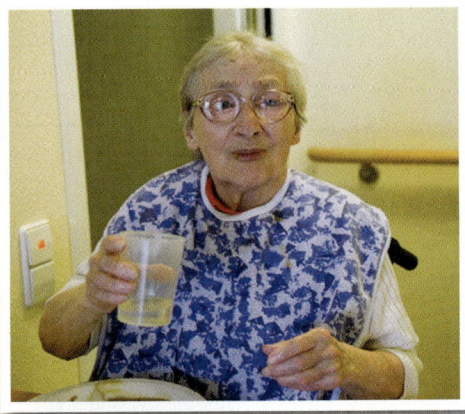

Theoretical Knowledge
knowing **why**

Bowel elimination is a normal process by which we eliminate waste products from our bodies. In this chapter you will come to understand concepts underlying the function of the gastrointestinal tract as well as factors that affect bowel elimination.

ABOUT THE KEY CONCEPTS

Bowel elimination is one of the overarching concepts in this chapter—the "hook" on which you hang your theoretical knowledge. The other key concept, **motility,** helps you to understand the processes that occur in normal elimination and in problems such as constipation and diarrhea. Other, more specific, concepts will enhance your understanding of bowel elimination. For example, when you grasp the concept of bowel diversion, you will see how it relates to various bowel elimination problems. As you study the chapter, identify the concepts and try to understand how they are connected. This will help you care for clients with any medical diagnosis affecting bowel elimination.

WHAT ARE THE ANATOMICAL STRUCTURES OF THE GASTROINTESTINAL TRACT?

The gastrointestinal (GI) tract is a smooth-muscle tube approximately 10 m (30 ft) long, running through the body from the mouth to the anus. Its major functions are to digest and absorb the nutrients present in food and to eliminate food waste products as feces. The structures of the GI tract are the upper GI tract, small intestine, large intestine, the rectum, and the anus (Fig. 29-1).

The Upper Gastrointestinal Tract

The upper GI tract contains the mouth, pharynx, esophagus, and stomach.

The Mouth is where mechanical digestion begins, with **mastication,** or chewing. Food is torn into small pieces, mashed, moistened with saliva, and formed into a bolus that is then swallowed into the esophagus. The mouth contains glands that secrete enzymes, such as ptyalin and salivary amylase, which begin the digestion of carbohydrates.

The Pharynx is the back part of the throat where food and air pass after chewing. To prevent choking and aspiration, a flap of connective tissue, called the **epiglottis,** closes over the trachea when food is swallowed.

The Esophagus is a tube of smooth muscle, which alternately contracts and relaxes in waves of **peristalsis** to push the bolus toward the stomach. The bolus travels the length of the esophagus (about 25 cm, or 10 in.) in about 15 seconds. The *cardiac sphincter* (also called the *gastroesophageal sphincter*) relaxes to allow the food to pass into the stomach. When the cardiac sphincter constricts, it prevents acidic stomach contents from flowing back into the esophagus.

The Stomach is a distensible sac that extends from the esophagus to the small intestine. The stomach stores food while it churns and mixes it, providing further mechanical breakdown. Chemical digestion continues in the stomach, which secretes hydrochloric acid (HCl), a protein-digesting enzyme called *pepsin,* and *gastric lipase,* an enzyme that begins

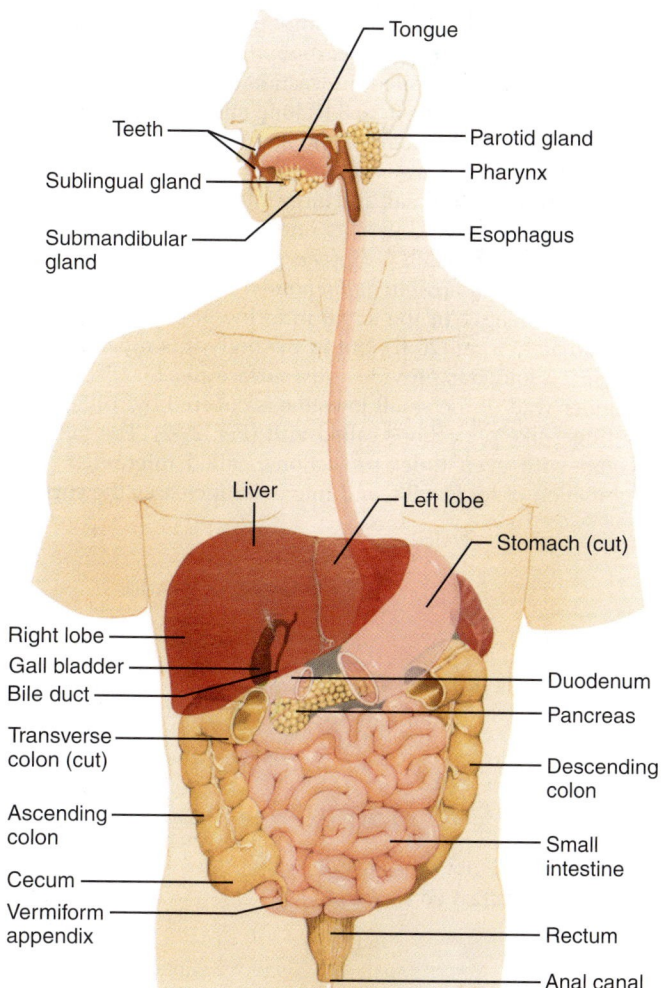

FIGURE 29-1 The gastrointestinal tract extends from the mouth to the anus. The major functions of the GI system are to digest and absorb the nutrients in food and to eliminate food waste products as feces.

the digestion of lipids. The stomach lining also secretes a mucous coating that protects the stomach from being corroded by HCl. Food remains in the stomach an average of 4 hours. Food leaves the stomach as a liquid, called **chyme.**

The Small Intestine

The small intestine is a folded, twisted, and coiled tube that connects the stomach and the large intestine. About 2.5 cm (1 in.) in diameter and approximately 6 m (20 ft) long if fully extended, it occupies most of the abdominal cavity. Most digestion and absorption of food occurs in the small intestine. Chyme travels through it slowly, by peristalsis. Peristalsis halts periodically to allow for absorption.

The small intestine consists of three segments: the duodenum, jejunum, and ileum.

- The **duodenum** is the first section of the small intestine. It is a C-shaped tube that branches off from the stomach, about 30 to 60 cm (1 to 2 ft) long. The duodenum processes chyme by mixing it and adding enzymes. The bile duct and main pancreatic duct both enter the small intestine at the level of the duodenum, providing bile from the liver and gallbladder to digest lipids and pancreatic enzymes to digest lipids, proteins, and carbohydrates.

- The **jejunum** is the coiled midsection of the small intestine. It is about 1.8 to 2.4 m (6 to 8 ft) long and forms the connection between the duodenum and ileum. Its major function is to absorb carbohydrates and proteins.
- The **ileum** joins the small and large intestine. It is responsible for absorption of fats; bile salts; and some vitamins, minerals, and water. **KEY POINT:** *However, nutrients are absorbed mainly in the duodenum and jejunum.*

The total length of the small intestine, if stretched out, is approximately 6 m (20 ft), but in the body it is much shorter because it is folded to provide a vast surface area for absorption. The inner wall of the small intestine is covered by millions of tiny finger-like projections called **villi** (Fig. 29-2). The villi are covered with even tinier projections, called **microvilli**. The combination of folds, villi, and microvilli increases the surface area of the small intestine greatly, facilitating absorption of nutrients.

The Large Intestine

The large intestine, also known as the **colon**, is larger in diameter than the small intestine (6.3 cm, or 2.5 in.) but shorter in length—about 1.5 to 1.8 m (5 to 6 ft). It extends from the ileum of the small intestine to the anus. It contains seven segments: the cecum, ascending colon, transverse colon, descending colon, sigmoid colon, rectum, and anus (Fig. 29-3).

- **The cecum.** Undigested food entering the first portion of the large intestine, the **cecum**, consists mostly of cellulose and water. The connection of the ileum to the cecum is controlled by the **ileocecal valve.** Under most conditions, the valve prevents backflow of chyme from the colon into the small intestine. The **appendix** is a small, finger-like appendage off the cecum. It is believed to be a **vestigial organ**—one whose significance has diminished over time—however, it is lined with lymphatic tissue and may play a role in immune function.
- **The next three segments,** the *ascending, transverse,* and *descending colon,* ring the small intestine. The **sigmoid colon** is a final small segment of bowel that twists medially and downward to connect with the rectum and anus.

Functions of the Colon The colon secretes mucus, which facilitates smooth passage of stool, and absorbs water, some vitamins, and minerals. Approximately 80% of the fluid that enters the colon is reabsorbed along its passage. Normal flora in the colon aid in the digestive process. These bacteria are responsible for producing vitamin K and several of the B vitamins.

The large intestine has two sets of muscles that give it a puckered appearance. Longitudinal muscles, known as **taenia**

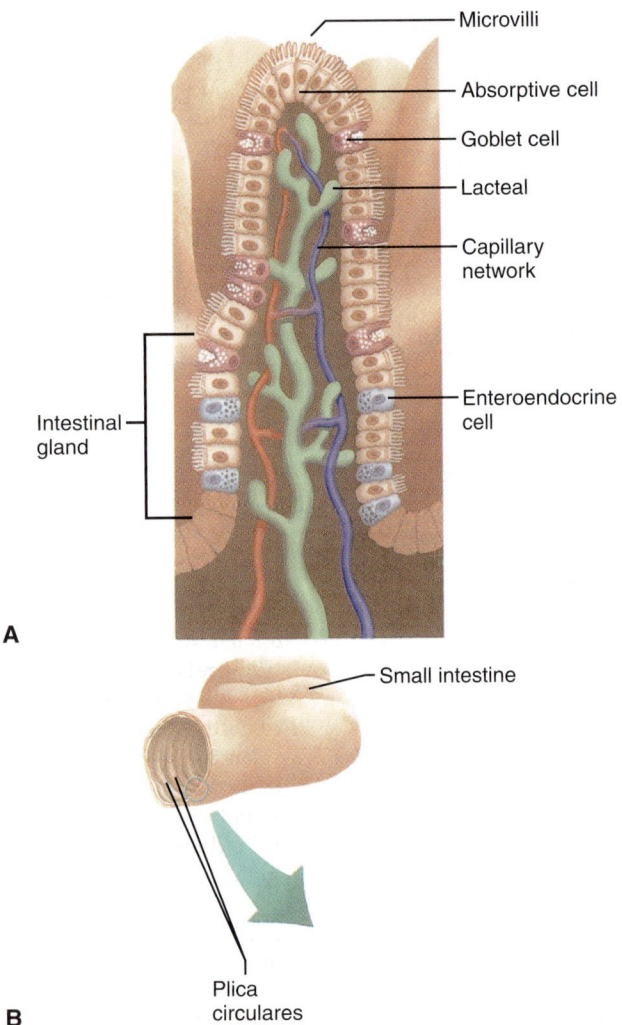

A

B

FIGURE 29-2 The small intestine is highly folded, providing a vast surface area for absorption of nutrients. The microvilli form a brush border, which is the site of most nutrient absorption. A. Microscopic view of a villus showing the internal structure. B. Section through the small intestine showing the plica circulares (circular folds) of the mucosa and submucosa.

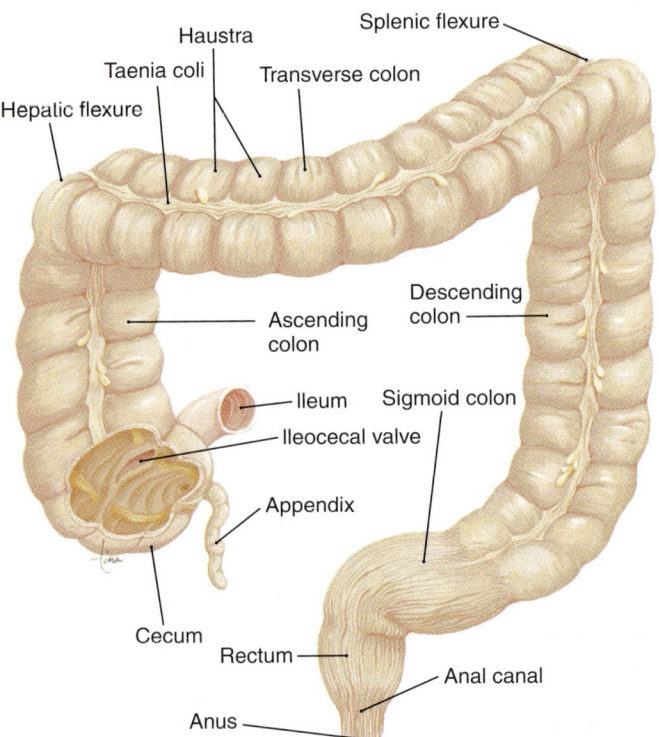

FIGURE 29-3 The large intestine shown in anterior view. The term *flexure* means a turn or bend.

coli, run lengthwise along the colon surface. Tension in these muscles gathers up the colon into pouched segments known as **haustra** all along its length (see Fig. 29-3). In addition, the colon wall contains circular muscles that, together with the taenia coli, cause the colon to expand and contract in length and width to achieve haustral churning, peristalsis, and mass peristalsis.

- **Haustral churning** moves digestive contents around within each haustra. This action promotes reabsorption of water.
- **Peristalsis** continues throughout the length of the large intestine, where it propels intestinal contents toward the rectum and anus.
- **Mass peristalsis** is a powerful contraction along a lengthy segment of bowel. It is facilitated by the **gastrocolic reflex,** which is triggered by food entering the stomach and small intestine. Mass movements usually occur only one to three times each day, and they are responsible for most of the propulsion of the contents in the transverse and sigmoid colon.

The Rectum and Anus

The **rectum** is approximately 15 cm (6 in.) long and is continuous with the **anus,** the last 2.5 cm (1 in.) of the colon. A highly vascular folded tube, the rectum is free of waste products until just before defecation.

The anus has two ring-like muscles that function as sphincters.

- The **internal sphincter** involuntarily relaxes and opens when stool is present in the rectum.
- The **external sphincter** is under voluntary control. Voluntary relaxation of the external sphincter allows stool to be expelled from the body (Fig. 29-4).

The anus is highly vascular. Chronic pressure on the veins within the anal canal, as with prolonged sitting or retained feces, can cause **hemorrhoids** (distended blood vessels within or protruding from the anus).

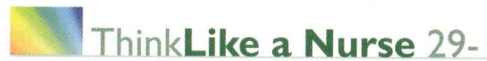

KnowledgeCheck 29-1

- What are the major functions of the small intestine and large intestine?
- How do the rectum and anus control elimination of feces from the body?

ThinkLike a Nurse 29-1

Based on your knowledge that hemorrhoids are dilated blood vessels in the anal canal, what symptoms would you expect a patient with hemorrhoids to exhibit?

HOW DOES THE BOWEL ELIMINATE WASTE?

As you have learned, reabsorption of water from chyme in the large intestine results in a semisolid mass known as **feces.** Feces are a mixture of fiber, undigested food, shed epithelial cells, inorganic material (e.g., calcium and phosphates), bacteria, and water. Small amounts of fat may be present.

Feces are usually brown because **bile salts,** which aid in the digestion of fat, are excreted in the feces. Bile is normally golden yellow, but the action of bacteria in the GI tract changes the color to brown. Bacteria are also responsible for the odor of feces.

Flatus, or gas, is formed in the digestive process. Some is swallowed air that accompanies the intake of food. A small portion diffuses from blood into the GI tract. However, most of the gas is created by bacterial fermentation in the colon.

The Process of Defecation

The process by which the bowel eliminates waste is called **defecation.** When fecal material reaches the rectum and causes it to distend, (1) stretch receptors are stimulated to start contraction of the sigmoid colon and rectal muscles, and (2) the internal anal sphincter relaxes. At the same time, sensory impulses transmitted to the central nervous system (CNS) produce a conscious urge to defecate. We respond to this signal by voluntarily contracting our diaphragm and abdominal muscles to increase downward pressure, while at the same time relaxing the external anal sphincter. These actions allow feces to be propelled through the anus. If we ignore the signal to defecate, the reflexive contractions ease for a few minutes, until mass peristalsis occurs again.

Valsalva Maneuver A person can increase the pressure to expel feces by contracting the abdominal muscles (straining) while maintaining a closed airway (e.g., holding the breath). This is called the **Valsalva maneuver.** Although it assists with the passage of stool, you should caution clients with heart disease, glaucoma, increased intracranial pressure, or a new surgical wound to avoid the Valsalva maneuver because it increases pressure within the abdominal cavity, raises blood pressure, and is associated with an increased risk for cardiac arrhythmias.

Normal Defecation Patterns

The sheer number of over-the-counter (OTC) products to treat "irregularity" suggests that bowel function problems are common. Nevertheless, many people avoid the topic of bowel elimination. As a result, patients may have unanswered questions about their bowel function and may turn to you for information.

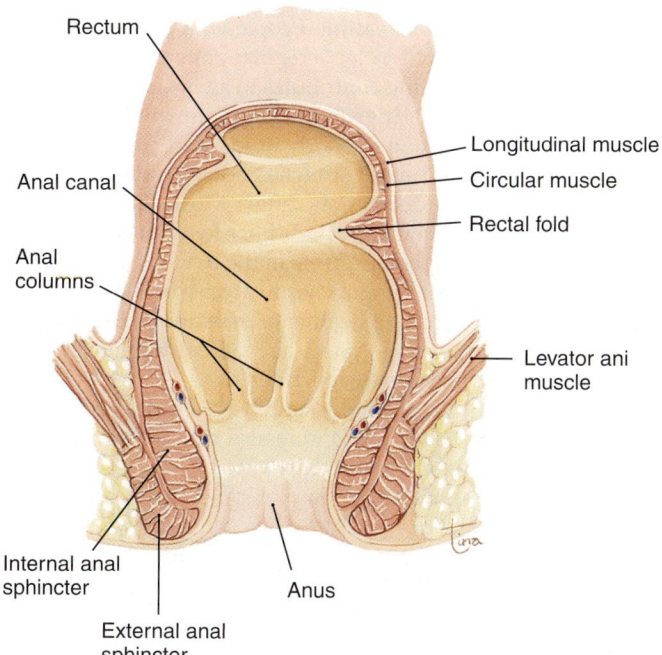

FIGURE 29-4 Internal and external anal sphincters shown in a frontal section through the lower rectum and anal canal.

Rectum

Anal canal

Anal columns

Internal anal sphincter

External anal sphincter

Anus

Longitudinal muscle

Circular muscle

Rectal fold

Levator ani muscle

"Normal" Function Part of the confusion about bowel function is that there is a wide range of "normal." The frequency of BMs may range from several times per day to once a week. **KEY POINT:** *As long as the person passes stools without excessive urgency (needing to rush to the toilet), with minimal effort and no straining, without blood loss, and without the use of laxatives, you can regard bowel function as normal.*

Normal Stool is a soft, formed semisolid, approximately 75% water and 25% solid when expelled.

- **If passage through the colon is slowed,** more water is reabsorbed from the feces. The stool becomes dry and hard, requiring more effort to pass.
- **If transit time through the colon is faster than normal,** less water is reabsorbed, and stools are watery.

Think**Like a Nurse** 29-2

- Based on your knowledge of normal bowel function, how would you describe Mrs. Zeno's (Meet Your Patient) bowel function? Is it normal or abnormal?
- What additional information, if any, do you need to know to answer this question?

WHAT FACTORS AFFECT BOWEL ELIMINATION?

Each person develops a bowel elimination pattern that is based on several factors, discussed in the sections immediately following.

Developmental Stage

Bowel elimination patterns change throughout the life span.

Infants During the first few days of life, the term newborn passes meconium through the anus. **Meconium** is green-black, tarry, sticky, and odorless. It is formed by swallowed mucus, hair, and amniotic fluid. Stools transition to a yellow-green color over the next few days. After that, breastfed babies pass golden yellow stools, whereas formula-fed babies pass tan stools. Initially babies defecate frequently, usually after each feeding. The stools tend to be watery while the large intestine is still immature. Gradually, normal flora develop in the colon, and stools become firmer and less frequent.

Children The ability to control defecation typically develops at about age 2 to 3 years of age. Toilet training requires neural and muscular control as well as conscious effort. The child must be aware of the urge to defecate, be able to maintain closure of the external anal sphincter while getting to the toilet, and be able to remove clothing. As children mature, they gradually learn to gain more control over defecation.

Adults The bowel pattern set in childhood normally continues into late adulthood if the client consumes adequate fiber and fluid and engages in regular physical activity. However, peristalsis, intestinal smooth muscle tone, perineal muscle tone, and sphincter control normally decrease with aging. These physiological processes can contribute to constipation among older adults, especially if they decrease their activity and fiber intake.

Personal and Sociocultural Factors

Refer to the accompanying iCare box Bowel Elimination.

Privacy and Time Privacy is important to most people, as is sufficient time to have a bowel movement without feeling the need to hurry.

- Clients working in fast-paced jobs may have difficulty even consciously recognizing the need to defecate, and some habitually ignore the need, promoting bowel dysfunction.

♥ iCare 29-1

Bowel Elimination

Rob has been an RN for 6 months. Gladys, 80 years old, is weakened and in need of assistance with her bladder and bowel routine; she is also at risk for falls. She comments that she has a grandson about Rob's age and seems slightly embarrassed that Rob must help her with her elimination needs. Rob is sensitive to her feelings and offers to get a female to assist her. She says, "Yes, please." A few days later, Gladys is getting stronger and can perform her bathroom routine independently, but she remains slightly unsteady on her feet. Rob walks her to the bathroom, makes sure she is safe, and then, while ensuring privacy, stays nearby just outside the door until she is finished. As Rob assists her back to her bed, Gladys thanks him for his good care. She says, "It's hard to depend on someone to take care of private things I've always done for myself. Thanks for being sensitive about that."

- Parents and caregivers of infants and toddlers may postpone their own toileting needs because of fear of leaving the children alone.
- Some clients are acutely embarrassed by the thought that anyone might realize they are having a bowel movement and will wait until they are entirely alone before even entering the bathroom.

Stress Have you ever heard the following phrase: "He puts his stress in his gut"? Stress has a major influence on motility of the GI tract. It may cause diarrhea or constipation, and it is a primary risk factor in the development of *irritable bowel syndrome,* a disorder associated with bloating, pain, and altered bowel function.

Nutrition, Hydration, and Activity Level

Foods and Fiber Regular intake of food promotes peristalsis.

- **A regular schedule for eating.** People who eat on a regular schedule are likely to develop a regular pattern of defecation, whereas irregular eating contributes to an irregular pattern.
- **Adequate intake of fiber.** Fiber promotes peristalsis and defecation. Bulky foods absorb fluids and increase stool mass. The increased mass stretches bowel walls, initiating peristalsis and the defecation reflex. Most people should have at least five servings of high-fiber foods each day.

Some foods have specific effects in the bowel. For example:

- The active bacteria in yogurt stimulate peristalsis, while at the same time promoting healing of intestinal infections.
- Low-fiber foods, such as pasta and other simple carbohydrates and lean meats, slow peristalsis.
- Foods such as broccoli, onions, and beans lead to excess gas in many people. Spicy foods may also cause gas as well as more frequent bowel movements.

Dietary Supplements Dietary supplements can also affect bowel function. For example:

- Calcium supplements may cause constipation.
- Magnesium loosens stools.
- Supplemental vitamin C softens stools and in high doses may cause diarrhea in sensitive clients.

Fluids A minimum of six to eight 8-ounce glasses (1,500 to 2,000 mL) of fluid per day is required to promote healthful bowel function.

- *Inadequate fluid intake or excessive fluid loss,* as in diarrhea or vomiting, slows peristalsis and leads to dry, hard stools that are difficult to pass (Fritz & Pitlick, 2012).

- *Excessive fluid intake* (especially beverages with high sugar content) may lead to rapid passage through the colon and soft or watery stools.
- *Different types of fluids* have varying effects on sensitive individuals. For instance, consuming large amounts of milk may cause constipation in some people. Coffee promotes peristalsis in many clients and may even cause loose stools in sensitive clients.

Activity Physical activity seems to stimulate peristalsis and bowel elimination. In addition, sedentary people are likely to have weaker abdominal muscles. Clients with health concerns that limit activity (e.g., shortness of breath, pain, or required bedrest) often experience constipation.

Medications

Many medications may affect peristalsis. All oral medicines have the potential to affect the function of the GI tract. Examples include the following:

- *Antacids,* often used for heartburn, neutralize stomach acid but may slow peristalsis.
- *Aspirin and other nonsteroidal anti-inflammatory drugs (NSAIDs),* such as naproxen and ibuprofen, irritate the stomach. Repeated use can lead to ulceration of the stomach or duodenum.
- *Antibiotics* given to combat infection decrease the normal flora in the colon. The result is often diarrhea. Bacterial populations can be maintained with supplements of probiotics (e.g., acidophilus) or daily consumption of yogurt (Salfi & Holt, 2012).
- *Iron,* a common mineral supplement, is available as an over-the-counter (OTC) medication and is often prescribed for the treatment of anemia. Iron has an astringent effect on the bowel and is notorious for causing constipation and changing stool color to black. It also causes nausea when taken when there is no food in the stomach.
- *Pain medications,* particularly opioids (narcotics), slow peristalsis and are associated with a high incidence of constipation.
- *Antimotility drugs,* such as diphenoxylate (Lomotil), may be used to treat diarrhea. They work by slowing peristalsis.
- *Laxatives* are used to treat constipation. In general, laxatives work by stimulating peristalsis (see Box 29-1). They are frequently abused by people who self-medicate with OTC drugs and so who may become dependent on them, requiring ever-increasing dosages until the intestine fails to work properly.

Surgery and Procedures

Clients undergoing anesthesia and surgery often experience sluggish bowel elimination. The delay in bowel elimination may be caused by a variety of circumstances:

Anesthesia General anesthesia (which renders the patient unconscious) and analgesics (administered preoperatively and postoperatively for pain) slow bowel motility. Spinal anesthesia and epidural anesthesia are less likely to cause this effect.

Stress Regardless of the type of anesthesia, most clients find surgery a stressful event. As you may recall from Chapter 12, if stress activates the general adaptation syndrome, autonomic nervous system and endocrine responses ensue. Among those responses is a slowing of peristalsis.

Manipulation of the Bowel During Surgery Abdominal or pelvic surgery in which the bowel is manipulated may result in a **paralytic ileus,** a cessation of bowel peristalsis.

- Although peristalsis halts, the bowel continues to produce secretions. The secretions remain stagnant, causing distention and discomfort.
- To decrease the complications of paralytic ileus, patients who have had bowel surgery typically have a nasogastric (NG) tube with low constant or intermittent suction. The NG tube removes secretions until peristalsis returns. To review insertion of an NG tube or management of a patient with an NG tube, refer to Procedure 28-2

Decreased Mobility After surgery, patients often experience discomfort that affects mobility. This further hinders GI motility and increases the risk for constipation.

Perineal Surgery Patients who have had surgical interventions involving the perineal region (e.g., an episiotomy after childbirth) may fear pain or that their sutures will "tear" or "break" during bowel elimination, and therefore they resist the urge to evacuate their bowel.

Anal Sphincter Surgery Patients who have had surgery that disrupts the anal sphincter may experience uncontrolled drainage after surgery.

BOX 29-1 ■ Types of Laxatives

- **Stool softeners** enable moisture and fat to penetrate the stool, thereby softening it and making it easier to pass. Effectiveness of stool softeners in relieving chronic constipation is being questioned, but they are still in use. *Example:* docusate sodium.
- **Osmotic laxatives** work by drawing water into the bowel from surrounding tissue, resulting in bowel distention. *Examples:* polyethylene glycol, lactulose.
- **Lubricant laxatives** coat the stool and the GI tract with a thin waterproof layer. Mineral oil is an example. Because the lubricant coats the entire GI tract, it may interfere with the absorption of nutrients. ✚ Mineral oil is potentially dangerous in debilitated patients. Inhaled droplets can lead to a form of pneumonia.
- **Stimulant laxatives** are bowel irritants. They irritate the intestinal wall, stimulating intense peristalsis. *Examples:* senna, bisacodyl, castor oil.

- **Bulking agents** are non-foods, high in fiber. They must be combined with sufficient fluid intake to be effective. The fiber attracts fluid into the colon, and the increased bulk of the stool stimulates the urge to evacuate. **KEY POINT:** *These are considered the safest form of laxative but may interfere with absorption of some medicines. They are the drug of choice for chronic constipation.* **Examples: *Metamucil, Citrucel, psyllium, FiberCon.***
- **Chloride channel activators** increase intestinal fluid and motility to help stool pass.
- **Combination laxatives** are laxatives that contain more than one type of laxative ingredient. The most common type is a combination stimulant laxative and stool softener.

Pregnancy

In early pregnancy, many women experience fluid loss due to "morning sickness"—periods of nausea and vomiting. As the pregnancy progresses, the growing uterus crowds and displaces the intestines and, along with the increased level of progesterone, slows intestinal motility. As a result, pregnant women often experience constipation, decreased appetite, and irregular food intake. In addition, the increasing pressure of the uterus and the increased blood volume of normal pregnancy increase the woman's risk for hemorrhoids.

ThinkLike a Nurse 29-3

- Review the case of Mrs. Zeno (Meet Your Patient). What factors may be affecting her bowel elimination?
- What additional information do you need?

Pathological Conditions

Several disorders affect bowel function. Among them are the following:

- Neurological disorders that affect innervation of the lower GI tract

---

PICOT

Constipation in Pregnancy

Situation: A 27-year-old pregnant client has a history of constipation, gas, and general abdominal discomfort after eating. She reports increasing her dietary intake of fluid and fiber, but with limited results. Focused assessment reveals hypoactive bowel sounds and a firm abdomen. The client is anxious about taking medication during pregnancy. The nurse wants to learn more about nonpharmacological interventions for constipation.

PICOT Components

P	Population/client	=	Pregnant women
I	Intervention/indicator	=	Increased physical activity
C	Comparator/control	=	Fiber and liquids only
O	Outcome	=	Relief from constipation
T	Time	=	During pregnancy

Searchable Question: Do _____(P) who receive _____(I), as compared to _____(C) demonstrate _____(O) during _____(T)?

Example of Evidence: The effect of hormones on the bowel, as well as the increased iron intake in prenatal vitamins, often causes early pregnancy constipation. The increasing size of the uterus and decreased maternal activity can further contribute to constipation. Many clients find relief with increased fiber and fluid intake. A commitment to daily exercise will also increase peristalsis, promoting fecal movement. The client on bedrest can also benefit with thigh-strengthening and ROM exercises.

Application to Practice: The nurse discusses with the client ways in which she can incorporate increased physical activity into her lifestyle during pregnancy.

Reference: Trottier, M., Erebara, A., & Bozzo, P. (2012). Treating constipation during pregnancy. *Canadian Family Physician, 58*(8), 836–838.

- Cognitive conditions that limit the ability to sense the urge to defecate
- Pain
- Immobility that leads to sluggish peristalsis
- Pathological conditions of the GI tract. Constipation and diarrhea are discussed in the Nursing Diagnosis section of the chapter.

The following are three common disorders that affect bowel function:

Food Allergies The National Institute of Allergy and Infectious Diseases (NIAID) characterizes a **food allergy** as a true immune system reaction prompted by the presence in the body of an allergenic food (NIAID, 2001, updated 2015).

- *Some common food allergens* include dairy products, egg whites, shellfish, gluten, peanuts and other nuts, citrus fruits, and soy.
- *Immune responses to foods* manifest as a variety of symptoms ranging from a mild rash to anaphylactic shock.
- *Common GI symptoms* suggesting food allergy include constipation; diarrhea; a red, blistering rash around the anus; abdominal discomfort; bloating; excessive gas; and intestinal bleeding (Bird, Lack, & Perry, 2015).

Food Intolerances In contrast to a food allergy, **food intolerance** is specifically linked to the GI system. It produces symptoms, such as GI discomfort, pain, gas, bloating, diarrhea, or constipation after the person consumes the food. Such symptoms can mimic those of a food allergy, but food intolerances are not caused by immune responses. An example is *lactose intolerance,* a deficiency of the enzyme lactase, which is responsible for the breakdown of milk sugar (lactose).

Diverticulosis When the colon must repeatedly move highly compacted fecal material, over time the longitudinal and circular muscles enlarge. This increases force on the mucosal tissues, causing them to "balloon" out between the muscles and to form small sac-like pouches in the mucosa, in which fecal matter becomes trapped. This is called **diverticulosis. Diverticulitis** is a condition in which the pouches become infected. Antibiotic therapy or surgery is required. People whose diets are low in fiber or consist mainly of refined foods are especially at risk for diverticulosis. Obesity and red meat intake are also risk factors (Humes, 2012).

KnowledgeCheck 29-2

- What is a normal defecation pattern?
- Identify the factors that affect bowel elimination.

WHAT IS A BOWEL DIVERSION?

Many pathologies affecting the GI tract can be treated with medication (e.g., laxatives, anti-inflammatory drugs). However, some conditions, such as cancer, ulcerations, trauma, or inadequate blood supply may require a **bowel diversion:** a surgically created opening for elimination of digestive waste products. A client with a bowel diversion does not eliminate via the anus. Instead, the **effluent** (output, fecal material) is expelled through a surgically created opening in the abdominal wall, called a **stoma** or **ostomy.** The effluent may range from liquid to solid, depending on the part of the bowel that is being diverted.

Bowel diversions may be temporary or permanent.

- *Temporary bowel diversions* may be done to allow part of the intestine to rest and heal. Once healing has occurred, surgical **reanastomosis** (reconnection) of the bowel is performed, and the patient once again has BMs from the anus.

- *Permanent bowel diversions* are performed if the bowel is necrotic (dead) or cannot be salvaged because of severe disease or trauma.

Ileostomy

An **ileostomy** brings a portion of the ileum through a surgical opening in the abdomen, bypassing the large intestine entirely. Because most of the water is absorbed from the feces in the large intestine, drainage at this level is liquid and continuous. The patient must wear an ostomy appliance at all times to collect the drainage.

Some variations of ileostomy are designed to control drainage more effectively and to cause less body image disturbance. However, many clients are not candidates for these procedures because of their underlying disease.

- A **Kock pouch,** or **continent ileostomy,** creates an internal pouch, or reservoir, to collect ileal drainage (Fig. 29-5A). To drain the pouch, the patient inserts a tube through the external stoma into the pouch several times per day. This alternative avoids continuous drainage, so the patient does not need to wear an ostomy appliance.
- A **total colectomy with ileoanal reservoir** is a surgical procedure in which the colon is removed, a pouch is created from the ileum, and the ileum is connected to the rectum (Fig. 29-5B). The patient evacuates the bowel on the commode in the usual manner. Although this procedure should result in continence of bowel elimination, the feces will still be liquid.

Colostomy

A **colostomy** is a surgical procedure that brings a portion of the colon through a surgical opening in the abdomen. The location of the colostomy determines the consistency of the feces eliminated as well as the need to wear an ostomy appliance (Fig. 29-6).

- *The closer the colostomy is to the* **ascending colon and the ileocecal valve** (between the small and large intestine) (see Fig. 29-3), the more liquid and continuous the drainage will be.
- In contrast, *a colostomy* **close to the sigmoid colon** will produce solid feces.
- *Colostomies* **near the rectum,** such as sigmoid colostomies, can often be controlled by diet and irrigation. As a result, the client may not need to wear an ostomy appliance to collect drainage.

A colostomy created in the transverse colon is usually temporary and may be either a double-barreled or loop colostomy.

- A **double-barreled colostomy** (Fig. 29-6C) has two separate stomas that externalize the bowel on both sides of the portion that has been removed. The proximal stoma is the functioning end that drains fecal material. The distal stoma may drain mucus and is sometimes called a mucous fistula.
- A **loop colostomy** (Fig. 29-7) consists of a segment of bowel brought out to the abdominal wall. The posterior wall of the bowel remains intact, but a plastic rod is wedged under the bowel to keep it from slipping back into the abdomen.

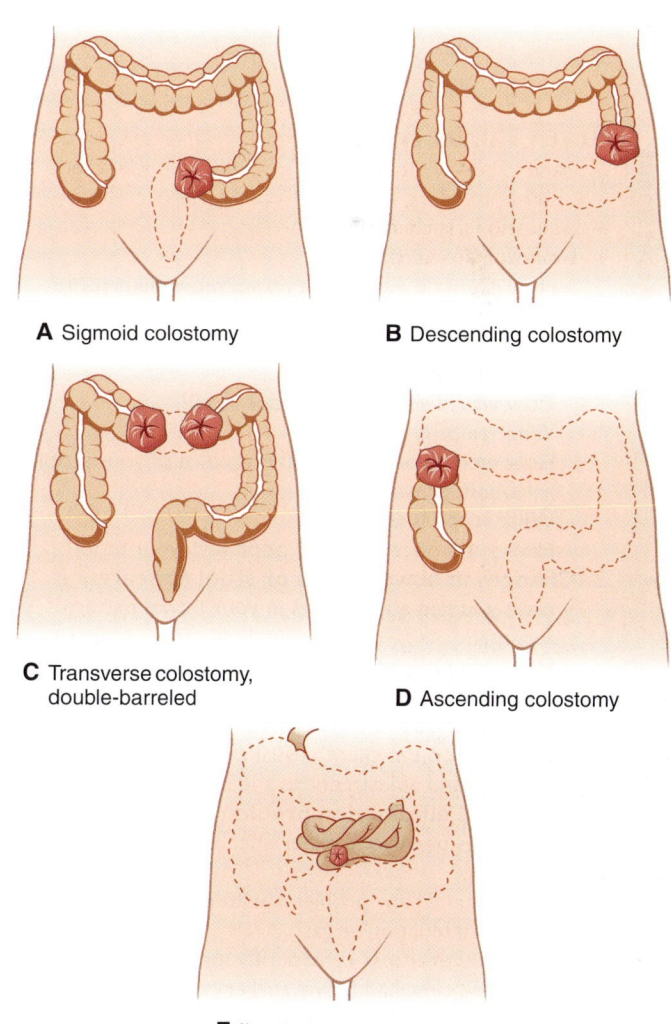

A Sigmoid colostomy   **B** Descending colostomy

C Transverse colostomy, double-barreled

D Ascending colostomy

E Ileostomy

FIGURE 29-6 A–E. Location of various bowel diversion ostomies. Shaded areas indicate sections of the bowel that are removed or being "rested."

FIGURE 29-5 Ileostomy variations. A. Continent ileostomy (Kock pouch). B. Ileoanal reservoir.

Small bowel

Abdominal wall

Stoma

Ileal pouch

A

Ileum

Ileoanal reservoir

Ileal-anal anastomosis

B

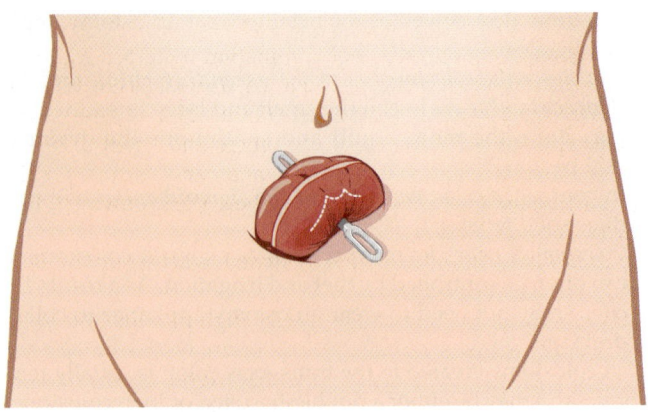

FIGURE 29-7 A loop colostomy.

The anterior wall is incised, and the mucosal surface is left visible and open to air. It, too, has a functioning proximal end and limited drainage from the distal end.

KnowledgeCheck 29-3

- What changes in bowel elimination are associated with constipation? With diarrhea?

- Why are bowel diversions performed?
- What determines the nature of the effluent from a bowel diversion?

PracticalKnowledge
knowing **how**

As a nurse, you will work collaboratively with the healthcare team to facilitate normal bowel function in well and ill clients. In the remainder of the chapter, we discuss teaching, monitoring, and assisting clients with bowel function.

ASSESSMENT NP

For a list of questions to use, as well as complete details of a focused physical assessment of bowel function see the accompanying Focused Assessment box, Bowel Elimination.

Focused Nursing History

Because bowel patterns vary, you will need a nursing history to determine what is normal for each client. As you interview clients, pay attention to their reactions to your questions. Many people are embarrassed about discussing bowel function. Tailor your assessment to the client's needs, and use language that

---

Focused Assessment

Bowel Elimination

Nursing History

Ask questions, such as the following:

1. **Normal bowel pattern**
   - How often do you have a bowel movement (BM)?
   - What time of day do you usually have a BM?
   - Do you follow any routines to help you have a BM?
2. **Appearance of stool**
   - How would you describe your stool?
   - What color is your stool?
   - How would you describe the texture of your stool—hard, soft, or watery?
   - What shape is the stool?
   - Have you noticed unusual odor with your stool?
3. **Changes in bowel habits or stool appearance**
   - Have you had any changes in your bowel pattern recently?
   - Have you noticed any changes in the appearance, texture, or odor of your stool?
4. **For clients with a bowel diversion,** you will also gather data on the client's usual care of the stoma, use of appliances, and adjustment to the ostomy.
5. **History of elimination problems**
   - What has been your experience with bowel elimination problems?
   - Have you had any problems with constipation, diarrhea, or severe bloating or gas?
   - Have you ever lost control of your bowels?
   - Have you ever had bowel surgery or diagnostic procedures of the digestive tract?
6. **Use of bowel elimination aids,** including diet, exercise, medications, and remedies
   - What aids, if any, do you use to help you have a BM?
   - What foods help you maintain your bowel pattern?

   - What foods do you avoid? What effect do these foods have on you?
   - What is your usual fluid intake over the course of a day?
   - What is your usual exercise pattern?
   - What medications are you taking? Have they had any effect on your bowel elimination pattern?
   - What is your current stress level? What effect does stress have on your bowel elimination pattern?

Physical Assessment

Examine the abdomen, rectum, and anus.
- Recall that in abdominal assessment, the order of the exam is inspection, auscultation, percussion, and palpation.
- Observe the size, shape, and contour of the abdomen and listen to bowel sounds.
- Percuss and palpate the abdomen for tenderness, presence of air or solid, and presence of masses.
- Inspect the anus for signs of hemorrhoids.
- Depending on the policies of your institution as well as your skill with assessment, you might also palpate the anus and rectum for the presence of stool or masses.
- When listening to bowel sounds, note the presence and timing of the sounds and the presence of any bruits. Note whether bowel sounds are normal, hyperactive, hypoactive, or absent.
- If, after listening for 3 to 5 minutes, you hear no bowel sounds, you should listen in several areas before describing them as absent.

  For a complete discussion of physical examination of the abdomen, rectum, and anus,

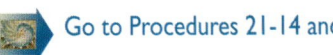 Go to Procedures 21-14 and 21-19.

makes her comfortable. Remember to ask about her medications because many have the potential to cause constipation (e.g., calcium and iron supplements). The following are examples of medications associated with constipation:

Antacids containing aluminum hydroxide or calcium carbonate

Anticholinergic drugs (e.g., belladonna)

Anticonvulsant drugs (e.g., phenytoin)

Antidiarrheals (e.g., loperamide)

Antihistamines (e.g., diphenhydramine)

Antiparkinsonian drugs (e.g., amantadine hydrochloride)

Antipsychotic drugs (e.g., chlorpromazine)

Calcium channel blockers (e.g., verapamil hydrochloride)

Diuretics (e.g., furosemide)

Iron supplements

Lithium

Nonsteroidal anti-inflammatory drugs (e.g., ibuprofen)

Opioids (e.g., morphine, codeine)

Sympathomimetics (e.g., ephedrine)

Tricyclic antidepressants (e.g., nortriptyline)

For clients with a bowel diversion, also gather data on the client's usual care of the stoma, use of appliances, and adjustment to the ostomy.

Focused Physical Assessment

Physical assessment for bowel elimination includes examination of the abdomen, rectum, and anus, as well as characteristics of normal and abnormal stool (Table 29-1). Observe the size, shape, and contour of the abdomen, and listen to bowel sounds. You might also palpate the anus and rectum for the presence of stool or masses. You may hear the following when auscultating the abdomen,

- *Normal bowel sounds* are high pitched, with approximately 5 to 15 gurgles every minute.
- *Hyperactive bowel sounds* are very high pitched and more frequent than normal. They may occur with small bowel obstruction and inflammatory disorders. They indicate hyperperistalsis, which can result in diarrhea.
- *Hypoactive bowel sounds* are low pitched, infrequent, and quiet. A decrease in bowel sounds indicates decreased peristalsis, which can result in constipation.
- *Absent bowel sounds.* If you hear no bowel sounds after listening in a quadrant for 3 to 5 minutes, you should listen in several areas before describing them as *absent*. Absent bowel sounds indicate a lack of intestinal activity, which may occur after abdominal surgery and may indicate a paralytic ileus.

Table 29-1 ▶ Normal Characteristics of Feces and Variations

STOOL CHARACTERISTIC	CONDITION	AGE-GROUP	DESCRIPTION
Frequency	Normal	Infants*	Bottle-fed—1 to 3 stools/day Breastfed—4 to 6 stools/day
		Adults	Daily; 2–3 BMs/wk
	Variations (Hypermotility)	Infants*	> 6 stools/day
		Adults	> 3 stools/day
	Variations (Hypomotility)	Infants*	Bottle-fed— < 1 stool every day or two Breastfed— < 1 stool/week
		Adults	< 1 stool/wk
Color	Normal	Infants*	Dark green (1st wk); then yellow
		Adults	Brown
	Variations		*Bile* pigment gives feces its brown color. Infant stools are yellow because of their rapid passage.
			White or clay-colored stool may indicate absence of bile (e.g., as in bile duct obstruction) or use of some antacids.
			Light brown stool may indicate diet high in milk products and low in meat.
			Pale, fatty stool may indicate malabsorption of fat.
			Black, tarry stool (**melena**) may indicate use of iron medications or upper GI bleeding; eating large quantities of red meat, spinach, and dark green vegetables may cause feces to be almost black.
			Red stool may indicate bleeding in lower intestinal tract or hemorrhoids.
			Stool darkens the longer it is left standing after defecation.

(Continued)

Table 29-1 ➤ Normal Characteristics of Feces and Variations—cont'd

STOOL CHARACTERISTIC	CONDITION	AGE-GROUP	DESCRIPTION
Quantity	Normal	Adults	Approximately 150 g/day
	Variations		Quantity varies with amount of food eaten, from 100 to 400 g per day.
Shape	Normal		Approximately the diameter of the rectum: about 2.5 cm (1 in.) in diameter
	Variations		Narrow, pencil-shaped stool may indicate intestinal obstruction or constriction or rapid peristalsis.
			Small, marble-shaped stool may indicate slow peristalsis, with longer time in the large intestine.
Consistency	Normal		Formed, soft, moist
	Variations		Consistency is related to gastric motility and is affected by food and fluid intake.
			Hard stool indicates constipation. The more time the stool spends in the large intestine, the more water is reabsorbed and the harder the stool. May also indicate dehydration.
			Liquid stool may indicate diarrhea; rapid peristalsis (e.g., from infection).
Odor	Normal		Pungent; affected by foods eaten
	Variations		Normal odor is created by putrefaction and fermentation in the lower GI tract. Odor is also influenced by the pH of the stool, which is normally neutral or slightly alkaline.
			Strong, foul odors may indicate blood in the stool, especially in the upper GI tract, or infection.

*All information about infant stool patterns applies after passage of meconium.

KnowledgeCheck 29-4

- What should you discuss with your client when performing a nursing history focused on bowel elimination?
- Describe the physical assessment you would perform for a client with constipation.

Diagnostic Tests

Several diagnostic tests may be performed to assess for bowel elimination problems (e.g., to screen for colorectal cancer, to diagnose diverticulosis). They may be classified as direct or indirect.

- **Indirect visualization studies** are radiographic views of the lower GI tract. The simplest of the tests is an abdominal flat plate, an anterior to posterior x-ray view of the abdomen used to detect gallstones, fecal impaction, and distended bowel.
- **Direct visualization studies** are used for diagnostic and treatment purposes. They are invasive procedures and are conducted by a gastroenterologist, who inserts various instruments (e.g., *endoscopes*) to examine the interior of the GI tract. The nurse's role during these studies is to prepare the patient for the test, function as an assistant, and provide aftercare.

For nursing care of patients undergoing such diagnostic tests, see the two Diagnostic Testing boxes: Indirect Visualization Studies of the Gastrointestinal Tract and Direct Visualization Studies of the Gastrointestinal Tract.

ThinkLike a Nurse 29-4

A client asks you why he must perform a bowel prep with a strong laxative before having a colonoscopy. How might you reply?

Laboratory Studies of Stool

Stool specimens may be analyzed to detect blood, infection, or parasitic infestation. A small sample is obtained and sent to the laboratory for analysis or analyzed at the bedside. To obtain a specimen from an infant or young child, you will collect freshly passed feces from a diaper.

Handling Stool Specimens

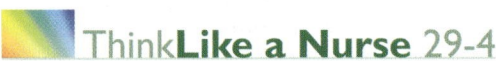 Wear clean gloves when you handle the container or manipulate stool specimens. Use tongue blades to transfer the stool specimen to the container provided by the lab. Do not contaminate the outside of the specimen container.

Diagnostic Testing

Indirect Visualization Studies of the Gastrointestinal tract

Abdominal Flat Plate

An anterior-to-posterior x-ray view of the abdomen used to detect gallstones, fecal impaction, and distended bowel. This test requires no preparation and no special post-test care.

Barium Enema (BE)

Radiological examination of the rectum, colon, and distal small bowel. A rectal tube is inserted into the rectum or an existing ostomy. Barium (a contrast medium) is instilled. The patient must retain the barium through several position changes while air is instilled and radiographs are obtained. The test is especially useful for visualizing polyps, diverticula, and tumors. In addition, it may be used to reduce certain obstructions. As a rule, patients are not sedated.

Preparation

➤ The test is invasive, so a signed informed consent is necessary.
➤ Patient instructions: Low-residue diet for several days prior to the procedure; consume only clear liquids the evening before the procedure; NPO for 8 hours before the test; possibly avoid dairy products that day.
➤ Administer a laxative, suppository, or cleansing enema the day before the test and cleansing enemas on the morning of the procedure (check agency policy). Enema administration is discussed in this chapter. For complete instructions for inserting a suppository, see Chapter 26, Procedure 26-6.

Post-Test Care

➤ The patient may have bloating and cramping after the test and will probably feel the need to empty her bowels as soon as the test is done.
➤ Instruct the client to resume food, fluids, and medications withheld before the procedure.
➤ Instruct the client to take a mild laxative and increase fluid intake (four glasses) to aid in elimination of barium (unless contraindicated). Barium can cause constipation for a few days.
➤ Explain that stools will be white or light colored for 2 to 3 days; if patient is unable to eliminate barium, she should call the physician.

Ultrasonography (Ultrasound)

Detects tissue abnormalities such as masses, cysts, edema, or stones. An ultrasound probe (a transducer) is moved over the skin surface of the abdomen. The probe emits a sound wave that abdominal tissue and organs reflect back based on their density. The sound waves may be transformed into images visible on a computer screen.

Computed Tomography (CT) Scan

Useful in diagnosis of many abdominal disorders. Examines body sections from different angles using a narrow x-ray beam and produces a three-dimensional picture of the area of the body being scanned. The patient needs to lie very still during the procedure. A CT scan may be enhanced by injecting contrast dye for improved visualization of circulatory function.

Preparation

If contrast dye is to be used:
➤ Determine that the patient is not allergic to contrast medium, iodine, or shellfish.
➤ Check blood urea nitrogen and creatinine levels to ensure adequate kidney function.
➤ Patients taking metformin (Glucophage) should discontinue it on the day of the test and withhold it for 48 hours after to prevent lactic acidosis.
➤ Restrict food and fluids for 6 to 8 hours if contrast medium is to be given.
➤ Sometimes the patient is asked to drink about 450 mL of a dilute barium solution 1 hour before the CT scan to distinguish GI from other abdominal organs.

During the Test

➤ Explain that the patient may feel nausea or warmth or experience a metallic taste or a transient headache after injection of contrast medium. Instruct the patient to take slow, deep breaths if this occurs.

Post-Test Care

➤ Patient may resume normal diet, activity, and medication.
➤ Renal function should be assessed before metformin (Glucophage) is restarted.
➤ The patient should increase fluid intake to help eliminate contrast medium.
➤ Diarrhea may occur after ingestion of oral contrast medium.
➤ Observe for delayed allergic reactions (e.g., hives, headache, nausea, vomiting) if contrast medium was used.

Magnetic Resonance Imaging (MRI)

Produces cross-sectional images of the body. MRI utilizes a strong magnetic field and radio waves. This type of diagnostic test does not use ionizing radiation, so it is free of the hazards of x-rays. MRIs are very sensitive and may be used to detect edema, hemorrhage, blood flow, infarcts, tumors, and infections in organ structures. When used, the contrast medium is noniodinated, administered intravenously to enhance contrast between normal and abnormal tissues. The patient must lie still in a narrow tube, sometimes for up to an hour.

Preparation

➤ Determine the presence of metal in the body, such as shrapnel or flecks of ferrous metal in the eye.
➤ Instruct the patient to remove all external metallic objects before entering the scanning room (e.g., jewelry, body piercing rings, eyeglasses, hairpins, credit cards).
➤ Food and fluids are not always restricted. The patient may be NPO for 4 to 6 hours before the exam.
➤ Have the patient void before the procedure.

Post-Test Care

➤ The patient can resume normal activity, medication, and diet.
➤ If a contrast medium was used, observe for delayed allergic reactions.

Source: Van Leeuwen, A., Poelhuis-Leth, D., & Bladh, M. (2015). *Davis's comprehensive handbook of laboratory and diagnostic tests with nursing implications* (6th ed.). Philadelphia, PA: F. A. Davis.

Direct Visualization Studies of the Gastrointestinal Tract

➤ These studies are invasive procedures; ensure that the patient has signed an informed consent.
➤ All of the tests require some degree of advance preparation, such as fasting. Check agency policy, as preparation may vary.
➤ Preparing the patient always includes telling him what he will experience and feel during the test.
➤ When the patient is sedated (e.g., with midazolam or diazepam), a crash cart must be in the room during the procedure and the patient monitored with pulse oximetry.
➤ All of the tests require teaching for aftercare.
➤ For all of these tests, explain that rectal bleeding is normal for a few days if polyps were removed or a biopsy was taken.

Esophagogastroduodenoscopy (EGD)

A *fiberoptic endoscope,* a long, flexible tube with a light and lens, is introduced through the mouth and advanced for direct visualization of the esophagus, stomach, and duodenum. The physician may also perform tissue biopsies or coagulate bleeding sites through the endoscope.

Preparation

➤ Instruct the patient to fast for 6 to 12 hours before the test (instructions usually are "NPO after midnight").
➤ Remove dentures and eyewear prior to the test.
➤ Because the tube is introduced through the mouth, patients often require sedation to limit gagging.

During the Test

➤ The patient will be sedated but awake.
➤ A local anesthetic will be sprayed into his mouth and throat to lessen the gag reflex.

Post-Test Care

➤ Check vital signs and gag reflex (per agency protocol).
➤ Keep the patient NPO until the gag reflex returns; then instruct him to eat lightly during the next 12 to 24 hours.
➤ Instruct the patient to resume normal activity, medications, and diet in 24 hours.
➤ Observe, and teach patient to observe, for Potential Complication: esophageal or bowel perforation—cyanosis, substernal or abdominal pain, vomiting blood, continuing difficulty swallowing, or black, tarry stools.
➤ Explain to the patient that he will have a sore throat and hoarseness for a few days. Suggest gargling with saltwater and using throat lozenges.
➤ Caution the patient to notify the physician immediately if he experiences severe pain, fever, difficulty breathing, or expectoration of blood.
➤ Inform the patient that belching, bloating, or flatulence is a result of introducing air into the intestine and will be temporary.

Sigmoidoscopy

A rigid metal scope or a flexible fiber-optic scope is used to visualize the anal canal, rectum, and sigmoid colon. The patient is usually not sedated. During the exam, the physician may perform a biopsy, remove polyps (small growths), or coagulate sources of bleeding in the area. This procedure is also used as a screen for colon cancer.

Preparation

➤ A light meal before the test may be allowed. For flexible sigmoidoscopy, the patient may be asked to follow a clear liquid diet for a day before the exam.
➤ Administer two commercially prepared, small-volume enemas before the test.
➤ For a flexible sigmoidoscopy, a strong laxative solution may also be prescribed.
➤ Have the patient void before the procedure.

During the Test

➤ Drape the patient for modesty.
➤ The patient may feel pressure, cramping, or the urge to defecate; encourage slow, deep breathing through the mouth to help alleviate the feeling.

Post-Test Care

➤ Observe for potential complication: bowel perforation (see discussion of EGD).
➤ The patient may resume normal activity.
➤ Explain that air was introduced into the intestines to distend them for better visibility and that this may cause gas pains or flatulence for a few hours.
➤ A small amount of blood in the first bowel movement is normal. Notify the physician of significant bleeding.

Fiber-Optic Colonoscopy

Provides direct visualization of the rectum, colon, entire large intestine, and distal small bowel. A flexible scope is inserted through the rectum and advanced to the cecum. Colonoscopy is useful in detecting lower GI disease. It is also often used for cancer screening instead of a sigmoidoscopy, because colonoscopy provides better visualization of the colon. This is the preferred test for clients with suspected problems above the level of the sigmoid colon.

Preparation

➤ The colon and rectum must be empty and clean so the physician can view the linings during the exam. Practitioners have different colon-cleansing routines to achieve this, such as the following:
  ➤ Instruct the patient to take strong cathartic and laxative (e.g., Dulcolax) tablets the day before the test and an enema on day of the test, until returns are clear.
➤ Instruct the patient to consume a clear liquid diet for 24 to 48 hours before test (nothing red or purple) and to remain NPO after midnight the night before the exam.
➤ The patient will be sedated before the test, so she may need someone to drive her home.

During the Test

➤ Position the patient on her side with knees flexed. Drape for modesty.
➤ Monitor vital signs.
➤ The patient may feel pressure, cramping, or the urge to defecate; encourage slow, deep breathing through the mouth to help alleviate the feeling.

Diagnostic Testing

Direct Visualization Studies of the Gastrointestinal Tract—cont'd

Post-Test Care

➤ Monitor vital signs (per agency protocol).
➤ Observe for Potential Complication: Bowel perforation (see discussion of EGD).
➤ Explain that air was introduced into the intestines to distend them for better visibility and that, as a result, the patient may experience gas pains or flatulence for a few hours.

➤ Instruct the patient to resume a normal diet when she has recovered from sedation.

Sources: American Cancer Society. (2011, revised 2016). Detailed guide: Colon and rectum cancer. Retrieved from http://www.cancer.org/acs/groups/cid/documents/webcontent/003096-pdf.pdf; Van Leeuwen, A., Poelhuis-Leth, D., & Bladh, M. (2015). *Davis's comprehensive handbook of laboratory and diagnostic tests with nursing implications* (6th ed.). Philadelphia, PA: F. A. Davis.

Except when testing for fecal occult blood (following), you will usually need approximately 2.5 cm (1 in.) of formed stool or 20 to 30 mL of liquid stool. If blood, mucus, or purulent material is present, be sure to include this with the sample. Transport the specimen to the laboratory as soon as possible, or consult the laboratory for appropriate storage. Usually you will need to refrigerate the specimen until it can be received in the lab.

Testing for Fecal Occult Blood

Blood from the GI tract may be visible to the eye or **occult** (hidden) especially when passed through the stool from higher up in the intestine. You can perform the test for occult blood at the bedside, although some institutions require that it be done in the laboratory. This is called a *guaiac* or *fecal occult blood* test. It requires use of a reagent that detects the presence of **peroxidase,** an enzyme present in hemoglobin. Only a small smear of stool is required. For home testing, remind patients to wash their hands before and after collecting stool. For the complete procedure, refer to Procedure 29-1.

Screening can detect colorectal polyps so they can be removed before becoming cancerous. Regular screening for colorectal cancer is key to preventing colorectal cancer. The U.S. Preventive Services Task Force (2014) recommends screening for colorectal cancer using stool for occult blood testing and sigmoidoscopy or colonoscopy beginning at age 50 (or at age 40 for high-risk patients who should also consider genetic testing) and until age 75 years.

Assessing for Pinworms

Pinworms (an intestinal parasite) are small, white, thread-like worms that spread through human-to-human transmission:

- By ingesting (swallowing) infectious pinworm eggs
- By entry through the anus (e.g., when eggs attach to a person's fingers and are transferred to the anal area by scratching or touching the anus)

Once present, the pinworms live in the cecum. They come to the anal area to deposit eggs during the night and migrate back up through the rectum during the day.

- In assessing a child, you can spread the buttocks while the child is sleeping and examine the anus to see whether any pinworms are visible to the naked eye.
- You can also test for the presence of the eggs with tape. In the morning, as soon as the patient awakens, press clear cellophane tape against the anal opening. Remove the tape immediately and place it adhesive side down on a slide.
- Alternatively, or in addition, insert a cotton-tipped swab gently into the rectum for not more than 2.5 cm (1 in.). Smear

the specimen on a slide for microscopic inspection for parasites and eggs.

- You may also check at night by using a flashlight. The test may need to be repeated on consecutive days.

ThinkLike a Nurse 29-5

You are reviewing a client's chart and note that the client was tested for fecal occult blood. The results are as follows:

3/10/18 negative for occult blood
3/11/18 no BM
3/12/18 no BM
3/13/18 no BM
3/14/18 positive for occult blood
3/15/18 negative for occult blood
3/16/18 negative for occult blood

What can you conclude? What questions do these findings raise?

ANALYSIS/NURSING DIAGNOSIS NP

Common NANDA-I nursing diagnoses related to bowel elimination include the following:

- *Bowel Incontinence* is a change in normal bowel habits characterized by involuntary passage of stool. It is more common among women and older adults. Other risk factors include neurological diseases, stroke, sphincter damage, and inflammatory bowel disease. (See the Example Problem: Bowel Incontinence, later in this chapter.)
- *Constipation.* Because frequency of bowel elimination varies, constipation is usually defined as a decrease in the frequency of bowel movements resulting in the passage of hard, dry stool. Constipation can be a temporary problem wherein symptoms resolve in a short time. Nearly everyone experiences constipation at some point.
- *Chronic constipation* typically lasts 3 months or longer and may persist for years. Unrelieved constipation may eventually result in **a fecal impaction,** in which dry, hard stools lodged in the rectum cannot be passed. (See the Example Problem: Constipation, later in the chapter.)
- *Risk for Constipation* is an appropriate diagnosis for clients at increased risk because of bedrest, medications such as opioids, or surgery. You might use this diagnosis for a client with a condition or taking medications known to decrease peristalsis.
- *Perceived Constipation* is an appropriate diagnosis for a client who makes a self-diagnosis of constipation and uses laxatives, suppositories, or enemas to ensure a daily bowel movement.

- *Diarrhea* is the passage of loose, unformed, or watery stools. (See the Example Problem: Diarrhea, later in the chapter.)
- *Dysfunctional Gastrointestinal Motility* is a broad label that encompasses increased, decreased, ineffective, or absent peristaltic activity within the GI system. If you use this label, you need to specify whether the GI motility is increased or decreased.
- *Toileting Self-Care* is impaired ability to perform or complete own toileting activities.

For NANDA-I definitions of these diagnoses, consult a nursing diagnosis handbook or

 Go to Davis Advantage, Resources, **Chapter 29, Alphabetical List of NANDA-I Diagnoses.**

Bowel elimination problems may also form the etiology of other nursing diagnoses and collaborative problems. Examples include the following:
- Social isolation r/t embarrassment secondary to bowel incontinence
- Potential Complication: Electrolyte imbalance secondary to diarrhea. Older adults, very young children, and infants are at especially high risk.
- Impaired Skin Integrity r/t irritating effects of feces secondary to diarrhea
- Anxiety r/t perceived need for a daily bowel movement
- Disturbed Body Image r/t bowel diversion

ThinkLike a Nurse 29-6

- What data do you have about Mrs. Zeno's (Meet Your Patient) bowel function?
- What else would you like to know about her bowel function? What other symptoms often accompany these cues?
- Which NANDA-I nursing diagnosis best describes this cue cluster?
- In addition to this nursing diagnosis, what other data in the scenario might also be contributing to her infrequent BMs?
- From the scenario data, how would you describe the etiology of Mrs. Zeno's problem?
- What questions do you still have about the etiology?

PLANNING OUTCOMES/EVALUATION NP

The general bowel elimination goal is that the patient will have soft, formed bowel movements regularly.

NOC standardized outcomes associated with bowel problems include:
- **For Bowel Incontinence:** Bowel Continence; Tissue Integrity: Skin and Mucous Membranes
- **For Constipation:** Bowel Elimination; Ostomy Self Care
- **For Perceived Constipation:** Bowel Elimination
- **For Diarrhea:** Bowel Elimination; Continence; Symptom Severity
- **For Dysfunctional GI Motility:** Bowel Elimination; Gastrointestinal Function

Note that Bowel Elimination is a useful outcome for most bowel problems.

When bowel elimination is the etiology, choose outcomes linked to the problem side of the diagnosis. For example, for Impaired Skin Integrity r/t irritating effects of diarrhea stool, you would probably find the relevant NOC outcomes under the diagnosis, Tissue Integrity: Skin and Oral Mucous Membranes.

Individualized goals/outcome statements depend on the nursing diagnosis. Because normal bowel elimination patterns are individualized, regularity is based on the individual's pattern. Examples include the following:

Resumes normal bowel pattern by (date).

Discusses his feelings about his colostomy.

PLANNING INTERVENTIONS/ IMPLEMENTATION NP

 ♥ iCare Bowel elimination is a normal physiological function. It is important for you to convey an attitude of acceptance and display professionalism when providing care for patients with bowel elimination problems.

A few examples of *NIC standardized interventions and activities* for patients with bowel elimination problems include: Bowel Incontinence Care, Bowel Management, Constipation/Impaction Management, Diarrhea Management, Bowel Management, and Teaching: Individual. For a more comprehensive list of NIC interventions for various nursing diagnoses, consult a nursing diagnosis handbook or

 Go to Davis Advantage, Resources, **Chapter 29, List of NIC Interventions.**

Specific nursing activities to promote normal bowel function and relieve elimination problems are found in the following sections. Both independent and dependent interventions are discussed.

Promoting Normal or Regular Defecation

There are six independent nursing activities for promoting regular defecation covered in the following sections: Provide privacy; assist with positioning; consider the timing of defecation; support the healthful intake of food and fluids; encourage exercise; and manage flatulence.

Provide Privacy

Try this exercise. Imagine that your class assignment for today is to stand in front of the classroom and describe to the class your normal pattern of defecation, including frequency, appearance, and other characteristics of the stool. How would you feel about that? Would you do it?

Although defecation is a normal physiological function, most patients consider it a very private matter. The following help to minimize embarrassment:
- *Take a matter-of-fact approach* to convey to patients that you are comfortable with this aspect of care.
- *Provide privacy* for your patient when discussing or providing care related to bowel elimination. When assisting a patient with bowel elimination, excuse visitors from the room, draw the dividing curtains in shared rooms, and close the door.
- *Control odors,* because many patients are embarrassed by the odor of bowel movements and therefore may ignore the urge to defecate. Using an aromatic spray or other odor-reducing product may help to reduce embarrassment.

Assist With Positioning

An upright seated or squatting position is the most comfortable for defecation and decreases the need to strain. See Procedure 29-2.
- When possible, assist the patient to the bathroom to use the toilet.
- Place a bedside commode next to the bed for patients who are unable to ambulate to the bathroom.

- A patient who must remain in bed should assume a semi-Fowler's position to use the bedpan. Patients who are unable to assume this position because of surgery, trauma, or other medical conditions must use supine or side-lying positions. These positions are unnatural for bowel elimination and place the patient at risk for constipation.
- Raise the siderails or provide an overhead trapeze so that the patient can grip them to maneuver on and off the bedpan.

Consider the Timing of Defecation

Recall that food entering the duodenum triggers mass peristalsis. As a result, the urge to defecate often occurs after meals.

- Advise patients not to ignore this urge, because doing so may result in constipation.
- For patients who are ambulatory, allow some free time after meals to use the restroom.
- Assist those who cannot toilet independently to ambulate to the bathroom or use the bedpan.
- **KEY POINT:** *Discuss with NAPs the need to offer assistance without waiting to be asked so that patients experience minimal delays.*

Support Healthful Intake of Food and Fluids

- **Diet Teaching.** Teach clients the importance of a balanced diet in promoting soft, formed, regular bowel movements.
- **Ample Fiber.** Encourage a daily intake of 25 to 30 g of fiber to attract water into the stool, and promote peristalsis. The diet should be rich in fresh fruits and vegetables (especially raw), whole-grain foods, flaxseeds, popcorn, dried beans, peas, and legumes. **KEY POINT:** *Adding fiber does not help to relieve* **opioid-induced** *constipation unless the patient's current intake is actually deficient.* In fact, excessive fiber might put the patient at risk for bowel obstruction due to the (1) opioid-induced decreased peristalsis, (2) delayed gastric emptying, and (3) prolonged intestinal transit time of the feces (Pitlick & Fritz, 2013).
- **Adequate Fluid.** Without adequate fluid intake, a high-fiber diet can actually cause constipation. Recommend a minimum intake of 1,500 mL of fluid per day to (1) keep stool soft and (2) aid in production of mucus to lubricate the colon. Ideally, a person should drink eight to ten 8-ounce glasses of fluid daily (2,000 to 2,400 mL).
- **Water Is Preferred.** Water is the preferred fluid because soda, coffee, and tea often contain caffeine or additives that promote diuresis. However, because the diuretic effect of these fluids is minimal, they are acceptable for clients who simply will not drink enough plain water.

Encourage Exercise

Physical activity increases peristalsis and promotes defecation.

- Encourage patients to exercise three to five times per week and to engage in daily walking or light activity.
- Assist patients to ambulate as soon as their condition permits. Even limited activity, such as getting out of bed or walking 10 feet, decreases the risk for constipation.
- Provide range-of-motion (ROM) exercises for patients who must remain on bedrest. Even passive ROM (the joints are moved through ROM by the nurse) promotes peristalsis. Chapter 33 provides additional information about activity and ROM exercises, if you need it.

  For clients who can assist with exercise, the following exercises promote abdominal and perineal strength:
- *Thigh strengthening.* Have the client slowly bring one knee up to his chest, briefly hold it, then lower the leg to the bed.

Repeat this pattern alternating legs. Encourage the client to perform this exercise several times per hour while he is awake.
- *Abdominal tightening.* Have the client tighten and hold the abdominal muscles for a count of five and then relax. This core exercise works the abdominal muscles used during defecation.

Manage Flatulence

Recall that flatus is a natural by-product of digestion. When gas is excessive or leads to complaints of abdominal distention, cramping, or discomfort, it is known as **flatulence.**

- Some people develop flatulence after eating gas-producing foods, such as beans, cabbage, cauliflower, onions, or highly spiced foods. For others, flatulence occurs when fiber intake is increased.
- Flatulence is one of the cluster of symptoms of irritable bowel syndrome.
- Constipation is often accompanied by flatulence because digestive by-products undergo prolonged fermentation in the colon.

  Use the following interventions to help clients manage flatulence:
- Teach clients to be aware of and avoid foods that trigger flatulence.
- Teach clients to follow self-care strategies (identified earlier) for maintaining regular bowel movements.
- Encourage patients who have had surgery with gaseous anesthesia to ambulate and perform bed exercises to stimulate peristalsis and the passage of gas.
- In severe cases, you may need to insert a rectal tube to aid in the elimination of flatus (see Procedure 29-5).

Teach Clients When to See a Primary Care Provider

Many GI symptoms are normal and do not require treatment. For example, everyone has excessive flatus and abdominal distention at some time—perhaps as a result of a high-fat, high-sugar meal. And it is common for bowel movements occasionally to become a little irregular. However, clients need to know when a symptom may be signaling a more serious condition.

> ✚ Teach clients to see their primary care provider for the following reasons if a symptom lasts longer than 3 weeks or is disabling:
> - Blood in the stool (unless they have hemorrhoids and this is not an unusual occurrence for them)
> - Severe stomach pain
> - Change in bowel habits
> - Unintended weight loss
> - Constipation that is not relieved after trying fiber, fluids, and exercise

KnowledgeCheck 29-5

Identify at least five independent nursing actions that you can take to encourage regular elimination in a well client.

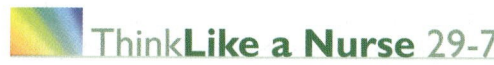

ThinkLike a Nurse 29-7

How could you facilitate regular bowel elimination for Mrs. Zeno (Meet Your Patient)? What information do you need?

INTERVENTIONS FOR EXAMPLE PROBLEM: DIARRHEA

Nursing interventions focus on treating the causes of the diarrhea, as well as monitoring and treating associated symptoms and defining characteristics. For more information about diarrhea, see the accompanying Example Problem: Diarrhea.

INTERVENTIONS FOR EXAMPLE PROBLEM: CONSTIPATION

Many of the nursing strategies to prevent and treat constipation are identical to the activities that promote regular bowel elimination.

- *Short-term constipation* is usually treated by lifestyle changes and may resolve without use of prescription medication. Many laxatives are readily available without prescription and are used by clients to treat actual or perceived constipation
- *Chronic constipation* usually involves some physiological dysfunction. When lifestyle modifications are ineffective in preventing and treating constipation, medications may be prescribed (see Box 29-1).
- *Fecal impaction* is the presence of a hardened, dry, fecal mass in the rectum. The impaction often blocks the passage of normal stool and sets up a vicious cycle of furthering hardening. Liquid stool may leak, seeping around the hardened mass, and the patient may report feelings of fullness, bloating, constipation, diminished appetite, and a change in bowel habits.

    Assessment: You can detect fecal impaction by digital examination of the rectum.

Treatment: Enemas; digital removal of stool

Prevention: Once the impaction has been removed, establish a bowel regimen to prevent recurrence of impactions.

For more complete information about caring for patients with constipation, refer to the Self-Care box Teaching Your Patient About Laxative Use and the accompanying Example Problem: Constipation.

Administering Enemas

An **enema** is the introduction of solution into the rectum to soften feces and distend or irritate the colon, in order to stimulate peristalsis and evacuation of feces. Responses to an enema are governed by the following conditions:

- The height of the solution container
- The speed of flow
- The concentration of the solution
- The resistance of the rectum.
    - Muscle tone and history of constipation or other bowel disorders determine the resistance of the rectum.
    - A client with a long history of constipation is more likely to be able to tolerate a large-volume enema, because the rectum and colon have become distended over time.
- Hypotonic and isotonic solutions are easier to retain.

    The primary care provider generally orders the specific type to administer to a patient (e.g., cleansing, retention, or return-flow). To learn how to administer various types of enemas, see Procedure 29-3.

Safe, Effective Nursing Care

Safe, Effective Nursing Care for Patients in Palliative Care

Competency: *Validate evidence-based research to incorporate in practice:* Incorporate into client care evidence-based findings.

Constipation is one of the most common problems in patients receiving palliative care and can cause extreme suffering and discomfort. While general principles of prevention should be followed, pharmacological treatment is often necessary. The combination of a softener and stimulant laxative is generally recommended, and the choice of laxatives should be made on an individual basis. Emphasis on evidence-based practice, quality improvement approaches, and further research is required to impact assessment, diagnosis, and management of constipation in palliative care.

Competency: *Provide safe quality client care:* Design a "Thinking, Caring, Doing" framework that incorporates a holistic approach to client care.

Recognize the patient or designee as the source of control and full partner in providing compassionate and coordinated care based on respect for the patient's preferences, values, and needs. The key is to strengthen the healthcare to include collaboration and improve health outcomes for patients.

Source: Pitlick, M., & Fritz, D. (2013). Evidence about the pharmacological management of constipation, Part 2: Implications for palliative care. *Home Healthcare Nurse, 31*(4), 207–216.

Self-Care

Teaching Your Patient About Laxative Use

Discuss the following topics with clients who have concerns about the frequency of their bowel movements or ask about laxatives:

1. The frequency of BMs may range from several times per day to once per week. As long as stools are passed without excessive urgency, with minimal effort and no straining, and without the use of laxatives, bowel function may be regarded as normal.
2. To maintain normal bowel function:
    - Eat a well-balanced diet that includes five servings of whole grains, fresh fruits, and vegetables.
    - Drink eight to ten 8-oz. glasses of fluid per day between 1900 and 2400.
    - Engage in daily exercise to stimulate peristalsis.
    - Set aside uninterrupted time after breakfast or dinner for using the toilet.
    - Do not ignore the urge to defecate.
    - Whenever there is a significant or prolonged change in bowel habits, report this to your healthcare provider.
3. If you are experiencing constipation, choose bulking agents, such as Metamucil or psyllium, to treat the problem rather than other over-the-counter laxatives. Be sure to drink plenty of water when using bulking agents.
4. Habitual laxative use, except for bulking agents, may cause reliance on medications for bowel elimination and, ironically, may lead to further constipation.

EXAMPLE PROBLEM: Diarrhea

Definition: Diarrhea is the passage of loose, unformed, or watery stools.
Chronic diarrhea: persists for more than 1 month.
Acute diarrhea: a response to infection or unusual foods.

Causes: Contaminated food, viral infection, dietary change, side effect of a medication or dietary supplement, psychosocial and behavioral factors.

Complications: Fluid and Electrolyte Imbalance (especially K+), Impaired Skin Integrity

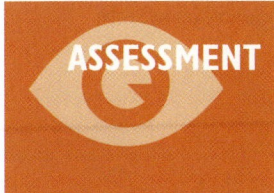

ASSESSMENT

Defining Characteristics

- Bowel pattern
- Dietary pattern (highly spiced foods, high-fat foods, greasy snacks, or large quantities of raw fruits and vegetables)
- Fever, nausea, vomiting, and abdominal pain (may indicate viral infection)
- Skin and mucous membranes
- Abdominal cramping

Risk Factors

- **KEY POINT:** *Infants, young children, and frail elderly are most vulnerable and may require hospitalization and IV fluid replacement therapy.*

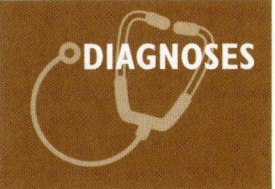

DIAGNOSES

Diarrhea
Dysfunctional Gastrointestinal Motility

Risk for Deficient Fluid Balance
Risk for Impaired Skin Integrity

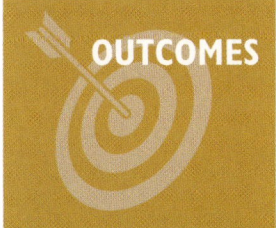

OUTCOMES

Resumes normal bowel pattern

Maintains fluid and electrolyte balance

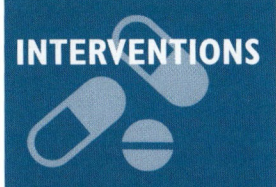

INTERVENTIONS

Preventive Interventions

- Teach hand hygiene; stress importance of washing often.
- Provide information about foods that can cause diarrhea (e.g., highly spiced, high-fat, large quantities of raw fruits and vegetables).
- Provide prompt hygiene care after any episodes of diarrhea.
- Review diet, fluid intake, and medicines. Work with the primary care provider to alter the above factors to encourage regular bowel movements.
- Plain yogurt and other probiotic foods consumed daily may help prevent diarrhea that is a response to antibiotics.

Monitoring Interventions

- Monitor stools (frequency, amount, color, consistency).
- Monitor fluid balance (I&O, weight, VS, skin turgor, mucous membranes).

- Monitor electrolyte levels.
- Monitor skin integrity (assess perineum for redness, irritation, and excoriation).

Treatment Interventions

- Provide, a clear liquid diet; electrolyte replacement fluids (e.g., Pedialyte), clear broth, gelatin, popsicles.
- Encourage your patient to sip liquids.
- Reduce the amount of fiber in the diet.
- Limit caffeine (e.g., coffee, tea, colas).
- Advise a BRAT diet if a child with diarrhea has an appetite (bananas, white rice, applesauce, and toast).
- Breastfed infants should continue on breast milk. It has a protective effect against enteritis.
- Resume normal diet gradually.

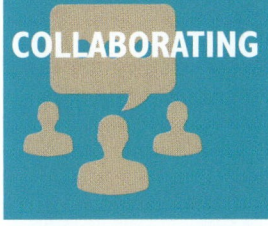

COLLABORATING

- *Antidiarrheal medications* (opiates [e.g., paregoric]) and opiate derivatives (e.g., loperamide); these act to slow peristalsis
  Side Effects: Drowsiness. Advise to use with caution.
- *Bismuth subsalicylate (Pepto-Bismol).* An OTC medication. Has antimicrobial and

antisecretory properties. Caution to avoid using without instruction from provider.
- Antidiarrheal drugs are not used in acute diarrhea. They are usually reserved for chronic diarrhea.

EXAMPLE PROBLEM: Constipation

Constipation: Decrease in the frequency of bowel movements accompanied by difficult or incomplete passage of stool and/or very hard, dry stool.

Short-term constipation: temporary, symptoms resolve in a short period of time.

Chronic constipation: lasts for 3 months; may persist for years.

Causes/Related Factors

Short-term Constipation: Lifestyle factors such as (1) decreased activity (e.g., prescribed bedrest),

(2) medications that slow peristalsis (e.g., opioids), (3) decreased fluid and fiber intake.

Long-term Constipation: In addition, physiological factors such as (1) dysfunctional anorectal musculature, (2) dysfunctional intestinal motility, (3) nervous system problems.

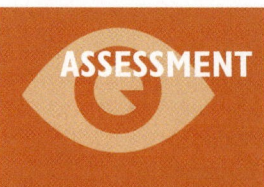

ASSESSMENT

- Bowel pattern
- Dietary pattern (low fiber, processed foods, poor or restricted fluid intake)
- Activity level
- Medications (opioids, laxatives) and polypharmacy
- Psychosocial and behavioral factors (ignoring the urge to defecate)
- Physiological factors
- Complications such as hemorrhoids or impaction (hardened, dry fecal mass)

- Screen older adults for risk factors, including a history of polypharmacy and taking laxatives.
- Other risk factors include impaired cognitive status, inadequate fluid intake, inadequate dietary fiber, reduced mobility, lack of privacy for toileting, and reliance on others for assistance.

Note: These risk factors are the same for all ages, but they are more likely for older adults.

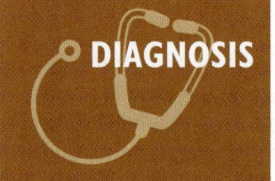

DIAGNOSIS

Constipation
Perceived Constipation

Risk for Constipation
Dysfunctional GI Motility

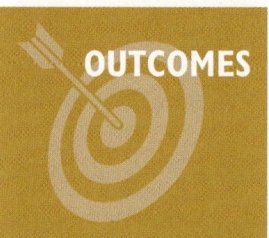

OUTCOMES

- Resumes normal bowel pattern
- Verbalizes importance of activity and balanced diet in promoting soft, formed, regular bowel movements

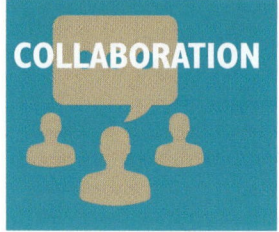

COLLABORATION

- Administer laxative as prescribed.

  - For older adults, osmotic laxatives (e.g., PEG and lactulose, bulking agents) have been found to be beneficial (Registered Nurses' Association of Ontario, 2011).

EXAMPLE PROBLEM: Constipation—cont'd

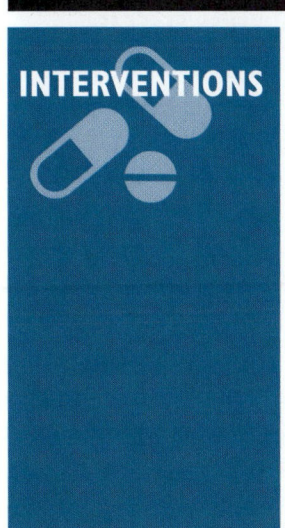

INTERVENTIONS

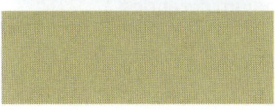

Nursing Treatments

- Encourage fluid intake: eight to ten 8-oz glasses/day; minimum should be 1,500 mL or 50 oz per day).
- Encourage the patient not to ignore the urge to defecate.
- Increase the intake of high-fiber foods if needed (normal adult RDA/AI is 25–38 g).
- Increase physical activity.
- Provide privacy for using the toilet.
- Allow the patient uninterrupted time for defecation, especially after meals, when mass peristalsis occurs.
- Assist the patient to a seated or squatting position whenever possible. A semi-Fowler's position is preferred for a client on bedrest.

Monitoring

- Monitor for anal fissures, hemorrhoids.
- Monitor for rectal ulcers, fecal seepage, and skin integrity.
- Monitor the pattern of BMs.
- Monitor for severe abdominal pain, which may indicate complications (impaction, obstruction, volvulus, bowel perforation).

Prevention

- Prevention measures are the same for all ages.
- However, for those unable to walk or who are restricted to bed, exercises such as trunk rotation, pelvic tilt, and leg lifts may be helpful.

Note: Also see the Self-Care box Teaching Your Patient About Laxative Use, and Procedures 29-3 (Administering an Enema) and 29-5 (Inserting a Rectal Tube).

Cleansing Enemas

Cleansing enemas promote removal of feces from the colon. They have the following uses:

- Treat severe constipation or impaction
- Clear the colon in preparation for visualization procedures, such as colonoscopy
- Empty the colon when starting a bowel-training program
- Clear the colon for surgeries of the lower GI tract and for some pelvic surgeries

"High" and "Low" Enemas A cleansing enema may be given "high" or "low." A "low" enema is given by standard procedure. A "high" enema attempts to clear as much of the large intestine as possible. With a "high" enema, the client receives initial instillation of the fluid in the left lateral position. The client then moves to the dorsal recumbent position and then the right lateral position for the remainder of the instillation. This turning process allows the fluid to follow the shape of the large intestine.

Cleansing enema solutions commonly are hypotonic and hypertonic solutions (see Table 29-2).

- **Hypotonic solutions** contain a large volume of fluid that is instilled into the rectum (500 to 1,000 mL for adults, 50 to 150 mL for infants).
- **Hypertonic solutions,** in contrast, are usually smaller in volume (90 to 120 mL, or 3 to 4 oz, for adults).
- **Isotonic solutions.** Refer to Table 29-2.

Retention Enemas

Retention enemas introduce a solution into the colon that is meant to be retained for a prolonged period. Consequently the volume is small, usually 90 to 120 mL (3 to 4 oz). The most common forms of retention enemas are:

- **Oil-retention enemas** instill 90 to 120 mL of oil into the rectum to soften stool and lubricate the rectum. This type of

enema may be used to assist a client to pass hard stool or before digital removal of stool.

- **Carminative enema** is a procedure in which 60 to 180 mL (2 to 6 oz) of solution are instilled into the rectum to help expel flatus and relieve bloating and distention. This procedure is used after abdominal or pelvic surgery when peristalsis is slow to return and the client experiences pressure from gas.
- **Medicated enemas** may be used to instill antibiotics to treat infections in the rectum or anus or to introduce anthelminthic agents for treatment of intestinal worms and parasites.
- **Nutritive enemas** administer fluid and nutrition through the rectum for patients who are dehydrated and frail. They are most commonly used in hospice care as a means to provide hydration for dying patients.

Return-Flow Enemas

A return-flow enema, known as a *Harris flush,* may be ordered to help a patient expel flatus and relieve abdominal distention. For adults, approximately 100 to 200 mL (3 to 7 oz) of tap water or saline is instilled into the rectum. See Procedure 29-3D to learn how to administer a return-flow enema.

Digital Removal of Stool

If fecal impaction does not respond to use of stool softeners and enemas, you will need to digitally remove feces from the rectum. Digital removal is accomplished by breaking up the hardened mass into pieces and manually extracting the pieces.

✚ Aside from discomfort, the pressure generated in the rectum may stimulate the vagus nerve, slowing the heart rate. For that reason, you must have a prescription from the primary care provider. For complete steps, see Procedure 29-4.

Table 29-2 ➤ Solutions Commonly Used in Enemas

SOLUTION	EXAMPLES	ACTION	TIME UNTIL BM	ADVERSE EFFECTS
Hypotonic	500–1,000 mL of tap water or saline, and soap 100–250 mL for infants	Large volume distends the colon, thereby stimulating peristalsis; leads to rapid evacuation of stool. Water also softens stool.	15 min	■ Fluid and electrolyte imbalance, especially water intoxication, is possible if enema is not expelled. ■ ✚ Large-volume solutions may be contraindicated in patients who have weakened intestinal walls.
Isotonic	500–1,000 mL of normal saline (0.9% NaCl solution)	Large volume distends the colon, thereby stimulating peristalsis; some softening of stool also occurs.	15 min	Fluid and electrolyte imbalance, especially sodium retention
Hypertonic	90–120 mL, or 3–4 oz, of sodium phosphate (e.g., Fleet) for adults; available as a commercially prepared solution	Attracts water into the colon, thereby causing distention and stimulating peristalsis and defecation.	Rapid acting: 5–10 min	Sodium retention ✚ Hypertonic solutions may be contraindicated for patients who tend to retain sodium or water (e.g., those with renal failure and congestive heart failure).
Oil	90–120 mL of mineral oil, cottonseed oil, or olive oil; available as a commercially prepared solution	Softens the feces, lubricates the rectum.	Varies widely. An oil-retention enema is often given 1–3 hr before a cleansing enema is administered.	
Soapsuds	Pure castile soap is added to tap water or saline.	Intestinal irritation stimulates peristalsis.	Varies.	Only pure castile soap is safe. Other soaps and detergents can cause bowel inflammation.
Carminative	For example, 1:2:3 "MGW" solution (e.g., 30 mL magnesium, 60 mL glycerin, and 90 mL water)	Provides relief from abdominal distention caused by flatus.		

Note: Solutions may be commercially prepared or prepared on the unit.

KnowledgeCheck 29-6

- Identify the types of enemas available for use.
- How do hypotonic and isotonic enemas differ from hypertonic enemas?
- What actions can you take to make the patient more comfortable when he receives an enema?

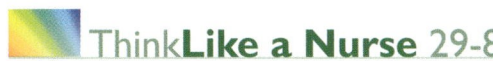ThinkLike a Nurse 29-8

Mrs. Zeno (Meet Your Patient) begins to pass liquid stool. What actions should you take? Explain your reasoning.

INTERVENTIONS FOR EXAMPLE PROBLEM: BOWEL INCONTINENCE

Clients with persistent bowel incontinence require special nursing care to prevent Impaired Skin Integrity because of the moisture and the activity of enzymes in the stool. In addition, bowel incontinence may be embarrassing. As clients worry about future episodes, anxiety escalates. For nursing care of patients with bowel incontinence, refer to these resources:

- Accompanying Example Problem: Bowel Incontinence.
- Clinical Insight 29-1 and Procedure 29-8.

 Go To Davis Advantage, Resources, Chapter 29, **Care Plan and Care Map.**

External Fecal Collection Devices

You may apply an external fecal incontinence pouch to protect perianal skin or to collect large fecal samples. This is a common approach for clients with uncontrolled diarrhea. The pouch collects fecal drainage, keeping feces away from the skin. Pouch systems vary widely. The equipment is similar to that used for patients with an ostomy, which is discussed later in the chapter. Refer to Procedure 29-8.

- **Advantages:** External collection systems can prevent skin breakdown, minimize odor, track output accurately, and enhance patient comfort.
- **Limitations:** They are not typically used for patients who are ambulatory, agitated, or active in bed because the device may be dislodged, causing skin breakdown.

Indwelling Fecal Drainage Devices

Indwelling fecal drainage devices are used to collect liquid stool from bedbound, immobilized ill patients. They consist of a soft, latex-free catheter and a collection bag (Fig. 29-8). The tube is inserted and a balloon on the end is filled with saline or water.

- *Advantages:* Internal devices protect perianal skin, protect caregivers from potentially infectious stool, and are thought to decrease urinary tract infections.
- *Disadvantages and Precautions:* They are approved by the U.S. Food and Drug Administration, but only for 29 consecutive days and not for pediatric patients. Other contraindications include patients who have severe hemorrhoids; recent bowel, rectal, or anal surgery or injury; rectal or anal tumors; or stricture or stenosis.

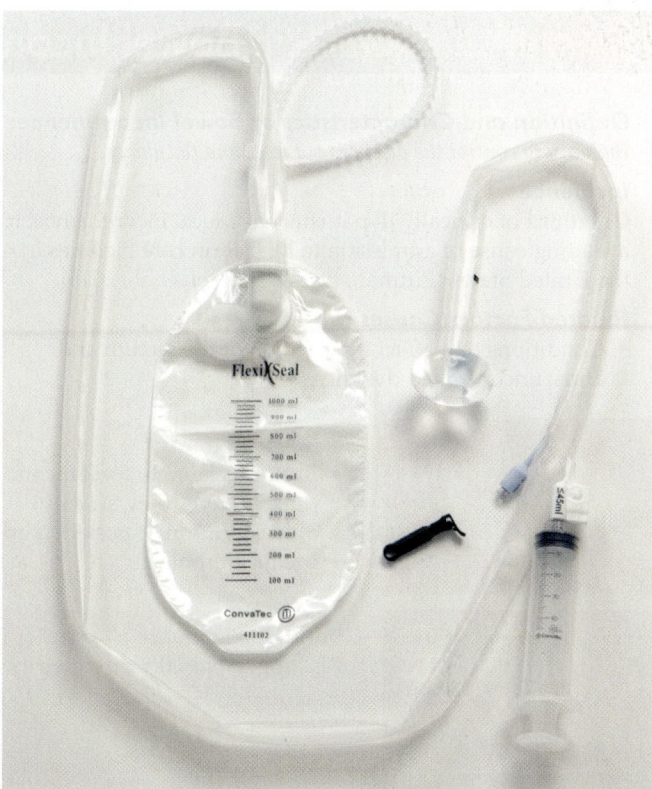

FIGURE 29-8 An indwelling fecal drainage device.

To learn more about placing and caring for a patient with an indwelling fecal drainage device, see Procedure 29-8B and Clinical Insight 29-1.

Bowel Training

A bowel-training program assists the patient to have regular, soft, formed stools. It is appropriate for clients who have chronic constipation, impaction, or bowel incontinence. Elements of a bowel-training program include the following:

- Plan the program with the patient and caregiver.
- Initiate a designated uninterrupted time for defecation, regardless of last BM or period of incontinence: usually after meals, especially in the morning.
- Provide privacy for the patient during the designated time.
- Develop a staged treatment plan if constipation develops. Usually additional fiber is added as a first measure. A stool softener is next, followed by a suppository such as bisacodyl (Dulcolax).
- Gradually increase fiber in the diet while monitoring consistency of the stool.
- Increase fluid intake to at least eight glasses of water per day, if not contraindicated.
- Regularly modify the plan based on the patient's response.

KnowledgeCheck 29-7

- What are the major patient care concerns associated with bowel incontinence?
- What are the elements of a bowel-training program?

EXAMPLE PROBLEM: Bowel Incontinence

Definition and Characteristics of Bowel Incontinence:
Inability to control the discharge of feces and flatulence.

Incidence
One-third of critically ill patients have fecal incontinence; it is a leading cause of admission to long-term care facilities in the United States (Pittman, Beeson, Carter, et al., 2015).

Related Factors/Causes
- Conditions that affect innervation of the rectum and anus; uncontrolled diarrhea
- Impaction resulting in leakage of stool
- Cognitive or emotional changes that alter the perception of the urge to defecate (e.g., dementia, low level of consciousness)
- Functional limitations (e.g., a client recognizes the need to defecate but cannot get to the toilet independently or on time; Toileting Self-Care Deficit)

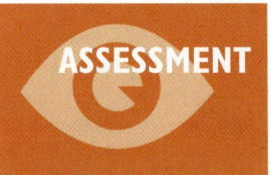 **ASSESSMENT**

- Bowel pattern
- Factors related to fecal incontinence (medications, diet, activity)
- Skin condition, especially perianal area
- Medical problems

- Psychosocial and behavioral factors (e.g., depression, caregiver problems)
- Other risk factors (e.g., smoking, underweight)

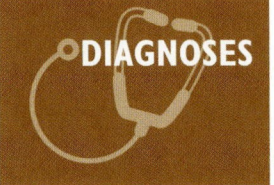 **DIAGNOSES**

Bowel Incontinence
Risk for Impaired Skin Integrity

Dysfunctional Gastrointestinal Motility: Increased

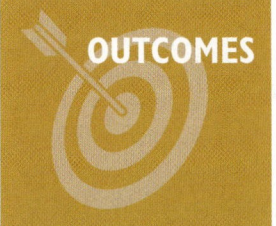 **OUTCOMES**

Resumes normal bowel pattern

Maintains skin integrity

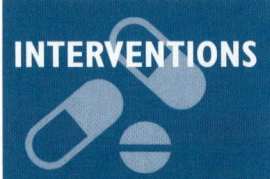 **INTERVENTIONS**

Monitoring
- Monitor pattern of BMs.
- Monitor for skin breakdown. Use moisture-barrier cream if redness or irritation is noted.

Treatments/Activities
- Provide the bedpan or assist the patient to the bathroom at regular intervals and at times BMs are most likely to occur.
- Change clothing and/or bed linens as soon as possible to prevent skin irritation and embarrassment.
- Provide prompt hygiene care after any episodes of incontinence. Keep the skin scrupulously clean.
- Use state-of-the-art skin protection products, such as perineal cleansers and skin barrier products.
- Review diet, fluid intake, activity, and medicines with patient.

Absorbent Products
- Consider absorbent pads and shields to keep from soiling clothing and linens. For large quantities, use adult incontinent garments. They may pull on like underwear or fasten like a diaper.
- Place moisture-resistant pads under the patient to help protect bed linens. Change the pad as soon as possible after defecation.

- ✚ Never place the plastic side of the pad next to the patient's body. This holds moisture next to the skin, which leads to irritation and breakdown.

- ♥ **iCare** • Never refer to incontinence pads as "diapers" when caring for adults or children who have been toilet trained. This inappropriate reference may cause embarrassment and lower the patient's self-esteem.

EXAMPLE PROBLEM: Bowel Incontinence—cont'd

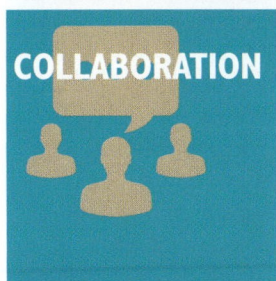

COLLABORATION

- Review diet, fluid intake, activity, and medicines. Work with the primary care provider to alter diet, fluids, and medications to encourage regular bowel movements.
- Consider a bowel-training program (explained later in the chapter; see the section Bowel Training).
- Use external or indwelling fecal collection devices to prevent drainage from soiling clothing.

KEY POINT: *Do not use external devices if skin is not intact because they will not seal tightly.*
- Research on patient outcomes of most of these methods is limited; they are discussed later in this chapter; also **see Procedure 29-8 and Clinical Insight 29-1.**

EVALUATION

- Monitor for changes in bowel pattern.
- Monitor skin integrity.

Caring for Patients With Bowel Diversions

Patients experience a variety of reactions to a bowel diversion, and each person has unique physical and psychological needs. Initially you will care for the ostomy, but the goal is for the patient to assume self-care.

Ongoing Assessments

Patients require thorough and ongoing monitoring of the stoma, output, and skin.

- **Assess the stoma.** A healthy stoma (Fig. 29-9) ranges in color from deep pink to brick red, regardless of the patient's skin color, and is shiny and moist. Pallor or a dusky blue color indicates ischemia, and a brown-black color indicates necrosis.

  Immediately after surgery, the stoma will be swollen and enlarged. As the inflammation subsides and healing occurs, the stoma will shrink. By 6 to 8 weeks, it will be at its permanent size. Stoma size varies according to the size of the person and the part of the bowel that was externalized (see Fig. 29-5). An ileostomy stoma is generally smaller than a colostomy stoma. The stoma will protrude above the level of the abdomen by approximately 1.3 to 2.5 cm (0.5 to 1 in.).

- **Assess the output.** Monitor the amount and type of drainage from the stoma. Output from an ileostomy stoma is liquid and contains digestive enzymes. An ostomy lower in the GI tract will have more solid output and fewer enzymes. The presence of enzymes in the effluent increases the likelihood of skin breakdown.

- **Assess the skin.** Pay close attention to the skin surrounding the stoma for signs of irritation, such as redness, tenderness, skin breakdown, and/or drainage. Skin breakdown may lead to infection, pain, and leakage.

Helping Patients Adapt to the Diversion

Patients experience a variety of reactions to a bowel diversion, and each person has unique needs. **KEY POINT:** *Initially you will care for the ostomy, but the goal is to have the patient assume self-care and resume a normal life.* The first step is for the patient to adjust to the presence of an ostomy. If the patient has been sick before the surgery and the ostomy leads to less pain or discomfort, the transition may be easier. Similarly, patients with continent ostomies may adapt more easily to their stoma.

Ostomy patients no longer have sphincter control, so they may need to modify their diet. You can promote adaptation by teaching the client about diet modifications. Box 29-2 discusses the effects of some foods on a patient with an ostomy.

With the exception of a temporary double-barreled colostomy, ostomy care is a lifelong task. In many hospitals and large communities, you can find an enterostomal therapy nurse to assist patients with their ongoing care and to provide consultation on ostomy appliances. Your attitude and willingness to discuss body changes will help your patient begin adapting. Clinical Insight 29-2 provides more information and guidelines for caring for patients with ostomies.

Colostomy Irrigation

Colostomy irrigation may occasionally be indicated as an intervention for constipation or in a select population of patients. Consult with the ostomy nurse and/or physician to see if colostomy irrigation is appropriate for your patient.

- Patients with an ostomy in the descending or sigmoid colon may use colostomy irrigation as a means to control bowel evacuation and possibly eliminate the need to wear an ostomy pouch.
- A stoma above the descending colon usually has liquid output that cannot be controlled. Therefore, it is not irrigated.

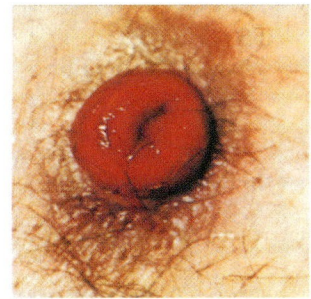

FIGURE 29-9 A healthy stoma is deep pink to brick red and shiny and moist.

Toward Evidence-Based Practice

Li, C. C., Rew, L., & Hwang, S. L. (2012). The relationship between spiritual well-being and psychosocial adjustment in Taiwanese patients with colorectal cancer and a colostomy. *Journal of Wound Ostomy & Continence Nursing, 39*(2), 161–169.

Participants were 45 Taiwanese patients, aged 42 to 83 years, who were diagnosed with colorectal cancer and underwent colostomy surgery. They completed a questionnaire that examined relationships among demographic and clinical characteristics, spiritual well-being, and psychosocial adjustment to the colostomy. Participants reported strong family relationships but poor adjustment in sexual relationships. Spiritual well-being was significantly associated with psychosocial adjustment and was found to play an important role for patients when faced with psychosocial adjustment related to a colostomy.

Poletto, D., & Silva, D. M. G. V. D. (2013). Living with intestinal stoma: The construction of autonomy for care. *Revista Latino-Americana de Enfermagem, 21*(2), 531–538.

Ten people who received a stoma, and their family members, participated in two semistructured interviews to investigate which care provided in the postoperative period played the largest role in promoting autonomy. The study identified common factors that influence the development of autonomy, including (1) the need to carry out stoma care; (2) receiving health support and care after discharge from hospital; (3) the family's support in developing autonomy; and (4) returning to daily activities and social reinsertion. The authors suggested that health professionals are fundamental to the process of developing autonomy by working as educators, supporting the achievement, and encouraging the care and the return to activities.

1. Based on these studies, write three nursing interventions you would use to help a patient accept and adapt to a stoma.

2. Suppose you wanted to know whether those interventions would be effective for patients with other medical conditions. For example, would the interventions that help clients adapt to a stoma help other clients to adapt to a different issue? Think of at least two health conditions for which you might want to perform the two studies just described. Explain your thinking.

 Go to Davis Advantage, Resources, Chapter 29, **Toward Evidence-Based Practice—Suggested Responses.**

BOX 29-2 ■ Teaching Dietary Changes Associated With an Ostomy

Note: These are only suggestions. Each person must, by trial and error, discover what works best for him.

General Guidelines for Patients

- Initially, you may be asked to follow a bland, low-residue or soft diet for a month or two to prevent obstructions and GI upsets. Advance the diet by adding one new food at a time.
- Eat three or more meals daily at regular times.
- Drink additional fluid to keep well hydrated. Those with colostomies need to compensate for the loss of the large intestine where fluid absorption occurs.
- Avoid chewing gum, as it may cause you to swallow air, causing a noisy stoma.
- Avoid foods that cause gas, odor, blockage, or loose stools. Eventually introduce them into your diet one at a time and be aware of their effects.
- Chew your food well to avoid blockage of the stoma.
- Avoid excessive weight gain.

Foods That May Cause Gas or Odor

Beverages: Alcohol, beer, carbonated beverages
Dairy: Milk, cheese, eggs, and other dairy
Fruits: Melons
Vegetables: Asparagus, beans, broccoli, Brussels sprouts, cabbage, cauliflower, cucumbers, garlic, onions, peas, radishes
Other foods: Fish, cod liver oil, nuts, peanut butter

Foods That May Help Control Gas or Odor

Buttermilk, yogurt
Cranberry juice
Parsley

High-Fiber Foods That May Cause Blockage

You can eat some of these foods (e.g., mushrooms, shrimp) if you cut them into small pieces and chew them very thoroughly.

As long as blockage does not occur, these foods should not necessarily be avoided, but used carefully.
- Foods with seeds (e.g., raspberries)
- Foods with tough skins (e.g., corn, dried fruits, pears, tomatoes)
- Mushrooms
- Nuts, popcorn
- Raw or minimally cooked fruits and vegetables (e.g., coleslaw, Chinese stir-fried vegetables, oranges, apple skins)
- Shrimp, lobster
- Stringy foods (e.g., celery, coconut, spinach, bean sprouts, green beans, orange pulp)

Foods That May Cause Loose Stools

Alcohol, beer, caffeine, chocolate, licorice
Milk
Baked beans, cooked cabbage, onions
Bran cereal, whole grains
Highly seasoned foods
Large meals
Prunes, raisins
Raw fruits and vegetables
KEY POINT: *Never restrict fluids in an effort to control diarrhea.*

Foods That May Alleviate Diarrhea

Bananas **R**ice **A**pplesauce **T**oast (BRAT)
Starchy foods (e.g., bread, potatoes)
Cheese and creamy peanut butter

Sources Lutz, C., & Przytulski, K. (2014). *Nutrition and diet therapy: Evidence-based applications* (6th ed.). Philadelphia, PA: F.A. Davis; United Ostomy Associations of America. (2005, updated 2011). Ostomates food reference chart. Retrieved from http://www.ostomy.org/uploaded/files/ostomy_info/food_ref_card.pdf?direct=1

Colostomy irrigation is similar in some respects to an enema. The nurse or patient inserts a flexible tube into the stoma and instills a traditional enema solution. The patient may use a special plastic sleeve over the stoma or an ostomy appliance to direct the output into the toilet. For the complete procedure, see Procedure 29-7.

KnowledgeCheck 29-8

- How can you help a patient adapt psychologically to living with a bowel diversion?
- What does a healthy stoma look like?
- Why is skin care around a stoma so important?

CLINICALREASONING

The questions and exercises in this section allow you to practice the kind of thinking you will use as a full-spectrum nurse. Critical-thinking questions usually have more than one correct answer, so we do not provide "correct answers" for these features. It is more important to develop your nursing judgment than to just cover content. You will learn by discussing the questions with your peers. If you are still unsure, see the Davis Advantage chapter resources for suggested responses.

Caring for the Nguyens

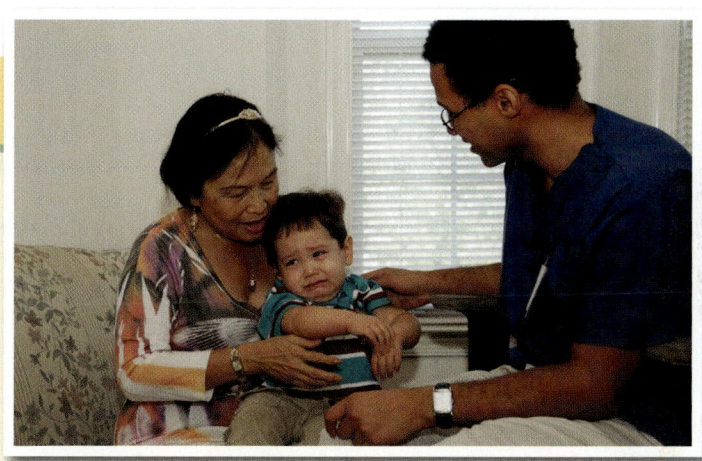

Yen Nyugen arrives at the family health center for a scheduled appointment, accompanied by her grandson, Kim Phan. Recently, Yen has been constipated and has had several episodes of bleeding with bowel movements (BMs). She has read that a change in bowel habits is a sign of colon cancer and is worried about that. She brought her grandson along because he is also having bowel problems. Kim's bowel habits are erratic. At times he has a soft BM. However, he has also had bouts of constipation and diarrhea. Yen would like advice on her grandson's elimination status. As a critical thinker, you will begin by obtaining accurate, credible information.

A. What history questions would be appropriate to ask Yen regarding her bowel concerns? What data do you need? How can you get the data? Are the data accurate? What information is important; what is not? Write some specific questions, just as you would ask them in an interview.

B. What physical assessments would you conduct for Yen to add to, and possibly to validate, your subjective data?

C. Now you must consider the context. What factors must you consider when gathering a history on Kim?

D. The family nurse practitioner (FNP) examines Yen and determines that she has external hemorrhoids that have been bleeding because of recent straining at stool. The FNP prescribes rectal suppositories to decrease

the swelling of the hemorrhoids and asks you to teach Yen about necessary lifestyle changes. What additional information will you need to gather to provide this teaching? Recall that you have already obtained a significant amount of information from the history questions. Again, think about context: Whatever the content of your teaching, Yen will be using that information to care for herself and her grandson in her home.

E. The FNP examines Kim and tells you that the examination is normal. Use your theoretical knowledge of bowel elimination and Kim's developmental stage to think of possible reasons for his erratic bowel pattern.

 Go to Davis Advantage, Resources, Chapter 29, **Caring for the Nguyens—Suggested Responses.**

Applying The **Full-Spectrum Nursing Model**

PATIENT SITUATION

Lucy Franklin is a frail elderly woman, a long-time resident in a long-term care facility. She can no longer communicate and lies in whatever position the NAPs place her in bed, seldom moving. She is very thin, does not eat or drink, and is being fed entirely through a gastrostomy tube. She is incontinent of both stool and urine and has recently started having copious diarrhea, probably from the tube feedings, but that has not been established definitely. The skin on Lucy's back, buttocks, and perineum is still intact, but it is quite red now. The healthcare team is considering various measures for controlling the diarrhea, but until that can be achieved, nurses want to protect her skin integrity.

THINKING

1. *Theoretical Knowledge:*
   a. Other than tube feedings, what else could be causing Lucy's diarrhea?
   b. In addition to Impaired Skin Integrity, what are some other risks associated with diarrhea?
   c. Why is fecal incontinence, especially with diarrhea, a risk factor for Impaired Skin Integrity?
2. *Critical Thinking:*
   a. *(Contextual Awareness):* What other factors in Lucy's situation do you think might make her even more vulnerable to Impaired Skin Integrity? If you do not yet have the theoretical knowledge you need, draw on your own experiences—and think carefully about everything you know about Lucy.
   b. *(Considering Alternatives):* A fecal incontinence pouch is being discussed as an intervention to preserve Lucy's skin integrity. Do you think it should be an external system or an internal system? Why?

DOING

3. *Practical Knowledge:*
   It has been decided that an external fecal collection system will be used. Describe the steps you will take to apply this system after you have made the necessary assessments.
4. *Nursing Process (Assessments):*
   What ongoing assessments will you need to make after the fecal collection system is applied?

CARING

5. *Self-Knowledge:*
   How comfortable would you be applying Lucy's fecal collection system? What aspects of the situation make you most uncomfortable?

 Go to Davis Advantage, Resources, Chapter 29, **Applying the Full-Spectrum Nursing Model—Suggested Responses.**

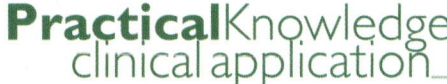
PracticalKnowledge
clinical application

CLINICAL INSIGHTS

Clinical Insight 29-1 ➤ **Caring for a Patient With an Indwelling Fecal Drainage Device**

A catheter is present in the rectum and is connected to a drainage tube and collection bag.

Nursing Goal 1: Prevent Injury to Rectal Sphincter and/or Rectal Mucosa.

- Do not add air or fluid to the balloon port of the catheter.
- Check the catheter frequently for kinks or obstructions.
- Monitor for signs of complications and notify the healthcare provider immediately if patient experiences rectal pain, rectal bleeding, and abdominal distention or pain.
- Monitor stool for change in consistency (solid or soft-formed stool cannot pass through the catheter and will cause an obstruction).
- How to discontinue the catheter:
  1. Attach a 60-mL syringe to the balloon inflation port and deflate the retention balloon by pulling back on the plunger.

2. Grasp the catheter as close to the patient as possible and slowly slide it out of the anus.
3. Dispose of the device accordance to the agency policy for disposal of medical waste.

Nursing Goal 2: Maintain Free Flow of Liquid Stool.

- Monitor the patient for changes in stool consistency. If the stool is no longer liquid and flowing, the device must be discontinued.
- Make sure the tubing and bag remain below the level of the patient.
- Irrigate the tube as often as necessary to maintain patency:
  1. Fill a 60-mL syringe with room-temperature tap water.
  2. Attach it to the irrigation port of the catheter and flush by depressing the plunger.
     Be sure you are using the irrigation port, NOT the balloon inflation port.

Clinical Insight 29-1 ➤ Caring for a Patient With an Indwelling Fecal Drainage Device—cont'd

3. Be sure to subtract the irrigation fluid from the stool volume to maintain an accurate record of intake and output.
■ Change the collection bag when it is three-fourths full.
4. Remove the collection bag from the tubing. Snap the cap onto the used bag and dispose of according to agency policy for medical waste.
5. Snap new collection bag securely onto the device.

Nursing Goal 3: Prevent Transmission of Pathogens to Others.

■ Follow the agency protocol for hand hygiene. Always wear clean procedure gloves when handling the fecal management device.
■ Monitor stool cultures and implement isolation protocols as indicated. If a stool sample is ordered, you may obtain it from the collection bag:
  1. If the collection bag is more than 24 hours old, place a new collection bag before obtaining sample.

2. Cut the collection bag at the bottom and transfer stool to an appropriate container for transport to the lab.
3. Apply a new collection bag to the connector at the end of the catheter.

Nursing Goal 4: Maintain Perineal Skin Integrity or Prevent Wounds from Being Contaminated by Stool.

■ Monitor insertion site for leakage and signs of infection.
■ If perineal wounds are present, keep clean and dry; notify the primary provider if signs of infection are present.
■ Perform perineal care according to agency policy.

Clinical Insight 29-2 ➤ Guidelines for Ostomy Care

Assess Stoma Appearance.

■ The stoma should be moist and red or pink.

■ ✚ Immediately report to the surgeon a stoma that is pale, dusky, or black in color; dry; or with sloughing tissues. These are signs of inadequate blood supply to, and possible necrosis of, the portion of intestine that has been externalized.

■ Protruding or retracted stomas will need special adjustments in wafer measurement and placement. It is normal for a new stoma to have yellow or blood-tinged mucus or dried blood on it.

Preserve Peristomal Skin.

■ Preserving peristomal skin is critical because skin excoriation may cause an ineffective seal between the wafer and the skin and leakage of effluent. This, in turn, causes more skin and tissue damage. Leakage may indicate the need for a different type of pouch system or sealant.
■ Use recommended moisture-proof barrier creams and skin care products.

Plan for and Change the Pouch as Scheduled.

■ Change the skin barrier pouch at times of lower effluent.
■ Avoid changing after meals, when the gastrocolic reflux increases chance of fecal effluent. Mucous secretion is normal.
■ Pouches are usually changed every 3 to 5 days, preferably before leakage occurs. Frequency also depends on the

type of stoma, the equipment used (e.g., one- or two-piece pouch), the effluent, the patient's preference, and the climate (i.e., pouches are changed more frequently during the summer).
■ To decrease skin irritation, avoid changing the entire system. In a one-piece or two-piece pouching system, change the skin barrier only every 3 to 7 days, never daily.

Assess the Patient's Self-care Ability.

■ Patients with poor vision may need to use magnification mirrors and yellow-tinted sunglasses to help reduce glare and improve contrast when they perform stoma care.
■ Patients with immobility or spinal cord injury may need equipment that has a longer pouch that the patient can easily empty independently when sitting.
■ Impaired dexterity or vision may warrant the use of a one-piece system or precut pouch and skin barrier, whereas a two-piece system may be better for patients who need to keep the skin barrier in place for several days and change just the pouch.
■ Patients who are blind can be taught to change their own equipment.

Determine Whether the Ostomy Should be Irrigated.

■ Consult a peristomal nurse or the primary care provider to determine whether an ostomy should be irrigated.

(Continued)

Clinical Insight 29-2 ➤ Guidelines for Ostomy Care—cont'd

- Many patients with left-end colostomies may be safely irrigated as a method of continence management. An ileostomy, however, drains liquid containing high concentrations of sodium, chloride, potassium, magnesium, and bicarbonate.

- Ileostomies should never be irrigated, except in cases of food blockage near the stomal outlet. Only a qualified person, such as an enterostomal therapy nurse, may perform a gentle lavage. For lavage, normal saline is preferred because excessive lavage could lead to a serious fluid and electrolyte imbalance.

Promote Psychological Adaptation.

- Be available to discuss the patient's reaction to the stoma. Your attitude and willingness to discuss the patient's body changes will help your patient begin adapting.
- Show acceptance when working with the patient and the stoma.
- Provide adequate ventilation and odor control when assessing the stoma or ostomy appliance.
- Provide ample time to explain stoma care and use of ostomy appliances. For most patients, this is a lifelong task; therefore, patient teaching is essential.

- Teach the client about diet modifications.
- Encourage patients to return to their usual activities as much as possible.
- Encourage patients to discuss intimacy issues associated with the ostomy. Use the PLISSIT model (in Chapter 34) bring up the subject, if necessary, and to convey to them that sexual functioning is an appropriate topic to discuss. You may wish to use the United Ostomy Associations of America's *Intimacy After Ostomy Surgery Guide*, or give it to the patient (Schuler, 2013).
- Refer the patient to the local ostomy association, if one is available. Most of the counselors are skillful because they, too, have ostomies. They are able to share practical and personal information based on their own experience with similar challenges. To find the local chapter consult your phone book, or

> Go to the **United Ostomy Associations of America** Web site at http://www.ostomy.org/

PROCEDURES

The procedures in this chapter will help you to provide care to patients who have problems with bowel elimination.

Procedure 29-1 ■ Testing Stool for Occult Blood

➤ For steps to follow in *all* procedures, refer to the Universal Steps for All Procedures found on the page facing the inside back cover.

Equipment

- Clean gloves
- Tongue blade or other wooden applicator
- Clean, dry collection container to place in the commode, or a clean, dry bedpan
- Facility-specific fecal occult blood test (FOBT) slide or test paper
- Developing solution

Delegation

You can delegate the collection and testing of a stool sample for occult blood to nursing assistive personnel (NAP) if the NAP has the necessary skills and the patient's condition is stable. Inform the NAP of any special considerations (e.g., the need to assist the patient with ambulation or the need for a bedpan). Instruct the NAP to inform you if there is visible blood in the stool and to show you the FOBT slide for evaluation of results when the test is complete.

Pre-Procedure Assessment

- Assess the patient's mobility status.
  Determines the patient's ability to participate in stool collection, the need for a bedpan or commode, and so forth.

- Assess the patient's dietary history for the past 24 to 48 hours.
  Some foods, such as red meat, chicken, fish, horseradish, turnips, or raw vegetables, may lead to a false-positive reading. Vitamin C in excess of 250 mg per day can produce a false-negative result (MedlinePlus, 2016).

- Assess medication history.
  If the patient is taking medications, such as salicylates, NSAIDs, iron, oxidizing drugs (e.g., iodine salts, boric acid), reserpine, corticosteroids, anticoagulants, colchicines, and high doses of vitamin C, consult with a physician. These medications may cause a false-positive reading. If possible, they will be discontinued for 7 days before the test. If the patient must have them, results must be interpreted taking them into consideration.

■ Assess for the presence of hemorrhoids.
Any source of blood may cause a false-positive result for intestinal bleeding.

■ If the patient is female, ask whether she is menstruating.

■ Check the expiration date on the developing solution for the FOBT test slide.

■ Assess the patient's or family's understanding of the need for the stool test.
Provides a baseline for health teaching.

> ➤ When performing the procedure, always identify your patient according to agency policy, using two identifiers, and be attentive to standard precautions, hand hygiene, patient safety and privacy, body mechanics, and documentation.

Procedure Steps

1. **Determine whether the test** will be done by the nurse at the point of care (e.g., in the home or at the bedside) or by lab personnel.
Because of the regulatory and billing practices in some settings, this test may be completed by lab personnel.

2. Gather the necessary testing supplies. Be sure you understand the directions for the testing kit you are using.
This procedure gives instructions for the FOBT slide method.

3. **Ask the patient to void** before collecting the stool specimen.
Helps prevent contaminating the stool with urine.

4. **Perform hand hygiene and don procedure gloves.**

5. **Place a clean, dry container** for the stool specimen into the toilet or bedside commode in such a manner that any urine falls into the toilet and the fecal specimen falls into the container. Obtain a clean, dry bedpan for a patient who is immobile.
Using a sample of stool that comes in contact with either urine or water may produce an inaccurate test result.

6. **Instruct the patient to defecate** into the container, or place the patient on the bedpan. Do not contaminate the specimen with toilet tissue.

7. **Once the specimen has been obtained** and the bedpan removed or the patient assisted to bed as necessary, perform hand hygiene and don clean procedure gloves.
Prevents the spread of intestinal bacteria.

8. **Explain the purpose of the test.** Explain to the patient that serial specimens may be needed.
Testing serial specimens decreases the chances of a false-negative finding.

9. **Open the specimen side** of the FOBT slide. With a tongue depressor or other applicator, collect a small sample of stool and spread it thinly onto one "window" of the FOBT slide.

10. **With a different applicator** or the opposite end of the tongue blade, collect a second small sample of stool from a different location in the large sample. Spread the second sample thinly onto the second "window" of the slide.
Reduces the possibility of a false negative result. ▼

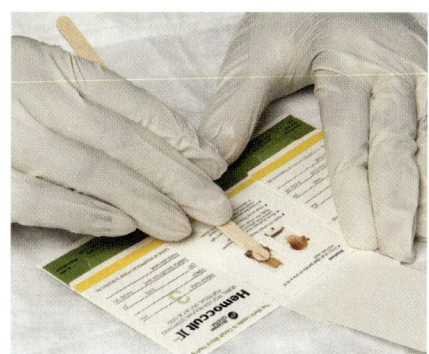

11. **Wrap the tongue depressor** in tissue and a paper towel; place it in a waste receptacle. Do not flush it.
Prevents transfer of microorganisms. Flushing would likely clog the plumbing.

12. **Close the FOBT slide.**
Prevents the transfer of microorganisms from the specimen smears on the slide.

13. **If the test is to be done by laboratory personnel,** transfer the specimen to a clean dry container, being careful not to contaminate the outside of the container with feces. Label the specimen in the presence of the patient according to agency policy, and place it into the proper receptacle for transportation to the lab.

14. **If you are to perform the test,** turn the slide over, and open the opposite side of the FOBT slide. Follow the directions on the package regarding the number of drops of the developing solution.
Ensures an accurate reading. ▼

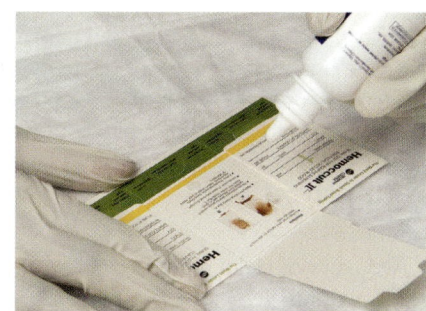

15. **Remove gloves and** perform hand hygiene.

(continued on next page)

Procedure 29–1 ■ Testing Stool for Occult Blood (continued)

Evaluation

- Observe the color of the paper inside the FOBT slide windows for 30 to 60 seconds.
- If the paper turns blue, consider the test for occult blood to be positive.

Patient Teaching

- Inform the patient of the reasons for performing the test.
- Explain the possible implications of a positive occult blood test, if one is obtained.

Home Care

- Determine the client's level of cognition and manual dexterity to assess his ability to follow instructions and physically perform the test.
- Explain necessary dietary and medication restrictions (see the Pre-Procedure Assessment section of this procedure).
- Instruct the client to collect the specimen in a clean, dry container. If an appropriate container is not available, the client may use the toilet.
- If defecating in the toilet, the client should flush it immediately prior to obtaining the sample. If commercial toilet bowl cleaners are in use, remove them from the tank, and flush twice. Then place rice paper (from the kit) directly on the water; it is okay to get it wet. When using the probe to take the stool sample, take the sample from any area of stool that is above the water line.
- Protect the slide from heat, light, and household chemicals.
- Home collection slides come in a kit, connected together as a set of three. Instruct the client not to tear them apart.
- Emphasize to the client that each sample should be from separate bowel movements on separate days.
- After all three specimens have been collected over the course of at least 3 days, store the slide in a paper envelope to air-dry.

- The client must place the slides in the special mailing pouch that comes with the slides, if they are to be sent back to the lab. The slides should be returned to the care provider or lab no later than 14 days after the first sample was collected. For additional instructions,

 Go to the **Hemoccult** Web site at http://www. hemoccultfobt.com/

Documentation

- Document the date and time of the specimen collection, both in the patient record and on the specimen container or FOBT kit.
- Note the appearance of the stool (e.g., color, odor) and the presence of blood, mucus, or other abnormal constituents.
- Note any rectal bleeding or discomfort during and after defecation.
- Document the test results on the appropriate agency form.
- Notify the appropriate care provider of the results.

Sample documentation

06/14/18   0915   *Specimen taken from 2 separate sections of yellowish-brown soft stool containing mucus. No rectal bleeding or discomfort with defecation. Specimen sent to lab; test results pending.* —————————————— *S. Hoeszle, RN*

Practice Resources

American Cancer Society (2016a); Gomella L., & Haist, S. (2006); The Joint Commission Accreditation Program (2016); Leggett, B. A., & Hewett, D. G. (2015); National Guideline Clearinghouse (2012); Siegel, J., Rhinehart, E., Jackson, M., et al. (2007).

Procedure 29–2 ■ Placing and Removing a Bedpan

➤ For steps to follow in *all* procedures, refer to the Universal Steps for All Procedures found on the page facing the inside back cover.

Equipment

- Bedpan
- Two pairs of clean gloves
- Toilet tissue
- Prepackaged disposable wipes
- Waterproof pad
- Bedpan cover

Delegation

You may delegate the placement and removal of a bedpan to the NAP after ensuring that the NAP has the necessary skills and that the patient's condition is stable. Complete the

following assessments, and inform the NAP of any special considerations (e.g., medical or surgical conditions that necessitate the use of a fracture pan, extra care with turning or required positioning based on medical condition).

Pre-Procedure Assessments

- Assess level of consciousness, ability to follow directions, mobility, and physical status.
  Helps determine the type of bedpan to use and whether one or two persons are needed to complete the procedure.

- Determine the patient's comfort level—note the presence of rectal or abdominal pain, hemorrhoids, or perianal irritation.
  Pain can cause difficulty with positioning and bearing down during defecation. Any unexplained pain should be evaluated by the primary care provider.

- Identify factors that will necessitate the use of a fracture pan (e.g., a fractured pelvis; total hip replacement; lower back surgery; presence of casts, splints, or braces on lower limbs; or obesity.)

- Auscultate bowel sounds, and palpate for distention if indicated.
  The colon when full with fecal matter is a rounded, firm mass. A smooth, round mass above the symphysis pubis is a distended bladder.

- Review the patient's chart to determine the need to obtain a stool specimen.
  Promotes efficiency by allowing you to obtain a specimen container before placing the patient on the bedpan.

Procedure 29–2A ■ Placing a Bedpan

➤ When performing the procedure, always identify your patient according to agency policy, using two identifiers, and be attentive to standard precautions, hand hygiene, patient safety and privacy, body mechanics, and documentation.

Procedure Steps

1. **Obtain the necessary supplies,** and take them to the patient's room. Warm the prepackaged disposable wipes and leave at the bedside for use during bedpan removal.
   The patient will need to wash her hands after using the bedpan.

2. **If the bedpan is metal,** place it under warm, running water for a few seconds. Then dry it, making sure the bedpan is not too hot.
   A warm bedpan allows the patient to be more comfortable and helps relax the anal sphincter. Most bedpans are made of disposable plastic.

3. **Raise the siderail** on the opposite side from where you are working.
   Prevents patient from falling out of bed and gives the patient something to hold onto while moving around in bed.

4. **Raise the bed to a comfortable height.**
   Allows you to use good body mechanics and prevents muscle strain.

5. **Prepare the patient** by folding down the covers to a point that will allow for placement of the bedpan and yet expose only as much of her body as necessary.
   Privacy facilitates elimination by promoting relaxation.

6. **Perform hand hygiene** and don clean procedure gloves.
   Prevents the spread of microorganisms via contact with urine or feces.

7. **Observe for the presence** of dressings, drains, intravenous fluids, and traction.
   These appliances may hinder the patient from assisting with the procedure and may create the need for assistance from another caregiver.

Procedure Variation: For the Patient Able to Move/Turn Independently in Bed

8. **Position the patient.**

Supine Position
   a. Lower the head of the bed, placing the patient in a supine position.
   b. Ask the patient to lift her hips. The patient may need to raise her knees to a flexed position, place her feet flat on the bed, and push up. You can also assist the patient to raise her hips by sliding a hand under the small of her back.

Semi-Fowler's Position
   c. Place the bed in a semi-Fowler's position.
   d. Ask the patient to raise her hips by pushing up on raised siderails or by using an overhead trapeze.

9. **Place the bedpan.**

Regular Bedpan
   a. Place the bedpan under the patient's buttocks so that the wide, rounded end is toward the back.
   Sliding the pan against the patient's skin may cause damage to the back.

Fracture Pan
   b. Place the wide, rounded end toward the front.

10. **Instruct or assist the patient** to lower her hips onto the bedpan. Move to step 16.

Procedure Variation for the Patient Unable to Move/Turn Independently

11. **Ask for help** from another healthcare worker if the patient's condition warrants.

12. **With the patient in the supine** position, lower the head of the bed.

13. **Assist the patient** to the side-lying position. Use a turn sheet, if necessary.

14. **Place the bedpan.**

Regular Bedpan
   a. Place the bedpan under the patient's buttocks so that the wide, rounded end is toward the back. Do not push the pan under the patient's buttocks. ▼

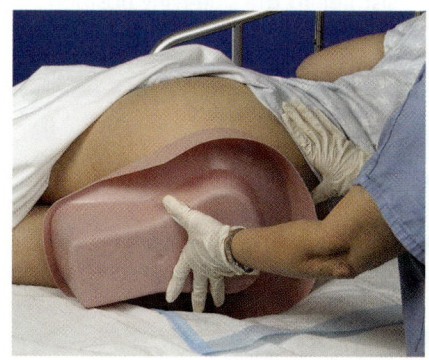

(continued on next page)

Procedure 29-2 ■ **Placing and Removing a Bedpan** (continued)

Fracture Pan

b. Place the wide, rounded end toward the front. ▼

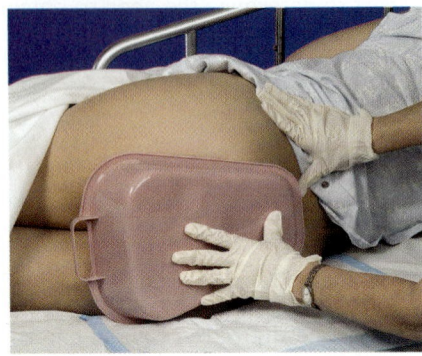

15. **Holding the bedpan in place,** slowly roll the patient back and onto the bedpan.

16. **Replace the covers;** raise the head of the bed to a position of comfort for the patient. Place a rolled towel, blanket, or small pillow under the sacrum (lumbar curve of the back).

17. **Place the call light** and toilet tissue within the patient's reach. Make certain that the bed is returned to its lowest position and that the upper siderails are raised.
Provides privacy, comfort, and safety.

18. **Remove your gloves and** perform hand hygiene.
Prevents the transmission of intestinal bacteria.

Procedure 29-2B ■ **Removing a Bedpan**

➤ When performing the procedure, always identify your patient according to agency policy, using two identifiers, and be attentive to standard precautions, hand hygiene, patient safety and privacy, body mechanics, and documentation.

Procedure Steps

1. **Don clean procedure gloves.** Open the prepackaged disposable wipes and place them near the work area.

2. **If the patient is immobile,** lower the head of the patient's bed. Pull down the covers only as far as needed to remove the bedpan.
Lowering the head of the bed is necessary only if the patient is immobile.

3. **Offer the patient toilet paper.** Assist patients who are unable to complete this task independently.

4. **Ask the patient to raise her hips.** Stabilize and remove the bedpan. If the patient is unable to raise her hips, stabilize the bedpan and assist her to the side-lying position.
Stabilizing the bedpan prevents spillage of contents.

5. **Cleanse the buttocks** with a warm, prepackaged wipes. Allow to air dry.
Provides comfort and hygiene and decreases the risk of skin irritation and breakdown.

6. **Replace covers and position** the patient for comfort. Offer the patient a clean wipe to cleanse her hands.
Encourages independence with personal hygiene and decreases transmission of bacteria.

7. **Empty the bedpan** into the patient's toilet. Measure the output if that is part of the treatment plan. Clean the bedpan, following facility-specific guidelines.
If there is no toilet in the patient's room, cover the bedpan and carry it to the nearest toilet or soiled utility room for emptying.

8. **Remove the soiled gloves** and perform hand hygiene.
Prevents transmission of infectious microorganisms.

? What if . . .

■ **Your patient is an older adult?**

Offer a bedpan at set intervals, perhaps in conjunction with a turning schedule. For elderly clients with limited mobility, you may wish to keep the bedpan readily available.
To minimize episodes of incontinence and/or falls. Trying to get out of bed to use the toilet is a common cause of falls.

Evaluation

■ Assess the amount and characteristics of any urine and/or stool.
■ Observe the skin on the perineum and buttocks for redness and breakdown.

Home Care

Teach the patient's family the steps of this procedure.

Documentation

■ Document the amount of urine or liquid stool voided if intake and output are being recorded.
■ Note the presence of any unusual characteristics of either stool or urine, and include in the nursing notes. If there are no unusual characteristics, document the passage of stool or urine in the graphic records.

Practice Resources

Ayello, E., & Sibbald, R. (2016); Balas, M., Casey, C., & Happ, M. (2016); Gray-Micelli, D. (2016); Siegel, J., Rhinehart, E., Jackson, M., et al. (2007).

 The videos, **Placing a Bedpan** and **Removing a Bedpan,** along with questions and suggested responses, are available on the **Davis's Nursing Skills Videos** Web site on Davis*Plus.*

Thinking About the Procedure

To practice applying clinical reasoning to this procedure,

Procedure 29-3 ■ Administering an Enema

➤ For steps to follow in *all* procedures, refer to the Universal Steps for All Procedures found on the page facing the inside back cover.

Equipment

- Enema administration container, correct enema solution, or prepackaged enema—depends on the type of enema ordered
  - *Enema kit:* This may be a grouping of supplies that includes a small plastic bucket or a 1-liter plastic bag with attached tubing, disposable toweling, lubricant, and castile soap.
  - *Prepackaged enema solution:* If a prepackaged enema (e.g., Fleets) is ordered, you may need to obtain the preparation from the pharmacy or central supply department.
- Prepackaged disposable wipes, and/or toilet tissue
- Bath blanket
- Waterproof pad
- Bedpan with cover or bedside commode, if needed
- Water-soluble lubricant
- Clean procedure gloves
- IV pole

Delegation

You may delegate this procedure to the NAP if the NAP is trained and the patient is stable. Complete the following assessments, and instruct the NAP about conditions under which the procedure should be stopped (e.g., severe abdominal pain occurs, bleeding is seen, or the patient is unable to retain the solution). Instruct the NAP to report the results of the enema and show you any stool that appears to be abnormal (e.g., containing blood or pus).

Pre-Procedure Assessments

- Assess for history of bowel disorders (e.g., diverticulitis, ulcerative colitis, recent bowel surgery, abdominal pain, abdominal distention, hemorrhoids).
  Some disorders put the patient at risk for complications, such as mucosal irritation or perforation. Abdominal pain along with

hypoactive bowel sounds and distention could indicate a bowel obstruction.

- Inspect the abdomen for distention.
  Establishes baseline for effectiveness of the enema.

- ✚ Review the patient's chart for the presence of increased intracranial pressure, glaucoma, or recent rectal or prostate surgery.
  An enema may cause the patient to strain, therefor increasing pressure on the brain or surgical incisions.

- Review lab results, paying particular attention to blood urea nitrogen (BUN), creatinine, and electrolytes.
  Hypertonic and hypotonic enemas have been linked to fluid and electrolyte changes. Phosphate enemas (Fleets) have been associated with hyperphosphatemia and hypocalcemia.

- Note the date and time of the patient's last bowel movement, recent bowel movement pattern, and bowel sounds.
  Establishes baseline for evaluating bowel function.

- Assess the patient's cognitive level and mobility.
  Determines the patient's ability to follow instructions and the need for placing him on a bedpan for the enema.

- Assess the patient's rectal sphincter control.
  Will determine whether you need to administer the enema with the patient on the bedpan. Also influences the amount of solution to instill.

- Assess for fecal impaction.
  May necessitate the need to obtain a prescription for a different type of enema.

(continued on next page)

Procedure 29-3 ■ Administering an Enema (continued)

Procedure 29-3A ■ Administering a Cleansing Enema

➤ When performing the procedure, always identify your patient according to agency policy, using two identifiers, and be attentive to standard precautions, hand hygiene, patient safety and privacy, body mechanics, and documentation.

Procedure Steps

1. **Before administering** a prescribed enema, explain the purpose of the enema and what the patient can expect (e.g., the patient will probably experience some cramping with a large-volume enema). Reassure the patient that you will be immediately available to help her to the restroom or bedpan.

2. **Place the bedpan** or commode nearby.
   So you can reach the bedpan during the procedure, or so the patient can easily get to the commode.

3. **Open the enema supplies or kit.** Attach the tubing to the enema pail, if you are using a pail.
   The 1-liter enema bag comes with pre-connected tubing.

4. **Close the clamp on the tubing,** and fill the container with 500 to 1,000 mL of warm solution. The water temperature should be lukewarm—105°F to 110°F (40°C to 43°C).

   ✚ Check the temperature with a bath thermometer. Never warm the enema solution in a microwave oven.

   a. For infants: Use 50 to 150 mL of solution.
   b. For toddlers: Use 250 to 350 mL of solution.
   c. For school-age children: Use 300 to 500 mL of solution.
      Cold solution causes intestinal cramping. Very hot solution can damage the intestinal mucosa. Use the correct amount of solution to decrease the necessity of repeating the procedure.

5. **Add castile soap** (or the soap solution used by your facility) to the fluid at this time if a soapsuds enema has been prescribed.
   Soap causes mucosal irritation, which stimulates peristalsis and defecation.

6. **Hang the container** on the IV pole. Holding the end of the tubing over a sink or waste can, open the clamp and slowly allow the tubing to prime (fill) with solution. Reclamp the tubing when the tubing is filled.
   Expresses air from the tubing. Air introduced into the bowel may cause intestinal distention and discomfort.

7. **Don clean procedure gloves.**
   Prevents the transmission of intestinal bacteria.

8. **Position the patient:** Ask the patient to turn, or assist the patient to turn, to a left side-lying position with the right knee flexed.
   Allows the enema solution to fill the rectum and lower intestine following the natural flow of gravity.

   a. If the patient has shortness of breath associated with a respiratory condition, elevate the head of the bed very slightly. Avoid the semi-Fowler's position.
      The semi-Fowler's position increases the likelihood that gravity will cause the solution to leak out.

   b. ✚ Do not administer the enema with the patient on the toilet. The curved rectal tubing can scrape the rectal wall.

   c. If the patient has poor sphincter control, position him on the bedpan in a comfortable dorsal recumbent position.
      He will not be able to retain all of the enema solution.

9. **Place the waterproof pad** under the patient's buttocks or hips.
   Prevents soiling of bed linens.

10. **Drape the patient** with the bath blanket, exposing only the buttocks and rectum. See Procedure 24-4 to review the procedure for draping.
    Promotes patient privacy.

11. **Depending on the patient's** mobility status, place the bedpan flat on the bed, directly beneath the rectum, up against the patient's buttocks.

12. **Lubricate the tip** of the enema tubing generously.
    Allows for ease of insertion, decreases patient discomfort, and helps prevent mucosal irritation.

13. **If necessary, lift the superior buttock** to expose the anus. Slowly and gently insert the tip of the tubing approximately 7 to 10 cm (3 to 4 in.) into the rectum. Have the patient take slow, deep breaths as you complete this step. If the tube does not pass with ease, do not force it. Infuse a small amount of fluid and then try again, inserting the tube slowly.
    Helps the patient to relax, provides additional lubrication, and decreases reflex tightening of the anal sphincter. ▼

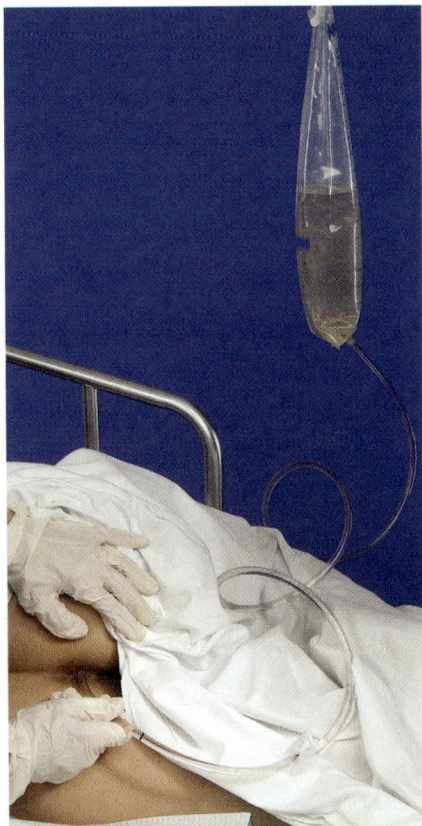

14. **Remove the container from the IV pole,** and hold it at the level of the patient's hips. Unclamp to begin instilling the solution.
    Lowering the container slows the force of the installation, decreasing pressure, cramping, discomfort, and reflex expulsion of the solution.

15. **Slowly raise the level** of the container, so that it is 30 to 45 cm (12 to 18 in.) above the level of the hips. Adjust the pole and re-hang the container. Continue a slow, steady instillation of the enema solution.
    The height of the container determines the speed of the flow. A slow, steady rate of infusion decreases cramping and increases the patient's ability to retain the solution.

16. **Continuously monitor the patient** for pain or discomfort. Assess his ability to retain the solution. If the patient has difficulty with retention, lower the level of the container, stop the flow for 15 to 30 seconds, and then resume the procedure.

➕ If the patient feels pain or you meet with resistance at any time during the procedure, stop and consult with the primary care provider.

17. **When the correct amount** of solution has been instilled, clamp the tubing, and slowly remove it from the rectum. If there is stool on the tubing, wrap the end of the tubing in a disposable wipe or toilet tissue until it can be rinsed or disposed of.
    Prevents transmission of pathogens.

18. **Clean the patient's rectal area,** recover the patient, and instruct him to hold the enema solution for approximately 5 to 15 minutes. Be certain the call light is within reach.
    - Retention of the enema solution will distend the bowel and increase the stimulus to defecate.
    - Leaving the solution in the bowel too long may result in fluid and electrolyte complications.
    - Retaining hypertonic solutions may result in dehydration related

to large amounts of fluids moving from the capillary bed into the bowel. Excessive retention of hypotonic solutions may cause fluid overload.

19. **Dispose of the enema supplies** or, if they are reusable, clean and store them in an appropriate location in the patient's room.
    Maintains a pleasant environment and helps prevent transfer of pathogens.

20. **Remove your gloves and perform hand hygiene.**
    Prevents transmission of intestinal pathogens.

21. **Depending on the patient's mobility,** assist him onto the bedpan, to the bedside commode, or to the toilet when he feels compelled to defecate. Perform hand hygiene and use clean procedure gloves as necessary.

22. **After the patient has defecated,** remove the bedpan or assist the patient to bed; inspect the stool for color, consistency, and quantity.

Procedure 29-3B ■ Administering a Prepackaged Enema

➤ When performing the procedure, always identify your patient according to agency policy, using two identifiers, and be attentive to standard precautions, hand hygiene, patient safety and privacy, body mechanics, and documentation.

Procedure Steps

1. **Open the prepackaged enema.** Remove the plastic cap from the container. Clip the tip of the container if it does not have a hole in it. The tip of the enema container comes prelubricated. However, you may need to add extra lubricant.
   Extra lubricant decreases discomfort and eases insertion of the tube into the rectum.

2. **Follow steps 7 through 13 of Procedure 29-3A** (regarding gloving, positioning, draping, and inserting the enema tip).

3. **Tilt the container slightly** and slowly roll and squeeze the container until all of the solution is instilled.

Ensures that the container empties completely and that an adequate amount of solution is instilled. ▼

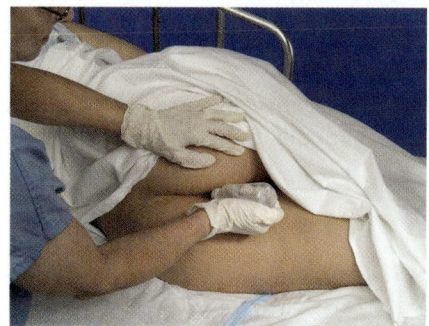

4. **Withdraw the container tip** from the rectum. Wipe the area with a disposable wipe or toilet tissue.
   Prevents transmission of pathogens.

5. **Cover the patient,** and instruct him to hold the enema solution for approximately 5 to 10 minutes. Be certain the call light is within reach.
   Retention of the enema solution will distend the bowel and increase the stimulus to defecate. Retaining the solution for longer than the prescribed time has been associated with dehydration and electrolyte imbalances.

6. **Dispose of the empty container.**
   Maintains a pleasant environment.

7. **Follow steps 19 through 21 of Procedure 29-3A** (regarding equipment disposal, assisting the patient, and observations of stool).

(continued on next page)

Procedure 29-3 ■ Administering an Enema (continued)

Procedure 29-3C ■ Administering an Oil-Retention Enema

➤ When performing the procedure, always identify your patient according to agency policy, using two identifiers, and be attentive to standard precautions, hand hygiene, patient safety and privacy, body mechanics, and documentation.

➤ *Note:* An oil-retention enema may be administered to help a client pass hard stool; it also may be administered before digital removal of stool; or it may be given at least 1 hour before a cleansing enema. See Procedure 29-4 for digital removal of stool.

Procedure Steps

1. **Obtain a commercial** oil-retention enema kit; these kits include a small rectal tube. If a commercial kit is not available, use a small tube and about 90 to 120 mL of the prescribed solution.
   A small tube allows for slower infusion, which minimizes cramping and thereby promotes retention.

2. ✚ **Warm the oil** to body temperature by running warm tap water over the container. Test a drop on your arm.
   If the oil is too cold, it will cause cramping and expulsion of the oil. If it is too warm, it may injure the patient.

3. **Follow steps 7 through 13 of Procedure 29-3A** (regarding gloving, positioning, draping, and inserting the enema tip).

4. **Instill the oil into the rectum.**
   Softens stool and lubricates the rectum for easier passage of stool.

5. **Withdraw the container tip** from the rectum. Wipe the area with a disposable wipe or toilet tissue.

6. **Cover the patient and instruct** him to retain the oil for at least 30 minutes.

7. **Follow steps 19 through 21 of Procedure 29-3A** (regarding equipment disposal, assisting the patient, and observations of stool).

Procedure 29-3D ■ Administering a Return-Flow Enema

➤ When performing the procedure, always identify your patient according to agency policy, using two identifiers, and be attentive to standard precautions, hand hygiene, patient safety and privacy, body mechanics, and documentation.

➤ *Note:* A return-flow enema (Harris flush) may be ordered to help a patient expel flatus and relieve abdominal distention.

Procedure Steps

1. **Obtain a rectal tube** and solution container (e.g., bag or canister).

2. **Prepare 100 to 200 mL** (for adults) of tap water or saline, the temperature should be lukewarm— 105°F to 110°F [40°C to 43°C].

3. **Follow steps 6 through 12 of Procedure 29-3A** (regarding gloving, positioning, draping, and inserting the enema tip).

4. **Instill all the solution** into the patient's rectum.

5. **Lower the tube and container** below the level of the rectum, and allow the solution to flow back into the container.

6. **Repeat this process** several times, or until the distention is relieved.

7. **Follow steps 19 through 21 of Procedure 29-3A** (regarding equipment disposal, assisting the patient, and observations of stool).

? What if . . .

- **The solution for a return-flow enema becomes thick with fecal matter?**

  Discard it and begin again with new solution.

Evaluation

- Observe the amount, color, and consistency of the stool.
- Evaluate the patient's tolerance of the procedure (e.g., amount of cramping, discomfort).
- Determine whether the prescriber's orders require subsequent enema administration.
- Some bowel exams require repeated enemas or enemas administered until the returns are "clear." For the latter, you will need to examine the return and determine whether stool particles are still present. "Clear" does not mean absence of color, but rather absence of stool particles and transparency of the liquid.

Patient Teaching

- Teach the patient that dependence on enemas can disrupt the normal process that stimulates defecation.
- Teach dietary and lifestyle changes that promote regular elimination (e.g., increased fluid intake, diet high in fiber, increased exercise).

Home Care

- Show the patient the box for a prepackaged enema and instruct him that he may purchase this type of enema at a local grocery or pharmacy.
- Assess the patient's ability to administer his own enema. If you determine that he will be unable to do so, encourage him to seek assistance and instruct the caregiver in the task.
- Teach the patient and caregiver proper hand washing. Encourage them to purchase nonsterile procedure gloves.
  Patients and caregivers may not be aware of the serious infections that can be caused by gram-negative intestinal bacteria.
- If the patient will be attempting to self-administer a cleansing enema, help him determine how and where to hang the container so that it is at the proper height.
- If a soapsuds enema is to be administered in the home setting, teach the patient which household soaps may be substituted for castile soap.
  Some soaps used in the home for cleaning purposes may be too harsh and irritating to the intestinal mucosa.

Documentation

- Document on the nursing notes the type of enema given and, if applicable, the amount of the solution instilled, patient's tolerance of the procedure, and characteristics and amount of stool.

- If the prescription is to administer enemas until the returns are clear, document the color of the return solution and the amount of stool seen.
- For prepackaged enemas, some facilities require documentation on the medication administration record (MAR) of the time given and the nurse's initials.

Sample Documentation

06/04/18   0825   Fleets enema administered (see MAR). Patient had no cramping; retained enema for 5 minutes. Passed moderate amount of solid, formed, brown stool with no mucus, but with a streak of blood on the surface. ———— R. Kline, RN

Thinking About the Procedure

To Practice applying critical reasoning to this procedure

 The video, **Administering a Cleansing Enema,** along with questions and suggested responses, is available on the *Davis's Nursing Skills Videos* Web site on DavisPlus.

Procedure 29-4 ■ Removing Stool Digitally

➤ For steps to follow in *all* procedures, refer to the Universal Steps for All Procedures found on the page facing the inside back cover.

Equipment

- Two pairs of clean procedure gloves
- Water-soluble lubricant (containing lidocaine, if agency policy permits)
- Bedpan and cover
- Prepackaged disposable wipes or moistened towelettes
- Bath blanket
- Waterproof pad

Delegation

This procedure should not be delegated to a NAP. Ongoing assessment of the patient by the professional nurse is required when stool is manually removed from the rectum. The nurse must monitor the patient for complications, such as bleeding and vagal nerve stimulation. Nursing judgment is necessary in determining the need to halt the procedure.

Pre-Procedure Assessments

- ✚ Assess the patient's baseline vital signs and history of heart disease. Be sure to monitor the patient's pulse before and during the procedure.
  Digital removal of stool can stimulate the vagus nerve, causing bradycardia. Patients who have a history of heart disease or dysrhythmia are at greater risk. You should check the physician order prior to administering.

- Assess the patient's white blood cell (WBC) count.
  If the patient has a compromised immune status as evidenced by a low WBC count, you should discuss this procedure with the primary care provider to evaluate the risks and benefits of the procedure.

- Assess the patient's cognitive level and mobility status.
  Determines the patient's ability to follow directions and turn in bed.

(continued on next page)

Procedure 29-4 ■ Removing Stool Digitally (continued)

- Determine the time of the patient's last bowel movement.
  The longer the stool remains in the lower bowel, the more water can be absorbed and the more likely it is that hard stool may form in the rectum.

- Assess the patient for history of fecal impaction.
  Can be a recurrent problem for immobile, disabled, or institutionalized patients.

- Assess stool consistency.
  Patients who are immobilized may become incontinent of watery stool. They may be able to pass small sections of hard stool or small quantities of watery stool. The latter, which may be intermittent or continuous, is a symptom of high colon impaction.

- Ask whether the patient experiences pain on defecation.
  Pain can cause the patient to suppress defecation.

- Assess the patient's pattern of bowel movements, diet, exercise, mobility status, and medications (e.g., iron supplements or narcotic analgesics).
  Determine whether any of these factors contribute to the problem and then add this information to the nursing care plan to help prevent recurrence.

- Assess bowel sounds and any abdominal distention.
  Peristalsis may be present without gastrointestinal patency, which creates distention. Abdominal distention can aggravate constipation.

Guidelines

- Prevention of fecal impaction is the best treatment, but if impaction has occurred, the stool must be removed. The procedure is both painful and embarrassing to your patient.
- An order from the healthcare practitioner may be necessary to perform digital disimpaction. Check your facility policy.
- Some practitioners may prescribe an oil-retention enema before the procedure to soften and moisten the stool, making removal easier.
- Many also advise that you follow digital removal of stool with either an oil-retention and/or tap water enemas. Enema(s) given after the procedure ensure the evacuation of stool that may not have been reached by digital removal.
- Trim and file your fingernails if they extend past the end of your fingertips.

> ➤ When performing the procedure, always identify your patient according to agency policy, using two identifiers, and be attentive to standard precautions, hand hygiene, patient safety and privacy, body mechanics, and documentation.

Procedure Steps

1. **Determine whether lubricant** containing lidocaine is to be used, and obtain the correct lubricant.
   May decrease rectal discomfort for the patient.

2. **Drape the patient** with the bath blanket. Go to Procedure 24-4 to review the procedure for draping. Assist him to turn on his left side, with his right knee flexed toward his head. Place the waterproof pad halfway beneath his left hip.
   Provides privacy and exposes the anus for visualization. The pad protects the bed from being soiled.

3. **Don clean procedure gloves.** Some sources recommend double-gloving.
   Prevents the transmission of intestinal bacteria.

4. **Expose the buttocks.** Place a clean, dry bedpan on the waterproof pad next to the buttocks in line with the rectum.

5. **Open the package of prepackaged disposable** wipes, or have toilet tissue ready to cleanse the rectal area when you complete the procedure.

6. **Generously lubricate either** the gloved forefinger and/or middle finger on your dominant hand.
   Helps prevent discomfort, pain, and mucosal injury.

7. **Slowly slide one lubricated finger** into the rectum. Observe for perianal irritation.
   The patient may need skin care to reduce pain during additional bowel evacuation. ▼

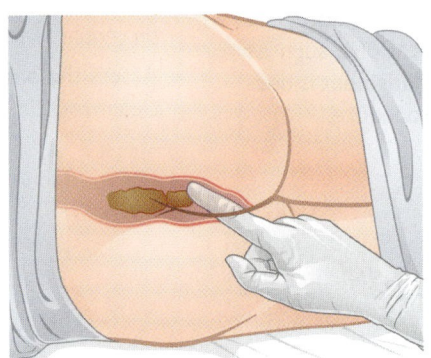

8. **Gently rotate your finger** around the mass and/or into the mass.
   Assists in determining the amount and texture of the fecal bulk.

9. **Begin to break the stool** into smaller pieces. At this point, you may insert a second finger and gently "slice" apart the stool, using a scissoring motion. Remove pieces of stool via the rectum as they become separated, and place them in the bedpan. ▼

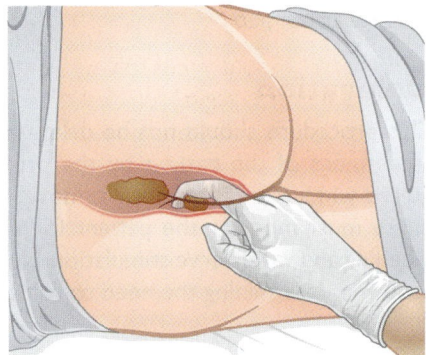

10. **As you proceed, instruct** the patient to take slow, deep breaths.
Helps the patient to relax his anal sphincter.

11. **Continue to manipulate** and remove pieces of stool, allowing the patient to rest at intervals. Reapply lubricant (containing lidocaine, if permitted) each time you reinsert your fingers.
Rest periods allow for assessment of and attention to the patient's comfort level and tolerance for the procedure.

12. ✚ **Assess the patient's heart rate** at regular intervals.
Bradycardia is a sign of vagal stimulation. Stop the procedure if the patient's heart rate falls or the rhythm changes from your initial assessment.

CAUTION: Some resources suggest that this procedure should be done in small steps (no more than four finger insertions in one session), giving a series of suppositories in between stool removal episodes.
Prevents patient fatigue and pain. Reduces the risk of injury to the rectal tissue and vagal stimulation.

13. **When removal of stool** is complete, cover the bedpan and set it aside. Use a prepackaged disposable wipe and/or toilet tissue to cleanse the rectal area.
Provides personal hygiene and decreases transmission of pathogens.

14. **Assist the patient to return** to a position of comfort. Note the color, amount, and consistency of the stool, and dispose of it properly.

15. **Remove your gloves and perform hand hygiene.**
Prevents transmission of intestinal pathogens.

? **What if . . .**

- **The patient is an infant?**
When treating infants with fecal impactions, avoid enemas and mineral oils. Glycerin suppositories may be used to soften the stool before removal.

Evaluation

- Determine whether evacuation of the retained stool was complete. Perform a rectal exam to assess for presence of stool.
- Reassess vital signs, and compare the results to the initial assessment. Continue to monitor for 1 hour for bradycardia.
- Assess bowel sounds.
- Palpate the abdomen for tenderness and firmness.
- Ask the patient whether he feels relief from rectal pressure or abdominal discomfort.

Patient Teaching

Retained stool is most often the result of poor dietary habits, lack of fluid intake, lack of exercise, inattentiveness to the urge to defecate, and laxative abuse. Focus patient teaching on lifestyle changes that facilitate a regular bowel elimination pattern.

Home Care

Home care should focus on preventing constipation that would require the digital removal of stool. Teach clients about high-fiber foods, adequate water intake, and the importance of exercise. Digital removal of stool may be necessary for some clients as part of a bowel-training program (e.g., patients who are paraplegic or quadriplegic). You can teach this procedure to the care provider in the home.

Documentation

- Document the bowel movement on the graphic record.
- Document the procedure and the patient's tolerance for the procedure in the nursing notes.
- Document the patient's pulse rate on the vital signs record.
- Document any unusual characteristics of the stool (e.g., black or green color, blood, or mucus).

Sample Documentation

07/11/18   1815   Impacted stool removed digitally. No perineal irritation noted. Removed moderate amount (approximately 6 oz [17 g]) dry, hard, gray-colored stool. Pulse 78 before removal; 84 after removal. Encouraged 8 oz fluids every hour. ————————— C. Byron, RNC

Practice Resources

National Guideline Clearinghouse (2014); McKay, S. L., Fravel, M., & Scanlon, C. (2012); Siegel, J., Rhinehart, E., Jackson, M., et al. (2007).

Procedure 29-5 ■ Inserting a Rectal Tube

➤ For steps to follow in *all* procedures, refer to the Universal Steps for All Procedures found on the page facing the inside back cover.

Equipment

- 22- to 34-French rectal tube for adults. Choose the size according to the size of the client. For children or petite adults, a smaller size tube (12- to 18-Fr) may be required.
- Water-soluble lubricant
- Procedure gloves
- Toilet paper
- Skin care items (e.g., soap, skin cleanser, disposable wipes)
- Collecting device (waterproof pad, graduated cylinder partially filled with water, a urine collection bag nicked at the top to vent)
- Paper tape
- Stool specimen container if needed

Pre-Procedure Assessments

- Obtain baseline vital signs.
- Auscultate bowel sounds; percuss for tympany.
- Observe and palpate the degree of abdominal distention.
- Ask whether the patient is passing any flatus.
- Assess discomfort caused by flatulence.
- Assess the condition of perianal tissues.
- Assess the history of cardiac disease.
  Insertion of a rectal tube can stimulate the vagus nerve, causing bradycardia.

➤ When performing the procedure, always identify your patient according to agency policy, using two identifiers, and be attentive to standard precautions, hand hygiene, patient safety and privacy, body mechanics, and documentation.

Procedure Steps

1. **Wear procedure gloves.**
   Follows standard precautions.

2. **Ask the patient to lift his hips** or roll from side to side to place a waterproof pad.
   Protects against soiling of linens.

3. **Attach a collecting device** to the end of the rectal tube: Tape a plastic bag or urine collection bag around the distal end of the rectal tube and vent the upper side of the bag.

   Alternatively, use one of these variations:

   - Insert the tube into the specimen container.
   - Place the end of the tube in a graduated container partially filled with water.
     Collects small pieces of stool expelled with flatus. Venting the plastic bag prevents overinflation and bursting the bag. An advantage of using water in the container is that gas generates bubbles, and you will be able to assess the effectiveness of the rectal tube based on the amount of bubbling in the container.

4. **Place patient in the left side-lying** position. Drape for privacy.
   Allows the tube to follow the normal curve of the rectum and sigmoid colon when inserted.

5. **Lubricate the tip of the rectal tube.**
   Prevents trauma to the rectal mucosa.

6. **Separate the buttocks** and ask the patient to take a deep breath. Gently insert the tube into the rectum.
   Adults: 10 to 12.5 cm (4 to 5 in.)
   Children: 5 to 10 cm (2 to 4 in.).
   Deep breaths relax the anal sphincter and ease tube insertion.

7. **For adults, tape the tube in place;** for children, hold it manually.

8. ✚ **Leave the rectal tube in place for 15 to 20 minutes.** If distention persists, you may reinsert the tube every 2 to 3 hours.
   Leaving the tube in place for more than 20 minutes may cause pressure necrosis of the mucosa; prolonged stimulation of the anal sphincter may result in loss of the neuromuscular response.

9. **Assist the patient to move** about in bed to promote gas expulsion. A knee–chest position is ideal.
   Because gas is lighter than fluid or solid, the position promotes passage of flatus. Unfortunately, many patients cannot tolerate this position.

10. **Remove the tube,** wipe the patient's buttocks with tissue, and assist to clean the rectal area as needed.
    Prevents transmission of microorganisms from feces; promotes patient comfort and skin integrity.

11. **Dispose of used equipment,** or clean it if it is to be reused. Follow agency procedures for cleaning.

Evaluation

- Evaluate the patient's response to the procedure (e.g., vital signs, fatigue).
- Assess abdominal distention and abdominal comfort.

Patient Teaching

- Teach the patient that chewing gum, sucking on hard candy, using a straw, smoking, and drinking carbonated beverages increase air swallowing and abdominal distention.
- Teach factors that promote normal elimination (e.g., exercise, increased fluid intake, adequate dietary fiber).

Documentation

Record the following:

- Date and time tube inserted
- Size of tube and characteristics of feces collected
- Abdominal distention before and after the procedure
- Pulse and respiratory rates before and after the procedure
- Tolerance of procedure and any complications
- Patient and family teaching

Procedure 29-6 ■ Changing an Ostomy Appliance

➤ For steps to follow in *all* procedures, refer to the Universal Steps for All Procedures found on the page facing the inside back cover.

➤ *Note:* Some pouches come with the wafer attached, some without. These instructions assume that the wafer is attached.

➤ *Note:* Also see Clinical Insight 29-2: Guidelines for Ostomy Care.

Equipment

- Ostomy pouch
  - One-piece pouch with the wafer attached, or a two-piece system with a separate wafer and pouch
  - Clamp for pouches with an opening at the bottom (a new clamp is not used each time; usually one clamp is packaged with each box of pouches)
- Skin care items per agency protocol or recommended by the enterostomal therapist (e.g., pH balanced skin cleanser, skin prep, skin barrier wipe, adhesive remover, adhesive paste, and stoma paste if needed to fill and smooth skin surface)
- Stoma measuring guide (or precut template)
- Scissors
- Pen or pencil
- Two pairs of clean procedure gloves
- Prepackaged disposable wipes
- Toilet tissue
- 4 in. × 4 in. gauze pad
- Bedpan or container for effluent (fecal material)
- Plastic bag (for disposal of used pouch)
- Plastic bag for disposal of other contaminated articles
- Waterproof pad
- Ostomy deodorant
- Hypoallergenic paper tape (optional) or ostomy belt
- Bath blanket ➤

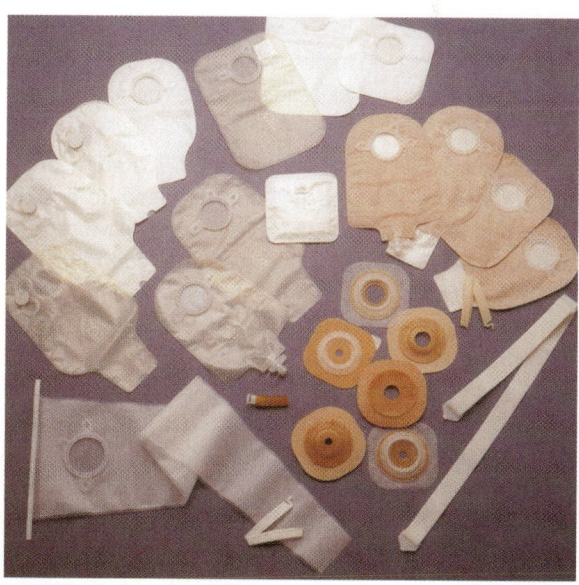

Delegation

During the immediate postoperative period, the professional nurse must assess the newly created stoma and peristomal skin area and use clinical judgment when changing a pouch. You may delegate to a NAP if it is a preexisting, stable stoma

(continued on next page)

Procedure 29-6 ■ Changing an Ostomy Appliance (continued)

and if you are sure the NAP is qualified to perform the task. If you do delegate this task, instruct the NAP to report any changes or unusual findings (e.g., changes in stoma color, swelling, peristomal redness, excoriation, deviations from expected amount) and color and consistency of drainage from the stoma.

Pre-Procedure Assessments

- Assess the type of stoma (e.g., ileostomy, colostomy, urostomy), number of stomas, and location on the abdomen (e.g., is the stoma near structures that will impact care?).
  Determines the type of pouch or system to use.

- Assess stoma color, shape, size, and/or length of protrusion or retraction; stoma construction (end, loop, double barrel); direction of stoma lumen; and discharge. Does the stoma lie flat or does it protrude?
  The stoma should be moist and red or pink. Alterations in stoma color (purple, black, or blue) may indicate poor circulation and possible necrosis and should be reported to the primary provider. Protruding or retracted stomas will need special adjustments in wafer measurement and placement. It is normal for a new stoma to have yellow or blood-tinged mucus or dried blood on it.

- Assess peristomal skin for redness, rash, irritation, or excoriation. Observe the existing skin barrier and pouch for leakage and length of time in place. You may have to remove the pouch to observe the stoma fully, depending on the type of pouch (i.e., if the pouch is opaque). Notify the provider or an ostomy specialist immediately if you note peristomal skin abnormalities.
  Preserving peristomal skin is critical because skin excoriation may cause an ineffective seal between the wafer and the skin and leakage of effluent. This in turn causes more skin and tissue damage. Leakage may indicate the need for a different type of pouch system or sealant.

- Determine the changing schedule for the pouch.
  Pouches are usually changed every 3 to 5 days, preferably before leakage occurs. Frequency also depends on the type of stoma, the equipment used (e.g., one- or two-piece pouch), the effluent, the patient's preference, and the climate (i.e., pouches are changed more frequently during the summer). To decrease skin irritation, avoid changing the entire system. In a one-piece or two-piece pouching system, change the skin barrier only every 3 to 7 days, never daily.

- Observe abdominal shape and incision, if present.
  Abdominal shape determines the proper placement of the pouch. Because of stomal and abdominal characteristics, some patients may need convexity in their ostomy pouching system to avoid leakage.

- Assess the patient's willingness to look at the stoma, touch the appliance, and discuss or participate in the task.
  May indicate a readiness or desire to learn.

- Assess the patient's condition and self-care ability. Consider vision, dexterity or mobility, and cognitive ability.
  Helps determine the best type of appliance to use.

- Auscultate for bowel sounds.
  Determines the presence of peristalsis.

- Observe for effluent from the stoma, and document your findings.
  Change the skin barrier pouch at times of lower effluent output. Avoid changing after meals, when the gastrocolic reflux increases chance of fecal effluent output. Mucous secretion is normal.

- Assess whether a new clamp will be needed or the one on the pouch can be used again.

- Consult a peristomal nurse or the primary care provider to determine whether an ostomy should be irrigated.
  Many patients with left-end colostomies may be safely irrigated as a method of continence management. An ileostomy, however, drains liquid containing high concentrations of sodium, chloride, potassium, magnesium, and bicarbonate.

- ✚ Ileostomies should never be irrigated, except in cases of food blockage near the stomal outlet. Only a qualified person, such as an enterostomal therapy nurse, may perform a gentle lavage.

➤ When performing the procedure, always identify your patient according to agency policy, using two identifiers, and be attentive to standard precautions, hand hygiene, patient safety and privacy, body mechanics, and documentation.

Procedure Steps

1. **Perform hand hygiene and don clean procedure gloves.**
   Prevents transmission of pathogens.

2. **Fold down the bed covers** to expose the ostomy site. Place a clean towel across the patient's abdomen under the existing pouch.
   Helps prevent spilling effluent onto the patient.

3. **Position the patient** so that no skinfolds occur along the line of the stoma.
   Ensures an adequate seal between the wafer and the skin, preventing leakage.

4. **If the present ostomy pouch** is drainable, empty it into the bedpan.
   Pouches should be drained when they are one-third to one-half full because the weight of the contents may dislodge the skin seal; ostomy drainage is irritating to the skin. The pouch also collects flatus, which needs to be expelled because it can disrupt the skin seal.

   a. To calculate the amount of output in milliliters for an ostomy with a liquid effluent (e.g., ileostomy or urostomy), use a graduated measuring container.

b. For pouches that you open by un-rolling them at the bottom, you must remove a clamp to empty the pouch. Save this clamp for reuse.

NOTE: Some pouches cannot be drained.

5. **Remove the appliance by applying a silicone-based** (hexamethyld-isiloxane) adhesive remover, with one hand as you press the skin away from the wafer barrier with your other hand. Avoid pulling the appliance straight off. Begin at the top and work downward. ▼

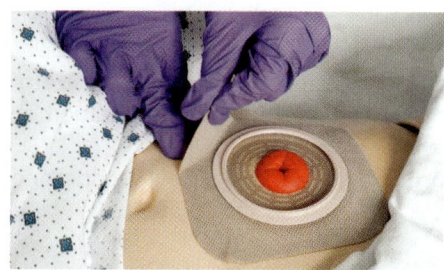

Silicone-based adhesive removers are preferred over alcohol- or oil-based products. Pulling the appliance from the skin tends to strip the loosely bound epidermal skin layers, making the skin more susceptible to moisture loss and irritation from effluent. Silicone-based products reduce the bind strength, whereas alcohol dissolves the adhesives; thus, alcohol may cause dryness and irritation. It also causes pain if the skin is not intact. Furthermore, if you use an oil-based solvent, the new pouch will not adhere to the oily skin.

6. **Place the old pouch and wafer** in the plastic bag for disposal. If the pouch is not a drainable one, dispose of it according to agency protocol.
Prevents transmission of infections caused by fecal bacteria.

7. **Inspect the stoma and peristomal** skin area for redness, rash, irritation, or excoriation (see Pre-Procedure Assessments).

8. **Remove your gloves and** perform hand hygiene.
Decreases the spread of intestinal bacteria.

9. **Don clean procedure gloves.**

10. **Cleanse the stoma** and surrounding skin using a skin-cleansing agent with a pH of 5.5 that is designed to both cleanse and moisturize the skin.
Removes old adhesive and any effluent that has leaked. Helps prevent skin irritation and/or breakdown and maintain skin moisture. Select cleansing agents that protect the stratum corneum lipids and proteins.

11. **Measure the size of the stoma.** You can accomplish this in several ways.
    a. Place a standard stoma measuring guide over the stoma.
    b. Reuse a previously cut template.
    c. Measure the stoma from side to side (approximating the circumference).
    The stoma may need to be remeasured frequently during the initial postoperative period because the size of the stoma may change as edema subsides. ▼

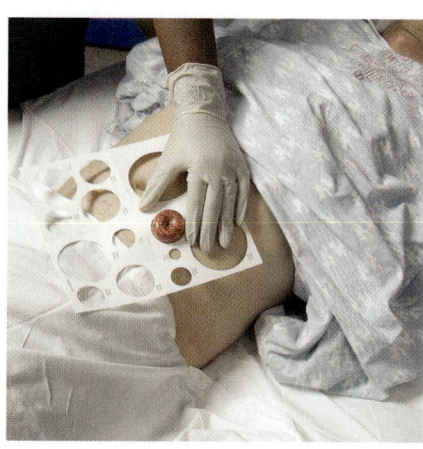

12. **Place a clean 4 in. × 4 in. gauze** pad over the stoma.
Gauze will absorb any leaking effluent, keeping the skin clean and dry during application of the new pouch.

13. **Trace the size of the opening** (obtained in step 11) onto the paper on the back of the new wafer. Cut the opening. The opening in the wafer should be approximately $1/16$ to $1/8$ in. (1.5 to 3 mm) larger than the circumference of the stoma. Holding the wafer between the palms of your hand to warm the adhesive ring.
Allows for skin movement with activity and prevents impaired circulation to the stoma. Warming the adhesive ring enhances the integrity of the seal by making the ring more "sticky" so that it will bond better with the skin.

14. **Apply ostomy skin care products** at this time using your clinical judgment, hospital protocol, or following the recommendations of the enterostomal therapist (e.g., wipe around stoma with skin prep, apply skin barrier powder or paste, or apply extra adhesive paste).
These products prevent or treat excoriated skin and/or ensure a tight seal between the wafer and the skin.

15. **Remove the gauze** from the stoma.

16. **Peel the paper off the wafer.** Center the wafer opening around the stoma and gently press it down. Make sure the bag is pointed toward the patient's feet. Press your hand firmly against the newly applied wafer and hold for 30 to 60 seconds.
Heat from the hand activates the adhesive ring, making it adhere better thus promoting optimal wear time. Some sources also suggest taping down the edges of the wafer.

17. **Remove your gloves and** perform hand hygiene.

18. **Return the patient** to a comfortable position.

19. **Dispose of the used ostomy pouch** following your facility's policy for biohazardous waste.

(continued on next page)

Procedure 29-6 ■ Changing an Ostomy Appliance (continued)

? What if . . .

■ **Your patient has a two-piece pouch?**

After applying the wafer around the stoma with a good seal (step 16), attach the bag following manufacturer's instructions.

■ **Your patient's ostomy uses an open-ended pouch?**

After applying the wafer securely around the stoma, fold the end of the pouch over the clamp and close the clamp, listening for a "click" to ensure that it is secure.

■ **When cleansing the stoma (step 7), you notice that the stoma is bleeding?**

Slight bleeding of the stoma is normal; report excessive bleeding to the primary care provider.

Evaluation

Make the following observations:

■ Characteristics of stoma: color, size, presence of edema, and shape
■ Presence of blisters, redness, or excoriation on peristomal skin
■ Amount and characteristics of effluent: color, odor, consistency
■ Whether the patient expressed a desire to participate in the task
■ Whether the patient demonstrated nonverbal cues that she is ready to learn about the task (e.g., looking at the stoma)

Patient Teaching

Patient teaching is aimed at preparing the patient to complete this skill at home. She (or a caregiver) will need to be instructed in how to complete all the steps of the procedure.

Home Care

■ Assess the patient's self-care ability and assist the client to establish a routine for changing the stoma wafer/pouch (see Clinical Insight 29-2). The client may need to stand in front of a mirror or sit to change her ostomy appliance if she is unable to view the stoma easily.

■ Teach the client that slight bleeding is normal when the stoma is washed.
■ The client should not use soaps and lotions containing oils. They decrease the adhesiveness of the wafer.
■ The appliance and wafer cannot be flushed down the toilet.
■ Teach the client to report changes in the color or size of the stoma and/or the presence of peristomal irritation or skin breakdown to the primary care provider.
■ Provide contact information for ostomy supply vendors and community support groups, such as Ostomates.

Documentation

Document the following:

■ Your assessment of the stoma and peristomal skin area
■ Patient's tolerance of the procedure
■ Type of appliance used, including the manufacturer and part number
■ Use of any special ostomy skin care products
■ Amount of liquid effluent (on the intake and output [I&O] portion of the graphics record)
■ Patient teaching and the degree to which the patient participated in the procedure

Sample EHR Documentation

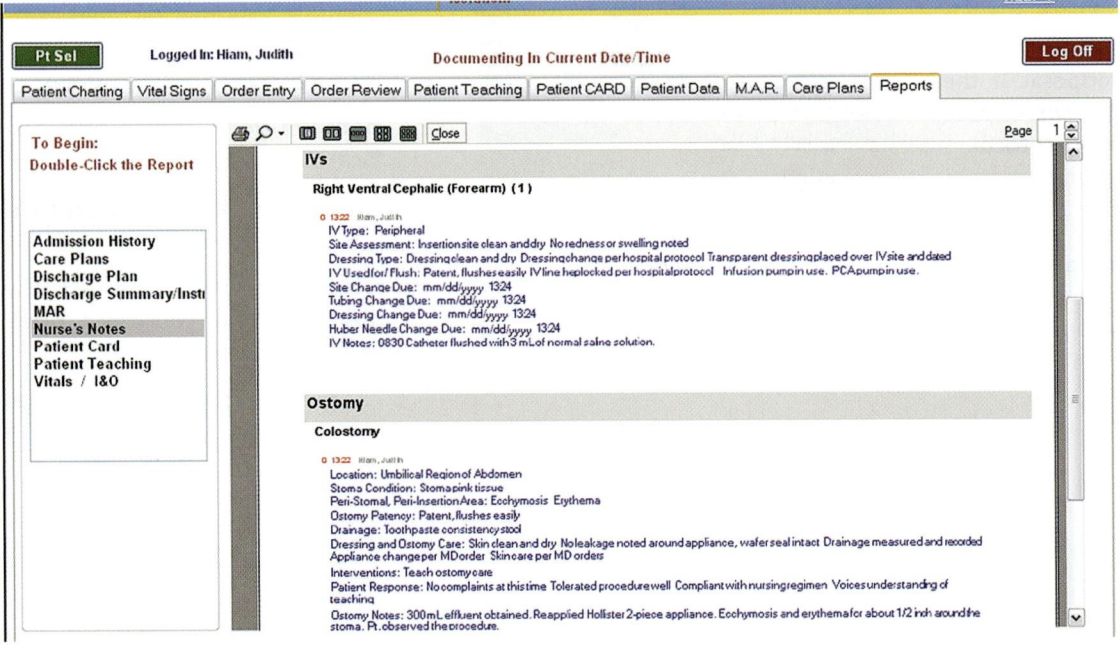

Practice Resources

Burch, J. (2014); Gray, M., Colwell, J. C., Doughty, D., et al. (2013); Tam, K. W., Lai, J. H., Chen, H. C., et al. (2014); Siegel, J., Rhinehart, E., Jackson, M., et al. (2007).

Thinking About the Procedure

To practice applying clinical reasoning to this procedure,

 The video, **Changing an Ostomy Appliance,** along with questions and suggested responses, is available on the ***Davis's Nursing Skills Videos*** Web site on Davis*Plus*.

Procedure 29-7 ■ Irrigating a Colostomy

➤ For steps to follow in all procedures, refer to the Universal Steps for All Procedures found on the inside back cover.

Equipment

- Irrigation equipment
  - One-piece system with a fluid container connected to tubing with cone or two-piece system with a container separate from tubing with cone
  - Irrigation sleeve; a sleeve without adhesive backing requires a belt to hold it in place
  - Clamp for a sleeve with an opening at the top
  - Prescribed irrigating solution (usually 500 to 1,000 mL warm tap water, 105°F to 110°F [40°C to 43°C])
- IV pole or other equipment to hang the irrigation container
- Chair
- Water-soluble lubricant
- Silicone-based adhesive remover
- Skin cleansers and barriers as recommended by your agency
- Toilet tissue
- Prepackaged disposable wipes
- Waterproof pad
- Two pairs of clean procedure gloves
- Toilet facilities that include a flushable toilet and a hook or some other device to hold the irrigation container; or bedpan or bedside commode (for patients with impaired mobility)
- New ostomy appliance and skin barrier or stoma cap cover
- Ostomy deodorant (optional)
- Plastic bag for disposal of the used pouch

Delegation

The initial irrigation of a newly created colostomy requires nursing judgment and clinical decision making. Initially, this procedure should not be delegated to the NAP, although in some situations it may be delegated to a licensed practical nurse (LPN), depending on agency policy.

Pre-Procedure Assessments

- Evaluate the defecation pattern (or absence) nature of stool, placement of stoma, abdominal distention, and nutritional pattern.
  Findings may indicate the need to irrigate to stimulate elimination function; consistency of stool varies along the length of the gastrointestinal (GI) tract.
- Identify the type of ostomy.
  Many patients with left-end colostomies may be safely irrigated as a method of continence management. However, do not irrigate an ileostomy.
- Assess the patient's usual bowel pattern.
  The purpose for irrigating a colostomy is to promote a regular pattern for bowel elimination.
- Assess for abdominal distention.
  Report distention to the primary care provider, as it may indicate excess gas or inflammation.
- Assess hydration.
  The colon may absorb some of the irrigation fluid if the patient is very dehydrated.
- Assess cognitive level and mobility status.
  Determines the necessity for a bedpan or bedside commode. Also determines whether patient teaching will be effective.
- Assess the patient's ability to maintain a sitting position.

(continued on next page)

Procedure 29-7 ■ Irrigating a Colostomy (continued)

➤ When performing the procedure, always identify your patient according to agency policy, using two identifiers, and be attentive to standard precautions, hand hygiene, patient safety and privacy, body mechanics, and documentation.

Procedure Steps

I. Place the IV pole near the location of the procedure (e.g., in the bathroom, next to the bedside commode, or next to the bed).
Allows you to work efficiently.

2. Assist the patient to the bathroom or commode, if possible. Ask the patient if she prefers to sit directly on the toilet or on a chair in front of it. If the patient must remain in bed, elevate the head of the bed.
Patients with impaired mobility can sit directly on or in front of the bedside commode, or they may remain in bed in the side-lying position.

3. Prepare the irrigation container
a. For two-piece systems, connect the tubing to the container. Clamp the tubing. Fill the container with 500 to 1,000 mL of warm tap water.

⊕ Water that is too cold will cause cramping, nausea, and discomfort. Water that is too hot will damage the intestinal mucosa.

NOTE: *Some ostomy resources suggest that using 1,000 mL of water will promote a more effective irrigation of the entire colon and decrease the necessity to irrigate more than once a day.*

4. Hang the solution container on the IV pole. Adjust the IV pole so that it reaches the height of the patient's shoulder (approximately 45 cm [18 in.], above the stoma).
The height of the container regulates the force of the flow.

5. Unclamp the tubing to prime it and allow it to fill.
Removes air from the tubing, preventing gas pains.

6. Perform hand hygiene and don clean procedure gloves.
Prevents the transmission of pathogens.

7. Remove the existing colostomy appliance (if the patient is wearing one) following the steps in Procedure 29-6.
Use of ostomy skin care preparations may be needed when you replace the pouch.

8. Dispose of the used colostomy appliance properly. Empty the contents into the bedpan or toilet, and discard the pouch in a moisture-proof (e.g., plastic) bag.
Prevents transmission of intestinal bacteria.

9. Assess the characteristics of the stoma and surrounding skin (see Clinical Insight 29-2).

10. Apply the colostomy irrigation sleeve, following the manufacturer's directions.
  ■ *If your patient is sitting on a toilet or bedside commode,* then the end of the sleeve should hang down past the patient's pubic area, but not down into the water. Place a waterproof pad under the sleeve over the patient's thighs.
  ■ *If your patient is in bed,* place the end of the sleeve into the bedpan.
  Prevents leakage and spilling of irrigation fluid and effluent.

11. Generously lubricate the cone at the end of the irrigation tubing with water-soluble lubricant.
Prevents irritation and damage to the stoma and intestinal lumen.

12. Open the top of the irrigation sleeve; insert the cone gently into the colostomy stoma, and hold it solidly in place.
Gentle insertion prevents damage to the mucosa. ➤

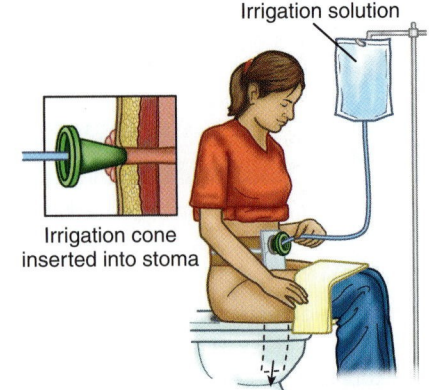

Irrigation solution

Irrigation cone inserted into stoma

13. Open the clamp on the tubing, and slowly begin the flow of water. The fluid should flow for about 10 to 15 minutes or as the patient can tolerate.
Proceeding slowly allows the patient to adjust to the distention of the bowel.

14. If the patient complains of discomfort, stop the flow for 15 to 30 seconds, and ask the patient take deep breaths.
Allows the patient to rest and adjust to the pressure of solution. Cramping may indicate that the bowel is ready to empty, the water is too cold, the flow is too fast, or the tube contains air.

15. When the correct amount of solution has instilled, clamp the tubing, and remove the cone from the stoma.

16. Wrap the end of the cone in toilet tissue or disposable wipe until you can clean or dispose of it properly.
Prevents transmission of intestinal bacteria.

17. Close the top of the irrigation sleeve with a clamp.
Prevents spillage of irrigation fluid and feces.

18. **Wait for evacuation to occur:**
    ■ *If the patient is sitting,* ask her to remain sitting until most of the irrigation fluid and bowel contents have evacuated. Alternatively, you can clamp the end of the sleeve and ask the patient to ambulate to stimulate complete evacuation of stool.
    ■ *If the patient is in bed,* massaging the abdomen may also help stimulate return.
    This should take about 30 minutes on average. You might wait for about an hour to be certain all the fecal material has been returned.

19. **When evacuation is complete,** open the top clamp, and rinse and remove the irrigation sleeve. Set it aside.
    The irrigation sleeve is reusable, but it should be rinsed promptly to make thorough cleansing easier in the following steps.

20. **Change gloves**

21. **Cleanse the stoma** and peristomal skin area with a warm prepackaged disposable wipe. Prep the skin and apply a new colostomy appliance, if the patient is wearing one, following the steps in Procedure 29-6. Otherwise, cover the stoma with a small gauze bandage.

22. **Clean the irrigation sleeve** with mild soap and water. Allow it to dry. Place the irrigation supplies in the proper place (e.g., in a plastic container or plastic bag).
    The irrigation sleeve is reusable, but it must be cleaned well to avoid odors and transmission of pathogens.

23. **Remove your gloves** and perform hand hygiene.
    Prevents healthcare-associated infections.

24. **Assist the patient** back to a position of comfort.

? What if . . .

■ **Your patient has a colostomy sleeve without an adhesive backing?**
Place the belt around the patient's waist, and attach the ends to the pouch flange on either side.

Evaluation

Observe the following:
■ Characteristics of the stool: color, amount, consistency
■ Signs of bleeding from stoma or bowel
■ Presence or absence of abdominal distention
■ Patient's tolerance of procedure (e.g., cramps, fatigue)
■ Patient's ability to participate in the irrigation

Patient Teaching

■ Teach the patient the purpose for the procedure.
■ Explain that using sufficient fluid will decrease the need for multiple irrigations during the day.
■ Teach the steps of the irrigation procedure to prepare the patient to complete the task at home.
■ Explain that it takes approximately 6 to 8 weeks to achieve bowel regulation with irrigations.

Home Care

■ Help the client determine where this procedure will be completed in the home setting.
■ Make sure the client has resources for purchasing the supplies for the irrigation. Provide contact information.
■ Help the client locate a place to hang the irrigation container. There may be a hook on the bathroom wall, for instance.
■ If the irrigating solution does not flow well, the client should:
  Check the tubing for kinks.
  Change the position of the cone.
  Put the container at a slightly higher level.
■ Explain and demonstrate how to care for the irrigation supplies (e.g., how to rinse and clean the sleeve and/or belt, if used).

Documentation

Document:
■ Your assessment of the stoma and peristomal area
■ The amount of irrigation solution used
■ The date and time that you performed the irrigation
■ Characteristics of the stool returned in the irrigation fluid
■ Patient teaching

Sample documentation

06/14/18   0830 AM   Ostomy irrigated with 750 ml warm tap water. Small amount of loose, formed, flakery stool returned in the fluid, with some undigested food apparent. No blood; very small amount of mucus. Stoma pink, peristomal area without redness. Explained procedure steps to patient as it was performed. Patient stated he will do some of the steps tomorrow. ————— C. Hiam, RNC

Practice Resources

Alverslid, I., Carlsson, E., Gylin, M., et al. (2012); Avent, Y. (2012); Bauer, C., Arnold-Long, M., & Kent, D. J. (2016); Cobb, M. D., Grant, M., Tallman, N. J., et al. (2015); Kent, D. J., Arnold- Long, M., & Bauer, C. (2015); Siegel, Rhinehart, Jackson, et al., and the Healthcare Infection Control Practices Advisory Committee, 2007.

Thinking About the Procdeure

To practice applying clinical reasoning to this procedure,

 The video, Irrigating a Colostomy, along with questions and suggested responses, is available on the ***Davis's Nursing Skills Videos*** website on DavisPlus.

Procedure 29-8 ■ **Placing Fecal Drainage Devices**

➤ For steps to follow in *all* procedures, refer to the Universal Steps for All Procedures found on the page facing the inside back cover.

Equipment

External Fecal Collection Device ▼

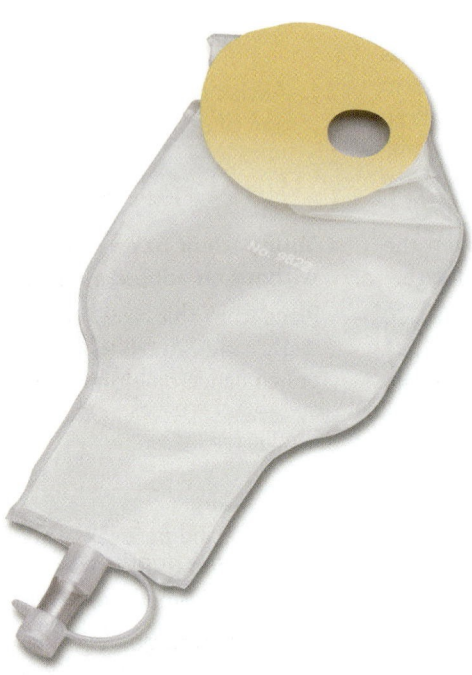

- pH-balanced soap and water or recommended skin cleanser
- Skin protection wipes (e.g., peristomal wipes to protect skin and improve adherence)
- Self-adhesive fecal containment device
- Procedure gloves
- Linen-saver pad
- Scissors

Internal Fecal Collection System

- Fecal device kit: Contains soft silicone catheter tube assembly, a syringe, and a collection bag.
- Water-soluble lubricant
- Approximately 100-mL container of filtered tap water or saline. (Follow the manufacturer's directions for amount and type of solution.)
- 500 mL of lukewarm irrigant (filtered tap water or saline)
- 60-mL luer-tip syringe and a catheter tip syringe (if not contained in the kit)
- Protective skin-care dressing (e.g., Stomahesive®, DuoDerm®)
- Tape
- Procedure gloves, mask, and goggles
- pH-balanced soap and water or recommended skin cleanser

- Scissors
- Linen-saver pad ▼

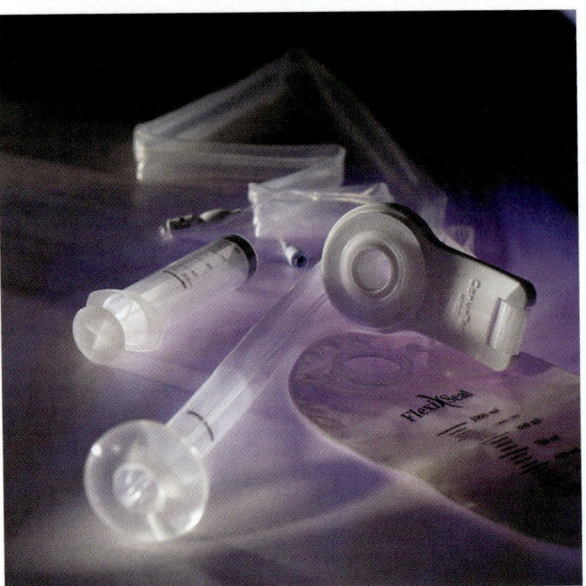

Delegation

Application of an external fecal collection system may be delegated to the NAP. Insertion of an internal fecal collection device is usually performed by a professional nurse, but may be delegated to an LPN depending on agency policy.

Pre-Procedure Assessments

- Assess the patient's bowel patterns.
  Fecal diversion is indicated when the patient is incontinent of liquid or semi-liquid stools (flowing).
- Assess for allergies to silicone. If the patient is sensitive or allergic to any of the materials in the device, it cannot be used.
- Inspect perirectal skin.
  External devices should not be used in patients with impaired skin integrity.

For Indwelling Devices, in Addition:

- Assess whether the patient has had a recent bowel movement.
  Patients who have not had a bowel movement for 2 or more days should be considered as having firm stool and will likely be given a bowel prep or enema before insertion of the indwelling device.
- Check for the presence of any indwelling anal or rectal device (e.g., thermometer for continuous temperature monitoring).
  The treatment plan may need to be changed. If suppositories or enemas are a part of the current treatment plan, collaborate with the prescriber as these medication delivery mechanisms will need to be changed.

- ⊕ Identify factors that increase your patient's risk for bleeding, including medications (anticoagulant and/or antiplatelet therapy) and lab results (prothrombin time, partial thromboplastin time, platelets).
Patients with an increased risk of bleeding should be monitored carefully.

- ⊕ Check the chart for contraindications to an indwelling fecal management system (e.g., proctitis, lacerations, rectal surgery in the past year, large or painful hemorrhoids).

If your patient has a history of any of these problems, contact the primary care provider immediately. You may elect to use an external device, but an internal fecal catheter is contraindicated.

- ⊕ Internal fecal catheters should not be used for children.

Procedure 29-8A ■ Applying an External Fecal Collection System

➤ When performing the procedure, always identify your patient according to agency policy, using two identifiers, and be attentive to standard precautions, hand hygiene, patient safety and privacy, body mechanics, and documentation.

1. **Recruit another nurse** or nursing assistant to help you. Assist the patient to a side-lying position and drape to expose the buttocks.
For successful application (without leakage) it is best to have one caregiver position the patient and a second person to apply the device.

2. **Don procedure gloves.**
Observes standard precautions.

3. **Cleanse the perineal area and dry well.** If perianal hair is present, trim it away.

4. **Wipe the area with skin protectant wipes.**
To obtain a leakproof seal, the device should be attached to clean, dry skin. The wipes protect the skin and improve adherence.

5. **Spread the buttocks apart** to expose the rectum.

6. **Remove the backing** from the adhesive on the fecal bag, then apply it, being careful to place the opening in the bag over the anus and to avoid gaps and creases.
Careful application helps to obtain a leak-proof seal.

7. **Release the buttocks.** Connect the fecal incontinence pouch to a drainage bag.

8. **Hang drainage bag** below patient.
To collect and promote gravity drainage of fecal material.

Procedure 29-8B ■ Inserting an Indwelling Fecal Drainage Device

➤ When performing the procedure, always identify your patient according to agency policy, using two identifiers, and be attentive to standard precautions, hand hygiene, patient safety and privacy, body mechanics, and documentation.

➤ Note: Because devices differ markedly, it is best to follow the manufacturer's instructions for placing the device. The following are generic instructions.

➤ Note: Also see Clinical Insight 29-1: Caring for a Patient With an Indwelling Fecal Drainage Device.

Procedure Steps

1. **Ensure that a primary care** provider has performed a digital rectal exam.
To assess for the presence of contraindications and to check sphincter tone. When sphincter tone is compromised, the patient may not be able to retain the device.

2. **Don procedure gloves, mask,** and goggles.
To protect from splatters when irrigating or disconnecting the device. Usually the devices are used for incontinence of loose, if not liquid, stool.

3. **Position the patient** in the left side-lying position.
Allows access to the rectum.

4. **Remove any indwelling device.**
The presence of a foreign body between the inflated balloon and rectum may damage rectal mucosa and a seal cannot be maintained.

5. **Depending on the type of device,** verify proper inflation and deflation of the intraluminal balloon. Attach the syringe, inflate with the recommended amount of air, deflate, and remove the syringe.

6. **Again depending on the device,** fill the retention cuff with 35 to 40 mL of water; disconnect syringe and check for leaks. After verifying function, slowly and completely aspirate all fluid from cuff and balloon and disconnect the syringe.

7. **Connect the indwelling tube** to the collection bag. Clamp and hang the bag lower than the level of the patient.

(continued on next page)

Procedure 29-8 ■ **Placing Fecal Drainage Devices** (continued)

8. **Some systems have an "introducer,"** which you must inflate with about 25 mL of air through a connector on the tube. Disconnect the syringe. ➤

9. **Insert your lubricated, gloved index** finger into the balloon cuff finger pocket (located above the position indicator line) and coat the balloon generously with lubricant.
This allows for digital guidance during insertion.

10. **Gently insert the balloon** end of the catheter through the anal sphincter until the balloon is beyond the anus and well inside the rectal vault.
This helps prevent accidental expulsion of the device.

11. **Inflate the retention cuff** with water or saline per the manufacturer's guidelines. Do not overfill. If the catheter will not accept the recommended amount of fluid, see the What if . . . ? section at the end of this procedure. ▼

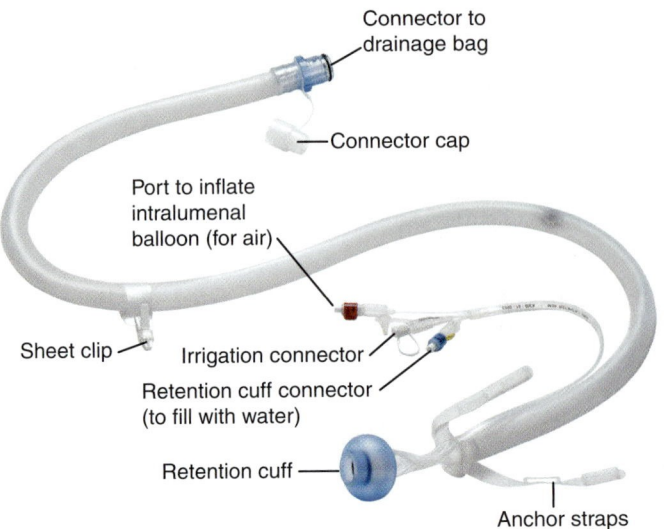

Connector to drainage bag

Connector cap

Port to inflate intralumenal balloon (for air)

Sheet clip

Irrigation connector

Retention cuff connector (to fill with water)

Retention cuff

Anchor straps

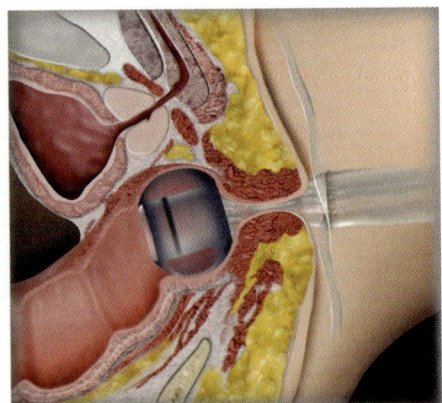

12. **Remove the syringe** from the inflation port and put gentle traction on the catheter.
To determine whether the balloon is securely in the rectum and appropriately positioned against the rectal floor.

13. **If you inflated an intraluminal** balloon or introducer in step 8, you must now completely aspirate the air from it.

➕ Do not leave an air-inflated intraluminal balloon inflated in an unattended patient.

An inflated balloon can cause tissue necrosis after a period of time.

14. **If the device has anchoring straps,** apply protective skin care dressing and tape one strap to each of the patient's buttocks.
Prevents internal migration of the tube and occlusion by twisting of the tube.

15. **Position the tubing along** the patient's leg, avoiding kinks and obstruction and position the collection bag lower than the patient.
Promotes flow of stool from the rectum to the collection bag.

? What if . . .

■ **When irrigating, the catheter will not accept the recommended amount of fluid?**

Deflate the balloon and reposition the catheter.
The catheter is probably not positioned correctly. Do not use more than the recommended amount of fluid, as this would result in excessive pressure on the rectal vault and may cause mucosal or sphincter damage.

■ **Rectal bleeding occurs with an internal fecal management device?**

Discontinue the device and notify the physician.
Bleeding may indicate pressure necrosis from the device.

Evaluation

■ Confirm catheter/bowel lumen patency by irrigating the bowel according to manufacturer's instructions and physician order. Regular irrigation is required to facilitate evacuation through most devices.
Stool needs to be of loose consistency to pass through the indwelling tube.

■ Assess how well the patient tolerated the procedure.
■ Note the color, consistency, and odor of stool.

■ Monitor the amount of stool in the collection bag. Change the fecal pouch at least every 72 hours (per protocol) and whenever there is evidence of leakage.
■ When the collection bag is approximately two-thirds full, change it to prevent it from getting too heavy.
■ Monitor for abdominal distention and pain.
■ Regularly assess that connections are secure and that the device is not leaking.

- In addition, for indwelling devices monitor:
  - Length of time the device is in place
    Not intended for use longer than 29 days.
  - Rectal bleeding
    May indicate tissue necrosis, bowel perforation, or fistula formation; device must be removed.

Documentation

- Date, time, and type of collection device used
- Your assessment of the perineal skin
- Patient's tolerance of the procedure
- Characteristics and amount of stool in the collection bag (output)
- Patient/family teaching

09/15/18　　1435　After prepping skin, an external fecal collection device was applied. Patient tolerated procedure well. Rationale for device was explained. Pt and family verbalized they will report leaking, pain, or discomfort. Device is draining large amounts of brown liquid stool, with no visible mucus or blood. ————————————— J. Smiley, RN

Practice Resources

Ayello, E., & Sibbald, R. (2016); Neilson, J., Avital, L., Willock, J., et al. (2014); Pittman, J., Beeson, T., Carter, B., et al. (2015); Siegel, J., Rhinehart, E., Jackson, M., et al. (2007); Wishin, J., Gallagher, T., & McCann, E. (2008); Wound, Ostomy and Continence Nurses Society (2003, updated 2010).

Thinking About the Procedure

To practice applying clinical reasoning to this procedure,

 The video, **Applying an External Fecal Collection System,** along with questions and suggested responses, is available on the **Davis's Nursing Skills Videos** Web site on Davis*Plus*.

 To explore learning resources for this chapter,

 Go to **www.DavisAdvantage.com** and find:

Answers and Suggested Responses for all questions in this chapter

Lists of NIC Interventions and NOC Outcomes

List of NANDA-I Diagnoses

Knowledge Map

Care Plan

Care Map

References and Bibliography

Concept Map

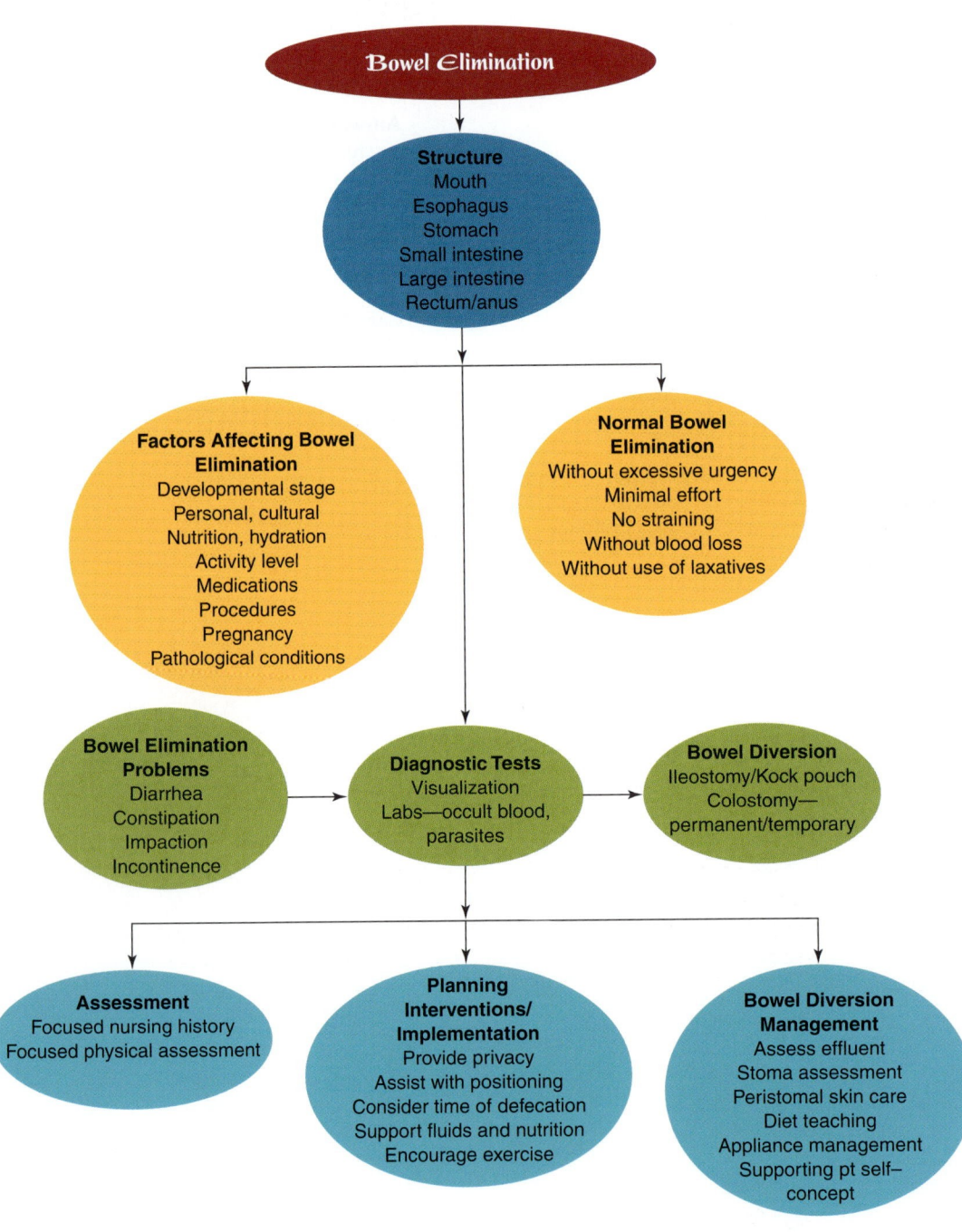

Bowel Elimination

Structure
Mouth
Esophagus
Stomach
Small intestine
Large intestine
Rectum/anus

**Factors Affecting Bowel
Elimination**
Developmental stage
Personal, cultural
Nutrition, hydration
Activity level
Medications
Procedures
Pregnancy
Pathological conditions

**Normal Bowel
Elimination**
Without excessive urgency
Minimal effort
No straining
Without blood loss
Without use of laxatives

**Bowel Elimination
Problems**
Diarrhea
Constipation
Impaction
Incontinence

Diagnostic Tests
Visualization
Labs—occult blood,
parasites

Bowel Diversion
Ileostomy/Kock pouch
Colostomy—
permanent/temporary

Assessment
Focused nursing history
Focused physical assessment

**Planning
Interventions/
Implementation**
Provide privacy
Assist with positioning
Consider time of defecation
Support fluids and nutrition
Encourage exercise

**Bowel Diversion
Management**
Assess effluent
Stoma assessment
Peristomal skin care
Diet teaching
Appliance management
Supporting pt self–
concept

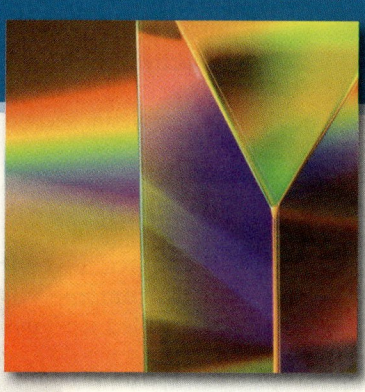

CHAPTER 30

Urinary Elimination

Learning Outcomes

After completing this chapter, you should be able to:

➤ Describe the normal structure and function of the organs in the urinary system.

➤ Describe the processes of urine formation and elimination.

➤ Discuss factors that affect urinary elimination.

➤ Conduct a nursing assessment and physical examination focused on urinary elimination.

➤ Accurately measure urine output.

➤ Perform procedures for collecting various types of urine specimens.

➤ List and describe diagnostic tests used in identifying urinary elimination problems.

➤ Discuss common elimination problems: urinary tract infection, urinary retention, and urinary incontinence.

➤ Identify nursing diagnoses associated with altered urinary elimination.

➤ Describe nursing interventions that promote normal urination.

➤ Provide care for clients experiencing urinary problems.

➤ Perform urinary catheterizations following accepted procedures.

➤ Discuss nursing care appropriate for clients who have a urinary diversion.

Key Concept

Urinary elimination

Related Concepts

See the Concept Map at the end of this chapter.

Example Problems

Urinary Incontinence

Urinary Retention

Urinary Tract Infection (UTI)

Meet Your Patient

During your assigned clinical experience at a local hospital, you are completing the admission process for Marlena, a 55-year-old woman who is complaining of frequent, painful urination and pain in her lower back. As you interview her, Marlena becomes embarrassed. "I really don't enjoy talking about this," she admits. When she asks to use the bathroom, you ask her to give you a midstream clean-catch urine sample. She returns with a small specimen of pink-colored, strong-smelling urine. "I have a strong urge to go and then I hardly have any urine. It burns like crazy when I urinate," she reports.

You close the door and interview Marlena in private about her usual urination pattern and current symptoms. Your calm approach and straightforward manner put her at ease. She confides that she is sexually active and that her symptoms began after spending the weekend with her new partner. You take her vital signs: oral temperature, 99.4°F (37.4°C); radial pulse, 88 beats/min; respiratory rate,

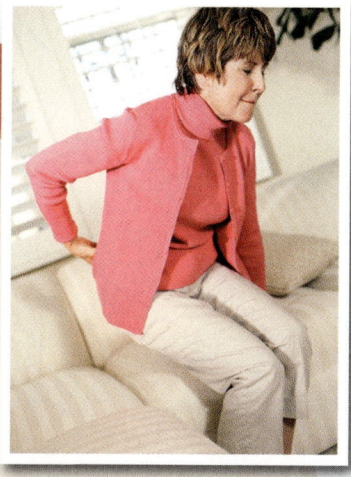

20 breaths/min; and blood pressure, 108/72 mm Hg.

The emergency department (ED) physician asks you to perform a dipstick urinalysis on the urine sample and to send the urine sample to the lab for culture and sensitivity. He says, "What do you think we need to do next?" How would you answer his question?

As you gain theoretical and practical knowledge of the concepts in this chapter, we will return to this case study to discuss how you might answer the physician's question and support Marlena's recovery. You will also have the opportunity to examine your feelings about giving care that patients may regard as personal or even embarrassing.

Theoretical Knowledge
knowing why

To support urinary health, you will need theoretical knowledge of the concepts associated with normal physiology of the urinary system, as well as other body systems that influence urinary function. Critical thinking and a good knowledge base will help you to care for patients with altered urinary elimination.

ABOUT THE KEY CONCEPTS

The key concept of **urinary elimination** is important because many of your nursing activities focus on promoting normal elimination. In order to best care for patients with urinary problems and provide holistic independent and collaborative interventions for them, you must understand the concepts involved in the formation and elimination of urine and how those processes may be altered.

HOW DOES THE URINARY SYSTEM WORK?

The body removes from food and fluids the nutrients necessary for essential bodily functions, such as physical activity, self-repair, and mental operations. The kidneys, ureters, bladder, and urethra help to excrete waste products left in the blood, and maintain a balance of chemicals and water (Fig. 30-1).

The Kidneys Filter and Regulate

Functions   Kidneys have the following functions:
- They filter metabolic wastes, toxins, excess ions, and water from the blood and excrete them as urine. If kidney function

is impaired, these substances reach toxic levels and damage body cells.
- They help to regulate blood volume, blood pressure, electrolyte levels, and acid–base balance by selectively reabsorbing water and other substances.
- Secondary functions are to produce erythropoietin, secrete the enzyme renin, and activate vitamin D_3.

Anatomy   The kidneys are **retroperitoneal** (located against the posterior abdominal wall behind the peritoneum). The average kidney weighs about 5 ounces and is the shape of a kidney bean (see Fig. 30-1).
- The outer layer, or **cortex,** of the kidney is composed of millions of microscopic functional units, called *nephrons* (Fig. 30-2).
- The inner layer, or **medulla,** consists of 8 to 10 wedge-shaped cones, called the *renal pyramids.* The renal pyramids are made up of bundles of collecting tubules.
- The innermost area is the **renal pelvis.**
- Funnel-shaped extensions known as **calyces** (singular: **calyx**) enclose the central portion of each renal pyramid and direct urine into the renal pelvis.

The Nephrons Form Urine

The **nephron** is the basic structural and functional unit of the kidney. Each nephron consists of:
- A **Bowman's capsule** (a double-walled hollow capsule), enclosing a **glomerulus** (a knotty ball of capillaries)
- A series of filtrating tubules
- A collecting duct

Together, these structures act as a microscopic filter, controlling the excretion and retention of fluids and solutes according to the body's moment-by-moment needs. Urine is formed by filtration, reabsorption, and secretion, which are discussed next.

Glomerular Filtration

Figure 30-3 summarizes the process of urine formation. The first step, **filtration,** occurs in the glomeruli. The renal arteries

FIGURE 30-1 The organs of the urinary system include the kidneys, ureters, bladder, and urethra.

Labels (Figure 30-1): Ribs; Aorta; Inferior vena cava; Left adrenal gland; Superior mesenteric artery; Left renal artery and vein; Left kidney; Left ureter; Left common iliac artery and vein; Lumbar vertebra; Pelvis; Sacrum; Opening of ureter; Trigone of bladder; Symphysis pubis; Urethra; Urinary bladder; Right ureter; Iliacus muscle; Psoas major muscle; Right kidney; Diaphragm

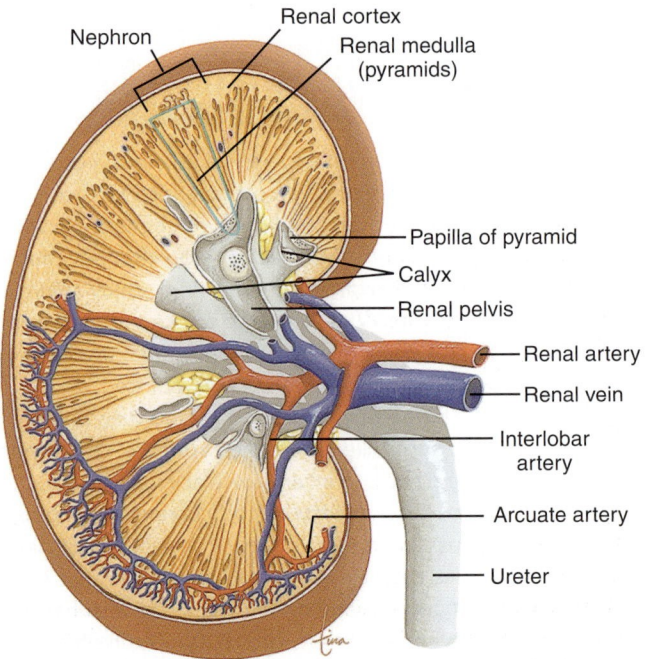

FIGURE 30-2 A cross section of the kidney, showing the renal cortex, medulla, pyramids, and calyces.

Labels (Figure 30-2): Nephron; Renal cortex; Renal medulla (pyramids); Papilla of pyramid; Calyx; Renal pelvis; Renal artery; Renal vein; Interlobar artery; Arcuate artery; Ureter

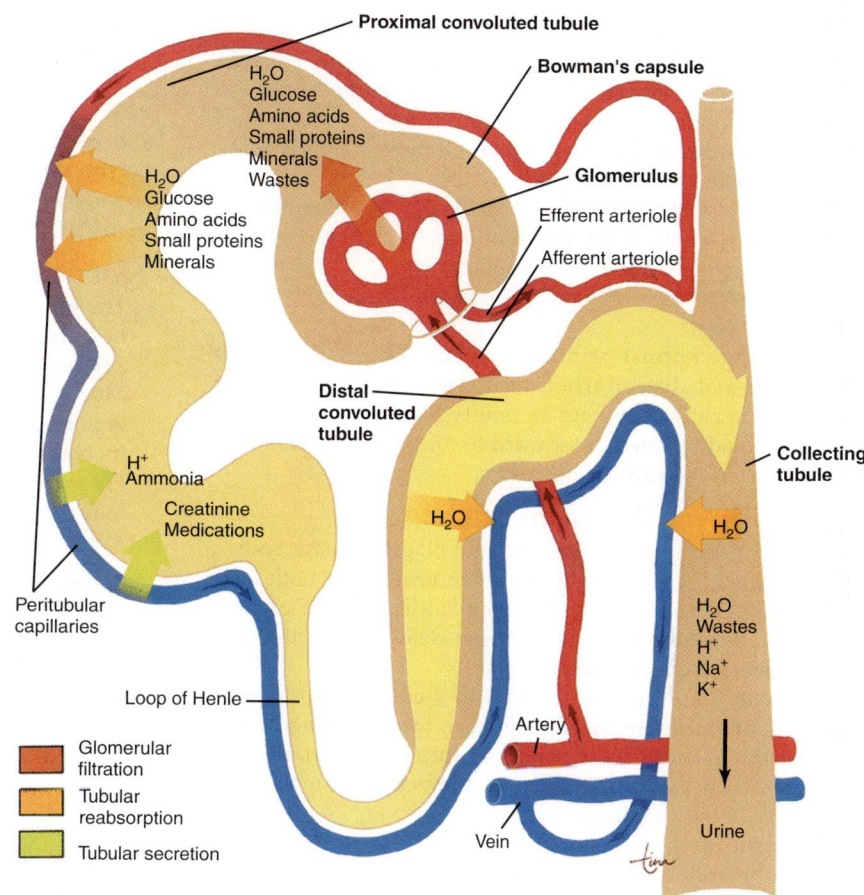

FIGURE 30-3 A schematic representation of the formation of urine.

bring blood to the kidneys and into the glomeruli. Blood pressure forces plasma, dissolved substances, and small proteins out of the porous glomeruli into Bowman's capsule to form a liquid called **filtrate.** The **glomerular filtration rate** is the amount of filtrate formed by the kidneys per minute.

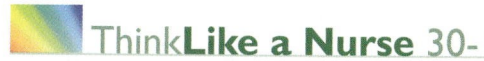Renal blood flow progressively decreases with aging, primarily because of changes to the micro–blood vessels to the kidney. This decline in glomerular filtration is the most important functional deficit of the kidneys caused by aging (Besdine, 2000, updated 2013).

Tubular Reabsorption
The filtrate moves from Bowman's capsule into a highly twisted tubule *(proximal convoluted tubule,* see Fig. 30-3). As the filtrate journeys through the tubule, the following occurs:
- *Peritubular capillaries* reabsorb 99% of the filtrate.
- *Collecting tubule*—Approximately 1% of filtrate returns, as urine, to the collecting tubule, which transports it into the ureters.
- *Distal and collecting tubules*—Wastes and toxins that remain in the blood after filtration are actively transported (reabsorbed) into the filtrate. Water and sodium are reabsorbed in these structures when antidiuretic hormone (ADH) and aldosterone are secreted.

When fluid in the body decreases (e.g., because of low fluid intake or excess fluid loss), the posterior pituitary gland secretes more ADH. This causes the distal and collecting tubules to reabsorb more water into the blood. At the same time, the adrenal cortex secretes more aldosterone, sodium

reabsorption increases, and water follows sodium back into the blood. This has the effect of maintaining normal fluid volume and blood pressure.

When water in the body increases (e.g., as in ingestion of excessive fluids), ADH is suppressed and the opposite effect occurs. Urine becomes dilute and water would be eliminated until its concentration returns to normal (Scanlon & Sanders, 2014).

Tubular Secretion
As blood flows through the peritubular capillaries:
- They remove (secrete) metabolic wastes (e.g., ammonia, creatinine, some medications) from the blood into the urine (filtrate).
- They secrete hydrogen ions (H^+), helping to maintain the normal pH of blood.

Think**Like a Nurse** 30-1

If a client is suffering from impaired kidney function, what signs and symptoms might you expect to see?

The Ureters Transport Urine
Each kidney has a ureter for urine transport from the renal pelvis to the urinary bladder (Fig. 30-1). A one-way valve at the opening between the ureter and the bladder allows urine to enter the bladder and prevents backflow **(reflux)** into the ureter.

The Urinary Bladder Stores Urine

The **urinary bladder** (see Fig. 30-1), a sac-like organ, receives urine from the ureters and holds it until discharged from the body. The bladder wall consists of four layers:

- *An innermost mucous membrane* seals off the remaining layers from exposure to urine.
- *A layer of connective tissue* supports the mucous membrane.
- *The detrusor muscle* is composed of three layers of longitudinal and circular smooth muscle fibers.
- *An outermost layer of fibrous connective tissue* covers the detrusor layer.

An average normal bladder can store 500 mL (1 pint) of urine, but it may distend when needed to a capacity twice that amount. You cannot palpate an empty bladder, but a full or distended bladder extends upward to form a pear shape that you can feel in the suprapubic region.

The Urethra Transports Urine

The **urethra** transports urine from the bladder to the body's exterior. The mucous membrane of the urethra (in both men and women) is continuous with the bladder and the ureters. Therefore, infection in the urethra can easily spread through the bladder and up into the kidneys.

- *In women,* the urethra is about 3 to 4 cm (1.5 in.) long; it opens at the **urinary meatus** between the clitoris and vaginal opening. Because the female urethra is so short, women are especially prone to urinary tract infection from microorganisms in the vagina and rectum.
- *In men,* the urethra extends about 20 cm (8 in.) from the bladder to the urinary meatus at the distal end of the penis. As it leaves the bladder, the male urethra passes through a surrounding gland known as the **prostate.** In addition to urine, the male urethra also carries semen.

KnowledgeCheck 30-1

- Identify the major structures of the urinary system.
- What are the functions of the kidneys?
- Briefly describe how urine is formed.
- What role do the ureters, bladder, and urethra play in urinary elimination?

HOW DOES URINARY ELIMINATION OCCUR?

Where the bladder connects to the urethra is a thickening of smooth muscle, called the **internal urethral sphincter.** When closed, the internal sphincter keeps urine from entering the urethra. The internal urethral sphincter is not under voluntary control. When the bladder contains 200 to 450 mL of urine (50 to 200 mL in children):

- Distention activates *stretch receptors* in the bladder wall.
- The stretch receptors send sensory impulses to the *voiding reflex center.*
- Those impulses cause the *detrusor muscle* to contract and the internal sphincter to relax for **voiding** (also called **urination** or **micturition).**
  - This triggers the conscious urge to void.
  - However, voiding may be voluntarily delayed by inhibiting release of the **external urethral sphincter.**
- *When the person is ready to urinate,* the brain signals the external urethral sphincter to relax, and urine flows out of the urethra. Further contraction of the detrusor muscle normally forces out any urine remaining in the bladder.

- *After the detrusor muscle relaxes,* the bladder begins to fill with urine again.

In addition to normal functioning of the bladder and urethra, control of urination requires that the brain, spinal cord, and nerves supplying the bladder and urethra be intact. The person must be aware of the need to urinate and able to respond by either inhibiting the reflex or by allowing the release of urine.

Normal Urination Patterns

- The kidneys produce about 50 to 60 mL of urine per hour, or 1,500 mL per day. Output may fluctuate by 1,000 mL to 2,000 mL.
- Most people void five or six times per day; even eight times is normal, depending on fluid intake. When fluid intake is increased, urination will be more frequent.
- Frequent urination is sometimes a sign of other medical problems, such as diabetes or urinary tract infection; whereas infrequent urination may indicate dehydration.

Characteristics of Normal Urine

Specific gravity is a measure of dissolved solutes in a solution. As the concentration of the urine solutes increases, specific gravity increases. The specific gravity of distilled water is 1.000 because there are no dissolved solutes. **KEY POINT:** *The normal specific gravity range for urine is 1.002 to 1.030.*

- *As fluid intake increases,* urine becomes dilute and lighter in color to almost clear as it approaches a specific gravity of 1.000.
- *If fluid intake is low or there have been fluid losses,* as with diarrhea or vomiting, the urine darkens as the specific gravity rises.

See Procedure 30-3B: Measuring Specific Gravity of Urine, at the end of this chapter.

 ThinkLike a Nurse 30-2

- How does Marlena's (Meet Your Patient) urinary elimination pattern differ from normal?
- What would you expect to find if you measured her specific gravity?
- Marlena's symptoms are suggestive of urinary tract infection. How might this be related to the fact that she is sexually active?

WHAT FACTORS AFFECT URINARY ELIMINATION?

Given the complex structure and physiology of the urinary organs, it isn't surprising that many variables affect their function.

Developmental Factors: Infants and Children

The normal specific gravity of a newborn's urine is 1.008. Over the first weeks of life, the urine becomes more concentrated, and the well-hydrated infant produces eight to ten wet diapers a day. Infants do not have voluntary control of voiding because neuromuscular functioning is immature.

The timing of toilet training is highly variable and is influenced by family and culture, as well as the presence of older children to model toileting behavior. In the United States, most parents begin toilet training when their child is between 18 and 36 months of age. Before toilet training can occur, toddlers must be able to control the external urethral sphincter, sense the urge to void, communicate their need to use the toilet, and remove their clothing.

- **Enuresis,** or occasional involuntary passage of urine, is normal in children, even in the early school years, especially when the child is intensely absorbed in an activity. Such events should be accepted calmly.

- **Nocturnal enuresis,** or nighttime bedwetting, occurs in about 5% in children aged 6 to 7 years (Brown, Pope, & Brown, 2011). Previously believed to be related to psychological factors, nocturnal enuresis is caused by an insufficient level of ADH. To manage nocturnal enuresis in children, see the accompanying Home Care box.

Developmental Factors: Older Adults

The size and functioning of the kidneys begin to decrease at about age 50, and by age 80 only about two-thirds of the functioning nephrons remain. This results in a decline in filtration rate, which affects the ability to dilute and concentrate urine, but does not normally create problems unless an illness alters fluid balance.

- When older adults lose fluids and electrolytes through vomiting and diarrhea, it is difficult for their kidneys to maintain acid–base and electrolyte balances.
- Chronic diseases such as arteriosclerosis, common in older adults, can reduce blood flow and impair renal function.
- Drug toxicity is a risk due to decreased kidney function.
    Other physiological changes include:
- Loss of elasticity in the bladder wall
- In women: Loss of abdominal and perineal muscle tone due to childbearing
- In men: Prostate gland enlargement
    Symptoms produced by physiological changes include:
- Nocturnal frequency of urine
- Bladder infections due to incomplete bladder emptying
- Leakage of urine
- Particularly in men, dribbling, urinary frequency, difficulty starting urination, and reduced force of the urinary stream

---

Managing Nocturnal Enuresis in Children

Home Care

Occasional wetting is normal in children even into the early school years. Children, especially older ones, can be embarrassed by nocturnal enuresis, or nighttime bedwetting. Stress of an illness or hospitalization can trigger episodes.

➤ Reassure parents that in most cases loving acceptance and passage of time provide the cure.
➤ Cover the mattress with plastic.
➤ Limit fluid intake in the evening.
➤ Wake the child to urinate just before the parents go to sleep.
➤ Use a bed alarm that wakens the child when wetting occurs. Over time, this conditioning may be effective; however, once the alarm is removed, the child may relapse into enuresis.
➤ If bedwetting persists after 10 to 12 years of age, the child should receive a thorough medical evaluation to rule out underlying disease processes.
➤ Parents should bathe the child in the morning rather than at bedtime to minimize urine odor.
➤ Medication can be effective for managing nocturnal enuresis in some children. It is helpful when the child is not sleeping at home.

Personal, Sociocultural, and Environmental Factors

Many people delay voiding while they are working or busy with other activities. This promotes urinary stasis and can lead to bladder infections. The following situations can also inhibit voiding: anxiety, lack of time, lack of privacy, loss of dignity, and cultural influences (e.g., modesty and toileting practices).

Nutrition, Hydration, and Activity Level

Caffeine acts as a diuretic and increases urine production. Consuming large amounts of alcohol impairs the release of antidiuretic hormone (ADH), resulting in increased production of urine. In contrast, a diet high in salt causes water retention and decreases urine production.

For most adults, pale to clear urine indicates adequate hydration. The kidneys conserve water when a person is dehydrated—for example, when fluid intake is inadequate. This causes the urine to be concentrated and low in volume. During prolonged periods of intense physical activity, especially in hot weather, the body loses sodium and other electrolytes rapidly through sweat, so electrolyte replacement beverages may be more beneficial than plain water in restoring fluids (Thompson & Manore, 2013).

Knowledge Check 30-2

- What quantity of urine in the bladder will stimulate the urge to void?
- Identify at least three indications for determining whether hydration is adequate and urine output is within normal limits.

Medications

Various medications are given specifically to affect urination—for example, by treating pain, increasing urination, relaxing smooth muscles, or causing urinary retention.

- **Analgesics.** Phenazopyridine hydrochloride (Pyridium) is used to treat bladder and urethral pain, burning, increased urination, and increased urge to urinate. This medication turns the urine a deep orange-red color.
- **Diuretics,** sometimes called "water pills," treat blood pressure, fluid retention, and edema by increasing elimination of urine. Diuretics are classified as thiazide, potassium-sparing, or loop-acting diuretics (Box 30-1).
- **Anticholinergics** promote urine retention by inhibiting involuntary contractions (spasms) of the bladder, increasing bladder capacity, and delaying the urge to void for people with urge incontinence. They may be given orally or transdermally. See Box 30-2 for a listing of the most common medications associated with urinary retention.
- **Antidepressants** (e.g., duloxetine, imipramine) reduce stress incontinence by relaxing bladder muscles. Some work by stimulating the nerve that controls the urethral sphincter.
- **Antispasmodics** help to stop bladder muscle contractions (that is, relax the bladder) and prevent urge incontinence. For example, propantheline bromide (Pro-Banthine) is prescribed to treat overactive bladder.
- **Muscarinic receptor antagonists** (e.g., tolterodine tartrate) block nerve receptors in the smooth muscle of the bladder. They control bladder contraction and reduce urinary frequency for people with overactive bladder and urge incontinence.
- **Estrogen** is used to improve the blood flow to the urethral tissues and increase thickness of mucosal and urethral tissues.

BOX 30-1 ■ Common Diuretic Classes

Thiazide diuretics are used to treat high blood pressure by reducing the amount of sodium and water in the body and dilating blood vessels.

Potassium-sparing diuretics reduce the amount of water in the body. Unlike other diuretic medicines, these do not cause potassium loss.

Loop-acting diuretics cause the kidneys to reabsorb less water. The increased urine excretion reduces the amount of water in the body and lowers blood pressure.

Medications that have significant interactions with diuretics include digoxin, antihypertensives, lithium, certain antidepressants (especially with thiazide or loop-acting diuretics), and the immunosuppressant cyclosporine, especially when the patient is taking a potassium-sparing diuretic.

Common side effects of diuretics include weakness, muscle cramps, skin rash, increased sensitivity to sunlight (with thiazide diuretics), dizziness, light-headedness, joint pain.

Estrogen is not approved by the U.S. Food and Drug Administration (FDA) for treatment of stress incontinence.

- **Botulinum toxin** injections control bladder spasms by relaxing the muscles. It has FDA approval for use in overactive bladder related to nerve damage, such as with spinal cord injury or multiple sclerosis.

  KEY POINT: *Some medications given for other than kidney conditions are nephrotoxic (damaging to the kidneys). These include some antibiotics, such as gentamicin and amphotericin B, and high doses or long-term use of aspirin and ibuprofen.*

Surgery and Anesthesia

Urinary Tract Surgeries can affect urinary solutes, normal urine characteristics, and the ability to pass urine normally. Manipulation of the urinary tract frequently leads to trauma, bleeding, or the introduction of bacteria into a normally sterile tract. Swelling after diagnostic or invasive procedures may cause urinary retention.

Surgery in the Pubic Area, Vagina, or Rectum is associated with a high incidence of trauma to the urinary organs; lower abdominal swelling; loss of pelvic muscle control; and increased pressure on the kidneys, ureters, or bladder.

Surgery on the Reproductive Organs, such as hysterectomy in women or transurethral resection of the prostate in men, usually requires the use of an indwelling catheter (tube) for draining the bladder postoperatively. The urine may be tinged red or pink after any invasive urinary tract surgery or procedure.

Anesthetic Agents can decrease blood pressure and glomerular filtration, thus decreasing urine formation. Spinal anesthesia decreases the patient's awareness of the need to void, which may lead to bladder distention.

Pathological Conditions

Disorders of the urinary system that affect urinary elimination include the following:

- Infection or inflammation of the bladder, ureters, or kidneys (For information about, and nursing care for, urinary tract infections [UTIs], see the accompanying Example Problem: Urinary Tract Infection [UTI].)
- **Renal calculi** (kidney stones) or tumors, which obstruct the normal flow of urine
- In older men, **hypertrophy** (excessive growth) of the prostate gland due to benign or cancerous lesions, which interferes with flow of urine from the bladder into the urethra

  Diseases involving other systems can indirectly affect urinary function, for example:
- *Cardiovascular and metabolic disorders* decrease blood flow through the glomeruli and thus impair filtration and urine production.
- *Nervous system* conditions that affect control of the urinary system organs will impair urinary elimination. After a stroke or spinal cord injury, for example, some patients may lose bladder control. **Neurogenic bladder** is an example of impaired neurological function. The person cannot perceive bladder fullness or control the urinary sphincters. The bladder becomes flaccid or spastic, causing frequent involuntary loss of urine.
- *Systemic infection,* especially when accompanied by a high fever, causes the kidneys to reabsorb and retain water.
- *Immobility and impaired communication* may interfere with the ability to get to the bathroom in time or to communicate the

---

BOX 30-2 ■ Medications Associated With Urinary Retention

Class	Use	Medication
Antihistamine	Treat allergy symptoms	fexofenadine (Allegra) diphenhydramine (Benadryl) chlorpheniramine (Chlor-Trimeton) cetirizine (Zyrtec)
Anticholinergics/antispasmodics	Treat stomach cramps, muscle spasms, and urinary incontinence	hyoscyamine (Levbid, Cystospaz, Gastrosed) oxybutynin (Ditropan, Oxytrol) tolterodine (Detrol) propantheline (Pro-Banthine)
Tricyclic antidepressants	Treat anxiety and depression	imipramine (Tofranil) amitriptyline (Elavil) nortriptyline (Aventyl)

Source: U.S. Department of Health and Human Services, National Institutes of Diabetes and Digestive and Kidney Diseases. (2014). *Urinary retention.* Retrieved from https://www.niddk.nih.gov/health-information/health-topics/urologic-disease/urinary-retention/Pages/facts.aspx

EXAMPLE PROBLEM: Urinary Tract Infection (UTI)

Definition: Infection in any part of the urinary system—kidneys, ureters, bladder, and urethra

Transmission: Microorganisms, usually *Escherichia coli* (*E. coli*), which normally live harmlessly in the colon, enter the urethra and begin to multiply, overwhelming the normal flora.

Types of UTIs
- **Urethritis**—infection limited to the urethra
- **Cystitis**—bladder infection caused by microbes within the urethra

- **Pyelonephritis**—infection that progresses upward to the ureters or kidneys
- **Catheter-associated UTIs**—In otherwise healthy patients, CAUTIs are often asymptomatic and likely to resolve spontaneously with the removal of the catheter.

Complications—UTIs can lead to prostatitis, epididymitis, cystitis, pyelonephritis, and gram-negative bacteremia, particularly in high-risk patients.

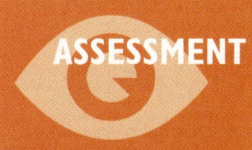
ASSESSMENT

Risk Factors
- **Sexual activity (women).** During intercourse, perineal pathogens (usually *E. coli*) may enter the urethra. Because a woman's urethra is short, pathogens can quickly enter the bladder.
- **Use of spermicidal contraceptive gel (women).** Spermicides reduce normal flora in the vagina, allowing pathogens to multiply.
- **Older women.** At menopause, estrogen loss leads to drying of the vaginal mucosa and urethra and a reduction in protective normal flora.
- **Pregnant women.** Hormone changes and pressure of the uterus on the bladder cause urinary stasis and stagnant urine—a good medium for bacterial growth.
- **Enlarged prostate (men).** Pressure from the prostate creates difficulty emptying the bladder, resulting in stagnant urine.
- **Kidney stones.** Renal calculi obstruct urine flow, creating stagnation and irritation of the urinary tract as they are passed.
- **Presence of an indwelling catheter.**
  - Pathogens may be introduced into the urethra during catheterization.
  - Failing to maintain a closed drainage system allows bacteria to enter the catheter, providing a pathway for bacteria.
  - The catheter irritates the urethral mucosa, creating a portal of entry for microbes.
  - The longer the catheter remains, the higher the risk of developing UTI.

- The urine collection bag is a closed system, acting as a reservoir for microorganisms.
- **Diabetes mellitus.** Glucose in the urine provides nutrients for bacteria to multiply.
- **Immunocompromised.** Neonates, the elderly, those receiving immunosuppressive drugs, people with a weakened immune system are less able to maintain a healthy balance of microbes in the urinary tract.
- **History of UTIs.** Previous UTIs suggest increased likelihood of recurrence because the urinary tract is colonized with pathogens.

Symptoms

Bladder spasms	Chills
Dysuria	Foul-smelling urine
Edema	Fever
Hematuria	Urinary frequency
Pain: back, sides, or under ribs	

Diagnostic Tests
- Midstream, clean-catch urine specimen—for culture
- Dipstick urine—for leukocytes, blood, estrace, and nitrates

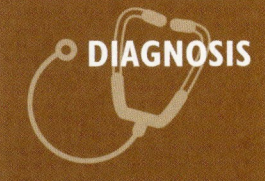
DIAGNOSIS

Risk for Infection   Acute Pain r/t UTI

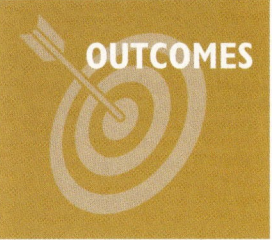
OUTCOMES

Resumes normal urinary pattern by [date].

(Continued)

EXAMPLE PROBLEM: Urinary Tract Infection (UTI)—cont'd

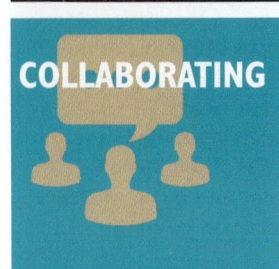

COLLABORATING

Prevention

- Length and type of antibiotic treatment depends on the location and severity of infection.
- Cystitis—oral antibiotics for 1 to 5 days
- Pyelonephritis—IV antibiotics followed by a course of oral antibiotics

- Preventive antibiotic treatment—not recommended; drug resistance develops easily
- Phenazopyridine to relieve burning and urgency for first 2 or 3 days of UTI
- Liberal fluid intake to flush out bacteria

---

need for assistance. This may result in urination in inappropriate settings or at inappropriate times.

■ *Cognitive changes* (e.g., brain changes or severe psychiatric conditions) that alter perception of the urge to void or ability to manage activities of daily living may lead to **incontinence** (involuntary loss of urine).

ThinkLike a Nurse 30-3

As you may have concluded, Marlena (Meet Your Patient) has a UTI. What additional history questions would you like to ask Marlena?

KnowledgeCheck 30-3

- What common medications increase the amount of urine voided?
- What types of medications are associated with urinary retention?
- What types of conditions or surgeries are associated with a high incidence of altered urination?

PracticalKnowledge
knowing **how**

As a nurse, you will monitor and assist clients with urinary elimination, teach them about bodily functions, and work collaboratively with the healthcare team to facilitate normal urinary function. Also see the Nursing Care Plan and the Care Map later in the chapter.

ASSESSMENT NP

To assess urinary elimination, you will use data from the nursing history, physical examination, and diagnostic and laboratory reports.

Nursing History

Because urination patterns vary among individuals, you will need a nursing history to determine what is normal for a particular person. **iCare** Pay attention to her reaction to your questions. Many people are embarrassed about discussing urination. Tailor your assessment to the client's needs, and use language that makes her comfortable. For specific questions, refer to the Focused Assessment box Urinary Elimination History Questions.

ThinkLike a Nurse 30-4

In the Meet Your Patient scenario, what additional physical assessments might you perform to complete this urinary tract assessment?

Physical Assessment

Physical assessment for urinary elimination includes examination of the kidneys, bladder, urethra, and skin surrounding the genitals, as appropriate. For a complete discussion of physical examination of the genitourinary system, see Chapter 21, Procedure 21-17 and Procedure 21-18. Also see the Focused Assessment box Guidelines for Physical Assessment for Urinary Elimination.

Common Diagnostic Procedures

Many diagnostic procedures of the urinary tract are performed in the operating room, procedures suite, or radiology department. Typically nurses prepare the client for the procedure, assist with specimen collection, deliver aftercare, and sometimes assist the physician.

Blood Studies Blood urea nitrogen (BUN) and creatinine levels are commonly measured to assess renal function and hydration. For normal ranges, see the Diagnostic Testing box Blood Studies: BUN and Creatinine.

Visualization Studies of the Urinary System Direct visualization studies tend to be invasive and, therefore, require a signed consent form. For associated pre- and post-procedure care of patients having these procedures, refer to the Diagnostic Testing box Studies of the Urinary System.

KnowledgeCheck 30-4

- What should you discuss with your client when performing a nursing history focused on urinary elimination?
- What are the key elements of a physical assessment for a client with urination problems?

ThinkLike a Nurse 30-5

After gathering a focused nursing history pertaining to urinary elimination, you check Marlena's vital signs: oral temperature 99.4°F (37.4°C); radial pulse, 88 beats/min; respiratory rate, 20 breaths/min; and blood pressure, 108/72 mm Hg. What other physical assessment findings might you expect?

Managing Urinary Incontinence

SENC Competencies: Patient Education, Health Promotion; Evidenced-Based Practice (Thinking, Doing, Caring)

Scenario

Dashondra Simms, RN, works in a urology practice. After participating in a radio interview to provide health information about urinary incontinence, many women call the urology practice to ask for help. Dashondra asks each woman how she manages her incontinence, where she obtains information, whether the condition has changed her quality of life, and whether she would be willing to participate in an incontinence support group. Her notes reveal a population with unmet healthcare needs. She decides to develop a patient-centered, evidence-based program to increase participants' knowledge and confidence about managing their incontinence.

First, Dashondra accesses the National Guideline Clearinghouse Web site to obtain evidence-based guidelines for incontinence management techniques. She searches databases such as MEDLINE and CINAHL for peer-reviewed studies that identify the psychosocial needs of patients and cultural or ethnic differences in managing incontinence. She also consults colleagues for practical strategies in managing this problem.

Dashondra asks women about the emotional impact of living with incontinence. They talk about the effects on their feelings of self-worth, dignity, and confidence. Self-image, sexuality, and their sense of freedom also emerged as specific issues. Dashondra asked what would be of value to them in an incontinence self-management program. They identified education about new treatments, a monthly support group meeting, an online forum for members, and phone, text, or e-mail access to Dashondra as desirable components of the program.

Think about it:
The following questions are for your own reflection or discussion with peers:
➤ How did Dashondra establish an evidence base for educating group members?
➤ How did she make the intervention patient centered?
➤ In what ways did Dashondra use information technology to help her design the program?
➤ How does Dashondra show caring for the women who experience incontinence participating in the study group?

Sources: Blanchette, K.A. (2012); National Guideline Clearinghouse (2013); National Institute for Health and Clinical Excellence (2013, updated 2015).

Urinary Elimination History Questions

Usual Urination Pattern

➤ How often do you urinate?
➤ Do you get up in the middle of the night to urinate?
➤ Do you have difficulty getting to the bathroom in time to urinate?
➤ Do you ever leak urine when you cough, laugh, or exercise?
➤ Do you ever leak urine on the way to the bathroom?
➤ Do you need to use pads or tissue in your underwear to catch urine?
➤ Do you have any difficulty starting to void?

Appearance of Urine

➤ How would you describe your urine?
➤ Have you noticed unusual odor with urination?

Changes in Urination Habits or Urine Appearance

➤ Have you experienced any recent changes in your voiding pattern?
➤ Has your urine changed in appearance or odor?

History of Urination Problems

➤ What has been your experience with urination problems?
➤ Have you had any urinary tract infections or kidney and bladder problems?

➤ Have you ever lost control of your urination?
➤ Have you ever had urinary tract surgery or diagnostic procedures?

Use of Urination Aids

➤ What aids, if any, do you use to help you urinate?
➤ What medications are you taking? Have they affected your urination pattern?

Lifestyle Questions

➤ Where is your bathroom located? Can you get to it easily?
➤ Can you manage your clothing when you go to the bathroom?
➤ How much fluid do you drink each day?
➤ How many caffeinated beverages do you drink?
➤ Do you smoke?
➤ Are you bothered with constipation?
➤ Do you do high-impact exercise (e.g., jogging)?

Presence of Urinary Diversions

➤ Have you ever had surgery of your urinary tract?
➤ If so, what and when?

For Infants and Young Children

➤ Has the child been toilet trained?
➤ What elimination routines have been established?

Guidelines for Physical Assessment for Urinary Elimination

THE KIDNEYS

The costovertebral (CV) angle is formed by the junction of the 12th rib and the spine on both sides of the back.

Technique	Rationale
Place one palm flat on the CV angle and lightly strike it with the closed fist of the other hand (see the accompanying figure).	You cannot usually palpate the kidneys. Instead, examine them by assessing for costovertebral angle tenderness (CVAT). If kidney inflammation is present, percussion of this angle produces pain.

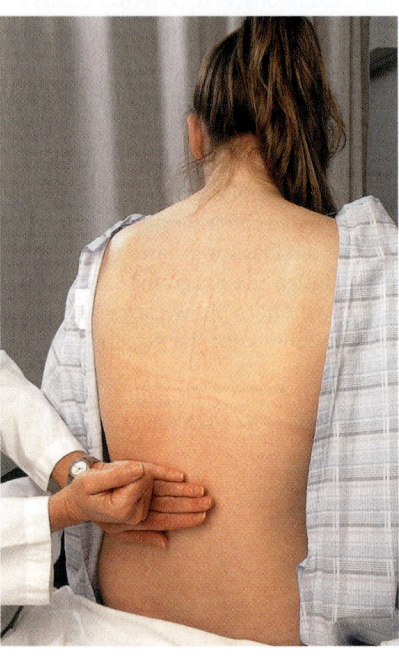

THE BLADDER

Inspect, palpate, and percuss the lower abdomen. Correlate your findings with data about the client's fluid intake and voiding.

➤ Inspect the lower abdomen.

➤ An empty bladder, or one with limited urine, is small and sits below the symphysis pubis. In contrast, a distended bladder rises above the symphysis pubis. If it is very distended, you may be able to see a rounded swelling above the symphysis pubis.

➤ Lightly palpate the lower abdomen to define the bladder margin. Observe the patient's response to palpation, noting signs of tenderness or discomfort.

➤ An empty bladder, or one with limited urine, will not be palpable.

➤ Percuss the area.

➤ A distended bladder produces a dull sound as opposed to the normal tympanic sound of intestinal air.

THE URETHRA

➤ Inspect the urethral orifice. Look for erythema, discharge, swelling, or odor.

➤ These are signs of infection, trauma, or inflammation.

THE PERINEAL AREA

➤ Frequently inspect skin color, condition, texture, turgor, and presence of urine or stool.

➤ Clients who have urine leakage or a urinary catheter are at risk for perineal skin problems. Ammonia in the urine may result in skin excoriation, skin breakdown, and subsequent infection. If both urine and stool are present on the skin, the likelihood of skin breakdown increases.

Diagnostic Testing

Blood Studies: BUN and Creatinine

Normal Ranges

Blood urea nitrogen (BUN)   8–20 mg/dL
Creatinine   0.5–1.1 mg/dL

Levels may be increased in:

➤ Renal failure
➤ Impaired renal perfusion
➤ Kidney infection or inflammation
➤ Kidney obstruction
➤ Dehydration

➤ Excessive protein intake
➤ Use of total parenteral nutrition (TPN)

Levels may be decreased in:

➤ Inadequate protein intake
➤ Malabsorption syndromes
➤ Liver disease

Source: Van Leeuwen, A., & Bladh, M. (2015). *Davis's comprehensive handbook of laboratory & diagnostic tests with nursing implications* (6th ed.). Philadelphia, PA: F.A. Davis.

Studies of the Urinary System

Direct Visualization Studies

Cystoscopy
Direct visualization of the urethra, bladder, and ureteral orifices by insertion of a scope. May be used to obtain biopsies and treat pathology of visualized areas.

Preparation
➤ Instruct the patient that the procedure is performed under general, spinal, or local anesthesia.
➤ Ensure that a signed consent form is on the chart.
➤ Restrict food and fluids for 8 hours before general anesthesia. For local anesthesia, allow only clear liquids for 8 hours before the procedure.

Post-Procedure Care
➤ Monitor vital signs and intake and output (I&O).
➤ Observe the characteristics of urine after the procedure.
➤ Encourage increased fluid intake.
➤ Report suprapubic or flank pain, chills, or difficulty urinating.

Cystometry
Done to determine whether a muscle or nerve problem is causing problems with how well the bladder holds or releases urine. A catheter is inserted into the bladder and a pressure probe into the rectum. A **cystometer** measures how much the bladder can hold and the pressure in the bladder. Sometimes a gas or contrast material is used.

Preparation
➤ Ensure a signed consent form is on the patient's health record.
➤ Explain that cooperation with positioning and activity is crucial.
➤ There are no food or fluid restrictions before the test.

Post-Procedure Care
➤ Monitor vital signs and I&O.
➤ Encourage increased fluid intake.
➤ Report suprapubic or flank pain, chills, or difficulty urinating.

Indirect Visualization Studies

Intravenous Pyelogram (IVP) and Retrograde Pyelogram
An IVP uses intravenous radiopaque contrast medium to visualize the kidneys, ureters, bladder, and renal pelvis. It evaluates renal function by analyzing flow of contrast over time.

A retrograde pyelogram uses radiopaque contrast medium to visualize the renal collecting system. Contrast media is injected via a ureteral catheter inserted through a cystoscope.

Preparation
➤ ✚ Assess for history of allergies. Radiopaque dyes can be highly allergenic for some patient; therefore, this test is contraindicated for patients with allergies to shellfish or iodinated dye.
➤ Ensure baseline BUN and creatinine results are available. IVP is contraindicated for patients in renal failure.
➤ Ensure that a signed consent form is on the chart.
➤ Restrict food and fluids for 8 hours prior to the procedure. Check agency protocols for specific guidelines, especially related to fluid intake.
➤ Some patients may require a laxative the evening before the surgery to clear the GI tract and improve visualization.
➤ Diabetic patients who take insulin make an adjustment to the insulin dose when fasting for this examination.
➤ Determine the patient is not pregnant, breastfeeding, or with an intrauterine device in place.
➤ Ask whether the patient has had an x-ray test using barium contrast material (such as a barium enema) or has taken a medication containing bismuth (e.g., Pepto-Bismol) in the 4 days prior to the test. These can affect the test results.
➤ Check for a history of bleeding disorders or whether the patient is taking any anticoagulant, aspirin, or other medications that affect blood clotting. It may be necessary to hold these medications prior to the procedure.

Post-Procedure Care
➤ Encourage increased fluid intake.
➤ Monitor vital signs and I&O.
➤ Observe for reactions to the contrast media: rash, nausea, hives.

Ultrasound
Using contrast media, computerized tomography (CT) scanning examines body sections from different angles using

(Continued)

Diagnostic Testing

Studies of the Urinary System—cont'd

a narrow x-ray beam to produce a three-dimensional picture of the area of the body being scanned.

Preparation
➤ Ensure a signed consent form is on the chart.
➤ There are no food or fluid restrictions with renal ultrasound. For a bladder ultrasound the patient need to drink 5 to 6 glasses of fluid 90 minutes before the procedure to ensure a full bladder.

Post-Procedure Care
➤ No special care is required.

Computerized Tomography
Using contrast media, a CT scan examines body sections from different angles using a narrow x-ray beam to produce a three-dimensional picture of the area of the body being scanned.

Preparation
➤ Obtain history of allergies. This test is contraindicated for patients with allergies to shellfish or iodinated dye.
➤ Ensure a signed consent form is on the chart.
➤ For a renal CT scan, food and fluids are usually restricted for 2 to 4 hours prior to the procedure.
➤ Remove all metal objects from the patient's body (e.g., eyeglasses, rings, safety pins).

Post-Procedure Care
➤ Monitor vital signs and I&O.
➤ Observe for reactions to the contrast media: rash, nausea, hives.

Renal Biopsy
Removal of a piece of kidney tissue for microscopic evaluation, usually done with ultrasound guidance.

Preparation
➤ Ensure baseline coagulation studies and hemoglobin results are available.
➤ Ensure a signed consent form is on the chart.
➤ NPO 6 to 8 hours prior to an open biopsy and at least 4 hours prior to a needle biopsy. Protocols may vary.
➤ Instruct the patient that sedation and/or pain medication may be given.

Post-Procedure Care
➤ Monitor vital signs and I&O.
➤ Bedrest for 6 to 24 hours as prescribed.
➤ Monitor biopsy site for bleeding.
➤ Monitor urine for presence of blood.

Source: Adapted from Van Leeuwen, A. M., Poelhuis-Leth, D., & Bladh, M. L. (2011). *Davis's comprehensive handbook of laboratory & diagnostic tests with nursing implications* (4th ed.). Philadelphia, PA: F. A. Davis.

Assessing the Urine

In addition to observations and diagnostic procedures already mentioned, assessment of the urine includes measuring urine output and conducting some bedside tests.

Interpreting Intake and Output (I&O) Data

The kidneys produce approximately 50 to 60 mL of urine per hour (1,500 mL per day). However, urinary output fluctuates depending on the following:
- Quantity of fluids the patient drinks
- Ability of the heart to circulate the blood
- Kidney functioning
- Ability of the patient to void the urine
- Amount of fluid being excreted (e.g., excessive sweating or significant vomiting and diarrhea)
- High fever can also contribute to reduced urine output.
- **KEY POINT:** *In order to interpret the meaning of fluid data, you must know the intake and output and the patient's relevant physical condition.*

   Examples:
   - If urine output is low, you might assume the patient's kidneys are not working properly. However, if his intake is also low, he may be dehydrated.
   - If his intake is high and output is low, this could mean his kidneys are not working well. However, it could also mean that his kidneys are producing urine but that he has urinary retention because something is obstructing flow.

   For information about and nursing care for Urinary Retention, see the accompanying Example Problem: Urinary Retention.

Measuring Intake and Output

Measuring urine output is an essential component of monitoring fluid status.
- **Record all fluids the patient drinks or receives intravenously.**
   - **Fluid intake:** oral fluids, semiliquid foods, ice chips, IV fluids, tube feedings, and irrigations instilled and not withdrawn immediately
   - **Fluid output:** urine output, gastrointestinal fluid loss (e.g., emesis), diarrhea, and drainage (e.g., from suction devices or wounds)
- **Ensure accuracy.** Explain to the client, family members, and caregivers that intake and output are being monitored. Post a sign at the bedside or on the door to the room as a reminder. When possible, have the client assist you with monitoring.
- **Perform I&O measurement.** You will usually total I&O at the end of each shift, as well as for each 24-hour period. In intensive care units, you may measure I&O hourly. Most healthcare agencies have standardized I&O forms, either a separate form or part of a flow sheet. See Figures 18-2 and 18-7.
- **Practice asepsis.** When handling urine, observe universal precautions, wear disposable procedure gloves, and avoid splashing the urine on yourself or objects in the room.

   Voided Urine The method you use to measure urine partially depends on the amount of help the patient needs with urination.
- **Ambulatory patients.** Inform them you are monitoring their I&O, and explain how they can help. Place a specimen "hat" (collection container) under the toilet seat to collect urine (Fig. 30-4), or have male clients void into a urinal. Periodically measure the output and empty the urine into the toilet.

EXAMPLE PROBLEM: Urinary Retention

Problem: Urinary Retention
Definition: Inability to completely empty the bladder

Complications: Urinary tract infections, bladder damage, kidney damage

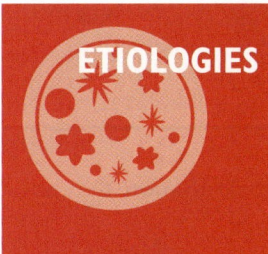

ETIOLOGIES

Assess for risk factors for Urinary Retention

- **Obstruction**—blockage of urinary outflow
- **Enlarged prostate**
- **Stones lodged in urethra** *strictures*
- **Scars from previous injury**
- **Tumors or blood clots in urinary system**
- **Fecal impaction**
- **Inflammation and swelling**

- **Infection or surgery** in the pelvic region
- **Neurological problems.** Spinal cord tumors or injury; herniated disk
- **Viral infections** involving perineal nerves
- **Medications, anesthesia**
- **Anxiety**
- **Stress leading to voluntary withholding of urination**

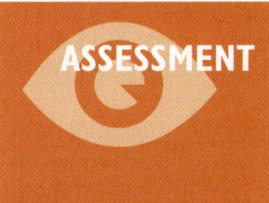

ASSESSMENT

Symptoms of Urinary Retention

Acute
- Urinary hesitancy, dribbling, or weak urine stream
- Urgent need to urinate
- Pain, discomfort, bloating in lower abdomen

Chronic
- Urinary frequency—urination 8+/day
- Trouble beginning a urine stream

- Weak or an interrupted stream
- Urgency, but with little stream
- Feels urination urge, even after voiding
- Mild, constant discomfort in lower abdomen

Note: Some may not have symptoms, increasing the likelihood of delaying treatment, leading to complications.

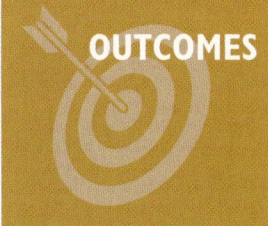

OUTCOMES

- Does not delay voiding.
- After voiding, states he feels he has emptied his bladder completely.

- Postvoiding residual volume < 150 m
- Bladder not palpable

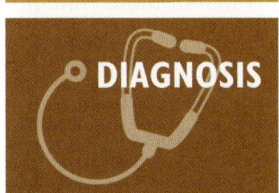

DIAGNOSIS

Acute Urinary Retention

Chronic Urinary Retention

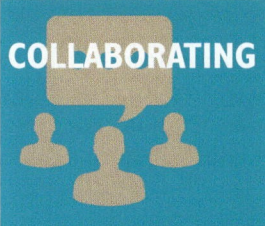

COLLABORATING

Medical Diagnosing
- Physical assessment
- Postvoid residual (PVR) measurement
- Cystoscopy
- CT scan
- Urodynamic tests
- Electromyography

Treatments
- **For mechanical obstruction** to urine flow: surgery, bladder drainage, urethral dilation, urethral stent
- **For loss of bladder tone:** Cholinergic medications stimulate contraction of detrusor muscle to trigger bladder emptying.
- **For poor bladder emptying:** Alpha-adrenergic antagonists reduce urethral resistance.

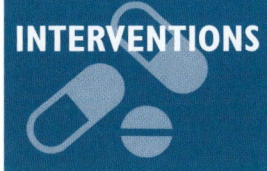

INTERVENTIONS

- Insert intermittent urinary catheter or patient self-catheterize as needed.
- Monitor for bladder distention (inspect and palpate).
- Measure PVR with bladder scanner.

- Apply heat to lower abdomen to relax the muscles near the bladder.
- Pour warm water over the perineum or sitz bath to stimulate voiding.

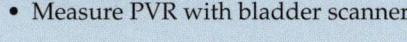

(Continued)

EXAMPLE PROBLEM: Urinary Retention—cont'd

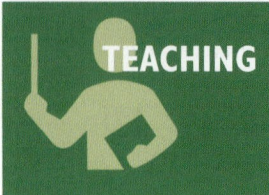
TEACHING

- Teach patient to use Credé's maneuver (manual pressure over the bladder)
- Advise the patient to contact a healthcare professional:
  - For urinary hesitancy, dribbling, or weak urine stream.
- For fever, vomiting, side or back pain, shaking chills, or passing little urine for 1 to 2 days.
- For blood in the urine, cloudy urine, frequency or urgency, or discharge from the penis or vagina.

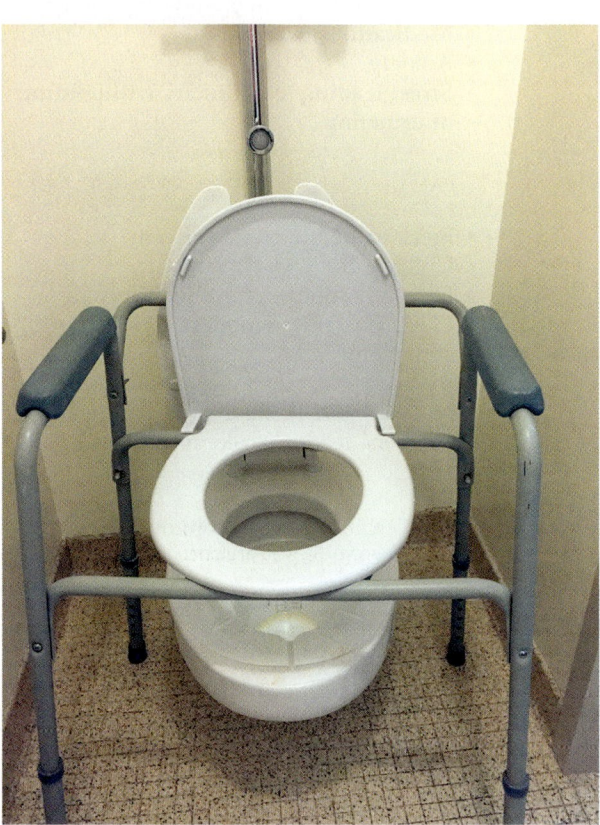

FIGURE 30-4 Toilet safety frame with urine collection container.

For clients who can assist with recording the I&O, provide a bedside clipboard. Older adults with poor balance weakness need support when using the commode. Provide a toilet safety frame that accommodates insertion of a urinary collection "hat."

- **Patients with mobility problems.** Use a bedpan or urinal to collect urine output. Male clients may void into a urinal while remaining in bed. Use a fracture pan for clients who have pelvis, lower back, or leg fractures, casts, splints, or braces. See Chapter 29, Procedure 29-2: Placing and Removing a Bedpan. For complete instructions for measuring urine output from a bedpan or urinal, see Procedure 30-1A.

Urine From a Catheter An indwelling urinary catheter is one that remains in the bladder for continuous drainage. It is held in place by a balloon that is inflated in the bladder above the detrusor muscle. Catheter insertion and ongoing care are discussed in the Planning Interventions/Implementation section of this chapter. Clients who require close monitoring of or hourly I&O will have a special collection bag with a measuring chamber. For complete instructions for measuring urine from

an indwelling catheter, see Procedure 30-1B, near the end of this chapter.

Obtaining Samples for Urine Studies

Many disorders of the urinary system can be assessed by examining urine. You will perform some of these tests at the bedside. For others, the specimen will be analyzed in the lab. The various types of urine samples are discussed in the following sections:

Freshly Voided Specimen

When collecting a urine sample, pour the urine into a specimen container labeled with the patient's name, the date, and the time of collection. Many facilities require packaging the container in a moisture-proof specimen-handling bag. Follow agency policy on additional packaging. Transport the specimen to the lab as soon as possible (according to agency policies). If there is a delay in transport, most agencies recommend refrigeration. To learn techniques for obtaining and measuring voided urine specimens, refer to Procedures 30-1 and 30-2, at the end of this chapter.

Clean-Catch Specimen

Many diagnostic tests require a clean-catch urine specimen. The client must cleanse the genitalia before voiding and collect the sample in midstream because the initial flow of urine may contain organisms from the urethral meatus, distal urethra, and perineum. A midstream sample is free of these contaminants. For the complete procedure, see Procedure 30-2A, at the end of this chapter.

Sterile Urine Specimen

A sterile urine specimen aids in determining the presence of a urinary tract infection. You can obtain a sterile urine specimen by inserting a catheter into the bladder or by withdrawing a sample from an indwelling catheter. Do not take the specimen from the collection bag because that urine may be several hours old.

✚ Never disconnect the catheter from the drainage tube to obtain a sample. Interrupting the system creates a portal of entry for pathogens, increasing the risk of contamination. For a discussion of the steps involved, see Procedure 30-2B, at the end of this chapter.

24-Hour Urine Collection

A 24-hour urine collection may be prescribed to evaluate some renal disorders by showing kidney function at different times of the day and night. For details about how to collect a 24-hour urine specimen, see Procedure 30-2C, at the end of this chapter.

Routine Urinalysis

A routine **urinalysis (UA)** is one of the most commonly prescribed laboratory tests. It is used as an overall screening test and as an aid to diagnosing renal, hepatic, and other diseases. Urinalysis requires a freshly voided sample.

Diagnostic Testing

Urinalysis

Characteristic	Expected Findings	Variations
Color	A freshly voided sample is pale yellow to deep amber.	Color is lighter, or even clear, if fluid intake is high or urine output is excessive. Color is darker as it becomes more concentrated (e.g., with decreased fluid intake or excessive fluid loss). Color is also affected by diet and medications.
pH	5.0–9.0, with an average of 6.0	Indicates kidneys' ability to help maintain balanced hydrogen ion concentration in the blood. The pH increases (more alkaline) if the client eats dairy products or citrus fruits or has a vegetarian diet. The pH decreases (more acidic) if the client eats a high-protein diet or consumes cranberry juice.
Specific gravity	1.002–1.030	This is a reflection of the kidney's ability to concentrate urine. Specific gravity rises with limited fluid intake, dehydration, and kidney disease. Specific gravity decreases as fluid intake increases.
Clarity	A freshly voided sample should be translucent. If the urine sits for a period of time, it will become cloudy.	Cloudiness in a freshly voided sample indicates the presence of other constituents in the urine: bacteria, red blood cells (RBCs), WBCs, sperm, prostatic fluid, or vaginal discharge.
Odor	Fresh urine has a scent.	Certain foods, such as garlic, onions, and asparagus, may give urine a distinctive odor. Bacteria give urine an ammonia-like odor. A sweet syrup odor may indicate a congenital metabolic disorder.
Protein	< 20 mg/day	Proteinuria is the most common indicator of renal disease. Protein is increased in diabetic nephropathy, glomerulonephritis, nephrosis, and toxemia of pregnancy. May be increased in benign proteinuria secondary to stress or physical exercise.
Glucose	Negative	Glucose is found in the urine with elevated blood sugars and diabetes.
Ketones	Negative	Presence of ketones indicates impaired carbohydrate metabolism (e.g., diabetes, fever, fasting, high-protein diets, starvation, vomiting, or the post-anesthesia period)
Hemoglobin	Negative on dipstick If RBCs are assessed via microscopic exam: < 5 per high-power field	Hemoglobin may be detected with infection of the urinary tract, disease of the bladder, glomerulonephritis, pyelonephritis, nephrolithiasis, hemolytic reactions, or trauma. May also be present in samples from women who are currently menstruating.
Bilirubin	Negative	Increased bilirubin occurs with liver disease.
Urobilinogen	Up to 1 mg/dL	Increased in cirrhosis, heart failure, liver disease, infectious mononucleosis, malaria, and pernicious anemia.
Nitrite	Negative	Increased in bacteriuria, presence of nitrite-forming bacteria.
Leukocyte esterase	Negative If WBCs are assessed via microscopic exam: < 5 per high-power field	Leukocytes are increased in bacterial infection, calculus formation, fungal or parasitic infection, glomerulonephritis, interstitial nephritis, or tumor.
Renal cells	None seen	Renal cells come from the lining of the collecting ducts. Their presence indicates damage to the tubular network.
Transitional cells	None seen	Transitional cells line the renal pelvis, ureter, bladder, and proximal urethra. Seen with infection, trauma, and malignancy.
Squamous cells	Rare	Typically insignificant: Squamous cells line the vagina and distal portion of the urethra.

(Continued)

Urinalysis—cont'd

Characteristic	Expected Findings	Variations
Casts	Rare hyaline; otherwise negative	Large numbers of *hyaline casts* are seen in renal disease, hypertension, diuretic use, and fever. *Granular casts* are seen in renal disease, viral infection, or lead intoxication.
Crystals	Absent in freshly voided sample	Crystals in the urine may indicate an old sample, stone formation in the urinary tract, gout, high dietary intake of oxalates, liver disease, or side effect of chemotherapy.
Bacteria, yeast, parasites	None seen	Microbes in the urine indicate an infection of the urinary tract.

Source: Adapted from Van Leeuwen, A., & Bladh, M. (2015). *Davis's comprehensive handbook of laboratory & diagnostic tests with nursing implications* (6th ed.). Philadelphia, PA: F.A. Davis.

Urinalysis techniques include "dipstick" testing and/or microscopic analysis. Dipstick testing is commonly performed at the bedside; microscopic examination is done in the lab. Box 30-3 contains several terms used to describe urine characteristics and quantity. For the expected findings and common variants of urinalysis, see the Diagnostic Testing box Urinalysis.

Bedside Testing (Dipstick)

Dipstick testing can determine pH and specific gravity and the presence of protein, glucose, ketones, and occult blood in the urine. Commercially prepared kits contain a reagent designed to detect a specific substance (e.g., glucose). The reagent may be a paper test strip, a fluid, or a tablet. When contacted by the urine, a chemical reaction causes a color change that you compare against a color chart (Fig. 30-5). For guidelines for dipstick testing and delegation of testing, see Procedure 30-3A, near the end of this chapter.

Specific Gravity

Specific gravity, an indicator of urine concentration, can be measured with a reagent strip. Specific gravity is usually tested in the laboratory, but it is a nursing responsibility in some

settings. For guidelines when testing urine specific gravity, see Procedure 30-3B.

For precise measurement of specific gravity, a **refractometer** might be used. A **refractometer** measures the extent to which a beam of light changes direction when it passes through the urine (the *refractive index*). If the concentration of solids is high, the light is refracted more. The method is quick and easy to perform and requires only a few drops of urine.

Knowledge Check 30-5

- Explain how to collect a clean-catch urine specimen.
- You are caring for a patient on a hospital unit from 0700 to 1200. Based on the following information, calculate the I&O and comment on your findings:
  Receiving IV fluid at 125 mL/hr
  0800 breakfast—4 oz juice, toast, scrambled eggs, 8 oz coffee
  0930—3 oz water
  0700 to 1200—wound drainage: 360 mL
  0700 to 1200—urine output per indwelling catheter: 180 mL

BOX 30-3 ■ Terms Associated With Urination

Acute renal failure (ARF): Acute rise in the serum creatinine level of 25% or more. May be caused by inadequate blood flow to the kidney, injury to the kidney glomeruli or tubules, or obstruction of kidney outflow.

Anuria: The absence of urine, or urine output of less than 100 mL in 24 hours. Often associated with kidney failure or congestive heart failure.

Dysuria: Painful or difficult urination. May be associated with infection, partial obstruction of the urinary tract, or medications that trigger urinary retention.

End-stage renal disease (ESRD): A chronic rise in serum creatinine levels associated with loss of kidney function that must be treated with dialysis or transplantation. Also known as chronic renal failure (CRF).

Enuresis: Involuntary loss of urine.

Frequency: The need to urinate at short intervals.

Hematuria: Blood in the urine. May be due to trauma, kidney stones, infection, or menstruation.

Oliguria: Urine output of less than 400 mL in 24 hours. For pediatric patients, oliguria is < 0.5–1.0 mL/kg per hour.

Nephropathy: A broad term meaning "disease of the kidney."

Nephrotoxic: A substance that damages kidney tissue. Some antibiotics (gentamicin, tobramycin, and amikacin), nonsteroidal anti-inflammatory drugs, lead, and contrast media have the potential to be nephrotoxic.

Nocturia: Frequent urination after going to bed. May be caused by excessive fluid intake or urinary tract and cardiovascular problems.

Nocturnal enuresis: Involuntary loss of urine while asleep.

Micturition: To start the stream of urine; to urinate; release urine from the bladder.

Pessary: An incontinence device that is inserted into the vagina to reduce organ prolapse or pressure on the bladder.

Polyuria: Excessive urination. May be caused by excessive hydration, diabetes mellitus, diabetes insipidus, or kidney disease.

Proteinuria: The presence of protein in the urine. May be a sign of infection or kidney disease.

Pyuria: Pus in the urine. May be caused by lesions or infection in the urinary tract.

Urgency: A sudden, almost uncontrollable need to urinate.

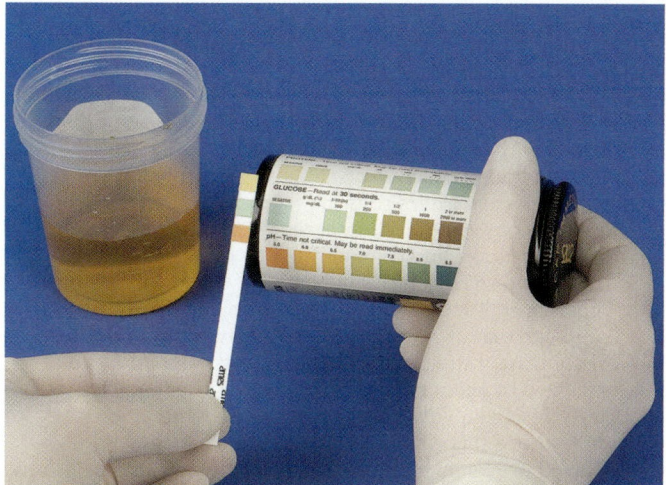

FIGURE 30-5 Commercial testing kits contain a reagent for a specific substance. A chemical reaction with the urine causes a color change that you interpret using a color chart.

ThinkLike a Nurse 30-6

- Why do you think the first voided urine is discarded at the start of a 24-hour urine collection?
- The following are the dipstick findings you obtained on the clean-catch specimen from Marlena (Meet Your Patient):

Characteristic	Result
pH	8.0
Specific gravity	1.030
Protein	Negative
Glucose	Negative
RBCs	Trace
Nitrite	+1
WBCs	+2
Bilirubin	Negative
Ketones	Negative
Urobilinogen	Negative

a. Identify the abnormal findings.
b. What would you expect the findings of her urine culture and sensitivity to demonstrate?

ANALYSIS/NURSING DIAGNOSIS NP

Urinary elimination problems are described by several nursing and medical diagnoses. NANDA-I diagnoses specific to urinary elimination include the following:

Infection, risk for
Urinary Elimination, impaired
Urinary Incontinence (functional, overflow, reflex, stress, urge, risk for urge)
Urinary Retention
Urinary Tract Injury, risk for

Urinary problems may also be the etiology of other nursing diagnoses, such as the following:

Anxiety r/t urinary urgency and recent episode of incontinence
Acute Pain r/t bladder spasms and urinary tract infection
Social Isolation r/t frequent periods of incontinence
Fluid Volume, risk for imbalanced

PLANNING OUTCOMES/EVALUATION NP

The general goal for urinary elimination is that patients will comfortably void approximately 1,500 mL of light yellow urine in 24 hours. Because normal urine elimination patterns vary, you must consider the individual's pattern, food and fluid intake, medications, and other factors, when setting target amounts.

NOC standardized outcomes for urinary problems, regardless of the specific problem, are the following: Kidney Function, Urinary Continence, Urinary Elimination, and Tissue Integrity: Skin & Mucous Membranes (because urinary elimination problems often place the patient at Risk for Impaired Skin Integrity).

Individualized goals/outcome statements you might use to evaluate the effectiveness of interventions for urinary problems include the following:

- Will discuss feelings about his urostomy.
- Will have no visible blood in urine after 2 days on antibiotics.
- Responds to the urge to void in a timely manner.
- Postvoiding residual volume is < 150 mL.

PLANNING INTERVENTIONS/IMPLEMENTATION NP

When Impaired Urination is the patient's problem, you might use NIC *standardized interventions,* such as the following examples.

Bladder Irrigation	Specimen Management
Environmental Management	Tube-Care: Urinary
Fluid Monitoring	Urinary Catheterization
Pelvic Muscle Exercise	Urinary Incontinence Care
Prompted Voiding	Urinary Retention Care
Self-Care Assistance: Toileting	

When Impaired Urination is the etiology of other problems, you might use NIC interventions such as Perineal Care, Self-Esteem Enhancement, and Skin Surveillance. The following are examples.

Diagnosis: Risk for Imbalanced Fluid Volume
NIC Intervention: Fluid Monitoring, Fluid Management

Diagnosis: Acute Pain r/t bladder spasms
NIC Intervention: Medication Administration

From your chosen intervention(s), select the activities that best meet individual patient needs and address problem etiologies.

Specific nursing activities for patients with elimination problems fall into the following categories:

- Promoting normal urination
- Preventing urinary tract infection
- Managing urinary retention
- Managing urinary incontinence
- Caring for patients who have urinary diversions

Promoting Normal Urination

As a nurse, you should have a repertoire of independent nursing activities (including the following) for promoting normal urination:

Provide Privacy

Although urination is a normal physiological process, most people consider it a private matter. ♥ **iCare** Provide privacy when discussing or providing care related to urination.

Excuse visitors from the room, draw the dividing curtains in shared rooms, and close the door to the room. Whenever possible, give the patient time alone to void. Do not, for example, hover outside the bathroom door asking, "Are you okay?" or "Are you finished yet?" Of course, if the client is weak and frail, you may need to remain with him. Taking a matter-of-fact approach confirms to patients that you are comfortable with this aspect of care.

Assist With Positioning

- **Most men stand to void** and may have difficulty voiding in other positions. Whenever possible, assist the patient to the bathroom and allow him to assume his preferred position. Alternatively, provide a bedside commode or urinal for the client

- **Women generally find an upright seated (semi-Fowler's) or squatting position** to be the most comfortable position for voiding. If a female patient must remain in bed, provide a bedpan. If the patient is very weak, you may need an assistant to help you position her on the bedpan, and you may need to stay with her to help her maintain her position on the bedpan. For the steps involved, see Chapter 29, Procedure 29-2: Placing and Removing a Bedpan.

Facilitate Toileting Routines

Most patients void on awakening, after meals or drinking a large volume of fluid, before bedtime, or, for some, during the night.

- Identify your patient's pattern and stick to it as much as possible.

- If you anticipate a change in the pattern for elimination, inform the patient. For example, if the patient is to receive a diuretic, explain that he will need to urinate more often. Similarly, if the patient is scheduled for a procedure or activity, inform him ahead of time so that he may empty his bladder before the activity begins.

- Assist all patients who have mobility problems and those who use the bedpan.

- Discuss with all nursing assistive personnel (NAP) the need to offer assistance so that patients experience minimal delays.

Promote Adequate Fluids and Nutrition

Adequate hydration promotes healthy urinary function and flushes the system of waste products. Most people should drink eight to ten 8-ounce glasses of fluid daily unless health problems limit the fluid. Unfortunately, many people do not meet the recommended intake. Water is the preferred fluid because soda, coffee, and tea often contain caffeine or additives that may cause diuresis and incontinence. However, the amount of fluid is more important than the type. If the patient will not or cannot drink water, provide the fluid he prefers. See Box 30-4 for strategies to increase your patient's fluid intake.

Assist With Hygiene

Urine is irritating to the skin. Therefore, perineal cleansing is an essential part of toileting hygiene. It may include pouring warm soapy water over the genitals while the patient is seated on the toilet, the bedside commode, or the bedpan. Be sure to rinse with warm water because soap is drying to the genital mucosa. Also offer a moist washcloth or towelette for washing hands after toileting.

You will need to provide perineal care because many patients are unable to do so for themselves. If the patient can ambulate to the bathroom, you merely need to assist with her usual cleansing

---

BOX 30-4 ■ Strategies to Increase Patients' Fluid Intake

- For patients with limited mobility, keep water or other liquids within easy reach.
- Remind young children or patients with cognitive or psychiatric disorders to drink fluids.
- For patients who have increased fluid needs, provide goals for intake and remind them to drink frequently.
- Many foods have a high fluid content. If the patient requires additional fluid for hydration, consider adding soup and watery foods, such as watermelon, to the diet. In contrast, if the patient requires fluid restriction, you will have to account for these foods in the fluid balance.
- Try offering liquids through a straw. Patients tend to drink more this way.
- Chilled drinks might be more appealing, particularly if the patient's mouth is dry. Offer beverages with ice if they are to be served cold.
- Provide good mouth care. Patients will often drink more readily if their mouth feels fresh.

---

routines. For further information, see Procedure 24-4: Providing Perineal Care.

Interventions for Example Problem: Urinary Tract Infection (UTI)

An important part of UTI care is prevention of UTIs. For more information about caring for patients with urinary tract infections, see the preceding Example Problem: Urinary Tract Infection (UTI).

KnowledgeCheck 30-6

- Identify activities that promote normal urination patterns.
- Write at least two nursing diagnostic statements for a patient with urinary frequency, burning, urgency, and a fever.

Interventions for Example Problem: Urinary Retention

Clients with a mechanical obstruction to urine flow are treated by surgery (e.g., resection of the prostate gland). Those with loss of bladder tone may be treated with medications. For independent nursing interventions, refer to the following discussion of Urinary Catheterization. Also see the Example Problem: Urinary Retention.

Urinary Catheterization

Catheterization is the introduction of a pliable tube (catheter) into the bladder, via the urethra, to allow drainage of urine. Urinary catheterization is performed to do the following:

- Obtain a sterile urine specimen.
- Drain the bladder for surgical or diagnostic purposes or when emptying is incomplete after urination.
- Prevent or treat bladder overdistention and urinary retention (e.g., after surgery) when other measures fail.
- Measure post-residual void (PVR) if a portable bladder ultrasound device is unavailable or if the results are inconclusive. PVR is measured to detect urinary retention or incontinence.
- Protect excoriated skin from contact with urine.
- Reduce the need for unnecessary movement of patients who are near death.

Risks and Complications Indwelling urinary catheterization is associated with *bacteriuria and urinary tract infection* because:

- A catheter provides a connection between the external environment and a normally sterile system, allowing entry of pathogens.
- When the patient has an indwelling catheter, microorganisms are no longer flushed from the urethra through voiding.

There is also the risk of *urethral injury* if the catheter is too large, is forced through strictures, inserted at an incorrect angle, or not well lubricated.

Self-Catheterization Patients with spinal cord injuries or neurological disorders use intermittent catheterization to drain the bladder and limit the risk of infection. Many actually perform **intermittent self-catheterization,** although caregivers may assist. Although you will use sterile technique for catheterization, most patients who self-catheterize use clean technique. In spite of this difference, intermittent catheterization carries a substantially lower risk of infection than does an indwelling catheter (Hooton, Bradley, Cardenas, et al., 2010).

The goals of intermittent self-catheterization are to (1) completely empty the bladder and (2) prevent urinary tract infections. See the Self-Care box Teaching Your Client About Clean, Intermittent Self-Catheterization (CISC).

Patient Teaching
- Teach patient to use Credé's maneuver (manual pressure over the bladder)
- Advise the patient to contact a healthcare professional:
  - For urinary hesitancy, dribbling, or weak urine stream
  - For fever, vomiting, side or back pain, shaking chills, or passing little urine for 1 to 2 days
  - For blood in the urine, cloudy urine, frequency or urgency, or discharge from the penis or vagina

---

Self-Care

Teaching Your Client About Clean, Intermittent Self-Catheterization (CISC)

In the home setting, CISC is a clean procedure rather than a sterile one. In teaching the steps of the procedure, consider the client's physical ability to reach the urethra and to manipulate the catheter and equipment (e.g., range of motion, fine motor skills, degree of sensation).

Procedure for Men

1. Try to void before catheterization. If you are unable to void or if the amount is less than 3 oz (or the amount specified by your healthcare provider), then insert the catheter.
2. Assemble the catheter, lubricant, and drainage receptacle.
3. Thoroughly wash your hands with soap and water; cleanse the penis and the urethral opening.
4. Lubricate the catheter to 6 in. (15 cm).
5. Stand over the toilet or assume a comfortable position (e.g., sitting on the toilet).
6. Hold the penis perpendicular (at a right angle) to the body.
7. Gently insert and advance the catheter.
8. When you meet resistance, at the level of the prostate, take deep breaths to try to relax, and advance the catheter.
9. When urine flow starts, advance the catheter 1 in. (2.5 cm) more; return the penis to its natural position; hold the catheter in place until the urine flow stops and bladder is empty.
10. Withdraw the catheter slowly in small increments to be sure the entire bladder empties.
11. Wash the catheter with soap and water, if it is reusable. Rinse and dry it well. If it is disposable, discard it immediately.
12. Store catheters in a clean, dry, secure place.
13. Record the amount of urine obtained.

Procedure for Women

1. Try to void before catheterization. If you are unable to void or if amount is less than 3 oz (or the amount specified by your healthcare provider), then insert catheter.
2. Assemble the catheter, lubricant, and drainage receptacle; a good light is important for women.
3. Thoroughly wash hands with soap and water; cleanse the labia and urethra with soap and water or with a moist towelette; rinse. Cleanse and rinse from front to back.
4. Lubricate the catheter to about 1 in. (2.5 cm).
5. Assume a comfortable position. Some women perform CISC standing up with one foot on the toilet.
6. Use a hand mirror to locate the urethral opening, which is between the clitoris and the vagina.
7. Spread the vaginal lips (labia) with the second and fourth fingers; use the middle finger to feel for the urethral opening.
8. Gently insert the catheter into the opening, guiding it upward toward the umbilicus (belly button). This is usually 2 or 3 in. (5 to 8 cm) past the urethral opening.
9. When urine flows, advance the catheter another 1 in. (2.5 cm); hold it in place until the urine stops and the bladder is empty.
10. Withdraw the catheter slowly in small increments to be sure the entire bladder empties.
11. If the catheter is reusable, wash it with soap and water; rinse and dry it well. If it is disposable, discard it immediately.
12. Store catheters in a clean, dry, secure place.
13. Record the amount of urine obtained.

Home Care

- Teach the client how to wash her hands before beginning.
- Encourage the client to drink 8 to 10 eight-oz glasses of fluid without caffeine each day to ensure a quantity of urine adequate to flush the bladder.
- Teach the client to report the signs and symptoms of urinary tract infection: burning, frequency, urgency, dull abdominal ache, fever, or malaise; urine that contains sediment or becomes cloudy; or burning on urination or a fever occurs. Older adults may experience confusion before the other signs and symptoms occur.
- Advise the client to contact a healthcare provider if there is bleeding, pain, or difficulty inserting the catheter.

(Continued)

Self-Care

Teaching Your Client About Clean, Intermittent Self-Catheterization (CISC)—cont'd

➤ Some CISC catheters can be reused; some are disposable.

➤ Catheterize as often as needed—perhaps every 2 to 3 hours at first.

➤ Discard a reusable catheter when it becomes difficult to clean or difficult to insert. A CISC catheter may be reused for 2 to 4 weeks.

➤ Soak the catheter in a white vinegar solution once a week to control odor and remove encrustation or deposits of mucus.

Source: Newman, D. K., & Willson, M. M. (2011). Review of intermittent catheterization and current best practices. *Urologic Nursing, 31*(1), 12–29, 48.

Types of Catheter Materials

There are several catheter types and materials from which to choose, depending on whether the patient requires catheterization for long-term or short-term use, has product sensitivity, or is at increased risk for infection.

- *Silver alloy*–coated catheters may reduce the risk of catheter-associated urinary tract infections for up to 14 days (Lam, Omar, Fisher, et al, 2014; Wound, Ostomy, and Continence Nurses Society, 2009). Silver-coated catheters are not routinely used for short-term catheterization because they are more costly than standard catheters.
- *Teflon-bonded latex*–coated catheters reduce friction and tissue irritation during insertion and while the catheter remains in place.
- *Polyvinyl chloride (PVC)* catheters are inexpensive and commonly used for intermittent catheterization. They are more rigid and therefore, less comfortable for indwelling use (WOCN, 2016).
- *Silicone catheters* are preferable to standard catheters for long-term catheterization. They cause less tissue irritation and prevent encrustation (Gould, Umscheid, Agarwal, et al., 2009). They are safe for patients with latex sensitivity.
- *Hydrogel-coated* catheters can be made of either latex or silicone. They cause less urethral trauma during insertion, resist encrustation, and can remain in place up to 12 weeks

(Turner & Dickens, 2011). This type of lubricant and/or antimicrobial coating helps prevent infection.

Types of Catheters

- A **straight catheter** is a single-lumen tube that is inserted for immediate drainage of the bladder (e.g., to obtain a sterile urine specimen, to measure PVR volume, or to relieve temporary bladder distention). After the bladder is empty or the sample obtained, the catheter is removed and the patient resumes voiding independently.
- An **indwelling catheter,** also known as a *Foley* or *retention catheter,* is used for continuous bladder drainage (e.g., when the bladder must be kept empty or when continuous urine measurement is needed). It is usually a double-lumen tube: one lumen is used for urine drainage, and the second lumen is used to inflate a balloon near the tip of the catheter. A triple-lumen indwelling catheter is used when the patient requires intermittent or continuous bladder irrigation. The inflated balloon holds the catheter in place at the neck of the bladder. The balloon is sized according to the volume of fluid used to inflate it. For most patients you will use a 5-mL balloon; for children, a 3-mL; and for achieving hemostasis after a prostatectomy, a 30-mL balloon. Figure 30-6 illustrates the different types of catheters.
- A **suprapubic catheter** is used for continuous urine drainage when the urethra must be bypassed (e.g., after gynecological surgery or where there is prostatic obstruction). It is inserted

---

Toward Evidence-Based Practice

Urinary catheter insertion is a common procedure and is a major cause of infection in hospitals.

Leis, J. A., Corpus C., Catt, B., et al. (2016). Medical directive for urinary catheter removal by nurses on general medical wards. *JAMA Internal Medicine, 176*(1), 113–115. doi:10.1001/jamainternmed.2015.6319

Researchers found that empowering nurses to remove urinary catheters that were no longer needed resulted in markedly reduced number of days patients used these catheters. In turn, reduced duration of catheterization reduced the risk of catheter-association urinary tract infection (CAUTI).

Meddings, J., Rogers, M. A., Krein, S. L., et al. (2014). Reducing unnecessary urinary catheter use and other strategies to prevent catheter-associated urinary tract infection: An integrative review. *BMJ of Quality and Safety, 23*(4), 277–289. doi:10.1136/bmjqs-2012-001774

Meddings et al. updated the evidence on prior research examining CAUTI prevention strategies. Reminders prompting removal of urinary catheters and routine stop orders reduced CAUTI rates by 53%. Antimicrobial catheters provided no significant benefit in preventing symptomatic CAUTIs.

Sutherland, T., McGrath, C., Liu, X., et al. (2015). A single-center multidisciplinary initiative to reduce catheter-associated infection rates: Quality and financial implications. *Health Care Manager, 34*(3), 218–224. doi:10.1097/HCM.0000000000000073

Researchers found that provider education and electronic documentation prompts led to a significant decrease in catheter utilization. Fewer catheter-days were followed by lower infection rates. However, when there was less emphasis on prevention goals, the rate of CAUTI increased.

Toward Evidence-Based Practice—cont'd

Plantier, G. M., Bosso, C. E., Azevedo, B. N., et al. (2015). Effect of chlorhexidine and urinary catheter infection prevention in a Brazilian coronary ICU. *Critical Care,* *19*(1), 80. doi:10.1186/cc14160

The use of chlorhexidine in the periprocedural antisepsis of urinary catheterization contributed to the decrease of urinary tract infections associated with long-term urinary catheterization in patients admitted to the coronary ICU.

Wilson, M., Wilde, M., Webb, M. L., et al. (2009). Nursing interventions to reduce the risk of catheter-associated urinary tract infection. Part 2: Staff education, monitoring, and care techniques. *Journal of Wound, Ostomy, and Continence Nursing,* *36*(2), 137–154. doi:10.1097/01.WON.0000347655.56851.04

Staff education for catheter management was found to reduce the incidence of CAUTI in patients managed by short-term, indwelling catheterization. Researchers also found evidence supporting the implementation of a hospital-wide program to ensure indwelling urinary catheters are used only when indicated and are promptly removed when not absolutely necessary.

1. Indwelling urinary catheters are an important cause of infection. In these four studies, what evidence-based practice strategies were shown to reduce the incidence of CAUTI?

2. Studies by Leis et al. (2016) found nurses' judgment for removing indwelling urinary catheters contributes to shorter duration of urinary catheterization. How might you assess your patient after removing the catheter?

3. Sutherland et al. (2015) and Wild et al. (2009) found that healthcare staff education led to reduced catheter-days and subsequently lower rates of CAUTI. In the educational session, the researchers suggested using indwelling urinary catheters for a duration as short as possible. What other questions might nurses ask about managing urinary catheterization to reduce the risk of infection?

 Go to Davis Advantage, Chapter Resources, Chapter 30, **Toward Evidence-Based Practice—Suggested Responses.**

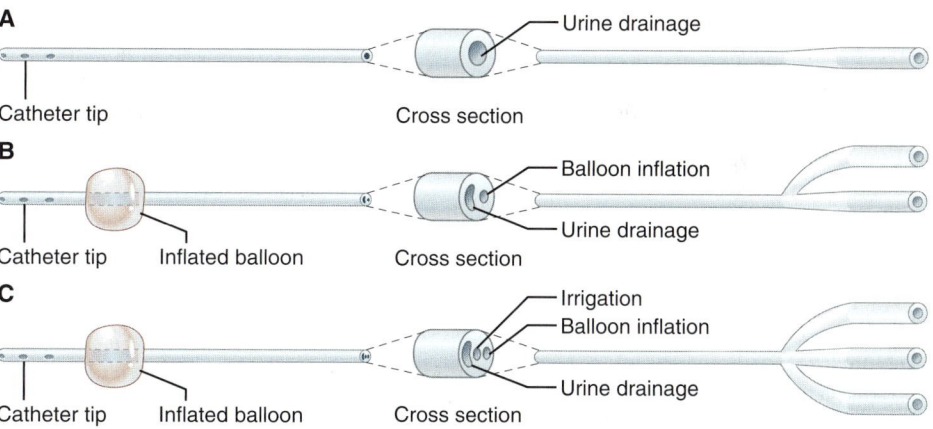

FIGURE 30-6 Types of catheters. A. A single-lumen catheter is used to obtain a urine sample or immediately drain the bladder. B. A double-lumen catheter is the most commonly used indwelling catheter. C. A triple-lumen catheter is inserted when the patient requires irrigation of the bladder.

through an incision above the symphysis pubis (Fig. 30-7). It may be sutured in place initially. Once the stoma tract has healed, a standard indwelling catheter is usually used and is held in place by inflation of the balloon.

Catheter Sizing

Catheters are sized by the *diameter* of the lumen; the larger the number, the larger the lumen. For example, 8- and 10-French (Fr) catheters are used for children; they are smaller in diameter than the 14- and 16-Fr catheters typically used for adults. Men usually need a larger lumen diameter (e.g., 18-Fr) than women. To minimize urethral trauma, use the smallest diameter catheter possible that provides proper drainage (Wald, Fink, Makic, et al., 2012). Catheters also come in different *lengths:* A 22-cm catheter is appropriate for women, whereas for men you will need a 40-cm catheter.

Supplies for Urinary Catheterization

The supplies used for inserting a catheter are usually prepackaged. Kits contain the most common catheter sizes, usually 12-, 14-, or 16-Fr. Pediatric kits contain 8- or 10-Fr catheters.

KnowledgeCheck 30-7

- Describe the difference between a catheter used for straight catheterization and one used for ongoing drainage.
- Why is intermittent catheterization preferred for patients who must be catheterized over lengthy periods of time?

Urinary Catheter Insertion

Always check for latex or Teflon and iodine allergies before performing a catheterization.

Most patients experience a sensation of pressure and some discomfort (but not pain) when a catheter is inserted. Explain that when the catheter is inserted it may feel as though the patient is voiding, but the urine is going into the tube, not on

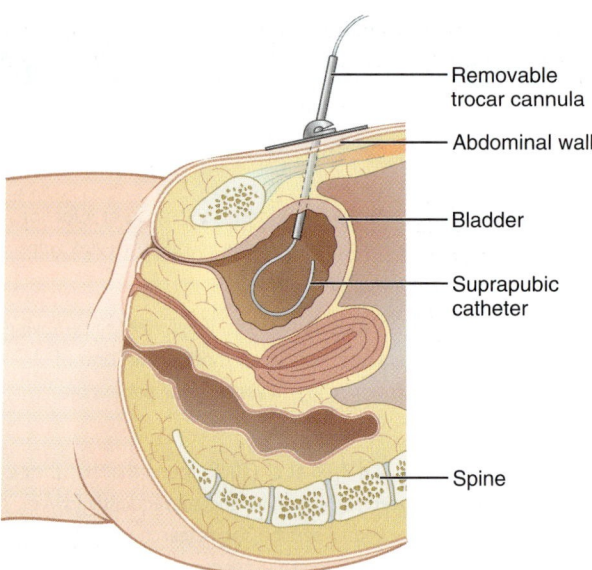

FIGURE 30-7 A suprapubic catheter drains urine from a surgically created opening into the bladder, bypassing the urethra.

the bed. If there is swelling or bleeding in the urinary tract, insertion may be painful.

♥ **iCare**   Many patients feel embarrassed during this procedure. A professional approach and privacy measures help relieve discomfort or distress. As you are preparing the patient for the procedure, offer to answer any questions he may have.

It may be difficult to visualize the urinary meatus in females. The following may help you:

- Lower the section of the bed called the knee gatch to better expose the urinary meatus.
- Place a firm cushion under the patient's buttocks to prevent her sinking into a soft mattress and obscuring visibility of the meatus.
- For women who are unable to assume a dorsal recumbent position, consider Sims' or a lateral position (Fig. 30-8).

Note that catheterization can injure the urethra if the catheter is too large, is forced through strictures, inserted at an incorrect angle, or not well lubricated.

➕ To reduce the risk of bacterial contamination, clean around the meatus and perineum before inserting or removing an indwelling urinary catheter; use aseptic technique and sterile equipment; perform strict and frequent catheter care; and maintain a closed system (Gould, Umscheid, Agarwal, et al., 2009). To learn how to insert

---

♥ **iCare 30-1**

Providing Warmth and Privacy During Urinary Catheterization

To prepare your female patient for urinary catheterization, you can show her that you care by wrapping her legs with a warmed blanket before exposure of her perineum. To read more about this technique,

 Go to Chapter 24, Procedure 24-4: Providing Perineal Care.

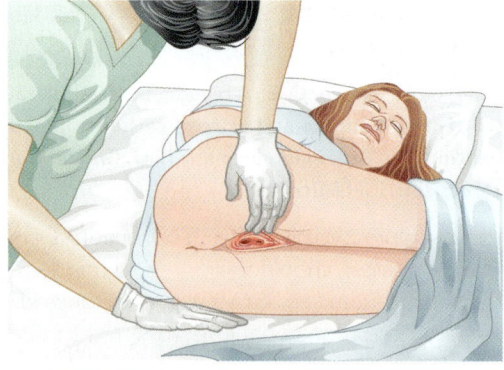

A

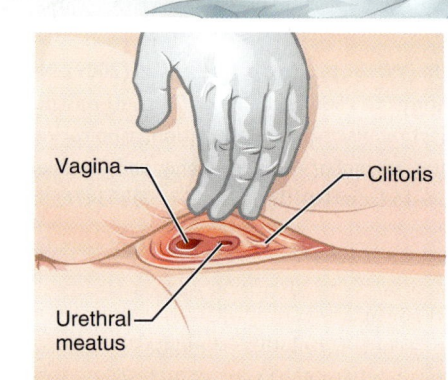

B

FIGURE 30-8 For women who cannot assume a dorsal recumbent position, you can use the side-lying position and lift the superior buttock to expose the urethral meatus.

straight and indwelling catheters, see Procedure 30-4, near the end of this chapter.

Caring for the Patient With an Indwelling Catheter

KEY POINT: *Remember above all, when providing care for a patient with an indwelling catheter, keep it closed, keep it flowing, and keep it clean* (Foley Catheter Care Guide, 2013; Wald, Fink, Makic, et al., 2012). *Best practice care is always to remove a urinary catheter as soon as it is no longer necessary.*

The goals of nursing care for a patient with an indwelling catheter are to:

- Prevent urinary tract infection
- Maintain free flow of urine
- Prevent transmission of infection
- Promote normal urine production
- Maintain skin and mucosal integrity

For in-depth guidelines when caring for a patient with an indwelling catheter, see Clinical Insight 30-1, later in the chapter.

Bladder Irrigation

You may perform an irrigation to maintain patency of a urinary catheter, to wash out the bladder (e.g., remove blood clots in the bladder after surgery), or to instill medications into the bladder.

- An *intermittent irrigation* is most commonly used for medication instillation.
- A *continuous irrigation* is used to maintain patency when blood, clots, or debris is anticipated.
- *Routine intermittent irrigations* (e.g., every shift, every week) are sometimes prescribed to ensure patency; however, these

should be avoided (Wound, Ostomy, and Continence Nurses Society, 2009).

A patient requiring a continuous irrigation should have a triple-lumen catheter in place: one lumen for injecting water into the balloon when the catheter is inserted, another for the irrigating solution to flow into the bladder, and a third for the solution and urine to flow out of the bladder.

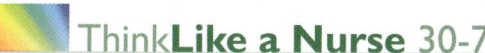 A double-lumen catheter system may need to be opened for irrigation and therefore creates a high risk for infection. Although "open" irrigation was used in the past, it is no longer recommended.

For complete bladder irrigation procedures, see Procedures 30-7A and 30-7B, at the end of this chapter.

Removing an Indwelling Catheter

Removing a urinary catheter is a simple task, but you must monitor patients carefully afterward. After removing the catheter:

- Note and record the time and amount of the first voiding and the appearance of the urine.
- Compare the patient's intake with output for the next 8 to 12 hours and palpate the bladder for distention. A portable bladder scanner may also be used to quantify the amount of any retained urine.
- Monitor regularly for bladder distention until normal voiding is reestablished. The catheter may have caused some edema of the urethra, which will interfere with voiding at first.

If a catheter is in place for several weeks, the bladder muscle loses tone and the patient may require bladder retraining. Agencies have differing procedures for this. One method is to begin clamping the catheter for certain periods of time (e.g., 1 to 4 hours) to allow the bladder to fill, and then releasing the clamp to allow urine to drain from the bladder. However, there is evidence stating that clamping is not necessary before removing the catheter (Gould, Umscheid, Agarwal, et al., 2009; Hadwen, 2011; Moon, Chun, & Lee, 2012).

For inpatients who have had a urinary catheter for a short time, you might remove the catheter late at night instead of in the morning. Patients tend to hold urine in the bladder for a longer period of time at night than in the morning.

For guidelines to follow when removing a retention catheter, see Procedure 30-6, at the end of this chapter.

KnowledgeCheck 30-8

- What actions should you take before inserting a catheter?
- When caring for a client with an indwelling catheter, you notice sandy particles around the urethral meatus. What should you do?
- How often should the urine collection bag be emptied?

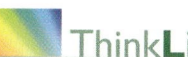 ThinkLike a Nurse 30-7

You are caring for a patient who had an indwelling catheter removed 12 hours ago. The patient has not voided. What action should you take?

Interventions for Example Problem: Urinary Incontinence

Because urinary incontinence is so prevalent, you are likely to be called on to deal with this problem in your practice. Most incontinence is managed with skin care and behavioral interventions, but medications are sometimes used. See accompanying Example Problem: Urinary Incontinence.

For ideas about home care management of urinary incontinence, see the Self-Care box Teaching Patients to Manage Urinary Incontinence.

ThinkLike a Nurse 30-8

- How do you feel about instructing patients about pelvic floor muscle exercises (PFME)? Do you think a woman should always be provided this instruction? Explain your thinking.
- What treatment options for incontinence have you seen used in your clinical experience? What options do you believe should be used more frequently? Less frequently? Explain your thinking.

Caring for a Patient With a Urinary Diversion

A patient with a urinary diversion requires physical and psychological care. Initially you will care for the ostomy. However, the long-term goals are for the patient to become comfortable with his changed body and to assume self-care.

What Are Urinary Diversions?

A **urinary diversion,** or **urostomy,** is a surgically created opening for elimination of urine. A patient with a urinary diversion does not eliminate urine via the urethra. Instead, urine bypasses the bladder and is expelled through the **stoma** or **ostomy.** The patient no longer has voluntary control of urination. Urine constantly flows through the stoma and is collected in a pouch the patient wears. Urostomies are used to treat patients who have urinary system defects or trauma. The primary risks associated with urinary diversions are infection and permanent kidney damage, which can occur from **hydronephrosis** (distention of the kidneys with urine, resulting from obstruction of the ureter). Four types of urinary diversions follow:

1. **Cutaneous ureterostomy.** This surgery reroutes the ureter(s) directly to the surface of the abdomen, forming a small stoma. This procedure has limited use because it provides a pathway for pathogens on the skin to enter the kidney. The stomas are small and difficult to fit with a collection appliance.

2. **Conventional urostomy (ileal conduit, Bricker's loop, ileal loop).** This is the most common type of urinary diversion (Fig. 30-9) because it is the simplest to perform surgically and eliminates the need for intermittent catheterization. The ureters are implanted into a loop of the ileum (the last segment of the small intestine) where urine drains freely into the stoma bag. The downside is urine can back up into the kidneys, causing infection or stone formation over time.

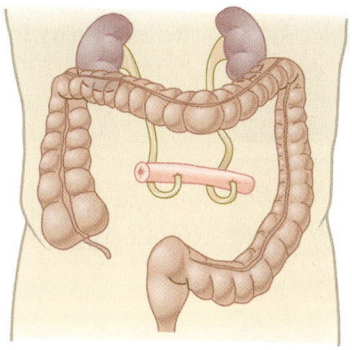

FIGURE 30-9 An ileal conduit is the most common urinary diversion.

EXAMPLE PROBLEM: Urinary Incontinence

Definition: Loss or lack of voluntary control over urination

Types and Causes of UI

Urge incontinence (overactive bladder)—Involuntary loss of urine with a strong urge to void

Stress Incontinence—Involuntary loss of urine with increased intra-abdominal pressure in the absence of an overactive bladder
Causes: Pregnancy, childbirth, obesity, chronic constipation and straining at stool, exercise, laughing, sneezing, coughing, lifting

Mixed incontinence—Combination of urge and stress incontinence

Unconscious (reflex) incontinence—Loss of urine when the person does not realize the bladder is full and has no urge to void
Causes: CNS disease, tissue damage from radiation, cystitis, bladder inflammation, or radical pelvic surgery

Functional incontinence—Untimely loss of urine with no urinary or neurological cause
Causes: Immobility, pain, external obstacles, or problems in thinking or communicating

Transient incontinence—Short-term incontinence expected to resolve spontaneously
Causes: UTI, medications (especially diuretics)

Overflow incontinence—Leakage of urine with a distended bladder
Causes: Fecal impaction, neurological disorders, enlarged prostate

Epidemiology—Who Is Affected?

- UI is common in older adults but is not a normal change of aging.
- Women are twice as likely as men to be affected.
- Current estimates may be low because providers often fail to ask specific questions about incontinence. Many people do not mention leakage of urine to healthcare providers because they are embarrassed, believe nothing can be done, or feel it's an inevitable condition that occurs with age.

Complications

- CAUTIs in healthy patients often resolve spontaneously with the removal of catheter.
- UI can lead to prostatitis, epididymitis, cystitis, pyelonephritis, gram-negative bacteremia.

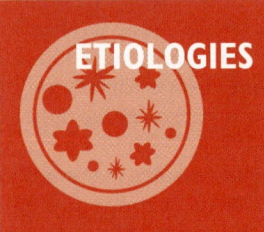
ETIOLOGIES

Risk Factors

Advanced age
Cigarette use
Diabetes
History of UTIs
Neurological disease (e.g., stroke)
Obesity

Reduced estrogen after menopause
Reduced mobility
Men: Benign prostatic hyperplasia (enlarged prostate) or to prostatectomy
Women: Childbirth, specifically to vaginal delivery, perimenopause

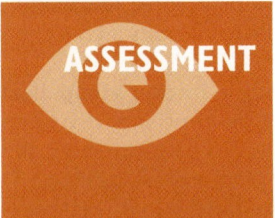
ASSESSMENT

Symptoms

Back pain, can be sides or under ribs	Edema	Pyuria
Foul smelling urine	Fever	Dysuria
Bladder spasms	Hematuria	Urinary frequency
Chills	Nausea, vomiting	Urgency

Diagnostic Tests

Midstream, clean-catch urine specimen for culture
Dipstick for leukocytes, blood, estrace, nitrates

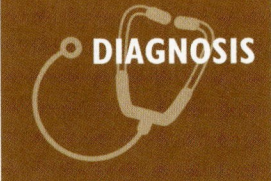
DIAGNOSIS

Functional Urinary Incontinence
Overflow Urinary Incontinence
Reflex Urinary Incontinence
Stress Urinary Incontinence

Urge Urinary Incontinence
Risk for Urge Urinary Incontinence
Risk for Infection
Acute Pain r/t UTI

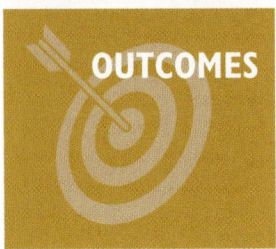
OUTCOMES

- Patient verbalizes improved quality of life, including capacity for physical activity and self-esteem.

- Patient's bladder holds increasingly greater volumes of urine.
- Interval between voidings increases.

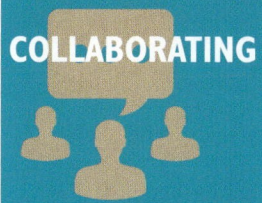
COLLABORATING

Treatments for Urinary Incontinence

- **Medications.** Topical estrogen for women with urogenital atrophy; anticholinergics for involuntary bladder contractions.
- **Incontinence devices,** such as a pessary, to prevent occasional leakage (e.g., during exercise).
- **Sacral nerve stimulation.** For those who have not responded to conservative treatment

Surgical Interventions

- **Sling procedures.** Lifts the urethra to relieve pressure.
- **Augmentation of the bladder.** Bladder is surgically enlarged to improve bladder size. Bowel is wrapped around the bladder neck to improve the squeezing action of the bladder.
- **Injection of bulking agents.** Collagen is injected alongside of the urethra. Lasts a period of years with few complications.
- **Sacral nerve stimulator.** A lead wire is placed near the sacral nerve; acts like a bladder pacemaker for better control of urge incontinence.
- **Prostate resection.** To relieve pressure of pelvic organs against the bladder.

Devices to Manage Urinary Incontinence

- **Incontinence pessary.** Placed in the vagina; relieves pressure of pelvic organs on the urethra. When used long term, monitor for vaginal infection and ulceration.
- **Vaginal weight training.** Small cone-shaped weight in the vagina for two 15-min periods per day. Contracts the pelvic floor muscles to keep the weight in the vagina.
- **External occlusive device.**
  - *Women:* Urethral meatus covering
  - *Men:* A penis clamp is a reusable, soft spongy rubber device used to control stress incontinence or dribbling urine, common with enlarged prostate.
- **Internal urethral meatus plug.** Disposable, single-use device for activities that cause stress incontinence; used by men and women.
- **Valved catheter.** Urine drained on a schedule.
- **Indwelling urethral catheter.** Last resort to control the flow of urine; protects perineal skin.
- **Bed alarm.** Wake the patient if incontinence occurs.
- **External collection device.** Condom catheters (urosheaths) for men with adequate bladder emptying and intact genital skin.

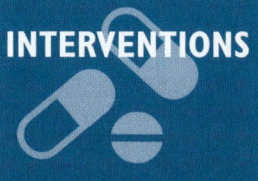
INTERVENTIONS

Bladder Training

- Record when emptying bladder (voiding diary).
- Distraction and relaxation strategies help inhibit the urge to void.
- Deep breathing, guided imagery, and pelvic floor contractions quiet the bladder.

Scheduled Voiding

- Timed voiding; habit retraining
- Must be mentally and physically capable of self-toileting

Pelvic Floor Muscle Rehabilitation Kegel Exercises

These strengthen by squeezing and relaxing as if stopping urination midstream.

Intermittent Self-Catheterization

A straight catheter to drain the bladder for overflow incontinence

Biofeedback

Electrodes on the abdomen provide feedback about the quality of perineal contraction.

Supportive Interventions

- Bedside commode, raised toilet seat, bedpan, and urinal make it easier to urinate independently.
- Men with UI can use a drip collector—a small pocket of padding worn over the penis, held in place with underwear.
- When continence cannot be achieved, consider use of absorbent products with waterproof coverings. ♥ **iCare** Under no circumstances should you refer to these as diapers. Reassure that incontinence is not shameful.

Perineal Skin Care

- Keep skin dry; clean using soap and warm water; rinse well.
- Apply barrier creams and antifungals, as prescribed.
- Use absorbent products for intractable UI.

Complementary Alternative Methods (CAM)

No CAM cures UI; may reduce symptoms. May try acupuncture or biofeedback.

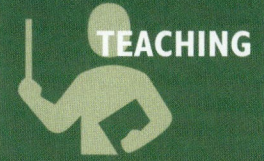
TEACHING

Refer to the Self-Care box Teaching Patients to Manage Urinary Incontinence.

Self-Care

Teaching Patients to Manage Urinary Incontinence

Most urinary incontinence (UI) is managed with skin care and behavioral interventions, but medications and other collaborative treatments are sometimes used.

Open Discussion About Incontinence

➤ Patients and families often do not raise the issue. Be direct and ask about continence using simple questions that are not embarrassing, such as, "Do you wear a pad to keep your clothes dry?" "Do you ever wet your clothing?"

➤ If you determine that the patient is incontinent, ask questions to identify the type of incontinence, such as, "Do you sometimes not make it to the toilet in time?" "Do you ever dribble urine when you sneeze or cough?"

➤ Encourage use of a bladder diary for 3 to 7 days, recording routine activities as well as atypical situations.

➤ **KEY POINT:** *Advise patients to contact a healthcare provider if:*
They have not been previously evaluated for incontinence.
The urinary stream is weak.
There is burning, fever, chills, pain, or passing little urine for 1 to 2 days.
Urine is cloudy or unusually foul smelling.
Discharge occurs from the penis or vagina.

➤ Advise patients to take prescribed diuretics early in the morning. Diuretics taken at night can cause nocturia and lead to interrupted sleep.

Lifestyle Modification

Make the following recommendations to patients:

➤ **Increase daily oral fluids** to 8 to 10 glasses (or 2,000 to 2,500 mL), as tolerated, to promote flushing of the bladder. *Limiting fluids has not been shown to be useful in preventing incontinence (Townsend, Jura, Curhan, et al., 2011) and increases the risk for UTIs, constipation, and dehydration (Lucas, Bedretdinova, Bosch, et al., 2014).*

➤ **Limit caffeine intake** to < 100 mg daily. This is about one cup of coffee or two 12-ounce cans of cola. *Caffeine is a diuretic and a bladder stimulant.*

➤ **Try limiting the intake** of alcohol, artificial sweeteners, spicy foods, and citrus fruits. *These are thought to irritate the bladder.*

➤ **Lose weight** (for persons, especially women, with a BMI > 30). *Weight reduction by as little as 5% to 10% alleviates incontinence symptoms (Rainsbury, Fabricius, & McLarty, 2011).*

➤ **Stop smoking.** *Smoking has been linked to stress UI and urge UI.*

➤ **Take prescribed diuretics early in the morning.** *Diuretics taken at night can cause nocturia and lead to interrupted sleep.*

➤ **Avoid constipation.** (See Chapter 29 for interventions to promote normal bowel elimination.) *Fecal impaction and chronic constipation, especially in older adults, are associated with increased risk of UI.*

➤ **Consider low-impact exercise.** *High-impact exercise (e.g., running, jumping rope) is associated with increased stress UI.*

Bladder Training

➤ Teach the mechanisms of urination.

➤ Teach distraction and relaxation strategies to help inhibit the urge to void. For example:
Instruct the patient to perform serial subtractions or become involved in an activity that requires concentration (e.g., a crossword puzzle) when she feels the urge to void.
Alternatively, the patient might perform several rapid pelvic floor muscle contractions to quiet the sensations from the bladder.
Other techniques include deep breathing and guided imagery.

➤ **Scheduled voiding** involves timed voiding and habit retraining. The patient must be mentally and physically capable of self-toileting.
Assist the patient to the toilet, commode, or bedpan on a timed schedule. Initially this may be every 2 hours or even more often.
As a pattern develops and the person gains greater control, increase the length of time between voidings.
Scheduled voiding is usually combined with other techniques, including lifestyle adjustments and pelvic floor muscle exercises.
Ask the patient to keep a daily record of her adherence to the schedule and of the number of incontinence episodes.
When the patient can adhere to the schedule comfortably, the voiding interval can be increased by 15 to 30 minutes.

Pelvic Floor Muscle Exercises (PFMEs)

Teach patients the following routine to strengthen pelvic floor muscles:

➤ Imagine that you are urinating and wish to stop the flow; also tighten your rectum as though you are trying to keep from passing gas. The muscles you contract are the pelvic floor muscles. ✚ Caution the patient against doing PFMEs while actually urinating because this may cause backflow of urine.

➤ You should feel your rectum tighten. Women may also feel the vagina tighten.
Do not tighten your abdomen—check by placing your hand lightly on your abdomen.
Do not contract the thigh and gluteal muscles.

➤ Hold each contraction for 5 to 10 seconds, then rest for 5 to 10 seconds. (Some people may be able to hold for only 3 seconds at first.) Count "one-and-two-and-three . . .". Keep contraction and relaxation times equal. For example, if you hold a contraction for 5 seconds, rest 5 seconds before the next one.

➤ Perform 10 to 15 PFMEs three times a day. Do not do all 30 to 45 exercises at one time; do them throughout the day.

➤ To help you remember to perform your exercises, associate them with an activity. For example, do PFMEs at every stoplight when you are in the car. Or do some PFMEs every time you go to the bathroom—but not while urinating.

Teaching Patients to Manage Urinary Incontinence—cont'd

Supportive Interventions

Supportive interventions focus on helping the patient reach the toilet and perform toileting self-care.

➤ Ask where the toilet is and whether the patient can get there easily. It may be useful to place a commode near where the patient spends most of his time. You may place

it on a large, absorbent, washable mat to absorb any urine that spills.

Sources: Dowling-Castronovo, A., & Bradway, C. (2012); Goode, P. S., Burgio, K. L., Richter, H. E., et al. (2010); Lucas, M. G., Bedretdinova, D., Bosch, J., et al. (2014).

3. **Continent urinary reservoir (ileal reservoir, Indiana pouch).** A continent urinary reservoir (Fig. 30-10) is similar to the ileal conduit, except urine drains into a pouch made from a portion of the large intestine. The stoma on the abdomen contains a valve to keep urine from leaking. The patient inserts a catheter into the stoma to drain urine through the valve. Unlike the ileal conduit, no external bag is needed; this means minimal risk of leaking and odor. A second valve prevents reflux of urine back into the kidneys.

4. **Neobladder.** A neobladder mimics the function of a urinary bladder. A portion of intestine is made into a pouch or reservoir that is connected to the urethra. Urine passes through the urethra, similar to the normal passage of urine.

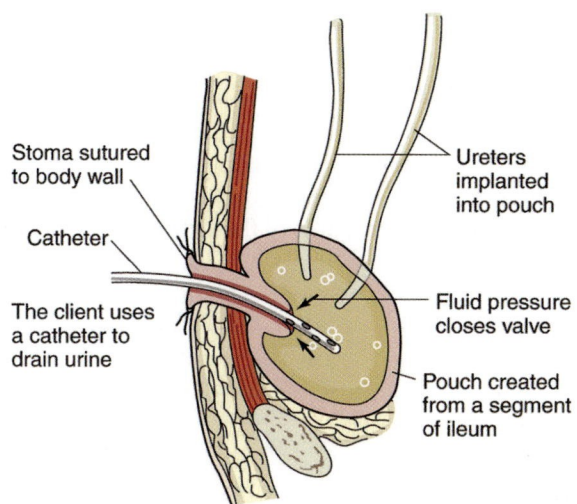

Stoma sutured to body wall
Catheter
The client uses a catheter to drain urine
Ureters implanted into pouch
Fluid pressure closes valve
Pouch created from a segment of ileum

FIGURE 30-10 A continent urostomy allows the client to manage urine without the need to wear an ostomy appliance.

The patient voids by bearing down or applying manual pressure over the bladder (Credé's maneuver), but may also need to perform intermittent self-catheterization to fully empty the bladder. This type of urinary reservoir requires no external stoma or bag. Urinary incontinence is fairly common after surgery, but typically resolves within the first 6 months.

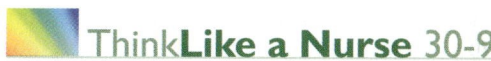

Think Like a Nurse 30-9

What challenges or problems do you think a patient with a urinary diversion might experience?

INTERVENTIONS/IMPLEMENTATION FOR PATIENTS WITH URINARY DIVERSIONS

Initially you may need to assist the patient with all aspects of his care after a urinary diversion. However, the long-term goal is for the patient to become comfortable with his changed body and to assume self-care.

Psychological Responses Patients experience a variety of reactions to the stoma. Patients with continent ostomies are usually more comfortable with their stoma because it offers control and avoids the embarrassment, odor, and inconvenience of urinary incontinence (UI). **KEY POINT:** *Your attitude and willingness to discuss the body changes associated with an ostomy will help your patient begin his adjustment.*

In many communities, local ostomy association counselors are available to visit patients, discuss the psychological changes associated with a urinary diversion, and help them with physical care of the stoma. Most counselors themselves have ostomies, so they can share practical and personal information and challenges with patients.

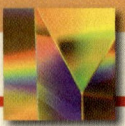

Nursing Care Plan

Client Data

Desmond Washington, a 69-year-old man, comes to the clinic 4 weeks after having a prostatectomy for prostate cancer. He had been discharged from the hospital on postoperative day 4 and went home with an indwelling urinary catheter. The catheter was removed at his last visit, 9 days after surgery.

Mr. Washington is meticulously groomed. He is friendly with other patients and chatty with the clinic personnel. In the exam room the nurse asks how he feels, he says, "I saw the sun come up today. I appreciate that more now. The good Lord has given me a new lease on life, and I intend to use it!" His nurse continues, "That's great, Mr. Washington. How have you been doing since the catheter was removed?" Mr. Washington's smile fades. He lowers his voice and says, "You know, I think that's the worst part of this whole thing. I hate wearing these diapers—they make me feel like an old man. I'm not ready for this."

The nurse continues, "Do you have *any* control of your urine?" Mr. Washington explains, "I may go for hours and stay dry, and then it seems for no reason, I wet myself. Yesterday, for example, I was sitting on the sofa watching the ball game. I got up to answer the doorbell, and all of a sudden, I felt wet. I hadn't even had anything to drink so I could stay dry through the afternoon. And if I cough? Forget it. Can something be done so I can hold my urine again?"

Nursing Diagnosis

Stress Urinary Incontinence related to disruption of the urinary sphincter and related pelvic muscles by surgery as evidenced by client report of involuntary loss of urine with increased intra-abdominal pressure.

NOC Outcomes	Individualized Goals/Expected Outcomes
Urinary Continence (0502) Urinary Elimination (0503)	*By the next visit, Mr. Washington will:* 1. Describe three things he can do that will help regain urinary continence. 2. Explain three interventions to cope with leaked urine. 3. Report that he is drinking adequate amounts of fluids during the day.

Nursing Interventions and Activities	Rationale

NIC Interventions	
Urinary Elimination Management (0590) Urinary Incontinence Care (0610)	

Nursing Activities

1. Obtain midstream voided urine specimen for urinalysis.	Urinary tract infection (UTI) can cause or worsen urinary incontinence (UI) (Goode, Burgio, Richter, et al., 2010; Lucas, Bedretdinova, Bosch, et al., 2014).
2. Identify factors that contribute to Mr. Washington's UI by using an incontinence diary for a minimum of 3 days, including variations in his usual activities.	Identifying activities or other factors that cause loss of urine control can guide specific interventions. A diary facilitates monitoring over time and can identify patterns that could otherwise be missed (Lucas, Bedretdinova, Bosch, et al., 2014; National Guideline Clearinghouse, 2013; Rainsbury, Fabricius, & McLarty, 2011; Shultz, 2012).
3. Use digital assessment to confirm pelvic floor muscle strength. Teach pelvic floor muscle exercises (PFMEs).	PFMEs strengthen pelvic muscles and enhance sphincter control. Some studies have shown that PFMEs increase UI without side effects in men who have undergone prostatectomy (Glazener, Boachie, Buckley, et al., 2011; Nahon & Adams, 2014; National Guideline Clearinghouse, 2013; Park & Kang, 2014; Rainsbury, Fabricius, & McLarty, 2011; Sighinolfi, Rivalta, Mofferdin, et al., 2009; Vaughan, Goode, Burgio, et al., 2011).

Nursing Care Plan (continued)

Nursing Activities

4. Use biofeedback when needed in conjunction with PFME training to help Mr. Washington isolate pelvic floor muscles.

   Biofeedback allows clients to receive auditory or visual (or both) cues when the proper muscles are contracted, so they learn what the proper muscle contraction feels like. Biofeedback also allows the nurse or therapist to objectively measure strength of contractions (Campbell, Glazener, Hunter, et al., 2012; Chernecky, & Berger, 2013; Herderschee, Hay-Smith, Herbison, et al., 2011; Lucas, Bedretdinova, Bosch, et al., 2014).

5. Teach timed voiding. Have Mr. Washington void on a schedule of every 2 hours.

   Voiding on a schedule of every 2 hours can reduce the amount of urine in the bladder, thus reducing the likelihood of leakage with activities of daily living (Lucas, Bedretdinova, Bosch, et al., 2014; Shultz, 2012).

6. Explain the need to drink adequate fluids and *not* limit fluids in an effort to prevent incontinence. Help Mr. Washington identify ways to drink a minimum of 1,500–2,000 mL/day.

   Adequate fluid intake is important to maintain dilute urine, which is less irritating to the bladder; to maintain systemic hydration; and to reduce the risk for constipation, which can contribute to UI (Rainsbury, Fabricius, & McLarty, 2011; Townsend, Jura, Curhan, et al., 2011).

7. Assist Mr. Washington in selecting appropriate absorbent products that collect urine strictly for temporary management while continence management is ongoing.

   Absorbent products should not be used as a long-term treatment for UI (National Guideline Clearinghouse, 2013). Proper absorbent garments and pads can collect and trap urine, keep skin clean and dry, reduce odor, and minimize the risk for skin breakdown (Lucas, Bedretdinova, Bosch, et al., 2014; National Institute for Health and Clinical Excellence, 2013, updated 2015).

8. Help Mr. Washington develop a personal hygiene routine that will maintain skin integrity.

   Conscientious skin care and good hygiene will reduce the risk of skin irritation and infection. Use warm (not hot) water and pat (don't scrub) the perineal area. A barrier cream will repel fluid and protect the skin from urine (Wound, Ostomy, and Continence Nurses Society, 2003).

9. Offer referral to a support group.

   Support groups provide a sense of community and enhance members' problem-solving skills. Mr. Washington may feel less embarrassment when he discovers that others share his problems.

10. Explain that urinary incontinence is common after prostatectomy, but that it may be only temporary.

    Urinary incontinence can be a troubling complication of prostatectomy for many men. Fortunately, it often resolves within 6 to 12 months after surgery (Glazener, Boachie, Bluckley, et al., 2011; Yu, Ko, & Sawatzky, 2008).

There are other treatment recommendations that are supported by research or have been identified anecdotally to be useful for some clients (Wound, Ostomy, and Continence Nurses Society, 2003). These include reducing caffeine consumption; eliminating bladder irritants, such as artificial sweeteners, spicy foods, and citrus from the diet; losing weight; and quitting smoking. In addition, it is important for nurses to understand the pathophysiology of urinary incontinence differs between men and women and that interventions that are successful in women may or may not be equally successful in men.

Evaluation

At the end of the visit, Mr. Washington said, "I didn't know there were things I could do about the leaking urine. Before surgery, all I cared about was getting rid of the cancer. I don't need a support group for me but maybe I'll lead one!" Mr. Washington had been placing folded paper towels in his underwear to collect urine because he thought absorbent products were too expensive, but with guidance from his nurse he identified products he could afford. He liked the fact that they would not be visible through his clothing.

At Mr. Washington's next visit, the nurse will review the initial collaborative goals and stated outcomes and perform a client assessment to determine whether the goals were reached in the stated time frame.

(continued)

Nursing Care Plan (continued)

Mr. Washington currently has a positive attitude and is focused on "beating" his cancer first and on managing complications of surgery second. As time passes, incontinence may persist and may become more frustrating for him once he is fully recovered from surgery. Mr. Washington initially declined referral to a support group, but he may be more interested in joining one in the future for help dealing with long-term consequences of prostatectomy.

References

Campbell, S. E., Glazener, C. M., Hunter, K. F., et al. (2012); Chernecky, C. C., & Berger, B. J. (2013); Glazener, C., Boachie, C., Bucklie, B., et al. (2011); Goode, P. S., Burgio, K. L., Richter, H. E., et al. (2010); Herderschee, R., Hay-Smith, E. C., Herbison, G. P., et al. (2011); Lucas, M. G., Bedretdinova, D., Bosch, J., et al. (2014); National Guideline Clearinghouse (2013); National Institute for Health and Clinical Excellence (2013); Rainsbury, P. G., Fabricius, M., & McLarty, E. (2011); Shultz, J. M. (2012); Sighinolfi, M. C., Rivalta, M., Mofferdin, A., et al. (2009); Townsend, M. K., Jura, Y. H., Curhan, G. C., et al. (2011); Vaughan, C. P., Goode, P. S., Burgio, K. L., et al. (2011); Wound, Ostomy, and Continence Nurses Society (2003); Yu, Ko, W. F., & Sawatzky, J. V. (2008).

Care Map

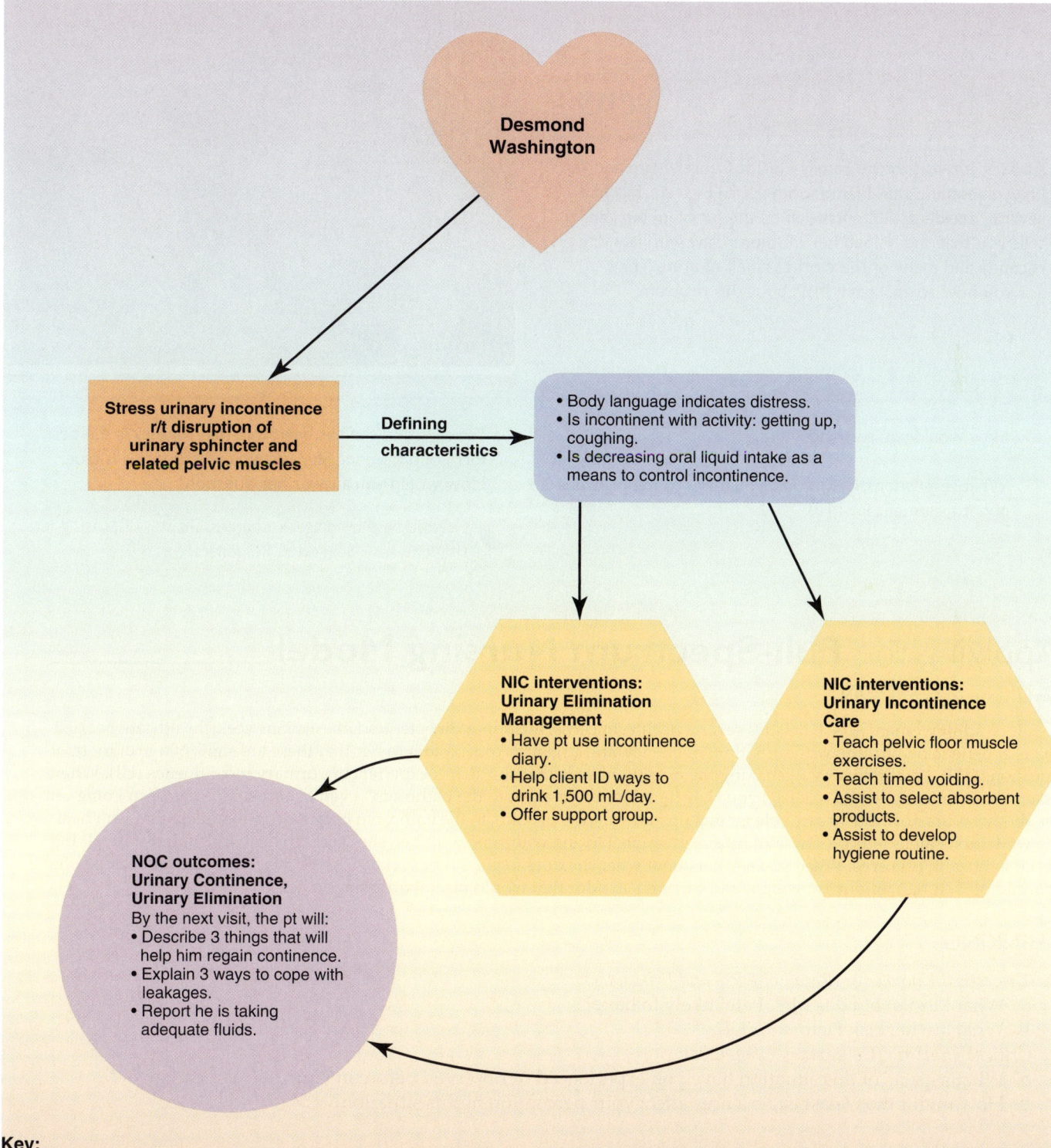

Desmond Washington

Stress urinary incontinence r/t disruption of urinary sphincter and related pelvic muscles

Defining characteristics

- Body language indicates distress.
- Is incontinent with activity: getting up, coughing.
- Is decreasing oral liquid intake as a means to control incontinence.

NIC interventions: Urinary Elimination Management
- Have pt use incontinence diary.
- Help client ID ways to drink 1,500 mL/day.
- Offer support group.

NIC interventions: Urinary Incontinence Care
- Teach pelvic floor muscle exercises.
- Teach timed voiding.
- Assist to select absorbent products.
- Assist to develop hygiene routine.

NOC outcomes: Urinary Continence, Urinary Elimination
By the next visit, the pt will:
- Describe 3 things that will help him regain continence.
- Explain 3 ways to cope with leakages.
- Report he is taking adequate fluids.

Key:
- Nursing diagnosis
- Defining characteristics
- NIC interventions and nursing activities
- NOC outcomes

CLINICALREASONING

The questions and exercises in this section allow you to practice the kind of thinking you will use as a full-spectrum nurse. Critical-thinking questions usually have more than one correct answer, so we do not provide "correct answers" for these features. It is more important to develop your nursing judgment than to just cover content. You will learn by discussing the questions with your peers. If you are still unsure, see the Davis Advantage chapter resources for suggested responses.

Caring for the Nguyens

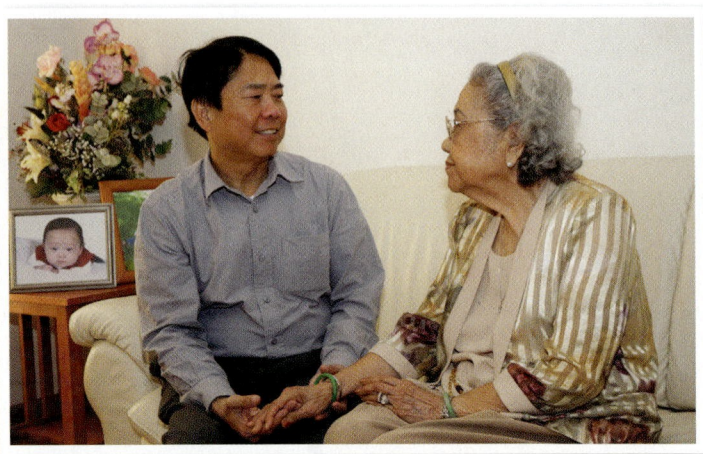

At a recent visit to the Family Health Center, Nam and Yen Nguyen confide that Nam's mother, Mai Nguyen, has had several "accidents." She has denied the problem but Yen tells you that she helped her mother-in-law with laundry recently and many of the clothes smell of urine. They ask you how to approach Mai about this problem.

A. How would you respond?

B. What suggestions, if any, could you make to the Nguyens about treatment for Mai?

C. Yen says that she has been told that surgery is the best form of treatment. She asks you whether this is true. How would you answer her question?

Go to Davis Advantage, Resources, **Chapter 30, Caring for the Nguyens—Suggested Responses.**

Applying the **Full-Spectrum Nursing Model**

PATIENT SITUATION

An older-adult woman, Mrs. Patel, has several health concerns, including diabetes and obesity. She seeks healthcare because she is experiencing burning with urination, frequency, and urgency. You explain to her that these are signs of a urinary tract infection (UTI). You discover while taking the nursing history that she also is experiencing urinary incontinence (UI). When asked about toileting habits, she tells you she often doesn't "make it to the bathroom" even at home. This has been going on for about 3 years now. She has trouble getting up and walking upstairs to the bathroom because of a foot ulcer that isn't healing well. Mrs. Patel's affect is flat with little expression. During your time with her, she seems to have little interest in talking about her health concerns. When you ask her about what she does to get out or socialize, she is hesitant to go far because she is afraid of wetting without knowing it and carrying an odor that would be embarrassing to her.

THINKING

1. *Theoretical Knowledge (Recall of Facts and Principles):*
   a. What kind(s) of UI is Mrs. Patel likely to have?
   b. What are her risk factors for UI?
2. *Critical Thinking (Contextual Awareness):*
   a. What aspects of this situation have you experienced or observed before in your role as a caregiver?
   b. How might those past experiences affect your perception in this situation?

DOING

3. *Practical Knowledge (Patient Teaching):*
   a. How could you encourage this woman to seek healthcare for managing her UI?
   b. What might you ask your patient to do in order to get a better idea of her bladder history and toileting habits?
   c. By looking at Mrs. Patel's bladder diary, you see a pattern suggestive of UI. What other behavioral strategies might you suggest to improve her ability to have control of her bladder?

CARING

4. *Self-Knowledge:*
   a. Have you ever personally experienced urinary urgency when you had trouble getting to the bathroom in time? Reflect on this experience and examine how you might feel if you were incontinent much of the time.
   b. In what way(s) can you show compassion for the patient who has UI?

PracticalKnowledge
clinical application

CLINICAL INSIGHTS

Clinical Insight 30-1 ➤ **Caring for a Patient With an Indwelling Catheter**

An indwelling catheter is connected to a drainage tube and collection bag, which constitute a closed system.

Goal 1: Prevent urinary tract infection.

- **Do not disconnect the tubing** or open the drainage system (e.g., to obtain specimens or measure the urine). A closed system minimizes the chance for pathogens to enter the system and infect the urinary tract.
- **Regularly check connections** between the catheter and drainage tubing and the drainage tube and collection bag. Loose connections cause leaks and serve as entry points for pathogens.
- **If the system becomes disconnected,** wipe the ends of both tubes with antiseptic (alcohol or chlorhexidine gluconate [CHG]–alcohol combination product) before reconnecting them.
- **After each bowel movement and if the catheter becomes soiled from drainage or feces,** cleanse it with mild soap and water, cleaning from the meatus outward. Rinse the catheter well and pat it dry. This removes the medium for growth of microorganisms.
- **Empty the collection bag at least every 8 hours** and more frequently if urine output is high. This prevents stagnation of urine.
- **Do not touch the spout to any surfaces** when emptying the collection bag. If the spout is accidentally contaminated, cleanse it with an antiseptic (alcohol or CHG–alcohol combination product).
- **Keep collection bag below the level of the bladder, but do not let it touch the floor** (see Goal 2). The floor is considered contaminated.
- **Teach the patient to report signs of UTI;** observe for cloudy, strong-smelling urine, chills, or fever.
- **Change the indwelling catheter only when necessary** (e.g., when sediment collects in the tubing or catheter or the urine does not drain well). Some agency policies specify that catheters be changed at specific intervals (e.g., monthly). However, this is not advisable because the more often a catheter is changed, the more likely an infection will develop.

Goal 2: Maintain free flow of urine.

Maintaining free flow of urine prevents backflow of urine into the bladder, which can cause bladder distension and injury. Stasis of urine also provides a medium for growth of microorganisms.

Note that some of the interventions in this section are the same as those for preventing infection (Goal 1).

- **Keep the tubing and bag below bladder level.** Never place the bag on the floor or the bed. This prevents backflow of stagnant urine into the bladder. Urine drains by gravity in this system.
- **If the collecting bag must be higher than the bladder** at any time, you must clamp the catheter. Clamping prevents backflow of stagnant urine into the bladder.
- **Frequently inspect the tubing to ensure that the urine flows freely.** Kinks, coils, or compression of the catheter or tubing may impede flow and cause backup into the bladder.
- **If urine is not flowing,** check to be sure the patient is not lying on the tubing.

Goal 3: Prevent transmission of infection.

- **Observe standard precautions** when providing catheter care.
- **Wear gloves when handling the catheter** or drainage system. Gloving prevents possible exposure to body fluids.
- **Always perform hand hygiene before and after providing care** to any patient, including one with an indwelling catheter.

Goal 4: Promote normal urine production.

Adequate urine production flushes pathogens out of the bladder, provides natural irrigation of the tubing, and prevents stasis of urine.

- **Encourage oral intake of at least 8 to 10 glasses** (approximately 2,000 to 2,500 mL) of fluid per day, unless contraindicated by other health problems (Turner &

(Continued)

Clinical Insight 30-1 ▶ **Caring for a Patient With an Indwelling Catheter—cont'd**

Dickens, 2011; Wound, Ostomy, and Continence Nurses Society, 2009). For patients who are unable to take oral liquid, provide an equivalent amount of parenteral or enteral fluids.

- **Monitor I&O at least every 8 hours** (more frequently if the patient is experiencing fluid and electrolyte imbalance).
- **For accurate determination of output,** empty the urine into a calibrated container.
  Volume markings on the urine collection bag are only approximate.
- **Observe the urine output for color and other** characteristics. Report evidence of blood, sediment, or infection to the primary care provider.
- **Encourage the patient to be active and out of bed** as much as possible.
  This promotes blood flow to the kidneys for better urinary function.

Goal 5: Maintain skin and mucosal integrity.

Perineal skin and mucosa can be irritated by feces and by movement or encrustation of the catheter.

- **Secure the tubing to the patient's thigh by applying a commercial catheter securement device,** such as

a catheter tube holder or a Velcro strap (or hypoallergenic tape if a securement device is unavailable).
Failure to secure the tubing may cause significant injury to the bladder neck and urethra. Although the inflated balloon holds the catheter in the bladder, you must secure the tubing to prevent traction on the bladder and urethral meatus.

- **Assist with routine hygiene care as needed.** Cleanse the area around the meatus with mild soap and filtered tap water or perineal wash solution daily, after each bowel movement, and more often if there is drainage or excessive sweating. Rinse well and pat dry.
  Routine hygiene care normally provides adequate cleanliness. Rinsing helps to avoid skin irritation by soap residue.
- **Avoid using powders or lotions in the perineal area.**
  Topical products can be irritating to the skin.
- **Monitor the urethral meatus and upper drainage tube.**
  Encrustation, as evidenced by sandy particles at the meatus, irritates the mucosa and signals a need to change the catheter.

Clinical Insight 30-2 ▶ **Caring for Patients With Urinary Diversions**

- **Perform a thorough assessment. KEY POINT:** *Be careful your facial expressions do not convey revulsion or disapproval when working with the patient and his stoma.*
- **Assess stoma appearance.** A healthy stoma ranges in color from deep pink to brick red, regardless of skin color, and is shiny and moist. ✚ Immediately document findings and report to the surgeon if the stoma is pale, dusky, or black. This often indicates inadequate blood supply.
- **Assess the skin surrounding the stoma for signs of irritation** (e.g., redness, tenderness, and skin breakdown).
  KEY POINT: *Skin care is critical. When the normally acid urine remains in contact with the skin, it becomes alkaline. Skin that becomes encrusted, macerated, and excoriated may lead to infection, pain, and leakage.*
- **Be certain that the collection device fits** snugly against the skin.
- **A moisture-proof skin barrier** is usually placed around the stoma to prevent maceration and irritation.
- **Barrier creams** may be prescribed for irritated skin—nystatin, if fungal infection develops.
- **Monitor the amount and type of drainage** from the stoma.
- **Empty the collection device frequently** during the day; connect it to a larger bag during the night.

- **Be available to discuss the patient's reaction** to the stoma.
- **Provide ample time** to explain stoma care and use of ostomy appliances.
  For most patients this is a lifelong task; therefore, patient teaching is essential.

Patients With a Continent Urinary Reservoir

Patients will also need instruction about catheterizing their reservoir to drain the urine. Once healed, the reservoir will need to be catheterized four or five times a day.

Patients With a Neobladder

- The patient will not have a stoma but will require bladder training once the postoperative retention catheter has been removed.
- Instruct the patient to perform pelvic floor muscle exercises three times a day and empty the bladder on a schedule, as often as every 2 hours initially. Once bladder capacity builds, he may increase the interval between voidings.
- The patient will need to relax the pelvic muscles and bear down to release urine from the bladder. He may also need to use **Credé's maneuver,** applying manual pressure over the bladder to promote emptying.
- If the patient is unable to fully empty the bladder with these techniques, he may need to perform intermittent self-catheterization.

PROCEDURES

Procedure 30-1 ■ Measuring Urine

➤ For steps to follow in *all* procedures, refer to Universal Steps for All Procedures found on the page facing the inside back cover.

Equipment

- Bedpan or urinal
- Clean procedure gloves
- Graduated container
- Toilet paper, as indicated
- Washcloth or towel
- Hand sanitizer for patient's hands

***Measuring Post-Void Residual Urine Volume (PVR)
With a Portable Bladder Scanner***

- Portable bladder scanning device
- Ultrasound gel
- Clean gloves
- Tissues
- Antiseptic swabs or wipes

Delegation

Measuring urine, including post-void residual volume (PVR) using a portable bladder scanner, may be delegated to specially trained nursing assistive personnel (NAP) in some facilities. However, you must be sure that the NAP knows how to perform the procedure correctly, including proper cleansing of the bedpan/urinal and the graduated container according to the facility's policies. Also complete the following assessments and instruct the NAP when to stop the procedure and seek assistance from the nurse, and to report the results immediately. In some instances, you may choose to perform the bladder scan to ensure accuracy and expedite any necessary treatment.

Pre-Procedure Assessments

- Cognitive status: Determine whether the patient can follow directions and complete this procedure on her own.
- Mobility status: Determine whether the patient can get out of the bed to use the toilet.
- Urinary status: Determine the patient's ability to control bladder function.
  For post-void residual urine volume: Determine the timing and amount of the last voiding.
- Palpate the bladder for distention.

NOTE: A bladder scan should be done as soon as possible after voiding and within no more than 10 to 15 minutes.

Procedure 30-1A ■ Measuring Urine Output From a Bedpan or Urinal

➤ When performing the procedure, always identify your patient according to agency policy, using two identifiers, and be attentive to standard precautions, hand hygiene, patient safety and privacy, body mechanics, and documentation.

Procedure Steps

1. **Wash your hands and don clean** procedure gloves.
   Prevents transmission of bacteria.

2. **Place a bedpan or urinal** by positioning the patient in a semi-Fowler's position with the legs slightly spread. For a male, place the urinal on the bed between his legs and insert (or ask him to insert) his penis in the urinal. For a female, raise the siderails or provide an overhead trapeze so that the patient will have grip holds to maneuver herself onto and off the bedpan.

3. **Remove the bedpan or urinal,** being careful not to spill the urine. Reposition the patient and transport the urine to the bathroom.

4. **While still wearing procedure gloves,** pour the urine into a graduated cylinder or calibrated measuring container.

5. **Ensure that the label** on the measuring device has the correct patient information (the label might be preprinted or bar coded). ✚ Do not use a measuring device for more than one patient.

6. **Place the measuring device** on a flat surface (e.g., shelf, table that is not used for food or personal care products) and read the amount at eye level.

7. **Observe the urine for color,** clarity, and odor.

8. **Discard the urine** in the toilet. If a specimen is required, transfer at least 30 mL of urine to the designated container.

9. **Clean the measuring container** and store in the patient's bathroom.

10. **Remove gloves.** Wash your hands.

11. **Record the time and volume** on the intake and output (I&O) record.

(continued on next page)

Procedure 30-1 ■ Measuring Urine (continued)

Procedure 30-1B ■ Measuring Urine From an Indwelling Catheter

➤ When performing the procedure, always identify your patient according to agency policy, using two identifiers, and be attentive to standard precautions, hand hygiene, patient safety and privacy, body mechanics, and documentation.

Procedure Steps

1. **Wearing clean gloves, place** the collection bag drainage spout inside a calibrated measuring container. Do not touch the spout to the inside of the container.
   Gloving prevents transmission of bacteria.

2. **Unclamp the drainage spout** and direct the flow of urine into the measuring device, still keeping the spout away from the sides of the container.
   Prevents contaminating the drainage spout. ➤

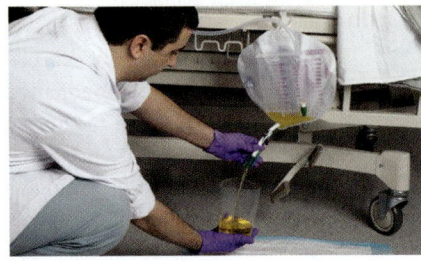

3. **Reclamp the spout** when the collection bag is empty.

4. **Wipe the drainage spout** with an alcohol pad and replace the spout into the slot on the collection bag.
   A clean spout reduces transmission of bacteria.

5. **Measure urine output** from the indwelling catheter at the end of each shift unless otherwise ordered. ▼

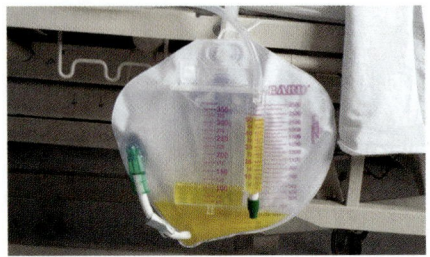

6. **Discard the urine** in the toilet.

7. **Remove gloves.** Wash your hands.

8. **Record the time and amount** on the I&O record; record urine color, clarity, and odor.

Procedure 30-1C ■ Measuring Post-Void Residual Urine Volume With a Portable Bladder Scanner

➤ When performing the procedure, always identify your patient according to agency policy, using two identifiers, and be attentive to standard precautions, hand hygiene, patient safety and privacy, body mechanics, and documentation.

Procedure Steps

1. **Perform hand hygiene** and apply clean gloves.
   Prevents transmission of bacteria.

2. **Assist the patient to a supine** position. Uncover only the patient's lower abdomen and suprapubic area.

3. **Clean the scanner head** with antiseptic wipes.
   Prevents transmission of microorganisms.

4. **Turn the scanner on.**

5. **Select the patient's gender** on the device. If a woman has had a hysterectomy, follow manufacturer's directions for gender selection. In some cases, you will select the MALE icon for a woman who has undergone hysterectomy.
   The device is calibrated to adjust for uterus and bladder anatomy.

6. **Palpate the symphysis pubis** and then apply an ample quantity of warmed ultrasound gel midline on the abdomen, approximately 2.5 to 4 cm (1 to 1.5 in.) above the symphysis pubis.
   Ensures proper transmission of the ultrasound. Warmth is for comfort.

7. **Position the scanner head in the gel** and aim it toward the bladder, pointing slightly downward toward the patient's coccyx.
   Proper placement allows for an accurate reading. ▼

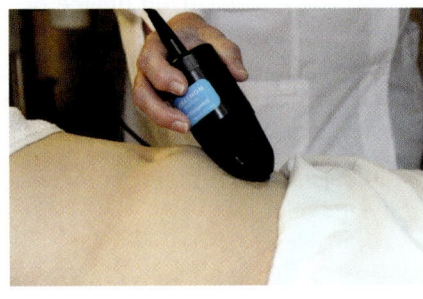

8. **Press and release the SCAN button.** Hold the scanner head steady until you hear the tone indicating that the scan is complete.

9. **Read the bladder volume measurement.** Repeat the scan several times to ensure accuracy.

   NOTE: Some scanners will also display an image of the bladder. The bladder image should be centered on the crossbars. If it is not, reposition the scanner head and repeat the scan.

   Taking several readings ensures maximum accuracy. ▼

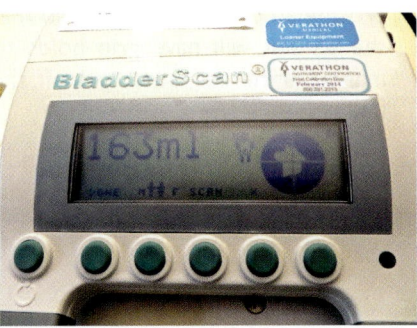

10. Press DONE when finished. Print the results by pressing PRINT. *A printout provides for accurate documentation and may, in some facilities, be added to the patient record.*

11. Wipe the gel from the patient's skin with tissue, cover the patient, and return him to a comfortable position.

12. Clean the scanner head with antiseptic. Remove gloves and perform hand hygiene.

? What if . . .

- **The provider orders hourly monitoring of the patient's urine output?**

Obtain a special collection bag with a small measuring chamber; document urine output on the I&O record every hour. Be sure that the cylinder does not overflow. Check the collection bag more frequently if the input is increased or if the patient has diuretic.

Evaluation

- Note any unusual characteristics of the urine (e.g., color, odor, presence of sediment or mucus).
- Note any difficulties with urination (e.g., pain, dribbling, hesitancy).
- Continue to monitor that urine is flowing freely and that the drainage bag is below the level of the bladder and not on the floor.
- Assess for bladder distention.
  Bladder distention indicates poor bladder emptying.

  NOTE: *If the facility has a bladder-scanning device, scan to determine whether there is residual urine.*

Patient Teaching

Instruct the patient and/or primary caregiver to document the intake and urine output on the I&O worksheet at the bedside.

Home Care

Teach the patient and/or the primary caregiver how to collect and measure urine and how to document intake and output on the I&O record.

Documentation

- Document urine volume and record the time and date the specimen was collected, per agency policy. You may chart specimen collection in the patient's health record (nurse's notes) or a graphic flow sheet, depending on the agency.
- Document the characteristics of the urine: color, odor, particulate matter, blood, clarity.

- Document any difficulty with voiding, pain or burning with urination, frequency, or difficulty starting the urine flow.
- For PVR, document the time and amount of the last void prior to the scan and the amount of residual urine. Attach a printout of the bladder scan to the patient record if agency policy requires.

Sample documentation

12/15/18   1500   Voided 75 mL of clear, yellow urine with no odor, blood, or mucus. Pt states that he still feels full. Bladder palpated just above level of symphysis pubis. Bladder scan performed— 350 mL of residual urine in bladder. Dr. Roy contacted and straight catheterization prescribed. ——————— S. Tran, RN

Practice Resources

Boyer, D. R., Steltzer, N., & Larrabee, J. H. (2009); Rigby, D., & Housami, F. A. (2009); Siegel, J. D., Rhinehart, E., Jackson, M., et al. (2007).

Thinking About the Procedures

To practice applying clinical reasoning to these procedures,

 The videos **Measuring Urine Output From a Bedpan or Urinal, Measuring Urine From an Indwelling Catheter,** and **Measuring Post-Void Residual Urine Volume (PVR) With a Portable Bladder Scanner,** along with questions and suggested responses, are available on the **Davis's *Nursing Skills Videos*** Web site on Davis*Plus*.

Procedure 30-2 ■ Obtaining a Urine Specimen for Testing

➤ For steps to follow in *all* procedures, refer to the Universal Steps for All Procedures found on the page facing the inside back cover.

Equipment

Collecting a Clean-Catch Urine Specimen

- Prepackaged collection kit
- If no kit is available:
  - Sterile specimen container
  - Antiseptic solution
  - Sterile cotton balls or 2 in. × 2 in. gauze pads
- Washcloth or towel
- Mild soap and water
- Two pairs of clean procedure gloves
- Patient identification labels
- Bedpan or bedside commode for an immobile patient

Obtaining a Sterile Urine Specimen From a Catheter

- Clean gloves
- Antiseptic swab
- Sterile specimen container with a lid
- Patient identification label
- Sterile syringe with a sterile 21- to 25-gauge needleless access device (a 5- to 10-mL syringe is usually sufficient)

Collecting a 24-Hour Urine Specimen

NOTE: *Some tests require using a double-storage container. Be sure to find out whether you need a double-storage container or preservative,*

and whether there are special instructions for collection of the sample.

- Basin and ice, possibly. Check with the laboratory to determine whether the specimen needs to be kept on ice.
- Large collection container

Delegation

You may delegate this procedure to the NAP if you are sure the NAP knows how to perform it correctly, including proper cleansing and maintaining sterility of the container. You must complete the pre-procedural assessments and instruct the NAP to report any abnormalities seen in the urine (e.g., blood, foul odor, mucus), as well as any complaints of dysuria by the patient. The NAP should bring the specimen to you for inspection.

Pre-Procedure Assessments

- Cognitive status: Determine whether the patient can follow directions and complete this procedure on her own.
- Mobility status
  The patient's mobility determines where the specimen will be collected (e.g., bed, commode, bedpan).
- Urinary status: Assess the ability to control urinary flow.
  To determine whether you can collect a specimen in this manner.

Procedure 30-2A ■ Collecting a Clean-Catch Urine Specimen

➤ When performing the procedure, always identify your patient according to agency policy, using two identifiers, and be attentive to standard precautions, hand hygiene, patient safety and privacy, body mechanics, and documentation.

Procedure Steps

1. **Don procedure gloves.** Wash the perineal area with periwash solution. Remove soiled gloves, perform hand hygiene, and apply new gloves.

2. **Cleanse, or instruct the patient** to cleanse, around the urinary meatus. Allow the area to dry.
   Cleansing prevents contamination of the specimen with surface bacteria.

3. **Remove soiled gloves,** perform hand hygiene, and don clean procedure gloves.

4. **Open the prepackaged kit** (if available), and remove the contents. Open the sterile specimen cup, being careful not to touch the inside of the lid or container, and place within easy reach. Make sure to place the lid with the inside surface facing upward.

5. **Cleanse the perineum and urethra:**

Variation for Women

a. Open the antiseptic towelette in the prepackaged kit. If there is no towelette, pour the antiseptic solution over the cotton balls.

b. To cleanse the perineum, wipe down one side of the meatus using one pad and discard it. Then wipe the other side with a second pad; discard. Wipe down the center over the urinary meatus with the third pad; then discard it. Clean the perineal area at least twice. Use each towelette or cotton ball only once.
   Following the "clean-to-dirty" principle decreases the likelihood of contamination of the specimen with feces. Antiseptic helps reduce the number of bacteria. ➤

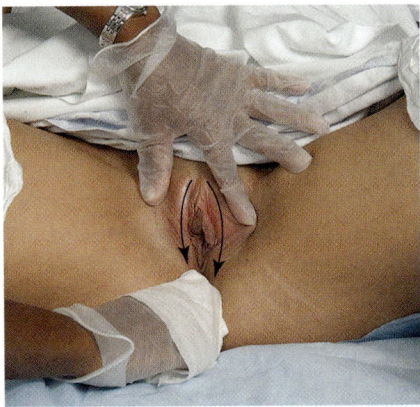

Variation for Men

c. If the penis is uncircumcised, retract the foreskin from the end of the penis.
   Allows for better access when cleansing the area around the meatus.

d. Use the towelette provided in the prepackaged kit or pour antiseptic solution over cotton balls. You might also use a 2 in. × 2 in. gauze pad soaked with povidone-iodine to cleanse the periurethral area.

➕ Before using an iodine-based solution, be sure to check the patient's health history for allergy to iodine.

e. With one hand, grasp the penis gently. With the other hand, cleanse the meatus in a circular motion from the meatus outward away from the urethral opening and cleanse for a few inches down the shaft of the penis. Repeat this cleansing two more times, using each towelette or cotton ball only once.

Cleansing the site in this manner helps prevent contaminating the specimen with bacteria.

f. Keep one hand in place to retract the foreskin (if uncircumcised), or to hold the penis (for a patient who is unable to assist).

6. **Pick up the sterile specimen container** and hold it near the meatus; instruct the patient to begin voiding.

For Men

a. Keep the foreskin retracted during voiding, if uncircumcised. If the patient is unable to assist, it will be necessary to hold the penis.

For Women

b. Separate and hold the labia apart, or have the patient do so.

To help keep bacteria from the foreskin (or labia) from contaminating the urine specimen.

7. **Allow a small stream of urine** to pass; and then without stopping the urine stream, place the specimen container into the stream, collecting approximately 30 to 60 mL. Check with the agency lab to determine how much urine to collect.

8. **Remove the container** from the stream, and allow the patient to finish emptying the bladder.

NOTE: For men, if the penis is uncircumcised, replace the foreskin over the glans when the procedure is finished.

9. **Carefully replace the container lid,** touching only the outside of the cap and container. Avoid touching the rim of the cup to the genital area. Do not get foreign matter (e.g., toilet paper, feces, pubic hair, menstrual blood) in the urine sample.

These measures maintain sterility of the specimen and prevent cross-contamination of others with urine.

10. **Label the container** with the correct patient information (labels may be preprinted or bar coded). Place the container in a facility-specific carrier (usually a plastic bag) for transport to the lab.

11. **Remove your gloves and wash** your hands. If the specimen has been obtained from a patient on a bedpan, leave your gloves on until you have removed, emptied, and stored the bedpan properly.

Hand hygiene and gloving prevent transmission of bacteria.

12. **Assist the patient back to bed,** or remove the bedpan or urinal, if applicable. (See Procedure 29-2 for instructions on removing a bedpan.)

13. **Transport the specimen** to the lab.

Delayed testing can cause inaccurate results (e.g., casts in the urine will break up if urine is allowed to sit for an extended time).

Procedure 30-2B ■ Obtaining a Sterile Urine Specimen From a Catheter

➤ When performing the procedure, always identify your patient according to agency policy, using two identifiers, and be attentive to standard precautions, hand hygiene, patient safety and privacy, body mechanics, and documentation.

Procedure Steps

1. **Don procedure gloves** and empty the drainage tube of urine.

2. **Clamp the drainage tube** below the level of the specimen port for 15 to 30 minutes to allow a fresh sample to collect. If the client's urine is flowing briskly, you may not need to clamp the catheter.

3. **Replace the contaminated** gloves with a sterile pair before scrubbing the specimen port with an antiseptic swab.

4. **Insert a needleless access device** with a 10-mL syringe into the specimen port and aspirate to withdraw the amount of urine you need. ➤

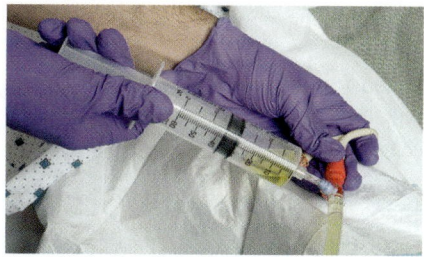

5. **Once you have the sample,** transfer the specimen into a sterile specimen container.

6. **Discard the needleless access** device and syringe in a safe container.

7. **Tightly cap the specimen container.**

8. **Remove the clamp** from the catheter.

➕ Be sure to unclamp the tubing of the urinary collection bag after you obtain the sample.

Urine backflow can cause bladder distention and lead to stasis-induced UTI.

9. **Label and package the specimen** with the correct patient identification according to agency policy. *To avoid a wrong-patient error.*

10. **Transport the specimen** to the lab. If immediate transport is not possible, refrigerate the sample.

➕ Never disconnect the catheter from the drainage tube to obtain a sample. Interrupting the system creates a portal of entry for pathogens, thereby increasing the risk of contamination.

(continued on next page)

Procedure 30-2 ■ Obtaining a Urine Specimen for Testing (continued)

Procedure 30-2C ■ Collecting a 24-Hour Urine Specimen

➤ When performing the procedure, always identify your patient according to agency policy, using two identifiers, and be attentive to standard precautions, hand hygiene, patient safety and privacy, body mechanics, and documentation.

Procedure Steps

1. **Use a large collection container** (usually supplied by the lab) and collect all urine voided in the 24-hour period. If you need to use more than one container during the 24-hour period, use one container at a time. When it is full, collect the urine in the next container. Occasionally you will be asked to collect each voiding in a separate container.

2. **To begin collection,** have patient void, and record the time.

   NOTE: Discard this first voiding.

   This marks the beginning of the urine collection period.

3. **Collect all urine voided** during the next 24 hours (e.g., if the first voiding was at 9:00 a.m. on Monday, collect all urine voided until 9:00 a.m. on Tuesday).

4. **Inform the patient and all staff** about the collection.

   Communication can help to prevent accidental discarding of urine.

5. **Post signs in prominent** locations, such as the patient's bathroom or entry door, to remind staff of the ongoing collection.

   KEY POINT: *It is essential none of the urine voided during the 24-hour period is accidentally discarded.*

6. **Apply a label on the specimen** with the patient's name, date, and time the test ended on your storage container.

? What if . . .

- **A urine culture is ordered on the specimen?**

  Be sure to list current antibiotic therapy on the laboratory request form. *This information is needed to determine sensitivity of the microorganisms.*

- **A clean-catch urine sample is needed for an immobile patient?**

  For the patient using a bedpan, raise the head of the bed to a semi-Fowler's position. *Facilitates correct direction of urine flow down into the specimen container you are holding. In addition, this is the anatomical position for voiding.*

Evaluation

- Note any unusual characteristics of the urine (e.g., color, odor, clarity, crystals, blood, mucus).
- Note any difficulties with urination (e.g., pain, burning, dribbling, difficulty beginning).

Patient Teaching

- Teach cognitively intact ambulatory patients to obtain a clean-catch specimen independently.
- For clean-catch and 24-hour urine specimen collection, teach the patient the steps of the procedure, focusing on how to maintain sterility of the specimen.
- Tell the patient to refrigerate a urine specimen for up to 24 hours until it can be transported to the lab. Instruct the patient to place the specimen in a plastic bag, separate it from food items, and label it appropriately.
- Explain that prepackaged antiseptic wipes cannot be flushed down the toilet.
- For clean-catch and 24-hour urine specimens, instruct a menstruating woman that perineal cleansing is especially important. The woman may use a tampon to prevent leakage during specimen collection. Instruct her to notify the lab that she is menstruating.

Documentation

- Document urine volume and the time and date that the specimen was collected per agency protocol. Some facilities use a Kardex® or flow sheet; others require documentation in nursing notes or electronic health records.
- Document the characteristics of the urine: color, odor, particulate matter, blood, clarity, or other qualities.
- Document any difficulty with voiding, including pain or burning with urination, frequency, or difficulty starting the urine flow.

Sample documentation

mm/dd/yyyy   0800   Order noted for clean-catch urine specimen. Explained to client the procedure for cleaning and obtaining urine specimen. Client stated, "I must clean my bottom from front to back using the toilet in here. Then begin to void and stop voiding. Void directly into this container." Assisted client to bedside commode. 100 mL of clear yellow urine without foul odor, blood, or particles collected. Pt denies difficulty voiding, pain, and burning. Urine container labeled per protocol and sent to laboratory. —————— L. Schaaf, RN

Mm/dd/yyyy   1000   Order noted for sterile urine specimen. Foley catheter clamped for 15 minutes. Port on Foley cleansed with antiseptic agent. 30 mL of pink-tinged urine without foul odor or sediment removed. Specimen labeled per protocol and sent to laboratory. —————— L. Schaaf, RN

Mm/dd/yyyy   1200   Order noted for 24-hour urine collection. Explained procedure to client. Client stated, "I will call you when I void. This first void will be flushed and the test will begin. During the test, I will void in the white hat that is in the commode. Then every time that I void, I will call you to empty the urine into the big container. The big container for the urine must be cold with ice." ————————— L. Schaaf, RN

Practice Resources

Dolan, V. J., & Cornish, N. E. (2013); Van Leeuwen, A. M., & Bladh, M. L. (2015).

Thinking About the Procedure

To practice applying clinical reasoning to Procedure 30-2B,

 The video **Obtaining a Sterile Urine Specimen From a Catheter,** along with questions and suggested responses, is available on the **Davis's** *Nursing Skills Videos* Web site on Davis*Plus.*

Procedure 30-3 ■ Testing Urine at the Bedside

➤ For steps to follow in *all* procedures, refer to the Universal Steps for All Procedures found on the page facing the inside back cover.

Equipment

Dipstick Testing

- Procedure gloves
- Dipstick testing kit

Refractometer Testing

- Refractometer
- Procedure gloves
- Distilled water
- Dropper
- Small urine sample

Delegation

You may delegate bedside urine testing to the NAP if you know that he has the knowledge and skill to perform the procedure. Ask the NAP to report the test results to you and to save the urine sample in case you should need to repeat the test.

Pre-Procedure Assessments

- Mobility status: To determine where the specimen will be collected (e.g., toilet, bedside commode, bedpan).
- Urinary status: Determine whether or not the patient has an indwelling urinary catheter.

Procedure 30-3A ■ Dipstick Testing of Urine

➤ When performing the procedure, always identify your patient according to agency policy, using two identifiers, and be attentive to standard precautions, hand hygiene, patient safety and privacy, body mechanics, and documentation.

Procedure Steps

1. **Read the instructions** on the diagnostic kit.

2. **Wash your hands** and don clean procedure gloves.

3. **Have the patient void** into the collection container or obtain urine from the indwelling urinary catheter. (See Procedures 30-1A and B for measuring urine.)

4. **Obtain a test strip from the kit,** dip it into the urine, and begin timing. Follow the manufacturer's directions regarding the time needed for the reagent to develop.

5. **Compare the results against the color** chart at the specified time. You will need good lighting to evaluate the results.

6. **Document the test results.**

Procedure 30-3B ■ Measuring Specific Gravity of Urine

➤ When performing the procedure, always identify your patient according to agency policy, using two identifiers, and be attentive to standard precautions, hand hygiene, patient safety and privacy, body mechanics, and documentation.

Procedure Steps

1. **Clean the equipment lens** with distilled water and dry with dry lens paper or a soft, nonabrasive cloth. *To ensure accurate results.*

2. **Calibrate the refractometer** before use, following the manufacturer's instructions. When calibrated, the refractometer should read 1.000.

3. **Perform hand hygiene** and don clean procedure gloves.

4. **Use fresh urine;** if you cannot perform the test within 1 hour, refrigerate the specimen.

5. **Wearing procedure gloves,** use the dropper to place one or two drops of urine on the prism surface (at the notched bottom of the cover).

6. **Hold the refractometer horizontally** and turn toward the light. Rotate the eyepiece until the scale is in focus.

(continued on next page)

Procedure 30-3 ▪ Testing Urine at the Bedside (continued)

7. **Read the scale** at the point where the dividing line between bright and dark fields crosses the scale. The scale reads from 1.000 to 1.035 in increments of 0.001.

8. **Record the results.**

9. **When you are finished,** dry the refractometer and add a drop of distilled water to cleanse the prism. Dry the equipment with lens paper.

? What if . . .

- **The diagnostic kit is outdated?**

  Contact the pharmacy and/or work with the patient's caregiver to obtain a valid kit.

Evaluation

- Characteristics of urine output (e.g., volume of output, color, clots, mucus)
- Abnormally concentrated or dilute urine

Patient Teaching

- Explain test procedures to the patient and the patient's caregiver and family members as indicated.

Home Care

- Teach the patient or caregiver the steps of the procedure.
- Tell the patient or caregiver that the urine must be tested within an hour or refrigerate the specimen to test later.
- Instruct the patient or caregiver that the specimen should be tested as ordered by the healthcare provider.
- Teach the patient or caregiver to record results on the flow sheet per agency protocol.

Documentation

- Document urine volume and the time and date that the specimen was collected per agency protocol (e.g., on a Kardex®, checklist, or nursing notes).

- Document the urine specific gravity and pH and note the presence of hemoglobin, glucose, ketones, protein, white blood cells, bilirubin, casts, crystals, and nitrites.
- Chart other characteristics of the urine: color, odor, clarity, particulate matter, gross blood, mucous shreds, or other qualities.
- Document any difficulty with voiding, including pain or burning with urination, frequency, or difficulty starting the urine flow.

Sample documentation

3/4/18   1515   Pt voided in bedside commode. Urine is straw-colored with sediment. No unusual odor, blood, or mucus evident. No hemoglobin, glucose, ketones, protein, WBC, bilirubin, casts, or crystal nitrates noted on urine dipstick. Specific gravity 1.015, pH 6.6, and 3+ protein noted. ——————— L. Schaaf, RN

Practice Resources

Ban, K. M., & Easter, J. S. (2014); Chernecky, C. C., & Berger, B. J. (2013); St. Jude Children's Research Hospital (2004a, 2004b).

Procedure 30-4 ▪ Inserting an Intermittent Urinary Catheter (Straight Catheter)

➤ For steps to follow in *all* procedures, refer to the Universal Steps for All Procedures found on the page facing the inside back cover.

Equipment

- Washcloth and towel
- Periwash solution
- Procedure gloves, at least two pairs
- Catheter insertion kit containing:
  - Sterile gloves
  - Urinary catheter
  - Antiseptic cleansing agent
  - Forceps
  - Cotton balls

- Sterile waterproof drapes
- Sterile lubricant
- Urine receptacle
- Specimen container
- Extra pair of sterile gloves and extra sterile catheter

  Obtaining extra supplies prevents the need to leave the bedside to obtain additional supplies should the gloves or catheter become contaminated.

- Bath blanket
- Procedure lamp or flashlight

■ Topical anesthetic gel (e.g., 2% lidocaine [Xylocaine]), according to agency policy and patient need ▼

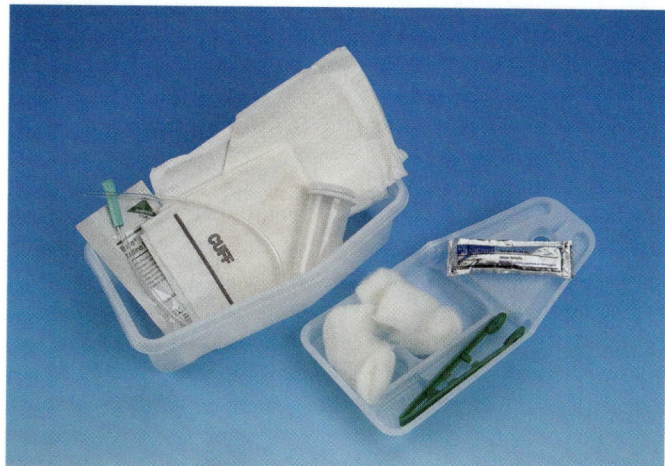

Straight catheter kit.

Delegation

In some institutions, NAPs undergo special training to learn this skill. In such instances, you may delegate this task to the NAP. However, you must complete the following assessments and instruct the NAP when to stop the procedure and what abnormal findings to report. You must from time to time supervise to ensure that the procedure is being performed correctly.

Pre-Procedure Assessments

■ Assess the patient's cognitive level.
To determine whether the patient will be able to follow instructions.

■ Assess for conditions that may impair the patient's ability to assume the necessary position.
To determine whether you will need assistance to help the patient maintain the correct position for catheter insertion.

■ Assess the presence and degree of bladder distension.
To establish a baseline against which to evaluate future data.

■ Determine time of last voiding or last catheterization.
To interpret the significance of the amount of urine obtained in this catheterization.

■ Assess the general body size of the patient and size of the urinary meatus.
To determine whether you need to choose a different size catheter.

■ ✚ Determine whether the patient has an allergy to iodine (if that is the antiseptic solution in the kit). If so, use a different solution.
■ Determine whether the patient is allergic to latex.
Many catheters are made of latex.

■ Note signs and symptoms of bladder infection (e.g., elevated temperature, urinary frequency, dysuria).
■ Note conditions (e.g., enlarged prostate in men) that may make it difficult to pass the catheter.
■ Assess the need for extra lighting.
It is sometimes difficult to visualize a woman's urinary meatus. Supplemental, direct lighting helps.

➤ When performing the procedure, always identify your patient according to agency policy, using two identifiers, and be attentive to standard precautions, hand hygiene, patient safety and privacy, body mechanics, and documentation.

➤ Note: Before starting the procedure, gather the appropriate supplies and prepare the patient. Explain to the patient the reason for the catheter insertion, the expected length of time the catheter will be needed, and the sensations he is likely to have.

Procedure Steps

➤ Note: The following steps are described for a female patient. If your patient is a male, refer to Procedure for Inserting an Intermittent Urinary Catheter (Straight Catheter) for a Male Patient, immediately following the Procedure Steps for females.

1. **If you are right-handed,** stand and work at the patient's right side; if you are left-handed, stand and work at the patient's left side.

2. **Place the patient in a supine** (dorsal recumbent) position to allow you to see the urinary meatus:
   a. Flex the patient's knees and place her feet flat on the bed (dorsal recumbent position).

   b. Instruct the patient to relax her thighs and allow them to rotate externally. Obtain help if patient is confused, unable to follow directions, or unable to hold her legs in correct position.
   The urinary meatus is sometimes difficult to visualize on women because it may resemble skinfolds or other anatomical landmarks in the area.

3. **Don clean procedure gloves.**

4. **Drape the patient.** Fold the blanket in a diamond shape, wrapping the corners around the patient's legs and folding the upper corner down over the perineum. (To review draping, see Procedure 24-4: Providing Perineal Care, in Chapter 24.)
   Providing privacy promotes comfort. ➤

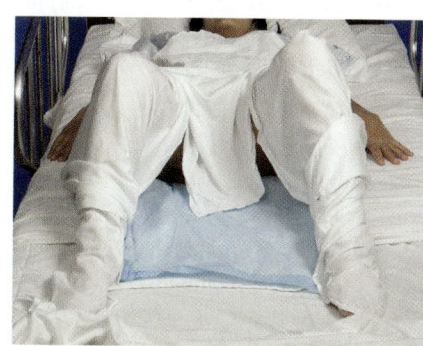

5. **Lift the corner of the privacy drape** to expose the perineum; position the procedure light to allow optimal visualization of the perineum, and then locate the urinary meatus.
   Locating the meatus during this step, especially if the patient is a woman, will help prevent delays at subsequent steps when it is important to maintain sterile technique.

(continued on next page)

Procedure 30-4 ■ **Inserting an Intermittent Urinary Catheter (Straight Catheter)** (continued)

6. **Cleanse the perineal area** with periwash solution; dry.

   Cleansing the perineum before inserting the catheter reduces the number of skin bacteria, thereby helping to prevent transmission of microorganisms into the bladder.

7. **Remove and discard gloves.** Perform hand hygiene.

   Prevents transmission of microorganisms.

8. **Organize your work area.**
   a. Arrange the bedside or overbed table within your reach.
   b. Open the sterile catheter kit according to directions and place it on the bedside or overbed table.
   c. Position a biohazard bag or other trash receptacle so that you will not have to reach across the sterile field (between the patient's legs) to dispose of soiled cotton balls and so forth (e.g., a trash can on the floor beside the bed, or a trash bag on the bed near, but not between, the patient's feet; or the outer wrapping of the catheter).

   Carrying contaminated objects above a sterile field can contaminate the field.

9. **Place sterile underpad** and drape as follows below.

   NOTE: This step assumes the waterproof drape is packed as the top item in the kit. If your kit is different, see "What if ..."

   The drapes provide sterile work surfaces and help prevent contaminating your gloves and sterile supplies.

   a. Place the sterile underpad: Remove the underpad from the kit carefully, allowing it to fall open as you remove it. Do not touch other kit items. Place it flat on the bed, shiny side down, and tuck the top edge under the buttocks, taking care to touch only the corners of the drape.
   b. Remove the sterile glove package, and don sterile gloves (see Procedure 22-7: Sterile Gloves, Open Method, in Chapter 22).

NOTE: Once you have donned the sterile gloves, you may touch items inside the catheter kit, arranging the supplies as needed.

   c. Place the fenestrated drape: This has a hole in the center. Pick up the drape, allowing it to unfold as you remove it, without touching any other objects from the kit. For women, place the drape over the perineum with the hole over the labia (see photos here and in step 11). ▼

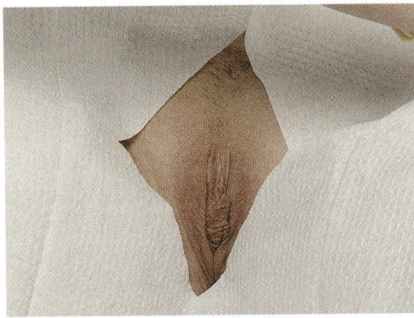

10. **Organize kit supplies on** the sterile field and prepare the supplies in the kit.
    a. Open the antiseptic package and pour antiseptic solution over the cotton balls.

    NOTE: Some kits contain a packet of sterile antiseptic swabs. Open the end of the packet where you feel the "stick"; leaving the swab portions covered by the packet.

    b. Lay the forceps near the cotton balls.
    c. Open the specimen container if you are to collect a specimen.
    d. Remove any unneeded supplies, such as the urine specimen container, from the urine collection basin.
    e. Remove the plastic wrapper from the catheter, if it is covered.
    f. Open the packet or uncap the syringe filled with sterile lubricant.
    g. Squeeze sterile lubricant into the kit tray; roll the catheter slowly in the lubricant. Lubricate the first 2.5 to 5 cm (1 to 2 in.) of the catheter. Leave the catheter

tip in sterile lubricant or on the sterile field until ready to use.

Lubrication allows for ease of insertion of the catheter. Prevents trauma to the mucosa.

   h. Touching only the box or sterile side of the wrapping, place the sterile catheter kit down onto the sterile field between the woman's legs or bedside.

   This allows you to reach supplies during catheter insertion. It also extends the sterile field created by the sterile underpad.

11. **Cleanse the urinary meatus.**
    a. To spread the labia: Place your nondominant hand above the labia, and with your thumb and forefinger spread the patient's labia, pulling up (or anteriorly) at the same time to expose the urinary meatus. Hold this position throughout the procedure—firm pressure is necessary. If the labia slip back over the urinary meatus, it is considered contaminated, and you will need to repeat the cleansing procedure.

    When a woman is supine, gravity may cause tissues above the meatus to fall downward and obscure the meatus from sight. Once placed on the patient's perineal area, your hand is considered contaminated.

    b. With your dominant hand, pick up a moistened cotton ball with the forceps and cleanse the perineal area, taking care not to contaminate your sterile glove.
       ■ Use one stroke and a new cotton ball for each area.
       ■ Wipe from front to back (clitoris to anus).
       ■ If there are five cotton balls or swabs: Wipe in this order: far labium majora, near labium majora, inside far labium, inside near labium, and directly down the center over the urinary meatus.
       ■ If there are only three cotton balls or swabs: Cleanse only

the inside far labium minora, inside near labium minora, and down the center of the urethral meatus.

- Discard the used cotton balls or swabs as you use them. Be careful not to move them across the open and sterile kit.
Because the urethra is close to the anus in female patients, thorough cleansing of the perineum is essential to reduce contamination of the catheter and prevent bacteria from being introduced into the urethra. Following the "clean-to-dirty" principle prevents recontamination of the cleansed area. ▼

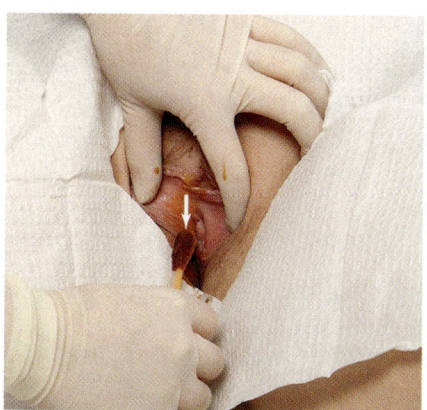

12. **Prepare the urine receptacle.** Place it 10 cm (4 in.) from the meatus (for women), between the patient's thighs (for men).
The end of the catheter will need to reach into the container to catch the draining urine.

13. **Insert the catheter.** ▼

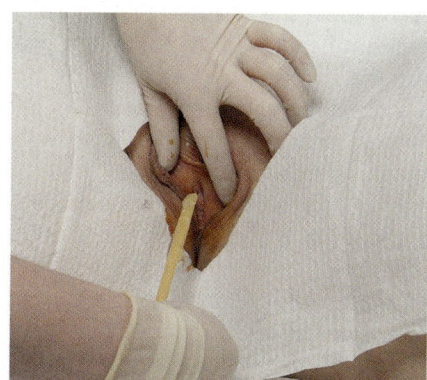

a. Grasp the catheter with your dominant hand, no more than 5 to 7.5 cm (2 to 3 in.) from the tip. Keep the rest of the catheter coiled in the palm of your hand. Slowly insert the end of the catheter into the meatus. Ask the patient to take slow, deep breaths until the initial discomfort has passed.
Bearing down helps relax the external sphincter and makes insertion easier and more comfortable. Holding the catheter close to the distal end will help to keep the tip stable and prevent it from being inserted into the vaginal opening. Deep breathing helps to relax the sphincters. Coiling the catheter in your hand keeps you from contaminating the catheter.

b. Ask the woman to bear down as though she is trying to void.

c. Continue inserting the catheter gently until urine flows, for a distance of 5 to 7.5 cm (2 to 3 in.). After you see urine, insert the catheter another 2.5 to 5 cm (1 to 2 in.).

d. ✚ If you feel slight resistance as the catheter goes through the sphincters, twist the catheter slightly or apply gentle pressure, but do not force the catheter while inserting it. You might need to remove it and cautiously attempt the insertion action again using a new catheter.

Forcing may damage mucosa. Insert the catheter more deeply after urine flow to be sure the catheter is well into the bladder so that the bladder can empty completely. The catheter might not advance while inserted when it is misplaced in the vagina or if there is a stricture within the urethra or sphincter spasm.

e. If the catheter touches the labia or unsterile linens, or if you inadvertently place it in the vagina, it is contaminated; you must insert a new, sterile catheter. Leave the contaminated catheter in the vagina while you are inserting the new one into the meatus.
Leaving the catheter in the incorrect location helps to serve as a visual landmark and helps you to avoid making the same mistake again.

14. **Manage the catheter** and or/urine collection device.
a. Continue to hold the catheter securely with your nondominant hand while the urine drains from the bladder.
Prevents the catheter from being expelled by bladder or urethral contractions.

b. If you are to collect a urine specimen, use your dominant hand to take the specimen container and put it into the flow of urine until you obtain the correct amount of urine. Cap the container, maintaining sterile technique. See Procedure 30-2B.

c. When the flow of urine has ceased and the bladder has been emptied, pinch the catheter and slowly withdraw it from the meatus. Discard the catheter in an appropriate receptacle.
Withdrawing slowly promotes adequate urinary drainage, preventing urinary stasis. Pinching prevents urine from dribbling out of the end of the catheter.

d. Remove the urine-filled receptacle and set it aside outside the patient care area so that is can be emptied when the procedure is finished.
Keeps it from spilling onto the bed.

15. **Cleanse and dry** the patient's perineal area as needed.
This removes residual antiseptic solution from the area, an especially important step if you used povidone-iodine (Betadine). Betadine left on intact healthy skin can cause irritation.

16. **Remove and discard disposable supplies** (e.g., drapes).

17. **Remove your gloves** and wash your hands.
Prevents transmission of bacteria.

18. **Return the patient to a position** of comfort.

(continued on next page)

Procedure 30-4 ■ Inserting an Intermittent Urinary Catheter (Straight Catheter) (continued)

Procedure Variation Inserting an Intermittent Urinary Catheter (Straight Catheter) for a Male Patient

Procedure Steps	Nursing Action
1. Position the patient.	Position the patient supine, legs straight and slightly apart.
2. Drape the patient.	Cover the patient's upper body with a blanket; fold bed sheets down to expose the penis.
3. Don procedure gloves and cleanse the perineum.	After donning procedure gloves, wash the penis and perineal area with perineal wash solution; dry. If you are using a topical anesthetic gel (e.g., Xylocaine), use a syringe (no needle) to insert it into the urethra now. Remove and discard gloves.
4. Organize the work area.	Perform hand hygiene before starting. Open the sterile catheter kit and place on overhead table without contaminating the inside of the wrap. Position a trash receptacle nearby.
5. Place the sterile underpad and sterile drape.	Remove underpad from the kit before donning sterile gloves. Place the drape shiny side down between or across the patient's thighs.
6. Don sterile gloves.	Remove the sterile glove package and don sterile gloves (see Procedure 23-7).
	NOTE: Once you are wearing the sterile gloves, you may touch items inside the catheter kit, arranging the supplies as needed.
7. Place the fenestrated drape.	Allow the fenestrated drape to fall open while removing it from the kit and without touching other kit items. Place the drape with the center hole over the penis.
8. Organize kit supplies on the sterile drape.	■ Open the antiseptic package and pour over cotton balls or use antiseptic swabs or wipes. ■ Open the sterile specimen container. ■ Remove any unneeded supplies. ■ Remove the wrapper from the catheter. ■ Touching only the kit or inside of the wrapping, place the sterile catheter kit down onto the sterile field between the patient's legs.
9. Lubricate the catheter.	■ Do not lubricate the catheter if you have already inserted a lubricant (lidocaine-based product) directly into the urethra. ■ If the lubricant comes in a packet, squeeze it into the kit tray and roll the catheter slowly in it to generously lubricate 12.5 to 17.5 cm (5 to 7 in.) of the catheter. Leave the catheter tip in sterile lubricant or on the sterile field until ready to use. ■ If your kit contains a prefilled syringe of lubricant, gently insert the tip of the syringe into the urethra and instill the lubricant.
10. Expose the urinary meatus.	■ With your nondominant hand, grasp the penis, taking care not to contaminate the surrounding drape. This glove is no longer sterile. ■ Hold the penis gently, but firmly, at a 90° angle to the body, exerting gentle traction. ■ If the penis is uncircumcised, retract the foreskin to fully expose the meatus. If the foreskin accidentally falls over meatus and does not remain retracted or if you drop the penis during cleansing, you must change gloves and repeat the cleansing procedure.
11. Cleanse the urinary meatus.	■ Continuing to hold the penis with your nondominant hand, hold the forceps in your dominant hand and pick up a cotton ball. Cleanse the glans in a series of circular motions, starting at the meatus and working partially down the shaft of the penis. ■ Repeat with at least two more cotton balls or swabs. Discard the cotton balls or swabs as they are used. Do not move them across the open sterile kit and field.
12. Prepare the urine receptacle.	■ Maintaining sterile technique, with your dominant hand place the plastic urine receptacle between the patient's thighs, close enough to the urinary meatus for the end of the catheter to rest inside the container as the urine drains. ■ Hold the catheter 5 to 7.5 cm (2 to 3 in.) from the tip with remainder coiled in the palm of the hand and the distal end of the catheter is in the plastic container.

Procedure Steps	**Nursing Action**
13. Insert the catheter into the urinary meatus.	■ Ask the patient to bear down as though trying to void; slowly insert the end of the catheter into the meatus. Instruct the patient to take slow, deep breaths until the initial discomfort has passed.
	If you feel resistance, withdraw the catheter. Do not force against resistance.
	■ Continue inserting the catheter to about 17.5 to 22.5 cm (7 to 9 in.) or until urine flows. After you see urine, insert the catheter another 2.5 to 5 cm (1 to 2 in.).
14. Collect a specimen if needed.	If a urine specimen is to be collected, continue to grasp the penis, and use your dominant hand to place the specimen container into the flow of urine; cap container using sterile technique.
15. Manage the catheter.	When urine flow stops and the bladder has been emptied, pinch the catheter and slowly withdraw it from the meatus. Replace the foreskin, if uncircumcised. Discard the catheter in an appropriate receptacle.
16. Finish the procedure.	Remove gloves and perform hand hygiene. Return patient to a comfortable position with call device within reach.

? What if . . .

■ **The sterile gloves are packed as the top item in the catheter kit?**

■ **A woman is unable to maintain a dorsal recumbent position?**

■ **The patient is having a menstrual period?**

■ **A man has an erection during the procedure?**

You will find instructions for all of these situations at the end of Procedure 30-5.

Evaluation

■ Note any difficulty with catheter insertion.

This can indicate structural problems, especially in an older male patient with an enlarged prostate gland.

■ Note the characteristics of the urine obtained (e.g., amount, color, odor, presence of sediment or mucus).

■ Assess and palpate for absence of bladder distention.

NOTE: Some facilities have a portable bladder-scanning device that will allow you to determine whether residual urine remains.

Palpating the bladder helps you to determine whether it has been emptied.

■ Record the patient's subjective statements.

■ Document if you collected a specimen and note the time it was sent to the lab.

■ In addition, some facilities require that you record the amount of saline used to inflate the balloon.

Practice Resources

Gould, C. V., Umscheid, C. A., Agarwal, R. K., et al. (2009); Herter, R., & Kazer, M. W. (2010); Newman, D. K., & Willson, M. M. (2011); Pratt, R., & Pellowe, C. (2010); Vahr, S., Cobussen-Boekhorst, H., Eikenboom, J., et al. (2013); Wound, Ostomy, and Continence Nurses Society (2009).

Thinking About the Procedure

To practice applying clinical reasoning to these procedures,

The video **Intermittent Urinary Catheterization**, along with questions and suggested responses, is available on the **Davis's Nursing Skills Videos** Web site on DavisPlus.

Documentation

■ Document the time and date of the procedure.

■ Document the size of catheter used.

■ Record the amount of urine obtained on the I&O portion of the graphics sheet. Record the color of urine, odor, presence of mucus, blood, and so on, in the nursing notes.

Procedure 30-5 ■ Inserting an Indwelling Urinary Catheter

➤ For steps to follow in *all* procedures, refer to the Universal Steps for All Procedures found on the page facing the inside back cover.

Equipment

- Washcloth and towel
- Periwash solution
- Procedure gloves, at least two pairs
- Catheter insertion kit containing:
  - Sterile gloves
  - A double-lumen or triple-lumen catheter with a balloon tip for inflation
  - Antiseptic cleansing agent
  - Forceps
  - Cotton balls
  - Sterile waterproof drapes
  - Sterile lubricant
  - Prefilled syringe with sterile water (to inflate the catheter balloon)
  - Urine collection bag with drainage tubing (often the tubing is preconnected to the catheter)
  - Specimen container
- Extra pair of sterile gloves and extra sterile catheter
  Obtaining extra supplies prevents the need to leave the bedside to obtain additional supplies should the gloves or catheter become contaminated.
- Bath blanket
- Procedure lamp or flashlight
- Topical anesthetic gel (e.g., 2% lidocaine [Xylocaine]), according to agency policy and patient need
- Commercial securement device (e.g., Velcro leg strap). If not available, use hypoallergenic tape.
- Safety pin and elastic band (if needed to secure tubing to the bed. You can usually use the clamp that is on the drainage tubing.

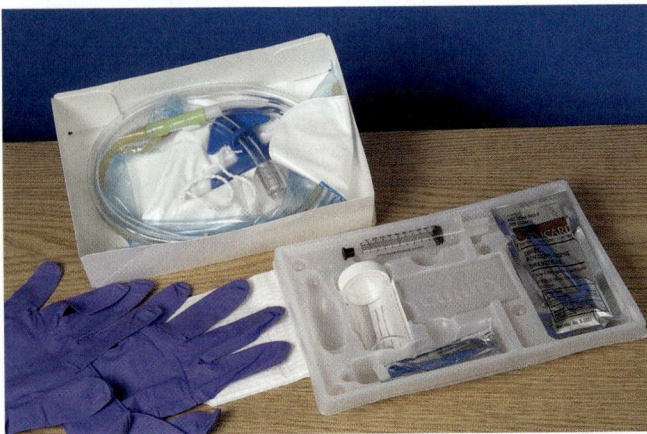

Indwelling catheter kit.

Delegation

In some institutions, NAPs undergo special training to learn this skill. In such instances, you may delegate this task to the NAP. However, you must complete the following assessments and instruct the NAP when to stop the procedure and what abnormal findings to report. You must from time to time supervise to ensure that the procedure is being performed correctly.

Pre-Procedure Assessments

- Assess the patient's cognitive level.
  To determine whether the patient will be able to follow instructions.
- Assess for conditions that may impair the patient's ability to assume the necessary position.
  To determine whether you will need assistance to help the patient maintain the correct position for catheter insertion.
- Assess the presence and degree of bladder distension.
  To establish a baseline against which to evaluate future data.
- Determine time of last voiding or last catheterization.
  To interpret the significance of the amount of urine obtained in this catheterization.
- Assess the general body size of the patient and size of the urinary meatus.
  To determine whether you need to choose a different size catheter.
- ✚ Determine whether the patient has an allergy to iodine (if that is the antiseptic solution in the kit). If so, use a different solution.
- Determine whether the patient is allergic to latex.
  Many catheters are made of latex.
- Note signs and symptoms of bladder infection (e.g., elevated temperature, urinary frequency, dysuria).
- Note conditions (e.g., enlarged prostate in men) that may make it difficult to pass the catheter.
- Assess the need for extra lighting.
  It is sometimes difficult to visualize a woman's urinary meatus. Supplemental, direct lighting helps.

➤ When performing the procedure, always identify your patient according to agency policy, using two identifiers, and be attentive to standard precautions, hand hygiene, patient safety and privacy, body mechanics, and documentation.

➤ *Note:* **The following steps are described for a male patient.** If your patient is a female, refer to the Procedure Variations for Women, immediately following the procedure steps.

Procedure Steps

1. **Place the patient supine** with legs straight and slightly apart. If the patient is confused, unable to follow directions, or unable to maintain correct position, obtain help with the procedure.

2. **If you are right-handed,** stand and work at the patient's right side; if you are left-handed, stand and work at the patient's left side.

3. **Drape the patient.** Cover the patient's upper body with a blanket; fold the bed sheets down to expose the penis.
   Preserves modesty and enhances a feeling of security while ensuring that you can expose the urinary meatus easily.

4. **Don clean procedure gloves.** Cleanse the penis and perineal area with antiseptic solution; dry.
   Cleansing the area reduces the risk of transmitting microbes into the bladder.

5. **If you are using topical anesthetic** gel, use a syringe (no needle) to insert it into the urethra now.
   This is frequently used for men to provide local anesthesia. You will need to wait at least 5 minutes for the gel to take effect before inserting the catheter.

6. **Remove and discard gloves.** Wash your hands.
   Helps prevent transmission of microbes.

7. **Organize your work area:**
   a. Arrange the bedside table or overbed table within your reach.
   b. Open the sterile catheter kit according to manufacturer's instructions and place it on the bedside table.
   c. Position a plastic bag or other trash receptacle so that you will not have to reach across the sterile field to dispose of soiled cotton balls and so forth (e.g., a

trash can on the floor beside the bed, or a trash bag or kit outer wrapper on the bed near, but not between, the patient's feet).
   Carrying contaminated objects above a sterile field can contaminate the field.

8. **Place the sterile waterproof underpad** and drape(s).

   NOTE: This step assumes the waterproof drape is packed as the top item in the kit. If your kit is different, see the "What if . . ." section.

   The drapes provide sterile work surfaces and help prevent contaminating your gloves and sterile supplies.

   a. Remove the underpad from the kit carefully, allowing it to fall open as you remove it. Do not touch other kit items. Drop the underpad across the patient's thighs, touching only the corners.
   b. Remove the sterile glove package and don sterile gloves (see Procedure 22-7, in Chapter 22).

   NOTE: Once you have donned the sterile gloves, you may touch any items inside the catheter kit, arranging the supplies as needed.

   c. Place the fenestrated drape. This has a hole in the center. Pick up the drape, allowing it to unfold as you remove it, without touching any other objects. Place it with the center hole over the penis.

9. **Organize the kit supplies** on the sterile field and prepare the supplies in the kit.
   a. Pour antiseptic solution, such as Betadine, over the cotton balls.

   NOTE: Some kits contain a packet of sterile antiseptic swabs. Open the end of the packet where you can feel the "stick," leaving the swabs covered by the remainder of the packet.

   b. Lay the forceps near the cotton balls.
   c. Open the specimen container, if you are to collect a specimen.
   d. Remove any unneeded supplies, such as the specimen container, from the kit. Remove the plastic wrapper from the catheter, if it is covered.
   e. Do not lubricate the catheter if you have already inserted a lubricant (Xylocaine gel) directly into the urethra. If you did not do that, be certain that the lubricant in the kit is packaged in a syringe rather than a packet.

Variation: **Lubricant in a Syringe**
If the sterile lubricant in the kit is packaged in a syringe, you will insert the lubricant into the urethra at Step 11.

Variation: **Lubricant in a Packet**
If the lubricant comes in a packet, squeeze the lubricant into the kit tray and roll the catheter slowly in the lubricant. Generously lubricate 12.5 to 17.5 cm (5 to 7 in.) of the catheter. Leave the catheter tip in sterile lubricant or on the sterile field until ready to use.

   f. Attach the sterile water-filled syringe to the balloon port of the catheter.
   g. Touching only the box or sterile side of the wrapping, place the sterile catheter kit down onto the sterile field on top of the man's thighs. You may, as an alternative, set up the sterile field between his legs.
   Placement of supplies in this manner allows you to reach supplies during catheter insertion.

   h. If the bedside bag is preconnected to the catheter itself, leave the bag on or near the sterile field until after the catheter is inserted.

(continued on next page)

Procedure 30-5 ■ **Inserting an Indwelling Urinary Catheter** (continued)

10. **Cleanse the urinary meatus.** Discard the used cotton balls as you use them, taking care not to move them across the open and sterile kit.
    Disposing of the used cotton balls reduces the risk for contaminating the sterile field. ▼

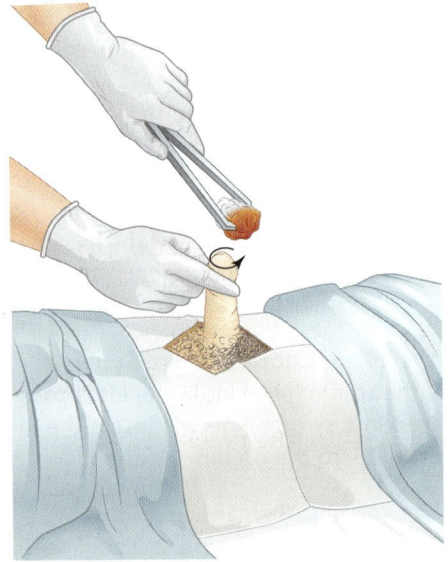

   a. With your nondominant hand, reach through the opening in the fenestrated drape and grasp the penis, taking care not to contaminate the surrounding drape. This glove is no longer sterile.
   b. Hold the penis gently, but firmly, at a 90° angle to the body, exerting gentle traction.
      Supporting the shaft with the fingers straightens the urethra, easing insertion of the catheter.
   c. If the penis is uncircumcised, retract the foreskin to fully expose the meatus. If the foreskin accidentally falls over the meatus or if you drop the penis during cleansing, you must repeat the cleansing procedure.
      Retracting the foreskin allows for full cleansing of the area.
   d. Continuing to hold the penis with your nondominant hand, hold the forceps in your dominant hand and pick up a cotton ball. Cleanse the glans in a series of circular motions, starting at the meatus and working partially down the shaft of the penis.

   e. Repeat with at least two more cotton balls or swabs. Discard cotton balls or swabs as they are used and do not move them across the open, sterile kit and field.
      Following the "clean-to-dirty" principle prevents recontamination of the cleansed area.
   f. Continue to grasp the penis with your nondominant hand during the next steps. This glove is no longer sterile.

11. **Instill lubricant** (if not done previously).

Lubricant Packaged in a Syringe
Before beginning the procedure, you should have made sure that the catheter kit contains a prefilled syringe of lubricant rather than a packet. Gently insert the tip of the prefilled syringe into the urethra and instill the lubricant (unless you have already inserted Xylocaine gel).

Lubricant Packaged in a Packet
If the kit contains only a single packet of lubricant and if no other kits are available, then make sure you have already lubricated 12.5 to 17.7 cm (5 to 7 in.) of the catheter. This is not the technique of choice.

12. **Insert the catheter.** ▼

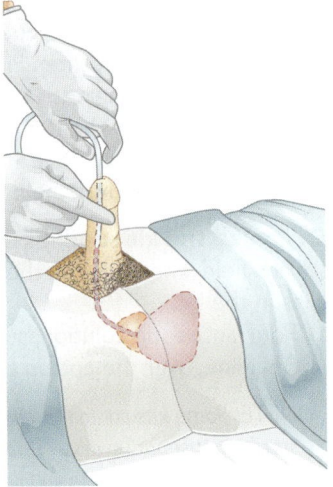

   a. With your dominant hand, stabilize the catheter before inserting it by holding the catheter approximately 7.5 cm (3 in.) from the proximal end. Keep the rest of the catheter coiled in the

palm of your hand if it is not already preconnected to the drainage tube.
   Coiling the catheter in your hand keeps you from contaminating the catheter. When you preconnect the drainage bag before you insert the catheter, you keep the urine from draining onto the bed. Frequently the catheter and drainage bag are connected by the manufacturer.

   b. With your nondominant hand, hold the penis gently but firmly at a 90° angle to the body, exerting gentle traction.
      Supporting the shaft with the fingers straightens the urethra, easing insertion of the catheter.
   c. Ask the patient to bear down as though trying to void; slowly insert the end of the catheter into the meatus. Ask the patient to take slow deep breaths until the initial discomfort has passed.
      These strategies help the patient relax the external sphincter, making insertion easier and more comfortable.
   d. Continue inserting the catheter to about 17 to 22.5 cm (7 to 9 in.) or until urine flows. You will feel slight resistance at the level of the external sphincter. Continue to advance to the bifurcation (Y connector).

   ✚ You will commonly feel resistance at the prostatic sphincter. Hold the catheter firmly against the sphincter until the resistance eases. Then advance it, but do not force it.

      Prevents compromised circulation and painful swelling.

13. **Manage the catheter.**
   a. Continue to hold the catheter securely with your nondominant hand to stabilize the catheter's position in the urethra. Use your other hand to pick up the saline or sterile water-filled syringe and inflate the catheter balloon slowly.
      Holding the catheter until the balloon is inflated reduces the chance of the catheter's being expelled by the bladder or urethral contractions.

The inflated balloon prevents the catheter from slipping out of the bladder. ▼

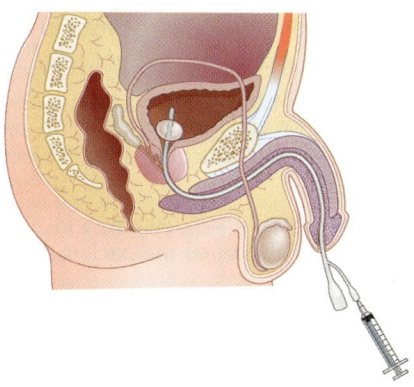

A. Catheter placement, male.

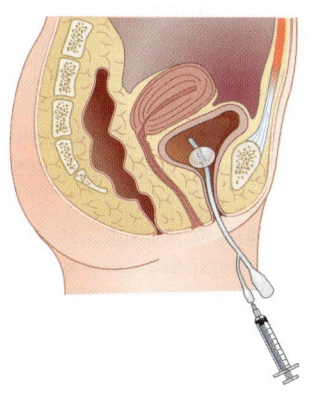

B. Catheter placement, female.

b. ✚ If the patient complains of pain on inflation of the balloon, withdraw the water from the balloon and reposition the catheter by advancing it 1 inch (2.5 cm). *Pain usually indicates that the balloon was in the urethra instead of in the bladder.*

c. After the balloon is inflated, pull back gently on the catheter until you feel resistance. Lower the penis and replace the foreskin. *Indicates that the balloon is correctly positioned at the neck of the bladder.*

14. **Connect the drainage bag** to the end of the catheter if it is not already preconnected. Hang the drainage bag on the side of the bed, below the level of the bladder. *Hanging the drainage bag below the bladder promotes adequate urinary drainage, preventing urinary stasis.*

15. **Using a commercial catheter** securement device (e.g., catheter tube holder of Velcro leg strap) if available, secure the catheter to the thigh or the abdomen. Otherwise, use hypoallergenic tape. *Prevents urethral irritation related to tugging or pulling of the catheter.*

16. **Cleanse the patient's penis** and perineal area as needed; dry. Cover the patient with a gown. *Removes residual antiseptic solution from the area, an especially important step if you used povidone iodine (Betadine), which is not commonly used for this procedure. Betadine left on intact healthy skin can cause irritation.*

17. **Remove and discard** disposable supplies (e.g., drapes).

18. **Remove your gloves** and discard them into biohazard receptacle. Perform hand hygiene.

19. **Return the patient** to a comfortable position.

Procedure Variation **Indwelling Catheter Insertion for a Female Patient**

Procedure Steps (Above)	Nursing Action
1. Position the patient.	Flex the patient's knees, and place her feet flat on the bed (dorsal recumbent position). Instruct the patient to relax her thighs and allow them to rotate externally.
	NOTE: Obtain help if the patient is confused, unable to follow directions, or unable to hold her legs in the correct position.
2. Drape the patient.	Fold the blanket in a diamond shape, wrapping the corners around the patient's legs and folding the upper corner down over the perineum (see Procedure 30-4).
3. Cleanse the perineal area.	▪ Don clean procedure gloves.
	▪ Lift the corner of the privacy drape to expose the perineum.
	▪ Position the procedure light to allow optimal visualization of the perineum and then locate the urinary meatus.
	▪ Cleanse the perineal area with antiseptic solution; dry.
	▪ Remove and discard gloves. Wash hands.
4. Organize the work area.	▪ Arrange the bedside table or overbed table within your reach. Open the sterile catheter kit according to the directions, and place it on the table.
	▪ Position a plastic bag or other trash receptacle so that you will not have to reach across the sterile field to dispose of soiled cotton balls and so forth.

(continued on next page)

Procedure 30-5 ■ Inserting an Indwelling Urinary Catheter (continued)

Procedure Steps (Above)

5. Apply the sterile underpad and fenestrated drape.

6. Organize the kit supplies on the sterile field.

7. Spread the labia and cleanse the urinary meatus.

8. Insert the catheter.

9. Manage the catheter.

10. Secure the catheter.

11. Finish up.

Nursing Action

- Remove the sterile underpad from the kit before donning sterile gloves. Be sure not to touch other kit items with bare hands. Touching only the corners, place the drape shiny side down under the patient's buttocks.
- Carefully remove the sterile glove package from the kit and put them on.
- Pick up the fenestrated drape; allow it to unfold without touching other objects; place over the perineum with the hole over the labia.

- Open the antiseptic packet and pour solution over the cotton balls, and position forceps nearby. Or if the kit comes with antiseptic swabs, open the packet so the sticks are convenient to grasp.
- Open the specimen container if a specimen is to be collected. Remove any unneeded supplies.
- Remove the plastic wrapper from the catheter, if it is covered. Squeeze the sterile lubricant into the kit tray. Roll the catheter slowly in the lubricant, being sure to generously lubricate the first 2.5 to 5 cm (1 to 2 in.) of the catheter. Leave the catheter tip in the sterile lubricant or on the sterile field until ready to use.
- Attach the sterile water-filled syringe to the balloon port of the catheter. Leave the syringe attached to the catheter.
- Touching only the box or sterile side of the wrapping, place the sterile catheter kit down onto the sterile field at the bedside. You may, as an alternative, set up the sterile field on the bed between her legs.

- Place your nondominant hand above the labia, and, with thumb and forefinger, spread the patient's labia, pulling up at the same time to expose the urinary meatus. Use firm pressure to hold this position throughout the procedure. If the labia accidentally slip back over the meatus during cleansing, repeat the procedure.
- Wipe from the clitoris to the anus, wiping in the order of: far labium majora, near labium majora, inside far labium, inside near labium, and directly down the center over the urinary meatus.
- Discard cotton balls or swabs as they are used; do not move them across the open, sterile kit and field. Use only one stroke and a new cotton ball or swab for each area.

Ask the woman to bear down as though she is trying to void. Grasp the catheter with your dominant hand, no more than 5 to 7.5 cm (2 to 3 in.) from the tip. Slowly insert the end of the catheter into the meatus. Ask the patient to take slow, deep breaths until the initial discomfort has passed.

- Continue inserting the catheter gently until urine flows, for a distance of 5 to 7.5 cm (2 to 3 in.). After you see urine, insert the catheter another 2.5 to 5 cm (1 to 2 in.).
- If the catheter touches the labia or unsterile linens, or if you inadvertently place it in the vagina, it is contaminated and you must insert a new, sterile catheter. Leave the contaminated catheter in the vagina while you are inserting the new one into the meatus.
- After urine flows, stabilize the catheter in the urethra with your nondominant hand; use the dominant hand to pick up the sterile water-filled syringe and inflate the catheter balloon.

- ✚ If the patient complains of pain when inflating the balloon, use a syringe to withdraw the water from the balloon. Then reposition the catheter by advancing it 2.5 cm (1 in.).

- Hang the drainage bag on the side of the bed below the level of the bladder.
- Using a commercial catheter securement device, if available, secure the catheter to the thigh.

Remove and discard disposable supplies. Remove and discard gloves. Perform hand hygiene. Return the patient to a comfortable position with call device within reach.

? What if . . .

- **The sterile gloves are packed as the top item in the catheter kit?**

  - Remove the sterile glove package and don sterile gloves (see Procedure 22-7 in Chapter 22).

    NOTE: Once you have donned the sterile gloves, you may touch any item inside the catheter kit, arranging the supplies as needed.

  - Place the sterile underpad: Grasp the edges of the sterile drape. Fold the entire edge down 5 to 7.5 cm (2 to 3 in.) and toward you, making a "cuff" to protect your gloves. Take care not to touch unsterile objects with your gloves or the drape.
  - *For women:* Carefully slide the drape under the patient's buttocks without contaminating your gloves. Ask the patient to raise her hips slightly if she can.
  - *For men:* Drop the sterile underpad across the thighs. ➤

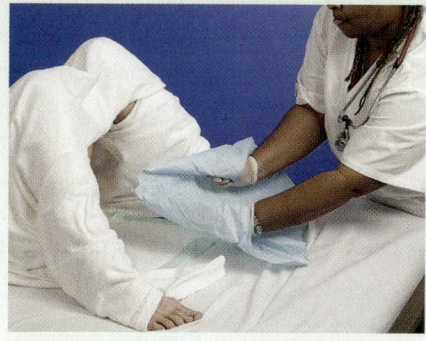

- **Continue with a fenestrated drape: Pick up the drape, allowing it to unfold as you remove it, without touching any objects. Protect sterility as you did with the underpad (preceding step).**

  - *For women:* Place the fenestrated drape over the perineum so that the hole is over the labia.
  - *For men:* Place the fenestrated drape so that the center hole is over the penis. You will pull the penis up and through the opening when cleansing the meatus.

- **A woman is unable to maintain a dorsal recumbent position?**

  Use Sims' position (side-lying with the upper leg flexed at the hip). Cover the rectal area.
  Prevents contamination from the rectal area to the urethra.

- **The patient is having a menstrual period?**

  Note on the lab form that the patient is having a menstrual period before sending a specimen for diagnostic testing.
  Blood in the urine from a menstrual period might lead to misinterpretation of the result.

- **A man has an erection during the procedure?**

  Treat the situation calmly. Take a break until the erection subsides. Never force the catheter.
  Forcing the catheter can cause urethral irritation or trauma.

Evaluation

- Note any difficulty with catheter insertion.
  This can indicate structural problems, especially in an older male patient with an enlarged prostate gland.
- Note the characteristics of the urine obtained (e.g., amount, color, odor, presence of sediment or mucus).
- Assess and palpate for absence of bladder distention.

  NOTE: Some facilities have a portable bladder-scanning device that will allow you to determine whether residual urine remains.

  Palpating the bladder helps you to determine whether it has been emptied.

- For indwelling catheters, continue to assess that drainage is not obstructed and that the drainage bag is below the level of the bladder

Home Care

For inserting indwelling catheters in the home, teach clients:
- When to change the catheter.
  Changing indwelling catheters at routine, fixed intervals is generally not recommended (Gould, Umscheid, Agarwal, et al., 2009). Clients should be taught to change catheters based on clinical indications, such as impaired urine drainage or encrustation.
- How to prevent catheter blockage (e.g., increase fluid intake, use bladder irrigation).
  Fluids increase the urine volume, helping to reduce the deposit of sediment or other particles in the tubing.

- To empty the drainage bag frequently and to keep the bag below the level of the bladder.
- How to prevent UTIs (e.g., use new silver/hydrogel-coated catheters, maintain a closed system, wash hands prior to handling catheter equipment, prevent blockage of urine outflow, adequate fluid intake [noncarbonated]).
- To take a shower rather than a bath to decrease the risk for UTIs.
- How to prevent discomfort at the urethra.
- Use of a leg bag.
- To eat foods that help acidify the urine: meat, eggs, cheese, prunes, cranberries, and whole grains.

Documentation

- Document the time and date of the procedure.
- Document the size of catheter used.
- Record the amount of urine obtained on the I&O portion of the graphics sheet. Record the color of urine, odor, presence of mucus, blood, and so on, in the nursing notes.
- Record the patient's subjective statements.
- Document if you collected a specimen, and note the time it was sent to the lab.
- In addition, some facilities require that you record the amount of saline used to inflate the balloon.

(continued on next page)

Procedure 30-5 ▪ **Inserting an Indwelling Urinary Catheter** (continued)

Sample documentation

3/4/18   1010   Order noted for insertion of indwelling catheter. Explained the procedure to Pt and reason for insertion. Pt verbalized understanding of the procedure and need for catheter. Placed Pt in a dorsal recumbent position with blankets to keep Pt warm and provide privacy. Perineal care completed. 14-Fr Foley catheter inserted using sterile technique per protocol. Foley draining dark yellow urine with sediment and foul odor. No mucus or blood noted in urine. Bladder is not distended. Client returned to semi-Fowler's position. No needs noted at this time. Reminded Pt to call nurse if there is any discomfort associated with urinary catheterization. Call light placed in Pt's dominant hand. ————————————— C. Chin, RN

Practice Resources

Gould, C. V., Umscheid, C. A., Agarwal, R. K., et al. (2009); Herter, R., & Kazer, M. W. (2010); Newman, D. K., & Wilson, M. M. (2011); Pratt, R., & Pellowe, C. (2010); Vahr, S., Cobussen-Boekhorst, H., Eikenboom, J., et al. (2013); Wound, Ostomy, and Continence Nurses Society (2009).

Thinking About the Procedure

To practice applying clinical reasoning to these procedures,

 The video **Indwelling Urinary Catheterization,** along with questions and suggested responses, is available on the **Davis's** *Nursing Skills Videos* Web site on Davis*Plus.*

Procedure 30-6 ▪ **Applying an External (Condom) Catheter**

➤ For steps to follow in *all* procedures, refer to the Universal Steps for All Procedures found on the page facing the inside back cover.

Equipment

- Condom catheter
- Two pairs of clean procedure gloves
- Washcloth and towel
- Basin of soap and water
- Bath blanket
- Urine collection bag (e.g., bedside drainage bag or leg bag)
- Disposable tape measure
- Skin prep (per agency policy)
- Scissors
- Commercial leg strap

Delegation

You may delegate the application of a condom catheter to the NAP once you have assessed the NAP's skill level and completed the following assessments. Instruct the NAP to report any alterations in the skin integrity along the shaft of the penis.

Pre-Procedure Assessments

- Assess the patient's cognitive status.
  Knowing whether the patient can follow directions helps you to determine how to approach the procedure and also to know whether the patient may be prone to pulling on the catheter.

- Assess pattern of voiding (e.g., degree, amount, and time of incontinence).
  Helps you to determine when the condom catheter should be applied.

- Assess the skin along the shaft of the penis, the glans, and the meatus (for swelling or excoriation).
  The condom catheter cannot be used on excoriated, irritated skin or over areas of impaired skin integrity.

- Note whether and how much the penis is retracted toward the body.
  There is an increased risk of nonadherence and leakage of urine in a patient with a retracted penis.

- Assess for neuropathy.
  Patients with neuropathies that affect sensation in the penis may not feel skin irritation from the condom catheter and will need to be assessed more frequently.

> ➤ When performing the procedure, always identify your patient according to agency policy, using two identifiers, and be attentive to standard precautions, hand hygiene, patient safety and privacy, body mechanics, and documentation.

Procedure Steps

1. **Determine appropriate size** of the external catheter by measuring the circumference of the penis using a disposable paper tape. Obtain a correctly sized catheter.

   A catheter that is too small impairs circulation. A catheter that is too large allows leakage of urine.

2. **Perform hand hygiene and** don procedure gloves.

   Hand hygiene and gloving prevent transmission of pathogens.

3. **Organize supplies** and prepare the leg bag or bedside drainage bag for attachment to the condom catheter by removing it from the packaging and placing the end of the connecting tubing near the perineal area.

4. **Position the patient** supine. If the patient has difficulty breathing, raise the head of the bed to 30°.

5. **Fold down the bed linen** to expose the penis, and drape the patient using the bath blanket.

   Covering the patient reduces patient embarrassment.

6. **Gently cleanse the penis** with soap and water. Rinse and dry it thoroughly. If the patient is uncircumcised, retract the foreskin, cleanse the glans, and replace the foreskin. Excess hair along the shaft of the penis may be carefully clipped off with the scissors.

   Cleansing the penis helps to prevent infection and increases adherence of the condom catheter to the shaft.

7. **Perform hand hygiene** and change procedure gloves.

8. **Apply skin prep** (if used by your agency) and allow it to dry.

   NOTE: Some external condom catheters require the placement of the special adhesive strip onto the penis before the application of the condom. Read the manufacturer's directions.

9. **Hold the penis** in your nondominant hand. With your dominant hand, place the condom catheter at the end of the penis and slowly unroll it along the shaft toward the patient's body. Leave 2.5 to 5 cm (1 to 2 in.) between the end of the penis and the drainage tube on the catheter.

   Unrolling in this manner helps to prevent irritation of the glans due to rubbing and allows for expansion of the penis if an erection were to occur. ▼

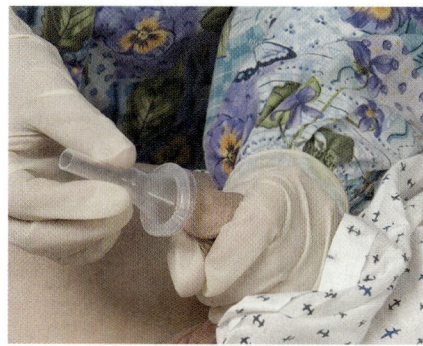

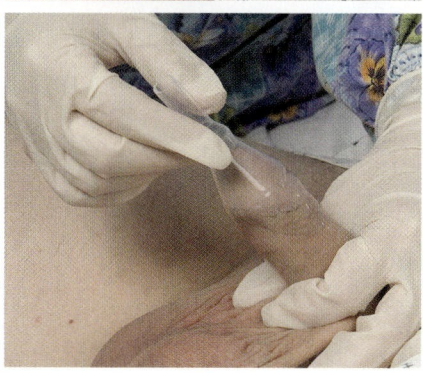

10. **Secure the condom** catheter in place on the penis.
    a. Ensure that the condom is not twisted.

       Twisting can obstruct urine flow.
    b. Do not use regular bandage or surgical dressing tape to hold an external condom catheter in place.

       Regular surgical dressing tape does not expand and could lead to decreased blood flow to the penis.

Catheter With Internal Adhesive

    c. Gently grasp the penis and compress so that the entire shaft comes in contact with the condom.

Catheter With External Adhesive Strip

    d. Wrap the strip around the outside of the condom in a spiral direction, taking care not to overlap the ends.

       Prevents constriction of blood flow to the penis.

11. **Assess the proximal end** of the condom catheter. If a large portion of the condom is still rolled above the adhesive strip, you may need to clip the roll.

    Clipping the roll helps prevent constriction of blood flow.

12. **Attach the tube end** of the condom catheter to a drainage system (e.g., a leg bag). Make sure there are no kinks in the tubing.

    Kinks impede the flow of urine. Urine that does not drain away from the meatus can cause irritation and skin breakdown and possibly cause the condom catheter to fall off.

13. **Secure the catheter tubing** to the patient's thigh using tape or a commercial leg strap. Hypoallergenic tape may be used if a commercial leg strap is unavailable. Follow agency protocol.

    Controls movement of the tubing and accidental pulling on the condom catheter. ▼

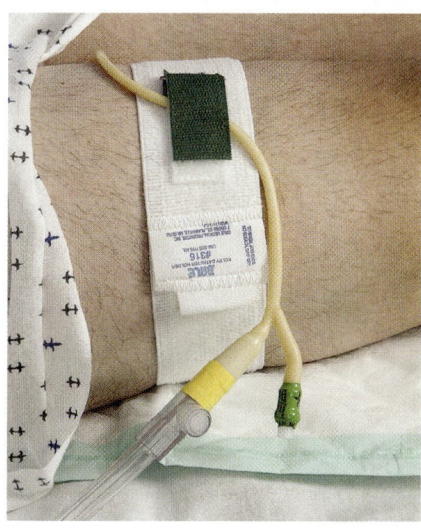

(continued on next page)

Procedure 30-6 ■ **Applying an External (Condom) Catheter** (continued)

14. Cover the patient and return him to a comfortable position. Raise the siderails and lower the bed.

15. Remove your gloves and wash your hands.

16. Change the condom daily or more often if needed.
This helps to prevent UTI and allows for inspection of the skin.

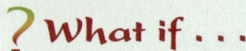 **? What if . . .**

■ **The urine flow becomes obstructed?**

Check the catheter and collecting tube for kinking; readjust if needed. If that does not solve the problem, irrigate the tubing (see Procedure 30-7). Replace the catheter and tubing, if necessary.

Evaluation

Within 30 minutes of condom application, assess for:
■ Urine flow (should not be obstructed).
■ Swelling or discoloration of the penis.
Swelling or discoloration might indicate that the condom is too tight.

Monitor:
■ The penis for circulatory changes.
■ Position and patency of the drainage tubing.
■ Characteristics of the urine (e.g., amount, color, odor, bleeding).
■ Patient comfort.
■ Leakage of urine.

Home Care

■ Clients and caregivers should wash their hands before and after any manipulation of the penis or apparatus.
■ Daily bag decontamination with a diluted (1:10) bleach solution has been found effective in reducing bacteria.
■ Teach the client and caregiver to recognize the signs and symptoms of skin irritation and excoriation, as well as the symptoms of a UTI.
■ Teach the client/caregiver to notify the care provider and discontinue use of the condom catheter if skin irritation or swelling occurs; if the urine becomes thick and cloudy, pink or red; if the urine has mucus in it; if no urine has drained from the catheter in 6 to 8 hours.
■ Change the external condom catheter every 24 hours. Use paper tape to secure the condom catheter to the inner thigh.
■ Keep the collecting bag below the level of the bladder and off the floor.

■ Empty the urine collection device.
■ Regularly empty the collection bag before it becomes completely full.
■ Never allow the draining spigot to come in contact with the nonsterile collecting container.
■ Disinfect the catheter–tubing junction before disconnecting them (if they must be disconnected).
■ Avoid disconnecting the catheter and drainage tube unless the catheter must be irrigated.

Documentation

■ Document the date and time of application of the external catheter in the nursing notes.
■ Note any unusual findings in your assessment of the skin on the penis.
■ Document characteristics of urine (e.g., color, odor, consistency, blood).

Practice Resources

Geng, V., Bonns, E., Eelen, P., et al. (2008); Wound, Ostomy, and Continence Nurses Society (n.d.).

Thinking About the Procedure

To practice applying clinical reasoning to this procedure,

 The video **Applying an External (Condom) Catheter,** along with questions and suggested responses, is available on the **Davis's *Nursing Skills Videos*** Web site on Davis*Plus*.

Procedure 30-7 ■ Removing an Indwelling Catheter

➤ For steps to follow in *all* procedures, refer to the Universal Steps for All Procedures found on the page facing the inside back cover.

Equipment

- Clean procedure gloves
- Syringe (5 to 30 mL, depending on balloon size)
- Towel or drape (as a receptacle for the catheter)
- Receptacle for the catheter (emesis basin)
- Hygiene supplies (washcloth, warm water, towel)

Delegation

In some institutions, unlicensed NAPs undergo special training to learn this skill. In such instances, you may delegate this task to the NAP. However, you must complete the following assessments and instruct the NAP about what abnormal findings to report.

Pre-Procedure Assessments

- **Assess the patient's cognitive level.**
  Knowing whether the patient can follow directions helps you to determine how to approach the procedure and also to know whether the patient may be prone to pulling on the catheter or your hands when you are removing the catheter.

- **Assess patient's ability to assume the necessary position.**
  Identifying limitations helps you to determine whether you will need assistance to help the patient maintain the position for catheter insertion.

- **Assess the condition of bladder** (e.g., distention), perineum, and meatus (e.g., color, swelling, crusting, drainage, lesion).
  This information helps you to establish a baseline for later assessment.

➤ When performing the procedure, always identify your patient according to agency policy, using two identifiers, and be attentive to standard precautions, hand hygiene, patient safety and privacy, body mechanics, and documentation.

Procedure Steps

1. **Gather the necessary supplies.**

2. **Tell the patient what you are about to do,** what she will feel, and that you will need to monitor her urination after removal.

3. **Perform hand hygiene** before and after removing the catheter.

4. **Wear clean procedure gloves** during the removal.
   Hand hygiene and gloving prevent transmission of bacteria.

5. **Explain that this** procedure is nearly always pain free.

6. **Instruct the patient** to assume a supine position (for males) or a dorsal recumbent position (for females).

7. **Place the catheter receptacle** near the patient (e.g., on the bed).

8. **Place a towel** or waterproof drape.

Variation, Female: Place the drape between the patient's legs and up by the urethral meatus.

Variation, Male: Place the drape on his thighs.
These methods preserve modesty and a feeling of security and prevent soiling of the linens.

9. **Obtain a sterile specimen** (see Procedure 30-2B), if needed. Some agencies require a culture and sensitivity test of the urine when an indwelling catheter is removed.

10. **Wash the perineum** with soapy filtered water or periwash prior to removal of the catheter.

11. **Remove the tape or device** securing the catheter to the patient.

12. **Deflate the balloon completely** by inserting a syringe into the balloon valve and allowing the balloon to self-deflate. Allow at least 30 seconds for the balloon to deflate.

    NOTE: Follow the manufacturer's directions for balloon deflation. If you must attempt aspiration, it should be done slowly and gently.

    Aspiration of the balloon may collapse the lumen and cause the formation of creases and ridges that may make removal of the catheter difficult (Wound, Ostomy, and Continence Nurses Society, 2009).

13. **Verify that the total fluid** volume has been removed by checking the balloon size written on the balloon port.

14. **Ask the patient to relax** and take a few deep breaths as you slowly withdraw the catheter from the urethra. Pinch the catheter while removing it.
    Deep breathing helps the patient to relax the sphincters.

15. **Wrap the catheter** in the towel or drape or place in the catheter receptacle.

16. **Again cleanse the perineal area** with warm filtered water or perineal wash solution on gauze pads or perineal disposable wipes. A mild soap may also be used. Be sure to rinse well if you use soap.
    Cleansing the perineum prevents transmission of bacteria. Soap is drying to the skin and mucosa.

17. **Measure the urine** and then empty it in the toilet; discard the catheter, drainage tube, and collection bag in the biohazard waste.

(continued on next page)

Procedure 30-7 ■ Removing an Indwelling Catheter (continued)

18. **Explain to the patient the need** to monitor the first few voidings after catheter removal. If the patient toilets independently, place a receptacle in the toilet or bedside commode. Ask him to notify the nurse when he voids and to save the urine.

19. **Remove and discard gloves;** perform hand hygiene.

20. **Record the procedure** (see Documentation, below).

21. **Return the patient to a position** of comfort.

? What if . . .

- **You cannot aspirate all the fluid from the balloon?**

  Do not pull on the catheter. Report to the charge nurse or the primary care provider before continuing the procedure.

  Pulling on the catheter could cause injury to the urethra.

Evaluation

- Observe for signs and symptoms of infection.

  Signs of a catheter-associated urinary tract infection include the presence of significant bacteriuria in a patient with signs or symptoms of a UTI such as fever, malaise, flank pain, dysuria, altered mental status, or hematuria.

- Observe the condition of the meatus.
- Monitor the next few voidings after removing the catheter.
- Assess the characteristics of the urine at the time the catheter is removed (color, amount, odor, and presence of blood). Then note the time of the first voiding and the amount voided.
- Compare voidings over the next 8 to 10 hours with the patient's intake.
- Monitor for bladder distention. A portable bladder-scanning device may be used to quantify any residual urine.

Patient Teaching

- Explain that you need to monitor the first few voidings after catheter removal to ensure that he does not have difficulty reestablishing bladder control.
- Teach the patient to notify you when he voids and to save the urine (if the patient toilets independently).

Home Care

For patients who will have catheters at home, teach the client and family the following:
- Steps for removing the catheter.
- To notify a healthcare provider if the client is unable to urinate within 8 hours after catheter removal, or if his abdomen becomes distended and painful.
- Signs and symptoms of a UTI.

  Signs and symptoms of a urinary tract infection develop rapidly.

- Increase fluid intake if not contraindicated by other health conditions.

  ✚ The client should never remove a catheter unless trained by a healthcare provider. Remove the catheter only when prescribed by the provider.

Documentation

- Date and time the catheter was removed
- Amount of urine (on the I&O portion of the graphics sheet).
- Characteristics of urine (e.g., color, odor, cloudiness, turbidity, or blood).
- The time the specimen was sent to the lab
- The amount of fluid removed from balloon, client response to removal of the Foley catheter, urine in drainage bag, and notification of first void
- Any unusual findings in your assessment of the perineum
- How the patient tolerated the procedure
- Patient teaching

Sample documentation

3/4/18   1010   Order noted for removal of indwelling catheter. Explained the procedure to patient. Pt stated, "I'm finally getting this thing out." Placed pt in a dorsal recumbent position with blanket to provide privacy. Perineal care completed. Allowed retention balloon to self-deflate, obtaining 10 mL of liquid. Removed catheter, using gentle pulling motion. Pt expressed no discomfort during removal. Perineal care again given. 250 mL of clear, yellow, strong-smelling urine noted in drainage bag. Instructed client to increase fluid intake, especially water, and to notify a nurse when she voids for the first time. ———— D. Drumpf, RN

Practice Resources

Geng, V., Cobussen-Boekhorst, H., Farrell, J., et al. (2012); Griffiths, R., & Fernandez, R. (2009); Hooton, T. M., Bradley, S. F., Cardenas, D. D., et al. (2010); Wound, Ostomy, and Continence Nurses Society (2009); Yates, A. (2008).

Thinking About the Procedure

To practice applying clinical reasoning to this procedure,

 The video **Removing an Indwelling Catheter,** along with questions and suggested responses, is available on the **Davis's** *Nursing Skills Videos* Web site on Davis*Plus*.

Procedure 30-8 ■ Irrigating the Bladder or Catheter

➤ For steps to follow in *all* procedures, refer to the Universal Steps for All Procedures found on the page facing the inside back cover.

Equipment

Intermittent Irrigation Through a Three-Way Catheter

- Bag of sterile irrigation solution
- Connecting tubing (to connect the bag to the irrigation port)
- IV pole
- Antiseptic swabs
- Bath blanket

Intermittent Irrigation via the Specimen Port Using a Syringe

- Sterile container
- Sterile 60-mL syringe with large-gauge needleless access device
- Two pairs of clean procedure gloves
- Antiseptic swabs or wipes

Continuous Bladder Irrigation

- Three-way (or triple-lumen) indwelling catheter in place
- Sterile irrigation solution at room temperature
- Connecting tubing
- Antiseptic swabs
- IV pole
- Bath blanket
- Measuring container
- Pair of clean procedure gloves

Delegation

Irrigation of an indwelling catheter requires nursing assessment and clinical decision making. Because of the high potential for UTI, you should not delegate this procedure to the NAP. Bladder/catheter irrigation may be delegated with supervision to qualified LPNs who are trained in the procedure.

Pre-Procedure Assessments

- Note the characteristics of the urine (e.g., amount, color, odor, presence of clots or mucus).
- Assess for the presence and degree of bladder distension.
  This information helps you to establish a baseline for assessment.
- Note patient complaints of discomfort.
- Assess the patient's cognitive status.
  To determine whether the patient can remain still during the procedure.
- Check the chart for the amount and type of sterile solution to use.
- Determine whether the irrigant is to remain in the bladder for any length of time.

Procedure 30-8A ■ Intermittent Bladder Irrigation

➤ When performing the procedure, always identify your patient according to agency policy, using two identifiers, and be attentive to standard precautions, hand hygiene, patient safety and privacy, body mechanics, and documentation.

NOTE: *This is the procedure for the closed methods of irrigation.* ✚ *The "open" method is no longer recommended. Because of the risk for infection, you should never disconnect the drainage tubing from the catheter.*

Procedure Steps

Procedure Variation Three-Way (Triple-Lumen) Indwelling Catheter

1. **Before starting bladder irrigation,** prepare the connection tubing and irrigation solution warmed to room temperature.
   a. Close the clamp on the connection tubing.
   b. Spike the tubing into the appropriate port on the irrigation solution bag, using aseptic technique.
   c. Invert the solution and hang it on an IV pole.

   d. Remove the protective cap from the distal end of the connection tubing. Hold the end of the tubing over the sink or trash receptacle. Open the roller clamp and allow the solution to fill the tubing. Be sure to keep the end sterile.
   e. Reclamp the roller on the tubing to stop the flow of irrigation solution.
   f. Recap the tubing.

2. **Perform hand hygiene.** And then don procedure gloves.
   To reduce the transmission of microbes.

3. **Position the patient supine.**

♥ **iCare** 4. **Drape the patient** so he is not exposed and only the connection port on the indwelling catheter is visible.
   Protects patient comfort and privacy.

5. **Before beginning the flow** of irrigation solution, empty any urine from the drainage bag, and perform hand hygiene. Document the volume on the I&O record.
   Starting the procedure with an empty draining bag gives you a baseline for correct calculation of true urine output during irrigation. The I&O record provides data for evaluating fluid balance and urinary system function.

6. **Scrub the irrigation port** with antiseptic swabs or wipes.
   To remove microorganisms and help prevent UTI.

7. **Connect the irrigation tubing** to the catheter port.

(continued on next page)

Procedure 30-8 ■ **Irrigating the Bladder or Catheter** (continued)

8. **Slowly open the roller clamp** on the irrigation tubing to the desired flow rate.
   Slow instillation prevents patient discomfort.

9. **Instill or irrigate** with the prescribed amount of irrigant. If the irrigant is to remain in the bladder for a certain time period, clamp the drainage tubing for that time.

10. **When the correct amount** of irrigant has been used and/or the goals of the irrigation have been met, close the roller clamp on the irrigation tubing, leaving the tubing connected to the catheter for use during the next irrigation.
    You can assess whether the goals of irrigation have been met by inspecting the color of the urine and assessing for clots, mucus, or blood. Clamping the drainage tubing prevents immediate outflow.

11. **Remove gloves,** perform hand hygiene, and return the patient to a position of comfort.

Procedure Variation **Two-Way Indwelling Catheter**

12. **Don clean procedure gloves.** Empty any urine currently found in the bedside drainage bag.
    Emptying the bag will ensure accurate output results.

13. **Perform hand hygiene** and then apply clean gloves.
    To prevent the transmission of microorganisms

14. **Drape the patient** so that only the specimen removal port on the drainage tubing is exposed. Place a sterile waterproof drape beneath the exposed port.
    Ensures patient privacy and prevents soiling of the bed linens.

♥ **iCare 15. Open the sterile irrigation** supplies. Pour approximately 100 mL of the irrigating solution, warmed to room temperature, into the sterile container, using aseptic technique.
Warm solution is more comfortable to the patient. Aseptic technique helps prevent UTI.

16. **Scrub all surfaces** of the specimen removal port with antiseptic swab.
    Cleaning the port reduces the risk of transmission of pathogens into the bladder.

17. **Draw up irrigation solution** into the syringe. Connect the syringe to the specimen port. For catheter irrigation, use a total of 30 to 40 mL; for bladder irrigation, the amount is usually 100 to 200 mL.

18. **Clamp or pinch the drainage** tubing distal to the specimen port.
    Clamping prevents irrigant from draining into the drainage bag instead of into the catheter and/or bladder.

19. **Inject the solution into the port.** Hold the specimen port slightly above the level of the bladder. If you meet resistance, have the patient turn slightly, and attempt a second time. If resistance continues, stop the procedure and notify the primary care provider.
    Holding the port above the level of the bladder enhances gravitational flow of irrigant into the bladder. Resistance might indicate trauma to the mucosa tissue or surgical site. ➤

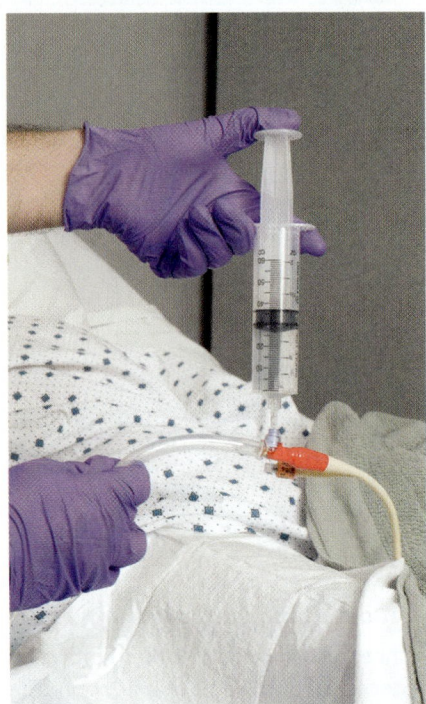

20. **When the irrigant has been** injected, remove syringe. Refill the syringe if necessary.

21. **Unclamp or release the drainage** tubing and allow the irrigant and urine to flow into the bedside drainage bag by gravity. (If the solution is to remain in the bladder for a prescribed time, leave the tubing clamped for that time period.)

22. **Repeat the procedure** as necessary until the prescribed amount has been instilled or until the goal of the irrigation is met (e.g., removal of clots and mucus, free-flowing urine).

23. **Remove gloves, perform hand hygiene,** and return the patient to a position of comfort with call device within reach.

Procedure 30-8B ■ Continuous Bladder Irrigation

➤ When performing the procedure, always identify your patient according to agency policy, using two identifiers, and be attentive to standard precautions, hand hygiene, patient safety and privacy, body mechanics, and documentation.

Procedure Steps

1. **If one is not already present,** insert a three-way (triple-lumen) indwelling catheter.
   A triple-lumen catheter provides an access for the irrigation solution without disrupting the sterile drainage unit.

2. **Prepare the irrigation fluid** and tubing by warming it to room temperature.
   a. Close the clamp on the connecting tubing.
      This prevents the introduction of microorganisms into the solution.
   b. Spike the tubing into the port on the irrigation solution container, using aseptic technique.
      Prevents introduction of microorganisms into the solution.
   c. Invert the container and hang it on the IV pole.
      The elevated bag allows the solution to flow by gravity.
   d. Remove the protective cap from the distal end of the connecting tubing. Hold the end of the tubing over a sink or other receptacle. Open the roll clamp slowly and allow the solution to fill the tubing completely. Recap the tubing.
      Priming the tubing flushes air from tubing, preventing bladder distension.

3. **Perform hand hygiene** and don clean procedure gloves.
   To prevent the spread of microorganisms.

4. **Place the patient supine** and drape her so that only the connection port on the indwelling catheter is visible.
   Provides privacy and expresses caring.

5. **Place a waterproof** drape under the irrigation port. Scrub the irrigation port with antiseptic swabs or wipes. Pinching the tubing and using aseptic technique, connect the end of the irrigation infusion tubing to the side port of the catheter.

6. **Before beginning the flow** of irrigation solution, empty any urine that is in the bedside drainage bag, and document the volume on the I&O record.
   Starting the procedure with an empty bag gives you a baseline for correct calculation of true urine output during irrigation. The I&O record provides data for evaluating urinary status.

7. **Cover the patient** and return him to a position of comfort with a call device within reach.

8. **Open the roller clamp** on the tubing and regulate the flow of the irrigation solution to meet the desired outcome for the irrigation.
   The goal of continuous bladder irrigation for patients who have had a transurethral resection of the prostate is to keep the urine light pink to clear. ▼

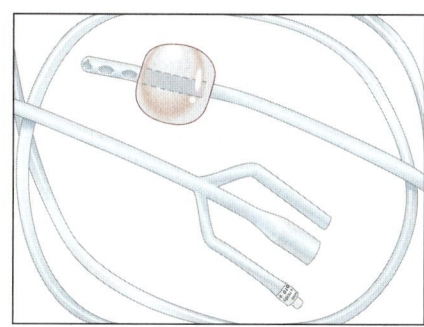

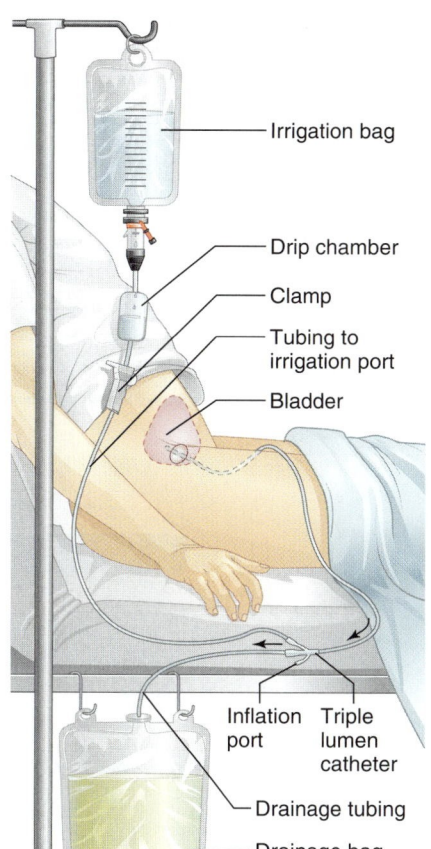

Irrigation bag

Drip chamber

Clamp

Tubing to irrigation port

Bladder

Inflation port | Triple lumen catheter

Drainage tubing

Drainage bag

9. **Discard used supplies.** Remove gloves and perform hand hygiene.

10. **Monitor the flow rate** for 1 to 2 minutes to ensure accuracy.
    Infusing irrigation fluid for a minute or two prevents rapid introduction of solution into the bladder, which would cause patient discomfort.

? What if . . .

- **The draining irrigant solution and/or urine appears to have red blood cells in it?**
  Stop the irrigation and report to the primary care provider.
  Increased red blood cells in the urine may indicate bladder irritation and possible trauma to the inner mucosal lining of the bladder.

- **You meet resistance when irrigating?**
  Ask the patient to turn slightly, and attempt a second time. If resistance continues, stop the procedure and notify the primary care provider.

(continued on next page)

Procedure 30-8 ■ Irrigating the Bladder or Catheter (continued)

Evaluation

- Note the flow rate of irrigant and/or inability to instill irrigant into the catheter.
- Note the characteristics of urine output (e.g., presence of output, color, amount, clots, mucus).
- Note patient report of discomfort (e.g., pain, spasms).
- Assess for development of bladder distention accompanied by lack of urine outflow. A portable bladder scanner may be used to quantify the amount of fluid retained in the bladder.

Home Care

For patients who will have continuous bladder irrigation at home, you will need to teach the family the necessary steps of the procedure. Also teach them to:

- Empty the urine collection device before beginning the procedure.
- Use strict aseptic technique when irrigating the bladder or catheter, and not disconnect the catheter and drainage tube.
- Irrigate the catheter using the closed method, which carries the least risk for introducing bacteria into the bladder. The catheter and drainage tubing should never be disconnected.
- Identify signs and symptoms of urinary retention and UTI.
- Wash their hands before and after any manipulation of the catheter site or apparatus.
- Be certain there are no kinks in the tubing to maintain unobstructed flow.
- For the syringe method, the patient will need access to syringes and needleless access devices and a process to dispose of them properly.

Documentation

Record the following:

- Date and time of procedure, type of irrigant, the total volume infused.
- Characteristics of the urine (e.g., color, odor, clarity, sediment, presence of clots or mucus).
- Evidence of catheter patency (e.g., flow of urine, absence of distention).

Sample documentation

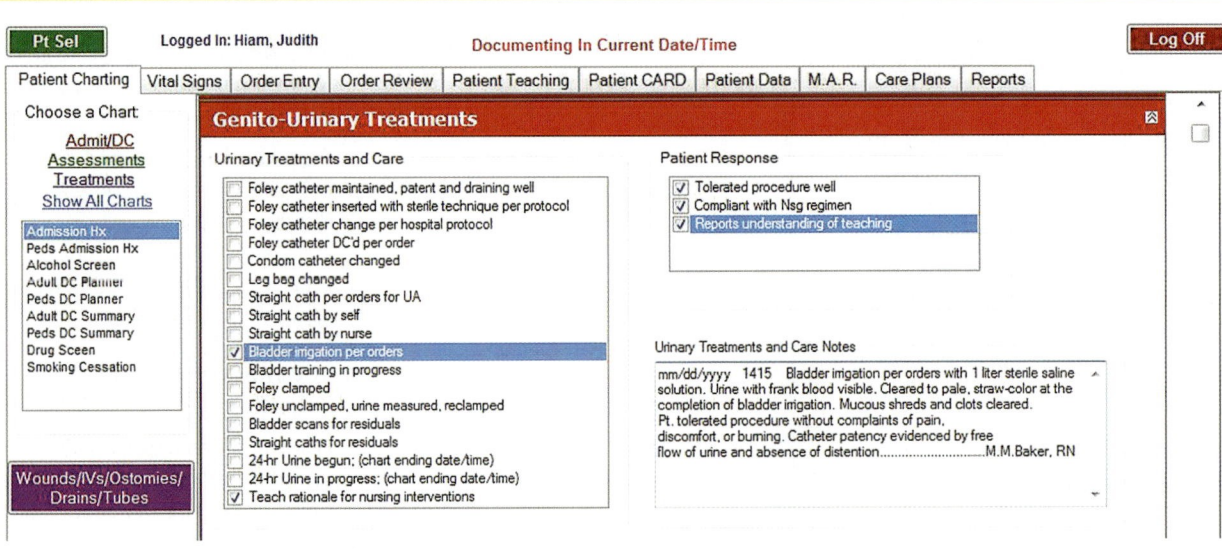

Practice Resources

Hagen, S., Sinclair, L., & Cross, S. (2010); Hooton, T. M., Bradley, S. F., Cardenas, D. D., et al. (2010); Wound, Ostomy, and Continence Nurses Society (2009).

Thinking About the Procedure

To practice applying clinical reasoning to this procedure,

 The videos **Intermittent Bladder Irrigation: Three-Way (Triple-Lumen) Indwelling Catheter, Intermittent Bladder Irrigation: Two-Way Indwelling Catheter,** and **Continuous Bladder Irrigation,** along with questions and suggested responses, is available on the **Davis's** *Nursing Skills Videos* Web site on Davis*Plus*.

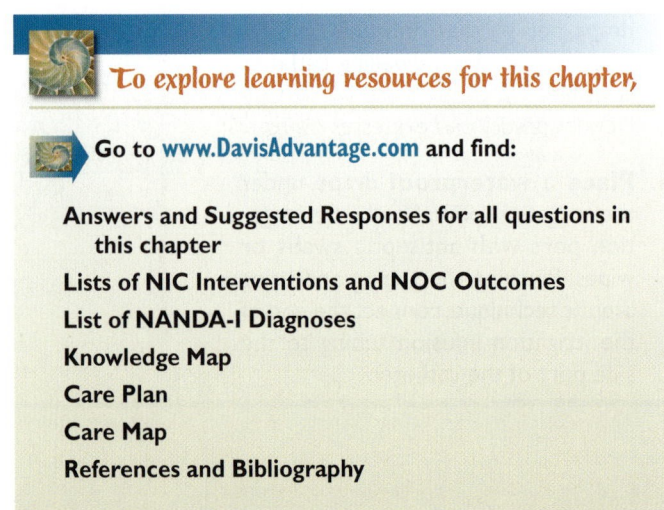

To explore learning resources for this chapter,

Go to **www.DavisAdvantage.com** and find:

Answers and Suggested Responses for all questions in this chapter

Lists of NIC Interventions and NOC Outcomes

List of NANDA-I Diagnoses

Knowledge Map

Care Plan

Care Map

References and Bibliography

Concept Map

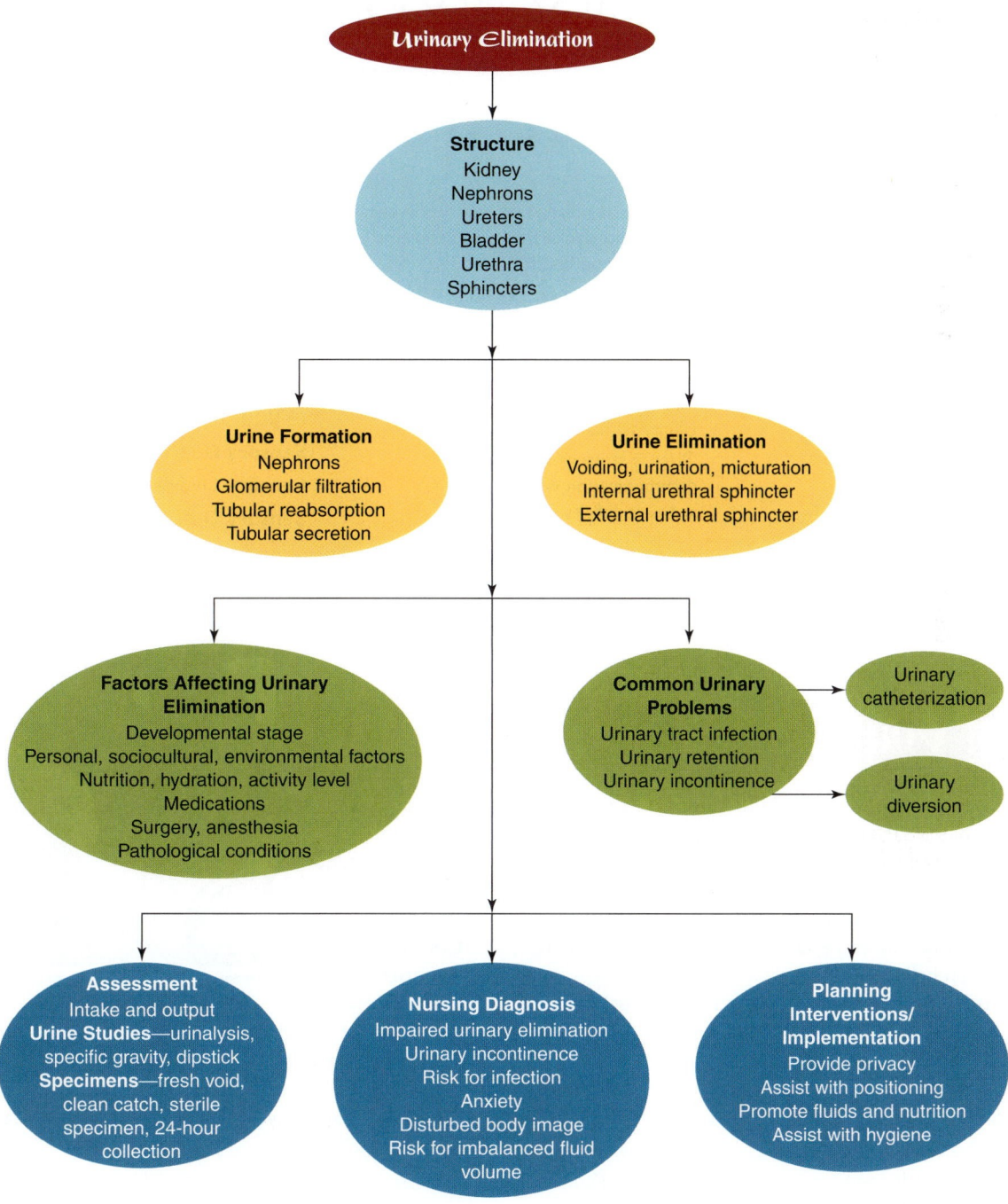

Urinary Elimination

Structure
Kidney
Nephrons
Ureters
Bladder
Urethra
Sphincters

Urine Formation
Nephrons
Glomerular filtration
Tubular reabsorption
Tubular secretion

Urine Elimination
Voiding, urination, micturation
Internal urethral sphincter
External urethral sphincter

Factors Affecting Urinary Elimination
Developmental stage
Personal, sociocultural, environmental factors
Nutrition, hydration, activity level
Medications
Surgery, anesthesia
Pathological conditions

Common Urinary Problems
Urinary tract infection
Urinary retention
Urinary incontinence

Urinary catheterization

Urinary diversion

Assessment
Intake and output
Urine Studies—urinalysis, specific gravity, dipstick
Specimens—fresh void, clean catch, sterile specimen, 24-hour collection

Nursing Diagnosis
Impaired urinary elimination
Urinary incontinence
Risk for infection
Anxiety
Disturbed body image
Risk for imbalanced fluid volume

Planning Interventions/ Implementation
Provide privacy
Assist with positioning
Promote fluids and nutrition
Assist with hygiene

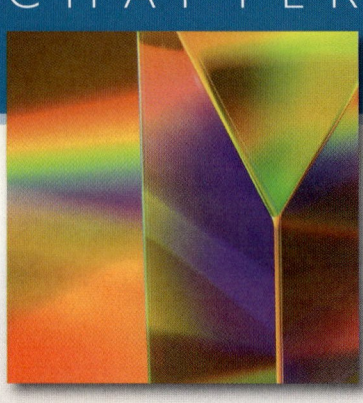

CHAPTER 31

Sensory Perception

Learning Outcomes

After completing this chapter, you should be able to:

➤ Identify the components of the sensory experience.

➤ Compare and contrast sensory deprivation and sensory overload.

➤ List factors placing clients at risk for altered sensory perception.

➤ Discuss the hazards of sensory deficits in vision, hearing, taste, smell, touch, and proprioception.

➤ Identify factors that affect sensory stimulation.

➤ Assess clients for signs and symptoms of altered sensory perception.

➤ State nursing diagnoses and outcomes appropriate for clients with problems of sensory perception.

➤ Plan and implement nursing interventions to prevent sensory deprivation and sensory overload.

➤ Plan and implement nursing interventions to meet the needs of clients with sensory deficits.

➤ Discuss strategies to enhance communication with clients with sensory deficits.

Key Concepts

Perception

Reception

Sensation

Related Concepts

See the Concept Map at the end of this chapter.

Example Problems

Sensory Deprivation

Sensory Overload

Sensory Deficits

Meet Your Patients

- Joshua is a 28-year-old patient in the intensive care unit (ICU). He had a car accident 3 weeks ago and has had several surgeries to repair a fractured femur, ruptured spleen, and intracranial bleeding. He was ventilated mechanically for 10 days and has had numerous invasive procedures. The nurses report that he is very confused and has been hallucinating.

- Richard is a 90-year-old man who has been a resident at a skilled nursing facility for 10 years. He has no visitors, never leaves his room, has no television or radio in the room, and no longer speaks. He does not respond to verbal or tactile stimulation. He lies in bed in a fetal position. When staff members try to move him, he moans and howls.

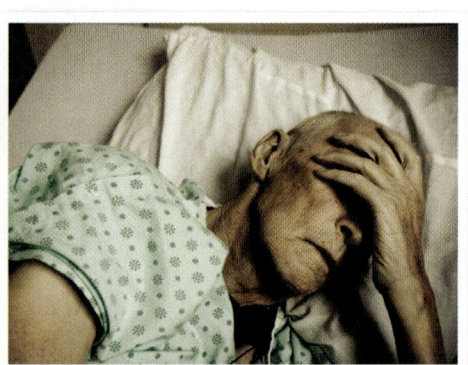

Consider how these patients are similar and how their care might overlap. It seems hard to imagine that these patients could have much in common. What similarities can you see? What differences? After you read this chapter, see if you answer these questions in the same way.

TheoreticalKnowledge
knowing why

We experience the world through our senses. Vision, hearing, smell, taste, touch, movement, and our sense of our body in space—all help us to interpret and interact with our environment in a meaningful way. To grow, develop, and function, we must be able to sense and respond to sensory input. As a nurse, you will likely care for patients with sensory deficits, regardless of the type of unit you work on.

- **Preexisting sensory deficit.** Many patients who are being treated for an unrelated condition also have a preexisting sensory deficit (e.g., you may need to teach self-injection to a diabetic client who is blind).
- **Sensory deficit caused by illness or medication.** Still other patients develop alterations in sensory function as a result of their illness or of medications they are taking.

The Joint Commission (2010) requires that you address the communication needs of patients with vision, speech, hearing, language, and cognitive impairments. This chapter will help you provide care for such patients.

ABOUT THE KEY CONCEPTS

To best meet patients' needs, you will need to understand how the concepts of **sensation, reception,** and **perception** influence their sensory experience. In this section, you will also learn about related concepts, including those needed to plan and implement care for sensory deprivation, overload, or deficits.

COMPONENTS OF THE SENSORY EXPERIENCE

The purpose of sensation is to allow the body to respond to changing situations and maintain homeostasis. A sensory experience involves four components in the nervous system: stimulus, reception, perception, and an arousal mechanism.

Stimulus

A **stimulus** may be a sight, sound, taste, touch, pain, or anything that stimulates a nerve receptor. The brain must receive and process it to make it meaningful.

Reception

Reception is the process of receiving stimuli from nerve endings in the skin and inside the body. A receptor converts a stimulus to a nerve impulse and transmits the impulse along sensory neurons to the central nervous system (CNS).

Adaptation Some receptors remain activated for as long as the stimulus is applied. However, most receptors *adapt* to stimuli; that is, their response declines with time. Adaptation explains why, over time, you become unaware of an unpleasant smell or the persistent hum of an air conditioner.

Specialized Receptors Receptors usually respond to only one type of stimulus. For example, taste buds in the mouth detect sweet, sour, salty, savory, or bitter, whereas receptors in the retina detect light rays. The following are examples of the many types of sensory receptors in the body:

- *Mechanoreceptors* in the skin and hair follicles detect touch, pressure, and vibration.
- *Hair cells* are receptors for hearing. Located in the cochlea of the ear, they detect sound waves. In the vestibular apparatus of the ear, receptors for equilibrium and balance also detect acceleration of the body and position of the head.
- *Thermoreceptors* in the skin detect variations in temperature.
- *Proprioceptors* in the skin, muscles, tendons, ligaments, and joint capsules coordinate input to enable us to sense the position of our body in space (proprioception).
- *Photoreceptors* located in the retina of the eyes detect visible light.
- *Chemoreceptors* for taste are located in our taste buds. *Olfactory receptors* (chemoreceptors for smell) are located in the epithelium of the nasal cavity.

Perception

Perception is the ability to interpret the impulses transmitted from the receptors and give meaning to the stimuli. When stimulated, the receptors generate nerve impulses that travel along neural pathways to the spinal cord and brain. They are then relayed to specialized locations in the brain where perception and awareness of the stimuli occurs (Fig. 31-1). For example, vision is perceived in the occipital lobes, hearing in the temporal lobes, and touch in the somatosensory area.

It is not possible to process all the stimuli that constantly bombard us, so the brain discards most sensory information as

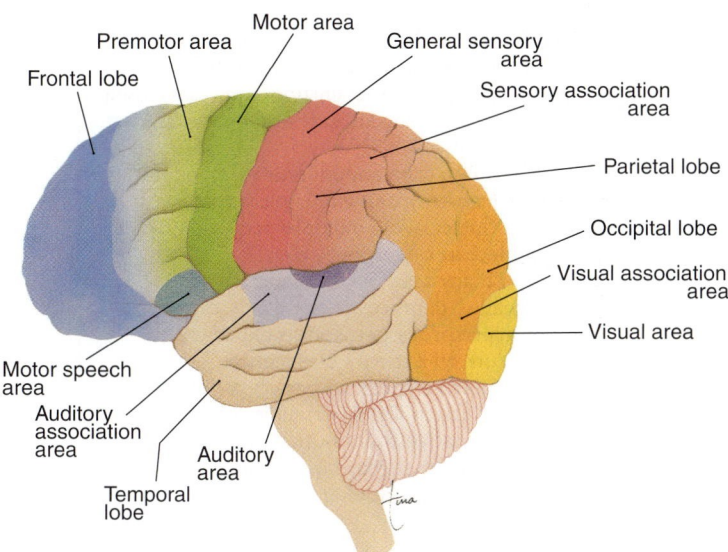

FIGURE 31-1 Special sensory areas of the brain receive and interpret stimuli from the sensory receptors.

irrelevant and unimportant. For example, you are usually unaware of your clothing touching your body. However, if you focus on it, you can feel it.

Perception of a stimulus is affected by *past experiences, knowledge,* and *attitude* as well as the following factors:
- *Location* of the receptors and pathway activated
- *Number* of receptors activated
- *Frequency* of action potentials generated (which varies according to the intensity of the stimulus)
- *Changes* in location, number, and frequency

Arousal Mechanism

For the central nervous system to perceive, interpret, and react to incoming stimuli, it must be *active*. The **reticular activating system (RAS),** located in the brainstem, controls consciousness and alertness. The neurons of the RAS make connections between the spinal cord, cerebellum, thalamus, and cerebral cortex. These connections relay visual, auditory, and other stimuli that help keep us awake, attentive, and observant.

Without such stimuli, the CNS becomes lethargic, and the person may lose consciousness. Anesthesia, sedatives, opioids, and some other drugs depress the RAS, as does a darkened, quiet environment. Not surprisingly, as you will learn in Chapter 35, sleep is regulated by the RAS (see Fig. 35-4). The following are two important points to consider:
- **The level of stimuli needed to maintain arousal varies.** Some people feel optimally alert in bright, noisy, fast-paced environments, whereas others prefer much lower levels of stimulation.
- **The brain adapts to constant stimuli,** such as a ticking clock. Thus, to maintain arousal, some variation in stimuli is required, such as different pieces of music or an ever-changing view.

Responding to Sensations

Once a stimulus is perceived, the brain either (1) discards it, (2) stores it in memory, or (3) sends impulses along motor pathways to various parts of the body (e.g., the muscles, the heart),

---

♥ iCare 31-1

Promoting Adaptation to the Hospital Environment

Changes in any aspect of the sensory experience can be unsettling for patients. Changes may involve sensory deprivation or sensory overload. Recognizing and addressing fear and anxiety exhibit a caring attitude and promote trust between patient and nurse.
- Approach a patient in a calm and reassuring manner.
- Promote a stress-free environment: Limit noise, adjust lighting, eliminate clutter, avoid multiple people gathering or tasks to complete at one time
- Assist persons with any assistive devices such as eyeglasses, eye shades, dentures, hearing aids, or gloves to facilitate optimal sensory perception experiences.
- Control temperature to patient's preference.
- Allow the patient time to speak and express concerns.
- Explore therapeutic touch if the person is receptive.
- Consider using alternative therapy, such as music therapy or pet therapy that may be soothing and comforting to the patient (Hooker, Freeman, & Stewart, 2002).

---

bringing about a response. Humans respond to sensations when they are alert and receptive to stimulation. For example, a fatigued new mother may wake up to the soft cry of her infant yet sleep through the persistent ringing of the doorbell. The response to a stimulus is based on the following factors:

Intensity An intense stimulus excites more receptors, leading to a stronger response. For example, a bright, glaring light can cause you to respond by squinting and shielding your eyes, whereas a dim light may cause little reaction.

Contrast Imagine being outside in cold, windy weather. If you enter an unheated garage, you instantly feel warmer because the building blocks the wind. If you then go inside a room with a blazing fireplace, you will need to take off layers of clothing rapidly because the contrast in temperature will make you feel hot.

Adaptation Often we take familiar stimuli for granted. Recall your first clinical experience. Did you notice the noise and activity on the unit? Nurses become accustomed to the noise, lights, activity, and even alarms and are able to "tune them out." These stimuli are all new to patients, so they notice them and may have difficulty resting.

Previous Experience with a stimulus affects ongoing responses to the same stimulus. Have you ever seen a patient scrunch her eyes, grit her teeth, or turn away from an injection before you are even ready to give it? This may mean that she has memory of a prior negative experience with injections.

KnowledgeCheck 31-1
- What is the difference between reception and perception?
- What are the four components of a sensory experience?
- What is the role of the reticular activating system in the sensory experience?

FACTORS AFFECTING SENSORY FUNCTION

This section will describe the effects of developmental variations, culture, illness and medications, stress, and personality and lifestyle.

Developmental Variations

Sensory perceptual abilities change throughout a person's life stages. In addition, the need and use for sensory stimulation differs throughout life.

Newborns
- Newborns can track objects and respond to light, but their *vision* is far less acute than that of older children and adults.
- Their *hearing* is especially acute at low frequencies.
- Newborns can discriminate among different *tastes,* and they prefer sweet over sour.
- They react to odors and seem to be able to discriminate between the *smell* of their own mother's breast milk and that of another woman.
- The sense of *touch* is keenly present at birth; the face, hands, and soles of the feet are the most sensitive (Polan & Taylor, 2015).

Infants Infants require sensory stimulation to grow and develop normally.
- *Tactile stimulation.* Through cuddling, feeding, and soothing, tactile stimulation creates a bond between infant and caregivers, provides comfort and pleasure, and teaches the infant about the external environment.

- *Auditory stimulation.* Exposure to voices, music, and ambient noise develops the auditory nervous system. By age 1 year, the child can discriminate between different sounds and often recognizes the source.
- *Visual stimulation.* Lights, colors, and contrast allow the infant to observe the world in which she lives.

Children and Adolescents

- *Vision.* In early childhood, visual acuity improves; full depth perception is achieved during the preschool period.
- *Hearing.* Although hearing is usually fully developed in young children, they may experience reversible hearing loss as a result of frequent ear infections and cerumen impaction.
- *Psychomotor skills.* In contrast to toddlers, who often lose their balance when walking, older children are sure and steady on their feet.
- *Social interaction.* During the school-age years and adolescence, children are developmentally driven toward peers, and the increased social interaction provides a wealth of sensory stimulation.

Adults and Older Adults
By early adulthood, senses function at their peak acuity, unless they are affected by illness or injury.

 As the adult ages, all of the senses are affected (see Table 31-1). Older adults experience a generalized decrease in the number of nerve conduction fibers, resulting in slower reflexes and delayed response to stimuli. Structural changes also occur in the aging eye and ear. Sensory decline with aging may cause withdrawal, depression, social isolation, and hallucinations. Keep in mind that aging is not the only cause of sensory deficits in older adults.

Culture
Culture affects the nature, type, and amount of interaction and stimulation with which people feel comfortable. People of different cultural backgrounds tend to prefer differing amounts of eye contact, personal space, and physical touch. For example, you consider how your hospitalized patient may need quiet time alone to rest. However, if he is accustomed to being surrounded by a large family, he may actually rest better in the midst of what seems like chaos to you. Use touch advisedly, however. For some people, it is comforting; for others, it may be an offensive stimulus.

Illness and Medications

- Neurological disorders, such as multiple sclerosis, slow the transmission of nerve impulses.
- Diseases that affect circulation (e.g., atherosclerosis) may impair function of the sensory receptors and the brain, thereby altering perception and response.
- Reduced or lack of oxygen (anoxia) harms and even destroys cells, causing widespread damage to the neurological system.

Table 31-1 ➤ Sensory Function Changes With Aging	
SENSE	**CHANGES ASSOCIATED WITH AGING**
Vision	▪ The vitreous humor becomes thinner and "floaters" appear in the visual field. ▪ The lens becomes discolored and opaque; the pupil becomes smaller. Therefore, less light reaches the retina, limiting vision. ▪ The lens becomes less flexible and less able to focus on near objects. ▪ The ciliary body contracts and the lens thickens, bringing loss of visual acuity, decreased ability to accommodate to distance and sudden changes in illumination, and decreased night vision. ▪ Peripheral vision decreases. ▪ Tear production decreases.
Hearing	▪ Cerumen becomes drier and more solid, creating hearing loss. ▪ Scarring may occur. ▪ Presbycusis (hearing loss of high-frequency tones) and diminished speech discrimination may occur.
Taste	▪ Taste buds atrophy and decrease in number, reducing the ability to perceive tastes, especially sweetness. ▪ Dry mouth may alter the sense of taste. ▪ Saliva production may decrease.
Smell	▪ Atrophy and loss of olfactory neurons decrease the ability to perceive smell (which may also alter the sense of taste).
Touch	▪ Loss of sensory nerve fibers and changes in the cerebral cortex decrease the ability to perceive light touch, pain, and temperature variations.
Kinesthesia	▪ Kinesthetic changes include a decrease in muscle fibers and diminished conduction speed of nerve fibers, resulting in slowed reaction time, decreased speed and power of muscle contractions, and impaired balance. ▪ There is an increased risk for falling.

- Some conditions affect specific sensory organs. For example:
  - *Diabetic retinopathy* is the leading cause of blindness among adults.
  - *Sickle cell disease,* like *diabetes,* causes new blood vessels to grow in the eye and pull on the retina, causing a retinal detachment.
  - *Hypertension* can also damage the retina of the eyes by hemorrhaging or depriving the retina with vital nourishment and oxygen.
  - *Toxoplasmosis* leads to vision loss; the infection may be acquired by the fetus during pregnancy, and throughout life.
- Physiological injury to the brain may occur from trauma, as follows:
  - *Closed head injury* (e.g., acute concussion) occurs when brain tissue is compressed from bleeding, bruising, fluid, or increased pressure inside the skull—for example, after a fall.
  - *Penetrating injury* occurs when a foreign object enters into the brain, resulting in damage to the brain tissue or structure.
- Medications that cross the blood brain barrier affect neurological or sensory function by damaging brain cells (Box 31-1). For example:
  - *Aspirin* and *furosemide* (Lasix) become ototoxic if taken for a long period of time and impair function of the auditory nerve.
  - *CNS depressants,* such as opioid analgesics and sedatives, blunt reception and perception of stimuli.

Stress

Physical illness, pain, hospitalization, tests, and surgery are all stressors that can lead to sensory overload—more stimuli than the person can handle. Joshua (Meet Your Patients) has been under tremendous physical and emotional stress as a result of his injuries and surgeries. His situation is one in which you might want to limit unnecessary stimuli (e.g., noise, lights, too many visitors).

BOX 31-1 ■ Medications That Cause Taste Disturbance

Numerous medications can cause a foul or metallic taste. This unpleasant side effect can result from medication taken orally, intramuscularly, or IV.

- Antibiotics (metronidazole, rifampin, clarithromycin, tetracycline)
- Anticonvulsants (phenytoin and carbamazepine)
- Antihistamines and decongestants
- Antihypertensive (captopril) and cardiac medications (angiotensin-converting enzyme inhibitors)
- Antiretroviral drugs (indinavir)
- Antithyroid medication
- Carbon anhydrase inhibitors, used to treat glaucoma (acetazolamide, methazolamide)
- Chemotherapy agents (procarbazine, vinblastine, vincristine, dacarbazine)
- Lithium carbonate
- Antipsychotics
- Antidepressants
- Statins
- Muscle relaxants (methocarbamol)

Personality and Lifestyle

Are you the kind of person who likes to have people around all the time? Do you thrive on noise and action? Or are you the kind of person who loves to curl up with a book and a cup of tea? Clients, too, vary in their personalities and lifestyles. Some people, by nature, like excitement, change, and stimulation; others prefer a more predictable and quiet life. Clients are at risk for sensory alterations if their previous level of stimuli does not match their current level. Health problems, a new environment, or loss of a partner can each create changes in stimuli.

KnowledgeCheck 31-2

- List five major factors that affect sensory function.
- Compare and contrast the sensory changes in childhood with those in older adulthood.

SENSORY ALTERATIONS

Humans are constantly striving to achieve **sensoristasis,** a state of optimal arousal. Sensory alterations occur when the body experiences meaningless or limited stimulation (**sensory deprivation**), excessive stimulation (**sensory overload**), or **sensory deficits.**

Example Problem: Sensory Deprivation

Sensory deprivation is common among hospitalized patients, elderly, and ill or injured people in the community. It occurs as a result of altered sensory reception in which the person does not receive and process adequate sensory input because of disruption or dysfunction with the nervous system, such as spinal cord injury, CNS disease, or brain damage. Deprived environments (isolation, immobility) can also lead to understimulation of the nervous system. See the Example Problem: Sensory Deprivation.

Example Problem: Sensory Overload

The complex sensory environment within the hospital can contribute to sensory overload. Monitor alarms, interruptions in rest and sleep by healthcare providers, medical therapies and procedures, patient care routines, and various odors, sounds, sights, and pain experiences can overwhelm the senses of patients in unfamiliar environments, such as the hospital. Sensory overload are described further in the Example Problem: Sensory Overload, later in the chapter.

KnowledgeCheck 31-3

- How does sensory deprivation occur?
- Identify five signs of sensory deprivation.
- How does sensory overload occur?
- Identify five signs of sensory overload.

ThinkLike a Nurse 31-1

Review the stories of Joshua and Richard (Meet Your Patients). How are these patients similar? What factors may have contributed to each patient's current concerns?

Example Problem: Sensory Deficits

Sensory deficits may stem from impaired reception, impaired perception, or both. Impaired vision and hearing are the two sensory deficits that you are most likely to encounter in

EXAMPLE PROBLEM: Sensory Deprivation

Definition: Sensory Deprivation is a state of RAS depression caused by a lack of meaningful input. When external stimuli are deficient, the remaining stimuli, such as distant noises, minor pain, and cold extremities, can become overly noticeable or distorted, filling in the "sensory gap" and causing the patient a level of distress that is greater than the intensity of the stimulus. **Complications** include depression, withdrawal, noncompliance, confusion, and ICU psychosis.

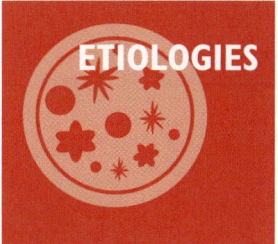

ETIOLOGIES

Risk Factors

- Impaired sensory reception (neurological injury, dementia, depression, sleep deprivation, CNS-depressant medications)
- Nerve or brain injury
- Restricted mobility
- Sensory deficits (blindness, deafness)

- Quiet, monotonous environment (homebound, disabled, and older people; hospitalized patients in isolation or private rooms)
- Unable to interpret language, social cues, and interactions

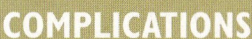

COMPLICATIONS

Depression
Withdrawal

Poor patient compliance
Confusion, ICU psychosis

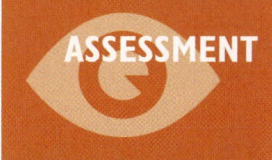

ASSESSMENT

Assess for symptoms of Sensory Deprivation:
- Irritability
- Reduced attention span
- Decreased problem-solving skills
- Drowsiness

- Preoccupation with somatic complaints
- Delusions, hallucinations
See the Focused Assessment box, Nursing History: Sensory Perceptual Status.

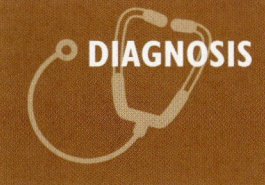

DIAGNOSIS

NANDA-I Diagnoses

- Ineffective Activity Planning
- Acute Confusion; Chronic Confusion
- Impaired Verbal Communication

- Decreased Diversional Activity
- Risk for Loneliness, Social isolation

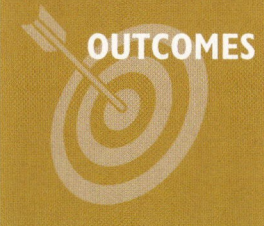

OUTCOMES

Individualized Outcome Statements

- Compensates for visual impairment by maximizing use of touch, smell, and hearing.
- Eats nutritious food even if taste is altered.

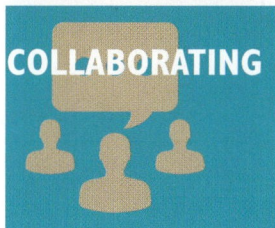

COLLABORATING

- Communicate the plan for care with caregivers and healthcare team.
- Monitor the use of sedatives.

- Music therapy, activities, physical therapy, speech therapy, nutritional therapy, and occupational therapy may all be valuable in the care of the client.

(Continued)

EXAMPLE PROBLEM: Sensory Deprivation—cont'd

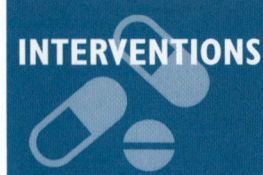

INTERVENTIONS

Visual Stimulation

- Help patient to put on clean eyeglasses when awake.
- Put personal items on the walls and place photos or flowers where the patient can see them.
- Open blinds during the day, except when patient is sleeping.

Auditory Stimulation

- Help the patient with a hearing aid to apply it whenever awake. Be sure it has working batteries and the alarm is set at an appropriate volume.
- When possible, move to a distraction-free area when communicating with the patient.

Olfactory Stimulation

- Offer pleasant smells or aromatherapy to help stimulate appetite.

Tactile Stimulation

- Use touch carefully in patient-care activities. People respond differently to physical contact.
- You might hold a patient's hand while talking or provide a back rub.
- Gentle hand massage may be calming.

Facilitating Communication

- Develop alternative methods of communication for the patient with aphasia; those who speak another language; or those who have difficulty hearing (communication board, mobile tablet, writing tools).
- Hang a message board in the room and ask family members to post photos, cards, or notes.
- Offer devices for messaging, electronic communication, and social media.

Promoting Adequate Sleep and Rest

- Schedule care to allow for uninterrupted periods of sleep and rest and to provide advance notice of what the client is to expect during the day.

Promoting Social Interaction

- Make regular contact with the patient. Introduce yourself and address the patient by name.
- Provide continuity of care by assigning the same staff whenever possible.
- Encourage patients to participate in scheduled activities.
- Assist acute care patient out of bed for meals or visitors.
- Encourage patients to leave their rooms when possible.
- Clients may play video games with others online.
- Ensure that a patient in isolation receives adequate stimulation from healthcare team, family members, or visitors.

Minimizing Anxiety & Confusion

- Place clock and calendar in patient's view.
- Encourage families to familiar objects from home.
- Introduce yourself and inform the patient of the plan for care with a calm, respectful approach.
- Explain all procedures and care.

Pet Therapy

Many facilities allow resident pets or pet visits to promote socialization, lower B/P, and reduce loneliness and pain.

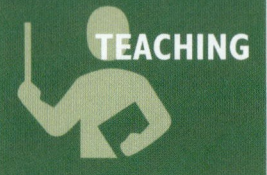

TEACHING

Teach during times when patient is able to concentrate.

Teach stress reduction techniques.

Complementary & Alternative Modalities (CAM)

Essential Oils

Aromatherapy is the use of naturally extracted aromatic essences from plants to balance, harmonize, and promote the health of body, mind, and spirit. It is a natural, noninvasive treatment system designed to affect the whole person, not just the symptom or disease. Essential oils are thought to work by promoting the body's natural ability to balance, regulate, heal, and maintain itself. Some oils may be used topically in certain situations (e.g., minor burns).

➤ **Eucalyptus, *Eucalyptus globulus* or *Eucalyptus radiata.*** Helpful in treating respiratory problems, such as coughs, colds, and asthma. Used to treat burns, wounds, and insect bites. Also helps to boost the immune system and relieve muscle tension.

➤ **Ylang-ylang, *Cananga odorata.*** Promotes relaxation and can reduce muscle tension. Good antidepressant. Used to counteract anxiety, hypertension, and stress.

➤ **Geranium, *Pelargonium graveolens.*** Helps to balance hormones in women. Can be both relaxing and uplifting, as well as an antidepressant. Used to control acne and oily skin.

➤ **Peppermint, *Mentha piperita.*** Used in treating headaches, sinusitis, vertigo, muscle aches, asthma, and digestive disorders such as slow digestion, indigestion, nausea, and flatulence.

➤ **Lavender, *Lavandula angustifolia.*** Relaxing; also useful in skin care and treating wounds and burns and relieving itching. Used to reduce asthma, labor pains, colic, anxiety, and dysmenorrhea.

➤ **Lemon, *Citrus limonum.*** Uplifting, yet relaxing. Helpful in treating wounds and infections and useful for house cleaning and deodorizing. Sometimes used to treat athlete's foot, colds, and warts.

➤ **Clary sage, *Salvia sclarea.*** Natural pain killer, helpful in treating amenorrhea and muscular aches and pains. Relaxing, and can help with insomnia. Used to balance hormones and treat sore throat, stress, and exhaustion.

➤ **Tea tree, *Melaleuca alternifolia.*** A natural antifungal oil, good for treating fungal infections including vaginal yeast infections, fungal infections, and ringworm. Used for insect bites, itching, and migraine. Also helps to boost the immune system.

➤ **Roman chamomile, *Anthemus nobilis.*** Relaxing; can help with sleeplessness and anxiety. Also good for muscle aches, arthritis, and tension. Useful in treating wounds and infection, insomnia, nausea, premenstrual syndrome (PMS), and earache.

➤ **Rosemary, *Rosmarinus officinalis.*** Uplifting and promotes mental stimulation. Also stimulating to the immune, circulatory, and digestive systems. Good for muscle aches and tension.

PICOT

Sensory Overload in the ICU

Situation: The nurse is caring for a client with an impulse control disorder who is admitted to the ICU after sustaining traumatic injuries from motorcycle accident. The client has a history of violent outbursts; the nursing team is meeting with a psychiatric social worker to develop an appropriate plan of care.

PICOT Components:

P	Population/patient	=	Hospitalized patients with impulse control disorder
I	Intervention/indicator	=	Sensory overload in ICU
C	Comparator/control	=	Patients without a psychiatric history
O	Outcome	=	Violent behavior
T	Time	=	During hospitalization

Searchable Question: Do _____ (P) who are _____ (I) demonstrate _____ (O) as compared to _____ (C) during _____ (T)?

Example of Evidence: Clients with a psychiatric history who are admitted to the acute medical facility pose special challenges for the nursing staff. Priorities include ensuring safety for this client and others, including healthcare staff. Initial assessment should focus on patterns and types of violent behavior, frequency, and characteristics of targeted victims. The nurse would also assess for triggers to agitation. In addition to collecting the client's psychiatric and medication history, the nurse would also be alert to potential highly stressful situations during hospitalization, such as sensory overload, that precipitate negative behaviors.

Practice Change: Healthcare staff will modify the environment to avoid exposing clients to excess sensory stimulation.

Sources: Flannery, R. B., Jr. (2005). Precipitants to psychiatric patient assaults on staff: Review of empirical findings, 1990–2003, and risk management implications. *Psychiatric Quarterly, 76*(4), 317–326. doi:10.1007/s11126-005-4965-y; National Institute of Neurological Disorders and Stroke. (2016, last updated). Traumatic brain injury: Hope through research. Retrieved from http://www.ninds.nih.gov/disorders/tbi/detail_tbi.htm.

nursing practice (Box 31-2 and Box 31-3). How many people do you know personally who wear glasses or contact lenses or who wear a hearing aid? You should know these facts about sensory deficit:

- A sudden onset of a deficit may lead to disorientation and anxiety.
- Gradual changes allow the person to adapt, often without even realizing the extent of the change.
- When there is a deficit in one sense, the other senses may become sharper to compensate (e.g., a person who is blind may develop more acute hearing).

Descriptions, complications, and interventions for six sensory deficits are discussed in the Example Problem: Sensory Deficits.

ThinkLike a Nurse 31-2

- Why do you think a person with impaired tactile perception is at risk for injury?
- Speculate about the possible nature of injuries that might occur.

Seizures

A **seizure** is the abrupt onset of disturbance in electrical activity in the brain—a group of neurons fires abnormally. This results in motor symptoms, such as rhythmic jerking of the limbs. In addition to motor symptoms, the person may have a decreased level of consciousness or a loss of consciousness. Symptoms and the duration of the seizure vary, depending on

---

BOX 31-2 ■ Common Visual Deficits

- **Myopia,** or *nearsightedness,* means that the patient is able to see close objects well but not distant objects. For example, a person with 20/200 vision can see an object from 20 feet away that a person with normal sight could see from a distance of 200 feet.
- **Hyperopia,** or *farsightedness,* implies that the eye sees distant objects well. A person with hyperopia may have 20/10 vision—he can see an object from 20 feet that a normal eye can see from 10 feet; however, near vision is impaired.
- **Presbyopia** is a change in vision associated with aging. The lens becomes less elastic and less able to accommodate to near objects. If you're older than age 40 years, there's a good chance you may be experiencing this problem.
- **Astigmatism** is caused by an irregular curvature of the cornea or lens that scatters light rays and blurs the image on the retina. The person has blurred vision with distortion.
- **Cataracts** are a clouding of the lens, resulting in blurred vision, sensitivity to glare, and image distortion. Can occur in one eye or both.

- **Glaucoma** is a type of vision loss caused by increased pressure in the anterior cavity of the eyeball that distorts the shape of the cornea and shifts the position of the lens, resulting in loss of peripheral vision. It can eventually lead to blindness. The most common type is open angle glaucoma.
- **Macular degeneration** is the loss of central vision due to damage to the macula lutea, the central portion of the retina. The leading cause of visual impairment in older adults, it is characterized by slow, progressive loss of central and near vision. It is usually present in both eyes. Risk factors include excessive sunlight exposure and smoking.
- **Strabismus,** or *crossed eyes,* in which one eye deviates from a fixed image, can cause permanent vision loss.
- **Retinopathy** (*disorders of the retina, e.g., inflammation*) occurs as a result of progressive, poorly controlled diabetes or hypertension. Both forms of damage to the retina can be treated with laser therapy.
- **Detached retina** is an ophthalmologic emergency. It can occur from trauma to the eye or failed recent cataract surgery. It presents as a curtain coming down across vision.

BOX 31-3 ■ Common Hearing Deficits

- **Conduction deafness** results when one of the structures that transmits vibrations is affected. It may be a temporary or permanent condition caused by infection of the middle ear, a punctured tympanic membrane, or arthritis of the auditory bones. Even cerumen impaction or a foreign object lodged in the ear canal can cause it. A hearing aid may be helpful for conduction deafness.
- **Sensorineural hearing loss** is a form of nerve deafness that occurs when there is damage to cranial nerve VIII or the receptors in the cochlea. It may result from ototoxic medications (e.g., gentamicin), trauma, hereditary causes, and bacterial or viral infections. Chronic exposure to loud noise may also lead to nerve and receptor impairment.
- **Presbycusis** is a progressive sensorineural loss associated with aging. The person experiences diminished ability to hear high-pitched sounds (e.g., s, z, sh, ch) and to distinguish sounds in a noisy environment. Presbycusis results from deterioration of the hair cells in the cochlea. Background noise further aggravates this type of hearing deficit. Hearing aids may not help sensorineural hearing loss.

- **Central deafness** results from damage to the auditory areas in the temporal lobes. Tumor, trauma, meningitis, or stroke in the temporal lobe may cause this.
- **Tinnitus** is a term used to describe ringing in the ears. Most tinnitus comes from damage to the endings of the nerve in the inner ear caused by trauma, Ménière's disease, hypertension, ear infection, medications, otosclerosis, or arthritic changes of the bones of the ear.
- **Impacted cerumen** is a condition in which earwax becomes tightly packed in the ear canal, blocking the canal. Patients with impacted cerumen may experience a feeling of fullness or pain, decreased hearing, or tinnitus.
- **Otosclerosis** is a hardening of the bones of the middle ear, especially the stapes. The stapes becomes fixed, leading to poor sound transmission to the inner ear. The cause of this disorder is unknown.
- **Otitis media** is a middle ear infection. It is a common childhood illness that may be caused by viruses or bacteria.

EXAMPLE PROBLEM: Sensory Deficits

Sensory Perception

Vision

Light rays on the retina trigger a nerve impulse that is transmitted to the visual area of the brain in the occipital region. See Box 31-2 for specific types of visual deficits.

Hearing

Sound waves entering the ear canal are converted to vibrations, and then they are transferred from the middle ear to inner ear. Vibrations cause hair cells in the cochlea to bend, generating impulses carried by cranial nerve (CN) VIII to the brain. The auditory region in the temporal lobes interprets sound and the direction it is coming from. See Box 31-3 for information about specific kinds of hearing problems.

Olfaction

Chemoreceptors generate impulses carried by olfactory nerve (CN I) into the olfactory area in the temporal lobes. Vaporized molecules can be detected from a distance; the sense of smell can serve as an early warning system for detection of smoke and noxious chemicals. Olfaction plays a role in memory, mood, and safety (see Fig. 31-2).

Gustation

Different types of taste buds are found in different areas of the tongue: sweet and salty (tip of tongue), sour (sides of tongue), bitter (back of tongue, soft palate), and savory (see Fig. 31-2). Taste buds generate nerve impulses that travel along the facial and glossopharyngeal nerves (CN VII and IX) to the taste area in the parietal–temporal cortex.

Tactile

The dermis contains receptors for cutaneous sensations of light touch, pressure, heat, cold, and pain. Information is transmitted to the sensory areas in the parietal lobes. The hands and face have the most receptors and the largest area in the sensory cortex. A person's ability to perceive touch is often measured in terms of *2-point discrimination*, which is perceiving 2 close but separate points of pressure. Discrimination on lips and fingertips is normally at points < 4 mm apart; it is wider on the torso, at > 2 cm.

Kinesthesia

Proprioceptors sense position and coordinates movement of head and body. Conscious muscle sense occurs in parietal lobes; unconscious in cerebellum.

ETIOLOGIES

Visual Deficit

Age-related changes, refractive errors, orbital trauma, cataracts, glaucoma, diabetic or hypertensive retinopathy, macular degeneration, stroke (see Box 31-2)

Gustatory Deficit

Medications; xerostomia (excessively dry mouth); low fluid intake; poor nutrition; poor oral hygiene; common cold; infections of the nose, sinuses, mouth, salivary glands; smoking; vitamin B_{12} or zinc deficiency; injury to mouth, nose, head (concussion) (see Box 31-1)

Olfactory Deficit

CN damage, tumor, or atherosclerosis; cocaine and tobacco use; concussion; zinc deficiency; inherited condition (nonpathological)

Hearing Deficit

Injury or disease in structures of ear, nerves, or brain (see Box 31-3)

Tactile Deficit

- Stroke, brain or spinal tumor or injury, peripheral nerve damage caused by diabetes,
- Guillain-Barré syndrome, chronic alcoholism, fracture, peripheral vascular disease

Kinesthetic Deficit

The vestibular apparatus of the inner ear has hair cells that detect rotation or body movement. Mismatch between the position or acceleration of the head and the visual field can result in motion sickness. Parkinson's disease, neurological disorders, tumors, medications; stroke; problems of the inner ear (Ménière's disease)

(Continued)

EXAMPLE PROBLEM: Sensory Deficits—cont'd

COMPLICATIONS

Visual Deficit

- Affects all ADLs and interpersonal interactions.
- Severely limited mobility

Hearing Deficit

- Impaired communication and social interaction
- Impaired ability to understand instructions
- Injury due to inability to hear warnings

Gustatory Deficit

Nutritional deficits and weight loss

Olfactory Deficit

Decreased appetite and nutritional deficits. When sense of smell is lost (anosmia), food doesn't taste the same.

Tactile Deficit

Failure to detect wounds and injury

ASSESSMENT

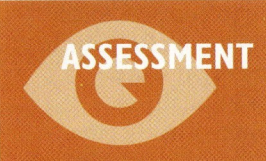

Refer to the Focused Assessment box, Nursing History: Sensory Perceptual Status and to the Focused Assessment box, Bedside Assessment of Sensory Function

OUTCOMES

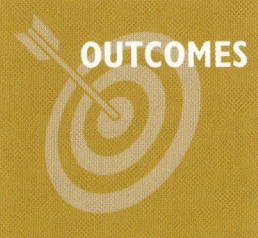

NOC Outcomes

Appetite
Sensory Function
Sensory Function: Hearing
Sensory Function: Proprioception
Sensory Function: Tactile
Coordinated Movement
Sensory Function: Taste and Smell
Sensory Function: Vision
Sensory Function: Cutaneous

NIC Interventions

Environmental Management Communication
   Enhancement: Hearing Deficit
Exercise Promotion: Strength Training
Exercise Therapy: Balance
Feeding
Nausea Management
Nutrition Management
Lower Extremity Monitoring
Peripheral Sensation Management

DIAGNOSES

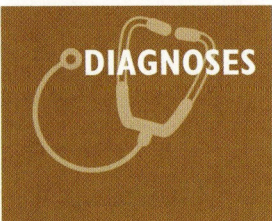

- Risk for Falls r/t visual impairment
- Risk for Injury r/t reduced tactile sensation
- Deficient Diversional Activity r/t hearing impairment
- Bathing Self-Care Deficit r/t kinesthetic impairment

- Feeding Self-Care Deficit r/t visual impairment
- Imbalanced Nutrition: Less Than Body Requirements r/t loss of appetite secondary to impaired taste

EXAMPLE PROBLEM: Sensory Deficits—cont'd

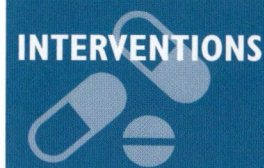

INTERVENTIONS

Refer also to the box Self-Care box Teaching Your Client About Sensory Perceptual Health.

Visual Deficit

- Keep the bed in a low position.
- Make sure eyeglasses are clean, in good repair, of proper prescription, and within reach; help patient put them on, if necessary.
- Offer magnifying lens, large-print, audio, Braille media.
- Use soft, diffuse lighting without glare.
- Provide an uncluttered environment. Orient patient to the room arrangement.
- Place call device, phone, self-care items within reach.

See Clinical Insight 31-2: Communicating With Visually Impaired Clients.

Auditory Deficit

- Inspect ear canals for cerumen impaction (common cause of conduction hearing loss). See Procedure 31-1 for otic irrigation procedure.
- Teach patients to use blinking alarm clocks, security alarms, smoke detectors.
- Ensure hearing aids batteries are charged; make sure audio is at a comfortable level; encourage wearing aids as needed.
- Use closed-captioning, voice control for mobile devices and computers.
- Provide written instructions.

See Clinical Insight 31-3: Communicating With Hearing-Impaired Clients.

Olfactory Deficit

- Check smoke detectors and replace batteries regularly.
- Teach patient not to rely on smell or taste to detect food spoilage; date foods, inspect before eating.
- Teach patient to arrange regular inspection and maintenance of gas appliances.
- Aromatherapy

Gustatory Deficit

- Check the fit of dentures or dental appliances. Weight changes may affect the fit and make it harder to eat.
- Perform frequent oral hygiene to encourage appetite and enhance the sense of taste.
- Assess for sores on the tongue, palate, and cheeks.
- Serve visually appealing meals. Vary food texture, color, temperature.
- Teach patient to eat foods one at a time or drink water between bites to enhance flavor.
- Use seasonings, salt substitutes, spices, or lemon to improve the taste of foods.

Kinesthetic Deficits

- Rhythmic movement (tai chi, dance, yoga)
- Aerobic exercise (running, cycling)
- Strength training (light weights)
- Flexibility activities (stretching)
- Balance conditioning (standing on one foot)
- Perform full ROM and, rotational movements.
- When helping the patient walk, ask which side patient prefers.

Tactile Deficit

- Nurses often use touch to express care and comfort. Use touch thoughtfully.
- If patient consents, brush hair, give a back rub, use touch when giving care.
- Use a bath thermometer to monitor water temperature and prevent burns.
- Change position often to relieve pressure on bony prominences.
- Use properly fitting shoes and socks.
- Report signs of impaired circulation (declining motor function, cool, gray-blue coloration).
- Inspect for wounds, abrasions, redness.
- Use a bed cradle; keep bed linens loose.
- Inspect for wounds, abrasions, and erythema.

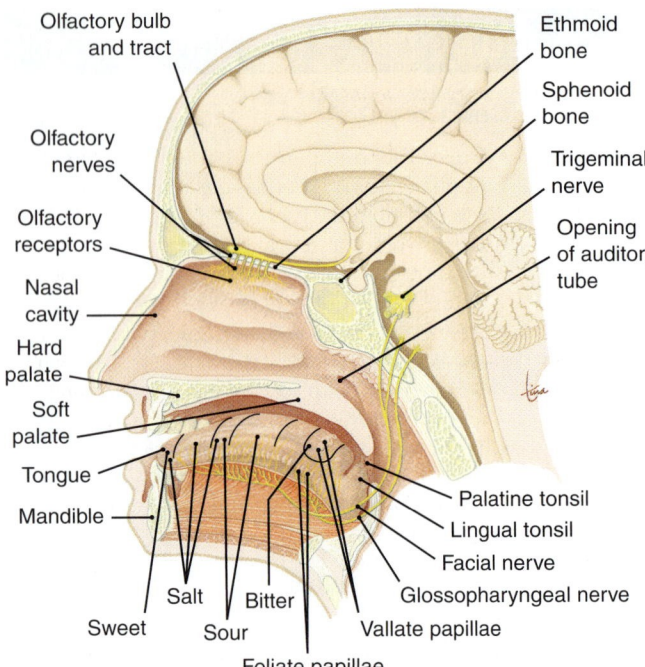

Olfactory bulb and tract
Olfactory nerves
Olfactory receptors
Nasal cavity
Hard palate
Soft palate
Tongue
Mandible
Sweet
Salt
Sour
Bitter
Foliate papillae
Ethmoid bone
Sphenoid bone
Trigeminal nerve
Opening of auditory tube
Palatine tonsil
Lingual tonsil
Facial nerve
Glossopharyngeal nerve
Vallate papillae

FIGURE 31-2 Structures for the senses of smell and taste.

the area of the brain affected. A seizure can last from a few seconds to more than 5 minutes; most last less than 3 minutes.

Types of Seizure Seizures are described as either generalized or partial. The difference between these types is in how and where they begin.

- **Primary generalized seizures** involve widespread electrical activity on both sides of the brain at once. Most commonly, this type is caused by hereditary factors and low levels of antiseizure medication.
- **Partial seizures** begin with electrical discharge from one side in a limited area of the brain.

Common triggers are ingesting mood-altering substances, infection in the brain or cerebral spinal fluid, tumor, head trauma, sleep deprivation, stress, illness, formation of the brain before birth, and hormone fluctuations. Sometimes no cause can be identified (Shafer & Sirven, 2014).

Incidence Seizures are not uncommon.

- Incidence is highest for those younger than age 10 or older than age 65 and higher among males than among females, especially in children.
- In 7 out of 10 people with seizures, no identifiable cause can be found.
- Children aged 3 months to 6 years may have a seizure when they have a high fever, especially when there is a family history of seizures.
- Three-quarters of children with seizures outgrow the events.

For guidelines regarding seizure precautions, see Clinical Insight 31-1.

KnowledgeCheck 31-4

- Discuss the difference between myopia and hyperopia.
- What is the difference between conduction deafness and nerve deafness?
- Identify three factors that may impair the sense of taste.

- How is the sense of smell triggered?
- What areas of the body have the greatest number of tactile receptors?
- What type of health concerns may be generated by kinesthetic deficits?

ThinkLike a Nurse 31-3

Imagine that you are experiencing sensory deficits. Which deficits would you find most challenging?

PracticalKnowledge
knowing **how**

As a nurse, you should always consider your client's sensory perceptual status. Sensory deficits, excess, and overload influence a person's safety and quality of life and may be especially troublesome for those in inpatient facilities.

ASSESSMENT NP

Assessment of sensory perception includes a history and physical exam to gather data about the following items (see Chapter 21):

- Factors affecting sensory perception (e.g., culture)
- Mental status, including mood, affect, cognition, and memory
- Level of consciousness
- Recent changes in sensory stimulation
- Use of sensory aids (e.g., glasses, contact lenses, hearing aids, canes, and walkers)
- The client's environment
- The support network
- Focused examination of vision, hearing, taste, smell, touch, and balance, ability to respond to stimulation, muscle tone, coordination

For instructions for specific topics, refer to the Focused Assessment box, Nursing History: Sensory Perceptual Status, and the Focused Assessment box, Bedside Assessment of Sensory Function.

- **Nursing Interview.** In your nursing interview, you will assess the client's usual and current state of sensory function, as well as gather a history of sensory problems and use of sensory aids.
- **Physical Assessment.** Physical assessment of sensory function requires assessment of the six senses. For guidelines, refer to Procedures 21-6, 21-7, and 21-16 in Chapter 21.

Assess Risk Factors for Impaired Sensory Perception

Perform a comprehensive assessment for any patient at increased risk for sensory alterations:

- Older adults
- People who are bedbound or homebound
- Patients in intensive care units
- Those with acute or chronic brain injury, limited mobility, or known sensory deficits, especially if the change has been acute

Routinely assess developmental level, health status, medications, stress and coping mechanisms, personality, history of head trauma, and lifestyle related to sensory alterations (see accompanying Focused Assessment boxes).

Focused Assessment

Nursing History: Sensory Perceptual Status

Ask questions such as the following:

Usual Sensory Function

- How would you rate your vision?
- How would you evaluate your ability to see objects up close or at a distance?
- Do you have any difficulty hearing conversations or listening to the radio or television?
- Have you experienced any difficulty locating sounds?
- Do you experience ringing or buzzing in your ears?
- Do you enjoy the taste of food?
- Do you notice any difficulty with your ability to smell?
- Are you experiencing any pain or discomfort?
- Do you have any areas of numbness or tingling on your body?
- Do you have any difficulty with sensing hot or cold?
- Describe your level of coordination.
- What medications are you taking? Have they had any effect on your vision, hearing, or sense of taste, smell, touch, or balance?
- What is your current stress level?
- What is your usual activity level?
- What is your preferred activity level?

Risk Factors for Impaired Sensory Function

- Developmental level (e.g., older adults)
- Health status (usual and current state of health, current health concerns, e.g., Ménière's disease), history of hospitalizations and surgeries)
- Medications (i.e., look up side effects to determine what, if any, effect the medications have on sensory function)
- Stress (current and usual stress level, major sources of stressors, usual coping mechanisms)
- Lifestyle (normal activity, noise, interaction levels, hobbies, and usual lifestyle)

History of Sensory Problems

- Have you experienced any problems with blurred vision, double vision, sensitivity to light, blind spots, objects moving in front of your eyes, or eye pain?
- Have you ever felt unable to follow a conversation because of difficulty hearing?
- Have you ever had problems with your ability to taste or smell?
- Have you ever had areas of numbness or tingling?
- Has anyone in your family ever been diagnosed with a stroke or circulation problem?
- Have you ever had episodes of confusion or disorientation?

Use of Sensory Aids, Including Diet, Exercise, Medications, and Remedies

- Does the client wear glasses or contact lenses at any time? If so, determine the following:
  When was the client's last eye exam?
  Are the glasses clean and in good repair? Are the glasses within easy reach?
  Are contact lenses in good condition? Is the client able to care for them?

- Does the client wear a hearing aid? If so, determine the following:
  Can the client hear adequately with the hearing aid in place?
  Are the batteries working?
  Is the hearing aid clean?
  How much help does the client need to place the aid in his ear?
- Does the client use a cane or walker? If so:
  Has the cane or walker been properly fitted to the client?
  How often does the client use the device when walking?
- What factors determine when the device will be used?

Assess Mental Status

- Assess behavior, appearance, response to stimuli, speech, memory, and judgment. If you need more specific instructions, see Procedure 21-16 and Questions for Evaluating Cognitive Status at the end of the procedure.
- For older adults, a tool called the Mini-Cog is especially useful (Borson, Scanlan, Brush, et al., 2000). It consists of three memory questions and instructions to draw a clock face.
- Assess level of orientation: Have the client tell you his name, the date, and his current location. If he can answer these questions correctly, describe him as "awake, alert, and oriented to person, place, and time" (AA&O×3).
- Assess level of consciousness:

Alert	Is the patient awake and aware of the environment and himself, speaking clearly, making eye contact?
Confused	Are actions and speech inappropriate?
Lethargic	Is speech slow or sluggish? Are mental processes and movements sluggish?
Obtunded	This is a low level of awareness and response to environment. Document it if it occurs.
Stuporous	This occurs when the patient can be aroused by vigorous stimulation but seems confused during periods of arousal.
Comatose	In this state, there is no spontaneous movement, no verbalization, and only nonpurposeful movement with stimulation (Huntley, 2008).

 Also see Chapter 21, **Procedure 21-16, Assessing the Sensory-Neurological System, including the Glasgow Coma Scale and Full Outline of UnResponsiveness Scale.**

Assess Support Network for Clients With Sensory Deficit

- Are there support persons to help the client by assuming chores he can no longer perform?
- Are there people who provide comfort to ease the client's distress about sensory losses?
- Who can provide sensory stimulation?
- Who can help reorient and calm the client?
- Does the client need help with transportation in order to maintain social contact?

Focused Assessment

Bedside Assessment of Sensory Function

Sense	Assessment Process
Vision	Use the Snellen chart, or have the client read a newspaper. Observe for squinting.
Hearing	Perform the whisper test. Inspect the ear canals for hardened cerumen. Observe client conversations. Are there frequent requests for repeating information or misunderstandings? How loud is the client's radio or television?
Smell	Ask the client to close his eyes and identify common smells (e.g., coffee, vanilla, cloves, tobacco).
Taste	Ask the client to close his eyes and identify common tastes (e.g., salt, lemon, sugar). Give water between tastes.
Tactile	With his eyes closed, touch the client with a wisp of cotton. Have him identify when you have touched him. Repeat this process with a sharp object, such as a needle. With his eyes closed, ask the client to identify where you are touching his body.
Kinesthesia	Have the client perform the Romberg test. See Procedure 21-7. Have the client perform alternating rapid motions, such as tapping heels or clapping. Observe the client's gait and movement.

Assess Mental Status

Sensory alterations may trigger changes in mental status and, conversely, altered mental status can interfere with sensory perception. Normal findings include an ability to express and explain realistic thoughts with clear speech, follow directions, listen, answer questions, and recall significant past events. In addition, you must specifically assess the client's level of orientation.

Chapter 21 presents additional discussion of mental status screening and orientation.

Assess Level of Consciousness

Level of consciousness is one indicator of cerebral function. It includes arousal (from alert to deeply comatose) and orientation (to time, place, person, and situation). An alert client will respond to auditory stimuli. If the client does not respond, progress to tactile and then painful stimuli (refer to Chapter 21). Remember, however, that if your client does not speak your language he may not respond to questions or commands.

KEY POINT: *If you are not using a coma scale, document your findings specifically and objectively in your nursing notes. Be sure to assess whether the patient is alert, confused, lethargic, obtunded, stuporous, or comatose.*

Assess the Environment

As part of your assessment, assess how the client is responding to the conditions of the environment. Consider how different the environment is for Joshua and Richard (Meet Your Patients). Joshua is in a crowded space with lights and noise 24 hours a day. He has had a number of invasive procedures and is most likely receiving pain medication. In contrast, Richard is in a quiet room with little exposure to light, noise, or touch. As Joshua's and Richard's situations demonstrate, a healthcare environment can have too many or too few stimuli.

■ **Compare your data about the patient's personality and lifestyle with the current environmental situation.** In healthcare facilities, patients are subjected to lights, noises, and odors that cause them anxiety. They may hear others who are crying out in pain. A patient whose home environment is quiet may become overwhelmed and develop sensory overload in a hospital setting. Even a patient used to a rapid-paced lifestyle may experience overload if he also feels pain, nausea, dizziness, or other symptoms of illness. Additionally, a patient used to competing demands on her time may have difficulty coping with confinement in the hospital environment.

■ **Assess the effect of the environment on sensory deficits.** For example, for a patient with age-related hearing changes, the background noise of the healthcare environment may make it difficult to hear higher-toned or low-volume voices. A patient with visual deficits or impaired balance will often modify his home environment to allow optimal function; however, when the patient hospitalized or moved to a long-term care facility, these aids may no longer be feasible. **KEY POINT:** *To assist the patient, you must determine which environmental factors make his deficits worse and which help to compensate.*

Assess the Support Network

Typically a support network is beneficial for a client with a sensory deficit or overload. Support persons may help the client to adapt to deficits by assuming tasks that the client can no longer perform or by providing comfort to the client so he is less impaired by the sensory losses.

Recall that Richard (Meet Your Patients) has no visitors. If Richard had more visitors, he would receive more stimulation and might have less sensory deprivation. Family members can also help clients who are confused from sensory alterations by reorienting and calming them.

KnowledgeCheck 31-5

■ Identify six areas you should assess for a client with known or suspected sensory alterations.

■ What factors must be evaluated when it is known that a client uses a sensory aid?

■ Identify at least two ways that you can assess vision and hearing deficits at the bedside.

ThinkLike a Nurse 31-4

How would you assess Joshua and Richard (Meet Your Patients) for sensory alterations? You may need to review the scenario at the beginning of the chapter to answer this question.

ANALYSIS/NURSING DIAGNOSIS NP

NANDA International (NANDA-I) (2017) identifies the following diagnostic labels that might be useful for patients with sensory-perception problems:

Acute Confusion
Chronic Confusion
Risk for Dry Eye
Impaired Memory
Unilateral Neglect

PLANNING OUTCOMES/EVALUATION NP

NOC standardized outcomes. Although NANDA-I has retired the diagnosis Disturbed Sensory Perception from the taxonomy, NOC still has outcomes for sensory-perceptual deficits. For some examples, see Outcomes in the Example Problem: Sensory Overload.

Individualized goals/outcomes statements you might write for a client with Disturbed Sensory Perception include the following:

- Compensates for visual impairment by maximizing the use of touch and hearing.
- Verbalizes the importance of eating nutritious foods, despite the fact they "taste funny."
- Demonstrates proper use of her hearing aid.
- Participates in at least one activity daily.

The outcomes focus your data collection; comparing the new data against the outcomes allows you to determine patient progress.

PLANNING INTERVENTIONS/ IMPLEMENTATION NP

NIC standardized interventions. Although NANDA-I has retired the diagnosis Disturbed Sensory Perception from the taxonomy, NIC still has interventions for sensory-perceptual deficits. The following are some examples:

For Sensory Deficits:
Communication Enhancement: Visual Deficit
Ear Care
Exercise Therapy: Balance
Nutrition Management
For Acute Confusion: Cognitive Stimulation, Reality Orientation
For Chronic Confusion: Anxiety Reduction, Dementia Management
For Impaired Memory: Memory Training, Neurologic Monitoring, Surveillance: Safety
For Unilateral Neglect: Self-Care Assistance, Unilateral Neglect Management

Specific, individualized nursing activities to address sensory perception problems are based on the nursing diagnosis chosen, especially on its etiology.

Promoting Optimal Sensory Function

Optimal sensory function requires periodic health screening along with early identification and treatment of health problems. Comprehensive healthcare is the ideal approach, because sensory problems are often related to other health disorders. For example, to protect the client's vision, a client with hypertension needs to have periodic eye examinations and to control his blood pressure. For information to teach your clients about vision and hearing, see the accompanying Self-Care box, Teaching Your Client About Sensory Perceptual Health, as well as the Example Problem: Sensory Deficits, earlier in the chapter.

ThinkLike a Nurse 31-5

Which of the strategies to treat sensory deprivation would be most appropriate for Richard (Meet Your Patients)?

ThinkLike a Nurse 31-6

Review the scenario of Joshua, the young ICU patient with sensory overload (Meet Your Patients). Provide a rationale for your choices. You may need to visit an ICU or talk with classmates who have been to an ICU to answer this question.

- Which strategies to prevent sensory overload would be most appropriate for an ICU patient?
- Which would be least likely to be successful or not feasible based on the setting?

KnowledgeCheck 31-6

- Identify three safety measures that may be used with clients with visual impairment.
- Identify three safety measures that may be used with clients with hearing impairment.

Caring for Patients With Confusion

Confusion interferes with the ability to interpret stimuli accurately. It can be temporary or permanent. Confusion is an aspect of both delirium and dementia.

- **Delirium** is an *acute, reversible state* of confusion caused by medications and a variety of physiological processes, such as hypoxia, metabolic disturbances, infection, or sensory alterations. It may be accompanied by changes in the level of consciousness.
- **Dementia** is a *chronic and progressive deterioration* in mental function caused by physical changes in the brain and is not associated with changing levels of consciousness.

Use the following suggestions for promoting patient orientation. Notice that some of the following interventions are similar to those for preventing sensory deficit.

Promote Orientation Introduce yourself and state the client's name each time you talk with him. Wear a readable (large, plain type) name tag to reinforce your introduction. Identify the day, date, and time as you interact. Provide visual clues to time, such as opening the drapes during the day and closing them at night and placing calendars and clocks where they are easy to see. Place personal objects, photos, and mementos in the immediate environment and discuss them with the client. Encourage the patient to participate in familiar activities, such as bathing.

Simplify Your Communications The patient cannot interpret stimuli accurately and may not understand what you say.

- Take an unhurried approach, allowing adequate time for the client to answer any questions you raise.
- Face the client and speak calmly, simply, and directly.

EXAMPLE PROBLEM: Sensory Overload

Definition:
Occurs when environmental and/or internal stimuli exceed a level more than the patient's sensory system can effectively process. This occurs when (1) the patient is unable to adapt to persistent, nonmeaningful stimuli and/or (2) the environment provides more stimuli than the patient can adjust to.

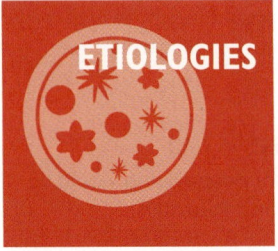

ETIOLOGIES

Risk Factors

- Physical discomfort and pain
- Unfamiliar hospital environment and familiar healthcare environment.
- Medications that stimulate the CNS contribute to overload (caffeine, weight-loss substances)
- Separation from loved ones
- Physical conditions that activate the CNS (hyperthyroidism)
- Neurological or psychiatric disorders (anxiety, psychosis, sensory integration disorder, ADHD)

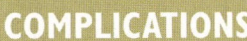

COMPLICATIONS

Lack of patient adherence with interventions
Distraction

Moodiness, anxiety
Restlessness, sleeplessness

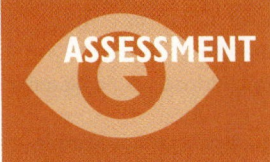

ASSESSMENT

- Irritability, anxiety, restlessness
- Reduced attention span
- Decreased problem-solving skills
- Drowsiness due to insomnia
- Muscle tension

- Inability to concentrate and focus
- Decreased ability to perform tasks
- Disorientation, confusion

Also refer to the Focused Assessment box, Nursing History: Sensory Perceptual Status.

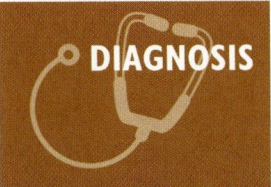

DIAGNOSIS

NANDA-I Nursing Diagnosis

Anxiety
Acute Confusion; Chronic Confusion
Ineffective Coping

Insomnia; Risk for Sleep Deprivation
Stress Overload

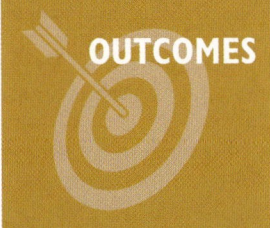

OUTCOMES

Effectively copes with excessive, environmental stimuli.

Reports adequate sleep and rest.

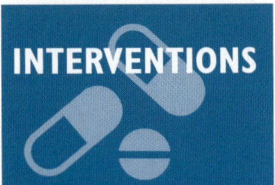

INTERVENTIONS

Control Visual Stimuli.

- Minimize unnecessary light.
- Instruct healthcare team to be aware of appropriate light levels, especially at night.
- Use a flashlight instead of turning on room lights.

Control Auditory Stimuli.

- Minimize unnecessary noise.
- Instruct NAPs to be aware of appropriate noise levels, especially at night.
- Speak using a calm and confident voice.
- Consider the use of earplugs for the patient.

Manage Olfactory Stimuli.

- Reduce noxious odors by promptly emptying commodes and bedpans, removing meal trays, using deodorant sprays, and keeping wounds covered.

Promote Sleep and Rest.

- Provide a quiet, restful environment to allow the patient optimal sleep.
- Establish a schedule for care that allows for uninterrupted periods of sleep and rest.

- Prevent interruptions during rest periods.

Minimize Stress.

- Observe the patient's reaction to environmental stimuli. Remove annoying or excessive stimuli when possible.
- Introduce yourself when meeting the patient; address him by name.
- Provide a calm presence: do not hurry with care or speak rapidly.
- Provide a private room, if possible, and limit visitors.
- Minimize nonessential tasks.
- Control pain and nausea with prescribed medications and other comfort measures.
- Provide relaxing music.
- Visualization and deep-breathing techniques.

Limit Screen Time.

- Choose programs to meet the patient's interests.
- Do not leave the TV or radio on continuously.
- Silence smartphone notification alerts.

Self-Care

Teaching Your Client About Sensory Perceptual Health

Vision

➤ Have regular eye examinations.
Infants and preschoolers—Screen at their routine office visits.
Young adults—Complete eye exam at least three times between the ages of 20 and 39.
At age 40—Have a baseline screening, and based on that information, the ophthalmologist will determine how frequently your eyes need to be reexamined.

 Age 65 and older—Complete eye exam every 1 to 2 years to check for cataracts and other eye conditions (American Academy of Ophthalmology, 2009). More recently, the U.S. Preventive Services Task Force (2016) concluded that the current evidence is insufficient to assess the balance of benefits and harms of screening for impaired visual acuity in older adults.

➤ If you are at risk for eye disease, have more frequent eye exams, regardless of your age—for example, if you (1) take steroids; (2) are of African ancestry; (3) have a family history of eye disease, diabetes, or high blood pressure; (4) or have any symptoms. Your ophthalmologist will recommend how often you should have an exam.
➤ Call your healthcare provider for prompt examination if you have eye pain, discharge, a change in vision, or bleeding.
➤ Have your prescriptions for glasses or contact lenses reviewed at each screening and updated if needed.
➤ Encourage sunglasses, visors, hats when outdoors.
➤ Be sure that visual screening is done at your child's elementary school. If not, consult your pediatrician or other care provider.
➤ Work with your primary healthcare provider to control conditions such as hypertension and diabetes.
➤ Clients with significant visual impairment should be evaluated for the ability to drive.
➤ Pregnant women should obtain early and adequate prenatal care to prevent the danger of premature birth and exposure to high-volume oxygen.
➤ Keep sharp or pointed tools (e.g., scissors) out of reach of infants, toddlers, and preschoolers.
➤ Teach children to stay away from activities that may cause projectiles, such as lawn mowing.

➤ Keep the child away from firearms and fireworks.
➤ Insist that your child use eye protection when playing sports such as tennis or baseball.
➤ Insist that children wear helmets when skating or riding bicycles and that teenagers wear helmets when riding motorcycles.
➤ For children who wear glasses, be sure the lenses are made of shatterproof safety glass.

Hearing

➤ Auditory screening is often performed in elementary school; however, most adults do not have their hearing screened regularly. If you work in an area with a high noise level, you should have your hearing checked regularly. Early detection may prevent hearing loss. However, the U.S. Preventive Services Task Force (2012) concludes that the evidence is insufficient to assess the balance of benefits and harms of screening for hearing loss in asymptomatic adults aged 50 years or older.
➤ If you are pregnant:
Obtain early prenatal care.
Avoid ototoxic drugs.
Be sure you are tested for syphilis and rubella (German measles).
Avoid anyone you suspect may have rubella.
➤ Children with frequent ear infections require evaluation to determine whether hearing loss has occurred.

 ➤ Middle and older adults may begin to experience difficulty distinguishing voices in a crowd or hearing the television or radio. These are indications of hearing loss and should be evaluated; you may need a hearing aid. Hearing loss is not a "natural part of aging."

Taste

Dental health is an important aspect of maintaining taste. Decayed teeth, gum disease, and other disorders of the mouth may affect the ability to taste. Have your teeth cleaned and examined at least yearly. You may need additional dental work to promote oral health.

■ Provide simple explanations for all care and treatments.
■ Use short sentences with few words: "It's bath time," rather than, "It is time now for you to have a bath and get ready for your visitors this evening when they come."
■ Do not offer too many choices because this further confuses an already confused patient.

Relieve Anxiety People with dementia are often anxious, worried, and fearful.

 Find ways to make the person feel more secure and comfortable before you focus on the content of your conversations.
■ Provide continuity of care. Establish a routine for care and assign the same caregivers each day when possible.
■ Gently hold or pat the patient's hand.

■ Realize that the person is probably distressed and is doing the best he can. Be affectionate, reassuring, and calm, even when things make no sense.
■ Try to respond to the person's feelings instead of the content of his words. This helps to reassure her. For example, if a woman is constantly searching for her husband, don't say, "Your husband is not here." Rather, say, "You must miss your husband," or "Tell me about your husband."
■ If the person has difficulty finding the right word, supply it for him unless it upsets him. This helps control his frustration.
■ If you do not understand what the patient is trying to say, ask him to point to it or describe it (e.g., "What does a zishmer look like?").
■ Consider using alternative therapy, such as music therapy.

Toward Evidence-Based Practice

Committee on the Public Health Dimensions of Cognitive Aging, Board on Health Sciences Policy; Blazer, D. G., Yaffe, K., & Liverman, C.T. (Eds.). (2015). *Cognitive aging: Progress in understanding and opportunities for action.* Institute of Medicine. Washington, DC: The National Academies Press.

The Institute of Medicine (IOM) supports the following actions for promoting cognitive health in individuals of all ages:

- Be physically active.
- Be intellectually active and seek opportunities to learn, remember, or solve problems.
- Engage in personal and social relationships and activities.
- Consume a healthy diet to avoid nutrient deficiency, although dietary supplements might not prevent cognitive decline.
- Reduce risk factors for cardiovascular disease, including hypertension, diabetes, and tobacco use.
- Avoid mind-altering medication, if possible.
- Get adequate sleep; seek treatment for sleep disorders, if needed.
- Avoid heavy alcohol consumption.

Williams, K., & Kemper, S. (2010). Exploring interventions to reduce cognitive decline in aging. *Journal of Psychosocial Nursing and Mental Health Services, 48*(5), 42–51. doi:10.3928/ 02793695-20100331-03

The authors investigated five factors likely to optimize brain health in an aging population:

1. Leisure activities demand short-term memory and reasoning skills that preserve cognitive performance.
2. People whose occupations involve complex and demanding thought processing and judgment benefit with some protection from cognitive decline.
3. Physical activity increases blood flow to the brain, enhances oxygen delivery, and preserves brain volume.
4. Meaningful relationships with family and the community protect the brain.
5. A balanced and nutritious diet likely preserves brain function.

More rigorous research is needed to validate the results.

Chew, E. Y., Clemons, T. E., Agron, E., et al. (2015). Effect of omega-3 fatty acids, lutein/zeaxanthin, or other nutrient supplementation on cognitive function. *JAMA, 314*(8), 791–801. doi:10.1001/jama.2015.9677

Some research suggests that dietary omega-3 fatty acids can protect brain health. Researchers at the National

Institutes of Health lacked evidence to support use of omega-3 supplements in reducing cognitive decline and Alzheimer's-related dementia in older persons.

Loveden, M. (2013). Lifestyle change and the prevention of cognitive decline and dementia. *Current Opinions in Psychiatry, 26*(3), 239–243. doi:10.1097/YCO.0b013e32835f4135

Researchers found (1) less cognitive decline and dementia in people who changed from a sedentary lifestyle to moderate physical activity; (2) no evidence to support the benefit of intellectual activities in reducing the incidence of dementia; and (3) dietary supplements improve brain performance when used to treat a nutritional deficiency, but are not likely to help prevent cognitive decline when the diet is adequate.

Sabia, S., Elbaz, A., Britton, A., et al. (2014). Alcohol consumption and cognitive decline in early old age. *Neurology, 82*(4), 332–339. doi:10.1212/WNL.0000000000000063

Researchers studying the effect of alcohol consumption during the middle age years on brain aging reported the following: (1) Men who consumed heavily (self-reported ≥ 36 g/day) experienced faster overall cognitive decline compared with light to moderate alcohol ingestion; (2) heavy alcohol intake (self-reported > 19 g/day) in women was also found to be harmful to short-term verbal memory, inductive reasoning, math tasks, and verbal fluency; and (3) moderate and light alcohol use was not found to be associated with cognitive decline in women.

1. When teaching clients about ways to protect brain health, what would strategies would you recommend?

2. Is there evidence to support the idea that a diet supplemented with omega-3 has benefit for reducing cognitive decline with aging?

3. Is there evidence to support intellectual activity as a way to prevent cognitive decline with aging?

4. What potential source of bias might there be in the Sabia, Elbaz, Britton et al. study regarding the relationship of midlife alcohol intake with cognitive aging?

 Go to Davis Advantage, Resources, Chapter 31, **Toward Evidence-Based Practice—Suggested Responses.**

Provide for Safety Recognize that the client's decision making may be poor. Maintain a safe environment. For example, store medications away from the patient's reach, keep doors and windows closed securely, and use bed or chair monitors to prevent wandering.

KnowledgeCheck 31-7

- What are the major concerns associated with loss of smell and taste?
- What safety measures should be taught to a client with tactile impairment?
- How can you best assist a client who is confused?

Caring for Patients With Altered Level of Consciousness

Consciousness is the state of being wakeful and aware of self, time, and the surroundings. **Unconsciousness** is an abnormal, neurological state resulting from disturbance of sensory perception to the extent that the patient is not aware of what is happening around him, is not responsive, and is not oriented. Unconscious patients are highly dependent on the nurse for patent airway, safety, nutrition and hydration, comfort, elimination, range of motion, skin care, sensory stimulation, and family support and education.

- **Safety measures are a priority.** Nurses' responsibility is to protect unconscious patients from injury, falls, and medical complications (aspiration, pneumonia, pressure ulcers, urinary retention). Keep the bed in low position when you are not at the bedside and keep the siderails up.

- **Eye care.** If the patient's blink reflex is absent or her eyes do not close totally, you may need to give frequent eye care to keep secretions from collecting along the lid margins. The eyes may be patched to prevent corneal drying, and lubricating eye drops may be ordered.
- **Oral care.** Such care is also important because the unconscious patient does not take fluids by mouth.
- **Pressure injury prevention.** Patients need frequent turning and positioning to prevent pressure injuries.

- **Immobility.** Range of motion is necessary for immobile patients to prevent muscle shortening and contractures.

Caring for Clients at Risk for Seizures

Seizures place the patient at high risk for injury from falls and airway obstruction. Institute seizure precautions for patients with any of the following:

- A new diagnosis of a seizure disorder or any seizure activity within the past 12 months
- Frequent seizure activity
- History of head trauma (including surgery) within the past 3 years
- Withdrawal of antiseizure medication or adjustment of the medication regimen.

KEY POINT: *The goal of seizure precautions is to protect the patient from injury and prevent serious complications.*

To protect patients who are at risk for seizures, pad the head, foot, and siderails of the bed, and place oral suction at the bedside.

If a seizure occurs, do not attempt to open the mouth and insert a padded tongue depressor, for the following reasons:

- This can result in airway obstruction by pushing the tongue back into the pharynx.
- The patient might bite your fingers.
- If you are anxious, you could break the patient's teeth trying to insert the depressor.
- You may need to perform suctioning after the episode to prevent aspiration of oral secretions.

For a comprehensive discussion of nursing care for patients with a seizure disorder, see Clinical Insight 31-1: Seizures: Safety, Care and Comfort.

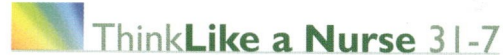

ThinkLike a Nurse 31-7

What types of interventions would be most appropriate for Joshua and Richard (Meet Your Patients)—that is, interventions for sensory deficits, sensory deprivation, sensory overload, or confusion?

CLINICALREASONING

The questions and exercises in this section allow you to practice the kind of thinking you will use as a full-spectrum nurse. Critical-thinking questions usually have more than one correct answer, so we do not provide "correct answers" for these features. It is more important to develop your nursing judgment than to just cover content. You will learn by discussing the questions with your peers. If you are still unsure, see the Davis Advantage chapter resources for suggested responses.

Caring for the Nguyens

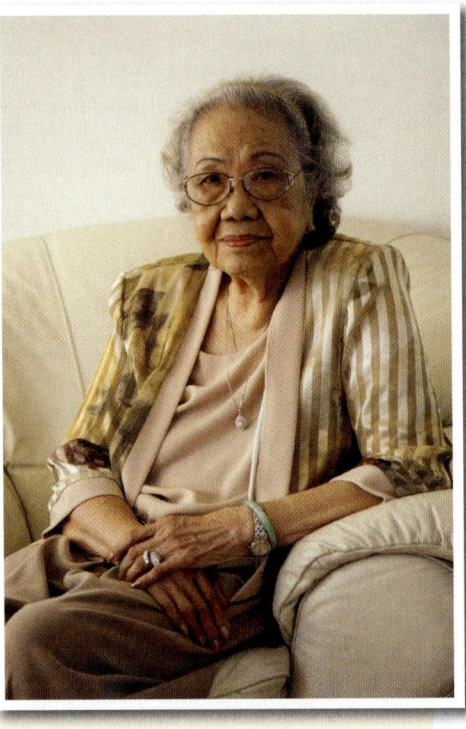

Mai Nguyen, Nam Nguyen's mother, has been experiencing blurred vision. At a recent ophthalmology appointment, she was told she has bilateral cataracts that will require surgical removal. She reports to the primary care clinic today, accompanied by Nam. Mai tells you, "I don't know what happened. I was pulling into a parking space at the grocery store, and the next thing you know, I hear this loud boom. I don't know how I did it, but I hit the car next to me. I just didn't see it."

Nam is very concerned and questions whether his mother should be allowed to drive. Mai is visibly upset.

"I don't want to hurt anyone, but I don't want to lose all my freedom." Nam insisted on this appointment to discuss his concerns.

A. What data will you need to gather from Mai and Nam?

B. What assessments will you need to perform?

C. How will cataract surgery most likely affect Mai? You will need to learn about the surgery and recovery to answer this question. Refer to a medical–surgical textbook, search the Web for "cataract surgery," or explore the following Web sites:
The National Eye Institute at https://www.nei.nih.gov
American Academy of Ophthalmology at http://www.aao.org/eye-health/diseases/what-is-cataract-surgery

D. What information would you offer to Mai and Nam?

➤ Go to Davis Advantage, Resources, Chapter 31, **Caring for the Nguyens—Suggested Responses.**

Applying the **Full-Spectrum Nursing Model**

PATIENT SITUATION

Clint Gossage is an 85-year-old man who lives at home alone. His wife moved to a nursing home a year ago. Although Mr. Gossage has many self-care deficits, he is still able to live at home with regular visits from a home health nurse and community services to help with some meals and bathing. When you visit him, you notice that he shouts when talking to you, looks at you intently when you speak, and constantly asks you to repeat what you say. You examine his external ear canal and note that there is some hardened cerumen in the canal. He is not wearing a hearing aid. The patient record reveals tympanic membrane scarring and a diagnosis of conductive hearing loss.

THINKING

1. *Theoretical Knowledge:* Describe the pathophysiology of conductive hearing loss.
2. *Critical Thinking (Considering Alternatives):* Based on your knowledge of conductive hearing loss and your assessment of Mr. Gossage, what is the first follow-up question you would ask him about his hearing?

DOING

3. *Practical Knowledge:* At a subsequent visit, you discover that Mr. Gossage has impacted cerumen in his left ear. After obtaining a medical order, you prepare to perform an otic irrigation. Refer to Procedure 31-1.
   a. To what temperature will you warm the solution?
   b. What position would you use for Mr. Gossage?
   c. Describe how you would place the tip of the syringe (or ear wash system) for irrigating.
   d. After the ear is cleared of cerumen and you have finished irrigating, what should you do next? And what position will you have Mr. Gossage assume when you do it?
4. *Nursing Process (Diagnosis):*
   a. Write a nursing diagnosis that focuses on Mr. Gossage's safety and that relates to hearing.
   b. Based on your nursing diagnosis, what safety measures would you recommend for Mr. Gossage's home? (Do not address the hearing aid issue here.)

CARING

5. *Ethical Knowledge:* Now think back to the first visit with Mr. Gossage. What are some reasons that he might not have been wearing a hearing aid? Consider physical changes associated with aging.

PracticalKnowledge:
clinical application

CLINICAL INSIGHTS

Clinical Insight 31-1 ▶ Seizure: Safety, Care, and Comfort

Before a Seizure Event (for at-risk patients)

- Explain to the patient the reasons for the precautions.
- If the patient has frequent or prolonged seizures, establish intravenous (IV) access. To provide a route to administer medications (e.g., diazepam [Valium]) in the event of a seizure. For intermittent episodes, you can use rectal diazepam (Diastat), lorazepam (Ativan), or midazolam (Versed).
- Obtain a bed with full-length siderails.
- Cover the headboard, footboard, and siderails with commercial pads or bath blankets. Tape the blankets in place. Padding protects the patient's limbs and head from injury if he has a seizure.
- Keep the rails raised and the bed in low position. To prevent falls and minimize injuries.
- Place oral or nasal suction equipment at the bedside. Test to be certain it is working.
- Place an airway at the bedside or tape to the wall, depending on your agency protocol.
- Make sure the family knows how to use a call device. To summon help in the event of a seizure.
- Assign the patient to a room close to the nurses' station. To allow closer monitoring.

- You may delegate to the nursing assistive personnel (NAP) the tasks of setting up seizure precautions.

When a Seizure Occurs

- If you are present when the patient reports having a pre-seizure aura, help him into bed, lower the head, and raise the siderails. Or if he is in another location, help him to the floor and put something soft under his head. To keep the head from being injured by hitting the floor.
- Provide privacy.
- Stay with the patient.
- You may insert an oral airway. To keep the tongue from blocking the airway.
- Don't put anything into the patient's mouth and don't force the airway in place. This might break the patient's teeth or cause other injury.
- Don't try to hold the jaw open or put your hands in the mouth. You may be bitten.
- Turn the patient on his side. This allows secretions to drain and the tongue to fall forward, keeping the airway patent.
- Loosen restrictive clothing.
- Move hard or sharp objects out of the way.

(Continued)

Clinical Insight 31-1 ▶ Seizure: Safety, Care, and Comfort—cont'd

- Do not try to restrain the patient or control his movements. This might cause muscle and joint injury to the patient.
- If the seizure is prolonged or hypoxemia is present, administer oxygen as needed. To avoid hypoxia during the event.
- Usually little nursing action is required beyond preventing physical injury and maintaining a patent airway. The exception is with status epilepticus, in which the patient has repeated seizures without regaining consciousness. In that event, notify a provider immediately.
- Observe the characteristics of the seizure: how it started, location and duration of motor activity type of movements (e.g., stiffening, jerking, twitching, loss of muscle tone), crying out, visual and auditory symptoms, tachycardia, pupil dilation, change in level of consciousness). Note the first symptom and how the seizure progressed. To help identify the area of the brain involved.
- You cannot delegate care of a patient who is having a seizure. Nursing assessments and interventions are required. You can ask the NAP to obtain help.
- Administer diazepam (Valium) as prescribed if the seizure is prolonged, typically more than 6 minutes.

After the Seizure

- Turn the patient on his side and apply suction, if needed. To allow secretions to drain and maintain a patent airway.
- Reorient and reassure the patient and make him comfortable. If the patient was incontinent, change bedding and clothing.

- Examine for injuries.
- Keep the room quiet and the lighting dim.
- Stay with the patient, as he may be sleepy or confused.
- Do not give any food or drink until the patient is fully conscious and alert.
- Monitor vital signs and mental status every 15 to 30 minutes for 2 hours. You can delegate this activity to a NAP.
- Observe post-seizure behavior: Evaluate muscle strength, ability to speak, memory, and orientation.
- Pad the siderails, if not already done.
- Ask the patient whether he experienced an aura and what activities preceded the seizure. The type of aura helps locate the area in the brain where the seizure originated.
- Document what happened and your post-procedure assessment.

Lifestyle Management

Sleep deprivation lowers the threshold for seizure activity. The patient should have sufficient rest and a healthy diet. Advise the patient to visit his primary care provider regularly and avoid excess alcohol and any drugs that may interact with seizure medications.

Practice Resource

Schachter, S. C., & Shafer, P. O. (2014).

Clinical Insight 31-2 ▶ Communicating With Visually Impaired Clients

The Joint Commission (2010) requires that institutions address the communication needs of patients with impaired vision.

- Introduce yourself when you enter the room.
- Call the client by her name so that she can be certain that you are addressing her.
- When you enter a room with a client who is visually impaired, describe the room, room layout, and activities that are occurring.
- Explain unfamiliar sounds, such as the paging system and monitor and pump alarms.
- If the client has limited vision, be sure to position yourself in the client's field of vision.

- Speak to the visually impaired person before you touch her so that she is prepared for your touch.
- Do not speak loudly unless the client has a hearing impairment.
- Let the client know when you are leaving the room.
- Use the words *see* and *look* as you would with a sighted person.
- Avoid expressions such as "over there" or "right here." Guide the client to the location or place her hand on the object.

Clinical Insight 31-3 ➤ **Communicating With Hearing-Impaired Clients**

Healthcare agencies should address the communication needs of those with vision, speech, hearing, language, and cognitive impairments (The Joint Commission, 2010).

Assess the Patient's Method of Receiving Speech.

■ If the patient wears a hearing aid, check to see that it is turned on.
■ If not, does the patient read lips or use sign language? Remember that only about ⅓ of spoken words can be understood by speech reading.
■ If possible, arrange a hearing evaluation for the client and construction of any required hearing aids.

Position Yourself and Minimize Noise.

■ Don't chew gum or eat while talking. Many clients use lipreading to help them interpret your speech.
■ Make sure you are clearly visible to the client before you start speaking. Use touch to get the client's attention.
■ Face the client directly; keep your hands away from your mouth.
■ If the hearing deficit is predominantly in one ear, move closer to the less affected ear.
■ Minimize environmental noise (e.g., turn off the television).

Send the Message.

■ Speak slowly and articulate clearly, in a natural way. Don't shout. Shouting distorts your words.

■ Don't drop your voice at the end of a sentence.
■ Use simple, plain language, but longer phrases (e.g., "Would you like for me to get you a drink of water?" instead of "Do you want a drink?")
■ Use gestures to provide visual cues (e.g., act out what you want the patient to do).
■ Use paper, pencil, or computer communication when necessary. Consider literacy skills.

Interpret the Client's Responses.

■ Observe the client's verbal responses, facial expressions, and body language for clues to understanding. An inappropriate response indicates misunderstanding.
■ Be aware the person may nod agreement or say yes even when she does not understand what is being said.
■ Confirm that the client understood you by asking her to repeat what you said, especially if you are giving specific information, such as a time or place. Many numbers and words sound alike (e.g., "fifteen" and "fifty," or "Prozac" and "Prograf").
■ If the person does not understand what you've said, rephrase your statement. Don't repeat the same words.

 For older adults: Use a low-pitched voice. The ability to hear high-pitched tones is lost first with aging.

PROCEDURES

Procedure 31-1 ■ **Performing Otic Irrigation**

➤ For steps to follow in *all* procedures, refer to the Universal Steps for All Procedures found on the page facing the inside back cover.

Equipment

■ A commercial ear wash or an ear irrigation system or an electronic jet ear irrigator.

 ✚ *Using a metal syringe is no longer recommended and is considered dangerous. An ear irrigation system is also preferred over an Asepto or bulb syringe because of the better ability to control pressure and remove cerumen (Harkin, n.d.).*

■ Asepto syringe or rubber bulb syringe (if an ear irrigation system is not available)
■ Irrigating solution (usually water, but may be an antiseptic solution), warmed to 98.6°F (37°C)
■ Bath towel and moisture-resistant towel

■ A headlight if one is available
■ Emesis basin
■ Otoscope
■ Cotton balls
■ Procedure gloves

Delegation

You must assess the client before performing this procedure and evaluate client responses during and after the procedure. The procedure requires knowledge of anatomy and physiology, use of an otoscope, and, sometimes, use of sterile technique. Therefore, you should not delegate otic irrigation to nursing assistive personnel (NAP).

(continued on next page)

Procedure 31-1 ■ **Performing Otic Irrigation** (continued)

Pre-Procedure Assessments

- Determine whether there are contraindications for ear irrigation.
  Contraindications include perforated or ruptured tympanic membrane, present or recent middle ear infection, prior surgery on the ear, cleft palate, previous pain on irrigation, acute inflammation of the ear canal, or very uncooperative patient.

- ✚ Assess the external ear for drainage. Do not irrigate the ears if drainage is present.
  Drainage from the ear may be a sign of rupture of the tympanic membrane.

- Assess the external ear for cerumen.
  Impacted cerumen is the most common reason for performing an ear irrigation.

- Assess the external ear canal for redness, swelling, or foreign objects; visualize the tympanic membrane. If a foreign object is present, attempt to remove it before irrigation.
  Establishes the baseline. If you irrigate with a foreign object in the ear, it may cause the object to swell and become more difficult to remove. Also, if you cannot visualize the tympanic membrane, it may be perforated; if so, otic irrigation is contraindicated.

- Assess for pain or hearing loss.
  Establishes the baseline. Cerumen blockage in the ear canal may result in a conductive hearing loss.

> ➤ When performing the procedure, always identify your patient according to agency policy, using two identifiers, and be attentive to standard precautions, hand hygiene, patient safety and privacy, body mechanics, and documentation.

Procedure Steps

1. **Warm the irrigating solution** to body temperature (98.6°F [37°C]) and fill the reservoir of the irrigator.
   Placing cool solutions in the ear can cause dizziness.

2. **Assemble the irrigator,** if necessary, and place a clean disposable tip on it.

3. **Assist the client into a sitting** or semi-reclined position, with the head tilted with the affected ear up. Explain what you are going to do.
   Positioning facilitates administering the solution and allows fluid to run along the roof of the ear canal. Knowing what to expect may decrease patient anxiety and improve his ability to cooperate during the procedure.

4. **Don gloves; put on the headlight.**
   The gloves are needed because of the risk of exposure to body fluids. The headlight facilitates direct vision.

5. **Drape the client** with a plastic drape, and place a towel on the client's shoulder on the side being irrigated. Ask the client to hold an emesis basin under his ear to collect the irrigating fluid that drains out of the ear.

NOTE: An emesis basin is not necessary if a comprehensive ear wash system is used.

Drape and towel protect the client's clothing.

6. **Set the irrigator pressure** to the minimum level. Let it run for 20 to 30 seconds to prime the tubing or nozzle before irrigation. (If you must use an Asepto or rubber bulb syringe, fill the syringe with about 50 mL of the irrigating solution and expel any remaining air.)

7. **Straighten the ear canal.**
   a. For a child younger than age 3 years, pull the pinna down and back.
   b. For older children and adults, pull the pinna upward and outward.
      Straightens the ear canal so that the solution can flow through the length of the canal.

8. **Instruct the client to notify you** if he experiences any pain or dizziness during the irrigation. Explain to the client that he may feel warmth, fullness, or pressure when the fluid reaches the tympanic membrane.
   Pain or dizziness may indicate a contraindication to the procedure.

9. **Place the tip of the nozzle** (or syringe) about 1 cm (½ in.) above the entrance of the ear canal, and direct the stream of irrigating solution gently along the top of the ear canal toward the back of the client's head.
   a. Do not occlude the ear canal with the nozzle.
   b. Instill the solution slowly.
   c. Allow the solution to flow out as it is instilled.
   d. Repeat these steps for 5 minutes or until you can see cerumen in the return solution.
      Directing the flow directly onto the tympanic membrane could injure the membrane. *Excessive pressure can cause discomfort and may even damage the tympanic membrane.* ▼

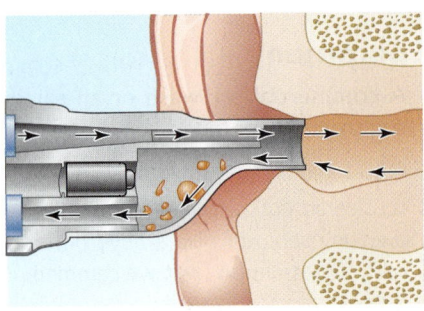

10. **Inspect the ear with an otoscope** to evaluate cerumen removal. See Procedure 21-7 if you need to review otoscopic examination.
    Allows visualization of the canal.

11. **Continue irrigating** until the examination indicates the canal is cleaned of cerumen and debris.
The irrigating solution will soften the cerumen, easing removal. Blocking the canal prevents the outward flow of the solution.

12. **Place a cotton ball loosely** in the ear canal and ask the client to lie on the side of the affected ear.
The cotton ball will absorb excess fluid that drains by gravity.

13. **Clean and disinfect the irrigator,** according to the manufacturer's instructions or agency protocols. Dispose of the disposable tips.

? What if . . .

■ **The cerumen is very hard or you have difficulty removing it?**
The irrigating solution will help soften it, so you may attempt again after 15 minutes.

■ **The patient is an infant or young child?**
Ask another caregiver to immobilize the child during the irrigation.

Evaluation

■ Observe the quantity and quality of ear cerumen you removed.
■ Observe the appearance of the ear canal.
■ Assess for complaints of pain or dizziness.
■ Assess for improvement in hearing acuity.
■ Reassess for drainage on the cotton ball.

Patient Teaching

■ Avoid use of cotton-tipped swabs.
They simply push cerumen deeper into the ear.

■ Keep the ear dry for a few days. Use cotton balls coated with petroleum jelly when bathing.
Exposure to a wet environment, such as a swimming pool, may increase the risk of bacterial or fungal infection. Petroleum jelly serves as a barrier to keep water from entering the ear.

■ Clean ears daily with washcloth, soap, and water. If earwax is a problem, over-the-counter preparations (oils) can be used to prevent wax buildup.

■ Notify the primary care provider if you experience ear pain, vertigo (dizziness), or "ringing in the ears."
Ear irrigation is an invasive procedure and may result in otitis media, trauma to the external meatus, vertigo, tinnitus, and perforation of the tympanic membrane, although this is not common.

Home Care

■ Provide the caregiver with instructions on ear care as stated above.
■ Teach parents that it is best to avoid irrigation in young children unless absolutely necessary. Oil- or water-based eardrops may be used to treat a wax problem in a child, applying the oil when the child is asleep.

■ Teach clients that ear candling is a not advisable. Candling consists of putting a hollow cone soaked in beeswax or paraffin in the ear and lighting the other end. The heat is supposed to draw out wax, but there is no evidence that it works. People using ear candles have burned themselves, blocked their ear canals with candle wax, and punctured their eardrums.

Documentation

■ Document the ear solution used, the quantity, character, and odor of cerumen or drainage.
■ Chart the condition of the ear canal and tympanic membrane after the irrigation.

Sample Documentation

3/1/16   1220   pt reported bilateral decreased hearing acuity. External ear canals occluded with dried cerumen. Irrigated with warm water using electronic ear irrigation system. Large amount of dry, brown cerumen removed with irrigation. External cannula and tympanic membrane intact after procedure with no report of pain, no bleeding, and no drainage. —————— N. Ephrain, RN

Practice Resources

Burtin, M., & Doree, C. (2009); Chau, J., Lee, D., & Lo, S. (2012); Harkin, H. (n.d.); Ratini, M. (2015); Van Wyk, F. C. (2016).

To explore learning resources for this chapter,

Go to **www.DavisAdvantage.com** and find:

Answers and Suggested Responses for all questions in this chapter

Lists of NIC Interventions and NOC Outcomes

List of NANDA-I Diagnoses

Knowledge Map

References and Bibliography

Concept Map

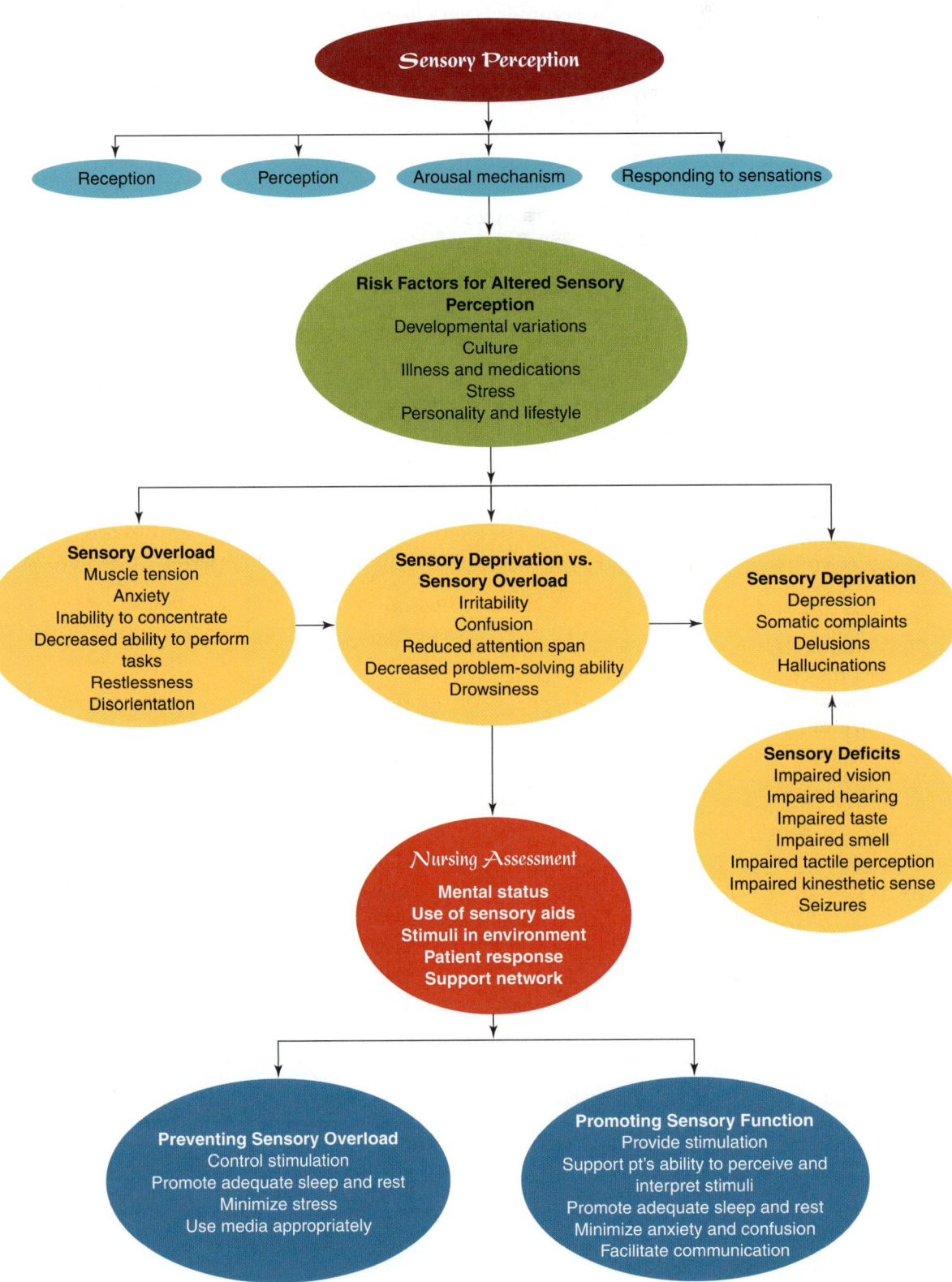

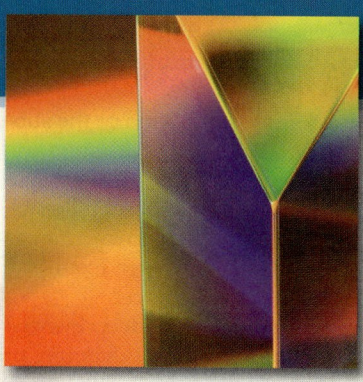 **32**

Pain

Learning Outcomes

After completing this chapter, you should be able to:

➤ Define *pain.*

➤ Classify pain according to origin, cause, duration, and quality.

➤ Describe the physiological changes that occur with pain.

➤ Discuss two physiological mechanisms involved in pain modulation.

➤ Discuss factors that influence pain.

➤ Identify the effect of unrelieved pain on each body system.

➤ Discuss nonpharmacological pain relief measures.

➤ Describe pharmacological pain relief measures, including nonopioid analgesics, opioid analgesics, and adjuvant analgesics.

➤ Describe chemical and surgical pain relief measures.

➤ Explain why pain should be considered the fifth vital sign.

➤ Identify the steps involved in creating a pain management program for a client.

➤ Individualize goals and interventions for clients with a nursing diagnosis of Acute Pain.

➤ Individualize goals and interventions for clients with a nursing diagnosis of Chronic Pain.

➤ Explain how to use a patient-controlled analgesia (PCA) system.

➤ Describe a method for evaluating the effectiveness of pain management.

Key Concepts

Pain

Pain management

Related Concepts

See the Concept Map at the end of this chapter.

Meet Your Patient

As a special experience, your instructor has arranged for you to spend a half day in the intensive care unit. Your patient today is a 23-year-old Asian woman who sustained chest and abdominal injuries in an automobile accident yesterday. Feeling apprehensive, you walk into the room with your clinical instructor to meet your patient, Ms. Eunice Chu Ling. She was taken to surgery during the night to have her spleen removed. She is intubated (i.e., she has an endotracheal tube in her airway that is connected to a ventilator) and has an intravenous line infusing and a chest tube on the left side that is draining bloody fluid. Her parents and siblings are in the room sitting rigidly in the chairs, smiling at you. Ms. Chu Ling is awake and grimacing. You want to ask her whether she is in pain, but she cannot speak.

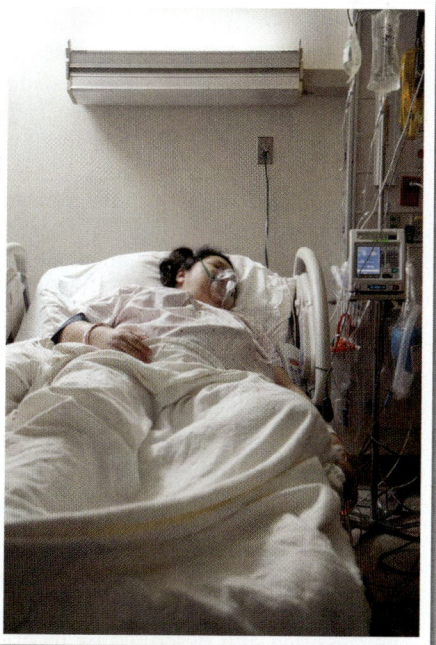

Theoretical Knowledge
knowing why

Pain is the most frequent reason people seek medical attention (National Institutes of Health, National Center for Complementary and Integrative Health, 2016). Most of the top 10 causes of death, such as heart disease, cancer, and chronic lower respiratory diseases, are associated with pain. As more people age and experience these chronic illnesses, you are likely to encounter more patients in pain. The following are some facts about the incidence of pain:

- More than one in four American adults experience pain lasting more than 24 hours or pain or discomfort that frequently disrupts sleep
- About one in three of all community-dwelling older adults reports pain that interferes with normal functioning.
- In spite of measures to relieve pain, more than half of all hospitalized patients die in moderate to severe pain.
- The most commonly reported types of pain are headaches, joint pain, and lower back and neck pain.

ABOUT THE KEY CONCEPTS

In this chapter, you will begin to understand the key concept of **pain**. Related concepts, such as **pain management, transduction, transmission, perception,** and **modulation** will help you to know what pain is and why it occurs; how to better assess it; and how to manage patients' experience with acute and chronic pain.

WHAT IS PAIN?

The following are two descriptions of pain:

- "**Pain** is an unpleasant sensory and emotional experience associated with actual or potential tissue damage, or described in terms of such damage" (Merskey & Bogduk, 1994, p. 971).
- **Pain** is "whatever the person says it is, and existing whenever the person says it does" (McCaffery, 1968, p. 95). In other words, pain is a subjective experience. Unlike a pulse or blood pressure, you cannot measure pain objectively. Furthermore, your expectations of your patients' pain will be influenced by your own values, ideals, and life experiences. As McCaffery's definition indicates, you will need to put aside your personal beliefs about pain and focus on the *patient's* experience.

The pain experience can significantly interfere with a person's quality of life and affect nearly every aspect of life. For example, severe pain can affect job performance, engagement in social activities, sexual intimacy, sleep and rest, ability to exercise, and ability to perform activities of daily living; thus, it can be destructive to both the patient and her family.

Although we usually think of pain in this negative context, pain is also protective, warning us of potential injury to the body. Pain can also prompt us to change our actions. After you have been working at the computer for a while, muscle pain may prompt you to get up and stretch; or the fear of pain with an injury inspires you to be more careful when handling sharp objects.

You will be able to manage pain more effectively if you can classify the type of pain the patient is experiencing. Pain can be classified and described by its origin, duration, pattern of occurrence, quality, intensity, and time since onset. Remember that patients often experience more than one kind of pain.

Origin of Pain

The origin of pain refers to the site where pain is felt and not necessarily the source of pain. The description of the quality and extent of the pain often serves as a strong clue to the cause.

Cutaneous or **superficial pain** arises in the skin or the subcutaneous tissue (e.g., a burn or an abrasion). Although the injury is superficial, it may cause significant short-term pain.

Deep somatic pain originates in the ligaments, tendons, nerves, blood vessels, and bones. Deep somatic pain is more diffuse than cutaneous pain and tends to last longer. Examples include fractures, sprains, arthritis, and bone cancer.

Visceral pain is caused by the stimulation of deep internal pain receptors, most often in the abdominal cavity, cranium, or thorax. Visceral pain may vary from local, achy discomfort to more widespread, intermittent, and crampy pain. Menstrual cramps, labor pain, gastrointestinal infections, bowel disorders, and organ cancers all produce visceral pain.

Radiating pain starts at the origin but extends to other locations. For instance, the pain of a severe sore throat may extend to the ears and head. Or the pain of gastroesophageal reflux ("heartburn") may radiate outward from the sternum to involve the entire upper thorax.

Referred pain occurs in an area that is distant from the original site. For example, the pain from a heart attack may be experienced down the left arm, through the back, or into the jaw. See Figure 32-1 for other examples of referred pain.

Phantom pain is pain that is perceived to originate from an area that has been surgically removed. Patients with amputated limbs may still perceive that the limb exists and experience burning, itching, and deep pain in that area.

Psychogenic pain refers to pain that is believed to arise from the mind. The patient perceives the pain despite the fact

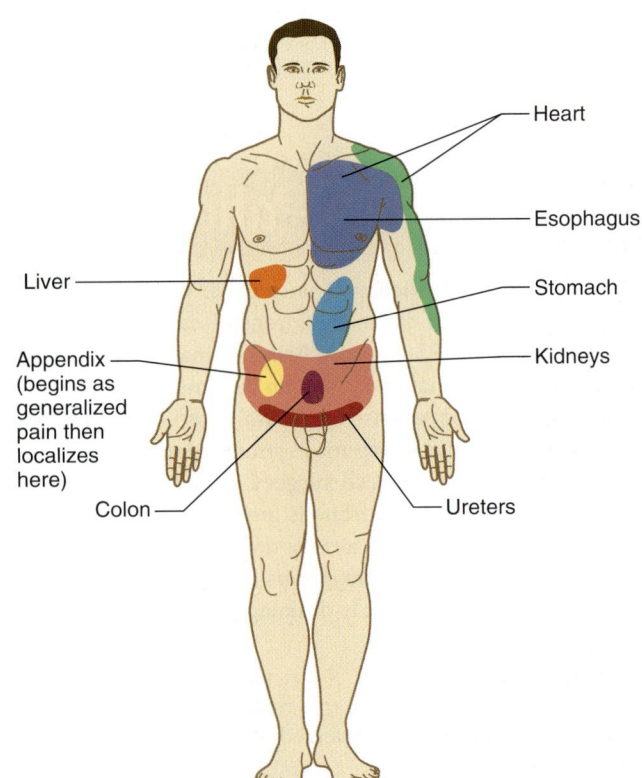

FIGURE 32-1 Most common areas of referred pain.

that no physical cause can be identified. Psychogenic pain can be just as severe as pain from a physical cause. See the discussion of somatoform pain disorder in Chapter 12, if you would like more information.

Cause of Pain

Physical pain is either nociceptive or neuropathic. These two types of pain differ in the way that they affect the patient as well as in how they are treated.

Nociceptive Pain is the most common type of pain. It occurs when pain receptors, which are called **nociceptors**, respond to stimuli that are potentially damaging, (e.g., noxious thermal, chemical, or mechanical stimuli). Nociceptive pain may occur as a result of trauma, surgery, or inflammation. It is most commonly described as aching. There are two types of nociceptive pain (described above): visceral and somatic

Neuropathic Pain is complex and often chronic pain that arises when injury to one or more nerves results in repeated transmission of pain signals even in the absence of painful stimuli. Neuropathic pain is described as burning, numbness, itching, and "pins and needles" prickling pain. The nerve injury may originate from any of a variety of conditions, such as injury to the lower back or hip, poorly controlled diabetes, a stroke, a tumor, alcoholism, amputation, or a viral infection (e.g., shingles). Some medications, such as chemotherapeutic agents, can trigger nerve damage that may cause neuropathic pain even after the medication is discontinued.

Duration of Pain

Acute pain has a short duration with rapid onset. It varies in intensity and may last up to 6 months (American Pain Society, 1994). This type of pain is most frequently associated with injury or surgery. It is protective in that it indicates potential or actual tissue damage. Although acute pain may absorb a patient's physical and emotional energy for a short time, it is helpful for the patient to know that it will usually resolve as the tissues heal.

Chronic (or **persistent**) **pain** lasts 3 to 6 months or longer and often interferes with daily activities. It can be related to a progressive disorder, or it can occur when there is no current tissue injury, as in neuropathic pain. Patients with chronic pain may experience periods of remission and exacerbation. It may lead to patient withdrawal, depression, anger, frustration, and dependence. Chronic pain is the second most feared aspect of cancer or other progressive diseases (American Geriatrics Society, Panel on Persistent Pain in Older Persons, 2009).

Intractable pain is both chronic and highly resistant to relief. This type of pain is especially frustrating for the patient and care provider. It should be treated with multiple methods of pain relief.

Quality of Pain

The words patients use to describe the quality of their pain help care providers to determine the probable cause and most effective treatment.

- **Pain quality** may be described as *sharp* or *dull, aching, throbbing, stabbing, burning, ripping, searing,* or *tingling.*
- **Pain periodicity** may be referred to as *episodic, intermittent,* or *constant.*
- **Pain intensity**, is described with a variety of terms, such as *mild, distracting, moderate, severe,* or *intolerable.*

KnowledgeCheck 32-1

How would you classify the pain that the following patients are experiencing?

- A patient with metastatic cancer
- A patient with back pain that was the result of an automobile injury a year ago
- A patient who had bowel surgery yesterday
- A patient with a fractured hip
- A patient who just had his leg amputated but feels as though the leg is still there
- A person who with an abrasion on her knee after a fall

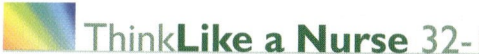

ThinkLike a Nurse 32-1

How would you expect a patient with neuropathic pain to appear?

WHAT HAPPENS WHEN SOMEONE HAS PAIN?

Review the story of Eunice Chu Ling in the Meet Your Patient scenario. Eunice was severely injured in an auto accident. She has had surgery and requires monitoring and invasive devices, such as a ventilator, a chest tube, and an IV line. You can see that she is restless and grimacing. Consider those aspects of Eunice's experience as we explore the physiology of pain.

Transduction

Pain-sensitive nociceptors (sensory nerve cell) are found in the skin, subcutaneous tissue, joints, walls of the arteries, and most internal organs. The skin has the highest density of nociceptors, and the internal organs the least. Painful stimuli prompt the release of substances that trigger release of inflammatory chemicals. These cause an injured area to become red, swollen, and hot. Inflammation is the most frequent cause of pain.

In a process called **transduction**, nociceptors become activated by the perception of mechanical, thermal, and chemical stimuli.

Mechanical stimuli are external forces that result in pressure or friction against the body. They involve stretching of body tissues (e.g., bleeding and swelling) and compression of tissues caused by the force of the trauma. Other types of mechanical stimuli are surgical incisions, friction or skin shearing (e.g., from sliding down in bed), or pressure from a mechanical device such as a cast or brace.

Thermal stimuli result from exposure to extreme heat or cold. If you've ever touched a hot object or suffered an earache when outdoors on a cold day without a hat, you have experienced pain from thermal stimuli.

Chemical stimuli can be internal or external. Lemon juice or any acidic substance on an open area in the skin causes sharp, sudden pain. This is an example of pain from *external* chemical stimuli. In contrast, the chest pain experienced during a myocardial infarction (heart attack) is caused by *internal* chemical stimuli, specifically, the chemical changes that result from tissue ischemia.

Transmission

Peripheral nerves carry the pain message to the dorsal horn of the spinal cord in a process known as **transmission** (Fig. 32-2). Pain messages are conducted to the spinal cord along either of two types of fibers:

- **A-delta fibers** are large-diameter myelinated fibers that transmit impulses at 6 to 32 meters per second. These fibers transmit *fast pain impulses* from acute, focused mechanical

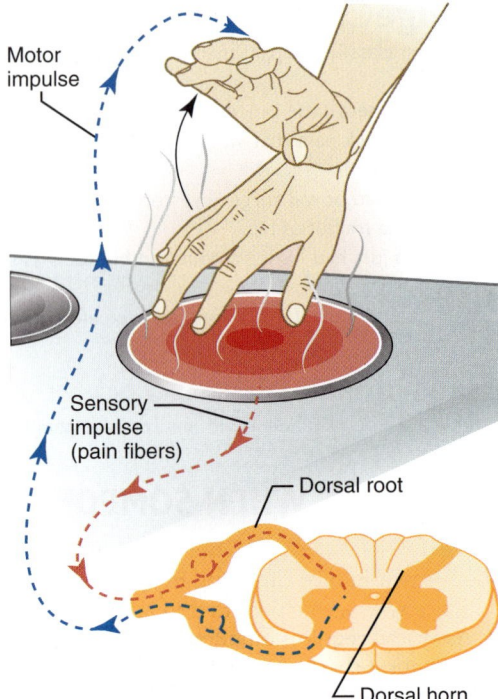

Motor impulse

Sensory impulse (pain fibers)

Dorsal root

Dorsal horn

FIGURE 32-2 After nociceptors are activated, pain is transmitted along A-delta fibers or C fibers to the dorsal horn of the spinal cord. From there, the pain message is sent to the brain for perception.

and thermal stimuli. For instance, when you bump your knee, the initial sharp pain is carried by A-delta fibers. Pleasurable stimuli to skin receptors (e.g., massage) also stimulate A-delta fibers.

- **C fibers** are smaller unmyelinated fibers that transmit *slow pain impulses,* that is, dull, diffuse pain impulses that travel at a slow rate. C fibers conduct pain from mechanical, thermal, and chemical stimuli. If you bump your knee, the lingering ache in the tissue will be carried by C fibers.

Pain transmission involves endogenous chemicals called **neurotransmitters.** Most pain impulses are sent to the thalamus of the brain, which acts as an integrating center to direct the impulses to three regions of the brain: (1) the somatosensory cortex perceives and interprets physical sensations; (2) the limbic system is involved in emotional reactions to stimuli; and (3) the frontal cortex is involved in thought and reason. The person now perceives pain.

Pain Perception

Perception involves the recognition and interpretation of pain in the frontal cortex. **Pain threshold** is the point at which the brain recognizes and defines a stimulus as pain. The number and intensity of stimuli necessary to produce pain, as well as the duration and characteristics of the pain produced, vary from patient to patient. Although the pain threshold usually remains fairly constant for an individual over time, repeated experience with pain can reduce a patient's threshold.

Pain tolerance is the duration or intensity of pain that a person can endure. This varies not only from person to person but also for the same person in different situations. For example, a mother donating a kidney to her child may not report

as much postoperative pain as if she had a kidney removed because it was cancerous. Extreme sensitivity to pain is called **hyperalgesia.**

Pain Modulation

A process called **modulation** changes the perception of pain by either facilitating or inhibiting pain signals through the endogenous analgesia system and the gate-control mechanism.

The Endogenous Analgesia System

In the **endogenous analgesia system,** neurons in the brainstem activate descending nerve fibers that conduct impulses back to the spinal column. These impulses trigger the release of endogenous opioids and other substances to block the continuing pain impulses and provide pain relief. **Endogenous opioids** are naturally occurring analgesic neurotransmitters that inhibit the transmission of pain impulses. Endogenous opioids bind to opiate receptor sites in the central and peripheral nervous system at four receptor sites, designated as mu (μ), kappa (κ), delta (δ), and sigma (σ). Each of the receptor sites has a different affinity for various pain medications. Nonpharmacological measures can also stimulate the endogenous analgesia system.

The Gate-Control Theory

Pain impulses can also be modulated at the spinal level. In explaining the mechanism of pain perception, the **gate-control theory of pain modulation** suggests that the perception of pain does not occur only by direct stimulation of *nociceptors* (pain-producing fibers). Instead, pain is perceived by the *interplay between two different kinds of fibers*—those that produce pain and those that inhibit pain.

- **C (small, slow) fibers.** As slow-pain impulses travel along C fibers from the periphery to the brain, they encounter a "gate" that either allows or blocks the transmission of pain to the brain. If the source of stimulation is nonpainful, the gate would be blocked to feeling pain. Likewise, noxious stimulation keeps the gate open to pain.
- **A-delta (large, fast) fibers.** Imagine that you've just hit your arm against a hard surface. Almost without thinking, you reach down and rub the area. That manual pressure stimulates skin receptors. These send sensory impulses along fast A-delta (large) fibers, which quickly excite inhibitory neurons at the "gate." The inhibitory neurons then block some of the pain signals being carried along the slower C fibers (Fig. 32-3). The gate-control theory is the basis for the use of transcutaneous electrical nerve stimulation (TENS) to relieve pain.

The following are some conditions and strategies are thought to open or close the gate. They are discussed in more depth later in the chapter.

- *Descending impulses from the brain,* including impulses related to mood or emotion, are also thought to open or close the gate. For this reason, medications for depression are sometimes used for patients with chronic pain.
- *Nonpharmacological therapies,* such as meditation, exercise, relaxation techniques, and laughter, may also compete with C fiber impulses and block the gate. These strategies are discussed later in this chapter.

In summary, on a purely physiological basis, pain is simply transduction, transmission, perception, and modulation. However, as we discuss next, our experience of pain involves far more than these four processes.

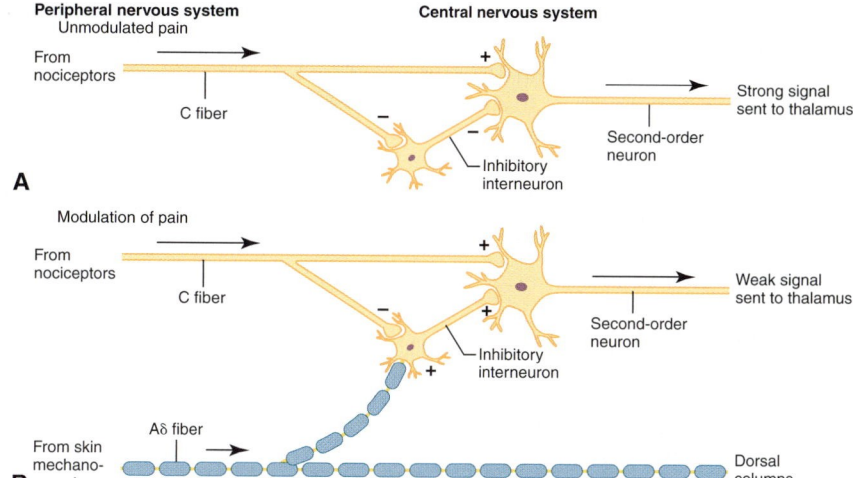

FIGURE 32-3 The gate-control theory of pain modulation. A. Normally, C fibers carrying slow-pain signals block inhibitory interneurons and transmit their signals across the synapse unimpeded. B. A-delta fibers carrying pleasurable signals (e.g., from touch) excite inhibitory interneurons, which then block the transmission of slow-pain signals (+ equals transmission, – equals no transmission).

KnowledgeCheck 32-2

- What must occur to generate pain?
- What are the four physiological steps involved in the pain process?

 ThinkLike a Nurse 32-2

Based on what you have learned about pain modulation, what nursing interventions might help Eunice (Meet Your Patient) be more comfortable?

WHAT FACTORS INFLUENCE PAIN?

Think back to the last time you experienced significant pain. Was it obvious to others that you were in pain? Were quiet? Withdrawn? Did you moan or cry out? Now recall Eunice Chu Ling's reaction. What accounts for these different responses to pain?

KEY POINT: *Pain is universal, yet each person experiences and responds to pain differently.* This demonstrates that pain is a complex phenomenon that influences and is influenced by emotions, previous experiences, age, sociocultural factors, communication, and cognitive impairments.

Emotions

People with pain do not experience one single emotional response. Instead, a multitude of feelings may overwhelm them and escalate their pain. Patients may enter a vicious cycle: Illness and pain trigger emotional reactions, and the emotional reactions exacerbate the pain. Rarely is pain purely physical or emotional. Instead, it is usually a combination of both. Interventions to relieve pain may relieve feelings of fear and helplessness, and interventions addressing these emotions (e.g., reflective listening) often aid in pain relief.

The most common emotions associated with pain are fear, frustration, anger, helplessness, and loneliness. In Meet Your Patient, imagine how Eunice Chu Ling must be feeling. How might her feelings affect and be affected by her pain?

Fear Some patients (e.g., Eunice) fear that their pain means their illness or injury is life threatening. Others fear their pain will eventually become intolerable. Many fear that if they ask for pain relief, they will be judged as weak or that they will become addicted to pain medications. Such fears can prolong or increase the patient's pain.

Confusion and Helplessness In addition to fear, Eunice is also probably experiencing confusion and helplessness. Depending on her role in the accident, she may also feel some guilt. When Eunice is by herself, she may experience loneliness or even a sense of abandonment.

Anxiety and Depression As you learned in Chapter 13, anxiety and depression are common in people who are ill or hospitalized. Anxiety is most often associated with acute pain, but the anticipation of pain may also trigger anxiety. Waiting for surgery or a procedure that you know will be painful offers plenty of time to think about the unpleasantness and to become anxious. In contrast, depression is most often linked with chronic pain, especially intractable pain.

Previous Pain Experience

Patients who have had numerous painful experiences may be more anxious about the prospect of experiencing pain and more sensitive to pain. This is especially an issue for those who require a series of surgeries or painful treatments. Patients who have had effective pain relief in the past are usually less fearful and are more confident they will achieve satisfactory pain relief.

 ThinkLike a Nurse 32-3

Imagine being in a situation similar to that of Eunice Chu Ling (Meet Your Patient). What emotions might you experience?

Developmental Stage

The behavior people exhibit when they have pain is strongly influenced by their stage of development.

Infants and Children Newborns in the first month of life are frequently subjected to painful procedures, with the most immature infants receiving the highest number of painful events. Newborns have the same sensitivity to pain as older infants and children, and preterm infants may have a greater sensitivity (McCaffery & Pasero, 1999).

Infants and small children usually respond to pain by crying loudly. However, in premature and term newborns, the pain does not always evoke detectable behavioral response. Indicators of pain in neonates may be subtle (e.g., mottling, poor feeding). As a result, even though an infant has a low pain score based on behavioral assessment tools, he may not be pain free (Keels, & Sethna; Committee on Fetus and Newborn, & Section on Anesthesiology and Pain Medicine, 2016; Slater, Cantarella, Franck, et al., 2008).

Older Adults Pain occurs in more than half of the geriatric population. In a recent review, 27 studies reported nearly three-fourths of nursing home residents have significant undertreated pain (Takai, Yamamoto-Mitani, Okamoto, et al., 2010).

- Some older adults may be unable to report pain because of cognitive impairment.
- Often their discomfort is evident only in nonverbal cues, such as grimacing, rapid blinking, withdrawal, labored breathing, altered gait, or decreased activity.
- Some older patients respond to pain in atypical ways, such as mental confusion or collapse (American Geriatrics Society, Panel on Persistent Pain in Older Persons, 2009; Flaherty, 2007, revised 2012).

Undertreated pain often leads to other problems that diminish the quality of life, such as social isolation, depression, sleep disturbances, and mobility-related problems.

Sociocultural Factors

We learn behaviors associated with pain through interactions with family (Shin & Kolanowski, 2010) and social support groups. Beliefs about the value of expressing pain or minimizing it are often tied to culture. As you care for clients of various backgrounds, you may notice patterns of pain behavior. Some patients may cry or moan when they are in pain, whereas some may be more stoic, viewing the expression of pain as a weakness. **KEY POINT:** *Do not assume that patients will react according to responses you have seen in others of the same ethnic or cultural group. Each patient and the response to pain are unique.* For example, do you respond to pain in exactly the same way as your parents and siblings?

- **Family and friends also have culturally influenced responses to the patient's pain.** From the Meet Your Patient scenario, recall how Eunice Chu Ling's family is responding. Although you may think it odd that they are smiling, they may be doing so because they want to make a favorable connection with you as the nurse responsible for providing care to Eunice.
- **Nurses, too, are affected by their culture.** Most nurses respond compassionately to those in pain. However, if you fail to recognize that pain is a unique, multidimensional experience, you may misjudge a patient's reaction to injury, surgery, or other discomforts. Disparities exist in the treatment of chronic pain among people of different sociocultural backgrounds. **KEY POINT:** *Nurses have a duty to provide culturally competent care and adequate pain control to every patient.*

Communication and Cognitive Impairments

One of your greatest challenges as a nurse will be caring for patients in pain who have impaired cognition or communication (e.g., from stroke or dementia, intubation, or limited command of language). Although people with dementia might not appear to be experiencing pain, there is no evidence they have less pain than others. Cognitively impaired adults are not less sensitive to pain but rather may fail to interpret sensations as painful. Or they might be unable to communicate their pain as effectively as others. Although they may not be able to recall their pain, they nonetheless still experience it (Horgas, Yoon, & Grall, 2012). These patients are at risk for underassessment of pain and inadequate pain relief (Baldridge & Andrasik, 2010;

Horgas, 2007, revised 2012). You will need to consider their behavioral cues as a form of self-report.

For most people, common nonverbal cues of pain include decreased activity, grimacing, frowning, crying, moaning, and irritability. Other less obvious indicators you may see in cognitively impaired patients include the following:

- Facial expressions (e.g., a sad or frightened expression, rapid eye blinking)
- Vocalizations (e.g., noisy breathing, profanity, verbally abusive language)
- Changes in physical activity (e.g., fidgeting, increased pacing or rocking, disruptive behavior)
- Changes in routines (e.g., refusing food, difficulty sleeping)
- Mental status changes (e.g., increased confusion, moodiness)
- Physiological cues, including elevated blood pressure, respiration, and pulse

KEY POINT: *It is important to know that the lack of these cues does not necessarily mean that pain is absent.*

KnowledgeCheck 32-3

- What are the most common emotional responses to pain?
- What factors influence behavioral responses to pain?

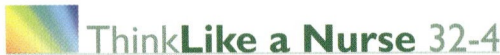

ThinkLike a Nurse 32-4

Eunice Chu Ling (Meet Your Patient) is unable to communicate verbally because of her intubation. She is grimacing in pain. After you medicate her for pain, how would you determine whether her pain has been relieved?

HOW DOES THE BODY REACT TO PAIN?

Pain triggers a variety of changes in the body.

- **The onset of acute pain activates the sympathetic nervous system.** As discussed in Chapter 12, this fight-or-flight (stress) response is protective. It minimizes blood loss, maintains perfusion to vital organs, prevents and fights infections, and promotes healing.
- **If the pain continues, the body adapts, and the parasympathetic nervous system takes over.** However, the pain receptors continue to transmit the pain message so that the person remains aware of the tissue damage. Again, this is largely protective; for example, the pain you feel for several days after you sprain your ankle reminds you to stay off it until it is fully healed.

The severity and duration of the pain significantly affect how the person continues to respond to it. Often the person is able to ignore mild pain, but pain that is severe and unrelieved can consume thoughts and change daily living patterns. Box 32-1 identifies common pain responses.

Unrelieved Pain

Unrelieved pain can produce harmful effects in various body systems.

Endocrine System Ongoing pain triggers excessive release of the hormones adrenocorticotropic hormone, cortisol, antidiuretic hormone (ADH), growth hormone, catecholamines, and glucagon. Insulin and testosterone levels decrease. These hormone shifts activate carbohydrate, protein, and fat catabolism (breakdown); hyperglycemia; and poor glucose use. The inflammatory process, combined with these endocrine and metabolic changes, can result in weight loss, tachycardia, fever, increased respiratory rate, and even death.

BOX 32-1 ■ Common Pain Responses

Physiological (Involuntary) Responses

Sympathetic Responses (Acute Pain)

Dilated blood vessels to the brain, increased alertness
Dilated pupils
Increased heart rate and force of contraction
Increased respiratory rate
Increased systolic blood pressure
Rapid speech
Pallor

Parasympathetic Responses (Deep or Prolonged Pain)

Changeable breathing patterns
Constricted pupils
Decreased pulse rate
Decreased systolic blood pressure, feeling faint, possible syncope
Slow, monotonous speech
Withdrawal

Behavioral Responses (Voluntary)

Agitation
Crying
Facial grimacing
Guarding the painful area
Moaning
Withdrawing from painful stimuli

Psychological (Affective) Responses

Anger
Anxiety
Depression
Exhaustion
Fear
Hopelessness
Irritability

Cardiovascular System Unrelieved pain leads to hypercoagulation (increased clotting) and an increase in heart rate, blood pressure, cardiac workload, and oxygen demand. The combination of hypercoagulation and increased cardiac workload may lead to unstable angina (chest pain), intracoronary thrombosis (clot formation in the vessels that supply the heart), and myocardial ischemia and infarction (heart attack).

Musculoskeletal System Unrelieved pain causes impaired muscle function, fatigue, and immobility. Poorly controlled pain can prevent the patient from performing activities of daily living and engaging in physical therapy.

Respiratory System Patients in pain tend to breathe shallowly—to limit thoracic and abdominal movement. This is called **splinting.** Splinting reduces tidal volume (air exchanged with each breath) and increases inspiratory and expiratory pressures. These changes can lead to pneumonia and atelectasis as well as underventilation (retained carbon dioxide, also called *hypercarbia*) and respiratory acidosis.

Genitourinary System Unrelieved pain causes release of excessive amounts of catecholamines, aldosterone, ADH, cortisol, angiotensin II, and prostaglandins. These hormones lead to decreased urinary output, urinary retention, fluid overload, hypokalemia, hypertension, and increased cardiac output.

Gastrointestinal (GI) System In response to pain, intestinal secretions and smooth muscle tone increase, and gastric emptying and motility decrease.

KnowledgeCheck 32-4

- What are the effects of untreated pain on each of the body systems?
- How might untreated pain affect the progress of a patient recovering from major illness?

PracticalKnowledge
knowing **how**

As discussed earlier, a person's *pain threshold* is the point at which that person perceives a stimulus as painful, whereas

pain tolerance is the amount of pain a person is willing or able to endure. Both differ greatly from person to person.

ASSESSMENT NP

To treat pain effectively, you must first understand the patient's perception of pain. Begin with a comprehensive pain history and assessment that includes the following:

- Pain location and quality
- Pain intensity
- Aggravating and alleviating factors
- Timing and duration
- Pain relief and expectations for how much pain is realistic
- Questions that reveal the patient's ability to perform activities of daily living
- Mobility
- Psychological/social factors (e.g., depression or substance abuse)

For a list of questions that are typically asked, see the Focused Assessment box Pain Assessment.

Also identify any knowledge deficits, fear of addiction, or any other fears or beliefs that may interfere with effective pain management. Focusing on the specific nature of pain enables you to plan the most useful interventions.

When pain is ongoing, the autonomic nervous system eventually adapts. When that happens, the outward signs of pain become less evident (Schneider, 2006–2007, Winter). You should make ongoing pain assessments regularly, as increases in pain may indicate change in condition or a need for more aggressive pain management.

You should accept the patient's self-report of pain, because it is the most reliable indicator of pain, even for those with mild cognitive impairment (Box 32-2) (Jacox, Carr, Payne, et al.; AHCPR, USDHHS, 1994). Health providers who fail to recognize the patient's ratings of pain intensity contribute to inadequate pain management.

Pain, the Fifth Vital Sign

The American Pain Society recommends assessing for pain as the fifth vital sign. That would mean asking patients to rate their pain intensity whenever you take a full set of vital

Focused Assessment

Pain Assessment

Taking a Pain History

Taking a pain history is the most effective way to perform an assessment. Each agency has a different assessment form for this history, but the questions typically will include the following:

Do you have pain now?

When did the pain begin?

Where is the pain located?

How do you rate your pain? (Use a pain scale.)

How would you describe your pain? Sharp? Dull? Achy? Burning?

How often do you have pain? Is it constant or intermittent?

Is there a rhythm or pattern to your pain?

What makes the pain better?

What makes it worse?

How many days this past week has pain interfered in your ability to do what you would like to do?

Does pain interfere with your ability to take care of yourself?

Does pain wake you up at night?

Does pain interrupt your concentration and reduce your ability to think clearly?

Have you experienced this type of pain in the past?

Do you have any other associated symptoms (such as nausea and vomiting) when you are experiencing pain?

Does pain prevent you from participating in pleasurable activities, hobbies, and socializing with friends?

Have you used any medications to treat the pain? If so, were they effective? How often do you need to take pain relievers?

What, if any, alternative treatments have you used for pain?

What past experiences or cultural factors, if any, influence the pain?

Observing for Nonverbal Indicators of Pain

Physiological (Involuntary) Responses

Sympathetic Responses (Acute Pain)

Increased systolic blood pressure

Increased heart rate and force of contraction

Increased respiratory rate

Dilated blood vessels to the brain, increased alertness

Dilated pupils

Rapid speech

Parasympathetic Responses (Deep or Prolonged Pain)

Decreased systolic blood pressure, possible syncope

Decreased pulse rate

Changeable breathing patterns

Withdrawal

Constricted pupils

Slow, monotonous speech

Behavioral Responses (Voluntary)

Withdrawing from painful stimuli

Moaning, crying, sighing, breathing heavily

Facial grimacing, frowning, fearful facial expression

Sleeping or eating poorly

Agitation, fidgeting

Guarding, bracing, rubbing, resisting certain movements

Psychological (Affective) Responses

Anxiety, irritability

Depression, hopelessness

Anger, fear

Exhaustion

Using Pain Scales

The most commonly used pain scales are the visual analog scale (VAS), the numerical rating scale (NRS), the simple descriptor scale (SDS), and the Wong-Baker FACES rating scale.

The Visual Analog Scale

The visual analog scale (VAS) is a 10-cm horizontal line in which "No pain" is written on the left side and "Worst pain imaginable" is written on the right. Patients point to a location on the line that reflects their current pain. Although this rating system is simple and quick, some patients have problems with the abstract nature of the scale.

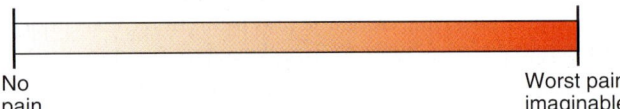

No pain   Worst pain
                                                 imaginable

The Numerical Rating Scale

The numerical rating scale (NRS) is a line numbered from 0 to 10. Zero indicates no pain at all, whereas a 10 indicates the worst possible pain. Patients choose a number from 0 to 10 to denote their level of pain. To use this scale, the patient must be able to count to 10. A scale of 0 to 5 may be more helpful for cognitively impaired patients.

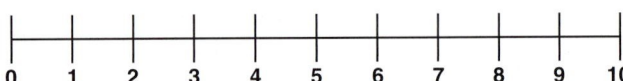

0   1   2   3   4   5   6   7   8   9   10

The Simple Descriptor Scale

The simple descriptor scale (SDS) is a list of adjectives that describe different levels of pain intensity. The simplest version of this scale uses the words mild, moderate, and severe. An SDS with many words is not recommended; it is time consuming to describe and may not be understood by many patients.

Pain Assessment—cont'd

The Wong-Baker FACES Pain Rating Scale
The FACES scale uses simple illustrations of faces to depict various levels of pain. It requires no numerical or reading

skill. Initially developed for use with children older than the age of 3, the scale also has proved to be extremely useful for adults with communication and cognitive impairments.

Wong-Baker FACES® Pain Rating Scale

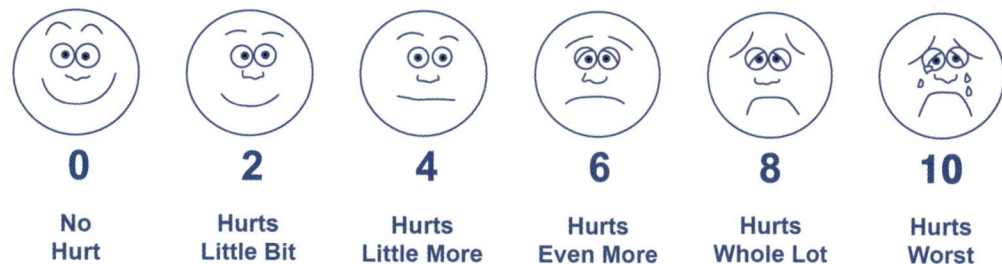

0	2	4	6	8	10
No Hurt	Hurts Little Bit	Hurts Little More	Hurts Even More	Hurts Whole Lot	Hurts Worst

©1983 Wong-Baker FACES Foundation. www.WongBakerFACES.org
Used with permission. Originally published in *Whaley & Wong's Nursing Care of Infants and Children.* ©Elsevier Inc.

Source: Hockenberry, M. J., Wilson, D., & Rogers, C. C. (2017). *Wong's essentials of pediatric nursing* (10th ed.). St. Louis, MO: Elsevier. Used with permission. Copyright Mosby.

 Go to the Wong-Baker FACES Foundation Web site at http://wongbakerfaces.org

Revised Faces Pain Scales

The Faces Pain Scale—Revised (FPS-R) is a self-report measure of pain intensity developed for children. It was adapted from the Faces Pain Scale to make it possible to score the sensation of pain using the widely accepted 0-to-10 metric. The use of grimacing can be more reflective

of the experience of pain than rating faces with smiles and tears.

Give direction for the person to score the chosen face 0, 2, 4, 6, 8, or 10 where 0 means *no pain* and 10 means *very much pain.* This scale is intended to measure how they feel inside, not how their face looks.

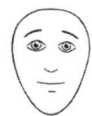 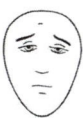 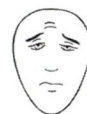 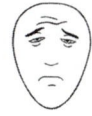 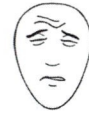 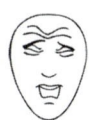

Sources: Bieri, D., Reeve, R., Champion, G. D., et al. (1990). The Faces Pain Scale for the self-assessment of the severity of pain experienced by children: Development, initial validation and preliminary investigation for ratio scale properties. *Pain, 41,* 139–150; Hicks, C. L., von Baeyer, C. L., Spafford, P., et al. (2001). The Faces Pain Scale—Revised: Toward a common metric in pediatric pain measurement. *Pain, 93,* 173–183. International Association of Pain. (2001). Faces Pain Scale—Revised (FPS-R). Retrieved May 1, 2017, from www.iasp-pain.org/FPS-R.

To see another FACES scales using photos of children of various ethnicities,

 Go to the OUCHER!™ Web site at http://www.oucher.org/

---

signs (Pasero, 1997). The goal is to provide a routine for assessing patient pain on a regular and ongoing basis. Some believe that frequent assessment has resulted in oversubscribing of opioids and thus has led to a recent rise in opioid abuse and overdose. **KEY POINT:** *Pain treatment strategies include not only prescribed analgesic, but also nonpharmacological options. Pain management should reflect a patient-centered approach that considers the risk and benefits of the strategy, including potential risk of dependency, abuse, and addiction.* Perform pain assessments routinely, but not limited to:

- On admission to a healthcare facility
- Before and after each potentially painful procedure or treatment
- When the patient is at rest, as well as when involved in a nursing activity
- Before you implement a pain management intervention, such as administering an analgesic drug, and 30 minutes after the intervention
- With each check of vital signs, if the pain is an actual or potential problem
- When the patient complains of pain

Culturally Competent Assessments

Three words—*pain, hurt,* and *ache*—seem to be used across many cultures to describe pain (American Geriatrics Society, Panel on Persistent Pain in Older Persons, 2009). You might

BOX 32-2 ■ Recommended Clinical Approach to Pain Assessment—Agency for Healthcare Policy and Research

Ask about pain regularly. **A**ssess pain systematically.
Believe the patient and family in their reports of pain and what relieves it.
Choose pain control options appropriate for the patient, family, and setting.
Deliver interventions in a timely, logical, coordinated fashion.
Empower patients and their families.
Enable patients to control pain management as much as possible.

Source: Jacox, A., Carr, D. B., Payne, R., et al., Agency for Healthcare Policy and Research, Public Health Service (AHCPR), U.S. Department of Health and Human Services. (1994). *The clinical practice guideline for the management of cancer pain (AHCPR Publication No. 94-0592).* Rockville, MD: Agency for Healthcare Research and Quality.

also use descriptions of *burning, itching,* and *cramping* when asking patients about their pain experience. If you work in an area where there are many non-English-speaking patients, you may benefit from pain assessment tools that have been translated into the languages you are most likely to encounter. The following are examples of the words for "pain" and "where" in various languages:

Spanish: dolor, donde?   Italian: dolore, dove?
French: douleur, ou?   German: Schmerz, wo?

Using Pain Scales

To help you assess the intensity of the pain as well as any changes in the pain, you can choose from among a variety of pain scales (see the Focused Assessment box Pain Assessment). Select a pain scale by considering the patient's age, level of education, language skills, eyesight, and developmental level. Once you choose a particular pain scale for a patient, use it consistently to prevent confusion and allow for comparison.

Assessing Pain in Infants and Children

You can assess pain in children through self-report, behavioral observation, or physiological measures. Be sure to ask parents about the child's usual stress signals and response to pain. With children, use art and play as a way to assess the child's coping with pain. Choose age-appropriate toys to engage the child in acting out feelings. You can also use a pain-rating scale consisting of simple illustrations of faces. When using a simple pain intensity scale, children can communicate the quality of pain before they are developmentally capable of indicating intensity.

Patients Who Are Difficult to Assess

- Patients who are under anesthesia or those receiving pancuronium bromide (Pavulon) are difficult to assess for pain.
- Those with brain injury may mimic pain-like behavior.
- Patients with Alzheimer's disease with severe cognitive and expressive deficits are also a challenge for assessing the extent of pain. It may not be possible to elicit a reliable self-report for

pain, and their behavioral cues might not be reflective of the pain experience either.

When using a pain scale for cognitively impaired patients, you must allow sufficient time for the patient to respond. There are many pain assessment tools. One example is the Pain Assessment in Advanced Dementia (PAINAD) Scale, a five-item observational tool, specifically geared to older adults with dementia (Table 32-1).

For patients who are difficult to assess, you will need to use the patient history and current environment to help you judge the intensity and quality of pain. Does the patient have an underlying painful condition? What is the likely source of pain? Are there physical signs that indicate that the patient has increased pain with movement? Nonverbal signs of pain become important cues for such patients.

Nonverbal Signs of Pain

In addition to the patient's verbal report of pain, you must recognize signal signals. Pay attention to the patient's physical signs and symptoms (see Box 32-1). You will see sympathetic nervous system responses if the pain is acute.

When assessing for nonverbal signs of pain, keep the following guidelines in mind:

- **Facial expression, posture, and body position are reliable indicators of the intensity of pain.** Basic and common facial expressions that signal pain are lowering the brow, wincing, clenching jaws, and closing eyelids (Horgas, 2007, revised 2012). Guarding a painful site or maintaining a tense position is also a sign of pain.
- **Changes in vital signs generally last only a short time.** The body seeks equilibrium; thus, after an hour or so, the vital signs typically return to baseline even though the patient may still be in pain. Continuous, severe pain may elevate the vital signs again from time to time, but they rarely remain elevated. **KEY POINT:** *Normal vital signs do not mean that the patient is free of pain.*
- **Patients may be in pain even if they don't "act like" they are.** Unfortunately, it has been well documented that healthcare professionals fail to assess pain and tend to underrate the pain that the patient is experiencing (American Geriatric Society, Panel on Persistent Pain in Older Persons, 2002; McCaffery & Pasero, 1999). They expect to see frowning, crying, or scowling. Patients who use laughter, distraction, or even sleep to cope with their pain are often undertreated. **KEY POINT:** *To assess pain accurately, you must ask your patients and then believe them.*
- **Use an interpreter if the patient speaks a different language.** Ask the interpreter to explain to the patient that it is important to manage pain and that you will be using a pain scale regularly to assess his pain. Have the interpreter translate and write out the explanation and directions for the pain scale so that you can refer to these when you assess your patient. With written directions, patients can point to a face or numeric line to tell you about their pain when no one is present to translate.
- **Some patients feel that they are being "bad" or "weak" if they express pain.** Such patients may withdraw or become stoic. It is important that you establish a trusting relationship with them. Convey your concern and acknowledge the person's pain. If the patient trusts you, she will feel free to verbalize thoughts and feelings.
- **Remember to assess for depression.** Depression is often overlooked and if it is not treated aggressively, pain management may be unsuccessful.

Safe, Effective Nursing Care

Assessing and Treating Pain in Cognitively Impaired Patients

Competency: Patient-Centered Care (Thinking, Doing, and Caring)

Scenario: Mr. Fagin, who has dementia, has been hospitalized for prostate cancer that has metastasized to his pelvis, femur, and ribs. Mr. Fagin seems confused and is loudly singing hymns and banging his hands against his table in rhythm. The nurse observes him carefully and asks him whether his bones hurt; he nods yes. She also asks Mrs. Fagin about her husband's usual responses to pain. Mrs. Fagin states that her husband has always been very religious and often sings hymns when upset. She says, "I can't stand to see him suffer." The nurse checks the medication administration record (MAR). While Mrs. Fagin speaks gently to her husband, the nurse administers an opioid analgesic. She documents the medication in the MAR, noting his behaviors prior to being medicated. Forty minutes later the nurse observes that his body and facial expression are relaxed, and he has stopped singing. Before leaving, the nurse asks Mr. and Mrs. Fagin whether they would like a visit from the hospital chaplain.

Think about it: A central nursing duty in the patient-centered care competency is alleviating pain and suffering.

1. How is Mr. Fagan's situation different from that of a patient with normal cognitive function?

2. What knowledge, skills, and attitudes did the nurse apply that demonstrate competency in pain management (and, therefore, in patient-centered care), particularly for the patient with dementia? As you think about it, consider the following:

> Why was it important to ask Mrs. Fagin about her husband's usual behavior?
> Was it appropriate to ask the Fagins whether they wanted a visit from the chaplain?
> How did the nurse show respect for the Fagins' preferences, values, and needs?
> Singing loudly doesn't seem to be an obvious indication of pain; what other factors let the nurse know Mr. Fagin was in pain?
> How is pain assessment modified for cognitively impaired patients?
> Do you see how the nurse recognized Mr. Fagin and his wife as full partners in care?

 Go to Davis Advantage, Resources, Chapter 32, **Safe, Effective Nursing Care—Suggested Responses.**

Table 32-1 ➤ Pain Assessment in Advanced Dementia (PAINAD) Scale

ITEMS	0	1	2	SCORE
Breathing independent of vocalization	Normal	Occasional labored breathing. Short period of hyperventilation.	Noisy labored breathing. Long period of hyperventilation. Cheyne-Stokes respirations.	
Negative vocalization	None	Occasional moan or groan. Low level speech with a negative or disapproving quality.	Repeated troubled calling out. Loud moaning or groaning. Crying.	
Facial expression	Smiling or inexpressive	Sad. Frightened. Frown.	Facial grimacing.	
Body language	Relaxed	Tense. Distressed pacing. Fidgeting.	Rigid. Fists clenched. Knees pulled up. Pulling or pushing away. Striking out.	
Consolability	No need to console	Distracted or reassured by voice or touch.	Unable to console, distract, or reassure.	
			TOTALS	

Source: Warden, V., Hurley, A.C., & Volicer, L. Development and psychometric evaluation of the Pain Assessment in Advanced Dementia (PAINAD) Scale. *Journal of the American Medical Directors Association,* 4(1), 9–15. Copyright 2003, with permission from American Medical Directors Association.

KnowledgeCheck 32-5

- How often should you assess the patient for pain, if pain is a potential problem for the patient?
- What are some of the common pain scales used?
- Who should determine whether the patient is in pain?

 Think**Like a Nurse** 32-5

What pain rating scale would you use to assess Eunice (Meet Your Patient)? Why?

ANALYSIS/NURSING DIAGNOSIS NP

Pain as Problem The following NANDA International (NANDA-I) labels are commonly used when pain is the focus of the problem:

- *Acute Pain.* Pain with an anticipated or actual duration of < 6 months.
- *Chronic Pain.* Pain with an anticipated or actual duration of > 6 months.

Notice that NANDA-I uses only duration, not speed of onset or severity, to differentiate between Acute Pain and Chronic Pain. When writing a pain nursing diagnosis, specify the location of the pain and any etiological or precipitating factors that you are aware of. For example:

Acute Pain (headache) related to changes of position and secondary to increased intracranial pressure.

Pain as Etiology Pain affects many areas of functioning. Therefore, it is often the etiology of other nursing diagnoses. The following are a few examples of such diagnoses.

- Self-Care Deficit (Bathing/Dressing/Feeding/Toileting)
- Impaired Walking
- Ineffective Sexuality Pattern
- Impaired Home Maintenance

The following are samples of diagnostic statements you might write for problems caused by pain:

- *Ineffective Airway Clearance* related to ineffective cough secondary to postsurgical incisional pain
- *Sleep Deprivation* related to chronic back pain of more than a year's duration

PLANNING OUTCOMES NP

The overall objective when working with a client in pain is to prevent pain or, if that is not possible, to reduce or eliminate it.

Examples of *NOC standardized outcomes* are:

- **For Acute Pain**—Pain Control, Pain Level, and Comfort Status: Physical
- **For Chronic Pain**—In addition to those for acute pain: Depression Level, and Pain: Disruptive Effects

Individualized goals/outcome statements you might write for a client with pain include the following:

- Within 15 minutes of PCA injection, reports pain is < 3 on a 0–10 scale.
- Reports that chronic pain does not prevent her from performing activities of daily living.
- Pain Control: Uses pain diary (4: Often demonstrated) (NOC)

PLANNING INTERVENTIONS/ IMPLEMENTATION NP

When planning care, remember the following:

- **Each situation is unique.** For example, one terminally ill patient may request complete relief of pain even if this leads to heavy sedation. Another patient with the same diagnosis and prognosis may prefer that the pain be kept at a just manageable level so he can interact with his family or complete unfinished business.
- **The most effective and least invasive method** of pain control is generally preferable.
- **Remember to include nonpharmacological interventions.**
- **The overall care of the patient depends on** the cause of the pain, whether pain is acute or chronic, and the patient's unique situation.
- **There are some nursing interventions and activities that address pain,** both acute and chronic, and regardless of its cause, despite the preceding statement.

NIC standardized interventions for Pain include the following examples:

> **For Acute Pain**—Analgesic Administration, Pain Management, Medication Management
>
> **For Chronic Pain**—Cognitive Restructuring, Pain Management, Coping Enhancement, Mood Management

Specific, individualized nursing activities (including focused assessments) for clients with Acute Pain and Chronic Pain include the following:

- Actively listen to the patient's reports of pain.
- Support the patient and family in maintaining an active role in treatment by including them as part of the pain management team.
- Provide prescribed analgesics promptly.
- Assess responses to analgesics and nonpharmacological measures, including level of sedation. Make assessments approximately 30 to 60 minutes after the administration of an oral medicine. Injectable medications work more quickly, so adjust the assessment time accordingly.
- Provide interventions to manage the side effects of medications.
- Reduce anxiety and fear by offering explanations about care and medications, by allowing the patient to be in control of his pain management, and by providing positive encouragement.
- Consult with the healthcare team about complex pain management issues.
- Alter the treatment if the pain is not adequately relieved.
- Delegate appropriate pain management strategies to NAPs. See Box 32-3 for a list of strategies that may be delegated to NAPs.

Nonpharmacological Pain Relief Measures

Integrating complementary therapies into a pain management plan can help ease chronic pain and reduce the need for drug therapy. According to a recent National Health Interview Survey, one-third of adults used some form of complementary alternative medicine (CAM) when confronted with pain or stress (Barnes, Bloom, & Nahin, 2008).

Nonpharmacological measures, such as exercise, meditation, visualization, and music therapy, can prompt the release of endogenous opioids. They offer an alternative for people with mild pain who do not wish to take medication for pain relief. They should be used as an adjunct to pharmacological therapies for patients with moderate to severe pain (Zeidan, Adler-Neal, Wells, et al., 2016).

Cutaneous Stimulation

Cutaneous stimulation is a pain relief method based on the gate-control theory. As discussed earlier, skin stimulation

BOX 32-3 ■ Pain Management Tasks That May Be Delegated to Nursing Assistive Personnel

Nursing assistive personnel (NAPs) may assist you in caring for patients with pain. However, you may never delegate the responsibility to assess the patient's pain, monitor the patient's response to pain management strategies, or evaluate the pain management plan. ♥ **iCare** The following acts of caring and comfort may be delegated:

- Repositioning, using pillows for support
- Back rub or massage
- Providing darkness and quiet in the room for sleep
- Reducing clutter in the patient's room
- Mouth care
- Soft music of the patient's preference
- Using distraction (talking or setting up a favorite game for the patient)

sends impulses along the large sensory fibers, which in turn excite inhibitory interneurons in the spinal cord to "close the gate." This process diminishes the patient's perception of pain. Cutaneous stimulation works best on pain that is localized and not diffuse.

TENS Units A **transcutaneous electrical nerve stimulator (TENS)** consists of electrode pads, connecting wire, and the stimulator. The pads are applied directly to the painful area, which is most often muscle and soft tissue. Once activated, the unit stimulates A-delta sensory fibers. A TENS unit can be worn intermittently or for long periods of time; pattern and intensity of the impulse can be adjusted depending on the type and location of the patient's pain.

PENS Units **Percutaneous electrical stimulation (PENS)** combines a TENS unit with needle probes percutaneously placed (through the skin) to stimulate peripheral sensory nerves. PENS is effective in short-term management of acute and chronic pain. PENS therapy in some patients promotes physical activity, increases the sense of well-being, reduces the use of nonopioid medication, and improves sleep.

Spinal Cord Stimulator Chronic neurological pain may be treated by a surgically implanted **spinal cord stimulator (SCS).** The SCS produces a tingly sensation that interferes with the perception of pain.

Acupuncture Application of extremely fine needles to specific sites in the body to relieve pain is called **acupuncture.** It is believed to stimulate the endogenous analgesia system. Acupuncture is documented to provide relief from joint pain (Manyanga, Froese, Zarychanski, et al., 2014) and dental discomfort. It is also used after surgery and chemotherapy to treat nausea. Acupuncture may lead to light-headedness, which may be a concern for patients who are at risk for falls. Assess these patients carefully after the treatment.

Acupressure Similar to acupuncture, from which it evolved, **acupressure** stimulates specific sites in the body. However, instead of needles, fingertips provide firm, gentle pressure over the various pressure points. This process may have a calming effect through the release of endorphins. Patients can be readily taught key points to stimulate so that they can self-administer acupressure at any time.

Massage and Myofascial Release Therapy Massage has been shown to be effective in reducing pain. By providing cutaneous stimulation and relaxing the muscles, **massage** helps to reduce pain. **Effleurage,** or the use of slow, long, guiding strokes, is used for obstetrical patients during labor and as back rubs for postsurgical patients. Massage requires little effort from the patient and may improve sleep. For most patients, superficial massage is soothing and relaxing, both mentally and physically. However, some patients do not like to be touched, and you should always obtain verbal permission before giving a massage.

Myofascial release, also called **active release therapy** (ART), is manual pressure applied between overused or injured muscles and nerves to loosen adhesions that develop from overuse. Adhesions can cause numbness and tingling and radiating pain and can limit muscle and joint movement. Some common conditions that can benefit from ART are tendonitis ("tennis elbow"), repetitive motion syndrome, back pain, plantar fasciitis, shin splints, and pulled muscles.

Application of Heat and Cold The application of cold causes vasoconstriction and can help prevent swelling and bleeding. Cold can be especially effective in reducing the amount of pain that occurs during procedures. Apply a cold pack to the site before and after a procedure to reduce pain. Heat promotes vasodilation and circulation, which speeds healing. Use caution with these methods, however, because the skin may be injured by extremes of either hot or cold.

✚ To safely use heat and cold:

- Avoid direct contact with the heating or cooling device. Cover the hot or cold pack with a washcloth, towel, or fitted sleeve.
- Apply heat or cold intermittently, for no more than 15 minutes at a time, to avoid tissue injury.
- Check the skin frequently for extreme redness, blistering, cyanosis (bluish color), or blanching (white color).
- If any of these occur, discontinue the treatment immediately and notify the provider.
- Take extra precautions when applying moist heat or cold, because the addition off moisture amplifies the intensity of the treatment.

Contralateral Stimulation Why does a patient experiencing pain in the right arm experience some relief when lotion is applied and rubbed into the left arm? The principle involved is called **contralateral stimulation**—stimulating the skin in an area opposite to the painful site. Stimulation may be in the form of scratching, rubbing, or applying heat or cold. This intervention is especially helpful if the affected area is painful to touch, under bandages, or in a cast. It has provided some relief to patients who have phantom pain after an amputation.

Oral Sucrose

Sucrose by mouth, alone or in combination with other analgesic measures, can be effective for pain control in newborns exposed to mild or moderately painful procedures (Keels & Sethna; Committee on Fetus and Newborn, & Section on Anesthesiology and Pain Medicine, 2016).

Immobilization

Immobilizing a painful body part (e.g., with splints) may offer some relief. It is particularly helpful with arthritic joints. You must remember to remove the splints at regular intervals so that the patient can exercise the area to strengthen the site and prevent further injury. Patients in severe pain have the tendency to immobilize a painful area by limiting its use.

Cognitive–Behavioral Interventions

Cognitive–behavioral therapy attempts to alter patterns of negative thoughts and to encourage more adaptive thoughts, emotions, and actions. It is used to decrease depression and anxiety, both of which play a role in pain. Cognitive therapy helps patients to deal with their pain by fostering a sense of control over their illness and decreasing feelings of helplessness.

Be sure to obtain consent before using these methods, because psychological or spiritual distress may occur if the method is inconsistent with the patient's belief system. Several of these interventions are discussed in more detail in Chapter 46. To read about holistic nursing, including complementary therapies,

 Go to Bonus Chapter 46, **Holistic Healing,** on Davis Advantage.

Distraction You can use **distraction** as a method of drawing the patient's attention away from the pain by focusing on something other than the pain. It is based on the belief that the brain can process only so much information at one time. When distraction works, the patient has only a peripheral awareness of pain. You may have responded to this strategy in the past. Have you ever had a headache or muscle pain go away when you became busy with other activities?

Distraction is most effective for mild to moderate pain and for brief periods of time (e.g., an injection). Distraction can be visual, tactile, intellectual, or auditory. The usefulness of the particular methods varies among patients.

- *Visual* tactics, such as watching a football game on TV, are effective distractions for some patients.
- *Tactile* distraction, such as massage, hugging a favorite toy, holding a loved one, or stroking a pet, is effective for other patients.
- *Intellectual* distractions include becoming engrossed in a crossword puzzle or playing a challenging game.
- *Auditory* distraction (music therapy) has been shown to reduce anxiety during acute or chronic pain. Mood and pain tolerance improve. Patients' self-reports show that pain is reduced and relaxation is achieved more easily. Physiological measures, such as respirations, heart rate, blood pressure, and muscle tension, also indicate a less intense pain experience (American Music Therapy Association, n.d.). Music should not be limited to adults; it can be used for infants and children as well.
- *Olfactory* stimulation works with the limbic system of the brain to substitute painful stimuli for more pleasant sensory experience. Soothing smells with aromatherapy using essential oils ease pain and anxiety especially for those suffering chronic pain.

Relaxation Techniques Relaxation techniques are especially useful for reducing chronic pain. In **sequential muscle relaxation,** or progressive relaxation, the person sits comfortably and tenses a group of muscles for 15 seconds and then relaxes the muscle while breathing out. After a brief rest, this sequence is repeated using another set of muscles. Patients often start at the facial muscles and work downward to the feet.

Guided Imagery Using directed words and music, this technique evokes positive, calm imaginary scenarios that leads to relaxation and a positive, focused state of mind.

Guided imagery is a holistic technique that creates harmony between the mind and body to promote feelings of well-being, elicit hope, and cope with pain.

Diaphragmatic Breathing Patients can be taught to use the diaphragm (large, dome-shaped muscle at the base of the lungs that is the most efficient muscle of breathing) to intentionally take slow, even breaths when inhaling and exhaling at the rate of five to eight breaths per minute. The technique invokes relaxation and improves tissue oxygenation for managing pain and promoting comfort.

Hypnosis Hypnosis involves the induction of a deeply relaxed state. Once the person is in this state, the hypnotist offers therapeutic suggestions to provide relief of symptoms. For example, the hypnotist may suggest to a patient with arthritis that the pain can be turned down, like the volume of a radio. Special training in hypnotherapy is required.

Therapeutic Touch (TT) This method was developed by nurses and derived from the ancient practice of laying on of hands. Despite its name, TT does not require physical contact. It focuses on the use of the hands to direct energy fields surrounding the body. Although research studies on its effect are not consistent, some patients become relaxed and require less pain medication after a TT session.

Humor For most people, laughter is enjoyable and indicates mental well-being. Humor has positive effects on a patient's physical and emotional health and may boost the immune system as well. It is especially helpful when used before a painful procedure because it lessens anxiety and serves as a form of distraction. Some institutions have humor carts and even humor rooms containing media, books, and playful items, such as bubbles, paints, and puppets. Humor is helpful for both children and adults, but it must always be in good taste and age appropriate. Involve the patient in choosing the humor material because what one person considers very funny another person may not.

Expressive Writing Journaling, blogging, and storytelling can help the patient cope with chronic pain. Some recommend structured writing sessions in which the patient describes stressful events for a specified period of time over consecutive days. Others benefit from frequent journaling in an informal way, expressing feelings, fears, or what comes to mind.

Animal Assisted Therapy Animals (typically dogs), trained to be obedient, calm, and comforting, provide therapeutic benefit to people with chronic pain (e.g., fibromyalgia) and other health problems (e.g., cancer). Patients' serum cortisol (stress hormone) levels decrease when they are exposed to therapy animals. In a study involving patients after knee replacement surgery, those with animal-assisted therapy postop required lower doses of pain medication and reported greater well-being after surgery (Havey, Vlasses, Vlasses, et al., 2014).

 Think**Like a Nurse** 32-6

What has been your experience with using nonpharmacological pain relief measures to manage your own pain? How would you incorporate these methods into your nursing practice?

Pharmacological Pain Relief Measures

Analgesics are classified into three groups: nonopioids, adjuvants, and opioids. The World Health Organization's (WHO) three-step ladder is often used to assist in the selection and titration of an analgesic (Fig. 32-4). Each step on the ladder represents severity of pain, by which the analgesic selection is determined.

- Choice of treatment is based on the level of pain the patient is experiencing. Patients in severe pain should start at the third step.
- If the patient's pain is not controlled, adjust by moving up the pain ladder.
- Titration is accomplished based on a valid and reliable assessment of pain and pain relief (Drew, Gordon, Renner, et al., 2014).
- Monitoring should be regular and continuous.
- To apply the ladder correctly, you need to know the interactions and side effects of all the drugs recommended on each step.

KEY POINT: *Analgesics work best if given before pain becomes too severe. "Keeping ahead of the pain" helps to maintain pain at an acceptable level allow patients to function optimally.* Nurses can achieve this by:

1. Determining the dosage that relieves pain at the desired level.
2. Assessing how long the first dose lasts.
3. Administering the next dose before the last dose wears off.

Around-the-clock dosing is believed to control pain better than prn (as needed) dosing (Pasero & McCaffery, 2011).

Nonopioid Analgesics

Nonopioid analgesics include a variety of medications that relieve mild to moderate pain, and chronic and acute pain. Many are available over the counter (e.g., acetaminophen, aspirin, ibuprofen, and naproxen). Most also reduce inflammation and fever.

The analgesic properties of nonopioid analgesics are often underestimated. Research indicates that standard doses of aspirin or acetaminophen may relieve as much pain as does low dose of the narcotic analgesics, oral meperidine, or oxycodone. Nevertheless, nonopioid analgesics are often compounded with opioids. This allows for a lower dose of opioid to be administered and reduces the incidence of side effects.

Nonsteroidal Anti-inflammatory Drugs The largest group of nonopioid analgesics is made up of nonsteroidal anti-inflammatory drugs (NSAIDs). These include aspirin and ibuprofen, as well as several others. NSAIDs act primarily in the peripheral tissues by interfering with the production of prostaglandins. Prostaglandins sensitize pain receptors and are involved with inflammation. Higher NSAID doses give longer duration of action rather than greater pain relief in the short term (McQuay, Derry, Eccleston, et al., 2012).

One of the most common side effects of NSAIDs is gastric irritation and bleeding. Because of the risk of GI bleeding, the long-term use of nonselective NSAIDs, such as naproxen, oxaprozin, and piroxicam, is generally not recommended in older adults. In addition, they can lead to renal failure, high blood pressure, and heart failure in geriatric patients (American Medical Directors Association, 2012, updated 2016).

- Taking NSAIDs with food, lowering the dose, or using enteric-coated pills can reduce the incidence of gastric irritation and bleeding.
- Some of the newer NSAIDs are less irritating to the GI tract, so they markedly decrease GI side effects. However, they are expensive and available only by prescription.
- Combining two NSAIDs is not often recommended because it increases the risks of side effects and may not be more effective.
- **Aspirin** is a unique NSAID. In addition to reducing inflammation, fever, and pain, it can inhibit platelet aggregation (clumping), the first step in clot formation. For that reason, NSAIDs, especially aspirin, should be used with caution in patients with impaired blood clotting, renal disease, and gastrointestinal bleeding or ulcers.
- Because it inhibits platelet aggregation, low-dose aspirin is prescribed to decrease the risk of myocardial infarction, stroke, and thrombophlebitis (a clot in the peripheral veins), all of which are all associated with platelet aggregation.
- Regular use of aspirin prolongs clotting time, so teach patients who use aspirin that they will bruise easily and will bleed more if cut.

Acetaminophen KEY POINT: *Unlike most nonopioid analgesics, acetaminophen has very little anti-inflammatory effect.* It does have analgesic and fever-reducing properties.

- Acetaminophen has fewer side effects and is probably the safest of the nonopioids.
- It does not affect platelet function, rarely causes gastrointestinal problems, and can be used in patients who are allergic to aspirin or other NSAIDs.
- However, even in recommended doses (up to a maximum of 4,000 mg daily), it can cause hepatotoxicity (liver toxicity) in patients with liver disease or those who heavily consume alcohol.

KnowledgeCheck 32-6

- How do NSAIDs induce pain relief?
- What is the main side effect of NSAIDs?
- In which patients are NSAIDs contraindicated?

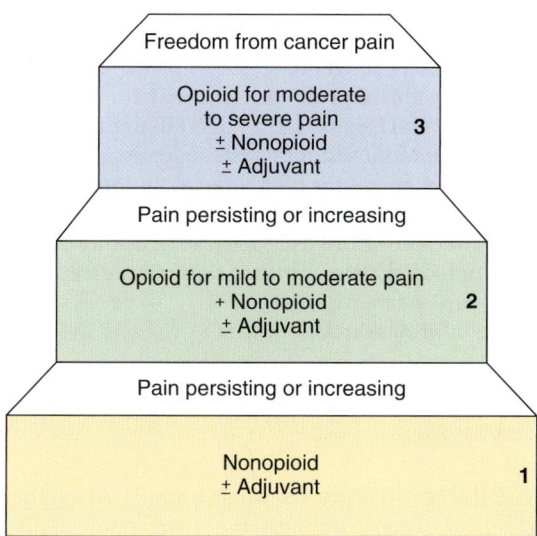

PAIN

FIGURE 32-4 The WHO three-step analgesic ladder.

Adjuvant Analgesics

Adjuvant analgesics reduce the amount of opioid the patient requires. Drugs in this category include anticonvulsants, antidepressants, local anesthetics, topical agents, psychostimulants, muscle relaxants, neuroleptics, corticosteroids, and others. It is used:

- As a primary therapy for mild pain
- In conjunction with opioids, for moderate to severe pain
- Especially by patients experiencing significant side effects from increased doses of opioids
- To manage neuropathic pain

Opioid Analgesics

Opioids are natural and synthetic compounds that relieve pain, although they vary in potency. To some degree, opioids work by binding with pain receptor sites to block pain impulses. The process of achieving pain relief is more complex than this, however. Opiate receptors include mu, delta, kappa, and sigma receptors; mu receptors are most effective in relieving pain.

- **Mu (μ) agonist opioids** stimulate mu receptors and are used for acute, chronic, and cancer pain. They include codeine, morphine, hydrocodone, hydromorphone, fentanyl, methadone, and oxycodone. This class of medication works for **breakthrough pain,** which is pain than occurs when the patient is already receiving an analgesic for pain control. Mu agonist opioids are used in that case for a rescue, extra, or catch-up dose.
  - Drugs used for breakthrough pain should have a rapid onset and short duration.
  - Whenever possible, use the same drug as that given for ongoing pain relief.
  - Increased dosing may be necessary for unrelieved pain.
  - There is no maximum daily dose limit and no "ceiling" to the level of analgesia from mu agonists so you can steadily increase the dose to achieve pain relief, as long as adverse effects do not occur.
- **Agonist–antagonists** are another group of opioids. These medications stimulate some opioid receptors but block others.
  - They are appropriate for moderate to severe acute pain.
  - They should not be given to patients taking mu agonists (e.g., morphine) because they may act as antagonists at the mu receptor sites and reduce or reverse the analgesia from the mu agonist.
  - Commonly used medications include *mixed agonist–antagonists,* such as pentazocine and nalbuphine, and *partial agonists,* such as buprenorphine.

Opioid Effectiveness The effectiveness of opioids for pain relief can vary depending on individual differences in metabolism. Body size has little to do with appropriate opioid dosing (D'Arcy, 2008b). For instance, a particular obese person may receive a therapeutic effect with the same dosage that effectively treats a frail, older adult.

Opioids are most effective for certain types of pain. For instance, visceral pain, which is more generalized, is most responsive to opioid treatment, whereas pain of neurological origin tends to be resistant to opioids, requiring that they be given as an adjunct to other therapies.

Patient Misconceptions About Opioids Although the American Society for Pain Management Nursing and the American Pain Society support safe medication practices with the appropriate use of prn range orders for opioid analgesics in the management of pain, some patients may be concerned about using opioids because they fear respiratory depression, drug tolerance, drug dependence, and addiction. To help them, you should understand the following concepts:

- **Respiratory depression** can be treated with naloxone (Narcan), an opioid antagonist.
- **Tolerance** to opioids can occur, but increasing the dose or changing the route of administration can correct that problem. Because of the problem of cross-tolerance, opioid rotation and new opioid compounds are used to produce better pain relief (D'Arcy, 2008b). Tolerance does not indicate addiction (Pasero & Portenoy, 2011)
- **Physical dependence** leads to withdrawal symptoms when the drug is removed abruptly; it can be prevented by decreasing the dose slowly over time. Physical dependence is not the same as addiction (Pasero & Portenoy, 2011)
- **Psychological dependence,** commonly called *addiction,* occurs in less than 1% of patients even after long-term prescribed use of opioids for pain. Thus, fear of addiction should not prevent patients from receiving opioids for appropriate pain relief (Oliver, Coggins, Compton, et al., 2012).

Screening for Abuse Potential Patients with chronic pain *can* become addicted to or abuse drugs. However, the addiction does not necessarily develop because of the opioid use, but because of each patient's tendencies toward abuse. Considering the prevalence of substance abuse in the general population, assessing the risk for abuse is particularly important for the patient with chronic, nonmalignant pain.

KEY POINT: *Healthcare professionals may fail to recognize substance abuse unless they actively screen for it. You can't rely on the normalcy of behavior to indicate opioid abuse. Random drug screening will show opioid use even when aberrant behavior is not evident.* Although you may be uncomfortable asking questions about alcohol and illicit drug use, gathering a reliable substance use history is important to provide a foundation for good pain management, especially for those with chronic pain. This history should include information on the pattern and amount of alcohol, narcotics, or recreational drug intake, because patients whose tolerance is high may require a higher dose of opioids. To screen for abuse, use validated risk assessment tools, such as the following:

- **Opioid Risk Tool (ORT).** This is a yes/no self-report designed to predict a patient's tendency for aberrant behaviors when prescribed opioid analgesia (Table 32-2).
- The **Screener and Opioid Assessment for Patients With Pain (SOAPP®).** This is more detailed than the ORT and is a highly reliable tool used for assessing patients experiencing chronic pain who might be helped with long-term opioid treatment.
- The **Current Opioid Misuse Measure (COMM™)** is used to identify opioid misuse among patients currently taking long-term opioid medication.

For more information about the SOAPP® and the COMM™,

 Go to the PainEDU.org Web site at http://www.painedu.org/soapp.asp

Side Effects of Opioids Most opioids share the same general side effects, although there are some differences among the specific drugs.

- *The most common side effects* are drowsiness, nausea, vomiting, and constipation. Some, such as drowsiness and nausea, improve after a few doses.

Table 32-2 ➤ Using the Opioid Risk Tool

MARK ANY CONDITIONS THAT APPLY		FEMALE	MALE
Is there a history of substance abuse in your family?	Alcohol	Yes / No	Yes / No
	Illegal drugs	Yes / No	Yes / No
	Other	Yes / No	Yes / No
Have you had a history of substance abuse?	Alcohol	Yes / No	Yes / No
	Illegal drugs	Yes / No	Yes / No
	Other	Yes / No	Yes / No
Are you between the ages of 16 and 34?		Yes / No	Yes / No
Have you ever been sexually abused?		Yes / No	Yes / No
Do you have a history of any of the following conditions?	Attention deficit disorder?	Yes / No	Yes / No
	Obsessive compulsive disorder?	Yes / No	Yes / No
	Bipolar disorder?	Yes / No	
	Schizophrenia?	Yes / No	
	Depression?	Yes / No	

Source: Adapted from Webster, L. R., & Webster, R. M. (2005). Predicting aberrant behaviors in opioid-treated patients: Preliminary validation of the Opioid Risk Tool. *Pain Medicine,* 6(6), 432–442. Permission obtained.

- *Large doses* may lead to respiratory depression and hypotension.
- *Other side effects* of opioids include difficulty with urination, dry mouth, sweating, tachycardia, palpitations, bradycardia, rashes, urticaria (hives), or pruritus (itching).
- *For strategies to prevent common side effects,* see Box 32-4.
- *Long-term use of opioid therapy* for chronic pain may increase the risk of serious harm with higher doses (Chou, Deyo, Devine, et al., 2014). Always assess the patient for level of alertness and respiratory status before you administer an opioid. Excessive sedation will precede respiratory depression.
- *Paradoxical reactions.* For some individuals, opioids may lead to a paradoxical increase in pain despite receiving increasing doses of opioids.
- *Sedation.* Most patients experience some degree of sedation at the beginning of opioid therapy or when the dose is increased. For postoperative patients who receive opioids, use oxygen saturation monitoring to assess for sedation and respiratory depression every 1 to 2 hours during the first 12 to 24 hours after surgery (Jarzyna, Jungquist, Pasero, et al., 2011). For an example of a sedation scale, see the Focused Assessment box Sedation Rating Scale.

KnowledgeCheck 32-7
- What are the most common side effects of opioids?
- Identify at least three things that you should monitor when administering opioids.
- What is the risk of addiction to opioids for patients with acute pain?

Equianalgesia Equianalgesia refers to the approximately equal analgesia that a variety of opioids will provide.

Equianalgesic dose calculations provide a starting point when changing (1) from one opioid to another or (2) from one route of administration to another. For example, in terms of the analgesic effect produced:
- A parenteral dose of 5 mg of morphine is equivalent to 60 mg of parenteral codeine or 100 mg of oral codeine.
- A parenteral dose of 5 mg morphine is the equivalent of 15 mg of oral morphine.

These doses are approximate and vary according to the number of doses, the variety of opioids the patient has received, and the needs of the patient.

Routes of Administration for Opioid Analgesics
Use the safest and least invasive route to administer opioids. See Box 32-5 for an overview of opioid administration routes.

Patient-Controlled Analgesia (PCA) Inadequate pain control in the past led to the use of routine PCA, which allows patients to self-administer medication for pain relief. Although PCA is most often delivered intravenously, analgesics can also be delivered by epidural, subcutaneous, and oral routes.

Intravenous PCA systems consists of an infusion pump, a syringe, IV tubing, and a trigger that the patient presses to self-administer a dose (Fig. 32-5). The pump must be programmed so that a dose can be administered frequently enough to manage the patient's pain effectively. Some providers order a low continuous rate of infusion that can be supplemented with patient-initiated doses. As a safeguard, have another nurse double-check the setup before patient use.

Most PCA pumps can be programmed with 1- or 4-hour maximum medication limits. If the patient reaches the limit set, the pump will automatically trigger a "lockout" even if the patient keeps pressing the button. Teach patients about this lockout feature; some may not activate the pump enough because they fear overdosing.

Sedation Rating Scale

Richmond Agitation–Sedation Scale

Score	Term	Description
+4	Combative	Overtly combative or violent; immediate danger to staff
+3	Very agitated	Pulls on or removes tube(s) or catheter(s) or has aggressive behavior toward staff
+2	Agitated	Frequent nonpurposeful movement or patient–ventilator dyssynchrony
+1	Restless	Anxious or apprehensive but movements not aggressive or vigorous
0	Alert and calm	
−1	Drowsy	Not fully alert, but has sustained (more than 10 seconds) awakening, with eye contact, to voice
−2	Light sedation	Briefly (less than 10 seconds) awakens with eye contact to voice
−3	Moderate sedation	Any movement (but no eye contact) to voice
−4	Deep sedation	No response to voice, but any movement to physical stimulation
−5	Unarousable	No response to voice or physical stimulation

Source: Sessler, C. N., Gosnell, M.S., Grap, M. J., et al. (2002). The Richmond Agitation–Sedation Scale: Validity and reliability in adult intensive care unit patients. *American Journal of Respiratory Critical Care Medicine, 166,* 1338–1344. doi:10.1164/rccm.2107138

BOX 32-4 ■ Preventing and Treating Side Effects From Opioids

Before deciding to add another medication to treat a side effect, consider changing the dose or frequency of the current opioid or changing to another opioid. You should also wait until after the peak effect of the first dose before giving another dose.

Side Effect: Constipation

- Add more fruits, vegetables, and fiber to the diet. *Keep in mind, though, that this does not help relieve opioid-induced constipation unless the patient's current fiber intake is deficient. Excessive fiber might even put the patient at risk for bowel obstruction due to the opioid-induced decreased peristalsis (refer to Chapter 29, as needed).*
- Increase exercise. Even walking short distances will help.
- Increase oral fluid intake to eight 8-oz glasses of water per day.
- If needed, administer stool softeners.
- If the above are not effective, administer a mild laxative.
- If constipation continues, soften stool with glycerin suppository and follow up with a soapsuds enema.

Side Effect: Nausea and Vomiting

- Reduce opioid dose by combining nonopioid or adjuvant drugs.
- Teach patients that nausea will usually subside after several doses.
- Premedicate or medicate consecutively with an antiemetic. Be aware this may increase sedation, depending on the antiemetic chosen.
- Teach relaxation techniques.

Side Effect: Pruritus

- Reduce opioid dose by combining with nonopioid or adjuvant drugs.
- Use cool packs, lotion, or topical anesthetics.

- Administer antihistamines, such as diphenhydramine (Benadryl). Be aware that this may increase sedation.
- Teach the patient that he can generally expect to develop a tolerance to pruritus.
- Use distraction techniques, which frequently work well.

Side Effect: Respiratory Depression

- Assess the patient's respiratory status *before* administering the opioid and frequently afterward.
- Reduce the opioid dose by combining with nonopioid or adjuvant drugs.
- Reduce the opioid dose by 25% when you observe signs of oversedation.
- If the patient is not responsive or is only minimally responsive, stop the opioid and administer an antagonist, such as naloxone (Narcan). After dosing with a narcotic antidote, reassess the patient for respiratory depression. *Naloxone is metabolized more quickly than opioids; therefore, repeat dosing might be needed.*

Side Effect: Drowsiness

- Assess the patient to ensure that the drowsiness is due to opioid administration and not from another cause.
- Teach the patient that drowsiness will generally subside after a few days as she develops tolerance.
- If analgesia is adequate, reduce the opioid by 25%.
- Discontinue all other nonessential CNS depressant medications.
- During the daytime, offer simple stimulants, such as caffeine.
- Offer a lower dose more frequently to decrease peak concentration.
- Consider another opioid or route of administration.

BOX 32-5 ■ Opioid Administration Routes

Oral

- Convenient and safe
- Generally produces steady analgesic levels
- The preferred route of administration unless rapid onset of analgesia is desired
- Includes medications that are swallowed but also includes sublingual, transmucosal, buccal, and gingival routes
- Use the oral route to relieve mild to severe pain.
- Oral patient-controlled analgesia (oral PCA) is being used in some hospitals to eliminate the delay between the patient's request for medication and the nurse's administration of it.

Nasal

- A mixed agonist–antagonist opioid, the mu (μ) agonist can be administered intranasally.
- A rich supply of blood to the nasal area provides the drug easy access to systemic circulation.
- This route may cause burning or stinging.

Transdermal

- Delivers a continuous release of drug for up to 72 hours
- A convenient alternative for a patient who requires constant opioid treatment for pain.
- Fentanyl (Duragesic) is commonly given as a transdermal patch.
- Use with care on patients who are febrile, because their increased temperature will increase absorption of the drug.
- Effective for ongoing pain relief but does not provide immediate relief
- Inform the patient and family about safe storage and proper disposal of transdermal patches. Proper dating and removing patches after the dose is complete can prevent confusion and dosing errors.

Rectal

- Suppositories are an excellent alternative to the oral route, especially in infants and young children.
- Effective when the patient is vomiting, has a gastrointestinal obstruction, or is at risk for aspiration of oral medications
- May be contraindicated in patients with neutropenia (low white blood cell count) or thrombopenia (low platelet count) because of the risk for rectal bleeding while inserting the suppository

Subcutaneous

- May be used for intermittent injections and continuous administration of opioids
- Continuous subcutaneous infusion (CSCI) of opioids is gaining popularity; hydromorphone and morphine are the drugs most commonly used.
- CSCI is appropriate for people who cannot tolerate oral opioids or who have dose-limiting side effects from oral administration (e.g., nausea) and who also have limited venous access.

- Absorption and distribution vary based on the injection site, medications, adiposity, age, patient's circulation, hepatic and renal status, and other health factors.
- Small portable medication pumps allow the patient to be mobile. However, some patients find this method painful and time consuming. You will need to teach patients and their families how to use the pumps, needles, syringes, and other equipment.
- Because of the small volume of drug (2 to 3 mL/hr) that can be absorbed, two sites may be needed if higher doses are required.

Intramuscular (IM)

- Often used for short-term pain relief postoperatively
- Not the preferred route of administration of pain medication because IM injections are painful, the onset of action is slow, and absorption is unreliable
- With repeated administration, sterile abscesses and fibrotic tissue can result.
- Should be avoided in children because they often refuse pain medication to avoid having an injection

Intravenous (IV)

- Produces immediate pain relief and is desirable for acute or escalating pain
- Most commonly used for short-term therapy and for hospitalized patients who can be monitored
- Used in the home care setting for patients with cancer and other pain who are unable to tolerate oral opioids
- Methods of IV delivery include continuous infusions, bolus, and patient-controlled analgesia (PCA).
- Patients using a continuous infusion can deliver a bolus for breakthrough pain or procedures such as wound care.
- Drawbacks to the IV route include the need for venous access and the need to maintain a patent line.
- Patients who previously used oral opioids may find the IV equipment cumbersome but they typically report less pain and fewer side effects than with the oral route.

Intra-articular

A pain pump is implanted into a joint during arthroscopic surgery to control postsurgical pain. A pain pump provides relief to patients by delivering continuous infusion of local anesthetic directly to the joint.

Intraspinal and Epidural Analgesics

- Intraspinal analgesia requires placement of a catheter in the subarachnoid space (for intrathecal analgesia) or the epidural space by an anesthesiologist or a certified registered nurse anesthetist.
- The epidural space (see figure in this box) is generally preferred because it poses less risk of complications, although they can occur (e.g., dural puncture, infection, hematoma, and nerve damage).

(Continued)

BOX 32-5 ■ Opioid Administration Routes—cont'd

- Placement of the catheter, as well as the type and concentration of medication, determines the area affected by the medication.
- Higher doses are needed for epidural than for intrathecal administration.

- The most commonly used opioids for epidural administration are morphine sulfate, fentanyl citrate, and hydromorphone.
- Local anesthetics are frequently combined with the opioids to reduce the total amount of drug necessary to produce analgesia.
- For nursing care activities associated with caring for a client with an epidural catheter for pain management, see Clinical Insight 32-1.

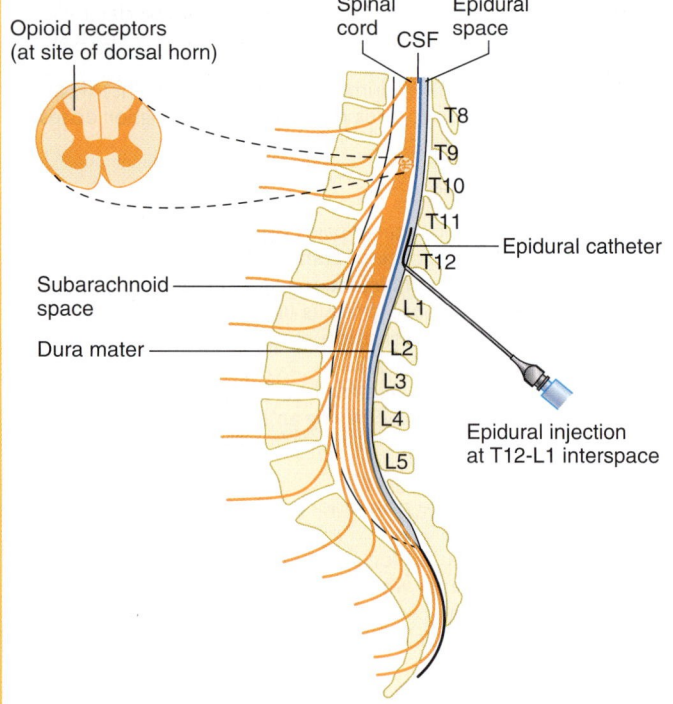

Labels in figure: Opioid receptors (at site of dorsal horn); Spinal cord; CSF; Epidural space; T8; T9; T10; T11; T12; Epidural catheter; Subarachnoid space; Dura mater; L1; L2; L3; L4; L5; Epidural injection at T12-L1 interspace

If you are educating the patient in the postoperative period, make sure she is alert enough to understand the directions and has been given a hearing aid or glasses, if needed. Encourage patients to administer a dose before potentially painful activities, such as walking or physical therapy.

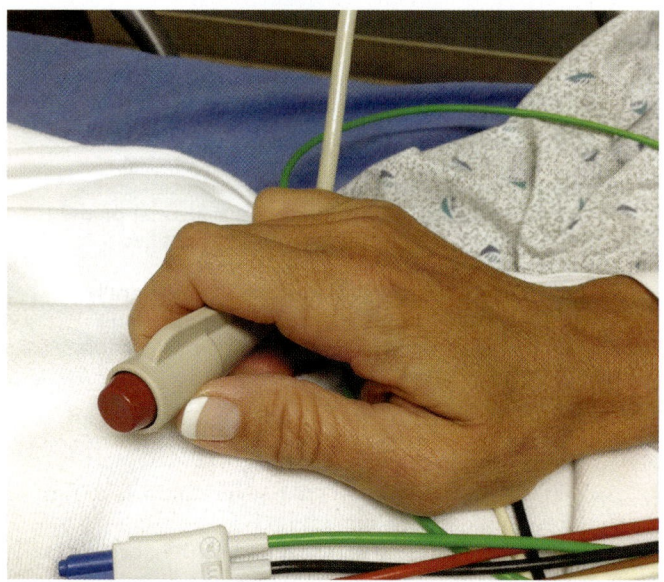

FIGURE 32-5 Dosing button for patient-controlled analgesia.

KEY POINT: *PCA pumps are contraindicated in patients who have limited ability to understand directions for use.*

For detailed instruction on using a PCA pump, see Procedure 32-1.

ThinkLike a Nurse 32-7

- What routes of opioid administration have you seen in your clinical rotation?
- What types of pain relief and side effects have you observed?
- What routes of administration would you like to see? Why?

Chemical Pain Relief Measures

Nerve blocks and **epidural injection** are types of regional anesthesia. An anesthetic agent is injected into or around the nerve or network of nerves *(plexus)* that supplies sensation to a specific part of the body. Nerve blocks may be used for short-term pain relief after surgical procedures or for long-term management of chronic pain. See Clinical Insight 32-1 to learn about caring for a patient with an epidural catheter.

Local anesthesia is the injection of anesthetics into relatively small areas of body tissues to numb the area. Short-acting agents (e.g., lidocaine) and long-acting agents (e.g., marcaine) may be used.

- Local anesthetics are injected into subcutaneous tissue for *minor surgical procedures.*
- They may also be injected into joints and muscle for *pain relief.*
- Pumps are commonly used to administer local anesthetics at surgical sites for *postoperative pain relief.*

Toward Evidence-Based Practice

Lambert, T. L., & Cata, D. M. (2014). The traditional method of oral as-needed pain medication delivery compared to an oral patient-controlled analgesia device following total knee arthroplasty. Orthopaedic Nursing, 33(4), 217–223. doi:10.1097/NOR.0000000000000065

Patients commonly experience a delay in receiving prn pain medication because of competing demands on nurses' time. For this reason, researchers wanted to know whether use of an oral patient-controlled analgesic device would benefit patients more than having to request pain relief doses from the nurse. Findings in postoperative orthopedic patients showed that those who could self-administer oral analgesics reported less pain with activity and physical therapy, improved mood, and better sleep and appetite.

Riemondy, S., Gonzales, L., Goskik, K., et al. (2014). Nurses' perceptions and attitudes toward use of oral patient-controlled analgesia. Pain Management Nursing, 17(2), 132–139. doi: http://dx.doi.org/10.1016/j.pmn.2016.02.051

Researchers found that patients were more favorable than nurses toward the use of patient-controlled oral analgesia (PCOA). Patients reported better pain control when they were able to self-administer medication. They found the electronic dispensing device for oral analgesics easy to use and also reported fewer restrictions in activity, sleep, and appetite due to pain compared with similar patients who needed to request medications from their nurses. However, some nurses perceived disruptions in their workflow using the new PCOA device, including operation of the device as well as staff and patient education, which required more of their time. Helping nurses develop a willingness to use the PCOA device may contribute to better pain control as well as greater patient satisfaction.

1. Discuss at least six possible benefits to patients using patient-controlled oral dosing of pain-relieving medication.

2. Discuss at least three benefits for nurses using patient-controlled oral dosing of pain-relieving medication.

3. Can you think of reasons why some nurses might resist using an electronic dispensing system for oral PCA? Include some of your own personal experiences or that of your preceptor or classmates.

 Go to Davis Advantage, Resources, Chapter 32, **Toward Evidence-Based Practice—Suggested Responses.**

Topical anesthesia involves applying a cream or ointment that typically contains lidocaine or benzocaine directly to the skin, mucous membranes, wounds, or burns. It is rapidly absorbed and provides pain relief for mild to moderate pain. Topical anesthetic cream or gel should be applied before vaccinating children to reduce pain associated with injection (Henderson, 2015) or circumcision.

Radiofrequency Ablation Therapy

Radiofrequency ablation therapy uses electromagnetic waves that travel at the speed of light to target nerves that carry pain impulses. This procedure is used to provide longer-term pain relief than that provided by injections of steroids, analgesics, and nerve blocks.

Surgical Interruption of Pain Conduction Pathways

Surgical interruption of pain conduction pathways results in permanent destruction of nerve pathways. It is used as a last resort for intractable pain. The various options depend on the type and location of pain.

- **Cordotomy** interrupts pain and temperature sensation below the tract that is severed. This is most frequently done for leg and trunk pain.
- **Rhizotomy** interrupts the anterior or posterior nerve route that is located between the ganglion and the cord. Anterior interruption is generally used to stop spastic movements that accompany paraplegia; posterior interruption eliminates pain in the area innervated. This procedure may be safely performed at any level along the spine but is most often used for head and neck pain produced by cancer.

- **Neurectomy** is used to eliminate intractable localized pain. The pathways of peripheral or cranial nerves are interrupted to block pain transmission.
- **Sympathectomy** severs the paths to the sympathetic division of the autonomic nervous system. This procedure is performed to improve vascular blood supply and eliminate vasospasm. It is used to treat the pain from vascular disorders, such as Raynaud's disease.

Surgical therapies disrupting pain pathways are not widely used because of advances in oral and transdermal opioid therapies.

KnowledgeCheck 32-8

- Identify three types of chemical pain relief measures.
- What type of patient might be suitable for surgical interruption of a pain pathway?

Misconceptions That Interfere With Pain Management

Pain is invisible to others but it exists when the patient says it does. It exists even when there are no sure signs of pain or an apparent cause.

Patients, caregivers, and clinicians sometimes have beliefs about pain or pain management strategies that interfere with the treatment plan. For instance:

- One older patient may fear that severe **pain is a sign of weakness** and try to endure it.
- Another might perceive **pain as a part of the normal physical declines** that accompany aging instead of an acute situation that requires treatment.

- An athlete might believe **"no pain, no gain,"** but actually, pain can signal a problem.
- One family member may worry that **pain medication may make the patient nonfunctional,** whereas others might **fear addiction to pain medication** even though non-narcotic analgesics are not addictive.

The beliefs of healthcare providers can also interfere with pain management. For example, nurses and other caregivers sometimes doubt the patient's report of pain because of the following:

- Most people don't have pain from that particular illness or procedure.
- There is no obvious, physical cause for the pain.
- The care providers are concerned about drug-seeking behavior and patient addiction.

As you care for patients in pain, remain open to the patient's description of pain and work with the patient and caregivers to provide pain control. Table 32-3 highlights some of the most common misconceptions about pain.

Managing Pain in Older Adults

Pain is common among older adults, especially those suffering from degenerative spine conditions, arthritis, nightly leg pain, or pain as a result of cancer. Pain management is especially difficult in older adults because:

- Most older adults have at least one chronic condition and take *multiple medications*. Adding analgesics to an already complex medication regimen increases the likelihood of drug interactions.
- *Drug distribution is altered in older patients* because of changes in blood flow to the organs, protein binding, and the difference in body composition.
- Older adults are at great risk for undertreatment of pain because they and their caregivers may be *reluctant to administer analgesics for fear of producing confusion, excessive sedation,* drug interactions, and respiratory depression (American Geriatrics Society, Panel on Persistent Pain in Older Persons, 2009).
- Healthcare providers often fail to recognize poor pain management because of the patient's *dementia, coexisting medical conditions, sensory impairment, or inability to verbally communicate* the quality or intensity of pain.

- With aging and declining renal and liver function, *the peak effect of medication is longer,* which *can lead to giving more pain-relieving medication than needed* (American Geriatrics Society, Panel on Persistent Pain in Older Persons, 2009).
- *Insufficient pain management can result in falls, poor sleep, delayed healing, reduced activity, prolonged hospitalization, anxiety, and poor quality of life* (Horgas, 2007, revised 2012).

Opioids
KEY POINT: *Persistent pain is not a normal part of aging and should not be ignored.* In light of increased cardiovascular risk and gastrointestinal toxicity in this population, the American Geriatrics Society recommends that older adults with moderate to severe pain or diminished quality of life due to pain should be considered for oral opioid therapy.

- The general rule is to start low and go slow, meaning to start with the lowest effective recommended dose and increase the dose slowly if needed (Kaye, Baluch, & Scott, 2010).

- ✚ Be aware that opioids in older adults increase the risk of falls.

Nonopioid Analgesics
- *Acetaminophen* is a first-line treatment for mild pain, particularly musculoskeletal pain, and is often used as an adjuvant therapy for older persons with recurring pain.
- *NSAIDs* are a good option for those with compromised kidney or liver function.
- **Gabapentin** has few side effects and can also be used in combination with non-opioid analgesics to relieve neuropathic pain.

ThinkLike a Nurse 32-8
Which groups of patients are most at risk for inadequate pain management?
- What can you do to assist each group?
- How do past pain experiences affect present pain experience?

Managing Postoperative Pain
Guidelines for the management of postoperative pain include some of the following interventions:
- Begin with a validated pain assessment tool to assess the patient's response to pain control measures.

Table 32-3 ▶ Common Misconceptions Among Patients and Caregivers About Pain	
FALLACY	**TRUTH**
The caregiver is more objective than the patient about the amount of pain experienced.	The patient's report is the "gold standard," and the patient is the authority.
You should wait until the pain is severe before taking medication.	You should take pain medication early and on a regular basis if pain is severe.
There is a significant danger of addiction to pain medications.	Patients in pain rarely become addicted to their pain medications.
Pain is a normal component of aging.	Pain is a symptom that something is wrong and should be treated.
Complaining of pain will label the person as a "bad patient."	The patient should report pain so that it can be treated.
Patients should have severe pain only if they have major surgery.	Even minor surgery and injury can produce severe pain.
Patients will have visible physical or behavioral signs if they are really in pain.	Even when patients are in severe pain, they may not exhibit physical or behavioral signs.

- Devise an individualized plan for pain control, depending on the procedure, underlying health, sensitivity to medication, and goals for pain control. Patients respond differently to treatment.
- Use a variety of analgesic medications and nonpharmacological techniques for their synergistic effect.
- Administer round-the-clock NSAIDs in addition to other pain control measures if not contraindicated. This helps to keep ahead of the pain.
- Oral opioids should be given in preference to IV opioids when possible. IM injection can cause additional pain. Plus, the absorption is unreliable postoperatively.
- Offer PCA when parenteral pain management is needed.
- Monitor for side effects of analgesics, including respiratory depression, hypotension, and allergic reaction (Chou, Gordon, de Leon-Casasola, et al., 2016).

Managing Pain in Patients With Substance Abuse or Active Addiction

It is important to differentiate between physical dependence—which is expected and treatable—and addiction. **Addiction** is a state of psychological dependence in which a person uses a drug compulsively and will engage in self-destructive behavior to obtain the drug. ♥ **iCare** When caring for clients with active addiction, try to remain nonjudgmental.

Properly managed, short-term medical use of opioid analgesic drugs is safe and rarely causes addiction. There is more risk of addiction if the patient has a personal or family history of drug abuse or mental illness (National Institutes of Health, National Institute on Drug Abuse, 2001, revised 2014). Nevertheless, substance abuse is a common problem among individuals from all backgrounds. Behaviors that indicate substance abuse or addiction include the following:

- Repeated requests for injections of an opioid or atypical high dosing when pain should normally be diminishing (e.g., after an injury or surgery)
- Refusal to try oral medication for pain relief
- "Doctor shopping"—moving from provider to provider in an effort to obtain multiple prescriptions for the drug(s) the person abuses
- "Pharmacy shopping"—using multiple pharmacies to dispense controlled substances

If you observe these signs, consult with pain management specialists as well as addiction and dependency professionals.

When analgesics are no longer needed, taper the dose to prevent withdrawal symptoms from occurring (Pasero & McCaffery, 2011). As a nurse, you will be in a position to help maintain the balance between providing adequate pain relief and protecting against inappropriate drug use.

For those at moderate risk for opioid abuse, maximize appropriate nonopioid medications and other nonpharmacological therapies to reduce pain. Do not substitute pain relievers with sedative medication (Oliver, Coggins, Compton, et al., 2012).

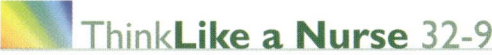
ThinkLike a Nurse 32-9

You are preparing to give your patient a bath. When you remove his bath equipment from under the bedside table, you find illicit drugs mixed in with the bath equipment. What would you do?

Pain Relief From Placebos

A **placebo** is any medication, procedure, or surgery that leads to analgesia or other desired outcome, even if lacking active substances or other actions that contribute to pain relief.

Clearly, placebos can relieve pain for some patients, but how they do so is not well understood. Theories include operant conditioning, faith, anxiety reduction, and endorphin release. **KEY POINT:** *Although use of placebos may be appropriate in clinical trials, they are not suitable for pain management* for the following reasons:

- When you administer a placebo to a particular patient, you risk inadequate pain relief. However, placebos can diminish pain in some people without the negative effects that other treatments impose. In classic studies done in the 1950s, 36% of patients demonstrated adequate pain relief from a placebo injection the day after abdominal surgery (Evans, 1974). However, there is no way to determine in advance which patients will experience pain relief.
- Even in the same patient, placebos may relieve pain at one time and not at another.
- Ethically, the most important reason for not using placebos is that their use involves deceit. If discovered, and it frequently is, the patient may lose trust in healthcare professionals.

Teaching the Patient and Family About Pain

Patients and caregivers tend to cope more effectively when they are well informed. Because pain can interfere with a patient's learning, be sure to include the patient's family in your teaching. If the patient is discharged from the facility with a prescription for opioids, you should discuss the following topics with the patient and family:

- The cause of the pain, if it is known
- The normal duration of the pain, if known (e.g., postoperative pain generally decreases every day as tissues heal)
- How to use the selected pain scale; ask for a demonstration of use
- The overall pain management plan
- Information about the analgesic prescribed—dose, interval, and route of administration
- If opioids are prescribed, explanation that the risk of addiction is extremely low
- Nonpharmacological ways to treat pain
- Side effects to assess
- The need to alter the treatment plan if relief is not achieved
- (Family) How to monitor for excessive sedation and to call the healthcare provider if pain relief is not adequate
- How to contact the healthcare team regarding side effects, missed doses, change in condition, or ineffective pain management

To improve patient comfort and satisfaction, educate patients about what they can expect for pain outcome and their options for managing pain. This helps involve patients in their care and helps to fine-tune pain management regimens (Bozimowski, 2012).

Documentation

Documentation may be narrative, in either nursing or interdisciplinary notes, or recorded on a pain management flow sheet. Although documentation varies from facility to facility, it typically reflects the entire spectrum of the nursing process:

- The expected outcome for pain management
- Patient's present pain level
- Patient's responses to any intervention for pain
- Adverse reactions that may have resulted from the analgesic
- Planned interventions to improve pain relief as needed

Typically, pain management flow sheets contain a column for time, pain ratings, and analgesic used, including dose and route, vital signs, and side effects. They are tailored to the patient population, the type of pain being monitored, and the clinical setting. For example, the pain flow sheet for a patient using an IV PCA pump would be more complex than a pain flow sheet for a patient taking oral medications at home. Documentation is important because typically pain recall is poor and patients often underestimate their pain after the fact. If pain is not adequately documented, there is no way to prove that it was accurately assessed.

EVALUATION

Evaluation is critical to pain management. Compare your findings with the expected outcomes to determine whether the pain management strategy is effective. Questions to ask include the following:

- Are the patient's pain scores consistently at or better than the desired level? Are they improving?
- Is the patient's behavior, mobility, range of motion, mood, and affect consistent with pain relief?
- What is the quality of the patient's life according to the patient's standards?

In addition to evaluating the extent of pain relief, you need to determine which interventions were or were not effective, as well as any adverse reactions to the interventions. Close examination of the patient's pain diary should provide most of the data you need for evaluation.

It is important to reassess the patient's pain regularly. An increase in pain may be a sign of inadequate pain management, but it could also be a sign of developing complications. Before changing the treatment plan, you should determine whether the plan was carried out correctly. If the healthcare team decides to make a change, remember to again evaluate the effect of the change. Do not assume the new intervention will provide adequate pain relief.

NURSING PROCESS IN ACTION

Mary Jean Thompson, 30 years old, was admitted to the hospital with severe abdominal pain and underwent an appendectomy yesterday. The physician has prescribed hydromorphone (Dilaudid) 2 mg tablet PO q 4–6 hr prn for pain. Ms. Thompson doesn't like the idea of taking pain medication and waits until she rates her pain a 9 or 10 on a scale of 0 to 10 before requesting an injection. Even after the medication, her pain never drops below a 7 on a scale of 0 to 10 and she is unwilling to turn or ambulate because of the pain.

When you perform your assessment, she tells you she does not want to be sedated. "I hate that groggy, drugged feeling. I'm willing to have some pain to avoid that." After you discuss the importance of pain management to aid in healing and the ability to participate in activities and therapy, Ms. Thompson states that she would like to have a pain score of 3 to 4 today. See the accompanying Pain Management Care Plan and Care Map for the nurse's application of nursing process for Ms. Thompson.

Pain Management: Nursing Care

Nursing Diagnosis: Acute Pain (surgical incision) related to possible inadequate analgesia (drug and dosing) because of reluctance to have IM injection, as manifested by not requesting medication until her pain is at a score of 9.

EXPECTED OUTCOMES	NURSING INTERVENTIONS	RATIONALE
On a scale of 0–10, the patient will verbalize pain relief at a score of 3 or below while in bed and 4 or below while ambulating at all times.	Assess and document the patient's verbal and nonverbal expressions of pain relief with each check of vital signs, with every procedure and ambulation, and when the patient is at rest.	Assessment is necessary to determine the effectiveness of the prescribed medications. Assessment and documentation are legal responsibilities for the nurse as well.
	Discuss with the prescriber the need to modify prescriptions if pain relief measures are ineffective. Recommend PCA.	Ineffective pain management will cause the patient increased stress and can lead to further complications because the patient will be unwilling to move.
	When you obtain new pain orders for a PCA morphine pump, educate the patient about the pump.	A patient using PCA requires instruction about safe use of the pump.
	Provide nonpharmacological interventions, such as a back rub or other techniques described in this chapter, before rest or sleep, with any exacerbation of pain, and after painful procedures such as ambulation.	Nonpharmacological interventions are synergistic and enhance the relief the opioid gives.
The patient will demonstrate pain relief by participating in ambulation and turning within 24 hours.	Teach the patient to press the PCA pump before activities.	Peak blood levels enable the patient to ambulate, cough and deep-breathe, and perform activities of daily living.

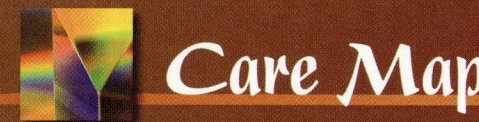

Care Map

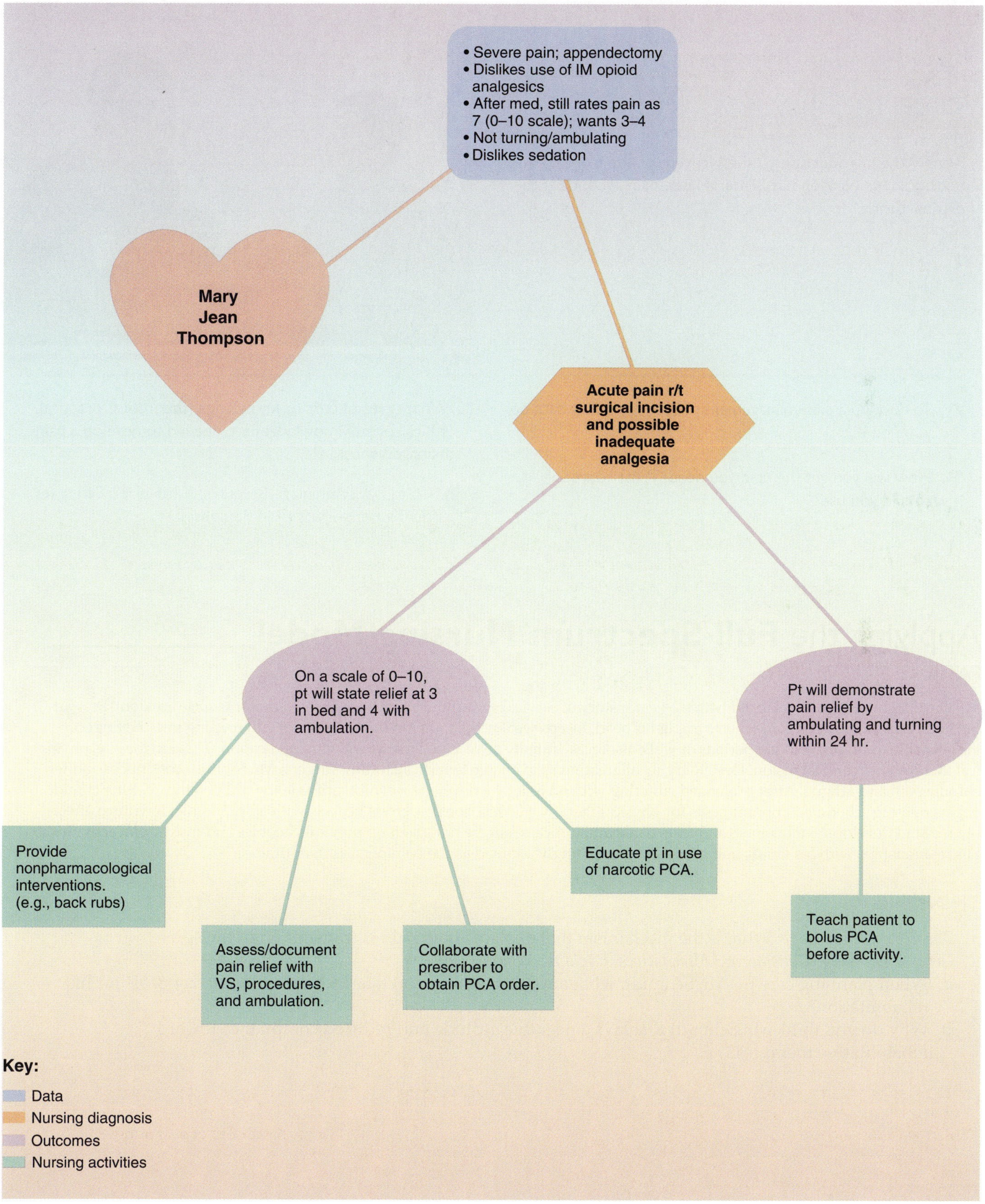

Data (blue box):
- Severe pain; appendectomy
- Dislikes use of IM opioid analgesics
- After med, still rates pain as 7 (0–10 scale); wants 3–4
- Not turning/ambulating
- Dislikes sedation

Mary Jean Thompson

Nursing diagnosis (orange hexagon):
Acute pain r/t surgical incision and possible inadequate analgesia

Outcomes (purple ovals):

On a scale of 0–10, pt will state relief at 3 in bed and 4 with ambulation.

Pt will demonstrate pain relief by ambulating and turning within 24 hr.

Nursing activities (green boxes):

Provide nonpharmacological interventions. (e.g., back rubs)

Assess/document pain relief with VS, procedures, and ambulation.

Collaborate with prescriber to obtain PCA order.

Educate pt in use of narcotic PCA.

Teach patient to bolus PCA before activity.

Key:
- Data
- Nursing diagnosis
- Outcomes
- Nursing activities

CLINICALREASONING

The questions and exercises in this section allow you to practice the kind of thinking you will use as a full-spectrum nurse. Critical-thinking questions usually have more than one correct answer, so we do not provide "correct answers" for these features. It is more important to develop your nursing judgment than to just cover content. You will learn by discussing the questions with your peers. If you are still unsure, see the Davis Advantage chapter resources for suggested responses.

Caring for the Nguyens

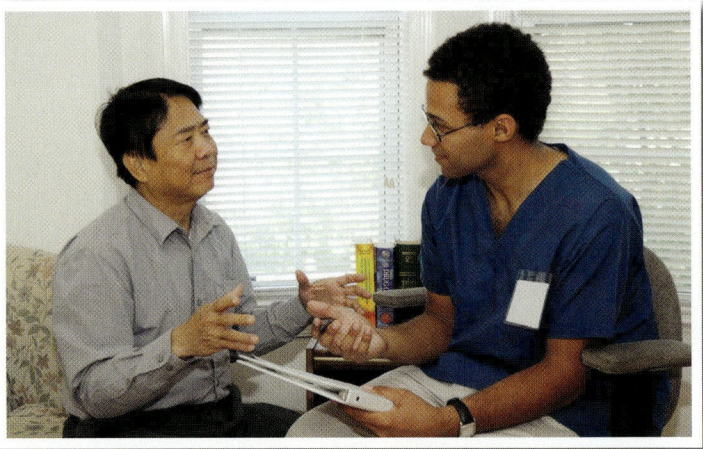

Review the introduction to the Nguyens at the front of the textbook. Mr. Nguyen has bilateral knee pain secondary to osteoarthritis.

A. To develop a pain-management plan, what patient data do you need?

B. How will you get the data you need? What sources should you use?

C. What types of nursing knowledge (theoretical, practical, ethical, or self-knowledge) are needed to develop a pain-management plan?

 Go to Davis Advantage, Resources, Chapter 32, **Caring for the Nguyens—Suggested Responses.**

Applying the **Full-Spectrum Nursing Model**

PATIENT SITUATION

Mr. Dieter Schmidt is a 48-year-old with a 2-year history of cervical spine injury that began after a motor vehicle accident. Presenting symptoms were neck pain when turning his head, biceps weakness, and pain down the arm with tingling into the fingertips. He is unable to sit for extended periods or walk distances. Initially he received treatment with medication, TENS to the site, physical therapy, and cervical fusion. Despite trying all treatments available to him, including surgery, Mr. Schmidt continues to suffer chronic pain and fatigue. After prolonged suffering with no relief, he develops a cynical attitude toward healthcare. Mr. Schmidt begins missing scheduled appointments for physical therapy. He describes the stress he feels with an economic downturn affecting his land development business and fears bankruptcy. As a result, he has given up previous hobbies and most social activities. His relationships with his family and friends are increasingly strained as the pain persists over time.

THINKING

1. *Theoretical Knowledge:* What is the mechanism that explains how pain is transmitted in the spine?
2. *Critical Thinking (Considering Alternatives, Deciding What to Do):*
    a. When planning care for Mr. Schmidt, what approach would you take in helping him to set goals for his rehabilitation?
    b. Why do you think Mr. Schmidt displays a negative attitude and reduced compliance toward rehabilitative therapies?

DOING

3. *Practical Knowledge:*
   a. *Nursing Process (Assessment):* What questions would you ask Mr. Schmidt to assess the impact of pain on his daily living and quality of life?
   b. *Nursing Process (Interventions):* In addition to drug therapy, what other measures might you teach your patient to perform for controlling pain and promoting comfort?

CARING

4. *Self-Knowledge:* Have you experienced chronic pain, such as back pain, fibromyalgia, arthritis, migraines, or that associated with sports injuries? If so, how has it affected your daily life? Has your pain affected your relationships? Has it interfered with your job or recreational activities? What other ways would you say chronic pain has reduced the quality of your life?

 Go to Davis Advantage, Resources, Chapter 32, **Applying the Full-Spectrum Nursing Model—Suggested Responses.**

PracticalKnowledge
clinical application

The following content provides the practical knowledge you will need to assist patients with pain control.

CLINICAL INSIGHTS

Clinical Insight 32-1 ➤ Caring for the Patient With an Epidural Catheter

Intraspinal analgesia is contraindicated in patients who received anticoagulant therapy or who have spinal defects, local or systemic infections, or increased intracranial pressure.

Monitoring

- Monitor for respiratory depression (every hour for the first 24 hr, then every 4 hr if the patient is stable).
- Monitor the site for leaking or drainage.
- Check connections for leaks. This can be fixed by carefully retightening connections. If the filter is cracked, replace with a new one using sterile technique.
- Assess for urine retention. Keep careful intake and output records. *Urinary retention is one side effect of epidural opioids.*
- Observe for signs of headache in the patient as a result of dural puncture. Treatment consists of bedrest, analgesics, and liberal hydration. Caffeine is also helpful and may be administered IV. If unresolved after 72 hours, patient might receive an epidural blood patch.
- Observe for signs of catheter migration: nausea, a decrease in blood pressure, and a loss of motor function without a recognizable cause.

Prevention

- Mark all epidural lines *clearly* for patient safety. *This line must not be confused with an arterial or venous catheter.*
- Ensure that the tape on the tubing connected to the patient is secure to prevent catheter migration.
- Use strict aseptic technique when changing tubing, including mask and sterile gloves for access and maintenance procedures.

Discontinuing the Catheter

- If you are specially trained to remove an epidural catheter, first loosen the tape securing the catheter. While wearing clean gloves, apply slow, steady pressure to withdraw the catheter. Inspect the catheter on removal. You must be able to see the tip of the catheter. If not, a portion of the catheter may still be lodged in the patient's epidural space. Notify the anesthesia team immediately of this finding.
- If the catheter cannot be withdrawn with minimal force, try repositioning the patient to the same position for removal as the patient was in during insertion of the catheter.
- Cleanse the insertion site and cover with a dry sterile dressing.

PROCEDURES

More and more, medication is being administered by patient-controlled analgesia. Although pump operation differs among manufacturers, you should understand in general how pumps work. Consult manufacturers' directions when you must use an unfamiliar pump.

Procedure 32-1 ■ Setting Up and Managing Patient-Controlled Analgesia by Pump

➤ For steps to follow in *all* procedures, refer to the Universal Steps for All Procedures found on the page facing the inside back cover.

Equipment

- PCA pump (infuser and central unit)
- Manufacturer's instructions for the pump
- Cartridge, syringe, or other type of sealed unit containing the medication
- Connecting tubing (to connect the PCA device to the patient's IV line)
- Maintenance IV supplies, as needed
- IV pole
- Antiseptic swab
- Flow sheet
- One pair of clean procedure gloves (if venipuncture is necessary)

Delegation

Because a narcotic medication is delivered intravenously to the patient, this procedure is outside the scope of practice of nursing assistive personnel (NAP) and should never be delegated. Furthermore, the NAP should not administer a dose for the patient, even if he asks her to do so. You can inform the NAP of expected side effects and ask her to report her observations to you.

Pre-Procedure Assessment

- Assess physical conditions that can affect respirations.
  Respiratory diseases (e.g., chronic obstructive pulmonary disease, obstructive sleep apnea, asthma) and conditions such as head injury and sleep apnea increase the risk for respiratory depression with opioid use (American Pain Society, 2016).

- Assess level of consciousness and cognitive level.
  Determines whether the patient will be able to follow directions for self-dosing.

- Review lab values reflecting liver and kidney function, such as blood urea nitrogen, creatinine, and liver enzymes.
  Narcotic analgesics are typically metabolized through the liver or kidneys.

- Assess the baseline respiratory rate, pulse, blood pressure, and oxygen saturation.
  A change in vital signs (e.g., hypotension, respiratory rate below 12) may indicate adverse responses to narcotic administration.

- Be aware of the patient's age and weight.
  Age is a factor when you are verifying the dose. Older patients and very young children are at increased risk for respiratory suppression, so they require lower doses. Pediatric doses are based on the child's weight.

- Assess the patient's baseline pain level using a standardized pain assessment tool or numeric scale ranging from 0 to 10.
- Assess the patient's manual dexterity.
  Patients with impaired fine motor control or upper extremity injury may not be able to operate the self-dosing mechanism.

- Review medications currently in use.
  The risk of respiratory suppression increases when a PCA pump is used in conjunction with other central nervous system (CNS) depressants, such as diazepam (Valium).

- ✚ Assess the extent of family involvement. Identify any family anxiety over the patient's pain. Reinforce that only the patient should use the PCA button.
  Only the patient should administer the medication. "PCA by proxy" (someone other than the patient pushing the dosing button) is a major factor contributing to adverse patient outcomes (D'Arcy, 2012).

➤ When performing the procedure, always identify your patient according to agency policy, using two identifiers, and be attentive to standard precautions, hand hygiene, patient safety and privacy, body mechanics, and documentation.

Procedure Steps

1. **Don clean procedure gloves** and initiate IV therapy if the patient does not currently have an IV solution infusing. Refer to Procedure 38-1 as needed.

2. **Obtain the medication** and double-check it with the original prescription. You may need to remove air from the vial by pushing the injector into the vial. Connect the PCA tubing to the vial (or cartridge).

   Some vials may not be completely filled with medication. Ejecting the air makes it faster to prime the connecting tubing.

3. ✚ **Double-check your dose** calculation with another nurse before starting the infusion or wasting medication. PCA settings for preventing unintended dosing include:

a. "On-demand" dose (the amount of drug to be delivered with each push of the button)

b. The "lockout" interval (the number of minutes allowed between each administration of an on-demand dose [e.g., q10 min]). Even if the patient pushes the button more frequently, the PCA pump will not administer a dose until the preset time between doses has been met.

c. Basal rate or continuous infusion (the amount of medication to be delivered automatically by the pump over 1 hour) should be used with caution. Giving the medication continuously without the patient having to push a button takes away some of the inherent safety of a PCA.

d. One-time "bolus" (or *loading*) dose, which you administer after setting up the pump

e. The 1-hour or 4-hour lockout interval (the maximum dose allowed in that time frame). For example, if the patient has a 4-mg on-demand dose with a 10-minute lockout interval, the patient can receive a maximum of six 4-mg doses per hour for a total of 24 mg/hr and a maximum dose of 96 mg in 4 hours.

NOTE: PCA prescriptions are usually written in milligrams; however, pump settings may be in milliliters. In such cases, you must verify the concentration (milligrams per milliliter) to set the pump correctly.

4. **Prime the tubing; then clamp** the tubing above the connector.
Priming prevents air from entering the pump and causing malfunction. Clamping prevents an accidental bolus of medication getting to the patient.

5. **Insert the cartridge or vial** injector into the pump, and lock the pump. Follow the manufacturer's instruction manual (e.g., some pumps can be set only if the door is closed and locked).
Depending on the pump, it may be a syringe, a cartridge, or other sealed container that can be "locked" into the pump. Locking the pump prevents unauthorized access to the opioid and dosing features.

6. **Turn the pump on, and set** the parameters according to the prescriptions and your calculations. The settings may include:
a. On demand
b. Lockout interval
c. Basal rate or continuous infusion—if applicable
d. The 1-hour or 4-hour lockout dosage limit
e. The one-time loading dose—if applicable

7. **Scrub the port on the IV** tubing closest to the patient, using alcohol or a chlorhexidine gluconate–alcohol product; then connect the PCA pump tubing.
Removes gross contamination and discourages growth of pathogens.

8. **Open the clamp and** administer the bolus (loading) dose if prescribed. Remain with the patient as the dose is delivered.
A loading dose is usually larger than the basal and on-demand doses because pain is likely to be more severe before the pump is initiated. Remaining with the patient allows you to observe for adverse effects.

9. **Close the pump door and lock** the machine with the key.

10. **Check for flashing lights** or alarms that may indicate the need to correct settings.

11. **Be sure to release tubing clamps** if you previously clamped the tubing; press the start button to begin pump operation.

12. **Ensure that the battery life** is sufficient or, preferably, that the pump in plugged into an appropriate electrical outlet.
To avoid battery failure.

13. **Place the control button** for on-demand doses within the patient's reach. Be sure the PCA cord is placed away from the call bell.
To avoid error in self dosing with PCA. ▼

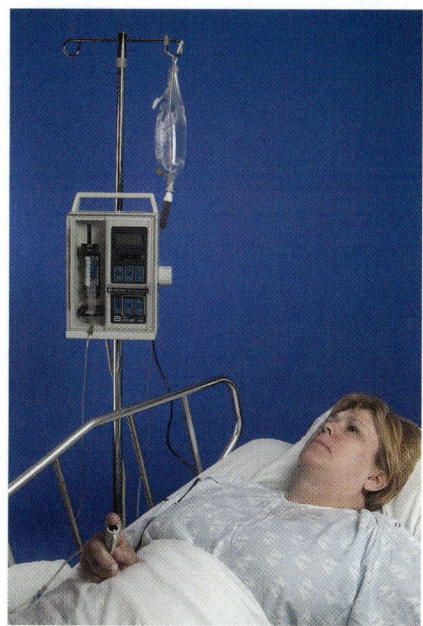

? **What if . . .**

■ **The patient cannot verbally communicate pain status?**

Use an alternate standardized pain tool, such as the FACES pain scale or a behavioral measure to determine pain level.
Pain assessment in patients who are uncommunicative may include behavioral or physiological indicators to assess and monitor the effectiveness of pain medication.

■ **The infusion infiltrates?**

Discontinue the IV and establish another IV site. Follow facility policy for application of cold or warm compresses to the infiltrated area. Assess pain level. You may need to contact the prescriber for a bolus dose if the IV has been interrupted for an extended period or the patient has insufficient pain relief.

(continued on next page)

Procedure 32–1 ■ **Setting Up and Managing Patient-Controlled Analgesia by Pump** (continued)

Evaluation

- Monitor the patient's pain level, sedation level, and respiratory rate at least every hour for the first 24 hours or according to facility policy after initiating PCA.
  Promotes the early detection of respiratory depression, oversedation, or inadequate pain control.

- Perform routine assessment of number and frequency of doses and pump settings per facility protocol.
- Check the IV site for redness, infiltration, or phlebitis.
- Check the IV tubing for patency (e.g., for kinks) to be sure the medication is infusing.

Patient Teaching

Patients who are candidates for use of PCA should be trained before surgery rather than in the immediate postoperative period, when the effects of anesthesia impair learning. Reinforce or teach the patient and family the following:

- Safe and correct use of the PCA pump
- The benefits of PCA for controlling pain
- The pump will deliver only the amount of medication prescribed. Pushing the button too many times will not result in overdosing.
- The patient cannot accidentally roll over on the button and unintentionally give additional medication.
- If pain is not being relieved, the patient should tell the nurse so adjustments can be made to the PCA.
- The pump will alarm when nearly empty, alerting nurses to change the syringe.
- The PCA button is to relieve pain—not to help the patient sleep.
- Signs and symptoms of allergic reaction and which ones to report
- How to rate pain using a standard pain scale
- The patient is the only one who may push the pain-dosing button. Explain why family members should not give "doses by proxy."

Documentation

You will usually document PCA initiation on a specialized checklist or flow sheet. Items to document include:

- Time the infusion was begun, including the drug, the patient demand dose, the loading dose, the basal dose if applicable, lockout interval, and hourly limit
- Patient's baseline pain level and evaluation of subsequent pain level performed at intervals determined by facility policy
- Baseline respiratory rate, pulse, blood pressure, and oxygen saturation; routine evaluation of subsequent vital signs performed at intervals determined by facility policy
- Sedation level
- Continuous monitoring of vital signs, level of consciousness, and pain status, as well as the dose and frequency of analgesic medications
- Unusual occurrences (e.g., oversedation, IV infiltration) in the nursing notes

Thinking About the Procedure

 The video **Setting Up and Managing Patient-Controlled Analgesia by Pump,** along with questions and suggested responses, is available on the **Davis's** *Nursing Skills Videos* Web site on Davis*Plus*.

 To explore learning resources for this chapter,

 Go to **www.DavisAdvantage.com** and find:

Answers and Suggested Responses for all questions in this chapter

Lists of NIC Interventions and NOC Outcomes

List of NANDA-I Diagnoses

Knowledge Map

Care Map

Care Plan

References and Bibliography

Concept Map

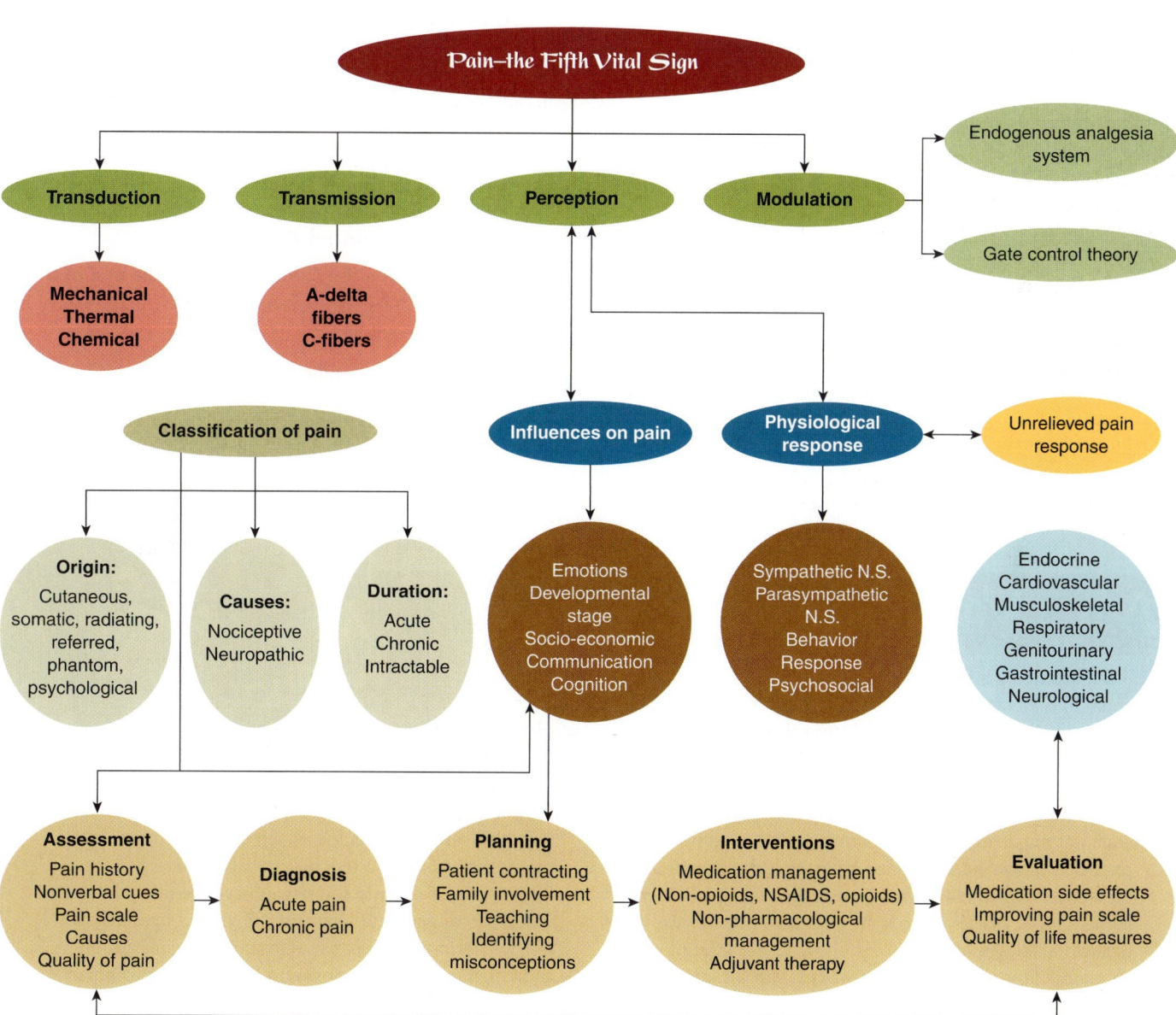

Pain–the Fifth Vital Sign

Transduction → **Mechanical Thermal Chemical**

Transmission → **A-delta fibers C-fibers**

Perception

Modulation → Endogenous analgesia system / Gate control theory

Classification of pain

- **Origin:** Cutaneous, somatic, radiating, referred, phantom, psychological
- **Causes:** Nociceptive Neuropathic
- **Duration:** Acute Chronic Intractable

Influences on pain → Emotions Developmental stage Socio-economic Communication Cognition

Physiological response → Sympathetic N.S. Parasympathetic N.S. Behavior Response Psychosocial

Unrelieved pain response → Endocrine Cardiovascular Musculoskeletal Respiratory Genitourinary Gastrointestinal Neurological

Assessment
Pain history
Nonverbal cues
Pain scale
Causes
Quality of pain

Diagnosis
Acute pain
Chronic pain

Planning
Patient contracting
Family involvement
Teaching
Identifying
misconceptions

Interventions
Medication management
(Non-opioids, NSAIDS, opioids)
Non-pharmacological
management
Adjuvant therapy

Evaluation
Medication side effects
Improving pain scale
Quality of life measures

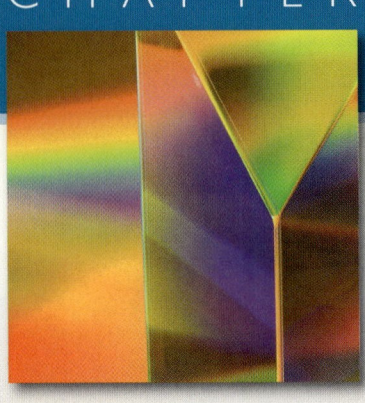

CHAPTER 33

Activity & Exercise

Learning Outcomes

After completing this chapter, you should be able to:

➤ Discuss the physiology of movement.

➤ Use proper body mechanics when providing patient care.

➤ Discuss the concept of fitness.

➤ Describe the five types of exercise discussed in this chapter.

➤ Compare the effects of exercise and immobility on the body.

➤ Describe the physical activity recommended for health promotion, cardiovascular fitness, and maintenance of healthy weight.

➤ Discuss factors that affect body alignment and activity.

➤ Demonstrate measures to prevent back injury associated with patient care.

➤ Identify patients who are at risk for immobility or activity intolerance.

➤ Develop a plan of care for patients with decreased activity tolerance.

➤ Implement care related to a patient's mobility problems.

Key Concepts

Fitness

Mobility

Physical activity

Related Concepts

See the Concept Map at the end of this chapter.

Example Problem

Immobility

Meet Your Patients

You are attending a health promotion series at the local hospital in order to fulfill your state's requirement for continuing nursing education. For the next 4 weeks, the topic is exercise. In the group, you meet the following people:

■ **Phillip Flanders.** Phillip is a 40-year-old accountant. He works long hours in an office setting doing work that is sedentary and requires concentration. Although he is not physically active, he often feels tired. He does not exercise regularly. Many of his friends have suggested that he begin some kind of exercise program to improve his energy and health. Phillip would like to learn how to get started with an overall fitness program that works with his job and family life. Before beginning, he makes an appointment with his primary care provider for a health evaluation.

■ **Peter Phan.** Peter is 28 years old and a marathon runner and triathlete. On average, he runs 35 miles per week and cycles at least twice per week. Peter has had plantar fasciitis in the past that was painful and caused him to miss exercising. Peter would like to learn what he can do to

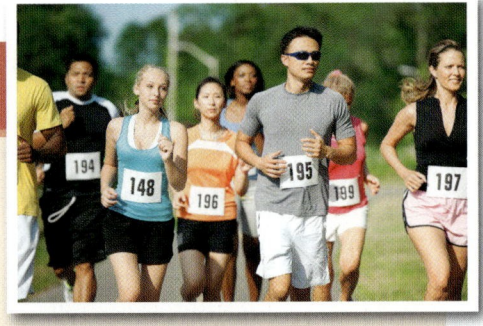

prevent other injuries.

■ **Helen Jillian.** Helen is 72 years old. She has hypertension and high cholesterol levels for which she takes four medications. She is 5 feet 1 inch tall and weighs 290 pounds. Recently she began having chest pain when starting a brisk walk. Her physician prescribed nitroglycerin for the chest pain, and after performing a thorough cardiac evaluation on her told her to enroll in the health promotion series and the cardio fitness program at the hospital. She does not understand why she is being asked to do these things because activity seems to trigger her chest pain.

In this chapter, you will find answers to each of these patient questions about activity and exercise. In addition, you will learn more about assisting patients with mobility problems.

Theoretical Knowledge
knowing **why**

Primitive nomadic people were active just meeting their daily needs. Tribes commonly journeyed to hunt for game; women were on foot gathering roots, fruits, and other edible plants. Survival depended on physical activity such as changing locations to find food or escape a dangerous situation. Later, the shift to an agricultural society reduced the need for most people to hunt and gather food. However, farming itself was hard work and people were physically active most of the year.

Today, with modern grocery distribution systems, we expend minimal energy to obtain food. In addition, there are many occupations in which people spend hours at a desk or in front of a computer screen. Many of today's leisure activities (watching television, playing video games) are also sedentary. Even though fitness equipment and health clubs are popular, the overall level of fitness in the United States is declining. Only about half of adolescents engage in moderate to vigorous activity on a regular basis. And fewer than a third achieve the recommended amount of physical activity needed for health and fitness. To get enough exercise, most people need to make a conscious effort to build exercise and activity into their lives. This chapter will help you to understand why that is important to help patients achieve activity and exercise goals.

ABOUT THE KEY CONCEPTS

Three concepts are widely used to describe human movement, mobility, physical activity, and exercise.
- **Mobility,** very simply, is body movement.
- **Fitness** (or physical fitness) is the ability to carry out activities of daily living with vigor and alertness, without undue fatigue, and with enough energy for leisure pursuits and to respond to emergencies (U.S. Department of Health and Human Services [USDHHS], 2008, updated 2011).
- **Physical activity** is bodily movement produced by the contraction of skeletal muscle that increases energy expenditure above a baseline level (USDHHS, 2008, updated 2011).
- *Exercise* is a subconcept of physical activity. It is planned, structured, and repetitive and purposeful for improving or maintaining physical fitness, physical performance, or health (Caspersen, Powell, & Christenson, 1985).

As you read this chapter, you will learn how the key concepts of activity, fitness, and mobility are related, and how they relate to subconcepts such as fitness, exercise, and body mechanics. Once you have a grasp of these concepts, you should be able to apply them to any patient, regardless of the health problem.

PHYSIOLOGY OF MOVEMENT

Activity and exercise require body movement **(mobility).** Mobility depends on the successful interaction among the skeleton, the muscles, and the nervous system.

Skeletal System

The skeletal system includes bones, cartilage, ligaments, and tendons. The **skeleton** forms the framework of the body, protects the internal organs, produces blood cells, and stores mineral salts (e.g., calcium) and fat.

Bones consist of a hard outer shell with a spongy interior (Fig. 33-1). There are 206 bones of various shapes in the human body:
Long bones—femur and humerus
Short bones—phalanges and metacarpals
Flat bones—sternum and cranial bones
Irregularly shaped bones—vertebrae and tarsal bones
The short, flat, and irregular bones contain red bone marrow that produces red blood cells.

Bones are composed of living tissue and are constantly building and remodeling. A delicate balance exists between the actions of the osteoblasts and the osteoclasts. **Osteoclasts** are specialized cells that function as housekeepers in the bone by breaking down old or damaged tissue. **Osteoblasts** repair damaged bone and build new bone to keep the skeleton strong.

Joints When two bones come close together **(articulate),** a joint is formed. Body movement occurs at the joints. Joints are classified based on the amount of movement they permit:
- **Synarthroses** are immovable joints (e.g., the sutures between the cranial bones). In youth, these joints have some flexibility to allow growth, but they gradually become rigid.
- **Amphiarthroses** allow for limited movement. Examples are the joints between the vertebrae and pubic bones.
- **Diarthroses,** or **synovial joints,** are freely movable because of the amount of space between the articulating bones. Synovial joints are filled with **synovial fluid,** and the joint surfaces of the articulating bones are covered with smooth **articular cartilage** (connective tissue found in the joints and skeleton). The synovial fluid and articular cartilage prevent friction as the bones move.

Cartilage, Ligaments, and Tendons serve as the interface between the skeleton and the muscles. **Ligaments** are fibrous tissues that connect most movable joints. Ligaments are flexible to allow freedom of movement, but tough so they do not yield under force of movement. **Tendons** are fibrous connective tissues that attach muscles to the bone. **Cartilage** is smooth, elastic, connective tissue that acts as a cushion around

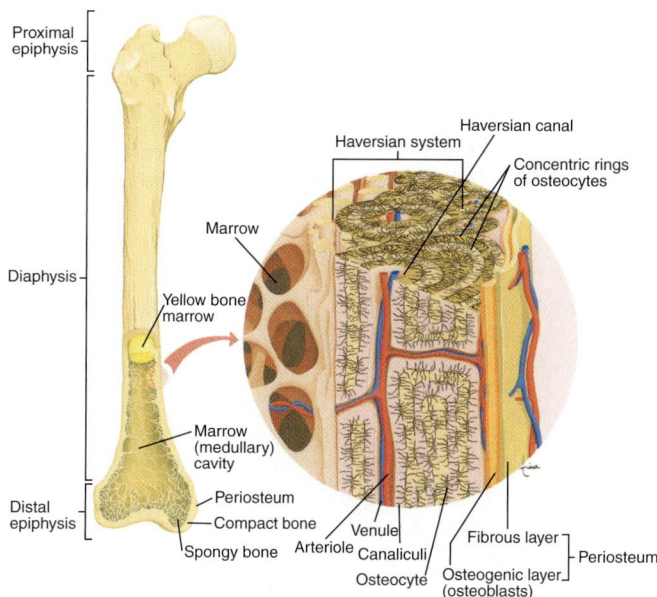

FIGURE 33-1 Bone is complex living tissue.

the joints and other parts of the body (rib cage, ear pinnae, nose, bronchial tubes, vertebral disks). Although cartilage is strong and flexible, it is relatively easy to damage.

Muscles

Muscles make up almost half of body weight. When they contract, they cause movement. The type of movement depends on the type of muscle: skeletal, smooth, or cardiac.

- **Skeletal muscles** move the skeleton.
- **Smooth muscle** occurs in the digestive tract and other hollow structures, such as the bladder and blood vessels. They produce movement of food through the digestive tract, urine through the urinary tract, and blood through the circulatory system.
- **Cardiac muscle** is a unique form of muscle that can contract spontaneously. It is responsible for the beating of the heart.

Muscles span a joint and attach by tendons to two different bones. They attach to bone at two points: (1) at **the *point of origin,*** to the more stationary bone, and (2) at the ***point of insertion,*** to the more movable bone. The "belly" (thickest part) of the muscle lies between these two points. When a skeletal muscle contracts, it shortens, thus causing one bone to move at the joint.

Muscles work in pairs. For example, the biceps brachii contracts to flex the forearm (bend the elbow joint). When the biceps contracts, the opposing muscle, the triceps brachii, relaxes. Similarly, contraction of the triceps is associated with relaxation of the biceps (Fig. 33-2).

Motor Nervous System

The motor nervous system controls the movement of the musculoskeletal system. Motor nerves are either autonomic or somatic.

- The **autonomic nervous system** consists of the sympathetic and parasympathetic nervous systems, which innervate involuntary muscles, such as the heart, blood vessels, and glands.
- The **somatic nervous system** innervates the voluntary skeletal muscles.

When you make a conscious decision to bend your elbow, the thought originates in the motor area of your cerebral cortex. The upper motor efferent nerves communicate with the lower motor neurons that conduct impulses to the muscles. When the muscle receives sufficient stimuli, it contracts the biceps as the triceps relaxes and moves the elbow.

Movement also occurs through reflex mechanisms. Common reflexes include the knee-jerk reflex and corneal reflex. Reflexes are discussed at length in Chapter 21.

A muscle contraction, whether conscious or reflexive, stimulates afferent nerves that convey information to the cerebral cortex and the cerebellum. This information helps control and coordinate movements.

KnowledgeCheck 33-1

- Name three purposes of the skeletal system.
- Identify three types of muscle.
- How do the muscles and the nerves interact?

BODY MECHANICS

Body mechanics is a term used to describe the way we move our bodies. It includes four components: body alignment, balance, coordination, and joint mobility. This chapter presents guidelines for good body mechanics and safe movement to prevent back injury. The following concepts cover healthy posture and alignment as well as problems with muscle mass, strength, or mobility. These concepts will be useful in patient teaching and safe patient handling.

Body Alignment

Body alignment, or **posture,** is an important aspect of body mechanics. Proper posture places the spine in a neutral (resting) position. There are four natural curves to the spine (Fig. 33-3). Proper posture maintains these natural curves because it allows

Scapula
Biceps (relaxed)
Radius
Triceps (contracted)
Ulna
Humerus
A
Extension
Biceps (contracted)
Triceps (relaxed)
B
Flexion

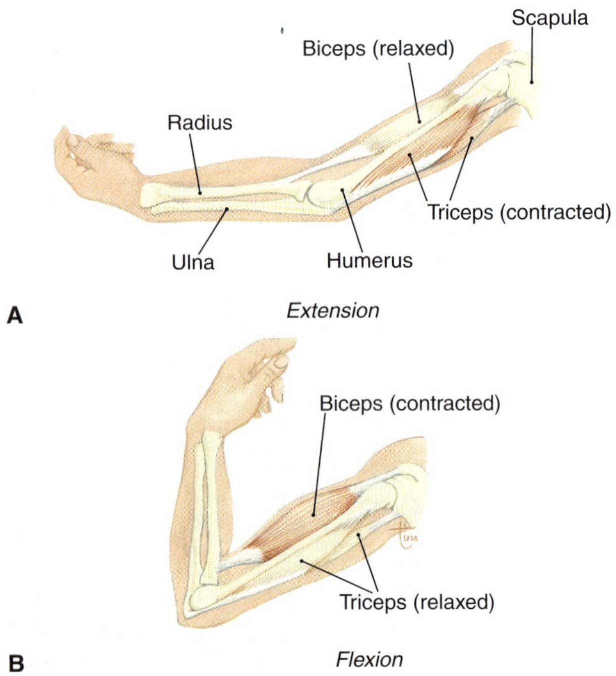

FIGURE 33-2 Antagonistic muscles. A. Extension of the forearm. B. Flexion of the forearm.

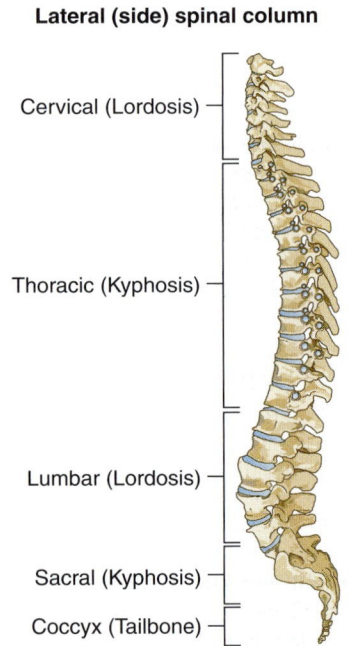

Lateral (side) spinal column
Cervical (Lordosis)
Thoracic (Kyphosis)
Lumbar (Lordosis)
Sacral (Kyphosis)
Coccyx (Tailbone)

FIGURE 33-3 There are four natural curves to the spine.

movement to occur with less stress and fatigue; the bones are aligned, and the muscles, joints, and ligaments can work at peak efficiency. Good posture contributes to the normal functioning of the nervous system and improves feelings of well-being (see the Self-Care box Tips to Maintain Proper Posture).

Balance

The body achieves balance when it is in alignment. For your body to be balanced, your line of gravity must pass through your center of gravity, and your center of gravity must be close to your base of support.

- The **line of gravity** is an imaginary vertical line drawn from the top of the head through the center of gravity.
- The **center of gravity** is the point around which mass is distributed. In the human body, the center of gravity is below the umbilicus at the top of the pelvis.
- The **base of support** is what holds the body up. The feet provide the base of support.

✚ To avoid injury when moving objects, place your center of gravity closest to your base of support and stand with your head erect, buttocks pulled in, abdominal muscles tight, chest high, shoulders pulled back, and feet wide apart (Fig. 33-4).

Use a wide stance, with feet apart and one foot forward when standing for a long time. **KEY POINT:** *The broader the base of support, the lower the center of gravity, and the easier it is to maintain balance.*

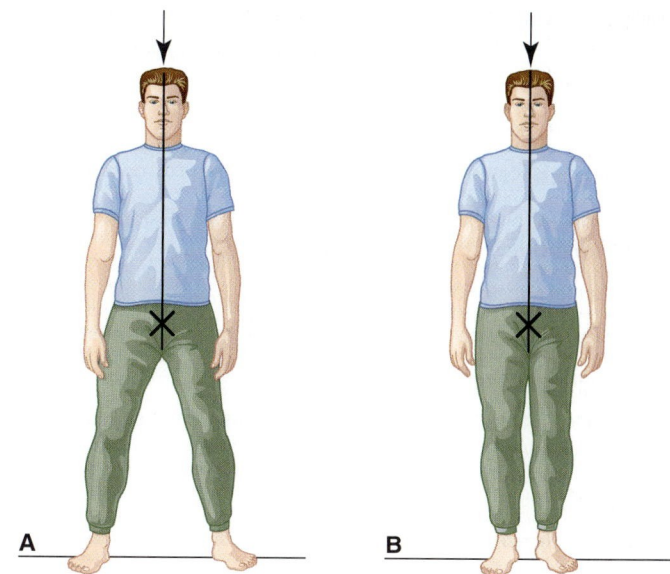

FIGURE 33-4 A. With a wide stance, the center of gravity (x) is closer to the base of support. B. With a narrow stance, the body is less stable.

Self-Care

Tips to Maintain Proper Posture

Most posture problems result from a combination of the following:

Accidents, injuries, and falls	Poor sleep support (mattress)
Careless sitting, standing, or sleeping habits	Poorly designed workspace
Excessive weight	Visual difficulties
Foot problems or improper shoes	Weak muscles or muscle imbalance
Occupational stress	Skeletal misalignment or malformation (e.g., scoliosis, kyphosis)

➤ Avoid standing in one position for a lengthy period. If you cannot change positions, elevate one foot on a stool or box and alternate foot placement frequently.
➤ Do not lock your knees when standing upright.
➤ Keep your stomach muscles tight to support your back.
➤ Do not bend forward at the waist or neck when you are working in a low position.
➤ When you are seated at your desk, work at a comfortable height.
➤ Do not wear high-heeled or platform shoes for long periods of time.
➤ Do not slump when you sit.
➤ Sit close to your work.
➤ Use a chair that supports your back in a slightly arched position.
➤ Sit with your feet flat on the floor and your knees below your hips.
➤ Sleep on a mattress that is firm but not extremely hard.

Coordination

Smooth movement requires coordination between the nervous system and the musculoskeletal system.

- **Cerebral cortex**—Initiates voluntary movement.
- **Cerebellum**—Coordinates movements; largely responsible for controlling *proprioception*, the awareness of posture, movement, and position sense.
- **Basal ganglia**—Located deep in the cerebrum, assist with coordination of movement.

Damage to the motor cortex, cerebellum, or basal ganglia affects coordination of movement. For example, a stroke affecting the motor cortex alters gait and changes posture.

Joint Mobility

Joint movement allows us to sit, stand, bend, walk, and perform other activities.

- **Range of motion (ROM)** is the maximum movement possible at a joint.
- **Active range of motion (AROM)** is movement of the joint performed by the individual without assistance.
- **Passive ROM (PROM)** involves moving joints through their ROM when the patient is unable to do so for himself.

Table 33-1 describes the movable joints and their range of motion.

Body Mechanics Guidelines

✚ **Principles of body mechanics** are the rules that allow you to move your body while reducing your risk for injury. Patient characteristics (e.g., obesity), as well as the patient care environment, make it difficult to rely on body mechanics alone to prevent injury. Think about it: A patient's weight is not evenly distributed. He might be combative, which makes moving the patient more difficult and increases the nurse's risk for back injury. For guidelines to help you assess patients' transfer abilities and use good body mechanics, see Clinical Insight 33-1.

(Text continued on page 1189)

Table 33-1 ➤ Range of Motion at the Joints

JOINT	ILLUSTRATION

Neck (Pivot Joint)

The joint is formed by a ring-like object that turns on a pivot. Motion is limited to rotation.

Flexion—Move the head from upright midline position to the chin, resting the head on the chest.

Normal Range: 45° from midline

Extension—Move the head from flexed to upright midline position.

Normal Range: 45° from midline

Hyperextension—Move the head from upright midline position to as far back as possible.

Normal Range: 10°

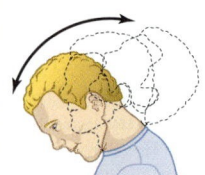

Lateral flexion—Tilt the head laterally from midline position toward the shoulder.

Normal Range: 40° from midline

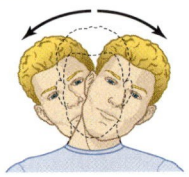

Rotation—Rotate the head in a circular motion from upright midline position to as far right or left as possible.

Normal Range: 180°

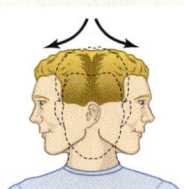

Shoulder (Ball-and-Socket Joint)

A rounded head (ball) fits into a cup-like structure (socket) to allow movement in all planes in addition to rotation.

Flexion—Raise the arm from a neutral position at the side to alongside the head.

Normal Range: 180°

Extension—Move the arm from flexed to a neutral position at the side of the body.

Normal Range: 180°

Hyperextension—Move the arm, keeping the elbow straight, from a neutral position at the side of the bed to behind the body.

Normal Range: 45°–60°

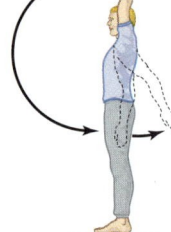

Abduction—Raise the arm laterally from a neutral position at the side of the body to a position at the side of the head, palm facing outward.

Normal Range: 180°

Adduction—Move the arm downward from a position beside the head to across the front of the body as far as possible.

Normal Range: 230°–320°

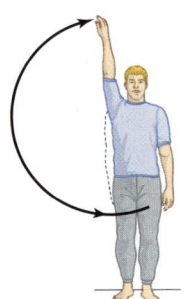

Table 33-1 ➤ Range of Motion at the Joints—cont'd

JOINT	ILLUSTRATION

Circumduction—Circle the arm from the shoulder.

Normal Range: 360°

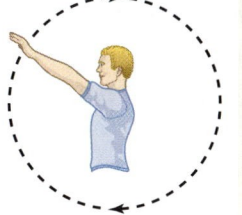

External rotation—Keeping arm held out to the side at shoulder level and bent to a right angle, fingers pointing down, move the arm upward so that the fingers point upward and are above the shoulder.

Normal Range: 90°

Internal rotation—Move the arm forward and down to return to the starting position, fingers pointing down.

Normal Range: 90°

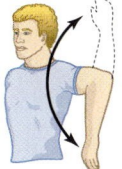

Elbow (Hinge Joint)

A convex surface fits into a cavity, allowing flexion and extension.

Flexion—Bend at the elbow to move the forearm from a straightened position up toward the shoulder.

Normal Range: 150°

Extension—Straighten the arm by bringing the lower arm forward and down.

Normal Range: 150°

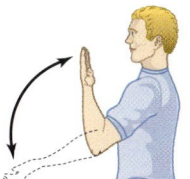

Rotation (for supination)—With the arm at the side, elbow bent, move the hand and forearm so that the palm is facing upward.

Normal Range: 70°–90°

Rotation (for pronation)—With the arm at the side, elbow bent, move the hand and forearm so that the palm is facing downward.

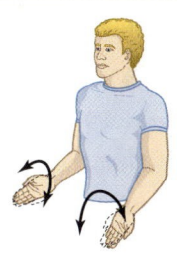

Wrist (Condyloid Joint)

An oval-shaped bone fits into an elliptical cavity to allow movement in two planes at right angles to each other.

Flexion—Bend the fingers of the hand toward the inner aspect of the forearm.

Normal Range: 80°–90°

Extension—Straighten the wrist so that it is on the same plane as the forearm.

Normal Range: 80°–90°

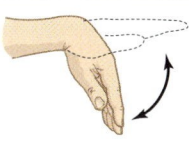

Hyperextension—Bend the wrist as far back as possible toward the outer aspect of the forearm.

Normal Range: 70°–90°

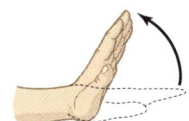

(Continued)

Table 33-1 ➤ Range of Motion at the Joints—cont'd

JOINT	ILLUSTRATION
Abduction (radial flexion)—With the hand supinated, bend each wrist laterally toward the thumb side. *Normal Range: 0–20°* **Adduction (ulnar flexion)**—With the hand supinated, bend each wrist laterally toward the fifth finger side. *Normal Range: 30°–50°*	
Hands and Fingers (Condyloid Joints: Interphalangeal Joints Are Hinges)	
Flexion—Bend the fingers into a fist. **Extension**—Straighten the fingers. *Normal Range: 90°* **Hyperextension**—Bend the fingers back. *Normal Range: 30°*	
Abduction—Spread the fingers apart. *Normal Range: 20°* **Adduction**—Bring the fingers together. *Normal Range: 20°*	
Thumb (Saddle Joint)	
One bone surface is concave in one direction and convex in the other. The other surface has the opposite construction so that the bones fit together. Movement occurs in two planes at right angles to each other.	
Flexion—Move the thumb across the palm of the hand toward the fifth finger. *Normal Range: 90°* **Extension**—Move the thumb laterally away from the fingers. *Normal Range: 90°*	
Opposition—Touch the thumb to the top of each finger of the same hand. *Normal Range: NA*	

Table 33-1 ➤ Range of Motion at the Joints—cont'd

JOINT	ILLUSTRATION

Hip (Ball-and-Socket Joint)

A rounded head (ball) fits into a cup-like structure (socket) to allow movement in all planes in addition to rotation.

Flexion—Move the leg forward and up.

  Normal Range: Knee extended 90°

Extension—Move the leg back down beside the other.

  Normal Range: Knee flexed 120°

Hyperextension—Move the leg back behind the body.

  Normal Range: 30°–50°

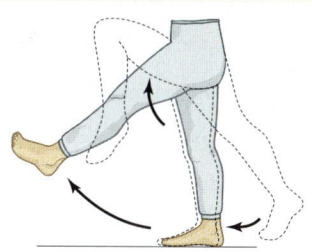

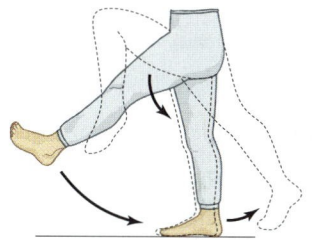

Abduction—Move the leg laterally.

  Normal Range: 45°–50°

Adduction—Sweep the leg inward across the midline.

  Normal Range: 20°–30° beyond the other leg

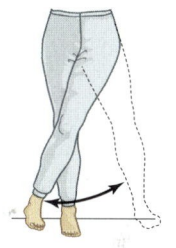

Circumduction—Circle the leg, keeping the knee straight.

  Normal Range: 360°

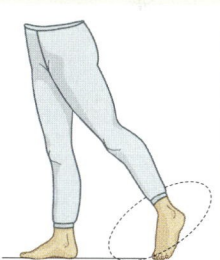

Internal rotation—Turn the foot and leg inward toward the other leg.

  Normal Range: 90°

External rotation—Turn the foot and leg outward, pointing the toes as far as possible away from the other leg.

  Normal Range: 90°

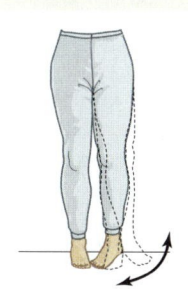

(Continued)

Table 33-1 ➤ Range of Motion at the Joints—cont'd

JOINT	ILLUSTRATION

Knee (Hinge Joint)

A convex surface fits into a cavity, allowing flexion and extension.

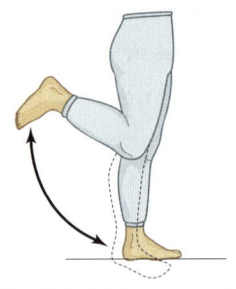

Flexion—Bend at the knee, bringing the heel back toward the buttocks.

Normal Range: 120°–130°

Extension—Straighten the knee, returning the leg to its original position.

Normal Range: 120°–130°

Ankle (Hinge Joint)

A convex surface fits into a cavity, allowing flexion and extension.

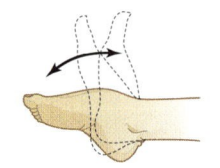

Extension (plantar flexion)—Point the toes and foot downward.

Normal Range: 45°–50°

Flexion (dorsiflexion)—Pull the toes and foot upward.

Normal Range: 20°

Foot (Gliding Joint)

Two flat plane surfaces move past each other.

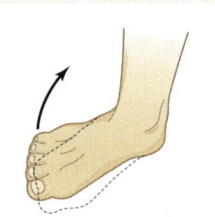

Eversion—Turn the sole of the foot laterally.

Inversion—Turn the sole of the foot medially.

Normal Range: 5°

Toes (Hinge Joint except intertarsal joints, which are Gliding Joints)

A convex surface fits into a cavity, allowing flexion and extension.

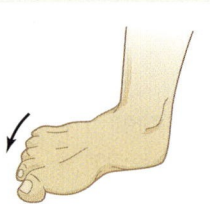

Flexion—Curl the toes downward.

Normal Range: 35°–60°

Extension—Straighten the toes.

Normal Range: 35°–60°

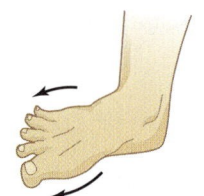

Abduction—Spread the toes apart.

Normal Range: 0°–15°

Adduction—Bring the toes together.

Normal Range: 0°–15°

JOINT	ILLUSTRATION

Table 33-1 ➤ Range of Motion at the Joints—cont'd

Trunk

Flexion—At the waist, bend forward toward the toes.

   Normal Range: 70°–90°

Extension—Straighten the trunk from the flexed position.

   Normal Range: 70°–90°

Hyperextension—Bend the trunk backward.

   Normal Range: 20°–30°

Lateral flexion—Bend the trunk to the side.

   Normal Range: 20°–40°

Rotation—Turn the upper body from side to side (twist at the waist).

   Normal Range: 30°–45°

KnowledgeCheck 33-2

- Identify the four components of body mechanics.
- Give at least five guidelines for good body mechanics.
- Define the following movements: abduction, adduction, flexion, extension, circumduction, internal rotation, supination, and pronation.

ThinkLike a Nurse 33-1

While you are attending the health promotion class, Helen Jillian (Meet Your Patients) develops chest pain and must be assisted to a wheelchair for transport to the emergency department.

- Based on what you know about body mechanics, how would you be able to assist Helen?
- What additional information do you need to know?

PHYSICAL ACTIVITY AND EXERCISE

Physical activity refers to bodily movement that results in energy. Physical activity can be grouped into two basic categories:

- **Baseline activity** refers to the light-intensity activities of daily living, such as standing, walking slowly, and lifting lightweight objects.
- **Exercise** (health-enhancing physical activity) is more than baseline to produce health-enhancing benefits. People who are physically fit are able to perform activities of daily living

with vigor and alertness and with enough energy to enjoy work and leisure activities (USDHHS, 2008, updated 2011).

Types of Exercise

Exercise may be classified by the type of muscle contraction it involves and according to whether it uses oxygen for energy.

Isometric Exercise involves muscle contraction without motion. These exercises are usually performed against an immovable surface or object, for example, pressing the hand against a wall. Each position is held for 6 to 8 seconds and repeated 5 to 10 times. Isometric training is effective for developing total strength of a muscle or group of muscles. It requires no special equipment, and there is little chance of injury. Patients who are bed bound can use this isometric exercise to maintain or regain muscle strength.

Isotonic Exercise involves movement of the joint during the muscle contraction. A classic example of an isotonic exercise is weight training with free weights. As the weight is moved throughout the ROM, the muscle shortens and lengthens. Calisthenics, such as pull-ups, push-ups, and planks, all of which use body weight as the resistance force, are also isotonic exercises.

Isokinetic Exercise is performed with specialized apparatuses that provide variable resistance to movement. Isokinetic exercise combines the best features of both isometrics and weight training by providing resistance at a constant, preset speed while the muscle moves through the full ROM. Machines available at health clubs and physical therapy departments are used for this form of exercise.

Aerobic Exercise occurs when the amount of oxygen taken into the body meets or exceeds the amount of oxygen required to perform the activity. Aerobic exercise uses large muscle groups, can be maintained continuously, and is rhythmic in nature. It increases the heart and respiratory rates, thereby providing exercise for the cardiovascular system while simultaneously exercising the skeletal muscles. Jogging, brisk walking, and cycling are common forms of aerobic exercise.

Anaerobic Exercise occurs when the amount of oxygen taken into the body does not meet the amount of oxygen required to perform the activity. Therefore, the muscles must obtain energy from metabolic pathways that do not use oxygen. Rapid, intense exercises such as lifting heavy objects and sprinting are examples of anaerobic exercise.

Planning and Evaluating a Fitness Program

A well-rounded fitness program focuses on flexibility, resistance training, and aerobic conditioning. The **mode** of exercise is the type of activity. Aerobic (endurance) and muscle-strengthening (resistance) physical activities both promote better health.

Flexibility Training Stretching before exercise helps warm up the muscles and prevents injury during exercise. Stretching after exercise cools the muscles and limits post-exercise stiffness.

As we get older, joints and muscles become stiffer. A regular flexibility program helps maintain mobility as the aging process progresses.

Resistance Training Movement against resistance increases muscular strength and endurance. Perhaps the most common type of resistance training is weight lifting.

Exercising for strength—increase the amount of resistance with each exercise (i.e., lift more weight).

Exercising for endurance—increase the number of repetitions with each exercise.

Aerobic Conditioning Fitness and body composition are improved by aerobic conditioning. Components of aerobic conditioning include intensity, duration, frequency, and mode. **Intensity** is how hard one is exercising. Box 33-1 describes three common tests used to evaluate exercise intensity.

Amount of Physical Activity **Duration** is the amount of time one is exercising. **Frequency** indicates how often one is exercising. See Box 33-2 for physical activity guidelines from the USDHHS.

Many people become discouraged because they don't see immediate results from their efforts. However, subtle changes occur long before the person sees changes in weight or shape. Instructional fitness videos, trainers, and group exercise make participation more engaging and also help to improve form and safety through demonstration of proper technique. Tips to help develop an exercise program are included in the Self-Care box Teaching Clients How to Set Up a Fitness Program.

Self-Care

Teaching Clients How to Set Up a Fitness Program

If you are older than 40, smoke or drink, are sedentary, are overweight, or have a chronic health condition, then you should have a medical evaluation before starting an exercise program.

Getting Started

➤ Choose a variety of exercises that you enjoy and feel comfortable doing, such as walking, biking, dancing, or a team sport.

➤ Find allies. Exercising with someone else can make it more fun. If you choose to exercise by yourself, pick a friend with whom you can discuss your exercise progress.

➤ Vary your routine. You may be less likely to become bored or injured.

➤ Choose a comfortable time of day.

➤ Don't get discouraged. It can take weeks or months before you notice some of the changes from exercise.

➤ Forget "no pain, no gain." Although a little soreness is normal after you first start exercising, pain isn't. Stop if you hurt.

➤ Make exercise fun. Find enjoyable things to do, such as taking a walk through the park or watching your favorite show while riding a stationary bike.

➤ Sign a contract committing yourself to exercise.

➤ Find an accountability partner. A fitness program is not only more enjoyable when shared with someone else but is also more successful with others for whom you are accountable.

➤ Keep a daily log of your activities.

➤ Think about joining a health club. The cost gives some people an incentive to exercise regularly.

Exercise Tips

➤ Warm up your muscles for 5 to 10 minutes before your main session of aerobic exercise.

➤ Maintain your exercise intensity for 30 to 45 minutes.

➤ Gradually decrease the intensity of your workout (cool down) and then stretch for 5 to 10 minutes at the end of your workout.

➤ Accumulate physical activity throughout the day. For example:

Take the stairs instead of the elevator.
Go for a walk during your coffee break or lunch period.
Walk all or part of the way to work.
Park your car at the far end of the parking lot.

➤ Wear good shock-absorbing footwear. Shoes that do not support your feet will cause stress on leg bones and the back and, over time, lead to injury.

➤ Alternate easy and hard exercise days, or alternate modes of exercise (e.g., alternate running, swimming, and biking).

➤ Take a day off periodically. The body needs a chance to rest and allow bones, joints, and muscles to rest and repair.

➤ To avoid becoming dehydrated, drink at least 8 ounces of fluid before the exercise, and then pause regularly during the exercise for more. If you are thirsty after the exercise session, drink until you feel satiated. Water is still the best liquid to drink during and after exercise. However, you can't rely on feeling thirsty as a reminder to replace fluid lost through sweating; one of nature's dirty tricks is that exercise suppresses thirst.

BOX 33-1 ▪ Tests for Determining Exercise Intensity

Target Heart Rate Method

In the target heart rate method, the target heart rate (THR) is calculated from an estimate of maximum heart rate. The estimated maximum heart rate is calculated using the following formula:

$$\text{Maximum heart rate} = 220 - \text{age}$$

The THR is calculated as a percentage of the maximum heart rate. Most persons can exercise at 60% to 80% of the maximum heart rate.

For example, consider a 50-year-old woman. Her maximum heart rate is 170 beats/min. To exercise at 75% intensity, her target heart rate is 128 beats/min.

$$\text{Maximum heart rate} = 220 - 50 = 170$$
$$\text{Target heart rate} = 0.75 \times 170 = 128$$

The person's heart rate during exercise should be 128 beats/min, excluding warm-up and cool-down.

Talk Test

The talk test evaluates exercise intensity based on the person's ability to talk while exercising. Short phrases interspersed with breaths or feeling like you can "just respond" is considered an appropriate level of exercise. If you are too short of breath to answer, the level of intensity is too high. An ability to carry on a conversation indicates that you are not exercising hard enough.

Borg Rate of Perceived Exertion Scale®

The Borg Rate of Perceived Exertion (RPE) Scale® is easy to use. The person who is exercising selects the rating based on how difficult the exercise feels at that time. The exerciser selects one of eight categories that best describes the intensity of activity. RPE ratings range from *No Exertion at All* to *Extremely Hard*. *Extremely Hard* is associated with exercise that corresponds to almost 100% of maximum heart rate. *Somewhat Hard* corresponds with 75% of maximum heart rate; this is the level you should encourage for most individuals.

Sources: Adapted from Borg, G. (1998). *Borg's perceived exertion and pain scales.* Stockholm, Sweden: Human Kinetics; Foster, C. (2004). "Talk test" measures exercise intensity. *Medicine & Science in Sports & Exercise, 36*(9), 1632–1636.

BOX 33-2 ▪ U.S. Department of Health and Human Services 2008 Physical Activity Guidelines for Americans

Children and Adolescents

- Engage in at least 1 hour of physical activity daily.
- Physical activity should be enjoyable. A variety of activities will improve adherence.
- Most activity should be aerobic, either of moderate or vigorous intensity.
- At least 3 days/week, children and teens should participate in vigorous-intensity exercise as well as muscle- and bone-strengthening physical activity.

Adults and Older Adults

- To gain substantial health benefits, get at least 150 min/week of moderate-intensity or 75 min/week of vigorous-intensity aerobic physical activity, or an equivalent combination of moderate- and vigorous-intensity aerobic activity. More frequent exercise (i.e., 300 min/week) is even more beneficial.
- Engage in aerobic activity throughout the week in episodes of at least 10 min. Longer periods of time provide additional benefits.
- For additional health benefits, perform moderate- or high-intensity muscle- and bone-strengthening activities on 2 or more days/week.

Specific to Older Adults

- Older adults unable to perform 150 min of moderate-intensity aerobic activity per week should be as physically active as abilities and conditions allow.

- Include exercises that maintain or improve balance and muscle strength.
- Walking is a good form of physical activity for those who can walk safely.

Adults, Children, and Adolescents With Disabilities

- Be as physically active as abilities allow with guidance from their healthcare provider.

Healthy Pregnant and Postpartum Women

- Consult with the healthcare provider regarding activity level throughout pregnancy. If the pregnancy or postpartum recovery is uncomplicated, then those who regularly engage in vigorous-intensity aerobic activity or in high amounts of activity can continue with this regimen.
- If not already engaged in vigorous-intensity physical activity, get at least 150 min of moderate-intensity aerobic activity per week, preferably spread throughout the week after consulting with healthcare provider.

Source: Adapted from U.S. Department of Health and Human Services. (2008, updated 2011). *Physical activity guidelines for Americans.* Retrieved from www.health.gov/paguidelines

Benefits of Regular Physical Activity

Regular exercise or other physical activity produces long-term health benefits, including a lower risk for early death, heart disease, stroke, type 2 diabetes, hypertension, hyperlipidemia, metabolic syndrome, colon and breast cancers, and depression. People with disabilities also benefit from physical activity (USDHHS, 2008, updated 2011).

 For older adults, walking is a good form of exercise and the risk of injury to joints is lower than other physical activities.

Brisk walking for as little as 30 minutes a day, when done consistently, promotes weight loss and maintenance of normal weight; lowers the risk of disability; reduces loss of bone density; and promotes better heart and lung function and muscular fitness.

Moderate-intensity walking helps to improve strength, balance, and muscle tone, all of which help to prevent falls and to improve overall physical stamina. It enhances psychological well-being, reduces depressive symptoms, and improves memory and mental clarity in older adults (Jitramontree, 2010; USDHHS, 2008, updated 2011). Along with a nutritious diet, social engagement, and mentally stimulating activities, physical activity is associated with a reduced risk of cognitive decline and Alzheimer's disease (National Institutes of Health, National Institute on Aging, 2011, updated 2016)

Risks Associated With Exercise

As a nurse, you can teach your clients realistically about the risks associated with exercise, helping them to exercise safely. Keep in mind that the benefits of exercise far outweigh the risks. Advise clients to follow the tips in the Self-Care box Teaching Your Patient How to Prevent Back Injury to help prevent injury.

Cardiac Injury Fear of triggering a cardiac event deters some people from exercising. However, physical activity is rarely life threatening, especially when compared with health risks related to sedentary lifestyle and a low level of fitness

Musculoskeletal Injury High-impact exercises may pose a risk for injury to bones, joints, and muscles. However, you can prevent most such injuries by ensuring proper body alignment as well as gradually increasing the activity level or varying activities. Weight lifting using correct form and appropriate weights markedly reduces the risk for injury

Dehydration Fluid and electrolyte loss occurs with prolonged exercise, high ambient temperatures, certain medication, and underlying health problems. Keep in mind that water is the best choice during and after most exercise. Some sports drinks contain glucose and electrolyte replacement for endurance activities or vigorous activity.

Temperature Regulation Problems

- **Hyperthermia** can occur when the person exercises in a hot climate. Hyperthermia is often accompanied by dehydration.
- **Heat exhaustion** is a potentially life-threatening event. Signs of heat exhaustion include light-headedness, nausea, headache, fatigue, hyperventilation, loss of concentration, abdominal cramps, elevated temperature, and cold, clammy skin.
- **Hypothermia** can occur when the person does not wear proper clothing or is exposed to cool water for an extended time. It is characterized by fatigue, confusion, and lack of coordination.

KnowledgeCheck 33-3

- Identify and describe four types of exercise.
- State the components of an exercise program.

ThinkLike a Nurse 33-2

- How would you address Helen Jillian's (Meet Your Patients) concerns about the risks associated with engaging in an exercise program?
- Peter Phan (Meet Your Patients) has experienced numerous injuries as a result of his exercise. Based on your knowledge of exercise, what questions would you like to ask Peter about his exercise program?

FACTORS AFFECTING MOBILITY AND ACTIVITY

Over recent decades with pervasive use of electronic devices for work, entertainment, and social contacts, people are generally more sedentary. In a study by the Physical Activity Council (2016), approximately 28% of Americans reported that in the previous calendar year they did not once participate in any of 104 listed physical activities (fitness, individual sports, team sports, outdoor sports, racquet sports, water sports, and winter sports). Those who would like to be more active report having someone to participate with as a strong motivator to begin a new activity. Others claimed their current health was a deterrent to engaging in exercise.

Developmental Stage

As expected, older adults were the least active but were the most likely participate in fitness activities rather than sporting or outdoor activities. See the accompanying Self-Care box for teaching your older adult patients about increasing physical activity and exercise.

Self-Care

✚ Teaching Your Patient How to Prevent Back Injury

- ➤ Poor posture is one of the main causes of back pain. Make a conscious effort to maintain good posture at all times.
- ➤ Use a firm mattress that provides adequate support.
- ➤ Sit with your knees slightly lower than your hips.
- ➤ If you must stand for a long period of time, flex your hip and raise one foot on a stool or object 6 to 8 inches off the ground. Periodically switch legs.
- ➤ Wear comfortable, low-heeled shoes. Avoid high heels as much as possible.
- ➤ Avoid restrictive clothing that inhibits your ability to use good body mechanics.
- ➤ Follow principles of body mechanics at all times (e.g., use wide base of support and do not lift with your back).
- ➤ Exercise regularly to maintain your optimal weight and strengthen the muscles of your body.
- ➤ Include abdominal exercises in your routine. Strong abdominal muscles help support the back.
- ➤ Avoid lifting excessive weight.
- ➤ Avoid exercises or movements that cause spinal flexion (e.g., toe-touches, sit-ups with knees extended), excessive flexion of the neck (e.g., abdominal crunches with neck curved to chest), or spinal rotation (twisting).

Self-Care

Teaching Older Adults About Activity and Exercise

What Kind of Physical Activity Should I Do?

➤ Get at least 30 minutes of *endurance* activity almost every day. Exercise that makes you breathe hard builds strength and staying power.

➤ Incorporate *resistance* into your exercise: Use resistance training with weights or isometric activity to build strength. Remember that you can do more and are less likely to fall when your muscles are strong.

➤ Do things to work on your *balance* (e.g., standing on one foot). This can help to prevent falls.

➤ Daily stretching will help you be more *flexible* and prevent injury.

When Should I Talk to My Doctor?

Almost anyone can do some type of physical activity, but before starting a new exercise program check with your healthcare provider if you experience any of the following:

➤ Any change in your health in the past 6 months
➤ Shortness of breath or dizziness
➤ Chest pain or pressure, or fluttering heart
➤ Joint pain or swelling
➤ Unexplained weight loss
➤ An infection with fever
➤ Eye problems
➤ Blood clot
➤ Hernia
➤ Recent hip surgery or joint injury

Source: Adapted from National Institutes of Health, National Institute on Aging. (2011, updated 2016). *Exercise and physical activity: Your everyday guide from the National Institute on Aging.* Retrieved from http://www.nia.nih.gov/HealthInformation/Publications/exercise.htm

Nutrition

- **Obesity** often leads to chronic health problems, which further reduce activity and contribute to further obesity. Movement becomes more difficult as body size increases. Joint and back injuries and osteoarthritis are more prevalent with obesity, which in turn reduces a person's ability to engage in physical activity for weight loss.
- **Chronic disease** may cause negative nitrogen balance—that is, inadequate protein stores to maintain or repair body tissue. Muscle wasting and fatigue occur, leading to reduced activity levels.

Lifestyle

Personal values about exercise and fitness determine when, or whether, exercise becomes part of a person's routine. Some people enjoy exercise. Others see it as pure drudgery or as "something I have to do." A person's culture and support system define what exercise the person is likely to accept. For example, swimming requires wearing a bathing suit; in some cultures, that may not be acceptable.

Environmental Factors

Environmental factors affecting exercise include the following:

- **Weather**—When it is cold, damp, or even hot and humid, people tend to avoid strenuous activity outside. Encourage patients to choose a variety of activities that they enjoy so they can be active, regardless of the weather.
- **Pollution**—When air quality is poor, suggest indoor activities to reduce exposure to allergens and pollutants.
- **Neighborhood conditions**—Crime and lack of parks are examples of conditions that influence attitudes about outside activities. Mall walking is a successful way to incorporate exercise into daily patterns when neighborhood conditions do not encourage activity.
- **Finances**—Joining a fitness center or engaging in sports might not be practical for some budgets. However, many activities, such as walking or playing basketball or tennis in the community park, are inexpensive or free.
- **Support system**—Family and friends who are active are likely to promote and support your efforts to exercise. Those who are sedentary may not encourage you to be more active or lose weight.

DISORDERS OF THE MUSCULOSKELETAL SYSTEM

Diseases and abnormalities in various body systems can negatively influence body alignment, balance, coordination, and joint mobility. In the next sections, we describe some disorders that can affect activity and exercise.

Congenital Anomalies of the Musculoskeletal System

The following are common congenital anomalies that affect appearance, motor function, and mobility:

- **Syndactylism** is the fusion of two or more fingers or toes. Most cases involving the hands are treated surgically at an early age to limit the effect on fine motor development.
- **Developmental dysplasia of the hip** is a congenital abnormality of the development of the femur, acetabulum, or both that shows as hip dislocation.
- **Foot deformities** such as clubfoot (talipes equinovarus) occur in about 4% of all newborns. Serial casts or surgery may be used to correct the defect and preserve function.
- **Scoliosis** is a lateral curvature of the spine. Scoliosis can result from congenital bone disorders, neuromuscular impairment, or trauma, but approximately two-thirds of cases have no known cause and are termed *idiopathic scoliosis*.

Diseases Related to Bone Formation or Metabolism

Bone formation abnormalities may be congenital or they may result from dietary deficiencies or bone disease.

- **Osteogenesis imperfecta (OI)** is a congenital disorder of bone and connective tissue that is characterized by brittle bones that fracture easily. Infants with OI are often born with fractures and continue to fracture with minimal trauma or even spontaneously. Prompt recognition and treatment of fractures help prevent deformities.
- **Achondroplasia,** or dwarfism, occurs when the bones ossify (harden) prematurely.
- **Paget's disease** is a metabolic bone disease in which increased bone loss results in pain, pathological fractures, and deformities. This disorder usually affects the skull, vertebrae, femur, and pelvis.

- **Vitamin D and calcium** are needed to form and maintain bone. Deficiencies lead to porous bones. In children, prolonged deficiencies (*rickets*) can cause the long bones of the legs to become bowed, retard growth, and lead to frequent fractures.

Diseases Affecting Joint Mobility

Diseases of the joints may be degenerative or inflammatory. Nursing activity for patients with joint mobility problems focuses on assisting with movement, providing comfort, and teaching about medications. If mobility is severely restricted, you will also assist patients with activities of daily living (ADLs).

Osteoarthritis (OA) is the most prevalent type of degenerative joint. **OA** involves a loss of articular cartilage in the joint, with pain and stiffness as the primary symptoms. Patients may also have decreased ROM and **crepitus,** a creaking or grating sound, with joint motion. Symptoms are aggravated by weight-bearing and joint use and are relieved by resting the affected joints. OA is more common in women, older adults, and people who are overweight.

Rheumatoid Arthritis (RA) is a systemic autoimmune disease involving chronic inflammation of the joints and surrounding connective tissue, frequently resulting in difficulty in performing ADLs. RA causes joint pain, deformity, and loss of function; patients may also experience fever, fatigue, weakness, and weight loss. RA occurs most frequently in the fingers, wrists, elbows, ankles, and knees. The illness usually begins in mid-life and more often in women. Unlike OA, RA does not improve with rest. Pain is most intense when the person arises from bed. Pain and joint deformities may so severely affect mobility that patients cannot care for themselves.

Ankylosing Spondylitis is a chronic inflammatory joint disease characterized by stiffening and fusion of the spine and sacroiliac joints. The inflammation occurs where the ligaments, tendons, and joint capsule insert into the bone. The disease usually develops in young adults, equally in men and women. Patients with ankylosing spondylitis have low back pain and stiffness and decreased ROM of the spine. The convex lumbar curve is lost, and the upper spine curve increases, causing kyphosis (see Chapter 21 for review).

Gout is an inflammatory response to high levels of uric acid. Crystals form in the synovial fluid, and small white nodules, or *tophi,* form in the subcutaneous tissues. Gout produces painful joints and severely limits activity during acute flare-ups. It usually affects the joint of the great toe, but can occur in feet, ankles, knees, hands, and wrists.

Problems Affecting Bone Integrity

Loss of bone integrity may occur from an imbalance in bone production, infection, or tumors.

Osteoporosis is a decrease in total bone density, which occurs when osteoclast activity outpaces that of the osteoblasts. The internal structure of the bone diminishes, and the bone collapses in on itself. Normally bone mass continues to increase up to the third decade of life. After age 30, bone loss begins. Women experience a rapid decline in bone mass at menopause. In men, a gradual loss continues. As bones become porous, they become weak, leading to vertebral collapse or fractures of the long bones of the arms and legs, spontaneously or with minimal trauma.

Genetics, body frame, menopausal status, chronic disease and lifestyle choices also contribute to osteoporosis. The most common risk factors for osteoporotic fracture are advanced age, low bone mineral density, and previous fracture as an adult. Smoking, low calcium and vitamin D intake, excess alcohol use, and sedentary lifestyle also increase the risk (National Institutes of Health, National Institute on Aging, 2012).

Osteomyelitis (infection of the bone) may develop after bone injury or surgery. It can be difficult and expensive to treat and can leave the patient with permanent disability. Bone contains microscopic channels that are impermeable to most of the natural defenses of the body. Once bacteria enter these channels, they multiply rapidly.

Bone Tumors may also affect form and function. Tumors in the bone cause considerable pain and severely limit activity. Nursing responsibilities for patients with osteomyelitis or bone tumors include collaborative treatments, patient education about the treatment plan, and providing comfort.

Trauma

Trauma may affect bones, ligaments, muscles, and joints.

- **Fractures,** or breaks in the bone, are one of the most common forms of trauma (see Fig. 33-5). Fractures are accompanied by tenderness at the site, loss of function, deformity of the area, and swelling of the surrounding tissues. However, x-ray is required for definitive diagnosis. The type and severity of fracture determine whether casting, traction, or surgical repair is necessary.
- **Sprains and strains** are more common than fractures.
  - A **sprain** is a stretch injury of a ligament that causes the ligament to tear. A partial tear can usually heal with rest, but a complete tear often requires surgery to stabilize the joint.
  - A **strain** is an injury to muscle caused by excessive stress on the muscle.

    Both strains and sprains cause pain at the site of injury, swelling, and loss of function. Because the signs and

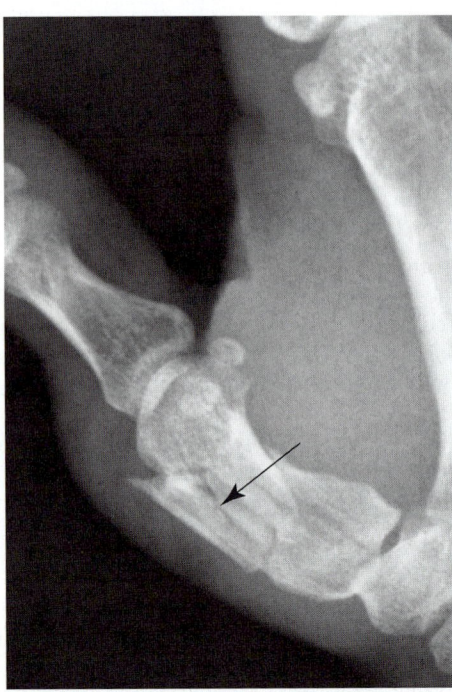

FIGURE 33-5 Fracture in hand occurring after traumatic injury.

symptoms are the same as those of a fracture, x-ray studies are used to distinguish these injuries. Initial treatment of fractures, sprains, and strains include rest, ice, compression, and elevation.

- **Stretching and tearing injuries** to the **meniscus** (cartilage under knee cap), lateral knee ligaments, and Achilles tendon are also common. Magnetic resonance imaging studies are done to determine the extent of injury. Rest and ice are necessary, but often surgical repair is needed to achieve full healing.

Disorders of the Central Nervous System

Any disorder that affects the motor centers of the brain or the transmission of nerve impulses will affect mobility. Examples include the following:

- Cerebrovascular accident (stroke)
- Head or spinal cord injury
- Multiple sclerosis (a disorder affecting nerve transmission)
- Myasthenia gravis (a disease caused by antibodies to the acetylcholine receptors at the neuromuscular junction)

Progressive degenerative disorders of the neurological system also affect mobility and coordination. For example, Parkinson's disease is a progressive degeneration of the basal ganglia that produces tremor, rigidity, and difficulty coordinating movement.

Diseases of Other Body Systems

Diseases affecting other body systems may affect mobility and activity tolerance, as in the following examples:

- *Respiratory disorders.* Any disorder that affects oxygenation limits exercise tolerance. Chronic obstructive pulmonary disease, asthma, and pneumonia are associated with shortness of breath, which becomes worse with increased activity.
- *Circulatory disorders.* Impaired arterial circulation limits oxygen delivery to the tissue. As activity increases, skeletal muscle pain develops. Impaired venous circulation causes leg swelling and discomfort, which are relieved by elevating the legs. As a result, patients may become relatively sedentary to relieve the pain and discomfort.
- *Fatigue.* Acute illnesses, such as influenza, produce fatigue during the acute illness and limit activity for short periods of time. Disorders that produce long-standing fatigue include anemia, anorexia nervosa, cancer, depression, and grief.
- *Bedrest.* For certain health conditions or after surgery, bedrest may be prescribed, though infrequently.

KnowledgeCheck 33-4

- In which age-groups are you more likely to see health concerns that affect mobility?
- What types of disorders limit activity or mobility?
- What are the signs and symptoms of a fracture?
- What is the difference between a strain and a sprain?

ThinkLike a Nurse 33-3

- Your teenage daughter complains when you ask her to take a calcium supplement and encourage her to exercise. What information should you provide so she understands why these measures are important?

- Phillip Flanders (Meet Your Patients) has never been involved in a regular exercise program. Phillip works as an accountant, and most of his friends are work associates. Phillip's siblings are overweight and do not exercise. Both of his parents died of heart disease. Many of Phillip's friends have suggested that he begin exercising to improve his energy level and health. What recommendations can you make to Phillip so that it will be more likely that he will start and then continue an exercise routine?

EXAMPLE PROBLEM: IMMOBILITY

Most people take their mobility for granted until illness, disease, or trauma affects their ability to move. Even short periods of immobility may be difficult. If you've ever had the flu or an illness that sent you to bed, you know that it can take several days to return to your pre-illness state, especially for older adults and people with underlying chronic illness. To learn about the effects of immobility on various body systems and about a few general interventions, refer to the Example Problem: Immobility.

KnowledgeCheck 33-5

- Identify the effects of immobility on the cardiovascular, musculoskeletal, and integumentary systems.
- Why might immobility be referred to as a stressor?
- What are three effects of immobility on the GI system?
- What changes in mood might be seen with immobility?

PracticalKnowledge
knowing how

As you have seen in the preceding sections, immobility can result in serious health consequences. In the remainder of the chapter, we discuss nursing actions to promote activity and exercise and eliminate the complications of immobility.

ASSESSMENT NP

Perform an assessment focused on mobility and physical activity for any patient who has musculoskeletal issues, is obese, has limited movement or range of motion, or is confined to bed or chair. As always, you will validate the nursing history data with physical examination. Box 33-3 defines a variety of terms used to describe problems with muscle mass, strength, or mobility. To help you with focused mobility assessments in the home, see the Home Care box Home Assessment for a Patient With Mobility Concerns.

Focused Nursing History

A nursing history focused on activity and exercise addresses usual activity, fitness goals, mobility problems, underlying health problems, lifestyle, and external factors. For questions to ask, see the accompanying Focused Assessment box.

When caring for patients with very limited activity, assessing the ability to perform activities of daily living (ADLs) or instrumental activities of daily living (IADLs) may be more appropriate. Recall that ADLs focus on hygiene, feeding, toileting, and transfer out of bed. In contrast, IADLs focus on tasks that are involved in helping a patient maintain independent living status. Assessment tools for ADLs and IADLs were presented in Chapter 3.

EXAMPLE PROBLEM: Immobility

PROBLEM

KEY POINT: *Prolonged immobilization causes physiological changes in almost every body system, as well as psychological changes.*

Muscles and Bones

- One of the first systems affected by immobility; 10% loss of muscle strength **(atrophy)** per week.
- Wasting of the gastrocnemius, soleus, and leg muscles that control flexion and extension of the hip, knee, and ankle.
- Joints become stiff.
- The strongest muscles (flexors) pull the joints, leading to contractures, or joint ankylosis.

Heart and Vessels

- Leads to ↑ cardiac and venous stasis.
- Heart rate and stroke volume ↑ to maintain blood pressure. But with immobility, cardiac reserves ↓, which means the heart is less able to respond to the body's demands.
- Without muscle activity, gravity causes blood to pool, which leads to edema. Fluid in the tissue is more prone to pressure injury.
- Leads to compression and injury of the small vessels in the legs and ↓ clearance of coagulation factors, causing blood to clot faster. Stasis, activation of clotting, and vessel injury *(Virchow's triad)* are associated with a ↑ risk for deep vein thrombosis (DVT) formation.
- Inactivates the baroreceptors involved with vasoconstriction and dilation; less able to regulate BP (orthostatic hypotension). Dizziness and light-headedness occur.

Lungs

- ↓ strength of all muscles, ↓ chest wall expansion, which affects ventilation.
- Shallow respirations; secretions pool in lungs.
- Pooled secretions block air passages and alveoli, ↓ air-gas exchange, and often lead to atelectasis (collapse of air sacs) or pneumonia.

Integumentary System

- Compresses capillaries; ↓ circulation causes pressure injury.

Metabolism

- ↑ serum lactic acid and ↓ ATP (energy).
- Metabolic rate drops; protein and glycogen synthesis ↓; fat stores ↑.
- Causes glucose intolerance; ↓ muscle mass.
- Triggers release of thyroid hormones, epinephrine, norepinephrine, ACTH from the pituitary gland, and aldosterone from the kidneys—same as stress response.
- Affects parathyroid function, calcium metabolism, and bone formation. The result is osteoporosis, calcium depletion in joints, and renal calculi (kidney stones) due to ↑ excretion of calcium.
- ↑ risk for fractures with minimal trauma.

Gastrointestinal System

- Slows peristalsis, leading to constipation, gas, and difficulty evacuating stool from the rectum. Paralytic ileus (cessation of peristalsis) can occur.
- Appetite diminishes and food digested more slowly, often leading to ↓ calorie intake.
- Muscle is broken down as a fuel source.

Genitourinary System

- Being supine inhibits drainage of urine from the kidney and bladder. Urine becomes stagnant—ideal environment for infection.
- ↑ calcium levels and stone formation.
- ↓ muscle tone leads to ↓ bladder tone, which leads to urinary retention.
- Many patients have difficulty voiding in a bedpan or urinal.

Psychological Effects

- Moodiness, depression, anxiety, hostility, disturbed sleep, apathy, poor body concept
- ↓ concentration, recall, and problem-solving
- Change in the ability to perform self-care

COMPLICATIONS

- Pressure injury
- Constipation
- Joint contracture
- Muscle weakness
- Balance problems
- DVT
- Pooling of secretions in lower lobes
- Orthostatic hypotension

EXAMPLE PROBLEM: Immobility—cont'd

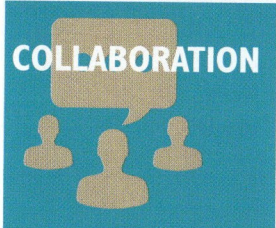

COLLABORATION

- Occupational therapy
- Physical therapy

- Wound specialist, as needed
- Dietician

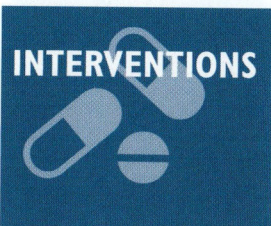

INTERVENTIONS

- Position the patient to allow for lung expansion and prevent atelectasis and pneumonia.
- Offer protein-rich diet to maintain muscle mass.
- Assist patient to standing position; assist with ambulation as tolerated.

- Use positioning devices to maintain body alignment. Prevent orthostatic hypotension by having patient sit on edge of bed before standing.
- Turn patient every 2 hours to prevent pressure on the skin and minimize edema.
- Encourage active and passive ROM.

BOX 33-3 ■ Terms Used to Describe Problems With Muscle Mass, Strength, or Mobility

Atrophy is a decrease in the size of muscle tissue due to lack of use or loss of innervation.

Clonus is spasmodic contraction of opposing muscles resulting in tremorous movement.

Flaccidity is a decrease or absence of muscle tone.

Hemiplegia is paralysis of one side of the body.

Hypertrophy is an increase in the size or bulk of a muscle or organ.

Paraplegia is paralysis of the lower portion of the trunk and both legs.

Paresis is partial or incomplete paralysis.

Paresthesia is numbness, tingling, or burning resulting from injury of the nerve(s) innervating the affected area.

Quadriplegia is paralysis of all four extremities.

Spasticity is a motor disorder characterized by increased muscle tone, exaggerated tendon jerks, and clonus.

Tremor is involuntary quivering movement of a body part.

Focused Physical Assessment

Important data to include in a physical assessment related to activity and exercise include vital signs, height, weight, body mass index, body alignment, joint function, gait, muscle strength, and activity tolerance. This section summarizes a few of these components. For a description of all the components, see the accompanying Focused Assessment box.

Before beginning the examination, be fully aware of the patient's mobility status and any restrictions in movement, pain, injury, or otherwise. As you move through the examination, observe for pain, inflammation and mobility limitations in all areas. For a thorough discussion of physical assessment of the musculoskeletal system, see Chapter 21.

Gait

The way a person moves communicates a great deal about his general state of health, mood, and risk for falls. You might want to assess abnormal gaits in patients with injury, neurological issues, or the following characteristics:

- **Antalgic gait**—limp to avoid pain when bearing weight on the affected side
- **Propulsive gait**—a stooped, rigid posture, with the head and neck bent forward; movement forward is by small, shuffling steps with involuntary acceleration; also known as festinating gait; common in Parkinson's disease
- **Scissors gait**—legs flexed slightly at the hips and knees with the thighs crossing in a scissors-like movement; common with cerebral palsy, stroke, or spinal tumor
- **Spastic gait**—a stiff, foot-dragging walk caused by one-sided, long-term muscle contraction; seen with cerebral palsy, head trauma, or brain tumor
- **Steppage gait**—an exaggerated motion of lifting the leg to avoid scraping the toes of a foot with footdrop (foot appears floppy with the toes pointing down); seen with Guillain-Barré syndrome
- **Waddling gait**—a distinctive rolling motion in which the opposite hip drops; seen in patients with muscular dystrophy or developmental dysplasia of the hip; characteristic gait in late pregnancy.

If you need additional information on gait, see the illustrations in Procedure 21-15.

Activity Tolerance

To promote the benefits of physical activity, people need to pace themselves during exercise, especially those who have been inactive. Health professionals can teach people to rate the perceived level of exertion and monitor target heart rate. Target heart rate requires a pulse check during exercises and staying within 50% to 85% of the maximum heart rate. To figure this out, take 220, subtract the person's age, and then multiply times 0.5 for a target heart rate for low-intensity exercise; or multiply times 0.85 for maximum heart rate during high-intensity exercise.

Assessing Activity and Exercise

Suggested History Questions

Usual Activity

Describe your typical daily activity level.

If the patient has very restricted activity, ask the following questions:

➤ Are you able to care for yourself in regard to hygiene, dressing, toileting, and getting out of bed?

➤ If the patient has ADL limitations: Who helps you with these daily activities?

If the patient does not indicate restricted activity, ask the following questions:

➤ What is your usual form of exercise?

➤ How often do you exercise?

➤ How long are your exercise sessions?

➤ How long have you been engaged in this type of activity?

➤ In what types of exercise or sports have you participated in the past?

➤ What has your activity level been over the past 10 years?

➤ Are you exercising more or less than in the past?

Fitness Goals

➤ What aspects of exercise do you enjoy? What aspects of exercise do you dislike?

➤ What do you think are the benefits of exercise?

➤ How do you schedule your exercise?

➤ What motivates you to exercise?

➤ What are your current fitness goals?

Mobility Concerns

➤ Do you have any pain or discomfort with activity?

➤ Do you avoid any activities because of pain, discomfort, shortness of breath, or chest pain?

If the patient answered yes to either question, describe the following:

➤ Type of problem

➤ Onset of concern

➤ Frequency of problem

➤ Activities that trigger and relieve problem

➤ Severity and type of symptoms

➤ Effect of problem on day-to-day activities

➤ Treatments used to alleviate problem and how they worked

Underlying Health Concerns

➤ Do you have any healthcare problem that affects your ability to engage in activity or exercise? If so, describe the problem and the effect.

➤ What medications do you take?

➤ Have you ever been told you have a bone problem? If so, what was the nature of the problem?

➤ Have you ever experienced a fracture, strain, or sprain? If so, where was the problem? When did it occur? How did it occur?

➤ Have you ever had weakness of the muscles or problems coordinating movement?

➤ Do you have any cardiac or respiratory problems that affect your ability to perform activities?

➤ Have you ever experienced anxiety or depression that affected your ability to participate in activities?

Lifestyle

What kind of work do you do?

Describe your typical work activities.

How many hours per week do you work?

What other commitments do you have (school, family, other obligations)?

External Factors

➤ Are there any restrictions in your home that limit your ability to be active?

➤ Do you feel you need an assistive device?

➤ Are you comfortable exercising outside your home or in your neighborhood?

Focused Physical Assessments for Activity and Body Alignment

With the patient standing, observe from the anterior, posterior, and lateral views. Check for the following:

➤ Shoulders and hips are level.

➤ Toes are pointed forward.

➤ The spine is straight, with no abnormal curvatures noted.

➤ The posture is not slumped.

Ask the patient to sit down; observe as he does so.

➤ Does he have difficulty lowering his torso?

➤ Can he control the movement?

➤ Is he able to get into this position with ease?

➤ When he sits, does he slump?

If the patient cannot stand or sit, assess his alignment in bed. Look for ability to move in bed, as well as the posture the patient maintains.

Joint Function

➤ Assessing joint function includes inspection and palpation of the joints and assessment of range of motion.

➤ Begin your assessment at the neck and systematically work your way through each of the joints.

➤ At each joint observe for swelling, erythema, asymmetry, or obvious deformity.

➤ Compare the size of the muscles above and below the joint and on each side of the body.

➤ Palpate the joint for temperature and crepitus. Warmth over a joint indicates inflammation or infection. Be sure to compare body temperature over several joints and right to left. **Crepitus** is a grating sensation when the joint is moved. It can often be heard as well as felt. Crepitus is associated with degenerative joint disease or arthritic changes in the joint.

➤ As you palpate the joint, move it through its range of motion.

Muscle Strength

➤ Assess muscle strength by having the patient push and then pull against your hands.

➤ Start at the neck, and test the strength of all major joints' range of motion.

➤ To see a nurse using a performing passive range-of-motion exercises,

Assessing Activity and Exercise—cont'd

 The video **Performing Passive Range of Motion Exercises,** along with questions and suggested responses, is available on the **Davis's *Nursing Skills Videos*** Web site on Davis*Plus.*

Gait

Gait is divided into two phases: stance and swing.

Stance—In the stance phase, the heel of one foot strikes the ground while the opposite foot pushes off and leaves the ground.

Swing—In the swing phase, the leg from behind moves in front of the body. When the right leg is in stance mode, the left leg is in swing mode.

You must observe the patient walking. Normal gait includes the following features:

➤ Head is erect, gaze forward.
➤ Heel strikes the ground before the toe.
➤ Opposite arm moves forward at the same time.
➤ Feet are dorsiflexed in the swing phase.
➤ Gait is coordinated and rhythmic.
➤ Weight is evenly distributed, with minimal swing from side to side.
➤ Movement starts and stops with ease.
➤ Movement is at a moderate pace.

If the patient uses an assistive device, such as a cane, crutch, or walker, pay attention to how he uses it. Ask the patient to ambulate a short distance with and without the device to determine how well the device is providing stability.

Activity Tolerance

➤ Assess and record vital signs before having the patient engage in 3 minutes of activity.

➤ Select an activity appropriate for the patient. For example, if the patient uses a walker, ask the patient to walk down the hallway. For a patient without obvious health limitations, consider asking her to run in place for 3 minutes.
➤ Observe the patient throughout the exercise. If she shows any signs of distress, stop the exercise, immediately take a set of vital signs, and repeat the vital signs every minute until they have returned to baseline.
➤ If the patient can exercise continuously for 3 minutes, assess the patient at the end of the 3-minute period and at 1-minute intervals. Note the change in heart rate, blood pressure, and respiratory rate.

This type of approach is not appropriate for patients who easily become short of breath, develop chest pain, or are very unsteady on their feet. Instead, for example, limit your assessment to determining the amount of assistance the patient needs to turn in bed or get out of bed.

Muscle Mass and Strength

➤ As you observe the patient, compare muscle mass on the right and left sides. If you notice an obvious discrepancy in size, measure the circumference of the limbs and compare.
➤ To assess strength, ask the patient to push against your hand with the hands and feet. Once again, compare both sides.

For guidelines for assessing mobility in the home, see the **Home Care box Home Assessment for a Patient With Mobility Concerns.**

Home Assessment for a Patient With Mobility Concerns

Assess the Environment

➤ Are there stairs or other obstacles that the patient must negotiate?
➤ What aspects of the home environment assist with patient care?
➤ What aspects of the home environment hinder patient care?
➤ What is the patient's history of falls or other mobility concerns?
➤ Would the patient benefit from assistive equipment (e.g., hospital bed, walker)?
➤ Can the patient negotiate the distance between the bedroom, bathroom, and kitchen?

Assess the Family's or Caregivers' Abilities and Needs

➤ Who is providing care?
➤ Is the available care sufficient to meet the patient's needs?
➤ Are additional support persons available to assist with care?

➤ Can the caregiver safely move the patient in bed or assist the patient out of bed?
➤ What are the health concerns or physical limitations of the caregivers?
➤ What is the backup plan if the family or caregiver can no longer meet the patient's needs?

Assess Resources

➤ What community resources are available to the patient or caregiver (e.g., Meals on Wheels, physical therapy, Visiting Nurses Association)?
➤ Are the patient and caregiver willing to use community resources?
➤ What services are provided by the patient's insurance?
➤ Can the patient or family afford private services? If so, what services are they interested in?

Effects of Teamwork and Collaboration on Activity and Exercise Outcomes

Chapter Key Concepts: Activity, Exercise (Thinking, Doing, Caring)

Competency: Teamwork and Collaboration; Patient-Centered Care

Scenario: Mr. Lee underwent surgery to repair a ruptured quadriceps tendon in his left leg. His discharge instructions provided general guidelines about wound care, signs and symptoms to report, and when to follow up with the surgeon.

At his 2-week post-op visit, Mr. Lee was making good progress. The surgeon gave him a prescription to begin physical therapy, telling him that the referred therapists knew his protocols. He also told Mr. Lee that he could drive and return to work, but that he should "listen to his body" and rest when he was tired or in pain. Mrs. Lee mentioned that the drive to work was 1 hour each way and wondered whether that was too much. After the surgeon left, the nurse removed the staples from the incision and talked to Mr. and Mrs. Lee about potential complications and how to perform wound care.

The next day, the physical therapist scheduled Mr. Lee for therapy on Mondays, Wednesdays, and Thursdays. During the first therapy session, Mr. Lee moaned with pain. On the second visit, Mrs. Lee remarked that his knee was very swollen but the therapist disagreed with her, noting that other patients had much more swelling than Mr. Lee had. One week later Mr. Lee, fearing something was wrong, went to the surgeon's office. He had a fever of 101°F and was in severe pain. The surgeon said, "Your knee is not damaged or infected, but it is very inflamed. You should not have scheduled back-to-back therapy sessions. You've been overdoing it."

Outcome: It was 2 weeks before Mr. Lee's pain, swelling, and fever subsided.

Think about it: Patient-centered care, teamwork, and collaboration are considered integral to patient safety and quality care. Reflect on this scenario, considering the following questions and concepts:

➤ How would you describe this team's functioning?
➤ What barriers to team functioning do you think might exist in this scenario?
➤ What could the office nurse have done to improve collaboration?
➤ How did teamwork and communication affect Mr. Lee's activity outcomes?
➤ Did the teamwork and communication affect his safety? If so, in what way?
➤ What system changes would you make to improve communication?
➤ Think about patient-centeredness. Did the team value Mrs. Lee's input (give examples)? How might outcomes have been different if Mrs. Lee had been recognized as a full partner in planning or providing care? Do you think quality, safety, costs, and patient satisfaction were affected?

KnowledgeCheck 33-6

- Describe a focused assessment for a patient experiencing mobility concerns.
- Identify the assessment methods (inspection, palpation, percussion, and auscultation) used when performing a physical examination focused on mobility concerns.

 ThinkLike a Nurse 33-4

Review the Meet Your Patients scenario. Which, if any, of the class participants requires a physical examination focused on mobility concerns? Explain your reasoning.

ANALYSIS/NURSING DIAGNOSIS NP

Nursing diagnoses that specifically describe activity and immobility problems include the following:

- *Activity Intolerance* is a state in which a patient has insufficient physical or psychological energy to carry out daily activities.
- *Impaired Physical Mobility* is limitation of independent purposeful movement of the body. Impaired Physical Mobility is a broad, general diagnosis. Use the following, more descriptive diagnoses when the patient has specific deficits: Impaired Bed Mobility, Impaired Walking, Impaired Wheelchair Mobility, and Impaired Transfer Ability.
- *Risk for Disuse Syndrome* exists when a patient's prescribed or unavoidable inactivity creates the risk for deterioration of other body systems.

- *Sedentary Lifestyle* is a habit of life that is characterized by a low physical activity level.
- Mobility problems may also be the etiology of other diagnoses. The following are examples:
  - Acute Pain r/t musculoskeletal injury
  - Risk for Injury r/t unsteady gait

Keep in mind that Immobility, especially bedrest, can be the etiology of problems in all body systems, as well as psychosocially.

To see a nursing care plan and care map for the diagnosis Impaired Physical Mobility,

 Go to Davis Advantage, Resources, Chapter 32, **Nursing Care Plan** and **Care Map**.

For a more comprehensive list of NANDA-I nursing diagnoses,

 Go to Davis Advantage, Resources, Chapter 33, List of NANDA-I Diagnoses.

PLANNING OUTCOMES/EVALUATION NP

NOC standardized outcomes for mobility diagnoses focus on energy maintenance, as well as mobility. They include:

For Energy Maintenance:

Activity Tolerance	Psychomotor Energy
Endurance	Rest
Energy Conservation	Sleep
Fatigue Level	

Standardized Language

NANDA-I Diagnoses

Nursing Diagnosis	Defining Characteristics	Etiologies
Activity Intolerance—A state in which a patient has insufficient physical or psychological energy to carry out daily activities	*Subjective:* fatigue, weakness, discomfort on exertion, dyspnea, and verbalization of no interest in activity *Objective:* changes in heart rate, blood pressure disproportionate to activity, dysrhythmias or evidence of ischemia on electrocardiogram (ECG), and pallor or cyanosis with activity	Conditions that affect tissue oxygenation (e.g., chronic obstructive pulmonary disease or cardiac disease) Conditions that produce fatigue, such as depression, prolonged immobility, bed rest, and sedentary lifestyle
Impaired Physical Mobility—Limitation of independent purposeful movement of the body (specify level of independence using a standardized functional scale)	*Subjective:* pain or discomfort with movement, exertional dyspnea *Objective:* limited ROM, limitations in fine or gross motor movement, lack of coordination with movement, unstable gait, decreased reaction time, postural instability, slowed movement, and difficulty performing ADLs	Neuromuscular, sensoriperceptual, or musculoskeletal impairment; malnutrition; obesity; deconditioning due to sedentary lifestyle; lack of knowledge about the importance of activity and exercise for maintenance of health; anxiety; cognitive impairment; discomfort; limited cardiovascular endurance; malnutrition, medications; pain; prescribed movement restrictions

Note: Impaired Physical Mobility is a broad, general diagnosis. Use the following, more descriptive diagnoses when the patient has specific deficits:

Impaired Bed Mobility	Impaired Walking	Sedentary Lifestyle
Impaired Wheelchair Mobility	Impaired Transfer Ability	

Note: Mobility problems may also be the etiology of other diagnoses. The following are examples:

➤ *Risk for Ineffective Peripheral Tissue Perfusion* (specify) r/t blood flow compromised by reduced mobility
➤ *Risk for Disuse Syndrome* occurs when there is a risk for deterioration of body systems due to musculoskeletal inactivity.
➤ Risk factors include prescribed bed rest, severe pain, altered level of consciousness, mechanical immobilization (traction), and paralysis.
➤ *Acute Pain* r/t musculoskeletal injury
➤ *Ineffective Health Maintenance* r/t prescribed bed rest
➤ *Risk for Injury* r/t unsteady gait
➤ *Self-Care Deficit (Bathing/Hygiene, Feeding, Dressing/Grooming, Toileting)* r/t Impaired Physical Mobility

---

For Mobility:

Ambulation	Immobility Consequences:
Ambulation: Wheelchair	Psycho-Cognitive
Body Positioning:	Joint Movement (specify)
Self-Initiated	
Coordinated Movement	Joint Movement: Passive
Immobility Consequences:	Mobility
Physiological	Transfer Performance

For a list of all NIC interventions for various nursing diagnoses,

 Go to Davis Advantage, Resources, Chapter 33, **Alphabetical List of NOC Outcomes and NIC Interventions.**

Individualized goals/outcome statements depend on the nursing diagnosis used. Because activity and exercise abilities are individualized, goals must consider the patient's current condition, expected condition changes, lifestyle, and values. Examples:

Will independently transfer to the wheelchair by [date].
Will discuss his feelings about his activity restrictions by [date].

PLANNING INTERVENTIONS/ IMPLEMENTATION NP

Because attitudes about fitness and activity vary widely, mobility is often a difficult topic. Some people are devastated by activity limitations caused by disease or treatment. Others are able to accept these changes. It is important for you to convey an attitude of acceptance about the patient's current activity level and provide care that helps the patient achieve his optimal level of function.

NIC standardized interventions and activities are found in the accompanying Standardized Language table Selected NIC Interventions for Mobility Diagnoses. Also,

 Go to Davis Advantage, Resources, Chapter 33, **List of NOC Outcomes and NIC Interventions.**

Individualized nursing activities to promote exercise and mobility are discussed in the remainder of the Planning Interventions/Implementation section, following.

Caring for Patients With Specific Diseases and Abnormalities

In addition, when caring for patients with specific diseases and abnormalities, you will need to add the following interventions:

▪ **For congenital anomalies**—Nursing responsibilities include early detection and referral for additional treatment and parent counseling.
▪ **For bone formation abnormalities**—Nursing responsibilities include collaborative treatments, providing comfort, and patient education to promote mobility. Also teach patients to consume a balanced diet that meets the minimum recommendations for vitamins and minerals.

Selected NIC Interventions for Mobility Diagnoses

Class: Activity and Exercise Management	Class: Immobility Management
Body Mechanics Promotion	Bed Rest Care
Energy Management	Cast Care: Maintenance
Exercise Promotion	Cast Care: Wet
Exercise Promotion: Strength Training	Physical Restraint
Exercise Promotion: Stretching	Positioning
Exercise Therapy: Ambulation	Positioning: Wheelchair
Exercise Therapy: Balance	Self-Care Assistance: Transfer
Exercise Therapy: Joint Mobility	Splinting
Exercise Therapy: Muscle Control	Traction/Immobilization Care
Teaching: Prescribed Activity/ Exercise	Transfer

Source: Bulechek, G., Butcher, H., Dochterman, J., et al. (Eds.). (2012). *Nursing interventions classification (NIC)* (6th ed.). St. Louis, MO: C.V. Mosby. Used with permission.

- **For joint mobility problems**—Nursing activities focus on providing comfort and teaching about medications. If mobility is severely restricted, you will also assist patients with ADLs.
- **For osteomyelitis or bone tumors**—Nursing activities include collaborative treatments, patient education about the treatment plan, and providing comfort.

Treating Osteoporosis The best treatment for osteoporosis is prevention. Teach adolescents and adults to eat a balanced diet high in calcium, fluoride, and other minerals and to start an exercise program they can continue throughout their lives.

- **Advise older women that weight-bearing exercise can help decrease the rate of bone loss, and advise them to ask their provider about medications to reduce bone mineral loss (National Osteoporosis Foundation, n.d.a).**
- The National Osteoporosis Foundation (n.d.b) recommends calcium intake for adults aged 50 and older to be 1,200 mg/day and vitamin D 800 to 1,000 IU daily to prevent bone loss. Phosphorus is another important bone mineral. But if there is a disproportionate amount of phosphorus compared with the amount of calcium in the diet, bone loss can occur.
- Urge people of all ages, but particularly postmenopausal women, to avoid smoking because tobacco reduces the absorption of calcium in the intestine. In addition, more than two drinks of alcohol per day decreases the matrix of the bone and reduces the body's ability to absorb calcium.

Promoting Exercise

Nurses are in an ideal role to encourage and educate people of all ages to be active for healthy living. Here are some common steps to help people attain and maintain fitness. Also see the Self-Care box Teaching Clients How to Set Up a Fitness Program.

- *Personalize the benefits of regular physical activity.* In other words, find out what motivates your patient. For instance, your patient might want to lose weight and improve his physical appearance. Yet another patient might be interested in improving the quality of sleep or overcoming periods of low energy during the day. Exercise also makes you feel happier, gives you more energy, boosts your self-confidence, calms your body to relieve stress, makes you more productive in your day, and can lead to a longer and healthier life.
- *Set personal goals for physical activity.* Simple, realistic goals tend to be best. Be sure to define them so they are specific and measurable.
- *Include a variety of activities to keep the patient from feeling bored.*
- *Remind your patient to recognize and appreciate success.*
- *Suggest strategies to achieve the patient's goals.* For instance, you might suggest a fitness program that is fun and entertaining. You can also inform your patient about ways to avoid joint injury or falls.
- *Provide encouragement.* Sometimes just the right approach is a positive, enthusiastic one. You might offer praise for taking steps toward health and fitness. Support from spouse, family members, friends, and coworkers can improve compliance and consistency.
- *Promote physical exercise as an enjoyable activity.*
- *Discuss barriers to regular activity and elicit ways to overcome those obstacles.*

People give various reasons for failing to develop a regular exercise program. See Box 33-4 for suggestions on dealing with such objections.

Teaching for Stress Relief How is your stress level? A high stress level can produce fatigue. Although you may view exercise as one more thing you don't have time for, exercise is energizing and can be used to relieve stress. For example, taking a brisk 20-minute walk during a break may allow you to continue working for several more hours. You can also use this technique when caring for patients. Hospitalized patients and family members often experience a great deal of stress. Helping the patient take a walk to the courtyard or instructing family members how to handle the wheelchair so they can take the patient out of the room often will help lessen some of the strain of illness and hospitalization.

♥ iCare 33-1

Activity & Exercise

Peter is caring for 82-year-old Mr. Brown, whose physician has ordered Mr. Brown to be out of bed at least three times daily and to ambulate at least 20 feet daily. Mr. Brown is hesitant to ambulate in the hallway because it takes him a while to do so, thinks he is a bother to the staff, and therefore has little to no motivation. During Peter's conversations with Mr. Brown he learns that he used to run track in high school. Peter develops signage on the unit to simulate a track with "mile markers" on the wall and floor and takes Mr. Brown for a walk slowly down one side of the hallway and back. This small innovative gesture fosters conversation on the unit among staff and leads to an increase in ambulation among other patients.

BOX 33-4 ■ Suggestions for Overcoming Objections to Exercise

Objection	Suggestion
"I hate to exercise."	Pick several activities that you enjoy.
"I burn out on exercise."	Plan ahead and build in rest days and varied activities.
"I am self-conscious about going to the gym and don't have the motivation to exercise by myself."	Find a friend to exercise with, or develop a reward system for yourself if you continue to exercise.
"I am too busy with work or family."	Develop a routine that you can do at lunchtime, or exercise *with* your family.
"I find exercise boring."	Change your routine frequently.
"Exercise hurts."	Make sure to exercise at your target heart rate, and plan a rest day after every weight-lifting session.
"I don't have time."	Schedule your exercise time. If need be, schedule several short 10- to 15-min sessions throughout the day.
"I have pain nearly all the time."	Take pain medication an hour or so before starting physical activity. If fatigue is the problem, try to arrange your schedule to keep a balance of rest and activity as well as avoid stimulants (e.g., caffeine or nicotine) that might interfere with the quality of sleep.
"I have difficulty getting around sometimes."	Stretch adequately before starting exercise, but not to overstretch joints. Walk on smooth, even surfaces.
"I am diabetic and have trouble with my feet. My vision is not very good, either."	Be sure shoes fit properly and the area is well lit.

Positioning Patients

Healthy people regularly shift position to maintain comfort. However, many patients are unable to move without assistance. They require a change of position at least every 2 hours to prevent skin breakdown, muscle discomfort, damage to superficial nerves and blood vessels, and contractures. Immobile people are more prone to pressure injury as a result of reduced circulation, impaired oxygen exchange to the tissues, and edema.

A firm mattress provides support to the patient's body and makes it easier to turn the patient (because he does not sink down into the mattress). Most hospital mattresses are firm. However, when you provide home care, you will find mattresses of various types and conditions. To provide additional support, you can place a large piece of plywood under a sagging mattress.

A clean, dry bed also makes it easier to turn the patient and decreases the risk of skin maceration or pressure injury formation. Bedding should provide coverage and warmth but not be tucked in so tightly as to restrict movement.

Protecting the Nurse's Back

Nurses are at risk for back and shoulder injury as a result of manual moving and repositioning of patients, residents, or clients. Rising obesity rates in the United States, aging of the workforce, and the shortage of nurses impact the physical demands on caregivers (Centers for Disease Control and Prevention, n.d., updated 2016).

✚ To protect yourself from back injury as you move patients, avoid manual lifting as much as possible. Some lifts and patient care tasks require multiple staff members to accomplish safely, and because low staffing makes this teamwork difficult, nurses often attempt these tasks alone (Waters, Nelson, Hughes, et al., 2009). Use assistive equipment and devices, as recommended by the American Nurses Association (2013), and always make sure you have adequate help. The amount of help you need depends on the size of the patient, the level of assistance the patient can offer, your size and strength, and the equipment or lines attached to the patient.

✚ Other measures to reduce the risk for injury for nurses include the following:

- Avoid slippery or wet surfaces during ambulation or moving patients.
- Remove physical obstructions (e.g., cabinets, toilets) when moving or transferring patients.
- Arrange a clutter-free environment that allows for free movement of equipment and personnel.
- Watch out for uneven floor surfaces or movable rugs.
- Lock wheels of furniture and equipment before moving patients.
- Avoid moving patients through too small a width to the entrance way.

Positioning Devices

Devices used to maintain body alignment, prevent contractures, and promote comfort are briefly discussed in the next sections. Positioning devices are commonly used to help minimize the risk for immobility. For guidelines on using common positioning devices, including hip abduction pillows, see Clinical Insight 33-2.

Adjustable Beds An adjustable bed, often referred to as a hospital bed, assumes a variety of positions. You can elevate or lower the head of the bed and elevate the foot of the bed. Often the bed breaks, or "gatches," at the knee to keep the patient from sliding down when the head is elevated. You can also adjust the height of the bed. You should raise the bed to waist height when providing care so that you can use proper body mechanics; place the bed in its lowest position before helping a patient get out of bed or if the patient is at risk for falling.

Several types of specialized beds are used in treating and preventing pressure injuries. These include alternating, low air loss, immersion (air-fluidized), and oscillating beds. The mattresses may be composed of air, water, or gel. With the advent of low-pressure specialized beds, circular and Stryker beds are now in limited use.

Pillows Pillows are the most common devices used to assist with positioning, provide support, and elevate body parts. They help position a patient by molding to the body and expanding the weight-bearing area. You will need a variety of sizes to position patients who are unconscious, paralyzed, or frail, or who have had surgery. To obtain the right size or type (abductor pillows), or if pillows are not available, you can use folded blankets or towels. Foam wedge pillows are useful for elevating the upper body when an adjustable bed is not available and for abducting the hips after hip surgery.

Siderails Most hospital beds are equipped with siderails. The rails may run the full length of each side of the bed or consist of an upper or lower rail on each side.

✚ Siderails are designed to ensure patient safety. They serve as a reminder that the patient should call for assistance before getting out of bed and provide a grip for the patient who is able to reposition himself in bed. Although siderails are designed to protect patients, they can be a source of injury. Patients can get tangled in the railing or fall between the bed and rail, and confused patients may injure themselves trying to climb over the rails.

Siderails may also be considered a form of restraint, so follow your agency's policy for use and be sure to discuss their purpose with patients and family. See Chapter 23 if you need to review restraint use.

Trapeze Bar A trapeze bar is a triangular-shaped device that is attached to an overhead bed frame (see Fig. 33-9). The patient can use the base of the triangle as a grip bar to move up in bed, turn, and pull up in preparation for getting out of bed or getting on and off the bedpan. Patients can use the trapeze to move about in bed and to exercise their upper extremities. Frail patients may not be able to use a trapeze bar because of the amount of effort it requires.

Other Positioning Devices When a person is supine, the toes tend to point downward toward the bed (footdrop), and the feet are in plantar flexion. Healthy people usually shift position throughout the night, so the foot and leg muscles are periodically contracted and relaxed. In contrast, the patient who is unable to move independently will experience a shortening of the gastrocnemius muscle and may have difficulty walking again if prolonged plantar flexion occurs.

■ *A footboard* is a device placed at the end of the bed to prevent footdrop and outward hip rotation, but it does not relieve heel pressure and can lead to pressure injury.

■ *Boots* made of spongy rubber with heel cutouts and ankle cushioning help prevent skin breakdown. Rigid heel-lift boots, in addition, help to prevent foot drop and external hip rotation. (Fig. 33-6). ✚ If any part of the boot is made of a latex product, be sure the patient does not have a latex allergy before applying.

■ *Trochanter rolls* prevent external hip rotation when the patient is in a supine position. They are made from tightly

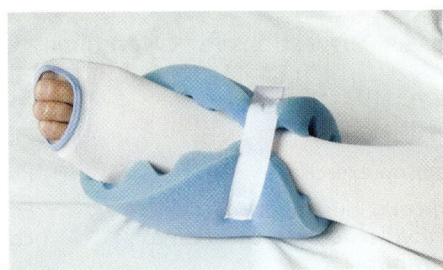

FIGURE 33-6 A foot-positioning boot is placed around the foot to help prevent pressure injury.

rolled towels, bath blankets, or foam pads. They are placed snugly adjacent to the hips and thighs to prevent external rotation of the hips (Fig. 33-7). To learn how to make them, see Clinical Insight 33-2.

■ *Hand and wrist splints* may be manufactured or fashioned from rolled washcloths. Often splints are custom made for patients. The purpose of splints is to hold the wrist and hand in natural position and prevent claw-hand deformities.

■ *Hand rolls* prevent hand contractures (Fig. 33-8). Some are commercially made. Otherwise, you can make a hand roll from a tightly rolled washcloth.

■ *Hip abduction pillows* prevent internal hip rotation and hip adduction when the patient is in a supine position (Fig. 33-9). Neutral positioning also prevents strain on hip ligaments. These wedge-shaped pieces of spongy material are used after femoral fracture, hip fracture, or surgery. Lateral indentations and straps that wrap around the patient's thighs hold the patient in the correct position.

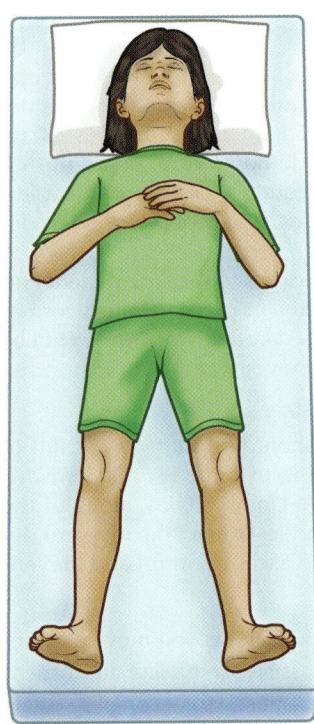 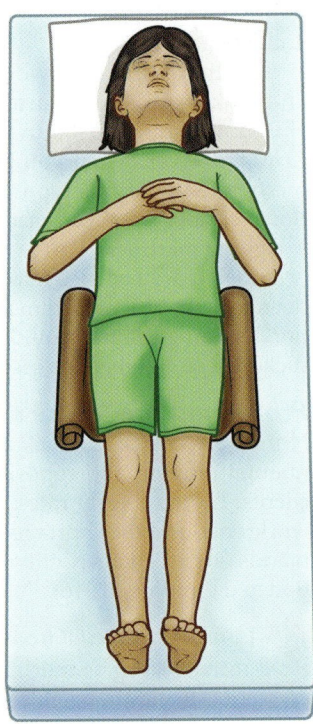

FIGURE 33-7 External rotation can occur without a trochanter roll.

Proper alignment using a trochanter roll.

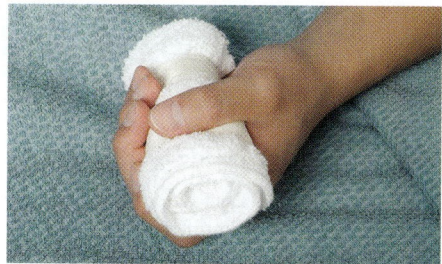

FIGURE 33-8 A hand roll maintains neutral position.

- *Foot cradles* are metal or plastic devices that are secured at the foot of the bed to hold bedding up off the toes and feet, allowing for free movement.
- *High-ankle footwear* may be used to prevent heel drop, but they do not reduce heel pressure. They do help in positioning hips and pelvis to prevent hip rotation.
- *Sandbags* are small fabric bags filled with sand. They are used in the same manner as pillows and trochanter rolls; however, they provide firmer support.

Positioning Techniques

In the next section we briefly describe the various ways to position patients. Table 33-2 illustrates these positions, identifies potential problems associated with them, and offers solutions to prevent the problems. The positions are also described and illustrated in Chapter 21, Table 21-1.

Fowler's Position is a semisitting position in which the head of the bed is elevated 45° to 60°. This position promotes

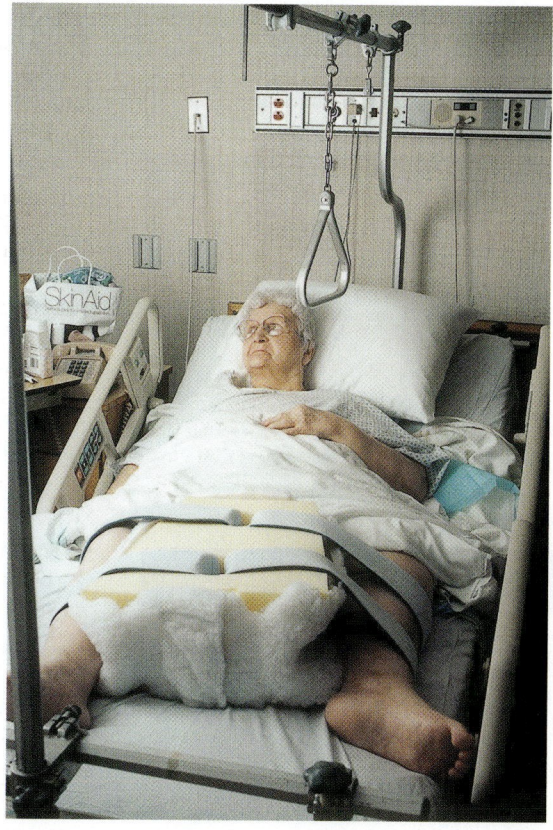

FIGURE 33-9 A hip abduction pillow prevents internal hip rotation and hip adduction when the patient is immobile in supine position.

Table 33-2 ➤ Positioning a Bed-Bound Patient

POSITION	POTENTIAL PROBLEM	SOLUTION
Fowler's	Hyperextension of the neck	Use a small pillow under the head and neck.
	Posterior flexion of the lumbar curvature	Use a firm mattress.
		Position the patient so that the angle of elevation begins at the hip.
	Dislocation of the shoulders	Position a pillow under the forearms to prevent pull on the shoulders.
	Flexion contracture of the fingers and abduction of the thumbs	Use hand splints if appropriate, or provide a large roll in the palm of the hand.
	Flexion contracture of the wrist and edema of the hands	Support the hands on pillows in alignment with the forearms.
	External rotation of the legs	Place sandbags or rolls alongside the trochanters and upper thighs.
	Hyperextension of the knees	Place a small pillow under the lower legs from the ankles to below the knees. Do this for short periods only; avoid pressure on the popliteal area.
	Footdrop	Use a footboard, positioning boot, or high-top sneakers to hold the foot in position.

(Continued)

Table 33-2 ➤ Positioning a Bed-Bound Patient—cont'd

POSITION	POTENTIAL PROBLEM	SOLUTION
Lateral 	Lateral flexion of the neck	Place a pillow under the head and neck to provide alignment.
	Internal rotation and adduction of the upper shoulder and limited respirations	Place a pillow under the upper arm and comfortably flex the lower arm.
	Internal rotation and adduction of the femur	Support the upper leg from groin to foot with pillows.
	Twisting of the spine	Align the shoulders with the hips.
	Flexion of the cervical spine	Place a pillow under the head and neck to provide alignment, unless drainage from the mouth is desired.
Prone 	Hyperextension of the lumbar curvature, pressure on the breasts in women or genitals in men, impaired respirations	Place a small pillow under the abdomen.
	Footdrop	Move the patient down in bed so the feet extend over the edge of the mattress, or place a small pillow under the shins so that the toes do not touch the bed.
	Lateral flexion of the neck	Place a pillow under the head and neck to provide alignment, unless drainage from the mouth is desired.
Sims' 	Internal rotation and adduction of the upper shoulder and limited respirations	Place a pillow under the upper arm and comfortably flex the arm at the elbow.
	Pressure on the shoulder and axilla of the inferior arm	Position the lower arm behind and away from the back.
	Twisting of the spine	Align the shoulders with the hips.
	Footdrop	Support the feet in dorsiflexion with sandbags.
	Hyperextension of the neck	Place a pillow under the head and neck to provide alignment.
Supine 	Internal rotation of the shoulders and extension of the elbows	Position the upper arms next to the body. Place pillows under the forearms and position the wrists in slight pronation.
	Flexion of fingers and abduction of the thumbs	Use hand splints if appropriate, or provide a large roll in the palm of the hand.
	Flexion of the lumbar curvature and hips	Provide a firm mattress, or place a small pillow under the lumbar curvature.
	External rotation of the legs	Place sandbags or rolls alongside the trochanters and upper thighs.
	Hyperextension of the knees	Place a small pillow under the lower legs from the ankles to below the knees.
	Footdrop	Use a footboard, cradle boots, or high-top sneakers to hold the feet in dorsiflexion.

respiratory function by lowering the diaphragm and allowing the greatest chest expansion. It is also an ideal position for some patients with cardiac dysfunction. Common variations include the following:

- **Semi-Fowler's position,** in which the head of the bed is elevated only 30°
- **High Fowler's position,** in which the head of the bed is elevated 90°
- **Orthopneic position,** in which the head of the bed is elevated 90° and an overbed table with a pillow on top is positioned in front of the patient (Fig. 33-10). Have the patient lean forward, resting his arms and head on the pillow. This position is helpful for a patient with shortness of breath.

Lateral Position is a side-lying position with the top hip and knee flexed and placed in front of the rest of the body. The lateral position creates pressure on the lower scapula, ilium, and trochanter but relieves pressure from the heels and sacrum.

- The **lateral recumbent position** is side-lying with legs in a straight line.
- The **oblique position** is an alternative to the lateral position that places less pressure on the trochanter. The patient turns on the side with the top hip and knee flexed; however, the top leg is placed behind the body (Fig. 33-11).

In Prone Position the patient lies on his abdomen with his head turned to one side. This is the only position that allows full extension of the hips and knees. It also allows secretions to drain freely from the mouth and thus is helpful for an unconscious patient. However, this is the most difficult position to move an unconscious or frail patient into because it requires the greatest amount of manipulation to position the patient appropriately. As a rule, you can use this position only for short periods of time.

- Avoid the prone position for patients with cardiac or respiratory difficulty because it inhibits chest wall expansion and, therefore, oxygenation.
- Avoid the prone position for patients with cervical or lumbar spine problems because it creates a significant lordosis (inward curving of the spine in the lower back) and rotation of the neck.

Sims' Position is a semiprone position. The lower arm is positioned behind the patient, and the upper arm is flexed. The upper leg is more flexed than the lower leg. Sims' position

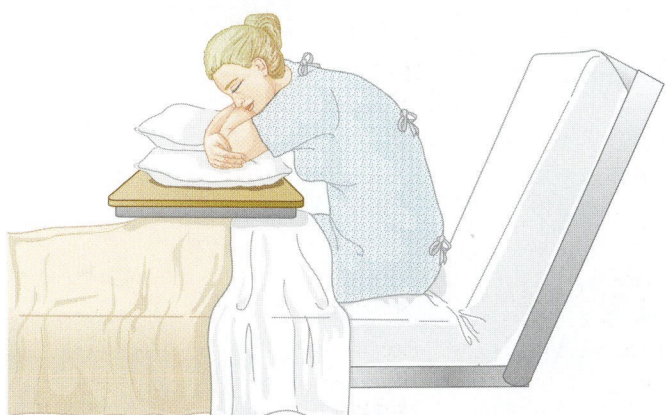

FIGURE 33-10 The orthopneic position is ideal for a patient with shortness of breath.

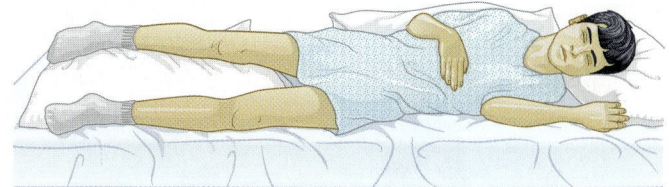

FIGURE 33-11 The oblique position is a modified lateral position that places less pressure on the trochanter.

facilitates drainage from the mouth and limits pressure on the trochanter and sacrum. This is an ideal position for administering an enema or a perineal procedure.

Supine Position, also known as the **dorsal recumbent position,** the patient lies on his back with head and shoulders elevated on a small pillow. The spine is aligned and the arms and hands comfortably rest at the side.

KnowledgeCheck 33-7

- Describe the following positions: Fowler's, lateral, prone, Sims', and supine.
- What is the advantage of the oblique position versus the lateral position?
- Identify and describe six positioning devices.
- What are three uses for siderails?

ThinkLike a Nurse 33-5

You are providing care for a young man who is recovering from Guillain-Barré syndrome, which produces a reversible paralysis after viral illness. He has been healthy until this present illness. How would you position this patient? Explain your reasoning.

Moving Patients in Bed

To position patients, you must be adept at moving and lifting them in bed. This involves positioning the patient in the length of the bed, as well as turning with as little friction and shearing on the skin as possible.

- **Moving Up in Bed.** Frail patients slide down in bed because of gravity and their inability to correct their position. Elevating the head of the bed accentuates the slide and places the patient in an awkward position. If the patient is light in weight or able to assist, you will be able to move her independently. For complete instructions, refer to Procedure 33-1A.
- **Turning in Bed.** This is the most important intervention to protect a patient's skin and prevent other complications of immobility. For efficient use of time, try to time turning to coincide with moving the patient up in bed. Pillows and other positioning devices help the patient maintain the new position. For a complete description, see Procedure 33-1B.
- **Logrolling.** Logrolling is a special turning technique used when the patient's spine must be kept in straight alignment. Logrolling moves the patient's body as a unit. For a complete description, see Procedure 33-1C.
- **Friction-Reducing Devices.** You can use one of a variety of friction-reducing devices when moving a patient in bed.
  - **Transfer roller sheets** are thin, low-friction fabric sheets that may be placed beneath the drawsheet to facilitate moving the patient in bed (Fig. 33-12).

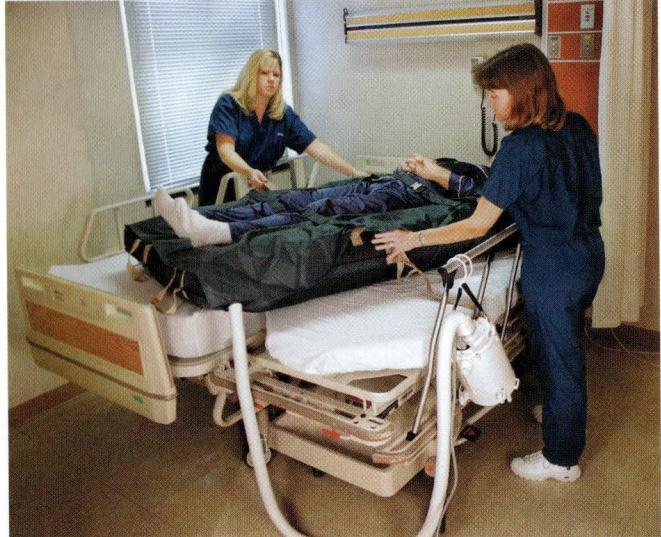

FIGURE 33-12 A transfer roller sheet reduces friction and facilitates movement.

- A **scoot sheet** is also a thin, low-friction fabric sheet that is often positioned under the drawsheet of the patient, but it is attached to a mechanical crank (Fig. 33-13). By turning the crank, a single person can move a patient up in bed. Transfer roller sheets are relatively inexpensive and are widely available on clinical units.
- A **roller tray** with disposable absorbent underpads can also be used to reduce low back stress when moving patients (Bacharach, Miller, & von Duvillard, 2016).

  If necessary, you can improvise a friction-reducing device by placing a large, clean, unused plastic bag under the drawsheet to help you move the patient. The plastic bag reduces drag and facilitates movement. However, unlike the thin fabric of transfer sheets, plastic allows moisture to pool under the patient. Consequently, you should remove the bag from under the drawsheet after moving the patient.

Transferring Patients Out of Bed

Stretchers and wheelchairs are used to transport patients between units and to tests or procedures. A stretcher is usually reserved for the patient who is weak or sedated or has a condition that does not permit transfer by wheelchair. In addition, you may transfer patients to a stationary chair to increase their general activity level. For detailed information about transferring patients in or out of bed, see Procedure 33-2.

A Transfer Board is a wood or plastic device designed to assist with moving patients. Using a transfer board reduces your risk of injury and promotes a smooth transfer. Place the board under the patient on the side to which he will be moved. It is best to use a drawsheet to slide the patient across the board (Fig. 33-14). Patients with long-standing mobility problems also use transfer boards to increase their independence.

A Mechanical Lift is a hydraulic device used to transfer patients. A fabric sling with chains or straps attaches to the lifting device (Fig. 33-15). Mechanical lift devices reduce the risk of back and musculoskeletal injury.

- Lifts are especially useful when providing care for obese and immobile patients.
- Lifts are often used in home care because they allow one person to transfer the patient safely.
- Most lifts position patients in a seated position and thus are ideal for assisting the patient into a chair.
- Others suspend the patient in a supine position; they may be used to transfer the patient from bed to stretcher or to suspend the patient while the bed is made.
- Many include scales that weigh the patient while he is suspended in the sling.
- Some are mounted on the ceiling to reduce caregiver back injuries and increase patient safety (see Fig. 33-16).
- **Standing assist devices** are mechanical lifts that help the patient move from a sitting to a standing position or support a patient in the standing position (Fig. 33-17). Specialized chairs and wheelchairs are also available. Each has a mechanical lift in the seat that rises to assist the patient to a standing position.

A Transfer Belt is a heavy belt several inches wide that is used to facilitate transfer or provide a secure mechanism to

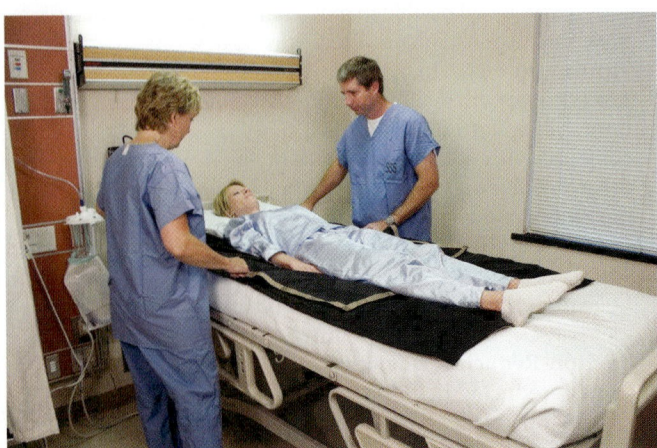

FIGURE 33-13 A scoot sheet allows a single person to move a patient up in bed.

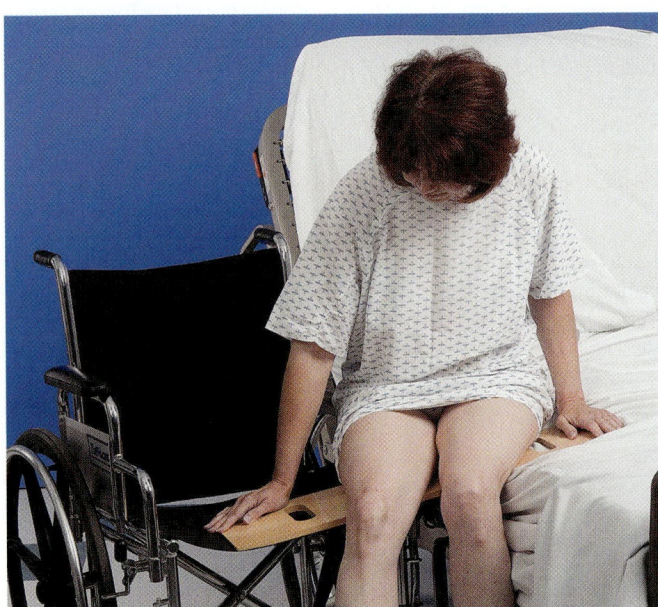

FIGURE 33-14 Transfer boards are used by patients with chronic mobility problems to increase their independence.

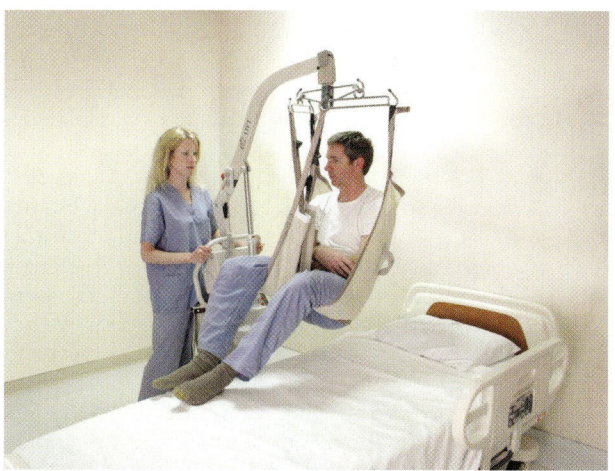

FIGURE 33-15 A mechanical lift is useful when providing care to patients with impaired mobility.

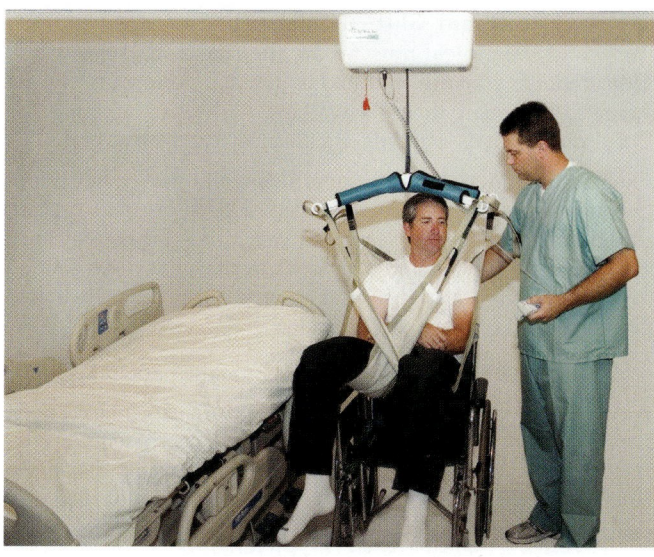

FIGURE 33-17 A mechanical lift with a sling chair is used to safely transfer an immobile patient into a wheelchair.

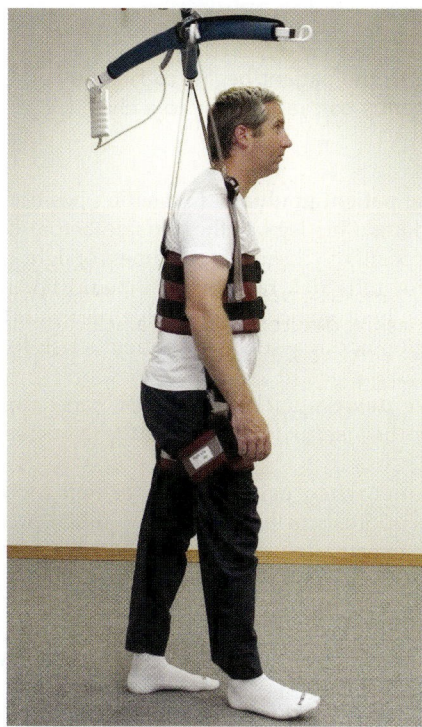

FIGURE 33-16 A ceiling-mounted mechanical lift is used to support patients in the standing position.

hold the patient when ambulating. Apply the belt around the patient's abdomen, close to the patient's center of gravity. The belt may have external grip holds, or you may grip the entire belt with your hand.

KnowledgeCheck 33-8

- What criteria determine whether your patient should be logrolled when he is repositioned?
- How often should you turn and reposition a patient?
- Identify the most appropriate device for the following activities:
    - Transferring an obese patient from a bed to a stretcher
    - Assisting an immobile patient to a recliner chair
    - Helping a weak patient from bed to chair

Performing Range-of-Motion Exercises

For patients with limited mobility, nursing interventions focus on preventing complications of disuse such as muscle atrophy, joint stiffness, and contractures.

- **Passive range of motion (PROM)** is movement of the joints through their range of motion by another person. Both AROM and PROM improve joint mobility, increase circulation to the area exercised, and help maintain function. However, AROM also improves muscle strength and tone, as well as respiratory and cardiac function. For an explanation of how to perform PROM, see Clinical Insight 33-3.
- **Active range of motion (AROM)** occurs when the patient independently moves his joints through flexion, extension, abduction, adduction, and circular rotation. Patients recovering from illness, injury, or surgery often perform AROM as a rehabilitation procedure. Movement with ADLs also helps to improve joint mobility, circulation, muscular strength and tone.
- **Continuous passive motion (CPM)** employs a device to gently flex and extend the knee joint. The CPM machine is often used after knee replacement or other knee procedures to allow the joint to improve range of motion, eliminate the problem of stiffness, and prevent the development of adhesions, which can limit motion further.

Assisting With Ambulation

Prolonged bedrest is no longer the standard of care. However, as a nurse, you will provide care to patients whose illnesses and injuries curtail their ability to walk and be active. This involves assisting patients with and preparing them for physical activity.

Physical Conditioning

Patients who have been confined to bed for more than a week or who have sustained major injury require conditioning before they are able to resume walking. The following conditioning exercises are summarized here. They are explained in detail in Clinical Insight 33-4.

Quadriceps and Gluteal Drills   The quadriceps muscle group and the gluteal muscles are the largest muscles of the body. Patients who are confined to bed can perform isometric exercises to prepare them for walking.

Arm Exercises   Patients use the biceps and triceps muscles when getting out of bed and for crutch walking. ✚ Be mindful of any upper body injury or musculoskeletal or other precautions that restrict arm movement or weight-bearing on the hands and wrists. If lymphedema is present in the upper extremities, do not encourage arm exercises or use of the trapeze, unless directed by the primary care provider.

Dangling   Use this position to prepare the patient to get up in a chair, to stand, or to ambulate. ✚ Patients who have been confined to bed frequently become light-headed or develop orthostatic hypotension when first getting up. Dangling allows the patient to experience being upright with limited risk of falling.

Preventing Orthostatic Hypotension   Some common approaches used for orthostatic problems include the following:

- Antiembolism stockings with compression wraps to prevent pooling of venous blood
- Abdominal binders
- Medication to control orthostatic hypotension

Patients with spinal cord injury experiencing autonomic dysfunctions need a high-backed reclining wheelchair so the back of the chair can be lowered (and someone might even have to lift up their legs for a few minutes) until blood pressure stabilizes. Tilt-table therapies are also used.

Daily Activities   Moving around in bed and performing ADLs exercise many of the muscle groups needed for ambulation. Getting up into a chair accustoms the patient to an upright posture and is an important predictor of success with ambulation.

Assisting the Patient to Walk

Before getting the patient out of bed, assess his readiness to walk. Also obtain the appropriate equipment and assistance.

✚ Move floor rugs and loose objects from the path of the patient and caregiver. Be sure the floor is not slippery. When possible, use a transfer belt. Have a chair or additional assistance available on the first few attempts at ambulation. If the patient becomes faint or begins to fall, do not attempt to hold him up by yourself. Instead, protect the patient as you guide him to a seated or lying position. Create a wide base of support, and project forward the hip closest to the patient. Help the patient slide down your leg as you call for help (Fig. 33-18). Protect the patient's head as his body descends.

To learn procedures for assisting with ambulation, see Procedures 33-3A and 33-3B.

🍁 **Assisting Older Adults**   When assisting an older adult to ambulate, find out how much assistance, if any, the patient typically requires and modify support as needed. Consider the following nursing interventions:

- **Observe constantly for weakness and fatigue.** Plan for periods of rest during ambulation, if needed. The older adult might become fatigued more quickly and recover more slowly when walking, especially if a heart or lung condition is present.

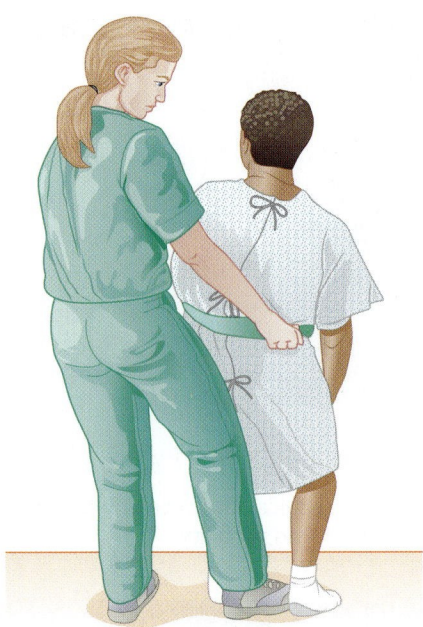

FIGURE 33-18 If the patient begins to fall, the nurse guides the patient gently to the floor or to a chair.

- **Move the patient gradually** to a sitting position and allow him to dangle his legs at the bedside before coming to a standing position. Observe for dizziness or light-headedness.
- **Assess for falls risk factors** (e.g., medications that cause dizziness; neurological or cognitive disorders). For more information about assessing a patient's risk for a fall, see Chapter 23.
- **Assistive devices** such as walkers, canes, and transfer belts can be useful for older adults who require more support.
- **Be cautious when using a transfer belt** for the patient with osteoporosis or back pain. Too much pressure from the belt can cause injury or pain.

KnowledgeCheck 33-9

- Identify four principles to be followed when performing PROM.
- Describe activities that can promote a patient's readiness for ambulation.
- What action should you take if a patient begins to fall when ambulating?

Mechanical Aids for Walking

Several kinds of aids are available to promote stability and independence when walking. Some patients consider the use of aids a sign of weakness or inconvenience and resist using them. However, most people dread loss of independence, so you can promote the use of walking aids by stressing their value in helping the person maintain independence. For instructions on sizing canes, walkers, and crutches, see Clinical Insight 33-5. For instructions on teaching patients to use these aids, refer to Clinical Insight 33-6.

Canes   The following are three basic types of canes (Fig. 33-19):

- **Single-ended cane with a half-circle handle**—ideal for the patient who needs minimal support and can negotiate stairs.

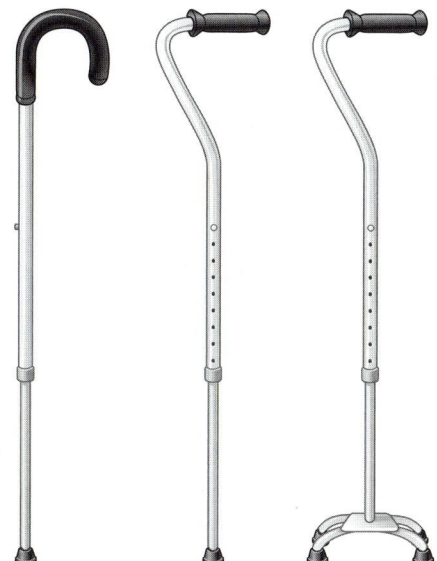

FIGURE 33-19 Three types of canes.

- **Single-ended cane with a straight handle**—ideal for the patient with hand weakness who has good balance.
- **Multiprong canes**—Most have three or four prongs; all types have a straight handle. These provide a wide base of support for patients with balance problems.

Walkers A walker is a lightweight metal frame device with four legs that provides a wide base of support as a patient ambulates (Fig. 33-20A). Various forms of walkers are available. Some models have wheels that allow the walker to be rolled forward; others have a seat that allows the patient to rest periodically (Fig. 33-20B). These walkers are best for patients whose mobility problems are related to fatigue or shortness of breath rather than gait instability.

Braces Braces support joints and muscles that cannot independently support the body's weight. They are most commonly used in the lower extremities. Physical medicine specialists usually fit the brace. Nursing responsibilities include assisting the patient into and out of the brace and monitoring the condition of the skin under the brace.

Crutches Crutches are commonly used for rehabilitation of an injured lower extremity. The purpose of using crutches is to limit or eliminate weight-bearing on the leg(s) by forcing the user to rely on strength in the arms and shoulders for support. Two forms of crutches are available.

- The *forearm support crutch* is more likely to be used by a patient with permanent limitations. It is usually constructed of lightweight aluminum with a handhold and a forearm support (Fig. 33-21A).
- *Axillary crutches* are for both short- and long-term use (Fig. 33-21B). Properly fitted axillary crutches support the body weight in the hands and arms, not the axilla. For guidelines on how to measure a patient for an axillary crutch, see Clinical Insight 33-5.

Crutch walking taxes the arms and hands and may cause discomfort to the axillae, arms, and palms where the patient is bearing weight. There are five basic crutch gaits: Two-point and four-point gait are used for partial weight-bearing, whereas three-point gait is used when weight-bearing must be avoided. Swing-to and swing-through are used when weight-bearing is permitted. See Clinical Insight 33-6 for gaits and teaching guidelines.

KnowledgeCheck 33-10

- What type of cane should a patient with significant balance problems use?
- When are forearm support crutches used?
- Identify five crutch gaits.

ThinkLike a Nurse 33-6

Discuss crutch walking with your peers and family. What instruction would facilitate the best understanding of proper crutch-walking technique?

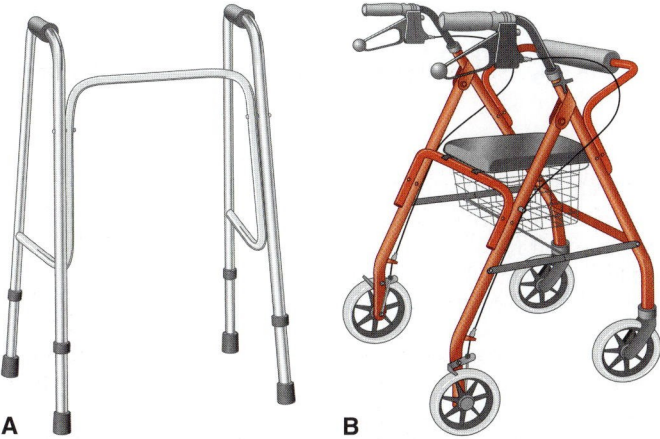

FIGURE 33-20 Walkers. A. The basic walker is picked up and advanced as the patient steps ahead. B. Some walkers have wheels and seats that allow the patient to rest periodically.

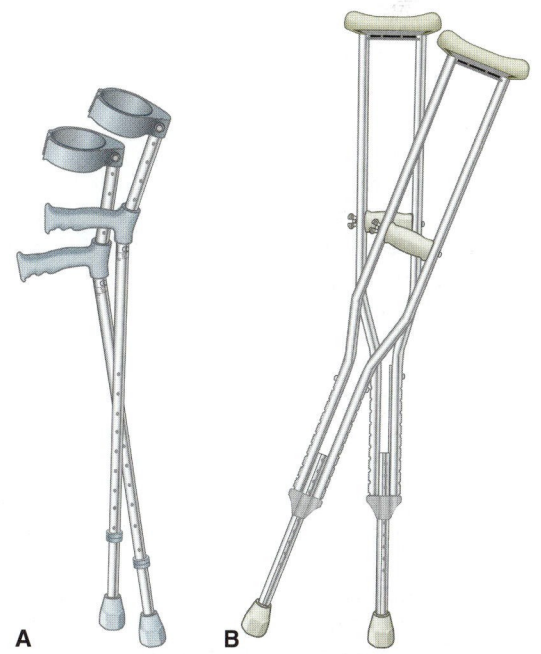

FIGURE 33-21 Crutches. A. Forearm support crutches. B. Axillary crutches.

CLINICALREASONING

The questions and exercises in this section allow you to practice the kind of thinking you will use as a full-spectrum nurse. Critical-thinking questions usually have more than one correct answer, so we do not provide "correct answers" for these features. It is more important to develop your nursing judgment than to just cover content. You will learn by discussing the questions with your peers. If you are still unsure, see the Davis Advantage chapter resources for suggested responses.

Caring for the Nguyens

As you may recall, Nam Nguyen has been advised to diet and exercise as part of the treatment plan for hypertension, type 2 diabetes mellitus, obesity, and osteoarthritis. Zach Miller's examination has revealed no other cardiovascular problems.

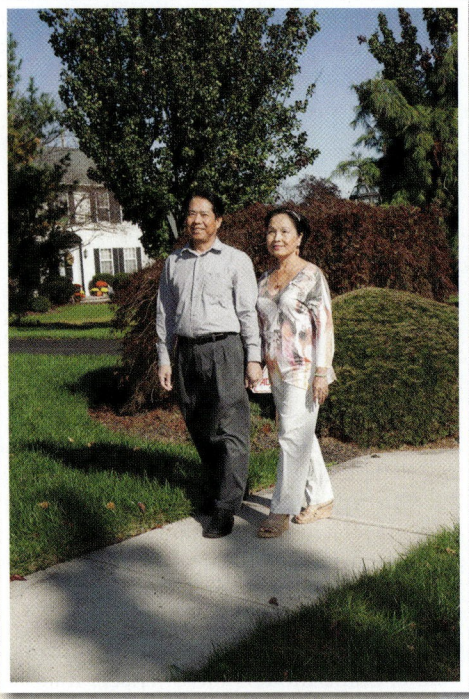

A. Design a fitness program for Nam. Describe the program in detail. Recall that Nam has been relatively sedentary.

B. Compare the type of program you would recommend for Nam with the type of program appropriate for his grandson, Kim.

C. What type of fitness program would be most appropriate for Mai Nguyen, Nam's mother? What additional information do you need to know to answer this question?

 Go to Davis Advantage, Resources, Chapter 33, **Caring for the Nguyens—Suggested Responses.**

Applying the **Full-Spectrum Nursing Model**_____

PATIENT SITUATION

Mr. Ronald Ornduff is a 72-year-old retired man who lives with his wife in a one-story home. He has excellent general health with no significant health problems. Ronald typically walks with a moderate to vigorous pace in his neighborhood or at the mall in the winter. He belongs to a health club and works out two or three times a week, walking on the treadmill, using the weight machines, or taking a basic conditioning class. Ronald considers himself fit and of an acceptable weight for his age. When going outdoors to pick up the morning paper, he slipped on a patch of ice and fell. You are now caring for him 2 days after hip surgery. He is experiencing pain and seems fearful his injury could be the beginning of a decline in his health.

THINKING

1. *Theoretical Knowledge:*
   a. Based on Ronald's age, physical condition, and activity level, make a rough estimate of the number of minutes per week of physical activity he should have after he recovers from surgery and resumes full mobility. What are the benefits of this physical activity?
   b. As a nurse planning the care for a patient after hip surgery, what complications of immobility should you assess for?

2. *Critical Thinking (Considering Alternatives):* What are some possible barriers to an older adult's participating in physical activity? What might you teach your patient to do to overcome those barriers?

DOING

3. *Practical Knowledge:*
  a. How might you position your patient after hip surgery?
  b. What equipment would you need to position your patient after surgery? Is there anything you can set up that will help your patient move around in bed when he can tolerate it?
  c. What type of physical activity would you recommend Ronald incorporate into his exercise plan after he experiences full recovery from his surgery? What benefit will these exercises provide?
  d. *Nursing Process (Diagnosis):* Write at least two nursing diagnoses for Ronald. Use just the data provided in the situation. Assume he is 2 days post-op.

CARING

4. *Self-Knowledge:* What would you be feeling if you were in Ronald's situation of being physically fit one day and suffering pain and immobility the next?
5. *Ethical Knowledge:* What are one or two things you would do to help Ronald feel cared for and cared about?

 Go to Davis Advantage, Resources, Chapter 33, **Applying the Full-Spectrum Nursing Model—Suggested Responses.**

PracticalKnowledge
clinical application

CLINICAL INSIGHTS

Clinical Insight 33-1 ➤ **Applying Principles of Body Mechanics**

Principles of body mechanics are the rules that enable you to move your body without causing injury. Use the following guidelines to decrease the risk of back and other injuries. Teach them to your patients as well.

✚ The American Nurses Association (n.d.) in its Handle With Care campaign, states you should use mechanical equipment (e.g., lift, transfer board) or get assistance for lifting and transferring whenever possible. Do not rely on body mechanics alone to prevent injury.

Account for Patient Factors

- **Assess patient dependency levels** and select equipment after determining the patient's ability to assist in the transfer. For patient safety, be aware of the patient's strength and ability to bear weight. Height and weight of the patient factor into how you transfer the patient safely.

Transferring Patients According to Dependency Level	
PATIENT LEVEL OF DEPENDENCE	**ASSISTIVE DEVICE**
Complete dependence (immobile; no assistance)	Mechanical lift with full sling
Extensive dependence (holds on to device but with minimal strength)	Mechanical lift with full sling or stand/assist lift
Moderate dependence (no patient assist for lifting from floor)	Mechanical lift with full sling, or if transfer is manual, more than one helper might be needed
Patient assists with limited mobility	Transfer belt or gait belt
Limited dependence	Stand/assist lift or friction-reducing device

Source: Adapted from American Nurses Association. (2013). *Safe patient handling and mobility: Interprofessional national standards.* Silver Spring, MD: Author.

(Continued)

Clinical Insight 33-1 ▸ Applying Principles of Body Mechanics—cont'd

Make Use of Inanimate Objects and Get Help When Possible

- **Raise the height of the bed and overbed table to waist level** when you are working with a patient.
- **Get help to move a heavy object** or patient. Assess the object or patient you are going to lift. If you have any doubt that you can do it by yourself, get help from a coworker.
- **Use assistive devices at all times** to limit the risk of back and musculoskeletal injury.
- **Maintain competency** in using all assistive and transfer devices.

Use Your Body Correctly

- **Use a wide base of support** (feet spread apart).
- **Minimize bending and twisting.** These movements increase the stress on the back. Instead, face the object or person and bend at the hips or squat.
- **Squat to lift heavy objects** from the floor. (Squatting lowers your center of gravity.) Push against the strong hip and thigh muscles to raise yourself to a standing position. Avoid bending at the waist.

- **Use the muscles in your legs** as the power for lifting. Bend your knees, keep your back straight, and lift smoothly. Repeat the same movements for setting the object down.
- **Keep objects close to your body** when you lift, move, or carry them. The closer an object is to the center of gravity, the greater the stability and the less strain on the back.
- **Use both hands and arms** when you lift, move, or carry heavy objects.
- **Do not stand on tiptoes to reach** an object. If you must use a ladder or stepstool to reach for an object, make sure it is stable and adequate to position your body close to the object.
- **Push, slide, or pull heavy objects** whenever possible rather than lifting.
- **Maintain a good grip** on the patient or object you are moving before attempting to move it.
- **When possible, keep your elbows bent** when you carry an object.
- **Work with smooth and even movements.** Avoid sudden or jerky motions.

Clinical Insight 33-2 ▸ Using Common Positioning Devices

Applying a Trochanter Roll

- Fold a towel or bath blanket lengthwise.
- Roll the towel or bath blanket tightly.
- Invert the roll. Turning the patient to one side, place the bath blanket or towel under the patient's hip and thigh. Repeat on the other side if needed.
- Roll the sheet or towel under until it is snug against the patient's hip and thigh. See Figure 33-7.

- Make sure the roll does not extend as far as the knee. *To avoid nerve compression and palsy that can lead to footdrop.*
- Alternately, you can place the patient on a sheet that has been folded so that the top edge is at the top of the hips, and the lower edge is about one-third the way down the thighs. Then place the rolled towels under the sheet and roll the sheet under tightly.

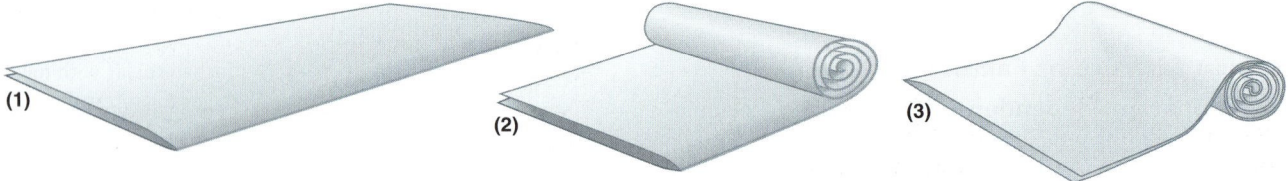

(1)   (2)   (3)

Applying Hand Rolls

- Place a rolled up washcloth or commercial hand roll in the patient's palm to maintain a neutral position. See Figure 33-8.
- Secure the strap, if present.
- Roll soft gauze around the hand and secure with nonallergenic, adhesive tape to keep it from falling out of the patient's hand.
- Place another roll in the patient's other hand, if needed.

Applying Hip Abduction Pillow

- Place the wedge-shaped, spongy pillow between the patient's legs when she is lying on her back. See Figure 33-9.
- Slide it toward the groin so it touches the legs all along the inside of the thigh.
- Place both upper legs in the pillow's lateral indentations.
- Secure the straps to prevent the pillow from slipping down the mattress.

Clinical Insight 33-2 ➤ Using Common Positioning Devices—cont'd

Applying Cradle Boots

- Open the slit on the top surface of the boot.
- Place the patient's heel in the round cutout for the heel. If the patient is positioned on her side, you may put the boot on the bottom foot.

- Support the flexed top foot with a pillow.
- Apply the boot to the other foot, as needed.
- Position the patient's legs in neutral alignment with slight flexion. See Figure 33-6.

Clinical Insight 33-3 ➤ Tips for Performing Passive Range-of-Motion Exercises

Passive range of motion (PROM) is the movement of the joints through their full range of motion by another person. Nurses frequently perform PROM to maintain joint mobility.

- **Explain the purpose of PROM.** You may also wish to teach family members and caregivers about the importance of ROM exercises and enlist their help in exercising the patient when they visit.
- **Observe the patient as you perform PROM.** You may need to perform the exercises in several short segments if the patient tires easily or experiences discomfort.
- **Support the patient's limb** above and below the joint that is to be exercised.
- **Move the joint in a slow, smooth, rhythmic manner.** Avoid fast movements; they may cause muscle spasm.

- **Never force a joint.** Some patients may have limited ROM. Move each joint to the point of resistance. This should not be painful.
- **Perform PROM** at least twice daily. Move each joint through ROM three to five times with each session. Consider incorporating PROM into care activities, for example, while bathing or turning the patient.
- **Return the joint to a neutral position** when exercise is complete.
- **Encourage active exercise** whenever possible.

 The video **Performing Passive Range-of-Motion Exercises**, along with questions and suggested responses, is available on the **Davis's *Nursing Skills Videos*** Web site on Davis*Plus*.

Clinical Insight 33-4 ➤ Assisting With Physical Conditioning Exercises to Prepare for Ambulation

Patients who have been confined to bed for more than a week or who have sustained major injury require conditioning before they resume walking. Conditioning exercises include the following.

Quadriceps and Gluteal Drills

- Ask the patient to tighten her thigh muscles by pushing downward with her knees and flexing her feet. Each leg may be done separately if moving both is contraindicated.
- Ask the patient to hold the position for a count of 5 and then relax.
- Repeat this process two to three times per hour during the waking hours.
- To exercise the gluteal muscles, ask the patient to pinch her buttocks together.
- Do this exercise when the patient exercises her quadriceps muscles.
- Instruct the patient not to hold her breath as she exercises.

Arm Exercises

- Install a trapeze bar on the patient's bed. Ask the patient to do pull-ups on the bar from a lying position. This exercises the biceps muscles.
- To exercise the triceps muscles, ask the patient to lift his upper body off the mattress by firmly pressing down with the palms.
- The patient can also do push-ups from a seated position at the side of the bed or from a stationary chair or wheelchair.

Dangling

- Dangling is a seated position at the side of the bed, feet resting on the floor.
- Provide a footstool if the patient's feet do not reach the floor.
- Assess for light-headedness or postural hypotension.
- Do not progress to ambulation until the patient is comfortable and stable in the dangling position.

(Continued)

Clinical Insight 33-4 ➤ Assisting With Physical Conditioning Exercises to Prepare for Ambulation—cont'd

Daily Activities

- Encourage your patient to be active in bed by repositioning and turning herself.
- Encourage the patient to get out of bed and into a chair before attempting to walk.

- Encourage the patient to perform as much of her activities of daily living (ADLs) as possible.
- ADLs exercise many of the muscle groups used in ambulation.

Clinical Insight 33-5 ➤ Sizing Walking Aids

Sizing Canes

- Ask the patient to stand erect and to place the cane tip 20 cm (4 in.) to the side of the foot.
- The top of the cane should reach the top of the hip joint so that the patient can hold the cane with her elbow flexed 30°.

Sizing Walkers

- Ask the patient to stand erect, holding onto the walker.
- The walker should extend from the floor to the hip joint so that the patient can comfortably hold the walker with 30° flexion of the elbow.

Sizing Crutches

To measure a patient for an axillary crutch, follow these guidelines:

- Ask the patient to lie down wearing the nonskid shoes that she will use when walking.
- Measure the distance between the heel and the anterior fold of the axilla, then add 2.5 cm (1 in.).
- Select a crutch that can be adjusted to this height.
- Have the patient stand and position the crutch tip 10 to 15 cm (4 to 6 in.) to the side of the heel. Adjust the axillary crutch pad three fingerbreadths below the axilla.
- Adjust the handgrips so that the patient can comfortably grasp the bar while the elbow is slightly flexed. The patient's axilla should not rest on the crutchpad.

Clinical Insight 33-6 ➤ Teaching Patients to Use Canes, Walkers, and Crutches

Canes

After ensuring the cane is the proper size (refer to Clinical Insight 33-5), instruct the patient to do the following:

- Hold the cane on the stronger side.
- Distribute weight evenly between the feet and cane.
- Advance the cane and weaker leg simultaneously, then bring the stronger leg through.
- Avoid leaning over or on the cane.
- Maintain the integrity of the rubber tip for traction.

Walkers

After ensuring the walker is the proper size (refer to Clinical Insight 33-5), instruct the patient to:

- Stand between the back legs of the walker. Do not stand too far behind the walker.
- Pick up the walker, and advance it as you step ahead. Do not advance it so far as to lose balance.
- If one leg is weaker, move it forward as the walker moves forward.
- Pick up, rather than slide, the walker (unless it has wheels).

Crutches

After ensuring the crutches are the proper size (refer to Clinical Insight 33-5), do the following:

- When first teaching crutch walking, instruct the patient to stand near a wall with a chair behind him. Help the patient to stand and grip the crutches. Ask the patient to sway from side to side on the crutches to become accustomed to weight-bearing by the arms.
- *Tripod position* is the basic crutch gait standing position. Place crutches 15 cm (6 in.) in front of the feet, with the crutch point 15 cm from the patient's center. In this position, a triangle is formed by the crutches and the body.
- Five crutch gaits exist (see accompanying chart): 2-point gait, 3-point gait, 4-point gait, swing-to gait, and swing-through gait.
- ✚ To teach the patient how to go up and down stairs, instruct him to lead with the unaffected leg when going up the stairs and to lead with the affected leg coming down the stairs. *Navigating stairs with crutches can be dangerous. When possible, have the patient practice this technique before discharge. When having a patient practice, the nurse should always stand below the patient on the stairs to prevent falling.*

Clinical Insight 33-6 ▶ Teaching Patients to Use Canes, Walkers, and Crutches—cont'd

NOTE: Read this table from bottom to top.

2-Point gait	3-Point gait	4-Point gait	Swing to	Swing through
• Partial weight bearing, both feet; faster, but less support than a 4-point gait	• Non-weight bearing; faster than a 4-point gait; can use with walker	• Partial weight bearing, both feet; patient must shift weight constantly	• Weight bearing, both feet; can use with walker	• Weight bearing; requires the most coordination and balance
4. Advance right foot and left crutch	**4.** Advance right foot	**4.** Advance right foot	**4.** Lift both feet; swing them forward, landing feet next to the crutches	**4.** Lift both feet; swing them forward, landing feet in front of the crutches
3. Advance left foot and right crutch	**3.** Advance left foot and both crutches	**3.** Advance left crutch	**3.** Advance both crutches	**3.** Advance both crutches
2. Advance right foot and left crutch	**2.** Advance right foot	**2.** Advance left foot	**2.** Lift both feet; swing them forward, landing feet next to the crutches	**2.** Lift both feet; swing them forward, landing feet in front of the crutches
1. Advance left foot and right crutch	**1.** Advance left foot and both crutches	**1.** Advance right crutch	**1.** Advance both crutches	**1.** Advance both crutches
Tripod position	Tripod position	Tripod position	Tripod position	Tripod position

Crutch gaits. The shaded area represents weight-bearing. The arrow shows movement.

PROCEDURES

In this section, you will learn about procedures and techniques for positioning, moving, turning, transferring, and ambulating patients safely. Although the American Nurses Association (2006) recommends that you use assistive equipment for all lifting and transferring, you may encounter situations in which equipment is not available or you do not have time to get it. In such situations, using good body mechanics may help you decrease the risk of injury to you and the patient.

Procedure 33-1 ■ Moving and Turning Patients in Bed

> ➤ For steps to follow in *all* procedures, refer to the Universal Steps for All Procedures found on the page facing the inside back cover.

Equipment

- Nonlatex gloves, if you may be exposed to body fluids
- Friction-reducing device, such as a transfer roller sheet or scoot sheet
- Pull or lift (draw) sheet
- Pillows, as needed

Delegation

You may ask nursing assistive personnel (NAP) to assist with moving a patient up in bed, turning a patient, or logrolling a patient after ensuring that the NAP has the necessary skills and that the patient's condition is stable. Complete the assessment, and inform the NAP of any special considerations when moving the patient.

Pre-Procedure Assessment

Assess the following:
- Level of comfort

If the patient is uncomfortable, you may need to administer an analgesic before moving.

- Level of consciousness, ability to follow directions, and ability to assist with the move
- Any restrictions in movement or position (ask the patient and check the provider's orders)
- Physical size of the patient and the assistive devices available
- The patient's medical diagnoses. Identify problems that may affect positioning (e.g., respiratory or cardiac problems, pain).
- Presence of equipment such as IV setups, pumps, or casts and what must be moved with the patient

The preceding assessments all help determine how many assistants and equipment you need, the patient's ability to assist in the procedure, and how to proceed with the move safely.

Procedure 33-1A ■ Moving a Patient Up in Bed

> ➤ When performing the procedure, always identify your patient according to agency policy, using two identifiers, and be attentive to standard precautions, hand hygiene, patient safety and privacy, body mechanics, and documentation.

Procedure Steps

KEY POINT: *Medicate the patient for pain, if needed, before moving the patient in bed.*

1. Lock the bed wheels. Lower the head of the bed and place the patient in a supine position. Position one nurse on each side of the bed. Lower the siderails on the "working" side of the bed. Raise the height of the bed to waist level.
These actions allows you to work with gravity and move the patient more easily while maintaining good body mechanics.

2. Ensure that a friction-reducing device, such as a transfer roller sheet, is in place under the drawsheet. If it is not in place, turn the patient from side to side to place the device under

the drawsheet. You can improvise this device by placing a clean, unused plastic bag or plastic film under the drawsheet.
A transfer roller sheet facilitates movement by reducing friction. This also helps to reduce back injury to the nurse.

NOTE: This procedure uses a transfer roller sheet. This device is inexpensive and readily available. Scoot sheets further reduce the risk of back and musculoskeletal injury; however, their availability varies. Having a second person to help move a patient up in bed is the safest approach for staff and patients. Also follow the guidelines in Clinical Insight 33-1.

3. Remove the pillow from under the patient's head. Place it at the head of the bed.

A pillow prevents patient from hitting his head on the head board.

4. Instruct the patient to fold his arms across his chest. If an overhead trapeze is in place, ask the patient to hold the trapeze with both hands if able. Have the patient bend his knees with feet flat on the bed.
This position facilitates the patient's assistance with the move.

5. Instruct the patient to flex his neck.
Protects the neck while moving.

6. With a nurse positioned on either side of the patient, grasp and roll the drawsheet close to the patient.

7. **Instruct the patient,** on the count of 3, to lift his trunk and push off with his heels toward the head of the bed.

8. **Stand as close as possible** to the client without twisting your back.

9. **Position your feet with a wide base** of support. Point your feet toward the direction of the move. Flex your knees and hips.
   Allows you to maintain proper body mechanics and prevents injury while moving the patient. ▼

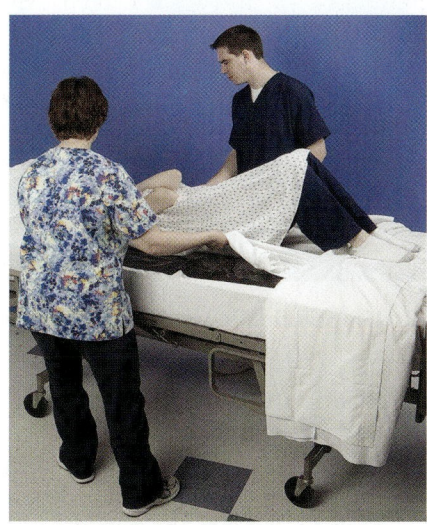

10. ✚ **Place your weight on your foot** nearest the foot of the bed. Count to 3, and shift your weight forward toward the head of the bed. Move along the patient's side instead of reaching. Use gentle rocking motions to reduce exertion.
    Shifting your weight allows you to use your momentum to move the patient, which helps protect your back from injury.

11. **Repeat until the patient** is positioned near the head of the bed. If you used a plastic bag or film to reduce friction, remove it now.
    Plastic is water impermeable, so it allows moisture to pool under the patient. This creates a risk for Impaired Skin Integrity.

12. **Straighten the drawsheet** and tuck it in tightly at the sides of the bed.
    A wrinkle-free sheet prevents uneven pressure, discomfort, and skin irritation.

13. **Place a pillow under** the patient's head and assist him to a comfortable position.
    Provides comfort and good body alignment.

14. ✚ **Place the bed in low position** and raise the siderail.
    Helps prevent falls.

15. **Place the call light** in a position where the patient can easily reach it.
    Allows patient to call for help, if needed.

Procedure Variation Use of an Approved Mechanical Lifting Device

16. **Lock the bed wheels.** Lower the head of the bed and place the patient in a supine position. Position at least one nurse on each side of the bed. Lower the siderails. Raise the height of the bed to waist level.

17. **Using the drawsheet, turn** the patient onto his side. Position the midline of the full body sling at the patient's back. Tightly roll the remaining half of the sling, and tuck the fabric under the drawsheet. ▼

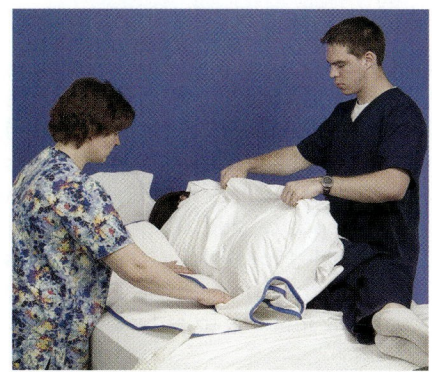

18. **With a second nurse positioned** on either side of the patient, use the drawsheet to turn the patient to the opposite side. Unroll the full body sling, and reposition the patient supine.

19. **Attach the sling** to the overbed lifting device or mechanical lift.

20. **Engage the lift** to raise the patient off the bed. Advance the lift toward the head of the bed until the patient is at the desired level. ▼

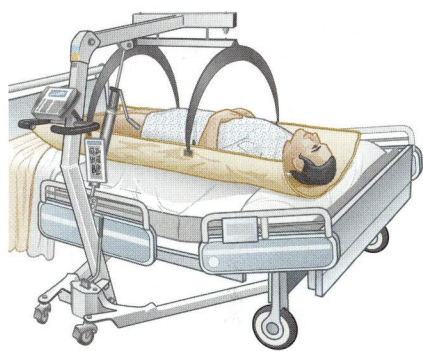

21. **Lower the lift** and turn the patient to the desired position. You may leave the sling in place for future movement, or you may remove it by turning the patient from side to side.

    NOTE: If a full body sling is not available, use a friction-reducing device, such as a transfer roller sheet, and at least three staff members.

(continued on next page)

Procedure 33-1 ■ Moving and Turning Patients in Bed (continued)

Procedure 33-1B ■ Turning a Patient in Bed

➤ When performing the procedure, always identify your patient according to agency policy, using two identifiers, and be attentive to standard precautions, hand hygiene, patient safety and privacy, body mechanics, and documentation.

➤ *Note:* This procedure describes the use of a transfer roller sheet. This device is inexpensive and readily available.

Procedure Steps

1. **Lock the bed wheels.** Lower the head of the bed and place the patient in a supine position. Position one nurse on each side of the bed. Lower the siderails. Raise the height of the bed to waist level.
   Lowering the siderails and raising the bed allow you to move the patient while maintaining good body mechanics and working with gravity to prevent injury.

2. **Position the patient for turning.**
   a. Remove the pillow from under the patient's head and place it at the head of the bed.
   b. Stand as close as possible to the client without twisting your back.
   c. Roll the patient side to side and place a friction-reducing device under the drawsheet. You can improvise this device by placing a large, clean plastic bag or plastic film under the drawsheet.
   d. Move the patient to the side of the bed you are turning him away from by rolling up the drawsheet close to the patient's body and pulling it.
   e. Align the patient's legs and head with the trunk.
   This allows you to position the patient in the center of the bed after turning. ▼

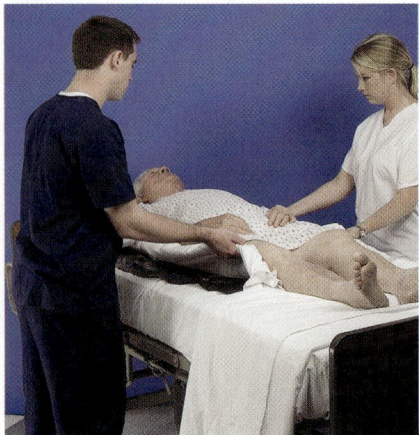

3. **Place the patient's near leg** and foot across the far leg (e.g., when turning the patient to his right, place his left leg over his right leg).

4. **Place the patient's near arm** (e.g., left when turning right) across his chest. And, position the patient's underneath arm up and away from his body.
   Positioning the patient's legs and his near arm facilitates turning. Abducting and rotating the other arm prevents it from being caught under the patient during the turn.

5. **Each nurse positions her feet** with a wide base of support with one foot forward of the other. Bend from the hips and place one hand on the drawsheet at the level of the patient's hip and the other at the level of the shoulder.
   A wide base of support allows you to maintain good body mechanics while performing the move.

6. **Instruct the patient** that the turn will occur on the count of 3.
   Counting coordinates and facilitates patient cooperation with the move.

7. **On the count of 3, flex** your knees and hips and shift your weight. The nurse positioned on the side toward which the patient will turn shifts his weight to the back foot. The nurse on the opposite side shifts her weight forward. Move along the patient's side instead of reaching. Use gentle rocking motions to reduce exertion.

Provides the best leverage to turn the patient. ▼

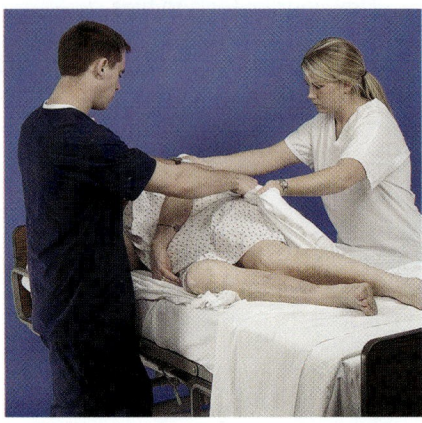

8. **If a plastic film is used,** remove it after you turn the patient.

9. **Position the dependent shoulder** forward. Place pillows behind the patient's back and between legs to maintain the patient in the lateral position. Replace the pillow under the patient's head.
   Positioning ensures that patient is not putting excess pressure on the inferior shoulder. Pillows help maintain good body alignment.

   See Table 33-2, Positioning a Bed-Bound Patient.

10. **Place the bed in low position** and raise the siderail.
    Helps ensure patient safety.

11. **Place the call light** in a position where the patient can easily reach it.
    Allows patient to call for help, if needed.

Procedure 33-1C ■ Logrolling a Patient

> ➤ When performing the procedure, always identify your patient according to agency policy, using two identifiers, and be attentive to standard precautions, hand hygiene, patient safety and privacy, body mechanics, and documentation.

Procedure Steps

1. **Lock the bed wheels.** Lower the head of the bed with the patient supine. Lower the siderail on the side where you are standing, but keep the opposite rail in the up position. Raise the height of the bed to waist level.
   Lowering the siderail and raising the bed allow you to move the patient while maintaining good body mechanics and working with gravity to prevent back injury.

2. **You should already have** a drawsheet with an underlying friction-reducing device, such as a transfer roller sheet, to move the patient to the side of the bed on which you are standing. (You can improvise this device by placing a clean, unused plastic bag or plastic film under the drawsheet.)

3. **Position one staff member** at the patient's head and shoulders; she is responsible for moving the head and neck as a unit. Position the other person at the patient's hips. If you need three staff members, position one at the shoulders, one at the waist, and the third at thigh level. One staff member must maintain the patient's head and neck in alignment. The other members assist with moving the rest of the body in alignment. ▼

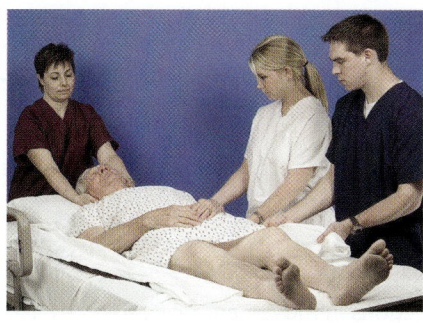

4. **Each nurse should position her** feet with a wide base of support with one foot slightly more forward than the other.
   Facilitates proper body mechanics and minimizes risk of injury to staff members.

5. **Use the drawsheet** or transfer sheet to move the patient to the side of the bed on which the nurses are standing. The move must be smooth so that the patient's head and hips are kept in alignment. Position the patient's head with a pillow.
   A transfer sheet maintains straight alignment of the spine.

6. **Instruct the patient to fold** his arms across his chest.

7. **Place a pillow** between the patient's knees.
   A pillow prevents internal rotation of the hip and spine with movement. Maintains straight alignment of the spine.

8. **Raise the siderail** and move to opposite side of the bed.
   Siderails keep the patient from falling out of bed.

9. **Lower the siderail** on the "new" side of the bed and face the patient. All nurses should position their feet with a wide base of support, with one foot forward of the other. Place your weight on the forward foot. Bend from the hips and position your hands evenly along the length of the drawsheet.
   Provides the best leverage to turn the patient while maintaining spine alignment. ▼

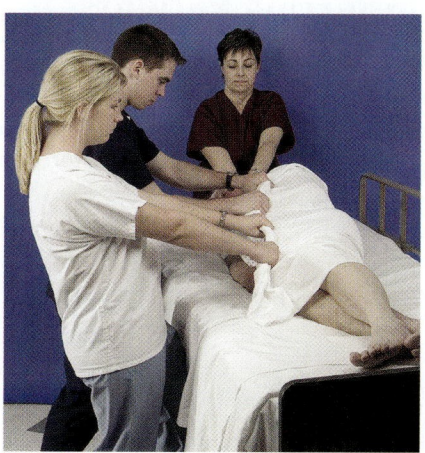

10. **All nurses flex their knees** and hips and shift their weight to the back foot on the count of 3. Be sure to support the head as the patient is rolled to his side.
    Allows you to maintain straight alignment and body mechanics while performing the move.

11. **Place pillows to maintain** the patient in the lateral position. See Table 33-2, Positioning a Bed-Bound Patient.
    A pillow provides support and maintains proper alignment.

12. **Place the bed in low position** and raise the siderail.

13. **Place the call light** in a position where the patient can easily reach it.
    Allows patient to call for help, if needed.

? What if . . .

- **Your facility has instituted a no-lift policy and you have to pull the patient up in bed?**

  Use assistive equipment such as friction-reducing devices, mechanical lifts, air-powered mattresses, and/or lateral transfer devices to help prevent work-related injuries.

- **Your patient is obese or unable to assist (totally dependent) and you need to lift him?**

  Minimize manual lifting in all cases and eliminate it where feasible. Therefore, follow facility recommendations/protocols and use approved devices. You should be familiar with the lift devices in your facility.

(continued on next page)

Procedure 33-1 ■ Moving and Turning Patients in Bed (continued)

■ **The patient has had a total hip replacement and you have to turn or logroll your patient?**

Maintain the affected leg in abduction by using a pillow or abduction wedge between the legs.
To ensure the hip will not become strained or dislocated during turning.

■ **The patient has a cast or is in traction and you have to turn or logroll your patient?**

Designate a person to assist in the turning by guiding the affected extremity.

■ **The patient has an external fixation device and you have to turn or logroll your patient?**

Secure the device in place to keep it from moving when lifting or moving the limb as needed.
By holding onto the device to secure it and keep it from moving, there is less movement of the healing bone, and therefore less trauma and pain.

Evaluation

■ Assess the patient's comfort level after the position change.
■ Assess body position and alignment after position change.
■ Assess skin for pressure areas.

Patient Teaching

■ Explain to the patient the importance of maintaining spine alignment.
■ Explain to the patient the importance of frequent position changes.
■ Instruct the patient to ask the nurse when she needs to be turned sooner than scheduled.
■ Teach the patient how she can assist with moving and turning.

Home Care

■ Instruct the family member or caregiver in the techniques for moving, turning, or logrolling the client.
■ Discuss the shearing effects on the skin from sliding down in bed (see Chapter 36).
■ Provide instruction on the importance of changing position and maintaining proper body alignment.

Documentation

Repositioning and turning patients are considered routine aspects of care and are not usually charted every time they are done. However, document in the nursing notes any problems with positioning the patient or any areas of skin breakdown. You might also chart turning as an intervention when charting to a specific problem. For example, if the patient has Impaired Skin Integrity, you might describe the skin and chart, "Position changed hourly." Some facilities have flow sheets on which you indicate by a checkmark each time a patient is repositioned.

Practice Resources

Centers for Disease Control and Prevention (n.d., updated 2016, 2012a); Collins, J. W., Nelson, A., & Sublet, V. (2006); Nelson, A., & Baptiste, A. S. (2004); Occupational Safety and Health Administration (2009); Waters, T. R., Nelson, A. N., Hughes, N., et al (2009).

 The videos **Moving a Patient Up in Bed, Moving a Patient Up in Bed Using a Mechanical Lifting Device, Turning a Patient in Bed,** and **Logrolling a Patient,** along with questions and suggested responses, are available on the **Davis's *Nursing Skills Videos*** Web site on Davis*Plus*.

Procedure 33-2 ■ Transferring Patients

➤ For steps to follow in *all* procedures, refer to the Universal Steps for All Procedures found on the page facing the inside back cover.

Equipment

■ Nonlatex gloves, if you may be exposed to body fluids
■ Transfer board (for transferring from bed to stretcher, and sometimes bed to chair)
■ Pull or lift (draw) sheet (for transfers)
■ Gait transfer belt (for dangling and transferring from bed to chair)

Delegation

You may ask the NAP to dangle, transfer a patient from bed to stretcher, or transfer a patient from bed to chair. Ensure that the NAP has the necessary skills and that the patient's condition is stable. Inform the NAP of any special considerations when dangling or transferring the patient and evaluate the patient after transfer.

Pre-Procedure Assessment

■ Assess for any restrictions in movement or position by asking the patient and checking the physician's orders.
■ Observe for the presence of equipment such as IV lines, drains, or catheters.
■ Assess possible side effects of medications (e.g., dizziness and sedation). Assess the patient's level of consciousness, ability to follow directions, and ability to assist with the move.
■ Assess the physical size of the patient and your own strength and ability to move the patient.

■ Before transferring a patient to a chair, assess the patient's tolerance of dangling.

The preceding assessments inform you about activity tolerance, readiness to get out of bed, and ability to participate in the transfer. They help you determine how many assistants you need, the appropriate transfer device, and how to proceed with the move while preventing injury and dislodging of equipment.

■ Assess vital sign and monitor for postural hypotension (light-headedness when sitting or standing up quickly from a recumbent position).

If the patient is at risk for postural hypotension, you may need to allow additional time for the patient to change position.

■ Assess the patient's level of comfort using a standardized pain scale.

If the patient is experiencing pain, you may need to administer an analgesic before moving.

Procedure 33-2A ■ Transferring a Patient From Bed to Stretcher

➤ When performing the procedure, always identify your patient according to agency policy, using two identifiers, and be attentive to standard precautions, hand hygiene, patient safety and privacy, body mechanics, and documentation.

Procedure Steps

1. **Lock the wheels on the bed.** Position the bed so that it is flat (if the patient can tolerate being supine) and at the height of the stretcher.
   Locking the wheels ensures client safety during the transfer. Having the bed flat helps prevent injury to staff, because the patient is easier to move.

2. **Lower the siderails** and position at least one nurse on each side of the bed. Move the patient to the side of the bed where the stretcher will be placed by rolling up the drawsheet close to the patient's body and pulling it toward the designated side. Align the patient's legs and head with her trunk.
   Positions patient to enable nurses to move her to the stretcher.

3. **Position the stretcher** next to the bed. Lock the stretcher wheels.
   Locking the wheels keeps the stretcher from moving during the transfer; prevents falls.

4. **Place the transfer board** against the patient's back.
   a. Place a friction-reducing device, such as a transfer roller sheet, over the transfer board. (You can improvise this device by placing a clean, unused plastic bag or plastic film under the drawsheet.)
   b. The nurse on the side opposite the stretcher uses the drawsheet to turn the patient away from the stretcher, while the other nurse places the transfer board against the patient's back halfway between bed and stretcher. Turn the

patient to her back and onto the transfer board.

Safely positions the transfer board under the patient, without friction. ▼

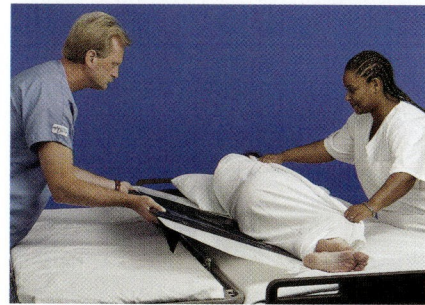

5. **Ensure the patient's feet** and shoulder are over the edge of the transfer board.
   To prevent injury to the patient from the edge of the board.

6. **Ask the patient raise her head** if able. Use the drawsheet to slide her across the transfer board onto the stretcher.
   Facilitates the move to the stretcher; prevents friction on patient's skin.

If Transferring a Patient From Bed to Stretcher With a Slipsheet

A slipsheet may be used instead of a transfer board. A slipsheet is a large, low-friction fabric that facilitates transfer. ▼

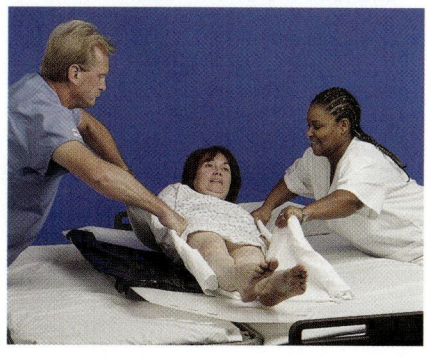

7. **With the drawsheet,** turn the patient to the side opposite where the stretcher will be placed.

8. **Position the midline of the slipsheet** under the patient. Roll the remaining half tightly and tuck it under the patient.

9. **Turn the patient back over to the** side near to the stretcher; pull the slipsheet through from under the patient.

10. **Place the patient supine** and lower the siderail on the side where the stretcher will be placed.

11. **Move the stretcher** next to the bed and lock the wheels on the stretcher.

12. **Position at least two nurses** on the far side of the stretcher. Using the slipsheet, pull the patient onto the stretcher. ▼

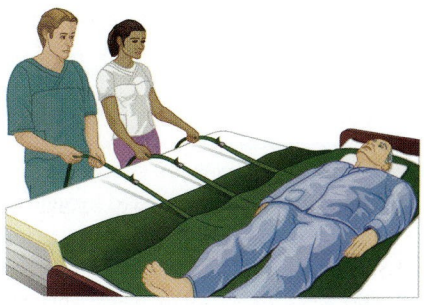

13. **Be sure to return the stretcher** to the locked position with the siderails raised for patient safety.

14. **Place the call light in reach** of the patient or position the patient where she can be seen by staff members at all times.

(continued on next page)

Procedure 33-2 ■ Transferring Patients (continued)

Procedure 33-2B ■ Dangling a Patient at the Side of the Bed

➤ When performing the procedure, always identify your patient according to agency policy, using two identifiers, and be attentive to standard precautions, hand hygiene, patient safety and privacy, body mechanics, and documentation.

Procedure Steps

1. ✚ **Lock the bed wheels.** Place the patient in a supine position and raise the head of the bed to 90°. Keep the siderail elevated on the side opposite where you are standing.
Locking the wheels prevents the bed from moving as you move the patient. Raising the head of the bed prepares the patient to be dangled and requires less effort from you to help the patient sit erect.

2. ✚ **Apply a gait transfer belt** to the patient at waist level. Be sure the belt is snug but not uncomfortable. You should be able to easily place your hand under the belt. Do not place it over the rib cage, as this could compromise breathing. You would not use a transfer belt after abdominal surgery or with other abdominal wound, colostomy, or internal organ contusion or other injury.

3. Place the bed in the low position.
Ensures patient safety and proper body mechanics.

4. **Instruct the patient to bend** his knees and turn the patient onto his side, if possible, keeping knees flexed.
Prepares the patient to be able to dangle his legs over side of bed.

5. **Stand at the side of the bed,** facing the patient and using a wide base of support. Place your foot closest to the head of the bed forward of the other foot. Lean forward, bending at the hips, with your knees flexed. Instruct the patient to use his arm to push off the bed.
Allows you to maintain proper body mechanics and prevents injury. ▼

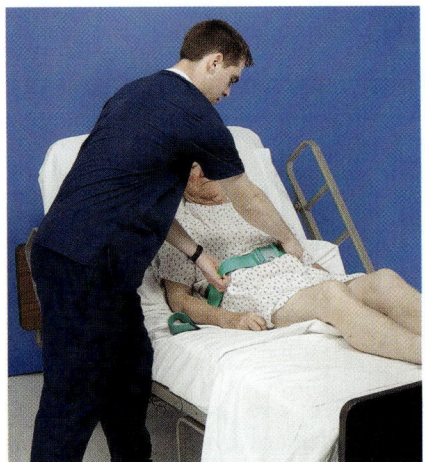

6. **Position your hands** on each side of the gait transfer belt.

7. **Rock onto your back foot** as you assist the patient toward you with the gait transfer belt, thereby moving the patient into a sitting position at the side of the bed.

Uses your body weight as leverage to reposition the patient, preventing injury to your back.. ▼

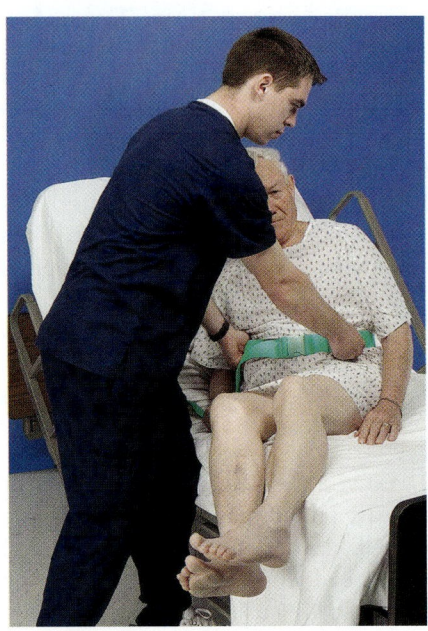

8. ✚ **Stay with the patient** as he dangles. Reassess comfort level and for dizziness.
Helps prevent falls.

Procedure 33-2C ■ Transferring a Patient From Bed to Chair

➤ When performing the procedure, always identify your patient according to agency policy, using two identifiers, and be attentive to standard precautions, hand hygiene, patient safety and privacy, body mechanics, and documentation.

Procedure Steps

1. ✚ **Position the chair** next to the bed. If possible, lock the chair.
Prevents the chair from moving during transfer. Ensures patient safety.

2. ✚ **Put nonskid footwear** on the patient.
Prevents the patient from slipping during transfer.

3. **Place the bed in a low position** and lock the bed wheels.
Prevents the bed from moving during the transfer. Low position allows patient to place feet firmly on the floor.

4. **Apply a transfer belt.**
Facilitates transfer of the patient to the chair and helps prevent back injury to the nurse.

5. **Assist the patient to dangle** at the side of the bed (see Procedure 33-2B). Be sure the patient doesn't need support before releasing him.

6. **Stand toward the bed,** facing the patient. Brace your feet and knees against the patient's legs. Pay particular attention to any known weakness. Bend your hips and knees, and, keeping your back straight, hold onto the transfer belt on both sides. If two

nurses are available to assist with the transfer, one nurse should be on each side of the patient.

Bracing provides stability. Bending the hips and knees allows you to use the major muscle groups and limit the risk of injury. Lifting the patient at waist level prevents injury to the arm or shoulder. ▼

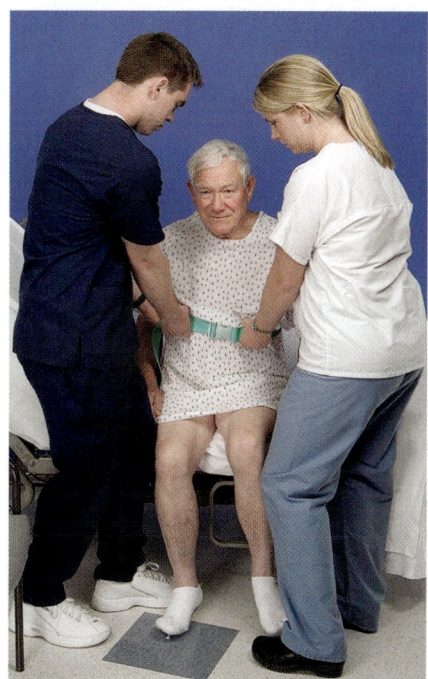

7. **Instruct the patient** to place his arms around you between the shoulders and waist (the location depends on your height and the height of the patient).
   Having the patient hold you on your trunk prevents injury to your neck.

8. **Ask the patient to stand** as you move to an upright position by straightening your legs and hips.
   Straightening your thighs and hips uses your large muscle groups and prevents injury to your back.

9. **Allow the patient to steady** himself for a moment. Ask whether he is feeling light-headed.
   Provides the patient an opportunity to rest before further movement. Allows you to evaluate his tolerance to activity and ability to maintain an upright posture before continuing.

10. **Instruct the patient to pivot** and turn with you toward the chair.
    Pivoting helps prevent twisting and straining the patient's back muscles.

11. **Assist the patient to position** himself in front of the chair. Have the patient flex his hips and knees, and as he lowers himself to the chair, reach for arms of the chair. Guide his motion while maintaining a firm hold on him and keeping your back straight.
    Maintains good body mechanics and balance and ensures patient safety. ▼

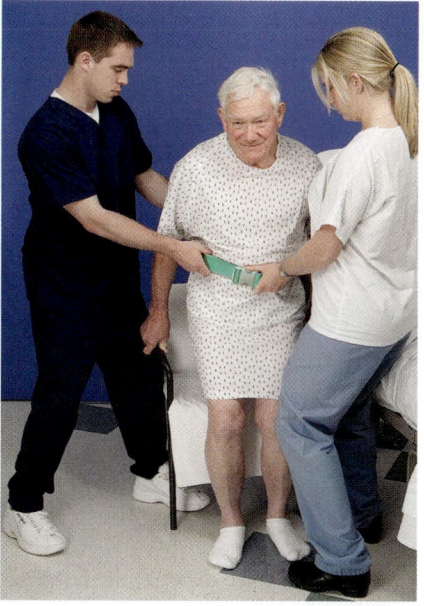

12. **Assist the patient** to a comfortable position in the chair.

13. **Provide a blanket** if needed for warmth or privacy.

14. **Place the call light in reach** of the patient or position the patient where he can be seen by staff members at all times.

? What if . . .

■ **The patient is obese?**

If the patient is obese or unable to assist, use a full body sling that allows the patient to assume a seated position. You may also use a powered standing assist lift, if one is available.

■ **The patient has had hip surgery (replacement or fracture repair)?**

When assisting the patient out of bed, raise the bed to a higher position, allowing the patient to exit the bed without acute hip flexion.
To avoid hip dislocation.

■ **The patient becomes dizzy during the transfer?**

Return the patient to sitting or recumbent position and assess his vital signs.

■ **The patient has a weaker side, for example, from a cerebrovascular accident or surgical procedure?**

Instruct the patient to exit the bed from his unaffected side. Stand on the patient's weaker side.
The stronger side should lead a transfer.

(continued on next page)

Procedure 33-2 ■ Transferring Patients (continued)

Evaluation

- Assess the level of patient participation in the transfer.
- Assess the patient's comfort level during the transfer and in the new position.
- Assess proper body position and alignment after his position change.
- Assess the patient's vital signs for postural hypotension after dangling or transferring to a chair.

Patient Teaching

- Explain the importance of frequent position changes and getting out of bed to avoid complications of immobility.

Home Care

- Instruct the family member or caregiver in the proper technique for assisting the client to dangle at the bedside or transfer to a chair.
- Provide instruction in the importance of changing position and maintaining proper body alignment.

Documentation

Patients are usually moved to a stretcher for transport to a test or procedure. The movement is a routine aspect of care and is not documented. When dangling or transferring a patient to a chair, document in the nursing notes how much assistance was required, the use of assistive devices, any problems with positioning the patient, how long the patient was out of bed, and how the patient tolerated the activity.

Practice Resources

Centers for Disease Control and Prevention (CDC) (n.d., updated 2016, 2012a); Collins, J. W., Nelson, A., & Sublet, V. (2006); Occupational Safety and Health Administration (2009); Waters, T. R., Nelson, A. N., Hughes, N., et al. (2009).

 The videos **Transferring a Patient from Bed to Stretcher, Dangling a Patient at the Side of the Bed,** and **Transferring a Patient From Bed to Chair,** along with questions and suggested responses, are available on the **Davis's _Nursing Skills Videos_** Web site on DavisPlus.

Procedure 33-3 ■ Assisting With Ambulation

➤ For steps to follow in _all_ procedures, refer to the Universal Steps for All Procedures found on the page facing the inside back cover.

Equipment

- Nonlatex gloves, if you may be exposed to body fluids
- Transfer belt
- Nonskid footwear

Delegation

You may ask nursing assistive personnel to assist with ambulation. Ensure that the NAP has the necessary skills and that the patient's condition is stable. Inform the NAP of any special considerations when assisting a patient with ambulation and evaluate the patient after the activity.

Pre-Procedure Assessment

- Assess for any restrictions in movement or position by asking the patient and checking the patient's health record.
- Observe for the presence of equipment such as IV lines, drains, or catheters.
- Assess possible side effects of medications (e.g., dizziness and sedation).
- Assess the patient's level of consciousness, ability to follow directions, and ability to assist with the move.

- Assess the physical size of the patient and your own strength and ability to move the patient.
- Assess the patient's tolerance when dangling before beginning to ambulate.
  The preceding assessments inform you about activity tolerance, readiness to get out of bed, and ability to participate in the transfer. They help you determine how many assistants you need, the appropriate transfer device, and how to proceed with the move while preventing injury and dislodging of equipment.

- Assess vital signs and monitor for postural hypotension.
  If the patient is at risk for postural hypotension, you may need to allow additional time for the patient to change position and plan for adequate help.

- Assess the patient's level of comfort using a standardized pain scale.
  If the patient is uncomfortable, you may need to administer an analgesic before moving.

- Assess for factors that may increase the risk of falls (elderly, muscle weakness, chronic disease, gait disturbance).
  Identifies patients at risk.

Procedure 33-3A ■ Assisting With Ambulation (One Nurse)

➤ When performing the procedure, always identify your patient according to agency policy, using two identifiers, and be attentive to standard precautions, hand hygiene, patient safety and privacy, body mechanics, and documentation.

Procedure Steps

1. **Put nonskid footwear** on the patient.
   Prevents the patient from slipping while transferring and ambulating.

2. **Place the bed in a low position** and lock the bed.
   Prevents the bed from moving during transfer. Makes it easier for the patient's feet to reach the floor.

3. **Apply the transfer belt.**
   Allows you to safely support the patient during the transfer and ambulation.

4. **Assist the patient to dangle** at the side of the bed (see Procedure 33-2B if you need to review).

5. **Face the patient.** Brace your feet and knees against the patient's feet and knees. Pay particular attention to any known weakness. Bend your hips and knees, and hold onto the transfer belt.
   Bracing provides stability of the patient's legs. Bending the hips and knees allows you to use the major muscle groups and limit injury. Lifting at the patient's waist level prevents injury to his arm or shoulder.

6. **Instruct the patient** to place his arms around you between the shoulders and waist (the location depends on your height and the height of the patient). Ask the patient to stand as you move to an upright position by straightening your legs and hips.
   Having the patient hold you on your trunk prevents injury to your neck. Straightening your thighs and hips uses your large muscle groups and promotes good body mechanics.

7. **Allow the patient to steady** himself for a moment.
   Allows the patient an opportunity to rest before further movement and to regain equilibrium before walking.

8. **Stand at the patient's side,** placing both hands on the transfer belt. If the patient is weak on one side, position yourself on the weaker side.
   By standing on the weaker side, the patient is freer to reach with the stronger arm and grip wall or bed rails with his strong-side hand and use the stronger side for strength and balance. This position also keeps you clear of a cane or other assistive device, which would be used on the strong side, and allows you to support the weaker side to prevent the patient from falling. ▼

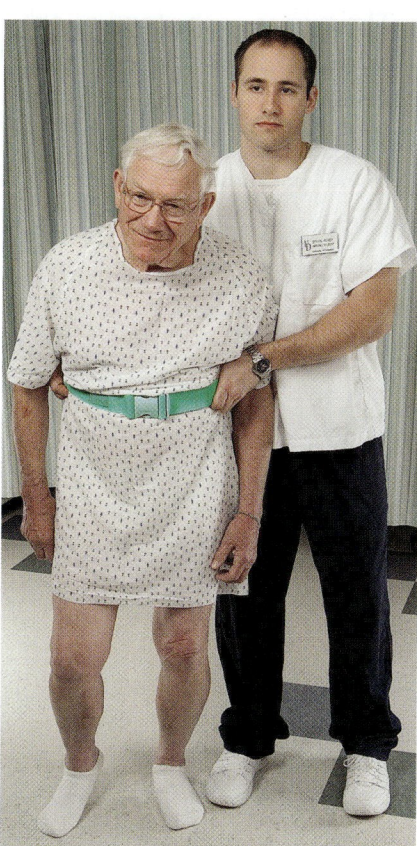

9. **Slowly guide the patient** forward. Observe for signs of fatigue or dizziness.
   Helps prevent falls.

10. **If the patient has an IV pole,** ask him to hold on to the pole on the side where you are standing. Assist the patient to advance the pole as you ambulate. Be sure the patient does not rely on the pole for support.
    Provides a grip for the patient and positions the IV pole near you so that you can assist the patient to move the pole. ▼

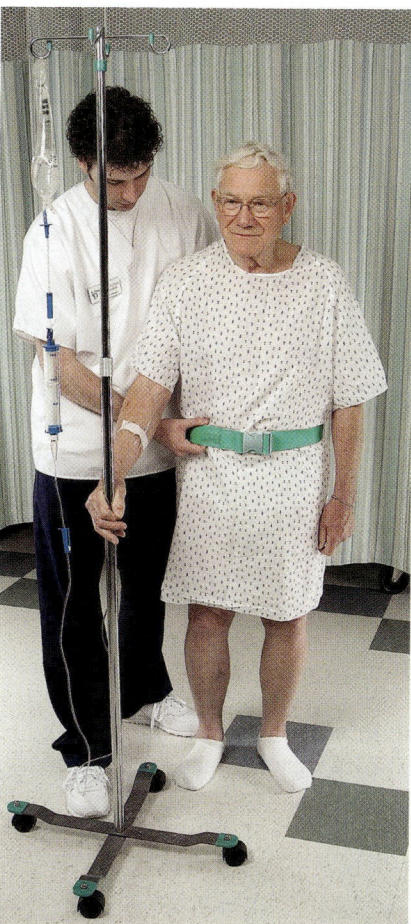

(continued on next page)

Procedure 33-3 ■ Assisting With Ambulation (continued)

Procedure 33-3B ■ Assisting With Ambulation (Two Nurses)

➤ When performing the procedure, always identify your patient according to agency policy, using two identifiers, and be attentive to standard precautions, hand hygiene, patient safety and privacy, body mechanics, and documentation.

Procedure Steps

1. **Put nonskid footwear** on the patient.
   Prevents the patient from slipping during the transfer and ambulation.

2. **Place the bed in low position** and lock the bed.
   Prevents the bed from moving during transfer and prevents the patient from falling.

3. **Apply the transfer belt.**
   Allows you to support client during transfer and ambulation.

4. **Assist the patient to dangle** at the side of the bed (see Procedure 33-2B, as needed).

5. **Each nurse should stand facing** the patient on opposite sides of the patient. Brace your feet and knees against the patient, paying particular attention to any known weakness. Bend from the hips and knees and hold onto the transfer belt.
   Bracing provides stability. Bending the hips and knees allows you to use the major muscle groups and limit injury. Lifting at the patient's waist level prevents injury to his arm or shoulder.

6. **Instruct the patient to place** his arms around each of you between the shoulders and waist (the location depends on your height and the height of the patient). Ask the patient to stand as each of you moves to an upright position by straightening your legs and hips.

7. **Allow the patient to steady** himself for a moment.
   Allows the patient an opportunity to rest before further movement and to regain equilibrium. Allows you to evaluate the patient's tolerance to activity and ability to maintain an upright posture before ambulating.

8. **The nurses each stand at** either side of the patient, grasping hold of the transfer belt. If no belt is available, the nurses grasp each other's arms at the patient's waist.
   Helps patient maintain an erect posture. ▼

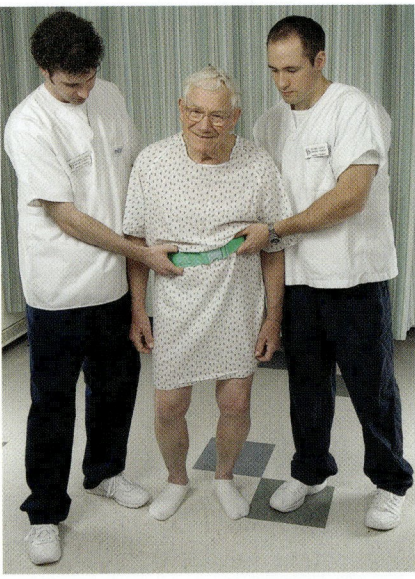

9. **Slowly guide the patient forward.** Observe for signs of fatigue or dizziness.
   Ensures client safety.

10. **If the patient has an IV pole,** one nurse advances the IV pole along the side of the patient by holding the pole with the outside hand. Remind the patient not to use the IV pole for support.
    Positions the IV pole out of the path of the patient. Because the IV pole is on rollers, it will not support the patient if he starts to fall.

? What if . . .

- **The patient has a weaker side (e.g., from a stroke or musculoskeletal injury)?**

  If the patient has weakness on one side, provide additional support but allow him to use that side as he is able.
  This will force him to use his weaker side.

Evaluation

- Assess the level of patient participation in the transfer.
- Assess patient comfort with ambulation.
- Assess posture and base of support.
- Assess vital signs for postural hypotension.

Patient Teaching

- Instruct the patient to inform you if he feels dizzy or weak.
- Explain the importance of ambulation to prevent complications of immobility.

Home Care

- Teach family members or caregivers how to assist the client with ambulation.
- Provide instruction on importance of ambulation.

Documentation

Document in the nursing notes how much assistance was required, any problems with ambulation, and the distance walked.

Sample documentation

11/11/18   0630   *pt assisted to ambulate to doorway in room. Required minimal assistance from one nurse. Placed in chair for 30 min and then assisted back to bed. Required maximum assist from two nurses to return to bed.* —————————— B. Bowen, RN

Practice Resources

Centers for Disease Control and Prevention (n.d., updated 2016, 2012a); Occupational Safety and Health Administration (2009); Waters, T. R., Nelson, A. N., Hughes, N., et al. (2009).

 The videos **Assisting with Ambulation (One Nurse)** and **Assisting with Ambulation (Two Nurses),** along with questions and suggested responses, are available on the **Davis's *Nursing Skills Videos*** Web site on Davis*Plus*.

 To explore learning resources for this chapter,

 Go to **www.DavisAdvantage.com** and find:

Answers and Suggested Responses for all questions in this chapter

Lists of NIC Interventions and NOC Outcomes

List of NANDA-I Diagnoses

Knowledge Map

Care Plan

Care Map

References and Bibliography

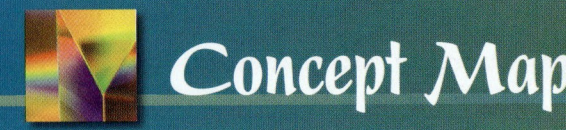

Concept Map

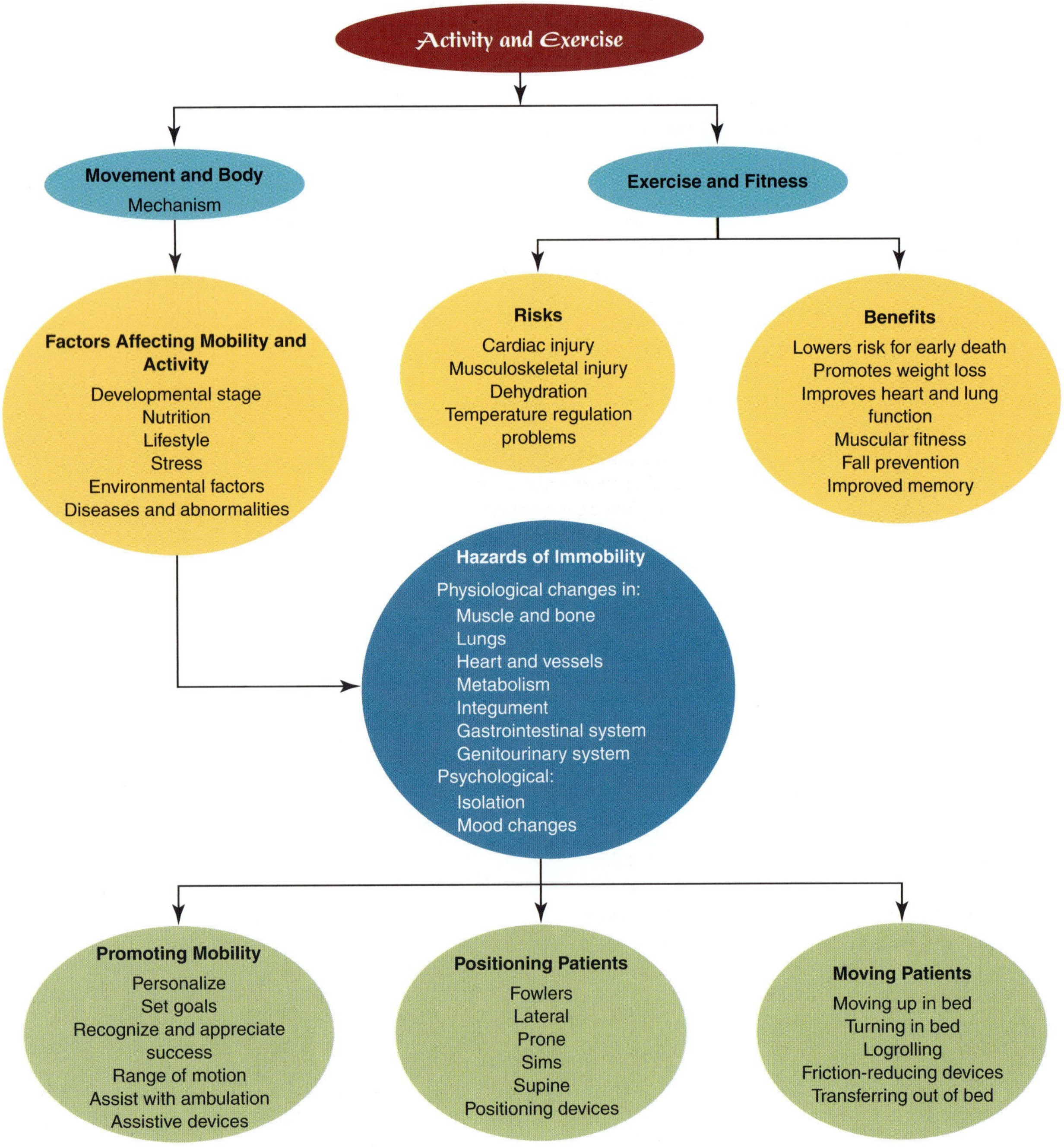

Activity and Exercise

Movement and Body Mechanism

Exercise and Fitness

Factors Affecting Mobility and Activity

Developmental stage
Nutrition
Lifestyle
Stress
Environmental factors
Diseases and abnormalities

Risks

Cardiac injury
Musculoskeletal injury
Dehydration
Temperature regulation problems

Benefits

Lowers risk for early death
Promotes weight loss
Improves heart and lung function
Muscular fitness
Fall prevention
Improved memory

Hazards of Immobility

Physiological changes in:
   Muscle and bone
   Lungs
   Heart and vessels
   Metabolism
   Integument
   Gastrointestinal system
   Genitourinary system
Psychological:
   Isolation
   Mood changes

Promoting Mobility

Personalize
Set goals
Recognize and appreciate
   success
Range of motion
Assist with ambulation
Assistive devices

Positioning Patients

Fowlers
Lateral
Prone
Sims
Supine
Positioning devices

Moving Patients

Moving up in bed
Turning in bed
Logrolling
Friction-reducing devices
Transferring out of bed

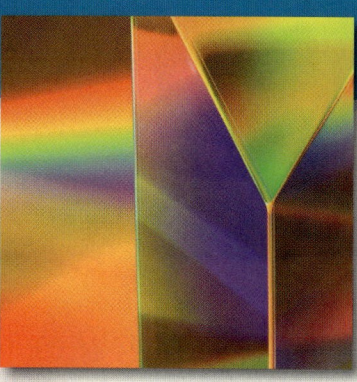

CHAPTER 34

Sexual Health

Learning Outcomes

After completing this chapter, you should be able to:

- Identify the female and male reproductive organs.
- Describe the physical, emotional, social, and spiritual aspects of human sexuality.
- Explain how gender, gender identity, and sexual orientation contribute to expression of sexuality throughout the life cycle.
- Differentiate between typical and atypical forms of sexual expression.
- Explore physical and psychological issues that affect sexuality and sexual functioning.
- Complete a sexual history as part of a comprehensive nursing assessment.

- State nursing diagnoses to describe sexuality problems.
- Explain how sexual health is challenged by high-risk sexual behaviors, sexually transmitted infections (STIs), menstrual problems, infertility, negative intimate relationships, sexual harassment, rape, and disorders of the sexual response cycle.
- Provide nursing interventions that enhance sexual well-being.
- Discuss strategies to increase your personal comfort and confidence in providing holistic nursing care.
- Describe approaches for dealing with inappropriate sexual behavior from patients or in the work environment.

Key Concepts

Sexual dysfunction

Sexual health

Sexuality

Related Concepts

See the Concept Map at the end of this chapter.

Meet Your Patients

- **Jocelyn Carter.** Two days after undergoing a fine-needle aspiration to evaluate a small breast mass, Ms. Carter's surgeon informed her that the mass was malignant. He recommended a mastectomy (removal of the breast). Today she arrives alone at the surgery registration area. You ask how she is feeling, and she tells you that the last week has been a whirlwind of activity. "I had to arrange child care, cancel a business trip, and organize the house so that I could take a few days off to have the surgery. My husband is working overseas this fall, so he couldn't be here to help me. Honestly, I don't know how I'm feeling. I haven't had time to think about it." A few minutes later, as she waits in the surgery holding area, she begins to cry. You hold her hand and ask whether she would like to talk. She asks you, "Do

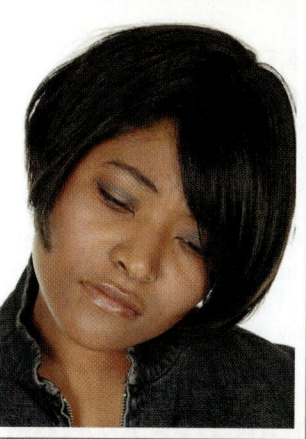

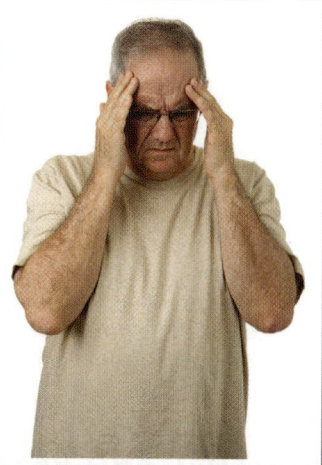

you think my husband will still want me? I'm afraid he will be turned off when he looks at me."

- **Gabriel Thomas.** Mr. Thomas comes to the outpatient clinic complaining of a throbbing headache over the past

(Continued)

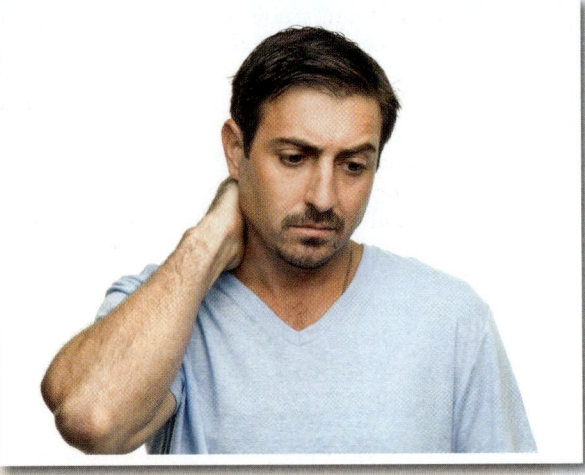

3 days. He explains that he has tried several over-the-counter medicines and has had no relief. You check his blood pressure and measure the reading at 240/130 mm Hg. When you ask whether he has ever been treated for high blood pressure, he replies, "Are you another one of these people trying to get me to take drugs that will ruin my sex life?"

- **Frank Thanee.** Mr. Thanee, who has heart disease, had a mitral valve replacement 3 days ago. He has been transferred to the cardiology floor for an additional day of hospitalization. His partner, Greg, has spent the past 3 days at the hospital and has just left to check on the apartment and feed their cat. Frank confides that he is worried about his parents' expected visit. "I've never been able to tell them about Greg. They wouldn't be able to understand it, never mind approve. I don't know how to handle this. What do you think I should do?"

Although each of these clients has a different medical diagnosis, all are experiencing a concern related to sexuality. In this chapter, we explore the relationship between health and sexuality, and the nurse's role in promoting sexual health.

Theoretical Knowledge
knowing why

When a baby is born, the first question the parents ask is, "Is it a boy or a girl?" In fact, many parents want to know the gender of their baby early in the pregnancy at the first sonogram. Hopes and dreams of future parent–child relationships (e.g., mother–daughter) often begin to form during the first months of pregnancy. As you will learn, sexuality encompasses much more than gender. It includes how we perceive ourselves, how we relate to others, and how we express ourselves as sexual beings.

ABOUT THE KEY CONCEPTS

Like many people, you may have been socialized to avoid talking openly about **sexuality.** As a nurse, though, you will find that you must discuss a variety of issues pertaining to sexuality that are vital for clients' optimal wellness. Some of these discussions may include **sexual dysfunctions,** infections, or behaviors. As you learn about concepts related to sexuality and sexual function, you will be challenged to confront and set aside your own biases to comfortably and competently address your clients' **sexual health** needs.

SEXUAL AND REPRODUCTIVE ANATOMY AND PHYSIOLOGY

The role of the reproductive system in human life extends far beyond its basic function of producing children. It influences body image, sexual desire, and sense of sexual identity. To explore human sexuality, you will need to understand the basics of reproductive anatomy and physiology.

Female Reproductive Organs

The female reproductive system consists of a pair of ovaries and fallopian tubes, the uterus, vagina, and external genital tissues (Fig. 34-1).

- **Ova** (eggs) are produced in the ovaries and travel through the **fallopian tubes** to the **uterus.** If fertilization occurs, the embryo embeds in the wall of the uterus for further development.
- The **vagina** is a muscular tube that receives sperm during sexual intercourse, allows the exit of menstrual flow if fertilization does not occur, and serves as a birth canal at the end of pregnancy.

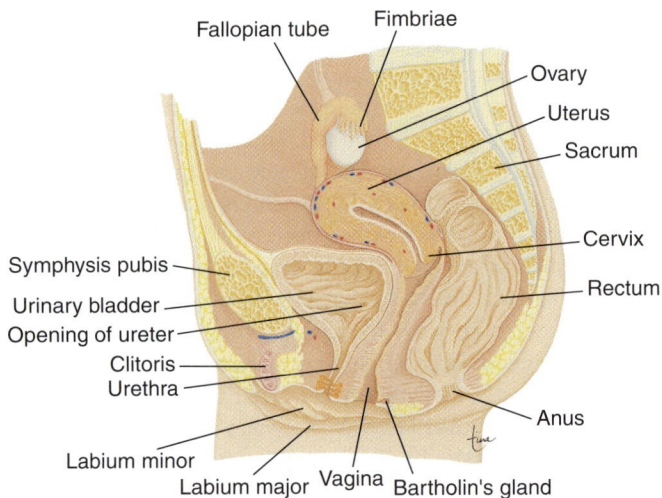

FIGURE 34-1 The female reproductive system.

- The external mons pubis and the external genitalia are a source of pleasurable sensations.
  - The **mons pubis** is a pad of fatty tissue over the symphysis pubis. It is covered with coarse hair and contains sensitive nerve endings.
  - The **external genitalia,** or **vulva,** consist of the clitoris, labia majora, labia minora, Bartholin's glands, urinary meatus, and vaginal introitus. The **clitoris** contains erectile tissue, blood vessels, and nerves. It is extremely sensitive and reacts to pleasurable stimuli. The **labia minora** also engorge and become sensitive during sexual stimulation. External genitalia organs such as the clitoris are protected by the **labia majora.**
- The **breasts** are important to female sexual arousal; in fact, some women can be brought to orgasm solely by caressing the breasts and nipples. The **mammary glands,** enclosed within the breasts, are also part of the reproductive system. Their function is to produce milk to provide nourishment for an infant after birth.

The Menstrual Cycle

Menstruation begins with puberty and involves hormone changes that prepare the body for pregnancy. The phases of the menstrual cycle are triggered by hormonal changes (Fig. 34-2).

- **Menstrual Phase**
  - Menstruation usually lasts 3 to 7 days, averaging 5 days.
  - The uterus sheds the endometrial lining and several ovarian follicles develop.
  - Follicle-stimulating hormone (FSH) from the anterior pituitary begins to increase, leading to a rise in estrogen levels.

- **Follicular Phase**
  - This phase begins on the first day of menstrual bleeding.
  - It is associated with growth of ovarian follicles and regrowth of the endometrium of the uterus.
  - This phase ends with **ovulation,** or release of the ovum from the mature follicle, around day 13 or 14 of the menstrual cycle.
  - Luteinizing hormone (LH) levels from the anterior pituitary rise, as does the estrogen level.
- **Ovulatory Phase**
  - A surge in LH and FSH occurs that lasts about 16 to 36 hours.
  - The follicle then ruptures and the egg is released for fertilization.
  - Estrogen peaks and progesterone rises, stimulating growth of the endometrium.
- **Luteal Phase**
  - If fertilization occurs, the endometrium thickens to support an embryo.
  - The pregnancy hormone, called chorionic gonadotropin, is produced. Pregnancy tests are based on detecting levels of this hormone.
  - If fertilization does not occur, progesterone levels drop, and menses begins.

Male Reproductive Organs

The male reproductive system consists of the testes and a series of ducts and glands that transport sperm.

- Sperm are produced in the **testes** and transported through the *epididymis, ductus deferens, ejaculatory duct,* and *urethra* (Fig. 34-3). Along the path, the **reproductive glands** (*seminal vesicles, prostate,* and *bulbourethral glands*) add secretions that mix with the sperm to produce semen.
- The **penis** functions in the urinary system to transport urine from the bladder to the outside of the body. It also has important functions in the reproductive system.
  - Within the penis are three sections of **erectile tissue:** the corpus cavernosum and sections of corpus spongiosum above and below the urethra.
  - During sexual arousal these erectile tissues fill with blood, making the penis erect.
- **Ejaculation** (the expulsion of semen) is brought about by peristalsis of the reproductive ducts and contraction of the prostate and muscles of the pelvic floor. With each ejaculation, approximately 100 million sperm cells are expelled in 2 to 4 mL of semen.

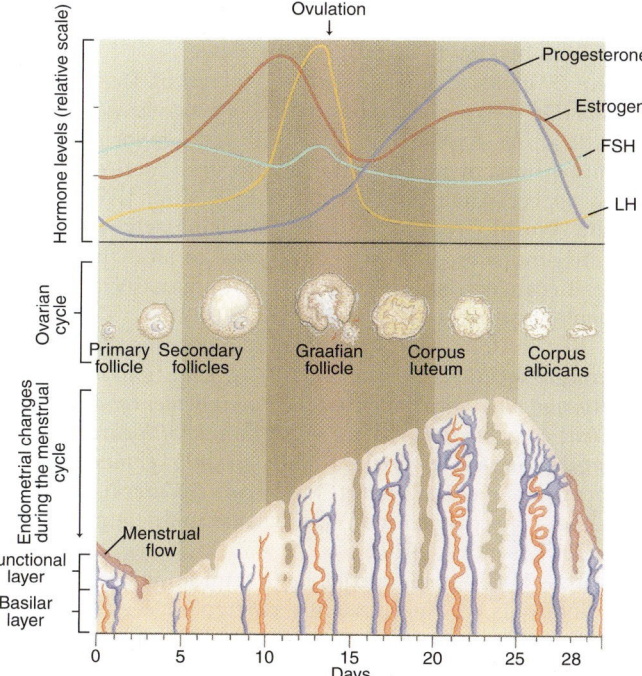

FIGURE 34-2 The menstrual cycle. Hormone levels and endometrial thickness throughout the cycle are shown.

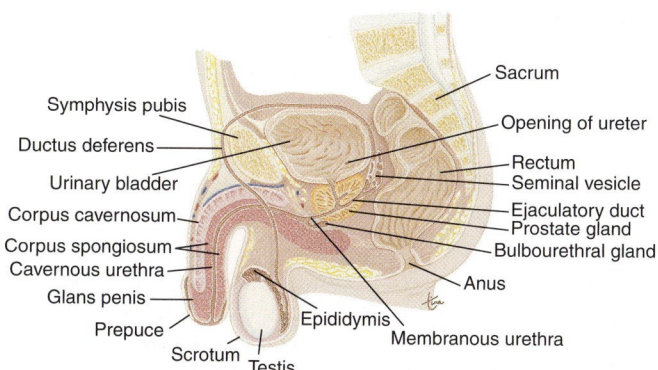

FIGURE 34-3 The male reproductive system.

KnowledgeCheck 34-1

- Identify the major structures of the female reproductive system.
- Summarize the phases of the menstrual cycle.
- Identify the major structures of the male reproductive system.

SEXUALITY

The World Health Organization (WHO) describes the following:

- **Sexuality** is a "central aspect of being human throughout life and encompasses sex, gender identities and roles, sexual orientation, eroticism, pleasure, intimacy and reproduction" (WHO, 2006, updated 2010).
- **Sexual identity** is a person's perception of his or her gender, gender identity, gender role, and sexual orientation. All of these are also a part of the person's overall self-concept (see Chapter 13 to review self-concept).

What Is Gender?

People often think of *sexuality* as a synonym for *sex*. This is inaccurate. In fact, even the word *sex* has multiple meanings. For example, *sex* is commonly used to describe intimate pleasurable activity or to indicate whether an individual is male or female. In this chapter, we use the term **gender** to indicate biological sex status (male or female) and follow WHO's definition of sexuality.

KEY POINT *Gender is determined at the moment of conception, when a sperm fertilizes an ovum. The ovum always provides an X chromosome.* The sperm may contribute either a second X chromosome, which results in a female offspring, or a Y chromosome, resulting in a male offspring (Fig. 34-4).

Gender Roles

Gender roles are the societal norms for gender-appropriate behavior. During the 1950s, the media portrayed the father-in-a-suit who went off to work to support his family. Mother, in her apron, spent the day cooking, cleaning, and caring for her perfect children and devoted husband. Even then, many Americans did not identify with this stereotype, and today it may seem unreal. But many of the values underlying those social norms remain embedded at some level within our contemporary culture (Fulcher & Coyle, 2011). Historically in Western culture,

- People expected men to be strong and to control their feelings. Boys received positive reinforcement for "masculine"

behaviors, such as competitiveness, and ridicule or teasing for showing emotions or being passive.

- Women were expected to be gentle and to express their feelings. In girls, "feminine" behaviors, such as cooperation, and passivity were reinforced, whereas assertiveness was often viewed as unacceptable aggression.

In the past 50 years, expectations regarding gender roles have changed and expanded. Women now perform jobs formerly thought to be "for men only" (e.g., physician, police officer); and men are entering professions once dominated by females (e.g., nursing, teaching).

Today, many parents encourage some **androgyny** in their children. The word *androgyny* is a combination of the Greek words for "male," *andro,* and "female," *gyn.* By one definition, *androgyny* refers to a blending of traditional masculine and feminine roles. It means that everyone has some skills, traits, and behaviors that may be classified as masculine and some that may be feminine. Androgyny is a positive trait in that it gives an individual greater adaptability in life situations.

ThinkLike a Nurse 34-1

- Provide at least three examples of nonconformity to traditional gender role expectations.
- As a parent, how might you encourage androgyny in your children, if you wished to do so?

Gender Identity

Gender identity, one component of sexual identity, is the image we have about ourselves as a man or woman. It is an internal experience: whether we "feel like" a woman or a man.

Gender identity emerges from environmental factors, developmental influences and societal norms (McCabe, McMillian, Padilla, et al., 2018).

- Gender Nonbinary or Gender Non-conforming. A person who does not identify with a gender (Wisner, 2018).
- **Transgender:** A person whose gender identity is not the same as his/her biological gender.
- The *Diagnostic and Statistical Manual of Mental Disorders (DSM-5)* replaced the concept of *gender identity disorder* with *gender dysphoria,* emphasized that gender nonconformity is not a mental disorder, and focused more on the clinical aspect (American Psychiatric Association [APA], 2013).
- **The World Health Organization** similarly reclassified transgender as gender incongruence to shift the focus to health care needs and minimize the stigma associated with a mental health classification (WHO, 2018).

    KEY POINT: *Although there are numerous and different terms associated with the concepts of gender and sexual identity, you must focus on providing nonjudgmental and quality client care. Barriers to care result from health care providers having limited awareness of the client's communication, social, and medical needs (Clark, Veale & Zaleski, 2018).*

    Other concepts commonly associated with gender identity include (Rosenthal, 2016):

- Transsexual is an older concept that traditionally referred to individuals who permanently change (or seek to change) their birth sex characteristics to that of the opposite gender by use medical interventions (e.g., surgery, hormones) and was later broadened to include those who were working toward living as a member of the sex opposite from that assigned at birth, irrespective of medical procedures undergone or planned (Moleiro & Pinto, 2015).
- KEY POINT: *The concept of transsexual may be viewed as derogatory and should be changed to trans woman or trans man.*

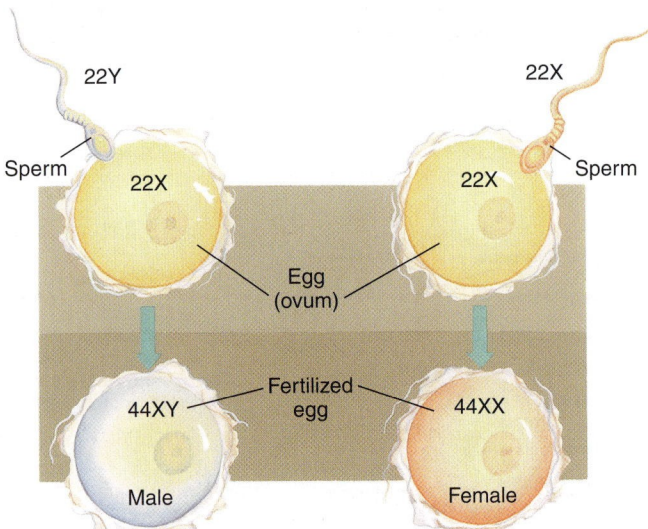

FIGURE 34-4 The woman provides the X chromosome and the may contribute either a second X chromosome, which results in a female offspring, or a Y chromosome, resulting in a male offspring.

♥ **iCare** *You should also ask the client what he or she prefers and communicate this to the healthcare team verbally and in the medical records to minimize repetitive questions to the client.*

- It is not uncommon for the trans individual to express dissatisfaction with his/her gender at an early age or have a preference for dress and play that is more typical of those of the nonbiological gender. The level of acceptance during the formative years can directly impact sexual health.

- Transition. The transitioning process from one's birth gender to the affirmed gender can range for social to medical choices. The social transition may include changing one's name, assuming the role of the affirmed gender, changing one's physical appearance through dress, cosmetics, and so on (Bizic, Jeftovic, Pusica, et al., 2018). To physically align one's body with the identified gender, various gender affirming treatments may be undertaken (e.g., hormonal therapy, gender reassignment surgery, mastectomy, oophorectomy) (Adriaansen, Perry, Perry, et. al, 2017). Transitioning requires therapeutic, and sometimes, extensive counseling to promote a successful social, emotional, role and physical transition.

- **Intersexed people** (formerly referred to as **hermaphrodites**) are born with ambiguous sexual organs. For example, the person may have female internal organs (ovaries, a uterus), but enlarged clitoral tissue resembling a penis. Initially, a developing embryo is in an **undifferentiated sexual state**—neither male nor female until about the seventh week of pregnancy when the gonads form into either testes or ovaries. A mutation of any of the genes during this process may result in altered genitalia. Parents must decide whether to have the child undergo surgery to make the assigned sex consistent with the physical appearance or to delay assignment and allow the child to choose at a later time.

- Genderqueer may describe a person whose identity is neither, both, or a combination of masculine and feminine characteristics or expressions.

KnowledgeCheck 34-2

- How is gender determined?
- Distinguish *gender*, *gender role*, and *gender identity*.
- What is *androgyny*?

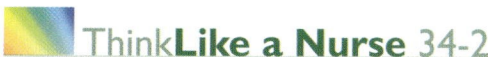 Think**Like a Nurse** 34-2

Do you believe that androgyny is a positive attribute? Explain your thinking

What Is Sexual Orientation?

Sexual orientation refers to the general tendency of a person to feel sexually attracted to people of a certain gender. Because most people in Western culture are thought to be **heterosexual** (sexually attracted to members of the opposite sex), heterosexuality is the predominant cultural expectation. However, in the mid-20th century, the research of Alfred C. Kinsey indicated that a population's sexual orientation falls on a bell curve, with the majority of people experiencing at least some attraction to people of the same gender (Kinsey, 1948/1998). Kinsey theorized that society influences people to sublimate homosexual feelings and choose exclusively heterosexual relationships.

Klein, Sepekoff, and Wolf (1985) described sexual orientation as an ongoing dynamic process, with people's gender-based inclinations changing over time. We do not fully understand what makes up sexual orientation or how it develops. With increasing research on the biological aspects of sexual orientation (Sanders,

Martin, Beecham, et al., 2015), more professionals are concluding that people come to "recognize" the object of their sexual desire rather than "choose" or "prefer" it. Therefore, *sexual orientation* is probably a more accurate term than *sexual preference*.

Heterosexuality

Heterosexuals are people who are sexually and emotionally attracted to members of the opposite sex. In informal discourse, people may refer to this segment of the population as *straight*. Although some heterosexuals may have had same-gender sexual thoughts or limited experiences during childhood, adolescence, or adulthood, they still consider themselves heterosexual and have relationships with people of the opposite gender.

Homosexuality

The focus of sexual attraction for **homosexuals** is a person of the same gender. Homosexuals may be referred to as *gay* men and *lesbian* women. Accurate prevalence statistics are difficult to obtain because most studies rely on self-report data. Same sex relationships, although not readily accepted by some religions are being integrated into the dominant culture. The landmark ruling by the U.S. Supreme Court has created a freedom of sexual expression in the lesbian, gay, bisexual, and transgender community and created legitimacy in relationships and marriage (*Obergefell v. Hodges,* 2015). More individuals from the LGBTQ community now share this aspect of their lives with employers, colleagues, family, and friends, as well as with researchers and pollsters. However, some may continue to hide this aspect of their life from others.

Bisexuality

A person who is **bisexual** is sexually and emotionally attracted to both males and females. This group is perhaps least understood and least accepted by both the heterosexual and homosexual communities and may experience feelings of isolation. Research shows that while bisexual individuals have poor mental health outcomes compared to their heterosexual counterparts, females have worse outcomes than males (Taylor, 2018).

Some bisexuals maintain stable and satisfying marriages because of their sustained sexual attraction to and amiable relationship with their spouse, as well as the importance they place on parenting; while others may experience difficulty in maintaining long-term monogamous relationships.

♥ **iCare** *It is important to conduct a thorough sexual health assessment and have an open, non-judgmental, caring attitude to fully ascertain the needs of your clients.*

Additional Concepts

Other concepts that describe sexual orientation include:

- Pansexual persons are attracted to other people regardless of their gender, biological sex, or gender identity.
- Polysexual persons are attracted to more than one gender or to a combinations of genders.
- Asexual persons usually do not feel a sexual attraction toward other people.

KnowledgeCheck 34-3

- What are the majority and minority sexual orientations in our culture?
- What is meant by transgender?

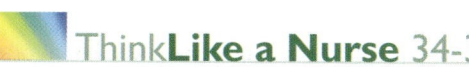 Think**Like a Nurse** 34-3

- What sexual orientations are you comfortable working with?
- Would you have difficulty working with a transsexual or other transgendered client?

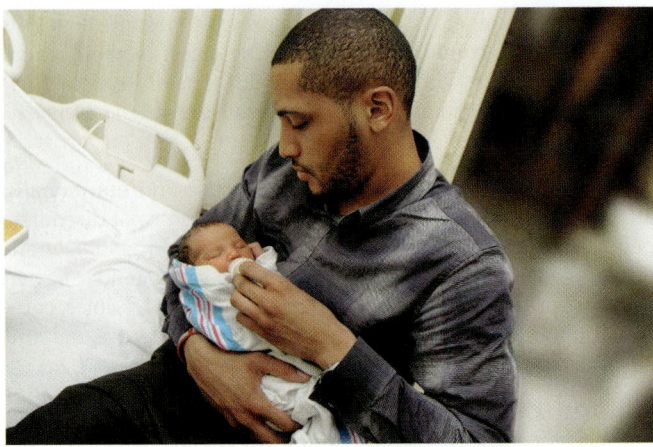

FIGURE 34-5 Parent–infant attachment occurs through daily contact and care through activities such as feeding, bathing, and holding.

give factual information without offering explanations beyond what the child asks.

School Age Through Puberty

The school-age child strongly identifies with the same-sex parent and has mostly same-sex friends. Through interaction at home, school, and other activities, children gain awareness of gender roles and emerging gender identity. From age 8 to 12 years, the child is in transition between childhood and puberty. Secondary sex characteristics become apparent.

- In females, breast buds form and pubic hair appears. For a significant number of girls, **menarche** (beginning of menstruation) occurs.
- Boys become more muscular, the voice deepens, facial and axillae hair develops, and the genitals begin to increase in size.
- The first attraction, either heterosexual or homosexual, may occur during this stage, and the child may begin to masturbate more frequently, but privately.
- For information on the Tanner stages of sexual development in boys and girls, see the tables in Procedures 21-17 and 21-18.

Many school-age children are curious and may ask explicit questions about sexual activity, reproduction, and sex roles. Parents and nurses should answer with facts and follow up with age-appropriate material. When children reach the age range of 10 to 12, parents should begin teaching them basic information about body changes, menstruation, sexual intercourse, and reproduction.

Adolescents

Adolescence is a time of heightened sexual interest and activity, primarily because of:

1. The hormonal changes accompanying puberty
2. Cultural emphasis on sex

Masturbation is common and a safe and comforting sexual activity that has neither interpersonal nor disease risks. However, some adolescents may encounter parental, cultural, or religious disapproval of masturbation. Further sexual exploration usually begins with kissing, moves on to fondling, and can lead to genital contact. This progression may occur over a period of years, or there may be an early initiation of oral, vaginal, or anal intercourse.

Incidence of Sexual Activity

- 18% of males had engaged in sexual intercourse by age 15, 44% by age 17, and 69% by age 19.

- Similarly, 13% of females had engaged in intercourse by age 15, 43% by age 17, and 68% by age 19 (Martinez & Abma, 2015).
- Despite the increasing frequency of sexual activity, the birth rate for adolescents and teenagers reached a historic low in 2013 (Martin, Hamilton, & Osterman, 2015).
- The incidence of oral sex is increasing in U.S. youths. Two-thirds of youths between the ages of 15 and 25 have engaged in oral sex (Copen, Chandra, & Martinez, 2012). Many teens believe that this behavior allows them to maintain their virginity and incorrectly assume that it carries no health risks.
- Sexuality education in the home and school dispels myths and prepares teens for adult roles. To make informed choices as they move toward adulthood, adolescents need information about body changes, interpersonal relationships, **contraception** (birth control), and preventing sexually transmitted infections (STIs).

To review physical changes of adolescence, see Chapters 9 and 21.

Young Adults

Traditionally, it was generally assumed that young adults would abstain from sexual intercourse until marriage. The husband and wife would become sexually active and start a family. Today, the age of first marriage is higher than in previous decades, and young adults engage more openly in sexual activity outside of marriage. Many young adults practice **serial monogamy,** in which the partners are mutually faithful but make no lifelong commitment. When the relationship ends, each partner usually enters another monogamous relationship.

During early adulthood, people define their sexual identity and resolve issues related to their sexual orientation and self-concept. As a part of sexual maturity, they develop an intimate relationship in which there is both communication and respect. Many people find a life partner during this period and make long-term plans, which often include parenting. However, some adults continue to struggle with their sexual identity, sexual orientation, or ability to form or commit to intimate relationships.

Young adults often wonder whether their sexual behaviors and responses are normal (e.g., "How often do most people have intercourse?" "Do other women have an orgasm every time they have sex?"). Information about birth control, prevention of STIs, sexual expression, and communication issues is still needed.

Middle Adults

In their middle years, adults experience life changes that may enhance physical and emotional intimacy. For many, their children are young adults who no longer rely on parental support, and the parents may have more privacy and time to spend together. However, new stressors may arise. In times of economic downturn, for example, middle adults are one of the groups most seriously affected. In addition, this may also be a time when physical changes and chronic diseases emerge that could affect sexual patterns.

Female Transitions Women transition through **menopause** (cessation of menstruation). Some are relieved that the prospect of childbearing has ended; others may mourn the loss of the ability to give birth. Normal physiological changes include decreased vaginal secretions and vaginal wall thinning, which result from decreased levels of estrogen and progesterone. These changes may result in painful intercourse and diminish a woman's desire for sexual activity.

Middle Adults

In their middle years, adults experience life changes that may enhance physical and emotional intimacy. For many, their children are young adults who no longer rely on parental support, and the parents may have more privacy and time to spend together. However, new stressors may arise. In times of economic downturn, for example, middle adults are one of the groups most seriously affected. In addition, this may also be a time when physical changes and chronic diseases emerge that could affect sexual patterns.

Female Transitions Women transition through **menopause** (cessation of menstruation). Some are relieved that the prospect of childbearing has ended; others may mourn the loss of the ability to give birth. Normal physiological changes include decreased vaginal secretions and vaginal wall thinning, which result from decreased levels of estrogen and progesterone. These changes may result in painful intercourse and diminish a woman's desire for sexual activity. Some women also experience hot flashes, sleep disturbances, and mood changes.

Male Transitions Because of the aging process or certain health conditions (e.g., type 2 diabetes or hypertension), men may experience erectile difficulty. They may perceive this problem as a threat to their masculinity and sexual attractiveness, and their self-image may suffer. Men also experience a decrease in the sex hormone testosterone. Many men remain fertile into old age, although sexual desire and the ability to achieve and maintain an erection decrease gradually with aging.

It may be a challenge for you to view middle adults as individuals who engage in and enjoy sexual relations. Patients of this age may remind you of your parents and thus it may be difficult for you to see them as persons who have sexual relationships. Holistic nursing care requires you to assess and formulate strategies to address their sexual concerns.

Older Adults

Most older adults are sexually active and regard sexuality as an important part of life. Little evidence exists to support the premise that age-related changes result in decreased sexual relationships (Delamater, 2010). A substantial number of men and women engage in vaginal intercourse, oral sex, and masturbation into their 80s and 90s (Delamater, 2010; Koh & Sewell, 2015; Taylor & Gosney, 2011). You should recognize that older adults have sexual needs (e.g., reassurance from a sexual partner or sexual stimulation) and sexual problems (e.g., lack of closeness).

Sexual problems are more likely to result from failing physical health and medication side effects than from age alone. For example, as noted earlier, men with diabetes are more likely to have difficulty achieving and maintaining an erection. Other obstacles for sexual expression include the following:

- Lack of a partner (especially for women)
- Lack of privacy (e.g., for those who live with family members or in a long-term care facility) (Bauer, McAuliffe, Nay, et al., 2013)

Some problems that may occur as a result of age-related changes include the following:

- **Postmenopausal women report less sexual stimulation and reduced desire,** so they tend to need more foreplay and direct clitoral stimulation for sexual enjoyment. They may have fewer orgasms or orgasms that are weaker in intensity. Nevertheless, some women "rediscover" sexual desire after menopause.
- **Older women may complain of pain during intercourse,** caused by loss of vaginal lubrication and vaginal thinning and dryness. You can help your patients by suggesting water-soluble lubricants to counteract dryness and enhance pleasurable sensations during sexual activity.
- **Some men report erectile difficulty** and need more time and more direct genital stimulation to achieve erection. It may take longer to ejaculate, and the orgasmic contractions may be less intense. When penetration is not possible (e.g., because of male erectile dysfunction [ED]), many couples find satisfaction with alternate forms of sexual stimulation and expression.

In the past, many healthcare providers have hesitated to offer sexual counseling out of fear that such intimate discussion might embarrass their patients. Older adults may also hesitate to discuss their sexual problems unless encouraged to do so. Address the topic as you would any other area (e.g., "We have discussed your medical needs and your dietary needs; let's now discuss your sexual needs"). Once you introduce the subject and people feel comfortable, they are usually eager for advice and solutions (American Geriatrics Society, updated 2012).

You can help aging clients to understand that sexual feelings do not necessarily disappear with age, and sexual expression need not stop. For example, sexual expression may include hugging, caressing, oral sex, and mutual manual stimulation. In addition, you may suggest ways to adapt coital positions to accommodate bodily changes, for example, when a partner is obese or has joint immobility.

KnowledgeCheck 34-4

- Why is it important to consider sexuality throughout the life cycle?
- What are the two major contributing factors to adolescents' heightened sexual interest and activity?
- What aspects of human sexuality are associated with young and middle adulthood?
- What challenges to sexuality may be found in the aging adult?

What Factors Affect Sexuality?

Various factors affect our attitudes toward sexuality, sexual behaviors, and intimate relationships. This section will help you to provide nonjudgmental, holistic care to people who have a wide range of values, lifestyles, and states of well-being.

Culture

Culture influences our ideas about gender role, gender identity, marriage, sexual expression, and social responsibilities. However, it is not unusual for people to be **ethnocentric**—that is, to see their own culture and sexual behaviors as the norm for all. Because the United States is a multicultural country, beliefs and practices related to human sexuality vary widely.

- Puritan and Victorian-era and later puritanical legacies have influenced many European Americans, some of whom consider sex to be "not nice," particularly if engaging in certain sexual activities or positions.
- African Americans are influenced by the dominant Anglo-Saxon culture as well as by their African heritage, history in America, and current economic and social situation. Marriage rates for African Americans are lower than for other ethnic groups, in part because of an unequal gender ratio (84 males per 100 females) (Hyde & DeLamater, 2013).
- Many Latinos have strong ties to the Roman Catholic Church and a tradition of rigidly defined gender roles. The norm in Hispanic culture is for the male to be given more freedom as a child, but he is expected to be a virile, responsible provider for his family as an adult. In contrast, the

female is typically raised to be more passive and obedient throughout her life.

- Asian Americans and Muslim Americans tend to be the most sexually conservative of the major U.S. cultural groups.

Culture determines what is acceptable and what is not. In some societies, **polygamy** (marriage to more than one partner) may be acceptable. Many cultures have special rites of passage at puberty, such as the Jewish bar mitzvah for boys and bat mitzvah for girls, or the vision quests in certain Native American cultures.

Female Genital Mutilation Generally, you should honor cultural practices unless they are harmful. An example of a harmful practice is **female genital mutilation** (formerly known as **female circumcision**), which is illegal in most countries but is still performed among certain tribes. In this procedure, the labia majora, labia minora, and clitoris are excised, and/or the vagina is sutured closed **(infibulation).** Infibulation may be done to ensure that the girl remains a virgin, whereas clitoral excision is meant to reduce sexual desire and ensure that the woman remains faithful to her husband. In addition to its psychosocial consequences, the procedure carries a high risk of infection and can cause the development of scar tissue that makes vaginal birth impossible.

The U.S. Congress passed a law in 1996 making female genital mutilation of girls younger than 18 a federal offense. The World Health Organization in 1997 and again in 2012, with the support of the United Nations, issued a statement to abolish the practice of female genital mutilation (WHO, 2010, updated 2014).

Religion

Religion also has a powerful influence on sexuality. Consider the following:

- Religious practices restricting premarital sex, birth control, homosexuality, abortion, extramarital relationships, and masturbation are common.
- Some religions restrict opposite gender healthcare providers and have rules about body coverings and modesty.
- Some religions even govern education about the structure and function of the human body.

The "sexual revolution" that began in the 1960s has led to permissive sexual values in the broader Western culture. When these values conflict with a person's traditional religious values, anxiety and sexual dysfunction may result. To review the influence of religion on health, see Chapter 16.

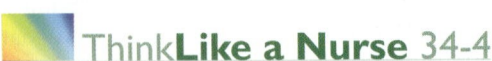

ThinkLike a Nurse 34-4

How have religion and culture influenced your views on sexuality?

Lifestyle

Life experiences encompass our interactions with others and the environment. Family, socioeconomic status, employment factors, and interpersonal relationships shape, but do not determine, our lifestyle. Consider the following examples:

- Having a beloved brother reveal to you that he is gay might alter your perception of homosexuality. Similarly, being raised by a lesbian couple might affect your view of gender roles.
- Being in an abusive relationship would affect your self-concept and might cause you to avoid intimacy in the future.

Lessons learned through day-to-day experiences create powerful impressions on our views and often modify cultural and religious influences.

Sexual Knowledge

Although sexuality and family life are part of the curriculum in many public schools, you cannot assume that young adults have adequate sexual knowledge. Community values play a large role in determining how sexuality is viewed and taught. Thus, even if a state mandates sex education, some schools may allow students to opt out with parenteral consent or may limit discussion on reproduction, STIs, birth control, intimacy, exploitive relationships, domestic abuse, or rape, believing that these topics are best addressed by the family or church. In addition, many children are home-schooled or taught in private or church-affiliated schools that do not allocate class time to sex education. **KEY POINT** *Do not let your clients' age, level of education, or life experiences lead you to make assumptions about their knowledge of sexuality.* For example, consider the following:

- A married person may not be sexually active.
- A woman with several children may not know what is involved in a pelvic exam or how conception occurs.
- A highly educated person may be uninformed regarding his body's structure and function.

It is difficult for most people to admit to a professional that they lack knowledge. Therefore, you must assess each client's knowledge and understanding of sexual terms. At times, you may need to use the vernacular or "street" terminology to be understood. You can then introduce medically specific terminology.

KnowledgeCheck 34-5

- What sexual knowledge would you expect an adult male with children to have?
- What sexual knowledge would you expect a nursing student to have?

Health and Illness

Sexuality involves body, mind, and spirit so it is not surprising that health status affects sexuality. For example, healthful nutrition and physical exercise are commonly reported to increase satisfaction in sexual relationships, whereas obesity and inactivity can undermine one's own feelings of attractiveness or one's attraction for one's partner. The importance of sexuality is readily apparent in the clinical setting. For example, the clients in the Meet Your Patients scenarios all expressed concerns related to their sexuality.

Physical Illness Diseases, injuries, and medical treatments may demand lifestyle changes in multiple areas, including sexual functioning. For example,

- *Heart disease or respiratory disease* may cause people to restrict sexual activity because of fatigue, dyspnea, or fear of overstressing the heart.
- *Diabetes mellitus* leads to neurological changes that may cause male erectile dysfunction; women may experience vaginal dryness and loss of orgasmic ability.
- *Mastectomy* (surgical removal of a breast) can have a significant influence on a woman's self-esteem and negatively impact sexuality

If a person becomes disabled while in a marriage or other committed relationship, the strain can threaten the partnership. In contrast, a person who is single or has a lifelong disability may experience difficulty establishing an intimate relationship because of physical limitations, social isolation, poor self-image, or discrimination.

A need for intimacy still exists even when people lose interest in sexual activities. Communication about sexual needs and desires may be difficult for couples, but as a nurse, you can support and facilitate discussions of your clients concerns. Holistic rehabilitation programs may offer comprehensive services and promote discussion regarding sexuality and relationship issues.

Mental Health Disorders Psychiatric disorders can lead to interpersonal disruptions and difficulty with sexual expression.

- A depressed person experiences significant loss of interest in activities that previously brought pleasure. Thus it is common for people with depression to avoid engaging in interpersonal activities, including sex.
- Conversely, a person with hypomania or mania may be preoccupied with pleasurable activities and increased sexual activity, as well as verbalization and acting out. Both extremes are disruptive to a relationship.
- For a person with psychosis, interpersonal relationships and sexual patterns are disrupted by lack of contact with reality or frank delusions.

Counseling for the couple is important when symptoms are controlled. During times of acute illness, it is vital that the client has medical and psychological support.

Medication Many medications used to treat health problems have unwelcome sexual side effects. Gabriel Thomas (Meet Your Patients) clearly illustrates the concern some clients have about commonly prescribed medications. Table 34-1 lists a number of medications and their effects on sexual function.

- **Medications may be prescribed to enhance sexual function,** particularly for men experiencing erectile dysfunction (ED), for example, those with diabetes mellitus or those who are taking beta-adrenergic blocking agents to treat high blood pressure. Three oral drugs are available for impotence: sildenafil, vardenafil, and tadalafil. These drugs generally work within 1 hour of administration, but have no effect without sexual stimulation. They increase blood flow to the corpus cavernosum of the penis.

- ✚ Sildenafil (Viagra) should be used with caution in patients with cardiovascular disease because of its vasodilation effects and is contraindicated in patients receiving nitrate drugs. Conduct a careful medication history and provide the appropriate patient teaching.

KnowledgeCheck 34-6

- Identify four factors associated with physical illness that may affect sexuality or sexual functioning.
- What determines our sexual attitudes?

SEXUAL HEALTH

The World Health Organization defines **sexual health** (a key concept in this chapter) as a state of physical, emotional, mental, and social well-being related to sexuality; it is not merely the absence of disease, dysfunction, or infirmity. Attaining and maintaining sexual health requires the following:

- A positive and respectful approach to sexuality and sexual relationships
- An openness and opportunity to have pleasurable and safe sexual experiences, free of coercion, discrimination, and violence
- The respected, protected, and fulfilled sexual rights of all persons (WHO, 2006, updated 2010).

To promote sexual health effectively, you will need theoretical knowledge about sexual responses, modes of sexual expression, and problems affecting sexuality.

ThinkLike a Nurse 34-5

Examine your own beliefs about sexuality. Identify areas of concern you have regarding sexuality. How do you think this will affect your ability to assist patients with sexual health concerns?

What Is the Sexual Response Cycle?

The **sexual response cycle** is the sequence of physiological events that occur when a person becomes sexually aroused. Based on research conducted in the 1950s, Masters and Johnson (1966) identified a four-stage sexual response: excitement, plateau, orgasm, and resolution (Fig. 34-6). Some scholars have suggested that a stage of desire be added to the original Masters and Johnson model. In some people, desire can either precede or follow excitement (Basson, 2001, 2008).

Table 34-1 ▶ Effects of Drugs on Sexual Function

MEDICATION	POSSIBLE EFFECT
Alcohol	In limited quantities, alcohol may enhance desire and function. However, heavy or chronic use may lead to decreased libido, orgasmic dysfunction, and erectile dysfunction.
Anti-anxiety agents	Decreased libido, delayed ejaculation
Anticonvulsants	Decreased libido, prolonged painful erections, difficulty achieving orgasm
Antidepressants	Decreased libido, difficulty achieving orgasm
	Bupropion (Wellbutrin) and trazodone (Desyrel) are least likely to cause sexual side effects.
Antihistamines	Decreased libido, decreased vaginal lubrication
Antihypertensives	Decreased libido, erectile dysfunction, delayed ejaculation
	Calcium channel blockers are least likely to cause sexual difficulties.
Chemotherapy	Fatigue, decreased libido
Opioids	Decreased libido, erectile dysfunction
Stimulants (cocaine, methamphetamines)	Initially, stimulants cause increased intensity of the sexual encounter; however, with continued use, sexual dysfunction develops.

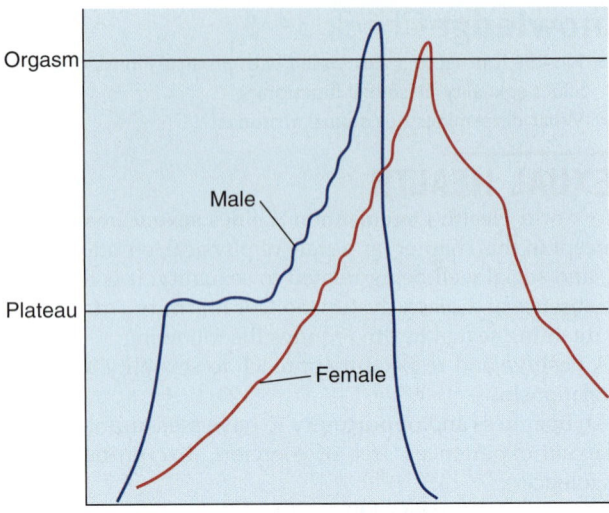

FIGURE 34-6 The sexual response cycle.

Although it is most intense in the genitals, **sexual response** is a total body response, involving many physiological changes (e.g., increased heart rate, flushing). The emotional and mental aspects of sexual activity are equally important to the person's satisfaction. The body has many **erogenous zones** (areas that cause sexual arousal when stimulated): the genitals, the skin, lips, ears, breasts, buttocks, and thighs. Table 34-2 shows normal physiological changes in sexual response that occur with aging.

Desire

Desire is a stage of varying length characterized by an interest in sexual intimacy. Desire occurs in the mind and is communicated verbally or through body language. This communication may be subtle and easily misread. Desire increases in proportion to the level of the sex hormones (e.g., a man with low testosterone is not as interested in sex). For women, desire reaches a peak each month near the time of ovulation, when estrogen levels are high. **Libido** is an individual's typical level of desire.

Toward Evidence-Based Practice

The sexual behaviors of older adults and the relationship between sexuality and quality of life in older adults are the subjects of ongoing research.

Penhollow, T. M., Young, M., & Denny, G. (2009). Predictors of quality of life, sexual intercourse, and sexual satisfaction in older adults. *American Journal of Health Education, 40*(1), 13–22.

This study attempted to identify aspects of sexuality that have the greatest influence on (1) sexual intercourse, (2) sexual satisfaction, and (3) overall quality of life of residents in a retirement community. Sexual self-confidence was found to be the single most important predictor of sexual intercourse and sexual satisfaction; for women, quality of life was also an important predictor. The following factors help to explain sexual satisfaction beyond the physical health:

- Cultural: Sexual acceptance and sexual priority
- Psychological: Sexual desire, sexual self-confidence, and control
- Social factors: Satisfaction in relationship and social life

Syme, M., Klonoff, E., Macera, C., et al. (2013). Predicting sexual decline and dissatisfaction among older adults: The role of partnered and individual physical and mental health factors. *Journals of Gerontology Series B: Psychological Sciences and Social Sciences, 68*(3), 323–332.

Researchers measured the concept of sexual unwellness in adults 63 to 68 years of ages. The majority of adults (64.2%) were sexually active at least once a month to once a day or more.

- Fatigue symptoms, history of diabetes, and poor spousal health were associated with a lack of sexual satisfaction and inability to maintain the sexual relationship.
- Gender differences revealed that women were more likely to report a lack of sexual satisfaction, which was usually partner related.

- For males, spousal support and good spousal health decreased the risk of unsatisfactory sexual relations.

Doll, G. (2013). Sexuality in nursing homes: Practice and policy. *Journal of Gerontological Nursing, 39*(7), 30–37.

Administrators or social workers in 91 nursing homes responded to a survey regarding sexual expressions of residents in nursing homes and residential care facilities. Results revealed that residents:

- Engaged in sexual talk (85%) (e.g., sexually explicit language, verbal propositioning)
- Demonstrated sexual acts (85%) (e.g., masturbation, fondling, intercourse)
- Formed romantic relationships (66%)
- Showed implied sexual acts (60%) (e.g., reading pornography).

The reactions of the nursing staff varied, from informing the supervisor (68.9%), trying to respectfully help the resident (51.1%), following the facility's policy (41%), and ignoring the issue (27.8%) to panic (20%).

1. What trend in the research about sexuality in older adults do you see?

2. In the Penhollow et al. study, what was the single most important factor influencing sexual satisfaction and quality of life, other than physical health? What additional factor was identified in the Syme et al. study? What do you think nurses can do to promote it?

3. Based on these studies, how do you think nurses can affect the quality of sexuality in older adults?

 Go to Davis Advantage, Resources, Chapter 33, **Toward Evidence-Based Practice—Suggested Responses.**

Table 34-2 ▶ Normal Physiological Changes in Sexual Response That Occur With Aging

SEXUAL RESPONSE STAGE	CHANGES IN WOMEN	CHANGES IN MEN
Desire	Decreased libido	Decreased libido
Excitement and plateau	Delayed nipple erection	Delayed nipple erection
	Reduced labial separation and swelling	Delayed and less-firm erection
	Reduced vaginal expansion	Longer excitement stage
	Reduced lubrication	Decreased pre-ejaculatory emissions
	Decreased elevation of the uterus	Reduced muscle tension
	Reduced muscle tension	Reduced lifting of the scrotum and testes
	Reduced vaginal tone (in those who have had multiple vaginal deliveries); results in less stimulation during intercourse	Shorter phase of impending orgasm
		May require more direct stimulation to achieve and maintain an erection
Orgasm	Reduced spread of sexual flush	Shorter ejaculation time
		Fewer ejaculatory contractions
		Reduced volume of ejaculate
Resolution	No cervical dilation	More rapid loss of erection
		Longer refractory period
		Nipple erection lasts longer after orgasm

Sources: Aging and the sexual response cycle. 2014). *SexInfo Online.* Retrieved from http://www.soc.ucsb.edu/sexinfo/article/aging-and-sexual-response-cycle-0; Cash, J., & Glass, C. (2015). *Adult-gerontology practice guidelines.* New York, NY: Springer; Ginsberg, T. (2010). Male sexuality. *Clinics in Geriatric Medicine, 26*(2), 185–195; Mauk, K. (2014). *Gerontological nursing: Competencies for care.* Burlington, MA: Jones & Bartlett Learning; Tsitouras, P. (2011). Male menopause: Just the facts. *Clinical Geriatrics, 19*(8), 28–32; Yee, L. (2010). Aging and sexuality. *Australian Family Physician, 39*(10), 718–721.

Sexual arousal (excitement) is desire that occurs with erotic stimuli such as sights, sounds, and fantasies. Desire can occur in anticipation of sexual activity or with physical stimulation.

What is considered "sexual" or "attractive" can vary greatly, because societal, cultural, and personal values influence the range of stimuli that provoke sexual desire. Desire may last only moments or be ongoing for years. Transient sexual thoughts are fleeting moments of desire that might be triggered by exposure to sexually explicit media or erotic thoughts, words, or actions.

Excitement

Excitement is the body's physical response to desire. During excitement the following bodily changes occur: heart rate, blood pressure, and respiratory rate increase; muscles tense **(myotonia);** nipples become erect; and genital and pelvic blood supply increases **(vasocongestion).**

- *In women,* vasocongestion leads to vaginal lubrication, swelling of the breasts, rise of the uterus, and swelling of the labia and clitoris.
- *In men,* erection begins as the penis increases in length and diameter. The testes rise closer to the body, and the scrotum thickens.

Excitement may lead to further sexual activity, but this is not inevitable. For both sexes, the person may lose and regain initial physical excitement many times without advancing to the next stage. Excitement may be communicated verbally or through body language.

Plateau

If stimulation continues, the person reaches the **plateau** phase. Plateau is associated with continued increases in pulse,

respiratory rate, blood pressure, and muscle tension. Some people flush around the face, neck, and chest in this phase. The person may achieve, lose, and regain the plateau phase several times without experiencing orgasm.

- *In women,* the areolae become firmer, the clitoris retracts into the clitoral hood, Bartholin's glands lubricate, and the lower vagina swells and narrows. With a male partner, the vagina tightens around the man's penis, increasing his sexual stimulation.
- *In men,* the ridge of the glans penis becomes more prominent, pre-ejaculate (two or three drops of fluid) is emitted, and the testes rise closer to the body.

Orgasm

Orgasm occurs at the peak of the plateau phase. At the moment of orgasm, the sexual tension that has been building is released. The heart rate, respiratory rate, and blood pressure reach their peak, and there is loss of voluntary muscle tone.

- *In women,* spinal cord reflexes cause powerful rhythmic contractions of the vagina, uterus, anus, and pelvic floor muscles; feelings of warmth spread through the pelvic area. The cervical canal dilates, allowing easy transport of the sperm to the uterus. Orgasm may last for a few seconds or up to nearly a minute.
- *In men,* spinal cord reflexes cause the urethra, anus, and pelvic floor muscles to contract, followed by **ejaculation** (the expelling of semen through the urethra). For men, orgasm usually lasts no more than 30 seconds.

The intensity of orgasm varies among individuals and in each individual from one sexual experience to another. Orgasm may involve intense spasm associated with intense focus on the sexual pleasure, or it may be signaled by as little as a sigh or subtle relaxation.

Resolution

Resolution is the period of time following orgasm. The muscles relax, and the body returns to its pre-excitement state.

- *Men*—Immediately after orgasm, men experience a **refractory period,** during which they cannot achieve an erection. The duration of this period varies among individuals and increases with age.
- *Women*—Woman experience no refractory period; they can either enter the resolution stage or return to the excitement or plateau stage immediately following orgasm.

KnowledgeCheck 34-7

Identify the phase of the sexual response cycle described in the following:

- This phase is reached if there is ongoing stimulation. This stage may be achieved, lost, and regained several times without the occurrence of orgasm.
- This stage occurs in the mind and may be communicated between potential sexual partners either verbally or through body language.
- This phase is associated with the release of sexual tension.

ThinkLike a Nurse 34-6

Critique the theory of Masters and Johnson, as represented in the preceding discussion of the sexual response cycle. How would you respond to the statement that the theory does not adequately address variation among individuals and even within an individual's sexual response?

What Are Some Forms of Sexual Expression?

People express their sexuality and gain sexual satisfaction in many different ways. Although opinions vary, a range of behaviors is socially acceptable and therefore considered "normal" by most people in our society. These behaviors are discussed in the following sections:

Developing Intimate Relationships

Developing intimate relationships involves a willingness to take risks and offer trust. Intimacy involves openness, mutual respect, caring, commitment, protection, honesty, and devotion. Although we often think of intimate relationships as sexual, they are not necessarily so. Furthermore, in our society, many sexual relationships occur without intimacy.

Fantasies and Erotic Dreams

Most men and women have sexual fantasies. They may be related to past experiences, dreams, or desires, or to stories heard, seen, or read. Sexual fantasies serve to increase self-esteem and sexual arousal and as an outlet to explore sexual desires. People in long-term monogamous relationships may fantasize to bring variety and excitement into a routine sexual encounter. Erotic dreams are common among both men and women. Nighttime or nocturnal orgasm may or may not occur with the dream.

Masturbation

Masturbation is self-stimulation of the genitals. Although there are many techniques, men typically stroke the shaft of the penis, and women typically stimulate the clitoris manually.

- Young children touch their genitals as a part of body exploration, but they quickly learn either that touching certain areas is not acceptable or that it should be done in private.
- Adolescents, particularly males, may masturbate frequently.
- Adults may masturbate for sexual release when a partner is not available or for variety in a partnered relationship.

Sex therapists often recommend masturbation as a means to resolve orgasm difficulties in women and ejaculatory problems in men. Religious and social taboos discouraging masturbation are common. Some people mistakenly believe that masturbation is harmful, causing acne, warts, blindness, or insanity. More commonly, masturbation is considered a "dirty," shameful, or perverted act.

Shared Touching

Mutual masturbation, or shared touching, may be an alternative to sexual intercourse. This is particularly appealing to individuals who seek to maintain virginity, decrease the risk of STIs, or have mobility or other physical problems that make intercourse difficult. Mutual masturbation is recognized as a form of safer sex because body fluids are not likely to be exchanged. This behavior can be satisfying because it allows for a significant level of sexual intimacy and for participants to experience orgasm.

Sexual Intercourse

Sexual intercourse and **coitus** are terms used to describe penile penetration of the vagina. People use a variety of positions for intercourse, depending on preference, mobility, cultural and religious influences, the relationship, and other personal beliefs. For some women, manual stimulation of the clitoris is also necessary to achieve orgasm. Partners typically do not reach orgasm at the same time, despite the romantic preoccupation with this phenomenon.

 Unprotected intercourse may lead to conception, so the couple should use some method of contraception if they want to avoid pregnancy. Because body fluids are exchanged, sexual intercourse may also lead to the transmission of infections. Using a lubricated latex condom decreases this risk but is not a foolproof measure to prevent STIs.

Oral–Genital Stimulation

Both heterosexual and homosexual couples practice oral–genital stimulation (oral sex). Couples in committed relationships may engage in it for sexual variety or as foreplay. Oral sex provides intimacy and cannot result in pregnancy. Many believe that their virginity status is protected. For the latter two reasons, oral sex has become more prevalent among adolescents. **KEY POINT** *Oral–genital contact may, however, lead to STIs.*

Cunnilingus is the oral stimulation of a woman's genitals. **Fellatio** is stimulation of the male genitals by a partner's mouth. Although swallowing semen is not a health issue, it may be a matter of personal preference whether the recipient ejaculates in the partner's mouth. Dental dams, plastic wrap, or latex condoms should be used to prevent the transmission of STIs.

Anal Stimulation and Anal Intercourse

Both homosexual and heterosexual couples engage in oral–anal stimulation (called **anilingus**). Objects for sexual stimulation, or the partner's finger, tongue, and mouth, may be used to stimulate the anus. **Anal intercourse** (also termed *sodomy*) is the insertion of the penis into the partner's rectum.

When a couple engages in anal intercourse, lubrication is essential to lessen the chance of tiny tears to the rectal mucosa or damage to the anal sphincter. A lubricated latex condom can be used to decrease the risk of STIs. The condom must be changed before vaginal penetration to avoid the transfer of *Escherichia coli* bacteria from the rectum to the vagina. Couples should follow the same precaution when using objects for sexual pleasure.

Celibacy

Celibacy, or *abstinence,* is a state in which a person refrains from sexual activity. Traditionally, a celibate is one who remains unmarried, often for religious reasons, and sublimates sexual desire through prayer, meditation, and service. Reasons some people choose to remain celibate include the following:

- Fear of or lack of desire for intimate relationships
- Childhood sexual trauma
- A developmental or physical disability that limits opportunities for meeting prospective partners, limits privacy, or interferes with the ability to communicate or act on desires
- The desire to focus energies elsewhere because of a low libido
- The need to regain balance after the loss of a relationship, whether through separation, divorce, or death

Married couples may be happily celibate. Others might be celibate after the loss of a relationship, whether through separation, divorce, or death, often feeling a considerable void.

Alternative Forms of Sexual Expression

The *DSM-5* (APA, 2013a) describes eight categories of **paraphilias,** or sexual deviation: exhibitionism disorder, fetishism disorder, frotteurism disorder, pedophilia disorder, sexual masochism disorder, sexual sadism disorder, transvestic disorder, and voyeurism disorder. Some people experience guilt, shame, and depression about their paraphilia, while others are distressed only by the societal disapproval, restrictions, and possible criminal charges associated with their mode of expression.

KnowledgeCheck 34-8

- What are aspects of an intimate relationship?
- Identify solitary types of sexual expression and those that may be conducted with a partner.

What Problems Affect Sexuality?

Sexual well-being is a complex mesh of physical, emotional, cognitive, social, and spiritual components. Therefore, it is not surprising that many people experience challenges to their sexual health. Difficulties can arise in loving, healthy relationships, as well as in dysfunctional relationships. Sexual dysfunction may be temporary, situational, or long standing.

Sexually Transmitted Infections

An STI may be caused by bacteria, viruses, fungi, or parasites. STIs spread through direct sexual contact with an open wound or with body fluids, such as semen, vaginal secretions, or blood that contains pathogens. **KEY POINT** *Contrary to myth, STIs are not transmitted by casual touching, coughing, or other indirect means.*

KEY POINT *Because many STIs have few or no initial symptoms, an infected person can transmit the infection without knowing it.*

STIs, including HIV, among older adults have increased, as many sexually active adults are exposed to the same risk factors as are their younger counterparts (Centers for Disease Control and Prevention, 2015c; Johnson, 2013). A sexual history should be a component of the assessment in older adults.

More than 20 different STIs have been identified and affect millions of men and women each year. STIs are **reportable** (or **notifiable) diseases:** those that have a significant effect on public health. When healthcare providers diagnose STIs, mandatory reporting laws require that the Centers for Disease Control and Prevention (CDC) be notified. Examples include the following STIs:

Chlamydia Trachomatis is the most commonly transmitted infection in the United States and is also known as the "silent infection" because the infected person may not have symptoms. Chlamydia can cause serious damage to a female's reproductive system if untreated. There were 1.4 million cases in 2014, which is a 2.8% increase from 2013 (CDC, 2015b).

Gonorrhea is caused by a bacterium and is common among sexually active teenagers and young adults. There were 350,000 cases in 2014, which is an increase of 5.1% from 2013 (CDC, 2015b).

Syphilis is caused by a bacterium that is transmitted from person to person by direct contact with the syphilis sore that can occur on the external genitalia, vagina, lips, mouth, anus, and in the rectum.

- Primary and secondary syphilis increased by 15.1% from 2013 to 2014, with 20,000 reported cases.
- Men account for more than 90% of cases.
- Men with known male partners represent 83% of the cases (CDC, 2015b).

Genital Human Papillomavirus, also called HPV, is the most common STI.

- Many people with HPV do not know they are infected, and in many instances the STI will go away without intervention.
- There are more than 40 types of HPV and it is possible for a person to contract more than one type.
- The HPV vaccine is recommended to minimize the chance of contracting HPV (CDC, 2016).

Nearly two-thirds of all STIs occur in people younger than 25 years.

To determine whether a patient has an STI, you must obtain a culture, that is, a swab of secretions from the genitals.

- Male—Insert the swab is into the urethral opening.
- Female—Use the swab to obtain secretions from near the cervix.
- A culture of the throat or rectum is obtained if the person has had oral or anal sex.

Many STIs can be treated fairly easily with antibiotics; however, if left untreated, they may cause serious problems. In women, the pathogens can travel up through the uterus into the fallopian tubes and cause pelvic inflammatory disease (PID). Untreated PID may cause sterility.

The best ways to prevent STIs are to practice abstinence or to participate only in a mutually monogamous sexual relationship with someone who has never had or is at a low risk for an STI. The following increase the risk for an STI:

- Unprotected sex
- More than one sexual partner
- Alcohol and drug use
- Sharing needles
- Nonadherence to the STI treatment regimen

To read about various STIs, their symptoms, treatment, and effect on sexual functioning, fertility, and childbearing, see Table 34-3.

Dysmenorrhea

Dysmenorrhea is painful menstruation caused by strong uterine contractions that lead to ischemia of the uterus.
- **Physical symptoms:** Cramping, lower abdominal pain, back and upper thigh pain, headache, vomiting, and diarrhea.
- **Treatments:** Bedrest, application of heat to the back and abdomen, and analgesics such as aspirin and other NSAIDs, for example, ibuprofen or naproxen.

Premenstrual Syndrome

Premenstrual syndrome (PMS) is characterized by physical and emotional changes occurring 3 to 14 days before the onset of the woman's menstrual period.
- **Physical symptoms:** Headaches, constipation, breast tenderness, and weight gain; associated with bloating, abdominal swelling, or swelling of the hands and feet.
- **Emotional and social symptoms:** Some women feel as though they are on an emotional roller coaster, with periods of depression, anxiety, irritability, tension, and an inability to concentrate. Some have difficulty maintaining social interactions because of severe emotional symptoms.

Table 34-3 ➤ Common Sexually Transmitted Infections (STIs)

Chlamydia

SYMPTOMS	TREATMENT AND LONG-TERM EFFECTS
Female: Usually asymptomatic **Male:** Occur 1–2 weeks after infection: thin, clear urethral discharge; mild discomfort with urination	*Treatment:* Antibiotics *Long-Term Effects* *Females:* Invasion of the uterus and fallopian tubes resulting in pelvic inflammatory disease (PID), which may lead to pain, sterility, and ectopic pregnancy *Pregnant women:* In utero transmission to fetus; newborn may have pneumonia; may be fatal *Males:* Epididymitis (may lead to sterility), proctitis (with anal intercourse)

Trichomoniasis

SYMPTOMS	TREATMENT AND LONG-TERM EFFECTS
Female: Cheesy, frothy, irritating, odorous vaginal discharge **Male:** Usually asymptomatic	*Treatment:* Amoebicide and antibiotic *Long-Term Effects* May be passed back and forth between partners if the male is not treated Untreated, it may damage cervical cells

Gonorrhea

SYMPTOMS	TREATMENT AND LONG-TERM EFFECTS
May be asymptomatic in both men and women **Female:** Usually no early symptoms **Male:** Thick white or yellowish urethral discharge, burning, frequent/painful urination	*Treatment:* Antibiotics **KEY POINT** Alert: *Some strains are becoming resistant.* *Long-Term Effects* *Females:* Invasion of the uterus and fallopian tubes resulting in PID, which may lead to pain, sterility, and ectopic pregnancy *Pregnant women:* Blindness and pneumonia in the newborn *Men:* Infertility, arthritis

Human papillomavirus (HPV)

SYMPTOMS	TREATMENT AND LONG-TERM EFFECTS
Female: Genital warts on the vulva, cervix, vaginal walls, anus, or mouth; cauliflower-like appearance **Male:** Genital warts on the urethra, shaft of the penis, scrotum, anus, or mouth; cauliflower-like appearance	*Treatment:* Antibiotics *Long-Term Effects* Warts appear months following genital contact. Greatest risk factor for cervical cancer. Associated with cancer of the penis and anus.

Table 34-3 ➤ Common Sexually Transmitted Infections (STIs)—cont'd

Genital herpes (HSV-2)

SYMPTOMS	TREATMENT AND LONG-TERM EFFECTS
Female: May be asymptomatic. Small, painful blisters on the genitals; pain with burst blisters as they become wet sores for several weeks; may include fever **Male:** Same as female	*Treatment* No cure Vaccine currently under investigation Antiviral (may minimize the duration and severity of an initial infection or later flare of symptoms; reduce the likelihood of transmission to a partner) *Long-Term Effects* Increased risk of HIV and cervical cancer Transmission to infant during vaginal delivery, with serious, even fatal sequelae Lifelong transmission risk, especially during flare-ups

Syphilis

SYMPTOMS	TREATMENT AND LONG-TERM EFFECTS
Female ■ *Primary Stage:* Chancre (painless, ulcer-like sore at site of contact; will disappear in about 14 days without treatment; cervical chancres will be undetected by the female) ■ *Secondary Stage:* Generalized, nonitchy, painless rash; sore throat; low-grade fever; aches and pains **Male** ■ *Primary Stage:* Chancre (painless, ulcer-like sore at site of contact, will disappear in about 14 days without treatment) ■ *Secondary Stage:* Generalized, nonitchy, painless rash; sore throat; low-grade fever; aches and pains	*Treatment:* Antibiotics *Long-Term Effects* If untreated: *Latent Stage:* Bacteria continue to attack internal organs. *Late (tertiary) Stage:* Damage to the heart, blood vessels, and central nervous system. May lead to death.

Hepatitis B (HBV)

SYMPTOMS	TREATMENT AND LONG-TERM EFFECTS
Female: May be asymptomatic Flu-like symptoms (low-grade fever, fatigue), decreased appetite, dark urine, and jaundice **Male:** May be asymptomatic Flu-like symptoms (low-grade fever, fatigue), decreased appetite, dark urine, and jaundice	*Treatment* Vaccine for prevention Rest, good nutrition Avoidance of alcohol and drugs *Long-Term Effects* Liver cancer Death

(Continued)

Table 34-3 ➤ Common Sexually Transmitted Infections (STIs)—cont'd

HIV

SYMPTOMS	TREATMENT AND LONG-TERM EFFECTS
Female: Asymptomatic carrier state	**Treatment**
Low T4 cell count	No cure (research is being conducted)
Weight loss, fatigue, diarrhea, fever	Viewed as a chronic disease with treatment
Vulnerability to bacterial, viral and fungal infections	Nucleoside inhibitors, nonnucleoside inhibitors, protease inhibitors
Male: Asymptomatic carrier state	**Long-Term Effects:** Opportunistic infections
Low T4 cell count	
Weight loss, fatigue, diarrhea, fever	
Vulnerability to bacterial, viral, and fungal infections	

- **Premenstrual dysphoric disorder (PMDD)** is a more severe form of menstrual cycle dysfunction in which women may become seriously depressed for a week or more before their periods.

    PMS is shorter, usually milder, and involves more physical symptoms than PMDD.

    A woman can suffer from both PMS and PMDD at the same time or may have one and not the other.

    Client teaching for PMS is discussed later in this chapter.

KnowledgeCheck 34-9

- Identify three methods to decrease the transmission of STIs.
- What are physical and emotional symptoms of premenstrual syndrome (PMS)?

Negative Intimate Relationships

Many relationships are sometimes satisfying and at other times less so—depending on a wide variety of factors such as stress, physical and mental illness, hormones, fatigue, distractions, low self-esteem, and financial pressures. Other reasons for negative intimate relationships (celibate or loveless union) include the following:

- Financial insecurity, social status, parenting obligations, or cultural or religious restrictions regarding divorce.
- **Domestic violence** (also called *intimate partner violence*), which may include neglect, physical and/or emotional intimidation, assault, and rape. Most often the woman is the victim, although this is not always so. The anger, domination, and physical violence of the partner lead to fear, intimidation, and submission in the victim. Often victims believe they deserve the abuse and may hesitate to admit the cause of their injuries, even in the hospital setting. Many abused women are either emotionally or financially dependent on their partner and believe staying in the relationship is their only option. If you wish to learn more about abuse and violence, see Chapters 9 and 10.

Sexual Harassment

- **Sexual harassment** occurs when a person in power makes unwanted sexual advances that implicitly or explicitly relate to the victim's employment, academic status, or success (e.g., sexual comments or behaviors, such as touching). Because of the power imbalance, the victim may keep silent and suffer physically and psychologically.
- **Sexual assault** includes contact with or without penetration, sexual touching of intimate parts, and any unwanted sexual activity.

    Sexual harassment may take two forms:

1. In *quid pro quo* cases, the employer makes the employee feel that she must engage in unwelcome sexual advances to maintain employment.
2. In *hostile environment* situations, the sexual advances are more subtle, but persistent, and create an intimidating environment.

Rape

Rape is a crime of violence rather than of sex. We discuss it here because it involves the sexual organs and usually has negative effects on the victim's sexuality. **Rape** is nonconsensual vaginal, anal, or oral penetration. It occurs through force, by the threat of bodily harm, or when the victim is incapable of giving consent. All 50 states consider rape, even within a marriage, to be a crime.

Incidence

- In 2014, there were 284,350 reported cases of rape (Truman & Langton, 2015).
- Victims of rape range from infants to older adults and may be either gender, although females are more likely to be victims.
- One in five women and 1 in 71 males reported being victims of rape (CDC, 2012e), with 37.4% of female victims' rape first occurring between the ages of 18 and 24 years.
- For females, perpetrators were primarily intimate partners (51%) and acquaintances (41%).
- For males, the majority of perpetrators were acquaintances; 15% were strangers (CDC, 2012e).
- People with developmental disabilities, especially mental retardation, are at twice the risk for sexual assault than the general population.

Types of Rape

- **Group rape** (gang) occurs when more than one person sexually assaults a victim. Group rape usually occurs when drugs and alcohol are involved.

PICOT

Sexuality, Dementia, and Competency

Situation: The adult children of a widow with early onset Alzheimer's disease are concerned about their mother's sexual advances directed at another resident at the assisted living facility. Although the residents are, legally, consenting adults, the children are concerned about their mother's judgment and sexual appropriateness.

PICOT Components:

P	Population/client	=	Adults with early onset Alzheimer's disease
I	Intervention/indicator	=	Nonpharmacological behavior modification
C	Comparator/control	=	No sexual relationships
O	Outcome	=	Appropriate, consensual sexual relationships
T	Time	=	Late adulthood

Searchable Question: Do _____(P) who receive/are exposed to _____(I) demonstrate _____(O) as compared to _____(C) during _____(T)?

Example of Evidence: All people have needs for intimacy, companionship, and touch. Clients with dementia pose a particularly difficult situation for both family and professionals, who may consider sexual behavior to be inappropriate, based on the elderly client's age, setting, situation, or health issues.

The central question for you to answer is whether the client is competent. The family and staff need to carefully and sensitively assess the following areas: Is the client's mental status suited to engaging in a consensual, sexual relationship? Who is initiating sexual contact? Is the client able to consent to sexual intimacy? Is the client aware of emotional and physical potential risks, such as the relationship ending? Is the sexual activity consistent with behavior the client exhibited prior to the onset of the dementia? Although there are no established treatment guidelines, various nonpharmacological plans may help to assure appropriate expression of sexuality.

Practice Change: After obtaining a thorough sexual assessment, the nurse may plan nonpharmacological behavior modification for the client to demonstrate appropriate sexual behaviors and meet the client's intimacy needs.

 Go to Davis Advantage, Resources, Chapter 34, **PICOT Box—Suggested Responses.**

Source: Joller, P., Gupta, N., Seitz, D. P., et al. (2013). Approach to inappropriate sexual behaviour in people with dementia. *Canadian Family Physician, 59*(3), 255–260.

- **Statutory rape** is sexual activity between an adult and a person under the "age of consent" (this ranges from 14 to 18 years of age, depending on state regulations). This charge may be filed even when the sex is consensual.
- **Date rape** is rape by an acquaintance when the assault occurs during an agreed-on social encounter. Although date rape is not a lesser violation, our society tends to blame the woman when date rape occurs

Why Many Rapes Go Unreported

Rape is an assault that involves significant psychological and physical injury; therefore, the police often become involved just because the victim requires medical attention. After a rape or other forms of sexual assault, care may be delayed for various reasons:

- Involvement of alcohol or drugs (particularly for teens)
- Fear of the assailant or fear of consequences to the assailant
- Knowledge of the low conviction rate for rapists
- Desire to avoid a trial; past sexual history
- Shame, embarrassment, and self-blame
- Wanting to "move on" and the wish to deny the event and its possible consequences

Effects of Rape

In addition to psychological and physiological trauma, the rape victim is at risk for STIs and pregnancy. Three-quarters or more of sexually assaulted teens experience post-traumatic stress disorder. **KEY POINT** *Referral to a local sexual assault support group is critical.* A **sexual assault nurse examiner** is a registered nurse who has received special training in the immediate care of sexual assault victims.

To learn about providing care for sexual assault victims, refer to Clinical Insight 34-1. Also see the accompanying iCare box.

♥ iCare 34-1

Sexual Health

The topic of sexual health is one of the most private topics a nurse can discuss with a person. Be compassionate, but take a matter-of-fact and accepting approach. Remember, the patient may want information but may not know how to bring up the topic. The following are tips for showing that you care:

- Confidentiality is paramount.
- Be available to listen. Sit down face-to-face, approach the topic unhurriedly, and make eye contact.
- Provide privacy and help the person feel comfortable. Pull the curtain, close the door.
- Be observant for both verbal and nonverbal cues that may indicate a concern.
- Be empathetic to the person's situation or concern, whatever it may be.
- Be cognizant of the fact that people can be very vulnerable when discussing sexual health topics.
- Be prepared to accept of a wide range of emotions, from withdrawal to outbursts of anger.

Sexual Response Cycle Disorders

Disorders in various stages of the sexual response cycle may affect desire, arousal, excitement, and orgasm.

Low Libido (hypoactive sexual desire) manifests as a significant decrease in or absence of sexual fantasies and sexual activity. Low libido may affect both men and women. It can be transient or long term. The person may experience low libido only with one particular partner, or the lack of desire can extend to all sexual activity. Persons with low libido may reluctantly engage in sexual encounters or avoid all sexual contact. However, once sexual activity has been initiated, the person is usually able to achieve orgasm.

Factors contributing to hypoactive sexual desire include the following:

- Sexual trauma
- Negative attitude toward sex
- Negative relationships
- Biological factors (e.g., hormone deficiencies, perimenopause)
- Side effects of various medications

Low sexual desire in both men and women sometimes responds positively to testosterone administration.

Arousal Disorders are experienced by both men and women. In women, arousal disorders manifest as minimal or absent pelvic congestion and vaginal lubrication, even though desire may be present.

- **Dyspareunia,** or painful intercourse, further reduces sexual desire. In women, it is often caused by vaginal dryness resulting from hormonal changes, the aging process, tampons, and medications including antihistamines. A water-based lubricant or saliva helps to resolve vaginal dryness. Other causes of female dyspareunia include vaginal or urinary tract infections, pelvic inflammatory disease, and endometriosis.

  Dyspareunia in men most commonly results from urinary tract infection or **phimosis,** a condition in which the foreskin of the penis is too tight. **Balanitis,** inflammation of the penis, is another cause of dyspareunia in men.

- **Vaginismus** is a rare female disorder affecting desire and arousal. It is characterized by intense involuntary contractions of the perineal muscles, which close the vaginal opening and prevent penile penetration. Vaginismus may be associated with psychological disorders (e.g., negative attitudes toward sex, history of sexual abuse/trauma) or physiological disorders (e.g., childbirth trauma).

- **Erectile dysfunction (ED)** is a sexual arousal disorder in men. Formerly known as *impotence,* ED is the persistent or recurring inability to achieve or to maintain an erection sufficient for satisfactory sexual performance. Causes of ED include the following:

  - Diseases of the blood vessels (e.g., hypertension, high cholesterol, or diabetes); this is the most common cause.
  - Neurological problems (e.g., spinal cord injury, Parkinson's disease, stroke).
  - Endocrine problems (diabetes).
  - Testosterone plays a minor role in erectile function and a major role in libido (desire).
  - Common psychological problems that contribute to ED include performance anxiety, childhood sexual abuse, relationship issues, or mental illness.
  - Some medications can also cause ED, such as antihistamines, antidepressants, antipsychotics, and antihypertensives.

Orgasmic Disorders are conditions with a delay in or absence of orgasm after a normal sexual excitement phase. Orgasmic disorder is more prevalent in younger women who have not had adequate sexual experience to learn how to reach orgasm. It is not unusual for a woman to require manual clitoral stimulation to reach orgasm because not all women can achieve orgasm through intercourse alone. Once a woman has had orgasms, it is uncommon for her to lose that ability unless there has been a sexual trauma, poor sexual communication, a conflicted sexual relationship, a mood disorder, a medical condition, or direct physiological effects from a drug.

Men, too, can experience orgasmic disorders. Some cannot achieve orgasm during intercourse but are able to reach orgasm through masturbation or manual or oral stimulation by their partner.

- **Premature ejaculation** occurs when the male reaches orgasm and ejaculates before, at the time of, or shortly after penetration. The disappointment of both partners may lead to issues with self-esteem, sexual avoidance, and ED. There are sexual techniques as well as medications that can help to delay ejaculation.

- **Retrograde ejaculation** occurs when the semen empties into the bladder instead of being ejaculated through the urethra. Normally this cannot occur because the internal bladder sphincter closes in the orgasmic phase. However, some medications, prostate surgery, and spinal cord injuries may lead to retrograde ejaculation, resulting in sterility.

KnowledgeCheck 34-10

- Identify three forms of sexual victimization.
- In which phases of the sexual response cycle can sexual dysfunction occur?

PracticalKnowledge
knowing **how**

You may find it difficult to gather information related to sexuality. Students and some nurses may be shy about talking about sexuality. They may also be concerned that the client will be embarrassed to talk openly about sexual topics because they are personal and private and can threaten a person's self-esteem. Including sexuality as a routine part of your nursing assessment reinforces the concept that sexuality is an integral part of life and provides an opportunity for much-needed client teaching on this topic.

ASSESSMENT NP

The extent to which you will assess a client's sexual health status varies. For example, a patient with a suspected STI requires a comprehensive health assessment and a focused sexual health assessment. Similarly, clients with illnesses that affect their sexual functioning should receive a full assessment. Jocelyn Carter (Meet Your Patients) is an example. Recall that chronic illness can have a profound effect on sexual functioning (e.g., recall Frank Thanee and Gabriel Thomas, also in the Meet Your Patients scenario). A focused sexual health assessment is needed in the following situations:

Pregnancy, infertility workup, request for birth control
Menstrual cycle irregularities or problems
Annual health visit or as part of a comprehensive physical examination
Unusual discharge from or change in genital organs
Urination problems
A known sexual problem (e.g., dyspareunia)
Illness, surgery, or drugs that may affect sexual function (e.g., arthritis, colostomy, antihypertensives)

Sexual History

Most healthcare facilities use a standard nursing assessment form. Some address sexuality in a comprehensive manner, but most have only a few superficial questions or nothing at all. You will need to be sensitive to your client's verbal and nonverbal cues to identify and explore relevant issues that are not on the form. For topics to include in a sexual history and for suggestions for questions to ask, see the accompanying Focused Assessment box Guidelines and Questions for Taking a Sexual History.

Tips for Taking a Sexual History When you are asking personal questions, always provide privacy. It is one thing to discuss blood pressure in the presence of family, but quite

another to discuss sexual health issues, which may threaten the very core of a relationship. For example, an 18-year-old man may not admit to having sex with another man when his father is present and a teenager may not want to discuss her STI in front of her mother. For guidelines and other suggestions, also see Clinical Insight 34-2, Guidelines for Taking a Sexual History.

Guidelines and Questions for Taking a Sexual History

Topics to Include in a Sexual History

The topics to include in the sexual history depend on the nature of the patient's concern. The following topics are most commonly included:
- Reproductive history
- Sexual self-concept
- History of sexually transmitted infections
- History of sexual dysfunction
- Present sexual functioning
- Other factors that affect sexuality, such as medications and diseases
- Signs or symptoms of sexual abuse (see Procedure 9-1: Assessing for Abuse)
- Knowledge level about sex, reproduction, and contraception

Tailor your assessment to meet the client's needs. For example, Frank Thanee (Meet Your Patients) is concerned about his family's reaction to his lifestyle and sexual orientation. In his situation, you would focus your assessment on his sexual self-concept, family relationships, present sexual functioning, and specific concerns about his heart and the impending family visit.

Questions to Ask Women

Menstrual Cycle
- How old were you when you started your menstrual periods?
- When was your last menstrual period?
- How often are your periods? How would you describe the flow? How long does your period last?
- Do you have any problems with your periods, such as cramping, breast pain, or heavy flow?
- Does your menstrual period ever prevent you from going to work or school or participating in the activities you enjoy?
- What products do you use during your period, such as tampons and pads? Do you ever use douches, either during your period or at other times?

Cancer Screening
- When was your last Pap smear?
- Have you ever had an abnormal Pap smear? If so, how was it treated?
- Have you received a vaccine for HPV?
- Do you examine your breasts? If so, how often?
- Have you noticed asymmetry, lumps, or masses in your breasts? If so, describe them and show me where they are.
- When was your last mammogram? What were the results?
- Is there any history of breast cancer in your family?

Childbearing History
- How many living children do you have?
- How many times have you been pregnant?
- Have you ever had a miscarriage? An abortion?
- How many of your births were preterm (prior to 38 weeks)? Term?

Sexual Activity
- How often do you typically have sexual intercourse per month?
- Are you satisfied with the frequency or quality of sexual activity?
- Is there anything in your life that prevents you from sexual activity?
- Do you have any difficulty achieving orgasm?
- Is sexual intercourse ever painful for you?
- Are you sexually attracted to women? Have you had oral or genital sexual intercourse with women?

Questions to Ask Men

Sexual Activity
- How many times a month do you typically have sexual intercourse?
- Do you have any difficulty achieving or maintaining an erection or orgasm?
- Are you satisfied with the firmness of your erection?
- Do you experience premature ejaculation or have difficulty achieving sexual orgasm?
- Are you sexually attracted to men? Have you had oral or anal intercourse with men?

Cancer Screening
- Have you been taught to examine your testicles? Do you practice testicular self-exam?
- Is there a history of testicular cancer in your family?

Questions to Ask Both Men and Women

Illnesses and Medications
- What types of illnesses have you been treated for in the past?
- Have you ever been hospitalized? Have you ever had surgery?
- What medications, herbal remedies, or over-the-counter medicines do you take?
- Has any medical treatment, surgery, or medication affected your sexual functioning?

Family Responsibilities
- Do you have children? If so, how many? How many are still at home? Dependent on you?

(Continued)

Focused Assessment

Guidelines and Questions for Taking a Sexual History—cont'd

➤ Are you responsible for other children or adults? (This question may reveal whether the person continues to care for an adult, disabled child, or grandchildren.)

Genitalia
➤ Have you noticed any redness, swelling, discharge, itching, or odor in your genital area?
➤ Have you noticed asymmetry, lumps, or masses in the genitals? If so, describe them and show me where they are.
➤ Have you ever been told you have a hernia?
➤ Have you ever had trauma to your genitals?
➤ Are you having any problems urinating?

Sexual Patterns
➤ Are you sexually active? If not, have you ever been?
➤ Do you have sex with men, women, or both?
➤ What types of sexual activity do you engage in? Oral, anal, or genital?
➤ How many partners do you currently have? How many partners have you had in the past 6 months?
➤ How would you describe your satisfaction with your current sexual relationship?
➤ What are your thoughts about how this procedure/illness may affect your sexual relationship?

➤ Have you experienced any recent changes in your sexual function—in your level of desire, your sexual activity, participation, or satisfaction?
➤ Do you have any concerns about your sexual function, including your level of desire, activity, participation, or satisfaction?

Contraception (as appropriate)
➤ Do you use birth control? If so, what type and how often?
➤ How satisfied are you with your method of contraception?

Sexually Transmitted Infections
➤ Have you ever been treated for an STI? If so, what type?
➤ Are you concerned about STIs or HIV?
➤ What precautions do you take to avoid STIs?

Abuse
➤ Have you ever been forced to have sex against your will?
➤ Have you ever been threatened or abused by a partner?
➤ Do you ever feel threatened by your partner?

For guidelines for your approach to taking a sexual history, see Clinical Insight 34-2.

Focused Physical Examination

Sexual health assessment includes a physical examination focused on the reproductive system. For detailed instructions about performing these examinations, see Procedure 21-17: Assessing the Male Genitourinary System and Procedure 21-18: Assessing the Female Genitourinary System, in Chapter 21.

KnowledgeCheck 34-11

What techniques can you use to increase comfort and communication during a sexual history assessment?

 ## ThinkLike a Nurse 34-7

Review the three case scenarios in the Meet Your Patients discussion. Consider the following questions for each client:
■ Would you be comfortable caring for and responding to each of these clients?
■ What topics, if any, that have been raised by these clients would be difficult for you to handle?
■ How would you answer each of the questions the clients asked in the scenario?

ANALYSIS/NURSING DIAGNOSIS NP

NANDA-I has two nursing diagnoses for describing sexual problems. The following discussion should help you differentiate between them:

Ineffective Sexuality Patterns Use this diagnosis when the patient expresses concerns about his own sexuality. Examples of such concerns might include conflict about sexual orientation, values conflicts, fear of acquiring an STI, lack of knowledge about how to adapt sexual techniques to altered body function, lack of privacy, not having a partner, or impaired relationship with the partner.

Sexual Dysfunction Use this label when there is an actual change in sexual function that the patient views as unsatisfying, unrewarding, or inadequate. This includes sexual response cycle disorders such as low libido, arousal disorders, orgasmic disorders, vaginismus, premature ejaculation, and erectile dysfunction. If these defining characteristics for Sexual Dysfunction do not seem to "fit" the client, then use the more general diagnosis of Ineffective Sexuality Patterns.

There is much overlap between these two NANDA-I diagnoses, so look closely at the client's defining characteristics. A defining characteristic of Ineffective Sexuality Pattern is that the patient reports difficulties or alterations in sexual behaviors or activities.

■ Jocelyn Carter (Meet Your Patients) is not actually experiencing problems with sexual satisfaction or performance. She is expressing a broader concern about her sexuality—about her future desirability as a sex partner. Therefore, the better diagnosis for her is Ineffective Sexuality Patterns.
■ The same is true for Gabriel Thomas (Meet Your Patients), who is expressing fear that he may have sexual problems in the future.

Sexual Dysfunction is the more specific diagnosis for physiological problems and for concerns about sexual performance. Thus it is best to use Sexual Dysfunction when the patient has one or more of the following defining characteristics:

Changes in achieving sexual satisfaction`
Change of interest toward others
Alteration in sexual satisfaction
Decrease in sexual desire
Change in sexual role
Seeking confirmation of desirability

Etiologies of Sexuality Diagnoses

Several nursing diagnoses may be the cause of sexuality problems. The following are the more common:

- *Activity Intolerance* and *Fatigue* (e.g., from cardiac or respiratory disease) may cause the person to alter his lifestyle, including sexual activity, to conserve energy. Lack of energy may decrease the person's interest in sex, or it may require a change in the mode of sexual expression.
- *Impaired Physical Mobility* (e.g., as occurs with arthritis or spinal cord injuries) may affect a person's ability to interact, meet potential partners, and perform sexually (e.g., assume certain positions, make certain movements).
- *Fear* that sexual activity may be dangerous can inhibit desire and the ability to perform (e.g., after heart surgery). This diagnosis may also apply to the client's partner, who may be afraid that sexual activity will hurt the client after surgery or hurt a pregnant partner or the baby.
- *Chronic Pain* may directly affect interpersonal relationships, interest in sex, or comfort during sexual intimacy. It may cause fatigue, indirectly affecting sexuality.
- *Chronic Low Self-Esteem* may result from chronic health problems and their consequences (e.g., loss of employment, inability to perform parenting roles). Sexual expression may also become a challenge, yet the intimacy and reassurance that accompany sexual encounters can be vital to self-esteem and a sense of wholeness.
- *Self-Care Deficits.* For clients who need assistance with activities of daily living—for example, with toileting—family or caretakers often find it difficult to accept and facilitate sexual relationships. When a person with a physical disability lives in a residential facility, lack of opportunity and privacy may interfere with sexual expression (Fig. 34-7).
- *Risk for Delayed Development.* Relationship challenges also exist for people who are developmentally disabled. Those with very low cognitive functioning are unable to seek out or understand sexual relationships. Unfortunately, this makes them vulnerable to sexual abuse. Sex education is vital for these individuals to help them understand body structure and function, relationship issues, and ways to avoid exploitation and abuse.

Sexuality problems can be the etiology of other nursing diagnoses, for example:

- *Disturbed Body Image* related to change in appearance secondary to orchiectomy (removal of a testicle)
- *Pain (during coitus)* related to inadequate vaginal lubrication secondary to aging
- *Fear* related to sexual abuse by others
- *Rape-Trauma Syndrome* (Note that you do not need an etiology for this nursing diagnosis. It is self-explanatory, as are most syndrome diagnoses.)

 Think**Like a Nurse** 34-8

Give a specific example (client situation) for each of the defining characteristics of Sexual Dysfunction listed in the preceding section.

PLANNING OUTCOMES/EVALUATION NP

NOC standardized outcomes associated with Ineffective Sexuality Patterns and Sexual Dysfunction include the following examples (Moorhead, Johnson, Maas, et al., 2013):

Abuse Recovery: Sexual	Role Performance
Body Image	Self-Esteem

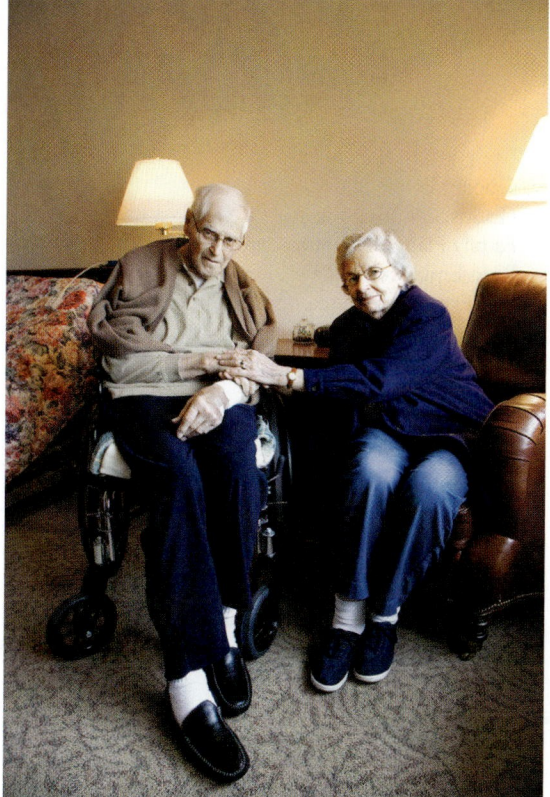

FIGURE 34-7 Adults with physical restrictions or those living within group settings such as skilled nursing care can maintain sexual relationships.

Physical Aging	Sexual Functioning
Risk Control: Sexually	Sexual Identity
Transmitted Diseases	

Individualized client outcomes and goals depend on the nursing diagnosis you identify. For Sexual Dysfunction and Ineffective Sexuality Patterns, you might write the following desired outcomes:

- Expresses comfort with sexual orientation.
- Describes plans for resolving values conflicts about extramarital sex (e.g., will talk to his minister).
- Describes techniques for preventing STIs.

The following are examples of outcomes that apply specifically to Sexual Dysfunction:

- Communicates sexual needs and preferences to partner.
- Describes ways to adapt positions for intercourse to accommodate painful knee joints.

PLANNING INTERVENTIONS/ IMPLEMENTATION NP

For *NIC standardized interventions* and selected nursing activities for sexuality, see the examples in the accompanying Standardized Language box Examples of NIC Interventions for Sexuality Problems.

Specific nursing activities for sexuality problems depend on the etiology of the problem and on the selected goals. Broadly speaking, nursing interventions involve teaching about sexual health and self-care, counseling for altered sexual functioning, and dealing with inappropriate sexual behavior.

Examples of NIC Interventions for Sexuality Problems

For Ineffective Sexuality Pattern:

Body Image Enhancement
Coping Enhancement
Counseling
Family Planning: Contraception
Role Enhancement
Self-Esteem Enhancement
Teaching: Safe Sex

For Sexual Dysfunction:

Abuse Protection Support
Behavior Management: Sexual
Infection Protection
Risk Identification
Sexual Counseling
Teaching: Sexuality

Source: Adapted from Bulechek, G., Butcher, H., Dochterman, J., et al. (Eds.). (2013). *Nursing interventions classification (NIC)* (6th ed.). St. Louis, MO: C.V. Mosby. Used with permission.

Those interventions are discussed in the following sections. You will also find a Nursing Care Plan and Care Map for Ineffective Sexuality Problems after the section Putting It All Together.

Teaching About Sexual Health

Before you begin teaching, take the time to get to know your client and find out what she already knows about sexuality. Take time to put the client at ease. When you develop rapport and trust, the client will be more likely to speak openly about sensitive or embarrassing topics, to retain what you teach, and

to feel free to ask questions. Offer to include the partner in the discussion if the client wishes. See Chapter 26 for a review of teaching and learning.

As part of teaching about sexual health, you should discuss prevention of STIs with all clients and discuss contraception with clients who are heterosexual or bisexual. Other common topics are presented in the next sections.

Teaching Children About Predators

The following contains important information you can teach parents and caregivers to do to reduce children's risk of sexual violence, predators, or other unhealthy exposure:

Set the Stage for Open Discussion

- Talk openly and directly with your child about her own development and sexuality. This establishes trust and makes it easier for the child to come to you when she has questions.
- Be open to your child's questions. Acting embarrassed discourages further conversation.
- Assure your child that she won't get in trouble for "tattling" on someone who asks her to keep a secret about sexual or touching encounters.
- Make discussion a natural part of growing up—don't save it "for later."

Know What's Going On

- Be involved in your child's everyday life and ask questions—that is, where he is, who he's with, what he's doing, what his closest friends are doing.
- Know the other adults your child is around. Go to your child's activities and get to know the adults involved.
- Know what he watches on TV, the iPod or iPad, and the computer, or what media games he plays.
- Locate computers in a central area in the home where you can monitor Internet use.
- Install a parental control to limit access to and monitor Web sites that would expose your child to sexual content or predators.
- Know whether sexual predators live near you. Check out the sexual predators registry in your area.

Application of Education and Evidence-Based Practice to Client Care

Chapter Key Concepts: Sexuality, Sexual health

Competencies: Provide Goal Directed, Client-Centered Care (Thinking, Doing, Caring); Validate Evidence-Based Research to Incorporate Into Client Care

Background: *Goal-directed, client-centered care* addresses the client's physical, psychosocial, and spiritual needs. This includes incorporating sexual health into your assessment.

The SENC competency of *goal-directed, client-centered care* directs that nurses provide education to foster informed decisions and involvement in care and to facilitate postdischarge health. Jocelyn Carter (Meet Your Patients) is expressing concern that postmastectomy, her husband will not find her attractive. In addition to measures to show caring (holding her hand, taking the time to listen to her), now is an opportunity to provide information on the effectiveness of postoperative cosmetic advances. This information can help to lessen the degree of loss she may feel.

The SENC competency of *validating evidence-based practice to incorporate into client care* involves keeping abreast of current research and applying findings to promote effective client outcomes. Research literature reveals that satisfaction with cosmetic outcomes was similar between women who had breast-conserving surgery and those who had mastectomy with reconstruction (Jagsi, Li, Morrow, et al., 2015). Ms. Carter may not focus on this information preoperatively, so you must include it in the nursing care plan so that other nurses can reinforce it. In addition, research shows that for women undergoing treatment for breast cancer, spouses are a significant source of support; however, to better support their wives, men need tailored information (Rowland & Metcalfe, 2014).

Think about it:

What other resources are available to promote Ms. Carter's sexual health?

- Establish curfew times and contingency communications if curfew is breached. Teach your child to use a code word that communicates he is in trouble.

  Just Say No
- Teach your child about body parts that are private and should not be touched or seen by others—except for medical reasons.
- Teach your child to firmly say no and get away if someone tries to touch or look at her in a way that makes her feel uncomfortable.
- Urge your child to tell you or another trusted adult if someone tries to touch or look at private areas or if the person tries to show the child his or her own private body parts.
- Teach your child never to get in the car with strangers and never go near a stranger's car for any reason.
- Always use a buddy system to prevent the child from being alone.
- Teach your child to yell, "Help! Stranger!" if anyone tries to follow her, either walking or in a car.
- Place limits on Internet use.
- Teach children not to disclose personal information in public settings or on the Internet, especially social networking sites.

Body Function and Reproduction

A person's age, experience, and educational level do not ensure knowledge of sexual functioning. Before you begin any teaching, explore your client's knowledge base by asking open-ended questions such as "What questions do you have about sex?"

Visual aids (e.g., a diagram of reproductive system anatomy) are helpful. For example, for pregnant clients, you could use drawings and charts illustrating fetal development. Most agencies provide handouts and brochures so that clients can review information at home.

As part of your general discussion on sexuality and bodily function, you may wish to discuss common myths and misconceptions about sex. The following list contains several statements about sex that provide a good starting point for discussion:

KEY POINT: *The following statements are all false.*
- You can't get pregnant the first time you have sex.
- You can't get pregnant if you're using a condom.
- You can tell the size of a man's penis by the size of his feet.
- You always have symptoms if you have an STI.
- Only "dirty" people have STIs. You will not get an STI if your partner practices good hygiene.
- People over age 70 don't have sex.
- A vaginal orgasm is better than a clitoral orgasm.
- If the relationship is good, the sexual partners will achieve simultaneous orgasm.
- It is not healthful to have intercourse during menstruation.
- The only normal position for intercourse is face-to-face. Anything else is deviant or at least "not nice."
- If a woman does not have an orgasm, she does not really love her partner. The same is true for a man.

Douching

Teach women that douching is unnecessary and is associated with significant risks. It can wash away the lactobacilli that clean the vagina and protect it from infection. Women who douche are at increased risk for some STIs and for PID (Gollub, Cyrus-Cameron, Armstrong, et al., 2013; Rew, 2009). Furthermore, douching is essentially useless as a method of contraception. Some women douche because they notice an odor. Reassure

them that this is normal during certain times of their menstrual cycle. If the odor doesn't disappear after perineal hygiene, they should see their healthcare provider.

Menstruation

- **Sexual activity during menstruation.** You may need to provide information to dispel myths about menstruation. For example, it is not dangerous to engage in sexual activity during menstruation. The bloody fluid is from the uterus, not the vagina, so intercourse will not harm the vagina. Actually, some women as well as men enjoy sex more during menstruation because the increased vascularity, warmth, and lubrication in the pelvic region increase their pleasurable sensations. An orgasm may relieve a woman's menstrual cramps. A protective pad placed under the woman's buttocks will protect the bed linen. A diaphragm can be used to prevent the flow from entering the vagina. Women who use a menstrual cup can also enjoy sex during menstruation without the excessive bloody fluid (Shihata & Brody, 2014; Ross, 2015).
- **Odor.** To prevent odor, women should use good perineal hygiene, bathe or shower every day, and change pads or tampons frequently. Advise women who use tampons to follow the manufacturer's directions for reducing the risk for toxic shock syndrome. Deodorized pads and tampons are not very effective and can cause irritation to the vulva and vagina. Another option is use of the menstrual cup, which decreases odor because, unlike with tampons, the bloody fluid is not exposed to air (Ross, 2015).
- **Cramping.** For mild cramping occurring before or during menses, aspirin and NSAIDs, such as ibuprofen or naproxen, are effective and can be taken unless contraindicated for other reasons. These drugs inhibit uterine contractions and also have analgesic properties. A warm bath or a heating pad may be comforting; lying supine also keeps the abdomen warm.

Premenstrual Syndrome

- **Nonpharmacological treatments.** You might suggest a variety of treatments, such as: getting adequate sleep; eating small, frequent meals; reducing dietary intake of sugar, caffeine, alcohol, and salt; taking vitamin and mineral supplements; and exercising.
- **Medications.** Selective serotonin reuptake-inhibiting drugs, such as fluoxetine (Prozac) and sertraline (Zoloft), are commonly being used as a front-line therapy for managing symptoms of PMS.

Menopause

Hormone replacement therapy (HRT) (estrogen-only, progestin-only, or combination) remains the most effective treatment to relieve symptoms of menopause, such as itching, dryness, discomfort with intercourse, hot flashes, sleep disturbances, and other symptoms.

- **Other benefits of HRT.** Prevention of loss of bone density in menopausal women, which leads to fewer hip fractures, is one benefit. HRT also reduces the risk of colorectal cancer. HRT can either increase or decrease risk of heart disease, depending on when hormone therapy is started; how long women remain on it; and individual differences.
- **Risks of HRT.** In a small number of women, the risks associated with long-term use include heart disease, blood clots, breast and ovarian cancers, and dementia. Therefore, consumers, healthcare providers, and third-party payors

have become more conservative in using HRT or reserving treatment for short-term use.

- **Teaching.** Teach women to discuss the risks and benefits of HRT with their primary care provider and inform them that there are some natural remedies and bioidentical therapies that may provide symptom relief (see the related CAM box).

Screening Exams

Breast self-examination and testicular sexual examinations are vital aspect of sexual health. For more information and for details about these assessments, see Chapters 9, 21, and 27.

Breast Exam Any change in how the breasts normally look and feel should be immediately reported to the healthcare provider. The American Cancer Society guidelines for screening are as follows (Oeffinger, Fontham, Etzioni, et al., 2015; Simon, 2015):

- At age 40—should discuss with their healthcare provider when to begin, and have the opportunity to begin, annual screening (qualified recommendation)
- Women with an average risk of breast cancer—undergo yearly mammography starting at age 45 years (strong recommendation)
- Aged 45 to 54 years—should be screened annually (qualified recommendation)
- Aged 55 years and older—should have mammograms every other year or have the opportunity to continue screening annually (qualified recommendation)
- Continue screening mammography as long as overall health is good and they have a life expectancy of 10 years or longer (qualified recommendation)
- Breast exams, either from a medical provider or self-exams, are no longer recommended.

Testicular Exam The American Cancer Society (2015) advises men that screening for testicular cancer should be a part of the annual cancer screening examination, unless certain risk factors are present (e.g., previous germ cell tumor in one testicle, family history, undescended testicle). A lump in the testicle

could be a sign of testicular cancer; however, some cancers may be at an advanced stage before symptoms are present. Although monthly examinations are a personal preference, checking for lumps after puberty is a good idea to detect change in the testicles.

Preventing Sexually Transmitted Infections

STIs are a worldwide health concern, and education is a key component of prevention.

- **KEY POINT** *The only absolutely safe sex is total avoidance of sexual activity with a partner.* However, most adults do not choose abstinence.
- The next safest sex occurs within a long-term, mutually monogamous relationship.
- Other safer sex practices involve the consistent, correct use of a condom and limiting the number of sexual partners.

Teach your clients the proper use of condoms (see Clinical Insight 34-3) and encourage them to discuss sexual feelings, activity, birth control, STIs, and safer sex with their partners or potential partners. If they are not comfortable talking about these topics, they need to consider whether it is wise to begin a sexual relationship. Planned Parenthood (n.d.) advocates the following behaviors for safer sex:

- Be honest about current sexual practices, sexual history, and sexual health concerns.
- Avoid the exchange of body fluids, including semen, blood, and vaginal secretions by correctly and consistently using latex barriers.
- Avoid contact with genital sores or growths.
- Have routine checkups for infection.
- Consult a healthcare provider for diagnosis and treatment of symptoms such as abnormal discharge from the vagina, penis, or rectum; a burning sensation with urination; sores in the genital area; or painful intercourse.
- Accept responsibility for your actions.

Also advise clients to choose a healthcare provider with whom they can comfortably discuss these issues. Freedom to speak frankly and openly about their sexual health concerns is important to health promotion. Assure them that testing, examination, and treatment for STIs are always confidential, but do explain mandatory reporting requirements.

Contraception

For clients who are heterosexual or bisexual, your sexual health teaching may include methods for preventing unwanted pregnancies. Several family planning strategies are available, each with advantages and disadvantages. Only abstinence and condom use can offer protection from STIs, although contraceptive sponges do offer some protection (see Box 34-1).

Counseling for Sexual Problems

The PLISSIT model was developed as a guideline for counseling for sexual problems (Annon, 1976). The first three PLISSIT steps have been successfully adapted to address sexual knowledge deficits, which you are qualified to assess and treat. The acronym PLISSIT represents the following:

*P*ermission. Permission means that you communicate an open, accepting attitude so that the client feels free to ask open-ended questions and express concerns and feelings and to engage in sexual behaviors with a consenting partner. For example, you might say, "Many women experience decreased vaginal lubrication after menopause. Tell me how well you have been lubricating."

Complementary & Alternative Modalities (CAM)

CAM for Perimenopausal Symptoms

Help, including hormone therapy, is available for perimenopause symptoms. In addition to finding a primary care provider with whom to discuss their symptoms, you might advise women to try the following:

- ➤ Eat a balanced diet, low in fat and rich in calcium.
- ➤ Use supplemental vitamins, if necessary.
- ➤ Take supplemental calcium and magnesium.
- ➤ Get adequate sleep.
- ➤ Exercise daily.
- ➤ Avoid tobacco use.
- ➤ Limit alcohol and caffeine.
- ➤ Drink plenty of water to counteract the drying effect of low estrogen levels.
- ➤ Use soy products (e.g., soy milk, tofu, and soy flour), which are rich in phytoestrogens that are converted during digestion to very weak estrogens.
- ➤ Try the herbal remedies red clover and black cohosh.
- ➤ Use natural progesterone cream, which is made from a yam root. Women usually apply a small amount of the cream for 12 days out of each month

BOX 34-1 ■ Methods of Contraception

Abstinence: No sexual intercourse. Only abstinence is considered 100% effective.

Fertility awareness (natural family planning, rhythm method): Intercourse only when a woman is thought to be in the infertile phase of her menstrual cycle. Has a relatively high failure rate.

Withdrawal (coitus interruptus): Removal of the penis from the vagina before ejaculation; relatively high failure rate in preventing pregnancy.

Male and female condoms: Relatively inexpensive; protect against STIs.

Spermicides: Jelly, creams, or foams placed in the vagina. Should be used with a barrier (condom) to effectively prevent pregnancy.

Contraceptive sponge: Inexpensive; can be inserted into the vagina up to 24 hours before intercourse.

Vaginal ring: Highly effective for preventing pregnancy; can be left in place for weeks to months (depending on type).

Oral contraceptives (birth control pills): Highly effective for preventing pregnancy; do not interfere with intercourse; regulate menstrual flow.

Depo-Provera injections: Highly effective for preventing pregnancy; lasts for 3 months.

Intrauterine device (IUD): A small piece of plastic that also may contain metal or a hormone: placed through the cervix into the uterus by a healthcare provider; highly effective for preventing pregnancy.

Diaphragm: Latex dome-shaped cup with a flexible rim that is inserted in the vagina and fits over the cervix; quite effective in preventing pregnancy if used properly with spermicide.

Cervical cup: Silicone cup shaped like a sailor's hat that is inserted into the vagina and fits over the cervix. Better fit in women who have not been pregnant or had vaginal deliveries. Quite effective in preventing pregnancy if used properly with spermicide.

Hormonal implant: Small rod(s) containing hormones that are inserted under the skin, usually in the back of upper arm. Safe, effective method; lasts for 3 years; can be removed at any time.

Female sterilization (tubal ligation): Effective for preventing pregnancy; may be reversible.

Male sterilization (vasectomy): Effective for preventing pregnancy; may be reversible in some cases.

Limited Information. Supplying limited information may include teaching about normal sexual functioning, expected changes in sexual functioning, medication side effects, and medical and surgical impacts on sexuality. For example, you might say, "Some women experience decreased vaginal lubrication because of decreased levels of certain hormones."

Specific Suggestions. You might make specific suggestions for self-care, as presented in this chapter. For example, you might say, "Some women find that using a water-soluble lubricant is helpful."

Intensive Therapy. If these interventions do not relieve the client's concerns, you should refer the client to someone with specialized knowledge of sexual health. For example, you might state, "I recommend that you discuss this with your gynecologist."

Dealing With Inappropriate Sexual Behavior

Nursing involves intimate contact. We see people disrobe, literally touch bodies, and discuss private topics. In most cases, clients recognize this as professional behavior associated with providing healthcare. Occasionally they may respond inappropriately. For example, a client may make sexually suggestive comments, request sexually related care that is not required (e.g., ask you to bathe his genitalia when he can do it adequately himself), disrobe or expose body parts that are not involved in the care delivered, or touch or grab you as you provide care. The following are the most common reasons for sexually inappropriate behaviors:

- Confusion
- Neurological disorders, especially those involving the frontal lobe
- Mental illness
- Poor impulse control

- Misinterpretation of nursing care
- Need to have power or control over others, especially when the client feels powerless in other aspects of his life
- Worries about sexual functioning
- Unrealistic view of nursing based on sexual stereotypes

If you believe a client is demonstrating inappropriate sexual behaviors, immediately tell the client that the behavior is inappropriate. Do not express anger, but use clear statements, such as, "I don't like your comments. They are inappropriate and make me feel uncomfortable. Please stop." Next, let the client know what behavior you expect. Be direct with your comments. If the client is exposing himself, let him know what you expect him to wear ("I expect you to keep your pajama pants on"). If the client is attempting to touch you, tell him, "Don't touch me." Refocus the client's attention to the care you are delivering ("Hold still now while I tape your IV"). If you are extremely uncomfortable or the client persists in the comments or actions, leave the room and report the incident to your faculty or the nurse assigned to the client. You may also wish to consider discussing the situation with the client while another person is in the room.

Sexual harassment is a unique form of inappropriate sexual behavior.

- If you believe you are being sexually harassed, you should confront your harasser and clearly state your concerns.
- If you feel unable to confront your harasser (e.g., if the harasser is a teacher or supervisor), keep a written record of the events and report your concerns to the worksite or school official in charge of personnel.

By law, all worksites and educational environments must have a written procedure for handling cases of sexual harassment. It will tell you how to file a grievance, what forms you need to use, to whom to report the incident, and details of the procedure for a hearing and resolution. For further information, see Chapter 44.

PUTTING IT ALL TOGETHER

Consider the three clients discussed in the Meet Your Patients scenario. Each situation illustrates how important sexual identity is to the sense of self. The clients are concerned about how their medical problem would affect their sexuality:

- Jocelyn Carter is worried about surgery will affect her relationship with her husband.
- Gabriel Thomas is concerned that blood pressure medications would impair his sexual abilities.
- Frank Thanee, recovering from open heart surgery, is focused on explaining his long-term same-sex relationship to his family.

The full-spectrum nursing model can help you to find the best approach when dealing with sexual health. In the following sections, we use the three clients from Meet Your Patients to illustrate how this works:

Thinking

Theoretical Knowledge A sound knowledge base enables you to teach and respond sensitively to all your clients. You will need theoretical knowledge about sexuality, the myths and taboos surrounding the subject, the effect of health concerns on sexual function and expression, and treatment of sexual health problems. What knowledge do you already have that would enable you to address Gabriel Thomas's concerns? What knowledge do you still need?

Critical Thinking To help Gabriel Thomas, you will need to focus on what he is experiencing and critically examine his concerns in light of what is known about hypertension and its treatment. You will need to prioritize your concerns about Mr. Thomas, balancing the need to control his blood pressure with his sexual requirements. Help him consider the consequences of various approaches, for example, by discussing alternative forms of sexual expression.

Doing

Practical Knowledge When dealing with sexuality, your verbal and nonverbal skills demonstrate to patients your comfort with sensitive topics. For example, suppose you responded to Jocelyn's question by telling her, "That's the least of your worries." How do you think she would feel? Now consider what might happen if you responded, "You must be worried about your sexual relationship. Tell me a little more about what you're feeling."

Nursing Process To help Mr. Thomas, you will need to assess his knowledge and concerns, clearly identify his problems (elevated blood pressure and Ineffective Sexuality Pattern), and develop a plan of care that is acceptable to him. When working with clients with sexual health concerns, tailor your approach to each individual's needs, just as you do in all areas of health.

♥ iCare Caring

Self-Knowledge To help clients identify and resolve sexual health concerns, you will need to examine your own beliefs and values. The self-knowledge gained from examining your own views on sexuality will help you to be open to your patients' sexual concerns. What are your beliefs about sex and sexuality? Are you uncomfortable around people whose sexual orientation is different from yours? Imagine how you would feel if Frank Thanee asked you for help with his family relationships.

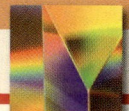 # Nursing Care Plan

Client Data

Emilio Juarez is a 50-year-old man hospitalized for cardiac monitoring after an acute myocardial infarction (MI; heart attack). He has no history of diabetes or hypertension. Mr. Juarez owns a computer software company and is active in the community (president of the Chamber of Commerce).

After dinner, Mr. Juarez's nurse sits down to teach Emilio and his wife, Luz, about the medications that he will be taking. She also begins to talk to them about a cardiac rehabilitation program. Mr. Juarez asks, "What do you mean by 'activity restriction'? Do I have to stop doing all the things I did before?" The nurse asks, "What things are you thinking about?" Mr. Juarez hesitates, then says, "Oh, like working in the yard, going up the stairs, and, you know, personal things." Mrs. Juarez immediately says, "There is no need to talk about that now. The most important thing is for my Emilio to feel better and get home—there is plenty of time for other things later." The nurse tells the Juarezes that many couples are anxious about resuming sexual activity after a heart attack and says, "I'd like to give you some information about that and answer any questions you might have."

Nursing Diagnosis

Ineffective Sexuality Patterns related to lack of knowledge about post-MI sexual activity and reluctance to ask questions, as evidenced by Mrs. Juarez's comment, "There is no need to talk about that now."

NOC Outcomes	Individualized Goals / Expected Outcomes
Sexual Identity (1207) Sexual Functioning (0119) Body Image (1200)	*By discharge, Mr. Juarez will:* 1. Be able to identify two resources he can use to learn more about sexual activity after myocardial infarction. 2. Commit to attending the cardiac rehabilitation classes offered at the hospital. *During and by the end of the cardiac rehabilitation program, Mr. Juarez will:* 1. Identify stressors in his life related to sexual activity. 2. Report a desire to resume sexual activity to pre-MI levels. 3. Resume previous sexual activity. 4. Discuss any problems encountered.

NIC Interventions/Activities	Rationale

NIC Interventions
Sexual counseling (5248)   Body image enhancement (5220)   Anxiety reduction (5820)

Nursing Activities	Rationale
1. Initiate discussions about sexual activity after MI, beginning with general, nonthreatening statements.	Clients and significant others are often too embarrassed to ask about sexual matters. The client's perception of his sexuality impacts personal and social behavior outside the bedroom (Svedberg, Johansson, Persson, et al., 2012). Lack of counseling and education on resuming sexual activity was associated with loss of sexual activity 1 year post–myocardial infarction (Lindau, Abramsohn, Kensey, et al., 2012). Clients should be reassured that after recovery from an MI, sexual activity presents no great risk of another MI ("Sex Generally Safe After Heart Attacks," 2013).

(continued)

Nursing Care Plan (continued)

Nursing Activities	Rationale
2. Allow Mr. Juarez to control the discussion of sexual matters.	The subject of sexual activity should be raised with patients within the context of cardiac rehabilitation (Paull, Arndt, Petkovski, et al., 2011). This shows respect for the client's privacy and his sexual being. Controlling what issues are discussed and when enhances self-esteem (Paull, Arndt, Petkovski, et al., 2011).
3. Listen carefully to Mr. Juarez's verbal and nonverbal expression of concerns.	Anxiety interferes with patients' return to sexual activity after an acute cardiovascular event (Lindau, Abramsohn, Gosch, et al., 2012). Some men may overtly express uninterest in discussing sexual matters; others avoid the topic by joking, avoiding eye contact, or brushing off concerns as not pressing. Commonly, men avoid verbalizing feelings in this area because of the personal nature and threats to masculine identity. Although depressive symptoms are more common in women after an MI and contribute to higher rates of rehospitalization, men also show depression (Lindau, Abramsohn, Gosch, et al., 2012; Mola, 2015).
4. Seek consultation from other members of the healthcare team as needed.	When nurses are uncomfortable talking about sexual matters and do not initiate the conversation, the client may think sexual activity is prohibited after MI. It is imperative that healthcare professionals incorporate sexuality into the plan of care to effectively meet the care needs of their clients (Parker & Yau, 2011; Paull, Arndt, Petkovski, et al., 2011).
5. Include Mrs. Juarez in counseling as much as possible, with Mr. Juarez's consent.	Marriage and close interpersonal relationships allow each member to support the other and alleviate negative effects of stress. The client and spouse may have different perceptions of recovery, anticipated needs, sexuality, and other uncertainties that must be addressed to minimize stress (Baird & Eliasziw, 2011).
6. Be clear about exploring the Juarezes' specific concerns and correct any misinformation.	Anxiety about sexual activity after MI often arises from misconceptions. Fewer than 1% of MIs occur during sexual activity ("Sex Generally Safe After Heart Attacks," 2013). There is no evidence suggesting that sexual activity poses a risk for sudden death ("Sex After Heart Attack," 2013). Regular exercise, such as in a cardiac rehab program, reduces the risk of MI from sexual activity. For some cardiac patients, sexual problems begin before a heart attack. Erectile dysfunction, the consistent inability to sustain an erection, affects more than 50% of men older than 60 and is a recognized symptom of cardiovascular disease. The typical period of maximum risk (which is still very low) is within 4 weeks of the MI (DeBusk, Drory, Goldstein, et al., 2000). Exercise training after acute MI improves cardiovascular efficiency and reduces myocardial oxygen demand during customary activities, including sexual activity. Erectogenic drugs, when used correctly, do not increase overall cardiovascular risk in patients after an MI (Kloner & Henderson, 2013).
7. Discuss the risks of using drugs for erectile dysfunction together with nitrates.	An unsafe drop in blood pressure can occur when erectile dysfunction medication is taken with nitrates (Kloner & Henderson, 2013). Men should be taught to contact their prescribers if they experience an erection lasting more than 4 hours or if a change in vision occurs.

Nursing Care Plan (continued)

Evaluation

After Mrs. Juarez left for the evening, the nurse returned to bring Mr. Juarez a medication. He said, "Thanks for bringing that up and for leaving the booklet. I love my wife, and I was worried. I sure didn't want to have another heart attack. She was embarrassed to let on that it is important to her, but we will be sure to make use of the rehab program." The nurse followed up later by giving the Juarezes a DVD that discusses sexual issues, which they can take home and watch in privacy and comfort when they are ready to do so.

References

Baird, D., & Eliasziw, M. (2011). Disparity in perceived illness intrusiveness and illness severity between cardiac patients and their spouses. *Journal of Cardiovascular Nursing, 26*(6), 481–486. doi:10.1097/JCN.0b013e3182092c11

DeBusk, R., Drory, Y., Goldstein, I., et al. (2000). Management of sexual dysfunction in patients with cardiovascular disease: Recommendations of the Princeton Consensus Panel. *American Journal of Cardiology, 86*(2), 175–181.

Kloner, R., & Henderson, L. (2013). Sexual dysfunction in patients with chronic angina pectoris. *American Journal of Cardiology, 111*(11), 1671–1676.

Lindau, S., Abramsohn, E., Gosch, K., et al. (2012). Patterns and loss of sexual activity in the year following hospitalization for acute myocardial infarction (a United States national multisite observational study). *American Journal of Cardiology, 109*(10), 1439–1444.

Mola, J. (2015). Erectile dysfunction in the older adult. *Urologic Nursing, 35*(2), 87–93.

Parashar, S., Rumsfeld, J. S., Reid, K. J., et al. (2008). Impact of depression on sex differences in outcome after myocardial infarction. *Circulation: Cardiovascular Quality and Outcomes, 2008*(2), 33–40.

Parker, M., & Yau, M. (2011). Sexuality in women with spinal cord injury. Occupational Therapy Australia, 24th National Conference and Exhibition, 29 June–1 July 2011 (#35501). *Australian Occupational Therapy Journal, 58*(Supp. 127).

Paull, G., Arndt, P., Petkovski, D., et al. (2011). Sexuality and chronic cardiovascular disease—a neglected area of practice: The role of the occupational therapist in a cardiac rehabilitation setting. Occupational Therapy Australia, 24th National Conference and Exhibition, 29 June–1 July 2011 (#35503). *Australian Occupational Therapy Journal, 58*(Supp. 127).

Sex after heart attack. (2013). *Harvard Health Letter, 37*(8), 5.

Sex generally safe after heart attacks. (2013) *Mayo Clinic Health Letter, 31*(4), 7.

Svedberg, P., Johansson, I., Persson, S., et al. (2012). Psychometric evaluation of the 25-Item Sex After MI Knowledge Test in a Swedish context. *Scandinavian Journal of Caring Science, 26*(1), 203–208.

Care Map

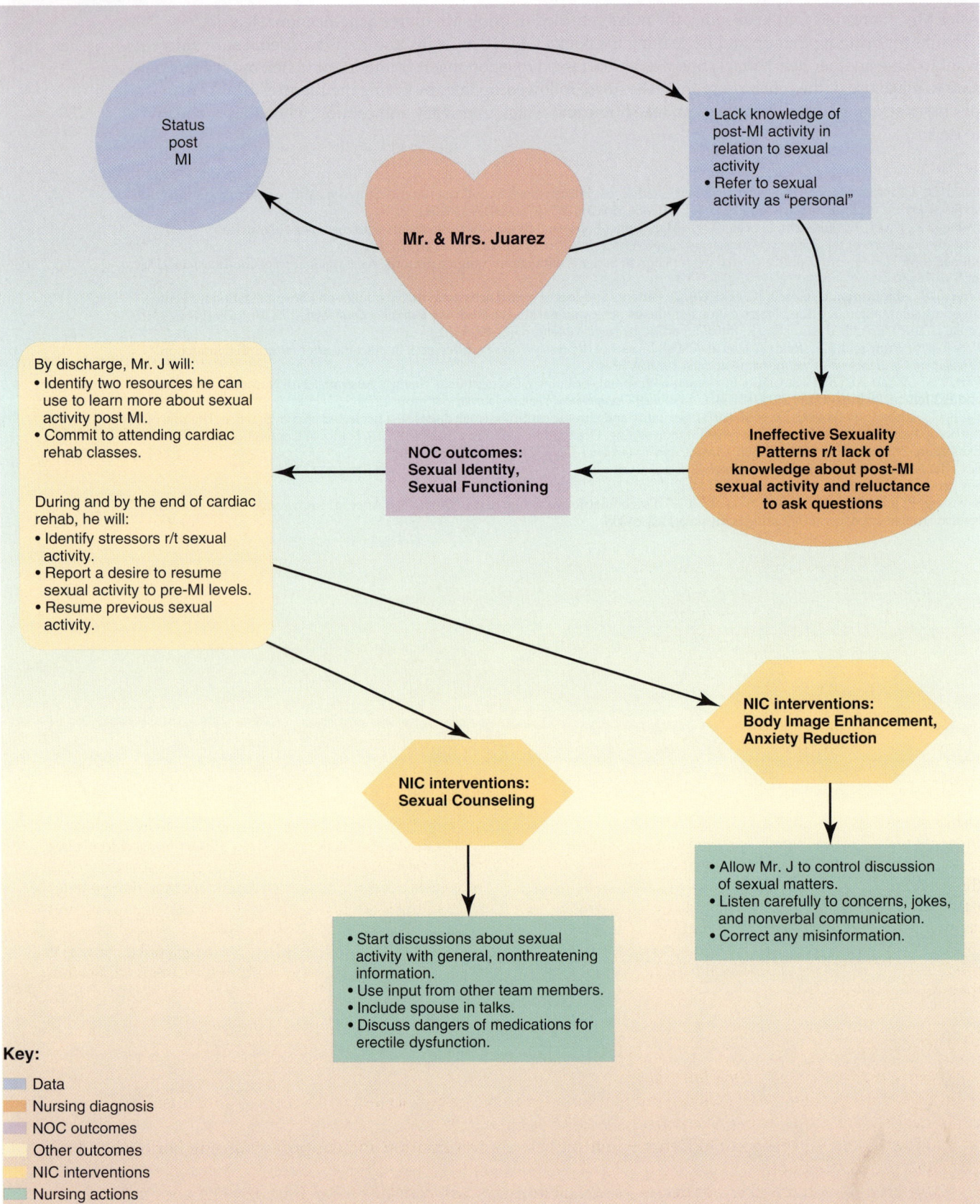

Status post MI

- Lack knowledge of post-MI activity in relation to sexual activity
- Refer to sexual activity as "personal"

Mr. & Mrs. Juarez

By discharge, Mr. J will:
- Identify two resources he can use to learn more about sexual activity post MI.
- Commit to attending cardiac rehab classes.

During and by the end of cardiac rehab, he will:
- Identify stressors r/t sexual activity.
- Report a desire to resume sexual activity to pre-MI levels.
- Resume previous sexual activity.

**NOC outcomes:
Sexual Identity,
Sexual Functioning**

Ineffective Sexuality Patterns r/t lack of knowledge about post-MI sexual activity and reluctance to ask questions

**NIC interventions:
Body Image Enhancement,
Anxiety Reduction**

**NIC interventions:
Sexual Counseling**

- Allow Mr. J to control discussion of sexual matters.
- Listen carefully to concerns, jokes, and nonverbal communication.
- Correct any misinformation.

- Start discussions about sexual activity with general, nonthreatening information.
- Use input from other team members.
- Include spouse in talks.
- Discuss dangers of medications for erectile dysfunction.

Key:
- Data
- Nursing diagnosis
- NOC outcomes
- Other outcomes
- NIC interventions
- Nursing actions

CLINICALREASONING

The questions and exercises in this section allow you to practice the kind of thinking you will use as a full-spectrum nurse. Critical-thinking questions usually have more than one correct answer, so we do not provide "correct answers" for these features. It is more important to develop your nursing judgment than to just cover content. You will learn by discussing the questions with your peers. If you are still unsure, see the Davis Advantage chapter resources for suggested responses.

Caring for the Nguyens

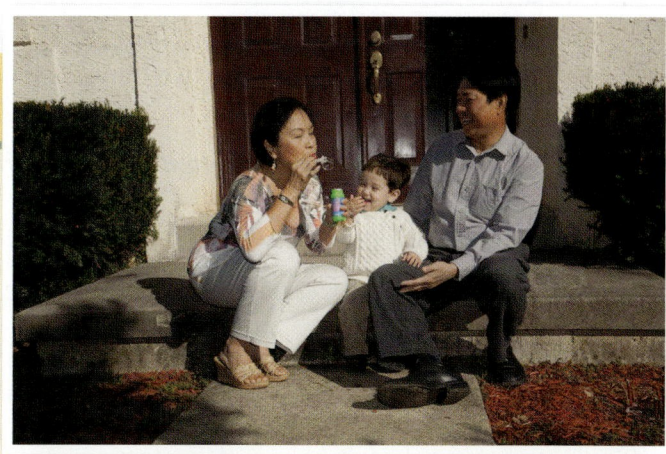

As you may recall, Nam and Yen Nguyen are raising their 3-year-old grandson, Kim. Kim has made friends with Dinh, another little boy at preschool. Kim has asked whether they can play together. Yen works at the preschool and knows Dinh and his family. She is unsure whether she should allow her grandson to play with Dinh because Yen is uncomfortable with the boy's family. Dinh was conceived via artificial insemination and is being raised by a lesbian couple. His parents are open about the relationship and shared the conception information with Yen voluntarily.

A. Yen calls the clinic to speak with you. She explains the situation and asks you whether you think it would be a problem to allow the children to play together. She is concerned that being around this family may be a bad influence on Kim. How would you respond?

B. Yen remains concerned and presses you for more information. She is concerned that Kim's interest in Dinh may indicate that Kim has homosexual tendencies. How would you address her concerns?

C. Yen admits that Nam does not agree with her. "He told me that sexual orientation is genetic." How would you react to this statement?

Go to Davis Advantage, Resources, Chapter 34, **Caring for the Nguyens—Suggested Responses.**

Applying the **Full-Spectrum Nursing Model**

PATIENT SITUATION

Debra is perimenopausal at age 52, and her husband, Roberto, is 59. She has been feeling tired in the afternoon and moody at times. At her annual women's health visit, Debra tells you that she feels a lower level of sexual desire than she used to. Debra says, "I chalk it up to being very busy at work and yet still having so many demands on my time and energy with care of our three kids and housework." Debra is physically active, exercising four times a week, and is in good general health. She takes no medication and is within 15 pounds of her normal weight. Debra still has her period, but the flow is very heavy and cramping is more uncomfortable than it ever had been.

Recently, Debra has noticed that Roberto has been taking longer to achieve an erection, and his erection is not as firm as it used to be. He is in general good health except for high blood pressure and high blood cholesterol levels. He takes medication for both conditions.

THINKING

1. *Theoretical Knowledge (Factual Information):*
   a. What are the common physical and emotional manifestations occurring with perimenopause?
2. *Critical Thinking (Analyzing Alternatives, Deciding What to Do):*
   a. How would you respond to Debra when she asks for information and support regarding her husband's erectile dysfunction?
   b. Debra asks you whether her desire for sexual intimacy will continue to decline after she goes through "the change of life." Describe in detail what you would tell her.

DOING

3. *Practical Knowledge:*
   a. What general topics would you explore with Debra to assess her sexual history?
   b. What questions would you ask Roberto to assess his sexual history?

CARING

4. *Self-Knowledge:* What might you be feeling if you were in Debra's situation?
5. *Ethical Knowledge:* What are one or two things you would do to help Debra and Roberto feel cared for and cared about?

 Go to Davis Advantage, Resources, Chapter 34, **Apply the Full-Spectrum Nursing Model—Suggested Responses.**

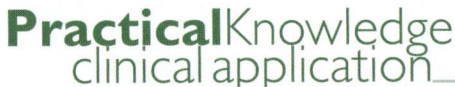

PracticalKnowledge
clinical application

CLINICAL INSIGHTS

Clinical Insight 34-1 ➤ **Providing Care After Sexual Assault**

- **Carefully collect information about the incident** and document findings in a fact-based manner, following your institution's protocol.
- **Be sensitive to the victim's fear, anxiety, and guilt** related to the event.
  Open discussion without communicating judgment or disapproval helps with fact finding for better care.
- **Assess the victim's emotional status,** including sexual identity, stress disorder, and risks for suicide and self-harm. Also discuss the potential for sexual and physical violence, including violence within relationships.
- **When collecting a nursing history for people with disabilities, be sure to screen for sexual violence.**
- **Administer prophylactic treatment** to patients who have been assaulted (vaginally, anally, or orally) to prevent sexually transmitted infections (STIs), such as chlamydia and gonorrhea. If there is a significant risk for HIV, prophylaxis may be prescribed within 72 hours of exposure.
- **Administer vaccines to prevent hepatitis B and human papillomavirus (HPV),** as prescribed and according to your agency's policy.

- **Administer emergency pregnancy prevention** (e.g., the "morning after" pill) to patients who have been vaginally assaulted even if penetration is uncertain, according to your agency's policy.
- **Document pregnancy status** with a urine or blood sample.
- **Teach follow-up care.** The victim should receive follow-up care within 1 week after the event to assess for healing of injuries and presence of STIs. Advise a female victim who has had vaginal penetration to obtain pregnancy testing again 2 weeks after the event.
- **Follow the current reporting requirements** for sexual assault in your state. Some states require reporting assault of children and adolescents, even if they do not consent to the reporting.
- **Know support services** available in your community for victims of abuse. Refer the victim to a sexual assault center for support, counseling, and additional information. Because of the long-term psychological and emotional consequences of sexual assault, most victims benefit from counseling.

Clinical Insight 34-2 ➤ **Guidelines for Taking a Sexual History**

1. **Provide privacy.**
   - Usually it is not enough merely to pull the curtains around the bed. Ask others who may be able to overhear private conversation behind the curtain to leave the room.
   - Talk to the client alone.
   - In some situations, it is also beneficial to talk to the partners as a unit, with the consent of both of course.
2. **Protect confidentiality.** Assure your client that information will not be shared with others, unless directly related to planning or delivering healthcare.
3. **Be relaxed in your approach** and allow the client time to fully answer your questions. Your manner and attitude are critical in putting the client at ease.
4. **Make eye contact.** Do not act embarrassed or allow your body language to show your discomfort.
5. **Avoid communication stoppers** such as:
   - "I'm only asking you these questions because I have to."
   - "I know that you probably won't want to tell me but ..."
   - "You're not having any sexual problems, are you?"
6. **Consider a more inviting opening** such as:
   - "Many people are embarrassed when asked questions about their sexuality, but whatever you tell me will remain confidential."
   - "Many people hesitate to talk about sexual problems. However, your sexual health is important to your overall health, and I would like to ask you a few questions about that."
7. **Be aware of verbal and nonverbal cues** that indicate concerns. Many people will cloak their concerns in comments such as, "I suppose that I won't need to worry about sexy lingerie any longer," or "Sex is for the young. I just have to accept that I'm sick and older now." Be careful that your response to such statements does not either negate or validate your patient's identity as a sexual being. Follow up with comments that encourage the client to provide more details (see Chapter 20 if you would like to review communication techniques).
8. **Realize the client may be embarrassed.** If the client is uncomfortable discussing topics about his own sexual health, reassure him by letting him know that some information, because of its private nature, may be difficult to discuss, but important.
9. **Encourage your client to use terminology that he is comfortable with.**
10. **Help the client feel comfortable.** Consider statements/questions such as the following:
    - "Most people wonder how this surgery [or illness] may affect their sexual functioning."
    - "Whenever these medications are suggested, there are questions about sexual side effects."
    - "Have you thought about the kinds of adaptations you may have to make in your sex life after this surgery/treatment/illness?"
11. **Begin with a less sensitive topic** such as "How is your relationship with your partner [spouse]?" Then you can move into more sensitive areas: "Many older women have some vaginal dryness that creates discomfort during intercourse. Do you have any concerns about this?"

Clinical Insight 34-3 ➤ Teaching Your Patient to Use a Condom

Using Male Condoms

The male condom is a sheath that covers the penis during sexual activity.

- Put the condom on before the penis touches the vagina, mouth, or anus.
- Inspect the package to ensure that the condom has not been damaged.
- Open the package without tearing the condom.
- Squeeze out the air at the tip of the condom and unroll it over the erect penis, leaving some space at the tip to collect the ejaculate.
- After sex, to avoid breaking the condom, hold the condom at the rim as the penis is withdrawn. Discard the condom. Wash your hands.
- Use a new condom if you want to have sex again.

Using Female Condoms

The female condom is a plastic pouch that fits inside the vagina so that all vaginal tissue is protected from contact with the penis. The condom is inserted with the inner ring placed high in the vagina near the cervix and the outer ring on the labia.

- Insert the condom before the penis touches the vagina.
- Inspect the package to ensure that the condom has not been damaged.

- Open the package without tearing the condom.
- Put the inner ring and pouch inside the vagina.
- Push the inner ring as far into the vagina as it will go.
- Ensure that the outer ring stays outside the vagina.
- If needed, add lubricant to the inside of the condom.
- After sex, gently pull out the condom and discard.

Do

- Do use latex condoms unless you or your partner are allergic to latex, or use polyurethane condoms.
- Do treat condoms gently and keep them out of the sun.
- Do use only water-based lubricants to reduce friction and prevent tearing.
- Do check the expiration date of the condom and packaging. Old condoms may be brittle and more likely to break.

Don't

- Don't store condoms in your wallet or other place where body heat can break down the latex.
- Don't use fingernails or teeth to open the condom wrapper; doing so can tear the condom.
- Don't reuse a condom.
- Don't use lotions or oils with condoms; these may cause breakage.

 To explore learning resources for this chapter,

 Go to www.DavisAdvantage.com and find:

Answers and Suggested Responses for all questions in this chapter

Lists of NIC Interventions and NOC Outcomes

List of NANDA-I Diagnoses

Knowledge Map

Care Plan

Care Map

References and Bibliography

Concept Map

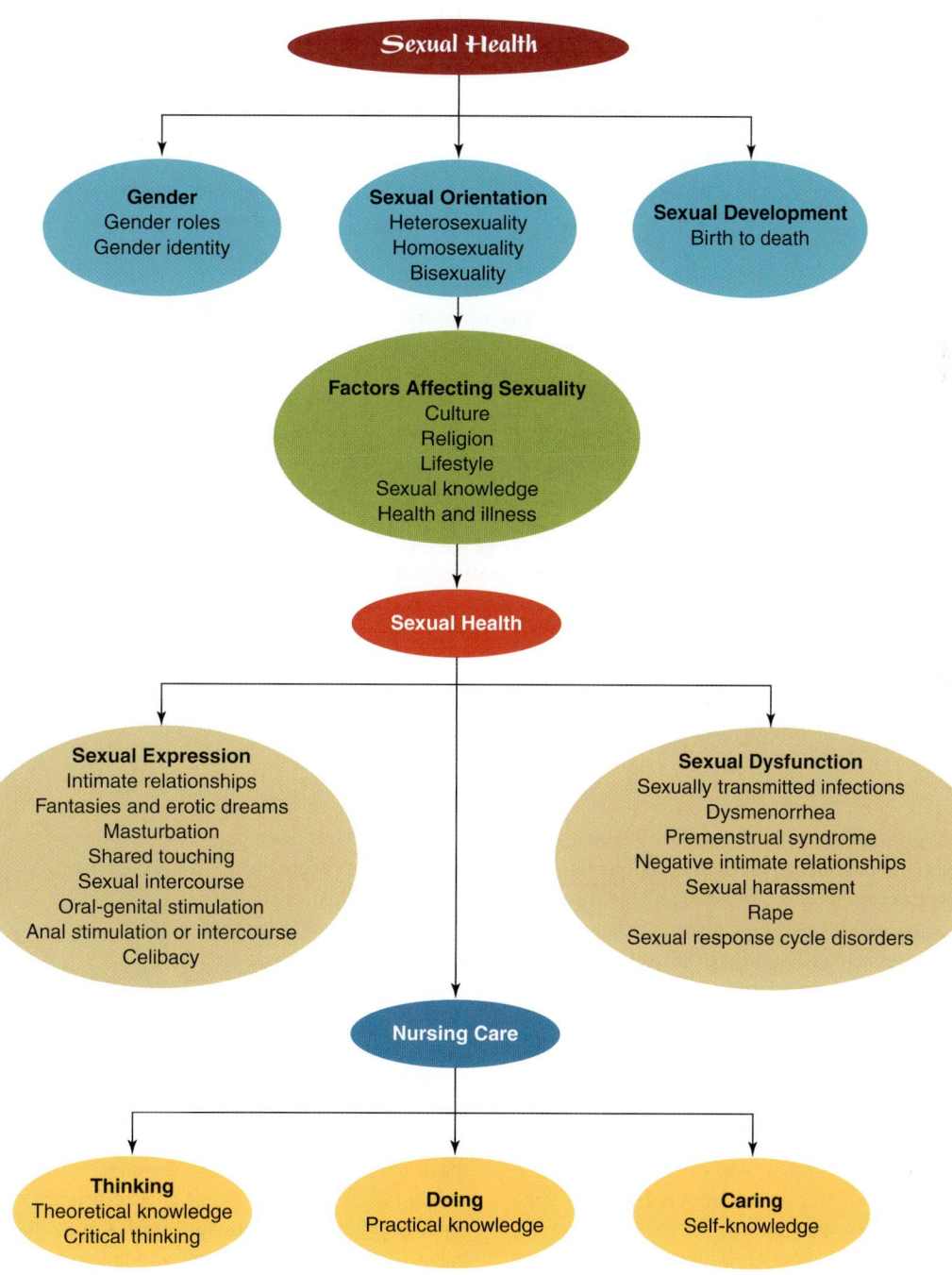

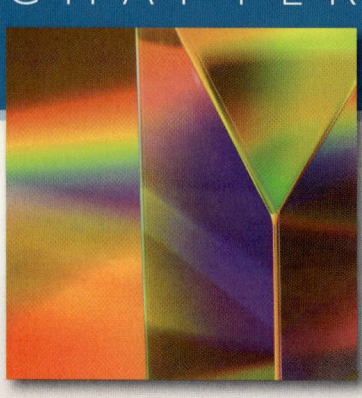

CHAPTER 35

Sleep & Rest

Learning Outcomes

After completing this chapter, you should be able to:

➤ Explain why rest and sleep are important.

➤ Describe the functions and physiology of sleep.

➤ Explain circadian rhythms and how they relate to sleep.

➤ Identify factors that influence rest and sleep.

➤ Discuss how sleep impacts physical, mental, and spiritual well-being.

➤ Describe nursing implications for age-related differences in the sleep cycle.

➤ Identify at least five common sleep disorders.

➤ Perform a comprehensive sleep assessment using appropriate interview questions, a sleep diary, and a sleep history.

➤ Formulate nursing diagnoses that identify sleep problems that may be treated through specific nursing interventions.

➤ Plan, implement, and evaluate nursing care related to specific nursing diagnoses addressing sleep problems.

Key Concepts

Rest

Sleep

Related Concepts

See the Concept Map at the end of this chapter.

Meet Your Patient

You are a nurse working on a surgical unit. Today you are meeting with Anne for preoperative teaching. She is scheduled for a complete hysterectomy next Monday. She has a secondary diagnosis of fibromyalgia, a chronic disorder characterized by widespread muscle pain and nonrestorative sleep.

Anne is a 49-year-old married woman with three children. She works full-time and manages the family with her husband. She says, "I'm a little nervous about the surgery, but I know I need it. But I haven't been sleeping well because of thinking about it." Anne tells you that she has actually had trouble sleeping for the past 20 years. "I take an Ambien pill, 10 milligrams, every night to help me sleep. Will I be able to get that in the hospital? I really can't sleep at all without it," explains Anne.

As you continue the interview, Anne explains that she suffered from physical and emotional abuse as a young woman and has had sleep problems ever since. She has been to counseling, but that did not improve her sleep. Recently her sleep has been even more troublesome. Aside from her upcoming

surgery, she has been coping with the recent death of her father. After meeting with Anne, you realize that sleep-promoting measures will be an important part of her nursing care while she is in the hospital.

What clues in Anne's situation would cause you to suspect that she will have difficulty sleeping while in the hospital? What characteristics of the hospital environment might interfere with Anne's sleep? You may not have enough theoretical knowledge and experience to feel confident about your answers to these questions, but use your present knowledge base and your life experiences to think about them.

Theoretical Knowledge
knowing **why**

Have you felt tired after waking up from a night's sleep? Have you ever been tired, but not sleepy, and, after relaxing a while, felt your normal energy return? How do you think sleep and rest are different? How are they alike?

ABOUT THE KEY CONCEPTS

In this chapter we will examine the concepts of rest and sleep, along with related concepts (e.g., stages of sleep, sleep disorders).

Rest is a condition in which the body is inactive or engaging in mild activity, after which the person feels refreshed. A person at rest is calm, at ease, relaxed, and free of anxiety and stress (Fig. 35-1). People rest by doing things that they find calming and relaxing.

Sleep is a cyclically occurring state of decreased motor activity and perception (Fig. 35-2). Body functions slow, and metabolism falls by 20% to 30%, so the body conserves energy. Sleep is characterized by altered consciousness: A sleeping person is unaware of the environment and responds selectively to external stimuli. For example, an alarm clock, bright light, or other meaningful stimuli usually awaken a sleeper, but everyday background noises and soft light do not.

Although necessary and beneficial, rest without sleep is inadequate. At rest, the body is disturbed by all exterior stimuli, whereas in sleep it is screened from them by altered consciousness. Thus, sleep restores the body; rest alone cannot do this.

WHY DO WE NEED TO SLEEP?

We spend more time sleeping than in any other single activity. So why is sleep so important? The reason is that sleep and rest are essential for physical, mental, and spiritual well-being. Think back to the last time you slept poorly. Remember the mental fogginess, the physical fatigue, the feeling of slight nausea? Poor quality or insufficient length of sleep for even one night can reduce mental performance, and long periods of sleep deprivation can result in stress-related illnesses (e.g., cardiac events) and injuries (e.g., sustained in an automobile accident).

- *Sleep affects almost every tissue in our bodies.* Sleep isn't essential just for the brain; it also affects growth and stress hormones, and even hormones that affect appetite and control

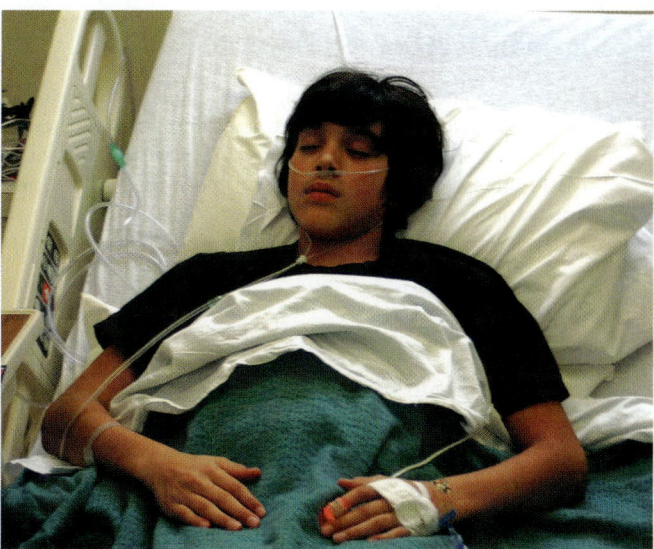

FIGURE 35-2 Boy sleeping in hospital setting.

body weight. Research also indicates that sleep strengthens the immune system (Cohen, Doyle, Alper, et al., 2009) and helps the body to fight infection. Lack of sleep increases the risk heart disease, stroke, infections (National Institutes of Health, 2013), and possibly even cancer (Hakin, Wang, Zhang, et al., 2014).

- *Sleep is an important regulator of energy metabolism.* Despite the fact that some regions of the brain are more active during sleep than when we are awake, total energy output is reduced during sleep, giving the body time for restoration and repair. Without sleep, the body is less able to tolerate glucose and yet responds with insulin resistance. Too little sleep is also linked to increased appetite through changes in the appetite control hormones, leptin and ghrelin. In addition, inadequate sleep leads to reduced energy expenditure, all of which can lead to obesity and type 2 diabetes (Broussard, Ehrmann, van Cauter, et al., 2012).

- *Sleep may also improve learning and adaptation.* It gives the individual a chance to mentally repeat and rehearse facts and situations before they are encountered in wakeful life. Some evidence suggests that sleep and dreaming may facilitate the storage of long-term memory, perhaps by assisting the brain in reorganizing and storing information (National Institutes of Health, 2010, reviewed 2012).

   Older adults have an even greater need for sleep to protect against the natural decline in cognitive function that comes with aging (Mander, Tao, Lu, et al., 2013).

- *Sleep also appears to reduce stress and anxiety,* improving our ability to cope and concentrate on activities of daily living. More sleep also reduces the body's sensitivity to pain (Roehrs, Harris, Randall, et al., 2012). Similarly, nonrestorative sleep contributes to widespread pain, which is common in older adults (McBeth, Lacey, & Wilkie, 2014).

- *Sleep/rest and illness are interrelated* (Fig. 35-3). Illness and injury increase the need to sleep and at the same time make it difficult to sleep. In turn, lack of sleep increases the susceptibility to illness by compromising the immune system. People who are ill or injured need more sleep to restore energy needed for tissue repair and healing. However, they often have difficulty resting because of pain and other symptoms of their illness.

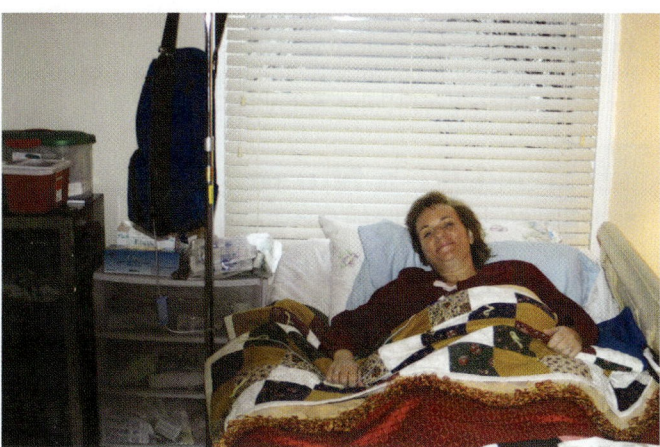

FIGURE 35-1 Woman receiving hospice care resting comfortably.

PICOT

Acupuncture for Neuropathic Pain

Situation: The nurse is caring for a client with peripheral neuropathy secondary to uncontrolled diabetes. The client is showing signs of daytime drowsiness, irritability, and restlessness. He states he has trouble sleeping but does not want to take medication for pain. He is willing to try alternative therapies.

PICOT Components

P	Population/client	=	Sleep-deprived adults with chronic pain
I	Intervention/indicator	=	Acupuncture
C	Comparator/control	=	No acupuncture
O	Outcome	=	Decreased pain and increased sleep
T	Time	=	(none needed)

Searchable Question

Do _____(P) who receive/are exposed to _____(I) demonstrate _____(O) as compared to _____(C)?

Example of Evidence: Persistent neuropathic pain can interfere with quality of life and impair sleep. It has been associated with depression, anxiety, and loss of sleep.

Acupuncture has been helpful in decreasing neuropathic pain. In one study, 77% of clients reported pain relief after six courses of acupuncture. Therefore, the client with neuropathic pain might use acupuncture to rest more comfortably and minimize the sleep disturbances that were impairing the sleep and rest cycle.

Application to Practice: The client who reports unsatisfactory sleep requires a more in-depth sleep history, including questions about the quality of sleep, sleep hygiene, napping, and bedtime routines. A complete medication and pain history should be obtained. As sleep disturbance may increase a patient's pain, the nurse may decide to explore with the healthcare team the possibility of suggesting acupuncture to a patient who is dealing with chronic pain.

 Go to Davis Advantage, Resources, **Chapter 35, PICOT—Suggested Responses.**

Source: Vinik, A. I., & Casellini, C. M. (2013). Guidelines in the management of diabetic nerve pain: Clinical utility of pregabalin. *Diabetes, Metabolic Syndrome, and Obesity, 6*, 57–78. doi:10.2147/DMSO.S24825

KnowledgeCheck 35-1

- Compare and contrast sleep and rest. How are they different? Alike?
- Why is promoting sleep an important nursing intervention?

ThinkLike a Nurse 35-1

What effect do you think surgery will have on your patient's sleep? Why?

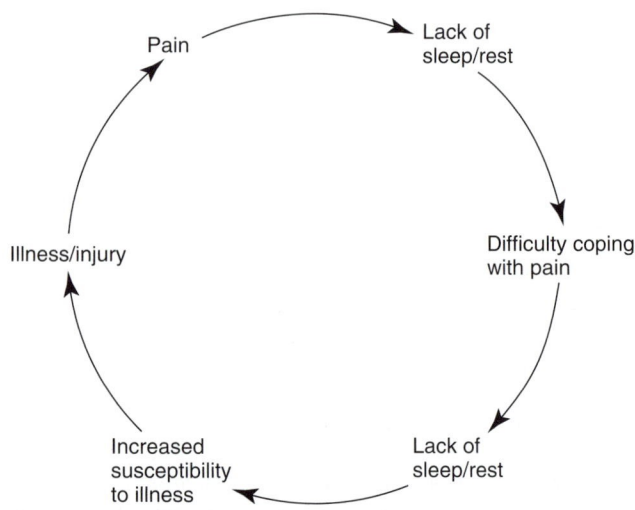

FIGURE 35-3 Relationship between sleep/rest and illness. Lack of sleep and rest increases susceptibility to illness. Likewise, the pain and stress of illness disturb sleep.

HOW MUCH SLEEP DO WE NEED?

Sleep needs vary widely among individuals. Some people are refreshed after napping for 15 or 20 minutes; others feel groggy; others cannot nap at all. Many people routinely awaken several times a night and do not report being tired, whereas others report fatigue, irritability, and loss of mental clarity if their sleep is even minimally interrupted. In most adults, sleep of 7 to 8 hours is fully restorative; however, there are wide individual variations. In some cultures, total sleep time is divided into an overnight sleep period and a midafternoon nap.

In spite of individual variations, different sleep patterns are characteristic of different age-groups (Table 35-1). For instance, older adults typically spend significantly less time sleeping but need more rest than do younger adults. They take longer to fall asleep, and their arousal periods during sleep are longer and more frequent. Frequent waking is commonly due to physical discomfort, anxiety, and nocturia (Polan & Taylor, 2015).

ThinkLike a Nurse 35-2

- How much sleep might you expect your patient, Anne (Meet Your Patient), to need in a normal night?
- How will a good night of sleep benefit Anne while she is in the hospital?
- If you were preparing for an important test, would it be better to stay up all night studying, or should you try to get a good night of sleep?
- How many hours of sleep do *you* need to feel rested and function well the next day? Compare notes with family members, friends, and classmates. Do they all need the same amount of sleep as you do?

Table 35-1 ➤ Average Sleep Requirements

AGE-GROUP	HOURS PER DAY
Newborns (birth–4 wk)	16–20
Infants (4 wk–1 yr)	14–16
Toddlers (1–3 yr)	12–14
Preschoolers (3–6 yr)	11–13
Middle and late childhood (6–12 yr)	10–11
Adolescents (12–18 yr)	8–9
Young adults (18–40 yr)	7–8
Middle-aged adults (40–65 yr)	7
Older adults (65 years and older)	5–7

Source: Adapted from: Centers for Disease Control and Prevention. (2015, updated). How much sleep do I need? Retrieved from http://www.cdc.gov/sleep/about_sleep/how_much_sleep.html

PHYSIOLOGY OF SLEEP

Our environment plays a role in the physiology of sleep, so we begin with an exploration of circadian rhythms, by which the body maintains synchrony with nature. **Synchrony** occurs when things happen, work, or develop at the same time, or on the same time scale, as something else.

How Do Circadian Rhythms Influence Sleep?

Do you feel sleepy at about the same time each night? Do you often awaken before the alarm clock goes off? If so, that's because the timing of sleep and waking is influenced by your circadian biorhythm. **Biorhythms** are "biological clocks" that are controlled within the body and synchronized with environmental factors (e.g., gravity, electromagnetic forces, light, darkness).

A **circadian rhythm** is a biorhythm based on the day–night pattern in a 24-hour cycle. It is regulated by a cluster of cells in the hypothalamus of the brainstem that respond to changing levels of light. Circadian rhythm affects our overall level of functioning; most people have a higher energy level in the daytime and less energy at night. However, some people are more alert and active in the morning, whereas others function at a higher level in the afternoon or evening.

Sleep quality is best when the time at which you go to sleep and wake up is in synchrony with your circadian rhythm. For this reason:

- *People who work evening and night shifts* can suffer significant sleep deprivation until their bodies adjust to the new pattern (see the accompanying Self-Care box).
- *Changing time zones* can also disrupt sleep–wake cycles and can thus be troublesome for people who travel frequently.
- *Hospitalization* can also interfere with a patient's circadian rhythm. Noises, lights, waking the patient for vital signs or medications, altered normal bedtime rituals, absence or presence of family members, recent losses, or fear of the unknown may compromise the patient's quality of sleep and the ability to fall and stay asleep (Meltzer, Davis, & Mindell, 2012).

Fatigue and Sleep Deprivation Among Healthcare Workers

Extended work hours and rotating shift work significantly increase fatigue and impair on-the-job performance and safety.

Impact of Fatigue

- ➤ Lapses in attention and memory; poor concentration
- ➤ Irritability
- ➤ Reduced motivation, apathy, and indifference
- ➤ Diminished reaction time
- ➤ Impaired judgment and decision making
- ➤ Altered communication
- ➤ More errors, needlestick and sharps injuries, and adverse events to patients

Fight Sleepiness on the Job

- ➤ Be honest with yourself about how you tolerate rotating shifts, night shifts, and longer shifts (e.g., 12 hours), and schedule accordingly. Plan rest days in between consecutive workdays.
- ➤ Engage in conversation with others, not just listen and nod.
- ➤ Do something that requires physical action periodically, even if it means just getting up and moving around.
- ➤ Take frequent breaks (e.g., every 1 to 2 hours) during the night shift, if possible.
- ➤ Be smart about your caffeine use; that is, don't take caffeine when you don't need it to stay awake, and avoid caffeine at the end of your shift before sleep.
- ➤ Practice good sleep hygiene measures during your off hours. See the Self-Care box Teaching Your Patients About Sleep Hygiene.

Source: Adapted from The Joint Commission. (2011). Health care worker fatigue and patient safety. *The Joint Commission Sentinel Event Alert, 48,* 1–4. Retrieved from http://www.jointcommission.org/assets/1/18/sea_48.pdf

ThinkLike a Nurse 35-3

What may upset Anne's (Meet Your Patient) circadian rhythm?

How Is Sleep Regulated?

The mechanisms of sleep are complex and poorly understood, but we know that centers in the lower part of the brain produce sleep by actively inhibiting wakefulness. As just noted, a major factor in regulating sleep is the amount of light received through the eyes. The increasing light of a dawning sky signals the hypothalamus (Fig. 35-4) to induce gradual arousal from sleep.

Reticular Activating System (RAS)   Another collection of nerve cell bodies within the brainstem, called the **reticular formation,** is responsible for maintaining wakefulness. The reticular formation is activated by stimuli from the cerebral cortex. Together, these reticular and cortical neurons are called the **RAS.** Neurotransmitters associated with excitatory and inhibitory sleep mechanisms include catecholamines, acetylcholine, serotonin, histamine, and prostaglandins.

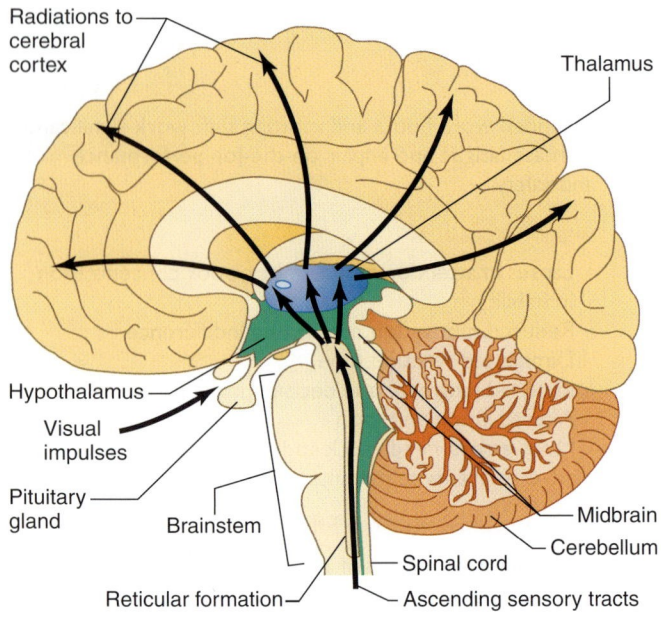

FIGURE 35-4 The reticular activating system works to regulate sleep and wakefulness.

An **electroencephalogram (EEG)** is used to record the electrical activity of the neurons in the brain. Electrical impulses are transmitted from the brain through electrodes attached to the scalp. These impulses create five different wave patterns, or *brain waves*. Figure 35-5 shows different types of brain waves during sleep:

- **Alpha waves** are high-frequency, medium-amplitude irregular waves. These occur in the drowsy stage.
- **Beta waves** are high-frequency, low-amplitude irregular waves. These occur during periods of wakefulness.
- **Delta waves** are low-frequency, high-amplitude regular waves common in deep sleep.
- **Theta waves** are high-amplitude waves that are common in children but rare in adults. These occur with delta waves when transitioning to a deeper sleep stage.
- **Spindles** or **K-complexes** are peaked, irregular waveforms that occur in the earlier phases of non–rapid eye movement sleep.

The EEG of a waking person differs greatly from that of a sleeping person. In general, the greater the brain activity, the more rapid the brain waves will be on the EEG.

- *While the person is awake*, brain waves are very rapid, irregular, and low in amplitude, mostly alpha and beta waves. Many neurons are firing at different intervals, at different times, and with different strengths.
- *When a person is relaxed* without intense stimulation of the senses, the EEG records mostly alpha activity.
- *During sleep* alpha waves disappear. They are replaced by slower, higher amplitude delta waves.

What Are the Stages of Sleep?

There are two distinct types of sleep, non–rapid eye movement (NREM) and rapid eye movement (REM. The body moves back and forth between them during the sleep cycle (Fig. 35-6).

NREM Sleep

NREM (non–rapid eye movement) sleep is generally the restful phase of sleep in which physiological function is slow. NREM sleep is also called slow-wave sleep because it is characterized

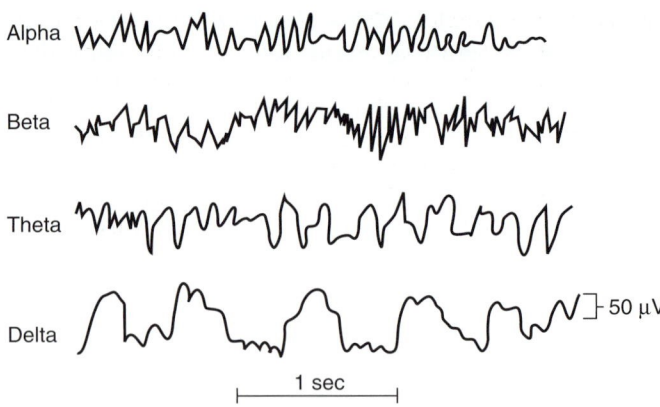

FIGURE 35-5 Four different types of brain waves.

by the presence of delta waves. NREM is divided into three stages, each deeper than the one preceding it. The parasympathetic branch of the autonomic nervous system becomes progressively more dominant during each stage of NREM sleep. During this phase, muscles relax; body temperature lowers; and heart rate, respirations, and blood pressure decrease.

REM Sleep

REM (rapid eye movement) sleep is essential for mental and emotional restoration. During REM sleep the brain becomes highly active and brain waves resemble those of a person who is fully awake. More spontaneous awakenings occur during this stage than any other. Loss of REM sleep impairs memory and learning. A person who is deprived of REM sleep for several nights will usually experience *REM rebound*—that is, spend a greater amount of time in REM sleep on successive nights, keeping the total amount of REM sleep constant over time.

Sleep Cycles

Cycling between REM and NREM sleep produces restorative rest. The American Academy of Sleep Medicine (2014a) identifies four stages of sleep (three NREM stages and the REM stage), based on brain activity and other physiological

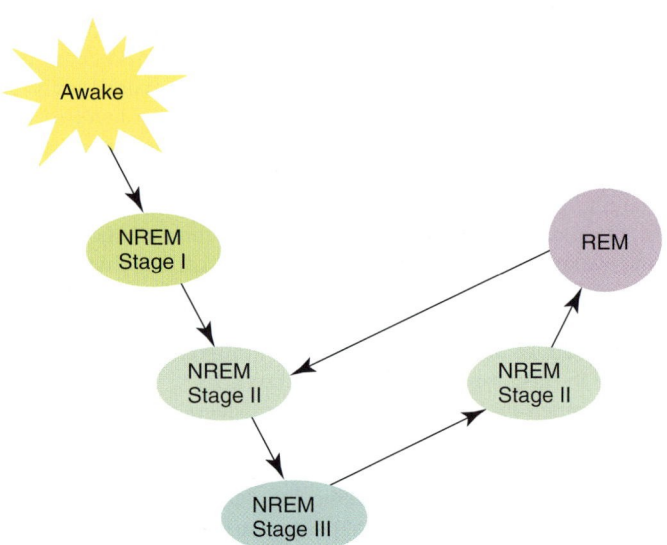

FIGURE 35-6 The normal adult sleep cycle. All but NREM stage I are repeated four or more times a night.

characteristics (Table 35-2). The NREM/REM sleep cycle repeats four to six times throughout the night, depending on the total amount of time spent sleeping (Fig. 35-6). Each cycle lasts about 90 to 100 minutes. The first REM period may last only about 20 minutes, but with each cycle, the REM period lengthens until, in the last cycle of a typical 8-hour sleep period, REM may last as long as 60 minutes. The amount of time spent in each sleep stage varies over the life span.

KnowledgeCheck 35-2

- List the five stages of sleep.
- Describe the progression of a typical sleep cycle for a young adult.
- Describe the physiological activity characteristic of each stage of sleep.
- What is the stage that must be "made up" if not enough time is spent in it?

Table 35-2 ► Characteristics of Stages of Sleep

Stage: W (Wakefulness)

Typical Brain Wave Type:	Characteristics:
Beta waves with some alpha waves	Ranges from full alertness to the early stages of drowsiness.
	Reading eye movements
	Eye blinks with eyes open or closed

Stage: NI (NREM)

Typical Brain Wave Type:	Characteristics:
Alpha waves with occasional low-frequency theta waves	Transition between wakefulness and sleep
	Slow eye movements
	Light sleep; can be awakened easily
	Relaxed but aware of surroundings
	Groggy, heavy lidded
	Regular, deep breathing; eyelids open and close slowly
	Account for about 5% of total sleep
	Dreams are not usually remembered

Stage: NII (NREM)

Typical Brain Wave Type:	Characteristics:
Theta waves, K-complexes, and sleep spindles	Light sleep
	Easily roused
	Temperature, heart rate, and blood pressure decreased slightly
	Accounts for about half of total sleep time

Stage: NIII (NREM)

Typical Brain Wave Type:	Characteristics:
Delta waves, sawtooth waves	Deep sleep
	Difficult to rouse; if awakened in this stage, may be confused
	Parasympathetic nervous system predominates: temperature, pulse, respirations, and blood pressure slow even more
	Skeletal muscles are very relaxed.
	Snoring may occur.
	Some dreaming may occur, but dreams are less vivid than those that occur in REM sleep. This sleep stage is especially important for restorative processes such as healing, growth, and tissue renewal.
	Makes up 20% to 25% of total sleep time

(Continued)

Table 35-2 ➤ Characteristics of Stages of Sleep—cont'd

	Stage: REM
Typical Brain Wave Type:	**Characteristics**
5–30 minutes (usually at least 20–30)	Highly active sleep with spontaneous awakenings
	Less restful than NREM sleep
	Eyes move rapidly and small muscles twitch.
	Essential for mental and emotional restoration
	Metabolism, temperature, pulse, and blood pressure increase.
	Pulse may be rapid and irregular.
	Apnea may occur.
	Gastric secretions increase.
	Deep-tendon reflexes are depressed.
	Dreaming occurs.
	If awakened, person will react normally.
	Accounts for about 25% of total sleep

ThinkLike a Nurse 35-4

- A physician has prescribed zolpidem tartrate for your patient, Anne (Meet Your Patient). This sedative/hypnotic (nonbarbiturate) is used as a short-term treatment for insomnia. Why do you think the doctor prescribed a sleeping medication even though she is physiologically and psychologically dependent on the medication?
- Anne will likely receive opioid analgesics after surgery. How do you think they will affect her sleep?

WHAT FACTORS AFFECT SLEEP?

People vary not only in the amount of sleep they need but also in their sleep patterns. **Sleep quality** is related to (1) the total amount of sleep, (2) how well the person slept, and (3) whether he obtained the needed amounts of NREM and REM. More than one-quarter of the U.S. population report occasionally not getting enough sleep, while nearly 10% experience chronic insomnia (Centers for Disease Control and Prevention, n.d., updated 2015).

Age

Age is an important factor affecting the duration of sleep (see Table 35-1). But sleep *patterns* are also affected by age. For instance:

- *Toddlers and preschoolers* often have trouble falling asleep, frequent awakenings, nightmares, and heavy snoring. They often have difficulty "winding down" after hectic activities in the late afternoon and early evening hours.
- *School-age children and adolescents* may suffer sleep disturbances related to stress, excitement, or social concerns, such as anticipating a school event or sports competition. Adolescents may not sleep well because of increased demands at school, or by staying up late to study, watch television, play video games, text, or participate in other social networking. They may stay out late with friends or use alcohol, nicotine, or drugs. Some teens consume caffeinated beverages that delay or disturb sleep. Most sleep with smartphones near their beds. The light produced by such devices disrupts circadian rhythms and suppresses naturally occurring melatonin, which results in difficulty falling asleep (Owens, Adolescent Sleep Work Group, & Committee on Adolescents, 2014).

- *College students* may stay up all night to cram for exams or may experience difficulty falling asleep or staying asleep because of worries about grades or future career choices. Many have a preference for a late-night schedule, yet have schedules requiring them to attend an 8:00 a.m. class.
- Some *young adults* may drive themselves too hard to succeed, prompting late nights at work or sleep loss due to hectic travel schedules or work-related stress. Others might not obtain enough sleep because of social and personal entertainment choices at night. Others might work an evening or night shift.
- Sleep for *parents of young children* is often interrupted. Breastfeeding mothers typically need to feed their infants one or more times each night until the infant begins to eat solid foods. Parents of toddlers often wake to care for a child who is having a nightmare, is ill, or needs to use the bathroom.
- *Middle-aged adults* may experience sleep difficulties because of the depression, anxiety, and tension that result from the stress and competing demands on time, such as work or family, the need to care for a parent, marital discord, worry about teenaged children, or financial problems. The lack of sleep compounds the problem, leading to reduced ability to cope and again contributing to further difficulty achieving quality sleep.
- *Menopausal women* may experience difficulty falling and staying asleep because of hormonal fluctuations. Obstructive sleep apnea (OSA) also plays a role in insufficient sleep.
- *Older adults* may suffer sleep disturbances because of the side effects of medications, underlying illnesses, depression, discomfort, nocturia, or pain. In addition, the levels of melatonin, the natural hormone that controls sleep, decline in the latter decades of life.

Lifestyle Factors

Lifestyle factors influencing sleep include work, exercise, nutrition, and use of medications and drugs.

Physical Activity If exercise occurs at least 2 hours before bedtime, it promotes sleep. Fatigue from a normal physically active day is thought to promote a restful night's sleep. However, the more tired a person is, the shorter the first period of REM sleep will be. Also, sedentary lifestyle can contribute to difficulty falling or staying asleep.

Diet Foods can either promote or interfere with sleep.

- A meal high in saturated fat near bedtime may interfere with sleep.
- Dietary L-tryptophan and adenosine are essential amino acids (meaning the body does not produce its own) found in milk, cheese, and animal products that may help to induce sleep by converting into serotonin.
- Carbohydrates seem to promote relaxation through their effects on brain serotonin levels. In general, satiation induces sleep.

Nicotine and Caffeine

- Central nervous system stimulants, such as nicotine and caffeine, interfere with sleep.
- Smokers tend to have more difficulty falling asleep and are more easily roused than nonsmokers. People who stop smoking often experience temporary sleep disturbances during the withdrawal period.
- Caffeine blocks adenosine and thereby inhibits sleep. However, individuals vary greatly in their sensitivity to caffeine.

Alcohol Consumption of alcohol, especially if heavy, disrupts REM and slow-wave sleep and may cause spontaneous awakenings with difficulty returning to sleep. It can prompt vivid dreams during REM sleep. Because alcohol is a diuretic, it can interrupt sleep by inducing nocturia.

Medications Many of the medications people take cause either sleeplessness or excessive grogginess and sedation. Medications to induce sleep (i.e., hypnotics) tend to increase the amount of sleep while decreasing the quality.

- Zolpidem tartrate promotes normal REM sleep and appears to influence sleep quality less than do other hypnotics.
- Amphetamines, tranquilizers, and antidepressants reduce the amount of REM sleep; barbiturates, in addition, interfere with NREM sleep.
- Opioids, such as morphine, suppress REM sleep and cause frequent awakening.
- Beta blockers are reported to cause sleep disorders and nightmares.

Illness

Illness increases the need for sleep and rest. At the same time, its associated mental and physical distress can cause sleep problems.

- **Disease symptoms,** such as fever, pain, nausea, and respiratory conditions (e.g., shortness of breath, dyspnea, sinus congestion), can also interfere with sleep.
- **Specific disease conditions** altering the quality of sleep include allergies, hyperthyroidism, and Parkinson's disease.
- **Fear of the unknown outcome** of an illness and **role changes** associated with hospitalization can cause anxiety.
- **Anxiety** increases gastric secretions, intestinal motility, heart rate, and respirations, all of which contribute to a restless night. Anxiety also stimulates the sympathetic nervous system, increasing the level of norepinephrine. This decreases stage III and REM sleep and leads to more awakenings. Depression may be associated either with too much sleep or with difficulty sleeping.

Environmental Factors

Environmental factors can promote or inhibit sleep. Some people need a cool room, whereas others need warmth. Some prefer heavy blankets, and others like to sleep with just a light sheet.

- **Noise**—Noise can also inhibit sleep, but a person can become habituated to noise over time and be less affected by it. Often loud noises are needed to awaken a person in NREM stage III and REM sleep. Any change in the usual environmental stimuli can affect sleep. Equipment noise, the muffled sounds of a busy medical–surgical unit, or the labored breathing or snoring of a roommate also can interfere with the patient's ability to sleep.
- **Light**—When people who are accustomed to sleeping in a dark room are hospitalized, they may have trouble falling asleep because of light outside their window or filtering into the room from the hallway. However, light can be therapeutic for some patients suffering from sleep problems. Exposure to bright light can alter circadian rhythms in some adults. Light therapy has not been shown to be effective in older adults with dementia living in skilled nursing facilities (Haesler, 2004).

KnowledgeCheck 35-3

- For each of the following patients, propose at least two factors that might affect sleep:
  A newborn in the neonatal intensive care unit
  A preschooler being treated for pneumonia
  An adolescent with cancer
  A breastfeeding mother of a newborn
  An elderly man who has fractured his hip
- Identify at least three types of environmental stimuli that can disturb sleep.

WHAT ARE SOME COMMON SLEEP DISORDERS?

Sleep disorders are classified by their signs and symptoms. The more common disorders fall into two groups:

- **Dyssomnias**—Difficulty falling or staying asleep, early awakening, or excessive sleepiness. Dyssomnias include insomnia, sleep–wake schedule (circadian) disorders, sleep apnea, restless legs syndrome, hypersomnia, and narcolepsy.
- **Parasomnias**—Patterns of waking behavior that appear during sleep (sleepwalking)

Insomnia

Insomnia as defined by the *Diagnostic and Statistical Manual,* 5th edition (DSM-5) is the predominant complaint of dissatisfaction with sleep quantity, associated with the inability to fall asleep, remain asleep, or go back to sleep.

- **The sleep disturbance causes significant distress** or social, occupational, academic, behavioral, and other functional impairment.
- **True insomnia occurs at least 3 nights per week and is present for 3 months** or longer, even when there is ample opportunity for sleep (American Psychiatric Association, 2013).
- **Sleep difficulty** may be *transient/short term* (less than a month) or *chronic* (longer than a month).

People with sleep difficulty usually report an insufficient quantity and quality of sleep and wake without feeling refreshed, even though they are often observed to sleep more than they perceive that they do.

Incidence Insomnia is the most common sleep disorder. It is more prevalent in women and in adults older than 60 years; those who suffer from chronic medical and psychiatric illness (e.g., depression, anxiety, hypertension, obesity, cancer, thyroid disorders); and shift workers (Budhiraja, Roth, Hudgel, et al., 2011; Institute of Medicine, 2006). In young adults, difficulties of sleep initiation are more common; in middle-aged and older adults, problems of maintaining sleep are more common (Chowla, Passaro, Park, et al., n.d., updated 2016).

Etiologies Insomnia also occurs as a side effect of medications (e.g., steroids, central adrenergic blockers, bronchodilating agents) or inadequate sleep hygiene (e.g., watching TV in bed, sleeping with smartphone nearby, drinking caffeine-containing beverages before bedtime).

Symptoms Daytime consequences of insomnia include symptoms of excessive daytime sleepiness, poor concentration, fatigue, lethargy, and irritability. Insomnia can also create an increased risk for depression, anxiety, and possibly cardiovascular disorders. Or it may be the presenting symptom of other primary sleep disorders, such as restless legs syndrome.

Treatment Primary care providers can diagnose and manage most cases of insomnia. Once underlying medical or psychiatric conditions have been identified and treated, a combination of behavioral and pharmacological therapy may be effective. The use of medication to induce sleep is controversial because some types can become habit forming, become less effective when taken continuously, and can have serious side effects. However, sedative–hypnotic treatment may be needed for short-term insomnia to relieve symptoms. It may also prevent the development of chronic insomnia.

Sleep–Wake Schedule (Circadian) Disorders

Abnormalities in sleep–wake schedules may be caused by rapid time-zone changes (jet lag), shift work, or a change in total sleep time from day to day. Symptoms include decreased vigilance, reduced ability to perform psychomotor tasks, and short sleep episodes *(microsleeps)* that the person is not aware of. People suffering a disruption in sleep–wake schedule can take several days to adjust their sleep pattern.

Restless Legs Syndrome (RLS)

Restless legs syndrome (RLS) is a disorder of the central nervous system characterized by an uncontrollable movement of the legs while resting or before sleep onset.

Incidence RLS tends to run in families. Children and young adults experience this condition, but it is especially common in older adults and is sometimes associated with low levels of iron (Armstrong, 2013; Ball & Caivano, 2008) and use of some antidepressants. It tends to be familial, more often occurring in women than in men.

Symptoms The unpleasant creeping, crawling, itching, tingling or burning sensations in the legs is relieved only by moving and stretching, which prevents the person from relaxing and falling asleep.

Management If RLS is severe, treatment may include **neuroleptic** agents and medication used to treat Parkinson's disease. People with RLS should avoid stimulants (e.g., caffeine). Other self-care measures include walking, massaging, stretching, heat or cold compresses, medication, vibration, and acupressure. Some people with severe symptoms might require anticonvulsant medication to control the

creeping and crawling sensation in the legs (National Sleep Foundation, n.d.a).

Sleep Deprivation

Sleep Deprivation is a NANDA-I nursing diagnosis. It is not actually a sleep disorder but rather, in NANDA-I terms, a human response to prolonged sleep disturbances (e.g., insomnia and parasomnias), involving NREM or REM deprivation, or both.

Defining Characteristics

- Persons experiencing sleep deprivation are likely to feel drowsy during the day or a have a general feeling of malaise. They have difficulty performing daily tasks; impaired cognitive processing, problem-solving, and decision making; restlessness, perceptual disorders, slowed reaction time, irritability; and somatic (body) complaints (e.g., hand tremors).
- If sleep deprivation is severe and prolonged, delusions, paranoia, and other psychotic behavior may occur.
- Going without sleep can weaken the body's protection against infection.

Etiologies Illness and hospital care are common causes of sleep deprivation, especially for patients in critical care units (CCUs). In CCUs, lights are on most of the time, and equipment noise, frequent treatments, and assessments all combine with the client's fragile physical condition to create sleep deprivation. Likewise, healthcare providers who work long and late hours or rotating day–night shifts experience serious fatigue that can lead to medical error, increased risk of occupational injury, and patient injury or death (The Joint Commission, 2011).

Hypersomnia

Hypersomnia is excessive sleeping, especially in the daytime. People with excessive daytime sleepiness doze, nap, or fall asleep at times and in situations when they need or wish to be awake and alert. Common causes of hypersomnia are sleep apnea, narcolepsy, and snoring; disorders of the central nervous system, kidney, or liver; and metabolic disorders (e.g., diabetic acidosis and hypothyroidism). Hypersomnia can also be a symptom of depression.

Sleep Apnea

Sleep apnea is a periodic interruption in breathing during sleep—an absence of air flow through the nose or mouth can potentially lead to serious health problems. Episodes may occur several or a hundred times a night and may last up to 1 minute or longer. During periods of apnea, the oxygen level in the blood drops, and the carbon dioxide level rises, often causing the person to wake up.

- **Symptoms and Complications.** Sleep apnea may result in cardiac dysrhythmias (irregularities) and increases in pulse and blood pressure. Many people with sleep apnea complain of unrefreshed sleep, fatigue and morning headache, and easily falling asleep during sedentary activity; however, some may experience mild sleep apnea without any symptoms (Epstein, Kristo, Strollo, et al., 2009). Untreated sleep apnea is associated with polycythemia, hypertension, angina, coronary artery disease, right-sided heart failure, stroke, impotence, depression, personality changes, and mood swings.
- **Diagnosis.** To definitively diagnose sleep apnea, a sleep study consisting of an EEG, monitoring of arterial oxygen saturation, and an electrocardiogram (ECG) is recommended.
- **Treatment.** Treatment depends on the type of apnea involved. The two main types of sleep apnea (obstructive and central) have different etiologies. Mixed apnea is a combination of the two main types.

Toward Evidence-Based Practice

Lee, J. A., Sunwoo, S., Kim, Y. S., et al. (2016). The effect of sleep quality on the development of type 2 diabetes in primary care patients. *Journal of Korean Medical Science*, 31(2), 240–246. Retrieved from https://doi.org/10.3346/jkms.2016.31.2.240

In a study of 563 patients in 22 family medicine clinics in Korea, researchers found that poor sleep quality was associated with a higher risk of diabetes after taking into account other factors (age, sex, body mass index, income, physical activity, and family history of diabetes).

Lowry, F. (2016, October). *Poor sleep linked to atherosclerosis in midlife women.* Presented at the North American Menopause Society (NAMS) annual meeting (Abstract S-16). Retrieved from http://www.medscape.com/viewarticle/870176?src=wnl_mdplsnews_161014_mscpedit_wir&uac=74261HR&impID=1215430&faf=1

In a study of 256 carotid arteries in peri- and postmenopausal women, shorter sleep time was associated with more plaque formation that can lead to atherosclerosis.

Roehrs, T. A., Harris, E., Randall, S., et al. (2012). Pain sensitivity and recovery from mild chronic sleep loss. *Sleep*, 35(12), 1667–1673. doi: http://dx.doi.org/10.5665/sleep.2240

With a small sample of healthy adults, investigators found that increased sleep time lessens daytime sleepiness and reduces pain sensitivity.

Paiva, T., Gaspar, T., & Matos, M. G. (2015). Sleep deprivation in adolescents: Correlations with health complaints and health-related quality of life. *Sleep Medicine*, 16(4), 521–527. Retrieved from http://dx.doi.org/10.1016/j.sleep.2014.10.010

In a study of 3,476 teens, 19% reported not getting enough sleep and 37.2% claimed to have sleep problems, especially with falling asleep. Shorter sleep duration occurred on weeknights. Adolescent girls had significantly more health complaints than did boys, particularly with headaches. Both groups perceived health-related quality of life to be reduced when sleep deprived.

1. Sleep deprivation produces detrimental effects for people of all ages. The studies included here show an association between poor sleep quality and health problems, such as type 2 diabetes, atherosclerosis, headaches, and pain sensitivity. In what other ways do you think sleep deprivation creates problems for the body?

2. Considering the deleterious consequences of sleep deprivation on physical and mental health, what questions might you ask your patients who report getting fewer than 6 hours of sleep per night?

3. People who are sleep deprived often report having lower quality of life. Describe your own personal experience with sleep deprivation.

 Go to Davis Advantage, Resources, Chapter 35, **Toward Evidence-Based Practice—Suggested Responses**.

Obstructive Sleep Apnea OSA is diagnosed clinically by reports of at least five witnessed breathing interruptions or awakenings due to gasping or choking events per hour (Epstein, Kristo, Strollo, et al., 2009). Typically the soft tissue of the pharynx and soft palate or other structures in the throat area (deviated nasal septum, enlarged tonsils) collapse and obstruct the airway during sleep, but the person continues to try to breathe. Although most often males over age 40, particularly if overweight, are affected by sleep apnea, the condition occurs in females of any age and weight.

- **Symptoms.** Sleeping partners often report that the person snores, snorts, grunts, or thrashes about during sleep. Also see symptoms of sleep apnea, preceding.
- **Management.** Treatment of OSA might involve surgery to remove obstruction within the airway. Other treatments include the following:

  Applying continuous positive airway pressure or bilevel positive airway pressure treatment. This is a device that delivers oxygen using forced air pressure and keeps the airways open.

  Oral appliance therapy to pull the tongue forward or adjust the space in the pharyngeal space.

  Advising the patient to avoid alcohol and smoking and lose excess weight (Epstein, Kristo, Strollo, et al., 2009).

Central Sleep Apnea Central sleep apnea (CSA) is a complete suspension of breathing resulting from a dysfunction in central respiratory control. Only about 10% of sleep apnea is central in origin. People with CSA tend to awaken during sleep and, therefore, experience daytime sleepiness.

Snoring

Although snoring is a hallmark sign of OSA, it does not necessarily indicate OSA. Snoring can significantly reduce the quality of sleep for the bed partner. Snoring results when the muscles at the back of the mouth relax during sleep, obstruct the airway, and vibrate with each breath. Obstruction is usually more pronounced when the person sleeps on his back. Many treatments have been invented to open the air passages, such as nose tapes or even surgery. Saline sprays, nose drops, and cortisone sprays are also used—all with mixed success.

Narcolepsy

Narcolepsy is a chronic disorder caused by the brain's inability to regulate sleep–wake cycles normally. The distinction between being asleep and being awake are blurred. At various times, the person with narcolepsy experiences a sudden, uncontrollable urge to sleep lasting from seconds to minutes, even though the person sleeps well at night. The person cannot avoid the sleep episodes but awakens easily.

Narcolepsy is characterized by:

- Sleepiness, slurred speech, slackening of the facial muscles, a feeling of impending weakness of the knees, paralysis, and hallucinations.
- Impaired performance during these microsleep episodes.
- Sleep episodes that come on suddenly, even while the person is alert and active.
- Awakening from episodes of unavoidable sleep feeling refreshed. Some people have other symptoms, such as **cataplexy,** a sudden loss of muscle tone usually triggered by an emotional event (e.g., laughter, surprise, or anger), but most only have hypersomnia.

People with narcolepsy do not tolerate irregular sleep–wake patterns, such as shift work, and have difficulty staying awake with passive activity, such as watching television. The condition is controlled by central nervous system stimulants, such as methylphenidate (Ritalin), with little evidence of tolerance, dependence, or abuse.

Some individuals suffer **pseudonarcolepsy,** which is characterized by involuntary episodes of sleep but is related to acute or chronic sleep deprivation. When the person is well rested, episodes resolve.

KnowledgeCheck 35-4

- What is the most common dyssomnia?
- What factors in the hospital may contribute to sleep deprivation in patients?
- What are the clinical signs of sleep deprivation?
- Why are sleeping pills not recommended for chronic insomnia?
- Why is snoring significant?

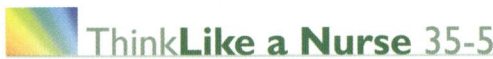

ThinkLike a Nurse 35-5

Compare and contrast insomnia and hypersomnia. How are they different? How are they alike?

Parasomnias

The parasomnias include sleepwalking, sleeptalking, bruxism, night terrors, REM sleep behavior disorders, and nocturnal enuresis.

Sleepwalking or *somnambulism,* occurs during stage III of NREM sleep, usually 1 to 2 hours after the person falls asleep. The sleeper leaves the bed and walks about, with little awareness of surroundings. He may perform what appear to be conscious motor activities (e.g., brush his teeth, make coffee), but does not wake up. The person is not aware of sleepwalking and has no memory of the event on awakening. The event may last 3 to 4 minutes or longer. Children sleepwalk more often than adults do. If the child does not outgrow the condition or serious safety risks exist, medication may be given to suppress the deepest stage III sleep. Stress, fatigue, and some drugs can trigger sleepwalking.

Sleeptalking occurs during NREM sleep, just before the REM stage. It does not usually interfere with the person's rest but may be disturbing to others.

Bruxism is grinding and clenching of the teeth and usually occurs during stage II NREM sleep. It can eventually erode tooth enamel and loosen the teeth. The noise can be disruptive to others.

Night Terrors are sudden arousals in which the person (often a child) is physically active, often hallucinatory, and expresses a strong emotion such as terror. Children experiencing night terrors typically cry or scream in fear, thrash about, and resist all attempts by their parents or other caregivers to hold or console them. The child appears to be fully awake, but she is not; in fact, children in the midst of night terrors are extremely difficult to awaken. Episodes may last from 10 to 30 minutes. The child typically returns to sleep without awakening and in the morning has no memory of the event. Unlike *nightmares* (unpleasant, frightening dreams), which occur during REM sleep, night terrors occur during stage III (deep NREM) sleep.

REM Sleep Behavior Disorders are associated with REM (or dreaming period) sleep, in which the sleeper violently acts out the dream. People have actually injured themselves or others without waking.

Nocturnal Enuresis, or *bedwetting,* is nighttime incontinence past the stage at which toilet training has been well established. It has incorrectly been associated with dreaming; however, most incidents occur during NREM sleep, during the first third of the night when the child is difficult to rouse. It may be distressing to the child and family because of the importance society places on continence, the inconvenience of keeping bed linens clean, and the misconception that the child is bedwetting to act out against parents. Because the great majority of children outgrow enuresis, the best strategy is patience (McCance & Huether, 2014). If the problem persists past age eight or ten, the child might require a full medical evaluation.

Secondary Sleep Disorders

Secondary sleep disorders occur when a disease causes alterations in sleep stages or in quantity and quality of sleep. The following are the most common causes:

- **Depression.** Depressed people may spend a great deal of time in bed. However, in general, they have difficulty falling asleep, experience less slow-wave (deep) sleep, spend less time in REM sleep, awaken early, and have less total sleep time.
- **Hyperthyroidism or hypothyroidism.** Hyperthyroidism increases metabolic rate, making it difficult for the person to fall asleep and causing an increase in stage III REM sleep. Hypothyroidism causes a decrease in stage III REM sleep.
- **Pain.** Both acute and chronic pain inhibit sleep, increase arousals during sleep, and cause longer waking intervals during the night.

Disorders That Are Provoked by Sleep

Sleep-provoked disorders are those that occur when signs and symptoms of the disease appear or become worse during sleep.

- **Coronary artery disease.** During REM sleep, dreams may increase heart rate and provoke angina and ECG changes.
- **Asthma.** People with asthma may experience bronchospasm during REM sleep. In adults, asthma attacks frequently occur during the night as the esophageal sphincter relaxes and reflux results. In children, they occur mostly during the latter two-thirds of the night, when there is less stage III sleep.
- **Chronic obstructive pulmonary disease (COPD).** Persons with COPD experience lowered oxygen tension and increased carbon dioxide retention during sleep, especially during REM sleep when neuromuscular control is normally depressed. This can result in pulmonary spasm and transient pulmonary hypertension.
- **Diabetes.** Blood glucose levels vary during sleep. Uncontrolled diabetes may profoundly affect the blood sugar level during sleep, when the person is not alert enough to deal

with it. Therefore, patients with uncontrolled diabetes may need to have blood glucose levels monitored during sleep.

- **Gastric and intestinal ulcers.** During REM sleep, people with duodenal ulcers secrete up to 20 times more gastric acid than do people who do not have duodenal ulcers. Peptic ulcers also contribute to increased acid, often producing nocturnal epigastric pain and sleep loss.
- **Epilepsy.** Seizures are sensitive to sleep patterns. Sleep deprivation can trigger seizures, increase their intensity, or cause seizures to last longer. Some forms of epilepsy are especially reactive to sleep cycles or transitions between sleep states (Schachter, Shafer, & Sirven, 2013).

KnowledgeCheck 35-5

- List and define at least three parasomnias.
- Describe ways in which depression can affect sleep.
- List two sleep-provoked disorders and explain how the sleep stage affects the disease.

PracticalKnowledge
knowing how

Because sleep enhances wellness and speeds recovery from illness, promoting sleep is an important independent nursing intervention. In the Practical Knowledge section, you will learn how to recognize signs of sleep disturbance, factors that interfere with patients' sleep, and specific measures to facilitate sleep for each client.

ASSESSMENT NP

It is important to assess usual sleep patterns and rituals for all patients who are being admitted to the hospital or seeking help for a sleep problem. A brief assessment for all patients should include questions about the following:

- Usual sleeping pattern
- Sleeping environment
- Bedtime routines/rituals
- Sleep aids
- Sleep changes or problems

KEY POINT: *You would conduct a more in-depth sleep assessment for patients who wake up at least three times a night; those who take more than 30 minutes to fall asleep; and if the difficulty falling or staying asleep has been ongoing for more than 30 days. A sleep study is recommended for unexplained daytime sleepiness (Qaseem, Dallas, Owens, et al., 2014).*

- A **sleep history** (self-report) includes in-depth questions about the person's usual times for sleep, preparation, preferences and routines, quality of sleep, napping habits (if any), and whether she wakes early and cannot return to sleep.
- A **sleep diary** provides very specific information on your patient's patterns of sleep. This allows you to identify trends in sleep/wakefulness and associate behaviors interfering with sleep. You will usually ask the patient to keep the diary for 14 days; remind him that it is important to be diligent in maintaining it. See the Focused Assessment box Questions for a Sleep History and Sleep Diary.

Focused Assessment

Questions for a Sleep History

A brief assessment for all patients should include questions about the following:

Usual Sleeping Pattern

- When do you go to sleep and wake up?
- How many hours do you sleep?
- Do you have a regular sleep schedule?
- How would you rate the quality of your sleep on a scale of 1 to 10, with 10 meaning "great"?
- Do you take a nap? If you do, for how long?
- How often do you waken during sleep, for example, to go to the bathroom?
- Do you feel adequately rested when you wake up?

Sleeping Environment

- Would you like a night-light?
- What room temperature do you prefer?
- What noise level do you prefer (for example, radio, television, absolute quiet)?

Bedtime Routines/Rituals

- What do you typically do in the hour before bedtime?
- What do you do to help you fall asleep?

Sleep Aids

- Do you need a special pillow or positioning aid?
- Do you take any sleep medications or other drugs, natural sleep aids, or homeopathic remedies that may affect sleep?

Sleep Changes or Problems

- Have your sleep patterns changed? If so, how?
- How often do you experience difficulty falling asleep? Staying asleep?
- Do you currently experience, or have you ever experienced, a sleep disorder (e.g., narcolepsy, insomnia)?
- Do you remember your dreams after you wake? Do you ever have night terrors? Do you sleepwalk?
- Do you ever experience an unpleasant creeping feeling, crawling, or tingling, relieved only by moving the legs at night?
- Do you snore? Does your own snoring or grunting ever wake you or anyone in the room?
- Do you wear a cap at night? Do you require oxygen at night? Do you require any other medical aid or therapy while you sleep?
- Do you grind your teeth while you sleep? Do you wear a dental appliance to prevent grinding?
- Do you experience any kind of pain that makes it difficult for you to fall asleep or stay asleep?
- Is there anything that I have not asked that might help you sleep while you are in the hospital (having surgery, receiving home care)?

If the client reports experiencing satisfactory sleep, that is an adequate assessment, and you merely need to support her usual sleep patterns and rituals. When you suspect a sleep problem, you will perform a more in-depth assessment, such as a detailed sleep history or have the patient keep a sleep diary.

Sleep Diary

A sleep diary provides specific information on the patient's sleep–wakefulness patterns over a long period. The diary is usually kept for 14 days and may include the following:

Note: If you work a night shift, in these questions adjust the time for sleep and waking accordingly.

Completed in the Morning

Time you went to bed:_____
Approximate time you fell asleep:_____
Times you woke during the night:_____
Times you fell back to sleep:_____
Time you woke up in the morning:_____
Did you feel refreshed upon wakening?_____
What did you eat or drink just before bedtime? _____

In what mental and physical activities did you engage in the 2 to 3 hours before bedtime?_____
Were you worried or anxious about anything when you went to bed?_____
Sleep medications you have taken:_____ Any repeated doses? _____ Times:_____

Completed in the Evening

How sleepy did you feel during the day?
_____ Sleepy; struggled to stay awake during the day
_____ Somewhat tired
_____ Fairly alert
_____ Wide awake
Any naps during the day? _____ If so, for how long? _____

Frequency of pain medication taken and times _____

Exercise during the day? _____ If so, for how long? _____ What time of the day? _____
Number of alcoholic drinks _____ What time? _____

Number of caffeinated drinks _____ What time? _____

Number of tobacco products _____ What time? _____

- An **actigraph** is an application on a mobile device or worn on the wrist that estimates a person's sleep and wake patterns, including time spent in various sleep stages.
- A **sleep study** is a test that observes what happens in the body during sleep. It is most useful in detecting sleep apnea and other sleep disorders, such as narcolepsy, night terrors, and periodic limb movement disorder.
- **Polysomnography,** one of the most common sleep studies performed in a sleep lab, records brain wave activity, eye movement, oxygen and carbon dioxide levels, vital signs, and body movements during the sleep phases. The American College of Physicians recommends polysomnography for anyone suspected to have OSA (Qaseem, Dallas, Owens, et al., 2014).

ANALYSIS/NURSING DIAGNOSIS NP

It is important to determine whether lack of sleep is a problem, a symptom of a problem, or is contributing to (etiology of) a different problem. For health promotion applications, use the NANDA-I diagnosis Readiness for Enhanced Sleep when a client has no particular sleep problem but wants to move to a higher level of functioning in the area of sleep.

Sleep as the Problem

When you focus on interventions to promote sleep, use the following NANDA-I labels on the problem side of the nursing diagnosis:

Insomnia—Use for patients who have a disruption in the amount of quality of sleep to the extent that it impairs functioning.

Sleep Deprivation—Use as the nursing diagnosis when the patient's amount, consistency, or quality of sleep is decreased over prolonged periods of time. Defining characteristics of Sleep Deprivation are more severe than those for Disturbed Sleep Pattern, so nursing activities may focus as much on relieving symptoms (e.g., confusion, paranoia) as on sleep promotion.

Disturbed Sleep Pattern—Use as the diagnosis when assessment data point to a time-limited sleep problem due to external factors (e.g., inability to sleep in the unfamiliar hospital environment).

Readiness for Enhanced Sleep—Use this diagnosis when a client without a sleep disorder desires improved quality or duration of sleep.

The problem should be one that can be treated by nursing therapy. Carefully describe the etiologies for sleep problems because they determine your interventions. To help you individualize goals, add modifying words to specify the type of sleep problem, as in these examples:

- Disturbed Sleep Pattern (difficulty falling and remaining asleep) related to noise of hospital environment and need for scheduled treatments
- Disturbed Sleep Pattern (premature awakening) related to sleeping aid dependence and lack of knowledge of nonpharmacological aids for insomnia
- Disturbed Sleep Pattern (excessive daytime sleeping) related to effects of biological aging and depression
- Disturbed Sleep Pattern (altered sleep–wake patterns) related to frequent rotations of shift and overtime

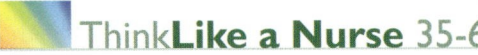

ThinkLike a Nurse 35-6

In the following nursing diagnoses, how do you think your interventions would be different for each diagnosis?
Disturbed Sleep Pattern related to:

- Changes in bedtime routines
- Exercising within 2 hours before sleep

- Drinking caffeinated beverages, eating chocolate, and drinking alcohol
- Emotional or physical pain
- Drug dependence or withdrawal
- Physical illness

Sleep Pattern as an Etiology

Disturbed Sleep Pattern and Sleep Deprivation affect many areas of functioning, so they often are the etiology of other nursing diagnoses, as in these examples:

- Risk for Injury or Falls related to sleepwalking (or REM sleep behavior disorder or narcolepsy)
- Fatigue (or Activity Intolerance) related to chronic insufficient quality or quantity of sleep (e.g., secondary to insomnia)
- Ineffective Coping related to decreased cognitive functioning and awareness, secondary to lack of sleep

Sleep Pattern as a Symptom

Difficulty sleeping may be one of the symptoms of another problem. For example, a client may have Spiritual Distress related to challenges to belief system *as manifested by nightmares, sleep disturbances,* and *verbalization of inner conflict about beliefs.* In this instance, you would focus on interventions for Spiritual Distress, assuming that the sleep pattern would improve as the Spiritual Distress is resolved. Other nursing diagnoses that may cause sleep loss include Anxiety, Chronic Sorrow, Death Anxiety, Decisional Conflict, Complicated Grieving, Diarrhea, Impaired Gas Exchange, Nausea, Pain, and Relocation Stress Syndrome.

KnowledgeCheck 35-6

- For a chronic, long-term sleep problem, would you use a diagnosis of Sleep Pattern Disturbance, Sleep Deprivation, or Readiness for Enhanced Sleep?
- Name at least two nursing diagnoses that might have a sleep problem as the etiology.
- Name at least one nursing diagnosis that might have a sleep problem as the defining characteristic.

PLANNING OUTCOMES/EVALUATION NP

NOC standardized outcomes linked to the NANDA-I sleep labels are as follows:

- Disturbed Sleep Pattern—Rest, Sleep, and Personal Well-Being
- Sleep Deprivation—Rest, Sleep, and Symptom Severity
- Insomnia—Concentration, Endurance, Fatigue Level, Mood Equilibrium, Personal Health Status, Personal Well-Being, Quality of Life, Rest, and Sleep

When sleep disturbances are the etiology of another nursing diagnosis, you will need to use the NOC outcomes associated with that diagnosis. For example:

Nursing diagnosis: Anxiety related to Sleep Deprivation
NOC outcomes for Anxiety: Anxiety Control, Coping

Individualized goals/outcome statements you might use to evaluate the success of interventions to promote sleep include the following:

- Verbalizes feeling rested or feeling less fatigue.
- Falls asleep within 30 minutes; sleeps 6 hours without awakening.
- Maintains a sleep–wake pattern that provides sufficient energy for the day's tasks.

- Demonstrates self-care behaviors that provide a healthy balance between rest and activity.
- Identifies stress-relieving rituals that enable falling asleep more easily.

PLANNING INTERVENTIONS/ IMPLEMENTATION NP

NIC standardized interventions for Sleep Deprivation, Sleep Pattern Disturbance, and Readiness for Enhanced Sleep include the following: Coping Enhancement, Energy Management, Environmental Management: Comfort, Relaxation Therapy, and Sleep Enhancement. Linkages have not yet been established for Insomnia.

Specific nursing activities for clients with sleep problems include:

- Scheduling nursing care to avoid interrupting sleep
- Supporting bedtime rituals and routines
- Other interventions described in the following sections.
  For a care plan and care map for Sleep Pattern Disturbance,

 Go to Davis Advantage, Resources, Chapter 35, **Care Plan** and **Care Map.**

Most people with sleep problems manage them at home by creating a restful environment, relaxing, avoiding distractions, and trying various sleep strategies without using sleep-inducing medication. Refer to the Self-Care box Teaching Your Patients About Sleep Hygiene.

♥ iCare 35-1

Promoting Sleep & Rest

Healthcare routines usually allow time for rest periods. Use nursing judgment to decide when a procedure must be done and when it is more important for your patient to sleep.

- Cluster care to avoid unnecessary interruptions in sleep and rest. Unless the patient is critically ill, do not wake him for morning vital signs if he is sleeping.
- You can often alter sleep routines; for example, you can allow the patient to sleep as long as he can in the morning and bring his breakfast later. Or if the care provider has prescribed sleep-inducing medication, give it early in the evening if he seems sleepy.
- Provide ear buds, eye masks, or soft music or white noise to help facilitate rest and sleep.
- Be mindful of little things you can do to promote sleep/rest. These include dimming lights, closing the door, being aware of voice levels, limiting overhead paging after hours, and servicing noisy equipment.
- Some patients need to rest after a procedure or after meals.
- If the person looks sleepy, give a prescribed sleep-inducing medication early to avoid waking him later in the evening.
- Keep the noise level to a minimum. Be aware that activities, conversation, and equipment, even outside the patient's room, can disrupt sleep.

Teaching Your Client About Sleep Hygiene

➤ **Follow a regular routine** for bedtime and morning awakenings.

➤ **Go to bed each night at the same time,** even on days you are off work.

➤ **If you cannot fall asleep in 30 minutes,** get up and do something nonstimulating, but avoid using the computer. The wavelengths of blue light emitted from the screen arouse the brain into a wakeful state. When you feel sleepy, go back to bed.

➤ **Use relaxation methods** to promote sleep: read a book, pray, or meditate.

➤ **Avoid going to bed angry or frustrated;** stay clear of emotional discussions before going to sleep.

➤ **Don't depend on sleeping aids;** be aware of the potential dangers of sleeping medications.

➤ **Use your bedroom only for sleep;** do not turn your bedroom into the family room.

➤ **Avoid caffeine, alcohol, tobacco products, and heavy meals** before going to sleep. Remember that some beverages and foods, such as black tea, chocolate, and cola, contain caffeine. Alcohol interferes with the transition to deeper phases of sleep. Heavy alcohol consumption can contribute to breathing impairment during the night.

➤ **Avoid eating carbohydrates** (e.g., crackers, cereal, or bread) before bed; they boost blood glucose levels, so a few hours later, the rapid drop in sugar will wake you.

➤ **Use aromatherapy** to relax.

➤ **If you take prescription drugs,** ask your prescriber or pharmacist about any possible side effects.

➤ **Use earplugs** to block out noise.

➤ **Walk or exercise in the early evening at least** 1 hour before going to sleep; doing so will raise your body temperature and tire your muscles. Even 15 minutes a day of exercise will give your body the activity and oxygen it needs to help you relax more and sleep better.

➤ **Take a warm bath** just before going to sleep. This will raise your body temperature and relax you to help you fall asleep more easily.

➤ **Avoid naps during the day,** unless you are an older adult who takes short "power naps." Daytime napping can lead to nighttime insomnia.

➤ **Don't try to "catch up" on sleep.** Rise at your regular time, even if you went to bed later than usual.

➤ **Try to keep your bedroom as dark as possible.** Even an illuminated bedroom clock is a source of light that can be distracting when trying to fall asleep. Either replace the clock or block the light with something.

➤ **Close your eyes and visualize something peaceful** when trying to fall asleep. Imagining your favorite, relaxing place where you find comfort or familiarity can relax you and help you get to sleep.

➤ **Try progressive relaxation** to fall asleep. Follow recorded instructions directing you in a sequence of relaxing certain muscle groups.

Create a Restful Environment

Many people find it difficult to sleep in an unfamiliar bed, even a comfortable one. Hospital beds are not noted for their luxury, but you can help make them more comfortable.

▪ Be sure the bed linens are tight on the bottom and loose on top to allow movement.

▪ Keep linens clean, dry, and free of irritants. Perspiration on the hospital gown or linens can lead to chill.

▪ Good body alignment also facilitates relaxation. Use extra pillows, a blanket from home, or any other item that may help the patient rest.

▪ Keep the room dark and quiet, unless the patient prefers a light.

▪ As much as possible, control the temperature of the room and provide good ventilation.

Promote Comfort

Pain, itching, and nausea may all be deterrents to rest and sleep in an ill person. Be sure to offer pain medications at scheduled times and before the patient's sleep time. Other comfort measures include providing a restful environment (see the preceding intervention) and offering appropriate snacks and beverages (see the Self-Care box Teaching Your Client About Sleep Hygiene). You might offer cool cloths or a back massage. For detailed instructions for back massage,

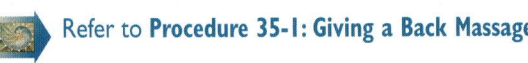 Refer to **Procedure 35-1: Giving a Back Massage.**

Promote Relaxation

Base your choice of relaxation strategies on your repertoire of techniques and on patient preference. Relaxation strategies may include a massage, a warm bath, or one of the following:

▪ *Guided imagery* can be used to help your patient move in his mind to a peaceful place, where relaxation is possible. You may ask the patient to picture the type of place that will soothe him. See Chapter 12 if you need to review.

▪ *Progressive muscle relaxation,* relaxing each muscle independently, moving from head to toe, may help to promote sleep.

▪ *Music therapy* has been shown to be effective in promoting relaxation. Some patients are distracted from worries while listening to music, whereas others may find music annoying. Slow, quiet music or a recording of forest or ocean sounds may be soothing.

For more details on relaxation strategies, you may wish to refer to **Bonus Chapter 46, Holistic Healing,** in your Davis Digital Version of the textbook.

Maintain Patient Safety

Guide sleepwalkers back to bed and remember that they startle easily, so be gentle. A person who sleepwalks needs protection from injury because the risk of falling is great. In the hospital setting, intravenous infusions, catheters, and nasogastric tubes can produce injury if they are pulled out of the body when the person gets out of bed.

Safe Sleep for Infants

✚ Infant suffocation is a common cause of death in infants and is often associated with sleep position and environment, such as the use of blankets, pillows, and infant positioners. The safest position for the first year of life is supine, and not on the side because they can roll forward onto their bellies. Babies should be placed on a firm sleep surface that is free of soft, loose objects and linens. They may share a room but not a bed. Commercial infant positioning devices are not recommended (American Academy of Pediatrics Task Force on Sudden Infant Death Syndrome; Moon, 2011; Centers for Disease Control and Prevention, 2012).

Administer and Teach About Sleep Medications

When considering sleep medications, it is important for the patient to understand the options, be aware of potential side effects, and know what questions to ask. Some medications are habit forming; others may have unpleasant side effects. Some natural or homeopathic aids can lead to rest and sleep. When patients first start taking prescription sleep aids, they should use caution during morning activities until they are sure how the drug affects them. Long-term effects of these medications are not known. **KEY POINT:** *As a general rule, they are not recommended for long-term use.*

Prescription Sleep-Inducing Medication

You should be familiar with the various prescription and non-prescription sleep medications your patients may be taking. Sleep medications are typically classified as a sedative/hypnotic (benzodiazepines and nonbenzodiazepines), anticonvulsant, or antidepressant.

Nonbenzodiazepines These have a short half-life; they are eliminated from the body quickly and do not cause daytime sleepiness. Examples are zolpidem tartrate and zaleplon.
- *Nonbenzodiazepines are selective,* meaning that they target specific receptors that are thought to be associated with sleep rather than depressing the entire central nervous system.
- *General side effects* include drowsiness, dizziness, fatigue, headache, and unpleasant taste.
- *Long-term effects* of these medications are not yet known, although an increased risk of fatal overdose has been reported.

Benzodiazepines This class of sedative/hypnotics is the first-line treatment for insomnia.
- *Benzodiazepines may be long-acting* or short-acting.
- *Long-acting medications* linger in the body and potentially cause daytime drowsiness. Older adults are particularly at risk for daytime sleepiness and dizziness.
- *The risk for rebound insomnia,* dependency, and tolerance, especially in older adults, is greater with this class of sleep-inducing drugs.
- *Benzodiazepines are potentially dangerous* when combined with alcohol and some medications.
- *Many benzodiazepines were originally formulated to treat anxiety.* Examples are diazepam, alprazolam, flurazepam, lorazepam, and triazolam.

Selective Melatonin Agonist This class regulates the sleep–wake cycle by targeting melatonin receptors. Ramelteon is used to treat insomnia that is associated with having trouble falling asleep. It is not designated as a controlled substance.

Barbiturates These sedative/hypnotics and anticonvulsants are rarely prescribed for insomnia because of the risk of addiction, abuse, and overdose. Examples are amobarbital, pentobarbital, and secobarbital.

Tricyclic Antidepressants At times, primary care providers prescribe antidepressants to promote sleep. Although none of these medicines is specifically approved by the U.S. Food and Drug Administration (FDA) for this purpose, they have shown clinical benefit for some people with insomnia who also suffer with depression. Examples are amitriptyline, doxepin, imipramine, and nortriptyline.

Nonprescription Sleep Medications

Nonprescription sleep medications usually contain an antihistamine, which may induce drowsiness that lasts into the next day. It is important to check the ingredient label of any over-the-counter (OTC) medication to see whether it contains an antihistamine. Advise clients that OTC sleep medications can interact with other medicines they may be taking, so they should consult their prescriber or pharmacist before using them. An example is diphenhydramine hydrochloride. Other nonprescription sleep aids include the following:
- *Melatonin.* Melatonin is a natural hormone produced by the pineal gland to modulate sleep. Products containing melatonin are widely sold as sleep aids; however, their effectiveness is controversial. Although approved by the FDA and generally safe for short-term use, melatonin is unregulated and varies in strength and purity across manufacturers. In addition, melatonin may interfere with anticoagulants, birth control pills, antidiabetic medication, and other drugs that suppress the immune system.
- *Herbal sleep aids.* Herbal remedies for sleep problems include chamomile tea, valerian root, hops, lavender, and passionflower. These herbal remedies have not undergone extensive testing for benefits and safety and have not been proved to be effective sleep aids.

KnowledgeCheck 35-7
- What is the classification of zolpidem tartrate? Why is it an especially desirable medication for sleep?
- What are two other classes of medications that are sometimes prescribed for sleep?
- Describe three independent nursing interventions to promote sleep.
- Why should people contact their prescriber before taking nonprescription sleep aids?

PUTTING IT ALL TOGETHER

Anne (Meet Your Patient) has arrived back on the surgical unit after her surgery. She has a urinary catheter, oxygen mask, IV line, and morphine by patient-controlled analgesia (PCA) for pain control. She is nauseated from the anesthesia and moaning in pain. Her husband, Eric, is at the bedside, looking worried. "With all this equipment and her moaning, is Anne going to be okay?" Eric asks. He tells you that Anne didn't sleep at all the night before surgery. "She didn't want to take a sleeping pill because we had to be at the hospital by 5:30 a.m.," he explains.

In your initial assessment Anne's vital signs are: BP, 118/74 mm Hg; pulse, 88 beats/min and regular; respirations, 26 breaths/min; T, 99.48°F; and oxygen saturation, 99%. Her lungs are clear, the dressing is dry and intact, and a small amount of light yellow urine is draining from the urinary catheter. The operating and recovery room notes indicate that

Anne has had nothing for pain in more than 90 minutes. The PCA is connected, but the pump administers analgesia only when manually triggered. Anne has been sedated and does not remember that she must push the button to obtain pain medication. You trigger a bolus of morphine and show Anne and Eric how the PCA works. You realize that she may not remember what you have taught her, but Eric assures you that he will be staying for the day and will reinforce your instruction.

Several minutes later Anne is calm. Her respirations have slowed to 20 breaths/min, and she is lightly snoring. Eric sighs in relief. "I guess she'll sleep for a while now," he says. You explain that she will sleep with the pain medication, but that "with the morphine she will wake frequently and not get much REM sleep—that's a type of sleep we all require for health."

You gathered data preoperatively from Anne about her sleep habits and routines. You are also aware that she has chronic sleep problems. In the nursing care plan, you have written the diagnosis: Disturbed Sleep Pattern related to pain (secondary to fibromyalgia), dependence on Ambien, anxiety, grief, stresses of surgery, and unfamiliar environment. You ask Eric to bring from home Anne's pillow and any personal items that are part of her usual bedtime ritual. Eric says, "She sometimes listens to music before bed," so you suggest that he also bring her favorite music.

After Eric returns from home with Anne's belongings, she is more alert and comfortable. She says she feels exhausted but not in pain. When you make your rounds, you explain that you would like to keep her usual bedtime routine and that she will be getting Ambien this evening. She is visibly relieved by your comments.

This scenario demonstrates full-spectrum nursing and shows how a nurse can make a difference for patients and their families by recognizing the need for sleep and providing appropriate interventions.

CLINICALREASONING

The questions and exercises in this section allow you to practice the kind of thinking you will use as a full-spectrum nurse. Critical-thinking questions usually have more than one correct answer, so we do not provide "correct answers" for these features. It is more important to develop your nursing judgment than to just cover content. You will learn by discussing the questions with your peers. If you are still unsure, see the Davis Advantage chapter resources for suggested responses.

Caring for the Nguyens

Yen Nguyen arrives at the clinic accompanied by her husband, Nam. She appears very tired. Nam tells you that she has been sleeping poorly. "She worries so much. She worries about Kim, our grandchild. She worries about our kids. Now she's worried about my mother. When we were going through that mammogram scare, she was even worse!"

Mrs. Nguyen shrugs her shoulders. "I can't help it. I'm like that. I've always been a worrier. But it's gotten worse lately. Now I worry and get so emotional. I lie in bed thinking about all this stuff and end up in tears. Then when I finally get to sleep, I wake up covered with sweat. I've tried extra soy for hot flashes, melatonin from the health food store, herbal tea, and even Benadryl—but nothing seems to work.

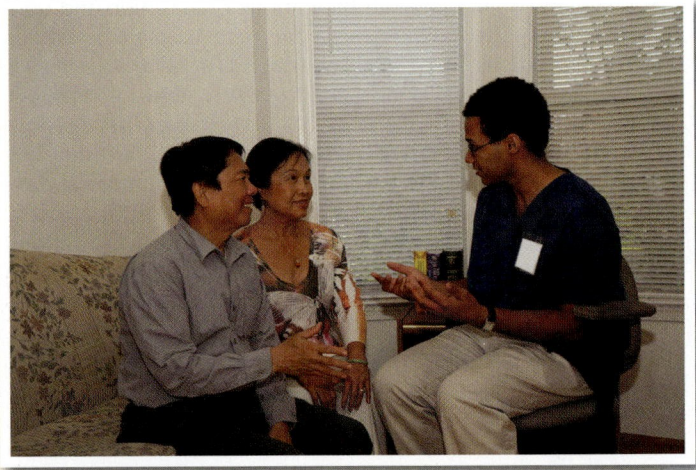

I'm so tired. But when I get up, I have to deal with all these little kids at work. They're bouncing all over the place and noisy. I just get so short-tempered with them. That's not like me. I can't take this anymore."

Caring for the Nyugens (continued)

A. *Patient data:* Clearly Mrs. Nguyen has a sleep problem. Underline the data that are defining characteristics (symptoms) of a sleep problem.

B. *Patient data:* Which data suggest ideas about the etiologies (causes) of Mrs. Nguyen's sleep problem?

C. *Nursing diagnosis:* Two NANDA-I sleep-related nursing diagnoses are Sleep Deprivation and Disturbed Sleep Pattern. You have already identified the patient's defining characteristics. Now, what *knowledge* do you need to decide which of these NANDA-I labels to use?

D. How could you obtain this knowledge?

E. Sleep Deprivation is defined as "prolonged periods of time without sleep" and Disturbed Sleep Pattern is defined as "time-limited disruption of sleep." Can you make the diagnoses on the basis of this knowledge? Why or why not?

F. Following are some of the defining characteristics for these two nursing diagnoses:

Disturbed Sleep Pattern	**Sleep Deprivation**
Change in activity level	Anxiety
Change in normal sleep pattern	Apathy
	Daytime drowsiness
Dissatisfaction with sleep	Decreased ability to function
Reports being awakened	
Reports no difficulty falling asleep	Hallucinations
	Hand tremors
Verbal complaints of not feeling well rested	Inability to concentrate
	Lethargy, listlessness, malaise
	Restlessness

Certainly there is some overlap between the two sets of symptoms. Nevertheless, which set seems to be a better fit for Mrs. Nguyen? Why?

G. Write a nursing diagnosis for Mrs. Nguyen.

 Go to Davis Advantage, Resources, Chapter 35, **Caring for the Nguyens—Suggested Responses.**

Applying the **Full-Spectrum Nursing Model**

PATIENT SITUATION

A 43-year-old healthy woman, Maria Lupe, is being seen for her annual women's health visit. She tells you she lies awake in bed for hours before falling asleep at night. Sometimes she falls asleep without problems but will wake up and then have trouble going back to sleep. After feeling as though she had been awake nearly all night, Maria wakes in the morning feeling exhausted. She tells you she feels tired all the time and can't seem to get things done during her time off because of her fatigue. Maria admits to feeling irritable with her coworkers and children. Because of her lack of rest, she doesn't have the desire to do things socially anymore.

THINKING

1. *Theoretical Knowledge:* The NANDA-I definition and defining characteristics of Insomnia differ slightly from the medical diagnosis of insomnia.
   a. What is insomnia, as defined medically (e.g., by the National Sleep Foundation)?
   b. What other health conditions might a medical diagnosis of insomnia be confused with?
   c. What factors either lead to or aggravate insomnia, as described medically?
2. *Critical Thinking (Contextual Awareness):*
   a. Obviously Maria has trouble sleeping. Based on the data you have, do you consider her difficulty sleeping significant enough to require consultation with her primary healthcare provider? Explain your thinking.

DOING

3. *Nursing Process (Assessments):*
   a. When conducting a sleep history for Maria, what questions would you ask her in order to (i) describe more fully her sleeping problem and (ii) identify the cause of her sleeping problem?
   b. What would you suggest Maria do to help you gain more information about her sleeping problem?
4. *Nursing Process (Nursing Diagnosis):* Based on the data in the Patient Situation, would you use a nursing diagnosis of Sleep Deprivation or Insomnia for Maria? Explain your thinking. Use a nursing diagnosis handbook, as needed, to compare the defining characteristics of the two diagnoses.
5. *Nursing Process (Interventions):* How might you help your patient manage her Insomnia other than using prescription medication? What might you suggest?

CARING

6. *Self-Knowledge:*
   a. Have you ever had trouble falling or staying asleep? How did you feel at the time and in the morning? Describe your experience.
   b. How might you provide better emotional care and support to your patient after recalling your own episodes of sleeping difficulty?

 Go to Davis Advantage, Resources, Chapter 35, **Applying the Full-Spectrum Nursing Model Suggested Responses.**

PracticalKnowledge
clinical application

Massage has therapeutic benefits. It promotes circulation, physical and emotional comfort, and sleep. It is an independent nursing activity, so offer a back rub whenever you can and teach and encourage NAPs to do so as well.

PROCEDURES

Procedure 35-1 ■ Giving a Back Massage

➤ For steps to follow in *all* procedures, refer to the Universal Steps for All Procedures found on the page facing the inside back cover.

Equipment
Skin care lotion

Delegation
You can delegate back massage to the NAP if the patient's condition and the NAP's skills allow. However, giving the back rub yourself provides an excellent opportunity to assess the patient, develop rapport, and provide emotional support.

Pre-Procedure Assessment
Check the skin for reddened areas or skin breakdown.

➤ When performing the procedure, always identify your patient according to agency policy, using two identifiers, and be attentive to standard precautions, hand hygiene, patient safety and privacy, body mechanics, and documentation.

Procedure Steps

1. **Warm the lotion** by placing the bottle in warm water.
   Cold lotion can cause muscle contraction; warming the lotion helps relax the muscles.

2. **Raise the bed to working height.**
   Prevents back strain of the nurse.

3. **Position the patient comfortably** on her side or prone.
   a. Untie the patient's gown and expose her back.
   b. Raise the siderail on the opposite side of the bed.
   c. Don procedure gloves.
      Siderails prevent the patient from falling off the bed when you turn her toward the side of the bed away from you.

   d. Wash the patient's back with warm water, if needed.
      Warm water will help relax the muscles while removing any sweat and soiling.

4. **Place lotion on your hands.**
   Placing the lotion directly on the back may cause the patient's muscles to tighten.

5. **Place your hands on either side** of the spine at the base of the neck. Using gentle, continuous pressure, rub down the length and then up the sides of the back.
   a. Repeat this motion several times.
   b. Never rub directly over the spine.
   The spine is a vulnerable area. ▼

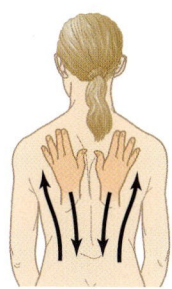

6. **Apply gentle thumb pressure** (using the fleshy part of your thumbs) on either side of the spine at the midback, pushing outward for about 2.5 cm (1 in.).
   a. Repeat from the midback to the base of the neck in a series of small, outward strokes.
   Strokes should be along the muscle length and not across the muscle to help stretch and relax it.
   b. Ask the patient whether the amount of pressure is comfortable. Be careful not to cause the patient discomfort, which might cause further muscle tightness.
   c. Always apply pressure away from the spine, not toward it.
   This gently stretches the muscles and helps prevent placing pressure on the spine.
   d. If you are unable to massage both sides at the same time, work on one side and then the other.
   Work as symmetrically as possible to increase muscle relaxation. ▼

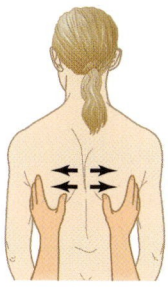

7. **Now go to the spots that felt** the tightest or that the patient states are tight. Work in small circles, using gentle thumb pressure.
   Small circular movements can help release muscle "knots" and relax tightened muscles. ▼

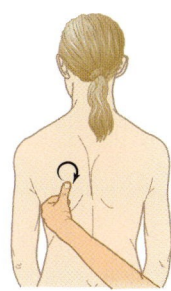

8. **Gently shake the scapulae.** Place your palm on one scapula, and gently shake it by quickly moving your palm back and forth. Repeat on the other side.
   Movement of the scapula decreases when muscles tighten; gently vibrating the scapula helps loosen the muscles. ▼

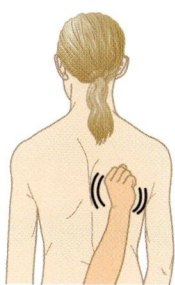

9. **Apply horizontal strokes** across the scapula, using your thumb. Using horizontal strokes from near the spine across the bottom of the scapula, push out all the way across the scapula from the spine. Move up and repeat until you have covered the entire scapula and top of the shoulder. Repeat on the other side.
   This movement helps loosen the trapezius muscle. ▼

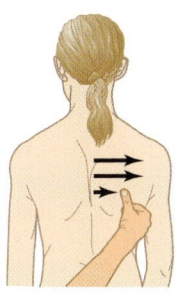

10. **If you find tender spots,** use the fleshy parts of your fingers in a small circular motion.

11. **Apply pressure in circles** using the heels of your hands down both sides of the spine. Beginning at the upper shoulder and working down to the lower back, apply pressure in medium-sized circles down the sides of the spine with the heels of your hands. Be cautious not to apply too much pressure. Assess patient for comfort.
    The circular motion helps relax tightened areas in the paraspinal muscles. ▼

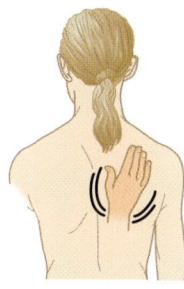

12. **Apply horizontal strokes** using the heels of your hands across the latissimus dorsi muscle. Using horizontal strokes from near the spine below the scapula, push out from the spine across to the ribs and work down across the lower back with the heels of your hands.
    This movement helps relax the latissimus dorsi muscle.

13. **Gently rub your hands up either side** of the spine from the base of the back to the base of the neck and then down the sides of the back. Repeat several times.
    Long strokes help increase circulation and promote relaxation of the back muscles.

    NOTE: *If you are unable to give a complete back massage, ask the patient where she is most uncomfortable and massage those areas. If the patient has general tightness, use the long strokes down each side of the spine and back up the sides.*

(continued on next page)

Procedure 35-1 ■ Giving a Back Massage (continued)

Evaluation

■ Assess the patient's report of comfort, relaxation, and how soon she falls asleep.

Documentation

This is a routine aspect of care and is usually documented on a flow sheet.

Practice Resources

Dosey, B. M., Keegan. L., Barrere, C., et al. (2012); Sports Injury Clinic (n.d.).

To explore learning resources for this chapter,

Go to www.DavisAdvantage.com and find:

Answers and Suggested Responses for all questions in this chapter

Lists of NIC Interventions and NOC Outcomes

List of NANDA-I Diagnoses

Knowledge Map

Care Plan

Care Map

References and Bibliography

Concept Map

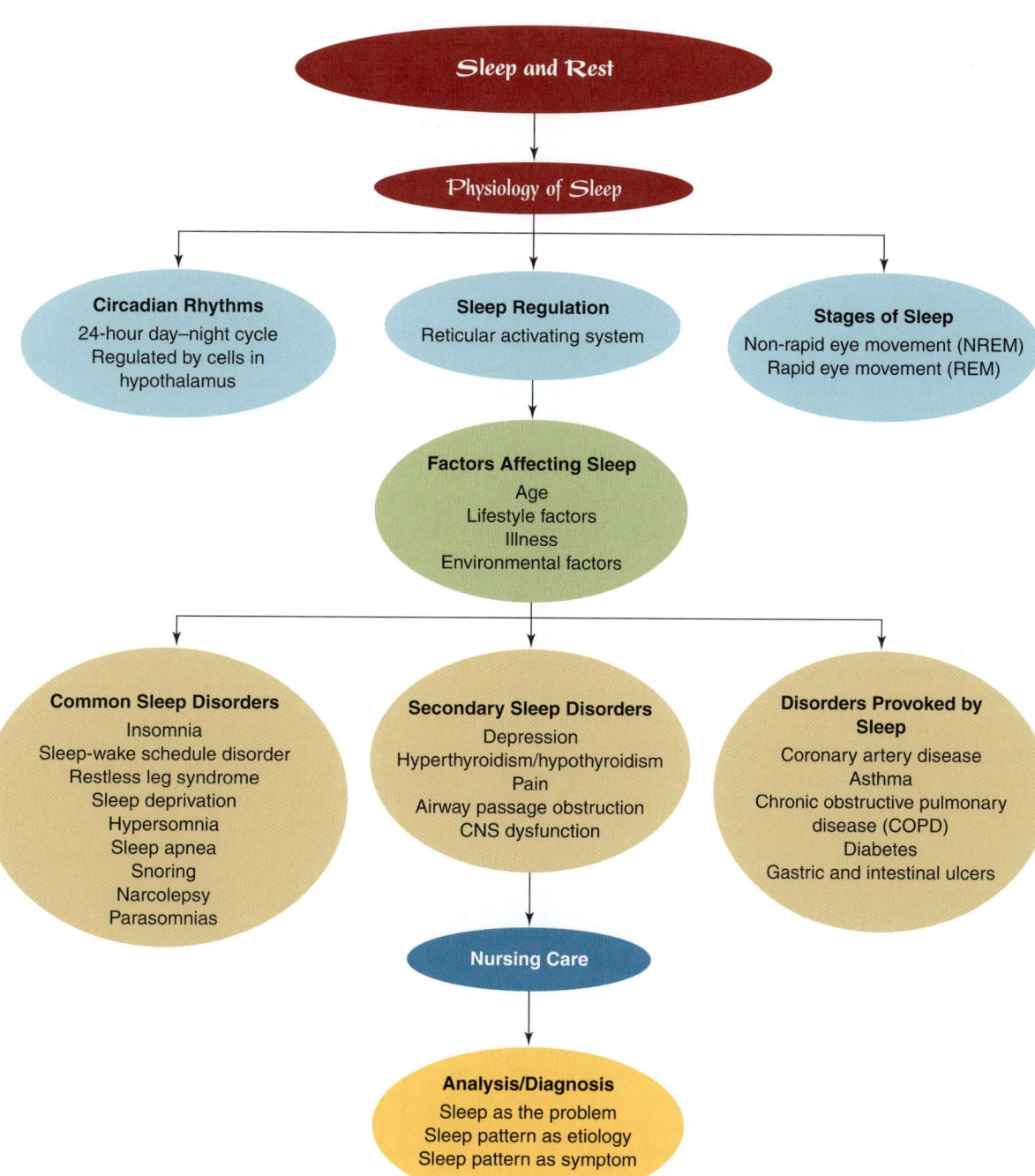

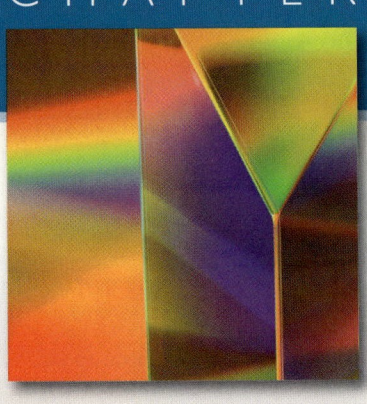

CHAPTER 36

Skin Integrity & Wound Healing

Learning Outcomes

After completing this chapter, you should be able to:

➤ Discuss the factors that affect skin integrity.

➤ Identify wounds based on accepted classification schemes.

➤ Describe the three phases of wound healing.

➤ Distinguish primary intention healing, secondary intention healing, and tertiary intention healing.

➤ Describe three types of wound drainage.

➤ Review the major complications of wound healing.

➤ Explain the factors involved in the development of pressure injury.

➤ Use the Braden scale to assess risk for pressure injury.

➤ Assess and categorize pressure injury based on the staging system.

➤ Provide nursing care that limits the risk of pressure injury development.

➤ Differentiate the kinds of chronic wounds.

➤ Accurately chart assessment of a wound.

➤ Demonstrate appropriate techniques for irrigating a wound.

➤ Describe care of a wound with a drain.

➤ Differentiate the five forms of wound débridement.

➤ Discuss the different kinds of tissue found in wounds.

➤ Discuss when and how to use absorbent, alginate, collagen, gauze dressings, transparent films, hydrocolloids, hydrogels, and foam and antimicrobial dressings.

➤ Describe guidelines to follow when applying heat or cold therapy.

➤ Demonstrate bandage and binder application.

Key Concepts

Skin integrity
Wound
Wound healing

Related Concepts

See the Concept Map at the end of this chapter.

Example Problem

Pressure Injury

Meet Your Patient

William Harmon is a 78-year-old man who fell and fractured his left hip 3 days ago. He underwent an open reduction and internal fixation of the left hip. Today is his second postoperative day. He is still bed bound and is unable to roll or pull himself up in bed.

Mr. Harmon's weight on admission was 140 lb (63.64 kg). His height is 73 in. His family reports that he has been steadily losing weight. He expresses little interest in eating and says he has been depressed since his wife died last year.

A large dressing covers the incision on Mr. Harmon's left hip. During your assessment, you loosen the dressing and see the staples are intact at the incision site and there is a

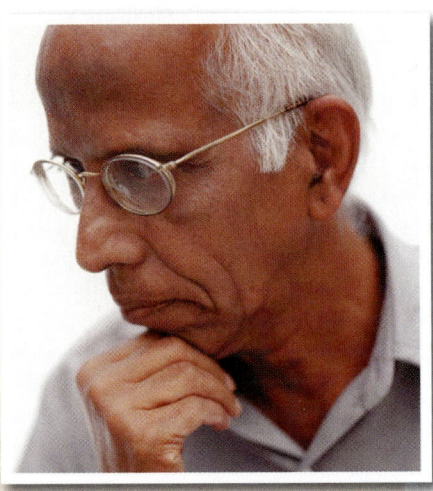

Meet Your Patient (continued)

minimal amount of serosanguineous drainage on the bandage. As you turn him in bed, you see a 10-cm by 6-cm reddened area on his coccyx and a 2-cm by 3-cm purple bruise-like area on his left heel. Mr. Harmon now has three wounds, an intentional surgical wound, and two

pressure injuries that have resulted from his impaired mobility. How will you care for each of these wounds? What factors contributed to each of the wounds and how will you promote healing?

Theoretical Knowledge
knowing **why**

The integumentary system consists of the skin, hair, nails, sweat glands, and the subcutaneous tissue below the skin. The skin is the largest organ of the body. The major functions of the skin include protection of the internal organs, unique identification of an individual, thermoregulation, metabolism of nutrients and metabolic waste products, and sensation.

ABOUT THE KEY CONCEPTS

For optimal function, **skin integrity** must be preserved—that is, all layers of the skin must be intact. A **wound** is a disruption in the normal skin integrity. It is easy to see how the concepts

of skin integrity and wound are related; they are opposites. You will use your knowledge of both these concepts as you protect your patients' skin and promote the physiological process of **wound healing.**

WHAT FACTORS AFFECT SKIN INTEGRITY?

To understand skin integrity, you need to understand the structure of the skin (Fig. 36-1).

Epidermis The **epidermis** is the outer portion of the skin. The epidermis is made up of four or five layers, of which the most important are the inner and outer layers.

- The **stratum corneum,** the outermost layer, is composed of numerous thicknesses of dead cells. Functioning as a barrier,

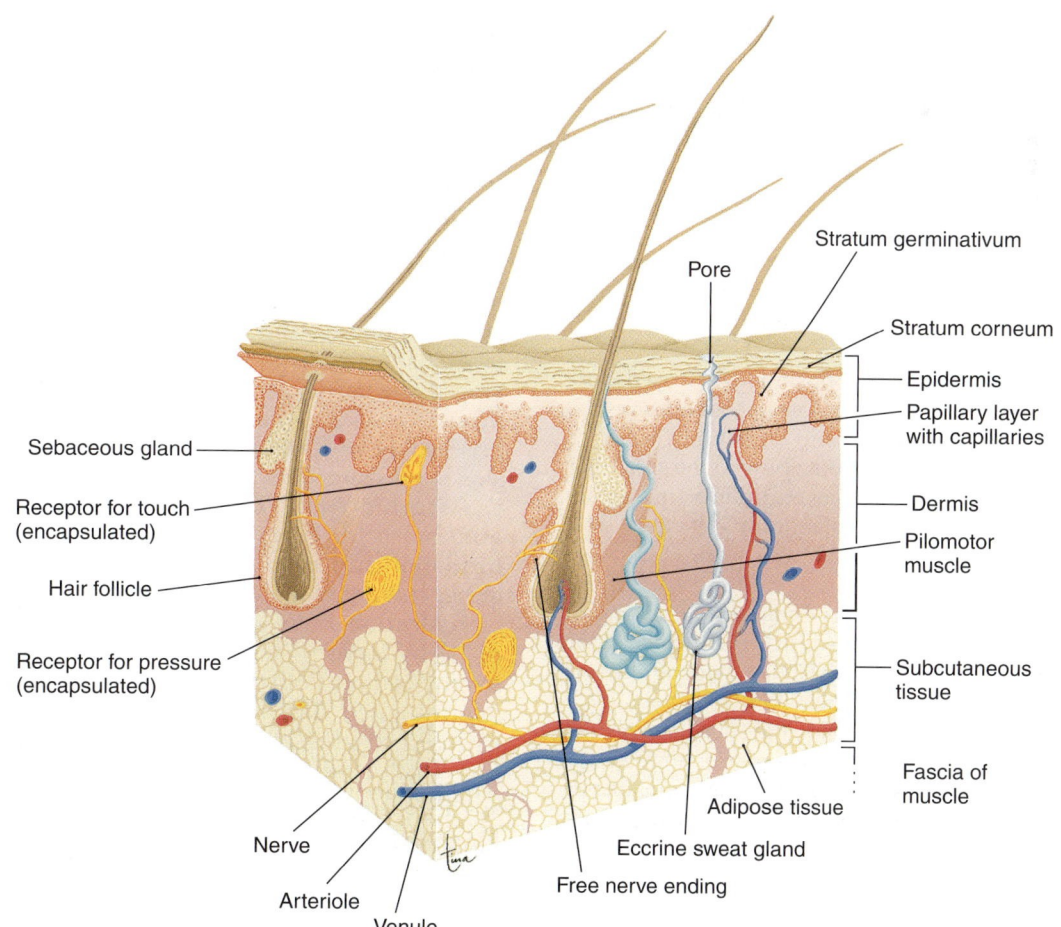

FIGURE 36-1 The structure of the skin.

it restricts water loss and prevents fluids, pathogens, and chemicals from entering the body.

- The **stratum germinativum,** the innermost layer of the epidermis, continually produces new cells, pushing the older cells toward the skin surface. In the dermal layer, the **keratinocytes** are protein-containing cells that give the skin strength and elasticity. Deeper in the epidermis are **melanocytes,** which produce melanin, a pigment that gives skin its color and provides protection from ultraviolet light. **Langerhans cells** are mobile. Their function is to phagocytize (engulf) foreign material and trigger an immune response.

Dermis The **dermis** lies below the epidermis and above the subcutaneous tissue. It is made of irregular fibrous connective tissue that provides strength and elasticity to the skin and is generously supplied with blood vessels. Within the dermis are sweat glands, sebaceous (oil) glands, ceruminous (wax) glands, hair and nail follicles, sensory receptors, elastin, and collagen.

Subcutaneous Tissue The **subcutaneous layer** is composed primarily of connective and adipose tissue. It provides insulation, protection, and a reserve of calories in the event of severe malnutrition. This layer varies in thickness in different body sites. Sex hormones, genetics, age, and nutrition also influence the distribution of subcutaneous tissue.

For optimal function, all layers of the skin must be intact. Breaks in the skin (e.g., surgical incisions, injuries) increase the risk of infection. In the following sections you will learn about factors that influence the ability to maintain intact skin and heal wounds (e.g., age).

Age-Related Variations

Age affects the condition and structure of the skin.

Infants and Children Infants are born with varying amounts of *vernix caseosa*, a creamy substance that protects their skin. Their skin is thinner and more permeable than that of adults, which predisposes infants to skin breakdown (e.g., diaper rash). The subcutaneous layer (brown fat) and sweat glands are not fully developed, especially for preterm infants. As a result, in the first few weeks of life thermoregulation is inadequate, and the infant must be swaddled to maintain body heat. The skin of infants and young children feels smooth, but as they are exposed to sun and other environmental elements, skin texture becomes coarser.

Adolescents and Adults Sex hormones released during puberty increase sebaceous and sweat gland activity, which leads to perspiration odor and sometimes acne. In women, high estrogen levels may contribute to the softening of connective tissue and cause striae and darkening of the skin, particularly on the face, areolae, nipples, vulva, and umbilicus, particularly in people with dark skin.

Older Adults As adults age, the activity of the sebaceous and sweat glands diminishes, resulting in drier skin. **Xerosis** (itchy, red, dry, scaly, cracked, or fissured skin) is a problem for up to 85% of older adults and can be a threat to the integrity of their skin.

Along with loss of lean body mass, the subcutaneous tissue layer thins, giving the individual a sharp, angular appearance if the patient is not overweight. The dermal layer loses elasticity as a result of changes in its collagen fibers. These changes make the skin prone to breakdown and prolong wound-healing time. Regeneration of healthy skin takes at least twice as long in an 80-year-old as in a 30-year-old.

In addition, many older adults have chronic diseases that interfere with healing. Diabetes, for instance, predisposes to

infection, and liver dysfunction interferes with synthesis of blood-clotting factors.

Impaired Mobility

A healthy person moves and shifts position unconsciously when he senses pressure or discomfort. However, for people who are unable to move independently, the weight of the body on the bed or chair causes an increase in pressure on the tissues. Impaired mobility, such as complete bedrest or conditions that limit activity (e.g., paralysis, extreme fatigue, high-risk pregnancy, sedation, casts, traction, and altered sensory perception) can cause injury to the skin.

KnowledgeCheck 36-1

- Identify the major functions of the skin.
- What is the function of the stratum corneum, the outermost layer of the skin?
- What is the function of the subcutaneous layer?
- What effect does aging have on skin?
- What effect does immobility have on skin?

Nutrition and Hydration

Adequate intake of protein, cholesterol, calories, fluid, vitamin C, and minerals is essential to maintaining skin integrity.

Protein Healthy skin depends on adequate protein levels to maintain the skin, repair minor defects, and preserve intravascular volume. As protein levels decline, minor defects cannot be repaired, fluid leaks from the vascular compartment of dependent areas, and **edema** (excess fluid in the tissues) develops. Edema decreases skin elasticity and interferes with the diffusion of oxygen to the cells. Therefore, the skin becomes prone to breakdown.

Cholesterol Low cholesterol levels predispose patients to skin breakdown and inhibit wound healing. Patients on low-fat tube feedings may experience deficiencies in cholesterol, fatty acids, and linoleic acid. Together, these fats aid in providing fuel for wound healing and maintain a waterproof barrier in the stratum corneum.

Calorie Intake If calorie intake is inadequate, the body uses proteins for energy **(catabolism);** they are then unavailable for building and maintenance functions **(anabolism)** (see Chapter 28 as needed). When undernutrition is prolonged, the person experiences weight loss, loss of subcutaneous tissue, and muscle atrophy. As a result, padding between the skin and the bones decreases, predisposing the skin to pressure injury.

Ascorbic Acid, Zinc, and Copper Vitamin C, or ascorbic acid, zinc, and copper are involved in the formation and maintenance of collagen. A deficiency of either can delay wound healing.

Hydration Poor skin turgor may occur as a result of dehydration, whereas edema may result from overhydration. Both dry, dehydrated skin and edematous, overhydrated skin are prone to injury, especially when exposed to pressure, shearing, friction, and moisture. For further discussion on fluid requirements, see Chapter 39.

Diminished Sensation or Cognition

If you've ever touched a hot surface and quickly pulled back your hand, you know the importance of tactile sensation. Clients with peripheral vascular disease, spinal cord injury, diabetes, cerebrovascular accident, trauma, or fractures often

PICOT

Situation: While caring for an emaciated patient after surgery, the nurse notes two new wounds on the patient's bony prominences. Pressure injury has developed secondary to the patient's immobility, friction, shear, and postoperative drainage.

PICOT Components:

P	Population/patient	=	Malnourished adults
I	Intervention/indicator	=	Nutritional supplements
C	Comparator/control	=	Diet without supplements
O	Outcome	=	Improved (or faster) healing time
T	Time	=	

Searchable Question: Do _____(P) who receive/are exposed to _____(I) demonstrate _____(O) as compared to _____(C) during _____(T)?

Example of Evidence: Protein intake has been associated with improved wound healing. To prevent pressure wounds, many acute and long-term care facilities recommend that patients' diets have increased protein content. To examine the effect of nutritional intervention in pressure injury care, researchers reviewed six clinical trials using oral nutritional supplementation enriched with arginine, vitamin C, and zinc for pressure injury care. Results showed pressure injury healing and reduced risk of developing pressure injury.

Practice Change: The nurse caring for patients at risk for pressure wounds needs to address the patients' nutritional needs, including a diet high in protein.

Sources: National Pressure Ulcer Advisory Panel, European Pressure Ulcer Advisory Panel, & Pan Pacific Pressure Injury Alliance (PPPIA). (2014). 2014 Guideline on prevention and treatment for pressure ulcers: Clinical practice guideline (2nd ed.). Emily Haesler (Ed.). Osborne Park, Australia: Cambridge Media.

have diminished tactile sense. They are therefore more prone to skin breakdown.

- *Clients with diminished sensation* are less able to sense a hot surface and would likely suffer a burn. A cut or wound in an area with limited sensation may go unnoticed and therefore untreated. They are also unable to feel pressure in an affected area. As a result, they may not shift position to relieve pressure over bony prominences or be aware that footwear or clothing are constricting.
- *Clients with impaired cognition* (i.e., Alzheimer's disease, dementia, altered level of consciousness) are at higher risk for pressure injury because they are not aware of the need to reposition. Cognitive impairment can be subtle and difficult to recognize. Talk to your patients' families or caregivers and review the patient's health history so that the plan of care can be adjusted.

Impaired Circulation

The vascular system brings oxygen-rich blood to the tissues and removes metabolic waste products.

- *Impaired arterial circulation* restricts activity, produces pain, and leads to muscle atrophy and thin tissue that can lead to ischemia and necrosis.

- *Impaired venous circulation* results in engorged tissues containing high levels of metabolic waste products that make the tissue susceptible to edema, ulceration, and breakdown.

  Both forms of circulatory impairment interfere with tissue metabolism and delay wound healing. **KEY POINT:** *Circulatory impairment is one of the main causes of chronic wounds.*

Medications

Any medication that causes pruritus (itching), dermatoses (rashes), photosensitivity, alopecia, or pigmentation changes can result in changes that impair skin integrity or delay healing (Fig. 36-2). The following are examples:

- *Blood pressure medications* decrease the amount of pressure required to occlude blood flow to an area, creating a risk for ischemia.
- *Anti-inflammatory medications,* such as over-the-counter NSAIDs (e.g., ibuprofen) and steroids (e.g., prednisone), inhibit wound healing.
- *Anticoagulants* (e.g., heparin, warfarin [Coumadin]) can lead to extravasation of blood into subcutaneous tissue. As a result, even minimal pressure or injury can cause a hematoma.
- *Chemotherapeutic agents* delay wound healing because of their cellular toxicity.
- *Certain antibiotics, psychotherapeutic drugs, and chemotherapy agents* increase sensitivity to sunlight, increasing the risk for sunburn.
- *Several herbal products,* such as those containing lavender and tea tree oil, cleanse the skin but also have a drying effect.

Moisture on the Skin

Excessive exposure to moisture leads to **maceration** (softening of the skin) and increases the likelihood of skin breakdown. Incontinence and fever are the most common sources of moisture. Bowel incontinence is particularly troublesome because feces contain digestive enzymes and microorganisms that can readily lead to **excoriation** (denuding) of superficial skin layers. This can lead to **moisture-associated skin damage (MASD), dermatitis** (inflammation of the skin), pressure injury, and infection.

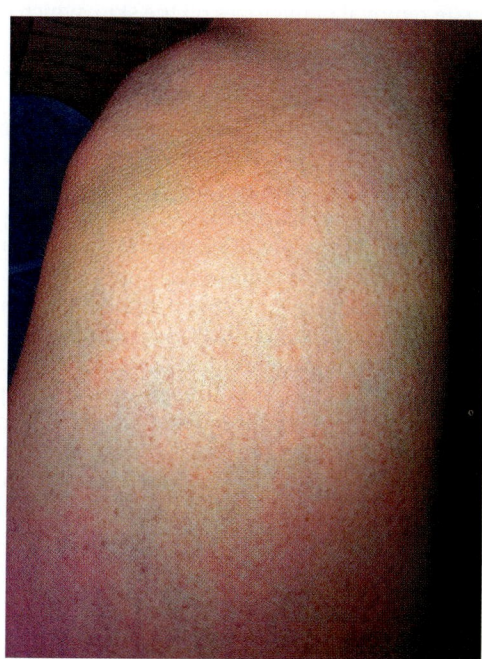

FIGURE 36-2 Skin reaction to medication.

Fever

Fever leads to sweating, which can cause maceration. Fever also increases the metabolic rate, thereby raising the tissue demand for oxygen. An increased oxygen demand is especially difficult to meet if there is circulatory impairment or pressure-induced tissue compression.

Contamination or Infection

- **Contamination** of a wound refers to the presence of microorganisms in the wound. **KEY POINT:** *All chronic wounds are considered contaminated.*
- **Colonization** occurs as bacteria begin to increase in number but are causing no harm. Wounds are colonized from the surrounding skin and local skin organisms, the external environment, and internal sources, usually from the mucous membranes of the gastrointestinal system. The acid nature of the skin keeps bacteria attached to the skin (Zulkowski, 2013).
- **Critical colonization** occurs when the bacteria begin to overwhelm the body's defenses. It may be detected by subtle signs, such as an increase in drainage, or by more pronounced signs, such as a new foul odor, a change in color of the wound bed, new tunneling of the wound, or absent or friable granulation tissue.
- **Infection** implies that the microorganisms are causing harm by releasing toxins, invading body tissues, and increasing the metabolic demand of the tissue. Infection of the skin makes it more vulnerable to breakdown and impedes healing of open wounds. If not stopped, bacteria can gain access to the systemic circulation.

Lifestyle

- *Tanning* exposes the skin to ultraviolet radiation, thereby increasing the risk for skin cancer as well as drying the skin.
- *Skin cleansing* that is either excessive or insufficient may impair skin integrity. Frequent bathing and use of soap remove skin oils and may lead to drying, which jeopardizes the skin's barrier function. Infrequent cleansing of the skin contributes to excessive oiliness, clogged sebaceous glands, and inadequate removal of microbes on the skin, which can then infect a wound or lesion.
- *Regular exercise* improves circulation, which is necessary for skin integrity and wound healing.
- *A nutritious diet* provides the nutrients needed to maintain skin integrity, as already discussed.
- *Smoking* compromises the oxygen supply to the tissues, making skin more prone to breakdown and delaying wound healing. It also interferes with vitamin C absorption, which is needed for collagen formation.
- *Body piercings and tattoos* present a risk for infection and scarring. Complications, which occur in about 20% of piercings, include local infections, sepsis, endocarditis, hepatitis, and toxic shock syndrome. Intraoral and perioral piercings can result in gingivitis, damage to teeth and gums, and choking. Advise patients to become informed about the procedure and about aftercare and to find reputable piercers.

KnowledgeCheck 36-2

- Identify the factors that affect skin integrity.
- What nutritional components are essential to maintain skin?

ThinkLike a Nurse 36-1

- Review the case of William Harmon (Meet Your Patient). What risks, if any, does Mr. Harmon have for skin breakdown or delayed healing?
- What additional information do you need to know to fully evaluate his risk?
- What risks do you have for impaired skin integrity? What actions can you take to protect your skin?

WOUNDS

Wounds are a disruption in the normal integrity of the skin. Wounds may be intentional, such as a surgical wound, or unintentional, such as a cut or a pressure injury.

Types of Wounds

Wounds are classified according to length of time the wound has existed, as well as the condition of the wound (e.g., contamination, severity).

Skin Integrity   The simplest wound classification system is based on the integrity of the skin.

- A **closed wound** exists when there are no breaks in the skin. Contusions (bruises) or tissue swelling from fractures are common closed wounds.
- An **open wound** occurs when there is a break in the skin or mucous membranes. Open wounds include abrasions, lacerations, puncture wounds, and surgical incisions. A compound fracture may also lead to an open wound caused by the projection of bone through the skin. Several open and closed wounds are described in Table 36-1.

Length of Time for Healing   The length of time for wound healing varies according to the skin integrity and the factors affecting it, discussed in the previous section.

- **Acute wounds** are expected to be of short duration. In a healthy person, these wounds heal spontaneously without complications through the three phases of wound healing (inflammation, proliferation, and maturation).
- **Chronic wounds** are wounds that exceed the expected length of recovery, usually because the natural healing progression has been interrupted or stalled because of infection, continued trauma, ischemia, or edema. Chronic wounds include pressure, arterial, venous, and diabetic ulcers. These wounds are frequently colonized with several types of bacteria, and healing is slow because of the underlying disease process. Unless the type of wound is properly diagnosed and the underlying disease process treated, a chronic wound may linger for months or years (Table 36-2).

Level of Contamination

- **Clean wounds** are uninfected wounds with minimal inflammation. They may be open or closed and do not involve the gastrointestinal, respiratory, or genitourinary tracts (these systems frequently harbor bacteria). There is very little risk of infection for a clean wound.
- **Clean-contaminated wounds** are surgical incisions that enter the gastrointestinal, respiratory, or genitourinary tracts. There is an increased risk of infection for these wounds, but there is no obvious infection.
- **Contaminated wounds** include open, traumatic wounds or surgical incisions in which a major break in asepsis occurred. The risk of infection is high for these wounds.
- **Infected wounds** are those in which the bacteria in the wound are above 100,000 organisms per gram of tissue.

Table 36-1 ➤ Types of Wounds

TYPE	DESCRIPTION
Abrasion	A scrape of the superficial layers of the skin; usually unintentional but may be performed intentionally for cosmetic purposes to smooth skin surfaces.
Abscess	A localized collection of pus resulting from invasion from a pyogenic bacterium or other pathogen; must be opened and drained to heal.
Contusion	A closed wound caused by blunt trauma; may be referred to as a bruise or an ecchymotic area.
Crushing	A wound caused by force leading to compression or disruption of tissues. Often associated with fracture. Usually there is minimal or no break in the skin.
Incision	An open, intentional wound caused by a sharp instrument.
Laceration	The skin or mucous membranes are torn open, resulting in a wound with jagged margins.
Penetrating	An open wound in which the agent causing the wound lodges in body tissue.
Puncture	An open wound caused by a sharp object. Often there is collapse of tissue around the entry point, making this wound prone to infection.
Tunnel	A wound with an entrance and exit site.

Table 36-2 ➤ Chronic Wounds

TYPE	ETIOLOGY	CHARACTERISTICS
Pressure injury	Caused by intense or prolonged pressure or pressure in combination with shear, resulting in tissue ischemia and injury.	Appearance depends on the stage or tissue layers involved. Pressure injury tends to be located over bony prominences. Can cause serious tissue damage.
Arterial ulcers	Blockage of arterial blood to an area (clot or stenosis of the arterioles) causes tissue necrosis.	■ Commonly found over the lower leg, especially the ankles, toes, side of the foot, and shin. ■ Ulcer appears "punched out," small and round with smooth borders. ■ Wound base is usually pale with or without necrotic tissue. ■ Surrounding skin is shiny, thin, and dry and is cool to touch. ■ Loss of hair in the surrounding area. ■ Delayed capillary refill time in the area. ■ Very painful, especially at night and with increased activity.
Venous stasis ulcers	Caused by incompetent venous valves, deep vein obstruction, or inadequate calf muscle function. Results in venous pooling, edema, and impaired circulation of the skin.	■ Usually located around the inner ankle or in the lower part of the calf. ■ Surrounding skin is reddened or brown and edematous. ■ Wounds are usually shallow, with irregular wound margins. The wound bed appears "ruddy" or "beefy" red and granular. ■ Drainage may be moderate to heavy depending on amount of edema. ■ Pain usually occurs with leg dependence and dressing changes.
Diabetic foot ulcer	Narrowing of the arteries, reduced oxygenation to the feet result in delayed wound healing and tissue necrosis.	■ Often painless. ■ Occurs mainly on the plantar surfaces and toes.

KEY POINT: *However, the presence of* **beta-hemolytic** **streptococci,** *in any number, is considered an infection.* Signs of wound infection include erythema and swelling around the wound, fever, foul odor, severe or increasing pain, large amount of drainage, or warmth of the surrounding soft tissue.

Depth of the Wound Wound depth is a major determinant of healing time: the deeper the wound, the longer the healing time.

- **Superficial wounds** involve only the epidermal layer of the skin. The injury is usually the result of friction, shearing, or burning.
- **Partial-thickness wounds** extend through the epidermis but not through the dermis.
- **Full-thickness wounds** extend into the subcutaneous tissue and beyond. The descriptor **penetrating** is sometimes added to indicate that the wound involves internal organs.

KnowledgeCheck 36-3

- Explain the difference between an acute and a chronic wound.
- Describe the wound categorization system based on the level of contamination.
- How does wound depth affect healing?

Wound Healing Process

All wounds heal through a physiological process in which epithelial, endothelial, and inflammatory cells, platelets, and fibroblasts migrate into the wound to bring about tissue repair and regeneration. The process is essentially the same regardless of the type of injury or the type of tissues involved.

Types of Healing

Wounds may heal by regeneration or by primary, secondary, or tertiary intention.

- **Regenerative/Epithelial Healing** takes place when a wound affects only the epidermis and dermis. No scar forms and the new (regenerated) epithelial and dermal cells form new skin that cannot be distinguished from the intact skin. Partial-thickness wounds heal by regeneration.
- **Primary (First) Intention Healing** occurs when a wound involves minimal or no tissue loss and has edges that are well approximated (closed) (Fig. 36-3A). Little scarring is expected. A clean surgical incision heals by this method. Even so, a scar is only 80% as strong as the original tissue.
- **Secondary Intention Healing** occurs when a wound (1) involves extensive tissue loss that prevents wound edges from approximating, or (2) should not be closed (e.g., because it is infected). Because the wound is left open, it heals from the inner layer to the surface by filling

Primary intention

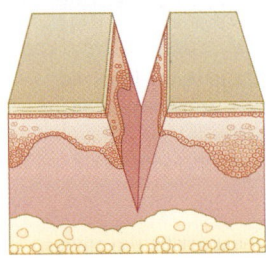 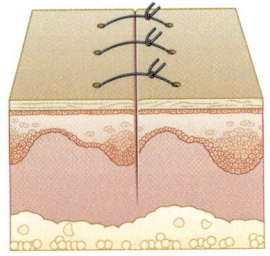 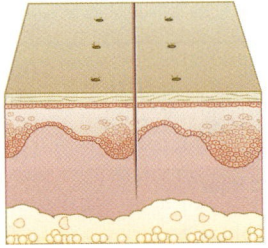

A Clean wound   Sutured early   Results in hairline scar

Secondary intention

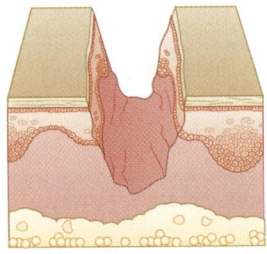 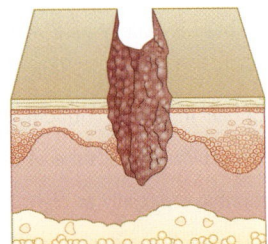 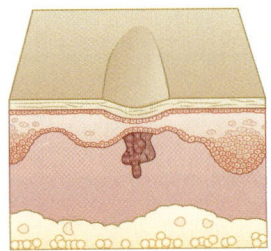

B Wound gaping and irregular   Granulation occurring   Epithelium fills in scar

Tertiary intention

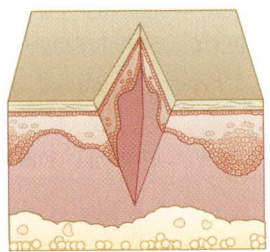 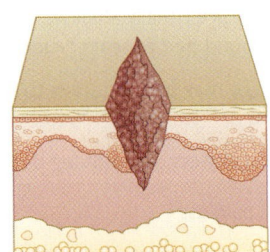 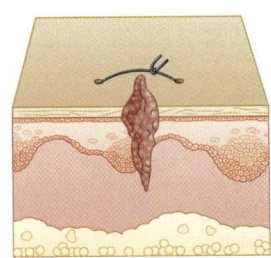

C Wound not sutured   Granulation partially fills in wound   Granulating tissue sutured together

FIGURE 36-3 A. In a wound with minimal tissue loss, the edges may be sutured together, resulting in rapid healing and minimal scarring. B. A wound that heals by secondary intention heals from the inner layer to the surface. Healing takes longer, and there is scarring. C. A wound that heals by tertiary intention is initially healed by secondary intention and later sutured.

in with beefy red **granulation tissue** (a form of connective tissue with an abundant blood supply) (Fig. 36-3B). Epithelial tissue may appear in the wound as small pink or pearl-like areas. Do not mistake this as a sign of infection. Wounds that heal by secondary intention heal more slowly, are more prone to infection, and develop more scar tissue.

- **Tertiary Intention Healing** (also called *delayed primary closure*) occurs when two surfaces of granulation tissue are brought together (Fig. 36-3C). This technique may be used when the wound is clean-contaminated or contaminated. Initially the wound is allowed to heal by secondary intention. When there is no evidence of edema, infection, or foreign matter, the wound edges are closed by bringing together the granulating tissue and suturing the surface. Such wounds require strict aseptic technique during all dressing changes because they are prone to infection. Tertiary intention healing creates less scarring than does secondary but more than primary intention healing.

Phases of Healing
Wound healing occurs in three stages (Fig. 36-4).

Inflammatory Phase—Cleansing This a phase that lasts from 1 to 5 days and consists of two major processes: hemostasis and inflammation.

- *Hemostasis.* At the time of injury, tissue and capillaries are destroyed, causing blood and plasma to leak into the wound. Area vessels constrict to limit blood loss. Platelets aggregate (clump together) to slow bleeding. At the same time, the clotting mechanism is activated to form a blood clot.
- *Inflammation.* The inflammatory reaction is characterized by edema, erythema, pain, temperature elevation, and migration of white blood cells into the wound tissues. Within 24 hours, macrophages begin engulfing bacteria **(phagocytosis)** and clearing debris. Along with plasma proteins and fibrin, they form a scab on the wound surface, which seals the wound and helps prevent microbial invasion.

Proliferative Phase—Granulation This phase occurs from days 5 to 21. Cells develop to fill the wound defect and resurface the skin. **Fibroblasts** (connective tissue cells) migrate to the wound where they form **collagen,** a protein substance that adds strength to the healing wound. New blood and lymph vessels sprout from the existing capillaries at the edge of the wound. The result is the formation of granulation tissue, a beefy red tissue that bleeds readily and is easily damaged. As the clot or scab is dissolved, epithelial cells begin to grow into the wound from surrounding healthy tissue and seal over the wound **(epithelialization).**

Maturation Phase—Epithelialization This phase, also known as *remodeling,* is the final phase of the healing process. It begins in the second or third week and continues even after the wound has closed. During the next 3 to 6 months, the initial collagen fibers that were laid in the wound bed during the proliferative phase are broken down and remodeled into an organized structure (e.g., scar tissue), increasing the tensile strength of the wound.

KnowledgeCheck 36-4
Identify the type of wound healing (primary, secondary, or tertiary intention):
- A wound that heals from inner layer to the surface
- A wound with approximated edges

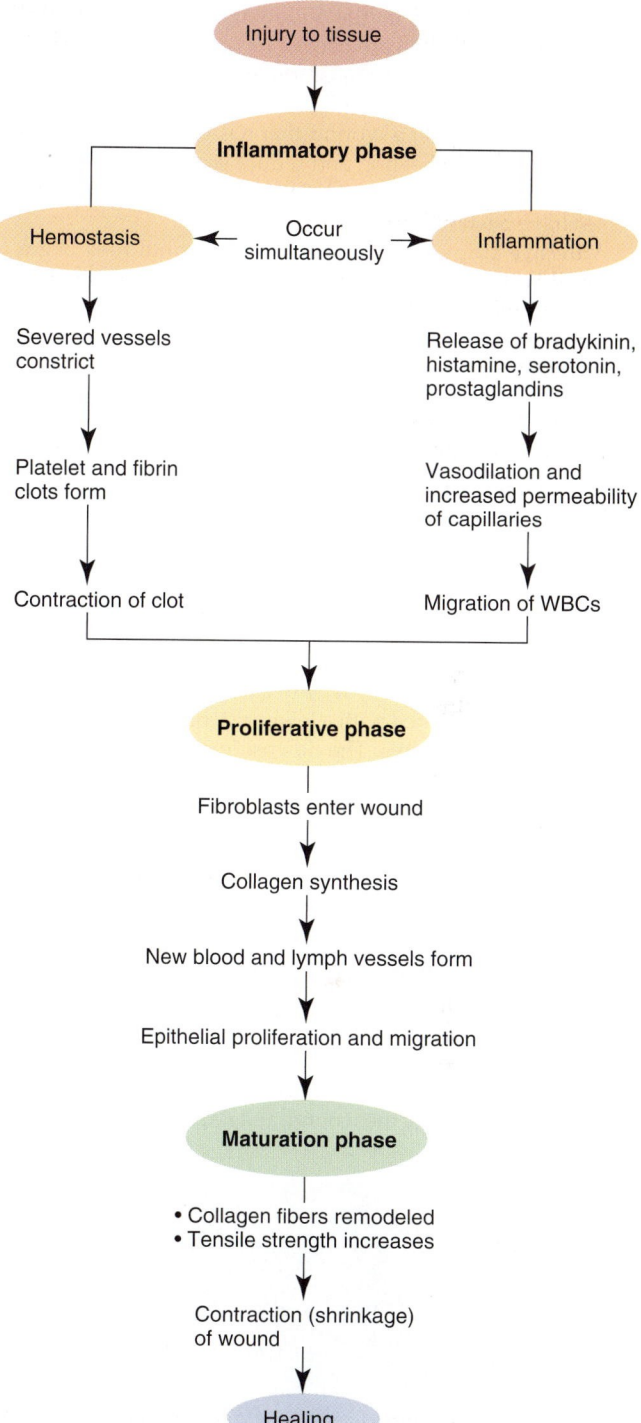

FIGURE 36-4 Stages in the wound healing process.

- A wound that heals by approximating two surfaces of granulation tissue
- A wound that is sutured and has minimal or no tissue loss

Wound Closures
Wounds that heal by primary and tertiary intention may be closed in several ways. The following are common choices.

Adhesive Strips In the following situations, adhesive strips (e.g., Steri-Strips) are used:

- Closing superficial low-tension wounds, such as skin tears or lacerations
- Closing the skin on a wound that has been closed subcutaneously to aid in healing and reduce scarring
- Giving additional support to a wound after sutures or staples have been removed

Adhesive strips are often kept in place until they begin to separate from the skin on their own. For complete instructions, see Procedure 36-9.

Sutures The traditional wound closures are sutures ("stitches"). Suturing creates small puncture wounds along the track of the laceration or incision. Several types of suture materials are available.

- *Absorbent sutures* are used deep in the tissues—for example, to close an organ or **anastomose** (connect) tissue. Because they are made of material that will gradually dissolve, there is no need to remove absorbent sutures.
- *Nonabsorbent sutures* are placed in superficial tissues and require removal, usually by the nurse. For complete steps, see Procedure 36-12A.

Surgical Staples Made of lightweight titanium, surgical staples provide a fast, easy way to close an incision (Fig. 36-5). They are also associated with a lower risk of infection and tissue reaction than are sutures. The downside of staples is that some wound edges are more difficult to align. The most common sites for wound stapling are arms, legs, abdomen, back, scalp, or bowel. Wounds on the hands, feet, neck, or face should not be stapled.

Surgical Glue This is safe for use in clean, low-tension wounds. It is an ideal wound closure method for skin tears.

Collaborative Wound Treatments

Collaborative treatments are necessary for wounds that will not heal despite aggressive care. Such treatments include the following:

- **Surgical options** such as extensive débridement, skin grafts, secondary closure of the wound, and flap techniques (partially

detached tissue placed over a wound) are used for complicated wounds.

- **Hyperbaric oxygen therapy (HBOT)** is the administration of 100% oxygen under pressure to a wound site. HBOT increases oxygen concentration in the tissue, stimulates the growth of new blood vessels, and improves white blood cell (WBC) action.
- **Platelet-derived growth factor** augments the inflammatory phase of wound healing and accelerates collagen formation in the wound.

Types of Wound Drainage

Drainage is the flow of fluids from a wound or cavity. It is often referred to as **exudate** and is fluid that oozes as a result of inflammation. Exudate may take several forms.

- **Serous exudate** is watery in consistency and contains very little cellular matter. Serous exudate consists of *serum*, the straw-colored fluid that separates out of blood when a clot is formed. Clean wounds typically drain serous exudate.
- **Sanguineous exudate** is bloody drainage. It indicates damage to capillaries. You will often see sanguineous exudate with deep wounds or wounds in highly vascular areas. Fresh bleeding produces bright red drainage, whereas older, dried blood is a darker, red-brown color.
- **Serosanguineous drainage** is a combination of bloody and serous drainage. It is most commonly seen in new wounds.
- **Purulent exudate** is thick, often malodorous, drainage that is seen in infected wounds. It contains pus, a protein-rich fluid filled with WBCs, bacteria, and cellular debris. It is commonly caused by infection from **pyogenic** (pus-forming) bacteria, such as streptococci or staphylococci. Normally, pus is yellow in color, although it may take on a blue-green color if the bacterium *Pseudomonas aeruginosa* is present.
- **Purosanguineous exudate** is red-tinged pus. It indicates that small vessels in the wound area have ruptured.

Complications of Wound Healing

Recall that wounds heal by moving through the phases of inflammation, proliferation, and maturation. At times, this process is interrupted by complications such as the following.

Hemorrhage

Hemorrhage implies a profuse or rapid loss of blood. Whenever a capillary network is interrupted or a blood vessel is severed, bleeding occurs. **Hemostasis** (cessation of bleeding) usually occurs within minutes of the injury. Hemostasis is delayed—and hemorrhage occurs—when large vessels are injured, a clotting disorder exists, or the client is on anticoagulant therapy. If bleeding begins again after initial hemostasis, something is probably wrong. Possible causes include a slipped suture, erosion of a blood vessel, a dislodged clot, or infection. The risk of hemorrhage is greatest in the first 24 to 48 hours following surgery or injury. Bleeding may be internal or external.

Internal Hemorrhage Swelling of the affected body part, pain, and changes in vital signs (i.e., decreased blood pressure, elevated pulse) may indicate internal bleeding. By *internal bleeding*, in this chapter we are referring to a **hematoma**, a red-blue collection of blood under the skin, which forms because of bleeding that cannot escape to the surface. A large hematoma causes pressure on surrounding

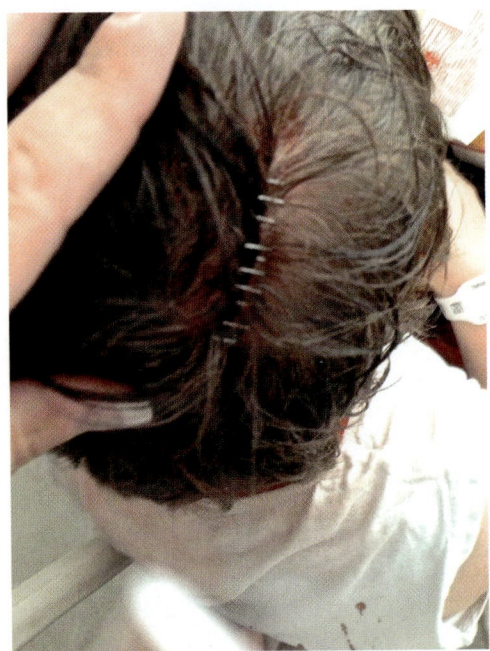

FIGURE 36-5 Surgical staples in the scalp.

tissues. If the hematoma is located near a major artery or vein, it may impede blood flow.

External Hemorrhage External hemorrhage is relatively easy to recognize. You will see bloody drainage on the dressings and in the wound drainage devices. When there is a brisk hemorrhage, blood often pools underneath the client as the dressings become saturated. To be sure that you are aware of the full extent of the bleeding, remember to look underneath the patient.

Infection

Microorganisms can be introduced to a wound during an injury, during surgery, or after surgery. Suspect infection if a wound fails to heal. Localized swelling, redness, heat, pain, fever (temperatures higher than 38°C [100.4°F]), foul-smelling or purulent drainage, or a change in the color of the drainage may also indicate infection.

- In a contaminated or traumatic wound, the symptoms are likely to occur within 2 to 3 days.
- In a clean surgical wound, you will usually not see signs and symptoms of an infection until the fourth or fifth postoperative day.
- Incisions that begin draining within 5 to 7 days of surgery are at risk for dehiscing.

Dehiscence

Rupture (separation) of one or more layers of a wound is called **dehiscence** (Fig. 36-6). Wound dehiscence is most likely to occur in the inflammatory phase of healing, before large amounts of collagen have been deposited in the wound to strengthen it. The most common causes of dehiscence are poor nutritional status, inadequate closure of the muscles, wound infection, or increased tension on the suture line (coughing, lifting an object). Obese clients are also more likely to experience dehiscence because fatty tissue does not heal readily and the patient's mass increases the strain on the suture line.

Dehiscence is usually associated with abdominal wounds. Patients often report feeling a "pop" or tear, especially with sudden straining from coughing, vomiting, or changing positions in bed. Usually there is an immediate increase in serosanguineous drainage. Nursing interventions include the following:

- Maintaining bedrest with the head of the bed elevated at 20° and the knees flexed.
- Applying a binder, if necessary, to prevent *evisceration*.
- Notifying the provider of the dehiscence.

Evisceration

Evisceration is total separation of the layers of a wound with internal viscera protruding through the incision (Fig. 36-7). **KEY POINT:** *This rare complication is a surgical emergency.* Immediately cover the wound with sterile towels or dressings soaked in sterile saline solution to prevent the organs from drying out and becoming contaminated with environmental bacteria. Have the patient stay in bed with knees bent to minimize strain on the incision. Do not put a binder on the patient. Notify the surgeon and ready the patient for surgery (see Chapter 40 for perioperative care).

Fistulas

A **fistula** is an abnormal passage connecting two body cavities or a cavity and the skin. Fistulas often result from infection or debris left in the wound. An abscess forms, which breaks down surrounding tissue and creates the abnormal passageway. Chronic drainage from the fistula may lead to skin breakdown and delayed wound healing. The most common sites of fistula formation are the gastrointestinal and genitourinary tracts. Figure 36-8 illustrates a fistula between the rectum and vagina.

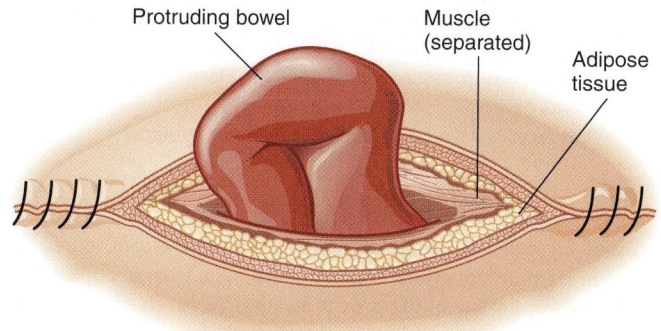

FIGURE 36-7 Evisceration is total separation of the layers of a wound with internal viscera protruding through the incision.

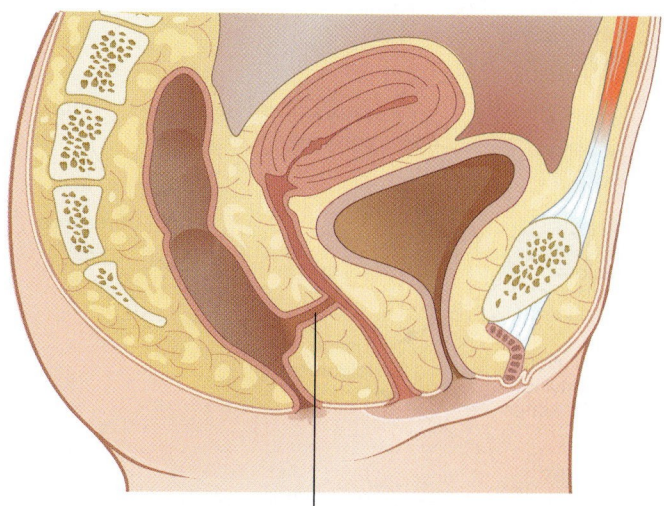

FIGURE 36-8 A fistula is an abnormal passage connecting two body cavities or a cavity and the skin. Fistulas are most common in the gastrointestinal and genitourinary tracts.

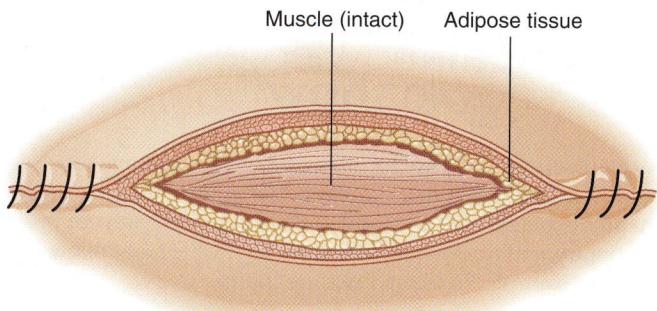

FIGURE 36-6 Dehiscence is separation of one or more layers of a wound. It is most common in the inflammatory phase of healing.

Knowledge Check 36-5

- Describe four types of wound closures.
- Identify five types of wound complications.
- Describe three signs of internal hemorrhage.
- Differentiate between dehiscence and evisceration.

 Think**Like a Nurse** 36-2

Recall the case of Mr. Harmon (Meet Your Patient). What form of wound healing (primary, secondary, or tertiary) is he undergoing? How long would you expect it to take before his wounds heal?

CHRONIC WOUNDS

A chronic wound is one that has not healed within the expected time frame. It has not moved through the repair process in an orderly fashion (inflammation, proliferation, maturation). Wounds that do not heal within 2 to 4 weeks may be considered chronic. Pressure injury is a type of chronic wound. To learn about pressure injury, see the Example Problem: Pressure Injury and Figures 36-9 and 36-10.

Knowledge Check 36-6

- What stage of pressure injury does Mr. Harmon (Meet Your Patient) have?
- What factors have contributed to its development?

 Think**Like a Nurse** 36-3

Based on your knowledge of the factors that have contributed to Mr. Harmon's pressure injury development, what actions may lead to healing of the pressure injury? *Note:* To answer this question, you do not need to know about wound care (e.g., irrigation) for a pressure injury.

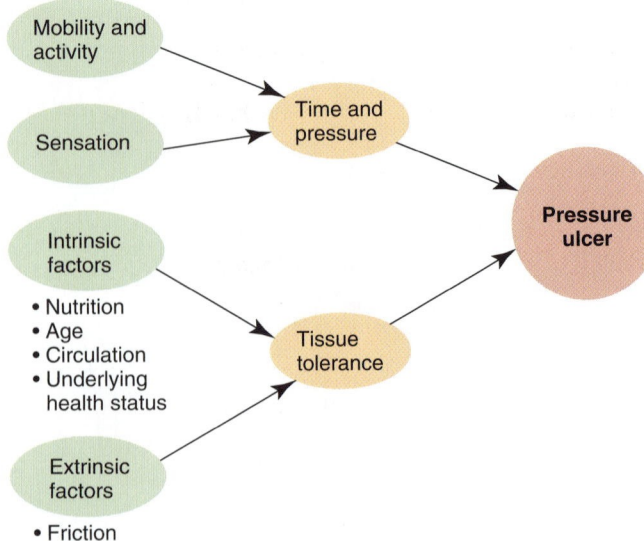

FIGURE 36-9 Several factors contribute to the development of pressure injury.

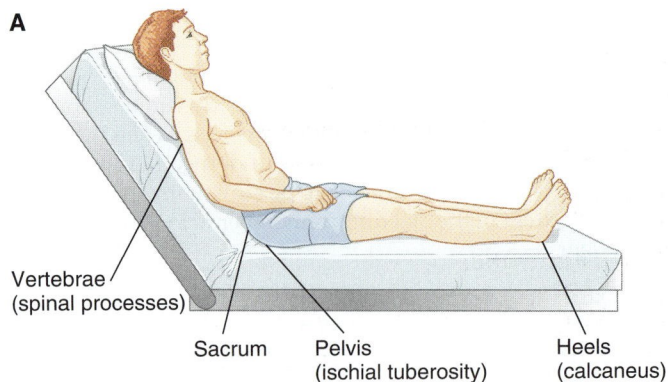

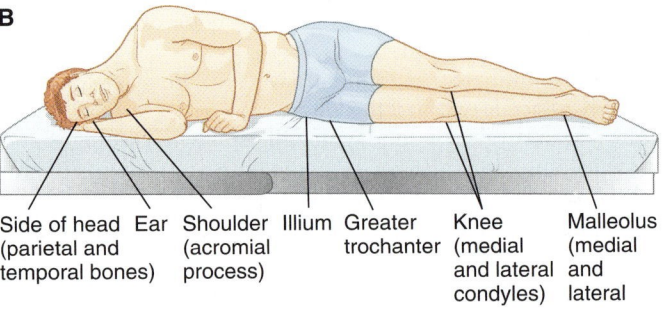

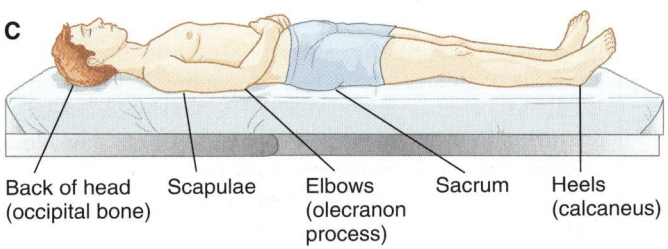

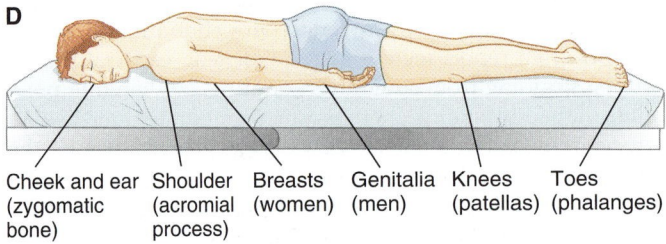

FIGURE 36-10 Most commonly, pressure injury develops over the bony prominences. A. Sitting. B. Lateral. C. Supine. D. Prone. (*Source:* Adapted from AHRQ Clinical Practice Guidelines.)

Practical Knowledge
knowing **how**

As a nurse, you will care for many patients who have wounds or who are at risk for skin breakdown. The remainder of the chapter explains how to maintain skin integrity, prevent pressure injury, and treat wounds; also see the PUSH tool (following) and the Example Problem: Pressure Injury.

ASSESSMENT NP

The National Pressure Ulcer Advisory Panel (NPUAP) recommends nurses perform a comprehensive wound assessment while identifying other health problems and their impact on

(Text continued on page 1306)

Focused Assessment

The PUSH Tool for Evaluation of Pressure Injury

PUSH Tool - Version 3.0

Patient Name:_____   Patient ID#:_____

Ulcer Location: _____   Date:_____

DIRECTIONS:

Observe and measure the pressure ulcer. Categorize the ulcer with respect to surface area, exudate, and type of wound tissue. Record a sub-score for each of these ulcer characteristics. Add the sub-scores to obtain the total score. A comparison of total scores measured over time provides an indication of the improvement or deterioration in pressure ulcer healing.

	0	1	2	3	4	5	Subscore
Length x Width	$0\ cm^2$	$<0.3\ cm^2$	$0.3 - 0.6\ cm^2$	$0.7 - 1.0\ cm^2$	$1.1 - 2.0\ cm^2$	$2.1 - 3.0\ cm^2$	
		6	7	8	9	10	
		$3.1 - 4.0\ cm^2$	$4.1 - 8.0\ cm^2$	$8.1 - 12.0\ cm^2$	$12.1 - 24.0\ cm^2$	$> 24\ cm^2$	
	0	1	2	3			Subscore
Exudate Amount	None	Light	Moderate	Heavy			
	0	1	2	3	4		Subscore
Tissue Type	Closed	Epithelial Tissue	Granulation Tissue	Slough	Necrotic Tissue		
							Total Score

Length x Width: Measure the greatest length (head to toe) and the greatest width (side to side) using a centimeter ruler. Multiply these two measurements (length • width) to obtain an estimate of surface area in square centimeters (cm^2). **Caveat**: Do not guess! Always use a centimeter ruler and always use the same method each time the ulcer is measured.

Exudate Amount: Estimate the amount of exudate (drainage) present after removal of the dressing and before applying any topical agent to the ulcer. Estimate the exudate (drainage) as none, light, moderate, or heavy.

Tissue Type: This refers to the types of tissue that are present in the wound (ulcer) bed. Score as a "4" if there is any necrotic tissue present. Score as a "3" if there is any amount of slough present and necrotic tissue is absent. Score as a "2" if the wound is clean and contains granulation tissue. A superficial wound that is reepithelializing is scored as a "1". When the wound is closed, score as a "0".

> **4 - Necrotic Tissue (Eschar):** black, brown, or tan tissue that adheres firmly to the wound bed or ulcer edges and may be either firmer or softer than surrounding skin.
> **3 - Slough:** yellow or white tissue that adheres to the ulcer bed in strings or thick clumps, or is mucinous.
> **2 - Granulation Tissue:** pink or beefy red tissue with a shiny, moist, granular appearance.
> **1 - Epithelial Tissue:** for superficial ulcers, new pink or shiny tissue (skin) that grows in from the edges or as islands on the ulcer surface.
> **0 - Closed/Resurfaced:** the wound is completely covered with epithelium (new skin).

Note: Refer to the NPUAP Website (www.npuap.org) for further information regarding development and use of the PUSH Tool.

(Continued)

The PUSH Tool for Evaluation of Pressure Injury—cont'd

PRESSURE ULCER HEALING CHART
(use a separate page for each pressure ulcer)

Patient Name:_____   Patient ID#:_____

Ulcer Location: _____   Date:_____

Directions: Observe and measure pressure ulcers at regular intervals using the PUSH Tool. Date and record PUSH Sub-scale and Total Scores on the Pressure Ulcer Healing Record below.

PRESSURE ULCER HEALING RECORD

DATE															
Length x Width															
Exudate Amount															
Tissue Type															
Total Score															

Graph the PUSH Total Score on the Pressure Ulcer Healing Graph below.

PRESSURE ULCER HEALING GRAPH

PUSH Total Score															
17															
16															
15															
14															
13															
12															
11															
10															
9															
8															
7															
6															
5															
4															
3															
2															
1															
Healed 0															
DATE:															

Version 3.0: 9/15/98
© National Pressure Ulcer Advisory Panel

Source: National Pressure Ulcer Advisory Panel. (1998). Pressure Ulcer Scale for Healing (PUSH) Tool, version 3.0. Retrieved from http://www.npuap. org/wp-content/uploads/2012/03/push3.pdf

EXAMPLE PROBLEM: Pressure Injury

Pressure Injury: Localized injury to the skin and underlying tissue usually over a bony prominence (Fig. 36-10). Formerly called *decubitus ulcers, pressure ulcers, bedsores.*

Stages
- Staged by degree of tissue involvement (Table 36-3).
- Become progressively shallow by filling with granulation tissue.
- Lose muscle, subcutaneous fat.
- Dermis not replaced.
- Healing ulcers are not "reverse" staged.

At Risk Patients
- Patients with poor circulation, such as those with diabetes, atherosclerosis, or low blood pressure
- Patients with reduced oxygen supply in the blood, such as those who use tobacco or are anemic
- Patients with limited mobility or reduced sensation to feel pressure points:
  → nerve damage
  → head injury, stroke, spinal cord injury
  → diabetes

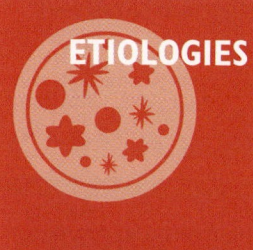
ETIOLOGIES

Contributing Factors

Unrelieved pressure in combination with (Fig. 36-9):
- Immobility
- Poor nutrition
- Fever
- Infection
- Dehydration
- Edema
- Impaired sensation (spinal cord injury, stroke)
- Pressure—Compresses small blood vessels, hindering blood flow and nutrient supply. Tissues become ischemic or damaged or die.
- **Shear**—When one layer of tissue slides horizontally over another, deforming adipose and muscle tissue, and reducing normal blood flow.
- **Friction**—When skin is moist, fragile, or dragged across a surface (e.g., moving patient up in bed).
- **Moisture**—Urine and feces macerate the skin.

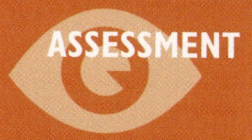
ASSESSMENT

Physical Findings

When ischemia first occurs, the skin over the area is pale and cool. When pressure is relieved (e.g., by turning the patient), vasodilation occurs, extra blood goes to the area, and the area flushes bright red **(reactive hyperemia).** If the redness does not disappear quickly, tissue damage has occurred.

Inspect Skin Daily

1. Skin care begins with regular inspection of the skin.
2. Ensure adequate light to detect subtle, early skin changes.
3. Check pressure points for erythema, tenderness, or edema.
4. Instruct caregivers how to detect early signs of skin problems.
5. In obese patient, breakdown occurs under breasts, in abdominal folds, and where skin contacts skin.

Assessing for and Evaluating Pressure Injury

- **Braden scale** rates sensory perception, moisture, activity, mobility, nutrition, friction, and sheer. The lower the score, the more likely the patient will develop a pressure injury. Braden Q is for children.
- **Norton scale** assesses risk based on the patient's physical condition, mental state, activity, mobility, and incontinence. A low score indicates risk for pressure injury.
- **PUSH tool** reports the progression of a pressure injury. Surface area, exudate, and type of wound tissue are scored and totaled. As the injured area heals, the total score falls. See the Focused Assessment box The PUSH Tool for Evaluation of Pressure Injury.

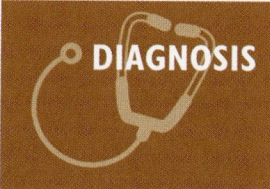
DIAGNOSIS

→ Impaired Skin Integrity, actual or risk for
→ Impaired Tissue Integrity, actual or risk for

→ Infection, actual or risk for
→ Pain
→ Body Image, alteration in

(Continued)

EXAMPLE PROBLEM: Pressure Injury—cont'd

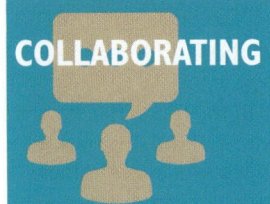

COLLABORATING

Adjunctive Wound Care Therapies

- **Electrical Stimulation.** Stimulates cellular growth through development of fibroblasts, new collagen; increases blood flow and tissue oxygenation.
- **Hyperbaric Oxygen Therapy.** High oxygen to accelerate healing.
- **Tissue Growth Factors.** Naturally occurring proteins that cause specific cells to grow and replicate; platelet-derived growth factor for chronic wound healing for diabetic and other nonhealing wounds; used for clean wounds without necrotic tissue and that have good blood supply.
- **Ultrasound.** Vibrations from the transducer create sound waves that pass into the tissue, causing it to vibrate and heat up. This stimulates movement of fluid within and between cells and aids in débridement and increases cell metabolism.
- **Bioengineered Skin Substitutes.** Aid in temporary or permanent closure of partial- and full-thickness wounds. Made of human epidermis or dermis, animal cells, or synthetic material.
- **Surgical** excision and débridement, skin graft, drains, and flaps close wounds and promote healing.

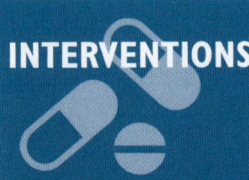

INTERVENTIONS

PREVENTION is the priority INTERVENTION!!

Pressure Injury Monitoring

- Reassess hospitalized patient daily, when transferred or discharged, and if condition changes;
- Reassess nursing home residents weekly for 1st 4 weeks; then quarterly; or if condition deteriorates.
- Monitor home patient with every visit. Inform the healthcare provider of patient's risk.
- Visual cues (stickers on charts, dots on ID bands) remind staff.

Manage Moisture.

Incontinence Care

- Provide skin care soon after each incontinence episode.
- Apply moisture barrier cream to protect perineal skin.
- Use absorbent products that wick moisture away from the skin.

Bathing

- Diaphoretic patient may need frequent bathing; sweat can irritate sensitive or injury-prone skin.
- Older adults don't usually require daily bathing due to ↓ sebaceous oil and sweat production.
- Gently bathe fragile skin, using a minimum of force and friction; washcloths can be abrasive.
- Use a mild, emollient cleansing soap only as needed; be sure to rinse thoroughly and gently pat the skin dry. Soaps remove oils from the skin. Use warm water; hot water dries the skin.

Lotion and Massage

- Use a gentle massaging motion to promote circulation and wound healing.
- Do not massage over bony prominences; can irritate the area and lead to tissue injury.

Linens

- Keep the linen soft, clean, dry, and free from wrinkles by changing it frequently.

Dressings

- **Hydrating Dressing.** Use hydrocolloid or foam dressings to reduce wound size. See Procedure 36-8.
- **Negative Pressure Wound Therapy.** Placed on a wound packed with foam or gauze dressings to create a vacuum. Subatmospheric pressure reduces edema from swollen tissues; promotes granulation tissue formation; removes exudate and infectious material. See Procedure 36-6.
- **Silver Dressing.** Acts as barrier to bacteria in wound bed; eliminates bacterial biofilms.
- **Transparent Dressing.** Apply the clear film or drape free of wrinkles. The occlusive dressing creates a seal to help create negative pressure within the wound. See Procedure 36-7.

Minimize Pressure.

Most patient who are at risk for pressure injury have mobility problems. Must provide frequent position changes to prevent tissue damage from ischemia.

EXAMPLE PROBLEM: Pressure Injury—cont'd

Turn and Reposition.

- At least every 2 hours; more often for fragile skin or little subcutaneous tissue. Every hour for chair-bound patient; teach patient to shift weight every 15 minutes.
- Place a turning schedule at the bedside so all caregivers can aid in the prevention strategy.
- Use the "rule of 30" to guide your positioning:
  Elevate the head of bed (HOB) 30° or less.
  When side-lying, position at a 30° to avoid direct pressure on the trochanter.
  If the HOB is up more than 30°, limit time in this position to minimize pressure and shear.
- Use lift devices or drawsheets, heel and elbow protectors, sleeves and stockings.

Support Surfaces

→ Specialty mattresses, integrated bed systems, mattress overlays—consist of air, gel, foam, water.
→ Various sizes and shapes for beds, chairs, exam and surgical tables.

- Redistribute pressure and moisture to prevent bacterial growth on the skin.
- Use products that raise the heels off the bed. Pillows may not redistribute the weight of patient's foot.
- Avoid donut-type devices. Use pressure-redistributing devices for chairs and wheelchairs.

Optimize Nutrition and Hydration.

Patients at risk: rapid weight loss, ↑ metabolic demands, limited intake, or ↓ serum albumin.

1. Monitor hydration status and offer water (if appropriate) whenever you reposition the patient
2. Provide adequate calories and protein (2 g/kg in an undernourished patient with a wound). Add protein or amino acid supplementation to reduce wound size.
3. Consider the consistency of the diet (soft diet for a patient who is frail or missing teeth).
4. Tube feeding or parenteral nutrition to supplement oral intake; dietary referral as needed.

Table 36-3 ► Staging Pressure Injury

STAGE	CLINICAL FINDINGS	DISCUSSION
Stage 1 Pressure Injury 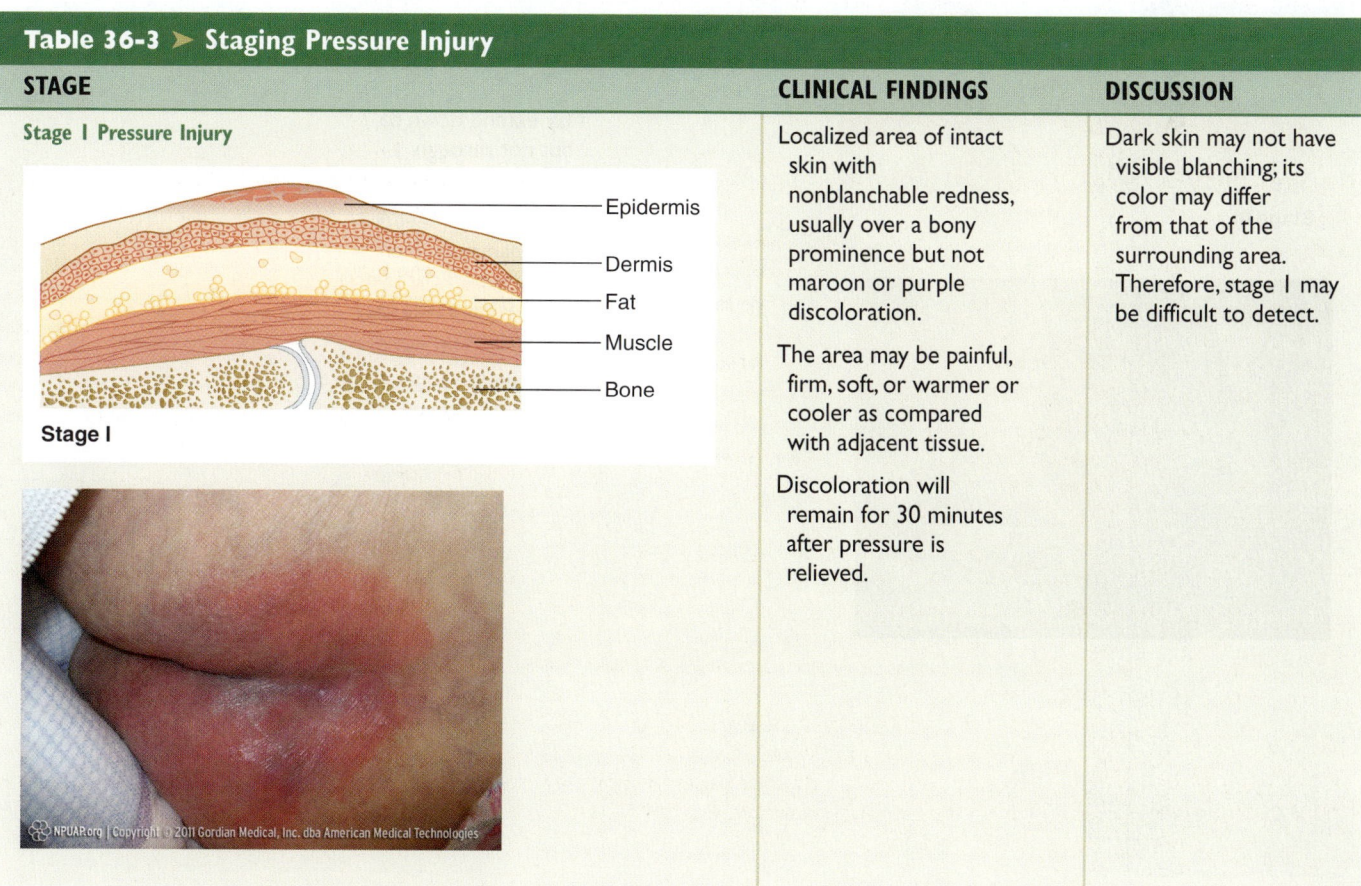 **Stage I**	Localized area of intact skin with nonblanchable redness, usually over a bony prominence but not maroon or purple discoloration. The area may be painful, firm, soft, or warmer or cooler as compared with adjacent tissue. Discoloration will remain for 30 minutes after pressure is relieved.	Dark skin may not have visible blanching; its color may differ from that of the surrounding area. Therefore, stage 1 may be difficult to detect.

Labels in illustration: Epidermis, Dermis, Fat, Muscle, Bone

NPUAP.org | Copyright © 2011 Gordian Medical, Inc. dba American Medical Technologies

(Continued)

Table 36-3 ➤ Staging Pressure Injury—cont'd

STAGE	CLINICAL FINDINGS	DISCUSSION
Stage 2 Pressure Injury **Stage II** NPUAP.org | Copyright © 2011 Gordian Medical, Inc. dba American Medical Technologies	Involves partial-thickness loss of dermis. Stage 2 pressure injury is open but shallow and with a red pink wound bed. There is no *slough* (tan, yellow, gray, green, or brown necrotic tissue). May also be an intact or open/ruptured serum-filled blister, or a shiny or dry shallow ulcer without slough or bruising.	Do not use this stage to describe skin tears, tape burns, perineal dermatitis, maceration, or excoriation. Do not mistake moisture-associated skin damage or fungal infections for Stage 2 pressure injury. Stage 2 pressure injury does not involve sloughing or bruising.
Stage 3 Pressure Injury **Stage III** NPUAP.org | Copyright © 2011 Gordian Medical, Inc. dba American Medical Technologies	A deep crater characterized by full-thickness skin loss with damage or necrosis of subcutaneous tissue. Adipose is visible. May extend down to, but not through, underlying fascia. Undermining (deeper-level damage under boggy superficial layers) of adjacent tissue may be present. Bone/tendon is not visible or directly palpable.	Some stage 3 pressure injury can be extremely deep when located in an area with significant adipose layers.

Table 36-3 ➤ Staging Pressure Injury—cont'd

STAGE	CLINICAL FINDINGS	DISCUSSION
Stage 4 Pressure Injury 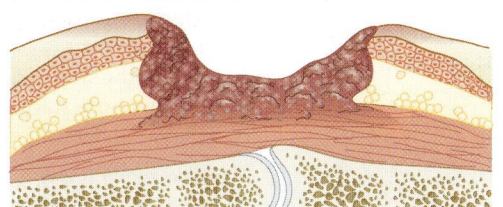 **Stage IV** 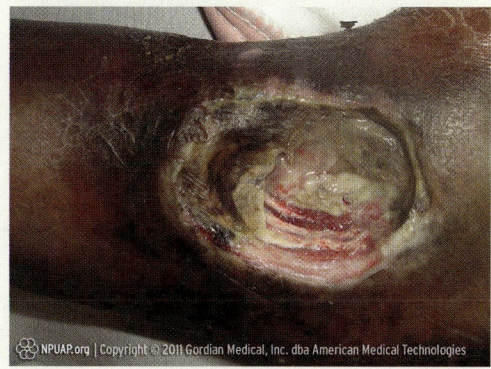	Involves full-thickness skin loss with extensive destruction, tissue necrosis, or damage to muscle, bone, or support structures. Exposed bone/tendon is visible or directly palpable. Slough or *eschar* (tan, black, or brown leathery necrotic tissue) may be present. Ebole (rolled edges), undermining, and sinus tracts (blind tracts underneath the epidermis) are common.	The depth of a stage 4 pressure injury varies by location. They can be shallow on the bridge of the nose, ear, occiput, and malleolus because these areas do not have subcutaneous tissue. Stage 4 injury can extend into muscle and supporting structures (e.g., fascia, tendon, or joint capsule). Often requires a full year to heal. Even once healed, the site remains at risk for future injury because the scar tissue is not as strong as the original tissue.
Deep Tissue Pressure Injury (DTI) 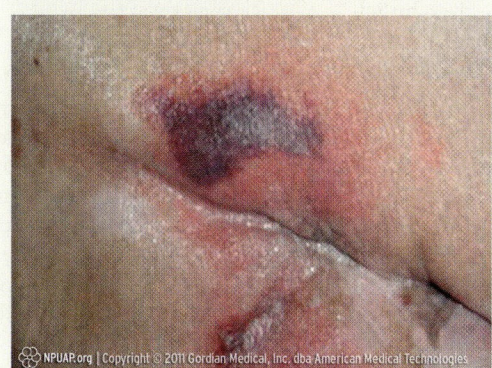	An area of skin that is intact but persistently discolored. It might be purplish or deep red, painful, or boggy, or have a blister. Pain and temperature change often come before skin color changes.	Occurs owing to damage of underlying soft tissue from pressure or shear. Findings can be subtle enough that often DTI is not recognized until after severe tissue damage has occurred. May heal or evolve further and become covered by thin eschar, rapidly exposing additional layers of tissue even with optimal treatment. In darker pigmented individuals, discoloration might go undetected.

(Continued)

Table 36-3 ► Staging Pressure Injury—cont'd

STAGE	CLINICAL FINDINGS	DISCUSSION
Unstageable Pressure Injury 	Involves full-thickness skin loss. The base of the wound is obscured by slough or eschar.	Until enough slough and/or eschar is removed to expose the base of the wound, the true depth, and therefore stage, cannot be determined. *Stable eschar* is dry, adherent, and intact without erythema or fluctuance. Do not remove or soften a stable eschar, as it serves as "the body's natural cover."

Source: Reprinted with permission. National Pressure Ulcer Advisory Panel. (2016a). NPUAP pressure injury stages. Retrieved from http://www.npuap.org/resources/educational-and-clinical-resources/npuap-pressure-injury-stages/

wound healing. Existing wounds require additional assessment. A thorough skin assessment includes a nursing history, physical examination, and diagnostic testing.

A comprehensive risk assessment tool enables you to evaluate the cumulative risk for pressure injury. Among the most commonly used are the Braden and Norton scales. Also, see Example Problem: Pressure Injury.

Focused Nursing History

To assess wound healing ability and the risk for skin breakdown, you will need to gather data on factors that affect skin integrity (discussed previously): age, mobility, nutrition, hydration, sensation, circulation, medications, moisture, lifestyle, underlying health and disease status, and the presence of microorganisms. Also consider the psychosocial issues related to coping with chronic wounds (Woo, 2011).

♥ **iCare** For instance, you will need to assess with care and compassion how the patient copes with the pain of a chronic wound, handles the loss of control and independence, is adapting to changes in body image, deals with the financial burden of caring for complex wounds, and adjusts to the social isolation that comes with impaired mobility and chronic illness. For history questions to help you assess these factors, see the Focused Assessment box History Questions for Skin and Wound Assessment.

ThinkLike a Nurse 36-4

Review the Braden scale (see the Focused Assessment box). Apply this risk assessment scale to Mr. Harmon (Meet Your Patient).
- What additional information, if any, do you need to complete these assessments?
- Calculate a Braden score based on Mr. Harmon's risk factors if he had also been incontinent of urine twice that day.

Focused Physical Examination

Inspect all areas of the body routinely. Evaluate the skin for color, integrity, temperature, texture, turgor, mobility, moisture, lesions, and hair distribution. Check pressure points for erythema, tenderness, or edema. Assess all bony prominences of individuals "at risk" for skin breakdown routinely. Include skin under special garments such as shoes, heel elevators, and antiembolism stockings. Also assess vulnerable pressure points for bed- or chair-bound patients. See Chapter 21 if you need more details on skin assessment.

Assessing Treated Wounds

All wounds require a focused assessment. Assessment frequency depends on the condition of the wound, the work setting, the patient's overall condition and underlying disease process, the type of wound, and the type of treatment used for the wound. If you are providing wound care, you will assess the wound with every treatment. For a wound assessment summary, see the Focused Assessment box Physical Examination: Wound Assessment. Assessment parameters include the following:

Location Describe the wound location in anatomical terms. For example, describe an incision from cardiac surgery as a midsternal incision extending from the manubrium to the xiphoid process. An accurate description of the location is important because:
- *Location influences the rate of healing.* Wounds in highly vascular regions, such as the scalp or hands, heal more rapidly than wounds in less vascular regions, such as the abdomen or a heel.
- *Location affects movement.* Wounds that can be readily stabilized heal more rapidly than those in areas that are affected by the constant stress of movement.
- *Location can give you clues to the wound etiology.* A wound over a bony prominence could be related to pressure, whereas one on the bottom of the foot could be a diabetic foot ulcer.

Type of Wound Look for the following information: Is it an acute wound? If the wound is sutured, examine the closure. Are the wound edges approximated (together)? Is there tension on any aspect of the wound? Are the stitches intact? Or is this a chronic wound?

BRADEN SCALE FOR PREDICTING PRESSURE SORE RISK

Patient's Name _____   Evaluator's Name _____   Date of Assessment _____

SENSORY PERCEPTION ability to respond meaningfully to pressure-related discomfort	**1. Completely Limited** Unresponsive (does not moan, flinch, or grasp) to painful stimuli, due to diminished level of consciousness or sedation. OR limited ability to feel pain over most of body.	**2. Very Limited** Responds only to painful stimuli. Cannot communicate discomfort except by moaning or restlessness OR has a sensory impairment which limits the ability to feel pain or discomfort over 1/2 of body.	**3. Slightly Limited** Responds to verbal commands, but cannot always communicate discomfort or the need to be turned. OR has some sensory impairment which limits ability to feel pain or discomfort in 1 or 2 extremities.	**4. No Impairment** Responds to verbal commands. Has no sensory deficit which would limit ability to feel or voice pain or discomfort.
MOISTURE degree to which skin is exposed to moisture	**1. Constantly Moist** Skin is kept moist almost constantly by perspiration, urine, etc. Dampness is detected every time patient is moved or turned.	**2. Very Moist** Skin is often, but not always moist. Linen must be changed at least once a shift.	**3. Occasionally Moist:** Skin is occasionally moist, requiring an extra linen change approximately once a day.	**4. Rarely Moist** Skin is usually dry, linen only requires changing at routine intervals.
ACTIVITY degree of physical activity	**1. Bedfast** Confined to bed.	**2. Chairfast** Ability to walk severely limited or non-existent. Cannot bear own weight and/or must be assisted into chair or wheelchair.	**3. Walks Occasionally** Walks occasionally during day, but for very short distances, with or without assistance. Spends majority of each shift in bed or chair.	**4. Walks Frequently** Walks outside room at least twice a day and inside room at least once every two hours during waking hours.
MOBILITY ability to change and control body position	**1. Completely Immobile** Does not make even slight changes in body or extremity position without assistance.	**2. Very Limited** Makes occasional slight changes in body or extremity position but unable to make frequent or significant changes independently.	**3. Slightly Limited** Makes frequent though slight changes in body or extremity position independently.	**4. No Limitation** Makes major and frequent changes in position without assistance.
NUTRITION usual food intake pattern	**1. Very Poor** Never eats a complete meal. Rarely eats more than 1/2 of any food offered. Eats 2 servings or less of protein (meat or dairy products) per day. Takes fluids poorly. Does not take a liquid dietary supplement OR is NPO and/or maintained on clear liquids or IVs for more than 5 days.	**2. Probably Inadequate** Rarely eats a complete meal and generally eats only about 1/2 of any food offered. Protein intake includes only 3 servings of meat or dairy products per day. Occasionally will take a dietary supplement. OR receives less than optimum amount of liquid diet or tube feeding.	**3. Adequate** Eats over half of most meals. Eats a total of 4 servings of protein (meat, dairy products per day. Occasionally will refuse a meal, but will usually take a supplement when offered OR is on a tube feeding or TPN regimen which probably meets most of nutritional needs.	**4. Excellent** Eats most of every meal. Never refuses a meal. Usually eats a total of 4 or more servings of meat and dairy products. Occasionally eats between meals. Does not require supplementation.
FRICTION & SHEAR	**1. Problem** Requires moderate to maximum assistance in moving. Complete lifting without sliding against sheets is impossible. Frequently slides down in bed or chair, requiring frequent repositioning with maximum assistance. Spasticity, contractures or agitation leads to almost constant friction.	**2. Potential Problem** Moves feebly or requires minimum assistance. During a move skin probably slides to some extent against sheets, chair, restraints or other devices. Maintains relatively good position in chair or bed most of the time but occasionally slides down.	**3. No Apparent Problem** Moves in bed and in chair independently and has sufficient muscle strength to lift up completely during move. Maintains good position in bed or chair.	

Total Score _____

© Copyright Barbara Braden and Nancy Bergstrom, 1988   All rights reserved

Source: U.S. Department of Health and Human Services. (1992). *Clinical practice guideline. Pressure ulcers in adults: Prediction and prevention* (PPPPUA Publication No. 92-0047, pp. 16–17). Rockville, MD: Public Health Service. Copyright © Barbara Braden and Nancy Bergstrom, 1988. Reprinted with permission.

The Norton Scale for Assessing Risk of Pressure Injury

Norton Scale for Assessing Risk of Pressure Ulcers

	Physical Condition	Mental Condition	Activity	Mobility	Incontinent	
	Good 4 Fair 3 Poor 2 Very bad 1	Alert 4 Apathetic 3 Confused 2 Stupor 1	Ambulant 4 Walk/help 3 Chair-bound 2 Bed 1	Full 4 Slightly limited 3 Very limited 2 Immobile 1	Not 4 Occasional 3 Usually/urine 2 Doubly 1	Total Score
Name/Date						

The Norton Scale uses five criteria to assess patients' risk for pressure ulcers. Scores of 14 or less indicate liability to ulcers; scores of <12 indicate very high risk.

Source: Norton, D., McLaren, R., & Exton-Smith, A. N. (1975). *An investigation of geriatric nursing problems in hospitals.* Edinburgh, Scotland: Churchill Livingstone. Used with permission.

History Questions for Skin and Wound Assessment

➤ What is your typical activity level?
➤ Do you ever use a wheelchair or mobile device to get around? Do you require assistance to get out of bed or a chair?
➤ Tell me about your usual diet.
➤ How much liquid do you drink each day?
➤ Do you have any areas of numbness and tingling?
➤ Have you had any recent changes in your skin?
➤ Do you have any sores or open areas? If so, how long have you had the wound?
➤ Have you ever had difficulty with wound healing?
➤ What kinds of health problems have you been experiencing?
➤ What medications—prescribed, herbal, or over the counter—are you taking?
➤ What is your typical hygiene routine?
➤ Do you ever lose control of your bladder or bowels?
➤ Do you smoke?
➤ How much time do you spend outdoors?
➤ Do you have diabetes? If so, how often do you check your feet? How often do you see a podiatrist? What is your average blood sugar?

Size The NPUAP recommends using a head-to-toe orientation for measuring wounds, the longest length head to toe, and the widest width side to side, perpendicular (90° angle) to length, encompassing the entire wound. Use serial photographs with grids showing the wound's dimensions, especially if the wound has an irregular border, to document the baseline and wound healing (European Pressure Ulcer Advisory Panel and NPUAP, 2014). To measure wound depth, gently insert a sterile cotton-tip applicator into the deepest part of the wound. Measure the applicator from the tip in the wound bed to the skin level.

Undermining or Tunneling Assess the wound edges for any undermining or tunneling. Pay close attention to any tissue that appears to have a separation either in tissue type or plane, as frequently tunnels may be found. Measure the depth and location of any undermining or tunneling using the face of a clock as a guide. If the top of the wound is 12:00 and the bottom of the wound is 6:00, for example, record "2 cm of undermining is present from 1:00 to 4:00" or "6 cm tunnel exists at the center of the wound tracking in the 3:00 direction."

Periwound Examine the skin surrounding the wound. Skin discoloration may indicate a hematoma or additional injury to the surrounding tissue. Look for the following:

- **Maceration** is caused by excessive moisture from pooled drainage on intact skin for periods of time or when a moist dressing is inappropriately applied, left on too long, or overlaps onto healthy skin. The skin may appear as pale and wrinkled or "pruned" and may flake and peel.
- **Undermining** (tunneling) will produce a boggy feel around the wound.
- **Crepitus** is gas trapped under the skin. If you palpate the surrounding skin and feel a crackling sensation, this is crepitus. Crepitus may be due to air leaking from the lung in a chest wound or may indicate the presence of gas-producing bacteria.
- **Erythema, swelling,** or other signs of irritation indicate that the surrounding tissue is in jeopardy.
- **Epiboly** is closed or rolled wound edges. Examine wound edges for epithelial tissue and contraction. Epiboly may

Focused Assessment

Physical Examination: Wound Assessment

All Wounds

Assess all wounds for the following:

Location

Describe the location of the wound in anatomical terms. For example, you would describe an incision from cardiac surgery as a midsternal incision extending from the manubrium to the xiphoid process.

Size

➤ Measure the length and width of the wound in centimeters.
➤ To measure wound depth, gently insert a sterile cotton-tip applicator into the deepest part of the wound. Measure the applicator from the skin level to the tip.
➤ If possible, use photo documentation, indicating the dimensions on the photo. This is especially useful in the case of a wound with an irregular border.

Appearance

Your description of the appearance of the wound should be very detailed. You must describe:
➤ *Type of wound* (open or closed)
➤ *If the wound is sutured,* examine the closure. Are the wound edges approximated? Is there tension on any aspect of the wound? Are the stitches intact?
➤ *The color of the wound.* Redness and inflammation for the first 2 to 3 days are normal, but erythema or swelling beyond that time may indicate infection.
➤ *Condition of the wound bed (in an open wound).* A beefy red, moist appearance is evidence of healing. A pale color or dry texture indicates a delay in healing.
➤ *Examine for necrosis, slough, and eschar.* Examine for a tunnel or sinus tract in the wound bed; if there is one, inspect and probe it for depth and characteristics.
➤ *The skin surrounding the wound.* Observe for skin discoloration, hematoma, or additional injury to the surrounding tissue. Observe for maceration, tunneling, crepitus, blistering, or erythema. Examine the edges of the wound for epithelial tissue and contraction. Look for undermining beneath the wound margins.

Drainage

➤ *Presence of drainage or exudate.* Describe the color, consistency, amount, and odor.
➤ *Assess the quantity of wound drainage* by weighing dressings before they are applied and again when they have been removed. The change in weight reflects the amount of drainage that they have absorbed.
➤ *If a drain is present,* measure the amount of fluid in the collection container.
➤ *Odor* may indicate fistula formation or contamination with bacteria. If a new odor develops, assess carefully for presence of a fistula.

Patient Responses

Ask your patients about pain, discomfort, or itching related to the wound or wound care.

Assessing an Untreated Wound

Your assessment should determine what, if any, additional professional support is necessary. Assess the following aspects as for treated wounds above: location, size, appearance, description of drainage, condition of wound margins, condition of surrounding skin, and effect of the wound on the patient. In addition, assess the following:
➤ *Bleeding.* If bleeding is profuse, apply direct pressure to the site. If bleeding continues after you apply pressure for 5 minutes or if blood is spurting from the wound, call the provider immediately.
➤ *Severity of the wound.* A gaping wound or a deep wound with fat, fascia, or muscle exposed will need additional care.
➤ *Last tetanus immunization.* Immunization should be given if (1) the last immunization was 10 years ago or longer, (2) the wound is contaminated with dirt or debris and the tetanus injection was given more than 5 years ago, or (3) it is uncertain when the patient last received an immunization.
➤ *Whether the wound was caused by a bite.* Determine whether the wound was caused by any type of bite, animal or human. A deep bite wound usually requires additional observation and/or antibiotics.
➤ *Pain.* Assess for pain. Any wound causing severe pain requires a comprehensive evaluation.
➤ *Numbness or loss of movement.* If any deficit is detected, the patient will need immediate evaluation.
➤ *Presence of chronic medical conditions.* Examples include diabetes, malnutrition, immunocompromise, a bleeding disorder. Patients with conditions that affect wound healing will need ongoing evaluation.

---

indicate that epithelial cells have moved down and rolled under the wound edges. Once the cells reach the wound bed, they will stall wound healing.
▪ **Slough** is usually soft, stringy, and pale yellow or gray.
▪ **Eschar,** also known as an *unstageable pressure injury,* is thick, hard, and black or brown.

Extent and Type of Tissue in Wound Base Assessment of the types of tissue and the percentage of each can give you an idea of the severity of the wound, treatment options, and/ or healing of the wound. Table 36-4 outlines different types of tissue you might see in a wound bed. **Viable** (living) tissue must be distinguished from nonviable tissue. Many wounds may have different types of tissue at the same time. Describe each type with percentages—for example, "80% of the wound bed contains granulation tissue and 20% remains necrotic." Granulation tissue is evidence of healing. A pale color or dry texture may indicate a delay in healing. Necrotic tissue of any type will delay wound healing and should be removed. The exception is stable eschar on a heel that is firmly attached to the healthy wound edges without signs of infection.

Improving Wound Care With Interprofessional Teams

Competency: Collaborate with the interdisciplinary

Interprofessional collaboration is essential to providing quality patient care and strengthening the healthcare system as a whole. The use of a team approach in treating both acute and chronic wounds, including diabetic foot ulcers, venous stasis ulcers, and pressure injury, has been the topic of research. Within this model, the patient remains central, with care efforts being provided based on patient needs and desires. The 2012 Institute of Medicine report identified honesty, discipline, creativity, humility, and curiosity as some of the personal values that must be held in order to have a high-functioning team.

The World Health Organization suggests a "wound navigator" as a wound care team leader. The navigator functions as a patient advocate, focusing on patient-perceived needs and involving the expertise of healthcare professionals. The wound navigator collaborates with other professionals to determine the best plan of care for each patient, using a referral and follow-up system. For example, the wound navigator could provide each patient a list of

care/service providers, including names and contact information, that are appropriate resources for the patient. Having easily accessible information about reliable care would lessen the burden on the patient.

Think about it.

➤ What considerations are important when building an interprofessional team?

➤ What practical challenges may need to be addressed within the context of a wound care team?

➤ How can technology play a role in effective implementation of wound care teams?

 Go to Davis Advantage, Resources, Chapter 36, **Safe, Effective Nursing Care—Suggested Responses.**

Source: Butcher, G., Corbett, L. Q., McGuiness, W., et al. (2014). Managing wounds as a team—Development of a universal model for the team approach to wound care (Z. Moore, Ed.). *International Journal of Integrated Care, 14*(6). doi:10.5334/ijic.1695

Table 36-4 ➤ Types of Tissue in the Wound Bed

TYPE OF TISSUE	DESCRIPTION	NURSING GOAL
Slough	Soft, moist, devitalized (necrotic) tissue; may be white, yellow, tan; may be stringy, loose, or adherent to bed.	Débride the wound.
Eschar	Necrotic tissue; dry, thick, leathery; may be black, brown, or gray depending on moisture level.	Débride the wound.
Granulation Tissue	Pink to red moist tissue; made of new blood vessels, connective tissue, and fibroblasts; surface is granular or pebble-like.	Cleanse, protect. Promote epithelialization.
Clean, Nongranulating	Absence of granulation tissue, but bed is pink, shiny, and smooth.	Cleanse, protect. Promote growth of healthy tissue.
Epithelial	Regenerating epidermis; may appear pink or pearly white as it crosses the wound bed; may begin as a ring around the wound or from epithelial cells lining hair follicles.	Cleanse, protect.

Drainage Determine whether exudate is present. If so, describe the amount, color, consistency, and odor. Compare changes in the exudate with the patient's previous status.

- *Amount.* Describe the amount as none, light, moderate, or heavy. Drainage amounts vary according to the type of wound (i.e., venous stasis ulcers usually produce more drainage than arterial ulcers).
- *Drains.* If a drain is present, measure the amount of fluid in the collection container.
- *Color.* Describe the color or consistency as serous or clear, serosanguineous, sanguineous, purulent, or seropurulent (composed of serum and pus).
- *Odor.* Describe odor as absent, faint, moderate, or strong.
  - Clean the wound of all exudate or foreign material before assessing for odor because odor characteristics vary depending on the wound moisture, organisms, amount of nonviable tissue, or types of dressings used.
  - Odor may indicate fistula formation or bacterial contamination. For example, if a patient has an abdominal wound

that was odorless but begins to smell of bile or feces, you should carefully assess for presence of a fistula.

Wound and Tissue Pain Routinely ask your patients about pain or discomfort related to the wound or wound care. You will need to develop a pain management plan if the patient is uncomfortable. Always take seriously the patient's complaint of pain, especially if there is a sudden increase. Pain is often an early symptom of infection—in the immunocompromised patient, pain may be the only symptom of infection.

Nutritional Status Screen and assess the nutritional status of each patient admitted with a pressure injury and whenever there is a change in the patient's condition. A referral to the dietitian for early assessment and intervention may be necessary if nutritional problems are present. Sufficient calories are needed for wound healing. This may involve adding oral supplemental meals, or even enteral or parenteral nutrition (Wound, Ostomy and Continence Nurses Society, 2010, revised 2016).

Assessing Untreated Wounds

For an untreated wound, make the same assessments as for a treated wound. Make additional assessments (e.g., for bleeding, pain, and numbness) that allow you to determine the immediate treatment needed. For a description of focused assessment for an untreated wound, see the Focused Assessment box Physical Examination: Wound Assessment.

Tetanus Immunization Determine whether the patient needs a tetanus immunization. Tetanus-prone wounds include compound fractures, gunshot wounds, crush injuries, burns, punctures, foreign object injuries, wounds contaminated with soil, and wounds neglected for more than 24 hours. An immunization should be given if:

- The last immunization was 10 or more years ago (Immunization Action Coalition, U.S. Department of Health and Human Services, Centers for Disease Control and Prevention [CDC], 2015; CDC, 2011)
- The wound is contaminated with dirt or debris or is a burn, and the most recent tetanus immunization was given more than 5 years ago
- It is uncertain when the patient last received an immunization

Laboratory Data

You should integrate laboratory data with your history and physical assessment findings. The most common laboratory assessments related to skin integrity are protein levels, complete blood count, erythrocyte sedimentation rate, glucose, thyroid and iron levels, coagulation studies, and wound cultures. To learn more about these tests and see the normal ranges, see the Diagnostic Testing box Tests for Assessing Wounds.

Diagnostic Testing

Tests for Assessing Wounds

Test	Normal Range	Comments
Leukocyte (WBC) count	4,500–11,000/mm³	Usually done as a part of a complete blood count (CBC) but may be ordered as an independent test. White blood cells (WBCs) may increase when a wound develops; continued elevation may signal infection. A low WBC count may delay wound healing. Leukocytes are responsible for an inflammatory reaction at the wound site, phagocytosis of bacteria and cellular debris, and the creation of antibodies.
Serum protein Serum albumin Serum prealbumin	6.0–8.0 g/dL 3.4–4.8 g/dL 12–42 mg/dL	Low serum levels indicate limited nutritional stores that delay wound healing or place the patient at high risk for pressure injury. Serum protein may be monitored as an indicator of the ability to heal a wound or prevent a pressure injury. Serum protein and albumin levels are closely related. However, both fluctuate slowly. A more accurate measure of a patient's immediate protein stores is reflected in the prealbumin level.
Erythrocyte sedimentation rate (ESR)	< 50 years old: 0–15 mm/hr; > 50 years old: 0–20 mm/hr	In the presence of an inflammatory and necrotic process, blood proteins are altered. This test indicates whether the RBCs stick together, become heavier, and settle at the bottom of a lab tube when held vertically.
Coagulation studies: Partial thromboplastin time, activated (aPTT)	Varies with respect to equipment and reagents used. Critical values: > 70 seconds or < 53 seconds	Prolonged coagulation times may result in excessive blood loss or ongoing bleeding in the wound bed. Shortened coagulation times increase the risk for blood clot formation problems, such as deep vein thrombosis, pulmonary embolus, or stroke.
Prothrombin time (clotting time)	Critical values: > 20 seconds (uncoagulated) or 3 times normal control (anticoagulated)	Altered coagulation may result from anticoagulant medications, a concurrent illness, trauma, or reaction to transfusions.
International normalized ratio (INR)	< 2.0 for patients not receiving anticoagulation therapy; 2.0–3.0 for those receiving coagulation therapy	A standardized test to evaluate clotting times, considered the gold standard.
Wound cultures	Negative; no growth of pathogens	Wound cultures may be prescribed to determine the types of bacteria present in the wound. Cultures may be obtained by swab, aspiration, or tissue biopsy. A positive culture may not indicate an infection as chronic wounds are colonized with bacteria.
Tissue biopsy	Negative; no growth of pathogens	Wounds are not considered infected unless the bacteria count exceeds 100,000 organisms per gram of tissue. Exception: The presence of beta-hemolytic streptococci in any number indicates infection.

Wound cultures may be ordered to determine the types of bacteria present. Local or systemic signs of infection, suddenly elevated glucose levels, pain in a neuropathic extremity, or lack of healing after 2 weeks in a clean wound may indicate the need for a wound culture. Cultures may be obtained by swab, aspiration, or tissue biopsy.

Swabbing The most common and most noninvasive method to obtain a culture is with a swab. Swab specimens have been shown to be acceptably accurate in representing bacteria counts biopsied from a wound (Mutluoglu, Uzun, Turhan, et al., 2012). The Wound, Ostomy and Continence Nurses Society (WOCN) (2016) recommends using swab cultures as a reasonable alternative to biopsy in the clinical setting. However, other recent studies refute this, claiming deep tissue biopsies are the most accurate way to detect infection (Aggarwal, Higuera, Deimemgian, et al., 2013). For the full procedure, see Procedure 36-1.

Needle Aspiration Needle aspiration of a wound involves insertion of a needle into the tissue to aspirate tissue fluid. Organisms present in the tissue fluid can then be detected. Needle aspiration is an invasive procedure. It is performed by a qualified professional trained to perform the procedure because of the risk of inadvertent needle damage to tissue and underlying structures.

Tissue Biopsy The most accurate method for culturing a chronic wound is **tissue biopsy.** It has long been considered the gold standard. Tissue is removed from the wound edge by a specially trained provider and sent to a pathology lab or other specialized diagnostic center. This is an invasive procedure. It creates a risk of sepsis, causes pain, and disrupts the wound bed, sometimes delaying healing.

KnowledgeCheck 36-7

- What should be included in a wound assessment?
- What is the preferred method of wound culture that may be performed by a registered nurse (RN)?
- Identify three types of laboratory data that may be associated with a delay in wound healing.

What Assessments Can I Delegate?

Initial assessment of a wound, as well as ongoing evaluation of a wound that requires treatment, must be done by the RN. You may delegate to nursing assistive personnel (NAP) inspection of the skin for evidence of skin breakdown. Instruct the NAP to notify you of redness, tissue warmth, or drainage that they observe during their care of the patient. You may also delegate turning and position changes to the NAP. You must provide them with the times for the turning and how they should position the patient at each turn. A turning chart at the bedside is helpful. Turning and movement prevent tissue damage from ischemia, thereby preventing pressure injury.

ANALYSIS/NURSING DIAGNOSIS NP

The following nursing diagnoses are appropriate for patients who are at risk for skin breakdown or for patients who have wounds.

- *Risk for Impaired Skin Integrity* is appropriate for patients who have one or more risk factors for skin breakdown (e.g., immobility, incontinence, extremes of age, impaired circulation, impaired sensation, undernutrition, emaciation). NANDA International recommends that you use a risk assessment tool (e.g., Norton or Braden scale) to identify these patients.

- *Impaired Skin Integrity* is appropriate for patients who have experienced damage to the epidermis or dermis—for example, patients who have superficial wounds or stage 1 or 2 pressure injury.

- *Impaired Tissue Integrity* is appropriate for patients with wounds that extend into the subcutaneous tissue, muscle, or bone. Use this diagnosis for patients with deep wounds or stage 3 or 4 pressure injury.

- *Risk for Impaired Tissue Integrity* is appropriate for clients with Impaired Skin Integrity who are at risk for delayed healing. For example, Mr. Harmon (Meet Your Patient) has a stage 1 pressure injury but is at risk for further progression of the injury because of his age, nutritional state, and the presence of another wound. Note that this is not a NANDA-I diagnosis; however, it is useful in the situation described.

Skin problems and wounds can be the etiology for other nursing diagnoses as well, for example:

- *Risk for Infection* is an appropriate diagnosis if the patient has a traumatic wound or is immunosuppressed, undernourished, or immobile.

- *Pain* is a diagnosis that may be used for patients who are experiencing discomfort from the wound or from the treatments required to heal the wound.

- *Disturbed Body Image* should be used if the patient is experiencing distress about the wound. Consider this diagnosis even if the patient is expected to make a complete recovery. Some patients experience extreme distress about wounds. You will certainly want to consider this diagnosis if the patient experiences an injury that is expected to result in disfigurement.

PLANNING OUTCOMES/EVALUATION NP

Examples of associated NOC standardized outcomes for skin and tissue integrity diagnoses, include the following:

    Infection
    Immobility Consequences: Physiological
    Nutritional Status: Food & Fluid Intake
    Tissue Integrity: Skin & Mucous Membranes
    Wound Healing: Secondary Intention

Individualized goals/outcome statements should address the need to maintain intact skin or heal the wound. For patients who have a diagnosis of Risk for Impaired Skin Integrity, you might write a goal such as the following, for example:

> *Maintains intact skin throughout treatment, as evidenced by good skin turgor with no erythema, edema, or breaks in the skin.*

For patients who have a wound (actual Impaired Skin Integrity or Impaired Tissue Integrity), you might write a goal such as the following:

> *Wound will heal by May 1, as evidenced by a progressive decrease in the size of the wound, a decrease in drainage from the wound, improvement in the condition of the surrounding skin, and no evidence of infection (erythema, purulent drainage, or odor).*

PLANNING INTERVENTIONS/ IMPLEMENTATION NP

Examples of NIC standardized interventions for skin and tissue integrity problems include the following:

Bedrest Care	Nutrition Management
Infection Protection	Positioning

Pressure Injury Prevention   Wound Care
Pressure Management   Wound Irrigation
Skin Surveillance

Specific nursing activities directed at maintaining skin integrity or healing wounds focus on preventing and treating pressure injury and other chronic wounds, providing wound care, applying heat and cold therapies, and providing patient teaching (see the accompanying Self-Care box). In the next section, we discuss these nursing therapeutic measures.

KnowledgeCheck 36-8

- Identify the major interventions for preventing pressure injury.
- What nursing diagnosis is most appropriate for a patient at risk for pressure injury development?

What Wound Care Competencies Do I Need?

Care planning to meet the complex, individualized needs of a patient with a chronic wound involves the entire multidisciplinary team (e.g., dietitians, infection control specialist, wound specialist). Your wound assessment will guide your choice of interventions, which depend on the nature of the wound. Consider these two examples:

- A patient with a diabetic foot ulcer must have all the pressure taken off that area because every step traumatizes healing tissues. The appropriate dressing must be selected; in addition, this patient will need to wear a special shoe that is specially made for patients with neuropathy.
- Patients with a venous stasis ulcer commonly wear compression garments (e.g., elastic hose, stocking, or multilayer compression wrap). These provide continuous pressure to the veins, which improves venous return and helps the ulcer to heal. ✚ Before applying elastic compression, be sure the limb is not increasing in edema. Lower extremity arterial disease must be ruled out before applying compression because it can compromise arterial circulation. Avoid thigh-high elastic stockings because they tend to roll and cause a tourniquet

effect (Institute for Clinical Systems Improvement [ICSI], 2012, reviewed 2014). See Procedure 40-2: Applying Antiembolism Stockings if you need more information.

Wound care is more than placing a dressing into a wound. It incorporates all of the strategies for preventing that wound, as well as treating it.

Cleansing Wounds

Cleansing removes exudate, slough, foreign materials, and microorganisms from the wound. This helps promote healthy tissue healing. Always clean a wound initially and with each dressing change. To cleanse a wound, gently pat the surface with gauze soaked with saline or other prescribed wound cleanser. If there is granulation tissue, be careful not to disrupt it.

Historically, antiseptic solutions, such as sodium hypochlorite (Dakin's solution), acetic acid, hydrogen peroxide, povidone-iodine, chlorhexidine, and alcohol, have been used to cleanse all types of wounds. ✚ However, some of these antiseptic solutions can damage granulating tissue and should not be used on healing tissue (WOCN, 2010, updated 2014). Clinical evidence suggests that polyhexanide/betaine may be nontoxic and effective in enhancing wound healing (Wilkins & Unverdorben, 2013). Antiseptic solutions should be reserved for new wounds, for those that are slow to heal, or for those in which the bacterial burden is more harmful than the solution itself.

The ideal solution should be isotonic; doesn't irritate or damage tissue; doesn't cause bleeding; and is easy to sterilize, inexpensive, and available.

- *Normal saline* is physiological, it is safe, and it will not harm injured or healing tissue. It will adequately cleanse most wounds if a sufficient amount is used to thoroughly flush the wound. *Note:* Normal saline should be used within 24 hours of opening the container to avoid bacterial growth within the solution.
- *Sterile water* and *distilled water* are clean, contain no additives, and are less expensive than normal saline. However, it is hypotonic, which means it can cause fluid shifts to damaged cells. When large volumes of sterile water are used, water toxicity to an open wound can occur.

Self-Care

Teaching Your Patient About Wounds

What Patient and Family Teaching Do I Need to Do?

Appearance of skin after unrelieved pressure
Skin care and hygiene for healthy & injured skin
Protection of the skin and prevention of pressure injury
Importance of adequate nutrition and hydration
Techniques for turning and positioning
Importance of frequent position changes
Use of pressure-redistributing devices
Skin changes that should be reported to healthcare
    professionals

Simple tips for taking care of wounds at home. If the wound is:

Wet → dry it
Open → cover it
Unclean → clean it
Necrotic → don't scrub it
Dry → moisten it (ICSI, 2008)

♥ iCare 36-1

Skin Integrity and Wound Healing

- *Scenario 1*—Mary is caring for Mrs. Skylar, a 62-year-old diabetic patient with venous stasis ulcers on her legs. Since developing these venous stasis ulcers, she has become very self-conscious and embarrassed about her legs. When taking Mrs. Skylar to x-ray, Mary covers her legs with a bath blanket for comfort and privacy. Mary was not only providing comfort and protecting privacy. She was also aware of Mrs. Skylar's feelings and cared enough to respond to them.
- *Scenario 2*—Mr. Robert Brown is an 18-year-old paraplegic who has developed a stage 4 sacral pressure ulcer with a foul odor. He is expecting some of his friends from school for a visit. Ken, his nurse, while nonchalantly cleaning up the room makes sure to remove the garbage liner with the old dressings in it. He also brings in some fresh-cut flowers and a cup of wet coffee grounds. Both the flowers and the coffee grounds are natural odor eliminators. Mr. Brown has a great visit with his friends from school.

- *Potable (drinkable) tap water* can also be used to cleanse wounds (WOCN, 2010, revised 2016) and is as effective as saline (Fernandez & Griffith, 2012a, 2012b). However, the decision to use tap water should be based on the nature and complexity of the wound and the patient's general condition, including the presence of comorbid conditions (e.g., diabetes) and immunological status (Watret & McLean, 2013).
- *Liquid or foam skin cleansers* that are pH balanced may be used to cleanse periwound skin or incontinence effluent. They are not for use in wounds.

KEY POINT: *The most important thing to remember is to use universal precautions to minimize the risk of cross-contamination when cleansing periwound or other nonwound skin.*

Irrigating Wounds

Nurses commonly use irrigation **(lavage)** to cleanse, hydrate, and assist with visual inspection of the wound. In addition, irrigation (1) facilitates progression from the inflammatory to the proliferative phase of healing and (2) helps prevent premature healing over an infected area of the wound. To flush cellular debris and surface pathogens from the wound bed, introduce the irrigation solution with a gentle amount of force. Ideal irrigation pressures range from 4 pounds per square inch (psi) to 15 psi. To remove material adhering to the wound bed use a 36-mL syringe attached to a 19-gauge angiocatheter to deliver the solution at approximately 8 psi (ICSI, 2012, reviewed 2014; Joanna Briggs Institute 2006, 2008a, 2008b, 2008c). Pressures above 15 psi increase the risk of driving bacteria into the tissues, as well as causing trauma to the wound bed.

Some agencies use a piston syringe for irrigation. Do not use a bulb syringe because it increases the risk of aspirating the drainage. Commercial irrigation systems are also available, such as whirlpool agitators, whirlpool hose sprayers, pressurized canisters, and pulsed lavages. ✚ Closely evaluate the amount of pressure they deliver before you use these devices. High-pressure irrigation systems (35 to 70 psi) may dislodge healing granulation tissue, especially in chronic wounds. High pressure can cause pain and also drive bacteria deeper into the wound compartment, leading to increased risk of infection (Gabriel & Schraga, 2015, updated).

Sterile technique is used for acute surgical wounds, wounds that have recently undergone sharp débridement, or when prescribed by the provider. Most wound irrigations use clean technique. For the complete steps, see Procedure 36-2.

Caring for Wounds With Drainage Devices

A variety of drains may be inserted into wounds to allow fluid and exudate to exit. Drains prevent excessive pressure from building up in the tissues. Drains are usually placed during a surgical procedure. Some are sutured into place, whereas others are simply placed into the cavity.

Types of Drains A **Penrose drain** is a flexible, flat latex tube that is placed in the wound bed but usually not sutured into place. A clip or pin may be attached to the drain at the insertion site to keep it from slipping into the wound. You may be asked to advance the drain by gradually removing it from the wound bed. For example, the surgeon may prescribe, "Advance the Penrose drain 6 mm (¼ in.) per day." Each day you will pull the drain out of the wound 6 mm (¼ in.) until the drain is finally removed. For complete guidelines, see Procedure 36-13.

Some drains are attached to a collection device, such as the Hemovac and Jackson-Pratt drains (Fig. 36-11). The provider may order a device to be "placed to suction." This means you will compress the device to create suction and facilitate removal of drainage (Fig. 36-12). For complete guidelines, see Procedure 36-14.

If a specific pressure is to be applied, some drains can be connected to wall suction. The provider will prescribe the amount of suction. For example: "Place Hemovac to 20 mm Hg suction at all times."

Nursing Activities for Maintaining Drains As a nurse you are responsible for monitoring wound drains. The provider will describe the number and type of drains present. Describe drain placement using the drain's position on a clock face. Consider the patient's head to be at the 12 o'clock position. Some patients have more than one drainage device in a wound. Label the drains numerically with a marker or by placing tape on the collection apparatus so that each caregiver provides consistent care.

- When removing dressings or irrigating wounds, be very careful to avoid dislodging the drain. Remember, many drains are not sutured in place.
- Monitor the amount and character of the drainage and record this information in your nursing notes as well as on the intake and output record.

Toward Evidence-Based Practice

Negative Pressure Wound Therapy

Webster, J., Scuffham, P., Stankiewicz, M., et al. (2014). Negative pressure wound therapy for skin grafts and surgical wounds healing by primary intention. *Cochrane Database of Systematic Reviews, 2014*(10). Art. No.: CD009261. doi:10.1002/14651858.CD009261.pub3

Researchers reviewed nine trials to assess the effects of negative pressure wound therapy (NPWT) on surgical wounds (primary closure, skin grafting, or flap closure) that are expected to heal by primary intention. Results showed that it is still unclear whether or not NPWT promotes faster healing and reduces complications associated with clean

surgery or grafts. Consider the normal healing process. How does NPWT assist with wound healing?

1. You are caring for a patient who has a new skin graft. What education would you provide to this patient regarding the use of NPWT?

2. NPWT has been prescribed for a patient. What nursing responsibilities are associated with initiating NPWT?

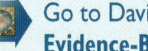 Go to Davis Advantage, Resources, Chapter 36, **Toward Evidence-Based Practice—Suggested Responses.**

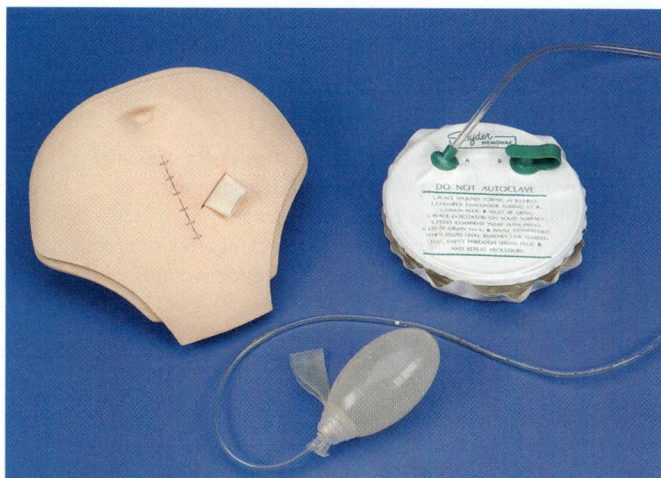

FIGURE 36-11 (Left) Penrose drain. (Center) Jackson-Pratt device. (Right) Hemovac drainage system.

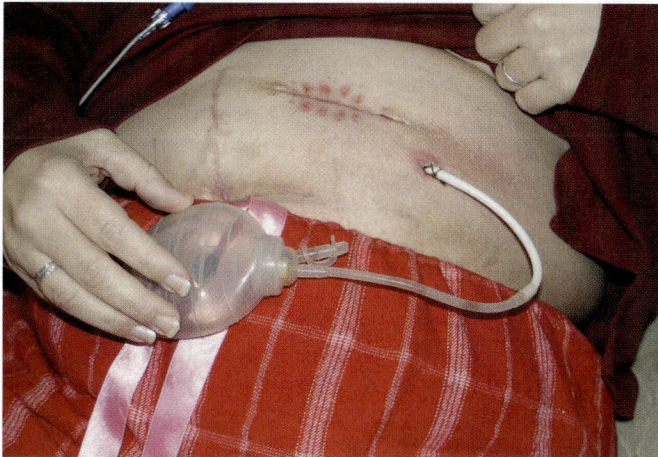

FIGURE 36-12 Compress the bulb of the Jackson-Pratt drain to create suction and remove wound drainage.

- Report to the provider any significant change in the amount or character of the drainage.
- If you suspect a drain is occluded, check the drain line from the insertion site to the collection device. Remove any kinks in the tubing. If this does not correct the problem, notify the provider of the blockage.
- You need to empty the collection apparatus at a designated volume to maintain suction. As the device fills, suction pressure decreases. If there is significant drainage, you may need to empty the device several times during your shift.

KnowledgeCheck 36-9

- Identify goals for wound care before applying a dressing to a wound.
- What solutions are used to cleanse a wound?
- How can you control the amount of force applied for wound irrigation?
- Identify three nursing responsibilities when caring for a client with a wound drain.

ThinkLike a Nurse 36-5

- Describe the percentage and type of tissue found in Mr. Harmon's (Meet Your Patient) wounds.
- What are the goals of treatment for each of Mr. Harmon's wounds?

Débriding a Wound

Débridement is the removal of devitalized tissue or foreign material from a wound. It also helps remove cells that are alive but not functioning **(senescent)** from the wound bed and edges. Removal of necrotic tissue, exudate, and infective material helps stimulate wound healing and prepare the wound bed for advanced therapies or biological agents. There are five types of débridement, following:

Sharp Débridement is the use of a sharp instrument, such as scalpel or scissors, to remove devitalized tissue. This method provides an immediate improvement of the wound bed and preserves granulation tissue. If a wound requires extensive débridement, it may be performed surgically. Stage 4 pressure injury extends into the bone, so a bone biopsy is often performed at the same time. The biopsy will detect osteomyelitis, the extension of the infection into the bone.

Mechanical Débridement may be performed via lavage (discussed in a preceding section), the use of wet-to-damp dressings, or hydrotherapy (whirlpool).

- **Wet-to-Dry Dressings** Coarse gauze is moistened with normal saline, packed into the wound, allowed to dry, and then removed. This form of debridement is now rarely used because it causes pain and provides only **nonselective debridement**. That is, it removes not only debris but also healthy granulation tissue.
- **Wet-to-Damp Dressings** Maintaining wet gauze (Procedure 36-5) helps with removal and reduces the pain. Moist wound healing speeds healing and often leads to less scarring than dry dressings and debridement. If changed in a timely manner (e.g., 2 or 3 times a day), the dressings will still be damp enough for removal. However, wounds that are too wet can become macerated, which can lead to further skin breakdown and infection.
- **Hydrotherapy or Whirlpool Treatments** are a vigorous form of nonselective débridement reserved for wounds with a large amount of nonviable tissue, such as burns. Hydrotherapy is usually performed in the physical therapy department once or twice per day. The wound is placed in a whirlpool containing tepid water for a prescribed amount of time (perhaps 5 to 15 minutes). The wound should not be exposed directly to the water jets. Risks include the following:
  - Increased risk for periwound maceration, contamination by waterborne infections, and cross-contamination; strict adherence to infection control measures is essential.
  - Vasodilation, which may increase edema and congestion, in patients with venous stasis; use hydrotherapy with caution.
  - Increased risk for burns in persons with diabetic neuropathies, because of a decrease in sensory abilities.

Enzymatic Débridement uses proteolytic agents to break down necrotic tissue without affecting viable tissue in the wound. To use an enzymatic product, clean the wound with normal saline, apply a thin layer of the cream, and cover with a moisture-retaining dressing. This may be done once or twice daily, depending on the product. Apply the product only to devitalized tissue because it might cause some local irritation.

Autolysis is the use of an occlusive, moisture-retaining dressing and the body's own enzymes and defense mechanisms to break down necrotic tissue. This process takes more time than the other techniques, but it is better tolerated. The procedure involves applying the dressing and observing the fluid that collects under it (wound fluid may be tan in color). The dressing is normally changed every 72 hours, or sooner if drainage breakthrough occurs. At that time, the wound is cleansed before a new dressing is applied. Observe the wound closely and regularly for signs of infection, such as an increase in pain or a foul odor. Autolysis is contraindicated in the presence of infection or immunosuppression.

Biotherapy or Maggot Débridement Therapy is the use of medical-grade larvae of the greenbottle fly to dissolve dead and infected tissue from wounds. The larvae secrete enzymes that liquefy dead tissue and create an alkaline environment. The enzymes are neutralized when they come in contact with normal tissue, so healthy tissue is unharmed. The larvae also digest bacteria from the wound. This therapy is effective and simple to use, though containing the larvae within the dressing can be problematic (Opletalova, Blaizot, Mourgeon, et al., 2012). Larvae are usually changed every 48 to 72 hours and disposed of as biohazardous medical waste.

♥ **iCare**   The use of maggots can be emotionally disturbing to both patients and nurses, so take this into consideration and discuss it with the patient.

Providing Moist Wound Healing

A physiological wound environment is one that maintains the right amount of moisture for cells to flourish. The skin maintains the necessary level of moisture by allowing water vapor to escape into the air around us in small amounts. With damage to the skin, body cells can dehydrate and die, so wound dressings must function as a barrier to water vapor loss.

Choosing a Dressing

When choosing a dressing, ask yourself whether it will achieve the purposes listed in the foregoing sections. Also consider how long the dressing should stay in place, how often it needs to be changed, and whether it can it be removed without damaging fragile skin or the wound itself (Table 36-5). The type of dressing used on a wound depends on the characteristics of the wound and the goals of treatment. The dressing of choice should:
- Prevent drying of the wound bed.
- Absorb drainage.
- Keep the surrounding tissue dry and intact.
- Protect from contamination and infection.
- Aid in hemostasis.
- Débride the wound.
- Eliminate dead space.
- Prevent heat loss.
- Splint the wound site.
- Provide comfort to the patient.
- Control odor.

Primary dressings are those that are placed in the wound bed and physically touch the wound. A **secondary dressing** is one that covers or holds a primary dressing in place. Many dressings can act as both, touching the wound bed and securing themselves to the wound with some type of adhesive. Figure 36-13 shows various sizes of gauze dressings. Figure 36-14 shows a transparent film dressing over an IV site.

There is no single "recipe" for healing a wound. Each wound must be treated and dressed individually based on the patient history and assessment. Many wound materials are available, and new products are continually introduced. Perform ongoing reassessment of your dressing choice every time

you assess the wound, modifying dressings and treatments as the wound evolves.

KnowledgeCheck 36-10
- What should you consider when choosing a dressing?
- Describe the five types of wound débridement.
- Identify the purposes of a wound dressing.
- Differentiate between the different categories of dressings.
- What types of dressings may be used for wounds with a large amount of exudate?
- What form of dressing is appropriate for a wound with an eschar that needs to be eliminated?

Securing Dressings

What you will use to secure a dressing depends on wound size, location, amount of drainage, frequency of dressing changes, patient's activity level, and type of dressings used. Tape, ties, bandages, secondary dressings, and binders are among the choices. Tape is most commonly used. It is available in several forms:
- **Adhesive tape** provides stability to a dressing. It is tough and durable and can be used if you need to apply pressure to a wound. It leaves a residue on the skin and can cause trauma to surrounding intact skin when it is removed. However, commercial adhesive removers are available to remove the residue and can be used to loosen tape as it is removed.
- **Foam tape** readily molds to the contours of the body and is ideal for dressings over joints.
- **Nonallergenic tape and paper tape** are best for sensitive skin. Ask patients whether they have any history of tape allergies or irritation, and use a tape that the patient has tolerated well in the past.

To tape a dressing, place strips of tape at the ends of the dressing, and space them evenly over the remainder of the dressing. To see the complete procedure, see Procedure 36-3: Taping a Dressing.

If a dressing requires frequent changes, you can use **Montgomery straps** with ties to secure the dressing (Fig. 36-15). Montgomery straps decrease the amount of pulling and irritation of skin around a wound. Apply the adhesive part of the straps to the skin at the ends of the dressing and at evenly spaced intervals. Lace the cloth ties between the straps to secure the dressing. Change the ties whenever they become soiled. Keep the straps in place until they begin to loosen from the skin.

Consider using thin hydrocolloids, low-adhesion foam dressings, or skin sealants under tape to also help prevent skin tears. For the fragile skin of older adults or infants, use porous tapes and avoid unnecessary tape use.

Controlling Infection

A wound provides a portal of entry or exit for microorganisms. When caring for patients with closed wounds, follow CDC Standard Precautions. For patients with open or draining wounds, follow CDC Tier Two: Contact Level Precautions in addition to Standard Precautions. See Chapter 22 and Clinical Insight 22-4: Following Transmission-Based Precautions.

The following nursing activities will also aid in preventing and controlling wound infections:

Asepsis Measures ✚ If the patient has an infection, place her in a private room or in a room with a patient who has an active infection caused by the same organism and no other infections.

Table 36-5 ▶ Types of Wound Dressings

DRESSING TYPE AND DESCRIPTION	USE	CAUTIONS	WOUND SIZE
Absorbent Dressings ■ Made from highly absorptive layers of fibers such as cellulose, cotton, or rayon. ■ May or may not have an adhesive border. See Procedure 36-4: Removing and Applying Dry Dressings and Procedure 36-5: Removing and Applying Wet-to-Damp Dressings.	■ Can be used as a primary or secondary dressing to manage drainage from partial- or full-thickness wounds. ■ Highly absorptive. Used for wounds with moderate to large amounts of drainage.	■ Do not use to pack undermining wounds. ■ Do not use if the wound is not draining. This can dry out the wound bed and damage tissue.	Moderate to large
Alginates ■ Fibers derived from brown seaweed and kelp. ■ Available in pad or rope form.	■ Very high absorbency (20 to 40 times their weight). ■ Promote a moist environment. ■ Facilitate autolytic débridement. ■ Ideal for wounds that have depth, tracts, tunneling, or undermining.	■ Will adhere to the wound bed if there is no drainage. ■ When the alginate comes in contact with exudate, a nonadhesive gel is created. Must irrigate this gel from the wound before placing the next dressing. ■ Allergy to seaweed or kelp.	Large
Antimicrobials (Antibiotic and Antifungal) ■ Available as ointments, impregnated gauzes, pads, gels, foams, hydrocolloids, and alginates. ■ Commonly contain silver and cadexomer iodine.	■ Reduce exudate and prevent infection by reducing bacteria in the wound. ■ Promote collagen deposition. ■ Can be used on partial- or full-thickness wounds, malodorous wounds with little to large amounts of drainage, or highly contaminated or infected wounds.	■ Allergy to antibiotic components or to iodine or silver.	Large
Collagens ■ Made from bovine (cow) or porcine (pig) sources and made into sheets, pads, powders, and gels.	■ Use with partial- and full-thickness and contaminated or infected wounds. ■ Absorb exudate. ■ Promote a moist wound bed for healing. ■ Stimulate wounds to produce collagen fibers and granulation tissue in the wound bed. ■ Do not stick to the wound bed and are easy to apply and remove.	**KEY POINT:** *If using porcine dressings, check that your patient has no religious practices that would forbid this use.*	Minimal to large

(Continued)

Table 36-5 ▶ Types of Wound Dressings—cont'd

DRESSING TYPE AND DESCRIPTION	USE	CAUTIONS	WOUND SIZE
Foams ▪ Made from semipermeable hydrophilic foam that forms an impermeable barrier over the wound. ▪ Made into wafers, rolls, and pillows; have film coverings; and are adhesive or nonadhesive.	▪ Absorbent; for wounds with moderate to heavy exudates. ▪ Thermal insulation. ▪ Promote a moist environment. ▪ Do not stick to wound bed. ▪ Used under compression. ▪ Protect friable periwound skin. ▪ Can be shaped around body contours. ▪ May be used in combination with alginates or films.	▪ Do not use with wounds that have tunneling or tracts. ▪ Not recommended for dry, desiccated wounds. ▪ May macerate periwound skin, if dressing becomes oversaturated.	Minimal to large
Gauze ▪ Simplest and most widely used dressings. ▪ Made of woven and nonwoven fibers of cotton, rayon, polyester, or a combination of these. ▪ Some are impregnated with antimicrobial agents, medications, or moisture, and others contain petrolatum to keep the wound moist.	▪ Cleansing ▪ Protection ▪ Used for packing large wounds, cavities, or tracts, deep or dirty wounds, or heavily draining wounds. ▪ Used in combination with amorphous hydrogels, saline, or medications. ▪ May be packed as sterile or nonsterile, in bulk or in smaller packages.	▪ Labor intensive. ▪ Can stick to wound tissue and damage new, regenerated cells with gauze removal. ▪ Does not ensure a moist wound environment, as they allow for fluid evaporation. ▪ May be applied incorrectly, as it must be fluffed to avoid pressure or overpacking of a wound. ▪ Dressing change interval is dependent on the amount of fluid saturation of the gauze. Frequent dressing changes disrupt the wound bed and cause the wound to become hypothermic (cold), which physiologically impairs cell growth for healing.	Large
Hydrocolloids ▪ Wafers, pastes, or powders that contain hydrophilic (water-loving) particles. See Procedure 36-8: Applying a Hydrating Dressing (Hydrocolloid or Hydrogel).	▪ Hydrophyllic particles interact with water to form a gel that keeps the wound moist. ▪ Provide a protective layer against friction/caustic agents and bacteria. Also reduce pain. ▪ Ideal for wounds with minimal exudates (e.g., partial thickness wounds, stage 2 pressure injury). ▪ Promote autolysis. ▪ Used under compression.	▪ Not the dressing of choice for wounds that require frequent dressing changes. ▪ Opaque. Do not allow the wound to be visualized. ▪ Not recommended for wounds surrounded by friable or sensitive skin (difficult to remove). ▪ Should not be used on infected wounds because they are impermeable to oxygen, moisture, and bacteria.	Light to moderate

Hydrogels

- Sheets, granules, or gels with a high water content, creating a jelly-like consistency that does not adhere to the wound bed.

See Procedure 36-8: Applying a Hydrating Dressing (Hydrocolloid or Hydrogel).

Uses:

- Mold to the shape of the body, making them useful for difficult areas, such as heels or between buttocks.
- Use around stomas to create an even surface on which to place the ostomy appliance.
- Do not require a secondary dressing.
- Enhance epithelialization to promote a moist environment.
- Rehydrate the wound bed.
- Promote autolysis.
- Soft, cooling texture promotes comfort.
- Soften slough or eschar in necrotic wounds.

Cautions:

- When an exudate comes in contact with the hydrocolloid material, it can produce an odor that might be confused with a malodorous wound. Clean the wound bed first before determining if it is malodorous.
- May facilitate the growth of anaerobic bacteria.
- Should not be used on wounds with tunneling or tracts because these wounds must be packed and allowed to drain. Wound should be shallow enough that the hydrocolloid touches the wound bed.
- Have limited absorptive capabilities (not practical for wounds with significant exudate). Require a secondary dressing.
- Easily macerate periwound skin due to high moisture content.

Exudate: Minimal

Skin sealants and moisture barriers

- Skin sealants—made from liquid transparent copolymer.
- Moisture barrier ointments—petrolatum, dimethicone, or zinc-based products that can be applied to skin to protect it from exudate, moisture, urine, and feces.

Uses:

- Simple and fast to use, and if needed should be used with each dressing change.
- Can be wiped or sprayed on skin to protect it from wound exudate and moisture, friction, and skin stripping from adhesives.
- Provide a barrier of protection over vulnerable skin from the effects of moisture and mechanical and chemical skin injury.

Cautions:

- Ointments impair the adhesion of wound dressings or tapes.

Exudate: Any

Transparent films
(See Fig. 36-14)

- Clear and semipermeable.

See Procedure 36-7: Applying and Removing a Transparent Film Dressing.

Uses:

- Promote a moist environment.
- Occlusive with oxygen permeability.
- Promote autolysis.
- Often used to dress IV sites.
- Prevent external bacterial contamination.
- Allow wound assessment without removing or disturbing the dressing.
- Can be placed over joints without inhibiting movement.

Cautions:

- If used over wounds that are draining, the tissues will become macerated.
- Adhere to the skin, so do not use them on friable skin.

Exudate: Minimal to none

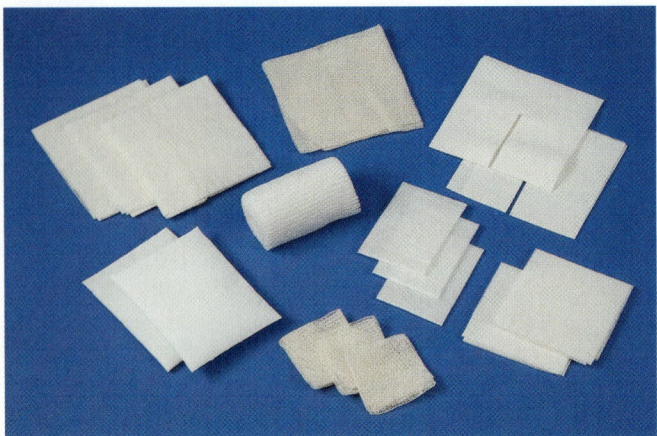

FIGURE 36-13 Gauze dressings are available in a variety of shapes and forms.

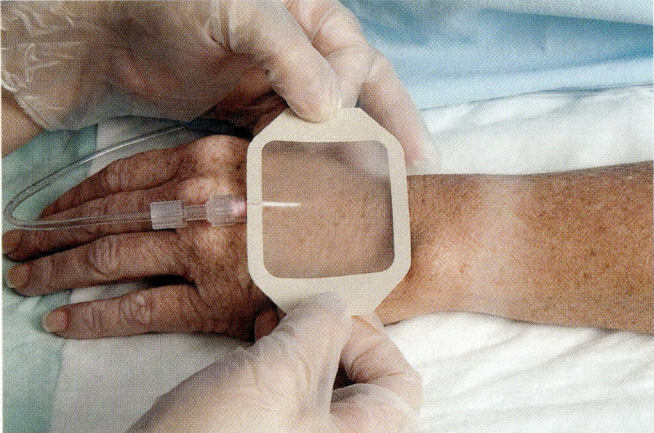

FIGURE 36-14 IV sites are commonly dressed with transparent film dressings.

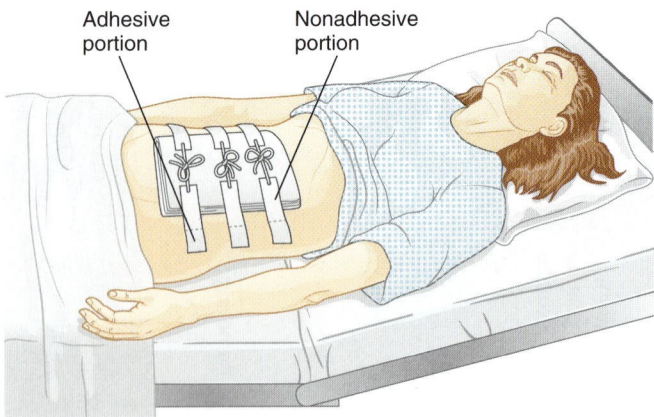

Adhesive portion   Nonadhesive portion

FIGURE 36-15 Montgomery straps with ties may be used to secure a dressing that requires frequent changing.

Follow any additional specific precautions for the microorganism identified. Most important, wash your hands frequently.

Use clean gloves when caring for the patient with a wound. Remove gloves and wash your hands before physical contact with another patient. Change your gloves after removing a soiled dressing and before applying a clean dressing.

If a patient has multiple wounds, treat the least contaminated wound first, then progress to the most contaminated. Wash your hands and change gloves between each wound.

Sharp Débridement   Use sterile instruments for sharp débridement. Monitor the patient for signs and symptoms of sepsis (e.g., fever, tachycardia, hypotension, and altered level of consciousness) after sharp débridement. Remember, only specially trained providers can do sharp débridement. **KEY POINT:** *Keep in mind there are reasons not to débride a wound. It is imperative not to remove eschar if the wound has poor circulation at the ulcer site. You would also leave alone a stable heel eschar. In addition, débridement would not benefit the patient who is critically unstable or with a grave prognosis (WOCN, 2010, revised 2016).*

Dressings and Supplies   Acute wounds may require sterile dressings. Use clean dressings for chronic wounds. However, even a chronic wound may require sterile dressings if the patient is immunocompromised. Carefully dispose of contaminated dressings in biohazard waste receptacles. Discard unused dressings if they become contaminated.

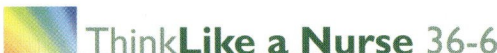 Store patient dressing supplies in a clean and dry area. Do not share supplies among patients. Access only the number of supplies you need for the dressing change. Do not touch the supply of dressings with gloves that have come in contact with the wound. Discard unused dressings if they have become contaminated.

ThinkLike a Nurse 36-6

What would be the best method to secure dressings for Mr. Harmon (Meet Your Patient)?

Supporting and Immobilizing Wounds

Binders and bandages are used to hold a dressing in place, apply pressure to a wound to impede hemorrhage, and support and immobilize an injured area, thereby promoting healing and comfort. Before applying a bandage or binder, determine the purpose of the application and assess the part being bandaged.

Binders

Binders may be used to keep a wound closed when there is danger of dehiscence, or to immobilize a body part to aid in the healing process. They are typically used on large areas of the body and are designed for a specific body part. They may be made of cloth or elasticized material and fasten with straps, pins, or Velcro. The most common binders are the following:

- A **triangular arm binder or sling** is used to support the upper extremities. Because commercial slings are readily available, you will rarely use a triangular sling.
- A **T-binder** is used to secure dressings or pads in the perineal area.
- An **abdominal binder** is used to provide support to the abdomen, for example, when there is an abdominal incision or an open abdominal wound healing by secondary intention. The binder decreases the risk of dehiscence.

To learn a procedure for applying binders, see Procedure 36-10.

Bandages

A bandage is a cloth, gauze, or elastic covering that is wrapped in place. They are packaged in rolls, individual packages for sterile technique, and various other forms.

- **Cloth bandages** are most commonly used as slings to immobilize an upper extremity or to hold large abdominal dressings in place.

- **Gauze** is the most frequently used type of bandage. It is available in many sizes and forms and readily conforms to the shape of the body. It may also be impregnated with medications for application to the skin or with plaster of Paris, which, when dried, hardens to form a cast.
- **Elastic bandages** are used to apply pressure and give support (e.g., to improve venous circulation in the legs). Ace bandages are the most common form of elasticized bandage.
- A **rolled bandage** is a continuous strip of material (gauze, stretchable gauze, or elastic webbing) that you unroll as you apply it to a body part. Rolled bandages come in various widths, commonly 1.5 to 7.5 cm (0.5 to 3 in.). Use a narrow width on small body parts, such as a finger, and wider bandages on arms and legs. To learn how to apply roller bandages, see Procedure 36-11.

Using Heat and Cold Therapy

Temperature-sensitive nerve endings respond readily to temperatures between 59°F and 113°F (15°C and 45°C). Response to heat or cold depends on the area being treated, the nature of the injury, duration of the treatment, patient age, physical condition, and the condition of the skin.

When heat or cold is first applied, the thermal receptors react strongly, and the person feels the temperature intensely. Over about 15 minutes, the receptors adapt to the new temperature, and the person notices it less. Caution clients not to change the temperature when this occurs because doing so can cause tissue injury. Monitor the patient especially carefully in the following situations:

- **Extremes of Age.** The very young and the very old are the least tolerant of heat and cold therapies.
- **Sensory Impairment.** Patients with sensory impairment are at increased risk for injury related to use of heat and cold therapy because they may not perceive temperature changes, burns, or ischemia.
- **Highly Vascular Areas.** Highly vascular areas, such as the fingers, hand, face, and perineum, are very sensitive to temperature changes and thus are at high risk for injury from heat and cold.
- **Application to a Large Area.** Application of cold or heat to a large body surface area decreases the patient's tolerance of the treatment. Application to a small area is best tolerated.
- **Injured Skin or Wounds.** Intact skin tolerates heat and cold therapy better than skin that has been injured or has open wounds.

Applying Heat Therapy Local application of heat is used to relieve stiffness and discomfort associated with musculoskeletal problems. It may also be used for patients with wounds. When heat is applied to a large area of the body, vasodilatation may cause a drop in blood pressure and a feeling of faintness. Warn patients to be alert for this effect if they will be administering heat at home. Heat therapy:

- Increases blood flow to an area through the mechanisms of vasodilatation, increased capillary permeability, and reduced blood viscosity. Increased blood flow brings oxygen and white blood cells to the wound and aids in the healing process.

- Promotes the delivery of nutrients and removal of waste products from the tissue.
- Promotes relaxation.

Either moist heat or dry heat may be used, depending on the patient situation and the goal of therapy.

- **Moist Heat.** Adding moisture to heat amplifies the intensity of the treatment. Moist heat can be applied in several forms, depending on the skin condition: a washcloth or towel compress, a gauze compress, or soaks and baths (Fig. 36-16).
- **Dry Heat.** Dry heat may be applied with electric heating pads, disposable hot packs, or hot water bags. *Electric heating pads* have the advantage of providing a constant temperature, but the risk of burns is high. *Aquathermia pads* (Fig. 36-17) may also be used for dry heat application. *Disposable hot packs and hot water bags or bottles* are also available.

For guidelines (including water temperatures) for applying moist and dry heat, see Clinical Insight 36-1.

Applying Cold Therapy The application of moist or dry cold causes vasoconstriction and decreases capillary permeability. It produces local anesthesia, reduces cell metabolism, increases blood viscosity, and decreases muscle tension. It also slows bacterial growth. The following are some uses for applications of cold:

- Prevent or limit edema.
- Reduce inflammation and pain.
- Reduce oxygen requirements.
- Help control bleeding.
- Treat fevers.

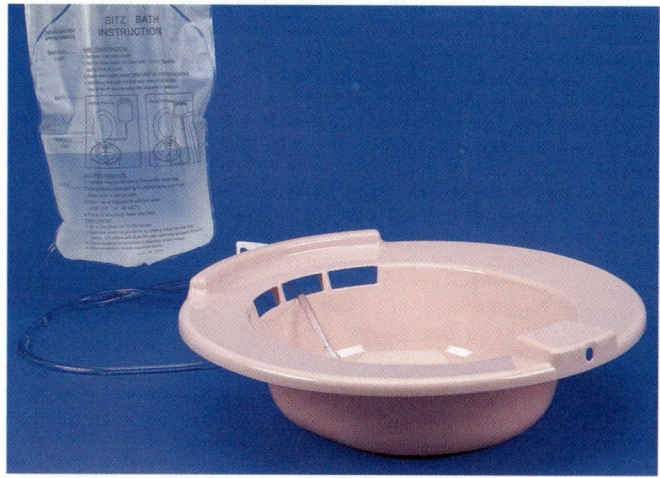

FIGURE 36-16 A sitz bath soaks the patient's perineal area.

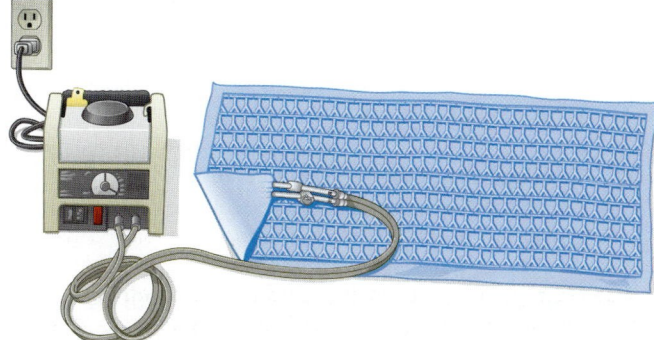

FIGURE 36-17 Aquapads circulate water in the interior of the pad to create a constant temperature.

- Treat musculoskeletal injuries (e.g., sprains, strains, fractures, and contusions).
- Prevent swelling after surgery (e.g., an ice bag may be applied to the perineum after childbirth; an ice collar may be applied to the throat after a tonsillectomy).

Applications of cold have the following side effects:

- *Elevated blood pressure* may be the result of resulting vasoconstriction.
- *Shivering* is a normal response to prolonged cold, as the body attempts to produce heat.
- *Tissue damage* may occur with because of impaired circulation that occurs with prolonged cold.

For guidelines in applying cold therapy, see Clinical Insight 36-2.

CLINICALREASONING

The questions and exercises in this section allow you to practice the kind of thinking you will use as a full-spectrum nurse. Critical-thinking questions usually have more than one correct answer, so we do not provide "correct answers" for these features. It is more important to develop your nursing judgment than to just cover content. You will learn by discussing the questions with your peers. If you are still unsure, see the Davis Advantage chapter resources for suggested responses.

KnowledgeCheck 36-11

- What is the effect of adding moisture to heat or cold treatments?
- How long should heat or cold be applied to an area?
- What precautions should you take before using heat or cold therapy?

CarePlanning & Mapping

For a Care Plan and Care Map for Impaired Skin Integrity,

 Go to Davis *Advantage*, Resources, Chapter 36, **Care Plan** and **Care Map.**

Caring for the Nguyens

Kim Phan, Nam and Yen Nguyen's 3-year-old grandchild, fell at the neighborhood playground. He has abrasions on his knees, a deep puncture wound on his left hand, and a laceration on his scalp. Mr. and Mrs. Nguyen bring him to the clinic for assessment. He is crying loudly and moving all extremities. No treatment has been given.

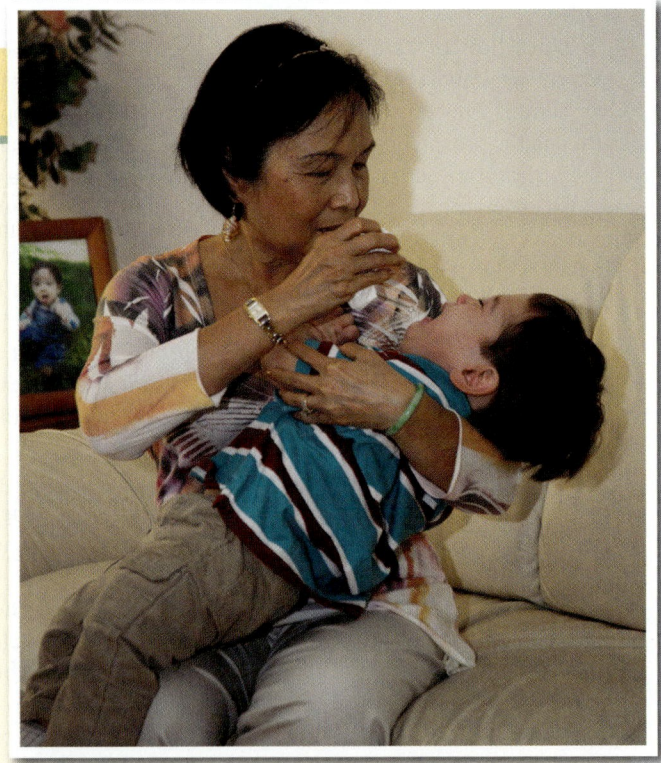

A. What should be your first course of action?

B. What kind of care will Kim need at the clinic?

C. You determine that the scalp laceration will need to be sutured. What actions should you take to prepare Kim for the suturing?

D. One week later, Kim arrives at the clinic with his grandmother to have the sutures removed. The scalp laceration is dried and healed. When you inspect his other wounds, you notice that his left knee is

erythematous and warm and painful to touch, and that there is a moderate amount of purulent drainage. What assessment questions should you ask?

E. Yen Nguyen tells you that Kim would not allow her to clean or dress the abraded knees. You cleanse his knee and remove several small pieces of gravel from the wound bed. The wound is yellow and malodorous. What kind of care will Yen need to provide to Kim to heal the left knee?

 Go to Davis Advantage, Resources, Chapter 36, **Caring for the Nguyens—Suggested Responses.**

Applying the **Full-Spectrum Nursing Model**_____

PATIENT SITUATION

Tio Santos is a 66-year-old obese man with diabetes and hypertension who is being seen for a wound on his right foot that doesn't seem to be healing. He injured his foot when repairing drywall at home. He is otherwise relatively sedentary at home. The wound is oozing, swollen, tender, and warm to the touch. Mr. Santos is now running a low-grade fever of 100.4°F at home. He tells you his foot is very painful, especially with any weight-bearing, and throbs when he is sitting or lying still. You measure the wound bed to be 6 cm × 4 cm and note purulent exudate at the distal edge. He is referred to an outpatient wound care center for treatment.

THINKING

1. *Theoretical Knowledge:*
   a. What is the Braden scale and why might it be used for Mr. Santos?
   b. What risk factors for delayed wound healing does Mr. Santos have?
2. *Critical Thinking (Considering Alternatives, Deciding What to Do):*
   a. To care for Mr. Santos's wound, should you use sterile gloves, clean nonsterile gloves, or no gloves? Explain your thinking.

DOING

3. *Practical Knowledge (Assessment):*
   a. What symptoms of infection does Mr. Santos have?
   b. To be certain the wound is infected, what would you need to know or do?

CARING

4. *Self-Knowledge:* Imagine you have had a wound on your foot for 6 weeks. It has not healed and you have all Mr. Santos's symptoms and, in fact, are in his situation. What would be the most troublesome symptom in your daily life? What would worry you the most?

 Go to Davis Advantage, Resources, Chapter 36, **Applying the Full-Spectrum Nursing Model—Suggested Responses.**

PracticalKnowledge
clinical application_____

As a nurse, you will care for many patients who have surgical or traumatic wounds, or who are at risk for impaired skin integrity. Nursing consists of thinking, doing, and caring. Therefore, you will need a good grasp of both the theoretical knowledge and practical knowledge about skin integrity and wound healing.

In this chapter, practical knowledge includes specific interventions and procedures directed at maintaining skin integrity and healing wounds. The following section will help you master the practical knowledge. It includes procedures for obtaining wound cultures, cleansing wounds, dressing wounds, placing and removing wound closures, managing wound drains, and applying binders and bandages. There are also Clinical Insights you can use for safely and effectively applying local heat and cold therapy.

CLINICAL INSIGHTS

Clinical Insight 36-1 ➤ **Applying Local Heat Therapy**

Preparation

- Determine whether there are any contraindications to the treatment, such as impaired circulation, bleeding, wound complications, or inability to tolerate the treatment.
- Explain the application and rationale to the patient.

Moist Heat (Irrigations, Compresses, Hot Soaks)

If skin is intact and heat is being applied for relaxation:

- Soak a washcloth or towel in warm water (105°F to 115°F [40°C to 46°C]) and wring out the excess before applying to the skin. Reapply and change water frequently to maintain a constant temperature.

   For open areas, use a sterile gauze compress, a soak, or a bath:

- **To make a compress,** soak gauze in the heated solution (105°F to 115°F [40°C to 46°C]) and then apply it to the wound. Usually, you will use sterile gloves, gauze, and solution. Reapply compresses or towels and change the water frequently to maintain a constant temperature.
- **For a soak,** you will need to immerse the affected area. Sterilized tubs are often used for this procedure. *Soaking helps cleanse a wound and remove encrusted material.*
- **A bath** is a modification of a soak. The most commonly used bath is a **sitz bath (Fig. 36-16),** which soaks the patient's perineal area. A special tub or chair may be used. Because of infection control concerns, disposable sitz baths are preferred. Check that the water temperature is from 105°F to 110°F (40°C to 43°C). Instruct the patient to soak for 15 minutes.

Dry Heat (Aquathermia Pads)

Aquathermia pads (also called K-pads) are plastic or vinyl pads that circulate water in the interior to create a constant temperature.

- Connect the pad via tubing to the electric heating unit, which constantly exchanges water that has been heated to the specified temperature.
- Fill the reservoir about two-thirds full of distilled water.
- Set the temperature control to 98°F to 105°F (37°F to 40.5°C).
- Cover the pad with a protective case and apply it to the body part.
  To prevent tissue injury.

Dry Heat: Disposable Hot Packs and Hot Water Bags or Bottles

➕ Hot water bags are common in home use but not in health-care agencies because of the danger of burns from improper use.

- Use water that is 115°F to 125°F (46°C to 52°C).
- Fill the bag about two-thirds full of warm tap water, expel the air from the bag, and close the top.
- Tip the bag upside down to test for leaking.
- Wrap the bag in a towel, and place it on the patient.

- ➕ Never place a heat source directly on the patient's skin. Burns can occur.

Dry Heat: Electric Heating Pads

- Be sure that the body part is dry or that the pad has a waterproof cover.

➕ Safety Precautions for Electric Heating Pads

- Do not use pins (e.g., to hold a cover in place) or other sharp objects on the pad.
  The pin could go through a wire and cause an electric shock.
- Tell the patient to report any discomfort during the treatment.
- For home use, warn the patient about the danger of burns from high settings. Use pads with a switch that cannot be turned up.
- Avoid direct contact with the heating device. Cover the heat source with a washcloth, towel, or fitted sleeve.
- Do not place the heating device (pad, bag) under the patient; place it over the body part.
  Helps prevent burns.
- Apply heat intermittently, leaving it on for no more than 15 minutes at a time in an area.
  This helps prevent tissue injury (e.g., burns, impaired circulation). It also makes the therapy more effective by preventing the rebound phenomenon:
- Check the skin frequently for extreme redness or blistering.
- Assess for hypotension and faintness. If they occur, discontinue the treatment. Have the patient lie down for several minutes, and check her blood pressure (BP). When the faint feeling passes, assist her to sit up slowly. Recheck the BP in the sitting position. If the BP remains low, encourage her to remain seated. If the patient is ambulatory, have her dangle her feet for several minutes before getting up.
- Caution patients to place the heating pad or device over the body area and never to lie on it.

Clinical Insight 36-2 ► Applying Local Cold Therapy

Preparation

- Determine whether there are any contraindications to the treatment, such as impaired circulation, bleeding, wound complications, or inability to tolerate the treatment.
- Explain the application and rationale to the patient.
- Assess for indications for cold application (e.g., fever above 104°F [40°C]). Measure the patient's temperature.

Cooling Baths

A cooling bath is often used to treat a high fever (above 104°F [40°C]). It promotes heat loss through conduction and vaporization.

- Prepare a pan of water with a temperature from 65°F to 90°F (18°C to 32°C).
- You may add a fan to increase heat loss if the temperature is markedly elevated.
- Slowly sponge the face, arms, legs, back, and buttocks with the cool water. Do not dry the areas; cover with a damp towel.
- Take about 30 minutes to complete the bath.
  Cooling the body too rapidly will cause shivering, which will increase heat production.
- You may also place ice bags or cold packs on the forehead in the axillae and the groin.
- Assess the patient constantly during a cooling bath.
  If the patient begins to shiver, the temperature may actually begin to rise.

Cold Compresses

- Apply a cool, damp cloth or towel to the body part.

- Renew the compress or cloth frequently.
  The temperature of the compress or cloth will rapidly rise toward body temperature.

Ice Collars, Ice Bags, Commercially Prepared Cold Packs, Aquapads

- You can make an ice bag out of a nonsterile glove or small plastic bag by filling it with ice chips and tying a knot in the top.
- Fill the ice bag with ice chips or an alcohol-based solution.
- Cover ice bags or packs with a towel or soft cover.
- Apply to the skin for a maximum of 15 minutes and then remove. You may reapply the cold pack in 1 hour.

✚ Safety Precautions for Cooling Devices

- Measure water temperature with a bath thermometer.
- Tell the patient to report any discomfort during the treatment.
- Avoid direct contact with the cooling device. Cover the cold pack with a washcloth, towel, or fitted sleeve.
- Apply cold intermittently, leaving it on for no more than 15 minutes at a time in an area.
  Helps to prevent tissue injury (e.g., impaired circulation). It also makes the therapy more effective by preventing the rebound phenomenon: At the time the cold reaches maximum therapeutic effect, the opposite effect (vasodilation) begins.
- Observe for tissue damage: bluish purple mottled appearance of the skin, numbness, and sometimes blisters and pain.
- Monitor for elevated blood pressure.

PROCEDURES

Procedure 36-1 ■ Obtaining a Wound Culture by Swab

➤ For steps to follow in *all* procedures, refer to the Universal Steps for All Procedures found on the page facing the inside back cover.

➤ *Note:* This procedure uses modified sterile technique because wound care is now usually performed using a clean approach rather than strict sterile technique.

Equipment

- Three pairs of clean nonsterile gloves
- Aerobic culturette tube with sterile calcium alginate or rayon swab
- Sterile 4 in. × 4 in. gauze in an impermeable tray or separate 4 × 4 packs and an impermeable barrier
- Sterile 0.9% (normal) saline solution for irrigation, warmed to body temperature when possible
  Cold solution lowers the temperature of the wound bed and slows the healing process.

- 35-mL syringe
- 19-gauge angiocatheter
- Gown and face shield
- Emesis basin
- Water-resistant disposable drapes

Delegation

This procedure requires knowledge of wound healing. It needs to be performed by a registered nurse (RN). Do not delegate this skill to nursing assistive personnel (NAP).

(continued on next page)

Procedure 36–1 ■ Obtaining a Wound Culture by Swab (continued)

Pre-Procedure Assessments

NOTE: *If the wound is covered when you begin, you will make these assessments once you remove the soiled dressing and after cleansing the wound.*

■ **Assess for pain.**

Wounds may be very painful, and wound irrigation may increase pain. Provide prescribed pain medication 30 minutes before performing the procedure, if indicated.

■ **Determine whether the wound requires sterile, modified sterile, or clean technique.**

Sterile technique is used for acute surgical wounds and for wounds that have undergone recent sharp débridement, or when the healthcare provider prescribes it. Chronic wounds are colonized with bacteria and may be cared for using clean technique, as in this procedure. To perform sterile wound irrigation, see Procedure 36-2.

■ **Assess the amount and type of tissue present in the wound bed.**

Granulating tissue is beefy red with a velvety appearance. It appears with the growth of new blood vessels and connective tissue. Pale pink tissue may indicate compromised blood supply to the wound bed. Necrotic tissue, which is black, brown, or yellow in appearance, is nonviable and inhibits healing. Only red granulating tissue should be swabbed for a culture.

■ **Assess the type and amount of exudate.**

Exudate may be a sign of infection.

■ **Assess the wound for odor.**

A foul odor may indicate infection. Cleanse wounds before you assess for odor because some dressings interact with wound drainage to produce an odor.

■ **Assess the tissue surrounding the wound edge.**

Surrounding tissue that is red, warm, and/or edematous may indicate infection.

➤ When performing the procedure, always identify your patient according to agency policy, using two identifiers, and be attentive to standard precautions, hand hygiene, patient safety and privacy, body mechanics, and documentation.

Procedure Steps

NOTE: *Steps are for aerobic culture, except as noted.*

1. **Place the patient** in a comfortable position that provides easy access to the wound and will allow the irrigation solution to flow freely from the wound with the assistance of gravity. Position a water-resistant disposable drape between the patient and the bed to protect the bedding from any possible runoff.

2. **After performing hand hygiene,** put on a gown, face shield, and clean gloves.

3. **Remove the soiled dressing.** Dispose of gloves and soiled dressing in a biohazard bag.

4. **Perform hand hygiene and again don clean gloves.**

   Soiled gloves are a source of contamination.

5. **Place an emesis basin** at the bottom of the wound to collect irrigation runoff. Avoid touching the wound with the basin.

Prevents contamination of wound from the emesis basin; protects linens from runoff.

6. **Using a 19-gauge angiocatheter, remove the metal stylet needle** and dispose into a sharps container. Attach the angiocatheter to a 35-mL syringe and fill with normal saline irrigation solution. Commercial irrigation kits containing a piston tip syringe may also be used. Their use is discussed in Procedure 36-2.

   Prevents contamination and needlestick injury. A 19-gauge angiocatheter with a 35-mL syringe provides 8 pounds per square inch (psi) of pressure and is effective for removing bacteria, necrotic tissue, exudate, and/or metabolic wastes.

7. **Holding the angiocatheter tip** 2 cm from the wound bed, gently irrigate the wound with a back-and-forth motion, moving from the superior aspect to the inferior aspect.

Irrigating from top to bottom prevents flow of contaminated solution over the cleansed area. ▼

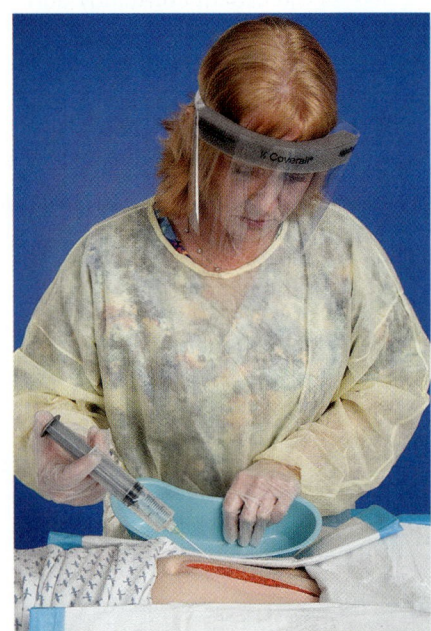

8. **Dispose of the syringe** and angiocatheter in the sharps container, and dispose of gloves in the biohazardous waste receptacle.

   Prevents contamination and needlestick injury.

9. **Obtain an aerobic culturette tube** with calcium alginate or rayon swab (not cotton tip) and twist the top of the tube to loosen the swab.
Swab specimens are not suitable for anaerobic culture. Culture for anaerobic organisms may be obtained in tissue biopsy or needle aspiration specimens only.

10. **Don clean nonsterile gloves after hand hygiene.** Locate an area of red, granulating tissue in the wound bed.

Using Levine Technique

a. Withdraw the swab from the culturette tube. Press the swab against the granulating area with sufficient pressure to express fluid from the wound tissue, and rotate the swab using a rolling motion.
Fluid from deeper within the wound bed is more indicative of the microbial colonization than culturing surface of a wound.

Using Z-Stroke Technique

b. Swab the wound from margin to margin in a 10-point, zigzag pattern, avoiding contact with the wound edge.
Provides a sampling in different areas of the wound bed. ▼

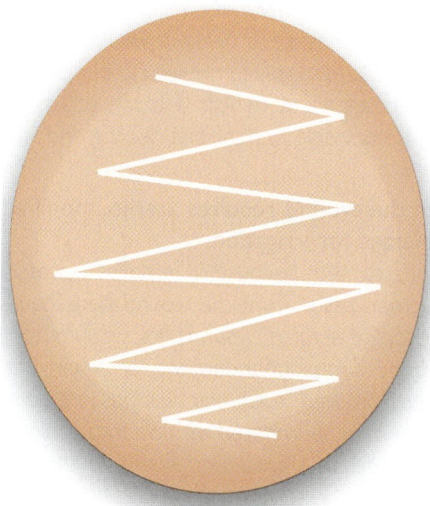

c. Do not allow the swab to touch anything other than the granulating area of the wound. Avoid wound edges.

d. Do not swab culture areas where slough or eschar is present.
These are areas of avascular or necrotic tissue and are contaminated with bacteria. Swab cultures detect only surface bacteria and are not a reliable means for diagnosing wound infection.

e. Do not roll the swab around in a pool of exudative material.
Pus is a collection of white blood cells that have already done their work, and includes the microorganisms that have already died. Obtaining a culture from this material would not produce reliable culture result. The culture specimen must be of "tissue" or "tissue fluid," not surface fluid or exudate.

f. Do not swab multiple sites with the same culturette. Use more than one culturette if several areas need to be cultured. ▼

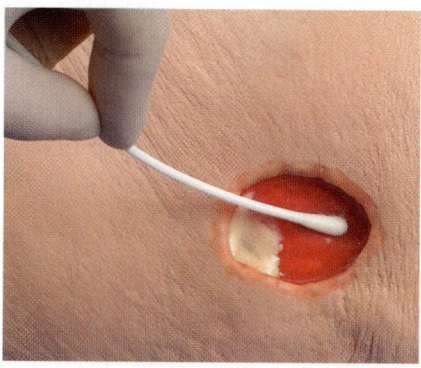

g. **Carefully insert the swab** back into the aerobic culturette tube, making sure it does not make contact with the opening of the tube upon reinsertion. Twist the cap to secure the tube.
Decreases risk of contamination; ensures that any microorganisms that grow in the culture are from the wound and were not introduced from the environment.

h. **Crush the ampule** of culture medium at the bottom of the tube. *NOTE: Inspect the culture tube to determine whether this step is required. In some systems it is not.*
The ampule contains medium for growth of microorganisms.

i. **Label the culturette tube** with the patient's name, patient identifier, birthdate, source of specimen, and date and time of collection.
Labeling ensures obtaining the results for the correct patient.

j. **Apply a clean dressing** to the wound, as needed.

k. **Arrange for transport** of the specimen for culture to the lab immediately. Do not refrigerate the specimen.

? What if . . .

■ **You determined this wound requires sterile technique?**

After removal of soiled dressing, apply sterile gloves for irrigating, obtaining culture, and applying new sterile dressing.
Sterile technique is used for acute surgical wounds and for wounds that have undergone recent, sharp débridement, or when the healthcare provider prescribes it.

■ **The culture tube is not sent to the lab within 72 hours?**

If the culture swab is not sent to the lab within 48 to 72 hours, it must be discarded. Be sure to check the policy within your institution.
The swab culture needs to be exposed to ideal laboratory conditions to allow microbial growth. If the culture sits on the unit too long, the culture medium might not produce reliable results. Most swab transport systems are validated for 48 to 72 hours after collection. However, if bacteria are suspected, the quicker the specimen is sent to the lab, the better.

■ **The wound care and culture supplies are kept on a common treatment cart?**

Common treatment carts should be left in the hall and not taken into individual rooms.
When a mobile cart is rolled into a room, it is a source for possible cross-contamination.

(continued on next page)

Procedure 36–1 ■ **Obtaining a Wound Culture by Swab** (continued)

Evaluation

- Assess the patient's pain level. Medicate according to prescriptions.
- Monitor lab reports for results of the swab culture.

Documentation

Document the following information (some agencies use a wound/skin flow sheet):

- Appearance and location of the wound and surrounding tissue. Note type, consistency and amount of exudate, and odor, if present, after irrigation.
- Patient's pain level before you obtained the culture
- If the patient has been medicated for pain, document the drug and dose used, time given, and patient response.
- Method by which the wound was cleansed before you obtained the swab culture

- Description of the area where the culture was obtained
- Dressing reapplied to wound, if applicable
- Education provided to the patient

Practice Resources

Baranoski, S., & Ayello, E. (2015); Benbow, M. (2010); Bonham, P.A. (2012); Cooper, R. (2010); Institute for Clinical Systems Improvement (2012); Levine, N. S., Lindberg, R. B., Mason, A. D., et al. (1976); McCulloch, J. M., & Kloth, L. C. (2010); Non, L. R. (2014, updated); Rushing, J. (2007).

Thinking About the Procedure

 The video **Obtaining a Wound by Swab,** along with questions and suggested responses, is available on the **Davis's** *Nursing Skills Videos* Web site on Davis*Plus*.

Procedure 36–2 ■ **Performing a Sterile Wound Irrigation**

➤ For steps to follow in *all* procedures, refer to the Universal Steps for All Procedures found on the page facing the inside back cover.

Equipment

- Nonsterile gloves
- Sterile gloves
- Gown and face shield
- Water-resistant, disposable drapes
- Tepid (body temperature) irrigation solution
  Cold solution lowers temperature of wound bed and slows the healing process.
- Sterile gauze
- Dressing supplies
- Biohazardous waste container
- Sterile impermeable barrier
- Sterile bowl

For Step 10A Variation:
- Sterile emesis basin
- 35-mL syringe
- 19-gauge angiocatheter (needle removed)

For Step 10B Variation:
- Sterile commercial irrigation kit containing a sterile basin and piston-tip syringe

Delegation

This is an invasive, sterile procedure that requires nursing assessment, judgment, evaluation, and teaching during the procedure. It requires knowledge of wound healing and should be performed by a registered nurse. Do not delegate this skill to nursing assistive personnel (NAP).

Pre-Procedure Assessments

NOTE: If the wound is covered when you begin, you will make these assessments when you remove the soiled dressing and after cleansing the wound.

- Assess the amount and type of tissue present in the wound bed.
  Granulating tissue is beefy red with a velvety appearance. It appears with the growth of new blood vessels and connective tissue. Pale pink tissue may indicate a delay in wound healing because of compromised blood supply to the wound bed or lack of proper nutrition. Necrotic tissue, which is black, brown, or yellow in appearance, is nonviable and inhibits healing and is a source of bacterial growth.

- Determine whether the wound requires sterile, modified sterile, or clean technique for irrigation.
  Irrigation helps wounds to heal because it removes bacteria, old drainage, and necrotic tissue from the wound bed. Sterile technique is used for acute surgical wounds, for wounds that have undergone recent sharp débridement, or when the healthcare provider has ordered it. Chronic wounds are colonized with bacteria and may be irrigated with clean technique. Irrigation using clean technique is presented in steps 1 through 8 of Procedure 36-1.

- Assess the wound for signs of infection (erythema, induration, amount and type of drainage).
  Exudate may be a sign of infection. Infected wounds require higher flow pressures for irrigation.

- **Assess the wound for odor.**
A foul odor may indicate infection. Cleanse wounds before you assess for odor, because some dressings interact with wound drainage to produce an odor.

- **Assess the tissue surrounding the wound edge.**
Surrounding tissue that is red, warm, and/or edematous may indicate infection. Tissue that is macerated (white and moist) indicates too much fluid is being held against the skin, usually from saturated dressings.*

- **Assess for pain and the need to premedicate.**
Wound irrigation may be very painful.

➤ When performing the procedure, always identify your patient according to agency policy, using two identifiers, and be attentive to standard precautions, hand hygiene, patient safety and privacy, body mechanics, and documentation.

Procedure Steps

1. **Administer pain medication** 30 minutes before the treatment, if necessary.

2. **Place the patient in a** comfortable position that provides easy access to the wound and will allow the irrigation solution to flow freely from the wound, with the assistance of gravity. Position a water-resistant disposable drape to protect the bedding from any possible runoff.

3. **After performing hand hygiene,** apply a gown, face shield, and clean nonsterile gloves.
Personal protective equipment provides a barrier against splattering that commonly occurs during wound irrigation.

4. **Remove the soiled dressing.** Dispose of gloves and soiled dressing in a biohazard bag.
Soiled dressings contain body fluids and other contaminants and should be treated as biohazardous waste.

5. **Set up a sterile field** on a clean, dry surface. Add the following supplies to the field depending on the type of solution and equipment to be used for irrigation:

   Sterile gauze

   Sterile bowl

   Dressing supplies

   A sterile commercial irrigation kit, *or* a 19-gauge angiocatheter, 35-mL syringe, and sterile emesis basin.
   Setting up a sterile field at bedside provides easy access to equipment for irrigation and reduces the risk for contamination when retrieving supplies after getting started. ▼

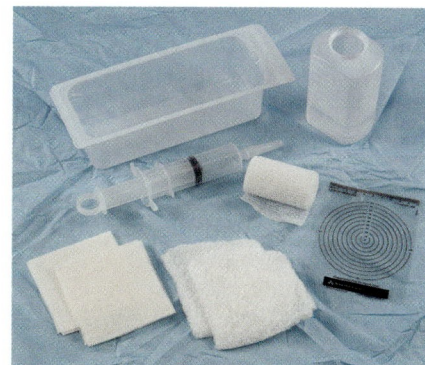

6. **Select irrigation solution** based on the wound assessment and goals of therapy. Sterile saline or sterile water is the solution of choice for irrigation, although commercial cleansers are increasingly used for irrigation for wounds with debris or in dirty, necrotic wounds.

   ✚ Do not use povidone-iodine (Betadine) if the patient has an iodine allergy.

   Cleansers contain surfactant (soap-like substance) that removes bacteria and cellular debris with less force and slow growth of bacteria, molds, and fungi. However, some antiseptic solutions can be harmful to healing tissues (e.g., hydrogen peroxide, acetic acid, povidone-iodine, bleach solutions, and sodium hypochlorite solutions [Dakin's solution]).

7. **Pour the tepid (room temperature)** irrigation solution into the sterile bowl.
Local cooling of wound tissues impairs healing. This can occur if you irrigate with refrigerated solutions and change dressings frequently.

8. **Don sterile gloves.**
Gloving maintains sterile technique.

9. **Place the sterile basin** at the bottom of the wound to collect irrigation runoff.

10. **Fill the irrigation syringe.**

If Using an Angiocatheter

   a. Attach the 19-gauge angiocatheter (with needle removed) to the 35-mL syringe and fill with the irrigation solution.
   A 19-gauge angiocatheter (with needle removed) and 35-mL syringe provides 8 psi of pressure and is effective for removing bacteria, necrotic tissue, exudate, and/or metabolic wastes.

If Using a Piston-Tip Syringe

   b. Fill a piston-tip syringe with irrigation solution.

11. **Gently irrigate the wound.** Holding the angiocatheter tip or syringe tip 2 cm from the wound bed and use a back-and-forth motion, moving from the superior aspect to the inferior aspect.
Irrigating from top to bottom prevents flow of contaminated solution over cleansed area. Irrigating a clean, noninfected wound with gentle low-pressure (8 psi) reduces disruption of the healthy, healing tissue. Irrigating an infected wound with higher flow (but < 15 psi) selectively débrides necrotic tissue while protecting healthy tissue. ➤

(continued on next page)

Procedure 36-2 ■ Performing a Sterile Wound Irrigation (continued)

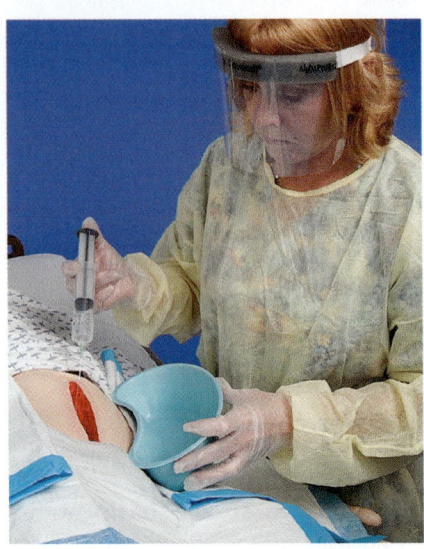

a. Ensure any undermining or tunneling is irrigated as well.

b. Repeat the irrigation until the solution returns clear.

Flushing removes exudate, debris, and some surface bacteria.

12. **Remove the basin** or sterile container from the base of the wound.

13. **Gently pat the skin surrounding** the wound dry with sterile gauze, beginning at the top of the wound and working downward.

Moisture on the surrounding tissue may lead to maceration and further breakdown of the wound margins.

14. **Dress the wound as prescribed.**

15. **Consider applying a waterproof** skin protectant around the wound if drainage is heavy.

Wound drainage contains irritating chemicals that can damage healthy tissues, especially at the wound edge and surrounding skin. Solutions used to keep the wound bed moist can also macerate or damage healthy skin if allowed to remain on intact skin.

16. **Dispose of the contaminated** irrigation fluid in a biohazardous receptacle.

Contaminated fluid should is biohazardous waste.

17. **Remove soiled drapes** from the patient area.

18. **Remove your gloves, face** shield, and gown. Dispose of these items into a biohazard collection container.

Contaminants from the irrigation may be present on these items, and they should also be considered biohazardous.

19. **Reposition the patient** to a comfortable position. Change any linen that may have become wet during the procedure.

20. **Wash your hands.**

Hand hygiene prevents cross-contamination and transmission of infectious organisms.

? What if . . .

- **The client has a wound covering a large area of the body?**

A general rule is that the larger the wound, the more solution needed to clean it.

The purpose of cleansing a wound is to remove bacteria and debris by flushing the wound.

- **Peroxide or another antiseptic solution is prescribed?**

First, identify the reason that the solution was ordered for the wound type. Then identify the length of time it is to be used. Weigh the benefit of using the solution with the potential risks to healing tissues. Finally, discuss any concerns with the healthcare provider.

Peroxide is indicated more for acute, traumatic wounds to remove dirt and other debris. Peroxide and other commercial antiseptics can damage fibroblasts and cause air embolism if used to forcefully irrigate or pack a tunneling wound. Fibroblasts produce collagen, the major structural protein of skin and healing tissues.

Evaluation

- Determine whether the patient remains comfortable. If not, medicate according to prescriptions.
- Reassess the wound at regular intervals.

Patient Teaching

- Answer any questions the patient may have.
- Teach the patient about the expected healing process.
- Inform the patient and caregiver about signs and symptoms of infection and the need to report these findings.

Home Care

- Wound irrigation is commonly done in the home. In most cases, clean technique is used in the home setting.
- Irrigation solutions, such as saline, can be made and stored up to 7 days if refrigerated.
- Review with the family proper disposal of contaminated supplies.

Documentation

Document the following information (many agencies use a wound/skin flow sheet):

- Appearance and location of the wound, size, tissue in wound base, periwound tissue, type and amount of exudate, and odor, if present, after irrigation
- The patient's pain level. If the patient has been medicated for pain, document the drug and dose used, time given, and patient response.
- Method by which the wound was cleansed
- Dressing reapplied to the wound, if applicable
- Education provided to the patient

Sample documentation

mm/dd/yyyy   0800   Dressing change to sacral wound using modified sterile technique due to saturation of old dressing with serious drainage. Patient premedicated with Lortab 5 mg PO 30 minutes prior to dressing change. Wound irrigated with normal saline using 19-gauge needleless angiocatheter and 35-cc syringe. Wound repacked with saline-moistened fluffed gauze and ABD to cover. Healing stage 4 pressure injury with 100% granulation tissue to the wound bed; 4 × 3.5 cm, with 1 cm of undermining at 6:00; copious serous drainage though no odor was noted. Periwound is slightly macerated; therefore, zinc-based barrier cream applied

for protection. Patient reported no pain with procedure. Will continue to monitor and change dressing as needed. ———————— L. Syzmanski, RN

Practice Resources

Fernandez, R., & Griffiths, R. (2012a, 2012b); Hess, C. T. (2013c); ICSI (2012, reviewed 2014); Myers, B. A. (2012); Rolstad, B. S., & Ovington, L. G. (2016); Wilkins, R. G., & Unverdorben, M. (2013); WOCN (2010, revised, 2016).

Procedure 36-3 ■ Taping a Dressing

➤ For steps to follow in *all* procedures, refer to the Universal Steps for All Procedures found on the page facing the inside back cover.

Equipment

- Nonsterile gloves
- Tape (cloth, plastic, foam, silk-like, etc.)

Delegation

As a nurse, you are responsible for assessing the wound and evaluating interventions. However, this procedure may be delegated to nursing assistive personnel (NAP).

Pre-Procedure Assessments

- Assess the degree of importance of the dressing.
  The more critical the dressing, the more adhesion will be required.

- Assess the characteristics of the dressing material, weight and conformability, and the device or tubing to be held.
  Heavier dressings require higher adhesion. Bulky dressings may need high conformability or greater adhesion.

- Assess the skin surface (i.e., dry, damp, diaphoretic, oily, hairy, edematous, fragile, or impaired skin integrity).
  Fragile skin may require less adhesion, whereas damp or oily skin may require higher adhesion.

- Assess the anticipated wear time.
  Tape adhesion gets stronger over time. Breathable tapes can be used longer. Occlusive plastic tapes build up moisture and are used when adhesion is intended for a shorter period of time.

- Assess the patient's history and current medical conditions.
  Review allergies or sensitivities to tapes. Review medical conditions that may be affected by adhesives.

- Assess for activity level of the patient and the anticipated length of time the dressing will be needed.
  The more active the patient is, the more adhesion will be required.

➤ When performing the procedure, always identify your patient according to agency policy, using two identifiers, and be attentive to standard precautions, hand hygiene, patient safety and privacy, body mechanics, and documentation.

Procedure Steps

1. **Perform hand hygiene.** Don gloves.

2. **Choose the type of tape** based on wound size, location, amount of drainage or edema, frequency of dressing changes, patient's activity level, and type of dressings used.
   Tapes come in many different adhesive types and backings. Select the tape based on individual characteristics.

   a. Choose tape of the width that is appropriate for the dressing. The larger the dressing, the wider the tape needed for securing.
   For example, a large abdominal dressing may require 3-inch tape,
   whereas a small incision on an extremity may need only ½-inch tape.

   b. Choose a tape that stretches if the area is at risk for distention, edema, hematoma formation, or movement.
   Skin distention under tape may cause blistering or skin tears.

3. **Tear strips that extend** approximately 1 to 1½ inches (2.5 to 4.0 cm) beyond the dressing, depending on the size of the dressing.
   To anchor the dressing to the skin.

4. **Place the tape perpendicular** to the incision.

   Fewer skin tension injuries occur with perpendicular taping.

   a. When taping over joints, apply the tape at a right angle to the direction of joint movement, or at a right angle to a body crease. For example, tape a shoulder or knee horizontally, not lengthwise.

   b. Apply tape with an even amount of tension on both sides, being careful not to pull at the edges.
   This reduces the risk of skin damage.

5. **Smooth tape in place** with your fingertips.
   To maximize the tape's adhesion to the skin surface.

(continued on next page)

Procedure 36-3 ■ Taping a Dressing (continued)

6. Replace tape if site becomes edematous or the skin is not intact. ▼

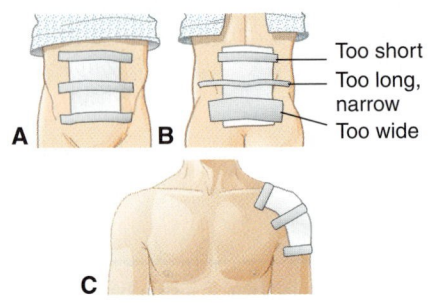

A   B

C

Too short
Too long, narrow
Too wide

? What if . . .

■ **The tape will not adhere to the patient's skin because of excess hair?**

Remove the hair with clippers or scissors. Do not shave the site with a razor.

Shaving can cause nicks or abrasions to the skin that could become a portal of entry for bacteria.

■ **The patient's skin is diaphoretic or excessively oily?**

Cleanse the skin with soap and water before the dressing change. Allow the skin to dry before applying the dressing and tape. You may also use polymer skin barriers to place a seal over the skin and allow the tape adhesive to adhere.

■ **The patient has fragile skin (e.g., is an older adult)?**

Use skin sealant preparations under adhesives. Use the least adhesive product possible.

The junction between the epidermis and dermis on the older adult is not as strong as it is in a younger person.

■ **The patient is allergic to tape adhesives?**

Use hypoallergenic products.

Circular wraps, ace bandages, or other such products may be used to secure dressings.

Evaluation

■ Verify type of tape that is appropriate for the patient and dressing.
■ Note whether the tape adheres comfortably to the skin.
■ Ensure that the patient verbalized understanding of the treatment.
■ Inspect the dressing daily for intactness, edema, or hematoma.

Patient Teaching

■ Teach the patient about the expected healing process.
■ Educate the patient about the purpose of the procedure.
■ Instruct the patient to keep the dressing dry.

Documentation

Document the following information (many agencies use a wound/skin flow sheet):
■ Type of dressing and tape applied
■ Location and characteristics of wound
■ Education given to patient

Sample documentation

02/16/2018   0815   Dressing applied to left hip incision using conformable cloth tape. Wound edges are well approximated with no drainage noted. Periwound skin is dry and intact without erythema, induration, or odor. Wound cleaned with normal saline using sterile technique. Educated patient about the purpose of the dressing and expected course for wound healing. Will continue to monitor. ————————— B. Hopkins, RN

Procedure 36-4 ■ Removing and Applying Dry Dressings

➤ For steps to follow in *all* procedures, refer to the Universal Steps for All Procedures found on the page facing the inside back cover.

➤ *Note:* This procedure uses clean technique because wound care is now usually performed using clean rather than sterile technique.

Equipment

■ Three pairs of clean nonsterile gloves
■ Normal saline solution for irrigation, warmed to body temperature when possible

Cold solution lowers the temperature of wound bed and slows the healing process.

■ Tray of sterile 4 in. × 4 in. gauze.
■ Sterile gauze for dressings
■ Tape
■ Adhesive removal pads

Delegation

This procedure requires knowledge of wound healing. It should be performed by a registered nurse. Do not delegate this skill.

Pre-Procedure Assessments

NOTE: When you begin, the wound will likely be covered with a dressing. You will make these assessments when you remove the soiled dressing and after cleansing the wound.

- Assess for pain at least 30 minutes before performing the procedure.
  Wounds may be very painful. Provide pain medication 30 minutes before performing the procedure, if needed, to allow the medication time to be distributed in target tissues. Changes in the quality or severity of pain are some symptoms linked with infection.

- Assess the type and amount of exudate.
  Exudate may be a sign of infection.

- Assess the wound for odor.
  A foul odor may indicate infection. Clean wounds before you assess for odor, because some dressings interact with wound drainage to produce an odor.

- Assess the tissue surrounding the wound edge.
  Surrounding tissue that is red, warm, and/or edematous may indicate infection.

- Determine the type of dressing needed.
  The type of dressing depends on the characteristics of the wound and the goal of treatment. Dry dressings are appropriate when there is no need to keep the wound bed moist, such as a wound healing by primary intention or a wound covered by eschar.

  ✚ *Removing a dry dressing can also interfere with wound healing by disrupting granulation tissue and can cause pain to the patient.*

➤ When performing the procedure, always identify your patient according to agency policy, using two identifiers, and be attentive to standard precautions, hand hygiene, patient safety and privacy, body mechanics, and documentation.

Procedure Steps for Removing the Dressing

1. **Place the patient in a** comfortable position that provides easy access to the wound.
   Provides for patient comfort and proper nurse body mechanics during dressing change.

2. **Perform hand hygiene** and don nonsterile procedure gloves.
   Hand washing is one of the most important measures for preventing infection transmission.

3. **Gently loosen the edges of the tape** of the old dressing at an angle parallel to the skin.
   a. Hold that edge with one hand and gently raise the edge until it is taut but not pulling on the skin.
   b. Using your other hand, push down on the exposed skin at the point where the tape and skin meet. Push the skin off of the tape. Adhesive remover pads are advised to help prevent tearing of fragile skin.
   The pull–push method will help prevent skin stripping from the adhesive and reduce discomfort and skin trauma as you remove the tape.

4. **Beginning at the edges** of the dressing, lift the dressing toward the center of the wound. If the dressing sticks, moisten it with normal saline before removing it completely.
   Moistening the dressing decreases the risk of bleeding and/or removal of granulating tissue.

5. **Assess the type and amount** of drainage on the soiled dressing.
   Allows for evaluation of wound healing. Purulent drainage is an indication of infection.

6. **Dispose of the soiled** dressing and gloves in a biohazard receptacle.
   Soiled dressings contain bodily fluids and other contaminants and should be disposed of as biohazardous waste.

7. **Remove the cover of a tray** of sterile 4 in. × 4 in. gauze. Moisten the gauze with sterile saline.
   The sterile container tray is impermeable and allows you to moisten the gauze while maintaining sterility. Gauze will not shed fibers into the wound (as do cotton balls). Fibers and any other foreign bodies in a wound promote inflammation and delay healing.

8. **Don clean nonsterile gloves.**

9. **Gather a gauze pad** by pulling the four corners up toward the middle. Use the center ball of the gauze to cleanse the wound.
   Forming a ball with the gauze pads prevents contamination of gloved hands during cleansing.

10. **Gently cleanse the wound** with the saline-moistened gauze by lightly wiping a section of the wound from the center toward the wound edge. Discard the gauze in a biohazard receptacle and repeat in the next section using a new piece of gauze with each wiping pass.
    Removes surface bacteria and exudate.

11. **Discard the gloves** and soiled gauze in a biohazard bag.

12. **Reassess wound** for size, color of tissue present, amount and type of exudate, and odor.

Procedure Steps for Applying Dry Dressing

13. **Wash your hands** or use an antiseptic hand rub for hand hygiene at the bedside.

14. **Open sterile gauze packages** on a clean, dry surface.
    Maintains sterility of gauze. ▼

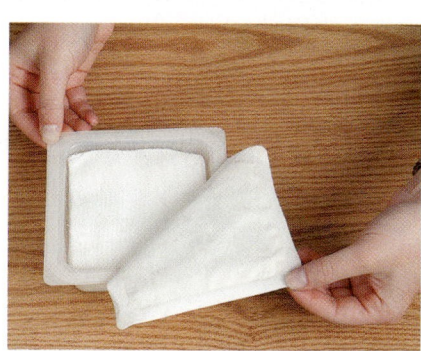

(continued on next page)

Procedure 36-4 ■ Removing and Applying Dry Dressings (continued)

15. **Don nonsterile procedure gloves.**

16. **Apply a layer of dry dressings** over the wound. If drainage is expected, use an additional layer of dressings.
    The first layer serves as a wick for drainage. A second layer is needed if increased absorption is required.

17. **Place strips of tape at the ends** of the dressing and evenly spaced over the remainder of the dressing. Use strips that are sufficiently long to secure the dressing in place. Tape the dressing around all edges, "window-paning," if appropriate.
    Edges remain taped down and dressing stays intact.

18. **Remove gloves** and discard them in a biohazard receptacle.

19. **Assist the patient** to a comfortable position.

? What if . . .

■ **Signs of infection are noted with wound assessment?**

Notify the healthcare provider. Cultures, wound care interventions, and potentially even antibiotics may be required.

■ **The wound is not approximated?**

Place the patient in a supine position, apply adhesive skin closures, and cover with sterile saline dressings. Notify primary healthcare provider.
This could indicate wound dehiscence.

■ **The skin surrounding the incision is not intact?**

Clean the area with sterile saline, dry thoroughly, and apply protective moisture barrier dressing. Consider using Montgomery straps.
Montgomery straps are useful when dressings must be changed frequently because they do not cause trauma to the skin.

■ **A drain or drainage tube is present?**

Always clean the drain site after cleaning the primary incision site.
Reduces the risk of cross-contamination.

Evaluation

■ Determine whether the dressing is clean, dry, and intact.
■ Verify that the patient experienced minimal discomfort during the procedure.

Patient Teaching

■ Teach the patient about the expected healing process.
■ Inform the patient and caregiver about the signs and symptoms of infection and the need to report these findings.

Home Care

■ Help the client to store dressings appropriately to keep them clean, for example, in a plastic container with a lid.
■ Teach the client or caregivers to dispose of contaminated dressings and gloves by double-bagging them in moisture-proof bags (e.g., plastic grocery bags).
■ Advise the client and family whether they can get the wound wet (e.g., during bathing). If it must be kept dry, demonstrate how to cover it with a waterproof barrier (e.g., a plastic bag).

Documentation

Sample documentation

10/22/2018   1420   Pt with no report of pain. Gauze dressing removed from lateral aspect of right forearm without difficulty. No drainage noted on gauze. Surrounding skin intact. Abrasion on right, lateral forearm cleansed with normal saline. Sterile gauze dressing reapplied to wound and anchored with cloth tape. Pt instructed to report any change at wound site, such as bleeding, drainage, or increase in pain. ——————— D. Enferma, RN

Practice Resource

Armstrong, D. G., & Meyer, A. J. (2013, updated 2016).

Thinking About the Procedure

 The video **Removing and Applying Dry Dressings,** along with questions and suggested responses, is available on the **Davis's *Nursing Skills Videos*** Web site on DavisPlus.

Procedure 36-5 ■ Removing and Applying Wet-to-Damp Dressings

➤ For steps to follow in *all* procedures, refer to the Universal Steps for All Procedures found on the page facing the inside back cover.

➤ *Note:* This procedure uses clean technique because wound care is now usually done using a clean or modified sterile approach rather than sterile technique. However, sterile technique is recommended for wounds that have recently had sharp débridement, have a drain, or are fresh surgical wounds; also used for patients with immunodeficiency.

Equipment

- Three pairs of clean nonsterile gloves
- Sterile or clean solution, typically normal saline or water, warmed to body temperature when possible.
  Cold solution reduces the temperature of the wound bed and slows the healing process.
- Water-resistant disposable drapes
- Sterile fine-mesh gauze in a tray for dressing
- Surgipad
- Tape or Montgomery straps
- Adhesive removal pads

Delegation

This is an invasive procedure that requires knowledge of wound healing. It should be performed by a registered nurse. Do not delegate this skill to nursing assistive personnel (NAP).

Pre-Procedure Assessment

NOTE: When you begin, the wound will likely be covered with a dressing. You will make these assessments when you remove the soiled dressing and after cleansing the wound.

- Assess the amount and type of tissue present in the wound bed.
  Granulating tissue is beefy red with a velvety appearance. It appears with the growth of new blood vessels and connective tissue. Pale pink tissue may indicate compromised blood supply to the wound bed. Necrotic tissue, which is black, brown, or yellow in appearance, is nonviable and inhibits healing.

- Assess the type and amount of exudate.
  Exudate may be a sign of infection.

- Assess the wound for odor.
  A foul odor may indicate infection. Clean wounds before you assess for odor, because some dressings interact with wound drainage to produce an odor.

- Assess the tissue surrounding the wound edge.
  Surrounding tissue that is red, warm, and/or edematous may indicate infection.

- Assess for pain.
  Wounds may be very painful. Assess for pain and provide prescribed pain medication 30 minutes before performing procedure, if needed. A change in the quality or intensity of pain may be a sign of infection.

➤ When performing the procedure, always identify your patient according to agency policy, using two identifiers, and be attentive to standard precautions, hand hygiene, patient safety and privacy, body mechanics, and documentation.

Procedure Steps for Removing the Wet-to-Damp Dressing

1. **Place the patient** in a comfortable position that provides easy access to the wound.
   Provides for patient comfort during dressing change.

2. **Perform hand hygiene** and don clean, nonsterile gloves.
   Hand washing complies with standard precautions, helping to prevent transfer of pathogens.

3. **Gently loosen the edges** of the tape of the old dressing. Hold that edge with one hand and gently raise the edge until it is taut, but not pulling on the skin. Using your other hand, push down on the exposed skin at the point where the tape and skin meet. Push the skin off of the tape. Use adhesive remover pads to avoid tearing fragile skin.
   The pull–push method will help prevent skin stripping from the adhesive and reduce discomfort and skin trauma as you remove the tape.

4. **Beginning with the top layer,** lift the dressing from the corner toward the center of the wound. If the dressing sticks, moisten it with normal saline or sterile water before completely removing it. Remove first from one side of the wound, first toward the wound and then from the other side. Continue to remove layers until you have removed the entire dressing.
   Moistening the dressing decreases the risk of bleeding and/or removal of granulating tissue. ▼

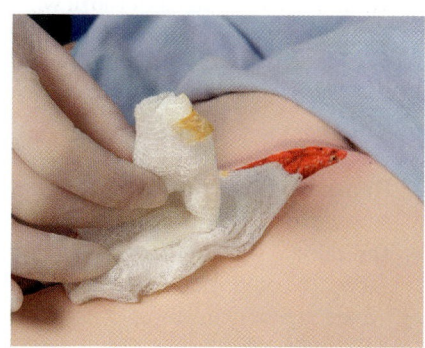

(continued on next page)

Procedure 36-5 ■ Removing and Applying Wet-to-Damp Dressings (continued)

5. **Assess the type and amount** of drainage present on the soiled dressing.
   Type of drainage is an indication of the stage of healing. Purulent drainage is an indication of infection.

6. **Dispose of the soiled dressing** and gloves in a biohazard container. Wash your hands.
   Soiled dressings contain body fluid contaminants and should be disposed of as biohazardous waste.

7. **Remove the cover of a tray** of sterile 4 in. × 4 in. gauze. Moisten the gauze with sterile saline or water.
   The sterile container tray is impermeable and allows you to moisten the gauze while maintaining sterility. Gauze will not shed fibers into the wound (as do cotton balls). Fibers and any other foreign bodies in a wound promote inflammation and delay healing.

8. **Don clean procedure gloves.**
   Avoids introducing microorganisms into the wound.

9. **Gather a gauze pad** by pulling the four corners up toward the middle. Use the center of the gauze to cleanse the wound.
   Prevents contamination of your gloves during wound cleansing.

10. **Using gauze moistened** with saline or filtered water gently wipe a section of the wound from the center toward the wound edge. Discard the gauze in a biohazard receptacle and repeat in the next section using a new piece of gauze with each wiping pass.
    Removes surface bacteria and exudate. Prevents transfer of microorganisms from the skin to the wound.

11. **Reassess the wound** for location, amount of tissue present, exudate, and odor.
    Allows for determination of most effective treatment and type of dressing.

12. **Discard the gloves** and soiled gauze into a biohazard bag. Perform hand hygiene.

Soiled gauze contains contaminants and should be disposed of as biohazardous waste.

Procedure Steps for Applying a Wet-to-Damp Dressing

13. **After establishing a sterile field** using a sterile impermeable barrier, open a sterile gauze pack tray and a surgipad. The amount of gauze you use depends on the size of the wound.
    Maintains sterile field and supplies.

14. **Moisten sterile gauze** with saline solution or sterile water for irrigation.

15. **Don clean nonsterile** gloves.

16. **Squeeze out excess moisture** from the gauze. Apply a single layer of moist, fine-mesh gauze to the wound. Be sure to place gauze in all depressions or crevices of the wound. You may need to use forceps or a cotton applicator to ensure that you fill deep depressions or sinus tracts with gauze. "Fluff" the mesh gauze before placing in the wound so as it dries it acts as a wick for any drainage.
    Maintains a moist environment for the wound bed. ▼

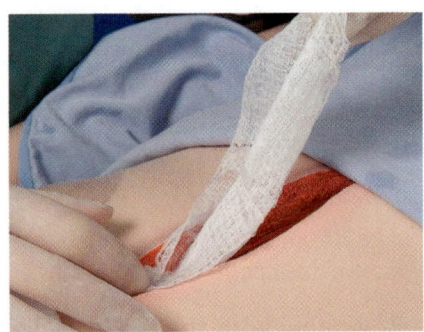

17. **Apply a secondary moist layer** over the first layer. Repeat this process until the wound is completely filled with moistened sterile gauze—but do not tightly pack the gauze into the wound. Do not extend the moist dressing onto the surrounding skin.

Packing the gauze tightly can restrict blood flow to the area. Moist dressings on the surrounding skin can cause maceration.

18. **Cover the moistened gauze** with a surgipad.
    Protects the wound from external contaminants. ▼

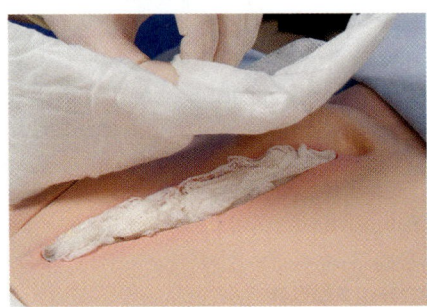

19. **Secure the dressing** with tape or Montgomery straps (see Fig. 36-15).
    Montgomery straps are useful when dressings must be frequently changed because they do not cause trauma to the skin.

20. **Dispose of gloves** and materials in the biohazard waste receptacle.

21. **Assist the patient** to a comfortable position.

? What if . . .

■ **Gauze becomes dry between dressing changes?**

Moisten dressings with sterile saline before removing them; change dressing more frequently; consider using a semi-occlusive dressing.

A moistened dressing, prevents débridement of granulating tissue, maintains a moist environment, and prevents tissue injury. Dressings that become too dry will injure healthy tissue and impair healing.

■ **The patient has multiple wounds?**

The most infected wound should be treated last. Remember to always change your gloves in between wound dressing changes.

The risk of cross-contamination is reduced when moving from clean to dirty and with fresh gloves.

Evaluation

- Evaluate whether the patient experiences pain with the procedure and afterward.
- Note whether the patient verbalizes understanding of the procedure.

Patient Teaching

- Teach the patient about the expected healing process.
- Inform the patient and caregiver about signs and symptoms of infection and the need to report these findings.

Home Care

- Help the client store dressings appropriately to keep them clean, for example, in a plastic container with a lid.
- Teach the client or caregivers to dispose of contaminated dressings and gloves by double-bagging them in moisture-proof bags (e.g., plastic grocery bags).
- Advise the client and family whether they can get the wound wet (e.g., during bathing). If it must be kept dry, demonstrate how to cover it with a waterproof barrier (e.g., a plastic bag).

Documentation

Document the following information (many agencies use a wound/skin flow sheet):

- Appearance and location of the wound, type and amount of exudate, and odor, if present, after cleansing
- The patient's pain level before and after the procedure
- Pain medication given including the dose, time, your name, and the patient's response
- Method of cleansing the wound
- Type of dressing applied to the wound
- Education provided to the patient
- Pressure relief measures, as applicable

Practice Resources

Bhimji, S. (n.d., updated 2013); Pieper, B. (2013); Wechter, D. G. (n.d., updated 2015); WOCN (2016).

Thinking About the Procedure

 The video **Removing and Applying Wet-to-Damp Dressings,** along with questions and suggested responses, is available on the **Davis's *Nursing Skills Videos*** Web site on Davis*Plus*.

Procedure 36-6 ■ Applying a Negative Pressure Wound Therapy (NPWT) Device

➤ For steps to follow in *all* procedures, refer to the Universal Steps for All Procedures found on the page facing the inside back cover.

Equipment

- Suction unit (pump)
- Collection canister with connecting tubing
- Open-pore reticulated polyurethane foam dressing
- Semipermeable transparent adhesive dressing
- Skin preparation product or sealant (skin prep)
- Sterile 4 in. × 4 in. gauze
- Clean nonsterile gloves
- Two pairs of sterile gloves (if using sterile technique)
- Sterile scissors (if using sterile technique)
- Waterproof pad
- Bath blanket
- Goggles or safety glasses, mask, and protective gown
- 10- to 20-mL irrigation syringe
- Normal saline for irrigation
- Emesis basis
- Biohazard bag for contaminated materials

Procedure 36-6A Open-Pore Reticulated Polyurethane Form Therapy

- GranuFoam (black), white or silver foam dressing
- Therapeutic regulated accurate care (TRAC) pad

Procedure 36-6B Gauze Dressing Application (i.e., Chariker-Jeter Dressing Method)

- Fenestrated drain
- Ostomy paste

Delegation

As a nurse, you are responsible for assessing the wound and evaluating interventions. You should not delegate application of a negative pressure wound therapy device to a NAP. However, you may ask the NAP to report to you any changes in the wound dressing, pressure in the unit, or alarms.

Pre-Procedure Assessments

- Assess the type of wound to be treated with negative pressure.

  Negative pressure wound therapy (NPWT) is used to promote wound healing by secondary or tertiary intention in acute, chronic, traumatic, and dehisced wounds; partial-thickness burns; or flaps and grafts. NPWT will prepare the wound bed for closure, reduce edema, promote granulation formation, and remove exudate and infective material.

- Determine whether there is any contraindication to use of a NPWT: nonenteric or unexplored fistulas; necrotic tissue with eschar; untreated osteomyelitis; malignancy in the wound or in exposed blood vessels, anastamosis sites, organs, or nerves.

- Assess patients for active or prolonged bleeding; patients who are on anticoagulant therapy or platelet aggregation inhibitors; or patients with infected, damaged, irradiated, or sutured blood vessels.

  Patients who are at increased risk for bleeding should be closely monitored. These conditions could be fatal if negative pressure is

(continued on next page)

Procedure 36-6 ■ Applying a Negative Pressure Wound Therapy (NPWT) Device (continued)

applied and bleeding is uncontrolled (exsanguination could occur). Notify the healthcare provider of these conditions.

■ **Assess the wound for bone fragments or sharp edges.**
When NPWT is activated, mechanical stress is placed on the wound. Sharp edges or bone may puncture protective barriers, vessels, or organs, causing injury, and bleeding, if uncontrolled, could be fatal.

■ **Assess the wound for infection.**
Monitor infected wounds closely, because they may require more frequent dressing changes than noninfected wounds.

■ **Assess the wound for size (length, width, and depth in centimeters); location and depth of undermining or tunneling; amount, character, and odor of drainage; type and percentage of tissue present in wound bed (granulation,** slough, fibrin, necrotic); and periwound condition (i.e., intact, denuded, erythema, induration, or maceration).
If no response or improvement in the wound condition occurs within 2 weeks, use of NPWT should be reevaluated.

■ **Assess the patient's nutritional status.**
Adequate protein stores are needed for wounds to heal. Evaluate the patient's albumin or prealbumin level before initiating therapy, as NPWT may deplete these levels and prevent healing.

■ **Assess for pain.**
Wound care is very painful. Wound pain that is inadequately treated can lead to wound bed hypoxia that impairs wound healing and increases infection rates. Wound pain also negatively affects the patient's quality of life.

➤ When performing the procedure, always identify your patient according to agency policy, using two identifiers, and be attentive to standard precautions, hand hygiene, patient safety and privacy, body mechanics, and documentation.

➤ *Note:* The success of NPWT partially depends on the training and expertise of the clinician. Allow adequate time for this procedure. Experienced nurses need at least 15 to 30 minutes. You will need more time if problems arise, and even more if you are a novice.

➤ *Note:* This procedure assumes you are performing the initial application of vacuum-assisted closure (VAC) therapy. If you are changing the dressing, first read the "What If . . ." section near the end of this procedure.

Procedure Steps

1. **Consider administering pain** medication before initiating negative pressure wound therapy.
   Allow sufficient time for the medication to take effect.

2. **Select the appropriate dressing** (per NPWT system used) to fill the entire wound cavity.
   Dressings should be placed directly against the wound surface to allow for equal suction/pressure throughout the wound bed.

3. **Obtain suction pump** unit as prescribed.
   Negative pressure wound therapy is provided by several different manufacturers. Use the unit and dressing method that is approved by your facility.

   a. Place the suction unit upright on a level surface.
   b. Remove the canister from the sterile package and insert it into the pump.
   c. Connect the tubing to the canister.
   d. Ensure the opposite end of the tubing remains clean before connecting with the tubing from the dressing.

   e. You may place the suction unit at the end of the bed or hang it on an IV pole.
   f. Do not place the unit on the floor. Ensure the unit is not knocked over, as drainage from the canister can back up and contaminate the pump's filter, blocking suction.

4. **Place the waterproof bag** or trash receptacle so you can reach it easily during the procedure.
   Convenient placement facilitates access to safe disposal of the dressing into a trash receptacle for biohazardous waste.

5. **Assist the patient** to a comfortable position that allows for easy access to the wound.
   Facilitates access to the wound site with less contamination and promotes good body mechanics for the nurse.

6. **Drape the patient** (use a bath blanket if needed) to expose only the wound area.
   Draping provides privacy and emotional comfort.

7. **Place a waterproof pad** as needed.
   An underpad protects the linens from moisture and drainage.

8. **Prepare a sterile or clean field** and add all supplies: gloves, scissors, irrigation supplies, gauze pad, selected wound dressings, tubing, and/or connectors.

9. **Don sterile or clean procedure gloves.** Use a gown and protective eyewear.
   Using sterile/aseptic versus clean technique is based on the wound type, physician preference, or facility protocol. A safe rule to follow is to use sterile gloves for a fresh noninfected wound and clean gloves for other wounds.

10. **Irrigate the wound** with 10 to 30 mL of sterile saline or other prescribed solution before all dressing changes. Use a 35-mL syringe and a 19-gauge angiocatheter (needle removed) to direct the flow of the irrigation fluid from the clean end toward the dirty end of the wound.
    Irrigation facilitates loosening of adherent tissue and removes debris and exudate while adhering to infection control principles of clean-to-dirty.

11. Remove the excess solution from the wound. Clean and dry the periwound skin with sterile gauze sponges, as needed. Consider a skin protectant around the wound edges.

Excess moisture predisposes skin to maceration and possible damage. Applying a skin protectant can assist the drape in sticking to the skin and protecting the skin when the drape is removed (i.e., from stripping of skin by the adhesive).

12. Remove soiled gloves and don new, sterile ones for the procedure.

Change gloves during patient care if the hands will move from a contaminated body site (e.g., perineal area or wound) to a clean body site.

13. To apply appropriate dressing per preferred negative pressure wound therapy unit, follow Procedure 36A or 36-6B.

Procedure 36-6A ■ Open-Pore Reticulated Polyurethane Foam Therapy (i.e., Vacuum-Assisted Closure [VAC])

> ➤ When performing the procedure, always identify your patient according to agency policy, using two identifiers, and be attentive to standard precautions, hand hygiene, patient safety and privacy, body mechanics, and documentation.

Begin with steps 1 through 13 at the beginning of Procedure 36-6. Then proceed as follows:

1. Select the appropriate foam dressing: black, white, or silver.

Black foam is sufficient for most wounds unless individual patient circumstances require white or silver. White foam is denser and will limit granulation formation. It may be used for painful or superficial wounds, tunneling/sinus tracts/undermining, or where granulation tissue growth needs to be limited. Silver dressings may act as a barrier to bacterial penetration in the wound bed. Silver may eradicate biofilms of colonized bacteria.

2. Cut the foam dressing to the appropriate size to fill the wound cavity. Do not cut the foam dressing over the wound. Rub the cut edges to remove any loose pieces.

If you cut the foam over the wound, particles may fall into the wound and create irritation. ▼

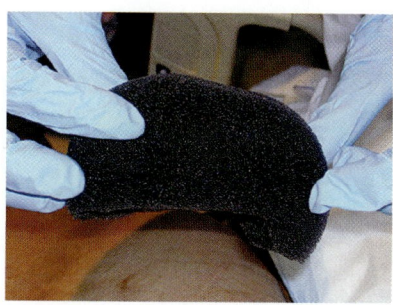

3. Gently place the foam dressing into the cavity without overlapping onto intact skin. Do not overfill the cavity or pack into deep crevices.

   a. **Do not place foam into blind/unexplored tunnels.**

   Forcing foam dressings into any area may damage tissue, alter the delivery of negative pressure, or hinder exudates or foam removal.

   b. **Do not allow foam dressing to overlap onto healthy skin.**

   Foam dressing becomes very wet during therapy and will macerate and damage intact skin.

   c. **If you use more than one piece,** note the total number of pieces that were placed into the wound so you can document them on the transparent dressing and in the patient record.

   An accurate record of the number of foam pieces is necessary to prevent retained material within the wound.

4. Apply a liquid skin preparation product to periwound, if needed.

Skin preps can protect the periwound skin from excess fluid, adhesive stripping, or other damage.

5. Apply transparent film/drape 3 to 5 cm (1 to 2 in.) from wound margins without pulling, stretching, or wrinkling the drape. Do not push down or compress foam while placing drape.

The occlusive dressing creates a seal to help create negative pressure within the wound. Tension from pulling, stretching, or wrinkling the dressing may lead to tissue injury. More pressure will be placed on the wound bed than necessary if you have flattened the foam before turning on the suction unit.

6. Avoid placing dressings that wrap all the way around an extremity. If necessary, place several smaller pieces of drape rather than one continuous piece.

When pressure is applied, a circumferential dressing may interfere with circulation, if wrapped too tightly.

7. Identify a site over the dressing for the suction track tubing apparatus.

8. Pinch up a piece of drape and cut at least a 2-cm round hole. Do not make a slit or X, as this may close off under pressure. ▼

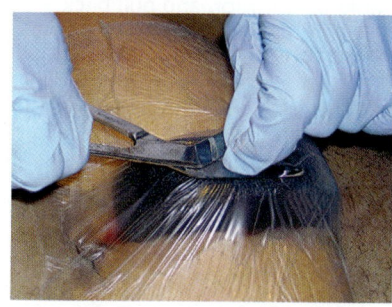

(continued on next page)

Procedure 36-6 ■ Applying a Negative Pressure Wound Therapy (NPWT) Device (continued)

9. **Place the track adhesive** and suction device directly over the hole in the drape and apply gentle pressure to secure.
Negative pressure removes excess wound exudate from the wound bed. ▼

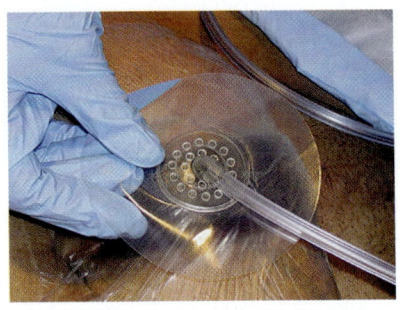

10. **Connect suction track tubing** to the canister tubing and open clamps. The canister is attached to a vacuum pump that provides either continuous or intermittent negative pressure, adjusted for the type of wound. Set suction to the prescribed pressure, which is typically in the range of −5 to −125 mm Hg

(adjustable pressures, depending on the particular device used).
Suction draws excess exudate away from the wound and into an evacuation container.

11. **Connect tubing from the dressing** to the suction track tubing going to the collection canister.
Allows for collection and measurement of drainage.

12. **Position the tubing** and connector away from bony prominences and skin creases.
Prevents pressure injury to the skin.

13. **Ensure clamps are open** on all tubing.

14. **Turn on power to the pump** and set to the prescribed therapy settings to initiate therapy.
Therapy should be maintained for at least 22 out of 24 hours daily. Alternate wound care should be considered if the vacuum cannot be tolerated for this length of time.

15. **Listen for audible leaks** and observe dressing collapse or wrinkling as pressure is applied to the wound bed.
With an adequate seal, the dressing will collapse almost immediately. Any leak (i.e., between the dressing and drape, around tubing, at skin crevices, or at tubing connection sites) will prevent collapse. ▼

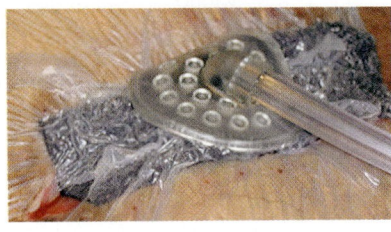

16. **Change the canister** at least once a week or when filled. Write the date on the canister.
This will help to know when it was changed last as well as how often it is being changed for fluid loss.

Procedure 36-6B ■ Gauze Dressing Application (i.e., Chariker-Jeter Method)

➤ When performing the procedure, always identify your patient according to agency policy, using two identifiers, and be attentive to standard precautions, hand hygiene, patient safety and privacy, body mechanics, and documentation.

Begin with steps 1 through 13, at the beginning of Procedure 36-6. Then proceed as follows:

1. **Measure the length of drain** from wound margin, starting with the first hole perforation and pull back 1 cm.

2. **Moisten gauze** with normal saline.

3. **Wrap or "sandwich" the drain** in the moistened gauze and place in the wound base. Tuck gauze into any undermining areas to ensure contact with the wound bed.

4. **Apply a strip or small amount** of ostomy paste 1 cm from the wound edge and secure the drain as needed.
Paste is occlusive and will help maintain a seal between the drain and the transparent film dressing. Paste that is too close to the wound edge can get sucked into the drain and occlude pressure.

5. **Apply liquid skin preparation** product to periwound, if needed. Extra drape, hydrocolloid, or transparent dressing may be used to protect fragile skin.
Skin preps can protect the periwound skin from excess fluid, adhesive stripping, or other damage.

6. **Apply transparent film** approximately 1.0 to 2.5 cm (1/2 to 1 in.) beyond the wound margin to intact skin. Pinch the film around the drain tubing to ensure a tight seal.

7. **Avoid wrapping dressings** around an extremity. If necessary, place several smaller pieces of drape rather than one continuous piece.
When pressure is applied, a circumferential dressing may interfere with circulation.

8. **Attach filter tubing** to the canister spout.

9. **Connect tubing** from the dressing to the evacuation tubing going to the collection canister.
Allows for collection and measurement of drainage. ▼

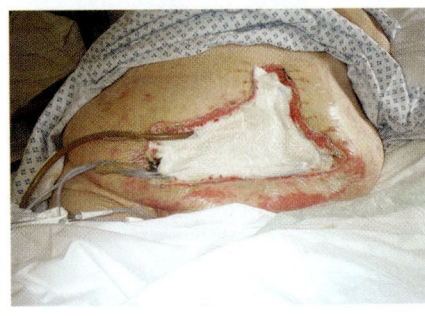

10. **Ensure clamps are open** on all tubing.

11. **Position the tubing** and connector away from bony prominences and skin creases.
Prevents pressure injury to the skin.

12. **Turn on power to pump** and set to the prescribed therapy settings to initiate therapy.
Therapy should be maintained for at least 22 out of 24 hours daily. Alternate wound care should be considered if suction cannot be tolerated for this length of time.

13. **Listen for audible leaks** and observe dressing collapse as pressure is applied to the wound bed.
With an adequate seal, the dressing will collapse almost immediately. Any leak (i.e., between the dressing and drape, around tubing, at skin crevices, or at tubing connection sites) will prevent collapse.

14. **Change the canister** at least once a week or when filled. Write the date on the canister.
This will help to know when it was changed last as well as how often it is being changed for fluid loss.

? What if . . .

- **You are changing the dressing instead of applying it for the first time?**

Follow the procedure steps below.
NOTE: Dressings should be changed every 48 to 72 hours.
Dressings left in the wound longer than the recommended time frame can become difficult to remove if tissue grows into the foam, or they can lead to infection or other adverse events.

a. Evaluate the need for analgesia.
b. Turn the suction pump unit off during the procedure.
c. Place a waterproof biohazard pad under the body part requiring the dressing change.

d. Perform hand hygiene and don sterile or clean gloves as appropriate.
e. Remove the transparent dressing using a push–pull method to gently pull up drape while pushing it slowly from the skin.
Separating the drape from the skin in this manner will decrease the risk of tape stripping.
f. Gently remove gauze or foam dressing. If dressing is difficult to remove, instill normal saline onto the dressing for 15 to 30 minutes.
Dressing removal can damage new granulation tissue if tissue has grown into the dressing.
g. Count all pieces of gauze or foam dressing that were removed to ensure none remains in the wound bed. Ensure no dressing is left in tunneled or undermined areas.
Dressings are not bioabsorbable and can abscess if left in the wound.
h. Discard soiled dressings in a biohazardous waste receptacle.
i. Start at the beginning of Procedure 36-6 and perform steps 1 through 13. Then, as instructed in step 13, follow either Procedure 36-6A or 36-6B.

- **After 2 weeks, you see that the wound is not improving?**

Consult with the healthcare provider or a wound care specialist. Average length of therapy is usually 4 to 6 weeks. Therapy should be discontinued if the wound shows no improvement in 1 to 2 consecutive weeks, the patient is unwilling or unable to follow the medical plan, or the goal of therapy has been met.
The longer a wound is open, the longer it takes to heal and places the patient at risk for complications. A steady decrease in wound size should be seen every week. If NPWT is not effective, alternate wound care should be evaluated.

- **You cannot find or remove a piece of foam?**

Notify the healthcare provider, as this may necessitate surgery.
The material could be retained in the patient and create an inflammatory response.

- **There is a foul odor when the dressing is removed?**

Clean the wound with normal saline to ensure odor is not emanating from the soiled dressing. If other signs of infection are present (i.e., fever, tenderness, redness, swelling, purulent drainage), notify the healthcare provider.

- **Suction cannot be maintained?**

Identify why the seal cannot be maintained. If the wound is very near the coccyx and gluteal fold, use a dollop of paste to help fill in the crack and maintain a seal. If the skin around the wound is moist, adhesive drape will not adhere to skin. Use a skin prep product or drape to protect the skin. If the tube is pulling away from the dressing or tension is being placed on the tube, anchor it with additional drape or tape several centimeters from the dressing or wound.

- **The canister is filling with blood?**

Immediately discontinue negative pressure therapy. The gauze or foam dressing will not stop the bleeding, so take measures to control bleeding (i.e., hold pressure on wound). Do not remove dressing until the treating healthcare provider is consulted.

- **Dressing does not collapse or the alarm sounds?**

a. Press firmly around the transparent dressing to seal.
b. Verify the machine is turned on and all clamps are open and tubing is not kinked.
c. Check tubing and drape for leaks. Listen for leaks with a stethoscope or by moving your hand around the wound margins while applying slight pressure.

(continued on next page)

Procedure 36-6 ■ Applying a Negative Pressure Wound Therapy (NPWT) Device (continued)

d. Additional small pieces of transparent dressing may be used to seal around hardware, skinfold, or creases.	e. Do not place multiple layers of drape or adhesive dressing. *Several layers may decrease the dressing's moisture vapor transmission rate, increasing the risk of maceration.*	f. Never leave foam in place without an adequate seal for more than 2 hours. If an adequate seal cannot be achieved in that time, remove the foam and apply a saline moistened gauze dressing.

Evaluation

- Note the patient's response to the procedure.
- Continue to monitor wound healing and changes in periwound tissues.
- Monitor dressing every 2 hours to ensure it is firm and collapsed in the wound bed while therapy is on.
- Monitor the seal of the dressing and pressure settings.
- Monitor for brisk or bright bleeding, evisceration or dehiscence, and symptoms of infection. These must be reported to the healthcare provider.

Home Care

- Refer the client to a home health agency for wound care.
- In limited circumstances, some patients or caregivers may be able to perform dressing changes. Determine their ability to perform dressing changes; teach and demonstrate as needed.
- Instruct the patient or family to visually check the dressing every 2 hours to ensure it is firm and collapsed in the wound bed.
- Review safety labeling, alarms, and pump instructions.
- Review conditions in which to seek medical care: bleeding, infection, unresolved alarms, or loss of suction.
- Review proper disposal of contaminated supplies.

Documentation

Document the following information:
- Date and time of dressing change
- Wound assessment: location of the wound, size (length, width, diameter), undermining or tunneling, amount and character of drainage, odor, wound bed including type and percentage of tissue seen, and periwound appearance
- Evaluation of therapy with evidence of healing
- Treatment selected: type of NPWT, type of gauze or foam, number of pieces placed in the wound

- Treatment settings: pressures, intermittent vs. continuous, or variable pressures
- Patient response to dressing change

Sample documentation for Procedure 36-6B: Chariker-Jeter Dressing Application

9/13/2018.   1010   Patient reported pain rating 5 on a scale of 1 to 10. Administered hydrocodone 5.0 mg PO for pain at 0815 before initiation of negative wound pressure therapy. See MAR. Stage 4 pressure injury to coccyx surgically débrided. Wound is 4 × 6 × 2 with no appreciable undermining. Wound bed is now clean of necrotic tissue with 100% pink tissue noted. Periwound has 2 cm of erythema to wound edges. Scant malodorous serosanguineous drainage. Using sterile technique, moistened saline gauze applied to wound bed with fenestrated drain. Ostomy paste applied at wound edge to assist in seal. Pump activated to 80 mm Hg continuous pressure. Patient rated pain in wound area as a 2 postprocedure. Plan: Begin dressing changes every 48 hours. ————————— L. Opperta, RN

Practice Resources

Bukovcan, P., Koller, J., Hajska, M., et al. (2016); Chariker, M. (2009); Gabriel, A., & Schraga, E. D. (2015, updated); McCulloch, J. M., & Kloth, L. C. (2010); National Pressure Ulcer Advisory Panel, European Pressure Ulcer Advisory Panel (2014); Pieper, B. (2013). Sullivan, N., Snyder, D. L., Tipton, K., et al. (2009, corrected).

Thinking About the Procedure

 The video **Open-Pore Reticulated Polyurethane Foam Therapy,** along with questions and suggested responses, is available on the **Davis's *Nursing Skills Videos*** Web site on Davis*Plus.*

Procedure 36-7 ■ Applying and Removing a Transparent Film Dressing

➤ For steps to follow in *all* procedures, refer to the Universal Steps for All Procedures found on the page facing the inside back cover.

Equipment

- Clean nonsterile gloves
- Sterile gauze
- Normal saline solution or specified cleansing agent, warmed to body temperature when possible
  Cold solution lowers the temperature of the wound bed and slows the healing process.
- Scissors (if needed)
- Liquid skin preparation (if needed)
- Transparent film dressing

Delegation

Because assessment of the wound and knowledge of clean technique are important, you should not delegate this procedure to a NAP.

Pre-Procedure Assessment

- Assess the area to determine whether a transparent film dressing is appropriate.

Transparent film dressings are indicated as primary dressings (dressings that touch the wound or area to be treated) to protect high-risk intact skin; for superficial or partial-thickness wounds that have little to no drainage (i.e., stage 1 or 2 pressure injury); and to assist in débriding eschar by autolysis. Films may be used as a secondary dressing to protect other types of dressings from bodily fluids (i.e., wounds near the perineum).

- Assess the wound to determine whether use of a transparent film is contraindicated.
  Films are contraindicated in third-degree burns, arterial ulcers, and infected wounds. Films should not be used to fill dead space.
- Determine the size of the wound.
  Film dressings are available in many sizes. Select the appropriate size based on wound measurements, allowing for a 2.5-cm (1-in.) perimeter of intact skin around the wound for the adhesive to stick.
- Assess the periwound area.
  Film dressings should be attached to intact skin. The adhesive is not waterproof and will not adhere to wet or moist skin.

➤ When performing the procedure, always identify your patient according to agency policy, using two identifiers, and be attentive to standard precautions, hand hygiene, patient safety and privacy, body mechanics, and documentation.

Procedure Steps

1. **Place the patient in a** comfortable position that provides easy access to the wound.

Procedure Steps for Applying the Dressing

2. **If a dressing is present, perform hand hygiene,** don clean nonsterile gloves, and remove the old dressing.

3. **Dispose of the soiled dressing** and gloves in the biohazard waste receptacle.
   Observe universal precautions, preventing transfer of pathogens.

4. **Don clean nonsterile gloves and** cleanse the skin surrounding the wound with normal saline or a mild cleansing agent. Be sure to rinse the skin well if you use a cleanser. Allow the skin to dry.
   Cleansing prepares the skin for application of the dressing. Skin must be dry for the dressing to adhere.

5. **Cleanse the wound** as prescribed or according to agency procedure.
   Cleansing of wounds removes bacteria and necrotic debris from wound beds.

6. **Consider placing a skin barrier** around the wound before transparent film dressing application.
   Skin sealants may be applied to skin before tape to protect fragile skin from tears or epidermal stripping.

7. **Remove the center backing liner** from the transparent film dressing. ▾

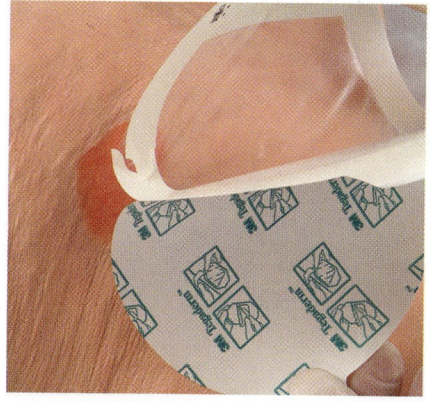

8. **Holding the dressing by the edges,** apply the transparent film to the wound without stretching or pulling the dressing or the skin.
   This reduces the risk of skin damage.

9. **Remove the edging liner** from the dressing.

10. **Gently smooth and secure** the dressing to skin.
    Allows the dressing to adhere fully to the patient's skin.

11. **Dispose of soiled equipment** and remove your gloves.

Procedure Steps for Removing the Dressing

Transparent film dressings are typically changed every 3 days. Change dressing sooner if drainage extends beyond the edges of the wound onto periwound skin. To remove the dressing, do the following:

12. **Grasp one edge of the film** dressing.

(continued on next page)

Procedure 36-7 ■ Applying and Removing a Transparent Film Dressing (continued)

13. **Gently lift the edge.**

14. **Stabilize the skin underneath** the elevated edge with your finger.
Stabilizing the skin as the adhesive is taken off will prevent epidermal stripping.

15. **With the other hand, slowly peel** the dressing back over itself, "low and slow," in the direction of hair growth. Use of an adhesive removal pad is recommended especially for sensitive skin.
Removing the dressing at an angle will increase the risk of pulling on the epidermis and causing mechanical trauma.

16. **As dressing is removed,** keep moving your finger as necessary to avoid newly exposed skin.

? What if . . .

■ **The adhesive will not adhere to the patient's skin because of excess hair?**

Hair may be removed with clippers/scissors. Do not shave the site with a razor.
Shaving can cause nicks or abrasions to the skin that could become a portal of entry for bacteria.

■ **The patient's skin is diaphoretic or excessively oily?**

Cleanse the skin with soap and water before the dressing change. Allow the skin to dry before continuing with the dressing. Also, polymer skin barriers may be used to place a seal over the skin and allow the tape adhesive to adhere.

■ **The patient has fragile skin (elderly patient)?**

Skin sealant preparations may be used under adhesives.
The junction between the epidermis and dermis on the older adult is not as strong as with a younger person. Less pressure or tension is needed to break those bonds and cause skin damage.

■ **The dressing sticks to itself before it can be applied?**

If a small portion of the dressing is stuck to itself, gently stretch or pull the edges in opposite directions. If a large portion is involved, throw the dressing away and start over.
Transparent dressings can be difficult to apply because they are polyurethane sheets coated on one side with an acrylic, hypoallergenic adhesive and are flimsy in nature, making them clumsy to work with at times.

■ **Purulent-appearing fluid has collected underneath the film dressing?**

This does not necessarily mean the wound is infected. Remove the dressing and clean the wound per policy. Select an alternate dressing that will be more absorptive.
Because films do not have absorptive capabilities, any drainage produced by the wound will pool underneath.

Evaluation

- Verify the transparent film dressing is appropriate for the wound.
- Determine whether the dressing adheres comfortably to skin.
- Ensure that patient verbalizes understanding of treatment.

Patient Teaching

- Teach the patient about the expected healing process.
- Teaching the patient about the use of transparent film dressings.
- Inform the patient and caregiver about signs and symptoms of infection and the need to report these findings.

Documentation

Document the following information (many agencies use a wound/skin flow sheet):

- Wound assessment: location of the wound, size (length × width × diameter), undermining or tunneling, amount and character of drainage, odor, wound bed including type and percentage of tissue seen, and periwound appearance
- Appearance and location of the wound, type and amount of exudate, and odor, if present, after cleansing
- The patient's pain level before the procedure. If the patient has been medicated for pain, document the drug and dose used, time given, and the patient's response to analgesia.
- Method of cleansing the wound and surrounding skin
- Type of dressing applied to the wound
- Education provided to the patient
- Preventive measures taken

Practice Resources

Association of periOperative Registered Nurses (2013); Bryant, R., & Nix, D. (2016).

Procedure 36-8 ■ Applying a Hydrating Dressing (Hydrocolloid or Hydrogel)

➤ For steps to follow in *all* procedures, refer to the Universal Steps for All Procedures found on the page facing the inside back cover.

Equipment

- Clean nonsterile gloves
- Hydrating dressing 3 to 4 cm (1.5 in.) larger than the wound
- Moisture-proof bag
  Obtain the following items, only if needed:
- Normal saline solution warmed to body temperature when possible
  Cold solution lowers the temperature of wound bed and slows the healing process.
- Emesis basin
- Sterile gauze for cleansing
- Disposable clippers or scissors (to trim hair or dressing)
- Skin prep
- Measuring device
- Tape

Delegation

This procedure requires knowledge of wound healing, dressings, and infection control and prevention. You should not delegate this procedure to a NAP.

Pre-Procedure Assessments

- Assess the area to determine whether a hydrating dressing is appropriate.
  Hydrating dressings are appropriate for wounds with small amounts of drainage. These dressings autolytically débride necrotic tissue from the wound bed. They may also be used to protect skin at risk for breakdown.
- Determine the size of the wound.
  Allows you to select a dressing of the appropriate size. Choosing a dressing size that extends beyond the ulcer ensures complete coverage.

➤ When performing the procedure, always identify your patient according to agency policy, using two identifiers, and be attentive to standard precautions, hand hygiene, patient safety and privacy, body mechanics, and documentation.

Procedure Steps

1. **Place the patient** in a comfortable position that provides easy access to the wound.
   Provides for patient comfort and proper nurse body mechanics during dressing change.

2. **If a dressing is present, perform hand hygiene,** don clean nonsterile gloves, and remove the old dressing.
   Prevents transfer of pathogens.

3. **Dispose of the soiled dressing** and gloves in the biohazard waste receptacle.
   Dressings may contain body fluids and other contaminants, so they must be disposed of in moisture-proof containers.

4. **Wash your hands.** Don nonsterile gloves and cleanse the skin surrounding the wound with normal saline or a mild cleansing agent. Be sure to rinse the skin well if you use a cleanser. Allow the skin to dry. Do not attempt to remove residue that is left on the skin from the old dressing.
   Cleansing and drying prepare the skin for application of the dressing.

Removing residue irritates the surrounding skin.

5. **Apply skin prep** to the area covered by tape.
   Skin prep protects intact skin from breakdown from tape removal.

6. **Cleanse the wound as directed.** Wound cleansing may be performed with clean or sterile technique, depending on the type of wound.
   Cleansing the wound removes microbes and necrotic debris from wound bed. Studies show using either saline or tap water is similarly effective for cleansing.

7. **Remove soiled gloves** and assess the condition of the wound. Note the size, location, type of tissue present, amount of exudate, and odor.
   Granulating tissue is beefy red with a velvety appearance. It appears with the growth of new blood vessels and connective tissue. Pale pink tissue may indicate compromised blood supply to the wound bed. Necrotic tissue, which is black, brown, or yellow in appearance, is nonviable and inhibits healing. A hydrocolloid dressing will interact with wound drainage to produce a thick, yellow gel that may have a foul

odor. Clean the wound before assessing for exudate and odor.

8. **With the backing still intact,** cut the hydrating dressing, if necessary, to the desired shape and size. Size the hydrocolloid dressing so it will extend 3 to 4 cm (1.5 in.) beyond the wound margin on all sides and cover all areas of nonintact skin.
   Provides complete coverage of the wound.

9. **Don clean nonsterile gloves** and remove the backing of the hydrocolloid dressing, starting at one edge. Place the exposed adhesive portion on the patient's skin. Position the dressing to cover the wound. ▼

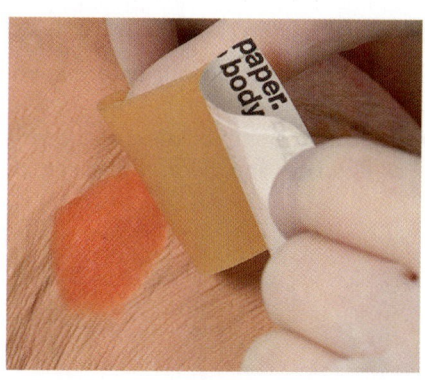

(continued on next page)

Procedure 36-8 ■ Applying a Hydrating Dressing (Hydrocolloid or Hydrogel) (continued)

10. Gradually peel away the remaining liner; smooth the hydrocolloid dressing onto the skin by placing your hand on top of dressing and holding in place for 1 minute.

Warmth helps the dressing adhere to the skin. ▼

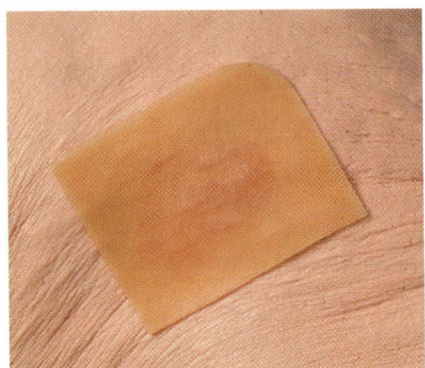

11. Assist the patient to a comfortable position, and remove your gloves. Wash your hands.

 What if . . .

■ **Signs of infection are noted?**

Notify healthcare provider. Cultures may be prescribed. A different type of dressing may be prescribed, as well.

■ **The surrounding skin is not intact?**

Choose a larger size hydrocolloid dressing to cover the nonintact area.

Document your observations and report new findings to the healthcare provider.

Evaluation

■ Verify that a hydrocolloid dressing is still appropriate for the wound.
■ Note whether the dressing adheres comfortably to the skin.
■ Ensure the patient verbalizes understanding of treatment.
■ Inspect the dressing daily. Change it if it becomes dislodged, leaks, or wrinkles or if it develops an odor.

Patient Teaching

■ Teach the patient about the expected healing process.
■ Inform the patient and caregiver about signs and symptoms of infection and the need to report these findings.

Home Care

■ Hydrating dressings may be required in the home setting. Teach caregivers to use the appropriate size and change the dressing if it begins to leak, develops an odor, or begins to separate from the skin.

Documentation

Document the following information (many agencies use wound care flow sheets):
■ Appearance and location of the wound, type and amount of exudate, and odor, if present, after cleansing. Include

wound measurements, if taken, and condition of surrounding skin
■ The patient's pain level before the procedure. If the patient has been medicated for pain, document the drug and dose used, time given, and patient response.
■ Method of cleansing the wound and surrounding skin
■ Type of dressing applied to the wound
■ Use of skin prep
■ Education provided to the patient

Sample documentation

Practice Resources

Bryant, R., & Nix, D. (2016); Dumville, J. C., O'Meara, S., Deshpande, S., et al. (2013); WOCN (2010, revised 2016).

Thinking About the Procedure

The video **Applying a Hydrating Dressing (Hydrocolloid or Hydrogel),** along with questions and suggested responses, is available on the **Davis's *Nursing Skills Videos*** Web site on *DavisPlus.*

Procedure 36-9 ■ Placing Skin Closures

➤ For steps to follow in *all* procedures, refer to the Universal Steps for All Procedures found on the page facing the inside back cover.

Equipment

- Adhesive skin closures
- Tincture of benzoin or skin protectant pads
- Forceps
- Normal saline
- Gauze
- Gloves (sterile if indicated)

Delegation

This procedure may be delegated to a NAP with the required training unless it is a new wound requiring sterile technique or has developed complications (e.g., dehiscence). Assessment of the incision line or wound is a licensed professional's responsibility and cannot be delegated.

Pre-Procedure Assessments

- Assess the type of wound to be closed.
  Adhesive closures are frequently used to keep surgical incisions well approximated. They may be used in conjunction with staples or sutures or following early staple/suture removal. Closures may be used to approximate the edges of lacerations or skin tears.

- Assess the wound for skin edge approximation.
  Wounds that are gaping or appear to have undermining should not be closed using adhesive closures.

- Assess the wound for drainage, amount, type, and odor.
  Wounds that are draining heavily might not be suitable for adhesive skin closures because the adhesive would not stick to the skin.

- Assess the periwound area or surrounding skin. Assessment should include skin color, texture, temperature, and integrity of the surrounding skin. Look for maceration (caused by heavy drainage), excoriation (from caustic effluent), stripping (from inappropriate adhesive removal), pustules, papules, or lesions.
  Adhesive closures should be placed only on intact skin.

- Assess the length of the wound, the location (over a joint), or whether edema may occur to determine the size of the skin closure used. Consider elastic skin closures if distention or movement is anticipated.
  Closures come in several different lengths, widths, and flexibility capabilities to meet elasticity and conformability needs.

➤ When performing the procedure, always identify your patient according to agency policy, using two identifiers, and be attentive to standard precautions, hand hygiene, patient safety and privacy, body mechanics, and documentation.

Procedure Steps

1. **Perform hand hygiene. Don clean nonsterile gloves.**
   Gloving prevents cross-contamination.

2. **Cleanse the skin** at least 5 cm (2 in.) around the wound with saline-moistened gauze. Pat the skin dry, allowing it to dry thoroughly.
   The skin surrounding the wound must be clean and dry in order for the strips to adhere.

3. **Apply a skin preparation product** and allow it to dry (or follow agency procedures). Avoid benzoin on fragile skin.
   Because the strips are prone to peeling off with moisture, benzoin enhances adhesion of the strips.

4. **Do not allow skin preparation** product to come into contact with the wound.
   It may impair healing.

5. **Peel back package tabs** to access the adhesive closures.

6. **Remove the card** from the package using modified sterile technique as necessary.
   Careful technique should be followed when applying to a surgical wound to minimize contamination and promote healing.

7. **Grasp end of the skin closure** with forceps or gloved hand and peel strip from the card at a 90° angle.
   Closures lifted at a lesser angle or directly back on themselves may "curl," complicating handling.

8. **Starting at the middle** of the wound, apply strips perpendicular to the wound, drawing the wound edges together. Apply closures without tension; do not stretch or strap closures.
   a. Apply half of the closure to the wound margin and press firmly in place.
   b. Using fingers or forceps, ensure skin edges are approximated.
   c. Press the free half firmly on the other side of the wound in a ladder fashion.
   d. Place the strips so that they extend at least 2 to 3 cm (¾ to 1 in.) on either side of the wound to ensure closure.
   e. Place the wound closure strips 3 mm (⅛ in.) apart along the wound. ▼

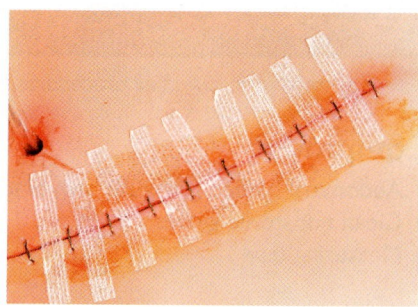

(continued on next page)

Procedure 36-9 ■ **Placing Skin Closures** (continued)

? What if . . .

■ **A flap of skin rolls up on the edges?**

Cleanse the wound with normal saline and reapproximate the edges of the skin flap with the intact epidermis. Apply skin closures across the flap.

■ **The skin around the wound is swollen?**

Apply skin closures without tension and reapply as swelling increases.

This prevents pulling on the skin that can delay healing or disrupt the approximated borders of the wound, which is more likely to lead to scarring.

■ **Edges are not accurately approximated or tension has been placed on the skin?**

Remove the closure over the affected area, peeling each side toward the wound, and reapply.

Use of adhesive products can cause superficial skin damage if the skin is stretched during application or with edema formation. Tension blisters are the most common problem associated with taping.

Evaluation

- Verify that skin closures are appropriate for the wound.
- Note whether the closures adhere comfortably to the skin.
- Ensure the patient verbalized understanding of the treatment.
- Inspect the wound daily. Lifted closure edges may be trimmed or closures replaced if less than half of the strip remains.

Patient Teaching

- Teach the patient about the expected healing process.
- Inform the patient or caregiver about signs and symptoms of infection and the need to report these findings.
- Instruct patients not to pull or tug on the strips. *Improper removal may damage the underlying skin or the wound itself.*
- Instruct patients that they do not need to keep the strips dry. They can bathe and shower as directed by the healthcare provider.
- Instruct the patient that adhesive strips are often kept in place until they begin to separate from the skin on their own.

Documentation

Sample documentation

02/08/2018   2040   *Skin closures applied to surgical incision along right forearm. Wound edges are well approximated with slight erythema noted 4 mm from incisional site. Periwound skin is dry and intact with no drainage, induration, or odor noted. Wound cleansed with normal saline using sterile technique. Patient educated on the purpose of the closures and expected time and course of healing. Will continue to monitor. ————————————— S. Wong, RN*

Practice Resource

Al-Mubarak, L., & Al-Haddab, M. (2013).

Thinking About the Procedure

 The video **Placing Skin Closures,** along with questions and suggested responses, is available on the **Davis's** *Nursing Skills Videos* Web site on *DavisPlus.*

Procedure 36-10 ■ **Applying Binders**

➤ For steps to follow in *all* procedures, refer to the Universal Steps for All Procedures found on the page facing the inside back cover.

Equipment

- Abdominal binder, triangular arm binder, or T-binder
- Clean nonsterile gloves
- Measuring tape

Delegation

This procedure may be delegated to a NAP. Assessment of the incision line or wound is a licensed professional's responsibility and cannot be delegated.

Pre-Procedure Assessments

- Assess the condition of the wound (if one is present). Note the amount and type of drainage. A wound must be dressed before it is bandaged; if there is a significant amount of exudate, you will need to apply a secondary dressing.
- Assess for pain and check the circulation of the underlying body parts before and after applying the binder. Look for cool, pale, or cyanotic skin; tingling; and numbness.
- Determine whether the patient or family has the skills to reapply the binder when necessary.

➤ When performing the procedure, always identify your patient according to agency policy, using two identifiers, and be attentive to standard precautions, hand hygiene, patient safety and privacy, body mechanics, and documentation.

➤ Observe steps 1 through 7, regardless of the type of binder you use.

Procedure Steps

1. **Choose a binder** of the proper size.

2. **Perform hand hygiene. Don non-sterile gloves.**

3. **Thoroughly clean and dry** the part to be covered.
   Moisture contributes to skin breakdown.

4. **Place the body part** in its natural comfortable position (e.g., with the joint slightly flexed) whenever possible.
   Prevents strain on ligaments and muscles.

5. **Pad between skin surfaces** (e.g., under the axilla) and over bony prominences.
   Prevents pressure and abrasion of the skin.

6. **Fasten from the bottom up,** especially for abdominal binders.

   ✚ Make sure the binder is secured with enough pressure to provide the needed support and control bleeding, but not so tightly that circulation is compromised or breathing impaired.

   Fastening from the bottom up gives upward support.

7. **Change binders** whenever they become soiled or wet.

   Proceed to step 8, 14, or 20, depending on the type of binder you are using.

Procedure Variation: Applying an Abdominal Binder

8. **Measure the patient** for the abdominal binder.
   a. Place the patient in supine position.
   b. With a measuring tape, encircle the abdomen at the level of the umbilicus. Note the measurement. This is the length of the binder. ▼

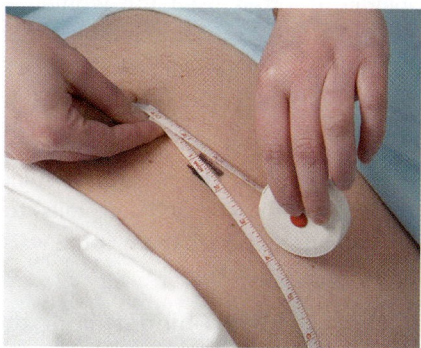

   c. Measure the distance from the costal margin to the top of the iliac crests. This is the width of the binder.
   d. Dispose of gloves and measuring tape and wash your hands.
   e. Based on the measurements, obtain an abdominal binder.

9. **Assist the patient to roll** to one side. Roll one end of the binder to the center mark. Place the rolled section of the abdominal binder underneath the patient. Position the binder appropriately between the costal margin and iliac crest.

10. **Make sure the binder** does not slip upward or downward.
    If the binder is positioned too high, it could impair lung expansion and gas exchange. If it is positioned too low, the binder will not provide adequate support.

11. **Assist the patient to turn** to the other side as you unroll the binder from underneath him. ✚ Pad any pressure areas or skin abrasions to avoid pressure injury.

12. **With your dominant hand, grasp the end of the binder** on the side furthest from you and steadily pull toward the center of the patient's abdomen. With your nondominant hand, grasp the end of binder closest to you and pull toward the center. Overlap the ends of the binder so that the hook and loop fasteners (e.g., Velcro) meet. ▼

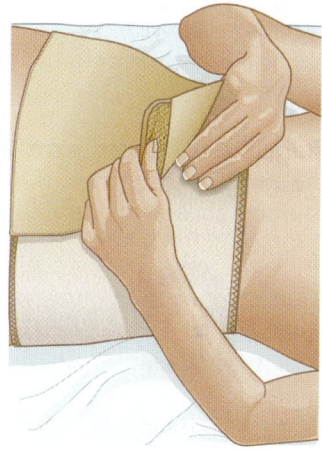

13. **Assess the abdominal binder** every 2 to 3 hours. Observe that the binder has not shifted up or down or compromised the patient's breathing. Remove it to assess the underlying skin and dressings. Change wound dressings if they are soiled, or as prescribed.

Procedure Variation Applying a Triangular Arm Binder

A triangular arm binder or sling is used to support the upper extremities. Obtain a commercial sling (consisting of a sleeve for the arm and a strap to go around the neck) or a triangular piece of fabric. To form a splint from a triangular cloth, follow these steps:

14. **Ask the patient to place** the affected arm in a natural position across the chest, elbow flexed slightly.
    Slight flexion prevents swelling of the hand and relieves pressure on the shoulder.

15. **Place one end of the triangle** over the shoulder of the uninjured arm and allow the triangle to fall open so that the elbow of the injured arm is at the apex of the triangle.

(continued on next page)

Procedure 36-10 ■ Applying Binders (continued)

16. **Move the sling** behind the injured arm.

17. **Pull up the lower corner** of the triangle over the injured arm to the shoulder of the injured arm.

18. **Tie the sling with a square knot** at the neck on the side of the arm requiring support.

A square knot will not slip and is easy to untie.

19. **Adjust the injured arm** within the sling.

To ensure patient comfort. ▼

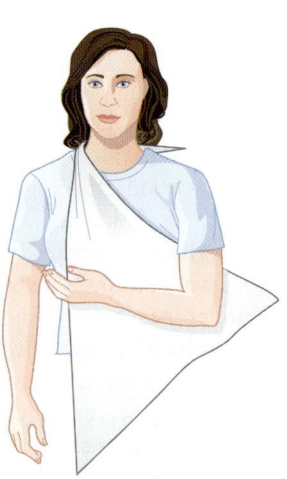

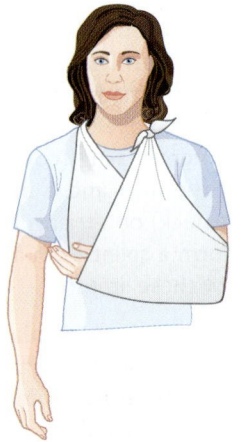

Procedure Variation **Applying a T-Binder**

A T-binder is used to secure dressings or pads in the perineal area. A single T-binder is often used for women. A double T-binder is most commonly used for men. To apply a T-binder, follow these steps:

20. **Position the waist tails** under the patient at the natural waistline. Bring the right and left tails together, and secure them at the waist with pins or clips.

21. **For a single T-binder,** bring the center tail up between the legs of the patient. Secure the tail at the waist with pins or clips. ▼

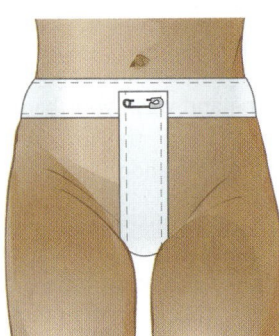

22. **For a double T-binder,** bring the tails up on either side of the penis. Secure the tail at the waist with pins or clips. ▼

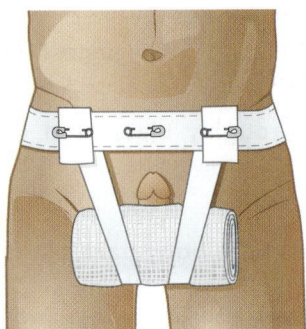

23. **Fasten the ties** at the waist using pins or clips.

? What if . . .

■ **The patient is obese?**

Obtain the appropriate size binder before applying. Do not try to position a binder that is too small for the patient.

A poorly fitting binder can constrict circulation, cause pressure points that can injure the skin, and can restrict movement of the chest for adequate breathing. A binder that is too tight is uncomfortable and will not provide the proper support of an incision or wound needed for healing.

Evaluation

■ Evaluate whether the patient's physical condition has changed since using the binder.

■ Assess circulation to be sure the binder is not secured too tightly. Check color, warmth, tingling, sensation, and capillary refill.

■ Assess the depth of breathing to be sure the binder is not restricting ventilation.

■ Check the skin under the binder to be sure there are no areas of irritation, pressure, or skin abrasion.

■ Assess incisions or wounds under the binder to be sure they are not bleeding and are healing properly.

■ Monitor comfort regularly.

■ Assess the client's ability to perform activities of daily living while wearing the binder.

Home Care

■ Teach the client and/or caregiver how to apply the binder in the proper position, snugly but not too tightly.

- Teach the family to inspect the site under the binder to be sure the skin is not pinched or with other points of pressure. This is especially crucial for older adults.
- Clean binders in warm, soapy water when soiled. Use a mesh laundry bag to keep the Velcro straps from catching other clothing in the washer. Air-dry thoroughly. Clients should have two binders at home—a clean one to wear while the other is laundered.
- Apply and remove binder to promote comfort and ensure good circulation. This also allows the patient and caregiver to inspect any incision or wound underneath.
- Binders for children at home could be decorated with permanent marking pens.
- Allow children to help with applying and removing the binder.

Documentation

Document the following information (many agencies use specialized wound care flow sheets):
- Appearance and location of the wound or incision under the binder, type and amount of exudates, and odor, if present, after cleansing
- Pain level before and after the procedure. If the patient has been medicated for pain, document the drug and dose used, time given, and patient response.
- Type of binder applied
- Date and time the binder was applied and removed
- Any change in the appearance of the wound or skin in contact with the binder
- Education provided to the patient

Procedure 36-11 ■ Applying Bandages

> For steps to follow in *all* procedures, refer to the Universal Steps for All Procedures found on the page facing the inside back cover.

Equipment

- Appropriate bandage dressing
- Clean nonsterile gloves (2 pairs)
- Gauze sponges
- Normal saline
- Primary dressing (as prescribed)
- Scissors
- Tape or metal closures

Delegation

This procedure may be delegated to a NAP who has the appropriate training. Assessment of the incision line or wound is a licensed professional's responsibility and cannot be delegated.

Pre-Procedure Assessment

- Determine the body part or area to be bandaged.
  This allows you to choose the correct width of gauze or elastic bandage to use.

- Assess the condition of the wound (if one is present). Assess the wound for size (length, width, and depth in centimeters); location and depth of undermining or tunneling; amount, character, and odor of drainage; type and percentage of tissue present in wound bed (granulation, slough, fibrin, necrotic); and periwound condition (intact, denuded, erythema, induration, or maceration).
  Wound dressings should be chosen based on the characteristics of the wound.

- Assess for pain and check the circulation of the underlying body parts before and after applying the bandage. Look for cool, pale, or cyanotic skin; tingling; and numbness.
  Circulation to an extremity can be compromised if the bandage is too tight or the extremity swells after application.

- Determine whether the client or family has the skills to reapply the bandage when necessary.
  Teaching might be needed for home care.

> When performing the procedure, always identify your patient according to agency policy, using two identifiers, and be attentive to standard precautions, hand hygiene, patient safety and privacy, body mechanics, and documentation.

Procedure Steps

Observe the following steps, regardless of the type of bandage you use:

1. **Choose a bandage** of the proper width. For example, use a 2.5-cm (1-in.) wide bandage for a finger, a 5-cm (2-in.) wide bandage for an arm, and a wider bandage for a leg.
   Prevents pressure and abrasion of the skin.

2. **Thoroughly clean and dry** the part to be covered. Use a nontoxic cleansing solution, such as normal saline.
   Cleaning the wound removes debris, exudates, and bacteria. Drainage and moisture on the skin contribute to irritation.

3. **Remove excess moisture** by gently patting the wound and surrounding skin with gauze sponge.
   Drainage and moisture contribute to skin breakdown.

4. **Stand facing the patient.**
   In this position you can wrap the bandage evenly in the proper direction.

5. **Bandage the body part** in a comfortable position (e.g., with the joint slightly flexed) whenever possible.
   This prevents strain on ligaments and muscles. Movement of the extremity (extension) may cause skin damage if the bandage is too tight or the extremity is not properly positioned.

6. **Always work from distal** to proximal (or peripheral to central).
   This improves venous return and helps to prevent edema.

(continued on next page)

Procedure 36–11 ■ Applying Bandages (continued)

7. **If a wound is present,** apply a primary dressing, as prescribed, over the wound.

   A primary dressing is any dressing that is placed first in the wound bed. It provides exudate absorption, holds medications in place, provides antimicrobial coverage, or maintains a moist wound bed.

8. **Apply the bandage** with enough pressure to provide the needed support, but do not bandage too tightly. Make sure circulation to the area is not compromised.

9. **If possible, leave the fingers** (if you are bandaging an arm) or toes (if you are bandaging a leg or foot) exposed so that you can assess the circulation to the extremity. Begin the wrap along the pad of the foot or hand, just under the first bend of the toes or fingers (metatarsal or metacarpal joints).

10. **Begin the wrap** with the bandage against the skin. Unwind the bandage as if rolling it over the extremity.
    This helps to keep the bandage snug against the skin.

11. **Pad bony prominences** before bandaging if there are pressure concerns.

12. **Change bandages** whenever they become soiled or wet from external sources (stool, urine, etc.) and internal sources (drainage that has wicked on the outer surface of the bandage).
    Wound drainage contains chemicals, enzymes, and bacteria that can damage fragile healing tissues.

13. **After bandaging, assess** circulation and comfort regularly.
    Proceed to step 14, 16, 19, 25, or 28, depending on the type of bandaging you are using.

Procedure Variation Circular Turns
Use this technique to wrap a finger or toe, or as an anchor at the beginning and end of another wrapping technique.

14. **With one hand, hold one end** of the bandage in place. With the other hand, encircle the body part two times with the bandage—the second wrap should partially cover the first wrap. Continue to wrap the body part by overlapping two-thirds of the width of the bandage.

15. **Secure the bandage** with tape or metal clips when you are finished, if circular turns are not being combined with another technique. ▼

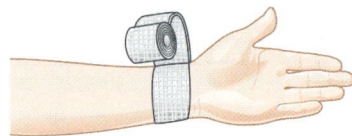

Procedure Variation Spiral Turns
Spiral turns are a variation of the circular turn technique. Spiral turns are most commonly used to wrap an extremity.

16. **Anchor the bandage** by making two circular turns—the second wrap completely covering the first one.

17. **Continue to wrap** the extremity by encircling the body part with each turn angled at approximately 30° so that you are overlapping the preceding wrap by two-thirds of the width of the bandage.

18. **Complete the wrap** by making two circular turns and securing the bandage with tape or metal clips. ▼

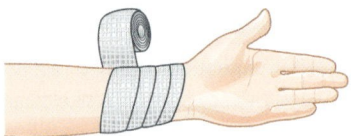

Procedure Variation Spiral Reverse Turns
Spiral reverse turns are used to bandage cylindrical body parts that are not uniform in size.

19. **Anchor the bandage** by making two circular turns.

20. **Bring the next wrap up** at a 30° angle.

21. **Place the thumb** of your nondominant hand on the wrap to hold the bandage. ▼

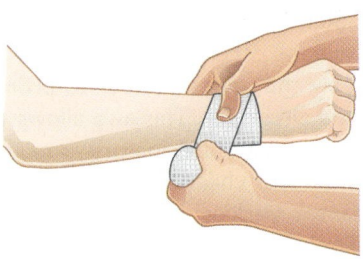

22. **Fold the bandage back on itself** and continue to wrap at a 30° angle in the opposite direction. ▼

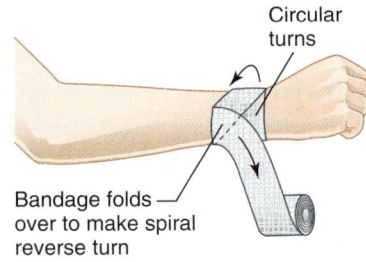

Circular turns

Bandage folds over to make spiral reverse turn

23. **Continue to wrap the bandage,** overlapping each turn by two-thirds. Align each bandage turn at the same position on the extremity. ▼

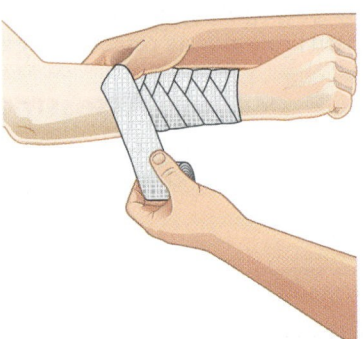

24. **Complete the wrap** by making two circular turns and securing the bandage with tape or metal clips.

Procedure Variation Figure-8 Turns
The figure-8 wrap is used on joints (e.g., ankle, elbow).

25. **Anchor the bandage** by making two circular turns.

26. Wrap the bandage by ascending above the joint and descending below the joint to form a figure 8. Continue to wrap the bandage, overlapping each turn by two-thirds. Align each bandage turn at the same position on the extremity. ▼

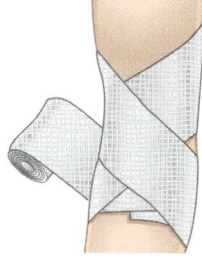

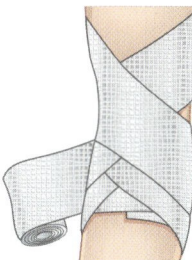

27. Complete the wrap by making two circular turns and securing the bandage with tape or metal clips.

Procedure Variation **Recurrent Turns**

28. Anchor the bandage by making two circular turns.

29. Fold the bandage back on itself; hold it against the body part with one hand. With the other hand, make a half turn perpendicular to the circle turns and central to the distal end being bandaged. ➤

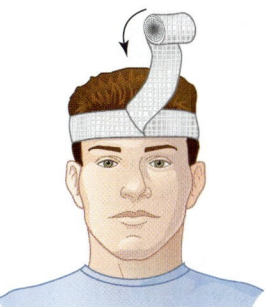

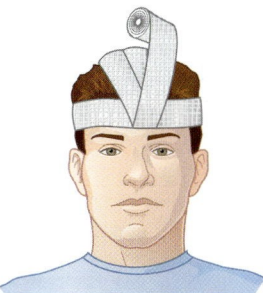

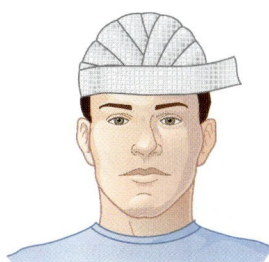

30. Hold the central turn with one hand and fold the bandage back on itself; bring it over the distal end of the body part to the right of the center, overlapping the center turn by two-thirds of the width of the bandage.

31. Next, hold the bandage at the center with one hand as you bring the bandage back over the end to

the left of center. Continue holding and folding the bandage back on itself, alternating right and left until the body part is covered. Overlap by two-thirds of the bandage width with each turn.

32. Start and return each turn to the midline or center of the body part and angle it slightly more each time to continue covering the body part.

33. Complete the bandage by making two circular turns and securing the bandage with tape or metal clips.

34. Assess circulation and comfort of the body part.

? What if . . .

■ **Drainage breaks through the outer bandage more frequently than expected?**

Determine the cause of the drainage if possible (i.e., is it blood or serum?). Increased drainage may be a sign of infection and should be evaluated. You might need to change the dressing more often or an alternate, more absorbent type of dressing may be needed.

Wound exudates can harm healing tissues. Dressings that are saturated should be changed as soon as possible to prevent prolonged moisture exposure or maceration.

Evaluation

■ Be sure the bandage is firmly wrapped without being too tight.
■ Check the circulation is not compromised to the area distal of the bandage.
■ Evaluate for numbness or pain around or distal to the bandaged area.

Patient Teaching

■ Teach the patient about the expected healing process.
■ Inform the patient and caregiver about signs and symptoms of infection and the need to report these findings.

■ Instruct the patient and family about signs of circulation problems and how to remove the bandage if needed.

Home Care

■ Refer the client to a home health agency for wound care.
■ Some clients or caregivers may be able to perform dressing changes. Determine the client and/or caregiver's ability to perform dressing changes; teach and demonstrate as needed.

(continued on next page)

Procedure 36–11 ■ Applying Bandages (continued)

Documentation

Many agencies use wound care flow sheets.

Sample EHR documentation

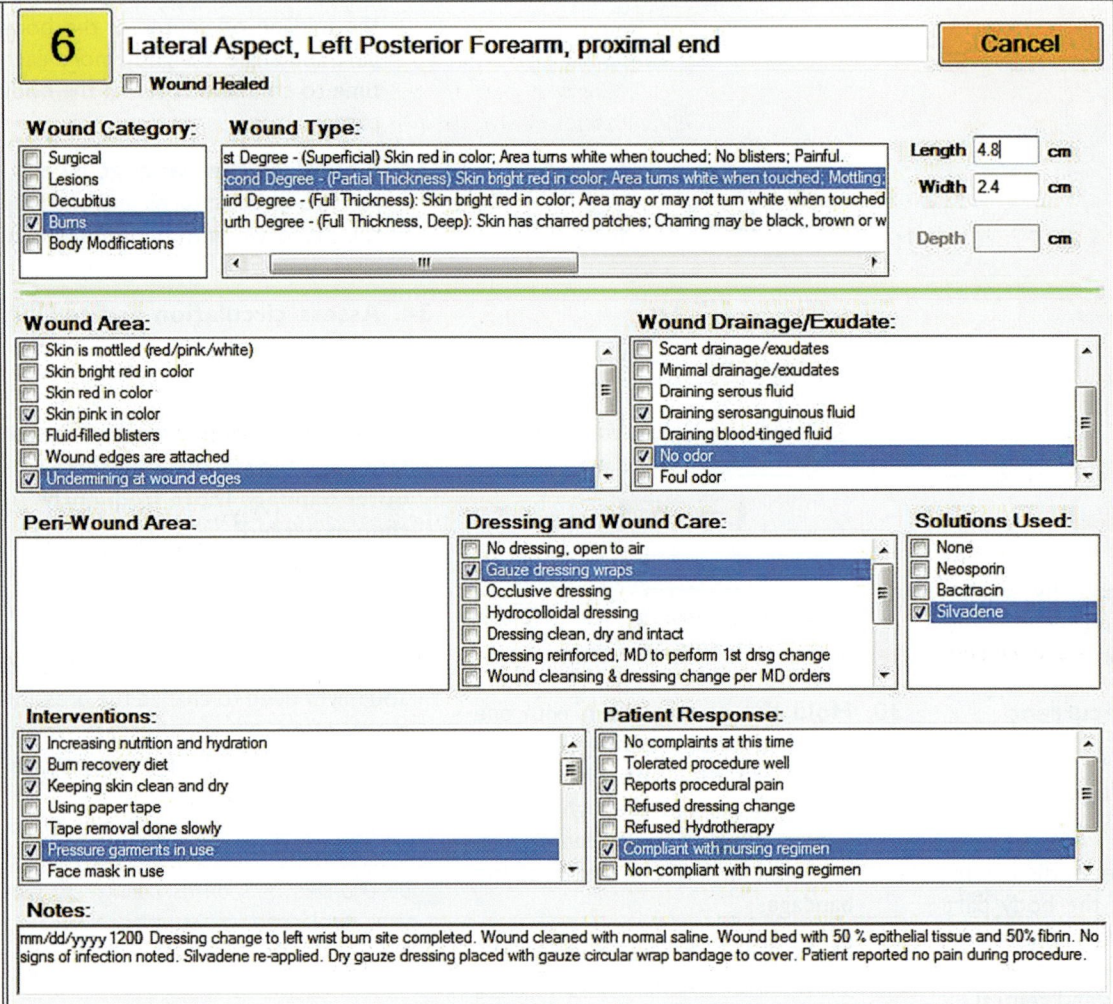

6	Lateral Aspect, Left Posterior Forearm, proximal end			Cancel

☐ Wound Healed

Wound Category:
- ☐ Surgical
- ☐ Lesions
- ☐ Decubitus
- ☑ Burns
- ☐ Body Modifications

Wound Type:
- st Degree - (Superficial) Skin red in color; Area turns white when touched; No blisters; Painful.
- cond Degree - (Partial Thickness) Skin bright red in color; Area turns white when touched; Mottling;
- ird Degree - (Full Thickness): Skin bright red in color; Area may or may not turn white when touched
- urth Degree - (Full Thickness, Deep): Skin has charred patches; Charring may be black, brown or w

Length 4.8 cm
Width 2.4 cm
Depth [ ] cm

Wound Area:
- ☐ Skin is mottled (red/pink/white)
- ☐ Skin bright red in color
- ☐ Skin red in color
- ☑ Skin pink in color
- ☐ Fluid-filled blisters
- ☐ Wound edges are attached
- ☑ Undermining at wound edges

Wound Drainage/Exudate:
- ☐ Scant drainage/exudates
- ☐ Minimal drainage/exudates
- ☐ Draining serous fluid
- ☑ Draining serosanguinous fluid
- ☐ Draining blood-tinged fluid
- ☑ No odor
- ☐ Foul odor

Peri-Wound Area:

Dressing and Wound Care:
- ☐ No dressing, open to air
- ☑ Gauze dressing wraps
- ☐ Occlusive dressing
- ☐ Hydrocolloidal dressing
- ☐ Dressing clean, dry and intact
- ☐ Dressing reinforced, MD to perform 1st drsg change
- ☐ Wound cleansing & dressing change per MD orders

Solutions Used:
- ☐ None
- ☐ Neosporin
- ☐ Bacitracin
- ☑ Silvadene

Interventions:
- ☑ Increasing nutrition and hydration
- ☑ Burn recovery diet
- ☑ Keeping skin clean and dry
- ☐ Using paper tape
- ☐ Tape removal done slowly
- ☑ Pressure garments in use
- ☐ Face mask in use

Patient Response:
- ☐ No complaints at this time
- ☐ Tolerated procedure well
- ☑ Reports procedural pain
- ☐ Refused dressing change
- ☐ Refused Hydrotherapy
- ☑ Compliant with nursing regimen
- ☐ Non-compliant with nursing regimen

Notes:
mm/dd/yyyy 1200 Dressing change to left wrist burn site completed. Wound cleaned with normal saline. Wound bed with 50 % epithelial tissue and 50% fibrin. No signs of infection noted. Silvadene re-applied. Dry gauze dressing placed with gauze circular wrap bandage to cover. Patient reported no pain during procedure.

Practice Resources

Bryant, R., & Nix, D. (2016); Le Badour, G., Bergeron, J. D., Bizjak, G., et al. (2012).

Thinking About the Procedure

 The video **Applying Bandages,** along with questions and suggested responses, is available on the **Davis's *Nursing Skills Videos*** Web site on Davis*Plus*.

Procedure 36-12 ■ Removing Sutures and Staples

➤ For steps to follow in *all* procedures, refer to the Universal Steps for All Procedures found on the page facing the inside back cover.

Equipment

- Nonsterile gloves
- Suture removal kit or sterile scissors and forceps (Procedure 36-12A)
- Staple remover (Procedure 36-12B)
- Gauze

Delegation

This procedure cannot be delegated to a NAP. Assessment of the incision line or wound is a registered nurse's responsibility

and cannot be delegated. The procedure requires assessment and judgment during removal and may require stopping the procedure if complications occur.

Pre-Procedure Assessment

- Assess staples to ensure none have rotated or turned instead of lying flat along the incision.

Procedure 36-12A ■ Removing Sutures

➤ When performing the procedure, always identify your patient according to agency policy, using two identifiers, and be attentive to standard precautions, hand hygiene, patient safety and privacy, body mechanics, and documentation.

Procedure Steps

1. **Obtain a suture removal kit.**

2. **Wash hands. Don nonsterile gloves.**

3. **Cleanse the wound** or suture line.

4. **Use the forceps** to pick up one end of the suture. ▼

Suture types

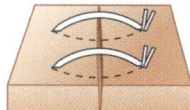
Plain interrupted

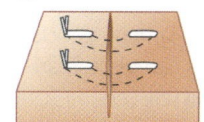
Mattress interrupted

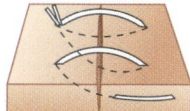
Plain continuous

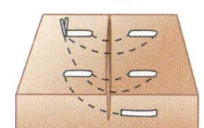
Mattress continuous

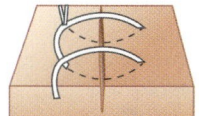
Blanket continuous

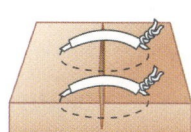
Retention

5. **Slide the small scissors** around the suture and cut near the skin. *This helps you avoid pulling the exposed portion of the suture through the underlying tissue.*

6. **With the forceps, gently pull** the suture in the direction of the knotted side to remove it. ▼

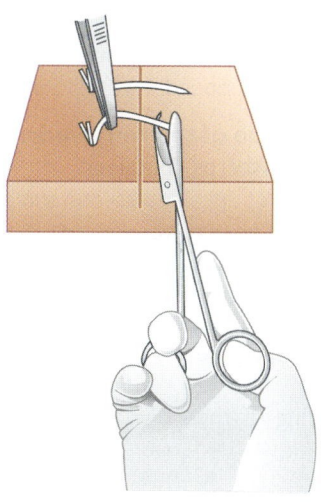
Removing interrupted sutures

7. **Apply a dressing** or adhesive skin closures if needed.

8. **Remove gloves** and dispose in proper biohazardous waste receptacle. Perform hand hygiene.

(continued on next page)

Procedure 36-12 ▪ Removing Sutures and Staples (continued)

Procedure 36-12B ▪ Removing Staples

1. **Wash hands.** Don nonsterile gloves.

2. **After cleansing the wound** or incision, position the staple remover so that the lower jaw is on the bottom.

3. **Place both tips of the lower jaw** of the remover under the staple. ▼

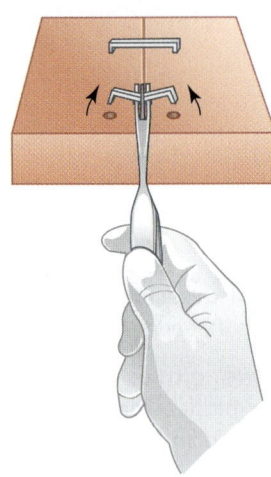

Removing staples

4. **Ensure the staple is** perpendicular to the plane of the skin. If not, reposition the staple with the tips of the lower jaw and apply gentle pressure, causing it to straighten the ends for easier removal.

5. **Lift slightly on the staple,** ensuring that it stays perpendicular to the skin.

6. **Continue to lift slightly** as you gently squeeze the handles together to close.
Spreads the ends of the staples apart, freeing them from the skin.

7. **Lift the reshaped staple** straight up from the skin.

8. **Remove alternate staples** and check the tension on the wound.

9. **If there is no significant pull** on the wound, remove the remaining staples.
Where there are a large number of staples over an area of stress (abdomen, legs), the remaining staples are often removed a day or two later after assuring the incision remains intact.

10. **Place the removed staples** on a piece of gauze.
Staples are small and can be easily lost. Keeping them in one place prevents this.

11. **Apply a dressing** or adhesive closures, if needed.

12. **Dispose of the removed staples** in the sharps container.
Ends of the staples are sharp and should be handled with care.

13. **Remove gloves and wash hands.**

? What if . . .

▪ **A staple gets stuck?**

Gently manipulate the staple with the remover until it is perpendicular to the skin.
When the skin is stapled, the edges of the staple are crimped to hold the incision together. For the staple to be removed, those edges must be reshaped and straightened. If one edge of the staple is reshaped and the other is not, continuing to remove it can cause pain and tissue trauma.

▪ **The incision needs a dressing once the staples or sutures have been removed?**

New surgical incisions should be covered with a sterile dressing the first 24 to 48 hours, but not necessarily after that time. Apply a dressing if you are concerned about soiling or per your institution's policy.
In a healing incision, epithelial resurfacing is complete in 24 to 48 hours. Though only a few cells thick, this epithelium is enough to keep the wound closed and provide a bacterial barrier.

Evaluation

▪ Note whether the incision is well approximated after the procedure.
▪ Ensure that the patient verbalized understanding of the treatment.
▪ Inspect the wound daily.

Patient Teaching

▪ Instruct the patient of signs and symptoms of wound infections (i.e., redness, drainage) and the need to report these findings.
▪ Instruct the patient that he may be able to shower once sutures or staples are removed, if approved by the healthcare provider.

Documentation

The following is an example (many agencies use wound care flow sheets):

Sample documentation

02/23/2018   1815   Staples removed from abdominal midline incision. Incision edges well approximated without erythema, drainage, or swelling. Dry dressing applied. Patient tolerated the procedure without discomfort. Discussed purpose of staple removal with patient. Will continue to monitor wound daily. ———————————— M. Dali, RN

Practice Resources

Al-Mubarak, L., & Al-Haddab, M. (2013); Hin-Lun, L., & Hon-Ping, C. (2012).

Procedure 36-13 ■ Shortening a Wound Drain

➤ For steps to follow in *all* procedures, refer to the Universal Steps for All Procedures found on the page facing the inside back cover.

Equipment
- Nonsterile gloves
- Sterile gloves
- Sterile scissors
- Two safety pins or other clips (sterile)
- Sterile gauze

Delegation

Assessment of the incision line or wound and the drain is a registered nurse's responsibility and cannot be delegated. This procedure should not be delegated to a NAP. The risk for accidently losing the drain into the body or pulling it out of the wound is too high.

Pre-Procedure Assessment

- Inspect the site around the drain, noting skin excoriation, tenderness, erythema, warmth to the touch, and drainage seeping from the wound.
  Could indicate a wound infection or irritation of the drain at the skin site. Excoriation can be the result of seeping drainage around the tube (e.g., if the tube diameter is not sufficient size to handle drainage output) or, more likely, an obstruction within the tubing.

- Assess the characteristics of the drainage, including color, volume of drainage, presence of blood, odor, pus, and any change in the type or amount of drainage through the tubing.
  A sudden decrease in drainage might indicate a blocked drain. Presence of fresh blood might be a sign of irritation within the wound. Pus and odor in the drainage could indicate wound infection.

- Check the suction apparatus to be sure it is functioning properly.
  A self-suction apparatus might need to be recompressed from time to time to maintain effective vacuum. Electric suction units can fail, delivering too much suction, which can lead to injury. Too little suction can contribute to insufficient drainage, which can lead to pressure on sutures if present, or cause the wound to become infected or heal more slowly.

➤ When performing the procedure, always identify your patient according to agency policy, using two identifiers, and be attentive to standard precautions, hand hygiene, patient safety and privacy, body mechanics, and documentation.

Procedure Steps

1. **Perform hand hygiene and don nonsterile gloves.** Remove wound dressings.

2. **Remove soiled gloves** and discard in a moisture-proof biohazard collection container. Perform hand hygiene.

3. **Open sterile supplies** (scissors, etc.).

4. **Don sterile gloves;** use sterile scissors to cut halfway through a sterile gauze dressing (for later use) or use a sterile precut drain dressing.

5. **If the drain is sutured in place,** use sterile scissors to cut the suture.

6. **Firmly grasp the full width** of the drain at the level of the skin and pull it out by the prescribed amount (e.g., 5 cm [2 in.]).

7. **Insert a sterile safety pin** through the drain at the level of the skin. Hold the drain tightly between your fingers and insert another pin above your fingers.
   The pin keeps the drain from disappearing into the wound. ▼

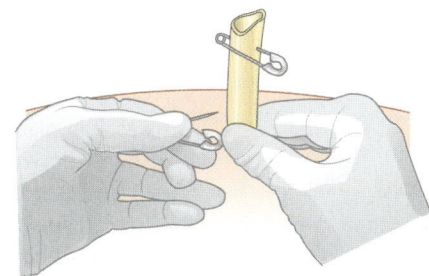

8. **Using sterile scissors, cut** the drain about 2.5 cm (1 in.) above the skin and pin. ▼

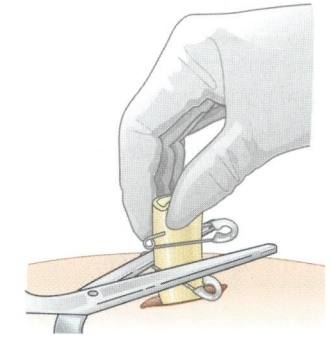

9. **Cleanse the wound,** using sterile gauze swabs and the prescribed cleaning solution. In some situations, you may use sterile forceps to manipulate the swabs.

10. **Apply precut sterile gauze** around the drain; then redress the wound. ▼

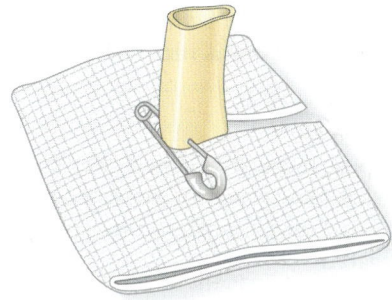

11. **Remove gloves** and discard in a biohazard container. Wash your hands.

12. **Leave the patient** in a safe and comfortable position.

(continued on next page)

Procedure 36-13 ■ Shortening a Wound Drain (continued)

? What if . . .

■ **You shorten the drain too much?**

Immediately notify the surgeon who placed the drain.

The drain will need to be evaluated to be sure it remains intact, which it mostly likely

will. Drainage tubing is secured under the skin surface and will probably not be dislodged with shortening.

Evaluation

■ Assess the local area of skin around the drain after manipulating it.
■ Note the patency of the drain after shortening it.
■ Be sure the drain is secure after shortening.
■ Evaluate for complications occurring related to shortening procedure.

Patient Teaching

■ Patients should not shorten their own drains. Consult a healthcare provider if concerned about the length of tubing or drains.

Documentation

■ Record the intervention.
■ Note the amount and characteristics of the drainage.

■ Document the appearance of the wound.
■ Note any complications that occur with shortening a drain (e.g., manipulation of tubing causes bleeding or drainage at the site).

Sample documentation

10/11/2018   0930   Penrose shortened 2.0 cm by post-op orders. Drain intact. Pt tolerated procedure without complication. ————————— M. Garcia, RN

Thinking About the Procedure

The video **Shortening a Wound Drain,** along with questions and suggested responses, is available on the **Davis's *Nursing Skills Videos*** Web site on DavisPlus.

Procedure 36-14 ■ Emptying a Closed-Wound Drainage System

➤ For steps to follow in *all* procedures, refer to the Universal Steps for All Procedures found on the page facing the inside back cover.

Equipment

■ Drainage container with graduated markings
■ Nonsterile gloves
■ Disposal sink for biomedical material
■ Biohazard disposal receptacle

Delegation

This procedure may be delegated to a NAP who is trained in the skill. Assessment of the wound and drainage characteristics is a licensed professional's responsibility and cannot be delegated.

Pre-Procedure Assessment

■ Assess the appearance of the drainage tube site and sutures, if in place.
■ Inspect for warmth, edema, redness, or pus where tubing penetrates the skin.
■ Check to be sure the closed-wound drainage system is securely fastened at the connections and within the wound.
■ Determine whether suction (electric, portable, or manual) is working properly.

➤ When performing the procedure, always identify your patient according to agency policy, using two identifiers, and be attentive to standard precautions, hand hygiene, patient safety and privacy, body mechanics, and documentation.

Procedure Steps

1. **Read the instructions** about the drainage device.
   Procedures vary among manufacturers and different systems.

2. **Don nonsterile gloves** and goggles or mask.

3. **Removes the drainage device** from the patient's gown.

The drainage device is often pinned to the patient's gown to prevent it from dislodging.

4. **Open the drainage port** and empty the drainage into a small graduated container. ▼

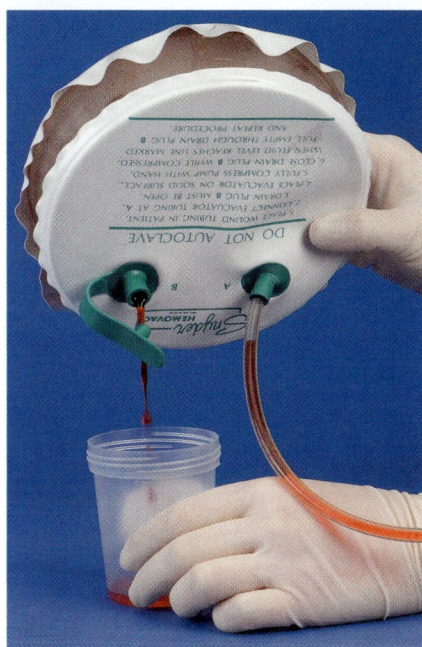

5. **With the port still open,** place the collection device on a firm, flat surface (e.g., the overbed table).

6. **Use the palm of one hand** to press down on the device and eject air from it. Do not stand directly over the air vent. Do not touch the drainage port.
It can splash or bubble.

7. **Use your other hand to scrub** the port and plug with an alcohol-based antiseptic or povidone-iodine swab (Betadine), if the patient is not allergic to iodine. ▼

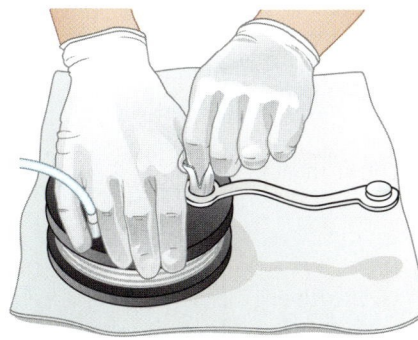

8. **Continuing to press down** on the device, replace the plug in the port. Do not touch the open port or the part of the plug that goes into the port.
Creates a constant, negative pressure vacuum to facilitate suction.

9. **Attach the drainage device** to the patient's gown.
Pinning keeps it secure and prevents it from accidentally dislodging.

10. **Measure the drainage** in the graduated container; discard drainage in the container for biohazardous material. Wash the graduated container. Do not stand in front of an air vent while doing so.
Forced air in the room can cause the drainage to splash or bubble, introducing biohazardous material into the environmental air.

11. **Remove your gloves.** Perform hand hygiene.

12. **Document** in the patient's record.

? What if . . .

■ **The wound drainage spills?**
Don nonsterile gloves and protective clothing. Keep people away from the spill area. If sharps are present, remove with forceps. Contain the spill with absorbent pads and place all used materials in a red biohazard bag. Use an approved disinfectant. When finished, place all materials including gloves and gowns in the bag and dispose of in the biohazard area.
Proper handling of contaminated biomedical materials is important to prevent transmission of infectious organisms.

Home Care
■ Teach family members who are emptying drainage systems at home to wear gloves and avoid touching the drainage port.

Documentation
■ Note the date and time the drainage system is emptied.
■ Record the volume lost. Report excess fluid loss to the healthcare provider.
■ Describe the appearance of drainage, including presence of blood or purulent material.

Sample documentation

03/12/2016   0750   Hemovac drained 18 mL serosanguineous fluid over 12 hours. No odor or purulent material noted at drainage site. ———— R. Ferretti, RN

Practice Resource
Wechter, D. G. (2016).

Thinking About the Procedure
The video **Emptying a Closed-Wound Drainage System,** along with questions and suggested responses, is available on the **Davis's *Nursing Skills Videos*** Web site on DavisPlus.

To explore learning resources for this chapter,

Go to **www.DavisAdvantage.com** and find:

Answers and Suggested Responses for all questions in this chapter
Lists of NIC Interventions and NOC Outcomes
List of NANDA-I Diagnoses
Knowledge Map
Care Plan
Care Map
References and Bibliography

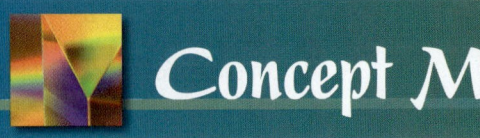

Concept Map

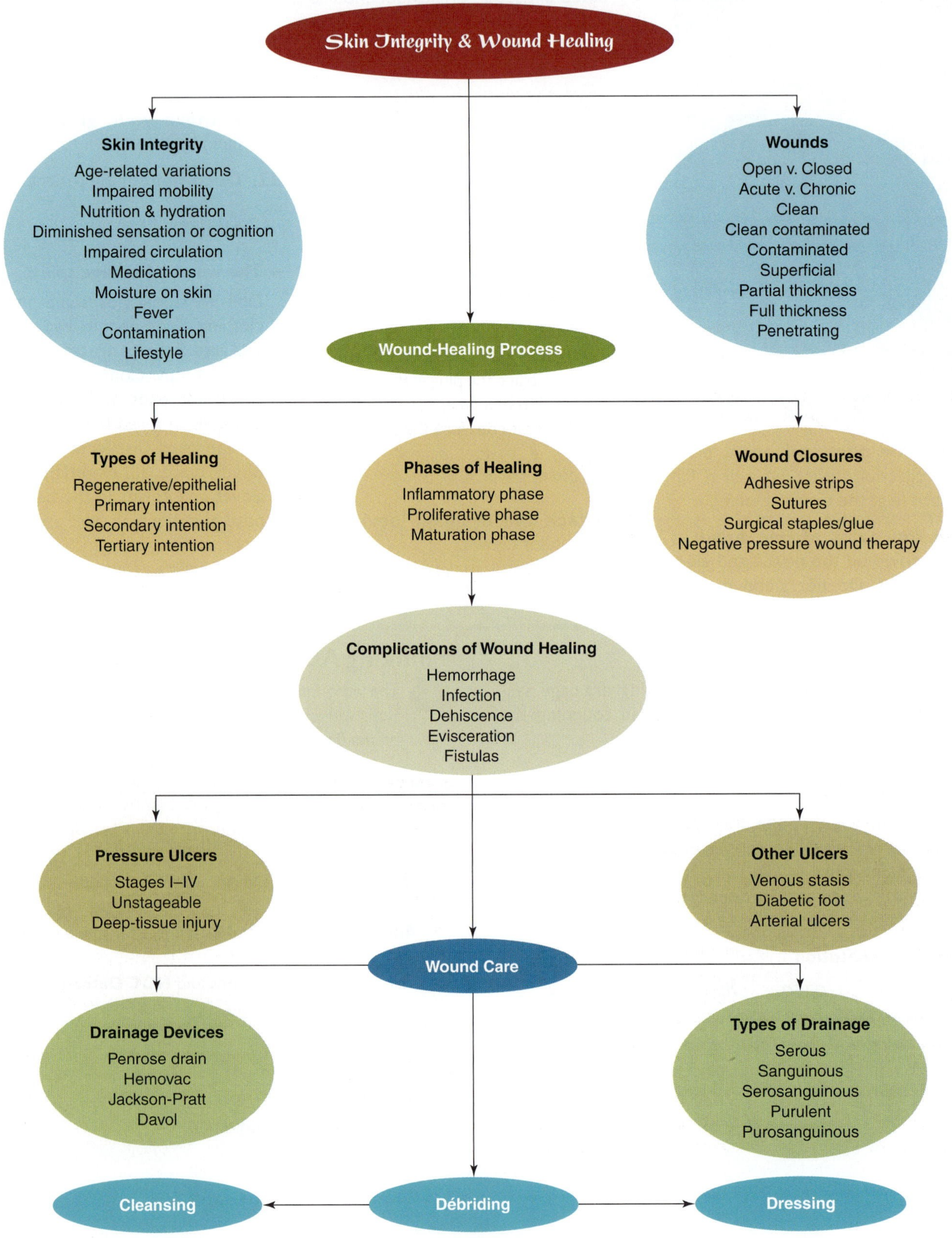

Skin Integrity & Wound Healing

Skin Integrity
Age-related variations
Impaired mobility
Nutrition & hydration
Diminished sensation or cognition
Impaired circulation
Medications
Moisture on skin
Fever
Contamination
Lifestyle

Wounds
Open v. Closed
Acute v. Chronic
Clean
Clean contaminated
Contaminated
Superficial
Partial thickness
Full thickness
Penetrating

Wound-Healing Process

Types of Healing
Regenerative/epithelial
Primary intention
Secondary intention
Tertiary intention

Phases of Healing
Inflammatory phase
Proliferative phase
Maturation phase

Wound Closures
Adhesive strips
Sutures
Surgical staples/glue
Negative pressure wound therapy

Complications of Wound Healing
Hemorrhage
Infection
Dehiscence
Evisceration
Fistulas

Pressure Ulcers
Stages I–IV
Unstageable
Deep-tissue injury

Other Ulcers
Venous stasis
Diabetic foot
Arterial ulcers

Wound Care

Drainage Devices
Penrose drain
Hemovac
Jackson-Pratt
Davol

Types of Drainage
Serous
Sanguinous
Serosanguinous
Purulent
Purosanguinous

Cleansing   **Débriding**   **Dressing**

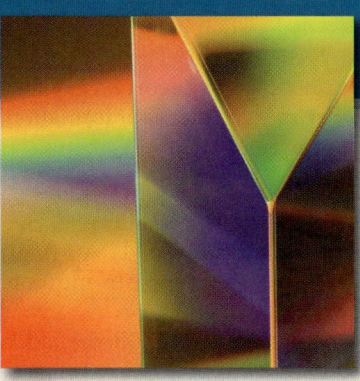

CHAPTER 37

Oxygenation

Learning Outcomes

After completing this chapter, you should be able to:

- ➤ Describe the structure and function of the respiratory system.
- ➤ Identify individual, environmental, and pathological factors that influence oxygenation.
- ➤ Assess oxygenation, breathing, and gas exchange.
- ➤ Interpret diagnostic testing related to oxygenation, breathing, and gas exchange.
- ➤ Develop nursing diagnoses related to oxygenation, breathing, and gas exchange.

- ➤ Plan outcomes and interventions for maintaining and improving oxygenation.
- ➤ Safely and correctly perform common nursing procedures related to oxygenation, breathing, and gas exchange.
- ➤ Evaluate adequacy of oxygenation, breathing, and gas exchange and modify nursing activities appropriately based on outcomes.
- ➤ Recognize medications used to enhance pulmonary function.

Key Concepts

Oxygenation
Respiration
Ventilation

Related Concepts

See the Concept Map at the end of this chapter.

Example Problems

Pneumonia
URI and Influenza

Meet Your Patients

In a pulmonary clinic, your student assignment is to (1) perform a focused assessment related to breathing and oxygenation, (2) perform common therapeutic interventions related to breathing and oxygenation, (3) identify desired outcomes and evaluate achievement of those outcomes, and (4) plan for follow-up and home-care needs. During of your clinical day, you care for the following clients:

- ■ **Mary** is a 4-year-old girl with a history of asthma. Her mother, Ms. Green, has brought her in because of an "asthma attack." Mary is sitting in her mother's lap and breathing rapidly through an open mouth. Her cough sounds congested and wheezy. The nurse practitioner has prescribed a nebulized treatment containing albuterol (Proventil) and ipratropium bromide (Atrovent).
- ■ **Mr. Chu** is a 78-year-old man complaining of cough, sore throat, fatigue, and weakness. His temperature is

100.4°F (38°C), pulse is 90 beats/min, respirations are 26 breaths/min, and blood pressure (BP) is 166/82 mm Hg.

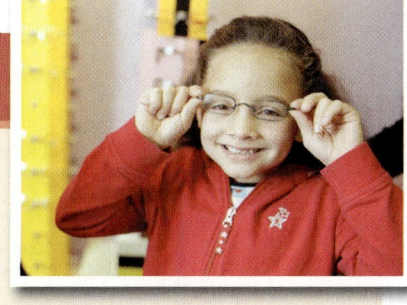

- ■ **William** is a 19-year-old male who has had a sudden onset of right-sided chest pain and shortness of breath. His chest x-ray revealed a right pneumothorax, and he is currently receiving 35% oxygen by face mask while waiting for an ambulance to transport him to the hospital for further evaluation.

Each of these patients is experiencing an oxygenation problem. In this chapter, you will learn a variety of assessment techniques and interventions to support breathing, oxygenation, and gas exchange for patients such as these.

Theoretical Knowledge
knowing **why**

The pulmonary, cardiovascular, musculoskeletal, and neurological systems work together to achieve oxygenation. The musculoskeletal and neurological systems regulate the movement of air into and out of the lungs. The lungs oxygenate the blood, and the heart circulates the blood throughout the body and back to the lungs. In this chapter, we focus on the pulmonary system; Chapter 38 presents the cardiovascular system. Remember, however, that the two systems work together. Changes in one system create changes in the other.

ABOUT THE KEY CONCEPTS

The concept of **oxygenation** refers to how well the cells, tissues, and organs of the body are supplied with oxygen. The concepts of **respiration** and **ventilation** are the two major processes that occur in the pulmonary system to oxygenate the blood. All of the problems and interventions in this chapter relate in some way to oxygenation, respiration, or ventilation. Knowledge of these concepts will help you to understand the rationale for interventions such as airway suctioning, oxygen, mechanical ventilation, and chest tubes.

THE PULMONARY SYSTEM

The pulmonary system has two major components: the *airway* and the *lungs*. The following presents a brief review of the anatomy and physiology of the pulmonary system and explains how breathing is controlled. For more in-depth information, consult anatomy and physiology texts.

The Airway

The airway consists of the nasal passages, mouth, pharynx, larynx, trachea, bronchi, and bronchioles (Fig. 37-1). Air flows through these structures into and out of the lungs. In addition, the airway structures do the following:

- *Moisten the air*—A moist mucous membrane lining adds water to inhaled air.
- *Warm the air*—Blood flowing through the vascular airway walls transfers body heat to the inhaled air.
- *Filter the air*—(1) Specialized cells in the lining of the airways secrete sticky mucus to trap foreign particles. (2) **Cilia,** tiny hair-like projections from the walls of the airways, move rhythmically to sweep trapped debris up and out of the airway.

Upper Airway Located above the larynx, the upper airway includes the nasal passages, mouth, and pharynx. The *pharynx* (throat) contains the openings to the esophagus and trachea. The *trachea* lies just in front of the esophagus. The

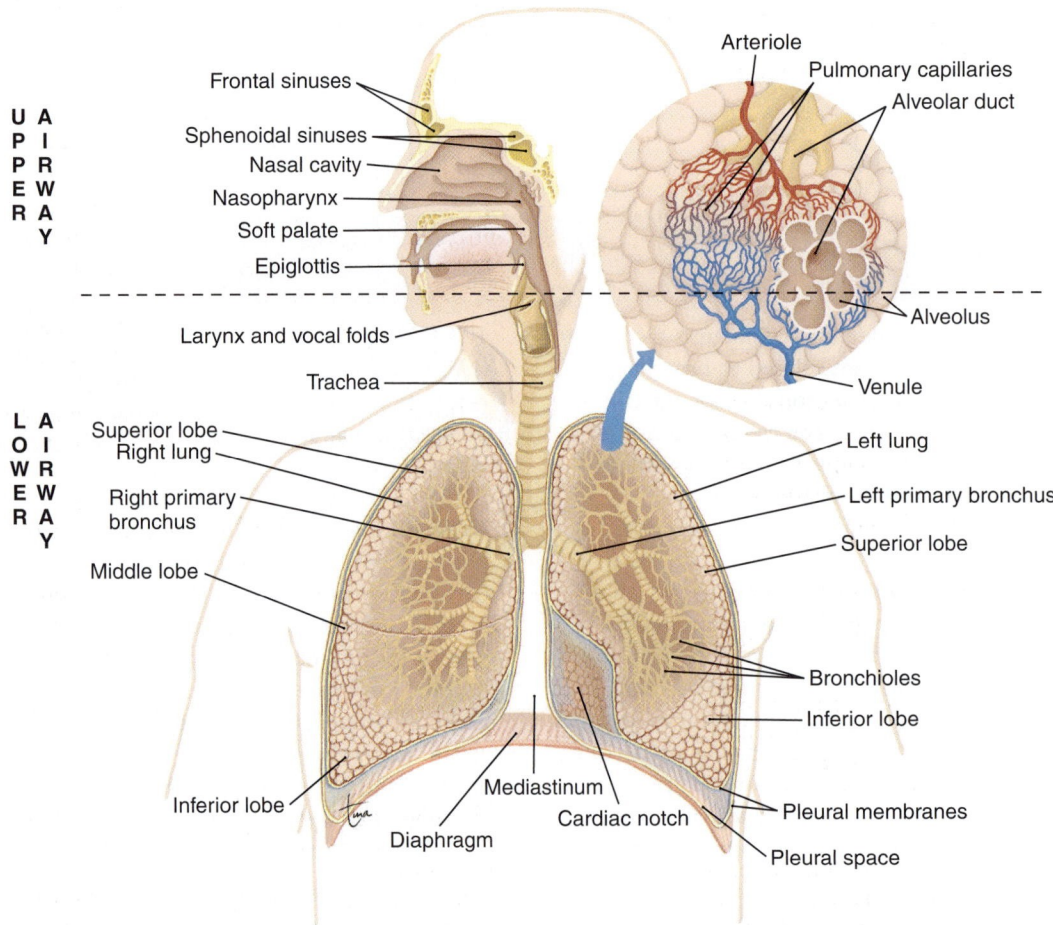

FIGURE 37-1 An anterior view of the respiratory system. The upper airway lies above the larynx. The lower airway, located below the larynx, is considered sterile.

epiglottis, a small flap of tissue superior to the larynx, closes off the trachea during swallowing so that food and fluids do not enter the lower airway. The epiglottis opens during breathing to allow air to move through the airway.

Lower Airway Located below the larynx, the lower airway includes the trachea, bronchi, and bronchioles. The lower airway is considered sterile. The **trachea,** sometimes called the *windpipe,* extends from the larynx to the point at which it divides to form the right and left mainstem bronchi. As the airways branch and become smaller, they have progressively thinner and less cartilage, until it disappears completely in the smaller bronchioles. Spasm of the layers of smooth muscle in the bronchi and bronchioles **(bronchospasm)** narrows the airway and obstructs airflow.

The Lungs

The *lungs* are soft, spongy, cone-shaped organs. They are separated by the **mediastinum,** which contains the heart and great vessels. The right lung has three lobes; the left lung has two lobes. The upper portion of each lung, the *apex,* extends upward above the clavicle. The lower portion of each lung, the *base,* rests on the diaphragm. **KEY POINT:** *Knowing the location of lung tissue beneath the chest wall helps you to perform a complete and accurate assessment of the lungs.*

The lungs are composed of millions of **alveoli**—tiny air sacs with thin walls surrounded by a fine network of capillaries. Gases (oxygen and carbon dioxide) easily pass back and forth between the alveoli and capillaries.

- *Type I alveolar cells* are the gas exchange cells.
- *Type II alveolar cells* produce **surfactant,** a lipoprotein that lowers the surface tension within alveoli to allow them to inflate during breathing.

See Figure 37-2 for an illustration of the alveolar structure.

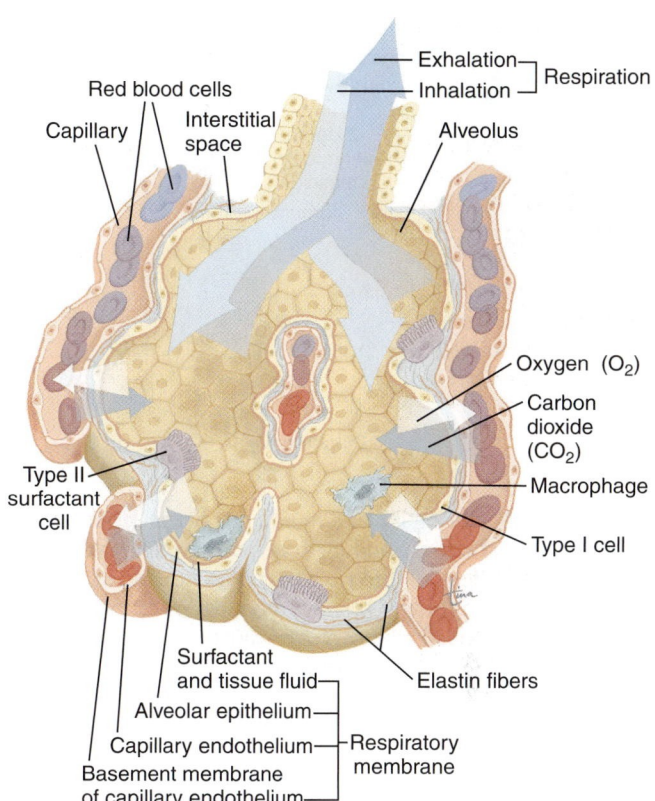

FIGURE 37-2 Alveolar structure showing type I and type II alveolar cells. Type I are the gas exchange cells. Type II produce surfactant.

KnowledgeCheck 37-1

- What happens to inhaled air in the airways? How does this occur?
- In which structures of the lung does gas exchange take place?
- What does surfactant do for alveoli?

 ## ThinkLike a Nurse 37-1

You are assigned to care for an adult patient who has a medical condition with which you are not familiar. You look it up and find that the condition causes a dramatic loss of surfactant. Based on your knowledge of the function of surfactant, what problems is this patient at high risk for developing?

WHAT ARE THE FUNCTIONS OF THE PULMONARY SYSTEM?

Two of the key concepts in this chapter are major processes that occur in the pulmonary system: ventilation and respiration. **Ventilation** is the movement of air into and out of the lungs through the act of breathing. **Respiration** is the exchange of the gases oxygen and carbon dioxide in the lungs.

Pulmonary Ventilation

Oxygenation of the blood, and ultimately of organs and tissues, depends on adequate ventilation. Ventilation must move enough air through the lungs to make adequate oxygen available to the alveoli. Ventilation is accomplished through cycles of inhalation and exhalation.

Inhalation is the expansion of the chest cavity and lungs to negative pressure inside the lungs and causes air to be drawn in through the nose or mouth and airways.

- The *diaphragm* is the major muscle of breathing. When it contracts with each inhalation, the chest cavity is pulled downward, pulling the lung bases downward with it.
- *Intercostal muscles,* the small muscles around the ribs, also contract on inhalation and pull the ribs outward, slightly expanding the chest cavity and lungs.
- The *pleural membrane* covering the lungs adheres ("sticks") to the pleural membrane lining the chest cavity, so the lungs expand.
- Lung expansion creates negative pressure and draws air in through the only opening to the outside, the trachea (Fig. 37-3A).

Exhalation occurs when the diaphragm and intercostal muscles relax, allowing the chest and lungs to return to their normal resting size (Fig. 37-3B). The reduction in size causes the pressure inside the chest and lungs to rise above atmospheric pressure, so air flows out of the lungs. Exhalation requires no energy or effort.

What Factors Affect Ventilation?

The adequacy of ventilation is affected by the rate and depth of respirations, lung compliance and elasticity, and airway resistance.

- **Respiratory rate and depth** are almost self-explanatory: **Rate** is how fast you breathe and **depth** is how much your lungs expand to take in air. These processes affect oxygen and carbon dioxide levels in the blood.

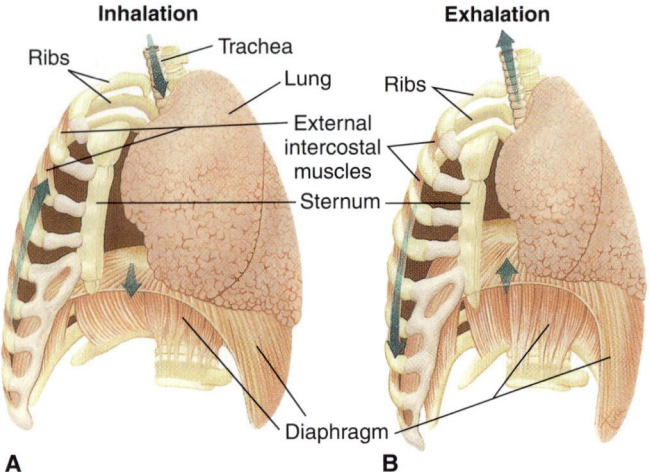

Inhalation

Ribs — Trachea — Lung
External intercostal muscles
Sternum

Exhalation

Ribs

Diaphragm

A   B

FIGURE 37-3 A. During inhalation, the diaphragm contracts, pulling the chest cavity and lung bases downward; the intercostal muscles pull the rib cage up and outward. B. In exhalation, the diaphragm relaxes, the lung bases move upward, and the ribs and intercostal muscles move down and in, resulting in lung compression.

- **Hyperventilation** occurs when a person breathes fast and deeply to move a large amount of air through the lungs, causing too much carbon dioxide to be removed by the alveoli. Mild hyperventilation can occur in response to **hypoxemia** (a low level of oxygen in the blood). When blood oxygen is low, ventilation increases to draw additional air (and oxygen) into the lungs. However, as ventilation increases, carbon dioxide levels fall. Severe hyperventilation is usually triggered by medication, central nervous system abnormalities, high altitude, heat, exercise, panic, fear, or anxiety.
- **Hypoventilation** occurs when a decreased rate or shallow breathing moves only a small amount of air into and out of the lungs. Hypoventilation can lead to hypoxemia because less air (carrying oxygen) reaches the alveoli. The concern is that hypoxemia will lead to **hypoxia** (an oxygen deficiency in the body tissues).
- **Lung compliance** refers to the ease of lung inflation. Normally the lungs inflate easily. Lung compliance is reduced by increased lung water (edema), loss of surfactant, or conditions that cause elastin fibers in the lungs to be replaced with scar tissue (collagen).
- **Lung elasticity** (or elastic recoil) refers to the tendency of the elastin fibers to return to their original position away from the chest wall after being stretched (think of stretching a rubber band, then letting go of it). Alveoli that have been overstretched, as with emphysema, lose their elastic recoil over time. This loss of elasticity allows the lungs to inflate easily but inhibits deflation, leaving stale air trapped in the alveoli.
- **Airway resistance** is the resistance to airflow within the airways. The larger the diameter of the airway, the more easily air moves through it. However, even small decreases in airway diameter (as might occur with secretions in the airway or mild bronchospasm) markedly increase airway resistance. Mary, the little girl with asthma (Meet Your Patients), is undoubtedly experiencing airway resistance.

KnowledgeCheck 37-2

- What is the difference between ventilation and respiration?
- Describe how the diaphragm, accessory muscles, and pressure changes within the lungs create inhalation and exhalation.
- How does hypoventilation affect risk for hypoxemia and hypoxia?

Respiration (Gas Exchange)

Respiration refers to gas exchange, that is, the oxygenation of blood and elimination of carbon dioxide in the lungs. Although nurses commonly use the term *respirations* to mean "breaths" in an assessment of vital signs, strictly speaking this is not accurate: **KEY POINT:** *You cannot measure gas exchange by counting breaths per minute. Gas exchange occurs at two equally essential levels:* **external** *(in the lungs) or* **internal** *(in other body tissues).*

External Respiration (Alveolar–capillary gas exchange)

occurs in the alveoli of the lungs. Oxygen (O_2) diffuses across the alveolar–capillary membrane into the blood of the pulmonary capillaries; carbon dioxide (CO_2) diffuses out of the blood and into the alveoli to be exhaled (Fig. 37-4).

- The *rate of diffusion* depends on the thickness of the membrane and the total surface of lung tissue available for gas exchange. Examples of conditions that slow diffusion are pleural effusion (fluid in the lungs), pneumothorax (lung collapse), and asthma (bronchospasms).
- If blood is not adequately oxygenated in the alveoli, hypoxemia (low blood-oxygen levels) occurs. Getting oxygen into the blood as it flows through the lungs is only the first step in oxygenation.

Internal Respiration (Capillary–Tissue Gas Exchange)

occurs in body organs and tissues. Oxygen diffuses from the blood through the capillary–cellular membrane into the tissue cells, where it is used for metabolism. From the cells, CO_2, a waste product of cellular metabolism, diffuses through the

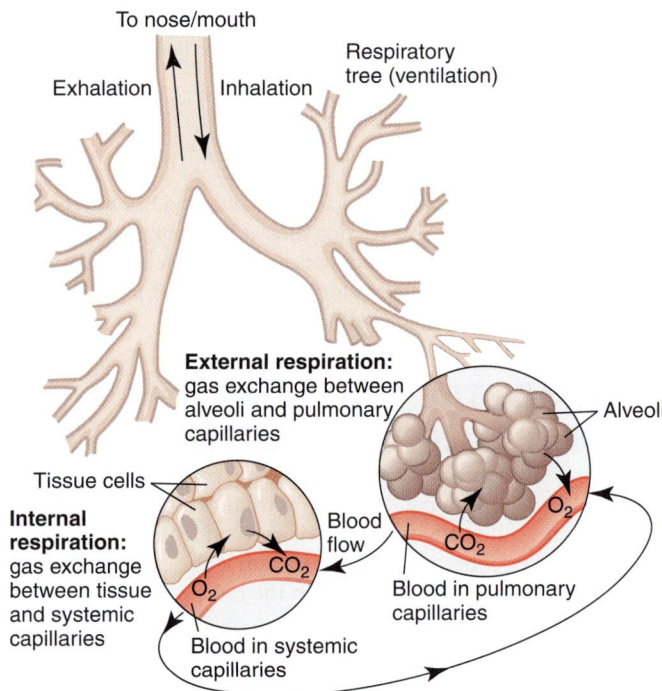

To nose/mouth

Exhalation   Inhalation

Respiratory tree (ventilation)

External respiration: gas exchange between alveoli and pulmonary capillaries

Alveoli

Tissue cells

Internal respiration: gas exchange between tissue and systemic capillaries

Blood flow

O_2 CO_2 O_2 CO_2

Blood in pulmonary capillaries

Blood in systemic capillaries

FIGURE 37-4 External respiration occurs at the alveolar–capillary membrane. Internal respiration occurs at the tissue–capillary membrane.

capillary–cellular membrane into the blood, which transports it to the lungs to be exhaled.

- Tissue oxygenation requires both adequate external respiration and adequate peripheral circulation. Limitations in either function may lead to hypoxia (oxygen deficiency in body tissues).
- In addition, if tissue cells are using more oxygen for metabolism than normal (e.g., during a high fever), hypoxia will occur unless more oxygen is made available to the tissues.

 ThinkLike a Nurse 37-2

William (Meet Your Patients) has a right pneumothorax. Which of the two factors affecting the rate of gas diffusion is causing William to be hypoxemic? If you do not know what a pneumothorax is, look it up.

How Is Breathing Controlled?

The respiratory centers in the brainstem control breathing using feedback from chemoreceptors and lung receptors. Voluntary control from the **motor cortex** can override the involuntary respiratory centers, but only temporarily. This allows a person to continue breathing while doing activities such as talking, singing, swallowing, whistling, and blowing.

- **Chemoreceptors,** located in the medulla of the brainstem, the carotid arteries, and the aorta, detect changes in blood pH, O_2, and CO_2 levels and send messages back to the central respiratory center in the brainstem. In response, the respiratory center increases or decreases ventilation to maintain normal blood levels of pH, O_2 (Po_2), and CO_2 (Pco_2). Normally the blood CO_2 level provides the primary stimulus to breathe.
  - High CO_2 levels stimulate breathing to eliminate the excess CO_2.
  - A secondary, though important, drive to breathe is hypoxemia. Low blood O_2 levels stimulate breathing to get more oxygen into the lungs.
- **Lung receptors,** located in the lung and chest wall, are sensitive to breathing patterns, lung expansion, lung compliance, airway resistance, and respiratory irritants. The respiratory center uses feedback from the lung receptors to adjust ventilation. For example, if the lung receptors sense respiratory irritants such as dust, cold air, or tobacco smoke, the respiratory center triggers airway constriction and a more rapid, shallow pattern of breathing.

KnowledgeCheck 37-3

- Describe two ways in which breathing is controlled.
- The level of which gas (oxygen or carbon dioxide) is the primary stimulant for breathing?

 ThinkLike a Nurse 37-3

A patient has adequate blood oxygen levels, based on a pulse oximeter reading of 98%. Can you conclude that organ and tissue oxygenation is adequate? Explain your thinking.

WHAT EXTERNAL FACTORS AFFECT PULMONARY FUNCTION?

Factors that influence pulmonary function include developmental stage, the environment, individual and lifestyle factors, medications, and pathophysiological states.

Developmental Stage

Normal development influences lung, heart, and circulatory function, all of which affect oxygenation. Developmental factors have less effect on function in young and middle adults than in older adults.

Infants

Premature infants (less than 35 weeks' gestation) do not have a fully developed alveolar surfactant system. Surfactant is the substance that keeps air sacs inflated for effective respiration. Therefore, premature infants are at high risk for **respiratory distress syndrome (RDS)**. RDS is characterized by widespread **atelectasis** (collapse of alveoli). The premature infant also has immature pulmonary circulation. Together with hypoventilation, this leads to hypercarbia (high CO_2 blood levels) and hypoxemia.

Infants born at term are also at risk for oxygenation problems (e.g., infection and airway obstruction) for the following reasons:

- Because the newborn's lower airway structures are immature and small, an infectious agent can spread rapidly.
- The infant's airways are quite narrow in diameter and, therefore, easily obstructed by edema, mucus, or a foreign body, such as meconium passed at birth.
- The central nervous system for preterm, and even some term, infants is immature, leading to periodic breathing patterns and apnea.
- In the first few months of life, the immune system is immature. Although at birth, infants enjoy the benefit of some maternal immunoglobulin circulating in their system, this protection is limited and not sufficient for fighting certain infections.
- By age 6 months, infants can grasp small objects and put them in their mouth. This new skill, combined with small airway diameter, puts them at risk for choking on small objects.

Toddlers

As the toddler's respiratory and immune systems mature, the risk for frequent and serious infections diminishes. However, *upper respiratory infections* (URIs) remain common because (1) the tonsils and adenoids are relatively large, predisposing to tonsillitis, and (2) many children are exposed to new infectious agents in preschool and day care. Most children recover from URIs without difficulty.

Toddlers actively explore the environment and often put objects in their mouths, which puts them at risk for:

- *Acquiring and transmitting infections* from toys and other objects.
- *Airway obstruction* from aspiration of small objects (e.g., candy, buttons, coins, peanuts, grapes). The toddler's airway is still relatively short and small and therefore easily obstructed.
- *Drowning* in very small amounts of water around the home (e.g., in a bucket of water or toilet bowl).

Preschool and School-Age Children

Preschool and school-age children have developed mature lungs, heart, and circulatory systems that can adapt to moderate stress and change. Healthy children typically have bouts of tonsillitis or URIs, which usually resolve without difficulty. Viral infections, such as croup and pneumonia, are common, especially in preschoolers and younger school-age children. Exercise-induced (and other) asthma is also a problem. Unfortunately, as early as middle school, children may begin social habits, such as tobacco use, that can have long-term adverse effects on oxygenation in both the pulmonary and cardiovascular systems.

Adolescents

In adolescence, the lungs develop adult characteristics. The average adolescent is developmentally at little risk for lung diseases. Some may, however, be developing behaviors and habits that can create risk throughout life.

- As do adults, young people often begin smoking for social reasons (e.g., peer pressure, advertising, desire to feel cool), but nicotine addiction perpetuates the habit.
- The use of e-cigarettes is becoming more common. Studies show that they do not deter smoking; rather, they contribute to nicotine addiction.
- Adolescents make fewer routine healthcare visits than do younger children, and as a result may not receive the recommended influenza vaccines.
- And finally, exercise-induced asthma is still a problem in this age-group.

Young, Middle, and Older Adults

Unhealthful practices (e.g., smoking and a lack of aerobic exercise) often continue from adolescence, or they may begin in, adulthood. About one in five U.S. adults is a cigarette smoker ("Vital Signs," 2011). About two-thirds of adults who smoke were regular smokers by their 18th birthday (U.S. Department of Health and Human Services, Public Health Service, 2014).

Changes in the respiratory system that begin in middle age may become significant when the person experiences stressors such as infection, surgery, anesthesia, and emotional problems. The number of cells and the efficiency of the organs decline in a subtle and progressive way as a person ages. Keep in mind, though, that endurance training and regular exercise minimize the rate of these changes. In fact, an older person who is physically conditioned by regular exercise may have better lung function than a younger adult who is not well conditioned.

Older adults tend to experience the following changes:

- *Reduced lung expansion and less alveolar inflation, especially in the bases of the lungs.* This is because (1) costal cartilage begins to calcify, reducing chest wall movement during breathing; (2) the lungs have less recoil ability; and (3) the alveoli lose elasticity.
- *Difficulty expelling mucus or foreign material* because of a less effective cough reflex, drier mucus, and fewer cilia in the airways.
- *Diminished ability to increase ventilation* when oxygenation demands increase (e.g., with exercise). As diaphragm strength decreases, vital capacity is reduced; therefore, exhalation becomes less efficient, causing progressive air trapping.
- *Declining immune response,* especially cell-mediated immunity, T-cell activity, and the inflammatory response.
- *Gastroesophageal reflux disease* is more common in older adults, creating a risk for aspirating stomach contents into the lungs. This may result in an inflammatory response.
- *Chemoreceptors* that control breathing respond more slowly to increased O_2 demand or rising levels of CO_2, making hypoxemia more likely when respiratory problems occur.

    All of these changes put older adults at risk for respiratory infections. URIs that would be mild and short lived in a younger person may quickly lead to pneumonia in an older adult.

Environment

This section will discusses environmental factors that affect oxygenation.

Stress The stress response stimulates the release of catecholamines from the sympathetic nervous system, resulting in (1) increased tendency of blood to clot (e.g., as in pulmonary embolus), and (2) suppression of the immune system and inflammatory response. A chronically suppressed immune and inflammatory response increases the risk for all infections, including respiratory.

For additional information on the effects of stress, see Chapter 12.

Allergic Reactions An **allergy** is a hypersensitivity, or overresponse, to an antigen. Pulmonary allergens include such things as dust, dust mites, cockroach particles, pollen, molds, newsprint, tobacco smoke, animal dander, and sometimes foods.

- **Hay fever** is an allergic reaction affecting the eyes, nose, and/or sinuses. It causes the release of *histamine,* which is largely responsible for accumulation of nasal fluid; swollen nasal membranes; nasal congestion; and itchy, swollen, watery eyes. Antihistamines are effective in combating hay fever.
- **Asthma** is an allergic reaction occurring in the bronchioles of the lungs. *Slow reacting substance of anaphylaxis* (SRS-A) is released, which causes bronchoconstriction and lower airway edema and spasms, making breathing difficult and ineffective. Because histamine is not a major factor in causing the asthmatic reaction, antihistamines have little effect in the treatment of asthma. Asthma is the most common serious chronic disease of childhood, and it can be life threatening.

Air Quality Air pollution triggers respiratory problems (e.g., lung cancer, carbon monoxide poisoning) that interfere with oxygenation. Even healthy people may experience headache, coughing, and other symptoms when exposed to air pollution. People with existing respiratory disease may become unable to function. Some sources of air pollution are natural (e.g., forest fires), but the most common and damaging sources result from human activities (e.g., automobile exhaust emissions). Indoor air pollutants include carbon monoxide, nitrogen oxides, radon, and suspended particles (e.g., dust, mold spores, aerosols, and tobacco smoke). Pollutants are most harmful to infants, toddlers, older adults, and people with heart or lung disease.

Altitude Atmospheric pressure falls from 760 mm Hg at sea level to 523 mm Hg at 10,000 feet. As the atmospheric pressure decreases, the partial pressure of oxygen also decreases. The decreased partial pressure makes it harder for the oxygen molecules to cross the alveolar membrane and get into the bloodstream and can cause hypoxemia and hypoxia. The percentage of molecules of oxygen in the air does not change with altitude, but the molecules are more spread out, so fewer are inhaled with each breath. If a person is suddenly exposed to low oxygen levels, arterial chemoreceptors stimulate ventilation, making more oxygen available in the alveoli and at the tissue level.

Over a long period, people who live at high altitudes undergo physiological changes that facilitate oxygenation, including an increase in the following:

- Ventilation, which brings more oxygen into the lungs
- Production of red blood cells (RBCs), which aids in the transport of oxygen to organs and tissues
- Lung volume and pulmonary vasculature, resulting in increased surface area for alveolar–capillary gas exchange
- Vascularity of body tissues allowing for improved oxygen delivery to the tissues

- Production of hemoglobin, which readily binds with oxygen so that the tissue cells can use oxygen even when oxygen pressure is low in the environment

Lifestyle

The following lifestyle factors affect oxygenation:

Pregnancy During pregnancy, oxygen demand increases dramatically. Maternal metabolism increases by approximately 15% during the last half of pregnancy, increasing the demand for O_2. At the same time, the enlarging uterus pushes upward against the diaphragm, limiting its downward movement. In response, the maternal respiratory rate increases in order to increase minute ventilation (amount of air moved into and out of the lungs in 1 minute) (Hall, 2015).

Occupational Hazards Occupational hazards may affect pulmonary function by irritating airways or causing cancer. Toxic agents may be categorized as follows:

- *Chemicals and their fumes* irritate the sensitive membranous lining of the lungs and airways and may lead to lung cancer or leukemia. Even common household cleaners can emit toxic fumes.
- *Products of combustion* (e.g., carbon monoxide) are known causes of lung cancer and chronic lung disease.
- *Microorganisms,* such as viruses, fungi, and mold, may lead to infections and precipitate asthma.
- *Fine particles* (e.g., coal dust and asbestos) suspended in the air can be inhaled into the smallest airways, causing irritation and toxic reactions, including cancer.

Nutrition The body needs an appropriate balance of proteins, carbohydrates, fats, and other nutrients for proper immune function. A healthy diet builds resistance to disease and infection, promotes normal cellular function and tissue repair, and maintains a healthy weight. Poor nutrition, especially in those with pulmonary disorders, can lead to loss of ventilatory muscle strength, making breathing more difficult.

Obesity is defined as a body mass index (BMI) above 30. Obesity causes certain health problems that affect pulmonary function. The following are two examples:

- *Respiratory infections.* Excess abdominal fat presses upward on the diaphragm, preventing full chest expansion, leading to hypoventilation and dyspnea on exertion. The risk for respiratory infection then increases because lower lung lobes are poorly ventilated and secretions not removed effectively.
- *Sleep apnea.* When the person lies down, chest expansion is limited even more. Excess neck girth and fat deposits in the upper airway often lead to obstructive sleep apnea, a condition characterized by daytime sleepiness, snoring, and periods of apnea lasting 10 to 120 seconds (Porth & Matfin, 2013).

Exercise Exercise increases metabolic demands. The body responds by increasing the heart rate and the rate and depth of breathing. Lack of exercise has the opposite effect. A sedentary lifestyle reduces the capacity to increase ventilation in response to exercise.

Substance Abuse People abuse various kinds of substances, including prescription medications.

- *Prescription medications.* Excess use or overdose of respiratory depressants, such as opioids, sedatives, anti-anxiety agents, and hypnotics, can cause hypoventilation, apnea, and respiratory failure, in some instances resulting in death.
- *Over-the-counter (OTC) medications* and other legally available products, such as alcohol, tobacco, caffeine, glue, aerosols, "bath salts" (a stimulant and hallucinogenic), and other inhalants, also have abuse potential and can be lethal.

Large amounts of alcohol, for example, depress respiratory and vasomotor centers of the brain.

- *Illicit drugs,* including stimulants (e.g., amphetamines, cocaine), hallucinogens (e.g., LSD, PCP), marijuana, and in some states "bath salts," also have adverse effects on the respiratory system. And of course, an overdose of these substances can depress respirations and increase the risk for aspiration.

Smoking

Tobacco smoke contains tiny particles of tar and approximately 200 known toxic chemicals, more than 60 of which are known to cause cancer. Tobacco smoke:

- Constricts bronchioles
- Increases fluid secretion into the airways
- Causes inflammation and swelling of the bronchial lining
- Paralyzes cilia

These effects lead to reduced airflow and increased production of secretions that are not easily removed from the airways. Lung inflammation stimulates the release of enzymes that break down elastin and other alveolar wall components. Continued smoking leads to chronic bronchitis, obstruction of bronchioles and alveolar walls, and emphysema. Cigarette smoking is estimated to be the cause of more than 80% of cases of lung cancer. **KEY POINT:** *The longer a person smokes and the more cigarettes he smokes, the greater the risk for cancer and other chronic lung diseases. (Centers for Disease Control and Prevention, n.d.c, reviewed 2016).*

Roughly one in five American adults smokes. However, once a person stops smoking, the body begins to repair the damage. In the first few days, the person will cough more as the cilia begin to clear the airways. Then the coughing subsides, and breathing becomes easier. Even long-time smokers can benefit from smoking cessation (Box 37-1).

Secondhand Smoke, also known as **environmental tobacco smoke (ETS),** is a general term for any smoke to which nonsmokers are exposed. There are two types of second-hand smoke:

- **Mainstream smoke** refers to the smoke that a smoker inhales and then exhales.
- **Side-stream smoke** refers to the smoke released from the burning tip of a cigarette, cigar, or pipe. Side-stream smoke has been found to account for about 85% of the ETS in a smoky room, so although it is no worse for you than mainstream smoke, it makes up the bulk of smoke that nonsmokers may encounter.

The Environmental Protection Agency classifies second-hand smoke as a Group A carcinogen, meaning it is a substance known to cause cancer in humans. There is no safe level of exposure to secondhand smoke. Even short exposure can make blood platelets stickier, causing damage to blood vessel lining and disturbing the heart rate. Secondhand smoke leads to death from cancer and health disease and has been linked to cerebral vascular accidents (stroke). Children younger than 18 months are especially vulnerable to lower respiratory tract infections related to secondhand smoke (American Lung Association, n.d.).

KnowledgeCheck 37-4

- What are the major risks to oxygenation related to developmental factors?
- What environmental and lifestyle factors that influence ventilation can be avoided or minimized?

BOX 37-1 ■ Health Effects of Smoking Cessation

- Life expectancy increases.
- Blood pressure and heart rate decrease.
- Circulation to the extremities improves within 2 hours.
- Carbon dioxide levels in the blood begin to drop within 4 hours.
- Oxygen levels in the blood begin to improve within 8 hours.
- Digestion improves.
- Coughing, congestion, and shortness of breath decrease.
- Overall energy increases.
- Lungs increase ability to clean themselves, thereby reducing the risk of infection.
- Risk of heart attack decreases and returns to that of a nonsmoker in 1 year.
- Risk of lung and other cancers, stroke, and chronic obstructive lung disease decreases.

KEY POINT: Healthy People 2020 (2010) *identified the goal of reducing illness, disability, and death related to tobacco use and secondhand smoke exposure by establishing policies to reduce exposure to secondhand smoke, increase the cost of tobacco, restrict tobacco advertising, and reduce illegal sales to minors.*

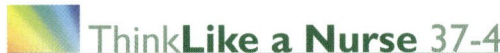

ThinkLike a Nurse 37-4

Review the Meet Your Patients scenario at the beginning of this chapter.

- Which patient(s) may be experiencing developmental, environmental, or lifestyle-related problems with oxygenation?
- Identify any additional information you need to know to answer this question.

Medications

Many drugs can interfere with pulmonary function by depressing respirations. Respiratory depressants generally act by depressing central nervous system (CNS) control of breathing or by weakening the muscles of breathing. They include general anesthetics, opioids (e.g., morphine), anti-anxiety drugs (e.g., diazepam), sedative-hypnotics (e.g., barbiturates), neuromuscular blocking agents, and magnesium sulfate. Drugs that block beta-2 adrenergic receptors (e.g., used to lower the blood pressure) have little effect on healthy lungs but can lead to serious bronchiole constriction in people with asthma.

Medications are also used to improve respiratory function. A few examples are bronchodilators, anti-inflammatory agents such as corticosteroids, cough suppressants, expectorants, and decongestants (see Table 37-1).

Table 37-1 ▶ Respiratory Medications that Promote Ventilation and Oxygenation

CLASS COMMENTS	ACTION	EXAMPLES AND COMMENTS
Bronchodilators	■ Relax the smooth muscles lining the airways. ■ Can be administered as oral or inhaled medicines.	Beta-2 adrenergic agonists Anticholinergics Methylxanthine
Respiratory Anti-Inflammatory Agents	■ Combat inflammation in the airways. ■ Important in treating and controlling respiratory conditions characterized by hypersensitive airways and airway inflammation (e.g., asthma).	Corticosteroids Cromolyn Leukotriene modifiers
Nasal Decongestants	■ Relieve stuffy, blocked nasal passages by constricting local blood vessels through stimulation of alpha-1 adrenergic nerve receptors in the vessels. ■ Although the desired effect is on the nasal mucosa, these medications can have systemic adrenergic effects causing elevated blood pressure, tachycardia, and palpitations, especially in those with a history of cardiovascular conditions.	Ephedrine Pseudoephedrine Phenylephrine
Antihistamines	■ Prevent the effects of histamine release. ■ Used to treat upper respiratory and nasal allergy symptoms.	Diphenhydramine Chlorpheniramine Brompheniramine Loratadine Fexofenadine Cetirizine
Cough Preparations	■ *Antitussives* (cough suppressants) reduce the frequency of an involuntary, hacking, nonproductive cough. ■ *Expectorants* help make coughing more productive. ■ The goal is to reduce the frequency of dry, unproductive coughing while making voluntary coughing more productive.	These agents are often found mixed together in one preparation to achieve both desirable effects with one medication.

WHAT PATHOPHYSIOLOGICAL CONDITIONS ALTER GAS EXCHANGE?

Poor exchange of oxygen and carbon dioxide at the alveolar–capillary membrane changes the levels of O_2 and CO_2 in the blood. Unchecked, it affects oxygenation in tissues and organs and can be life threatening. Box 37-2 describes some alterations in gas exchange.

Alterations in gas exchange are caused by infections, as well as a number of disorders that affect the structure, function, and regulation of the pulmonary and cardiovascular systems. Because it is difficult to separate pulmonary and cardiovascular causes and effects, both are included in the following discussion of pulmonary disorders. For a thorough description of these diseases and pathological conditions, consult a medical–surgical nursing text.

KnowledgeCheck 37-5

- What are some indirect indicators of tissue oxygenation?
- How are hyperventilation and hypoventilation related to carbon dioxide levels?
- What are the effects of carbon dioxide levels on the nervous system?

 ThinkLike a Nurse 37-5

You are assessing a very anxious young man who looks frightened and is complaining of having trouble breathing. His respiratory rate is 32 breaths/min and deep. He states his fingers and hands are numb.

- What is the most likely cause?
- What blood levels would help you clarify what is going on?

Respiratory Infections

Respiratory infections are any infection of the sinuses, throat, airways, or lungs. Respiratory infections are one of the main reasons why people visit their primary care provider. The common cold is the most widespread. Respiratory infections are usually caused by viruses, but can be caused by bacteria.

Example Problem: URI and Influenza

Upper respiratory infections (URIs) are among the most common causes of short-term disability in the United States. Diagnosis is difficult because many other conditions begin with cold-like symptoms (e.g., allergies, measles, and pneumonia). Colds are more common in children and tend to be less frequent in adults. They are rarely dangerous to healthy adults and children. The following are some URIs:

- **The common cold**—nonspecific upper respiratory infections caused by viruses.
- **Rhinosinusitis**—inflammation of the nasal mucosa and sinus cavities. Differentiating viral from bacterial sinusitis cannot be done on the basis of clinical findings alone.
- **Pharyngitis**—sore throat. Pharyngitis may be viral or bacterial. "Strep" throat, caused by *Streptococcus pyogenes*, is the most common cause of infectious pharyngitis. It cannot be differentiated from a viral sore throat by any one sign or symptom, so pharyngeal cultures or rapid antigen tests are conducted.
- **Influenza**—is usually more severe than the common cold and often involves the lower airways—although some types may not. Most flu fatalities occur in children under age 2 and older adults, especially the frail elderly.
  See the Example Problem: URI and Influenza.

Infections of the Lower Airways

Lower respiratory tract infections (including acute bronchitis, pneumonia, and tuberculosis) occur more often in children, older adults, and those with impaired immunity or lung function.

Respiratory Syncytial Virus (RSV) can affect the upper respiratory tract and the lower airways. Healthy people usually recover from RSV infection in 1 or 2 weeks. However, RSV can be severe in infants, young children, and older adults. Almost all children have had an RSV infection by the age of

---

BOX 37-2 ■ Alterations in Gas Exchange

Hypoxemia—Low arterial blood oxygen levels.
Etiology: Poor oxygen diffusion across the alveolar–capillary membrane into the blood (ineffective external respiration) as a result of lung or pulmonary circulation disorders. Hypoventilation predisposes to the development of hypoxemia and may lead to hypoxia.
Comments: Even if the blood is adequately oxygenated, hypoxia may still occur in the organs and tissues because of poor circulation.

Hypoxia—Inadequate oxygenation of organs and tissues.
Etiology: Either hypoxemia or circulatory disorders.
Comments: The effects of hypoxia depend on the organs affected. For example:
- Hypoxic central nervous system tissue causes abnormal brain functioning (e.g., altered level of consciousness).
- Hypoxic renal tissue causes abnormal kidney functioning (e.g., poor urine output).
- Hypoxic limb tissue results in abnormal muscle functioning (e.g., muscle weakness and pain with exercise).

Hypercarbia (hypercapnia)—An excess of dissolved CO_2 in the blood.
Etiology: Hypoventilation is caused by abnormalities affecting the lungs or chest cavity or by neuromuscular abnormalities that interfere with normal breathing. Hypercarbia can occur suddenly, as in acute airway obstruction or drug overdose, or chronically, as in chronic lung disease.
Comments: Very high blood levels of CO_2 have an anesthetic effect on the nervous system and can lead to somnolence progressing to coma and death, a syndrome known as carbon dioxide narcosis.

Hypocarbia (hypocapnia)—A low level of dissolved CO_2 in the blood. In most cases (except high altitude), blood O_2 levels remain normal.
Etiology: Hyperventilation.
Comments: Severe hypocarbia stimulates the nervous system, leading to muscle twitching or spasm (especially in the hands and feet) and numbness and tingling in the face and lips.

EXAMPLE PROBLEM: URI and Influenza

Definition: Infection of the upper airways. URIs and influenza are caused by viruses.

Symptoms
- Cold-like symptoms: stuffy nose, sore throat, cough, sneezing, tearing, and a mild fever

- In addition to cold-like symptoms, the person with influenza may experience headache, muscle pain, fatigue, weakness, exhaustion, and high fever.
- **KEY POINT:** *The flu virus is highly contagious.*

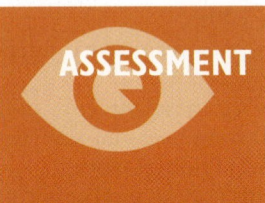
ASSESSMENT

- Assess for risk factors (e.g., contact with an infected person within the past 72 hours).
- Ask about immunization for influenza.
- Assess for history of fever and chills, hoarseness, laryngitis, sore throat, rhinitis, or rhinorrhea.
- Inspect the patient's throat for redness of the soft palate, tonsils, and pharynx.

- Palpate for enlargement of the anterior cervical lymph nodes.
- Assess for an increase in patient temperature.
- Assess for respiratory rate, which may be increased.
- Auscultate the patient's lungs.

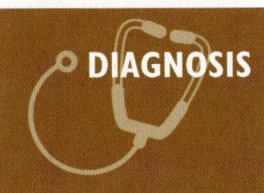
DIAGNOSIS

KEY POINT: *URIs and influenza begin with similar symptoms. It is important to distinguish between them because antiviral medications are available for the flu; they are not effective for colds.*

NANDA-I Diagnoses
- **Ineffective Airway Clearance** related to tracheobronchial and nasal secretions

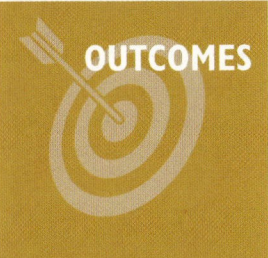
OUTCOMES

NOC Outcomes
- Discomfort Level
- Respiratory Status: Airway Patency
- Rest
- Vital Signs

Individualized Goals
- Patient will be free of infection as demonstrated by:
  - Breath sounds clear to auscultation

- Abating cough
- Respiratory status parameters with optimal air exchange
- Temperature < 99.0°F

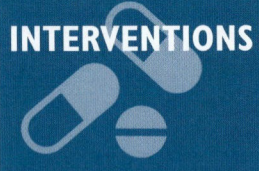
INTERVENTIONS

Influenza: KEY POINT: Prevention Is Key. *The most effective strategy for preventing influenza is annual vaccination. The Centers for Disease Control and Prevention has recently recommended universal vaccination—that is, that all people aged 6 months and older receive annual influenza vaccination.*
- Encourage fluid intake.
- Encourage rest.
- Administer medications (antipyretics, antibiotics, antiviral agents) as ordered.
- Instruct patient to take prescription medications as ordered.

- ▪ ✚ Teach clients that antibiotics should be used only as prescribed for diagnosed bacterial infections. This includes taking the full course of prescribed antibiotics, even if symptoms are no longer present. Antibiotics are not without risks, and they are not effective for treating the common cold. Do not pressure clinicians for prescriptions, and do not take antibiotics from previous prescriptions.

Colds: Teach patient and family members how to avoid infection.
- Avoid others who are sick.
- Avoid close contact with others, such as hugging, kissing, or shaking hands.
- Move away from people before coughing or sneezing.
- Cough and sneeze into a tissue and then throw it away, or cough and sneeze into your upper shirt sleeve, completely covering your mouth and nose.
- Wash your hands after coughing, sneezing, or blowing your nose.
- Disinfect frequently touched surfaces and objects such as toys and doorknobs.
- Practice healthy behaviors:
  - Balanced diet
  - Adequate rest
  - Daily exercise

EVALUATION

- Monitor for improved respiratory status.
- Monitor body temperature.

- Monitor for complications (dehydration, pneumonia).

2 years (Centers for Disease Control and Prevention, 2008b). It is spread by airborne droplets and by direct and indirect contact with infected persons, and can survive on hard surfaces for many hours.

Acute Bronchitis is an infection of the bronchi, causing bronchial irritation and inflammation and leading to coughing and mild airway obstruction. The bronchi are inflamed, but with no evidence of pneumonia, common cold, or asthma. Bronchitis may be viral or bacterial. Symptoms include fever, cough, chills, malaise, and chest wall pain from coughing. In bacterial infections, the cough is productive, with yellow to green sputum. In viral infections, the cough is nonproductive and aggravated by cold, dry, or dusty air and may cause prolonged bouts of continuous coughing.

Tuberculosis (TB) is an infection caused by the acid-fast bacillus *Mycobacterium tuberculosis*. Although TB is commonly thought of as a respiratory disease, infection may occur anywhere in the body. Historically, TB was a major cause of death and disability in North America. TB was almost eradicated after 1950 because of the use of effective antibiotics. However, the incidence is rising again because of (1) the growing number of drug-resistant strains and (2) the number of people with compromised immune responses (related to aging and disease).

- **Transmission and infection.** Pulmonary TB is transmitted via airborne droplets, which may occur in overcrowded, poorly ventilated living conditions. Once inhaled into the lungs, the TB bacteria are usually walled off through the inflammatory response into granulomatous lesions. Immunity develops, and the bacteria either can remain walled off and dormant or can escape and cause active tuberculosis, especially in someone with impaired immunity.
- **Symptoms.** Common signs and symptoms include fatigue, weight loss, anorexia, night sweats, and blood-tinged sputum.
- **Diagnosis.** TB diagnosis is made via sputum cultures or chest x-ray changes.
- **Collaborative treatment.** Medications are the cornerstone of tuberculosis treatment. Treating TB takes much longer than treating other types of bacterial infections; antibiotics must be taken for at least 6 to 9 months. The exact drugs and length of treatment depend on age, overall health, possible drug resistance, the form of TB (latent or active), and the infection's location in the body.

Pneumonia is an infection of the lungs caused by bacteria, fungi, viruses, or rarely parasites. It occurs more often during winter months and often follows a recent upper respiratory tract infection or influenza. For more information, refer to the Example Problem: Pneumonia.

Other Disorders Affecting Gas Exchange

In addition to respiratory infections, gas exchange may be altered by disorders in the pulmonary system, the pulmonary circulation, the central nervous system, and the neuromuscular system.

Pulmonary System Abnormalities

The following is a brief discussion of various pulmonary system abnormalities that can lead to alterations in gas exchange:

Structural Abnormalities Structural abnormalities include anything that restricts or limits the free movement of the chest wall (e.g., fractured ribs, kyphosis), interruptions in the chest cavity that inhibit inflation of the lungs (e.g., pneumothorax), or a collection of fluid (blood, lymph, pus) in the pleural space that inhibits lung expansion.

Airway Inflammation and Obstruction Allergic reactions (e.g., asthma) or irritation from smoke or other irritants may cause airway inflammation. Obstruction may be mechanical, as with a foreign object or bolus of food, or due to spasm (e.g., laryngospasm). Swollen tonsils and a swollen epiglottis may also cause obstruction.

Alveolar–Capillary Membrane Disorders These disorders are characterized by a change in the consistency of the lung tissue, especially at the alveolar level. The alveoli become stiff and difficult to ventilate, and gas exchange is impaired. Pulmonary edema, acute respiratory distress syndrome, and pulmonary fibrosis are examples.

Atelectasis Anything that reduces ventilation (e.g., tumor, obstructed airway) can cause atelectasis, or alveolar collapse.

Pulmonary Circulation Abnormalities

For gas exchange to occur in the alveoli, there must be adequate blood flow through the pulmonary circulation. The most common causes of impaired pulmonary circulation are pulmonary embolus and pulmonary hypertension.

- A **pulmonary embolus** is obstruction of pulmonary arterial circulation by a foreign substance (e.g., a blood clot, air, or fat).
- **Pulmonary hypertension** is elevated pressure within the pulmonary arterial system. High pressure increases the workload of the heart. Over time, this causes right-sided heart failure, with a reduced amount of blood pumped into the pulmonary circulation. You will learn about the difference between right-sided and left-sided heart failure in a medical–surgical nursing course.

Central Nervous System Abnormalities

Any condition that injures or alters the function of the CNS can interfere with the regulation of breathing and, therefore, gas exchange.

- Trauma and stroke (cerebrovascular accident) are the most commonly seen CNS problems in adults.
- Spinal cord injuries interfere with nerve transmission between the brain and the area below the level of the injury and may, for example, limit diaphragm function.
- Immature breathing patterns, such as apnea or periodic breathing, are common in preterm and term infants.

Neuromuscular Abnormalities

Neuromuscular abnormalities can affect gas exchange by interfering with the regulation of breathing or by limiting movement of the muscles involved with breathing. Trauma, stroke, and medications are the most common causes. Neuromuscular disorders that affect the nerves involved in breathing can also depress respiratory function (e.g., Guillain-Barré syndrome, amyotrophic lateral sclerosis, and myasthenia gravis).

KnowledgeCheck 37-6

- Identify four pathophysiological conditions that affect pulmonary function. How are they similar? How are they different?
- What types of injuries are most likely to cause oxygenation problems?

EXAMPLE PROBLEM: Pneumonia

Definition: Infection of the lungs caused by bacteria, fungi, or viruses

Characteristics/Symptoms: Cough, malaise, pleural pain from coughing, discolored sputum, fever, chills, dyspnea, elevated WBC counts

KEY POINT: *Pneumonia is a leading cause of infectious death in the United States, with a mortality rate of about 50% in people older than age 65.*

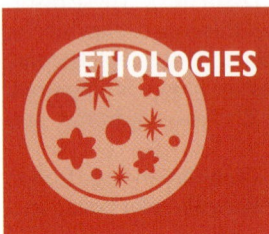 **ETIOLOGIES**

Transmission: Organisms gain entry to the lungs (1) through the air (after being expelled by coughing, sneezing, or talking); (2) from contaminated respiratory equipment; (3) from spreading to the lung via the blood; (3) or from the nose and throat.

Pathophysiology: Full-scale inflammatory response triggers edema in the small airways and deposits debris and exudate in the alveoli. The affected area of the lung becomes **consolidated** (solid rather than air filled).

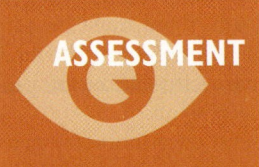 **ASSESSMENT**

- Obtain history of:
  - Immunization
  - Fever and chills, cough, pleural pain, discolored sputum, dyspnea, shortness of breath, malaise
- Auscultate the lungs.
- Diagnostic tests:
  - Blood tests
  - Chest x-ray

- Sputum culture
- Pulse oximetry
- Observe sputum for color, consistency, amount.
- Observe for and describe any cough.
- Obtain the temperature (may be elevated).
- Observe for increased respiratry rate and difficulty breathing.

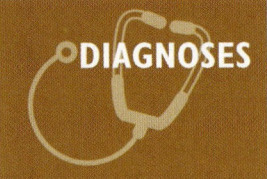 **DIAGNOSES**

Impaired gas exchange

Ineffective breathing pattern

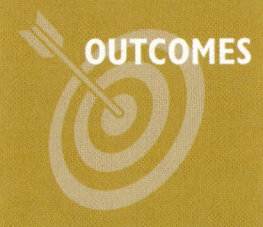 **OUTCOMES**

- Demonstrates adequate oxygenation (activity tolerance, O_2 saturation, mucous membrane color).
- Respiratory rate and depth at baseline

- Temperature ≤ 99°F (37°C)
- Lungs clear to auscultation

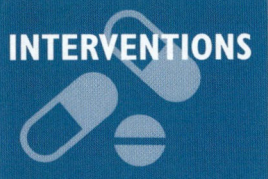 **INTERVENTIONS**

- Humidity, to moisten inhaled air
- Hydration, to thin secretions
- Rest, to conserve body energy stores
- Position patient for ease of breathing.
- Pulmonary hygiene (deep breathing, coughing, and chest percussion and vibration), to move secretions out of the airways

  Note: Also see the section "Prevent Healthcare-Associated Pneumonia"

Prevention

Immunization for high-risk groups including the following (CDC, 2012a):
- Adults aged 65 years or older
- Children younger than age 5 years

- Children aged 6 through 18 years who have certain medical conditions
- People aged 2 through 64 years who have chronic illnesses (e.g., those with heart disease, diabetes, pulmonary disease, alcoholism, HIV infection) or lowered resistance to infection
- Adults aged 19 through 64 years who have asthma or are smokers

EXAMPLE PROBLEM: Pneumonia—cont'd

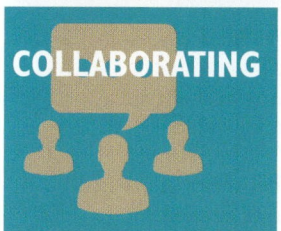

COLLABORATING

- Antipyretics, for fever
- Expectorants, to enhance mobilization of secretions

- Curative therapy includes appropriate anti-infective agents
- Oxygen therapy, if needed

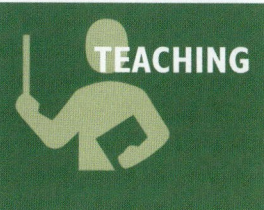

TEACHING

- Avoid infection.
- Eat well-balanced meals.
- Get adequate rest.
- Exercise.
- Avoid smoking.
- Avoid others with upper respiratory infections.

- Get prompt treatment for early symptoms.
- Drink large amounts of fluids to thin secretions and replace fluid loss.
- Avoid spread of infections by washing hands and properly disposing of tissues.
- Wash hands frequently.

ThinkLike a Nurse 37-6

You are the nursing supervisor on the night shift in a small community hospital. At the beginning of the shift, you have only one critical care bed available. During your shift, you receive calls for assistance on the following patients:

- Patient A has burns on her face, scalp, and chest and is coughing up sputum with black streaks.
- Patient B has pneumonia and has suddenly become confused.
- Patient C is short of breath and complaining that he can't breathe. His skin is cool and moist, and he is coughing up clear sputum with small bubbles in it.

Which patient would you admit to the critical care bed? Why?

♥ iCare 37-1

Oxygenation

- Experiencing **inadequate oxygenation** is very frightening. Anxiety, fear, and panic can set in very quickly.
- Use a calm and confident approach when performing interventions to promote optimal respiratory function.
- Provide emotional support and comfort during episodes of deoxygenation to help alleviate fear.
- Sit down and look the patient in the eye. Speak calmly and keep the patient informed of what you are doing— for example, *Mr. Brown, I realize you are having trouble breathing right now, but you have had a nebulizer treatment. I am here with you. Let's take some deep breaths together and relax. I will recheck your respiratory status and oxygenation level in a few minutes.*
- Hold the person's hand, practice therapeutic touch, and sit with him while providing interventions.

PracticalKnowledge knowing **how**

In the remainder of the chapter, we discuss focused respiratory assessment and the nursing activities to maximize ventilation and gas exchange. In Chapter 19, the section "Respirations" provides information about assessing respirations. Also see Procedure 19-5: Assessing Respirations.

ASSESSMENT NP

An evaluation of oxygenation includes a history and physical examination to assess lung, heart, and circulatory function. This chapter focuses on the respiratory system. The order of data collection and the priorities of assessment vary with the patient's condition and the purpose of the assessment. For example:

- For someone in obvious respiratory distress, the immediate assessment focus is to ask simple questions about current symptoms while performing a quick examination to determine adequacy of breathing, circulation, and oxygenation.
- For a healthy person, assessment for risk of respiratory disease might include more extensive questions about occupation, smoking habits, and living environment; a medical history; and an extensive physical examination.

For a complete focused respiratory assessment, you will need to identify risk factors, perform a physical examination, and be familiar with certain diagnostic tests.

Assessing for Risk Factors

The health history should include questions about the presence of risk factors that affect lung and airway function. Topics to assess include demographic data, health history, respiratory history, cardiovascular history, environmental history, and lifestyle. For a detailed list of interview questions for each of these topics, see the Focused Assessment box Oxygenation.

Focused Assessment

Oxygenation

Part I. Questions to Assess Risk for Impaired Oxygenation

Demographic Data
➤ What is your age?
➤ Where do you live?
➤ What is your occupation?

Health History
➤ What healthcare problems are you currently being treated for?
➤ Have you ever been hospitalized or had surgery? If so, when and for what reason?
➤ Do you have a history of allergies or asthma?
➤ What medications do you currently take?
➤ What over-the-counter medications or alternative treatments do you use? What do you use them for?

Respiratory History
➤ Have you ever been diagnosed with a respiratory problem? If so, what was the diagnosis? When was the diagnosis made?
➤ Have you noticed any changes in your breathing?
➤ How often do you cough?
➤ When you do cough, is it productive?
➤ What do the secretions you cough up look like and smell like?
➤ How much sputum do you produce?
➤ How do you treat your cough? What effect did it have?
➤ Do you ever wheeze or feel short of breath?
➤ What causes you to wheeze or feel short of breath?
➤ Do body positions affect your breathing pattern?
➤ What position do you lie in when you sleep? Do you use more than one pillow?
➤ Do you ever wake up short of breath?

Environmental History
➤ Are there pets in the house?
➤ What response, if any, do you have to pets, dust, pollen, or plants?
➤ Are you exposed to smoke or fumes in the home and workplace?
➤ Are you exposed to respiratory irritants such as asbestos, chemicals, coal dust, fungus, molds, or soot in the home or workplace?
➤ What type of heating, air-conditioning, or air-filtering system do you have in the home or workplace?

Lifestyle
➤ What is your current stress level? What are your major sources of stress?
➤ What is your usual diet? Is your current diet typical, or have you recently changed your eating habits?
➤ What is your usual activity level?
➤ What level of activity makes you feel short of breath?
➤ Do you smoke now, or have you ever smoked?
➤ If you smoke, how many packs per day and for how many years have you smoked?
➤ Do you smoke marijuana or use other substances?

Part II. Focused Physical Examination

Pulmonary System
➤ *Inspect* to observe respiratory patterns, signs of respiratory distress, chest structures and movement, skin and mucous membrane color, presence or absence of edema, sputum characteristics, and overall general appearance.
➤ *Palpate* skin temperature and areas of tenderness.
➤ *Percuss* over the lung fields (for consolidation or excess air pockets).
➤ *Auscultate* breath sounds and vascular sounds.
➤ *Assess breathing patterns:* eupnea, tachypnea, bradypnea, apnea, Kussmaul's respirations, Biot's respirations, and Cheyne-Stokes respirations.
➤ *Assess cough and related symptoms:*
  Nasal congestion, sneezing, water eyes, and nasal discharge suggest allergies.
  Fever, chest congestion, noisy breath sounds, sputum production suggest a URI.
  Dyspnea, chest tightness, and wheezing suggest airway obstruction (e.g., asthma).
➤ *Assess sputum* for appearance, color, odor, amount, and timing.
➤ *Obtain sputum samples* as needed.
➤ *Assess respiratory effort.* Breathing should be effortless. Observe for shortness of breath, dyspnea, nasal flaring, head bobbing, retractions, use of accessory muscles during inspiration, grunting, needing to sit upright to breathe, paroxysmal nocturnal dyspnea, conversational dyspnea, stridor, and wheezing.

KEY POINT: *Ask all patients, not just those with oxygenation problems, whether they use tobacco and document their tobacco-use status regularly.*

Physical Examination

You will use all four examination techniques to assess respiratory function:

■ *Inspect* to observe respiratory patterns, signs of respiratory distress, chest structures and movement, skin and mucous membrane color, presence or absence of edema, sputum characteristics, and overall general appearance. Refer to Chapter 21 to review the details of inspecting the skin and mucous membranes. Also see Procedure 21-2: Assessing the Skin and Procedure 21-12: Assessing the Chest and Lungs.

■ *Palpate* pulses, skin temperature, heart pulsations through the chest wall, and areas of tenderness.

■ *Percuss* over the lung fields to screen for areas of consolidation or excess air pockets in the lungs.

■ *Auscultate* breath sounds, heart sounds, and vascular sounds. For a step-by-step discussion of how to assess the chest and lungs, refer to Procedure 21-12: Assessing the Chest and Lungs.

You may also need to monitor oxygenation and ventilation with pulse oximetry and capnography.

Pain Recall that pain alters the rate and depth of respirations. Often patients in pain breathe shallowly and are at risk for atelectasis. Regularly assess all patients for pain. Once you have medicated the patient, reassess breath sounds and encourage the patient to breathe deeply and cough.

Assessing Breathing Patterns

Assess for normal and altered breathing patterns. Most irregular breathing patterns are the result of brain injury or the effects of drugs on the brain. Irregular patterns are described following; they are illustrated in Table 19-5.

- **Eupnea**—Normal breathing; rate about 12 to 20 breaths/minute.
- **Tachypnea**—Fast, shallow breathing; more than 24 breaths/minute. Generally caused by hypoxemia or increased oxygen demand (e.g., exercise). Rapid, shallow respirations draw limited air into the alveoli and may result in hypoventilation.
- **Bradypnea**—Slow respirations (fewer than 10 breaths/minute). Bradypnea may cause poor gas exchange. Causes include sedative and opioid medications and neuromuscular dysfunction.
- **Kussmaul's respirations**—Regular but increased in rate and abnormally deep respirations. These may be a compensatory mechanism for metabolic disorders that lower blood pH, as well as a form of hyperventilation caused by fear, anxiety, or panic.
- **Biot's respirations**—Irregular respirations of variable depth (usually shallow), alternating with periods of apnea. This pattern is often associated with damage to the medullary respiratory center or high intracranial pressure as a result of brain injury.
- **Cheyne-Stokes respirations**—Gradual increase in depth of respirations, followed by a gradual decrease in depth, then a period of apnea. This pattern is often associated with damage to the medullary respiratory center or high intracranial pressure as a result of brain injury.
- **Apnea**—Absence of breathing. Respiratory arrest requires immediate cardiopulmonary resuscitation.

Assessing Respiratory Effort/Dyspnea

A patient experiencing shortness of breath or dyspnea requires a thorough assessment. However, you must take care not to increase his respiratory effort. Use closed questions that the patient can answer with yes, no, or only a few words. Ask whether the shortness of breath began suddenly or gradually, how severe it is right now, and whether it is getting better or worse. At the same time, observe for or ask about the signs of increased respiratory effort discussed below. Note that these signs are most easily visible in infants and small children.

- **Nasal flaring**—The visible enlargement of the nostrils with inhalation. It helps reduce resistance to airflow in the nose and keep the nasal passages open to take in more air.
- **Retractions**—The visible "pulling in" of intercostal, supraclavicular, and subcostal tissue, caused by excessive negative pressures generated in the chest to try to increase the depth of inhalation
- **Use of accessory muscles** during inspiration—The patient may use the intercostals, abdominal muscles, and muscles of the neck and shoulders when there is an increased demand for oxygen or problems with ventilation.
- **Grunting**—Noisy, difficult breathing. It is caused by forced expiration against a closed glottis and by involuntary muscle contraction during expiration to help keep alveoli open and enhance gas exchange

- **Body positioning** to facilitate respirations—The patient usually finds an upright posture the most comfortable. In the upright position, gravity pulls the abdominal organs down and allows the diaphragm more room to contract. Most patients with dyspnea cannot tolerate lying down. *Orthopnea* is the term used to describe difficulty breathing when lying down. Ask how the patient usually sleeps. Some patients may report sleeping in a recliner or chair.
- **Paroxysmal nocturnal dyspnea**—Sudden awakening caused by shortness of breath that begins during sleep. The patient feels panic and extreme dyspnea and must sit upright to ease breathing.
- **Conversational dyspnea**—The inability to speak complete sentences without stopping to breathe. The more frequently the patient pauses when speaking, the more severe the dyspnea.
- **Stridor**—A high-pitched, harsh, crowing, inspiratory sound caused by partial obstruction of the larynx or trachea. You can hear it without a stethoscope. ✚ Partial airway obstruction can easily become complete airway obstruction. Therefore, the patient with stridor needs immediate care.
- **Wheezing**—A musical sound produced by air passing through partially obstructed small airways. It is often heard in patients with asthma and lung congestion.
- ✚ **Diminished or absent breath sounds**—In a patient experiencing dyspnea these are signs of worsening ventilation and oxygenation. Oxygen therapy and measures to restore adequate ventilation may be required.

Assessing Cough

Everyone coughs from time to time to remove small amounts of mucus and debris from the airways. Coughing is a normal protective response to respiratory irritants (e.g., cigarette smoke, irritating fumes, dust particles) or when food or fluid accidentally enters the airways. If a cough persists, is recurring, or is productive, it may indicate ongoing or recurring airway irritation. **KEY POINT:** *Advise patients to obtain medical evaluation for a cough that lasts more than 3 weeks and cannot be explained.*

Assess the Type of Cough

- Is it dry, productive, or hacking? A cough is described as **productive** if it raises sputum (mucus and debris) up from the airways.
- When does the cough occur and how long has the patient been coughing?
- What makes it worse? What seems to help it?
- What has been used to treat the cough, and what were the effects?

Assess for Other Clinical Findings Associated With a Cough This helps determine its cause.

- *Allergies.* A cough associated with nasal congestion, sneezing, or watery eyes or nose discharge is most likely the result of allergies and may be successfully treated with OTC remedies.
- *URI.* A cough occurring with fever, chest congestion, noisy breath sounds, and sputum production is more likely to be caused by a URI, which may require antibiotics.
- *Airway obstruction/constriction.* A cough associated with dyspnea, chest tightness, and wheezing may be caused by an airway obstruction disorder such as asthma, which requires corticosteroids and bronchodilating medications.

Assess the Sputum Observe sputum appearance, odor, amount, and timing.

- **Sputum Appearance and Odor** provide valuable *clues* about the cause and significance of a cough (see Box 37-3).
- **Sputum Amount** can vary from a teaspoon to pints. In general, sputum production increases with the severity of the underlying condition. However, limited sputum production does not always indicate that the problem is minor, because excess mucus and debris may be trapped in the airways, causing the patient to be unable to cough it up and out of the body.
- **Sputum Timing** Sputum production ranges from constant to once per day. Tobacco smokers often have a "morning cough," which helps clear their airways of mucus and debris accumulated overnight. In contrast, someone with a URI is more likely to produce sputum throughout the day.

KnowledgeCheck 37-7

- What areas should you include in a nursing history for a patient with oxygenation concerns who is undergoing a comprehensive assessment?
- When is a cough significant? What aspects of a cough should be assessed?
- Identify at least five signs that you may observe in a patient experiencing dyspnea.
- A patient has a respiratory rate of 30 breaths/min that is rhythmic and moderate in depth. What term would you use to describe this breathing pattern?

ThinkLike a Nurse 37-7

Review the patients presented in the Meet Your Patients scenario.

- Which patients are experiencing respiratory distress? Identify the signs of distress in these patients.
- Which patients require a comprehensive assessment, and which patients will need a rapid assessment and immediate treatment because of the severity of their symptoms?

BOX 37-3 ■ Significance of Sputum Appearance and Odor

Color/Appearance	Significance
White or clear	Usually present in viral infections (e.g., common cold, viral bronchitis), often requiring only supportive care
Yellow or green	A sign of infection
Black	Caused by coal dust, smoke, or soot inhalation
Rust colored	Associated with pneumococcal pneumonia, tuberculosis, and possibly the presence of blood
Hemoptysis	The coughing up of blood or bloody sputum. It may range from small streaks of blood to large amounts of frank blood.
Pink and frothy	Associated with pulmonary edema
Foul-smelling sputum	Bacterial infection (e.g., pneumonia, lung abscess).

Diagnostic Testing

Diagnostic testing helps clinicians identify the causes of impaired oxygenation and monitor patient responses to treatment. You will need to assist with and be familiar with the results of the tests of respiratory function. We discuss several of these tests in the next sections. For others, see the Diagnostic Testing box Tests Related to Oxygenation.

Obtaining Sputum Samples

You may need to collect sputum samples. Sputum is examined microscopically and cultured in the lab to identify organisms and test for sensitivity to different anti-infective agents. To learn a procedure for collecting sputum specimens, refer to Procedure 37-1.

Skin Testing

Tuberculin Skin Testing is widely used to detect exposure and antibody formation to the tubercle bacillus. Annual screening is recommended for low-income populations, residents in congregate living conditions (e.g., dormitories, correctional facilities), immigrants from countries with a high prevalence of tuberculosis (TB), and healthcare workers. For the skin test to be effective, you must administer the antigen intradermally, not subcutaneously. Read the test site 48 to 72 hours after administration.

A *positive skin test* is defined as an area of **induration** (hardness) at the test site. The size of the induration that indicates a positive result depends on risk factors. Patients with positive TB skin tests must undergo further testing (chest x-ray study and sputum cultures) to determine whether they have merely been exposed to disease or whether they have active disease. See the Diagnostic Testing box Reading a Tuberculin Skin Test Result.

Allergy Testing uses skin testing to identify antigens that may cause hypersensitivity reactions in susceptible individuals. Testing is performed by scratching antigen samples onto the skin. The area is then observed over time for allergic skin reactions. Skin testing is performed in facilities with resuscitation equipment and personnel trained in its use, because life-threatening airway obstruction sometimes occurs in response to the allergens.

Pulse Oximetry

Pulse oximetry is a noninvasive estimate of arterial blood oxygen saturation (SaO_2). **SaO_2** reflects the percentage of hemoglobin molecules carrying oxygen. The normal value is 95% to 100%. Values below 94% are considered abnormal in healthy people and should be investigated to determine the cause. Well-oxygenated hemoglobin and deoxygenated hemoglobin in the circulating red blood cells absorb light differently. Using a light-emitting diode (LED), the oximeter is able to detect this difference and calculate the percentage of oxygenated hemoglobin.

Pulse oximetry is simple to perform, provides a rapid reading, and can be used intermittently or continuously. Frequency of measurement depends on the clinical condition of the patient. Recent recommendations are that pulse oximetry can be used to screen newborns for critical congenital heart disease (American Academy of Pediatrics, 2011; Manja, Mathew, Carrion, et al., 2015).

For tips to assure accuracy, refer to Clinical Insight 37-1. For the complete procedure, see Procedure 37-2.

Capnography

Capnography measures the carbon dioxide (CO_2) in inhaled and exhaled air. Capnography directly measures ventilation

Tests Related to Oxygenation

Test	Purpose
Angiogram	A contrast dye is injected into a vein, and serial films are taken to assess patency of the vessels.
Arterial blood gases (ABGs)	An analysis of arterial blood that evaluates the effectiveness of gas exchange.
Bronchoscopy	Insertion of a flexible endoscope to examine the larynx, trachea, and bronchial tree.
Chest x-ray study (CXR)	Provides an anterior–posterior or lateral view of the heart and lungs, shows tissue density (e.g., to evaluate size, masses, fluid).
Hemoglobin (Hb)	A serum measurement that affects the oxygen carrying capacity of the blood. May be measured separately or as part of a complete blood count.
Pulmonary function studies	A series of tests to detect lung volume and capacity.
Sputum culture	A microscopic evaluation of the sputum.
Thoracentesis	Insertion of a large-bore needle through the chest wall into the pleural space to obtain fluid specimens, to instill medication, or to drain accumulations of fluid.
Throat culture	A swab of the pharynx or tonsils is performed to assess pathogens present in the pharynx.
Ventilation–perfusion scan	Used to assess for pulmonary embolus, this scan entails injection of a radioactive substance that allows blood flow to the lungs to be evaluated. A second substance is inhaled that maps out oxygen distribution in the lungs.
White blood cell (WBC) count	A serum measure to assess for the presence of infection.

Diagnostic Testing

Reading a Tuberculin Skin Test Result

Size of Induration	Considered Positive for
5 mm	➤ People who have had recent close contact with someone with active TB ➤ People who have HIV or risk factors for HIV ➤ People with previous history of TB ➤ IV drug users known to be HIV negative
> 10 mm	➤ People with medical conditions that increase the risk of progressing from latent TB to active TB (e.g., diabetes mellitus, use of steroids, chronic renal failure, some malignancies) ➤ Residents and employees of high-risk congregate settings: prisons, skilled nursing facilities and other long-term facilities, healthcare facilities, and homeless shelters ➤ Foreign-born persons recently arrived (i.e., within the past 5 yr) from countries having a high incidence of TB ➤ Low-income groups ➤ Children younger than age 4 yr or exposed to adults in high-risk categories
> 15 mm	➤ People who do not meet any of the above criteria

Diagnostic Testing

and indirectly measures the partial pressure of CO_2 in the arterial blood. Normally the difference between arterial blood and expired CO_2 is very small.

- One method is to use a device that displays the results digitally and prints out a graph showing CO_2 at various times in the breathing cycle. As a beam of infrared light passes through a sample of respiratory gases, more or less of it is absorbed depending on the amount of CO_2 present.
- A second method is a naso-buccal sensor (Fig. 37-5) designed to collect expiratory gas immediately at the airway opening both at the nose and mouth. To perform the measurement, a sample of gas is transmitted from the patient to the monitor (Fig. 37-6). For each respiratory cycle, the capnogram is displayed on the monitor.

Capnography is often used with pulse oximetry because:
- It provides information about ventilation because it shows accumulation or depletion of CO_2, whereas pulse oximetry reflects only oxygenation of the blood.
- Capnography is a more reliable indicator of respiratory depression than is pulse oximetry.

A few of the many situations in which capnography is used include the following: when a patient is receiving opioids, during general anesthesia, and for adjusting parameter settings in mechanically ventilated patients.

CO_2 detectors, although they do measure carbon dioxide, are different from capnography. They use chemically treated paper that changes color when exposed to CO_2. They do not give exact readings but can measure only a range of values.

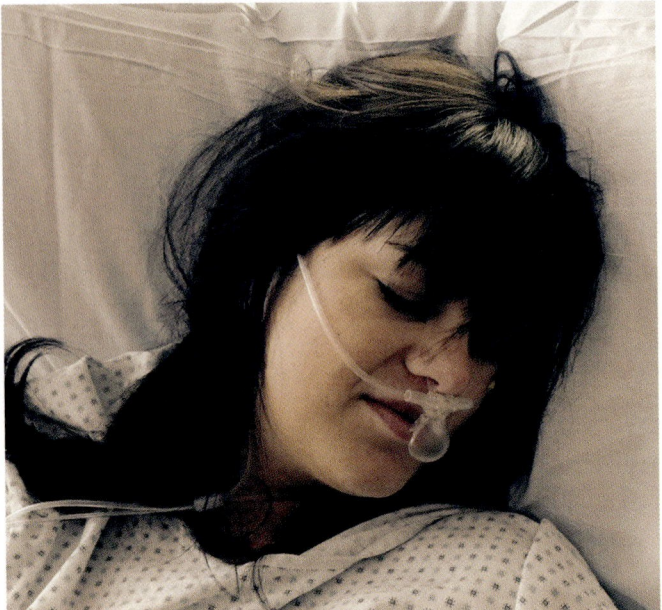

FIGURE 37-5 Naso-buccal sensor.

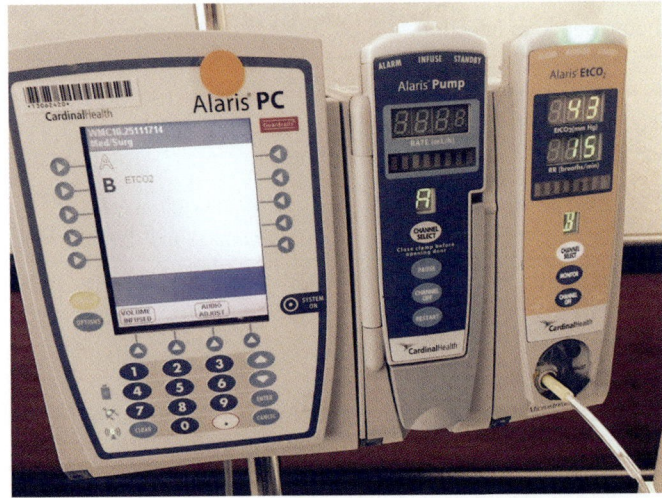

FIGURE 37-6 Naso-buccal sensor monitor. Module B (far right) enables continuous respiratory monitoring, including End Tidal CO_2 (EtCO$_2$) and respiratory rate (RR) via a nasobuccal sensor monitor.

Spirometry

Spirometry is a measure of air that moves into and out of the lungs. To describe the events of pulmonary ventilation, the air in the lungs is divided into four volumes and four capacities. Normal lung volumes and capacities vary with body size, age, and exercise. Men, large people, and athletes have greater lung volume and capacity for ventilation. For a summary of this information, see the Diagnostic Testing box Lung Volumes and Capacities.

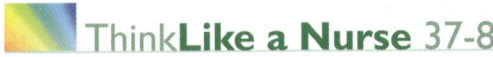

ThinkLike a Nurse 37-8

You hear a pulse oximeter alarm sound in a nearby patient room and find it reading 75%.

- What observations should you make?
- What actions should you take?

Arterial Blood Gases

Arterial blood gas (ABG) analysis measures the levels of oxygen and carbon dioxide in arterial blood. ABG analysis measures pH, partial pressure of oxygen (Po$_2$), partial pressure of carbon dioxide (Pco$_2$), saturation of oxygen (SaO$_2$), and bicarbonate (HCO$_3$) level. Here, we discuss only Po$_2$ and Pco$_2$. For a more thorough discussion of arterial blood gas values, see Chapter 39.

A blood sample is obtained from an artery (usually the brachial, radial, or femoral), either by arterial puncture or by withdrawal from an existing arterial line. Arteries are located deep under the skin and alongside nerves, making needle insertion painful. Nurses in critical care units routinely draw ABGs and monitor patients with invasive arterial monitoring; however, you may care for patients on medical–surgical units, or even outpatients, who will undergo periodic ABG evaluation.

Understanding Arterial Blood Oxygen Three values are important when assessing the degree to which the tissues are receiving oxygen:

- **Hemoglobin** is the iron-containing pigment of red blood cells that as *oxyhemoglobin* carries oxygen in the blood.
- **Po$_2$ (partial pressure of oxygen)** is the amount of oxygen available to combine with hemoglobin to make oxyhemoglobin.
- **SaO$_2$ (saturation of oxygen)** reflects oxygen that is actually bound to hemoglobin.

At sea level, the normal Po$_2$ range in arterial blood is 80 to 100 mm Hg. After tissues have extracted oxygen from arterial blood and the blood enters the veins to return to the heart, the venous blood Po$_2$ has fallen to around 40 mm Hg. The SaO$_2$, along with the Po$_2$ and hemoglobin level, indicates the degree to which the tissues are receiving oxygen. Small changes in SaO$_2$ are associated with large changes in Po$_2$. For blood gas values, refer to the Diagnostic Testing box Arterial Blood Gas Values: Evaluating Adequacy of Oxygenation.

To fully interpret Po$_2$ and SaO$_2$ values, you need to know the percentage of oxygen in the air the patient is inhaling. This is known as the **fraction of inspired oxygen, or Fio$_2$.** At sea level, atmospheric air (commonly known as *room air*) is 21% oxygen (Fio$_2$ = 21%). The norms quoted for Po$_2$ and SaO$_2$ are based on an Fio$_2$ of 21%.

- If a healthy patient receives 100% oxygen for a few minutes, the arterial Po$_2$ would rise to 500 to 600 mm Hg, and the SaO$_2$ would remain at 100%. The reason is that the SaO$_2$ measures the oxygen *bound to hemoglobin*—and of course the hemoglobin cannot be "filled" with oxygen to more than 100% capacity.
- When gas exchange is impaired as a result of disease or injury, Po$_2$ and SaO$_2$ levels fall. However, they can be kept at normal levels if supplemental oxygen is given.

Measuring Arterial Blood Carbon Dioxide The partial pressure of carbon dioxide (Pco$_2$) is a measure of the CO_2 dissolved in the blood. Normal arterial Pco$_2$ is 35 to 45 mm Hg. Carbon dioxide readily diffuses across the alveolar–capillary membrane in the lungs even when there are obstacles such as alveolar fluid or thickened membranes. As a result, Pco$_2$ levels remain normal until a severe disorder interferes with all gas exchange. Once in the alveoli, the amount of carbon dioxide exhaled from the lungs is directly influenced by how well air is moving into and out of the lungs (ventilation).

- **Hypocarbia.** When a person hyperventilates, he exhales large amounts of CO_2, causing arterial Pco$_2$ values to fall. Hyperventilation brings more oxygen into the lungs, so unless it is

Lung Volumes and Capacities

The norms presented in this table are based on averages for a young adult man. The following are measured by spirometry:

Title	Definition	Significance
Tidal volume (V_T)	The amount of air moved into and out of the lungs with each normal breath. Normally around 500 mL.	In a healthy state, V_T increases when oxygen demand increases. Diseases that restrict lung inflation, create muscular weakness, or paralyze the diaphragm limit the ability of the body to increase tidal volume. When such disorders become severe, V_T will fall too low to support even resting oxygen demands.
Inspiratory reserve volume (IRV)	The maximum amount of air that can be inhaled above and beyond the normal tidal volume. Ranges from 2,000 to 3,000 mL.	IRV determines how much the tidal volume can increase when oxygen demands increase.
Expiratory reserve volume (ERV)	The maximum extra amount of air that can be forcefully exhaled after the end of a normal tidal expiration. Ranges from 1,000 to 1,500 mL.	Some diseases (e.g., emphysema) cause collapse of alveoli and airways, which traps extra air in the lungs. This "trapped" air cannot be exhaled and lowers ERV.
Residual volume (RV)	The amount of air remaining in the lungs after the most forceful exhalation. Ranges from 1,000 to 1,500 mL.	Diseases that reduce ERV lead to an increase in RV. As more air is trapped in the lungs and cannot be exhaled even with forceful attempts (ERV), it becomes part of the residual volume that is never completely exhaled.
Inspiratory capacity (IC)	The combination of the tidal volume and inspiratory reserve volume (V_T + IRV). Ranges from 2,500 to 3,500 mL.	This is the amount of air that can be inhaled with maximum effort. It reflects the capacity one has to inhale deeply.
Functional residual capacity (FRC)	The combination of expiratory reserve volume and residual volume (ERV + RV). Ranges from 2,000 to 3,000 mL. Exhalation of additional air requires effort to force more air out.	This is the amount of air that stays in the lungs at the end of a normal passive, quiet exhalation. Disorders that cause air trapping increase the FRC.
Vital capacity (VC)	The combination of inspiratory reserve volume and expiratory reserve volume (IRV + ERV). Ranges from 3,000 to 4,500 mL.	This is the maximum amount of air that can be forcefully exhaled after filling the lungs to their maximum level with the deepest possible inspiratory effort.

Arterial Blood Gas Values: Evaluating Adequacy of Oxygenation

SaO_2	Arterial Po_2	Comment
95%–100%	80–100 mm Hg	Normal arterial values in healthy people.
90%	60 mm Hg	Po_2 > 60 mm Hg is required to sustain life and activity. This level is **not** normal in healthy people.
75%	40 mm Hg	Normal venous values; **a life-threatening arterial value** in anyone.

triggered by hypoxemia, oxygen levels (P_{O_2}) usually remain normal.

- **Hypercarbia.** Conversely, in hypoventilation less CO_2 moves into the alveoli for exhalation, leaving more CO_2 in the arterial blood. This causes P_{CO_2} values to rise. High P_{CO_2} levels (hypercarbia) suppress the respiratory drive, have an anesthetic effect on the nervous system, and can be toxic. Hypoventilation severe enough to cause hypercarbia is usually associated with hypoxemia because not enough oxygen is inhaled.

KnowledgeCheck 37-8

- What does a pulse oximetry reading tell you?
- What is the relationship between arterial P_{O_2} and S_{aO_2} levels?
- Identify normal P_{O_2}, S_{aO_2}, and P_{CO_2} levels.
- What effect does ventilation have on arterial P_{CO_2}?
- How is P_{CO_2} related to oxygenation?

ThinkLike a Nurse 37-9

You are caring for two patients, both of whom have a P_{O_2} of 95 mm Hg and an S_{aO_2} of 99%. Do they have similar lung function? Explain your answer.

Peak Flow Monitoring

Peak expiratory flow rate (PEFR) measures the amount of air that can be exhaled with forcible effort. Patients with asthma use PEFR monitoring to detect subtle changes in their condition, often before symptoms occur. A peak flow meter is used to monitor these changes (Fig. 37-7). Peak flow is expressed in liters per minute. Treatment protocols describe the use and frequency of medications based on individualized peak flow rates. The Home Care box Home Use of a Peak Flow Meter describes self-monitoring.

ANALYSIS/NURSING DIAGNOSIS NP

Alterations in pulmonary function may be nursing diagnoses, etiologies of other problems, or merely symptoms of other problems. In analyzing the assessment data, you must determine which. For example, suppose a patient is breathing shallowly and slowly. The pulmonary problem might be one of the following:

- **A nursing diagnosis:** *Ineffective Breathing Pattern (hypoventilation)* r/t pain secondary to rib fractures. In this case, you would provide pain relief; the desired outcome is that the patient will have effective (normal) ventilation. To sees a nursing care plan and care map for Ineffective Breathing Pattern,

 Go to Davis Advantage, Resources, Chapter 37, **Care Plan** and **Care Map.**

- **An etiology:** Risk for Ineffective Cerebral Tissue Perfusion r/t *Ineffective Breathing Pattern (hypoventilation).* In this case, you might address the etiology by administering oxygen; the desired outcome would be effective cerebral perfusion, evidenced by normal speech and alertness.
- **A symptom:** Decreased Intracranial Adaptive capacity r/t brain injury, *as manifested by Ineffective Breathing Pattern (hypoventilation),* and baseline ICP ≤ 10 mm Hg. In this situation, you would, of course, support ventilation (the symptom) until the problem subsides. However, the primary interventions would be directed toward the head trauma

---

Home Use of a Peak Flow Meter

Home Care

People with asthma are often asked to monitor their peak flow readings at home and to compare their current readings with their baseline "personal best."
➤ Teach patients that to get an accurate reading, they need to take a deep breath and forcefully exhale.
➤ Teach patients to take a series of three readings and record the highest reading.
➤ Teach patients to maintain or adjust their medication according to their highest reading. They should follow the color-coded treatment protocols prescribed by their physician. These are individualized for each patient. Notice that these correspond to the color-coded markers on their peak flow meter.

Green = All clear: Baseline peak flow—*Peak flow is within 80% to 100% of personal best baseline.*
    Treatment protocol calls for routine medication use.

Yellow = Caution: Peak flow is 50% to 80% of usual or "normal" rate. *Said another way, there is a 20% to 50% reduction in peak flow—This reading signals the onset of airway changes.*
    Treatment protocols usually specify an increase in the dosage of maintenance medications, use of rescue therapies (e.g., fast-acting bronchodilators), or a call to the healthcare provider. These measures are designed to reverse acute exacerbations before they become severe.

Red = Medical alert: Peak flow is less than 50% of personal best baseline. *Severe reduction in peak flow.*
    Treatment protocols usually specify immediate treatment with rescue medications and to seek emergency treatment if symptoms do not improve.

Source: Adapted from American Lung Association. (2016). Measuring your peak flow rate. Retrieved from http://www.lung.org/lung-health-and-diseases/lung-disease-lookup/asthma/living-with-asthma/managing-asthma/measuring-your-peak-flow-rate.html

---

and increased intracranial pressure (ICP). Once these etiologies were corrected, the hypoventilation would disappear. The goal would be normal intracranial pressure, evidenced in part by a normal breathing pattern.

Problems of Ventilation and Gas Exchange Five NANDA International (NANDA-I) diagnoses directly describe problems with ventilation and gas exchange. Use these diagnoses when they are the central problem and you intend to use interventions to eliminate the cause of the problem.

- *Ineffective Airway Clearance* is the inability to maintain a clear airway.
- *Ineffective Breathing Pattern* is used to describe inadequate ventilation, such as hypoventilation, hyperventilation, tachypnea, or bradypnea.
- *Impaired Gas Exchange* is the appropriate diagnosis if the patient is ventilating adequately but diffusion of gases across the alveolar–capillary membrane is impaired.
- *Impaired Spontaneous Ventilation* describes a condition in which a patient, as a result of decreased energy reserves, is unable to maintain breathing adequate to support life.

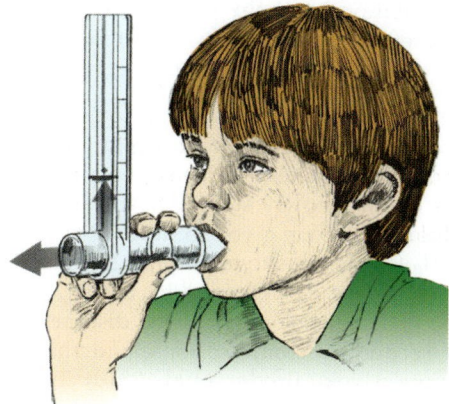

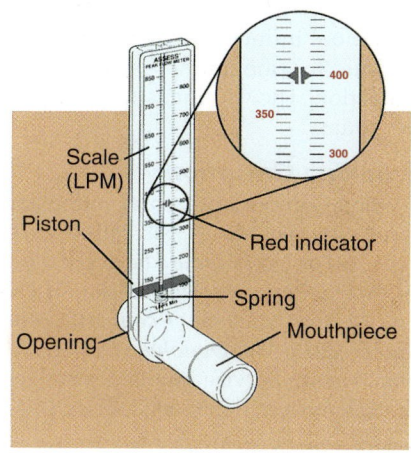

Scale (LPM)

Piston

Opening

Red indicator

Spring

Mouthpiece

400

350

300

FIGURE 37-7 A patient with asthma using a peak flow meter to monitor peak expiratory flow rate (PEFR).

- *Dysfunctional Ventilatory Weaning Response* represents a specific situation in which a patient who is being mechanically ventilated cannot adjust to lower levels of ventilator support, prolonging the ventilatory weaning process.
- *Risk for Aspiration* should be used when there is a risk for secretions, solids, or fluids entering into tracheobronchial passages (e.g., for patients who have had head or neck surgery or who have a reduced level of consciousness).

PLANNING OUTCOMES/EVALUATION NP

NOC standardized outcomes appropriate for patients with pulmonary function problems include, for example:

Aspiration Prevention
Mechanical Ventilation Weaning Response: Adult
Respiratory Status: Airway Patency
Respiratory Status: Gas Exchange
Respiratory Status: Ventilation
Swallowing Status
Vital Signs

These provide a general guide for care planning. Depending on individual patient needs, other NOC outcomes or NIC interventions may also be appropriate.

Individualized goals/outcome statements depend on the nursing diagnosis you identify. For diagnoses related to gas exchange, the following are examples of goals you might write:

Expectorates secretions effectively
No dyspnea or shortness of breath
Lungs clear; no adventitious sounds present

PLANNING INTERVENTIONS/ IMPLEMENTATION NP

NIC standardized interventions related to oxygenation are found in the Respiratory Management category. They focus on maintaining a patent airway and promoting gas exchange, and include Airway Management, Airway Suction, Cough Enhancement, Oxygen Therapy, and Respiratory Monitoring.

Specific nursing interventions for patients with oxygenation problems include health promotion, prevention, and treatment activities. They are discussed in the sections that follow.

Administering Respiratory Medications

Respiratory medications promote ventilation and oxygenation by their effects on the respiratory system itself. Some need a prescription; others do not. Medications are also used to improve respiratory function. A few examples include bronchodilators and anti-inflammatory agents such as corticosteroids, cough suppressants, expectorants, and decongestants.

See the accompanying Self-Care box Cough and Cold Medicines: Tips for Parents for assistance in administering such medications to children. Also refer to the accompanying CAM box for some common alternative cold remedies.

Self-Care

Cough and Cold Medicines: Tips for Parents

➤ Do not give children medicines labeled for adults only.
➤ Do not give OTC cough and cold remedies to children younger than age 4 years. There is a risk of serious and even life-threatening side effects.
➤ The safety and effectiveness of OTC cough and cold remedies for children aged 2 through 11 years is still in question. It is not certain they are safe, and they may not be effective.
➤ Read labels! Some labels are marked "Do not use for children under age 4."
➤ Choose medications with safety caps. Close caps tightly and store out of sight and reach of children.
➤ Do not give more than one medicine with the same active ingredient. Check the "active ingredients" on the label. Your child could be harmed by getting too much of the ingredient.
➤ Carefully follow the directions on the label for how to use the medicine. Overuse or misuse can cause serious side effects (e.g., drowsiness, breathing problems, and seizures).
➤ Measure carefully. Do not use household spoons because they come in different sizes.
➤ Understand that OTC medicines do not cure the cold or cough. They only treat symptoms such as runny nose, congestion, fever, and aches. They do not shorten the length of time your child is sick.

Source: Centers for Disease Control and Prevention. (2010b). For parents: Young children and adverse drug events. Medication Safety Program. Retrieved from http://www.cdc.gov/MedicationSafety/parents_childrenAdverseDrugEvents.html; U.S. Food and Drug Administration. (2013, updated 2015). Using over-the-counter cough and cold products in children. Retrieved from http://www.fda.gov/ForConsumers/ConsumerUpdates/ucm048515

Common Cold Remedies

➤ Cold care products containing *Pelargonium sidoides,* an extract of the South African geranium, may reduce the intensity of the common cold. However, more evidence is needed (Ross, 2012). In the United States, Zucol products are one example.

➤ ✚ Honey is more effective than dextromethorphan in children with nocturnal cough (Oduwole, Meremikwu, Oyo-Ita, et al., 2014). However, avoid giving honey to children younger than the age of 1 year because it is a reservoir of *Clostridium botulinum* spores and may cause botulism in infants.

➤ Vitamin C in daily doses of 200 mg or more has not been found to prevent colds, but it did reduce the length and severity of symptoms. Be aware that in amounts of 2,000 mg, it may cause diarrhea and gas (Hemilä & Chalker, 2013).

➤ A systematic review of research studies found there is no evidence that echinacea preparations are effective for preventing and treating the common cold (Karsch-Völk, Barrett, & Linde, 2015).

➤ Although lab studies are preliminary, elderberry *(Sambucus nigra),* an herb, has been found to help combat viruses, specifically influenza. It is thought to strengthen the immune system and keep the flu virus from adhering to cells (Mousa, 2017).

Promoting Optimal Respiratory Function

Deep, regular breathing promotes ventilation and optimizes gas exchange. Other interventions to promote optimal respiratory function include preventing URIs, performing immunizations, supporting smoking cessation, preventing and treating pneumonia, positioning, providing incentive spirometry, and preventing aspiration.

Prevent Healthcare-Associated Pneumonia

Healthcare-associated pneumonia (HCAP) is pneumonia that is contracted by a patient in a hospital or inpatient facility. It is often caused by bacteria other than *Streptococcus pneumoniae,* which is the organism involved in most cases of pneumonia. HCAP tends to be more complicated and to have a higher mortality rate than community-acquired pneumonia. Guidelines for preventing healthcare-associated pneumonia include following standard precautions for hand hygiene and gloving.

- ✚ Wear gloves for handling respiratory secretions or objects contaminated with respiratory secretions of all patients.
- Change gloves and decontaminate hands:
  - Between contacts with different patients
  - After handling respiratory secretions or contaminated objects and before contact with another patient, object, or environmental surface
  - Between contacts with a contaminated body site and the respiratory tract or respiratory device on the same patient (Sickbert-Bennett, DiBiase, Willis, et al., 2016)

For interventions to help prevent ventilator-associated pneumonia, refer to "Caring for a Patient Requiring Mechanical Ventilation" and Procedure 37-10, later in this chapter.

Promote Immunization

The most effective strategy for preventing influenza is annual vaccination. Vaccines are developed annually to closely match the major known strains of the virus that have evolved. Immunizations given to healthy young adults are 70% to 90% effective. Though less effective in preventing the disease in older adults, immunization decreases the severity of the disease, the development of secondary complications, and the incidence of death (Fiore, Uyeki, Broder, et al., 2010). The Centers for Disease Control and Prevention continues to recommend universal vaccination—that is, all people aged 6 months and older receive annual influenza vaccination. People who are most susceptible to pneumonia should be immunized against the infection. The vaccine is recommended annually for high-risk groups.

Support Smoking Cessation

Smoking cessation is important in preventing and treating all respiratory problems, including URIs, influenza, and pneumonia. **KEY POINT:** All *patients should be asked whether they use tobacco, and their tobacco-use status should be documented regularly (e.g., by chart stickers or computer prompts) (Fiore, Jorenby, & Baker, 2016; Ma, Donohue, DeNofrio, et al., 2016).* The U.S. Public Health Service guidelines suggest the "5A's" model for treating tobacco dependence (Box 37-4) (Fiore, Jaén, Baker, et al., 2008).

Motivational counseling includes discussion about the connection between tobacco use and current health status, the risks of continued tobacco use, the rewards of quitting, anticipated barriers to quitting, and strategies for addressing barriers. It may also be important to refer the person to a tobacco cessation program. Most smokers are not able to quit "cold turkey."

Combining medication and counseling is more effective than either used alone. Encourage patients to contact their

---

BOX 37-4 ■ The 5A's for Treating Tobacco Dependence

Ask about tobacco use and document tobacco use status for every patient at every visit.

Advise to quit. Use a clear, strong, personalized approach to urge the patient to quit.

Assess willingness to make a quit attempt at this time.

Assist in a quit attempt. If the patient is willing, refer for counseling and medication. If the patient is not willing to quit at this time, provide interventions designed to increase future quit attempts.

Arrange follow-up. If the patient is willing to quit, make follow-up contacts beginning the first week after the quit date. If the patient is not willing to quit at this time, address tobacco dependence and willingness to quit at the next clinic (or other) visit.

Source: Adapted from Fiore, M., Jaén, C., Baker, T., et al. (2008). *Treating tobacco use and dependence: 2008 update.* Clinical Practice Guideline. Rockville, MD: U.S. Department of Health and Human Services. Public Health Service.

primary care provider for nicotine replacement therapy or other medications (e.g., antidepressants, clonidine) to treat tobacco dependence. For pregnant women, smokeless tobacco users, light smokers, and adolescents, medications may be contraindicated or may lack evidence of effectiveness (Stead & Lancaster, 2012; U.S. Preventive Services Task Force, 2015).

Box 37-1 highlights some of the benefits of smoking cessation. Share these and smoking cessation tips with patients (Self-Care box Smoking Cessation Tips).

Position for Maximum Ventilation

An upright or elevated position pulls abdominal organs down, allowing maximum diaphragm excursion and lung expansion. Therefore, this intervention is applicable to almost all respiratory problems, including UTIs, influenza, and pneumonia.

- If the patient is short of breath, provide an overbed table to lean forward on. Patients with impaired respiratory function adopt a tripod position to allow maximum expansion. They may need to rest their arms on an overbed table.
- When the patient is lying on her side, provide pillows to support the upper arm.
- Assist with frequent position changes to keep all areas of the lungs well ventilated, and ambulate as often as possible without creating fatigue.

Assist With Incentive Spirometry

Incentive spirometers are designed to encourage patients to take deep breaths by reaching a goal-directed volume of air. It is usually reserved for patients at risk for developing atelectasis or pneumonia (e.g., patients who have had abdominal, chest, or pelvic surgery; are on prolonged bedrest; or have a history of respiratory problems). Incentive spirometers offer various visual cues (such as elevation of a ball or piston) to show patients whether they are inhaling deeply enough.

As a registered nurse (RN), you can delegate incentive spirometry coaching to licensed practical nurses (LPNs) and qualified nursing assistive personnel (NAP). However, you are responsible for ensuring that incentive spirometry is carried out correctly and at required frequencies. You must also evaluate patient responses, airway clearance, and ventilation. See Figure 40-6 and the Self-Care box Teaching Your Patient About Incentive Spirometry in Chapter 40.

Take Aspiration Precautions

Aspiration is a risk for patients with a decreased level of consciousness, diminished gag or cough reflex, or difficulty with swallowing. Preventing aspiration requires you to have practical knowledge about positioning, enteral and oral feedings, and administering medications. For guidelines to use with at risk patients, see Clinical Insight 37-2: Guidelines for Preventing Aspiration. Many of the guidelines involve basic care and can be delegated to qualified LPNs and NAPs. **KEY POINT:** *The RN is responsible for monitoring for aspiration.* Record in the nursing notes any preventive measures taken.

KnowledgeCheck 37-9

Identify at least three nursing interventions to promote optimal respiratory function in a hospitalized patient with chronic lung disease.

ThinkLike a Nurse 37-10

- Review the Meet Your Patients scenario. For which of these patients should you recommend annual flu or pneumonia immunizations? Why?
- A 24-year-old nursing student has no previous hospitalizations or known chronic health problems, takes no medications, and has no current respiratory symptoms. On routine purified protein derivative testing (tuberculin skin testing), the student has an area of induration measuring 5 mm. How would you interpret these results?

Mobilizing Secretions

Coughing promotes deep inhalation and forceful expulsion of secretions. Interventions that help enhance coughing and mobilize secretions include deep breathing, coughing exercises, and hydration. Mobilizing secretions is useful for many respiratory conditions, including UTIs, influenza, and pneumonia.

Self-Care

Smoking Cessation Tips

➤ Identify several personal reasons to quit smoking, such as "I'll live longer and be able to spend more time with my children and grandchildren" or "My father died of lung cancer. He really suffered. I have no desire to experience that."

➤ Make a list of things you enjoy doing. Choose one of these items as a reward for not smoking.

➤ Before smoking, ask yourself, "What can I do instead of smoking this cigarette?"

➤ Identify friends who do not smoke and plan to spend time with them.

➤ Have carrot sticks, celery, gum, or sunflower seeds available to chew instead of smoking a cigarette. These also help you cope with the increased hunger you may feel.

➤ Learn several relaxation techniques, such as meditation or visualization, to help you through the stress of quitting.

➤ Use positive affirmations daily. "I can successfully quit smoking. I am no longer a smoker."

➤ Tell several supportive people of your plan to quit. Ask them to help you be successful.

➤ Plan a time to quit. Choose a time that will not require many additional demands on you.

➤ Talk with friends and coworkers who have successfully quit smoking.

➤ Save the money you would have spent on cigarettes. Treat yourself to an activity or event with the money you have saved.

➤ Tell your healthcare providers that you would like to quit smoking.

➤ When you feel a craving to smoke, breathe deeply, find something to distract yourself, or call a supportive person.

➤ To help cope with irritability, use relaxation exercises or deep breathing; take a hot bath; or do something else you enjoy.

➤ Participate in a structured smoking cessation program, if possible.

➤ Consider asking your healthcare provider about nicotine-replacement therapy such as gum or patches.

Teach Deep Breathing and Coughing

Deep breathing promotes ventilation and gas exchange. Coughing after deep breathing mobilizes secretions, which keeps airways and alveoli open and provides greater surface area for gas exchange. This intervention is important, for example, in treating pneumonia and preventing stasis pneumonia postoperatively. For information about teaching patients to deep-breathe and cough, see Procedure 37-1A.

Alter this procedure for patients with chronic lung disease. Have the patient exhale through pursed lips and cough throughout expiration in several short bursts to avoid high expiratory pressures, which collapse diseased airways.

Maintain Hydration

The following activities are important to keep pulmonary secretions thin and mobile (e.g., in infections such as influenza and pneumonia):

- *Maintain systemic hydration.* Encourage oral fluid intake as much as possible. Supplement oral intake by intravenous fluid administration if the patient cannot ingest adequate amounts of fluid. For guidelines to use in teaching patients to maintain hydration, refer to the Self-Care box Teaching Patients to Prevent Fluid and Electrolyte Imbalances, in Chapter 39.
- *Humidify inhaled air.* Use humidification devices or nebulizers. A **humidifier** is a device that delivers small water droplets from a reservoir. Small humidifiers filled with sterile distilled water are attached to oxygen delivery systems to moisten the dry oxygen and keep secretions thin and mobile. A **nebulizer** is a device that turns liquids into an aerosol mist that can be inhaled directly into the lungs. Nebulizers are often used to deliver medications to the lungs, but they can also be used to deliver moisture to the airways and lungs. See "Administering Respiratory Inhalations" in Chapter 25, and Figure 25-11. Also refer to Clinical Insight 37-3: Oxygen Therapy Safety Precautions.

Perform Chest Physiotherapy

Chest physiotherapy moves secretions to the large, central airways for expectoration or suctioning (Fig. 37-8). It involves postural drainage, chest percussion, and chest vibration. In many institutions, respiratory therapists routinely perform chest physiotherapy. For a detailed description of chest physiotherapy, see Procedure 37-3.

- *Postural drainage* is the use of positioning to promote drainage from the lungs. Postural drainage uses gravity to drain the lungs, so you will place the affected area in an uppermost position so that secretions will drain down toward the large, central airways. For example, if the patient has pneumonia of the right lower lobe, you would place her on her left side and elevate the foot of the bed to allow the right lower lobe to drain.
- *Chest percussion and chest vibration* are used in conjunction with postural drainage to loosen and mobilize secretions. Have the patient assume the desired drainage position for 10 to 15 minutes before percussing and vibrating. **Chest percussion** is the rhythmic clapping of the chest wall using cupped hands. **Chest vibration** is the vibration of the chest wall with the palms of the hands.

ThinkLike a Nurse 37-11

Your patient has pneumonia in the right lower lobe. She is mildly dyspneic with any activity. Strategize how you would perform chest physiotherapy on this patient. What activities would you consider to make this procedure more tolerable for the patient?

Providing Oxygen Therapy

Oxygen therapy provides oxygen at concentrations greater than the level found in room air. Room air contains only about 21% oxygen. Because oxygen is a medication, it requires a medical prescription for dosage (concentration) and route. Many agencies have protocols with standing orders for oxygen administration in an emergency. (Note that oxygen therapy may be needed for pneumonia.) Oxygen is supplied in several different ways:

- *Wall outlets* connected to a large central tank of oxygen are usually provided in healthcare facilities.
- *Compressed O_2 in portable tanks* may also be available.
- *Liquid oxygen units* are often used for home oxygen therapy (Fig. 37-9).
- An *oxygen concentrator* removes nitrogen from room air and concentrates O_2. It requires a battery pack or electrical outlet

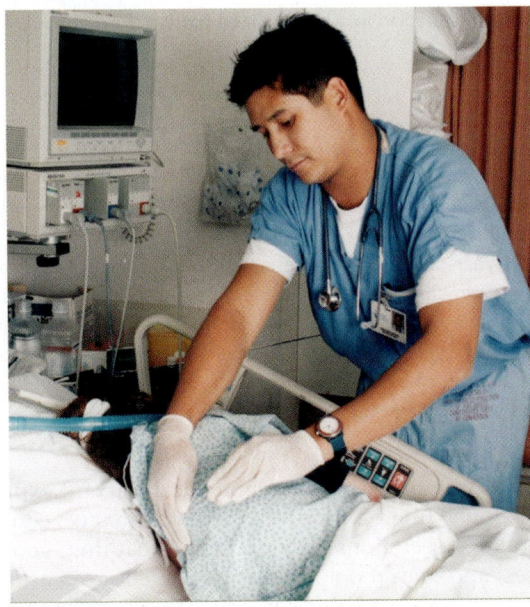

FIGURE 37-8 Patient receiving chest physiotherapy.

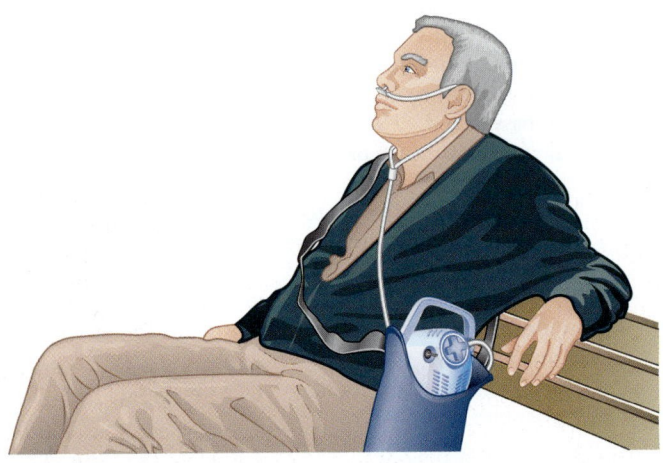

FIGURE 37-9 Liquid oxygen units are small and portable. They are ideal for home use.

for power. These devices eliminate the need for buying oxygen cylinders, relieving clients' anxiety about running out of oxygen. However, they are expensive, noisy, and not portable; moreover, the client must still have backup oxygen in case of a power failure.

To learn how to administer oxygen to patients, refer to Procedure 37-4.

Oxygen Hazards

The following risks are associated with oxygen therapy. Refer to Procedure 37-4 for guidelines to minimize these risks.

- ✚ *Oxygen toxicity can develop* when O_2 concentrations of more than 50% are administered for longer than 48 to 72 hours. Prolonged use of high O_2 concentrations reduces surfactant production, which leads to alveolar collapse and reduced lung elasticity.
- *Oxygen supports combustion,* although it does not burn. High concentrations of oxygen will turn a small spark or fire into a large fire. Fire prevention precautions must be used near oxygen delivery systems.
- *Oxygen tanks contain oxygen under pressure.* If the tank ruptures or falls, compressed oxygen shoots forcefully from the tank, turning it into an unguided missile. Oxygen tanks have been known to hurtle through walls when ruptured.

Transtracheal Oxygen Delivery

A **tracheostomy** is a surgical opening into the trachea through the neck. It may be permanent or temporary. Air inhaled through a tracheostomy bypasses the upper airway, which normally warms and moistens air before it reaches the lower airway. Oxygen may be delivered through the tracheostomy via a collar or an adapter.

KnowledgeCheck 37-10

- Why is oxygen humidified?
- Name the appropriate oxygen delivery method that is appropriate for the following patients:
  A patient prescribed to receive 2 L/min of oxygen
  A patient who complains of being claustrophobic and requires low-flow humidified oxygen
  A patient with chronic obstructive pulmonary disease with an order for oxygen at an FIO_2 of 24%
  A patient who wants to avoid intubation but requires an FIO_2 of 100%

Using Artificial Airways

Artificial airways provide an open airway for patients who have or who are at risk for airway obstruction. Airways may be placed into the pharynx or deeper, into the trachea.

Pharyngeal Airways

Pharyngeal airways provide an open air passage by holding the tongue away from the back of the pharynx. When artificial airways are properly placed, air can flow around and through them, and suction catheters can be passed through them. Pharyngeal airways may be placed through the mouth or the nose.

- **Oropharyngeal airways** are C-shaped, hard plastic devices inserted through the mouth into the pharynx. To select the appropriate size, hold the airway next to the patient's face. The length of the airway should extend from the front of the teeth to the end of the jawline. If it is *too short*, it will not keep the tongue pulled forward; if it is *too long*, it may push

the epiglottis against the laryngeal opening and completely obstruct the airway

- **Nasopharyngeal airways** are flexible rubber tubes that are inserted through a nostril into the pharynx. Patients who are semiconscious can tolerate nasal airways because they do not stimulate the gag reflex. Nasopharyngeal airways are available in a variety of pediatric and adult sizes. To learn about sizing and inserting a nasopharyngeal airway, refer to Procedure 37-13.

Endotracheal Airways

Patients who cannot breathe effectively because of airway obstruction or respiratory or cardiac failure need an airway inserted directly into the trachea. **Endotracheal airways** are pliable tubes inserted into the trachea through the following routes:

Orotracheal tube—the mouth
Nasotracheal tube—the nose
Tracheostomy tube—an opening directly into the trachea

There are several types of tracheostomy tubes made of various materials. They may be cuffed or uncuffed and may have a single or double lumen.

- A cuffed tube is used for patients who are being ventilated or who have difficulty swallowing.
- For self-care at home, a tube with an inner cannula is preferred because the inner tube can be removed and cleaned to avoid tube occlusion, primarily because of accumulation of secretions in the airway.

Because tracheostomy tubes bypass the upper airway, the patient inhales air directly into the lower airway without humidification, filtering, or warming. For this reason, devices that warm and humidify inhaled air are used with endotracheal airways. Figure 37-10A illustrates the parts of an endotracheal tube. Figure 37-10B shows the placement of an orotracheal

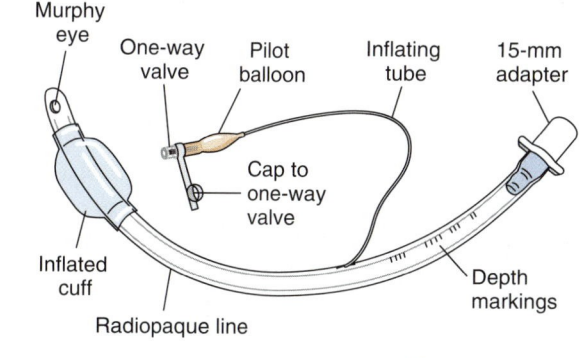

A

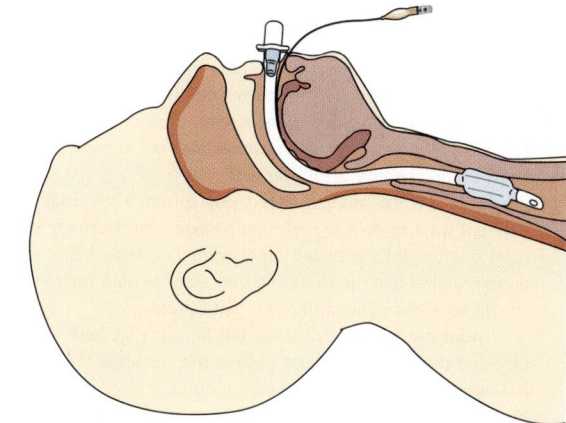

B

FIGURE 37-10 A. An endotracheal tube. B. Placement of an orotracheal tube.

tube. Nursing responsibilities related to endotracheal airways are to assist in their insertion, maintain stabilization, and provide routine suctioning and management.

Assisting With Endotracheal Airway Insertion

Insertion of endotracheal airways is within the scope of practice of certain specially trained nurses (e.g., nurse anesthetist). As a nurse in general practice, you will assist with insertion by gathering equipment and preparing the patient. On most units, you will find intubation equipment in the resuscitation cart. Intubation must often be done quickly, in response to a temporary decline in the patient's respiratory function during a procedure. See Clinical Insight 37-4 for guidelines for assisting with and managing endotracheal airways.

Managing Endotracheal and Tracheostomy Tubes

Managing endotracheal and tracheostomy tubes generally requires the expertise of a respiratory therapist or an RN, but you can delegate this activity to specially trained and skilled LPNs, especially in critical care areas. Once the ostomy is well healed, the airway will not collapse if the tracheostomy tube is dislodged. This means a NAP, or even the patient, can reinsert it if necessary. Many patients with permanent tracheostomies perform self-care at home.

Evidence is still mixed about whether to use sterile or clean gloves when performing endotracheal care. The following are the different levels of asepsis currently in use for tracheostomy care:

- **Sterile technique** is the use of a sterile suction catheter and other supplies with sterile gloves. For new tracheostomies, most facilities use sterile technique. However, some use sterile technique only for patients who have increased susceptibility to infection.
- **Modified sterile technique** is use of a sterile suction catheter and supplies but with nonsterile procedure gloves. For healed tracheostomies, and in many institutions for

all tracheostomies, the trend is toward a modified sterile technique.

- **Clean technique** is use of a clean catheter and clean hands or nonsterile gloves. The portion of the catheter that will be inserted in the tracheostomy tube is protected to avoid contact with unclean surfaces. Clean technique is the usual method in the home setting. Anyone who is not a family member and anyone concerned about acquiring an infection should wear nonsterile procedure gloves, even in the home setting.

You should follow the procedure used in your healthcare facility or school. To learn a procedure and guidelines for tracheostomy care, respectively, see Procedure 37-6 and Clinical Insight 37-4.

KnowledgeCheck 37-11

- In what circumstances would you use an oropharyngeal airway? A nasopharyngeal airway?
- What facts should you record if a patient is intubated?
- Describe seven interventions associated with caring for a patient with an endotracheal tube.

Suctioning Airways

Airways are suctioned to remove secretions and maintain patency. Signs that indicate the need for suctioning include agitation, gurgling sounds during respiration, restlessness, labored respirations, decreased oxygen saturation (SaO_2), increased heart and respiratory rates, and adventitious breath sounds on auscultation. Although suctioning helps remove secretions, it also removes air from the airways and causes the patient's O_2 levels to fall. As a result, suctioning must be done quickly and is often accompanied by supplemental oxygen. Suctioning can also irritate mucous membranes if done too frequently.

Safe, Effective Nursing Care

Removing Barriers to Patient and Family Involvement in Care

Patient-Centered Care (Thinking, Doing, Caring)

Scenario: Mrs. Yablonski, a 66-year-old former smoker, has recently had a permanent tracheostomy but can speak using an electromechanical device. She needs to learn how to suction herself and change the tracheotomy dressing. For 3 days in a row, different nurses have tried to explain how to perform the care. Each time she became tearful and frustrated. The nurse manager speaks with her to identify problems that may be occurring. Mrs. Yablonski cites several issues:

> Sometimes it's me. I may just feel too overwhelmed or I may just not have any energy. But the nurses don't always ask me if I feel well enough to learn. None of them really knows me, and they don't take enough time with me. And sometimes my nurse would rather just do it herself and get it over with.
>
> There are too many nurses trying to teach me. They tell me different ways to do it or make me go over what I already know, so I get confused. I try to tell them what I already know or what another nurse told me to do, but they want to do it their way. They should have this all written down somewhere.
>
> I want my husband to learn, but he can't be here during the day, and that's the only time anyone tries to show me how to do it. I asked the doctor about learning about it later on in his office but he didn't want to talk about it. He said the nurses here would teach me.

Thinking: Including patients or their significant others as equal partners in care is the foundation of patient-centered care. Think about the following questions:

- What barriers to participating in her own care does Mrs. Yablonski identify? Would they be applicable to other patients?
- How is team communication affecting this situation?
- Does Mrs. Yablonski see herself as a valuable partner in her care?
- What might the effects be if Mrs. Yablonski felt more empowered?
- Does she seem to have a conflict regarding how much care she wants to take over? If so, how should her nurse manage the conflict?
- What are the potential negative outcomes if Mrs. Yablonski goes home before she masters her tracheostomy care?
- What can the nurse manager do to make Mrs. Yablonski's care more patient centered?

Source: Kozin, E., Straton, J., & Kapo, J. (2012). Tracheostomy care. *Journal of Palliative Medicine, 15*(3), 359–360.

Suction catheters may be open tipped or "whistle tipped" (Fig. 37-11A and B). Most suction catheters have a port on the side, over which you place your thumb to control the suction. A Yankauer tube (Fig. 37-11C) is a rigid device for suctioning the oral cavity.

Both respiratory therapists and nurses are responsible for suctioning and tracheostomy care. The respiratory therapist and the nurse should keep each other informed of changes in the patient's condition. Airway suctioning is usually performed by RNs and LPNs, but not by NAPs. NAPs may use a Yankauer tube to suction the oral cavity as part of maintaining hygiene and preventing aspiration of oral secretions.

Suctioning the Upper Airway

Pharyngeal suctioning is performed to prevent oral and nasal secretions from entering the lower airway when the patient is too weak to cough up secretions. Suctioning the pharynx triggers a cough, which helps loosen and mobilize secretions. The patient's condition determines whether you suction the pharynx through the mouth or nose. Most patients find oropharyngeal suctioning more comfortable than the nasal approach. However, if the patient is unable to cooperate and automatically bites down when anything is placed in his mouth or if the jaw is wired, use a nasal approach. To learn how to suction the pharynx, refer to Procedure 37-9.

Suctioning the Lower Airway

In tracheal suctioning, a catheter is passed beyond the pharynx into the trachea to remove secretions from the lower airways. The catheter may be inserted through the mouth, nose, or an endotracheal airway. In the healthcare setting, deep tracheal suctioning is a sterile procedure.

Orotracheal or Nasotracheal (NT) Approach
When suctioning through the nose or mouth, insert the catheter into the pharynx and advance it into the trachea during inspiration. This prevents the catheter from entering the esophagus and causing the patient to gag or vomit. When the suction catheter enters the trachea, it will stimulate coughing. Except in an emergency, NT suctioning should be done through a nasopharyngeal airway. For complete procedure steps, see Procedure 37-8.

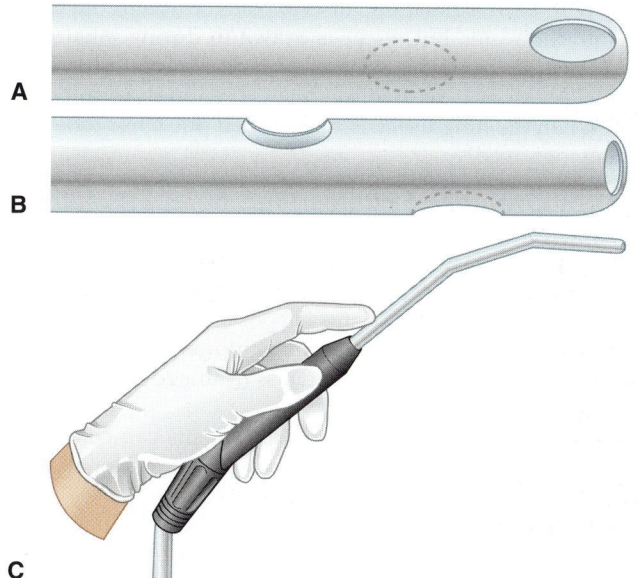

FIGURE 37-11 A. Whistle-tipped suction catheter. B. Open-tipped suction catheter. C. Yankauer (oral) suction tube.

Endotracheal or Tracheostomy Approach
An endotracheal or tracheostomy tube provides a direct path into the trachea. To suction, insert the catheter through the artificial airway into the trachea. You do not need to insert the catheter as far into a tracheostomy tube because you are bypassing the long upper airway. Before suctioning, make sure the airway is secured so it is not dislodged by coughing or suctioning. You will find instructions for this skill in Procedure 37-7.

KnowledgeCheck 37-12

- Describe the difference between pharyngeal and tracheal suctioning.
- How can you ensure that the suction catheter enters the trachea and not the esophagus?

Caring for a Patient Requiring Mechanical Ventilation

A **mechanical ventilator** is a machine that assists a patient to breathe. The patient is intubated before he is connected to the ventilator. The endotracheal tube or tracheostomy tube is connected by oxygen tubing to the ventilator. Mechanical ventilation is indicated for acute or chronic respiratory failure and may be a short- or long-term therapy.

- **Negative pressure ventilators** consist of shells that fit externally around the chest. Negative pressure generated inside the shell pulls the chest outward and forces the patient to inhale air, similar to normal breathing. These ventilators are rarely used for acutely ill patients, but they are occasionally used for chronic conditions, for example, in patients with muscle weakness from neuromuscular disease.
- **Positive pressure ventilators** (also called mechanical ventilation), the most widely used type, require the patient to have an artificial airway (Fig. 37-12). Positive pressure ventilation carries risks, including *barotrauma* (injury to the airways due to pressure changes) and decreased cardiac output as the positive pressure in the chest decreases venous return to the heart.

To care for a patient receiving mechanical ventilation you will need to be familiar with the types of ventilators in use. You need a thorough understanding of the ventilator, its settings, and how to troubleshoot problems. In the event of a malfunction, if the repair is not readily obvious, manually ventilate the patient with an Ambu bag (resuscitation bag) connected to supplemental oxygen while a colleague troubleshoots the problem. Procedure 37-10 describes care of patients requiring mechanical ventilation, including ventilator terminology and delegation of care.

Patients being mechanically ventilated, even for a short period, are at high risk for developing *ventilator-associated pneumonia (VAP)*. VAP is associated with high mortality rates. Procedure 37-10 includes guidelines for nursing interventions to help prevent VAP. For ventilator terminology, refer to Table 37-2.

Caring for a Patient Requiring Chest Tubes

Normally there is negative pressure in the pleural space and only a thin layer of fluid between the lung and chest wall membranes.

- **Hemothorax**—Accumulation of fluid and blood in the pleural space interferes with lung expansion, ventilation, and gas exchange.

Toward Evidence-Based Practice

Rello, J., Afonso, E., Lisboa, T., et al. (2012). A care bundle approach for prevention of ventilator-associated pneumonia. *Clinical Microbiology and Infection, 19*(4), 363–369.

In this study, patients in three adult intensive care units (ICUs) were intubated and mechanically ventilated. Nurses implemented a ventilator-associated pneumonia (VAP) bundle (which includes elevating the head of the bed to 30° and practicing good hand hygiene, as well as other interventions). There was a significant reduction in VAP related to hand hygiene, intra-cuff pressure control, oral hygiene, and sedation. In addition, there was a reduction of ICU length of stay (from 10 to 6 days) and duration of mechanical ventilation (from 8 to 4 days).

Kelly, D. M. (2012). *The organization of critical care nursing and outcomes of mechanically ventilated older adults* (Doctoral dissertation). Retrieved from http://repository.upenn.edu/dissertations/AAI3542907

This multistate analysis examined the organization of critical care nursing and outcomes of 56,826 mechanically ventilated ICU patients cared for in 303 hospitals. Critical care nurse staffing, the practice environment, proportion of bachelor's prepared (BSN) nurses, and proportion of specialty certified nurses were the critical care nursing measures. Healthcare-associated infections were less likely to occur when staffing and resources in the critical care unit were higher, with a greater proportion of BSN prepared nurses and a better practice environment.

Mateoso, J., Gonzalez, N., Sadaba, M., et al. (2011). Nursing care in the prevention of ventilator-associated pneumonia. *Enfermería Intensiva, 22*(1), 22–30.

Researchers observed and described the care of 26 patients with more than 24 hours of invasive mechanical ventilation. They reported good nursing compliance with established protocols for oral hygiene, oropharyngeal suction, turning of patients, and patient tolerance of enteral nutrition. Incidence of VAP was low and well within internationally established ranges. They concluded, nevertheless, that incidence of VAP could be further reduced with better control of endotracheal tube cuff pressures and by elevating the head of the bed to between 30° and 45°.

1. Based on these study findings, list at least two interventions a staff nurse could do to help prevent VAP.

2. Which study might you use to convince a hospital administrator to hire more nurses?

 Go to Davis Advantage, Resources, Chapter 37, **Toward Evidence-Based Practice—Suggested Responses.**

- **Pneumothorax**—Air in the pleural space creates positive pressure, causing lung tissue to collapse.

The purpose of a chest-drainage system is to make room for the lungs to fully expand. This is done by removing air and fluid from the pleural space. A valve in the line or a water-sealed compartment prevents reentry of air and fluid. A chest-drainage system is composed of a chest tube inserted into the pleural space and a drainage collection system. The system usually is attached to some form of suction.

Flow of air and fluid must be in one direction: from the patient to the collection system. Think of the chest tube as an extension of the pleural space. To provide negative pressure within the chest tube, the open end of the tube is placed under water. With each exhalation, air is expelled through the chest tube into the water, but no air is drawn in during inhalation (Fig. 37-13). Once all air is expelled from the pleural space, negative pressure is reestablished and the lung can fully expand. When the lung tissue is reexpanded, the chest tube can be safely removed.

Types of Drainage Systems

Various chest drainage systems are available, including the older, reusable glass, three-bottle, water-seal system. However, you will most often use a disposable system. These are more compact and lightweight. Disposable systems may be water seal or dry seal and may or may not use suction. To learn how to set up disposable chest drainage systems, see Procedure 37-11.

Water-Seal Systems Water-seal systems can consist of one, two, or three chambers (or bottles, in the traditional glass bottle system).

- **A one-chamber device** is the simplest chest drainage system. The chest tube connects to one drainage chamber, which serves as both a collector and a water seal. This system can handle only small volumes of fluid or air. As fluid drains through the chest tube, it raises the fluid level in the

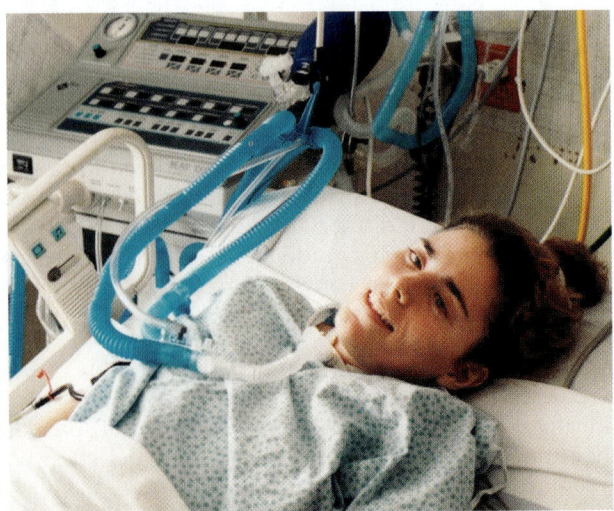

FIGURE 37-12 A patient connected to a ventilator via tracheostomy.

Table 37-2 ➤ Ventilator Terminology

TERM	EXPLANATION
Fio$_2$	Fraction of inspired oxygen
Modes of Ventilation	Describes the setting on the ventilator that assists the patient to breathe. Can be controlled (CMV), intermittent mandatory (IMV), or synchronized intermittent mandatory (SIMV).
Tidal Volume	Amount of air delivered from the ventilator with each breath
Assist-Control Mode—also known as Continuous Mechanical Ventilation (CMV)	The preset number of breaths per minute delivered by the machine. If the patient is able to initiate breaths, the machine will deliver a breath when the patient begins to inspire. If the patient is unable to breathe on his own, the machine will deliver the preset number of breaths in a rhythmic fashion.
Intermittent Mandatory Ventilation	A ventilator setting that delivers a minimum number of breaths per minute if the patient does not ventilate independently.
Synchronized Intermittent Mandatory Ventilation (SIMV)	A ventilator setting that delivers a minimum number of ventilations per minute if the patient does not ventilate independently. The ventilator breaths are synchronized with the patient's breaths. This mode is used for weaning patients from the ventilator.
Pressure Support	Provides positive pressure on inspiration to decrease the workload of breathing.
Continuous Positive Airway Pressure (CPAP)	Provides positive pressure during inspiration and expiration to keep alveoli open in a spontaneously breathing patient.
Positive End Expiratory Pressure (PEEP)	Provides positive pressure on expiration to keep airways open for patients on CMV or SIMV mode ventilation.

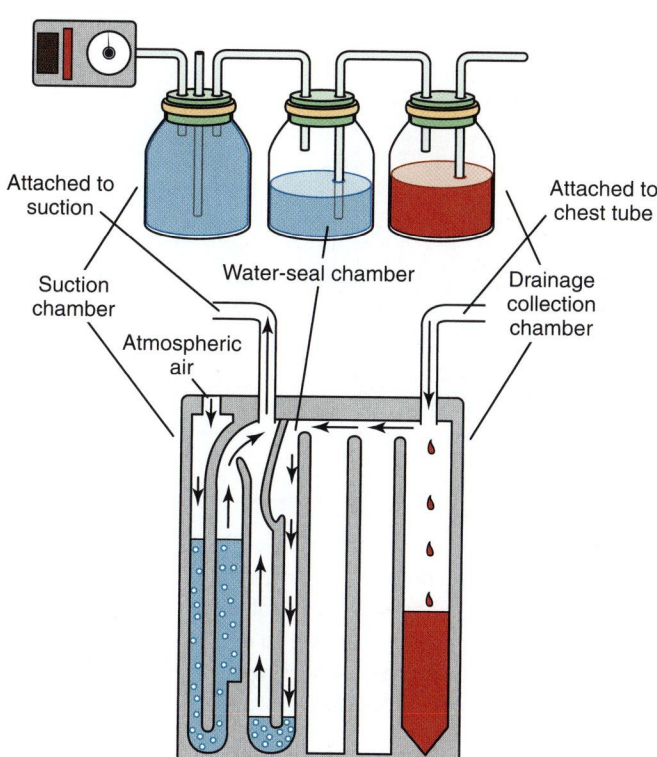

FIGURE 37-13 A disposable chest drainage system.

Labels on figure: Attached to suction; Suction chamber; Water-seal chamber; Atmospheric air; Attached to chest tube; Drainage collection chamber

chamber, making it harder for the patient to exhale. It is important that the device not be tipped over because the vent tube would no longer be below water and air would enter the pleural space.

- **A two-chamber system** has one chamber that connects directly with the chest tube and serves as a collection bottle. The second chamber serves as the water seal; it maintains negative pressure as air flows through it. Because the chest drainage never enters the water-seal chamber, you can measure the amount of drainage more accurately. The two-chamber system can handle large amounts of fluid drainage, but its design can still contribute to labored breathing.

- **A three-chamber system** adds a third chamber, which connects to the water-seal chamber and placed to suction (Fig. 37-14). This creates controlled negative pressure within the system. The suction control chamber has three vent tubes: one connected to suction, one connected to the water seal chamber, and a long middle tube with one end open to air at the top. The amount of sterile water in the suction chamber determines the maximum suction possible within the system. Suction pressure is expressed in centimeters of water.

For proper functioning, adjust the suction regulator to create gentle bubbling in the suction control bottle.

Dry-Seal Systems Dry-seal systems are fairly new. They are one-piece devices with three chambers: fluid collection, dry seal, and dry suction control. They do not use water in the suction chamber, relying instead on a mechanical automatic control valve (ACV) and an air leak monitor. The valve allows air to pass out of the patient and prevents it from returning to

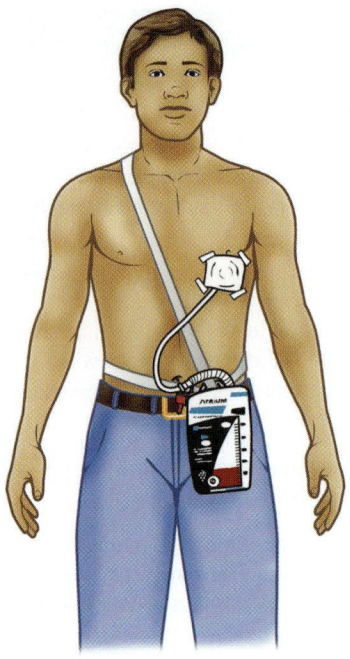

FIGURE 37-14 A one-chamber, dry-seal, portable chest drainage system.

the patient—even if the system is knocked over. Pressure is set by adjusting the rotary suction dial. The ACV keeps the pressure constant by adjusting to changes in air leaks and fluctuations in the suction source.

Portable Systems Portable or mobile systems consist of a single, dry-seal chamber attached to the patient's chest tube (see Fig. 37-14). It drains by gravity but can be connected to wall suction. Portable systems improve ambulation and reduce the risk of deep vein thrombosis and pulmonary embolism. They are thought to decrease the length of time a patient must stay in the hospital. The collection chamber holds a maximum of 500 mL, so portable systems are not practical for patients whose drainage is more than 500 mL daily. To learn how to set up disposable chest drainage systems, see Procedure 37-11. For guidelines to help you manage care for patients with chest tubes, see Clinical Insight 37-5.

KnowledgeCheck 37-13

- What is the purpose of mechanical ventilation?
- Why is a chest tube inserted?
- What is the advantage of a three-chamber system (compared with a one-chamber or two-chamber system)?
- How does a portable chest drainage system compare with a water-seal drainage system?

CLINICALREASONING

The questions and exercises in this section allow you to practice the kind of thinking you will use as a full-spectrum nurse. Critical-thinking questions usually have more than one correct answer, so we do not provide "correct answers" for these features. It is more important to develop your nursing judgment than to just cover content. You will learn by discussing the questions with your peers. If you are still unsure, see the Davis Advantage chapter resources for suggested responses.

Caring for the Nguyens

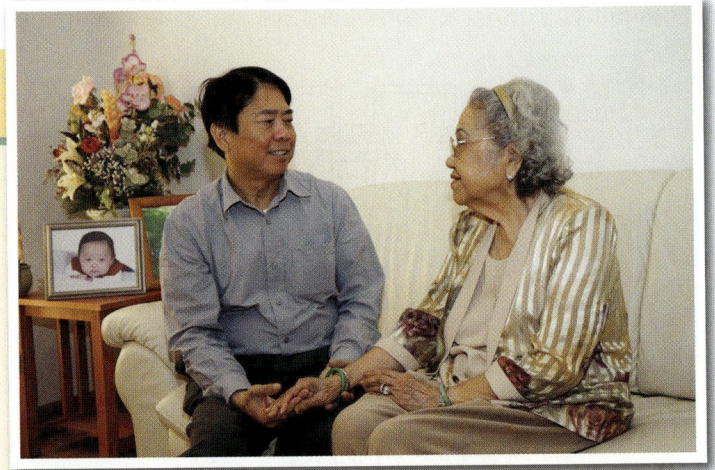

Mai Nguyen, Nam's 76-year-old mother, has been complaining of fatigue and a persistent cough for approximately 2 weeks. Nam has brought his mother to the family clinic where you are a nurse. Mrs. Nguyen appears disheveled. Her clothes are rumpled and her hair is tousled. Normally she appears at the clinic dressed neatly and wearing makeup. She has a hard time signing in at the desk and tells the receptionist she has a 1:00 p.m. appointment, but it is 9:00 a.m. Mrs. Nguyen's vital signs are as follows: BP, 142/90 mm Hg; pulse, 94 beats/min and regular; respirations, 24 breaths/min and labored; temperature, 99.6°F (37.5°C) oral.

A. What additional assessment data would be useful to gather at this time?

B. During her visit at the clinic, you notice that Mrs. Nguyen is very confused. Her weight has dropped 7 pounds since her visit last month, her mucous membranes are dry, and she is dyspneic with any activity. She is diagnosed with pneumonia. Because of her rapid decline, Mrs. Nguyen is admitted to the hospital to receive intravenous antibiotics. At the hospital, her initial pulse oximetry reading is 90%, and she is unable to cough up secretions. Write the most appropriate nursing diagnosis to focus interventions for Mrs. Nguyen.

Caring for the Nguyens (continued)

C. What actions should you anticipate taking?

D. The hospitalist (hospital-based physician) writes prescriptions for IV fluids, antibiotics, suction prn, and continuous pulse oximetry. What additional prescriptions will you need to provide care for Mrs. Nguyen? What therapy would you suggest?

E. Mrs. Nguyen requires suctioning to help remove secretions. She has a weak cough and crackles and rhonchi throughout all lung fields. There are few secretions in her oropharynx,

and she bites down on the catheter. What technique would you use to suction her? Explain your choice.

F. After 4 days in the hospital, Mrs. Nguyen is discharged to home. She asks the hospital nurse, "What can I do to make sure I never get that sick again?" How would you answer this question?

 Go to Davis Advantage, Resources, Chapter 37, **Caring for the Nguyens—Suggested Responses.**

Applying the **Full-Spectrum Nursing Model**_____

PATIENT SITUATION

Haley, a 15-year-old female high school student, was admitted to the hospital with shortness of breath and right-sided chest pain when breathing. She states that she has had "the flu" for 3 days. She has a history of asthma since age 6, and she smokes a half pack of cigarettes a day. Both her parents are heavy smokers. An IV was initiated, and she is receiving 800 mg of vancomycin (an antibiotic) intravenously every 12 hours. She is not on oxygen therapy, but receives 10 incentive spirometer treatments per hour while awake. Her heart rate is 80 beats/min, respiratory rate 24 breaths/min, and blood pressure 110/70 mm Hg. Her skin is pale but warm, and capillary refill time is 2 seconds. She has no clubbing of the fingers. She is urinating approximately 400 mL of clear yellow urine every 8 hours and maintaining a normal bowel elimination pattern. Laboratory results are:

Red blood cell count (RBCs): 3.56×10^6 (3.56 million/mm³)
White blood cell count (WBCs): 11,800/mm³
Hemoglobin: 11.2 g/dL
Hematocrit: 32.7%

Haley says, "I feel really tired and too weak to even pick up a glass of water." Her cough produces white, thick sputum. Sputum culture on admission confirms a diagnosis of streptococcal pneumonia.

THINKING

1. *Theoretical Knowledge:*
   a. According to the Centers for Disease Control and Prevention, should Haley have received a pneumonia immunization? Why or why not?
   b. What is clubbing of the fingers? You may wish to refer to Chapter 21 for review or to a medical–surgical nursing text.
2. *Critical Thinking (Analyzing Assumptions):*
   Why is it a positive finding for Haley that she does not have clubbed fingers?

DOING

3. *Practical Knowledge:*
   Twenty-four hours after the antibiotics were started, Haley's respiratory status becomes worse. She says, "It's so hard to breathe." It is decided to begin administering oxygen. Another sputum culture is prescribed. You are to collect a sputum specimen from the patient.
   a. What position should Haley assume for this procedure?
   b. What kind of protective clothing do you need for this procedure?
   c. You remove the lid from the specimen container. When you hand it to Haley, she touches the inside of the container with her fingers. What should you do?
   d. What would you tell Haley to do in order to expectorate the sputum specimen?
4. *Nursing Process (Assessment):*
   In the admission data, what important information is missing with regard to her respiratory status?

CARING

5. *Self-Knowledge:*
   Describe one or two patient care experiences you might draw upon to help you in caring for Haley. In what ways were those patients similar to Haley and how might that help you?
6. *Ethical Knowledge:*
   After you finish collecting the sputum specimen, what do you think Haley's biggest concern is right now?

 Go to Davis Advantage, Resources, Chapter 37, **Applying the Full-Spectrum Nursing Model—Suggested Responses.**

PracticalKnowledge:
clinical application

The Clinical Insights and Procedures in this section will help you acquire the skills to safely provide for clients' oxygenation needs.

CLINICAL INSIGHTS

Clinical Insight 37-1 ➤ **Tips for Obtaining Accurate Pulse Oximetry Readings**

Patient Movement. A *nailbed* is the most common site to place the probe. However, a tremor, twitch, shivering, or movement in bed can make pulse oximetry readings inaccurate. If the patient is unable to cooperate or control his movement, try using an ear probe or nasal sensor.

Acrylic Fingernails and Nail Polish. If the patient has acrylic nails, place the probe on a toe or earlobe. Many facilities stock individually packaged nail polish remover pads to remove nail polish before placing the probe.
Nail polish or acrylic nails may interfere with signal transmission, causing inaccurate SaO_2 measurement. However, a recent study found that nail polish did not cause a clinically significant change in readings in healthy people (Chan, Chan, & Chan, 2013).

Dirt and Skin Oils. Dirt and oils on the site can interfere with passage of light waves.

Poor Perfusion. A low reading may result from poor perfusion of the area where the probe is placed.
- A bent elbow, for example, may cause a slight decrease in circulation to the nailbed. If SaO_2 results are crucial to the patient's plan of care, use the earlobe to minimize the effect of movement on the reading.
- Keep the extremities warm to obtain a more accurate reading.
  Vasoconstriction due to cool extremities may also limit circulation.

- If poor perfusion is related to a disease process, use the earlobe or nose as the monitoring site.

Lighting. Bright fluorescent lighting may influence the accuracy of the reading. Dim the lights or cover the probe with bed covers or a towel to reduce error.

Anemia, Carbon Monoxide, Intravascular Dyes, and Dark Skin Color. These must be considered when interpreting oximetry readings. Because these factors cannot be controlled, watch for trend changes in the readings.

Equipment Function. Look for a displayed waveform; a reading is meaningless without the waveform. If there is a weak signal or no signal, check the patient's vital signs. If vital signs are satisfactory, check the circulation to the site. If that is satisfactory, check equipment connections.

Accuracy of the Reading. If there is an instantaneous change in saturation (e.g., from 99% to 82%), suspect an error. This is not physiologically possible. For any suspected inaccuracy, check the reading using the equipment on a healthy person. If it seems accurate, check the patient's medications and check for history of circulatory disorders; also check the items listed above. When in doubt, rely on your clinical judgment more than the reading from the machine.

Clinical Insight 37-2 ➤ Guidelines for Preventing Aspiration

 To prevent aspiration, use the following guidelines:

For At Risk Patients

Position the unconscious patient on his side to protect the airway.

Request medications in elixir or liquid form.

Break or crush pills, when appropriate.

Keep a suction setup available for routine and emergency use.

If the patient is intubated, keep the endotracheal or tracheostomy cuff inflated and suction above the cuff before deflating the cuff.

Do not offer food or fluids if the patient is heavily sedated or in the initial recovery phase of anesthesia.

Enteral Feedings

Check the placement of the nasogastric tube before you administer enteral feedings.

Check gastric residual volume before administering the next enteral feeding. Hold the feeding if the residual volume is high. (*Note:* The amount of acceptable residual volume depends on the amount and frequency of feedings.)

If the patient is receiving continuous tube feedings, the head of the bed must remain elevated.

See Procedure 28-3 for step-by-step instructions for administering feedings through gastric and enteric tubes.

Oral Feedings

Position the patient upright or with the head of the bed elevated for feedings or meal.

Be sure the head of bed remains elevated for at least 30 minutes after each feeding or meal.

Offer small, frequent meals.

Avoid thin liquids, or use thickening agents.

Offer foods or liquids that can be formed into a bolus before they are swallowed.

Cut food into small pieces.

Clinical Insight 37-3 ➤ Oxygen Therapy Safety Precautions

- Post signs indicating that oxygen is in use.
- Do not permit smoking near oxygen delivery systems.
- Ensure that three-pronged plugs are used for electrical devices (to prevent sparks).
- Allow no open flames (e.g., candles) near oxygen.
- Do not use electrical equipment with frayed wires or loose connections.

- Do not use petroleum products, aerosol products, and products containing acetone where oxygen is in use. (These are flammable substances that are easily ignited.)
- Secure oxygen tanks to rigid stands.
- Secure portable oxygen cylinders in holders or carriers provided.

Clinical Insight 37-4 ➤ Caring for Patients With Endotracheal Airways

Assisting With Endotracheal Airway Insertion

- **Gather equipment.** You will need an oxygen source and a bag (e.g., Ambu or nonrebreather bag) to inflate the lungs, a laryngoscope, endotracheal tubes of various sizes, water-soluble lubricant, a syringe to inflate the cuff, and tape to secure the tube in place.
- **Keep suction at the bedside** to clear the mouth and airway if secretions are obstructing your view of the cords.
- **You will need a surgical tray** if a tracheostomy is performed to create the direct opening into the trachea.
- **Remain calm and explain** to the patient that the airway will enable him to breathe effectively.
- **Once the airway is in place, listen to breath sounds** to establish that both lungs are ventilated.

- **Reassess breath sounds periodically.** After the airway is inserted, record the type and size, as well as the patient's response to the procedure.
- **Expect that a portable chest x-ray will be prescribed** to confirm correct placement.

Managing and Monitoring Endotracheal Airways

The following are activities associated with the care of all types of endotracheal airways.

- Have emergency equipment, including a duplicate tracheostomy kit, extra cannula, and suction setup, immediately available for reintubation if the tube should become dislodged.

(Continued)

Clinical Insight 37-4 ➤ **Caring for Patients With Endotracheal Airways—cont'd**

- **Keep an extra cannula at the bedside,** as patients may accidentally decannulate.
- **Secure the endotracheal tube** with ties, Velcro tapes, or a commercial holder to prevent accidental displacement.

- **Provide tracheostomy care every 4 to 8 hours** (Mitchell, Hussey, Setzen, et al., 2013).
- **Secure the orotracheal tube** to the opposite side of the mouth with each change of tape or ties to prevent skin erosion and breakdown.
- **Inspect skin around the tube** or tracheal stoma for redness, swelling, drainage, or irritation at least every 8 hours.
- **Provide skin care** around the tube and tape or holder at least daily.
- **Perform regular oral care.**
- **Inflate the cuff of the tube with a minimal occlusive volume and monitor cuff pressures** to prevent pressure necrosis inside the trachea. (This is a joint responsibility with the respiratory therapist.) Maximum acceptable tube cuff pressure is 25 mm Hg. The following is a method for checking for minimal occluding volume:
  1. Place stethoscope on patient's neck over the carotid pulse.
  2. Attach a 10-mL syringe to the pilot balloon of the inflated cuff.

  3. Remove air from the cuff (1 mL at a time) until you hear a slight leak at the peak of inspiration.
  4. When you hear the leak, inject 1 mL of air back into the cuff.
- **Monitor and document cuff pressure** once per shift and when the tube is changed or repositioned.
- **Note the centimeter reference marking** on the endotracheal tube to monitor for possible displacement.
- **Minimize pulling and traction** on the artificial airway by supporting all tubing connected to the airway and using flexible catheter mounts and swivels.
- **Remind conscious patients not to pull on the airway.**
- **Use a bite block between the teeth** to prevent the patient from occluding an orotracheal tube.
- **Provide 100% humidification** of inspired air. Check the oxygen setup regularly.
- **Routine saline instillation** to thin secretions is no longer recommended.
- **Ensure adequate hydration** with oral or IV fluids to keep the mucosa moist and thin secretions.
- **Suction the airway when** secretions collect. Remember, the patient probably can't cough effectively to clear secretions.

Clinical Insight 37-5 ➤ **Managing Chest Tubes**

Monitor breathing, gas exchange, and drainage.

- **Frequently assess breathing patterns, breathing effort, and breath sounds.**
- **Assess mental status, heart rate and rhythm, and pulse oximetry readings.**
  These reflect adequacy of oxygenation.
- **Monitor character, color, and amount of chest drainage.** Immediately report sudden or large increases in drainage or new onset of bright red blood, along with an assessment of the patient's condition at that time.
  Drainage is usually greatest when the chest tube is initially inserted and decreases as the lung reexpands. The chest drainage unit (CDU) must be replaced when the drainage compartment is almost full.

Prevent complications or intervene if they occur.

- **Observe the dressing at least every 4 hours.** Make sure that the chest dressing around the tube insertion site is occlusive (e.g., not wet or loose). Usually, petroleum gauze is wrapped around the insertion site to ensure occlusion.

- **Inspect for excessive, abnormal, or foul-smelling drainage.**
  This may indicate hemorrhage or infection.
- **Palpate around the dressing for *subcutaneous emphysema*** (air in the subcutaneous tissues).
  This may be caused by an incomplete seal at the chest tube insertion site.
- **Assess for pain;** medicate as needed.
- **Reposition the patient every 2 hours** and use pillows to keep the patient's weight off the chest tube.
  To prevent occlusion of the tube, to promote drainage, and to preserve skin integrity.
- **Encourage the patient to use the arm on the affected side.** Assist with range-of-motion exercises, if necessary.
  To maintain joint mobility.
- ✚ **Recollapse of the lung can occur** because of loss of negative pressure within the system. This is commonly caused by air leaks, disconnections, or breaks or cracks of the bottles or chambers. If any of these occur, immediately place the disconnected end nearest the patient into a bottle of sterile water or saline.

Clinical Insight 37-5 ➤ Managing Chest Tubes—cont'd

■ ✚ **Do not clamp the chest tube.** Doing so can lead to a **tension pneumothorax.** Clamp chest tubes only for changing the drainage system. Limit the clamp time and monitor respiratory status constantly until the clamp is removed.

■ ✚ **If the tube is accidentally pulled out,** immediately cover the wound with a dry, sterile dressing. Listen for air leaking out of the site. If you can hear air, tape the dressing loosely so that you do not occlude the site.
If air cannot escape from the chest, a tension pneumothorax will occur, eventually compromising cardiovascular function.

Promote Lung Reexpansion

■ **Encourage the patient to be as active as his condition permits.**
Chest drainage systems are bulky, but with disposable systems, some patients can still get out of bed and ambulate but will need assistance to protect and monitor the system and the patient.

■ **Instruct the patient to perform deep breathing and coughing every 2 hours,** unless contraindicated. Assist the patient to sit upright and splint the chest with a pillow or the hands, and provide analgesia as needed.
These interventions help to minimize discomfort.

Key Points for Managing a One-Bottle System

■ **Keep the intake tube below the fluid level in the drainage bottle.**
To prevent drawing air into the pleural space with inhalation.

■ **Maintain the tubing about 2 cm below the water level.** As tubing length below the water increases, more effort is required to exhale.

■ **Take precautions to see that the bottle is not accidentally tipped over,** uncovering the long vent tube and allowing air to enter the pleural space.

Maintain the drainage system.

For All Types of CDUs:

■ **Make sure the drainage system is located below the insertion site.**
If the drainage system is higher than the insertion site, fluid may flow back into the pleural cavity, compromising the patient's respiratory status.

■ **Regularly inspect tubing** to ensure that connections are airtight and tubing is not kinked or occluded.
Kinks in the drainage tubing increase pressure in the pleural cavity and prevent fluid drainage.

■ **Monitor drainage.**
Blood or purulent matter can occlude the tubing.

■ **Inspect the air vent in the drainage system** to make sure it is patent.
If air builds up in the pleural cavity, pneumothorax may occur.

■ **Monitor to ensure the system is maintaining consistent negative pressure levels.**

■ ✚ **Do not "milk" or strip the tubing.**
*Doing so can create excess negative pressure and damage lung tissue. **Always be sure to verify operation** through the users' manual or with the product's vendor. Most systems will have some type of check system to ensure that the system is operating correctly.*

■ **To transport or ambulate a patient:** (1) Keep the CDU upright below chest level; (2) disconnect the CDU from suction source and make sure the air vent is open.
Water-Seal Drainage Systems:

■ **Take precautions that the CDU is not tipped over** (e.g., tape it to the floor).

■ **Observe for *tidaling*** (fluctuations in the water-seal chamber's fluid level that correspond with respiration). The level will increase on inspiration and decrease on exhalation. This will be opposite for a patient on a mechanical ventilator.

■ **Bubbling in the bottom of the water-seal chamber indicates an air leak.** When this occurs, check for poor tubing connections. A small amount of bubbling right after insertion or with exhalation or cough is normal.

■ **Check the water in the suction control chamber;** replace as needed.
The water can evaporate.

■ ✚ **If the chest tube disconnects from the drainage unit,** establish a temporary water seal by immersing the open end of the chest tube in a bottle of sterile water to a depth of 2 cm until a new system can be connected. Cleanse the end of the patient connector on the drain system with alcohol and reconnect it if it has not been contaminated. If the patient connector on the drain system is contaminated, you must initiate a new CDU.

Dry-Seal Drainage Systems:

■ **Inspect the air vent in the drainage system** to make sure it is patent.
The air vent must remain patent to allow air to escape. If air builds up in the pleural cavity, pneumothorax may occur.

■ **Check the indicators on the CDU to be certain that suction is operating properly.**
A dry chest drainage system doesn't use water in the suction chamber. A valve inside the regulator continuously balances the forces of suction and the atmosphere. The valve automatically responds and adjusts to changes in patient air leaks and fluctuations in suction source vacuum to deliver accurate suction to the patient. Pressure can be set from -10 cm H_2O to -40 cm H_2O by adjusting the rotary dry suction dial.

■ **Observe for bubbling.**
If the water in a dry-seal CDU is bubbling, it means there is an air leak.

PROCEDURES

Procedure 37-1 ■ Collecting a Sputum Specimen

> ➤ For steps to follow in *all* procedures, refer to the Universal Steps for All Procedures found on the page facing the inside back cover.

Equipment

For all sputum specimens, you will need a patient identification label, a completed laboratory requisition form, and a small plastic bag with a biohazard label (or container designated by the agency) for delivering the specimen to the laboratory. Depending on how you obtain the specimen, you also need the following:

Procedure 37-1A: Obtaining an Expectorated Specimen

- Sterile specimen container with lid
- Procedure gloves
- Glass of water
- Emesis basin
- Tissues
- Pillow (if abdominal or chest incision is present)

Procedure 37-1B: Obtaining a Specimen by Suction

- Sterile suction catheter or sterile suction kit
- Suction device (portable or wall)
- Sterile gloves
- Protective eyewear
- Inline sputum specimen container or trap
- Sterile saline solution
- Oxygen therapy equipment, if indicated
- Linen-saver pad or towel

Delegation

You can delegate collection of an expectorated sputum specimen to a nursing assistive personnel (NAP) who has been adequately trained in performing the skill. Assess the patient's respiratory status first; if the patient's condition is unstable, do not delegate the procedure. Do not delegate obtaining a specimen by tracheal suctioning.

Pre-Procedure Assessment

- Assess the patient's comprehension of the procedure.
  Understanding allays anxiety and promotes cooperation.

- Assess breath sounds; respiratory rate, depth, and pattern; skin and nailbed color; and tissue perfusion.
  You may need to delay sputum collection if the patient is in respiratory distress.

- Assess ability to deep-breathe, cough, and expectorate.
  If the patient is unable to deep-breathe, cough, and expectorate, suctioning may be necessary to obtain an adequate sputum specimen.

- Determine when the patient last ate or had a tube feeding, especially for a specimen obtained by suction.
  Specimen collection should be delayed for 1 to 2 hours after eating because the procedure may cause vomiting, which creates a risk for aspiration of stomach contents.

- If suctioning is required to obtain the specimen, check for factors such as anticoagulant therapy, bleeding disorders, or low platelet count.
  These factors place the patient at risk for bleeding when the suction catheter is introduced.

> ➤ When performing the procedure, always identify your patient according to agency policy, using two identifiers, and be attentive to standard precautions, hand hygiene, patient safety and privacy, body mechanics, and documentation.

Procedure Steps

1. **Verify the medical prescription** for type of sputum analysis.
   The type of sputum specimen determines the number of specimens required and the time of day the specimen should be collected. For example, specimens to confirm tuberculosis typically require three consecutive morning samples.

2. **Position the patient** according to the required specimen collection technique.
   a. *For an expectorated specimen,* assist the patient to high or semi-Fowler's position or to a sitting position at the edge of the bed.

   b. *For a suctioned specimen,* position the patient in high or semi-Fowler's position.
   These positions facilitate insertion of the suction catheter and the ability to cough. They also promote lung expansion and prevent aspiration should the patient vomit during the procedure.

3. **Drape a towel or linen-saver pad** over the patient's chest. Ask the patient to rinse his mouth and gargle with water.
   A towel or pad protects the patient's gown from soiling during specimen collection. Rinsing the mouth removes flora that may contaminate the specimen; however, evidence is not conclusive on this point.

4. **If the patient has an abdominal or chest incision,** have the patient splint the incision with a pillow.
   Splinting the incision decreases discomfort when the patient coughs. Splinting the incision decreases discomfort when the patient coughs.

Procedure 37-1A ■ Collecting an Expectorated Sputum Specimen

Procedure Steps

Follow steps 1 through 4, preceding.

5. **Provide the patient with the specimen container.** Advise the patient to avoid touching the inside of the container. If you must hold the container for the patient, first don procedure gloves.
The inside of the container must remain sterile. Wear gloves because you may come in contact with secretions or airborne bacteria when the patient coughs and expectorates. ▼

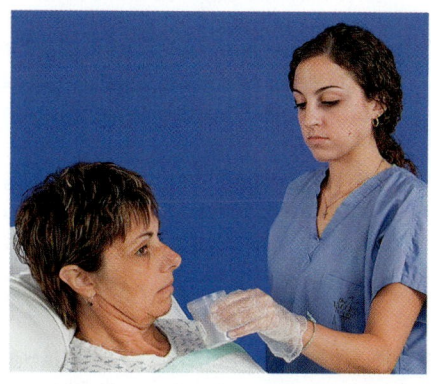

6. **Ask the patient to breathe deeply** for three or four breaths, and then ask him after a full inhalation to hold his breath and then cough.

Deep breathing opens airways and stimulates the cough reflex. Coughing after a full inhalation creates enough force to mobilize secretions through the airways and into the pharynx.

7. **Instruct the patient to expectorate** the secretions directly into the specimen container.
Prevents specimen contamination from outside organisms.

8. **Tell the patient to repeat deep breathing** and coughing until an adequate sample is obtained.
Typically 5 to 10 mL of sputum is required to ensure adequate sputum analysis.

9. **Don procedure gloves,** if you are not already wearing them; cover the specimen container with the lid immediately after the specimen is collected.
Gloves protect you in the event the patient's coughing has contaminated the outside of the container. Covering the container immediately prevents spread of microorganisms.

10. **After the patient expectorates,** offer tissues and provide mouth care.
Promotes patient comfort.

11. **Label the specimen container** with a patient identification label that contains the name of the test and collection date and time.
Correctly identifying the specimen ensures accurate diagnosis and treatment.

12. **Place the specimen in a plastic bag** with a biohazard label. Attach a completed laboratory requisition form.
The plastic bag protects healthcare workers from exposure to microorganisms. Completing the laboratory requisition form ensures proper processing of the specimen.

13. **Send the specimen to the laboratory** immediately, or refrigerate it if transport might be delayed.
If bacterial cultures are delayed, contaminating organisms may grow, producing false culture results and possibly inappropriate treatment.

Procedure 37-1B ■ Collecting a Suctioned Sputum Specimen

Procedure Steps

Follow steps 1 through 4, preceding.

5. **Administer oxygen** to the patient, if indicated.
Suctioning may cause hypoxemia.

6. **Prepare the suction device** and make sure it is functioning properly.

7. **Don protective eyewear.**
   ■ Protects your eyes from splattering of secretions during suctioning.

8. **Attach the suction tubing** to the male adapter of the inline sputum specimen container. ➤

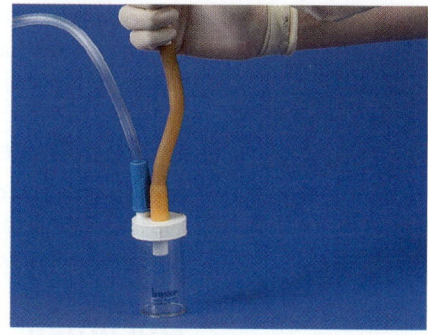

9. **Don sterile gloves.**
Protects the patient's sterile airways from contamination by outside organisms.

10. **Attach the sterile suction** to the flexible tubing on the sputum specimen container. The hand that touches the specimen container is no longer sterile.
Ensures that the sputum specimen goes directly into the specimen container instead of the suction tubing. ▼

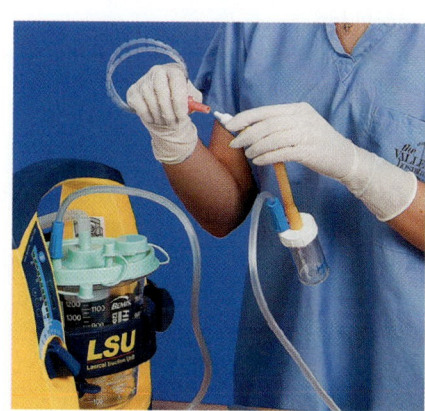

(continued on next page)

Procedure 37-1 ▪ **Collecting a Sputum Specimen** (continued)

11. Lubricate the suction catheter with sterile saline solution.
Lubrication eases insertion and prevents trauma to mucosa.

12. Insert the tip of the suction catheter gently through the nasopharynx, endotracheal tube, or tracheostomy tube. Advance the tip into the trachea (see Procedure 37-6 or Procedure 37-8).
Gentle insertion prevents airway trauma.

13. When the patient begins coughing, apply suction by placing your finger over the suction control port for 5 to 10 seconds to collect the specimen.
Applying suction for longer than 10 seconds can cause hypoxia.

14. If an adequate specimen (5 to 10 mL) is not obtained, allow the patient to rest for 1 or 2 minutes and then repeat the procedure. Administer oxygen to the patient at this time, if indicated.
Allowing the patient to rest and administering oxygen prevent hypoxia. You must assess your patient continually during this procedure to ensure patient safety and respiratory status.

15. When you have collected an adequate specimen, discontinue suction, then gently remove the suction catheter.
Applying suction during catheter removal can damage the airway mucosa.

16. Remove the suction catheter from the specimen container, and dispose of the catheter in the appropriate container.
Disposal of contaminated supplies prevents the spread of infection.

17. Remove the suction tubing from the specimen container, and connect the rubber tubing on the specimen container to the plastic adapter. ▼

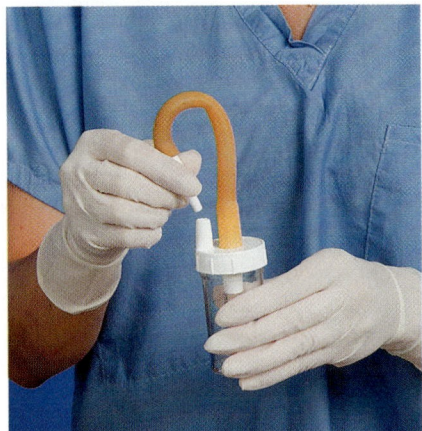

18. If sputum comes in contact with the outside of the specimen container, clean the outside with a disinfectant, according to agency policy.
Prevents spread of infection to staff members who must handle the specimen.

19. Label the specimen container with patient identification, the name of the test, and collection date and time.
Correctly identifying the specimen ensures accurate diagnosis and treatment.

20. Place the specimen in a plastic bag with a biohazard label. Attach a completed laboratory requisition form.
Placing the specimen in a plastic bag protects healthcare workers from exposure to microorganisms. Completing the laboratory requisition form ensures proper processing of the specimen.

21. Send the specimen to the laboratory immediately, or refrigerate it if transport might be delayed.
If bacterial cultures are delayed, contaminating organisms may grow, producing false culture results and possibly inappropriate treatment.

Evaluation

▪ Evaluate the patient's respiratory status during and after the procedure, especially if suctioning was necessary.
▪ Examine the color, consistency, and odor of the sputum specimen.
▪ Promptly report laboratory results to the primary care provider.
▪ Evaluate the patient's understanding of the procedure and test results.

Patient Teaching

▪ Explain proper collection techniques to avoid specimen contamination.
▪ Show the patient proper coughing techniques to ensure an adequate specimen.

▪ Explain the importance of avoiding mouthwash before the procedure, as it may alter laboratory results.
▪ If the patient has an incision, show him how to splint his incision to avoid discomfort during coughing and expectoration.

Home Care

Explain how to collect an expectorated sputum specimen and the importance of sending the specimen to the laboratory immediately after collection.

Documentation

▪ Record the date and time the specimen was collected, the method of collection, and the type of specimen ordered.
▪ Note the amount, color, consistency, and odor of the specimen.
▪ Document the patient's tolerance of the procedure.

Sample documentation

06/05/18   0700   Patient suctioned via tracheostomy. Sputum specimen obtained and sent for acid-fast bacillus (AFB) analysis. Specimen contained 15 ml of yellow, tenacious, odorless sputum. Patient became short of breath with suctioning. 100% O_2 administered via tracheostomy hood for 10 minutes after suctioning. Shortness of breath abated with treatment. O_2 returned to 40%. ——————————— S. Ryan, RN

Practice Resources

Centers for Disease Control and Prevention (n.d.a); Texas Department of State Health Services, Laboratory Services Section Home (2009, updated 2014).

Procedure 37-2 ■ Monitoring Pulse Oximetry (Arterial Oxygen Saturation)

➤ For steps to follow in *all* procedures, refer to the Universal Steps for All Procedures found on the page facing the inside back cover

Equipment

- Nail polish remover, if necessary
- Oximeter and probe sensor appropriate for patient age, size, and weight and for the desired location

Delegation

Because it is noninvasive and simple to perform, the registered nurse (RN) can delegate application of the pulse oximeter probe and measurement of arterial oxygen saturation (SaO_2) to a NAP or licensed practical nurse (LPN) who is adequately trained to perform the skill. Inform the NAP or LPN how often to take measurements, and instruct them to notify you immediately if SaO_2 falls below 95%. Although this procedure can be delegated, it is the responsibility of the RN to interpret the results, assess the patient, and notify the primary care provider.

Pre-Procedure Assessment

- Assess the patient's need for SaO_2 monitoring: low hemoglobin level; confusion, decreased level of consciousness, or respiratory distress; or risk factors, such as heart or pulmonary disease, recovering from anesthesia, or ventilator dependent.
  SaO_2 monitoring helps detect oxygenation problems early. Monitoring is especially important in patients with risk factors. Patients with underlying pulmonary disease may be accustomed to low oxygen saturation levels, so you may need to adjust the lower limit alarm and, if you have delegated the procedure, the level for notification for these patients.

- Assess the patient's respiratory status, including breath sounds; respiratory rate, depth, and pattern; tissue perfusion; SaO_2; and skin and nailbed color.
  Assessment findings may suggest a decrease in oxygen saturation and validate oximetry readings.

- Determine the optimal location for the oximeter probe sensor, for example, the fingertip, earlobe, forehead, or bridge of the nose. Check the capillary refill and pulse at the pulse closest to the site.
  To ensure accurate monitoring, choose a site that has adequate circulation, is free of artificial nails, and contains no moisture. Clinical Insight 37-1 offers suggestions on site placement based on patient factors.

- Assess for factors that may interfere with pulse oximetry measurement, such as hypotension, hypothermia, and tremors.
  The sensor requires adequate circulation to recognize hemoglobin molecules that absorb the emitted light. Tremors may produce artifact that may be misinterpreted by the oximeter, causing false readings.

- Check patient history for allergy to adhesive.
  An allergic reaction may occur if an adhesive-backed disposable probe sensor is used in a patient with a history of allergy to adhesives.

➤ When performing the procedure, always identify your patient according to agency policy, using two identifiers, and be attentive to standard precautions, hand hygiene, patient safety and privacy, body mechanics, and documentation.

➤ *Note:* This procedure explains how to apply a pulse oximeter. Refer to Clinical Insight 37-1 for tips for obtaining accurate pulse oximetry readings.

Procedure Steps

1. **Choose a sensor appropriate** for the patient's age, size, and weight and for the desired location.
   - If the patient is allergic to adhesive, use a clip-on probe sensor.
   - If the patient's peripheral circulation is compromised, use a nasal sensor.
     An appropriate type of sensor is more comfortable for the patient and ensures accurate readings.

2. **Prepare the site** by cleansing and drying it. If the finger is the desired location, remove nail polish or an acrylic nail, if present.
   Dirt and skin oils on the site can interfere with passage of light waves. Nail

(continued on next page)

Procedure 37-2 ■ Monitoring Pulse Oximetry (Arterial Oxygen Saturation) (continued)

polish or acrylic nails may interfere with signal transmission, causing inaccurate SaO₂ measurement. However, a recent study found that nail polish did not cause a clinically significant change in readings in healthy people (Chan, Chan, & Chan, 2013).

3. Remove the protective backing if you are using a disposable probe sensor that contains adhesive.

4. Attach the probe sensor to the chosen site. Make sure the photodetector and LEDs on the probe sensor face each other. Most probe sensors contain markings to facilitate correct placement.

When Using a Clip-on Probe Sensor

If you are using a clip-on probe sensor, warn the patient that he may feel a pinching sensation. Choose the site based on the status of circulation to the extremity and patient movement.

Inadequate circulation to the site and artifact caused by motion may alter SaO₂ results. The photodetector diodes and LEDs must be properly placed to ensure accurate readings.

5. Connect the sensor probe to the oximeter and turn it on. Check the

pulse rate displayed on the oximeter to see whether it correlates with the patient's radial pulse. (Be sure the pulse oximeter is plugged in to an electrical socket.)

Correlation between the oximeter pulse display and the patient's radial pulse confirms accurate readings.

6. Read the SaO₂ measurement on the digital display when it reaches a constant value, usually in 10 to 30 seconds, but may take up to 2 minutes.

The oximeter requires time to detect the pulse, calculate oxygen saturation, and register an accurate reading. ▼

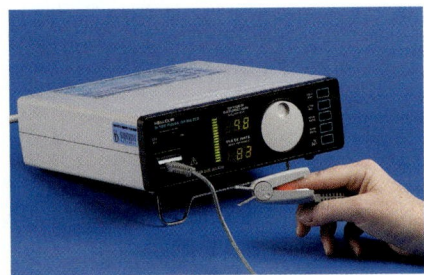

7. Set and turn on the alarm limits for SaO₂ and pulse rate, according to the manufacturer's instructions, patient condition, and agency policy if continuous monitoring is necessary.

Alarms must be set at appropriate levels to signify when SaO₂ or pulse rate falls below predetermined levels. Alarms help ensure prompt recognition and treatment of hypoxia.

8. Obtain readings as prescribed or indicated by the patient's respiratory status.

Some agencies require a prescription for pulse oximetry to ensure reimbursement.

9. Rotate the site if continuous monitoring is indicated.

For an Adhesive Probe Sensor

Rotate the site every 4 hours.

For a Clip-on Probe Sensor

Rotate the site every 2 hours.

Probe sensors and prolonged pressure may irritate the skin; rotating the site prevents skin breakdown.

10. Remove the probe sensor and turn off the oximeter when monitoring is no longer necessary.

Some oximeters are battery powered; leaving them on after use depletes the battery.

Evaluation

- Evaluate the patient's understanding of the procedure and the obtained values.
- Compare pulse oximetry results with the patient's clinical presentation.
- Evaluate the effectiveness of therapy by comparing SaO₂ results before, during, and after treatment.
- Assess the site every 4 hours if you are using an adhesive probe sensor or every 2 hours if you are using a clip-on probe sensor.

Patient Teaching

- Demonstrate the procedure to the patient and caregiver, especially if the patient will be continuing pulse oximetry at home.
- Explain to the patient and caregiver the significance of SaO₂ results.
- Discuss the signs and symptoms of hypoxia (confusion, restlessness, shortness of breath, dyspnea, cyanosis, and somnolence) with the patient and caregiver.

Home Care

- Explain where to obtain a pulse oximeter.
- Tell the client and caregiver when to notify the primary provider of abnormal results or signs and symptoms of hypoxia.
- Help the client identify risk factors that decrease SaO₂ levels.

Documentation

- Record the date and time of each pulse oximetry reading obtained. Most agencies use a flow sheet if frequent monitoring is necessary.
- Document whether readings are intermittent or continuous.
- If readings are continuous, record alarm parameters.
- Chart the patient's vital signs and SaO₂ results and indicate whether the patient is breathing room air or receiving oxygen therapy. For oxygen therapy, note the oxygen concentration and the mode of delivery.
- Document acute decreases in SaO₂, any precipitating factors, treatment interventions, and the patient's response.

Sample Documentation

July 1, 2018   0300   Stated "short of breath."
Crackles throughout lung fields. BP 140/92, apical
pulse 110 beats/min, resp rate 32 breaths/min. Pulse
oximetry applied to left index finger, and SaO₂ 88% on
room air. Placed on O₂ at 4 L/min via nasal cannula.
Dr. Jones notified. ——————— Kate Jackson, RNC

Practice Resources

American Association of Critical-Care Nurses (2010); Bunker, D. L. J., Kumar, R., Martin, A., et al. (2014); Chan, E. D., Chan, M. M., & Chan, M. M. (2013); Jones, M., Olorvida, E., Monger, K., et al. (2015).

Thinking About the Procedure

 The video **Administering Oxygen,** along with questions and suggested responses, is available on the **Davis's *Nursing Skills Videos*** Web site on Davis*Plus*.

Procedure 37-3 ■ Performing Percussion, Vibration, and Postural Drainage

➤ For steps to follow in all procedures, refer to the Universal Steps for All Procedures found on the page facing the inside back cover.

Equipment

- Bed capable of being placed in the Trendelenburg position
- Pillows
- Patient gown
- Facial tissues
- Emesis basin
- Sputum specimen container, if needed
- Suction equipment, if needed
- Stethoscope

Delegation

You should assess the patient to determine the need for the procedure and to evaluate whether the patient can tolerate it. You must perform the initial procedure, but you can delegate subsequent treatments to a respiratory therapist or NAP who is adequately trained. Instruct the respiratory therapist or NAP to report any changes in the patient's condition immediately. The RN is responsible for ongoing assessment and monitoring of airway clearance and respiratory status.

Pre-Procedure Assessment

- Check the patient's chest x-ray results.
  Identifies which lung fields require treatment.

- Assess the patient's respiratory status, including respiratory rate, depth, and rhythm; breath sounds; color; and pulse oximetry results.
  Determines the need for and effectiveness of percussion, vibration, and postural drainage.

- Determine when the patient has last eaten.
  Postural drainage should not be performed for at least 2 hours after meals to prevent nausea, vomiting, and aspiration.

- Assess for dysrhythmias, coagulopathy (a defect in blood clotting), hypertension, and pain or tenderness in the chest area being treated.
  If any of these are present, the procedure should be avoided because it might worsen these conditions.

➤ When performing the procedure, always identify your patient according to agency policy, using two identifiers, and be attentive to standard precautions, hand hygiene, patient safety and privacy, body mechanics, and documentation.

Procedure Steps

1. **Help the patient assume the appropriate position,** based on the lung field that requires drainage.
   Helps mobilize secretions in the affected lung field by gravity.

   a. *Apical areas of the upper lobes.* Ask the patient to sit at the edge of the bed, if possible. If needed, place a pillow at the base of the spine for support. If the patient is not able to sit at the edge of the bed, use high Fowler's position. ▼

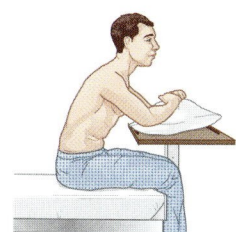

   b. *Posterior section of the upper lobes.* Position supine with a pillow under the hips and knees flexed. Have the patient rotate slightly away from the side that requires drainage. ▼

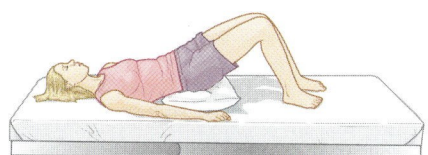

(continued on next page)

Procedure 37-3 ■ **Performing Percussion, Vibration, and Postural Drainage** (continued)

c. *Middle or lower lobes.* Place the bed in the Trendelenburg position. Position the patient in Sims' position. To drain the left lung, position the patient on his right side. For the right lung, position the patient on his left side. ▼

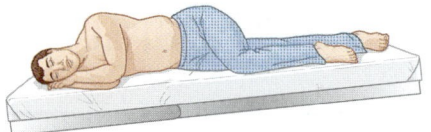

d. *Posterior lower lobes.* Keeping the bed flat, position the patient prone with a pillow under her stomach. ▼

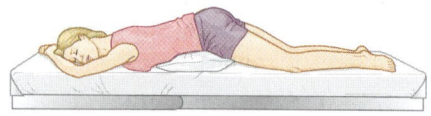

2. **Have the patient remain** in the desired position for 10 to 15 minutes, if tolerated.
   Allows adequate drainage of secretions by gravity from the desired lung field.

3. **Perform percussion** over the affected lung area while the patient is in the desired drainage position.
   Loosens and mobilizes secretions.

   a. Instruct the patient to breathe deeply and slowly.
      Relaxation helps the patient tolerate the procedure.

   b. Place a towel over the patient's skin or cover with the patient's gown the area to be percussed.
      Protects the skin and promotes patient privacy and comfort.

   c. ✚ Avoid clapping over bony prominences, female breasts, or tender areas of the chest.
      Percussing over these areas may cause discomfort and compromise tissue integrity.

d. Cup your hands, keeping your fingers flexed and your thumbs pressed against your index fingers.
   Cupping your hands promotes patient comfort during percussion.

e. Place your cupped hands over the lung area that requires drainage.

f. Percuss the lung area for 1 to 3 minutes by alternately striking your cupped hands rhythmically against the patient. ▼

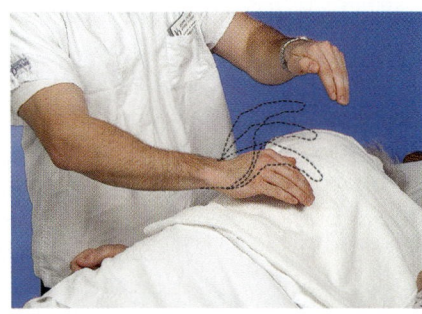

4. **Perform vibrations** while the patient remains in the desired drainage position. ▼

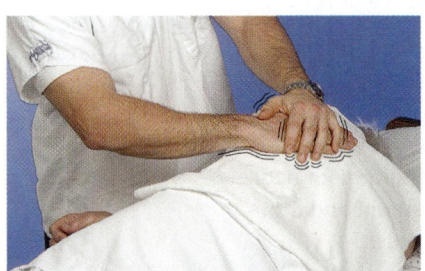

a. Place the flat surface of one hand over the lung area that requires vibration. Place your other hand on top of that hand at a right angle.
   Using the flat surfaces of the hands provides a large surface area to transmit vibrations through the chest. Placing one hand on top of the other provides better leverage for vibrating.

b. Instruct the patient to inhale slowly and deeply.
   Promotes relaxation and lung expansion.

c. Instruct the patient to make a "fff" or "sss" sound as she exhales.

d. As the patient exhales, press your fingers and palms firmly against her chest wall.
   Vibrating during exhalation enhances the downward movement of the rib cage that occurs during exhalation.

e. Push down, and gently vibrate with your hands over the lung area.
   Vibration helps mobilize secretions.

f. Continue performing vibrations for three exhalations.

5. **After performing postural drainage,** percussion, and vibration, allow the patient to sit up. Ask her to cough at the end of a deep inspiration. Suction the patient if she is unable to expectorate secretions. If a sputum specimen is needed, collect it in a specimen container.
   Coughing helps clear the airway of secretions.

6. **Repeat steps 1 through 5** for each lung field that requires treatment. The entire treatment should not exceed 60 minutes.
   Treating for longer than 60 minutes fatigues the patient.

7. **Provide mouth care.**
   Cleanses the mouth of secretions and promotes patient comfort.

Evaluation

- Evaluate the effectiveness of percussion, vibration, and postural drainage.
- Auscultate breath sounds every 2 to 4 hours, as indicated.
- Monitor pulse oximetry and arterial blood gas (ABG) results.
- Evaluate the need for further treatments.

Patient Teaching

- Demonstrate percussion, vibration, and postural drainage if the patient will be continuing it at home.
- Reinforce the importance of immediately reporting shortness of breath or any difficulty breathing.
- Explain the importance of drinking fluids to help thin and mobilize secretions.
- Teach coughing and deep-breathing exercises.

Home Care

- Be sure the client family/caregiver knows how often the procedure should be done. There should be a prescription from the primary care provider.
- Most clients will not have a bed that can be placed in the Trendelenburg position.
- Demonstrate how to position the client with hips elevated on pillows, higher than the chest, or, if the client is able, to assume a knee–chest position.
- Provide the client and caregiver with contact information of healthcare personnel who can be reached for advice or emergencies.

Documentation

- Document the date and time you performed percussion, vibration, and postural drainage.
- Note the positions used for postural drainage and the length of time the patient maintained each position.
- Note the anatomical locations in which you performed percussion and vibration.
- Document the patient's tolerance of the procedure, as well as any complications and the nursing interventions you used to treat the complication.
- Document the amount, color, odor, and consistency of sputum you obtained during the procedure and whether you sent a sputum specimen to the lab.

Sample documentation

June 15, 2018   Percussion and vibration done over Right lower lobe. Expectorated 10 mL thick, yellow, odorless mucus. Specimen to lab. BP 142/78, HR 98 bpm, respirations 24/min. Few crackles auscultated over Right lung base, SaO_2 98% on 2 L/minute nasal cannula. ———————————— Jeffrey Fine, RN

Practice Resources

Bilton, D. (2012); *Lippincott nursing procedures* (2015).

Procedure 37-4 ■ Administering Oxygen

➤ For steps to follow in all procedures, refer to the Universal Steps for All Procedures found on the page facing the inside back cover.

Equipment

- Oxygen source
- Flow meter
- Oxygen tubing
- Nasal cannula, oxygen mask, or face tent
- Prefilled humidification device

Delegation

The RN is responsible for assessing respiratory function and initiating and monitoring response to oxygen therapy. However, you may delegate reapplication and maintenance of oxygen therapy (e.g., adjusting the face mask) to appropriately trained assistive personnel when necessary.

Pre-Procedure Assessment

- Assess the patient's understanding of oxygen therapy.
- Assessment of the patient's respiratory status; includes respiratory rate, depth, and rhythm; breath sounds; color; capillary refill and pulse oximetry results.
  Determines the need for further treatment and effectiveness of oxygen therapy.
- Assess nares for patency (if a nasal cannula is being used) and behind the ears for signs of skin breakdown.

(continued on next page)

Procedure 37-4 ■ Administering Oxygen (continued)

➤ When performing the procedure, always identify your patient according to agency policy, using two identifiers, and be attentive to standard precautions, hand hygiene, patient safety and privacy, body mechanics, and documentation.

➤ *Note:* Oxygen requires a medical prescription. In an emergency, administer oxygen to prevent respiratory distress, then notify the primary care provider for a prescription.

Procedure Steps

➕ Also use Clinical Insight 37-3: Oxygen Therapy Safety Precautions.

1. Attach the flow meter to the wall oxygen source (in the photo, the green meter on the wall). ▼

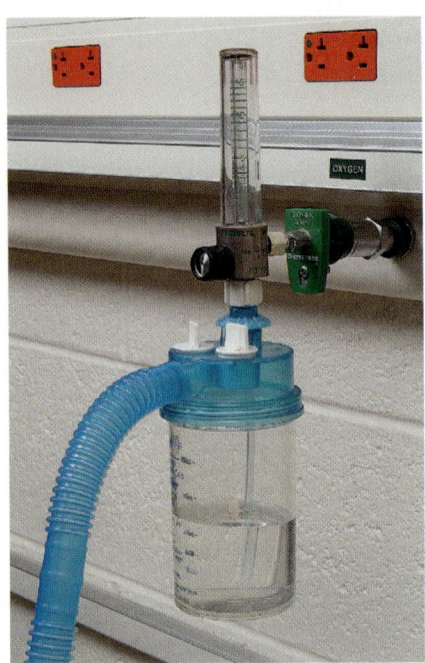

If Using a Portable Oxygen Tank
Attach the flow meter to the tank if it is not already connected. Once tubing is attached to the portable tank, check the amount of oxygen in the tank by looking at the meter.

The flow meter regulates the amount of oxygen delivered per minute. ▼

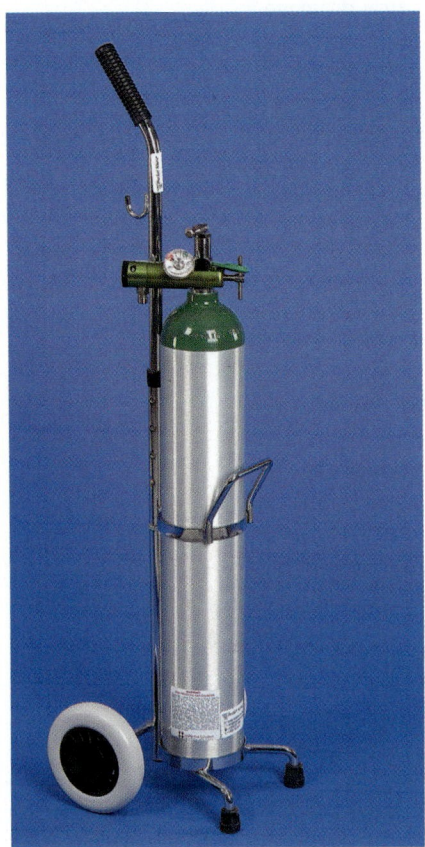

2. Assemble the oxygen equipment. (See the table at the end of this procedure for various oxygen delivery devices.)

3. Attach the humidifier to the flow meter. The humidifier is simply a small plastic container containing normal saline. If you are not using a humidifier, attach the adapter to the flow meter.
The humidifier adds moisture in with the oxygen, which can dry the nasal or oral cavity.

4. Turn on the oxygen at the flow meter and adjust the prescribed flow rate.

Nasal Cannula
Follow steps 1 through 4.

5. Attach the nasal cannula tubing to the humidifier or the adapter.

6. Place the nasal prongs in the patient's nares—prongs curved downward—and then place the tubing around each ear.
Properly positions the device for optimal oxygen delivery.

7. Use the slide adjustment device to tighten the cannula in place under the patient's chin. It must fit securely, but not too tightly. Then proceed to step 12.
The nasal cannula must fit securely to maximize the amount of oxygen inhaled by the patient. A good fit minimizes the amount of oxygen lost around the prongs. ▼

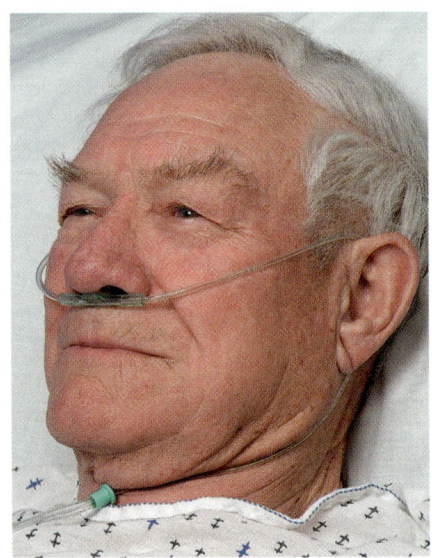

Face Mask

Follow steps 1 through 4.

8. **Gently place the face mask** on the patient's face, applying it from the bridge of the nose to under the chin.

9. **Secure the elastic band** around the back of the patient's head. Make sure the mask fits snugly but comfortably. Then proceed to step 12.

   The mask must fit snugly so that oxygen cannot escape around the edges of the mask. If the mask is too tight, it may cause skin breakdown. ▼

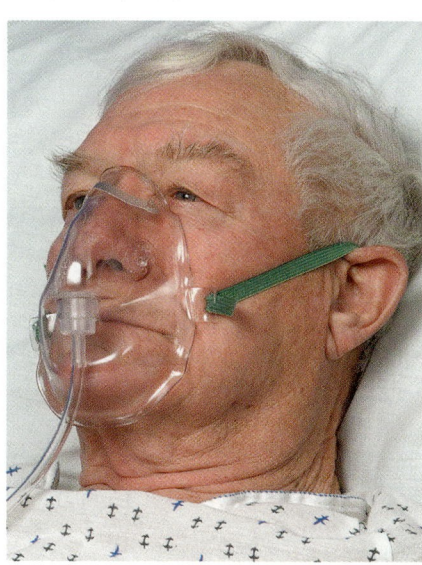

Face Tent

Follow steps 1 through 4.

10. **Gently place the face tent** in front of the patient's face, making sure that it fits under the chin.

11. **Secure the elastic band** around the back of the patient's head.

   To keep the face tent in place. ▼

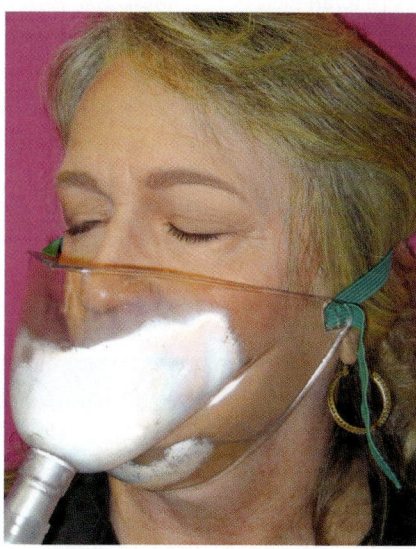

12. **Double-check that the oxygen** equipment is set up correctly and functioning properly.

   Ensures that the oxygen is delivered at the prescribed rate. Oxygen delivered at an incorrect rate can cause patient injury.

13. **Assess the patient's respiratory status** before leaving the bedside.

   To be certain it is safe to leave the patient.

Evaluation

- Assess respiratory rate, depth, and effort.
- Auscultate breath sounds before leaving the bedside, then monitor every 2 to 4 hours, and as indicated.
- Monitor pulse oximetry until respiratory status improves.
- Monitor ABG results if prescribed.
- Evaluate for skin breakdown, paying close attention to areas behind the ears, cheekbones, and under the chin—areas that are in contact with the oxygen delivery system.
- Notify the primary provider of respiratory status, oxygen, and response and any additional prescriptions needed.

Patient Teaching

- Demonstrate oxygen administration to the patient and caregiver if the patient will be continuing oxygen therapy at home. Allow for time to answer questions, and return demonstration of attaching and placing oxygen on.
- Explain the importance of immediately reporting shortness of breath or any difficulty breathing to the nursing staff before discharge. If the patient is at home, he will need to report the difficulty to the home health and/or primary care provider, and, if needed, to call 911.

Home Care

- Explain to the family and caregiver where to obtain oxygen equipment and what services are available. Make sure they choose a supplier who has 24-hour emergency services.
- Instruct the client and caregiver about oxygen therapy and its use, as well as safety measures that they must institute. Safety measures include keeping oxygen away from items that may cause ignition such as lighters, cigarettes, fireplaces, and heaters.
- To demonstrate the oxygen is on, the client can hold nasal prongs on the side of the cheek to feel air flow or over a glass of water to see air moving the water.
- Teach the client and caregiver to clean the nasal cannula or face mask with soap and warm water when it becomes soiled, and allow the mask to air-dry.
- Provide the client and caregiver with contact information of healthcare personnel who can be reached for advice or emergencies.
- Explain the importance of immediately reporting shortness of breath or any difficulty breathing to the home health and/or primary care provider and, if needed, to call 911.

(continued on next page)

Procedure 37-4 ■ Administering Oxygen (continued)

- In the home, liquid oxygen and oxygen concentrators are more commonly used than portable oxygen tanks. Liquid oxygen may be kept in small, portable containers; an oxygen concentrator removes nitrogen from room air and concentrates O_2. It requires a battery pack or electrical outlet for power. Oxygen concentrators can deliver flow up to 4 liters per minute (L/min) to create an FIO_2 of approximately 36%. Concentrations are higher at lower flow rates (e.g., an FIO_2 of 95% at 1 L/min).

Documentation

- Document the date, time, and reason oxygen therapy was initiated.
- Note the type of oxygen delivery system used, the amount of oxygen administered, and the patient's response to oxygen therapy.

- Document vital signs, pulse oximetry values, breath sounds, skin color, and respiratory effort.

Sample documentation

12/14/18   2015   Patient developed acute shortness of breath. RR 36/min & labored, P = 126 beats/min, and BP 212/110 mm Hg. Pulse ox 80% on room air. Crackles and expiratory wheezes auscultated throughout both lungs. Dr. Chow notified of patient's condition. Partial rebreather mask @ 10 L/min and Lasix 40 mg IV prescribed and administered. Pulse ox on partial rebreather = 90%. ————S. Peters, RN

Practice Resource

Lippincott nursing procedures (2015).

Oxygen Delivery Systems

DELIVERY METHOD	FIO₂	DISCUSSION	NURSING RESPONSIBILITIES
Nasal cannula.	1 L/min = 24% 2 L/min = 28% 3 L/min = 32% 4 L/min = 36% 5 L/min = 40% 6 L/min = 44%	■ Relatively comfortable. ■ Patients can eat, talk, and cough with a nasal cannula in place. ■ Works best if the patient breathes through his nose.	■ Check frequently that the prongs are in the patient's nose. ■ Assess for dryness of the nasal mucosa. ■ Humidify flow at rates above 3 L/min (flow rates > 3 L/min) are drying. ■ Encourage the patient to take slow, deep breaths, so he will inhale more oxygen and less room air.
Simple face mask: A clear, flexible mask that covers the nose and mouth and delivers oxygen flow into the mask.	5–10 L/min = 40%–60% FIO₂	■ Requires flow rates greater than 5 L/min to prevent accumulation and rebreathing of exhaled CO₂ from within the mask. ■ Masks are not easily tolerated because they fit tightly and keep heat from radiating from the face, making patients feel hot. ■ Talking is muffled by the mask, and it must be removed for the patient to eat or drink.	■ Place face mask securely over the mouth and nose. ■ Elastic straps fit around the head to hold the mask in place. Place the straps well above the ears to prevent skin irritation and breakdown. ■ Place gauze or other soft material beneath the straps to prevent irritation. ■ Check the skin around the mask frequently. ■ Check the skin over the ears where the mask strap rubs. ■ Encourage the patient to take slow, deep breaths, so he will inhale more oxygen and less room air.

Oxygen Delivery Systems—cont'd

DELIVERY METHOD	FIO_2	DISCUSSION	NURSING RESPONSIBILITIES
Partial rebreather mask: Uses the reservoir bag to capture some exhaled gas for rebreathing.	6–15 L/min = 50%–90% FIO_2	■ Allows higher FIO_2 levels to be delivered because O_2 is collected in the reservoir bag for inhalation. ■ Exhalation ports allow most exhaled air to escape. ■ Several types are available. ■ Can deliver an FIO_2 above 50% at flow rates of 6–15 L/min. ■ Patient rebreathes some exhaled air along with O_2.	■ Maintain the flow at a high enough rate to prevent the reservoir bag from collapsing during inhalation. ■ Encourage the patient to take slow, deep breaths, so he will inhale more oxygen and less room air.
Nonrebreather mask: A type of reservoir bag mask; a valve keeps exhaled air from entering the reservoir bag.	6–15 L/min = 70%–100% FIO_2	■ Contains only O_2, which allows higher FIO_2 delivery. An FIO_2 of 70%–100% can be delivered at flow rates of 6–15 L/min. ■ This mask is the only external device capable of delivering an FIO_2 of 100% (in practice, it is rare to achieve a concentration over 75% because the mask does not seal perfectly with the face).	■ Maintain the flow at a rate high enough to keep the reservoir at least one-third to one-half full during inhalation. ■ Be sure the mask fits snugly so the patient will breathe in less room air.
Venturi mask: A cone-shaped adapter that serves as a mixing valve to control the amount of O_2 and room air that flows through the mask.	24%–50% FIO_2	■ The cone-shaped adapter at the base of the mask allows a precise FIO_2 to be delivered. This is very useful for patients with chronic lung disease. ■ Exhalation ports keep CO_2 buildup to a minimum.	■ The adapter indicates the required oxygen flow rate needed to deliver the desired FIO_2. Ensure that flow is set at the rate specified to deliver the FIO_2 desired.

(continued on next page)

Procedure 37-4 ■ Administering Oxygen (continued)

Oxygen Delivery Systems—cont'd

DELIVERY METHOD	FiO$_2$	DISCUSSION	NURSING RESPONSIBILITIES
 Face tent: A large, open plastic mask that fits under the chin. It is open at the top and is held in place with an elastic band around the head.	8–12 L/min = 30%–55% FiO$_2$	■ Less reliable than a face mask for delivering precise FiO$_2$ levels. ■ Allows moderate- to high-density aerosol delivery for humidification. ■ Patients who feel claustrophobic in a face mask often tolerate a face tent.	■ Check the skin over the ears where the mask strap rubs.
 Tracheostomy collar: A small, cup-shaped device that fits over the tracheostomy opening and is held in place with elastic straps around the neck.	4–10 L/min = 24%–100%	■ It is possible to deliver both high FiO$_2$ and high humidity with a tracheostomy collar. ■ Large-bore tubing is used to deliver humidification to the trachea; however, water frequently condenses inside the tubing and can be accidentally drained into the tracheostomy. Usually, a water trap of some sort is placed in the tubing to prevent this problem.	■ Watch for water accumulation in the tubing.
 T-piece: A T-shaped plastic piece; the bottom of the T fits directly and tightly onto the tracheostomy tube.	4–10 L/min = 24%–100% FiO$_2$	■ Oxygen and humidity are delivered into one side of the T and exhaled through the other side.	■ Take care that the oxygen delivery tubing does not pull on the T-piece, which can dislodge the tracheostomy tube and create an airway emergency.

Thinking About the Procedure

 The video **Administering Oxygen,** along with questions and suggested responses, is available on the **Davis's** *Nursing Skills Videos* Web site on Davis*Plus.*

Procedure 37-5 ■ Performing Tracheostomy Care Using Modified Sterile Technique

➤ For steps to follow in all procedures, refer to the Universal Steps for All Procedures found on the inside back cover.

- Also refer to Clinical Insight 37-4.
- Recall that the basic differences in sterile and modified sterile technique are that modified sterile technique uses nonsterile procedure gloves and tap water.

Equipment

- Tracheostomy suction equipment (see Procedure 37-6)
- Tracheostomy care kit or the following sterile supplies: several cotton-tipped applicators, two basins, a brush, sterile 4 in. × 4 in. gauze pads, sterile precut tracheostomy dressing
- Two pairs of nonsterile gloves (for sterile technique, use sterile gloves)
- Disposable inner cannula that is the same size as the tracheostomy, if available. Most tracheostomy tubes have disposable inner cannulas.
- Distilled or filtered water if agency policy allows (for sterile technique, use sterile normal saline solution)
- Hydrogen peroxide for cleaning of reusable inner cannula only
- Roll of twill tape or hook and loop fastener (Velcro) tracheostomy holder
- Bandage scissors
- Towel or linen-saver pad
- Overbed table
- Face shield and protective gown
- For modified sterile technique: disposable prepackaged wipes, or washcloth and distilled water and soap.

✚ Use only the sterile precut dressing, or open and refold a 4 in. × 4 in. gauze pad into a V-shape. Do not cut 4 in. × 4 in. gauze, and do not use cotton-filled gauze squares. The patient may aspirate the cotton or gauze fibers.

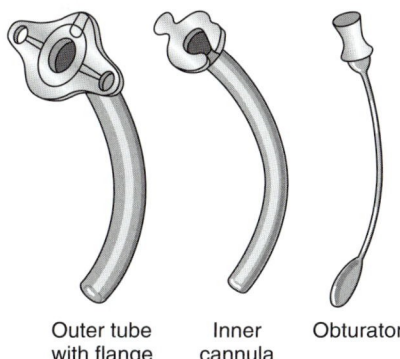

A. Nondisposable tracheostomy equipment.

Outer tube with flange   Inner cannula   Obturator

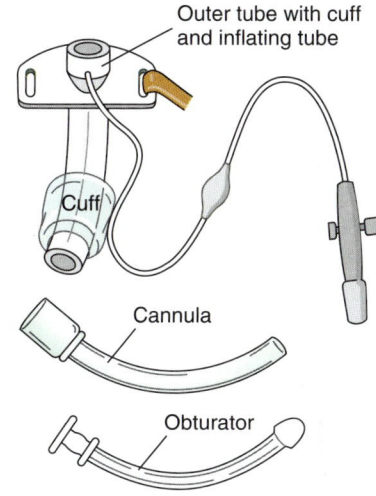

B. Disposable tracheostomy equipment.

Outer tube with cuff and inflating tube
Cuff
Cannula
Obturator

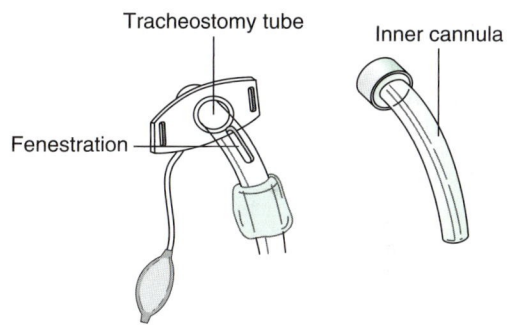

C. Fenestrated tracheostomy equipment.

Tracheostomy tube   Inner cannula
Fenestration

Delegation

In acute care settings and with new tracheostomies, you should not delegate this procedure to the NAP. For long-standing and well-healed tracheostomies, you can safely delegate care to a NAP or LPN who is adequately trained to perform the skill. This varies by state. In some states, only RNs can perform tracheostomy care. If you are not familiar with your state's nurse practice act, contact your state board of nursing.

(continued on next page)

Procedure 37-5 ■ Performing Tracheostomy Care Using Modified Sterile Technique (continued)

Pre-Procedure Assessment

- Assess the patient's respiratory status, including respiratory rate, depth, and rhythm; breath sounds; color; and pulse oximetry results.

  Helps determine whether the patient can tolerate tracheostomy care.

- Assess the tracheostomy site for drainage, redness, or swelling.

  Drainage, redness, or swelling may indicate infection.

- Determine when the patient last ate.

  It is best to schedule this procedure at least 3 hours after a meal to decrease the risk of the patient vomiting and aspirating stomach contents.

> ➤ When performing the procedure, always identify your patient according to agency policy, using two identifiers, and be attentive to standard precautions, hand hygiene, patient safety and privacy, body mechanics, and documentation.

Procedure Steps

1. **Position the patient** in semi-Fowler's position and place a towel or linen-saver pad over the patient's chest.

   A semi-Fowler's position promotes lung expansion and prevents back strain for the nurse. A towel or linen-saver pad prevents soiling of the patient's gown.

2. **Don clean procedure gloves, gown, and face shield or mask.**

3. **Hyperoxygenate the patient,** as needed, and suction the tracheostomy (see Procedure 37-6 or 37-7)

   Suctioning clears the tracheostomy of secretions that could occlude the outer cannula after the inner cannula is removed for care.

For a Passy–Muir Valve

Remove the Passy–Muir valve (PMV) before suctioning the patient to prepare for tracheostomy care. (A PMV is a device that is used to enable the patient with a tracheostomy to speak. It is attached to the end of the inner cannula at the tracheostomy site.)

4. **Remove and discard** the soiled tracheostomy dressing in the appropriate receptacle, and then remove and discard your gloves. Perform hand hygiene.

5. **Place the tracheostomy care equipment** on the overbed table and prepare the equipment, keeping all supplies and equipment sterile.

   Ensures efficiency and helps prevent contamination during tracheostomy care.

   a. *Disposable inner cannula*—Pour filtered tap water or normal saline solution into the two sterile containers (per agency policy).

   b. *Reusable inner cannula*—Pour hydrogen peroxide into one of the sterile solution containers, and pour filtered tap water or normal saline solution into the other one. If the inner cannula is not disposable, use hydrogen peroxide to clean only the inner cannula. Use filtered tap water to rinse the inner cannula and clean the faceplate and tracheostomy site.

   Steps c through g apply to both types of cannula.

   c. Obtain and open a package of disposable prepackaged wipes for cleaning the skin around the tracheostomy site.

   d. Open one cotton-tipped applicator package. Wet the applicators with filtered tap water or normal saline solution.

   Prepares the applicators for cleaning the exposed surface of the outer cannula and the stoma site located under the faceplate of the tracheostomy tube, respectively.

   e. Open the package containing a new disposable inner cannula.

   Allows for quick replacement of the inner cannula.

   f. Open the package of Velcro tracheostomy ties, or cut a length of twill tape long enough to go around the patient's neck two times. Make sure to cut end of the tape on an angle.

   Allows for quick stabilization of the tracheostomy tube, preventing dislodgement. Cutting the twill tape on an angle allows for easy insertion through the faceplate eyelets.

   g. Position a biohazard bag within reach.

   Allows you to dispose of contaminated supplies safely as you use them without leaving the patient or interrupting the procedure.

6. **Don clean procedure gloves.** Consider your dominant hand to be clean and handle supplies with that hand only.

7. **For patients receiving oxygen:** With your nondominant hand, remove the oxygen or humidification source. Attach the oxygen source to the outer cannula, if possible. If not possible, have the respiratory therapist set up oxygen blow-by to use while you are cleaning the reusable inner cannula.

   Prevents oxygen desaturation in the patient during the procedure.

8. **Unlock and remove the inner cannula** with your nondominant hand and care for it accordingly.

For a Disposable Inner Cannula

   a. Dispose of the inner cannula in the biohazard receptacle according to agency policy. You should never clean and reuse a disposable inner cannula.

   Prevents contamination by bacteria contained in the inner cannula.

   b. With your dominant hand, insert the new inner cannula into the patient's tracheostomy in the direction of the curvature. Following the manufacturer's instructions, lock the inner cannula in place securely to prevent it from dislodging. Remember to keep your dominant hand clean.

For a Reusable Inner Cannula

c. If a reusable inner cannula was used, place the inner cannula into the basin filled with hydrogen peroxide.

Hydrogen peroxide helps loosen tenacious (sticky) secretions.

d. Pick up the reusable inner cannula from the container of hydrogen peroxide with your nondominant hand and scrub it with the sterile nylon brush, using your dominant hand. ▼

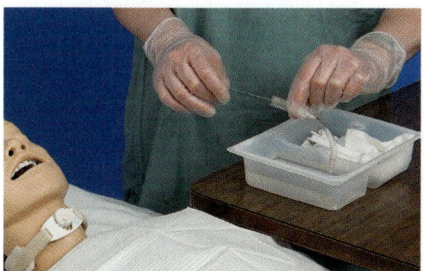

e. Immerse the inner cannula in the container of filtered tap water and agitate it until it is rinsed thoroughly.

Immersing the inner cannula in filtered tap water and agitating it removes the hydrogen peroxide and debris from the inner cannula, minimizing tissue irritation.

f. Shake the cannula to remove water.

Removes excess fluid so the patient does not aspirate it when you reinsert the cannula.

g. With your dominant (clean) hand, reinsert the inner cannula into the patient's tracheostomy in the direction of the curvature. Following the manufacturer's instructions, lock the inner cannula in place securely to prevent it from dislodging. Remember to keep your dominant hand clean.

For a Passy–Muir Valve

h. Swish the PMV in warm tap water with mild soap.

i. Rinse the PMV thoroughly in warm filtered tap water.

j. **KEY POINT:** *DO NOT use hot water, peroxide, bleach, vinegar, alcohol, brushes, or cotton-tipped applicators to clean PMV, as this could damage the valve.*

k. Shake the PMV to remove excess fluid. If you are going to store the valve, be sure to air-dry the valve before placing it in a storage container.

Removes moisture, which can promote bacterial growth.

l. Set the PMV aside on clean surface to be replaced when the inner cannula is replaced.

For Patients Receiving Oxygen

m. Remove the humidification or oxygen source from the outer cannula, if indicated, using your nondominant hand.

n. Reinsert the inner cannula into the patient's tracheostomy in the direction of the curvature.

o. Following the manufacturer's instructions, lock the inner cannula in place securely. Remember to keep dominant hand clean.

Lock the inner cannula in place securely to prevent it from dislodging.

p. Reattach the humidification or oxygen source, if indicated.

Provides the patient with needed humidity or oxygen and prevents oxygen desaturation.

9. **Clean the stoma under the faceplate** with cotton-tipped applicators saturated with filtered tap water or normal saline solution, using a circular motion from the stoma site outward. Use each applicator only once, and then discard it.

Prevents contamination of the cleaned area. ▼

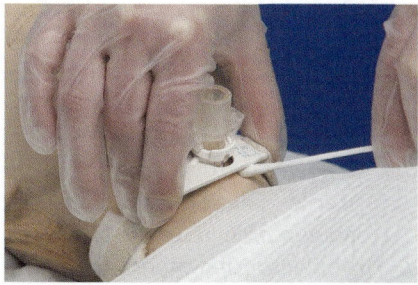

10. **Clean the top surface of the faceplate** and the skin around it with the prepackaged wipe or gauze pads saturated with filtered tap water or normal saline solution. Use each wipe or gauze pad only once and then discard it.

Removes secretions that provide a medium for microbial growth; prevents contamination of cleaned areas.

11. **Dry the skin and outer cannula** surfaces by patting them lightly with the remaining dry gauze pad.

Clean, dry skin is needed to avoid skin breakdown and removes moisture, which can promote bacterial growth around the stoma site.

To finish the procedure, skip to steps 12 through 17 of Procedure 37-5B.

Procedure 37-5B ■ Performing Tracheostomy Care Using Sterile Technique

Procedure Steps

1. **Position the patient** in semi-Fowler's position and place a towel or linen-saver pad over the patient's chest.

A semi-Fowler's position promotes lung expansion and prevents back strain for the nurse. A towel or linen-saver pad prevents soiling of the patient's gown.

2. **Don clean procedure gloves.**

3. **Hyperoxygenate the patient,** as needed, and suction the tracheostomy (see Procedure 37-6 or 37-7)

Suctioning clears the tracheostomy of secretions that could occlude the outer canula after the inner cannula is removed for care.

For a Passy–Muir Valve

Remove the Passy–Muir valve (PMV) before suctioning the patient to prepare for tracheostomy care. (A PMV is a device that is used to enable the patient with a tracheostomy to speak. It is attached to the end of the inner cannula at the tracheostomy site.)

4. **Remove and discard** the soiled tracheostomy dressing in the appropriate receptacle, and then remove and discard your gloves. Perform hand hygiene.

(continued on next page)

Procedure 37-5 ■ **Performing Tracheostomy Care Using Modified Sterile Technique** (continued)

5. **Place the tracheostomy care equipment** on the overbed table and prepare the equipment, keeping all supplies and equipment sterile.
Ensures efficiency and helps prevent contamination during tracheostomy care.

   a. *Disposable inner cannula*—Pour sterile normal saline solution into the two sterile containers (per agency policy).

   b. *Reusable inner cannula*—Pour hydrogen peroxide into one of the sterile solution containers and pour sterile normal saline solution into the other one. If the inner cannula is not disposable, use hydrogen peroxide to clean only the inner cannula. Use sterile normal saline to rinse the inner cannula and clean the faceplate and tracheostomy site.

   Steps c through g apply to both types of cannula.

   c. Obtain and open two 4 in. × 4 in. sterile gauze packages. Wet the gauze in one package with sterile normal saline solution, and keep the second package dry.
   You will use the second package of gauze to dry the skin around the tracheostomy site after cleaning.

   d. Open one cotton-tipped applicator package. Wet the applicators with sterile normal saline solution.
   Prepares the applicators for cleaning the exposed surface of the outer cannula and the stoma site located under the faceplate of the tracheostomy tube, respectively.

   e. Open the package containing a new disposable inner cannula.
   Allows for quick replacement of the inner cannula.

   f. Open the package of Velcro tracheostomy ties, or cut a length of twill tape long enough to go around the patient's neck two times. Make sure to cut end of the tape on an angle.
   Allows for quick stabilization of the tracheostomy tube, preventing dislodgement. Cutting the twill tape on an angle allows for easy insertion through the faceplate eyelets.

   g. Position a biohazard bag within reach.
   Allows you to dispose of contaminated supplies safely as you use them without leaving the patient or interrupting the procedure.

6. **Don sterile gloves. Consider your dominant hand sterile and your nondominant hand clean (nonsterile).** Handle the sterile supplies with the dominant hand only.

7. **For patients receiving oxygen:** With your nondominant (nonsterile) hand, remove the oxygen or humidification source. Attach the oxygen source to the outer cannula, if possible. If not possible, have the respiratory therapist set up oxygen blow-by to use while you are cleaning the reusable inner cannula.
Prevents oxygen desaturation in the patient during the procedure.

8. **Unlock and remove the inner cannula** with your nondominant (nonsterile) hand and care for it accordingly.

   For a Disposable Inner Cannula

   a. Dispose of the inner cannula in the biohazard receptacle according to agency policy. You should never clean and reuse a disposable inner cannula.
   Prevents contamination by bacteria contained in the inner cannula.

   b. With your dominant hand (sterile), insert the new inner cannula into the patient's tracheostomy in the direction of the curvature. Following the manufacturer's instructions, lock the inner cannula in place securely to prevent it from dislodging. Remember to keep your dominant hand sterile.

   For a Reusable Inner Cannula

   c. If a reusable inner cannula was used, place the inner cannula into the basin filled with hydrogen peroxide.
   Hydrogen peroxide helps loosen tenacious (sticky) secretions.

   d. Pick up the reusable inner cannula from the container of hydrogen

peroxide with your nondominant hand and scrub it with the sterile nylon brush, using your dominant (sterile) hand.

   e. Immerse the inner cannula in the container of sterile normal saline solution and agitate it until it is rinsed thoroughly.
   Immersing the inner cannula in sterile saline solution and agitating it removes the hydrogen peroxide and debris from the inner cannula, minimizing tissue irritation.

   f. Tap the inner cannula against the side of the container to remove water.
   Removes excess fluid so the patient does not aspirate it when you reinsert the cannula.

   g. With your dominant (sterile) hand, reinsert the inner cannula into the patient's tracheostomy in the direction of the curvature. Following the manufacturer's instructions, lock the inner cannula in place securely to prevent it from dislodging. Remember to keep your dominant hand clean.

   For a Passy–Muir Valve

   h. Swish the PMV in warm tap water with mild soap.

   i. Rinse the PMV thoroughly in warm filtered tap water.

   j. DO NOT use hot water, peroxide, bleach, vinegar, alcohol, brushes, or cotton-tipped applicators to clean PMV, as this could damage the valve.

   k. Shake the PMV to remove excess fluid. If you are going to store the valve, be sure to air-dry the valve before placing it in a storage container.
   Removes moisture, which can promote bacterial growth.

   l. Set the PMV aside on clean surface to be replaced when the inner cannula is replaced.

   For Patients Receiving Oxygen

   m. Remove the humidification or oxygen source from the outer cannula, if indicated, using your nondominant hand.

n. Using your dominant (sterile) hand, reinsert the inner cannula into the patient's tracheostomy in the direction of the curvature.

o. Following the manufacturer's instructions, lock the inner cannula in place securely. Remember to keep dominant hand clean.

Lock the inner cannula in place securely to prevent it from dislodging.

p. Reattach the humidification or oxygen source, if indicated.

Provides the patient with needed humidity or oxygen and prevents oxygen desaturation.

9. **Clean the stoma under the faceplate** with cotton-tipped applicators saturated with sterile normal saline solution, using a circular motion from the stoma site outward. Use each applicator only once and then discard it.

Prevents contamination of the cleaned area.

10. **Clean the top surface of the faceplate** and the skin around it with the gauze pads saturated sterile normal saline solution. Use each wipe or gauze pad only once, and then discard it.

Removes secretions that provide a medium for microbial growth; prevents contamination of cleaned areas.

11. **Dry the skin and outer cannula** surfaces by patting them lightly with the remaining dry gauze pad.

Clean, dry skin is needed to avoid skin breakdown and removes moisture, which can promote bacterial growth around the stoma site.

The following steps apply to both modified sterile and sterile technique:

12. ✚ **Seek assistance from another** staff member to help with changing the tracheostomy stabilizers. *Prevents accidental dislodging should the patient begin coughing during the procedure.*

13. **Remove soiled tracheostomy stabilizers.**

Removing a Soiled Velcro Tracheostomy Holder

a. With an assistant stabilizing the tracheostomy tube, disengage the Velcro on both sides of the soiled holder and remove it gently from the eyes of the faceplate. Discard the Velcro holder in the nearest biohazard receptacle.

Removing the soiled holder promotes hygiene and prevents the spread of infection.

Removing Soiled Twill Tape Tracheostomy Ties

b. With an assistant stabilizing the tracheostomy tube, cut the soiled tracheostomy ties using bandage scissors. *Do not* cut the tube of the tracheostomy balloon (if you do, the tracheostomy tube must be replaced). Remove the ties gently from the eyes of the faceplate and discard them in the nearest biohazard receptacle.

The tracheostomy balloon helps stabilize the tracheostomy in the trachea and prevents an air leak. Cutting the tube to the balloon prevents the balloon from holding air. Removing the soiled holder promotes hygiene and prevents the spread of infection.

14. **Ask the patient to flex his neck,** or, if he is unable, ask the assistant to hold the patient's head forward, and apply new tracheostomy ties.

Flexing the neck provides the same neck circumference as when the patient coughs and thus ensures you do not place and secure the tracheostomy stabilizers too tightly.

Using a Velcro Tracheostomy Holder

a. Unfasten the Velcro. Thread one end of the tracheostomy holder through the eyelet of the faceplate and fasten it.

b. Bring the holder around the back of the patient's neck.

The holder must be placed around the patient's neck to adequately secure the tracheostomy.

c. Thread the remaining end of the tracheostomy holder through the empty eyelet of the faceplate

and fasten the Velcro, making sure that the holder fits securely. ▼

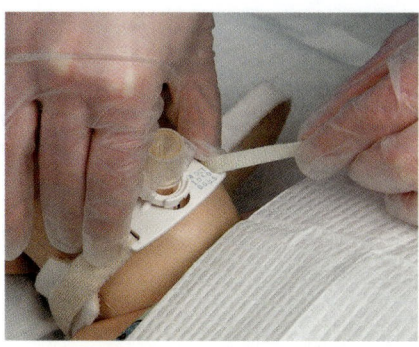

d. ✚ Place one finger under the holder to make sure that the holder is securing the tracheostomy effectively but isn't too tight.

Securing the tracheostomy too tightly might place pressure on the jugular veins, interfere with coughing, or cause necrosis at the tracheostomy insertion site.

Using Twill Tape

e. Thread one end of the twill tape into one of the eyelets on the tracheostomy faceplate.

f. Continue to thread the twill tape through the eyelet, bringing both ends of the tape together.

g. Bring both ends of the twill tape around the back of the patient's neck.

To adequately secure the tracheostomy.

h. Thread the end of the twill tape that is closest to the patient's neck through the back of the eyelet on the faceplate.

i. Have your assistant place one finger under the twill tape while you tie the two ends together in a square knot.

Ensures you do not secure the tracheostomy too tightly.

j. Place one finger under the holder to make sure that the holder is securing the tracheostomy effectively but isn't too tight.

See step 14d.

15. **Don a new pair of sterile gloves** (after removing gloves and performing hand hygiene).

(continued on next page)

Procedure 37–5 ■ **Performing Tracheostomy Care Using Modified Sterile Technique** (continued)

16. Insert a precut, sterile tracheostomy dressing under the faceplate and new tracheostomy stabilizers or fold a 4 in. × 4 in. gauze pad into a V shape (below). ▼

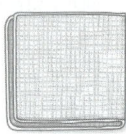

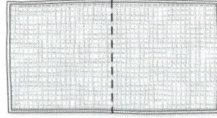

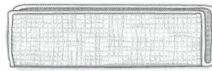

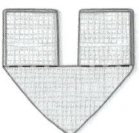

The new dressing absorbs secretions and prevents skin breakdown under the faceplate. Never cut the gauze to make a dressing because lint and fibers from the cut edge could enter the trachea and cause respiratory distress. ▼

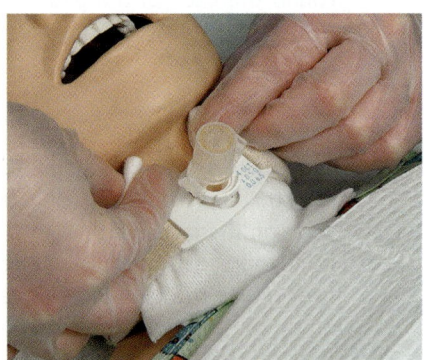

17. Dispose of the used equipment in the appropriate biohazard receptacle according to agency policy.
Helps prevent cross-contamination.

❓ What if . . .

■ **Your patient begins coughing?**

a. If the tracheostomy is still secured with ties or Velcro holder, wait to continue tracheostomy care until coughing has ended.

b. If tracheostomy is unsecured, stabilize the tube so that it does not become dislodged being careful not to press too hard on the site. Continue with tracheostomy care when the patient finishes coughing.
Pressing too hard at the tracheostomy site will stimulate the coughing reflex.

c. If coughing continues, suspend tracheostomy care and suction the patient to remove any retained secretions.
Retained secretions may cause increased airway irritation and coughing. Removing secretions will reduce this irritation.

■ **You do not have an assistant to hold the cannula in place while you replace the soiled tracheostomy ties?**

✚ Never cut the soiled tape before applying the clean tape. Always place the new tape/holders, be certain the tracheostomy is secured, and then cut off the soiled tape or holder.

■ **The tracheostomy tube becomes dislodged?**

a. To prevent this, plan ahead and always have another staff member with you to secure the tracheostomy tube while you change the tracheostomy ties or Velcro holder.

b. If the tracheostomy tube slips out slightly but is still in the trachea site, gently push it back into the stoma and secure it.
The pilot balloon will help to keep the tracheostomy tube from completely dislodging.

c. If the tracheostomy tube becomes completely dislodged, stay with the patient and ask your assistant to call for the respiratory therapist or trained person in your facility to insert a new tracheostomy tube.

■ **At step 9, there are crusts around the stoma when you are cleaning the stoma?**

Remove the crusts with a cotton-tipped swab soaked in hydrogen peroxide, then rinse with a swab soaked in filtered tap water or normal saline. Have the patient hold his breath while you remove crusts so he does not inhale them.

Evaluation

■ Assess the area around the stoma site for signs of skin breakdown.
■ Evaluate the patient's tolerance of the procedure. Note whether there were any signs of respiratory distress.

Patient Teaching

■ Explain to the patient and his family that bloody secretions are normal for 2 to 3 days after tracheostomy tube insertion or for 24 hours after a tracheostomy tube change.
■ Tell the patient and/or family to inform the nurse immediately if the tracheostomy tube becomes dislodged.

■ Teach tracheostomy care to the patient and caregiver if the tracheostomy is expected to remain long term.

Home Care

■ Clean, rather than sterile, technique can be used for tracheostomy care if the tracheostomy is more than 1 month old.
■ Instruct the client and caregiver about home oxygen therapy and suctioning, if necessary.
■ Demonstrate tracheostomy care to the caregiver and ask for a return demonstration.
■ Provide the client and caregiver with information about where to obtain tracheostomy care supplies.

- Supply the client and caregiver with contact information of healthcare personnel who can be reached for advice or emergencies.
- Recommend ways of adding moisture to the air, with a goal of maintaining a relative humidity of 50% (e.g., a large humidifier, house plants, wearing damp gauze over the stoma, closing the bathroom door and turning on the hot water to fill the room with steam).
- The stoma should be cleaned using clean technique at least twice daily (or more often, depending on the amount of secretions).
- Stress good hand washing before and after doing any part of tracheostomy care.
- Remind client and caregiver not to use cotton or gauze.
  These can leave fibers that may get into the airway and increase the incidence of infection.

Documentation

- Document the date and time you performed tracheostomy care.
- Record the color, amount, consistency, and odor of secretions.
- Record the condition of the stoma and skin around the stoma site; note the presence of drainage, redness, or swelling.
- Document respiratory status, including respiratory rate, depth, and pattern; skin color; and breath sounds.
- Document the patient's tolerance of the procedure.
- If problems arose, document any interventions that were necessary.

Sample documentation

NOTE: Because this is only a partial computer screen, it may not show all the information you would need to record about the patient. ▼

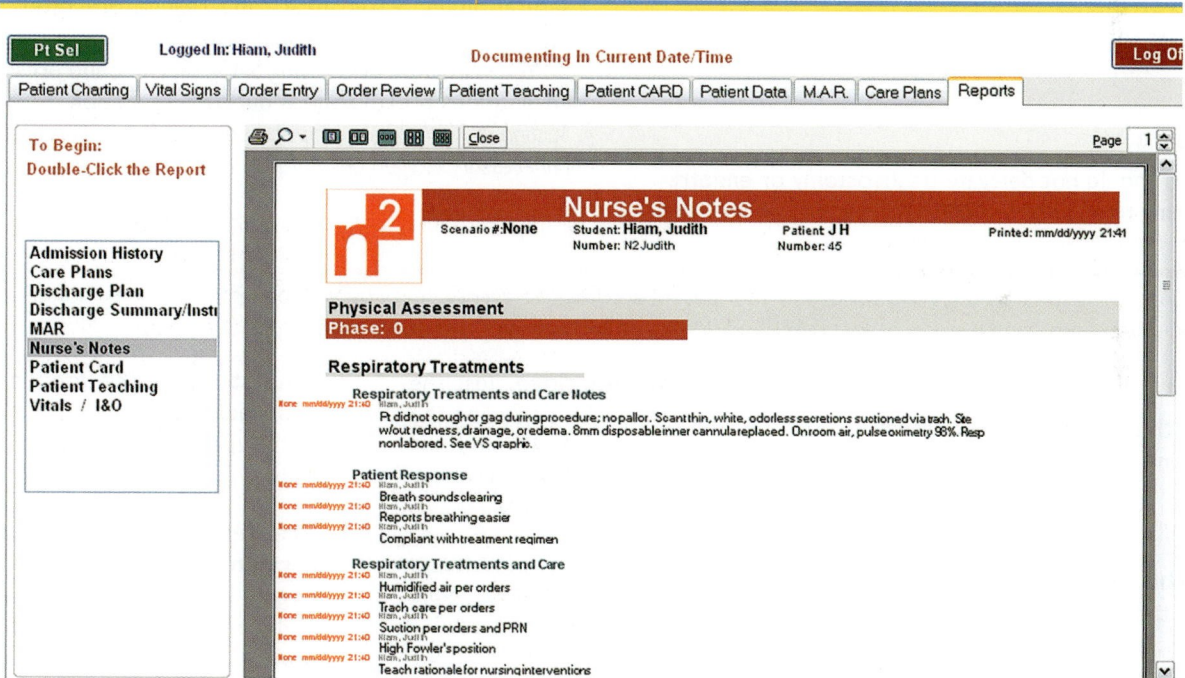

Practice Resources

Barnett, M. (2012); Johnston, J., Davis, S., & Sherman, J. (n.d., updated 2016); Kozin, E., Straton, J., & Kapo, J. (2012); Mitchell, R. B., Hussey, H. M., Setzen, G., et al. (2013); National Guideline Clearinghouse (2011); Siddiqui, J., Sherren, P. B., & Birchall, M. A. (2013); Siegel, J., Rhinehart, E., Jackson, M., et al. (2007).

Thinking About the Procedure

 The video **Performing Tracheostomy Care Using Sterile Technique,** along with questions and suggested responses, is available on the **Davis's** *Nursing Skills Videos* Web site on *DavisPlus*.

Procedure 37-6 ■ Performing Tracheostomy or Endotracheal Suctioning (Open System)

➤ For steps to follow in *all* procedures, refer to the Universal Steps for All Procedures found on the page facing the inside back cover.

Equipment

- Portable or wall suction device with tubing and a collection canister
- Linen-saver pad or towel
- Resuscitation bag connected to oxygen source
- Sterile suction catheter kit: adults: 12- to 18-Fr, children: 8- to 10-Fr, infants: 5- to 8-Fr
- If a kit isn't available, collect the following: sterile gloves, sterile suction catheter of the appropriate size, and a sterile container.
- Pour-bottle of sterile, normal saline solution
- Sterile basin or container for fluids
- Prefilled 10-mL containers of normal saline solution
- Face shield or goggles
- Sterile gloves (or procedure gloves; follow agency policy)
- Protective gown

Delegation

As a rule, you should not delegate tracheostomy or endotracheal suctioning to an LPN or NAP, because both procedures require professional-level theoretical knowledge, assessment skills, and problem-solving ability. However, if the patient has a permanent tracheostomy tube and will require long-term care, you can delegate care to trained personnel. Refer to individual state board of nursing for rules on delegating this procedure.

Pre-Procedure Assessment

- Assess the patient's respiratory status, including rate, depth, and rhythm; breath sounds; color; and pulse oximetry results.
- Assess for signs that indicate the need for suctioning: restlessness, cyanosis, labored respirations, decreased oxygen saturation, increased heart and respiratory rates, visible secretions in the airway, increased peak airway pressures on the ventilator, decreasing SaO_2 or PaO_2, and presence of adventitious breath sounds during auscultation.

Suctioning should be performed only when necessary to prevent unnecessary oxygen desaturation and tissue trauma.

➤ When performing the procedure, always identify your patient according to agency policy, using two identifiers, and be attentive to standard precautions, hand hygiene, patient safety and privacy, body mechanics, and documentation.

Procedure Steps

1. **Position the patient** in semi-Fowler's position, unless contraindicated.
   Promotes lung expansion and oxygenation.

2. **Place the linen-saver pad** or towel on the patient's chest.
   Prevents soiling of the patient's gown during suctioning.

3. **Don face shield or googles.**

4. **Turn on the wall suction** or portable suction machine, and adjust the pressure regulator according to agency policy, using the lowest possible suction pressure. Typically, this is:
   Adults: 100 to 150 mm Hg
   Children: 100 to 120 mm Hg
   Infants: 50 to 95 mm Hg
   Using the appropriate pressure prevents tissue trauma and ensures successful suctioning. Higher pressures are associated with hypoxemia, tissue trauma, and atelectasis, yet do not improve removal of secretions

5. **Don a nonsterile glove.** Test the suction equipment by occluding the connection tubing. Remove and discard the glove. Perform hand hygiene.
   Ensures proper functioning before you insert suction catheter.

6. **Remove and discard glove.** Perform hand hygiene.

7. **Open the suction catheter kit** or (if a kit isn't available) the gathered equipment. Maintain sterility of the inside of the suction kit or the gathered equipment.
   This prevents contaminating the upper airway when you introduce the suction catheter.

8. **Don gloves.** Follow agency policy, as some guidelines allow for clean nonsterile rather than sterile procedure gloves. Consider your dominant hand clean and your nondominant hand contaminated.

9. **Pour sterile saline** into the sterile container.
   Sterile saline is used to clear the suction catheter of secretions after suctioning.

10. **Premeasure the catheter insertion distance** for 0.5 to 1 cm (¼ to ½ in.) past the distal end of the endotracheal tube (ETT); the ETT normally sits between 3 and 7 cm (1 to 2¾ in.) above the carina.

11. **Don sterile gloves.** Consider your dominant hand sterile and your nondominant hand unsterile.

12. **Pick up the suction catheter** with your dominant hand and attach it to the connection tubing. Do not touch the connection tubing with your sterile glove.
    Prepares the suction catheter for use.

13. **Put the tip of the suction catheter** into the sterile container of normal saline solution and suction a small amount of normal saline solution through the suction catheter. Apply suction by placing a finger over the suction control port of the suction catheter.

Lubricates the catheter and helps ensure that the suction equipment is functioning properly. Sterile saline is necessary to clear the suction of secretions after suctioning. The outside of the saline container is not sterile; it would contaminate your dominant hand.

14. **If the patient is receiving oxygen,** hyperoxygenate the patient according to agency policy. If the patient does not require oxygen, you do not need to hyperoxygenate.

Helps prevent hypoxia and related complications (cardiac arrhythmias, seizures, arrest) during suctioning. Suctioning clears secretions, but it also removes oxygen from airways.

If the Patient Requires Mechanical Ventilation

a. Press the 100% O_2 button on the ventilator. Some agencies require the nurse to manually hyperoxygenate the patient; follow agency policy.

Ventilators typically have a button that allows you to hyperoxygenate the patient for a total of 2 minutes. Once this time period elapses, the ventilator automatically resumes its previous settings.

If the Patient Does Not Require Mechanical Ventilation

b. Obtain the assistance of a second provider.

c. Have your partner attach the resuscitation bag to the tracheostomy or endotracheal tube, and hyperoxygenate the patient by compressing the resuscitation bag three to five times as the patient inhales. Remove the resuscitation bag, and place it next to the patient when you are finished.

You must perform hyperoxygenation manually if the patient does not require mechanical ventilation. ➤

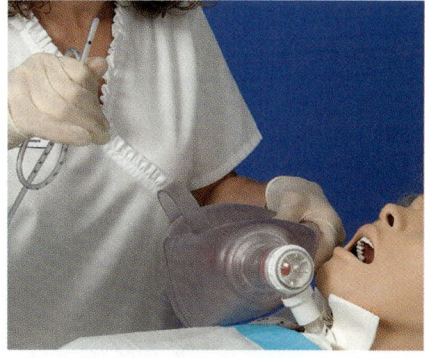

15. **Perform suctioning.**

a. Lubricate the suction catheter tip with the normal saline solution.

Lubrication eases passage of the suction catheter through the endotracheal tube or tracheostomy tube.

b. Using your dominant hand, gently but quickly insert the suction catheter into the endotracheal tube or tracheostomy tube. ▼

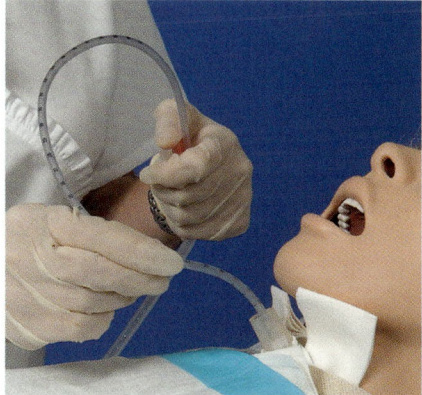

c. ✚ Advance the suction catheter, with suction off, gently aiming downward and being careful not to force the catheter. Insert to the premeasured length: no farther than the **carina tracheae** (the ridge at the lower end of the trachea that separates the openings of the two mainstem bronchi); do not insert more than 6 in. (15 cm) and do not force against any resistance.

Forcing the catheter during insertion may cause tissue trauma.

d. Apply suction while you withdraw the catheter; rotate the catheter (roll it between your thumb and forefinger) as you remove it. Make sure to apply suction for no longer than 15 seconds.

Applying suction for longer than 15 seconds causes hypoxia and may cause tissue trauma.

16. **Repeat suctioning as needed.**

Several passes with the suction catheter may be needed to clear the airway of secretions.

a. Allow at least 30-second intervals between suctioning.

b. Hyperoxygenate the patient between each pass.

c. Limit total suctioning time to 5 minutes.

17. **Coil the suction catheter** in your dominant hand (alternatively, wrap it around your dominant hand). Pull the sterile (or clean) glove off over the coiled catheter. Discard the glove containing the catheter in a fluid-resistant receptacle designated by your agency.

Prevents contaminating the environment with secretions.

18. **Replace the oxygen source** if it was removed during suctioning.

To prevent hypoxia.

19. **Using your nondominant hand,** clear the connecting tubing of secretions by placing the tip into the container of sterile saline.

Prepares the tubing for later reuse.

20. **Turn off the** suction units (and the oxygen, if appropriate).

21. Remove glove from nondominant hand, perform hand hygiene and don clean procedure gloves.

22. **Provide mouth care.**

23. **Reposition the patient.**

Promotes comfort and prevents skin breakdown.

? What if . . .

■ **The patient has a cuffed tracheostomy tube?**

Check to see that it is properly inflated before suctioning. Usually this is 20 to 25 mm Hg or less, but follow the manufacturer's instructions and use a cuff manometer. See Clinical Insight 37-4 to learn how to check cuff inflation.

(continued on next page)

Procedure 37-6 ■ Performing Tracheostomy or Endotracheal Suctioning (Open System) (continued)

Evaluation

- Assess the color, amount, and consistency of secretions.
- Evaluate the patient's tolerance of the procedure (e.g., were there signs of respiratory distress during the procedure)?
- Evaluate the effectiveness of the procedure by comparing breath sounds, vital signs, and pulse oximetry before and after suctioning.

Patient Teaching

- Teach the patient and caregiver how to perform suctioning if the patient will be discharged with an artificial airway. Make sure they can successfully provide a return demonstration.
- Teach the caregiver strategies for managing the patient's airway at home.

Home Care

- Provide the family and caregiver information about where to obtain suction equipment, contact information for healthcare personnel who can be reached for advice or emergencies, and information about home oxygen therapy.
- Guidelines recommend clean technique for home care and for repeated catheter use as long as the catheter is still clear.
- Teach the family and caregiver how to clean catheters for reuse (soak in hot, soapy water; rinse inside and out with clean water; air-dry; store in a dry container).

Documentation

Document the following:

- Date, time, and reason you performed suctioning
- The size of the suction catheter you used
- Amount, color, consistency, and odor of secretions
- Patient's respiratory status before and after the procedure
- Patient's tolerance of the procedure
- Any complications that occurred as a result of the procedure and interventions you made in response

Sample documentation

Sept. 18, 2018   0900   Pulse ox 93%, VS elevated, upper airway rhonchi auscultated. Hyperoxygenated with 100% O₂; suctioned moderate amount thick, yellow mucus with #12-Fr suction catheter. After procedure lungs clear, pulse ox 98%, VS WNL. ——— Jackie Estes, RN

Practice Resources

American Association for Respiratory Care (2010); Sole, M. L., Bennett, M., & Ashworth, S. (2015).

Thinking About the Procedure

 The video **Performing Endotracheal Suctioning (Open System),** along with questions and suggested responses, is available on the **Davis's *Nursing Skills Videos*** Web site on **Davis*Plus.***

Procedure 37-7 ■ Performing Tracheostomy or Endotracheal Suctioning (Inline Closed System)

> ➤ For steps to follow in *all* procedures, refer to the Universal Steps for All Procedures found on the page facing the inside back cover.

Equipment

For the once-a-day steps: Procedure gloves and inline suction catheter
   When suctioning: Sterile normal saline ▼

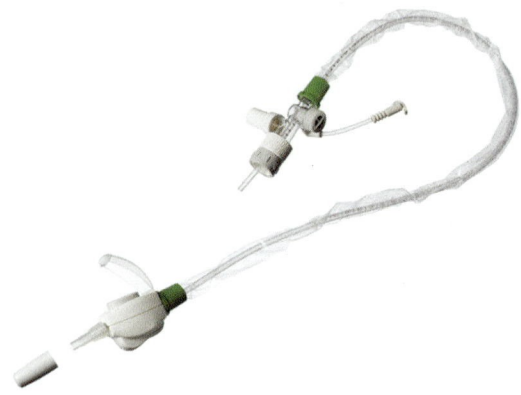

Delegation

As a rule, you should not delegate tracheostomy or endotracheal suctioning to an LPN or NAP, because both procedures require professional-level theoretical knowledge, assessment skills, and problem-solving ability. Refer to the individual state board of nursing for rules on delegating this procedure.

Pre-Procedure Assessment

- Assess respiratory status, including respiratory rate, depth, and rhythm; breath sounds; color; and pulse oximetry results.
- Assess for restlessness, cyanosis, labored respirations, decreased oxygen saturation, increased heart and respiratory rates, visible secretions in the airway, and the presence of adventitious breath sounds during auscultation.

These assessments help determine whether the patient requires suctioning. Suctioning should be performed only when necessary to prevent unnecessary oxygen desaturation and tissue trauma.

> ➤ When performing the procedure, always identify your patient according to agency policy, using two identifiers, and be attentive to standard precautions, hand hygiene, patient safety and privacy, body mechanics, and documentation.

> ➤ *Note:* This procedure uses modified sterile technique.

Daily Procedure Steps

1. An inline suction unit is available only for patients on a mechanical ventilator. Most agencies require the respiratory therapy department to set up the inline suction equipment. If this is not the agency policy, you may need to perform these steps once per day. Open the inline suction catheter package, using sterile technique.

2. Remove the adapter on the ventilator tubing.

3. Attach the inline suction catheter equipment to the ventilator tubing.

4. Reconnect the adapter on the ventilator tubing.

5. Attach the other end of the inline suction catheter to the connection tubing placed to suction.

Suctioning Procedure Steps

1. **Place the patient in semi-Fowler's** position, unless contraindicated.
   The suction catheter is contained within a sterile unit.

2. **Don clean procedure gloves.**
   You do not need to wear sterile gloves.

3. **Place a linen-saver pad** or towel on the patient's chest.

4. **If a lock is present** on the suction control port, unlock it.

5. **Turn on the wall suction** or portable suction machine and adjust the pressure regulator according to agency policy or provider's prescription.
   Using the appropriate pressure prevents tissue trauma and ensures successful suctioning.

6. **Pick up the catheter** with your dominant hand and use your non-dominant hand for the suction port.
   Using the dominant hand improves dexterity.

7. **Unlock the inline catheter** and gently insert the suction catheter into the airway by maneuvering the catheter within the sterile sleeve. ▼

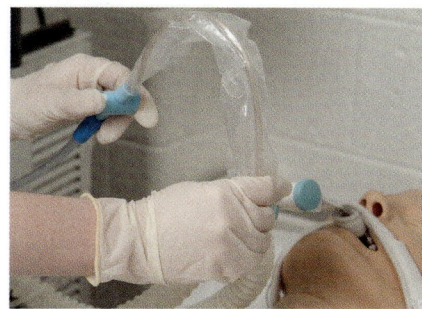

8. ✚ **Advance the suction catheter** into the airway, being careful not to force the catheter. Ask the patient to take slow, deep breaths if she can cooperate. Advance the catheter to the predetermined and premarked distance. Do not apply suction while advancing.
   Forcing the catheter during insertion may cause airway trauma.

9. **Apply suction** by depressing the button over the suction control port as you withdraw the catheter. Apply suction for no longer than 15 seconds.
   Applying suction for longer than 15 seconds causes hypoxia and may cause tissue trauma.

10. **Withdraw the inline suction** catheter completely into the sleeve. The indicator line on the catheter should appear through the sleeve.
    The indicator line is a safety mechanism designed to make sure the suction catheter is withdrawn completely to prevent airway obstruction.

11. **Attach the prefilled, 10-mL** container of normal saline solution to the saline port located on the inline equipment.
    Provides a flush solution to clear the suction catheter of secretions.

12. **Squeeze the 10-mL container** while applying suction.
    Clears the catheter of secretions, preparing the catheter for repeat use. If allowed to remain in the catheter or suction line, secretions may dry and harden, reducing line suction efficiency.

13. **Lock the suction regulator port.**
    Prevents you from inadvertently applying suction.

? What if . . .

■ **The patient experiences a dysrhythmia?**

Stop suctioning and hyperoxygenate the patient. If a further attempt at suctioning promotes a dysrhythmia, notify the medical care provider.

For Evaluation, Patient Teaching, and Documentation, see Procedure 37-6. Typically, you would not be doing inline suctioning in the home.

Thinking About the Procedure

 The video **Performing Endotracheal Suctioning (Inline Closed System),** along with questions and suggested responses, is available on the **Davis's** *Nursing Skills Videos* Web site on Davis*Plus.*

Practice Resources

National Guideline Clearinghouse (2011); Parker, L. C. (2014); Restrepo, R. D., Brown, J. M., & Hughes, J. M. (2010).

Procedure 37-8 ■ Performing Orotracheal and Nasotracheal Suctioning (Open System)

➤ For steps to follow in *all* procedures, refer to the Universal Steps for All Procedures found on the page facing the inside back cover.

➤ *Note:* This procedure uses modified sterile technique. Although the oropharynx and nasopharynx are not sterile, you should keep the suction catheter free from other contaminants as much as possible. Some facilities do use sterile gloves for this procedure

Equipment

- Portable or wall suction device with connection tubing and a collection canister
- Linen-saver pad or towel
- Sterile, flexible, multiple-eyed suction catheter kit (12- to 18-Fr for adults, 8- to 10-Fr for children, and 5- to 8-Fr for infants). If a kit isn't available, collect the following: clean procedure gloves, sterile suction catheter of the appropriate size, and a sterile container for fluids.
- Pour-bottle of sterile water or normal saline solution
- Face shield or goggles and gown
- Water-soluble lubricant for NT suctioning
- Sputum trap, if a specimen is needed
- Nasopharyngeal airway when frequent NT suctioning is required
- Resuscitation bag with mask

Delegation

You should not delegate orotracheal and nasotracheal suctioning to an LPN or NAP, because these procedures require professional-level theoretical knowledge, assessment skills, and problem-solving ability.

Pre-Procedure Assessment

- Assess respiratory status, including respiratory rate, depth, and rhythm; breath sounds; skin color; and pulse oximetry results.
- Assess for signs that indicate the need for suctioning: gurgling sounds during respiration; restlessness, labored respirations; decreased oxygen saturation; increased heart and respiratory rates; and the presence of adventitious breath sounds during auscultation.

Suctioning removes oxygen from airways and can cause tissue trauma. It should be done only when essential (i.e., only when less invasive techniques have proved unsuccessful and when the secretions are causing physiological deterioration and/or distress).

- Assess the effectiveness of the cough.

➤ When performing the procedure, always identify your patient according to agency policy, using two identifiers, and be attentive to standard precautions, hand hygiene, patient safety and privacy, body mechanics, and documentation.

Procedure Steps

1. Position the patient.

For Orotracheal Suctioning

  a. Position the patient in semi-Fowler's position, with the head turned to face you.

For Nasotracheal Suctioning

  b. Position the patient in semi-Fowler's position, with his neck hyperextended, unless contraindicated.

    Hyperextending the neck makes it easier to insert the suction catheter. Upright position helps to prevent back strain.

2. Place the linen-saver pad or towel on the patient's chest.

Prevents soiling of the patient's gown during suctioning.

3. Put on a face shield or goggles and gown.

Protects you from contamination with secretions that may splash during suctioning.

4. Turn on the wall suction or portable suction machine, and adjust the pressure regulator according to agency policy. Guidelines from the American Association for Respiratory Care specify:

Adults: 100 to 150 mm Hg
Children: 100 to 120 mm Hg
Infants: 80 to 100 mm Hg
Neonates: 60 to 80 mm Hg

The suction regulator must be set appropriately to prevent tissue trauma and hypoxia and yet remove secretions effectively.

5. Don a procedure glove and test the suction equipment by occluding the connection tubing. Discard the glove and perform hand hygiene.

Testing the equipment ensures proper functioning before you insert the catheter in the patient's airway.

6. Open the suction catheter kit or, if a kit isn't available, the gathered equipment.

Nasal approach: If you are using the nasal approach, open the water-soluble lubricant and, preferably, a nasopharyngeal airway.

7. Don clean nonsterile gloves. Consider your dominant hand clean and your nondominant hand contaminated.

Keeping the dominant hand sterile prevents contaminating the upper airways with a anon sterile suction catheter. This is a modified sterile suction technique because the catheter enters the trachea via nose or the mouth, which are not sterile. However, take care to keep the catheter free from other contamination.

If Using Sterile Technique
Don sterile gloves. Consider dominant hand sterile and your nondominant hand unsterile. Alternatively, put a sterile glove on your dominant hand and a nonsterile glove on your nondominant hand.

NOTE: if you consider both hands sterile (i.e., for sterile technique), you must remove the cap from the sterile water before donning gloves.

8. **Pour sterile saline into** the sterile container, using your nondominant hand.
   Sterile saline will be used to clear the suction catheter of secretions after suctioning.

9. **Pick up the suction catheter** with your dominant hand and attach it to the connection tubing, maintaining sterility of your hand and the catheter.
   Prepares the suction catheter for use.

10. **Put the tip of the suction catheter** into the sterile container of normal saline solution, and suction a small amount of normal saline solution through the suction catheter. Apply suction by placing a finger over the suction control port of the suction catheter.
    Lubricates the catheter and helps ensure that the suction equipment is functioning properly.

11. **Ask the patient to take several slow,** deep breaths. If the patient's oxygen saturation is < 94%, or if he is in any distress, you may need to give supplemental oxygen before, during and after suctioning. See Procedure 37-4.
    Promotes relaxation and helps hyperoxygenate the patient before suctioning.

12. **Using your nondominant hand,** remove the oxygen delivery device, if present (for the nasal suctioning only).

For Oral Approach, Patient Receiving Nasal Oxygen
   a. If the patient is receiving nasal oxygen and you are performing orotracheal suctioning, you do not need to remove the oxygen source.

For Nasal Approach, Patient Receiving Nasal Oxygen
   b. Remove the nasal oxygen and place the nasal cannula in the patient's mouth. See Procedure 37-4.
   Placing the cannula in the patient's mouth makes it easier to access the nares for suctioning while still delivery oxygen to the patient (orally).

13. **Premeasure to approximate the depth** you should insert the suction catheter. For adults, insert the catheter about 15 cm (6 in.) for an oral approach and 20 cm (8 in.) for a nasal approach. Be careful not to contaminate the catheter while you measure.
    Prevents trauma at the carina and ensures suctioning of the full length of the trachea.

Oral Approach
   a. Measure the distance between the edge of the patient's mouth to the tip of the earlobe and down to the bottom of the neck. ▼

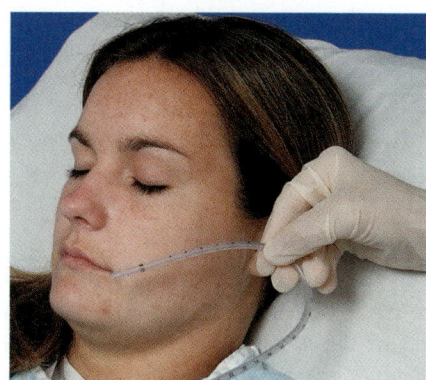

For Nasal Approach
   b. Measure the distance from the tip of the nose to the tip of the earlobe and down to the bottom of the neck.

   c. Insert nasopharyngeal airway gently into the nostril, with the bevel toward the septum (center of the nose), advance the airway straight in, following floor of the nose. See Procedure 37-13.
   Do not force nasopharyngeal airway into the nostril as this may cause unnecessary edema and trauma.

14. **Lubricate and insert** the suction catheter.
    Lubrication makes it easier to pass a suction catheter through the nares.

For Orotracheal Suctioning
   a. Lubricate the suction catheter tip with normal saline solution.
   b. Using your dominant hand, gently but quickly insert the suction catheter along the side of the patient's mouth or through the endotracheal tube into the oropharynx.
   Quick insertion along the side of the mouth prevents gagging.
   c. When the patient inhales, advance the suction catheter to the predetermined distance, being careful not to force the catheter.
   Advancing the suction catheter when the patient inhales ensures that the catheter enters the trachea rather than the esophagus. Forcing the catheter during insertion may cause tissue trauma.

For Nasotracheal Suctioning
   d. Lubricate the catheter tip with the water-soluble lubricant.
   Water-soluble lubricant is preferred because it will dissolve if it accidentally enters the lungs, whereas an oil-based lubricant (e.g., petroleum jelly) won't dissolve in the respiratory tract and causes complications if it enters the lungs.
   e. Using your dominant hand, gently but quickly insert the suction catheter into the naris and down to the pharynx. When the patient inhales, advance the suction catheter, gently aiming downward to the predetermined distance, being careful not to force the catheter.

(continued on next page)

Procedure 37-8 ■ Performing Orotracheal and Nasotracheal Suctioning (Open System) (continued)

Ensures that the catheter enters the trachea. Forcing the catheter during insertion may cause tissue trauma.

15. **Place a finger or thumb over** the suction control port of the catheter.
Apply suction while you withdraw the catheter, using a continuous rotating motion. Apply suction for no longer than 15 seconds.
Using a continuous rotating motion and suctioning while withdrawing the catheter prevents trauma to any one area of the airway. Limiting suctioning to less than 15 seconds prevents hypoxia. ▼

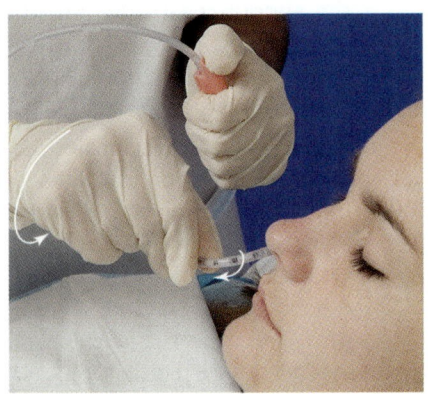

16. **After you withdraw the catheter,** clear it by placing the tip of the catheter into the container of sterile saline and applying suction. ➤

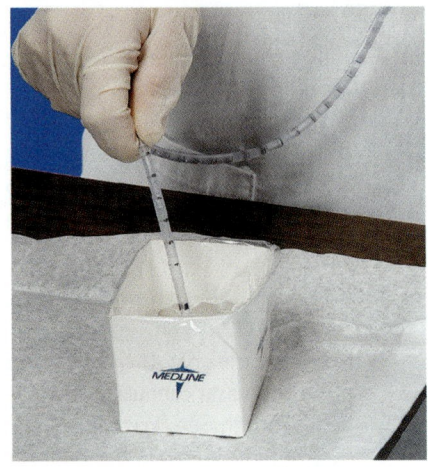

17. **Lubricate the catheter** and repeat suctioning as needed, allowing intervals of at least 30 seconds between suctioning. Reapply oxygen between suctioning efforts, if required.
Several passes with the suction catheter may be needed to clear the airway of secretions. Total suctioning time should be limited to 5 minutes, however, to prevent trauma and hypoxia.

18. **Replace the oxygen source.**
Prevents hypoxia.

19. **Coil the suction catheter** in your dominant hand (alternatively, wrap it around your dominant hand). Hold the catheter while you pull the sterile glove off over it. Discard the glove containing the catheter in a biohazard receptacle (e.g., bag) designated by your agency.

These actions prevent contaminating the environment with secretions.

20. **Using your nondominant hand,** clear the connecting tubing of secretions by placing the tip into the container of sterile saline.

21. **Dispose of equipment** and make sure new suction supplies are readily available for future suctioning.
The patient may require suctioning at any time, so equipment must be readily available.

22. **Remove glove from nondominant** hand and perform hand hygiene.

23. **Don clean procedure gloves** and provide mouth care.
Promotes patient comfort and clears the mouth of any secretions the patient may have expectorated.

24. **Assist the patient** to a comfortable position, and allow him to rest.
Comfort and rest help the patient recover from the stress of suctioning.

? What if . . .

■ **The patient's oxygen saturation is less than 94%, or he is in any distress?**
Administer supplemental oxygen before, during, and after suctioning. Notify the patient's primary provider if the patient does not respond to additional oxygen.

Evaluation

■ Assess the color, consistency, and amount of secretions.
■ Evaluate the patient's tolerance of the procedure. Note whether there were signs of respiratory distress during suctioning.
■ Evaluate the effectiveness of the procedure by comparing breath sounds, vital signs, and pulse oximetry or blood gas data before and after the procedure.

Patient Teaching

■ Explain the importance of administering supplemental oxygen or taking several deep breaths before suctioning.
■ Inform the patient that coughing typically increases with suctioning.

■ Demonstrate orotracheal or nasotracheal suctioning to the caregiver, and ask for a return demonstration if suctioning will be required at home.

Home Care

■ Instruct the family and caregiver about where to obtain suction equipment.
■ Provide the client and caregiver with contact information of healthcare personnel who can be reached for advice or emergencies.
■ Explain that the procedure can be performed using clean technique instead of sterile technique in the home.

- Instruct the caregiver that suction catheters can be cleaned for reuse by washing them with soapy water and then boiling them for 10 minutes. After they are cleaned, rinse the catheters with normal saline solution or tap water.
- Instruct the caregiver to change the secretion collection container every 24 hours, or clean it according to home-care agency guidelines every 24 hours.

Documentation

- Document the date, time, and reason you performed suctioning.
- Note the suction technique you used and the catheter size.
- Note the color, consistency, and odor of secretions.
- Document the patient's respiratory status before and after the procedure.
- Document the patient's tolerance of the procedure and any complications that occurred as a result of the procedure.
- Document any interventions you performed to address complications that occurred.

Sample documentation

July 31, 2018   0930   O₂ sat 89% on room air, bilateral rhonchi to bases auscultated, unproductive cough, heart rate 90, RR-18. Assistant nurse recruited for manual ventilation. Client placed in semi-Fowler's position, hyperventilated for 1 minute to 100% O₂ sat, oropharyngeal suctioning performed using sterile technique, resulting in moderate amounts of white, tenacious, yellow-tinged secretions. Improved breath sound with diminished rhonchi auscultated, O₂ sat at 97% on room air, heart rate 78, RR-14. Client smiles when asked how he feels. Bed in low position, call light and fluids in reach. ———————— Kelton Jones, RN

Practice Resources

American Association for Respiratory Care (2010); American Red Cross (2011); Barnett, M. (2012); Restrepo, R. D., Brown, J. M., & Hughes, J. M. (2010).

Procedure 37-9 ■ Performing Upper Airway Suctioning

➤ For steps to follow in *all* procedures, refer to the Universal Steps for All Procedures found on the page facing the inside back cover.

➤ *Note:* Upper airway suctioning may be done via the oropharyngeal or nasopharyngeal route. However, nasal suction is usually required only to improve oxygenation in infants because most adult airway obstruction occurs in the mouth and oropharynx.

- ✚ Vigorous nasal suction can induce epistaxis (nosebleed) and further complicate an already difficult airway.

Equipment

- Portable or wall suction device with connection tubing and a collection canister
- Linen-saver pad or towel
- Sterile suction catheter kit (12- to 18-Fr for adults, 8- to 10-Fr for children, and 5- to 8-Fr for infants). If a kit isn't available, collect the following: sterile suction catheter of the appropriate size and a sterile container. If you plan to suction both the oropharynx and the nasopharynx, you need a separate sterile catheter for each.
- Yankauer device can be used for oropharyngeal suction.
- Pour-bottle of sterile normal saline solution
- Sterile basin or other container for fluids
- Face shield or goggles and gown
- Procedure gloves
- Water-soluble lubricant for nasopharyngeal suctioning
- Sputum trap, if a specimen is needed
- Biohazard bag

Delegation

Do not delegate oropharyngeal and nasopharyngeal suctioning to an LPN or NAP, because these procedures require professional-level theoretical knowledge, assessment skills, and problem-solving ability. However, the NAP (and the client or family) can use a Yankauer tube to suction the oral cavity because there is less risk for trauma to mucosa than with oro- or nasopharyngeal suctioning.

Pre-Procedure Assessment

- Assess respiratory status, including rate, depth, and rhythm; breath sounds; color; and pulse oximetry results. Note signs that indicate the need for suctioning: restlessness, cyanosis, labored respirations, decreased oxygen saturation, increased heart and respiratory rates, visible secretions in the airway, and the presence of adventitious breath sounds during auscultation.

You must be certain the patient requires suctioning. Suctioning should be performed only when necessary to prevent unnecessary oxygen desaturation and tissue trauma.

(continued on next page)

Procedure 37-9 ■ **Performing Upper Airway Suctioning** (continued)

> ➤ When performing the procedure, always identify your patient according to agency policy, using two identifiers, and be attentive to standard precautions, hand hygiene, patient safety and privacy, body mechanics, and documentation.

> ➤ *Note:* This procedure describes modified sterile technique: sterile supplies with clean procedure gloves. Although the oropharynx and nasopharynx are not sterile, you should keep the suction catheter free from other contaminants as much as possible. Some facilities require sterile gloves for this procedure.

Procedure Steps

1. **Position the patient.** Explain that suctioning may stimulate coughing or gagging, but that coughing helps mobilize secretions.

For Oropharyngeal Suctioning

Position the patient in a semi-Fowler's or high Fowler's position, with his head turned toward you.
Facilitates insertion of the suction catheter and prevents straining your back. Also promotes lung expansion and effective coughing.

For Nasopharyngeal Suctioning

Position the patient in semi-Fowler's or high Fowler's position with his neck hyperextended, unless contraindicated.

2. **Place the linen-saver pad or towel** on the patient's chest.
Prevents soiling of the patient's gown during suctioning.

3. **Put on a face shield or goggles and gown.**
Protects you from contamination with secretions that may splash during suctioning. Not all guidelines specify wearing a gown for this procedure.

4. **Turn on the wall suction** or portable suction machine, and adjust the pressure regulator according to agency policy, typically:
Adults: 100 to 150 mm Hg
Children: 100 to 120 mm Hg
Infants: 50 to 95 mm Hg
The suction regulator must be set appropriately to prevent tissue trauma and hypoxia and to function effectively to remove secretions. Higher pressures are associated with hypoxemia, tissue trauma, and atelectasis, yet do not improve removal of secretions.

5. **Test the suction equipment** by occluding the connection tubing.
Ensures proper functioning before use.

6. **Open the suction catheter kit** or the gathered equipment. If you are using the nasal approach, open the water-soluble lubricant.

7. **Don procedure gloves;** consider (and keep) your dominant hand clean; consider your nondominant hand to be contaminated.
This is not a sterile suction procedure but care should be taken to keep the suction catheter free from other contaminants. Keeping the dominant hand clean prevents contaminating the upper airways with an unclean suction catheter.

8. **Pour sterile saline** into the sterile container, using your nondominant hand.
Sterile saline is necessary to clear the suction catheter of secretions after suctioning. The outside of the saline container is not sterile; it would contaminate your dominant hand.

9. **Pick up the suction catheter** with your dominant hand, and use your other hand to hold the connection tubing (to suction) while you attach it.

10. **Put the tip of the suction catheter** into the sterile container of normal saline solution, and suction a small amount of normal saline solution through the suction catheter. Apply suction by placing a finger over the suction control port. When using a Yankauer-type device, the suction is continuous and there is no port to occlude.
Ensures that the suction equipment is functioning properly. If you need to see a Yankauer device, see Figure 37-11.

11. **Approximate the depth** to which you will insert the suction catheter.

For Oropharyngeal Suctioning

Measure the distance between the edge of the patient's mouth and the tip of the patient's earlobe.
Determines the proper distance you should insert the suction catheter for oropharyngeal suctioning.

For Nasopharyngeal Suctioning

Measure the distance between the tip of the patient's nose and the tip of the patient's earlobe.
Helps determine the correct distance to insert the suction catheter for nasopharyngeal suctioning.

12. **Using your nondominant hand,** remove the oxygen delivery device, if present (for nasopharyngeal suctioning only). Have the patient take several slow, deep breaths.
Deep breathing helps to hyperoxygenate the patient and helps prevent hypoxia during suctioning.

13. **Lubricate and insert the suction catheter.**

For Oropharyngeal Suctioning
   a. Lubricate the catheter tip with the normal saline solution.
   b. Using your dominant hand, gently but quickly insert the suction catheter along the side of the patient's mouth into the oropharynx.
   Inserting the suction catheter along the side of the mouth prevents gagging. ▼

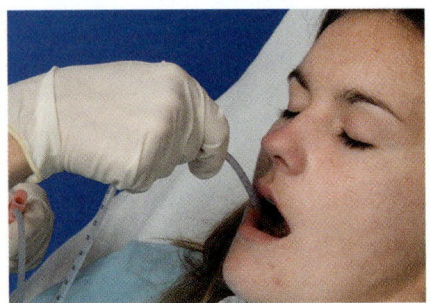

c. Advance the suction catheter quickly to the premeasured distance—usually 7.5 to 10 cm (3 to 4 in.) in the adult—being careful not to force the catheter.
Ensures that the suction catheter will reach the pharynx. Forcing the catheter during insertion may cause tissue trauma.

For Nasopharyngeal Suctioning

d. Lubricate the catheter tip with the water-soluble lubricant.
Eases passage of the suction catheter through the naris. Water-soluble lubricant is preferred because it will dissolve if it accidentally enters the lungs, whereas an oil-based lubricant (e.g., petroleum jelly or lotion) will not dissolve in the respiratory tract and causes complications if it enters the lungs.

e. Using your dominant hand, gently but quickly insert the suction catheter into the naris.
Prevents trauma to the naris. ▼

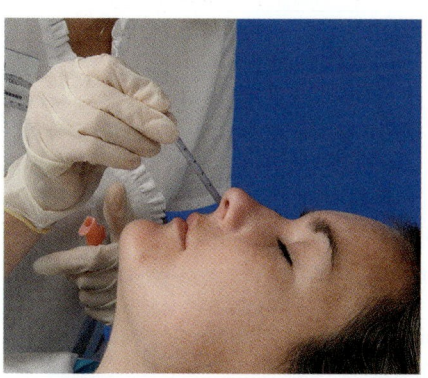

f. Advance the suction catheter, aiming downward to the premeasured distance—usually 13 to 15 cm (5 to 6 in.) in the adult—and being careful not to force the catheter. If you meet resistance, you may need to try the other naris.
Advancing the suction catheter the premeasured distance ensures that the suction catheter will reach the pharynx. Forcing the catheter during insertion may cause tissue trauma.

14. **Place a finger or thumb over** the suction control port of the suction catheter and start suctioning the patient. Apply suction as you withdraw the catheter, using a continuous rotating motion.

✚ Limit suctioning to 10 to 15 sec.
Using a continuous rotating motion while withdrawing the catheter prevents trauma to any one area of the airway. Limiting suctioning to less than 10 to 15 seconds prevents hypoxia.

15. **After you withdraw the catheter,** clear it by placing the tip of the catheter into the container of sterile saline and applying suction.
Ensures patency of the catheter for repeat suctioning.

16. **Lubricate the catheter and repeat** suctioning as needed, allowing at least 20-second intervals between suctioning. Limit total suctioning time to 5 minutes.
Several passes with the suction catheter may be needed to clear the airway of secretions. The total suctioning time should be limited to 5 minutes, however, to prevent hypoxia and trauma to the mucosal membranes.

For Nasopharyngeal Suctioning

Each time you repeat suction, alternate nares.
Prevents trauma that would occur if you used only one naris.

17. **Coil the suction catheter** in your dominant hand. Pull the sterile glove off over the coiled catheter. (Alternatively, wrap the catheter around your dominant, gloved hand, and hold the catheter as you remove the glove over it.) Discard the glove containing the catheter in a biohazard receptacle designated by your agency.
Coiling the catheter inside the glove prevents contamination with secretions.

18. **Using your nondominant hand,** clear the connecting tubing of secretions by placing the tip into the container of sterile saline.
Ensures patency and prepares the equipment for future use.

19. **Dispose of equipment** in biohazard waste container/bag and make sure new suction supplies are readily available for future suctioning needs.
The patient may require suctioning at any time, so equipment must be readily available.

20. **Provide mouth care.**
Promotes patient comfort and clears the mouth of any secretions the patient may have expectorated.

21. **Discard your other glove** and remaining supplies.

22. **Position the patient** in a comfortable position and allow him to rest.
Promoting comfort and allowing for a period of rest helps the patient recover from suctioning, which may be very tiring.

? What if . . .

■ **The patient's oxygen saturation is less than 94%, or he is in any distress?**

You may need to administer supplemental oxygen before, during, and after suctioning. See Procedure 37-4.

(continued on next page)

Procedure 37-9 ■ Performing Upper Airway Suctioning (continued)

Evaluation

- Assess the color, consistency, and amount of secretions.
- Evaluate the patient's tolerance of the procedure. Note whether there were signs of respiratory distress during the procedure.
- Evaluate the effectiveness of the procedure by comparing breath sounds, vital signs, and pulse oximetry before and after the procedure.

Patient Teaching

- Explain the importance of administering supplemental oxygen to the patient before suctioning.
- Inform the patient that coughing typically increases with suctioning.
- Demonstrate oropharyngeal or nasopharyngeal suctioning to the caregiver and ask for a return demonstration if suctioning will be required at home.

Home Care

- Instruct the family and caregiver where to obtain suction equipment.
- Provide the client and caregiver with contact information for healthcare personnel who can be reached for advice or emergencies.
- Explain that the procedure can be performed using clean technique instead of sterile technique in the home setting.
- Instruct the caregiver that suction catheters can be cleaned for reuse by washing them with soapy water and then boiling them for 10 minutes. After they are cleaned, rinse the catheters with normal saline solution or tap water.
- Teach to change the secretion collection container every 24 hours, or clean it according to home-care agency guidelines every 24 hours.

Documentation

- Document the date, time, and reason you performed suctioning.
- Note the suction technique you used and the catheter size.
- Note color, consistency, and odor of secretions.
- Document the patient's respiratory status before and after the procedure.
- Document the patient's tolerance of the procedure and any complications that occurred as a result of the procedure, with resulting interventions.

Sample documentation

3/15/18   2200   Resp. labored, rate 28 breaths/min. Pulse oximetry on room air 92%. Breath sounds with rhonchi scattered throughout. Gurgling audible in upper airways. Patient unable to mobilize secretions with coughing. Suctioned by nasopharyngeal route using a 14-Fr. catheter. Approximately 30 mL thin, tan, odorless secretions obtained. After suctioning, resp. nonlabored, rate 20 breaths/min, and lungs clear on auscultation, with no gurgling audible. Pulse oximetry 96%. Patient tolerated procedure with no difficulty. ———————— C. F. Hiam, RN

Practice Resources

McGrath, B. A., Bates, L., Atkinson, D., et al. (2012); Siegel, J., Rhinehart, E., Jackson, M., et al. (2007); Sole, M. L., Bennett, M., & Ashworth, S. (2015); Sole, M. L., Penoyer, D. A., Bennett, M., et al. (2011).

Thinking About the Procedure

 The video **Performing Upper Airway Suctioning: Oropharyngeal,** along with questions and suggested responses, is available on the **Davis's *Nursing Skills Videos*** Web site on Davis*Plus*.

Procedure 37-10 ■ Caring for Patients Requiring Mechanical Ventilation

> For steps to follow in *all* procedures, refer to the Universal Steps for All Procedures found on the page facing the inside back cover.

Equipment

- Two oxygen sources
- Air source that provides 50 pounds per square inch (psi)
- Mechanical ventilator
- Humidification device
- Ventilator tubing, connectors, and adaptors
- Condensation collection device
- Inline thermometer
- Resuscitation bag with oxygen connection tubing
- Pulse oximetry device
- Procedure gloves, protective gown, and eye covering
- Sterile gloves if you will perform suctioning
- Suction equipment (possibly)
- Sterile water for the humidifier. Some guidelines also recommend sterile water for rinsing the mouth.

Delegation

Care of a mechanically ventilated patient requires advanced knowledge of pulmonary anatomy and physiology and should not be delegated to assistive personnel. In critical care settings, specially trained LPNs may provide care, but the RN is responsible for ensuring that procedures are implemented safely and effectively. RNs also provide ongoing assessment of the patient's ventilatory and oxygenation status. Patients requiring long-term ventilation are often cared for at home or in specialized long-term care units, where LPNs and family members may provide care.

Pre-Procedure Assessment

- Review the health record to make sure that mechanical ventilation is included in the options outlined in the patient's advance directive.
  The patient may not wish to pursue mechanical ventilation as a care option. If a patient who does not wish to be ventilated mechanically is currently on a ventilator, consult your hospital ethics committee.

- If the patient's condition allows, assess his understanding of mechanical ventilation therapy.
  Understanding helps allay the patient's anxiety and promotes cooperation.

- Assess respiratory status, including rate, depth, and rhythm; breath sounds; color; and pulse oximetry results.
  Confirms the need for mechanical ventilation.

- Assess the oral cavity for bleeding, inflammation, odor, and presence of yeast or plaque.
  May indicate the need for more frequent oral care or for referral.

- Blood will probably be drawn for an ABG analysis
  To establish a baseline and, after that, to monitor response to therapy.

> ➤ When performing the procedure, always identify your patient according to agency policy, using two identifiers, and be attentive to standard precautions, hand hygiene, patient safety and privacy, body mechanics, and documentation.

> ➤ Refer to Table 37-2 if you need to review ventilator terminology.

Procedure Steps

Initial Ventilator Setup

1. **Prepare the resuscitation bag.**
   The resuscitation bag should be readily available to provide ventilation in the event of an emergency. ▼

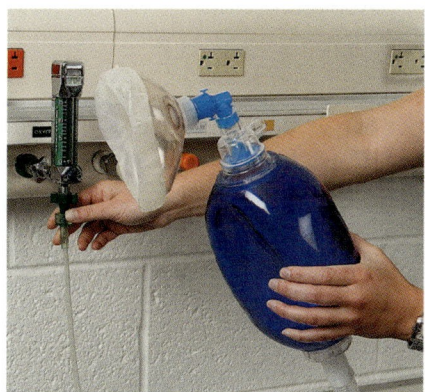

  a. Attach a flow meter to one of the oxygen sources.
   To help regulate and adjust oxygen flow.

  b. Attach an adapter to the flow meter and connect the oxygen tubing to the adapter.

  c. Turn on the oxygen and adjust the flow rate

2. **Respiratory therapists** are responsible for setting up mechanical ventilation in most agencies because they are specially trained. If you must assume the responsibility, refer to the manufacturer's instructions.

3. **Plug the ventilator** into a grounded electrical outlet and turn it on.

4. **Verify ventilator settings** and adjust as medically prescribed.
   Ventilator settings must be individualized according to the patient's need for respiratory support. Incorrect settings may cause harm (e.g., hypoxia or barotrauma) to the patient. ▼

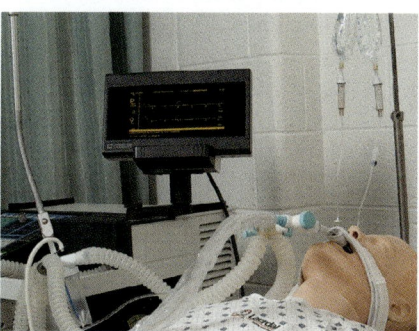

5. **Make sure that ventilator alarm** limits are set appropriately.
   Inappropriately set alarm limits can result in harm to the patient.

6. **Make sure the humidifier** is filled with sterile distilled water.

7. **Don gloves, gown, and eye** protection if you have not already done so.

8. **Attach the ventilator tubing** to the endotracheal tube or tracheostomy tube.

9. **Place the ventilator tubing** in the securing device.
   Prevents dislodging the endotracheal tube or tracheostomy when the patient moves.

10. **Attach a capnographic device,** if available.
    To measure levels of carbon dioxide. These data are used to confirm placement of the endotracheal tube and disconnection from or malfunction of the ventilator. Oxygen levels alone are not sufficient for the ventilated patient.

11. **Prepare the inline (closed) suction** equipment (see Procedure 37-7).
    Suctioning equipment should be readily available when the patient requires suctioning. Closed catheters are recommended to prevent ventilator-associated pneumonia.

(continued on next page)

Procedure 37-10 ■ Caring for Patients Requiring Mechanical Ventilation (continued)

After Initial Ventilator Setup

12. Check respiratory status and ABGs about 30 minutes after setup. Also check whenever there are changes in the ventilator settings and as the patient's condition indicates.
To be certain the patient is being adequately ventilated and not experiencing oxygen toxicity.

13. Check the ventilator tubing frequently for condensation. Drain the fluid into a collection device, or briefly disconnect the patient from the ventilator and empty the tubing into a waste receptacle, according to agency policy.

✚ Never drain the fluid into the humidifier.
Condensation in the ventilator tubing can cause resistance to airflow. Moreover, the patient can aspirate it. The fluid should not be drained into the humidifier because the patient's secretions may have contaminated it.

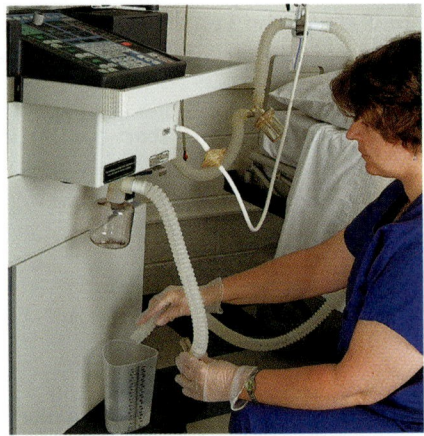

14. ✚ **Maintain the patient in** a semirecumbent position (head of bed elevated 30° to 45°). This is extremely important.
To promote lung expansion, reduce gastric reflux, and prevent ventilator-associated pneumonia.

15. Check ventilator and humidifier settings regularly.

16. Check the inline thermometer.
To ensure that the air being delivered to the patient is close to the body temperature to prevent scalding of the mucosal tissue or cooling the patient (core temperature).

17. Provide the patient with an alternative form of communication, such as a letter board or white board.
A patient being mechanically ventilated is unable to speak, which can produce extreme anxiety. The patient must have a way to express her needs and concerns.

18. Reposition the patient regularly (every 1 to 2 hours), being careful not to pull on the ventilator tubing.
Repositioning protects skin integrity. However, pulling on the tubing creates pain. Patient comfort promotes relaxation, which improves the effectiveness of the ventilator.

19. Keep the patient's lips moistened with a cool, damp cloth and water-based lubricant and provide regular antiseptic oral care. A recommended regimen includes the following:
- Brush the teeth twice a day for 3 to 4 minutes.
- Use a soft toothbrush.
- Rinse mouth with sterile water, according to agency policy.
- Moisturize oral mucosa and lips every 2 to 4 hours.
- Use a chlorhexidine gluconate (0.12%) rinse twice a day during the perioperative period for patients who undergo cardiac surgery (adult patients).

- Use mouthwash twice a day for adult patients (American Association of Critical-Care Nurses, 2008).
Mouth care provides comfort and preserves integrity of the mucous membranes. Patients being mechanically ventilated, even for a short period, are at high risk for developing ventilator-associated pneumonia (VAP). VAP is not uncommon, and it is associated with high mortality rates. This regimen is thought to help prevent VAP.

20. Make sure the call light is always within reach, and answer call light and ventilator alarms promptly.
Provides the patient with immediate access to help if a breathing problem occurs; reassures the patient and thus relieves anxiety.

21. Monitor the tracheostomy tube for proper cuff inflation (usually 20 to 25 mm Hg); see Clinical Insight 37-5.

22. Check for gastric distention and take measures to prevent aspiration.
Aspiration creates high risk for pneumonia.

23. Clean, disinfect, or change ventilator tubing and equipment according to agency policy.
There is no good evidence to indicate how often this should be done. Research so far indicates that tubing and equipment should not be "routinely" changed for infection control purposes (Han & Liu, 2010).

24. Give sedatives or anti-anxiety drugs as prescribed.

Evaluation

- After mechanical ventilation is instituted, assess for chest expansion and auscultate for bilateral breath sounds.
- Evaluate the patient's tolerance of mechanical ventilation. Verify that the patient is being adequately ventilated and that she is breathing in synchrony with the ventilator.
- Auscultate breath sounds every 2 to 4 hours, according to agency policy.
- When monitoring vital signs, count spontaneous breaths as well as those delivered by the ventilator.
- Monitor continuous pulse oximetry, capnography, and ABGs.

Patient Teaching

- Explain mechanical ventilation to the patient and her family. Include information about the alarms they will hear.
- Demonstrate an alternative form of communication to the patient and family.
- When appropriate, explain the weaning process to the patient and family.
- If the patient requires mechanical ventilation after discharge, make arrangements for a home ventilator and teach the patient and caregiver how to use it.

Home Care

- Consult with your facility discharge planning program and/or case management for discharge plans.
- Explain to the family and caregiver where to obtain a home ventilator, resuscitation bag, and oxygen equipment and what services are available. Make sure they choose a supplier who has 24-hour emergency services available.
- Help the client and caregiver devise a backup plan for ventilating the client in the event of a power failure.
- Tell the caregiver to notify the utility company and area emergency personnel that the client is being maintained on a ventilator at home.

- Instruct the client and caregiver about oxygen therapy and its use, as well as safety measures that they must institute.
- Teach the client and caregiver to clean the ventilator tubing with soap and warm water when it becomes soiled.
- Provide the client and caregiver with contact information of healthcare personnel who can be reached for advice or emergencies.

Documentation

- Document the date and time mechanical ventilation was initiated.
- Note the type of ventilator used and the prescribed settings used.
- Document the client's response to mechanical ventilation, including vital signs, breath sounds, ease of breathing, pulse oximetry, intake and output, skin color, and ABG and chest x-ray results.

Sample documentation

02/26/18   0800   Patient found difficult to arouse. Dr. Henry made aware. ABG obtained; results included: pH 7.28; PCO₂ 78 mm Hg; PO₂ 48 mm Hg. Dr. Henry in to evaluate patient. Anesthesia called to intubate patient. Medicated with Versed 5 mg IV and intubated orally with a 7.5-Fr ET tube. Connected to mechanical ventilator: TV 700 mL; FIO₂ 80%, respiratory rate 14 breaths/min. Portable chest x-ray confirms ideal placement of ET tube as well as white-out of both lung fields. ABGs to be obtained in 30 min. Pulse oximetry 90% since being placed on ventilator. ———————— L. Houck, RN

Practice Resources

American Association of Critical-Care Nurses (2008, 2010); El-Rabbany, M., Zaghlol, N., Bhandari, M., et al. (2015); Feider, L. L., Mitchell, P., & Bridges, E. (2010); Grap, M. J., Munro, C. L., & Gardner, M. (2016); Maselli, D., & Restrepo, M. (2011).

Procedure 37-11 ■ Setting Up Disposable Chest Drainage Systems

➤ For steps to follow in *all* procedures, refer to the Universal Steps for All Procedures found on the page facing the inside back cover.

Equipment

- Two disposable closed drainage systems
- Chest tube insertion kit (common tube size for adults is 36-Fr). Should contain povidone-iodine, local anesthetic, syringe, needles, drapes, scalpel, suture, sterile drape, chest tube, connecting tubing, and necessary instruments.
- 5-in-1 or Y-connector for two chest tubes, if not contained in insertion kit
- Sterile water (for water-seal system)
- Two rubber-tipped hemostats
- Sterile gloves, masks, and sterile gowns

- Dressings: sterile 4 in. × 4 in. gauze dressings, precut drain dressings, petroleum (or other recommended) gauze dressings, and large drainage dressings
- Tape: 2-in. silk tape, 1-in. silk tape (or nylon banding system)

For disposable dry-seal systems:

- 50-mL syringe and 45 mL of sterile water or saline. Some dry-seal chest drainage units (CDUs) include these.

(continued on next page)

Procedure 37-11 ■ Setting Up Disposable Chest Drainage Systems (continued)

Delegation

Some agencies permit only registered nurses in the critical care units to perform dressing changes. The physician must perform dressing changes on other units. You should not delegate this procedure because it requires advanced knowledge of pulmonary anatomy and physiology. As needed, teach the LPN and NAP how to safely provide care for the patient with chest tubes. Instruct them to notify an RN immediately if the chest drainage system becomes disconnected, the chest tube becomes dislodged, sudden bleeding occurs, or the patient develops respiratory distress.

Pre-Procedure Assessment

- Ensure that the patient has venous access.
- Assess vital signs.

- Assess the level of consciousness, orientation, responsiveness, anxiety, and restlessness.
  These indicate hypoxemia.

- Assess the patient's knowledge of chest tube therapy.
  Understanding helps allay fears and anxiety.

- Assess cardiac status; respiratory rate, depth, and rhythm; breath sounds; skin color; pulse oximetry; and ABG results.
  Provides a baseline for comparison after chest tube insertion. Evaluates chest tube functioning afterward.

> ➤ When performing the procedure, always identify your patient according to agency policy, using two identifiers, and be attentive to standard precautions, hand hygiene, patient safety and privacy, body mechanics, and documentation.

Steps for Preparing the CDU

1. **Obtain and prepare the prescribed** chest drainage unit (CDU). ▼

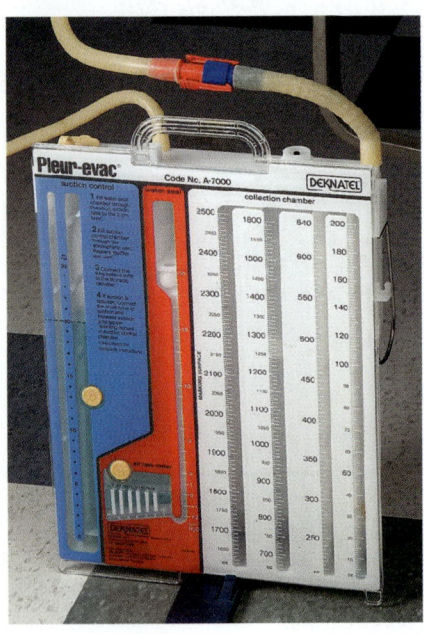

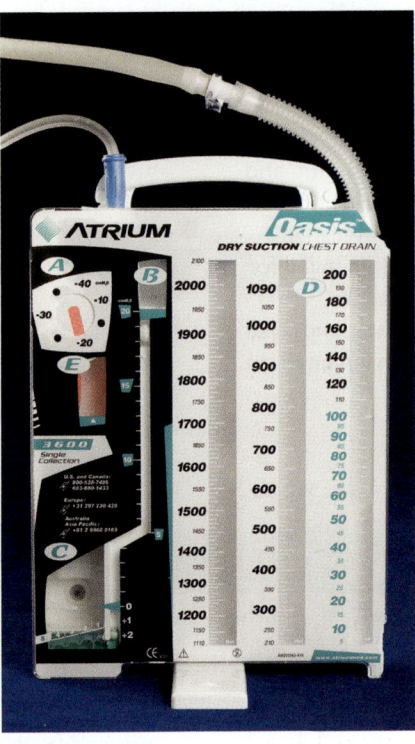

Procedure Variation for a Disposable Water-Seal CDU Without Suction

2. **Remove the cover** on the water-seal chamber and, using the funnel provided, fill the second (water-seal) chamber with sterile water or normal saline. Fill the chamber to the 2-cm mark, or as indicated. (Note that some systems come prefilled.)
   The water-seal chamber allows air to exit from the pleural space during exhalation and prevents air from entering the pleural space during inspiration.

3. **Place the chest drainage unit (CDU)** upright, usually on the floor, and at least 30 cm (1 ft) below the patient's chest level.

4. **Replace the cover** on the water-seal chamber.
   Protects the chamber from contamination.

> ➤ Go to step 13.

Procedure Variation for a Disposable Water-Seal CDU With Suction

5. **Remove the cover on the** water-seal chamber. If it is not a prefilled system, use a syringe or the funnel provided to fill the water-seal chamber (second chamber) with sterile water or normal saline to the 2-cm mark.

   The water-seal chamber allows air to exit from the pleural space during exhalation and prevents air from entering the pleural space during inspiration.

6. **Add sterile water or normal saline** solution to the suction control chamber in the amount prescribed, typically 20 cm (7 in.). Place the CDU upright, usually on the floor, and at least 30 cm (1 ft) below the patient's chest level.

   Suction is regulated by the weight of fluid in the suction control chamber.

7. **Attach the tubing** from the suction control chamber to the suction source tubing. Turn on the wall (or other) suction source. A wall suction of –80 cm H_2O is common.

➤ Go to step 13.

Procedure Variation for a Disposable Dry-Seal CDU With Suction

8. **Remove the nonsterile outer** protective bag and the sterile inner wrapper following agency policy.

9. **Place the CDU upright,** usually on the floor, and at least 30 cm (1 ft) below the patient's chest level. Some CDUs have hangers for hanging at the bedside.

10. **If suction will be required,** attach the tubing from the suction control chamber to the connecting tubing attached to the suction source.

11. **Fill a syringe with 45 mL** of sterile water or saline (follow agency policy and the manufacturer's recommendation for type of fluid), or use the small bottle of sterile fluid in the CDU package. Fill the air leak monitor on the CDU by injecting the fluid via the needleless injection port on the back until it reaches the fill line.

    Once filled, the water may become colored for improved visibility of air leaks. Bubbles in this section of the CDU indicate an air leak.

➤ Go to step 13.

Procedure Variation for a Heimlich Valve

12. **When a patient has little or no** drainage and does not require suction, the chest tube may be connected to a Heimlich valve instead of a CDU. These valves are attached to the end of the chest tube and allow one-way flow of air out of the chest tube. They contain "flutter" leaflets that allow air to exit but not reenter the pleural space. These valves can also be used for emergency transport until a chest drainage system is available.

➤ Go to step 13.

Steps for Inserting and Connecting the Chest Tube

NOTE: The remaining steps apply to all the preceding variations.

13. **Position the patient** according to the indicated insertion site.
    - For removing air: second intercostal space at the midclavicular line
    - For fluid drainage: on the midaxillary line in the fifth or sixth intercostal space.

14. **Open the chest tube insertion** tray and set up the sterile field. Using sterile technique, drop any necessary supplies on the field (e.g., 4 in. × 4 in. split gauze dressing, petroleum or other recommended gauze, syringes).

15. **Don a mask, gown, and sterile gloves** and organize the supplies you will need for dressing the chest tube insertion site.

Protective clothing prevents contamination of the surgical site and protects you from splashing.

16. **Provide support to the patient** while the physician prepares the sterile field, anesthetizes the patient, and inserts and sutures the chest tube.

17. **As soon as the chest tube** is inserted, attach it to the CDU tubing, using a connector.

    Usually the nurse holds the nonsterile tubing that leads to the collection chamber and the physician attaches the sterile chest tube to it. Immediately attaching the chest tube to the drainage system prevents air from entering the pleural cavity.

18. **If suction is prescribed, adjust** the CDU suction to the level the clinician specifies, usually –20 cm H_2O. Also adjust the wall (or other) suction source, usually to –80 cm H_2O.

For Water-Seal Drainage Unit

Adjust the suction source (e.g., wall suction) until gentle bubbling occurs in the suction control chamber. When the tube is functioning properly, the height of the fluid level in the drainage tube fluctuates with the respiratory cycle.

NOTE: Increasing suction at the suction source increases airflow through the system and creates more bubbling, but it does not increase the amount of suction placed on the chest cavity.

For a Dry-Seal Drainage Unit

Adjust the CDU suction (e.g., to –20 cm H_2O) by turning the suction control dial on the CDU. Adjust the wall (or portable) suction pressure to –80 mm Hg or greater until the display on the suction-control chamber confirms adequate suction.

If Suction Is Not Prescribed

Leave the suction tubing on the drainage system open to maintain negative pressure. Follow the manufacturer's directions on the CDU, as models will differ.

(continued on next page)

Procedure 37-11 ■ Setting Up Disposable Chest Drainage Systems (continued)

Steps for Dressing the Chest Tube

19. When the chest tube is functioning properly, the physician or nurse practitioner will suture it in place. Then don a new pair of sterile gloves. Using sterile technique, wrap petroleum, saline soaked, or other recommended gauze around the chest tube at the insertion site. (*Note:* Sometimes the physician dresses the site.)

Theoretically, the moistened gauze creates a seal that prevents air from leaking around the site. However, continued use of petroleum gauze or ointments can macerate the skin, so they should be used with caution. Recent research suggests that saline-soaked or even dry gauze may be preferable to petroleum gauze; follow your agency policy.

20. Place a precut, sterile split-drain dressing over the petroleum gauze.
Absorbs drainage from the insertion site, thereby reducing skin irritation and possible breakdown. ▼

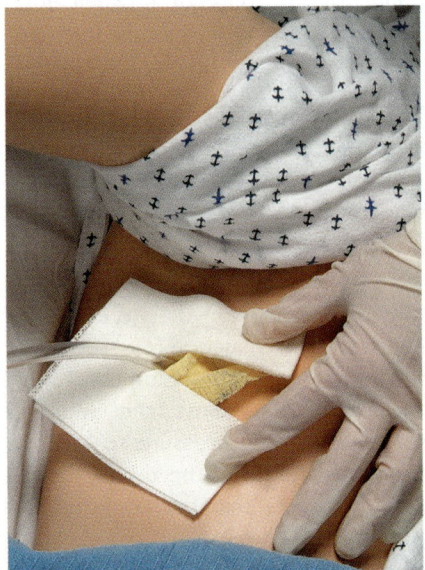

21. Place a second sterile, precut drain dressing over the first drain dressing with the opening facing in the opposite direction from the first.
The second drain dressing helps secure the first drain dressing and provides reinforcement against drainage.

22. Place a large drainage dressing (e.g., ABD) over the two precut drain dressings.

NOTE: Some guidelines recommend that instead of large amounts of tape and padding, a transparent dressing be used. This minimizes moisture collection around the site, allows nurses to inspect for leakage or infection, and does not restrict chest wall movement. Follow your agency's policy.

The large dressing covers the insertion site, protecting it from outside sources of infection.

23. Secure the dressing in place with wide tape, making sure to cover the dressing completely.
Creates an occlusive dressing that protects the chest tube from becoming dislodged and provides a seal over the insertion site, protecting it from outside sources of infection.

24. Date, time, and initial the dressing.
Informs other staff members when the dressing change was completed and by whom.

25. ✚ Using the spiral taping technique, wrap 1-in. silk tape around the chest tube, starting above the connector and continuing below the connector. Reverse your wrapping by taping back up the tubing (using the spiral technique) until the wrapping is above the connector. The CDU may come with locking connections or bands; if so, use those.

Ensures a tight connection between the two tubings, thereby preventing an air leak at the connection site. ▼

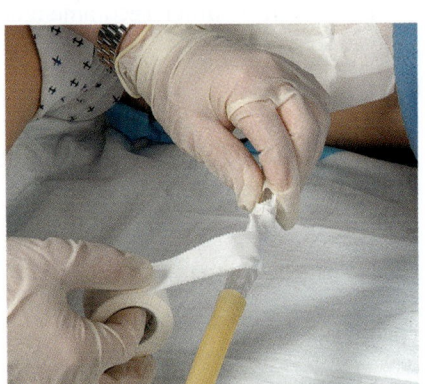

26. Cut an 8-in.-long piece of 2-in. tape. Loop one end around the top portion of the drainage tube and secure the remaining end of the tape to the chest tube dressing.
Prevents pulling at the chest tube site when the patient moves.

27. Make sure the drainage tubing lies with no kinks from the chest tube to the drainage chamber.
Facilitates drainage and prevents fluid from accumulating in the pleural cavity. ▼

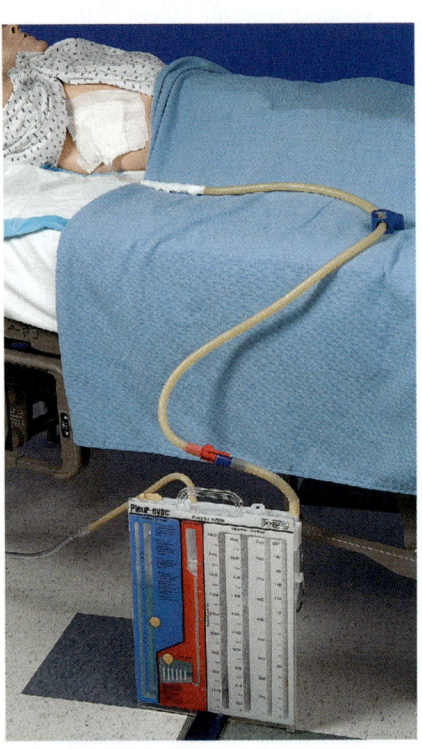

28. Prepare the patient for a portable chest x-ray.
A chest x-ray should be performed after the chest tube is inserted to ensure proper placement.

29. ✚ **Institute safety measures.**
  a. Place two rubber-tipped clamps at the patient's bedside for special situations.
  Rubber-tip clamps are used to clamp the chest tube to check for an air leak, to change the drainage system, and to assess whether the chest tube can be safely removed.

b. Place a petroleum gauze dressing at the bedside.

In case the chest tube becomes dislodged. Placing a petroleum gauze dressing over the insertion site keeps air from entering the pleural cavity.

c. Keep a spare disposable drainage system at the patient's bedside.

To use in case the drainage system in use is accidentally upended or the drainage collection chamber becomes filled.

30. Position the patient for comfort, as indicated, but with the head of the bed elevated to at least 30°.

- If the patient received a chest tube to relieve a pneumothorax, the preferred position is semi-Fowler's position.
- If the chest tube was inserted to promote fluid drainage, high Fowler's position is recommended.

Evaluation

- Evaluate tolerance to the chest tube insertion. Determine whether the respiratory status has changed.
- Auscultate breath sounds every 2 hours.
- Check chest drainage every 15 minutes for the first 2 hours, and then check as prescribed. Observe type, color, and amount.
- Monitor the chest tube insertion site for drainage and subcutaneous emphysema at least every 4 hours.
  Crepitus is a sign that air is leaking into the subcutaneous tissues. Drainage is a sign that fluid is leaking around the insertion site. Both may indicate a compromise in tube patency.
- Confirm chest tube patency and determine whether bleeding is present.
- Monitor intake and output every 8 hours.
- Check laboratory values to evaluate blood loss and oxygenation.
- Check the disposable chest drainage system for the presence of an air leak
  An air leak indicates that air is leaking from the chest and a tight seal has not yet formed over the site of injury.

Patient Teaching

- Teach the patient and family about chest tube insertion.
- Explain the importance of immediately reporting chest pain, shortness of breath, or tube dislodgement.

Home Care

- Explain to the client and caregiver how to care for the chest tube at home.
- Provide the client and caregiver with contact information should problems with the chest tube arise.

Documentation

- Assessment findings before, during, and after chest tube insertion (e.g., vital signs, breath sounds, cardiac status, pulse oximetry)
- Date and time of the chest tube insertion
- Name of the clinician who performed the procedure

- The location of the insertion site, the size of the chest tube, the type of drainage system, and the amount of suction applied, if any
- Any medications the patient received during the procedure
- Color and amount of drainage
- Chest tube output on the intake and output portion of the documentation record (often a flow sheet)
- Patient's tolerance of the procedure
- Presence of subcutaneous emphysema or air leak, if any
- Complications and any interventions preformed as a result of the complications
- Chest x-ray findings

Sample Documentation

8/25/18   0230.   Patient presented with acute shortness of breath, pulse ox 84%, respirations 40 breaths/min and shallow, heart rate 132 beats/min. BP 188/100 mm Hg. Breath sounds absent on right side. Patient received morphine sulfate 4 mg IVP. #36-Fr chest tube placed by Dr. Phan under sterile conditions in right anterior chest, midclavicular line, above the 2nd ICS. Chest tube attached to 20 cm of water pressure. Small air leak present, no crepitus. Portable chest x-ray obtained after procedure, revealed chest tube in good placement and right lung reexpanded. Vital signs post insertion: pulse ox 94%; BP 153/90 mm Hg, heart rate 100 beats/min and respiratory rate 24 breaths/min. Breath sounds audible bilaterally. —————— Pennie Bowen, RNC

Practice Resources

Kane, C. J., York, N. L., & Minton, L. A. (2013); Maliakal, M. (2013); Siegel, J., Rhinehart, E., Jackson, M., et al. (2007).

Thinking About the Procedure

The videos **Disposable Chest Drainage Systems: Setting Up** and **Disposable Chest Drainage Systems: Connecting & Dressing,** along with questions and suggested responses, are available on the **Davis's** *Nursing Skills Videos* Web site on *DavisPlus.*

Procedure 37-12 ■ Inserting an Oropharyngeal Airway

> ➤ For steps to follow in *all* procedures, refer to the Universal Steps for All Procedures found on the page facing the inside back cover.

✚ The American Heart Association guidelines (2015b) direct that you should insert an oropharyngeal airway only if you are trained in its use.

Equipment

- Oral airways in a variety of sizes
- Tongue blade
- Procedure gloves
- Suction equipment
- Resuscitation bag and oxygen source (depending on the patient's status)
- Padded tongue blade

Delegation

You should not delegate this procedure because it requires specialized knowledge, training, and assessment skills.

Pre-Procedure Assessments

- Determine the appropriate airway size by placing the airway on the outside of the patient's cheek. The length of the airway should extend from the front teeth to the end of the jaw line.
- Assess respiratory status (e.g., breath sounds, respiratory rate and effort, skin color, pulse oximetry findings).
  Findings confirm the need for the airway and provide a baseline for evaluating the effectiveness of the intervention.
- Assess for contraindications (e.g., patient is conscious or semiconscious; patient has loose teeth or recent oral surgery).
  An oropharyngeal airway may stimulate the gag reflex, causing vomiting or laryngospasm in a conscious patient.

> ➤ When performing the procedure, always identify your patient according to agency policy, using two identifiers, and be attentive to standard precautions, hand hygiene, patient safety and privacy, body mechanics, and documentation.

Procedure Steps

1. **Perform hand hygiene and don** clean procedure gloves.
   Helps prevent transfer of microorganisms from the patient.

2. **Explain the procedure** to the patient, even if he appears to be unresponsive.
   Recall that hearing is the last sense lost, so the patient may be able to hear you. Information may help relieve the patient's anxiety, if present.

3. **Clear the mouth of any debris** or secretions. You may need to suction the mouth.

4. **Place the patient in supine** or semi-Fowler's position. Hyperextend the neck, unless contraindicated.
   Mild hyperextension allows the airway to slide naturally toward the pharynx.

5. **Gently open the mouth.** Remove dentures, if present.
   Dentures may cause further airway obstruction.

Tongue Blade Technique
Open the patient's mouth and use the blade to depress the tongue.

Crossed Fingers Technique
Place your thumb on the lower teeth. Cross your index finger over your thumb and place the finger on the upper teeth. Push the teeth apart.

6. **You may need to hold** the tongue down with a tongue blade as you insert the airway.

7. **Insert the airway** into the mouth in the upside-down position (inner curve of the C faces upward toward the nose).

Prevents pushing the tongue toward the pharynx. ▼

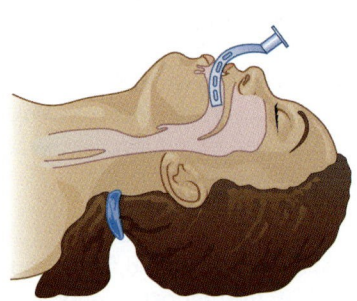

8. As the airway approaches the posterior wall of the pharynx, rotate the airway 180° so that the ends of the C turn downward over the back of the tongue. Continue to insert the airway until the front flange is flush with the lips. ▼

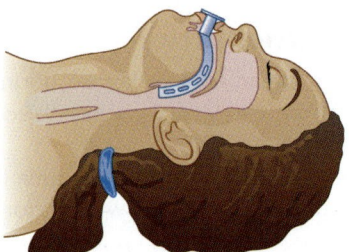

9. Keep the patient's head tilted slightly back and the chin elevated.
This position helps the oropharyngeal airway to function optimally.

10. Do not tape the airway in place.
You may need to remove the airway quickly for suctioning. Untaping would delay airway removal, increasing the risk of aspiration.

11. Position the patient on her side.
To minimize the risk of aspiration.

12. Provide oral hygiene at least every 2 to 4 hours. Remove and cleanse the airway at that time; use hydrogen peroxide and then rinse with water.

? What if . . .

- **After inserting the airway, respirations are absent or inadequate?**

Use a mouth-to-mask technique, a handheld resuscitation bag, or an oxygen-powered breathing device to ventilate the patient. Have someone call for help.

Evaluation

- After inserting the airway, verify patency by auscultating for bilateral breath sounds.
- Check for bleeding or tooth damage in the mouth.
May be caused by airway insertion, especially if it must be done rapidly.
- Check to be certain the patient's lips and tongue are not caught between the teeth and the airway.
Prevents trauma to the soft tissues.
- Monitor the airway position frequently.
Ensures correct placement.
- Continually reassess the need for the airway. Remove it when the patient begins to cough or gag.
- Frequently assess oral mucous membranes when you remove the airway for care.
Prolonged airway use can cause tissue irritation or ulceration.

- Keep suction available at the bedside. Suction the oropharynx as needed by inserting the suction catheter alongside the airway.

Documentation
Document the following:
- Date and time of airway insertion
- Type and size of airway (oropharyngeal or nasopharyngeal)
- Assessments before and after the procedure, including breath sounds and focused respiratory assessment
- Any suctioning performed
- Patient's tolerance of the procedure
- Adverse reactions and interventions taken

Practice Resources
American Association of Critical-Care Nurses (2010); American Heart Association (2015a, 2015b); Walls, R., & Murphy, M. (2012).

Procedure 37-13 ■ Inserting a Nasopharyngeal Airway

➤ For steps to follow in *all* procedures, refer to the Universal Steps for All Procedures found on the page facing the inside back cover.

✚ The American Heart Association guidelines (2015b) direct that you should insert a nasopharyngeal airway only if you are trained in its use.

Equipment
- Nasopharyngeal airway of the correct size
- Tongue blade
- Procedure gloves
- Water-soluble lubricant
- Penlight
- Suction equipment
- Resuscitation bag and oxygen source (depending on the patient's status)

Delegation
You should not delegate this procedure because it requires specialized knowledge, training, and assessment skills. Commonly, this procedure is performed by a respiratory therapist.

Pre-Procedure Assessments
- Determine the appropriate airway size: (1) Measure the diameter of the patient's nostril and use an airway that is slightly smaller than that; and (2) measure the distance from the tip of the patient's nose to the earlobe and use an airway about 2.5 cm (1 in.) longer than that measurement. Airways are sized by their internal diameter. Generally, the larger the internal diameter, the longer the tube. Airways are available in a variety of pediatric and adult sizes:
Small adult: 6 to 7 mm
Medium adult: 7 to 8 mm
Large adult: 8 to 9 mm
- Assess respiratory status (e.g., breath sounds, respiratory rate and effort, skin color, pulse oximetry findings).
Findings confirm the need for the airway and provide a baseline for evaluating the effectiveness of the intervention.
- Assess for contraindications (e.g., anticoagulant therapy, hemorrhagic disorder, nasopharyngeal deformity, sepsis).
Up to 30% of patients experience airway bleeding after insertion of a nasopharyngeal airway.

(continued on next page)

Procedure 37–13 ■ Inserting a Nasopharyngeal Airway (continued)

➤ When performing the procedure, always identify your patient according to agency policy, using two identifiers, and be attentive to standard precautions, hand hygiene, patient safety and privacy, body mechanics, and documentation.

Procedure Steps

1. **Perform hand hygiene** and don procedure gloves.
   Helps prevent transfer of microorganisms from the patient.

2. **Position the patient** in semi-Fowler's position. Explain the procedure to the patient.
   A semi-Fowler's position facilitates airway insertions. Explaining may alleviate anxiety, enabling the patient to cooperate more with the procedure.

3. **Validate that the airway size** is correct. Hold the airway next to the patient's face. The length of the airway should extend from the nares to the end of the jawline below the ear.

4. **Lubricate the airway** with water-soluble lubricant.
   Prevents trauma to mucosa during insertion.

5. **Tilt the patient's head backward** to hyperextend the neck. Then push up the tip of the nose and gently insert the tip of the airway into the nose.

6. **Advance the airway** along the floor of the nostril into the posterior pharynx behind the tongue—until the outer flange rests on the nostril. If you meet resistance, rotate the tube slightly to enhance passage. Do not force against resistance.
   Forcing the tube can cause tissue trauma and airway kinking.

7. **Have the patient open** her mouth. Depress the tongue with a tongue blade and inspect the pharynx for proper placement of the tube tip. Use a penlight, if necessary, for better visualization.
   When the tube is fully inserted, the outer flange of the tube should rest on the nostril, and only the tip of the tube should be visible at the top of the posterior pharynx. ▼

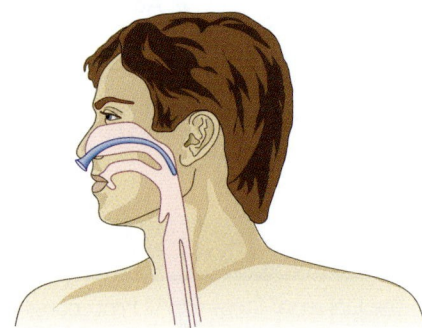

8. **Check for correct placement** and function: Close the patient's mouth and place your finger close to the tube's opening to feel for air exchange.

9. **Auscultate the lungs** for the presence of bilateral breath sounds.

10. **Remove the airway** at least every 8 hours to check nasal mucous membranes for ulceration or irritation. Clean the airway at this time: Place in a basin, rinse with hydrogen peroxide, then rinse with water. Use a pipe cleaner to remove secretions, if necessary. Reinsert the airway in the other nostril.
    To avoid skin and mucous membrane irritation and breakdown and to prevent infection

? What if . . .

■ **After you insert the airway, the patient coughs, gags, vomits, or has laryngospasm?**

The tube may be too long. If the tip extends beyond the top of the posterior pharynx, remove it and insert a shorter one.

Evaluation

■ Assess respiratory rate and effort.
■ Assess breath sounds.
■ Observe for bleeding of nasal mucosa; suction as necessary.
■ If the patient is receiving artificial ventilation, monitor for gastric distention and hypoventilation.
■ Provide frequent oral and nares care; assess the skin around the nostril.

Documentation

■ Date and time of airway insertion
■ Type and size of airway (oropharyngeal or nasopharyngeal)
■ Assessments before and after the procedure, including breath sounds, focused respiratory assessment, and condition of the mucous membranes
■ Any suctioning performed
■ Patient's tolerance of the procedure
■ Adverse reactions and interventions taken
■ Removal of the airway, cleaning, and replacement in the other nostril

Practice Resources

American Association of Critical-Care Nurses (2008); American Heart Association (2015a, 2015b); Bullard, D., Brothers, K., Davis, C., et al. (2012); Walls, R., & Murphy, M. (2012).

To explore learning resources for this chapter,

Go to **www.DavisAdvantage.com** and find:

Answers and Suggested Responses for all questions in this chapter

Lists of NIC Interventions and NOC Outcomes

List of NANDA-I Diagnoses

Knowledge Map

Care Plan

Care Map

References and Bibliography

Concept Map

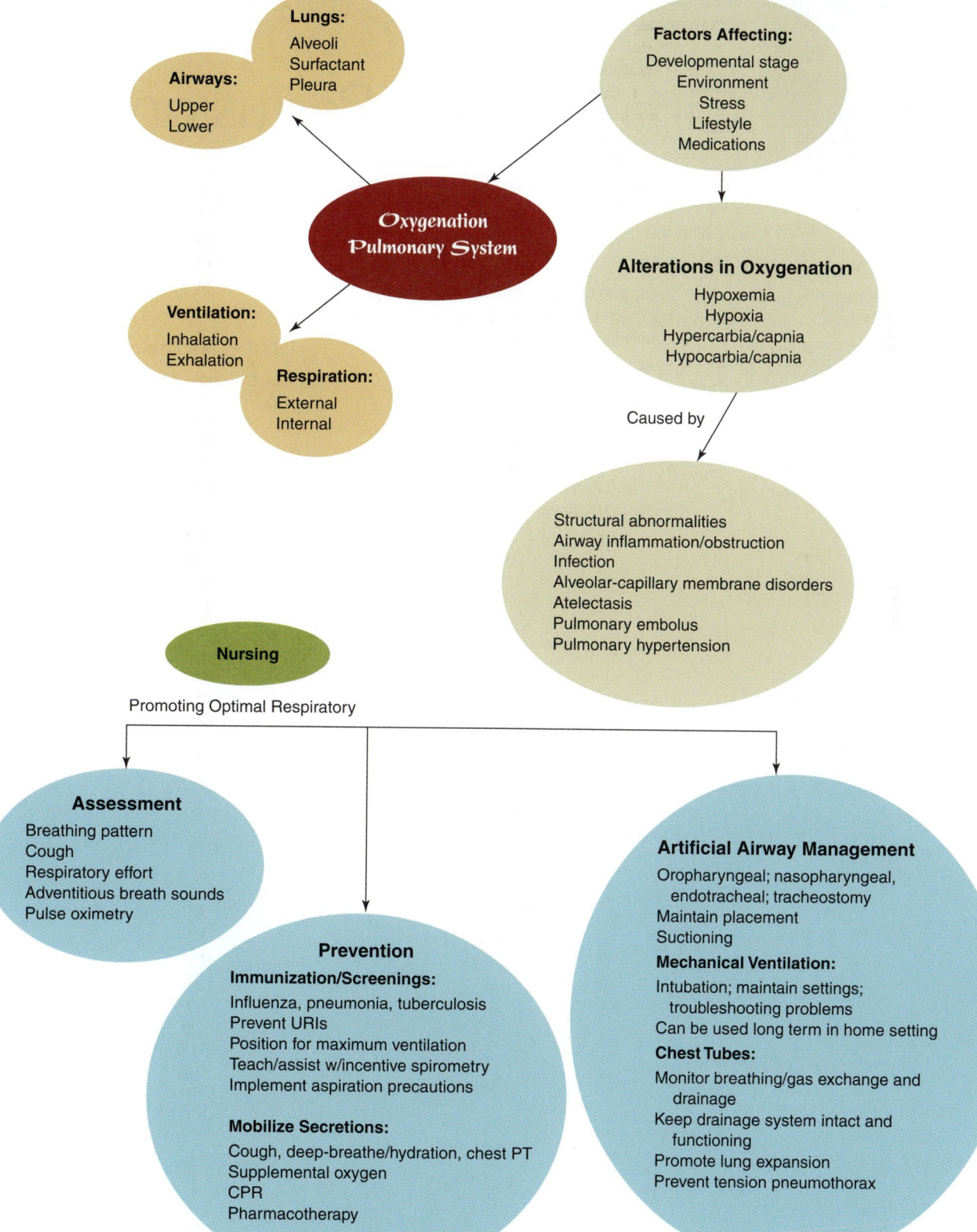

Lungs:
Alveoli
Surfactant
Pleura

Airways:
Upper
Lower

Factors Affecting:
Developmental stage
Environment
Stress
Lifestyle
Medications

Oxygenation Pulmonary System

Alterations in Oxygenation
Hypoxemia
Hypoxia
Hypercarbia/capnia
Hypocarbia/capnia

Ventilation:
Inhalation
Exhalation

Respiration:
External
Internal

Caused by

Structural abnormalities
Airway inflammation/obstruction
Infection
Alveolar-capillary membrane disorders
Atelectasis
Pulmonary embolus
Pulmonary hypertension

Nursing

Promoting Optimal Respiratory

Assessment
Breathing pattern
Cough
Respiratory effort
Adventitious breath sounds
Pulse oximetry

Prevention

Immunization/Screenings:
Influenza, pneumonia, tuberculosis
Prevent URIs
Position for maximum ventilation
Teach/assist w/incentive spirometry
Implement aspiration precautions

Mobilize Secretions:
Cough, deep-breathe/hydration, chest PT
Supplemental oxygen
CPR
Pharmacotherapy

Artificial Airway Management

Oropharyngeal; nasopharyngeal,
   endotracheal; tracheostomy
Maintain placement
Suctioning

Mechanical Ventilation:

Intubation; maintain settings;
   troubleshooting problems
Can be used long term in home setting

Chest Tubes:

Monitor breathing/gas exchange and
   drainage
Keep drainage system intact and
   functioning
Promote lung expansion
Prevent tension pneumothorax

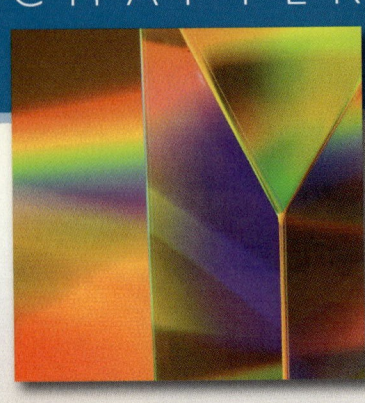

CHAPTER 38

Circulation & Perfusion

Learning Outcomes

After completing this chapter, you should be able to:

- ➤ Describe the structure and function of the cardiovascular system.
- ➤ Identify individual, environmental, and pathological factors that influence circulation and perfusion.
- ➤ Assess circulation and perfusion.
- ➤ Interpret diagnostic testing related to circulation and perfusion.
- ➤ Develop nursing diagnoses related to circulation and perfusion.
- ➤ Safely and correctly perform common nursing procedures related to circulation and perfusion.
- ➤ Evaluate adequacy of circulation and perfusion and modify nursing activities appropriately based on outcomes.
- ➤ Provide measures to promote peripheral circulation.
- ➤ Recognize medications used to enhance cardiovascular function.

Key Concepts

Circulation
Perfusion

Related Concepts

See the Concept Map at the end of this chapter.

Meet Your Patient

You are scheduled for a clinical placement in the urgent care clinic. Your assignment is to (1) perform a focused assessment related to circulation, (2) perform common therapeutic interventions related to circulation, (3) identify desired outcomes and evaluate achievement of those outcomes, and (4) plan for follow-up and home-care needs. One of your clients is Ms. Saunders, a 55-year-old accountant. She says she has been extremely tired, easily becomes short of breath, and is unable to complete her chores without frequent rest breaks. She is pale and moves slowly. Her vital signs are as follows: temperature, 98.4°F (36.7°C); pulse, 86 beats/min; respirations, 24 breaths/min and unlabored; BP, 136/78 mm Hg; and pulse oximetry, 98% on room air. She is now waiting for her lab results, which include a complete blood count (CBC).

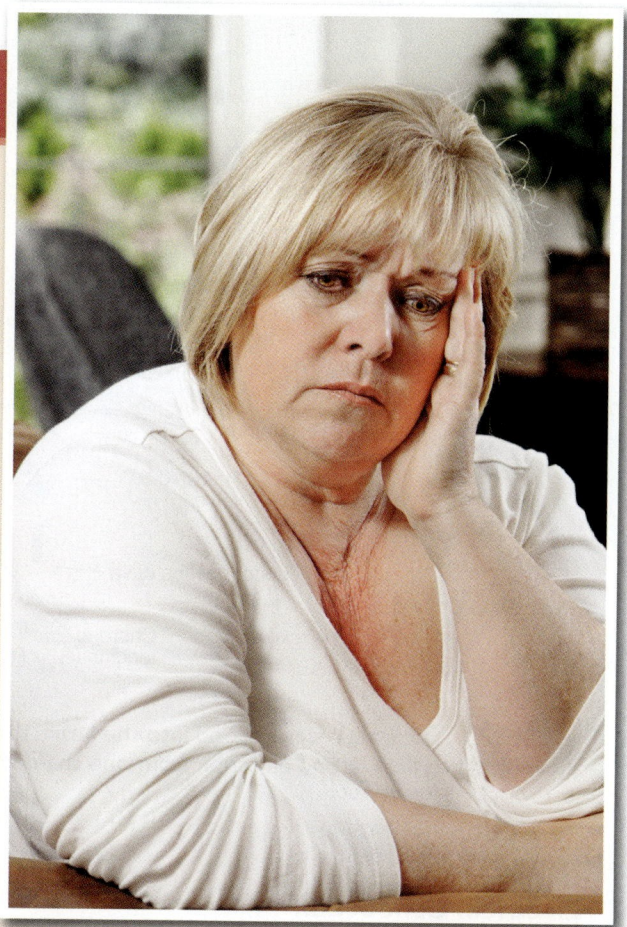

Theoretical Knowledge
knowing why

As you have you have already learned in Chapter 37, the pulmonary, cardiovascular, musculoskeletal, and neurological systems work together to achieve oxygenation. The lungs oxygenate the blood, and the heart circulates the blood throughout the body and back to the lungs. The circulatory system transports oxygenated blood throughout the body to meet the needs. Changes in one system create changes in the other. Theoretical knowledge in this chapter consists of the structures, functions, regulation, and factors that affect cardiovascular function.

ABOUT THE KEY CONCEPTS

The concept of **circulation** refers to flow of blood throughout the heart and blood vessels. **Perfusion** describes blood flow to a capillary bed to provide nutrients and oxygen to tissues and organs. Although the distinction between these two concepts is subtle, they go hand in hand in explaining how a healthy circulatory system contributes to healthy functioning of every body organ.

STRUCTURES OF THE CARDIOVASCULAR SYSTEM

The structures of the cardiovascular system are the heart, the systemic and pulmonary blood vessels, and the coronary arteries.

The Heart

The heart is a four-chambered muscular organ encased in the **pericardium** (a sac of connective tissue) located inside the chest cavity. The two thin-walled **atria** receive blood into the heart, and the two thick-walled **ventricles** pump blood out of the heart. Valves between the heart chambers open widely to allow blood to flow easily and without turbulence from one chamber to another, and the valves close tightly to prevent backflow of blood. The **base,** or broadest side of the heart, which houses the atria, faces upward. The **apex,** or tip of the heart, which houses the ventricles, faces downward (Fig. 38-1).

A strong, efficient heartbeat keeps blood flowing through the vascular system.

- Deoxygenated blood from organs and tissues flows through the venous system into the right side of the heart and then into the pulmonary circulation.
- At the alveolar–capillary membrane, external gas exchange occurs.
- The newly oxygenated blood then flows from the lungs into the left side of the heart and out into the arterial circulation.

The Cardiac Cycle

The **cardiac cycle** is the sequence of mechanical events that occurs during a single heartbeat. Very simply, it is the simultaneous contraction of the two atria, followed a fraction of a second later by the simultaneous contraction of the ventricles. The electrical activity of the myocardium regulates the cardiac cycle (Fig. 38-2).

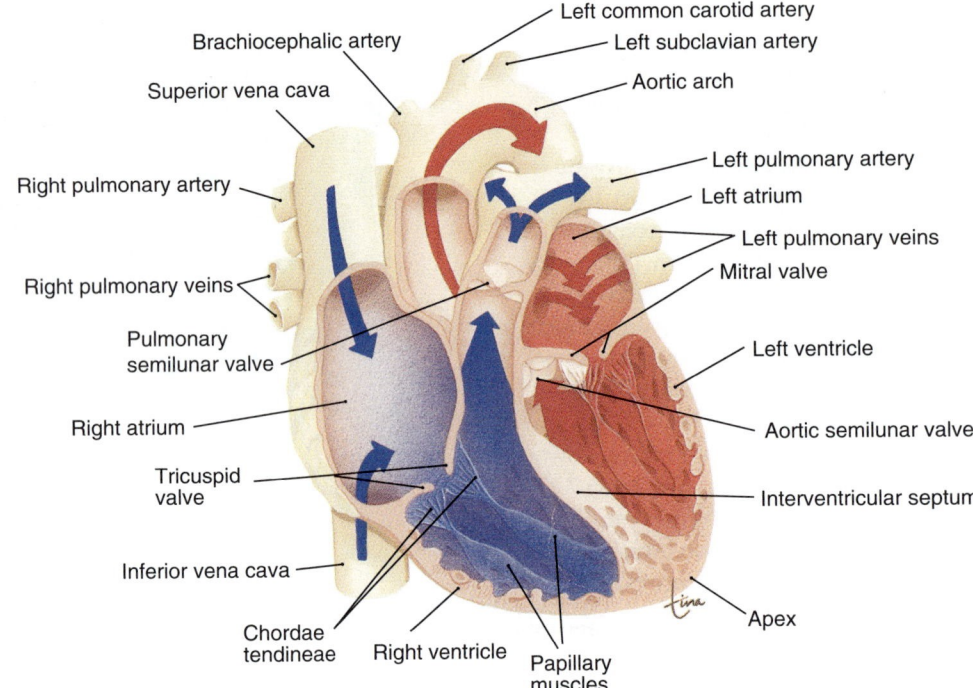

Brachiocephalic artery
Superior vena cava
Right pulmonary artery
Right pulmonary veins
Pulmonary semilunar valve
Right atrium
Tricuspid valve
Inferior vena cava
Chordae tendineae
Right ventricle
Papillary muscles

Left common carotid artery
Left subclavian artery
Aortic arch
Left pulmonary artery
Left atrium
Left pulmonary veins
Mitral valve
Left ventricle
Aortic semilunar valve
Interventricular septum
Apex

FIGURE 38-1 The atria receive blood into the heart; the ventricles pump blood out of the heart. Valves between the chambers allow blood to flow in one direction from one chamber to another without backflow.

Electrical Conduction

The heart contains specialized areas of nerve tissue that initiate electrical impulses without external nervous system stimulation.

- The **sinoatrial (SA) node** acts as the pacemaker. Located in the right atrium, it initiates an impulse that triggers each heartbeat. The impulse travels rapidly down the atrial conduction system so that both atria contract as a unit.
- At the **atrioventricular (AV) node,** there is a slight delay. From the AV node, impulses pass into the left and right *bundles of His* and into the *Purkinje fibers* to the ventricles.

In this way, myocardial fibers are electrically stimulated almost simultaneously to create a unified cardiac muscle contraction strong enough to pump blood out of a heart chamber. This spontaneous rhythm of the heart is called **automaticity.** If there are defects in this electrical system, impulses travel more slowly through the heart and some areas contract before others. This can lead to ineffective heart pumping and decreased cardiac output.

Normally, the SA node initiates a rate of 60 to 100 beats/min, depending on the body's oxygen needs. If the SA node fails, the AV node can take over as the pacemaker, but it generally triggers a slower heart rate. If both the SA and AV nodes fail, the conduction fibers can initiate impulses. Ventricular conduction generates a very slow rate, usually less than 40 beats/min; however, this can be lifesaving if no other node or fiber is initiating an impulse.

Systemic and Pulmonary Blood Vessels

The vascular system is composed of three types of vessels: arteries, veins, and capillaries. All vessels are lined with a smooth endothelial layer that promotes nonturbulent blood flow and prevents platelets from sticking to the sides of the walls and beginning a clot.

- **Arteries** have thick, elastic walls that allow them to stretch during cardiac contraction **(systole)** and to recoil when the heart relaxes **(diastole).**
- **Arterioles** are smaller branches of arteries. They are primarily smooth muscle and thinner than arteries. Under control by the sympathetic nervous system, the arterioles constrict or dilate to vary the amount of blood flowing into capillaries and help maintain blood pressure.
- **Capillaries** are microscopic vessels, created as arterioles branch into smaller and smaller vessels. Capillaries connect the arterial and venous systems and carry blood from arterioles to venules. Because they are only one cell thick, capillaries facilitate the exchange of gases, nutrients, and wastes between the tissue cells and the blood. Billions of capillaries provide blood flow to every cell in the body.
- The **venous system** returns the deoxygenated blood to the heart. **Veins** and **venules** have thin, muscular, but inelastic walls that collapse easily. These walls contract or relax in response to feedback from the sympathetic nervous system: When blood volume is low, the veins contract to provide a smaller space for smaller volume of blood; when blood volume is high, veins relax and enlarge to accommodate increased volume of blood. Think of the venous system as a holding tank for fluctuations in blood volume.

The Coronary Arteries

The heart has its own blood supply through the coronary arteries (Fig. 38-3). The coronary sinus (not shown), located just above the aortic valve, fills with blood during diastole. From the coronary sinus, blood flows into the two main coronary arteries, which branch into several sections to supply the

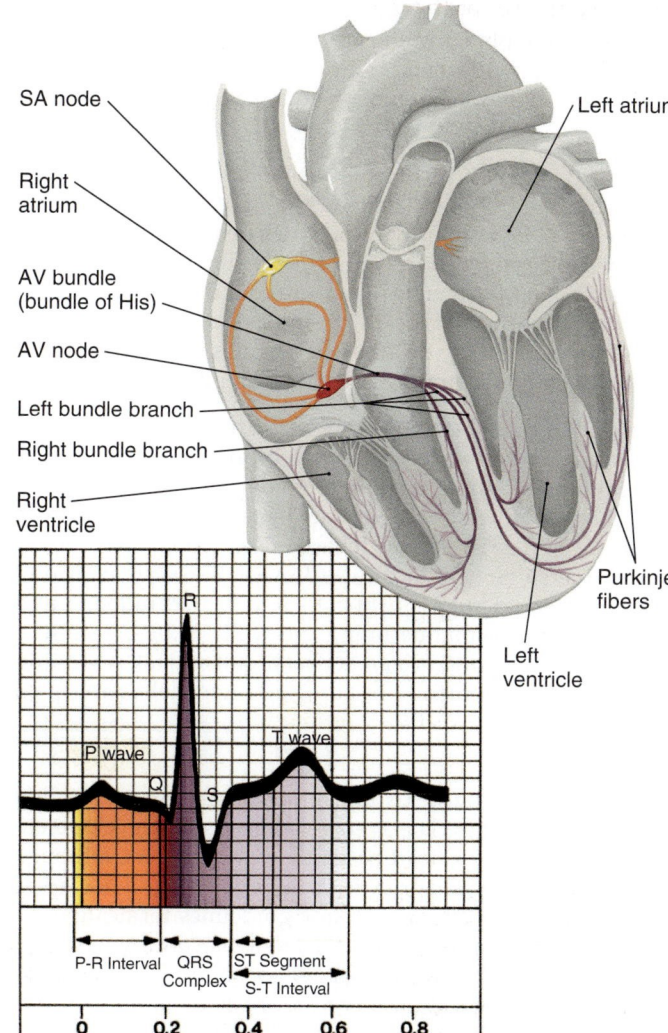

FIGURE 38-2 Conduction pathway of the heart. Anterior view of the interior of the heart. The electrocardiogram tracing is one of a normal heartbeat. See text for description.

heart muscle with blood. The coronary arteries are the only arteries in the body that fill during diastole.

KnowledgeCheck 38-1

- Describe *oxygenation* and *perfusion*.
- Trace the path of normal electrical impulses in the heart.
- How do the walls of arteries, veins, and capillaries differ?
- What is the importance of diastole to perfusion of the heart?

ThinkLike a Nurse 38-1

Your patient has a condition that has caused the mitral valve to become stiff with only a narrow opening for blood flow. What type of problems related to circulation would you anticipate in this patient?

TRANSPORTATION OF OXYGEN AND CARBON DIOXIDE

The cardiovascular system circulates oxygenated blood to organs and tissues and returns deoxygenated blood to the heart. Maintaining this blood flow requires adequate

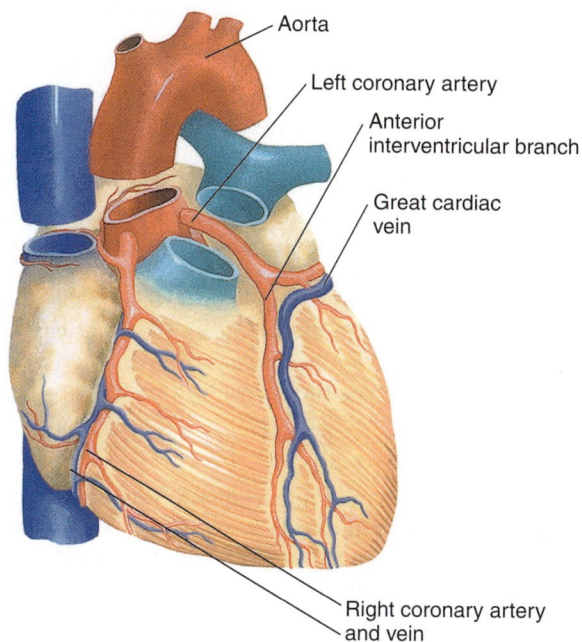

FIGURE 38-3 Coronary vessels in anterior view. The pulmonary artery has been cut to show the left coronary artery emerging from the ascending aorta.

circulation and effective regulation of cardiovascular function.

A full 97% of blood oxygen is bound to hemoglobin, the iron-containing protein in red blood cells; only 3% is in a dissolved state. At the tissue level, O_2 leaves the hemoglobin, becomes dissolved in the blood, and passes through the capillary membrane into the tissues. Only the dissolved form of O_2 can pass through capillary membranes. Hemoglobin thereby serves as a reservoir for oxygen until it is needed in the dissolved state.

Carbon dioxide is a waste product of normal aerobic tissue metabolism. Carbon dioxide can be carried in the blood in three ways: About 7% of CO_2 is dissolved in plasma, 23% attaches to hemoglobin, and 70% is converted into bicarbonate ions. However, CO_2 diffuses through cellular and alveolar–capillary membranes only in its dissolved state. The CO_2 bound to hemoglobin eventually detaches and becomes dissolved in the plasma for diffusion into the alveoli of the lungs. The bicarbonate ions in the plasma are converted back to CO_2, which becomes dissolved, diffuses into the alveoli, and is exhaled.

REGULATION OF CARDIOVASCULAR FUNCTION

Cardiovascular function is regulated by the autonomic nervous system and by control centers in the brainstem.

Autonomic Nervous System

The autonomic nervous system regulates cardiovascular function through its influence on cardiac rate and muscle contractility, as well as vascular tone.

Heart Through branches at the thoracic level of the spinal cord, *sympathetic fibers* stimulate the heart to beat faster and contract more strongly. *Parasympathetic fibers* innervate the heart through the vagus nerve. Parasympathetic stimulation results in a slowed heart rate, but it does not influence myocardial contractility.

Vascular System All blood vessels are innervated by *sympathetic fibers* that maintain them in a constant baseline state of partial contraction (**tone**). Vascular tone maintains blood pressure and blood flow even when a person is resting or asleep. Sympathetic stimulation above and beyond baseline tone varies in response to body needs. Increased sympathetic stimulation causes constriction of some vessels (e.g., skin, gastrointestinal tract, and kidneys) and dilation of other vessels (skeletal muscle). This shunts blood flow to the skeletal muscles for a fight-or-flight response. The *parasympathetic nervous system* has no significant control over blood vessels. For more complete information, consult an anatomy and physiology text.

Brainstem Centers

The brainstem centers integrate feedback from baroreceptors and chemoreceptors in the body to regulate cardiac function and blood pressure. The *vasomotor center* controls sympathetic stimulation of the heart and vascular system. The *cardioinhibitory center* controls parasympathetic slowing of the heart rate.

Baroreceptors located in the walls of the heart and blood vessels are sensitive to pressure changes. The aortic arch and carotid artery baroreceptors are particularly important in the regulation of heart rate and vascular tone. When baroreceptors sense even a small drop in pressure, they send messages to the brainstem centers to stimulate the sympathetic nervous system to increase heart rate and induce vasoconstriction. This mechanism allows us to change positions and maintain blood pressure.

Chemoreceptors located in the aortic arch and the carotid arteries are sensitive to changes in blood pH, oxygen levels, and carbon dioxide levels. Their main function is to regulate ventilation, but they also send information to the vasomotor center in response to lack of oxygen. The vasomotor center responds by activating sympathetic stimulation.

KnowledgeCheck 38-2

- How are oxygen and carbon dioxide transported in the blood?
- How is the cardiovascular system regulated?
- Does poor peripheral perfusion increase the risk for hypoxemia (a low level of oxygen in the blood)?

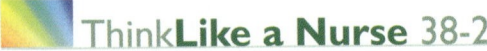

ThinkLike a Nurse 38-2

You are assigned the care of a 4-year-old girl, Mary, with a history of asthma. She is receiving a nebulized treatment containing albuterol and ipratropium bromide. These medications stimulate the sympathetic nervous system.

- What cardiovascular side effects can you anticipate?
- How might these side effects affect oxygenation?
- What do you need to know about the patient's history to safely administer the drugs?

FACTORS INFLUENCING CARDIOVASCULAR FUNCTION

Similar to respiratory function, cardiovascular function is influenced by developmental stage, environment, lifestyle, substance abuse, medications, and pathophysiological conditions.

Developmental Stage

Normal development influences heart and circulatory function. Developmental factors exert more of an influence on infants and older adults than on young and middle adults.

Infants

Successful transition from life inside the uterus to the extrauterine environment depends on critical physiological changes that occur at birth. Prior to delivery, the fetus uses the placenta for gas and nutrient exchange. Fetal circulation bypasses the lungs. When the umbilical cord is clamped and the newborn takes the first breath, the resistance in the pulmonary vessels then markedly decreases. The lungs inflate, and blood circulates without shunting as it did during fetal life.

Preschool and School-Age Children

The heart and circulatory systems of preschool and school-age children are mature enough to adapt to moderate stress and change. However, even school-age children sometimes begin social habits, such as tobacco use, that can have long-term adverse effects on the cardiovascular system. A diet high in fats and sugars contributes to hyperlipidemia and the beginning of plaque lining the walls of blood vessels. Processed foods contain a great deal of salt and fat, which can contribute to high blood pressure and high cholesterol, even in children.

Adolescents

In adolescence, the heart and blood components develop adult characteristics. The average adolescent is developmentally at little risk for heart or circulatory disorders, although some athletes can be at risk for collapse and sudden cardiac dysrhythmia that is familial. New guidelines for health professionals performing sports assessments call for thorough investigation of the family history for fainting, collapse, or sudden death. Some adolescents adopt behaviors and habits that can create risk throughout life. For example:

- *Tobacco use*—87% of adults who use tobacco were regular smokers by their 18th birthday, and almost half of middle and high school students reported using two or more tobacco products on one or more of the 30 days preceding the survey (American Lung Association, 2016; U.S. Department of Health and Human Services, 2014).
- *Obesity*—Although obesity rates have fallen among preschoolers, the overall incidence of childhood obesity in the United States has risen to epidemic levels. As a result, some adolescents exhibit signs of cardiovascular disease (e.g., high blood levels of lipids and cholesterol, a known factor in the development of high blood pressure, heart disease, and blockages in the arteries of the heart).

Young and Middle Adults

Lifestyle in young and middle adulthood can create cardiac risk factors.

- *Poor nutrition*—Some adults become "too busy" to prepare and eat nourishing foods, or more often simply prefer the taste of high-fat, high-sugar foods.
- *Lack of exercise*—A sedentary lifestyle and lack of aerobic exercise contribute to cardiovascular disorders in this group.
- *Substance abuse*—Tobacco use is a risk factor for cardiovascular disorders. Crack cocaine and methamphetamine abuse can lead to sudden cardiac failure.
- *Family history* of cardiovascular disease is yet another risk factor for this age-group.

Older Adults

Cardiac efficiency gradually declines as the heart muscle loses contractile strength and heart valves become thicker and more rigid. The peripheral vessels become less elastic, which creates more resistance to ejection of blood from the heart. As a result of these changes, the heart becomes less able to respond to increased oxygen demands, and it needs longer recovery times after responding. For example, in response to exercise, an older adult's heart rate does not increase as much as a younger person's, but it does remain elevated longer. Thus, older adults have lower exercise tolerance, need more rest after exercise, and are more prone to orthostatic hypotension. Keep in mind, though, that endurance training and regular exercise slow the rate of these changes. In fact, an older person who is physically conditioned by regular exercise may have better heart and circulatory function than a younger adult who is not well conditioned.

Environment

Environmental factors, such as stress, allergic reactions and air quality, altitude, and temperature, affect cardiovascular function.

Stress

The stress response stimulates release of catecholamines from the sympathetic nervous system. This results in increased heart rate and contractility, vasoconstriction, and increased tendency of blood to clot. Sustained stimulation of the sympathetic nervous system can lead to cardiovascular disease. In addition, a chronically suppressed immune and inflammatory response increases the risk for all infections. For additional information on the effects of stress, see Chapter 12.

Allergic Reactions and Air Quality

An **allergy** is a hypersensitivity, or overresponse, to an antigen. Inflammatory substances released during an allergic response (e.g., histamine, protease) cause the following cardiovascular events:
- Blood vessels dilate in areas affected (which increases blood flow to the areas).
- Eosinophils and neutrophils are attracted to the reaction site.
- Local tissues are damaged by protease.
- Capillaries become more permeable, resulting in fluid leak into tissues.
- Local (e.g., vascular) smooth muscle cells contract.

Altitude

Oxygen pressure falls proportionally with increased altitude (to review, refer to Chapter 37), making more oxygen available in the alveoli and at the tissue level. Over the long term, people who live at high altitudes undergo physiological changes that facilitate oxygenation. Among the cardiopulmonary changes are the following:
- Increased production of red blood cells
- Increased vascularity of body tissues
- Increased ability of tissue cells to use oxygen even when atmospheric oxygen pressure is low

Heat and Cold

Heat generally causes vasodilation, which increases cardiac output and oxygenation. However, heat also increases metabolism. As a result, people are naturally more sedentary in hot weather.

Cold slows cell metabolism, reducing O_2 demand. It also causes vasoconstriction and slows the heart rate. Induced hypothermia is used in some surgical procedures. As another example, victims of cold-water near drowning have been revived after long periods of time, in part because of the reduced O_2 demands associated with hypothermia. Prolonged exposure to cold causes frostbite, loss of hypothalamic temperature regulation, and death.

Lifestyle

Lifestyle factors that affect cardiovascular function include pregnancy, nutrition, obesity, exercise, tobacco use, and substance abuse.

Pregnancy

During pregnancy, oxygen demand increases dramatically as a result of the needs of the fetus. Therefore, there is an approximate 15% increase in maternal metabolism during the last half of pregnancy. To compensate, the mother's blood volume increases by 30%. The woman requires additional iron to produce this blood as well as to meet fetal requirements. Failure to meet these iron demands can result in maternal anemia, reducing tissue oxygenation to the mother and fetus.

Nutrition

The body needs an appropriate balance of proteins, carbohydrates, fats, and other nutrients for proper immune function, resistance to disease and infection, normal cellular function and tissue repair, and maintenance of a healthy weight. A diet high in saturated fat predisposes to atherosclerosis, coronary artery disease, and hypertension, all of which can compromise circulation and oxygenation. A low-fat, low-cholesterol, low-sodium diet is considered "heart healthy." Vitamins, minerals (especially iron), and protein are important to prevent anemia, which reduces blood-oxygen–carrying capacity. Green tea consumption has been associated with reduced mortality due to cardiovascular disease (Kokubo, Iso, Saito, et al., 2013).

Obesity

Obesity is a body mass index (BMI) above 30 (see Chapter 28). Obesity causes multiple health problems, many of which affect the heart and circulation. Obesity increases the risk of developing atherosclerosis and hypertension. Excess fat stores in and around the heart itself reduce its effectiveness as a pump. At the same time, the workload of the heart is increased by the need to perfuse the excess body tissues.

Exercise

Exercise improves blood circulation and delivery of oxygen to tissues and cells. It also increases metabolic demands. The body responds by increasing the heart rate and the rate and depth of breathing. Like skeletal muscles, the heart muscle is strengthened with regular aerobic exercise. As the heart becomes stronger, it becomes a more efficient pump. As a result, resting heart rate is slower because a higher heart rate is not required to maintain cardiac output. Lack of exercise has the opposite effect. A sedentary lifestyle reduces the efficiency of the heart and the capacity to increase ventilation in response to exercise.

Tobacco Use

Tobacco use is a major risk factor in several chronic cardiovascular conditions: stroke, peripheral arterial disease, aortic aneurysm, and heart disease. Smoking has been shown to cause atherosclerosis (fatty buildups in the arteries), hypertension, and decreased high-density lipoprotein (HDL) (good) cholesterol—all of which lead to coronary heart disease and heart attack.

- The risk of coronary artery disease is four times higher in cigarette smokers than in nonsmokers.
- Cigarette smoking doubles a person's risk for stroke.
- Older adults who smoke have a 73% higher chance of developing heart failure than nonsmokers.
- Former smokers' risks are related to how long they have smoked.

Even light smoking increases the risk of sudden cardiac death. Cigar and pipe smoking are also implicated, but not to the extent of cigarettes (American Heart Association, 2016).

Substance Abuse

Substances that people abuse include over-the-counter and prescription medications, commonly available commercial products, and illegal substances.

- Large amounts of alcohol depress respiratory, cardiac, and vasomotor centers of the brain. Chronic alcohol abuse causes fatty infiltration of the heart muscle, thrombi in the coronary arteries, heart enlargement, and dysrhythmias, all of which can ultimately lead to heart failure.

- Illicit drugs, including stimulants (e.g., methamphetamine, cocaine), hallucinogens (e.g., LSD [acid], mescaline [buttons]), and cannabinoids (e.g., marijuana), also have adverse effects on the cardiovascular system (e.g., links to myocardial dysfunction, dysrhythmias, endocarditis, and aortic dissection).

Medications

Various types of medication are used therapeutically to improve cardiac output and tissue oxygenation. They act to slow the heart rate or reduce the force of myocardial contraction; ease the workload of the heart; dilate blood vessels and reduce blood pressure in the pulmonary circulation and systemically; rid the body of excess fluid accumulation; and block abnormal heart rhythms (American Heart Association, 2011a, updated 2016). See Table 38-1.

Aspirin   An aspirin regimen can help prevent cardiovascular disease. Aspirin blocks the production of prostaglandin, a hormone-like substance that activates the formation of blood clots, signals an injury, and triggers pain. This helps reduce the risk of heart attack or stroke from clot-blocked arteries, decreases pain and inflammation, and reduces the short-term risk of death among people suffering from heart attacks. Daily aspirin is recommended for men ages

Table 38-1 ➤ Medications That Promote Circulation

CLASS	ACTION	EXAMPLES AND COMMENTS
Vasodilators	■ Enhance cardiac output, providing increased blood flow and oxygenation to organs and tissues. ■ Cause vessel dilation, which eases workload of the heart. ■ Control blood pressure. ■ Treat heart failure.	Angiotensin-converting enzyme (ACE) inhibitors Angiotensin II receptor blockers Nitrates
Beta-adrenergic Blockers	■ Block norepinephrine and epinephrine (adrenaline) ■ Reduce the workload of the heart and oxygen consumption. ■ Control abnormal heart rhythms (dysrhythmias) by slowing conduction through the AV node. ■ Control blood pressure.	Beta$_1$-selective: atenolol, metoprolol Nonselective: carvedilol, metoprolol, propranolol
Calcium Channel Blockers	■ Block the flow of calcium into the cells of the heart and blood vessels. ■ Decrease blood pressure. ■ Reduce the strength of myocardial contraction; slow heart rate. ■ Dilate the arteries and arterioles.	Nifedipine
Positive Inotropic Agents	■ Improve the effectiveness of the heart's pumping action without creating excess cardiac workload and oxygen demand. ■ Reduce the heart muscle cells' ability to trigger their own contractions (automaticity). ■ Dilate blood vessels.	Cardiac glycosides: digoxin Phosphodiesterase (PDE) inhibitors: PDE3 inhibitors (congestive heart failure) PDE5 inhibitors (erectile dysfunction)

Table 38-1 ➤ Medications That Promote Circulation—cont'd		
CLASS	**ACTION**	**EXAMPLES AND COMMENTS**
Diuretics	■ Remove sodium and water from the body through urine. ■ Reduce the volume of circulating blood. ■ Prevent accumulation of fluid in the pulmonary circulation and body tissues.	Thiazide diuretics: hydrochlorothiazide (HCTZ), metolazone Loop diuretics: furosemide Potassium-sparing diuretics: spironolactone Bumetanide Metolazone Triamterene

45 to 79 years to reduce risk of myocardial infarction (MI) and for women ages 55 to 79 years to reduce risk of ischemic stroke (U.S. Preventive Services Task Force [USPSTF], 2016).

KnowledgeCheck 38-3

- What changes occur in the cardiovascular system with aging?
- How does smoking affect the cardiovascular system?

Pathophysiological Conditions

Alterations in circulation and perfusion at the tissue or cellular level may be life threatening, particularly when hypoxemia and acidosis occur. Refer to Chapter 37 to review the effect of poor oxygenation on body systems.

Cardiovascular Abnormalities

Alterations in gas exchange are caused by a number of disorders that affect the structure, function, and regulation of the cardiovascular system. Cardiovascular abnormalities interfere with the flow of oxygenated blood to organs and tissues and continue to be the number one cause of death for adults in the United States (Centers for Disease Control and Prevention, 2014). Major abnormalities are as follows:

- **Heart failure** occurs when the heart becomes an inefficient pump and is unable to meet the body's demands. Blood is oxygenated when it passes through the lungs, but it is not well circulated to the organs and tissues. Impaired circulation leads to systemic and pulmonary edema, which further impairs gas exchange.
  - *Right-sided heart failure* occurs when the right ventricle does not pump sufficient amounts of blood to the lungs for oxygenation, and blood backs up into the peripheral veins.
  - *Left-sided heart failure* occurs when the left ventricle does not pump sufficient amounts of blood to body organs and tissues.

Both right-sided and left-sided heart failure reduce the amount of oxygenated blood available to organs and tissues, resulting in fatigue and organ dysfunction. **KEY POINT:** *Because the right and left ventricles are part of one circuit, failure of one side of the heart eventually leads to failure of the other side.*

- **Cardiomyopathy** is a heart muscle disorder that results in heart enlargement and impaired cardiac contractility. **Primary cardiomyopathy** results from genetic or noncardiovascular

causes, whereas **secondary cardiomyopathy** results from another cardiovascular disease. Secondary cardiomyopathy occurs as previously normal heart muscle enlarges to compensate for increased workload.

- **Cardiac ischemia** occurs when oxygen requirements of the heart are unmet. Prolonged ischemia leads to myocardial infarction (MI) as parts of the heart *necrose* (die) from inadequate oxygen. **Angina pectoris** is transient chest pain due to myocardial ischemia. The tissue becomes injured but does not necrose.
  - **Stable angina** is a predictable pattern of ischemic chest pain that is precipitated by known triggers (e.g., activity, large meal, temperature extremes, cigarette smoking, stimulants, sexual activity, strong emotion, circadian rhythm patterns). It is alleviated by rest and medications.
  - **Unstable angina** (sometimes called preinfarction angina or crescendo angina) is ischemic chest pain that has worsened in frequency, severity, or duration and is not relieved by usual measures. When untreated, it may lead to myocardial infarction.
- **Coronary artery disease,** a leading cause of cardiac ischemia, is a condition in which plaque builds up inside the coronary arteries. Plaque narrows the arteries, reducing blood flow to the heart muscle and making it more likely that clots will form and block the arteries.
- **Dysrhythmias** (alterations in heart rate or rhythm) can lower cardiac output, decrease tissue oxygenation, and increase the risk of stroke.
- **Heart valve abnormalities** create turbulent flow, leading to a decrease in cardiac output and compromised tissue oxygenation. Often there is an audible murmur. The valves most commonly affected are the mitral and aortic valves.
  - **Valve stenosis** (narrowing) refers to blood flow through a narrow, constricted opening. Pumping blood through a narrow valve increases the workload of the heart and leads to hypertrophy of the chamber that precedes the stenotic valve. The chamber receiving blood through a stenotic valve can be underfilled.
  - **Valve incompetence** (failure to close tightly) refers to incomplete closure of a valve, resulting in regurgitation of blood into the chamber from which it came. Regurgitation causes distention and increased work for the chamber ejecting blood. This chamber can become weak and ineffective as a pump. The chamber receiving blood through an incompetent valve can be underfilled.

Peripheral Vascular Abnormalities

Disorders of peripheral blood vessels impair blood flow to and from organs and tissues.

- *Arterial abnormalities* disrupt flow of oxygenated blood to tissues. When arterial blood flow is compromised, signs and symptoms include pallor, pain, weak or absent pulses, poor capillary refill, cool skin, and tissue dysfunction.
- *Venous abnormalities* disrupt blood return to the heart. Clinical signs of compromised venous blood flow include edema, brown skin discoloration, and tissue dysfunction (e.g., stasis ulcers).

Oxygen Transport Abnormalities

Even if the heart is functioning well and arterial blood flow is intact, tissues can become hypoxic if the blood is unable to carry adequate amounts of oxygen. The most common causes are anemia and carbon monoxide poisoning. **Anemia** is an abnormally low level of red blood cells, hemoglobin, or both. **Carbon monoxide** is a colorless, odorless gas produced by the combustion of flammable materials and fuels. When inhaled, carbon monoxide binds tightly to hemoglobin at the oxygen receptor sites, making it impossible for hemoglobin to carry oxygen.

PracticalKnowledge
knowing **how**

Nursing care for patients with cardiovascular problems is directed at assessing for and maximizing the effectiveness of the heart and circulatory system.

ASSESSMENT NP

Although this section focuses on cardiovascular assessments, evaluation of overall circulation and perfusion status includes a history and examination that gather information about lung, heart, and circulatory function. **KEY POINT:** *The patient's condition and the purpose of the assessment determine your priorities for assessment and the order in which you gather information.* For example:

- For someone with a cardiac emergency, the immediate assessment focus would be to ask simple questions about current symptoms while performing a quick examination to determine adequacy of circulation, perfusion, and oxygenation.
- The assessment for risk of coronary artery disease in a healthy individual might include more extensive questions about occupation and smoking habits, a medical history, and an extensive physical examination.

You will need information about the patient's past and present cardiovascular signs and symptoms, risk factors, medications, activity level, tolerance of activity, and lifestyle factors that affect cardiovascular functioning.

Assessing for Risk Factors

One aspect of improving cardiovascular health and quality of life is prevention, detection, and treatment of risk factors for heart attack and stroke (*Healthy People 2020*, 2010, updated 2016). A health history related to cardiovascular functioning includes questions about the presence of risk factors that affect the heart, and peripheral vascular function. Topics to assess include the following:

- Demographic data
- Health history
- Family history
- Respiratory history
- Cardiovascular history
- Environmental history
- Lifestyle

Anxiety   You should also assess the patient's level of anxiety. Patients with cardiac or respiratory problems are almost certain to be anxious, and anxiety interferes with achieving good outcomes for these patients. Pay close attention to verbal cues because heart rate and blood pressure changes may not be useful in assessing acutely ill patients for anxiety (Van Beek, Mingels, Voshaar, et al., 2012). For a detailed list of interview questions for each of these topics, see the Focused Assessment box Assessing Circulation.

Physical Examination

Start the physical exam by obtaining the patient's height and weight. BMI and waist circumference indicate obesity, which is a major risk factor for cardiovascular disease. Assessment of heart and peripheral vessels includes inspection, palpation, and auscultation (and occasionally percussion). Use inspection to observe for signs of distress (e.g., chest pain), skin and mucous membrane color, presence or absence of edema, and overall general appearance. Palpate pulses, skin temperature, edema, heart pulsations through the chest wall, and areas of tenderness. Auscultate heart sounds, vascular sounds, and blood pressure. Auscultate the lungs because adventitious sounds, such as rales, may signal decreased cardiac output. For a step-by-step discussion of how to assess the heart and vascular system, see Procedure 21-13: Assessing the Heart and Vascular System. Also see the accompanying Focused Assessment box, Assessing Circulation.

Assess Pain

If a patient has chest pain, evaluate it immediately because chest pain is the most common heart attack symptom. Ask the patient to describe the pain and its location, duration, frequency, and radiation. Chest pain may also be caused by musculoskeletal or respiratory conditions, for example, a fractured rib or *pleuritis* (inflammation in the pleural space). **KEY POINT:** *You can differentiate cardiac pain because it usually occurs in the center or on the left side of the chest and radiates to the left arm (most often in men). The pain typically lasts several minutes; it may subside and then return. Some women have milder chest pain, sometimes none at all. They are more likely than men to experience other symptoms, such as jaw or back pain, nausea, fatigue, and shortness of breath. Cardiac pain typically does not change with inhalation or exhalation.* Ask the client to rate the pain on a scale of 0 to 10, with 0 representing no pain and 10 representing the worst pain possible. See Chapter 32 for pain assessment, as needed.

Patients experiencing chest pain are likely to be fearful—most people are aware that chest pain may signal a heart attack. You need to work quickly but calmly to instill confidence in the patient. If the person is experiencing a cardiac event, anxiety and stress can make it worse by increasing oxygen consumption, thereby extending hypoxic damage to the heart.

When assessing for a clot in the veins (deep vein thrombosis [DVT]), deep under the muscles of the leg, you will assess for pain, warmth, redness, and swelling of the leg. **KEY POINT:** **Homan's sign** *(pulling toes forward)* and **Pratt's sign** *(squeezing calf to trigger pain) have not been found to be reliable in diagnosing DVT.* However, these signs may help confirm DVT when also considering the clinical signs of DVT, as well as the results of more accurate and specific diagnostic tests, such as ultrasound or venography (Naib & Salih, 2013).

Focused Assessment

Assessing Circulation

Part I. Questions to Assess Risk for Impaired Circulation

Demographic Data
➤ What is your age?
➤ Where do you live?
➤ What is your occupation?

Health History
➤ Do you have current health problems? Describe.
➤ Do you have past health problems? Describe.
➤ Have you ever been hospitalized or had surgery? If so, when and for what reason?
➤ Do you take medication for your heart, blood pressure, cholesterol, erectile dysfunction, diabetes, breathing difficulty, or other conditions?
➤ Do you have chronic fatigue, heartburn, anxiety, swelling of the ankles, difficulty breathing, chest discomfort, palpitations, dizziness or fainting spells, dental problems, pain in the calf when walking that stops with rest, chronic cough or wheezing, shortness of breath, or unexplained weight loss?
➤ Do you take over-the-counter products such as vitamins, supplements, aspirin?
➤ What else do you want to tell me about your physical or mental health history?

Family History
➤ Did your father or a brother develop coronary artery disease or have a heart attack before the age of 55?
➤ Did you mother or sister develop coronary artery disease or have a heart attack before the age of 65?

Cardiovascular History
➤ Have you ever had or been diagnosed with a heart attack, angina, coronary artery disease, peripheral artery disease, stroke, aortic aneurysm?
➤ Do you have high or low blood pressure? Do you feel dizzy if you stand up quickly?
➤ Have you ever had chest pain? If so, describe the circumstances? What was done to relieve the symptoms? What measures do you take to prevent the pain?
➤ Do you become easily fatigued or feel your heart rate is rapid? Do you ever feel heart palpitations?
➤ Do you have pain in your legs when you are walking uphill or walking for a long time?
➤ Do you experience cold hands and feet? If so, how often?
➤ Do you have pain or tingling in your feet or toes with exercise? Do they feel numb when you are at rest? Does the pain worsen when your leg is elevated and/or improve when you dangle your legs over the side of the bed?

➤ Do you have pain in your leg, foot, or toes that is so severe that shoes or the weight of a sheet at night is painful?
➤ If you are male, do you experience impotence?
➤ Do you have ulcers that do not heal?

Nutrition History
➤ In a typical day, how many servings of whole grains, fruits, vegetables, dairy products, eggs, nuts, and red meat or fish do you eat or drink per day?
➤ How many meals per week do you east fast food or other high-fat food?
➤ How many meals per week do you eat out? Where?
➤ How many times per day do you add salt or eat salty foods?
➤ How many times per week do you skip a meal?
➤ Do you have diabetes or prediabetes? Are you a normal weight?

Lifestyle and Health Promotion Activities
➤ What is your current stress level? What are your major sources of stress? How do you relieve stress?
➤ What is your usual diet? Is your current diet typical, or have you recently changed your eating habits?
➤ What is your usual activity level? Do you exercise regularly? If so, how many minutes per week of moderate to vigorous physical activity do you get?
➤ Do you check your lipid profile (cholesterol and triglycerides) and blood sugar (fasting blood sugar and hemoglobin A_{1c}) on a regular basis?
➤ Do you smoke now, or have you ever smoked? If you smoke, how many packs per day and for how many years have you smoked?
➤ Do you use crack cocaine or other illicit substances?

Part II. Focused Physical Examination

Cardiovascular System
➤ Review Procedure 21-13: Assessing the Heart and Vascular System.
➤ *Inspect the neck* for carotid and jugular pulsations. Palpate each carotid separately. Auscultate the carotid arteries and jugular veins for bruits and hums.
➤ *Inspect the precordium* for pulsations. Palpate for pulsations, lifts, heaves, and thrills. Auscultate for heart sounds.
➤ *Assess peripheral circulation.* Palpate peripheral pulses, assess skin color and temperature, note hair distribution on extremities. Inspect for skin ulcers and edema of the feet and ankles.
➤ *Inspect* for venous valve competence.
➤ *Perform the capillary refill test* anywhere you note signs of diminished blood flow.

Assess Fatigue

Fatigue is a subjective experience. The patient feels tired and lacks endurance. Fatigue is a common symptom of various oxygenation problems, including anemia and heart failure. Ask your patient to rate his fatigue on a 0 to 10 scale, as you do for pain.

Assess Dyspnea

Dyspnea (shortness of breath) is discussed in Chapter 37 in relation to respiratory conditions. Recall that dyspnea is a sign of hypoxia, which can be associated with cardiovascular diseases and anemia, as well as with respiratory problems. As with pain, dyspnea provokes anxiety.

Assess Peripheral Circulation

Even if the lungs and heart are functioning well, pathology in the arteries and veins can interfere with tissue perfusion.

- Palpate the peripheral pulses, assess skin color and temperature, and note the distribution of hair on the extremities. Weak pulses, cool feet, lack of hair, and shiny skin on lower legs and feet usually accompany peripheral vascular disease.
- Look for skin ulcers that often accompany severe venous or arterial disease.
- Check for edema of the feet and ankles; this is one symptom of heart failure.

KnowledgeCheck 38-4

Why would you auscultate the lungs as a part of your assessment of cardiac function?

Providing Safe Clinical Monitoring

Chapter Key Concepts: Circulation, Perfusion

Competencies: (1) Embrace/Incorporate technological advances: Use technology to deliver safe, effective care. (2) Collaborate with the interdisciplinary healthcare team: Function as an essential member of the healthcare team (Thinking, Doing).

Because of reported safety issues that have been identified with the clinical monitoring of patients, The Joint Commission has asked hospitals to analyze the safety of hospital-based monitoring devices. Keep in mind that telemetry monitoring is not in and of itself a lifesaving intervention, but it is known to improve mortality in certain conditions in which cardiac dysrhythmia is possible or likely. As a telemetry nurse, you may be asked to participate in evaluating and identifying techniques/processes to avoid medical/nursing errors in the delivery of client care.

Several initiatives have been implemented to improve the safety of cardiac monitoring for patients including the following:

➤ Updated hospital-specific procedures to include escalation, team empowerment, alarm management for daily operations
➤ Standardized training course mandatory for all telemetry technicians and telemetry unit nurses (including competency testing)
➤ Four-week preceptor-supervised unit orientation mandatory for all new telemetry nurses with skills checklist completion
➤ Quarterly lethal arrhythmia drills on all shifts
➤ Maximum ratio of monitored patients to telemetry technicians
➤ Telemetry policy to emphasize medically indicated telemetry use

Source: Whalen, D. A., Covelle, P. M., Piepenbrink, J. C., et al. (2014). Novel approach to cardiac alarm management on telemetry units. *Journal of Cardiovascular Nursing, 29*(5), E13–E22.

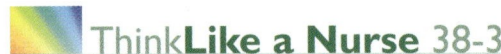

ThinkLike a Nurse 38-3

Why might it be more difficult to recognize a heart attack in a woman than in a man?

Diagnostic Testing

Diagnostic testing helps clinicians identify the causes of cardiovascular symptoms and monitor patient responses to treatment. We discuss several of these tests in the next sections. For others, see the Diagnostic Testing box Tests Related to Circulation.

Tests of Blood Oxygenation

Pulse oximetry, capnography, and arterial blood gases are discussed in the Diagnostic Testing box in Chapter 37. You should understand, though, that results from all of those tests are pertinent to cardiac conditions. **KEY POINT:** *Remember: The heart and lungs work together to provide oxygenation; a problem in one creates a problem in the other.* See Chapter 37, Procedure 37-2, and Clinical Insight 37-1.

To review (and use in clinical assignments) arterial blood gas values, see the section Interpreting ABGs and Table 39-6.

Laboratory Testing

Cholesterol, lipid panel, C-reactive protein (CRP), and glucose testing are a valuable part of cardiovascular risk assessment. The National Heart, Lung, and Blood Institute (NHLBI) (2013) recommends testing total cholesterol, high density lipoproteins (HDL), low-density lipoprotein (LDL), and triglyceride levels every 5 years for adults over age 20. For adults with total cholesterol greater than 200 mg/dL, a fasting measurement is recommended. In the past, providers relied on specific ranges for LDL and HDL. These ranges are no longer used; rather LDL levels are considered as one factor of many in evaluating cardiovascular risk. Glucose testing is indicated, particularly for those at risk for metabolic syndrome, which includes heart disease. **KEY POINT:** *The CRP appears to be the most reliable marker for arterial inflammation currently available.*

Screening for Children An Expert Panel appointed by the NHLBI (2013) recommended aggressive cholesterol screening for all children, regardless of family history. The panel recommends:

- Select lipid screening between the ages of 9 and 11 years followed by another full lipid screening test between 18 and 21 years of age.
- Measuring fasting glucose levels to test for diabetes in children 10 years of age (or at the onset of puberty) who are overweight with other risk factors, including a family history, for type 2 diabetes mellitus.

Cardiac Monitoring

Cardiac monitoring is the continuous monitoring of the **electrocardiogram (ECG),** a rendering of the electrical activity of the heart. Three to five electrodes placed on the skin of the chest display a waveform on a monitor screen or printout (Fig. 38-4). In contrast to cardiac monitoring, *electrocardiography* uses 12 "leads" (views of the heart). These are done by specially trained nurses or technicians.

The ECG illustrates electrical activity, but not mechanical activity. In other words, the ECG reflects what the nerves are telling the heart muscle to do, but not what the heart muscle is actually doing in response.

The purposes of cardiac monitoring are to:

- Identify the patient's baseline rhythm and rate.
- Recognize significant changes in the baseline rhythm and rate.

Diagnostic Testing

Tests Related to Circulation

Test	Purpose
Angiogram	A contrast dye is injected into a vein, and serial films are taken to assess patency of the vessels.
Arterial blood gases (ABGs)	An analysis of arterial blood that evaluates the effectiveness of gas exchange and perfusion.
Cardiac catheterization	A catheter is passed into the heart to assess pressures, blood flow, and the size and patency of chambers.
Chest x-ray study (CXR)	Provides an anterior–posterior or lateral view of the heart and lungs, shows tissue density (e.g., to evaluate size, masses, fluid).
Cholesterol, lipid profile	Indicates risk for cardiovascular disease long term.
Creatine kinase-MB (CK-MB)	The MB isoenzyme is present only in the heart muscle. A serum measurement of the MB band is used to detect a myocardial infarction (MI). Levels rise with an acute MI.
Echocardiogram	An ultrasound evaluation of the heart that examines heart function and blood flow.
Electrocardiogram (ECG)	Electrodes placed on the extremities and chest wall conduct electrical activity from the heart. ECG illustrates heart rate, rhythm, and size and helps evaluate heart damage.
Hemoglobin (Hb)	A serum measurement that affects the oxygen carrying capacity of the blood. May be measured separately or as part of a complete blood count.
Holter monitor	A continuous ECG tracing used to correlate symptoms and cardiac activity. Typically the tracing lasts 48 hours to 7 days.
Magnetic resonance	This is an MRI exam of the blood vessels. Unlike a traditional angiography, there is no **angiography (MRA)** tube (catheter) placed into the body. MRA is noninvasive.
Technetium scan	Technetium 99m sestamibi is injected intravenously. Approximately 90 to 120 minutes later, the heart is scanned. Areas of myocardial damage appear as "hot spots" on the scan.
Treadmill test	Evaluates the effect of exercise on the heart and circulation via continuous ECG and vital sign monitoring during exercise.
Troponin	A serum evaluation of a complex of proteins is used to detect myocardial infarction (MI). Levels of these contractile proteins remain elevated for up to 7 days after MI.
Ultrasound (Doppler)	A transducer, which directs high frequency sound waves to the artery or vein, is used to examine blood flow. A normal result shows no areas of narrowing or closure in the blood vessels.
Venography	Using dye and x-ray technology, a narrow tube (catheter) is inserted into a large vein to identify any blood clots or unusual narrowing or blockage of venous blood flow.
VQ scan	Used to detect a blood clot in the lungs.

- Recognize lethal dysrhythmias that require immediate intervention.

The USPSTF (2012) recommends against screening with resting or exercise ECG for the prediction of coronary heart disease (CHD) events in asymptomatic adults at low risk for CHD events. The current evidence is insufficient to balance the benefits and harms of screening for the prediction of CHD events.

Cardiac Cycle The ECG reading illustrates the complete cardiac cycle. Each part of the ECG complex has been given a letter to identify it: **P, Q, R, S, T,** and sometimes **U.**

- The **P wave** represents the firing of the SA node and conduction of the impulse through the atria. In the healthy heart, this leads to atrial contraction.
- The **QRS complex** represents *ventricular depolarization* and leads to ventricular contraction.
- The **T wave** represents the return of the ventricles to an electrical resting state so they can be stimulated again (*ventricular repolarization*). The atria also repolarize, but they do so during the time of ventricular depolarization; thus, they are obscured by the QRS complex and cannot be seen on the ECG complex.

- The **U wave** is not always seen on the ECG, but may be detected with electrolyte imbalance, such as hypokalemia or hypercalcemia. U waves sometimes occur in response to certain medication (e.g., digitalis, epinephrine). Inverted U wave may occur with ischemia to the cardiac muscle.

Cardiac Rhythms Dysrhythmias (abnormal heart rhythms) can be broadly categorized according to type as follows:

Tachydysrhythmias—Rates > 100 beats/min
Bradydysrhythmias—Rates < 60 beats/min
Ectopy—Extra beats

Within each of those categories, dysrhythmias can be further classified by their site of origin:

Supraventricular—Above the ventricles
Junctional—Within the AV node
Ventricular—In the ventricles

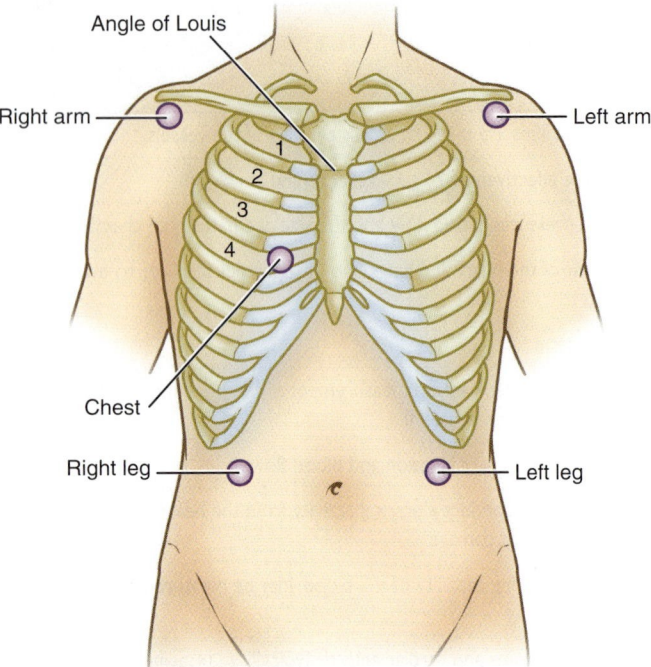

Angle of Louis

Right arm

Left arm

1
2
3
4

Chest

Right leg

Left leg

FIGURE 38-4 Electrodes placed for continuous cardiac monitoring.

Note that a tachy- or bradydysrhythmia depends on the patient's baseline heart rate. Some people have a low resting heart rate (fewer than 60 beats/min) without distress. Keep this in mind before assuming that the heart rate is abnormal.

All dysrhythmias have the potential to decrease cardiac output, resulting in hypotension and tissue hypoxia. Skill in identifying cardiac rhythms (both normal and abnormal) requires study and experience and is beyond the scope of this chapter. For the complete procedure, see Procedure 38-1.

KnowledgeCheck 38-5

- What do the P wave, QRS complex, and T and U waves of an ECG complex represent?
- What kind of dysrhythmia would describe a heart rate of 140 beats/min that originates in the ventricles?

ANALYSIS/NURSING DIAGNOSIS NP

Several nursing diagnoses address impaired circulation and tissue or organ hypoxia. They are briefly discussed below.

- *Decreased Cardiac Output* is the appropriate diagnosis when the heart is unable to pump adequate amounts of blood to meet the metabolic demands of the body. Definitive interventions for this problem are collaborative.
- *Risk for Decreased Cardiac Tissue Perfusion* is appropriate for a patient who has no symptoms of decreased cardiac perfusion, but has risk factors such as elevated C-reactive protein, cardiac surgery, taking birth control pills, hyperlipidemia, and substance abuse.
- *Risk for Ineffective Cerebral Tissue Perfusion* is appropriate for a patient who is at risk for experiencing poor perfusion to the brain, (e.g., a patient with a brain tumor, certain heart problems, embolism, substance abuse).

- *Ineffective Peripheral Tissue Perfusion* is appropriate for a patient experiencing poor perfusion to the arms and/or legs (e.g., peripheral arterial disease (PAD) or DVT).
- *Risk for Shock* should be used for patients who have inadequate blood flow to body tissues that may lead to life-threatening cellular dysfunction (e.g., patients with sepsis and hypovolemia).

Cardiovascular functioning can also be the etiology of other nursing diagnoses, such as the following examples:

- Risk for Activity Intolerance related to decreased oxygen-carrying capacity of the blood secondary to anemia
- Acute Pain secondary to myocardial ischemia
- Anxiety related to shortness of breath
- Death Anxiety related to diagnosis of myocardial infarction (heart attack)
- Ineffective Coping related to hospitalization for oxygenation impairment

PLANNING OUTCOMES/EVALUATION NP

NOC standardized outcomes and evaluation criteria related to cardiovascular status are included in NOC Domain II: Physiologic Health, in the Cardiopulmonary class. For examples of NOC outcomes and NIC interventions for selected oxygenation nursing diagnoses, see Table 38-2.

Individualized goals/outcome statements depend on the nursing diagnosis you identify. For diagnoses related to cardiac function or circulation, the following are examples of goals you might write the following:

- No dyspnea or shortness of breath
- Heart rate in expected range
- Peripheral pulses strong and equal bilaterally
- Brisk capillary refill

PLANNING INTERVENTIONS/ IMPLEMENTATION NP

NIC standardized interventions related to the cardiovascular system are found in NIC Domain 2: Complex Physiological Interventions, in the subcategory of Tissue Perfusion Management. Tissue Perfusion Management focuses on optimizing circulation. These provide a general care planning guide. Depending on individual patient needs, other NIC interventions may also be appropriate.

♥ iCare 38-1

Circulation

- Cardiovascular function is influenced by many factors including developmental, environmental, lifestyle, substance abuse, medications, and pathophysiological conditions.
- As a caring nurse, always maintain a nonjudgmental attitude when interacting with persons with cardiovascular problems, especially when lifestyle and substance abuse are contributing factors. Never, ever think or say, "Well, you did this to yourself."
- Do not judge. Rather, display caring behaviors through the interpersonal process. See that your actions express dignity and respect for others, positive communication, and finally, professional knowledge and skills.
- If the patient perceives that you care, a trusting relationship will develop, wherein patient teaching can occur and be received.

Table 38-2 ➤ Examples of NOC Outcomes and NIC Interventions Linked to Circulation Diagnoses

NURSING DIAGNOSIS	NOC OUTCOMES	NIC INTERVENTIONS
Activity Intolerance (could also be related to Pulmonary Functioning)	Activity Tolerance Energy Conservation Self-Care: Activities of Daily Living (ADL)	Energy Management Exercise Promotion: Strength Training Self-Care Assistance
Decreased Cardiac Output	Blood Loss Severity Cardiac Pump Effectiveness Circulation Status Tissue Perfusion: Cardiac Tissue Perfusion: Abdominal, Cerebral, Pulmonary, Peripheral Vital Signs	Bleeding Reduction Cardiac Care Cerebral Perfusion Promotion Circulatory Care: Arterial or Venous Insufficiency Fluid and Electrolyte Management Hemodynamic Regulation Intravenous Therapy Shock Management
Ineffective Peripheral Tissue Perfusion	Circulation Status Fluid Overload Severity Sensory Function: Tactile Tissue Integrity: Skin & Mucous Membranes	Circulatory Care (Arterial and Venous Insufficiency) Fluid Management Peripheral Sensation Management Skin Surveillance
Risk for Ineffective Cerebral Tissue Perfusion	Circulation Status Electrolyte & Acid/Base Balance Cognition Fluid Balance Neurological Status: Consciousness Kidney Function Tissue Perfusion: Abdominal Organs	Cerebral Perfusion Promotion Neurologic Monitoring Hypovolemia Management Fluid/Electrolyte Management Circulatory Care (Arterial and Venous Insufficiency) Circulatory Precautions Hemodialysis Therapy

Sources: Bulechek, G., Butcher, H., Dochterman, J., et al. (Eds.). (2012). *Nursing interventions classification (NIC)* (6th ed.). St. Louis, MO: C.V. Mosby; Johnson, M., Moorhead, S., Bulechek, G., et al. (2012). *NOC and NIC linkages to NANDA-I and clinical conditions.* St. Louis, MO: C.V. Mosby; Moorhead, S., Johnson, M., Maas, M., et al. (Eds.). (2012). *Nursing outcomes classification (NOC)* (5th ed.). St. Louis, MO: C.V. Mosby. Used with permission.

Specific nursing interventions for patients with cardiovascular problems focus on relieving anxiety, promoting circulation, administering medications, and performing cardiopulmonary resuscitation (CPR).

Manage Anxiety

Anxiety activates the sympathetic nervous system and triggers the stress response. Hormone changes occur, including the release of aldosterone, which promotes fluid retention and increases blood pressure. The heart rate and contraction force increase, peripheral and visceral vessels constrict, and the blood clots more readily. All of these factors make a cardiac or vascular condition more serious. Therefore, anxiety reduction is a priority intervention.

You will, of course, need to intervene first to prevent life-threatening situations. However, strive to implement the following:

- Try not to appear rushed.
- Speak calmly and quietly to the patient and to those around you.
- Do not leave the patient alone.
- Provide clear factual information and keep the patient and family informed about treatments being given.
- Many patients are reassured by the presence of a family member. Make that happen if you can.

If you need a review of detailed information about assessments and interventions for anxious patients, see Chapter 13.

Promote Circulation

Adequate circulation ensures that oxygenated blood reaches tissues and organs and that venous blood returns to the heart. Important nursing interventions are to promote venous return and peripheral arterial circulation and to prevent clot formation.

Promote Venous Return

Measures that promote venous return increase the flow of blood back to the vena cava and the right side of the heart.

- Elevate the patient's legs above the level of the heart. Gravity promotes venous return from the feet and legs.
- If a recliner is available, have the patient sit in one that elevates the legs rather than sitting upright in a chair with legs elevated on a stool. Flexion of the hips, legs, and knees constricts the veins and slows venous blood flow.
- Teach patients to avoid sitting with the legs crossed; doing so interferes with blood flow.
- Encourage and support early and frequent ambulation (e.g., after surgery). Contraction of the muscles in the legs moves venous blood upward against gravity.
- Encourage or provide range-of-motion (ROM) exercises, which increase venous blood flow through rhythmic massaging of the veins by the active muscles (see Chapter 33 to review ROM).
- Apply compression devices. **Antiembolism stockings (TED hose)** are elastic stockings that compress superficial leg veins and promote venous return. **Sequential compression devices (SCDs),** also called *pneumatic compression devices,* are cuffs that surround the legs and alternately inflate and deflate to promote venous return to the heart. Antiembolism stockings and SCDs are frequently used in perioperative patients to promote venous return and prevent clot formation (Woo & Cowie, 2013). See Chapter 40 for further discussion and instructions on how to apply these stockings and appropriate follow-up care. See Procedure 40-2: Applying Antiembolism Stockings.

Promote Peripheral Arterial Circulation

Peripheral arterial disease, usually found in the legs and feet, occurs when tissues don't receive enough blood flow to keep up with the demand for oxygen. It is caused by the buildup of fatty deposits and plaque within the arteries (atherosclerosis). When arteries that supply blood to the legs are narrowed, leg pain occurs, especially with walking. This is called **intermittent claudication.** As the blood flow becomes more restricted, pain occurs at rest, as well as numbness or a cold feeling to the leg or foot, especially on one side; weak pulse; change in color; hair loss or shiny skin on the legs; sores that won't heal; and erectile dysfunction in men. Teach the patient and family the following:

- Patients with poor peripheral circulation need to quit using tobacco because smoking restricts blood flow.
- When circulation is poor, it is especially important to take good care of the feet and prevent injury to the feet. Even dry, cracked skin can result in a sore and become infected. Patients need to wear well-fitting shoes with smooth, dry socks.
- Regular exercise improves circulation and oxygen delivery to body tissue.
- Medication might be needed to control blood pressure, control pain, lower cholesterol, prevent clots, and control blood sugar if the patient has diabetes.

- Angioplasty using a mesh stent or graft bypass surgery might be necessary to create a new path for blood flow to go around the damaged area of the blood vessel.

When treated properly, new collateral blood vessels can form, allowing blood to circulate around the damaged area.

Prevent Clot Formation

A **thrombus** is a stationary clot adhering to the wall of a vessel. Clots can form after injury to vessels or in response to hypercoagulability. An **embolus** is a clot that travels in the bloodstream.

Anticoagulant Therapy Patients at high risk for thrombus formation may be prescribed anticoagulant medications to help prevent abnormal clot formation. Anticoagulant medications include heparin and warfarin sodium. Newer anticoagulants (e.g., dabigatran, apixaban, and rivaroxaban) work by inhibiting thrombin or factor X in the clotting chain. They have the advantage of not requiring tests of blood levels. However, unlike heparin and warfarin, they have no specific antidote.

> ✚ Hospitalized patients are at particularly high risk for clot formation and may develop an asymptomatic DVT and die of pulmonary embolism even before the diagnosis is suspected. For this reason, The Joint Commission (2013) identified anticoagulant therapy as the "number one patient safety practice" for hospitalized patients.

Other Nursing Activities Of course, all the strategies to promote venous return also help prevent clot formation.

- **Turn patients frequently;** teach patients to change positions frequently. This prevents vessel injury from prolonged pressure in one position.
- **Use scrupulous sterile technique** for intravenous therapy. This prevents infection that can damage the vessel lumens.
- **Be sure IV medications are adequately diluted.** This prevents chemical irritation of veins.
- **Promote adequate hydration** (i.e., monitor intake and output, assess hydration, manage fluid intake, teach patients to drink plenty of fluids). Unless contraindicated, adult fluid intake should be approximately 2,000 mL per day to keep urine output at about 1,500 mL per day. Adequate hydration keeps respiratory secretions thin but also keeps the blood from becoming viscous ("thick"). Viscous blood clots more readily.
- **Promote smoking cessation.** Nicotine increases the risk for thrombus formation because of its constricting effects on vessel walls.

Administer Cardiovascular Medications

Cardiovascular medications are used to enhance cardiac output, thus providing increased blood flow and oxygenation to organs and tissues. They include the following:

- *Vasodilators* cause vessel dilation, which eases the work of the heart. Vasodilating agents include angiotensin-converting enzyme (ACE) inhibitors, angiotensin II receptor blockers, and nitrates.
  - *Drugs that dilate arterioles* decrease the resistance against which the heart pumps (afterload).
  - *Drugs that dilate veins* decrease venous return to the heart (preload).

  KEY POINT: *Vasodilators can cause hypotension, especially when the person rises from a sitting or lying position. Be sure to warn patients of this effect, monitor the* *patient's blood pressure, and observe for symptoms of hypotension.*

- **Beta-adrenergic agents** block stimulation of beta receptors, which are located primarily in the heart, lungs, and blood vessels. Beta$_1$-selective agents are used to treat angina, acute myocardial infarction, and congestive heart failure (CHF). They decrease heart rate, slow conduction through the AV node, and decrease myocardial oxygen demand by reducing myocardial contractility.
- **Diuretics** increase removal of sodium and water from the body by increasing urine output. In patients with CHF, diuretics are used to reduce the volume of circulating blood and prevent accumulation of fluid in the pulmonary circulation.
- **Positive inotropes** increase cardiac contractility. They are used therapeutically to make the heart a more effective pump. The goal is to improve pumping effectiveness without creating excess heart work and oxygen demand. The two main classes of positive inotropes are cardiac glycosides and phosphodiesterase inhibitors.
- **Anticholesterol medications (statins)** are a class of drugs that protect against coronary artery disease by lowering the level of triglycerides and reduce the production of cholesterol by the liver. Statins block the liver enzyme that is responsible for making cholesterol. Statins are used for those who have an elevated LDL cholesterol level. For primary prevention, recent guidelines recommend their use for all persons, even with a normal level, if they have diabetes or a high risk of cardiovascular disease (Ray, Kastelein, Boekholdt, et al., 2014; Stone, Robinson, Lichtenstein, et al., 2014).

Cardiopulmonary Resuscitation

You must be prepared to perform *cardiopulmonary resuscitation (CPR)* in the event your patient experiences a respiratory, cardiac, or cardiopulmonary arrest.

- **Cardiac arrest** is the cessation of heart function. Signs of cardiac arrest are pale, cool, grayish skin; absence of femoral or carotid pulses; apnea; and pupil dilation. **KEY POINT:** *In the event of cardiac arrest, you have only 4 to 6 minutes before the brain is damaged by lack of oxygen.*
- **Respiratory (pulmonary) arrest** is cessation of breathing. It can be caused by a blocked airway or occur after a cardiac arrest; it may be sudden or preceded by increasingly labored breathing.

CPR procedures are regularly updated as new knowledge is gained. The American Heart Association provides training sessions for healthcare professionals to become certified in CPR. This is a prerequisite for employment and clinical practice. **KEY POINT:** *We recommend that you obtain CPR training*

Toward Evidence-Based Practice

Mizuno, J., & Monteiro, H. L. (2012). An assessment of a sequence of yoga exercises to patients with arterial hypertension. *Journal of Bodywork and Movement Therapies, 17*(1), 35–41.

This study describes the effects of a yoga sequence on patients with hypertension. Thirty-three volunteers participated in the study (control = 16, yoga = 17) for 4 months. Blood pressure measurements and cardiac and respiratory rates were collected monthly. The yoga group showed a significant reduction of systolic blood pressure and heart and respiratory rates ($p < 0.05$). The authors concluded that yoga exercises should be implemented as a means of complementary nonpharmacological control of blood pressure in patients with hypertension.

Begum, M. N. (2013). To evaluate the effect of yoga on moderate degree hypertension and lipid profile. *National Journal of Integrated Research in Medicine, 4*(3), 109–114.

Sixty patients (30 females and 30 males) aged 40 to 60 years, with moderate degree hypertension, were trained in asanas (postures), pranayama (breathing exercise), and relaxation techniques for 6 months. Blood pressure; serum total cholesterol; LDL, VLDL, and HDL cholesterol; and total triglycerides were measured at the beginning and at the end of the study. The results demonstrated that yoga practice in patients with moderate degree hypertension leads to a decrease in blood pressure and lipid profile within a period of 6 months.

Deepa, T., Sethu, G., & Thirrunavukkarasu, N. (2012). Effect of yoga and meditation on mild to moderate essential hypertensives. *Journal of Clinical and Diagnostic Research, 6*(1), 21–26.

This study evaluated the effect of yoga and meditation on mild to moderate essential hypertensive patients. Patients were divided into two groups: (1) 15 patients treated with antihypertensive drugs along with yoga and (2) 15 patients with antihypertensive drugs alone. Yoga was practiced for 45 minutes daily in the morning and again in the evening. The study showed a significant decrease of mean blood pressure after 3 months of yoga, suggesting that yoga can be used as adjunctive treatment with drug therapy for those with mild and moderate hypertension.

These three studies demonstrate that yoga may be a complementary therapy for use in patients with hypertension. Using what you know about yoga,

---

1. What may be some reasons for patients not participating in this type of exercise?

2. What strategies can you use to motivate patients to practice yoga?

 Go to Davis Advantage, Resources, Chapter 38, **Toward Evidence-Based Practice—Suggested Responses.**

from certified professionals. However, if you are already trained and just want to review the procedure,

 Go to the Highlights of the 2015 American Heart Association Guidelines Update for CPR and ECC at http://eccguidelines.heart.org/wp-content/uploads/2015/10/2015-AHA-Guidelines-Highlights-English.pdf

Key points of the most recent guidelines *for trained professionals* include the following:
- Focus on effective, uninterrupted chest compressions.
- Push hard, push fast in the center of the chest.
- Administer about 100 compressions per minute.
- Perform 30 compressions to 2 breaths—for all victims except newborns.
- Give breath over 1 second and make the chest rise visibly (American Heart Association, 2015; Dumas, Rea, Fahrenbruch, et al., 2013).

In-Hospital Arrests

All agencies have procedures (called a Code Blue in many agencies) for announcing cardiac or respiratory arrest; in acute care facilities there is usually an emergency alert system in the patient rooms. In the event of an arrest:
1. Activate the alert system (e.g., by pulling down a handle) to summon a code team trained in CPR.
2. Begin CPR immediately after activating the alert, as it will take a few minutes for the code team to arrive. Use a defibrillator as soon as one is available.
   - *For an automatic external defibrillator* (AED), follow the visual and audio prompts from the AED.
   - *For a manual defibrillator,* use a dose of 2 joules/kg for the first shock and a dose of 4 J/kg for the second and subsequent shocks.

   KEY POINT: *Before beginning CPR, you are responsible for knowing whether your patient has an advance directive stating whether or not he would want CPR.*

Hands-Only™ CPR

The American Heart Association (2011a, updated 2016) recommends different responses for laypersons, first responders, and CPR-trained professionals. The goal of these changes is to make it easier to learn, remember, and perform CPR.
- **Hands-Only™ CPR,** using compressions only, is recommended for people who see an adult collapse suddenly in the community.
- **Traditional CPR,** which combines breaths and compressions should be used only for:
   Adults found already unconscious and not breathing normally
   Victims of drowning or collapse due to breathing problems
   All infants and children

See the Self-Care box Teaching Your Client Hands-Only™ CPR for a detailed description of CPR that you can teach to lay persons.

KnowledgeCheck 38-6
- Identify three strategies that prevent clot formation.
- How do diuretics affect oxygenation?

Self-Care

Teaching Your Client Hands-Only™ CPR for a Single Rescuer, Adult Victim Collapse

Witnessed Collapse

If you see an adult suddenly collapse in an "out-of-hospital" setting:
1. Call 911 (or send someone to do that).
2. Push hard and fast in the center of the chest (100 pumps per minute).
3. Continue until help arrives.

For an Unwitnessed Collapse of an Adult Victim:

1. Establish unresponsiveness (ask, "Are you okay?").
2. Call 911 (or send someone to do it).
3. Obtain an AED, if possible.
4. Start traditional CPR, if you know how, while waiting for the AED.

Traditional CPR

1. When the AED arrives, turn it on for rhythm analysis.
2. After turning on the AED, open the airway (tilt the head, lift the chin).
3. Check for breathing.
4. Give two rescue breaths (each 1 second long). Look for chest movement, listen for breathing, and feel for air coming from the mouth or nose.
5. Administer one shock and wait for the AED to tell you what to do next.
6. When the AED says to continue CPR, start alternating 30 compressions with 2 breaths. Continue until help arrives. Stop only to check the AED for rhythm.

   KEY POINT: *The most important action is to deliver uninterrupted, hard and fast chest compressions.*

Source: American Heart Association. (2011b). Hands Only™ CPR. Retrieved from http://handsonlycpr.eisenberginc.com/

CLINICALREASONING

The questions and exercises in this section allow you to practice the kind of thinking you will use as a full-spectrum nurse. Critical-thinking questions usually have more than one correct answer, so we do not provide "correct answers" for these features. It is more important to develop your nursing judgment than to just cover content. You will learn by discussing the questions with your peers. If you are still unsure, see the Davis Advantage chapter resources for suggested responses.

Caring for the Nguyens

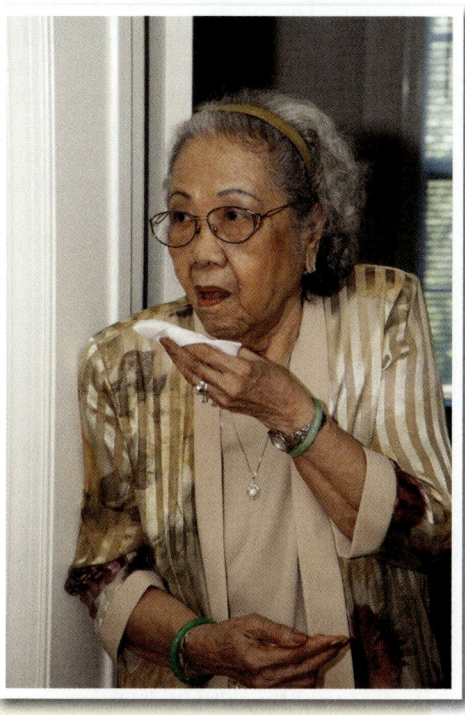

Mai Nguyen, Nam's 76-year-old mother, has been complaining she feels tired all the time, as though she just can't do what she normally does. She describes having a hard time catching her breath as she walks up stairs and goes about her day. Nam has noticed that his mother's ankles are more swollen than he has ever seen them. He schedules an appointment for his mother at the family clinic where you are the nurse. Mrs. Nguyen appears pale and not her usual energetic self. Nam tells you that his mom is "not right" and seems to be confused about things at home, which is not like her. She has a history of chronic congestive heart failure.

A. What additional health history data would be useful to gather at this time?

B. During her visit at the clinic, you observe that Mai has a cough. She spits a small amount of pink, frothy mucus into a tissue. Mrs. Nguyen's vital signs are as follows: BP, 142/90 mm Hg; pulse, 96 beats/min and with some irregular beats; respirations, 38 breaths/min and shallow; temperature, 97.8°F (36.5°C) oral.
  - Which of these symptoms and vital signs is/are not within normal limits?
  - For each abnormal finding, explain why you think it is occurring.

C. You decide to include a nursing diagnosis of Acute Confusion in Mrs. Nguyen's plan of care.
  - What symptoms does she have that support this nursing diagnosis?

- What physiological changes are causing these symptoms?

D. In addition to angiotensin-converting enzyme (ACE) inhibitor, beta blocker, diuretic, and digoxin, what additional therapies do you anticipate the physician will prescribe?

E. Mrs. Nguyen asks you, "What can I do to make sure I never get this sick again?" How would you answer this question?

 Go to Davis Advantage, Resources, Chapter 38, **Caring for the Nguyens—Suggested Responses.**

Applying the **Full-Spectrum Nursing Model**_____

PATIENT SITUATION

Margarita, a 62-year-old Director of Management Technology for a large company, was admitted to the hospital with shortness of breath, sudden and intense fatigue, and intense chest pressure that she describes as feeling like a steel band tightening around her rib cage. She reports the pain moved up to her jaw. The pain began suddenly but lasted approximately 5 to 7 minutes. During the episode, her husband tells you that Margarita acted as though she had a feeling of doom.

Margarita also has a history of sudden onset neck pain that seems to be triggered by heightened stress at work. Margarita is pale and clammy. She states she feels nauseated and has burning in her epigastric area. Her heart rate is 80 beats/min; respiratory rate, 12 breaths/min; and BP, 168/92 mm Hg. Skin is pale but warm, and capillary refill time is 4 seconds. Height is 5 ft 4 in. Weight is 156 lb. Body mass index (BMI) is 29.2. Waist circumference is 36 in.

The health history includes type 2 diabetes mellitus, high blood pressure, and tobacco use (half a pack of cigarettes a day). Margarita's mother had a heart attack in her 50s.

Lab work prior to admission:

Fasting lipids: Total cholesterol 288 mg/dL, LDL 148 mg/dL, HDH 44 mg/dL, triglycerides 222 mg/dL

Serum glucose: 244 mg/dL

hs-CRP: 3.1 mg/dL

THINKING

1. *Theoretical Knowledge:*
   a. What predisposing factors increase Margarita's risk for myocardial infarction?
   b. What does it mean to have infarcted myocardial tissue?
2. *Critical Thinking (Analyzing Assumptions):*
   Based on your knowledge of vascular causes of myocardial infarction, what are the most likely causes in this patient?

DOING

3. *Practical Knowledge:*
   After your patient's vital signs are stable and her pain is controlled, the emergency physician prescribes further diagnostic testing to determine the extent of damage to her heart.
   a. What tests would you expect your patient to have?
   b. You attempt to adhere electrodes for cardiac monitoring to Margarita's chest. The ECG tracing shows a great deal of artifact rather than a clear ECG tracing. What should you do to obtain an accurate tracing?
   c. You notice your patient is experiencing multiple "runs" of aberrant heartbeats. What should you do in response to the abnormal ECG tracing?
4. *Nursing Process (Assessment):*
   In the admission data, what important information is missing with regard to her cardiac status?

CARING

5. *Self-Knowledge:*
   Describe a personal experience involving someone in your own family or a friend who experienced a life-threatening event. How did you feel when your loved one was faced with a potentially life-altering heart condition? How might you draw upon this experience to help you in caring for Margarita?
6. *Ethical Knowledge:*
   a. After Margarita is finished with the last diagnostic test, what do you think her biggest concern is likely to be?
   b. Margarita tells you that she does not want anyone to know she has a heart problem. Yet her husband wants to tell other family members. How do you best respond to her concerns for privacy?

 Go to Davis Advantage, Resources, Chapter 38, **Applying the Full-Spectrum Nursing Model—Suggested Responses**.

PracticalKnowledge:
clinical application_____

In this section, you will find a procedure for supporting circulation and perfusion. As you perform the procedure, apply the theoretical knowledge you obtained in the preceding material. The registered nurse is responsible for assessing patients' circulation and perfusion and their responses to procedures.

PROCEDURES

Procedure 38-1 ■ Performing Cardiac Monitoring

➤ For steps to follow in *all* procedures, refer to the Universal Steps for All Procedures found on the page facing the inside back cover.

Equipment

- Alcohol pads
- Gauze dressing
- Washcloth
- Shaving supplies or scissors, if necessary
- Disposable electrodes

For Hardwire Monitoring, Add:

- Cardiac monitor
- Cable with lead wires
- Safety pin
- 1-in. tape

For Telemetry, Add:

- Transmitter with lead wires (with a new battery inserted before each use)
- Pouch to carry transmitter

Delegation

You should not delegate this procedure to the licensed practical nurse or nursing assistive personnel because it requires knowledge of anatomy, physiology, and advanced assessment techniques.

Pre-Procedure Assessment

- Assess cardiovascular status, including heart sounds, pulse rate, and blood pressure, and check for the presence of pain.
- Assess skin integrity of the chest before applying electrodes.
  Skin lesions contraindicate the application of leads to the affected area.
- Assess for history of dysrhythmias.
  Early recognition of dysrhythmias allows for prompt treatment, which improves patient outcomes.

➤ When performing the procedure, always identify your patient according to agency policy, using two identifiers, and be attentive to standard precautions, hand hygiene, patient safety and privacy, body mechanics, and documentation.

Procedure Steps

1. **Prepare the monitoring equipment.**

For Hardwire Monitoring

a. Plug the cardiac monitor into an electrical outlet and turn it on.
   Allows the monitor to warm up while you prepare the patient for monitoring.

b. Connect the cable with lead wires into the monitor.
   The cable and lead wires must be properly connected to the monitor to obtain an accurate ECG tracing. Most are color coded.

For Telemetry Monitoring

c. Insert a new battery into the transmitter.
   A new battery should be inserted with each use to ensure transmitter function.

d. Turn on the transmitter.
   Tests the unit to make sure the battery is functional.

e. Connect the lead wires to the transmitter, if they are not permanently attached. Be sure to attach each one to its correct outlet.
   The lead wires must be properly connected to the transmitter to obtain an accurate ECG tracing.

2. **Expose the patient's chest** and identify electrode sites based on the monitoring system being used and the patient's anatomy. Gently rub the placement sites with a washcloth or gauze pad until the skin reddens slightly.
   The monitoring system will dictate lead placement. Sites over soft tissues or close to bone provide accurate waveforms; sites over bony prominences, thick muscles, and skinfolds can produce artifact. ➤

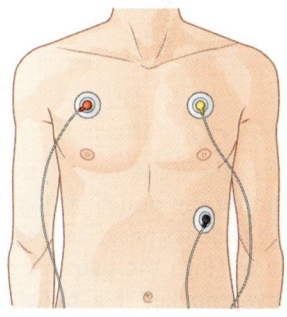

3. **If the patient's chest has dense hair,** shave or clip the hair with scissors at each electrode site.
   Hair may interfere with electrical contact, preventing accurate ECG waveform transmission.

4. **With an alcohol pad,** clean the areas chosen for electrode placement and allow them to dry.
   Alcohol removes oil on the skin that may prevent the electrodes from adhering.

(continued on next page)

Procedure 38-1 ■ **Performing Cardiac Monitoring** (continued)

5. Remove the electrode backing and make sure the gel is moist. Discard the electrode if the gel is dry. The number of electrodes needed depends on the monitoring system being used. It will be three to five electrodes.
A dry electrode will not conduct electrical activity.

6. Attach the lead wires to the electrodes by snapping or clipping them in place.

7. Apply the electrode to the site by pressing it firmly. Repeat with the remaining electrodes.
Pressing the electrode firmly creates a tight seal, which ensures electrical contact.

8. Secure the monitoring equipment.

For Hardwire Monitoring

a. Wrap a piece of 1-in. tape around the cable and secure it to the patient's gown with a safety pin.
Secures the cable so leads are not disconnected with patient movement.

For Telemetry Monitoring

b. Place the transmitter in the pouch and tie the pouch strings around the patient's neck. Place the transmitter into the patient's robe or gown pocket if a pouch is not available.
Allows the patient independence with ambulation.

9. Check the patient's ECG tracing on the monitor. If necessary, adjust the gain on the monitor to increase the waveform size.
The ECG tracing should be of adequate size to accurately assess all of the waveform components.

For Telemetry Monitoring

You may need to call a monitoring room to verify ECG tracing and rhythm.

10. Set the upper and lower heart rate alarm limits according to agency policy or patient condition and turn them on.

11. Obtain a rhythm strip by pressing the "record" button.
You must obtain a rhythm strip to document the patient's cardiac rhythm. ▼

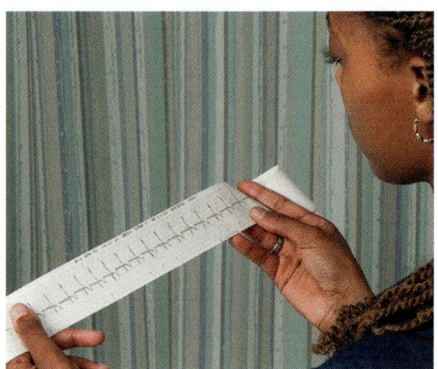

For Hardwire Monitoring

a. Press the "record" button on the bedside monitor.
The "record" button, located on the monitor at the bedside, allows you to print a rhythm strip immediately when cardiac symptoms occur.

For Telemetry Monitoring

b. Press the "record" button on the transmitter of the telemetry unit, or call the monitoring room to have the ECG trip printed.
The "record" button on the telemetry transmitter allows you or the patient to print a rhythm strip immediately when cardiac symptoms occur.

12. Interpret the rhythm strip and mount it appropriately (e.g., with transparent tape) in the patient's chart.
Provides a permanent record of the patient's heart activity; identifies abnormalities in the patient's rhythm.

? What if . . .

■ **The patient is diaphoretic?**

Remove electrodes, clean the area with alcohol, allow the area to dry, and then reapply electrodes.
To obtain an accurate ECG tracing.

■ **The patient is receiving a cardiac medication?**

Print a strip before giving medication and after giving medication. You may also need to call the telemetry station to have the ECG monitored.
To assess and monitor effects of medication.

■ **You are not getting a good reading on the monitor?**

Recheck the leads; replace leads or move leads if necessary.

Evaluation

■ Evaluate changes in the patient's cardiac rhythm.
■ Check skin integrity and replace the electrodes at least every 24 hours.
Avoids skin irritation at the electrode sites. In addition, the gel begins to dry, so replacement ensures an adequate waveform.

■ Tell the patient being monitored by telemetry to remove the transmitter before showering. Ask the patient to inform you before removing it.
■ Discuss home telemetry monitoring with the patient and caregiver if the patient requires telemetry monitoring after discharge.

Patient Teaching

■ Explain the rationale for cardiac monitoring.
■ Teach the patient that if he experiences symptoms (e.g., shortness of breath, chest pain, dizziness, palpitations) he should notify the nurse immediately so a rhythm strip can be recorded.

Home Care

■ Evaluate the patient's and caregiver's ability to continue telemetry monitoring at home with help from an outside agency.
■ Help the patient and caregiver contact the home-care agency to arrange for home telemetry monitoring.

- Explain to the caregiver and patient that the emergency medical service will be notified by the monitoring agency if a dysrhythmia develops.
- Instruct the caregiver and patient about proper lead placement and the need to rotate electrode sites to prevent skin breakdown.

Documentation

- Document the date and time that monitoring was instituted.
- Note the monitoring lead selected.
- Document a rhythm strip every 8 hours and with changes in the patient's condition according to agency policy. Label the rhythm strip (if the monitor does not label it for you) with the date, time, patient's name, and room number. Indicate on the strip when symptoms and treatment interventions occurred.
- Document the patient's response to treatment.

Practice Resources

Hancock, E. W., Deal, B. J., Mirvis, D. M., et al. (2009); Lieberman, K. (2008); Morrison, L. J., Neumar, R. W., Zimmerman, J. L., et al. (2013).

To explore learning resources for this chapter,

Go to **www.DavisAdvantage.com** and find:

Answers and Suggested Responses for all questions in this chapter

Lists of NIC Interventions and NOC Outcomes

List of NANDA-I Diagnoses

Knowledge Map

References and Bibliography

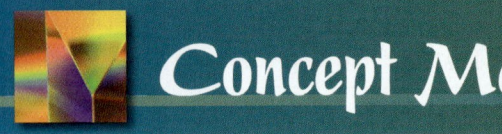

Concept Map

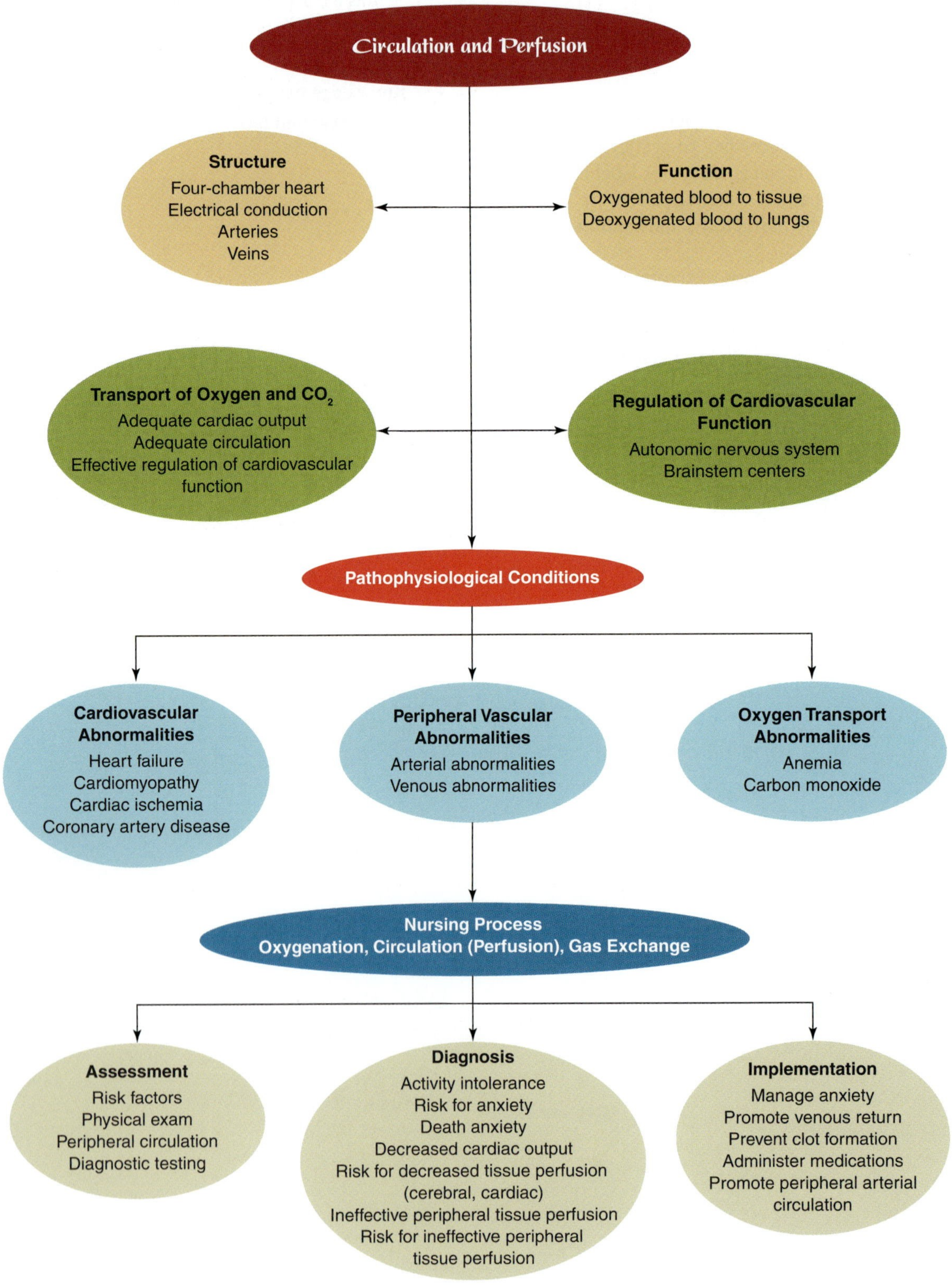

Circulation and Perfusion

Structure

Four-chamber heart
Electrical conduction
Arteries
Veins

Function

Oxygenated blood to tissue
Deoxygenated blood to lungs

Transport of Oxygen and CO$_2$

Adequate cardiac output
Adequate circulation
Effective regulation of cardiovascular
function

**Regulation of Cardiovascular
Function**

Autonomic nervous system
Brainstem centers

Pathophysiological Conditions

**Cardiovascular
Abnormalities**

Heart failure
Cardiomyopathy
Cardiac ischemia
Coronary artery disease

**Peripheral Vascular
Abnormalities**

Arterial abnormalities
Venous abnormalities

**Oxygen Transport
Abnormalities**

Anemia
Carbon monoxide

**Nursing Process
Oxygenation, Circulation (Perfusion), Gas Exchange**

Assessment

Risk factors
Physical exam
Peripheral circulation
Diagnostic testing

Diagnosis

Activity intolerance
Risk for anxiety
Death anxiety
Decreased cardiac output
Risk for decreased tissue perfusion
(cerebral, cardiac)
Ineffective peripheral tissue perfusion
Risk for ineffective peripheral
tissue perfusion

Implementation

Manage anxiety
Promote venous return
Prevent clot formation
Administer medications
Promote peripheral arterial
circulation

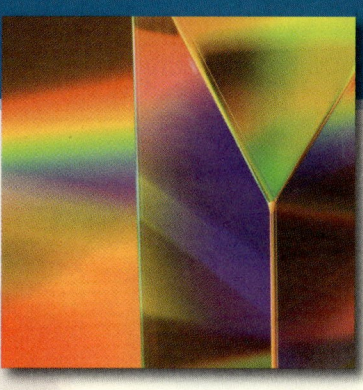

CHAPTER 39

Fluids, Electrolytes, & Acid–Base Balance

Learning Outcomes

After completing this chapter, you should be able to:

- ▶ Identify the fluid compartments within the body.
- ▶ Describe the location and function of the major electrolytes of the body.
- ▶ Differentiate between active and passive transport, osmosis, diffusion, and filtration.
- ▶ Describe the body mechanisms for maintaining fluid and electrolyte balance.
- ▶ Summarize the major fluid and electrolyte balance disorders.
- ▶ Compare and contrast respiratory and metabolic acidosis and alkalosis.
- ▶ Describe compensatory mechanisms for acid–base imbalances.
- ▶ Apply the nursing process to clients with fluid, electrolyte, and acid–base imbalances.

Key Concepts

Acid–base balance

Electrolyte balance

Fluid balance

Related Concepts

See the Concept Map at the end of this chapter.

Example Problems

Fluid, Electrolyte, and Acid–Base Imbalances

Meet Your Patients

Your instructor assigned you to care for Jackson LaGuardia, a 60-year-old man with end-stage renal disease. You arrived at the hospital to review his chart to provide care the following day. On the unit, the charge nurse informs you that Mr. LaGuardia is still in the emergency department (ED) waiting to be admitted to the medical–surgical unit. You go to the ED to review his chart, gather data, and introduce yourself as a student nurse.

The ED charge nurse tells you that five members of the LaGuardia family have all come to the hospital complaining of nausea, vomiting, and diarrhea related to severe gastroenteritis, a viral intestinal disorder. The family members include the following:

- ■ 8-month-old Jason, grandson of Jackson
- ■ 26-year-old Susanna, Jackson's daughter and Jason's mother

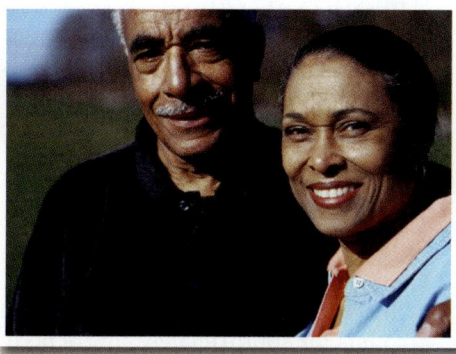

- ■ 58-year-old Gemma, Jackson's wife
- ■ 60-year-old Jackson
- ■ 82-year-old Martha, Jackson's mother

Jason, Jackson, and Martha are being admitted to the hospital. However, Susanna and Gemma have been asked to follow up tomorrow in the urgent care clinic. As you prepare for your clinical day, you think, "If they all have the same disorder, why are only three family members being admitted? What makes these patients different?" In this chapter, we follow the LaGuardias and answer those questions

Theoretical Knowledge
knowing **why**

When we are healthy, the fluid and chemical state of our bodies is in balance. However, illness can disturb this balance. In this chapter, we examine how fluid, electrolyte, and acid–base balances are maintained and what happens when there are disturbances in each of these areas.

ABOUT THE KEY CONCEPTS

The concepts of **fluid balance** and **electrolyte balance** are intricately related. Usually, when one electrolyte changes, so does another, and often with fluid shifts that can lead to dysfunction and disease. Likewise, disruption of **acid–base balance** can impact overall body functioning. The pH balance (acidity and alkalinity) has a profound effect on overall health.

BODY FLUIDS AND SOLUTES

Body fluid is essential for proper functioning of the body organs. It is made up primarily of water and contains *gases* (e.g., carbon dioxide and oxygen) and *solid substances,* called **solutes,** that dissolve in body fluids. Solutes are of two types:

- **Electrolytes**—substances (e.g., sodium, potassium) that develop an electrical charge when dissolved in water
- **Nonelectrolytes**—substances (e.g., glucose, urea) that do not conduct electricity

Total body water content varies with the number of fat cells, age, and sex (see Table 39-1). Women have less body fluid than do men because they have proportionately more body fat. Likewise, obese people have less body fluid proportionately than do those of lean build.

Body fluids perform several important functions:

- Maintain blood volume.
- Regulate body temperature.
- Transport material to and from cells.
- Serve as a medium for cellular metabolism.
- Assist with digestion of food.
- Serve as a medium for excreting waste.

What Are the Body Fluids Compartments?

Most body fluid is contained within two compartments. Figure 39-1 illustrates the distribution of body fluids.

Intracellular Fluid (ICF) is contained within the cells. It accounts for approximately 40% of body weight and is essential for cell function and metabolism.

Extracellular Fluid (ECF) is found outside the cells. ECF carries water, electrolytes, nutrients, and oxygen to the cells and removes the waste products of cellular metabolism. It accounts for 20% of body weight and exists in three main locations in the body:

- **Interstitial fluid** lies in the spaces between the body cells. Excess fluid within the interstitial space is called *edema.*
- **Intravascular fluid** is the plasma within the blood. Its main function is to transport blood cells.
- **Transcellular fluid** includes specialized fluids that are contained in body spaces (e.g., cerebrospinal, pleural, peritoneal, and synovial fluid) and digestive juices.

Third Spacing Certain conditions cause fluid to move into an area that makes it physiologically unavailable, such as into the peritoneal space (in *ascites*), the pericardial space (with *pericardial effusion*), or into the *vesicles* (blisters) with a burn wound.

Table 39-1 ➤ Total Body Fluid in Relation to Sex and Age

AGE	TOTAL BODY FLUID (% OF BODY WEIGHT)
Full-Term Newborn	70%–80%
1 Year Old	64%
Young Adult	Men: 60%
	Women: 50%–55%
Middle Adult	Men: 55%
	Women: 45%–50%
Older Adult	Men: 50%
	Women: 45%

This type of fluid movement is known as **third spacing** because fluid is literally trapped in a third compartment—not within interstitial (cells) or the intravascular spaces (blood vessels).

What Electrolytes Are Present in Body Fluids?

In addition to water, body fluid is composed of oxygen, carbon dioxide, dissolved nutrients, metabolic waste products, and electrolytes. **Electrolytes** are substances that carry an electrical charge, either positive or negative:

Cations carry a positive charge.

Anions carry a negative charge.

Electrolytes are measured in milliequivalents per liter (mEq/L) of water or milligrams per 100 mL (mg/100 mL or mg/dL). Note that 1 dL, or deciliter, equals 100 mL. **KEY POINT: Milliequivalent** *is a measure of chemical combining power,* whereas **milligram** *is a weight measure.*

The composition of body fluids varies between compartments:

- **In the ICF,** the major cations are *potassium* and *magnesium.* The major anion is *phosphate.* Other electrolytes are present, but to a lesser degree.
- **In the ECF,** the major electrolytes are *sodium, chloride,* and *bicarbonate. Albumin* is also present in the ECF, mostly in the intravascular fluid. Gastric and intestinal secretions (transcellular fluids) also contain electrolytes.

Severe electrolyte imbalances can occur if electrolytes move into a compartment they do not normally occupy or if they are lost in excess amounts from the body through perspiration, wounds, injury, or illness.

Knowledge Check 39-1

- Define *solute, electrolyte, intracellular fluid, extracellular fluid, cation,* and *anion.*
- Identify the major electrolytes in the ICF and ECF.

Think Like a Nurse 39-1

- Based on the information presented in the Meet Your Patients scenario, rank the members of the LaGuardia family based on total body water content.
- Does this information help you understand which family members were admitted to the hospital?

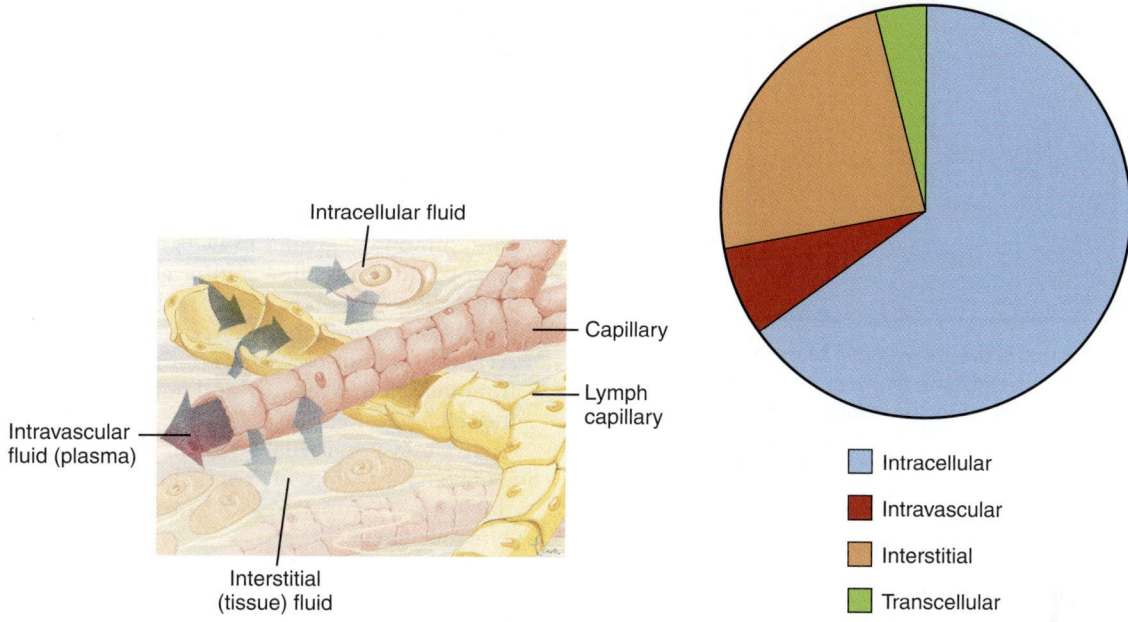

FIGURE 39-1 Normal distribution of body fluids. Transcellular fluid includes specialized fluids such as cerebrospinal and peritoneal fluids and digestive juices.

How Do Fluids and Electrolytes Move in the Body?

The selectively permeable membranes of cells and capillaries separate ICF and ECF (see Fig. 39-1). Fluid and electrolytes move across these membranes by passive and active mechanisms.

- In **active transport,** movement of fluid and solutes requires energy.
- **Passive transport** requires no energy. The three passive transport systems are osmosis, diffusion, and filtration.

Osmosis

Osmosis involves movement of water (or other pure solute) across a membrane from an area of a less concentrated solution to an area of more concentrated solution. Water moves across the membrane to dilute the higher concentration of solutes (Fig. 39-2). **Solutes** (substance dissolved in body fluids) may be crystalloids or colloids.

> **Crystalloids** are solutes that readily dissolve (e.g., electrolytes).
> **Colloids** are larger molecules that do not dissolve readily (e.g., proteins).
> **Osmolality** (or **tonicity**) refers to the concentration of

solutes providing pressure in body fluid. **Osmols** refers to the number of particles of solute per kilogram of water and is expressed as milliosmoles per kilogram (mOsm/kg). *Sodium is the greatest determinant of serum osmolality; potassium is the greatest determinant of intracellular osmolality. Glucose and urea also contribute to osmolality in the ICF and ECF.*

- An **isotonic solution** is of the same osmolality as blood; thus, no osmosis will occur. *Isotonic fluids are often given by intravenous (IV) infusion if blood volume is low because the fluid will remain in the vascular space.*
- A **hypotonic solution** is of lower osmolality than blood. *When a hypotonic solution is infused, water moves by osmosis from the vascular system into the cells.*
- A **hypertonic solution** contains a higher concentration of solutes than does blood. *When a hypertonic solution is infused, water moves by osmosis from the cells into the ECF.*

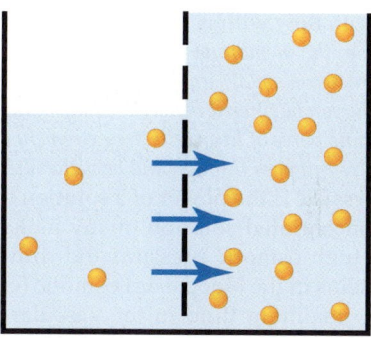

FIGURE 39-2 Osmosis is the movement of water across a membrane from a less concentrated solution to a more concentrated solution.

Diffusion

Diffusion is a passive process by which molecules of a solute move through a cell membrane from an area of higher concentration to an area of lower concentration. Movement occurs (Fig. 39-3) until the concentrations are equivalent on both sides of the membrane.

> *For example, if you add cream to a cup of coffee, the cream is initially concentrated in the area where poured. However, very soon the cream becomes evenly dispersed throughout the coffee. If you stir the coffee, the cream disperses even more quickly.*

Fluids within the human body work on a similar principle; body movement speeds the diffusion of molecules. The rate of diffusion varies according to size of the molecules, concentration of the solution, and temperature of the solution:

- *Small molecules* move more rapidly than larger molecules.
- *Large differences in concentration* require a longer period of time to reach equilibration.
- *Higher temperatures* cause molecules to move faster, so that diffusion occurs more rapidly.

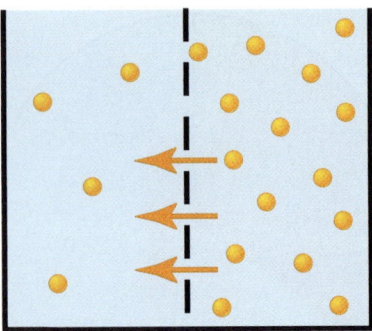

FIGURE 39-3 Diffusion is the movement of molecules of a solute through a cell membrane from an area of higher concentration to an area of lower concentration.

Filtration

Filtration is the movement of both water and smaller particles from an area of high pressure to one of low pressure (Fig. 39-4).

- **Hydrostatic pressure** is the force created by fluid within a closed system and is responsible for normal circulation of blood. Blood flows from the high-pressure arterial system to the lower pressure capillaries and veins. As fluid (plasma) moves through the capillary membrane, only solutes of a certain size can flow with it.

  For example, the membrane pores of Bowman's capsule in the kidneys are very small, and only albumin, the smallest of the proteins, can be filtered through the membrane. By contrast, the membrane pores of liver cells are extremely large, so a variety of solutes can pass through and be metabolized.

- **Osmotic pressure** is the power of a solution to draw water. A highly concentrated solution (many molecules in solution) has a high osmotic pressure and draws water. The plasma proteins in the blood exert osmotic (colloidal) pressure to help maintain fluid in the vascular space. When hydrostatic pressure exceeds osmotic pressure, fluid leaves the vessels.

- **Filtration pressure** is the net pressure created when hydrostatic pressure exceeds osmotic pressure. This pressure difference is the force that moves fluid and solutes. For example, the hydrostatic pressure is higher at the arteriole end of the capillary and lower at the venous end; thus, blood is forced out at the arteriole in and returned at the venule side.

Active Transport

Active transport occurs when molecules (e.g., electrolytes) move across cell membranes against a concentration gradient (from an area of low concentration to an area of high concentration). Active transport requires energy expenditure (Fig. 39-5).

- *Adenosine triphosphate* (ATP) is released from the cell to enable certain substances to acquire the energy needed to pass through the cell membrane. For example, sodium concentration is greater in ECF; therefore, sodium tends to enter by diffusion into the intracellular compartment.
- The *sodium-potassium pump,* which is located on the cell membrane, offsets the tendency of ATP. In the presence of ATP, the sodium-potassium pump actively moves sodium from the cell into the ECF and potassium from the ECF into the cell.

Active transport is vital for maintaining the unique composition of both the extracellular and intracellular compartments.

Table 39-2 summarizes the processes of fluid and electrolyte movement.

KnowledgeCheck 39-2

For each of the following, identify the appropriate mechanism: osmosis, diffusion, filtration, or active transport:

- Molecules move across a membrane to equalize concentration.
- Fluid moves across a membrane to equalize concentration.
- Molecules move against a concentration gradient.
- Molecules move to equalize pressure.

How Does the Body Regulate Fluids?

A balance between fluid intake and output is essential to maintain homeostasis. Excesses or deficits of intake or output can lead to severe disorders.

Fluid Intake

You have undoubtedly been told to drink 8 to 10 glasses of water per day or 1,920 to 2,400 mL of fluid. The Institute of Medicine (IOM) (2004), however, recommends a total fluid intake of 2,700 mL per day for women and 3,700 mL per day for men. Further, the IOM states that we should obtain 80% of this intake from drinking fluids and the remaining 20% from food and cellular metabolism of foods. Prolonged exercise and heat exposure increase the requirements. The IOM did not set an upper limit on fluid intake. A daily intake of 1,500 to 2,000 mL of noncaffeinated fluids will maintain hydration in older adults (Miller, 2012).

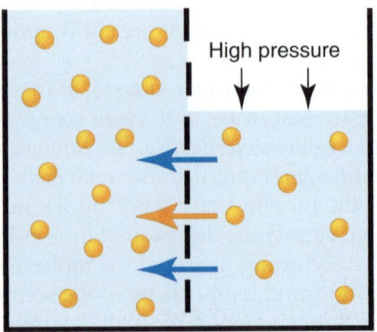

FIGURE 39-4 Filtration is the movement of water and smaller particles from an area of high pressure to an area of low pressure.

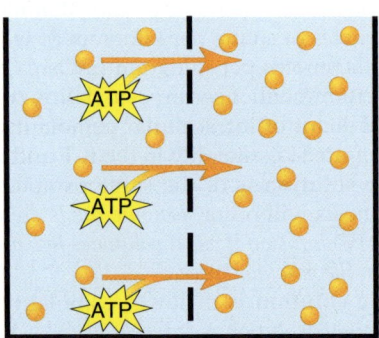

FIGURE 39-5 Active transport is the movement of electrolytes against a concentration gradient. For the movement to occur, active transport requires energy expenditure.

Table 39-2 ▶ Processes of Fluid and Electrolyte Movement

PROCESS	WHAT MOVES	FROM AREA OF	TO AREA OF
Diffusion	Molecules (solute)	High concentration	Low concentration
Active transport	Molecules (solute)	Low concentration	High concentration
Osmosis	Water	Low concentration	High concentration
Filtration	Water and small particles	High pressure	Low pressure

Thirst is the major regulator of fluid intake. Changes in plasma osmolality signal the thirst center in the hypothalamus, which leads to the urge to drink.

- *Situations that increase plasma osmolality (thereby promoting thirst)* include excessive fluid loss, excessive sodium intake, and decreased fluid intake.
- *Situations that inhibit the thirst mechanism* include a high intake of fluids, fluid retention, excessive IV infusion of hypotonic solutions, and low sodium intake.

Fluid Output

Fluid loss occurs throughout the day, creating a constant need to replenish fluid. In a healthy state, fluid losses are equivalent to fluid intake.

- **Sensible fluid loss** is measurable and/or perceived (e.g., urine, diarrhea, ostomy, and gastric drainage).
- **Insensible fluid loss** is loss that we do not perceive and is not easily measured, but accounts for about 900 mL per day. It occurs primarily by diffusion and evaporation through the skin, but also from the lungs. Insensible loss increases with open wounds, burns, or other breaks in the protective layer of the skin.

 The following are common sources of fluid loss:

- *Urine* (1,500 mL/day). Urine accounts for the greatest amount of fluid loss. Urine output varies according to intake and activity, but should remain at least 30 to 50 mL/hour. The volume of urine increases as intake increases, and it decreases to compensate for other fluid losses (e.g., vomiting and excessive perspiration).
- *Feces* (100 to 200 mL/day). Soft stools contain more water than hard stools. As stool frequency increases, water loss also increases.
- *Skin* (about 600 mL/day). Fever, exercise, and some disease processes increase metabolic activity and heat production, leading to increased fluid loss.
  - *Sensible (perceived) loss* through the skin occurs through perspiration. Perspiration varies based on temperature, skeletal muscle activity, and metabolic activity.
  - *Insensible loss* through the skin occurs through evaporation.
- *Lungs* (about 300 mL/day). Insensible loss occurs through the lungs as water is exhaled with each breath. An increase in respiratory rate increases the amount of fluid lost.

Hormonal Regulation

The kidneys are the principal regulator of fluid and electrolyte balance. The following hormones are involved:

Antidiuretic Hormone Pressure sensors in the vascular system stimulate or inhibit the release of **antidiuretic hormone (ADH)** from the pituitary gland. ADH causes the kidneys to retain fluid. If fluid volume within the vascular system is low, fluid pressures within the system decrease, and more ADH is released. If fluid volume (and therefore pressure) increases, less ADH is released, and the kidneys eliminate more fluid. ADH is also produced in response to a rise in serum osmolality, fever, pain, stress, and some opioids.

Renin–Angiotensin System When extracellular (i.e., intravascular) fluid volume is decreased, receptors in the glomeruli respond to the decreased perfusion of the kidneys by releasing renin. **Renin** is an enzyme responsible for the chain of reactions that converts angiotensinogen to angiotensin II. **Angiotensin II** acts on the nephrons to retain sodium and water and directs the adrenal cortex to release aldosterone.

Aldosterone When aldosterone is released, it stimulates the distal tubules of the kidneys to reabsorb sodium and excrete potassium. Sodium reabsorption results in passive reabsorption of water, thereby increasing plasma volume and improving kidney perfusion. When fluid excess is present, renin is not released and this process stops.

Other Hormones Other hormones affect fluid and electrolyte balance by their effect on certain organs of the body:

- *Thyroid hormone* affects fluid volume by influencing cardiac output. An increase in thyroid hormone causes an increase in cardiac output, thereby increasing glomerular filtration rate and urine output. A decrease has the opposite effect.
- *Atrial natriuretic peptide (ANP), brain natriuretic peptide (BNP), and C-type natriuretic peptide (CNP)* are important in renal and cardiovascular regulation of fluid maintenance. **Natriuresis** (natriuretic) is the discharge of sodium through urine. All three of these peptides are produced by heart cells; in addition, BNP is also released from the brain. In clinical practice, BNP can be measured in the serum to help determine presence of heart failure with fluid excess and to distinguish heart failure from pulmonary edema. The test can be performed at the bedside.

Think**Like a Nurse** 39-2

Apply the information on fluid balance to the LaGuardia family (Meet Your Patients). What have you learned that helps you explain why some family members require hospitalization? What additional information do you need to be able to predict each person's fluid balance?

How Does the Body Regulate Electrolytes?

To maintain health, the body must balance electrolyte losses and intake. For example, potassium lost through diarrhea and vomiting must be replaced by dietary potassium or potassium supplements. Table 39-3 provides information about the function, regulation, and food sources of major

Table 39-3 ➤ Major Electrolytes

ELECTROLYTE	FUNCTION	REGULATION	SOURCES
Sodium (Na⁺) Major cation in the ECF *Normal serum level is 135–145 mEq/L	Regulates fluid volume. Helps maintain blood volume. Interacts with calcium to maintain muscle contraction. Stimulates conduction of nerve impulses.	Moves by active transport across cell membranes. Regulated by aldosterone and ADH levels. Reabsorbed and excreted through the kidneys. Minimal loss through perspiration and feces. Low sodium may be caused by excess water intake.	Table salt, soy sauce, cured pork, cheese, milk, processed foods, canned products, and foods preserved with salt.
Potassium (K⁺) Major cation in the ICF Normal serum level is 3.5–5 mEq/L	Maintains ICF osmolality. Regulates conduction of cardiac rhythm. Transmits electrical impulses in multiple body systems. Assists with acid–base balance.	Regulated by aldosterone. Excreted and conserved through the kidneys. Lost through vomiting and diarrhea. Loss triggered by many diuretics.	Common food sources include bananas, oranges, apricots, figs, dates, carrots, potatoes, tomatoes, spinach, dairy products, and meats.
Calcium (Ca²⁺) Most abundant electrolyte in the body Normal serum level is 8.5–10.5 mg/dL	Promotes transmission of nerve impulses. Major component of bone and teeth. Regulates muscle contractions. Maintains cardiac automaticity. Essential factor in the formation of blood clots. Catalyst for many cellular activities.	Combines with phosphorus to form the mineral salts of the teeth and bones. Calcium and phosphorus levels are inversely proportional. Parathyroid hormone (PTH) stimulates release of calcium from bones and reabsorption from kidneys and intestines. Calcitonin (from the thyroid) blocks bone breakdown and lowers calcium levels. Absorption is stimulated by vitamin D.	See Table 39-4 for average daily requirements. Common food sources include milk, milk products, dark green leafy vegetables, and salmon, as well as calcium-fortified foods such as breads and cereals.
Magnesium (Mg²⁺) Present in skeleton and ICF; second most abundant cation in ICF Normal serum level is 1.6–2.6 mEq/L	Involved in protein and carbohydrate metabolism. Necessary for protein and DNA synthesis within the cell. Maintains normal intracellular levels of potassium. Involved in electrical activity in nerve and muscle membranes, including the heart.	Ingested in the diet and absorbed through the small intestine. Excreted by kidneys. Loss may be triggered by diuretics, poorly controlled diabetes mellitus, and excess alcohol intake.	Average daily requirement is 18–30 mEq. Found in most foods, but high levels are present in green vegetables, cereal grains, and nuts.

Table 39-3 ➤ Major Electrolytes—cont'd

ELECTROLYTE	FUNCTION	REGULATION	SOURCES
	May have a role in regulating blood pressure and may influence the release and activity of insulin (Crawford & Harris, 2011a; Institute of Medicine, 2004).		
Chloride (Cl⁻) Major anion in the ECF Normal serum level is 95–105 mEq/L	Works with Na⁺ to maintain osmotic pressure between fluid compartments. Essential for production of HCl for gastric secretions. Functions as buffer in oxygen–carbon dioxide exchange in RBCs. Assists with acid–base balance.	Reabsorbed and excreted through the kidneys along with sodium. Levels increase and decrease simultaneously with sodium levels. Regulated by aldosterone and ADH levels. Deficits lead to potassium deficits; potassium deficits lead to chloride deficits.	Found in foods high in sodium.
Phosphate (PO₄⁻) Major anion in the ICF Normal serum level is 2.5–4.5 mg/dL	Serves as a catalyst for many intracellular activities. Promotes muscle and nerve action. Assists with acid–base balance. Important for cell division and transmission of hereditary traits.	Combines with calcium to form the mineral salts of the teeth and bones. Calcium and phosphorus levels are inversely proportional. Regulated by PTH; has inverse response to calcium. Excreted and reabsorbed by the kidneys.	Foods high in phosphorus are meat, fish, poultry, milk products, carbonated beverages, and legumes. Readily available in body as a result of metabolism.
Bicarbonate (HCO₃⁻) Major buffer in the body In ECF and ICF Normal serum level is 22–26 mEq/L	Maintains acid–base balance by functioning as the primary buffer in the body. Levels rise and fall to maintain pH.	Lost through diarrhea, diuretics, renal insufficiency. Excess possible if person ingests quantities of acid neutralizers.	Present in acid neutralizers (e.g., sodium bicarbonate).

*Note that normal ranges may differ among references and in different laboratories.
ADH = antidiuretic hormone; ECF = extracellular fluid; ICF = intracellular fluid; PTH = parathyroid hormone; RBC = red blood cell.

electrolytes in the body. Maintenance of normal serum electrolyte levels also depends on dietary intake, as well as various body regulatory mechanisms, discussed in the remainder of this section.

Sodium (Na⁺)

Sodium is the major cation in the ECF. Its primary function is to regulate fluid volume. When sodium is reabsorbed in the kidney, water and potassium are also reabsorbed, thereby maintaining ECF volume. Adults should limit the intake of salt to 2,300 mg/day (U.S. Department of Health and Human Services, U.S. Department of Agriculture, 2015). People who are especially sensitive to the blood pressure–raising effects of salt are advised to limit salt intake to 1,500 mg/day. This includes people (including children) with a chronic disease (e.g., hypertension, diabetes, chronic kidney disease), African Americans, and those older than age 51. This limitation applies to nearly half of the U.S. population.

Potassium (K⁺)

Potassium is the major cation of the ICF and a key electrolyte in cellular metabolism. Only 2% of body potassium is found in the extracellular fluid. *The Dietary Guidelines for Americans, 2015–2020* recommends that adults consume at least 4,700 mg/day. However, most people do not consume enough potassium. Moderate potassium deficiency is associated with increases in blood pressure, salt sensitivity, risk of kidney stones, and risk of bone turnover (U.S. Department of Health and Human Services, U.S. Department of Agriculture, 2015). Low intake of dietary potassium is associated with increased risk of stroke.

In a healthy person, a high potassium intake does not result in hyperkalemia because the kidneys efficiently eliminate excess dietary potassium. However, potassium should come from one's diet (e.g., fruit, vegetables) rather than from supplements (Bhatt, 2016).

Calcium (Ca²⁺)

Calcium is responsible for bone health and neuromuscular and cardiac function and is an essential factor in blood clotting. About 99% of body calcium is located in the bones and teeth. The remaining 1% circulates in the blood and affects system functions. Because calcium is so vital for cardiac and muscle function, serum levels are tightly regulated. As serum levels drop, calcium leaches from the bones into the blood to compensate.

Although calcium requirements are highest during childhood, adolescence, pregnancy, and breastfeeding, it should be a regular component of the diet throughout the life span (see Table 39-4). Most Americans do not include the recommended amount of calcium in their diets. Prolonged insufficient dietary intake can cause bone loss that leads to osteoporosis. People over the age of 50 are susceptible to osteoporosis, which can lead to fractures. You should teach patients that most calcium should be obtained from naturally calcium-rich foods, such as dairy products; however, calcium-fortified foods and calcium supplements can be used as a secondary source.

Magnesium (Mg²⁺)

Magnesium is a mineral used in more than 300 biochemical reactions in the body. Like calcium, only about 1% of magnesium is found in the blood. The remaining 99% is divided between the ICF and bone (in combination with calcium and phosphorus). Although magnesium deficiency is rare, you may find low levels in individuals who have a high alcohol intake. Some malabsorption disorders may also cause magnesium depletion.

Chloride (Cl⁻)

Chloride is the most abundant anion in the extracellular fluid. It is usually bound with other ions, especially sodium or potassium (e.g., as sodium chloride, or salt). A healthy adult between the ages of 19 and 50 should consume 2.3 grams of chloride each day along with 1.5 grams of sodium to replace daily losses and maintain serum blood levels (Baker, 2015; IOM, 2004).

Phosphorus (Phosphate [PO₄⁻])

Phosphate in the ECF is known as **phosphorus.** Most phosphorus in the body is combined with oxygen, forming **phosphate**—mostly bound with calcium in teeth and bones as calcium phosphate.

Phosphate is the most abundant *intracellular* anion. Phosphate and calcium exist in an inverse relationship; as one increases, the other one decreases. As a result, high blood phosphate levels decrease the movement of calcium from the bones.

Bicarbonate (HCO₃⁻)

Bicarbonate is present in both ICF and ECF. The kidneys regulate extracellular bicarbonate to maintain acid–base balance. When serum levels rise, the kidneys excrete excess bicarbonate. If serum levels are low, the kidneys conserve bicarbonate. Bicarbonate is not consumed in the diet but is produced by the body to meet current needs.

KnowledgeCheck 39-3

- Identify the major functions of sodium, potassium, calcium, magnesium, chloride, phosphate, and bicarbonate.
- What are the major concerns associated with sodium and potassium intake?
- Identify at least five potassium-rich foods.
- Identify the ideal calcium intakes for each member of the LaGuardia family (Meet Your Patients).

ThinkLike a Nurse 39-3

Based on the information you have learned about the major electrolytes of the body, which electrolytes are most likely to be out of balance in members of the LaGuardia family. Explain your answer.

How Is Acid–Base Balance Regulated?

Acids and bases are formed in the body as part of normal metabolic processes.

- An **acid** is any compound that contains hydrogen ions (H⁺) that can be released. For this reason, acids are referred to as *cation donors* (a **cation** is a positively charged particle). A common strong acid is hydrochloric acid (HCl), which is present in gastric secretions.
- A **base** or **alkali** is a compound that combines with (accepts) hydrogen ions in solution. Therefore, bases are referred to as *cation acceptors*. A strong base has a tendency to bind hydrogen ions, whereas a weak base binds only a small portion of the available hydrogen ions.

pH Measurement The amount of acid or base present in a solution is measured as **pH.** The pH is reported on a scale of 1 to 14: 1 to 6.9 is acidic, 7 is neutral, and 7.1 to 14 is basic, or alkaline. The stronger an *acid* is, the lower the pH will be. In contrast, a strong *base* has a high pH. The pH is a *logarithmic* scale. For example, a pH of 4 is 10 times more acidic than a pH of 5. The body functions normally within a narrow range of pH values.

- *Normal serum pH*—Arterial blood and tissue fluid normally have a pH of 7.35 to 7.45; therefore, they are slightly alkaline.
- *A serum pH below 7.30 or above 7.52* alters enzymatic activity and creates myocardial irritability.
- *A serum pH below 6.9 or above 7.8* is usually fatal.

Three complex mechanisms maintain acid–base balance: (1) buffers, (2) respiratory control of carbon dioxide, and (3) renal regulation of bicarbonate (HCO₃⁻).

Buffers

Buffer systems prevent wide swings in pH. A **buffer system** consists of a weak acid and a weak base. Buffer molecules keep strong acids or bases from altering the pH either by absorbing or releasing free hydrogen ions.

Carbonic Acid–Sodium Bicarbonate System KEY POINT: *Carbonic acid (H₂CO₃) and sodium bicarbonate (NaHCO₃) buffer almost 90% of metabolic processes in the ECF.* Blood and tissue fluids depend on this buffer system to maintain a relatively constant pH. During normal metabolism, blood and tissue fluids tend to become acidic; therefore, more sodium bicarbonate is required than carbonic acid.

- *The usual ratio of NaHCO₃ to H₂CO₃ is 20:1.* As long as this ratio is maintained, the pH remains within its normal range.

Table 39-4 ➤ Recommended Daily Allowances (RDA) for Calcium and Vitamin D*

AGE	CALCIUM (MILLIGRAMS)	VITAMIN D* (INTERNATIONAL UNITS)
Birth to 6 months	200	400
6–12 months	260	400
1–3 years	700	600
4–8 years	1,000	600
9–13 years	1,300	600
14–18 years	1,300	600
19–30 years	1,000	600
31–50 years	1,000	600
51–70 years, males	1,000	600
51–70 years, females	1,200	600
Older than 70 years	1,200	800
Pregnant or Lactating Women		
18 years or younger pregnant or lactating	1,300	600
19–50 years	1,000	600

*Adequate intake of Vitamin D is necessary for absorption of calcium.
Source: National Institutes of Health, Office of Dietary Supplements. (2016). *Calcium, dietary supplement fact sheet.* Retrieved from https://ods.od.nih.gov/factsheets/Calcium-HealthProfessional/#h2; U.S. Department of Health and Human Services, U.S. Department of Agriculture. (2015). *Dietary guidelines for Americans, 2015–2020* (8th ed.). Retrieved from https://health.gov/dietaryguidelines/2015/resources/2015-2020_Dietary_Guidelines.pdf

- *If bicarbonate is depleted* while neutralizing a strong acid, the pH may drop below 7.35, resulting in a condition called **acidosis.**
- *If carbonic acid is depleted* (by adding a strong base to extracellular fluid), the pH may rise above 7.45, resulting in a condition called **alkalosis.**

Phosphate System The phosphate system helps regulate acid–base balance in intracellular fluids. The phosphate system works in the same way as the bicarbonate system but converts *alkaline* sodium phosphate (Na_2HPO_4) to *acid* sodium phosphate (NaH_2PO_4).

Protein System Plasma proteins and the globin portion of hemoglobin (in red blood cells) contain chemical groups that can either combine with or free up hydrogen ions. This system helps buffer intracellular fluid and plasma to maintain pH balance.

Respiratory Mechanisms

KEY POINT: *The lungs are the second line of defense to restore normal pH.* They control the body's carbonic acid supply via carbon dioxide retention or removal to maintain the 20:1 ratio of base to acid.

- *When the serum pH is too acidic (pH is low),* the lungs remove carbon dioxide through rapid, deep breathing. This reduces the amount of carbon dioxide available to make carbonic acid.
- *When the serum pH is too alkaline (pH is high),* the lungs try to conserve carbon dioxide through shallow respirations.

Renal Mechanisms

KEY POINT: *The last line of defense is the kidneys, which regulate the concentration of plasma bicarbonate.* They can neutralize more acid or base than either the respiratory system or the chemical buffers.

- *If the serum pH is too acidic,* the kidneys conserve additional bicarbonate to neutralize the acid.
- *If the serum pH is too alkaline,* the kidneys excrete additional bicarbonate to lower the amount of base and thereby decrease the pH.
- The kidneys also buffer pH by forming acids and ammonium (a base).

Compensation Although the renal system is very effective at altering pH, it is slow. It may take up to 3 days to return the pH to normal limits. This process is known as **compensation.** The pH returns to normal, but the carbon dioxide or bicarbonate level is abnormal. Over time, or when the original problem is corrected, these levels also return to normal.

KnowledgeCheck 39-4

- Briefly describe the three mechanisms used to maintain pH.
- Rank in order the acid–base balance mechanisms from the most rapidly acting to the slowest acting.

IMBALANCES: FLUID, ELECTROLYTE, AND ACID–BASE

Illness or disease may lead to imbalances of fluid, electrolytes, or pH. These are discussed in the next sections. The Practical Knowledge section, later in this chapter, presents some interventions to correct these imbalances.

Example Problem: Fluid Imbalances

Fluid imbalances involve a deficit or excess in fluid volume or an alteration in distribution among the fluid compartments. Concepts used to describe fluid imbalances are *hypovolemia* (fluid deficit) and *hypervolemia* (fluid excess) (*hypo* = low, *vol* = volume, *emia* pertains to blood).

Deficient Fluid Volume

Deficient fluid volume (hypovolemia) occurs when there is a proportional loss of fluid and electrolytes from the ECF from various causes (e.g., surgery, trauma, uterine rupture).

Dehydration

Dehydration describes a state of negative fluid balance in which there is a loss of water (*hydro* = water) from the intracellular, extracellular, or intravascular spaces. Dehydration can be categorized by three causes:

1. *Insufficient fluid intake* (e.g., as may occur with depression, sedation, or alcohol abuse)
2. *Excessive fluid loss* (e.g., bleeding, diarrhea, vomiting)
3. *Fluid shifts* (e.g., intravascular fluid leak into body tissues, burns)

The first symptom of dehydration is thirst. Patients usually respond by drinking liquids. If the patient is unable to drink, if fluids are not provided, or if blood loss exceeds replacement fluids (e.g., hemorrhage), a fluid deficit occurs. At that point, the heart rate increases and the blood vessels constrict. This increases the blood pressure to help circulate the remaining fluid to meet the body's fluid demands.

Continuing Fluid Loss (Hypovolemic Shock)

As volume loss continues, the heart pumps faster but less powerfully, resulting in a rapid, weak pulse and orthostatic hypotension. This is known as **hypovolemic shock.** Water is pulled from the interstitial spaces and the ICF into the vascular system, resulting in dry skin and mucous membranes, decreased skin and tongue turgor, decreased urine output, and flat neck veins. Patients complain of muscle weakness, fatigue, and feeling warm. Temperature increases because the body is

 less able to cool itself through perspiration. However, body temperature in older adults may not be elevated above normal.

Assessing for and Preventing Deficient Fluid Volume

Check for the early symptoms of dehydration, mentioned previously. Assess the blood pressure when the patient is lying, sitting, and standing. A drop in the systolic blood pressure (BP) (from lying to sitting or standing) of 20 mm Hg or more is called **orthostatic hypotension.** Low fluid volume is only one of its causes. Other assessments include the following:

- **KEY POINT:** *Weight is a sensitive measure of fluid loss. A sudden loss of body weight of 5% is clinically significant, severe at 8%, and usually fatal at 15%.*
- Blood urea nitrogen (BUN)-to-creatinine ratio and hematocrit are elevated because there is less water in proportion to the solid substances.
- Urine specific gravity increases as the kidneys attempt to conserve water, resulting in more concentrated urine.

Patients at highest risk for dehydration are older adults, infants, children, and any patients with conditions associated with fluid loss (e.g., diabetes insipidus, vomiting, diarrhea, fever). See the Planning Interventions/Implementation section for ways to facilitate intake and provide parenteral fluids.

Excess Fluid Volume (Hypervolemia)

Excessive retention of sodium and water in the ECF increases osmotic pressure and causes fluid to shift from the cells into

the ECF. **Excess fluid volume** (hypervolemia) can result from excessive salt intake, disease affecting kidney or liver function, or poor pumping action of the heart.

- **Signs of Fluid Overload**—Elevated blood pressure, bounding pulse, increased shallow respirations, and cool pale skin; neck veins may become distended. **Edema** occurs when excess ECF accumulates in the tissues, especially in dependent areas; rapid weight gain also occurs.

  In severe fluid overload, the patient develops moist crackles in the lungs, dyspnea, and **ascites** (excess peritoneal fluid). Hemodilution causes BUN, hematocrit, and specific gravity of the urine to decrease.
- **Preventing Fluid Overload**—Monitor intake and output and carefully regulate intravenous infusions, using electronic pumps. See Planning Interventions/Implementation section for additional measures.

KnowledgeCheck 39-5

- Define *deficient fluid volume* and *excess fluid volume.*
- Identify the signs and symptoms of deficient fluid volume and excess fluid volume.
- Describe dehydration and hypervolemia.

Example Problem: Electrolyte Imbalances

Any electrolyte may become imbalanced. Table 39-5 discusses the common causes, signs and symptoms, and treatment of sodium, potassium, calcium, magnesium, and phosphate imbalances.

We can apply the information in Table 39-5 to the LaGuardia family (Meet Your Patients). Jackson LaGuardia has renal disease and is at risk for electrolyte imbalances. Now he is experiencing nausea, vomiting, and diarrhea. This will further aggravate the imbalance of potassium and sodium. He requires careful monitoring of all of his electrolytes and may need fluid replacement (rehydration). He is a candidate for admission to the hospital. The remaining family members are likely to be experiencing sodium, potassium, and fluid deficits.

ThinkLike a Nurse 39-4

Martha LaGuardia (Meet Your Patients) is taking the following medications: atenolol 50 mg daily at bedtime, alendronate sodium 10 mg daily, furosemide 20 mg every morning, and calcium carbonate 500 mg three times per day. Using your reference books, look up her prescribed medications. Given that Ms. LaGuardia is now experiencing nausea and vomiting, she may be at risk for developing medication-related side effects and problems. Which medications may cause problems? What problems might they cause? Explain why.

Example Problem: Acid–Base Imbalances

The two broad types of acid–base imbalance are acidosis and alkalosis:

- **Acidosis** occurs when the serum pH falls below 7.35.
- **Alkalosis** occurs when the serum pH increases above 7.45 (Fig. 39-6).

  Arterial blood gases (ABGs) are used to monitor acid–base balance. **ABG analysis** measures pH, partial pressure of oxygen (P_{O_2}), partial pressure of carbon dioxide (P_{CO_2}), saturation of

Table 39-5 ➤ Electrolyte Imbalances

DISORDER	COMMON CAUSES	SIGNS AND SYMPTOMS	TREATMENT
Hyponatremia $Na^+ < 135$ mEq/L	Diuretics GI fluid loss Adrenal insufficiency Excessive intake of hypotonic solutions, such as water or D_5W IV fluids Syndrome of inappropriate ADH	Anorexia, nausea, and vomiting Weakness Lethargy Confusion Muscle cramps or twitching Seizures	Monitor I&O. Monitor sodium level. Increase oral sodium intake. Administer IV saline infusion and take seizure precautions, if severe.

Hypernatremia $Na^+ > 145$ mEq/L	Excessive sodium intake
	
	Water deprivation
	
	Increased water loss through profuse sweating, heat stroke, or diabetes insipidus
	
	Administration of hypertonic tube feeding
		Thirst
		
		Elevated temperature
		
		Dry mouth and sticky mucous membranes
		
		If severe:
		  Hallucinations
		  Irritability
		  Lethargy
		  Seizures
			Monitor I&O.
			
			Monitor sodium level.
			
			Monitor vital signs and level of consciousness.
			
			Restrict sodium in the diet.
			
			Beware of hidden sodium in foods and medications.
			
			Increase water intake.
			
			Administer IV solutions that do not contain sodium.

Hypokalemia $K^+ < 3.5$ mEq/L	Diuretics GI fluid loss through vomiting, gastric suction, or diarrhea Steroid administration Hyperaldosteronism Anorexia or bulimia	Fatigue Anorexia, nausea, and vomiting Muscle weakness Decreased GI motility Dysrhythmias Paresthesia Flat T wave on ECG Increased sensitivity to digitalis	Monitor I&O. Monitor potassium level. If the client is taking digoxin, monitor pulse and observe for toxicity. Encourage intake of foods rich in potassium. Administer potassium supplements. ➕ (*Note:* IV supplements must be well diluted and administered into a central vein slowly.)
Hyperkalemia $K^+ > 5.0$ mEq/L	Renal failure Potassium-sparing diuretics Hypoaldosteronism High potassium intake coupled with renal insufficiency Acidosis Major trauma Hemolyzed serum sample produces pseudohyperkalemia	Muscle weakness Dysrhythmias Flaccid paralysis Intestinal colic Tall T waves on ECG	Monitor I&O. Monitor potassium level. Caution about potassium-rich food intake in patients with elevated creatinine levels.
Hypocalcemia $Ca^{2+} < 8.5$ mg/dL	Hypoparathyroidism Malabsorption Pancreatitis	Diarrhea Numbness and tingling of extremities	Monitor I&O. Monitor serum calcium.

(Continued)

Table 39-5 ➤ Electrolyte Imbalances—cont'd

DISORDER	COMMON CAUSES	SIGNS AND SYMPTOMS	TREATMENT
	Alkalosis Vitamin D deficiency	Muscle cramps Tetany Convulsions Laryngeal spasms Cardiac irritability *Positive Trousseau's and Chvostek's signs	Encourage increased calcium intake. Administer calcium supplements. If severe, monitor patency of airway, institute seizure and safety precautions, and administer parenteral calcium.
Hypercalcemia Ca^{2+} > 10.5 mg/dL	Hyperparathyroidism Malignant bone disease Prolonged immobilization Excess calcium supplementation Thiazide diuretics	Muscle weakness Constipation Anorexia, nausea, and vomiting Polyuria and polydipsia Kidney stones Bizarre behavior Bradycardia	Monitor I&O. Encourage fluid intake to prevent stone formation. Encourage fiber to prevent constipation. Eliminate calcium supplements and limit calcium-rich foods. Avoid calcium-based antacids. Renal dialysis may be required.
Hypomagnesemia Mg^{2+} < 1.6 mEq/L	Chronic alcoholism Malabsorption Diabetic ketoacidosis Prolonged gastric suction	Neuromuscular irritability Disorientation Mood changes Dysrhythmias Increased sensitivity to digitalis	Monitor I&O. Encourage foods high in magnesium. Avoid alcohol intake. If the client is taking digoxin, monitor pulse and observe for toxicity.
Hypermagnesemia Mg^{2+} > 2.6 mEq/L	Renal failure Adrenal insufficiency Excess replacement	Flushing and warmth of skin Hypotension Drowsiness, lethargy Hypoactive reflexes Depressed respirations Bradycardia	Monitor vital signs and airway. Monitor reflexes. Avoid magnesium-based antacids and laxatives. Restrict dietary intake of foods high in magnesium.
Hypophosphatemia PO_4^- < 2.5 mg/dL	Refeeding after starvation Alcohol withdrawal Diabetic ketoacidosis Respiratory acidosis	Paresthesia Joint stiffness Seizures Cardiomyopathy Impaired tissue oxygenation	Monitor serum phosphorus level. Monitor calcium levels as phosphate is replaced. Start TPN slowly to avoid drops in phosphate.
Hyperphosphatemia PO_4^- > 4.5 mg/dL	Renal failure Hyperthyroidism Chemotherapy Excess use of phosphate-based laxative	Short term: tetany symptoms—tingling of extremities and cramping Long term: Calcification in soft tissue	Monitor serum phosphorus level. Monitor for tetany. If severe, administer aluminum hydroxide with meals to bind phosphorus.

*See Clinical Insight 39-1.
ADH = antidiuretic hormone; ECG = electrocardiogram; GI = gastrointestinal; I&O = intake and output; TPN = total parenteral nutrition.
Source: Van Leeuwen, A., & Bladh, M. (2015). *Davis's comprehensive handbook of laboratory & diagnostic tests with nursing implications* (6th ed.). Philadelphia, PA: F.A. Davis.

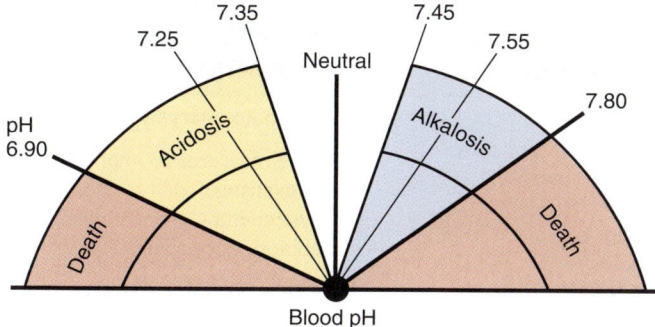

FIGURE 39-6 The pH scale ranges from 1 to 14. Normal blood pH is 7.35 to 7.45.

oxygen (SaO_2), and bicarbonate (HCO_3^-) level. **KEY POINT:** *Acid–base balance is reflected by the pH, PcO_2, and HCO_3 values.*

- *A respiratory disturbance alters the carbonic acid portion of the buffering system, and the resulting imbalance is labeled* **respiratory acidosis** *or* **respiratory alkalosis**.
- *A metabolic disturbance alters the bicarbonate portion of the buffering system, so the resulting imbalance would be labeled as* **metabolic acidosis** *or* **metabolic alkalosis**.

Metabolic and respiratory problems can coexist, resulting in disturbances of both sides of the buffering system. Compensatory mechanisms may also produce both bicarbonate and carbon dioxide abnormalities.

Interpreting ABGs

To determine acid–base balance, you must examine the ABG results. The pH, PcO_2, and HCO_3^- values are of primary importance (Table 39-6). The partial pressure of oxygen (PO_2) and saturation of oxygen (SaO_2) are also part of the ABG result, but they affect tissue oxygenation (also see Chapter 36). Table 39-7 describes the causes, manifestations, ABG results, and treatments of acid–base imbalances. Use the following steps to interpret acid–base balance of blood:

Step 1: Examine the pH. *Is it acidotic, alkalotic, or normal?*

- If the pH is low (< 7.35), the blood is *acidic*.
- If the pH is high (> 7.45), the blood is *alkalotic*.
- If the pH is between 7.35 and 7.45, the blood is *normal*.

KEY POINT: *Don't forget that neutral pH is 7.4. This will be very important when we discuss compensation.*

Step 2: Check the amount of carbon dioxide in the blood (PcO_2). *Is there too little or too much?*

- If PcO_2 is < 35 mm Hg—there is too little acid in the blood (*respiratory alkalosis*).
- If PcO_2 is > 45 mm Hg—there is too much acid in the blood (*respiratory acidosis*).
- If PcO_2 is 35 to 45 mm Hg—the cause for the *abnormal pH is not respiratory*.

Step 3: Think about the bicarbonate level (HCO_3). *Is there too little or too much?*

- If HCO_3 is < 22 mEq/L—there is too little base in the blood (*metabolic acidosis*).
- If HCO_3 is > 26 mEq/L—there is too much base in the blood (*metabolic alkalosis*).
- If HCO_3 is 22 to 26 mEq/L—the cause for the *abnormal pH is not metabolic*.

UNCOMPENSATED ABG	pH	$Paco_2$	HCO_3
Respiratory acidosis	↓	↑	normal
Respiratory alkalosis	↑	↓	normal
Metabolic acidosis	↓	normal	↓
Metabolic alkalosis	↑	normal	↑

Step 4: Is there compensation? *If so, is it partially or fully?*

Now let's look at what happens when the acid–base imbalance continues for a period of time.

KEY POINT: *The body will naturally try to correct the unhealthy situation by using the lungs and kidneys to buffer the abnormality and return the pH into a normal range.*

- **If breathing is the reason** *for the abnormal pH, then the kidneys will pick up the slack and try to improve the situation.*
- **If the problem is metabolic,** *then breathing (either faster and deeper or slower and more shallow) is the answer.*

Table 39-6 ➤ Using ABGs To Assess Acid–Base Balance

EXPLANATION OF CHANGES	ABG COMPONENT	NORMAL RANGE	ACIDOSIS	ALKALOSIS
Indicates acidosis, alkalosis, or normal acid–base balance.	pH	7.35–7.45 (7.4 is "neutral")	Low	High
Carbon dioxide ("acid"). Signals respiratory cause.	PcO_2	35–45 mm Hg	High	Low
Sodium bicarbonate ("base"). Signals metabolic cause.	HCO_3^-	22–26 mEq/L	Low	High

Table 39-7 ➤ Acid–Base Imbalances

DISORDER	CLINICAL MANIFESTATIONS	INTERVENTIONS
Respiratory Acidosis May be caused by conditions or medications that impair gas exchange at the alveolar–capillary membrane, depressed respiratory rate and depth, or injury to the respiratory center in the brain.	*Acute:* Increased pulse and respiratory rate Headache, dizziness Confusion, decreased level of consciousness (LOC) Muscle twitching *Chronic:* Weakness Headache	Provide pulmonary hygiene. Institute measures to improve gas exchange, such as chest physiotherapy, bronchodilators, antibiotics possible. Provide supplemental oxygen. Maintain hydration.
Respiratory Alkalosis May be caused by hyperventilation resulting from anxiety, fever, sepsis, thyrotoxicosis, lesion in the respiratory center in the brain, or excessive ventilation with a mechanical ventilator.	Confusion, difficulty focusing Headache Tingling Palpitations Tremors	If caused by anxiety, encourage the patient to relax and breathe slowly. For other causes: Identify and treat the underlying disorder.
Metabolic Acidosis May be caused by retained acids in the blood resulting from renal impairment, poorly controlled diabetes mellitus, or starvation. Conditions that decrease bicarbonate, such as excessive GI loss, will also trigger metabolic acidosis. May be caused by excessive intake of acids, which may occur with aspirin poisoning, or by prolonged infusion of chloride-containing IV fluids.	Headache Confusion, drowsiness Weakness Peripheral vasodilatation Nausea and vomiting Kussmaul's breathing (rapid and deep) Frequently associated with hyperkalemia	Treatment is directed at correcting the underlying problem. Bicarbonate may be ordered.
Metabolic Alkalosis May be caused by excessive acid loss due to vomiting or gastric suction, use of potassium-wasting diuretics, hypokalemia, excess bicarbonate intake, or hyperaldosteronism.	Dizziness Tingling of extremities Hypertonic muscles Decreased respiratory rate and depth	Treatment is directed at correcting the underlying problem. Treatment often includes administration of NaCl-rich fluids.

No Compensation If the pH is abnormal, no compensation has occurred. The following example shows a low pH level and a high level of carbon dioxide. This is respiratory acidosis with no compensation.

$$pH = 7.30, P_{CO_2} = 50 \text{ mm Hg}, HCO_3^- = 24 \text{ mEq/L}$$

Partial Compensation If the *pH and one ABG component are abnormal*, the *second ABG* value is starting to change, and the *pH is moving toward normal*, then partial compensation is taking place. Consider the following example of *partially compensated respiratory acidosis:*

$$pH = 7.32, P_{CO_2} = 50 \text{ mm Hg}, HCO_3^- = 28 \text{ mEq/L}$$

In this example, although the pH is increasing, it is still acidotic, and the P_{CO_2} remains high. Note that the HCO_3 is increasing to alkalosis to bring the pH closer to normal.

PARTIAL COMPENSATION	pH	Paco₂	HCO₃
Respiratory acidosis	↓	↑	↑
Respiratory alkalosis	↑	↓	↓
Metabolic acidosis	↓	↓	↓
Metabolic alkalosis	↑	↑	↑

Full Compensation Full compensation occurs when the *pH returns to normal range* and *both other ABG components are abnormal*. The initial causal component is still abnormal, and the second ABG component (that had the normal values) has changed enough to return the pH to normal. Note in the blood gas below, the pH is now in the normal range and the P_{CO_2} is still high. But the HCO_3 is now also high; it has moved enough to raise the pH into the normal range. The problem is now *fully compensated respiratory acidosis.*

$$pH = 7.35, Pco_2 = 50 \text{ mm Hg}, HCO_3^- = 30 \text{ mEq/L}$$

FULL COMPENSATION	pH	Paco$_2$	HCO$_3$
Respiratory acidosis	Normal, but < 7.35	↑	↑
Respiratory alkalosis	Normal, but > 7.45	↓	↓
Metabolic acidosis	Normal, but < 7.35	↓	↓
Metabolic alkalosis	Normal, but > 7.45	↑	↑

KnowledgeCheck 39-6

Interpret the following ABG results:

pH = 7.53   Pco_2 = 26 mm Hg   HCO$_3^-$ = 22 mEq/L
pH = 7.40   Pco_2 = 39 mm Hg   HCO$_3^-$ = 25 mEq/L
pH = 7.30   Pco_2 = 70 mm Hg   HCO$_3^-$ = 30 mEq/L
pH = 7.48   Pco_2 = 46 mm Hg   HCO$_3^-$ = 30 mEq/L

PracticalKnowledge
knowing **how**

In the remainder of this chapter, you will learn to apply theoretical knowledge of fluids, electrolytes, and acid–base balance to patient care.

ASSESSMENT NP

The purposes of a focused assessment for the Example Problem: Fluid, Electrolyte, and Acid–Base Imbalances are to identify clients at risk for or already experiencing imbalances, to identify the nature of the disorder, and to evaluate responses to treatments. The assessment includes a focused nursing history, a physical assessment, and a review of pertinent laboratory tests.

- **A focused nursing history** for fluids, electrolytes, and acid–base balance includes questions about demographic data, past medical history, current health concerns, food and fluid intake, fluid elimination, medications, and lifestyle (see the accompanying Focused Assessment box for complete guidelines).
- **A focused physical assessment** requires you to correlate physical assessment data with the nursing history and laboratory studies (see the accompanying Focused Assessment box).

KnowledgeCheck 39-7

- Identify 10 physical assessment components that can be used to monitor fluid, electrolyte, and acid–base balance (refer to the Focused Assessment box).
- What aspects should be evaluated in a nursing history focused on fluid, electrolyte, and acid–base balance?

Early Treatment of Metabolic Acidosis

Situation: Several family members are being seen in the emergency department for suspected food poisoning. The grandfather, who has chronic kidney disease (CKD), is diagnosed with metabolic acidosis and admitted for treatment. The nurse wonders about the rationale for the treatments the patient receives.

PICOT Components:

P	Population/client	=	Patients with CKD
I	Intervention/indicator	=	Early metabolic acidosis treatment
C	Comparator/control	=	Late or no treatment for metabolic acidosis
O	Outcome	=	Reduced muscle wasting
T	Time	=	The course of the disease

Searchable Question: Do _____(P) who receive/are exposed to _____(I), as compared to _____(C), demonstrate _____(O) during _____(T)?

Example of Evidence: The kidneys regulate fluid, electrolyte, and acid–base homeostasis. When these balances are altered, a client with CKD commonly develops chronic metabolic acidosis. This can lead to acceleration of the CKD, muscle wasting, development of bone disease, resistance to insulin, and increased mortality. Metabolic acidosis can be treated early in renal disease with oral medications or the addition of bases to dialysate. This helps maintain a normal plasma bicarbonate level and prevent chronic CKD.

Practice Change: The nurse acquired new knowledge of the importance of early treatment of CKD and its potential for preventing muscle wasting and other CKD complications.

Sources: Campbell, D., & Weir, M. (2015). Defining, treating and understanding chronic kidney disease—a complex disorder. *Journal of Clinical Hypertension, 17*(7), 514–527; Kraut, J., & Madias, N. (2011). Consequences and therapy of the metabolic acidosis of chronic kidney disease. *Pediatric Nephrology, 26*(1), 19–28.

ThinkLike a Nurse 39-5

What vital sign changes would you expect to find when assessing Jackson LaGuardia (Meet Your Patients)?

Laboratory Studies

Several laboratory tests are performed to evaluate fluid, electrolyte, and acid–base status.

Complete Blood Count Fluid status is reflected in a **complete blood count (CBC),** which is a measure of red blood cells (RBCs), white blood cells (WBCs), and platelets. Included in the CBC is the hematocrit, a measure of the percentage of RBCs in whole blood.

- *As fluid levels decrease,* the hematocrit increases (because the percentage of blood made up by cells increases).
- *As fluid levels increase,* the hematocrit falls.

Assessing Fluids, Electrolytes, and Acid–Base Balance

Nursing History

Demographic Data
Age, gender, height, weight, body mass index

Past Medical History
➤ Have you ever been hospitalized or had surgery? If so, when and for what reason?
➤ For what healthcare problems are you currently being treated?
➤ Have you ever been diagnosed with kidney disease, high blood pressure, diabetes, or thyroid or parathyroid problems?

Current Health Concerns
➤ What symptoms are you currently experiencing?
➤ Have you recently experienced any of the following symptoms?

Excessive thirst	Difficulty breathing
Fever	Swelling of your hands, feet, or ankles
Excessive perspiration	
Nausea, vomiting, or diarrhea	Dizziness or feeling faint
	Muscle weakness
Dry skin or mucous membranes	Excessive fatigue
	Numbness, tingling, or cramping sensations
Dark, concentrated urine	
Limited amounts of urine	

➤ Is your weight stable? Have you had any recent changes in your weight?
➤ Do you believe you have any problems with fluid loss?

Food and Fluid Intake
➤ How much fluid do you usually drink in a 24-hour period?
➤ Do you believe you drink adequate amounts of fluid?
➤ Describe your usual diet.
➤ Have you recently changed your diet or fluid intake?
➤ Are you following a special diet?
➤ Have you ever been placed on a restricted diet?
➤ Have you experienced any recent changes in your appetite or thirst?
➤ Do you salt your food?
➤ Do you ever use a salt substitute?

Fluid Elimination
➤ How often do you urinate in a 24-hour period? Has that changed recently?
➤ How often do you get up during the night to urinate?
➤ Have you noticed any recent changes in the amount or appearance of your urine?
➤ How often do you experience vomiting, diarrhea, or constipation? Describe your experience.
➤ Do you have any wounds? If so, where are they and how did they happen? What is the color of drainage and how much drainage are you experiencing?
➤ Do you have any breaks in your skin? If so, describe the problem and show me the area.

Medications
➤ What prescribed medications do you currently take?
➤ What over-the-counter medications or alternative treatments do you use? Why do you use them?
➤ How often do you take laxatives or antacids?
➤ What vitamins, herbals, or supplements do you take?

Lifestyle
➤ What is your usual activity level?
➤ What type of exercise do you engage in? How often?
➤ How much fluid do you consume before, during, and after exercise?
➤ Do you drink alcohol? If so, how much do you consume in a day, a week?
➤ Do you smoke? If so, how much? For how long?
➤ Do you use any illegal medications or drugs?

Physical Assessments

Skin
Assess the skin for the following:
➤ Color and temperature may be cues to the presence of fever and circulation status.
➤ Moisture content offers some indication of fluid status. A diaphoretic client is losing fluid at a faster rate than a client with dry skin. Dry, scaling skin may indicate a fluid deficit. Any breaks in the skin are potential areas for fluid loss.
➤ Turgor varies with age, weight, and skin condition but does offer information on fluid status. Pinch the skin over the sternum. Normally skin immediately returns to its usual position. In fluid volume deficit or malnutrition the skin may remain "tented" for a period of time before returning to its original position. You must, however, correlate skin turgor with context and other clinical signs. For example, the skin loses elasticity with aging, so clients older than age 65 often have decreased turgor, which is normal for them.
➤ Edema in dependent areas is a cue for fluid volume excess. In an ambulatory client, assess the lower extremities and hands. In a bedridden client, edema will shift as the client is turned.
➤ To grade edema (on a scale +1 to +4, +1 represents minimal edema and +4 represents the most severe edema).

Mucous Membranes
➤ Inspect the tongue and buccal mucosa. Mouth breathing alone usually does not change these areas.
➤ Assess tongue turgor in all age-groups because it is not affected by age.
➤ Assess the color, moisture, and continuity of the mucous membranes
➤ Dry, cracked, or dull mucous membranes are signs of fluid volume deficit.

Cardiovascular System
➤ Assess vital signs (see later section).
➤ Pulse and blood pressure are affected by fluid and electrolyte status.
➤ If you suspect fluid volume deficit, assess for orthostatic hypotension:
  ➤ Assess blood pressure while client is lying or sitting.
  ➤ Have the client rise to a seated or standing position, and reassess the blood pressure (BP).
  ➤ A drop in systolic BP of > 15 mm Hg is a sign of orthostatic hypotension.
➤ Check capillary refill. Delayed capillary refill is a sign of fluid volume deficit; rapid capillary refill indicates adequate circulation and volume. If capillary refill is delayed, evaluate feet and hands bilaterally. Delays in just one area indicate impaired circulation to the extremity rather than volume changes.

Assessing Fluids, Electrolytes, and Acid–Base Balance—cont'd

➤ Assess venous filling by observing the jugular and hand veins. Flat jugular or hand veins indicate low fluid volume. Distended vessels are a sign of overload.

➤ Assess peripheral edema (discussed above).

Respiratory System

➤ Assess respiratory rate, depth, and pattern. The respiratory system rapidly responds to changes in pH. Similarly, alterations in gas exchange at the alveolar–capillary membrane may trigger pH changes.

➤ Assess breath sounds. Crackles or moist rales may indicate fluid overload. Areas of consolidation indicate impaired gas exchange.

Neurological System

➤ Assess level of consciousness and orientation.

➤ Assess neuromuscular irritability.

➤ Assess energy level and fatigue.

➤ Assess reflexes.

For specific neurological cues to alterations in fluid, electrolyte, or acid–base balance, see **Tables 39-5** and **39-7.**

Vital Signs

➤ Temperature. An elevated body temperature increases the loss of body fluids.

In hypernatremia, body temperature elevates because less fluid is available for sweating.

In uncomplicated fluid volume deficit, body temperature decreases.

➤ Pulse:

  ➤ Tachycardia is an early sign of fluid volume deficit.

  ➤ Pulse rate is affected by fluid status and some electrolytes (primarily sodium, potassium, calcium, and magnesium).

  ➤ Dysrhythmias are seen with potassium and magnesium imbalances.

The pulse volume is directly affected by fluid status. As fluid volume increases, the pulse volume also increases.

Similarly, a drop in fluid volume leads to a drop in pulse volume.

➤ Respiratory rate. Alterations in respiratory rate may cause acid–base imbalances or be associated with compensation for a metabolic disorder.

➤ Blood pressure:

  ➤ Assess for orthostatic hypotension (a drop in the systolic BP from lying or sitting to standing positions greater or equal to 20 mm Hg).

  ➤ Blood pressure rises and falls with fluid volume.

  ➤ Blood pressure is elevated by hypernatremia and fluid volume excess.

  ➤ Respiratory acidosis causes increased heart rate, resulting in BP elevation.

  ➤ High potassium intake may lower blood pressure.

Daily Weights

➤ Are an accurate method of assessing fluid status.

➤ Use the same balanced scale each day to monitor fluid status accurately.

➤ Weigh the client at the same time of day, making sure that the client is wearing the same amount of clothing.

➤ Each kilogram (2.2 lb) of weight is equivalent to 1 liter (1,000 mL) of fluid.

➤ For clients undergoing hemodialysis (blood cleansing through an artificial kidney), weigh the client before and after dialysis treatments. Many lose 3 to 4 kg (6.6 to 8.8 lb) after several hours of dialysis.

➤ You may institute weight monitoring as an independent nursing prescription, which can be delegated to an assistive personnel.

➤ Important when it is impractical or impossible to measure I&O accurately (breastfeeding intake, incontinence, draining wounds).

Fluid Intake and Output

See Clinical Insight 39-2.

Serum Electrolytes Venous blood samples are taken to measure sodium, potassium, chloride, and bicarbonate levels. In many labs, a basic metabolic panel also includes calcium, glucose, and the BUN/creatinine ratio, which are sensitive measures of fluid status and kidney function.

Serum Osmolality A measure of the solute concentration of the blood is **serum osmolality,** expressed as milliosmoles per kilogram (mOsm/kg). Changes in serum osmolality usually indicate alterations in sodium levels, because sodium is the greatest determinant of serum osmolality. Glucose and urea also contribute. Serum osmolality may be directly measured with venous blood, or estimated by doubling the serum sodium level.

■ In *fluid volume deficit,* serum osmolality rises.

■ In *fluid volume excess,* serum osmolality decreases.

Urine Osmolality The solute concentration of urine is measured by **urine osmolality.** The body excretes nitrogenous wastes and electrolytes. As a result, urine osmolality is substantially higher than serum levels.

■ *Fluid volume deficit* increases urine osmolality.

■ *Fluid volume excess* decreases urine osmolality.

This test may call for a 24-hour urine specimen, or for discarding the first morning specimen and collecting a clean-catch specimen 2 hours later.

Urinalysis The routine screening **urinalysis** includes a measure of urine pH and specific gravity. **KEY POINT:** *Urine pH normally ranges from 5.0 to 9.0, with an average of 6.0.*

■ *Urine pH*

  ■ Urine becomes *more acidic* in fluid volume deficit, acidosis, or starvation.

  ■ Urine becomes *more alkaline* with alkalosis.

■ *Specific gravity* rises and falls in opposition to fluid status.

  ■ A *low specific gravity* occurs when fluid is plentiful.

  ■ *Specific gravity* increases when fluid levels decrease and urine becomes more concentrated.

For a procedure for testing specific gravity of urine, see Procedure 30-3B: Measuring Specific Gravity of Urine (Refractometer) in Chapter 30.

Arterial Blood Gases Interpretation of ABGs was discussed earlier in this chapter. For a list of lab values for ABGs, refer to the Diagnostic Testing box Assessing Fluid, Electrolyte, and Acid–Base Balances.

Assessing Fluid, Electrolyte, and Acid–Base Balances

Venous Blood Sample | Normal Ranges

Venous Blood Sample	Normal Ranges
Sodium	135–145 mEq/L
Potassium	3.5–5 mEq/L
Chloride	97–107 mEq/L
Bicarbonate	22–26 mEq/L
BUN	10–31 mg/dL
Creatinine	0.5–1.2 mg/dL
Serum osmolality	275–295 mOsm/kg
Urine osmolality	250–900 mOsm/kg
Hematocrit	43%–49% in men
	38%–44% in menstruating women

Freshly Voided Urine Sample

pH	5.0–9.0
Specific gravity	1.001–1.029

Arterial Blood Sample

pH	7.35–7.45
P_{CO_2}	35–45 mm Hg
HCO_3^-	22–26 mEq/L

ANALYSIS/NURSING DIAGNOSIS NP

Nursing diagnoses directly related to fluid include Deficient Fluid Volume [isotonic], Excess Fluid Volume, Risk for Deficient Fluid Volume, and Risk for Imbalanced Fluid Volume.

Nursing diagnoses directly related to electrolyte or acid–base imbalances include Impaired Gas Exchange and Risk for Electrolyte Imbalance.

Imbalances (e.g., dehydration, metabolic acidosis, respiratory alkalosis) may also be etiologies of other nursing diagnoses. Below are a few examples:

- Activity Intolerance related to excess fluid and electrolyte loss through Diarrhea
- Impaired Oral Mucous Membrane Integrity related to Deficient Fluid Volume
- Decreased Cardiac Output related to hypovolemia

PLANNING OUTCOMES/EVALUATION NP

The overall goal for a client experiencing the Example Problem: Fluid, Electrolytes, and Acid–Base Imbalances is to restore balance.

NOC standardized outcomes for describing fluid and electrolyte status include:

Electrolyte & Acid/Base Balance—Balance of electrolytes and nonelectrolytes in the intracellular and extracellular compartments of the body

Electrolyte Balance—Concentration of serum ions necessary to maintain equilibrium among electrolytes

Fluid Balance—Water balance in the intracellular and extracellular compartments of the body

Fluid Overload Severity—Severity of signs and symptoms of excess intracellular and extracellular fluids

Hydration—Adequate water in the intracellular and extracellular compartments of the body

Individualized goals/outcome statements you might write for a client include the following examples:

- Maintains fluid balance, as evidenced by balanced 24-hour intake and output; good skin and tongue turgor; blood pressure and heart rate within normal limits; and no adventitious breath sounds.
- Electrolyte balance restored, as evidenced by alertness and cognitive orientation and no muscle cramping, seizures, or electrocardiogram changes.
- Drinks at least 2,500 mL in 24 hours.
- Urine specific gravity within normal limits.

PLANNING INTERVENTIONS/ IMPLEMENTATION NP

Examples of *NIC standardized interventions* related to the Example Problem: Fluid, Electrolyte, and Acid–Base Imbalances include the following:

Acid–Base Management—Promotion of acid–base balance and prevention of complications resulting from acid–base imbalance

Electrolyte Management—Promotion of electrolyte balance, prevention of complications resulting from abnormal or undesired serum electrolyte levels

Fluid Management—Promotion of fluid balance and prevention of complications resulting from abnormal or undesired fluid levels

Fluid/Electrolyte Management—Regulation and prevention of complications from altered fluid and/or electrolytes levels.

There are, of course, *specific* interventions for each type of fluid, acid–base, or electrolyte imbalance, for example:

Acid–Base Management: Metabolic Acidosis
Electrolyte Management: Hypernatremia
Fluid Management: Dehydration

Overall, nursing care focuses on preventing imbalances, modifying oral intake, providing parenteral fluids, and transfusing blood products as discussed in this chapter.

♥ iCare 39-1

Fluids, Electrolytes, and Acid–Base Balance

- Because an alteration in fluids, electrolytes, and acid–base balance encompasses such a wide variety of disease processes, nurses must possess keen assessment skills.
- Constant observation of a person's weight, laboratory values, eating habits/choices, and bowel and bladder habits is essential to proper care and management.
- Consideration of the patient's cultural and religious beliefs concerning fluids and artificial feeding should be explored and honored at all times. You may be involved in some of these conversations with patients/families. You are obligated to share their beliefs with other members of the healthcare team in order to provide a unified approach and to respect the patient's wishes—especially if it involves the withholding of fluids/feedings. If appropriate, you can suggest a palliative care consultation to help patients/families and teams.

PREVENTING FLUID AND ELECTROLYTE IMBALANCES

It is better to prevent imbalances than to treat them. Use the data obtained from your assessment to plan with your client to avoid imbalances. Common strategies are listed in the accompanying Self-Care box Teaching Patients to Prevent Fluid and Electrolyte Imbalances.

Dietary Changes

To promote fluid and electrolyte balance, most people need to limit their sodium intake and increase their dietary potassium and calcium. Some may need oral electrolyte supplements as well. Teach clients to eat foods rich in potassium and calcium daily, to avoid sodium-rich foods (e.g., processed foods), and to read food labels to identify the percentage of each (see Chapter 28 to review foods, as needed).

Oral Electrolyte Supplements

Many clients are unable to correct electrolyte disturbances with dietary changes alone. This is especially true for clients who have food intolerances, who rely on prepared meals, or who live in group settings. Such clients may need oral

supplements to meet their daily dietary requirements. Potassium and calcium are among the most common supplements. 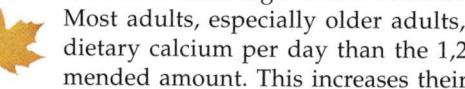 Most adults, especially older adults, consume less dietary calcium per day than the 1,200-mg recommended amount. This increases their risk of osteoporosis and fractures. Calcium supplements come in tablet, liquid, and chewable forms. Potassium supplements are available in pill and liquid forms. Many supplements have an unpleasant taste. To promote patient compliance, see suggested nursing activities in the Self-Care box Taking Oral Electrolyte Supplements.

KnowledgeCheck 39-8

- Identify laboratory tests that monitor fluid, electrolyte, and acid–base balance.
- Give at least five strategies to prevent fluid and electrolyte imbalance.

Modifying Oral Fluid Intake

Clients experiencing fluid imbalances may need to restrict or increase their daily oral intake to correct the underlying disorder.

Teaching Patients to Prevent Fluid and Electrolyte Imbalances

- ➤ Teach the client about usual fluid needs and circumstances that increase fluid needs: high environmental temperature, fever, gastrointestinal fluid loss, or draining wounds. Base your teaching on the client's current intake and the changes required to meet fluid goals.
- ➤ Identify medications or conditions that place the client at risk for imbalances. For example, if the client is receiving a potassium-wasting diuretic, she will need to increase potassium intake, either by taking a supplement or by altering the diet.

Also teach clients to do the following:

- ➤ Drink at least eight to ten 8-ounce glasses of water per day unless your healthcare provider has told you to limit fluids.
- ➤ Healthy adults use thirst as a guide to fluid intake. However, adults older than age 50 may have diminished thirst sensation and cannot depend solely on thirst for fluid replacement.
- ➤ Colorless urine is also a guide to adequate hydration, whereas darker urine is associated with dehydration. You can also use a urine color chart to monitor hydration.

- ➤ Limit consumption of fluids high in salt, sugar, caffeine, or alcohol.
- ➤ Vigorous exercise may delay the thirst mechanism. Athletes should become accustomed to consuming fluids at regular intervals during training sessions and competition so that they do not experience dehydration.
- ➤ Drink water before, during, and after strenuous exercise.
- ➤ Avoid routine use of laxatives, antacids, weight-loss products, or enemas. These products may cause imbalances of fluids and electrolytes such as sodium and potassium.
- ➤ Weigh yourself daily if fluid balance is critical or if you are experiencing excessive loss or gain.
- ➤ Contact a health professional if there is a sudden change of weight, decreased urine output, swelling in dependent areas (e.g., hands and feet), shortness of breath, or dizziness.
- ➤ Contact a healthcare provider if you experience prolonged vomiting, diarrhea, or inability to tolerate liquids or food.
- ➤ Eat a well-balanced diet, including dairy products rich in calcium.

Taking Oral Electrolyte Supplements

- ➤ Encourage clients to take potassium supplements with juice to mask the taste.
- ➤ Teach clients to take supplements as prescribed to maintain electrolyte balance.
- ➤ Remind clients that supplements are medications and should be viewed as part of the treatment plan.
- ➤ If the client's medications are altered, review the continued need for supplements.

- ➤ Caution clients that salt substitutes contain potassium. If the client has been advised to use salt substitutes, evaluate the need for potassium supplements.
- ➤ Encourage clients who take calcium supplements to consume at least 2,500 mL of fluid per day to avoid constipation and reduce the risk of kidney stone formation.

Facilitating Fluid Intake

Clients with actual or potential fluid volume deficit may need to increase their fluid intake. Whenever possible, clients should take fluids by mouth. You may provide replacement through a nasogastric or feeding tube if the client is unable to meet his needs independently but can tolerate fluids in the gastrointestinal tract. Parenteral fluid replacement is used only when enteral replacement cannot meet the client's fluid needs (for review, see Chapter 28).

To increase fluid successfully, you must first establish the desired amount of fluid intake for the client. The daily fluid goal reflects the client's current fluid balance and underlying condition. For example, if a prescription for a dehydrated client reads, "Force fluids: 2,500 mL oral fluids per 24 hours," you can use this to develop a fluid schedule. Typically, people drink more fluid during the day and early evening, when they are more likely to be active, and less in the late evening to avoid sleep interruption. Thus, an example of a fluid distribution is:

  0700 to 1500—1,300 mL
  1500 to 2300—1,000 mL
  2300 to 0700—200 mL

Strategies to increase fluid intake include the following:

- Assess the client's fluid preferences.
- Offer a variety of fluids throughout the day on a regular schedule. Vary hot and cold liquids, and offer a choice of juices and other drinks each time you are at the bedside.
- Instruct nursing assistive personnel to make "fluids rounds" to offer and help with oral fluids.
- Break daily goals into hourly amounts. For example, in the preceding example, in the 8 hours between 0700 and 1500 have the patient drink 150 mL of fluid every hour.
- Provide a cup with milliliter markings so that the patient will know how much he is drinking.
- Always have fluid readily available for the patient. Keep a pitcher of water at the bedside.
- Encourage family members participate in offering fluids and tracking the patient's fluid intake.
- Schedule procedures to minimize the length of time the patient must fast.

Facilitating Fluid Restriction

Patients may need to limit fluids for a variety of reasons (e.g., impaired cardiovascular, liver, or renal function). To facilitate fluid restrictions effectively, teach patients and caregivers the reason for the restriction and the amount of fluid allowed per shift. Fluid restrictions usually include *all* forms of intake. For example, a prescription might read, "Limit total fluid intake to 1,500 mL per 24 hours." If the patient is receiving IV antibiotics in 75 mL of fluids four times per day, you must include this 300 mL as a part of the total fluids. You can distribute the remaining 1,200 mL of oral intake as 800 mL on the day shift and 400 mL on the night shift. Strategies to restrict fluid intake include the following:

- Do not offer liquids with meals. Reserve liquids for between meals.
- Limit intake of foods that increase thirst (e.g., dry, salty, or spicy).
- Keep liquids away from the bedside; offer ice chips to help quench thirst.
- Provide frequent oral hygiene.
- Provide diversional activities for the patient.

PARENTERAL REPLACEMENT OF FLUIDS AND ELECTROLYTES

When fluid loss is severe or the client cannot tolerate oral or tube feedings, fluid volume is replaced parenterally.

- **Parenteral** refers to any route other than through the alimentary canal (passage from the mouth to the anus).
- **Intravenous (IV) therapy** is the administration of fluids, electrolytes, medications, or nutrients by the venous route. IV fluids are used to:
  - Expand intravascular volume.
  - Correct an underlying imbalance in fluids or electrolytes.
  - Compensate for an ongoing problem that is affecting either fluid or electrolytes.

Martha LaGuardia (Meet Your Patients) is being treated in the ED for gastroenteritis. She is experiencing fluid loss from vomiting and diarrhea, complicated by her use of a diuretic. IV therapy will provide fluids to expand her intravascular volume and to maintain hydration. It will also provide electrolyte replacement based on her laboratory studies. Mrs. LaGuardia will receive IV fluids and electrolytes until she can meet her needs orally. Other members of the LaGuardia family are experiencing fluid losses and should increase their fluid intake, but may not need IV fluid replacement. When fluid balance is fragile, or the client cannot tolerate oral fluids, replacement may be supervised in an inpatient setting.

When initiating and maintaining intravenous infusions, always use careful aseptic technique. Remember that the IV catheter provides a portal of entry for pathogens directly into the bloodstream. You should know that Medicare will not reimburse a hospital for the expenses (e.g., antibiotics, extra hospital days) caused by catheter-related infections that occur during hospitalization. Excellent nursing technique can reduce IV catheter-associated infections.

Types of Intravenous Solutions

Solutions, including IV fluids, are classified according to how they compare with the osmolality of blood serum. To review: IV fluids are these classified as isotonic, hypotonic, and hypertonic solutions. To help you remember, here is a somewhat oversimplified summary. When infused:

- *Isotonic* fluids *remain in* the intravascular compartment.
- *Hypotonic* fluids *pull body water out* of the intravascular compartment.
- *Hypertonic* fluids *pull body water into* the intravascular compartment.

Isotonic Fluids

Normal blood serum osmolality is 275 to 295 mOsm/kg. Isotonic solutions have similar tonicity (250 to 375 mOsm/L). Therefore, when infused, they remain inside the blood vessels. **KEY POINT:** *As a result, isotonic fluids are useful for clients with hypotension or hypovolemia.* Commonly prescribed isotonic fluids are the following:

- 0.9% sodium chloride (0.9% NaCl), also called *normal saline (NS)*
- Lactated Ringer's (LR)

The solution 5% dextrose in water (D_5W) may be classified as both isotonic and hypotonic. It is isotonic in the bag, but is not prescribed for isotonic use because after (rapid) metabolism, it is hypotonic in the body.

✚ Clients at risk for fluid volume excess (e.g., congestive heart failure) must be closely monitored when they receive isotonic fluid replacement, because they may easily develop fluid overload.

Hypotonic Fluids

The osmolality of a hypotonic solution is less than that of serum (less than 250 mOsm/L). Therefore, when infused, these solutions pull body water from the intravascular compartment into the interstitial fluid compartment. As the interstitial fluid is diluted, its osmolarity decreases, drawing water into the adjacent cells. **KEY POINT:** *Hypotonic fluid is used for hyperglycemic conditions, such as diabetic ketoacidosis, in which high serum glucose draws fluid out of the cells and into the vascular and interstitial compartments.* Examples of hypotonic fluids include:

- 5% dextrose in water (D_5W). Recall that D_5W is isotonic in the bag, with an osmolality of 253 mOsm/L, but becomes hypotonic in the body.
- 0.45% NaCl (½ normal saline)
- 0.33% NaCl
- 0.2% NaCl

✚ Administer hypotonic fluids carefully to prevent a sudden fluid shift from the intravascular space to the cells. Never give hypotonic solutions to patients at risk for increased intracranial pressure because they can cause or worsen cerebral edema.

Hypertonic Fluids

The osmolality of hypertonic fluids is higher than that of serum. When administered, they pull fluids and electrolytes from the intracellular and interstitial compartments into the intravascular compartment. **KEY POINT:** *Hypertonic fluids can help stabilize blood pressure, increase urine output, and reduce edema. Volume expanders (e.g., dextran and serum albumin) are hypertonic and are used to increase blood volume following severe loss of blood or plasma, such as in major burns or hemorrhage.* Following are examples of hypertonic fluids:

- D_5 0.9% NaCl (D_5 NS)
- D_5 0.45% NaCl (D_5 ½ NS)
- D_5 lactated Ringer's
- 3% NaCl and 5% NaCl—highly hypertonic; used only in critical situations
- 10% dextrose in water ($D_{10}W$)
- $D_{20}W$—used as an osmotic diuretic to promote diuresis

Peripheral Vascular Access Devices

Intravenous therapy requires placement of a vascular access device. You will choose the type of device based on the client's condition, type of fluid that will be infused, and the anticipated length of treatment.

KEY POINT: *IV catheters (and needles) are sized by their diameter, which is called the gauge. The smaller the diameter is, the larger the gauge will be (e.g., a 16-gauge catheter is larger than a 21-gauge catheter).* Therefore, the smaller the gauge, the more rapidly fluid can be delivered. Various types of catheters are used to access peripheral veins, including the following:

Over-the-Needle Catheters are also called an angiocatheters (**angiocaths**) (Fig. 39-7A). A polyurethane or Teflon catheter is threaded over a metal stylet (needle). You pierce the skin and vein with the needle, advance the catheter into the

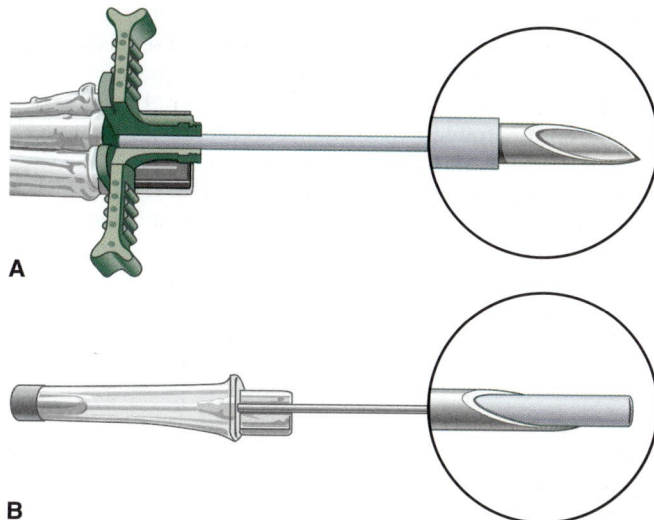

FIGURE 39-7 Typical IV access devices. A. An over-the-needle catheter. B. An inside-the-needle catheter.

vein, and remove (or retract) the metal needle. In most cases, the plastic catheter is less than 7.5 cm (3 in.) in length. This type of access device is ideal for brief therapy. ✚ However, you cannot give highly irritating or hyperosmolar solutions through this type of catheter because it may cause severe damage to the vein.

An Inside-the-Needle Catheter is similar to an over-the-needle catheter; however, the polyurethane or Teflon catheter lies inside the metal needle (Fig. 39-7B). After you advance the catheter into the vein, you withdraw the needle.

A Butterfly Needle is also called a *scalp vein needle* or *wing-tipped catheter*. It is a short, beveled metal needle with flexible plastic flaps attached to the shaft (Fig. 39-8). You can pinch the flaps and hold them tightly together to facilitate insertion. After insertion, flatten them out and tape them against the skin to prevent dislodgement during the infusion process.

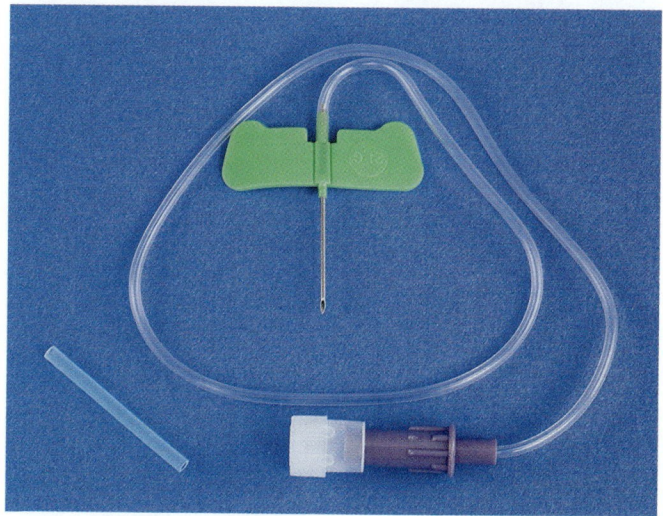

FIGURE 39-8 The butterfly needle is commonly used for intermittent or short-term therapy for children and infants.

These needles are commonly used for intermittent or short-term therapy for children and infants or for single-dose medications and drawing blood. Because the inflexible metal needle remains in the vein, a butterfly needle is more likely than a plastic catheter to **infiltrate** (damage the vein and allow fluid to leak into the interstitial spaces).

A Midline Peripheral Catheter (midline VAD) is a flexible IV catheter, typically inserted into the antecubital fossa and then advanced into the larger vessels of the upper arm for greater hemodilution. It can be used for a longer period of time than a shorter, over-the-needle catheter—typically 1 to 4 weeks. A midline catheter is still considered a peripheral line, so you cannot administer highly osmolar and irritating solutions through it.

➕ It is essential to distinguish a midline VAD from a peripherally placed central line (PICC). Because visual identification is not sufficient for identification, the *type* of VAD must be marked on the dressing label. If you are uncertain about the catheter type, consult the patient's health record.

➕ In response to the Needlestick Safety and Prevention Act passed by Congress in 2000, the Occupational Safety and Health Administration (OSHA) requires the use of "needleless" systems (OSHA, 2011). If you find you must use an older, nonsafety device without the safety features to prevent accidental "sticks," do not attempt to recap the needle after removing it from the vein.

A Peripheral Intravenous Lock (e.g., saline lock, prn adapter, heparin lock) establishes a venous route for clients whose condition may change rapidly or who may require intermittent infusion therapy. A peripheral IV catheter or butterfly wing-tipped catheter is inserted into a vein, and the hub is capped with a lock port (Fig. 39-9). Patency of the lock is maintained by injecting normal saline or a dilute heparin solution, depending on agency policy. See Procedure 39-6.

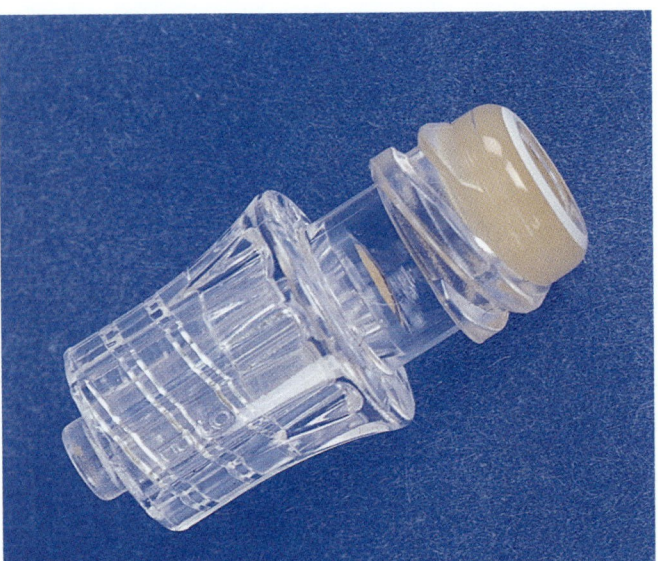

FIGURE 39-9 A peripheral intravenous lock establishes a venous route as a precautionary measure for clients whose condition may change rapidly or who may require intermittent infusion therapy.

Central Venous Access Devices

A **central venous access device (CVAD)** is an intravenous line inserted into a major vein. Typically, the subclavian or internal jugular vein is used. Using surgical asepsis, a catheter is advanced from the insertion site into the superior vena cava. You will likely care for patients with central lines and you may assist with inserting them. To learn how to care for patients with central lines, see Clinical Insight 39-4, Procedure 39-5, and Procedure 39-9.

Advantages of Central Lines include the following:

- A central vein can accommodate highly irritating and hyperosmolar solutions because the blood and solution mix rapidly at the infusion site.
- Central veins are accessible even if the patient is experiencing severe fluid depletion.
- Some types of central lines may also be used to monitor central venous pressure.
- Central lines can be left in longer than peripheral IVs, ranging from a week to long term, depending on the type of central line used.
- Nutrition can be given parenterally.
- Phlebitis, extravasation, and infiltration are less likely to occur with central lines.
- Central lines with extra ports allow you to withdraw blood to use for laboratory tests.

Disadvantages of Central Lines include the following:

- Practitioners must have specialized training to insert the catheter.
- Patient consent is required. Placement is treated as a minor surgical procedure.
- Placement must be confirmed by radiography.
- Placement and dressing changes require strict sterile technique.
- Several risks are possible (e.g., sepsis, air embolus, ventricular dysrhythmia if the catheter floats to the right side of the heart; pneumothorax when placed though the subclavian vein).

Preventing Line-Associated Infections of the Blood

KEY POINT: *To help prevent central venous catheter (CVC)–related infections, The Joint Commission recommends the following set of measures:*

- **Education and training**—regarding proper infection control measures to prevent intravascular catheter-related infections. Encourage patients to report any changes or new discomfort in their catheter site.
- **Hand hygiene**—Wearing gloves does not make hand washing unnecessary.
- **Full barrier precautions for insertion**—Includes sterile drape for patient, hat, mask, and sterile gown and gloves.
- **Chlorhexidine skin antisepsis**—Use 2% chlorhexidine gluconate in 70% isopropyl alcohol to prep the insertion site.
- **Optimal catheter site selection**—The subclavian vein has the lowest rate of infection. The femoral vein should be avoided if possible.
- **Type of catheter**—To reduce the risk of catheter-related infection, the catheter with the fewest number of ports or lumens needed to manage the patient is best.
- **Daily review of lines**—The CVC should be removed as soon as it is no longer necessary. Risk of infection is closely related to the length of time the CVC is in place (Agency for Healthcare Research and Quality, 2014; Centers for Disease Control and Prevention, 2016; Marschall, Mermel, Fakih, et al., 2014).

Types of Central Venous Catheters

There are four types of CVADs: peripherally inserted central catheters, nontunneled CVCs, tunneled CVCs, and implanted ports.

Peripherally Inserted Central Catheters (PICC lines)

PICCs are long, soft, flexible catheters inserted at the antecubital fossa through the basilic or cephalic vein of the arm. The catheter is then advanced into the superior vena cava (Fig. 39-10). A qualified provider performs the insertion. PICC lines are most commonly used for prolonged IV antibiotic therapy, parenteral nutrition, and chemotherapy. **KEY POINT:** *A PICC line is intended for intermediate to long-term use and does not need to be replaced unless the site appears infected or the catheter is no longer patent.*

Nontunneled Central Venous Catheters
are inserted by a qualified provider through the skin into the jugular, subclavian, and, occasionally, femoral veins. They are sutured in place. These are often referred to as single-, double-, triple-, or quadruple-lumen catheters, depending on the number of ports in the line (Fig. 39-11). **KEY POINT:** *These CVADs are intended for shorter use than a PICC line (less than 6 weeks) and should not be routinely replaced.*

Blood can be drawn from a nontunneled CVAD for diagnostic studies or use to measure central venous pressure (CVP) to obtain information on blood volume. ✚ If parenteral nutrition or blood is running in a port, do not use that same port for blood draws.

> *Example:* Imagine that you have patient who needs two different kinds of IV fluid, parenteral nutrition, and frequent blood draws for lab tests. He has fragile peripheral veins and is at high risk for infection. With a multiple-lumen central catheter, the patient needs only one insertion site. You can infuse both fluids and the parenteral nutrition fluids, and still reserve one port for drawing blood. The patient has less risk for the catheter to become dislodged or infiltrate, or for phlebitis to develop.

Tunneled Central Venous Catheters **KEY POINT:**
Tunneled CVCs are intended for long-term use. The catheter is

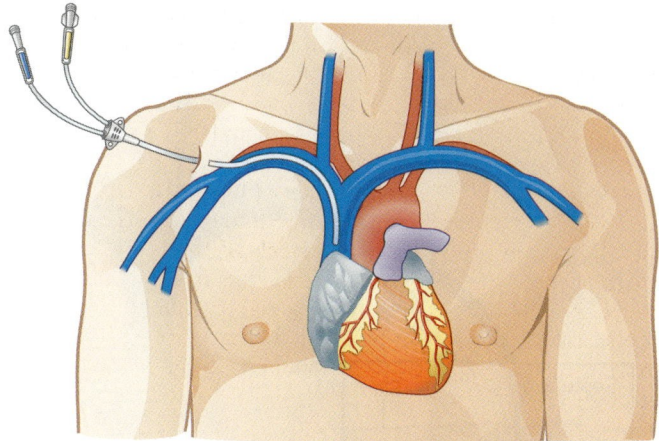

FIGURE 39-11 Nontunneled central venous catheters are inserted into the jugular, subclavian, and, occasionally, femoral veins.

inserted by a surgeon through a 7.5- to 15-cm (3- to 6-in.) subcutaneous tunnel in the chest wall and then into the jugular or subclavian vein (Fig. 39-12). One end of the catheter comes out through the skin and is sutured in place, with the sutures removed when fibrosis has developed around the catheter, or it can be secured with an IV-securing device. CVCs are tunneled through the skin rather than through a vein and, therefore, have a lower the risk of infection.

Implanted Ports
are devices made of a radiopaque silicone catheter and a plastic or stainless steel injection port with a self-sealing silicone-rubber septum. The catheter enters the internal jugular vein in the neck, and it may be tunneled or untunneled to a completely implanted subcutaneous reservoir (port) in the upper chest (Fig. 39-13). **KEY POINT:** *Implanted ports are also intended for long-term use.* Implanted ports are placed by surgeons and only specially trained nurses are allowed to access an implanted port because of the risk of infiltration into the tissue if the needle placement is not correct.

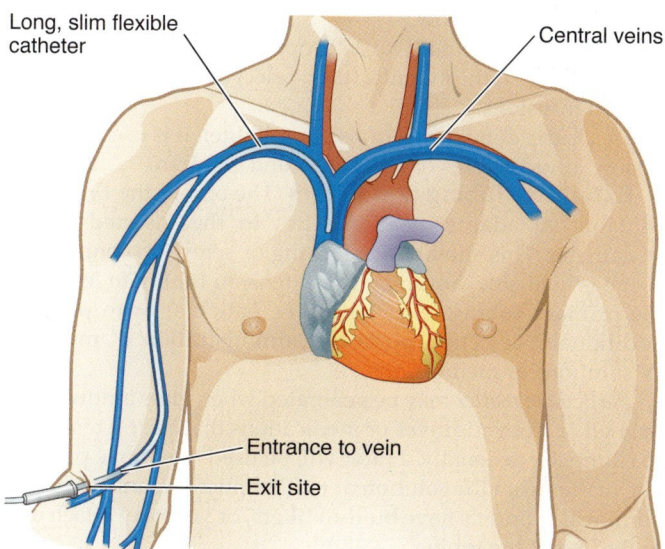

Long, slim flexible catheter — Central veins — Entrance to vein — Exit site

FIGURE 39-10 A PICC line is a long, soft, flexible catheter inserted through a vein in the arm and threaded into a central vessel.

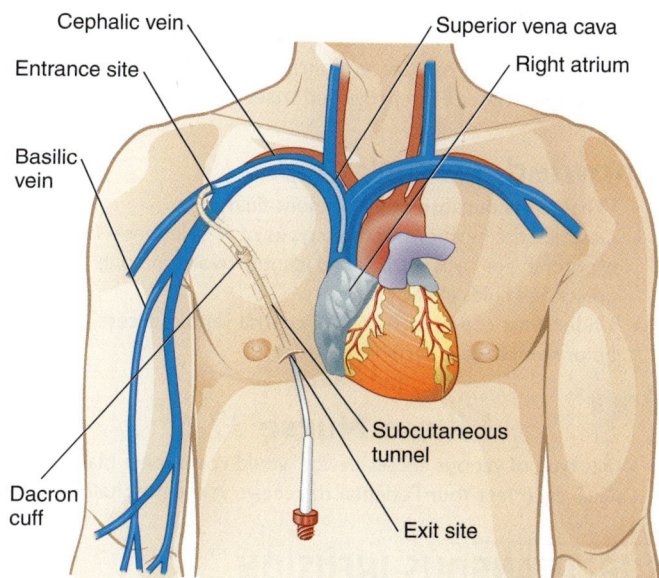

Cephalic vein — Entrance site — Basilic vein — Dacron cuff — Superior vena cava — Right atrium — Subcutaneous tunnel — Exit site

FIGURE 39-12 A tunneled central venous catheter is inserted through subcutaneous tissue in the chest wall into the jugular or subclavian vein.

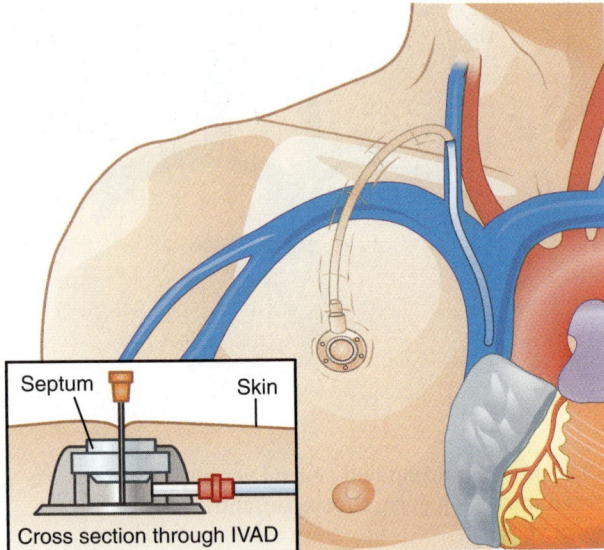

Septum   Skin

Cross section through IVAD

FIGURE 39-13 An implanted venous access port (IVAD) is a CVAD that enters the internal jugular vein in the neck but is tunneled to a completely implanted subcutaneous reservoir (port) in the upper chest.

✚ Avoid taking blood pressures or drawing blood in the extremity on the side of the chest where the implanted port has been placed.

Intraosseous Devices

Designed for immediate access (within seconds) and short-term use (less than 24 hours), intraosseous (IO) access devices are used to administer fluids when a peripheral catheter cannot be inserted or when a central line insertion is not advisable—especially in emergency situations. IOs are placed into the matrix of a bone. The venous sinusoids in the matrix can quickly absorb fluids to send to the central circulation. The most common access site is the proximal tibia in both children and adults. The sternum and the head of the humerus can also be used in adults. Osteomyelitis is a rare complication, occurring in fewer than 1% of cases. Contraindications for IO use include obesity, fracture, recent surgery, infection, or evidence of poor circulation at the proposed insertion site.

KnowledgeCheck 39-9

- What is the purpose of intravenous fluids?
- Describe the functions of three types of IV solutions—isotonic, hypotonic, and hypertonic—and identify two commonly prescribed fluids in each category.
- Under what conditions would a central venous access device be preferable to a peripheral device?

ThinkLike a Nurse 39-6

What type of venous access device would you expect Martha LaGuardia (Meet Your Patients) to receive in the hospital? Why?

SUBCUTANEOUS INFUSION

Subcutaneous infusions are an alternate method to administer medications, continuous fluids, or nutrition. They have been widely used in home-based therapy with palliative care patients. Advantages of subcutaneous infusions are low cost, ease of use, and low infection and complication rates (Gabriel, 2014; Thomas

& Barclay, 2015). Typical sites for infusions include thighs, abdomen, back, and arms (Fig. 39-14).

Starting an Intravenous Infusion

To start an IV infusion, you will need to gather equipment and supplies, set up the solution and administration set, select a venipuncture site, and perform the venipuncture.

Obtain Equipment and Supplies

Venipuncture supplies and IV infusion equipment are sterile, prepackaged, and disposable. They vary among manufacturers, so familiarize yourself with what is available in your facility. Set up the solution and administration set before performing the venipuncture.

IV Catheter Select the catheter with the smallest diameter and the shortest length that will accommodate the prescribed therapy. Nurses commonly use a 20- or 22-gauge catheter for adult peripheral infusions. A 20-gauge needle will accommodate adult blood transfusions. You will need the larger 16- or 18-gauge needle for rapid infusions, viscous (thick) fluids, or surgical or trauma patients. The smaller 24-gauge needle is used in geriatric and neonates. The following are infusion rates catheters of different gauges are expected to deliver (Masoorli, 2012):

18 gauge	4,000 mL/hr
20 gauge	3,500 mL/hr
22 gauge	2,000 mL/hr
24 gauge	1,500 mL/hr

Administration Set (Infusion Kit) The administration set connects the fluid container to the catheter inserted in the patient. The set consists of tubing with a plastic insertion spike, a drip chamber, a roller clamp to regulate the flow, an injection port, and a catheter adapter (hub) (Fig. 39-15).

✚ Both ends of the infusion set (the spike and the hub) must remain sterile. Remove the protective caps just before use. Avoid touching the spike and hub when connecting the tubing to the solution container and the IV catheter in the patient's vein.

The drip chamber is calibrated to allow a predictable amount of fluid to be delivered in each drop. The drop factor is indicated on the package. A roller clamp on the tubing controls the rate of flow.

- A *macrodrip* delivers 10 to 20 drops per milliliter of solution, depending on the manufacturer. Select a macrodrip for most adult infusions.
- A *microdrip* delivers 60 drops per milliliter. It is used for very slow infusion rates or for infants and children.

Extension Tubing and Filters The end of the IV tubing contains an adapter that attaches to the inserted sterile IV catheter. This should be a locking or screw-on connection, if one is available. You may use extension tubing to lengthen the primary tubing (e.g., for active patients) or to provide additional Y-injection ports for administration of multiple IV solutions or medications.

Particulate matter may be generated when glass ampules are opened or from additives or medications that have a tendency to clump. Occasionally, a filter will be used to remove particulate matter from the solution or to filter microorganisms. Some administration sets have built-in filters, or you may attach one to the end of the tubing.

Injection Port Use the injection port to administer a secondary IV fluid or medication (see Chapter 25, Procedures 25-15: Administering Medications to Intravenous Fluids, 25-16: Administering IV Push Medications, and 25-17: Administering Medication by Intermittent Infusion).

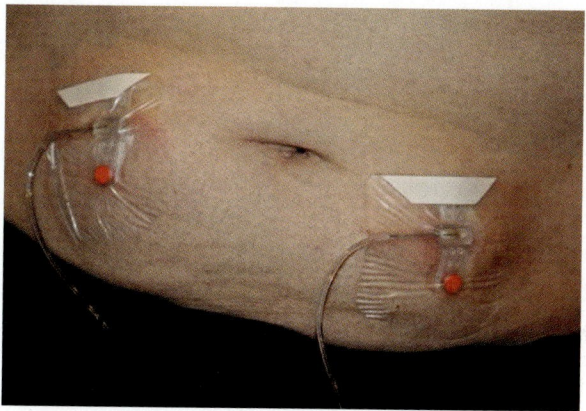

FIGURE 39-14 Subcutaneous infusions of medications, continuous fluids, or nutrition are widely used in home palliative care.

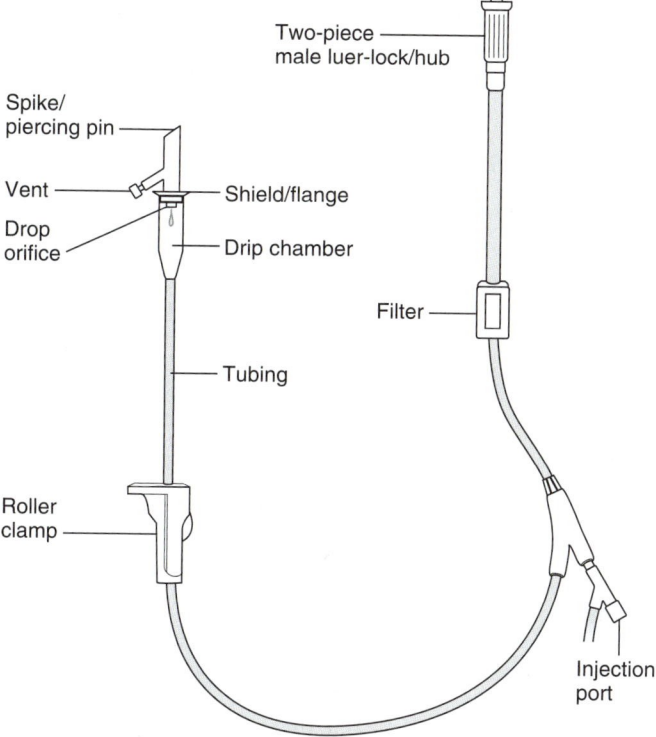

FIGURE 39-15 A basic administration set, or infusion kit.

Solutions Inspect the solution container to be certain that it contains the desired fluid, the fluid is clear, the bag is intact, and the solution has not expired. Most IV fluid containers are plastic, but a few are glass. Fluids for continuous infusions are packed in 1-L or 500-mL bags. Smaller bags (50 mL, 100 mL, and 250 mL) are used for intermittent infusions, such as antibiotics or other medications. Plastic containers collapse as fluid infuses, so you can use a nonvented administration set. Glass bottles do not collapse and therefore require a vented administration set.

Select a Peripheral Intravenous Site

To select a venipuncture site, consider the following factors:
- *Age.* For adults, you will usually use veins in the hand or arm; for infants, veins in the scalp or dorsum of the foot.

- *Type of solution.* For hypertonic solutions, viscous solutions, or irritating medications, use a large vein to cause the least amount of trauma.
- *Speed of infusion.* The faster the rate, the larger the vein and the larger the IV catheter you will need. Use the largest vein available, keeping other selection criteria in mind.
- *Duration of infusion therapy.* To prevent bacterial colonization and phlebitis, some guidelines recommend changing short peripheral IV catheters every 72 to 96 hours (Centers for Disease Control and Prevention, 2011a), whereas others recommend changing it as clinically indicated (Infusion Nurses Society, 2011). You should know and follow your institution's policy.
- *Presence of disease or previous surgery.* For example, avoid areas with scarring or impaired circulation.

For more detailed guidelines for selecting an insertion site, see Clinical Insight 39-3.

Perform Venipuncture

For a successful venipuncture, you need to be able to visualize or palpate the vein before attempting to insert the catheter. Use a vein viewer, if available, to aid in locating the vein. These instruments use infrared light and camera technology to project the patient's superficial veins onto the skin surface. Refer to Procedure 39-1 for additional suggestion on locating a vein, stabilizing the vein, the angle of insertion, and related techniques.

KEY POINT: *If you are not successful with the venipuncture, you can make a second attempt above the initial site or in the opposite extremity. But do not make more than two attempts to start an IV on a patient. Get help from a more experienced colleague.*

Regulating and Maintaining an Intravenous Infusion

Intravenous fluids can flow by gravity or be regulated by an electronic infusion control device (pump). You are responsible for maintaining the correct rate of flow and for monitoring the client's response to the infusion. Many factors can influence the flow rate of an IV solution, especially when using gravity flow.
- *Height of the solution container.* The greater the distance is between the height of the container and the patient's heart, the faster the rate of flow. Check the flow rate each time the client or IV solution is repositioned to ensure that it is correct.
- *Client position.* Pressure on the IV site decreases flow. If an IV is infusing in the right arm and the patient is positioned on his right side, the pressure on the right arm will be greater than if the client were positioned supine or on his left side.
- *Blood pressure.* As blood pressure rises, more force is required to infuse into the vein.
- *Internal diameter of the IV catheter.* The smaller the diameter (that is, the higher the gauge), the more you must open the roller clamp to achieve the flow rate desired.
- *Condition of the catheter and tubing.* If the catheter is dislodged from the vein, flow may stop entirely or continue at a slowed rate. A knot or kink at any point in the tubing will slow flow.

Gravity Flow

Most IV fluids are administered by a volume-control pump. However, you may still encounter instances when you will need to regulate the rate with the roller clamp on the tubing. You should check gravity infusion rates hourly and adjust the flow as needed. ✚ If the fluid is running too slowly, do not attempt to catch up by administering extra fluid rapidly. If the fluid is running too fast, slow the rate and assess the client for signs of fluid volume excess.

If the client is ambulatory, attach the fluid container to a pole with wheels. Instruct the client to keep the solution container above the infusion site and to avoid pulling on the tubing or the infusion site. Procedure 39-2 describes how to regulate a gravity-flow IV.

Volume-Control Set

A volume-control set (e.g., Buretrol, Soluset, Volutrol) is another method for regulating an IV infusion (see Fig. 25-31). You will drain a small amount of fluid from the larger IV solution container into the volume-control container. Typically, the volume placed in the volume-control container is equal to the prescribed hourly infusion rate. The rate is regulated in the same way as other administration sets (the drip factor is usually 60 gtts/mL [60 drops/mL]); however, the maximum amount of fluid that can enter a patient is limited to the volume in the volume-control set. An advantage of this system is that medications can be added to the volume-control set and diluted with IV fluid for intermittent administration.

You may use this type of equipment when the client is at risk for fluid volume excess and for infants and children, who require close supervision of fluid intake. However, more often the policy will be to use an infusion pump for continuous infusions for such patients. To learn or review how to use a volume-control set, see Procedure 25-17C: Using a Volume-Control Administration Set in Chapter 25.

Infusion Pump

If you are using an electronic volume-control device (pump), the machine will maintain the infusion rate that you program into it. Most infusion pumps sound an alarm when the fluid bag is almost empty, when air is in the line, or when there is resistance to flow. Infusion control devices save time and prevent accidental delivery of large amounts of fluid. They do not, however, excuse you from regularly monitoring the flow rate and assessing the needle insertion site.

✚ You should know that absence of an alarm does not mean there is no problem. For example, if the IV is infiltrated, the pump may keep infusing fluid into the tissues.

To find out more about how to regulate an IV using an infusion pump, see Procedure 39-3.

KnowledgeCheck 39-10

- What factors should you consider when selecting an insertion site for a peripheral IV line?
- What are the preferred locations for peripheral IV lines?
- What equipment is needed when inserting an IV and starting an IV infusion?
- Identify three ways to regulate the flow rate of IV fluid.

Calculating Flow Rates

As you already know, intravenous administration sets are sized as microdrips (delivers 60 gtts/mL) or macrodrips (delivers 10 to 20 gtts/mL). To begin, you need to know the prescribed infusion rate and the flow rate of the administration set in drops per minute. See Box 39-1 to learn how to calculate flow rates.

BOX 39-1 ■ Calculating IV Flow Rates

Microdrips = 60 drops/mL
Macrodrips = 10 to 20 drops/mL

You need to know drops per minute: the prescribed infusion rate and the flow rate of the administration set.
1. Multiply the hourly rate (number of mL to be infused in 60 minutes) by the drop factor (in drops per milliliter) to obtain the total drops per hour.
2. Then divide by 60 to get the drip rate in drops per minute. For example, an hourly rate of 100 mL multiplied by 15 drops per milliliter and divided by 60 equals the drip rate. Therefore, the drip rate equals 25 drops per minute.

Use this formula to calculate flow:

$$\frac{\text{Hourly rate in mL} \times \text{drop factor (drops/mL)}}{60 \text{ minutes}} = \text{drip rate}$$

Example Calculation

$$\frac{100 \text{ (mL per hour)} \times 15 \text{ (gtts/mL)}}{60 \text{ minutes}} = 25 \text{ gtts/min}$$

Managing Multiple Lines

When a patient has multiple IV solutions and multiple lines, you must label each line to identify what is infusing in it. Label the IV tubing close to the catheter so that it is easy to see which fluid is infusing the line. This is especially true when using double- and triple-lumen catheters. Multiple lines are often used because solutions are not compatible with each other.

✚ You can never infuse blood, parenteral nutrition, or lipids through a line with anything else, and you can never draw blood samples from these lines.

- **Record the name of each line in your nursing notes and the intake form.** For peripheral IVs, use RA for right arm, LA for left arm, and so on, and designate a number for each site because there may be more than one line or site in each arm (e.g., RA-1, RA-2, LA-1). If the lines are in separate arms, it may seem unnecessary to give each one a number; however, over the course of therapy, some lines may need to be discontinued and new ones started.
- **For multiport central lines, label each port, in addition to recording in the nursing notes.** For example, with a triple-lumen central catheter, you might have named each lumen as proximal, mid, and distal, or CVAD-1, CVAD-2, CVAD-3. The finished labeling and nursing record may indicate "CVAD-1—TPN; CVAD-2—D₅ ½ NS; CVAD-3—insulin."

✚ Always keep the lines untangled and know where your main IV fluid is (e.g., the D₅-½ NS), so that if a crisis occurs or intermittent infusions are needed, you can quickly identify the correct solution and tubing for use.

Complications of Intravenous Therapy

Complications at the IV site include infiltration, extravasation, infection, thrombus, and thrombophlebitis.
- Inserting an IV catheter breaks the body's first line of defense (the skin) and provides a portal of entry for microorganisms.
- In addition, trauma roughens the vein wall and predisposes the person to platelet clumping and thrombus formation.

Minimize this effect by swiftly piercing the skin and anchoring the catheter and tubing to reduce tissue trauma.

Systemic complications occur less frequently than do local complications but may be life threatening. They include fluid volume excess, sepsis, and embolus. Table 39-8 describes potential complications of IV therapy, and Clinical Insight 39-5 discusses managing infiltration and extravasation.

Changing Intravenous Solutions, Tubing, and Dressings

Follow practice guidelines and agency policies for changing IV solutions, tubing, and dressings. As with IV insertion, use meticulous aseptic technique.

Changing IV Solutions Hang a new container of fluid when the present container is nearly empty, but fluid still

Table 39-8 ▶ Complications of Intravenous Therapy

COMPLICATION	CAUSES	SIGNS AND SYMPTOMS	NURSING RESPONSE
Local Complications			
Hematoma—a localized mass of blood outside the blood vessel	Nicking the vein during an unsuccessful insertion, discontinuing an IV line without holding pressure over the site, or applying a tourniquet too tightly above a previously attempted venipuncture site	Ecchymosis, localized mass, discomfort	Be gentle with venipuncture technique. Apply pressure when discontinuing an IV.
*****Infiltration**—the seepage of nonvesicant solution or medication into surrounding tissues	IV catheter dislodges or the tip penetrates the vessel wall	Slowed or stopped flow Swelling, tenderness, pallor, hardness, and coolness at the site The patient may report a burning sensation in the area	Stop the infusion immediately. Restart the IV infusion in a different vein, higher in the extremity or in another extremity. Elevate the affected arm on a pillow to promote absorption of excess fluid.
*****Extravasation**—seepage of a vesicant substance into the tissues. (A *vesicant* is a solution that causes the formation of blisters and subsequent tissue sloughing and necrosis.)	IV catheter dislodges, or the tip penetrates the vessel wall	Slowed or stopped flow Pain, burning, and swelling at IV site, blanching and coolness of the surrounding skin Blistering is a late sign If extravasation resulted from vasoconstricting medication may see necrosis (death) of dermis	Treatment depends on the severity of the infiltration. Stop the IV infusion immediately. Administer an antidote, if one is available. (Antidotes alter the pH, alter DNA binding, neutralize the drug, or dilute the extravasated drug.) Apply cold compresses, and elevate the extremity.
Phlebitis—inflammation of the vein	May be due to mechanical irritation, infusion of solutions that are irritating to the vessel, or sepsis Dextrose solutions, potassium chloride, antibiotics, and vitamin C are associated with a higher risk of phlebitis Trauma to the vessel, compression of the line by client movement, or a low flow rate	Redness, pain, and warmth at the site; local swelling; palpable cord along the vein; sluggish infusion rate; and elevated temperature Slowed or stopped infusion, localized warmth at the site, inability to restart flow of IV	Discontinue the IV infusion and restart in a new location. Initially, apply cold compresses to the site if the site is warm and tender. Thereafter, use warm compresses. Assess for circulatory impairment. Consult the primary care provider if there is streaking or erythema along the vein or a palpable cord.

(Continued)

Table 39-8 ▶ Complications of Intravenous Therapy—cont'd

COMPLICATION	CAUSES	SIGNS AND SYMPTOMS	NURSING RESPONSE
			Prevention measures: Use the smallest catheter practical (usually 22-gauge or 24-gauge thin-walled catheter). Use polyurethane catheters instead of Teflon. Stabilize and secure the catheter to minimize movement in the vein. Rotate the site at least every 96 hours.
Thrombophlebitis— thrombosis and inflammation	Use of veins in the legs for infusion, use of a hypertonic or highly acidic solution; can be a result of untreated phlebitis	Sluggish flow rate, edema, tender and cord-like veins, warmth, and erythema at site	Discontinue the IV infusion and restart in the opposite extremity, using all new equipment. Apply warm, moist compresses. Consult the primary care provider.
Local infection— mic-robial c ontamination of the cannula or IV site	Using poor technique when inserting the catheter, leaving the catheter in place for longer than 96 hours, or direct contamination	Redness, swelling, exudate, elevated temperature	Remove the IV line. Apply a sterile dressing over the site. Administer antibiotics, if necessary.
Nerve injury— a nerve is inadvertently injured during venipuncture (direct) or is compressed	Using veins on inner surface of the wrist and forearm; not anchoring the vein for puncture; using a large needle; advancing the needle across instead of with the vein; "probing" (excessive redirection of the needle at insertion); inserting too deeply and through the back wall of the vein; too many venipuncture attempts; infiltration; extravasation; tourniquet too tight or left on too long	*Direct injury*—sharp, acute pain at the site or up and down the arm; pins and needles or electric shock sensation; pain, numbness, or tingling in fingers; pain that persists after the needle is removed *Compression injury*—pain and tingling typically appear 24 to 96 hours after venipuncture	Do not make more than 2 venipuncture attempts. *If patient complains of symptoms:* Stop the procedure and withdraw the catheter. Apply pressure to prevent hematoma. Report to the supervisor and provider. Do not start a new IV in the affected arm. Treat infiltration if it occurs. **Fasciotomy** (incisions around the area to let blood or fluid seep out) is the usual treatment, or fluid may be expressed.
Systemic Complications			
Septicemia— the presence of microorganisms or their toxic products in the circulatory system	A break in aseptic technique, or contaminated IV solution	Fluctuating fever, chills, tachycardia, confusion, hypotension, altered mental status, elevated WBC count	Discontinue the IV infusion immediately. Consult the primary care provider.

Table 39-8 ➤ Complications of Intravenous Therapy—cont'd

COMPLICATION	CAUSES	SIGNS AND SYMPTOMS	NURSING RESPONSE
			Treatment often involves antibiotics, fluids, and medications to support vital signs.
Fluid overload	Infusing excessive amounts of IV fluids or administering fluid too rapidly	Weight gain, edema, hypertension, shortness of breath, crackles, distended neck veins	Slow the IV flow rate. Place the client in high-Fowler's position. Monitor vital signs. Administer oxygen, if needed. If severe, diuretics may be ordered.
Air embolus—a rare complication involving the introduction of air into the vascular system	Loose connections, adding a new IV bag to a line that has run dry without clearing the line of air, air in tubing cassette of infusion pump	Palpitations, chest pain, light-headedness, dyspnea, cough, hypotension, tachycardia, sudden change in mental status	Call for help. Place client in Trendelenburg position on the left side. Administer oxygen. Have emergency equipment available.
Catheter embolus—a piece of catheter breaks off and travels through the vascular system	Reinserting a catheter used in an unsuccessful insertion; removing and reinserting a stylet, causing shearing of the catheter; placing the catheter in a joint flexion	Sharp, sudden pain at IV site, jagged catheter end on removal, dyspnea, chest pain, tachycardia, hypotension	Apply a tourniquet above the site. Notify the provider and radiologist. Start a new IV line. Prepare the patient for radiographic examination.

*For more information about interventions for infiltration and extravasation, see Clinical Insight 39-5.
Source: Phillips, L., & Gorski, L. (2014). *Manual of IV therapeutics* (6th ed.). Philadelphia, PA: F.A. Davis.

remains at the appropriate level in the drip chamber. The infusion rate dictates how often you need to change the IV solution. For example, a liter of IV fluid infusing at 125 mL/hr must be changed every 8 hours; a liter infusing at 50 mL/hr will hang for 20 hours. Evidence-based practice does not provide an exact length of time that an IV solution can hang before it has to be changed (Centers for Disease Control and Prevention, 2011a); therefore, you should follow your agency's policy. For full instructions on the procedure for changing solutions, tubing, and dressings, see Procedures 39-4A, 39-4B, and 39-5.

Changing Administration Sets The Infusion Nurses Society (2011) and the Centers for Disease Control and Prevention (2011b) recommend that primary and secondary administration sets be changed no more frequently than 96 hours, but at least every 7 days; primary intermittent administration sets should be changed every 24 hours. This guideline applies to administration sets that are continuously used and the patient is not receiving blood, blood products, or fat emulsions.

Administration sets used for parenteral nutrition are exposed to intravenous fat emulsions and should be changed

every 24 hours; non-lipid-containing parenteral nutrition solutions should be changed every 96 hours (Infusion Nurses Society, 2011).

KEY POINT: *As a rule, if you start an IV at a new site, use a new administration set. Reusing a set from a previous site increases the risk of contamination.*

Changing IV Dressings Change peripheral IV dressings routinely when the catheter is replaced, or as clinically indicated (e.g., when the dressing becomes damp, soiled, or loose) (Centers for Disease Control and Prevention, 2011b). For central venous catheters (CVCs), the Infusion Nurses Society (2011) recommends the following:

- *For short-term CVCs,* the dressing at the site must be changed every 2 days for gauze dressings and every 7 days for transparent dressing. In pediatric patients, if the risk of dislodging the catheter is high, the dressing can be left in place.
- *For tunneled or implanted sites,* unless soiled or loose, a transparent dressing is changed no more than once a week until the insertion site has healed.
- *For long-term cuffed and tunneled CVS with well-healed sites,* no recommendations are made. You should follow your

agency's policy for dressing changes on these sites. In home care, the dressing may be left in place for 1 week.

- Change any dressing, regardless of site, when it becomes soiled, damp, or loosened.

KEY POINT: *It is best to dress both central and peripheral lines with transparent semipermeable dressings. These dressings allow direct visualization of the site between dressing changes, permit evaporation of moisture, and provide a secure anchor for the catheter.* You may still sometimes see tape securing a catheter at the insertion site; however, the use of a *catheter stabilization device* is preferred over tape or sutures (Infusion Nurses Society, 2011; Marschall, Mermel, Fakih, 2014).

Converting to a Peripheral Intravenous Lock

The terms *peripheral lock, saline lock,* and *prn adapter* are used interchangeably. Recall that you may need a peripheral IV lock (PIV) for intermittent infusions or for venous access for emergencies. Also, when clients do not need the additional fluids provided by a constant infusion of solution, a peripheral infusion can be easily converted to a peripheral lock. To do this, you simply remove the tubing from the IV catheter and replace it with a sterile injection cap (see Fig. 39-9). Some IV locks also contain a short segment of tubing. The Infusion Nurses Society (2011) recommends that 0.9% sodium chloride be used to flush the peripheral IV lock.

- Each time you give a medication through the lock, you will need to disinfect and flush the lock before and after you administer the medication.
- A PIV should also be flushed and locked at least every 12 hours when not in use.

Discontinuing an Intravenous Line

Discontinue the IV line and IV catheter when IV fluids and medications are no longer needed or if the integrity of the line is compromised. Inspect the catheter to ensure that it is intact when you remove it. For complete steps to remove an IV catheter, see Procedure 39-7.

KnowledgeCheck 39-11

- A prescription reads, "5% dextrose in water/ 0.45% saline solution (D$_5$ ½ NS) with 20 mEq KCl; infuse 1 liter in 5 hours." Calculate the hourly rate and the drip rate using (1) a macrodrip administration set with 15 gtts/mL and (2) a microdrip set.
- Describe the difference between infiltration and extravasation as a complication of IV therapy.
- In general, how often are administration sets changed on peripheral IV lines? How often are administration sets changed when TPN is infused?

REPLACEMENT OF BLOOD AND BLOOD PRODUCTS

Intravenous fluids can replace fluid volume, but they do not restore oxygen-carrying capacity or replace clotting factors. Blood products are infused when the patient has experience significant blood loss, diminished oxygen carrying capacity, or a deficiency in one of the blood components. The American Association of Blood Banks (AABB) estimates that 6.8 million volunteers donate blood each year; a total of 13.6 million units of whole blood and red blood cells was donated in 2013 (AABB, n.d.).

Each unit of donated blood is separated into multiple components, such as red blood cells, plasma, platelets, and clotting factors. Thus, one unit of donated blood may be used in the care of four clients. To be eligible to donate blood, a person must be in good health (no cold or flu, uncontrolled hypertension, or diabetes), be at least age 16 years (although some states permit younger people, with parental consent, to donate), and weigh at least 110 pounds. In addition, each potential donor is screened for travel to certain countries and for a variety of disorders, such as hepatitis, HIV, and Creutzfeldt-Jakob disease (the human form of "mad cow" disease).

Blood Groups

Human blood is classified into four main groups (A, B, AB, and O) based on the presence or absence of certain antigens and antibodies. You inherit the blood group you belong to from your parents. See Table 39-9 for a description of blood groups. Patients must receive only blood that is compatible with their own blood group to prevent a fatal hemolytic reaction (Table 39-9).

An additional antigen, known as Rh factor, is also important with blood typing. If the antigen is present, you are referred to as Rh-positive (Rh$^+$). If it is absent, you are Rh-negative (Rh$^-$). Thus, you can belong to one of the following eight groups:

A Rh$^+$ B Rh$^+$ AB Rh$^+$ O Rh$^+$
A Rh$^-$ B Rh$^-$ AB Rh$^-$ O Rh$^-$

Blood Typing and Crossmatching

Once blood is donated, several tests are performed on the sample. First, the sample is tested for ABO group (blood type) and Rh type (positive or negative), as well as for any unexpected red blood cell antibodies that may cause problems in a recipient. Screening tests assess for evidence of donor infection with hepatitis B and C viruses, HIV, human T-lymphotropic viruses, West Nile virus, and syphilis. If all disease screens are negative, the blood is acceptable for transfusion and is placed in the pool of available products.

When a potential donor is identified, crossmatching is performed. **Crossmatching** identifies possible minor antigens that will affect the compatibility of the donor blood in the recipient. RBCs from the donor blood are mixed with plasma from the potential recipient. A reagent is added, and the sample is observed for clumping or agglutination. If no clumping is observed, the risk of transfusion reaction is low, and it is considered safe to transfuse the sample of blood. Table 39-9 summarizes blood group matching.

- **KEY POINT:** *People with blood group O are considered universal donors because of the absence of antigens, whereas people with blood group AB are considered universal recipients because of the absence of plasma antibodies.*
- People who are Rh$^+$ may receive blood with or without Rh factor. However, people who are Rh$^-$ may receive only Rh$^-$ blood.

When possible, **autologous** (self-donated) units of blood are given instead of blood from a donor. This negates the risk of a mismatch or exposure to undetected disease. The patient's blood is usually collected in the preoperative weeks for possible transfusion during elective surgery. Autologous donation is most often done with orthopedic, cardiac, and vascular surgeries. The process of donating autologous blood stimulates the bone marrow to produce new blood cells. Given adequate time for recovery, the collected cells may be wholly or partially replaced prior to surgery.

Table 39-9 ▸ Blood Groupings for Transfusions

BLOOD GROUP	ANTIGENS	ANTIBODIES	CAN GIVE BLOOD TO	CAN RECEIVE BLOOD FROM
AB	A and B	None	AB	AB, A, B, and O
A	A	B	A and AB	A and O
B	B	A	B and AB	B and O
O	None	A and B	AB, A, B, and O	O

Blood Products

Several blood products are available for transfusion:
- *Whole blood* contains RBCs, WBCs, and platelets suspended in plasma.
- *Red blood cells* are prepared from whole blood by removing the plasma. RBCs can raise the client's hematocrit and hemoglobin levels while minimizing an increase in volume. RBCs are available for transfusion as packed RBCs (PRBCs).
- *Plasma* is the liquid portion of the blood. It is 90% water and makes up about 55% of blood volume. Plasma may be transfused whole or may be separated into specific products, such as albumin, clotting factor concentrates, and immune globulins.
- *Platelets* help the clotting process by sticking to the lining of blood vessels. Units of platelets are prepared by using a centrifuge to separate the platelet-rich plasma from the donated unit of whole blood. The platelet-rich plasma is then centrifuged again to further concentrate the platelets. Platelets are used to treat clients who have a shortage of platelets or have abnormal platelet function.
- *White blood cells (WBCs)*, specifically granulocytes, can be collected by centrifugation of whole blood. They are transfused within 24 hours after collection and are used for infections that are unresponsive to antibiotic therapy.
- *Plasma derivatives* are concentrates of specific plasma proteins prepared from many units of plasma. Plasma derivatives include a variety of clotting factors, immune globulins, and albumin.

Initiating a Transfusion

✚ It is critical to identify the patient and the blood product when transfusing blood. Before beginning a transfusion, verify the written prescription for the blood product. Some patients will refuse a blood transfusion because of cultural, religious, or other beliefs. Be ready to discuss with them any available alternatives to whole blood administration.

Obtain a set of vital signs 5 to 15 minutes before initiating the infusion. If the patient's temperature is elevated, inform the primary care provider before hanging the transfusion. Most patients experience a minor elevation in temperature after a transfusion is given. A preexisting elevated temperature may exacerbate this response. As a result, premedication may be prescribed.

Toward Evidence-Based Practice

Sullivan, K., Vu, T., Richardson, G., et al. (2015). Evaluating the frequency of vital sign monitoring during blood transfusion: An evidence-based practice initiative. *Clinical Journal of Oncology Nursing, 19*(5), 516–520.

Researchers evaluated the literature to identify evidence-based guidelines on the frequency of monitoring vital signs for cancer patients receiving blood products. Results indicated that obtaining a baseline reading and assessing the vital signs within 15 minutes of initiating the transfusion and again at the completion of the infusion were effective in detecting symptoms of transfusion reactions in cancer patients. The findings resulted in a revision to policy on blood transfusion and reaction policy.

Menendez, J., & Edwards, B. (2016). Early identification of acute hemolytic transfusion reactions: Realistic implications for best practice in patient monitoring. *MEDSURG Nursing, 25*(2), 88–90, 109.

After analyzing data from case studies involving transfusion reactions, a transfusion-monitoring program was initiated at a medical center. The goal was to develop an evidence-based patient-monitoring protocol for patients receiving blood transfusions. The team implemented a process that involved obtaining a baseline assessment and continuous monitoring during the first 15 minutes of the transfusion, followed by a two-nurse analysis of vital signs and assessment for indicators of a transfusion reaction. A patient assessment then occurred every hour until the transfusion was completed.

1. Based on these studies, how do you see that nurses can affect institution policy and procedure?

2. What factors must be considered when implementing new changes in practice?

 Go to Davis Advantage, Resources, Chapter 39, **Applying the Full-Spectrum Nursing Model—Suggested Responses.**

Inspect the IV site to be sure it is patent before hanging the blood product. Nurses commonly use a 20-gauge catheter to infuse blood—and a larger size for rapid flow rates. There is evidence that a 22-gauge catheter can be used in adults without damage to the red blood cells (Infusion Nurses Society, 2011). Certainly, for children and the frail elderly, you will need a smaller, 22- or 24-gauge catheter. For the complete procedure for initiating and monitoring a blood transfusion and managing a transfusion reaction, see Procedures 39-8A and 39-8B.

Transfusion Reactions

Even though you use perfect technique, transfusion reactions can and do occur. Five types of reaction are possible: allergic, bacterial, febrile, or hemolytic reactions and circulatory overload. Table 39-10 describes each of these reactions. To help prevent transfusion reactions, be extremely careful in identifying the patient and the blood, start the transfusion slowly, remain with the patient for the first 5 minutes of the transfusion, and assess again at 15 minutes (see Procedure 39-8).

KnowledgeCheck 39-12

- Identify the eight potential blood types.
- Describe the types of blood products that are available for transfusion.
- Identify and describe types of transfusion reactions.

Table 39-10 ➤ Transfusion Reactions

TYPE OF REACTION	SIGNS AND SYMPTOMS	NURSING RESPONSIBILITIES
Allergic—allergy to blood being transfused	Flushing, itching, wheezing, urticaria (hives); anaphylaxis, if severe	Stop the transfusion. Replace with a saline infusion. Notify the provider immediately. Administer prescribed antihistamine.
Bacterial—contamination of the blood	Fever, chills, vomiting, diarrhea, hypertension	Stop the transfusion. Replace with a saline infusion. Notify the provider. Administer antibiotics as ordered. Treat symptoms.
Febrile—temperature elevation due to sensitivity to WBCs, plasma proteins, or platelets	Fever, chills, warm, flushed skin, aches	Stop the transfusion. Replace with a saline infusion. Notify the provider. Treat symptoms.
Hemolytic reactions—destruction of RBCs as a result of infusing incompatible blood; occurs in 1 in 600,000 transfusions	Fever, chills, dyspnea, chest pain, tachycardia, hypotension; can be fatal	Stop the transfusion immediately. Replace with a saline infusion. Notify the provider immediately. Send the remaining blood, including tubing and filter; a sample of venous blood; and the first voided urine to the lab for analysis. Treat shock.
Circulatory overload—administering too great a volume or too rapidly	Persistent cough, crackles, hypertension, distended neck veins	Slow or stop the transfusion. Monitor vital signs. Place the client upright. Notify the provider.

CLINICALREASONING

The questions and exercises in this section allow you to practice the kind of thinking you will use as a full-spectrum nurse. Critical-thinking questions usually have more than one correct answer, so we do not provide "correct answers" for these features. It is more important to develop your nursing judgment than to just cover content. You will learn by discussing the questions with your peers. If you are still unsure, see the Davis Advantage chapter resources for suggested responses.

Caring for the Nguyens

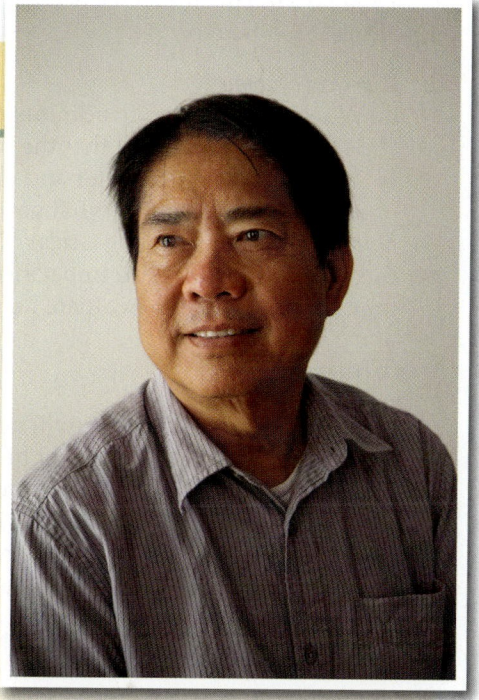

Nam Nguyen has been prescribed the following medicines:

Lisinopril 20 mg PO daily
Hydrochlorothiazide 25 mg PO daily in the a.m.
Metformin 500 mg PO before breakfast and lunch

Today he had blood drawn for analysis. Following are the electrolyte panel results:

Sodium	136 mEq/L
Potassium	3.0 mEq/L
Chloride	96 mEq/L
Bicarbonate	24 mEq/L
BUN	18 mg/dL
Creatinine	0.8 mg/dL

A. Review the lab results. Compare Nam's lab work with the established norms for these values. Based on the lab results, what kind of assessment questions would be appropriate to ask Nam?

B. Use your pharmacology text to review Nam's medications. Which, if any, of these medicines might be contributing to Nam's lab results?

C. What teaching would be appropriate for Nam?

Go to Davis Advantage, Resources, Chapter 39, **Caring for the Nguyens—Suggested Responses.**

Applying the **Full-Spectrum Nursing Model**

PATIENT SITUATION

Darlene Malone, age 42, has been admitted to the emergency department with complaints of fatigue, extreme weakness, and heart palpitations. She says she has not seen a healthcare provider in nearly 10 years. Suddenly, she slumps and falls over. She is not breathing, has no pulse, and does not respond to verbal stimuli. She is resuscitated with CPR and IV epinephrine, and an endotracheal tube is placed. STAT lab results show a potassium level of 7.7 mEq/L, BUN of 102 mg/dL, and creatinine of 5 mg/dL. A physician diagnoses acute renal failure. Among other interventions, an IV is started to administer 10% calcium chloride solution, 1,000 mg, by slow IV push to counteract the toxic effects of hyperkalemia on the cell membranes. The nurse used a 20-gauge over-the-needle catheter in Ms. Malone's right cephalic vein, about 5 cm (2 in.) above her wrist.

THINKING

1. *Theoretical Knowledge:*
   a. Which lab results are abnormal? Are they high or low?
   b. Which lab results directly reflect her renal failure?
   c. What term correctly describes serum potassium of 7.7 mEq/L?

2. *Critical Thinking (Considering Alternatives):*
   a. What do you think is causing Ms. Malone to have hyperkalemia? You should be able to think this through and make a reasonable guess even if you have not studied pathophysiology.
   b. Ms. Malone is to be given 50 mEq of sodium bicarbonate by slow IV push for an acid–base imbalance that is often associated with hyperkalemia. Which imbalance do you think would be treated with sodium bicarbonate: metabolic acidosis or metabolic alkalosis?

DOING

3. *Practical Knowledge:*
   a. When you prepare to administer the sodium bicarbonate (in question 2b), you notice that the IV infusion is barely flowing and that the insertion site is swollen and pale. What is the first thing you should do?
   b. You aspirate the catheter and do not obtain a blood return. Ms. Malone absolutely must have this medication. Describe what you would do in the order you would do it.
4. *Nursing Process (Planning Goals):* The NOC outcome best suited to evaluating Ms. Malone's hyperkalemia is Electrolyte & Acid–Base Imbalance. Based on the function of this electrolyte, what is the primary indicator that you could use to evaluate her goal achievement for this problem?

CARING

5. *Self-Knowledge:* Ms. Malone will need dialysis to replace her inadequate renal function and control her serum potassium level. It is likely that her renal failure was brought on by years of illegal drug abuse. She has never held a full-time job and has not worked at all for the past 7 years. Her dialysis treatments will need to be paid for by Medicaid, which is funded by tax dollars. How do you feel about this—specifically, how do you feel about the issues of (a) a person's responsibility for her own health and (b) compassion for people who cannot afford to pay for healthcare? Focus on your own feelings, not on issues of what "should" be done.

 Go to Davis Advantage, Resources, Chapter 39, **Applying the Full-Spectrum Nursing Model—Suggested Responses.**

PracticalKnowledge:
clinical application

CLINICAL INSIGHTS

Clinical Insight 39-1 ➤ **Assessing for Trousseau's and Chvostek's Signs**

Positive Trousseau's and Chvostek's signs are signs of hypocalcemia. To check for these signs, follow these instructions:

Trousseau's Sign

Inflate a blood pressure cuff above systolic pressure. Flexion of the wrist and hand constitutes a positive sign.

Chvostek's Sign

Tap the face in front of the ear and below the zygomatic bone (cheek bone). Facial twitching constitutes a positive sign.

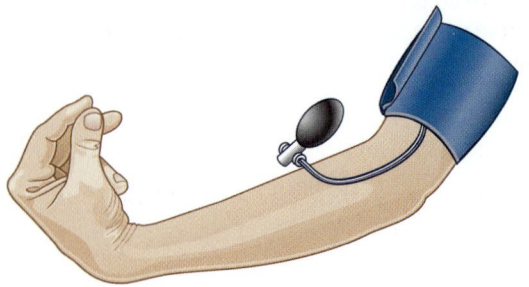

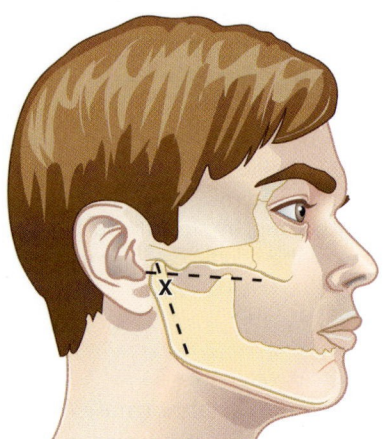

Clinical Insight 39-2 ➤ Guidelines for Measuring Intake and Output (I&O)

General Guidelines

Assessing

- Identify factors that can affect the patient's fluid intake or output (e.g., surgery, medical condition, or medications such as diuretics).
- Measure all fluids the patient consumes or excretes.
- Enlist the patient's help in keeping track of I&O if she is able.
- If you delegate the task of recording intake and output:
  - Be sure the assistive person understands its importance and knows how to perform the procedure correctly.
  - Be certain to evaluate the totals and the fluid sources. A patient or NAP can collect the data, but an RN must make the assessments.
- For accuracy, use a graduated container and hold it at eye level when measuring fluids.

Recording

- You will usually record measurements on a bedside I&O form and transfer the 8-hr total to a graphic sheet or the 24-hr I&O on the patient's record. You may sometimes need hourly measurements. See Chapter 18, "Intake and Output Records," and Figure 18-7.
- Document your findings in milliliters (mL). Describe any fluid restrictions and the patient's compliance with them.

Measuring Intake

It is most accurate to premeasure fluids before they are consumed. However, if that is not possible, you can use the following estimates:

Equivalents

1 oz = 30 mL
1 teaspoon = 5 mL
1 tablespoon = 15 mL
1 home measuring cup of fluid = 8 oz (240 mL)
1 pint of fluid = 16 oz (480 mL)
1 quart of fluid = 32 oz (960 mL)

Various Containers

Record ice chips as fluid at half their volume (1 cup ice = ½ cup fluid)
Bowl (soup) = 180 mL
Creamer (small) = 30 mL
Custard cup = 100 mL
Drinking cup = 180 mL
Coffee mug = 240 mL
Gelatin cup = 100 mL
Ice cream serving = 120 mL
Juice glass = 120 mL
Paper cup, large = 200 mL

Paper cup, small = 120 mL
Water glass = 200 mL
Water pitcher = 1,000 mL

Examples of Fast-Food Drinks

Child-size drink = 12 oz
Small drink = 16 oz
Medium drink = 21 oz
Large drink = 32 oz

Assessing

- Fluid intake includes the following:
  Oral fluids, including the liquid in prepared foods
  Soups
  Everything that melts into liquid at room temperature (e.g., gelatin, custard, ice cream, and ice)
  Liquid medications and fluids used to take tablets or capsules
  IV fluids
  Enteral or parenteral nutrition fluids
  Instillations into the gastrointestinal tract
  Bladder irrigations
- Measure oral fluids according to agency policy.
- For increased accuracy, use a graduated cup to measure and record fluid amounts before the patient consumes them. Subtract from the total any fluid that the patient throws away or saves for future consumption.
- Wash the measuring cup after each use, except after measuring water.
- Measure and teach the patient to measure and record the amount of fluid he drinks with each meal, with medicine, and between meals.
- In the home, cups come in many different sizes, so do the following:
  Use a measuring cup to measure how much the drinking cups and glasses hold.
  Always use the same drinking cup or glass.
  Explain that the labels on cans and bottles will help to determine precise fluid amounts.

Recording

- At least every 8 hours, record the type and amount of all fluids the patient has received and indicate the route (oral, parenteral, rectal, or enteric tube).
- Record all forms of intake Including blood and blood products

Measuring Output

Assessing

- Refer to Procedure 30-1: Measuring Urine to review how to measure urine.

(Continued)

Clinical Insight 39-2 ➤ Guidelines for Measuring Intake and Output (I&O)—cont'd

Fluid output includes everything that leaves the body in fluid form: urine, watery stool, vomitus, wound drainage, surgical drains, NG tubes, chest tubes, and any fluid aspirated from a body cavity.

- Use a calibrated container to measure fluids. Observe it at eye level and take the reading at the bottom of the fluid meniscus.
- Use a different graduated container for each patient; clean after use.
- Teach the patient to keep toilet paper out of the urine for accurate measurement.
- If irrigating an NG tube or the bladder, measure the amount instilled and subtract it from total output.
- You will need to empty wound drains or other devices to measure this volume.
- If a wound is draining, but the fluid is not collected in a drainage device, you may measure the amount of fluid lost by weighing dressings before and after they are applied. If measuring the exact volume is not crucial, you may evaluate the degree of saturation of the dressing.

Recording

- Record the type, route, and amount of all fluids the patient loses.
- Insensible fluid losses can't be easily quantified. However, unusual losses (e.g., saturated dressing, excessive perspiration, rapid breathing patterns, and large burn areas) should be objectively described in narrative charting.

Tips for Analyzing I&O

- Measure and record all intake and output.
- Determine if output is more or less than intake.
- Evaluate trends over for a period of 24 to 48 hours.
- To identify problems, when evaluating total urine output, ask how many times the patient voided. For example, was a total of 300 mL obtained from 2 voids or from 10 voids of 30 mL each?
- Evaluate patterns and values outside the normal range (e.g., frequent voiding, infrequent voiding), keeping in mind the normal range for 24-hour intake and output.
- The amount of output is important, but consider color, color changes, and odor.
- Analyze intake and output holistically. Take into account the patient's usual pattern and amounts, age, medical problem, and type of surgical procedure.
- You must correlate I&O with daily weights to accurately determine overall fluid status (Collins & Claros, 2011; Crawford & Harris, 2012b; Shepherd, 2011).

Clinical Insight 39-3 ➤ Guidelines for Selecting a Peripheral Venipuncture Site

- As a general rule, select the most distal vein on an upper extremity.
- If available, use visualization technologies such as portable ultrasound or imaging devices.
  This minimizes the number of needlesticks the patient must undergo.
- For adults, you will usually use veins in the hand or arm; for infants, veins in the scalp or dorsum of the foot can also be used.
- If possible, select a vein on the patient's nondominant hand or arm.
  Helps to preserve functional ability.

- Look for a vein that has a firm, round appearance with a relatively straight pathway. Do not use a red, hot, or hard vein.
- Avoid veins that are highly visible; they tend to roll.
- The cephalic vein of the arm is one of the best veins to use because it is relatively large, and the forearm provides a natural splint
- The dorsal veins of the hand are easy to access and are splinted by the metacarpals, but these veins are often quite small and fragile.

Clinical Insight 39-3 ➤ **Guidelines for Selecting a Peripheral Venipuncture Site—cont'd**

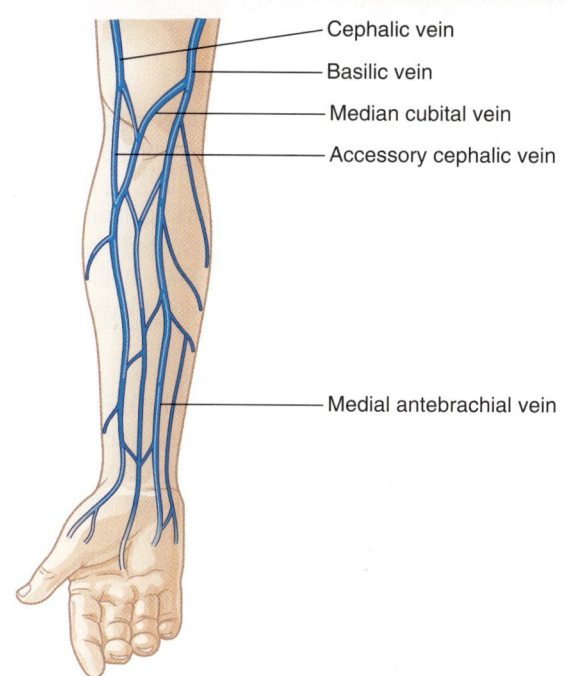

- Cephalic vein
- Basilic vein
- Median cubital vein
- Accessory cephalic vein
- Medial antebrachial vein

Superficial veins of the forearm

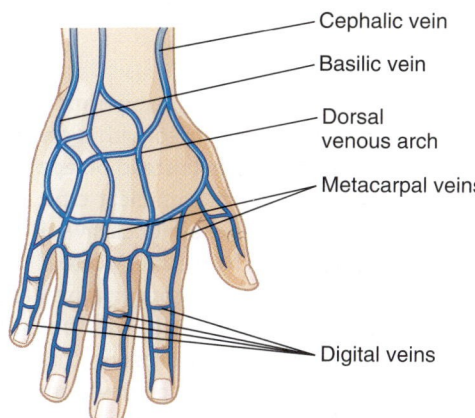

- Cephalic vein
- Basilic vein
- Dorsal venous arch
- Metacarpal veins
- Digital veins

Superficial veins of the hand

- Avoid the antecubital veins if possible. If the patient flexes her arm, the IV catheter may become displaced, so you would probably need to splint her elbow to prevent that. Furthermore, if a PICC line is needed at a later time, you will still have the antecubital veins available for it.
- For these situations, you need to use the largest vein available, keeping other selection criteria in mind:
  - Hypertonic solutions, viscous solutions, or irritating medications
  - Rapid rates (also require a larger IV catheter)
- If the infusion is to be ongoing, begin the infusion with the best lowest vein and move proximal to the previous site (toward the heart) for subsequent insertions. Peripheral IV catheters are routinely changed at 96-hour intervals, but at least every 7 days. If you start the next IV below an already used site (i.e., to change the site or after a failed attempt at insertion), fluid may leak from the old site.

- Avoid areas at which the vein crosses over joints. If you must use such an area, splint the joint to limit movement. *Splinting the joint helps preserve the vein for use, but it limits functional ability.*
- Avoid areas with scarring, or with impaired circulation or neurological status (e.g., the affected arm following a mastectomy; an area with signs of infection, previous infiltration, or thrombosis; an arm with an arteriovenous fistula [shunt for dialysis]; or the affected side after cerebrovascular accident [stroke, brain attack]). If you must use such an area, first obtain a medical prescription.
- Do not use veins in the legs and feet unless there is no other option. *Peripheral circulation may not be adequate in the lower limbs, so there is increased danger of thrombus formation. In adults, this location also interferes with mobility. Foot veins may be used for infants if the IV is taped securely.*

Clinical Insight 39-4 ➤ Caring for Patients With a Central Venous Access Device (CVAD): CVC and PICC

✚ Asepsis

- Use good hand hygiene and follow agency protocols for site care.
  To protect yourself and the patient.
- Use strict aseptic technique when manipulating injection ports, catheter hub and extension legs, needleless connectors, insertion site, and dressing. This includes sterile gloves and supplies, mask, and in some agencies a mask for the patient.
  To minimize line contamination and infection.
- Scrub injection ports, extension legs, and catheter hubs vigorously for at least 15 seconds, preferably with 70% alcohol or 2% chlorhexidine preparation, before accessing them.
- Appropriate antiseptics include alcohol and chlorhexidine gluconate (CHG). Do not use povidone-iodine and tincture of iodine to scrub ports unless there is some reason alcohol or CHG-alcohol combination products can't be used.
- Do not apply organic solvents, such as acetone or acetone-based products, to the skin before insertion of a catheter or during dressing changes.

Assessments

- ✚ Check the patient record for radiographic confirmation of correct tip location before beginning prescribed therapies.

- Inspect catheter–skin junction sites through the transparent dressing and palpate for tenderness daily. Do not remove transparent dressing except when dressing change is required. If site is dressed with gauze, remove it to inspect the site.
  A high-risk route of infection is via migration of skin organisms at the insertion site into the cutaneous catheter tract, with colonization of the catheter tip.
- Observe for excessive bleeding at the insertion site.
  You may need to obtain a prescription for a topical hemostatic agent and use with a pressure dressing.
- If symptoms of infection occur (e.g., fever without obvious cause; redness, edema, induration, exudates, or tenderness at the site), remove the dressing and inspect the site directly. Anticipate that blood cultures will be needed from both the peripheral site and the central catheter.
- Be aware that risk of infection is higher with femoral catheters and with multilumen catheters.
  Multilumen catheters require more manipulation, which encourages more colonization and bacterial growth within the catheter lumen.
- Assess for compromised catheter integrity (wet dressing; kinked, cracked, or leaking external catheter).
- Inspect catheter connections and pump function, including flow rate.
- Observe for symptoms of catheter migration to the right atrium or ventricle (i.e., mid- to lower sternal pain, dysrhythmias).

- If there are signs of complications, notify the medical provider.
- Assess the patient daily for indications that the CVC or PICC line is still needed.
  CVCs or PICC line should be removed as soon as possible because the infection rate is closely related to the length of time the catheter is in place.

Maintenance Interventions

- The site should be covered with a semipermeable transparent dressing, the catheter secured with a sterile commercially manufactured stabilizer (instead of tape), and the lumens anchored near the ports with clear tape.
- Keep dressings dry, intact, and air occlusive. Protocols generally require a dressing change every 5 to 7 days unless the integrity of the dressing is compromised (e.g., it is damp, loosened, or soiled) or if the site must be examined (e.g., because of pain or odor). A dressing change every 2 days is required for a gauze and tape dressing.
- Perform site care with each dressing change. Cleanse the catheter–skin junction with an appropriate antiseptic solution, apply a sterile stabilizer, and apply a new sterile dressing.
- Manipulate the catheter hub as little as possible.
  To minimize catheter movement, phlebitis, and contamination of the line. Less catheter manipulation is associated with fewer bloodstream infections.
- Flush catheters before and after any infusions or per agency protocol. This may be every 12 to 24 hours when not in use.
  - Flush volume should be twice the volume of the catheter and add-on devices (consult package label).
  - Use a syringe size recommended by the catheter manufacturer (10 mL is the smallest size recommended because of the pressure generated).
  - Type of flush solution depends on agency policy (saline versus heparin).
  - Use single-use, labeled syringes of flush solution to prevent cross-contamination.
  - If you have trouble flushing, the catheter may be kinked or malpositioned, the inline filter may be clogged, or a clamp may need to be released. You can correct these problems.
- ✚ Never flush against resistance.

  The catheter might be clogged and you would risk dislodging a small clot. This could also rupture the catheter.

- ✚ If the patient has a PICC line, take blood pressures on the alternate arm.

  Using the arm with the PICC can cause bleeding at the site, thrombus formation, retrograde blood flow, and increased risk of catheter occlusion.

Clinical Insight 39-4 ➤ Caring for Patients With a Central Venous Access Device (CVAD): CVC and PICC—cont'd

- If the patient is receiving parenteral nutrition, reserve and label one lumen just for that purpose.

Documentation

- Document routine assessments and the condition of the catheter–skin junction site. When site care is given, also document the patient's response and any actions taken to correct or prevent adverse reactions.

Related Information

For information about dressing changes, refer to Procedure 39-5B: Central Line Dressings.

For information about administering medications through a CVAD, see Procedure 25-18: Administering Medication Through a Central Venous Access Device.

Practice Resources

Centers for Disease Control and Prevention (2016); Infusion Nurses Society (2011); Institute for Healthcare Improvement (2012); Marschall, J., Mermel, L., Fakih, M., et al. (2014).

Clinical Insight 39-5 ➤ Managing Infiltration and Extravasation

- At the first sign or symptom of infiltration or extravasation, stop the IV. Symptoms include slowed or stopped flow, swelling, tenderness, pallor, hardness, and coolness at the site.
- The patient may report a burning sensation in the area.

For a Central Venous Access Device: CVC or PICC:

- Clamp and cap the catheter hub.
- Do not remove the catheter.
- Follow agency policy when you suspect infiltration or extravasation.
- If the patient has an implanted port, aspirate, remove the port access needle, and apply a dressing.
- Notify the provider who inserted the catheter, who may order an x-ray to help determine the cause of the problem.

For a Short Peripheral Catheter:

- Disconnect the tubing from the catheter hub; attach a 3- to 5-mL syringe and try to aspirate fluid from the catheter lumen. Use aseptic technique.
- Photograph the site to create a record of its condition, if agency policy allows.
- Wearing gloves, remove the catheter and hold a dry gauze pad over the site to stop the bleeding. Apply a dry dressing. Do not apply excessive pressure to the site.
- If you are to start a new IV, start it on the other arm, if possible. If it is not possible, start it in a more proximal location on the same arm.
- Measure the circumference of the arm and compare it with the opposite arm.
- Assess capillary refill, sensation, and motion distal to the infiltrated site.

- Apply cold or warm compresses depending on which fluid has escaped into the tissues.
  - For alkaloids (e.g., vincristine) and epipodophyllotoxins (e.g., etoposide), use heat.
  - For hypertonic fluids or medications, use cold.
  - For isotonic or hypotonic fluids or medications, choose either heat or cold, or alternate them, based on patient comfort.
- Apply compresses for 15 to 30 minutes every 4 to 6 hours; continue for 24 to 48 hours.
- Estimate the volume of fluid that escaped into the tissues; notify the prescriber.
- Some medications leaked into the surrounding tissue can cause damage and even necrosis. For instance, when dopamine extravasates, you might need to give a prescribed amount of antidote (e.g., regitine injected subcutaneously) as well as hydrocortisone and an anti-inflammatory to minimize tissue damage. Be sure to check the protocol at your facility.
- Elevate the extremity and advise the patient to rest.
- Document all fluids and medications involved, equipment being used (e.g., pump), size and type of the catheter, description of the site (including location, size, and color), methods used to assess the site before administering the fluids (e.g., aspiration), patient's signs and symptoms, interventions, notifications, and patient teaching.
- Complete an occurrence (incident) report as required by your facility.

Practice Resources

Gahart, B., & Nazareno, A. (2016); Masoorli, S. (2012).

PROCEDURES

To prevent, identify, and treat fluid, electrolyte, and acid–base problems, you will need to be skilled at initiating and managing intravenous infusions of fluids and blood, performing focused history and physical assessments, and interpreting arterial blood gas (ABG) values. When performing the procedures, apply the concepts and other theoretical knowledge you have learned.

Procedure 39-1 ■ Initiating a Peripheral Intravenous Infusion

> ➤ For steps to follow in *all* procedures, refer to the Universal Steps for All Procedures found on the page facing the inside back cover.

Equipment

- IV solution
- Administration set or IV lock and injection caps. (For a glass solution container, use vented tubing; for a plastic container, you may use either vented or nonvented tubing.)
- Extension tubing with or without saline lock.
- Appropriately sized intravenous (IV) catheter
- Prefilled syringe to prime extension tubing.
- Clean, unsterile gloves
- Scissors
- Antiseptic swabs that contain solutions such as chlorhexidine (preferred by the Centers for Disease Control and Prevention [CDC], 2011a) or 70% alcohol wipes.
- Tourniquet (non-latex, if available)
- Sterile manufactured catheter stabilization device or ½-in. tape.
- 2 in. × 2 in. sterile gauze, and/or transparent semipermeable occlusive dressing
- 1-in. nonallergenic tape, preferably clear
- Labels, time tape
- Linen-saver pad
- Arm board, if necessary

Delegation

In some states and agencies you can delegate peripheral IV catheter insertion to a licensed practical nurse (LPN) who is adequately trained in the skill.

Pre-Procedure Assessment

- Assess the patient's need for IV therapy by checking vital signs, laboratory values, urine output, skin turgor, breath sounds, and the condition of mucous membranes.
- Check for any situations that may contraindicate administering the prescribed fluids to the patient.
- Assess for allergy to tape.
- Assess the veins on the arms and hands for a potential insertion site.
  The upper extremities are preferred because of better blood flow, easier access, and less potential for complications than in other locations.
- Check the medical record for factors such as anticoagulant therapy, bleeding disorders, or low platelet count.
  These factors place the patient at risk of bleeding during IV catheter insertion.

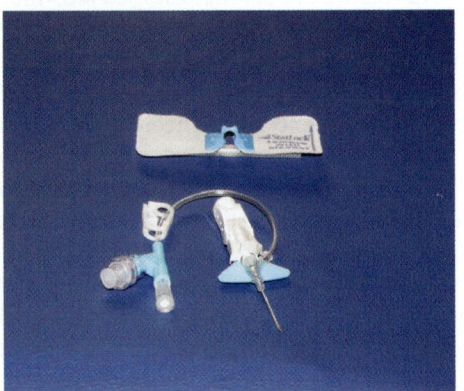

➤ When performing the procedure, always identify your patient according to agency policy, using two identifiers, and be attentive to standard precautions, hand hygiene, patient safety and privacy, body mechanics, and documentation.

Procedure Steps

✚ NOTE: *Maintain scrupulous aseptic technique throughout this procedure.*
Any microorganisms introduced can cause infection at the site, which could quickly migrate into the bloodstream and cause sepsis.

1. **Place the patient in** a comfortable position, the bed at a comfortable working height, and supplies within reach. Explain the procedure to the patient.
   Makes the procedure safer and easier and decreases the risk for the nurse to develop back problems from improper body mechanics.

2. **Prepare the IV solution** and administration set or IV lock.
   a. Following the "rights" of medication administration, check the IV solution to make sure that you have the proper solution with the prescribed additives.
      IV solution is considered medication, and you should check it carefully to avoid administration and compatibility errors.
   b. Check the expiration date on the IV solution. Do not use IV solution after the expiration date
   c. Check the IV solution for discoloration or particulate matter.
      Indicates contamination and should not be used.
   d. Label the IV solution container with the patient's name, date, and your initials. Place a time tape on the solution container with the prescribed infusion rate, time the infusion begins, and the time it is to be completed.
      Policies govern when solution containers, administration sets, dressings, and IV catheters all need to be changed to avoid complications such as infection. Although not all agencies require a time tape, labeling infusion rates on the solution containers in this manner will alert others and makes it easy to see at a glance whether the solution is infusing on time. ➤

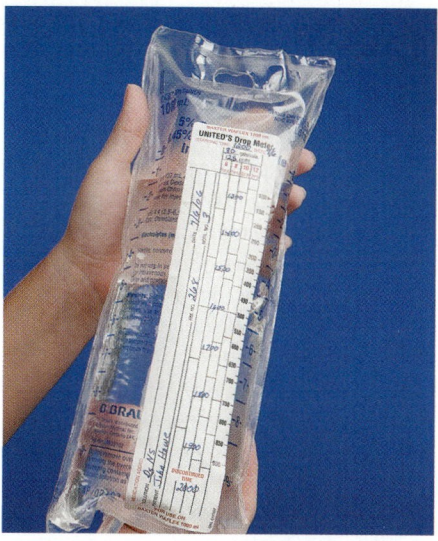

e. Take the administration set from the package and close the roller clamp by rolling it downward. Label the tubing with the date and time.
   Ensures that fluid does not flow through inadvertently after the bag is spiked.
f. Remove the protective cover from the solution container port.
g. Remove the protective cover from the spike on the IV administration set, keeping the spike sterile. Insert the spike into the port of the solution container. ▼

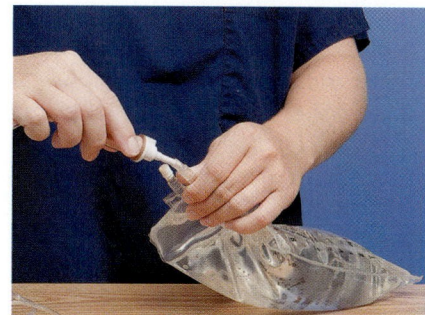

When Using a Glass Bottle
Clean the rubber stopper on the top of the bottle with an alcohol pad. Then insert the spike of the administration set through the stopper.
   h. Be certain the tubing is clamped. Hang the IV solution container on an IV pole.
      Clamping prevents leakage of fluid.

i. Lightly compress the drip chamber, and allow it to fill up halfway.
   Overfilling the drip chamber will impair your ability to see the drips and adequately regulate the IV flow rate. ▼

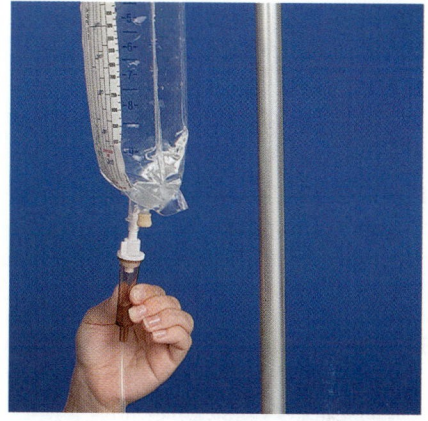

When Not Using Extension Tubing
Prime the tubing by opening the roller clamp and allowing the fluid to slowly fill the tubing. When tubing is filled, close the clamp.

When Using Extension Tubing
Either attach it to the end of the administration set now and prime it with the rest of the IV line or prime it separately, as follows:
   j. Scrub the injection port of the extension tubing with an alcohol pad and let it dry.
   k. Attach a flush syringe filled with normal saline to the injection port or to the non-luer-lock end and slowly push the fluid through the tubing until completely primed. (Consult packaging instructions for the amount of saline needed to flush the tubing.)
   l. Leave flush syringe attached to the extension tubing.
      IV extension tubing makes it easier to convert an IV to a saline lock without disturbing the IV dressing and catheter. Manipulation of the IV catheter increases the risk of complications such as phlebitis, inflammation, infection, and infiltration.

(continued on next page)

Procedure 39–1 ■ **Initiating a Peripheral Intravenous Infusion** (continued)

m. Inspect the tubing for air. If air bubbles remain in the tubing, flick the tubing with a fingertip to mobilize them into the drip chamber. Recap the end of the tubing firmly.
Air in the tubing creates the potential for air embolism.

3. **Place a linen-saver pad** under the patient's arm.
Protects the bed from soiling during venipuncture.

4. **Place the patient's arm** in a dependent position.
Gravity helps fill and dilate the vein, making venipuncture easier.

5. **Apply a tourniquet** 10 to 20 cm (4 to 8 in.) above the selected site. Palpate the radial pulse. If no pulse is present, loosen the tourniquet, and reapply it with less tension.
Occluding the arterial flow diminishes venous filling, making venipuncture difficult.

6. **Locate a vein for inserting the IV** catheter. Select the best most distal vein on the hand or arm. Check with the medical provider before using an arm or hand that contains a dialysis graft or fistula, or the affected arm of a patient who has undergone a mastectomy. See Clinical Insight 39-3 for more guidelines.
Choose the most distal veins on the hand or arm so that you can perform subsequent venipunctures proximal to the previous site. This preserves veins for long-term therapy and prevents extravasation of fluid and medicines.

7. **Palpate the vein and press it** downward, making sure that it rebounds quickly. If the vein is not adequately dilated, ask the patient to open and close his fist; apply heat (e.g., a warm towel, a warming mitt); lightly tap the vein site; or stroke the extremity from distal to proximal, beginning below the selected venipuncture site. If available in your agency, use an infrared or other visualization device to assist in locating a vein.

These maneuvers bring blood to the local area to dilate the vein, making it easier to locate and making venipuncture easier.

8. **Loosen the tourniquet.** If excessive hair is present at the venipuncture site, clip it with scissors.
Loosening the tourniquet restores blood flow and allows for patient comfort while preparing for venipuncture. Clipping the hair helps the dressings to adhere after catheter insertion. Shaving is not recommended because it may abrade the skin, providing a portal of entry for pathogens.

9. **Don clean nonsterile gloves.**
Provides protection from inadvertent exposure to blood. Note that some nurses don gloves routinely, even when preparing supplies and equipment. However, there is no risk for coming in contact with body fluids before this step, so strictly speaking, CDC standard precautions require gloves only from this step forward.

10. **Select an IV catheter** appropriate for the size of the vein, the solution to be infused, and the expected duration of therapy. Using aseptic technique, open the package touching only the outside of it.
Reduces the risk of extravasation and phlebitis. Always use the smallest diameter and shortest catheter that will deliver the desired solution flow. For most adults this will be a 20- to 24-gauge to minimize venous irritation and promote blood flow around the catheter. Aseptic handling reduces the risk of infection.

11. **Gently reapply the tourniquet** and scrub the site, using an antiseptic swab that contains chlorhexidine gluconate (preferred, CDC, 2011a); if this is not available, use 70% alcohol wipes. Cleanse for 30 seconds, using friction.
Removes microorganisms from the skin so that they do not enter the venous system during venipuncture. Working "clean to dirty," or from the venipuncture site

outward, avoids moving microorganisms toward the puncture site. ▼

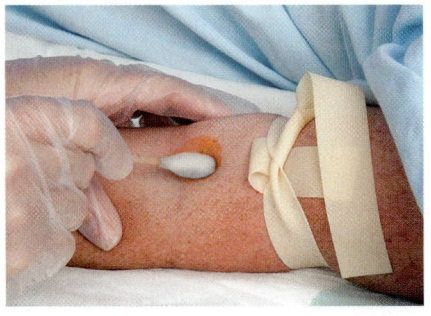

12. **Allow the antiseptic to air-dry.** Do not fan.
The antiseptic promotes adherence of the dressing. Fanning can cause contamination of the skin.

13. **Pick up the catheter and inspect the tip.**
There should be no burrs (rough spots, ridges) on the needle or peeling of the catheter material.

14. **Inform the patient** that you are about to insert the catheter and that it may be uncomfortable.
Keeping the patient informed promotes cooperation and lessens anxiety.

Procedure Variation If Using a Wing-Tipped Catheter (Butterfly)

15. **Grasp the catheter by the wings,** using the thumb and forefinger of your dominant hand, making sure that the bevel is up. Remove the protective cap from the needle.
Stabilizes the catheter for insertion. Inserting the needle bevel up makes it less likely that you will pierce both vein walls (go "through" the vein) as well as making piercing the skin less painful for the patient. ▼

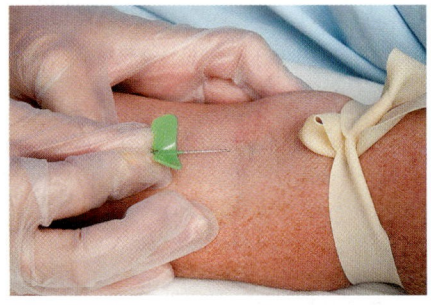

Procedure Variation If Using an Over-the-Needle Catheter

16. **Grasp the catheter** by the hub, using the thumb and forefinger of your dominant hand, making sure that the bevel is up.

    See Wing-Tipped Catheter rationale, preceding. ▼

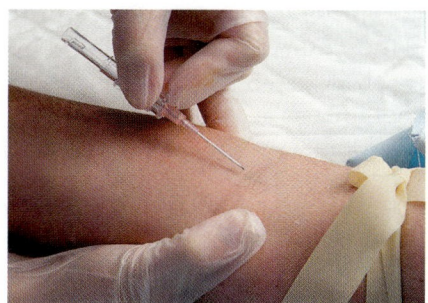

17. **Using your nondominant hand,** stabilize the vein by continuously pulling the skin taut below the puncture area (pull downward toward the hand or fingers). Do not press too hard and make sure not to contaminate the insertion site.

    Stabilizing the vein eases insertion and prevents damage to the underside of the vein as well as preventing the vein from rolling. Pressing too hard compresses blood flow in the vein and causes it to collapse. ▼

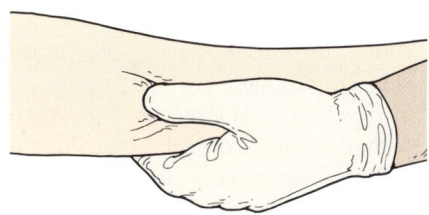

18. **Holding the catheter** at a 30° to 45° angle, pierce the skin directly over the vein. Penetrate all layers of the vein with one quick, smooth motion.

    A 30° to 45° angle allows you to pierce the skin without inadvertently passing through the vein and allows backflow of blood into the catheter.

19. **Look for a flashback of blood** into the chamber of the catheter or the tubing of the winged catheter.

    The flashback of blood indicates that the vein has been entered, but only by the needle when using an over-the-needle catheter.

20. **Lower the angle of the catheter** and needle to skin level and advance them into the vein.

For a Wing-Tipped Catheter
Fully advance the catheter.

For an Over-the-Needle Catheter
Still maintaining traction on the skin with your nondominant hand, hold the catheter hub with your thumb and middle finger and use your index finger to advance the catheter to at least half of its length before you begin withdrawing the needle. When a steady backflow of blood occurs, partially withdraw the needle while advancing the catheter fully into the vein. For an animated illustration of an over-the-needle IV catheter,

Withdrawing the needle too early will result in the catheter not fully entering the vein, only the needle. There will be no bleeding from the catheter and infiltration will occur when starting the IV solution. The patient will also experience pain. ▼

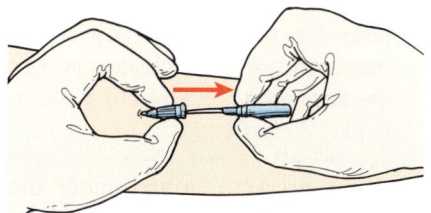

21. **While holding the catheter** in place with one hand, release the tourniquet and remove or retract the needle.

For an Over-the-Needle Catheter
Hold the catheter in place by placing light pressure on the catheter, away from the hub and venipuncture site.

➕ Never attempt to reinsert the needle after it is withdrawn. This can damage the catheter and even cause bits of it to break off within the vein.

For a Winged Needle
Place a finger lightly on the same area plus a finger farther along the vein away from the needle so the needle does not go through the vein.

Releasing the tourniquet restores full circulation to the patient's extremity and prevents injury. Placing light pressure on the catheter or vein minimizes bleeding from the catheter or needle while you complete the procedure.

22. **Quickly connect** the administration set to the IV catheter, using aseptic technique.

    To minimize bleeding and prevent infection. ▼

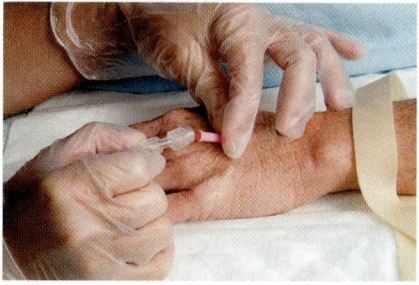

If Using a Peripheral IV Lock
Once the lock is connected, flush with normal saline and then disconnect the flush. A common amount is 1 to 2 mL, but tubing varies, so check package instructions for the exact amount needed.

Flushing the catheter both clears it and keeps it sterile.

23. **While still stabilizing** the catheter, slowly open the roller clamp. Observe that flow is achieved. Adjust the drip to the prescribed flow rate.

24. **Secure the connection** between the tubing and the catheter. Many sets have luer-lock connections, so no further securing is needed. If not using luer-lock tubing, clasping devices and threaded devices can be used. Do not use tape.

    Secure the connection to prevent separation of tubing from the hub.

➕ Taping is not recommended because the junction is not visible under tape; therefore, the tubing could separate from the catheter without being discovered, possibly leading to air embolism, bleeding, or infection.

25. **Stabilize the catheter.** Use an agency-approved device. Catheter stabilization devices include manufactured devices (such as StatLok) or tape.

When Stabilizing With Tape
Place a narrow (¼-in.) strip of tape under the catheter hub and crisscross the ends over the hub to form a chevron. Apply tape only to the catheter hub, not to the

(continued on next page)

Procedure 39-1 ■ **Initiating a Peripheral Intravenous Infusion** (continued)

catheter itself, and do not apply tape directly to the site where the catheter enters the skin.

Luer-locks are designed to prevent accidental disengagement of tubing and catheter; they do not stabilize the catheter. Catheter stabilization is important to minimize catheter movement and help prevent complications such as phlebitis, inflammation, infiltration, and infection.

26. **Dress the site,** following agency policy. If needed, clean the site with an antiseptic swab and allow it to dry before applying the dressing.

If Using a Transparent Dressing (Preferred)

a. Open the package containing the dressing. Remove the protective backing from the dressing, making sure not to touch the sterile surface.

b. Cover the insertion site and the hub or winged portion of the catheter with the dressing. Do not cover the junction with the administration tubing. ▼

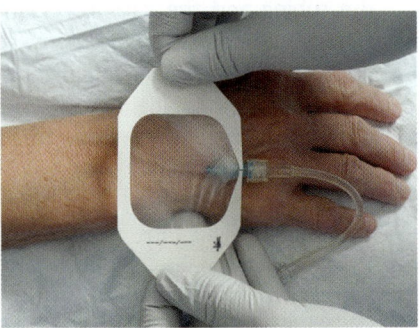

c. Gently pinch the transparent dressing around the catheter hub to secure the hub further. Smooth the remainder of the dressing so that it adheres to the skin. ▼

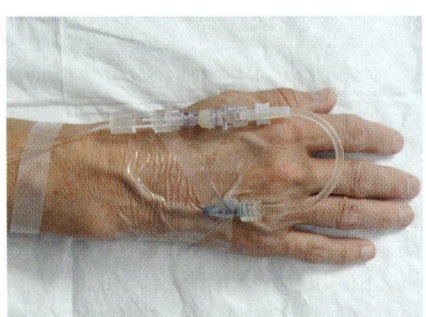

If You Must Use a Gauze Dressing

a. Fold a 2 in. × 2 in. sterile gauze dressing in half, cover it with 1-in. tape (about 3 in. long).

b. Place under the tubing/hub junction and press down on the tape.
Raises hub off the skin and prevents pressure on the skin.

c. Place a sterile gauze pad over the insertion site and catheter hub—but not over the catheter–hub junction.

d. Secure all edges with tape.

27. **Label the dressing** with the date and time of insertion, catheter size, and your initials.
A label lets nurses see at a glance how long the dressing has been in place.

28. **Secure the IV administration** tubing by looping and taping the tubing to the skin.
Helps prevent the IV catheter from becoming dislodged and decreases movement of the catheter, thereby decreasing the risk of phlebitis, inflammation, and infiltration.

29. **Place an arm board** under the joint and secure it with tape, if the insertion site is located near a joint.
An arm board stabilizes the joint and helps prevent the catheter from becoming dislodged. However, avoid inserting an IV near a joint when possible, as there is increased potential for movement of the IV catheter, leading to an increased risk of complications. IVs placed in the antecubital fossa are difficult to assess for infiltration. Arm boards are not widely used because of the high acuity of inpatients, many of whom have central lines instead of peripheral IVs.

30. **Dispose of all supplies,** including sharps, into appropriate receptacles; raise the siderail; lower the bed; and be sure the patient call system is within reach. Wash your hands.
Prevents infection and ensure patient and staff safety.

? *What if . . .*

■ **The patient is an older adult?**

Do not scrub skin too vigorously.
This can damage fragile surface tissue, creating a portal for pathogens.

Use a softer tourniquet and do not apply tightly; for well-dilated veins, do not use one at all.
This decreases the risk of rupture of fragile veins.

Use the smallest catheter possible to meet the infusion needs.
Insert the needle at an almost flat angle (10° to 20°).
In most older adults, veins are close to the skin surface.

Before penetrating the skin, apply traction to the vein below the insertion site.
Makes it easier and less painful for the needle to enter the skin.

Insert the catheter on top of the vein; do not use the side access technique.
If bleeding occurs, hold gentle pressure longer than for younger patients.
A clot may take longer to form.

■ **The patient is an infant younger than 2 months old?**

Allow the antiseptic to air-dry on the skin. Do not fan.
Increases the antiseptic's effectiveness; promotes patient comfort on puncture of the skin; promotes adherence of dressing. Fanning increases exposure to airborne microbes.

■ ✚ **The patient is allergic to iodine or shellfish?**

Use 70% alcohol or chlorhexidine for 30 seconds to cleanse the site, not povidone-iodine or iodine.

- **You are not successful with the first venipuncture attempt?**

  Use a new cannula and make a second attempt on the other arm or, if that is not possible, higher up on the same arm. Do not make more than two attempts to start an IV without seeking assistance.

- **When you insert the needle and catheter and connect the tubing, you see bright red blood quickly appear and start to advance up the tubing?**

  You may have inadvertently entered an artery. If this occurs, remove the catheter and apply direct pressure for at least 5 minutes. Notify the primary care provider. Monitor the extremity distal to the insertion site for pulses, color, and temperature.

Evaluation

- Monitor the IV site and flow rate regularly (many agency standards require hourly) while IV fluid is infusing. Check for signs of infiltration, inflammation, and phlebitis.
- Monitor the patient's tolerance of IV therapy by auscultating breath sounds and monitoring vital signs, urine output, laboratory values, and neck vein distention. Report to the primary provider any signs of fluid overload, such as crackles, edema, shortness of breath, diminished urine output, increased blood pressure, increased heart rate with bounding pulse, and distended neck veins. Fluid overload can lead to pulmonary edema and heart failure.

Patient Teaching

- Instruct the patient about IV therapy.
- Teach the patient the importance of notifying staff immediately if the catheter or administration set becomes dislodged; the insertion site becomes tender, red, or swollen; or the patient notices moisture or fluid leakage.
- Explain the desired and adverse effects of IV therapy and tell the patient to notify staff if he develops discomfort or breathing difficulty.
- Teach the patient measures to avoid dislodging the catheter.

Home Care

- Explain home IV therapy to the client and caregiver and teach them how to identify complications.

- Provide the client with the name and phone numbers of people to contact in case problems arise with the catheter site or if there is a change in level of comfort.

Documentation

- Date and time of insertion, gauge and type of catheter, number of attempts, and location of the insertion site
- Tourniquet use (or nonuse)
- Blood return in catheter; whether the IV flushes, type and amount of flush solution used
- Dressing and tape type used
- Method of securing or stabilizing the IV line
- Type and rate of the IV fluid infusing
- Patient's tolerance of the procedure, any adverse reactions to the insertion or IV therapy, and the interventions required
- Patient teaching
- Often, IV care is documented on a flow sheet. Fluids infused are documented on the intake and output (I&O) record as well.

Practice Resources

Barclay, L., & Nghiem, H. (2011); Camp-Sorrel, D. (2010); Centers for Disease Control and Prevention (2011a); Infusion Nurses Society (2011); Masoorli, S. (2012); Shlamovitz, G. (2015a, updated).

Thinking About the Procedure

The video **Initiating a Peripheral Intravenous Infusion,** along with questions and suggested responses, is available on the **Davis's *Nursing Skills Videos*** Web site on Davis*Plus.*

Procedure 39-2 ■ Regulating the IV Flow Rate

> For steps to follow in *all* procedures, refer to the Universal Steps for All Procedures found on the page facing the inside back cover.

Equipment

- IV solution hanging on an IV pole and attached to an administration set
- Watch with a second hand or digital seconds
- Time tape

Delegation

Refer to your state nurse practice act and agency policy regarding delegation of this task to an LPN.

Pre-Procedure Assessment

- Assess the IV catheter for patency and date of insertion before starting the infusion and then regularly (many agencies specify hourly) while the IV fluid infuses.

  Decreases risk of complications related to incorrect infusion rate, expired infusion solution, tubing, or catheter dwell time.

- Assess the IV site for signs of phlebitis, infiltration, infection, or inflammation.

  You must change the IV catheter before regulating the flow rate if any of these complications occur.

(continued on next page)

Procedure 39-2 ■ **Regulating the IV Flow Rate** (continued)

- Confirm the patient's need for IV therapy by verifying the order and checking laboratory values, urine output, vital signs, and breath sounds.

Ensures that the patient still needs IV fluids and that the solution is correct. Laboratory values and assessment findings monitor the IV treatment plan. IV therapy creates a risk for fluid overload.

➤ When performing the procedure, always identify your patient according to agency policy, using two identifiers, and be attentive to standard precautions, hand hygiene, patient safety and privacy, body mechanics, and documentation.

Procedure Steps

1. **Follow all the "checks" and "rights"** of medication administration, including verifying the prescription. Check the solution to make sure that you have the proper IV fluid hanging with the prescribed additives, and that there is no discoloration of or particles or crystallization in the fluid. Also verify the infusion rate.

   IV solution is considered medication, and you should check it carefully to avoid administration and compatibility errors. Do not simply pull a bag of fluid from a shelf assuming that the shelf is labeled properly, as bags are often misplaced and this is a potential source of error.

2. **Calculate the hourly rate** if it is not specified in the order. Divide the volume to be infused by the number of hours it is to be infused. For example, if the physician prescribes 1,000 mL to run over the course of 4 hours, the infusion rate is 250 mL/hr.

   You must carefully calculate the infusion rate to ensure that the patient receives the correct volume of fluid.

   NOTE: If you are using a volume-control pump, you can omit steps 3 and 4.

3. **Calculate the drip rate** by multiplying the number of milliliters to be infused in 60 minutes by the drop factor in drops [gtts]/per milliliter; then divide by 60 minutes:

$$\frac{\text{Hourly rate in mL} \times (\text{gtts/mL})}{60 \text{ minutes}} = \text{drip rate}$$

   For example, an hourly rate of 100 mL multiplied by 15 gtts/mL and divided by 60 minutes equals 25. Therefore, the drip rate equals 25 gtts/minute. Each

administration set has a drip factor that is determined by the manufacturer. The **drip factor** *is the number of drops necessary to deliver 1 mL of solution. Micro-drip tubing has a drip factor of 60 gtts/mL; blood administration tubing typically has a drip factor of 10 gtts/mL; macrodrip tubing has a drip factor of 15 gtts/mL.*

4. **Verify your calculations.**
   To prevent dosage errors, either have a second person verify your calculations or check them a second time yourself.

5. **Apply a time tape** when hanging a new bag to the IV solution container next to the volume markings. Mark the time tape with the time that the infusion was started. Continue to mark 1-hour intervals on the time tape until you reach the bottom of the container.
   The time tape allows all nurses to accurately monitor the rate of administration.

6. **Open the roller clamp** so that IV fluid begins to flow (when hanging a new bag).
   The roller clamp must be opened to allow the flow of fluid.

7. **Set the rate.**

For Gravity Drip
Using a watch placed next to the drip chamber, count the number of drops entering the drip chamber in 1 minute. Adjust the roller clamp by increasing or decreasing the flow until you achieve the prescribed drip rate.
Timing the drip rate for 1 minute helps to accurately achieve the correct drip rate and having the watch next to what you are counting will ensure that you do not miss seeing any drops. ➤

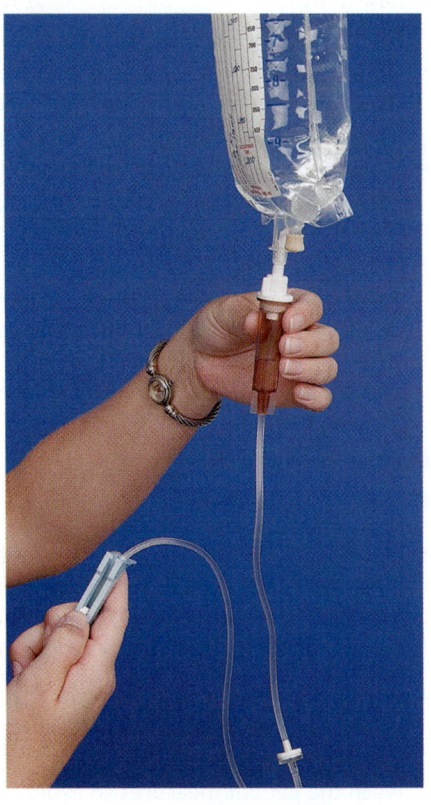

For a Volume-Control Pump
Program the ordered rate into the pump.
IV solution is considered a medication and must infuse at the prescribed rate.

8. **Monitor manually regulated** infusion rates closely for the 15 minutes after you begin an infusion; then monitor at least hourly by counting drops per minute or reading the numbers on the pumps.
   Changes in the patient's position may speed up or slow down the infusion rate; frequent monitoring of the infusion rate ensures that the correct volume of fluid infuses over the correct length of time.

? What if . . .

- **The prescription for the IV flow rate changes?**

  Recalculate the new flow rate and adjust the drops/minute to obtain the desired new flow rate. Also, remove the old time tape and place a new time tape with the new rate of infusion.

- **When you check the rate, you discover that the IV has been running too slowly for the past hour?**

  Adjust to the correct rate, but do not attempt to catch up by adjusting the flow to a rate higher than prescribed. *Too rapid IV infusion can lead to fluid overload for patients with congestive heart failure or other cardiopulmonary problems.*

- **When you check the rate, you discover that the IV has been running too fast for the past hour?**

  Slow the rate and assess the patient for signs of fluid volume excess.

Evaluation

- Evaluate the patient's response to IV therapy by checking for signs of excessive or deficient fluid volume.
- Evaluate the IV site for signs of infiltration, inflammation, infection, and phlebitis.
- Check laboratory studies to help evaluate the effectiveness of IV therapy.
- Monitor for correct IV rate at least hourly.
- Evaluate the tubing for kinks or for patient lying on the tubing.
  Kinked tubing will interfere with the flow rate.

Patient Teaching

- Explain the desired and adverse effects of IV therapy.
- Discuss the importance of notifying staff immediately if the catheter or administration set becomes dislodged; if the insertion site becomes tender, red, or swollen; if the patient notices moisture or fluid leakage; or if he has difficulty breathing.
- Teach safety measures if the patient is permitted to ambulate while the IV is infusing.

Home Care

- Explain home IV therapy to the client and caregiver and teach them how to identify complications.
- Provide the client and caregiver with the name and phone numbers of people to contact in case problems arise with the catheter, insertion site, or level of comfort.

Documentation

Often IV care is documented on a flow sheet and includes the following:

- Date and time the infusion was started
- Type of IV fluid, rate of infusion, and IV catheter site
- Whether rate is manual or pump controlled
- Patient's tolerance of IV therapy, any complications, and the interventions taken
- Document the volume infused on the I&O record.

Practice Resources

Infusion Nurses Society (2011); Phillips, L., & Gorski, L. (2014); Shlamovitz, G. (2015a, updated).

Procedure 39-3 ■ Setting Up and Using Volume-Control Pumps

➤ For steps to follow in *all* procedures, refer to the Universal Steps for All Procedures found on the page facing the inside back cover.

Equipment

- Nonsterile gloves
- Alcohol wipes or chlorhexidine/alcohol antiseptic product
- Volume-control pump and IV pole
- Administration set appropriate for the pump
- IV fluid or medicated solution
- Tape for IV fluid solution time tape

Delegation

You can delegate the task of setting up a volume-control pump to an LPN who is specially trained in IV therapy, if covered by the agency's policy. Do not delegate this task to nursing assistive personnel (NAP). Do, however, instruct the NAP to notify you of any pump alarms that sound.

Pre-Procedure Assessment

- Confirm the patient's need for IV therapy by checking vital signs, laboratory values, urine output, skin turgor, breath sounds, and the moisture of mucous membranes.
  IV therapy creates a risk for fluid overload and electrolyte imbalance, which may be revealed by assessment data.

- Assess the existing IV catheter for patency.
  Occlusion of the IV catheter prevents the infusion of IV fluid. If not patent, you will need to change the IV.

- Assess the IV site hourly for signs of phlebitis, infiltration, infection and inflammation.
  Complications of IV therapy retard the therapeutic benefit of the fluids, as well as increase medical concerns and treatment cost for the patient. You must change the IV catheter and site if any of these complications occur.

(continued on next page)

Procedure 39-3 ■ Setting Up and Using Volume-Control Pumps (continued)

> ➤ When performing the procedure, always identify your patient according to agency policy, using two identifiers, and be attentive to standard precautions, hand hygiene, patient safety and privacy, body mechanics, and documentation.

Procedure Steps

1. Calculate the infusion rate by dividing the volume to be infused by the number of hours it is to be infused. For example, if the order states 1,000 mL to run over 8 hours, divide 1,000 mL by 8 hours to determine the infusion rate of 125 mL/hr.
This ensures that the patient receives the correct dose. Pumps are usually programmed in milliliters per hour instead of drops per minute.

2. Verify your calculations.
To prevent dosage errors, either ask a second person to verify your calculations or check them a second time yourself.

3. Attach the pump to the IV pole and plug it in the nearest electrical outlet.

✚ Check to be sure that the infusion pump has a safety sticker on it and that the cord and plug are intact.

Volume-control pumps need regular maintenance checks. Using an electrical outlet saves battery power if needed for transport or electrical outage. As with gravity flow, the IV solution container needs to remain above the pump to prevent occlusion and for proper drainage of the container. ▼

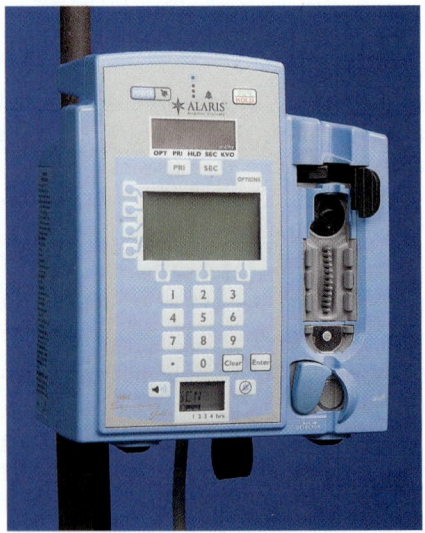

4. Take the administration set from the package and close the clamp on it.
To prevent inadvertent loss of fluid.

5. Attach a filter to the end of the administration set, if required.
Filters are sometimes used to filter minute particles from the solution.

6. Remove the protective covers and spike the port of the solution container with the administration set, maintaining sterility. Label the IV tubing and solution container with the date and time and place a time tape on the solution container. Hang the container on the IV pole.
Labeling the administration set with the date and time informs the nursing staff when the administration set should be changed. The time tape allows you, and other nurses, to see at a glance whether the correct volume is infusing.

7. Compress the drip chamber of the administration set and allow it to fill halfway. Consult the manufacturer's instructions for setup, as pumps differ. (On older gravity pumps, place the electronic eye on the drip chamber between the fluid level and the origin of the drop.)
Prepares the administration set for priming and prevents air from entering the tubing with the solution. Infusion pumps compress the tubing to move fluid; they measure the amount internally. On older gravity-type pumps, an electronic eye counts the number of drops to ensure the proper rate.

8. Prime the administration set with fluid by opening the roller clamp and allowing the fluid to flow slowly through the tubing. Close the clamp.
Priming removes air from the tubing to prevent air embolus.

9. Inspect the tubing for air. If air bubbles remain in the tubing, flick the tubing with a fingertip to mobilize the bubbles into the drip chamber.
Air bubbles in the administration tubing interrupt flow and they can cause air emboli, which can be dangerous to the patient if they accumulate in the circulation.

10. Turn on the pump and load the administration tubing into the pump according to the manufacturer's instructions.

NOTE: This process differs among manufacturers. ▼

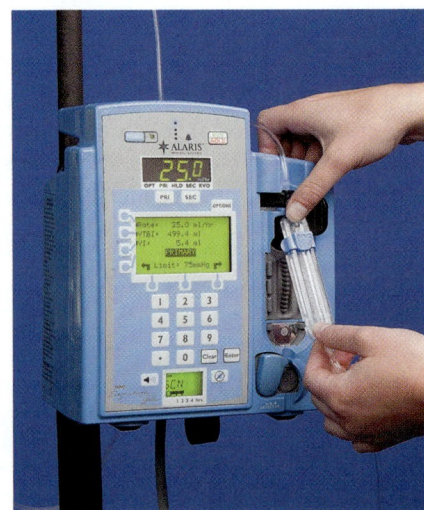

11. Program the pump with the prescribed information: total hours, infusion rate (hourly rate), and the volume to be infused (usually the total amount in the IV bag). *Note: Some pumps have only total hours and volume to infuse and do not have a feature that allows you to program in the infusion rate.* ➤

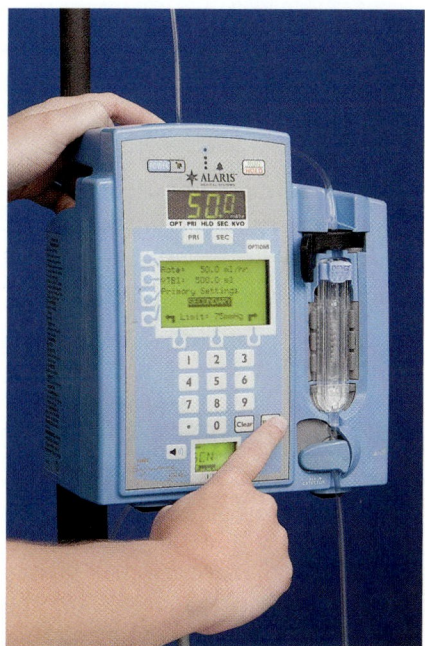

12. Don clean nonsterile gloves (per agency policy), check the IV site for patency, and scrub all surfaces of the primary line injection port or needleless connector, including the threads, with an antiseptic pad for at least 15 seconds. Allow it to dry.

Clean nonsterile gloves protect from exposure to body fluids when you connect the tubing to the IV catheter or port. Scrubbing the port helps prevent infection.

13. Connect the administration set adapter to the injection port, keeping the connecting ends sterile.

Aseptic technique decreases the risk for contamination.

14. Unclamp the administration set tubing (open the roller clamp all the way) and press the start button on the pump.

Allows the IV fluid to flow through the administration set.

15. Make sure the alarms are turned on and audible.

The alarms must be functioning so that the pump can alert you of problems, such as kinks, air in the tubing, or catheter occlusion.

KEY POINT: *Do not depend completely on the pump alarms to indicate IV patency. Pumps can infuse fluid, even if the line is clogged or infiltrated into the surrounding tissue.*

16. Check the pump regularly to make sure the correct volume is infusing. Checks are commonly done hourly.

Infusion pumps sometimes malfunction, so frequent monitoring is essential.

17. At the end of your shift (or at the time specified by your healthcare facility), clear the pump of the volume infused and record the volume on the patient's I&O form.

This helps the oncoming shift accurately monitor the fluid infused during their shift.

? What if . . .

- **You later find the IV free flowing and not running via the pump setting?**

Immediately slow the IV fluid down. At the same time, begin assessing the patient: vital signs, mental awareness, lung sounds, pulse oximetry. Depending on the type of fluid running, you may need to make other assessments. Calculate the amount of IV fluid actually infused compared with the prescribed amount. Notify the provider and write out an occurrence report. If the pump is malfunctioning, set it aside, label it as "not working," and notify biomedical engineering so they can repair it.

Labeling the pump will prevent others from using it, until it can be repaired.

Evaluation

- Monitor the correct functioning of the pump regularly, perhaps hourly.
- Assess the IV site hourly for signs of phlebitis, infiltration, infection, and inflammation.

Complications of IV therapy interfere with the therapeutic benefit of the fluids and increase medical concerns, and treatment costs for the patient. You must change the IV catheter and document if any of these complications occur.

Patient Teaching

- Explain use of the IV infusion pump to the patient.
- Teach the patient the importance of notifying staff immediately if the infusion pump alarm sounds; the catheter or administration set becomes dislodged; the insertion site becomes tender, red, or swollen; or the dressing becomes wet.
- Teach the patient safety measures if he is able to ambulate while the infusion pump is in use.

Home Care

- Explain home IV infusion pump use to the client and caregiver and teach them how to identify complications. Most home infusion pumps are smaller than institutional pumps.
- Provide the client with the name and phone numbers of people to contact in case problems arise with the catheter, insertion site, IV infusion pump, or other equipment.

Documentation

- Type and volume of IV fluid infusing, along with the infusion rate
- Use of the infusion pump, and patient's tolerance of IV therapy
- Any complications of IV therapy and the interventions taken
- Document volume infused on the patient's I&O record and/or an IV flow sheet.

(continued on next page)

Procedure 39-3 ■ Setting Up and Using Volume-Control Pumps (continued)

Sample documentation

07/26/16   0600   Patient admitted from the ED with dehydration. NSS infusing at 250 mL/hr via infusion pump through an 18-gauge catheter. No signs of infiltration. No tenderness, redness, or swelling at the insertion site. Temp 102.6°F orally. HR 118 beats/min, RR 24 breaths/min, and BP 90/46 ———— R. Brill, RN

Practice Resources

Cummings, K., & McGowan, R. (2011); Phillips, L., & Gorski, L. (2014).

Thinking About the Procedure

 The video **Setting Up and Using Volume-Control Pumps,** along with questions and suggested responses, is available on the **Davis's *Nursing Skills Videos*** Web site on Davis*Plus.*

Procedure 39-4 ■ Changing IV Solutions and Tubing

➤ For steps to follow in *all* procedures, refer to the Universal Steps for All Procedures found on the page facing the inside back cover.

Equipment

- Nonsterile gloves
- Administration set
- IV solution
- IV pole
- Antiseptic swabs that contain solutions such as 70% alcohol or 2% chlorhexidine (chlorhexidine is not recommended in infants younger than age 2 months). You may use iodine-based products if alcohol or chlorhexidine is contraindicated and the patient is not allergic to iodine.
- 1-in. nonallergenic tape
- Time tape
- Watch with a second hand or digital seconds

Delegation

You can delegate the tasks of changing IV solutions and tubing to an LPN who is specially trained in IV therapy. The task should not be delegated to a NAP. However, do instruct the NAP to notify you of any problems that occur with IV therapy, such as the disconnecting of the administration set; catheter dislodging; or complaints of pain, swelling, or redness at the insertion site.

Pre-Procedure Assessments

- Assess the IV catheter for patency before changing the solution container or administration set.
- Assess the IV site for signs of phlebitis, infiltration, infection, or inflammation.
  If any of these complications occur, discontinue the IV and start a new IV at a different site.
- Check IV catheter insertion date.
  IV catheters are replaced per agency guidelines, which are based on the CDC recommendations of changing a peripheral IV site when clinically indicated (e.g., signs of phlebitis, infiltration, irritation).

Procedure 39-4A ■ Changing the IV Solution

➤ When performing the procedure, always identify your patient according to agency policy, using two identifiers, and be attentive to standard precautions, hand hygiene, patient safety and privacy, body mechanics, and documentation.

Procedure Steps

1. **Following the rights** of medication administration, prepare and label your next container of IV solution at least 1 hour before the present infusion is scheduled to finish.
   Preparing the next IV solution container reduces the risk of the present container running dry, thereby causing clots to form that would occlude the catheter.

2. **Close the roller clamp** on the infusing administration set.
   Prevents air from entering the tubing while changing the IV solution container.

3. **Wearing clean nonsterile gloves,** remove the old IV solution container from the IV pole. Remove the spike from the bag, keeping the spike sterile.
   The spike must remain sterile to prevent contamination of the new IV fluid. Clean nonsterile gloves protect you from exposure to body fluids.

4. **Remove the protective cover** from the new IV solution container port.

5. **Place the spike into the port** of the new solution container.

For a Glass Bottle

First scrub the rubber stopper on the top of the bottle with an antiseptic pad, then insert the spike of the administration set through the rubber stopper.

Cleansing the stopper removes particulate matter and microbes.

6. **Hang the IV solution** container on the IV pole.
   Allows the fluid to infuse by gravity.

7. **Inspect the tubing** to be sure that it is free of air bubbles and the drip chamber remains half-filled. Flick the tubing with a finger to mobilize the bubbles into the drip chamber.
   Prevents air from entering the system as the new solution is hung. If the drip chamber becomes too full, it will be difficult to impossible to count the drip rate properly and regulate the IV.

8. **Open the roller clamp** and adjust the drip rate, as prescribed.

IV solution is considered a medication and must infuse at the prescribed rate for therapeutic effect and to prevent fluid overload.

9. **Affix the time tape** to the new IV solution container, if practiced within your agency. Mark the tape with the time the infusion was started and mark 1-hour intervals on the tape until you reach the bottom of the container.

The time tape allows you and other nurses to monitor the rate of administration easily.

10. **Dispose of used supplies** into appropriate receptacles, according to agency policy in line with CDC guidelines.

Procedure 39-4B ■ Changing the IV Administration Tubing and Solution

➤ When performing the procedure, always identify your patient according to agency policy, using two identifiers, and be attentive to standard precautions, hand hygiene, patient safety and privacy, body mechanics, and documentation.

Procedure Steps

1. **Prepare the IV solution** and tubing as you would when initiating a new IV. (See Procedure 39-1, step 2.)

2. **Hang the new administration** set on the IV pole.

3. **Close the roller clamp** on the old administration set.
Stops the flow of fluid from the old container.

4. **Disconnect the old tubing.**
   a. Wearing clean nonsterile gloves, place a sterile swab under the catheter hub.
   The swab absorbs any leakage from the catheter hub when you disconnect the tubing.

   b. Apply pressure to the vein about 3 inches above the insertion site, using the fourth or fifth finger of your nondominant hand. Hold the catheter hub firmly with the thumb and index finger of that hand, but do not apply downward pressure.
   Prevents blood from leaking out of the catheter during the tubing change. Holding the hub firmly keeps the catheter from moving about and traumatizing the vein.

   c. Then carefully remove the device securing the connection between the catheter and tubing. This may be as simple as unscrewing a luer-lock. The connection should not be covered by tape, but if it is, remove it so you can access the connection.

5. **Remove the protective cover** from the distal end of the new administration set.
Cover keeps the distal end sterile until you are ready to connect it to the IV catheter.

6. **Continue to stabilize the IV** catheter with your nondominant hand while applying pressure over the vein. ▼

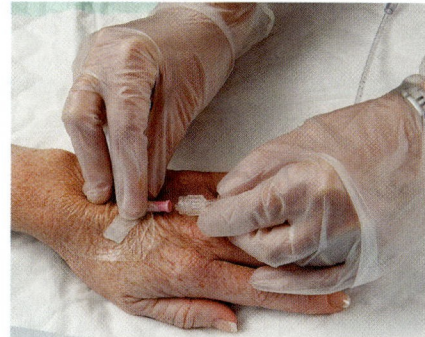

7. **Gently disengage the used** tubing from the IV catheter, and place it in a basin or other receptacle. Quickly insert the new tubing into the catheter hub.
The CDC recommends IV tubing should be changed at 96-hour intervals, but at least every 7 days, depending on agency policy and solution. Certain solutions (e.g., blood, blood products, fat emulsions) require more frequent tubing changes. Change it quickly to prevent microorganisms from entering the IV catheter.

8. **Open the roller clamp** on the new administration set and allow the IV solution to infuse.
This clears the IV catheter of blood, preventing catheter occlusion.

9. **Program and turn on** the volume-control pump. Or, for a gravity drip, use the roller clamp to adjust the flow to the prescribed rate.
IV solution is considered a medication and must infuse at the prescribed rate.

10. **Cleanse the IV site** and secure the IV catheter and tubing connection.

Removes microorganisms and media for growth, helps preserve the integrity of the intact line, and prevents air and microorganisms from entering the line.

11. **Loop and tape tubing** to patient's skin.
Helps minimize catheter movement, which contributes to phlebitis.

12. **Label tubing and solution** with date, initials, rate, and time tape.
Alerts staff to when tubing and solution was changed and to when they will need to be changed again to decrease the incidence of infection.

13. **Dispose of used supplies** in appropriate receptacles according to agency policy in line with CDC guidelines.

? What if . . .

■ **The drip chamber becomes too full (over half) so that drops cannot be adequately counted?**

Close the roller clamp, invert the bag or bottle, and squeeze the excess fluid back into the bag/bottle.

■ **The tubing will not separate from the catheter connection when you attempt to disconnect it?**

If the lock does not twist off, gently try using a hemostat ("mosquito" clamp) to twist the lock. Do not lock the hemostat; merely use it lightly as a grip. After the lock is off, if the tubing will not separate, use the hemostat to gently twist the tubing back and forth. If the catheter needs to be stabilized, wear a sterile glove or use a sterile hemostat.

(continued on next page)

Procedure 39-4 ■ Changing IV Solutions and Tubing (continued)

Evaluation

- Assess the IV insertion site for signs of infiltration, inflammation, infection, and phlebitis.
- Evaluate the effectiveness of IV therapy by assessing the patient's hydration status or expected effect of the intravenous medication/solution.
- Monitor the IV rate regularly (usually hourly).

Patient Teaching

- Discuss the importance of notifying staff immediately if the catheter or administration set becomes dislodged; if the insertion site becomes tender, red, or swollen; or if the IV dressing becomes wet.

Home Care

- Explain home IV therapy to the client and caregiver and teach them how to identify complications.
- Obtain a return demonstration to ensure the caregiver is able to perform fluid and tubing changes, when necessary.

Documentation

- Fluid and tubing changes are usually documented on a flow sheet.
- Document the date and time the IV fluid and tubing were changed, type of IV fluid and rate of infusion, and the location and condition of the IV catheter insertion site.
- Document any complications of IV therapy and the interventions taken.

Sample documentation

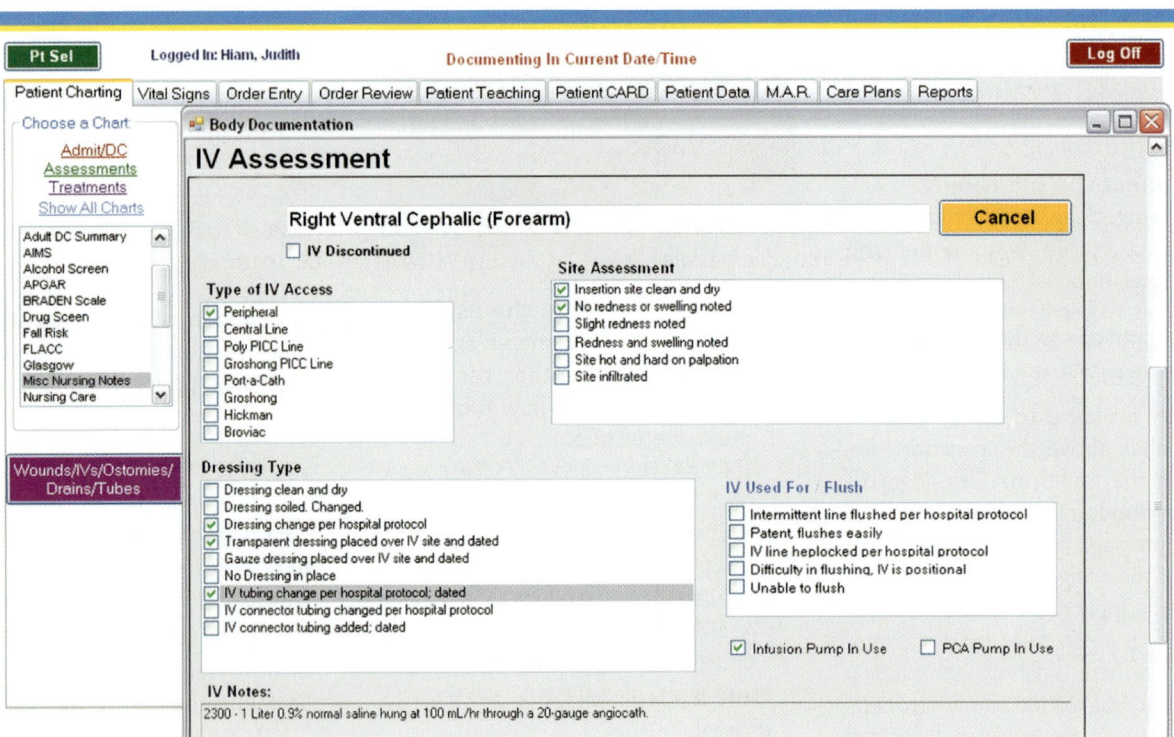

Practice Resources

Centers for Disease Control and Prevention (2011b, 2016); Infusion Nurses Society (2011); Phillips, L., & Gorski, L. (2014).

Procedure 39-5 ■ Changing IV Dressings

➤ For steps to follow in *all* procedures, refer to the Universal Steps for All Procedures found on the page facing the inside back cover. For this procedure, also refer to Clinical Insights 22-1 through 22-4 if you need to review information about medical and surgical asepsis.

Equipment

Peripheral IV Dressings

- Clean nonsterile gloves
- Sterile transparent semipermeable dressing or dressing specified by institution
- Antiseptic swabs: alcohol or chlorhexidine

  (NOTE: Use iodine-based products only if the preferred antiseptics cannot be used. Chlorhexidine is not recommended in infants younger than age 2 months.)

- 1-inch nonallergenic tape or manufactured stabilization device

Central Line Dressings

- Clean nonsterile gloves
- Central line dressing kit. It should include sterile gloves, a mask, a sterile transparent semipermeable dressing, sterile tape, an antimicrobial agent, and a sterile catheter stabilization device. If it does not, obtain them.

  NOTE: It is acceptable to use povidone-iodine followed by alcohol as the antimicrobial if the preferred chlorhexidine is contraindicated.

- A sponge containing the antimicrobial agent chlorhexidine gluconate may be used as a part of the dressing, as well.
  To reduce the risk for catheter-related infection

- Mask for patient (possibly)

  NOTE: Some institutions do not include this in their procedure and a few patients cannot tolerate wearing a mask.

Delegation

You can delegate the tasks of changing dressings to an LPN who is specially trained in IV therapy. The task should not be delegated to a NAP. Do, however, instruct the NAP to notify you of any problems that occur with dressing such as soiling, blood, leakage, or loosening.

Pre-Procedure Assessments

- Assess the IV catheter for patency before changing the dressing.
  Ensure that the IV is still working properly.

- Assess the IV site for signs of phlebitis, infiltration, infection, or inflammation.
  If any of these complications exist, the current IV will need to be discontinued and a new IV started.

- Assess for allergy to tape.
- Assess IV catheter start date.
  IV catheters are replaced per agency guidelines, which are based on the CDC recommendations of changing a peripheral IV site at 96-hour intervals, but at least every 7 days. Changing more often than recommended actually increases the risk of infection.

Procedure 39-5A ■ Peripheral IV Dressings

➤ When performing the procedure, always identify your patient according to agency policy, using two identifiers, and be attentive to standard precautions, hand hygiene, patient safety and privacy, body mechanics, and documentation.

➤ Note: This procedure is usually performed at the same time the IV tubing is changed because the old dressing may need to be removed to do that. The CDC recommends that dressing be changed when damp, loosened, or visibly soiled. You should follow your agency's policy.

Procedure Steps

1. **Wearing clean nonsterile gloves,** stabilize the catheter with your nondominant hand, avoiding direct pressure on the catheter/hub junction, and carefully remove and discard the dressing and the catheter stabilization device.
   Remove the dressing gently to avoid dislodging the catheter.

2. **Inspect the insertion site.** Look for erythema and drainage and note any tenderness. Remove procedure gloves and perform hand hygiene.
   If signs of infection, phlebitis, or infiltration are present, you must remove the IV catheter.

3. **Don a clean pair of nonsterile gloves.**

4. **Cleanse the insertion site** and then allow the antiseptic to dry on the skin. Do not fan.

If Using Chlorhexidine

Apply using a back-and-forth motion and friction for at least 30 seconds. (Avoid using chlorhexidine in infants younger than age 2 months.)

If Using Alcohol or 2% Tincture of Iodine

Using a circular motion, start at the insertion site and work outward 2 to 3 inches. Do not go back over any cleansed area.

Removes microorganisms from the skin to minimize the risk of their entering the venipuncture site. Allowing the antiseptic to dry increases its effectiveness.

5. **Perform hand hygiene** and change procedure gloves. Apply a new sterile catheter stabilization device and dressing. For illustrations, see Procedure 39-1.

If Using a Transparent Dressing

a. Open the package containing the sterile, semipermeable, transparent dressing. Remove the protective backing from the dressing, making sure not to touch the sterile surface.

(continued on next page)

Procedure 39-5 ■ Changing IV Dressings (continued)

b. Cover the insertion site and the hub or winged portion of the catheter with the dressing. Do not cover the junction with the tubing of the administration set.

c. Gently pinch the transparent dressing around the catheter hub to secure the hub. Smooth the remainder of the dressing so that it adheres to the skin.
Pinching the dressing around the hub prevents pressure of the hub on the underlying skin.

If Using a Gauze Dressing

d. Fold a 2 in. × 2 in. sterile gauze dressing in half, cover it with 1-in. tape (about 3 in. long).

e. Place under the tubing/hub junction and press down on the tape.
Raises the hub to prevent pressure on the skin.

f. Place a sterile gauze pad over the insertion site and catheter hub—but not over the catheter/hub junction

g. Secure all edges with tape.

6. **Secure the connection between** the catheter and the tubing, but do not cover the catheter-tubing junction with tape.
Securing the connection helps maintain a closed system and prevents entry of microorganisms. You should not cover the junction with tape because removing the tape may interfere with your ability to disconnect the tubing from the hub quickly, should you need to do so. Removing tape requires much manipulation; the more the catheter is manipulated, the higher the risk for infection.

7. **Secure the IV administration** tubing by looping and taping the tubing to the skin.
Looping the tubing provides slack to prevent the IV catheter from becoming dislodged.

8. **Label the dressing with the date** and time of insertion, catheter size,

and the date the dressing was changed and your initials.
Peripheral IV catheters should be replaced as clinically indicated (e.g. phlebitis, infiltration, irritation) to prevent complications. Labeling the dressing with the date and time of insertion helps communicate to other nurses the date of the IV insertion and dressing change.

9. **Discard all supplies** in the appropriate containers according to agency policy in line with CDC guidelines.

? What if . . .

- **The patient is immunocompromised? Or the peripheral midline catheter must be in the same site for an extended time?**

Use sterile gloves and a mask when changing the dressing and giving site care.

Thinking About the Procedure

The video **Peripheral IV Dressings,** along with questions and suggested responses, is available on the **Davis's *Nursing Skills Videos*** Web site on DavisPlus.

Procedure 39-5B ■ Central Line Dressings

➤ When performing the procedure, always identify your patient according to agency policy, using two identifiers, and be attentive to standard precautions, hand hygiene, patient safety and privacy, body mechanics, and documentation.

➤ *Note:* This procedure focuses on dressing change. Refer to Clinical Insight 39-4 for assessments and maintenance of CVCs.

Procedure Steps

1. **Obtain a sterile central line** dressing kit (or equivalent supplies if there is no kit) and mask for the patient, if one is needed.
Because central lines have direct access to the central circulation, the risk of systemic infection is greater. Therefore, the procedure uses aseptic technique. All supplies must be sterile.

2. **Place the patient** in a semi-Fowler's position, if tolerated. Lower the siderail and adjust the bed to working height.
Semi-Fowler's position and bed adjustments facilitate site cleansing and dressing application and reduce strain on the nurse's back.

3. **Explain the procedure** and ask the patient to turn his head to the opposite side from the insertion site. If he cannot cooperate, place a mask on the patient.
Explanation may reduce anxiety and enhance cooperation; turning helps prevent contamination of the insertion site.

4. **Put on your mask and clean nonsterile gloves**. Carefully remove the old dressing and catheter stabilization device, if present.

5. **Inspect the site** for signs and symptoms of infection and other complications.
If a complication is suspected, notify the person who placed the central line.

6. **Remove and discard your gloves,** along with the soiled dressing. Wash your hands.

7. **Set up a sterile field** and open the dressing kit.
To prevent contamination of the insertion site and the sterile supplies.

8. **Don the sterile gloves** contained in the kit and arrange sterile supplies as needed.

9. **Scrub the insertion site** and surrounding skin with an antiseptic swab.

If Using Chlorhexidine
Use a back-and-forth motion with friction and scrub for at least 30 seconds.

If Using Povidone-Iodine and Alcohol
The kit should contain three swabs of each. Beginning with a povidone-iodine swab, start at the insertion site and work outward several inches. Repeat with the other two povidone-iodine swabs. Then, using the same method, clean with the three alcohol swabs. With each swab, do not "go back over" an area you have just cleaned with that swab.
To rid the site of any potential infectious microorganisms, start at insertion site and work outward.

10. **Scrub the sutures (if any)** and the catheter from insertion site to the hub or bifurcation for at least 15 seconds with an alcohol swab or chlorhexidine/alcohol antiseptic product.

11. **Allow the site to dry**—do not fan.
    Allows the antiseptic time to work completely and allows the dressing to stick properly. Povidone-iodine requires 1 minute to air-dry completely; chlorhexidine requires 30 seconds.

12. **Apply the transparent dressing** that comes in the kit.

If You Place Gauze Under the Catheter Hub
You may first place a small piece of folded sterile gauze under the catheter hub.
To reduce pressure on the skin under the hub.

If Chlorhexidine Gluconate Sponge Is Part of the Dressing
Apply the sponge directly over the catheter insertion site, ensuring that the sponge is in full contact with the skin. Then apply the transparent dressing over the sponge.
Reduces the risk for catheter-related infection, especially in units with high infection rates or in high-risk patients (CDC, 2016; Marschall, Mermel, Fakih, et al. (2014).

13. **Apply a new catheter** stabilization device, if one is used.

14. **Remove the drape** if you used one.

15. **Loop the catheter gently** and secure it with tape to the skin.

Avoid securing it to the dressing. Or, depending on type of CVC, place a piece of clear tape across the ends of the catheter lumens, near but not on the hubs.
Ensures that accidental tugging on the catheter does not dislodge the catheter. Do not cover the hubs, as you may need to access them.

16. **Label the dressing** with the date changed, time, and your initials.
    Alerts staff to when the next dressing change will be due.

17. **Dispose of supplies** into the appropriate receptacles according to agency policy in line with CDC guidelines.

18. **Place the patient in** a comfortable position, raise the siderail, and be sure the call light is accessible.

19. **Remove your mask and gloves** and the patient's mask.

Thinking About the Procedure

 The video **Central Line Dressings,** along with questions and suggested responses, is available on the **Davis's Nursing Skills Videos** Web site on Davis*Plus.*

Procedure 39-5C ■ PICC Line Dressings

➤ When performing the procedure, always identify your patient according to agency policy, using two identifiers, and be attentive to standard precautions, hand hygiene, patient safety and privacy, body mechanics, and documentation.

Procedure Steps

1. **Obtain a sterile PICC** (central) line dressing kit (or equivalent supplies if there is no kit) and mask for the patient, if one is needed.
   Because central lines have direct access to the central circulation, the risk of systemic infection is greater. Therefore, this procedure uses aseptic technique, even though the insertion site is peripheral. All supplies must be sterile.

2. **Place the patient in a semi-Fowler's position,** if tolerated. Lower the siderail and adjust the bed to working height.
   Semi-Fowler's position and bed adjustments facilitate site cleansing and dressing application and reduce strain on the nurse's back.

3. **Explain the procedure** and ask the patient to turn his head to the opposite side from the insertion site. If the patient cannot cooperate, place a mask on him, if consistent with agency policy.
   Explanation may reduce anxiety and enhance cooperation; turning helps prevent contamination of the insertion site from nasal and oral airborne secretions.

4. **Inspect the site** for signs and symptoms of infection and catheter migration.

5. **Put on your mask and clean nonsterile gloves** and carefully remove the old dressing by pulling toward the insertion site and

catheter stabilization device, if present. Discard your gloves with the dressing.
The mask helps prevent contamination of the insertion site from the nurse's nasal and oral airborne secretions. Pulling toward the insertion site minimizes the possibility of dislodging the catheter.

6. **Perform hand hygiene,** open the kit, and remove and don the sterile gloves.

7. **Unfold drape and establish** your sterile field. Transfer items from kit to your sterile field.
   Ensures that strict sterile technique is maintained.

(continued on next page)

Procedure 39-5 ■ Changing IV Dressings (continued)

8. **Use a sterile tape measure** to compare the external length of the PICC with the baseline insertion length (if consistent with agency's policy).
   Detects catheter migration, which may indicate that the PICC line is not in the correct location.

9. **Scrub the insertion site** and surrounding skin with an antiseptic solution. Ensure that blood or encrustations are removed from the site and catheter. (Refer to Procedure 39-5B: Central Line Dressings, steps 9 and 10.)

10. **If using a chlorhexidine sponge** as part of the dressing, apply it directly over the insertion site and ensure that it is in direct contact with the skin.
    Minimizes the proliferation of microorganisms.

11. **Allow the site to air-dry.**

12. **Apply a commercial stabilization** device, if applicable.

13. **Apply a transparent dressing** over catheter site. ▼

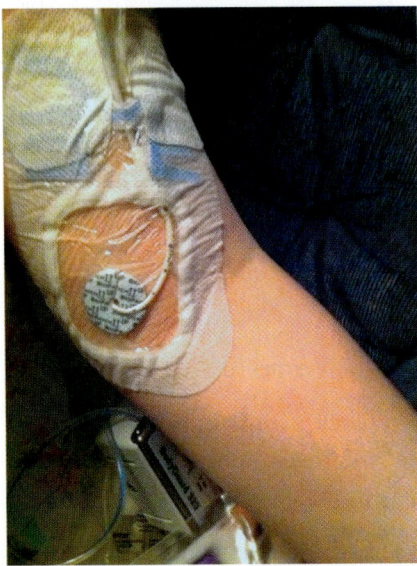

14. **Label the dressing** with the date, time, and your initials.

Used to identify the next scheduled dressing change.

15. **Loop and anchor the catheter;** secure it with tape.
    Reduces the risk of accidental dislodgement.

16. **Place the patient** in a comfortable position, raise the siderails, and place the call light so it is accessible to patient.

17. **Dispose of used supplies** in the appropriate receptacles according to agency policy and consistent with CDC guidelines.

Evaluation

- Evaluate the IV insertion site and surrounding tissue for signs of infiltration, inflammation, infection, and phlebitis.
- Monitor the dressing for dampness, blood, soiling, or loosening.
  If these occur, the dressing must be changed.

Patient Teaching

- Explain the importance of notifying staff if the IV dressing becomes soiled, dampened, or loosened.
- Remind the patient to notify staff immediately for bleeding, pain, or swelling around the catheter or dressing area or discomfort in the hand, arm, or shoulder on the same side as the catheter.

Home Care

- Explain home IV therapy to the client and caregiver and teach them how to identify complications.
- Obtain a return demonstration by the client or caregiver to ensure competent performance of fluid, tubing, and dressing changes when necessary.

Documentation

Sample documentation

mm/dd/yyyy   2300   new transparent semipermeable dressing applied over PICC insertion site in left forearm. No redness, tenderness, swelling, or exudate at the site. ——————— Mary Ramirez, RNC

Practice Resources

Centers for Disease Control and Prevention (2011a, 2016); Hadaway, L. (2010); Infusion Nurses Society (2011); Institute for Healthcare Improvement (2012); The Joint Commission (2012); Marschall, J., Mermel, L., Fakih, M., et al. (2014); Moureau, N., & Chopra, V. (2016).

Thinking About the Procedure

The video **PICC Line Dressings,** along with questions and suggested responses, is available on the **Davis's *Nursing Skills Videos*** Web site on DavisPlus.

Procedure 39-6 ■ Converting a Primary Line to a Peripheral IV Lock

> For steps to follow in *all* procedures, refer to the Universal Steps for All Procedures found on the page facing the inside back cover.

Equipment

- Clean nonsterile gloves
- Peripheral intermittent IV lock adapter
- Two syringes containing saline solution (one syringe with dilute heparin solution, if required by agency policy)
- Linen-saver pad
- Transparent semipermeable dressing
- Alcohol or chlorhexidine/alcohol or other antiseptic swab

Delegation

You can delegate the task of converting a primary IV line to an intermittent lock device to an LPN who is specially trained in IV therapy. The task should not be delegated to a NAP. However, you should instruct the NAP to notify you of any problems with the intermittent lock device, such as dislodging of the catheter or client complaints of pain, swelling, or redness at the insertion site.

Pre-Procedure Assessment

- Assess the patient's readiness to have the IV fluid discontinued (e.g., tolerating oral fluids, adequate urine output, and laboratory values within normal limits).
  If the patient's condition indicates that he still requires IV fluids, notify the primary care provider and do not discontinue the IV line.
- Assess for allergy to tape.
- Assess the IV site for signs of phlebitis, infiltration, extravasation, or infection.
  If complications are present or the IV has been in place longer than 96 hours or at least 7 days, remove the IV catheter instead of converting it to an intermittent lock.

> When performing the procedure, always identify your patient according to agency policy, using two identifiers, and be attentive to standard precautions, hand hygiene, patient safety and privacy, body mechanics, and documentation.

> Maintain sterility of supplies and equipment (e.g., do not touch catheter opening or ends of the IV lock; keep flush syringe connector sterile).

Procedure Steps

1. **Help the client assume** a comfortable position that provides access to the IV site.
   Promotes cooperation and facilitates your ability to perform the procedure.

2. **Lower siderails, raise the bed** to working height, and place linen-saver pad under extremity with the IV.
   Protects linens from blood and fluid that might leak from the vessel during catheter removal and ensures good body mechanics.

3. **Don clean nonsterile gloves.** Remove the IV lock from the package and flush the adapter with the first syringe of saline or dilute heparin, according to agency policy. Place the lock back loosely inside the sterile package, keeping it sterile. **Continue with step 5.**
   Removes air from the lock. >

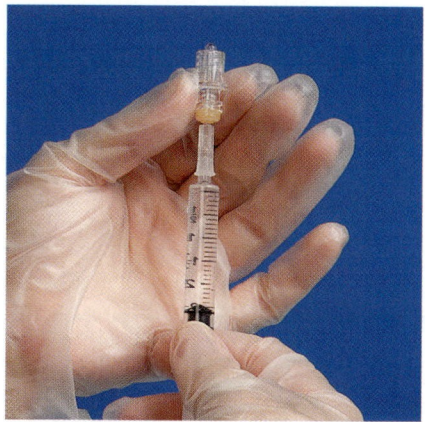

For Primary Tubing Set-Up With Extension Tubing With a Lock
Merely discontinue the IV solution and disconnect the primary tubing from the extension tubing with lock. Then, flush extension tubing per agency policy and **skip to step 13.**

4. **Carefully remove the IV dressing** and the tape that is securing the tubing.
   Provides access to the IV catheter.

5. **Close the roller clamp** on the administration set.
   Prevents loss of IV fluid during the procedure.

6. **With the side of your** nondominant hand, apply pressure over the vein just above the insertion site but not directly on the catheter/hub junction. At the same time, stabilize the catheter hub with your thumb and forefinger.
   Applying pressure over the vein stops blood from flowing from the catheter as you change the administration tubing.

7. **Gently disengage the used tubing** from the IV catheter. If the tubing does not separate from the catheter, see the "What If . . ." section at the end of step 13.

8. **Quickly insert the lock adapter** into the IV catheter and turn it to lock it in place.
   Insert the adapter quickly to prevent bleeding from the IV catheter. ▼

(continued on next page)

Procedure 39-6 ■ Converting a Primary Line to a Peripheral IV Lock (continued)

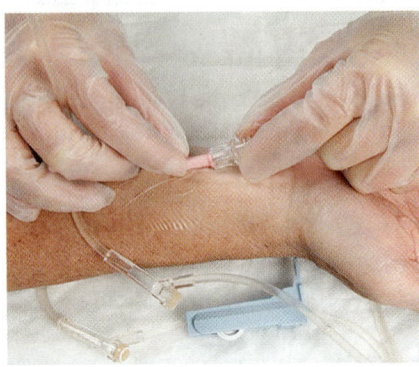

9. Scrub the injection port of the adapter with an antiseptic pad.
Cleaning the port with antiseptic helps prevent contamination by microorganisms when the adapter is flushed.

10. Insert the second syringe containing saline or dilute heparin into the injection port of the adapter. Flush the catheter using the method recommended in your agency (e.g., push-stop-push or a slow, steady push).
Some experts recommend a turbulence (push-stop-push method) based on the theory that turbulence ensures patency of the IV catheter by clearing the catheter and helping prevent reflux of blood back into the catheter. Others believe this method has undesired effects and recommend, instead, a steady, slow push. There is no evidence to support the turbulence theory

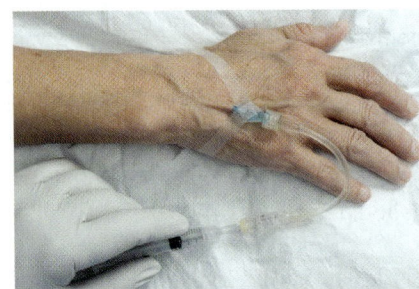

(Infusion Nurses Society, 2011). In the meantime, follow agency policy regarding the flushing technique. ▼

11. Using aseptic technique, cover the insertion site and catheter hub with a sterile transparent semipermeable dressing. Do not cover the junction of the catheter hub and the IV lock. See Procedure 39-5A for review of dressings.
Secures the IV catheter and prevents contamination of the site.

12. Label the dressing with the date changed and your initials.

13. Discard used supplies into appropriate receptacles according to agency policy in line with CDC guidelines.
Discarding used equipment properly keeps the healthcare environment safe.

? What if . . .

■ **At step 7, the tubing will not separate from the catheter?**

First, if it is a luer-lock connection, be sure you have twisted the luer-lock "open." If so, place a hemostat ("mosquito" clamp) on the IV tubing and gently twist back and forth to loosen the connection. Then if the IV tubing still does not come loose, use the hemostat to gently twist the lock back and forth to loosen the connection. Do not lock the hemostat; merely use it lightly as a grip.
Use of hemostat may help loosen tubing from the catheter, but placement is critical so that the IV catheter and connector are not damaged.

■ **At step 7, the IV catheter becomes dislodged while trying to disconnect the tubing?**

If you can see as much as three-fourths of the catheter emerging from the site, you must remove it and start a new IV at a different site.
Trying to readvance the catheter might cause it to pierce through the vein as well as increase the risk of infection from reinserting a catheter that is no longer sterile. It also causes tissue trauma and increases the risk of phlebitis from catheter manipulation.

Evaluation

- Assess the patency of the catheter before each use according to institutional policy. Patency check and flushing are usually done every 8 to 24 hours.
- Evaluate the patient's tolerance to intermittent IV therapy.
- Inspect the insertion site for signs of complications.

Patient Teaching

Explain the importance of notifying staff if the IV site becomes red, painful, or swollen; or if the dressing becomes soiled, damp, or loosened (indicating that the catheter has become dislodged or the connection is loose). Include the family in the teaching, as the patient may not be able to assess his own IV therapy.

Home Care

- Explain home use of the intermittent lock to the patient and caregiver. Teach them how to flush the catheter before and after administering prescribed medications.

- Provide the patient and caregiver with the name and phone numbers of people to contact in case problems arise with the catheter or insertion site.

Documentation

- Chart the date and time the IV line was converted to an intermittent lock device.
- Note the size and location of the catheter, as well as the type and amount of flush solution used.
- Record on the I&O record the amount of IV fluid infused.
- Document the condition of the IV site and any complications noted.
- Often, IV care is documented on a flow sheet or the electronic patient record.

Practice Resources

Centers for Disease Control and Prevention (2011); Goossens, G. (2015); Hadaway, L. (2010); Infusion Nurses Society (2011); Kordzadeh, A., Austin, T., & Panayiotopoulos, Y. (2013).

Procedure 39-7 ■ Discontinuing a Peripheral IV

➤ For steps to follow in *all* procedures, refer to the Universal Steps for All Procedures found on the page facing the inside back cover.

Equipment
- Clean nonsterile gloves
- Sterile 2 in. × 2 in. gauze dressings
- 1-in. tape or transparent semipermeable dressing
- Linen-saver pad

Delegation
You can delegate the task of discontinuing an IV to an LPN who is specially trained in IV therapy. The task should not be delegated to a NAP. However, you should instruct the NAP to notify you of any bleeding from the insertion site.

Pre-Procedure Assessment
- Assess the patient's readiness to have the IV fluid discontinued and verify the order. For example, determine whether he is tolerating oral fluids and has adequate urine output and whether laboratory values are within normal limits.
  If the patient's condition indicates that he still requires IV fluids, notify the physician and do not discontinue the IV line.

➤ When performing the procedure, always identify your patient according to agency policy, using two identifiers, and be attentive to standard precautions, hand hygiene, patient safety and privacy, body mechanics, and documentation.

Procedure Steps

1. **Assist the client to a comfortable position** and raise the bed to working height.
   Helps ensure patient cooperation with the procedure; supports good body mechanics for the nurse.

2. **Place a linen-saver pad** under the extremity with the IV.
   Protects linens from blood and fluid that might leak from the vein during catheter removal.

3. **Don clean nonsterile gloves** and close the roller clamp on the administration set.
   Closing the roller prevents IV fluid from spilling onto the bed or client during catheter removal. Procedure gloves protect you from body fluid exposure.

4. **Carefully remove the IV dressing,** catheter stabilization device, and the tape that is securing the tubing.
   Removing tape and dressings can be painful especially if over hair or sensitive or thin skin.

If the IV Is Running Through an Extension Tubing or a Saline Lock
Disconnect the administration set tubing and close the slide clamp on the extension tubing.

5. **Scrub the catheter–skin junction** with an alcohol prep pad or chlorhexidine/alcohol antiseptic product for at least 15 seconds.
   Removes microorganisms from the skin entry site.

6. **Apply a sterile 2 in. × 2 in. gauze** pad above the IV insertion site and gently remove the catheter, directing it straight along the vein. Do not press down on the gauze pad while removing the catheter.
   Directing the catheter along the vein prevents vein injury while you are removing the catheter. ▼

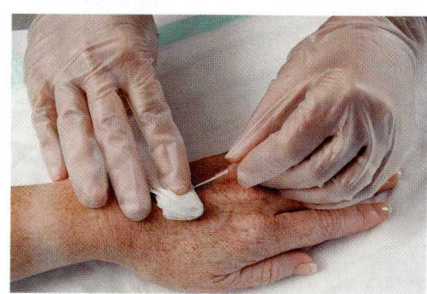

7. **Immediately apply firm pressure** with the gauze pad over the insertion site. Hold pressure for 1 to 3 minutes; hold longer if bleeding persists.
   This typically stops bleeding by hastening clot formation.

8. **Remove the soiled 2 in. × 2 in.** gauze pad and replace it with a sterile 2 in. × 2 in. gauze pad folded over to form a pressure dressing. Secure it with 1-in. tape or a transparent semipermeable dressing.
   Protects the site from contamination.

9. **Return the bed to a low position.** Discard all supplies in the appropriate receptacles according to agency policy in line with CDC guidelines.

Evaluation
- Assess the integrity of the removed catheter; compare the length with the original insertion length to ensure the entire catheter is removed. If a catheter defect is noted, report to the manufacturer and regulatory agencies and complete an incident report according to agency policy.
- Evaluate the patient's response to oral fluids after IV therapy is discontinued.
- Monitor for changes in the patient's condition to assess whether IV therapy should be reestablished.

(continued on next page)

Procedure 39-7 ■ Discontinuing a Peripheral IV (continued)

Patient Teaching

- Instruct the client and family to notify staff if bleeding or discomfort occurs at the insertion site.
- Teach the importance of drinking adequate amounts of fluid, within the prescribed treatment plan, to prevent dehydration. (Some patients have fluid restrictions.)

Documentation

Sample documentation

mm/dd/yyyy   2100   RA#2, 22-gauge catheter discontinued. Site without redness, swelling, tenderness, or exudates. Pressure applied to site for 3 minutes. Bleeding stopped and sterile 2 in. × 2 in. gauze dressing applied. Informed patient to notify staff if bleeding or discomfort occurs. ——— S. Horowitz, RN.

Practice Resources

Centers for Disease Control and Prevention (2011a); Infusion Nurses Society (2011).

Thinking About the Procedure

The video **Discontinuing a Peripheral IV,** along with questions and suggested responses, is available on the **Davis's *Nursing Skills Videos* Web site on Davis*Plus.***

Procedure 39-8 ■ Administering a Blood Transfusion

➤ For steps to follow in *all* procedures, refer to the Universal Steps for All Procedures found on the page facing the inside back cover.

Equipment

- Clean nonsterile gloves
- Blood product
- Normal saline IV solution, 250 mL

  KEY POINT: *Normal saline solution is the only solution that is compatible with blood products; other IV solutions cause hemolysis of blood cells.*

- Blood administration set (with a 200-micrometer filter and luer-lock connection). If there is no filter on the tubing, you must attach one.
- IV pole
- Watch with a second hand or digital seconds
- Thermometer
- Blood pressure cuff with sphygmomanometer
- Stethoscope

Delegation

Do not delegate this procedure to the LPN or NAP, because blood product administration requires advanced assessment and critical-thinking skills. The LPN and NAP can assist by monitoring vital signs. Instruct both about the complications associated with blood product administration, and instruct them to inform you if any occur.

Pre-Procedure Assessment

- Confirm the patient's need for blood products by assessing vital signs, urine output, and laboratory studies.
  Blood products may cause life-threatening complications; therefore, they should be administered only when needed.

- Check the patient's history for previous blood transfusions and reactions and verify her blood type.
  If the patient has a history of a blood transfusion reaction, precautions must be taken before she receives additional transfusions. For example, she may need premedication with acetaminophen, a corticosteroid, and diphenhydramine; specially treated blood products; and the use of a specialized administration set with greater filtering capabilities.

- Assess patency of the existing IV catheter and make sure that it is the proper size for blood product administration.
  Nurses often use a 20-gauge catheter for blood administration. However, for routine transfusion, a 22-gauge or even a 24-gauge catheter can be used. You would need an 18- or 20-gauge catheter when large amounts of blood must be transfused rapidly. The primary consideration should be the size of the patient's veins and not an arbitrary catheter size.

- Assess for allergy to tape.

Procedure 39-8A ■ Administering Blood and Blood Products

➤ When performing the procedure, always identify your patient according to agency policy, using two identifiers, and be attentive to standard precautions, hand hygiene, patient safety and privacy, body mechanics, and documentation.

Procedure Steps

1. **Verify that informed consent** has been obtained.
   Informed consent is required for blood product administration, as for any invasive or risk-bearing procedure.

2. **Verify the medical prescription,** noting the indication, rate of infusion, and any medications. If there are any pretransfusion medications, administer them as prescribed.
   Helps prevent administration errors.

3. **Obtain a blood administration set** and 250 mL of IV normal saline solution, or as prescribed. Some agencies may require a flush with normal saline between infusions.

4. **Obtain infusion pump,** if possible, and blood warmer, if necessary
Having all supplies and equipment on hand minimizes delays in starting the transfusion.

5. **Obtain the blood product** from the blood bank, according to your institution's policy. Wear clean nonsterile gloves whenever handling blood products.
Some blood banks require a pickup slip that verifies the presence of a functioning IV catheter, signed informed consent, and a prescription, because blood must be discarded after it has been out of refrigeration for 30 minutes.

6. **Verify that the blood product** matches the prescription. Inspect the blood. If you note any of the following abnormalities, return the blood to the blood bank and obtain a new bag:
   a. Pink plasma indicates hemolysis.
   b. The red cells should be red, not purple or black.
   c. There should be no large clots visible.
   d. There should be no leakage.

7. **Verify the patient and blood** product identification with another qualified staff member (as deemed by your institution).
Only one of the staff members is required by The Joint Commission to be qualified to administer blood products; however, agency policies may specify those requirements.
   a. Use two patient coidentifiers (e.g., ask the patient to tell you her full name and date of birth) and compare it with the name and date of birth located on the blood bank form and patient ID band.
   Allowing the patient to confirm her identity and comparing the information against the blood bank form is a safety measure to ensure that the correct patient is receiving the correct blood product.
   b. Compare the patient name and hospital identification number on the patient's identification bracelet with the patient name and hospital identification number on the blood bank form attached to the blood product.

Verifies that the correct patient is receiving the correct blood product.
   c. Compare the unit identification number located on the blood bank form with the identification number printed on the blood product container.
   Verifies that the blood bank has dispensed the correct blood product. ▼

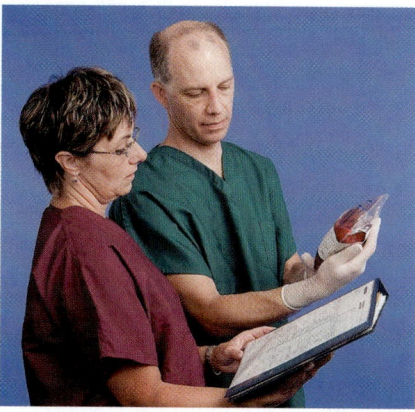

   d. Compare the patient's blood type listed on the blood bank form with the blood type listed on the blood product container.
   Verifies that the blood type of the product matches the patient's blood type.
   e. If all verifications are in agreement, both staff members should sign the blood bank form attached to the blood product container.

   ✚ Contact the blood bank immediately if any discrepancies occur during the identification process. If there are any discrepancies, do not administer the blood product.
   Signing the blood bank form confirms that the blood product was identified and verified by two qualified staff members.

   f. Document on the blood bank form the date and time that the transfusion was started.
   Blood cannot be infused past the expiration time; documenting the start time alerts the nurse of the expiration time.
   g. Make sure that the blood bank form remains attached to the

blood product container until administration is complete.
Ensures product identity should a transfusion reaction occur.

8. **Remove the blood administration set** from the package and label the tubing with the date and time. Then, close all clamps on the administration set.
Labeling the administration set with the date and time informs the nursing staff when the administration set should be changed.

9. **Remove the protective covers** from the normal saline solution container port and from one of the spikes located on the "Y" of the blood product administration set. Place the spike into the port of the solution container.

10. **Hang the normal saline solution** container on the IV pole. Refer to the photo in step 16.

11. **Compress the drip chamber** of the administration set and allow it to fill halfway.
Prevents air from entering the tubing with the solution.

12. **Open the roller clamp** and prime the administration set tubing with normal saline.
Removes air from the tubing.

13. **Close the roller clamp.** Inspect the tubing for air. If air bubbles are in the tubing, flick the tubing with a fingertip to mobilize the bubbles up into the drip chamber.
Air bubbles in the administration tubing can cause an air embolus.

14. **Gently invert the blood** product container several times, but do not shake the bag.
Mixes the blood product with the preservatives that are added to the container without causing trauma (lysis) to the cells.

15. **Hang the blood product bag** on the IV pole and thread the line through the infusion pump.
Enables the blood to flow by gravity.

(continued on next page)

Procedure 39-8 ■ Administering a Blood Transfusion (continued)

16. Remove the protective covers from the blood spike on the blood tubing and the blood product port. Carefully spike the blood product container through the port.
Prevents inadvertent puncturing of the container. ▼

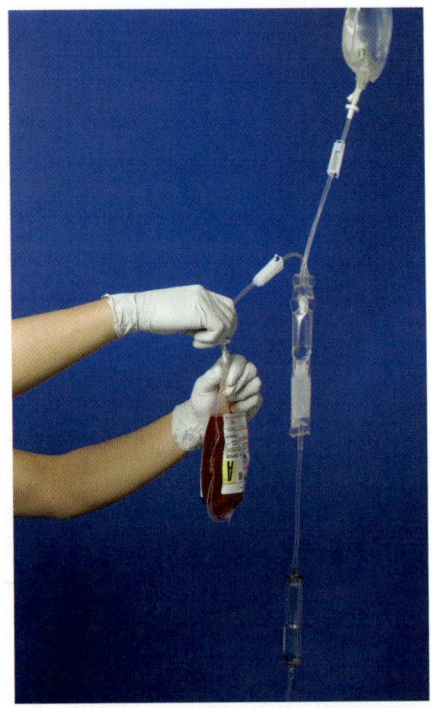

17. Obtain and record the patient's vital signs, including temperature, pulse, and blood pressure, before beginning the transfusion.
Establishes a baseline to help monitor for transfusion reactions.

18. Using aseptic technique, attach the distal end of the administration set to the IV catheter.
Prevents contamination of the IV catheter and administration set.

19. Slowly open the roller clamp closest to the blood product.
Allows the blood product to slowly fill that side of the "Y" of the administration set tubing.

20. Set the infusion rate. Start the rate slowly until 50 mL have infused; if there is no reaction, set it to prescribed rate.
A unit of blood cannot hang for more than 4 hours (some guidelines say 6 hours); otherwise, bacterial growth may occur.

For a Volume-Control Infusion Pump
Program the rate. Push "Start." Start the rate slowly until 50 mL have infused; if there is no reaction, set it to the prescribed rate.

For Gravity Flow
Using the roller clamp, adjust the drip rate. Keep in mind that blood administration sets have a drip factor of 10 gtts/mL.

NOTE: *When using a 24-gauge needle, you will usually (but not always) use gravity infusion instead of a pump.*

Forcing red blood cells through a smaller size catheter could result in some cell damage. Allowing the blood to flow by gravity allows time for the cells to change shape as they naturally do when flowing through small capillaries. However, only pumps that have been approved for blood transfusions should be used, because they prevent hemolysis.

21. Remain with the patient during the first 5 minutes and then obtain vital signs.
Most severe blood transfusion reactions occur during the transfusion of the initial 50 mL of blood.

22. Ensure that the patient's call device is readily available and have her alert you immediately of any signs or symptoms of a transfusion reaction, such as back pain, chills, itching, or shortness of breath.
If the patient alerts you immediately, you should be able to stop the transfusion in time to prevent serious complications.

23. Obtain vital signs again in 15 minutes (follow agency procedures), then again in 30 minutes, and then hourly while the transfusion infuses. Blood and blood product infusions must be completed within 4 to 6 hours.
Frequent monitoring alerts you to detect early signs of transfusion reaction or fluid overload.

24. After the unit has infused, close the roller clamp to the blood product container and open the roller clamp to the normal saline solution to flush the administration set with normal saline solution.
Flushing the tubing with normal saline solution clears the tubing of any blood and avoids wasting any of the blood product.

25. Close the roller clamp to the normal saline and then disconnect the blood administration set from the IV catheter, if an additional unit of blood has not been prescribed.

26. If another unit of blood is required, you may hang the second unit with the same administration set. However, administration sets and add-on filters need to be changed every 4 hours.
The same administration set can be used for two units of blood or per agency policy.

27. Discard the empty blood container and administration set in a biohazard receptacle, according to your institution's policy.
Promotes a safer healthcare environment.

? What if . . .

■ **Two individuals are not available to verify that the blood and the patient are a match, and the blood must be hung now?**

In this instance, if it is available, an automated identification technology (e.g., bar coding) may be used.

Procedure 39-8B ▪ Managing a Transfusion Reaction

➤ When performing the procedure, always identify your patient according to agency policy, using two identifiers, and be attentive to standard precautions, hand hygiene, patient safety and privacy, body mechanics, and documentation.

Procedure Steps

1. ✚ If signs or symptoms of a transfusion reaction occur, stop the transfusion immediately. Do not flush the tubing.
   Flushing the tubing causes the patient to receive the blood that remains in the tubing.

2. **Disconnect the administration set** from the IV catheter. Call for help. Obtain vital signs, and auscultate heart and breath sounds.
   Severe transfusion reactions may cause respiratory distress and shock; early recognition and treatment improve patient outcomes.

3. **Maintain patency of the IV** catheter by hanging a new infusion of normal saline solution, using new tubing.
   Maintaining a patent IV catheter with normal saline solution provides IV access

in which emergency medication can be administered if necessary.

4. **Notify the primary provider** as soon as you have stopped the blood, assessed the patient, and hung the new normal saline solution.

5. **Place the administration set** and blood product container, with the blood bank form attached, inside a biohazard bag. Send the bag to the blood bank immediately.
   The remainder of the blood must be sent to the blood bank, where it can be analyzed to help determine the cause of the reaction.

6. **Obtain blood** (in the extremity opposite the transfusion site) and urine specimens according to your institution's policy.
   Blood banks typically require (a) a specimen for a type and crossmatch to compare with the pretransfusion type and

crossmatch, (b) a specimen for free hemoglobin, and (c) a specimen for serum bilirubin level. A urine sample should also be sent to check for hemoglobinurinia, a sign of acute hemolytic reactions.

7. **Continue to monitor vital signs** frequently, at least every 15 minutes.
   To quickly detect worsening of the patient's condition.

8. **Administer medications** as prescribed.
   Medications will vary depending on the type of transfusion reaction.

? What if . . .

■ **At step 3, you do not have a new bag of normal saline to hang?**

Clamp the normal saline line until you can obtain a new bag of normal saline, then disconnect the old normal saline. Do this as quickly as possible.
Preserves the patency of the IV catheter.

Evaluation

■ Evaluate the patient's response to the blood transfusion by checking for changes in blood pressure and oxygenation, improvement in color, or signs of fluid overload.
■ Monitor for signs and symptoms of transfusion reaction.
■ Assess the IV insertion site for signs of infiltration, phlebitis, infection, or inflammation.
■ Monitor laboratory studies, such as complete blood count, to help evaluate the effectiveness of therapy and/or transfusion reaction.

Patient Teaching

■ Explain the signs and symptoms of transfusion reactions and tell the client and family to notify staff immediately should they occur.
■ Warn the client or family to notify staff immediately if tenderness, redness, or swelling occurs at the IV catheter insertion site.
■ Explain the importance of notifying staff immediately if the administration set becomes disconnected from the IV catheter or the IV catheter becomes dislodged.

Documentation

■ Chart the date, time, and reason the transfusion was started.

■ Document transfusion vital signs according to institution policy (many institutions have a special form for transfusion vital signs).
■ Record the amount of blood transfused on the I&O record.
■ Chart any complications and the interventions taken.

Sample documentation

10/26/2018   0600, 1 unit (250 mL)   PRBCs was hung at 0300 and infused through 20-gauge catheter in LA, for Hbg 8.3 mg/dL. Pretransfusion vital signs: T 98.9°F, BP 100/68 mm Hg, HR 114 beats/min, and RR 22 breaths/min. See frequent vital sign sheet for other transfusion vital signs. Breath sounds remained clear throughout the transfusion. No evidence of reaction. Post-transfusion lab due at 1200. ——— L. Gilmore, RN

Practice Resources

American Association of Blood Banks (n.d.); Infusion Nurses Society (2011); The Joint Commission (2011); Kessler, C. (2013); Tolich, D., Blackmur, S., Stahorsky, K., et al. (2013).

Thinking About the Procedure

 The video **Administering Blood and Blood Products,** along with questions and suggested responses, is available on the Davis's ***Nursing Skills Videos*** Web site on DavisPlus.

Procedure 39-9 ■ Assisting With Percutaneous Central Venous Catheter Placement

➤ For steps to follow in *all* procedures, refer to the Universal Steps for All Procedures found on the page facing the inside back cover.

Equipment

- Sterile gloves (two or three pairs)
- Masks, hats, barrier gowns
- 10-mL vials of normal saline (three or four)
- Syringes with 1-in. needle (two or three)
- 25-gauge ⅝-in. and 18-gauge 1½-in. needles (two or three of each)
- Central venous catheter (CVC) kit containing an introducer, antiseptic solution/swabs, sterile drapes, 10-mL syringe, 1% or 2% Xylocaine (lidocaine) without epinephrine, suture, sterile scissors and needle holder, CVC kit (single lumen or multilumen)
- Injection caps
- Alcohol wipes

Delegation

Do not delegate this procedure because complex assessment and support skills are needed. The nurse must be alert to changes in the patient's condition and signs of developing complications. CVC placement at the bedside is associated with pneumothorax, hemothorax, cardiac tamponade, and air emboli.

Pre-Procedure Assessments

- Obtain baseline vital signs.
- Verify that informed consent has been given.
- Assess for allergy to tape.

➤ When performing the procedure, always identify your patient according to agency policy, using two identifiers, and be attentive to standard precautions, hand hygiene, patient safety and privacy, body mechanics, and documentation.

Procedure Steps

1. **Explain the procedure** to the patient.
   To relieve anxiety and increase the patient's ability to cooperate with the procedure.

2. **Verify informed consent** and obtain vital signs.

3. **Gather supplies and perform** meticulous hand hygiene.
   Promotes efficiency; removes contaminants to help prevent infection.

4. **Set up the sterile field** and add supplies. Position the table so it is easily accessible by the physician or advanced practice nurse (APN) during the procedure.
   Promotes efficiency and makes the procedure faster and therefore less burdensome for the patient.

5. **Position the patient** to facilitate the procedure, usually in the Trendelenburg position with a rolled towel between the shoulders.
   To prevent air embolism and dilate neck veins.

6. **Offer mask, gown, and sterile gloves** (and possibly hat, depending on agency policy) to the physician or APN after she performs hand hygiene.
   Maximum barrier precautions are required for central line placement.

7. **Don mask and then sterile gloves.**
   To prevent contamination of sterile areas and of the insertion site as you cleanse it. Don mask first to keep gloves sterile.

8. **Prep the marked site** with 2% chlorhexidine gluconate in 70% alcohol applicators, using a friction scrub.
   a. Use a back-and-forth motion to scrub an area at least 20 to 25 cm (8 to 10 in.) in diameter. Do not go back over an area with the same applicator.
   b. Repeat with three applicators. Total scrub should take at least 30 seconds (2 minutes for a moist site such as the femoral vein).
   c. Allow site to air-dry completely (about 2 minutes). Never wipe or blot dry.
   Insertion kits and agency policies may vary. Follow agency policy. If it

does not conform to evidence-based guidelines, work for policy change.

9. **Drape the insertion site** with a large sterile drape, exposing only the prepared skin area. Use other large drapes to cover the patient from head to toe. If your agency does not have a policy that the patient wears a mask, have the patient turn his head in the opposite direction from insertion site.
   Creates a sterile field and decreases the chance of contamination by the patient's exhalations. Turning the head to the opposite side also helps to make it easier to advance the catheter when it passes through the subclavian site.

10. **Observe while the physician** or APN performs the following steps:
    a. Anesthetizes the area with lidocaine.
    b. Primes the central venous catheter with saline.
    c. Performs venipuncture with the insertion needle (in the internal jugular or subclavian site). The femoral site may be used in

emergencies, but it is associated with a higher rate of complications than other sites.

d. Attaches a syringe to the needle and aspirates for blood.
To ensure the needle is in the vein.

e. After obtaining blood return, removes syringe from the needle and inserts a guidewire through the needle.
The guidewire guides the flexible catheter into the vein.

f. Aspirates all air out of the catheter lumens and then flushes them with normal saline.
To reduce the risk of air embolism.

g. Places injection caps on each lumen.
To prevent blood loss and maintain sterility of the lumens

h. Sutures the catheter in place.
To minimize movement and prevent catheter migration (in or out).

11. Apply sterile transparent dressing over the site after the physician or APN is finished.

Minimizes contamination of the site. The most common route of infection is via migration of skin organisms at the insertion site into the cutaneous catheter tract with colonization of the catheter tip. Transparent dressing allows for observation of the site without removing the dressing and manipulating the catheter.

12. If there are clamps on the lumens, close them.

13. Place tape over the lumens near the ends, but not on the injection caps.
To minimize movement of the catheter that increases the risk of dislodgement.

14. Remove sterile drape and assist the patient to a comfortable position.

15. Dispose of used supplies and equipment in the appropriate receptacles according to agency policy in line with CDC guidelines.

16. Remove and dispose of mask and gloves. Perform hand hygiene.
Observes standard precaution guidelines.

Guidelines

- The patient and all staff in the room should wear a mask.
- A health professional who has received appropriate education (e.g., a nurse) should observe the CVC insertion to ensure that aseptic technique is maintained.
- This person should stop the procedure if aseptic technique errors are made.
- A central line checklist should be used during the procedure. You may be responsible for auditing the procedure and completing the checklist.

? What if . . .

- **In step 9, a large sterile drape is not available?**

Use two small drapes to cover the patient from head to toe.
Evidence-based guidelines advise maximal barrier precautions for insertion of CVCs.

Evaluation

- Obtain vital signs.
- Auscultate the lungs and assess for respiratory distress, sharp chest pain, and coughing. Monitor for 24 hours for these signs.
To detect pneumothorax or cardiac tamponade.

- Obtain a chest x-ray.
To verify correct location of catheter tip in the distal third of the superior vena cava, as well as absence of thorax and cardiac puncture.

- Assess the patient daily to determine continuing need for the CVC.
Risk of infection is closely related to the length of time the CVC is in place.

- For further evaluation and follow-up, refer to Clinical Insight 39-4 and Procedure 39-5B.

Documentation

- Date and time of catheter insertion
- Catheter type and size
- Site location
- Assessments and interventions performed at insertion and immediately after

- Patient's tolerance of procedure (subjective and objective data)
- X-ray verification of catheter placement

Practice Resources

Centers for Disease Control and Prevention (2011a, 2016); Dumont, C., & Nesselrodt, D. (2012); Infusion Nurses Society (2011); Institute for Healthcare Improvement (2012); Moureau, N., & Chopra, V. (2016).

To explore learning resources for this chapter,

Go to **www.DavisAdvantage.com** and find:

Answers and Suggested Responses for all questions in this chapter

Lists of NIC Interventions and NOC Outcomes

List of NANDA-I Diagnoses

Knowledge Map

Care Plan

Care Map

References and Bibliography

Concept Map

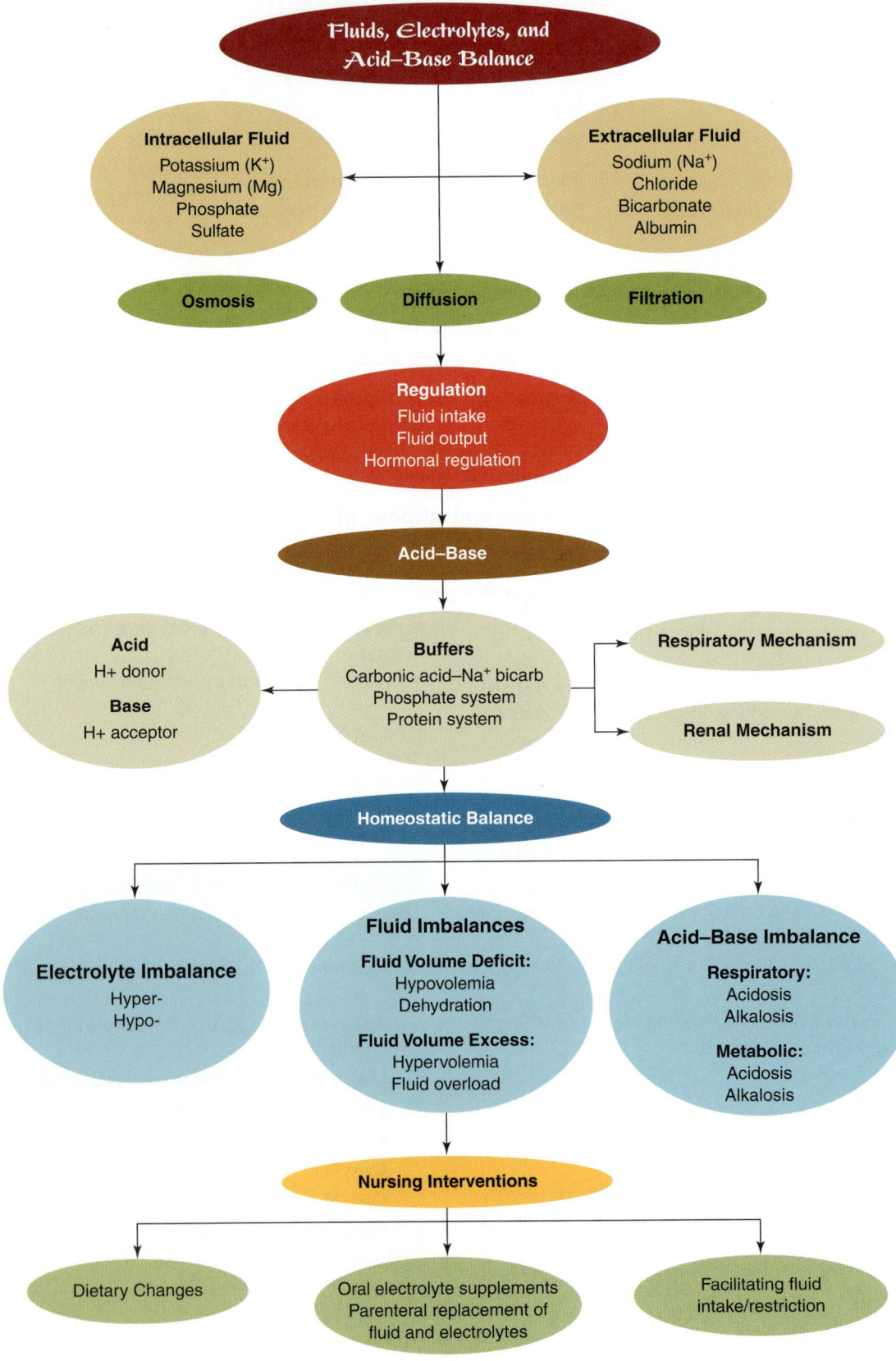

Fluids, Electrolytes, and Acid–Base Balance

Intracellular Fluid
Potassium (K⁺)
Magnesium (Mg)
Phosphate
Sulfate

Extracellular Fluid
Sodium (Na⁺)
Chloride
Bicarbonate
Albumin

Osmosis

Diffusion

Filtration

Regulation
Fluid intake
Fluid output
Hormonal regulation

Acid–Base

Acid
H+ donor

Base
H+ acceptor

Buffers
Carbonic acid–Na⁺ bicarb
Phosphate system
Protein system

Respiratory Mechanism

Renal Mechanism

Homeostatic Balance

Electrolyte Imbalance
Hyper-
Hypo-

Fluid Imbalances
Fluid Volume Deficit:
Hypovolemia
Dehydration
Fluid Volume Excess:
Hypervolemia
Fluid overload

Acid–Base Imbalance
Respiratory:
Acidosis
Alkalosis
Metabolic:
Acidosis
Alkalosis

Nursing Interventions

Dietary Changes

Oral electrolyte supplements
Parenteral replacement of
fluid and electrolytes

Facilitating fluid
intake/restriction

The Context for Nurses' Work

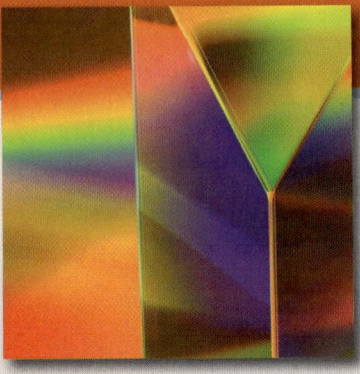

CHAPTER 40

Perioperative Nursing

Learning Outcomes

After completing this chapter, you should be able to:

➤ Discuss the importance of perioperative safety.

➤ Name and differentiate the three phases of the perioperative period.

➤ Describe the ways in which surgeries can be classified.

➤ Discuss factors that affect the degree of risk of surgery.

➤ Describe nursing actions associated with the preoperative phase, including physical preparations for surgery, preoperative teaching, and surgical consent forms.

➤ Compare and contrast the roles of the circulating nurse and the scrub nurse.

➤ Compare and contrast general anesthesia, local anesthesia, regional anesthesia, and conscious sedation.

➤ Discuss common nursing interventions during the intraoperative phase, including skin preparation, positioning for surgery, and intraoperative safety measures.

➤ Describe nursing assessments appropriate for surgical clients on admission to the nursing unit.

➤ Provide nursing care to prevent postoperative complications, including application of sequential compression devices, use of incentive spirometry, and management of gastric suction.

➤ Use nursing diagnoses appropriately to describe a patient's unique needs during the preoperative, intraoperative, and postoperative periods.

Key Concepts

Intraoperative care
Perioperative nursing
Postoperative care
Preoperative care

Related Concepts

See the Concept Map at the end of this chapter.

Meet Your Patient

Nishad Singh is a 68-year-old man who came to the emergency department (ED) with sudden onset of rectal bleeding. He tells the ED nurse, "I've been real tired and dragging for several months. This morning I felt a little worse than usual. When I went to the bathroom, there was a lot of blood. I've never had that before, and it scared me. I've had to go to the bathroom a couple times this morning, and it's all blood." The ED nurse collects the following data:
BP: 138/88 mm Hg
Pulse: 104 beats/min and regular
Respiratory rate: 20 breaths/min
Temperature: 36.7°C (98.0°F)
Oxygen saturation: 98%

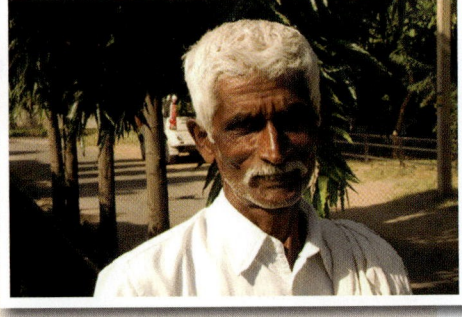

The ED nurse assesses that Mr. Singh is mildly anxious. His breath sounds are clear, but his abdomen is tender in the left lower quadrant. The nurse draws blood to be sent to the lab. While they are waiting for the lab results, Mr. Singh tells the nurse, "My stomach is cramping down low, and I need to go to the bathroom." She provides him with a bedpan. He passes approximately 200 mL of bright red blood with a small amount of fecal material. He becomes sweaty and light-headed after the BM.

Meet Your Patient (continued)

The nurse rechecks his vital signs and notes that his BP is now 120/76 mm Hg and that his pulse is up to 120 beats/min. The nurse shows the ED physician the bloody bowel movement and updates him on the change in vital signs. When the ED physician examines Mr. Singh, he tells Mr. Singh that he will need to be admitted to the hospital for further evaluation of the bleeding.

You are the nurse assigned to care for Mr. Singh on the medical–surgical unit. Mr. Singh has been sent from the ED directly to radiology for a computed tomography scan of

his abdomen. The scan reveals a tumor in the sigmoid colon. Since leaving the ED, Mr. Singh has had three more bloody bowel movements. His blood pressure is 100/72 mm Hg, and his pulse rate is now 134 beats/min. The physician prescribes a bolus of 1,000 mL of lactated Ringer's solution and a unit of packed red blood cells as soon as it is available. Mr. Singh is scheduled for colon resection surgery, which will occur as soon as the surgical team can be assembled and the room prepared.

ABOUT THE KEY CONCEPTS

The overarching concept for this chapter is **perioperative nursing**, which includes the key concepts of **preoperative, intraoperative**, and **postoperative care**. To help you understand and remember those concepts, we discuss how to prepare a client for surgery and the activities that occur before, during, and after surgery as we follow Mr. Singh (Meet Your Patient) through his perioperative experience. We will present definitions and examples of the key concepts, as well as numerous subconcepts that relate to each other in various ways. We begin with perioperative nursing.

PERIOPERATIVE NURSING

Perioperative nursing involves the care of clients before, during, and after surgery and some other invasive procedures. Historically, perioperative nursing practice was called "operating room nursing" and was limited to transferring patients into and out of operating rooms and handing instruments to surgeons during surgical procedures. Now nurses in all phases of the operative experience actively provide and manage care, teach, and study the care of perioperative patients.

The Association of periOperative Registered Nurses (AORN) is a highly organized and influential specialty organization within the nursing profession. AORN's *Guidelines for Perioperative Practice* (2009, revised 2014) keep perioperative nurses up to date on current practice. For additional information about AORN,

 Go to the **AORN Web site** at http://www.aorn.org/

Perioperative Safety

An important aspect of perioperative nursing is to help prevent complications of surgery. Hand hygiene is an important component of perioperative prevention (Box 40-1).

Preventable perioperative errors cause 10% of surgery-related deaths, have an unfavorable financial impact on healthcare institutions, and result in physical and emotional harm to patients (Agency for Healthcare Research and Quality, 2008). Various government and private organizations, including the following, stress the importance of patient safety:

- *The Association of periOperative Registered Nurses (AORN, 2009, revised 2014).* Perioperative Safety is one of the three domains under which AORN organizes its perioperative

BOX 40-1 ■ Recommended Practices for Hand Hygiene

- Perform hand hygiene:
  Immediately before and after each patient contact
  After removing gloves. Wearing gloves does not substitute for hand hygiene.
  Any time you may have come in contact with blood or potentially infectious substances
  Before and after eating
  After using the restroom
- Remove rings, watches, and bracelets before performing hand hygiene.
- It is preferable that you do not wear rings. They have been associated with a significant increase in skin microorganism count.
- Keep fingernails short and clean. They should not extend beyond the fingertips.
- Replace nail polish when it is chipped or at least every 4 days.
- Do not wear artificial nails. Fungal growth often occurs under them.
- Be certain there are no lesions or breaks in skin integrity on your hands.
- For hand washing and handrub procedures, see Procedure 22-1, Hand Hygiene, in Chapter 22.

Sources: Adapted from AORN. (2009, revised 2014). Guidelines for perioperative practice. Denver, CO: Author; Boyce, J., & Pittet, D. (2002). Guideline for hand hygiene in health-care settings. Recommendations of the Healthcare Infection Control Practices Advisory Committee and the HICPAC/SHEA/APIC/IDSA Hand Hygiene Task Force. Morbidity and Mortality Weekly Report (MMWR), 51(RR16), 1–44. Retrieved from http://www.cdc.gov/mmwr/pdf/rr/rr5116.pdf; Siegel, J., Rhinehart, E., Jackson, M., et al.; Healthcare Infection Control Practices Advisory Committee. (2007). 2007 guideline for isolation precautions: Preventing transmission of infectious agents in healthcare settings. Retrieved from http://www.cdc.gov/hicpac/2007IP/2007isolationPrecautions.html

patient outcomes. Specific safety outcomes include prevention of injury and freedom from infection.
- *The Joint Commission (2016).* The Joint Commission's 2016 National Patient Safety Goals applicable to surgery include preventing infection, improving the accuracy of patient

identification, using medication safely, and performing a time-out immediately before starting procedures.

- *The National Priorities Partnership (NPP, 2011).* The NPP National Quality Forum established a national priority that includes the aims of achieving better care, providing improved health for people and communities, and making quality care more affordable. One of its six national priorities and goals is making care safer by reducing harm caused in the delivery of care.
- *The Institute for Healthcare Improvement (IHI, n.d., 2011).* This independent, not-for-profit organization works to reduce morbidity and death in American healthcare, including perioperative care. One goal of its 100,000 Lives Campaign and its 5 Million Lives Campaign was to reduce surgical complications and, specifically, surgical infections. To see the entire list of IHI recommendations (IHI, 2011),

 Go to the **IHI Web site** at http://www.ihi.org

"Never Events"

"Never events" are serious and costly errors resulting in severe consequences for the patient, and that are mostly preventable. Believing these events are reasonably preventable and should never happen in a hospital, Medicare no longer reimburses institutions for care related to such complications (Centers for Medicare & Medicaid Services, 2006, updated 2011). Several of the "never events" (also called *serious reportable events*) are also targeted by the national organizations listed earlier. Among the never events important to perioperative care are:

- Surgery on the wrong body part
- Surgery on the wrong patient
- Wrong surgery on a patient
- Deep vein thrombosis (DVT) or pulmonary embolism (PE) after total knee or hip replacement
- Foreign body left in a patient after surgery (e.g., sponge, clip for draping)
- Surgical site infections after certain elective procedures (e.g., after bariatric surgery for obesity). AORN, The Joint Commission, National Priorities Partnership, and IHI extend that to include all infections. The Centers for Disease Control and Prevention targets certain antimicrobial-resistant bacterial infections.

You will see those themes recur in the Theoretical and Practical Knowledge sections in the remainder of this chapter.

PREOPERATIVE CARE

The **preoperative phase** begins with the client's decision to have surgery and ends with he enters the operating room. The length of the preoperative period and the extent of the patient teaching depend on the type of surgery to be done and the patient's overall health status.

Theoretical Knowledge
knowing **why**

Nursing care during the preoperative phase focuses on identifying existing health concerns, planning for intraoperative and postoperative needs, and providing preoperative teaching. Preoperative nursing care is delivered in a variety of settings. More than two-thirds of surgeries in the United States are performed in outpatient settings, such as endoscopy suites,

---

♥ iCare 40-1

Perioperative Care

- Perioperative nursing is a specialized area of nursing with specific, established standards of care. A caring nurse strives to integrate those standards into the nursing process and to apply standards to each patient in a caring manner.
- Caring nurses ensure that a person is cognitively and psychologically prepared for surgery.
- Caring nurses advocate for patients. An example is stopping the line and placing a HOLD on surgery when a person identifies an error or a risk in a process or in the surgical procedure. This exhibits *200% accountability* and embraces *high reliability* behaviors. You can do this by saying to others, *"I have a concern"; "We need to stop and verify"; "I am uncomfortable proceeding";* or even stronger language: *"I cannot send Ms. Brown until the surgeon comes back up and reviews her surgical procedure with her again; she clearly does not understand."*

KEY POINT: *Preventing errors and "never events" is everyone's responsibility.*

---

physicians' offices, and ambulatory surgery centers (Cullen, Hall, & Golosinskiy, 2009).

How Are Surgeries Classified?

Knowing the type of surgery helps you to identify the patient's perioperative needs and plan patient care. Surgeries can be classified by body system, purpose, level of urgency, and acuity. The classifications often overlap.

By Body System

The body system classification is useful for determining the postoperative risk of infection. For example, surgical incisions that enter the gastrointestinal, respiratory, or genitourinary tract have a higher risk for infection than does surgery of other body systems. However, if an organ ruptures or surgery is required to repair a penetrating injury, the risk of infection is very high regardless of the body system involved. Mr. Singh (Meet Your Patient) will have surgery of the gastrointestinal system.

By Purpose

See whether you can identify which of the following purposes describes Mr. Singh's (Meet Your Patient) surgery:

- **Ablative surgery** involves removal of a diseased body part. For example, a cholecystectomy removes a diseased gallbladder.
- **Diagnostic (exploratory) surgery** is done to confirm or rule out a diagnosis. Examples include biopsy and invasive tests, such as a cardiac catheterization.
- **Palliative surgery** is performed to relieve discomfort or other disease symptoms without producing a cure. Examples include nerve root destruction for chronic pain.
- **Reconstructive surgery** is performed to restore function, for example, rotator cuff repair (repair of a torn ligament).
- **Cosmetic surgery** is done to improve appearance (e.g., face-lift).
- **Transplant surgery** replaces a malfunctioning body part, tissue, or organ. Joint replacements and organ replacement procedures are included in this category.
- **Procurement surgery** is related to transplant surgery. An organ or tissue is harvested from someone pronounced brain dead for transplantation into another person.

By Degree of Urgency

Based on the following definitions, how would you describe the degree of urgency for Mr. Singh's surgery?

- **Emergency surgery** requires transport to the operating suite as soon as possible to preserve the patient's life or function. The surgical team is summoned and preparations are made rapidly. Internal hemorrhage, rupture of an organ, and trauma are common causes of emergency surgery.
- **Urgent surgery** is scheduled within 24 to 48 hours to alleviate symptoms, repair a body part, or restore function. Removal of a cancerous breast and internal fixation of a fracture are examples.
- **Elective surgery** is performed when surgery is the recommended course of action, but the condition is not time sensitive. The client may delay surgery to gather information, consider options, or organize care for the family. Examples include repair of a torn ligament and removal of rectal polyps.

By Degree of Risk

♥ **iCare** There is an adage concerning surgery: "The only minor surgery is someone else's surgery." This statement reflects the anxiety that often accompanies anticipating a surgical procedure. Nevertheless, surgery is defined as major or minor based on the degree of seriousness or risk associated with the procedure. The degree of risk varies with the condition of the client, as well as with the type of surgery and anesthesia.

- **Major surgery** is associated with a high degree of risk, for example, the potential for significant blood loss, a prolonged or complicated procedure, surgery involving vital organs, or a high risk for postoperative complications. Some examples of major procedures are coronary artery bypass graft, nephrectomy (removal of a kidney), and colon resection.
- **Minor surgery,** often performed on an outpatient basis, involves little risk and usually has few complications. Examples include breast biopsy and inguinal hernia repair.

What Factors Affect Surgical Risk?

The patient's age, general health, and personal habits can contribute to increased surgical risk during any surgical procedure.

Age The very young and very old are at greatest risk during surgical procedures.

- *Infants* have the following risk factors:
  - Limited ability to regulate temperature.
  - Immature immune, cardiovascular, liver, and renal systems.
  - Increased risk for infection.
  - Increased risk for excess fluid volume, and deficient volume. Even minor blood loss may represent a substantial portion of an infant's total blood volume.
  - Infants may have difficulty calming. They are unable to understand what is happening, so you cannot use verbal reassurance and explanations to comfort them.
- *Toddlers* understand simple explanations but may be anxious about separation from parents or caregivers. Many fear the dark.
- *Preschoolers* fear damage to body parts. Fear of pain or of needles is common for children of any age.
- *Teens* might fear disfigurement resulting from scars.
- *Young adults* commonly are anxious about the costs associated with hospitalization or surgery.

- *Older adults* are at increased risk because they have less physiological reserve and often have comorbid conditions (other illness not related to the surgery). Many of the physiological changes of aging predispose older adults to increased risk. Among these changes are decreased kidney function, diminished immune function, decreased bone and lean body mass, increased peripheral vascular resistance, decreased cardiac output, decreased cough reflex, and increased time required for wound healing.

Type of Wound Both preexisting wounds (e.g., from trauma) and the wounds (incisions) created by the surgical procedure can pose a risk for infection (Table 40-1). Risk to the patient increases along with the risk for or presence of infection. Which type of wound will Mr. Singh (Meet Your Patient) have immediately after surgery?

Preexisting Conditions The ideal surgical candidate is a healthy young adult who takes no medications. Unfortunately, many surgical clients have underlying acute or chronic disorders that increase surgical risk (Box 40-2). See the accompanying PICOT box.

Table 40-1 ▸ Wound Type and Potential for Infection

WOUND TYPE	WOUND CHARACTERISTICS	EXAMPLES OF SURGERY ASSOCIATED WITH THE WOUND
Clean Wounds	Uninfected; minimal inflammation; little risk of infection AND Surgery does not involve the gastrointestinal, respiratory, or genitourinary tract.	Face-lift, cataract surgery, joint replacement, breast biopsy, tonsillectomy
Clean-Contaminated Wounds	Not infected, but carry increased risk for infection	Surgical incisions that enter the gastrointestinal, respiratory, or genitourinary tract.
Contaminated Wounds	Not infected, but carry high risk for infection	Surgery to repair trauma to open wounds, such as compound fractures; surgery in which a major break in surgical asepsis occurred.
Infected Wounds	Evidence of infection, such as purulent drainage, necrotic tissue, or bacterial counts above 100,000 organisms per gram of tissue	A postoperative surgical incision of any type that has evidence of infection.

BOX 40-2 ■ Preexisting Conditions That Increase Surgical Risk

Acute Conditions

Acute infections tax the patient's energy and physiological reserves, increasing the risk for various postoperative complications.

Upper respiratory tract infections are associated with increased risk of postoperative pneumonia, especially if the patient receives a general anesthetic.

Chronic Conditions

Cardiovascular diseases (such as hypertension, congestive heart failure, and myocardial infarction) affect the ability of the heart to work as an efficient pump. If these disorders are well controlled (e.g., with blood pressure medications or cardiotonic medications), risk is limited.

Chronic respiratory disorders (such as emphysema, asthma, or bronchitis) decrease pulmonary function, increase the risk of respiratory infection, and may be exacerbated (made worse) by general anesthesia.

Coagulation disorders delay clotting and increase blood loss, placing the patient at risk for hemorrhage and hypovolemic shock. In contrast, a hypercoagulation state increases the risk of stroke, embolism, or intravascular clotting.

Diabetes mellitus delays wound healing and increases the risk of infection and cardiovascular disorders associated with diabetes.

Liver disease affects the body's ability to metabolize amino acids, carbohydrates, and fat; to manufacture prothrombin for clotting; and to detoxify medications. Therefore, the patient is at increased risk for poor wound healing, hemorrhage, and toxic reactions to anesthetics and medications.

Neurological disorders (such as paralysis or spinal cord injury) increase the risk for vasomotor instability and thus create the potential for wide swings in blood pressure. In addition, patients with seizure disorders are more likely to have a seizure in the perioperative period.

Nutritional disorders can affect surgical outcomes. Patients who are malnourished or obese are at risk for delayed wound healing, infection, and fatigue. Obese clients are also more prone to cardiovascular disorders and impaired pulmonary function.

Renal disease affects the patient's ability to excrete many medications, including anesthetic agents. It also affects the body's ability to regulate fluid and electrolytes.

PICOT

Older Adults, Comorbidity, and Risk for Surgical Site Infection

Situation: The student is caring for an elderly patient who is 4 days postoperative after a colon resection. The abdominal incision is reddened, with purulent yellow drainage on the dressing. The patient has a history of chronic obstructive pulmonary disease (COPD), and obesity (body mass index of 31).

PICOT Components

P	Population/patient	=	Older adults
I	Intervention/indicator	=	Chronic disease and comorbidity
C	Comparator/control	=	No health problems
O	Outcome	=	Increased risk of incision infection
T	Time	=	After surgery

Searchable Question

Do _____ (P) who receive/are exposed to _____ (I), as compared to _____ (C), demonstrate _____ (O) during _____ (T)?

Example of Evidence: Surgical site infections (SSIs) account for roughly 11% of healthcare-acquired infections in patients aged 65 and older. Older people who experience SSIs tend to have a worse clinical outcome than do younger adults. Researchers evaluated cases of elderly patients with SSIs and identified several independent predictors of surgical site infections. These include obesity, COPD, congestive heart failure, American Society of Anesthesiologists grade of ≥ 3, wound class > 2, and socioeconomic factors.

Application to Practice: Patients with these risk factors can be identified preoperatively, and nursing care adjusted to decrease the potential for SSIs.

Source: Agodi, A., Quattrocchi, A., Barchitta, M., et al. (2015). Risk of surgical site infection in older patients in a cohort survey: Targets for quality improvement in antibiotic prophylaxis. *International Surgery,* 100(3), 473–479.

Mental Status Patients with altered cognition, from either physical or mental illness, may be unable to understand preoperative instructions or give informed consent for surgical procedures. They may also require medications (e.g., antipsychotic agents) that interact with anesthetics and analgesics. Surgery and anesthesia may aggravate preexisting dementia, confusion, and disorientation.

Medications Both prescribed and over-the-counter medications may increase surgical risk (Box 40-3). For example, patients who self-prescribe high doses of vitamin E may be at increased risk for bleeding. Certain herbal and alternative medications can have the following effects:

- Increase the risk for cardiac dysrhythmias secondary to potassium loss.

- Interfere with metabolism of anesthetics because of their effects on the liver.
- Increase the potential for excessive bleeding.
- Decrease cerebral blood flow.
- Cause hypertension.
- Increase the effects of opioids and sympathetic nervous system stimulants.

Personal Habits The following are some reasons why substance abuse can increase surgical risk.

- Smoking affects pulmonary function.
- Long-term alcohol use contributes to liver disease, increasing the risk for bleeding.
- Alcohol and other drugs interact with anesthetic agents and medications to create adverse effects.

BOX 40-3 ■ Medications That Increase Surgical Risk

Antibiotics	May potentiate the action of anesthetic agents.
Anticoagulants	Increase risk for bleeding.
Antidysrhythmics	May impair cardiac function during anesthesia.
Antihypertensives	Increase the risk for hypotension during surgery; may interact with anesthetic agents to cause bradycardia and impaired circulation.
Aspirin	Increases risk for bleeding.
Corticosteroids	Delay wound healing and increase risk for infection.
Diuretics	Alter fluid and electrolyte balance (especially potassium balance).
Opioids	Increase the risk of respiratory depression.
NSAIDs	Inhibit platelet aggregation, increasing the risk for bleeding.
Tranquilizers	Increase the risk of respiratory depression.

■ Habitual substance abusers may have a cross-tolerance to anesthetic and analgesic agents, causing them to need higher than normal doses.

Allergies Patients may be allergic to medications such as antibiotics (e.g., penicillin) and analgesics (e.g., codeine), tape, latex, and solutions used in surgery. Reactions range from unpleasant to life threatening.

KnowledgeCheck 40-1

- Define *preoperative phase*.
- What are four ways surgeries can be classified?
- What factors affect surgical risk?

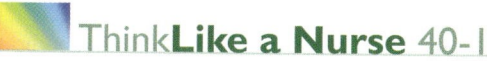

ThinkLike a Nurse 40-1

How would you evaluate Mr. Singh's (Meet Your Patient) surgical risk? What additional information do you need to answer this question?

PracticalKnowledge knowing **how**

The nursing focus in the preoperative phase is to prepare the patient for surgery. You will use the nursing process to identify any unique nursing diagnoses a patient might have. However, many preoperative nursing interventions are routine preventive measures that you will use for *all* surgical patients.

Perioperative Nursing Data Set

The Perioperative Nursing Data Set (PNDS) is a standardized vocabulary specifically designed to describe the care of perioperative patients. It is recognized by the American Nurses Association. The latest update of PNDS reflects the nursing process, including nursing assessment, diagnoses, identified nursing-sensitive outcomes, nursing interventions, and implementation and evaluation. The PNDS promotes better communication among nurses and other healthcare providers, increases visibility of nursing interventions, improves patient care, and standardizes a way to evaluate nursing care outcomes (Petersen & Kleiner, 2011).

In this chapter, we continue to use the NANDA-I, NOC, and NIC standardized languages, to which you have already been introduced in previous chapters.

Perioperative Patient-Focused Model The PNDS is derived from the AORN's Perioperative Patient-Focused model. The patient is at the center of the model and is the focus of care. The perioperative nurse intervenes within the context of the healthcare system to assist the patient throughout the perioperative experience to achieve outcomes in the Health System domain and the Patient-Centered domains (which include Safety, Physiological Responses to Surgery, and Behavioral Responses to Surgery).

The Health System domain refers to the system in which perioperative care is given. It involves administrative and structural elements necessary for successful surgical outcomes—for example, equipment, supplies, staff, and policies (AORN, 2009, revised 2014).

ASSESSMENT NP

For patient safety, data must be correct and complete. To prevent omission of important information, most organizations have developed a preoperative checklist. Although the forms may vary at each institution, the areas for assessment are the same and are discussed in the sections that follow.

Focused Nursing History

It is essential to determine whether the client is physiologically, cognitively, and psychologically prepared for the intraoperative and postoperative phases of surgery. For a complete and accurate nursing history, collect assessment data from the client, significant others, medical records, and other members of the healthcare team. Include the following topics in your preoperative assessment: health history, physical status, allergies, medications (including herbal products and over-the-counter medications), mental status, knowledge and understanding of the surgery and anesthesia, cultural and spiritual factors, access to social resources, coping strategies, and use of alcohol and drugs. It is also important to elicit patients' values and expressed needs (see the accompanying Safe, Effective Nursing Care box). For an example of a preoperative assessment form developed by the AORN, see the Focused Assessment box Example of a Preoperative Checklist (AORN).

Additional assessments may be needed if the client is undergoing outpatient surgery or has a planned short stay after surgery (see the Home Care box Preoperative Assessment for the Surgical Client Who Will Be Discharged to Home).

Focused Physical Assessment

If you identify risk factors from the nursing history, focus on those aspects during your brief head-to-toe physical assessment. For example, if the patient states she had a cough last week, perform a focused assessment of the ear, nose, throat, and lungs to determine how the cough may affect the patient's risk. If the patient has lower airway congestion, as evidenced by rhonchi and productive cough, communicate these findings to the surgeon and the anesthesia team; if a general anesthetic is planned, it may be necessary to delay the surgery.

Focused Assessment

Example of a Perioperative Checklist (AORN)

| **AORN _SAMPLE_ Preoperative Assessment Form**
(Facility Name and Address)

NOTE: _This record is a sample only. Clinical records should be customized to incorporate data fields that represent the setting, facility, procedure, and patient. Reproductions and variations are encouraged, provided credit is given to AORN._

Date:_____ | Addressograph

(Patient Information:
name, age, gender, medical record number, date) |

Structural Data:

Admitted via:
- ☐ Ambulatory   ☐ Wheelchair   ☐ Stretcher
- ☐ Other assistive devices:_____

Admitted from:
- ☐ Home   ☐ Transferring hospital
- ☐ Acute rehab facility   ☐ Extended/skilled care facility

Date of preoperative assessment:_____

Planned procedure:_____

Language(s) spoken: ☐ English ☐ Spanish ☐ Other:_____

☐ Patient's records, belongings, valuables secured (I115)
  Belonging inventory: ☐ Watch   ☐ Jewelry
  ☐ Contacts/glasses   ☐ Dentures/partial(s)   ☐ Hearing aid

Identity confirmed (I26):   ☐ Yes   ☐ No

Advance directive signed: ☐ Yes   ☐ No
  Location:_____

Operative procedure, surgical site, and
laterality verified (I143):   ☐ Yes   ☐ No

Consent for planned procedures verified (I124):
                                  ☐ Yes   ☐ No

NPO status verified (I138):   ☐ Yes   ☐ No
  Since: (date/time)_____

Preadmission testing
- ☐ CBC_____   ☐ Urinalysis_____
- ☐ Potassium level_____   ☐ EKG_____
- ☐ CXR_____   ☐ Pregnancy test:_____
- ☐ Type and cross   # of units:_____

Nursing Data Elements:

General health status: (check when present)
- ☐ Diabetes   ☐ Cancer   ☐ Obesity   ☐ Pregnancy
- ☐ Hematologic disorders (anemia, sickle cell disease or conditions)

☐ Vital signs:
  Temperature:_____   Pulse:_____   BP:_____
  Respirations:_____   Height:_____   Weight:_____

☐ Allergies verified (note type of reaction) (I123)
  Latex allergy: ☐ Yes   ☐ No
  Medications: ☐ Yes:_____   ☐ No
              _____
              _____
  Food: ☐ Yes:_____   ☐ No
         _____

☐ Daily medications (prescription, OTC, vitamins, alternative medication, herbal remedies, chemotherapy):
  _____
  _____
  _____
  Medications taken day of surgery:_____

☐ Alcohol/Drug social use:_____

☐ **Neurologic assessment:** ☐ Alert and oriented
  ☐ Speech intact   ☐ Follows simple commands
  ☐ Risk of falls   ☐ History of seizures
  LOC: ☐ Alert/oriented ☐ Drowsy   ☐ Sedated
       ☐ Asleep   ☐ Unresponsive ☐ Disoriented
       ☐ Other:_____

☐ **Sensory assessment:**
  ☐ No limitations   ☐ Hearing impairment   ☐ Visual impairment

☐ **Cardiovascular assessment:**
- ☐ Pacemaker   ☐ Implanted defibrillator
- ☐ Chest pain
- ☐ Peripheral edema: Location:_____
- ☐ DVT/PE risk:
  ☐ None ☐ Low ☐ Med ☐ High
  _____
  _____

☐ **Respiratory assessment:**
- ☐ Tracheotomy
- ☐ Intubated
- ☐ Chest tube
- Respirations: ☐ Regular   ☐ Labored
- Smoking history   ☐ Yes   ☐ No
  Packs/day:_____ Years smoked:_____
  Quit date:_____
- ☐ Cough   ☐ Cold symptoms
- ☐ Current or recent respiratory infection
- ☐ Preexisting respiratory problems (specify):
  _____
  _____

☐ **Musculoskeletal assessment:**
- ☐ No limitations
- ☐ Paralysis
- ☐ Traction
- ☐ Limited ROM
- ☐ Amputation:_____
- ☐ Prosthesis:_____

Focused Assessment

Example of a Perioperative Checklist (AORN)—cont'd

Nursing Data Elements (continued):

☐ **Skin assessment:**
  ☐ Cool ☐ Warm ☐ Intact
  ☐ Dry ☐ Moist
  ☐ Body jewelry removed
  ☐ Makeup removed
  ☐ Tattoos: _____
  ☐ Rash:_____
  ☐ Bruises: _____
  ☐ Wounds: _____
  ☐ Ostomy:_____
  ☐ Catheter/Drain: _____
  ☐ Venous access device: _____

☐ **Gastrointestinal assessment:**
  Last bowel movement (date/time):_____
  Usual diet: _____
  _____

  Recent unexplained weight loss
  ☐ Yes: Amount:_____ Time frame:_____
  ☐ No
  Problems chewing or swallowing
  ☐ Yes ☐ No
  Special needs:
  ☐ Chewing ☐ Swallowing
  ☐ Appetite ☐ Diet preferences

☐ **Genitourinary/Gynecology assessment:**
  ☐ Voided on call to OR
    Time:_____ Amount:_____
  ☐ Urinary catheter: Amount in bag:_____
  ☐ Urinary incontinence

☐ **Psychosocial assessment:**
  ☐ Calm/relaxed ☐ Anxious ☐ Talkative
  ☐ Crying ☐ Restless ☐ Withdrawn
  ☐ Other:_____
  ☐ Concerns regarding surgery or hospitalization:
  _____
  ☐ Religious/cultural concerns/requests:
  _____
  ☐ Receives help from:
    ☐ Children ☐ Support person
    ☐ Other (specify):
  _____
  ☐ Patient cares for:
    ☐ Children: Ages:_____
    ☐ Self ☐ Spouse
    ☐ Other (specify):
  _____

☐ Determine level of knowledge (I135):
  ☐ Barriers to learning:_____
  ☐ Motivation to learn
    ☐ excellent ☐ average ☐ limited

☐ Abuse screening
  Have you ever felt threatened verbally,
  emotionally, or physically in any of your
  relationships?
  ☐ Yes ☐ No
  Have you been hit, slapped, kicked, or other-
  wise physically hurt by an intimate partner?
  ☐ Yes ☐ No
  Are you afraid of your partner or anyone you
  live with?
  ☐ Yes ☐ No
  If yes, describe and make appropriate referral

☐ **Pain assessment**
  ☐ Instructed on use of pain scale
  ☐ Pain assessment (0-10): _____
    Location: _____

☐ **Discharge planning**
  Will require assistance after discharge
  ☐ Yes ☐ No
  Discharge plan:
  ☐ Home
  ☐ Home nursing service
  ☐ Short-term care facility
  ☐ Extended care facility
  ☐ Other:_____

  Individual who will escort patient home:
  Name: _____
  Phone number: _____
  Relationship: _____

Comments:
_____
_____
_____
_____
_____

Preoperative nursing diagnoses
☐ Anxiety/fear (X4)
☐ Therapeutic regimen management ineffective (X33)
☐ Deficient knowledge (X30)
☐ Risk for injury (X29)
☐ Pain (X38)
☐ Other:_____

Comments:

RN Signature:
X

Safe, Effective Nursing Care

Surgical Team Communication

Key Concepts: Perioperative Nursing, Preoperative Care, Intraoperative Care, Postoperative Care

SENC Competency: Provide goal-directed, client-centered care

Eliciting each patient's values, preferences, and expressed needs as part of the focused nursing history will assist you in providing goal-directed, client-centered care. You can then communicate patient values, preferences, and expressed needs to other members of the healthcare team to assure patient-centered care with sensitivity and respect for the diversity of individual patients.

SENC Competency: Collaborate with the interdisciplinary healthcare team

To provide for effective collaboration within nursing and interdisciplinary teams, nurses must engage in open communication, mutual respect, and shared decision to ensure safe and effective patient care. Two-minute briefings just before surgery, led by the attending surgeon using a standardized format, have been found to improve communication and reduce delays and wrong-site surgery (Lee, 2016). Surgical briefings encourage team members to talk when there is no problem, so they are more likely to speak up when they have misgivings when problems occur (Berger, Greenberg, & Bilimoria, 2015).

Home Care

Preoperative Assessment for the Surgical Client Who Will Be Discharged to Home

The type of surgery, the client's condition, and the support system determine whether it is safe to discharge a client to home after surgery. Your assessment should focus on the following questions:

➤ What kind of care will be needed?

➤ Is the client able to take care of himself? If not, who is available to assist with care?

➤ Does the caregiver have the necessary skills to provide care?

➤ If not, can these skills be taught before the client is discharged?

➤ What features in the home environment will facilitate the client's progress? What features will inhibit progress? For example, can the client get to the bathroom? Can the client negotiate the stairs in the house?

➤ How will the client be followed after discharge? That is, how soon should he visit his physician? Will he receive home nursing care?

For all patients, assess risk factors for thrombophlebitis, as venous thrombus is one of the never events that are important to prevent. For additional details on a brief bedside physical assessment, see Procedure 21-20 in Chapter 21.

Recent guidelines state that optimal preoperative assessment of older adults include the following:

- Cognitive ability
- Capacity to understand the surgery

- Nutritional status
- Risk factors for postoperative delirium and pulmonary complications
- Patient's treatment goals and expectations
- Family and social support system
- Depression
- Cardiac status
- Functional status
- History of falls
- Detailed medication history, including polypharmacy
- Baseline frailty score
- Diagnostic tests specific to elderly patients (Chow, Ko, Rosenthal, et al., n.d.)

Diagnostic Testing

Preoperative screening tests are usually prescribed before surgical procedures. The type of testing depends on the patient's age, health history, and facility policies.

- **CBC, UA, and ECG.** Most institutions require a complete blood count and urinalysis, and an electrocardiogram for patients older than age 50.
- **Routine chest x-ray is *not* recommended** for all patients prior to surgery. Chest radiology incurs extra costs to the healthcare system and exposes patients to small risks from radiation exposure (National Guideline Clearinghouse, 2016).

Patients with chronic health problems may require additional testing. See the accompanying Diagnostic Testing box Common Preoperative Screening Tests.

KnowledgeCheck 40-2

- List the information you should gather in the preoperative nursing history.
- What type of physical assessment is performed as part of the preoperative assessment?
- What laboratory tests are most commonly prescribed before surgery?

ThinkLike a Nurse 40-2

- What factors will affect your preoperative assessment of Mr. Singh (Meet Your Patient)?
- Describe how you might perform the assessment as well as provide physical care. What modifications, if any, should you make in his assessment?

ANALYSIS/NURSING DIAGNOSIS NP

As you learned in Chapter 4, nursing diagnoses describe the individualized needs of patients. However, preoperative patients share a common set of needs, regardless of their individual differences and the type of surgery they are to have. Consider the following examples:

- All preoperative patients need preoperative teaching, so it's not necessary to write a nursing diagnosis of Deficient Knowledge for every patient. Agency protocols or critical pathways will almost certainly mandate teaching.
- Almost all surgical patients have at least mild anxiety, and many of your routine actions will help to relieve anxiety, so there is no need to always include a diagnosis of Anxiety.

  KEY POINT: *Do not put any nursing diagnosis on the care plan unless you plan to address it with something other than the routine preoperative interventions.*

Diagnostic Testing

Common Preoperative Screening Tests

Test	Uses
Urinalysis	To detect urinary tract infections (UTIs) and the presence of glucose or protein in the urine, which may indicate poorly controlled diabetes or renal disease
Complete blood count (CBC)	To detect irregularities in hemoglobin (Hgb) and hematocrit (Hct). A low Hgb level is an indication of anemia, which may place the client at risk if significant blood loss occurs.
	Measures white blood cell (WBC) count as an indicator of immune function
	Measures platelet count, which affects clotting ability
Electrocardiogram (ECG)	To detect cardiac dysrhythmias and other cardiac pathology
Chest x-ray examination	To detect underlying pulmonary disease; also to reveal heart size, as an indicator of heart function
Blood type and crossmatch	To identify blood type in the event that blood transfusion becomes necessary
Serum electrolytes	To detect sodium, potassium, chloride, magnesium, calcium, and pH imbalances, which affect cardiac and other organ function and fluid balance
Fasting blood sugar	To detect diabetes or poorly controlled diabetes
Comprehensive metabolic panel	Includes electrolytes, blood glucose, liver function tests (alanine aminotransferase, aspartate aminotransferase), serum albumin and protein, and renal function tests (blood urea nitrogen and creatinine); used to detect underlying health problems that may affect surgical risk or outcome

Individualized Nursing Diagnoses

Individualized nursing diagnoses for the preoperative patient evolve from your assessment. You should identify an actual nursing diagnosis only if the patient has the defining characteristics for it. **KEY POINT:** *Identify risk (potential) diagnoses only if the patient has an underlying condition that places him at higher risk than the average surgical patient.*

The following NANDA-I nursing diagnoses may be useful for certain preoperative patients:

- *Anxiety* may be mild, moderate, severe, or at panic level. In the preoperative client, anxiety may be related to the current change in health status or due to concerns about being unable to provide care for loved ones. Make this diagnosis only if the client has symptoms such as restlessness, trembling, increased pulse, and other defining characteristics.
- *Fear* is a common reaction to surgery. Fear may be related to the unknown outcome of the surgery, to learning the diagnosis after a diagnostic procedure, and to the prospect of pain during and after surgery. Fear and Anxiety share several defining characteristics. Many of the routine preoperative interventions help to address Fear. Use this nursing diagnosis only if more than routine interventions are needed.
- *Ineffective airway clearance* may be used for patients who have a preexisting health problem, such as bronchitis or emphysema.
- *Disturbed Sleep Pattern* often results from anxiety about the upcoming surgery.
- *Ineffective Coping* may be appropriate for a patient with extreme anxiety and concerns about the outcomes of the surgery.
- *Latex Allergic Reaction* is appropriate for patients who have a known allergy to latex.
- *Risk for Latex Allergic Reaction* is appropriate for patients who have had multiple surgeries or urinary catheterizations;

are in professions with daily exposure to latex; have a history of asthma; or are allergic to bananas, avocados, kiwi, chestnuts, or poinsettia plants. Do not use it routinely for all patients.

- *Deficient Knowledge.* As you know, you do not usually need a Deficient Knowledge diagnosis. If you believe the patient may not learn, or that the information is too complex to remember, then identify the problem likely to result from the Deficient Knowledge. For example:

  Ineffective Health Management related to Deficient Knowledge of postoperative medications and office visits

  Risk for Surgical Site Infection related to Deficient Knowledge of wound care and asepsis

Special Risks for Older Adults. Older adults, especially those older than age 70 and the frail elderly, are likely to need some individualized nursing diagnoses. They present unique risks not only because they often have other illnesses, but also because of certain physiological changes that accompany aging. For example, older adults metabolize anesthetic agents differently from the way younger adults do (see Table 40-2), so they may experience Confusion or Impaired Gas Exchange.

ThinkLike a Nurse 40-3

Which, if any, of the preceding nursing diagnoses would be most appropriate for Mr. Singh (Meet Your Patient)? Do not use the potential complications in Table 40-2. Explain your reasoning.

PLANNING OUTCOMES/EVALUATION NP

The overall nursing goal in the preoperative phase is to prepare the patient adequately for surgery and to deliver him to the operating suite in the best condition possible. Outcomes that provide evidence of achieving this goal, and that are

Table 40-2 ➤ Special Risks for Older Adults

RISK FACTORS	POTENTIAL COMPLICATIONS (PC) AND NURSING DIAGNOSES
Most older adults have at least some degree of coronary artery disease.	▪ PC: Hypotension ▪ Risk for Falls secondary to postural hypotension
Delirium is one of the most common surgical complications in older adults. Predisposing factors include being older than 75 years, preoperative hyperglycemia or hypoglycemia, psychological distress, preoperative cognitive impairment, inadequate nutrition, and functional impairment (Brooks, 2012).	▪ PC: Delirium ▪ Acute Confusion ▪ Chronic Confusion
Age-related respiratory changes, such as decreased chest wall compliance, forced vital capacity, and diaphragmatic strength	▪ PC: Pneumonia ▪ PC: Atelectasis ▪ Impaired Gas Exchange ▪ Ineffective Airway Clearance
Age-related skin changes: Dry, fragile skin; decreased turgor and elasticity	▪ Risk for Impaired Skin Integrity ▪ Risk for Impaired Tissue Integrity
Age-related musculoskeletal changes: Decreased bone mass and muscle fiber mass	▪ Risk for Impaired Physical Mobility ▪ Risk for Falls
Comorbidities of the central nervous system are more common in older adults. Some conditions may be aggravated by surgery and anesthesia.	▪ PC: Dementia ▪ Risk for Acute Confusion
Age-related decrease in gastrointestinal motility	▪ PC: Ileus ▪ Risk for Aspiration secondary to vomiting
Age-related decreases in genitourinary function: decreased bladder tone, elasticity, and tone; decreased renal function	▪ PC: Side effects of medications ▪ PC: Renal complications ▪ PC: Urinary tract infection ▪ Risk for Impaired Skin Integrity r/t urinary incontinence

appropriate for nearly all preoperative patients, are that the patient:

- Is able to describe his surgical procedure in a basic manner.
- Provides informed consent.
- When asked, states what he can expect in the postoperative period.
- States he has very little anxiety.

    Associated NOC outcomes for the preoperative nursing client depend, of course, on the nursing diagnoses you identify. For outcomes and goals using NOC terminology for the diagnoses Anxiety, Fear, Deficient Knowledge, and Disturbed Sleep Pattern, and for *individualized goals/outcome statements* you might write for those diagnoses, refer to Table 40-3.

PLANNING INTERVENTIONS/ IMPLEMENTATION NP

For *NIC standardized interventions* and nursing activities designed to achieve the expected outcomes for the nursing diagnoses of Anxiety, Fear, Deficient Knowledge, and Disturbed Sleep Pattern, refer to Table 40-3.

    Many preoperative nursing activities are routine interventions to be used for *all* preoperative patients, regardless of

their nursing diagnoses. NIC has a special Perioperative Care domain (category) for such interventions. The following are the preoperative NIC interventions in that domain:

- *Preoperative Coordination:* Facilitating preadmission diagnostic testing and preparation of the surgical patient. (Activity example: Notify the physician of abnormal diagnostic test results.)
- *Surgical Preparation:* Providing care to a patient immediately before surgery and verifying required procedures/ tests and documentation in the clinical record. (Activity example: Complete the preoperative checklist.)
- *Teaching: Preoperative:* Assisting a patient to understand and mentally prepare for surgery and the postoperative recovery period. (Activity example: Correct unrealistic expectations of the surgery, as appropriate.)

    The following sections explain in more detail how to carry out interventions that are "routine" in that they are performed for all preoperative patients.

Confirm That Surgical Consent Has Been Obtained

Before a surgical procedure is performed, professional standards and the law require the surgeon to obtain the patient's informed consent. The signed consent form verifies that the

Table 40-3 ➤ Preoperative Patients: Selected Standardized Nursing Diagnoses, Outcomes, and Interventions

SELECTED NOC OUTCOMES AND GOALS USING NOC INDICATORS	SELECTED NIC INTERVENTIONS AND NURSING ACTIVITIES (*Note:* Interventions and activities marked with an asterisk (*) are routinely performed for ALL surgery patients.)

Nursing Diagnosis: Anxiety related to change in health status

NOC Outcomes: Anxiety Level Anxiety Self-Control *NOC Goals:* Patient will exhibit: ■ (5) No restlessness ■ (4) Only mild muscle and facial tension ■ (4) Only mild difficulty concentrating ■ (5) No increased blood pressure, pulse rate, or respiratory rate ■ (5) No physical signs of anxiety such as: dilated pupils, sweating, and dizziness ■ (3) Moderate verbalized anxiety	**Anxiety Reduction** ■ Use a calm, reassuring approach.* ■ Explain all procedures, including sensations likely to be experienced during the surgical procedure.* ■ Seek to understand the patient's perspective of the situation. ■ Provide accurate factual information about the surgery.* ■ Discuss common feelings and concerns that patients have about surgery. This helps the patient feel supported and less anxious.*
Individualized Goals: ■ Identifies symptoms that are indicators of her anxiety. ■ Communicates need for assistance.	**Calming Technique** ■ Maintain eye contact with patient.* ■ Maintain calm, deliberate manner.* ■ Encourage slow, purposeful deep breathing. **Presence** ■ Stay with the patient and provide assurance of safety and security during periods of anxiety. ■ Listen to the patient's concerns.* ■ Administer medications as appropriate to reduce anxiety.

Nursing Diagnosis: Fear related to unknown outcome of surgery and fear of pain that may result

NOC Outcomes: Fear Level Fear Self-Control *NOC Goals:* ■ (5) Exhibits no restlessness or irritability. ■ (5) Reports no difficulty concentrating. ■ (5) No physical signs of fear: increased BP, radial pulse rate, respiratory rate, sweating, dilated pupils, pale skin ■ (5) No verbalized fear ■ (5) No crying *Individualized Goals:* ■ Does not exhibit physical signs of fear (e.g., pupil dilation; dry mouth; increased BP, pulse and respiratory rate). ■ Reports understanding of pain control measures to be used during and after surgery.	**Anxiety Reduction** See Anxiety diagnosis. **Coping Enhancement** ■ Assist the patient in developing an objective appraisal of the event ■ Evaluate the patient's decision-making ability.* ■ Encourage the use of spiritual resources, if desired. **Preparatory Sensory Information** ■ Identify the typical sensations (what will be seen, felt, smelled, tasted, heard) the majority of patients describe as associated with each aspect of the procedure/treatment.* ■ Personalize the information by using personal pronouns.* **Security Enhancement** ■ Explain all tests and procedures to the patient/family.* ■ Assist the patient to use coping responses that have been successful in the past.

(Continued)

Table 40-3 ➤ Preoperative Patients: Selected Standardized Nursing Diagnoses, Outcomes, and Interventions—cont'd

SELECTED NOC OUTCOMES AND GOALS USING NOC INDICATORS	SELECTED NIC INTERVENTIONS AND NURSING ACTIVITIES (*Note:* Interventions and activities marked with an asterisk (*) are routinely performed for ALL surgery patients.)

Nursing Diagnosis: Deficient Knowledge of preoperative procedures and postoperative expectations

Knowledge-Related Diagnoses (e.g., Ineffective Health Management, Risk for Infection)

NOC Outcomes: Knowledge: Disease Process Knowledge: Treatment Regimen *NOC Goals:* Provides: ■ (3) Moderate description of specific disease process ■ (4) Substantial description of strategies to minimize disease progression ■ (4) Substantial description of signs and symptoms of disease complications *Individualized Goals:* ■ Verbalizes rationale for pre- and postoperative interventions. ■ Describes or demonstrates postoperative expectations (i.e., deep breathing, turning/position changes).	**Teaching: Preoperative** ■ Inform the patient/significant others how long surgery is expected to last.* ■ Determine the patient's previous surgical experiences and level of knowledge related to surgery.* ■ Provide time for the patient to ask questions and discuss concerns.* ■ Instruct the patient or caregiver how to participate in the care.* ■ Describe preoperative routines (e.g., anesthesia, diet, bowel preparation, tests/labs, voiding, skin preparation, IV therapy, clothing, family waiting area, transportation to operating room).* ■ Describe any preoperative medications, the effects these will have on the patient, and the rationale for using them.* ■ Inform significant others of the place to wait for the results of the surgery.* ■ Introduce the patient to perioperative staff as appropriate.* ■ Discuss possible pain control measures.* ■ Describe postoperative routines/equipment (e.g., medications, respiratory treatments, tubes, machines, support hose, surgical dressings, ambulation, diet, family visitation) and explain their purpose.* ■ Instruct the patient in postoperative deep-breathing exercises, splinting incision, coughing.* ■ Reinforce information provided by other healthcare team members, as appropriate.* ■ Include the family/significant others [in the teaching-learning process] as appropriate.*

Nursing Diagnosis: Disturbed Sleep Pattern related to anxiety about the upcoming surgery

NOC Outcome: Sleep *NOC Goals:* ■ (4) Mild interrupted sleep ■ (5) Hours of sleep (at least 5 hr/24 hr), not compromised ■ (4) Sleeps through the night consistently, mildly compromised. *Individualized Goals:* ■ Reports minimal compromise in hours of sleep and sleep pattern. ■ No difficulty falling and staying asleep reported or observed.	**Sleep Enhancement** ■ Determine the patient's usual sleep-activity pattern.* ■ Determine effects of patient's current medications on sleep pattern.* ■ Adjust environment (lighting, noise, temperature, etc.) to promote sleep.* ■ Demonstrate and explain the procedure for progressive muscle relaxation. ■ Administer medication to promote sleep, as appropriate.

Sources: Bulechek, G. M., Butcher, H. K., Dochterman, J. M., et al. (Eds.). (2013). *Nursing interventions classification (NIC)* (6th ed.). St. Louis, MO: C.V. Mosby; Moorhead, S., Johnson, M., Maas, M., et al. (Eds.). (2013). *Nursing outcomes classification (NOC)* (5th ed.). St. Louis, MO: C.V. Mosby; *Nursing Diagnoses—Definitions and Classification 2018–2020.* © 2010 NANDA International, ISBN 978-1-62623-929-6. Used by arrangement with the Thieme Group, Stuttgart/New York.

surgeon and patient have communicated adequately about the surgery (Dale, Rothrock, & McEwen, 2014). Once signed and witnessed, the consent form is part of the patient's record and accompanies him to the operating room. **KEY POINT:** *The surgeon is responsible for (1) giving the patient the necessary information and (2) determining the patient's competence to make an informed decision about the surgery. You are responsible for verifying that the surgical consent form is signed and witnessed.*

The following two sections are about the "mechanics" of consent. They describe the contents of a consent form is and the processes of obtaining a patient's signature.

What Is a Surgical Consent Form?

A **surgical consent form** includes the following information (The Joint Commission, 2010):

- The type of surgery being performed
- The name and qualifications of the person performing the surgery (e.g., Jason Esmar, MD) and the primary practitioner for the patient's care and treatment
- A statement that the risks and benefits of surgery, as well as reasonable alternatives, have been explained to the patient
- A statement of the relevant risks, benefits, and side effects of the alternatives
- The likelihood of achieving goals
- A statement that the patient has the right to refuse surgery or withdraw consent at any time
- When indicated, any limitations on the confidentiality of information about the patient

How Do I Obtain a Signature?

Often you will obtain the patient's signature and document on the preoperative checklist that you have done so. As a patient advocate, you should:

- **Verify.** First verify with the patient that the physician has explained the procedure and answered all his questions: Ask the patient to state what he was told during the consent process.
- **Notify and delay, if necessary.** If the patient has questions or if you have any questions about the patient's competence, notify the surgeon and delay sending the patient to surgery.
- **Document.** Be sure to document these conversations, and document in the nursing notes that the surgeon was notified of any additional questions or concerns.

What Is Informed Consent?

A signature on a form implies consent. However, you must be certain that the signature represents *informed* consent. **KEY POINT: Informed consent** *requires that the patient understood the communication and was not coerced (pressured) to consent.* There are two important requirements:

- The patient must be alert, rational, mentally competent, and not sedated when he signs.
- The information must be given to him in a language and vocabulary that he can understand.

Patients who are unconscious or have a mental disability; who have been judged insane; who cannot read, write, or hear; and those under the influence of sedative drugs or alcohol are generally not competent to give consent (Buppert, 2012). In most states a family member, conservator, or legal guardian may give consent for the procedure.

Informed consent helps protect patients from having a surgery they do not understand or want. The *signed document* protects the healthcare agency and workers from later claims that the patient did not consent to have the procedure. If you would like more information on *informed* consent, see Chapters 43 and 44.

KnowledgeCheck 40-3

- Who is responsible for obtaining informed consent for the surgical procedure?
- What are the nursing responsibilities related to informed consent?

Provide Preoperative Teaching

Preoperative teaching prepares the patient for the surgical experience, allays fears, and decreases the risks of postoperative complications. See Chapter 26 as needed to review patient teaching.

What to Teach

The content of the teaching plan should focus on:

- What will happen before, during, and after surgery
- How the patient or caregiver can participate in the care
- Common feelings and concerns that patients have about surgery. This helps the patient feel supported and less anxious.
- What patients and families can do to prevent surgical site infection (The Joint Commission, 2016). Teach patients the content in the Self-Care box Teaching Patients How to Help Prevent Surgical Site Infections.

The type of surgery influences the content of your teaching. For example, if the patient is scheduled for an outpatient knee

---

Self-Care

Teaching Patients How to Help Prevent Surgical Site Infections

Before Surgery

➤ If you smoke, stop. Those who smoke are more likely to get infections.
➤ Discuss your health problems with your surgeon (e.g., diabetes, allergies). These can affect incision healing.
➤ Ask your surgeon whether you should have antibiotics before surgery.
➤ Don't shave near where you will have surgery. Not all procedures require hair removal, but if they do, it should be done with electric clippers. If someone starts to use a razor to shave you, speak up.

After Surgery

➤ Be sure family and friends wash their hands or use alcohol-based hand rub before and after they visit you.
➤ When anyone examines you or checks your incision, ask them if they have washed their hands (or used alcohol-based handrub).
➤ Wash your hands before and after caring for your own incision.
➤ Do not allow family and friends to touch your incision or the surgical dressing.
➤ Be sure you know how to care for your incision before you go home.
➤ If you have fever or redness, pain, or drainage at the surgery site, call your physician right away.

Source: Adapted from Centers for Disease Control and Prevention. (n.d.) (updated 2016). Having surgery? What you should know before you go. Retrieved from http://www.cdc.gov/features/SafeSurgery/

arthroscopy (visualization of the joint) under spinal anesthesia, the teaching plan needs to describe the procedure and the anticipated discharge of the patient within hours after surgery. This is different from the teaching for a patient who will have cardiac surgery and spend a number of days in the hospital. **KEY POINT:** *In general, preoperative teaching should focus on explaining what will happen before, during, and after surgery.* You will find specific teaching content in the Preoperative Teaching interventions for Deficient Knowledge in Table 40-3. Also refer to Clinical Insight 40-1. For the complete steps of deep breathing, coughing, moving in bed, and leg exercises, see Procedure 40-1.

How to Teach

You can use written instructions, video presentations, phone contact, or face-to-face discussion to provide preoperative teaching. Teach in a language that the patient understands and at a level that is easily understood. Use terms the patient understands clearly; that is, avoid medical jargon. See Chapter 26 if you need to review patient teaching techniques and information about health literacy.

Obtain an interpreter for translation if the patient speaks a language that you do not speak. When possible, avoid using family members as translators in order to protect the patient's privacy or avoid a bias in translation (see Chapter 15 if you need more information about language differences).

Teaching Children Include family members in the teaching as much as possible and as much as desired by the patient, especially if the patient is a child or dependent adult. Play is an effective way for children to learn (e.g., have the child give medicine to her doll with an empty syringe or listen to its "heart" with your stethoscope). Simple language is a must! For example, you'd say to a young child, "Lie on your tummy, please."

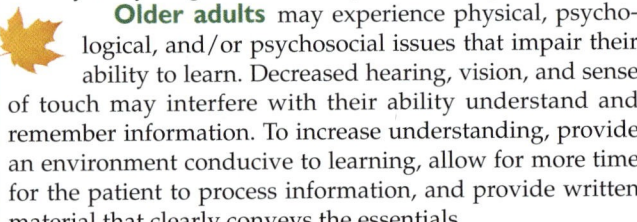 **Older adults** may experience physical, psychological, and/or psychosocial issues that impair their ability to learn. Decreased hearing, vision, and sense of touch may interfere with their ability understand and remember information. To increase understanding, provide an environment conducive to learning, allow for more time for the patient to process information, and provide written material that clearly conveys the essentials.

When to Teach

For elective surgery, many patients have a scheduled preoperative assessment about a week before the surgery. The session may include preoperative testing, an appointment with the anesthesia staff, signing the consent form, and planned preoperative teaching.

Patients undergoing emergency surgery usually require extensive physical care preoperatively. You may need to give IV fluids, transfuse blood, treat for pain, and administer many medications, as in the case of Mr. Singh (Meet Your Patient). This means that you may have limited time for preoperative teaching. However, you should always teach the patient as much as possible to prepare him for the surgical experience.

Prepare the Patient Physically for Surgery

Physical preparation of the patient for surgery involves several nursing concerns:

Maintaining Normothermia Recent evidence-based guidelines stress that maintaining a normal body temperature helps produce good surgical outcomes (Levin, Wright, Pecoraro, et al., 2016; Rightmyer & Singbartl, 2016). Compared with normothermic patients, hypothermic patients have more frequent wound infections, cardiac complications, and blood transfusions. Hypothermic patients feel uncomfortable, and shivering raises oxygen consumption by about 40%.

- The patient's core temperature should be measured 1 to 2 hours before the start of anesthesia, and either continuously or every 15 minutes during surgery.
- Active prewarming before induction of general anesthesia has been found to be effective in preventing perioperative hypothermia. Prewarming, with forced-air warming gowns or mattresses, should last for 10 to 30 minutes.

Nutritional Status Anxiety and anesthesia reduce gastrointestinal motility. To decrease the risk of nausea and vomiting, patients usually fast, taking no food or liquids (NPO) for 8 hours before surgery. Stress to patients and family the importance of fasting (for the prescribed length of time) to avoid the danger of aspiration.

You should know, though, that years of evidence support shorter fasting times than you will see used in most institutions. The American Society of Anesthesiologists preoperative fasting guidelines for healthy patients, recommends ingesting clear liquids up to 2 hours before surgery—and even a light meal up to 6 hours before surgery (Lambert & Carey, 2015; "Practice Guidelines for Preoperative Fasting," 2011).

Skin Preparation Preoperative whole-body bathing or showering is considered good clinical practice to make the skin as clean as possible prior to surgery in order to reduce the number of bacteria on the skin, especially at the site of incision. Patients should bathe or shower with either soap or an antiseptic (e.g., 4% chlorhexidine gluconate, Betadine) the evening before surgery and the morning of the surgery (National Guideline Clearinghouse, 2014; World Health Organization, 2016). Final skin preparation and hair removal, if done, should be completed before taking the patient into the surgical suite.

Bowel Preparation Enemas are now used primarily for surgical procedures of the colon, not for all surgeries. To empty the colon of feces, patients are asked to consume a low-residue diet for several days before surgery and are given a regimen of medications and/or enemas to clear the bowel. Stress the importance of adhering to the regimen to limit the risk of contaminating the operative site with feces.

Urinary Elimination Indwelling catheters are not routinely inserted for surgery. Catheterization may be prescribed if it is important to keep the bladder empty during surgery, if fluid status is being carefully monitored, or if the surgery is expected to last for a prolonged period of time.

✚ If a catheter is not prescribed, have the patient void before receiving preoperative medications. The patient could fall if he gets out of bed after being sedated or given opioids for pain.

Preoperative Medications The anesthesiologist may prescribe preoperative medications to relax the patient, reduce respiratory secretions, or reduce the risk of vomiting and aspiration (Table 40-4). The medication is prescribed at a prearranged time (e.g., at 0615) or it may be prescribed to give "on call." You will give an on-call medication when the surgical suite staff notifies you it is time to do so.

Antibiotics are often administered prophylactically to help prevent postoperative infection before:

- Clean surgery involving the placement of a prosthesis or implant
- Clean-contaminated surgery
- Contaminated surgery

Table 40-4 ➤ Preoperative Medications

TYPE OF MEDICATION	USE	EXAMPLES
Antibiotics	Reduce the microbial burden of intraoperative contamination to a level that cannot overwhelm host defenses	Cephalosporins (e.g., cefazolin, cefoxitin), clindamycin, vancomycin
Anticholinergics (e.g., phenothiazines)	Reduce oral and pulmonary secretions, prevent laryngospasms, prevent bradycardia	Atropine chlorpromazine, scopolamine, glycopyrrolate
Anxiolytics (e.g., benzodiazepines)	Control anxiety, calming	Alprazolam, clonazepam, diazepam, lorazepam, midazolam
Antihistamines	Provide sedation and antiemetic effects	Hydroxyzine, diphenhydramine
Barbiturates	Provide sedation without significant cardiopulmonary depression	Secobarbital, pentobarbital
H₂ Receptor Antagonists	Reduce gastric acidity	Cimetidine, ranitidine
Hypnotics	Provide sedation and increase the duration of sleep	Temazepam
Neuroleptics	Provide sedative, antiemetic, and anticonvulsant effects	Droperidol, fentanyl
Opioid Analgesics	Provide pain relief and sedation; induce anesthesia	Fentanyl, meperidine, morphine

You will usually administer the antibiotic intravenously, timed so that a bactericidal concentration of the drug will be present in serum and tissues by the time the incision is made (usually within 60 minutes preceding incision, just as the patient is going to the surgical suite) (National Guideline Clearinghouse, 1999, revised 2013). Antibiotics may, instead, be given at the start of anesthesia and repeated if the surgery is longer than the duration of the antibiotic.

Routine Medications Many routine medications are held (not administered) on the day of surgery. For example, an insulin-dependent diabetic patient may be instructed to hold her morning injection or administer half of the normal dose. The patient needs less insulin because her NPO status will keep her blood sugar lower than usual. The anesthesiologist will monitor the blood sugar in the operating room and give additional insulin if needed. Some patients may be instructed to stop routine medications several days before surgery. For example, a client receiving warfarin for anticoagulation may need to stop the medication 7 days before surgery.

Prostheses Before being transported to the operating suite, the patient must remove all artificial body parts, such as dentures, artificial limbs, or contact lenses. Wigs, eyeglasses, makeup, and jewelry must also be removed.

Antiembolism Stockings These are also referred to as *thromboembolic disorder hose* (or "T.E.D. hose"). They are elastic stockings that compress the veins of the legs and increase venous return to the heart (Fig. 40-1). They may be applied preoperatively to prevent venous pooling during surgery and decrease the risk of thrombus formation. Along with prophylactic medications (antithrombotics), antiembolism stockings aid in the prevention of DVT and PE. However, hospitals are increasingly using sequential compression devices and anticoagulation therapy, instead of elastic

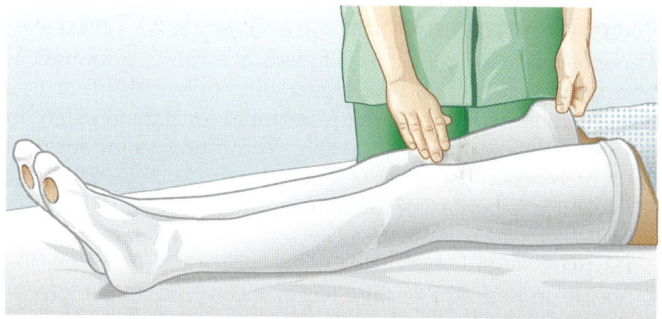

FIGURE 40-1 Antiembolism stockings compress the veins of the legs and increase venous return to the heart.

stockings, to prevent DVT (Perry, Borchert, Burke, et al., 2012, reviewed 2014).

Older adults and those with risk factors for venous thromboembolism are most in need of antiembolism stockings. Risk factors include the following conditions (Association of periOperative Registered Nurses, 2009, revised 2014):

- Venous stasis (such as occurs with bedrest, lengthy surgery, varicose veins, and heart failure)
- Vascular wall injury, which initiates clotting (e.g., surgery, IV catheter, irritating IV drugs, prior deep vein thrombus, smoking)
- Hypercoagulability (e.g., estrogen therapy, oral contraceptive use, cancer, dehydration, pregnancy)

Older adults may be at higher risk for DVT because they have more than one of these risk factors. Safety measures to prevent DVT in older adults include range-of-motion exercises and applying antiembolism stockings to prevent pooling of blood in the extremities (Bashaw & Scott, 2012)

Antiembolism stockings may extend from foot to knee, or foot to thigh, although the Institute for Clinical Systems Improvement suggests that thigh-high stockings be avoided because of their tendency to roll and restrict circulation (Perry, Borchert, Burke, et al., 2012). Some stockings have an opening at the toes that allows you to assess circulation in the feet. Stockings must be sized and applied correctly in order to be effective (see Procedure 40-2). Stockings are contraindicated for some patients (e.g., those with peripheral arterial disease) (National Guideline Clearinghouse, 2007, revised 2015).

Take Measures to Prevent Wrong Patient, Wrong Site, Wrong Surgery

The following safety measures will help prevent patient misidentification and wrong-site surgery (The Joint Commission, 2016):

- Use a preoperative checklist to confirm that appropriate documents are available and the appropriate activities have been performed.
- Verify the patient's identity before the patient leaves the preoperative area.
- Mark the surgical site before surgery. Use a permanent marker so that your marks will not be removed by the surgical skin prep, and involve the patient in the marking process.
- Take a time-out with all team members before starting the procedure (see "Perioperative Safety," near the beginning of this chapter).

Communicate With the Surgical Team

The most common root cause of medical errors is communication failure (Berger, Greenberg, & Bilimoria, 2015). For this reason, good communication is essential for patient safety in perioperative care. For successful communication, surgical team members must:

- Receive a summary of the plan of care (e.g., a short briefing by the surgeon) and develop a shared understanding of the plan.
- Speak up and be assertive with concerns about the procedure or decisions.
- Ask questions to clarify confusion.
- Acknowledge that they have heard and understood.
- Ask for and provide feedback (e.g., read back) on critical information.
- Use standard terminology (e.g., checklists). In one study, implementation of the World Health Organization's (WHO) Surgical Safety Checklist was associated with a reduction in morbidity and length of in-hospital stay and reduction in mortality (Mayer, Sevdalis, Rout, et al., 2016).

Two-minute briefings just before surgery, led by the attending surgeon using a standardized format, have been found to improve communication and reduce delays and wrong-site surgery (Lee, 2016). Surgical briefings encourage team members to talk when there is no problem, so they are more likely to speak up when they have misgivings or when problems occur (Berger, Greenberg, & Bilimoria, 2015).

KnowledgeCheck 40-4
- Identify topics that should be discussed in preoperative teaching.
- Describe the typical physical preparation of a client undergoing surgery.

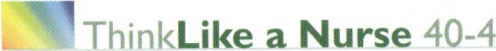

ThinkLike a Nurse 40-4
- What aspects of preoperative teaching should you stress when caring for Mr. Singh (Meet Your Patient)?
- A bowel preparation is typically part of preoperative preparation for a client having colon surgery. Do you think this will be part of Mr. Singh's physical preparation? Why or why not?

Transfer to the Operative Suite

Once you have completed your preoperative care, the patient is ready for transport by stretcher to the operative area, usually to the surgical holding area (Fig. 40-2). Attend to the following:

- *Preoperative checklist and patient's chart*—Must accompany the patient.
- *Valuables*—Lock these up according to agency policy, or have the patient's family keep them.
- *Glasses, hearing aid*—Occasionally, especially if the patient has a significant sensory deficit, the patient can wear his hearing aid or glasses to the surgical suite. You will need to arrange this in advance with the surgical staff or anesthesia team.

Children are often permitted to bring a favorite toy with them to the operating room (OR) to provide comfort. They may fear being separated from their parents, so arrange for parents to spend time with the child immediately before the surgery and as soon as possible afterward. Keep the parents informed and let them know what to expect.

Prepare the Postoperative Room

If you transfer the patient to the surgical suite from a nursing unit in the hospital, you should prepare the room for the patient's return after surgery. Put clean linens on the bed and arrange the supplies and equipment you will need. Raise the bed to stretcher height and lock the wheels.

INTRAOPERATIVE CARE

The **intraoperative phase** begins when the patient enters the operating suite and ends when she is admitted to the postanesthesia care unit.

TheoreticalKnowledge
knowing why

To provide intraoperative care, you will need theoretical knowledge of the roles of the various members of the intraoperative team and of the different types of anesthesia that are used.

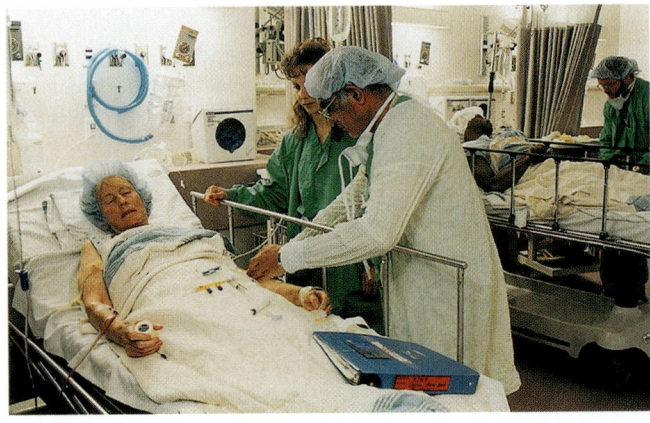

FIGURE 40-2 Surgical holding area.

Operative Personnel

The personnel who attend the client during the surgical procedure are called the *intraoperative team*. The team is divided into members who must use sterile technique and those who use clean technique (see Chapter 22 if you need to review medical and surgical asepsis). During the intraoperative phase, registered nurses can function as the scrub nurse, circulating nurse, or registered nurse first assistant. Each of these roles contributes to the safe care of surgical clients.

Sterile Team Members of the sterile intraoperative team include the surgeon, surgical assistant, and scrub person. Before beginning the surgery, they perform a surgical scrub of the hands and arms, dry with sterile towels, and don sterile gowns and gloves. To review these procedures, see Chapter 22.

- The **scrub nurse** can be an RN, LVN/LPN, or a surgical technician. The scrub nurse sets up the sterile field, prepares the surgical instruments, assists with the sterile draping of the patient, anticipates and responds to the surgeon's needs, and maintains the integrity of the sterile field.

- A **registered nurse first assistant (RNFA)** is an RN with additional education and training in surgical technique. The RNFA serves as an assistant to the surgeon, a role that has historically been filled by physicians. The RNFA may be employed by the surgeon or the hospital.

Sterile team members are the only persons allowed to enter the sterile field. Creation of the operative field is explained in Clinical Insight 40-2.

Clean Team Team members who abide by clean technique (medical asepsis) include the anesthesiologist or nurse anesthetist, the circulating RN, biomedical technicians, and radiology technicians. **KEY POINT:** *These personnel never enter the sterile field, but instead function around and beyond it.*

Either an **anesthesiologist** or a **nurse anesthetist (CRNA)** induces amnesia, analgesia, and muscle relaxation or paralysis with anesthesia. His role is to continuously monitor and evaluate the patient's responses to the anesthetic agent and the surgical procedure. CRNAs administer more than half of all anesthetics in the United States.

The **circulating nurse** is an RN who applies the nursing process to coordinate all activities in the operating room. He is a client advocate who continuously monitors the client and the sterile field. The circulating nurse maintains a safe, comfortable environment; communicates with appropriate personnel outside the operating room; and responds to emergencies. An important aspect of the circulating nurse's role is to attend to the patient during the induction of anesthesia.

KnowledgeCheck 40-5

- Identify the intraoperative nursing roles that are part of the sterile intraoperative team and those that are part of the clean intraoperative team.
- Which nursing roles are always held by a registered nurse?

Toward Evidence-Based Practice

| Dixon, J. L., Mukhopadhyay, D., Hunt, J., et al. (2016). **Enhancing surgical safety using digital multimedia technology.** *The American Journal of Surgery, 211*(6), 1095–1098.

The researchers investigated whether incorporating digital and video multimedia components improved surgical time-out performance of a surgical safety checklist. The multimedia system included the four critical elements of a time-out (staff member introduction, patient identification, description of the procedure and laterality to be performed, and clarification of key patient safety components) but was further enhanced with a patient video stating name, date of birth, surgical procedure and laterality, along with team member visualization of the signed consent. All the time-out components were streamed to the wall monitor present in the operating room. The surgical team in its entirety was able to visualize all time-out components and follow along as a group. Findings indicated that a multimedia time-out improves performance of key safety elements and enhances team communication.

| Mainthia, R., Lockney, T., Zotov, A., et al. (2012). **Novel use of electronic whiteboard in the operating room increases surgical team compliance with pre-incision safety practices.** *Surgery, 151*(5), 660–666.

In this study, the researcher used an electronic checklist system displayed on a white board in the operating room to observe whether its use improves and sustains surgical

team compliance with the pre-incision time-out. The safety whiteboard was visible to the entire team and was referenced during the pre-incision time-out. As each item was announced, the circulator nurse checked a box in the nursing documentation application. At the end of the checklist, the whiteboard noted "time-out complete." These strategies culminated in a significant increase in in time-out procedural compliance.

Imagine that you are the OR nurse manager and that the incidence of wrong-site surgery in your hospital is higher than the national average. You want to introduce some changes in the OR, and are considering introducing new technology. You are trying to decide the type of technology to implement that would ultimately improve surgical outcomes. In practice, you would have more studies to rely on, but pretend in this instance that you must base your decision on just the two studies described here.

1. What conclusions can you make based on the findings of the two studies?

2. How can the findings of the studies be used to improve outcomes in your population?

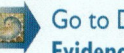 Go to Davis Advantage, Resources, Chapter 40, **Toward Evidence-Based Practice—Suggested Responses.**

Types of Anesthesia

During surgery, anesthesia is used to obtain **analgesia** (control of pain), muscle relaxation or paralysis, and **amnesia** (memory loss). Anesthesia is classified as general, conscious sedation, or regional.

General Anesthesia

General anesthesia produces rapid unconsciousness and loss of sensation. The anesthesiologist or nurse anesthetist administers inhaled and intravenous medications that depress the patient's central nervous system and relax the musculature. Muscle relaxants, paralyzing agents, narcotics, barbiturates, and inhaled gases are some of the agents used during general anesthesia.

Advantages of General Anesthesia

- The patient is unconscious, so she experiences no anxiety that might affect cardiac and respiratory functioning.
- The muscles are relaxed, so the patient remains completely motionless during the surgical procedure.
- Anesthesia can be adjusted to accommodate age, physical condition, and the length of the procedure. For example, an older adult may require less anesthetic than anticipated; if so, the anesthetist can decrease the dosage without interrupting the procedure.
- If surgical complications occur, the anesthesia can be continued for longer than originally planned.

Disadvantages of General Anesthesia

- The respiratory and circulatory muscles are depressed, so mechanical ventilation is needed while the patient is under the effects of the anesthetic agent(s). These effects predispose the patient to pneumonia and thrombophlebitis in the postoperative period.
- General anesthesia creates a risk for death, heart attack, stroke, and malignant hyperthermia. **Malignant hyperthermia** is a rare, often fatal, metabolic condition that can occur during the use of muscle relaxants and inhalation anesthesia. Metabolism increases in the skeletal muscles and they become rigid. The temperature rises rapidly. Predisposition to this condition is inherited.
- Frequent minor complaints after general anesthesia include sore throat (from intubation), nausea and vomiting (from relaxation of gastrointestinal smooth muscle), headache, uncontrollable shivering, and confusion.

Conscious Sedation

Conscious sedation provides intravenous sedation and analgesia without producing unconsciousness. During conscious sedation, the patient may feel sleepy but is aware of his surroundings, can be easily aroused by touch or speech, and can talk with the surgical team. Nevertheless, blood pressure, heart rate, respiratory rate, and oxygen saturation are monitored, and the patient usually receives oxygen via nasal cannula during the procedure. Because of the amnesic effect of many of the medications, the patient may not recall aspects of the procedure afterward. Conscious sedation is used for procedures such as bronchoscopy and cosmetic surgery.

Advantages: Pain and anxiety are adequately controlled without the risks of general anesthesia. Recovery is rapid.

Disadvantages: Not practical for highly anxious patients.

Regional Anesthesia

Regional anesthesia prevents pain by interrupting nerve impulses to and from the area of the procedure. The patient remains alert but is numb in the involved area. Regional anesthesia may be administered by infiltration of the surgical site and surrounding tissue with local anesthetics, such as lidocaine or bupivacaine. These medications may also be injected into and around specific nerves to depress the sensory, motor, and/or sympathetic impulses of a limited area of the body.

Advantages: Low in cost, simple to administer, and requires a minimal recovery period. It is especially suitable for minor ambulatory procedures.

Disadvantages: May not be practical if the patient is highly anxious or if adequate pain control cannot be achieved. Many patients are apprehensive about being able to see and hear the procedure.

Techniques for achieving regional anesthesia are discussed, following:

Peripheral Nerve Block   A **nerve block** is the injection of an anesthetic into and around a nerve or group of nerves (e.g., the facial nerve).

A **Bier (intravenous) block** is a technique in which the anesthetist places a tourniquet on an arm or leg and then injects a local anesthetic agent intravenously below the level of the tourniquet. The tourniquet is maintained at a pressure that limits venous return but continues to allow arterial circulation. The patient feels no pain in the extremity as long as the tourniquet is in place.

Advantages of Bier Block:

- Onset and recovery time are both rapid.
- The tourniquet decreases bleeding during the surgical procedure and prevents systemic absorption of the local anesthetic.

Disadvantages of Bier Block:

- When the procedure is finished, the tourniquet is deflated, and there is potential for systemic absorption of the anesthetic.
- To prevent tissue damage, the tourniquet must not be left in place for more than 2 hours.

Spinal Anesthesia   is the injection of an anesthetic into the cerebrospinal fluid (CSF) in the subarachnoid space (Fig. 40-3A). This injection blocks sensation and movement below the level of the injection. Spinal anesthesia is often used for surgical procedures in the lower abdomen, pelvis, and lower extremities. This technique allows the patient to remain conscious during the procedure and usually does not depress respirations.

Occasionally a higher level of spinal anesthesia is achieved than intended—that is, the medication may migrate upward in the spinal fluid. This can depress respirations and cardiac rate. Placing the patient in Fowler's position may prevent respiratory paralysis.

Side effects of spinal anesthesia include hypotension, nausea, vomiting, urinary retention, and headache from leakage of CSF. A headache after spinal anesthesia must be closely monitored and may require additional treatment by the anesthesia staff.

The blood pressure may also decrease suddenly as a result of pervasive vasodilation—the anesthesia blocks the sympathetic vasomotor nerves, which normally maintain muscle tone in peripheral blood vessels. Patients with these complications often require ventilation and support of blood pressure during surgery, so they must be carefully monitored during surgery and in the recovery period.

Epidural Anesthesia   requires insertion of a thin catheter into the epidural space (Fig. 40-3B). Anesthetic agents are

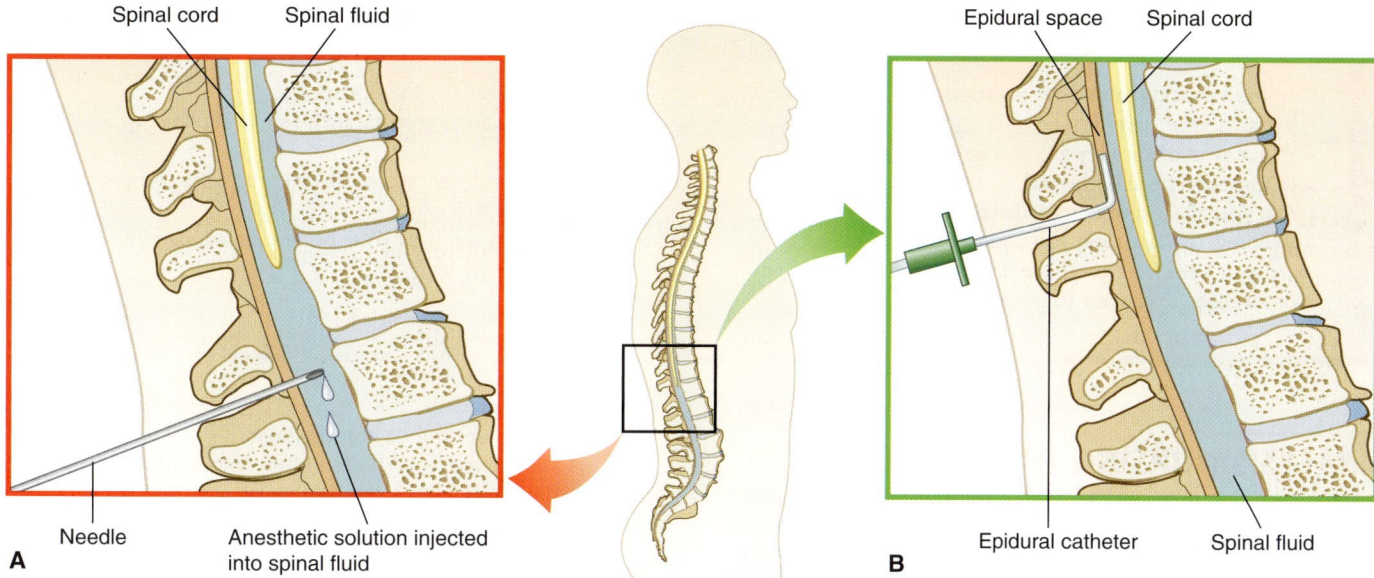

FIGURE 40-3   A. Spinal anesthesia is the injection of a local anesthetic into the subarachnoid space to block sensation and movement. B. Continuous epidural anesthesia can be used to provide postoperative analgesia.

infused through the catheter to produce loss of sensation. Epidural anesthesia can be used as a surgical anesthetic and to provide postoperative analgesia. Advantages and disadvantages of epidural anesthesia are similar to those of spinal anesthesia.

- Epidural anesthesia is safer than spinal anesthesia because the anesthetic does not enter the subarachnoid space and the depth of anesthesia is not as great.
- Drugs used for epidural administration are of a higher concentration than those for spinal administration; if the medication is inadvertently injected too deeply (into the subarachnoid space), hypotension and respiratory paralysis occur, and temporary mechanical ventilation is necessary.
- Epidural anesthesia is ideal for obstetrics procedures (e.g., cesarean birth or pain control with vaginal birth) because the mother is awake to bond with the newborn, and her mobility is limited for only a short time.

Local Anesthesia

Local anesthesia produces loss of pain sensation at the desired site (e.g., a wound to be sutured, a skin growth to be removed). It is typically used for minor procedures. However, after finishing a major surgery, the surgeon may infiltrate the operative area with local anesthetics to provide postoperative pain relief. Local anesthetics may be applied topically or injected. A **topical anesthetic** is applied directly to the skin and mucous membranes. Lidocaine and benzocaine are commonly used because they are rapidly absorbed and rapid acting.

KnowledgeCheck 40-6

- What is the purpose of anesthesia?
- Under what type(s) of anesthesia does the client remain conscious?

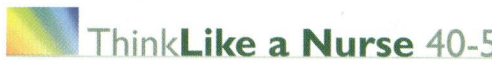ThinkLike a Nurse 40-5

What form of anesthesia is Mr. Singh (Meet Your Patient) most likely to receive? Why?

PracticalKnowledge knowing **how**

When a patient arrives in the surgical suite the nurse verifies the information on the preoperative checklist and assesses the patient. The nursing focus is on safe and successful completion of the surgery.

ASSESSMENT NP

The circulating nurse greets the client in the preoperative holding area and performs a brief assessment by doing the following:

- Verify that the surgical consent has been signed and witnessed and that the preoperative checklist is complete.
- Assess the client's anxiety level and physical condition.
- Measure the vital signs; examine the surgical site; and inspect IV lines, drainage tubes, and catheters. Often the circulating nurse or the anesthetist starts an IV line in the holding area if one is not already present.
- Give preoperative medication in the holding area, if prescribed.
- Monitor vital signs often, or even continuously, during the intraoperative period.

For common interview questions to use in the intraoperative period, see the accompanying Focused Assessment box Intraoperative Care Questionnaire.

In addition to the checklist completed in the preoperative period, the surgery team will also probably complete a surgical safety checklist. The World Health Organization Surgical Safety Checklist covers the three phases of a surgical procedure, commonly referred to as "sign in," "time-out," and "sign out." The three phases of the checklist are reviewed by the checklist coordinator, who verbally checks that each element was done. The goal of using a surgical checklist is to enhance communication, teamwork, and safety by addressing key activities that occur as part of the perioperative process (WHO, 2009). Refer to the Focused Assessment box Example of a Surgical Safety Checklist.

Focused Assessment

Intraoperative Care Questionnaire

Common nursing interview questions include the following:
➤ What is your name?
➤ What type of surgery are you going to have today?
➤ Is someone here with you?
➤ Are you allergic to any medications, latex, or tape?
➤ When is the last time you had anything to eat or drink?
➤ Do you have false teeth, contact lenses, or any other prostheses that need to be removed?

➤ Have you taken any medications today?
➤ Do you have any implants, such as metal plates or a pacemaker?
➤ Do you have any scratches, bruises, or other wounds on your body at this time?
➤ Are there any parts of your body that are painful, such as a stiff shoulder or leg?

ANALYSIS/NURSING DIAGNOSIS NP

As in the preoperative phase, most intraoperative nursing care consists of standard activities to be used for all patients. Most intraoperative patients, regardless of the surgery, have the following potential complications (collaborative problems) of surgery and anesthesia:

- Potential complications of surgery:
  Hypothermia
  Fluid and electrolyte imbalance
  Excessive bleeding or hemorrhage
  Musculoskeletal injury secondary to positioning
- Potential complications of anesthesia:
  Aspiration
  Vasomotor instability (and resultant hypotension and diminished peripheral perfusion)
  Respiratory depression
  Cardiovascular compromise
  Except in unusual circumstances (e.g., a patient in poor nutritional status, a frail elderly patient), you may not need to

Focused Assessment

World Health Organization Surgical Safety Checklist.

Surgical Safety Checklist

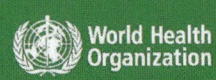

World Health Organization | Patient Safety
A World Alliance for Safer Health Care

Before induction of anaesthesia	Before skin incision	Before patient leaves operating room
(with at least nurse and anaesthetist)	(with nurse, anaesthetist and surgeon)	(with nurse, anaesthetist and surgeon)

Before induction of anaesthesia
(with at least nurse and anaesthetist)

Has the patient confirmed his/her identity, site, procedure, and consent?
☐ Yes

Is the site marked?
☐ Yes
☐ Not applicable

Is the anaesthesia machine and medication check complete?
☐ Yes

Is the pulse oximeter on the patient and functioning?
☐ Yes

Does the patient have a:

Known allergy?
☐ No
☐ Yes

Difficult airway or aspiration risk?
☐ No
☐ Yes, and equipment/assistance available

Risk of >500ml blood loss (7ml/kg in children)?
☐ No
☐ Yes, and two IVs/central access and fluids planned

Before skin incision
(with nurse, anaesthetist and surgeon)

☐ **Confirm all team members have introduced themselves by name and role.**

☐ **Confirm the patient's name, procedure, and where the incision will be made.**

Has antibiotic prophylaxis been given within the last 60 minutes?
☐ Yes
☐ Not applicable

Anticipated Critical Events

To Surgeon:
☐ What are the critical or non-routine steps?
☐ How long will the case take?
☐ What is the anticipated blood loss?

To Anaesthetist:
☐ Are there any patient-specific concerns?

To Nursing Team:
☐ Has sterility (including indicator results) been confirmed?
☐ Are there equipment issues or any concerns?

Is essential imaging displayed?
☐ Yes
☐ Not applicable

Before patient leaves operating room
(with nurse, anaesthetist and surgeon)

Nurse Verbally Confirms:
☐ The name of the procedure
☐ Completion of instrument, sponge and needle counts
☐ Specimen labelling (read specimen labels aloud, including patient name)
☐ Whether there are any equipment problems to be addressed

To Surgeon, Anaesthetist and Nurse:
☐ What are the key concerns for recovery and management of this patient?

This checklist is not intended to be comprehensive. Additions and modifications to fit local practice are encouraged.   Revised 1 / 2009   © WHO, 2009

Source: Reprinted with permission from the World Health Organization. Retrieved from http://whqlibdoc.who.int/publications/2009/9789241598590_eng_Checklist.pdf

identify nursing diagnoses for a patient because the standardized care addresses all the potential complications. However, for nurses who prefer to organize care according to nursing diagnoses, the following potential diagnoses apply to most patients having major surgery:

- *Perioperative Hypothermia* related to exposure in cool environment and administration of cool IV fluids. This applies especially to very young, very old, and very thin patients.
- *Risk for Aspiration* related to depressed respirations and reflexes. For patients who have weak muscles for coughing or a poor gag reflex, this diagnosis is especially relevant.
- *Risk for Imbalanced Fluid Volume* related to NPO status and blood loss from surgery. Some patients are at higher than normal risk, for example, patients with renal or cardiac problems.
- *Risk for Perioperative Positioning Injury* related to patient factors such as edema, emaciation, obesity, and sensory perceptual disturbances secondary to anesthesia.

Use the following nursing diagnoses only if the patient has the necessary defining characteristics or risk factors. Do not use them routinely for all patients.

- *Risk for Latex Allergic Reaction* related to multiple exposures (e.g., multiple surgeries, catheterizations) or history of related allergies
- *Latex Allergic Reaction* (needs no etiology)

PLANNING OUTCOMES/EVALUATION NP

The overarching goals in the intraoperative phase are that the patient will:

Be free from injury.
Remain physiologically stable.
Experience optimal surgical outcomes.

For *associated NOC standardized outcomes* for intraoperative patients, along with examples of goals created with NOC indicators and scales, refer to Table 40-5. Notice that the goals are appropriate for nearly all surgical patients.

Individualized goals/outcome statements are formulated from the patient's nursing diagnoses. The following are examples:

- Maintains body temperature within the normal range.
- Has clear lung sounds and patent airway.
- Has urine output of at least 30 mL/hr.
- Will have no skin, tissue, or neuromuscular injury as a result of positioning.
- Will not acquire healthcare-related infection.

PLANNING INTERVENTIONS/ IMPLEMENTATION NP

Intraoperative care focuses on maintaining a safe environment and assisting the surgery team to provide appropriate care for the client. The nurse anesthetist manages the interventions for most of the patient's potential problems, for example, fluid volume status, airway protection, and vital signs monitoring.

NIC standardized interventions for the intraoperative period come from the domain of Perioperative Care. They include interventions for all intraoperative patients, regardless of their individual nursing diagnoses. One intervention, Anesthesia Administration, must be performed by an anesthesiologist or nurse anesthetist. The nurse assists in implementing a number of interventions:

- Anesthesia Administration
- Autotransfusion
- Infection Control: Intraoperative

Table 40-5 ▶ Intraoperative Patients: Selected Standardized Nursing Diagnoses, Outcomes, and Interventions	
NOC OUTCOMES AND INDICATORS	**NIC INTERVENTIONS AND ACTIVITIES** (*Note:* Interventions and activities marked with an asterisk (*) are routinely performed for ALL surgery patients.)
Nursing diagnosis: Risk for Aspiration related to depressed respirations and reflexes secondary to anesthesia	
Collaborative problem: Potential Complication of anesthesia: Aspiration	
Comments: This is especially relevant for patients who have weak muscles for coughing or a poor gag reflex.	
NOC Outcome: Respiratory Status: Airway Patency **NOC Goal:** - (5) No choking or adventitious breath sounds	**Artificial Airway Management*** - Institute endotracheal suctioning, as appropriate.* **Aspiration Precautions*** - Monitor pulmonary status.* - Keep suction setup available.* - Maintain an airway.* **Sedation Management*** - Ensure that emergency resuscitation equipment is readily available, specifically source to deliver 100% O_2, emergency medications, and a defibrillator.* - Initiate an IV line. - Ensure availability of and administer antagonists as appropriate, per physician's order or protocol. **Vomiting Management*** - Position to prevent aspiration.

(Continued)

Table 40-5 ➤ Intraoperative Patients: Selected Standardized Nursing Diagnoses, Outcomes, and Interventions—cont'd

NOC OUTCOMES AND INDICATORS	NIC INTERVENTIONS AND ACTIVITIES (*Note:* Interventions and activities marked with an asterisk (*) are routinely performed for ALL surgery patients.)

Nursing diagnosis: Risk for Perioperative Hypothermia related to exposure in cool environment and administration of cool IV fluids

Collaborative problem: Potential Complication of surgery and anesthesia: hyperthermia, hypothermia, malignant hyperthermia

Comments: Applies especially to very young, very old, and very thin patients

NOC OUTCOMES AND INDICATORS	NIC INTERVENTIONS AND ACTIVITIES
NOC Outcome: Thermoregulation *NOC Goals:* ■ (5) No hyperthermia ■ (5) No hypothermia ■ (4) Mild increased (or decreased) skin temperature	**Temperature Regulation: Intraoperative*** ■ Begin warming preoperatively and continue during intraoperative phase.* ■ Adjust operating room temperature for therapeutic effect.* ■ Apply head covering.* ■ Cover exposed body parts.* ■ Warm or cool all irrigating, IV, and skin preparation solutions, as appropriate.* ■ Continuously monitor the patient's temperature.* ■ Cover patient with heated blanket for transport to postanesthesia care unit.* **Malignant Hyperthermia Precautions*** ■ Maintain emergency equipment for malignant hyperthermia, per protocol, in operative areas.* ■ Notify anesthesiologist and surgeon of patient history.* ■ Provide a cooling blanket.* **Vital Signs Monitoring*** ■ Monitor blood pressure, pulse, temperature, and respiratory status, as appropriate.* ■ Monitor skin color, temperature, and moistness.*

Nursing diagnosis: Risk for Imbalanced Fluid Volume related to NPO status and blood loss from surgery.

Collaborative problem: Potential complication of surgery: Fluid and electrolyte imbalance

Comments: Clients undergoing surgery are at risk for vascular, cellular, and/or intracellular dehydration. Patients with renal or cardiac problems are at higher than normal risk for fluid and electrolyte imbalance.

NOC OUTCOMES AND INDICATORS	NIC INTERVENTIONS AND ACTIVITIES
NOC Outcomes: Blood Loss Severity Fluid Balance Urinary Elimination Vital Signs *NOC Goals:* ■ (4) Systolic and diastolic blood pressures, mild deviation from normal range ■ (5) Mean arterial pressure not compromised ■ (5) Central venous pressure not compromised ■ (5) Pulmonary wedge pressure not compromised ■ (4) Peripheral pulses mildly compromised ■ (4) 24-hr intake and output balance mildly compromised	**Fluid Management*** ■ Maintain accurate intake and output record.* ■ Insert urinary catheter, if appropriate.* ■ Administer IV therapy, as prescribed.* ■ Monitor hemodynamic status, including CVP, MAP, PAP, and PCWP, if available.* ■ Prepare for administration of blood products (e.g., check blood with patient identification and prepare infusion setup), as appropriate.* **Fluid Monitoring*** ■ Determine possible risk factors for fluid imbalance (e.g., renal pathologies, liver dysfunction).* ■ Monitor color, quantity, and specific gravity of urine.* ■ Monitor for distended neck veins, crackles in the lungs, peripheral edema, and weight gain.*

Table 40-5 ➤ Intraoperative Patients: Selected Standardized Nursing Diagnoses, Outcomes, and Interventions—cont'd

NOC OUTCOMES AND INDICATORS	NIC INTERVENTIONS AND ACTIVITIES (*Note:* Interventions and activities marked with an asterisk (*) are routinely performed for ALL surgery patients.)
■ (5) Adventitious breath sounds not present	■ Monitor blood pressure, heart rate, and respiratory status.*
■ (5) Neck vein distension not present	■ Monitor serum and urine electrolyte values.*
■ (5) Peripheral edema not present	**Intravenous (IV) Therapy***
	■ Monitor IV flow rate and IV site during infusion.*
	■ Monitor for IV patency before administration of IV medication.*

Nursing diagnosis: Risk for Latex Allergic Reaction; or **Latex Allergic Reaction** related to multiple previous exposures to latex

Comments: Use these diagnoses only if the patient has the necessary defining characteristics or risk factors. Do not use them routinely for all patients.

NOC Outcomes: Immune Hypersensitivity Response Symptom Severity *NOC Goals:* ■ (5) No localized inflammatory responses ■ (5) Respiratory, cardiac, renal, and neurological functions not compromised	**Latex Precautions (Intraoperative)** ■ Place allergy band on patient [if not already done preoperatively]. ■ Record allergy or risk in patient's medical record [or check to see that it was done].* ■ Post sign indicating latex precautions. ■ Survey environment and remove latex products. ■ Monitor latex-free environment. ■ Report information to physician, pharmacist, and other care providers, as indicated. **Latex Precautions (Preoperative)*** ■ Question patient or appropriate other about history of neural tube defect (e.g., myelomeningocele) or congenital urological condition (e.g., extrophy of the bladder).* ■ Question patient or appropriate other about systemic reactions to natural rubber latex (e.g., facial or scleral edema, tearing eyes, urticaria, rhinitis, and wheezing).* ■ Question patient or appropriate other about allergies to foods such as bananas, kiwi, avocado, mango, and chestnuts.*

Nursing diagnosis: Risk for Perioperative Positioning Injury related to patient factors such as edema, emaciation, obesity, and sensory perceptual disturbances secondary to anesthesia

Collaborative problem: Potential complication of surgery: Neuromuscular, skeletal, or skin injury

NOC Outcomes: Circulation Status Mobility Neurological Status Physical Injury Severity Tissue Perfusion: Peripheral *NOC Goals:* ■ (4) PaO_2 mild deviation from normal range ■ (4) $PaCO_2$ mild deviation from normal range ■ (4) Pallor and dependent rubor mild ■ (5) Joint movement not compromised ■ (5) Spinal sensory/motor function not compromised ■ (5) Central motor control not compromised	**Circulatory Precautions*** ■ Perform a comprehensive appraisal of peripheral circulation (e.g., check peripheral pulses, edema, capillary refill, color, and temperature of extremity).* **Positioning: Intraoperative*** ■ Use assistive devices for immobilization.* ■ Lock wheels of stretcher and operating room bed.* ■ Use an adequate number of personnel to transfer patient.* ■ Support the head and neck during transfer.* ■ Immobilize or support any body part, as appropriate.* ■ Maintain patient's proper body alignment.* ■ Apply padding to bony prominences.* ■ Apply safety strap and arm restraint, as needed.* ■ Record position and devices used.*

(Continued)

Table 40-5 ➤ Intraoperative Patients: Selected Standardized Nursing Diagnoses, Outcomes, and Interventions—cont'd

NOC OUTCOMES AND INDICATORS	NIC INTERVENTIONS AND ACTIVITIES (*Note:* Interventions and activities marked with an asterisk (*) are routinely performed for ALL surgery patients.)
■ (5) No burns, bruises, extremity or back sprains, impaired mobility ■ (4) Capillary refill (fingers and toes) mild deviation from normal range ■ (5) No numbness ■ (5) All pulses no deviation from normal range ■ (5) Skin integrity not compromised	**Surgical Precautions**** ■ Verify surgical site.* ■ Verify client's blood type.* ■ Verify that there is blood on reserve.* ■ Verify client's identity.* ■ Verify patient's allergies.* ■ Check ground isolation monitor.* ■ Verify the correct functioning of equipment.* ■ Check suction for adequate pressure and complete assembly of canisters, tubing, and catheters.* ■ Count sponges, sharps, and instruments before, during, and after surgery, per agency policy; record results of counts.* ■ Provide an electrosurgical unit, grounding pad, and active electrode, as appropriate.* ■ Verify the integrity of electrical cords.* ■ Verify the proper functioning of electrosurgical unit.* ■ Verify that the client is not in contact with metal.* ■ Check for the presence of implants, pacemakers, and metal prostheses pacemakers contraindicating use of electrosurgical cautery.* ■ Verify the patient's skin integrity at site of [electrocautery] grounding pad.* ■ Verify that skin prep solutions are nonflammable.* ■ Adjust coagulation and cutting currents, as instructed by physician or per agency policy.* ■ Inspect the patient's skin for injury [at conclusion of procedure].* ■ (non-NIC) Monitor sterile technique throughout procedure.*

Sources: Bulechek, G. M., Butcher, H. K., Dochterman, J. M., et al. (Eds.). (2013). *Nursing interventions classification (NIC)* (6th ed.). St. Louis, MO: C.V. Mosby; Moorhead, S., Johnson, M., Maas, M., et al. (Eds.). (2013). *Nursing outcomes classification (NOC)* (5th ed.). St. Louis, MO: C.V. Mosby; *Nursing Diagnoses—Definitions and Classification 2018–2020.* © 2010 NANDA International, ISBN 978-1-62623-929-6. Used by arrangement with the Thieme Group, Stuttgart/New York.

■ Positioning: Intraoperative
■ Surgical Assistance
■ Surgical Precautions
■ Surgical Preparation
■ Temperature Regulation: Intraoperative

For *NIC standardized interventions* for specific intraoperative nursing diagnoses, refer to Table 40-5. Notice, however, that most of the interventions apply to all surgical patients and are subsumed by (or fall under) the preceding NIC Perioperative Care interventions. As in all of healthcare, you should be always mindful of using hand hygiene. Sterile asepsis is an important focus in the intraoperative period; you can review that in Chapter 22.

The following sections explain in more detail how to carry out "routine" interventions, such as providing skin preparation, positioning, and intraoperative safety measures.

KEY POINT: *"Routine" in this context means that the activities are planned and performed for all patients. Nursing interventions are* **never** *routine in the general sense; they must always be performed with thought and skill.*

Skin Preparation

Surgical skin preparation reduces the risk of postoperative wound infection by reducing the microbial count at the operative site. Skin preparation may begin in the preoperative phase, when the client cleanses the skin with an antimicrobial solution the evening before and the morning of surgery. The intraoperative nurse provides additional skin preparation as follows:

■ **Assess the skin for signs of infection, rash, or other skin irritation.** Document the condition of the skin on the intraoperative record.

- **Remove hair from the site only if necessary.** Historically, the surgical site was always shaved. Now, however, you will remove hair only if there is a large amount of it in the area of the surgery or if the surgeon specifies a preference for hair removal. Hair removal increases the risk of abrasions or nicks in the skin, which provide a portal of entry for bacteria. If you do remove hair, you will likely do it in the preoperative holding area immediately before surgery to reduce the time for bacterial growth. Use clippers or depilatory cream to trim hair because they are less likely than a razor to cause skin irritation (Allegranzi, Bischoff, de Jonge, et al., 2016).

- **Cleanse the surgical site.** In the operative suite, skin preparation precedes draping of the client. Using sterile technique, cleanse the surgical site and a generous part of surrounding area with the recommended anti-infective solution. Povidone-iodine (Betadine) is commonly used for the scrub; then the skin is painted with Betadine solution. ✚ If the client is allergic to iodine, use an alternative preparation solution.

Positioning

The position of the patient in the OR is determined by the surgical site, access to the patient's airway, the need to monitor vital signs, comfort, and safety. A position that is ideal for accessing the surgical site may not be used if any of the other factors are compromised. If the patient has preexisting injuries or discomfort, factor this information into the decision about how to position. For example, a patient with chronic cervical spine pain may be positioned using a neck roll.

The patient is usually positioned after anesthesia has begun. Use straps, wedges, pillows, and surgical table attachments to maintain the position during the surgery. To prevent shearing, lift—do not slide—the patient into position. In many cases, the surgical team assists with positioning.

The circulating nurse is responsible for preventing positioning injuries. Surgical patients often spend 3 to 4 hours, or even longer, in the same position. This places them at risk for pressure ulcer formation. Some anesthetic agents decrease tissue perfusion, further increasing the patient's risk for sustaining positioning injuries. Padding bony prominences is one measure to protect the client during surgery. For nursing interventions to address the NANDA-I diagnosis Risk for Perioperative Positioning Injury, see Table 40-5.

Intraoperative Safety Measures

Just before starting any surgical or invasive procedure, you should conduct a final verification process to confirm the correct patient, procedure, and site (The Joint Commission, 2016). The circulating nurse is responsible for a variety of other measures that protect the patient in the intraoperative phase. These measures are briefly explained here.

- **Assist the scrub nurse to prepare and maintain the sterile field.** The circulating nurse gathers surgical supplies and equipment for use during surgery. She works with the scrub nurse to transfer the supplies to the sterile field.

- **Provide supplies and materials during surgery.** If additional supplies are needed during surgery, the circulating nurse obtains them and opens them onto the sterile field. Supplies may include dressings, surgical equipment, medications, irrigating solutions, or sutures.

- **Monitor intake and output of the client.** Together with the anesthetist, the circulating nurse monitors the fluid infused, urine output, drainage, and blood loss.

- **Handle specimens.** The circulating nurse handles specimens and sends them to the lab or pathology for evaluation after the surgery is complete. The surgeon may sometimes obtain a tissue sample that must be analyzed during the operative procedure. The circulator receives the specimen, coordinates with the pathologist to review the sample, and reports the pathology findings to the surgeon.

- **Perform sponge, sharps, and instrument counts.** ✚ The circulating nurse and the scrub nurse count the supplies that are added to the sterile field. As the surgery comes to an end, a repeat count is performed to ensure that no instruments, sponges, or sharps are left inside the client. A retained sponge can lead to infection and additional surgeries.

A major surgery, such as a heart surgery, can use several hundred sponges. Once soaked in blood, sponges can blend in with the body cavity and be difficult to see. Some agencies are now using sponges with barcodes, which the nurse scans before and after use. The system alerts the surgical team if a sponge is left behind. In another system, the surgical team relies on chip-embedded sponges with radiofrequency identification technology to count sponges and locate any that are left behind.

- **Document the care provided and the client's response to care on the surgical record.** This is usually a graphic or a checklist form, perhaps with some space for narrative notes about anything the form does not address.

KnowledgeCheck 40-7

- What activities is the circulating nurse responsible for in the surgical suite prior to the skin incision?
- Describe six intraoperative safety measures performed by the circulating nurse.

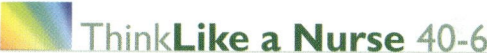

ThinkLike a Nurse 40-6

What special concerns, if any, may affect Mr. Singh (Meet Your Patient) during the intraoperative phase of care?

POSTOPERATIVE CARE

The postoperative phase begins when the client enters the postanesthesia care unit and ends when he has healed from the surgical procedure. This phase consists of two parts: recovery from anesthesia and recovery from surgery.

TheoreticalKnowledge
knowing why

When the surgical procedure is complete, members of the surgical team prepare the client for transfer to the postanesthesia care unit (PACU), also called the recovery room (Fig. 40-4).

Recovery From Anesthesia

The first postoperative phase is often known as the *postanesthesia phase* or the *immediate postoperative phase*. When the surgery is completed, the surgical team moves the client from the operating table to a bed (or gurney) for transport to the PACU. During this period, the client is at high risk for respiratory and cardiovascular compromise. As a precaution, the anesthetist and the circulating nurse accompany the client and attend to his needs during transport. They are also

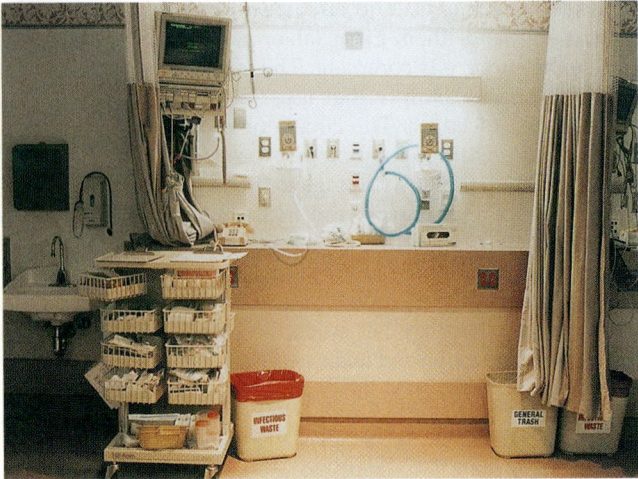

FIGURE 40-4 Postanesthesia care unit.

responsible for giving a comprehensive report to the PACU nurse.

The PACU, located near the OR, is typically an open unit that allows nurses to observe clients easily. PACU nurses have specialized education and experience in caring for postoperative clients. Commonly, nurses working in the PACU have experience in critical care. The PACU nurse receives a comprehensive report from the anesthesia provider and circulating nurse (Box 40-4).

Recovery From Surgery

The second phase of postoperative care begins when the patient is discharged from the PACU and admitted to the surgical nursing unit. The patient is transported to the surgical unit only after he has recovered from anesthesia and his condition is stable. The goal of this phase is to facilitate healing and prevent postoperative complications.

PracticalKnowledge
knowing **how**

The next sections discuss nursing care associated with both phases of postoperative care.

BOX 40-4 ■ Information Contained in the Report From the Surgical Suite

- Procedure performed
- Type of anesthesia
- Medications administered in the surgical suite
- Duration of the procedure and anesthesia
- Postoperative vital signs
- Pulse oximetry values
- Allergies
- Lab values
- Estimated blood loss
- Fluid intake and output, including urine, stool, gastric losses
- Preoperative mobility status, skin integrity, and sensory perception abilities
- Surgical complications
- Presence of tubes, drains, catheters
- Existing IV lines
- Postoperative prescriptions

Nursing Care in the Postanesthesia Care Unit

The PACU nurse performs a quick, focused initial assessment of the surgical patient in the presence of the anesthesia provider and circulating nurse. After that, she assesses the patient every 5 to 15 minutes. AORN (2009, revised 2014) has identified the essential elements of assessment in the PACU. For that information, refer to the Focused Assessment box Postanesthesia Assessments: Essential Elements.

> An unconscious client is usually positioned on his side to help maintain an open airway. This decreases the likelihood of aspirating mucus or saliva by allowing it to drain out instead of back into the throat. Elevating the superior arm on a pillow allows for good chest expansion so the patient can breathe deeply and expand the lungs fully.

Focused Assessment

Postanesthesia Assessment: Essential Elements

AORN (2009, revised 2014) has identified the essential elements of assessment in the PACU.
➤ **Vital signs**
   ➤ Blood pressure, cuff or arterial
   ➤ Respiratory rate, respiratory competence, and breath sounds
   ➤ Respiratory adequacy, including skin color and condition
   ➤ Temperature (record type of measurement used, e.g., skin, tympanic, oral)
   ➤ Pulse (apical and peripheral)
   ➤ Oxygen saturation (e.g., pulse oximeter reading)
➤ **Peripheral circulation** (postoperative tissue perfusion), for example, peripheral pulses and sensation at extremities
➤ **Neurological status,** including pupil response and intracranial pressure (if indicated)
➤ **Mental status:** Level of consciousness, alertness, lucidity, orientation
➤ **Intravenous therapy:** Patency, location of sites, rates of solution(s), and/or blood products infusing
➤ **Allergies and sensitivities**
➤ **Pain**
➤ **Motor abilities,** including return of sensory and motor control in areas affected by local or regional anesthetics
➤ **Skin integrity**
➤ **Temperature regulation**
➤ **Positioning**
➤ **Surgical incision site,** including condition of suture line(s) if visible
➤ **Nausea and vomiting**
➤ **Fluid and electrolyte balance**
➤ **Safety needs** (e.g., siderails raised)
➤ **Central venous pressure (CVP), pulmonary wedge pressure**
➤ **Airway:** patency, presence of artificial airway, mechanical ventilator settings
➤ **Condition of dressing(s)**
➤ **Drainage:** Type, patency, and amount and type of drainage from dressings, tubes, and catheters

NIC: Postanesthesia Care. The only postoperative intervention from NIC's Perioperative Care category is Postanesthesia Care. Postanesthesia Care encompasses the preceding assessments and adds measures such as providing for safety and administering oxygen. Many patients arrive in the PACU with an artificial airway or endotracheal tube in place. The patient remains in the PACU until the PACU nurse determines that he has recovered from the effects of anesthesia (Box 40-5) and is able to maintain his own airway. She then removes the airway and transfers the patient to the surgical unit.

Postoperative Nursing Care on the Surgical Unit

The assigned nurse admits the patient to the surgical unit. If the patient is transported by gurney, assist him to the bed. As soon as the patient has arrived, perform an assessment and listen to a summary report from the PACU nurse (see Box 40-4).

ASSESSMENT NP

The initial postoperative assessment is identical to the assessment performed by the PACU nurse. However, the patient has undergone a period of stabilization since surgery, so the frequency of assessment can be less than in the PACU, where the patient was assessed every 5 to 15 minutes. You may increase the frequency if the patient's condition changes. Of course, agency protocols vary, but a common pattern is to assess the patient:

> On arrival to the nursing unit
> Every 15 minutes for the first hour

> Every 30 minutes for the next 2 hours
> Every hour for the next 4 hours
> Then every 4 hours

KnowledgeCheck 40-8

- What are the two phases of the postoperative phase of care?
- How often is a patient typically assessed after surgery?
- What assessments are made in the postoperative phase?

ANALYSIS/NURSING DIAGNOSIS NP

If healing proceeds normally and no complications develop, most postoperative patients have a common set of collaborative problems (Table 40-6), regardless of the type of surgery they underwent. You will not need to write potential ("risk for") nursing diagnoses, except in special situations (e.g., patients with comorbid conditions such as diabetes or asthma).

Potential Nursing Diagnoses Write potential nursing diagnoses (instead of collaborative problems) only if a patient has a higher risk for the problem than the average surgical patient. For example, you might use:

- *Risk for Ineffective Peripheral Tissue Perfusion* for patients who have a history of peripheral arterial disease or cardiac insufficiency.
- *Risk for Deficient Fluid Volume* for patients who have lost a large amount of blood in surgery or who are dehydrated on admission.
- *Risk for Ineffective Breathing Pattern* for patients with weak accessory muscles for breathing, with a decreased level of consciousness, or with a respiratory condition such as emphysema.
- *Risk for Surgical Site Infection* for patients who have compromised immune status or who may not be capable of managing their own wound care at home.

Actual Nursing Diagnoses Of course, you will use a nursing diagnosis whenever a problem becomes actual instead of merely potential. Nursing diagnoses will vary based on the surgical procedure and the client situation. There is usually no need for a *Deficient Knowledge* diagnosis because patient teaching is a routine intervention for all postoperative patients.

A common postoperative nursing diagnosis is Acute Pain. Examples of two common postoperative nursing diagnoses you might formulate are:

- *Delayed Surgical Recovery.* This is appropriate when the patient requires more days to recover than the anticipated length of stay for the surgery.
- *Acute Pain.* There are independent nursing interventions to relieve pain (e.g., teaching the patient to splint the incision). However, they do not usually provide adequate relief in the early post-op period. You will nearly always need to administer analgesics, which require a medical prescription.

Other nursing diagnoses and etiologies that may occur postoperatively, include the following:

- *Activity Intolerance* r/t pain, manipulation of tissues in the surgical procedure, stressors of surgery
- *Anxiety* r/t change in health status, unfamiliar (hospital) environment

---

BOX 40-5 ■ Evidence of Recovery From Anesthesia

Airway—The patient is able to maintain a patent airway independently and to deep-breathe, cough, and expectorate secretions.

Level of consciousness—The patient is conscious and easily reoriented. Often patients will drift off to sleep between arousals; however, they easily reorient and are generally aware of circumstances and surroundings.

Vital signs—Vital signs are stable and within an acceptable range. The blood pressure may be markedly different from that taken during the immediate preoperative measures, because BP is often elevated preoperatively. This can also be due to anxiety, pain, and not administering routine BP medications because of NPO status. The patient may require medication to control pain or BP before he can be discharged from the PACU.

Mobility and sensation—The patient is able to move all extremities that he could move preoperatively. The patient regains movement and sensation once spinal or epidural anesthesia has worn off.

Fluid balance (I&O)—The patient is urinating at least 30 mL/hr and is in relative fluid balance. Consider blood loss, urine output, gastric drainage, and emesis when calculating fluid balance.

Dressings and drains—Dressings are dry and intact, or wound drainage is considered appropriate for the procedure. The patient should have no overt signs of excessive blood or fluid loss before he is transferred to the surgical unit.

Table 40-6 ➤ Potential Postoperative Complications (Collaborative Problems)

RESPIRATORY SYSTEM

PC: Aspiration Pneumonia—Airway inflammation caused by inhaling gastric secretions (especially hydrochloric acid from the stomach) because of absent gag reflex secondary to anesthesia

Clinical Signs	*Interventions for Prevention and Early Detection*
Cough, fever, elevated WBC, decreased or absent breath sounds, decreased oxygen saturation (SaO₂), tachypnea, dyspnea, blood-tinged sputum.	*Preoperative:* Institute NPO for at least 8 hours prior to surgery. *Postoperative:* Continue NPO until intestinal motility returns; carefully monitor sedated patient and place in side-lying position.

PC: Atelectasis—Collapse of alveoli due to hypoventilation, airways blocked by mucous plugs, opioid analgesics, immobility

Clinical Signs	*Interventions for Prevention and Early Detection*
Decreased or absent breath sounds, noisy respirations, decreased O₂ saturation (SaO₂), chest asymmetry, sternal retractions, accessory muscle use, trachea deviated from midline, fever, tachypnea, dyspnea, tachycardia, diaphoresis, pleural pain, increased restlessness, anxiety	▪ Monitor for clinical signs (Column 3). ▪ Monitor rate, rhythm, depth, and effort of respirations. ▪ Monitor ability to cough effectively. ▪ Determine need for suctioning by listening for crackles and rhonchi over major airways. ▪ Suction, as needed. Auscultate lung sounds after suctioning and other respiratory treatments to determine effectiveness. ▪ Encourage deep breathing, coughing, moving in bed, ambulation, use of incentive spirometry. ▪ See interventions for NIC category Respiratory Monitoring.

PC: Pneumonia—Inflammation of the alveoli due to infection with bacteria or viruses, toxins, or irritants. Caused by hypoventilation secondary to anesthesia and opioid analgesics, and by poor cough effort as a result of aging or weakness.

Clinical Signs	*Interventions for Prevention and Early Detection*
Productive cough with blood-tinged or purulent sputum, fever, elevated WBC, decreased or absent breath sounds, decreased SaO₂, chest pain, tachypnea, dyspnea	▪ Monitor for clinical signs. ▪ Encourage and assist with deep breathing, coughing, moving in bed, ambulation, use of incentive spirometry.

PC: Pulmonary Embolus—A clot that occludes blood flow to a portion of the lungs; usually a result of clot formation in the lower extremities, which breaks loose and migrates to the lungs. May also be due to venous injuries, hypercoagulable state, use of high-dose estrogen, preexisting circulatory disorders.

Clinical Signs	*Interventions for Prevention and Early Detection*
Sudden onset of dyspnea, shortness of breath, chest pain, hypotension, tachycardia, decreased SaO₂, cyanosis	▪ Prevent thrombophlebitis: Encourage and assist with leg exercises, ambulation, antiembolism stockings, sequential compression devices, hydration. See Procedures 40-2 and 40-3. ▪ If thrombophlebitis occurs, position and immobilize the limb; do not massage calves.

CARDIOVASCULAR SYSTEM

PC: Thrombophlebitis—Blood clot and inflammation of a vein or artery, usually in the legs. Results from increased coagulability and venous stasis due to immobility during and after surgery.

Clinical Signs	*Interventions for Prevention and Early Detection*
Superficial: Vein is red, hard, and hot to touch. *Deep:* Limb is pale and edematous; aching, cramping in limb; Homans' sign (pain in calf when foot is dorsiflexed).	Refer to Pulmonary Embolus actions, above.

Table 40-6 ➤ Potential Postoperative Complications (Collaborative Problems)—cont'd

CARDIOVASCULAR SYSTEM

PC: Embolus—Movement of a thrombus or foreign body from its original location.

- Movement in the arterial system results in symptoms in the area affected (e.g., cerebrovascular accident, myocardial infarction, or loss of circulation to an area).

- In the venous system, often results in pulmonary embolus (see Pulmonary Embolus, above).

Clinical Signs	*Interventions for Prevention and Early Detection*
See Pulmonary Embolus, above. For arterial emboli, symptoms depend on the location.	■ Monitor for clinical signs. ■ Prevent thrombophlebitis. If thrombophlebitis occurs, position and immobilize the limb. ■ Do not massage calves.

PC: Hemorrhage—Bleeding may be internal or external. May be caused by slipped ligature, uncontrolled bleeder, or infection.

Clinical Signs	*Interventions for Prevention and Early Detection*
If external: Dressings saturated with bright red blood; increased output in drains or chest tubes *If internal:* Increased pain, increasing abdominal girth, ecchymosis or swelling around incision, tachycardia, hypotension	Frequently monitor vital signs, dressings, and wound drainage.

PC: Hypovolemia—Decreased blood volume. May be due to blood loss during and after surgery; dehydration; or excess loss through vomiting, diarrhea, or drains.

Clinical Signs	*Interventions for Prevention and Early Detection*
Hypotension, tachycardia, decreased urine output, fatigue, thirst, dehydration	■ Monitor vital signs and I&O. ■ Insert urinary catheter, if appropriate. ■ Monitor skin color, temperature, and moistness; central and peripheral cyanosis. ■ Identify possible causes of changes in vital signs. ■ Administer IV therapy as prescribed. ■ Promote oral intake when tolerated. ■ Prepare to administer blood or blood products, as prescribed.

GASTROINTESTINAL SYSTEM

PC: Nausea and Vomiting—Stomach upset or vomiting related to pain, anxiety, anesthesia, medications, or oral intake before peristalsis returns

Clinical Signs	*Interventions for Prevention and Early Detection*
Vomiting, retching, stated nausea	■ Have patient remain NPO until return of bowel sounds. ■ Advance diet slowly. ■ Treat pain.

PC: Abdominal Distention (Tympanites)—Excess gas within the intestines; may be due to a slow return of peristalsis or from handling of the intestines during surgery.

Clinical Signs	*Interventions for Prevention and Early Detection*
Abdominal discomfort, bloating, hypoactive or absent bowel sounds	■ Encourage and assist to move in bed and ambulate. ■ Maintain NPO until return of bowel sounds; avoid drinking with a straw. ■ Provide fluids at room temperature.

(Continued)

Table 40-6 ▶ Potential Postoperative Complications (Collaborative Problems)—cont'd

GASTROINTESTINAL SYSTEM

PC: Constipation—A decrease in the frequency of bowel movements, resulting in the passage of hard stool. Usually related to use of opioids, immobility, inadequate fluid intake, or low-fiber diet.

Clinical Signs	Interventions for Prevention and Early Detection
Abdominal discomfort, bloating, hypoactive or absent bowel sounds	Encourage and assist the patient to move in bed, ambulate, and increase fluid and fiber intake after bowel sounds return.

PC: Ileus—Loss of the forward flow of intestinal contents due to decreased peristalsis secondary to anesthesia, handling of the intestines during surgery, electrolyte imbalances, infection, or ischemic bowel

Clinical Signs	Interventions for Prevention and Early Detection
Abdominal pain, distention, absent bowel sounds, vomiting	There are few independent preventive measures. Observe for symptoms; notify the surgeon.

GENITOURINARY SYSTEM

PC: Renal Failure—Decreased or absent urine output due to hypovolemia, shock, or toxic reaction to medications

Clinical Signs	Interventions for Prevention and Early Detection
Urine output < 30 mL/hr; rising BUN and creatinine levels	Carefully monitor I&O and lab values.

PC: Urinary Retention—Accumulation of urine in the bladder. May result from poor muscle tone as a result of anesthesia and anticholinergic medications, handling of tissues during surgery, or inflammation in the pelvic region.

Clinical Signs	Interventions for Prevention and Early Detection
Bladder distention, suprapubic pain, diminished urine output or output less than fluid intake, inability to void or small, frequent voidings, hypertension, restlessness	■ Monitor for clinical signs. ■ Provide privacy and adequate time to urinate. ■ Catheterize if needed.

PC: Urinary Tract Infection—Infection in the urinary tract related to catheterization, stagnant urine in the bladder secondary to immobility or anticholinergic medications, or instrumentation of the urinary tract

Clinical Signs	Interventions for Prevention and Early Detection
Urinary frequency, suprapubic discomfort, burning on urination, cloudy urine	■ Monitor for clinical signs. ■ Monitor I&O. ■ Use aseptic technique with catheterization and perineal care. ■ Provide adequate IV and oral fluids.

SURGICAL INCISION

PC: Dehiscence—Separation of one or more layers of the wound due to poor nutritional status, obesity or other strain on suture line, inadequate closure of the muscles, or wound infection

Clinical Signs	Interventions for Prevention and Early Detection
A pop or tearing sensation, especially with sudden straining from coughing, vomiting, or changing positions in bed. Usually an immediate increase in serosanguineous drainage occurs.	■ Provide adequate nutrition. ■ Use binders to support the incision. ■ Have client avoid strain. ■ Monitor for infection.

PC: Evisceration—Protrusion of organs or tissues through the separated incision. For causes, see Dehiscence, above.

Clinical Signs	Interventions for Prevention and Early Detection
Visible protrusion of organs through incision	Same as for Dehiscence.

PC: Wound Infection—Inflammation or drainage from a wound due to growth of microorganisms secondary to inadequate aseptic technique or pathogens already present in surgical area.

Table 40-6 ➤ Potential Postoperative Complications (Collaborative Problems)—cont'd

SURGICAL INCISION

Clinical Signs	*Interventions for Prevention and Early Detection*
Localized swelling, redness, heat, pain, fever > 100.4°F (38°C), foul-smelling drainage, or a change in the color of the drainage	■ Effective skin prep in preoperative period ■ Surgical scrub according to guidelines in the intraoperative period ■ Monitor for systemic and localized signs and symptoms of infection. ■ Inspect incision and drain areas for redness and extreme warmth. ■ Inspect surgical dressings for drainage and odor. ■ Monitor vital signs, especially temperature. ■ Maintain aseptic nontouch technique with surgical dressing changes. ■ Use and teach good hand hygiene. ■ Use sterile saline for wound cleansing up to 48 hours post-op (National Institute for Health and Clinical Excellence, 2008, updated 2014). ■ See interventions for NIC category Infection Protection. ■ Limit the number of visitors, as appropriate. ■ Obtain cultures as needed. ■ Encourage sufficient nutritional and fluid intake. ■ Teach client about signs of infection.

■ *Nausea* r/t manipulation of gastrointestinal tract; decreased peristalsis secondary to anesthesia

■ *Constipation* r/t decreased activity, decreased food or fluid intake, decreased peristalsis secondary to anesthesia, pain medication

■ *Urinary Retention* r/t anesthesia, preoperative medications (anticholinergics), pain, fear, unfamiliar surroundings, client's position

■ *Delayed Surgical Recovery* (etiologies will vary with pathology)

PLANNING OUTCOMES/EVALUATION NP

A comprehensive plan of care for common postoperative nursing diagnoses includes NOC standardized outcomes as well as individualized goals. Because of shortened hospital stays, the postoperative period now extends well past the patient's discharge from the hospital. Often, especially for those who have had major or complex procedures, a home health nurse continues to follow the patient at home to facilitate a smoother transition through the postoperative process.

Examples of *NOC standardized outcomes and individualized goals* for the postoperative period include:

Activity Tolerance	Hydration
Ambulation	Nausea and Vomiting Severity
Anxiety Level	Pain Control; Pain Level
Blood Loss Severity	Post-Procedure Recovery
Bowel Elimination	Urinary Elimination
Circulation Status	Wound Healing: Primary Intention
Energy Conservation	

For other NOC outcomes,

 Go to Davis Advantage, Resources, Chapter 40, **List of NOC Outcomes and NIC Interventions.**

PLANNING INTERVENTIONS/ IMPLEMENTATION NP

Most postoperative interventions focus on prevention and early detection of potential complications (collaborative problems). Many such interventions are done as a part of the preoperative teaching. Interventions for collaborative problems are described in Table 40-6. Nursing diagnoses are included in Table 40-7. To see other *NIC interventions,*

 Go to Davis Advantage, Resources, Chapter 40, **List of NOC Outcomes and NIC Interventions.**

Specific nursing activities should be designed to relieve identified nursing diagnoses. In the next sections, we discuss pain management, routine postoperative teaching, and the use of sequential compression devices.

Pain Management

The primary goal of postoperative pain management is to minimize the dose of medications (to lessen side effects) while

Table 40-7 ➤ Selected Standardized Nursing Diagnoses, Outcomes, and Interventions for Postoperative Patients

OUTCOMES AND GOALS	NURSING INTERVENTIONS AND ACTIVITIES

Nursing Diagnosis: **Activity Intolerance** r/t pain and the surgical procedure and stressors of surgery

OUTCOMES AND GOALS	NURSING INTERVENTIONS AND ACTIVITIES
NOC Outcomes: Activity Tolerance Endurance Energy Conservation Psychomotor Energy **NOC Goals:** ■ O₂ saturation, heart rate, respiratory rate, systolic and diastolic blood pressure not compromised with activity ■ Ease of breathing with activity not compromised ■ Walking pace and distance not compromised ■ Ease of performing activities of daily living (ADLs) not compromised ■ Ability to speak with physical activity not compromised ■ Energy restored after rest, not compromised ■ Uses naps to restore energy, often demonstrated. ■ Exhibits concentration, consistently demonstrated.	**NIC Interventions:** Activity Therapy Energy Management Exercise Promotion: Strength Training **Nursing Activities:** ■ Collaborate with other disciplines to plan and monitor activity program as appropriate. ■ Assist to choose appropriate activities. ■ Assist to focus on strengths rather than weaknesses. ■ Assist to identify activity preferences. ■ Instruct the client and family how to perform desired activities. ■ Refer to community centers, programs as appropriate. ■ Arrange physical activities to reduce competition for oxygen supply to vital body functions (e.g., avoid activity immediately after meals). ■ Avoid care activities during scheduled rest periods. ■ Assist to sit on side of bed ("dangle"), if unable to transfer or walk. ■ Monitor location and nature of pain during activity. ■ Teach activity organization and time management techniques to prevent fatigue.

Nursing Diagnosis: **Acute Pain** r/t (1) inflammation or injury in the surgical area (2) abdominal distention secondary to decreased peristalsis (3) muscle pain secondary to positioning and tension

OUTCOMES AND GOALS	NURSING INTERVENTIONS AND ACTIVITIES
NOC Outcomes: Pain Level Pain Control **NOC Goals:** ■ Consistently rates pain as controlled. ■ No moaning or crying ■ No facial expressions of pain ■ Describes causal factors. ■ Uses preventive measures. ■ Uses nonanalgesic relief measures. ■ Uses analgesics as recommended. ■ Reports changes in symptoms to a health professional. **Other Goals:** ■ No guarding of incision	**NIC Interventions:** Analgesic Administration Pain Management Patient-Controlled Analgesia (PCA) Assistance **Nursing Activities:** ■ Assess location, characteristics, onset, duration, frequency, quality, and intensity of pain and predisposing factors. ■ Observe for nonverbal discomfort cues. ■ Assure the client of analgesic availability. ■ Consider cultural influences of responses to pain. ■ Utilize developmentally appropriate assessment method. ■ Determine necessary frequency of pain assessment and formulate pain assessment plan. ■ Control environmental factors that may contribute to the client's response. ■ Provide information about the pain, such as causes of the pain, how long it will last, and anticipated discomforts from procedures (e.g., teach the client to splint incision when ambulating).

Table 40-7 ▶ Selected Standardized Nursing Diagnoses, Outcomes, and Interventions for Postoperative Patients—cont'd	
OUTCOMES AND GOALS	**NURSING INTERVENTIONS AND ACTIVITIES**

OUTCOMES AND GOALS	NURSING INTERVENTIONS AND ACTIVITIES
	■ Provide optimal pain relief with analgesics as appropriate.
	■ Implement PCA as appropriate.
	■ Intervene before pain becomes severe.
	■ Medicate before activity to increase participation.
	■ Teach nonpharmacological pain relief measures (e.g., visualization, progressive muscle relaxation).
	■ Utilize multidisciplinary approach to pain management.

Nursing Diagnosis: **Anxiety** r/t change in health status, hospital environment

OUTCOMES AND GOALS	NURSING INTERVENTIONS AND ACTIVITIES
NOC Outcomes: Anxiety Level Anxiety Self-Control *NOC Goals:* ■ Consistently uses effective coping strategies. ■ Often seeks information to reduce anxiety. ■ Consistently uses relaxation techniques to reduce anxiety. ■ Often maintains concentration. ■ Verbalizes that anxiety is mild. ■ Minimal restlessness, hand wringing, muscle tension, facial tension, difficulty concentrating. Minimal changes in vital signs; no dilated pupils, sweating or dizziness ■ Controls anxiety response consistently.	*NIC Intervention:* Anxiety Reduction *Nursing Activities:* ■ Use calm, reassuring approach. ■ Observe for verbal and nonverbal signs of anxiety. ■ Explain all procedures and activities. ■ Provide information concerning diagnosis, treatment, prognosis. ■ Administer back rub or neck rub as appropriate. ■ Listen attentively. ■ Create trusting atmosphere. ■ Assist the client to identify stressful situations. ■ Assist the client to recognize that she is anxious. ■ Assess the client's ability to make decisions. ■ Encourage verbalization of feelings, perceptions, and fears related to the surgical procedure. ■ Encourage family visits if these ease the client's stress. ■ Support use of appropriate defense mechanisms. ■ Instruct the client in use of relaxation techniques.

Nursing Diagnosis: **Nausea** r/t manipulation of gastrointestinal tract, decreased peristalsis secondary to anesthesia

OUTCOMES AND GOALS	NURSING INTERVENTIONS AND ACTIVITIES
NOC Outcomes: Nausea & Vomiting Control Nausea & Vomiting: Disruptive Effects Nausea & Vomiting Severity Nutritional Status: Food & Fluid Intake *NOC Goals:* ■ No nausea, or intensity only mild ■ Reports nausea, retching, and vomiting controlled. ■ Mild or no intolerance of odors ■ Mild or no intolerance of movement ■ Recognizes onset of nausea. ■ Recognizes precipitating stimuli. ■ Frequency, intensity, and distress of nausea are mild. ■ Uses preventive measures often. ■ Only mild decrease in food and fluid intake	*NIC Interventions:* Nausea Management Medication Management *Nursing Activities:* ■ Provide information about the cause of nausea and vomiting and the expected duration. ■ Provide information about the goals, effects, and possible side effects of treatment with antiemetics. ■ Describe the limited role of administering parenteral fluids to prevent dehydration and to administer supplemental electrolytes (e.g., potassium). ■ Encourage the client to monitor own nausea experience, including use of a symptom diary. ■ Encourage the client to learn strategies for managing own nausea. ■ Perform complete assessment including frequency, duration, severity, and precipitating factors.

(Continued)

Table 40-7 ➤ Selected Standardized Nursing Diagnoses, Outcomes, and Interventions for Postoperative Patients—cont'd

OUTCOMES AND GOALS	NURSING INTERVENTIONS AND ACTIVITIES
■ No weight loss ■ Reports bothersome side effects from antiemetics. ■ Reports failure of antiemetic treatment.	■ Observe for nonverbal cues of discomfort. ■ Evaluate past experiences with nausea. ■ Identify strategies that have been successful in relieving nausea. ■ Discuss relaxation and distraction techniques if anxiety is suspected of playing a role (e.g., guided imagery, self-hypnosis, biofeedback, music therapy). ■ Encourage frequent oral hygiene unless it stimulates nausea. Keep tissues and water to rinse the mouth nearby. ■ Give cold, clear, odorless foods, as appropriate. ■ Encourage the client to eat high-carbohydrate and low-fat foods and to eat small, frequent meals. ■ Drink cola, but not too cold; suck on an ice cube, sorbet, or a piece of frozen fruit. ■ Have the client sit in an upright position for 30 to 45 min after eating. ■ Control odors and unpleasant visual stimuli in the room. ■ Administer antiemetic medications. ■ Refer to a dietician as needed.

Nursing Diagnosis: Constipation r/t decreased activity, decreased food or fluid intake, decreased peristalsis secondary to anesthesia, pain medication

NOC Outcome: Bowel Elimination **NOC Goals:** ■ Elimination pattern not compromised ■ Reports ease of stool passage not compromised. ■ Bowel sounds not compromised ■ Muscle tone to evacuate stool not compromised ■ Passes soft, formed stool in amount appropriate for diet. ■ No pain with passage of stool **Other:** ■ Bloating not present	**NIC interventions:** Bowel Management Constipation/Impaction Management **Nursing activities:** ■ Monitor for signs and symptoms of constipation. ■ Note date of last bowel movement. ■ Monitor bowel sounds. ■ Monitor frequency, consistency, shape, volume, and color of bowel movements. ■ Teach the client about specific foods that assist promotion of bowel regularity. ■ Insert a rectal suppository, enema, or irrigation, as needed. ■ Evaluate medication profile for GI side effects (e.g., narcotic analgesics). ■ Give warm liquids after meals. ■ Instruct the client in foods high in fiber.

Nursing Diagnosis: Urinary Retention r/t anesthesia, preoperative medications (anticholinergics), pain, fear, unfamiliar surroundings, client's position

NOC Outcome: Urinary Elimination **NOC Goals:** ■ Empties bladder completely. ■ Fluid intake not compromised ■ No hesitancy with urination	**NIC Interventions:** Urinary Retention Care Urinary Catheterization **Nursing Activities:** ■ Perform comprehensive urinary assessment (fluid intake, urinary output, voiding pattern, cognitive function, preexisting urinary problems).

Table 40-7 ➤ Selected Standardized Nursing Diagnoses, Outcomes, and Interventions for Postoperative Patients—cont'd

OUTCOMES AND GOALS	NURSING INTERVENTIONS AND ACTIVITIES
Other: ■ Bladder not palpable ■ Reports subjective feeling of empty bladder. ■ 24-hr intake and output balanced	■ Provide privacy for elimination. ■ Use power of suggestion (run water, flush toilet). ■ Provide ample time (at least 10 minutes) for client to empty bladder. ■ Use spirits of wintergreen in bedpan or urinal. ■ Insert urinary catheter as appropriate. ■ Use percussion and palpation to estimate degree of bladder distention. ■ Catheterize for post-voiding residual as appropriate.

Nursing Diagnosis: **Delayed Surgical Recovery** (etiologies will vary with pathology)

■ *Note:* This diagnosis is broad and encompasses some of the other diagnoses. If the client has Delayed Surgical Recovery, you will not, for example, need a diagnosis of Nausea on the plan of care.

■ This diagnosis is appropriate when the patient requires more days to recover than the anticipated length of stay for the surgery.

NOC Outcomes: Post-Procedure Recovery Wound Healing: Primary Intention Ambulation Blood Loss Severity Endurance Hydration Infection Severity Nausea & Vomiting Severity Pain Level *NOC Goals:* ■ Systolic BP within 20 mm Hg of baseline ■ Ambulation tolerance in normal range ■ No nausea, vomiting, shivering ■ Only mild pain *Other:* ■ Ready for discharge within prescribed length of stay for surgery performed ■ No postoperative complications (e.g., bleeding, infection, delayed wound healing, pneumonia)	*NIC Interventions:* Embolus Precautions Exercise Therapy: Ambulation Incision Site Care Nutrition Management Pain Management Self-Care Assistance *Nursing Activities:* ■ Monitor for postoperative complications. ■ Monitor the healing process in the incision site. ■ Provide incision care as needed. ■ Teach the client and family how to care for the incision. ■ Facilitate early ambulation postoperatively. ■ Encourage increased intake of protein, iron, and vitamin C, as appropriate. ■ Determine, in collaboration with the dietician as appropriate, number of calories and type of nutrients needed to meet nutrition requirements. ■ Select and implement a variety of measures (e.g., pharmacological, nonpharmacological, interpersonal) to facilitate pain relief, as appropriate. ■ Teach principles of pain management. ■ Encourage independence, but intervene when the client is unable to perform.

Sources: Bulechek, G. M., Butcher, H. K., Dochterman, J. M., et al. (Eds.). (2013). *Nursing interventions classification (NIC)* (6th ed.). St. Louis, MO: C.V. Mosby; Moorhead, S., Johnson, M., Maas, M., et al. (Eds.). (2013). *Nursing outcomes classification (NOC)* (5th ed.). St. Louis, MO: C.V. Mosby; *Nursing Diagnoses—Definitions and Classification 2018–2020.* © 2010 NANDA International, ISBN 978-1-62623-929-6. Used by arrangement with the Thieme Group, Stuttgart/New York.

still providing adequate pain management. **KEY POINT:** *Keep in mind that no one drug is likely to work for every person with pain.*

Pain control should be individualized, with consideration of medical, psychological, and physical condition; age; level of fear or anxiety; surgical procedure; personal preference; and response to care. Alternative methods of pain relief may be initiated for patients who are at increased risk for analgesia-related complications or side effects (see the CAM box).

A multidisciplinary team approach should be used to formulate a plan for pain relief, particularly in complicated patients, such as those who have medical comorbidities. Potential benefits, possible adverse events, and patient preferences must be weighed in order to decide which pain relief method to use

Benefits of adequate pain management are early mobilization, shorter hospital stay, reduced hospital costs, and increased patient satisfaction.

Postoperatively, a patient usually receives analgesics via more than one route. For example, in the immediate postoperative period, the patient may receive intravenous or epidural medications, progress to oral opioids in a day or two, and then move to nonopioid analgesics (e.g., acetaminophen).

Providing sufficient pain control for older adults can be a challenge. Because of concerns about impaired cognition, medical comorbidities, drug interactions, and problems with appropriate dosing, many older adults may be undermedicated and experience unnecessary pain (García, Duggan, McCullough, et al., 2015).

For a complete discussion of types of pain relief, refer to the section "Routes of Administration for Opioid Analgesics" in Chapter 32. Also, refer to Procedure 32-1: Setting Up and Managing Patient-Controlled Analgesia by Pump and Clinical Insight 32-2: Nursing Care of the Patient With an Epidural Catheter.

Single-Use, Continuous-Flow Pump   One recent development is a single-use pain relief pump that administers a continuous, regulated flow of local anesthetic through a thin catheter directly into the patient's surgical site. A dressing

Complementary & Alternative Modalities (CAM)

Acupuncture for Acute Postoperative Pain, Anxiety, and Tension

Mallory, Croghan, Sandhu, and colleagues (2015) collected data from 20 adult breast cancer patients undergoing mastectomy and/or breast reconstruction. All of the patients received acupuncture in addition to the usual pain management during postoperative days one through discharge. They reported significantly improved symptoms of postoperative pain, anxiety, and tension.

holds the tubing in place, and the pump can be carried in a small bag and used after the patient returns home. It reduces the need for opioids, thus reducing complications such as nausea, vomiting, and respiratory depression. It is said to hasten ambulation and the return to normal activities. Depending on the type of pump, it is filled with 65 to 750 mL of medication and can remain in place for up to 5 days, depending on the amount of anesthetic included (Fig. 40-5).

Postoperative Teaching

Teaching is especially important postoperatively because most patients must perform quite a bit of self-care. Postoperative

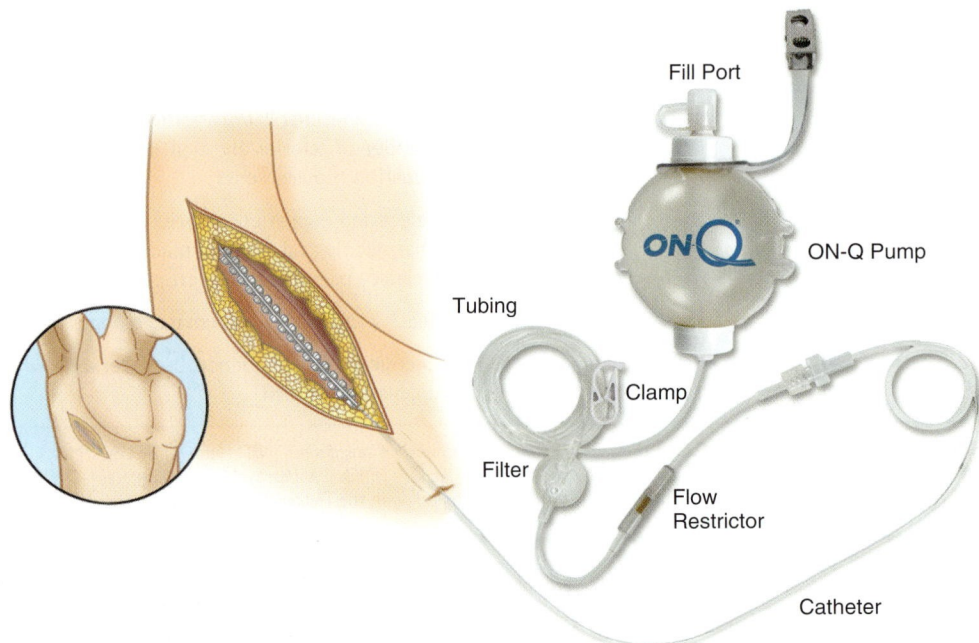

FIGURE 40-5 A single-use pain relief pump delivers a local anesthetic directly into the patient's surgical site.

teaching should reinforce content taught preoperatively. Also teach the patient about the applicable topics in the Self-Care box Postoperative Patient Teaching Topics.

- To use time efficiently, try to do some teaching each time you are at the bedside for other care.
- Be sure the patient is comfortable but alert.
- Do not attempt teaching when the patient is in pain, needs to void, or is drowsy from opioid analgesics.

Incentive Spirometry

Incentive spirometry may be prescribed for patients who are at high risk for atelectasis and pneumonia (e.g., the patient has a history of lung problems or smoking or will experience a prolonged period of inactivity). This treatment facilitates deep breathing, increases lung volume, and promotes coughing to clear mucus from the respiratory tree. The equipment varies in appearance, but all devices include a gauge to monitor the patient's progress visibly (Fig. 40-6).

If incentive spirometry is prescribed postoperatively, explain its use to the patient (see the Self-Care box Teaching Your Patient About Incentive Spirometry). If you know in advance that the patient will be using an incentive spirometer postoperatively, include its use in your preoperative teaching.

Postoperative Patient Teaching Topics

➤ Postoperative treatment regimen (e.g., dressing changes, exercises), including rationale for the treatments
➤ Self-management of the treatment regimen
➤ Expected results and effects of the surgery
➤ The prescribed diet and how to select foods on the diet
➤ Prescribed activity
➤ Signs and symptoms of complications that require the patient to notify the surgeon or primary care provider
➤ Return office or clinic visits
➤ Lifestyle changes that may be needed
➤ Community resources available (e.g., Reach for Recovery)

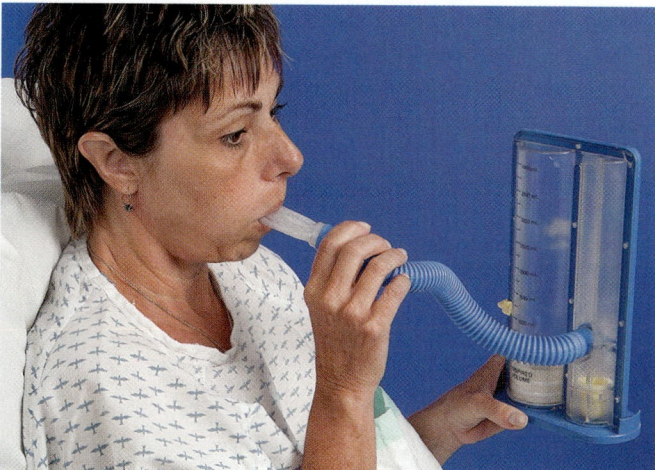

FIGURE 40-6 Incentive spirometry facilitates lung expansion and coughing to clear mucus from airways.

Teaching Your Patient About Incentive Spirometry

➤ Explain to the patient that the machine will enable him to monitor the depth of his breathing.
➤ Patients with abdominal or chest incisions may require pain medication to use the incentive spirometer.
➤ Assist the patient to an upright position in the bed or chair.
➤ Instruct the patient to do the following:
   1. Breathe out normally.
   2. Place the mouthpiece in the mouth and create a seal with the lips.
   3. Breathe in slowly and as deeply as possible through the mouthpiece. Monitor the depth of inspiration by viewing the gauge. (Establish goals for the patient so that progress can be monitored.)
   4. Hold your breath as long as possible, at least to a slow count of 3.
   5. Remove the mouthpiece from your mouth and exhale.
   6. Rest for a few seconds
   7. Repeat this process 10 times every hour while awake, if possible.
   8. After each set of 10 deep breaths, cough to be sure lungs are clear. Support any incision when coughing by holding a pillow firmly against it.

Antiembolism Stockings and Sequential Compression Devices

More than half of hospitalized patients are at risk for venous thromboembolism, and surgical patients seem to be at higher risk than medical patients. Preventive measures include anticoagulant medications (so-called blood thinners), postoperative exercises, and antiembolism stockings.

Antiembolism Stockings were discussed previously as a preoperative care intervention in preparing the patient physically for surgery. Encourage postoperative patients to ambulate as soon and as often as possible to promote peripheral circulation and prevent thrombophlebitis. **KEY POINT:** *Antiembolism stockings are not a substitute for activity.* To learn how to apply antiembolism stockings, see Procedure 40-2.

Sequential Compression Devices (SCDs) may be prescribed in addition to antiembolism stockings for patients at high risk for thrombophlebitis. The SCD is a plastic sleeve with chambers. The sleeve is wrapped around the patient's legs and connected to an air pump that provides sequential pressure to the chambers of the plastic sleeve. Starting at the ankle, the first chamber is inflated. When the second chamber inflates, the first chamber deflates, and so on. SCDs apply brief pressure to each segment of the leg. The pressure compresses the veins and promotes venous return to the heart. To learn to apply SCDs, refer to Procedure 40-3.

Gastrointestinal Suction

Patients having certain surgeries, such as a procedure to relieve a bowel obstruction, are at high risk for abdominal distention. In addition to causing pain, abdominal distention can increase postoperative respiratory problems, place a strain on suture lines, and interfere with wound closure. Such patients will return from surgery with a nasogastric (NG) or nasointestinal tube in place for gastric or intestinal decompression. If prolonged intestinal decompression is anticipated, a gastrostomy may be performed instead of using an NG tube.

Decompression tubes are typically connected to either intermittent or continuous suction to collect excess fluid and gas. Suction is continued until peristalsis resumes, bowel sounds are audible, and the patient is passing flatus. While suction is in place, the patient remains NPO. To review insertion and care of NG and nasoenteric tubes, see Chapter 29. To learn how to manage gastrointestinal suction, see Procedure 40-4.

KnowledgeCheck 40-9

- Identify six potential postoperative complications.
- Why are sequential compression devices used?

CLINICALREASONING

The questions and exercises in this section allow you to practice the kind of thinking you will use as a full-spectrum nurse. Critical-thinking questions usually have more than one correct answer, so we do not provide "correct answers" for these features. It is more important to develop your nursing judgment than to just cover content. You will learn by discussing the questions with your peers. If you are still unsure, see the Davis Advantage chapter resources for suggested responses.

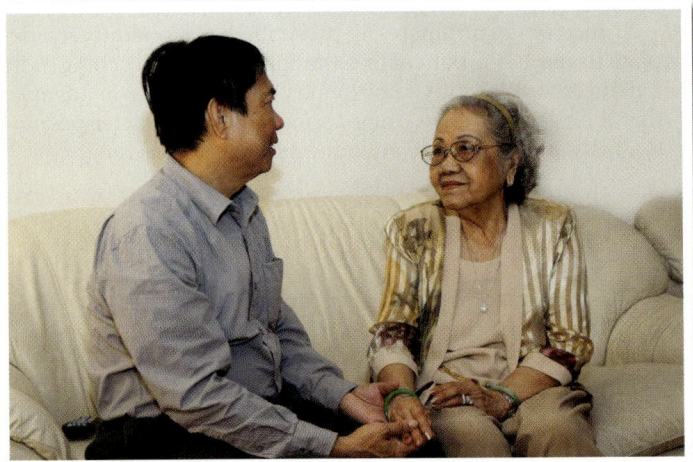

Caring for the Nguyens

Mai Nguyen, the 76-year-old mother of Nam Nguyen, has been experiencing blurred vision and decreased visual acuity. A local ophthalmologist diagnosed bilateral cataracts and has recommended cataract removal in the left eye, with insertion of an intraocular lens. He told Mai Nguyen to schedule the surgery "at your convenience" and explained that the surgery would be performed on an outpatient basis. The ophthalmologist gave Mai Nguyen the following list of activities to prepare for the surgery:

- Schedule a date for your surgery. My receptionist will set up a time for your surgery. All surgeries are performed at Western Medical Center Same-Day Surgery Department.
- Please arrange to be seen by your primary care provider 1 to 2 weeks prior to the surgery to receive clearance for surgery.

- Make an appointment with the Preoperative Center at Western Medical Center Same-Day Surgery Department 1 to 2 days before surgery.
- Arrange to have a ride to and from the surgery.

A. What preoperative testing is Mrs. Nguyen likely to undergo? Explain your rationale.

B. The preoperative list states that the client must be seen by the primary care provider to receive clearance for surgery. Why is this an essential part of the preoperative period?

C. What theoretical knowledge do you need to perform preoperative teaching for Mai Nguyen? How could you obtain that information? Be specific about your sources.

D. What content would you include in Mrs. Nguyen's preoperative teaching?

E. The ophthalmologist has planned anesthesia via conscious sedation. What factors, if any, might keep Mrs. Nguyen from receiving this form of anesthesia? What additional information do you need to answer this question?

 Go to Davis Advantage, Resources, Chapter 40, **Caring for the Nguyens—Suggested Responses.**

Applying the **Full-Spectrum Nursing Model**_____

PATIENT SITUATION

Recall Nishad Singh (Meet Your Patient). He is a 68-year-old man who came to the emergency department (ED) with sudden onset of rectal bleeding. He had been "tired and dragging for several months." The ED nurse identified nursing diagnoses of Mild Anxiety, Pain, and Risk for Bleeding. Preoperatively, his vital signs were as follows:

BP: 138/88 mm Hg

Pulse: 104 beats/min and regular; 120 beats/min; 134 beats/min

Respiratory rate: 20 breaths/min

Temperature: 36.7°C (98.0°F)

Oxygen saturation: 98%

Mr. Singh was admitted to the hospital, where he received an IV of 1,000 mL of lactated Ringer's solution and a unit of packed red blood cells. He was to undergo emergency colon resection surgery; however, a left hemicolectomy including the sigmoid colon and the anus was required. He spent 4 hours in the PACU, until his vital signs stabilized. Mr. Singh now has a colostomy high in his descending colon, with a stoma on his left abdomen slightly superior to the level of his umbilicus. He also has an abdominal incision that was made for exploration. On the next day after the surgery, the surgeon informed Mr. Singh that he has widespread adenocarcinoma (cancer) of the colon with metastasis to the liver. The nurse has identified these four nursing diagnoses (among others):

Deficient Knowledge (colostomy care) r/t lack of prior experience and no preparation prior to surgery

Fear r/t diagnosis of colon cancer, liver metastasis, and possible terminal illness

Pain secondary to surgical incision and manipulation of abdominal organs during the surgical procedure

Risk for Impaired Skin Integrity r/t irritation from fecal drainage and ostomy pouch

THINKING

1. *Theoretical Knowledge:*
   a. What is a left hemicolectomy? If you do not know the answer, consult an appropriate reference.
   b. What does "metastasis to the liver" mean? If you do not know the answer, consult an appropriate reference.
2. *Critical Thinking (Inquiry):*
   a. Why might Mr. Singh have needed a colostomy instead of having his transverse colon reconnected to the remaining lower colon or rectum? State the reference you used to answer this question.
   b. Why do you think Mr. Singh has a colostomy above the level of the umbilicus and not lower down in his abdomen? State the reference you used to answer this question.

DOING

3. *Practical Knowledge:* Mr. Singh returned from surgery with knee-high antiembolism stockings.
   a. You notice that the stockings have slid down and become wrinkled between his knees and ankles. After you straighten them and pull them up, the tops reach to about 7.6 cm (3 in.) below Mr. Singh's knees. What does this probably mean, and what should you do?
   b. Which of the following instructions should you give when delegating care of Mr. Singh's antiembolism stockings to the nursing assistant? (Mr. Singh's stockings have closed toes.)
      - Remove the stockings and bathe and dry the legs every 8 to 12 hours.
      - Massage the legs after removing Mr. Singh's stockings.
      - Before reapplying stockings, report the presence of any lesions, sores, or redness of the lower extremities.
      - Instruct the patient to remain supine for at least 15 minutes after removing the stockings.
      - Make sure there are no wrinkles in the stockings once they have been applied.
      - Tug gently on the end of the stocking to create a small space between the end of the toes and the stocking.
4. *Nursing Process (Nursing Diagnosis):* List Mr. Singh's four nursing diagnoses in order of priority. List the highest priority first. Explain how you decided the priorities.

CARING

5. *Self-Knowledge:*
   a. If you were assigned to care for Mr. Singh today, what aspect of care would you feel best prepared to give? Explain your thinking.
   b. What aspect of Mr. Singh's care would you be most uncomfortable providing? Explain your thinking.
6. *Ethical Knowledge:* You want to provide culturally competent care. What is the first thing you will need to do in order to address Mr. Singh's cultural needs? Review Chapter 15 if you need to.

 Go to Davis Advantage, Resources, Chapter 40, **Applying the Full Spectrum Nursing Model—Suggested Responses.**

Practical knowledge:
clinical insights & procedures

Perioperative nursing care includes procedures and techniques designed for prevention and early detection of complications. Recall that full-spectrum nursing involves thinking, doing, and caring—all are equally important in perioperative care.

CLINICAL INSIGHTS

Clinical Insight 40-1 ➤ **Preoperative Teaching**

Explain What to Expect Before Surgery.

- Explain the planned preoperative testing—lab tests, x-ray studies, ECG, and so on.
- Discuss skin preparation, including preoperative wash with an antibacterial product if this is included in the treatment plan.
- Discuss prescribed preoperative medications.
- Outline activities that will occur before surgery, such as insertion of an IV, placement of a urinary catheter, or cardiac monitoring.
- Review the preoperative restriction of fluid and food.
- Tell the patient that a member of the anesthesia team will speak with him about the proposed anesthesia before surgery.
- If the patient is having surgery on the gastrointestinal (GI) tract, explain that an additional bowel prep may be ordered (e.g., a low-residue diet beginning 1 week before surgery and a liquid diet for the 48 hours preceding surgery). Patients having GI surgery also may have enemas before surgery.
- Explain the need to remove jewelry, makeup, hearing aids, glasses, contact lenses, and any removable dental prostheses before being transported to the operating suite. It is best to have a family member take valuable belongings home for safekeeping.
- Give the patient and family a tentative schedule for the operative day, including the time to arrive at the hospital or surgery center.

Explain What to Expect in the Operative Suite.

- Inform the patient and family where relatives may wait during surgery.

- Describe the operating room and the activities that the patient may anticipate there.
- Describe the types of people who may be present in the operative suite. This is particularly important if the patient is not receiving a general anesthetic.
- Explain that the anesthesiologist or nurse anesthetist will monitor the patient and is responsible for keeping him comfortable with medications throughout the entire procedure.
- Describe the activities that may occur in the preoperative holding area.

Explain What to Expect After Surgery.

- Explain that the patient will initially be cared for in the postanesthesia care unit. After a period of observation, he will be transferred to the surgical unit. Note that some patients may be transferred directly to a critical care unit after surgery. If this is expected, inform the patient and family preoperatively.
- Family may visit after the patient has been admitted and assessed on the surgical unit.
- Tell the patient what to expect in terms of dressings, equipment, and monitoring devices.
- Describe the types of assessments that will be performed.
- Explain that pain medication will be given to keep the patient comfortable. If he experiences pain, he should tell the nursing staff.
- Discuss the usual progression of recovery, including activity level, deep breathing, coughing, leg exercises, and dietary intake.
- Discuss the anticipated length of stay.
- Teach the patient how to move into and out of bed after surgery.

Clinical Insight 40-1 ➤ Preoperative Teaching—cont'd

■ Teach the importance of deep breathing and coughing, especially after general anesthesia. Demonstrate how to splint the incision to facilitate deep breathing and coughing. Refer to Procedure 40-1.

■ Teach and emphasize the importance of leg exercises to minimize the risk of thrombus formation. Refer to Procedure 40-1.

■ If decreased activity or prolonged bedrest is anticipated, explain the use of antiembolism stockings or sequential compression devices. Refer to Procedure 40-2.
  Note: If the patient is to be discharged the day of surgery, inform him in advance about what to wear to the facility and explain that he must arrange for a responsible adult to drive him home.

Clinical Insight 40-2 ➤ Creating an Operative Field

■ A nonsterile team member (usually the circulating nurse) performs a surgical prep, using a scrub agent and "paint," to cleanse the operative site. Antiseptic agents must be approved by the U.S. Food and Drug Administration and approved by the agency's infection control professional. Chlorhexidine and povidone-iodine solutions are most commonly used.

■ The **operative field** encompasses the patient and the immediate surrounding area.

■ Creation of the sterile field proceeds as follows:
  ■ Don head covering and shoe covers before entering the surgical suite.
  ■ Perform a surgical scrub.

■ Don sterile gown, gloves, and other surgical attire (e.g., mask).

■ Cover the area surrounding the operative site with sterile drapes so that only the patient's operative area is exposed.

■ Place sterile draping over the remainder of the patient's body.

■ In most cases, suspend a vertical drape at neck level so the client's head and airway are accessible to the anesthesiologist or nurse anesthetist (who is not sterile). For neurosurgery, even the head is draped, and the anesthesiologist or nurse anesthetist sits to the side of the head.

PROCEDURES

Procedure 40-1 ■ Teaching a Patient to Deep-Breathe, Cough, Move in Bed, and Perform Leg Exercises

➤ For steps to follow in *all* procedures, refer to the Universal Steps for All Procedures found on the page facing the inside back cover.

Equipment

For Teaching Deep Breathing and Coughing:

■ Folded blanket or a pillow (if teaching will include splinting of a surgical incision site)
■ Tissues

For Moving in Bed:

■ Small pillow or folded blanket
■ Pillows

Delegation

A registered nurse (RN) should perform the initial teaching. You may delegate reinforcement of the teaching to a licensed vocational/practical nurse (LVN/LPN) or nursing assistive personnel (NAP).

Pre-Procedure Assessments

■ Assess cognitive level and level of consciousness.
  Helps assess the patient's ability to understand and follow directions and select the appropriate teaching method.

■ Assess pain level.
  Even preoperatively, pain must be well controlled to ensure full patient participation.

■ Determine whether the surgical procedure and/or a physical disability will limit the patient's participation.
  For example, a fractured arm that has not yet been repaired will impair the patient's ability to hold a pillow for splinting.

■ Determine whether the surgical procedure may entail special exercises or equipment. In addition, assess for any special equipment, such as braces, slings, or abductor wedges, that may be needed when turning a patient in bed.

(continued on next page)

Procedure 40–1 ■ Teaching a Patient to Deep-Breathe, Cough, Move in Bed, and Perform Leg Exercises (continued)

✚ *Knee and hip surgeries often involve special exercises or equipment postoperatively. Consult the surgeon before teaching leg exercises. Spinal and neurological surgeries often limit movement in the postoperative period. For example, some spinal surgeries require the patient to logroll (move from head to toe as one unit). Some neurological procedures require limiting the amount of time the patient's head of bed is above 30°. Identify these restrictions preoperatively and inform the patient and family about them during your teaching session.*

- Assess the patient's belief about the ability of the surgical incision to remain intact.

  This is a common fear. If the patient believes that the incision will not stay together when he coughs or moves, he is less likely to comply.

Procedure 40–1A ■ Teaching a Patient to Deep-Breathe and Cough

➤ When performing the procedure, always identify your patient according to agency policy, using two identifiers, and be attentive to standard precautions, hand hygiene, patient safety and privacy, body mechanics, and documentation.

Deep breathing and coughing expand the lungs, improve ventilation, promote gas exchange, and help prevent atelectasis and pneumonia. Coughing after deep breathing mobilizes secretions, which keeps airways and alveoli open and provides greater surface area for gas exchange.

Procedure Steps

1. **Assist the patient to a Fowler's or semi-Fowler's position,** with the shoulders relaxed.
   Allows for best chest and lung expansion.

2. **Assist the patient who will have a chest or abdominal incision** to practice splinting the site with a folded blanket or pillow.
   Counterpressure supports the incision and decreases pain. ▼

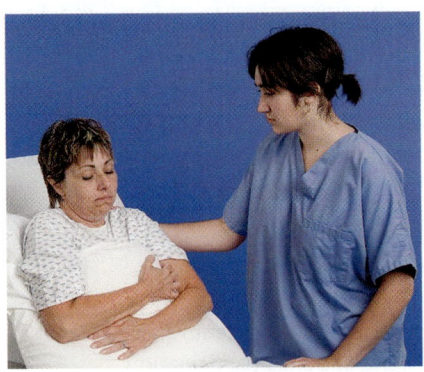

3. **Teach the patient diaphragmatic/deep breathing.** Tell the patient to:
   a. Place her hands anteriorly, along the lower end of the rib cage. The tips of the third fingers should touch at the midline.
   b. Slowly take a deep breath in through the nose. Tell the patient that she should feel her chest expanding as the diaphragm moves down.
   c. Hold her breath for 2 to 5 seconds.
      Stimulates surfactant production and helps prevent alveolar collapse.
   d. Slowly and completely exhale the breath through her mouth.

4. **Teach the patient to cough** in conjunction with diaphragmatic breathing. Instruct her to:
   a. Complete two or three cycles of diaphragmatic breathing.

   b. On the next breath in, have the patient lean forward and cough rapidly, through an open mouth, using the muscles of the abdomen, thighs, and buttocks. Cough several times on that breath.
      This information helps the patient to distinguish coughing from merely clearing her throat.

For a Patient Experiencing Weakness

If the patient is too weak to perform this maneuver, have the patient inhale deeply, bend forward slightly, and perform three or four "huffs" against an open glottis to move secretions forward.

Procedure 40-1B ■ Teaching a Patient to Move in Bed

➤ When performing the procedure, always identify your patient according to agency policy, using two identifiers, and be attentive to standard precautions, hand hygiene, patient safety and privacy, body mechanics, and documentation.

Moving in bed promotes blood circulation, stimulates respiratory function, and helps mobilize gas in the intestines.

Procedure Steps

1. **Start with the patient in the supine position,** bedrails up. Then instruct the patient as follows.

2. **To turn to the left side:** Bend the right leg, sliding the foot flat along the bed and flexing the knee.
   Enables the patient to push herself over to the opposite side.

3. **Reach the right arm across the chest** and grasp the opposite bedrail.
   Helps the patient to turn, reduces the need to use the abdominal muscles for turning, and minimizes incision pain.

4. **Breathe deeply and practice splinting** any potential abdominal or chest incisions. Assist the patient to practice as needed.
   Facilitates comfort during movement.

5. **Pull on the bedrail** while pushing off with the right foot.
   Assists patient to turn to the left. ▼

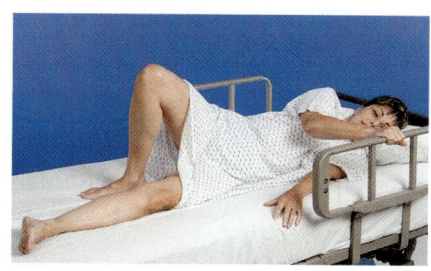

6. **If the patient cannot maintain** this position independently, place a folded pillow or blanket along her back for support.

7. **Teach the patient to change** positions every 2 hours, repeating the turning process with the opposite arm and leg. For a patient who needs pillows placed for support, you will need to assist with turning.

Procedure 40-1C ■ Teaching Leg Exercises

➤ When performing the procedure, always identify your patient according to agency policy, using two identifiers, and be attentive to standard precautions, hand hygiene, patient safety and privacy, body mechanics, and documentation.

Leg exercises flex and extend the leg muscles to increase peripheral circulation and help prevent thrombus formation. Thrombus formation is a common postoperative complication.

Procedure Steps

1. **Instruct the patient to lie supine** in the bed.

   NOTE: *Although these exercises can be done when the patient is up in a chair, the therapeutic effect will be diminished by the effects of gravity.*

2. **Perform ankle circles.** Instruct the patient to:
   a. Start with one foot in the dorsi-flexed position.
   b. Slowly rotate the ankle clockwise.
   c. After three rotations, repeat the procedure in a counterclockwise direction.

   d. Repeat this exercise at least three times in each direction, then switch and exercise the other ankle. ▼

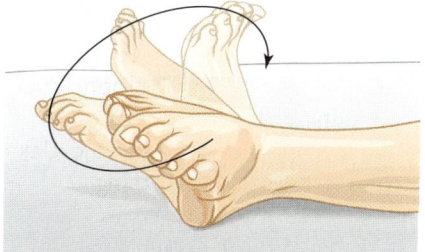

3. **Perform ankle pumps.** Instruct the patient to:
   a. Start with one foot, leg extended.
   b. Point the toe until her foot is plantar flexed.
   c. Pull the toes back toward her head until the foot is dorsiflexed; at the same time, press the back of the knee into the bed.
   d. Make sure she feels a pull, or a stretch, in the calf.

   e. Repeat the alternation between plantar and dorsiflexion several times.
   f. Repeat the cycle with the other foot.

4. **Perform leg exercises.** Instruct the patient to:
   a. Lie supine in the bed.
   b. Slowly begin bending the knee, sliding the sole of the foot along the bed until the knee is in a flexed position. ▼

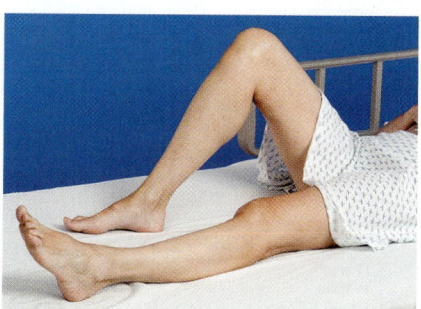

(continued on next page)

Procedure 40–1 ■ Teaching a Patient to Deep-Breathe, Cough, Move in Bed, and Perform Leg Exercises (continued)

c. Reverse the motion, extending the knee until the leg is once again flat on the bed. ▼

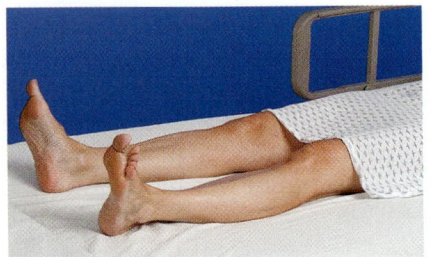

d. Repeat several times.
e. Repeat using the opposite leg.

? What if . . .

■ **The patient has had knee, hip, or back surgery?**

Leg exercises may be contraindicated in patients having knee, hip, or back surgery. Check the surgeon's prescriptions and/or collaborate with the physical therapist.

■ **The patient has had nasal, ophthalmic, or neurological surgery?**

Coughing and deep-breathing exercises are contraindicated.

To avoid increasing intracranial pressure.

Evaluation

Make sure that the patient performs correctly a return demonstration of the procedures taught.

Documentation

In many healthcare facilities, checklists and charts have special areas in which to document patient teaching. Documentation should identify the person who completed the teaching, the person to whom the procedures were taught, what procedures were taught, and whether the patient understood the teaching. Also include the name and type of any printed materials given.

Sample electronic documentation

Note that because this is just one screen of a documentation system, not all of the information is visible. For example, you cannot see the date or the name of the nurse.

Practice Resources

Cao, C., & Zhang, L. (2015); Vancouver Coastal Health (2014).

Thinking About the Procedure

The videos **Teaching a Patient to Deep-Breathe and Cough, Teaching a Patient to Move in Bed,** and **Teaching Leg Exercises,** along with questions and suggested responses, are available on the **Davis's *Nursing Skills Videos*** Web site on Davis*Plus*.

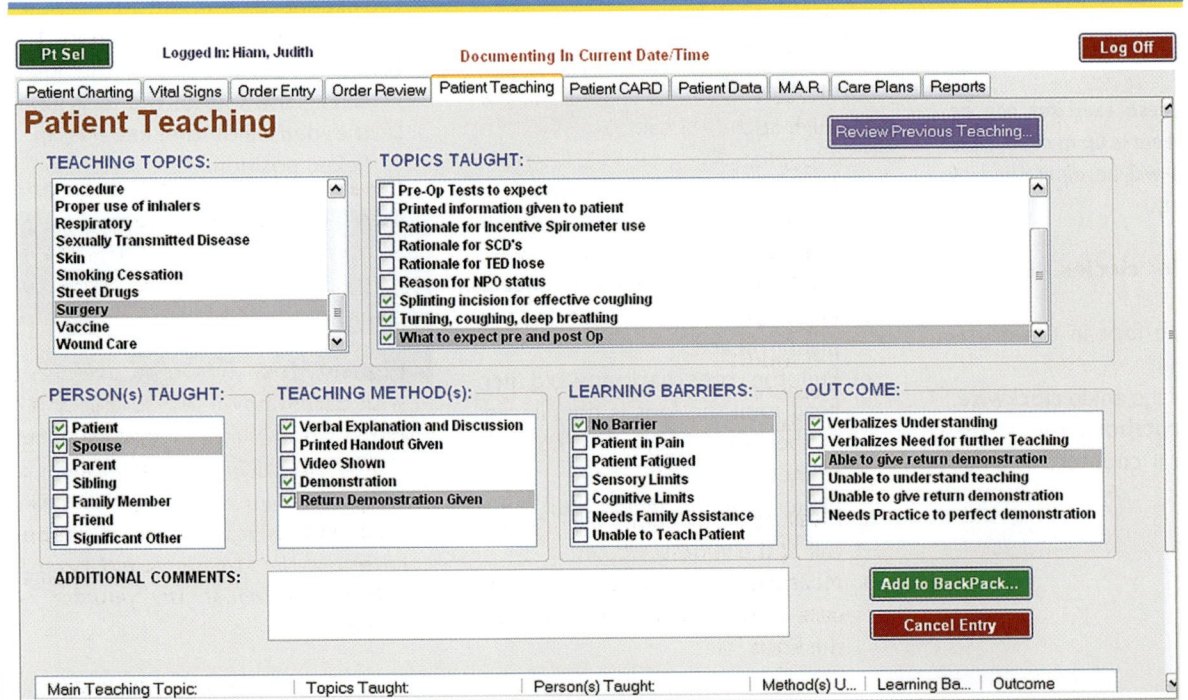

Procedure 40-2 ■ Applying Antiembolism Stockings

➤ For steps to follow in *all* procedures, refer to the Universal Steps for All Procedures found on the page facing the inside back cover.

Equipment

- Measuring tape
- Antiembolism stockings
- Disposable wipes or washcloth and towel (if needed to cleanse legs)
- Talcum powder (optional: check manufacturer's recommendations)

Delegation

You can delegate application of antiembolism stockings to nursing assistive personnel who have been trained in the task. Instruct the NAP as follows:

- Report the presence of any abnormalities on the lower extremities, such as lesions, sores, or redness, before applying the stockings.
- Instruct the patient to maintain a recumbent position for at least 15 minutes before applying the stockings.
- Do not massage the legs.
- Make sure there are no wrinkles in the stockings once they have been applied.

Pre-Procedure Assessment

- Assess the level of consciousness and cognitive ability.
  If the patient is unconscious or confused, you will need to call for assistance to hold and stabilize the lower extremities as you apply the stockings.
- Assess for signs and symptoms of severe peripheral arterial disease, such as weak or absent pulses, discoloration or cyanosis, or gangrene.
  Antiembolism stockings should not be used in patients with any of these findings because they compress the vessels and, therefore, further impede the already compromised arterial flow.
- Assess skin condition. Note any lesions, dermatitis, or major edema, as evidenced by shiny, taut skin.
  If skin is overstretched by edema, antiembolism stockings may irritate or worsen skin conditions and cause skin breakdown.
- Note the patient's position and length of time she has been in that position.
  Place the patient supine for at least 15 minutes before stocking application. This prevents trapping of pooled venous blood.

➤ When performing the procedure, always identify your patient according to agency policy using two identifiers, and be attentive to standard precautions, hand hygiene, patient safety and privacy, body mechanics, and documentation.

➤ If possible, apply stockings in the morning, before the patient gets out of bed. This prevents venous distention and edema that occur when the patient is sitting or standing.

Procedure Steps

1. Measure the patient's lower extremity to obtain the correct size stocking. This is critical to their effectiveness

Stockings must be sized correctly in order to apply the correct amounts of pressure at the ankle, mid-calf, and upper thigh. If they are not tight enough, they will not improve venous return effectively. If they are too tight, they may compress the veins and impair circulation to the skin. ▼

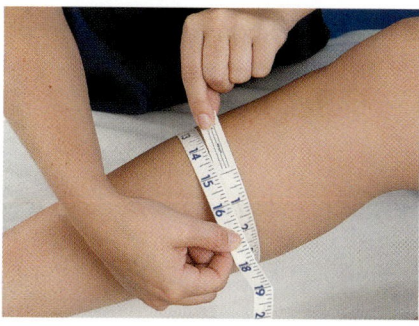

For Thigh-High Stockings

✚ NOTE: Thigh-high elastic stockings have not been proved to be more effective in preventing thromboembolism than knee-high ones, and should probably be avoided because of the tendency to roll and have a tourniquet effect (Perry, Borchert, Burke, et al., 2012, reviewed 2014).

a. Measure the circumference of the thigh at the gluteal fold.
   The manufacturer of T.E.D. brand stockings recommends that thigh-high stockings not be applied if the thigh circumference exceeds 82 cm (32 in.). Use knee-high stockings instead.

b. Measure the calf circumference at the widest section.

c. Measure the distance from the gluteal fold to the base of the heel.

Knee-High Stockings

a. Measure the circumference of the calf at the widest section.

b. Measure the distance from the base of the heel to the middle of the knee joint.

Evidence is not conclusive, but increasingly supports the use of knee-high instead of thigh-high hose.

2. Assist the patient to a supine position and instruct him to maintain that position for at least 15 minutes before you apply the stockings.
Prevents trapping of pooled venous blood by the antiembolism stockings.

3. Cleanse the patient's legs and feet if necessary. Dry well.
Removing surface dirt and bacteria will decrease the likelihood of infection and odor.

4. Lightly dust the legs and feet with talcum powder if desired and if recommended by the manufacturer.
KEY POINT: *Do not use powder if the patient is or is likely to become diaphoretic. Powder eases the application of the stockings, but perspiration will cause the powder to clump.*

(continued on next page)

Procedure 40-2 ■ Applying Antiembolism Stockings (continued)

5. **Holding one stocking at the top cuff** in your dominant hand, slide your nondominant arm down and into the stocking until your hand reaches the heel of the stocking.

6. **Grasp the center of the heel** with your hand inside the stocking, and then slowly turn the stocking inside out to the level of the heel with your other hand.
   The elastic in the stockings is very strong; this method is the easiest way to fit it over the foot and calf. ▼

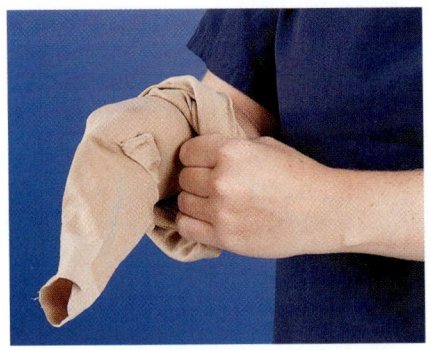

7. **Ask the patient to point his toes** as you grasp the turned foot of the stocking and ease it onto his foot and heel (like putting on a sock). Center the patient's heel in the heel of the stocking.
   Ensures that the pressure of the stocking is over the correct anatomical areas.

8. **Gradually pull the remainder** of the stocking up and over the leg, turning it right side out as you proceed. Be certain the stocking is straight. ▼

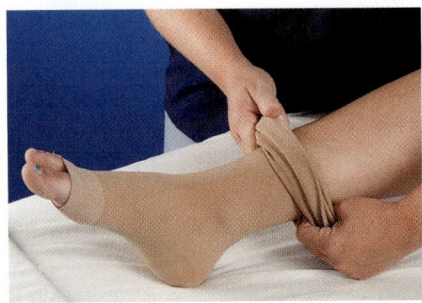

Knee-High Stockings
Pull up to 2.5 to 5 cm (1 to 2 in.) below the knee

Thigh-High Stockings
Pull up to the gluteal fold of the thigh, rotating inward so the gusset is centered over the femoral artery, slightly toward the inside of the leg.
Stockings apply varying amounts of compression between ankle, calf, and thigh areas. Keeping the stocking straight ensures that the pressure occurs over the correct areas.

9. **Smooth out any excess material;** keep stockings free of wrinkles and bunching.

Decreases the risk of skin breakdown and areas of potentially dangerous constriction.

10. **When using stockings with** closed toes, tug gently on the end of the stocking over the toes to create a small space between the end of the toes and the stocking.
    Prevents compression of small vessels in the toes which may impede circulation.

11. **Repeat the procedure** on the other leg.

12. **Remove the stockings** and bathe and dry the legs daily.

13. **Launder the stockings** at least every 3 days; dry them on a flat surface.
    Soiled stockings can irritate the skin; dry flat to prevent stretching.

? What if . . .

■ **Both legs do not measure the same?**

Order two different sizes of stockings and use one from each package to make two pairs.

Evaluation
■ Evaluate patient comfort.
  Severe, continuous discomfort may indicate that the stockings are the wrong size.
■ Check the stockings for wrinkles and/or rolling down at the top, especially when sitting.
  Wrinkles and rolling down can cause skin breakdown and areas of constriction.
■ Evaluate and monitor skin condition.
  Elastic stockings should be removed for 20 to 30 minutes every 8 to 12 hours to allow you to inspect the patient's skin and evaluate the adequacy of his circulation.
■ Evaluate the patient's ability to ambulate.
  It is important to reduce the time the patient is immobile due to pain, sedation, mechanical ventilation, and so on.

■ Remeasure the legs regularly.
  To prevent complications related to swelling and weight gain.

Home Care
■ Teach the client and/or caregiver to apply the stockings.
■ Encourage the client to have two pairs of stockings on hand so that one pair can be used while the other is being laundered.
■ Instruct the client to follow the manufacturer's directions for washing the stockings.
■ Teach the client not to roll down the tops of the stockings.

Documentation
■ Document leg measurements and size of the stockings used to provide a baseline.

- Document the time and date applied.
- Note the condition of the skin, including any abnormalities.

Sample electronic documentation

Note that because this is just one screen of a documentation system, not all of the information is visible. For example, you cannot see the date or the name of the nurse.

Practice Resources

American Association of Critical-Care Nurses (2016); National Guideline Clearinghouse (2007, revised 2015); Wade, R., Sideris, E., Paton, F., et al. (2015).

Thinking About the Procedure

 The video **Applying Antiembolism Stockings,** along with questions and suggested responses, is available on the **Davis's *Nursing Skills Videos*** Web site on Davis*Plus*.

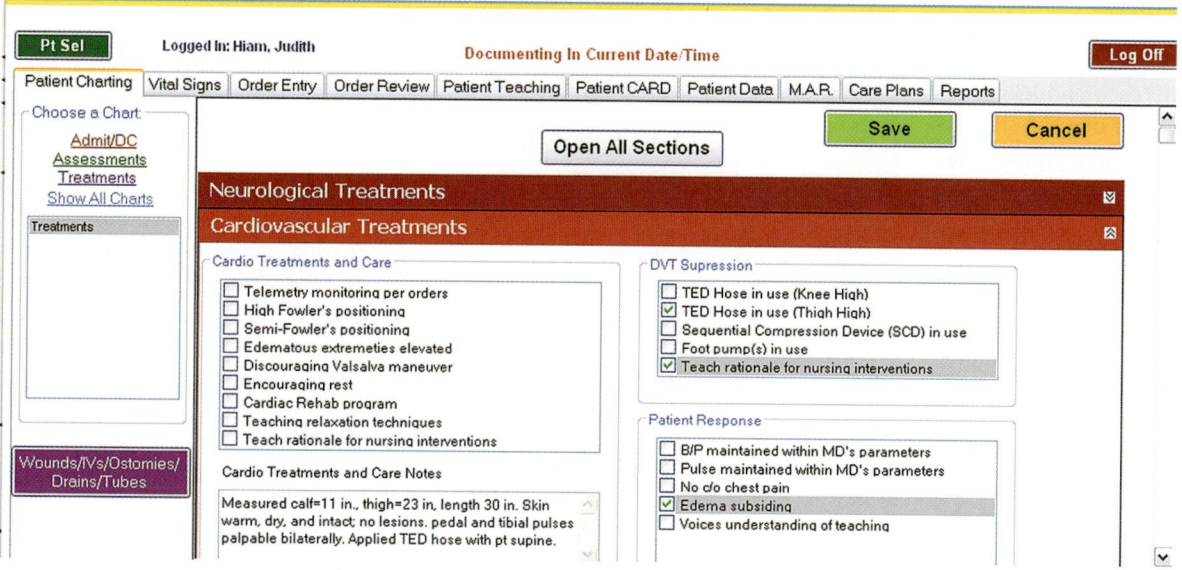

Procedure 40-3 ■ Applying Sequential Compression Devices

➤ For steps to follow in *all* procedures, refer to the Universal Steps for All Procedures found on the page facing the inside back cover.

Equipment

NOTE: Sequential compression devices may be referred to by several different brand names, including SCDS (sequential compression decompression stockings), Flowtrons, and PAS (pneumatic air stockings).

- Compression pump, motor, or machine
- Connecting tubing, if applicable (In some devices, the tubing is preconnected to the sleeves.)
- Compression sleeve (knee-high or thigh-high, depending on the order and the type of device)
- Elastic stockings (if also prescribed)
- Disposable wipes or washcloth and towel as needed to cleanse the lower extremities
- Measuring tape

Delegation

You may delegate the application of the sequential compression device to a NAP who has had training in that task. Instruct the NAP to report any redness, irritation, or open areas on the lower extremities. SCDS should not be removed for long periods of time because they are needed to support the patient's peripheral circulation.

✚ Instruct the NAP to ensure that all cords and connecting tubing are in a place that will not create a fall risk for the patient or visitors.

Pre-Procedure Assessment

- Assess cognitive level and level of consciousness.
  Patients with altered cognition may be at higher risk for falls related to the presence of the connecting tubing and attachment to the compression pump. Patients who are unconscious will not be able to report a device that is creating too much pressure.
- Assess signs and symptoms of severe peripheral arterial disease, such as weak or absent pulses, discoloration or cyanosis, or gangrene.
  Increased compression of vessels by the sequential device may further impede arterial flow.
- Assess skin condition. Note lesions, dermatitis, or major edema, as evidenced by shiny, taut skin.
  If skin is overstretched by edema, the sequential compression sleeve may irritate or worsen skin conditions and cause skin breakdown.

(continued on next page)

Procedure 40–3 ■ Applying Sequential Compression Devices (continued)

> When performing the procedure, always identify your patient according to agency policy, using two identifiers, and be attentive to standard precautions, hand hygiene, patient safety and privacy, body mechanics, and documentation.

Procedure Steps

1. **Position the patient supine.**
   Prevents venous pooling. Allows for easier application of the compression sleeve.

2. **For thigh-high SCD sleeves,** measure the circumference and length of both thighs to ensure that the sleeves are of the proper size. Follow the manufacturer's instructions.

3. **Cleanse the lower extremities,** if necessary.
   Remove surface dirt and/or bacteria, decreasing the likelihood of infection and odor.

4. **Apply elastic stockings if they have been** prescribed in conjunction with the sequential compression device, following the steps in Procedure 40-2.

5. ✚ **Place the compression device** pump in a location near an electrical outlet so that the cord will not pose a fall risk. Plug in the pump.

   NOTE: Many compression pumps come equipped with hangers so you can hang the device at the bottom of the patient's bed.

6. **Apply the compression sleeve.** ▼

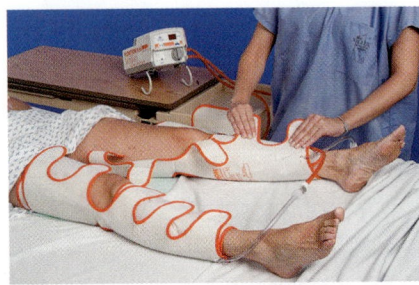

For Flowtron Brand (available in knee-length only):

   a. Open the Velcro fasteners on the sleeve.
   b. Place the sleeve under the lower leg below the knee with the "air bladder" side down on the bed.
   c. Bring the ends of the sleeve up and wrap them around the lower leg, leaving one to two fingerbreadths of space between the leg and the sleeve.
   Prevents excess pressure and overcompression.

For SCDS/PAS Brands

   a. Open the Velcro fasteners on the sleeve.

   b. Place the sleeve under the leg, ensuring that the knee opening is at the level of the knee joint and that the fastener will close on the anterior surface.
   Ensures that compression occurs over the correct structures. Prevents restricted range of motion of the knee joint.

   c. Bring the ends of the sleeve up and wrap them around the leg, leaving one to two fingerbreadths of space between the leg and the sleeve.
   Prevents excess pressure and overcompression.

7. **Connect the sleeve** to the compression pump.

8. **Turn the pump on** and, if applicable, set the compression pressure on the pump device to the manufacturer's recommended setting.

   NOTE: In some facilities, the compression pressure amount is preset and can be changed only by the central supply/ equipment department.

Evaluation

After applying the device, make the following ongoing assessments:
- Inflation and deflation of the sleeve
  Ensures that the device is actually working.
- Kinking or pinching of the connecting tubing
  Interferes with inflation of sleeves and may cause overheating or malfunction of the unit.
- Circulation, sensation, and motion of the foot, including skin color, pulses, temperature, capillary refill, motion, and sensation
- Patient comfort
  Increasing discomfort may indicate excess or incorrect pressure.
- Skin condition. Remove the compression sleeves at intervals so that you can inspect skin and evaluate the adequacy of circulation.

   NOTE: If elastic stockings are being used in conjunction with the sequential compression device, follow the recommendations in Procedure 40-2.

- Signs and symptoms of deep vein thrombosis
  Even with sequential compression device therapy, a patient can still develop thrombi.

Patient Teaching

✚ Teach the patient to call for assistance when disconnecting the tubing from the compression pump in order to ambulate.
Prevents patient falls. The SCD tubing is a tripping hazard, and injuries from falls involving SCDS are likely to be more severe than injuries associated with general patient falls (Johnston & Davis, 2008).

Documentation

- Document the date and time you applied the device.
- Note the type and size (if applicable) of the compression sleeve used.
- Document the skin condition, including any abnormalities.

Sample documentation:

11/11/18   1100   Knee-high SCD applied per order. Skin warm, dry, and intact at time of application. Peripheral pulses palpable. Pt's wife instructed on use of SCD. Pt unresponsive. No evidence of discomfort, no grimace or movement with application. ———————S. Bee, RN

Practice Resources

Johnston, J., & Davis, M. (2008); Nelson, E. A., Mani, R., Thomas, K., et al. (2011); Sadaghianloo, N., & Dardik, A. (2016).

Thinking About the Procedure

 The video **Applying Sequential Compression Devices,** along with questions and suggested responses, is available on the **Davis's** *Nursing Skills Videos* Web site on DavisPlus.

Procedure 40-4 ■ Managing Gastric Suction

➤ For steps to follow in *all* procedures, refer to the Universal Steps for All Procedures found on the page facing the inside back cover.

Equipment

Procedure 40-4A: Initial Equipment Setup

- Nonsterile procedure gloves
- Suction source (either a portable machine or piped-in wall source)
- Suction container and tubing
- Stopcock (to connect the NG tube to suction tubing)

Procedure 40-4B: Emptying the Suction Container

- Clean nonsterile procedure gloves
- Graduated container
  To measure gastric output when emptying the suction container. Not needed if suction canister is marked for measuring.
- Alcohol wipes or chlorhexidine/alcohol antiseptic product

Procedure 40-4C: Irrigating the Nasogastric Tubing

- Nonsterile procedure gloves
- Irrigating set (basin and bulb syringe or catheter-tipped syringe)
- Normal saline irrigant (unless another irrigant is prescribed)
- Linen-saver pads

Procedure 40-4D: Providing Comfort Measures

- Nonsterile procedure gloves
- Emesis basin, cup, and water for mouth care
- Water-soluble lubricant
- Cotton-tip applicators
- Tissues or damp washcloth

NOTE: *This procedure assumes an NG or other enteric tube is already in place and that its correct placement has already been verified. If you need to insert an NG tube or check placement, refer to*

Chapter 28. Tubes for gastric decompression are typically large-lumen tubes such as a Salem sump or Levin tube. See the table at the end of this procedure for more information about tubes. ▼

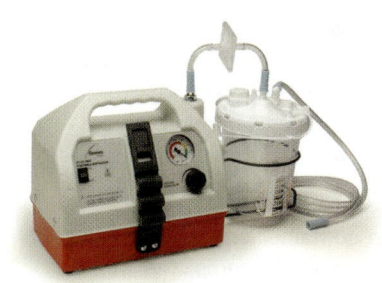

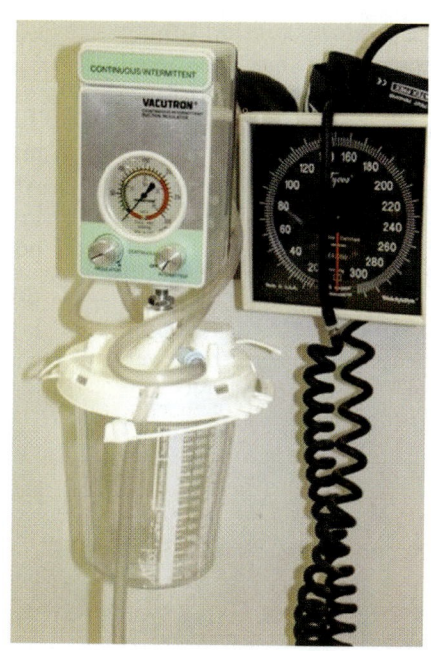

(continued on next page)

Procedure 40-4 ■ Managing Gastric Suction (continued)

Delegation

A registered nurse should do the initial setup and any subsequent irrigation. You may delegate a NAP to empty and measure drainage and perform comfort measures. You must monitor equipment functioning and the patient's responses to the decompression. Instruct the NAP about observations that should be reported to you.

Pre-Procedure Assessments

■ Determine that the NG tube has been inserted and placement has been verified.

■ Verify the prescriber's order for type of tube and whether it is to be placed to suction or a drainage bag; also verify the type of suction to be used (low, high, continuous, intermittent).

■ Auscultate for bowel sounds.

■ Assess the patient's ability to cooperate with the procedure and understand explanations.

■ Refer to the Evaluation section of this procedure. This procedure assumes an NG tube is already in place, so assessments are ongoing.

Procedure 40-4A ■ Initial Equipment Setup

➤ When performing the procedure, always identify your patient according to agency policy, using two identifiers, and be attentive to standard precautions, hand hygiene, patient safety and privacy, body mechanics, and documentation.

Procedure Steps

1. **Place the collection container** in the holder (on the portable suction machine or on the wall). Plug the power cord into a grounded outlet if using a portable suction machine.

2. **Connect the short tubing** between the container and the suction source. In some systems, the port will be marked "vacuum."

3. **Connect the long suction tubing** to the container (it may be marked "patient"); if a stopcock is available, connect it to the open end nearest the patient.

4. **Don clean nonsterile procedure gloves.**
   Helps prevent transfer of microorganisms.

5. **After the nasogastric (NG) tube** has been inserted and placement verified, attach the end of the NG tube to the suction tubing.
   See Chapter 28 to review importance of tube placement. You must be certain the NG tube is in the stomach, not in the esophagus or airways.

6. **If using a double lumen** catheter (e.g., Salem sump), instill 10 to 20 mL of air into the vent lumen to make sure it is patent. This should create a soft hissing sound.

7. **Secure the NG tube** to the client's nose and gown (see Chapter 28 to review).
   Minimizes movement of the tube, helping to prevent irritation of the nares or other insertion site, as well as helping to keep the tube from migrating up out of the stomach.

8. **Turn on the suction source** to the prescribed amount. In an emergency when there is no order, always use low suction. Open the stopcock—note the direction of the arrows.

9. **Observe that drainage appears** in the collection container.
   It may take up to 5 minutes for air to be removed from the canister before the stomach contents will drain. ➤

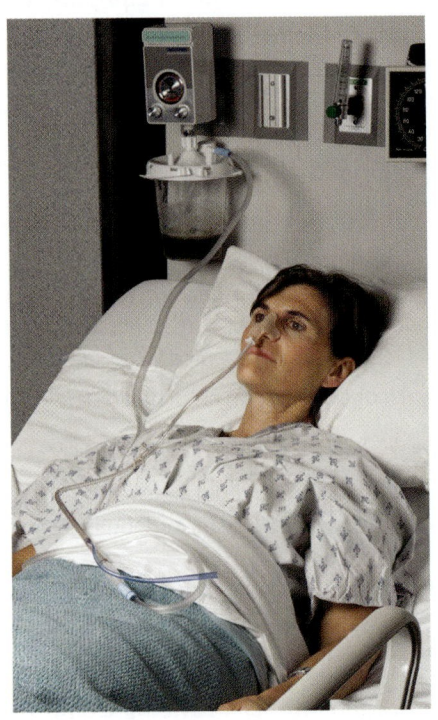

Procedure 40-4B ■ Emptying the Suction Container

➤ When performing the procedure, always identify your patient according to agency policy, using two identifiers, and be attentive to standard precautions, hand hygiene, patient safety and privacy, body mechanics, and documentation.

1. **Don clean nonsterile gloves.**
   Limits the transfer of microorganisms; protects your hands from contact with body secretions.

2. **Turn off the suction source** and close the stopcock on the tubing (or clamp the tubing, if there is no stopcock).

   Prevents suction flow during emptying of the container.

3. **Empty the suction canister.**

For a Suction Container that is Marked with Measurements.

Note the amount, color, and odor of the contents. Empty and rinse the container.

For a Suction Container that is not Marked Incrementally.

Remove the cap from the lid of the suction container and pour the drainage into a graduated measuring container. Note color, odor, and amount. Empty and rinse the container.

A container with graduated markings enables you to monitor intake and output

(I&O) accurately. Rinsing removes organic material that could be a reservoir for microorganisms.

4. **Wipe the port of the suction** container with an alcohol wipe. Place the suction container back in its holder and close the stopper on the lid.

5. **Turn on the suction source** to the prescribed amount. Note the direction of the arrows and turn the stopcock to the "On" position. If there is no stopcock, unclamp the tubing.

6. **Observe for proper functioning** of the suction and patency of the tubing.
   Prevents complications that would result in malfunction.

7. **Remove and discard gloves.** Perform hand hygiene.

Procedure 40-4C ■ Irrigating the Nasogastric Tubing

➤ When performing the procedure, always identify your patient according to agency policy, using two identifiers, and be attentive to standard precautions, hand hygiene, patient safety and privacy, body mechanics, and documentation.

1. **Place a linen-saver pad** on the bed under the NG tube.

2. **Open the irrigation set** and pour saline into the basin.
   Water is not used because it may cause electrolyte imbalances.

3. Place patient at a 30° to 45° elevation (unless contraindicated or not tolerated)
   This position helps avoid gastric reflux of irrigant.

4. **Don clean procedure gloves.**
   Limits the transfer of microorganisms; protects your hands from contact with body secretions.

5. **Check for correct placement** of the NG tube, using at least two bedside methods (see Chapter 28 as needed).
   Prevents accidental instillation of irrigant into the airways.

6. **Fill the syringe with 10 to 20 mL** of saline and place it on the linen-saver pad.

7. **Clamp the NG tube** or turn off the stopcock connecting to the suction tubing. Then disconnect the NG tube from the suction tubing.
   Prevents backflow of drainage and soiling of linens and clothing.

8. **Hold the drainage tubing up** until suction clears it. Then lay it on the linen-saver pad or hook it over the suction machine.
   Keeps secretions from soiling the bed linens or clothing.

9. **Turn off the suction machine.**

10. **Unclamp the NG tube** or turn on the stopcock.

11. **Unpin the NG tube** (or remove tape) from the patient's clothing.

12. **Attach the syringe and instill the irrigant** slowly into the NG tube. Do not force the solution. Be careful not to instill fluid into the air vent.
    Clears the NG tube of gastric contents to keep it patent and helps keep the tube from adhering to the gastric mucosa. Partially digested food, clotted blood, or tissue debris may clog the tube and prevent effective drainage.

13. **Lower the end of the NG tube** and then release the syringe bulb (or depending on the type of syringe, pull back the plunger) to withdraw fluid. Instill and withdraw until fluid flows in and out freely.
    Uses the force of gravity with negative pressure to withdraw instilled fluid and gastric contents.

For a Double-Lumen NG Tube

Draw 30 mL of air into the syringe and inject it into the "pigtail" (the smaller-bore tube). Follow agency policy for this.
This clears the air-vent tube of any secretions. It must be patent in order to equalize pressure and prevent gastric tissue trauma at the drainage ports. The air also keeps the tube from draining fluid out of the stomach by capillary action.

14. **Reclamp the NG tube** or turn off the stopcock.
    Prevents backflow of drainage.

15. **Reconnect the NG tube** to the suction tube. Then release the clamp or turn on the stopcock.

16. **Reattach the NG tube** to the patient's clothing (with a pin or tape—see Chapter 28 as needed).
    Prevents pulling on and irritating the patient's nostril.

17. **Provide comfort measures** (e.g., mouth care).

18. **Remove and discard gloves.** Perform hand hygiene.

(continued on next page)

Procedure 40-4 ■ Managing Gastric Suction (continued)

Procedure 40-4D ■ Providing Comfort Measures

➤ When performing the procedure, always identify your patient according to agency policy, using two identifiers, and be attentive to standard precautions, hand hygiene, patient safety and privacy, body mechanics, and documentation.

1. **Don clean nonsterile procedure gloves.**

2. **Provide mouth care** (see Procedures 24-6, 24-7, and 24-8 if you need to review). Use mouthwash as desired. Avoid using lemon-glycerin swabs. Apply water-soluble lubricant to the lips if they become dry and crusty.
   The patient most likely has a dry mouth from not receiving oral intake and from mouth breathing. Lemon-glycerin swabs cause even more drying of tissues.

3. **Remove nasal secretions** with a tissue or a damp washcloth. Moisten a cotton-tip applicator and wipe the inside of each nostril. If secretions are encrusted, moisten the applicator with hydrogen peroxide, then follow with an applicator moistened with water.
   To soften, dissolve, and remove secretions and prevent tissue irritation.

4. **Apply a small amount of** water-soluble lubricant to the inside of each nostril.
   Soothes and softens dried skin. Avoid petroleum-based lubricants, as complications may occur if they are inhaled.

5. **Check that the tape or tube fixation** device is secure. If it is not, replace it (see Procedure 28-2 as needed).
   Prevents irritation of the nasal skin and mucosa. Helps prevent migration of the NG tube from the stomach.

? What if . . .

■ **Resistance is met when you irrigate the NG tube?**

Check the tubing for kinks or evidence of obstruction. Have the patient to turn to the left side.
Turning to one side changes the position of the distal tip of the NG tube.

■ **The patient complains that the NG tube is pulling against her nostril?**

The tube may not be properly anchored to her clothing. Reattach the safety pin (or tape) closer to the nose so that there is more slack in the tube.

■ **The NG tube causes excoriation of the nares?**

Remove the tape or fixation device from the nose. Remove the residual adhesive from the skin. Apply skin sealant and anchor the tube so that the adhesive touches in a different place on the skin. Keep the excoriated areas clean and dry.

■ **The NG tube does not drain?**

Check tubing for kinks or blockage. Check the suction apparatus. If the collection container is higher than the patient's abdomen, lower it. If these aspects are working properly, irrigate the tube (see Procedure 40-4C, preceding). If the tube still is not draining and the patient is uncomfortable, document and notify the primary care provider. Encourage the patient to relax and breathe slowly through her nose. If the patient has abdominal distention, pain, or vomiting, notify the provider immediately.

✚ If the container is too high, the negative pressure of low suction may not be enough to overcome the force of gravity. Abdominal distention, pain, or vomiting may mean the system is not working. Continued distention creates undue strain on the suture line. You should notify the care provider of these symptoms even when the mechanical aspects of the suction seem in working order.

Gastric Decompression Tubes

TYPE	LUMEN(S)	USE	MANAGEMENT	DISCUSSION
Levin	1, unvented	Decompression, feedings, or irrigation	Use low intermittent suction; may require irrigation.	If the tube opening(s) rest(s) against the gastric mucosa, the suction may irritate or injure the tissue.
Salem Sump	2	Decompression, suction, gastric lavage	Vented. May use high continuous suction.	The air vent helps keep the tube away from the gastric mucosa during suction.
Sengsten–Blakemore	3	Decompression; treatment of active bleeding from esophageal or gastric varices	Use low intermittent suction.	Gastric or esophageal balloons hold the tube in place.

Gastric Decompression Tubes—cont'd				
TYPE	**LUMEN(S)**	**USE**	**MANAGEMENT**	**DISCUSSION**
Cantor	1, unvented	Decompression	Use intermittent suction.	Distal end is weighted with a balloon. Used in bowel obstruction. Rarely used because of the hazard posed by the mercury in the weighted balloon.
Miller–Abbott	2	Decompression	Use intermittent suction.	Distal end weighted with a balloon. Used in bowel obstruction. Rarely used because it contains mercury in the weighted balloon.
Ewald or Other Very Large-Bore Tube	May be passed orally for emergency evacuation of stomach contents to prevent absorption of ingested medications, poisons, or products. A piston tip syringe is placed on the end of the tube for manual suction. Typically, the stomach is washed repeatedly with saline and all contents are withdrawn. Because of its large diameter, this type of tube is not tolerated by patients who are alert, and is not left in place after lavage is completed.			
Weighted Small-Bore Tubes (e.g., Keofeed)	For feedings only. Suction collapses the tube.			

Evaluation and Maintenance

- Periodically assess placement of the tube by a combination of methods (i.e., checking pH of aspirate, listening over the stomach with a stethoscope while injecting air into the tube, and reviewing radiographic reports). See Chapter 28 for review, as needed.
- Monitor patency of the tube and the effectiveness of the suction. Check tube connections.
- Monitor patient comfort (e.g., sore throat).
  The continuing presence of a tube in the nose and throat is bothersome to patients. The major nuisance is the pressure of the tube against the internal mucous membranes, irritating the nostril, pharynx, and esophagus.
- Auscultate for bowel sounds; turn off suction while auscultating.
  Bowel sounds indicate the return of peristalsis and the success of gastric decompression. You may hear the sound of the suction apparatus and misinterpret it as bowel sounds.
- Monitor for gastric distention, vomiting, and abdominal pain.
  These symptoms probably indicate the suction is not working effectively. See the "What if . . ." section, preceding.
- Examine skin and mucous membranes around the insertion site (e.g., nares, abdomen).
- Follow agency policy or the primary care provider's prescription for irrigation of the gastric tube. It is common to irrigate with 10 to 30 mL of normal saline every 3 to 4 hours.
- Monitor the color of the drainage (should be green to gold). If there is blood in the drainage, notify the primary care provider.

- For clients undergoing prolonged GI suction, observe for signs and symptoms of hyponatremia and hypokalemia (i.e., fatigue, lethargy, confusion, seizures, muscle weakness, paresthesia, and cardiac dysrhythmias). Review lab results and report any symptoms to the primary care provider.
- Assess the patient's ability to move about in bed while attached to the suction source.

Patient Teaching

- Instruct the patient to notify you of any discomfort and not to tug on or try to reposition the NG tube if it becomes uncomfortable.
- Instruct the patient to notify you if feeling nauseated.
  This could mean the tube is blocked and not draining effectively.

Home Care

Gastric suction is usually performed in a hospital. If the client is to go home with gastric suction (e.g., a terminally ill person who has a bowel obstruction and wants to be in her own home), teach the family how to use the device before the person is discharged. Also arrange for home healthcare.

Documentation

- Record all drainage as output on the I&O record.
- Record the time, type, and volume of irrigations and the drainage returned.
- Be sure to include irrigation fluids as input on the I&O record.
- Note color, odor, and consistency of drainage.
- Document emotional and physical responses to NG intubation.

(continued on next page)

Procedure 40–4 ■ Managing Gastric Suction (continued)

- Document any evidence of tube or equipment malfunction.
- Document epigastric pain, discomfort, distention, or vomiting.

Practice Resources

Allied Healthcare Products (n.d.); *Best Practices: Evidence-Based Nursing Procedures* (2007); National Guideline Clearinghouse (2009, revised 2011).

Thinking About the Procedure

 The videos **Managing Gastric Suction: Initial Equipment Setup, Managing Gastric Suction: Emptying the Suction Container,** and **Managing Gastric Suction: Irrigating the Nasogastric Tubing,** along with questions and suggested responses, are available on the **Davis's *Nursing Skills Videos*** Web site on Davis*Plus* **Davis's *Nursing Skills Videos*** Web site on Davis*Plus*.

 To explore learning resources for this chapter,

 Go to www.DavisAdvantage.com and find:

Answers and Suggested Responses for all questions in this chapter

Lists of NIC Interventions and NOC Outcomes

List of NANDA-I Diagnoses

Knowledge Map

Care Plan

Care Map

References and Bibliography

Concept Map

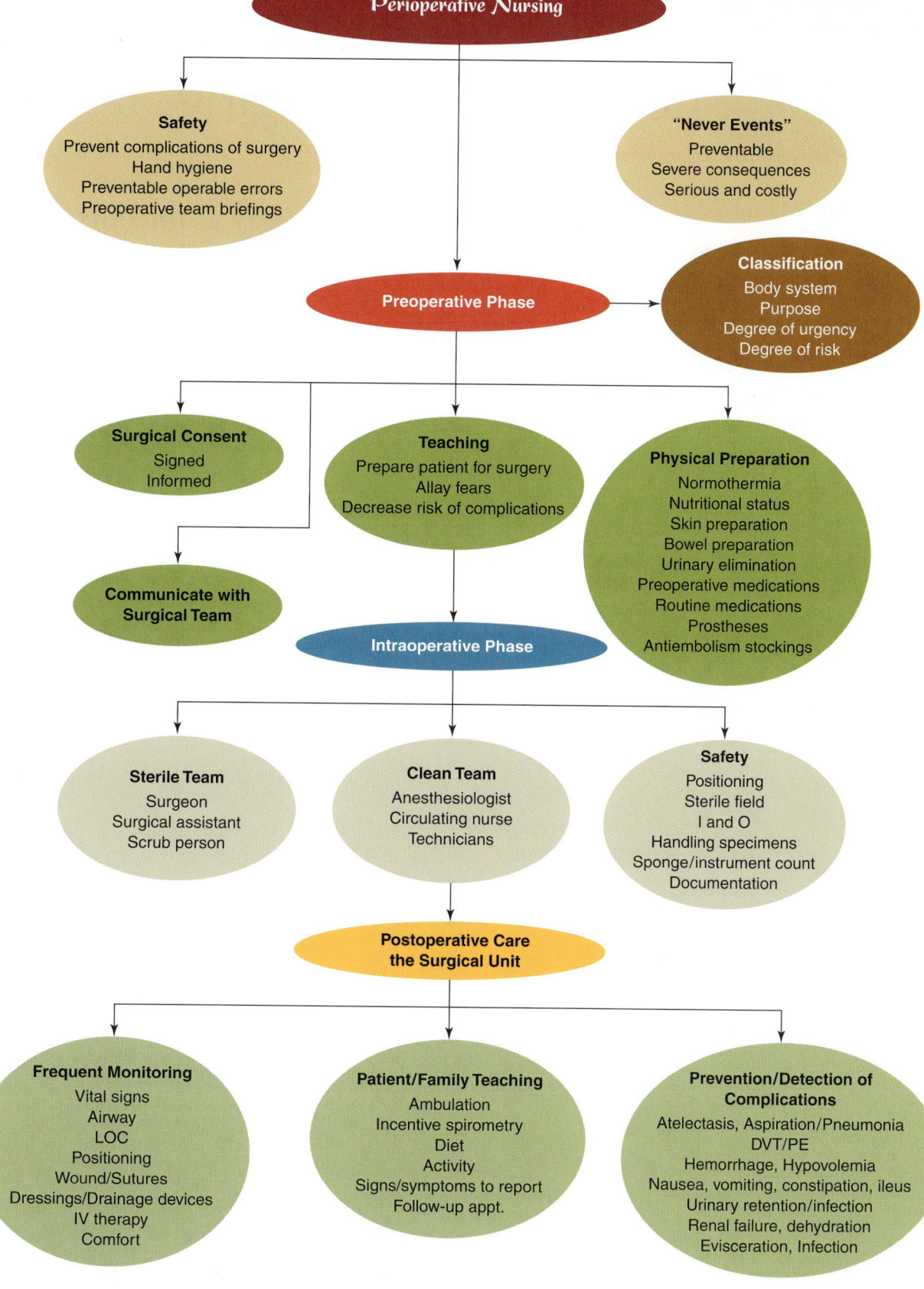

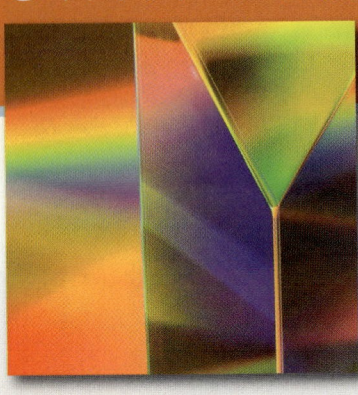

CHAPTER 41

Leading & Managing

Learning Outcomes

After completing this chapter, you should be able to:

➤ Distinguish between leadership, followership, and management.

➤ Compare and contrast authoritarian, democratic, and laissez-faire leadership styles.

➤ Explain the differences between transactional and transformational theories.

➤ Discuss the qualities, behaviors, and strategies that contribute to effective leadership and followership.

➤ Discuss the qualities and activities that contribute to effective management.

➤ Explain how a SWOT analysis and a SOAR analysis are used in leading and managing.

➤ Discuss the qualities of preceptors and mentors.

➤ Describe the challenges presented to nurse managers by the economy and the nursing labor market.

➤ Describe several ways to empower nurses.

➤ Discuss the importance of effective communication skills to nurse leaders and managers.

➤ Describe the change process, including methods to decrease resistance to change.

➤ Describe the major concepts of conflict, conflict resolution, and informal negotiation.

➤ Describe the major concepts of safe and effective delegation.

➤ Establish short- and long-term personal and career goals.

➤ Develop effective time management strategies.

Key Concepts

Change
Followership
Leadership
Management

Related Concepts

See the Concept Map at the end of this chapter.

Portions of this chapter were taken from Weiss, S., & Tappen, R. (2014). *Essentials of nursing leadership and management* (6th ed.). Philadelphia, PA: F. A. Davis. Used with permission.

Meet Your Peer

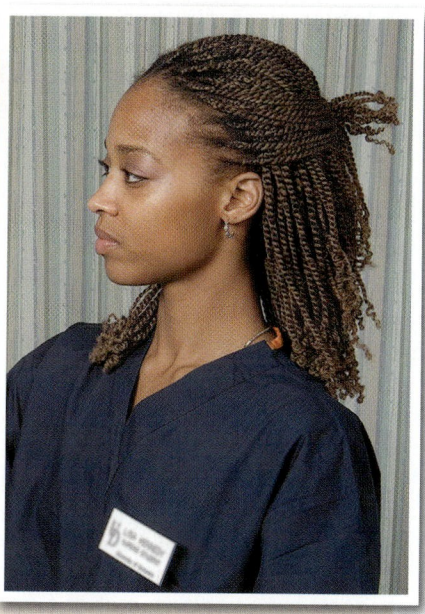

Mary is a student in a nursing program. She considers herself a "pretty good test-taker" and has a GPA of 3.4. She received her first test grade in the Nursing Fundamentals class, and it was a C. Mary is sure that she will never pass this course and that her dream of becoming a nurse will vanish. When discussing the test with her classmates, she realized there are several other disappointed students who have been used to making As and Bs on exams. The nursing exams seem different, because they not only ask students to recall memorized material but also apply what they have learned. Mary decides to get the group together and plan some strategies for study groups. She asks the instructor whether she will meet with them and review their plan to ensure they are on the right track. In so doing, Mary has exhibited some leadership qualities.

Theoretical Knowledge
knowing why

In this chapter, we discuss the challenges to nurses as they lead and manage others in organizations and healthcare environments. The theoretical knowledge you will need to begin professional practice includes an understanding of change, conflict, delegation, and time-management principles.

ABOUT THE KEY CONCEPTS

Have you ever heard the phrase "Not every good leader can manage, and not every good manager can lead"? This chapter differentiates between the key concepts of leadership and management. To lead and manage effectively, you will also need to grasp and apply the key concepts of **leadership, management, followership,** and **change,** as well as the subconcepts of power, empowerment, conflict resolution, delegation, and time management. As you study each of those concepts, think about how they relate to leadership and management.

WHAT IS LEADERSHIP?

You may be thinking, "I just started in my nursing program. How can you expect me to be a leader now?" Although you do need time to learn how nurses function in a work environment, you can begin to assume some leadership skills as a student. **KEY POINT:** *The essence of leadership is the ability to influence other people and motivate action toward a common goal.* Effective leaders enable people to move "in the same direction, toward the same destination, at the same speed, not because they have been forced to, but because they want to" (Lansdale, 2002, p. 63; Gonzalez, 2012). A leader in healthcare has three primary tasks:

- Set direction (i.e., help people develop vision, a mission, goals, and purpose).
- Build commitment (i.e., help people develop motivation, team spirit, and teamwork; inspire others to act).

- Confront challenges that arise from innovation, change, and turbulence (Grindel, 2016; Porter-O'Grady & Malloch, 2014).

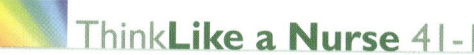

Think Like a Nurse 41-1

1. Think of a goal your class might have. Obviously, each student wants to develop the skills necessary to provide excellent client care and learn the theory content to pass the course and continue in the program. What other goals might you have as a group? As a leader, how might you help the group meet their goals?
2. Brainstorm with your peers to identify some shared goals of professional nurses.

Leadership Theories

How does a person become a leader? What type of leader is most effective? Despite much research on these questions, no theory has yet emerged as the clear answer. The reason may be that different situations require different qualities and behaviors. Let's look now at some of the best-known leadership theories, beginning with some of the early ones.

Trait Theories Early leadership research attempted to identify the qualities, or traits, that distinguish a leader from a nonleader. The traits most often identified are intelligence, initiative, self-confidence, high self-esteem, emotional stability, willingness to take risks, and ability to tolerate the consequences of taking risks (Northouse, 2015; White & Lippitt, 1960). **KEY POINT:** *Although leadership may come more naturally to some than to others, almost anyone can gain the necessary knowledge and skills to be a leader in certain areas.*

Behavioral Theories Leadership is viewed as a personality trait under behavior theories. The focus is on what the leader does. One influential theory identifies three styles used by leaders (Northouse, 2015; White & Lippitt, 1960).

- **Authoritarian Leadership.** This type of leadership, also called *autocratic, directive,* or *controlling,* is an efficient way to achieve high productivity when a group needs lots of direction (Marquis & Huston, 2014). The **authoritarian**

leader gives direction, makes the final decisions, and bears most of the responsibility for the outcomes. For example, when a decision needs to be made, an authoritarian leader would say, "I've given this a great deal of thought and decided this is the way we're going to solve our problem." When used with skilled workers or over a long time, this style can inhibit creativity and motivation. Authoritarian leadership may be either punitive or kind and compassionate.

- **Democratic Leadership.** Also called a *participative leader,* the **democratic leader** shares the planning, decision making, and responsibility for outcomes with other members of the group. This type of leader tends to provide guidance rather than control. Although viewed as less efficient, group output tends to be of high quality. It is more flexible and fosters motivation and creativity.

- **Laissez-Faire Leadership.** Also called *permissive* or *nondirective* leadership, laissez-faire leadership gives followers control in the decision-making process. A **laissez-faire leader** has a relatively inactive style and intervenes only when goals have not been met or a problem arises (Zineldin & Hytter, 2012). Some mature individuals thrive under laissez-faire leadership because they need little guidance. However, followers who look to the leader for direction may become confused and frustrated with no specified goal, guidance, or direction. The laissez-faire leader offers little feedback and support to followers and postpones or fails to make decisions, which leads to poor quality and inefficient work output. Mature, skilled workers may thrive under this type of leader.

KnowledgeCheck 41-1

- Identify the three common styles of leadership in the behavioral theories of leadership.
- Discuss the type of follower who would benefit from each style of leadership.

Task Versus Relationship Theories Another important distinction in leadership style is the one between a task focus and a relationship focus (Blake, Mouton, & Tapper, 1981; Bortoluzzi, Caporale, & Palese, 2014). Some leaders emphasize the tasks (e.g., keeping the nursing station neat, getting charting done) and fail to realize the importance of interpersonal relationships (e.g., healthcare team treating one another with respect) on employee morale and productivity. Others focus on the interpersonal aspects and ignore the quality of job performance. The most effective leader is able to balance the two, attending to both the task and the relationship aspects of working together.

Emotional Intelligence Theory (EI) focuses on the ability of leaders to manage their emotions and of those of their followers (Grindel, 2016). These leaders possess the following traits:

- *Empathy*—Able to make emotional connections with others.
- *Self-awareness*—Recognize and understand their own emotions.
- *Self-management*—Control their personal emotions.
- *Relationship management*—Use self-emotions to successfully interact with and manage others. Ability to build trust, respect, and cooperation within the team (Sadri, 2012).
- *Social awareness*—Accurately assess and respond to the emotions of others. Ability to listen and accurately interpret unspoken emotions.

Situational Theories People and leadership situations are far more complex than the early theories recognized. Instead of assuming one approach works in all situations, situational theories emphasize that it is important to (1) understand all of the factors that affect a particular group of people in a particular environment, and (2) vary the type of leadership to meet the needs of the rapidly changing situations (Giltinane, 2013).

KEY POINT: *Adaptability is the key to the situational approach.* For example, a nurse who is in charge of a code situation must give clear, direct instructions in a calm, confident manner. Conversely, a nurse who develops a policy regarding nurse to client ratios will need to elicit input from the staff.

Transformational Theories Situational theories do not address meaning, inspiration, and vision, which are the distinguishing features of transformational leadership theory. Transformational leaders aspire to meet the self-actualization needs of their followers. People need a sense of purpose and vision that goes beyond good interpersonal relationships or the reward for a job well done (Giltinane, 2013; Grindel, 2016).

Transformational leaders engage and empower others to accomplish the mission, creating feelings of loyalty, trust, inspiration, and satisfaction. They create a supportive climate, listen, and act as a coach and mentor. Followers become motivated to go beyond their own self-interests for the good of the group or organization, often accomplishing more than what would normally be expected of them (Doody & Doody, 2012). This is especially true in nursing. Caring for people, sick or well, is the goal of our profession. Most of us chose nursing for our vision: to do something for the good of humankind. Our nursing leaders empower us toward achieving that vision.

The American Nurses Credentialing Center's (ANCC) Magnet Model is a framework to achieve excellence in nursing practice. It recognizes transformational leadership as an essential component of the model (ANCC, 2015). Leaders in Magnet organizations are expected to demonstrate the transformational qualities listed in Table 41-1.

Transactional Theories assume that people are motivated by reward and punishment and that they work best within a clear chain of command and a structured environment. The structure usually includes position descriptions, policies and procedures, and formal systems of discipline. The traditional employer–employee relationship exemplifies transactional, wherein workers are rewarded with a salary and benefits for performance of their duties and disciplined for nonperformance. Leaders may be tasked oriented, enforce rules, and provide guidance to workers. When the demand for a skill—or for workers of a specific type—is greater than the supply, the usual rewards may not be sufficient, and other types of leadership are more effective.

ThinkLike a Nurse 41-2

- Observe a nurse in one of the healthcare agencies at which you are doing a clinical rotation. What leadership qualities and behaviors do you see the nurse exhibiting?
- How do these behaviors help in planning nursing care?

WHAT IS MANAGEMENT?

Whereas leaders may or may not have official appointments to the position, managers are usually formally designated. A **manager** is an employee of an organization who has the power, authority, and responsibility for enforcing decisions,

Table 41-1 ▶ Contrast of Traits in Transactional and Transformational Leadership

TRANSACTIONAL LEADERSHIP	TRANSFORMATIONAL LEADERSHIP
Directive	Participative
Top down	Bottom up
Information	Conversation
Hierarchical communication	Matrix communication
Event oriented	Future oriented
Task focused	Overall experience focused
Directed	Facilitated
Rigid	Flexible
Here and now	Visions for the future
Traditional	Contemporary
Rules	Risk taking
Control	Creativity
Individual performance	Team and relationships
Responsibility	Accountability

Source: Used with permission of Patricia Davis, RN, DNP, MS, NEA-BC, CNL; Concord, CA.

planning, organizing, coordinating, and directing the work of others. Every nurse should be a good leader and a good follower; however, not everyone can or should be a manager. As you read further, you may notice that management overlaps a great deal with the content on leadership. That is because managers have leadership responsibilities and exhibit varying styles of leadership. **KEY POINT:** *Not all leaders should be managers, but all managers should be leaders.*

As a registered nurse (RN), you will manage groups of clients, and will be responsible for supervising nursing assistants, licensed practical nurses, and ancillary staff. You may be interested to know that the NCLEX-RN® Testing Plan has an entire section devoted to management of care, which is about organizing and delivering (managing) care to the client. Even as a staff nurse, you will be a manager of care.

Management Theories

Although there are many management theories, the two major schools of thought in management are (1) scientific management, which emphasizes the task aspects of managing people, and (2) the human relations approach to management, with emphasis on the relationship aspects.

Scientific Management Almost 100 years ago, Frederick Taylor argued that most jobs could be done more efficiently if they were thoroughly analyzed (Locke, 1982). Given a properly designed task and sufficient incentive to get the work done, workers would be more productive because repetition promotes efficiency. For example, Taylor encouraged paying people "by the piece," that is, by the number of "widgets" made rather than by the number of hours worked (Taylor, 1911/2011). This encourages workers to get the most quality work done in the least amount of time. In healthcare, the equivalent would be to pay for the number of tasks completed (e.g., IVs started; clients bathed).

Human Relations–Based Management McGregor's (1960) Theory X and Theory Y are good examples of the difference between scientific management and human relationships.

- **Theory X.** Managers believe that most people do not want to work very hard and that the manager's job is to make sure that they do work hard. Per Theory X, a manager needs to use strict rules, constant supervision, and the threat of punishment (e.g., reprimands, withheld raises, and threats of job loss) to create industrious, conscientious workers. Theory X is similar to scientific management.
- **Theory Y.** Managers believe that work itself can be motivating, that people want to do their jobs well, and that they will work hard if their managers provide a supportive atmosphere. A Theory Y manager emphasizes guidance over control, development rather than close supervision, and reward over punishment.

A Theory Y nurse manager is human-relations oriented. He is concerned with keeping staff morale as high as possible, assuming that satisfied, motivated staff will do the best work. Such a manager would make an effort to work out conflicts and promote mutual understanding among the staff to provide an atmosphere in which people can do their best work.

Servant Leadership Despite its name, servant leadership applies more to supervisors and administrators than to nurses in staff positions. This type of leader assumes the role to selflessly serve others, cultivates a culture of trust, seeks diverse opinions, and works to develop other leaders (Brown & Bryant, 2015). He is committed to improving the way each employee is treated at work, removing barriers, making the work easier, and providing employees with whatever they need to provide quality client care. The servant leadership manager believes people have value as people, not just as workers and places the employee first.

Qualities of an Effective Manager

Two-thirds of people who leave their jobs say the main reason was an ineffective or incompetent manager (Ripper, 2013). Given the high costs associated with orientation of new employees, nurse managers are challenged to retain staff nurses. Effective leadership styles of nurse managers and administrators can enhance staff nurse retention (Blake, Leach, Robbins, et al., 2013). An effective nurse manager has the following combination of qualities: None of the qualities alone is enough.

- **Leadership.** Effective managers must understand people, leadership, and power. They must have competencies in emotional intelligence, staff and client advocacy, communication, and collaboration (Cleary, Horsfall, Jackson, et al., 2013; Grindel, 2016).
- **Clinical Expertise.** Nurse managers need a strong knowledge base, acquired through clinical experiences, education, training, and professional development, to ensure clients receives quality care (Grindel, 2016). They readily respond to clinical situations and promote professional accountability.
- **Business Sense.** Nurse managers must be knowledgeable of practice structures (lines of authority), budgets, and how the cost of nursing services aligns within the overall hospital

and unit budgets (Grindel, 2016). They analyze the time needed to provide client care, the effectiveness of care, reimbursement rated, and revenue sources (private insurance, government subsidy, or self-pay). This requires knowledge of budgeting, staffing, and measuring outcomes, most of which are beyond the scope of this textbook.

Activities of an Effective Manager

Mintzberg (1989) divides the manager's activities into three categories: interpersonal, decisional, and informational. Weiss and Tappen (2014) build on that work.

Interpersonal Activities

Interpersonal activities are important to both leaders and managers. In fact, they are important to everyone! From the beginning of your nursing education, you will have many opportunities to develop positive working relationships with members of other disciplines and units within the organization. Can you see how Mary (Meet Your Peer) would need interpersonal skills to accomplish her goals?

Interpersonal activities of managers include the following:

- *Networking.* Managers must clearly articulate nurses' roles in and value to the institution.
- *Conflict negotiation and resolution.* For example, conflict may arise on a unit over work schedules, especially on holidays.
- *Advocacy.* Managers must advocate for and support staff to upper level management.
- *Employee development.* This includes providing for continuing learning and upgrading employees' skills.
- *Rewards and punishments.* Examples include salary increases, time off, and praise.
- *Coaching.* The goal is to help the employee do a better job through learning. Some managers use a directive approach ("Let me show you how to do this"). Others use a nondirective approach ("How do you think we can improve our outcomes?").

Decisional Activities

Nurse managers must make decisions to enhance unit efficiency, retain personnel, improve client outcomes, and promote interdisciplinary collaboration. Decisions made include the following:

- *Employee evaluation,* including conducting formal performance appraisals
- *Resource allocation* (e.g., budgeting and how to use available funds wisely)
- *Hiring and terminating* employees
- *Planning* for future changes (e.g., in budgets or client populations)
- *Job analysis and redesign* (e. g., improve efficiency)
- *Unit-based decisions* (e.g., staffing policies, space utilization, interdisciplinary collaboration)

See if you can identify the decisions Mary (Meet Your Peer) made.

Informational Responsibilities

Managers also have informational responsibilities and roles, including the following:

- *Spokesperson.* Nurse managers relay information from administration to staff members and speak with administration on behalf of staff members.
- *Monitor.* Nurse managers monitor the activities of their units or departments (e.g., the number of clients seen, length of stay), as well as the staff (e.g., absenteeism) and the budget (e.g., money spent).

- *Public Relations.* Nurse managers share information with clients, staff members, and employers, for example, regarding new developments in healthcare and policy changes.

What kinds of information do you think Mary (Meet Your Peer) would need to communicate to the students interested in forming a study group?

KnowledgeCheck 41-2

- How is transformational leadership different from the other theories of leadership?
- Define *manager*.
- In McGregor's management theory, which is more like scientific management: Theory X or Theory Y?

HOW CAN I PREPARE TO BECOME A LEADER AND MANAGER?

Besides learning the role of the RN, you should begin to look at the skills employers think you need to be ready to work for them. Along with passing the NCLEX-RN examination to obtain nursing licensure, employers cite the skills listed in Box 41-1 as desirable in job candidates (Ghannadian, 2013; Villarreal, 2002). These skills will assist you as you progress through your nursing program and will also make your adjustment to the RN role much easier. Note that leaders and managers also use these skills in the performance of their responsibilities. It is not too early to begin to develop your abilities in these areas.

One of the first steps in identifying what skills you already possess and which you need to develop is to do a brief SWOT analysis. A SWOT (strengths, weaknesses, opportunities, threats) analysis plan, borrowed from the corporate world, can guide you through an analysis of your own internal strengths and weaknesses and reveal external opportunities and threats that may help or hinder your leadership and management skills (Orr, 2013). Your SWOT analysis may include the factors listed as examples in Table 41-2, but certainly you will have others.

You might prefer to use the SOAR (strengths, opportunities, aspirations, results) strategic planning model to help you prepare to become a leader and manager (Table 41-3). This model can be used to analyze any type of situation and create a plan to achieve personal and professional goals. With this

---

BOX 41-1 ■ Desirable Job Candidate Skills

- Ability to adapt equipment to serve user needs
- Ability to assume responsibility
- Ability to teach others
- Computer knowledge
- Critical-thinking and analytical skills
- Interpersonal skills
- Flexibility to adjust action in relation to others
- Leadership abilities
- Motivation, initiative, and flexibility
- Oral and written communication skills
- Organizational skills
- Problem-solving and decision-making abilities
- Proficiency in field of study or technical competence
- Self-discipline
- Teamwork ability
- Willingness to work hard

Table 41-2 ▶ SWOT Analysis Plan—Examples

STRENGTHS	WEAKNESSES	OPPORTUNITIES	THREATS
Relevant work experience	Poor communication and people skills	Changes in healthcare	Changes in healthcare
Advanced education	Underdeveloped organizational skills	Availability of mentors and preceptors	Lack of time
Good communication and people skills	Poor time management skills	Variety of experiences in clinical rotations	Competition from other students and other nursing programs
Computer skills	Difficulty adapting to change; inflexibility	Many leadership and management resources and self-learning programs available	

SWOT = Strengths, Weaknesses, Opportunities, Threats

Table 41-3 ▶ SOAR Strategic Planning

THE PROCESS: HOW TO SOAR	THE SOAR REPORT OR SUMMARY
To SOAR: Inquire, imagine, innovate, and inspire.	Use SOAR to report or tell your story.
Inquiry: Internal analysis of strengths and external analysis of opportunities.	**Strengths.** My (or the group's) strengths are . . . (Examples of strengths may be a supportive environment, individual strengths, a product that others need, etc.)
Imagination: Co-create vision, values, and mission. Imagine desired outcomes. Imagine the best pathway to achieve the outcomes.	**Opportunities.** My values are . . . (e.g., dedication, quality). As I imagine the future, my vision (for myself, for our group) is . . . (e.g., to become a transformational manager on a nursing unit).
Innovation: Create initiatives, strategies, structures, and systems. Create plans for tactics.	**Aspirations.** Here is how I believe I (or we) can achieve the desired outcomes . . .
Inspiration: Inspire action-oriented activities that achieve results. Implement a plan for continuous improvement.	**Results.** To achieve your desired outcomes, you must be motivated (and possibly need to inspire others) to take the necessary actions.

SOAR = Strengths, Opportunities, Aspirations, Results
Source: Adapted from Stavros, J., Cooperrider, D., & Kelley, D. (2009). SOAR: A new approach to strategic planning. In P. Holman, T. Devane, S. Dady, et al. (Eds.), *The change handbook: The definitive resource on today's best methods for engaging whole systems* (pp. 268–285). San Francisco, CA: Berrett-Koehler.

model, you would use inquiry, imagination, and innovation while focusing on strengths, opportunities, aspirations, and results (Stavros & Cole, 2013).

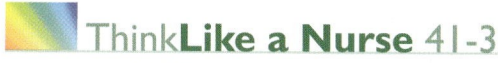

ThinkLike a Nurse 41-3

Stop and think! Take some time to personalize the SWOT analysis in Table 41-2. What weaknesses do you need to minimize, or which strengths do you need to develop as you begin to develop your leadership and management skills?

How Can Mentors and Preceptors Help Me?

There are two aspects to consider as you get ready to become a leader and manager. The first part consists of developing self. The second part is a combination of developing self and developing others: mentorship and preceptorship. A **mentor** is someone more experienced who provides career development assistance, such as coaching, sponsoring advancement, providing challenging assignments, protecting protégés from adversity, and promoting positive visibility. Mentors provide guidance to new students or recent graduates as they continue in the profession. They offer a constructive example as a role model to novices. Mentors can also fulfill psychosocial roles, such as personal support, friendship, acceptance, role modeling, and counseling. ✚ You should always use sound judgment when following the advice of others. Do not blindly engage in behaviors or actions because others are engaging in them.

Many organizations have preceptors for new employees. A preceptor is an experienced nurse who provides practical teaching and guidance for a student or new employee. As a student, you may be assigned an RN preceptor in your clinical rotations (Fig. 41-1). You may work with a preceptor to provide client care as a student and as a new nurse. In many instances, the preceptor will become your mentor. However, the mentor role is much more encompassing than the preceptor role. The mentor relationship is a voluntary one and is built on mutual respect and development of the mentee. Box 41-2 identifies responsibilities of the mentor and mentee in this relationship.

You should look for a competent mentor in the nursing program right now—someone to guide you as you grow into your professional role. A student who has already completed several semesters and appears to be a leader is a good choice. In some programs, you may be assigned a student preceptor while you are in the program. Although this student may or may not become your mentor, you will need to have leadership and management skills to work effectively together.

Will you assume the role of preceptor or mentor while you are still in school? We hope your response is yes. As you

progress in the program, remember the feelings of uncertainly and anxiety that you may now have, and volunteer to mentor another new student. Through the mentoring process, you can continue to develop yourself as a leader. Mentoring and precepting are part of your professional responsibilities, as the American Nurses Association (ANA) Standard of Nursing Practice 11, Leadership, (2015) states:

The registered nurse mentors colleagues for the advancement of nursing practice and the profession to enhance safe, quality health care. (p. 75)

How Will Leadership Grow in My Nursing Career?

As you begin your nursing clinical experiences, your nursing instructor will supervise most of your decisions. As you continue to develop your knowledge and skills, you will begin working more as a member of the team. You will be expected to work with clients' family members and the multidisciplinary healthcare team. You will prioritize interventions in providing care to clients. You may go to community agencies and network with groups. To be successful in your continued role development as a nurse, you must work on perfecting the skills discussed in this chapter.

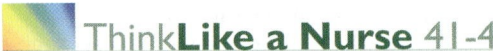

KnowledgeCheck 41-3

- Identify four skills that employers cite as desirable in job candidates.
- Identify three responsibilities of a mentor and three responsibilities of a mentee.

ThinkLike a Nurse 41-4

Think about how you are working with your peers now. What mentor responsibilities are you exhibiting? Is there someone who is already mentoring you? If so, what qualities does this person exhibit?

WHAT IS FOLLOWERSHIP?

Leadership and followership are two separate concepts and roles that are complementary, not competitive. Great leaders can create successful followers, and great followers create successful leaders. No one person can have the best strategy, have the clearest vision, or identify the most effective approaches to solve problems. All participants need to be recognized as full partners in the organizational venture. If we define **followers** as individuals who take another person as a role model and

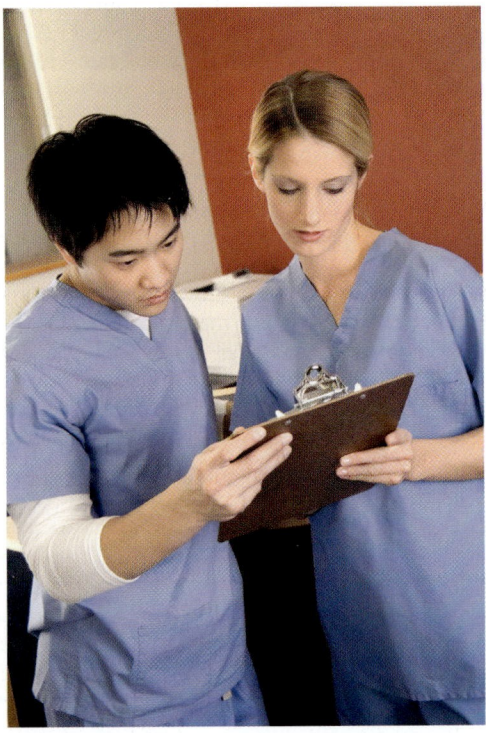

FIGURE 41-1 Nurse precepting a new graduate.

BOX 41-2 ■ Mentor and Mentee Responsibilities

Mentor Responsibilities

- Demonstrate excellent communication and listening skills.
- Be sensitive to the needs of nurses, clients, and the workplace.
- Encourage excellence in others.
- Share and provide counsel.
- Exhibit good decision-making skills.
- Demonstrate an understanding of power and politics.
- Demonstrate trustworthiness.

Mentee Responsibilities

- Demonstrate eagerness to learn.
- Participate actively in the relationship by keeping all appointments and commitments.
- Seek feedback and use it to modify behaviors.
- Demonstrate flexibility and an ability to change.
- Be open in the relationship with the mentor.
- Demonstrate an ability to move toward independence.
- Evaluate choices and outcomes.

Source: Weiss, S., & Tappen, R. (2014). *Essentials of nursing leadership and management* (6th ed.). Philadelphia, PA: F.A. Davis.

who act in accordance with, imitate, support, and advocate the ideas and opinions of another (Grossman & Valiga, 2012), then we can define **followership** as the willingness to work with others toward accomplishing the group mission. This term also refers to those who show a high degree of teamwork and build cohesion among the group (Thomas & Berg, 2014).

An *organization* is a community of many leaders and many followers, frequently changing places depending on the activity that is occurring. Blindly following a leader without question or taking a passive role in one's work or professional organization will do little to advance the profession, promote individual growth, or achieve quality client care. To participate fully and provide significant feedback, followers need to demonstrate important qualities and behaviors (Grossman & Valiga, 2012; Hoption, 2014):

- Suggest ways to improve client care.
- If you discover a problem, inform your team leader right away and propose a solution if you can. If it is not accepted, your job is then to support—not undermine—the leader and continue to seek an effective solution.
- Listen carefully and reflect on what the leader or manager says.
- Be truthful. Give honest feedback and constructive criticism, even if it means politely challenging the leader's ideas. Suggest alternative courses of action.
- If you feel you must have a "heated" discussion with the leader, do so privately. When you disagree, explain why.
- Freely invest your interest and energy in your work and in finding best solutions for the group.
- Function independently; be a self-starter; take on extra tasks without being asked.
- Be innovative, creative, and actively involved.
- Be responsible and hold up your end of the bargain; accept responsibility when it is offered.
- Be supportive of new ideas and directions suggested by others, but think critically about ideas that are proposed. Seek information so you can see the larger picture.
- Don't gossip. Present situations objectively.
- Think and act as a team; be cooperative and collaborative.
- Draw on and complement one another's and the leader's specialties, strengths, and areas of expertise.
- Work on behalf of the organization and the mutually agreed on vision and goals.
- Continue to learn as much as you can about your specialty area; share what you learn with others.
- Know your own strengths and what can be your unique contributions to the effort.
- Know how to assume the role of the leader when necessary.
- Have a positive sense of self-worth and a "can do" attitude.
- Take care of yourself and your family. If you and they are unhappy, your job performance will suffer.

WHAT ARE THE CHALLENGES TO BEING AN EFFECTIVE LEADER AND MANAGER?

Even after you have developed the skills necessary to become an effective leader or manager, challenges exist in the healthcare environment. These challenges include the economic climate of healthcare and the nursing labor market.

Economic Climate of Healthcare

For many years, decisions about care were based primarily on providing the best quality care, whatever the cost. More recently, however, healthcare providers are pressured to seek methods of care delivery that achieve quality outcomes at lower cost. This economic perspective is rooted in three fundamental observations:

1. *Resources are scarce.* The scarcity of resources means that three decisions must be made:

   How much do we spend on healthcare services. And what do those services consist of?

   How will those healthcare services be produced?

   How should, or can, we distribute healthcare? In other words, how are services apportioned within the population?

2. *Resources have alternative uses.* Because resources are limited, a choice to spend resources in one area eliminates the allocation of those same resources for another use. If, for example, we wish to have more nursing homes in the community, then we must be willing to accept fewer hospitals or less housing, education, or other uses of those same resources. In healthcare, an expanded program of immunization may mean limiting care for certain age-groups.

3. *Individuals want different things or have different preferences.* Some people choose alternative treatment modalities such as acupuncture, herbal therapy, or massage therapy rather than traditional healthcare. The assumption exists that preferences for products and services can be influenced—hence, the extensive marketing of healthcare services.

Nursing Labor Market

The number of registered nurses employed in the nurse workforce in the United States is at 3.1 million (Kaiser Family Foundation, 2016) and continues to grow. There are 61% registered nurses employed in hospitals (Bureau of Labor Statistics, U.S. Department of Labor, 2015). More than half of RNs work at least 40 hours a week in their principal position, and another 24% work 32 to 39 hours per week (U.S. Department of Health and Human Services, 2013).

The Bureau of Labor Statistics predicted there would be more than 1 million vacant positions for registered nurses by 2020 (Robert Wood Johnson Foundation, 2013). The need for nurses is expected to increase even more dramatically as the baby boomers reach their 60s, 70s, and beyond. From now until 2030, the population aged 65 and older will double. The questions are (1) whether there will be enough nurses available to fill those jobs, and (2) even if nurses are available, whether it will be economically feasible for organizations to hire as many as they need. The Affordable Care Act has increased the demand for advanced practice registered nurse practitioners.

Historical trends show that cost control and demand for nursing services will impact nurse staffing patterns, the model of care, and professional nursing practice. These changes will affect you, the nurse. Regardless of the changes, healthcare system changes will likely demand that the RN lead and manage personnel delivering client care while maintaining fiscal responsibility. Even though government and other agencies heavily regulate healthcare, it is a big business. You must juggle the needs of your clients with the needs of the organization. From time to time, think about how we might do that.

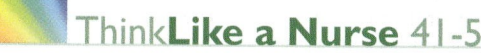 Think**Like a Nurse** 41-5

Identify changes in your community that will affect you as you embark upon your nursing career. What will you do to prepare for these changes?

WHAT ARE POWER AND EMPOWERMENT?

The leadership and management techniques discussed so far will help you to achieve your goals. However, there are times when your attempts to influence others are overwhelmed by other forces or individuals. Where does this power come from? Who has it? Who does not?

Although people at the top have most of the *authority* in an organization, they do not have all of the *power*. In fact, people at the bottom of the hierarchy also have some power. **Power** is the ability of a person to get things done and is created through both formal and informal systems (Laschinger, Wong, Cummings, et al., 2014). Power may be use to facilitate growth and productivity within an organization or can be the basis for stagnation and decreased morale.

Sources of Power

Various sources of power are available to nurses, depending on the situation:

- **Positional/legitimate:** A person's authority is derived from her location in the organization's hierarchy. The person at the top has the most power.
- **Referent:** Informal power created through relationships with people within the organization. Power is acquired through the person's ability to influence and gain other's respect.
- **Reward:** The ability of an individual to control or allocate incentives (e.g., promotion, salary increases, recognition, or other benefits).
- **Expertise:** "Knowledge is power" (Bacon, 1597, quoted in Fitton, 1997, p. 150). The person's expertise and analytical skills are deemed critical to the organization.
- **Coercion:** The power to control others through threats or discipline. The person has the authority to enforce standards, policies, and procedures.

Let's look at the types of power available to various groups in a healthcare organization.

Managers have reward power; they reward people with salary increases, promotions, and recognition. They can also use coercion to provide structure and order or to impose economic or psychological pain based on their authority to evaluate and fire people.

Clients at first appear to be relatively powerless in a healthcare organization. However, an organization would eventually cease to exist without clients. They reward healthcare workers by praising them or cause discomfort by complaining about them to supervisors.

Registered nurses have expert, legitimate, and coercion power. They delegate responsibilities to licensed practical nurses (LPNs), nursing assistive personnel (NAPs), and other staff by virtue of their position in the hierarchy and the state's nurse practice act. Nurses are essential to the operation of most healthcare organizations and could cause considerable disruption if they refused to work. They must also ensure others are performing their roles and act if there are deviations from the standards of practice.

Nurses have always had the power of information, or expertise. For example, Florence Nightingale showed very graphically in the 1800s that wherever her nurses were, far fewer patients died; and wherever they were not, far more died. Think of the power of that information. Immediately people were saying, "What would you like, Miss Nightingale?

Would you like more money? Would you like a school of nursing? What else can we do for you?" (Fralic, 2000, p. 340). She had solid data. She knew how to collect, interpret, and distribute the data in terms of things that people valued (Stanley & Sherratt, 2010).

Assistants and Technicians may appear to have less power because of their position in an organization's "top-down" hierarchy. Imagine, though, how the work of the healthcare organization would grind to a halt if all the nursing assistants failed to appear one morning. Therefore, they have both expertise and coercive power.

KnowledgeCheck 41-4

What are the sources of power available to nurses?

Sources of Empowerment

How can nurses, either individually or collectively, maximize their power and increase their feelings of empowerment? To answer this question, you should first distinguish between the concepts of power and empowerment. Recall that *power* is the ability of the person to get things done. **Empowerment** is a psychological state: a feeling that one has been given the power to solve problems, take initiatives, and exercise autonomy. **KEY POINT:** *Given these definitions, it is possible to be powerful and yet not feel empowered. Power refers to action, and empowerment refers to feelings. Both are of interest to nursing leaders and managers.*

Feeling empowered includes the following:

- **Self-determination:** Feeling free to decide how to do your work
- **Meaning:** Caring about your work, enjoying it, and taking it seriously
- **Competence:** Confidence in your ability to do your work well
- **Impact:** Feeling that people listen to your ideas, that you can make a difference

Nurses, like most people, want to have some power and to feel empowered, valued, and respected. Organizations that foster empowerment provided employees with access to information, support systems, required resources to do their job, and the opportunity to learn and grow (Laschinger, Wong, Cummings, et al., 2014). You will feel a sense of empowerment in settings that ensure: (1) manageable, reasonable work assignments; (2) reward, recognition, and appreciation for a job well done; and (3) fair, consistent treatment of all staff.

Enhancing Expertise

Not all empowerment comes from others. You are empowered to some degree by your own professional knowledge and competence. Following are some ways in which you can enhance your competence, thereby increasing your own sense of empowerment:

- **Actively participate** in interdisciplinary team conferences, client-centered conferences, and clinical or governance committees on your unit.
- **Enhance your expertise** by attending continuing education activities. This might include local, regional, national, and international conferences sponsored by nursing organizations.
- **Participate in nursing research projects** or use evidence-based practice guidelines, current nursing journals, and books to make decisions regarding your nursing practice.

- **Discuss with colleagues** how to handle a difficult clinical situation and observe the practices of experienced nurses or other providers. Do not be afraid to ask questions.
- **Continue your education by** earning additional degrees and certifications in nursing.

Although you have just begun your nursing career, it is not too early to begin thinking of ways to become empowered.

Sharing Expertise

You also become empowered by sharing with others your knowledge and experience. This means not only using your knowledge to improve your own practice but also communicating what you have learned to other students and, later, to your colleagues in nursing. It also means informing and demonstrating to your instructors and supervisors that you have enhanced your professional competence. You can share your knowledge with your clients, empowering them as well. As you gain expertise in a clinical area or skill set, you can share it by writing an article for publication.

PracticalKnowledge
knowing **how**

As a leader or manager, you will need to get people to work together to make things happen. To do so, you will need to communicate effectively, delegate, deal with conflict and change, and manage your time appropriately. These can be thought of as skills or processes (or practical knowledge).

COMMUNICATING

Leaders use communication to develop relationships with other people and to engage and support these relationships. Some view communication as a circular process that is affected by many factors. This means the activity is continuous and mutually interdependent, and influenced by the behaviors of each communicator. You need to use active listening to pick up all levels of meaning in a communication. Surface listening, or inattention, often causes a misinterpretation of the message. Your attitude influences what you hear and how you interpret the message. Communication skills are taught extensively in Chapter 20, if you need to review them now.

To effectively manage client care, it is important to keep the lines of communication open to various individuals (other nurses, interdisciplinary team, client family members). Trust and sincerity enhance communication. Congruence (agreement) between your words and your deeds promotes trust. If you are viewed as trustworthy and sincere, others will be more likely to ask questions, seek clarification, and accept your leadership when they are uncertain of something.

A leader is responsible for providing frequent evaluative feedback. Done poorly, evaluation can be stressful, even injurious. Done well, it promotes professional growth and employee satisfaction. Evaluative feedback is important because it:

- **Reinforces constructive behavior.** Positive feedback lets people know which behaviors are most productive and encourages them to continue the behaviors.

Safe, Effective Nursing Care

The Effect of Authority Gradients on Teamwork and Client Safety

Chapter Key Concept: Management, Leadership, Followership

Competencies: Collaborate with the interdisciplinary healthcare team; Provide safe, quality client care

Teamwork and collaboration are influenced by the psychological distance a team member feels between himself and others higher up in the team structure. This is called the *authority gradient*. The greater the authority gradient, the less likely a person is to feel part of a team, question those in authority, or communicate concerns. Research shows that a high authority gradient will impede essential communication that will protect clients from harm. Minimizing the authority gradient has been shown to improve communication, which reduces errors and promotes better client outcomes.

The authority gradient between providers and nurses is very steep and is reinforced by tradition, individual personalities, providers' attitudes, and, at times, nurses' fears of being incorrect. Observe the differences in the authority gradients between experienced nurses and other members of the healthcare team in highly collaborative practice areas (e.g., emergency departments, intensive care units) and new nurses or student nurses.

Team Briefings: To flatten these gradients, team briefings should be an expected routine. Briefings promote clear, effective communication and include introductions all around, review of the client's problems and the treatment plan, and specific requests by providers for input. Briefings create a shared understanding and foster an environment in which team members can and do speak up about any concerns.

Individual Skills: Individually, you can develop your communication skills, adopt an attitude of collaboration, and learn more about how to become a capable team member. To begin this process, consider the following questions and suggested responses:

➤ What are your strengths and weaknesses as a team member? How can you better function as an essential member of the healthcare team?

➤ How can you gain the confidence to question a provider's order or assert your perspective on a client's treatment plan? What do you consider assertive communication?

➤ Are you succinct when you communicate? What structured communication style can you adopt to keep your comments and requests clear?

Sources: Friedman, Z., Hayter, M., Everett, T., et al. (2015). Power and conflict: The effect of a superior's interpersonal behavior on trainees' ability to challenge authority during a simulated airway emergency. *Anaesthesia, 70*(10), 1119–1129; Marx, M. (2014). Examining the structural challenges to communication as experienced by nurse managers in two US hospital settings. *Journal of Nursing Management, 22*(8), 964–973; St. Pierre, M., Scholler, A., Strembski, D., et al. (2012). Do residents and nurses communicate relevant concerns? Simulation study on the influence of the authority gradient. *Der Anaesthesist, 61*(10), 857–866. doi:10.1007/s00101-012-2086-1

- *Discourages unproductive behavior.* Constructive feedback prompts the person to correct inappropriate behavior.
- *Provides recognition.* Praise is an excellent motivator.

DELEGATING

An important aspect of leadership and management is learning how use the nursing process to delegate. This is an essential nursing skill to ensure safe and quality client care. To properly delegate:

- *Assess and diagnose.* You must assess each client's needs before assigning the client to particular team member.
- *Plan goals and interventions.* Set client-specific goals and identify the interventions required to achieve these goals. Mentally identify which staff member is best suited for the task or activities before delegating helps to prevent problems later.
- *Implement.* Next, determine which personnel have the knowledge and skills to care for the client and assign the tasks to the appropriate person.
- *Evaluate.* You are still accountable to oversee care and ensure client care needs have been met. Establish timelines for feedback during the day. This enables all personnel review their care and what still need to be completed. If you must give negative feedback, do so privately.

You will find an extended discussion of delegation in Chapter 7. You might also find helpful the American Nurses Association and National Council of the State Boards of Nursing's (NCSBN) (n.d.) joint statement on delegation and a decision tree to promote proper delegation. For use of the checklist *Five Rights of Delegation* (NCSBN, 2009), see Box 7-2 in Chapter 7.

A manager must first determine the mix of personnel (RN, LVN/LPN, or NAP) required to deliver care on a unit before being able to delegate tasks to individuals. By looking at the needs of each client, you can make an educated decision about which staff members have the appropriate education and skill to deliver safe, quality care.

What If I Lack the Experience to Delegate?

The added responsibility of delegation often causes discomfort for new graduates. You may be accustomed to providing total care for one or more clients but lack the experience of organizing care for groups of clients with other team members. To overcome your discomfort, you need to observe how more experienced nurses delegate to others. Working with a preceptor will also give you experience in delegation.

Become familiar with nursing professional organization guidelines. The ANA has specified that RNs may not delegate the following tasks (Neuman, 2010):

- Initial nursing assessment; follow-up assessments if nursing judgment is indicated
- Nursing diagnosis
- Decisions and judgments about outcomes
- Formulation and approval of a client plan of care
- Interventions that require professional nursing knowledge, decisions, or skills
- Decisions and judgments necessary for the evaluation of client care

The ANA (2002, 2007) issued a position statement on the use of nursing assistive personnel. The list includes direct and indirect client care that may be delegated to NAPs (Box 41-3). Various other nursing personnel can also be used to meet client care needs (Fig. 41-2).

BOX 41-3 ■ Examples of Care That May Be Delegated to Nursing Assistive Personnel

Direct Client Care Activities

- Assisting with activities of daily living: feeding, drinking, ambulating, grooming, toileting, dressing
- Assisting with socializing
- Taking vital signs

Indirect Client Care Activities

- Providing a clean, safe environment
- Providing transport for noncritical clients
- Assisting with stocking nursing units
- Providing messenger and delivery services
- Making beds
- Ordering supplies

What Are the Concerns About Delegating?

Today's healthcare environment requires nurses to delegate. Many nurses voice concerns about the personal risk to their licensure if they delegate inappropriately. The courts have usually ruled that nurses are not liable for the negligence of other workers, provided that the nurse delegated appropriately. State boards of nursing view delegation as within the scope of nursing practice. If you would like further discussion of the legal aspects of delegation, see Chapter 44.

KEY POINT: *Nurses have also expressed concern over the effects of delegation on the quality of client care. When you delegate, you control the delegation. You decide to whom and what you will delegate. Remember you must ensure that the delegation process results in quality client care.*

KnowledgeCheck 41-5

Explain the relationship of delegation and the nursing process.

MANAGING CHANGE

Change is a naturally occurring phenomenon, a part of everyone's life. Every day, we have new experiences, meet new people, and learn new things. We grow up, leave home, graduate from college, begin a new career and, perhaps, a new family as well. Some of these changes are milestones in our lives, ones for which we have prepared and anticipated for some time. Others are entirely unexpected—sometimes welcome and sometimes not. Many are exciting, leading us to new opportunities and challenges. When change occurs too rapidly or comes with high demands, it can make us very uncomfortable.

The Comfort Zone

The basic stages of the change process are unfreezing, change, and refreezing (Lewin, 1951; Shirey, 2013). Figure 41-3 shows the relationship among those stages and the following concepts of comfort zone, the discomfort associated with change, and the establishing of a new comfort zone.

Let's assume that your daily routine was basically stable before you started your nursing program. You took care of the family or worked during the day and took a class or two each term. You knew what to expect and how to deal with whatever problems arose. In other words, you were operating within

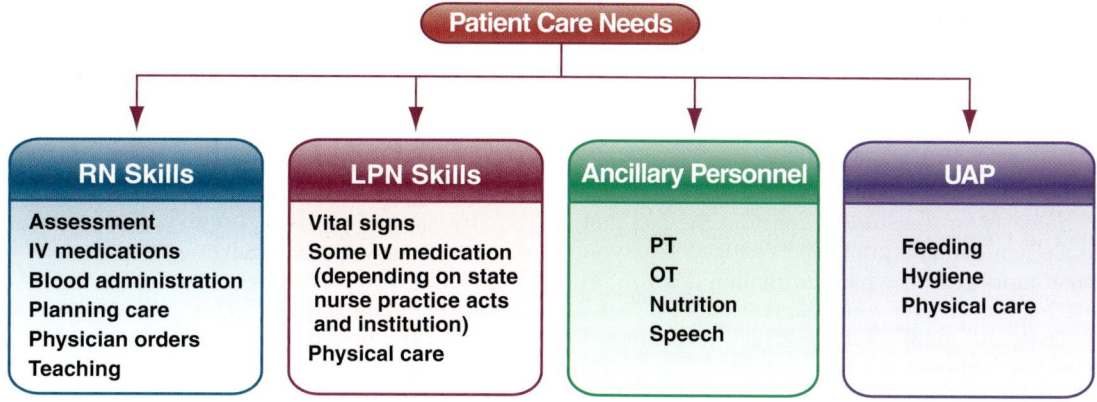

FIGURE 41-2 Patient care needs.

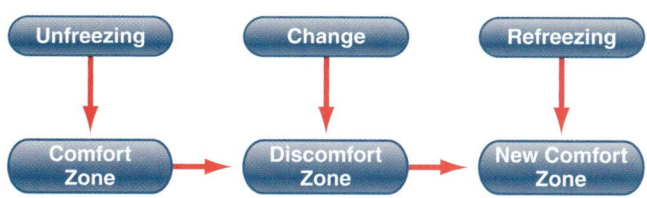

FIGURE 41-3 The change process.

your "comfort zone" (Farrell & Broude, 1987; Lapp, 2002; Ryder, 2013). A big change is likely to move you out of your comfort zone into disequilibrium, possibly into discomfort. Now you may be juggling changes in finances, child-care arrangements, and planning options for your future career. This first stage in the change process is called *unfreezing*. You are moving out of your comfort zone.

Resistance to Change

People resist change for a variety of reasons. For example, you may find that that you can manage the change in class schedule, but that the child-care arrangements are more difficult. Resistance to change (and *unfreezing*) comes from three major sources: technical concerns, psychosocial needs, and threats to a person's position and power. For a student, so-called technical concerns may involve practical issues related to transportation to school or work, getting children to school, or managing household responsibilities.

Recall in Maslow's (1970) hierarchy of needs theory, the more basic needs (e.g., physiological and safety needs) must be at least partially met before a person is motivated to seek fulfillment of the higher-order needs. Once status, power, and influence are gained within families and organizations, they are hard to give up. You may be the one in charge in the family or work situation, yet be a novice in the nursing program.

Recognizing Resistance

It is easy to recognize resistance to a change when it is directly expressed. When a person says to you, "That's not a very good idea," or "I will quit if I can't get better grades," or "There's no way I'm going to do that," there is no doubt that you are meeting resistance. When resistance is less direct, however, you may not recognize it unless you know what to look for.

Resistance may be active or passive.

- **Active resistance** can take the form of aggressive actions or outright refusals to comply, negative communications designed to demean the idea or the person who suggested it,

quoting existing rules that make the change difficult to implement, or organizing others to resist the change.
- **Passive resistance** involves avoidance, such as canceling meetings to discuss implementing the change; being "too busy" to implement the change; or agreeing to the change, but citing numerous barriers to it.

ThinkLike a Nurse 41-6

Recall one change that you have experienced that was put into effect by a command, new rule, policy, or law

- What effects did this change have on your life (e.g., work, school, home)?
- How did the command make you feel?
- What would have made this change easier for you?

Lowering Resistance

KEY POINT: *A change that is welcomed by one group may be strongly resisted by another group. Resistance to change is affected by the leadership approach and the type of organizational structure.*

You can use various approaches to lower people's resistance to change. Strategies fall into four categories: commanding, change/sharing information, refuting currently held beliefs, and providing psychological safety (Weiss & Tappen, 2014).

Commanding Change Obviously, the quickest way to implement change, if you have the authority to do so, is to issue a command. Dictating change is not necessarily the best strategy, but it is sometimes necessary when the change must be made quickly. Commanding a change may not be effective if there are ways for people to resist, for example, when:

- Passive resistance can undermine the change.
- High motivational levels are necessary to make the change successful.
- People can refuse to implement the change without negative consequences.

Sharing Information Much resistance is simply the result of misunderstandings about a proposed change. Sharing information is usually an effective way to reduce uncertainty and ease transition. Information about the change can be shared on a one-to-one basis, in group meetings, or through written materials distributed as printed matter or by electronic means. For you, as a student, it is important that any changes in the program are communicated to you without delay. You should also communicate any changes in your plans to the appropriate people (e.g., other students, nurse team leader, instructor). You should treat client resistance to change in the same manner. The more information you provide the client, the more likely she will be to cooperate with the change.

Refuting Currently Held Beliefs You can sometimes increase a person's willingness to change simply by providing evidence that his actions or beliefs are inadequate, incorrect, or inefficient. For example, a client may enter the hospital recalling horror stories from friends and family, but may then find that there was no basis for the stories. Consider the fact that your ideas about the nursing program have changed since you first began. What happened, or what information did you receive, that caused you to change your beliefs?

Providing Psychological Safety When a proposed change threatens basic human needs in some way, reducing that threat can lower resistance. This leaves people feeling more comfortable about the change. Although each situation poses different kinds of threats and requires different actions to reduce them, Box 41-4 identifies common strategies to help increase psychological safety and reduce resistance to change.

Implementing the Change

In planning for change, you will already have asked yourself these questions:

> What is the purpose of this change? What are we trying to accomplish?
>
> Is the change necessary?
>
> Is the change technically correct?
>
> Will the change work?
>
> Is there a better way to do this?

After employing some unfreezing strategies (e.g., making the status quo unfavorable), you are ready to make the change that has been so carefully planned. In addition to employing strategies to lower resistance, increase motivation, and help people work well together, consider the following factors related to change:

- **Magnitude of the Change.** Is this a major change that affects almost everything people do, or is it a minor one with little impact on what people do every day?

- **Complexity of the Change.** Is this a difficult change to make? Does it require much new knowledge or skills or both? How long will it take for people to acquire the necessary knowledge and/or skills?

- **Pace of the Change.** How urgent is this change? Can it be done gradually, or must it be implemented all at once?

- **Stress Level of Those Involved.** What is the current stress level of the people involved in this change? Is this the only change that is taking place, or is it just one of many changes taking place? How stressful are these changes? How can I help people keep their stress levels within tolerable bounds?

As indicated earlier, some discomfort is likely to occur with almost any change, but it is important to keep it within tolerable limits. You need enough pressure to get people to pay attention to the change process, but not so much that they are overstressed by it. In other words, you want to raise the heat enough to get them moving, but not so high that they boil over (Battilana & Casciaro, 2013).

Integrating the Change

Integrating the change is the last step. After change is made, it is important to make sure that everyone has moved into a new comfort zone. Ask yourself:

- Is the change well integrated into everyday operations?
- Are people comfortable with it now?
- Is it well accepted and perceived as valuable? If not, why not? What can be done to increase acceptance?
- Is there any residual resistance that could still undermine full integration of the change? If there is, how can this resistance be overcome?

Change "sticks" when, instead of being the new way to do something, it has become "the way we always do things around here" (Kotter, 1999, p. 18; Dean, 2013). Change is an inevitable part of living and working. Your leadership can influence how people respond to change, the amount of stress it causes, and the amount of resistance it provokes. Handled well, most changes can become opportunities for professional growth and development rather than just additional stressors for students, nurses, and their clients.

CONFLICT

Nursing education and healthcare settings bring together people of different ages, genders, income levels, statuses, ethnic groups, educational levels, lifestyles, and professions. They share the goal of maintaining clients' health. Differences of opinion over how to best accomplish goals are a normal part of working with people of various skill levels, backgrounds, and cultures. Each unique individual brings different experiences, beliefs, values, and habits to interactions with others. These differences are a natural part of our being unique individuals and members of different segments of our society. Various pressures and demands in the classroom, clinical setting, and workplace can create problems and conflicts. Any or all of these can interfere with the ability to work together.

Conflicts Occur at All Levels

Conflicts can occur at any level and involve any number of people, including your boss, subordinates, peers, clients, or client families.

- **On the individual level,** they can occur between two people working together on a classroom or clinical project,

---

BOX 41-4 ■ Common Strategies to Increase Psychological Safety and Reduce Resistance to Change

- Point out similarities between old and new procedures.
- Suggest ways in which the change can provide new opportunities and challenges.
- Allow time for learning and practice of any new procedures, if possible, before a change is implemented.
- Recognize the competence and skill of the people involved.
- Involve as many people as possible in both the design and implementation of the change.
- Express approval of people's concern for providing the best care possible.
- Express the value of each individual's and group's contributions in general and to the proposed change.
- Provide a climate of trust and acceptance in which mistakes can be made without negative consequences for individuals.
- If possible, provide assurance that no one will lose his or her position because of the change.
- Provide opportunities for people to express their feelings and ask questions about the proposed change.

Toward Evidence-Based Practice

Siddiqui, Z., Zuccarelli, R., Durkin, N., et al. (2015). Changes in patient satisfaction related to hospital renovation: Experience with a new clinical building. *Journal of Hospital Medicine, 10*(3), 165–171. doi:10.1002/jhm.2297

Researchers noted that, contrary to previously believed assertions, patients could distinguish between positive renovations to the hospital physical environment and satisfaction with patient care. Although renovations were associated with improved room- and visitor-related satisfaction, there was not a corresponding improvement in satisfaction with clinical providers. Thus, even with renovations to client care areas, measures of patient satisfaction should include the quality of care given by healthcare providers.

Shattell, M., Bartlett, R., Beres, K., et al. (2015). How patients and nurses experience an open versus an enclosed nursing station on an inpatient psychiatric unit. *Journal of the American Psychiatric Nurses Association, 21*(6), 398–405.

Researchers investigated nurses' and patients' perceptions of the inpatient environment both before and after the removal of a Plexiglas enclosure at the nurses' station. Nurses viewed it as important to ensure confidentiality and a concentrated workspace, but also noted its limitations in communicating with patients. Not surprisingly, patients preferred no enclosure and felt more freedom, safety, and connection with the nurses after its removal. The results support the findings from Southard, Jarrell and Shattell (2012) that likewise showed no statistically significant difference in patient or staff perceptions when the enclosure was removed. Conclusions from this study indicated that the focus of administrators should focus on other aspects of allocation of resources (e.g., staffing) rather than solely on nursing station redesigns.

Lake Health TriPoint Medical Center, Concord Township, Ohio. Results and data collected on new acute care hospital using state-of-the-art digital hospital design include the following (Gardiner, 2012):

- A 20% to 30% reduction in operating costs resulted from custom air-handling units and integrated controls

solutions that delivered the desired temperature and humidity to both critical and noncritical spaces. The sustainable design also increased additional usable floor space.
- A long-term contingency emergency preparedness plan was developed that would minimize the amount of time the hospital would be out of service and would quickly restore productivity in operating rooms.

Paoli Hospital, Paoli, Pennsylvania. Results collected on a new patient pavilion found that (Nash & Taylor, 2011):

- Patients felt the design features (e.g., private rooms, décor, increased room size, larger windows and natural light, and rooms with window views) positively affect their hospital experience. Patient satisfaction scores increased significantly.
- Staff felt the design features (e.g., materials, temperature, and noise) provide patient privacy and improve everyday work tasks except access to staff break rooms.
- The rate of patient falls per 1,000 patient days was reduced by nearly 10% in the new pavilion, with an 86% reduction in the rate of falls with injury. Key features of the redesign included location of nurses' work areas and visibility of the patient by the staff.
- Medication errors decreased by 19%. Design strategies included placing medications in a box outside each patient room with a closed door to minimize distractions during medication preparation.

1. Imagine you are a nurse manager about to present at a budget meeting your ideas for why it would be effective in terms of costs and client satisfaction to remodel the clinic lobby, including the addition of skylights, plants, and a small fountain. List your rationale and discuss which studies support your recommendations.

2. In addition to remodeling designs, what others factors should be the focus of managers and leaders during renovations?

 Go to Davis Advantage, Resources, Chapter 41, **Toward Evidence-Based Practice—Suggested Responses**.

---

between two people in different departments, or even between a staff member and a client or a client's family member.
- *On the group level,* conflict can occur between two or more teams, departments, or professional groups (e.g., nurses and case managers may conflict over who is responsible for discharge planning).
- *On the organizational level,* conflicts can occur between two or more hospitals, health agencies, or community organizations.

"Win-Win" Resolutions
Some people think about problems and conflicts in the same way as they think about a football game or tennis match: Someone must win, and someone must lose. There are problems, however, with this thought process:
- In healthcare, our aim should be to work together more effectively, not to defeat the other party.
- The people who lose are likely to feel bad about it. As a result, they may spend their time and energy preparing to win the next round rather than on their work.

♥ **iCare 41-1**

Leading and Managing

Every nurse possesses a degree of leadership and has the ability to influence other people. You are all change agents in the variety of different healthcare arenas that exist today and must recognize and embrace your sources of power and use them in a positive manner.

Ask, "What can I contribute?" "What am I comfortable doing at this point in my career?"

- Can I speak up for safety?
- Can I attend a safety huddle?
- Can I report not only actual errors but near misses too?
- Do I feel comfortable calling a fellow nurse or doctor out on poor hygiene practice?

- Will I start attending my own department meeting?
- Can I join a committee of interest? Falls Committee? Safety Committee? Staffing and Scheduling? Patient Satisfaction?

The answer to all of the listed questions is YES, YOU CAN!

- Empowerment, delegation, prioritization, managing change, effective time management, and conflict resolution are all skills that you are responsible for.
- Remember: Not all leaders can be managers and not all managers can be leaders.
- You should find mentors, ask questions, explore strengths and weaknesses, embrace new opportunities, reflect often on performance, and remember to always support others.

- A tie (neither side wins nor loses) may be just a stalemate; no one has won or lost, but the problem is also still there and no gain is achieved.

So the answer to the question, "Win, lose, or draw?" is, "None of the above." Instead, a win-win result, in which both sides gain some benefit, is the best resolution. People address conflict in various ways. Some avoid it, some make immediate decisions, others use an analysis approach.

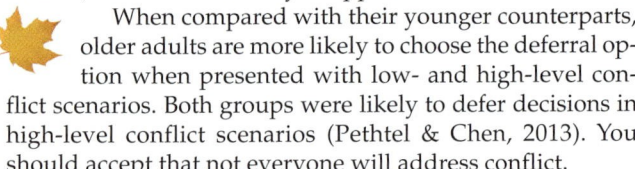 When compared with their younger counterparts, older adults are more likely to choose the deferral option when presented with low- and high-level conflict scenarios. Both groups were likely to defer decisions in high-level conflict scenarios (Pethtel & Chen, 2013). You should accept that not everyone will address conflict.

Conflict Resolution

When differences and disagreements first arise, problem-solving may be sufficient. If the situation has already developed into a full-blown conflict, however, formal or informal negotiation of a settlement may be necessary. Using a problem-solving process, the goal is to find a solution that satisfies everyone involved.

Step 1. Identify the Problem or Issue. Ask people what they want (Hagemann & Stroope, 2012). Sometimes, if the issue is not a highly charged or highly political one, it is easy to identify the real issue or problem. At other times, however, some discussion and exploration of the issues are necessary before the real problem emerges.

It would be easier if what people are saying were always obvious; however, they do not clearly label all their essential thoughts. Moreover, not all knowledgeable people agree about answers to important questions (Browne & Kelly, 2010). Even though this is ideal, it may not happen. People are often vague about their real concern; sometimes they are genuinely uncertain about what the real problem is. Emotional involvement may further cloud the issue. All of this must be sorted out so that the problem is clearly identified and a solution can be sought.

Step 2. Generate Possible Solutions. Here creativity is especially important. As a leader, begin the process of trying to find new, creative solutions. It is natural for people to try to repeat something that worked well for them in the past, but solutions that were previously successful may not work in the future. Instead, encourage people to spend some time searching for innovative solutions. Think outside the box for new and better ways to handle things.

Step 3. Evaluate Suggested Solutions. An open-minded, objective evaluation of each suggestion is needed, but you may find that this is not always easy to accomplish. When a group engages in problem-solving, it is sometimes difficult to separate the suggestion from its source. For example, in a team situation, the status of the person who made the suggestion may influence whether the suggestion is judged to be useful. Judge the suggestion on its merits, not its source.

Step 4. Choose the Best Solution. Choose the solution that is most likely to work—one that will give you the best results with the fewest negative effects. You may have to combine suggestions to get the best solution.

Step 5. Implement the Solution Chosen. The true test of any solution is how well it works when applied. Once a solution has been implemented, it is important to give it time to work. Impatience may lead you to prematurely abandon a good solution.

Step 6. Evaluate—Is the Problem Resolved? Not every problem is resolved successfully on the first attempt. If the problem has not been resolved, look at why the chosen solution did not work. You then need to resume the process with even greater attention to identifying the real problem and how it can be successfully resolved.

Informal Negotiation

If problem-solving does not resolve the conflict, you may have to move on to the next step—informal negotiation. The following steps may prove useful:

1. **Clarify the situation in your own mind.**
   What am I trying to achieve?
   What is the environment in which I am operating?
   What problems am I likely to encounter?
   What do both sides want?
2. **Set the stage.**
   This may involve confronting the two parties or groups with their behavior toward one another, making direct statements designed to open communication and challenge them to seek resolution of the situation.
3. **Conduct the negotiation.**
   Manage the emotions.
   Set the ground rules.
   Clarify the problem.
   Make your opening move.
4. **Continue with offers and counteroffers.**
5. **Agree on the resolution of the conflict.**

Conflict is inevitable within any large or diverse group of people who are trying to work together over an extended time. However, it does not have to be destructive, and it does not even have to be a negative experience if everyone handles it skillfully. In fact, conflict can stimulate people to learn more about one another and how to work together in more effective ways. Resolution of a conflict, when it is done well, can improve relationships, lead to more creative methods of problem-solving, and improve productivity.

TIME MANAGEMENT

Many of the personal management and workplace organizational skills focus on time management and scheduling. Although new nurses may have the required job skills, many lack personal management skills, specifically time management. You might be able to handle conflict and change, delegate appropriately, and have strong leadership skills. But if you can't organize and manage your time, you will never gain your full potential.

Many nurses "punch a time clock" that records the minute they enter and leave work. Management accepts very few excuses for tardiness. Timesheets and schedules are part of nurses' lives. We are expected to follow precisely set schedules and meet deadlines for virtually everything we do, from distributing medications to charting on time. Many agencies analyze computer-generated data to determine the time spent on various activities. Consider how you can use the following suggestions to improve your time management:

Setting Your Own Goals

It is difficult to decide how to spend your time, because there are so many things that need time. A good first step is to get an overview of the situation. Then ask yourself, "What are my goals?" Goals help clarify what you want and give you energy, direction, and focus. Once you know where you want to go, set priorities. This is not an easy task. In Lewis Carroll's *Alice's Adventures in Wonderland* (1865/2010), the child heroine, Alice, becomes lost and asks for help from a fantasy creature, the Cheshire Cat. They have this conversation:

> *"Would you tell me please, which way I ought to go from here?" asked Alice.*
> *"That depends a good deal on where you want to go to," said the Cat.*
> *"I don't care where," said Alice.*
> *"Then it doesn't matter which way you go," said the Cat.*

How can you get somewhere if you do not know where you want to go? It is important to explore your personal and career goals. This can help you make decisions about the future. You can apply these ideas to daily activities as well as to career decisions. Spend some time thinking about what you want to accomplish over a given period of time.

To help organize your time, you need to set both short- and long-term goals. **Short-term goals** are those you wish to accomplish within the near future (e.g., organizing your day to participate in a study group). **Long-term goals** are those you wish to complete in the future. A good question to ask is, "What do I see myself doing 5 years from now?" It may be getting an advanced nursing degree. Every choice you make requires a different allocation of time.

Organizing Your Work

Many healthcare professionals are linear, fast-tempo, achievement-oriented people. However, working at a rapid pace is not necessarily the same as being efficient or effective. You can spend much energy rushing around while actually achieving very little.

To "manage" time, you need a measure of skill to efficiently meet client care needs during your nursing shift. Organizing your work can eliminate extra steps or serious delays in finishing. It can also reduce the amount of time you spend doing things that are neither productive nor satisfying. As you begin your nursing program, you may care for only one or two clients. However, you will need to develop time management skills to meet the expectation of handling a workload of caring for five to six clients. The following are some suggestions:

Time Inventory To begin managing your time, you need to develop a clear understanding of how you use your time. A personal time inventory helps you estimate how much time you spend in typical activities. Keeping the inventory for a week gives a fairly accurate estimate of how you spend your time. It also helps to identify "time wasters." Set up a time log and enter your activities every half hour. You may be surprised to see the pattern that emerges when you review these data. Observational data revealed that nurses spent less time on directed client care activities than they self-reported (Gholizadeh, Janati, Nadimi, et al., 2014). Various studies have indicated that nurses spend about 25% of their time on documentation and 30% to 45% of their time on patient care (Hendrich, Chow, Skierczynski, et al., 2008; Robert Wood Johnson Foundation, 2009; Stowkowski, 2013).

Energy Use Work on the most difficult tasks when you have the most energy. This lessens frustration later in the day, when you may be more tired and less efficient. Consider your energy levels when beginning a big task. Start when levels are high and not at, say, 4 p.m., if that is when you find yourself winding down. For example, if you are a "morning person," plan your demanding work in the morning. If you get energy spurts later in the morning or early afternoon, plan to work on larger or heavier tasks at that time. Of course, this choice is not always within your control. Many nursing tasks are based on a schedule. If the wound care is due at 1 p.m., you must carry out the task then. Analyze your work to determine which tasks are fixed and what you can manipulate to match your energy.

Lists and Schedules Make a "to do" list and prioritize the tasks in order of importance. Determine when each must be completed and how much time it will require. If you find yourself postponing an item for several days, either give it top priority the next day or drop it from the list altogether.

Daily Worksheet To help organize your day, provide yourself with reminders of when various tasks need to be done. Without some type of schedule, you are more likely to drift through a day or shift from one activity to another in a disorganized fashion. The risk in using schedules, however, is that the more they divide the day into discrete segments, the more they fragment the work and discourage a holistic approach. Use the schedule as an organizational tool, but focus on your clients.

Say "No" Take control to avoid time wasters. It is important to prevent endless activities and other people controlling you. Learn when to say no. Learn to say, "I would really like to help you; can it wait until I finish this?" Or, "I am sorry, I won't be able to help you with that."

Delegate See previous discussions on delegation.

Do Not Multitask Studies show that people who do many things at once are not likely to do any of them well. Finish one task, then move on to the next one.

Streamline Your Work Many tasks cannot be eliminated or delegated, but they can be done more efficiently. Here are three wise sayings in time management:

- "Work smarter, not harder." This should appeal to nurses facing increasing demands on time (Box 41-5).

BOX 41-5 ■ Work Smarter, Not Harder

- Gather materials, such as bed linens, for all of your patients at one time. As you go to each room, leave the linen so that it will be there when you need it.
- While giving a bed bath or providing other personal care, perform some of the aspects of the physical assessment, such as taking vital signs, skin assessment, and parts of the neurological and musculoskeletal assessment.
- If a client does not "look right," do not ignore your instincts. The patient is probably having a problem.
- Prevention is always a good idea. If you are not sure about a treatment or medication, ask before you proceed. It is usually less time consuming to prevent a problem than it is to resolve one.
- When you set aside time for a specific task that has a high priority, stick to your schedule and complete it.
- Do not allow interruptions while you are completing any tasks (e.g., paperwork, medication administration). Focus on the task at hand.

- "Never handle a piece of paper more than once." This relates to client care as well as office work and schoolwork. In other words, handle an issue now rather than putting it off until later.
- "A stitch in time saves nine." Preventive action saves time and effort in the long run.

Plan Ahead Take a few minutes at the beginning of your shift to organize your patient's supplies for the day or whatever you need to do to avoid retracing your steps.

Components of Time Management

Time can be your best friend or your worst enemy. Nursing requires that you perform numerous activities within what often seems to be a short period of time, so learn how to make the most of your day. Finally, remember that you should set aside 8 hours for sleep and a few more for personal or leisure time (time off). Use Table 41-4 to help you to review the necessary components of time management.

KnowledgeCheck 41-6

- List the steps of conflict resolution.
- List several suggestions for organizing your work.
- State one "wise saying" to guide you in streamlining your work.

PUTTING IT ALL TOGETHER

You are just beginning your journey toward becoming a nurse. Undoubtedly you will want to function well within your organization and provide high-quality patient care. Begin now to

---

Table 41-4 ► Components of Time Management	
ACTION	**EXAMPLES**
Prioritize	List tasks in order of importance.
	Remember that some tasks must be done at specific times, whereas others can be done at any time.
	Emergencies take precedence.
	Identify events you control and events others control.
	Use critical-thinking skills to assign priorities.
Question	
■ Effectiveness	■ Did the task produce the desired outcome?
■ Efficiency	■ How can I accomplish the plan with the least expenditure of time? Is there a way to break this down into simpler tasks?
■ Efficacy	■ Do I have the skill and ability to obtain the desired effect?
Recheck	Mentally and physically recheck an unfinished or delegated task.
Practice self-reliance	Identify tasks that are within your control and those that are not.
	Use critical-thinking skills and adaptability to revise priorities.
	"Go with the flow."
Treat	Treat yourself to a break when you can.
	Treat yourself to time off.
	Treat yourself to an educational experience: Commit yourself to excellence.
	Treat others with courtesy and respect.

examine and work on your own strengths and weaknesses. As you work with your classmates, your instructors, and the clinical facilities, focus on developing the traits of a good leader. You will soon recognize that conflict and change are a normal part of life and your clinical practice, so learn to become proactive as issues arise. You will observe how "real" nurses delegate and manage their time. Learn from their examples and adopt useful practices. Watch for opportunities to be mentored and make time to mentor others. **KEY POINT:** *Above all, remember that you may be the most important person in the life of your patient during the time you are with him or her—a very big responsibility, but one you will meet with honor and courage.*

CLINICALREASONING

The questions and exercises in this section allow you to practice the kind of thinking you will use as a full-spectrum nurse. Critical-thinking questions usually have more than one correct answer, so we do not provide "correct answers" for these features. It is more important to develop your nursing judgment than to just cover content. You will learn by discussing the questions with your peers. If you are still unsure, see the Davis Advantage chapter resources for suggested responses.

Caring for the Nguyens

Anh Chu, Nam's aunt, is scheduled for outpatient cataract surgery later this week at the local hospital. Nam reports to the clinic wishing to discuss the plan for his aunt's surgery "with whoever is the boss." Nam is concerned that his aunt will not be staying at the hospital. "She's having surgery. I don't understand this! She's 78 years old. She's going to need help. This doesn't make sense. You have to change things. It won't be safe to do this as planned."

Nam tells you he has discussed his concerns with the ophthalmologist. He tells you that the ophthalmologist told him he was "overreacting. We always do it this way. You just don't understand." Nam is visibly upset. He believes that his aunt is receiving inadequate care. He appeals to you to help him take care of his aunt. "This is where Aunt Chu gets her care. You know her. You have to change this."

Anh Chu has been seen at the family clinic several times over the past few years. She takes a medication for osteoporosis and has been counseled about the need for exercise and weight loss. She has also begun to experience problems with "accidents," that is, urine leakage. She has never had surgery in the past, and her only hospitalizations have been for childbirth. Ms. Chu's husband recently passed away, and she has been living alone since then.

A. Devise a plan to resolve this conflict with Nam.

 Go to Davis Advantage, Resources, Chapter 41, **Caring for the Nguyens—Suggested Responses.**

Applying the **Full-Spectrum Nursing Model**

ORGANIZATIONAL SITUATION

A small, not-for-profit hospice center in a small community has received a generous memorial gift from the family of a client who recently died. The family asked only that the money be "put to the best possible use." Everyone in the facility has an opinion about the best use for the money.

The administrator wants to renovate their old, run-down headquarters. The financial officer wants to put the money in the bank "for a rainy day." The chaplain wants to add a small chapel to the building. The nurses want to create a food bank to help the poorest of their clients. The social workers want to buy a van to transport clients to healthcare providers. The staff has agreed that all the ideas have merit and all the needs are important. Unfortunately, there is enough money to fund only one of them.

The more the staff members discuss how to use this gift, the more insistent each group becomes about defending its own idea. At the last meeting, it is clear that some are becoming angry and frustrated. A shouting match even occurs between the administrator and the financial officer.

THINKING

1. *Theoretical Knowledge:*
   Which is appropriate at this point, a problem-solving approach or informal negotiation? Explain your answer.

DOING

2. *Practical Knowledge:*
   If you were to conduct the informal negotiation, list the steps of the plan you would follow.

CARING

3. *Self-Knowledge:*
   Which idea do you think has the most merit? Why did you select the one you did?
4. *Ethical Knowledge:*
   Which groups or individuals seem to demonstrate the value of caring for clients? Explain your thinking.

 Go to Davis Advantage, Resources, Chapter 41, **Applying the Full-Spectrum Nursing Model—Suggested Responses.**

 To explore learning resources for this chapter,

 Go to **www.DavisAdvantage.com** and find:

Answers and Suggested Responses for all questions in this chapter

Lists of NIC Interventions and NOC Outcomes

List of NANDA-I Diagnoses

Knowledge Map

References and Bibliography

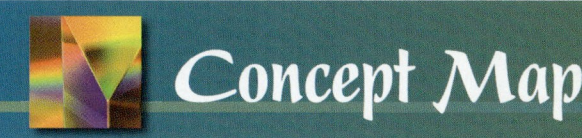
Leadership and Management

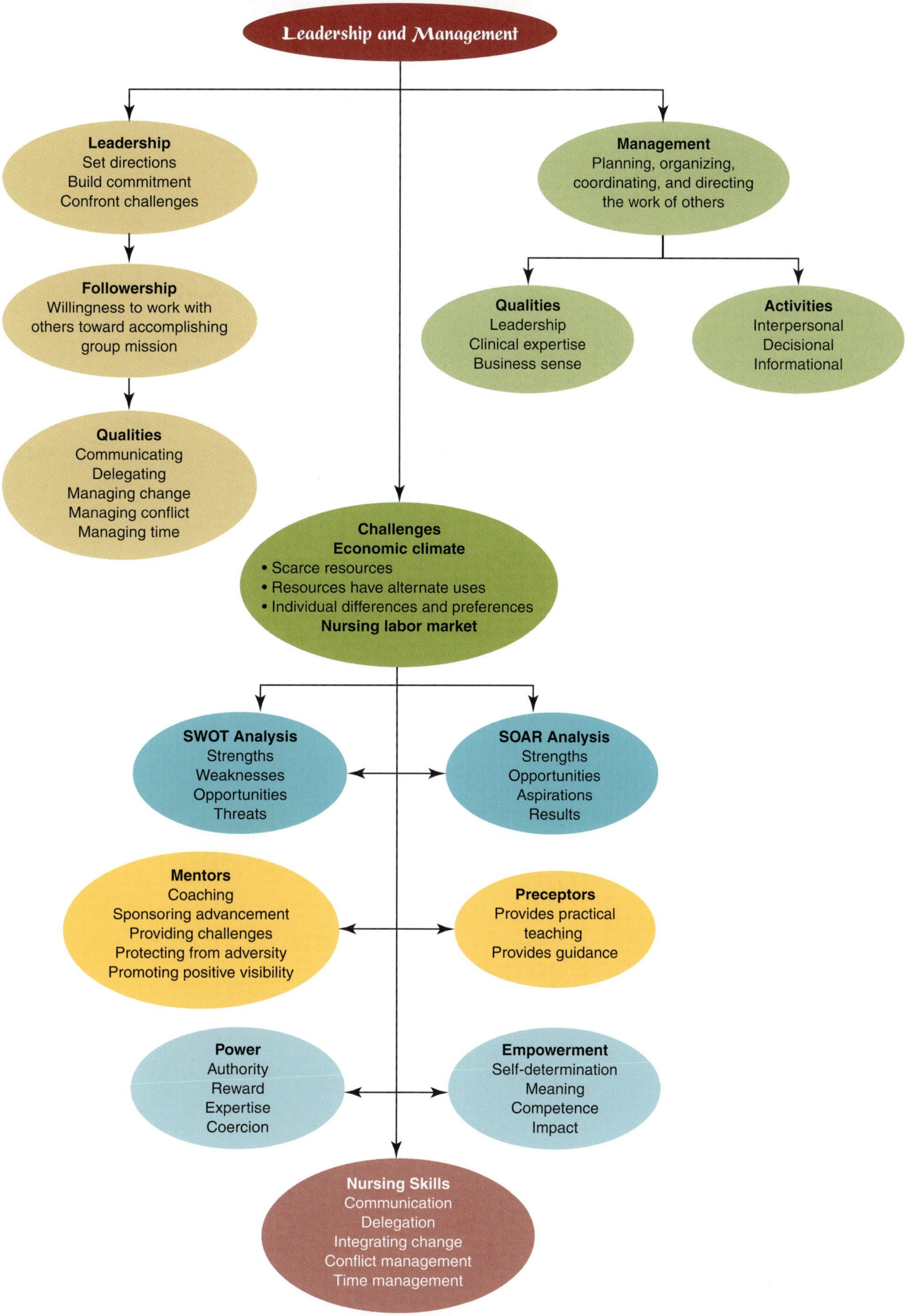

Leadership
Set directions
Build commitment
Confront challenges

Management
Planning, organizing, coordinating, and directing the work of others

Followership
Willingness to work with others toward accomplishing group mission

Qualities
Leadership
Clinical expertise
Business sense

Activities
Interpersonal
Decisional
Informational

Qualities
Communicating
Delegating
Managing change
Managing conflict
Managing time

Challenges
Economic climate
• Scarce resources
• Resources have alternate uses
• Individual differences and preferences
Nursing labor market

SWOT Analysis
Strengths
Weaknesses
Opportunities
Threats

SOAR Analysis
Strengths
Opportunities
Aspirations
Results

Mentors
Coaching
Sponsoring advancement
Providing challenges
Protecting from adversity
Promoting positive visibility

Preceptors
Provides practical teaching
Provides guidance

Power
Authority
Reward
Expertise
Coercion

Empowerment
Self-determination
Meaning
Competence
Impact

Nursing Skills
Communication
Delegation
Integrating change
Conflict management
Time management

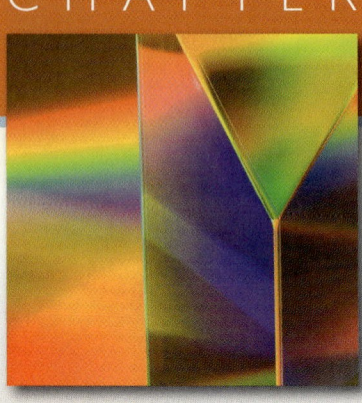

Community & Home Health Nursing

Learning Outcomes

After completing this chapter, you should be able to:

➤ Define the meaning of community.

➤ Identify at least four factors by which you can recognize a healthy community.

➤ Discuss factors that create vulnerability for a population.

➤ Compare and contrast community-based care, community health nursing, public health nursing, and community-oriented nursing.

➤ Distinguish between primary, secondary, and tertiary interventions in regard to a community health scenario.

➤ Discuss at least three strategies that nurses use to gather community data.

➤ Describe the roles of nurses in the community setting.

➤ Identify the primary goals of home care.

➤ Describe ways in which home healthcare differs from hospital nursing.

➤ Categorize the various agencies that deliver home healthcare according to purpose, client served, and funding source.

➤ Describe how the nurse's emphasis differs in hospice nursing compared with home health nursing.

➤ List at least four criteria clients must meet for home care costs to be reimbursed by Medicare.

➤ Outline the steps required to prepare for a home visit, including considerations for the nurse's safety.

➤ Explain the role of the nurse in helping clients and families manage medications and treatments in the home setting.

➤ Describe how infection control measures differ in the home and in the hospital.

➤ State two important safety concerns in home care that arise out of The Joint Commission 2016 home care safety goals.

➤ Describe the nurse's role in treating caregiver strain.

➤ Apply the nursing process to the care of patients in the home and community.

➤ Use standardized nursing language taxonomies (NANDA-I, NOC, NIC, Omaha, and CCC) to describe care planning in community and home care.

Key Concepts

Community nursing

Home healthcare

Population

Related Concepts

See the Concept Map at the end of this chapter.

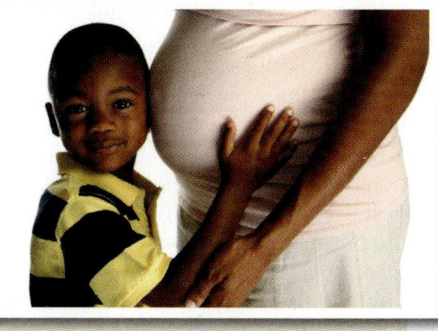

Meet Your Patients

Your Neighbor, Tanya

You are nearing completion of your fundamentals course. One night the telephone rings. It is your neighbor Tanya. Her 5-year-old son, Jacob, came home from kindergarten with a letter from the school nurse stating that a classmate was ill with HINI influenza and that all the students in the class had been exposed to the disease. Tanya is concerned about the risks to Jacob and the rest of the family. She is 8 months pregnant, and the family has no health insurance. She says, "You are a nursing student; do you know what I should do or where I might go for assistance?"

Although you are flattered that Tanya has consulted you, you need to consider whether you have the expertise to answer her questions. This situation requires knowledge of many aspects of nursing (e.g., immunizations, pregnancy, microbiology, pathophysiology). Though you may not have all of the information you need to answer her questions, you should be able to help your neighbor resolve her concerns. You will need to consider the following questions:

- What is going on in the situation that may influence the outcome?
- Who should be involved to improve the outcome?
- What theoretical knowledge do I need to answer Tanya's questions? Where would I find this information?
- What additional data do I need to collect from Tanya?
- What suggestions and/or referrals should I offer to Tanya?

Your Patients, the Escobars

Flora Escobar is 78 years old. She lives at home with her husband, Roland, also age 78. Both enjoyed good health until Roland was hospitalized for a cerebrovascular accident (a stroke) 3 weeks ago. He then spent 2 weeks in a skilled nursing facility. He returned home yesterday and will be followed by the local home health agency for physical therapy and nursing care.

At your initial visit, Mrs. Escobar greets you at the door. She is a petite woman who looks exhausted. Her apron pockets are stuffed with pill bottles. The hallway is partially blocked with a bedside commode, walker, and tray table. Mr. Escobar, wearing pajamas and a robe, is in a hospital bed in the living room. He is a tall, stocky man who is sitting up in bed but is slumped and leaning to the left.

After introducing yourself, you ask an open-ended question to build rapport: "How have things been going since you came home yesterday?" Mrs. Escobar sighs, and says, "I'm worried that I'm doing things wrong. I have a hard time helping him move. He is so much bigger than I am, and I don't want to hurt him. He is frustrated with me, but he has difficulty telling me what he needs." Tears fill Mrs. Escobar's eyes. Her husband turns away to avoid eye contact with you. To refocus their attention, you suggest that you go over some information and then begin to look at what additional services might be helpful.

Imagine how stressed Mrs. Escobar must feel. How do you think you could best help this family? In this chapter, as you read the section on home health nursing, you should find it easier to answer those questions.

Theoretical Knowledge
knowing why

The U.S. population is aging rapidly and the number of older adults is expected to double by 2050. At the same time, hospital stays have become shorter in an effort to reduce healthcare costs. As a result, community-based healthcare, including home nursing care, is rapidly expanding. Perhaps your career path will lead you to caring for clients in one of the many community healthcare settings, including clients' own homes. In this chapter, you will learn about communities and community and home nursing care and explore the roles, interventions, and career opportunities for nurses who work in communities.

ABOUT THE KEY CONCEPTS

In this chapter, you will learn about the concepts of **community nursing** and **home healthcare** and how different **populations** have unique healthcare needs. You will learn how these concepts are related to each other and to subconcepts such as public health nursing, vulnerable populations, and home visits.

UNDERSTANDING THE CONCEPT OF COMMUNITY

The word **community** comes from the Latin *communis*, meaning the "gift or fellowship of common relations and feelings." Historically and now, the notion of community suggests a general sense of selflessness, sharing, relationship, and doing good that comes from working together. Most members of a community share a common language, certain rituals, and special customs.

In contrast to community, we tend to think of a **population** as a certain geographic region. But the word *population* has other meanings as well:

- It can mean the group of people of a particular race or class in a specified place (e.g., "There are 1,500 Latino people living in Edwards County").
- It can also mean *any* group of people subject to statistical or other study (e.g., all the homeless people in Edwards

County, or all the pregnant adolescents living in Edwards County).

The U.S. Bureau of the Census (n.d.) conducts a survey and count of the American people (the population of the United States) every 10 years, most recently in 2010. When the census is completed, the U.S. Census Bureau groups the data into sections of 1,500 to 8,000 people, known as **census tracts.** The area of individual census tracts varies according to the density of the population. In urban centers, a census tract covers a small area. Rural census tracts are large. Census tracts are useful to public officials and market analysts, as well as anyone else—including community nurses—who studies the characteristics and concerns of smaller sections of people.

Maps and census tracts show the *geopolitical* boundaries of a community. But as we noted earlier, a community can also be a group of people with a common purpose. They may live in different geographic areas, but they have a "sense of belonging" to their group (community). For a comparison of geopolitical boundaries and census tracts, see Figure 42-1.

An **aggregate** is a group of individuals with at least one shared characteristic, either personal or environmental. For example, a community health nurse may work with a class of high school girls to reduce the incidence of adolescent pregnancy. The shared characteristics of this aggregate are that they are female and of childbearing age and attend a particular school. As another example, the nursing students in your school are an aggregate. What characteristics and goals do you share?

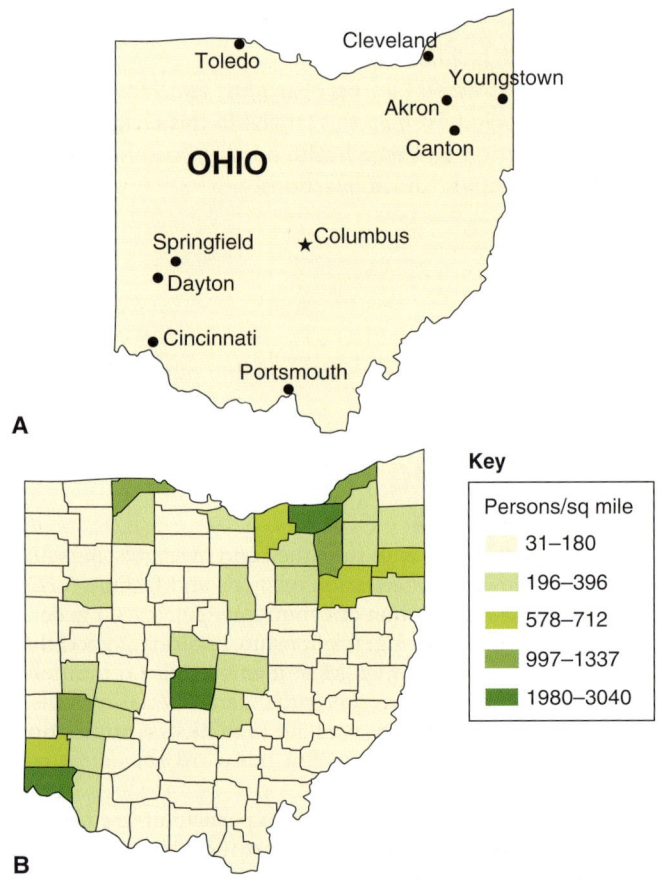

FIGURE 42-1 A. Illustrates political boundaries. B. Shows density using census tract data.

Key

Persons/sq mile

	31–180
	196–396
	578–712
	997–1337
	1980–3040

KnowledgeCheck 42-1

- Give several examples of a community.
- How is a population different from a community?

ThinkLike a Nurse 42-1

- Why might the boundaries of a census tract change every 10 years?
- How could you figure out what census tract you live or go to school in?

What Are the Components of a Community?

To understand a particular community and its needs, you will need information about its three components: the concepts of structure, status, and process.

   Structure refers to the general characteristics of a community.
- **Demographic data:** For example, gender, age, ethnicity, and educational and income levels
- **Data about healthcare services:** For example, number of primary care providers or emergency care facilities in the area
   Status describes the biological, emotional, and social outcome components of a community.
- **Biological data:** Morbidity (illness) and mortality (death) rates, life expectancy ratios, and risk factor profiles for the respective age-groups within a community
- **Emotional data:** General indications of mental health and consumer satisfaction survey results about various aspects of the community as compared with other locales
- **Social data:** Crime rates, citizenship involvement in community-wide activities, and general functioning levels of the community members
   Process describes the overall effectiveness level of the community. For example:
- Do the members of the community perceive that they are part of a group with common purpose, values, or interests?
- What is the extent of interaction among community members?
- Does the community have an established forum for conflict resolution?

What Makes a Community Healthy?

As with individuals, the meaning and perception of health varies among aggregates. For nurses, it is important to understand what a particular community defines (and values) as health rather than relying on personal definitions.

When determining what makes a community healthy, the national consensus paper *Healthy People 2020* provides useful guidelines. That document is based on the understanding that many of the health problems of Americans were preventable. *Healthy People 2020* identifies leading indicators for measuring the health of our nation (U.S. Department of Health and Human Services, n.d.a). Some examples include:

Physical activity	Mental health
Overweight and obesity	Injury and violence
Tobacco use	Environmental quality
Substance abuse	Immunizations
Sexual behavior	Access to healthcare

The four overarching goals of the *Healthy People 2020* initiative are to:
1. Attain high-quality, longer lives free of preventable disease, disability, injury, and premature death
2. Achieve health equity, eliminate health disparities, and improve the health of all groups

3. Create social and physical environments that promote good health for all
4. Promote quality of life, healthy development, and healthy behaviors across all life stages

These aggregate goals are to be achieved through promoting healthy behaviors, increasing access to quality healthcare, and strengthening community health resources. For more information,

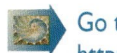 Go to the **Healthy People 2020 Web site,** at http://www.healthypeople.gov

KnowledgeCheck 42-2

- What makes up the *structure* of a community?
- What is community *status*?
- What is community *process*?
- Use the guidelines from *Healthy People 2020* to compile a list of several characteristics that make a community healthy.

What Makes a Population Vulnerable?

The concept of **vulnerable population** is defined as an aggregate that is at increased risk of adverse health outcomes. Members of vulnerable populations have a higher probability of developing health problems than do members of the general population. Because of their increased risk, vulnerable populations are a major focus of community health efforts. Vulnerability involves multiple factors:

- **Limited Economic Resources.** Income is a major predictor of health risk. People with higher incomes typically have greater access to health services and greater selection of providers, treatment options, and location of health services. In contrast, the more limited a person's income is, the more limited her healthcare options will be. Many persons with low income forgo preventive care and seek healthcare only when they are very ill.
- **Limited Social Resources.** Friends and family are valuable resources to help a person deal with day-to-day stress and demands of an illness. They can provide feedback, listen to concerns, and offer emotional and physical assistance. Unfortunately, not everyone has social resources. Older adults who live alone and people with mental illness are examples of groups at increased risk because of social isolation.
- **Extremes of Age.** The very young and the very old are less able to adapt to physiological stress and are at increased risk of disease. They are more prone to infections and may not be able to protect themselves against environmental hazards, such as cold or heat. These age-groups are also more often living in poverty.
- **Chronic Disease and Obesity.** People who have chronic diseases are at greater risk of health problems. For example, people with obesity are at increased risk of heart disease, diabetes, impaired mobility, joint pain, and other complications. People with diabetes are at risk of blindness, impaired wound healing, kidney failure, poor peripheral circulation, heart disease, and other complications.
- **History of Abuse or Trauma.** People who have experienced abuse or traumatic events often feel they have limited control over their health and circumstances. They may feel powerless or hopeless and be unable to take actions that promote health or lead to early treatment of illness. Abuse and trauma also stress a person's ability to cope, placing him at risk for physical and mental health problems.

Other vulnerable populations include people who are poor or homeless, migrant workers, people with disabilities, premature infants, women with a high-risk pregnancy and pregnant adolescents, people with communicable disease, people who abuse substances, members of certain ethnic/racial groups, and the untreated mentally ill.

UNDERSTANDING THE CONCEPT OF COMMUNITY-BASED NURSING

A community can be either a *site* for healthcare delivery or a *recipient* of healthcare services. As the technological advances of the past 30 years have escalated the costs of delivering health services, efforts to lower costs have resulted in a move back to more community-based care, including complementary and alternative care.

Community-based care refers to healthcare or rehabilitative services performed in clinics, offices, mobile care units, and other facilities in the community—rather than in acute care settings, such as hospitals (although acute care settings also exist within the community). For example, many surgeries and diagnostic procedures are performed in privately owned surgical centers, health clinics, and physicians' offices rather than in hospitals. Extended care facilities, or nursing homes, commonly provide rehabilitative care for patients after acute traumatic injuries as well as continuous skilled care for older adults and people with chronic illness. The following sections describe three approaches to community-based nursing.

Community Health Nursing

Although many people use the terms community health nursing and public health nursing interchangeably, they are not identical. **Community health nursing** focuses on how the health of individuals, families, and groups affects the community as a whole. Community health nurses strive to promote, protect, preserve, and maintain the health of the population through the delivery of personal health services to individuals, families, and groups.

Example: A community health nurse may work in a prenatal clinic providing healthcare for low-income women. The nurse provides a direct service to each pregnant woman. By improving the health of the mother and baby—who are members of the community—the overall health of the community is also supported.

Public Health Nursing

Public health nursing focuses on the community as a whole and the eventual effect of the community's health status on the health of individuals, families, and groups. The goal of public health is to prevent individual disease and disability, in addition to promoting and protecting the overall health of the community. Today's public health nurses functioning in a health promotion role must possess skills such as community assessment, cultural competence, program planning, communication, financial planning and management, leadership, systems thinking, and policy development.

Example: A public health nurse may be employed by a county health department to provide surveillance services to monitor for tuberculosis (TB). The nurse helps to protect the entire community by screening for TB at the local school, by testing high-risk individuals for TB, and by identifying and tracking clients with active disease to ensure that they complete the prescribed 6- to 9-month medication regimen.

Because public health focuses on large-scale programs for the entire community, government-based agencies often provide these services. The U.S. Public Health Service is an example of a public health agency within the federal government. Examples of successful public health programs are human papillomavirus (HPV) immunizations for adolescents, smoking cessation programs for healthcare workers, motor vehicle and infant car-seat safety instruction, and obesity prevention programs for children.

Community-Oriented Nursing

Community-oriented nursing combines components of community and public health. It focuses on health promotion, illness prevention, early detection, and treatment provided within the community setting. The practice is evidence-based and collaborative with other community health disciplines. The approach is a comprehensive look at the individual, family, group, and community at large.

Example: A nurse with a community-oriented approach might work in an adolescent prenatal program. The nurse provides individual care at the local clinic 2 days per week. While at the clinic, she gathers data from adolescents about the schools they attend as well as their knowledge of birth control, pregnancy, and childbirth. On the remaining 3 days, she:

- Meets with school officials to identify pregnant teens who need prenatal care.
- Teaches a class about sexuality in the local high school
- Works with teachers to identify strategies to keep pregnant teens in school.
- Provides parenting education to adolescents who have children.
- Advocates changing a bus route so that teens can easily get to the local clinic.

Each aspect of care allows the nurse to gather more data about the needs of the individuals and the community as a whole.

Figure 42-2 provides a schematic of the relationship of the three community-based nursing approaches identified in this section.

KnowledgeCheck 42-3

- What is the distinction between an aggregate population and a vulnerable population?

♥ **iCare 42-1**

Community Health Nursing: Getting Involved

While currently working at a home healthcare agency in an urban area, Kyra observes an apparent lack of commitment to preventive care among patients she is caring for and their family members. After reflecting on what she can do to help the greater community, Kyra volunteers to help with a traveling health fair campaign to provide blood pressure, blood sugar, cholesterol, and body weight screenings. Kyra has such a good experience providing community healthcare at the health fair that she is able to interest other nurses in her agency, who then join the campaign.

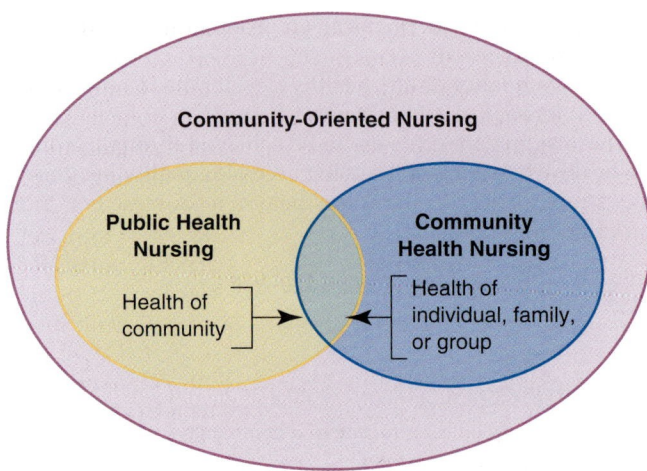

FIGURE 42-2 Schematic relationship of community nursing approaches.

- Identify practice differences between a community-based nurse and an acute care nurse.
- How is public health nursing different from community health nursing? How is it the same?
- How is community-oriented nursing related to community health nursing and public health nursing?

 Think**Like a Nurse** 42-2

Review the scenario of Tanya and Jacob (Meet Your Patients). Which form of community-based nursing would be most appropriate to address their concerns?

Who Were Some Pioneers of Community Nursing?

The following are some of the most notable people who have contributed to the development of community-based nursing care:

- *Florence Nightingale*—Established the importance of promoting health by manipulating the environment (e.g., light, warmth, sanitation, cleanliness) and nursing the whole person.
- *Lillian Wald*—Known as the first community health nurse; founded the first visiting nurses' association in New York.
- *Clara Barton*—Founder of the American Red Cross.
- *Margaret Sanger*—Founded the International Planned Parenthood Federation. Pioneered the use of family planning and birth control education.

WORKING WITHIN COMMUNITIES

Community nurses' roles vary depending on the community and its identified needs. Community nursing care is holistic and serves a large, client population. Therefore, one of the most effective nursing interventions is **empowerment**. This means assisting the client (individual or community) to recognize and use available resources to achieve or maintain the desired level of health, achieve autonomy, and maintain positive self-esteem.

What Are the Roles of Community Nurses?

Community health nurses function as client advocates, educators, collaborators, counselors, and case managers. All of these roles require excellent written and oral communication skills.

Client Advocate The effective community health nurse consistently supports the identified or expressed concerns of the client and/or community. As a community health nurse, you can effect change by getting involved in your local student nurses' association, professional nursing organizations, school board, and citizen committees, or by attending council meetings.

Educator Because community nursing focuses on wellness and disease prevention, much of what the nurse does involves education—of individual clients, groups of people (aggregates) at risk of disease, politicians, or a community. Be aware of the stage of development, educational level, and learning style of the community group you plan to educate. The most effective educational programs are concise; provide relevant, practical information; and can be easily incorporated into the learner's daily routine. For more information about teaching clients, see Chapter 26.

Collaborator A primary role of a community health nurse is to serve as a collaborator.

Example: A community health nurse is concerned about poor compliance with recommended immunization schedules for 2-year-olds in her local community. After surveying some of the parents, the nurse discovers that the clinic's operating hours are limited and the automated call routing system is frustrating for people trying to set up an appointment; the clinic does not offer online scheduling. The nurse also discovers clinics do not e-mail or text reminders to clients, nor follow up to reschedule missed appointments. The nurse schedules a meeting of clinic staff, practice managers, and patients to resolve these issues. At the meeting, some larger issues are revealed, such as the insufficient number of Medicaid providers to serve the community, and the failure of state Medicaid agencies to reimburse the providers adequately and in a timely manner.

Partnerships and coalitions can effectively address common concerns among different communities, as well as those within a single community.

Counselor Once you have established rapport with a group, members may consult you about a variety of health-related and non-health-related concerns. Be careful to offer counsel only within your scope of practice and make recommendations that are practical yet meet the needs of the community. You may need only to serve as a witness to the group's concerns. Allowing clients to discuss or work through issues empowers them and fosters self-reliance.

Case Manager Community nurses commonly make referrals to or collaborate with various health and social agencies. Be aware when referring clients to these resources that agency policies and financing change frequently. Also, because community agencies often operate on grants and time-limited funding, a program that is available at one time may be dissolved at another. As a community health nurse, you will need to remain informed about the community services in your area.

Example: A local group has established a healthcare program at a minimal charge for low-income families. Providers and nurses volunteer their time to provide the care. Pharmaceutical representatives donate the medical supplies and routine medications. Local specialists (e.g., surgeons) provide services to those with complex or specialized needs. However, in such a clinic the appointment times fill up quickly, and often clients must wait more than a month or two for an appointment. Before enrolling families

in the program, you would need to be aware of these limitations and share this information with clients.

KnowledgeCheck 42-4

Give an example of a nursing activity involved in each of the following community health roles: educator, advocate, case manager, counselor, and collaborator.

How Are Community Nursing Interventions Classified?

There are three basic levels of care in which nursing interventions can be classified: primary, secondary, and tertiary. Most community-oriented nursing practices are aimed at the primary (prevention) level.

Primary Interventions

The goal of **primary (first-level) interventions** is to promote health and prevent disease. Primary interventions include educating, collaborating, and civic involvement. Examples are:

- **Educating** susceptible individuals with no known disease process. For example, a nurse may educate women of childbearing age to wear insect repellent when in a location where mosquitos potentially carrying Zika virus might be.
- **Collaborating** with local agencies to provide clean and secure temporary housing for migrant farm workers.
- **Lobbying** elected representatives for a ban on smoking in restaurants and other public places.

Secondary Interventions

Secondary (second-level) interventions aim to reduce the impact of the disease process by early detection and treatment. For example, a community health nurse may screen a sexually active adolescent girl for hepatitis B and/or HPV. She has known risk factors for sexually transmitted infection (STI) but no apparent disease symptoms. The nurse will also teach the client how to protect herself from STIs, hepatitis B, and HIV in the future. Other examples of secondary interventions include providing outreach screening programs offering mammography, scoliosis screening, lipid testing, and prostate-specific antigen testing for prostate cancer (Fig. 42-3).

Tertiary Interventions

The goal of **tertiary (third-level) interventions** is to halt disease progression and/or restore client functioning to the

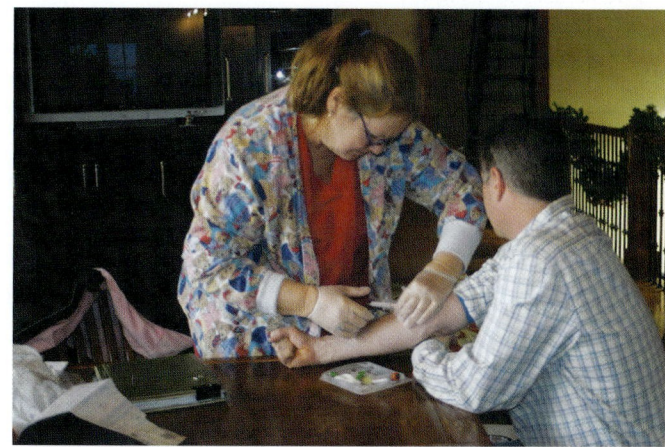

FIGURE 42-3 Secondary interventions. Early detection of heart disease with lipid screening.

Safe, Effective Nursing Care

Promoting Patient-Centered Care in Community Health

Chapter Key Concept: Community Nursing

Competency: Patient-Centered Care (Thinking, Doing, and Caring)

Scenario: Nurses at a healthcare clinic note an increased number of Hispanic clients seeking services. To best serve this growing community, one of the nurses researches healthcare issues affecting urban Hispanic populations. Latino men are more likely to be diagnosed with late-stage prostate cancer and to die of the disease than non-Latino men. Clinic staff plan to develop a flyer about prostate cancer screening, directed at Hispanic men aged 50 and older. The nurse asks the community outreach healthcare educator what cultural norms might influence health behaviors. He says that some Latino men view seeking healthcare as a sign of weakness. He explains *machismo* and *caballerismo,* concepts of manliness in the Latino culture that value courage, honor, and dignity. This means that for many Latino men, a digital rectal exam would be emasculating, embarrassing, and an affront to dignity.

The nurse searches the literature for more information and learns that some Hispanic men feel healthcare providers do not understand their culture and do not take time to develop a relationship with them. After synthesizing the literature, the nurses decided to adopt the following strategies:

➤ They will create educational materials that will be available in Spanish.

➤ Educational materials will specifically address culture-based fears that the exam is a threat to manliness.

➤ To reach the men (who tend to avoid healthcare), nurses will educate the women in the family. They believe the women will then encourage their men to get screened.

➤ The nurses will use community leaders, public service announcements, and churches to spread information.

Think about it:

Reflect on the following questions. You might want to discuss them with your peers.

➤ In what ways did the nurses make the planned educational materials patient- centered?

➤ How could the nurses evaluate the patient-centeredness of the educational materials? What information would they need? Where might they obtain the information?

➤ Patient-centered care often correlates to improvements in care. How can the clinic staff evaluate improvements in the healthcare of Latino men in their community after the educational campaign? Consider the following questions in your answer.

➤ What goals are reasonable for this educational effort?

➤ What assessments would be used to determine effectiveness?

Source: Agency for Healthcare Research and Quality. (2011, December). Human factors challenges in home health care: Research activities, 376. Rockville, MD: Author.; Purnell, L. D. (2014). Guide to culturally competent healthcare (3rd ed.). Philadelphia, PA: F.A. Davis.

pre-disease state. The disease process is clinically apparent and client debilitation, including death, is likely without intervention. Tertiary-level interventions require the nurse to **collaborate** with members of other healthcare providers to provide treatment. For example, a student may report to a school nurse that she has been involved in unprotected sexual activities.

- The school nurse may refer the student to the public health clinic for a pelvic exam and lab testing to detect STI, and hepatitis B, HPV, and HIV screening. The student has an abnormal Pap smear, showing cells suggestive of HPV exposure.
- The clinic nurse, in collaboration with the provider, administers medical treatment.
- There is no cure for HPV, so the teen also needs to learn how to prevent the spread of the disease to others; get immunized with the HPV vaccine; and obtain regular Pap and pelvic exams to detect cervical cancer and other STIs.

ThinkLike a Nurse 42-3

What level of intervention is required to address the concerns of Tanya and Jacob (Meet Your Patients)? Discuss your response.

KnowledgeCheck 42-5

For each of the nursing actions listed, identify the level of the nursing intervention as *primary, secondary,* or *tertiary.*

- Taking a client's blood pressure at a health fair
- Administering insulin to an older adult at an extended care facility
- Teaching second grade students to wash their hands correctly

What Career Opportunities Are Available for Community-Based Nurses?

The following are only a few of the many career opportunities for those who want to practice community-based nursing:

School Nursing

Nursing practice in the school setting began when educators realized that children with health problems had more difficulty learning. The core focus is keeping students healthy and in school as school attendance is essential for academic success (American Academy of Pediatrics, 2016). School nurses:

- Provide direct care for children with chronic health conditions such as asthma, attention deficit disorder, and diabetes.
- Help children who need routine procedures, such as catheterization, during the school day.
- Perform vision and hearing screenings.
- Administer prescribed medication.
- Ensure that age-appropriate immunizations are documented.
- May offer health education on topics such as nutrition, physical activity, and sexual and reproductive health.
- Serve as role models for students who lack parental support or who are struggling with peer pressure.

For the most part, a school nurse is autonomous and must be capable of prioritizing and making decisions (American Nurses Association and the National Association of School Nurses, 2011).

Occupational Health

Occupational health nurses work primarily in industrial or corporate settings. Their work includes the following:

- Provide health promotion programs for employees and their families in an effort to reduce absentee hours, increase productivity, and reduce illness and complications.
- Complete required medical documentation for disability claims or occupational hazardous events.
- Conduct new-hire and annual screenings.
- Provide care to injured or ill workers.
- Obtain random drug testing.
- File workers' compensation claims.

To reduce costs, some industries contract a staffing agency to provide trained occupational health nurses. Nursing autonomy and responsibility vary with the employer and the negotiated contract.

Parish Nursing

Parish nursing is a specialized area of nursing practice that focuses on the promotion of health within the context of the values, beliefs, and practices of a faith community. The parish nurse acts as health educator and personal health counselor, increasing awareness of the interrelationship between lifestyle, personal habits, attitudes, and spiritual beliefs. The nurse develops support groups, trains volunteers, and provides community referrals as needed. The level of autonomy and responsibility of parish nurses varies, depending on the faith community setting.

Nursing in Correctional Facilities

Corrections nurses deliver healthcare within the criminal justice system, for example, in juvenile detention, substance abuse treatment facilities, and prisons. The nurse provides primary care services to people of all ages in an unbiased and nonjudgmental manner (American Nurses Association, 2013a). Correctional facilities employ providers and nurse practitioners who conduct routine examinations and acute and chronic healthcare on a scheduled or as-needed basis. They administer medication, perform intake assessments, deliver triage care, and perform other primary care services as needed. The nurse may also perform occupational health duties for facility staff. For personal safety, nurses must meet certain physical requirements and complete special weapons training before working in most correctional facilities. Nurses have a high level of autonomy in most correctional or substance rehabilitation facilities and are commonly involved in policy decisions involved inmate healthcare.

Public Health Clinics

Many community nurses practice within local and state departments of health, including public health clinics. Large cities tend to have nurses who specialize (immunizations, prenatal health, school health, or epidemiological survey). Smaller communities may have fewer nurses (or full-time equivalents) providing broader services. The autonomy and scope of practice of public health nurses are often limited by the philosophy of the political administration and availability of funding.

Disaster Services Nursing

A disaster is any event or catastrophe inflicting widespread loss of life, diminution of health, and destruction of property. Features characterizing a disaster typically involve unpredictability, urgency, threat, speed, and uncertainty. They may develop as sudden-onset or slow-onset.

- *Human-generated disasters* might be the result of chemical spills, war, or acts such as a terrorist attack, causing harm or fear.
- *Technological disasters* cause damage or disruption on a large scale (e.g., computer systems failure, mass power outage, explosion, or hazardous substance exposure).
- *Natural or ecological disasters* include hurricanes, earthquakes, floods, or even environmental degradation, such as deforestation.
- *Biological disaster* may involve exposure to pathogenic microorganism, toxin, or other bioactive substance (e.g., an outbreak of endemic disease or plant contagion).

Community-oriented nursing emphasizes community assessment and education to reduce the number of casualties when disasters occur and to achieve the best possible level of health for the people and community involved in a disaster (Box 42-1).

Disasters affect the health status of a community by:

- Leading to premature death, illness, or injury.
- Disrupting healthcare services offered within the community.
- Causing environmental issues, such as outbreaks of communicable disease or food/water-borne illness.
- Causing shortages of safe food and drinking water.
- Burdening other healthcare systems when displaced populations shift to a host community for basic needs (Veenema, 2013).

In large-scale disasters, a nurse's duties may include:

- Rapidly assessing the overall situation and that of individual victims.
- Triaging care and initiating lifesaving measures first.
- Adapting nursing skills to the disaster situation, considering available equipment, supplies, and personnel.
- Evaluating the safety of the environment and remove health hazards.
- Providing leadership in coordinating care, assigning priorities for care, and transporting victims.
- Preventing further injury or illness.
- Providing compassionate support to victims and their families.

KEY POINT. *Good Samaritan laws protect nurses when volunteering—in any state—as long as actions are reasonable.*

International Nursing

Nurses working internationally commonly provide relief services after a natural or human-caused disaster. They may also offer health or human aid services through a medical clinic,

---

BOX 42-1 ■ What You Should Do During a Disaster Event

- Remain calm and be patient.
- Follow the advice of local emergency officials.
- Listen to the radio, watch television, or consult the Internet for news and instructions.
- If the disaster occurs near you, check for injuries. Give first aid and get help for seriously injured people.
- If the disaster occurs near your home while you are there, check for damage using a flashlight. Do not light matches or candles or turn on electrical switches. Check for fires, fire hazards, and other household hazards. Sniff for gas leaks, starting at the water heater. If you smell gas or suspect a leak, turn off the main gas valve, open windows, and get everyone outside quickly.
- Turn off any other damaged utilities.
- Confine or secure your pets.
- Contact your family contact.
- Check on your neighbors, especially those who are older or disabled.

faith-based mission, orphanage, or international relief program. International nursing requires a high level of autonomy, flexibility, and ingenuity, depending on community needs and available resources. Common problems affecting the health of international communities are poor sanitation, contaminated food and water, waste management, limited or dangerous transportation, communicable disease, parasitic infections, cultural practices, and limited education. Nurses working globally commonly treat people with malnutrition, dehydration, mosquito- and other insect-related illnesses, parasitic infestation, hepatitis, and HIV, to name a few (Fig. 42-4). Because of poor access to healthcare and limited or no resources to pay for medication, many people do not receive adequate healthcare.

Think**Like a Nurse** 42-4

Increase your self-knowledge: Assume you are going to be a community-based nurse. Of the many career opportunities available, which work do you think you would rather do? Explain why.

PracticalKnowledge
knowing **how**

The American Nurses Association, in the *Standards of Community Health Nursing* (1986) (Box 42-2), describes the goal of community health nursing as the promotion and preservation of the health of the community population as a whole, defined groups, families, and individuals. Community nursing care should be delivered in a practical, culturally sensitive manner (Kulbok, Thatcher, Park, et al., 2012).

ASSESSMENT NP

The nursing process follows the same steps you have studied in the previous chapters but uses different forms and different language when your client is a community. Community assessment is usually ongoing and requires the nurse to collaborate with and compile information from a variety of sources. The assessment approach is based on the type of community, the purpose of the assessment, and personal

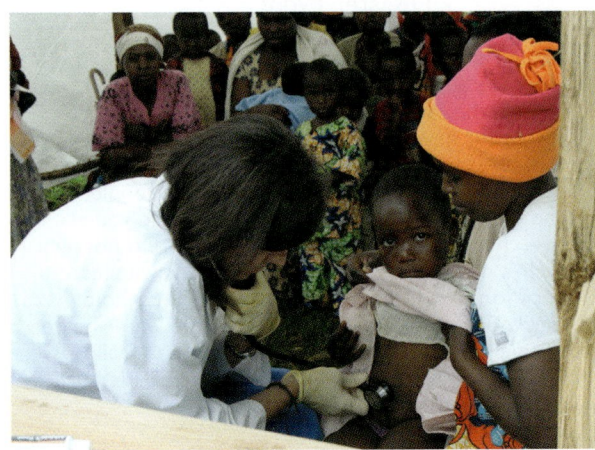

FIGURE 42-4 International nursing. Health and nutrition program for women and children at an African health clinic.

BOX 42-2 ■ American Nurses Association Standards of Community Health Nursing Practice

Standard 1: Theory. The nurse applies theoretical concepts as a basis for decisions in practice.
Standard 2: Data collection. The nurse systematically collects data that are comprehensive and accurate.
Standard 3: Diagnosis. The nurse analyzes data collected about the community, family, and individuals to determine diagnosis.
Standard 4: Planning. At each level of prevention, the nurse develops plans that specify nursing actions unique to the client's needs.
Standard 5: Intervention. The nurse, guided by the plan, intervenes to promote, maintain, or restore health; to prevent illness; and to effect rehabilitation.
Standard 6: Evaluation. The nurse evaluates the responses of the community, family, and individual to interventions to determine progress toward goal achievement and to revise the database, diagnosis, and plan.
Standard 7: Quality assurance and professional development. The nurse participates in peer review and other means of evaluation to ensure the quality of nursing practice. The nurse assumes responsibility for professional development and contributes to the professional growth of others.
Standard 8: Interdisciplinary collaboration. The nurse collaborates with other healthcare providers, professionals, and community representatives in assessing, planning, implementing, and evaluating programs for community health.
Standard 9: Research. The nurse contributes to theory and practice in community health nursing through research.

Source: American Nurses Association. (1986). *Standards of community health nursing practice.* Washington, DC: Author.

---

preference. Most beginning students elect to assess a geopolitical community because the data are more readily available than data from aggregate groups. Therefore, we focus on the geopolitical community assessment procedure.

Windshield Survey   Community assessment usually begins with a windshield survey. A **windshield survey** is performed while physically present in the area. It is similar to general observation of the individual client in that it provides an overview and allows you to see the community in its natural state. As you observe, make note of the condition of buildings and public facilities; residences; religious facilities; streets and sewers; modes of transportation; lighting; outward signs of poverty, crime, or violence; pollution; waste disposal; and other signs of the well-being of the community. Protective services, such as police and fire services, should be included. You may need to repeat the survey over time at different times of the day, month, or year to get an accurate picture of the community. For more reliable survey results, observers should be trained.

- Begin by describing the neighborhood and the people you see in the community.
- Remain objective in your observations; avoid using personal opinions and biases.
- Route your course prior to conducting the visit.

- Record your findings as soon as possible after your survey.
- Document the observation with photographs and videography when possible.

Databases and Public Records You can also obtain data from publicly available resources, such as birth records, marriage licenses, local news publications, and community Internet sites. Internet search engines can help you obtain demographic information, morbidity and mortality data, vital statistics, educational levels, criminal activity, political leadership issues, and/or information about community resources.

Client Perceptions You will also gather information about how individuals in the community perceive the community and its state of health. Through community gatherings and informal conversations, you can assess a cross section of the population. This is not only an important part of your assessment, but also an excellent way to establish rapport, convey your concerns, and develop a working relationship with key community members.

ANALYSIS/NURSING DIAGNOSIS NP

After a thorough assessment, you will analyze the complete set of data and compile a list of community strengths and limitations. Work with the community to develop a list of their priorities, considering needs identified by the client and based on availability of funding and political feasibility.

The NANDA-International Taxonomy

In community practice, you need nursing diagnoses that describe the health status of individuals, families, groups, and entire communities. Recall from Chapter 4 that the NANDA-I taxonomy of nursing diagnoses can be used in any nursing setting or specialty. You would simply add the term *community* to other NANDA-I labels when creating a community-based diagnosis: for example, Decisional Conflict (Community) related to safety needs of the homeless population. In addition, the NANDA-I taxonomy includes three diagnoses that specifically describe the health status of a community:

- Deficient Community Health
- Ineffective Community Coping
- Readiness for Enhanced Community Coping

The Omaha Problem Classification System

The Omaha System is a problem-solving model for community health practice, education, and research. The taxonomy consists of *diagnostic labels* organized into four *domains* (categories), along with two sets of *modifiers*. The problem labels in the environment domain are especially useful in community nursing. For the complete problem classification scheme,

 Go to the **Omaha System Web site,** at http://www.omahasystem.org

To create a diagnostic statement, choose an appropriate label and add a modifier to it from each of the two sets in the accompanying Standardized Language box. For a community-based diagnosis, you would add "group" as the modifier. See the accompanying Standardized Language box Omaha System: Domains and Examples of Problem Labels.

PLANNING OUTCOMES/EVALUATION NP

In the community you will need to write goals and outcomes for aggregates. The *Healthy People 2020* goals, for example, are aggregate goals.

Standardized Language

Omaha System: Domains and Examples of Problem Labels

Environmental Domain—The material resources, physical surroundings, and substances both internal and external to the client, home, neighborhood, and broader community

Problem (Diagnosis) Labels: Income, Sanitation, Residence, Neighborhood/Workplace Safety

Psychosocial Domain—Patterns of behavior, communication, relationships, and development.

Problem (Diagnosis) Labels: Social Contact, Role Change, Interpersonal Relationships, Spirituality, Grief, Mental Health, Sexuality, Caretaking/Parenting, Neglect, Abuse

Physiological Domain—Functional status of processes that maintain life.

Problem (Diagnosis) Labels: Hearing, Vision, Oral Health, Speech and Language, Pain, Respiration, Digestion-Hydration, Communicable/Infectious Condition

Health Related Behaviors Domain—Activities that maintain or promote wellness, promote recovery, or maximize rehabilitation potential.

Problem (Diagnosis) Labels: Nutrition, Personal Hygiene, Prescribed Medication Regimen, Sleep and Rest Patterns, Family Planning, Physical Activity

Problem Modifiers

Set 1—Health Promotion, Potential Deficit, Deficit
Set 2—Family, Individual, Group*

_____
*Martin and Scheet (1992, p. 67) suggest that Group be added to these modifiers.
Source: Martin, K. S., & Scheet, N. J. (1992). *The Omaha system: Applications for community health nursing* (pp. 67–74). Philadelphia, PA: W. B. Saunders. Used with permission; Omaha System (2016). *Solving clinical data-information: Problem rating scale for outcomes.* Retrieved from http://www.omahasystem.org

---

Nursing Outcome Classification (NOC)

Use these NOC labels in the Community Health domain to write goals by adding the appropriate NOC indicators and scales (Moorhead, Johnson, Maas, et al., 2013).

- Community Competence
- Community Disaster Readiness
- Community Disaster Response
- Community Health Status
- Community Health Status: Immunity
- Community Risk Control: Chronic Disease
- Community Risk Control: Communicable Disease
- Community Risk Control: Lead Exposure
- Community Risk Control: Violence
- Community Violence Level

Omaha System Outcomes

Using the Omaha system, you will develop goals/outcomes from the nursing diagnosis. Recall that all nursing diagnoses are identified as *individual, family,* or *group;* so a group nursing diagnosis will automatically indicate a group goal. The Omaha system uses a 5-point Problem Rating Scale for Outcomes that describes what you expect to achieve in terms of the client's *knowledge, behavior, and status.* For example, for the diagnosis Deficit in Group Workplace Safety, you would might create the following group goals:

Knowledge	(4) Adequate knowledge of workplace safety
Behavior	(4) Usually appropriate group safety behaviors
Status	(4) Minimal signs/symptoms (e.g., few accidents or injuries)

PLANNING INTERVENTIONS/ IMPLEMENTATION NP

As a community health nurse, you will need interventions to promote and preserve the health of individuals, aggregates, and communities. Both NIC and the Omaha system provide standardized vocabularies for aggregate interventions.

The Nursing Interventions Classification (NIC)

The NIC taxonomy includes 18 interventions specifically designed for community health. See the accompanying box, below.

The Omaha Intervention Taxonomy

The Omaha system taxonomy provides four "intervention categories" you can use in community-oriented nursing practice:

- **Health Teaching, Guidance, and Counseling**—Primary prevention activities that include giving information; anticipating client problems; encouraging client action and responsibility for self-care; and assisting with coping, decision making, and problem-solving.
- **Treatments and Procedures**—Secondary interventions directed toward preventing disease, identifying risk factors and early signs and symptoms, and decreasing or alleviating signs and symptoms.
- **Case Management**—A tertiary intervention that includes coordination, advocacy, and referral.

- **Surveillance**—Includes detection, measurement, critical analysis, and monitoring to indicate client status in relation to a given condition or phenomenon.

To write an intervention statement, you must:

1. Combine one of those four "categories" with one of the 75 "targets" (objects of the nursing interventions), such as bowel care and nutrition.
2. Then add patient-specific information to individualize the nursing order.

To see the entire set of intervention targets,

 Go to the **Omaha System Web site,** at http://www. omahasystem.org/shminter.htm

You will notice that the targets can be used for individuals as well as groups. It is the designation of the nursing diagnosis as *individual, family,* or *group* that determines this. For examples of Omaha interventions statements, see the accompanying Standardized Language box Omaha System: Intervention Categories and Examples of Targets.

APPLYING THE NURSING PROCESS IN COMMUNITY-BASED CARE

Community assessment and care planning may at first seem different from what you have been doing for individual patients. But it does follow the same problem-solving process:

Scenario: As a nurse employed by a local immunization clinic, you have been hired into a new position created by federal and state grant monies to investigate why immunization levels are low among 2-year-olds in Census Tract 15. You would begin with an assessment.

1. **Gather data about the community.**
   - *Define the community.* For instance, determine the physical boundaries of Census Tract 15, a geopolitical community.
   - *Learn the community.* Start interacting with the community to build rapport. Begin the ongoing assessment by

---

Standardized Language

NIC Community Health Classes and Interventions

Class: Community Health Promotion—Interventions that promote the health of the whole community

Interventions:
Case Management
Community Health Development
Fiscal Resource Management
Health Education
Health Policy Monitoring
Immunization/Vaccination Management
Program Development
Social Marketing

Class: Community Risk Management—Interventions that assist in detecting or preventing health risks to the whole community

Interventions:
Bioterrorism Preparedness
Community Disaster Preparedness
Communicable Disease Management
Environmental Management: Community
Environmental Management: Worker Safety
Environmental Risk Protection
Health Screening
Risk Identification
Surveillance: Community
Vehicle Safety Promotion

Source: Bulechek, G. M., Butcher, H. K., Dochterman, J. M., et al. (Eds.). (2013). *Nursing interventions classification (NIC)* (6th ed.). St. Louis, MO: C.V. Mosby. Used with permission from Elsevier Science.

Standardized Language

Omaha System: Intervention Categories and Examples of Targets

Categories

I. Health Teaching, Guidance, and Counseling
II. Treatments and Procedures
III. Case Management
IV. Surveillance

Examples of Targets

Anatomy/physiology
Behavior modification
Communication
Discipline
Feeding procedures
Homemaking
Substance use
Wellness

Examples of Aggregate Targets

Caretaking/parenting skills
Day care/respite
Durable medical equipment
Education
Employment
Environment
Finances
Housing
Legal system
Transportation
Other community resource

Examples of Nursing Intervention Statements

Treatments and Procedures (II): Feeding procedures (Demonstrate to Mrs. Adams how to feed Mr. Adams at the next visit.)

Surveillance (IV): Feeding procedures (After teaching, observe a feeding. Monitor for choking.)

Source: Omaha System. (2016, updated). *Solving the clinical data-information scheme: Intervention scheme.* Retrieved from http://www.omahasystem.org/interventionscheme.html

---

conducting windshield surveys, searching for information through reputable databases, and talking with community members.

■ *Focus the data collection.* Focus on the information that will help you determine possible causes of low immunization rates. In this case, the priority problem has already been defined by the financing agency.

ThinkLike a Nurse 42-5

What data would you want to look at? What are possible reasons for low immunization rates?

2. **Analyze the Data.** Examine the characteristics of the families failing to provide immediate immunization for children, including:
    ■ Family demographics
    ■ Age of children
    ■ Number of immunizations needed and the cost
    ■ Beliefs about negative effects of vaccines
    ■ Availability of transportation
    ■ Public sites providing vaccinations
    ■ Overall continuity of general healthcare for children

Assume that after working with the community for 6 months, you have spoken at parenting classes about the need to vaccinate children. Several community members have told you they thought their child had already received all necessary immunizations or that their healthcare provider had said to wait until they have better insurance. You would need to arrange a meeting with the local providers to discuss low immunization status. They explain that many vaccinations are too expensive to provide based on the reimbursement they receive from government funding sources.

3. **Plan care.** Your next move is to do some planning. Using the Omaha system, you could generate a care plan to address some of the issues raised by community members and physicians.

4. **Evaluate results and follow up.** Community assessment is never complete because the community is constantly changing. However, you need to define the identified needs and desired outcomes during a given period of time, based on best data available at the time of collection. In this case, you would share with local healthcare providers, the health department, and local health policy committee your approach to addressing the factors suspected of contributing to poor immunization compliance. An important part of your role as a community health nurse is to continue to monitor and evaluate the data and provide updates to the appropriate groups.

Now that you have some understanding of community healthcare, the rest of the chapter focuses on a specific type of community nursing: delivering healthcare in the patient's home.

TheoreticalKnowledge
knowing why

UNDERSTANDING THE CONCEPT OF HOME HEALTHCARE

Recall that community-based healthcare refers to services performed outside of acute care settings. Home healthcare is one such service. **Home healthcare** is the delivery of health-related services in the client's home. Home healthcare is appropriate when a client needs ongoing care that exceeds the abilities of friends and family, as in the following situations:

- To serve as a backup for safety or additional assessment

  - For older adults who need ongoing care but want to avoid moving to a skilled nursing facility

- For people of any age who require home-care service when they require support services for acute illness, injury, or surgery (e.g., insulin management, IV therapy, oxygen support)
- For ongoing care of chronically ill adults and children to avoid hospitalization (chemotherapy)
- For support of patients with terminal illness (medication, nutrition)

Goals of Home Healthcare

Nurses provide home care to clients with complex, chronic, or terminal illness. The primary goals in home healthcare are that (1) the client's self-care ability and independence will improve and (2) caregivers gain the ability to assist the client with ongoing health needs.

This approach may be different from what you have experienced in other clinical settings. For example, as the nurse in the Meet Your Patients scenario, you would help the couple manage Mr. Escobar's care independently at home. Initially you might show Mrs. Escobar how to administer medications and explain their function, and demonstrate strategies for moving and turning Mr. Escobar. However, your goal would be for her to progress to managing these tasks independently.

Distinctive Features of Home Healthcare

Home health nursing differs from hospital nursing in several ways; for example:

1. **The hospital environment is controlled.** Surfaces are regularly disinfected; supplies are stocked; and foods, medications, and other therapies are readily available. Computers are conveniently located, making patient information easily accessible.
2. **The hospital nurse can consult almost immediately with a team of healthcare providers** (i.e., other nurses, the primary care provider, various therapists, social workers, a pastoral care provider, and even a business office staff).

In contrast, when you are in a patient's home, surprisingly little is within your control. The home may be spotless or filthy, food plentiful or scarce, and supplies readily available or unreliable. The television or music may be loud; a dog may be barking; or young children may interrupt your interactions with the client or caregiver. Nursing care in the home is different from inpatient settings in the following ways:

- You are a guest in the client's home. The client and family determine whether they are willing to let you enter the home to deliver care.
- You are responsible for making the assessments and determining whether to advise the primary care provider of client changes.
- You must bring all necessary supplies or arrange to have them delivered ahead of time.
- You must be able to distinguish between skilled services, which are eligible for reimbursement from Medicare, and homemaker services.
  - **Skilled services** are services that must be performed or supervised by a licensed healthcare professional (Box 42-3).
  - **Homemaker services** (e.g., cleaning, meal preparation) are reimbursed to clients only if the principal reason for

---

BOX 42-3 ■ Skilled Nursing Services

Medicare defines skilled nursing care as services and care that can be done safely and correctly only by a licensed registered or practical nurse. The services must be reasonable and necessary for the treatment of the illness or injury.

- Patient assessment
- Ongoing monitoring of patient status
- Management and coordination of the patient's plan of care
- Evaluation of response to medications or treatment
- Medication instruction
- Teaching patients or caregivers to provide care or therapies
- Disease-related teaching (e.g., diabetes education)
- Complex tasks, such as injections, insertion of urinary catheters, infusion therapy, wound care, tube feedings, or ventilator management

---

home care is a skilled service. These services are provided by home health aides.

- You must be more self-sufficient and function independently. Often there are no other team members immediately available for support, assistance, or consultation.
- You must be aware of and comfortable with the family observing you as you provide care.
- You will need to adapt to varying family relationships and some home environments that are difficult or even dysfunctional.
- You will need to encourage the family to help in providing care and in taking over care when you leave the home. Be aware that overburdened caregivers may need your help as much as does the client.
- You must preplan your visit by figuring out the directions to sites in advance and arranging appointments efficiently.
- Your personal safety may be more of a concern when making home visits. You must always be aware of the environment around you and alert to possible dangers.
- Things do not always go as planned in a less controlled home environment, so you will need to be flexible and learn to modify your plan.

One advantage of home healthcare is that it allows you to expand your understanding of the concept of *client*. The home setting is a window into the client's life, through which you can see his personal environment: how he lives, eats, and makes daily choices for health and welfare of himself and others within the home. The photos, mementos, personal belongings, and other things the client values and cherishes make cultural beliefs and practices more visible. These items provide clues to his lifestyle, strengths, resources, and motivation.

KEY POINT: *Home health nursing also differs from community healthcare. Community health nurses provide care for individuals, families, and groups with an emphasis on population-based care. In contrast, home health nursing focuses on the individual and his support system.*

KnowledgeCheck 42-6

Identify at least four skilled services that may be provided in the home.

WHO PROVIDES HOME HEALTHCARE?

Home healthcare is provided by a variety of healthcare professionals employed by or working in cooperation with home healthcare agencies.

Home Health Agencies

Home health agencies coordinate the services of various professionals and paraprofessionals. The various types of agencies may be categorized by purpose, by type of client served, or by funding source.

Purpose   In this category, direct care agencies are the most common.

- **Direct care agencies** focus on direct client interaction by providing skilled care, associated therapies and health services, home health aides, and chore workers, and delivery of respite care.
- **Respite care,** a specific type of direct care agency, provides relief for family caregivers.
- **Indirect service agencies** also play a vital role in home healthcare. Examples include pharmaceutical and infusion companies and suppliers of durable medical equipment.
- **Durable medical equipment (DME)** is reusable equipment (e.g., walkers, wheelchairs, apnea monitors). Medicare pays for some, but not all, such devices. It is expensive, so before ordering it, be sure the DME is covered or the client can pay for it.

Type of Client Served   An important specialty home service agency is hospice care. This may be a separate agency or a division of a home health agency. Still other agencies specialize in caring for patients with complex diseases, such as AIDS, or ventilator-dependent clients, or patients of a certain age-group (services for older adults or chronically ill children).

Funding Source   Agencies may take on many forms based on funding source, profit or nonprofit status, and relationship with other healthcare organizations.

- **Public agencies** are official or governmental agencies organized at the city, county, state, or national level. They are usually funded by taxes, along with reimbursement from insurance companies. The local health department is a good example of a public agency. Health departments focus chiefly on community needs, although they often also offer some home health services, especially when tracking clients in some of their disease management programs.
- **Voluntary agencies** are prominent in the delivery of home healthcare. These agencies are normally governed by a board of directors and funded by donations, endowments, and third-party (insurance) reimbursement. Many **hospice organizations** (groups that provide care for people who are frail, terminally ill, dying, or not expected to improve) are voluntary organizations.
- **Proprietary organizations** are corporate or privately owned businesses that provide services for profit. These agencies receive payment from insurance companies but also accept private-pay clients. Proprietary organizations may provide traditional home health services as well as private-duty care and other services that assist individuals to remain independent.
- **Hospital-based agencies** are an extension of the services provided by a hospital. Clients who no longer meet the criteria for continued hospitalization may be transferred to home care for continued services. A benefit of this type of home health agency is in the ease of transition between hospital and home.

Home Health Nurses

To succeed in home healthcare, you must have the ability to work independently and collaboratively, be flexible and resourceful, and adapt to different home environments and family interactions. Home health nurses provide a broad range of services to clients of all ages. Communication is crucial in home care because of the need to establish good rapport with the client and family, as well as other members of the healthcare team. Roles include the following.

Direct Care Provider   As a direct care provider, you may administer medications, dress wounds, provide stoma care, or perform other skilled, complex tasks.

Educator   Recall that the goal of home healthcare is to promote self-care. Your focus will be to help the client or family take over the care. You must be able to clearly explain the care required, the rationale for it, and how to safely perform the care. This requires patience, skill, and repetition.

Client Advocate   In home care, the client and family are directly in charge of the plan of care. As client advocate, you support the client's right to make healthcare decisions yet protect the client from harm if he is unable to make decisions. In the event family members disagree with the client's choices, remember that as the client's advocate, you must ensure that his intentions are respected and his rights upheld. You must also advocate for client services, for example, securing additional home health support to avoid hospitalization. Or based on your assessment of the client and discussion with the client and family, you might advocate for another level of service, such as referral to hospice or placement in the hospital.

Care Coordinator   In this role, you will need to gather data at an initial visit and develop a plan of care that addresses the client's needs. Your plan may require you to make additional visits as well as specify and perhaps arrange delivery of therapies and services by other professionals in the home.

KnowledgeCheck 42-7

What roles does the nurse assume in home care? List and describe them.

Hospice Nurses

As you learned in Chapter 17, **hospice nursing** focuses on care of patients who are dying or whose condition is not expected to improve. "Considered the model for quality compassionate care for people facing a life-limiting illness, hospice provides expert medical care, pain management, and emotional and spiritual support expressly tailored to the patient's needs and wishes" (National Hospice and Palliative Care Organization, 2014, p. 3).

Hospice services are provided in the patient's home, in the hospital, in nursing homes, and in homes specifically designed for end-of-life care. The goal of hospice care is to promote comfort and quality of life. Because the client is not expected to recover, the focus of home hospice care is quite different from traditional home care. More than promoting self-care and independence, hospice care focuses on providing comfort and managing symptoms (Table 42-1).

As a direct care provider, the hospice nurse assesses the client's condition and monitors responses to interventions aimed at relieving distress. As an educator, the hospice nurse teaches the client and family how to adjust medications and care to control pain and other symptoms. The roles of communicator and client advocate assume prime importance as the

Table 42-1 ➤ Home Healthcare and Home Hospice Care		
	HOME HEALTHCARE	**HOME HOSPICE CARE**
Purpose	Promote self-care and independence	Promote comfort and quality of life
Focus of nursing interventions	Teach caregivers to assist the client with ongoing health needs and activities of daily living (ADLs)	Reduce pain, provide comfort, manage symptoms, support caregivers

client's condition deteriorates. The nurse shares these roles with the family and other home caregivers. If you need more information on hospice care, see Chapter 17.

WHO PAYS FOR HOME HEALTHCARE?

Medicare, Medicaid, private insurance, government-mandated insurance, and individual payments (private pay) help pay for home-care services. Medicare and Medicaid are the largest payers for home healthcare.

Medicare Reimbursement

Medicare is a federally funded healthcare system designed to provide health coverage for persons who are older than 65 years and younger people who are disabled or diagnosed with end-stage renal disease or amyotrophic lateral sclerosis (ALS) (Social Security Administration, 2016). Reimbursement by Medicare for home care depends on the following, strictly applied criteria:

- *The client must need skilled care.* See Box 42-3. Other services may also be provided, but the primary purpose for establishing care must be based on a skilled care need. This means that Medicare will not pay for personal care such as bathing and dressing when this is the only care the client needs.
- *The client must be homebound.* This means (1) the client must have a condition that restricts the ability to leave the home, and (2) leaving the home requires special assistance, transportation, or supportive devices.
- *The client must require nursing care that is part-time and intermittent.* This means Medicare will pay for a limited number of hours per day or days per week that the client can get skilled nursing care or home health aide services.
- *The plan of care must be authorized by the physician and re-certified every 62 days.* For the client to continue to receive care, there must be evidence of continued need that remains acute.
- *The care must be medically necessary and reasonable.* The plan of care must address the client's health concerns and have clearly delineated outcomes. The expectations of the patient must be reasonable.
- *Medicare will pay only for interventions identified on the treatment plan.* The payer may periodically request patient health records to verify that the care was given.
- *The home health agency must be approved by Medicare.* An agency must show that it meets the Medicare definitions and requirements to become Medicare certified.

Medicaid is a program sponsored jointly by the federal government and the states to provide services to people whose income is below a mandated level. In many states, the criteria for reimbursement are the same as those required by Medicare. However, each state at present determines what services will be part of its medical assistance plan.

Private Insurance and Self-Payment

Private insurance companies may also offer home health services. The type and extent of covered services are specified in each separate insurance plan. Many people require assistance in the home but do not meet criteria for reimbursement from Medicare, Medicaid, or their private insurer. Frequently, older clients require home health assistance but may not need skilled services. For example, they may need assistance with grocery shopping, meal planning and preparation, or transportation. Services are billed directly to the client.

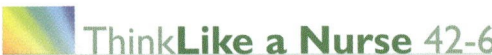

ThinkLike a Nurse 42-6

Review the scenario focused on Mr. Escobar (Meet Your Patients). What members of the home health team may be required to provide care? Why?

WHAT IS THE FUTURE OF HOME HEALTHCARE?

Healthcare analysts have predicted several changes in home care during the next few decades:

- **Increased need for home healthcare.** Considering the growing number of older adults in the United States, it is more cost effective to provide healthcare in the home than in an inpatient setting.
- **Increased use of the home for hospice care.** Public acceptance of the home as a place of comfort and care, as well as concerns about the cost of inpatient care, has increased the number of persons who choose this compassionate option for end-of-life and palliative care.
- **Increased technology.** Technological advances, such as online resources or telemedicine consultation, make it safer and more affordable to deliver complex care in the home and allow home health nurses to deliver information and provide support (Bradford, Armfield, Young, et al., 2013). Computerized monitoring and documentation allow home health agencies to better coordinate care, receive needed supplies, and manage costs.
- **Continued research.** Research is needed in strategies to improve the effectiveness of care, identify predictors of need for rehospitalization, and integrate home care into overall community-based services.

HOW ARE CLIENTS REFERRED TO HOME HEALTHCARE?

Referrals to home healthcare come from a variety of sources. However, for home care to begin, there must be a medical prescription and a physician-approved treatment plan.

Hospital-based agencies have a built-in referral base. If the primary provider or nursing staff determine that the client would benefit from home health services, they refer the patient to the agency while he is still hospitalized.

Many agencies have *intake coordinators* who work in the hospital and review clients for suitability of services, gathering information from the chart, the client, the family, and the hospital team. Home services are arranged before discharge from an inpatient facility. Ideally, a discharge planner gathers information, secures the prescription from the provider, and sets up home care for the patient. In some smaller hospitals, this task falls to the staff nurse providing predischarge care.

Referrals may also come from doctors, nurses, primary care offices and clinics, mental health workers, and other healthcare providers in the community, as well as directly from families and clients. Most home health agencies evaluate clients to determine whether they are eligible for services that are reimbursable by insurance. They may also offer services that the client may pay for independently.

PracticalKnowledge
knowing **how**

As a home healthcare nurse, your days will vary. Normally your caseload will be contained within a limited geographic boundary, so that you can schedule your visits efficiently, spending less time driving to visits, and have more time for delivering care. If you want to envision what it would be like to be a home health nurse, you need only to look at the list of services Medicare recognizes as skilled; see Box 42-3.

HOW DO I MAKE A HOME VISIT?
The home visit has three phases: preparation before the visit, nursing care during the visit, and evaluation after the visit.

Before the Visit
First review the client's chart and referral form to determine why you are making the visit. You may also need to review material about the client's health problem, medications, or treatment plan. Then you can begin to plan for the visit. What supplies will you need? What teaching materials will you need? What are the goals of the visit? Does the agency require additional client information, such as insurance data, to provide care? The agency will probably have a set of forms (e.g., HIPAA privacy forms, billing information) for you to complete during the first visit. Be sure you have those with you.

➕ Before the visit you will need directions to the home, and you will need to determine whether there are safety concerns. Contact the client to notify him of the planned date and time of the visit and to determine whether his health status has changed since the referral was made. This will allow you to bring additional equipment or personnel along if needed.

Prepare Supplies
Home health nurses usually bring an equipment bag (Fig. 42-5) with supplies geared to the needs of the clients in the nurse's caseload.
- Hand-washing supplies (e.g., soap or antibacterial handrub, paper towels)
- Stethoscope
- Sphygmomanometers (with cuffs in a variety of sizes)

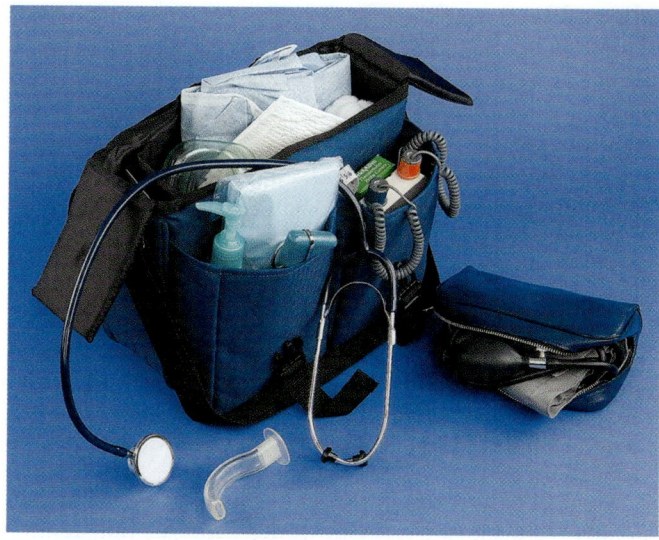

FIGURE 42-5 The home health nursing bag contains some standard items but is usually customized according to the requirements of the clients in the nurse's caseload.

- Thermometers (oral and rectal)
- Small equipment (scissors, forceps, penlight, staple remover)
- Tape measure (with plastic coating that can be cleaned, or several disposable ones)
- Full, protective gown
- Gloves, sterile and clean
- An assortment of gauze dressings, tape, scissors, cotton balls
- Occupational Safety and Health Administration (OSHA) supplies: N95 respirator, face masks, protective eyewear, disinfectant spray, disposable gowns to protect clothing
- A variety of syringes and safety needles (this varies widely among agencies)
- Venipuncture supplies
- Airway and resuscitation mask
- Tablet or laptop with electronic health record
- Specific supplies as needed (IV therapy, ostomy supplies, urinary catheter kit, wound care, etc.)

You may need other supplies, such as medications, a scale, and a transfer belt, depending on the requirements of the clients in your caseload. If the client needs frequent dressing changes or supplies for treatments (e.g., tube feedings), it is best to have the supplies delivered directly to the client's house to reduce the number of materials you must carry. Note that in some states nurses are not permitted to carry medications because of safety concerns. You will need to check on the rules that apply to your state.

Provide for Your Safety

➕ As you drive to the home, begin to make your assessment. Locate the stores, hospital, and community resources. What is the overall character of the neighborhood? Does this appear to be a safe neighborhood? What are the conditions of the approach to the home?

Safety for yourself and the client is an essential consideration even more so when you enter someone's home. You should provide your agency with your patient care schedule for the day and a tracking device to identify your location if case you need to summon for help. For suggestions about the safe delivery of home healthcare, see Clinical Insight 42-1.

KnowledgeCheck 42-8

What are the major tasks that must be completed before making a home visit?

At the Visit

When you arrive at the home, you must remember this is the client's domain. Knock or ring the doorbell and wait to be invited in. Introduce yourself to the client and family. Be respectful of their home, as well as their beliefs, values, practices, and cultural preferences.

The first few minutes of the initial visit set the tone for the relationship between client, family, nurse, and agency. This is your opportunity to develop rapport and trust. Introducing yourself, waiting for permission to enter, and treating the client and family members with respect are ways to help to establish rapport.

You should also offer your card or identification badge to identify yourself and provide contact information for the home health agency. Generally, agencies provide clients with information packets that include the client's bill of rights, client responsibilities, billing information, information on the frequency and duration of services, how to reach the agency, and the date and time of the next visit.

As you do all this, you also gather data. Who answered your questions? What is the relationship between the caregiver and the client? How do they interact? What other people live there? What is the condition of the home? If this is an initial visit, you may need to verify or complete client data on the referral form. In the hospital, admissions personnel usually gather admitting data and obtain consent for treatment. In home care, you need to collect and document this information.

At a home visit, you might do a variety of things, such as performing physical care; drawing blood samples for lab work; checking weight; administering medication, IV fluid, or tube feedings; providing wound or ostomy care; or whatever else may be needed.

ThinkLike a Nurse 42-7

Review the case of Mr. Escobar (Meet Your Patients). What information did you gain from the first few minutes of the visit?

- Both Mr. and Mrs. Escobar are in need of nursing interventions. However, this is your agency's first home visit to them, and you have other clients you must visit today, so you will need to prioritize. What must the home health nurse do during the initial visit to a client?
- In addition to completing your assessment and talking about a plan of care with the Escobars, what do you think is the single most important thing you can do for them today? Explain your thinking.
- When Mrs. Escobar meets you at the door and brings you into the living room, you notice a large German shepherd dog lying beside Mr. Escobar's bed. Mrs. Escobar says, "Stay, King"; and then to you, "Roland likes having him nearby." What should you do?

After the Visit

After you leave the home, there is still a lot of work for you to do. Often you will need to complete the documentation for the visit. In Chapter 18, you learned about documentation techniques, various forms of charting, and legal aspects of documentation. In home care all of these rules apply; however, some aspects of home-care documentation are unique.

Home health agencies use Medicare's Outcome and Assessment Information Set (OASIS) to record initial assessment data. To continue to provide needed services to the client, you must include in your documentation (1) evidence of homebound status and (2) evidence of continued need for skilled care. Other post-visit activities include ordering supplies needed for the next visit, making referrals to additional services (e.g., occupational therapy), coordinating care among the various services, and scheduling the next visit.

NURSING PROCESS IN HOME CARE

The nursing process moves through the same phases in all patient care settings. The difference in home care is that you must use forms structured to satisfy Medicare and other insurance requirements. Nevertheless, you need to assess the client, the family, the home, and the community to identify health problems. You will work from a plan of care prescribed by a medical provider, but individualize it with suitable nursing diagnoses and interventions.

ASSESSMENT NP

Typically, a full assessment requires multiple visits. On the initial visit, you need to perform an assessment to establish a baseline and determine the type of care required. This assessment includes the following:

- Health history
- Pertinent family and social history
- Review of all medications—prescribed, over the counter, and alternative
- Mental status
- Functional ability
- Availability of family, informal support, and caregivers
- Nutritional status
- Assessment of the home environment

Medicare requires home health agencies to collect specific information for all Medicare clients they serve. The OASIS data must be collected at the start of care, with each recertification (every 60 days), and at the termination of care. Medicare uses these data to determine the effectiveness of care and to monitor client outcomes. In addition to the required OASIS information, many agencies use other assessment tools created specifically for their needs. If you would like to see an OASIS form,

 Go to http://www.oasisanswers.com/downloads/SAMPLE_FORMS_OAI_Manual_2008.pdf

It is also important to assess the needs of the caregivers—the family members, friends, and support system in the home. To be successful in home care, you must work with and support the caregivers. Take time at each visit to speak with them, making sure to include them in your assessment, plan of care, and teaching. Assessment of the caregivers often allows you to determine what services are needed in the home. Caregivers, especially older adults, may have health problems of their own that affect their ability to provide care for another.

ANALYSIS/NURSING DIAGNOSIS NP

As in any setting, the nursing diagnoses are based on the client's responses to illness and care. As a home healthcare nurse, you will work with clients with numerous medical and nursing diagnoses. Two frequently used nursing diagnoses are Caregiver Role Strain and Deficient Knowledge.

Caregiver Role Strain and Risk for Caregiver Role Strain These diagnoses are appropriate for those for whom the burden of caregiving has become, or is at risk of becoming, overwhelming. Providing care to a loved one at home can be a challenge, especially when finances don't allow a family to hire home health aides. Around-the-clock caregiving duties can lead to physical exhaustion, social isolation, resentment, sadness, or depression. In addition, the demands of caring for the client can interfere with other responsibilities.

Common signs of caregiver role strain include difficulty adjusting to role changes, fatigue, isolation, depression, and difficulty in performing routine care for the client.

Deficient Knowledge Client and family teaching is especially important in home care because most of the caregiving is performed by the client and significant others. You will spend much of your time teaching them the skills necessary for self-care (e.g., how to administer insulin, how to manage the oxygen equipment). Recall that to be eligible for home nursing care, clients must require skilled nursing care. Client education is a service for which Medicare and other insurers will reimburse. You must include a Deficient Knowledge diagnosis on the care plan to ensure the client's continued eligibility and reimbursement for the service.

Safety and Risk for Infection are also key concerns in the home. These are thoroughly discussed in Chapters 23 and 22, respectively. Infection control measures in the home are also presented in the section "Infection Control in the Home," later in this chapter. Associated diagnoses include Impaired Home Maintenance, Risk for Falls, Risk for Infection, and Risk for Poisoning.

KEY POINT: *In other chapters, we caution against indiscriminate use of the Deficient Knowledge diagnosis. However, an exception must be made for home care because of Medicare regulations.*

KnowledgeCheck 42-9

- Why are the first few minutes of the initial visit so important?
- Identify five things that should be assessed at an initial home visit.

ThinkLike a Nurse 42-8

- Based on the information in the scenario, what nursing diagnoses might Mr. Escobar (Meet Your Patients) have? There may not be enough data to make definite diagnoses, but what probable diagnoses are there for which you would want to gather confirming data? Do not include potential diagnoses, such as Risk for Imbalanced Nutrition.
- Mr. Escobar has a potential problem, Risk for Falls. What are two interventions you would probably be able to do today to reduce his risk for falls?
- What, if any, evidence of caregiver strain does Mrs. Escobar exhibit?

Standardized Terminology for Home Health Nursing Diagnoses

Various disciplines, including nursing, have developed classifications of common terminology (also called taxonomies, vocabularies, and standardized languages) for describing their work and for planning, communicating, and documenting care. You are familiar with the NANDA-I taxonomy of nursing diagnoses; however, home-care nurses more

commonly use the Clinical Care Classification (CCC) because it is closely related to the OASIS reporting forms required by Medicare.

The CCC contains standardized and coded nursing diagnostic categories that are especially applicable to home healthcare. The CCC coding structure and framework system is relevant to home care in the following ways:

- Parallels the steps of the nursing process
- Links the CCC diagnoses to nursing interventions and client outcomes
- Standardizes the terminology for client care within clinical information systems
- Facilitates nursing documentation at the point of care
- Provides a structure for planning resources needed for client and community care
- Quantifies the nursing workload to optimize productivity
- Defines client outcomes for quality care
- Provides quantitative data for research (Saba, 1994, 2004, 2012).

The system uses care components that represent the functional, health behavior, physiological, and psychological patterns of patient care. Common CCC nursing diagnoses used in the home include:

Activities of Daily Living (ADLs) Alteration
Caregiver Role Strain
Family Processes Alteration
Home Maintenance Alteration
Knowledge Deficit
Physical Mobility Impairment
Self-Care Deficit

For complete information on the CCC and complete lists of diagnoses, outcomes, and interventions,

 Go to the **Clinical Care Classification Web site,** at http://www.sabacare.com

PLANNING OUTCOMES/EVALUATION NP

Clinical Care Classification (CCC) Each CCC Nursing Diagnosis requires an Expected Outcome, which is the anticipated goal of the nursing actions planned to care for the patient's condition (Saba, 2012). To formulate a goal/outcome in the CCC system, attach one of the three CCC "modifiers" (*improve, stabilize, deteriorate*) to the diagnosis.

- The outcome describes the *desired* client health status.
- To evaluate client progress, you again use one of the three modifiers to describe the client's *actual* health status.
- The following is an example:

CCC nursing diagnosis:	Knowledge Deficit
Goal/expected outcome:	Knowledge Deficit, Improve
Actual status on evaluation:	Knowledge Deficit, Stabilized

Medicare requires that the client's status be evaluated and coded as improved, stabilized, or deteriorated, the same as the CCC system. In your nursing notes, you would include additional narratives to support your evaluation.

Nursing Outcomes Classification (NOC) can also be used in home health nursing (Moorhead, Johnson, Maas, et al., 2013). A few of the outcomes that pertain to home and families are:

Caregiver Home Care Readiness	Family Coping
Caregiver Performance: Direct Care	Family Functioning

Caregiver Physical Health   Family Resiliency
Caregiver Stressors   Family Support During
                               Treatment

To prepare the client and family for self-care, inform them of the needs you have identified and involve them in setting goals and planning care. They may be able to identify strategies to solve problems or to help you identify needs that are not apparent.

PLANNING INTERVENTIONS/ IMPLEMENTATION NP

Medicare requires that the provider-prescribed plan of care include the following, as applicable:

- Parameters for notifying the primary provider of changes in vital signs and other clinical findings
- Diabetic foot care, including education
- Falls prevention interventions
- Depression interventions
- Interventions to monitor and treat pain
- Interventions to prevent pressure injury
- Pressure injury treatments

Once the plan of care has been agreed on, you will document it and forward it to the client's physician for certification. At the first visit, you will determine the specific skilled care required and make referrals to other required services such as physical, occupational, or speech therapy; social services; nutritional support; or home health aide services.

Standardized Nursing Interventions

The CCC system is commonly used in planning and recording home care, but the NIC taxonomy is also an option.

CCC Nursing Interventions An intervention consists of a label (e.g., Activity Care) and a definition (e.g., Actions performed to carry out physiological or psychological daily activities). In addition to the label, you must specify the type of intervention action from among *four qualifiers:*

   Assess/Monitor/Evaluate/Observe
   Care/Perform/Provide/Assist
   Teach/Educate/Instruct/Supervise
   Manage/Refer/Contact/Notify

The CCC nursing interventions include only skilled services because this type of service is the only type of care reimbursed by Medicare and most insurers in home health. In the Meet Your Patients scenario, Mrs. Escobar is clearly experiencing Caregiver Strain. This is a nursing diagnosis under the Care Component of Coping. Several interventions are possible, for example:

   Coping Support: Actions to sustain a person dealing with responsibilities, problems, or difficulties
      Assess for Caregiver Strain.
      Provide (perform) emotional support.
      Refer to community services: caregiver support groups, Meals on Wheels, and respite care services.

You can see the entire list of interventions on the previously cited CCC Web site (sabacare.com).

NIC Interventions for Home Health The Nursing Interventions Classification (NIC) may also be used in home health nursing (Bulechek, Butcher, Dochterman, et al., 2013). A few of the interventions that pertain to home and families are:

Caregiver Support   Family Support
Family Integrity Promotion   Home Maintenance
                             Assistance

Family Involvement   Respite Care
   Promotion

Assisting With Medication Management

✚ The Joint Commission One of The Joint Commission 2016 safety goals for home care is to use medications safely. This includes:

- Preventing errors with look-alike and sound-alike medications
- Educating patients about anticoagulant therapy
- Keeping a list and reconciling medications when a client transfers from one agency to another

The Joint Commission also advises nurses to diligently compare those medications the patient is already taking with new ones to be given in the home. Ensure that your patients know about medications they take at home. Recommend they keep a complete list of medications, including dosing, in a safe place, in the event of an emergency. They should also bring a complete and updated list every time they visit a healthcare provider.

Nonadherence Some patients, particularly older adults, have visual and motor deficits that limit their ability to read labels and manipulate bottle caps, syringes, and so on. Other reasons for noncompliance include lack of outward symptoms, inability to tolerate side effects, pain, forgetfulness, low motivation, and impaired mental capacity. **KEY POINT:** *Always investigate the patient's reasons for nonadherence so that you can take appropriate actions.*

Teaching Skills You may need to teach clients and caregivers skills, such as measuring dosages, giving injections, and managing intravenous therapy. Or they may need tips on how to help clients with difficulty swallowing take oral medications. For example, for some clients, pills may be crushed and mixed in a small amount of applesauce or pudding.

Older Adults Involve family members in the care of the older adult as needed, including giving medication. Older adults and caregivers may have difficulty remembering when to take their pills, which ones to take, and even whether they have already taken them.

- *Medication Organizer*—Suggest they use a medication organizer with a compartment for each day of the week. You may need to prepare a week's worth of oral medications for them during your visits.
- *Drug Cards*—To help them remember which drug is used for each of their illnesses or symptoms, write the medical condition, names of medication, and doses, and how and when to take the medication on a large card. Then use clear tape to attach a sample of each drug next to its name on the card.

✚ Safe Disposal Because improper disposal of medication may end up in the local drinking water supply, it is important for clients to be informed about how to safely dispose of medications in the home:

- Return unwanted or expired prescription and over-the-counter drugs to a drug take-back program.
- Some counties offer household hazardous waste collection days where drugs are accepted at a local collection location.
- Expired or unwanted prescription and over-the-counter drugs should never be flushed down the toilet or drain unless the label or accompanying patient information specifies that it is safe to do so.

For more information about ways to properly discard medication, see the Home Care box Preventing Poisoning in the Home, in Chapter 23.

Infection Control in the Home

The Joint Commission safety goals for home care include reducing the risk of healthcare-associated infections. In the hospital, you have ready access to supplies that facilitate infection control. The home presents unique challenges.

Hand hygiene is one of the most important home interventions to prevent the transmission of infection. You will need to follow standard precautions but recognize how to modify infection control techniques for the home environment. For suggestions to help you maintain infection control during a home visit, see Clinical Insight 42-2.

Homes and conditions vary widely. Do not assume that a client lives in clean surroundings or that water and electricity are readily available. Some people with limited financial resources, especially in urban environments, live in single-room occupancy hotels (SROs). Residents of SROs live in a small room with shared bath and shower areas. To provide optimal care, you need to bring infection control supplies and personal protective equipment to the visit or order them to be delivered to the home.

Barrier Precautions

✚ The reason you implement barrier precautions in the home setting differs from use in hospital practice. As a rule, you will use gowns, gloves, and masks in home care to protect yourself rather than the patient. You will need to use standard precautions, but will usually need a mask primarily when caring for clients who have pulmonary tuberculosis, airborne pathogens, or multidrug-resistant infections. Such organisms may be transmitted to other home-care patients through inanimate objects or hands, so use appropriate barrier precautions (Lescure, Locher, Eveillard, et al., 2009). See Chapter 22 if you need to review infection control.

Clean and Sterile Technique

Infection control in home care is different in many ways from that in acute care. In acute care, the patient is exposed to invasive interventions and environmental risks, including other patients and contaminated inanimate objects. Generally, patients have developed some resistance to the microorganisms in their own homes and are less likely to acquire infections there than in the hospital environment. You may find differences in how you handle home infusion therapy, urinary tract care, respiratory care, wound care, and enteral therapy. It is safe, in many instances, to replace sterile with clean technique, as in some of the following examples:

- **Intravenous therapy.** Sterile practices should be the same at home as in the hospital because of the associated risk for sepsis with IV therapy.
- **Subcutaneous injections.** Many patients must give themselves repeated injections (e.g., insulin), perhaps several each day. Supplies for home use are expensive. Insurance may or may not cover the cost, or the person may not have insurance. Therefore, although manufacturers recommend that disposable syringes and needles be used only once and discarded in a puncture-proof container, it is safest to do that, some people find it practical to reuse needles and

Toward Evidence-Based Practice

Shang, J., Larson, E., Liu, J., et al. (2015). Infection in home health care: Results from national Outcome and Assessment Information Set data. *American Journal of Infection Control, 5*(1), 454–459. Retrieved from http://dx.doi.org/10.1016/j.ajic.2014.12.017

Researchers examined the problem of infection in home healthcare (HHC). Using national OASIS data of nearly 200,000 patients from 8,255 HHC agencies, they found that 3.5% of HHC clients developed infection requiring hospitalization or emergency care. Infections included urinary tract infection, intravenous catheter–related infection, wound infection, or deterioration. Infection rates varied between agencies.

Shang, J., Ma, C., Poghosyan, L., et al. (2015). The prevalence of infections and patient risk factors in home health care: A systematic review. *American Journal of Infection Control, 42*(5), 479–484. Retrieved from http://dx.doi.org/10.1016/j.ajic.2013.12.018

Patients in the home healthcare (HHC) setting are at a higher risk for infection for many reasons: the uncontrolled home environment, increased use of indwelling devices, and complexity of illnesses now cared for outside of acute care facilities. Researchers comparing risk factors for infections from 25 clinical studies found that patients receiving home parenteral nutrition treatments had higher infection rates than did patients receiving other types of home infusion therapy. They recommend that HHC agencies (1) use a monitoring and reporting system for identifying patients at risk for infection; (2) customize patient education to improve infection control practices in the home; and (3) improve communication among HHC agencies when an infection rate exceeds a threshold level.

1. What are some of the patient-related factors that are likely to be related to higher infection rates in the home setting?

2. What might be some other HHC factors that could contribute to a less effective control of infection in the home setting?

3. What are at least three other possible research-related explanations for the wide variation in infection rates between the different studies?

4. What are some ideas you have to improve the effectiveness of infection control practices in the home setting in which you might work?

 Go to Davis Advantage, Resources, Chapter 42, **Toward Evidence-Based Practice—Suggested Responses.**

Using CAM for Preventing Illness

Goodyear, N. (2016). Increasing delivery of healthcare at home and the importance of hygiene. *Perspectives in Public Health, 13(4), 208–209.* doi:10.1177/1757913916642964

Immunocompromised, ill, elderly, and very young patients in the home setting are very susceptible to infection. They require meticulous hygiene of hands, surfaces, and food handling. Various natural products, such as vinegar, tea tree oils, and castile soap, are popular alternatives to traditional or commercial solutions for cleaning or disinfection. Although these products can be effective antimicrobial agents, some cause dermatitis, respiratory irritation, and other health hazards.

Ask your patients what natural products they are using for cleansing and handwashing. Teach them about the various products, and to observe for the side effects that may occur.

syringes. For guidelines for teaching patients about this, see Clinical Insight 25-2: Reusing Needles and Syringes: Home Care.

- **Urinary catheters.** Clients and family typically use clean, rather than sterile, gloves to perform catheterization. In the home, clients frequently interrupt the drainage system to empty a leg bag or to change or disinfect the drainage bag. They may also disinfect and reuse urinary catheters.
- **Respiratory care.** As an example, tracheostomy care in the home is nearly always performed using clean, not sterile, technique.
- **Wound care.** Procedures for wound care should be based on the potential for contamination and infection. Usually clean technique is adequate. For example, a surgical site that is primarily closed and has no drains should be low risk for home-care-acquired infection. However, if the incision has drains or is open, the risk for infection increases, and your wound-care procedures must address the risk. Also, you do not need to arbitrarily "always" discard irrigation fluids at set intervals (e.g., every 24 hours). Order for them, or guide caregivers to buy, small containers (e.g., no more than 500 mL) that can be used up in two or three visits. Teach them how to avoid contaminating the fluids (e.g., how to handle the cap, always recap the bottle, and store the bottle away from children and pets).

- **Enteral therapy.** Emphasize the need to refrigerate the feedings after opening and store solutions until expiration. Teach caregivers to keep the kitchen appliances, enteral supplies, and utensils used in preparation meticulously clean.

KnowledgeCheck 42-10

Identify three infection control supplies that you should bring in your nursing bag on a home health visit.

Safety in the Home

The following two The Joint Commission 2016 home-care safety goals are important to keep in mind:

- ✚ *Reduce the risk of client harm resulting from falls.* Assess the client and the home for risk factors (e.g., dimly lit stairs, loose rugs, clutter on the floors) and teach caregivers falls reduction measures. Educate the patient concerning the potential for their medications to make them feel weak, dizzy, or sleepy. You will find extensive discussion of falls prevention in Chapter 24 if you need more information about that.
- *Identify risks associated with oxygen therapy.* Be certain the home has working smoke detectors, fire extinguishers, and a fire safety plan. Assess the client and family's ability to understand and comply with fire prevention activities and report any concerns to the physician.

Supporting Caregivers

Even when the client is receiving in-home care from an agency, it is not usually around-the-clock care. If the client cannot perform self-care, most of the duties fall to family members. One study found that even with short-term services, family caregivers provided three-fourths of the care of homebound patients. Half of the caregivers said they were not adequately prepared to provide full patient care when it was time for home health services to be discontinued. And at all stages, they expressed significant isolation, anxiety, and depression (Levine, Albert, Hokenstad, et al., 2006).

Unrelieved caregiving duties are physically and emotionally taxing. Caregivers may become depressed, physically exhausted, isolated from friends, and neglectful of their own health. There is some evidence to indicate that caregiver support and training workshops can relieve depression, reduce the perceived burden of caregiving, and better prepare the caregivers for their role. However, the most improvement in adaptation to the caregiver role was shown by those with more independent lives and social support (Huynh-Hohnbaum, Villa, Aranda, et al., 2008). See Box 42-4 for suggestions to help caregivers.

BOX 42-4 ■ Ways to Help Caregivers

Provide a listening ear. Encourage caregivers to talk about what they do and how they feel, and listen actively to their concerns. Find time to focus on the caregiver's needs rather than on those of the care recipient.
Give positive feedback and validate their importance to the client's health.
Help the caregiver identify people who may be able to help, for example, family members living outside the home, neighbors, church members, community support groups.

Talk with family and friends, if the caregiver wishes. Teach them how to support the caregiver, for example, by telephoning regularly, visiting, sending cards, or staying with the client for a few hours (or days) so the caregiver can rest or take a vacation. Encourage them to listen to the caregiver without giving advice and to help her feel appreciated (e.g., "I really appreciate all you do for Dad").
Arrange for a home health aide, if possible. This relieves the caregiver of housekeeping and grocery shopping.

BOX 42-4 ■ Ways to Help Caregivers—cont'd

Remind family members and significant others to take care of themselves. Explain that their health is important both to them and to the patient. Even the most devoted and self-sacrificing person may understand when you explain, "You must take care of yourself so that you are able to take care of your loved one."

- Stress the need for the person to eat nutritious meals. Arrange for meals to be delivered to the home, if needed.
- Encourage the caregiver to rest as much as possible, perhaps while the home health aide is there; or ask family members and friends to take turns staying an hour or two with the patient while the caregiver rests or "gets away." Help contact those offering respite care and make a schedule, if needed.
- Stress the need for the caregivers to take some time for themselves, even if it is just an hour alone or coffee with a friend.
- Encourage caregivers to take a vacation, if they can afford it, even if the getaway is close to home or for a

short time. Reassure them that competent help can be obtained and that it is okay to delegate caregiving to others for a while.

- Some agencies offer respite for caregivers. The client is admitted to a skilled care unit for 2 or 3 days so the caregiver can have a break.

Encourage the caregiver to maintain spiritual connections, for example, to take time to go to church. Or ask the spiritual adviser to visit the home.

Communicate medical updates about the client—lab results, new treatment plans, and so on.

Help the family understand the goals of care and solve problems when needed.

Teach the family what to expect with regard to medications, treatments, and signs of approaching death. If family members know what is normal, they will be less likely to panic or fear the inevitable.

Follow up with other healthcare team members promptly if the family has questions that are outside your scope of practice.

CLINICALREASONING

The questions and exercises in this section allow you to practice the kind of thinking you will use as a full-spectrum nurse. Critical-thinking questions usually have more than one correct answer, so we do not provide "correct answers" for these features. It is more important to develop your nursing judgment than to just cover content. You will learn by discussing the questions with your peers. If you are still unsure, see the Davis Advantage chapter resources for suggested responses.

Caring for the Nguyens

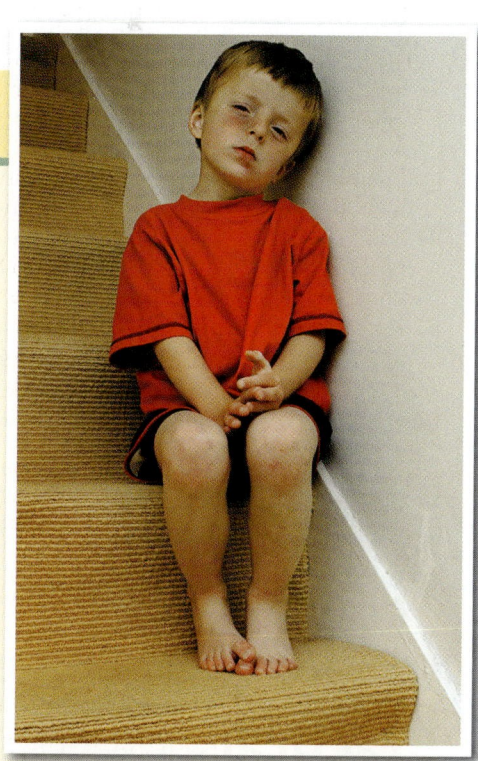

Yen Nguyen works as preschool teacher in her community. Andre is a 4-year-old boy in her class. Over the past few months, she has noticed that Andre has many bruises in various stages of healing. He seems withdrawn and does not interact much with the other children. She is concerned that Andre might be a victim of child abuse, but she is reluctant to make that accusation, especially because her assistant doesn't seem to have noticed anything amiss.

Mrs. Nguyen talks to her husband, Nam, about her concerns: "I'm worried about a child at school, but I'm afraid to say anything. What if I'm wrong? I'd probably lose my job. But if I'm right and I don't say anything, I could still lose my job, and this boy could be hurt even worse." Nam suggests that she contact the clinic nurse at the Family Medicine Center for confidential advice on how to proceed.

(Continued)

Caring for the Nyugens (continued)

A. Imagine that you are the clinic nurse. Use the full-spectrum nursing model to identify at least 10 questions that you would need to answer to investigate Yen's concerns further.

B. *Self-knowledge:* What personal values do you have that would affect the way you handle this situation? Explain.

C. *Ethical knowledge:* What is the most important ethical issue in this situation? That is, what is the most important goal? Note that there may be several moral and legal issues, but you are being asked to identify the *most* important one. Note also that we are not asking you

what the nurse *can* do, but rather what the nurse ideally *should* do.

D. You share the questions you have with Yen. She believes that there is a real need to investigate child abuse. You advise her to call the local child protective services (CPS) agency. Based on your knowledge of community and public health nursing, what aspects of the community health role will the nurse from CPS use as she investigates this situation?

 Go to Davis Advantage, Resources, Chapter 42, **Caring for the Nguyens—Suggested Responses.**

Applying the **Full-Spectrum Nursing Model**_____
PATIENT SITUATION

While honeymooning in the Caribbean, Lorenzo and Elvia learn that the area has infected *Aedes aegypti* mosquitos, which can spread the Zika virus. Later she learns that she conceived when traveling to this area and seeks healthcare for her first trimester pregnancy in south Florida. The couple is concerned about the possibility of contracting Zika virus.

THINKING

1. *Theoretical Knowledge:*
  a. How is Zika virus spread?
  b. What symptoms would Elvia show if she has the Zika infection?
2. *Critical Thinking (Contextual Awareness):*
  Why is it important to detect and treat Zika infection in women of childbearing age?

DOING

3. *Nursing Process (Assessment):*
  How might you assess the extent of the problem of Zika virus infection within the southern Florida community (Dade County)?
4. *Practical Knowledge:*
  a. As the Community Health nurse, you design a *primary* intervention program to prevent women of childbearing age to acquire Zika virus infection during pregnancy. What might you do for this program?
  b. What *secondary* interventions would you include in your patient education?

CARING

5. *Self-Knowledge:*
  a. When showing compassion for your client, what information about her pregnancy might you offer?
  b. How would you feel if you were exposed to the Zika virus during your first trimester of pregnancy?

 Go to Davis Advantage, Resources, Chapter 42, **Applying the Full-Spectrum Nursing Model—Suggested Responses.**

PracticalKnowledge:
clinical application_____

CLINICAL INSIGHTS

Clinical Insight 42-1 ➤ **Safety Considerations in Home Care**

✚ Before the Visit

- **Plan ahead.** Know where you are headed. Use a map or global positioning system for navigation. Contact the client or family for directions if it is unclear where you are headed. File a visit plan with your office each day.
- **Dress in appropriate clothing** as determined by your agency. Wear a nametag clearly identifying you and the agency. Wear comfortable shoes.
- **Carry a cell phone** and keep it close at hand for emergency aid if you feel threatened during the visit. Check to be sure it is charged. Program 911 in case of emergency.
- **Do not carry a purse,** multiple credit cards, or excess cash. Instead, use a waist or fanny pack and conceal it under clothing. Carry enough money for emergency transportation, telephone numbers for clients and home health agency, and emergency contact information.
- **Keep your car in good repair** and always have enough gasoline in the tank or electrical charge for the vehicle. Be prepared for inclement weather and always carry an emergency car safety pack.
- **Do not get out of your car for any reason if driving in an area that might not be safe.** Carjacking involves minor car impact ("fender bender") as a strategy to get a person to exit the vehicle, leaving her vulnerable for attack, assault, or theft.
- **Observe your surroundings** as you drive to the visit. Notice the location of emergency services, local gas stations, and public places if help is required.
- **Carry mace, pepper spray, or other items to aid in self-defense** in situations in which you feel threatened.
- **Park as close to your destination as possible.** If possible, park your car facing the direction you wish to go when you leave. Never enter dead-end streets or alleys.
- **Lock the car. Leave no valuables in sight.**
- **Prepare your bag while you are still in the car.**
- **Carry your bag on one arm. In the opposite hand, carry your keys.** Always have them ready. You may need them if you decide to exit quickly. You can use keys to defend yourself by placing the pointed ends of the keys between your fingers.
- **Walk directly to the client's house.** Walk in the middle of the sidewalk. Use common walkways. Avoid isolated and poorly lighted areas. Do not take shortcuts.
- **Knock or ring the doorbell before entering.** Never enter without being invited. If there is no answer at the door, call the patient using your cell phone.
- **If for any reason you feel that the neighborhood is unsafe, do not get out of the car.** Instead, leave the area immediately and contact your agency.

At the Visit

- **Introduce yourself** and clearly identify your agency. Show your name badge.

- **Sit where you have access to an exit.** When you enter the home, observe all exits.
- **Notice who is present in the home. Request introductions.** This information is useful for planning care as well as for ensuring safety.
- **Leave immediately if you suspect substance use,** drug dealing, or drunken behavior.
- **Leave immediately if there is a violent domestic argument or any other aggressive behavior.** Do not attempt to intervene. When you return to your car, use your cell phone to dial 911 or drive to a safe location to place the call.
- **Request that animals be kept in another room** while you make your visit.
- **If weapons are visible, request that they be put away** immediately. Leave the home if this request is not met.
- **If household members interfere with the visit,** discuss the problem with the client. You may need to arrange a time to visit when other household members are not present.

After the Visit

- **Continue to observe the safety precautions** you used when getting to the visit. Do not let down your guard as you return to your car.
- **If you are in an unsafe neighborhood or poorly lighted area, leave immediately.** Keep your mobile phone within reach in case you need to call for help. Do not stop to use the phone or consult driving directions until you are in a secure area.
- **Inform your agency** if you believe the home or neighborhood is potentially hazardous.
- **Request a security escort service** if future visits are required.
- **Document your assessments** and the care delivered.
- **Report abuse** if you suspect it in the home.

Other

The preceding tips focus on avoiding harm inflicted by others. However, you also need to protect yourself from infection and accidental injury, as you would in a hospital (see Clinical Insight 42-2).

- Use safe lifting techniques, especially because in the home setting you might have to improvise more than you would in the hospital. There will probably not be others with you to assist with patient transfer, ambulation, or lifting. Mechanical lifts are likely not available.
- Improper needle disposal in the home puts you at risk for injury and serious infection. Loose sharps should never be thrown away in household trash containers, toilets, or recycling bins. Used sharps should be immediately placed in a sharps disposal container. If a sharps container is not available, use a puncture- and leak-resistant plastic household container, such as a laundry detergent bottle or empty milk jug.

Clinical Insight 42-2 ➤ Infection Control in the Home

The following suggestions can help you maintain infection control during a home visit.

Hand Hygiene

- Keep antibacterial cleanser and OSHA-approved protective equipment in your nursing bag.
- Perform hand hygiene using soap and warm water or an antibacterial handrub at the beginning and end of each visit and before and after any treatment.
- If the home conditions are very dirty or your hands become grossly soiled, wash your hands with soap and warm water as soon as possible after (if not during) the visit.

Supplies

- In homes in which hygiene and sanitation may be a problem, limit the supplies you bring into the home. For example, leave your nursing bag in the car and bring only the supplies you need for the visit.
- Some infection control experts believe the "bag technique" (i.e., placing a newspaper under the nursing bag before placing it on a surface) is not routinely needed, but should be used when home conditions warrant. If you use items from your nursing bag during the visit, always clean them with an approved antibacterial wipe before placing them back into your bag.
- If necessary, use a 1:10 dilution of chlorine bleach in water to disinfect surfaces or equipment in the home. Some equipment may need to be disinfected by boiling in a covered pan of water for 15 to 20 minutes. Do not boil plastic or rubber items.
- You can disinfect hard plastic items by wrapping them with a wet paper towel and placing them in a zippered plastic bag. Microwave the entire bag on high for 10 minutes.

Biohazard and Sharps Disposal

- Flush wound irrigation or potentially contaminated liquids down the toilet while wearing gloves and any other appropriate protective equipment.
- Double-bag dressings, equipment, or disposable supplies that have been contaminated with body secretions to prevent leakage. The bags should be labeled *Biohazard*.
- ✚ Carry small biohazard sharps containers. Place syringes and sharps in the container without recapping. If clients or family must use syringes or sharps, you may wish to leave a sharps container in the home. An alternative solution is to have them use a metal coffee can with lid or a thick plastic milk jug with lid.

Client Teaching

- Provide instruction on home cleanliness, hygiene, hand washing, and food preparation and instructions to avoid contact with persons who are ill, as needed.
- If the client is immunocompromised, teach the signs and symptoms of infection and the process for immediate notification of the primary care provider.

Special Situations

- If the patient has a multidrug-resistant infection or pulmonary tuberculosis, use appropriate barrier precautions. Leave reusable equipment (e.g., stethoscope, blood pressure cuff) in the home; if possible, schedule these clients as the last appointment of the day.

 To explore learning resources for this chapter,

 Go to www.DavisAdvantage.com and find:

Answers and Suggested Responses for all questions in this chapter

Lists of NIC Interventions and NOC Outcomes

List of NANDA-I Diagnoses

Knowledge Map

Care Plan

Care Map

References and Bibliography

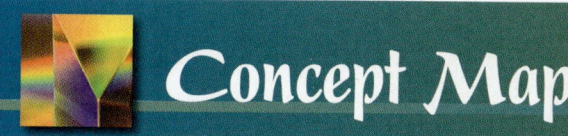

Concept Map

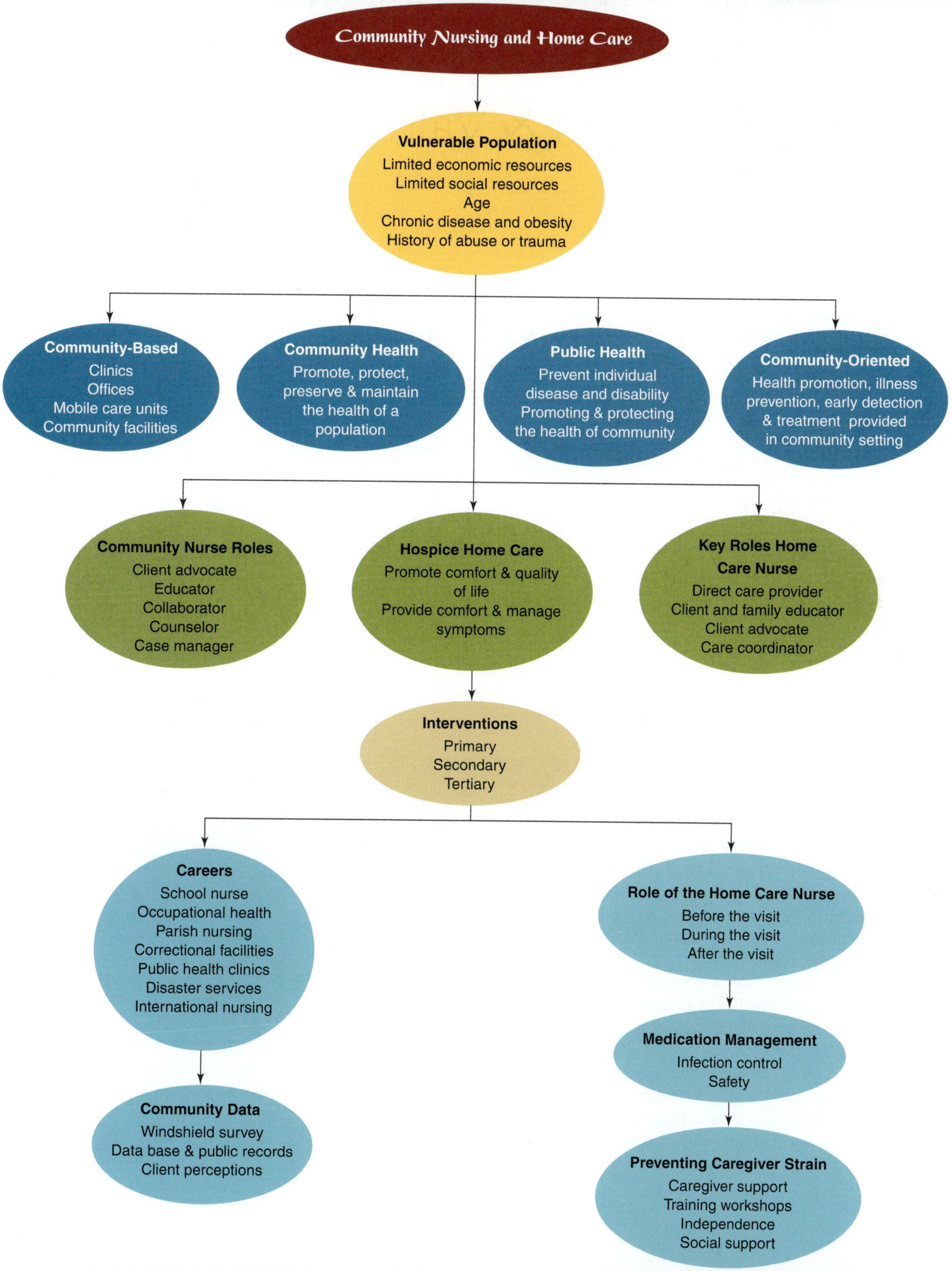

Community Nursing and Home Care

Vulnerable Population
Limited economic resources
Limited social resources
Age
Chronic disease and obesity
History of abuse or trauma

Community-Based
Clinics
Offices
Mobile care units
Community facilities

Community Health
Promote, protect,
preserve & maintain
the health of a
population

Public Health
Prevent individual
disease and disability
Promoting & protecting
the health of community

Community-Oriented
Health promotion, illness
prevention, early detection
& treatment provided
in community setting

Community Nurse Roles
Client advocate
Educator
Collaborator
Counselor
Case manager

Hospice Home Care
Promote comfort & quality
of life
Provide comfort & manage
symptoms

**Key Roles Home
Care Nurse**
Direct care provider
Client and family educator
Client advocate
Care coordinator

Interventions
Primary
Secondary
Tertiary

Careers
School nurse
Occupational health
Parish nursing
Correctional facilities
Public health clinics
Disaster services
International nursing

Role of the Home Care Nurse
Before the visit
During the visit
After the visit

Medication Management
Infection control
Safety

Community Data
Windshield survey
Data base & public records
Client perceptions

Preventing Caregiver Strain
Caregiver support
Training workshops
Independence
Social support

CHAPTER 43

Ethics & Values

Learning Outcomes

After completing this chapter, you should be able to:

- ► Differentiate between *morals, ethics, bioethics,* and *nursing ethics.*
- ► Discuss what is meant by *ethical agency.*
- ► Identify at least four factors that contribute to the frequency of nurses' moral problems.
- ► Differentiate personal values and morality from professional values.
- ► Explain how developmental stages, values, ethical frameworks, professional guidelines, and ethical principles affect moral decisions.
- ► Describe five major ethical principles that are used in reasoning about healthcare.
- ► Compare and contrast four ethical frameworks: consequentialism (e.g., utilitarianism), deontology, an ethics of care, and feminist ethics.
- ► Identify the ethical issues and moral principles involved in a given ethical situation.
- ► Describe a systematic approach to resolving ethical dilemmas.
- ► Discuss the concept of an integrity-producing compromise.
- ► Describe the nurse's obligations in ethical decisions.
- ► Discuss the role of the nurse as client advocate in ethical situations.
- ► Apply the steps identified in the MORAL model to make ethical decisions.

Key Concepts

Morals
Nursing ethics
Values

Related Concepts

See the Concept Map at the end of this chapter.

Example Problems

Moral Distress
Whistleblowing

Meet Your Patient

Angie and Edward Frese and their two teenage children are a close and loving family with a large network of family and friends. Their son, Alan, 15 years old, has just been severely injured in a high school soccer game. At the hospital, Angie and Edward are told that Alan has multiple bone fractures and active internal bleeding.

The surgeon informs the distressed parents that Alan will need a blood transfusion to survive. Although genuinely devastated, the parents adamantly refuse to consent to a lifesaving blood transfusion, stating they are Jehovah's Witnesses and that receiving blood is against their religious beliefs. The surgeon asks you, Alan's nurse, to convince the parents to change their minds right away. You talk with the couple, but they continue to refuse a blood transfusion. You immediately contact your charge nurse. Try to answer the following critical-thinking questions about Alan and his parents. You may not have the experience or theoretical knowledge to answer them all—you will acquire that in this chapter and in Chapter 44—but do your best based on the background you have.

- Do the Freses have the right to refuse a blood transfusion for their son based on their religious beliefs?
- Do you think the fact that Alan is a minor (under 18 years old) may make a difference in this situation?
- What actions do you think the charge nurse should take?
- Can an ethical conflict such as this be resolved to everyone's satisfaction?

Theoretical Knowledge
knowing why

The theoretical knowledge you will need to begin professional practice includes an understanding of the nature of morals and ethics (and especially nursing ethics) and basic information about factors that affect ethical decisions (i.e., values, moral frameworks, professional guidelines, and ethical principles).

ABOUT THE KEY CONCEPTS

Nursing ethics, morals, and **values** are key concepts in this chapter because everything in the chapter is related to those concepts in some way—as you will discover. The subconcepts of *advocacy* and *compromise,* for example, are intimately integrated in the implementation of nursing ethics in clinical practice. Remember to use the key concepts to help you organize chapter content in your mind. As you read, try to understand how each subconcept you encounter relates to nursing ethics, morals, and values.

ETHICS AND MORALS

The terms *ethics* and *morals* have similar meanings, but they are different concepts. In modern theory, **morals** refers to private, personal, or group standards of right and wrong (e.g., "In general, it is wrong to steal"). **Ethics** answers the question "What should I do in a given situation?" (e.g., "Is it wrong to steal food to feed your children?").

Morals are learned from external influences and communicated through various systems (e.g., religious, political, educational, societal). **Moral behavior** is that which is consistent with customs or traditions based on the external influence (such as religious beliefs). A person whose behavior is inconsistent with traditional notions of right and wrong is labeled as immoral. Consider the conversation between two nurses discussing a teenager who assaulted and robbed a wheelchair-bound 92-year-old female:

Nurse A: "I cannot believe someone would be so heartless as to attack an innocent, helpless elderly woman."

Nurse B: "I agree—that person is immoral. Absolutely no morals."

You may agree with this, because you have been taught to respect and protect older adults. Morals are linked to a person's character and often determine how we treat others. Another example is the "Golden Rule," which states that you should treat others as you wish to be treated.

- Can you think of another example of moral behavior that you may have learned as a child?
- Can you identify any morals that are evident in the scenario about Alan at the beginning of the chapter?
- How do his parents' morals influence Alan's care?

Ethics in contrast, is the study of a system of moral principles and standards, or the process of using them to decide your conduct and actions. Ethics helps us to decide what is right or wrong and what actions should be taken in certain circumstances. Whereas a nurse's *moral code* would find the act of driving under the influence thoughtless and reprehensible, his *ethics* as a nurse would require him to provide care to the driver for the injuries received in the motor vehicle accident. In the case of Alan and his family (Meet Your Patient), the ethical decision making is quite different from the moral perspective of Alan's parents. The parents believe a blood transfusion is morally wrong; this fits with their religious beliefs. The surgeon and the nurse, however, believe withholding blood from Alan would be unethical.

Ethics and the Law How are laws related to ethics and morals? In some situations, there is a fine line between law and ethics. Think about the following:

- *Law:* It is illegal to drive faster than the speed limit.
    Situation: A child is bleeding profusely and may have cut an artery. The driver drives very fast and even drives through a red light.
    Question: Was that illegal? Was it immoral?
- *Law:* In the United States, it is legal in certain situations to have an abortion.
    Fact: Although everyone would have to agree that the act is legal, people are about evenly divided about whether abortion is moral.

The adage "Courts are ill equipped to deal with ethical issues" reflects the difficulty of trying to decide a case on a continuum of right and wrong (ethics) versus applying strict legal principles (law). Although ethics is rooted in the religious, political, customs, and other values of a society, you should be able to see now that ethics is not the same as law, religion, institutional practices, or customs. An action that is legal or customary may not be morally right or ethically justifiable. The same holds true of religion. You cannot assume that an accepted practice of a certain religion is an ethical practice in every situation.

What Is Nursing Ethics?

Bioethics refers to the application of ethical principles to every aspect of healthcare. Bioethics is concerned with every area of healthcare, including direct care of patients, allocation of resources, utilization of staff, and medical and nursing research. **Nursing ethics** is a subset of bioethics. It refers to ethical questions that arise out of nursing practice. The first things to come to your mind may be dramatic questions such as, "Should we turn off the ventilator and allow this patient to die?" and "Should this baby have surgery even though his quality of life will probably never be good?" In reality, you may have some input, but the patient, physician, and family will make the final decision in such situations. As a nurse, you are responsible for deciding the nature and extent of your own involvement in each situation, and you must support patients who are making ethical decisions or perhaps coping with the results of decisions made by others. Consider the following true story, paraphrased from Curtin and Flaherty (1982, pp. 3–4):

A woman took her 6-year-old son to the emergency department (ED) to have a scalp laceration sutured. On the way to the hospital, she tried to calm him by telling him that the doctors would "numb" him and "no one would hurt him" on purpose. On arrival, they were placed in a cubicle next to another little boy who was awaiting treatment for a similar laceration. His father was also trying to reassure his son.

In the cubicle of the father and son, a nurse roughly cleansed the cut with no explanation or words of comfort. The provider came and sutured the laceration without a word and without waiting for the local anesthetic to take effect. The boy screamed in pain and terror the whole time. The woman was horrified, and her son was scared. But when the same nurse approached the woman and her son, she was kind and gentle. The same provider carefully injected a local anesthetic and waited for it to take effect before suturing.

Why do you think there was such difference in the treatment? Was it because the man and boy appeared to be of lower socioeconomic status? Was it the presence of a father rather than a mother? Was it because the father and son were from a minority group and the woman and son were not? Regardless of why it happened, what makes this case important? After all, both boys received medical treatment; both incisions will heal; no one's life or health was threatened; no life-and-death decisions were made. But notice that the first child's humanity and dignity were violated, and the actions were not fair. **KEY POINT:** *This case is a perfect example of nursing ethics: questions that have to do with the nurse's actions, not the actions of others. The nurse did not need a medical prescription or permission from hospital administration to act ethically.*

In the Meet Your Patient scenario, you, as the nurse, are not responsible for deciding the broad questions: "Is blood transfusion right or wrong?" or "Do the parents have a right to refuse blood transfusion?" Your decision is, "What should *I* do? Should I try to persuade the parents to change their minds, as the surgeon directs, or not?" That is the *nursing ethics* question. And in that scenario, you will need to deal with the effects of the final decision on Alan. He may be frightened; he may be angry; he may die. The nurse is there for patients' most human and vulnerable moments.

Why Should Nurses Study Ethics?

This section will help you understand the many reasons why nurses should study ethics.

- *You will frequently encounter ethical problems in your work.* You will be prepared to make an informed decision, knowledgeable of the ethical issues involved. The most difficult question you will face as a nurse will not be "How do I do this?" but "Should I do this?"
- *Ethics is central to nursing.* Commitment to caring for other human beings supports the claim that nursing is a moral art (Butts & Rich, 2015). Caring for the sick, promoting health, and practicing with care and compassion are central values in nursing.
- *Multidisciplinary input is important.* Many healthcare facilities have an ethics committee to address complex ethical issues. The committee is composed of providers, nurses, clergy, social workers, therapists, case managers, attorneys, and so on, depending on the issues. Multidisciplinary input becomes increasingly important to adequately evaluate the complex ethical issues.
- *Ethical knowledge is necessary for professional competence.* Being a professional includes being accountable to others in the profession for the ethical conduct of your work. Using professional expertise for social good is one hallmark of a profession. Therefore, to conduct our work well and have it stand the test of public scrutiny, we need to be clear about the ethics of our work.
- *Ethical reasoning is necessary for nursing credibility among other disciplines.* For your opinion to be valued by others, you must be able to clearly express your ethical position in a logical way. You must be able to (1) understand your own values as they relate to basic morality and (2) use ethical reasoning to articulate your moral position.
- *Ethical proficiency is essential for providing holistic care.* Nurses care for the whole person—that includes providing support for spiritual and moral concerns.
- *Nurses have a responsibility to be advocates for patients.* **Advocacy** is the communication and defense of the rights and interests of another. Since the 1960s, schools have socialized nurses to include client advocacy in their role conceptions. The American Nurses Association (ANA) Code of Ethics for Nurses (2015a), provision 3, states: "The nurse promotes, advocates for and protects the rights, health and safety of the patient."

Advocacy includes protecting patients' legal or moral rights (e.g., taking appropriate action when the actions of a provider jeopardize the patient's rights or best interests). You can also advocate for patients in everyday practice, for example, by contacting a provider to request a new prescription when a pain medication is not effective. To advocate for patients, you must know the ethical issues and your resources and communicate the patient's wishes.

- *Studying ethics will help you to make better decisions.* Most ethical nursing problems have more than one acceptable answer. Each situation is unique in its details—for example, the people differ in how they evaluate what is and is not beneficial for themselves. The study of ethics prepares you to analyze ethical dilemmas from multiple perspectives rather than relying entirely on your personal values, intuition, and emotions. Practice in analyzing dilemmas will help you to become an informed decision maker, capable of understanding the perspectives of everyone in a situation—for example, why the Freses (Meet Your Patient) are refusing a blood transfusion.

KnowledgeCheck 43-1

- Define *morals* and give an example that is not in the text.
- Define *ethics* and give an example that is not in the text.
- How is bioethics different from ethics?
- Why do nurses need to study ethics?

What Is Ethical Agency?

Moral or **ethical agency** for nurses is the ability to base their practice on professional standards of ethical conduct and to participate in ethical decision making. Simply stated, it means that nurses have choices and are responsible for their actions. An ethical agent must be able to do the following:

- Perceive the difference between right and wrong.
- Understand abstract ethical principles.
- Reason and apply ethical principles to make decisions, weigh alternatives, and plan sound ways to achieve goals.
- Decide and choose freely.
- Act according to choice (this assumes both the power and the capability to act).

Moral Distress

When situational constraints prevent nurses from acting on their moral decisions, **moral distress** may occur. Said another way, moral distress can occur when nurses are unable to act as moral agents. See the Example Problem: Moral Distress.

Whistleblowing

Nurses experience **moral outrage** when they perceive that others are behaving immorally (Wilkinson, 1987/1988). Moral outrage is similar to moral distress, except that in cases

EXAMPLE PROBLEM: Moral Distress

Diagnosis: Response to the inability to carry out one's chosen ethical/moral decision/action

Defining Characteristics

Mental anguish and/or physical pain experienced based on involvement in a moral situation. Feelings of frustration, anger, emotional exhaustion.

Etiology

Nurse feels morally responsible for an outcome or client, identifies an acceptable course of action, but is unable to implement the chosen intervention, based on real or perceived constraints (Rushton, 2013; Wilkinson, 1987/1988). It is a compromise of one's values or moral agency.

    Internal Constraints: Relationships with others (e.g., providers, colleagues, client, family members); lack of skills, confidence, and courage; fear; concerns about perceptions of others

    External Constraints: Time, power imbalances, lack of institutional support, policies and procedures, threat of lawsuits, regulatory directives (American Association of Critical-Care Nurses, 2004).

Note: Moral distress research has been conducted mainly with nurses as subjects. However, NANDA-I has accepted a nursing diagnosis for use with patients.

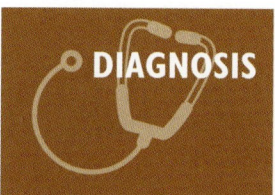

DIAGNOSIS

Moral Distress

Response to the inability to carry out one's chosen ethical/moral decision/action.

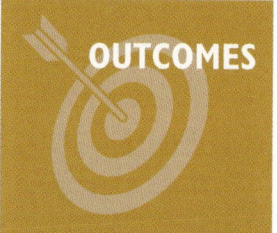

OUTCOMES

- Decreased anxiety level
- Lack of fear
- Psychospiritual comfort status
- Spiritual health
- Preservation of personal autonomy and integrity
- Relief from frustration and anger

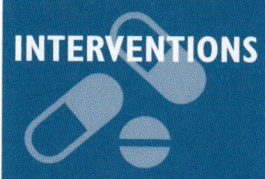

INTERVENTIONS

Note: These interventions focus on nurses experiencing moral distress.

- Recognize the source of the moral distress.
- Understand your values, thoughts, and beliefs.
- Reflect on your values that are threatened in the situation. Are these personal or professional values?
- Engage in values clarification.
- Self-manage emotions; discuss with a mentor if you are having difficulty.
- Make decisions based on reasoned choices.
- Discuss the basis for your decision with members of the interprofessional team, client, and family members. Be sure to express it logically and clearly and with controlled emotions.
- View the situation from the other perspective. Identify reasons that support this perspective. This helps to ensure that you have a comprehensive knowledge of factors that led to the other person's decision.

- Engage with personal and professional resources to resolve intrapersonal conflicts that occur when decisions are made that are contrary to your selected choice.
- Accept that clients have the right to make decisions that they feel best adhere to their values and beliefs. Treat them with kindness and respect and show compassion. The client is also experiencing some type of loss in these situations.
- Make a commitment to care for self.
- Acknowledge your feelings and seek support sources, separate personal from professional.
- Engage in self-care activities (e.g., exercise, meditation, reflection, recreational activities, adequate sleep; balanced diet).
- Seek spiritual guidance and support.
- Develop a network of supportive interprofessional colleagues.
- Seek counseling for unresolved feelings or development of moral outrage (anger directed toward others).

Toward Evidence-Based Practice

Peters, K., Luck, L., Hutchinson, M., et al. (2011). The emotional sequelae of whistleblowing: Findings from a qualitative study. *Journal of Clinical Nursing, 20*(19/20), 2907–2014.

Fourteen nurses who were either whistleblowers or the subject of a whistleblowing episode identified persistent, severe emotional distress after the incident because of a lack of social support and an unwelcoming work environment. Three major themes emerged from their interviews: (1) feelings of overwhelming distress, sadness, and depression; (2) physical symptoms associated with anxiety, insomnia, and hypervigilance; and (3) pervasive thoughts about the situation, resulting in nightmares and constant stress. Although moral distress may cause nurses to become whistleblowers, the act itself can create long-lasting emotional distress.

Mansbach, A., Ziedenberg, H., & Bachner, Y. (2013). Nursing students' willingness to blow the whistle. *Nurse Education Today, 33*(1), 69–72. doi:10.1016/j.nedt.2012.01.008

Researchers used an equally divided sample of undergraduate nursing students and experienced nurses to compare each group's willingness to blow the whistle to ensure safe, quality patient care. Each group responded to two vignettes—one describing a candidate for a supervisor's position who used a forged degree to meet the educational qualifications and the second related to a manager who planned to misuse pediatric funds to buy lavish furniture for her office. Both groups reported a willingness to blow the whistle; however, the nursing students reported a greater willingness to blow the whistle, even though their perception of the severity of the misconduct was lower than the experienced nurses.

1. What type of moral situation (for the nurse) is best illustrated by the Peters et al. study: moral distress or whistleblowing? Explain your reasoning.

2. How does the Peters et al. study impact your thoughts of becoming a whistleblower?

3. What factors do you think would contribute to greater readiness of the nursing students to blow the whistle to promote client safety in the Mansbach et al. study?

---

of moral outrage, nurses do not participate in the act. Therefore, they do not believe that they are responsible for doing wrong, but that they are powerless to prevent others from doing so (Burkhardt & Nathaniel, 2014; O'Mara, Jackson, Batson, et al., 2011). A nurse may respond to moral outrage by "blowing the whistle" (see Example Problem: Whistleblowing). Whistleblowing is difficult in the case of an impaired colleague.

Impaired Nursing Practice

Impaired nursing practice occurs when the nurse's ability to perform the essential nursing functions is diminished by chemical dependence on drugs or alcohol or by mental illness. Impairment is a threat to clients and the impaired nurse may have difficulty being accountable to herself or assessing her self-competence. Nurses are required to report impaired nurses to their nursing leadership. The Code of Ethics for Nurses (ANA, 2015a) guides that advocacy includes supporting nurses who return to practice after receiving the appropriate assistance and treatment for substance abuse.

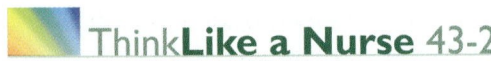 ThinkLike a Nurse 43-2

Consider the five components of ethical agency. To what extent do you believe nurses possess those abilities? Explain your thinking.

KnowledgeCheck 43-2

- Define *ethical agency*.
- What five abilities must be present for ethical agency to exist?
- List at least three constraints that can keep nurses from carrying out their ethical decisions.

What Are Some Sources of Ethical Problems for Nurses?

Factors that contribute to the frequency of nurses' ethical problems include societal factors, the nature of nursing work, and the nature of the nursing profession itself.

Societal Factors

This section discusses how some ethical problems for nurses are created by the ever-changing nature of our dynamic, multicultural society.

Increased Consumer Awareness　Historically, sick people sought the advice of a physician without question. Now, the Internet has increased consumer awareness and the availability of information. People are more actively involved in healthcare decisions. Providers are now expected to share knowledge with clients, defend treatment choices different from those found on the Internet, and obtain truly informed consent for treatments.

Technological Advances　New technology creates new ethical issues. For example, in vitro fertilization and embryo transfer methods raise questions about the ownership of embryos that are not implanted into a uterus. If implanted without the father's consent, what child support obligations exist? Other ethical questions include the right to a late-term abortion when amniocentesis reveals fetal defects, human embryonic stem cell research, costs versus quality of life for ventilator-dependent patients, and security of electronic healthcare records.

Multicultural Population　We live in a multicultural, multifaith society. You cannot assume that your values and beliefs are similar to those of your patients, other providers, and colleagues. You will need to respect a variety of belief systems and serve as a patient advocate even when the patient's value system is

EXAMPLE PROBLEM: Whistleblowing

Definition: A whistleblower is a person who reveals information about practices of others that are perceived as wrong, fraudulent, corrupt, illegal, or a detriment to the health, safety, and welfare of the clients they serve.

Risks and Consequences
- Nurses must carefully weigh their ethical obligations to advocate for clients against their obligations to the employer.

- Whistleblowing can have harmful and long-lasting effects on the nurses' personal and professional lives. The impact can be loss of employment, fear of physical violence, and rejection by colleagues (Delk, 2013; Jackson, Peters, Andrews, et al., 2010).

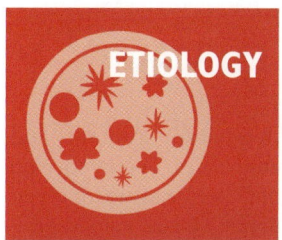
ETIOLOGY

- **Moral outrage** occurs when unresolved moral distress leads to anger, disgust, and powerlessness (Rushton, 2013). The anger or outrage is directed toward individuals or groups perceived as responsible for the wrongdoings, acts, or policies that created the threat to one's personal and/or professional integrity, values, or beliefs (Burkhardt & Nathaniel, 2014; Rushton 2013; Wilkinson, 1987/1988).
- A nurse may respond to moral outrage by becoming a **whistleblower.**

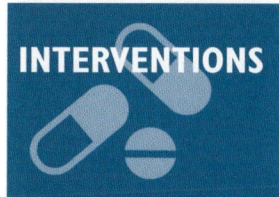
INTERVENTIONS

Actions

To determine whether to **ACT** or **THINK:**
Assess the nature of the action, the likelihood of immediate harm, and the accuracy and completeness of your data.
- In some situations, you will **ACT** by immediately reporting situations that involve an immediate threat to the health, safety, and well-being of others.
- In other situations, **THINK.**
Talk with an attorney or other legal representative. Whistleblowing laws must be strictly followed.
Have concrete and credible evidence of the violation or wrongdoing.
Institute a survival plan if your job is put in jeopardy or you are fired.
Note the nature and consequences of the problem—its type, severity, and potential impact. Weigh the risks against the benefits.
Know your reporting options and support systems that can correct the problems.

Rationale

THE ANA CODE OF ETHICS, Provision 3.5, Protection of Patient Health and Safety by Acting on Questionable Practice, guides the need to support nurses who become whistleblowers:

"All nurses have a responsibility to assist whistleblowers who identify potentially questionable practices that are factually supported in order to reduce the risk of reprisal against the reporting nurse" (ANA, 2015a, p. 12).

---

strikingly different from your own. There are nursing theories that can help you recognize various cultural values, for example, Leininger's (2002) theory of Cultural Care Diversity and Universality (for a review, see Chapters 8 and 15).

Cost Containment The emphasis on reducing health-care costs creates many ethically questionable situations. For example:

- Clients are being sent home from the hospital while they still require considerable nursing care. On being discharged, they may discover that insurance payments are limited for services outside the hospital, including specialists, home care, and medical supplies (e.g., bandages, walkers).
- In efforts to contain costs, healthcare agencies have increased the number of clients each nurse is assigned. You will undoubtedly find yourself in situations in which fewer nurses are available than clients' acuity requires. You will

have to decide how far you will stretch your own resources to maintain clients' safety.

The Nature of Nursing Work

Ethical problems exist in all kinds of work. However, the nature of nursing work can create unique ethical problems.

Nurses' Ethical Problems Nurses' ethical problems are immediate, serious, and frequent. In the classroom, you have the luxury to leave questions unsettled. In the real world, you must always decide: Either you take action, or you do not. For a nurse, deciding *not* to act is, in effect, an act. For example, suppose the family wishes a patient to have aggressive resuscitation efforts (to code); however, you know the patient does not wish to be "coded." When the patient's heart stops, whether or not you know the "right" thing to do, you must immediately decide to code or not code. If you wait too long to ponder the ethical issues, the patient may die. If you do not decide, the effect is the same as though you had decided it was wrong to code.

Nurses' Unique Position In Healthcare Organizations   Nurses have multiple obligations and relationships that can create conflicting loyalties:

- They are *employees* (with a relationship with the agency) and *professionals* (with a special relationship with clients and interprofessional team members).
- Nurses are expected to follow the provider's prescriptions for client care, although the provider is not the nurse's employer.
- In addition, in most organizations providers are higher on the power and status hierarchy than are nurses.

Ethical dilemmas arise when nurses experience conflicts in their loyalties to clients, families, providers, employers, and other nurses. Consider the following example: A patient wants to know his test results, but the provider is reluctant to tell him. What are the conflicting loyalties? Should the nurse give the client the information? There are two options, tell or don't tell:

Tell. By telling the test results, the nurse would honor the principle of autonomy and fulfill her obligation to the patient. But this might harm the client's relationship with the provider, which is important to the patient's medical well-being. Furthermore, if the nurse tells the patient his test results, it may create problems between the provider and the employer (e.g., the hospital). In addition, this action may violate hospital policies and, therefore, harm the nurse's relationship with the hospital.

Don't tell. The nurse could preserve the patient–physician relationship by not telling the test results to the patient. This choice does not honor her relationship with the patient. If the nurse withholds this information, the patient may find out anyway and be angry at the provider, the nurse, and the hospital.

According to professional ethics, your first allegiance is to the patient. However, the patient's needs often conflict with institutional policies, family desires, or even state laws. There may also be conflicts in your relationships with the patient and his family. You can see an example of this in the Meet Your Patient scenario, wherein the nurse finds it impossible to honor the parents' autonomy and at the same time advocate for Alan. You may also encounter this type of conflict when a patient does not want any heroic measures and wishes only to die peacefully, but the family has not accepted the imminent death and are insisting on full resuscitation.

The Nature of the Nursing Profession

Some ethical problems arise because of value conflicts and a lack of clarity within the nursing profession. We have unresolved questions about the nature, scope, and goals of our practice, as well as our professional values. In most of the following examples, we value both of the opposites. We would not wish to give up either one, but specific situations require us to choose between them. That can be a source of discomfort.

- *Caring versus time spent with clients.* Nursing values caring, humanistic care, and nurse–client relationships—but nurses now spend less time at the bedside than ever before. One reason is understaffing and heavier client loads, but there are other factors: the use of technology; the need for careful documentation; and the nursing emphasis on leading, managing, and delegating instead of hands-on client care.

- *Autonomy versus escaping hard choices.* On one hand, we believe that nurses should have an equal status with other healthcare professionals—on the other hand, many nurses are uncomfortable making the hard choices and prefer to "let the provider decide."

- *Higher pay versus cost-effectiveness.* Most nurses believe we deserve higher pay—yet we claim nurses are cost effective because we work less expensively than the primary providers.

- *Professionalism versus caring.* We claim the nurse is a professional, citing critical thinking, knowledge, and management skills, yet we emphasize caring, with the nurse at the bedside offering comfort and doing hands-on tasks.

WHAT FACTORS AFFECT ETHICAL DECISIONS?

By now, you should have an idea of the nature of morals and ethics and of the need to study nursing ethics. Focus now on some basic theoretical knowledge about factors that are involved in making ethical decisions: developmental stages, values, ethical frameworks, ethical principles, and professional guidelines. As you learn about each of these concepts, consider how it affects ethical decision making.

Developmental Stage

A person's stage of moral development affects the way he reasons about moral issues. We learn and internalize our morals throughout the life span, beginning in childhood.

Kohlberg's research (1968, 1981) found that children go through a sequence of moral reasoning ability, proceeding through several stages (see the section "Moral Development Theory: Kohlberg" in Chapter 9 for an in-depth description of the stages).

- Stage I—Moral reasoning is based on personal interest and avoiding punishment.
- Stage II—Principles focus on pleasing others and following rules.
- Stage III—Moral principles are based on universal and impartial principles of justice. This is the final level; it occurs in adulthood.

The stages overlap. Kohlberg found that more than half of a person's thinking reflects the stage he is in, and the remainder reflects the stage he is leaving or the stage into which he is moving. Some people never achieve Kohlberg's highest levels, yet progression through the stages is always forward, never backward, except in extreme trauma; people do not skip stages.

Gilligan challenged Kohlberg's perspective of moral development, citing it as being male biased (1993). Gilligan's research found that girls develop morally by paying attention to community and to relationships, whereas boys tend to process dilemmas through more abstract ideals or principles. If you need a review of Gilligan's three stages—caring for oneself, caring for others, and caring for self and others—refer to Chapter 9.

Values, Attitudes, and Beliefs

Your values are entangled in all ethical situations because they influence what you think and do. This is important to know because your values unconsciously influence your moral judgment. If asked, could you identify your values and explain how they affect your views about right and wrong in a given situation? If so, that's a great beginning. If not, you will learn more as you move through this section.

What Are Values? A **value** is a belief you have about the worth of something; it serves as a principle or a standard that influences your decision making.

- Values are ideals, beliefs, customs, modes of conduct, qualities, or goals that are highly prized or preferred by individuals, groups, or society. You can value an idea, a person, a way of doing things, or even an object (e.g., money).
- People express their values through behaviors, feelings, knowledge, and decisions. For example, the nurse who values compassion will interact with patients in a sensitive, caring manner.
- Your **value set** is your "list" of values. It gives direction for your life and forms a basis for behavior.
- Your **value system** is your value set ranked from most important to least important. Your value system begins to emerge shortly after birth and continues throughout your life, as various sources (parents, teachers, religious figures, peers, and so on) influence your values.
- The total number of values a person has is rather small. The number of significant ones is even smaller, but these are the ones that have a consistent and predictable impact on your actions (e.g., love, freedom, responsibility, and so on).
- Values are highly individualized.
- Values can vary and change with new experiences and thoughtful consideration. As you progress through your study of nursing, you will incorporate the professional values associated with the practice of a registered nurse (e.g., caring, compassion, human dignity). You may experience role conflict when your values are different from practice expectations.

KnowledgeCheck 43-3

- What are values?
- What are three characteristics of values?

ThinkLike a Nurse 43-3

- Think about what you value personally in your own life. What are the five ideals, principles, or things that are most important to you?
- Now refer to Chapter 15, where you were asked to list five ideals, principles, or things that were most important to you. What did you list then? Is your list any different now that you have gained some clinical experience and theoretical knowledge?

What Are Attitudes? **Attitudes** are mental dispositions or feelings toward a person, object, or idea. They can be cognitive (thinking), affective (feeling), and behavioral (doing). Attitudes are our way of responding to situations or things. Let's say you have a positive *attitude* about cleanliness—that is, you may think it is a good thing (e.g., "The floor is clean; that's nice"). But if you *value* cleanliness, you would be willing to scrub the floor. You would also wash your hands at appropriate times, bathe regularly, and teach others about hygiene.

What Are Beliefs? A **belief** is something that one accepts as true (e.g., "I believe that germs cause disease and washing my hands will remove the germs").

- Beliefs are sometimes based on faith and sometimes on facts.
- A belief may or may not be true.
  - Our beliefs can be altered by acquiring knowledge and experiences. Research shows that nursing students' attitudes toward and beliefs about older

adults changed when they spent quality time with older adults and were given the appropriate geriatric assessment tools. The students' misperceptions were replaced with an understanding of the unique needs, abilities, and desires of geriatric patients (Potter, Clarke, Hackett, et al., 2013).

- Beliefs may or may not involve values. Consider the following statements of belief:

  "I believe the Earth is round." (Does not involve a value)

  "Working hard to achieve goals is important to me; therefore, I believe that I must work during the summer to save money for college." (Involves a value)

How Are Values and Ethics Related? Values and morals are learned in conscious and unconscious ways and become a part of your makeup. When we evaluate right and wrong, or good and bad, we are using moral judgment. Therefore, our individual preferences (values) of right or wrong become our moral values. Whether or not you are aware of it, your values shape the manner in which you make ethical decisions in your nursing practice (Burkhardt & Nathaniel, 2014; Butts & Rich, 2015). Values, beliefs, and behaviors are all related.

KEY POINT: *It is important to clarify the influence of your values each time you enter into a situation in which you are called on to be objective in your decision making.*

ThinkLike a Nurse 43-4

- Think about Alan and his family (Meet Your Patient). What do you think were the values of Alan's parents that influenced their behavior at the hospital? First, identify their behaviors specifically. Then speculate about the values underlying each behavior.
- How do you think values can influence health?

KnowledgeCheck 43-4

- Define *belief*; give a new example.
- Define *attitude*; give a new example.

Professional Versus Personal Values

Your **personal value system** is a set of values that you have reflected on and chosen that will help you to lead a good life (Doherty & Purtilo, 2015). You have internalized some *societal values* and have come to perceive them as your own (e.g., good manners; saying "please" and "thank you"). In addition, you probably have some *personal values* (e.g., friendship, fairness, creativity) that are important to you but may or may not be important to society at large.

As you move forward in your profession, you will integrate what you learn and experience and form **professional values,** such as those identified by the American Association of Colleges of Nursing (AACN). Many of these will simply expand your personal values (e.g., caring, veracity). For definitions of the AACN professional values and a list of other nursing values, see Table 43-1.

Personal and professional values are not always congruent. Consider the following situation:

Alexandra Jensen is a 17-year-old pregnant woman who is admitted to your ambulatory surgical center for a voluntary termination of an early pregnancy. You are assigned to complete her preoperative care. Imagine that your personal value is that you do not believe women should have abortions. Yet, your professional value is guided by the ANA standards of professional practice, which state that the nurse provides holistic care that considers "norms and values, health and

Table 43-1 ➤ American Association of Colleges of Nursing (AACN) and Other Professional Nursing Values and Behaviors

American Association of Colleges of Nursing (AACN) Values	
Altruism	Concern for the welfare and well-being of others. Altruism is reflected by the nurse's concern for the welfare of patients, other nurses, and other healthcare providers. Includes patient advocacy.
Autonomy	The right to self-determination—to choose and act on that choice. Every competent person has the right to decide his own course of action.
Human Dignity	Respect for the inherent worth and uniqueness of individuals and populations.
Integrity	Acting in accordance with an appropriate code of ethics and accepted standards of practice. Includes honesty.
Social Justice	Upholding moral, legal, and humanistic principles. Treating others fairly regardless of race, age, citizenship, economic status, disability, or sexual orientation. This value is reflected in professional practice when the nurse works to ensure equal treatment under the law and equal access to quality healthcare.

Additional professional values frequently cited for nursing include the following:

- Aesthetics (qualities of objects or people that are pleasing)
- Caring
- Competence, excellence (skill, knowledge, performance of nursing work)
- Diversity
- Education (basic and lifelong continuing education for nurses)
- Equality (having the same rights, privileges, or status)
- Excellence
- Freedom (capacity to choose)
- Holism
- Loyalty (feeling of duty or attachment to other nurses)
- Service (commitment to work useful to others)
- Truth (faithfulness to fact or reality)

Sources: American Association of Colleges of Nursing. (2008). *The essentials of baccalaureate education for professional nursing practice.* Washington, DC: Author. Retrieved from http://www.aacn.nche.edu/Education/pdf/BaccEssentials08.pdf; Jameton, A. (1984). *Nursing practice: The ethical issues.* Englewood Cliffs, NJ: Prentice Hall; National League for Nursing. (2007). *Core values.* Retrieved from http://www.nln.org/about/core-values; Paquin, S. (2011). Social justice advocacy in nursing: What is it? How do we get there? *Creative Nursing, 17*(2), 63–67; Park, M. (2009). The legal basis of nursing ethics education. *Journal of Nursing Law, 13*(4), 106–113.

illness perspectives and practices, customs, behaviors, and beliefs of the healthcare consumer" (ANA, 2015b, p. 16).

- How might you feel in the situation just described?
- Do you think that your personal and professional values need to be compatible in order for you to be a competent nurse?
- Do you think that you should have the absolute right to refuse to participate in a situation (such as the one involving Alexandra) that may violate your personal values?

How Are Values Transmitted?

Think about how values are transmitted to children (e.g., modeling, rewards, punishment). Table 43-2 outlines the methods of value transmission. Research supports the reciprocal transmission of values between parents and adolescents, which is enhanced in the presence of a receptive and supportive parent (Pinquart & Silbereisen, 2004). Another study found when adolescents' basic needs (i.e., for autonomy, competence, and relatedness) were satisfied within the home, their values were more aligned with the maternal values (Lekes, Joussemet, Koestner, et al., 2011).

Nursing students develop professional values through education and clinical experiences. Research highlights that professional values occur in a long continuum that requires the clinical application of theoretical principles and values is transmitted via the role-modeling behaviors of instructors (Parandeh,

Khaghanizade, Mohammadi, et al., 2014). In addition, early childhood cultural values help to shape students' professional values.

What Is Value Neutrality?

You have probably been taught that nurses need to be nonjudgmental in working with their patients. As a nurse, you do have a duty to provide the best care to patients. You should not assume that your personal values are right, and you should not judge patients' values as right or wrong on the basis of whether they agree with your value system. Think back to the discussion regarding Alexandra, who was seeking to terminate her pregnancy. A nurse who does not believe that women should have abortions could still provide competent nursing care to Alexandra even though his personal values about abortion are different from Alexandra's.

Value neutrality means that we attempt to understand our own values regarding an issue and to know when to put them aside, if necessary, to become nonjudgmental when providing care to clients. However, many ethicists and some healthcare providers believe it is not possible to achieve value neutrality. Further, they say it is not even desirable because it obligates healthcare providers to suppress their own deepest moral and religious beliefs (Balch, 2006; Clark, 2006;). It requires significant insight to recognize how your value-laden perspective impacts your perceptions and thus conclusion about a situation.

Table 43-2 ➤ Modes of Value Transmission

MODE	DESCRIPTION	RESULTS
Modeling	Children learn values from a variety of role models (parents, peers, rock stars, significant others) by observation.	Modeling can lead to socially acceptable or unacceptable behaviors.
Moralizing	"This way is the only way." Children are taught a complete set of values in an authoritarian approach. If the child does not conform, the parent may inflict guilt and fear on him.	This approach by parents, teachers, church leaders, and other authority figures may make it difficult for young people to make independent choices because they have no experience selecting values that are good for them.
Laissez-faire	"Doing your own thing." Children are allowed to explore differing sets of values on their own with little guidance or discipline.	This may lead to conflict and confusion on the part of the child.
Reward and punishment	The child's behavior is controlled by offering rewards for certain valued behaviors and punishing the child who fails to comply.	Rewards can strengthen behavior, whereas physical punishment may teach that violence is an acceptable behavior.
Responsible choice	A balance of freedom and restriction allows children to select the values, explore new behaviors, and experience the consequences.	Having choices can result in personal satisfaction and parental support.

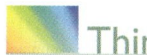 Think**Like a Nurse** 43-5

- Name some other examples of societal values.
- What groups and social experiences have helped to form your values?
- Examine your personal values to see whether they match the ANA Standards of Professional Practice. Examine whether or not you share those values

Knowledge Check 43-5

- What is the difference between personal and professional values?
- What is an example of professional values?
- What are some other types of values?
- What are some ways that values can be transmitted?
- What is value neutrality?

Ethical Frameworks

Ethical (or **moral**) **frameworks** are systems of thought (theories) that are the basis for the differing perspectives people have in ethical situations. Many of these frameworks are rooted in ancient works, for example, those of the Greek philosophers Plato and Aristotle.

There is no single "best" theory that will provide the one "true" answer to an ethical problem because each one will provide a different perspective. Using more than one framework to analyze a situation enables you to perform a more comprehensive analysis of the problem. **KEY POINT:** *No matter how well you know the theories, they will not provide the "right" answers for what to do in a specific patient situation. They merely offer a lens through which you can examine an ethical problem.* See Chapter 8 to review the purposes and use of theories.

What Is Consequentialism?

In **consequentialist** theories, the rightness or wrongness of an action depends on the consequences of the act rather than on the act itself. **Utilitarianism,** the most familiar consequentialist theory, asserts that the value of an action is determined by its usefulness. The **principle of utility** states that an act must result in the greatest good (positive benefit) for the greatest number of people. Any act can then become the ethical choice if it delivers "good" results. In healthcare, the principle of "first, do no harm" is consequentialist in nature. Because of this principle, we are concerned with weighing the risks and benefits of our care (e.g., a medication may kill cancer cells, but side effects may harm the patient's quality of life).

Using utilitarianism to address an ethical problem requires you to engage in a **risk-benefit analysis.**

- *Evaluate every alternative action* for its potential outcomes, both positive (pros) and negative (cons)—similar to a technique you may already use when making other decisions.
- *Then select the action* that results in the most benefits for the greatest number of people involved in the situation.

The following is an example of utilitarian reasoning: The practice of triage is used in a disaster when emergency workers sort patients to determine who will be treated first or who will receive the limited resources (e.g., oxygen or intravenous therapy). If a victim has little potential for survival, he may receive comfort care, or his treatment may be postponed to allow the healthcare team to treat those victims with the greatest potential to survive (i.e., "benefit the greatest number").

 Think**Like a Nurse** 43-6

- Describe a time in your life when you used consequentialism to resolve a difficult situation.
- What types of clinical dilemmas might best be resolved using this model?

What Is Deontology?

Unlike the utilitarian theory, **deontology** uses rules, principles, and standards to determine whether an action is right or wrong. The consequences of the act are not the major considerations.

There are a variety of deontological theories; however, they share the following similar principles:

Rights and Duties Major concepts derived from deontological frameworks are rights (e.g., the right to freedom, the right of self-determination) and duties (obligations). Nurses have a duty to help others and accept their decisions even if they produce some bad consequences.

Treat People as Ends and Never as Means This means that the person is more important than the goal you may be trying to accomplish. Can you imagine the ethical concerns created if research subjects were exposed to some amount of risk (e.g., a new surgical procedure) to find a drug or treatment that will benefit many other people?

Ethical Rules and Principles An analysis of a situation to determine which actions are right or wrong uses ethical rules and principles, such as justice, autonomy, doing good, and doing no harm. These principles come from universal values that underlie all major religions and are regarded as unchanging and absolute.

The Categorical Imperative This principle, established by the philosopher Immanuel Kant (1724–1804), states that one should act only if the action is based on a principle that is universal—or in other words, if you believe that everyone should act in the same way in a similar situation.

Additional Considerations The following are two issues that may arise when using a deontology framework:

- **Conflict of Universal Principles.** Sometimes you must choose between conflicting universal principles. It is not always clear which principle to follow. Allowing Alan's parents (Meet Your Patient) to withhold their consent for him to receive blood honors the principle of autonomy, but their decision may interfere with a right: Alan's right to life. Can you see that it might be difficult to decide which is the appropriate principle to honor?
- **Evaluating motives.** In deontology, it is important to consider motives. It is one thing for Alan's parents to refuse a blood transfusion because they are honoring a religious principle; it would be quite another thing if they refused the transfusion because they stood to inherit a large trust fund left to Alan by his grandfather. Motives may place more weight on one of the conflicting universal principles over the other and make a decision clearer. Unfortunately, motives are sometimes difficult to determine.

KEY POINT: *As a nurse, you will always need to consider the consequences of your actions; you will almost never be able to decide only on the basis of principles and rules.*

KnowledgeCheck 43-6

- Describe utilitarianism.
- Define *deontology*.

What Is Feminist Ethics?

Feminist ethics is based on the belief that traditional ethical models provide a mostly masculine perspective and that they devalue the moral experience of women (Butts & Rich, 2015). Virtues such as love, relationships, caring, nurturing, and sympathy are more relevant, but are rarely seen in traditional theories that focus on abstract principles such as fairness, justice and rights. Feminist ethical reasoning uses relationships and stories rather than universal principles. Feminists argue that being influenced by relationships is positive and should not be lessened by an attempt at objectivity, which is seen as impossible to achieve.

Feminist theories do use principles and consequences, but they also ask you to look at gendered, cultural, and socially diverse issues in the ethical situations, especially those involving women (Green, 2012). Let's look at an example that shows how the issue of gender influences the reasoning process. A group is deciding whether to allocate federally funded healthcare resources either to younger people or to older adults. Feminist reasoning might say that, all other considerations being equal:

- In the United States, older women outnumber older men.
- Older women tend to be poorer and are more likely to be alone than are men.
- Therefore, if healthcare for older adults were to be rationed, it would negatively affect women more than men.
- Thus, more healthcare resources should be allocated to older adults, especially women.

What Is an Ethics of Care?

An **ethics-of-care** nursing philosophy directs attention to the specific situations of individual clients, viewed within the context of their life narrative. You would ask: "What is the story of this person's life? What is going on right now in his life? And what does that have to do with the morality of the action I'm considering?" Care theories (which grew out of feminist ethics) integrate the notion that caring is a natural human quality with the commitment and responsibility that you assume by entering into a helping profession (Lachman, 2012). Care is not viewed as an obligation (deontology, utilitarianism), but as a responsibility based on your relationship with the person (Lachman, 2012). An ethics of care emphasizes the role of feelings, but also includes some of the principles that are part of traditional ethics, such as *autonomy* (self-determination) or *beneficence* (doing good).

Using an ethics-of-care perspective, you would ask the question, "How do I best care for this client?" Consider the guidance provided by the ANA Code of Ethics as you plan your care. Some aspects of care include the ability and duty to appreciate, understand, and even share the client's pain or condition. The following guidance is derived from an ethics-of-care philosophy (Edwards, 2011; Lachman, 2012; Vanlaere & Gastman, 2011):

- Caring is viewed as a central responsibility for nurses.
- Knowing the client's story promotes dignity and respect for the client as a person.
- Your relationship and professional competence allow you to meet the client's needs.
- You should cultivate a habit of care that includes virtues such as kindness, attentiveness, empathy, compassion, and reliability.

The following is a question that reflects this model of reasoning: Should we provide free medical care to the homeless? A person with an ethics-of-care perspective would probably say yes, even though that might not, for example, provide the greatest good for the greatest number of people. Ethics-of-care models provide a refreshingly new perspective on ethical situations. As you gain more clinical experience, revisit these philosophies and reflect on how they apply to your nursing practice.

KnowledgeCheck 43-7

- How does feminist ethics affect ethical decision making?
- What do the ethics-of-care philosophies emphasize?

Ethical Concepts and Principles

Remember from Chapter 8 that theories are made up of concepts and principles. The same is true for moral theories. Ethical concepts and principles are useful in client care discussions because they provide a common language for healthcare professionals to identify the issues. Even if people disagree about which action is right in a situation, they can agree on which principles apply. Agreement "in principle" can provide common ground for a compromise or other resolution of the problem. The following ethical principles are used in healthcare:

Autonomy

Autonomy refers to a person's right to choose and ability to act on that choice. It is based on respect for human dignity.

- You demonstrate respect for autonomy when you:
  - Treat clients with consideration.
  - Believe clients' stories about the course and symptoms of their illnesses.
  - Protect those who are unable to decide for themselves.
  - Protect privacy and confidentiality.
- You honor autonomy when you respect the client's or surrogate decision maker's right to decide, without judgment, even when you believe those choices are not in the client's best interest.

In the Meet Your Patient scenario, if you considered autonomy to be the most important principle in the situation, you would respect Alan's parents' decision to refuse blood products for their son. If respect for autonomy were not your dominant ethical principle, you would probably try to persuade them to change their minds.

Informed Consent   The principle of autonomy incorporates informed consent—the right of competent patients to decide whether to agree to a proposed treatment. **KEY POINT:** *Remember this general nursing principle: "Every competent adult has the right to accept or refuse treatment and should be provided all the information needed to make an informed decision."*

To ensure truly informed consent, patients need to know the diagnosis and related information, the recommended treatment, alternative treatment options, the risks and benefits associated with each, and the providers involved in the treatment regimen. The nurse's role is to verify that the patient understands and to obtain her signature. **KEY POINT:** *The nurse should notify the provider if the patient does not understand the treatment before obtaining her signature.*

To promote autonomy, you should educate clients and encourage them to formulate advance directives to ensure they have a voice in their long-term treatment. Advance directives (e.g., living will, durable power of attorney for healthcare) allow adults while they are competent to make decisions about their healthcare that will guide their care when they are no longer able to do so on their own.

Privacy and Confidentiality   The principles of privacy and confidentiality support the principle of autonomy. An autonomous person has control over the collection of, use of, and access to her personal information. Clients share sensitive information with nurses that they would not share with others, based on the nurse-client relationship. To maintain that trust you should:

- Discuss information relevant to client care in approved areas (conference rooms, bedside) and not in areas where others can overhear you (e.g., hallways, cafeterias, elevators).
- Share information with team members who have a need to know based on their involvement in the client care.
- Obtain the client's consent before providing information to family members or friends.

- Do not post pictures of clients on social media sites. Even inadvertently capturing patients in photographs has led to harsh disciplinary actions against the nurse.
  KEY POINT: *A person who knowingly violates the privacy and confidentiality requirements of the Health Insurance Portability and Accountability Act (HIPAA) can face imprisonment of 1 to 10 years and a monetary fine of $50,000 to $250,000, depending on motive.*

If you would like more information about privacy and confidentiality, see Chapters 18 and 44.

Nonmaleficence

The principle of **nonmaleficence** is the twofold duty to (1) do no harm and to (2) prevent harm. It encompasses actual harm, risk of harm and intentional and unintentional harm. Both the physicians' Hippocratic Oath and the nurses' Nightingale Pledge state that care providers have a duty to cause no harm to patients.

When you are careful to prevent medication errors or use an ambulation belt for assisting patients to walk, you honor the nonmaleficence principle.

In nursing it is rare to find intentional harm, but unintentional harm does occur as a result of incompetence or failure to adhere to each component of the nursing process (Beauchamp & Childress, 2012).

Nonmaleficence requires that you *think critically* and *identify the potential risks and benefits* in the treatment plan. You should then analyze whether the treatment causes more harm than good.

- **Risk of harm is not always clear.** Suppose you are about to get a client out of bed for the first time after surgery to prevent postoperative complications such as pneumonia and thrombophlebitis. However, the risks, in terms of excessive pain or unintentional damage to the operative site, may be less clear.
- **Weighing risks and benefits is a value-laden exercise.** Who determines whether pain is excessive—you or the client? To honor the principle of nonmaleficence in this situation, you would need to premedicate the client and carefully assess his pain during ambulation.

Respect for Dignity   This is an essential value in nursing. Respect for dignity refers to the nurse's respect for the intrinsic worth of the person, regardless of age, race, religion, medical condition, or any other factor. You must recognize that clients are vulnerable and not exploit their vulnerability for personal gain. Avoid inappropriate sexual or romantic relationships or other breaches of professional boundaries. To learn more about professional boundaries, search online for National Council of State Boards of Nursing Web site, look for the publication *A Nurse's Guide to Professional Boundaries,* or

 Go to **https://www.ncsbn.org/ProfessionalBoundaries_Complete.pdf**

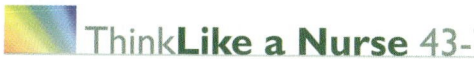 Think**Like a Nurse** 43-7

Think about the Meet Your Patient scenario in terms of nonmaleficence. The parents refuse to allow a blood transfusion. You, the nurse, have tried to persuade them to change their minds. You do not need to decide what you ought to do—just analyze the situation in terms of the risks.

- What is it that creates the risk for harm to Alan?
- What is the risk for harm to Alan's parents because of the nurse's actions?

Beneficence

Beneficence is the duty to do or promote good. You can think of this principle as being on a continuum with nonmaleficence. At one end of the continuum is beneficence, the duty to bring about positive good; at the other end is the duty to do no harm. The following examples illustrate the duties in priority order:

- *Do no harm.* (Don't push the man into the river.)
- *Prevent harm* when you can. (If the man is getting dangerously close to the river's edge, warn him that he is about to fall into the river.)
- *Remove harm* when it is being inflicted. (If you see a struggle and someone is trying to push the man into the river, interfere and try to stop it if you can do so without undue harm to yourself.)
- *Bring about positive good.* (If the man has fallen in the river, jump in and try to save him, or toss him a lifeline and call 911 if you can't swim.)

When weighing the risks and benefits of an action, you are actually balancing nonmaleficence with beneficence. Keep in mind that clients, family members, and health professionals may identify benefits and harms differently. A benefit to one may represent a burden to another. For example, in Meet Your Patient, you may see a blood transfusion as a benefit to Alan, but to the parents it may represent harm. Doing good very much depends on the context and the rights of the person for whom the action is being taken.

Paternalism   Although viewed by some as beneficence, **paternalism** (treating others like children) can have negative outcomes. For example, you will lose the client's trust if you coerce the client to act based on what think you know is best, rather than what the client wishes. Saying to a client, "Trust us; we know what is best for you to do in this situation," may seem to be beneficent because you are trying to support the client and relieve anxiety. But it is actually paternalistic behavior that lacks respect for the patient's autonomy (and therefore represents harm).

Fidelity

Fidelity (faithfulness) is the duty to keep promises. It is a basic part of every nurse–client relationship. Sometimes the promises are of major significance, such as promising not to share certain information with members of the healthcare team. At other times, it may be a promise to come back to provide a requested item or check the effectiveness of a pain medication.

In practice, you will often find that competing tasks prevent you from being able to deliver something exactly as you have promised. Instead of "I'll be right back with your medication," you might say, "I'll get back with your medication as quickly as I can" or "I must go help another patient, but I'll get your medication as quickly as I can."

KEY POINT: *The duty to keep a promise is the same regardless of its level of importance. Make promises in a thoughtful, careful manner to maximize the likelihood that you can keep them.*

Veracity

Veracity is the duty to tell the truth. This seems straightforward, but there are times when veracity presents a challenge.

For example, should you tell the truth when you know that it might cause harm to the client? Would it be appropriate to tell a lie to relieve extreme client anxiety?

Most nurses would agree that it isn't hard to tell the truth, but at times it may be very hard to determine how *much* of the truth to tell.

For example, healthcare professionals may feel uncomfortable giving families "bad news." So instead of saying, "Your father has a fatal illness and is unlikely to live for more than a month," they may say, "Your father is very ill, but we will do everything we possibly can for him."

In this, as in most situations, the risk of losing client trust outweighs any benefit of withholding some of the truth.

Although you always presume the value of telling the truth, there may be times when you are justified to withhold information. In the United States, we tend to place a high value on autonomy. However, in some cultures, families go to great lengths to protect a dying family member from the harsh truth of his prognosis, and the client himself may not wish to know. In such a situation, you need to be culturally sensitive so that your care incorporates the family's values and not the dominant cultural values. **KEY POINT:** *Always consider the context.*

 ## ThinkLike a Nurse 43-8

Review the Meet Your Patient scenario. Alan will not survive without a blood transfusion, yet his parents refuse to allow one. He asks the nurse, "Am I going to die?" You do not need to decide which response is best here; just write an example that illustrates each of the following. What might the nurse say if she wishes to:

- Tell Alan the truth?
- Withhold or partially disclose the truth?
- Answer with an untruth?

Justice

Justice is the obligation to be fair. It implies equal treatment of all clients. Questions of justice will become a part of your everyday experience in client care, from deciding how to allocate your time among clients to larger decisions, such as how to allocate limited healthcare resources. Justice can be distributive, compensatory, or procedural in focus.

Distributive Justice requires fair distribution of both benefits and burdens (Butts & Rich, 2015). It is especially relevant to healthcare, as in the following issues:

- **Allocating Resources.** Distributive justice questions come up when more than one person or group competes for the same resources (e.g., human organs for transplantation). How do we decide which patient should receive an available organ? Is an 18-year-old more deserving of a kidney than a 75-year-old? Is a person with liver disease due to alcoholism less deserving of a liver than someone with liver disease not caused by alcoholism? The decision of who should live and who may die is never an easy one. In the United States, a national committee sets criteria for how organs will be distributed so the standard of justice can be considered.
- **Fair Access to Care.** Access to care is a specific kind of healthcare resource. The principle of distributive justice holds that all should have equal access to healthcare. As nurses from the baby boomer generation retire, there may be fewer nurses to care for aging clients at a time when national healthcare dollars are stretched thin. How will the nation decide where to spend the limited dollars? How will nurse managers decide how to provide adequate care if they do not have enough staff nurses? The ability to develop sound

criteria on which to allocate resources is the challenge of distributive justice.

Compensatory Justice focuses on making amends for wrongs that have been done to individuals or groups. Malpractice suits consider this type of justice when they decide how much money to award a victim for being harmed. The goal is to make the person "whole."

Procedural Justice is important in processes that require ranking or ordering (Landwehr, 2013). For example, institutional policies are written to ensure that the same procedures apply to all clients or employees in the same way (e.g., visiting hours, working on holidays, sick leave). Can you think of an example of procedural justice that you have experienced during your nursing education?

ThinkLike a Nurse 43-9

Look again at the emergency department situation described in "What Is Nursing Ethics?" at the beginning of this chapter. In this scenario, two little boys were treated for lacerations. Which principle of justice was violated: distributive, compensatory, or procedural? Explain your thinking.

KnowledgeCheck 43-8

Provide the definition of each of the six ethical principles.

Professional Guidelines

You should consult professional guidelines when making ethical decisions. Healthcare professionals have an obligation to society to be competent in their field; to allow only qualified persons entry into the profession; to discipline members of the profession who do not practice at an acceptable level; to do no harm; and to use high moral and ethical standards to resolve dilemmas (Husted, Husted, & Scotto, 2015; Landwehr, 2013). You can find ethical standards for nurses in codes of ethics, standards of practice, statements of clients' rights, and various laws.

Nursing Codes of Ethics

Professional codes of ethics are formal statements of a group's expectations and standards for professional behavior generally accepted by members of the profession. Codes of ethics set forth ideal behaviors, but they are only as effective as the behaviors of the nurses who live up to the codes. The purposes of a nursing code of ethics are to:

- Inform the public about the profession's minimum standards.
- Demonstrate nursing's commitment to the public it serves.
- Outline major ethical considerations of nursing.
- Provide general guidelines for professional behavior.
- Guide the profession's self-regulating functions.
- Remind us of the special responsibility we assume in caring for the sick.

Nursing codes are not legally binding. However, they often exceed legal obligations. In most states, the state board of nursing uses the nursing code of ethics as the standard against which to evaluate a nurse's ethical behavior. The board has the legal authority to censure or reprimand the nurse who does not practice within the boundaries of ethical practice. The following two nursing organizations have long had codes to guide nurses' ethical decision making. The codes differ in specific details, but they are based on similar principles.

International Council of Nurses (ICN) The ICN adopted its *Code of Ethics for Nurses* as "a guide for action based on social values and needs" (ICN, 2012, revised) and serves as the standard for nurses worldwide. It stresses respect for human rights, including cultural rights, the right to life and choice, the right to dignity, and the right to be treated with respect. The Code of Ethics is designed to guide nurses in everyday choices, and supports their refusal to participate in activities that conflict with caring and healing. If you wish to see the revised code, you can search for *The ICN Code of Ethics for Nurses,* or

 Go to the ICN Web site at http://www.icn.ch/images/stories/documents/about/icncode_english.pdf

The American Nurses Association The ANA revised its Code of Ethics for Nurses in 2015a (Box 43-1). It "establishes the ethical standard for the profession" and serves as a "guide for nurses to use in ethical analysis and decision making" (p. vii). The code has nine provisions, followed by interpretive statements to explain what is meant by each provision. If you would like more information about the ANA Code for Nurses,

 Go to the ANA Web site at http://www.nursingworld.org/codeofethics

---

> **BOX 43-1** ■ American Nurses Association Code of Ethics for Nurses
>
> 1. The nurse practices with compassion and respect for the inherent dignity, worth, and unique attributes of every person.
> 2. The nurse's primary commitment is to the patient, whether an individual, family, group, community, or population.
> 3. The nurse promotes, advocates for, and protects the rights, health, and safety of the patient.
> 4. The nurse has authority, accountability, and responsibility for nursing practice; makes decisions; and takes action consistent with the obligation to promote health and to provide optimal care.
> 5. The nurse owes the same duties to self as to others, including the responsibility to promote health and safety, preserve wholeness of character and integrity, maintain competence, and continue personal and professional growth.
> 6. The nurse, through individual and collective effort, establishes, maintains, and improves the ethical environment of the work setting and conditions of employment that are conducive to safe, quality health care.
> 7. The nurse, in all roles and settings, advances the profession through research and scholarly inquiry, professional standards development, and the generation of both nursing and health policy.
> 8. The nurse collaborates with other health professionals and the public to protect human rights, promote health diplomacy, and reduce health disparities.
> 9. The profession of nursing, collectively through its professional organizations, must articulate nursing values, maintain the integrity of the profession, and integrate principles of social justice into nursing and health policy.
>
> *Source:* Reprinted with permission from American Nurses Association. (2015a). *Code of ethics for nurses with interpretive statements.* Silver Spring, MD: Nursebooks.org.

ANA Standards of Care

In addition to its Code of Ethics, the ANA sets standards for all aspects of clinical practice. In *Nursing: Scope and Standards of Practice* (2015b), standard 7 focuses on ethical practice. This standard (see Box 43-2) directs nurses to practice within the parameters described in the Code of Ethics for Nurses. Standard 7 speaks to the nurse's responsibilities to patients and directs nurses to contribute to the establishment and maintenance of an ethical environment.

BOX 43-2 ■ American Nurses Association Standards of Professional Performance Standard 7. Ethics

Definition: The registered nurse practices ethically

Measurement Criteria

The registered nurse:

■ Integrates the Code of Ethics for Nurses with Interpretive Statements (ANA, 2015a) to guide nursing practice and articulate the moral foundation of nursing.
■ Practices with compassion and respect for the inherent dignity, worth, and unique attributes of all people.
■ Advocates for healthcare consumers' rights to informed decision-making and self-determination.
■ Seeks guidance in situations where the rights of the individual conflict with public health guidelines.
■ Endorses the understanding that the primary commitment is to the healthcare consumer regardless of setting or situation.
■ Maintains therapeutic relationships and professional boundaries.
■ Advocates for the rights, health, and safety of the healthcare consumer and others.
■ Safeguards the privacy and confidentiality of healthcare consumers, others, and their data and information within ethical, legal, and regulatory parameters.
■ Demonstrates professional accountability and responsibility for nursing practice.
■ Maintains competence through continued personal and professional development.
■ Demonstrates a commitment to self-reflection and self-care.
■ Integrates principles of social justice into nursing and policy.
■ Contributes to the establishment and maintenance of an ethical environment that is conducive to safe, quality health care.
■ Advances the profession through scholarly inquiry, professional standards development, and the generation of policy.
■ Collaborates with other health professionals and the public to protect human rights, promote health diplomacy, enhance cultural sensitivity and congruence, and reduce health disparities.
■ Articulates nursing values to maintain personal integrity and the integrity of the profession.

Source: Excerpted from American Nurses Association. (2015b). *Nursing: Scope and standards of practice* (3rd ed.). Silver Spring, MD: Author.

The Patient Care Partnership

When patients are admitted to hospitals or to extended care facilities, they are entitled to specific rights in terms of their treatment—the right to:

■ Make their own decisions.
■ Be active partners in the treatment process.
■ Be treated with dignity and respect.

Because rights are rooted in values, and because values are derived from culture, patient rights are different throughout the world. The American Hospital Association published the *Patient Care Partnership* (2003). Instead of using "rights" language, this document is written in terms of patient expectations and responsibilities. The *Patient Care Partnership* encourages healthcare providers to be more aware of the need to treat patients in an ethical manner and to protect their rights (Box 43-3).

The Joint Commission Accreditation Standards

The Joint Commission standards contain sections on organizational ethics and individual rights. The section on organizational ethics requires ethical behavior in care, treatment, services, and business practices. The patient's values, preferences, need for information, and other factors that promote autonomy must be considered in her plan of care. It includes a statement about the need to provide for meeting patient needs in the event care must be denied in the institution. In meeting the patient's needs, you must also consider the organization's legal responsibility.

BOX 43-3 ■ American Hospital Association: The Patient Care Partnership

Patients, when hospitalized, should expect the following:

■ High-quality care, including the right to know the identity of caregivers
■ A clean, safe environment, including safety, freedom from abuse and neglect, and discussion of any changes in care
■ Respect for healthcare goals, values, and spiritual beliefs
■ To be involved in making decisions about their care and treatment. This includes receiving information about: Health condition and treatments
  The benefits and risks of treatments, and whether a treatment is experimental or part of a research study
  What the patient and family will need to do regarding treatment follow-up after leaving the hospital
■ Information about the right to make decisions and to refuse care, including advance directives and counselors or chaplains available to help with decision making
■ Protection of privacy and confidentiality
■ Help reviewing the bill and filing insurance claims
■ Preparation and information when leaving the hospital, including:
  Identification of sources for follow-up care and whether the hospital has a financial interest in any of the referrals
  Coordination of hospital activities with caregivers outside the hospital
  Information and training about the self-care the person will need at home

Source: Excerpted and adapted from American Hospital Association. (2003). *Patient care partnership: Understanding expectations, rights and responsibilities.* Chicago, IL: Author.

KnowledgeCheck 43-9

- How would the nurse use a professional guideline or code of ethics to assist in the ethical decision-making process?
- What are some examples of such resources?

ETHICAL ISSUES IN HEALTHCARE

As a nurse, you are likely to encounter several ethical issues that occur in healthcare. For example, ethical questions arise in the following situations:

Abortion

Acquired immune deficiency syndrome (AIDS)

Advance directives

Allocation of healthcare goods and services

Compelling unwanted treatment

Confidentiality and privacy (e.g., reporting gunshot wounds and child abuse)

Do Not Attempt Resuscitation (DNAR) / Allow Natural Death (AND) orders

Euthanasia, assisted suicide, aid in dying, extraordinary (heroic) measures to prolong life

Informed consent

Organ transplantation

Reproductive technology (e.g., in-vitro fertilization, surrogate mothering, sex preselection)

Withdrawing or withholding life-sustaining treatments (e.g., ventilators, artificial nutrition, hydration)

Extended discussion of those specific issues is best handled in an ethics text or an ethics course. They are beyond the scope of a fundamentals text.

PracticalKnowledge
knowing **how**

To fulfill your professional obligations for ethical practice, you will need practical knowledge of the processes of values clarification, ethical decision making, patient advocacy, and integrity-producing compromise.

ASSESSMENT/ANALYSIS/DIAGNOSIS NP

A holistic, comprehensive client assessment will help you establish the context in which ethical decisions are made. For clients struggling with ethical issues, the following diagnoses of may apply:

- **Decisional Conflict**—Use this label when the patient is uncertain about which course of action to take. The patient may verbalize distress and uncertainty; may delay decision making; may show physical signs of distress (e.g., increased heart rate); and may question moral rules, values, and personal beliefs.
- **Moral Distress**—Use this label when the patient has made a moral decision but is unable to carry out the chosen action. Cues include expressions of powerlessness, guilt, frustration, anxiety, self-doubt, and fear.

  NANDA-I also lists other diagnoses in the Value/Belief/Action Congruence class, including Impaired Religiosity, Readiness for Enhanced Religiosity, Risk for Impaired Religiosity, Powerlessness, Risk for Powerlessness, Spiritual Distress, Risk for Spiritual Distress, and Readiness for Enhanced Spiritual Well-Being.

VALUES CLARIFICATION

Values clarification refers to the process of becoming conscious of and naming one's values (Burkhardt & Nathaniel, 2014). If you are clear about your values, you will be able to make good decisions and to avoid imposing your values on others. Because each person has his own unique values set, it is important that you appreciate how others' values influence their decisions. Clarifying values should be a positive process of growth that results in more awareness, empathy, and insight (Peate, Watts, & Wakefield, 2013; Roberts, 2012). **KEY POINT:** *A values clarification process does not tell you what your values ought to be; it merely helps you discover what they are.* Values change over time, so you may need to repeat the process more than once in your lifetime.

How Can I Clarify My Values?

As a nurse, you will need to examine your values regarding life, death, wellness, and illness. A good place to start is to think about situations in which you may be uncomfortable, such as caring for a patient who molested a 5-year-old child, an unwed adolescent mother who is pregnant for the second time in 11 months, or parents such as the Freses (Meet Your Patient), who refuse treatment for a child because of religious beliefs. Ask yourself questions such as:

- Could I take care of this person?
- Does this bother me?
- What would I do if confronted with such a situation?
- Could I provide the same quality care as for my other clients?

How Can I Help Clients to Clarify Their Values?

Some clients may exhibit behaviors that indicate that their values are not clear. Consider this example:

> Jon White is the Chief Executive Officer of a large healthcare facility. Jon has had two myocardial infarctions (heart attacks) in the past 5 years. He also has hypercholesterolemia (high cholesterol) and hypertension (high blood pressure). Jon's physician has prescribed a heart medicine, low-dose aspirin, and medications to control his hypertension and cholesterol. Jon has repeatedly been taught about his diet, medications, and activity. He insists he is compliant. Jon's wife tells you that he has stopped exercising and is eating whatever he wants, including saturated fats. Jon tells her it is okay to eat what he wants because he is taking a "cholesterol-buster" pill.

The following behaviors may indicate that a client needs values clarification:

- Ignoring the advice of a health professional
- Client's words not consistent with his actions
- Numerous admissions for the same problem
- Uncertainty or confusion about which action to take

Which of those behaviors did Jon exhibit? To help Jon clarify his values, you might ask him to list the three things that are most important to him in life. Or you could help him work through the steps in Table 43-3 (choosing, prizing, and acting).

KnowledgeCheck 43-10

- What does the term *values clarification* mean?
- What are the steps in values clarification?

Table 43-3 ➤ Values Clarification	
STEP AND DESCRIPTION	**QUESTIONS TO ASK YOUR PATIENT**
Choosing (cognitive)	
Beliefs are chosen: Freely (allows you to cherish your choice) From alternatives After considering all consequences (ensures that the alternative is right for you)	Do (did) you have any choice about what you do? Do you have any control over what happens? What have you decided to do? Can you list some alternative actions? What are your options? What could you do instead of …? What do you think will happen if you do that? What will you gain by doing that? What is the disadvantage of doing that?
Prizing (affective)	
Beliefs and behaviors that are chosen are prized: With pride (feeling good about your choice) With public affirmation	How do you feel about your decision? People sometimes feel good after making such a decision. Others feel pressured. How is it for you? How do you intend to tell your family (friends) about this decision? What will you say to your spouse (friends, family)? When will you announce your decision to …?
Acting (behavioral)	
Beliefs are acted on: By incorporating the choice into one's own behavior With consistency and repetition	Try to determine whether the client will act on the decision: ■ How do you think your spouse (significant other) will react when you do that? ■ When will you actually carry out this decision? ■ Try to predict consistent behavior by asking: How many times in the past have you …? What kind of schedule have you worked out? How often and when will you …?

Source: Adapted from Raths, L. E., Harmin, M., & Simon, S. B. (1978). *Values and teaching: Working with values in the classroom.* Columbus, OH: Merrill.

ETHICAL DECISION MAKING

Decision models used in bioethics do not offer easy decisions, but they do provide a guiding structure to follow to help you arrive at the best answer in specific situations. Decision models can help you decide on a course of action even if they do not tell you absolutely that the action is right or wrong.

How Can I Recognize Ethical Issues? We have said it is important to be aware of the ethical issues in client care situations, but how can you recognize them? **KEY POINT:** *The key is that there is usually a conflict:*

■ About the right action to take
■ Between the duties and obligations of healthcare professionals (or they are unclear)

■ Between the needs and interests of an individual and a group of clients
■ Between what the family wants and what the client wants or needs
■ Between the family and health professionals
■ Between ethical principles or values (e.g., autonomy versus nonmaleficence, as in the Meet Your Patient scenario)

Problem or Dilemma?

In the best of all possible worlds, you could easily apply ethical principles and decide what to do. However, often in moral situations one ethical principle is in conflict with another equally important principle. It is also possible for an ethical framework to produce more than one acceptable option. An **ethical dilemma** is a situation in which a choice must be made between two equally undesirable actions. There is no clearly right or wrong option. Such situations are emotionally painful for everyone in the situation, as you can see from the Meet Your Patient scenario. If you support Alan's parents' right to refuse a blood transfusion, you honor the principle of autonomy, but at the expense of the principle of nonmaleficence, which says we should prevent harm to Alan.

Fortunately, not all moral problems are dilemmas nor are they all complex and difficult. You may only occasionally confront a true dilemma, but are more likely to encounter ethical questions or problems. For example, you can easily answer: "Should I take the patient's morphine to relieve my back pain?" Only problems that pose a question between competing and equally valuable interests are true dilemmas.

Ethical behavior and decision making do not deal only with dilemmas. They really involve choosing to be ethical in the everyday aspects of your practice: for example, treating colleagues and patients with respect, not passing up a room when you see a patient crying, or helping out a new graduate who is frustrated and anxious. The "What Is Nursing Ethics?" scenario about the two little boys in the emergency department is more representative of everyday ethics than is the Meet Your Patient scenario.

How Do I Work Through an Ethical Problem?

Once you have identified an ethical problem, a decision model can help you logically decide the best action to take. Still, in the case of a true ethical dilemma, you will probably not be comfortable with any course of action, no matter how logically you think it through.

Ethical decision-making models will help you carefully consider several perspectives, guide your reasoning, and explain the reasons for your final action. Each approach may produce a different solution. One of the easiest to remember and use is the MORAL model. This model has been credited to two different authors: Thiroux (1977) and Crisham (in Scott, 1985). The letters MORAL will remind you of the steps in this model, which is described in the following section. To use the model in clinical settings, see Clinical Insight 43-1.

First, Use Problem-Solving

As a first step in ethical decision making, use the nursing process approach to describe the problem and alternative approaches:

- *Assessment—What are the relevant facts?* Alan needs a blood transfusion to survive. Both you and the surgeon have tried to persuade the parents to consent, but they still refuse. The parents' religion prohibits blood transfusions. Alan is 15 years old (a minor), so you cannot administer a transfusion without his parents' consent.
- *Analysis/Diagnosis—Identify the problem; state the conflict.* There is a values conflict: The healthcare professionals value preserving physical life; the parents place more value on preserving the soul. There is an ethical dilemma, as well: If no transfusion is given, you violate the principle of nonmaleficence (harm to Alan); if you somehow coerce the parents to consent, you have violated the principle of autonomy (respect for their values and their freedom to choose). So the decision to be made is whether to (1) follow the parents' wishes, (2) find a legal way to transfuse without their consent, or (3) find some compromise that will work.

Next, Use the MORAL Model

Now use the MORAL model to come up with alternative solutions for the Frese family

M—Massage the Dilemma

1. *First identify and define the issues in the dilemma, and consider the values and options of all the major players:* Mr. and Mrs. Frese, Alan, the surgeon, possibly a member of the clergy, and you (the nurse). You have already identified the values in the problem-solving approach: physical life versus spiritual life. You and the surgeon also value the principles of autonomy and nonmaleficence

2. *Then identify the information gaps.* In massaging the situation, you should ask yourself:
   - Do I fully understand the situation that is causing the need for blood?
   - How much time is available to make this decision—is there time for the parents to discuss this with their congregational elders?
   - Does the surgeon have any treatment that could be used to stabilize Alan while the parents discuss the situation?
   - Does the physician know that the family members are Jehovah's Witnesses?
   - Do Alan's parents fully understand the nature of Alan's physical emergency?
   - In the Freses' religious view, what is the consequence of receiving blood?
   - Do they understand what might happen if blood is not administered (i.e., do they understand the consequence of their action or inaction)?
   - Is this what Alan would want? Has Alan expressed in the past what he feels about blood transfusions? Have they ever had family discussions when other young Jehovah's Witnesses have been faced with such a decision? Where did Alan stand in those discussions?
   - How is this situation like other situations they have experienced in their lives?
   - Have they thought about their opposing duties: the duty to uphold their religious values and the duty to protect their son from harm?
   - Has everyone's voice been heard?
   - Have the parents contacted their congregational elders and discussed the situation?
   - What emotions are coming into play in this situation?
   - How is this decision affecting the parents as individuals? Are they in agreement on the issue, or is there dissension? If there is dissension, are both sides being supported fairly?
   - Is there some common ground between what the surgeon wants and what the parents feel they need to do to uphold their religious convictions?

O—Outline the Options

At this step in the MORAL model, you (or the charge nurse or a member of the ethics committee) should outline all of the options to all parties, including those that are less realistic and conflicting. You might ask a member of the ethics committee or the hospital chaplain to help the family and the doctor understand the opposing viewpoints.

The surgeon needs to outline the state of emergency that exists for Alan and to explain what the limited medical options are: to transfuse blood or, if no blood is given, what other treatments are available (e.g., volume enhancers). The surgeon will need to say how soon the decision must be made based on

Alan's condition. He should clearly, and with as little emotion as possible, explain the consequences of each action to the parents. He should also state whether one administration of blood will likely fix the situation or whether continued administration may be required.

The family (or congregational elders) should explain for the doctor and nurse the basis for their refusal to consent and what they believe the consequence would be if blood were given.

R—Resolve the Dilemma

Now carefully review the issues and options. Apply basic ethical principles. If you can, also look at the situation using alternate ethical frameworks.

- **Autonomy.** By their refusal to give consent, the Freses are exercising their autonomy. How far will we go to honor their autonomy?
- **Beneficence and Nonmaleficence.** How are we defining "good" (beneficence) and "harm" (nonmaleficence) in this situation? The surgeon defines "good" as Alan's receiving the needed blood. He defines "harm" as the outcome for Alan without the blood, even if he uses a less effective alternative. Alan's parents would define "good" as following their religious mandates and making sure their son will remain pure in the eyes of God. They might explain that a Jehovah's Witness who willingly accepts a blood transfusion might forfeit his or her eternal life. The Freses might believe the taking of blood to be more harmful than death, because that would affect Alan's eternal life, not just his physical life.
- **Fidelity.** The surgeon is being loyal (exhibiting fidelity) to the principles of medicine and evidence-based practice, which mandate the administration of the blood. To the parents, their loyalty to their religious principles to ensure that Alan has eternal life may be more important than the loss of the physical life itself.
- **Veracity.** The principle of veracity holds that the surgeon should not exaggerate the need for the blood, and he should be honest with the parents in terms of the consequences of the alternative actions. Another question of veracity involves the parents: Are they being honest with each other regarding their feelings?

Your role as a nurse is to be an advocate for the client and the family. Talk with the family and their religious representative, if available, about what they see as their opposing duties: the duty to uphold their religious values and the duty to protect their son from physical harm. Explain to the surgeon the reasoned position of Alan's parents, if you can do so.

KEY POINT: *Ensure that everyone's viewpoint has been respected and considered. This may be as important as the final decision that is reached. In this and other difficult situations, always look for the opportunity for a good compromise (discussed later in this chapter).*

A—Act by Applying the Chosen Option

This step is the first one that actually requires action. The hospital is bound to follow the parents' decision because Alan is a minor. However, if there is time, many agencies might refer this situation to the hospital ethics committee. The hospital might also ask a legal court authority to resolve the situation. If an emergency requires an immediate decision, the only *legal* action is to follow the parents' decision, whether or not you consider it the best *moral* action.

♥ **iCare**   Whatever happens, Alan's parents will need emotional support. If they decide to refuse the blood transfusion, you must remain nonjudgmental in supporting them, even if you do not agree with their decision. If they, or

the courts, decide that the blood will be given, they may need even more support. They may feel overwhelming guilt and may fear that Alan will be forever burdened with guilt at the realization that the medical care violated church doctrine. If family support is not present, you could volunteer to call in extended family, friends, and church members if they wish. They will need a quiet, private place to await the outcome of the treatment.

L—Look Back and Evaluate

This phase calls for evaluation of the entire process, not just the consequence of the decided action:

- How well did the process work? Were processes in place for the dilemma to be discussed respectfully without undue delay in treatment?
- Were all parties' expectations realistic?
- How are all of the affected parties feeling now (doctor, parents, family, Alan, you)? Regardless of the outcome of the decision, do all involved feel they had a voice and their views were respected?
- How well did you do in the situation? Did you act as an effective advocate for the rights of Alan and his parents? Did the power and authority of the provider or hospital in the situation unduly influence you?
- Were policies and procedures in place to guide you in the process of working out this situation?
- Has anything changed since the dilemma came to light? Has a greater good been achieved for future situations? Have future situations been made easier as a result of the things learned in this situation? Has any aspect of this ethical decision now become a universal policy at the institution?
- Are further actions required in terms of this or like situations?

Look for a Good Compromise

Even if you believe you know the right thing to do, others may not agree with you, or there may be constraints that prevent you from doing it. For example, in the case of Alan, even if you decided the right thing to do is to give him a blood transfusion, (1) his parents do not agree with you, and (2) the law says you cannot do so without his parents' consent. This will happen often—much more often than a true dilemma, in which you cannot *decide* the right thing to do. No matter how well we work together, there will always be ethical problems and disagreements. Many cases are full of complexity and uncertainty, and sometimes the price of acting on your beliefs is extremely high. For example, what might have happened if the surgeon had infused blood without the Freses' consent? What might have happened if you had refused to talk to the parents as the surgeon asked you?

Many times, it will be possible to reach a "good" compromise. A **good compromise** is one that preserves the integrity of all parties. This means that:

- **The discussions are carried out in a spirit of mutual respect**—all viewpoints are respected and considered.
- **The compromise solution itself is ethically sound;** that is, you should be able to provide a principles-based rationale for the compromise, as well as for each of the opposing positions. In the case of Alan and his parents, there probably is no compromise position between "give blood" and "don't give blood." Perhaps the parents would agree to one, but no more than one, transfusion; but that is hard to justify ethically. If one transfusion is acceptable (to honor nonmaleficence), why not two or three? If two transfusions are against their religious beliefs, why would

one be acceptable? Nevertheless, in many other cases compromise is possible.

So how do you compromise without losing moral integrity? To begin, you must realize there is more at stake than the issue itself ("Is a blood transfusion right or wrong?"). There are some things that are inherently good in compromising.

- **First, it is never good to settle things by force** (as you would if you got a court order to transfuse Alan without his parents' consent). You have probably heard the old saying "Might doesn't make right." A compromise can preserve the rights of the less powerful party in a disagreement.
- **Keeping peace on a nursing unit is good for both the nurses and clients.** When there is upheaval and moral suffering, care quality throughout the unit can suffer. A compromise can bring peace.
- **There is intrinsic good in taking part in a process in which we must try to see things from others' points of view.** It may make us more open minded, more creative, and less judgmental.
- **Keep in mind that most issues do contain room for reasonable differences of opinion.** In the Meet Your Patient scenario, can you see that both sides are people of good will who have ethical reasons to justify their opinion? There is also often room for doubt, on your own part, about the morally best action to take.
- **A compromise may achieve mutual respect.** It is a significant thing to reach a settlement in which each party feels assured of the other's respect for its seriousness and sincerity.

Given all those ideas, a person of good will might want to re-examine and back away from a very strong opinion. Remember, sometimes your position isn't all that strong, and the other position isn't all that weak (as in the case of Alan). There is also always the chance that you may have made an error in your reasoning or have not completely understood some facts of the case. Ethical disputes can be settled only if you are willing to engage in discussion and admit that the other people might have a point! There may be cases in which you cannot compromise (perhaps Alan's case is one), but don't listen to people who say, "You can never reach agreement on ethical issues. They are too complex." It is possible to achieve integrity-producing compromises, and in nursing, it is often necessary.

What Are My Obligations in Ethical Situations?

As you can see, in making ethical decisions nurses rarely act alone. Usually you will be one of several healthcare professionals and family members who will jointly arrive at the best decision. Your role when an ethical decision is needed includes the following:

- *Be aware of and sensitive to issues,* so you can identify them when they arise. Educate yourself—attend workshops, read, and talk to other nurses.
- *Assume responsibility for your own ethical actions.* Even if you do not have the "last word" about what happens to a client or about what others do, you are always responsible for your own actions in every situation.
- *Function as a team member* when ethical problems arise. Realize you should have input—no one profession has full ethical expertise—and realize that your input can be valuable.
- *Support the client and family members* while they are making the decision and afterward. Listen, ask questions, and provide unbiased information. Be helpful without being too directive or judgmental.

- *Support clients who are not being allowed to decide.* For example, in the Meet Your Patient scenario, you would want to be sure Alan's wishes were considered, if possible. However, if the parents insist on deciding for him, against his wishes, he may need a great deal of emotional support.
- *Use and participate in institutional ethics committees* if you are given the opportunity.
- *Most important, advocate for your client.* You may need to balance your client's autonomy with the wishes of family members or the responsibilities of other healthcare professionals to the client. As an advocate, you may find yourself in conflict with other team members or family members, or have a different ethical perspective.
- *Continually strive to improve your ethical decision making.*

Use and Participate in Institutional Ethics Committees

There is no easy way to decide which principle should outrank another principle, or which person's values are best in a given situation. For this reason, many healthcare institutions have ethics committees. These interdisciplinary committees typically include nurses, doctors, clergy, ethicists, and lay representatives. Ethics committees develop guidelines and policies, provide education and counseling, and, in the case of ethical dilemmas, review the case and provide a forum for the expression of the diverse perspectives of those involved. Ethics committees usually follow one of three models when discussing a dilemma: the autonomy model, the patient benefit model, and the social justice model.

Autonomy Model This model is useful when the patient is competent to decide and emphasizes client autonomy and choice. For example, if this committee knew Alan's (Meet Your Patient) wishes, they might be inclined to try to persuade his parents to do as Alan wants.

Patient Benefit Model This model assists in decision making for the incompetent patient by using substituted judgment (i.e., what the patient would want for himself if he were capable of making these issues known). If Alan is unconscious and cannot say what he wants, this committee would probably ask Alan's parents, family, and friends, "What do you think Alan would want? Have you ever heard him talk about a situation such as this?"

Social Justice Model This model focuses more on broad social issues involving the entire institution rather than on a single client issue (Yoder-Wise, 2014). Such a committee might consider whether, in general, an institution should seek a legal order to act against the wishes of the parents. Or the committee members might discuss whether supporting parents' religious beliefs in this instance would have implications for supporting other types of religious beliefs in future cases.

KnowledgeCheck 43-11

- Define *ethical dilemma.*
- How can you recognize an ethical problem?
- What is an integrity-producing compromise?
- What are the functions of an ethics committee?
- What does the mnemonic *MORAL* stand for?

Be a Client Advocate

The role of an advocate is to safeguard clients against abuse and violation of their rights. When you think of the rights and values described in the *Patient Care Partnership* and in nursing codes of ethics, you can see how this role is important. Be aware that advocacy in clinical practice is less about the client's legal rights and ethical theory, and more about such seemingly "routine" measures as obtaining a new prescription when an analgesic is ineffective, even if it does mean telephoning the prescriber for the third time during your shift. The advocacy role requires you to be respectful, considerate, courageous, persistent, and concerned with justice.

Why do you think advocacy is so important? Why can't clients do these things for themselves? The following are some of the reasons:

You Have Special Knowledge That the Client Does Not Have Diseases, treatments, and the healthcare system are so complex that when clients become ill, they may not have the energy to deal with the complexity, even if they have the necessary knowledge. You may need to help them to "jump through the necessary hoops" to get what they need. When clients' rights are denied or when they do not have the ability to exert their rights, nurses have a responsibility to step in. Advocacy is essential in ensuring client rights are protected.

Your Professional Role Includes Defending Clients' Autonomous Decisions The ANA Code of Ethics requires you to be a client advocate (see Boxes 43-1 and 43-2). You will be called on to defend your client's autonomous decisions even if you do not agree with them and even if they conflict with the opinions of others healthcare providers. You may find yourself the sole supporter of a client's right to choose the direction of his care.

You Have a Special Relationship With Clients You may find that you are able to obtain information about a client that is not available to other professionals. In general, nurses interact with clients over longer time intervals and are involved in very personal activities, especially in inpatient settings. They often become the most trusted caregivers. Details about family life, coping styles, personal preferences, fears, and insecurities are more likely to be discussed during the time involved in nursing interventions than in the brief minutes of interaction when a provider makes rounds.

In addition, clients may perceive less social distance between themselves and the nurse and, therefore, feel freer to confide in them. The nurses' point of view can be a valuable asset to resolving an ethical problem satisfactorily. Of course, many providers have long-standing relationships with their clients; however, this does not negate the importance of the nurse's input, which may provide a different perspective.

Your Role as an Advocate Is to Inform, Support, and Communicate You should inform competent clients of their rights and provide the information they need to make informed decisions. Then you must remain objective and support them in the decisions they make. If others are not respecting client choices, you will need to intervene. This may simply be a matter of conveying information and clarifying the client's wishes to family or healthcare professionals (e.g., "I know how hard it is for you to let him go, but your dad says he has made peace and is ready to die. His treatments make him feel even more ill, and he simply does not want to fight anymore"). Advocacy may require you to arrange for the client to consult with a religious leader or an attorney for advice and support, or may require you to consult an institutional ethics committee.

You Should Inform Clients About Advance Directives Advocacy includes asking clients whether they have an advance directive and educating them on their significance. Kossman (2014) found that completion of advance directives increased when providers asked culturally sensitive questions and educated clients on advance directives. However, advance directives needed to be detailed to ensure adherence to the clients' wishes. Even people who have an advance directive may not understand the statements they have checked in the boxes on the form. Take the time to review the form with your clients. See Chapters 17 and 44 if you need further discussion on advance directives. For guidelines that will help you to function effectively as an advocate, see Clinical Insight 43-2: Guidelines for Advocacy.

Improve Your Ethical Decision Making

Research has found that when faced with ethical dilemmas, nurses tended to use conventions (e.g., rules, procedures) as criteria for decision making rather than clients' personal needs and well-being (Dierckx de Casterlé, Izumi, Godfrey, et al., 2008). A full-spectrum nurse must move from the conventional (rules-bound) to the post-conventional (reasoning) stage of moral development. The following suggestions can provide guidance:

- **Use Theoretical Knowledge.** Review nursing and other literature for discussion of cases and experiences of other nurses. This will give you a broader view of the problems you may confront and the strategies for managing them. Become familiar with the codes of ethics, the *Patient Care Partnership*, and ethical frameworks and principles.
- **Use Self-Knowledge.** Examine your personal value system. Explore the influences of your religion, cultural beliefs, and personal experiences. This will help you to recognize your comfort zone with specific ethical issues.
- **Use Practical Knowledge.** While you are still a student, ask to attend either ethical rounds or an ethics committee meeting. As a graduate nurse, to gain insight into ethical situations at your institution, volunteer to serve on the ethics committee or participate in nursing ethics rounds.
- **Consult Reliable Sources.** Attend ethics education programs and discuss issues with healthcare providers, attorneys, ethicists, and clergy to obtain the perspectives of others.
- **Share.** Regularly engage in discussions with the staff on your unit to determine differences in value systems and to collaborate proactively to identify methods to effectively resolve ethical dilemmas. When faced with a difficult ethical decision, seek guidance and support from peers, coworkers, and teachers.
- **Evaluate.** After a situation is resolved, evaluate your decision and the effects of your actions. You should be able to learn from even the worst decision. And when everything goes well, you can file your strategies away to use in similar future situations.

KnowledgeCheck 43-12

- What are three reasons why clients may need a nurse advocate?
- Briefly describe the nurse's role as a client advocate.

CLINICALREASONING

The questions and exercises in this section allow you to practice the kind of thinking you will use as a full-spectrum nurse. Critical-thinking questions usually have more than one correct answer, so we do not provide "correct answers" for these features. It is more important to develop your nursing judgment than to just cover content. You will learn by discussing the questions with your peers. If you are still unsure, see the Davis Advantage chapter resources for suggested responses.

Caring for the Nguyens

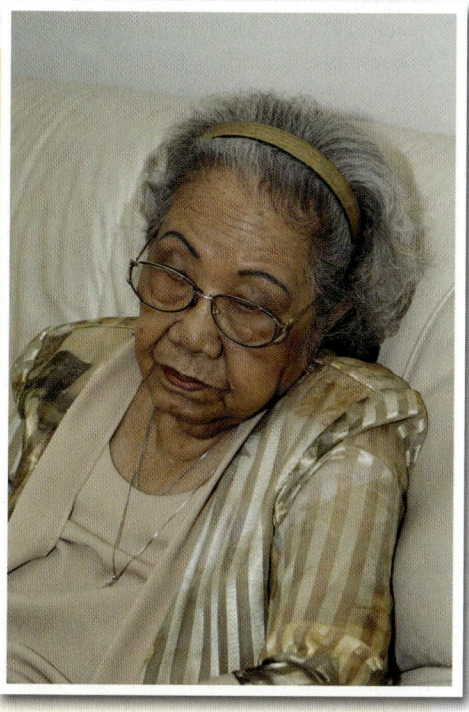

Mai Nguyen, Nam Nguyen's mother, has hypertension. She is forgetful about taking her medicines. Since her husband died, she has experienced periods of depression. When asked about her medicines she often replies, "It doesn't really matter since my husband died. If I die, what difference will it make?"

Mai Nguyen was scheduled to have lunch with friends but did not arrive. When her friends called the house, they got no answer. At the end of lunch, one of Mai's friends decided to call Nam to inform him of her concerns about his mother. Nam found his mother unresponsive on the kitchen floor. He called 911, and she was brought to the hospital by ambulance. At the hospital, the emergency department (ED) doctor tells Nam that his mother has had a massive stroke (brain attack) brought on by uncontrolled hypertension. He asks Nam whether Mrs. Nguyen has an advance directive. She does not. The provider asks Nam to consider what level of care to offer his mother. He tells Nam that comprehensive treatment would include intubation, mechanical ventilation, and tube feeding support. The provider feels it is unlikely that she will experience significant recovery from this stroke.

Nam tells you, "I want everything done for my mother. I lost my father this year, and I'm not going to lose her, too." Yen, Nam's wife, reminds you that Mai has been depressed since her husband died and has expressed a desire to die. Because Nam and Yen are not in agreement about the course of action, no decision is communicated. Mai Nguyen's condition continues to deteriorate, and the ED provider feels he must intubate her, place her on a ventilator, and admit her to the ICU according to hospital protocol.

A. You are aware of Mai's statements and her poor compliance with treatment. What, if any, concerns do you have about this course of action?

B. Mai continues to decline. Nam is informed that the "only thing keeping your mother alive is the ventilator and IV medicines." Do you consider this heroic treatment?

C. How would you approach Mr. Nguyen to speak with him about how he is feeling?

D. Nam and Yen have asked to meet with the team providing care to Mai. They announce that they would like all the "heroic measures to end." They request that Mai be allowed to die. Could you participate in this care? With what actions would you be comfortable? With what actions would you be uncomfortable?

 Go to Davis Advantage, Resources, Chapter 43, **Caring for the Nguyens—Suggested Responses.**

Applying the **Full-Spectrum Nursing Model**_____

PRACTICE SITUATION

Read the following summary of the Kothari and Kirschner article:

> Kothari, S., & Kirschner, K. (2006). Abandoning the Golden Rule: The problem with "putting ourselves in the patient's place." *Topics in Stroke Rehabilitation, 13*(4), 68–73.

A large body of evidence documents the difficulties healthcare professionals have in predicting what their patient believes or wishes. These difficulties extend from the predictions of:

- Very specific patient wishes, such as for life-sustaining therapies
- More global assessments of patients' lives as a whole (e.g., their quality of life)

One explanation for this phenomenon is that healthcare professionals, either consciously or unconsciously, adopt "Golden Rule thinking." This refers to our attempts to understand another person's situation by imagining what we would believe or want under similar circumstances, in other words, "putting ourselves in the patient's place."

Although Golden Rule thinking would seem to be a promising strategy, studies show that it actually results in inaccurate presumptions of a patient's wishes or beliefs. These presumptions, in turn, have significant clinical and ethical implications. That is, they cause healthcare professionals and families to make decisions for the patient that are, in reality, *not* what the patient would want. The thinking goes:

> I should put myself in the patient's place.
> If I were the patient, I would want X.
> Therefore, the patient probably wants X.
> Because the patient probably wants X, we will do X.

This thinking process can have different results: (1) The patient really does want X, so you have met his needs. (2) The patient really wanted Y, so you did not meet his needs.

THINKING

1. *Theoretical Knowledge:* What is the Golden Rule, or what does it say?
2. *Critical Thinking (Inquiry):* What is one thing that could be done ahead of time to prevent the need for Golden Rule thinking? Explain why that would work.

DOING

3. *Nursing Process (Assessment):* If you do not know what the patient would want, instead of thinking what *you* would want, how might you get an idea of what the patient might want?

CARING

4. *Self-Knowledge:* What is your earliest memory of being taught the Golden Rule?
5. *Ethical Knowledge:* Which ethical principle does the Golden Rule seem to try to follow: autonomy, nonmaleficence/beneficence, fidelity, veracity, or justice?

PracticalKnowledge: clinical application

CLINICAL INSIGHTS

Clinical Insight 43-1 ► Using the MORAL Model for Ethical Decision Making

- **M—Massage the dilemma.** Identify and define the issues in the dilemma. Consider the options of all the major players in the dilemma and their value systems. This includes patients, family members, nurses, physicians, religious representatives, and other interdisciplinary healthcare members. Identify the information gaps.
- **O—Outline the options.** Examine all the options, including those that are less realistic and conflicting. This stage is designed only for considering options and not for making final decisions.
- **R—Resolve the dilemma.** Review issues and options, applying basic principles of ethics to each option. Decide the best option based on the views of all those concerned in the dilemma.

- **A—Act by applying the chosen option.** This step is usually the most difficult because it requires actual implementation, whereas the previous steps allow only for dialogue and discussion.
- **L—Look back and evaluate.** Reflect on the entire process and evaluate all steps, including the implementation. No process is complete without thorough evaluation. Ensure that those involved are able to follow through on the final option. If not, a second decision may be required and the process must begin again at the first step.

Practice Resources

Badruddin, S. (2016); Tschundin, V. (2003); Yoder-Wise, P. (2014).

Clinical Insight 43-2 ► Guidelines for Advocacy

The following principles will help you to function effectively as an advocate:

- **Keep the ethical principle of patient autonomy always in mind.**
- **Know and document the facts** of the case.
- **Know the arguments** of those who oppose the patient. Use role-playing to develop a strategy for responding to the arguments.
- **Have a sound base of support for your actions.** Be familiar with any policies or laws that apply.
- **Form a coalition of allies,** if you can. Get consultation. Communicate, inform, and clarify their collaborative roles.
- **Intervene high enough in the hierarchy** to get the job done. If the difficulty is with a physician or an organizational policy, merely going to the charge nurse will not

be enough. You will need to communicate with nurse administrators or other agency administrators.
- **Demonstrate to the system** how it is defeating its own goals (e.g., for patient care).
- **Avoid getting into a power struggle** if possible (use the preceding steps first). If you must, decide how far you need to go and whether you are willing to go that far. You will need to enlist people with more power in the system than you have (e.g., family members, physicians, administrators).
- **Be aware of client vulnerability.** When possible, avoid confrontation. If there is risk for the client (as in a power contest), be sure the client is aware of his risks and possible gains; then let him choose how far to take the situation.
- **Have alternative actions.** Assess risks realistically. Weigh them against potential gains.

To explore learning resources for this chapter,

Go to www.DavisAdvantage.com and find:

Answers and Suggested Responses for all questions in this chapter

Lists of NIC Interventions and NOC Outcomes

List of NANDA-I Diagnoses

Knowledge Map

References and Bibliography

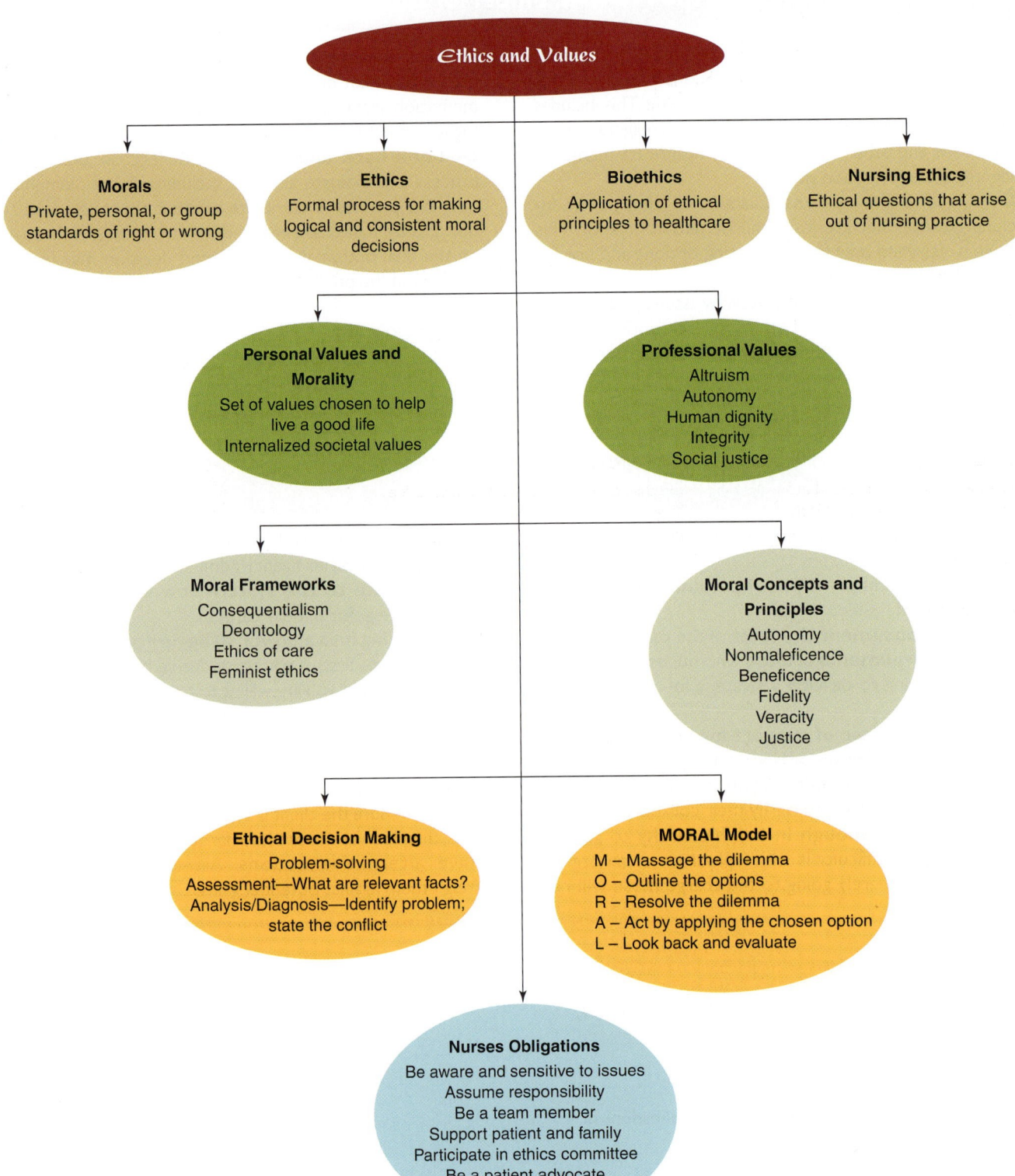

Concept Map

Ethics and Values

Morals
Private, personal, or group standards of right or wrong

Ethics
Formal process for making logical and consistent moral decisions

Bioethics
Application of ethical principles to healthcare

Nursing Ethics
Ethical questions that arise out of nursing practice

Personal Values and Morality
Set of values chosen to help live a good life
Internalized societal values

Professional Values
Altruism
Autonomy
Human dignity
Integrity
Social justice

Moral Frameworks
Consequentialism
Deontology
Ethics of care
Feminist ethics

Moral Concepts and Principles
Autonomy
Nonmaleficence
Beneficence
Fidelity
Veracity
Justice

Ethical Decision Making
Problem-solving
Assessment—What are relevant facts?
Analysis/Diagnosis—Identify problem; state the conflict

MORAL Model
M – Massage the dilemma
O – Outline the options
R – Resolve the dilemma
A – Act by applying the chosen option
L – Look back and evaluate

Nurses Obligations
Be aware and sensitive to issues
Assume responsibility
Be a team member
Support patient and family
Participate in ethics committee
Be a patient advocate

CHAPTER 44

Legal Accountability

Learning Outcomes

After completing this chapter, you should be able to:

➤ Identify four basic sources of law.

➤ Discuss direct implications of the Nurses' Bill of Rights to practice.

➤ Relate the impact of the Health Insurance Portability and Accountability Act (HIPAA) to patient rights and protections.

➤ Discuss the effects of the Patient Self-Determination Act (PSDA) on healthcare practices.

➤ Describe accommodations that conform to the Americans With Disabilities Act (ADA).

➤ Apply state mandatory reporting laws to patient care situations.

➤ Apply the concepts of Good Samaritan laws to nurses' actions.

➤ Identify seven rights of nurses within the healthcare workplace.

➤ Discuss how nurse practice acts provide the foundation for nursing practice.

➤ Explain disciplinary actions for unacceptable nursing decisions or actions.

➤ Discuss basic principles of criminal law that affect nursing practice.

➤ Compare and contrast intentional and unintentional torts.

➤ Discuss common causes of malpractice litigation.

➤ Describe the phases of the litigation process in a nursing malpractice case.

➤ Identify strategies to minimize liability in nursing practice.

Key Concepts

Law

Liability

Malpractice

Related Concepts

See the Concept Map at the end of this chapter.

Disclaimer: The material contained in this chapter is intended to convey information on topics of interest to nursing students. Although prepared by a nurse attorney, this chapter should not be used as a substitute for legal counseling. No one should act on the information contained in this chapter without professional guidance. These materials should not be considered legal advice or a legal opinion.

Meet Your Nurse Role Model

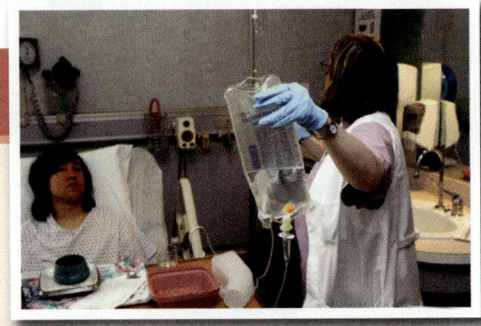

A nurse with 3 years of experience on a medical–surgical unit arrives at work and discovers that two of her colleagues called in sick, including the charge nurse. The nursing supervisor informs her that she will need to assume the charge nurse role, in addition to assuming care for three clients. Feeling frustrated, the nurse ponders whether she should just quit and find another job, but then decides to accept the assignment. Two hours into the shift, one of her clients begins to experience complications, requiring blood glucose checks every 2 hours and frequent monitoring. In addition, one of the nurses becomes ill and is replaced by a float nurse from the labor and delivery unit. The nurse contacts the nursing supervisor and requests additional assistance, but is told no other nurse is available and that the supervisor is involved with an emergency situation on another unit. The nurse begins to analyze this situation from a legal perspective to determine the best course of action.

- Should the nurse have accepted the assignment? If yes, what factors should the nurse have considered before accepting the assignment?
- If the nurse should not have accepted the assignment, could she have been charged with abandonment?
- How should the nurse handle this situation?

Theoretical Knowledge
knowing why

In clinical practice, nurses are often confronted with situations that present legal issues. You must have an understanding of the legal guidelines governing nursing practice to protect yourself, your patients, your colleagues, and your employers. The theoretical knowledge in this chapter, combined with the critical thinking model in Chapter 2, will help you to answer questions related to the Meet Your Nurse Role Model scenario.

ABOUT THE KEY CONCEPTS

- The concept of **law** can be described as a binding practice, rule, or code of conduct that guides appropriate actions and defensible decisions of an individual or a group. Laws protect society by establishing acceptable patterns of behaviors and are enforceable by a controlling authority.
- **Liability** means that the person is financially or legally responsible for something. Nurses are legally responsible for their own actions and this legal responsibility cannot be delegated—this is the basis for liability in nursing practice.
- **Malpractice** is one source of legal liability. It means that a professional person has failed to act in a reasonable and prudent manner. If someone is harmed, the professional may be held liable.

WHAT ARE THE SOURCES AND TYPES OF LAW?

The U.S. Constitution establishes three branches of government: executive, legislative, and judicial. Each branch has specified authority, designed to equalize power among the three and to provide a system of checks and balances. Laws are derived primarily from four sources: (1) the Constitution, (2) statutes, (3) administrative bodies, and (4) the courts (Table 44-1).

Constitutional Law A **constitution** is a system of fundamental laws and principles that prescribes the nature, functions, and limits of a government.

- *The U.S. Constitution is the superior law of the land and applies to all states throughout the United States.* The U.S. Constitution limits the powers of the federal government and gives each state the power to govern itself and to pass laws to promote the health, welfare, order, and security of its citizens (police power).
- *Each state has a similar structure that likewise establishes the governing system for the state, its cities, and municipalities.* Thus, all state and federal laws must be consistent with the U.S. Constitution. Any law that conflicts with the Constitution is considered invalid or void.
- If you would like to see the seven Articles of the Constitution,

 Go to **http://www.senate.gov/civics/constitution_item/ constitution.htm**

Statutory Law A **statute** is a law passed by the federal Congress or by a state legislative body. Congress passes laws for the benefit of society as a whole, whereas states use their police power to pass laws to ensure the general health, safety, and welfare of their citizens. Nurse practice acts (NPAs) are examples of statutory law. NPAs, passed by the legislative body of each state, are regulations that govern the profession of nursing.

Administrative Law Formally defined, **administrative law** refers to the laws that govern the activities of administrative agencies. These agencies are created at the federal level by Congress and at the state level by its legislative bodies. As applied to nursing, within each state's nurse practice act the legislative body created a board of nursing to enforce the NPA. The board of nursing creates rules and regulations that define and expand on the provisions in the NPA necessary to ensure compliance with its statutory mission—to regulate the practice of nursing.

Table 44-1 ➤ Branches of Government and Sources of Law

Branches of Government		
	EXAMPLES	**DESCRIPTION**
Executive	The President of the United States, Attorney General, Secretary of State, state governors	Authority to execute and/or enforce laws.
Legislative	Congress (House of Representatives + Senate)	Make or formulate laws.
Judicial	U.S. Supreme Court; state and local courts	Interpret statutory law and decide cases and controversies.
Type/Source of Law		
	EXAMPLE	**QUESTION POSED**
Constitutional Law	Freedom of speech	Can an employer prevent internationally educated nurses from speaking in their native language in the work environment?
Statutory Law	Definition of nursing	What is the nurse's scope of practice (duties and responsibilities)?
Administrative Law	Delegation and supervision	Is the registered nurse legally responsible for tasks or assignments delegated to other nurses?
Common Law	Affirmative duty	Does a registered nurse have a responsibility to exercise an independent judgment to prevent harm to patients?

Common (Judicial) Law A compilation of laws made by judges or courts is known as **common law.** Also referred to as *case law,* common law is based on common customs and traditions. It comes from legal principles and guidelines that judges use to determine the outcome of legal cases.

WHAT LAWS AND REGULATIONS GUIDE NURSING PRACTICE?

As a professional nurse, you will need to understand the various laws and regulations that guide nursing practice. Laws and regulations at the federal and state levels have a direct impact on nurses' actions and decisions.

Federal Law

Several federal statutes have direct implications for professional nursing practice. Many NPAs require nurses to have knowledge of federal laws such as the following:

Bill of Rights

The first 10 Amendments to the U.S. Constitution are known as the *Bill of Rights.* The Bill of Rights clearly identifies, and in many ways limits, the role of government in individuals' lives. Many of these rights have direct implications for healthcare, including the rights of nurses and of patients. For example, protecting patients' privacy rights is a fundamental role of the professional nurse that is derived from the Fourth Amendment to the U.S. Constitution. If you would like to review all the amendments in the Bill of Rights, you can search the Web or in your browser,

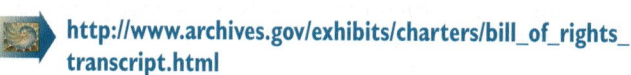
http://www.archives.gov/exhibits/charters/bill_of_rights_transcript.html

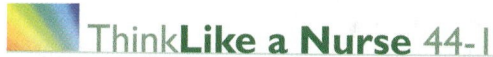
Think Like a Nurse 44-1

- Develop a scenario illustrating how a nurse might protect a client's right to privacy.
- What is one thing a nurse can do to respect a client's property rights?

Health Insurance Portability and Accountability Act (HIPAA)

The Health Insurance Portability and Accountability Act (HIPAA) was passed by Congress in 1996 to:
- Protect health insurance benefits for workers who lose or change their jobs.
- Protect coverage to persons with preexisting medical conditions.
- Establish standards to protect the privacy of personal health information.

Under HIPAA rules, healthcare agencies and their employees must take steps to ensure the confidentiality of the patient information and medical records. Nurses and other healthcare providers must protect the patient's right to privacy by not sharing patient information with unauthorized individuals. In addition, HIPAA allows patients to see, make corrections to, and obtain copies of their medical records. The cases in the following box highlights the importance of understanding and complying with the safeguards created under HIPAA.

Case: Violation of a Patient's Privacy

- A nursing assistant spent 8 days in jail after being convicted of invasion of personal property for posting

(Continued)

graphic photos of elderly and disabled patients on Facebook.

- Several emergency room nurses were fired after painting the face of an unconscious obese patient with charcoal, making unprofessional comments, and taking pictures of him with their cell phones.
- A man who received the registration face sheets of patients admitted to the hospital from the manager of the hospital's trauma unit and provided them to personal injury attorneys was sentenced to 33 months in federal prison for violation of HIPAA.

Health Information Technology for Economic and Clinical Health (HITECH) Act

Under the HITECH Act data breach notification provision, healthcare agencies are required to notify clients of breaches without unreasonable delay and by no longer than 60 days. In addition, its enhanced enforcement provisions increase civil penalties for breaches caused by willful neglect up to $250,000, with a maximum penalty of $1.5 million for repeated or uncorrected violations. Posting client information online can trigger HITECH violations.

Case: Posting Patient Information on Social Media

A certified nursing assistant (CNA) was charged with voyeurism after posting on her Facebook page a picture of a patient's buttocks after he had had a bowel movement. As required by the HITECH Act, her coworkers reported the breach after seeing it on social media. The CNA was terminated and lost her license.

Emergency Medical Treatment and Labor Act (EMTALA)

The Emergency Medical Treatment and Labor Act (EMTALA) requires healthcare facilities to provide emergency medical treatment to patients who seek healthcare in the emergency department (ED), regardless of their ability to pay, legal status, or citizenship status. The obligation is for the medical facility to provide medical screening to determine whether an emergency exists and to stabilize the patient before transferring him or her to another healthcare facility.

Case: EMTALA

A client presented to the ED with complaints of chest pain. Per protocol, the triage nurse obtained information about the onset and severity of the pain and medications taken by the client. She then completed a focused history and assessment, obtained a pulse oximeter reading, and ordered an electrocardiogram and lab work. She reported the results to the ED provider, who consulted a cardiologist. The client initiated a lawsuit, alleging he suffered heart damage because of a delay in treatment. Ruling in favor of the hospital and nurse, the court noted that the care received via protocol was the same as that of any client with similar complaints (*Byrne v. Chester Co. Hospital*, 2013).

ThinkLike a Nurse 44-2

A 54-year-old uninsured and unemployed woman arrives at the emergency department of a small private hospital complaining of chest pain and nausea. The triage nurse calls the on-call provider, who instructs the nurse to send the client to the county hospital several blocks away. The nurse assesses the client and contacts her supervisor, who tells her to call the medical chief of staff and inform him that the client is in need of emergency treatment.

- Discuss whether the nurse's action was appropriate or inappropriate.

Patient Self-Determination Act (PSDA)

The Patient Self-Determination Act (PSDA) of 1991 recognizes the client's right to make decisions regarding his own healthcare, based on the information provided to him by the healthcare provider, regarding the medical or surgical treatment options available, the benefits, risks, and alternatives. Box 44-1 describes agency and healthcare workers' responsibilities under the PSDA.

There are two types of legal written advance directives: the living will and the durable power of attorney for healthcare.

- A **living will** is prepared by an alert and oriented (competent) individual and gives directions to others about the person's wishes regarding life-prolonging treatments if he becomes unable to make those decisions. As a legal document, the living will's requirements may vary from state to state. However, language common in the living will gives the person the opportunity to specify treatment in numerous areas (Box 44-2).
- A **durable power of attorney (DPOA)** for healthcare identifies a person (called *the surrogate decision maker*) who will make healthcare decisions in the event the client is unable to do so. The surrogate has the right to make the medical decisions for as long as the person is not able to do so for himself (is incompetent).

Case: Durable Power of Attorney (DPOA)

Mr. Green was in a coma as a result of head trauma experienced in a motor vehicle accident. In his DPOA, he had designated his brother, Joey, as his surrogate. Although Mr. Green was married with two adult children, Joey was

---

BOX 44-1 ■ The Patient Self-Determination Act

The Patient Self-Determination Act requires healthcare facilities to:

- Provide written information to each client regarding the right to make decisions, including the right to accept or to refuse medical treatment, and the right to make advance directives.
- Document in the client's medical record the presence or absence of advance directives.
- Provide education to the staff, healthcare providers, and community on advance directives.
- Follow state law as it relates to advance directives.
- Treat everyone the same regardless of the presence or absence of advance directives (facilities may not discriminate).

BOX 44-2 ▪ Sample Living Will Language

If I am in a terminal condition, irreversible coma, or in a persistent vegetative state, my wishes are as follows:

I ☐ **do** ☐ **do not** want to be in or taken to a hospital.

I ☐ **do** ☐ **do not** want pain medications to keep me comfortable.

I ☐ **do** ☐ **do not** want cardiac resuscitation, including drugs and electrical shock.

I ☐ **do** ☐ **do not** want mechanical respiration/artificial respiration.

I ☐ **do** ☐ **do not** want tube feeding or any other artificial or invasive form of nutrition (food).

I ☐ **do** ☐ **do not** want hydration (water), via tube or intravenously.

I ☐ **do** ☐ **do not** want blood or blood products.

I ☐ **do** ☐ **do not** want any form of surgery or invasive diagnostic tests.

I ☐ **do** ☐ **do not** want renal dialysis.

I ☐ **do** ☐ **do not** want antibiotics.

the person legally recognized to make decisions regarding Mr. Green's healthcare. Two weeks later, Mr. Green came out of the coma and regained the ability to make decisions. At that point, Mr. Green no longer required Joey as a surrogate.

The American Nurses Association (ANA, 2016) highlighted the nurse's role in advance care planning and counseling in a position statement. As a nurse, you have the following responsibilities:

▪ Listen to patients to identify their concerns, expectations, and hopes regarding end-of-life care.

▪ Review patients' documented preferences upon admission to healthcare facilities.

▪ Recognize that advance care planning is a continual process and not a one-time execution of documents.

▪ Encourage patient and family participation in healthcare decisions about advance directives and end-of-life decisions.

You might want to ask the following questions about advance directives as a part of the nursing admission assessment:

▪ What is your understanding of an advance directive, including the living will and durable power of attorney for healthcare?

▪ Do you have an advance care directive? If so, do you have a copy with you?

▪ If you don't have an advance care directive, do you wish to initiate one?

▪ Who will make your healthcare decisions if you are unable to do so? Have you discussed your end-of-life choices with this person, significant others, and your provider?

Case: Durable Power of Attorney (DPOA)

Mrs. Terri Schiavo collapsed in her Florida home in 1990 after a suspected potassium imbalance secondary to bulimia and was without oxygen for about 5 minutes. She suffered severe brain damage. Terri Schiavo did not have a living will. According to Florida law, her husband became her legal guardian, and thus the decision maker regarding her medical treatments. In November 1992, Mr. Schiavo won a medical malpractice lawsuit for $1 million from her physician on the theory that he failed to diagnose Mrs. Schiavo's bulimia.

In 2000, Mr. Schiavo petitioned the court to have her feeding tube removed. Her parents opposed the action. During the next 5 years, extensive legal battles ensued. Finally, the court ruled in favor of removing the feeding tube. Mrs. Schiavo died on March 31, 2005. It was lack of a living will that (1) allowed this situation to go on for so long and (2) made it impossible to know for sure what Terri Schiavo would have wanted. It's all guesswork without a documented living will (Shepard, 2009).

Americans With Disabilities Act (ADA)

The Americans With Disabilities Act (ADA) of 1990 provides protection against discrimination of individuals with disabilities. A person has a **disability** if he has a physical or mental impairment that substantially limits one or more major life activities, has a record of such impairment, or is regarded as having an impairment (ADA Amendments Act of 2008). In general, the ADA says that employers must provide reasonable accommodations within the work setting to allow employees with disabilities to perform their jobs.

Case: ADA Accommodations

▪ A nurse with a substance abuse addiction was caught using illegal drugs. She was allowed to return to work after rehabilitation. Her employer had a policy that provided employees with a last-chance agreement. When the nurse returned to work, she was reassigned to a job that did not require her to dispense medication. She was given periodic drug tests.

▪ A nurse with fibromyalgia syndrome was provided accommodations to help her overcome extreme fatigue and pain at work. She switched from evening to day shift to better regulate her sleep pattern, eliminated working two consecutive 12-hour shifts, and changed from full-time to part-time employment status.

▪ A nurse with insulin-dependent diabetes had difficulty maintaining glucose control. Her employer provided consistent times for breaks and lunch and privacy to check blood sugar levels and administer insulin as needed.

▪ A nurse with osteoarthritis in both knees was unable to perform her duties in the birthing center. A reassignment to the only vacant position, as a scheduler, which entailed a pay cut, was a reasonable accommodation (Job Accommodation Network, n.d.).

KnowledgeCheck 44-1

▪ Which federal law requires healthcare agencies to provide clients with information about advance directives?

▪ Which federal law ensures that clients can receive emergency treatment regardless of their ability to pay?

▪ What protections are provided to clients by the Department of Health and Human Services "privacy rule" of HIPAA?

State Laws

In addition to federal law, many states have laws that directly impact nurses' actions and behaviors. These include mandatory reporting laws, Good Samaritan laws, nurse practice acts, and medical malpractice statutes.

Mandatory Reporting Laws

The law in various states requires healthcare workers to report communicable diseases. You also have a duty to report physical, sexual, or emotional abuse or neglect of vulnerable individuals (e.g., children, older adults, the mentally ill), whether you suspect it or have actual evidence of it. The intent is to protect people who cannot protect themselves and to protect society against the spread of communicable diseases. Since the mandatory reporting laws vary from state to state, you should be familiar with the law in your state.

- Mandatory reporting laws also protect you when reporting abuse. In most instances, the identity of the reporter is kept confidential.
- If you fail to report certain communicable diseases, or child abuse, you can be charged for criminal misdemeanor or be subject to disciplinary action by the board of nursing.
- The duty to takes priority over the patient's right to privacy. Therefore, if you report abuse or neglect, you cannot be charged with violating a patient's right to privacy (e.g., under HIPAA).

Case: Mandatory Reporting

A high school principal and superintendent were arrested and charged with failure to report child abuse for allegedly failing to notify the Department for Children and Families of a student allegation of inappropriate touching by a teacher. State law mandates that allegations of child abuse be reported within 24 hours after allegations are brought (Wellington, 2013).

Good Samaritan Laws

Good Samaritan laws are designed to protect from liability those who provide emergency care to someone who is in need of medical services. To successfully use the Good Samaritan defense, the following elements must be present:

- Care was provided in an emergency situation.
- Person(s) providing the care did not cause the emergency or injury.
- Care was provided in a reasonably competent manner.
- Care provided must be voluntary (not paid or eligible for payment).
- Person receiving care did not object to receiving care.

In addition, nurses should follow these guidelines to ensure their protection by Good Samaritan laws:

- Call 911, or have someone else call, as soon as you can.
- Do not leave the person unless you transfer care to an equally competent professional.
- Place the person under the care of emergency personnel or other qualified healthcare professionals as soon as possible and follow their instructions.
- Do not accept money or any other form of compensation for the services provided.

Good Samaritan laws vary from state to state. You should be familiar with the law in your state. A typical case involving Good Samaritan laws is as follows:

Case: Good Samaritan

A registered nurse (RN) is leaving the hospital after working a 12-hour shift when she witnesses a single-person motor vehicle accident. She calls 911, stops, and approaches the accident scene, where she smells gasoline. Fearing that the car will explode, she pulls the accident victim from the car, places him flat on the ground, and assesses his injuries. She puts pressure on his bleeding femoral artery and stays with him until the ambulance arrives. The victim has spinal cord injuries and sues the nurse for removing him from the car. The nurse is protected from liability by the Good Samaritan law.

Nurses working in healthcare environments may not be protected by Good Samaritan laws if they already have a responsibility to provide care to those in need.

Case: Good Samaritan

The court denied the Good Samaritan defense for two physicians who were sued for malpractice. The physicians were salaried employees of a college of medicine that contracted with a community health clinic to provide backup emergency services for medically complex cases. The college of medicine received a fixed amount of money from the clinic for such services. The two physicians were called to assist with a complicated delivery that resulted in the death of an infant from injuries received during birth. One physician billed the clinic for her services and the court ruled that based on the relationship, the physician rendered emergency services for a fee. The other physician deviated from policy and did not submit a bill. However, the court ruled that a provider who is eligible for payment is not protected from liability under the Good Samaritan doctrine simply because he does not bill for his services (*Rodas v. Seidlin*, 2011).

Nurse Practice Acts

Nurse practice acts (NPAs) are statutory laws passed by each state's legislative body that define the practice of nursing. Nurse practice acts are designed to:

- Regulate nursing practice to protect the health, safety, and welfare of the general public.
- Define the scope of nursing practice.
- Approve programs providing pre-licensure nursing education to students.

The components of NPAs are discussed in more detail later in the chapter.

Medical Malpractice Statutes

Medical malpractice refers to a lawsuit brought against a healthcare provider for damages (e.g., money) when there has been death of, injury to, or other loss to the person being treated. Laws governing medical malpractice vary from state to state, primarily regarding the time frame for bringing a lawsuit (statute of limitations) and the amount of monetary compensation allowed. To protect themselves from personal losses, many healthcare providers purchase malpractice insurance, which provides them with an attorney to defend against the claim and pay the damages (money) awarded to the claimant by a judge or jury. Malpractice is discussed in more detail later in this chapter.

Other Guidelines for Practice

In addition to federal and state laws, other practice guidelines may define what constitutes reasonable and prudent nursing care.

Institutional Policies and Procedures

Institutional policies and procedures usually are more specific and detailed than standards set by professional organizations. They describe care that is reasonable, appropriate, and expected in the context of that facility. You must be familiar with these policies and procedures because they can be used as evidence of a violation of a standard of care if you failed to follow them. Healthcare facilities should not have policies and procedures that conflict with the nurse practice act, professional standards of practice, the ANA Code of Ethics for Nurses, or other documents that guide nursing practice. If you encounter any conflicts, or if a policy is not working well, you should bring the matter to your supervisor's attention and/or contact the board of nursing in your state for advice.

American Nurses Association Code of Ethics

The **ANA Code of Ethics for Nurses** (2015a) describes the standards of professional responsibility for nurses and provides insight into ethical and acceptable behavior. It describes nurses' obligations for safe, compassionate, nondiscriminatory, and quality care, while defining commitments to self, the client, the employer, and the profession.

The Code of Ethics is not a law, and therefore a nurse would not be charged with criminal offenses for violating the code's provisions. In many situations, there is a fine line between what is legal and what is ethical. When confronted with a situation, to avoid legal jeopardy you should ask yourself, "Is there a law that relates to this situation?" If the answer is yes, you should understand the guidance provided by the law. If you cannot follow the law in good conscience, talk with your supervisor or seek legal advice. If there is no law, or if it seems immoral or unethical to you, ask, "What guidance is provided under the Code of Ethics?" Your action should then be consistent with the code, if at all possible. The ANA code guarantees the client the right to dignity, privacy, and safety, and that the nurse will:

- Be accountable and competent.
- Use informed judgment.
- Maintain employment conditions conducive to quality client care.
- Protect the client from misinformation and misrepresentation.
- Collaborate with other healthcare professions to meet the client's healthcare needs.

A nurse who violates a provision of the code of ethics may have to defend her action to the state board of nursing. Also, in a malpractice suit, courts may look to these codes to judge whether the nurse's action was at the level expected by the profession. However, you must understand that the code will not likely protect you if you break a law or fail to follow agency policies, even if you believe the law to be immoral. If you need more information on nursing codes of ethics, see Chapter 43.

Patient Care Partnership (PCP)

The **Patient Care Partnership** replaced the American Hospital Association's Patient Bill of Rights. The PCP brochure is available in eight languages. It explains in detail to patients that during hospitalization, they should expect:

- High-quality care
- A clean and safe environment
- Involvement in care
- Protection of privacy
- Help when leaving the hospital
- Help with billing claims

Like the ANA Code of Ethics, these rights are not necessarily legally binding, but they can provide evidence by which to judge whether the client's care and environment met reasonable and appropriate standards. For more information on the Patient Care Partnership, see Box 43-3.

American Nurses Association Nurses' Bill of Rights

The **Nurses' Bill of Rights** is a policy statement adopted by the ANA to identify the seven conditions that nurses should expect from their workplace that are necessary for sound professional practice. It provides a framework for employers to understand what nurses need for a safe work environment and to support nurses as they address such issues as unsafe staffing, workplace violence, and mandatory overtime (ANA, n.d.a). The Nurses' Bill of Rights highlights that nurses have the right to:

- Practice in a manner that fulfills their obligations to society and to those who receive nursing care.
- Practice in environments that allow them to act in accordance with professional standards and legally authorized scopes of practice.
- A work environment that supports and facilitates ethical practice as defined by the Code of Ethics for Nurses.
- Freely and openly advocate for themselves and their clients, without fear of retribution.
- Fair compensation for their work, consistent with their knowledge, experience, and professional responsibilities.
- A work environment that is safe for themselves and for their clients.
- Negotiate the conditions of their employment, either as individuals or collectively, in all practice settings.

American Nurses Association Standards of Practice

The ANA (2015c) Standards of Practice has three components:

1. *Professional standards of care* that incorporate the nursing process in the diagnostic, intervention, and evaluation aspects of client care
2. *Professional performance standards* that identify the various role functions of the nurse in direct client care, quality of practice, ethics, education, communication, research, leadership, collaboration, resource management, collegiality, and environmental health
3. *Practice guidelines* for the various specialty areas that are developed by professional organizations (e.g., American Association of Critical-Care Nurses).

If you need to review the ANA Standards of Clinical Nursing Practice, refer to Chapter 1, Table 1-3. Standards establish the minimum level of competency for nurses. Nurses are expected to follow the standards that apply to their specialty areas.

ThinkLike a Nurse 44-3

Recall the Meet Your Nurse Role Model scenario. Would the nurse have done the right thing if she had decided not to accept the assignment and leave the facility immediately?

- What standards, guidelines, and laws would apply to determine whether the nurse's behavior was in accordance with standards of practice?
- Which statements in the ANA Nurses' Bill of Rights might the nurse use to justify her actions?

Nurse Practice Acts

As you have learned, nurse practice acts (NPAs) contain a provision that creates and empowers a state board of nursing to regulate the practice of nursing in that state. All 50 states, the District of Columbia, and the four U.S. territories have established boards of nursing. Although NPAs can vary from state to state, they all have common components, because states used ANA guidelines in developing their regulations. A state's nurse practice act usually includes the following:

- The authority of the board of nursing, its composition, and powers
- A definition of *nursing* and the boundaries of nursing practice
- Standards for the approval of nursing education programs
- Requirements for licensure of nurses
- Grounds for disciplinary action against a nurse's license

Case: Nurse Practice Act

Mejonus X Institute advertised an associate degree nursing program that could be completed in 12 months at a cost of $44,000. You are interested in the program, but are not sure whether the program is legitimate. Your initial investigation of the program should start with the state board of nursing, which approves nursing education programs. A list of approved nursing programs can usually be found on the state board of nursing Web site in many states.

Requirements for Licensure

Perhaps the most important function of state boards of nursing is establishing and enforcing the requirements for licensure. Unlicensed health providers pose a danger to the health, safety, and welfare of the general public because they have not met the specified standards to ensure a minimum level of competency to enter the nursing profession. In most states, the applicant for licensure must:

- Graduate from an approved or accredited nursing program.
- Meet the established character criteria.
- Undergo a criminal background check and fingerprinting.
- Pass the NCLEX-RN or -PN exam.
- Pay an application fee.
- Meet additional state requirements (e.g., a jurisprudence examination in Texas).

Case: Applicant for Licensure With a Criminal Conviction

An RN applicant for licensure was convicted 3 years earlier of a misdemeanor theft. He was sentenced to 12 months in jail, with 11 months of the sentence suspended; 2 years of probation; 180 hours of community service; and $1,200 in fines. The board of nursing approved his application for licensure by examination and reprimanded him for the criminal conviction.

Special Cases of Licensure

To protect the public, licensing is meant to ensure to practicing nurses have met the minimum competencies set by the state.

Mutual Recognition Model (MRM) / Multistate Licensure Compact Certain states, through a multistate agreement, allow nurses whose primary state of residency is in a compact state to practice in other compact states without obtaining a new license. You must obtain licensure "by endorsement" if you change your state of residency to another compact state or if your state of residency is not a member of the compact. To be *licensed by endorsement,* you do not have to retake the NCLEX examination, but must apply to the new state and fulfill any of that state's application requirements such as fingerprinting, background check, transcripts, and fees.

Case: Multistate Compact

Roberto is a clinical nurse residing in Overland Park, Kansas (his primary state of residency), and originally licensed in the state of Kansas after passing the NCLEX-RN. He is now employed at the Children's Hospital on the other side of the state line in Missouri. Roberto is required to maintain active licensure in the state where he was employed. He received an RN licensure by endorsement in the state of Missouri by meeting the requirements of the Missouri State Board of Nursing, but did not have to retake the NCLEX-RN.

Government/Military Personnel Another special case of licensure involves nurses employed by the military, Veterans Administration, Public Health Service, or other entities of the federal government. These nurses may practice in other states without obtaining a new license as long as they are practicing within the scope of their employment.

Case: Special Case of Licensure

Jane was a clinical nurse in the U.S. Air Force Reserve. She was licensed in the state of Texas, but is assigned to a military hospital in Nevada for her 2-week annual military tour. Jane will not need to obtain a license in the state of Nevada to practice at the military hospital.

Scope of Practice

The scope of nursing practice is found in the definition of nursing at the various levels. Nurses must be familiar with the definition of their level of *nursing* to appropriately plan and implement care that is consistent with their scope of practice. **KEY POINT:** *A nurse who practices outside the scope of practice can be charged with violation of the nurse practice act.*

Nurse practice acts vary slightly state by state. However, in most states, the licensed practical nurse's (LPN) scope of practice is limited in assessment privileges and interpretation of clinical data. Typically, LPN/LVNs do not have authority to alter nursing care plans. The following landmark case should make clear that no one, including an employer or physician, can increase a nurse's legal scope of practice:

Case: Scope of Practice

A physician delegated to an LPN the task of administering a polio booster to a 2-year-old boy. The nurse put the boy over her knee and proceeded to give the injection. The boy moved and the needle broke off in his buttocks, where it remained for 9 months despite attempts to surgically remove it. Since the Washington State Nurse Practice Act at that time did not allow LPNs to give injections, the nurse was in violation of the nurse practice act by performing a task that was outside of her legal limits (*Barber v. Reinking*, 1966).

Disciplinary Actions

The state board of nursing can take disciplinary actions against your license for violation of the NPA.

What Is the Process? A disciplinary action usually involves some or all of the following:

- The process begins with a complaint from an individual, employer, or professional organization that the nurse has engaged in unprofessional conduct.
- The complaint is then assigned to an investigator to determine its legitimacy or validity.
  - If the investigator decides the complaint is invalid or does not constitute a violation of the NPA, it will be dismissed.
  - If the complaint may violate the NPA, the investigator gathers additional information by contacting the nurse, interviewing witnesses, and reviewing documents and records.
- The case may be heard by the board of nursing members, who will decide whether there was a violation of the NPA and the appropriate punishment. To fulfill the due process requirements of the Fourteenth Amendment, the board of nursing must provide you with:

  Notice of the charges against you

  Evidence that supports the charges

  A *hearing* in which you have the opportunity to cross-examine the witnesses and to present your own evidence and witnesses

- If you are not satisfied with the board's actions and punishment, you can appeal your case to the appropriate state court.
- At every stage during the disciplinary process, you have the right to have an attorney present. Questions that you should ask a potential attorney include the following: (1) How many of your cases were in the area of administrative law and procedures? (2) How many times have you represented clients in front of professional boards, such as the board of nursing?

What Constitutes Unprofessional Conduct? The following are a few examples of actions that may constitute unprofessional conduct:

- Acting outside your scope of practice
- Accepting duties or responsibilities for which you are not prepared or competent
- Inaccurately recording, falsifying, or altering patient or agency records.
- Causing intentional or careless physical abuse or harm to a client, including unreasonable use of restraint, isolation, or medication; threatening or frightening patients; verbal abuse; sexual abuse, misconduct, or exploitation
- Violating the patient's confidentiality
- Failing to take appropriate action to safeguard a patient from incompetent practice of another nurse (e.g., reporting to the state board of nursing)
- Diverting drugs, supplies, or property of any patient or agency
- Using a false or assumed name or impersonating another person licensed by the board (Kansas State Board of Nursing, 1993, last amended 2007)

ThinkLike a Nurse 44-4

A registered nurse was assigned to care for a 76-year-old client who had a stroke (brain attack). On entering the room, the nurse found the client surrounded by 10 family members. The nurse requested the family members leave the room so she could conduct her initial assessment and perform any related treatments. They did so. The nurse provided care in a professional, unhurried, and gentle manner. As she was leaving, the client said, "Thank you. You are a wonderful nurse." Later, the nursing supervisor told her the client told his family members that the nurse had spoken harshly to him and had yanked his arms. The family stated they would file a complaint with the hospital administrator and the board of nursing.

- Are there grounds for disciplinary actions?
- What should the nurse do?

KnowledgeCheck 44-2

How does each of the following protect clients?

- The Patient Care Partnership (PCP)
- Nursing codes of ethics
- Mandatory reporting laws

Credentialing

Many healthcare disciplines, including nursing, use a voluntary form of self-regulation called **credentialing.** In the legal sense, credentialing includes accreditation and certification. Having credentials implies that the person or agency has met higher standards than the minimum required (e.g., licensure).

Accreditation Most nursing boards require that a nursing program be **accredited** by an agency recognized by the Department of Education (e.g., Accreditation Commission for Education in Nursing or the Commission on Collegiate Nursing Education). This helps to ensure students receive education that meets the minimum standard for quality client care. Similarly, The Joint Commission accredits healthcare facilities that meet established standards focused on safe, appropriate, and quality client care.

Certification Another form of credentialing is **certification.** Through certification and licensing, the board identifies nurses who are qualified for advanced practice (e.g., clinical nurse specialists, midwives, and nurse practitioners) or for certification in a subspecialty, such as emergency nursing or pediatric nursing. In some states, the board establishes the criteria for certification, including (1) educational preparation, (2) clinical experience, and (3) certification by other professional organizations. In other states, the nurse may obtain an advanced practice license only if she is first certified by a national organization, such as the American Nurses Credentialing Corporation or a specialty organization.

WHAT IS CRIMINAL LAW?

Criminal law deals with wrongs or offenses against society. It may result in prosecution (legal action) by the state or federal government for engaging in behavior that constitutes a crime. A **crime** is a violation of a law as defined by a legislative body. The legislature also specifies the punishments for the crime. State-level criminal laws vary from state to state. There are two "levels" of crimes: misdemeanors and felonies. The primary difference is the possible punishment.

- A **felony** is a crime punishable by more than 1 year in jail (e.g., murder, assisted suicide, rape/sexual assault, stealing drugs and equipment, felony abuse). A person convicted of a felony loses the right to vote, hold public office, serve on a jury, and possess firearms. The person may also lose any professional license.
- A **misdemeanor,** compared with a felony, is a minor charge. Misdemeanors involve less than a year in jail. They include crimes such as assault, battery, and petty theft. You may also lose your nursing license if you are convicted of a misdemeanor that involves crimes against persons or that can cause harm to others.

The defendant in a criminal case has the right to an attorney and the right to remain silent, which means he does not have to answer questions during interrogation. If you are arrested, you should ask for an attorney and not answer any questions without your attorney present. The defendant also has a right to a jury trial.

An emerging issue in the nursing profession is whether nurses who accidentally cause harm to clients should be charged with criminal offenses (e.g., a client dies after a nurse accidentally administers the wrong drug). In the past, these cases have been dealt with under civil law and by the board of nursing. Now state prosecutors are beginning to bring felony and misdemeanor charges against these nurses.

Case: Criminal Law

Several clients complained that their pain medication was not working. An investigation revealed that, with one exception, all clients who received pain medication from the assigned nurse had similar complaints. When confronted, the nurse admitted to stealing the clients' pain medication and giving them saline. She also admitted to using other nurses' passwords to steal narcotics. The nurse was terminated and reported to the board of nursing. She refused to enroll in an impaired nurse's program. Her license was revoked after a hearing. She also faced criminal charges for theft of controlled substances.

Case: Criminal Law

Joan, RN, was arrested for stealing computer equipment and wound supplies from the hospital that were valued at $55,000. She was charged with grand larceny, a felony. Two weeks before her trial, she entered into a plea deal that reduced the charge to a misdemeanor with probation for 6 months and reimbursement to the hospital of $55,000.

WHAT IS CIVIL LAW?

In contrast to criminal law, in which the state or federal government brings charges against a person, **civil law** involves a dispute between individuals or entities. A settlement in civil law often results in the guilty party paying monetary damages. Two types of civil law are contract law and tort law.

- **Contract law** involves a written or oral agreement between two parties in which one party accepts an offer made by the other party to perform (or not perform) certain acts in exchange for something of value. A breach of contract occurs if either party does not comply with the terms of the agreement. An employment contract is one example.
- **Tort law,** in comparison, deals with wrongs done to one person by another person that do not involve contracts. A tort is a civil wrong and there are three types of tort: quasi-intentional torts, intentional torts, and unintentional torts.

What Are Quasi-intentional Torts?

Quasi-intentional torts involve actions that injure a person's reputation. The overall concept for these torts is defamation of character. All four of the following essential elements of defamation of character must be present. The communication (written or oral) about the person:

- Was false.
- Was made to another person or persons.
- Caused the defamed person to experience shame and ridicule and had a negative impact on the person's reputation.
- Was made as a statement of fact rather than as an opinion.

Libel is the written or published form of defamation of character. **Slander** is the spoken or verbal form of defamation of character.

A person is not guilty of defamation of character if the statement made about the other person is true or if the person has the protection of a "privilege," such as reporting possible child abuse.

Case: Quasi-intentional Torts

The nursing supervisor calls you into a conference room and states, "I know that you have been stealing (diverting) narcotics from the unit and injecting yourself with it while at work. It shows, because your work is sloppy and you are falsifying your documentation. You are a poor excuse for a nurse." Before you can defend yourself, the supervisor turns and leaves. The statements are not true. Nurses in the conference room try to console you. The supervisor committed slander.

What Are Intentional Torts?

An **intentional tort** is an action taken by one person with the intent to harm another person. The harm does not have to be violent, hostile, or cause a significant amount of pain or distress to the other person. The person must have merely intended to cause harm or known the action would bring about the harm.

Intentional torts may also be prosecuted under criminal law. For example, a nurse who is sued for malpractice in civil court may also be charged with a homicide if a client died because of the nurse's intentional actions. Intentional torts most commonly encountered in nursing are assault, battery, false imprisonment, and invasion of privacy.

Assault

An **assault** occurs when a nurse intentionally places a client in immediate fear of personal violence or offensive contact. An assault must include words expressing an intention to cause harm and some type of action. For example, a nurse has committed an assault if she says to the client, "I will slap you" and raises her hand as if to strike the client. The combination of the words and action causes the client to believe the threat will be carried out.

Battery

A **battery** is committed when (1) an offensive or harmful physical contact is made to the client without his consent, or (2) there is unauthorized touching of a person's body by another person. To avoid charges of battery, always obtain informed consent before providing certain treatments. On admission to healthcare facilities, clients sign a general consent form, which usually covers routine aspects of nursing care, such as vital signs and patient assessments. However, when performing any invasive procedure, such as insertion of central venous catheters, you should always explain the procedure to the client and obtain his consent before beginning.

Case: Battery—Withdrawal of Consent During the Procedure

A client having blood drawn experienced severe pain and requested the technician to stop while he was attempting to fill a second vial of blood. The technician continued and filled the second vial. Ruling in favor of the technician, the court noted that the client did not allege that stopping the treatment was feasible and without harm. No battery is committed if, at the client's request, the procedure cannot be stopped without creating harm (*Pallacovitch v. Waterbury Hosp.*, 2012).

Assault and Battery

An **assault and battery** occurs when there is the intent to cause a person fear combined with an offensive or harmful contact.

Case: Assault and Battery

A client admitted for an elective surgical procedure complained that the automatic blood pressure cuff was causing her extreme pain and demanded it be removed. The nurse did not immediately remove the cuff as requested by the client. The nurse was guilty of a battery, but not assault, because there was no evidence that the nurse intended to create or cause fear or pain (*Coulter v. Thomas*, 2000).

False Imprisonment

False imprisonment is the restraining of a person without proper legal authorization. It includes any type of unjustified restriction on a person's freedom of movement—for example, when nurses restrain clients without their permission. False imprisonment can involve the use of physical restraints (e.g., vest or wrist restraints) or chemical restraints (e.g., sedatives or opioids). You may restrain clients who pose an immediate threat to themselves or others. However, you must immediately obtain the proper authorization to continue the restraint.

Against Medical Advice (AMA) If a competent client wishes to leave the healthcare facility, you should contact the nursing supervisor and the primary care provider. The client must be informed of the risks associated with leaving and given the choice to stay and receive treatment or to sign out against medical advice (AMA). You need to be aware of the hospital policy and procedures on AMA discharges.

Invasion of Privacy

Invasion of privacy violates a person's right to be left alone. The law recognizes that a person's personal life should not be opened up for public scrutiny and the person has the right to freedom from unwanted interference in her private affairs. A person has the right to:

- Have her private information protected.
- Not be falsely portrayed or intentionally misrepresented in character, beliefs, or actions.
- Be free from unwanted intrusion (spying, eavesdropping).

Examples of violating right to privacy include discussing clients in public places (e.g., elevators, cafeterias), photographing clients without their permission, providing information to news media without consent, searching a client's personal belongings without permission, and releasing medical information without the client's consent.

Fraud

Fraud is the false representation of significant facts by words or by conduct. It can occur through making false statements, falsifying documentation, or concealing information that should have been disclosed. It is intentionally misleading or deceiving another person to act (or not act) for the personal gain of the one committing the fraud.

Case: Fraud

A home health nurse was terminated from her salaried position after she refused to falsify Medicare documentation. She was instructed to bill clients for more visits than actually occurred, alter care records to prolong a client's eligibility for home services, and admit a nonhomebound client to homebound therapy (*Admore v. Nurse Connection, Inc.*, 2009). An award of damages and attorney fees in her favor was upheld by the court of appeals (*Nurse Connection, Inc. v. Admore*, 2010).

What Are Unintentional Torts?

The most common type of unintentional tort involving health-care professionals is negligence or malpractice.

- **Negligence** is the failure to use ordinary or reasonable care or the failure to act in a reasonable and prudent (careful) manner.
- **Malpractice** has a similar definition, but applies only to professionals, such as nurses and physicians. It is defined as the failure of a professional person to act in a reasonable and prudent manner. A malpractice lawsuit may occur when such actions cause injury or death to the client. The person bringing the lawsuit is the **plaintiff** and the person who must defend against the lawsuit is the **defendant.**

Malpractice/Negligence Liability

To win and recover damages (money) in a malpractice lawsuit, the plaintiff must prove four elements (duty, breach of duty, causation, and damages). The elements must be proved by a **"preponderance of the evidence,"** meaning with enough evidence to tip the scale in his favor.

Duty The nurse–client relationship creates this legal obligation. A **duty** forms when the client is assigned to the nurse or seeks treatment from the nurse, or when the nurse observes another person doing something that could harm the client.

Breach of Duty A **breach of duty** occurs when the nurse fails to meet standards of care. Attorneys look to the following sources of information to identify the standards of care and to determine what a reasonable and prudent (careful) nurse would have done in the situation: the NPA, job descriptions, hospital policies and procedures, textbooks, professional standards and guidelines developed by professional organizations, and the nursing codes of ethics.

The plaintiff's attorney will usually hire an **expert witness** who is a nurse with advanced education or experience. The purpose of that witness is to educate the judge and jury on the local practice of nursing and how the nurse's actions or omissions failed to meet acceptable practice standards for nurses. The defendant's attorney may hire an expert to testify that the nurse, based on the circumstances, adhered to standards of practice.

Causation The breach of duty or deviation from acceptable standards of care by the nurse must be the direct and proximate cause of the injury suffered by the client. Causation is usually established based on the testimony of experts (e.g., healthcare providers) who can clearly show the connection between the nurse's action or omission and the resulting client injury.

Case: Causation

A nurse forgot to change the client's dressing at the scheduled time, but changed it 3 hours later. The hospital policy reads that nurses must administer medications or perform prescribed treatments within 30 minutes before or 30 minutes after the scheduled time. The client did not experience any harm or infection. In this case, there were both the existence of a duty and a breach of duty, but the breach of duty did not cause any harm or injury to the client. Therefore, if a malpractice action had been brought, the plaintiff did not have any compensable injuries. Nurses are encouraged to promptly report medication and treatment errors so that actions can be taken to prevent and/or minimize injury to the client.

Damages In civil cases, the remedy for the harm the client suffered is money. The judge or jury will award the plaintiff money to compensate him for pain and suffering, lost wages, additional medical bills, and other losses. In some cases, the plaintiff may be awarded punitive damages (not paid by insurance companies) for grossly negligent or wrongful behavior by the healthcare provider.

Case: Damages

The client began to bleed excessively after a nonemergency cesarean section delivery. The nursing staff notified the provider of the bleeding, decreased blood pressure and oxygen level, and increased heart rate. The client had surgery to repair a uterine laceration and returned to the recovery room, where additional blood products and fundal massage were prescribed. The client's blood pressure and oxygen remained low, despite the repair. The provider indicated that nurses had not notified him that the client's pulse rate was high and the blood pressure and blood oxygen content remained low. He admitted that he had not read the monitor. The nurses also did not notify the provider of the client's readings because they assumed he reviewed and interpreted the monitor readings each time he visited the client. Two hours after being admitted to the recovery room, the client arrested, was resuscitated, but suffered severe brain damage. She died 6 months later when mechanical ventilation was removed.

Analysis of the case:

Duty: Based on the nurse–client relationship

Breach of Duty: Failure to communicate to the provider; failure to intervene to counteract the client's deteriorating condition

Causation: Appropriate medical care was not provided based on the client's signs and symptoms.

Damages: A settlement was reached with a present value of about $1.35 million.

(Nurses Service Organization, 2013a).

KnowledgeCheck 44-3

- Distinguish negligence from malpractice.
- Distinguish civil law from criminal law.
- Under which type of law (constitutional, statutory, administrative, or common law) does each of the following fall?
  A defendant claiming the right not to incriminate himself under the Fifth Amendment
  A nurse having her license revoked by the state board of nursing
  The wording of a state nurse practice act
- Define *plaintiff* and *defendant* in the context of civil law.

ThinkLike a Nurse 44-5

- Give one nursing example of each: negligence, malpractice, damages.
- Can you think of one nonfraudulent example of a nurse being untruthful with a client? Do you think that the circumstances described in your example make the untruthfulness justifiable?
- Can you think of an example of a nurse committing assault, other than the one given in the text?

Toward Evidence-Based Practice

Patient's fall: Court sees evidence of faulty nursing assessment of patient's injuries. (2015). *Legal Eagle Eye Newsletter for the Nursing Profession, 23*(7). Retrieved from http://www.nursinglaw.com/fall-injury-assessment.pdf

A 69-year-old client was admitted to a rehabilitation unit after back surgery. She was assessed as a high fall risk and required a two-person transfer. She was also on anticoagulant (blood-thinning) therapy. On the day she fell, the client was found on the floor after she attempted to get back into bed without assistance. X-rays did not reveal any fractures. The next day the nurses assessed purple bruising on the client's right buttocks. The second day after the fall, the client was found pale and with labored breathing. She died the next day at an acute care hospital as a result of retroperitoneal hemorrhage. The expert witness testimony focused on the client care after the fall, although the fall precautions were inadequate (*Nexion v. Townsend,* 2015).

1. What components of the nursing process were not followed in this case?

Patient's fall: Safe patient transfers require nursing assessment and care planning. (2013). *Legal Eagle Eye Newsletter for the Nursing Profession, 21*(8). Retrieved from http://www.nursinglaw.com/patient-fall-nursing-assessment.pdf

An 85-year-old client with left-side paralysis and a history of falls was being assisted out of bed by a CNA. The client suffered a fractured leg when she either fell or was assisted to the floor. The nursing facility argued that the physical therapy department determined the guidelines for client transfers. The client was not prescribed a mechanical lift, a gait belt, or a two-person transfer. A nursing expert witness

testified that the nurses should have assessed the client as needing a mechanical lift. Rejecting the facility's argument, the court ruled that the legal standard of care for a nurse is not determined by physical therapists. The facility cannot control the standard of care applicable to its caregiving employees (*Hill v. Fairfield Nursing & Rehabilitation,* 2013).

2. What should the nurse have done in this case to address conflicts between facility policies and standards governing nursing practice?

Nurses Service Organization. (2013c). Woman falls while home health nurse is weighing her—fractured leg, surgery, rehab and need for continuing care—$791,573 verdict. Retrieved from http://www.nso.com/case-studies/casestudy-article/315.jsp

A 74-year-old patient was receiving home healthcare services after a total knee replacement. The nurse instructed the patient to stand on a scale in the bathroom to obtain her weight. The patient fell and broke the fibula and tibia in one leg. Her injuries required additional surgery, hospitalizations, and continuing 24-hour home care. She sued the nurse, alleging a breach of duty by not providing her with proper support given her unstable balance and weighing her in a confined space. The jury rejected the nurse's defense that proper support was given and weighing her in the bathroom was reasonable.

3. In this case, what was the basis for the jury's decision that the client's injury was the result of the nurse's negligence?

 Go to Davis Advantage, Resources, Chapter 44, **Toward Evidence-Based Practice—Suggested Responses.**

Vicarious Liability

You are legally accountable for your actions or inactions. This is a common legal principle that should guide your behavior. It means that you can be sued for behavior or omissions that deviate from acceptable standards. In certain circumstances, the law will assign liability to a person or entity that did not directly cause the injury, but with whom you have a specific kind of relationship. This type of liability is known as **vicarious** or **substituted liability.** The types of vicarious liability existing under common law are discussed in the following:

Captain of the Ship This principle applies to situations in which a physician (e.g., surgeon or obstetrician) is held liable for the negligence of another healthcare provider. *Captain of the ship* usually applies to surgical suite situations. Many states no longer recognize it as protection for the nurse because the nurse is still liable for her own actions.

Borrowed Servant Doctrine This doctrine relieves the primary employer of liability for the actions or omission of its employee when the employee was borrowed by another person. In theory, the borrower becomes liable for the actions

of the employee. This would apply, for example, to agency nurses.

Respondeat Superior This Latin term means "let the master answer." The employer must answer for the negligent acts or omissions of its employees who are functioning within the scope of their employment. For example, the hospital can be sued for a medication error made by a labor and delivery nurse working within the scope of her practice.

KnowledgeCheck 44-4

- Define these terms: *assault, battery, fraud, slander, libel, negligence, malpractice.*
- State the four elements of malpractice.

LITIGATION IN CIVIL CLAIMS

Litigation is the formal process wherein the legal issues, rights, and duties between the parties are heard and decided (adjudicated). The litigation process follows the stages explained in what follows.

Pleading and Pretrial Motions

The litigation process starts when the plaintiff files a complaint. A **complaint** is a legal document outlining how another person has harmed the plaintiff. Once the case is filed with the court, the complaint is served on (delivered to) the defendant. The complaint identifies the plaintiff, the specific allegations and time frame, the standards allegedly breached (e.g., behaviors or omissions), the persons (defendants) involved, and the harm suffered.

If you are served with a complaint, you must immediately notify your employer. In addition, if you have malpractice insurance, you must also notify your insurance company. You will need an attorney to defend you. Your attorney has a specified time frame within which to file an *answer* (response) to the complaint. The answer addresses each of the allegations (unproven accusations). As a defendant, you should not contact the plaintiff or the plaintiff's attorney or discuss the case with coworkers or friends. The facility's risk manager and your attorney will advise you. You should fully cooperate and be honest in all your answers.

Discovery Phase

The discovery process allows for both parties to gather facts and evidence about the case that can be used at trial. Discovery is designed to make sure there are no "surprises" during the trial. Attorneys may obtain discovery through written questions **(interrogatories),** requests for documents and other evidence, and **depositions** (attorneys orally question parties to the lawsuit under oath, as though they were testifying in court). You may be *deposed* (questioned) as either a fact witness, a party to the lawsuit (defendant), or an expert witness. A *fact witness* is someone who was present when the incident occurred, whereas the *defendant* will testify about the care provided and the actions taken.

Depositions may occur several years after the incident, so you may not remember specific information. You should prepare for the deposition by reviewing the medical records and any other evidence that may exist regarding the lawsuit. During the deposition, listen to your attorney, do not volunteer information, take your time before answering each question, and provide only objective information. Always tell the truth, but base your answers on facts; do not speculate. If your attorney objects to any question, immediately stop and do not provide an answer unless directed to do so by your attorney.

Alternative Dispute Resolution

Lawyers and involved parties usually try to resolve disputes before going to trial. The three most common methods of alternative dispute resolution are as follows:

- **Negotiation** takes place informally between the lawyers for the plaintiff and the defendant in an attempt to settle the case prior to trial.
- **Mediation** is the attempt to resolve the dispute using a neutral third party. The primary role of the mediator is to help the parties focus on the issues and to facilitate communication to identify what is needed to reach a resolution.
- **Arbitration** involves a third party making a decision after formally hearing the evidence and information from both parties.

Trial Process

If the dispute cannot be resolved and is not dismissed by the court during pretrial motions, the case goes to trial. A jury usually hears malpractice cases. After hearing the evidence presented by plaintiff and defendant and reviewing submitted documents, the judge or jury makes a decision, which is either dismissal or the award of damages.

Appeal

After the judge or jury has made a decision, either party has the opportunity to present post-trial motions, move for a new trial, or appeal the verdict and/or damages to a court of appeals. The court of appeals will review the transcript and documents from the trial and determine whether errors (e.g., improper evidence allowed) were made during that trial that resulted in an unfair verdict. The verdict can be upheld or dismissed, in part or in whole, and the case sent back to the trial court with special instructions.

KnowledgeCheck 44-5

- Identify the phases of the trial process.
- How is arbitration different from mediation?

PracticalKnowledge knowing **how**

To decrease your chances of being involved in a malpractice suit, you should know the most common causes of malpractice claims and some practical preventive actions you can take. Keep in mind that causes are often difficult to categorize because they overlap; an error usually results from interlocking causes.

WHAT ARE THE MOST COMMON MALPRACTICE CLAIMS?

Nurses must use the nursing process to provide safe and efficient care to patients. The most common causes of nursing malpractice claims (Box 44-3) can be categorized according to where they fall in the nursing process: failure to assess and diagnose, failure to plan, failure to implement, and failure to evaluate (O'Keefe, 2001; Reising, 2012).

Failure to Assess and Diagnose

As the first step in the nursing process, the failure to conduct an adequate assessment and failure to analyze the data and make correct nursing diagnoses can lead to incorrect actions, no action, or improper delegation.

Case: Failure to Assess and Diagnose

A 67-year-old client had an epidural catheter inserted for pain management following a total knee replacement. After successful treatment of an episode of hypotension in the postanesthesia care unit, he was transferred to the medical–surgical unit. The registered nurses assessed the client and delegated direct care to an LPN, although this was denied by the LPN. Three hours later, the client experienced nausea and vomiting. The client was found cyanotic and unresponsive 10 minutes later and subsequently died of anoxic encephalopathy. Many facts were disputed among the numerous codefendants and documentation was poor (Nurses Service Organization, 2012).

Excessive Self-Disclosure—Discussing personal problems or intimate details with the client
Flirtation—Communication that is sexual in nature or reveals personal attraction between client and nurse
Secretive Behavior—When the nurse is defensive or guarded about the interaction between client and nurse
"Super Nurse" Attitude—The nurse who acts as though she is the only one who understands and can meet the client's needs
Excessive Attention to Client—When the nurse spends much more time with a particular client than is required by his needs. Personal gifts, off-duty visits, or trading assignments are signs of boundary violation.
Unclear Communication—When only part of the story is told about client care. The client might repeatedly seek out the nurse, even when not assigned to his care.

Source: Used with permission from the National Council of State Boards of Nursing. (2014a). *A nurse's guide to professional boundaries.* Retrieved from https://www.ncsbn.org/ProfessionalBoundaries_Complete.pdf

Safe and competent assessment and diagnosis practices require the nurse to:
- Perform an admission assessment. This duty cannot be delegated to a nursing assistant.
- Analyze the assessment data to clearly identify problems.
- Apply theoretical knowledge to ensure a correct diagnosis. The presenting signs and symptoms should be consistent with the disease process or medical problem. Remember that the nursing diagnosis consists of Patient Response r/t Etiology.
- Report the symptoms to the appropriate provider and carry out the standard nursing care and prescribed interventions when assessment reveals adverse symptoms.
- Conduct frequent, focused assessments until the end of the shift or until the problem is resolved.

Failure to Plan

ANA standards specifically require nurses to formulate a plan of care. The plan of care may be written or unwritten, depending on state regulations. Safe and competent practices in this category require the nurse to:
- Know the correct approach to treat client actual or potential problems.
- Have the theoretical knowledge base to successfully plan nursing care for clients.
- Develop a plan of care that is individualized to the client.
- Develop a plan that is consistent with standards of treatments acceptable for the given diagnosis or problem.

Failure to Implement a Plan of Care

Implementation is the nursing process step in which the nurse performs the care or nursing interventions. Failure to implement encompasses a variety of actions, such as:
- **Failure to respond,** for example, to a client's specific symptoms or request for care.
- **Failure to educate** by not answering questions, not teaching self-care measures, or not explaining procedures or equipment adequately on discharge

- **Failure to follow standards of care and institutional policies and procedures:** Most often this failure occurs as medication errors and failure to follow a provider's prescriptions; failure to use equipment responsibly; and may be the result of understaffing and inexperience
- **Failure to notify a provider in a timely manner** when a client's condition warrants action.
- **Failure to act as an advocate,** to intervene to prevent harm to a client by other healthcare provides or significant others, or failure to report impaired nursing practice.

Failure to Evaluate

Evaluation is the last step in the nursing process. It requires you to make a judgment about how well your interventions have succeeded in addressing the client's problems. The duty to evaluate requires an ongoing cycle of the following:
- *Observing for changes after interventions and treatments.* You must know the expected outcomes and side effects of

---

Safe, Effective Nursing Care

The Use of the Nursing Process to Provide Legally Safe Nursing Care

Key Concepts: Malpractice, Negligence, Liability

SENC Competency: Provide safe quality client care (Thinking, Doing, Caring)

Background: At one time, nurses were not held liable for client injuries because they were perceived as "only following the physician's orders." Nurses were not viewed as educated, knowledgeable professionals. Many doctrines (e.g., captain of the ship, borrowed servant) provided nurses a shield of protection from being held accountable for their negligent actions. This view began to erode when the court ruled that nurses owe an "independent duty" of care to the client (*NKC Hosps, Inc. v. Anthony,* 1993).

The concept of providing legally safe, quality actions began to emerge in the education of nursing students and as expectations for practicing nurses. **KEY POINT:** *The nursing process is viewed as a critical-thinking tool that if correctly used will minimize errors in client care. It seamlessly aligns with the "Thinking, Caring, Doing" model that is designed to provide a holistic approach to client care.*

Think About It: Reflect on the stages of the nursing process and how they are related to safe, effective care.
- Assessment is the first stage of the nursing process. *Why is assessment essential to ensuring the client receives the appropriate care?*
- Analysis/Diagnosis is the second stage of the nursing process; planning involves formulating outcomes identifying interventions to achieve them. *How do the analysis/diagnosis and planning stages align with the "thinking" concept?*
- Implementation is the process of taking the actions identified in planning. It includes documenting the actions and the client's responses. *What aspects of the "Thinking, Caring, Doing" model are incorporated in this stage of the nursing process?*
- Evaluation is the determination of whether the client goals have been achieved. *How is this stage used to evaluate the potential liability of client care?*

medications and treatments, so you can accurately interpret and document anticipated and adverse responses.

- *Recognizing significance of the change.* For example, if Mr. Adkins's blood pressure (BP) is usually 140/88, a change to 150/90 after exercise would not be significant for him. But for Mrs. Jonas, whose BP is usually 100/64, a change to 150/90 would be cause for concern.
- *Documenting or reporting symptoms to the appropriate person.* If a change is significant, you have a legal duty to report the change to the appropriate provider and to document this change in the appropriate medical record.
- *Following up on client responses to nursing interventions.* This requires you to know the expected outcomes and side effects of medications and treatments.

KnowledgeCheck 44-6

- State the four requirements of the nurse's duty to assess.
- State four ways in which the nurse may fail to implement a plan of care.
- Give one example of the duty to advocate for a client.
- List the four components of the nurse's legal duty to evaluate.

HOW CAN YOU MINIMIZE YOUR MALPRACTICE RISKS?

The best way to minimize your risk of malpractice is to practice in a safe and competent manner. You must have the appropriate body of theoretical knowledge, as well as familiarity with your state's NPA and your agency's policies and procedures. **KEY POINT:** *Ignorance of the law and of practice standards is no excuse for failing to comply with the law, and it is no defense in a malpractice suit.* You will find discussion of other helpful suggestions in the remainder of this chapter and in Clinical Insight 44-1.

Use the Nursing Process and Follow Professional Standards of Care

The nursing process provides you with a systematic approach to client care and is the legally acceptable model of decision making in nursing practice. Your documentation should reveal that you have assessed, diagnosed, planned, implemented, and evaluated care based on current and acceptable standards.

Avoid Medication and Treatment Errors

Medication errors are among the most common healthcare errors. To administer medications accurately, you must know the rationale for administering the drug, safe dosage ranges, side effects of the medications, and relevant information to teach the client about the medication. To prevent medication errors, you should:

- Follow the "rights of medication administration" (see Chapter 26).
- Investigate any client concerns before giving the medication (e.g., the client might say, "Is this a new medication? I have not taken this one before").
- Question prescriptions that are incomplete or that seem inappropriate.
- Make sure equipment used to administer drugs is working properly.
- Use the correct technique to provide client treatment (e.g., maintain a sterile field during wound care to prevent an infection).

For tips to help you use equipment properly and safely, refer to Clinical Insight 44-2.

♥ iCare 44-1

Honoring Safety and Confidentiality

Jon is a newly graduated RN. He is taking care of Mr. Belvidere, who has been admitted with a stroke. It is an extremely busy day on the unit and Jon is behind on his morning medication pass. One of the senior nurses casually says to Jon, "If you're behind, why don't you prepare the medications and just ask the CNA, Mark, to administer them? He is really thorough, I trust him to give medications, and he has been doing this for a long time." Jon feels uncomfortable with this practice because he knows that as a licensed professional it is his responsibility to administer the medications.

Jon asks to speak to the senior nurse privately and tells her that what she is doing violates safe medication and legal practices and places the patient in danger. The nurse is initially upset that Jon called her out on this behavior, but then thanks him for coming to her first to address it privately. In the spirit of transparency, she discusses the past actions with her manager. As a result, the charge nurse and the nurse manager provide an in-service presentation as a refresher about legal responsibilities related to medication administration.

As a caring nurse, Jon was aware of his responsibility for Mr. Belvidere's safety and cared enough to take action to effect change. He was also considerate of the senior nurse when he spoke to her privately about the matter.

Report and Document

For every suggestion for minimizing malpractice risk, add the reminder "Document what happened." Remember the adage "If it isn't documented, it wasn't done." If you are ever required to appear in court, the client record may be the only proof you have of the care you gave. It is unlawful to make false entries or destroy entries in medical records, but do carefully record in detail all care you provide.

Cases: Documentation Can Make a Difference

The plaintiff alleged that the nurse had violated numerous standards of practice including the failure to properly assess the client, failure to properly monitor vital signs and in-take and output, and failure to recognize and respond to signs and symptoms of sepsis. A settlement was reached for $706,250. Weaknesses in documentation revealed that the client's blood pressure was not documented until day 14 of home care, and evidence of infection—wound appearance and size, amount and appearance of drainage—was not consistently documented by the nurses caring for the client (Nurses Service Organization, n.d.).

In contrast, a verdict was rendered in favor of a nurse accused of failure to properly assess and monitor an impaired, restrained client and to provide proper care in a safe environment. The client suffered severe burns over 25% of his body when the bed linen ignited as he attempted to burn off the restraints with a lighter. Strengths in documentation showed that the nurse monitored and assessed the client every 15 minutes as prescribed, missing one time to care for a critical client. The assessment findings at each check were fully documented in the client's medical records (Nurses Service Organization, 2013b).

Charting

KEY POINT: *A basic principle of charting is that a third person should be able to read your documentation and form a mental picture of your client and the care provided during your shift.* Record all interactions with clients, as well as any refusal of or noncompliance with treatment. Document telephone conversations with primary care providers, including time, content of the conversation, and the action you took. Document the facts; do not editorialize (e.g., do not write, "I could not check on the patient as often as prescribed because we were understaffed"). Refer to Chapter 18 for a review of your documentation responsibilities and use the mnemonic F-A-C-T–U-A-L as a reminder when charting.

F—Your information must be **factual** and objective. Don't document your opinions.

A—You must be **accurate:** For example, record the vital signs accurately.

C—Your information must be **complete:** Don't omit any important information.

T—You must be **timely:** Document care as soon as possible after doing it; don't wait until the end of your shift and then try to remember everything that happened.

U—You must always document **unusual occurrences.**

A—You must document your **assessment data** and the plan of care.

L—Remember that the client's chart is a **legal record** and is subpoenaed in a malpractice case.

Incident Reports

If a standard of care is breached or an unusual incident occurs (e.g., a visitor or client falls or is injured), you should complete an **incident report** (also called *variance report* or *occurrence report*). These reports are used, in part, for quality improvement in the agency and should not be used to discipline staff members or be placed in employees' files. The goal is to prevent the incident from occurring again.

In many states, an incident report is not made available as a part of discovery in litigation. It becomes discoverable (available to the plaintiff) if it is mentioned in the medical records. **KEY POINT:** *You can prevent an otherwise confidential report from becoming evidence by not writing "Incident report completed" in the patient record.*

When reporting an incident, be sure to clearly identify the client, date, time, and location. Briefly describe the incident in factual terms. Use the exact words of the client or persons involved and put the information in quotes. Do not speculate, draw conclusions, or place blame. Identify any witnesses to the event or equipment involved. For example:

1900	Demerol 50 mg given intramuscularly. Provider prescribed: Demerol 15 mg.
1930	Client's respirations: 8 breaths/min; BP 100/60; skin pale
2000	Called Dr. Smith. Prescription for naloxone (Narcan) 1 mg IV STAT
2005	Narcan given as prescribed. Resp 12 breaths/min, BP 118/70

In this example, you should be prepared to discuss the 30-minute delay between the client's findings and contacting the provider. The standard of care would require that the provider be notified immediately. Chapter 18 presents additional information on occurrence (incident) reports.

Obtain Informed Consent

Informed consent is the client's permission to receive any and all types of care with full knowledge of the risks, benefits, costs, and alternatives. For hospital admission and for invasive or specialized treatments or diagnostic procedures, the consent must be written and signed by the client or his legal guardian. The law provides for implied or assumed consent in emergency situations; therefore, written consent is not necessary in an emergency if experts would agree that there was an immediate threat to the client's life or health.

Elements of Consent

To be legally valid, the informed consent should fulfill the following requirements:

- **Completeness.** Healthcare consumers need adequate information to make educated decisions regarding their treatment. Be sure they get information on the nature of the procedure, risks, benefits, post-procedure care and considerations, and treatment alternatives.

- **Clarity and Comprehension.** Language should be at the appropriate educational level so the client (or his surrogate decision maker) can understand the explanation. Always ask the client to describe in his own words the procedure to which he is consenting. If the client asks, "What will the doctor do during surgery?" you would be aware that the client does not understand the nature of the surgery. You should contact the surgeon.

- **Voluntariness.** The client must be free to accept or reject the treatment. He must not be pressured or coerced to give consent. There must be no actual or implied threat by anyone to force the client into having the surgery (e.g., "Mom, if you don't let them do this, I'm never coming back to see you"). Otherwise, the consent is not valid.

- **Competence.** The person must have the ability to understand the information and make a choice about the particular situation (e.g., the ability to decide what clothing to wear does not necessarily mean that the person is competent to decide whether to have surgery). If the person is confused and disoriented, you should contact the case manager or your supervisor for guidance. State law identifies the order of individuals who can make decisions for individuals who are judged incompetent. It is usually the spouse, then parents, then sisters and brothers, and so on. If the person does not have relatives, the court will appoint a legal guardian to make healthcare decisions.

Generally speaking, a competent adult has the legal right to consent to or refuse any treatment. However, this right does not always extend to situations in which an adult is making the decision for a minor. A court sometimes will authorize treatment of a child against his parents' wishes. In some states, a minor who is married or living independently is considered emancipated and can make his/her own healthcare decisions.

The Nurse's Role

As a nurse, your legal role regarding written consent is to collaborate with the primary provider, usually a physician or advanced practice nurse. **KEY POINT:** *You may witness a client's signature on a consent form, but you are not legally responsible for explaining the treatments and options, or for evaluating whether the provider has adequately explained them. You must, however, determine that the elements of a valid informed* *consent are in place, communicate the client's needs for more information to the care provider, and provide feedback if the client wishes to change her consent.*

Be sure you have the client's informal, verbal consent for nursing interventions that you perform (e.g., urinary catheterization). Coming to the agency for healthcare implies that the client consents to usual treatment, such as injections and vital signs. However, you should explain all procedures to the client before their implementation. If the client objects, identify the reasons for the refusal, correct any misinformation, and explain the benefits of the treatment. If the patient still objects or refuses, do not proceed; contact the primary care provider.

In addition to state statutes, case law, and agency policy, The Joint Commission standards provide valuable guidance regarding informed participation in decision making. See Chapter 43 for discussion of informed consent from an ethical perspective.

Case: Breakdown in Informed Consent

A pulmonologist expected an interventional radiologist to obtain informed consent for placement of a chest tube to drain fluid from around the heart of a client with congestive heart failure. Because of the client's confused state, the nurses contacted the client's daughter to obtain consent, explaining that the procedure was "no big deal." The daughter agreed and the nurses completed the telephonic consent form and placed it in the chart. No healthcare provider explained the benefits, risks, or alternatives. During the procedure, the client suffered one of the risks of the procedure (punctured aorta), necessitating emergency surgery. The client's condition deteriorated after the surgery and she died 18 months later. The court ruled that the failure to obtain informed consent was a basis for a lawsuit (*Gonsalves v. Sharp,* 2013).

Maintain Patient Safety

Falls are by far the most common incident reported in hospitals and long-term care facilities. On admission to the facility, all clients should be assessed for risks of falls and "fall precautions" should be instituted when needed. Simply raising the siderails on the bed is not enough to prevent falls. You may still be found negligent if the client falls because he called for help and no one came to assist him out of bed, or if the call device was not placed within the client's reach and he was unable to call for assistance. Several useful tools have been developed for assessing falls. See Chapter 23 for information about meeting clients' safety needs, including falls and use of restraints. For falls risk tools, see Figures 23-1 and 23-2 and the section "Assessing for Example Problem: Falls" in Chapter 23.

Maintain Confidentiality and Privacy

Always maintain client confidentiality unless directed by law to do otherwise (e.g., when a client is threatening to harm someone). Family members and significant others do not have an automatic right to information about the client. For example, parents do not have an automatic right to see the medical records of their adult child or minor child who is married or emancipated. Of course, you need to discuss clients' medical conditions with other health team members, but you should not chat about the client's personal life or talk about the client in the breakroom. **KEY POINT:** *You should discuss the patient's health status with those who have a need to know (those involved in the patient's care).*

Confidentiality of Client Records is another aspect of privacy (e.g., do not leave a client's health record in locations that are accessible to visitors or nonauthorized staff). Do not give information about clients over the phone unless the agency has a system that enables you to know that you are speaking to a person authorized by the client. If you require advice about maintaining confidentiality of electronic records, see Bonus Chapter 45 and the section "Electronic Health Record Systems" in Chapter 18.

Provide Education and Counseling

Part of your role as a nurse is to provide information to clients and caregivers about their illness, medications, and other treatments. This helps to fulfill informed consent requirements and involve clients in their own healthcare. Make sure the client understands, retains the knowledge, and can demonstrate any skills. Ask the patient to repeat instructions to you or to provide a return demonstration of a skill, such as self-injection of insulin. To reinforce understanding, always review written information with the client. Refer to Chapter 26 for more information on teaching patients.

Delegate According to Guidelines

As a nurse, you are expected to properly delegate to ensure clients receive timely and quality care. This involves implementing the five rights of delegation: delegating the *right task* to the *right person,* under the *right circumstances,* using the *right directions and communication,* and practicing the *right supervision and evaluation.* To do this safely, you (the delegator) must know the education background, knowledge, experience, and physical and emotional capability of those to whom you delegate *(delegatee).* You must also know the scope of practice of the delegatee as determined by the state board of nursing. In addition, you must consider the condition and requirements of the client. The registered nurse should not delegate to LPNs or nursing assistive personnel (NAPs) clients who:

- Require complex care.
- Are unpredictable.
- Require nursing judgment.
- Involve a high level of interaction.

When delegating, be sure the delegatee understands the assignment. The Case box Failure to Assess and Diagnose identifies numerous breakdowns in the delegation process. The duty to delegate has a corresponding duty to supervise the care and evaluate the outcome. For example, if you assign an LPN to provide direct care for a new postoperative client, you should obtain hourly updates on the client's status. If you need to review specific guidelines for delegating, see Chapter 7.

Accept Assignments for Which You Are Qualified

As a nurse, when you accept an assignment, you must consider whether the assignment is within your level of education, experience, and physical and emotional capability. The refusal to accept an assignment does not mean that you have abandoned the client. Your duty to the patient begins once you accept the assignment. **KEY POINT:** *You are legally responsible for the assignment that you accept. If your assignment becomes overwhelming and unmanageable, immediately contact the charge nurse or nursing supervisor for assistance.*

Nursing supervisors have a duty to ensure adequate staffing and patient coverage. This means that you must report to the nurse in charge when leaving the client care unit. Failure to do this may result in charges of patient abandonment. A nurse should never leave the client care unit without making certain there is another nurse available to provide care to the client. This does not mean that you must work overtime (e.g., a double shift), as long as you follow established policies and procedures, which will include giving notice and explaining your reasoning (e.g., that you are too fatigued to provide safe care).

If you work a double shift or if a unit is understaffed, you are still liable for any malpractice that you commit. Unfortunately, being "busy" and overwhelmed is not a defense for error. In addition, you have the duty to tell supervisors that staffing is inadequate; be sure to do it in writing. You should know and follow agency policy on how to address short-staff issues.

Participate in Continuing Education

As a nurse, you have a duty to participate in ongoing education in your area of practice and to keep up with new laws, equipment, treatments, and procedures. Be sure to obtain documentation of your attendance. In some states, continuing education is mandatory for license renewal. In states where it is not mandatory, other standards of care still require that you obtain the education and training necessary to implement current nursing procedures and practices. In malpractice cases, the nurse's competency in providing nursing care is frequently an issue.

Observe Professional Boundaries

Nurses must be careful to maintain professional boundaries, not only with the client but also with other healthcare providers. Do not accept gifts from clients or encourage attempts to have close personal relationships outside the healthcare setting. Violations of professional boundaries may be physical, sexual, emotional, or financial in nature. Cues to possible overstepped boundaries are listed in Box 44-3.

If you would like more specific information on professional boundaries,

Go to the **National Council on State Boards of Nursing Web site,** at **https://www.ncsbn.org/ProfessionalBoundaries_Complete.pdf**

Sexual Harassment Be aware of and report the behaviors of staff members who commit sexual harassment. **Sexual harassment** involves the use of power over people lower in the power structure of the organization. It is defined as "unwelcome sexual advances, requests for sexual favors, and other verbal or physical conduct of a sexual nature" if submission fits one of the following criteria:
1. Is a condition of employment
2. Interferes with job performance
3. Is the basis for employment decisions
4. Creates a hostile and intimidating work environment (Equal Employment Opportunity Commission, n.d.).

If you witness or experience sexual harassment, your first step is to consult the agency's sexual harassment policy. Every agency receiving federal funding must have such a policy in place. It will tell you how to file a grievance, what forms you need to use, to whom the incident is reported, and what the procedure is for hearing and resolution.

Observe Mandatory Reporting Regulations

As noted earlier in the chapter, most states have laws requiring the nurse to report communicable diseases, known or suspected abuse of patients, and impaired or unsafe professional practice. When you observe violations of the state's licensing regulations, you have a professional and legal responsibility to report them to the appropriate authority. The "authority" varies among states; it may be your immediate supervisor, the board of nursing, or a peer assistance program. See the section "Mandatory Reporting Laws," earlier in the chapter, and the following discussion of reportable situations.

Impaired Nurses

Nurses who come to work under the influence of alcohol or mind-altering substances pose a danger to the health, safety, and welfare of the clients. You have a legal obligation to protect clients from impaired nurses. Always pay attention to the possibility of a coworker using or stealing narcotics. Impaired nurses account for a major percentage of disciplinary actions against nurses. The board of nursing in many states has programs that provide monitoring and support to nurses with substance addictions who seek help as an alternative to disciplinary actions against their license. See Box 44-4 for signs of chemical dependence in the workplace. To determine the magnitude of the problem in your state, go to the state board of nursing's Web site and click on or search for *disciplinary actions*.

Unauthorized Practice

Your employer will require you to submit verification of current licensure in the state where you are working. If your license expires and you continue to practice nursing, you can be charged with unauthorized practice of nursing. You must report any unauthorized practice of nursing, which means reporting persons practicing nursing without a proper license. In addition, you must know the scope of practice for yourself, LPNs/LVNs and nursing assistive personnel to ensure practice within their professional boundaries. For example, unlicensed personnel cannot perform the initial patient assessment on a newly admitted patient.

Abuse and Communicable Diseases

State laws require you to report known or suspected child, elder, and spousal abuse, and communicable disease. Because state laws may vary, you need to be familiar with them to know what and to whom to report in your area. If you are working for a healthcare agency when you suspect abuse, always report it to your supervisor. If you need to review signs of abuse, see Procedure 9-1: Assessing for Abuse.

Other Safeguards for Nurses

In addition to the Good Samaritan laws and the ANA Nurses' Bill of Rights (previously discussed), safe harbor laws and professional liability insurance offer some legal protection for nurses.

Safe Harbor Laws

Safe harbor laws, found in the nurse practice act or other state laws, provide for exceptions to certain laws. They protect you from being suspended, terminated, disciplined, or discriminated against for refusing to do (or not do) something you believe would be harmful to a client. Under these laws, you also have a right to ask for peer review of either the situation or directives that you believe would violate the nurse practice act. You must follow the guidelines required under the safe harbor provisions.

BOX 44-4 ■ Signs of Potential Chemical Dependence in the Workplace

Absenteeism

- Frequent unscheduled absences with improbable excuses
- Frequent late arrivals or early departures
- Absences after payday or days off
- Higher than average absences for cold, flu, and minor illnesses

Absent "On the Job"

- Long shift breaks
- Brief, unexplained absences from the nursing unit
- "Locked door syndrome" (excessively long use of the restroom)
- Frequent visits to Occupational Health Services for illness on the job

Difficulty Concentrating

- Errors, particularly involving medication or with taking and transcribing verbal prescriptions
- Omitted, illogical, incomplete, or illegible documentation
- Taking more time to carry out assignments than is expected given the nurse's skill and experience
- Deterioration of handwriting during the shift
- Overlooking the signs of client's deteriorating condition

Inconsistent Work Patterns

- Alternating periods of high and low efficiency
- Minimal or substandard work compared with that of peers
- Frequent requests for help with client assignments
- Altered judgment in client care decisions

Physical or Emotional Problems

- Nervousness, excessive sweating, tremors of the hands
- Physical or emotional condition changes during shift
- Deteriorating personal appearance, grooming, and hygiene
- Weight gain or loss

Decreasing Efficiency

- Omitting treatments, making bad decisions; showing poor judgment related to client care
- Requests to be changed to a less supervised shift (e.g., night or weekend shifts)

Poor Relationships on the Job

- Mood swings, from isolation to angry outbursts
- Uncooperativeness
- Avoidance of contact with supervisors
- Client complaints of irritability, roughness, or verbal abuse
- Lethargy or hyperactivity
- Emotional hypersensitivity
- Isolation from others

Medication-Centered Problems

- Excessive use of prn psychoactive medications or narcotics recorded for clients
- Increased waste or breakage of controlled substances
- Missing drugs, unaccounted-for doses
- Omission of dates or times from narcotic sign-out sheets
- Client complaints about lack of pain relief

Personal Life Interferes With Job

- Frequent or excessively long phone calls
- Visitors or unexplained errands during work shift
- Legal problems
- Increased number of accidents

Source: Georgia Nurses Association. (n.d.). What is chemical dependent. Retrieved from http://www.georgianurses.org/?page=ChemicalDependent; Thomas, C., & Siela, D. (2011). The impaired nurse: Would you know what to do if you suspected substance abuse? *American Nurse Today, 6*(8). Retrieved from https://www.americannursetoday.com/the-impaired-nurse-would-you-know-what-to-do-if-you-suspected-substance-abuse/

Case: Prepping a Patient for a Surgical Procedure

The nurse cannot find documentation in the client's medical record for informed consent. Knowing her legal role in informed consent, she refuses to assist with treatment when the client has not given informed consent. Safe harbor laws protect her from dismissal for denying the surgeon's request for her to obtain informed consent.

Professional Liability Insurance

If you are sued for malpractice, the insurance company pays for the attorney's fees and for any judgment or settlement, up to the policy limits. You should carefully review your insurance policy because most insurance policies have **exclusions** (items not covered by the policy). If the client's claim arises out of excluded activities, the insurance company will not pay for the costs of litigation and damages. The following are examples of exclusions:

- Sexual abuse of a client, assault and battery, and other intentional torts
- Injury caused while the nurse is under the influence of drugs or alcohol
- Criminal activity

- Behaviors/actions that can lead to an award of punitive damages (damages awarded to punish the defendant for egregious acts or omissions)

Types of Coverage   There are two types of malpractice coverage:

- **Occurrence-type insurance** is most often recommended for nurses, because this policy covers malpractice claims for any injury or damage that occurred during the time the policy was in force, regardless of when the claim was reported and the lawsuit occurred.
- **Claims-made insurance,** in contrast, covers only those claims in which the negligent action or omission occurred and the claim was filed or reported during the policy period. To maintain coverage under a claims-made policy after it has lapsed or been canceled, some insurers will offer "tail" insurance. You should consult an attorney to decide which type of policy is best for you.

As a rule, if you work for a hospital or other institution, you will be covered by the institution's insurance. However, it covers you only while you are working within the scope of your employment. For example, you would not be covered during the one day a week that you volunteer at a free clinic. Some legal experts recommend that you purchase individual liability insurance in addition to the coverage provided by your employer. Again, consult an attorney before making a decision.

ThinkLike a Nurse 44-6

Susan, RN, was employed by Landold Nursing Service and assigned to Alvalup Hospital from June 1, 2014, to May 30, 2015. Susan carried her own professional liability claims-made policy during this time. She decided to attend real estate school and not renew her policy. On August 10, 2016, a medical malpractice claim was filed against Susan.

■ Based on this scenario, would Susan have coverage under her policy?

■ What kind of policy should she have obtained to have coverage for the claim made against her?

Student Responsibilities   As a student, you are held to the same standards of care as are licensed nurses. You must be familiar not only with your state's standards of practice but also with the policies and procedures in the agency in which you have your clinical experiences. Your instructor is responsible for making assignments that are within your areas of competence and is also responsible for providing clinical supervision. However, this does not release you from your own legal responsibilities. To help protect yourself and your clients:

■ Prepare carefully for each clinical experience.

■ Never attempt a procedure or make a judgment about which you feel unsure. If you lack the theoretical or practical knowledge for an assignment, notify your clinical instructor immediately.

■ Notify your instructor or a staff nurse if your client's condition changes significantly.

■ Unless otherwise arranged, take instructions only from your clinical instructor.

Your nursing school may require you to carry personal professional liability insurance. The school's policy will cover you only for the nursing care you give in your educational experiences. If you are employed as a nursing assistant, for example, the school's policy will not provide coverage for you at work. Furthermore, you are legally permitted to perform only the procedures contained in your job description. For example, even though you administer injections in your student role, you are not licensed to do so in your role as a nursing assistant.

SUMMARY

Ethical and legal issues are a major source of conflict for nursing practice. This chapter discusses only the legal aspects of the major issues. See Chapter 43 for ethical considerations. It is important to be clear in your mind that what is *legal* and what is *ethical* are not always the same thing. On the one hand, an act may be legal (e.g., abortion) even if it is considered unethical by some. On the other hand, you may believe an action (e.g., assisted suicide) is ethically necessary, but the law may forbid it. You should be aware of the legal consequences of your ethical decisions.

CLINICALREASONING

The questions and exercises in this section allow you to practice the kind of thinking you will use as a full-spectrum nurse. Critical-thinking questions usually have more than one correct answer, so we do not provide "correct answers" for these features. It is more important to develop your nursing judgment than to just cover content. You will learn by discussing the questions with your peers. If you are still unsure, see the Davis Advantage chapter resources for suggested responses.

Caring for the Nguyens

Nam and Yen Nguyen have requested an appointment with you, the nurse at the Family Medicine Clinic, to discuss advance directives. Their experience with Nam's mother, Mai, has created concerns about end-of-life care.

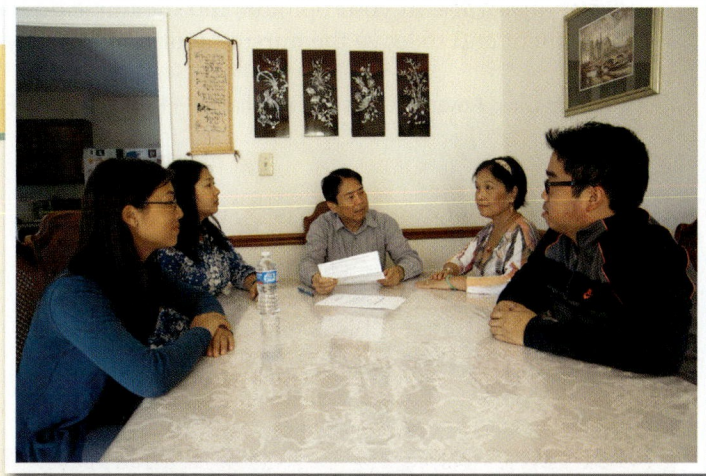

A. Nam asks you, "Do you think it's appropriate to create an advance directive at my age?" How would you respond?

B. Nam tells you that he believes in "natural death." He states, "I don't want extraordinary measures, and I never want to be resuscitated." Yen responds that she is extremely uncomfortable with blanket statements about treatment. "If he got hit by a car or had some

accident I would want you to do everything in your power to treat him. I couldn't carry out his wishes," she states. What actions should you take to help Nam and Yen resolve this discrepancy?

 Go to Davis Advantage, Resources, Chapter 44, **Caring for the Nguyens—Suggested Responses.**

Applying the **Full-Spectrum Nursing Model**_____

CLIENT SITUATION

A nurse employed by a temporary agency is assigned to a neurology unit for a 12-hour shift. On arrival, she discovers that the registered nurse (RN) assigned for the shift called in sick, leaving her with two nursing assistive personnel (NAPs) to provide client care and administer medication, including controlled substances. The nursing supervisor informs her that she will be responsible for the unit with 22 clients, 12 of whom are acutely ill and require close observation and frequent care. The nursing supervisor is not available to work on the unit and has no additional RNs to provide client care. The nurse decides not to accept the assignment, to report the decision and reasons to her agency supervisor, and to leave the neurology unit immediately before starting the shift.

THINKING

1. *Theoretical Knowledge:*
   a. In addition to protecting her nursing license, what other factors should the nurse have considered in deciding whether to stay on or leave the unit?
   b. Because the nurse decided not to accept the assignment, would this have been considered abandonment?
   c. What standards, guidelines, and laws would apply to determine whether the nurse's behavior was in accordance with standards of practice?
2. *Critical Thinking (Contextual Awareness):*
   a. Which statements in the ANA Nurses' Bill of Rights should the nurse have considered before deciding whether to accept the assignment?
   b. What factors in this situation could create legal problems for the nurse?

DOING

3. *Nursing Process (Planning/Intervention):* The nurse's action (leaving the unit) might be viewed, under some laws in some situations, as abandonment of clients. What are some alternative actions the nurse might have taken to avoid that risk?

CARING

4. *Self-Knowledge:* Have you ever been in a situation in which you felt a moral obligation to help, yet knew you would be in over your head? Describe your experience.
5. *Ethical Knowledge:* In your opinion, did the nurse do the right thing when she decided not to accept the assignment and to leave the nursing unit immediately? Explain your thinking.

 Go to Davis Advantage, Resources, Chapter 44, **Applying the Full-Spectrum Nursing Model—Suggested Responses.**

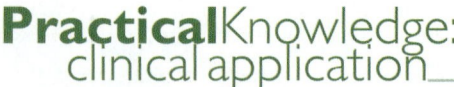

PracticalKnowledge:
clinical application_____

CLINICAL INSIGHTS

Clinical Insight 44-1 ▶ **Tips for Avoiding Malpractice**

Client Relationships

- **Develop open, honest, respectful, and caring relationships** with patients and families. Patients are less likely to sue if they feel that you were caring and professional.

- **Maintain client privacy and confidentiality.**
- **Recognize "problem" clients.** Try to identify the basic problem or complaint and intervene to resolve it. Angry clients who feel mistreated are more likely to bring a malpractice lawsuit.

Clinical Insight 44-1 ➤ Tips for Avoiding Malpractice—cont'd

Professional Interactions

- **Don't blame or criticize other healthcare providers** in the presence of clients (e.g., "Sorry you didn't get your pain medication. The night shift was a little short-staffed last night").
- **Don't make statements that may appear to be an admission of guilt** (e.g., "Omigosh, I forgot to shut off that IV!"). Errors should not be included on the client's health record, but instead recorded in an incident report.

Client Assessments

- **Perform timely assessments and recognize significant assessment cues;** notify primary care providers of changes in the client's condition or client complaints.
- **Recognize significant assessment cues** and notify primary care providers of changes in the client's condition or client complaints.
- **Use the proper chain of command** to ensure appropriate and timely care when the primary healthcare provider is not available (Banford & Budake, 2012).
- **Perform falls risk assessments,** document, and take measures to ensure client safety. Falls are a common cause of client injury.

Documentation

- **Careful, thorough documentation** is the best defense if a lawsuit does occur:
  - Use and document all steps of the nursing process.
  - Be especially thorough when documenting care for patients who will not comply with treatments or who complain a lot.

- Courts assume that if care is not documented, it was not given.
- **Document the time and content of telephone conversations with other healthcare providers.**
- **Send copies only,** never originals, of records and reports requested by other professionals.

Competent Practice

- **Know and follow applicable laws:** (1) federal and state laws, (2) your state's nurse practice act (perform only the activities within your scope of practice and competence).
- **Know and follow agency policies and procedures.**
- **Know and follow standards of care** set forth in the state nurse practice act, by professional organizations, in professional literature, by agency policy, and so on.
- **Stay competent in your area of practice;** for example, attend continuing education, webinars, and in-service programs to improve your knowledge and skills.
- **Don't accept a clinical assignment that you think you are not competent to perform.** Evaluate your assignment with your supervisor if there is a question.

Medication Administration

- **Follow the "rights" of medication administration** (see Chapter 25).
- **Follow medical prescriptions,** but clarify them as needed. Do not implement a questionable prescription or one you do not understand.

Practice Resources
Austin, S. (2008); Banford, E., & Budake, A. (2012); Reising, D. (2012).

Clinical Insight 44-2 ➤ Using Equipment Safely

The following will help you to ensure proper and safe use of equipment:
1. Obtain appropriate training on equipment use.
2. Follow the healthcare agency's protocols, policies, and procedures on the use of the equipment.
3. Follow the manufacturer's operating instructions.
4. Be sure medical equipment has been properly inspected.
5. Perform safety checks regularly and before each use.
6. Position and use equipment properly during treatment.
7. Know how the equipment functions; be alert to signs that it is not working properly.

8. Make sure rooms are not cluttered with equipment.
9. Follow agency policies regarding equipment brought from the client's home (e.g., hair dryers, electric shavers, radios); usually these should be inspected for proper grounding and safe cords.
10. Remove and label equipment that is malfunctioning to prevent others from using it until it can be repaired or replaced.

Practice Resource
Mattox, E. (2012).

Clinical Insight 44-3 ➤ Guidelines for Documenting Care

To be accurate and complete, your reporting and documentation of client care must address the following:

1. Client status (e.g., symptoms and responses to treatments)
2. The nursing care given
3. Providers' prescriptions
4. Medications and treatments
5. Client responses
6. Consultations with other members of the healthcare team regarding client status

You might find the 5 C's mnemonic helpful for documenting care. Charting should be:

Complete
Clear
Correct
Comprehensive
Chronological

Practice Resources

Arnold, P. (2012); Austin, S. (2011); Helm, A. (2003, pp. 1–33).

To explore learning resources for this chapter,

Go to www.DavisAdvantage.com and find:

Answers and Suggested Responses for all questions in this chapter
Lists of **NIC Interventions** and **NOC Outcomes**
List of **NANDA-I Diagnoses**
Knowledge Map
Care Plan
Care Map
References and Bibliography

Concept Map

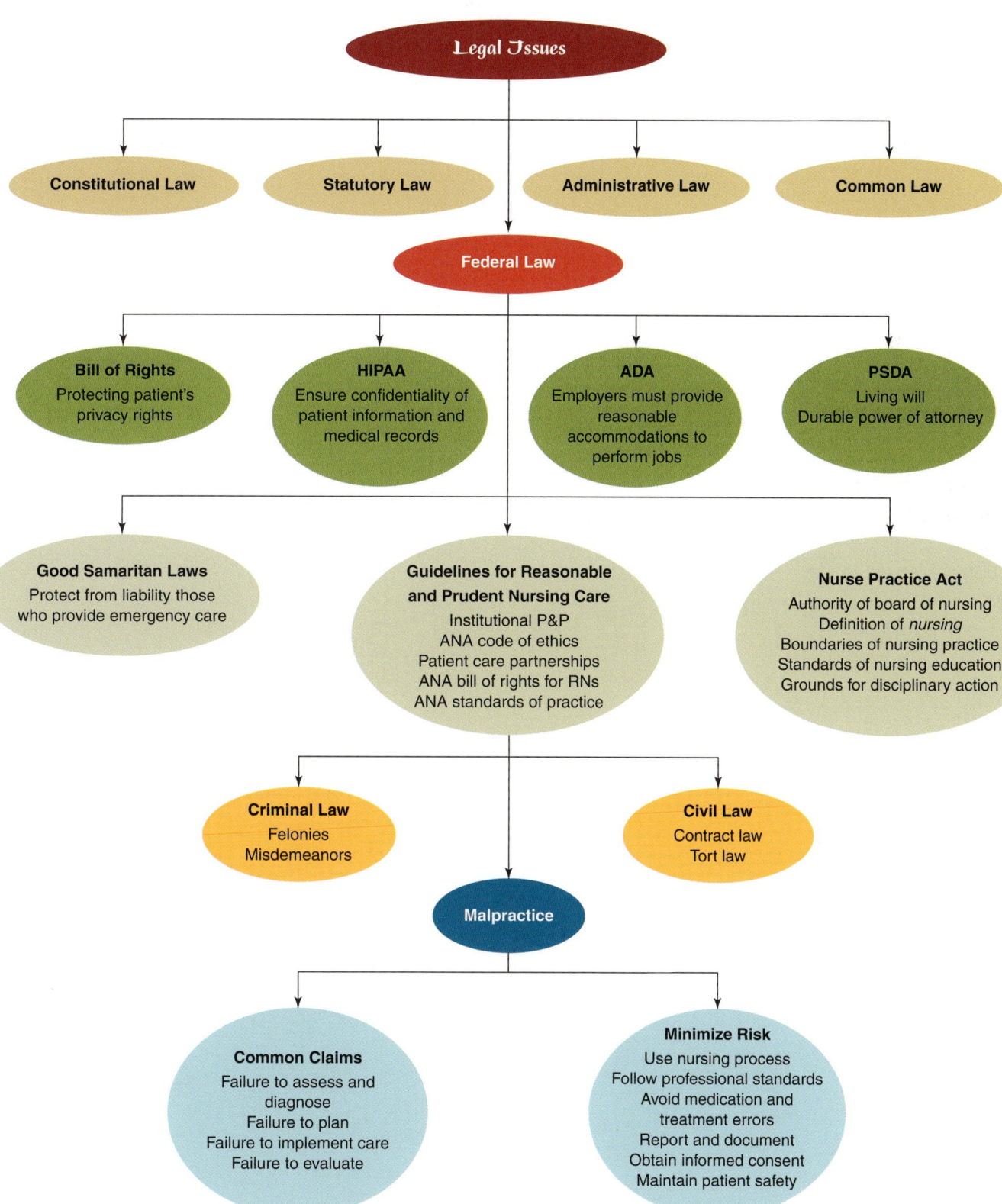

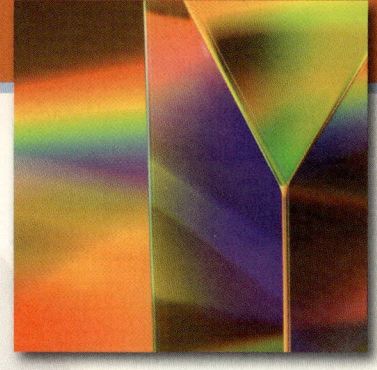

Illustration Credits

*Note: Unless cited below, text credits appear within the text

CHAPTER 1

Nurses Make a Difference 1-1: The National Library of Medicine

Nurses Make a Difference 1-2: © BananaStock

Figure 1-1: Courtesy of the National Library of Medicine

Figure 1-2: © Stephen Mahar, www.photos.com

Figure 1-3: © Cynthia Farmer, www.photos.com

Figures 1-4 and 1-5: © DNY59. istockphoto.com

Figure 1-6: © Penn State Nursing Magazine. Used with permission.

CHAPTER 2

Meet Your Patient: Royalty-Free/Corbis

Figures 2-1–2-3: From Wilkinson, J. M., Treas, L. S., Barnett, K. L., & Smith, M. H. (2016). *Fundamentals of nursing.* Philadelphia: F.A. Davis Company. Used with permission.

CHAPTER 3

Meet Your Patient: Everyday Faces, Photo Copyright Photodisc.

Figure 3-1: From Wilkinson, J. M., Treas, L. S., Barnett, K. L., & Smith, M. H. (2016). *Fundamentals of nursing.* Philadelphia: F.A. Davis Company. Used with permission.

Figure 3-2: From Wilkinson, J. M. (2011). *Nursing process and critical thinking* (5th ed.). Upper Saddle River, NJ: Pearson Education, Inc. Used with permission.

Figure 3-4: Courtesy Shore Memorial Hospital, Somers Point, New Jersey

CHAPTER 4

Meet Your Patient: Photo © BananaStock

Figures 4-1–4-5: From Wilkinson, J. M., Treas, L. S., Barnett, K. L., & Smith, M. H. (2016). *Fundamentals of nursing.* Philadelphia: F.A. Davis Company. Used with permission.

Figure 4-6: Adapted from Maslow, A. (1971). *The farther reaches of human nature.* New York: Viking Press; and Maslow, A., & Lowery, R. (Eds.). (1998). *Toward a psychology of being* (3rd ed.). New York: Wiley & Sons.

CHAPTER 5

Meet Your Patient: Ryan McVay/Photodisc/PunchStock

Figure 5.1: From Wilkinson, J. M., Treas, L. S., Barnett, K. L., & Smith, M. H. (2016). *Fundamentals of nursing.* Philadelphia: F.A. Davis Company. Used with permission.

Figure 5-2: Adapted from Genesis Medical Center, Davenport, Iowa

Figure 5-3: From the Hospital of the University of Pennsylvania, Philadelphia, Pennsylvania

CHAPTER 6

Meet Your Patient: Ryan McVay/Photodisc/PunchStock

Figures 6-1 and 6-3: From Wilkinson, J. M., Treas, L. S., Barnett, K. L., & Smith, M. H. (2016). *Fundamentals of nursing.* Philadelphia: F.A. Davis Company. Used with permission.

Figure 6-2: Courtesy Fain, J. A. (2003). *Reading, understanding, and applying nursing research: A text and workbook* (2nd ed., p. 82). Philadelphia: F.A. Davis Company.

Figure 6-4: Copyright © Ergo Partners, L.C. All rights reserved. Use with permission.

CHAPTER 7

Meet Your Patients: Thinkstock/Getty Images

Figure 7-1: From Wilkinson, J. M., Treas, L. S., Barnett, K. L., & Smith, M. H. (2016). *Fundamentals of nursing.* Philadelphia: F.A. Davis Company. Used with permission.

Figure 7-2: Courtesy Ergo Partners, L.C., Boulder, Colorado. Used with permission.

CHAPTER 8

Meet Your Patient: From Wilkinson, J. M., Treas, L. S., Barnett, K. L., & Smith, M. H. (2016). *Fundamentals of nursing.* Philadelphia: F.A. Davis Company. Used with permission.

Figure 8-2: Courtesy Jean Watson

Figures 8-3 and 8-4: From Wilkinson, J. M., Treas, L. S., Barnett, K. L., & Smith, M. H. (2016). *Fundamentals of nursing.* Philadelphia: F.A. Davis Company. Used with permission.

Figure 8-5: Adapted from Maslow, A. (1970). *The farther reaches of human nature.* New York: Viking Press; and Maslow, A., & Lowery, R. (Eds.). (1998). *Toward a psychology of being* (3rd ed.). New York: Wiley & Sons.

CHAPTER 9

Meet Your Patient: Photodisc Blue/Getty Images

Figures 9-1, 9-2, 9-4: From Dillon, P. M. (2007). *Nursing health assessment: A critical thinking case studies approach* (2nd ed.). Philadelphia: F.A. Davis Company.

Figure 9-3: Polan, E., & Taylor, D. (2007). *Journey across the lifespan* (3rd ed.). Philadelphia: F.A. Davis Company.

Figure 9-5: People Images/iStockphoto.com

Figure 9-6: © Robert Dant, www.istockphoto.com

Figure 9-7: © PunchStock

Figure 9-8: Photodisc Red/Getty Images, Scott T. Baxter

Figure 9-9: Everyday Faces, Photodisc

Figure 9-10: Photodisc Green/Getty Images, Anderson Ross

Figure 9-11: From Wilkinson, J. M., Treas, L. S., Barnett, K. L., & Smith, M. H. (2016). *Fundamentals of nursing.* Philadelphia: F.A. Davis Company. Used with permission.

CHAPTER 10

Meet Your Patient: © Silvia Jansen, www.istockphoto.com

Figure 10-1: U.S. Census Bureau, The Next Four Decades, The Older Population in the United States: 2010 to 2050, p. 2. Retrieved from http://www.census.gov/prod/2010pubs/p25-1138.pdf

Figure 10-2: Photodisc/Getty Images

Figure 10-3: Courtesy of V. Pempusheski, PhD, RN, FAAN

CHAPTER 11

Meet Your Patient: © iStockphoto.com

Figure 11-1: From Wilkinson, J. M., Treas, L. S., Barnett, K. L., & Smith, M. H. (2016). *Fundamentals of nursing.* Philadelphia: F.A. Davis Company. Used with permission.

Figure 11-2: Adapted from Dunn, H. L. (1959). High level wellness for man and society. *American Journal of Public Health, 49*(6), 786–788.

Figure 11-3: Source: Adapted from Neuman, B. (1995). The Neuman systems model. In N. Neuman, *The Neuman systems model* (3rd ed.). Norwalk, CT: Appleton & Lange.

Figure 11-4: Senior Lifestyles, Photodisc

Figures 11-5 and 11-6: Fishermen's Hospital, Marathon, Florida. Used with permission.

Clinical Insight 11-1: From Wilkinson, J. M., Treas, L. S., Barnett, K. L., & Smith, M. H. (2016). *Fundamentals of nursing.* Philadelphia: F.A. Davis Company. Used with permission.

CHAPTER 12

Meet Your Patient: © Digital Vision

Figures 12-1, 12-2, 12-4, 12-6: From Wilkinson, J. M., Treas, L. S., Barnett, K. L., & Smith, M. H. (2016). *Fundamentals of nursing.* Philadelphia: F.A. Davis Company. Used with permission.

Figures 12-3 and 12-5: From Scanlon, V., & Sanders, T. (2014). *Essentials of anatomy and physiology* (7th ed.). Philadelphia: F.A. Davis Company.

CHAPTER 13

Meet Your Patient, Figures 13-1–13-4: From Wilkinson, J. M., Treas, L. S., Barnett, K. L., & Smith, M. H. (2016). *Fundamentals of nursing.* Philadelphia: F.A. Davis Company. Used with permission.

Figure 13-5: Townsend, M. C. (2009). *Psychiatric mental health nursing: Concepts of care* (5th ed., p. 248). Philadelphia: F.A. Davis Company.

CHAPTER 14

Meet Your Patient, Figures 14-1, 14-2, 14-5: © Getty Images

Figure 14-3: © Punchstock, Photodisc

Figure 14-4: © Kali9, iStockphoto.com

Figure 14-6: From Dillon, P. M. (2007). *Nursing health assessment: A critical thinking case studies approach* (2nd ed.). Philadelphia: F.A. Davis Company.

CHAPTER 15

Meet Your Patient: © Braclark, iStockphoto.com

Figure 15-2: © Rich Lindle, iStockphoto.com

Figures 15-3, 15-6, 15-7: From Wilkinson, J. M., Treas, L. S., Barnett, K. L., & Smith, M. H. (2016). *Fundamentals of nursing.* Philadelphia: F.A. Davis Company. Used with permission.

Figure 15-4: © JerryPDX, iStockphoto.com

Figure 15-5: © 2010 Jupiterimages collection

CHAPTER 16

Meet Your Patient: © Photodisc, Senior Lifestyles

Figure 16-1: © Fotosearch.com

Figure 16-2: From Corbis Images

Figure 16-3: Courtesy of Barbara Proud

Figure 16-4: Adapted from Millspaugh, C. D. (2005). Assessment and response to spiritual pain: Part II. *Journal of Palliative Medicine, 8*(6), 1110–1117.

Figure 16-5: Courtesy of Jonas Ngirinshuti

CHAPTER 17

Meer Your Patient: Bananastock

Figure 17-1: © Gina Guarnieri, www.istockphoto.com

Clinical Insight 17-3: From Wilkinson, J. M., Treas, L. S., Barnett, K. L., & Smith, M. H. (2016). *Fundamentals of nursing.* Philadelphia: F.A. Davis Company. Used with permission.

CHAPTER 18

Meet Your Patient: © Getty Images

Figures 18-1, 18-6, 18-7, 18-10: From Wilkinson, J. M., Treas, L. S., Barnett, K. L., & Smith, M. H. (2016). *Fundamentals of nursing.* Philadelphia: F.A. Davis Company. Used with permission.

Figures 18-2, 18-3, 18-5, 18-8, 18-9: Courtesy of Cerner Corporation, Kansas City, Missouri

CHAPTER 19

Meet Your Patient: Photo © BananaStock

Figures 19-1–19-12: From Wilkinson, J. M., Treas, L. S., Barnett, K. L., & Smith, M. H. (2016). *Fundamentals of nursing.* Philadelphia: F.A. Davis Company. Used with permission.

Home Care box: © Omron Healthcare, Inc.

Procedures 19-1 (A–F), 19-2 (A–H)–19-6: From Wilkinson, J. M., Treas, L. S., Barnett, K. L., & Smith, M. H. (2016). *Fundamentals of nursing.* Philadelphia: F.A. Davis Company. Used with permission.

CHAPTER 20

Meet Your Patient: www.iStockphoto.com
Figures 20-1–20-5: From Wilkinson, J. M., Treas, L. S., Barnett, K. L., & Smith, M. H. (2016). *Fundamentals of nursing*. Philadelphia: F.A. Davis Company. Used with permission.

CHAPTER 21

Figures 21-5B, 21-7; Box figures 21-1–21-17; Procedure figures 21-4-1, 21-4-2, 21-6-1–21-6-3, 21-11-4, 21-11-5, 21-12-2, 21-14-1B, 21-14-3, 21-19-1: From Wilkinson, J. M., Treas, L. S., Barnett, K. L., & Smith, M. H. (2016). *Fundamentals of nursing*. Philadelphia: F.A. Davis Company. Used with permission.

Figures 21-1–21-4, 21-6, 21-8–21-11; Box figures 21-18–21-23; Table figures 21-1–21-8; Procedure figures 21-2-1–21-2-3, 21-4-3, 21-4-5, 21-5-1–21-5-4, 21-6-5–21-6-9, 21-6-13–21-6-16, 21-7-1, 21-7-2, 21-7-4, 21-7-5, 21-7-8–21-7-10, 21-8-1–21-8-4, 21-9-1–9-3, 21-10-1, 21-10-2, 21-11-1–21-11-3, 21-12-3–12-6, 21-13-1–13-5, 21-14-1A, 21-14-2, 21-14-4–21-14-7, 21-15-1–21-15-30, 21-16-1–21-16-14, 21-17-1–17-5, 21-18-1–21-18-3: From Dillon, P. M. (2007). *Nursing health assessment: A critical thinking case studies approach* (2nd ed.). Philadelphia: F.A. Davis Company.

Figure 21-5A, Procedure figures 21-6-4, 21-12-1: From Scanlon, V. C., & Sanders, T. (2003). *Essentials of anatomy & physiology* (4th ed.). Philadelphia, F.A. Davis Company.

Procedure figure 21-4-4: From Goldsmith, L. A., Tharp, M. D., & Lazarus, G. (1997). *Adult and pediatric dermatology: A color guide to diagnosis and treatment*. Philadelphia: F.A. Davis Company.

Procedure figures 21-7-3, 21-7-6, 21-7-7: Courtesy of Ann Marie Ramsey, RN, MSN, CPNP

Procedure figure 21-9-4: Courtesy Robert A. Levine, DDS, and Sheryl Radin, DDS

Procedure figures 21-9-5, 21-9-8, 21-9-9: Courtesy of Tina S. Liang, DMD

Procedure figure 21-9-7: Courtesy of MCP-Hahneman University Department of Dermatology, Philadelphia, Pennsylvania

Figures 21-1–21-4, 21-6, 21-8–21-11; Describing Skin Lesions, Clinical Insight 21-1A and B; Clinical Insight 21-3 (all figures); Procedure 21-2B (step 7 [Malignant Melanoma]); Documentation; Procedure 21-5 (all figures); Procedure 21-6 (steps 3–8 [all figures]); Procedure 21-7 (steps 1–3e, 5 [Weber Test], and 6); Procedure 21-10 (all figures); Procedure 21-13 (steps 1b, c, and 2 [adapted]); Procedure 21-14 (step 7c, Deep Palpation Techniques [1, 2]); Procedure 21-15 (steps 1c [1] [2], 1d, 2 [all], 6c [1], and 6c [2]): From Dillon, P. M. (2007). *Nursing health assessment: A critical thinking case studies approach* (2nd ed.). Philadelphia: F.A. Davis Company.

Procedure figures 21-6-10–21-6-12: Courtesy Will's Eye Institute, Philadelphia

CHAPTER 22

Meet Your Patient: www.istockphoto.com
Figures 22-1, 22-4, 22-5, all Procedure figures except 22-2-1: From Wilkinson, J. M., Treas, L. S., Barnett, K. L., & Smith, M. H. (2016). *Fundamentals of nursing*. Philadelphia: F.A. Davis Company. Used with permission.

Figures 22-2 and 21-3: From Scanlon, V. C., & Sanders, T. (2003). *Essentials of anatomy and physiology* (4th ed.). Philadelphia: F.A. Davis Company.

Procedure figure 22-2-1: Courtesy of Moldex-Metric, Inc. Culver City, California

CHAPTER 23

Meet Your Patient: © Jay Freis/Digital Vision/ Getty Images
Figure 23-1; Box figures 23-1–23-3; Table figure 23-1; Procedure figures 23-2-1, 23-2-2–21-2-5: From Wilkinson, J. M., Treas, L. S., Barnett, K. L., & Smith, M. H. (2016). *Fundamentals of nursing*. Philadelphia: F.A. Davis Company. Used with permission.

Figure 23-2: Dr. Louise P. de Courval © CLSC Cote-des-Neiges, McGill University

Figure 23-3: © www.istockphoto.com

Procedure figures 23-1-3 and 23-1-4: Courtesy of Smart Caregiver Fall Prevention and Anti-wandering Products

CHAPTER 24

Meet Your Patient: Getty Images
Figures 24-1, 24-5, 24-6–24-8; Self-Care 24-3; Clinical Insight 24-1 (all); Procedure 24-1 (steps 4, 5b, 7c, 9f, 10b, and 10d); Procedure 24-2 (step 5b); Procedure 24-3 (Equipment); Procedure 24-4 (steps 3c, 3f); Procedure 24-5 (Pre-assessment, steps 6 and 12); Procedure 24-6 (steps 10 and 11a, b, and c); Procedure 24-7 (steps 1a, b, and 7); Procedure 24-8 (Equipment, step 5a); Procedure 24-9 (step 10); Procedure 24-9c (What if . . .); Procedure 24-10 (step 4); Procedure 24-11 (step 4c); Procedure 24-12 (all figures); Procedure 24-13 (all figures); Procedure 24-14 (all figures): From Wilkinson, J. M., Treas, L. S., Barnett, K. L., & Smith, M. H. (2016). *Fundamentals of nursing*. Philadelphia: F.A. Davis Company. Used with permission.

Figure 24-2: Courtesy of Invacare Corporation

Figures 24-3 and 24-4: From Dillon, P. M. (2007). *Nursing health assessment: A critical thinking case studies approach* (2nd ed.). Philadelphia: F.A. Davis Company.

CHAPTER 25

Meet Your Patient; Figures 25-1–25-11, 25-14–25-21, 25-24–25-26; Medication Guidelines (step 12b); Procedure 25-1 (steps 1h, 2e, 2f, and 7); Procedure 25-2 (steps 6, 8, and 11); Procedure 25-2A (step 6c); Procedure 25-3 (step 6a and b); Procedure 25-4 (step 4b and c); Procedure 25-5 (steps 3, 6c and j); Procedure 25-6 (step 9a, c); Procedure 25-7A (step 4); Procedure 27-7D (step 5); Procedure 25-8 (steps 7 and 11); Procedure 25-9 (Equipment); Procedure 25-9A (steps 2, 4a and b); Procedure 25-9B (steps 6a–9); Procedure 25-9C (steps 2, 4, and 5); Procedure 25-9E (step 5); Procedure 25-10 (Equipment 2 and 3, steps 3, and 3a, b, c); Procedure 25-10B (steps 2–5); Procedure 25-11 (Equipment, step 11); Procedure 25-12 (step 1b); Procedure 25-13A (steps 3 and 4); Procedure 25-13B (step 2); Procedure 25-13C (step 4); Procedure 25-14B (steps 8 and 11); Procedure 25-15A (steps 6 and 8); Procedure 25-15B (step 5); Procedure 25-16 (step 5); Procedure 25-16B (steps 9 and 12); Procedure 25-16C (step 7); Procedure 25-17 (step 8); Procedure 25-17B (step 7); Procedure 25-17C (step 6); Clinical Insight 25-3 (all); Clinical Insight 25-4 (step 6); Clinical Insight 25-5 (steps 6 and 7); Clinical Insight 25-6: From Wilkinson, J. M., Treas, L. S.,

Barnett, K. L., & Smith, M. H. (2016). *Fundamentals of nursing.* Philadelphia: F.A. Davis Company. Used with permission.

Figure 25-16: From http://www.hospira.com/GlobalPages/concactus.aspx. Used with permission.

Figure 25-18: Courtesy of Medi-Dose, Inc./EPS, Inc., Ivyland, Pennsylvania

Figure 25-27: Courtesy of pfm medical ag

Figure 25-30, Procedure figure 25-17A-1: Courtesy of Dr. Donna Clarren and Dr. Brian Oxhorn, Roseman College of Nursing

Procedure figure 25-10-1: From Ingenious Technologies, Corp, Osprey, Florida

CHAPTER 26

Meet Your Patient: Photo © BananaStock

Figures 26-2 and 26-2: From Wilkinson, J. M., Treas, L. S., Barnett, K. L., & Smith, M. H. (2016). *Fundamentals of nursing.* Philadelphia: F.A. Davis Company. Used with permission.

Figure 26-4: From Scanlon, V. C., & Sanders, T. (2003). *Essentials of anatomy and physiology* (4th ed.). Philadelphia: F.A. Davis Company.

Figure 26-5: Courtesy Merck & Co., Inc. #994795(1)-05-COZ

CHAPTER 27

Meet Your Peer: © Thomas Eyedesign, www.istockphoto.com

Figures 27-1, 27-2, 27-3: From Wilkinson, J. M., Treas, L. S., Barnett, K. L., & Smith, M. H. (2016). *Fundamentals of nursing.* Philadelphia: F.A. Davis Company. Used with permission.

CHAPTER 28

Figures 28-5, 28-7; Clinical Insight 28-3; Clinical Insight 28-5; Procedure 28-1 (steps 10g, 13, and 16); Procedure 28-2 (steps 3, 13, and 20e); Procedure 28-3 (steps 11 and 18): From Wilkinson, J. M., Treas, L. S., Barnett, K. L., & Smith, M. H. (2016). *Fundamentals of nursing.* Philadelphia: F.A. Davis Company. Used with permission.

Figure 28-1: USDA Choosemyplate.gov

Figure 28-2: USFDA 2004

Figure 28-3: Source: Vegan Resource Group. www.vrg.org. Text by Reed Mangels, PhD, RD

Design by Lindsey Siferd.

Figures 28-4 and 28-6: Courtesy of Covidien

Clinical Insight 28-2A and B: From Lutz, C., & Przytulski, K. (2006). *Nutrition and diet therapy* (4th ed.). Philadelphia: F.A. Davis Company.

Procedure 28-2 (step 11): From Scanlon, V. C., & Sanders, T. (2003). *Essentials of anatomy and physiology* (4th ed.). Philadelphia: F.A. Davis Company.

Procedure figures 28-2-5 and 28-5-1: Courtesy Dale Medical Products, Inc., Plainville, Massachusetts

Procedure figure 3A-1: Nestle Healthcare Nutrition Inc.

CHAPTER 29

Meet Your Patient: © The Linke, www.istockphoto.com

Figures 29-1–29-5: From Scanlon, V., & Sanders, T. (2014). *Essentials of anatomy and physiology* (7th ed.). Philadelphia: F.A. Davis Company.

Figure 29-6, all Procedure figures not courtesy of Hollister Inc.: From Wilkinson, J. M., Treas, L. S., Barnett, K. L., & Smith, M. H. (2016). *Fundamentals of nursing.* Philadelphia: F.A. Davis Company. Used with permission.

Figure 29-8: Courtesy of ConvaTec Inc., Skillman, New Jersey

Figure 29-9, Procedure figures 29-6-1, 29-8-1, 29-8-2, 29-8B-1, 29-8B-2: Courtesy of Hollister Incorporated, Libertyville, Illinois

CHAPTER 30

Meet Your Patient: © BananaStock

Figures 30-1: From Scanlon, V., & Sanders, T. (2014). *Essentials of anatomy and physiology* (7th ed.). Philadelphia: F.A. Davis Company.

Figures 30-2, 30-3, 30-5–30-10, all Procedure figures: From Wilkinson, J. M., Treas, L. S., Barnett, K. L., & Smith, M. H. (2016). *Fundamentals of nursing.* Philadelphia: F.A. Davis Company. Used with permission.

Box figure 30-1: From Dillon, P. M. (2007). *Nursing health assessment: A critical thinking case studies approach* (2nd ed.). Philadelphia, F.A. Davis Company.

CHAPTER 31

Meet Your Patient: © Aguru, www.istockphoto.com

Figures 31-1 and 31-2: From Scanlon, V., & Sanders, T. (2014). *Essentials of anatomy and physiology* (7th ed.). Philadelphia: F.A. Davis Company.

Procedure figure 31-1-1: From Wilkinson, J. M., Treas, L. S., Barnett, K. L., & Smith, M. H. (2016). *Fundamentals of nursing.* Philadelphia: F.A. Davis Company. Used with permission.

CHAPTER 32

Meet Your Patient: © Jason Doiy, www.istockphoto.com

Box figure 32-1: From Wilkinson, J. M., Treas, L. S., Barnett, K. L., & Smith, M. H. (2016). *Fundamentals of nursing.* Philadelphia: F.A. Davis Company. Used with permission.

Figures 32-1–32-3, 32-5, Box figures: From Wilkinson, J. W., & Treas, L. (2011). *Fundamentals of nursing* (2nd ed.). Philadelphia: F.A. Davis Company.

Wong Baker FACES Scale: © 1983 Wong-Baker FACES Foundation. www.WongBakerFACES.org. Used with permission. Originally published in Whaley & Wong's Nursing Care of Infants and Children. © Elsevier Inc.

Faces pain scale sources: Hicks, C. L., von Baeyer, C. L., Spafford, P., et al. (2001). The Faces Pain Scale–Revised: Toward a common metric in pediatric pain measurement. *Pain, 93,* 173–183; Bieri, D., Reeve, R., Champion, G. D., et al. (1990). The Faces Pain Scale for the self-assessment of the severity of pain experienced by children: Development, initial validation and preliminary investigation for ratio scale properties. *Pain, 41,* 139–150.

CHAPTER 33

Meet Your Patient: © Christopher Futcher, www.istockphoto.com

Figures 33-1 and 33-2: From Scanlon, V., & Sanders, T. (2014). *Essentials of anatomy and physiology* (7th ed.). Philadelphia: F.A. Davis Company.

Figures 33-3, 33-4–33-8, 33-10, 33-11, 33-14, 33-18–33-21, Table figures, Procedure figures: From Wilkinson, J. M.,

Treas, L. S., Barnett, K. L., & Smith, M. H. (2016). *Fundamentals of nursing*. Philadelphia: F.A. Davis Company. Used with permission.

Figures 33-9, 33-11–33-13, 33-15–33-17: Courtesy EZ Way, Inc., Clarinda, Iowa

Figure 33-9 Clinical Insight (Hip Abduction): From Williams, L., & Hopper, P. (2015). *Understanding medical surgical nursing* (5th ed.). Philadelphia: F.A. Davis Company.

CHAPTER 34

Meet Your Patients, Figures 34-5, 34-7: www.istockphoto.com

Figures 34-1–34-4, 34-6: From Wilkinson, J. M., Treas, L. S., Barnett, K. L., & Smith, M. H. (2016). *Fundamentals of nursing*. Philadelphia: F.A. Davis Company. Used with permission.

CHAPTER 35

Meet Your Patient: © Diane Diederich, www.istockphoto.com

Figures 35-1–35-4, all Procedure figures: From Wilkinson, J. M., Treas, L. S., Barnett, K. L., & Smith, M. H. (2016). *Fundamentals of nursing*. Philadelphia: F.A. Davis Company. Used with permission.

Figure 35-5: From Guyton, A. C., & Hall, J. E. (2006). *Medical physiology* (10th ed.). Philadelphia: W.B. Saunders. Used with permission.

CHAPTER 36

Meet Your Patient: From Photodisc, Everyday Faces

Figure 36-1: From Scanlon, V., & Sanders, T. (2014). *Essentials of anatomy and physiology* (7th ed.). Philadelphia: F.A. Davis Company.

Figure 36-10: Adapted from AHRQ Clinical Practice Guidelines.

Table figures 36-2, 36-4, 36-6, 36-8, 36-10: From The National Pressure Ulcer Advisory Panel

Procedure 36-6A figures: From Rhoads, J., & Meeker, B. J. (2008). *Davis's guide to clinical nursing skills*. Philadelphia: F.A. Davis Company.

Procedure figure 36-6B-1: From Talley Group Limited

Figure 36-8: Adapted from AHRQ Clinical Practice Guidelines

Figures 36-4, 36-6–36-9, 36-11, 36-12, 36-14–36-16, all other Procedure figures: From Wilkinson, J. M., Treas, L. S., Barnett, K. L., & Smith, M. H. (2016). *Fundamentals of nursing*. Philadelphia: F.A. Davis Company. Used with permission.

CHAPTER 37

Meet Your Patient: © BananaStock

Figures 37-1–37-3: From Scanlon, V., & Sanders, T. (2014). *Essentials of anatomy and physiology* (7th ed.). Philadelphia: F.A. Davis Company.

Figures 37-8, 37-10, 37-12–37-14: From Williams, L., & Hopper, P. (2007). *Understanding medical surgical nursing* (2nd ed.). Philadelphia: F.A. Davis Company.

Procedure figure 37-7-1: © Unomedical a/s, used with permission.

Figures 37-7, 37-9, 37-11, Table figures, all other Procedure figures: From Wilkinson, J. M., Treas, L. S., Barnett, K. L.,

& Smith, M. H. (2016). *Fundamentals of nursing*. Philadelphia: F.A. Davis Company. Used with permission.

CHAPTER 38

Meet Your Patient: www.istockphoto.com

Figures 38-1 and 38-2: From Scanlon, V., & Sanders, T. (2014). *Essentials of anatomy and physiology* (7th ed.). Philadelphia: F.A. Davis Company.

Figures 38-3, 38-4, Procedure figures: From Wilkinson, J. M., Treas, L. S., Barnett, K. L., & Smith, M. H. (2016). *Fundamentals of nursing*. Philadelphia: F.A. Davis Company. Used with permission.

CHAPTER 39

Meet Your Patient: Getty Images, Photodisc

Figure 39-1: Adapted from Scanlon, V., & Sanders, T. (2014). *Essentials of anatomy and physiology* (7th ed.). Philadelphia: F.A. Davis Company.

Figures 39-2–39-5, 39-7–39-13, 39-15, all Procedure and Clinical Insight figures: From Wilkinson, J. M., Treas, L. S., Barnett, K. L., & Smith, M. H. (2016). *Fundamentals of nursing*. Philadelphia: F.A. Davis Company. Used with permission.

CHAPTER 40

Meet Your Patient: © Vikram Raghuvanshi, www.istockphoto.com

Figures 40-1, 40-3, 40-6, all Procedure figures except 40-1: From Wilkinson, J. M., Treas, L. S., Barnett, K. L., & Smith, M. H. (2016). *Fundamentals of nursing*. Philadelphia: F.A. Davis Company. Used with permission.

Figures 40-2, 40-4: From Williams, L., & Hopper, P. (2015). *Understanding medical surgical nursing* (5th ed.). Philadelphia: F.A. Davis Company.

Procedure figure 40-1: Courtesy of Allied Healthcare Products, St. Louis, Missouri

Figure 40-5: Used with permission from Kimberly-Clark Worldwide, Inc.

CHAPTER 41

Meet Your Patient: © Photo Euphoria, www.istockphoto.com

Figure 41-1: www.iStockPhoto.com

Figure 41-3: Based on Farrell, K., & Broude, C. (1987). *Winning the change game: How to implement information systems with fewer headaches and bigger paybacks*. Los Angeles: Breakthrough Enterprises; and Lewin, K. (1951). *Field theory in social science: Selected theoretical papers*. New York: Harper & Row.

CHAPTER 42

Meet Your Patient: © Photo Euphoria, www.istockphoto.com

Figures 42-2–42-5: From Wilkinson, J. M., Treas, L. S., Barnett, K. L., & Smith, M. H. (2016). *Fundamentals of nursing*. Philadelphia: F.A. Davis Company. Used with permission.

CHAPTER 43

Meet Your Patient: © Nathan Watkins, www.istockphoto.com

CHAPTER 44

Meet Your Patient: © ntmw, www.istockphoto.com www.istockphoto.com

CHAPTER 45

Meet Your Patient, Figures 45-3, 45-4: www. iStockphoto.com

Figure 45-1: Adapted from Engelbardt, S., & Nelson, R. *Health care informatics: An interdisciplinary approach.* Copyright 2002. With permission from Elsevier.

Figure 45-2: Used with permission from Doctors Telehealth Network. http://www.doctorstelehealthnetwork.net/index-6.html

CHAPTER 46

Meet Your Patient: © Monkey Business Images, www. shutterstock.com

Figure 46-5: From the National Institutes of Health

Figure 46-6: Dean Mitchell, www.istockphoto.com

INDEX

Note: Page numbers followed by *f* refer to figures; page numbers followed by *t* refer to tables; page numbers followed by *b* refer to boxes; page numbers followed by *p* refer to procedures; page numbers followed by "e" refer to bonus chapter content available in eBook on DavisAdvantage.com.

Universal Steps for All Procedures:

You should consider the following nursing activities to be a part of every procedure.

Before Approaching a Patient

- Check the medical order or obtain an order, if necessary.
- Refer to agency protocols unless you already know them.
- Get a signed, informed consent, if needed.
- Wash your hands. Follow agency policy and CDC guidelines for hand hygiene.
- Gather the necessary supplies and equipment.
- Obtain assistance from another healthcare worker, if it will be needed (e.g., to lift a patient).

Preparing the Patient

- Identify the patient using two identifiers (e.g., read the wrist band and ask the patient to state his or her name).
- Explain the procedure to the patient: What you will do, what the patient will feel, and what he or she is expected to do (e.g., "You will need to lie very still.")
- Provide privacy. For example, ask visitors to step out of the room, draw bed curtains, and close the door.
- Position the bed or treatment table to a working level; lower the near siderail.
- Make any relevant assessments (e.g., take vital signs) to ensure that the patient (1) still requires the procedure and (2) is able to tolerate it.

During the Procedure

- Wash your hands before touching the patient, before gloving, and after removing gloves. Wash them again before leaving the room.
- Maintain correct body mechanics.
- Continue to observe the patient while performing the procedure steps.

After the Procedure

- Evaluate the patient's response to the procedure.
- Leave the patient in a comfortable, safe position, with the call light within reach.
- If the patient is in bed, return the bed to its original position and raise the siderail (if the patient requires this precaution).
- Document that the procedure was done; document the patient's responses.
- Dispose of supplies and materials according to agency policy.

Remember:

All procedures are "rules of thumb." Patient care can be altered by medical orders, agency policies, and individual patient needs

Everything you do requires nursing judgment!